P9-BJF-404

Sleisenger & Fordtran's

Gastrointestinal and Liver Disease

Sleisenger & Fordtran's

Gastrointestinal and Liver Disease

Pathophysiology/Diagnosis/Management

7th Edition

Mark Feldman, MD
William O. Tschumy, Jr., M.D. Chair of Internal Medicine
Presbyterian Hospital of Dallas
Clinical Professor of Internal Medicine
University of Texas Southwestern Medical School
Dallas, Texas

Lawrence S. Friedman, MD
Professor of Medicine
Harvard Medical School
Physician, Gastrointestinal Unit
Chief, Walter Bauer Firm (Medical Services)
Massachusetts General Hospital
Boston, Massachusetts

Marvin H. Sleisenger, MD
Professor of Medicine, Emeritus
University of California, San Francisco, School of Medicine
Distinguished Physician
Department of Veterans Affairs Medical Center
San Francisco, California

Volume 2

SAUNDERS
An Imprint of Elsevier Science
Philadelphia London New York St. Louis Sydney Toronto

SAUNDERS
An Imprint of Elsevier Science

The Curtis Center
Independence Square West
Philadelphia, Pennsylvania 19106

SLEISENGER AND FORDTRAN'S GASTROINTESTINAL AND LIVER DISEASE **ISBN 0-7216-8973-6**

Notice

Gastroenterology is an ever-changing field. Standard safety precautions must be followed, but as new research and clinical experience broaden our knowledge, changes in treatment and drug therapy may become necessary or appropriate. Readers are advised to check the most current product information provided by the manufacturer of each drug to be administered to verify the recommended dose, the method and duration of administration, and contraindications. It is the responsibility of the treating physician, relying on experience and knowledge of the patient, to determine dosages and the best treatment for each individual patient. Neither the Publisher nor the editors assumes any liability for any injury and/or damage to persons or property arising from this publication.

THE PUBLISHER

Library of Congress Cataloging-in-Publication Data

Sleisenger & Fordtran's gastrointestinal and liver disease: pathophysiology, diagnosis, management / [edited by] Mark Feldman, Lawrence S. Friedman, Marvin H. Sleisenger.—7th ed.
p. ; cm.
Includes bibliographical references and index.
ISBN 0-7216-8973-6
1. Gastrointestinal system—Diseases. 2. Liver—Diseases. I. Title: Gastrointestinal and liver disease. II. Title: Sleisenger and Fordtran's gastrointestinal and liver disease. III. Feldman, Mark IV. Friedman, Lawrence S. (Lawrence Samuel) V. Sleisenger, Marvin H.
[DNLM: 1. Gastrointestinal Diseases. 2. Liver Diseases. WI 140 S632 2002]
RC801 .G384 2002
616.3′3—dc21 2002021046

Acquisitions Editor: Sue Hodgson
Developmental Editor: Melissa Dudlick
Project Manager: Peter Faber
Book Designer: Marie Gardocky Clifton

Printed in China.

Last digit is the print number: 9 8 7 6 5 4 3 2 1

The Editors dedicate the Seventh Edition of this textbook to the late John H. Walsh, MD, in recognition of his enormous contributions to gastroenterology in general and to Gastrointestinal and Liver Disease *in particular. Dr. Walsh contributed outstanding treatises on gastrointestinal hormones and transmitters for each of the first six editions of this book. He was also a valued advisor to and friend of the Editors, and we sorely miss him.*

We also dedicate this edition to our parents: Mildred and the late Jerome Feldman; the late Maurice and Esther Friedman; and the late Celia Levin, Louis Levin, and Abraham Sleisenger.

MARK FELDMAN, MD
LAWRENCE S. FRIEDMAN, MD
MARVIN H. SLEISENGER, MD

CONTRIBUTORS

Jane M. Andrews, MBBS, PhD, FRACP
Senior Research Fellow, Department of Medicine, Adelaide University; Consultant Gastroenterologist, Department of Gastroenterology, Hepatology, and General Medicine, Royal Adelaide Hospital, Adelaide, South Australia, Australia
Small Intestinal Motor Physiology

Paul Angulo, MD
Associate Professor of Medicine, Mayo Medical School; Senior Associate Consultant, Division of Gastroenterology and Hepatology, Mayo Clinic and Foundation, Rochester, Minnesota
Primary Biliary Cirrhosis

Thomas Anthony, MD
Associate Professor, Department of Surgery, University of Texas Southwestern Medical Center, Dallas, Texas
Gastrointestinal Carcinoid Tumors and the Carcinoid Syndrome

John E. Antoine, MD
Professor of Radiation Oncology, University of Texas Southwestern Medical Center; Chief, Radiation Oncology Service, Dallas Veterans Administration Medical Center, Dallas, Texas
Radiation Enteritis

Bruce R. Bacon, MD
James F. King, MD, Endowed Chair in Gastroenterology; Professor of Internal Medicine; Director, Division of Gastroenterology and Hepatology, St. Louis University School of Medicine, St. Louis, Missouri
Hereditary Hemochromatosis

William F. Balistreri, MD
Director, Division of Gastroenterology, Hepatology, and Nutrition, Children's Hospital Medical Center, Cincinnati, Ohio
Inherited Metabolic Disorders of the Liver

John G. Bartlett, MD
Professor of Medicine, Johns Hopkins University School of Medicine; Chief, Division of Infectious Diseases, Johns Hopkins Hospital, Baltimore, Maryland
Pseudomembranous Enterocolitis and Antibiotic-Associated Diarrhea

Nathan M. Bass, MD, PhD
Professor of Medicine, University of California, San Francisco, School of Medicine; Medical Director, Liver Transplant Program, University of California, San Francisco, Hospitals, San Francisco, California
Sclerosing Cholangitis and Recurrent Pyogenic Cholangitis; Portal Hypertension and Variceal Bleeding

Marina Berenguer, MD
Hospital Universitario La Fe, Servicio de Medicina Digestiva, Valencia, Spain
Viral Hepatitis

Patricia C. Bergen, MD
Associate Professor of Surgery, University of Texas Southwestern Medical School; Active Staff, Zale Lipshy University Hospital, Parkland Memorial Hospital, and Veterans Administration North Texas Healthcare System, Dallas, Texas
Intestinal Obstruction and Ileus

Lyman E. Bilhartz, MD, FACP
Professor of Internal Medicine, University of Texas Southwestern Medical Center; Attending Physician, Parkland Hospital and Zale Lipshy University Hospital, Dallas, Texas
Gallstone Disease and Its Complications; Acalculous Cholecystitis, Cholesterolosis, Adenomyomatosis, and Polyps of the Gallbladder

David Blumberg, MD
Assistant Professor of Surgery, University of Pittsburgh School of Medicine, Pittsburgh, Pennsylvania
Other Diseases of the Colon and Rectum

Scott J. Boley, MD
Professor of Surgery and Pediatrics, Albert Einstein College of Medicine; Emeritus Chief of Pediatric Surgery, Montefiore Medical Center, Bronx, New York
Intestinal Ischemia

Lawrence J. Brandt, MD
Professor of Medicine and Surgery, Albert Einstein College of Medicine; Chief of Gastroenterology, Montefiore Medical Center, Bronx, New York
Intestinal Ischemia; Vascular Lesions of the Gastrointestinal Tract

Robert S. Bresalier, MD
Professor of Medicine, and Chairman, Department of Gastrointestinal Medicine and Nutrition, The University of Texas MD Anderson Cancer Center, Houston, Texas
Malignant Neoplasms of the Large Intestine

Robert S. Britton, PhD
Associate Research Professor of Internal Medicine, Division of Gastroenterology and Hepatology, St. Louis University School of Medicine, St. Louis, Missouri
Hereditary Hemochromatosis

Simon J. Brookes, PhD
Senior Lecturer, Department of Human Physiology, School of Medicine, Faculty of Health Sciences, Flinders University; Senior Research Fellow, National Health and Medical Research Council of Australia, Adelaide, South Australia, Australia
Motility of the Large Intestine

William R. Brugge,, MD
Associate Professor of Medicine, Harvard Medical School; Director, Gastrointestinal Endoscopy, Massachusetts General Hospital, Boston, Massachusetts
Assistant Editor (Imaging)

J. Steven Burdick, MD
Associate Professor of Medicine, Division of Gastroenterology, University of Texas Southwestern Medical School; Director of Endoscopy and Gastroenterology, Parkland Memorial Hospital, Dallas, Texas
Anatomy, Histology, Embryology, and Developmental Anomalies of the Pancreas

Julie G. Champine, MD
Associate Professor of Radiology, University of Texas Southwestern Medical Center; Medical Director of Radiology, Parkland Memorial Hospital, Dallas, Texas
Abdominal Abscesses and Gastrointestinal Fistulas

Suresh T. Chari, MD
Assistant Professor of Medicine, Mayo Medical School; Consultant, Division of Gastroenterology and Hepatology, Mayo Clinic, Rochester, Minnesota
Acute Pancreatitis

Tsu-Yi Chuang
Professor of Dermatology Clinical Research, Indiana University School of Medicine, Indianapolis, Indiana
Oral Disease and Oral-Cutaneous Manifestations of Gastrointestinal and Liver Disease

Raymond T. Chung, MD
Assistant Professor of Medicine, Harvard Medical School; Medical Director, Liver Transplant Program, and Director, Hepatology Service, Massachusetts General Hospital, Boston, Massachusetts
Liver Abscess and Bacterial, Parasitic, Fungal, and Granulomatous Liver Disease

Ray E. Clouse, MD
Professor of Medicine and Psychiatry, Washington University School of Medicine; Physician, Barnes-Jewish Hospital, St. Louis, Missouri
Esophageal Motor and Sensory Function and Motor Disorders of the Esophagus

Robert H. Collins, Jr., MD
Associate Professor, University of Texas Southwestern Medical School; Director, Bone Marrow Transplantation, Dallas, Texas
Gastrointestinal Lymphomas, Including Immunoproliferative Small Intestinal Disease

Ian J. Cook, MD (Syd), FRACP
Associate Professor of Medicine, University of New South Wales; Head, Gastroenterology Department, St. George Hospital, Sydney, New South Wales, Australia
Motility of the Large Intestine

Diane W. Cox, PhD, FCCMG
Professor and Chair, Department of Medical Genetics, University of Alberta; Director, Medical Genetic Services, Northern Alberta; Child Health Program, Capital Health Authority, Edmonton, Alberta, Canada
Wilson Disease

Byron Cryer, MD
Associate Professor of Medicine, University of Texas Southwestern Medical School; Staff Physician, Gastroenterology Section, Dallas Veterans Administration Medical Center, Dallas, Texas
Nonsteroidal Anti-Inflammatory Drug Injury

Albert J. Czaja, MD
Professor of Medicine, Mayo Medical School; Consultant, Gastroenterology and Hepatology, Mayo Clinic, Rochester, Minnesota
Autoimmune Hepatitis

Timothy J. Davern, MD
Adjunct Assistant Professor of Medicine, University of California, San Francisco, School of Medicine, San Francisco, California
Biochemical Liver Tests

Marta L. Davila, MD
Assistant Professor of Medicine, Stanford University School of Medicine, Stanford, California
Complications of Gastrointestinal Endoscopy

Rene Davila, MD
Assistant Professor of Medicine, Gastroenterology, and Hepatology, The University of Tennessee Health Science Center, Memphis, Tennessee
Pregnancy-Related Hepatic and Gastrointestinal Disorders

Paul A. Dawson, PhD
Associate Professor of Internal Medicine, Section of Gastroenterology, Wake Forest University School of Medicine, Winston-Salem, North Carolina
Bile Secretion and the Enterohepatic Circulation of Bile Acids

Margo A. Denke, MD, FACP, FACE
Professor of Medicine, University of Texas Southwestern Medical School; Attending Physician, Veterans Affairs Medical Center, Parkland Memorial Hospital, Zale Lipshy University Hospital, and St. Paul Medical Center, Dallas, Texas
Anorexia Nervosa, Bulimia Nervosa, and Obesity

John Dent, MBBChir, PhD
Clinical Professor of Medicine, Department of Medicine, Adelaide University; Director of Gastroenterology, Hepatology, and General Medicine, Royal Adelaide Hospital, Adelaide, South Australia, Australia
Small Intestinal Motor Physiology

Nicholas E. Diamant, MDCM
Professor of Medicine and Physiology, University of Toronto; Attending Physician, Toronto Western Hospital, Division of The University Health Network, Toronto, Ontario, Canada
Esophageal Motor and Sensory Function and Motor Disorders of the Esophagus

Anna Mae Diehl, MD
Professor of Medicine, Johns Hopkins University School of Medicine; Staff, Division of Digestive Diseases, Johns Hopkins Hospital, Baltimore, Maryland
Nonalcoholic Fatty Liver Disease

Eugene P. DiMagno, MD
Professor of Medicine, Mayo School of Medicine; Consultant, Division of Gastroenterology and Hepatology, Mayo Clinic, Rochester, Minnesota
Acute Pancreatitis

Douglas A. Drossman, MD
Professor of Medicine and Psychiatry, Co-Director, Center for Functional Gastrointestinal and Motility Disorders, Division of Digestive Diseases, University of North Carolina at Chapel Hill School of Medicine, Chapel Hill, North Carolina.
Chronic Abdominal Pain (With Emphasis on Functional Abdominal Pain Syndrome); A Biopsychosocial Understanding of Gastrointestinal Illness and Disease

David E. Elliott, MD, PhD
Associate Professor of Medicine, University of Iowa School of Medicine; University of Iowa Hospitals and Clinics, Iowa City, Iowa
Intestinal Infections by Parasitic Worms

Grace H. Elta, MD
Professor of Medicine, University of Michigan School of Medicine, Ann Arbor, Michigan
Motility and Dysmotility of the Biliary Tract and Sphincter of Oddi

Geoffrey C. Farrell, MD, FRACP
Robert W. Storr Professor of Hepatic Medicine, University of Sydney; Director, Storr Liver Unit, Westmead Millennium Institute, Westmead Hospital, Westmead, New South Wales, Australia
Liver Disease Caused by Drugs, Anesthetics, and Toxins

James J. Farrell, MD
Faculty, Division of Digestive Diseases, University of California, Los Angeles, School of Medicine, Los Angeles, California
Digestion and Absorption of Nutrients and Vitamins

Richard J. Farrell, MD, MRCPI
Assistant Professor of Medicine, Harvard Medical School; Associate Physician, Division of Gastroenterology, Beth Israel Deaconess Medical Center, Boston, Massachusetts
Celiac Sprue and Refractory Sprue

Michael J. G. Farthing, DSc(Med), MD, FRCP
Executive Dean and Professor of Medicine, University of Glasgow Faculty of Medicine, Glasgow, Scotland
Tropical Malabsorption and Tropical Diarrhea

Mark Feldman, MD, FACP
Clinical Professor of Internal Medicine, University of Texas Southwestern Medical School; William O. Tschumy, Jr., M.D. Chair of Internal Medicine, Presbyterian Hospital of Dallas, Dallas, Texas
Gastric Secretion; Gastritis and Other Gastropathies

Carlos Fernández-del Castillo, MD
Associate Professor of Surgery, Harvard Medical School; Associate Visiting Surgeon, Massachusetts General Hospital, Boston, Masschusetts
Pancreatic Cancer, Cystic Pancreatic Neoplasms, and Other Nonendocrine Pancreatic Tumors

J. Gregory Fitz, MD
Waterman Professor of Medicine, University of Colorado Health Sciences Center; Head, Division of Gastroenterology and Hepatology, University of Colorado Health Sciences Center, Denver, Colorado
Hepatic Encephalopathy, Hepatopulmonary Syndromes, Hepatorenal Syndrome, Coagulopathy, and Endocrine Complications of Liver Disease

David E. Fleischer, MD
Professor of Medicine, Mayo School of Medicine; Chair, Division of Gastroenterology and Hepatology, Mayo Clinic Scottsdale, Scottsdale, Arizona
Esophageal Tumors

Chris E. Forsmark, MD
Associate Professor of Medicine, Chief of Endoscopy, Division of Gastroenterology, Hepatology, and Nutrition, University of Florida, Gainesville, Florida
Chronic Pancreatitis

Ronald Fried, MD
Staff Physician, University Hospital, Basel, Switzerland
Proctitis and Sexually Transmissible Intestinal Disease

Lawrence S. Friedman, MD
Professor of Medicine, Harvard Medical School; Physician, Gastrointestinal Unit, and Chief, Walter Bauer Firm (Medical Services), Massachusetts General Hospital, Boston, Massachusetts
A Short Treatise on Bowel Sounds; Liver Abscess and Bacterial, Parasitic, Fungal, and Granulomatous Liver Disease

Cheryl E. Gariepy, MD
Assistant Professor of Pediatrics, University of Michigan School of Medicine, Ann Arbor, Michigan
Anatomy, Histology, Embryology, and Developmental Anomalies of the Small and Large Intestine

Gregory G. Ginsberg, MD
Associate Professor of Medicine, University of Pennsylvania School of Medicine; Director of Endoscopic Services, Gastroenterology Division, Hospital of the University of Pennsylvania, Philadelphia, Pennsylvania
Foreign Bodies and Bezoars; Esophageal Tumors

Robert E. Glasgow, MD
Assistant Professor, Department of Surgery, University of Utah Health Sciences Center, Salt Lake City, Utah
Abdominal Pain, Including the Acute Abdomen; Surgical Management of Gallstone Disease and Postoperative Complications

Sherwood L. Gorbach, MD
Professor of Medicine, Family Medicine, and Community Health, Tufts University School of Medicine; Attending Physician, New England Medical Center and St. Elizabeth's Medical Center, Boston, Massachusetts
Infectious Diarrhea and Bacterial Food Poisoning

David Y. Graham, MD
Professor of Medicine and Molecular Virology and Microbiology, Baylor College of Medicine; Chief of Gastroenterology, Veterans Affairs Medical Center, Houston, Texas
Helicobacter pylori

David A. Greenwald, MD
Associate Professor of Medicine, Albert Einstein College of Medicine; Attending Physician and Fellowship Program Director, Division of Gastroenterology, Montefiore Medical Center, Bronx, New York
Vascular Lesions of the Gastrointestinal Tract

Clark R. Gregg, MD
Professor of Internal Medicine, University of Texas Southwestern Medical School; Chief, Medical Service, Veterans Affairs North Texas Health Care System, Dallas, Texas
Enteric Bacterial Flora and Small Bowel Bacterial Overgrowth Syndrome

Richard L. Guerrant, MD
Professor of Medicine and Chief, Division of Geographic and International Medicine, University of Virginia, Charlottesville, Virginia
Intestinal Protozoa

Davidson H. Hamer, MD
Assistant Professor of Medicine and Nutrition, Tufts University School of Medicine; Adjunct Assistant Professor of International Health, Boston University School of Public Health; Director, Traveler's Health Service, and Attending Physician, New England Medical Center, Boston, Massachusetts
Infectious Diarrhea and Bacterial Food Poisoning

Heinz F. Hammer, MD
Associate Professor of Internal Medicine, University of Graz, Department of Internal Medicine, Division of Gastroenterology and Hepatology, Graz, Austria
Maldigestion and Malabsorption

William Harford, MD
Professor of Internal Medicine, University of Texas Southwestern Medical School; Chief, Gastrointestinal Endoscopy, Veterans Affairs North Texas Health Care System, Dallas, Texas
Diverticula of the Hypopharynx, Esophagus, Stomach, Jejunum, and Ileum; Abdominal Hernias and Their Complications, Including Gastric Volvulus

Christoph Högenauer, MD
Fellow in Gastroenterology, Department of Internal Medicine, Division of Gastroenterology, University of Graz, Graz, Austria
Maldigestion and Malabsorption

Jay D. Horton, MD
Assistant Professor of Internal Medicine and Molecular Genetics, University of Texas Southwestern Medical Center, Dallas, Texas
Gallstone Disease and Its Complications

Tracy Hull, MD
Staff Surgeon, Colon and Rectal Surgery, and Director, Anal Physiology Section, The Cleveland Clinic Foundation, Cleveland, Ohio
Examination and Diseases of the Anorectum

Christopher D. Huston, MD
Division of Infectious Diseases, University of Virginia, Charlottesville, Virginia
Intestinal Protozoa

Steven H. Itzkowitz, MD
Dr. Burrill B. Crohn Professor of Medicine, Mount Sinai School of Medicine; Director, Dr. Henry D. Janowitz Division of Gastroenterology, Mount Sinai Hospital, New York City, New York
Colonic Polyps and Polyposis Syndromes

Robert T. Jensen, MD
Chief, Digestive Diseases Branch, National Institutes of Health, Bethesda, Maryland
Pancreatic Endocrine Tumors

Khursheed N. Jeejeebhoy, MBBS, PhD, FRCPC
Professor, University of Toronto; Director, Nutrition and Digestive Disease Program, St. Michael's Hospital, Toronto, Ontario, Canada
The Malnourished Patient: Nutritional Assessment and Management

Derek P. Jewell, DPhil, FRCP, F Med Sci
Professor of Gastroenterology, University of Oxford; Consultant Physician, John Radcliffe Hospital, Oxford, United Kingdom
Ulcerative Colitis

Rohan Jeyarajah, MD, FACS
Assistant Professor, Departments of Surgery and Internal Medicine, University of Texas Southwestern Medical Center; Attending Surgeon, Parkland Memorial Hospital, Zale Lipshy University Hospital, and Veterans Administration Medical Center, Dallas, Texas
Diverticula of the Hypopharynx, Esophagus, Stomach, Jejunum, and Ileum; Abdominal Hernias and Their Complications, Including Gastric Volvulus

Ramon E. Jimenez, MD
Fellow in Surgical Oncology, Memorial Sloan-Kettering Cancer Center, New York, New York
Pancreatic Cancer, Cystic Pancreatic Neoplasms, and Other Nonendocrine Pancreatic Tumors

Daniel B. Jones, MD, FACS
Assistant Professor, Department of Surgery, University of Texas Southwestern Medical Center; Director, Southwestern Center for Minimally Invasive Surgery, University of Texas Southwestern Medical Center, Dallas, Texas
Current Role of Surgery in Peptic Ulcer Disease

Peter J. Kahrilas, MD
Marquardt Professor of Medicine, Northwestern University Medical School; Chief, Gastroenterology and Hepatology, Northwestern Memorial Hospital, Chicago, Illinois
Gastroesophageal Reflux Disease and Its Complications, Including Barrett's Metaplasia

David J. Kearney, MD
Assistant Professor of Medicine, University of Washington School of Medicine; Staff Physician, Veterans Administration Puget Sound Health Care System, Seattle, Washington
Esophageal Disorders Caused by Infection, Systemic Illness, Medications, Radiation, and Trauma

Emmet B. Keeffe, MD
Professor of Medicine, Stanford University School of Medicine; Chief of Hepatology and Co-Director, Liver Transplant Program, Stanford University Medical Center, Stanford, California
Complications of Gastrointestinal Endoscopy

David J. Keljo, MD, PhD
Visiting Associate Professor of Pediatrics, University of Pittsburgh School of Medicine; Attending Pediatric Gastroenterologist, Children's Hospital of Pittsburgh, Pittsburgh, Pennsylvania
Anatomy, Histology, Embryology, and Developmental Anomalies of the Small and Large Intestine

Ciarán P. Kelly, MD
Associate Professor of Medicine, Harvard Medical School; Associate Physician, Division of Gastroenterology, Beth Israel Deaconess Medical Center, Boston, Massachusetts
Celiac Sprue and Refractory Sprue

Michael C. Kew, PhD, MD, DSc
Dora Dart Professor of Medicine, University of the Witwatersrand Medical School; Director, MRC/CAMSA/ University Molecular Hepatology Research Unit; Consultant Hepatologist, Johannesburg Academic and Baragwanath Hospitals; Honorary Research Associate, South African Institute for Medical Research, Johannesburg, South Africa
Hepatic Tumors and Cysts

David D. Kim, MD
Senior Gastroenterology Fellow, University of California, San Francisco, San Francisco, California
Gastrointestinal Manifestations of Systemic Disease

Karen E. Kim, MD
Assistant Professor of Clinical Medicine, University of Chicago; Director, Colorectal Cancer Prevention Clinic, Chicago, Illinois
Protein-Losing Gastroenteropathy

Lawrence T. Kim, MD
Assistant Professor of Surgery and of Cell Biology and Neuroscience, University of Texas Southwestern Medical Center; Assistant Chief, Surgical Service, Veterans Administration North Texas Health Care System, Dallas, Texas
Gastrointestinal Carcinoid Tumors and the Carcinoid Syndrome

Samuel Klein, MD
William H. Danforth Professor of Medicine and Nutritional Science; Director, Center for Human Nutrition, Washington University School of Medicine, St. Louis, Missouri
The Malnourished Patient: Nutritional Assessment and Management; Enteral and Parenteral Nutrition; Assistant Editor (Nutrition)

Theodore J. Koh, MD
Assistant Professor of Medicine, University of Massachusetts Medical School, Worcester, Massachusetts
Tumors of the Stomach

Braden Kuo, MD
Instructor in Medicine, Harvard Medical School; Assistant Physician, Gastrointestinal Unit (Medical Services), Massachusetts General Hospital, Boston, Massachusetts
A Short Treatise on Bowel Sounds

Jeanne M. LaBerge, MD
Professor of Radiology, University of California, San Francisco, School of Medicine; Interventional Radiologist, Moffitt-Long and Mount Zion Hospital, San Francisco, California
Endoscopic and Radiologic Treatment of Biliary Disease

John R. Lake, MD
Professor of Medicine and Surgery, University of Minnesota School of Medicine; Department of Medicine, Fairview University Medical Center, Minneapolis, Minnesota
Gastrointestinal Complications of Solid Organ and Hematopoietic Cell Transplantation

Edward L. Lee, MD
Professor of Pathology, University of Texas Southwestern Medical Center; Chief of Pathology and Laboratory Medicine Service, Department of Veterans Affairs Medical Center, Dallas, Texas
Gastritis and Other Gastropathies; Assistant Editor (Pathology)

Makau Lee, MD, PhD
Clinical Professor of Medicine, University of Mississippi Medical Center, Jackson, Mississippi
Nausea and Vomiting

John E. Lennard-Jones, MD, DSc(Hon), FRCP, FRCS
Emeritus Professor of Gastroenterology, University of London, London; Emeritus Consultant Gastroenterologist, St. Mark's Hospital, Harrow, England
Constipation

Mike A. Leonis, MD, PhD
Fellow in Pediatric Gastroenterology, Hepatology, and Nutrition, Children's Hospital Medical Center, Cincinnati Ohio
Inherited Metabolic Disorders of the Liver

Michael D. Levitt, MD
A.C.O.S. Research, Minneapolis Veterans Affairs Medical Center; Professor of Medicine, University of Minnesota School of Medicine, Minneapolis, Minnesota
Intestinal Gas

Rodger A. Liddle, MD
Professor of Medicine, Duke University School of Medicine; Chief, Division of Gastroenterology, Duke University Medical Center, Durham, North Carolina
Gastrointestinal Hormones and Neurotransmitters

Steven D. Lidofsky, MD, PhD
Associate Professor of Medicine and Pharmacology, University of Vermont College of Medicine; Director of Hepatology, Fletcher-Allen Health Care, Burlington, Vermont
Jaundice; Acute Liver Failure

Keith D. Lillemoe, MD
Professor and Vice-Chairman, Department of Surgery, Johns Hopkins University School of Medicine; Deputy Director, Department of Surgery, Johns Hopkins Hospital, Baltimore, Maryland
Tumors of the Gallbladder, Bile Ducts, and Ampulla

Keith D. Lindor, MD
Professor of Medicine, Mayo Medical School; Chair, Division of Gastroenterology and Hepatology, and Consultant, Division of Gastroenterology and Hepatology, Mayo Clinic and Foundation, Rochester, Minnesota
Primary Biliary Cirrhosis

Peter M. Loeb, MD
Clinical Professor of Medicine, University of Texas Southwestern Medical School; Chief of Gastroenterology, Director of Gastroenterology Laboratory, Presbyterian Hospital of Dallas, Dallas, Texas
Caustic Injury to the Upper Gastrointestinal Tract

John D. Long, MD
Assistant Professor of Medicine, University of Cincinnati College of Medicine; Director, Gastrointestinal Clinic, University Hospital, Cincinnati, Ohio
Anatomy, Histology, Embryology, and Developmental Anomalies of the Esophagus

David J. Magee, MD
Assistant Professor, Division of Gastroenterology, University of Texas Southwestern Medical Center, Dallas, Texas
Anatomy, Histology, Embryology, and Developmental Anomalies of the Pancreas

Uma Mahadevan, MD
Assistant Clinical Professor of Medicine, University of California, San Francisco, School of Medicine; Director of Clinical Research, Inflammatory Bowel Disease Center, Mount Zion Hospital, San Francisco, California
Sclerosing Cholangitis and Recurrent Pyogenic Cholangitis

Jacquelyn J. Maher, MD
Associate Professor of Medicine, University of California, San Francisco, School of Medicine; Attending Physician in Medicine and Gastroenterology, San Francisco General Hospital, San Francisco, California
Alcoholic Liver Disease

Matthias Maiwald, MD
Visiting Scholar, Department of Microbiology and Immunology, Stanford University School of Medicine, Stanford, California
Whipple's Disease

Arshad Malik, MD
Fellow, University of Texas Southwestern Medical Center, Dallas, Texas
Short Bowel Syndrome

Paul Martin, MD
Professor of Medicine, University of California, Los Angeles, School of Medicine; Medical Director, Liver Transplant Program, Cedars Sinai Medical Center, Los Angeles, California
Liver Transplantation

Elizabeth J. McConnell, MD
Assistant Professor of Surgery, Mayo School of Medicine; Senior Associate Consultant, Mayo Clinic Scottsdale, Scottsdale, Arizona
Megacolon: Congenital and Acquired

George B. McDonald, MD
Professor of Medicine, University of Washington School of Medicine; Head, Gastroenterology/Hepatology Section, Fred Hutchinson Cancer Research Center, Seattle, Washington
Esophageal Disorders Caused by Infection, Systemic Illness, Medications, Radiation, and Trauma

Kenneth R. McQuaid, MD
Professor of Clinical Medicine, University of California, San Francisco, School of Medicine; Director of Endoscopy, Veterans Affairs Medical Center, San Francisco, California
Dyspepsia

Joseph P. Minei, MD
Associate Professor of Surgery, Chief, Section of Trauma and Critical Care, Division of Burn, Trauma, and Critical Care, University of Texas Southwestern Medical Center; Medical Director of Trauma Services, Surgeon-in-Chief, Parkland Health and Hospital System, Dallas, Texas
Abdominal Abscesses and Gastrointestinal Fistulas

Ginat W. Mirowski
Assistant Professor, Department of Dermatology, Oral Pathology, Medicine, and Radiology, Indiana University School of Medicine, Indianapolis, Indiana
Oral Disease and Oral-Cutaneous Manifestations of Gastrointestinal and Liver Disease

Sean J. Mulvihill, MD
Professor and Chairman, Department of Surgery, University of Utah Health Sciences Center, Salt Lake City, Utah
Abdominal Pain, Including the Acute Abdomen; Surgical Management of Gallstone Disease and Postoperative Complications

Nam P. Nguyen, MD
Clinical Assistant Professor, University of Texas Southwestern Medical Center; Radiation Oncologist, Dallas Veterans Administration Medical Center, Dallas, Texas
Radiation Enteritis

Jeffrey A. Norton, MD
Department of Surgery, University of California, San Francisco; Chief, Surgical Service, San Francisco Veterans Affairs Medical Center, San Francisco, California
Pancreatic Endocrine Tumors

Michael J. Nunez, MD
Department of Internal Medicine, Division of Gastroenterology, Presbyterian Hospital of Dallas, Dallas, Texas
Caustic Injury to the Upper Gastrointestinal Tract

Roy C. Orlando, MD
Professor of Medicine and Physiology, Tulane University Medical School; Chief, Gastroenterology and Hepatology, Tulane University Medical Center, New Orleans, Louisiana
Anatomy, Histology, Embryology, and Developmental Anomalies of the Esophagus

James W. Ostroff, MD
Clinical Professor of Medicine and Pediatrics, University of California, San Francisco, School of Medicine; Director, Endoscopy Unit and Gastrointestinal Consultation Service, Moffitt-Long and Mount Zion Hospital, San Francisco, California
Endoscopic and Radiologic Treatment of Biliary Disease

Stephen J. Pandol, MD
Professor of Medicine, University of California, Los Angeles, School of Medicine; Staff Physician, Veterans Administration Greater Los Angeles Health Care System, Los Angeles, California
Pancreatic Physiology and Secretory Testing

John E. Pandolfino, MD
Assistant Professor, Northwestern University Medical School; Attending Physician, Northwestern Memorial Hospital, Chicago, Illinois
Gastroesophageal Reflux Disease and Its Complications, Including Barrett's Metaplasia

Lisa Ann Panzini, MD
Assistant Clinical Professor of Medicine, Yale University School of Medicine; Connecticut Gastroenterology Consultants, PC, New Haven, Connecticut
Isolated and Diffuse Ulcers of the Small Intestine

Gustav Paumgartner, MD
Professor of Medicine, Department of Medicine II, Klinikum Grosshadern, University of Munich, Munich, Germany
Nonsurgical Management of Gallstone Disease

John H. Pemberton, MD
Professor of Surgery, Mayo Graduate School of Medicine; Consultant, Colon and Rectal Surgery, Mayo Clinic and Mayo Foundation, Rochester, Minnesota
Ileostomy and Its Alternatives; Megacolon: Congenital and Acquired

Walter L. Peterson, MD
Professor of Medicine, University of Texas Southwestern Medical Center; Staff Physician, Department of Veterans Affairs Medical Center, Dallas, Texas
Helicobacter pylori

Patrick R. Pfau, MD

Assistant Professor of Medicine, University of Wisconsin Medical School; Division of Gastroenterology, University of Wisconsin Hospital and Clinic, Madison, Wisconsin
Foreign Bodies and Bezoars

Sidney F. Phillips, MD

Professor of Medicine, Mayo Graduate School of Medicine; Mayo Clinic and Mayo Foundation, Rochester, Minnesota
Ileostomy and Its Alternatives

Joseph R. Pisegna, MD

Associate Professor, Department of Medicine, University of California, Los Angeles, School of Medicine; Chief, Division of Gastroenterology and Hepatology, Veterans Administration Greater Los Angeles Healthcare System, Los Angeles, California
Zollinger-Ellison Syndrome and Other Hypersecretory States

Daniel K. Podolsky, MD

Mallinckrodt Professor of Medicine, Harvard Medical School; Chief, Gastrointestinal Unit, Massachusetts General Hospital, Boston, Massachusetts
Cellular Growth and Neoplasia

Fred Poordad, MD

Assistant Professor of Medicine, University of California, Los Angeles, School of Medicine; Hepatologist, Cedars Sinai Medical Center, Los Angeles, California
Nonalcoholic Fatty Liver Disease

Deborah D. Proctor, MD

Associate Professor of Medicine, Section of Digestive Diseases, Department of Internal Medicine, Yale University School of Medicine; Attending Physician, Yale-New Haven Hospital, New Haven, Connecticut
Isolated and Diffuse Ulcers of the Small Intestine

Eamonn M. M. Quigley, MD, FRCP, FACP, FRCPI, FACG

Professor of Medicine and Human Physiology, Head of the Medical School, National University of Ireland; Consultant Physician and Gastroenterologist, Cork University Hospital, Cork, Ireland
Gastric Motor and Sensory Function, and Motor Disorders of the Stomach

Nicholas W. Read, MA, MD, FRCP

Professor of Integrated Medicine, Institute of General Practice, University of Sheffield; Consultant Gastroenterologist and Psychoanalytical Psychotherapist, Northern General Hospital, Sheffield, United Kingdom
Irritable Bowel Syndrome

Carol A. Redel, MD

Assistant Professor of Pediatrics, University of Texas Southwestern Medical School; Attending Physician, Pediatric Gastroenterology, Children's Medical Center of Dallas, Dallas, Texas
Anatomy, Histology, Embryology, and Developmental Anomalies of the Stomach and Duodenum

Robert V. Rege, MD, FACS

Professor and Chairman, Department of Surgery, University of Texas Southwestern Medical School, Dallas, Texas
Current Role of Surgery in Peptic Ulcer Disease

David A. Relman, MD

Associate Professor of Medicine, Microbiology, and Immunology, Stanford University School of Medicine, Stanford; Staff Physician, Veterans Affairs Palo Alto Health Care System, Palo Alto, California
Whipple's Disease

Joel E. Richter, MD

Chairman, Department of Gastroenterology, Cleveland Clinic Foundation; Professor of Medicine, The Cleveland Clinic Foundation Health Center of the Ohio State University, Cleveland, Ohio
Dysphagia, Odynophagia, Heartburn, and Other Esophageal Symptoms

Caroline A. Riely, MD

Professor of Medicine and Pediatrics, University of Tennessee School of Medicine, Memphis, Tennessee
Pregnancy-Related Hepatic and Gastrointestinal Disorders

Eve A. Roberts, MD, FRCPC

Professor of Pediatrics, Medicine, and Pharmacology, Division of Gastroenterology and Nutrition, The Hospital for Sick Children, Toronto, Ontario, Canada
Wilson Disease

Don C. Rockey, MD

Associate Professor of Medicine, Duke University School of Medicine; Director, Liver Center, Duke University Medical Center, Durham, North Carolina
Gastrointestinal Bleeding

Hugo R. Rosen, MD

Associate Professor of Medicine, Molecular Microbiology, and Immunology, Portland Veterans Administration Medical Center; Medical Director, Liver Transplantation Program, Portland, Oregon
Liver Transplantation

Deborah C. Rubin, MD

Associate Professor of Medicine, Washington University School of Medicine, St. Louis, Missouri
Enteral and Parenteral Nutrition

Bruce A. Runyon, MD

Professor of Medicine, University of Southern California, Los Angeles, School of Medicine, Los Angeles; Chief, Liver Unit, Rancho Los Amigos Medical Center, Downey, California
Ascites and Spontaneous Bacterial Peritonitis; Surgical Peritonitis and Other Diseases of the Peritoneum, Mesentery, Omentum, and Diaphragm

Anil K. Rustgi, MD

T. Grier Miller Associate Professor of Medicine and Genetics, University of Pennsylvania School of Medicine; Chief of Gastroenterology, University of Pennsylvania, Philadelphia, Pennsylvania
Cellular Growth and Neoplasia; Small Intestinal Neoplasms

James C. Ryan, MD
Associate Professor, University of California, San Francisco, School of Medicine, San Francisco, California
Gastrointestinal Manifestations of Systemic Disease

Hugh A. Sampson, MD
Professor of Pediatrics and Biomedical Sciences, Mount Sinai School of Medicine, New York University; Director, General Clinical Research Center, and Chief, Pediatric Allergy and Immunology, Mount Sinai Hospital, New York, New York
Food Allergies

Bruce E. Sands, MD, SM(Epidem)
Assistant Professor of Medicine, Harvard Medical School; Assistant in Medicine and Director, Clinical Research, Gastrointestinal Unit, Massachusetts General Hospital, Boston, Massachusetts
Crohn's Disease

George A. Sarosi, Jr., MD
Assistant Professor, Department of Surgery, University of Texas Southwestern Medical School; Staff Surgeon, Dallas Veterans Affairs Medical Center, Dallas, Texas
Appendicitis

R. Balfour Sartor, MD
Professor of Medicine, Microbiology, and Immunology, University of North Carolina at Chapel Hill School of Medicine; Director, Multidisciplinary Center for IBD Research and Treatment, University of North Carolina, Chapel Hill, North Carolina
Mucosal Immunology and Mechanisms of Gastrointestinal Inflammation

Daniel F. Schafer, MD
Associate Professor of Medicine, Department of Internal Medicine, University of Nebraska School of Medicine; Adult Hepatologist, University of Nebraska Medical Center, Omaha, Nebraska
Vascular Diseases of the Liver

Bruce F. Scharschmidt, MD
Adjunct Professor of Medicine, University of California, San Francisco, School of Medicine, San Francisco; Vice President, Clinical Development, Chiron Corporation, Emeryville, California
Biochemical Liver Tests; Consulting Editor

Lawrence R. Schiller, MD
Clinical Professor of Internal Medicine, University of Texas Southwestern Medical Center; Program Director, Gastroenterology Fellowship, Baylor University Medical Center, Dallas, Texas
Diarrhea; Fecal Incontinence

Michael D. Schuffler, MD
Professor, Department of Medicine, University of Washington School of Medicine; Chief of Gastroenterology, PacMed Clinics, Seattle, Washington
Chronic Intestinal Pseudo-Obstruction

Joseph H. Sellin, MD
Professor of Medicine and Integrative Biology; Director, Division of Gastroenterology, Hepatology, and Nutrition; Director, Gastroenterology Fellowship Training Program, The University of Texas Medical School–Houston; Director, Gastroenterology Service, Memorial Hermann Hospital; Director, Gastroenterology Service, Lyndon Baines Johnson General Hospital, Houston, Texas
Diarrhea; Intestinal Electrolyte Absorption and Secretion

Michael A. Shetzline, MD, PhD
Assistant Professor of Medicine, Duke University School of Medicine, Durham, North Carolina
Gastrointestinal Hormones and Neurotransmitters

G. Thomas Shires III, MD
Clinical Professor of Surgery, University of Texas Southwestern Medical Center; Chairman, Surgical Services, Presbyterian Hospital of Dallas, Dallas, Texas
Diverticular Disease of the Colon

Clifford L. Simmang, MD, MS
Associate Professor of Surgery, University of Texas Southwestern Medical Center; Attending Surgeon, Parkland Memorial Hospital and Zale Lipshy University Hospital, Dallas, Texas
Diverticular Disease of the Colon

Taylor A. Sohn, MD
Resident, General Surgery, Johns Hopkins Medical Institutions, Baltimore, Maryland
Tumors of the Gallbladder, Bile Ducts, and Ampulla

Michael F. Sorrell, MD
Robert L. Grissan Professor, University of Nebraska College of Medicine; Hepatologist, Department of Internal Medicine, University of Nebraska Medical Center, Omaha, Nebraska
Vascular Diseases of the Liver

Stuart Jon Spechler, MD
Professor of Medicine and Berta M. and Cecil O. Patterson Chair in Gastroenterology, University of Texas Southwestern Medical Center; Chief, Division of Gastroenterology, Dallas Veterans Administration Medical Center, Dallas, Texas
Peptic Ulcer Disease and Its Complications

Andrew Stolz, MD
Associate Professor of Medicine, Keck School of Medicine, University of Southern California, Los Angeles, California
Liver Physiology and Metabolic Function

Fabrizis L. Suarez, MD, PhD
Adjunct Assistant Professor, School of Allied Medical Professions, The Ohio State University; Associate Director, Medical Affairs Medical Nutrition, Ross Product Division, Abbott Laboratories, Columbus, Ohio
Intestinal Gas

José Such, MD
Consultant, Liver Unit, Hospital General Universitario, Alicante, Spain
Surgical Peritonitis and Other Diseases of the Peritoneum, Mesentery, Omentum, and Diaphragm

Frederick J. Suchy, MD
Herbert H. Lehman Professor and Chair, Department of Pediatrics, Mount Sinai School of Medicine, New York University; Pediatrician-in-Chief, Mount Sinai Hospital, New York, New York
Anatomy, Histology, Embryology, Developmental Anomalies, and Pediatric Disorders of the Biliary Tract

Christina Surawicz, MD
Professor of Medicine, University of Washington School of Medicine; Section Chief, Gastroenterology, Harborview Medical Center, Seattle, Washington
Proctitis and Sexually Transmissible Intestinal Disease

Nicholas J. Talley, MD, PhD
Professor of Medicine, University of Sydney; Head, Division of Medicine, Nepean Hospital, Penrith, New South Wales, Australia
Eosinophilic Gastroenteritis

Dwain L. Thiele, MD
Professor of Internal Medicine, Vice-Chief, Division of Digestive and Liver Diseases and Chief of Hepatology, University of Texas Southwestern Medical Center; Chief of Liver Diseases Service, Parkland Health and Hospital System; Attending Physician, Zale Lipshy University Hospital, Dallas, Texas
Hepatic Manifestations of Systemic Disease and Other Disorders of the Liver

Phillip P. Toskes, MD
Professor of Internal Medicine and Chairman, Department of Medicine, University of Florida College of Medicine, Gainesville, Florida
Enteric Bacterial Flora and Small Bowel Bacterial Overgrowth Syndrome

Richard H. Turnage, MD
Professor and Chair, Department of Surgery, Louisiana State University School of Medicine, Shreveport, Louisiana
Appendicitis; Intestinal Obstruction and Ileus

Axel von Herbay, MD
Lecturer, Institute of Pathology, University of Heidelberg, Heidelberg, Germany
Whipple's Disease

Arnold Wald, MD
Professor of Medicine, University of Pittsburgh School of Medicine; Associate Chief for Education and Training, Division of Gastroenterology, Hepatology, and Nutrition Support, University of Pittsburgh Medical Center, Pittsburgh, Pennsylvania
Other Diseases of the Colon and Rectum

Timothy C. Wang, MD
Gladys Smith Martin Professor of Medicine, Chief, Division of Digestive Diseases and Nutrition, University of Massachusetts Memorial Medical School, Worcester, Massachusetts
Tumors of the Stomach

Ian R. Wanless, MD, FRCPC
Professor of Pathology, University of Toronto; Staff Pathologist, Toronto General Hospital, Toronto, Ontario, Canada
Anatomy, Histology, Embryology, and Developmental Anomalies of the Liver

Sally Weisdorf-Schindele, MD
Associate Professor, Pediatric Gastroenterology, Hepatology, and Nutrition, University of Minnesota School of Medicine; Pediatric Gastroenterology, Hepatology, and Nutrition, University/Fairview Medical Center, Minneapolis, Minnesota
Gastrointestinal Complications of Solid Organ and Hematopoietic Cell Transplantation

Henrik Westergaard, MD
Professor of Internal Medicine, University of Texas Southwestern Medical Center, Dallas, Texas
Short Bowel Syndrome

David C. Whitcomb, MD, PhD
University of Pittsburgh Medical Center, Pittsburgh, Pennsylvania
Hereditary and Childhood Disorders of the Pancreas, Including Cystic Fibrosis

C. Mel Wilcox, MD
Professor of Medicine and Director, Division of Gastroenterology and Hepatology, University of Alabama at Birmingham, Birmingham, Alabama
Gastrointestinal Consequences of Infection with Human Immunodeficiency Virus

Teresa L. Wright, MD
Professor of Medicine, University of California, San Francisco, School of Medicine; Chief, Gastroenterology Section, Veterans Administration Medical Center, San Francisco, California
Viral Hepatitis

Francis Y. Yao, MD
Associate Clinical Professor of Medicine, University of California, San Francisco, School of Medicine; Associate Medical Director, Liver Transplant Program, University of California, San Francisco, Hospitals, San Francisco, California
Portal Hypertension and Variceal Bleeding

Hal F. Yee, Jr., MD, PhD
Assistant Professor of Medicine and Physiology, University of California, Los Angeles, School of Medicine; Attending Physician, University of California, Los Angeles, Medical Center and Greater Los Angeles Veterans Affairs Healthcare System, Los Angeles, California
Acute Liver Failure

FOREWORD

I consider it an enormous honor to be writing the foreword to this the seventh edition of Sleisenger and Fordtran's *Gastrointestinal and Liver Disease*. Those asked to write forewords to earlier editions included Franz Ingelfinger and Tom Almy. These two giants were, in Dean Acheson's words, "present at the conception" of modern, science-based gastroenterology. I was lucky enough to be "present at the conception" of the first modern, science-based textbook of gastroenterology. Marvin Sleisenger and John Fordtran, who trained with Tom Almy and Franz Ingelfinger, respectively, invited experts concerned with virtually every aspect of gastrointestinal and biliary tract disease to put together the first edition of *Gastrointestinal Disease: Pathophysiology, Diagnosis, and Management*. And what a wonderful textbook it turned out to be! It was well organized and contained authoritative, up-to-date chapters describing both scientific advances and clinical features. The scope of the book and the quality of its content assured its immediate, wholehearted, and widespread acceptance.

As they produced the next five editions, the editors refused to stand still and take the book's continuing success for granted. Instead, they kept to the task of changing with the times while sustaining excellence. More and more illustrations were added to demonstrate histologic, radiologic, and endoscopic abnormalities. Experts were recruited who came from disciplines outside traditional gastroenterology but whose interests were relevant to gastrointestinal function and disease. The scope of the book was broadened to include a section on liver disease, an entirely appropriate expansion because meaningful practice of gastroenterology is not possible without adequate knowledge of liver disease, just as the practice of hepatology requires an understanding of diseases of the gastrointestinal and biliary tracts.

And now 30 years after this remarkable textbook began, here comes the seventh edition. The tradition of excellence continues in this edition with its concise coverage of relevant basic science and pathophysiology, its meticulous, judicious chapters on disease, and—most important—the careful editing, organization, referencing, and indexing that make a textbook easy to use. Happily, I continue to see among the array of outstanding authors experts outside the mainstream of gastroenterology, such as David Relman in microbiology and John Bartlett and Sherwood Gorbach in infectious disease, to name but three. The inclusion of authorities from other disciplines adds an important dimension. The editors have further strengthened the book by increasing the number and improving the quality of diagnostic images—whether they be radiologic, endoscopic, or pathologic—that are of ever-increasing importance to gastroenterologists.

Readers will no doubt continue to use the seventh edition much as they have in the past. Practitioners will review chapters to answer questions about their patients or to prepare a talk for their colleagues. Academic gastroenterologists will bring themselves up to date in areas outside their own specific expertise and will frequently refer to the book at conferences and when supervising the work of fellows, residents, or medical students. Trainees and students of course will depend on the book, as they always have, to provide information for themselves and documentation they can use in case presentations. Of the many people who will be using the book, I envy most the students who'll be opening it for the first time to discover the astonishing world of digestive diseases. What a marvelous journey they're about to begin!

Robert M. Donaldson, Jr., MD
David Paige Smith Professor of Medicine Emeritus
Yale University School of Medicine

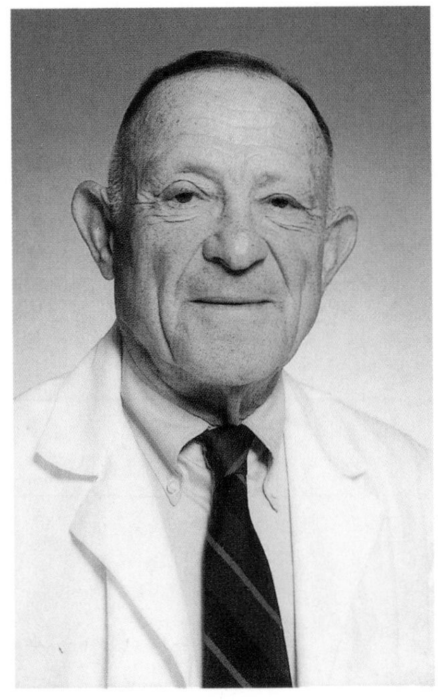

Marvin H. Sleisenger, MD
Editions 1–7

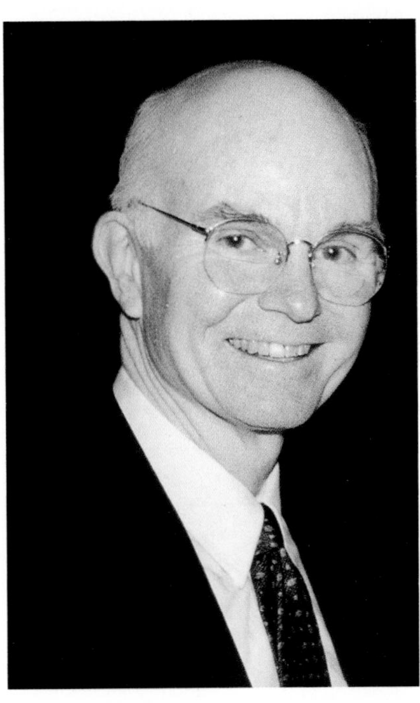

John S. Fordtran, MD
Editions 1–5

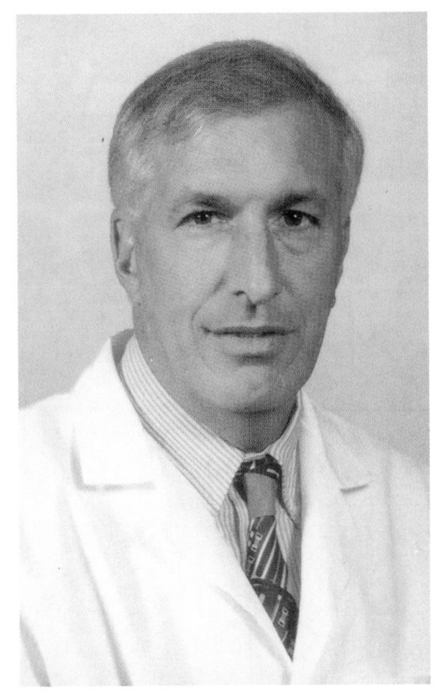

Mark Feldman, MD
Editions 5–7

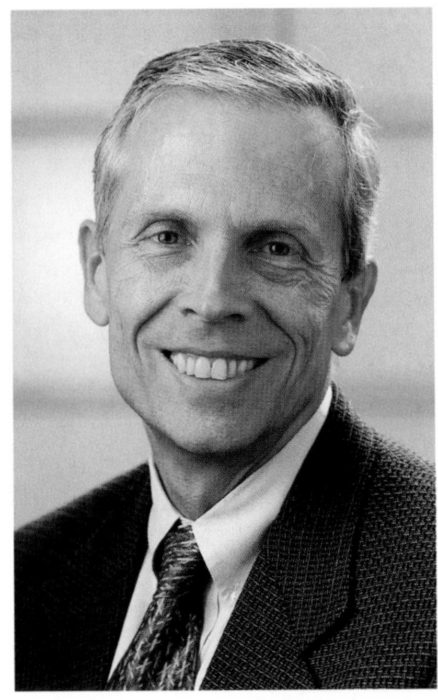

Bruce F. Scharschmidt, MD
Editions 5, 6

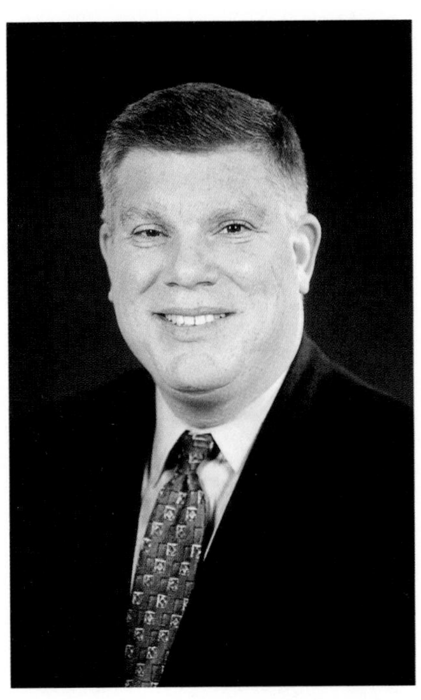

Lawrence S. Friedman, MD
Edition 7

PREFACE

The seventh edition of *Gastrointestinal and Liver Disease*, like its predecessors, is a comprehensive and authoritative textbook intended for gastroenterologists, trainees in gastroenterology, primary care physicians, residents in medicine and surgery, and medical students. The goal remains to produce a state-of-the-art, user-friendly textbook that covers disorders of the gastrointestinal tract, biliary tree, pancreas, and liver, as well as the related topics of nutrition and peritoneal disorders. Inclusion of a section on liver disease in the sixth edition was well received, and just as liver disease is integral to the practice of gastroenterology, so it has become integral to this textbook.

Considerable time and effort have been invested in improving and refining the seventh edition. A new editor, Lawrence S. Friedman, has replaced Bruce Scharschmidt, whose contributions to the fifth and sixth editions of the book and whose assistance in planning the seventh edition are gratefully acknowledged. As in the past, the editors have made a thorough and comprehensive review of the sixth edition, with the assistance of colleagues, fellows, and residents at our respective institutions, to correct deficiencies and eliminate redundancies. Because the practice of gastroenterology depends greatly on visual interpretation of endoscopic images, radiographs, and pathology specimens, a notable addition to the seventh edition is the designation of William R. Brugge as Imaging Editor and William Lee as Pathology Editor. Dr. Brugge reviewed endoscopic and radiographic figures submitted by authors to be certain that they were of the highest possible quality and, when appropriate, provided examples from his personal collection or other sources. Dr. Lee did the same for all submitted gross pathology illustrations and photomicrographs. As a result, the figures in this edition of the textbook are of exceptionally high quality and clarity. In addition, over 100 photographs that were submitted in color have been placed directly (in color) into the relevant chapters, rather than in a separate section of color plates or in a companion atlas, as was done in the sixth edition. The editors are confident that this arrangement will provide convenience and clarity for the reader.

Many aspects of the seventh edition will be familiar to the readers of previous editions. Section One deals with the Biology of the Gastrointestinal Tract and Liver with new up-to-date contributions on hormones and neurotransmitters by Dr. Liddle and on immunology and inflammation of the gastrointestinal tract by Dr. Sartor. Section Two on the Approach to Patients with Symptoms and Signs, which was reinstituted in the sixth edition, has been retained (with the addition of a short "treatise" on the history and significance of bowel sounds by Drs. Kuo and Friedman), as has Section Three on Nutrition and Gastroenterology, for which Samuel Klein again served as consulting editor. Section Four consists of Topics Involving Multiple Organs, including authoritative chapters on diverticula of the esophagus, stomach, and small bowel as well as on hernias and volvulus of the gastrointestinal tract by Drs. Harford and Jeyarajah. Sections Five through Eleven contain the chapters dealing with the broad spectrum of diseases of the esophagus, stomach and duodenum, pancreas, biliary tract, liver, small and large intestines, vascular disorders of the gut, and disorders of the peritoneum, mesentery, omentum, and diaphragm. Overall, nearly one third of the authors are new to this edition. There are now separate chapters on acute pancreatitis by Drs. DiMagno and Chari and chronic pancreatitis by Dr. Forsmark. In addition, there are separate chapters on protozoal intestinal diseases by Drs. Huston and Guerrant and on intestinal infections by worms, flukes, and other nonprotozoal parasites by Dr. Elliot. Finally, there is an eloquent concluding section on psychosocial factors in gastrointestinal disease by Dr. Drossman.

Successful features from previous editions have been retained. At the start of each chapter is a mini-outline with page citations. Each major section also contains a listing of the chapters with page citations in that section. High quality glossy paper continues to be used, and the text is amply illustrated with figures, tables, and algorithms. Chapters are appropriately cross-referenced, and the index remains extensive and useful for locating material quickly.

The seventh edition of this classic textbook remains true to the spirit of the first edition published nearly 30 years ago, namely, a critical overview of the state of gastrointestinal practice and its scientific underpinnings by eminent authorities in their respective fields. The book is truly international in scope, with authors from 11 different countries. Celebrating 30 years of excellence, this textbook remains the definitive resource for anyone involved in the care of patients with gastrointestinal and hepatic disorders.

MARK FELDMAN, MD
LAWRENCE S. FRIEDMAN, MD
MARVIN H. SLEISENGER, MD

ACKNOWLEDGMENTS

The Editors of the Seventh Edition are most grateful to more than 100 contributing authors from around the globe whose scholarship and clinical experience fill its pages. The editors also appreciate the support of our professional colleagues in Dallas, Boston, and San Francisco.

Vicky Robertson, Tracy Cooper, Hildreth Curran, and Rita Burns provided outstanding administrative support. The Editors have also greatly benefited from the contributions of the professional staff at Saunders, particularly Richard Zorab and Sue Hodgson, Melissa Dudlick, Marjory Fraser, Carol DiBerardino, and Angela Holt. We also acknowledge the valuable assistance provided by our two Assistant Editors, Edward Lee for Pathology and William Brugge for Imaging, and to Mukesh Harisinghani, who assisted Dr. Brugge. As in the sixth edition, Dr. Samuel Klein helped us immensely with the Nutrition chapters.

We are especially grateful for the constant encouragement and understanding of our wives, Barbara Feldman, Mary Jo Cappuccilli, and Lenore Sleisenger, and of our children, Matthew, Elizabeth, Daniel, and Lindsay Feldman; Matthew Friedman; and Thomas Sleisenger.

MARK FELDMAN, MD
LAWRENCE S. FRIEDMAN, MD
MARVIN H. SLEISENGER, MD

CONTENTS

Volume 1

Section One
BIOLOGY OF THE GASTROINTESTINAL TRACT AND LIVER

Section Two

APPROACH TO PATIENTS WITH SYMPTOMS AND SIGNS

Section Three
NUTRITION IN GASTROENTEROLOGY

Section Four
TOPICS INVOLVING MULTIPLE ORGANS

Section Five
ESOPHAGUS

Section Six

STOMACH AND DUODENUM

Section Seven

PANCREAS

Section Eight

BILIARY TRACT

Volume 2

Section Nine
LIVER

Section Ten
SMALL AND LARGE INTESTINE

Section Eleven
VASCULATURE AND SUPPORTING STRUCTURES

Section Twelve

PSYCHOSOCIAL FACTORS IN GASTROINTESTINAL DISEASE

Section Nine

LIVER

Chapter 62

Anatomy, Histology, Embryology, and Developmental Anomalies of the Liver

Ian R. Wanless

The knowledge of normal morphology is basic to the understanding of pathologic processes and the secure practice of hepatobiliary surgery. This chapter is a brief introduction to anatomy of the human liver and its variations. More detailed expositions can be found elsewhere.[1–4] Embryology of the liver is reviewed in Chapter 52.

SURFACE ANATOMY

The normal liver occupies the right upper quadrant, extending from the 5th intercostal space in the midclavicular line to the right costal margin. The lower margin of the liver descends below the costal margin during inspiration. The median liver weight is 1800 g in men and 1400 g in women.[5, 6]

Transcutaneous liver biopsies commonly are obtained in the midaxillary line through the 3rd interspace below the upper limit of liver dullness during full expiration. This usually is in the 9th intercostal space.

The superior, anterior, and right lateral surfaces of the liver are smooth and convex, fitting against the diaphragm. The posterior surface has indentations from the colon, right kidney, and duodenum on the right lobe and the stomach on the left lobe (Fig. 62–1).

The fibrous capsule on the posterior aspect of the liver reflects onto the diaphragm and posterior abdominal wall and leaves a "bare area" where the liver is in continuity with the retroperitoneum. The liver is supported by the peritoneal reflections that form the coronary ligaments, the right and left triangular ligaments, and the falciform ligament (see Fig. 62–1). The lower free edge of the falciform ligament contains the round ligament, which is composed largely of the obliterated umbilical vein. The falciform ligament joins the anterior surface of the liver to the diaphragm. Superiorly, the falciform ligament joins the peritoneal reflections to the left of the vena cava.

The hepatoduodenal ligament connects the liver to the superior part of the duodenum. The free margin of this ligament contains the hepatic artery, portal vein, bile duct, nerves, and lymphatic vessels. These structures connect with the liver in the transverse portal fissure. The caudate lobe of the liver is posterior and the quadrate lobe is anterior to this fissure. The quadrate lobe is further demarcated on the right by the gallbladder and on the left by the umbilical fissure.

SEGMENTAL ANATOMY

The liver classically has been divided into left and right lobes by the location of the falciform ligament. Because this location does not correspond to the internal subdivisions of the liver, a more functional nomenclature was developed by Hjortso and Couinaud on the basis of the distribution of vessels and ducts within the liver.[7, 8] In this nomenclature, the line extending between the vena cava and the gallbladder (Cantlie's line) demarcates the right and left livers (or hemilivers), each with independent vascular and duct supplies. This line marks a relatively bloodless plane that is of use to the surgeon. The liver can be further divided into eight segments, each containing a pedicle of portal vessels and ducts and drained by hepatic veins situated in the planes (called *scissura*) between the segments[7] (Fig. 62–2). Because branching of the left portal vein is irregular, Strasberg has recommended that the segments be defined by the divisions of the arteries or ducts.[8]

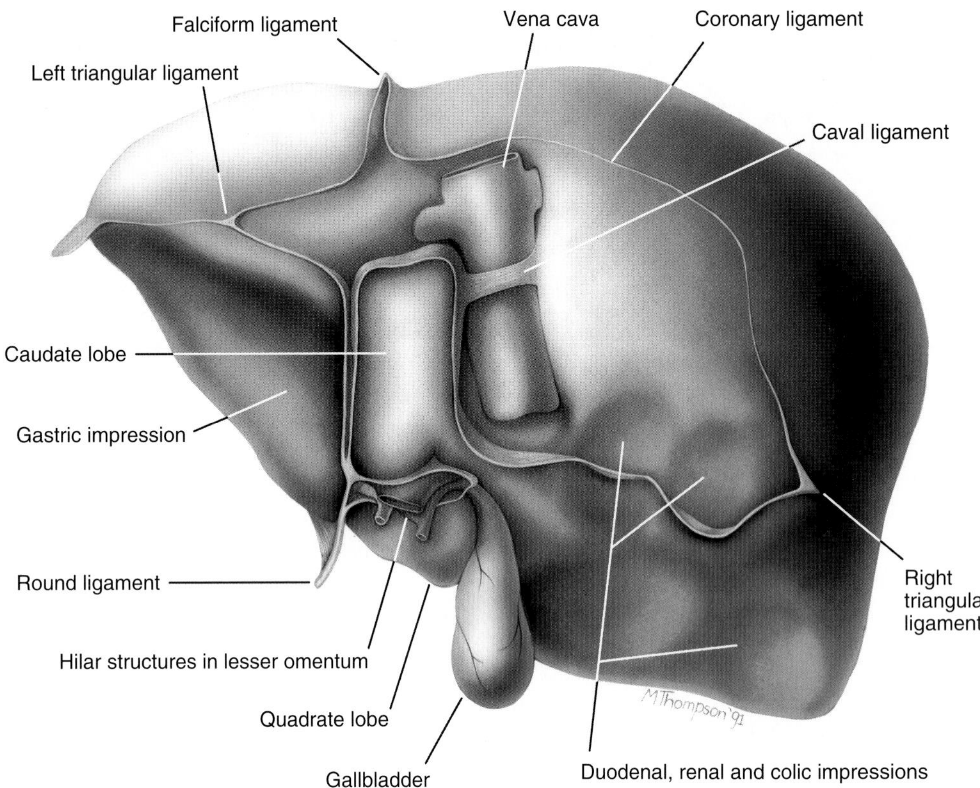

Figure 62–1. Posterior view of the liver. The shape of the liver is determined by molding against adjacent organs. At the porta hepatis, the common bile duct lies to the right, the hepatic artery to the left, and the portal vein to the rear. Variations in the location of the artery are frequent.

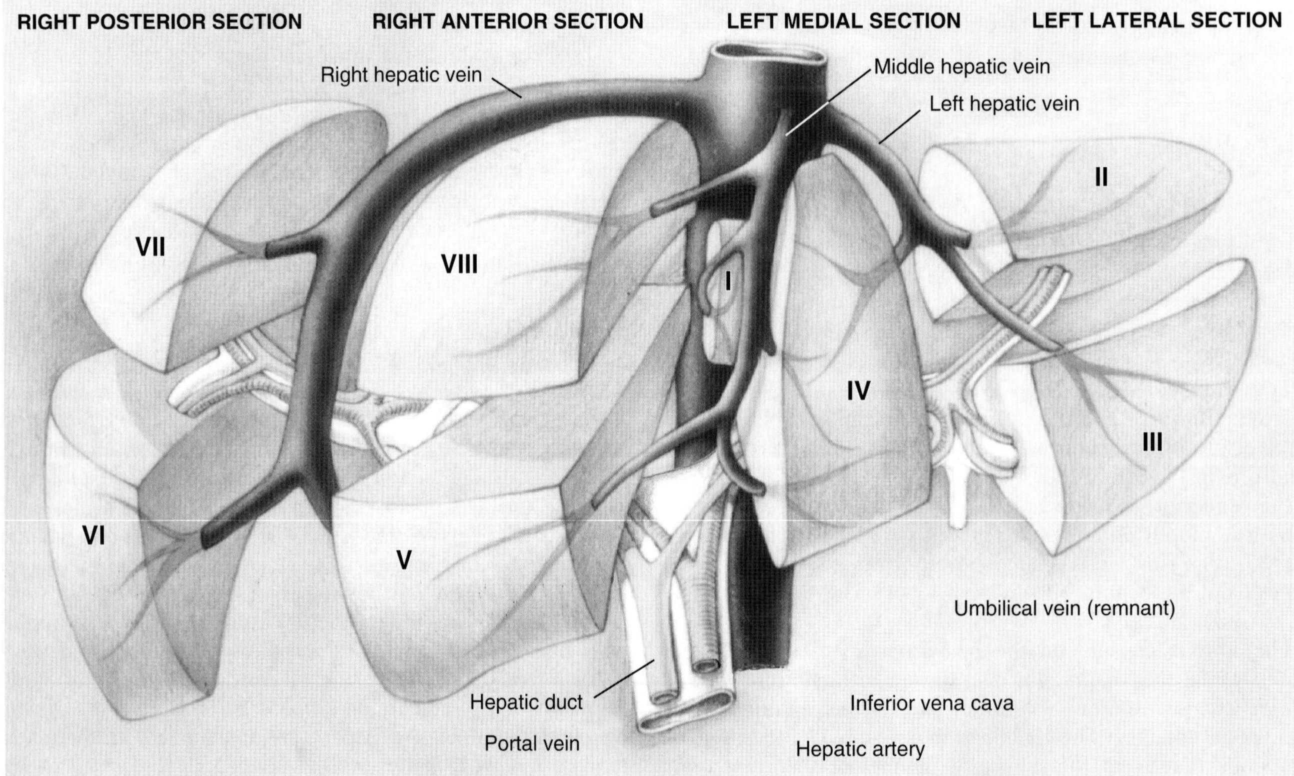

Figure 62–2. Diagram of the functional segments using the nomenclature of Couinaud. For explanation, see text. Segment 1 (not shown) is the caudate lobe (see Fig. 83–6). (From Wanless, IR: Physioanatomic considerations. *In* Schiff L, Schiff ER [eds]: Schiff's Diseases of the Liver, 8th ed. Philadelphia, JB Lippincott, 1999, p 3.)

The segments usually have no surface fissures to allow their accurate identification. The left hemiliver is composed of the classic left lobe plus the caudate lobe and the quadrate lobe and its superior extension. There is considerable individual variation in the location of the segments, especially in the right hemiliver.[9, 10]

The common resections, using the Strasberg nomenclature, are right hemihepatectomy (segments 5 to 8, or right hepatectomy, right hepatic lobectomy), right trisectionectomy (segments 4 to 8, or right lobectomy, trisegmentectomy of Starzl), left hemihepatectomy (segments 1 to 4, or left hepatectomy, left hepatic lobectomy), and left lateral sectionectomy (segments 1 to 3, or left lobectomy, left lateral segmentectomy).[7, 8]

VARIATIONS IN SURFACE ANATOMY

An elongation of the right lobe (Riedel's lobe) can be mistaken for hepatomegaly. This anomaly and minor variations in the shape of the liver explain why clinical estimation of liver size correlates poorly with more objective measures.

Deep fissures may demarcate supernumerary lobes. Rarely, the left lobe is attached to the right lobe by a narrow pedicle. Accessory livers may be found in the ligaments or mesentery or on the surface of the gallbladder, spleen, or adrenals.

Atrophy of the left lobe is usually an acquired abnormality resulting from thrombosis of the portal or hepatic veins.[11] Coarse lobulations (hepar lobatum) are a result of obliterative lesions in large and medium-sized vessels, typically after invasion by neoplasms[12] or in syphilis (see Chapter 69).

LARGE VESSELS OF THE LIVER

Portal Veins

The portal vein normally supplies 70% of the blood flow to the hepatic parenchyma. The portal vein receives almost all of the blood flow from the digestive tract between the proximal stomach and upper rectum as well as from the spleen, pancreas, and gallbladder (Fig. 62–3). The splenic and superior mesenteric veins join behind the pancreas to form the portal vein. The splenic vein sits in a groove of the pancreas and receives the short gastric veins, pancreatic veins, left gastroepiploic vein, and inferior mesenteric vein. The portal vein receives the superior pancreaticoduodenal vein and the left gastric (coronary) vein. The superior mesenteric vein receives the inferior pancreaticoduodenal vein and the right gastroepiploic vein. There is some variation in the veins draining into the portal system.

The portal trunk bifurcates in the portal fissure. The left branch has a transverse segment that turns caudally to form the umbilical portion, which terminates in the obliterated umbilical vein. The left portal vein supplies the quadrate, caudate, and left lobes of the liver. The right portal vein usually receives the cystic vein.

The periductal venous plexus is a collection of variable veins that arise from the pancreas, duodenum, and stomach. The plexus runs along the common bile duct and drains into the perihilar segments of liver or into large branches of the portal vein.[13] This periductal plexus may explain some ex-

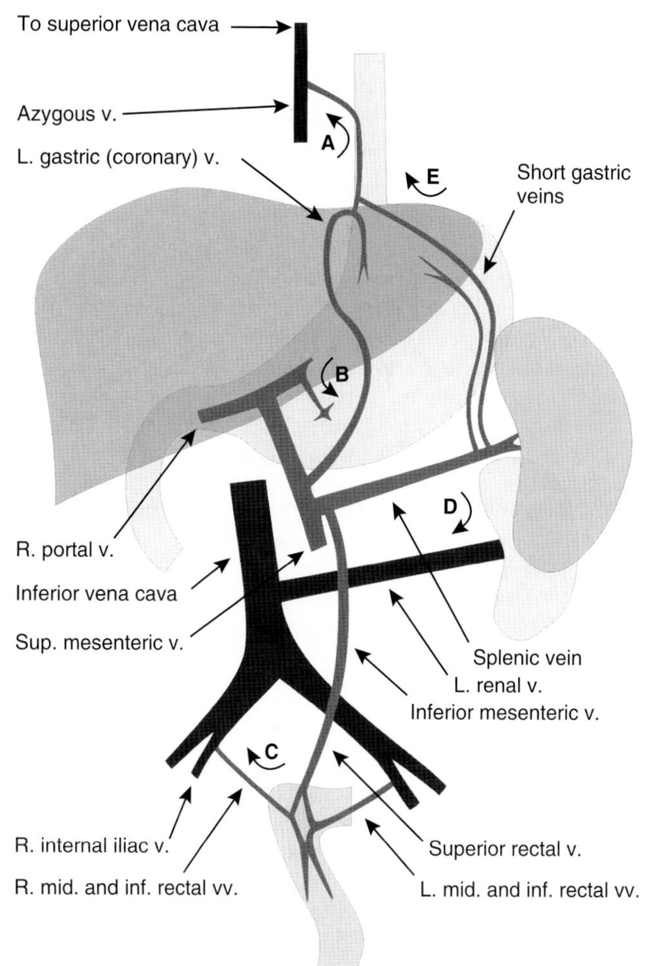

Figure 62–3. Diagram of portal circulation. The most important sites for the potential development of portosystemic collaterals are shown. *A*, Esophageal submucosal veins, which are supplied by the left gastric vein and drain into the superior vena cava via the azygous vein. *B*, Paraumbilical veins, which are supplied by the umbilical portion of the left portal vein and drain into abdominal wall veins near the umbilicus. These veins may form a caput medusae at the umbilicus. *C*, Rectal submucosal veins, which are supplied by the inferior mesenteric vein through the superior rectal vein and drain into the internal iliac veins through the middle rectal veins. *D*, Splenorenal shunts, which are created spontaneously or surgically.

amples of focal fatty change and focal fatty sparing because of the variable concentration of insulin delivered to the perihilar parenchyma.[14]

Anomalies of the Portal Venous System

Anomalies of the portal venous system are uncommon. A portion of the right liver may be supplied by a branch of the left portal vein.[15] The ductus venosus usually closes shortly after birth. Persistent ductus venosus prevents the normal development of the portal vein, thereby leading to hypoplasia of the intrahepatic branches, nodular hyperplasia of the liver, and hyperammonemia; atrial septal defect has been associated.[16]

Atresia or agenesis of the portal vein may be congenital (and often associated with anomalies of the systemic vasculature)[17, 18] or a result of neonatal omphalitis or portal vein thrombosis. Portal vein thrombosis may lead to remodeling of the liver, recognized as nodular hyperplasia or atrophy of the left lobe.[19] Aneurysm of the portal trunk or intrahepatic branches can occur.[20]

Hepatic Veins

There are three main hepatic veins. In 80% of persons the middle and left hepatic veins join before entering the vena cava. The major veins divide at acute angles into branches of equal diameter to form an axial tree that receives smaller tributaries at right angles. Anastomoses are commonly found between branches of the hepatic veins.

Several additional veins, including those from the caudate lobe, drain directly into the vena cava. The caudate veins usually remain patent when thrombosis affects the main hepatic veins in Budd-Chiari syndrome, thereby allowing the caudate lobe to undergo compensatory hyperplasia.[21] Webs commonly develop in the hepatic veins and vena cava after thrombosis.[22] Rarely, venous webs are congenital malformations.

Hepatic Arteries

The common hepatic artery arises from the celiac artery, ascends in front of the portal vein, usually to the left and behind the bile duct, and gives off the left and right hepatic arteries. The gallbladder is supplied by one or two cystic arteries that arise from the right hepatic artery.

Although the left and right hepatic arteries are end-arteries, they often anastomose within the hilar tissues.[15] There are also abundant collateral channels between branches of the celiac axis and branches of the superior mesenteric artery.[23] Anomalies in these large arteries are frequent. The right hepatic artery may arise from the superior mesenteric artery, and the left hepatic artery may arise from the left gastric artery.[23, 24]

Although arterial ligation is usually well tolerated in persons with normal liver function,[25] the cirrhotic liver is highly dependent on arterial flow because of marked loss of portal vein perfusion. Loss of arterial perfusion after liver transplantation is often followed by ischemic stricturing of the bile duct near the hilum,[26] possibly because of ligation of potential collaterals during extirpation of the donor liver.

Hepatic Collateral Circulation

When portal vein blood flow is impeded by cirrhosis or thrombosis of portal or hepatic veins, dilated collateral veins are found at many sites (see Fig. 62–3). These collaterals are prone to rupture, especially in the submucosa of the esophagus and stomach and less often in the colon and at colostomy sites. The surgeon encounters collateral veins at additional sites, especially in various hepatic ligaments, retroperitoneal attachments of other abdominal organs, both sides of the diaphragm and the lesser omentum, and near the bladder and rectum. These veins drain into the systemic circuit mainly via the azygous, renal, adrenal, and inferior hemorrhoidal veins. Dilated paraumbilical veins arise from the umbilical portion of the left portal vein, extend to the umbilicus via the round ligament, and connect with epigastric and internal mammary veins to produce umbilical and abdominal wall varices. Within the cirrhotic liver, there is significant collateral flow in small veins that connect branches of the portal and hepatic veins.[27]

LYMPH VESSELS

Hepatic lymph forms in the connective tissue spaces beneath the sinusoidal endothelial cells (space of Disse), in portal tracts, and around hepatic veins.[28] Recognizable lymphatic vessels are found in small portal tracts and the walls of small hepatic veins. These vessels drain to lymph nodes of the hilum and vena cava, respectively. Additional lymphatics in the liver capsule drain to various ligaments, across the diaphragm to esophageal and xiphisternal nodes, and along the bile duct. The frequent occurrence of pleural effusion in the presence of massive ascites may be explained by lymph flow in transdiaphragmatic lymphatics.

NERVE SUPPLY

The liver has a rich sympathetic and parasympathetic innervation.[29, 30] Fibers derive from lower thoracic ganglia, the celiac plexus, the vagi, and the right phrenic nerve to form the plexuses about the hepatic artery, portal vein, and bile duct. The arteries are innervated mainly by sympathetic fibers. The bile ducts are innervated by both sympathetic and parasympathetic fibers. Unmyelinated sympathetic fibers send branches to individual hepatocytes.

The denervated state of the transplanted liver persists for years,[31] but this does not affect liver function significantly.[32]

BILIARY SYSTEM

The common bile duct is usually located anterior to the portal vein and anterior and to the right of the hepatic artery. There is considerable variation in the position of the duct relative to the vessels and in the branching pattern at the hilum, but intrahepatic bile ducts closely follow the course of intrahepatic portal veins and arteries within the portal tracts.[33]

The common hepatic duct and common bile duct normally have a luminal diameter of 4 to 6 mm. Lobar ducts measure 2 to 4 mm. Segmental bile ducts measure between 0.4 and 0.8 mm in diameter. All of these large ducts have columnar epithelium supported by a well-defined sheath of collagen.[34] Medium-sized (septal) ducts measure 0.1 to 0.4 mm and also have columnar epithelium. Small (interlobular) ducts measure less than 0.1 mm and have cuboidal epithelium. Terminal bile ducts are the smallest biliary radicals to be accompanied by arteries. Bile ductules connect the terminal ducts to the canals of Hering. The canals of Hering connect ductules to hepatocellular canaliculi.

The canals of Hering are composed of both hepatocytes and cholangiocytes and can be identified by cytokeratin 19 staining in the proximal third of the acinus or choleohepaton (see later).[35] There has been renewed interest in the duct of Hering, which has been identified as the site of hepatic stem cells.[4, 36] Bone marrow–derived stem cells are believed to home to this site. Stem cells are believed to be capable of differentiating into either hepatocytes or duct cells, depending on the nature of local stimuli.

The large intrahepatic and all extrahepatic ducts are accompanied by periductal glands and rarely by ectopic pancreatic acinar tissue.[37]

Anatomic Variations of the Biliary System

There is considerable variation in the extrahepatic and primary intrahepatic branches of the biliary tree, which can provide surprises for the surgeon[33, 38] (see Chapter 52). Large ducts from one side of the liver may drain into the opposite lobar duct. The cystic duct may drain into the right hepatic duct. The common bile duct may be short or absent, with the right and left ducts joining just before their entry into the duodenum. Medium-sized ducts often anastomose between lobes, sometimes providing spontaneous relief of obstruction after ligation. The ducts of Luschka are ducts in the gallbladder bed that, if transected during cholecystectomy, may leak bile into the peritoneal cavity.[39]

Choledochal cyst is a focal dilation of the biliary tree; Caroli's disease is a subtype of choledochal cyst characterized by diffuse intrahepatic dilation. These conditions may present with cholangitis, abscesses, jaundice, or cirrhosis. Common bile duct dilation is commonly seen after cholecystectomy and is sometimes a feature of polycystic liver disease.[40]

Atresia of the large bile ducts is one of the most common causes of cirrhosis in children (see Chapter 52). Hypoplasia and atresia are often associated with other anomalies and may thus be a congenital malformation. It is possible that acquired infections also may cause atresia.

Periductal glands are prone to inflammation and the formation of retention cysts,[37] which are usually incidental findings but rarely obstruct the bile ducts at the bifurcation.[41]

MICROANATOMY

Hepatocytes are polyhedral with a central spherical nucleus. They are arranged in plates that are one cell thick and have blood-filled sinusoids on each side. The cytoplasmic membrane has specialized domains that provide a canalicular region on the lateral walls and numerous microvilli on the sinusoidal (basolateral) surfaces. The canalicular domains of adjacent hepatocytes are bound together by tight junctions to form bile canaliculi that coalesce and ultimately drain into ducts within portal tracts. The sinusoidal surface is covered with a layer of endothelial cells to enclose the extravascular space of Disse. Within this space are liver-associated lymphocytes and stellate (fat-storing) cells. The stellate cells normally contain numerous droplets of vitamin A ester. When activated by various cytokines, stellate cells lose their fat droplets and function as the principal hepatic fibroblasts. Kupffer cells are the hepatic macrophages that reside in the sinusoids and have pseudopodia anchored to subendothelial structures.

Hepatic sinusoids differ from systemic capillaries in that the endothelial cells are fenestrated and subendothelial stromal material is scanty, thereby permitting passage of large macromolecules including lipoproteins. The sinusoidal walls are supported by a delicate network of collagen fibers that stains with the reticulin stain.

Normal and abnormal ultrastructure is discussed in detail in other reviews.[1, 42]

Sinusoidal Pathology

During the development of cirrhosis the sinusoids acquire some features of systemic capillaries; the space of Disse becomes widened with collagen, basement membrane material is deposited, endothelial fenestrations become smaller and less numerous, and hepatocellular microvilli are effaced. These changes likely reduce transport across the sinusoidal walls.

Weakening of reticulin fibers may predispose to the rupture of sinusoidal walls and the formation of blood-filled cysts, a condition known as *peliosis hepatis*.[19]

Organization of Hepatic Parenchyma: The Acinus and the Lobule

The organization of the hepatic parenchyma has been conceptualized in two contrasting models: the acinus and the lobule[43] (Fig. 62–4). Terminal portal veins interdigitate with the terminal hepatic venules, with sinusoids bridging the gaps between these vessels. The terminal hepatic venules can be considered as being the center of a lobule or the periphery of several acini. The conceptual advantage of the acinus is that the blood supply of a small portion of parenchyma and the bile duct draining that parenchyma reside in the same portal triad. Thus, "structural, circulatory, and functional unity is established in this small clump of parenchyma."[3] In contrast, the classic lobule is supplied by several separate portal vein branches, each of which also supplies adjacent lobules.

Portal vein blood actually is distributed by numerous small inlet venules, thereby giving a portal supply that is more diffuse and less granular than pictured by the original description of the acinus.[44] Thus, acini appear to be subsumed as components of a hedge rather than as individual grapes on a vine.

A smaller conical subunit has been described, the hepatic microcirculatory subunit (HMS).[45] Each HMS is defined by its portal supply from a single inlet venule. Each venule is usually paired with a single ductule. The HMS is a structural unit that includes two functional compartments, the choleon and the hepaton, that reside in a common space. The choleon is composed of hepatocytes from which the bile produced drains into a canal of Hering. The hepaton is composed of the hepatocytes supplied by a single inlet venule. Although the notion of a choleohepaton is conceptually attractive, collateral blood flow between subunits may relegate functional unity to larger units that are the size of acini or primary lobules.

In normal human liver there are no sharp demarcations between adjacent subdivisions, so that acini are difficult to visualize. However, acini become evident in pathologic conditions such as nodular regenerative hyperplasia, in which there is a pruning of the portal venous supply. As with a

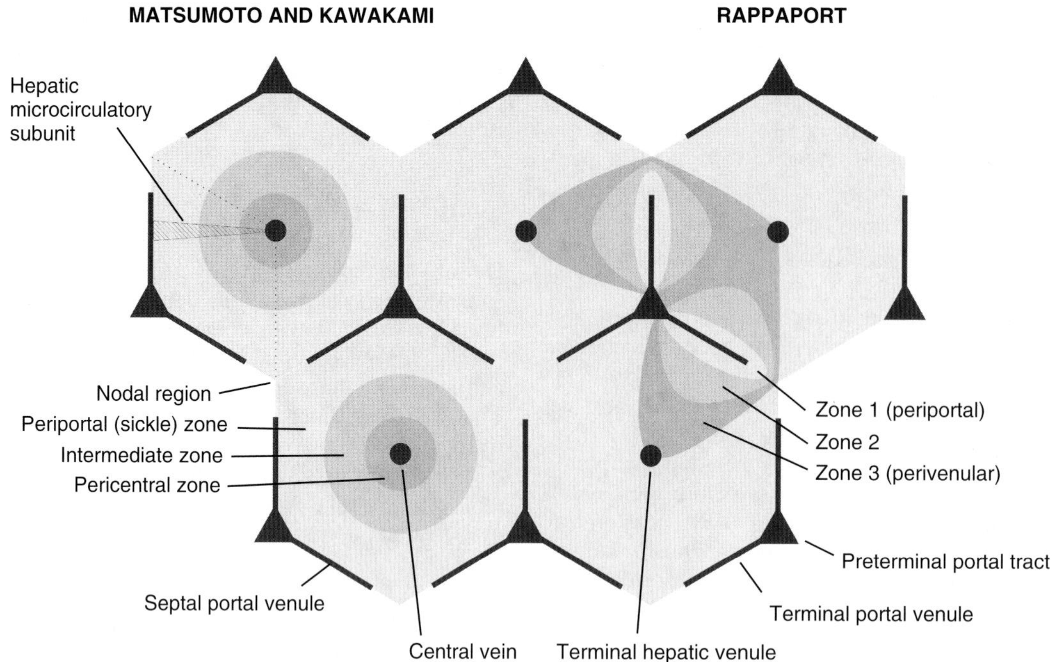

Figure 62–4. The acinar structure of the hepatic microcirculation, as conceived by Rappaport[43] and modified by Matsumoto and Kawakami.[44] In both models, the margins of the shaded zones represent planes of equal blood pressure (isobars), oxygen content, or other characteristics. Periportal tissue (zone 1) receives blood that is higher in oxygen content than perivenular (zone 3) tissue. The models differ in the shape of the isobars surrounding terminal portal venules. The acinus is bulb shaped, and the classic lobule is composed of several wedge-shaped portions (called primary lobules, indicated by *dotted lines, upper left*), which have cylindrical (*sickle-shaped*) isobars. The hepatic microcirculatory subunit is the smallest functional unit in which there is the potential for countercurrent flow, shown as a hatched wedge (*left*).

hedge, when individual portal units are pruned, the remaining units undergo hyperplasia to form an array of spherical units, revealing the underlying acinar structure.

Regardless of how one visualizes the vascular arrangements, hepatocytes close to the portal supply (acinar zone 1) are adapted to an environment that is rich in oxygen and nutrients. Cells more distant from the portal supply (acinar zones 2 and 3) have a different enzymatic phenotype and respond differently to hypoxia and toxin exposure.[3, 29, 46, 47]

Hepatic Microcirculation

The terminal portal twigs supply sinusoids directly and give a constant but sluggish blood flow.[3] The arteries form a peribiliary plexus that surrounds and nourishes small bile ducts. The efferent flow from this plexus drains into terminal portal venules and proximal (zone 1) sinusoids. Some arterioles drain directly into zone 1 sinusoids. The artery gives a pulsatile but small-volume flow that appears to enhance sinusoidal flow, especially in periods of reactive arterial flow, such as the postprandial state. Arterial flow varies inversely with portal vein flow.[48] Local control of the microcirculation may depend on arteriolar sphincters and, at the sinusoidal level, by the state of contraction of endothelial cells and stellate cells.[30]

Microcirculation in Chronic Liver Disease

After hepatocellular necrosis, the sinusoidal stroma is normally repopulated with hepatocytes. If regeneration is delayed, usually because vessels are obstructed, the stroma becomes fibrotic and cannot support hepatocellular regeneration. The affected acini become extinct and are replaced by a focal scar. When numerous acini become extinct, the fibrotic and regenerative changes are recognized as cirrhosis.[49] In cirrhosis, small portal and hepatic veins are markedly reduced in number,[50] thereby leading to increased intrahepatic resistance and portal hypertension. The cirrhotic liver is predisposed to secondary thrombotic events, unrelated to the original etiology, that lead to the progression of tissue extinction and increased clinical morbidity.[51]

REFERENCES

1. MacSween RNM, Desmet VJ, Roskams T, Scothorne RJ: Developmental anatomy and normal structure. In MacSween RNM, Burt AD, Portmann BC, et al (eds): Pathology of the Liver, 4th ed. Edinburgh, Churchill Livingstone, 2002, p 107.
2. Ishak KG, Sharp HL: Developmental abnormalities and liver disease in childhood. In MacSween RNM, Burt AD, Portmann BC, et al (eds): Pathology of the Liver, 4th ed. Edinburgh, Churchill Livingstone, 2002, p 107.
3. Wanless IR: Physioanatomic considerations. In Schiff L, Schiff ER (eds): Schiff's Diseases of the Liver, 8th ed. Philadelphia, JB Lippincott, 1999, p 3.
4. Saxena R, Theise ND, Crawford JM: Microanatomy of the human liver—exploring the hidden interfaces. Hepatology 30:1339, 1999.
5. Furbank RA: Conversion data, normal values, nomograms, and other standards. In Simpson K (ed): Modern Trends in Forensic Medicine. New York, Appleton-Century-Crofts, 1967, p 344.
6. Ludwig J: Current Methods of Autopsy Practice. Philadelphia, WB Saunders, 1972.
7. Bismuth H, Chiche L: Surgical anatomy and anatomical surgery of the

liver. In Blumgart LH (eds): Surgery of the Liver and Biliary Tract, 2nd ed. Edinburgh, Churchill Livingstone, 1994, p 3.

8. Strasberg SM: Terminology of liver anatomy and liver resections: Coming to grips with hepatic Babel. J Am Coll Surg 184:413, 1997.
9. van Leeuwen MS, Noordzij J, Fernandez MA, et al: Portal venous and segmental anatomy of the right hemiliver: Observations based on three-dimensional spiral CT renderings. AJR Am J Roentgenol 163:1395, 1994.
10. Fasel JHD, Selle D, Everetsz CJG, et al: Segmental anatomy of the liver: Poor correlation with CT. Radiology 206:151, 1998.
11. Benz EJ, Baggenstoss AH, Wollaeger EE: Atrophy of the left lobe of the liver. Arch Pathol 53:315, 1952.
12. Qizilbash A, Kontozoglou T, Sianos J, Scully K: Hepar lobatum associated with chemotherapy and metastatic breast cancer. Arch Pathol Lab Med 111:58, 1987.
13. Couinaud C: The parabiliary venous system. Surg Radiol Anat 10:311, 1988.
14. Battaglia DM, Wanless IR, Brady AP, Mackenzie RL: Intrahepatic sequestered segment of liver presenting as focal fatty change. Am J Gastroenterol 90:238, 1995.
15. Madding GF, Kennedy PA: Trauma of the liver. In Calne RY (ed): Liver Surgery with Operative Color Illustrations. Philadelphia, WB Saunders, 1982, p 5.
16. Wanless IR, Lentz JS, Roberts EA: Partial nodular transformation of liver in an adult with persistent ductus venosus. Arch Pathol Lab Med 109:427, 1985.
17. Odievre M, Pige G, Alagille D: Congenital abnormalities associated with extrahepatic portal hypertension. Arch Dis Child 52:383, 1977.
18. Komatsu S, Nagino M, Hayakawa N, et al: Congenital absence of portal venous system associated with a large inferior mesenteric-caval shunt: A case report. Hepatogastroenterology 42:286, 1995.
19. Wanless IR: Vascular disorders. In MacSween RNM, Burt AD, Portmann BC, et al (eds): Pathology of the Liver, 4th ed. Edinburgh, Churchill Livingstone, 2002, p 539.
20. Itoh Y, Kawasaki T, Nishikawa H, et al: A case of extrahepatic portal vein aneurysm accompanying lupoid hepatitis. J Clin Ultrasound 23: 374, 1995.
21. Tavill AS, Wood EJ, Creel L, et al: The Budd-Chiari syndrome: Correlation between hepatic scintigraphy and the clinical, radiological, and pathological findings in 19 cases of hepatic venous outflow obstruction. Gastroenterology 68:509, 1975.
22. Kage M, Arakawa M, Kojiro M, Okuda K: Histopathology of membranous obstruction of the inferior vena cava in the Budd-Chiari syndrome. Gastroenterology 102:2081, 1992.
23. Michels NA: Newer anatomy of liver—variant blood supply and collateral circulation. JAMA 172:125, 1960.
24. Bengmark S, Rosengren K: Angiographic study of the collateral circulation to the liver after ligation of the hepatic artery in man. Am J Surg 119:620, 1970.
25. Brittain RS, Marchioro TL, Hermann G, et al: Accidental hepatic artery ligation in humans. Am J Surg 107:822, 1964.
26. Hesselink EJ, Slooff MJ, Schuur KH, et al: Consequences of hepatic artery pathology after orthotopic liver transplantation. Transplant Proc 19:2476, 1987.
27. Popper H, Elias H, Petty DE: Vascular pattern of the cirrhotic liver. Am J Clin Pathol 22:717, 1952.
28. Trutmann M, Sasse D: The lymphatics of the liver. Anat Embryol 190: 201, 1994.
29. Sasse D, Spornitz UM, Maly IP: Liver architecture. Enzyme 46:8, 1992.
30. McCuskey RS, Reilly FD: Hepatic microvasculature: Dynamic structure and its regulation. Semin Liver Dis 13:1, 1993.
31. Kjaer M, Jurlander J, Keiding S, et al: No reinnervation of hepatic sympathetic nerves after liver transplantation in human subjects. J Hepatol 20:97, 1994.
32. Lindfeldt J, Balkan B, Vandijk G, et al: Influence of periarterial hepatic denervation on the glycemic response to exercise in rats. J Autonom Nerv Syst 44:45, 1993.
33. Smadja C, Blumgart LH: The biliary tract and the anatomy of biliary exposure. In Blumgart LH (ed): Surgery of the Liver and Biliary Tract. Edinburgh, Churchill Livingstone, 1988, p 11.
34. Nakanuma Y, Hoso M, Sanzen T, Sasaki M: Microstructure and development of the normal and pathologic biliary tract in humans, including blood supply. Microsc Res Tech 38:552, 1997.
35. Theise ND, Saxena R, Portmann BC, et al: The canals of Hering and hepatic stem cells in humans. Hepatology 30:1425, 1999.
36. Theise ND, Nimmakayalu M, Gardner R, et al: Liver from bone marrow in humans. Hepatology 32:11, 2000.
37. Terada T, Nakanuma Y, Kakita A: Pathologic observations of intrahepatic peribiliary glands in 1000 consecutive autopsy livers: Heterotopic pancreas in the liver. Gastroenterology 98:1333, 1990.
38. Prinz RA, Howell HS, Pickleman JR: Surgical significance of extrahepatic biliary tree anomalies. Am J Surg 131:755, 1976.
39. Braghetto I, Bastias J, Csendes A, Debandi A: Intraperitoneal bile collections after laparoscopic cholecystectomy: Causes, clinical presentation, diagnosis, and treatment. Surg Endosc 14:1037, 2000.
40. Terada T, Nakanuma Y: Congenital biliary dilatation in autosomal dominant adult polycystic disease of the liver and kidneys. Arch Pathol Lab Med 112:1113, 1988.
41. Wanless IR, Zahradnik J, Heathcote EJ: Hepatic cysts of periductal gland origin presenting as obstructive jaundice. Gastroenterology 93: 894, 1987.
42. Phillips MJ, Poucell S, Patterson J, Valencia P: The Liver: An Atlas and Text of Ultrastructural Pathology. New York, Raven Press, 1987.
43. Rappaport AM, Wanless IR: Physioanatomic considerations. In Schiff L, Schiff ER (eds): Diseases of the Liver, 7th ed. Philadelphia, JB Lippincott, 1993, p 1.
44. Matsumoto T, Kawakami M: The unit-concept of hepatic parenchyma: A reexamination based on angioarchitectural studies. Acta Pathol Jpn 32(Suppl 2):285, 1982.
45. Ekataksin W, Wake K: New concepts in biliary and vascular anatomy of the liver. In Boyer J, Ockner RK (eds): Progress in Liver Diseases. Philadelphia, WB Saunders, 1997, p 1.
46. Lamers WH, Hilberts A, Furt E, et al: Hepatic enzymic zonation: A reevaluation of the concept of the liver acinus. Hepatology 10:72, 1989.
47. Jungermann K, Kietzmann T: Oxygen: Modulator of metabolic zonation and disease of the liver. Hepatology 31:255, 2000.
48. Lautt WW: Relationship between hepatic blood flow and overall metabolism: The hepatic arterial buffer response. Fed Proc 42:1662, 1983.
49. Wanless IR: Vascular disorders. In MacSween RNM, Burt AD, Portman BC, et al (eds): Pathology of the Liver, 4th ed. Edinburgh, Churchill Livingstone, 2002, pp. 539–573.
50. Popper H: Pathologic aspects of cirrhosis. Am J Pathol 87:228, 1977.
51. Wanless IR, Wong F, Blendis LM, et al: Hepatic and portal vein thrombosis in cirrhosis: Possible role in development of parenchymal extinction and portal hypertension. Hepatology 21:1238, 1995.

Chapter 63

LIVER PHYSIOLOGY AND METABOLIC FUNCTION

Andrew Stolz

The liver is the second largest organ in the body and serves a key function in critical metabolic pathways and synthetic functions. It is strategically situated to perform these diverse metabolic functions because it is the first organ to receive a nutrient-enriched blood supply from the portal system. The unique vascular structure of the liver provides unparalleled access to nutrients and xenobiotics absorbed from the intestinal lumen. Processing and redistribution of metabolic fuels such as glucose and fatty acids are thus a major responsibility of the liver. The liver also contains a host of biochemical pathways for the modification and detoxification of compounds absorbed from the small intestine.

Acute or chronic liver injury can reduce the metabolic and synthetic capabilities of the liver, thereby resulting in diverse clinical disorders. With the advent of liver transplantation, more patients with end-stage chronic liver diseases are surviving. In this chapter, the discussion is focused on the specific pathways of biotransformation of endogenous compounds for metabolic needs as well as their associated clinical implications.

HEPATIC ARCHITECTURE

The hepatic architecture is ideally suited for the liver's diverse metabolic functions[1] (see Chapter 62). The liver has two distinct vascular beds that receive systemic arterial blood and pooled venous drainage from the portal system. Hepatic vascular drainage is mediated by a central vein (terminal venule) that drains perpendicular to the distal sinusoidal drainage. The fundamental unit in the liver is the hepatic acinus, which can be visualized as a central vein comprising a hub and four to six portal triads representing the rim of a wheel, as illustrated in Figure 63–1. In the acinar model, hepatocytes that abut the hepatic central vein form the pericentral zone. Functional differences exist in pericentral hepatocytes as compared with hepatocytes that surround the hepatic portal triad, referred to as the *periportal zone.* These two populations of cells exhibit different synthetic capabilities, expressions of biotransformation enzymes, and patterns of susceptibility to liver injury (see Chapter 73). The precise factors that regulate this differential expression of hepatic functions in these two zones remain unknown. However, differences in local environment resulting from relative hypoxia in the pericentral cells compared with the periportal hepatocytes or from nutrient depletion of sinusoidal blood are potential contributors to variations in hepatocyte function.[2]

The urea cycle and synthesis of glutamine illustrate how compartmentalization of hepatic metabolic pathways in different zones leads to efficient utilization of metabolic byproducts.[2, 3] Ammonia is converted to urea by the concerted activity of urea cycle enzymes in the liver. This high-capacity, low-affinity system is located predominately in the periportal and central zones of the liver acinus. These same populations of cells also are the principal sites of ammonium generation as a by-product of amino acid metabolism. Glutamine synthesis utilizes ammonium and is catalyzed by glutamine synthetase, which is expressed exclusively in hepatocytes lining the pericentral vein. Pericentral hepatocytes thus scavenge ammonium and convert it to glutamine, thereby eliminating toxic ammonium from the systemic circulation.[3]

Hepatocytes are polarized epithelial cells that are bounded by three distinct membrane domains: (1) the sinusoidal or

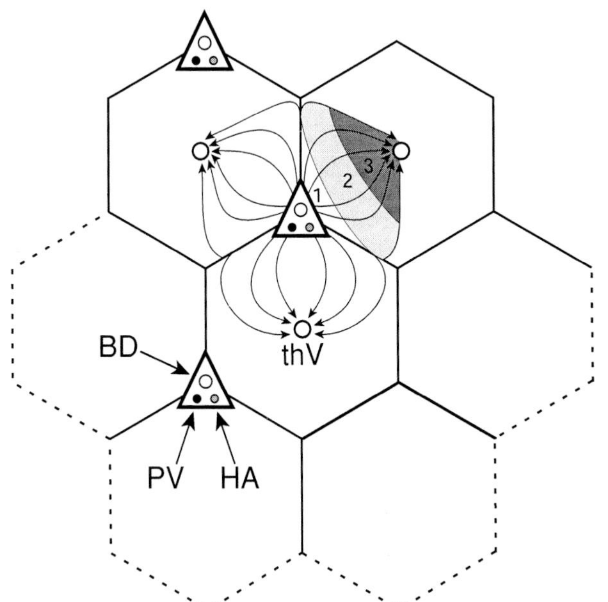

Figure 63–1. Acinar organization of the liver. A model of the structural and functional features of the liver acinus. Portal regions are identified as triangles containing bile ducts (BD), hepatic artery (HA), and portal vein (PV). Blood flow *(arrows)* is perpendicular to the portal triad and drains into the terminal hepatic vein (thV). The periportal zone (1), midzonal region (2), and pericentral zone (3) are illustrated within the hepatic acinus. (Modified from Katz N, Jungermann K: Metabolic heterogeneity of the liver. In Tavoloni N, Berk PD [eds]: Hepatic Transport and Bile Secretion: Physiology and Pathophysiology. New York, Raven Press Ltd, 1992, p 55.)

basolateral membrane, which abuts the sinusoidal space; (2) the apical, or canalicular, membrane, that circumscribes the canaliculus, the earliest component of the biliary drainage system; and (3) the lateral hepatic membrane between adjacent hepatocytes.[4–6] Tight junction complexes between neighboring hepatocytes separate the sinusoidal space from the bile canaliculi. Disruption of tight junctions can permit regurgitation of biliary solutes into the bloodstream.

The liver's unique sinusoidal structure is well suited for the bidirectional transfer of a variety of solutes, including macromolecules, across the sinusoidal membrane. The low pressure allows blood to percolate slowly through the sinusoids and hepatic acinus. Fenestrae within the sinusoidal endothelium and the absence of a basement membrane permit direct contact of the portal blood with the hepatic sinusoidal surface in the subsinusoidal vascular space, referred to as the *space of Disse*. Microvilli on the hepatic sinusoidal plasma membrane further facilitate interchange of nutrients between sinusoidal blood and hepatocytes.

Nonparenchymal cells in the liver serve other important physiologic roles and participate in the hepatic response to injury and inflammation. In addition to endothelial cells that line the sinusoids, the sinusoidal space includes macrophage-derived Kupffer cells, which are phagocytic cells and important mediators of the hepatic inflammatory response. The stellate cell, also known as *lipocyte, fat storage cell,* or *Ito cell,* is identified phenotypically by its high lipid content and is the major site for vitamin A storage. The stellate cell is the major cell type responsible for synthesis of extracellular collagen and is a critical component of the fibrogenic response to liver injury (see Chapter 71). Activation of stellate cells to a myofibroblast-like state is associated with collagen gene expression, reduction of intracellular vitamin A content, and profound morphologic changes. Regulation of stellate cell activation is an important early event in hepatic fibrosis and cirrhosis formation. New strategies for the prevention of hepatic fibrosis may involve inhibition of this activation pathway.

EXCRETORY PATHWAY

The liver's ability to biotransform xenobiotics and endogenous compounds is predicated on the transport capability of the sinusoidal membrane.[7–9] The liver expresses a large number of functionally interrelated sinusoidal transport proteins that facilitate movement of these compounds to and from the hepatic interior.[7, 8]

Transport proteins can be divided into different classes, depending on energy sources used to promote uptake. Transporters that require consumption of adenosine triphosphate (ATP) are considered primary active transporters, whereas secondary active transporters use the existing electrochemical gradient to drive uptake or efflux. A host of sinusoidal transporters have been identified by molecular cloning technique. Some of them are unique to the liver, such as the sodium-dependent bile acid transporter (NTCP).[9, 10] Receptor-mediated endocytosis, passive diffusion, and transcellular transport associated with intracellular binding proteins or vesicles are also important in the uptake and intracellular trafficking of diverse compounds. Association of nutrient-absorbed lipophilic compounds such as tocopherol or fat-soluble vitamins with lipoproteins is another means for the delivery of hydrophobic compounds to the liver.

A different group of membrane transporters is found at the canalicular membrane domain. Many of these transporters mediate the secretion of native or biotransformed metabolites from the hepatocyte into bile. The ATP-binding cassette proteins (ABCs) represent a large family of transport proteins that share a common nucleotide-binding domain. Different members of the ABC supergene family are expressed in the canaliculus and involved in biliary secretion. Specific family members identified by their ABC nomenclature and their substrates include members of the multidrug resistance (MDR) gene family (ABC B gene family) such as MDR 1 (ABC B1) (organic cation), MDR 2 (ABC B4) (phospholipids), bile salt export pump, (BSEP, ABC B11) (bile salts), specific MDR protein gene family members (MRP) (ABC C gene family) including MRP 2 (ABC C2) (organic anions such as bilirubin), and likely other ABC proteins as well.[8, 9] The cystic fibrosis transmembrane conductance regulator (CFTR) (ABC C7) is expressed in the apical membrane of bile duct cells and appears to play an important role in ductular secretion.

Metabolites biotransformed in the liver may be excreted directly through bile into the intestinal lumen and then outside the body. Alternatively, metabolites may efflux across the basolateral membrane into blood for elimination by the kidney, lung, and skin. The excretory role of the liver becomes apparent during cholestasis, in which diminished hepatic excretory capability dominates the clinical presentation. Clinical features of cholestatic syndromes are jaundice, pruritus, and cutaneous xanthoma, with elevated serum levels of cholesterol, alkaline phosphatase, total bilirubin, and serum bile acids (see Chapters 14 and 64).

INTRODUCTION TO LIVER METABOLISM

A major responsibility of the liver is to provide a continual source of energy for the entire body. The liver's ability to store and modulate the availability of systemic nutrients is regulated by numerous local factors and the requirements of peripheral organs for energy sources.[11] Hepatic metabolic function is subject to hormonal modulation by endocrine organs, such as the pancreas, adrenal gland, and thyroid, as well as to neuronal regulation. The liver regulates nutrient flux during periods of nutrient absorption (meals), when absorbed nutrients are metabolized, modified for storage in the liver and fatty tissue, or made available to the remaining organs as sources of energy metabolism, and during nonabsorptive periods (fasting), when metabolic requirements need to be maintained from stored fuel sources or by synthesis.

The regulation of these metabolic pathways involves complex interactions among the nutrient content of the blood, end-products of nutrient metabolism that are present in the blood and represent precursors for hepatic synthesis, and hormonal regulation. The following discussion summarizes the metabolism of carbohydrates and fatty acids (Fig. 63–2), the major classes of nutrients, the metabolism of lipoproteins, and the clinical manifestations of metabolic disorders associated with liver disease (Table 63–1). Detailed reviews of hepatic metabolism are available elsewhere.[12–20]

CARBOHYDRATE METABOLISM

Glucose is the primary nutrient source for the brain, erythrocytes, muscle, and renal cortex. The liver serves a key role in maintaining total carbohydrate stores because of its ability to store glycogen and synthesize glucose from precursors.[12, 21, 22]

The liver is the major site of gluconeogenesis from precursors. Glucose synthesis involves nonoxidative metabolic products of glucose (pyruvate and lactate), which are generated predominantly by red blood cells (RBCs), and amino acid precursors, which are provided predominantly by muscle tissue during extensive periods of starvation or exercise. Maintaining adequate circulating levels of glucose is essential for the central nervous system, which normally uses glucose as its major metabolic fuel. After fasting for 24 to 48 hours, the brain is able to utilize ketones as a metabolic fuel, thereby reducing its glucose requirement by 50% to 70%, in turn significantly reducing the need for gluconeogenesis by the liver.[16]

Regulation of Intrahepatic Glucose Concentration

Glucose is a central component of the metabolic pathway because it can be converted to amino acids, fatty acids, or glycogen, the major storage form of glucose. Glucose enters the liver by the glucose transporter-2, a member of the facilitative glucose transport gene family, with an apparent Michaelis constant Km of 60 mmol.[23] Glucose transporter-2 activity is independent of metabolic conditions or insulin levels and is thereby different from other glucose transporters, which are regulated by insulin through vesicular insertion into or removal from the basolateral membrane. Glucose transporter-2 facilitates diffusion of the hydrophilic glucose across the sinusoidal plasma membrane and is capable of promoting glucose uptake from or efflux to the sinusoidal space, which is of critical importance during fasting conditions.[24] The high Km of glucose transporter-2 is well above the peak glucose levels detected during meals or renal transport capacity, thereby ensuring continuous uptake of glucose by the liver. The low-affinity, high-capacity characteristics of the glucose transporter-2 mean that intrahepatic glucose concentration is determined by the circulating concentration of glucose, which is regulated by glucokinase activity (see "Formation of Glucose-6-Phosphate" later). The glucose transporter-1, present in the brain and erythrocytes, has a Km of 10 to 20 μmol and is also present in pericentral hepatocytes. The selective location of this low-capacity, high-affinity glucose transporter permits uptake of glucose by pericentral hepatocytes when the circulating glucose concentration is low.[2] During fasting, glucose transporter-1 expression is increased, presumably to enhance glucose uptake.

Glucose homeostasis is maintained in the hepatocyte by interdependent cyclic pathways that serve as branch points for the metabolic pathways of glucose metabolism. These interlinking pathways are regulated and efficiently integrated by multiple signals that prevent competing pathways from operating at the same time.[13, 25] Figure 63–2 illustrates these pathways and the modulating influences that direct metabolic flux of glucose and other carbohydrates such as fructose. The rapid conversion of glucose to glucose-6-phosphate (glucose-6-P) efficiently reduces the glucose concentration within the hepatocyte, thereby regulating the concentration gradient that promotes either glucose uptake or efflux by the hepatocyte. The reader is referred to References 12, 17, 19, and 20 for a more detailed review.

Glucose-6-P is a nodal branch point compound that can enter three independent metabolic pathways: (1) synthesis of glycogen, which can be mobilized rapidly during fasting; (2) anaerobic glycolysis by means of the Embden-Meyerhof pathway, in which generated pyruvate or lactate is a substrate for the tricarboxylic acid (Krebs cycle) in mitochondria; or (3) the pentose-phosphate shunt, which generates reducing equivalents necessary for anaerobic glycolysis and fatty acid synthesis and which is regulated by the activity of mitochondrial glucose-6-P dehydrogenase.[16, 17, 26, 27]

Formation of Glucose-6-Phosphate

Phosphorylation of glucose is mediated by two distinct members of the hexokinase gene family. Hexokinase is capable of phosphorylating several different hexose substrates (including glucose), whereas glucokinase (GK), also referred to as *hexokinase type 4* or *D*, is expressed predominantly in the liver and pancreas and is specific for glucose.[28] In contrast with other hexokinases, GK has a high Km (5 to 10 mmol vs. 0.2 mmol) for glucose and is not inhibited by the end-product of the reaction. The relative activity of GK

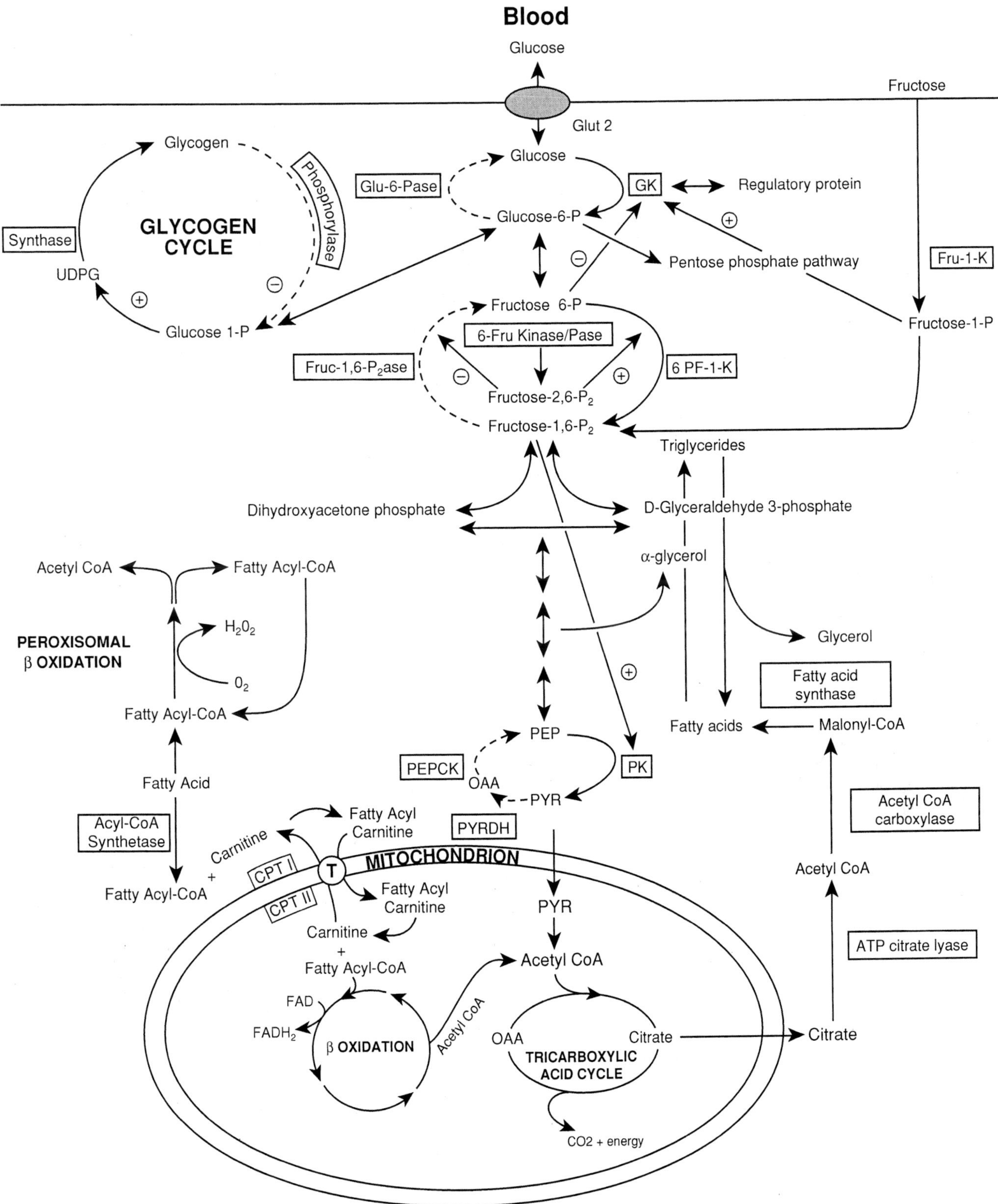

Figure 63–2. Hepatic carbohydrate and lipid metabolism. Gluconeogenic pathways are identified by dashed lines. GK, glucokinase; Glu-6-Pase, glucose-6-phosphatase; 6-Fru Kinase/Pase, 6-phosphofructo-2-kinase/fructose-2,6-bisphosphatase; Fructose 6-P, fructose-6-phosphate; 6 PF-1-K, 6-phosphofructo-1-kinase; Fruc-1,6-P_2ase, fructose-1,6-biphosphatase; PK, pyruvate kinase; PEPCK, phosphoenol pyruvate carboxykinase; CPT, carnitine palmitoyltransferase; Glut 2, glucose transporter 2; T, carnitine: acylcarnitine transferase; PEP, phosphoenol pyruvate; FAD, flavine adenine dinucleotide; PYR, pyruvate; OAA, oxaloacetate; UDPG, uridine diphosphate glucose. (Data from references 12, 16, 21, and 27.)

Table 63–1 | **Clinical Manifestations of Metabolic Disorders Associated with Liver Diseases**

LIVER DISEASES	METABOLIC ABNORMALITIES	CLINICAL MANIFESTATIONS
Glycogen storage diseases	Absence of glucose-6-phosphatase activity	Hepatomegaly resulting from glycogen storage; associated with hepatic adenoma and carcinoma formation; hypoglycemia
Alcoholic liver disease	Hypertriglyceridemia, hyperglycemia, hypoglycemia	Hepatomegaly resulting from fatty liver
Chronic cholestatic syndromes (primary biliary cirrhosis, primary sclerosing cholangitis, pediatric cholestatic syndromes)	Hypertriglyceridemia, hypercholesterolemia, lipoprotein-Y and lipoprotein-X	Jaundice, pruritus, xanthoma, neurologic disorders associated with vitamin E deficiency

determines the hepatic uptake of glucose from the sinusoidal blood. Increased GK activity reduces the free glucose concentration and promotes hepatic glucose extraction. GK can thus be considered to be the major regulator of hepatic glucose uptake because it is not inhibited by end-product or limited by glucose concentration and because the glucose transporter-2 merely facilitates bidirectional glucose transport.

GK expression is activated by insulin and inhibited by glucagon, which mediates its effect by increasing cyclic adenosine monophosphate (cAMP) levels in the cell.[16, 19–21] Some rare cases of non–insulin-dependent diabetes presenting in young adults are associated with mutations in the GK gene and support an important role for GK in glucose homeostasis.[28] GK activity also is inhibited by interaction with a negative regulatory protein, the activity of which is enhanced by fructose 6-phosphate (fructose 6-P) and inhibited by low levels of fructose-1-phosphate (fructose 1-P). Thus, fructose levels serve to modulate the activity of GK by regulating the relative inhibitory activity of the GK regulatory protein.[29] Binding of the regulatory protein in the presence of fructose 6-P leads to a complex of higher molecular weight with a reduction in catalytic activity and inhibition of glucose binding to GK. The regulation of GK by fructose is thought to prevent futile cycling between glucose and glucose-6-P that consumes ATP. Starvation decreases GK, thereby further reducing futile recycling and promoting efflux of glucose from the hepatocyte.

The conversion of glucose-6-P to glucose is catalyzed by glucose-6-phosphatase (glu-6-Pase), a multisubunit microsomal enzyme with an active site that faces the lumen of the endoplasmic reticulum (ER).[12, 30, 31] Glucose-6-P needs to traverse the ER membrane and enter the lumen to be dephosphorylated. Absence of glu-6-Pase is responsible for type Ia glycogen storage disease (see Chapter 65).[30] Glucose-6-P transport is mediated by a microsomal transport protein, which when defective causes type Ib glycogen storage disease. Other microsomal glucose transport proteins may also exist. As expected, glu-6-Pase activity is increased by starvation or diabetes mellitus, causing net flux of glucose out of the liver and into the sinusoidal space by the bidirectional glucose transporter-2.

Glucose-6-P can either be stored as glycogen or enter the pentose monophosphate shunt that generates the reduced form of nicotinamide dinucleotide phosphate (NADPH). The other possible metabolic fate of glucose-6-P is conversion to fructose 6-P, which can enter the fructose 6-P–fructose 1,6-diphosphate (fructose-1,6-P_2) pathway. Fructose-1,6-P_2 modulates the activity of pyruvate kinase (PK), which can affect substrate cycling in the subsequent pyruvate (PYR)–phosphoenol pyruvate (PEP) pathway. These opposing enzyme reactions regulate the formation of gluconeogenesis precursors and glycolysis.

The relative production of fructose 6-P and fructose-1,6-P_2 is regulated by the opposing action of 6-phosphofructo-1-phosphokinase (6-PK-1-K) and fructose-1,6-bisphosphatase (fruc-1,6$_2$Pase).[12, 17, 21, 27] Within this cycle is a unique enzyme: 6-phosphofructo-2-kinase/fructose-2,6-biphosphotase (6-fru kinase/Pase). This enzyme, which combines the properties of both a 6-PF-2K and its corresponding phosphorylase enzyme activity, produces the regulatory product fructose-2,6-P_2. Fructose-2,6-P_2 is a potent activator of 6-PF-1-K and inhibitor of fruc-1,6$_2$Pase. Moreover, it favors the formation of the fructose-1,6-P_2 product. This enzyme, which is regulated by both hormonal and nutrient regulations, serves as another modulator of glucose metabolism. During starvation, when fructose-2,6-P_2 levels are low, gluconeogenesis is enhanced. On the other hand, high levels found during refeeding and insulin administration promote glycolysis and fatty acid synthesis.

6-Fru kinase/Pase is a homodimer with distinct kinase and phosphatase catalytic protein domains as well as a regulatory cAMP-dependent phosphorylation site. The enzyme is dephosphorylated predominantly by phosphatase 2A. The phosphorylation status of the enzyme is regulated both by the cAMP-dependent kinase site and phosphatase activity. Formation of fructose-2,6-P_2 increases kinase activity, which in turn stimulates the activity of 6-PF-1-K and inhibits fruc-1,6-P_2ase, thereby increasing the concentration of fructose-1,6-P_2. Fructose-2,6-P_2 is the most potent stimulator of 6-PF-1-K. It can counter the inhibitor effect of ATP and thereby increase the affinity of the enzyme for the substrate, fructose 6-P. This pathway favors glycolysis and lipogenesis by increasing the concentration of PYR, which can be further metabolized in the mitochondrion to citrate. Citrate, by way of the citrate acid cycle, can then be converted to fatty acid, which is a more concentrated and efficient form of energy storage.

From fructose-1,6-P_2, a sequential series of four biochemical reactions leads to formation of PEP with generation of eight molecules of ATP.[11, 19, 20] PEP can then be metabolized into PYR as part of the third regulatory cycle in glucose metabolism. Pyruvate kinase, which transforms PEP to PYR, generates two ATP molecules. PYR is another nodal branch point in the metabolic pathway in which PYR can undergo further metabolism in the mitochondrion to form acetyl coenzyme A (acetyl-CoA). Thereafter, it can undergo aerobic metabolism by the tricarboxylic acid cycle.[11, 19, 20] In this pathway, PYR may be metabolized ultimately to water and carbon dioxide, with the production of 15 molecules of ATP per molecule of PYR. Other products of the tricarboxcylic acid cycle are also precursors for fatty acid (citrate) or amino acids by means of oxaloacetate formation. Fructose-1,6-P_2 is also an inducer of PK.[27] In the reverse reaction, PYR is metabolized to oxaloacetate, which is a precursor for the amino acid L-aspartate. Oxaloacetate is converted by the energy-dependent activity of phosphoenolpyruvate carboxykinase (PEPCK), an important regulator of gluconeogenesis.

PEPCK is potently regulated at the transcriptional level by both cAMP and insulin and has been used as a model for nutrient-regulated gene expression.[16, 27] Insulin is able to inhibit PEPCK gene transcription rapidly in the presence of protein synthetic inhibitors by a presumed transcription-dependent mechanism. PEPCK is activated at the transcriptional level during fasting or in diabetes mellitus.

Hepatic Metabolism of Other Carbohydrates

In addition to glucose itself, two other major carbohydrates that participate in glucose metabolism are fructose and galactose. The important disaccharide lactose, which is present in high concentration in the milk of humans (7%) and cows (5%), is a rich source of galactose. Galactose can be converted to glucose-6-P, after which it can be utilized for glycogen synthesis; or it can be oxidized further to form PYR or acetyl-CoA for additional energy generation or use in fatty acid synthesis.[11] Galactose is initially phosphorylated by galactokinase to form galactose-1-P. In the presence of uridine diphosphate glucose (UDPG), it can then undergo metabolism by uridyltransferase to form UDP-galactose and glucose-1-phosphate (glucose-1-P) (not shown in Figure 63–2). Galactose is not a substrate for hexokinase activity. UDP-galactose can be epimerized by UDP-glucose-4-epimerase to form UDP-glucose, which is a precursor for glucose-1-P. In this way, glucose-1-P can be converted to glucose-6-P and participate in the same glycolytic pathway as the native glucose.

Fructose is the second most abundant carbohydrate in the Western diet, especially since the introduction of high fructose corn syrups in 1967.[32] Fructose is absorbed in the intestinal lumen by a sodium-independent carrier distinct from the intestinal glucose transporter. It is converted to fructose-1-phosphate (fructose-1-P) by a liver associated fructokinase (Fru-1-K) using either ATP or guanine triphosphate (GTP) as a cofactor. The fructose-1-P product acts as a positive inducer of GK activity by removing the inhibitory regulatory protein. Fructose-1-P cannot enter the glucogenic pathway but is further metabolized by fructose-1-phosphate aldolase to form two trioses, dihydroxylacetone phosphate and glyceraldehyde-3-phosphate. Dihydroxylacetone phosphate may be isomerized to glyceraldehyde phosphate and enter the glycolytic pathway, or it may be reduced to glyceraldehyde-3-phosphate and provide the glycerol backbone for triacylglycerol and phospholipids. Glyceraldehyde-3-phosphate may be combined with dihydroxylacetone phosphate by aldolase B to ultimately form fructose-1,6-P_2. At this juncture, depending on the metabolic requirements of the liver, fructose-1,6-P_2 can undergo gluconeogenesis and potential glycogen synthesis or participate in glycolysis, ultimately resulting in the formation of lactate. Because fructose enters into the carbohydrate cycle at the second regulatory step, fructose is a better substrate for lipogenesis in the liver than is glucose. Hereditary fructose intolerance is caused by a deficiency of aldolase B in liver, kidney, and small intestine that results in the excess build-up of fructose-1-P. Liver and renal dysfunction develop in patients with this disease. Treatment consists of avoidance of sucrose and fructose in the diet.[19]

Glycogen Formation

Hepatic glycogen is the main storage site for the glucose-dependent organs in the body (erythrocytes, retina, and renal medulla) and for the brain, a glucose-preferential organ.[14] By gluconeogenesis, the liver is able to produce up to 240 mg of glucose a day, which is approximately twice the metabolic needs of the retina, RBCs, and brain. The liver can store up to an approximately 2-day supply of glucose in the form of glycogen, before gluconeogenesis occurs using either the glucose itself or the glucose precursor lactate. Lactate is the three-carbon end-product of anaerobic glucose metabolism and is part of the Cori cycle.[11, 15, 17, 33] The three-carbon precursors generated by anaerobic metabolism from muscle, intestine, liver, or RBCs may account for up to 50% of the glycogen pool formed during nonabsorptive states. Alanine, another major glucose precursor, is generated by the catabolism of muscle proteins and is a major cause of muscle wasting during prolonged fasting. Glycogen stored in muscle is utilized locally and cannot be exported out of the cell for use by other tissues because it lacks glu-6-Pase. The relative contribution of each of the precursors for glycogen synthesis depends on the person's nutritional status, amount and route of glucose administration (oral vs. intravenous), and hormonal regulation.

Glycogen synthesis and breakdown is regulated by a cascade of enzymes that allows rapid switching between these opposing activities. This enzyme cascade is regulated by the amounts of local nutrients and hormonal alterations when rapid availability of glucose may be required.[11, 19, 20] Glycogen phosphorylase is required to break down subunits of glycogen, and glycogen synthase is required to add glucose to the expanding glycogen storage chain. These enzymes exist in active and inactive forms, referred to as synthase D (inhibited) and synthase I (activated), and phosphorylase A (active) and phosphorylase B (inactive), and are regulated by their phosphorylation status.[15] Phosphorylation induces phosphorylase A, the active form of glycogen phosphorylase that promotes glycogen breakdown. Synthase I promotes the addition of UDPG to glycogen and is activated by its dephosphorylation. Activation of synthase D to I is caused by phosphatase activity that occurs after phosphorylase A has been converted to its inactive form, phosphorylase B. This enzyme system operates as an effective on-off switch for glycogen metabolism. In addition to regulation by phosphorylation status, both enzymes are regulated by the allosteric effects of glucose, glucose-6-P, and glycogen. Glucose and glucose-6-P are both allosteric inducers of synthase enzyme activity. When glucose binds to phosphorylase A, the enzyme can be converted to its inactive form, phosphorylase B.

Glycogen constitutes approximately 10% of liver weight and exists as aggregates with an average molecular weight of 1×10^8. It is initially formed by the unique autocatalytic activity of tyrosine glucosyltransferase at codon 194 (tyrosine).[22, 34] Additional carbohydrates are added by the activity of glycogen synthase, which elongates the glycogen chain utilizing UDPG as the carbohydrate unit (not shown in Fig. 63–2). Glycogen synthase in combination with branching enzymes allows additional glucose chains to be added. As the chain grows, glycogenin is released from the growing chain by debranching enzymes, allowing it to initiate a new glycogen molecule.

Glycogen exists as two distinct populations consisting of proglycogen, with a molecular weight of approximately 400,000, and macroglycogen, with a molecular weight of 1×10^7. These two populations reside in equilibrium with each other, depending on the relative activities of enzymes favoring proglycogen formation (phosphorylase and debranching enzymes) and those favoring glycogenin formation (branching enzymes). The ability of glycogenin to initiate the formation of glycogen also may be a critical factor in carbohydrate metabolism in the liver cell. The existence of these two distinct populations of glycogen permits subtle control of glucose homeostasis and provides a pool of readily accessible glucose. The relative contribution of these two pools could have an important physiologic role in disease states such as diabetes mellitus.

Regulation of Glycolytic-Gluconeogenic Pathways

Regulation of the three interdependent glycolytic-gluconeogenic pathways represents an integration of multiple factors, including hormonal signals and the relative availability of nutrient substrates. Insulin is the predominant hormone that induces the messenger RNA (mRNA) for the genes that encode the glycolytic enzymes and represses the transcriptional regulation of the metabolic enzymes responsible for gluconeogenesis. The actions of insulin are inhibited by those hormones, such as glucagon, catecholamines, corticosteroids, and growth hormones, that increase cellular cAMP levels and increase expression of the gluconeogenic pathway. In addition to transcriptional regulation, post-transcriptional stabilization or degradation contributes to the relative abundance of specific enzymes.[12, 21, 27] The individual enzymes in these interrelated pathways may be regulated at the post-translational level by protein modification, such as phosphorylation, or by enzyme activity. They also can be altered by either end-product inhibition or allosteric modulation involving the end-products of other metabolic pathways. Glucose and fructose are also important modulators of enzyme activity, by either directly inhibiting enzyme activity or modulating enzyme activity through allosteric effects.

In fed animals, high activity of GK, 6-PF-1-K, and PK induced by insulin favors formation of PYR, with low activity for PEPCK and other gluconeogenic enzymes. At the beginning of a fasting period, plasma insulin levels begin to fall, thereby removing the inhibition of the gluconeogenic enzymes, PEPCK and fruc-1,6-P_2ase. Levels of glucagon and other α-adrenergic agonists are also elevated in the early fasting period, thereby increasing intracellular cAMP levels. Increased cAMP levels inactivate 6-PK-2 kinase activity and activate fruc-2,6-Pase, causing decreased concentration of fructose-2,6-P_2. This leads to activation of fruc-1,6_2Pase with a net increase in gluconeogenesis. After a prolonged fast, gluconeogenesis is further stimulated by increased substrate supply and alterations in the concentration of various enzymes. Because most of these enzymes are in their phosphorylated state, minimal acute changes in gluconeogenic flux can occur. With refeeding or administration of insulin, a prolonged period (hours) is necessary to reverse gluconeogenic flux by the inhibition of PEPCK and fruc-1,6-P_2ase activity and induction of de novo synthesis of the enzymes of the glycolytic pathway.[12, 21, 27]

Carbohydrate Metabolism in Cirrhotic Patients

Patients with cirrhosis have an increased frequency of hyperglycemia associated with increased serum insulin levels.[35, 36] Multiple abnormalities in glucose metabolism and elevated serum levels of hormones are implicated in this impaired glucose metabolism. Cirrhotic patients have an increased basal metabolic rate and preferentially utilize fatty acids as an energy source. Hyperglycemia in cirrhotic patients has been explained by decreased absorption of glucose by muscle and reduced glycogen storage in liver and muscle. The changes lead to resistance to insulin, which in turn leads to increased serum levels of insulin. Other potential contributors to relative insulin resistance are increased serum levels of fatty acids (which can inhibit glucose uptake by muscle), altered second messenger activity after insulin binds to its receptor, and increased serum concentrations of cytokines resulting from elevated serum levels of endotoxin. Increased levels of glucagon and catecholamines also may be contributing factors. The net result is impaired nonoxidative utilization of glucose with decreased storage of glycogen and impaired uptake of glucose by muscle, thereby causing a relative insulin-resistant state similar to that found in patients with diabetes and obesity.

SYNTHESIS AND METABOLISM OF FATTY ACIDS

Fatty acids play an important role as an energy source for the liver as well as a storage form of fuel within and outside the liver.[11] Oxidation of fatty acids to carbon dioxide and water yields the highest ATP production of any metabolic fuel, and fatty acids are thus the most efficient long-term storage form of energy. In addition, most organs are capable of utilizing fatty acids as a fuel.[19, 20, 37, 38] The production and metabolism of fatty acids are regulated by multiple factors, with the liver playing a central role in regulating the body's total fatty acid needs. Excess glucose can be converted to fatty acid for future use and stored in distal sites such as adipose tissue and delivered by lipoproteins (see "Lipid Transport" later). Fatty acids also may undergo beta oxidation in two distinct subcellular components—the mitochondria and peroxisomes—with different physiologic consequences.[18, 39, 40] The regulation of fatty acid synthesis and the ultimate transport of fatty acids to other organs in association with lipoproteins constitute another central role of the liver in governing the metabolic needs of the entire body.

Fatty Acid Synthesis

Fatty acid synthesis is highly complex because of the various physiologic functions that fatty acids perform. In addition to their use as an efficient form of energy storage, fatty acids are constituent parts of various cellular structural components such as membranes. Furthermore, they are involved in regulatory functions in intracellular communication, Golgi function, and anchoring of membrane proteins as well as their own synthesis.[41] Fatty acid synthesis occurs in the cytosol and is regulated closely by the availability of precursors.[11, 19] The fatty acid chain increases until an appropriate length has been achieved, and the fatty acid is then esterified with glycerol to form triglycerides. These newly formed triglycerides can be transported by lipoproteins to distal sites for storage and use. In situations of excess carbohydrates, pyruvate can be converted to acetyl-CoA by the mitochondrial pyruvate dehydrogenase complex to serve as fatty acid precursors, although lipogenesis from carbohydrates consumes about 25% of the energy contained in the carbohydrates.

Malonyl-CoA is the source of acetyl-CoA, which forms the basic subunit of the developing fatty acid carbon chain. The availability of acetyl-CoA is a major limiting factor in fatty acid synthesis.[41] Acetyl-CoA is synthesized predominately in mitochondria and is derived from carbohydrate metabolism, but a small fraction may come from amino acids.[11, 19, 20] Acetyl-CoA cannot traverse the mitochondrial membrane and is condensed with oxaloacetate to form citrate, which can be exported outside the mitochondria by a mitochondrial antiport system. Citrate is then cleaved to provide oxaloacetate and acetyl-CoA by the cytosolic ATP citrate lyase, referred to as the *citrate cleavage enzyme*. The activity of citrate lyase and the transport of citrate out of the mitochondrion and into the cytosol are important regulatory sites of fatty acid synthesis. Acetyl-CoA is converted to malonyl-CoA by the action of acetyl-CoA carboxylase, which is the first step in fatty acid synthesis. Acetyl-CoA carboxylase is the key enzyme in regulating fatty acid synthesis, because it provides the necessary building blocks for elongation of the fatty acid carbon chain.[41]

Malonyl-CoA is utilized by a set of enzymatic activities contained within a single peptide chain that comprises the remarkable fatty acid synthase system.[11, 18–20] Fatty acid synthesis occurs in a series of catalytic steps in which the malonyl-CoA substrate is bound to acyl carrier protein (ACP) by means of a sulfhydryl group. Catalytic activity is contained within two distinct domains that catalyze a sequential series of condensation, reduction, dehydrogenation, and reduction, which constitute the fatty acid synthetic cycle (not shown in Fig. 63–2). Two NADPH molecules are required for each two-carbon unit that is added to the growing fatty acid chain. After completion of the first cycle, the 4-carbon butyl group is transferred from ACP to a peripheral thiol, thus allowing it to accept the next malonyl-CoA group to restart the entire cycle. The cycle continues for another six or seven rounds until a carbon-16 (palmitate) or carbon-18 (stearate) fatty acid is synthesized. Fatty acid-CoA is then released and used for other metabolic pathways.

Further elongation of the fatty acid chain can occur either in the mitochondrion or within the microsomal membrane.[11, 18–20] In the mitochondrion, fatty acid elongation occurs by reversal of some enzymatic reactions involved in beta oxidation. The first step is mediated by enoyl-CoA reductase, which is not part of the beta oxidation system (see "Beta Oxidation of Fatty Acids" later). Low mitochondrial activity of these enzymes suggests that microsomal-mediated elongation may be the preferred site for this metabolic pathway. Microsomal elongation utilizes malonyl-CoA to increase the size of fatty acyl-CoA in a process that involves four separate enzymatic reactions. The elongation ability of microsomes is tissue dependent and serves the needs of specific organs, such as the synthesis of 22- and 24-carbon fatty acids required for myelin formation in the nervous system.

Beta Oxidation of Fatty Acids

Beta oxidation of fatty acids provides a significant fuel source for multiple organs, including the liver. End-products of fatty acid oxidation may include ketone formation, which may be overwhelmingly produced in the absence of insulin (diabetic ketoacidosis). Ketones are formed as an end-product of acetyl-CoA and acetoacetyl-CoA.[11] Acetyl-CoA is produced extensively during beta oxidation of fatty acids that occurs in two distinct subcellular locations: the peroxisome and mitochondrion. In addition, sufficient amounts of nicotinamide adenine dinucleotide (NAD) or nicotinamide adenine dinucleotide phosphate (NADP) are required for fatty acid beta oxidation.

Inherent in both fatty acid synthesis and beta oxidation is the trafficking of substrates between mitochondria and cytosol. The mitochondrion is enveloped in distinct inner and outer membrane structures that are impermeable to most molecules greater than 1000 daltons. Selective mitochondrial transport systems permit shuttling of substrates that are required for either fatty acid synthesis or beta oxidation in different locations in the cell.[11] Regulation of the transport of products to be metabolized in the mitochondrion, or of precursors that are generated from compounds within the mitochondrion and are required for synthesis of fatty acids or glucose in the cytosol, provides an exquisite means of coordinating metabolic pathways through the cell. This strategy prevents metabolic pathways from entering into futile cycles of synthesis and degradation and allows the regulation of key transport systems by nodal compounds.[18–20]

Mitochondrial Beta Oxidation

The first step in fatty acid beta oxidation in the mitochondrion is the translocation of fatty acids across the mitochondrion in preparation for fatty acid oxidation and ketone formation. Fatty acids are translocated by first undergoing fatty acyl-CoA formation by the activity of distinct fatty acyl-CoA synthetases with specific substrate specificities for short-, medium-, and long-chain fatty acids in the mitochondrial outer membrane.[11, 18, 19, 41, 42] Fatty acyl-CoA is then conjugated with carnitine and catalyzed by carnitine palmitoyltransferase I located within the mitochondrial membrane to form fatty acylcarnitine. Fatty acylcarnitine is then translocated into the mitochondrion by a fatty acylcarnitine:carnitine translocase, an integral inner membrane protein, in exchange for free carnitine.[43] Within the mitochondrion, a reverse reaction mediated by carnitine palmitoyltransferase II releases fatty acyl-CoA, which is now a substrate for beta oxidation. The first step that is unique to beta oxidation is formation of *trans*-enol fatty acid, which is generated by acyl-CoA dehydrogenase. Acyl-CoA dehydrogenase transfers two electrons to flavin adenine dinucleotide (FAD), which then transfers them to the electron transport chain in the mitochondrion. 3-Keto fatty acyl-Co then undergoes a series of sequential reactions to acetyl-CoA and fatty acyl-CoA, which undergo another round of beta oxidation (not shown in Fig. 63–2). Acetyl-CoA can enter the tricarboxylic acid cycle, thus generating 12 ATP, or it can enter the 3-hydroxyl methyl glutaryl-CoA cycle to form ketone bodies. Only mitochondria in the liver are capable of forming ketone bodies. Regulation of mitochondrial beta oxidation lies with fatty acylcarnitine formation, which is catalyzed by carnitine palmitoyltransferase I.[43] Malonyl-CoA, the basic subunit of fatty acid synthesis, is a potent inhibitor of carnitine palmitoyltransferase I, thereby preventing beta oxidation and fatty acid synthesis from occurring concurrently.

Peroxisomal Oxidation of Fatty Acids

In addition to beta oxidation of fatty acids in mitochondria, another site for beta oxidation of fatty acids is peroxisomes.[18, 39, 40] The metabolic pathway in peroxisomes possesses certain unique features that differentiate it from its mitochondrial counterpart. The relative contribution of peroxisomes to beta oxidation is dependent on the length of the fatty acid chain and administration of recognized peroxisomal inducers. The mitochondrion has a much greater capacity than peroxisomes for beta oxidation of fatty acids. In both pathways, fatty acids must be converted to fatty acyl-CoA that utilizes an ATP. In contrast to the mitochondrion, initial fatty acyl-CoA formation within the peroxisome does not require fatty acyl carnitine formation for entry into the peroxisomes. This difference may provide a means of differentially regulating fatty acid beta oxidation.

During the next metabolic step in which *trans*-enoyl fatty acyl-CoA is formed, another significant difference occurs in the peroxisomes as compared to mitochondria. Two electrons produced by this step are transferred to FAD to form $FADH_2$, which is then transferred directly to oxygen to form hydrogen peroxide. Hydrogen peroxide is detoxified by catalase to form water and oxygen. In the mitochondrion, electrons are delivered to the mitochondrial electron transport system that ultimately generates water and ATP. The significance of this difference lies in both loss of ATP production and generation of hydrogen peroxide in the peroxisomes, which in the presence of transitional metals can yield toxic hydroxyl radicals and can thus promote lipid peroxidation and oxidant injury. NADH generated in subsequent reactions needs to be removed from the peroxisomes, whereas, in mitochondria, NADH can enter the electron transport cycle and generate additional ATP molecules. Peroxisomal enzymes can metabolize only long-chain fatty acids with a minimal chain length of 10 carbons and a maximal length of 24 carbons. As in mitochondria, beta oxidation in peroxisomes proceeds similarly by 2-carbon acetyl-CoA cleavage until octanoyl-CoA is formed. Octanoyl is then combined with carnitine to form fatty acyl carnitine, which can be transported by the mitochondrial inner membrane transporter and undergo completion of beta oxidation. Acyl-CoA formed in peroxisomes by beta oxidation of fatty acids can diffuse out of the peroxisomes after formation of acetyl carnitine.[19] The regulation of peroxisomal metabolism of fatty acids appears to be solely at the level of substrate availability, which may be regulated by a family of soluble fatty acid binding proteins present in the cytosol of all cells.

The physiologic function of peroxisomal beta oxidation is unknown. The ability of peroxisomes to beta oxidize long-chain fatty acids is unique, and thus peroxisomes play an important role in long-chain fatty acid metabolism. The peroxisomal pathway provides a supply of acetyl-CoA that does not require citrate formation and that can be used in fatty acid synthesis. However, because the initial electron transfer is not coupled to the mitochondrial electron transport system, peroxisomal fatty acid oxidation is less efficient than mitochondrial beta oxidation and may provide a means of eliminating fatty acids with energy loss. Peroxisomes are induced by a large number of hypolipidemic agents, such as clofibrate. The relative contribution of peroxisomal fatty acid beta oxidation can increase fivefold to tenfold when induced by partially hydrogenated fish oils and hypolipidemic agent. Because peroxisomal beta oxidation produces less ATP than does beta oxidation in mitochondria, a relative increase in peroxisomal fatty acid beta oxidation can lead to a reduction in lipid mass and weight loss. This pathway also provides a means of generating hydrogen peroxide, which can be used by catalase for the oxidation of substrates such as ethanol.[40]

Alcoholic Liver Disease and Fatty Acid Metabolism

Increased fatty acid synthesis and steatosis that is predominately macrovesicular with a pericentral distribution are well-recognized features of chronic alcoholic liver injury (see Chapter 71). These complications occur when alcohol forms a large percentage of the total caloric intake in an alcoholic and are biochemical consequences of ethanol metabolism.[44] Metabolism of ethanol can cause increased triglyceride synthesis and decreases in very-low-density lipoprotein (VLDL) synthesis and fatty acid beta oxidation. Alteration in the redox potential with excess NADH produced by ethanol metabolism is one of the major contributors to increased hepatic lipid synthesis. An increase in the NADH/NAD ratio favors formation of α-glycerol phosphate, which promotes triglyceride formation. An increase in NADH may also promote fatty acid synthesis because this pathway can utilize excess reducing equivalents. A decrease in NAD in the mitochondria may limit fatty acid beta oxidation that could contribute to fatty acid accumulation.[45] Ethanol may also directly increase the esterification pathway, further leading to increases in triglyceride synthesis.

LIPID TRANSPORT

The liver serves a central role in the synthesis of fatty acid for storage in distal sites and the trafficking of lipids within

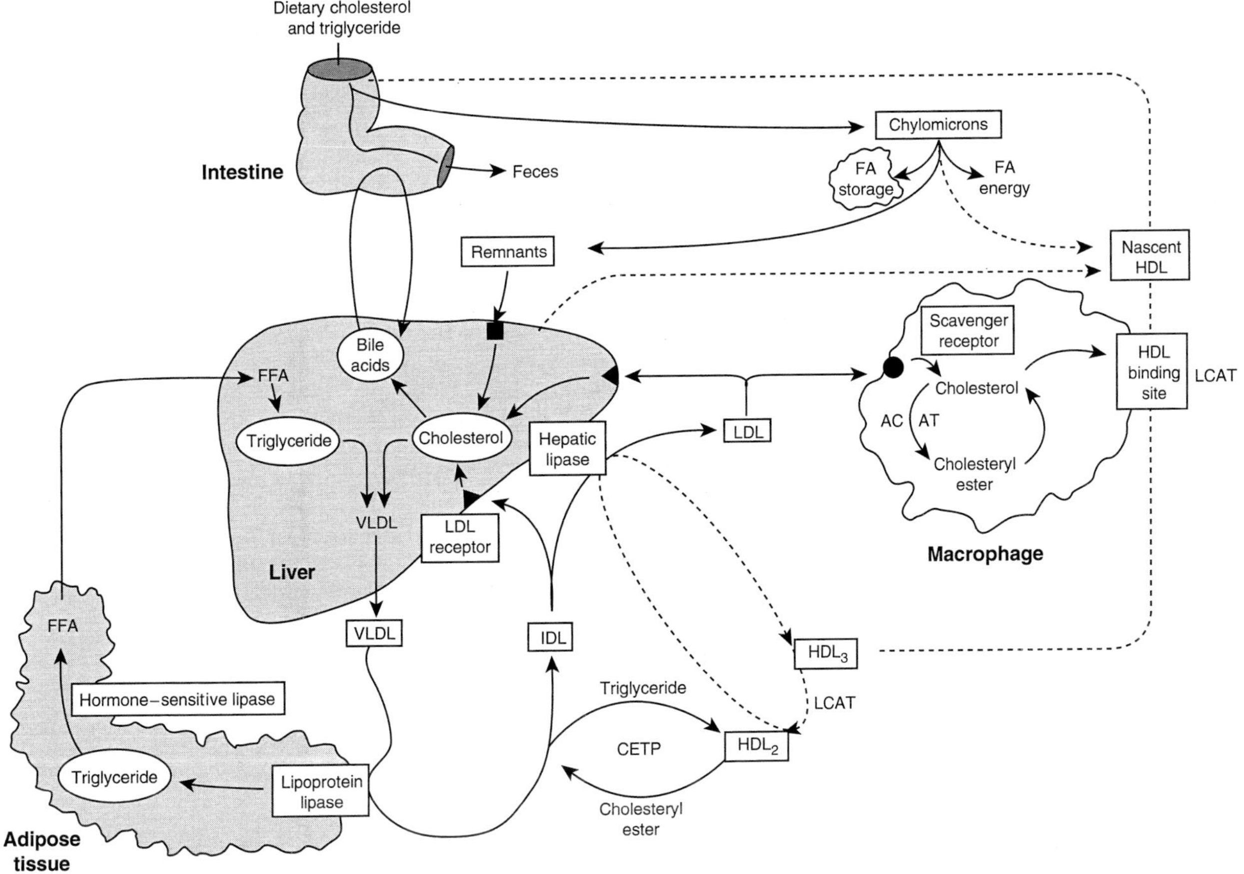

Figure 63–3. Lipoprotein metabolism. FFA, free fatty acids; ACAT, acylcholesterol acyltransferase; CETP, cholesteryl ester transfer protein; LCAT, lecithin-cholesterol acyltransferase; FA, fatty acids; LDL, low-density lipoproteins; HDL, high-density lipoproteins; VLDL, very-low-density lipoproteins. (Modified from Shepherd J: Lipoprotein metabolism. An overview. Drugs 47(Suppl 2):2, 1994.)

the body. For lipids to be transferred between different locations within the circulation, the liver synthesizes and extracts a large number of apolipoproteins. Apolipoprotein (apo), in combination with triglycerides, phospholipids, cholesterol and its esters, and lecithins, constitutes circulating lipoproteins. In addition to these protein and lipid synthesizing functions, the liver expresses cell surface receptors for circulating lipoproteins and modulates intravascular levels of these important macromolecules. A brief review of lipoprotein trafficking and the central role that the liver plays is summarized in this section and depicted in Figure 63–3. Detailed reviews are available elsewhere.[46–52]

Classification of Major Lipoproteins

Lipoproteins were originally classified by their buoyancy on a sucrose density gradient into five major categories listed in increasing density: chylomicrons, VLDL, low-density lipoproteins (LDL), intermediate-density lipoproteins (IDL), and high-density lipoproteins (HDL). Density differences in these particles are caused by differences in both the content and amount of specific lipids and the percentage of protein present within these lipoprotein fractions. As more lipid is extracted, the relative protein contribution increases, leading to increased density.[47] Individual lipoproteins also contain different classes of apolipoproteins that serve specific functions. Specific apolipoproteins may bind to lipids to retain them, assist in the transfer or metabolism of lipids by enzymes in serum or lining endothelial walls, or act as targets for specific lipoprotein receptors necessary for uptake by target tissues. The contents of lipoproteins are in a constant dynamic flux between delivery of lipids and cholesterol to cells, transfer to other lipoproteins (mediated by lipid transfer proteins), and catalysis by lipolytic enzymes. Triglycerides are the major lipids contained in chylomicrons and VLDL. They are the energy source for peripheral tissues and components of cellular membrane structures. Cholesterol constitutes the major lipid in LDL and HDL.

Cholesterol, unlike triglycerides, is not used as a fuel source but as a structural component of membranes and as precursors for steroid hormones. Trafficking of cholesterol is usually in the form of cholesteryl ester, which is generated in the serum by the activity of lecithin-cholesterol acyltransferase (LCAT) (see "High-Density Lipoproteins" later). Tangier's disease, a rare autosomal recessive disorder characterized by the accumulation of cholesteryl esters in reticuloendothelial cells, including the tonsils, thymus, and lymph nodes, as well as liver, spleen, and gallbladder in combination with the near absence of serum HDL cholesterol, is now recognized to be caused by mutations in the ABC A1 transporter, a new member of the ABC supergene family.[53] This same gene is responsible for familial HDL deficiency. Affected patients classically present with enlarged, orange-colored tonsils and have a fourfold to sixfold increased risk of atherosclerotic heart disease. Although the precise function of the transporter is not completely known, its location at the plasma membrane suggests that it mediates the active transport of cholesterol across the plasma membrane, possibly acting as a "flippase" that transports cholesterol from the inner to the outer leaflet of the plasma membrane.[53, 54] Once at the outer membrane surface, cholesteryl ester can be transferred to apolipoprotein as described in "Hepatic Transport of Lipids" later.

Major Classes of Apolipoproteins

Lipoproteins are the circulating complex of lipids with apolipoproteins. A description of the major apolipoproteins, their associated lipoproteins, and their metabolic function follows.[47]

The major apolipoproteins associated with triglyceride transport are apoB-100, which is synthesized in the liver, and apoB-48, which is synthesized in the intestine.[55] Both mRNAs are transcribed off the same gene. In the intestine of humans, apoB-48 undergoes a unique post-transcriptional RNA editing process in which a specific nonsense mutation is generated by cytidine deamination, resulting in a truncated protein approximately 48% of the size of the native protein in the liver.[56] ApoB-100 is essential for secretion of VLDL by the liver and serves as the binding protein for the LDL receptor present throughout the body. This LDL receptor binding domain is not contained within the apoB-48 fragment.[49, 57]

ApoC is synthesized predominately in the liver with minor expression in the intestine and other organs and is composed of three different proteins responsible for distinct metabolic functions. The genes for apoC-I and apoC-II are located on chromosome 19 in close proximity to that for apoE, whereas the gene for apoC-III is located next to the gene for apoA-I on chromosome 11.[54] The function of apoC-I is unknown. It is a small component of VLDL, HDL, and IDL. ApoC-II is present in VLDL, IDL, HDL, and chylomicrons and is an essential activator of lipoprotein lipase (LPL) (see "Intestinal Lipoprotein Metabolism" later). Persons lacking apoC-II have hypertriglyceridemia. ApoC-III is present in IDL, HDL, and chylomicrons and may be an inhibitor of LPL activity (see "Intestinal Lipoprotein Metabolism" later). All apoC proteins can inhibit the removal of chylomicrons or chylomicron remnants by the liver.[46, 54]

ApoE is synthesized in the liver and is found on all lipoproteins. ApoE is important for removal of lipoprotein remnants in the serum, can bind to LDL and other membrane proteins, and is important for targeting lipoproteins to specific receptors on peripheral cells. Three major alleles for apoE gene exist (ε2, ε3, and ε4), with the ε3 allele being the most abundant and ε2/ε3 genotype being the most frequent. Each allele possesses a different ability to bind to the LDL receptor. Absence of apoE can cause significant elevation of chylomicrons and VLDL remnants by reducing their clearance and is associated with an increased risk of atherosclerosis.[51, 58]

ApoE plays a particularly important role in the transport of lipids in the central nervous system. It is synthesized and secreted predominately by astrocytes and macrophages, and its synthesis is increased after injury.[59] Nonesterified cholesterol released after neuronal injury is re-esterified and then transported by apoE to those neurons undergoing reparation and reinnervation. In addition to its lipid transport abilities, apoE has been postulated to have antioxidant activity or to function as a modulator of neurotrophic factors. Studies have demonstrated a strong association between the apoE ε4 genotype and risk for the development of nonfamilial Alzheimer's disease. This association is based on the relative prevalence of the apoE ε4 genotype in patients with Alzheimer's disease, as compared with nonafflicted members of the same ethnic groups, as well as an increased frequency in sporadic early-onset Alzheimer's disease in persons without other mutations in amyloid precursor proteins. Inheritance of a single ε4 allele is associated with a 6- to 8-year earlier onset of disease as compared to inheritance of the ε3/ε3 genotype.[60] The explanation for this association is unknown; a proposed mechanism is the ability of apoE ε4 protein to form insoluble beta amyloid from soluble proteins, in contrast to other major apoE proteins.[59, 60]

ApoA-I is the major component of HDL lipoproteins. ApoA-I can exist in a lipidated or delipidated state; lipid-poor apoA-I functions as an acceptor of cell membrane cholesterol. ApoA-I and -II are synthesized in the liver and intestine as preproproteins. ApoA-I is a key activator of LCAT, which enhances cholesterol esterification in the plasma (see "High-Density Lipoproteins" later). The absence of a specific, conserved region in apoA-I protein causes loss of LCAT activation by apoA-I. ApoA-II is also present in HDL. ApoA-IV is a minor constituent synthesized in the intestine.[61]

Lipolytic Enzymes and Lipid Transport Proteins

Lipoprotein lipase is synthesized in fat and muscle cells, from where it traverses endothelial cells and binds to the luminal surface of the capillary bed.[46, 62] Found in adipose, lung, and muscle tissues, LPL promotes lipolysis of triglycerides present in VLDL, chylomicrons, or HDL. Regulation of LPL involves multiple stimuli, including fasting, fatty acids, hormones, and catecholamines. Patients with absent LPL activity because of homozygous mutations present with severe hypertriglyceridemia in childhood (type I hyperlipidemia) and pancreatitis. Hepatic triglyceride lipase (HTGL) is a member of the same lipase gene family as LPL and is synthesized in the liver. It binds to the luminal surface of hepatic endothelial cells, is involved in lipolysis of VLDL or IDL, and thus plays a major role in LDL formation. HDL may be another substrate for its activity. The relative roles of these two lipases have been assessed in animal studies in which the effects of antiserum that blocks specific lipases can be measured and in human and animal models in which a deficiency in one activity exists. Absence of LPL leads to accumulation of large particles containing both apoB-100 and apoB-48, with almost complete absence of smaller apoB-containing lipoprotein. Inhibition of HTGL results in accumulation of VLDL and IDL, with the enrichment of HDL in triglycerides.

Within the serum, lipid exchange between particles is facilitated by the activity of LCAT and cholesteryl ester transfer protein (CETP).[46, 47, 63, 64] LCAT is synthesized in the liver, and apoA-I is a cofactor for the activity of LCAT. CETP is synthesized predominantly in the liver and circulates in association with HDL. CETP mediates the exchange of cholesteryl esters from HDL with triglycerides from chylomicrons or VLDL. The activity of LCAT in combination with the lipid transfer proteins, CETP and phospholipid transfer protein (PLTP), is essential for the transfer of cholesterol from nonhepatic tissue to the liver[65] (see "High-Density Lipoproteins" later).

Intestinal Lipoprotein Metabolism

Fatty acids and cholesterol absorbed during meals are assimilated and modified within the enterocyte and excreted as chylomicron particles. Fatty acids are formed into triglycerides, and cholesterol is esterified and packaged into nascent chylomicrons composed of predominately triglycerides (85% to 92%), phospholipids (6% to 12%), cholesteryl ester (1% to 3%), fat-soluble vitamins, and the following apolipoproteins (1% to 3%): apoB-48, apoA-I, apoA-II, and apoA-IV.[66] Nascent chylomicrons enter into interstitial space and drain into the vascular compartment via the lymphatic system through the thoracic duct. In the interstitial space, they acquire apoC-II, which allows activation of LPL, thereby promoting triglyceride release. Release of triglycerides may be reduced by acquisition of apoC-III, which may inhibit LPL activity. Addition of apoE is critical for targeting of the chylomicron remnant, which can then be taken up by hepatocytes through the chylomicron remnant receptor.

Chylomicron remnants that are enriched in cholesteryl esters (by extraction of intestinal-derived triglycerides by peripheral tissues) are taken up by a hepatocyte membrane transporter that recognizes a binding domain on the apoE protein, such as LDL, LDL-related protein (LRP), and other members of the LDL receptor family (see "Lipoprotein Receptors" later).[58] These membrane receptors target delivery of the chylomicron remnants to lysosomes, where they are degraded. Persons who express an apoE with a mutated domain exhibit decreased clearance of chylomicron remnants. An important action of this pathway is the bidirectional trafficking of fatty acids to peripheral tissue and transport of cholesterol to the liver from peripheral sources. The activity of LPL is also critical for the release of fatty acid, and the activity of LPL is continually modified in response to the requirements of local tissue as well as hormonal regulation.

This lipid transport process allows triglycerides derived from dietary sources to be delivered to tissues in exchange for cholesteryl esters and phospholipids. These products are delivered to the liver for bile acid or membrane synthesis, biliary excretion of cholesterol, or redistribution of phospholipids to other tissues.[64, 67, 68] Under normal conditions, these pathways provide a means for the excretion of excess cholesterol or phospholipids by the liver and are an integral part of reverse cholesterol transport. When chylomicron excretion is delayed, as when LPL activity is reduced or apoC-II levels are decreased, chylomicron remnants that accumulate in the serum may be taken up by endothelial cells or macrophages, which transform into foamy cells, the precursors of fatty streak and atheroma formation. Increased VLDL secretion resulting from excess fatty acid absorption can also compete with the chylomicron remnant uptake system.

Hepatic Lipid Metabolism

The liver functions as the hub for receiving fatty acids and cholesterol from the diet and peripheral tissues, packaging them into lipoprotein complexes, and releasing the complexes into the circulation. Fatty acids released from adipocytes by the action of intracellular hormone-sensitive lipase are bound to serum albumin and transported to other tissues including the liver, where they are used for synthesis of phospholipids and triglycerides.[69] The liver is capable of synthesizing fatty acids from low-molecular-weight precursors, whereas cholesterol synthesis is regulated by the rate-limiting enzyme 3-hydroxyl-3-methylglutaryl coenzyme A reductase (HMG-CoA reductase). Lipids are exported from the liver by VLDL particles, which are the major carrier of plasma triglycerides during nonabsorptive states.[11, 70, 71] Lipids may be stored temporarily in the liver as fat droplets (or, in the case of cholesterol, as cholesteryl esters), excreted directly into bile, or metabolized into bile acids. The liver is the major site of sterol excretion from the body and is the site of bile acid synthesis.

The coordinated input, synthesis, and excretion of sterols require complex regulation of multiple enzymatic pathways. Bile acids play a critical role in modulating these enzyme activities and undergo a unique enterohepatic circulation (see Chapter 54).[9] Bile acids are recirculated 20 to 30 times per day via the enterohepatic circulation, which requires the activity of specific transmembrane transporters at both the apical and basolateral domains as well as intracellular binding proteins of hepatocytes and enterocytes.[72] In the terminal ileum, a unique sodium-dependent bile acid transporter prevents loss of bile acids in the stool.[73] Bile acids also play an important role in micellization of fats for intestinal absorption and as a coactivator of bile acid–dependent lipase activity. Bile acids are an important direct regulator of bile acid synthesis and HMG-CoA reductase activity, the rate-limiting enzyme in cholesterol synthesis.[67] The discovery that a member of the sterol nuclear receptor family, farnesoid X receptor (FXR), can specifically bind to and be activated by bile salts provides a specific pathway by which bile salts can regulate gene expression. FXR dimerizes with the retinoid X receptor (RXR) transcription factor (see "Vitamin A" later) and can modulate gene expression of key bile salt transporters, such as NTCP, BSEP, and intestinal bile acid transporter (IBAT), as well as cholesterol-7α-hydroxylase.[74, 75]

Hepatic Transport of Lipids

Lipid transport by the liver has an important regulatory influence on total lipid metabolism of the organism and movement of lipids to the peripheral tissues. In this section, hepatic transport of lipoproteins is examined by dividing them into apoB-containing lipoproteins (VLDL, LDL, and IDL) and apoA-containing lipoprotein, HDL.

ApoB Lipoproteins

In the fasting state, VLDLs, which are synthesized in the liver and composed of the complete apoB-100, replace chylomicrons as the major transporter for triglycerides. The constituents of VLDL are triglycerides, which are either taken up by the liver from endogenous sources or derived from the lipolysis of fatty acid stores; cholesteryl esters, either exogenous or endogenously synthesized; and phospholipids.

VLDL synthesis is coupled tightly to fatty acid synthesis and storage and regulated by a complex interplay of dietary and hormonal factors.[70, 76–78] During fasting, fatty acids in VLDL result predominantly from hormone-sensitive lipase action in the adipocyte, whereas after a meal, dietary fatty acids form the majority of VLDL content. Fatty acid uptake into the liver may be mediated by passive diffusion, although studies have identified a sinusoidal fatty acid transport protein in liver and adipocyte membrane fractions. Once inside the liver, fatty acids may bind to the abundant 12-kd fatty acid binding protein gene family, the purpose of which may be to direct intracellular trafficking of fatty acids to specific subcellular targets, such as smooth ER for VLDL synthesis or peroxisomes for beta oxidation. Fatty acid binding proteins are transcriptionally regulated by peroxisomal proliferating agents and hypolipidemic agents, suggesting an important function in global lipid metabolism.

ApoB-100 is the predominant transport carrier; apoC-I, C-II, C-III, and apoE arise from other lipoproteins within the serum. The regulation of apoB-100 synthesis is an intense area of investigation, because it may be an important regulator of VLDL secretion. Although the precise mechanisms are unknown, apoB-100 synthesis, along with VLDL secretion, appears to be predicated on the availability of cotransported lipids and sterols in the smooth ER; levels of apoB-100 may change dramatically without alterations in apoB-100 mRNA levels.[51, 70, 78, 79] ApoB-100 is synthesized in the smooth ER, where it interacts with newly synthesized triglycerides and cholesteryl esters that enter the ER by specific membrane transporters. The apoB and its associated lipids are translocated into the lumen, transported through the Golgi apparatus, and secreted into the sinusoidal space.[80] If these components are not available, apoB-100 undergoes a degradative pathway in the ER, whereas in the presence of abundant triglycerides, apoB is synthesized and rapidly appears in VLDL. In tissue culture studies, addition of cholesterol to the media enhances apoB synthesis and VLDL secretion, suggesting that cholesterol, like triglycerides, can regulate apoB synthesis. Thus, short-term changes in apoB and VLDL secretion are regulated post-translationally by substrate availability rather than by changes in gene transcription. The size and structure of VLDL vary and presumably are modified to meet various metabolic demands. During periods of low triglyceride levels, the liver secretes smaller IDL-like particles or even LDL-type particles.

Once outside of the liver, VLDL is acted on by LPL to form smaller and denser particles called *IDL*. The particles eventually become LDL. This transformation from IDL to LDL requires the activity of both LPL and HTGL. Conversion of IDL to LDL requires the activity of apoE. Conversion of VLDL to LDL involves LPL hydrolysis of triglycerides and accumulation of cholesteryl ester from other lipoproteins, predominantly HDL, with release of apoC to HDL. Following these modifications, LDL is composed almost entirely of apoB. LDL is subsequently removed from the circulation by LDL receptors in the liver and peripheral tissues. Not all VLDL is converted directly to LDL; subpopulations of VLDL that begin as large VLDL undergo lipolysis with removal of IDL by the LDL receptor.

High-Density Lipoproteins

The other major class of lipoproteins excreted by the liver is HDL, in which the apoA family of lipoproteins predominates.[61, 63, 64] HDL appears to have a protective role against atherosclerosis, because elevated HDL cholesterol levels are associated with a reduced incidence of coronary artery disease. HDL comprises the largest number of lipoproteins in the circulation because of their small size. HDL is a heterogeneous population of lipoproteins that can be separated by sophisticated analytical centrifugation techniques.

Nascent HDL is formed in the liver and intestine by lipolysis from VLDL and chylomicrons, with modification by peripheral tissue. The major protein constituents of HDL are apoA-I and apoA-II, with minor amounts of apoA-IV, the apoCs, apoE, and others.[81] In humans, apoA-I is synthesized in the liver and intestine as a preproapolipoprotein of 267 amino acids and secreted as a 249-amino acid propeptide that is cleaved by a serum protease to form the mature 243-amino acid protein. Some apoA-I is secreted with chylomicrons, which explains its elevated levels in postprandial serum. Nascent lipoprotein complexes (containing apoA) that appear as discoid particles can be transformed into HDL particles in the serum by the action of LCAT and the lipid transfer proteins, CETP and PLTP. This conversion of discoid particles to HDL is dependent on LCAT activity, as demonstrated in patients with LCAT deficiency.

Within the HDL group of lipoproteins, the HDL_3 subclass is particularly important because of its ability to participate in reverse cholesterol transfer. These cholesterol-poor particles are able to deliver cholesterol extracted from peripheral membranes and provide a substrate for serum LCAT activity. Cholesteryl esters formed by LCAT are extremely hydrophobic and move into the core of the lipoprotein complex, thereby providing space on the surface of the lipoprotein for extraction of additional cholesterol from cell membranes. This complex enlarges with increasing amounts of cholesteryl esters, which are able to accommodate apoC-II and C-III, thereby resulting in HDL_2 formation. CETP removes esterified cholesterol out of HDL in exchange for triglycerides, which are eventually hydrolyzed by HTGL, thereby regenerating small HDL. Acquisition of apoC-II also promotes activity of LPL, thereby increasing lipolysis.[65]

The movement of apolipoproteins between HDL and chylomicrons allows the recycling of lipids and proteins between these two pools. Cholesterol and phospholipids are also transferred to the chylomicrons as triglycerides are released by LPL activity to local tissues. As the remnant is further processed, apoC-II and apoC-III, phospholipids, and cholesterol are transferred back to HDL. Triglycerides that are transferred from VLDL and chylomicrons to HDL are more accessible to lipolysis by endothelial-based lipases because of their smaller size. With the removal of triglycerides, these particles revert to HDL_3 and apoC-II, after which apoC-II and apoE recycle to chylomicrons and VLDL.

Lipoprotein Receptors

The major classes of lipoprotein receptors include the LDL receptor, chylomicron remnant receptor, HDL receptor, and scavenger receptor. These receptors are part of the larger LDL supergene family, which shares four major structural features: (1) cysteine-rich complement-type repeats; (2) epidermal growth factor precursor-like repeats; (3) a transmembrane domain; and (4) a cytoplasmic domain.[82] A brief review of the major subclasses follows.[48, 49, 51, 57]

LDL Receptor

The LDL receptor is the prototypic member of the LDL supergene family and exists as an oligomeric, surface glycoprotein that plays a pivotal role in LDL clearance and cholesterol homeostasis. This receptor binds ligand on the surface of cells, after which the ligand-receptor complex is internalized by receptor-mediated endocytosis. Ligand and receptor dissociate in acidic endosomal vesicles, after which ligand is delivered to lysosomes for degradation. LDL receptor is present on all cell types; however, the liver expresses approximately 70% of the total body pool of LDL receptors. LDL receptor recognizes apoB-100 but not apoB-48 and apoE. Chylomicron remnants containing apoE, VLDL, LDL, IDL, and HDL all can be taken up by the LDL receptor. Approximately two thirds of LDL are cleared by this receptor. Absence of this functional receptor caused by homozygous mutations occurs in approximately 1 in 1 million persons and is associated with accelerated atherosclerosis appearing in childhood (familial hypercholesterolemia). LDL receptors are highly conserved among species.

VLDL Receptor

The VLDL receptor was identified by its high-sequence homology to the LDL receptor. The complementary DNA and genomic structure are very similar but are expressed in different locations; the majority of VLDL receptors are expressed in extrahepatic tissues such as heart, muscle, and fat. Unlike the LDL receptor, the VLDL receptor cannot bind to apoB. Thus, this receptor may serve specifically to take up triglyceride-rich apoE containing lipoproteins, such as VLDL or IDL, for fatty acid metabolism.[82, 83]

Chylomicron Receptor

Chylomicron remnants are removed from the circulation exclusively by the liver. The ability of these large complexes to penetrate the unique sinusoidal vascular space is believed to play a major role in this selective hepatic removal. Chylomicron remnants containing apoE are substrates for LDL receptor–mediated uptake only after removal of triglycerides by hydrolysis.[64] The existence of an LDL-independent chylomicron receptor is indicated by normal chylomicron remnant removal in humans and rabbits deficient in the LDL receptor.

Studies suggest that the multifunctional, α_2-macroglobulin/LDL–related protein (LRP) is the chylomicron remnant receptor.[84] This protein is a member of the LDL receptor gene family. LRP is considerably larger than LDL and is present in liver, brain, and muscle. In tissue culture studies, LRP is able to transport chylomicron remnants containing apoE and, like the LDL receptor, internalize the lipoprotein complex via endocytosis. Animals made selectively deficient in LRP in the liver have absent chylomicron remnant uptake, confirming that LRP is the major chylomicron remnant receptor.[83, 85] Unlike LDL, LRP is able to bind to a large number of diverse unrelated ligands such as lipoprotein, proteinase-inhibitor complex, and protein-lipid complex.

HDL Receptor

The existence of an HDL receptor is based on identification of high-affinity HDL binding protein in the plasma membrane of many cells, including hepatocytes, macrophages, adrenal cells, and adipocytes.[64] These receptors appear to recognize specific apoA present in HDL particles. Unlike the LDL receptor, in which apolipoprotein complex is internalized by endocytosis, the HDL receptor allows only selective delivery of lipids to and from the HDL lipoprotein without internalization and destruction of the lipoprotein. Thus, this receptor system facilitates the transfer of cholesterol from the plasma membrane to the HDL lipoprotein and is implicated in the process of reverse cholesterol transport. HDL receptor is now recognized to be a class B scavenger receptor, referred to as *SR-B1*.[81] Scavenger receptors mediate binding of chemically modified lipoproteins, including acetylated and oxidized LDL. These receptors are most abundantly expressed in the liver, ovary, and adrenal glands, organs previously shown to be the principal sites of cholesterol uptake from HDL in vivo. At these sites, cholesterol is utilized either for generation of steroid hormones or biliary excretion.

LDL Scavenger Receptor

The existence of an LDL scavenger receptor was first recognized when accumulated LDL cholesterol was found in certain cell types in LDL receptor–deficient patients.[64] Ligands for this receptor include natural products, such as endotoxin, polyanionic lipids, and LDL, in which some of the free lysine residues have been chemically modified. These membrane receptors may exist in two forms, both trimeric, which differ in the presence of a carboxyl terminal cysteine-rich region, and are integral membrane glycoproteins located in macrophages, endothelial cell, and Kuppfer cells in the liver. Oxidized LDL can be recognized by the scavenger receptor but are poorly metabolized in the macrophage, leading to accumulation of cholesteryl esters within the cell. Monocytes also can be induced to express the scavenger receptor, which can be found routinely in lipid-enriched atherosclerotic lesions.

LIVER DISEASE AND LIPID ABNORMALITIES

The association of lipid abnormalities with liver disease is well recognized.[11, 86, 87] In chronic liver disease, abnormalities in serum lipoprotein can result from multiple defects, including decreased synthesis of lipoproteins, decreased clearance of lipoprotein complexes by the liver, and regurgitation of biliary content into the serum. The most common lipid abnormality is hypertriglyceridemia (250 to 500 mg/dL), which is found in chronic liver disease of multiple causes (viral or alcoholic) and tends to resolve when the liver disease improves. Excess alcohol ingestion is associated with dyslipoproteinemia, especially hypertriglyceridemia. Hypertriglyceridemia may be caused by a combination of increased fatty acid synthesis and decreased beta oxidation of fatty acids, owing to excess NADH generated by alcohol metabolism. Moderate alcohol ingestion is associated with increased levels of HDL_3, which may explain the reduced risk of atherosclerosis in alcoholics.[86] The specific effect of alcohol on changes in the serum lipid profile may be difficult to dissociate from toxic injury to the liver. Careful assessment of serum lipoprotein profiles in relationship to the Child-Turcotte score in cirrhotic patients has revealed a significant and progressive decrease in LDL, HDL, and total serum cholesterol levels in patients with Child-Turcotte class C as compared with class A cirrhosis. Patients with chronic hepatitis also have decreases in LDL, HDL, and total serum cholesterol levels as compared with normal controls, whereas no differences have been found in serum VLDL cholesterol levels. Serum cholesterol levels in noncholestatic liver disease may be useful prognostic markers.[88]

Cholestatic disorders present with a distinct dyslipoproteinemia pattern.[87] This is not surprising because biliary excretion is rich in cholesterol, phospholipids, and lecithin. Total serum cholesterol and lipid levels are usually elevated in these patients and can be associated with xanthoma formation in prolonged conditions, such as primary biliary cirrhosis. Serum triglyceride levels also may be elevated. Within the LDL fraction of cholestatic serum, three distinct lipoproteins can be identified and are labeled β_2-lipoprotein (triglyceride rich), also known as lipoprotein Y (LP-Y), lipoprotein X (LP-X), and normal LDL. LP-Y appears to be a remnant of a triglyceride-rich lipoprotein that is distinct from IDL. Cholestatic patients with elevated triglycerides often have clear serum because most of the triglycerides are contained in LP-Y and LDL. LP-X is a complex composed of equimolar amounts of excess phospholipid and cholesterol in combination with albumin and certain members of the apoC family. This complex can be detected on serum agar gel electrophoresis by its delayed migration as compared to other lipoproteins. The action of MDR3 (ABC B4), with its phospholipid flippase activity, is essential for LP-X formation; mice lacking the murine homologue, mdr2, are unable to form LP-X during cholestasis caused by complete bile duct obstruction.[89] Altered lipid metabolism resulting from regurgitation of biliary phospholipids into serum has been implicated as a major contributor to dyslipoproteinemia in cholestatic conditions.

In chronic parenchymal liver disease, decreased concentration of serum cholesteryl esters is a common finding, suggesting a decrease in LCAT activity because of impaired hepatic synthesis. Some authors hypothesize that most of the dyslipoproteinemia in chronic liver disease is caused by decreased LCAT activity. Alternatively, decreased activity may be caused by reduced apoC-II levels or release of cholesteryl ester hydrolase from damaged hepatocytes, with conversion of cholesteryl esters to cholesterol. Chronic dyslipoproteinemia in these patients can also lead to alterations in cellular membrane lipids, resulting in formation of abnormal RBCs, such as echinocytes, and alterations in membrane function with potential pathophysiologic consequences.

SERUM PROTEINS SYNTHESIZED BY THE LIVER

In addition to its role in the metabolism of lipids and carbohydrates, the synthetic capability of the liver is routinely assessed by measurement of serum proteins. The liver is the major site for the synthesis of serum proteins involved in coagulation and transport, such as albumin and iron binding, and of protease inhibitors. Alterations in the serum levels of these proteins may be caused by hepatic insufficiency, genetic mutations within specific serum proteins, or specific liver diseases, such as reduced ceruloplasmin levels in Wilson disease.

The liver is the major site for synthesis of acute-phase reactants, a widely diverse group of proteins that are expressed routinely during acute and chronic systemic inflammation. These proteins are assumed to play an important role in the host defense against tissue damage and infection. Fibrinogen aids in clot formation, and antiproteases serve to protect normal cells from proteases that are released from necrotic tissues. The hormonal mediators responsible for the profound activation of gene transcription in the liver in response to acute, systemic inflammatory diseases include interleukin-6, tumor necrosis factor-α, glucocorticoids, and interferon-γ. The major proteins synthesized by the liver and their postulated functions are listed in Table 63–2. A brief review of major classes of serum proteins associated with liver disease follows.

Vitamin K–Dependent Blood Coagulation Proteins

The liver synthesizes blood coagulation factors, including factor II (prothrombin), factor VII, factor IX, and factor X (which form part of the coagulant pathway), as well as protein C and protein S (which act together to inactivate the activated forms of factor VIII and factor V complexes) (see Chapter 79). All these proteins undergo a unique, vitamin K–dependent post-translational modification involving gamma-carboxylation of specific glutamic acid residues, which is essential for normal activity. Protein Z is another gamma-carboxylated protein whose function is unknown. All the procoagulants share a homologous amino-terminal end containing the glutamic acid residues that undergo gamma-carboxylation and that enable these proteins to bind calcium.[90–92] These modified glutamic acid residues bind to divalent cations such as calcium and subsequently to phospholipid or plasma membrane, which is required for their activation. These proteins are secreted into serum as proenzymes, which are then activated to form serine proteases that function in the coagulation cascade.

Biosynthesis of Gamma-Carboxylated Glutamic Acid

Post-translational modification of glutamic acids is mediated by a series of enzymes that require vitamin K as a cofactor

Table 63–2 | **Serum Proteins Produced by the Liver**

PROTEIN	MOLECULAR WEIGHT	FUNCTION	ASSOCIATION WITH LIVER DISEASE	ACUTE-PHASE RESPONSE
Albumin	66,500	Binding protein, osmotic regulator	Decreased in chronic liver disease	Decreased
Alpha fetoprotein	66,300	Binding protein	Increased in hepatocellular carcinoma	Decreased
α_1-antitrypsin (α_1-AT)	54,000	Inhibitor of elastin	Missense mutations associated with liver disease	Increased
Ceruloplasmin	132,000	Ferroxidase	Decreased in Wilson disease	Increased
Fibrinogen	340,00	Precursor to fibrin in homeostasis, wound healing	Decreased in chronic liver disease	Increased
Transferrin	79,500	Iron-binding protein	Increased in iron deficiency	Decreased
Complement C 3	185,000	Complement pathway		Increased
Complement C 4	200,000	Complement pathway		Increased
α_1-Acid glycoprotein (orosomucoid)	40,000	Inhibits proliferating response of peripheral lymphocytes to mitogens		Increased
α_1-Antichymotrypsin	68,000	Inhibits chymotrypsin-like serine proteinase		Increased
Haptoglobin	Protein complex approximately 100,000	Binds hemoglobin released by hemolysis		Increased
C-reactive protein	118,000	Binds foreign pathogens and damaged cells to initiate their elimination		Increased
Serum amyloid A	9,000	Unknown function		Increased
Ferritin	450,000	Intracellular iron storage	Increased in hemochromatosis	Increased

Data from references 148 and 149.

along with molecular oxygen, carbon dioxide, and NADPH. The process involves two enzymatic reactions in which the glutamic residue is first carboxylated by a vitamin K–dependent carboxylase, during which the vitamin K cofactor (naphthohydroquinone) is converted to 2,3-epoxide vitamin K, which is catalyzed by a multiprotein complex associated with the microsomal membrane. The second step involves reduction of the 2,3-epoxide vitamin K. Multiple microsomal or cytosolic reductases can reduce the 2,3-epoxide vitamin K to replenish the vitamin K cofactor. The action of the oral anticoagulant warfarin (Coumadin) is mediated by inhibition of the reduction of vitamin K epoxide, thereby impairing the necessary replacement of vitamin K.[90–92]

Abnormal coagulation associated with chronic liver disease is usually caused by a combination of factors, including reduced synthesis of functional clotting factors and impaired reticuloendothelial function.[93, 94] Reticuloendothelial cells of the liver regulate coagulation by clearance of activated clotting or fibrinolytic factors, such as activation complexes, and end-products of the conversion of fibrinogen to fibrin. Abnormalities in both platelet number and function also are associated with chronic liver disease and can contribute to hemostatic defects routinely found with chronic liver disease.

Vitamin K deficiency also can develop in patients with long-standing cholestatic syndromes who are unable to absorb fat-soluble vitamins, including vitamin K.[95] Clotting dysfunction in these patients improves with vitamin K supplementation. During acute hepatitis and chronic cirrhosis, noncarboxylated, nonfunctional forms of the vitamin K–dependent clotting factors accumulate in serum and can be identified by immunologic methods or functional testing. Treatment with vitamin K in this setting is unable to correct the defect, which results from impaired post-translational modification and not from a relative absence of vitamin K. Elevated levels of non–γ-carboxylated prothrombin (des-γ-carboxylated prothrombin) and other coagulation factors have been detected in up to 91% of patients with hepatocellular carcinoma and are attributed to the inability of the tumor to gamma-carboxylate prothrombin adequately.[92, 96] In more than two thirds of these patients, levels are in excess of 300 ng/mL, which far exceed the normal levels found in cirrhosis and acute hepatitis. Resection of hepatocellular tumors in patients with elevated levels of des-γ-carboxylated prothrombin is associated with a decrease in serum levels, which increase again with tumor recurrence. Des-γ-carboxylated prothrombin constitutes a potential serum marker for hepatocellular carcinoma, along with alpha fetoprotein (see Chapter 81).[96]

α_1-Antitrypsin

α_1-Antitrypsin (α_1-AT) is a hepatic secretory glycoprotein that is a member of the serpin serine protease inhibitor family (see Chapter 65). Contrary to its designation, the predominant targets of this inhibitor are macrophage-derived elastase, the major target of which is pulmonary elastin, as well as cathepsin and proteinase 3.[97] α_1-AT inhibits protease activity by occupying the active site for the targeted substrate of the specific serine protease; it is also an acute phase reactant. Absent or reduced α_1-AT activity is manifested clinically by chronic destruction of the lung parenchyma with the early onset of emphysema. The protein is found normally in the lung and can be detected in monocytes and macrophages. More than 95% of serum α_1-AT is synthesized by the liver, as evidenced by correction of α_1-AT deficiency following orthotopic liver transplantation.

Different isoforms of α_1-AT have been classified by their migration patterns on starch gel electrophoresis, although the recent molecular identification of specific DNA mutations has greatly expanded the number of different isoforms. Using the electrophoretic separation technique, the normal protein is designated as the M isoform, with two common deficiencies designated as the Z allele, in which a single mutation results in a substitution of lysine for glutamate at codon 342, and the S allele, a valine-for-glutamate substitution at position 264. Gene deletion and specific nonsense, missense, or abnormal splicing mutations all are responsible for reduced or absent production of the protein. Patients with the null allele produce no α_1-AT but do not develop liver disease.[97]

The liver disease associated with α_1-AT deficiency is variable and depends on the molecular consequence of the missense point mutations and host factors. Recent studies demonstrate that specific point mutations can alter normal processing of the protein in the ER, thereby promoting oligomerization between adjacent proteins and leading to formation of protein aggregates that eventually cause obstruction of the secretory pathway.[98] The formation of these aggregates is associated with accumulation of abnormal protein that causes hepatocellular injury. Thus, unlike the pulmonary disease, which results from a lack of sufficient antiproteolytic activity, the liver disease is caused by retention of excess protein aggregates composed of α_1-AT.

Variation in the processing of α_1-AT in the ER has been implicated as the reason that patients with the same α_1-AT mutation may present with a spectrum of liver injury ranging from none to severe. Teckman and colleagues described the reduced clearance of abnormally folded α_1-AT in the fibroblasts of patients with and without liver disease but with the same α_1-AT mutation, thereby providing strong supportive evidence for intrinsic differences in protein processing.[99] In the ER, folding of nascent proteins is facilitated by chaperones to ensure the proper conformation required for functional activity. Proteins that fail to fold properly are retained in the ER and ultimately degraded, a sequence that occurs infrequently with normal α_1-AT. In patients with certain α_1-AT mutations, missense mutations can promote aggregation of adjacent nascent proteins, which are then recognized to be misfolded and are selected for degradation, leading to reduced serum levels of α_1-AT. Liver disease is hypothesized to develop in persons in whom the normal clearance and degradation pathways are overwhelmed, either because of a genetic factor or increased synthesis of α_1-AT with excessive oligomerization and eventual obstruction within the ER. Recent studies suggest that small "chemical chaperone" molecules such as 4-phenylbutryic acid (PBA) can enhance the clearance activity of ER, thereby providing a potential strategy to augment endoplasmic clearance of retained proteins.[100] Treatment with oral PBA was shown to increase serum levels of mutated α_1-AT in a transgenic mouse model, proving the potential feasibility of using this strategy to treat patients with α_1-AT deficiency.

Ceruloplasmin

Ceruloplasmin is another acute phase protein that is an important diagnostic tool for the detection of Wilson disease, also referred to as *hepatolenticular degeneration* (see Chapter 67). This glycosylated serum protein with a molecular weight of 132 kd normally contains six copper molecules and accounts for greater than 95% of serum copper. The gene for ceruloplasmin is transcriptionally up-regulated, like those for other acute phase reactants by trauma or systemic inflammatory response. Decreased serum levels of ceruloplasmin are found in patients with Wilson disease because of inadequate incorporation of copper during its biosynthesis, leading to secretion of an unstable apoceruloplasmin that is rapidly degraded. Ceruloplasmin does not function as a serum copper binding protein but rather as a serum ferroxidase that promotes oxidation of ferrous to ferric iron and is necessary for its incorporation into apotransferrin. This oxidation ultimately promotes mobilization of intracellular iron stores. Consistent with this proposed function is the development in copper-deficient animals of anemia that is unresponsive to iron but corrects with copper replacement. Recently, a patient with aceruloplasminemia caused by a frame-shift mutation was found to exhibit abnormal iron metabolism associated with late-onset neurologic defects and increased intracellular iron stores in the basal ganglia, further confirming the role of ceruloplasmin in iron metabolism.[101, 102] Ceruloplasmin ferroxidase activity may be necessary for movement of iron from intracellular stores to extracellular transferritin. Patients lacking this activity may present with iron deficiency and increased intracellular iron stores.

The gene defect in Wilson disease results from a mutation in a putative ATP-dependent copper transport protein similar to that responsible for Menkes disease.[103] Reduced activity of this transporter is responsible for impaired incorporation of copper into ceruloplasmin and absent biliary copper secretion, although its precise function is incompletely understood. For a more complete discussion of Wilson disease, see Chapter 67.

Serum Albumin

Serum albumin, the predominant serum binding protein, is used routinely to assess the synthetic function of the liver. The absolute serum level of albumin reflects not only hepatic synthesis, but also volume of distribution; availability of amino acid precursors; and loss into urine, peritoneum, pleural cavities, or intestinal lumen and from the skin.[104] In the presence of portal hypertension and ascites, an increased volume of distribution may contribute to low serum levels despite increased synthetic rates. Albumin functions as a nonspecific carrier protein that binds fatty acids, bile acids, and numerous endogenous and exogenous compounds. It also provides serum oncotic pressure that opposes hydrostatic pressure. A rare genetic disorder manifested by the absence of serum albumin has been identified with minimal clinical sequelae.[105] Affected patients have increased levels of gamma globulins that compensate for albumin in providing oncotic pressure. Hepatic synthetic rates of albumin are regulated in part by the serum oncotic pressure, as demonstrated both in isolated hepatocytes and an isolated perfused rat liver model.[106, 107] Patients with elevated serum immunoglobulin levels also may have low serum albumin levels, possibly to compensate for increased serum oncotic pressure contributed by the excess immunoglobulins.[108]

Alpha Fetoprotein

Alpha fetoprotein and albumin evolve from a common ancestral gene and share significant sequence homology and similar genomic organization.[109] Alpha fetoprotein serves a function in the developing organism similar to that of albumin in the adult and is postulated to bind fatty acids. Alpha fetoprotein is entirely replaced by serum albumin at the end of the first year of life. During liver regeneration, as in acute viral hepatitis, and in hepatocellular carcinoma, serum alpha fetoprotein levels may be elevated. Serum values greater than 400 ng/mL are almost exclusively associated with hepatocellular carcinoma. Serum alpha fetoprotein may be used in the appropriate clinical setting to screen patients for potential hepatocellular carcinoma or to follow patients after resection or treatment of hepatocellular carcinoma (see Chapter 81).

Iron Storage and Binding Proteins

Iron storage and binding proteins are used routinely for the identification and assessment of hemochromatosis, a common genetic disorder associated with multisystemic disease in advanced cases (see Chapter 66).[110, 111] The ability to identify the genotype of persons with hereditary hemochromatosis has led to re-evaluation of the role of iron studies in the diagnosis of hemochromatosis. Because hemochromatosis can be treated easily by phlebotomy, it is essential for persons to be identified before permanent iron-induced injury occurs. Definitive assessment of the body's iron stores involves either direct quantification of hepatic iron or histologic staining of liver biopsy samples for iron. The liver contains approximately 10% of total body iron stores, predominantly bound to ferritin within hepatocytes. Iron stored in the liver can be exchanged with iron bound to transferrin, which can be exchanged with iron in peripheral tissues. In iron overload syndromes, the liver is the main site of excess iron storage. See Chapter 66 for additional information.

Iron is carried in the serum by transferrin, which binds to the transferrin receptor on the sinusoidal plasma membrane of hepatocytes and other cells. Iron bound to transferrin is taken up by peripheral tissues, especially proliferating or malignant cells. The receptor-transferrin complex then undergoes receptor-mediated endocytosis, where it enters into acidic endosomal space that releases iron from the transferrin. Iron is then dispersed within the cell to be used in multiple proteins or stored bound to ferritin. The receptor-transferrin complex is then recycled back to the plasma membrane, where it is released from the receptor in the nonacidic extracellular environment.

Iron Storage

Iron is stored in all cells in association with ferritin, a microcrystalline core of magnetically ordered, polymeric, ferric oxyhydroxide phosphate. Each ferritin particle may contain from 2500 to 4000 molecules of iron, and iron may comprise up to one third of the molecular weight of the iron-ferritin complex. Release of iron from ferritin requires reduction from the ferric to the ferrous state. Ascorbate can increase the mobilization of iron, and supplemental vitamin C should be avoided by patients with iron storage disorders.

Iron is now known to regulate the translation of a number of iron-related proteins at the mRNA level by a combination of a *cis*-acting RNA sequence, referred to as an iso-RNA response element. Specific RNA-binding proteins, the iso-RNA regulatory peptides, which are aconitase homologues, regulate translation of these genes.[112] Iron interacts with these regulatory peptides to regulate the coordinated expression of critical genes, including those for ferritin, transferritin, transferrin receptor, and divalent metal transporter 1 (DMT-1, the apical iron transporters expressed in the duodenum), as well as gene products that utilize oxygen, such as enzymes involved in heme synthesis. In addition to iron, this pathway is regulated by oxygen tension, nitrous oxide, hydrogen peroxide, and inhibitors of the protein kinase C pathway. Increasing intracellular concentrations of iron can lead to either release of a repressor protein, which results in increased translation of the mRNA, or release of a peptide that promotes degradation of the mRNA. For example, increased cellular iron results in increased translation of ferritin mRNA, thereby promoting storage of iron, with decreased transferrin receptor mRNA, leading to reduced uptake of iron. The net effect of this common regulatory mechanism is the rapid, orchestrated response of a cascade of iron-responsive genes in individual cells depending on their needs.

FAT-SOLUBLE VITAMINS

Absorption of fat-soluble vitamins depends on adequate fatty acid micellization in the intestine by sufficient amounts of bile acids in bile. Prolonged cholestasis can lead to fat malabsorption and subsequent deficiency of fat-soluble vitamins. In addition, the liver mediates the total body metabolism of fat-soluble vitamins.[95] Table 63–3 summarizes the functions of fat-soluble vitamins and their associated abnormalities in patients with liver diseases.

Vitamin A

Vitamin A belongs to the retinoid family of chemicals that are members of natural and synthetic analogs of retinols and the provitamin A carotenoids.[95, 113, 114] The all-*trans* and 9-*cis* isomers of retinoic acid mediate their effects by interacting with members of the ligand-dependent transcription factors RXR α, β, and γ and retinoid alpha receptors (RAR) α, β, and γ. These transcription factors form homodimers or heterodimers among themselves or with other transcription factors and interact with specific *cis*-acting elements of genes to regulate their expression. These proteins mediate transcriptional activity of vitamin A, which plays a critical role both in embryonic development and in gene regulation of multiple adult genes.

Retinoids and provitamin A carotenoids are absorbed from the gastrointestinal tract and can be metabolized to retinol (vitamin A alcohol) by the action of intraluminal

Table 63–3 | **Fat-Soluble Vitamins**

VITAMIN	FUNCTION	ASSOCIATED ABNORMALITIES IN PATIENTS WITH LIVER DISEASE
A	Activator of gene expression by RXR and RAR transcription factors. Important for embryonic development and regulation of adult genes	Vitamin A toxicity can lead to microvesicular fat, cirrhosis; hepatotoxicity potentiated in alcoholic liver disease
D	Regulation of calcium and phosphate homeostasis	Rickets caused by vitamin D deficiency in childhood cholestatic diseases
K	Posttranslational gamma-carboxylation of glutamic residues in coagulant and anticoagulant pathways and osteocalcin	Cholestatic liver disease can lead to fat malabsorption and vitamin K deficiency
E	Antioxidant residing in cellular membranes throughout the body	Chronic cholestatic syndromes can lead to secondary neurologic impairment due to long-standing vitamin E deficiency; mutations in cytosolic tocopherol-binding protein associated with selective vitamin E deficiency

RAR, retinoid alpha receptor; RXR, ligand-dependent transcription factor.

organism and enterocytes. Foods that are rich in these compounds, including dairy products, internal organs, yellow and leafy green vegetables, and fruits, may be lacking in the diets of children or alcoholics. Vitamin A forms mixed micelles containing retinol, carotenoids, sterols, and phospholipids, which are taken up by passive diffusion across the enterocyte membrane. Approximately 80% of the vitamin A consumed is absorbed, and approximately 30% to 50% of the absorbed vitamin A is excreted within 1 week as oxidized or biotransformed product. The remainder is stored in the liver for future use.

In the liver and intestine, retinols undergo a complex metabolic pathway and trafficking, mediated and regulated by specific intracellular and extracellular binding proteins. Within cells, retinols and retinals are bound by cytosolic retinol binding protein-I (CRBP-I). In the intestine, provitamin A carotenoids are absorbed directly and converted into retinaldehyde (vitamin A aldehyde), a substrate for microsomal retinaldehyde reductase, to form retinol. A second cytosolic retinol binding protein (CRBP-II), expressed exclusively in the intestine of adults, appears to enhance the activity of microsomal retinaldehyde reductase. This protein can bind both retinol and retinaldehyde and appears to play a critical role in directing enterocyte processing of retinoids. Absence of CRBP-I in mice leads to reduced storage and a shortened half-life of retinoids, suggesting that CRBP-I plays a critical role in net retinoid metabolism.[115]

Once retinoids are formed into retinols, they are esterified with long-chain fatty acids by the action of lecithin-to-retinol acyltransferase (LRAT). CRBP-II also is required for the activity of LRAT. Retinols are exported as retinyl esters with palmitate or other fatty acids, packaged within chylomicrons, and released into the lymphatic drainage. In the absence of CRBP, acyl-CoA-to-retinal acyltransferase (ARAT) can also esterify retinol, but this is a minor pathway. Retinol esters remain in the chylomicron remnant and are deposited in the liver, which is the major storage site of the body. Retinoids are stored predominantly as retinyl ester in nonparenchymal stellate cells, also referred to as *Ito cells*, with the remainder stored in hepatocytes in lipid droplets. Kidney and adrenal glands are also minor storage sites.

Retinyl esters are metabolized to retinol by a bile salt–dependent and bile salt–independent esterase activity in the liver and then transferred to stellate cells bound to serum retinol–binding protein (RBP), a 21-kd protein that comigrates in serum with transthyretin (prealbumin), a tetramer that also binds thyroid hormone. Retinol may also be re-esterified and stored in hepatocytes. RBP is expressed solely in the liver, and its release into the circulation is dependent on an adequate supply of retinol. During retinol-deficient states, RBP accumulates in the liver with no change in steady-state mRNA levels, indicating that post-translational regulation is responsible for altered serum levels. Retinyl esters are formed by the activity of hepatic LRAT, through which retinol is bound by CRBP-I. Relative storage of retinol between parenchymal cells and stellate cells is dependent on total body retinol status. In depleted states, retinols are stored in the liver, whereas during repleted states, the majority of retinols are stored in lipid droplet in the stellate cells. Stellate cells and hepatocytes contain CRBP-I as well as cellular retinoic acid binding protein-I (CRABP-I). CRABP-I and CRBP-II have high affinities for retinoic acid, the key ligand for the RXR and RAR transcription factors, and in concert with CRBPs, maintain intracellular levels of these two important classes of retinoids.[116]

Hepatotoxicity of Vitamin A

Oversupplementation with vitamin A, including nonprescription vitamin supplements, especially in the setting of chronic alcoholic liver disease, is associated with hepatotoxicity.[117, 118] Chronic vitamin A toxicity can present with hair loss, localized erythema, exopthalmos, and thickened epithelium with fatty infiltration of the liver and heart, as demonstrated in animal studies. The toxic manifestation of fatty liver in both alcoholic and vitamin A–associated liver injury suggests a common pathway. Reduced vitamin A levels were found in rats fed alcohol and vitamin A, despite normal serum concentrations of RBP and vitamin A, suggesting that activation of stellate cells with loss of vitamin A storage may be responsible for decreased hepatic stores. Vitamin A may also disrupt mitochondrial membranes, thereby causing cellular damage. Activation of microsomal enzymes by alcohol and alterations in cellular reducing equivalents by metabolism of ethanol may be contributing factors to the well-recognized potentiation by alcohol of vitamin A hepatotoxicity. Elderly persons also may be at increased risk of vitamin A hepatotoxicity because of an age-associated decrease in clearance and metabolism.[119] The possibility of illicit use of vitamin supplements must be considered in patients with chronic liver disease who are at increased risk of vitamin A–associated hepatotoxicity.

Vitamin D

Vitamin D_2 (ergocalciferol) is a fat-soluble vitamin that is present in fortified milk products, egg yolk, fish liver, and fish liver oil. Its intestinal absorption depends on adequate micelle formation and requires bile acids. The other major source of vitamin D is the result of photochemical, cutaneous production of vitamin D_3 (cholecalciferol), which is generated by exposure of 7-dehydrocholesterol to ultraviolet irradiation.[95, 120, 121] Vitamin D_2 is absorbed through enterocytes, packaged in chylomicrons, and taken up by the liver in chylomicron remnants. Vitamin D_3 that is photosynthesized in the skin is bound in serum by vitamin D–binding protein and is taken up by the liver, where it undergoes additional biotransformation. Vitamin D–binding protein as well as serum albumin probably also mediates the transport of the hydroxylated metabolites in the serum. Reduced serum levels of vitamin D–binding protein have been found in patients with chronic liver disease.

In the liver, vitamin D is hydroxylated to form 25-hydroxyl vitamin D by a microsomal P-450 NADPH oxidase that requires molecular oxygen, NADPH, and magnesium.[121] Amino acid sequence analysis of the purified protein has demonstrated the same amino-terminal end amino acid sequence as in cytochrome P-4502C11, which is expressed preferentially in male liver microsomes. A low-affinity, high-capacity mitochondrial enzyme, sterol-27-hydroxylase, is also capable of hydroxylating vitamin D at the 25 position. This is the same enzyme that is deficient in, and the cause of, cerebrotendinous xanthomatosis. The kidney and intestine are other organs in which 25-hydroxylation occurs. 25-Hydroxyl vitamin D then undergoes hydroxylation at the first position to form its most potent metabolite in the kidney.

In chronic cholestatic syndromes such as primary biliary cirrhosis, impaired vitamin D absorption may contribute to the debilitating metabolic bone disease that in adults is predominantly osteoporosis.[122, 123] When vitamin D is deficient, supplemental vitamin D can ameliorate the rickets associated with chronic cholestatic conditions in children.[95] In addition, fatty acid malabsorption can contribute to calcium malabsorption when excess, unabsorbed fatty acids present in the intestinal lumen bind to intraluminal calcium. However, there is no correlation between vitamin D deficiency and metabolic bone disease. The metabolic bone disease associated with cholestatic disorders may be caused, in part, by augmentation of known risk factors associated with the development of osteoporosis, such as cigarette smoking and menopause.

Vitamin D supplementation does not benefit the severe osteoporosis associated with chronic liver disease. In these cases, excess reabsorption of bone and poor mineralization of osteoid are the primary causes of osteopenia. Improvements in bone mass have been demonstrated in patients with primary biliary cirrhosis who have undergone liver transplantation, although the mechanism of improvement is still unknown. Thus, vitamin D deficiency is not a major cause of metabolic bone disease associated with chronic cholestatic syndromes in adults.

Vitamin E

The term *vitamin E* is used to describe eight related compounds called the *tocopherols* and *tocotrienols*.[95] These compounds consist of a substituted hydroxylated chromanol ring linked to an isoprenoid side chain. The most active member is the stereoisomer D-alpha-tocopherol. The common food groups that contain vitamin E are oils derived from grains, plants, and vegetables. Vitamin E is a potent antioxidant that serves a unique role in protecting membrane structures against lipid peroxidation and free radical formation.[124] The hydrophobic property of vitamin E allows it to be embedded within cellular membranes, where it can donate electrons, thereby preventing formation of lipid peroxides. Oxidized vitamin E can be reduced by chemical reaction with ascorbate, glutathione, or cysteine. Ascorbate can be reduced by a monodehydroascorbate reductase in the cytosol, thereby regenerating the antioxidant.

All classes of tocopherol are taken up by enterocytes and require intestinal solubilization by bile acids. Twenty percent to 40% of ingested tocopherol is taken up by passive diffusion into enterocytes, where alpha- and gamma-tocopherol are packaged into chylomicrons and excreted into lymph.[125, 126] During conversion of chylomicrons to chylomicron remnants, a portion of the tocopherols are transferred to LDL and HDL, whereby they are distributed to other tissues. Most tocopherol is taken up by hepatocytes by way of the chylomicron remnant receptor. In the liver, selective retention of the D-alpha-tocopherol isoform occurs; gamma-tocopherol is either metabolized or excreted into bile. Retained D-alpha-tocopherol is then packaged with VLDL, secreted into the plasma for redistribution to other lipoproteins, and delivered to peripheral tissue.

The molecular mechanisms responsible for the selective hepatic sorting of D-alpha-tocopherol are not completely understood, but a recently identified cytosolic vitamin E–binding protein plays a major role. A rare homozygous recessive disorder was identified in children presenting with severe neurologic symptoms caused by selective vitamin E deficiency in the absence of a generalized cholestatic syndrome. These patients were able to absorb tocopherol after an oral challenge but failed to synthesize VLDL containing vitamin E.[125, 126] By positional cloning techniques, the disease gene locus was localized to the same chromosomal region encoding a recently characterized cytosolic, tocopherol-binding protein.[127] In these patients, nonsense mutations within the gene were identified, indicating that loss of selective hepatic retention of D-alpha-tocopherol is dependent on this protein.

In chronic cholestatic syndromes, especially those affecting children, chronic vitamin E deficiency can lead to severe neurologic disorders manifested initially by decreased deep tendon reflexes and ataxia caused by spinocerebellar dysfunction.[128] Peripheral neuropathy, dysarthria, decreased proprioception and vibratory sensation, myopathy, and retinitis pigmentosa with progressive visual field constriction also can develop. Anemia related to vitamin E deficiency also can occur, but only in children. Oral vitamin E supplementation is able to prevent these complications. Treatment with supplemental vitamin E has been proposed to reduce oxidant-induced liver injury, which is implicated in alcoholic liver injury and metabolic liver diseases such as Wilson disease, hemochromatosis, and tyrosinemia. In one study, serum aminotransferase levels decreased in obese children with steatohepatitis when they were treated with supplemental vitamin E and increased after cessation of therapy.[129] Vitamin E deficiency should be sought in all patients with long-standing cholestatic syndromes associated with fat malabsorption or abetalipoproteinemia, because oral supplementation can correct these disorders. Failure to treat affected persons can lead to permanent neurologic disability.

Vitamin K

Vitamin K is a fat-soluble vitamin that requires adequate micelle formation for absorption in the intestinal tract.[92, 95] Cholestatic syndromes with decreased bile flow are associated with impaired vitamin K absorption. Osteocalcin, a low-molecular-weight protein secreted by bone osteoblasts, is the other major gamma-carboxylated protein dependent on vitamin K for its synthesis, in addition to the coagulation proteins.[93]

There are two predominant forms of vitamin K in the diet: phylloquinone (vitamin K_1), which is found in green vegetables, and menaquinone, which is formed by the bacterial metabolism of phylloquinone. Intestinal absorption of both forms of vitamin K requires micelle formation. Phylloquinone is taken up from the intestine by an active transport process, whereas menaquinone is absorbed by nontransport, passive diffusion.[90, 91] Water-soluble synthetic vitamin K, known as *menadione,* is also used to treat vitamin K deficiency. Menadione is absorbed by passive diffusion and is distributed through the body, whereas phylloquinone is incorporated into chylomicrons and taken up by the liver with chylomicron remnants.

HEPATIC REGENERATION

The liver possesses the unique capacity to undergo rapid regeneration and replacement.[130] During acute toxic injury caused by acetaminophen or acute viral hepatitis, temporary support of the patient until the liver is able to regenerate is the mainstay of therapy. This unique regenerative capacity has engendered a great deal of interest in determining the responsible biochemical and molecular mechanisms. The eventual hope is that by understanding the regulation of this process, new therapeutic strategies can be developed for the treatment of acute and chronic liver disease. The liver's capacity to regulate its own growth is evident in liver transplantation, in which the size of the donor organ either expands or diminishes with time, as appropriate to the size of the patient. This regenerative ability of the liver is also evident in the successful use of single-lobe liver transplantation in children.[130, 131] The ability of the liver to regulate its size is dependent on signals generated outside of the liver, such as hormonal or metabolic signals, as well as internal signals generated within the liver.

Liver regeneration is associated with proliferation of hepatocytes sufficient to generate a critical mass necessary to maintain normal liver function. Sequential studies in a 70% partial hepatectomy rat model have determined the peak timing of DNA synthesis and cell growth for both hepatocytes and nonparenchymal cells.[132, 133] During acute regeneration, more than 30% to 50% of remaining hepatocytes undergo cell division. Detailed analyses in this animal model have determined the sequence of activation of various genes and identified unique genes that are highly expressed during the initial phase of liver regeneration. As expected, these genes encode a wide variety of proteins, including membrane receptors, transcription factors, tyrosine phosphatases and kinases, and metabolic enzymes. Induction of growth factors is another important feature that predates the increase in DNA synthesis. Using partial hepatectomy and knock-out mouse models lacking specific cytokines, a sequential series of gene expression patterns have been characterized that initiate the rapid proliferation of hepatocytes and the eventual cessation of cell growth, leading to replacement of the resected liver. In this cascade, a sequential combination of key cytokines and growth factors is necessary to initiate rapid proliferation and to prevent the alternative pathway of apoptosis (see "Apoptosis" later). This process also requires complex restoration of the extracellular matrix, which is necessary for the appropriate orientation of hepatocytes in relation to nonparenchymal cells.

The major hepatic growth factors identified during acute hepatic regeneration are epidermal growth factor (EGF), which can bind to the EGF receptor and the transforming growth factor-α (TGF-α) receptor, and hepatocyte growth factor (HGF), which binds to its receptor, the cellular homologue of the *met* oncogene. HGF is a heterodimeric glycoprotein composed of 64-kd and 32-kd peptides produced as a single proprotein by nonparenchymal cells.[130, 132] Levels of mRNA are increased 12 to 24 hours after surgical resection in a rat animal model. Elevated levels of HGF have been detected in the serum of patients with fulminant hepatic failure, suggesting that HGF also plays an important role in regeneration of human liver.

When infused in a normal rat, however, EGF and HGF do not cause hepatocyte replication. The lack of response to growth factors in the normal liver indicates that liver regeneration involves a two-step process in which the initial signals induced by liver resection trigger a set of early-response genes that primes hepatocytes to respond to various growth factors. Hepatocytes move from their resting G_0 stage in the cell cycle into the G_1 phase, where they are committed to undergo proliferation, which is the hallmark of the hepatocyte response in the partial hepatectomy model of liver regeneration. The mediators for the priming of the hepatocytes are unknown, but they are believed to include reactive oxygen species generated in part as a consequence of the acute metabolic needs necessary to compensate for the immediate loss of hepatic function. This process then starts a cascade of responses that leads ultimately to increased expression of growth-promoting factors such as TGF-α or HGF and enhanced sensitivity of hepatocytes to their actions. The increased metabolic activity caused by the acute loss of hepatic function leads to increased TNF-α and Il-6 expression associated with increased production of reactive oxygen species in the mitochondria, resulting in the activation of the NF-κB pathway along with other transcription factors. Early immediate genes are also expressed, leading to transition of hepatocytes from the resting stage of the cell cycle to active proliferation. This compensatory hyperplasia is accompanied by activation of typical cell-cycle expressed genes. Ultimately, restitution of hepatic function leads to the return of hepatocytes to their quiescent G_0 resting state. Immediate induction of c-jun and the NF-κB pathway after partial hepatectomy suggests that these are crucial transcription factors that mediate hepatic regeneration. Absence of either c-jun or a component of NF-κB complex in mice leads to embryonic death and immature liver development, confirming the essential role of these factors in liver organogenesis.[134, 135]

APOPTOSIS

The other major pathway involved in the attainment and remodeling of the liver is apoptosis, or programmed cell death.[136–138] This pathway also has been implicated in acute and chronic liver disease.[139] Apoptosis allows the remodeling of tissues during organogenesis, elimination of senescent cells, and noninflammatory removal of severely damaged cells in which extensive injury precludes their adequate restoration. Tremendous progress has been made in defining the molecular features of this pathway, and the reader is referred to detailed reviews of this rapidly evolving field[138–142] (see also Chapter 3). In the apoptotic pathway, cells undergo discrete morphologic changes, including cell rounding with chromatin condensation and nuclear chromatin digestion, with little disruption of cell membranes and internal organelles. The cells eventually disintegrate into small fragments containing parts of the condensed nuclei and are phagocytized by macrophages. Unlike cytotoxic cell injury, apoptotic cell death is associated with little or no inflammation.

The apoptotic pathway can be broadly divided into three phases: initiation, execution, and termination. Numerous signals can initiate apoptosis depending on the target cell and include withdrawal of key growth factors, ultraviolet or gamma irradiation, chemotherapeutic agents, reactive oxygen intermediates, or activation of so-called "death receptors" on the plasma membrane surface. In the liver, the role of the Fas/Apo 1 antigen and its ligand has been closely examined as a prime example of this last pathway. Fas/Apo 1 antigen is a member of the TNF receptor gene family, which consists of single-spanning, transmembrane receptors. Binding of the Fas/Apo 1 receptor by ligand or agnostic monoclonal antibody results in trimerization of the receptor and activation of the apoptotic pathway, resulting in massive hepatocellular necrosis exhibiting characteristic pathologic features of apoptosis.[143] A specific cytosolic protein domain within the Fas receptor, referred to as the *death domain,* is required to initiate apoptosis. Transgenic mice in which the Fas antigen has been mutated by homologous recombination develop progressively enlarging livers with an increased number of hepatocytes, suggesting that the Fas antigen mediated process is critical for the routine removal of senescent hepatocytes.[144]

In addition to activators of apoptotic pathways, inhibitors of this process have been identified. Bcl-2, originally identified in B-cell lymphomas, is the best characterized inhibitor of apoptosis and is a member of a family of related proteins that may either inhibit or activate apoptosis.[145] These proteins can form either homodimers or heterodimers and, depending on their composition, can either protect against or induce apoptosis. Bcl-2 is inserted into the outer mitochondrial membranes and nuclear envelope, with a portion also residing within the ER. Bcl-2 can inhibit the mitochondrial permeability, which is associated with release of cytochrome C, a potent signal that activates a cascade of proteolytic enzymes referred to as the *caspases.* These proteolytic enzymes are key components of the executionary phase of the apoptotic process. Overexpression of Bcl-2 inhibits apoptosis in many experimental models, including oxidant-induced apoptosis in fibroblasts and cytokine withdrawal in a cytokine-dependent cell line. The ability of Bcl-2 to block apoptosis from different signals indicates that it is inhibiting activation of a late event in the apoptotic pathway. In liver, Bcl-2 is normally expressed in cholangiocytes of the small bile ducts and endothelial cells but not in hepatocytes. Transgenic mice that overexpress *Bcl-2* in hepatocytes are protected against Fas-mediated massive hepatic necrosis as compared to nontransgenic animals.[146] Other antiapoptotic proteins also act by inhibiting activation of the caspase cascade, thereby inactivating the executionary phase of the pathway.

In human liver disease, the presence of "Councilman bodies" on histologic evaluation is the morphologic evidence of apoptosis. Normally, few apoptotic cells are seen because apoptosis in the liver is rare due to the long half-life of normal hepatocytes. Activation of the apoptotic pathway has been implicated in viral hepatitis and in autoimmune, cholestatic, alcoholic, and drug-induced liver injury. When large numbers of hepatocytes die by apoptosis, the normal phagocytic removal of these cells may be overwhelmed, resulting in the histologic appearance of necrotic cell death with infiltration by inflammatory cells. The activation of the apoptotic pathway in chronic liver disease is predicted to play a key role in liver injury.

REFERENCES

1. McCuskey RS: The hepatic microvascular system. In Arias IM (ed): The Liver: Biology and Pathobiology, 3rd ed. New York, Raven Press, 1994, p 1089.
2. Gumucio JJ, Bilir BM, Moseley RH, et al: The biology of the liver cell plate. In Arias IM (ed): The Liver: Biology and Pathobiology, 3rd ed. New York, Raven Press, 1994, p 1143.
3. Haussinger D, Gerok W: Metabolism of amino acids and ammonia. In Thurman RG, Kauffman FC, Jungermann K (eds): Regulation of Hepatic Metabolism. New York, Plenum, 1986, p 253.
4. Petzinger E: Transport of organic anions in the liver: An update on bile acid, fatty acid, monocarboxylate, anionic amino acid, cholephilic organic anion, and anionic drug transport. Rev Physiol Biochem Pharmacol 123:47, 1994.
5. LeBlanc GA: Hepatic vectorial transport of xenobiotics. Chem Biol Interact 90:101, 1994.
6. Nathanson MH, Boyer JL: Mechanisms and regulation of bile secretion. Hepatology 14:551, 1991.
7. Muller M, Jansen PL: Molecular aspects of hepatobiliary transport. Am J Physiol 272:G1285, 1997.
8. Lecureur V, Courtois A, Payen L, et al: Expression and regulation of hepatic drug and bile acid transporters. Toxicology 153:203, 2000.
9. Bahar RJ, Stolz A: Bile acid transport. Gastroenterol Clin North Am 28:27, 1999.
10. Hagenbuch B, Stieger B, Foguet M, et al: Functional expression cloning and characterization of the hepatocyte Na+/bile acid cotransport system. Proc Natl Acad Sci U S A 88:10629, 1991.
11. Seifter S, Englard S: Energy metabolism. In Arias IM (ed): The Liver: Biology and Pathobiology, 3rd ed. New York, Raven Press, 1994, p 323.
12. Pilkis SJ, Granner DK: Molecular physiology of the regulation of hepatic gluconeogenesis and glycolysis. Annu Rev Physiol 54:885, 1992.
13. Van Schaftingen E: Glycolysis revisited. Diabetologia 36:581, 1993.

14. McGarry JD, Kuwajima M, Newgard CB, et al: From dietary glucose to liver glycogen: The full circle round. Annu Rev Nutr 7:51, 1987.
15. Radziuk J, Pye S, Zhang Z: Substrates and the regulation of hepatic glycogen metabolism. Adv Exp Med Biol 334:235, 1993.
16. Felber JP, Golay A: Regulation of nutrient metabolism and energy expenditure. Metabolism 44:4, 1995.
17. Foster DW: Banting Lecture 1984: From glycogen to ketones—and back. Diabetes 33:1188, 1984.
18. Bremer J, Osmundsen H: Fatty acid oxidation and its regulation. In Numa S (ed): Fatty Acid Metabolism and Its Regulation. Amsterdam, Elsevier, 1984, p 113.
19. Mathews CK, van Holde KE: Biochemistry. Redwood City, CA, Benjamin/Cummings, 1990, pp 431–466.
20. Davidson VL, Sittman DB: Biochemistry, 3rd ed. Philadelphia, Harwal, 1994.
21. Granner D, Pilkis S: The genes of hepatic glucose metabolism. J Biol Chem 265:10173, 1990.
22. Alonso MD, Lomako J, Lomako WM, et al: A new look at the biogenesis of glycogen. FASEB J 9:1126, 1995.
23. Pessin JE, Bell GI: Mammalian facilitative glucose transporter family: Structure and molecular regulation. Annu Rev Physiol 54:911, 1992.
24. Nordlie RC, Foster JD, Lange AJ: Regulation of glucose production by the liver. Annu Rev Nutr 19:379, 1999.
25. Cherrington AD, Stevenson RW, Steiner KE, et al: Insulin, glucagon, and glucose as regulators of hepatic glucose uptake and production in vivo. Diabetes Metab Rev 3:307, 1987.
26. Kletzien RF, Harris PK, Foellmi LA: Glucose-6-phosphate dehydrogenase: A "housekeeping" enzyme subject to tissue-specific regulation by hormones, nutrients, and oxidant stress. FASEB J 8:174, 1994.
27. Vaulont S, Kahn A: Transcriptional control of metabolic regulation genes by carbohydrates. FASEB J 8:28, 1994.
28. Matschinsky FM: Glucokinase as glucose sensor and metabolic signal generator in pancreatic beta-cells and hepatocytes. Diabetes 39:647, 1990.
29. Van Schaftingen E, Detheux M, Veiga da Cunha M: Short-term control of glucokinase activity: Role of a regulatory protein. FASEB J 8: 414, 1994.
30. Burchell A: Hepatic microsomal glucose transport. Biochem Soc Trans 22:658, 1994.
31. Burchell A, Allan BB, Hume R: Glucose-6-phosphatase proteins of the endoplasmic reticulum. Mol Membr Biol 11:217, 1994.
32. Hallfrisch J: Metabolic effects of dietary fructose. FASEB J 4:2652, 1990.
33. Youn JH, Bergman RN: Enhancement of hepatic glycogen by gluconeogenic precursors: Substrate flux or metabolic control? Am J Physiol 258:E899, 1990.
34. Kurland IJ, Pilkis SJ: Indirect versus direct routes of hepatic glycogen synthesis. FASEB J 3:2277, 1989.
35. Petrides AS, DeFronzo RA: Glucose metabolism in cirrhosis: A review with some perspectives for the future. Diabetes Metab Rev 5: 691, 1989.
36. Nolte W, Hartmann H, Ramadori G: Glucose metabolism and liver cirrhosis. Exp Clin Endocrinol Diabetes 103:63, 1995.
37. Girard J, Perdereau D, Foufelle F, et al: Regulation of lipogenic enzyme gene expression by nutrients and hormones. FASEB J 8:36, 1994.
38. Coppack SW, Jensen MD, Miles JM: In vivo regulation of lipolysis in humans. J Lipid Res 35:177, 1994.
39. Osmundsen H, Bremer J, Pedersen JI: Metabolic aspects of peroxisomal beta-oxidation. Biochim Biophys Acta 1085:141, 1991.
40. Lazarow PB: Peroxisomes. In Arias IM (ed): The Liver: Biology and Pathobiology, 3rd ed. New York, Raven Press, 1994, p 292.
41. Kim KH, Tae HJ: Pattern and regulation of acetyl-CoA carboxylase gene expression. J Nutr 124:1273S, 1994.
42. Kerner J, Hoppel d: Fatty acid import into mitochondria. Biochim Biophys Acta 1486:1, 2001.
43. Bremer J: The role of carnitine in intracellular metabolism. J Clin Chem Clin Biochem 28:297, 1990.
44. Eaton S, Record CO, Bartlett K: Multiple biochemical effects in the pathogenesis of alcoholic fatty liver. Eur J Clin Invest 27:719, 1997.
45. Lieber CS: Biochemical factors in alcoholic liver disease. Semin Liver Dis 13:136, 1993.
46. Ginsberg HN: Lipoprotein metabolism and its relationship to atherosclerosis. Med Clin North Am 78:1, 1994.
47. Dixon JL, Ginsberg HN: Hepatic synthesis of lipoproteins and apolipoproteins. Semin Liver Dis 12:364, 1992.
48. Havel RJ: Functional activities of hepatic lipoprotein receptors. Annu Rev Physiol 48:119, 1986.
49. Havel RJ, Hamilton RL: Hepatocytic lipoprotein receptors and intracellular lipoprotein catabolism. Hepatology 8:1689, 1988.
50. Hoeg JM, Brewer HBJ: Human lipoprotein metabolism and the liver. Prog Liver Dis 8:51, 1986.
51. Glickman RM, Sabesin SM: Lipoprotein metabolism. In Arias IM (ed): The Liver: Biology and Pathobiology, 3rd ed. New York, Raven Press, 1994, p 391.
52. Shepherd J: Lipoprotein metabolism: An overview. Drugs 47(Suppl 2): 1, 1994.
53. Oram JF: Tangier disease and ABCA1. Biochim Biophys Acta 1529: 321, 2000.
54. Jong MC, Hofker MH, Havekes LM: Role of ApoCs in lipoprotein metabolism: Functional differences between ApoC1, ApoC2, and ApoC3. Arterioscler Thromb Vasc Biol 19:472, 1999.
55. Green PH, Glickman RM: Intestinal lipoprotein metabolism. J Lipid Res 22:1153, 1981.
56. Teng B, Burant CF, Davidson NO: Molecular cloning of an apolipoprotein B messenger RNA editing protein. Science 260:1816, 1993.
57. DeVilliers WJS, Coetzee GA, Van Der Westhuyzen DR: Lipoprotein receptors. In Schettler G, Habenicht AJR (eds): Principles and Treatment of Lipoprotein Disorders. Berlin, Germany, Springer-Verlag, 1994, p 53.
58. Mahley RW, Ji ZS: Remnant lipoprotein metabolism: Key pathways involving cell-surface heparan sulfate proteoglycans and apolipoprotein E. J Lipid Res 40:1, 1999.
59. Strittmatter WJ, Roses AD: Apolipoprotein E and Alzheimer disease. Proc Natl Acad Sci U S A 92:4725, 1995.
60. Saunders AM, Trowers MK, Shimkets RA, et al: The role of apolipoprotein E in Alzheimer's disease: Pharmacogenomic target selection. Biochim Biophys Acta 1502:85, 2000.
61. Tall AR: Plasma high-density lipoproteins: Metabolism and relationship to atherogenesis. J Clin Invest 86:379, 1990.
62. Ameis D, Greten H, Schotz Md: Hepatic and plasma lipases. Semin Liver Dis 12:397, 1992.
63. Fielding CJ, Fielding PE: Molecular physiology of reverse cholesterol transport. J Lipid Res 36:211, 1995.
64. Fielding CJ: Lipoprotein receptors, plasma cholesterol metabolism, and the regulation of cellular free cholesterol concentration. FASEB J 6: 3162, 1992.
65. Bruce C, Chouinard RA, Tall AR: Plasma lipid transfer proteins, high-density lipoproteins, and reverse cholesterol transport. Annu Rev Nutr 18:297, 1998.
66. Hussain MM: A proposed model for the assembly of chylomicrons. Atherosclerosis 148:1, 2000.
67. Spady DK, Woollett LA, Dietschy JM: Regulation of plasma LDL-cholesterol levels by dietary cholesterol and fatty acids. Annu Rev Nutr 13:355, 1993.
68. Barth CA: Regulation and interaction of cholesterol, bile salt, and lipoprotein synthesis in liver. Klin Wochenschr 61:1163, 1983.
69. Yeaman SJ: Hormone-sensitive lipase—a multipurpose enzyme in lipid metabolism. Biochim Biophys Acta 1052:128, 1990.
70. Gibbons GF: Assembly and secretion of hepatic very-low-density lipoprotein. Biochem J 268:1, 1990.
71. Gibbons GF, Wiggins D: The enzymology of hepatic very-low-density lipoprotein assembly. Biochem Soc Trans 23:495, 1995.
72. Meier PJ: Molecular mechanisms of hepatic bile salt transport from sinusoidal blood into bile. Am J Physiol 269:G801, 1995.
73. Wong MH, Oelkers P, Craddock AL, et al: Expression cloning and characterization of the hamster ileal sodium-dependent bile acid transporter. J Biol Chem 269:1340, 1994.
74. Sinal CJ, Tohkin M, Miyata M, et al: Targeted disruption of the nuclear receptor FXR/BAR impairs bile acid and lipid homeostasis. Cell 102:731, 2000.
75. Lu TT, Makishima M, Repa JJ, et al: Molecular basis for feedback regulation of bile acid synthesis by nuclear receptors. Mol Cell 6:507, 2000.
76. Sniderman AD, Cianflone K: Substrate delivery as a determinant of hepatic apoB secretion. Arterioscler Thromb 13:629, 1993.
77. Yao Z, McLeod RS: Synthesis and secretion of hepatic apolipoprotein B–containing lipoproteins. Biochim Biophys Acta 1212:152, 1994.
78. Dixon JL, Ginsberg HN: Regulation of hepatic secretion of apolipoprotein B–containing lipoproteins: Information obtained from cultured liver cells. J Lipid Res 34:167, 1993.

79. Vance JE, Vance DE: Lipoprotein assembly and secretion by hepatocytes. Annu Rev Nutr 10:337, 1990.
80. Davis RA: Cell and molecular biology of the assembly and secretion of apolipoprotein B–containing lipoproteins by the liver. Biochim Biophys Acta 1440:1, 1999.
81. Krieger M: Charting the fate of the "good cholesterol": Identification and characterization of the high-density lipoprotein receptor SR-BI. Annu Rev Biochem 68:523, 1999.
82. Hussain MM, Strickland DK, Bakillah A: The mammalian low-density lipoprotein receptor family. Annu Rev Nutr 19:141, 1999.
83. Willnow TE: The low-density lipoprotein receptor gene family: Multiple roles in lipid metabolism. J Mol Med 77:306, 1999.
84. Strickland DK, Kounnas MZ, Argraves WS. LDL receptor–related protein: A multiligand receptor for lipoprotein and proteinase catabolism. FASEB J 9:890, 1995.
85. Rohlmann A, Gotthardt M, Hammer RE, et al: Inducible inactivation of hepatic LRP gene by cre-mediated recombination confirms role of LRP in clearance of chylomicron remnants. J Clin Invest 101:689, 1998.
86. Chait A, Brunzell JD: Acquired hyperlipidemia (secondary dyslipoproteinemias). Endocrinol Metab Clin North Am 19:259, 1990.
87. Miller JP: Dyslipoproteinaemia of liver disease. Baillieres Clin Endocrinol Metab 4:807, 1990.
88. Cicognani C, Malavolti M, Morselli-Labate AM, et al: Serum lipid and lipoprotein patterns in patients with liver cirrhosis and chronic active hepatitis. Arch Intern Med 157:792, 1997.
89. Elferink RP, Ottenhoff R, van Marle J, et al: Class III P-glycoproteins mediate the formation of lipoprotein X in the mouse. J Clin Invest 102:1749, 1998.
90. Suttie JW: Vitamin K–dependent carboxylase. Annu Rev Biochem 54: 459, 1985.
91. Suttie JW: Recent advances in hepatic vitamin K metabolism and function. Hepatology 7:367, 1987.
92. Furie BC, Furie B: Vitamin K–dependent blood coagulation proteins. In Arias IM (ed): The Liver: Biology and Pathobiology, 3rd ed. New York, Raven Press, 1994, p 1217.
93. Mammen EF: Coagulation abnormalities in liver disease. Hematol Oncol Clin North Am 6:1247, 1992.
94. Mammen EF: Coagulation defects in liver disease. Med Clin North Am 78:545, 1994.
95. Sokol RJ: Fat-soluble vitamins and their importance in patients with cholestatic liver diseases. Gastroenterol Clin North Am 23:673, 1994.
96. Weitz IC, Liebman HA: Des-gamma-carboxy (abnormal) prothrombin and hepatocellular carcinoma: A critical review. Hepatology 18:990, 1993.
97. Sifers RN, Finegold MJ, Woo SLd: α_1-Antitrypsin: Molecular defects. In Arias IM (ed): The Liver: Biology and Pathobiology, 3rd ed. New York, Raven Press, 1994, p 1357.
98. Lomas DA, Evans DL, Finch JT, et al: The mechanism of Z α_1-antitrypsin accumulation in the liver. Nature 357:605, 1992.
99. Teckman JH, Qu D, Perlmutter DH: Molecular pathogenesis of liver disease in α_1-antitrypsin deficiency. Hepatology 24:1504, 1996.
100. Burrows JA, Willis LK, Perlmutter DH: Chemical chaperones mediate increased secretion of mutant α_1-antitrypsin (α_1-AT) Z: A potential pharmacological strategy for prevention of liver injury and emphysema in α_1-AT deficiency. Proc Natl Acad Sci U S A 97:1796, 2000.
101. Harris ZL, Takahashi Y, Miyajima H, et al: Aceruloplasminemia: Molecular characterization of this disorder of iron metabolism. Proc Natl Acad Sci U S A 92:2539, 1995.
102. Gitlin JD: Aceruloplasminemia. Pediatr Res 44:271, 1998.
103. Bull PC, Thomas GR, Rommens JM, et al: The Wilson disease gene is a putative copper transporting P-type ATPase similar to the Menkes gene. Nat Genet 5:327, 1993.
104. Rothschild MA, Oratz M, Schreiber SS: Serum albumin. Hepatology 8:385, 1988.
105. Watkins S, Madison J, Galliano M, et al: Analbuminemia: Three cases resulting from different point mutations in the albumin gene. Proc Natl Acad Sci U S A 91:9417, 1994.
106. Pietrangelo A, Panduro A, Chowdhury JR, et al: Albumin gene expression is down-regulated by albumin or macromolecule infusion in the rat. J Clin Invest 89:1755, 1992.
107. Pietrangelo A, Shafritz DA: Homeostatic regulation of hepatocyte nuclear transcription factor 1 expression in cultured hepatoma cells. Proc Natl Acad Sci U S A 91:182, 1994.
108. Keshgegian AA: Hypoalbuminemia associated with diffuse hypergammaglobulinemia in chronic diseases: Lack of diagnostic specificity. Am J Clin Pathol 81:477, 1984.
109. Taketa K: Alpha-fetoprotein: Reevaluation in hepatology. Hepatology 12:1420, 1990.
110. Young SP, Aisen P" The liver and iron. In Arias IM (ed): The Liver: Biology and Pathobiology, 3rd ed. New York, Raven Press, 1994, p 597.
111. Irie S, Tavassoli M: Transferrin-mediated cellular iron uptake. Am J Med Sci 293:103, 1987.
112. Theil EC, Eisenstein RS: Combinatorial mRNA regulation: Iron regulatory proteins and iso-iron-responsive elements (Iso-IREs). J Biol Chem 275:40659, 2000.
113. Blaner WS: Retinoid (vitamin A) metabolism and the liver. In Arias IM (ed): The Liver: Biology and Pathobiology, 3rd ed. New York, Raven Press, 1994, p 529.
114. Goodman DS: Vitamin A and retinoids in health and disease. N Engl J Med 310:1023, 1984.
115. Ghyselinck NB, Bavik C, Sapin V, et al: Cellular retinol-binding protein I is essential for vitamin A homeostasis. EMBO J 18:4903, 1999.
116. Napoli JL: Interactions of retinoid binding proteins and enzymes in retinoid metabolism. Biochim Biophys Acta 1440:139, 1999.
117. Hathcock JN, Hattan DG, Jenkins MY, et al: Evaluation of vitamin A toxicity. Am J Clin Nutr 52:183, 1990.
118. Iatrogenic liver disease from vitamin A. Nutr Rev 49:309, 1991.
119. Russell RM: The vitamin A spectrum: From deficiency to toxicity. Am J Clin Nutr 71:878, 2000.
120. Holick MF: Vitamin D: Photobiology, metabolism, and clinical application. In Arias IM (ed): The Liver: Biology and Pathobiology, 3rd ed. New York, Raven Press, 1994, p 543.
121. Okuda K, Usui E, Ohyama Y: Recent progress in enzymology and molecular biology of enzymes involved in vitamin D metabolism. J Lipid Res 36:1641, 1995.
122. Compston JE: Hepatic osteodystrophy: Vitamin D metabolism in patients with liver disease. Gut 27:1073, 1986.
123. Lindor KD: Management of osteopenia of liver disease with special emphasis on primary biliary cirrhosis. Semin Liver Dis 13:367, 1993.
124. Parker RS: Dietary and biochemical aspects of vitamin E. Adv Food Nutr Res 33:157, 1989.
125. Traber MG, Sokol RJ, Burton GW, et al: Impaired ability of patients with familial isolated vitamin E deficiency to incorporate alpha-tocopherol into lipoproteins secreted by the liver. J Clin Invest 85:397, 1990.
126. Traber MG, Sokol RJ, Kohlschutter A, et al: Impaired discrimination between stereoisomers of alpha-tocopherol in patients with familial isolated vitamin E deficiency. J Lipid Res 34:201, 1993.
127. Ouahchi K, Arita M, Kayden H, et al: Ataxia with isolated vitamin E deficiency is caused by mutations in the alpha-tocopherol transfer protein. Nat Genet 9:141, 1995.
128. Morrow MJ: Neurologic complications of vitamin E deficiency: Case report and review of the literature. Bull Clin Neurosci 50:53, 1985.
129. Lavine JE: Vitamin E treatment of nonalcoholic steatohepatitis in children: A pilot study. J Pediatr 136:734, 2000.
130. Fausto N, Webber EM: Liver regeneration. In Arias IM (ed): The Liver: Biology and Pathobiology, 3rd ed. New York, Raven Press, 1994, p 1059.
131. Steer CJ: Liver regeneration. FASEB J 9:1396, 1995.
132. Michalopoulos GK: Liver regeneration: Molecular mechanisms of growth control. FASEB J 4:176, 1990.
133. Fausto N, Laird AD, Webber EM: Liver regeneration: II. Role of growth factors and cytokines in hepatic regeneration. FASEB J 9: 1527, 1995.
134. Beg AA, Sha WC, Bronson RT, et al: Embryonic lethality and liver degeneration in mice lacking the RelA component of NF-kappa B. Nature 376:167, 1995.
135. Hilberg F, Aguzzi A, Howells N, et al: c-jun is essential for normal mouse development and hepatogenesis Nature 365:179, 1993.
136. Wyllie AH: Apoptosis and the regulation of cell numbers in normal and neoplastic tissues: An overview. Cancer Metast Rev 11:95, 1992.
137. Ellis RE, Yuan JY, Horvitz HR: Mechanisms and functions of cell death. Annu Rev Cell Biol 7:663, 1991.
138. Kaplowitz N: Mechanisms of liver cell injury. J Hepatol 32:39, 2000.
139. Rust C, Gores GJ: Apoptosis and liver disease. Am J Med 108:567, 2000.
140. Schmitz I, Kirchhoff S, Krammer PH: Regulation of death receptor–mediated apoptosis pathways. Int J Biochem Cell Biol 32:1123, 2000.

141. Thornberry NA, Lazebnik Y: Caspases: Enemies within. Science 281: 1312, 1998.
142. Green DR: Apoptotic pathways: The roads to ruin. Cell 94:695, 1998.
143. Ogasawara J, Watanabe Fukunaga R, Adachi M, et al: Lethal effect of the anti-Fas antibody in mice. Nature 364:806, 1993.
144. Adachi M, Suematsu S, Kondo T, et al: Targeted mutation in the Fas gene causes hyperplasia in peripheral lymphoid organs and liver. Nat Genet 11:294, 1995.
145. Hockenbery DM: bcl-2, a novel regulator of cell death. Bioessays 17: 631, 1995.
146. Lacronique V, Mignon A, Fabre M, et al: Bcl-2 protects from lethal hepatic apoptosis induced by an anti-Fas antibody in mice. Nat Med 2:80, 1996.
147. Katz N, Jungermann K: Metabolic heterogeneity of the liver. In Tavoloni N, Berk PD (eds): Hepatic Transport and Bile Secretion: Physiology and Pathophysiology. New York, Raven Press, 1993, p 55.
148. Putnam FW: Progress in plasma proteins. In Putnam FW (ed): The Plasma Proteins: Structure, Function, and Genetic Control. Orlando, Academic Press, 1984, p 45.
149. Kushner I, Mackiewicz A: The acute-phase response: An overview. In Mackiewicz A, Kushner I, Baumann H (eds): Acute-Phase Proteins. Boca Raton, FL, CRC Press, 1993, p 3.

Chapter 64

Biochemical Liver Tests

Timothy J. Davern and Bruce F. Scharschmidt

"Liver function tests are no more infallible than the people who use them."

A. M. Snell[1]

The liver performs a diverse array of biochemical, synthetic, and excretory functions, and, as a result, no single biochemical test is capable of providing an accurate global assessment of hepatic function. Biochemical liver tests have limited sensitivity and specificity, do not all reflect liver function as the common misnomer "liver function tests" implies, and provide limited information regarding the presence or severity of complications of liver disease, such as portal hypertension, which can be life-threatening. Interpretation of biochemical liver tests, therefore, should be done in concert with a careful history and physical examination to assess the likelihood of significant liver disease as well as its severity and possible etiology.[2]

Despite these limitations, different types of liver disease are often associated with distinct patterns of biochemical abnormalities. Recognition of these characteristic patterns is critical to guide further clinical evaluation, biochemical testing for disease-specific markers, radiologic imaging, and liver biopsy. This chapter summarizes the biochemical basis of commonly used liver tests, defines the patterns of abnormalities characteristic of various liver disorders, outlines approaches to the selection and interpretation of serum biochemical liver tests, and briefly summarizes information regarding the potential utility of so-called "quantitative" liver function tests. For a comprehensive review of the biochemistry of these and other tests, some of historical interest only, interested readers are referred to dedicated monographs.[3, 4]

BIOCHEMICAL LIVER TESTS

Commonly used liver tests and their clinical significance are summarized in Table 64–1.[5] Tests that assess hepatocellular necrosis, cholestasis, and hepatic synthetic capacity are discussed separately later. Note, the term *necrosis* as used here refers to hepatocellular damage in general, not to a specific pathologic or pathophysiologic process.

Markers of Hepatocellular Necrosis

Aminotransferases

The aminotransferases include aspartate aminotransferase (AST, formerly SGOT, or serum glutamic oxaloacetic transaminase) and alanine aminotransferase (ALT, formerly SGPT, or serum glutamic pyruvic transaminase). They participate in gluconeogenesis by catalyzing the transfer of amino groups from aspartic acid or alanine to ketoglutaric acid to produce oxaloacetic acid and pyruvic acid, respectively. ALT is a cytosolic enzyme, whereas AST is present as both cytosolic and mitochondrial isoenzymes. Elevation of the activity of these enzymes in serum is believed to be the result of leakage from damaged cells and thus reflects hepatocyte injury. These enzymes are elevated in many forms of liver disease, especially those that are associated with significant hepatocyte necrosis, such as acute viral hepatitis and chemical or ischemic injury.

It is important to note that ALT is relatively liver-specific, whereas AST is found in skeletal and cardiac muscle, kidney, brain, pancreas, and blood cells, in addition to hepatocytes. Therefore, the hepatic origin of an isolated AST elevation should be confirmed by obtaining an ALT, and an isolated or disproportionate elevation of the AST should prompt a search for extrahepatic sources, in particular myocardial or skeletal muscle injury. For example, vigorous physical activity, such as long-distance running or weight lifting, may increase the serum AST level severalfold. However, in rare cases, elevation of both AST and ALT may reflect muscle disease or injury (e.g., muscular dystrophy, myositis).[6–8]

AST/ALT RATIO. The ratio of serum AST to ALT may be useful in differential diagnosis. In most forms of acute liver injury, this ratio is less than or equal to 1, whereas in alcoholic hepatitis the ratio is characteristically greater than 2. This elevated ratio may result in part from pyridoxine deficiency, which frequently complicates chronic alcoholism. Pyridoxyl 5′-phosphate is a required coenzyme for both aminotransferases; however, AST appears to have a higher affinity for this cofactor. Repletion of pyridoxine usually increases serum ALT in this setting and reduces the AST/ALT

Table 64–1 | **Clinical Significance of Common Liver Tests**

TEST (Normal Range)	BASIS OF ABNORMALITY	ASSOCIATED LIVER DISEASES	EXTRAHEPATIC SOURCES
Aminotransferases (10–55 U/L, 0.17–0.92 μkat/L for ALT, 10–40 U/L, 0.17–0.67 μkat/L for AST)	Leakage from damaged tissue	Modest elevations—many types of liver disease Marked elevations—hepatitis (viral, autoimmune, toxic, and ischemic) AST/ALT > 2 with the value of each less than 300 U suggests alcoholic liver disease or cirrhosis of any etiology	ALT, relatively specific for hepatocyte necrosis AST, muscle (skeletal and cardiac), kidney, brain, pancreas, red blood cells
Alkaline phosphatase (45–115 U/L, 0.75–1.92 μkat/L)	Overproduction and leakage into serum	Modest elevations—many types of liver disease Marked elevations—extra- and intrahepatic cholestasis, diffuse infiltrating disease (e.g., tumor, MAC), occasionally alcoholic hepatitis	Bone growth or disease (e.g., tumor, fracture, Paget's disease), placenta, intestine, tumors
Gammaglutamyl transpeptidase (0–30 U/L, 0–0.50 μkat/L)	?Overproduction and leakage into serum	Same as for alkaline phosphatase; induced by ethanol, drugs GGTP/AP >2.5 suggests (but not diagnostic of) alcoholic liver disease	Kidney, spleen, pancreas, heart, lung, brain
5′-Nucleotidase (0–11 U/L, 0.02–0.18 μkat/L)	?Overproduction and leakage into serum	Same as for alkaline phosphatase	Found in many tissues but serum elevation relatively specific for liver disease
Bilirubin (0.0–1.0 mg/dL, 0–17 μmol/L)	Decreased hepatic clearance	Modest elevations—many types of liver disease Marked elevations—extra- and intrahepatic bile duct obstruction, alcoholic, drug-induced or viral hepatitis, inherited hyperbilirubinemia	Increased breakdown of hemoglobin (resulting from hemolysis, ineffective erythropoiesis, resorption of hematoma) or myoglobin (resulting from muscle injury)
Prothrombin time (10.9–12.5 sec) or International Normalized Ratio (INR) (0.9–1.2)	Decreased synthetic capacity	Acute or chronic liver failure (unresponsive to vitamin K) Biliary obstruction (usually responsive to vitamin K administration)	Vitamin K deficiency (secondary to malabsorption, malnutrition, antibiotics), consumptive coagulopathy
Albumin (4.0–6.0 g/dL, 40–60 g/L)	Decreased synthesis ?Increased catabolism	Chronic liver failure	Decreased in nephrotic syndrome, protein-losing enteropathy, vascular leak, malnutrition, malignancy, and inflammatory states

The normal values given are for adult men and will vary, depending on the methodology used for the test.
ALT, alanine aminotranferase; AP, alkaline phosphatase; AST, aspartate transaminase; GGTP, gammaglutamyl transpeptidase; MAC, *Mycobacterium avian* complex.

ratio to approximately 1. In addition to pyridoxine deficiency, there are likely other as yet incompletely understood reasons for the characteristic AST/ALT ratio of greater than 2 in alcoholic hepatitis (see Chapter 71). By comparison, in nonalcoholic steatohepatitis (NASH), which can be indistinguishable histologically from alcoholic hepatitis, the AST/ALT ratio is almost always less than or equal to 1 in the absence of cirrhosis.[9] A second, much less common disorder characterized by disproportionate elevation of the AST relative to ALT is acute Wilson disease (see Chapter 67). An AST/ALT greater than 4 in the appropriate clinical setting is highly suggestive, albeit not diagnostic, of fulminant Wilsonian hepatitis.[10, 11]

As with other liver tests, the AST/ALT ratio must be interpreted in the light of clinical information. For example, a ratio exceeding 1 occurs in the absence of alcoholic injury in patients with cirrhosis from any type of chronic liver disease.[12] Indeed, if alcohol abuse can be excluded, an AST/ALT greater than 1 in a patient with known liver disease may suggest the presence of cirrhosis. Measurement of the mitochondrial isoenzyme of AST has shown promise as a marker of occult alcohol use, but this test is not readily available and further study is necessary to define its clinical utility.[13]

AST AND ALT LEVELS. Modest elevations of the serum aminotransferase levels (<500 U/L) are found in a wide variety of liver diseases. In the absence of other disorders, the aminotransferase levels are typically less than 300 U/L in patients with alcoholic hepatitis or biliary obstruction. However, dramatic though transient rises in these enzymes may occasionally occur immediately after acute biliary obstruction.[14] In addition, when other insults, such as viral or acetaminophen-induced liver injury, are superimposed on alcoholic liver disease, serum aminotransferase activity often exceeds 1000 U/L, but the characteristic AST/ALT ratio is usually preserved. Extreme aminotransferase elevations (>2000 U/L) have a relatively restricted differential diagnosis, discussed later. It is surprising that the degree of aminotransferase elevation correlates poorly with the extent of hepatocyte necrosis, as determined by liver biopsy, and is not predictive of outcome in acute hepatitis. Indeed, a rapid fall in aminotransferase levels in association with a rising bilirubin and prothrombin time portends a poor prognosis in patients with acute liver failure (see Chapter 80).

Although the aminotransferases are fairly sensitive indicators of hepatocellular necrosis and, in fact, are commonly employed as screening tests for occult viral hepatitis in blood donors, levels are frequently normal or nearly normal in patients with advanced cirrhosis in the absence of significant ongoing liver injury, as with chronic hepatitis, hereditary hemochromatosis, methotrexate use, and a previous jejunoileal bypass. Azotemia may falsely lower the serum AST concentration. Conversely, AST rarely may exist in serum as a macroenzyme complex with albumin, thereby resulting in persistent elevation of the serum AST activity.[15]

Lactate Dehydrogenase

Lactate dehydrogenase (LDH) has a wide tissue distribution, and elevated serum levels are seen with skeletal or cardiac muscle injury, hemolysis, stroke, and renal infarction, in addition to acute and chronic liver disease. Because of this nonspecificity, LDH rarely adds useful information to that obtained from the aminotransferase levels alone. Uncommon situations in which serum LDH levels may be useful diagnostically include the massive but transient serum elevation of LDH characteristic of ischemic hepatitis and the sustained LDH elevation, accompanied by elevation of the alkaline phosphatase level, that suggests malignant infiltration of the liver.

Markers of Cholestasis

Alkaline Phosphatase

Alkaline phosphatase (AP) comprises a group of enzymes present in a variety of tissues, including liver, bone, intestine, kidney, placenta, leukocytes, and various neoplasms. The physiologic roles of AP enzymes are generally unclear, but AP production tends to increase in tissues undergoing metabolic stimulation. Thus, AP serum activity during adolescence is up to three times higher than that in adults because of rapid bone growth; it also rises during late pregnancy because of placental growth and metabolism.[16] Bone and liver are the major sources of serum AP, although persons with blood groups O and B may have an elevated serum AP level derived from the small bowel, particularly after a fatty meal. This occurrence provides the rationale for obtaining fasting measurements of AP. Patients with chronic renal failure also may have elevations of the intestinal isoform of AP, and the serum AP level rarely may be elevated on a genetic basis without overt liver disease.

Hepatic AP is normally present on the apical (i.e., canalicular) domain of the hepatocyte plasma membrane and in the luminal domain of bile duct epithelium. Elevation of AP in the setting of liver disease results from increased synthesis and release of the enzyme into serum rather than from impaired biliary secretion.[17] Bile acids, which are retained in cholestatic liver disease, may solubilize the hepatocyte plasma membrane and facilitate the release of AP. Because elevation of AP in serum requires synthesis of new enzyme, AP may not become elevated for a day or two following acute biliary obstruction. Moreover, because the half-life of serum AP is approximately 1 week, the level in serum may remain elevated for several days after resolution of biliary obstruction.

Levels of AP up to three times normal are relatively nonspecific and occur in various liver diseases. Striking elevations of AP are seen predominantly with infiltrative hepatic disorders (for example, primary or metastatic tumor) or biliary obstruction, either within the liver (e.g., primary biliary cirrhosis, PBC) or in the extrahepatic biliary tree. Elevation of serum AP with hepatic infiltration likely results from compression of small, intrahepatic bile ducts. It is important to note that the AP level may be elevated in the setting of focal intrahepatic duct obstruction from a tumor, whereas the serum bilirubin level is typically normal in this setting. Although fairly sensitive, serum AP is occasionally normal despite extensive hepatic metastasis or, rarely, despite documented large duct obstruction.[18] The level of AP cannot be used to distinguish reliably between intra- and extrahepatic duct obstruction or hepatic infiltration. For example, identical levels can be seen with strategically located hepatic metastases, obstructing choledocholithiasis, and PBC. Rarely, the AP level may be elevated in the setting of malignancy, without identifiable liver or bone involvement. This so-called "Regan isoenzyme" is biochemically distinct from liver AP and has been identified in association with a variety of different cancers (e.g., lung neoplasms). Another explanation for elevation of the serum AP in a patient with cancer is a nonspecific hepatitis that has been reported in association with Hodgkin's disease and renal cell carcinoma without demonstrable direct liver involvement. Elevation of AP is seen commonly in neonatal liver disease of various causes (see Chapter 65).

Gamma Glutamyl Transpeptidase

Hepatic gamma glutamyl transpeptidase (GGTP) is derived from hepatocytes and biliary epithelia but, like AP, GGTP is found in many extrahepatic tissues, including the kidney, spleen, pancreas, heart, lung, and brain. However, it is not found in appreciable quantities in bone, and it is thus helpful in confirming the hepatic origin of an elevated AP level. The normal serum GGTP level is significantly higher in infants than in adults. Both benign recurrent intrahepatic cholestasis (BRIC) and Byler's syndrome, rare cholestatic liver diseases that often present in infancy, are characterized by elevation of the serum AP without an elevated GGTP (see Chapter 65). Thus, serum GGTP should be measured in all pediatric patients with cholestatic liver disease. GGTP is a microsomal enzyme and is therefore inducible by alcohol and drugs including most anticonvulsants and warfarin. Indeed, a GGTP/AP ratio of greater than 2.5 has been reported to be suggestive of alcohol abuse (see Chapter 71). However, more than one third of habitual consumers of alcohol (>80 g/day) have normal serum GGTP levels, and the enzyme often does not rise during alcohol binges.[19] Thus the value of GGTP for assessing surreptitious alcohol use is limited.

5′-Nucleotidase

5′-Nucleotidase (5′NT) is found in many tissues, including liver, cardiac muscle, brain, blood vessels, and pancreas.

Despite this widespread tissue distribution, significant serum elevations of 5′NT are found almost exclusively in the setting of liver disease. Within the liver, this enzyme is located both in the hepatocyte sinusoidal and canalicular plasma membranes. The enzyme has a sensitivity comparable to that of AP in detecting biliary obstruction, hepatic infiltration, and cholestasis but may exhibit kinetics that are different from those of both AP and GGTP, with levels rising several days after experimental bile duct ligation.[20] Thus, 5′NT may occasionally be normal with acute elevations of the other two enzymes and may be less useful than the GGTP as a test to confirm the hepatic origin of an elevated AP.

Bilirubin

Bilirubin is an organic anion that is derived primarily from the catabolism of hemoglobin. The metabolism and measurement of bilirubin and diagnostic approach to the jaundiced patient are reviewed in detail in Chapter 14 and will be discussed only briefly here. Serum bilirubin consists of two major forms, a water-soluble, conjugated, "direct" fraction and a lipid-soluble, unconjugated, "indirect" fraction. The normal serum concentration of bilirubin is less than 1 mg/dL (18 μmol/L). The serum bilirubin level is normally almost entirely unconjugated when measured with sensitive techniques and reflects a balance between the rates of production and hepatobiliary excretion. Production of bilirubin is accelerated by hemolysis, ineffective erythropoiesis, resorption of a hematoma, or, rarely, muscle injury, all of which may result in unconjugated hyperbilirubinemia. Impaired biliary excretion, as occurs in parenchymal liver disease or biliary tract obstruction, characteristically results in a conjugated hyperbilirubinemia. Bilirubin in the urine is always in a conjugated form and thus indicative of hepatobiliary disease, because the unconjugated form is bound to albumin and is not filtered by the normal glomerulus.

UNCONJUGATED HYPERBILIRUBINEMIA. Unconjugated hyperbilirubinemia (i.e., indirect bilirubin fraction >85% of the total serum bilirubin) results from either increased bilirubin production or inherited or acquired defects in hepatic uptake or conjugation (see Chapter 14 and Table 14–1 and Table 14–2). The diagnosis of hemolysis rests on a careful history (e.g., history of anemia, recent blood transfusions, medications) and standard screening tests (i.e., complete blood count, peripheral blood smear, reticulocyte count, LDH, and haptoglobin). If hemolysis is suggested by these screening tests, a specific cause may be ascertained by more specialized testing (e.g., Coombs' test, glucose-6-phosphate dehydrogenase [G6PD] assay, hemoglobin electrophoresis). Of note, chronic hemolysis cannot account for a sustained elevation of serum bilirubin to concentrations greater than 5 mg/dL in the presence of normal hepatic function.[3, 4]

CONJUGATED HYPERBILIRUBINEMIA. Conjugated hyperbilirubinemia (i.e., direct bilirubin fraction > 50% of the total serum bilirubin) occurs as a result of inherited or acquired defects in hepatic excretion, the rate-limiting step in bilirubin metabolism, and subsequent regurgitation of conjugated bilirubin from hepatocytes into the serum. Although measurement of the conjugated fraction does not reliably distinguish biliary obstruction from parenchymal liver disease,[21] the magnitude of the bilirubin elevation may be useful prognostically in patients with alcoholic hepatitis, primary biliary cirrhosis, and acute liver failure. Because conjugated bilirubin is cleared by the kidney, serum concentrations of bilirubin rarely exceed 30 mg/dL in the absence of hemolysis or renal failure.

A fraction of circulating conjugated bilirubin found in the setting of prolonged cholestasis (the delta fraction) is tightly bound to albumin, does not appear in the urine, but still reacts directly with the diazo reagent used for measurement of bilirubin (see Chapter 14).[22] This phenomenon may explain the occasional paradox of a patient with parenchymal liver disease who has a modest elevation in the direct-reacting serum bilirubin level but little or no bilirubinuria, as well as the tendency of bilirubinuria to disappear before hyperbilirubinemia resolves in patients with resolving liver disease. It also may contribute to the tendency of hyperbilirubinemia to resolve more slowly than other biochemical parameters of liver injury.

Bile Acids

Bile acids are organic anions synthesized from cholesterol exclusively in the liver (see Chapters 54 and 63). Although several studies suggest that measurement of the serum bile acid concentration is a sensitive marker of liver disease, there is little evidence that its determination offers any advantage over conventional biochemical tests for early detection of liver disease.[23, 24] Moreover, the utility of serum bile acid measurements in assessing prognosis in acute or chronic liver disease is uncertain, and such measurements are not widely used.

Markers of Hepatic Synthetic Capacity

Prothrombin Time

The liver plays a crucial role in hemostasis. All the major coagulation factors are synthesized in hepatocytes, except factor VIII, which is made in vascular endothelium and reticuloendothelial cells. The prothrombin time (PT) measures the rate of conversion of prothrombin to thrombin and reflects the activity of several of the factors involved in the extrinsic coagulation pathway, including factors II, V, VII, and X. Vitamin K is required for the gamma-carboxylation of factors II, VII, IX, and X, which is essential for the normal function of these factors. The differential diagnosis of an elevated PT includes vitamin K deficiency (caused by malnutrition, malabsorption, or antibiotic use), warfarin administration (which interferes with the vitamin K–dependent gamma-carboxylation), consumptive coagulopathy (e.g., disseminated intravascular coagulation [DIC]), rare congenital deficiencies, and liver disease. DIC usually can be distinguished from liver disease as a cause of a prolonged PT by measurement of the level of factor VIII, which is decreased in DIC and normal or increased in liver disease.[25] Prolongation of the PT may occur in decompensated liver disease with hepatocellular dysfunction and in chronic cholestatic disease with concomitant fat malabsorption and vitamin K deficiency, and these can be distinguished by measurement of factor V, which is not affected by vitamin K. Alternatively, vitamin K replacement (10 mg SQ) should reduce a prolonged PT secondary to vitamin K deficiency by at least

30% within 24 hours and is used more commonly than measurement of factor V. Because of the short half-life of some of the coagulation factors measured by the PT (i.e., approximately 6 hours for factor VII), changes in the PT, and in factor VII levels in particular, are useful in monitoring hepatic synthetic function in patients with acute liver disease.[26] Of note, the International Normalized Ratio (INR), which is the preferred test to monitor patients on anticoagulation because of its standardization and reproducibility, appears to offer no advantage over the PT in patients with liver disease.[27, 28]

Albumin

Approximately 10 g of albumin is synthesized and secreted by hepatocytes each day. With progressive parenchymal liver disease, albumin synthetic capacity decreases and its serum concentration falls. However, the serum albumin concentration reflects a variety of extrahepatic factors, including nutritional and volume status, vascular integrity, catabolism, hormonal factors, and loss in the urine or stool, and thus a low serum albumin level is not specific for liver disease. In addition, because the serum half-life of albumin is approximately 20 days, serum albumin measurements are less useful than PT in assessing hepatic synthetic function in patients with acute liver disease. Despite these limitations, the serum albumin concentration does correlate with prognosis in chronic liver disease. Prealbumin, which is also synthesized by the liver, has a much shorter half-life than albumin and has been used by some investigators to assess the severity of acute liver failure. However, like albumin, a low serum concentration of prealbumin is not specific for liver disease, and its measurement has not found widespread use in the United States.

CHARACTERISTIC BIOCHEMICAL PATTERNS: INTERPRETATION AND APPROACH

Certain characteristic patterns of the biochemical tests can be useful in differential diagnosis. The general patterns, outlined in Table 64–2, include hepatocellular necrosis, cholestasis, and infiltration. Not all patients fit neatly into one of these broad categories; many present with biochemical features of more than one group. Nonetheless, recognition of the predominant pattern, in the context of the clinical history and physical examination, is often helpful in guiding further evaluation.

Hepatocellular Necrosis

The hallmark of hepatocellular necrosis is elevation of the aminotransferase levels. The magnitude and tempo of the elevation may be useful diagnostically, especially when the elevations are dramatic, in which case the differential diagnosis is relatively narrow.

Marked Aminotransferase Elevation

Striking elevations of the aminotransferase levels (i.e., >2000 U/L) are seen almost exclusively with drug- or toxin-induced hepatic injury, ischemic liver injury, and acute viral hepatitis. There are rare exceptions to this rule. For example, an occasional patient with acute obstructing choledocholithiasis may present with extreme aminotransferase elevations, sometimes greater than 2000 U/L, associated initially with minimal elevations of serum AP and bilirubin levels. However, the presenting clinical features (e.g., right upper quadrant pain often with nausea and vomiting) and evolving biochemical pattern (e.g., precipitous fall in aminotransferases over 1 to 2 days accompanied by a rise in AP and bilirubin levels) usually suggest the diagnosis of acute biliary obstruction. In addition, autoimmune hepatitis and giant cell hepatitis rarely may be associated with massive aminotransferase elevations. Extreme aminotransferase elevations in autoimmune hepatitis are associated with aggressive disease and a poor prognosis without treatment.[29]

Liver injury from ischemia can usually be differentiated from viral hepatitis or toxin- and drug-induced liver disease by the clinical history as well as the time course of the aminotransferase elevation. Figure 64–1 depicts changes in aminotransferase activities over time for idealized cases of ischemic, toxic, and viral hepatitis (see Chapters 68, 70, and

Table 64–2 | **General Patterns of Biochemical Liver Tests***

TEST	TYPE OF LIVER DISEASE: Hepatocellular Necrosis			Biliary Obstruction		Hepatic Infiltration
Causative agent	Toxin/ischemia	Viral	Alcohol	Complete	Partial	
Examples	Acetaminophen or shock liver	Hepatitis A or B	—	Pancreatic carcinoma	Hilar tumor, PSC	Primary or metastatic carcinoma, TB, sarcoid, amyloidosis
Aminotransferases	50–100×	5–50×	2–5×	1–5×†	1–5×†	1–3×
Alkaline phosphatase	1–3×	1–3×	1–10×	2–20×	2–10×	1–20×
Bilirubin	1–5×	1–30×	1–30×	1–30×	1–5×	1–5× (often normal)
Prothrombin time	Prolonged and unresponsive to vitamin K in severe disease			Often prolonged and responsive to parenteral vitamin K		Usually normal
Albumin	Decreased in subacute/chronic disease			Usually normal; decreased in advanced disease (i.e., cirrhosis)		Usually normal

*Illustrative disorders for each category are included.

†Rapid onset of complete biliary obstruction (e.g., secondary to choledocholithiasis) rarely may result in massive (20–50x normal), but transient, elevation of the aminotransferases.

PSC, primary sclerosing cholangitis; TB, tuberculosis; x, times normal serum concentration.

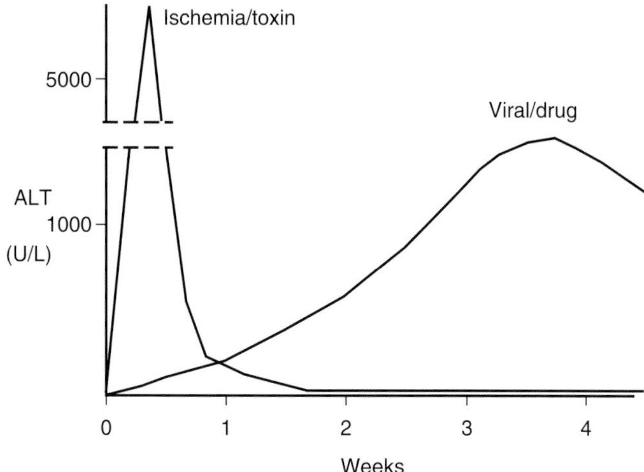

Figure 64–1. Time course of alanine aminotransferase (ALT) elevations characteristic of ischemic or toxic liver injury (typically abrupt and relatively brief), compared with viral hepatitis or drug injury (typically lasting many days to weeks).

73). Ischemic hepatitis, or "shock liver," is the result of acute hepatic circulatory insufficiency that typically occurs in the setting of serious illness, such as acute or chronic heart failure, myocardial infarction, arrhythmias, sepsis, extensive burns, severe trauma, or heat stroke.[30] It is interesting that hypotension is often not documented before the abnormal liver tests are recognized.[31] The characteristic biochemical pattern is a sudden, massive (often over 2000 U/L) elevation in the aminotransferase levels, which return to normal within 1 week. There often is a subsequent mild and transient increase in the serum levels of bilirubin and AP. The PT is rarely prolonged more than 3 seconds. Associated extreme elevations of the lactate dehydrogenase (LDH) (i.e., often >5000 U/L), not usually seen in viral hepatitis, and transient renal insufficiency, if present, also are suggestive of ischemic hepatitis.[32] Despite the magnitude of the aminotransferase elevation, ischemic hepatitis is usually subclinical. Only rare cases of acute liver failure attributed to circulatory failure alone have been reported. Prognosis is largely determined by the underlying circulatory disorder rather than the presence of liver dysfunction per se, and management consists of improving circulatory dynamics promptly.

The diagnosis of drug- or toxin-induced hepatitis relies on a high index of suspicion and careful history taking (see Chapter 73). Indeed, drug-induced hepatotoxicity is so common that it should be considered in all patients with abnormal biochemical liver tests. The duration of aminotransferase elevation varies depending on the inciting agent but is, in general, more prolonged than with ischemic hepatitis. The presence of fever, rash, and eosinophilia, which may occur in some forms of drug-induced liver injury (e.g., halothane hepatitis) is helpful in the diagnosis, but these signs are absent in liver disease caused by most drugs. For example, hepatotoxicity caused by acetaminophen, the most common cause of severe drug-induced liver disease in Western countries, is not associated with signs of allergy. Doses of acetaminophen greater than 10 to 12 grams are usually required to produce significant liver injury in previously healthy persons, but much lower doses may cause severe liver injury in the setting of chronic alcohol consumption or prolonged fasting. Other drugs or toxins associated with severe hepatocellular necrosis and massive aminotransferase elevations include halothane (and, less commonly, other inhalational anesthetics) and solvents such as carbon tetrachloride.

Acute viral hepatitis is a common cause of massive aminotransferase elevation. The magnitude of the aminotransferase elevation with viral hepatitis is usually less, and the time course longer, than that associated with ischemic or acute drug- or toxin-induced liver injury. All the well-characterized hepatotropic viruses (A–E) can cause acute hepatitis (see Chapter 68). The diagnosis of acute viral hepatitis rests on the clinical history of epidemiologic risk factors, such as ingestion of raw shellfish for hepatitis A, intravenous drug-use for hepatitis B, C, and D, and travel to endemic areas for hepatitis E, and can be confirmed with serologic testing.

Moderate Persistent Aminotranferase Elevation

Moderate aminotransferase elevations of 250 to 1000 U/L have much less diagnostic specificity than do massive elevations. Indeed, almost any type of liver disease may be associated with aminotransferase elevations in this range; viral and drug-induced hepatitis are probably the most common causes. Other diagnostic considerations include autoimmune hepatitis, Wilson disease, and alpha-1 antitrypsin deficiency. Over-the-counter medications, such as nonsteroidal anti-inflammatory drugs, may result in asymptomatic hepatotoxicity in some persons that is characterized by mild-to-moderate elevations of serum aminotransferase levels. Illicit drug use, especially of cocaine and metamphetamines, is also frequently associated with moderate, usually transient elevations of the aminotransferases. In addition to the hepatotropic viruses, the herpes viruses (Epstein-Barr, cytomegalovirus, and herpes simplex virus) may cause hepatitis with moderate elevations of the aminotransferases.

Mild Persistent Aminotransferase Elevation

Almost any type of liver disease characterized by modest hepatic inflammation and necrosis can produce low-level aminotransferase elevations. Steatosis, drugs, alcohol, chronic viral hepatitis, cirrhosis, various causes of cholestasis, neoplasms, and hemochromatosis are potential causes of mild (i.e., <250 U/L) elevations of the aminotransferases. Nonalcoholic fatty liver disease is probably the most common cause in this category (see Chapter 72). Alcohol use and hepatitis C are also common causes of mild persistent aminotransferase elevations.

Cholestasis

Cholestasis is a generic term referring to an impairment in bile flow and is characterized biochemically by greater elevation in the serum AP or conjugated bilirubin levels than in the aminotransferase levels. Elevation of both AP and bilirubin, although relatively nonspecific, is seen most commonly with biliary tract obstruction (see Table 64–2) caused, for example, by strategically located metastases that impinge on bile ducts. Various forms of hepatitis, especially alcoholic hepatitis and occasionally hepatitis A, and some drugs, such as oral contraceptives, also may present with this pattern.[33] Biochemical patterns that may be useful diagnostically are discussed here.

Disproportionate Rise in Alkaline Phosphatase

The two major diagnostic considerations in patients with an elevated AP without significant hyperbilirubinemia include partial biliary obstruction and hepatic infiltration. Partial biliary obstruction may result from choledocholithiasis or biliary strictures that involve small intrahepatic ducts, as occurs with recurrent pyogenic cholangitis or primary sclerosing cholangitis, or occasionally from malignant obstruction of only the left or right ductal system near the ductal bifurcation (a Klatskin tumor). The nearly normal serum levels of bilirubin in such patients presumably reflect the high capacity of hepatocytes in uninvolved areas of the liver to secrete the daily bilirubin load. A stone that produces intermittent (ball-valve) obstruction of the common bile duct may result in an identical pattern, as may early primary biliary cirrhosis. Hepatic infiltration with primary or metastatic cancer, amyloid, mycobacteria, or other granulomatous disorders (e.g., sarcoidosis) characteristically results in an elevated AP level without jaundice until advanced stages. Drug-induced cholestasis, particularly from anabolic steroids, estrogens, and psychiatric medications (e.g., antipsychotics), also may have this biochemical pattern. Finally, severe extrahepatic bacterial infection, although often associated with a moderate conjugated hyperbilirubinemia, rarely may cause a disproportionate elevation of the alkaline phosphatase level[34]; the pathogenesis of this pattern is not entirely clear.

The diagnostic approach to patients with a disproportionate elevation of the fasting serum AP is relatively straightforward (Fig. 64–2). First, the hepatic origin of the AP elevation should be verified by demonstrating an elevation of either the GGTP or 5′-NT. If the AP is of hepatic origin, an imaging test, such as abdominal computed tomography (CT) or ultrasonography, should be used to look for dilated intrahepatic ducts and the presence of liver masses. If ductal dilation is present, or if the clinical suspicion of biliary obstruction remains high despite negative initial imaging studies, either endoscopic retrograde cholangiopancreatography, magnetic resonance cholangiopancreatography, or percutaneous transhepatic cholangiography can be used to define the location and nature of the obstruction. The relative merits of these procedures are discussed in Chapter 14. If a focal mass is present, ultrasound- or CT-guided aspiration cytology or biopsy may be indicated. If neither obstruction nor a focal mass is seen, an antimitochondrial antibody test should be ordered, especially in a middle-aged female patient, to look for primary biliary cirrhosis. If drug-induced cholestasis is a consideration, the drug(s) should be discontinued and the AP repeated at regular intervals to document resolution of cholestasis. Percutaneous liver biopsy may be necessary to evaluate such patients further and to look for an infiltrating disorder. However, as many as one third of patients with an isolated elevation of the liver isoform of AP will have no evidence of liver disease after an extensive investigation, including liver biopsy.[35]

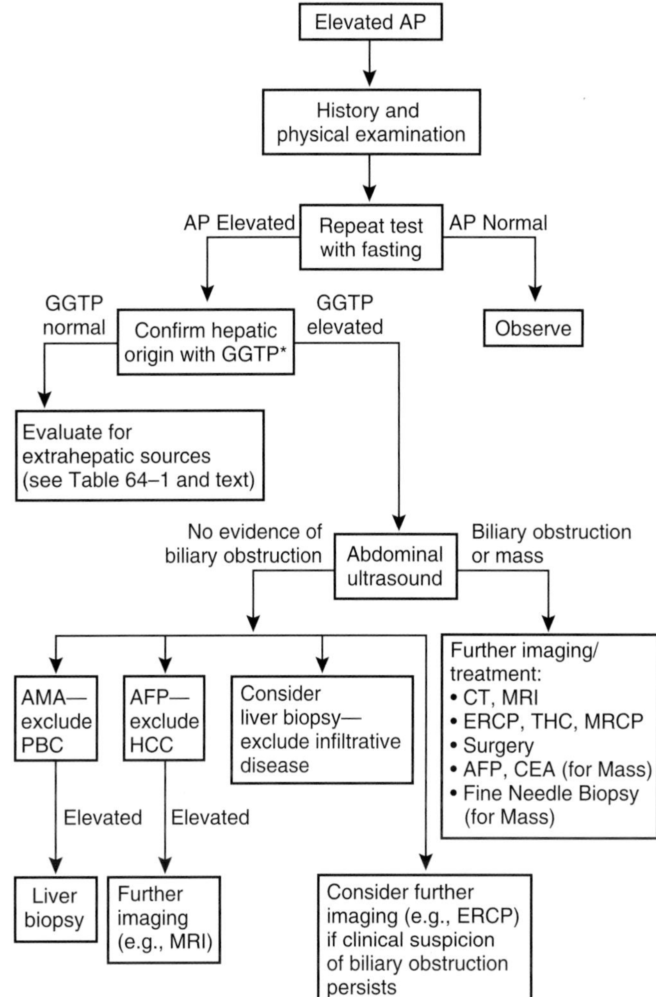

Figure 64–2. Evaluation of isolated alkaline phosphatase (AP) elevation. Clinical history-taking should focus on excluding extrahepatic sources of AP (e.g., symptoms of bone disease, pregnancy), medication use, symptoms of biliary colic, and cholestasis (e.g., pruritus). The physical examination should focus on detection of stigmata of chronic liver disease (e.g., splenomegaly) as well as signs of chronic cholestasis (e.g., excoriations).

AFP, alpha fetoprotein; AMA, antimitochondrial antibodies; CEA, carcinoembryonic antigen; ERCP, endoscopic retrograde cholangiopancreatography; GGTP, gamma glutamyl transpeptidase; HCC, hepatocellular carcinoma; MRCP, magnetic resonance cholangiopancreatography; MRI, magnetic resonance imaging; PBC, primary biliary cirrhosis; THC, transhepatic cholangiography.

Disproportionate Rise in Bilirubin Compared with Alkaline Phosphatase

The first step in evaluating patients with this biochemical pattern is to determine whether the bilirubinemia is primarily conjugated or unconjugated. A disproportionate rise of the conjugated bilirubin compared with AP has little diagnostic specificity and can be seen with a variety of causes of liver disease (e.g., alcohol, drugs, viral hepatitis) as well as rare inherited disorders (e.g., Dubin-Johnson and Rotor's syndromes—see Chapter 14). Disproportionate elevation of unconjugated serum bilirubin compared with AP is caused by inherited or acquired defects in hepatic uptake or conjugation (e.g., Gilbert's syndrome) or hemolysis that occurs either coincidentally with or as a manifestation of some forms of liver disease, such as acute Wilson disease. Gilbert's syndrome is a common, benign disorder of bilirubin conjugation characterized by an intermittent, mild, unconjugated bilirubinemia (indirect bilirubin of 2 to 5 mg/dL) that is exacerbated by fasting and ameliorated by treatment with phenobarbital (both of which provide diagnostic clues to the disorder). The disproportionate elevation of unconjugated serum bilirubin compared with AP in fulminant Wilson disease results from both hemolysis and a depression in serum AP activity. Although the reason why the serum AP is low in this setting is unclear, hemolysis in Wilson disease is thought to result from rapid release of excess copper into the bloodstream with resulting lysis of erythrocytes.[36, 37] Significant hemolysis often is seen in patients who discontinue chelating therapy abruptly but also can be seen in patients presenting with Wilson disease for the first time (see Chapter 67).

Isolated Rise in GGTP

GGTP is inducible by alcohol and drugs, including most anticonvulsants and warfarin. In patients with an elevated GGTP but normal AP level and normal levels of other routine liver tests, a careful medication history and a quantitative assessment of alcohol intake will usually explain the laboratory findings. No further evaluation is usually necessary, although documenting a normal GGTP after a period of abstinence from alcohol or withdrawal of an offending medication, if possible, is reassuring.

Elevated Alkaline Phosphatase with Normal GGTP

The most common explanation for an AP elevation with a normal GGTP (or 5′-NT) level is rapid bone growth (e.g., in children), bone disease (e.g., Paget's disease), or pregnancy. Certain rare liver disorders also are characterized by this pattern: Byler's syndrome, benign recurrent intrahepatic cholestasis (BRIC), and hereditary defects of bile acid synthesis (see Chapters 54 and 65). Byler's syndrome is a lethal autosomal recessive cholestatic disease that was first described in an Amish kindred. The pathogenesis of the disorder is unclear, and orthotopic liver transplantation remains the only available therapy.[38] BRIC is an idiopathic familial syndrome characterized by recurrent, self-limited episodes of intrahepatic cholestasis, which may last several months and often are associated with flulike symptoms and abdominal pain. Elevation of the AP and bilirubin with near-normal aminotransferase and GGTP levels is typical. The gene responsible for both Byler's syndrome and BRIC has been localized to the chromosome 18q.[39] The reason for the normal GGTP level and for the defects in bile acid synthesis in these two cholestatic disorders is unknown, but failure of hepatocytes to secrete bile acids into the canaliculus may be involved.[38]

FREQUENTLY ENCOUNTERED CLINICAL PROBLEMS

The appropriate interpretation of biochemical liver tests in the context of a carefully obtained clinical history and physical examination should lead to the correct diagnosis or, at least, help guide decisions regarding further evaluation of the selected common and often challenging clinical scenarios that are summarized next.

Asymptomatic Aminotransferase Elevations

The incidental discovery of asymptomatic patients with mild-to-moderate elevations of the aminotransferase levels represents a common clinical problem.[40] Blood donors, screened in the past with serum ALT in the United States, account for many of these patients.[41] Because the prevalence of liver disease is low in volunteer blood donors, the majority of these abnormalities do not indicate serious liver disease. To illustrate, if the prevalence of liver disease is assumed to be 1% in blood donors and the normal range of serum ALT and AST levels is assumed to include 95% of the normal population, then less than 20% of patients with abnormal values would be anticipated to have liver disease. Thus, a careful approach to the evaluation of these patients is warranted in order to avoid unnecessary cost, inconvenience, discomfort, or risk to the patient. In general, the finding of an elevated aminotransferase level, especially when minimal, should lead to retesting before extensive evaluation.[40] With a persistent aminotransferase elevation, the higher the elevation, the less likely it is to represent a false-positive result and the more likely it is to reflect significant underlying liver disease. Likewise, concomitant abnormalities in the other biochemical liver tests, such as bilirubin and AP, increase the likelihood of liver disease.

The reported etiology of mild serum aminotransferase elevations in asymptomatic patients varies depending on geography and patient selection. For example, hepatitis B, schistosomiasis, and malaria are common causes of elevated serum aminotransferases in the Far East, Egypt, and Africa, respectively, but are rare causes in most Western countries. Similarly, chronic (presumably autoimmune) hepatitis accounted for asymptomatic aminotransferase elevation in almost three quarters of patients reported from a center in the United States with expertise in autoimmune liver disease, whereas this diagnosis was made in only 10% to 20% of patients in other large studies.[42] In most Western countries, hepatic steatosis (which may be present in patients who are only modestly overweight), drug-induced liver disease, and alcohol-related liver disease are among the most common causes of an asymptomatic aminotransferase elevation. Other common explanations include chronic viral hepatitis and nonhepatic causes such as muscle injury (although muscle injury results in an isolated serum AST elevation more often than elevations of both AST and ALT). Metabolic liver diseases, especially hemochromatosis and alpha-1 antitrypsin deficiency, accounted for 7% of patients with an aminotransferase elevation in one study, whereas drug-induced hepatitis was the apparent explanation in approximately 5% of patients in another large study.[43, 44]

The evaluation of asymptomatic patients with serum aminotransferase elevations should be guided by the clinical history, physical examination, and nature of the test abnormalities (Fig. 64–3). History-taking should focus on use of prescription and over-the-counter medications and alcohol, occupational exposures to hepatotoxins, risk factors for viral hepatitis, and a family history of liver disease. The physical examination should focus on detection of signs of chronic liver disease, such as splenomegaly, ascites, and cutaneous stigmata of chronic liver disease (e.g., spider angiomata) and should include a general assessment of body habitus (e.g., obesity). Repeat testing is essential in asymptomatic patients without risk factors for and signs of liver disease. For example, approximately one third of blood donors with asymptomatic aminotransferase elevations have only a single elevation of the serum ALT on longitudinal follow-up.[41] Obtaining medical records or a history of blood donation that entailed ALT testing is useful in determining the chronicity of the problem. Patients with an isolated AST elevation should be evaluated for extrahepatic sources of this enzyme, particularly muscle.[40] Patients with occult celiac sprue or adrenocortical insufficiency (Addison's disease) as a cause of otherwise unexplained aminotransferase elevations have been described, and these disorders should be considered when more common explanations have been excluded.[45, 46]

The diagnostic evaluation of patients with elevated aminotransferase levels should focus on detecting potentially treatable conditions. Thus, iron studies should be obtained routinely to address the possibility of hemochromatosis, whereas urinary copper quantitation and a serum ceruloplasmin level are appropriate in younger patients to detect Wilson disease. Markers of autoimmune liver disease should be considered in young female patients with persistent aminotranferase elevations (see Chapter 75). Serologic studies for hepatitis B and C should be obtained, because many patients with hepatitis C and even hepatitis B lack conventional risk factors for hepatitis. Although rare, most patients also should be tested for alpha-1 antitrypsin deficiency (see Chapter 65).

All patients with persistent aminotransferase elevations of uncertain etiology should be advised to discontinue unnecessary medications and abstain from alcohol. Abstinence from alcohol for several weeks often lowers the AST to the normal range if the elevation is caused by alcohol. Similarly, discontinuation of drugs responsible for hepatotoxicity usually results in relatively rapid improvement in liver biochemistries, although exceptions to this general rule have been reported.[47] Weight loss is advisable in overweight patients or if imaging studies suggest fatty liver, because the biochemical abnormalities associated with hepatic steatosis may improve, and the risks, cost, and discomfort of further evaluation, especially liver biopsy, may be avoided.[48] If these interventions have little or no effect and aminotransferase levels remain elevated (more than 1.5 times the upper limit of normal) over 6 to 12 months in the absence of a discernible cause, a liver biopsy should be considered.

Differentiating Intrahepatic Cholestasis from Obstruction

Differentiating intrahepatic cholestasis from biliary obstruction is crucial in the management of patients with cholestasis. Although accurate differentiation of so-called "medical" from "surgical" cholestasis is not possible with routine biochemical liver tests, the clinical history and physical examination in conjunction with the biochemical tests permit accurate diagnosis in most cases. Indirect or direct imaging of the biliary tree and possibly liver biopsy are ultimately necessary for precise diagnosis (see Chapter 14).

Assessing Operative Risk

Assessing operative risk in patients with liver disease is a challenging task that has been reviewed recently.[49] The he-

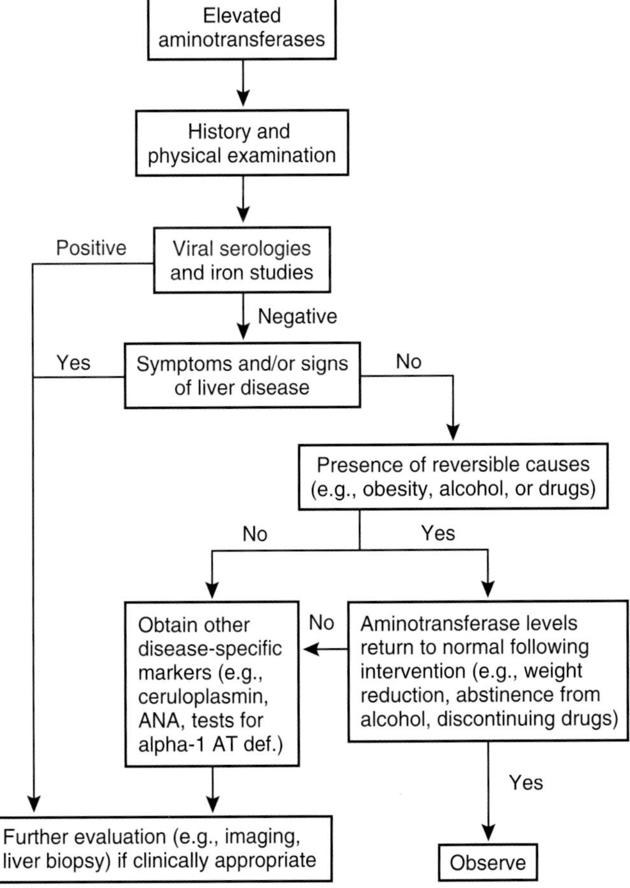

Figure 64–3. Evaluation of mild but sustained aminotransferase elevations. The algorithm assumes elevation of both aspartate and alanine aminotransferases, making a nonhepatic source unlikely. Clinical history-taking should focus on risk factors for viral hepatitis, medication, alcohol and illicit drug use, recent weight gain, and a family history of liver disease. The physical examination should focus on the detection of stigmata of chronic liver disease (e.g., splenomegaly, cutaneous spiders), Kayser-Fleischer ring (especially in young patients), and extrahepatic disease that could contribute to elevated aminotransferases (e.g., signs of right-sided heart failure). See text for further details. ANA, antinuclear antibodies; α1-AT def., alpha-1 antitrypsin deficiency.

modynamic changes that occur during surgery, in part secondary to anesthesia and bleeding, may have a profoundly detrimental effect on the function of an already compromised liver. The lack of large, prospective trials assessing the risks of surgery in patients with liver disease makes firm recommendations difficult. What can be stated with confidence is that patients with active or decompensated liver disease, whether acute or chronic, have a higher frequency of postoperative complications and mortality. This is particularly true with certain types of surgery, including hepatic resection, biliary surgery, gastric surgery, colectomy, and cardiac surgery, but elective surgery of any kind should be avoided in patients with acute hepatitis, severe chronic hepatitis, and decompensated cirrhosis. In addition, in patients with abnormal liver biochemistries discovered incidentally during a preoperative evaluation, it is prudent to postpone elective surgery until the cause, stage, and course of the liver disease can be ascertained.

For patients with established cirrhosis, the Child-Turcotte-Pugh (CTP) scoring classification, which was originally devised to predict the prognosis of patients with liver disease who were undergoing portosystemic shunt surgery, also appears to be useful in predicting prognosis in other types of surgery (Table 64–3). In one recent retrospective study of 92 patients with cirrhosis who underwent abdominal surgery, the mortality rate was 10% for Child's class A patients, 30% for class B patients, and 82% for class C patients.[50] The CTP classification also correlates with the frequency of postoperative complications such as renal failure, hepatic encephalopathy, bleeding, infection, intractable ascites, and worsening liver failure.

In general, for patients with well-compensated cirrhosis (i.e., a normal bilirubin, albumin, prothrombin time, and nutritional status and no evidence of ascites or encephalopathy), operative risk appears to be increased only modestly, whereas in those with decompensated or active liver disease, the risks of surgery are significant.[49] In these patients, surgery should be avoided if possible or postponed until the risks of surgery are reduced (e.g., by portal decompression; see Chapter 77) or liver transplantation (see Chapter 83). If surgery is essential, meticulous preoperative preparation, intraoperative management, and postoperative care, including optimization of nutritional and fluid status, correction of coagulopathy, and avoidance of hypotension, nephrotoxins, and drugs that may exacerbate liver injury or encephalopathy (e.g., sedatives) are critical.

Table 64–3 | **Child-Turcotte-Pugh Scoring System to Assess Severity of Liver Disease**

CLINICAL AND LABORATORY MEASUREMENTS	POINTS SCORED FOR INCREASING ABNORMALITY		
	1	2	3
Encephalopathy (grade)	None	1–2	3–4
Ascites	None	Mild (or controlled by diuretics)	At least moderate despite diuretic treatment
Prothrombin time (seconds prolonged)	<4	4–6	>6
[Or INR	<1.7	1.7–2.3	>2.3]
Albumin (g/dL)	>3.5	2.8–3.5	<2.8
Bilirubin (mg/dL)	<2	2–3	>3
Grade (A): 5–6, grade (B): 7–9, grade (C): 10–15			

INR, International Normalized Ratio.

Screening for Drug Hepatotoxicity

Many commonly prescribed drugs have the potential to cause liver damage (see Chapter 73). Hepatotoxicity is usually idiosyncratic and impossible to predict in the individual patient. Some drugs, such as methotrexate (MTX) and isoniazid (INH), cause a more predictable hepatotoxicity. The goal of screening patients who are taking potentially hepatotoxic drugs is to detect hepatic injury before the onset of irreversible liver damage. However, the efficacy of screening for drug hepatotoxicity is controversial, in part because of the poor predictive value of biochemical liver tests for significant drug-induced liver injury. For example, at least 10% of patients taking INH develop modest elevations of the serum aminotransferases, but usually these levels return to normal despite continued use of the drug. Conversely, significant hepatic fibrosis, and even cirrhosis, has been reported to occur in patients taking methotrexate despite persistently normal liver tests. Finally, the onset of liver injury may be abrupt, so that periodic screening for hepatotoxicity is not useful. Precise and well-supported recommendations on screening for hepatotoxicity are not available for most drugs. For most patients taking INH, routine screening is probably unnecessary in the absence of symptoms of hepatitis. Recommendations for screening in patients on MTX are listed in Chapter 73, Table 73–8. Other drugs for which screening is often employed and is potentially useful but for which no formal recommendations are available include lovastatin (and other lipid-lowering drugs), valproate, pyrazinamide, ketoconazole, dantrolene, tacrine, and synthetic retinoids (e.g., isotretinoin).

Assessing Prognosis

The biochemical tests of liver disease, especially the markers of hepatic synthetic function and bilirubin, are useful for predicting prognosis in certain settings. For example, prolongation of the PT and elevation of the serum bilirubin level are associated with a poor prognosis in nonacetaminophen-related acute hepatic failure (see Chapter 80).[26] Both tests are also predictive of early mortality from severe alcoholic hepatitis and are thus useful in deciding whether glucocorticoid therapy is likely to be beneficial (see Chapter 71).[51] Prognosis in PBC correlates directly with the serum bilirubin level, and a composite score derived from the serum bilirubin, prothrombin time, serum albumin, patient's age, and severity of fluid retention is useful in assessing prognosis (see Chapter 76).[52] For many liver diseases, however, prognosis is more variable and difficult to predict using the conventional biochemical liver tests. Moreover, these tests often become abnormal only late in the course of the liver disease when complications are likely to occur.

The ability to determine functional liver mass, and thus a

Table 64–4 | **Model for End-Stage Liver Disease (MELD) to Assess Severity of Liver Disease**

PROGNOSTIC FACTOR	REGRESSION COEFFICIENT
Serum creatinine (Log_e value)	0.957
Serum bilirubin (Log_e value)	0.378
INR (Log_e value)	1.120
Etiology*	0.643

*For etiology, use 0 for alcohol-related liver disease or cholestatic liver disease and 1 for all other causes. Using these regression coefficients, the risk score is calculated with this formula: $R = 0.957 \times Log_e(\text{creatinine mg/dL}) + 0.378 \times Log_e(\text{bilirubin mg/dL}) + 1.120 \times Log_e(\text{INR}) + 0.643 \times (\text{etiology})$. An automated program for calculation of the MELD score and prognosis is available on the World Wide Web (http://www.mayo.edu/int-med/gi/model/mayomodl-5.htm).
INR, International Normalized Ratio.

patient's prognosis, accurately is becoming increasingly important as waiting times for orthotopic liver transplantation lengthen. Currently, transplant priority status is primarily determined by CTP score, although a new model, the Model for End-Stage Liver Disease (MELD) (Table 64–4), based on INR, serum bilirubin, and serum creatinine, as well as the etiology of liver disease, is likely to replace the CTP score for this purpose in the near future (see Chapter 83).[53] The MELD model has been used successfully to predict early mortality following transjugular intrahepatic portosystemic shunt (TIPS) in diverse patient populations and has several advantages over the CTP score for predicting survival. The CTP score relies on prognostic factors, such as ascites and encephalopathy, that are graded subjectively and divides patients into low, intermediate, and high risk without quantifying expected survival. More importantly, the CTP score does not discriminate among patients with advanced liver disease (Child's class C).[54] For example, two patients with cirrhosis, one with a serum bilirubin level of 3.5 mg/dL and the other with a serum bilirubin level of 28 mg/dL, may have the same CPT score but clearly different prognoses. The MELD model takes into account such differences and thus may be more useful in assessing expected survival in patients with end-stage liver disease.

QUANTITATIVE TESTS OF LIVER FUNCTION

Because of the shortcomings of the biochemical liver tests, attention has been directed toward the development of more sensitive and quantitative (and thus less subjective) tests that reflect liver function more accurately at a given point in time in an individual patient. Several of these so-called quantitative liver function tests are summarized in Table 64–5.[55] Despite claims that these tests are superior to conventional biochemical tests in establishing the presence of liver disease and predicting prognosis, their use generally has been limited to specialized research centers.

Several factors have prevented widespread adoption of these tests: they are more expensive, invasive, cumbersome, and time- and labor-intensive than the conventional biochemical tests. In addition, it is unclear whether these tests are superior to scoring systems based on conventional laboratory parameters (e.g., CPT, MELD scores) in predicting survival or life-threatening complications.[56] Well-controlled,

Table 64–5 | **Quantitative Liver Function Tests**

TEST	DESCRIPTION*	COMMENTS†
Indocyanine green clearance (ICG)	Concentration of dye, which is taken up almost exclusively by hepatocytes and excreted unchanged into the bile, is measured photometrically in blood samples taken at regular intervals following a bolus intravenous injection (0.5 mg/kg). Clearance of the dye decreases with loss of hepatocyte mass	May help predict death in patients with primary biliary cirrhosis and outcome after orthotopic liver transplantation Not useful for measuring hepatic blood flow in patients with liver disease Rare anaphylaxis reported
Galactose elimination capacity (GEC)	Metabolism of intravenously administered galactose (0.5 g/kg) is measured with serial blood samples collected 20–50 minutes following intravenous injection	May predict death in primary biliary cirrhosis and outcome in chronic hepatitis Safe, although large volume of fluid required No drug interactions
Aminopyrine breath test (ABT)	Radioactivity ($^{14}CO_2$) is measured in breath at 15-min intervals for 2 hr following oral or intravenous administration of ^{14}C-labeled methyl aminopyrine	May predict death and histology in chronic hepatitis Safety not established Radioactivity exposure required
Antipyrine clearance	Metabolite of antipyrine is measured in saliva 24 hr following oral administration (15 mg/kg)	Time-consuming to perform Safety not established Drug interactions may influence results
Monoethylglycinexylidide (MEGX)	Lidocaine metabolite is measured in blood sample 15 min after intravenous administration (1 mg/kg)	May predict death and complications before and after orthotopic liver transplantation May predict donor liver function
Caffeine clearance	Caffeine metabolites are measured in saliva samples over 24 hr following oral administration (280 mg)	Safe Drug interactions Relatively easy to perform

*As typically performed; variations may exist.
†Utility not clearly established for any of the tests listed.

prospective trials comparing quantitative liver function tests to conventional biochemical tests (used, of course, in conjunction with clinical assessment) are needed to define the role of these quantitative tests in the management of patients with liver disease.

REFERENCES

1. Henley KS, Schmidt FW, Schmidt E: Newer diagnostic tests in liver disease. In Popper H, Schaffner F (eds): Progress in Liver Diseases, Vol 1. New York, Grune & Stratton, 1961, p 216.
2. Sackett DLHR, Guyatt GH, Tugwell P: Clinical Epidemiology: A Basic Science for Clinical Medicine. Boston, Little, Brown, 1991.
3. Friedman LS, Martin P, Munoz SJ: Liver function tests and the objective evaluation of the patient with liver disease. In Zakim D, Boyer TD (eds): Hepatology: A Textbook of Liver Disease, Vol 1. Philadelpia, WB Saunders, 1996, pp 791–833.
4. Pratt DS, Kaplan MM: Laboratory tests. In Schiff ER, Sorrell MF, Maddrey WC (eds): Schiff's Diseases of the Liver, Vol 1. Philadelphia, Lippincott-Raven, 1999, pp 205–244.
5. Kratz A, Lewandrowski KB: Case records of the Massachusetts General Hospital. Weekly clinicopathological exercises. Normal reference laboratory values. N Engl J Med 339:1063–1072, 1998.
6. Begum T, Oliver MR, Kornberg AJ, Dennett X: Elevated aminotransferase as a presenting finding in a patient with occult muscle disease. J Paediatr Child Health 36:189–190, 2000.
7. Zamora S, Adams C, Butzner JD, et al: Elevated aminotransferase activity as an indication of muscular dystrophy: Case reports and review of the literature. Can J Gastroenterol 10:389–393, 1996.
8. Helfgott SM, Karlson E, Beckman E: Misinterpretation of serum transaminase elevation in "occult" myositis. Am J Med 95:447–449, 1993.
9. Sorbi D, Boynton J, Lindor KD: The ratio of aspartate aminotransferase to alanine aminotransferase: Potential value in differentiating nonalcoholic steatohepatitis from alcoholic liver disease. Am J Gastroenterol 94:1018–1022, 1999.
10. Berman DHLR, Gavaler JS, Cadoff EM, et al: Clinical differentiation of fulminant wilsonian hepatitis from other causes of hepatic failure. Gastroenterology 100:1129–1134, 1991.
11. Sallie R, Katsiyiannakis L, Baldwin D, et al: Failure of simple biochemical indexes to reliably differentiate fulminant Wilson's disease from other causes of fulminant liver failure. Hepatology 16:1206–1211, 1992.
12. Williams AL, Hoofnagle JH: Ratio of serum aspartate to alanine aminotransferase in chronic hepatitis. Relationship to cirrhosis. Gastroenterology 95:734–739, 1988.
13. Nalpas B, Vassault A, Charpin S, et al: Serum mitochondrial aspartate aminotransferase as a marker of chronic alcoholism: Diagnostic value and interpretation in a liver unit. Hepatology 6:608–614, 1986.
14. Fortson WC, Tedesco FJ, Starnes EC, et al: Marked elevation of serum transaminase activity associated with extrahepatic biliary tract disease. J Clin Gastroenterol 7:502–505, 1985.
15. Litin SC, O'Brien JF, Pruett S, et al: Macroenzyme as a cause of unexplained elevation of aspartate aminotransferase. Mayo Clin Proc 62:681–687, 1987.
16. Bacq Y, Zarka O, Bréchot JF, et al: Liver function tests in normal pregnancy: A prospective study of 103 pregnant women and 103 matched controls. Hepatology 23:1030–1034, 1996.
17. Seetharam S, Sussman NL, Komoda T, et al: The mechanism of elevated alkaline phosphatase activity after bile duct ligation in the rat. Hepatology 6:374–380, 1986.
18. McGarrity TJ, Samuels T, Wilson FA: An analysis of imaging studies and liver function tests to detect hepatic neoplasia. Dig Dis Sci 32: 1113–1137, 1987.
19. Penn R, Worthington DJ: Is serum gamma-glutamyltransferase a misleading test? Br Med J 286:531–535, 1983.
20. Reichling JJ, Kaplan MM: Clinical use of serum enzymes in liver disease. Dig Dis Sci 33:1601–1614, 1988.
21. Scharschmidt BF, Blanckaert N, Farina FA, et al: Measurement of serum bilirubin and its mono- and diconjugates: Application to patients with hepatobiliary disease. Gut 23:643–649, 1982.
22. Weiss JS, Gautam A, Lauff JJ, et al: The clinical importance of a protein-bound fraction of serum bilirubin in patients with hyperbilirubinemia. N Engl J Med 309:147–150, 1983.
23. Ferraris R, Colombatti G, Fiorentini MT, et al: Diagnostic value of serum bile acids and routine liver function tests in hepatobiliary diseases. Sensitivity, specificity, and predictive value. Dig Dis Sci 28:129–136, 1983.
24. Hofmann AF: The aminopyrine demethylation breath test and the serum bile acid level: Nominated but not yet elected to join the common liver tests. Hepatology 2:512–517, 1982.
25. Mammen EF: Coagulation defects in liver disease. Med Clin North Am 78:545–554, 1994.
26. O'Grady JG, Alexander GJ, Hayllar KM, et al: Early indicators of prognosis in fulminant hepatic failure. Gastroenterology 97:439–445, 1989.
27. Kovacs MJ, Wong A, MacKinnon K, et al: Assessment of the validity of the INR system for patients with liver impairment. Thromb Haemost 71:727–730, 1994.
28. Denson KW, Reed SV, Haddon ME: Validity of the INR system for patients with liver impairment. Thromb Haemost 73:162, 1995.
29. Davis GL, Czaja AJ, Baggenstoss AH, et al: Prognostic and therapeutic implications of extreme serum aminotransferase elevation in chronic active hepatitis. Mayo Clin Proc 57:303–309, 1982.
30. Rawson JS, Achord JL: Shock liver. South Med J 78:1421–1425, 1985.
31. Gibson PR, Dudley FJ: Ischemic hepatitis: Clinical features, diagnosis and prognosis. Aust N Z J Med 14:822–825, 1984.
32. Gitlin N, Serio KM: Ischemic hepatitis: Widening horizons. Am J Gastroenterol 87:831–836, 1992.
33. Gordon SC, Reddy KR, Schiff L, et al: Prolonged intrahepatic cholestasis secondary to acute hepatitis A. Ann Intern Med 101:635–637, 1984.
34. Fang MH, Ginsberg AL, Dobbins WOD: Marked elevation in serum alkaline phosphatase activity as a manifestation of systemic infection. Gastroenterology 78:592–597, 1980.
35. Brensilver HL, Kaplan MM: Significance of elevated liver alkaline phosphatase in serum. Gastroenterology 68:1556–1562, 1975.
36. Shaver WA, Bhatt H, Combes B: Low serum alkaline phosphatase activity in Wilson's disease. Hepatology 6:859–863, 1986.
37. Willson RA, Clayson KJ, Leon S: Unmeasurable serum alkaline phosphatase activity in Wilson's disease associated with fulminant hepatic failure and hemolysis. Hepatology 7:613–615, 1987.
38. Jacquemin E, Dumont M, Bernard O, et al: Evidence for defective primary bile acid secretion in children with progressive familial intrahepatic cholestasis (Byler disease). Eur J Pediatr 153:424–428, 1994.
39. Carlton VE, Knisely AS, Freimer NB: Mapping of a locus for progressive familial intrahepatic cholestasis (Byler disease) to 18q21-q22, the benign recurrent intrahepatic cholestasis region. Hum Mol Genet 4: 1049–1053, 1995.
40. Pratt DS, Kaplan MM: Evaluation of abnormal liver-enzyme results in asymptomatic patients. N Eng J Med 342:1266–1271, 2000.
41. Friedman LS, Dienstag JL, Watkins E, et al: Evaluation of blood donors with elevated serum alanine aminotransferase levels. Ann Intern Med 107:137–144, 1987.
42. Hay JE, Czaja AJ, Rakela J, et al: The nature of unexplained chronic aminotransferase elevations of a mild to moderate degree in asymptomatic patients [see comments]. Hepatology 9:193–197, 1989.
43. Hultcrantz R, Glaumann H, Lindberg G, et al: Liver investigation in 149 asymptomatic patients with moderately elevated activities of serum aminotransferases. Scand J Gastroenterol 21:109–113, 1986.
44. Van Ness MM, Diehl AM: Is liver biopsy useful in the evaluation of patients with chronically elevated liver enzymes? Ann Intern Med 111: 473–478, 1989.
45. Boulton R, Hamilton MI, Dhillon AP, et al: Subclinical Addison's disease: A cause of persistent abnormalities in transaminase values. Gastroenterology 109:1324–1327, 1995.
46. Bardella MT, Vecchi M, Conte D, et al: Chronic unexplained hypertransaminasemia may be caused by occult celiac disease. Hepatology 29:654–657, 1999.
47. Murphy EJ, Davern TJ, Shakil AO, et al: Troglitazone-induced fulminant hepatic failure. Acute Liver Failure Study Group. Dig Dis Sci 45: 549–553, 2000.
48. Palmer M, Schaffner F: Effect of weight reduction on hepatic abnormalities in overweight patients. Gastroenterology 99:1408–1413, 1990.
49. Friedman LS: The risk of surgery in patients with liver disease. Hepatology 29:1617–1623, 1999.
50. Mansour A, Watson W, Shayani V, et al: Abdominal operations in patients with cirrhosis: Still a major surgical challenge. Surgery 122: 730–735, 1997; discussion 735–736.

51. Ramond MJ, Poynard T, Rueff B, et al: A randomized trial of prednisolone in patients with severe alcoholic hepatitis. N Engl J Med 326: 507–512, 1992.
52. Dickson ER, Grambsch PM, Fleming TR, et al: Prognosis in primary biliary cirrhosis: Model for decision making. Hepatology 10:1–7, 1989.
53. Malinchoc M, Kamath PS, Gordon FD, et al: A model to predict poor survival in patients undergoing transjugular intrahepatic portosystemic shunts. Hepatology 31:864–871, 2000.
54. Conn HO: A peek at the Child-Turcotte classification. Hepatology 1: 673–674, 1981.
55. Jalan R, Hayes PC: Review article: Quantitative tests of liver function. Aliment Pharmacol Ther 9:263–270, 1995.
56. Albers I, Hartmann H, Bircher J, et al: Superiority of the Child-Pugh classification to quantitative liver function tests for assessing prognosis of liver cirrhosis. Scand J Gastroenterol 24:269–276, 1989.

Chapter 65

Inherited Metabolic Disorders of the Liver

Mike A. Leonis and William F. Balistreri

Inborn errors of metabolism encompass a vast variety of maladies with varied presentations and pathophysiology. Metabolic liver disease may present as an acute, life-threatening illness in the neonatal period or may be manifested as chronic liver disease, presenting in adolescence or adulthood, and progress to liver failure, cirrhosis, or hepatocellular carcinoma. In one review of 37 transplant centers in the United States, 5.3% of all liver transplantations were performed because of complications resulting from metabolic liver disease.[1] When the pediatric population alone is analyzed, this percentage is significantly higher. At the authors' institution, more than 20% of the liver transplants performed over a 9-year period were for complications of metabolic liver disease.[2] Liver transplantation has become a life-saving measure for many of these patients; however, new *nontransplant* treatment options have become available that may help alleviate the donor shortage.[3]

The diverse presenting symptoms of metabolic liver disease are listed in Table 65–1. Metabolic liver diseases in young patients may mimic other illnesses such as acute infections or intoxications. In contrast, older patients with metabolic liver disease may present with symptoms of chronic disease. Because metabolic diseases can resemble multiple other maladies, a high index of suspicion is required.

An infant presenting with cholestasis should undergo an evaluation for metabolic liver disease. (The approach to the patient with jaundice is discussed in depth in Chapter 14.) Any patient with progressive neuromuscular disease, developmental delays, or regression of developmental milestones also requires evaluation. Metabolic liver disease should be an immediate consideration for patients with elevations in serum aminotransferase levels, hepatomegaly, acidosis, hypoglycemia, ascites, bleeding diathesis, hyperammonemia, coma, recurrent vomiting, or failure to thrive.

A detailed history can often raise the possibility of the diagnosis and help direct the investigation. A family history of consanguinity, multiple miscarriages, or early infant deaths may be an indication of a metabolic derangement. Close relatives with undiagnosed liver disease, progressive neurologic or muscle disease, or undiagnosed developmental delays should also raise suspicion. A careful dietary history is important in identifying the nature of the illness; introduction of certain foods may correlate with the onset of symptoms, as in patients with urea cycle enzyme defects, galactosemia, or fructosemia. A history of specific dietary aversions also may be revealing.[4]

Recommended screening tests, which should direct further diagnostic work-up, are listed in Table 65–2. Because patients with metabolic liver disease often present with acute or recurrent symptoms, it is of utmost importance for the physician to obtain the diagnostic studies as soon as possible. The laboratory values for many of these illnesses may normalize between acute episodes. Serum and urine should always be saved and frozen if needed for definitive studies. A liver biopsy also can be a valuable diagnostic tool. If a metabolic liver disease is suspected, it is important to save a frozen segment of the biopsy specimen and consider an electron microscopic study to look at the subcellular organelles, which may have typical changes in some of these disorders.

α_1-ANTITRYPSIN DEFICIENCY

Deficiency of α_1-antitrypsin (α_1-AT) is the most common metabolic disease affecting the liver. It is transmitted in an autosomal recessive fashion with codominant expression. The prevalence is highest in the northern European white population, in whom the incidence of homozygous deficiency is 1 in 1500 persons.[5] In the white population of the United States, the incidence is closer to 1 in 1800 to 2000 live births. The incidence in the black, Hispanic, and Asian populations is much lower.

Pathophysiology

α_1-Antitrypsin, a member of the serpin family of protease inhibitors, binds with and promotes the degradation of serine proteases, most importantly neutrophil elastase, in the serum and tissues. The serine proteases, which are produced in cells throughout the body, are responsible for triggering inflammatory cascades and activation of complement and ultimately are controlled by the serpin inhibitor proteins. α_1-AT is normally responsible for more than 90% of antielastase activity in alveolar lavage fluid, and this activity results from formation of a tight 1:1 complex with elastase. Once formed, this complex binds to the serpin-enzyme complex (SEC) receptor on hepatocytes, as well as to the low-density lipoprotein receptor-related protein, both of which contribute to clearance of the α_1-AT:elastase complex from the circulation.[6, 7]

The α_1-AT gene has been localized to chromosome 14q31-32.3. α_1-AT alleles show codominant expression of the protease inhibitor (Pi) gene product. Allelic variants are determined by electrophoretic methods, with the normal allelic representation being PiMM. The most common pathologic form, which causes both liver and lung disease, is the PiZZ variant, which produces α_1-ATZ protein. This variant represents a replacement of glutamine with a lysine residue at position 342 in α_1-ATZ. The serum α_1-AT activity level in persons with PiZZ is less than 15% of normal.[8] There are more than 75 structural variants of α_1-AT; however, most are of no clinical significance or are extremely rare.[3, 5]

α_1-AT is produced almost exclusively in the hepatocyte in the rough endoplasmic reticulum (ER) and is targeted to the secretory pathway via the Golgi apparatus. Structural misfolding and polymerization of α_1-ATZ cause this protein to be retained in the ER, with subsequent failure of progression through the secretory pathway. Abnormal polymerization of other members of the serpin superfamily, such as C1 inhibitor, antithrombin III, and α_1-antichymotrypsin, is also likely to be the basis of the corresponding diseases associated with deficiency of these proteins, which leads to angioedema, thrombosis, and chronic obstructive pulmonary disease, respectively.[9] In addition, there is diminished degradation of α_1-ATZ in the ER. Studies suggest that the rate of intracellular degradation may be genetically determined and may influence the expression of disease, because α_1-ATZ appears to be degraded more slowly in the ER of certain persons with PiZZ who are susceptible to liver disease than in those who are not susceptible.[10] The interaction of α_1-ATZ with the molecular chaperone calnexin triggers the polyubiquitination of calnexin and subsequent degradation of α_1-ATZ:calnexin complexes by proteasomes. Both ubiquitin-dependent and ubiquitin-independent mechanisms have been found to be involved in the degradation of α_1-ATZ.[11] Alternatively, failure to interact with calnexin in the first place may account for decreased degradation of α_1-ATZ in some susceptible persons.[10]

The pathophysiology of liver injury resulting from the retention and accumulation of α_1-ATZ in the ER in α_1-AT deficiency is unclear. Two distinct signaling pathways, the *unfolded protein* response and the *endoplasmic reticulum overload* state, are activated by the retention of proteins in the ER, and both can influence the transcriptional regulation of genes that may further drive pathologic processes within the cell. Either or both pathways may be involved in the pathophysiology of α_1-AT deficiency.[5]

α_1-AT production is stimulated by increased serum elastase levels and by the binding of the α_1-AT–elastase complex to the SEC receptor in the hepatocyte.[5] Release of α_1-AT also may be stimulated by stress, injury, pregnancy, or neoplasia; α_1-AT is considered to be a hepatic acute phase reactant. Because these factors can influence production of α_1-AT, even in patients with PiZZ, the diagnosis of α_1-AT deficiency should be based on phenotype analysis and not solely on the α_1-AT level.

Table 65–1 | **Presenting Features of Metabolic Liver Disease**

SYMPTOMS	SIGNS
Hyperammonemic symptoms	Short stature
Hypoglycemic symptoms	Dysmorphic features
Acidosis	Unusual odors
Coagulopathy	Cataracts
Ketosis	Hepatomegaly
Acute liver failure	Splenomegaly
Recurrent vomiting	Cardiac dysfunction
Growth failure	Ascites
Neurologic or motor skill deterioration	Abdominal distention
Coma	Hypotonia
Seizures	Jaundice
Developmental delay	Cholestasis
	Bruises
	Rickets

Table 65–2 | **Screening Laboratory Tests for Metabolic Liver Disease**

Serum electrolytes
Anion gap
Serum glucose
Serum ammonia
Serum amino acids
Urine organic acids
Urine orotic acid
Serum aminotransferases
Serum albumin
Fractionated bilirubin levels
Serum alkaline phosphatase
Serum γ-glutamyl transpeptidase
Coagulation profile
Serum lactate*
Serum pyruvate*
Uric acid*
Urine for reducing substances
Serum ferritin
Peripheral blood smear, to evaluate for hemolysis
Save specimens of serum and urine obtained during acute episodes for later studies

*Indicated in patients who are acidotic or have neurologic symptoms.

Clinical Features

Eight percent to 12% of newborns with α_1-AT deficiency (PiZZ) present with cholestasis, whereas an additional 3% to 7% of older children present with other clinical evidence of liver disease.[5, 12] Although up to 50% of affected infants have elevated serum aminotransferase levels at age 3 months, most are clinically asymptomatic.[12] Presenting symptoms of neonatal hepatic involvement can include jaundice, slow weight gain, irritability, lethargy, acholic stools, or a bleeding diathesis. Later presentation can include abdominal distention, hepatosplenomegaly, ascites, or an upper gastrointestinal bleed secondary to esophageal varices.[5] Emphysema develops in all persons with null α_1-AT phenotypes by age 20 to 30 years, whereas liver disease develops in none of them.[13] Relatively small increases in plasma levels in α_1-AT are needed to inhibit destructive proteolysis in deficient persons. Persons with variants associated with a 60% to 70% reduction in plasma α_1-AT levels do not appear to have an increased frequency of destructive lung disease. The prognosis of patients with liver disease presenting in infancy secondary to α_1-AT deficiency (PiZZ) is variable; not all patients progress to end-stage liver disease.

Of 200,000 Swedish infants screened for α_1-AT deficiency, 184 were found to have abnormal allelic forms of α_1-AT (127 were PiZZ, 2 were PiZnull, 54 were PiSZ, and 1 was PiSnull), and 6 died in early childhood (5 with PiZZ and 1 with PiSZ), although only 2 died from cirrhosis.[14] Twelve percent to 15% of these patients with α_1-AT deficiency had clinically apparent liver disease during childhood. Of the 150 patients who underwent evaluation at 16 and 18 years of life, none had clinical signs of liver disease. Elevations of serum aminotransferase or gamma glutamyl transpeptidase levels were found in less than 20% of patients with PiZZ and less than 15% of those with PiSZ. Only 2 patients (one PiSZ and the other PiZnull) had abnormal liver tests at both visits.[14]

Some patients with α_1-AT deficiency progress to cirrhosis. One study demonstrated that of all PiZZ patients, regardless of age at autopsy, 37% had histologic evidence of cirrhosis.[15] A strong correlation has been demonstrated between homozygous α_1-AT deficiency and primary liver cancers, including hepatocellular carcinoma and cholangiocarcinoma, especially in male patients over age 50 years.[16, 17] The diagnosis of α_1-AT deficiency should be considered in any patient presenting with a noninfectious chronic hepatitis, hepatosplenomegaly, cirrhosis, portal hypertension, or primary liver cancer.

Histology

Histopathologic features of α_1-AT deficiency change as the patient ages. In infancy the liver biopsy may show a paucity of bile duct, intracellular cholestasis with or without giant cell transformation, mild inflammatory changes or steatosis, and few characteristic periodic acid–Schiff (PAS)-positive, diastase-resistant globules. These inclusions are most prominent in periportal hepatocytes but also may be seen in Kupffer cells. Immunohistochemistry with monoclonal antibody to α_1-ATZ also can be performed to verify the diagnosis.[17] As the patient ages, the histologic changes may resolve completely or progress to chronic hepatitis or cirrhosis.[18] It is unclear why some patients progress to severe liver disease while others remain asymptomatic, but multivariant sources of the liver damage are likely.

Diagnosis

The diagnosis of α_1-AT deficiency, as stated earlier, should be made by phenotype analysis rather than α_1-AT level alone. However, an apparently normal PiMM phenotype does not exclude the possibility of α_1-AT deficiency associated with intracellular accumulation of aberrantly folded protein; the prognosis with respect to liver disease in these rarer phenotypes is less clear than in those with PiZZ phenotypes.[5] A liver biopsy, although not always indicated, should confirm the diagnosis.

Treatment

The initial treatment of the patient with α_1-AT deficiency is symptomatic. It has been suggested that breast-feeding until the end of the first year of life may decrease the manifestations of cholestatic liver disease, as may administration of ursodeoxycholic acid. The importance of the use of fat-soluble vitamins, when indicated, adequate nutrition, and counseling regarding the avoidance of smoking and secondhand smoke cannot be overemphasized. The role of neonatal screening for α_1-AT deficiency is still unsettled, although there appears to be a positive impact on smoking practices in patients diagnosed at an early age.[19] If effective therapy becomes available for liver disease, neonatal screening would be even more useful in possibly avoiding liver transplantation.

Orthotopic liver transplantation (OLT) has been employed as a treatment for patients who have progressed to end-stage liver disease, and α_1-AT deficiency is the most common metabolic liver disease for which transplantation is performed. In addition to replacing the injured organ, transplantation corrects the metabolic defect, thereby avoiding progression of systemic disease.

Replacement therapy of deficient α_1-AT has been considered as a treatment for lung disease and has been shown to increase the antineutrophil elastase activity in bronchoalveolar lavage fluid. In studies to date, improvements in lung function have been minimal, although survival rates in patients receiving replacement therapy are improved.[20] The impact of this therapy on α_1-AT deficiency–associated liver disease is as yet unclear.

Other treatment options are being investigated. The most promising approaches involve the use of medicinal agents to influence the stability and secretion rates of α_1-ATZ within the ER. Chemical chaperones such as phenylbutyric acid (an agent already approved for use in patients with urea cycle defects) and glucosidase and mannosidase inhibitors markedly increase the secretion of α_1-ATZ in both in vitro and in vivo experimental models of α_1-AT deficiency.[21, 22] There also appears to be a dramatic increase in α_1-ATZ blood levels after treatment of mice transgenic for the α_1-ATZ gene with phenylbutyric acid. This approach has the potential to be efficacious in humans, because mutant α_1-ATZ retains approximately 80% of normal antielastase activity, and relatively small increases in plasma α_1-ATZ levels are needed to inhibit destructive proteolysis caused by α_1-AT deficiency.[21, 23]

Deficiency of α_1-AT is one of many diseases for which reconstitution of the normal genotype through gene therapy is being attempted. Long-term expression of human α_1-AT from murine liver has been achieved using a hydrodynamics-based intravenous transfection procedure.[24] A ribozyme construct with targeted destruction of mutant α_1-ATZ RNA and expression of a modified, but otherwise normal, α_1-AT gene also has been effective in correcting the disease phenotype in an in vitro model of α_1-AT deficiency.[25] These results are promising first steps in the goal of achieving successful gene therapy for this disease.

GLYCOGEN STORAGE DISEASE

More than 10 distinct disorders of glycogen metabolism have been described in the literature; however, this chapter includes a discussion of only the three inborn errors associated with liver disease: glycogen storage disease (GSD) types I, III, and IV.[4, 26] Other GSDs may demonstrate hepatomegaly or microscopic changes in liver histology, but their clinical impact on liver disease is less significant. The overall incidence of GSD is estimated to range from 1 in 50,000 to 1 in 100,000.

Glycogen metabolism occurs in many tissues, but the areas of most clinical importance are the muscle and liver (see Chapter 63). The body uses glycogen as a storage system for glucose and as a ready reserve for times of systemic glucose requirement. Glycogen is comprised of long-chain glucose molecules arranged in a 1,4 linkage; 8% to 10% of the glucose molecules are attached in a 1,6 linkage to form branching chains. This structure allows for efficient storage of glucose while minimizing the impact on intracellular osmolality. The substrates for glycogen synthesis, glucose-6-phosphate (G6P) and glucose-1-phosphate (G1P), are derived from several pathways, including fructose and galactose metabolism, gluconeogenesis, and glycogenolysis (Fig. 65–1). By the action of uridine diphosphate glucose (UDPG) pyrophosphorylase and glycogen synthase, G1P is metabolized to UDPG and glycogen, sequentially. The 1,4 linkages can be converted to 1,6 linkages by the actions of branching enzymes. Amylo-1,6-glucosidase is a debranching enzyme that can release 8% to 10% of the glucose stored in glycogen. The remaining glucose is released as G1P, by the action of phosphorylase *a*, which is converted to G6P by phosphoglucomutase. Phosphorylase has an active *(a)* and an inactive *(b)* form; protein kinase is responsible for the conversion of phosphorylase *b* to *a*. Protein kinase is stimulated by epinephrine, glucagon and fasting, thereby increasing glycogenolysis. High levels of glucose influence the conversion back to phosphorylase *b*, thereby decreasing glycogenolysis. Glycogen synthase also consists of active (*a*) and inactive (*b*) forms. Phosphorylase *a* inhibits the conversion to glycogen synthase *a*, thereby decreasing glycogen synthesis. High levels of glycogen also can favor the formation of glycogen synthase *b*.[26, 27]

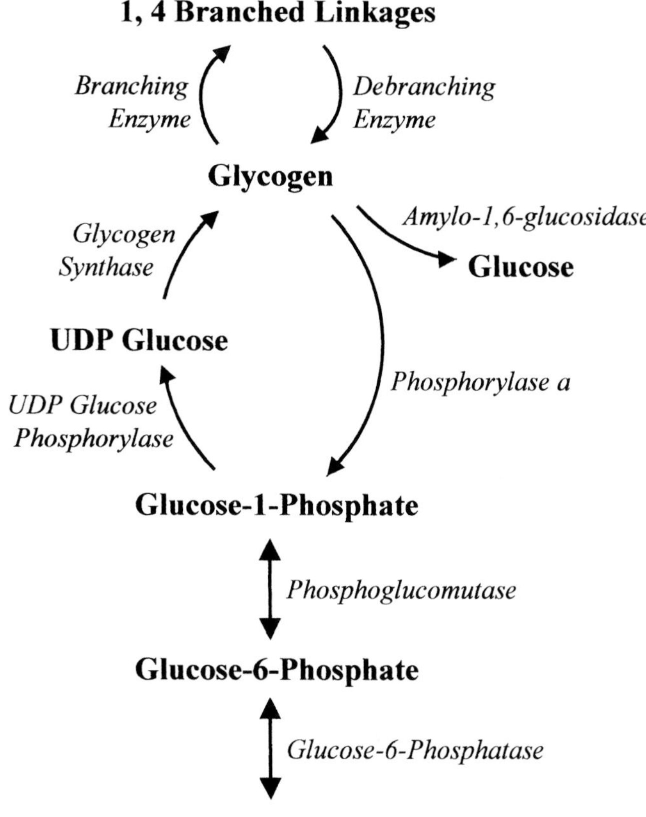

Figure 65–1. The biosynthetic pathway of glycogen synthesis and glycogenolysis.

Type I

Glycogen storage disease type I, resulting from the deficiency of glucose-6-phosphatase activity, is the most common of the errors in glycogen metabolism and the most investigated. For the effective functioning of this enzyme, located in the ER, three transport functions are required: the transport of the substrate G6P into, and both products—glucose and phosphate—out of the lumen of the ER. Previous studies posited at least three subtypes of GSD type I: IA, caused by the complete absence of the catalytic activity of the phosphatase; IB, caused by deficient G6P transport into the ER; and IC, associated with deficient transport of phosphate out of the ER. Cloning of the genes for glucose-6-phosphatase and the G6P translocase, and mutational analysis of patients previously classified as GSD types IA, IB, or IC show that there are only two subtypes of GSD type I, IA and IB, that account for all patients examined and that patients classified previously as type IC universally have genetic defects in the G6P transporter (GSD type IB).[28–30] The clinical phenotype with respect to liver disease is similar in both IA and non-IA forms; however, patients with GSD type IB can have significant neutropenia and impaired phagocytic function and are prone to recurrent episodes of severe bacterial infections and Crohn's-like intestinal disease.[31]

Clinical Features

The main presenting symptoms of GSD type I are profound hypoglycemia, hepatomegaly, and growth failure. Most patients present in infancy with this clinical picture. They also may have metabolic acidosis or hypoglycemic seizures. Disruption of the function of glucose-6-phosphatase inhibits the utilization of glucose from several mechanisms: gluconeogenesis, glycogenolysis, and the metabolism of fructose or galactose. This inability to release stored glucose leads to hypoglycemia in the fasting state, from 90 to 180 minutes after the last ingested glucose. Lactate metabolism and glycolytic pathways are then used for energy.

Physical signs invariably include hepatomegaly, usually with a normal-sized spleen. Patients with long-standing, poorly controlled disease exhibit short stature and growth failure; they may be prone to adiposity. Delayed bone age with osteopenia or osteoporosis has been described. Xanthoma can appear after puberty and localize to the elbows, knees, buttocks, or nasal septum, the latter leading to epistaxis.

Several other metabolic derangements can be seen. Lactic acid levels can reach four to eight times normal; the accompanying metabolic acidosis may manifest as muscle weakness, hyperventilation, malaise, headache, or recurrent fever. Uric acid levels are consistently elevated, whereas serum adenosine triphosphate (ATP) and phosphorus levels are low, secondary to an increase in purine synthesis and the inability to release phosphorus from G6P. Complications of hyperuricemia such as gout, arthritis, or progressive nephropathy may occur. Nephromegaly and hypertension are often evident secondary to the increased glycogen deposition. Renal failure requiring dialysis and transplantation has been reported. As a result of the hypoglycemia, affected patients have chronically increased serum levels of glucagon with depressed levels of insulin. Hyperlipidemia is a common feature, with triglyceride levels reaching 4000 to 6000 mg/dL (45 to 68 mmol/L) and cholesterol levels approaching 400 to 600 mg/dL (10 to 15 mmol/L). The formation of glucose by means of gluconeogenesis and glycogenolysis is blocked, and carbohydrates are converted to lactic acid, an early step in glycolysis, which increases fatty acid synthesis and raises the concentration of glycerol-3-phosphate, thereby favoring the formation of triglycerides. The low insulin:glucose ratio also leads to abundant release of free fatty acids and glycerol from adipose tissue.

Hepatic Involvement

Hepatic involvement may be identified initially by hepatomegaly, which is caused by vastly increased glycogen storage in the liver and a large degree of fatty infiltration. These patients demonstrate mild elevations in serum aminotransferase levels and generally do not progress to cirrhosis or liver failure.[4, 27] By age 15, most patients develop hepatic adenomas; however, adenomas have been described in patients as young as 3 years of age. With age, adenomas tend to increase in both size and number, and there are reports of the transformation of an adenoma to hepatocellular carcinoma.[32] Serum alpha fetoprotein levels are unreliable markers for the presence of carcinoma. Several theories have been advanced as to the pathogenesis of the adenomas, but the most commonly discussed is the chronic stimulation of hepatocytes by the imbalance in glucagon and insulin that exists in patients with uncontrolled disease.[32] After receiving adequate nutritional therapy for GSD type I, some patients demonstrate regression and disappearance of hepatic adenomas, but this is not always the case, and the course is unpredictable.[33]

If patients with GSD type I are undiagnosed or undertreated, death may occur. Death is usually secondary to hypoglycemia, seizures, metabolic acidosis, hepatocellular carcinoma, or, as in the case of patients with GSD type IB, sepsis from neutropenia. Granulocyte-macrophage colony-stimulating factor has been used with success to prevent bacterial infections in GSD type 1B.[34]

Diagnosis

The most accurate diagnostic measure is direct enzyme analysis performed on fresh liver tissue. Fasting glucose and lactate levels, a glucagon response test, or response to fructose or galactose administration (patients with GSD type I do not show the expected rise in serum glucose concentration after administration of these substances) often provide supportive evidence but may not yield a definitive diagnosis.[27] DNA analysis–based approaches to diagnosis, integrating biochemical features and the presence or absence of persistent neutropenia, have been proposed and may provide an alternative approach to diagnosis that avoids liver biopsy.[29]

Treatment

Historically, the first intervention attempted to treat GSD type I was surgical portal diversion shunting. Routing the portal blood supply to the systemic circulation was done in an attempt to deliver ingested glucose to the tissues before hepatic processing. This treatment provided satisfactory results and restored normal glucose control to many patients; however, others still required nutritional supplementation to maintain metabolic control and normal growth. Direct surgical complications and shunt occlusion also occurred in younger patients.[27]

Nutritional supplementation then became the mainstay of therapy and consisted initially of intravenous glucose administration throughout the night, with advancement to intragastric, continuous feedings of various formulas. It was determined that if the serum glucose levels were maintained above 70 mg/dL, metabolic control could be sustained. Soon dietary regimens of frequent, high-carbohydrate daytime feedings and continuous nighttime drip feedings were shown to provide good metabolic control and lead to normalized growth and development.[35] In the 1980s, a different feeding strategy was shown to be successful. Oral administration of uncooked cornstarch, a complex polymer, was shown to allow slow, continuous release of glucose because of the action of pancreatic amylase. Ingestion of cornstarch throughout the day has eased the dietary restriction on some patients and freed others from the requirement for a night-time drip. A dose of 2 g/kg every 6 hours (6 to 8 mg/kg/min) has been suggested; however, alternative regimens have been implemented successfully. Patients treated in this manner show a tendency toward obesity, so dietary management, including maintenance of adequate protein intake, needs continued observation after therapy has been initiated. Because of the relative lack of pancreatic amylase in infants and toddlers, there is limited experience in the use of this therapy in patients younger than 2 years of age.[35]

For infants, once the diagnosis is confirmed, a formula that does not contain fructose or galactose should be prescribed. Frequent daytime feedings and continuous nocturnal administration are required. The rate of delivery required to maintain euglycemia has been shown to be 8 to 9 mg/kg/min.[36] Morning feedings should be given quickly after discontinuation of the drip to avoid hypoglycemia. As solids are introduced, high-carbohydrate foods should be emphasized. These patients require special attention during acute illnesses that may affect intake or metabolism because they can become hypoglycemic quickly.

Liver transplantation has successfully corrected the metabolic error in patients with GSD type I and allowed catch-up growth, even into the 3rd decade.[37] As survival is extended because of aggressive medical management, these patients may demonstrate signs of other systemic complications such as progressive kidney disease, cardiovascular disease, and malignancy.[34]

Type III

GSD type III, resulting from a deficiency of amylo-1,6-glucosidase debranching enzyme, leads to the accumulation of limit dextrin units that restrict glucose release. Affected patients have a clinically milder course than those with GSD type I and are able to fast for longer periods. However, in infancy the two syndromes may be indistinguishable. Patients with GSD type III still have effective mechanisms for gluconeogenesis, which leads to a more stable clinical pattern as the patient ages. There are two main subtypes of GSD type III: type IIIA affects both liver and muscle and accounts for 80% of patients with GSD type III, and type IIIB affects the liver only (and accounts for 15% of patients). The molecular basis for tissue-specific expression of the enzyme is unknown, although there appear to be subtype-specific mutations in the gene for debranching enzyme, a finding that may make diagnosis by genotype analysis worthwhile.[38]

Clinical Features

Persons with GSD type III typically exhibit hypoglycemia, hepatomegaly, and growth failure. Liver enlargement results from increased glycogen deposition, not fatty infiltration. The liver may show fibrotic septa, which rarely lead to frank cirrhosis and liver failure. Serum lactate and uric acid levels tend to be normal, with only moderate increases in serum aminotransferase levels until advanced liver disease is present. Hyperlipidemia may be present but is not as pronounced as in GSD type I. Patients have normal responses to fructose and galactose loading.

Patients with GSD type III may display muscle involvement. Progressive weakness, which worsens with activity, and muscle wasting are seen. Nephromegaly is not seen, but cardiomegaly may be present. The diagnosis can be made by direct enzyme analysis of muscle or liver tissue.[27] Hepatic adenomas can develop, although less frequently than in patients with GSD type I disease.[33] Cirrhosis leading to hepatocellular carcinoma in affected patients has been reported.[39]

Treatment

A high-protein, low-carbohydrate diet has been suggested to normalize metabolic activity, ensure normal growth, normalize muscle function, and minimize hepatomegaly. This diet provides adequate substrates for gluconeogenesis while decreasing the need for glycogen storage. Patients with refractory hypoglycemia or persistent hepatomegaly may require a nighttime drip or cornstarch therapy.[35]

Type IV

Deficiency of the branching enzyme is seen in the rare syndrome of GSD type IV, also known as *amylopectinosis*. Glycogen and amylopectin accumulate in hepatocytes. The onset of symptoms is typically between the ages of 3 and 15 months. Symptoms can include failure to thrive, abdominal distention, hepatomegaly, and various gastrointestinal complaints. Signs of liver disease predominate later in the course of the disease. One half of these patients also demonstrate abnormal neuromuscular development with hypotonia, atrophy, and decreased deep tendon reflexes. A severe form of GSD type IV, which presents as early-onset fetal hydrops, has been reported in several instances; in addition, there are milder nonprogressive presentations of hepatic disease in GSD type IV that do not lead to cirrhosis or have skeletal muscle or neurologic involvement.[40] Genotype-phenotype analysis of the brancher enzyme gene with respect to the 3 forms of GSD type IV have been initiated.[41]

Hypoglycemia is relatively uncommon in GSD type IV; patients have normal responses to fructose/galactose challenges but varied responses to epinephrine.[27] Serum lactate and pyruvate levels are normal, and aminotransferase levels are only moderately elevated until more severe liver involvement becomes apparent. Progressive macronodular cirrhosis is present with an abundance of PAS-positive deposits in hepatocytes. Cirrhosis may progress to liver failure, and adenomas and hepatocellular carcinoma may develop rarely.[42]

The diagnosis of GSD type IV is made by direct enzyme analysis of liver tissue. Most patients die within the first 3 years of life if the disease is left untreated. Diets high in protein and low in carbohydrate have been associated with improved growth but have shown little impact on liver involvement. Liver transplantation has been used successfully and results in both correction of the metabolic error and normal growth, but amylopectin deposits may persist in the heart (with progressive cardiomyopathy) and leukocytes of affected patients as well.[43]

CONGENITAL DISORDERS OF GLYCOSYLATION

Congenital disorders of glycosylation (CDG), formerly known as *carbohydrate-deficient glycoprotein syndromes*, comprise a group of inherited defects in asparagine *(N)*-linked glycosylation that produce a wide spectrum of clinical abnormalities. Glycosylation of proteins serves many purposes, ranging from facilitation of proper conformational folding and protection from degradation, to proper targeting to either the secretory or lysosomal sorting pathways. *N*-

linked glycosylation is complex and involves multiple enzymatic steps and subcellular compartments, from the endoplasmic reticulum to the Golgi apparatus. Secretory glycoproteins with altered carbohydrate moieties in CDG include coagulation factors, albumin and other binding proteins, growth hormone, insulin, and thyroxine-binding globulin.[4, 44]

Four types of CDG have been delineated based on isoelectric focusing of serum transferrin, which serves as a marker protein for the disease phenotype. The first type comprises two subtypes; *CDG type 1a* is caused by a defect in phosphomannomutase (PMM), an enzyme that converts mannose-6-phosphate to mannose-1-phosphate (Fig. 65–2).[4, 44] Patients typically have severe neurologic abnormalities (ataxia, marked psychomotor delay, and progressive peripheral neuropathy), dysmorphism (inverted nipples, abnormal fat distribution, and esotropia), diarrhea with failure to thrive, heart dysfunction, and hepatic steatosis. Patients with *CDG type 1b* have a defect in phosphomannose isomerase (PMI), which converts fructose-6-phosphate to mannose-6-phosphate.[45, 46] Patients with CDG type 1b do not have the severe neurologic symptoms seen in patients with CDG type 1a, perhaps because maternally derived mannose is a sufficient source for protein glycosylation during fetal nervous system development.[47] However, patients do manifest intractable diarrhea, protein-losing enteropathy, intestinal lymphangiectasia, and congenital hepatic fibrosis. Patients with CDG type 1b also can develop severe hypoglycemia and cyclic vomiting.[47, 48] Limited preliminary experience in treating patients with CDG type 1b with dietary mannose has been encouraging.[45] For both subtypes Ia and Ib, serum aminotransferase levels are usually only mildly elevated.

The biochemical and clinical features of the remaining types of CDG are characterized less well. The defect in CDG type II is in Golgi-localized *N*-acetylglucosaminyltransferase; patients have marked dysmorphic features and severe developmental retardation. Patients with CDG type III and type IV have similar, severe neurologic features, which are

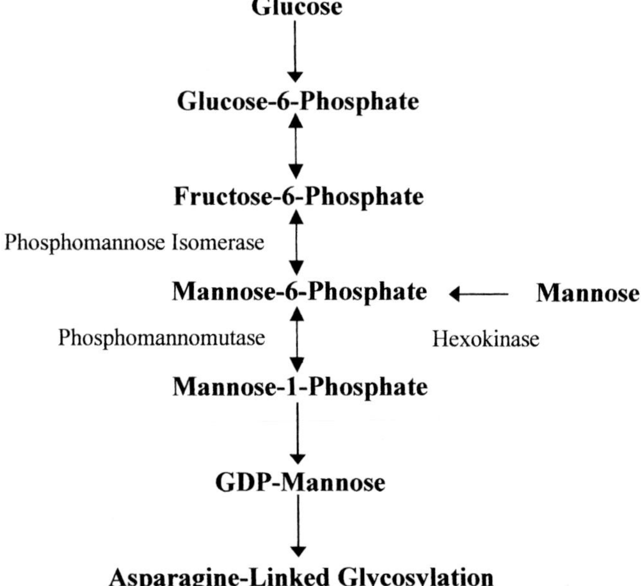

Figure 65–2. Pathway of mannose metabolism.

distinct from those noted in patients with CDG types I and II.

Hepatic dysfunction is usually mild in CDG and usually does not lead to symptoms. Mild steatosis and fibrosis typically are seen on light microscopy; on electron microscopy, lysosomal vacuoles with concentric electron-dense membranes and variable electron-lucent and electron-dense material are noted. Patients uncommonly progress to liver failure, with micronodular cirrhosis at autopsy.

Any patient with unexplained congenital hepatic fibrosis, protein-losing enteropathy, or a procoagulant tendency should be evaluated for the possibility of CDG. An initial screening of serum transferrin by isoelectric focusing should be performed, followed by confirmatory enzymatic analysis in fibroblasts, leukocytes, or liver tissue.[43]

PORPHYRIAS

The clinical syndromes of the porphyrias were first described in the 1800s. This diverse group of metabolic derangements stems from errors in the synthesis of heme, with many forms associated with primary expression in the liver or direct hepatic toxicity. In this section, the pathway for heme synthesis and the diseases associated with enzyme deficiencies along this pathway are reviewed.

Pathophysiology

Heme synthesis occurs in both the liver (15% to 20%) and the bone marrow (75% to 80%). The metabolic pathways are essentially the same for the two tissues, but synthetic control may differ. Here, the focus of the discussion is on hepatic synthesis (Fig. 65–3). In the mitochondria, glycine and succinyl CoA, under the influence of 5-aminolevulinic acid (ALA) synthase and its cofactor pyridoxine, form ALA. This is the rate-limiting step in hepatic heme synthesis and the only step that requires a cofactor. ALA synthase activity is decreased by the end product of the pathway, heme, and increased by substances that induce hepatic cytochrome P-450.

ALA then diffuses into the cytosol, where two molecules combine by the action of ALA dehydratase to form porphobilinogen (PBG). Four units of PBG combine in a linear manner to form hydroxymethylbilane (HMB) by the action of PBG deaminase. HMB may cyclize spontaneously to form uroporphyrinogen I, an inactive metabolite, or may be converted to uroporphyrinogen III by the action of uroporphyrinogen III cosynthase. Uroporphyrinogen carboxylase then converts uroporphyrinogen III to coproporphyrinogen III, which returns to the mitochondria for further metabolism. Coproporphyrinogen oxidase converts coproporphyrinogen to protoporphyrinogen IX, which becomes protoporphyrin IX by the action of protoporphyrinogen oxidase. In the final step of the pathway, ferrochelatase adds the ferrous iron to create heme.[49] Protoporphyrin is the only true porphyrin in the pathway, but the porphyrinogens quickly oxidize to their corresponding porphyrin on exposure to oxygen. Porphyrins readily absorb light in the 400- to 410-nm range and can emit an intense fluorescence.

The porphyrias usually are classified either by the site of

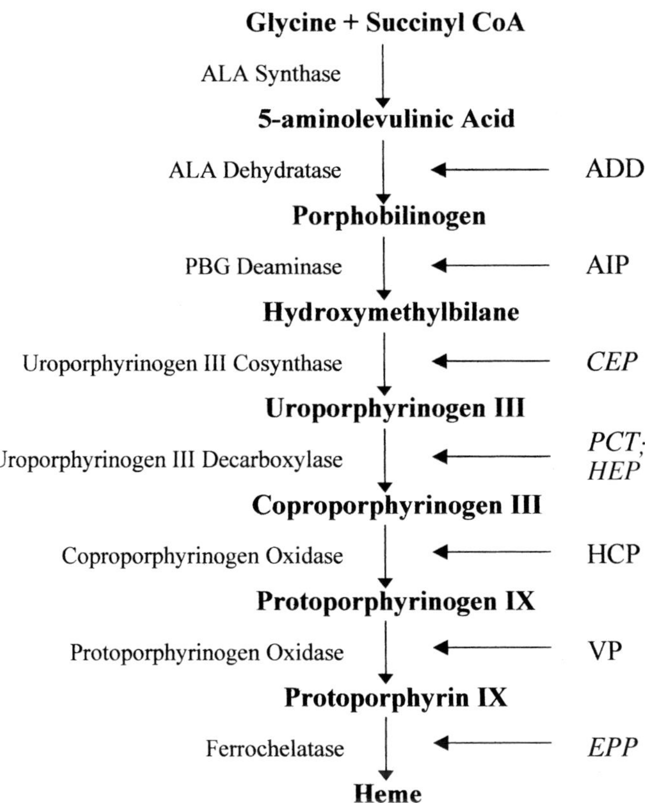

Figure 65–3. Pathway of heme synthesis. The locations of enzymatic deficiency in the various porphyrias are noted. *Italicized,* cutaneous porphyrias; normal type, acute porphyrias. (ADD, aminolevulinic acid dehydratase deficiency; AIP, acute intermittent porphyria; ALA, 5-aminolevulinic acid; CEP, congenital erythropoietic porphyria; EPP, erythropoietic protoporphyria; HCP, hereditary coproporphyria; HEP, hepatoerythropoietic porphyria; PBG, porphobilinogen; PCT, porphyria cutanea tarda; VP, variegate porphyria.)

major biochemical abnormality or the clinical features (Table 65–3). In five of the porphyrias the liver is the major site of expression, in two others both the liver and bone marrow are involved, and in one only is the bone marrow alone involved. The porphyrias are divided clinically into those that are acute, with dramatic and potentially life-threatening neurologic symptoms, and those with only cutaneous symptoms. Clinical features alone are usually not specific enough to confirm a diagnosis or distinguish among the various forms, and correct interpretation of biochemical tests is necessary for precise diagnosis and management.

The Acute Porphyrias

The term *acute porphyria* refers to the nature of the neurologic attacks, which are recurrent, dramatic, and life threatening. These attacks appear to be related to the overproduction and excretion of ALA and PBG. Both the serum and tissue levels of these products have been shown to be elevated during the acute neurologic attacks. ALA and PBG have been shown experimentally to elicit neurotoxic reactions, most likely because of their structural similarity to γ-aminobutyric acid (GABA), a major inhibitory neurotransmitter in the central nervous system.[49]

The symptoms and signs of the neurologic crises may vary. Abdominal pain is present in more than 90% of patients, followed in frequency by tachycardia and dark urine in about 80% of patients.[50] Other features include constipation, extremity pain, paresthesias, nausea, vomiting, urinary retention, hypertension, peripheral sensory deficits (often in a "bathing trunk" distribution), and weakness leading to ascending paralysis or quadriplegia. Neuropsychiatric features may include hysteria, depression, psychosis, confusion, hal-

Table 65–3 | **The Porphyrias**

	ENZYMATIC DEFECT	MODE OF INHERITANCE	CLINICAL FINDINGS	SITE OF EXPRESSION	MAJOR BIOCHEMICAL FINDINGS
Acute Porphyrias					
ALA dehydratase deficiency	ALA dehydratase	Autosomal recessive	Neurologic	Liver	Urine: ALA
Acute intermittent porphyria	PBG deaminase	Autosomal dominant	Neurologic	Liver	Urine: ALA < PBG
Hereditary coproporphyria	Coproporphyrinogen oxidase	Autosomal dominant	Neurologic, cutaneous	Liver	Urine: ALA > PBG, coproporphyrin Stool: coproporphyrin
Variegate porphyria	Protoporphyrinogen oxidase	Autosomal dominant	Neurologic, cutaneous	Liver	Urine: ALA > PBG, coproporphyrin Stool: coproporphyrin, protoporphyrinogen
Cutaneous Porphyrias					
Porphyria cutanea tarda	Uroporphyrinogen III decarboxylase	Autosomal dominant or acquired	Cutaneous	Liver	Urine: uroporphyrin, 7-carboxylate porphyrin Stool: isocoproporphyrin
Hepatoerythropoietic porphyria	Uroporphyrinogen III decarboxylase	Autosomal recessive	Cutaneous	Liver, bone marrow	Urine: Uroporphyrin, 7-carboxylate porphyrin Stool: isocoproporphyrin
Erythropoietic protoporphyria	Ferrochelatase	Autosomal dominant	Cutaneous, rarely neurologic	Liver, bone marrow	Urine: none Stool: protoporphyrin, coproporphyrin
Congenital erythropoietic porphyria	Uroporphyrinogen III cosynthase	Autosomal recessive	Cutaneous	Bone marrow	Urine and stool: coproporphyrin I

ALA, 5-aminolevulinic acid; PBG, porphobilinogen.

lucinations, seizures, or coma, although there is little evidence that chronic psychiatric illness is produced.[49, 51] The disease is clinically latent in 65% to 80% of patients, in whom symptoms never develop.

The acute episodes are about five times as common in women as in men. Episodes may be precipitated by many factors, most commonly drugs, alcohol ingestion, and smoking.[50] Glucocorticoids, sex hormones, and medications that stimulate the hepatic cytochrome P-450 system, perhaps by increasing the requirements for heme production, are often identified as precipitants. This finding may explain why many patients present during, and rarely before, puberty.[49] Other inciting factors include fasting, infections, and pregnancy; some women report increased problems during the luteal phase of their menstrual cycles.[49]

Acute intermittent porphyria (AIP) is the most common of the acute porphyrias and occurs in approximately 5 to 10 in 100,000 people and as many as 1 in 500 patients with psychiatric disorders.[51] Inheritance is autosomal dominant with incomplete penetrance. PBG deaminase activity is approximately 50% of normal in affected persons. The main manifestations are derangements in the autonomic nervous system. Excretion of PGB and ALA (PGB > ALA) in dark urine is common during attacks; however, levels may be normal during asymptomatic periods and in prepubertal patients.

Inheritance of both *hereditary coproporphyria* (HCP) and *variegate coproporphyria* (VP) is autosomal dominant with variable penetrance, and enzyme activity is 50%; patients with HCP lack coproporphyrinogen oxidase and patients with VP lack protoporphyrinogen oxidase. VP is more common in South Africa than elsewhere. Although HCP and VP give rise to neurologic symptoms similar to those of AIP, cutaneous lesions also occur and predominate in VP.[50] Patients with either disorder excrete high levels of ALA and PBG in the urine; however, as opposed to AIP, affected patients excrete more ALA than PGB. Fecal coproporphyrin is increased in both, whereas in VP fecal protoporphyrin also is increased.

ALA dehydratase deficiency is a rare, autosomal recessive syndrome with enzyme activity of less than 3%. Carriers demonstrate enzyme activity of 50% but are asymptomatic. Affected patients have severe, recurrent neurologic attacks that may be life threatening. They excrete large amounts of ALA in the urine. There exists one report of successful liver transplantation with complete resolution of symptoms in a patient with ALA dehydratase deficiency.[52]

The overall survival for patients with acute porphyria is good. Treatment is based on avoidance of drugs and other precipitating factors. Generous administration of fluid and glucose is recommended during the acute attacks to elicit a "glucose effect" to decrease ALA synthase activity. Intravenous administration of hematin, a congener of heme, has been shown to decrease the drive for heme synthesis and its abnormal by-products. Hematin also can have a dramatic effect on the neurologic symptoms, especially if given early in an attack.[53] Women in whom symptoms are affected by the phases of their menstrual cycle may improve while taking oral contraceptives. Orthotopic liver transplantation (OLT) has been attempted for several of the porphyrias, with mixed results.[52]

The Cutaneous Porphyrias

The cutaneous porphyrias differ from the porphyrias previously discussed in that they exhibit little or no neurologic symptoms. In these illnesses, the excess porphyrins or porphyrinogens are deposited in the upper dermal capillary walls and basement membrane zone. By absorbing light in the 400- to 410-nm wavelength range, these compounds react with molecular oxygen to form reactive oxygen species that can cause tissue damage in several ways: peroxidation of lysosomal and plasma membrane lipids, crosslinking of membrane proteins, free radical reactions, and activation of complement. Lysosomal damage is a main mechanism of injury in all the cutaneous porphyrias except protoporphyria, in which the mitochondria are affected more severely.[47]

The typical skin lesions are vesicles and bullae in the areas exposed to light and heat from skin fragility. Scarring, infection, pigment changes, and hypertrichosis can follow. Repeated bullae formation and infection can lead to severe mutilation.[54]

Because of the wavelengths absorbed by the porphyrins, affected patients are at risk for damage not only by sunlight but also by household and fluorescent lights. Special sunscreen lotions must be used to block rays in the 400- to 410-nm range. Patients must also be cautioned to minimize skin trauma as much as possible; early treatment of skin infections can decrease scarring. Special screens for indoor lighting also have been developed. Use of these screens may be especially important for exposure to operating room lighting, because some patients have had severe and lethal internal burns during surgery, a special concern for those going on to liver transplantation.[55]

Porphyria cutanea tarda (PCT) is the most common porphyria and typically involves a 50% reduction in activity of the enzyme uroporphyrinogen decarboxylase. Patients usually present after 20 years of age. PCT is not a single monogenic disorder, and there are at least two types. Type I, comprising 80% of patients, is a sporadic form with enzyme deficiency restricted to the liver, and type II, comprising about 20% of patients, is familial but with an unclear inheritance pattern.[56] Symptoms develop in less than 10% of patients with type II PTC. An acquired form of PCT also exists. Acquired PCT is strongly associated with high alcohol intake, estrogen therapy, and systemic illnesses including systemic lupus erythematosus, diabetes mellitus, chronic renal failure, and acquired immunodeficiency syndrome. Patients usually do not show signs of clinical liver disease, apart from elevated serum aminotransferase levels. On liver biopsy, 80% of patients have siderosis, and 15% have cirrhosis. Most have evidence of iron overload as well.[56]

Initial treatment of PCT is to remove any offending agent. Historically, the treatment has been phlebotomy to decrease the iron overload and siderosis. Phlebotomy may lead to relief of cutaneous symptoms in 4 to 6 months. Chloroquine complexes with and aids the intracellular release and excretion of uroporphyrin, but caution is required during chloroquine therapy because the drug is potentially hepatotoxic.[54]

Hepatoerythropoietic porphyria (HEP) is a rare form of porphyria with a pathogenesis similar to that of PCT. HEP appears to result from homozygous uroporphyrinogen decarboxylase deficiency, which yields less than 10% of normal enzyme activity. The cutaneous lesions, which resemble those of PCT, are typically more severe and mutilating. The disease usually presents in the first year of life, and as the patient ages, the dermatologic manifestations may subside, but liver disease, a nonspecific hepatitis, worsens. Treatment strategies for HEP are similar to, but have not been as successful as, those for PCT.

Congenital erythropoietic porphyria (CEP) is another rare form of porphyria that mainly affects the erythropoietic tissue. It results from the autosomal recessive–transmitted deficiency of uroporphyrinogen III cosynthase. Affected persons typically present in the first year of life with blistering, disfiguring skin lesions in exposed areas. Infants may present with pink urine and photosensitivity. As patients age, erythrodontia, a red or brownish discoloration of the teeth, is seen frequently and is pathognomonic.

CEP can be distinguished clinically from HEP by the presence of a Coombs' negative hemolytic anemia of variable severity; some patients may have severe anemia. Splenomegaly is common. Therapy consists of limiting exposure to sunlight, avoiding skin trauma, and use of beta-carotene.[57] Splenectomy, which increases the life span of red blood cells and decreases the erythropoietic drive, is effective in many patients. Frequent blood transfusions or hematin infusions inhibit the stimulus for heme production and decrease or eliminate the cutaneous manifestations of the disease.[57] Bone marrow transplantation in severely affected patients has proven curative.[57, 58]

Erythropoietic protoporphyria (EPP) is the second most common porphyria. Inheritance is also autosomal dominant with variable penetrance. The activity of the enzyme ferrochelatase, the final step in the heme pathway, is 20% to 50% in affected persons. Bone marrow is the predominant source of excess protoporphyrin, with a variable contribution from the liver and other tissues. The principal clinical manifestation is photosensitivity, which may present in infancy and is caused by the exquisite photoreactivity of protoporphyrin that circulates in the dermal blood vessels. Exposure of skin to light can lead quickly to a wide spectrum of symptoms (e.g., itching, burning, or pain) and subsequently to scars and lichenification of the skin. Vesicles are rare. Patients may have a mild hypochromic, microcytic anemia.

Clinical liver disease resulting from progressive hepatic accumulation of protoporphyrin develops in 5% to 10% of patients with EPP. Liver disease typically occurs after 30 years of age but has been described in children. The liver appears black and nodular. Of 57 patients with EPP followed over 20 years, 50% had normal serum aminotransferase levels and normal liver histology, and of the remainder, 7 had cirrhosis. Liver failure, which can progress rapidly, developed in 2.[59] Liver disease is not believed to be directly secondary to alcohol consumption, viral infections, or external toxins; however, these insults can worsen liver function.[45] Genetic heterogeneity in the ferrochelatase gene has been noted in multiple studies and among those patients requiring liver transplantation.[60]

As in the other cutaneous porphyrias, limiting light exposure and using appropriate sunscreens are important. Transfusions, hematin, charcoal, and cholestyramine all have demonstrated clinical benefit, but long-term resolution has not been shown.[56] OLT has been accomplished in patients with end-stage liver disease, with mixed results; the erythropoietic defect persists.[61, 62] Therefore, liver transplantation must be considered to be symptomatic therapy, except in the case of acute liver failure, in light of the high risk of recurrent disease in the graft and the added risk of intraoperative photodynamic injury to internal organs.[55, 61] Combined bone marrow and liver transplantation may be an option in the future.

Hepatic Complications of Porphyria

Hepatic involvement is variable; in general, the acute porphyrias may be associated with elevated serum aminotransferase and bile acids levels, which are accentuated during the acute episodes. However, liver biopsy may show fatty changes and iron deposition. Although these changes are minor, patients with acute porphyria are at increased risk of developing hepatocellular carcinoma.[63]

PCT and HEP are associated with hepatic complications more commonly than the other porphyrias; findings include enlarged livers with fatty infiltration, inflammatory changes, and granulomatous changes. Siderosis and fibrosis may lead to cirrhosis and liver failure. The risk of hepatocellular carcinoma is increased only slightly in these patients. The liver injury in CEP is similar.[47]

The diagnosis of porphyria should be considered in patients with recurrent bouts of severe abdominal pain, dark urine, constipation, and neuropsychiatric disturbances or in patients with typical dermatologic findings. To differentiate among the porphyrias, a 24-hour urine collection should be sent for quantitation of ALA and PBG (as well as other porphyrins); sodium bicarbonate should be added to the specimen to prevent degradation of PBG. Rapid spot tests for PBG in urine samples can be performed, although these tests are less reliable. Additional studies on urine, stool, or erythrocytes may need to be sent to referral laboratories to establish the diagnosis.

TYROSINEMIA

There are four known human diseases involving enzymatic deficiencies in the catabolic pathway for the amino acid tyrosine: alkaptonuria and hereditary tyrosinemia types I, II, and III. Although all of the enzymes involved in this pathway are found in the liver, only hereditary tyrosinemia type I (HTI) leads to progressive liver dysfunction. Formerly known as *hepatorenal tyrosinemia,* HTI also affects other organ systems, in particular the kidneys and peripheral nerves. Recent advances in our understanding of the pathophysiology of the disease and new treatment options, such as an inhibitor of an early step in the degradation pathway, have altered the clinical course dramatically for affected persons.

HTI is an autosomal recessive–transmitted disease with a worldwide incidence of about 1 in 100,000. The incidence is much greater in some areas such as northern Europe (1 in 8000) and the Saguenay-Lac-St. Jean region of Quebec, Canada (1 in 1846), where a founder effect has been documented.[4, 64]

Pathophysiology

The pathway for tyrosine metabolism is shown in Figure 65–4. The enzymatic defect in patients with tyrosinemia has been identified as the final step in the degradation process, fumarylacetate hydrolase (FAH); the gene for FAH has been localized to chromosome 15. FAH deficiency leads to accumulation of the upstream metabolites fumarylacetoacetate (FAA) and maleylacetoacetate, which are then converted to the toxic intermediates succinylacetoacetate (SAA) and succinylacetone (SA). FAA has been shown to deplete blood and liver of glutathione,[65] the consequence of which may be augmentation of the mutagenic potential of FAA.[66] SA, likely via direct modification of amino acids in enzyme active sites, is an inhibitor of the degradation of δ-aminolevulinic acid (δ-ALA) to porphobilinogen and also inhibits DNA ligase activity in fibroblasts isolated from patients with HTI.[67] Over time, the combined effects of elevated FAA and SA levels on the integrity of DNA and cellular repair mechanisms may account for increased chromosomal breakage observed in fibroblasts isolated from patients with HTI[68] as well as an increased risk of hepatocellular carcinoma (HCC) in patients with HTI.

Clinical Features

Patients with tyrosinemia (HTI) present either acutely with liver failure or with chronic disease, with or without hepatocellular carcinoma. In the *acute* form, patients manifest liver disease in the first 6 months of life; symptoms may include those associated with hepatic synthetic dysfunction, such as hypoglycemia, ascites, jaundice, and a bleeding diathesis, as well as anorexia, vomiting, and irritability.[69] Laboratory studies show elevated serum aminotransferase, γ-glutamyl transpeptidase, and bilirubin levels, and decreased levels of coagulation factors. Serum tyrosine, methionine, and alpha fetoprotein levels are elevated substantially. Analysis of the urine reveals phosphaturia, glucosuria, hyperaminoaciduria, renal acidosis, and elevated excretion of δ-ALA and phenolic acids. The acute form of HTI is usually fatal within the first 2 years of life. In a multicenter study, Van Spronsen and associates showed that 77% of patients with tyrosinemia presented before the age of 6 months. The 1- and 2-year survival rates were 38% and 29%, respectively, if they presented between 0 and 2 months, and 74% and 74%, respectively, if they presented between 2 and 6 months. Survival rates for both time intervals increased to 96% if the onset of symptoms occurred after age 6 months. The cause of death was usually recurrent bleeding and liver failure (35 of 47 deaths); however, hepatocellular carcinoma (7 of 47) and neurologic crisis (3 of 47) accounted for some deaths.[69]

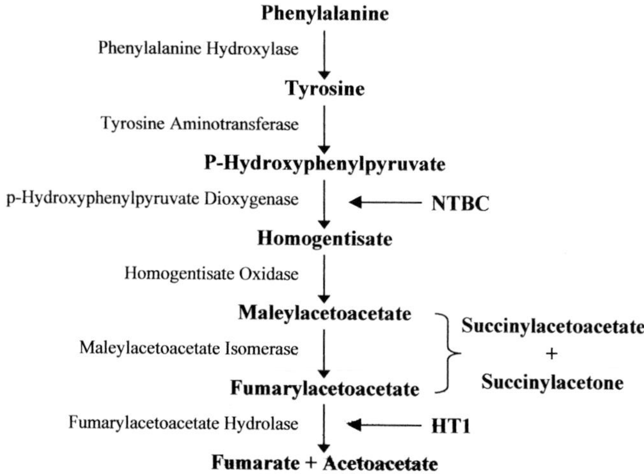

Figure 65–4. Pathway of tyrosine metabolism. The location of the enzymatic defect in hereditary tyrosinemia type I and the site of action of NTBC are noted. (HTI, hereditary tyrosinemia; NTBC, 1-(2-nitro-4-trifluoro-methylbenzoyl)-1,3-cyclohexanedione.)

Patients with the *chronic* form of HTI classically show similar but milder symptoms than those who present acutely. They usually present after 1 year of age with hepatomegaly, rickets, nephromegaly, and growth retardation. These patients also are likely to have neurologic problems and hepatocellular carcinoma.

The histologic changes differ between the acute and chronic forms of the disease.[4] Acutely, the liver may appear enlarged with a pale, nodular pattern or may be shrunken, firm, and brown. There may be micronodular cirrhosis, fibrous septa, bile duct proliferation and plugging, steatosis, pseudoacinar and nodular formations, and giant cell transformations. Variable amounts of FAH enzyme activity have been found in liver tissue from some patients with HTI, as a result of spontaneous reversion of FAH gene mutations.[70] Analysis of mutations in the FAH gene in 13 unrelated families with HTI revealed no predominant mutation type in the affected families and no correlation between genotype and phenotype.[71]

In the chronic form of tyrosinemia, the liver appears enlarged, coarse, and nodular. On biopsy, micronodular and macronodular cirrhosis may be present, as may steatosis, fibrous septa, and a mild lymphoplasmacytic infiltrate. Cholestasis is less pronounced than in the acute form of HTI. Large or small cell dysplasia may be present, reflecting premalignant changes. Because of the nodular changes noted in patients with tyrosinemia, identification of progression to hepatocellular carcinoma can be difficult. Because the serum alpha fetoprotein level is elevated before hepatocellular carcinoma has developed, the test is not helpful in the diagnosis. It has been proposed that the visualization of both low- and high-attenuation nodules on computed tomographic (CT) scan is highly suggestive of hepatocellular carcinoma.[72]

Renal involvement is nearly universal in patients with tyrosinemia. Minimal symptoms include decreased glomerular filtration rate, proximal renal tubular dysfunction, nephromegaly, phosphaturia (which is responsible for the development of rickets), glucosuria, and aminoaciduria. It is believed that the toxic metabolites SA and SAA may have a direct effect on kidney function. Some patients progress to renal failure and require renal transplantation.[73, 74]

The neurologic manifestations may be the most concerning feature for the older patient with tyrosinemia. More than 40% of patients experience porphyria-like symptoms.[75] In a study of 20 children with 104 neurologic crises, the most common symptoms were pain (96%), hypertonia (76%), vomiting and ileus (69%), weakness (29%), and diarrhea (12%). Eight of 104 crises required mechanical ventilation. The neurologic crises have been considered to be frequent causes of death.[69] The onset of a neurologic crisis may not be associated with worsening liver disease. It is believed that blockage of the degradation of δ-ALA by SA is responsible for the neurotoxicity.

Diagnosis

The diagnosis of tyrosinemia should be suspected in any child with neonatal liver disease or a bleeding diathesis or in any child older than 1 year of age with undiagnosed liver disease or rickets. The diagnosis is suggested by increased serum levels of tyrosine, methionine, phenylalanine, and alpha fetoprotein. Elevated serum and urine SA and urine δ-ALA levels are regarded as pathognomonic for tyrosinemia. The diagnosis can be confirmed with an assay for FAH using lymphocytes, erythrocytes, or liver tissue.

Treatment

Historically, the treatment of tyrosinemia has been dietary management, based on the restriction of tyrosine and phenylalanine. Dietary restriction has been shown to reverse the renal damage and improve the metabolic bone disease; however, the liver disease progresses. Nevertheless, an adequate intake of these amino acids is necessary to ensure normal growth and development. Few long-term studies are available on the long-term outcome with strict dietary management alone.

OLT has become a mainstay therapy for patients with tyrosinemia. The transplant corrects the phenotype and normalizes FAH activity and liver function. Additionally, the biochemical profiles normalize and kidney disease improves, with a rapid improvement in glomerular filtration rate, tubular acidosis, and hypercalcemia in most patients. Abnormal renal size and architecture persist after liver transplantation,[76] and many patients continue to excrete SA despite normal serum values.[74]

In 1992, Lindstedt and associates published data regarding the treatment of tyrosinemia with the herbicide 2- (2-nitro-4-trifluro-methybenzoyl)-1,3-cyclohexanedione (NTBC).[77] Recently, Holme and Lindstedt published the results of a large long-term study of 220 patients with HTI who were treated with this agent for 7 years.[78] NTBC is a potent inhibitor of 4-hydroxyphenylpyruvate dioxygenase, one of the initial steps in tyrosine metabolism. It was postulated that blocking the degradation of tyrosine to the downstream toxic metabolites (i.e., FAA, SA, and SAA) would lead to improved hepatic function. Preliminary results were encouraging, and treated patients exhibited increased liver synthetic function as reflected by a decreased prothrombin time, decreased serum aminotransferase levels, and reduction in liver parenchymal heterogenicity and nodules on CT. There also is a decrease in alpha fetoprotein levels, renal tubular dysfunction, and δ-ALA levels.[3, 107] Long-term results showed continued improvement in all parameters noted earlier, as well as a decreased risk of the early development of hepatocellular carcinoma in patients who started therapy and were free of hepatocellular carcinoma before the age of 2 years. Because the frequency of hepatocellular carcinoma in patients older than 2 years was 18% in the survey of Van Spronsen and colleagues,[69] the finding that hepatocellular carcinoma did not develop in any patient older than age 2 years who started treatment before age 2 indicates that NTBC may prevent the early development of hepatocellular carcinoma.[78] Thus, therapy with NTBC significantly improves the clinical course of patients treated at an early age. For patients in whom therapy is initiated at a later age, NTBC offers a palliative benefit, and the risk of hepatocellular carcinoma is still high in these patients. No patient withdrew from the study because of adverse side effects of the drug. However, transient thrombocytopenia or neutropenia as well as ocular symptoms suggestive of corneal irritation have been noted rarely.

UREA CYCLE DEFECTS

Although the syndromes related to the urea cycle defects are not associated with significant liver disease, the basic genetic defect is located within the liver, and the manifestations can mimic other metabolic liver diseases. The urea cycle consists of five enzymes that, through several steps, process ammonia derived from amino acid metabolism to urea. Genetic defects in each of the enzymes have been reported, and the overall incidence of urea cycle defects has been estimated at 1 in 20,000 to 1 in 30,000.[79]

Pathophysiology

The steps of the urea cycle are illustrated in Figure 65–5. Carbamyl phosphate synthetase (CPS) I forms carbamyl phosphate from ammonium and bicarbonate. This step requires *N*-acetyl glutamate as a cofactor. Ornithine transcarbamylase (OTC) combines carbamyl phosphate with ornithine to form citrulline. A second nitrogen enters the cycle as

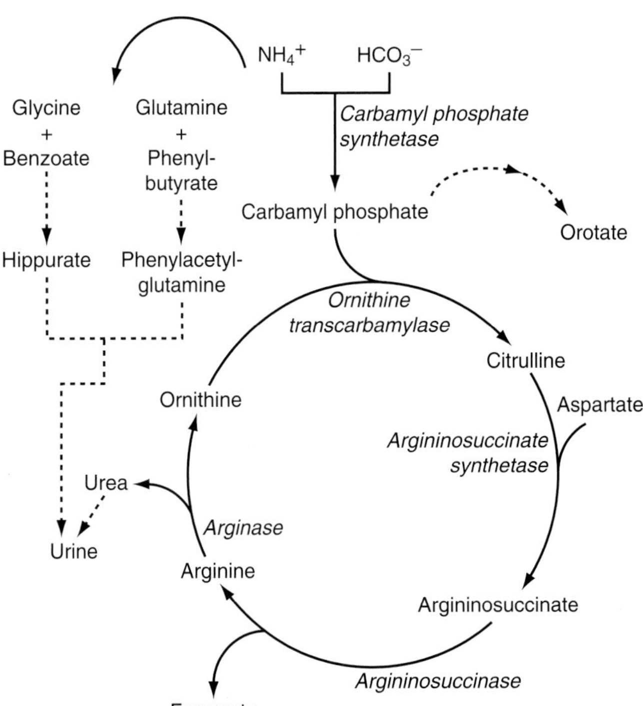

Figure 65–5. The urea cycle. Alternative pathways for waste-nitrogen disposal used therapeutically are also illustrated.

aspartate, which combines with citrulline by the action of argininosuccinate synthetase (AS) to form argininosuccinate. Argininosuccinate is converted to arginine and fumarate by argininosuccinase, or argininosuccinate lyase (AL). Arginase then catalyzes the breakdown of arginine to urea and ornithine in the final step of the pathway. CPS II, through the pyrimidine synthetic pathway, leads to the formation of orotic acid. Excess carbamyl phosphate can be used by this pathway if there is a block distal to OTC in the metabolic pathway. Excess nitrogen in the form of amino acids can be shunted to alternative pathways for waste nitrogen excretion by the medicinal use of sodium benzoate and sodium phenylacetate, which lead to the generation of hippurate and phenylacetylglutamine, respectively.

Enzymatic defects have been identified in all five steps of the urea cycle. Deficiency of four of these enzymes is transmitted autosomal recessively, whereas OTC deficiency is transmitted as an X-linked trait. More than 140 different mutations have been found in the gene giving rise to OTC deficiency, the most common urea cycle defect.[80] Numerous defects in the other enzymes of the cycle have been characterized as well.

A urea cycle defect has two main biochemical consequences: arginine becomes an essential amino acid (except in arginase deficiency), and nitrogen accumulates in a variety of molecules, some of which can lead to deleterious toxic effects.[79]

Clinical Features

The spectra of clinical presentations in patients with any of the urea cycle defects are virtually identical; these disorders usually present as acute life-threatening events in the neonatal period. Late-onset adult presentations also have been described. Neonates usually do not have any associated perinatal risk factors.[81] Affected infants initially appear normal for the first 24 to 72 hours of life as they are exposed to their first feeding. This feeding provides the initial protein load that fosters ammonia production. Symptoms include irritability, poor feeding, vomiting, lethargy, hypotonia, seizures, coma, and hyperventilation, all secondary to the hyperammonemia.[79] Initially, neonates are often mistakenly diagnosed as having sepsis, which delays diagnostic laboratory testing.[81] Plasma ammonia levels should be drawn whenever a workup for sepsis is initiated in a neonate; levels in patients with urea cycle defects may reach greater than 2000 μmol/L (3400 μg/dL), with normal being 50 μmol/L (85 μg/dL) or less. Blood gas analysis shows respiratory alkalosis secondary to the hyperventilation caused by the effects of ammonia on the central nervous system. Blood urea nitrogen levels are typically low but can be elevated during times of dehydration or hypoperfusion. Serum levels of liver enzymes are usually normal or minimally elevated, and liver function is relatively unaffected. Severe hepatomegaly can occur in early-onset forms of AL deficiency.[79]

As stated earlier, more than 60% of patients present in the neonatal period; the rest are diagnosed at variable times from infancy to adulthood. Male patients with OTC deficiency and a varied phenotypic presentation have been diagnosed as late as 40 years of age. As many as 10% of female carriers of OTC deficiency can show varied symptoms, which may be severe and fatal, although most female carriers have no symptoms or report only nausea following high-protein meals.[82] Late-onset CPS deficiency also has been described,[83] and the adult form of AS deficiency is relatively common in Japan.[84]

Symptoms and signs of late-onset urea cycle defects, especially OTC and CPS deficiencies, include episodic irritability, lethargy, or vomiting; self-induced avoidance of protein such as milk, eggs, and meats; and short stature or growth delays. Neurologic symptoms, which also can be episodic, include ataxia, developmental delays, behavioral abnormalities, combativeness, biting, confusion, hallucinations, headaches, dizziness, visual impairments, diplopia, anorexia, and seizures. Acute hyperammonemic episodes can resemble Reye's syndrome.[79] These hyperammonemic episodes can be precipitated by high-protein meals, viral or bacterial infections, medications, trauma, or surgery. Infants may present on weaning from breast milk and the introduction of the higher protein content of infant formulas. There are reports of women presenting in the postpartum period with acute decompensation and death from either OTC or CPS deficiency.[85, 86]

Diagnosis

To diagnose errors of the urea cycle promptly, a high index of suspicion is required. Symptoms can mimic those of other acute neonatal problems such as infections or pulmonary or cardiac disease. Presentations later in life can mimic other behavioral, psychiatric, or developmental disorders. An elevated serum ammonia level with normal serum aminotransferase levels and without metabolic acidosis may be the first clue. Therefore, if these diagnoses are considered, the following laboratory tests should be obtained: serum ammonia, arterial blood gases, urine organic acids, serum amino acids, and urinary orotic acid. Table 65–4 reviews the expected laboratory results. Urinary organic acid profiles are typically

Table 65–4 | **Laboratory Values in Urea Cycle Defects**

	PLASMA NH_3	CITRULLINE (SERUM)	ARGININO-SUCCINATE (URINE OR SERUM)	OROTIC ACID (URINE)	ARGININE/ ORNITHINE (SERUM)
Carbamyl phosphate synthase deficiency	↑–↑↑↑	↓	↓	↓	↓
Ornithine transcarbamylase deficiency	↑–↑↑↑	↓	↓	↑↑	↓
Argininosuccinate synthase deficiency	↑–↑↑↑	↑↑↑	↓	Normal–↑	↓
Argininosuccinase deficiency	↑–↑↑↑	↑↑↑	↑↑↑	Normal–↑	↓
Arginase deficiency	↑	↑↑	↑↑	Normal–↑	↑↑

normal in defects of the urea cycle. The plasma amino acid profile is distinctive with abnormal levels of arginine, ornithine, and citrulline. Citrulline levels are barely detectable in OTC or CPS deficiencies but markedly elevated in AS and AL deficiencies. Distinguishing AS from AL deficiency can be made by finding argininosuccinic acid in the plasma and urine of patients with AL deficiency. OTC deficiency is distinguished from CPS deficiency by the excessive urinary excretion of orotic acid.[79, 87] Direct enzyme analysis can be performed and can be useful in late-onset or partial deficiencies presenting in adulthood. Prenatal enzyme and genetic linkage analysis can be done in families of known carriers.[88, 89] It has been shown that early neonatal diagnosis leads to improved survival.[90] The allopurinol loading test leads to excretion of orotic acid in amounts 10-fold to 20-fold greater than normal in heterozygote female carriers of OTC deficiency; however, the test is nonspecific and needs to be interpreted with caution, because it can be positive in some patients with mitochondrial disease or defects in pyrimidine metabolism.[87] Liver histology typically shows minimal fatty infiltration.

Treatment

All external protein intake should be discontinued in infants with urea cycle defects who present acutely. Serum ammonia levels should be restored to normal. Hemodialysis is often required, but exchange transfusions and peritoneal dialysis are ineffective. Alternative pathways for waste nitrogen disposal should be employed, specifically intravenous administration of sodium benzoate and sodium phenylacetate. Levels of arginine, carnitine, and long-chain fatty acids are usually low and should be supplemented.[91] Once the patient stabilizes, low levels of dietary protein, 0.5 to 1.0 gm/kg, may be introduced, with progressive increases as tolerated to provide sufficient protein for growth and tissue repair, while minimizing urea production. Long-term therapy and protein restriction are then tailored to each patient; those with a severe disorder may need essential amino acids to supplement their protein intake. Oral phenylbutyrate can be substituted for phenylacetate to improve palatability.

The outcome of patients who present with hyperammonemic coma and delayed diagnosis is poor. The level of ammonia at the time of the first hyperammonemic episode is a rough guide to the eventual neurodevelopmental outcome.[92] The sooner the hyperammonemia is treated and the correct diagnosis is made, the better the long-term survival, although for patients who survive the neonatal period, the median survival without OLT is less than 4 years and is associated with severe developmental delay and neurologic morbidity.[81] With optimal dietary and medical management, patients may still have repeated hyperammonemic crises, often during intercurrent viral infections. Symptomatic OTC heterozygote females benefit as well from therapy and have fewer hyperammonemic episodes and a reduced risk of further cognitive decline.[93]

Patients with a urea cycle defect and a deterioration or lack of improvement despite therapy have undergone OLT successfully, with normalization of enzyme activity and ammonia levels and the ability to tolerate a normal diet.[94, 95] If OLT is considered, it should be done before neurologic damage is permanent. In a retrospective study of 16 pediatric patients who underwent liver transplantation for urea cycle defects, the neurologic status failed to improve following transplantation. The metabolic condition of the patients normalized completely, however, and in no patient did the neurologic status worsen after transplantation. For patients without severe neurologic compromise before transplantation, this therapeutic approach is obviously worthwhile. In addition, it is likely that the annual cost of care for this group of patients will be reduced dramatically following OLT.[95] The importance of identifying the deleterious mutation in patients with a urea cycle defect will likely be increasingly important, not only as a means of allowing carrier testing and prenatal diagnosis but also in treatment decisions. For example, patients with the most severe mutations of OTC deficiency (e.g., abolished enzyme activity) may benefit preferentially from immediate OLT to prevent severe mental retardation or death, whereas those with milder mutations may be managed better medically using dietary restrictions and ammonia scavengers to allow for growth before possible OLT.[80]

Murine models of urea cycle defects have been developed, and an adenoviral-mediated correction of a murine model of OTC deficiency has been achieved.[96] However, successful protocols have not yet been developed for humans. Indeed, gene therapy initiatives are currently on hold because of concerns that toxicity was unexpectedly excessive in one of the initial trials undertaken to evaluate the adenoviral-mediated correction of partial OTC deficiency in humans.[97]

Arginase Deficiency

There are at least two forms of arginase activity in humans: arginase I (AI) predominates in the liver and red blood cells, and arginase II (AII) is found predominantly in kidney and prostate. Arginase deficiency involving AI is the least common of the urea cycle defects. Hyperammonemia is atypical in affected persons, but hyperammonemic coma and death have been reported. The clinical disorder is unique compared with the other urea cycle defects and is characterized by indolent deterioration of the cortex and pyramidal tracts, leading to progressive dementia and psychomotor retardation, spastic diplegia progressing to quadriplegia, seizures, and growth failure. The syndrome is often confused with cerebral palsy.

Laboratory studies may reveal elevated arginine levels, mild hyperammonemia, and a mild increase in urine orotic acid levels. Variable amounts of urea are still produced in these patients secondary to the compensatory elevated expression of AII in the kidneys, which likely results in a less severe clinical disorder.[98] The diagnosis is confirmed by enzymatic analysis, which can be performed prenatally on cord blood samples. Treatment consists of protein restriction and, when needed, medical therapy with sodium phenylbutyrate.[79]

BILE ACID SYNTHESIS AND TRANSPORT DEFECTS

The pathways for bile acid synthesis and transport within the hepatobiliary system are complex, involving several enzymes and transport processes located in multiple subcellular fractions of the hepatocyte (see Chapter 54). In the past 30 years, with the aid of technologic advancements in molecular biology and mass spectrometry, several different inborn errors in bile acid synthesis and transport have been identified as a cause of clinical disease. The definition and classification of these disorders have improved, particularly in the clinically heterogeneous subset of patients comprising *progressive familial intrahepatic cholestasis* (PFIC) syndromes. For some of these disorders, this progress had led to dramatic advancements in often life-saving therapy.[99]

The diagnosis of PFIC is imprecise; the accepted criteria include (1) the presence of chronic, unremitting intrahepatic cholestasis; (2) exclusion of identifiable metabolic or anatomic disorders; and (3) characteristic clinical, biochemical, and histologic features.[100, 101] Other symptoms and signs include severe pruritus, hepatomegaly, wheezing and cough, short stature, delayed sexual development, fat-soluble vitamin deficiency, and cholelithiasis.[101] Affected patients exhibit severe and progressive intrahepatic cholestasis, usually presenting within the first few months of life, and often progress to cirrhosis and end-stage liver disease by the 2nd decade of life. Patients with PFIC syndromes have been found to have defects in bile acid synthetic and transport processes.

Some patients previously believed to have idiopathic neonatal hepatitis and those having previously undiagnosed familial hepatitis syndromes may now be diagnosed accurately as having a form of PFIC.[99] It has been estimated that 1% to 2.5% of patients with idiopathic cholestasis may have defects in bile acid metabolism and transport.[102] Table 65–5 lists the known errors of primary and secondary bile acid synthesis and transport.

Table 65–5 | **Inborn Errors of Bile Acid Synthesis and Transport**

Defective bile acid synthesis
Primary defects
Cerebrotendinous xanthomatosis (27-hydroxylase deficiency)
3β-hydroxy-ΔC_{27}-steroid dehydrogenase/isomerase deficiency
Δ^4-3-oxosteroid 5β-reductase deficiency
C_{24}-steroid-7α-hydroxylase deficiency
Secondary defects (due to organelle damage)
Peroxisomal biogenesis disorders (PBD)
Zellweger's syndrome
Neonatal adrenoleukodystrophy
Infantile Refsum's disease
Zellweger-like syndrome
Rhizomelic chondrodysplasia punctata
Other
Hyperpipecolic acidemia
Leber's congenital amaurosis
Disorders with loss of single peroxisomal function
X-linked adrenoleukodystrophy
Thiolase deficiency (Pseudo-Zellweger's syndrome)
Bifunctional protein deficiency
Acyl-CoA oxidase deficiency
Hyperoxaluria type I
Acatalasemia
Adult Refsum's disease
Generalized hepatic synthetic dysfunction
Acute liver failure (multiple causes)
Tyrosinemia
Neonatal iron storage disease
Defective bile acid transport
PFIC type 1
FIC1 defect
Byler's disease
Benign recurrent intrahepatic cholestasis (BRIC) syndrome
Greenland familial cholestasis
PFIC type 2: BSEP deficiency
PFIC type 3: MDR3 deficiency
Other
North American Indian childhood cirrhosis
Cholestasis-lymphedema syndrome (Aagenaes' syndrome)
Alagille syndrome

BSEP, bile salt export pump; MDR, multidrug resistance; PFIC, progressive familial intrahepatic cholestasis.

Modified from Balistreri WF: Inborn errors of bile acid biosynthesis: Clinical and therapeutic aspects. In Hoffmann EF, et al (eds): Bile Acids in Gastroenterology. London, Kluwer, 1995, pp 333–335; and Balistreri WF: Liver disease in infancy and childhood. In Schiff ER, et al (eds): Schiff's Diseases of the Liver, 8th ed. Philadelphia, Lippincott-Raven, 1999, pp 1357–1512.

Bile Acid Synthesis Defects

Bile acid synthetic pathways are discussed in detail in Chapter 54. The most common enzyme deficiencies are described here; all can be diagnosed by mass spectrometry of the urine or serum. General principles of therapy rely on the hypothesis that inborn errors of bile acid biosynthesis lead to underproduction of normal trophic and choleretic primary bile acids and overproduction of hepatotoxic primitive bile acid metabolites.[99]

Cerebrotendinous xanthomatosis (CTX), *C_{27}-steroid-27-hydroxylase deficiency,* is characterized by bilateral juvenile cataracts and chronic diarrhea, followed by progressive neurologic dysfunction, hypercholesterolemia, atherosclerosis, and deposition of cholesterol and cholestanol in tissues.[99, 102] CTX should be treated with chenodeoxycholic acid. A series of 5 children with CTX showed dramatic improvement in biochemical and electroencephalographic abnormalities and resolution of diarrhea on this therapy. In addition, no further delay in motor development was noted, and 3 patients showed an improved intelligence quotient.[103] Patients with *3β-hydroxy-C_{27}-steroid dehydrogenase/isomerase* (3β-HSD) deficiency may present with cholestatic symptoms of pruritus, jaundice, hepatomegaly, steatorrhea, and fat-soluble vitamin deficiencies. Δ^4-3-Oxosteroid 5β-reductase deficiency also leads to neonatal cholestasis but rapidly progresses to liver failure with hepatic and synthetic dysfunction. Both conditions have been treated with a primary bile acid (i.e., chenodeoxycholic acid for 3β-HSD deficiency and cholic acid for 5β-reductase deficiency) and ursodeoxycholic acid supplementation.[99, 104] Chenodeoxycholic acid and cholic acid bypass the enzymatic block and provide negative feedback to earlier steps in the synthetic pathways, and ursodeoxycholic acid displaces toxic bile acid metabolites and serves as a hepatobiliary cytoprotectant. Other known disorders result from deficiencies in 25-hydroxylase and C_{24}-steroid-7α-hydroxylase and in amidation.[99]

Many peroxisomopathies have been described; these disorders are associated with multiple abnormalities and up to 50 wide-ranging biochemical defects.[105] They are diagnosed by a combination of specialized tests, such as a test for very-long-chain fatty acids (VLCFA) and ultrastructural analysis of tissue biopsies. Peroxisomes are responsible for β-oxidation in the final steps of bile acid synthesis to yield the primary bile acids cholic acid and chenodeoxycholic acid. These disorders can be divided into two groups: disorders of peroxisome assembly, which cause multiple abnormalities, and disorders of single proteins, which result in limited dysfunction (see Table 65–5).[105–107] The first group includes *peroxisome biogenesis disorders* (PBDs), which are grouped because they share similar clinical and biochemical features without distinctive features or boundaries between phenotypes, and *rhizomelic chondrodysplasia punctata* (RCDP), which is characterized by severe rhizomelic shortening of the limbs, severe skeletal abnormalities, cataracts, and facial abnormalities. PBDs include disorders such as *Zellweger's syndrome* (ZS), with the most severe clinical abnormalities and neonatal adrenoleukodystrophy, and infantile Refsum's disease, with the mildest features.[106]

ZS is a primary disorder of peroxisome biogenesis. The multiple features of ZS include distinctive dysmorphic features (hypertelorism, large anterior fontanelle, deformed earlobes), neonatal hypotonia, impaired hearing, retinopathy, cataracts, seizures, and skeletal changes. Hepatomegaly is frequent, and the progressive liver disease that develops in ZS is similar to that identified in other errors of bile acid synthesis.[108]

Peroxisome biogenesis involves more than 13 genes and requires the targeting and importation of cytosolic proteins, aided by peroxins (encoded by *PEX* genes), into the peroxisomal membrane and matrix.[105, 107] Importation of proteins fated for the peroxisomal matrix requires guidance from one of two peroxisome-targeting signals, PTS1 or PTS2.[105] Patients with PBD and RCDP display defects in the importation of proteins that use PTS1 and PTS2, respectively.[109] In infantile Refsum's disease, there is a temperature-sensitive block in peroxisomal biogenesis, which for 4 of 6 patients with IRD was caused by a temperature-sensitive defect in a protein, PEX1p, that is required for receptor-mediated importation of PTS1-containing proteins.[107] Genotype-phenotype correlations have yet to be established for the transport of peroxisomal membrane proteins, which involves a process separate from that described earlier for matrix proteins.[105]

The most common disorder of peroxisomes, X-linked adrenoleukodystrophy (X-ALD), is included in the *second* grouping of peroxisomopathies and results from a defect in the peroxisomal adrenoleukodystrophy protein (ALDP), which is a member of the adenosine triphosphate binding cassette (ABC) superfamily of membrane transporters. Phenylbutyrate induces expression of a protein related to ALDP, thereby leading to correction of VLCFA beta oxidation and an increase in the number of peroxisomes in fibroblasts isolated from patients with X-ALD and in vivo in the X-ALD transgenic knock-out mouse. These findings suggest that this drug may play a future role in the therapy of patients with X-ALD.[110]

Historically, the treatment for ZS has been supportive, with most patients not surviving the first year of life. The goals of medical therapy have been to improve nutrition and growth, control central nervous system symptoms, and limit progression of liver disease. Treatment with primary bile acids has been shown to improve biochemical tests and histology and to increase growth and improve neurologic symptoms.[111] In an uncontrolled study, the use of docosahexaenoic acid (DHA) led to improved myelination in patients with peroxisomal disorders; however, the use of DHA currently should be limited to controlled clinical trials.[106, 112]

Bile Acid Transport Defects

Byler's syndrome (or PFIC type 1) was first described in 1965 in an Amish kindred descended from Jacob Byler. Children with similar clinical features, but unrelated to the Byler family, are said to have Byler's syndrome (e.g., PFIC type 2 or type 3) and are genotypically distinct from those with the original Byler's syndrome. Byler's syndrome is caused by mutations in a single gene (*FIC1*) located on chromosome 18q21. *F1C1* encodes a P-type adenosine triphosphatase involved in ATP-dependent aminophospholipid transport and is expressed in many organs in addition to the liver and intestine. Defects in *FIC1* also have been found in patients with benign recurrent intrahepatic cholestasis (BRIC), which, as the name implies, gives rise to recurrent episodes of intrahepatic cholestasis beginning in childhood or adulthood that can last for days to months and then resolve spontaneously without causing detectable lasting liver damage.[113] Patients with Greenland familial cholestasis also have been reported to have defects in the *FIC1* gene.[114] In all three conditions, serum gamma glutamyl transpeptidase (GGTP) and cholesterol levels are normal or mildly elevated, and levels of bile acids are elevated in the serum and low in the bile. Serum aminotransferase and bilirubin levels are elevated as well. Impaired bile acid transport in the intestine may account for the striking malabsorption and diarrhea manifested by some patients with PFIC type 1; these intestinal clinical features do not resolve following liver transplantation in these patients.[113] That sweat electrolyte concentrations are frequently abnormal in patients with PFIC type 1 and the *FIC1* gene is expressed widely in epithelium suggests that the F1C1 protein acts globally at sites of secretion and absorption.[113] On electron microscopic evaluation of liver tissue from patients with PFIC type 1, characteristic coarse, granular bile deposits are seen in the canaliculus ("Byler's bile").

A second subset of patients with intrahepatic cholestasis (PFIC type 2) also have low serum GGTP and elevated bile acid levels. On routine histology of the liver early in the disease, a nonspecific giant cell hepatitis is found, and on electron microscopy, amorphous bile deposits are seen in the canaliculi. The disease-causing gene for PFIC type 2 maps to chromosome 2q24 and encodes for an ABC protein that serves as the canalicular bile salt export pump (BSEP).[115]

Yet another subset, PFIC type 3, comprises patients with high serum levels of GGTP and bile acids, as well as bile ductular proliferation on routine microscopy. The defect in PFIC type 3 has been localized to chromosome 7q21 and is caused by mutations in the *MDR3* gene, which encodes for a phosphatidylserine translocase located on the canalicular membrane.[116] MDR3 deficiency is thought to lead to decreased excretion of cytoprotective biliary phospholipids, leaving an increased pool of cytotoxic biliary bile salts that give rise to subsequent bile duct damage and proliferation and release of GGTP into the serum. Heterozygous carriers of a mutation in *MDR3* have been found in a group of female patients with familial intrahepatic cholestasis of pregnancy, which likely leads to a genetic predisposition that requires the coexistence of other nongenetic factors for full expression of this disease.[117, 118]

Other chronic cholestatic diseases, such as North American Indian childhood cirrhosis and cholestasis-lymphedema syndrome (Aagenaes' syndrome), are at the early stages of investigations at the molecular genetic level; the disease-causing loci for both conditions have recently been linked to chromosomes 16q22 and 15q, respectively, suggesting that these two diseases are genetically distinct from *FIC1*, BSEP, and MDR3 mutations.[119, 120] Additional series of patients with "PFIC-like" syndromes have been reported but have not been characterized beyond the clinical level.[121, 122]

Medical treatment of patients with PFIC as a group with phenobarbital, cholestyramine, opioid antagonists, rifampin, or phototherapy has been largely ineffective. Therapy with ursodeoxycholic acid may be effective in relieving pruritus and improving biochemical parameters in up to 50% of patients, regardless of GGTP level.[123] Surgical alternatives such as ileal exclusion or partial external biliary diversion have given satisfactory symptomatic relief to some patients by decreasing the bile acid pool and pruritus. The long-term outcome of six pediatric patients treated with partial biliary diversion has been reported, with marked improvement in pruritus and growth after this procedure.[124] If all else fails, OLT has been shown to normalize bile acid synthesis and growth in selected patients.[125]

CYSTIC FIBROSIS

Cystic fibrosis (CF) is discussed in detail in Chapter 47; here, a brief discussion of the *hepatic complications* seen in this multisystemic disorder is presented. Liver disease can be the presenting symptom of CF in the newborn, and CF-associated liver disease has been associated with meconium ileus syndrome. Although CF has been identified in less than 2% of patients with neonatal cholestasis, the diagnosis should be considered in any infant with neonatal cholestasis.[4, 126]

Liver disease may become more prevalent as the mean age of survival for patients with CF increases; however, liver involvement is not universal and seems to peak during the adolescent years.[127] Up to 30% of patients may have clinical or symptomatic liver disease after the neonatal period.[128]

The diagnosis of significant liver disease in this patient population can be difficult because the presenting signs are subtle. Hepatomegaly, present in approximately 30% of patients, has been shown to correlate well with the presence of cirrhosis and is often the first finding of liver disease. Liver biochemical test results may remain relatively normal despite histologic evidence of cirrhosis. Needle biopsy of the liver can be helpful; however, because of focal distribution, sampling error may occur. Ultrasonography can detect biliary stones and bile duct or hepatic vein dilatation and permits Doppler flow study of the hepatic vasculature.[128]

Hepatobiliary diseases noted in patients with CF can be grouped into three categories (Table 65–6). The pathognomonic lesion of CF, focal biliary cirrhosis (FCC), presumably results from defective function of the cystic fibrosis gene product, which is expressed in bile duct cells. Obstruction of small bile ducts leads to chronic inflammatory changes, bile duct proliferation, and portal fibrosis. At autopsy, FCC has been identified in 25% to 30% of patients older than 1 year of age.[129] Progression to multilobular biliary cirrhosis occurs in approximately 10% of patients with CF and leads to typical symptoms of portal hypertension such as splenomegaly and variceal bleeding.[128] Hepatic steatosis also develops in roughly one half of patients but does not appear to correlate with outcome. Biliary abnormalities range from microgallbladder, which is largely asymptomatic and found in up to 20% of patients, to cholelithiasis and cholangiocarcinoma.[4]

Treatment of patients with CF with ursodeoxycholic acid improves the biochemical indices of liver injury; however, conclusive evidence that the drug halts the progression to cirrhosis is not yet available.[128, 130] Portosystemic shunts can be effective treatment for patients with portal hypertension. OLT is rarely needed for end-stage liver disease but has been performed successfully for patients with portal hypertension and stable pulmonary function.[131]

Table 65–6 | **Spectrum of Hepatobiliary Disease in Patients with Cystic Fibrosis**

Lesions Specific to Cystic Fibrosis
Hepatic
Focal biliary cirrhosis with inspissation
Multilobular biliary cirrhosis with inspissation
Biliary
Microgallbladder
Mucous hyperplasia of gallbladder
Mucocoele
Lesions Secondary to Extrahepatic Disease
Lesions associated with cardiopulmonary disease
Centrilobular necrosis
Cirrhosis
Lesions associated with pancreatic disease
Pancreatic duct sludge (obstruction)
Pancreatic fibrosis (leading to bile duct compression/stricture)
Lesions that Occur with a Higher Frequency in Patients with Cystic Fibrosis
Hepatic
Fatty liver
Neonatal cholestasis
Drug hepatotoxicity
Endotoxemia
Viral hepatitis
Biliary
Sclerosing cholangitis
Biliary sludge
Cholelithiasis
Cholangiocarcinoma

From Balistreri WF: Liver disease in infancy and childhood. In Schiff ER, et al (eds): Schiff's Diseases of the Liver, 8th ed. Philadelphia, Lippincott-Raven, 1999, p 1379.

MITOCHONDRIAL LIVER DISEASES

Over the past decade, an increasing number of liver diseases have been attributed to defects in mitochondrial function. In addition to previously characterized defects of mitochondrial enzymes involved in the urea cycle or energy metabolism, several mitochondrial hepatopathies have been delineated that involve respiratory chain/oxidative phosphorylation/electron transport defects or alterations in mitochondrial DNA (mtDNA) composition. The mitochondrial genome is especially vulnerable to oxidative injury not only because of its spatial relationship to the respiratory chain but also because of its lack of protective histones or an adequate excision and recombination repair system. Mitochondrial DNA is inherited almost entirely from the maternal ovum; therefore, primary mitochondrial deficiencies usually are inherited in a dominant fashion. Normal mtDNA and mutant mtDNA are present in varying amounts in a given cell, because of the large number of mitochondria and multiple copies of mtDNA in a mitochondrion. This *heteroplasmy* for mitochondrial DNA mutations can often lead to mixed involvement of organs throughout the body.[132] Heterogeneity of clinical features can lead to a delayed or missed diagnosis and can confound therapeutic decision-making, for example, with respect to the merits of OLT.

Neonatal liver failure has been reported in association with *cytochrome c oxidase deficiency*. The key features of this disorder are lactic acidemia and an elevated ratio of serum lactate to pyruvate. Infants with *Alpers' disease* (progressive neuronal degeneration in childhood with liver disease ascribed to mitochondrial dysfunction) have vomiting, hypotonia, seizures, and liver failure often beginning by age 6 months. Frequently, the liver disease is unsuspected clinically and evident late in the course of the disease. Alternatively, in *mtDNA depletion syndrome*, hypoglycemia, acidosis, and liver failure develop early in infancy, and neurologic abnormalities are less prominent. Other multisystemic mitochondrial diseases with significant liver involvement include *Pearson's marrow-pancreas syndrome* and *chronic diarrhea and intestinal pseudo-obstruction with liver involvement*; these syndromes are still in the early stages of characterization.[132]

The diagnosis of a mitochondrial respiratory chain defect should be considered in patients with liver disease and unexplained neuromuscular symptoms, including a seizure disorder, involvement of seemingly unrelated organ systems, or a rapidly progressive course.[132] In about 80% of patients symptoms appear early in life, before age 2 years.[133]

Liver biopsy specimens typically show macrovesicular and microvesicular steatosis, with increased density and occasional swelling of mitochondria on electron microscopy. Immunohistochemical techniques are being used more frequently (e.g., to diagnose cytochrome c oxidase deficiency). Direct measurement of the enzymatic activity of the respiratory chain electron transport protein complexes can be performed on frozen tissue from the organ that expresses the clinical disease, although skin fibroblasts and lymphocytes also may be of help. Few academic centers around the world can perform the assays for mitochondrial respiration (polarographic studies) or mtDNA analysis at this time.

There is no effective therapy for respiratory chain disorders that alters the course of the disease. Several strategies have been proposed to delay the progression of these diseases, including the use of antioxidants such as vitamin E or ascorbic acid, as well as carnitine or succinate supplementation, but the use of these agents is experimental at this time.[132]

REFERENCES

1. Kilpe VE, Krakauer H, Wren RE: An analysis of liver transplant experience from 37 transplant centers as reported to medicare. Transplantation 56:554, 1993.
2. Alonso MH, Ryckman Fd: Current concepts in pediatric liver transplant. Semin Liver Dis 18:295–307, 1998.
3. Teckman J, Perlmutter DH: Conceptual advances in the pathogenesis and treatment of childhood metabolic liver disease. Gastroenterology 108:1263, 1995.
4. Balistreri WF: Liver disease in infancy and childhood. In Schiff ER, Sorrell MF, Maddrey WC (eds): Schiff's Diseases of the Liver, 8th ed. Philadelphia, Lippincott-Raven, 1999, pp 1357–1512.
5. Perlmutter DH: Alpha$_1$-antitrypsin deficiency. In Schiff ER, Sorrell MF, Maddrey WC (eds): Schiff's Diseases of the Liver, 8th ed. Philadelphia, Lippincott-Raven, 1999, pp 1131–1150.
6. Perlmutter DH, Joslin G, Nelson P, et al: Endocytosis and degradation of α_1-antitrypsin-proteinase complexes is mediated by the SEC receptor. J Biol Chem 265:16713–16716, 1990.
7. Kounnas MZ, Church FC, Argraves WS, et al: Cellular internalization and degradation of antithrombin III-thrombin, heparin cofactor II-thrombin, and α_1-antitrypsin-trypsin complexes is mediated by the low-density lipoprotein receptor-related protein. J Biol Chem 271: 6523–6529, 1996.
8. Pittschieler K: Heterozygoses and liver involvement. Acta Paediatr Suppl 393:21, 1994.
9. Lomas DA: Loop-sheet polymerization: The mechanism of α_1-antitrypsin deficiency. Respir Med 94:S3–S6, 2000.
10. Wu Y, Whirtman I, Molmenti E, et al: A lag in intracellular degradation of mutant α_1-antitrypsin correlates with the liver disease phenotype in homozygous PiZZ α_1-antitrypsin deficiency. Proc Natl Acad Sci U S A 91:9014–9018, 1994.
11. Teckman JH, Gilmore R, Perlmutter DH: Role of ubiquitin in proteasomal degradation of mutant α_1-antitrypsin Z in the endoplasmic reticulum. Am J Physiol Gastrointest Liver Physiol 278:G39–G48, 2000.
12. Mowat AP: α_1-Antitrypsin deficiency (PiZZ): Features of liver involvement in childhood. Acta Paediatr Suppl 393:13, 1994.
13. Brantly M, Lee JH, Hildesheim J, et al: α_1-Antitrypsin gene mutation hot spot associated with the formation of a retained and degraded null variant. Am J Respir Cell Mol Biol 16:225–231, 1997.
14. Sveger T, Eriksson S: The liver in adolescents with α_1-antitrypsin deficiency. Hepatology 22:514–517, 1995.
15. Sveger T: Liver disease in α_1-antitrypsin deficiency detected by screening of 200,000 infants. N Engl J Med 294:1316, 1976.
16. Eriksson S: α_1-Antitrypsin deficiency and liver cirrhosis in adults: An analysis of 35 Swedish autopsied cases. Acta Med Scand 221:461, 1987.
17. Zhou H, Fischer HP: Liver carcinoma in PiZ α_1-antitrypsin deficiency. Am J Surg Pathol 22:742–748, 1998.
18. Poley JR: Malignant liver disease in α_1-antitrypsin deficiency. Acta Paediatr Suppl 393:27, 1994.
19. Thelin T, Sveger T, McNeil TF: Primary prevention in a high-risk group: Smoking habits in adolescents with homozygous α_1-antitrypsin deficiency (ATD). Acta Paediatr 85:1207–1212, 1996.
20. Dirksen A, Dijkman JH, Madsen F, et al: A randomized clinical trial of α_1-antitrypsin augmentation therapy. Am J Respir Crit Care Med 160:1468–1472, 1999.
21. Burrows JA, Willis LK, Perlmutter DH: Chemical chaperones mediate increased secretion of mutant α_1-antitrypsin (α_1-AT) Z: A potential pharmacological strategy for prevention of liver injury and emphysema in α_1-AT deficiency. Proc Natl Acad Sci U S A 97:1796–1801, 2000.
22. Marcus NY, Perlmutter DH: Glucosidase and mannosidase inhibitors mediate increased secretion of mutant α_1-antitrypsin Z. J Biol Chem 275:1987–1992, 2000.
23. Campbell EJ, Campbell MA, Boukedes SS, et al: Quantum proteolysis by neutrophils: Implications for pulmonary emphysema in α_1-antitrypsin deficiency. J Clin Invest 104:337–344, 1999.
24. Zhang G, Song YK, Liu D: Long-term expression of human α_1-antitrypsin gene in mouse liver achieved by intravenous administration of plasmid DNA using a hydrodynamics-based procedure. Gene Ther 7:1344–1349, 2000.
25. Ozaki I, Zern MA, Liu S, et al: Ribozyme-mediated specific gene replacement of the α_1-antitrypsin gene in human hepatoma cells. J Hepatol 31:53–60, 1999.
26. Woldsdorf JI, Holm IA, Weinstein DA: Glycogen storage diseases: Phenotypic, genetic, and biochemical characteristics, and therapy. Endocrin Metab Clin 28:801–823, 1999.
27. Grishan FK, Ballew M: Inborn errors of carbohydrate metabolism. In Suchy FJ (ed): Liver Disease in Children. St. Louis, Mosby–Yearbook, 1994, p 720.
28. Veiga-da-Cunha M, Gerin I, Van Schaftingen E: How many forms of glycogen storage disease type I? Eur J Pediatr 159:314–318, 2000.
29. Rake JP, ten Berge AM, Visser G, et al: Glycogen storage disease type Ia: Recent experience with mutation analysis—a summary of mutations reported in the literature and a newly developed diagnostic flowchart. Eur J Pediatr 159:322–330, 2000.
30. Veiga-da-Cunha M, Gerin I, Chen YT, et al: The putative glucose-6-phosphate translocase gene is mutated in essentially all cases of glycogen storage disease type I non-A. Eur J Hum Genet 7:717–723, 1999.
31. Garty BZ, Douglas SD, Danon YL: Immune deficiency in glycogen storage disease type IB. Isr J Med Sci 32:1276–1281, 1996.
32. Bianchi L: Glycogen storage disease type I and hepatocellular tumours. Eur J Pediatr 152(Suppl 1):S63–S70, 1993.

33. Labrune P, Trische P, Duvaltier I, et al: Hepatocellular adenomas in glycogen storage disease type I and III: A series of 43 patients and review of the literature. J Pediatr Gastroenterol Nutr 24:276–279, 1997.
34. Talente GM, Coleman RA, Alter C, et al: Glycogen storage disease in adults. Ann Intern Med 120:218, 1994.
35. Goldberg T, Slonim AE: Nutritional therapy for glycogen storage diseases. J Am Diet Assoc 93:1423, 1993.
36. Schwenk WF, Haymond MW: Optimal rate of enteral glucose administration in children with glycogen storage disease type I. N Engl J Med 314:682, 1986.
37. Matern D, Starzl TE, Arnaout W, et al: Liver transplantation for glycogen storage disease types I, III, and IV. Eur J Pediatr 158(Suppl 2):S43–S48, 1999.
38. Fukuda T, Sutie H, Ito H: Novel mutations in two Japanese cases of glycogen storage disease type IIIa and a review of the literature of the molecular basis of glycogen storage disease type III. J Inherit Metab Dis 23:95–106, 2000.
39. Haagsma EB, Smit GP, Niezen-Koning TE, et al: Type IIIb glycogen storage disease associated with end-stage cirrhosis and hepatocellular carcinoma. The Liver Transplant Group. Hepatology 25:537–540, 1997.
40. Cox PM, Brueton LA, Murphy KW, et al: Early-onset fetal hydrops and muscle degeneration in siblings due to a novel variant of type IV glycogenosis. Am J Med Genet 86:187–193, 1999.
41. McConkie-Rosell A, Wilson C, Piccoli DA, et al: Clinical and laboratory findings in four patients with the non-progressive hepatic form of type IV glycogen storage disease. J Inherit Metab Dis 19:51–58, 1996.
42. de Moor RA, Schweizer JJ, van Hoek B, et al: Hepatocellular carcinoma in glycogen storage disease type IV. Arch Dis Child 82:479–480, 2000.
43. Rosenthal P, Podesta L, Grier R, et al: Failure of liver transplantation to diminish cardiac deposits of amylopectin and leukocyte inclusions in type IV glycogen storage disease. Liver Transplant Surg 1:373–376, 1995.
44. Gordon N: Carbohydrate-deficient glycoprotein syndromes. Postgrad Med J 76:145–149, 2000.
45. Niehues R, Hasilik M, Alton G, et al: Carbohydrate-deficient glycoprotein syndrome type Ib: Phosphomannose isomerase deficiency and mannose therapy. J Clin Invest 101:1414–1420, 1998.
46. Jaeken J, Matthijs G, Saudubray JM, et al: Phosphomannose isomerase deficiency: A carbohydrate-deficient glycoprotein syndrome with hepatic-intestinal presentation. Am J Hum Genet 62:1535–1539, 1998.
47. Babovic-Vuksanovic D, Patterson MC, Schwenk WF, et al: Severe hypoglycemia as a presenting symptom of carbohydrate-deficient glycoprotein syndrome. J Pediatr 135:775–781, 1999.
48. De Koning TJ, Dorland L, Nikkels P, et al: Phosphomannose isomerase deficiency with cyclic vomiting and congenital hepatic fibrosis. J Inherit Metab Dis 21(Suppl 12):96, 1998.
49. Bloomer JR: The porphyrias. In Schiff ER, Sorrell MF, Maddrey WC (eds): Schiff's Diseases of the Liver, 8th ed. Philadelphia, Lippincott-Raven, 1999, pp 1151–1178.
50. Elder GH, Hift RJ, Meissner PN: The acute porphyrias. Lancet 349: 1613–1617, 1997.
51. Crimlisk HL: The little imitator: Porphyria—a neuropsychiatric disorder. J Neurol Neurosurg Psychiatry 62:319–328, 1997.
52. Thunell S, Henrichson A, Floderus Y, et al: Liver transplantation in a boy with acute porphyria due to aminolaevulinate dehydratase deficiency. Eur J Clin Chem Clin Biochem 30:599, 1992.
53. Mustajoki P, Nordmann Y: Early administration of heme arginate for acute porphyria attacks. Arch Intern Med 153:2004–2008, 1993.
54. Murphy GM: The cutaneous porphyrias: A review. Br J Dermatol 140:573–581, 1999.
55. Meerman L, Verwer R, Slooff MJ, et al: Perioperative measures during liver transplantation for erythropoietic protoporphyria. Transplantation 57:155–158, 1994.
56. Elder GH: Porphyria cutanea tarda. Semin Liver Dis 18:67–75, 1998.
57. Fritsch C, Lang K, Bolsen K, et al: Congenital erythropoietic porphyria. Skin Pharmacol Appl Skin Physiol 11:347–357, 1998.
58. Thomas C, Ged C, Nordmann Y, et al: Correction of congenital erythropoietic porphyria by bone marrow transplantation. J Pediatr 129:453–456, 1996.
59. Doss MO, Frank M: Hepatobiliary implication and complications in protoporphyria, a 20-year study. Clin Biochem 22:223–229, 1989.
60. Bloomer J, Bruzzone C, Zhu L, et al: Molecular defects in ferrochelatase in patients with protoporphyria requiring liver transplantation. J Clin Invest 102:107–114, 1998.
61. Meerman L, Haagsma EB, Gouw AS, et al: Long-term follow-up after liver transplantation for erythropoietic protoporphyria. Eur J Gastroenterol Hepatol 11:431–438, 1999.
62. Cox TM, Alexander GJ, Sarkany RP, et al: Protoporphyria. Semin Liver Dis 18:85–89, 1998.
63. Andant C, Puy H, Faivre J, et al: Acute hepatic porphyria and primary liver cancer. N Engl J Med 338:1853–1854, 1998.
64. De Braekeleer M, Larochelle JL: Genetic epidemiology of hereditary tyrosinemia in Quebec and in Saguenay-Lac-St.-Jean. Am J Hum Genet 47:302–307, 1990.
65. Stoner E, Starkman H, Wellner D, et al: Biochemical studies of a patient with hereditary hepatorenal tyrosinemia: Evidence of glutathione deficiency. Pediatr Res 18:1332–1336, 1984.
66. Jorquera R, Tanguay RM: The mutagenicity of the tyrosine metabolite, fumarylacetoacetate, is enhanced by glutathione depletion. Biochem Biophys Res Commun 232:42, 1997.
67. Prieto-Alamo MJ, Laval F: Deficient DNA-ligase activity in the metabolic disease tyrosinemia type I. Proc Natl Acad Sci U S A 95: 12614–12618, 1998.
68. Gilbert-Barness E, Barness LA, Meisner LF, et al: Chromosomal instability in hereditary tyrosinemia type I. Pediatr Pathol 10:243–252, 1990.
69. Van Spronsen FJ, Thomasse Y, Smit GP, et al: Hereditary tyrosinemia: A new clinical classification with difference in prognosis on dietary treatment. Hepatology 20:1187, 1994.
70. Kvittingen EA, Rootwelt H, Berger R, et al: Self-induced correction of the genetic defect in tyrosinemia type I. J Clin Invest 94:1657–1661, 1994.
71. Ploos van Amstel JK, Bergman AJ, van Beurden EA, et al: Hereditary tyrosinemia type 1: Novel missense, nonsense and splice consensus mutations in the human fumarylacetoacetate hydrolase gene—variability of the genotype-phenotype relationship. Hum Genet 97:51–59, 1996.
72. Macvicar D, Dicks-Mreaux C, Leonald JV, et al: Hepatic imaging with computed tomography of chronic tyrosinaemia type I. Br J Radiol 63:605, 1990.
73. Kvittingen EA, Talseth T, Halvorsen S, et al: Renal failure in adult patients with hereditary tyrosinemia type I. J Inherit Metab Dis 14:53, 1991.
74. Paradis K, Weber A, Seidman EG, et al: Liver transplantation for hereditary tyrosinemia: The Quebec experience. Am J Hum Genet 47: 338, 1990.
75. Mitchell G, Larochelle J, Lambert M, et al: Neurologic crisis in hereditary tyrosinemia. N Engl J Med 322:432, 1990.
76. Forget S, Patriquim HB, Dubois J, et al: The kidney in children with tyrosinemia: Sonographic, CT, and biochemical findings. Pediatr Radiol 29:104–108, 1999.
77. Lindstedt S, Holme E, Lock EA, et al: Treatment of hereditary tyrosinaemia type I by inhibition of 4 hydroxyphenylpyruvate dioxygenase. Lancet 340:813–817, 1992.
78. Holme E, Lindstedt S: Tyrosinaemia type I and NTBC (2-[2-nitro-4-trifluoromethylbenzoyl]-1,3-cyclohexanedione). J Inherit Metab Dis 21: 507–517, 1998.
79. Brusilow SW, Horwich AL: Urea cycle enzymes. In Schriver CR, Beaudet AL, Sly WS, et al (eds): The Metabolic and Molecular Basis of Inherited Disease, 7th ed. New York, McGraw-Hill, 1995, pp 1187–1232.
80. Tuchman M, Morizono H, Rajagopal BS, et al: The biochemical and molecular spectrum of ornithine transcarbamylase deficiency. J Inherit Metab Dis 21(Suppl 1):40–58, 1998.
81. Maestri NE, Clissold D, Brusilow SW, et al: Neonatal onset ornithine transcarbamylase deficiency: A retrospective analysis. J Pediatr 134: 268–272, 1999.
82. Maestri NE, Lord C, Glynn M, et al: The phenotype of ostensibly healthy women who are carriers for ornithine transcarbamylase deficiency. Medicine 77:389–397, 1998.
83. Lo WD, Sloan HR, Sotos JF, et al: Late clinical presentation of partial carbamyl phosphate synthetase I deficiency. Am J Dis Child 147:267–269, 1993.
84. Kobayashi K, Shaheen N, Kumashiro R, et al: A search for the primary abnormality in adult-onset type II citrullinemia. Am J Hum Genet 53:1024–1030, 1993.

85. Wong LJ, Craigen WJ, O'Brien WE: Postpartum coma and death due to carbamoyl-phosphate synthetase I deficiency. Ann Intern Med 120: 216–217, 1994.
86. Arn PH, Hauser ER, Thomas GH, et al: Hyperammonemia in women with a mutation at the ornithine carbamoyltransferase locus: A cause of postpartum coma. N Engl J Med 322:1652–1655, 1990.
87. Bonham JR, Guthrie P, Downing M, et al: The allopurinol load test lacks specificity for primary urea cycle defects but may indicate unrecognized mitochondrial disease. J Inherit Metab Dis 22:174–184, 1999.
88. Kamoun P, Fensom AH, Shin YS, et al: Prenatal diagnosis of the urea cycle diseases: A survey of the European cases. Am J Med Genet 55: 247–250, 1995.
89. Bale AE: Prenatal diagnosis of ornithine transcarbamylase deficiency. Prenat Diagn 19:1052–1054, 1999.
90. Maestri NE, Hauser ER, Bartholomew D, et al: Prospective treatment of urea cycle disorders. J Pediatr 119:923–928, 1991.
91. Sanjurjo P, Ruiz JI, Montejo M: Inborn errors of metabolism with a protein-restricted diet: Effect on polyunsaturated fatty acids. J Inherit Metab Dis 20:783–789, 1997.
92. Uchino T, Endo F, Matsuda IJ: Neurodevelopmental outcome of long-term therapy of urea cycle disorders in Japan. J Inherit Metab Dis 21(Suppl 1):151–159, 1998.
93. Maestri NE, Brusilow SW, Clissold DB, et al: Long-term treatment of girls with ornithine transcarbamylase deficiency. N Engl J Med 335: 855–859, 1996.
94. Jan D, Poggi F, Jouvet P, et al: Definitive cure of hyperammonemia by liver transplantation in urea cycle defects: Report of three cases. Transplant Proc 26:188, 1994.
95. Whitington PF, Alonso EM, Boyle JT, et al: Liver transplantation for the treatment of urea cycle disorders. J Inherit Metab Dis 21(Suppl 1): 112–118, 1998.
96. Batshaw ML, Robinson MB, Ye X, et al: Correction of ureagenesis after gene transfer in an animal model and after liver transplantation in humans with ornithine transcarbamylase deficiency. Pediatr Res 46: 588–593, 1999.
97. Marshall E: Gene therapy on trial. Science 288:951–957, 2000.
98. Iyer R, Jenkinson CP, Vockley JG, et al: The human arginases and arginase deficiency. J Inherit Metab Dis 21(Suppl 1):86–100, 1998.
99. Balistreri WF: Inborn errors of bile acid biosynthesis and transport. Gastroenterol Clin North Am 28:145–171, 1999.
100. Bezerra JA, Balistreri WF: Intrahepatic cholestasis: Order out of chaos. Gastroenterology 117:1496–1498, 1999.
101. Whitington PF, Freese DK, Alonso EM, et al: Clinical and biochemical findings in progressive familial intrahepatic cholestasis. J Pediatr Gastroenterol Nutr 18:134–141, 1994.
102. Setchell KDR, O'Connell N: Inborn errors of bile acid metabolism. In Suchy FJ (ed): Liver Disease in Children. St. Louis, Mosby–Yearbook, 1994, p 835.
103. van Heijst AF, Verrips A, Wever RA, et al: Treatment and follow-up of children with cerebrotendinous xanthomatosis. Eur J Pediatr 157: 313–316, 1998.
104. Witzleben CL, Piccoli DA, Setchell KD: Case 3: A new category of causes of intrahepatic cholestasis. Pediatr Pathol 12:269–274, 1992.
105. Raymond GV: Peroxisomal disorders. Curr Opin Pediatr 11:572–576, 1999.
106. Noetzel MJ: Fish oil and myelin: Cautious optimism for treatment of children with disorders of peroxisome biogenesis. Neurology 51:5–7, 1998.
107. Imamura A, Tamura S, Shimozawa N, et al: Temperature-sensitive mutation in *PEX*1 moderates the phenotypes of peroxisome deficiency disorders. Hum Mol Genet 7:2089–2094, 1998.
108. Brown FR III, Voigt R, Singh AK, et al: Peroxisomal disorders: Neurodevelopmental and biochemical aspects. Am J Dis Child 147: 617–626, 1993.
109. Moser HW: Genotype-phenotype correlations in peroxisomal disorders. Dev Brain Dys 10:282–292, 1999.
110. Kemp S, Wei HM, Lu JF, et al: Gene redundancy and pharmacological gene therapy: Implications for X-linked adrenoleukodystrophy. Nature Med 4:1261–1268, 1998.
111. Setchell KD, Bragetti P, Zimmer-Mechemias L, et al: Oral bile acid treatment and the patient with Zellweger syndrome. Hepatology 15: 198–207, 1992.
112. Martinez M, Vazquez E: MRI evidence that docosahexaenoic acid ethyl ester improves myelination in generalized peroxisomal disorders. Neurology 51:26–32, 1998.
113. Bull LN, van Eijk MJ, Pawlikowska L, et al: A gene encoding a P-type ATPase mutated in two forms of hereditary cholestasis. Nature Genet 18:219–224, 1998.
114. Klomp LW, Bull LN, Knisely AS, et al: Greenland familial cholestasis is caused by a missense mutation in FIC1. Hepatology 32:430A, 2000.
115. Strautnieks SS, Bull LN, Knisely AS, et al: A gene encoding a liver-specific ABC transporter is mutated in progressive familial intrahepatic cholestasis. Nature Genet 20:233–238, 1998.
116. De Vree JM, Jacquemin E, Sturm E, et al: Mutations in the *MDR3* gene cause progressive familial intrahepatic cholestasis. Proc Natl Acad Sci U S A 95:282–287, 1998.
117. Jacquemin E, Cresteil D, Manouvrier S, et al: Heterozygous non-sense mutation of the *MDR3* gene in familial intrahepatic cholestasis of pregnancy. Lancet 353:210–211, 1999.
118. Dixon PH, Weerasekera N, Linton KJ, et al: Heterozygous MDR3 missense mutations associated with intrahepatic cholestasis of pregnancy: Evidence for a defect in protein trafficking. Hum Mol Genet 9: 1209–1217, 2000.
119. Betard C, Rasquin-Wever A, Brewer C, et al: Localization of a recessive gene for North American Indian childhood cirrhosis to chromosome region 16q22 and identification of a shared haplotype. Am J Hum Genet 67:222–228, 2000.
120. Bull LN, Roche E, Song EJ, et al: Genetic mapping of the locus for cholestasis-lymphedema syndrome (Aagenaes syndrome). Hepatology 32:297A, 2000.
121. Kocak N, Gurakan F, Yuce A, et al: Nonsyndromic paucity of interlobular bile ducts: Clinical and laboratory findings of 10 cases. J. Pediatr Gastroenterol Nutr 24:44–48, 1997.
122. Naveh Y, Bassan L, Rosenthal E, et al: Cholestasis among the Arab population in Israel. J Pediatr Gastroenterol Nutr 24:548–554, 1997.
123. Jacquemin E, Hermans D, Myara A, et al: Ursodeoxycholic acid therapy in pediatric patients with progressive familial intrahepatic cholestasis. Hepatology 25:519–523, 1997.
124. Ng VL, Ryckman FC, Porta G, et al: Long-term outcome after partial external biliary diversion for intractable pruritus in patients with intrahepatic cholestasis. J Pediatr Gastroenterol Nutr 30:152–156, 2000.
125. Soubrane O, Gauthier F, De Victor D, et al: Orthotopic liver transplantation for Byler disease. Transplantation 50:804, 1990.
126. Lykavieris P, Bernard O, Hadchouel M: Neonatal cholestasis as the presenting feature in cystic fibrosis. Arch Dis Child 75:67–70, 1996.
127. Lindblad A, Glaumann H, Straudvik B: Natural history of liver disease in cystic fibrosis. Hepatology 30:1151–1158, 1999.
128. Sokol RJ, Durie PR: Recommendation for management of liver and biliary tract disease in cystic fibrosis. J Pediatr Gastroenterol Nutr 28: S1–S13, 1999.
129. Colombo C, Apostolo MG, Assaisso M, et al: Liver disease in cystic fibrosis. Neth J Med 41:119, 1992.
130. Narkewicz MR, Smith D, Gregory C, et al: Effect of ursodeoxycholic acid therapy on hepatic function in children with intrahepatic cholestasis. J Pediatr Gastroenterol Nutr 26:49–55, 1998.
131. Noble-Jamieson G, Valente J, Barnes ND, et al: Liver transplantation for hepatic cirrhosis in cystic fibrosis. Arch Dis Child 71:349–352, 1994.
132. Sokol RJ, Treem WR: Mitochondria and childhood liver diseases. J Pediatr Gastroenterol Nutr 28:4–16, 1999.
133. Munnich A, Rotig A, Chretien D, et al: Clinical presentation of mitochondrial disorders in childhood. J Inherit Metab Dis 19:521–527, 1996.

HEREDITARY HEMOCHROMATOSIS

Chapter 66

Bruce R. Bacon and Robert S. Britton

Trousseau was the first to describe a case of hemochromatosis in the French pathology literature in 1865.[1] Almost 25 years later, in 1889, von Recklinghausen, in the German literature, was the first to use the term *hemochromatosis*, based on the thinking that the disease was a blood disorder that caused increased skin pigmentation.[1] In 1935, Sheldon, a geriatrician, published a description of all 311 cases of the disease that had been reported in the world's medical literature to that time, including several from his own records. His conclusions were borne out over subsequent years. Sheldon realized that hemochromatosis was an inborn error of iron metabolism and that all the pathologic manifestations of the disease were caused by increased iron deposition in the affected organs.[1]

In the 1960s, a controversy developed when MacDonald suggested that hemochromatosis was a nutritional disorder associated with alcoholism.[2] This theory was dispelled in 1976 by the seminal work of Simon and coworkers, who demonstrated that the gene for hereditary hemochromatosis (HH) was linked to the human leukocyte antigen (HLA) region on the short arm of chromosome 6, thus confirming the genetic origin of the disease.[3] The benefit of early diagnosis on survival was clearly shown in a classic paper by Niederau and colleagues, who demonstrated that, if HH is identified before the development of cirrhosis or diabetes, survival is equivalent to that of an age- and gender-matched population.[4] Several population surveys have shown that the frequency of the homozygous disease ranges from 1 in 100 to 1 in 400 in white populations in several areas of the world.[5]

In 1996, the gene for HH, called *HFE*, was identified, thereby allowing genetic testing for the two major mutations (C282Y, H63D) that are responsible for HH.[6] Subsequently, numerous clinical and pathophysiologic studies have led to improved diagnosis, better family screening, and new insights into normal and abnormal iron homeostasis. HH is a common autosomal recessive disorder of iron metabolism; if it is diagnosed early and treated appropriately, affected persons can have a normal life span.

CAUSES OF IRON OVERLOAD

Hereditary hemochromatosis (also called genetic hemochromatosis) is the term used for the inherited disease of iron overload that is *HFE*-related and that is characterized by an inappropriately elevated rate of intestinal iron absorption. The older terms *primary* or *idiopathic hemochromatosis* should no longer be used. The primary genetic defect lies in the regulation of intestinal absorption of iron; additionally, there is an abnormality in the reticuloendothelial metabolism of iron that results in preferential sparing of reticuloendothelial stores of iron. The liver is the principal recipient of the majority of the absorbed iron, and the liver is always involved in HH.

Persons who absorb excessive amounts of iron as a result of an underlying cause other than the *HFE*-related inherited defect have *secondary iron overload*.[7] Examples of secondary iron overload include disorders of ineffective erythropoiesis, some cases of liver disease, increased oral intake of iron, and the rare condition of congenital atransferrinemia. Both HH and the various causes of secondary iron overload should be distinguished from *parenteral iron overload*, which is always iatrogenic and which leads to iron deposition that is found initially in the reticuloendothelial system. In patients with ineffective erythropoiesis who require red blood cell transfusions, parenchymal and reticuloendothelial iron overload coexist, because such persons have a stimulus to increased iron absorption and they receive iron in the form of red blood cell transfusions. A syndrome of *neonatal iron overload* that appears to be distinct from any of the aforementioned disorders has been described.[8] Family studies have failed to show an *HFE*-related form of hemochromatosis in these infants.

Finally, other inherited forms of iron overload that are not *HFE*-related but that result in increased iron absorption have been described. These forms include *juvenile hemochromatosis*,[9] *African iron overload*,[10] iron overload resulting from a mutation in transferrin receptor 2,[11] and an inherited abnormality of iron overload in a three-generation pedigree from Italy.[12] Juvenile hemochromatosis is characterized by rapid iron accumulation and is linked genetically to chromosome 1.[9] African iron overload (formerly known as Bantu hemosiderosis) is characterized by an increase in iron absorption aggravated by the ingestion of large amounts of iron in beer that is home-brewed in steel drums.[10] Disorders of iron overload resulting from mutations in additional genes that regulate iron metabolism may also exist.

PATHOPHYSIOLOGY

The pathophysiologic mechanisms involved in HH can be categorized into three main areas: (1) the function of the HFE protein; (2) the increased intestinal absorption of dietary iron; and (3) iron-induced tissue injury and fibrogenesis. Studies of the structure and function of the HFE protein have been a direct consequence of the cloning of the *HFE* gene. The *HFE* gene encodes a 343-amino acid protein consisting of a 22-amino acid signal peptide, a large extracellular domain, a single transmembrane domain, and a short cytoplasmic tail.[6] The extracellular domain of the HFE protein consists of three loops ($\alpha 1$, $\alpha 2$, and $\alpha 3$), with intramolecular disulfide bonds within the second and third loops. The structure of the HFE protein is similar to that of other major histocompatibility complex (MHC) class I proteins, but HFE protein does not participate in antigen presentation.[13] However, like MHC class I molecules, HFE protein is physically associated with β_2-microglobulin (β_2m).

The major mutation responsible for HH results in the substitution of tyrosine for cysteine at amino acid 282 in the $\alpha 3$ loop (C282Y) and abolishes the disulfide bond in this domain.[6] Loss of this disulfide bond interferes with the interaction of HFE protein with β_2m, and the C282Y mutant protein demonstrates decreased presentation at the cell surface, increased retention in the endoplasmic reticulum, and accelerated degradation.[14] The HH-like phenotype of β_2m-knockout mice provides independent evidence of the importance of the HFE protein-β_2m association for normal HFE protein function.[15] A second mutation associated with HH results in the change of a histidine to an aspartate at position 63 in the $\alpha 1$ chain (H63D), but the functional consequences of this amino acid change on HFE protein are unclear.

Transgenic methodology has provided important information about the consequences of *HFE* gene disruption in the whole animal. Like patients with HH, *HFE*-knockout mice manifest increased hepatic iron levels, elevated transferrin saturation, increased intestinal iron absorption, and relative sparing of iron loading in reticuloendothelial cells.[16–18]

The first identified mechanistic link between HFE protein and cellular iron metabolism was the observation that HFE protein forms a complex with the transferrin receptor (TfR). The physical association of HFE protein with TfR has been observed in cultured cells and in duodenal crypt enterocytes, the site of regulation of dietary iron absorption. Studies examining the stoichiometry of the HFE protein-TfR complex in vitro have provided evidence for both a 1:2 and a 2:2 HFE:TfR monomer relationship,[19] but the precise stoichiometry of HFE protein, TfR, and diferric transferrin at the cell membrane is unknown. The observation that HFE protein and TfR are physically associated has led to a number of investigations on the effect of HFE protein on TfR-mediated iron uptake and cellular iron status.[20] These studies have yielded conflicting results concerning the effects of HFE protein on cellular iron metabolism, and more research is required to resolve this issue, especially in important sites of iron metabolism, such as the duodenum and the reticuloendothelial system.

The primary disorder in HH is an increased rate of intestinal iron absorption relative to body iron stores.[5] The sensing of the body's iron status is thought to occur in the duodenal crypt cells, which subsequently influence the level

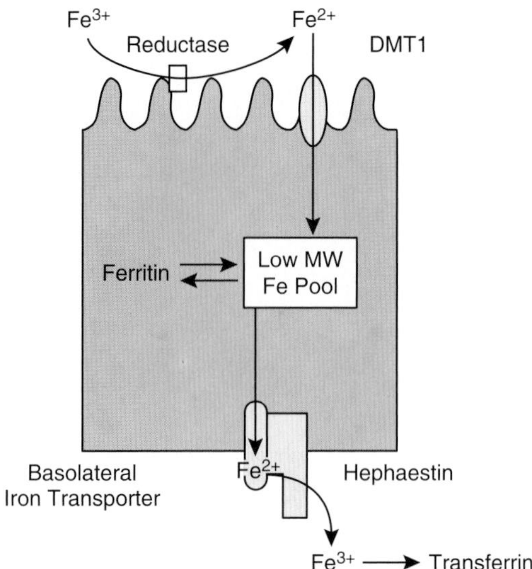

Figure 66–1. Iron absorption pathway in duodenal villus enterocytes. The iron transport protein DMT1 is located on the apical surface of these cells, and its mRNA expression is increased in patients with hereditary hemochromatosis.[26] On the basolateral surface, an iron transporter termed ferroportin1 and a ferroxidase, hephaestin, play important roles in the efflux of iron from villus cells, but their regulation in hereditary hemochromatosis is not yet known. MW, molecular weight.

of dietary iron absorption when these cells differentiate into absorptive enterocytes and migrate to the villus tip.[21] HFE protein is highly expressed in the crypt (but not villus) cells of the duodenum, where it is physically associated with TfR.[22] Dietary iron absorption at the villus tip occurs via the iron transport protein divalent metal transporter-1 (DMT1).[23] This protein is upregulated in iron deficiency via an increase in mRNA levels. Taken together, these observations have led to the proposal[22, 24, 25] that normal HFE protein acts to facilitate the uptake of plasma iron by the TfR-mediated pathway in duodenal crypt cells and that mutant HFE protein lacks this facilitating effect. Functional loss of HFE protein would thereby decrease the regulatory iron pool in crypt cells and increase the binding of iron regulatory protein to iron-responsive elements in certain mRNAs, including the one encoding the iron transport protein DMT1. The result is the increased expression of DMT1 (and perhaps other proteins involved in basolateral iron transport[20] such as ferroportin1 and hephaestin) in daughter villus enterocytes and increased dietary iron absorption (Fig. 66–1). This hypothesis is supported by the demonstration of increased DMT1 mRNA levels in the duodenum of both HFE-knockout mice[24] and patients with HH.[26] Ultimately, testing this working hypothesis for the effect of HFE protein on intestinal iron absorption will require investigation of the consequences of *HFE* mutation on iron homeostasis in the duodenal crypt cell.

The final major pathophysiologic mechanism that should be considered in HH is related to the causes of liver damage in iron overload. In patients with advanced HH, the principal pathologic findings are hepatic fibrosis and cirrhosis. In experimental hepatic iron overload, iron-dependent lipid peroxidation has been identified, and membrane-dependent functions of mitochondria, microsomes, and lysosomes are abnormal when hepatic iron concentrations reach levels at which lipid peroxidation occurs.[27] Finally, a relationship between iron-induced lipid peroxidation and fibrosis has been shown in several studies.[28, 29] One hypothesis is that iron-induced lipid peroxidation occurs in hepatocytes and results in hepatocellular injury or death. Kupffer cells may become activated after the phagocytosis of injured iron-loaded hepatocytes, thereby producing profibrogenic cytokines such as transforming growth factor-β. In turn, these cytokines stimulate hepatic stellate cells to produce increased amounts of collagen, thereby leading to pathologic fibrosis.[28, 29]

Studies of iron-induced tissue damage in organs other than the liver, such as the heart, pancreas, and endocrine glands, have been limited. Studies in myocardial cells have shown functional abnormalities resulting from iron-induced peroxidation.[30]

CLINICAL MANIFESTATIONS

Currently, many patients with HH come to medical attention without any symptoms or physical findings. They are identified as homozygous relatives of probands who are detected by family screening studies or by serum iron studies performed as part of a routine screening blood chemistry panel (Table 66–1).[31, 32] Nonetheless, it is important to appreciate the typical clinical manifestations that may be present in patients with symptomatic disease. Most patients with symptomatic HH are 40 to 50 years of age at the time of diagnosis. Although the defective gene is distributed equally between men and women, most clinical series have identified more men than women, with ratios ranging from 8:1 to 2:1. Thus, the frequency of HH in females is often underestimated when based solely on phenotypic expression, most likely because of iron loss from normal menses and childbirth.

In symptomatic patients, the most common presenting symptoms are weakness, lethargy, arthralgias, abdominal pain, and loss of libido or potency in men.[4, 33] On physical examination, hepatomegaly is found in the majority of patients; splenomegaly and other complications of chronic liver disease, including ascites, edema, and jaundice, may be present. The frequency of diabetes has decreased as a result of earlier diagnosis and is typically not seen in the absence of cirrhosis. The characteristic but subtle bronzed or slate-gray skin pigmentation of HH may be detected by an astute clinician. The degree of organ damage and severity of symptoms are usually related to the degree of iron loading. When patients are identified prospectively by either family screening or population screening, the proportion of patients who are asymptomatic increases dramatically.

All patients with HH have increased hepatic iron stores, but the degree of iron loading is often not high enough to cause liver damage. In the late 1960s, cirrhosis was found in over 50% of patients with a diagnosis of HH[4]; more recent studies since 1985 have identified cirrhosis in only 5% to 10% of patients.[31, 32] Two recent population screening studies from Western Australia[34] and San Diego[35] identified 59 patients with HH, only 1 of whom had cirrhosis. Elevations in serum aminotransferase levels are usually mild and are present in 30% to 50% of patients. With regular phlebotomy and depletion of excess iron stores, liver enzyme abnormalities typically revert to normal. When HH is diagnosed and treated before the development of fibrosis or cirrhosis, long-term hepatic complications do not occur. However, when HH is detected after cirrhosis has developed, hepatocellular carcinoma can occur, even after successful phlebotomy,[36] thus emphasizing the importance of early diagnosis and treatment. Finally, patients with HH may have nonspecific right upper quadrant abdominal pain that most likely is caused by hepatic capsular distention.

Other clinical manifestations of HH relate to the degree of iron loading in nonhepatic organs. In older series, diabetes was a common complication of pancreatic iron loading,[4] but in more recent series of patients diagnosed earlier in the course, diabetes has rarely been present.[31, 32] Other endocri-

Table 66–1 | **Clinical Manifestations of Hereditary Hemochromatosis**

VARIABLE	NIEDERAU ET AL[4]	ADAMS ET AL[31]	BACON AND SADIQ[32]
How patients were identified	Symptomatic index cases, family screening	Family screening by HLA-typing	Screening chemistry panels, family screening
Time period	1959–1983	Before 1990	1990–1995
Number of patients	163	37	40
Men	145	19	26
Women	18	18	14
Mean Age (yr)	46	Men: 49 Women: 53	Men: 46 Women: 47
Range (yr)	18–77	11–79	23–73
Symptoms (%)			
Asymptomatic	9	46	73
Weakness or lethargy	83	19	25
Abdominal pain	58	3	3
Arthralgias	43	40	13
Loss of libido, impotence (% of men)	38	32	12
Findings (%)			
Cirrhosis	69	3	13*
Hepatomegaly	83	3	13
Skin pigmentation	75	9	5
Clinical diabetes	55	11	5
Abnormal liver enzymes	62	27	33

*Five of forty patients had cirrhosis, but one had concomitant chronic hepatitis C, and one had alcoholic liver disease.

nologic abnormalities include loss of libido and impotence in men, owing to both primary testicular failure and gonadotropin insufficiency caused by the effects of iron on pituitary function.[37] Hypothyroidism has been described in patients with HH, but adrenal function is typically normal. Other endocrinologic effects can result from the complications of cirrhosis. Cardiac manifestations are now rare because patients are diagnosed earlier than in the past. Cardiomyopathy, atrial and ventricular dysrhythmias, and congestive heart failure can occur.[38] The arthropathy of HH is characterized most commonly by changes in the second and third metacarpophalangeal joints, including joint space narrowing, chondrocalcinosis, subchondral cyst formation, osteopenia, and swelling of the joints.[4, 33, 39] Unfortunately, the arthritic symptoms of HH usually do not improve with phlebotomy. The skin pigmentation of HH can be subtle and characterized by either a bronze discoloration caused by a predominant deposition of melanin or a gray pigmentation caused by deposition of iron in the basal layers of the epidermis.[33] The risk of certain infections is increased (although still rare) in iron-loaded patients, including those caused by *Vibrio vulnificus, Listeria monocytogenes, Yersinia enterocolitica,* and *Yersinia pseudotuberculosis.*

Table 66–2 | **Representative Iron Measurements in Patients with Hereditary Hemochromatosis**

	NORMAL	HEREDITARY HEMOCHROMATOSIS
Serum		
Iron		
(μg/dL)	60–180	180–300
(μmol/L)	11–32	32–54
Transferrin saturation (%)	20–50	55–100
Ferritin		
Men (ng/mL; μg/L)	20–200	300–3000
Women (ng/mL; μg/L)	15–150	250–3000
Liver		
Iron staining	0, 1+	3+, 4+
Iron concentration		
(μg/g dry weight)	300–1500	3000–30,000
(μmol/g dry weight)	5–27	53–536
Iron index		
(μmol/g dry wt ÷ age in years)	<1.1	>1.9

DIAGNOSIS

The requirements for diagnosis of HH have changed since the availability of *HFE* mutation analysis. However, as in the past, a high index of suspicion is required, and abnormal results of laboratory tests (liver enzymes, screening iron studies) should not be ignored. If the diagnosis of HH is a possibility, then serum iron studies (see later) along with *HFE* mutation analysis should be obtained. With the advent of genetic testing, the need for liver biopsy has diminished. The diagnosis of HH should be considered in patients with symptoms seen in HH (most commonly fatigue, malaise, right upper quadrant abdominal pain, and arthralgias), symptoms of chronic liver disease, diabetes, and congestive heart failure. Many of these symptoms are nonspecific or are related to other common diseases, and HH is frequently not considered when symptomatic patients are first encountered.

In the early 1990s, most patients with HH were discovered because of screening blood chemistries obtained as part of routine health maintenance or for some other unassociated reason.[32] Many commercial laboratories had added iron and total iron binding capacity (TIBC) with a calculated transferrin saturation (iron ÷ TIBC x 100%) to their panel of screening serum chemistries. Thus, many patients inadvertently had a transferrin saturation (TS) obtained even though it was not specifically ordered. In one series, 62% of patients with newly identified HH between 1990 and 1995 were found to have come to medical attention in this way.[32] Another 14% were identified by screening of family members of a known proband. Thus, as many as 75% of patients came to medical attention because of screening laboratory tests; the majority of these patients were asymptomatic and had no physical findings, and the frequency of end-stage complications of HH such as cirrhosis and diabetes was much lower than that found in earlier series of patients who presented with symptoms of the disease.[32] However, in 1998, the Health Care Finance Administration (HCFA) stopped providing reimbursement for screening tests of any kind, and fewer American patients are now identified because of routine screening.

Once HH has been considered, the diagnosis is relatively straightforward. A serum iron and TIBC or transferrin level with calculation of the TS along with a serum ferritin level should be obtained in the fasting state (Table 66–2). Over 50% of patients have transiently elevated serum iron levels after eating, and if the blood sample is not drawn in the fasting state, the TS can be elevated in the absence of increased iron stores. In addition to an increased serum iron level after meals, there is a diurnal variation in serum iron concentration. For these reasons, blood should be drawn for serum iron studies from fasting patients in the morning. A TS of greater than 45% is the earliest phenotypic manifestation of HH; as a result, TS is more sensitive and specific than the serum ferritin level, which can be normal in young persons with HH or elevated for a variety of reasons other than HH, including various types of necroinflammatory liver disease (e.g., chronic viral hepatitis, alcoholic liver disease, nonalcoholic fatty liver disease), certain malignancies, and other inflammatory conditions.

In most cases, a person with an elevated ferritin level but a normal TS and another inflammatory disorder does not have HH. On the other hand, an elevated TS with a normal ferritin level in a young person does not exclude HH. A recent large population screening study from San Diego demonstrated that 1 in 237 persons is homozygous for the C282Y mutation in *HFE* but only 64% of these homozygotes have a TS greater than 45%.[35] These findings indicate that the proportion of nonexpressing C282Y homozygotes is much higher than had previously been recognized.

The combination of an elevated TS level and an elevated ferritin level in an otherwise healthy person has a sensitivity rate of 93% for HH.[40] In someone older than age 35 years, the combination of a normal ferritin level and a normal TS has a negative predictive accuracy of 97%, indicating that there is only a 3% chance of missing a diagnosis of HH in a patient of this age or older with normal iron studies.[40] These conclusions were based on a study using HLA-typing to

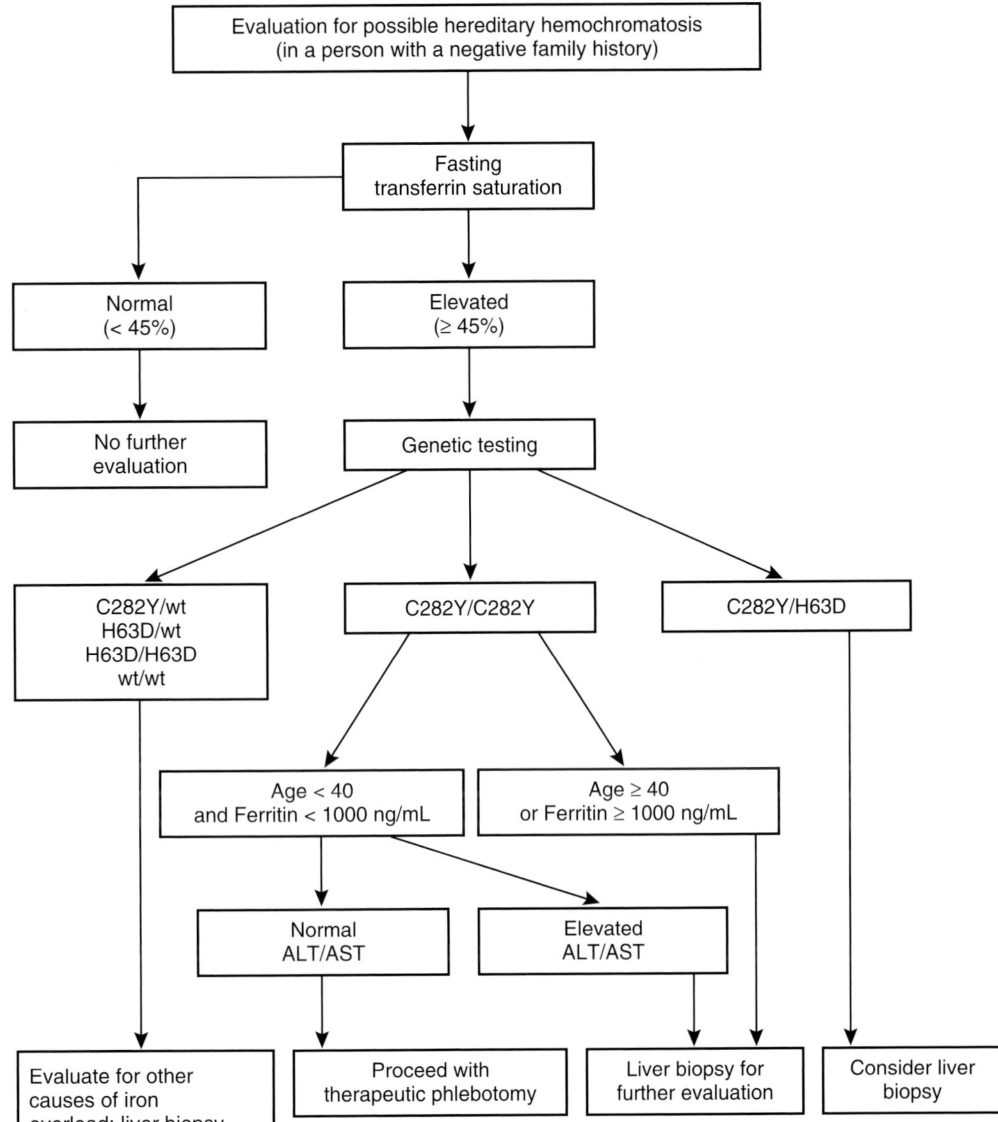

Figure 66–2. An algorithm for the evaluation of persons with possible hereditary hemochromatosis.[41] ALT, alanine aminotransferase; AST, aspartate aminotransferase; wt, wild type.

identify young siblings of affected probands; thus, they will need to be confirmed in population studies using genetic testing.

Once abnormal serum iron studies have been determined in the appropriate setting, the next test that should be performed is *HFE* mutation analysis. If the patient is a C282Y homozygote or a compound heterozygote (C282Y/H63D), is less than 40 years of age, has a serum ferritin level of less than 1000 ng/mL, and has normal liver enzymes and no evidence of hepatomegaly, then there is no need for a liver biopsy.[41–43] With the advent of genetic testing, liver biopsy is performed only to assess the degree of damage (if any) to the liver. When liver biopsy is performed, sufficient tissue for histopathologic evaluation and for biochemical measurement of the hepatic iron concentration (HIC) should be obtained. An algorithm has been proposed for evaluating persons with possible HH and determining who should undergo liver biopsy (Fig. 66–2).[41]

When liver biopsy is performed, the Perls' Prussian blue stain is used for the determination and localization of storage iron. Iron stores are typically found in a periportal distribution in hepatocytes, with little or no iron found in Kupffer cells (Fig. 66–3; see also Color Fig. 66–3*B*).[44] In patients with a higher HIC, iron distribution becomes panlobular, and storage iron can be seen in Kupffer cells and in bile duct cells. Grade 1 or 2 Perls' Prussian blue staining can be seen in normal liver or in patients with early HH, confirmed by *HFE* mutation analysis. Grade 3 stainable iron can occasionally be seen in alcoholic cirrhosis but correlates poorly with HIC in this setting. In the absence of other disorders, grade 3 to grade 4 stainable iron is consistent with HH. In addition to histochemical staining, biochemical iron measurement is important (see Table 66–2). Typically, patients with HH who present with symptoms will have an HIC of greater than 10,000 μg/g (dry weight) (normal <1500 μg/g), and levels may be 30,000 μg/g or higher. In uncomplicated HH, fibrosis and cirrhosis usually are not seen until the HIC exceeds 20,000 μg/g.[45] In patients with both HH and other

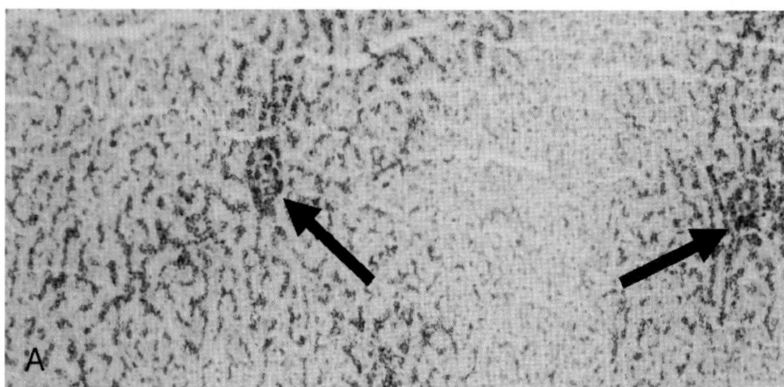

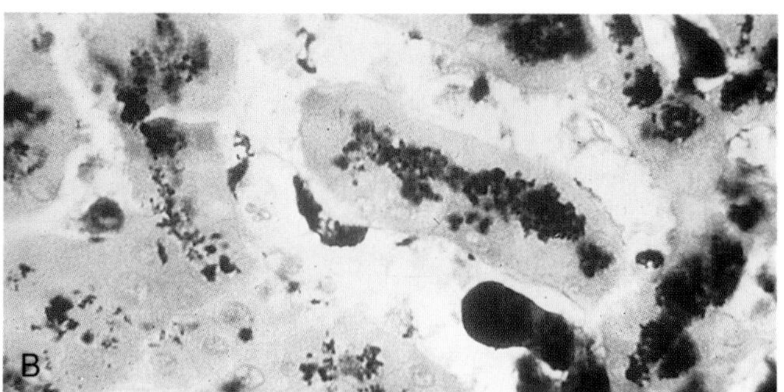

Figure 66–3. Histology of hereditary hemochromatosis. *A*, This liver biopsy specimen is from a 47-year-old woman who presented with a transferrin saturation of 63% and a serum ferritin level of 590 ng/mL. The hepatic iron concentration was 9840 μg/g, with a calculated hepatic iron index of 3.7. At low power, iron deposition is seen to be much greater in the periportal zone (acinar zone 1) *(arrows)* than in the centrilobular zone (acinar zone 3). Perls' Prussian blue stain, magnification × 100. (Courtesy of E. M. Brunt, MD). *B*, At a higher power of a specimen from another patient with hereditary hemochromatosis, iron deposition is seen to be in hepatocytes arranged in cords and not in reticuloendothelial (Kupffer) cells that line the intervening sinusoids. In patients with higher hepatic iron concentrations, iron deposition becomes panlobular, and storage iron can be in Kupffer cells and bile duct cells. Perls' Prussian blue stain. (Courtesy of Edward Lee, MD.)

forms of chronic liver disease, such as alcoholic liver disease or chronic viral hepatitis, increased fibrosis or cirrhosis can occur at a much lower HIC.[46, 47] In asymptomatic or younger patients with early HH, the HIC will be increased to a lesser degree, and levels often are much less than 10,000 μg/g.

A frequent diagnostic dilemma occurs when it is not clear whether a patient has liver disease with abnormal iron studies or HH with abnormal liver enzymes. In this setting, *HFE* mutation analysis is extremely useful. If the patient is a C282Y homozygote or a compound heterozygote (C282Y/H63D), then the iron loading is most likely due predominantly to the genetic abnormality. On the other hand, if the patient has underlying liver disease and is a C282Y heterozygote, an H63D heterozygote, or an H63D homozygote, or has neither mutation, then the iron loading is most likely due to the underlying liver disease, perhaps with a minor component due to the *HFE* genotype. In the past, the hepatic iron index (HIC in μmoles/g ÷ the patient's age in years) was useful for distinguishing HH from secondary iron overload.[45] With the advent of *HFE* mutation analysis, the value of the hepatic iron index has diminished.

Computed tomography, magnetic resonance imaging, and magnetic susceptibility testing have all been proposed as techniques to quantify HIC without the need for a liver biopsy. However, computed tomography and magnetic resonance imaging are usually not reliable in early HH in mildly iron-loaded persons, and magnetic susceptibility is available only as a research tool. The usefulness of these modalities has diminished since *HFE* mutation analysis became available.

TREATMENT AND PROGNOSIS

The treatment of HH is relatively straightforward and simple, because most patients can be treated with routine therapeutic phlebotomy (Table 66–3). Ideally, diagnosis and initiation of treatment should begin before the development of fibrosis or cirrhosis. If treatment is initiated before cirrhosis develops, the patient will have a normal life span. Each unit of whole blood (500 mL) contains approximately 200 to 250 mg of iron, depending on the hemoglobin level; therefore, homozygotes who have 10 to 20 g of excess storage iron will require extended phlebotomy regimens (40 to 80 units). Most patients can tolerate weekly phlebotomy of 1 unit of whole blood, and, occasionally, younger patients can tolerate the removal of 2 or 3 units per week. Some older patients or occasionally patients with a coexistent underlying hematologic disorder resulting in anemia can tolerate phlebotomy of only 0.5 unit per week or every other week. The iron-chelating drug deferoxamine is used in patients with HH who have cardiac manifestations or who cannot tolerate phlebotomy. Although not absolutely necessary, it is useful to obtain a TS and ferritin level every 2 to 3 months to predict the eventual return to normal iron stores.[33] Typically, the serum ferritin level will fall progressively as iron stores decrease, whereas TS usually remains elevated until just before normal iron stores are reached. In uncomplicated patients, the ferritin level will drop about 30 ng/mL for each unit of blood removed. Once the iron stores have reached a low normal level, the ferritin level should be less than 50 ng/mL, with a TS of less than 50%. At this point, maintenance phlebotomy every 2 to 3 months will be required in most patients. The rate of reaccumulation of iron varies among persons, and some patients may require regular phlebotomy at more or less frequent intervals.

The prognosis of patients with HH has been improved significantly by therapeutic phlebotomy.[4, 48, 49] Life expectancy is reduced in patients who present with cirrhosis or diabetes, and there is an increased risk of death from hepatocellular carcinoma in patients with HH. Hepatocellular cancer is usually seen only in patients who already have cirrho-

Table 66–3 | **Treatment of Hereditary Hemochromatosis**

Perform weekly phlebotomy of 500 mL (1 unit) of whole blood until hematocrit value drops below 37%
Check transferrin saturation and ferritin levels at 2- to 3-month intervals to monitor response (optional)
Once iron stores are depleted (ferritin: <50 ng/mL; transferrin saturation: <50%), proceed to maintenance phlebotomy of 1 unit of whole blood every 2 to 3 months

sis. Reversal of fibrosis or established cirrhosis typically does not occur with phlebotomy; however, as many as 30% of patients may have some reduction in the degree of fibrosis if they are treated aggressively. Unfortunately, neither arthritis nor hypogonadism improves. Management of diabetes may become easier after removal of iron. The value of screening for hepatocellular carcinoma in cirrhotic HH patients is controversial, because the cost-effectiveness of the screening regimens has not been validated; however, most authorities recommend an abdominal ultrasound and a serum α-fetoprotein level every 6 months in patients with HH and cirrhosis.

When diagnosis and treatment of HH are delayed and complications of end-stage liver disease develop, orthotopic liver transplantation may be an option. Although the experience with orthotopic liver transplantation for HH is limited, the existing data indicate that the mortality rate is higher for transplantation for HH than for other causes of end-stage liver disease.[50, 51] The increased mortality relates to iron overload, whether caused by HH or secondary iron overload in conjunction with another liver disease such as chronic hepatitis C or alcoholic liver disease. In fact, only approximately 10% of patients with iron overload in the setting of end-stage liver disease are C282Y homozygotes.[52] Therefore, when iron overload is recognized, it should be treated to decrease the rate of post-transplantation mortality.

Post-transplant deaths are usually related to infectious or cardiac complications.[52, 53] Unfortunately, HH or secondary iron overload often is not diagnosed before transplantation. Moreover, one series has shown a high frequency of primary liver cancer diagnosed incidentally at the time of transplantation.[50] Another factor that may account for the increase in post-transplantation mortality rates for HH is the extent of iron deposition in extrahepatic sites in previously undiagnosed and untreated patients. A high index of suspicion for iron overload in patients with end-stage liver disease should lead to improved diagnosis and allow for prompt institution of either phlebotomy or iron-chelation therapy before transplantation. It is anticipated that improved management will reduce post-transplantation complications and improve long-term survival.

FAMILY SCREENING

Once a proband with HH has been identified and therapy initiated, there is still a responsibility to the patient's family. For asymptomatic C282Y homozygotes and compound heterozygotes (C282Y/H63D) identified by *HFE* mutation analysis within a sibship, there is no need for liver biopsy. In this setting, it is reasonable to proceed to therapeutic phlebotomy, reserving liver biopsy for those patients in whom a question of another underlying liver disease may exist. Persons who are C282Y heterozygotes are not at risk of progressive iron overload. If the spouse of a C282Y homozygote is a C282Y heterozygote, there is a 50% chance that a child of the couple will be homozygous for C282Y. *HFE* mutation analysis in children can eliminate the need for subsequent serum iron testing if a genotype of C282Y/C282Y or C282Y/H63D is not found, although the possibility of genetic discrimination and stigmatization must be acknowledged and considered. In children who are C282Y homozygotes or compound heterozygotes, ferritin levels should be measured yearly and phlebotomy instituted when ferritin levels become elevated.

REFERENCES

1. Bacon BR: Joseph H. Sheldon and hereditary hemochromatosis: Historical highlights. J Lab Clin Med 113:761, 1989.
2. MacDonald RA: Hemochromatosis and Hemosiderosis. Springfield, IL, Charles C Thomas, 1964.
3. Simon M, Bourel M, Fauchet R, et al: Association of HLA-A_3 and HLA-B_{14} antigens with idiopathic hemochromatosis. Gut 17:332, 1976.
4. Niederau C, Fischer R, Sonnenberg A, et al: Survival and causes of death in cirrhotic and noncirrhotic patients with primary hemochromatosis. N Engl J Med 313:1265, 1985.
5. Bacon BR, Powell LW, Adams PC, et al: Molecular medicine and hemochromatosis: At the crossroads. Gastroenterology 116:193, 1999.
6. Feder JN, Gnirke A, Thomas W, et al: A novel MHC class 1-like gene is mutated in patients with hereditary haemochromatosis. Nat Genet 13: 339, 1996.
7. Pippard MJ: Secondary iron overload. In Brock JH, Halliday JW, Pippard MJ, et al (eds): Iron Metabolism in Health and Disease. Philadelphia, WB Saunders, 1994, p 271.
8. Knisely AS: Neonatal hemochromatosis. Adv Pediatr 39:383, 1992.
9. Roetto A, Totaro A, Cazzola M, et al: Juvenile hemochromatosis locus maps to chromosome 1q. Am J Hum Genet 64:1388, 1999.
10. Gordeuk VR, Mukubi J, Hasstedt J, et al: Iron overload in Africa—interaction between a gene and dietary iron content. N Engl J Med 326: 95, 1992.
11. Camaschella C, Roetto A, Cali A, et al: The gene TFR2 is mutated in a new type of haemochromatosis mapping to 7q22. Nat Genet 25:14, 2000.
12. Pietrangelo A, Montosi G, Totaro A, et al: Hereditary hemochromatosis in adults without pathogenic mutations in the hemochromatosis gene. N Engl J Med 341:725, 1999.
13. Lebron JA, Bennett MJ, Vaughn DE, et al: Crystal structure of the hemochromatosis protein HFE and characterization of its interaction with transferrin receptor. Cell 93:111, 1998.
14. Waheed A, Parkkila S, Zhou XY, et al: Hereditary hemochromatosis: Effects of C282Y and H63D mutations on association with β2-microglobulin, intracellular processing, and cell surface expression of the HFE protein in COS-7 cells. Proc Natl Acad Sci USA 94:12384, 1997.
15. de Sousa M, Reimao R, Lacerda R, et al: Iron overload in β2-microglobulin-deficient mice. Immunol Lett 39:105, 1994.
16. Zhou XY, Tomatsu S, Fleming RE, et al: HFE gene knockout produces mouse model of hereditary hemochromatosis. Proc Natl Acad Sci USA 95:2492, 1998.
17. Bahram S, Gilfillan S, Kuhn LC, et al: Experimental hemochromatosis due to MHC class I HFE deficiency: Immune status and iron metabolism. Proc Natl Acad Sci USA 96:13312, 1999.
18. Levy JE, Montross LK, Cohen DE, et al: The C282Y mutation causing hereditary hemochromatosis does not produce a null allele. Blood 94:9, 1999.
19. Bennett MJ, Lebron JA, Bjorkman PJ: Crystal structure of the hereditary haemochromatosis protein HFE complexed with transferrin receptor. Nature 403:46, 2000.
20. Roy CN, Enns CA: Iron homeostasis: New tales from the crypt. Blood 96:4020, 2000.
21. Anderson GJ: Control of iron absorption. J Gastroenterol Hepatol 11: 1030, 1996.
22. Waheed A, Parkkila S, Saarnio J, et al: Association of HFE protein with transferrin receptor in crypt enterocytes of human duodenum. Proc Natl Acad Sci USA 96:1579, 1999.
23. Andrews NC: Disorders of iron metabolism. N Engl J Med 341:1986, 1999.
24. Fleming RE, Migas MC, Zhou X, et al: Mechanism of increased iron absorption in murine model of hereditary hemochromatosis: Increased duodenal expression of the iron transporter DMT1. Proc Natl Acad Sci USA 96:3143, 1999.
25. Kuhn LC: Iron overload: Molecular clues to its cause. Trends Biochem Sci 24:164, 1999.
26. Zoller H, Pietrangelo A, Vogel W, Weiss G: Duodenal metal-trans-

porter (DMT1, NRAMP-2) expression in patients with hereditary haemochromatosis. Lancet 353:2120, 1999.
27. Bacon BR, Britton RS: The pathology of hepatic iron overload: A free radical-mediated process? Hepatology 11:127, 1990.
28. Britton RS, Bacon BR: Role of free radicals in liver diseases and hepatic fibrosis. Hepatogastroenterology 41:343, 1994.
29. Pietrangelo A: Iron, oxidative stress and liver fibrogenesis. J Hepatol 28(Suppl 1):8, 1998.
30. Hershko C, Link G, Cabantchik I: Pathophysiology of iron overload. Ann N Y Acad Sci 850:191, 1998.
31. Adams PC, Kertesz AE, Valberg LS: Clinical presentation of hemochromatosis: A changing scene. Am J Med 90:445, 1991.
32. Bacon BR, Sadiq SA: Hereditary hemochromatosis: Presentation and diagnosis in the 1990s. Am J Gastroenterol 92:784, 1997.
33. Edwards CQ, Cartwright GE, Skolnick MH, et al: Homozygosity for hemochromatosis: Clinical manifestations. Ann Intern Med 93:511, 1980.
34. Olynyk JK, Cullen DJ, Aquilia S, et al: A population-based study of the clinical expression of the hemochromatosis gene. N Engl J Med 341:718, 1999.
35. Beutler E, Felitti V, Gelbart T, Ho N: The effect of HFE genotypes on measurements of iron overload in patients attending a health appraisal clinic. Ann Intern Med 133:329, 2000.
36. Deugnier YM, Guyader D, Crantook L, et al: Primary liver cancer in genetic hemochromatosis: A clinical, pathological, and pathogenetic study of 54 cases. Gastroenterology 104:228, 1992.
37. Lufkin EG, Baldus WP, Bergstralh EJ, et al: Influence of phlebotomy treatment on abnormal hypothalamic-pituitary function in genetic hemochromatosis. Mayo Clin Proc 62:473, 1987.
38. Olson LJ, Edwards WD, Holmes DR, et al: Endomyocardial biopsy in hemochromatosis: Clinicopathologic correlates in six cases. J Am Coll Cardiol 13:116, 1989.
39. Shumacher HR: Articular cartilage in the degenerative arthropathy of hemochromatosis. Arthritis Rheum 25:1460, 1982.
40. Bassett ML, Halliday JW, Ferris RA, et al: Diagnosis of hemochromatosis in young subjects: Predictive accuracy of biochemical screening tests. Gastroenterology 87:628, 1984.
41. Bacon BR, Olynyk JK, Brunt EM, et al: *HFE* genotype in patients with hemochromatosis and other liver diseases. Ann Intern Med 130:953, 1999.
42. Guyader D, Jacquelinet C, Moirand R, et al: Noninvasive prediction of fibrosis in C282Y homozygous hemochromatosis. Gastroenterology 115:929, 1998.
43. Powell LW: Hereditary hemochromatosis. Pathology 32:24, 2000.
44. Brunt EM, Olynyk JK, Britton RS, et al: Histological evaluation of iron in liver biopsies: Relationship to *HFE* mutations. Am J Gastroenterol 95:1788, 2000.
45. Bassett ML, Halliday JW, Powell LW: Value of hepatic iron measurements in early hemochromatosis and determination of the critical iron level associated with fibrosis. Hepatology 6:24, 1986.
46. LeSage GD, Baldus WP, Fairbanks VF, et al: Hemochromatosis: Genetic or alcohol-induced? Gastroenterology 84:1471, 1983.
47. Bonkovsky HL, Banner BF, Rothman AL: Iron and chronic viral hepatitis. Hepatology 25:759, 1997.
48. Adams PC, Speechley M, Kertesz AE: Long-term survival analysis in hereditary hemochromatosis. Gastroenterology 101:368, 1991.
49. Niederau C, Fischer R, Pürschel A, et al: Long-term survival in patients with hereditary hemochromatosis. Gastroenterology 110:1107, 1996.
50. Kowdley KV, Hassanein T, Kaur S, et al: Primary liver cancer and survival in patients undergoing liver transplantation for hemochromatosis. Liver Transpl Surg 1:237, 1995.
51. Poulos JE, Bacon BR: Transplantation for hemochromatosis. Dig Dis 14:316, 1996.
52. Brandhagen DJ, Alvarez W, Therneau TM, et al: Iron overload in cirrhosis: *HFE* genotypes and outcome after liver transplantation Hepatology 31:456, 2000.
53. Tung BY, Farrell FJ, McCashland TM, et al: Long-term follow-up after liver transplantation in patients with hepatic iron overload. Liver Transpl Surg 5:369, 1999.

Chapter 67

Wilson Disease

Diane W. Cox and Eve A. Roberts

Copper, a component of several essential enzymes, is toxic to tissues when present in excess. Dietary intake of copper generally exceeds the trace amount required, and mechanisms to control influx and efflux from cells must maintain an appropriate balance. Two disorders of copper transport are known: Menkes disease, an X-linked defect in transport of copper from the intestine, and Wilson disease, an autosomal recessive disorder of copper overload. Wilson disease was first described in 1912 by Kinnear Wilson as a familial disorder characterized by progressive, lethal neurologic disease with chronic liver disease and a corneal abnormality, the Kayser-Fleischer ring.[1] He also observed that some younger siblings of typical patients died of severe liver disease without developing neurologic abnormalities. In Wilson disease, inadequate biliary copper excretion leads to copper accumulation in the liver, brain, kidney, and cornea. The incidence in most populations is approximately 1 in 30,000.

THE COPPER PATHWAY

Dietary copper is absorbed in the upper intestine and binds to the serum protein albumin. Albumin and trace amounts of copper-histidine transport copper to a variety of tissues; most is transported to the liver. Transcuprein and ceruloplasmin also may be involved in transport. Trace amounts of copper are required for essential enzymes that affect connective tissue and elastin cross-linking (lysyl oxidase), free radical scavenging (superoxide dismutase), electron transfer (cytochrome oxidase), pigment production (tyrosinase), and neurotransmission (dopamine β-mono-oxygenase). Copper in hepatocytes and in other cells is bound to metallochaperones, which are low-molecular-weight proteins that each deliver copper to a specific target molecule.[2]

In the liver, copper is incorporated into apoceruloplasmin to form ceruloplasmin (also called holoceruloplasmin). More than 90% of the copper in plasma is an integral part of ceruloplasmin, an α2-glycoprotein containing 6 molecules of copper, with a molecular weight of 132 kD. The normal serum concentration of ceruloplasmin in adults, measured by immunochemical or enzymatic techniques, is 200 to 350 mg/L; the level is very low at birth and rises to 300 to 500 mg/L in the first years of life. Ceruloplasmin is an acute-phase protein and is elevated by inflammatory hepatic disease, pregnancy, or the use of exogenous estrogen. The majority of ingested copper is excreted via the bile; a small fraction is excreted in urine. When tissues such as the intestine or liver are overloaded with copper, metallothioneins are induced. These are low-molecular-weight, cysteine-rich proteins that sequester copper in a nontoxic form. The normal pathway of copper transport is shown in Figure 67–1.

THE BASIC MOLECULAR DEFECT

Our understanding of the basic defect in Wilson disease has increased dramatically with the cloning of the genes for X-linked Menkes disease and for Wilson disease.[3, 4] The gene for Menkes disease (*ATP7A*), which was cloned by using a chromosomal breakpoint in an affected female, was found to be related to bacterial copper resistance genes. Cloning of the Wilson disease gene (*ATP7B*) was accomplished by a combination of conventional linkage analysis,[5] physical mapping of the relevant region of chromosome 13q14, and recognition that the gene has high homology with the Menkes disease gene.[3, 4] The coding region of the gene is 4.1 kb in length, with mRNA of about 8 kb. The product is a membrane P-type adenosine triphosphatase (ATPase) that consists of 1443 amino acid residues and has a molecular mass of 160 kD. There are predicted to be six copper-binding motifs, a phosphorylation motif, an ATP-binding region, and eight transmembrane motifs[3] (Fig. 67–2). All functionally important regions are conserved in bacteria and yeast.

Although the gene for Menkes disease is expressed in many tissues, including muscle, kidney, heart, and intestine, the gene for Wilson disease is expressed predominantly in the liver and kidney, with minor expression in the brain, lungs, and placenta. Studies in cultured cells show localization of the protein in the trans-Golgi network, with trafficking from the trans-Golgi network to cytoplasmic vesicles in the presence of increased copper.[6] The protein is found at the apical membrane in hepatocytes, consistent with its proposed function of facilitating excretion of copper via bile.[7] Mutations in the *ATP7A* gene result in retention of copper in the liver as well as impaired incorporation of copper into ceruloplasmin.

The Long-Evans cinnamon (LEC) rat and the toxic milk (tx) mouse have mutations in their homologous *Atp7B* genes and are thus suitable models for the study of disease mechanisms and therapy.[8, 9]

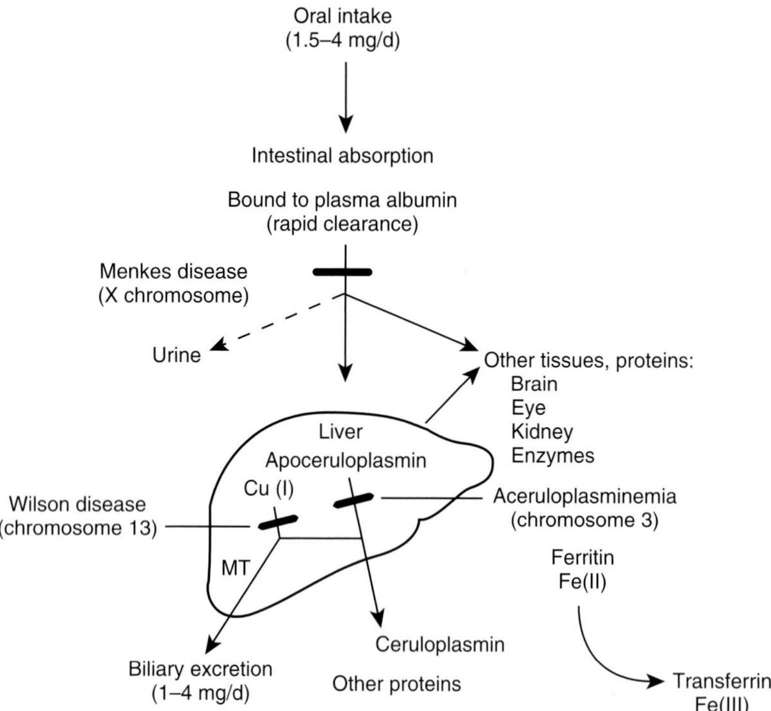

Figure 67–1. Simplified overview of the pathways for copper ion transport. MT, metallothioneins. (Modified from Cox DW: Genes of the copper pathway. Am J Hum Genet 56:828, 1995.)

CLINICAL FEATURES

The clinical presentation of Wilson disease is extremely variable. The age at onset of symptoms is usually from 6 to 40 years. Wilson disease with hepatic involvement has been identified in patients less than 5 years old and even for the first time in patients older than 50 years of age. The presentation may be as chronic or fulminant liver disease, a progressive neurologic disorder without clinically prominent hepatic dysfunction, isolated acute hemolysis, or psychiatric illness. Clinical variability occasionally makes confirmation of the diagnosis difficult.

Hepatic Presentation

The hepatic presentation of Wilson disease is more common in children than in adult patients. Wilson disease should be considered as a possible diagnosis in any child, symptomatic or not, with hepatomegaly, persistently elevated serum aminotransferase levels, or evidence of fatty liver. Symptoms may be vague and nonspecific, such as fatigue, anorexia, or abdominal pain. Occasionally patients present with a self-limited clinical illness resembling acute hepatitis, with malaise, anorexia, nausea, jaundice, elevated serum aminotransferase levels, and abnormal coagulation tests. Some patients

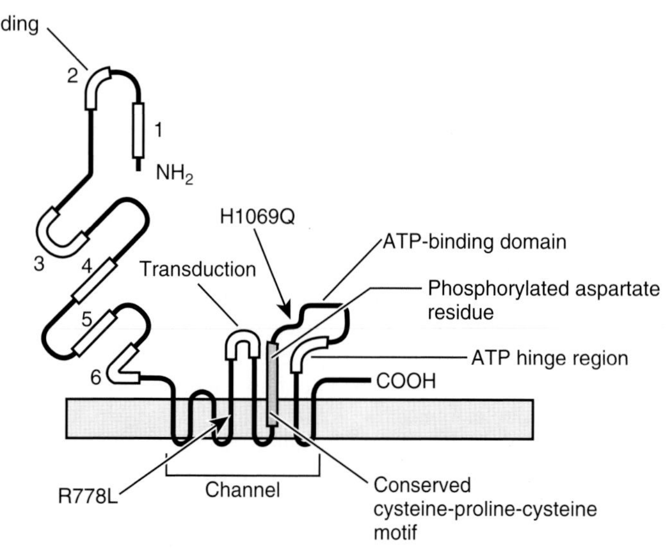

Figure 67–2. A model of the predicted product of the Wilson disease gene. The functional domains conserved in the Menkes disease gene are indicated. Two common missense mutations (*arrows*) are shown: H1069Q and R778L (see text). Numerous mutations occur in functionally important regions: transmembrane (particularly Tm 4) and the ATP-binding domain. (Model modified from Bull PC, Cox DW: Wilson disease and Menkes disease: New handles on heavy-metal transport. Trends Genet 10:246, 1994.)

have a history of self-limited jaundice, apparently caused by unexplained hemolysis. Patients may present with severe, established chronic liver disease characterized by hepatomegaly, ascites, congestive splenomegaly, a low serum albumin level, and persistently abnormal coagulation tests. Some patients have isolated splenomegaly without hepatomegaly. Many of these findings relate to portal hypertension as a consequence of Wilson disease rather than to the metabolic disorder itself.

Wilson disease may present in children and young adults with clinical liver disease indistinguishable from autoimmune hepatitis (previously called *chronic active hepatitis*).[10] As in autoimmune hepatitis, patients may seem to have an acute illness. Fatigue, malaise, arthropathy, and rashes may occur; laboratory findings include elevated serum aminotransferase levels, a greatly increased serum immunoglobulin (Ig) G concentration, and positive nonspecific autoantibodies such as antinuclear antibody and antismooth muscle (antiactin) antibody. Wilson disease must be specifically ruled out, because the treatment of the two diseases is entirely different. With appropriate treatment, the long-term outlook for patients with Wilson disease manifesting as autoimmune hepatitis appears to be favorable even if cirrhosis is present.

Wilson disease may present as fulminant hepatic failure, with severe coagulopathy and encephalopathy.[11] Acute intravascular hemolysis is usually present. Renal failure may develop. Because the patient typically has not been suspected to have underlying liver disease, fulminant viral hepatitis is usually the working diagnosis. Unlike fulminant viral hepatitis, fulminant Wilson disease is usually characterized by disproportionately low serum aminotransferase levels (usually much less than 1500 U/L) from the onset of clinically apparent disease. Serum levels of alkaline phosphatase are in the normal range or even low for age, and the serum bilirubin level is often disproportionately elevated as a result of hemolysis.[12] However, simple biochemical indices are not specific.[13] Slit-lamp examination may reveal Kayser-Fleischer rings. Urinary copper excretion is greatly elevated. These patients do not respond well to chelation treatment and require urgent liver transplantation. This presentation of Wilson disease is more common than initially supposed, and these patients account for a significant proportion of liver transplant recipients each year.

Recurrent bouts of hemolysis may predispose to the development of gallstones. Cirrhosis, if present, may be a further predisposing factor. Children with unexplained cholelithiasis, particularly with small bilirubinate stones, should be tested for Wilson disease. Unlike other types of chronic liver disease, Wilson disease is rarely complicated by hepatocellular carcinoma.

In patients who have predominantly hepatic disease, evidence of subtle neurologic involvement often can be found. Mood disturbance (mainly depression, but sometimes impulsive or neurotic behavior), changes in school performance or handwriting, and clumsiness may be identified by careful direct questioning. A soft whispery voice (hypophonia) is another early feature of neurologic involvement.

Neurologic Presentation

The neurologic presentation of Wilson disease tends to occur in the second and third decades or later but has been reported in children as young as 6 to 10 years old. Patients with a neurologic presentation usually have hepatic involvement, albeit often asymptomatic. Neurologic involvement follows two main patterns: movement disorder or rigid dystonia.[14] Movement disorders tend to occur earlier and include tremors, poor coordination, and loss of fine motor control. Spastic dystonic disorders generally develop later, with masklike facies, rigidity, and gait disturbance as well as pseudobulbar involvement, such as dysarthria, drooling, and swallowing difficulty. Intellect is not impaired.

Psychiatric Presentation

As many as 20% of patients may present with purely psychiatric symptoms.[15] These symptoms are highly variable, although depression is common. Neurotic behavior such as phobias or compulsive behaviors have been reported; aggressive or antisocial behavior may occur.

Ocular Signs

The classic Kayser-Fleischer ring, which is found at the limbus, is caused by copper deposition in Descemet's membrane in the cornea. Copper is actually distributed throughout the cornea, but fluid streaming favors accumulation in this layer, especially at the superior and inferior poles, and eventually circumferentially around the iris. Kayser-Fleischer rings are visible on direct inspection only when the iris pigmentation is light and copper deposition is heavy. A careful slit-lamp examination is mandatory. Copper deposition in the lens ("sunflower cataract"), which does not interfere with vision, may be seen on slit-lamp examination and, like Kayser-Fleischer rings, disappears on chelation therapy. Kayser-Fleischer rings may be absent in 15% to 50% of patients with exclusively hepatic involvement and in presymptomatic patients. Most patients with a neurologic or psychiatric presentation of Wilson disease will have Kayser-Fleischer rings; only 5% do not. Kayser-Fleischer rings are not specific for Wilson disease. They may be found in patients with other types of chronic liver disease, usually with a prominent cholestatic component, such as primary biliary cirrhosis, primary sclerosing cholangitis, autoimmune hepatitis, or familial cholestatic syndromes. Kayser-Fleischer rings have also been reported in patients with non-hepatic diseases.

Involvement of Other Systems

Wilson disease can be accompanied by various extrahepatic disorders besides neurologic disease. Episodes of hemolytic anemia can result from the sudden release of copper into the blood. Renal disease, mainly Fanconi syndrome, may be prominent. Findings include microscopic hematuria, aminoaciduria, phosphaturia, and defective acidification of the urine. Nephrolithiasis also has been reported. Arthritis affecting mainly the large joints may occur as a result of synovial copper accumulation. Other musculoskeletal problems include osteoporosis and osteochondritis dissecans. Vitamin D–resistant rickets may develop as a result of the renal damage. Copper deposition in the heart can lead to cardiomyopathy or cardiac arrhythmias. Sudden death in Wilson disease has been attributed to cardiac involvement but is rare. Copper deposition in skeletal muscle can cause rhabdomyolysis. Endocrine disorders also can occur. Hypoparathyroidism has been attributed to copper deposition. Amenorrhea and testicular problems appear to be caused by Wilson disease itself, not as a consequence of cirrhosis. Pancreatitis, possibly resulting from copper deposition in the pancreas, also may occur.

PATHOLOGY

In the earliest stages, before cirrhosis develops, histologic findings in the liver include steatosis, focal necrosis, glycogenated nuclei in hepatocytes, and sometimes apoptotic bodies. As parenchymal damage progresses, possibly by repeated episodes of lobular necrosis, periportal fibrosis develops. Cirrhosis is usually macronodular but may be micronodular.

Early in the disease, hepatocellular copper is bound mainly to metallothionein and distributed diffusely in the cytoplasm of hepatocytes; therefore, histochemical stains for copper are frequently negative. As the disease progresses, copper exceeds the metallothionein capacity and is deposited in lysosomes. These lysosomal aggregates of copper can be detected by special staining techniques for copper or copper-binding protein (such as rubeanic acid or orcein). Copper is usually distributed throughout the lobule or nodule, but in the cirrhotic liver some areas may have no stainable copper at all. If the clinical presentation mimics autoimmune hepatitis, the liver biopsy reveals classic histologic features of chronic hepatitis, such as interface hepatitis (piecemeal necrosis). Inflammation may be severe. Mallory's stain for hyalin may be positive, and hepatocellular copper accumulation may be detected. In the fulminant hepatic failure presentation of Wilson disease, histologic examination confirms preexisting liver disease. Cirrhosis may be present. Parenchymal copper is mainly in Kupffer cells rather than in hepatocytes.

Changes in hepatocellular mitochondria, identified by electron microscopy, are an important feature in Wilson disease.[16] The mitochondria vary in size; dense bodies in mitochondria may be increased in number. The most striking change is dilation of the tips of the mitochondrial cristae as a result of separation of the inner and outer membranes of the cristae so that the intercristal space is widened to an irregular cystic shape. If only the tip of the crest is dilated, the crest resembles a tennis racquet. This finding, although not absolutely specific, can be helpful diagnostically, even in quite young and minimally affected patients. Involvement of hepatocytes may not be uniform so that abnormalities may be found in some hepatocytes in some lobules and not in others. The mitochondrial changes are probably a consequence of oxidative damage from excessive liver copper.

DIAGNOSIS

The patient with the classic combination of chronic liver disease, tremor or dystonia, and Kayser-Fleischer rings is readily diagnosed on clinical grounds, but such patients are uncommon. Suggestive clinical symptoms are often the main prerequisite for diagnosing Wilson disease, and laboratory investigations may provide confirmation. Kayser-Fleischer rings should be sought through a careful slit-lamp examination, repeated if necessary. Lack of Kayser-Fleischer rings does not exclude the diagnosis of Wilson disease. Routine liver biochemical tests usually yield abnormal results, with mild to moderate elevations of serum aminotransferase levels. Serum alanine aminotransferase (ALT) levels may be much lower than aspartate aminotransferase (AST) levels, which possibly reflects damage to hepatocyte mitochondria.

Two major disturbances of copper disposition in Wilson disease are a reduction in the rate of incorporation of copper into ceruloplasmin and a decrease in biliary excretion of copper. A summary of biochemical features in Wilson disease in comparison with normal persons is shown in Table 67–1. Typically, more than 95% of patients have been considered to have a low ceruloplasmin concentration, but a much larger proportion of patients with liver manifestations can have ceruloplasmin concentrations within the normal range.[17] In these patients, hepatic inflammation may be sufficient to elevate serum ceruloplasmin levels. The increased normal range in young children also must be considered. The explanation for a normal ceruloplasmin may also lie in part in the method of measuring the ceruloplasmin concentration. Immunologic methods, which are commonly used in routine laboratories, measure both apoceruloplasmin and holoceruloplasmin. The former can form a significant portion of the ceruloplasmin in patients with Wilson disease. Therefore, immunologic methods typically overestimate the true amount of holoceruloplasmin in plasma. The oxidase assay, although technically less convenient in automated laboratories, provides a more reliable measure of ceruloplasmin.

A low serum level of ceruloplasmin does not necessarily indicate Wilson disease, because synthesis can be reduced in other types of chronic liver disease. Intestinal malabsorption, nephrosis, and malnutrition also can cause a reduction in the serum concentration of ceruloplasmin. Furthermore, low ceruloplasmin concentrations are found in at least 10% of heterozygotes for Wilson disease. Almost complete absence of ceruloplasmin is also seen in hereditary aceruloplasminemia, a rare recessive condition that is associated with neurologic, retinal, and pancreatic degeneration as a result of iron accumulation in the brain, retina, and pancreas.[18, 19] Anemia and an increase in the plasma ferritin level are observed. Excessive iron storage could be mistaken for hereditary hemochromatosis. The rare occurrence of aceruloplasminemia has confirmed the important function of ceruloplasmin as a

Table 67–1 | **Biochemical Parameters in Patients with Wilson Disease and in Normal Adults**

	WILSON DISEASE*	NORMAL ADULTS
Serum ceruloplasmin (mg/L)†	0–200	200–350
Serum copper (μg/L)	190–640	700–1520
(μmol/L)†	3–10	11–24
Urinary copper (μg/d)	100–1000	<40
(μmol/d)†	>1.6	<0.6
Liver copper (μg/g dry weight)	>200	20–50

*In all assays, there is overlap with heterozygotes in some cases.
†SI units.

ferroxidase that oxidizes iron for transport from ferritin to transferrin, a function proposed in the late 1960s. A targeted disruption of the ceruloplasmin gene in a mouse model has confirmed the critical role of ceruloplasmin in transporting iron out of cells.[20] Theoretically, patients undergoing rigorous, prolonged chelation therapy could show these effects if ceruloplasmin oxidase activity is reduced to undetectable levels, but this possibility remains to be confirmed.

The serum copper concentration is low, in parallel with the low serum ceruloplasmin level, in most patients with Wilson disease. The serum nonceruloplasmin-bound copper concentration is elevated. This concentration can be estimated by subtracting the amount of copper associated with ceruloplasmin from the total serum copper level. The amount of ceruloplasmin-bound copper (in micrograms per liter) is estimated by multiplying serum ceruloplasmin, in milligrams per liter, by 3.15 (the amount of copper in micrograms per milligram of ceruloplasmin). If the total serum copper is reported in micromoles per liter, it is converted to micrograms per liter by multiplying that value by 63.5, the molecular weight of copper. In normal persons the nonceruloplasmin-bound copper concentration is approximately 50 to 100 μg/L. In Wilson disease, the concentration is more than 200 μg/L, and even ten times higher in the presence of fulminant liver failure and intravascular hemolysis. The usefulness of this calculation is highly dependent on the accuracy of the copper and ceruloplasmin measurements.

Serum uric acid and phosphate concentrations may be low, reflecting renal tubular dysfunction in patients with untreated Wilson disease. Urinalysis may show microscopic hematuria; if possible, aminoaciduria, phosphaturia, and proteinuria should be quantified. Studies of urinary copper excretion, preferably three separate 24-hour collections, are also useful for diagnosis. It is critically important to ensure that the collection is complete and that precautions are taken against contamination with copper in the collection process. The basal 24-hour urinary copper excretion rate is elevated. Presymptomatic patients may not necessarily have an increased daily urinary copper excretion; however, even borderline elevations merit further investigation. Heterozygotes usually have a normal 24-hour urinary copper excretion rate, although the level may be borderline abnormal in some cases. A provocative test of urinary copper excretion in which penicillamine (500 mg orally every 12 hours) is given while a 24-hour urinary collection is obtained sometimes provides useful information.[21] Although a normal person may excrete as much as twenty times the baseline level after penicillamine administration, a patient with Wilson disease will excrete considerably more. Martins da Costa and colleagues in Mowat's group have shown that after a penicillamine challenge, urinary excretion of 25 μmoles or more of copper per 24 hours is diagnostic of Wilson disease; they suggest that this test is more reliable than measurement of hepatic tissue content of copper.[21] In fact, when one biochemical assay result is borderline, others tend to be borderline as well.

Hepatic tissue copper concentration, usually measured by neutron activation analysis or atomic absorption spectrometry, may provide important diagnostic information. A hepatic copper content greater than 250 μg per g of dry weight is considered diagnostic of Wilson disease. The copper concentration is typically ten or more times the value found in normal persons. Liver biopsy samples must be collected without extraneous copper contamination, and the reference range must be adjusted for the biopsy needle used.[22] In early stages of Wilson disease, when copper is distributed diffusely in the liver cell cytoplasm, this measurement may clearly indicate hepatic copper overload. In later stages of hepatic Wilson disease, the measurement of hepatic copper is less reliable, because copper is distributed unequally in the liver.[23] However, liver biopsy may not be safe in such patients because of coagulopathy or ascites, and therefore this diagnostic parameter may not be available. Some patients with Wilson disease have a hepatic tissue copper concentration intermediate between normal and definitely elevated (between 100 and 250 μg per g of dry weight). Some heterozygotes have similar moderate elevations of the liver tissue copper concentration. An elevated hepatic copper concentration is not specific: patients with chronic cholestasis or diseases such as Indian childhood cirrhosis may have elevated hepatic copper levels.

The impaired incorporation of copper into ceruloplasmin has been measured using radioactive isotopes (^{64}Cu, ^{67}Cu) or a stable isotope (^{65}Cu). Patients with Wilson disease show little or no incorporation of radiolabeled copper into total plasma, or into the ceruloplasmin component, following an oral or intravenous dose of radiocopper. Incorporation of copper into ceruloplasmin is not always reliable in distinguishing presymptomatic heterozygotes from homozygous patients. Some heterozygotes show no incorporation of copper into ceruloplasmin and are therefore indistinguishable from presymptomatic patients.[24] This test, although demonstrating a characteristic feature of Wilson disease that can be diagnostic, is seldom used at present and will become unnecessary as molecular diagnosis becomes more readily available.

In view of the number of diagnostic tests, some prioritization is required. Minimum diagnostic criteria for Wilson disease applicable to all patients are difficult to establish. In the presence of chronic liver disease (indicated by hepatomegaly or biochemical abnormalities) or a typical neurologic presentation, the combination of low serum ceruloplasmin and elevated basal 24-hour urinary copper excretion levels is highly suggestive of Wilson disease. Results of measuring 24-hour urinary copper excretion after penicillamine administration may be so definitive that the diagnosis is no longer in doubt. Typical ocular findings complete the clinical diagnosis. A percutaneous liver biopsy still has merit for assessing the severity of liver damage and measuring parenchymal copper concentration, which is considered by some to be the sine qua non for diagnosis. However, this procedure, if hazardous, may have to be deferred or delayed. Other clinical entities in the differential diagnosis must be excluded. In the patient who does not have classic manifestations, extensive studies must be pursued meticulously, but ultimately a gene mutation analysis may be the only convincing diagnostic procedure.

Mutation Analysis

More than 200 mutations in the gene for Wilson disease have been detected by single-strand conformation polymorphism analysis, sequencing of each of the 21 exons, or both.[4, 25, 26] Mutation analysis, however, can be clinically useful even now. At least two typical features, clinical or biochemical, usually should be present before mutation analysis is initiated.

The identification of one mutation is usually adequate to confirm the diagnosis, if typical clinical symptoms are present. Various ethnic groups have different specific mutations. The common histidine1069glutamine (His1069Gln) mutation[4] is present at least in the heterozygous state in 35% to 75% of affected Europeans, with the higher number being relevant only for eastern Europe. Exon 8 of the gene is particularly rich in mutations in European populations, and depending on the age of onset, at least one mutation can be identified in 50% to 60% of patients tested for His1069Gln. The mutation arginine778leucine is common in Chinese populations.[25] Japanese and Mediterranean populations have no mutation present in high frequency, so mutation detection is more difficult in these populations. In some populations, particularly those with ethnic homogeneity, mutation testing strategies can identify the mutations in more than 90% of patients, as in Sardinians, in whom the disease frequency is 1 in 7000 live births.[27]

Gene deletions, duplications, nonsense mutations, and splice site mutations would be predicted to prevent almost completely the formation of the gene product and thus produce a severe defect. This prediction is true to some extent, and the onset of liver disease has been reported as early as 3 years of age in a patient with a severe gene defect that was predicted to abolish the gene product.[28] The common His1069Gln mutation[4] tends to be associated with neurologic disease and later onset; however, this mutation has been reported in homozygotes as young as 9 years of age with hepatic disease. The position of this and other missense mutations (amino acid substitutions) is shown in Figure 67–2. Most patients are compound heterozygotes and carry two different mutations of the gene. As a result, correlation of clinical features with specific mutations is difficult, because homozygosity for a single mutation is relatively infrequent. If the patient is clinically normal, has only slight clinical evidence of the disease, or is an older symptomatic patient, the possibility exists that the patient is actually a heterozygote. However, up to now, heterozygotes have not been known to become clinically affected or require treatment.

With the possibility of confirming a diagnosis of Wilson disease by direct identification of mutations, it is becoming clear that the spectrum of manifestations of Wilson disease is even wider than might have been recognized previously. No individual biochemical test is reliable for the identification of patients. In some cases, even all combinations of tests prove inadequate for a diagnosis. For example, Kayser-Fleischer rings, which were once thought to occur inevitably in the presence of neurologic symptoms, are not necessarily present even in conjunction with well-established neurologic symptoms. The ceruloplasmin concentration, which was thought to be reduced in a great majority of patients, may be normal in a major proportion of patients with hepatic manifestations of Wilson disease. The use of molecular tests in patients with any clinical symptoms of the disease may become routine in the near future and is already feasible in some populations.

Presymptomatic Diagnosis of Siblings

Genetic markers that closely flank the gene for Wilson disease are important for presymptomatic diagnosis of siblings of a known patient, when the patient and parents are available for testing. The most useful markers for the study of this and other diseases are those that can be tested with polymerase chain reaction methodology. The commonly used genetic markers are stretches of dinucleotides or trinucleotides that show enough variability in the normal population that most parents within any one family will carry different alleles for the marker. This variability allows the disease gene to be tracked as it segregates within families, as shown in Figure 67–3. It is important that informative markers flank the gene, because rarely an erroneous diagnosis may result if markers on only one side of the gene are informative and a recombinant event has occurred close to the gene. The combination of markers, or haplotype, reliably indicates the genetic status within the family. According to marker studies, occasional persons who are considered as a result of

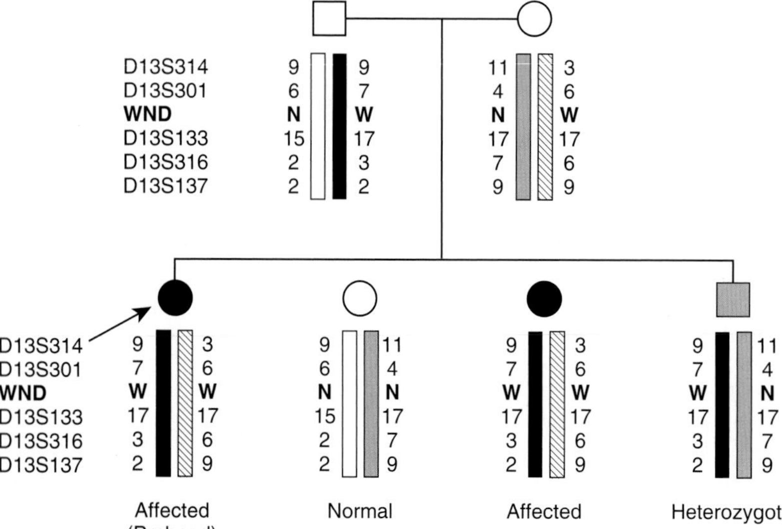

Figure 67–3. Diagnostic use of polymorphic DNA markers for siblings of a confirmed patient, mostly dinucleotide repeats, in a pedigree. DNA markers are listed in centromeric to telomeric order. Three markers are usually sufficient for an unambiguous result: D13S314, D13S301, and D13S316. Numbers represent alleles of each marker listed. The proband is shown as a filled circle (*arrow*). Results indicate the genotype of each sibling, with one confirmed as a presymptomatic patient.

biochemical testing to have a high probability of being presymptomatic patients have been shown to be heterozygotes.[24] Overt symptoms of Wilson disease have not been reported to develop in heterozygotes. Therefore, confirmation of the genotype is highly recommended before treatment is initiated. If heterozygotes are found to accumulate copper stores later in life, they may need to be evaluated further for signs of copper overload.

In the absence of marker analysis, screening should include a physical examination, liver biochemical tests, serum copper and ceruloplasmin levels, 24-hour urinary copper measurement, and careful slit-lamp examination. Children who are 6 years old or younger and who appear not to be affected should be rechecked at intervals over the next 5 to 10 years. However, genetic screening, with the use of flanking markers, is the most reliable way to identify affected siblings when the patient's DNA is available, and in some cases testing for the specific mutation will be possible.

TREATMENT

There are three generally recognized treatments for Wilson disease: penicillamine, trien (trientine), and zinc (Table 67–2).[29] Chelation with tetrathiomolybdate is a relatively new, and still experimental, option. With effective chelator treatment, most patients live normal, healthy lives. Early treatment is critical, and the outcome is best for patients in whom the disease is diagnosed and treatment begun when the disease is presymptomatic. However, whether routine institution of chelator therapy in infancy is advantageous remains unknown. Likewise, the potential role for gene transfer therapy remains uncertain. Although drug treatment simply to interfere with absorption of dietary copper is now rarely used, most patients should eliminate copper-rich foods from their diet. These foods include organ meats, shellfish, nuts, chocolate, and mushrooms. Vegetarians require specific dietary counseling. If there is reason to believe that the patient's drinking water is high in copper, the water should be analyzed, and a copper-removing device may be needed in the plumbing system.

Penicillamine, introduced in 1956 by J. M. Walshe, is effective in most patients with Wilson disease. The drug, which is the sulfhydryl-containing amino acid cysteine substituted with two methyl groups, greatly increases urinary excretion of copper. Studies in the LEC rat model indicate that penicillamine inhibits the accumulation of copper in hepatocellular lysosomes and, once accumulated, solubilizes copper for mobilization from these particles, but not from cytoplasmic metallothioneins.[30] In addition to its chelating action, penicillamine inhibits collagen cross-linking and has some immunosuppressant properties. The neurologic status of patients with mainly neurologic symptoms may worsen initially after penicillamine treatment is started; most, but not all, such patients recover with continued use of penicillamine. Some patients experience a febrile reaction with rash and proteinuria within 7 to 10 days of beginning treatment. Although penicillamine can be restarted slowly, along with glucocorticoids, changing to an alternative chelator may be safer.

Although effective, penicillamine can have extremely serious adverse side effects. Adverse reactions involving the skin include various types of rashes, pemphigus, and elastosis perforans serpiginosa. Other side effects vary from minor (loss of taste, gastrointestinal upset, and arthralgias) to severe (proteinuria, leukopenia, and thrombocytopenia). Aplastic anemia occurs rarely but does not always reverse when penicillamine is stopped. Nephrotic syndrome, Goodpasture syndrome, myasthenia syndrome, and a systemic disease resembling lupus erythematosus all have been reported. These severe side effects require immediate discontinuation of penicillamine and use of a different chelator. Some side effect of penicillamine that necessitates a change of treatment develops in up to 30% of patients with Wilson disease.[31] It is not yet apparent whether life-long treatment with penicillamine is free of adverse consequences. Patients who have taken penicillamine for 30 to 40 years may have chronic skin changes with loss of elastic tissue. Whether the antifibrotic effect weakens other connective tissues is not known. Chronic depletion of other trace metals may occur and may not be entirely benign.

Trientine, or triethylene tetramine dihydrochloride (2,2,2-tetramine), known by its official short name "trien," was also

Table 67–2 | **Approach to Treatment in Wilson Disease**

DRUG	DOSE*	MONITOR EFFICACY	MONITOR SIDE EFFECTS
Penicillamine (+ pyridoxine, 25 mg/day)	Initial: 1–1.5 g/day (adults) *or* 20 mg/kg/day (children), divided bid or tid Maintenance: 0.75–1 g/day as needed to maintain cupruresis	24-hr urinary copper: 500–800 μg (8 μmol)/day as target; estimated nonceruloplasmin-bound copper <100 μg/L	Complete blood count; urinalysis; examine skin
Trien†	Initial: 1–1.2 g/day divided bid or tid‡ Maintenance: Same	Same as for penicillamine	Complete blood count; iron studies
Zinc	Initial: 50 mg elemental zinc tid (adults)§ Maintenance: Titrate dose against efficacy monitoring data‖	24-hr urinary copper 200–400 μg (3 μmol)/day as target; estimated nonceruloplasmin-bound copper <100 μg/L	Serum Zn

*All medications should be taken at least 1 hr before or after mealtime if possible, but adjustments to the timing of the dose may be required to enhance compliance.
†Requires refrigeration.
‡Children's dose of Trien not established (approximately 20 mg/kg/day).
§Children's dose of zinc not yet established.
‖The 24-hr urinary copper excretion reflects total body copper load and thus can be used to monitor zinc treatment even though zinc does not cause cupruresis; some groups prefer to use the estimated nonceruloplasmin-bound copper determination.

introduced by J. M. Walshe and is the usual second-line treatment for patients who are intolerant of penicillamine.[32, 33] Trien differs chemically from penicillamine by its lack of sulfhydryl groups. Copper is chelated by forming a stable complex with the four constituent nitrogens in a planar ring. Trien increases urinary copper excretion and may interfere with intestinal absorption of copper. Trien is a less potent chelator than penicillamine, but this difference is not clinically important. Trien produces little significant toxicity in patients with Wilson disease except for occasional gastritis and iron deficiency, apparently by chelating dietary iron. Bone marrow suppression is extremely rare. Adverse effects of penicillamine resolve and do not recur during treatment with trien.[34] Neurologic worsening after beginning treatment with trien has rarely been reported.

Oral zinc, described for therapy by T. U. Hoogenraad and colleagues in 1979, is a newer treatment modality in North America.[35] The mechanism of action is entirely different from that of the chelators. In pharmacologic doses, zinc interferes with the absorption of copper from the gastrointestinal tract and increases copper excretion in the stools. The postulated mechanism of action is that excess zinc induces metallothionein production in enterocytes. Metallothionein, which has a greater affinity for copper than for zinc, preferentially binds copper from the intestinal contents. Once bound, the copper is not absorbed but is lost in the feces as enterocytes are shed in normal turnover.[36]

Problems with zinc therapy include gastritis, which is a common side effect, and uncertainty about dosing. Using zinc salts other than the sulfate may minimize gastritis. Food interferes with the effectiveness of zinc, and some investigators recommend that no food be taken for 1 hour before or after the zinc dose. However, this dosing regimen tends to increase the severity of gastritis and may be sufficiently inconvenient to compromise compliance, for example, in adolescents. An alternative approach is to be less rigorous about avoiding zinc at meal times but to titrate the dose against the serum nonceruloplasmin-bound copper concentration. There appear to be few adverse side effects of zinc. Rare patients have been reported to experience a deterioration in hepatic Wilson disease when started on zinc. Zinc may have immunosuppressant effects and reduce leukocyte chemotaxis. Studies in rats suggest possible interference with bone formation. The long-term effectiveness and adverse side effects of zinc require further investigation. However, present data indicate that zinc is effective maintenance therapy and has low toxicity.[37]

Ammonium tetrathiomolybdate may be especially suitable for treatment of severe neurologic Wilson disease because, unlike penicillamine, it is not associated with early neurologic deterioration.[38] Tetrathiomolybdate interferes with copper absorption from the intestine and binds to plasma copper with high affinity. Unlike penicillamine, tetrathiomolybdate has been found in LEC rats to remove copper from metallothionein at low doses; at higher doses, an insoluble copper complex is deposited in the liver.[39] Although the drug is regarded as nontoxic, bone marrow suppression is a noteworthy adverse effect. Little is known about where mobilized copper and molybdate might be deposited. Dose, length of treatment, and long-term side effects will require careful study. Such a potent copper-binding drug could, in fact, produce copper deficiency.

Antioxidants may be a useful adjunct in preventing tissue damage. Studies in copper-loaded animals and in patients with Wilson disease indicate that copper enhances free radical production in tissues and that this effect may be an important cause of liver damage.[40] Oxidative damage could also be enhanced by low plasma α-tocopherol and ascorbate levels, which have been reported in patients with untreated Wilson disease.[41, 42] Oxyradical damage may be reflected in reports of an increased rate of mutations in the p53 tumor suppressor gene and increased activity of nitric oxide synthase in the livers of patients with Wilson disease.[43] Antioxidants such as α-tocopherol may be important adjuncts in the treatment of Wilson disease by preventing and reversing liver damage, particularly in patients with severe hepatic decompensation.

Family screening is an important preventive measure. Because the best outcome is associated with treatment begun in the presymptomatic period, screening of the patient's siblings is mandatory when Wilson disease is diagnosed. The recommended approach has been described earlier.

PROGNOSIS

Patients with Wilson disease are generally regarded as having a good prognosis if the disease is diagnosed promptly and treated consistently. An asymptomatic sibling who is diagnosed on biochemical or genetic grounds before any sign of clinical impairment can be recognized has the best outlook. Patients with early hepatic disease have a generally favorable prognosis as long as treatment is consistent and well tolerated.[31, 44] Severe neurologic disease may not resolve entirely on treatment.

The role of liver transplantation in Wilson disease is limited (see also Chapter 83). Fulminant hepatic failure in Wilson disease necessitates liver transplantation. Some patients with severe liver disease that is unresponsive to drug therapy may also require early transplantation, although the potential for rescue by antioxidants has not been well explored. Liver transplantation may improve severe neurologic disease, but experience is limited.[45, 46] Transplantation should be reserved for patients with severe, decompensated liver disease that is unresponsive to therapy or those with fulminant hepatic failure.[46–48] Living-related donor liver transplantation from a heterozygous relative has been performed successfully, based on an average follow-up of 30 months,[49] with the assumption that heterozygotes are not at risk for disease.

Patients who stop chelation treatment have a poor prognosis. New neurologic abnormalities such as dysarthria may develop. Rapidly progressive hepatic decompensation has been observed an average of 3 years or less but as early as 8 months after treatment is stopped. The liver damage is usually refractory to reinstitution of chelator therapy. These patients require liver transplantation.

The quality of life in patients with Wilson disease may be compromised by drug toxicity. Anecdotal observations suggest that damage to collagen may accrue over decades in patients maintained indefinitely on penicillamine, but the risk has not been adequately assessed. Deficiencies in trace metals may develop with the use of any chelator, although it is not yet clear whether these deficiencies are clinically important. Abnormal iron metabolism, leading to hepatic iron overload and anemia, can be predicted if ceruloplasmin oxidase activity is reduced to zero.

REFERENCES

1. Wilson SAK: Progressive lenticular degeneration: A familial nervous disease associated with cirrhosis of the liver. Brain 34:295, 1912.
2. Valentine JS, Gralla EB: Delivering copper inside yeast and human cells. Science 278:817, 1997.
3. Bull PC, Thomas GR, Rommens JM, et al: The Wilson disease gene is a putative copper transporting P-type ATPase similar to the Menkes gene [erratum in Nat Genet 6:214, 1994]. Nat Genet 5:327, 1993.
4. Tanzi RE, Petrukhin KE, Chernov I, et al: The Wilson disease gene is a copper-transporting ATPase with homology to the Menkes disease gene. Nat Genet 5:344, 1993.
5. Frydman M, Bonne-Tamir B, Farrer LA, et al: Assignment of the gene for Wilson disease to chromosome 13: Linkage to the esterase D locus. Proc Natl Acad Sci USA 82:1819, 1985.
6. Hung IH, Suzuki M, Yamaguchi Y, et al: Biochemical characterization of the Wilson disease protein and functional expression in the yeast *Saccharomyces cerevisiae*. J Biol Chem 272:21461, 1997.
7. Schaefer M, Roelofsen H, Wolters H, et al: Localization of the Wilson's disease protein in human liver. Gastroenterology 117:1380, 1999.
8. Wu J, Forbes JR, Chen HS, et al: The LEC rat has a deletion in the copper transporting ATPase gene homologous to the Wilson disease gene. Nat Genet 7:541, 1994.
9. Theophilos MB, Cox DW, Mercer JF: The toxic milk mouse is a murine model of Wilson disease. Hum Molec Genet 5:1619, 1996.
10. Schilsky ML, Scheinberg IH, Sternlieb I: Prognosis of Wilsonian chronic active hepatitis. Gastroenterology 100:762, 1991.
11. McCullough AJ, Fleming CR, Thistle JL: Diagnosis of Wilson's disease presenting as fulminant hepatic failure. Gastroenterology 84:161, 1983.
12. Hoshino T, Kumasaka K, Kawano K: Low serum alkaline phosphatase activity associated with severe Wilson's disease. Is the breakdown of alkaline phosphatase molecules caused by reactive oxygen species? Clin Chim Acta 238:91, 1995.
13. Sallie R, Katsiyiannakis L, Baldwin D: Failure of simple biochemical indexes to reliably differentiate fulminant Wilson's disease from other causes of fulminant liver failure. Hepatology 16:1206, 1992.
14. Oder W, Prayer L, Grimm G: Wilson's disease: Evidence of subgroups derived from clinical findings and brain lesions. Neurology 43:120, 1993.
15. Dening TR, Berrios GE: Wilson's disease; Psychiatric symptoms in 195 cases. Arch Gen Psychiatry 46:1126, 1989.
16. Sternlieb I: Mitochondrial and fatty changes in hepatocytes of patients with Wilson's disease. Gastroenterology 5:354, 1968.
17. Steindl P, Ferenci P, Dienes HP, et al: Wilson's disease in patients with liver disease: A diagnostic challenge. Gastroenterology 113:212, 1998.
18. Yoshida K, Furihata K, Takeda S, et al: A mutation in the ceruloplasmin gene is associated with systemic hemosiderosis in humans. Nat Genet 9:267, 1995.
19. Harris ZL, Takahashi Y, Miyajima H, et al: Aceruloplasminemia: Molecular characterization of this disorder of iron metabolism. Proc Natl Acad Sci USA 92:2539, 1995.
20. Harris ZL, Durley AP, Man TK, et al: Targeted gene disruption reveals an essential role for ceruloplasmin in cellular iron efflux. Proc Natl Acad Sci USA 96:10812, 1999.
21. Martin da Costa C, Baldwin D, Portmann B, et al: Value of urinary copper excretion after penicillamine challenge in the diagnosis of Wilson's disease. Hepatology 15:609, 1992.
22. Ludwig J, Moyer TP, Rakela J: The liver biopsy diagnosis of Wilson's disease. Methods in pathology. Am J Clin Pathol 102:443, 1994.
23. Faa G, Nurchi V, Demelia L, et al: Uneven hepatic copper distribution in Wilson's disease. J Hepatol 22:303, 1995.
24. Lyon TD, Fell GS, Gaffney D, et al: Use of a stable copper isotope (65Cu) in the differential diagnosis of Wilson's disease. Clin Sci 88: 727, 1995.
25. Thomas GR, Forbes JR, Roberts EA, et al: The Wilson disease gene: Spectrum of mutations and their consequences. Nat Genet 9:210, 1995.
26. Loudianos G, Dessi V, Lovicu M, et al: Mutation analysis in patients of Mediterranean descent with Wilson disease: Identification of 19 novel mutations. J Med Genet 36:833, 1999.
27. Loudianos G, Dessi V, Lovicu M, et al: Molecular characterization of Wilson disease in the Sardinian population—evidence of a founder effect. Hum Mutat 14:294, 1999.
28. Wilson DC, Phillips MJ, Cox DW, et al: Severe hepatic Wilson's disease in preschool-aged children. J Pediatr 137:719, 2000.
29. Brewer GJ, Yuzbasiyan-Gurkan V: Wilson disease. Medicine 71:139, 1992.
30. Klein D, Lichtmannegger J, Heinzmann U, et al: Dissolution of copper-rich granules in hepatic lysosomes by D-penicillamine prevents the development of fulminant hepatitis in Long-Evans cinnamon rats. J Hepatol 32:193, 2000.
31. Walshe JM: Wilson's disease presenting with features of hepatic dysfunction: A clinical analysis of eighty-seven patients. Q J Med 70:253, 1989.
32. Walshe JM: Treatment of Wilson's disease with trientine (triethylenetetramine) dihydrochloride. Lancet 1:643, 1982.
33. Dubois RS, Rodgerson DG, Hambridge KM: Treatment of Wilson's disease with triethylene tetramine hydrochloride (trientine). J Pediatr Gastroenterol Nutr 10:77, 1990.
34. Scheinberg IH, Jaffe ME, Sternlieb I: The use of trientine in preventing the effects of interrupting penicillamine therapy in Wilson's disease. N Engl J Med 317:209, 1987.
35. Hoogenraad TU, Van Haltum J, Van der Hamer CJA: Management of Wilson's disease with zinc sulphate. J Neurol Sci 77:137, 1987.
36. Yuzbasiyan-Gurkan V, Grider A, Nostrant T, et al: Treatment of Wilson's disease with zinc: X. Intestinal metallothionein induction. J Lab Clin Med 120:380, 1992.
37. Brewer GJ, Dick RD, Johnson VD, et al: Treatment of Wilson's disease with zinc: XV. Long-term follow-up studies. J Lab Clin Med 132: 264, 1998.
38. Brewer GJ, Dick RD, Johnson V, et al: Treatment of Wilson's disease with ammonium tetrathiomolybdate. I. Initial therapy in 17 neurologically affected patients. Arch Neurol 51:545, 1994.
39. Ogra Y, Suzuki KT: Targeting of tetrathiomolybdate on the copper accumulating in the liver of LEC rats. J Inorg Biochem 70:49, 1998.
40. Sokol RJ, Twedt D, McKim JM, et al: Oxidant injury to hepatic mitochondria in patients with Wilson's disease and Bedlington terriers with copper toxicosis. Gastroenterology 107:1788, 1994.
41. von Herbay A, de Groot H, Hegi U, et al: Low vitamin E content in plasma of patients with alcoholic liver disease, hemochromatosis and Wilson's disease. J Hepatol 20:41, 1994.
42. Ogihara H, Ogihara T, Miki M, et al: Plasma copper and antioxidant status in Wilson's disease. Pediatr Res 37:219, 1995.
43. Hussain SP, Raja K, Amstad PA, et al: Increased p53 mutation load in nontumorous human liver of Wilson disease and hemochromatosis: Oxyradical overload diseases. Proc Natl Acad Sci USA 97:12770, 2000.
44. Stremmel W, Meyerrose KW, Niederau C, et al: Wilson disease: Clinical presentation, treatment and survival. Ann Intern Med 115:720, 1991.
45. Mason AL, Marsh W, Alpers DH: Intractable neurological Wilson's disease treated with orthotopic liver transplantation. Dig Dis Sci 23: 373, 1993.
46. Bellary S, Hassanein T, Van Thiel DH: Liver transplantation for Wilson's disease. J Hepatol 23:373, 1995.
47. Rela M, Heaton ND, Vougas V, et al: Orthotopic liver transplantation for hepatic complications of Wilson's disease. Br J Surg 80:909, 1993.
48. Schilsky ML, Scheinberg IH, Sternlieb I: Liver transplantation for Wilson's disease: Indications and outcome. Hepatology 19:583, 1994.
49. Asonuma K, Inomata Y, Kasahara M, et al: Living related liver transplantation from heterozygote genetic carriers to children with Wilson's disease. Pediatr Transplant 3:201, 1999.

Chapter 68

Viral Hepatitis

Marina Berenguer and Teresa L. Wright

The past three decades have seen enormous advances in our understanding of viruses that are either associated with or cause liver disease in man. These advances have been the result of concerted efforts by virologists, immunologists, and clinicians. Five viruses have been identified that produce liver disease as their major clinical manifestation: four are RNA viruses, one is a DNA virus. Two recently discovered RNA viruses, initially thought to be hepatotropic, do not cause liver disease. Along with advances in our understanding of the liver disease associated with infection with these viruses has been an appreciation of clinical disease outside the liver. Knowledge of the mechanism of replication of these viruses has largely depended on the availability of suitable cell culture systems and animal models. These systems have also been enormously important in the identification and testing of new drugs. Understanding the host immune response to infection is critical to understanding the mechanism of clearance of a virus after acute infection, the failure of viral clearance in persistent infection, and the pathogenesis of liver disease associated with chronic infection. This chapter reviews the virology, epidemiology, immunology, clinical manifestations, and treatment of the major hepatitis viruses that have been associated with liver disease in humans.

HEPATITIS A VIRUS

Virology

Classification

Hepatitis A virus (HAV) is a hepatotropic virus that recently has been assigned to a separate genus—*Hepatovirus*—within the Picornaviridae family (Table 68–1).[1] Features that distinguish hepatoviruses from other picornaviruses include their tropism for the liver, exceptional stability, unique capsid structure with very small VP4, characteristic RNA structure within the 5′ nontranslated region of the genome, and low level of genetic relatedness to other picornaviruses.[2]

Structure

HAV is a 27 to 32 nm diameter, icosahedral-shaped, nonenveloped virus, first visualized in 1973 with electron microscopy in fecal samples of volunteers in whom hepatitis developed after infection with HAV.[3] Both "full" and "empty" particles can be identified with electron microscopy, but the particles are indistinguishable antigenically.

Table 68–1 | **Virology of Hepatitis Agents**

CHARACTERISTIC	HAV	HBV	HCV	HDV	HEV
Family	Picornaviridae	Hepadnaviridae	Flaviviridae	Viroid	Caliciviridae/Flaviviridae/alpha super group
Size	27–32 nm	42 nm	55 nm	35 nm	32 nm
Shape	Icosahedral	Spherical	Spherical	Spherical	Icosahedral
Envelope	No	Yes	Yes	Yes (HBsAg)	No
Genome	7.5 kb	3.2 kb	9.4 kb	1.7 kb	7.5 kb
Genome type	ssRNA	partially dsDNA	ssRNA	ssRNA	ssRNA
Antibodies	IgG, IgM anti-HAV	anti-HBs; IgG, IgM anti-HBc	anti-HCV; directed against c100-3; c22-3 c33c; 5-1-1	IgG, IgM anti-HDV	IgG, IgM anti-HEV

dsDNA, double-stranded DNA; HAV, hepatitis A virus; HBV, hepatitis B virus; HCV, hepatitis C virus; HDV, hepatitis D virus; HEV, hepatitis E virus; ssRNA, single-stranded RNA.

Genomic Organization

This positive-strand RNA virus, 7474 nucleotides long, is divided into three regions: 1) 5′ noncoding or untranslated region (UTR) of 743 nucleotides, which contains an internal ribosomal entry site; 2) a single long, open reading frame (ORF) of 6681 nucleotides, which encodes a long polypeptide of 2227 amino acids; and 3) a short 3′ noncoding region of 63 nucleotides, which terminates as a polyadenylated tract of variable length (Fig. 68–1). The RNA genome acts as a messenger directing the translation of a single polyprotein that is cleaved by the 3C proteinase into eleven structural and nonstructural proteins (see Fig. 68–1). The structural protein-encoding region P1 yields four capsid proteins (VP1, VP2, VP3, VP4), while nonstructural protein-encoding regions P2 and P3 yield three and four nonstructural proteins, respectively, including the 5′ terminal protein (VPg), a protease (3C), and an RNA-dependent RNA polymerase (3D).[2, 4] A VP0 peptide can also be detected in immature virions; VP0 is cleaved to form VP4 and VP2.

Studies from different geographical areas have shown that there are at least four distinct genotypes of human HAV that differ from each other by 15% to 20% of the nucleotides within the P1 region of the genome.[2] Genotypes have been numbered in order of discovery. Most human HAVs belong to genotypes I and III. Despite their epidemiologic interest, no significant differences in biologic or antigenic properties have been found among the different human HAV genotypes, and only one serotype exists, so that infection with one strain confers immunity to the other strains. The single immunodominant epitope is conformationally dependent, with involvement of VP3 and VP1. It is therefore detectable in intact virions and natural empty capsids but not in isolated structural proteins.[5, 6]

Replication

Study of the pathogenesis of HAV infection has been aided by the use of animal models and tissue culture. Humans and specific nonhuman primates (marmosets, tamarins, chimpanzees) are the only natural hosts of HAV. Infection in the latter generally produces mild disease with biochemical and histologic changes similar to those in humans.[7]

Slow growth and absence of cytopathic effects lead to the establishment of a persistent, nonlytic infection in different cell lines. Wild-type virus replicates poorly in cell culture. Efficient replication in tissue culture specimens of primate origin requires a number of passages to achieve adaptation of the human virus to growth.[8] Several cell culture–adapted HAV strains with an attenuated ability to cause disease yet with the ability to maintain immunogenicity have been used for the production of both attenuated live and formalin-inactivated HAV vaccines.

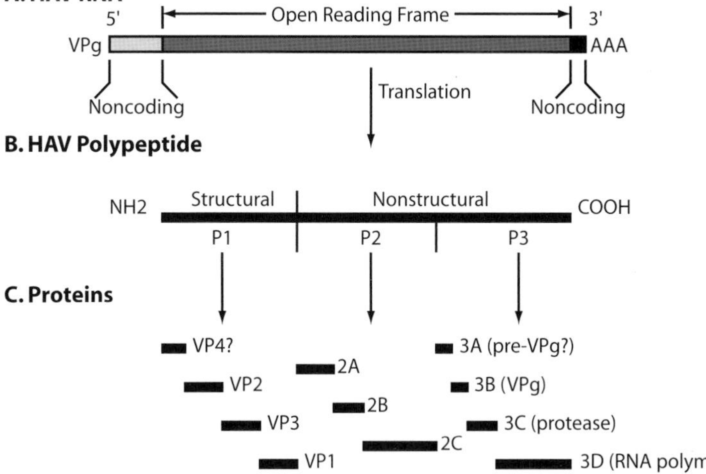

Figure 68–1. Genomic organization of HAV. (From Lavine JE, Bull FG, Millward-Sadler GH, et al: Acute viral hepatitis. In Millward-Sadler GH, Wright R, Arthur MJP [eds]: Wright's Liver and Biliary Disease, 3rd ed. London, WB Saunders, 1992, pp 679–786.)

Immunofluorescence of liver tissue shows that hepatitis A virus antigen (HAVAg) is located diffusely throughout the cytoplasm of the hepatocyte but not in the nucleus. HAV replication can be inhibited in cell culture by addition of α-interferon, ribavirin, amantadine, and 2-deoxy-D-glucose.

Data regarding replication of the virus within the gastrointestinal epithelium are conflicting. Recent studies support HAV replication within crypt cells of the small intestine.[9]

Epidemiology

Infectious Cycle

Infection with HAV generally occurs through the oral route (Table 68–2). Once absorbed in the intestine, the virus reaches the liver through the portal vein. A mucin-like glycoprotein has been identified in cultured cells as the cellular receptor for the virus. Hepatocyte replication takes place in the cytoplasm, in which antigenic detection is possible 1 to 2 weeks after inoculation and persists up to 8 weeks. New virions are either excreted via bile to the intestine or released into the systemic circulation. Shedding of the virus through the apical canalicular surface of infected Coco 2 cells can be blocked by brefeldin A, which also inhibits HAV replication.[9] The typical shedding of infectious virus in feces begins within the second week of incubation, increases until the prodromic phase, and declines once jaundice develops. Infectious virus may be identified in feces up to 2 weeks after jaundice occurs. Although chronic fecal shedding has not been described, it may continue for months in neonates, and reactivation may occur with relapsing hepatitis.

Transmission

The major mode of transmission is person to person via the fecal-oral route. HAV is shed into the stool in high titers, and because it is relatively resistant to degradation by environmental conditions, the virus is spread easily within a population, with a very high attack rate (70%–90% of those exposed become infected). The secondary attack rate is approximately 15% to 20%, with a progressive increase in the number of cases until a maximum is reached within 2 to 3 months. This situation is more likely to occur when there is close contact and difficulty in maintaining adequate hygiene, as in daycare centers, institutions for the mentally handicapped, and army camps.[10]

Fecally contaminated food or water is also an important mode of spread. Consumption of contaminated uncooked or undercooked food, such as shellfish, and less frequently foods that are contaminated during food preparation or after cooking by an infected food handler has led to outbreaks of disease that affect large numbers of people. Contamination of water supplies may occur in areas with inadequate sewage disposal systems. In developing countries, waterborne transmission likely leads to widespread infection at an early age.[10]

Because the period of viremia is generally short (1–2 weeks) and the concentration of virus in blood is relatively low, transmission through nonsterile needle sharing occurs only rarely. Transmission of HAV via bloodborne biologic

Table 68–2 | **Clinical Features of Hepatitis Agents**

FEATURE	HAV	HBV	HCV	HDV	HEV
Transmission					
Oral	Common	Not likely	No	No	Common
Percutaneous	Rare	Common	Common	Common	Unknown
Sexual	No	Common	Yes, rare	Yes, rare	No
Perinatal	No	Common	Yes, low frequency	No	Yes, unknown frequency
Incubation period (days)	15–49 (average = 25)	60–180	14–160	21–45	15–60
Clinical illness at presentation	5% pediatric, 70%–80% adults	10%–15%	5%–10%	10%, higher with superinfection	70–80% in adults
Jaundice	Adults 30% Children <5%	5%–20%	5%–10%	Unknown	Common
Fulminant	<1%	<1%	Rare	2%–7.5%	<1%, up to 30% in pregnancy
Diagnostic tests					
Acute infection	IgM anti-HAV	HBsAg, IgM anti-HBc	HCV RNA (anti-HCV)	IgM anti-HDV	IgG anti-HEV (seroconversion)
Chronic infection	Not applicable	HBsAg, IgG anti-HBc	Anti-HCV (EIA) RIBA, HCV RNA	IgG anti-HDV	Not applicable
Immunity	IgG anti-HAV	IgG anti-HBc, anti-HBs	Unknown	Not applicable	Not applicable
Case-fatality rate	0.1%–2.7%	1%–3%	1%–2%	<1% coinfection >5% superinfection	0.5%–4% 1.5%–21% in pregnant women
Chronic infection	None	<5% adults >90% infants	80%–90%	Superinfection ~80% Coinfection ≤5%	None

HAV, hepatitis A virus; HBV, hepatitis B virus; HCV, hepatitis C virus; HDV, hepatitis D virus; HEV, hepatitis E virus.

products inactivated with solvent and detergent treatments has been described.[11]

Incidence and Prevalence

HAV has a worldwide distribution and is considered the most common cause of viral hepatitis. Prevalence data based on the presence of anti-HAV have provided important information on the epidemiology of hepatitis A infection. The prevalence of infection is related to the quality of the water supply, level of sanitation, and age of the population. Although HAV has been a reportable disease for decades, incidence data are unreliable because the disease is frequently mild and hence unrecognized, making under-reporting likely.

Three different patterns of prevalence are recognized (Table 68–3). In countries with poor sanitary conditions, HAV infection is highly endemic. Household crowding, poor levels of sanitation, and inadequate water supplies contribute to the propagation of infection within communities in countries such as Africa, Asia, and Central and South America. Most persons become infected within the first few years of life and are asymptomatic; hence, reported rates of infection are low.[10] By the age of 10 years, the majority in the community are immune, and the prevalence of protective antibodies to HAV in adults approaches 100%.[10] In areas of intermediate endemism (Eastern Europe, republics of former Soviet Union, parts of the Americas and Asia), sanitary conditions are variable, and some children escape infection in early childhood.[10] Hence, the peak rates of clinically apparent infection occur in older children and adolescents, and because infection is likely to be symptomatic in this group, reported disease rates may be higher in regions of intermediate endemism than in high-endemic areas. In intermediate-endemic countries, anti-HAV seroprevalence in adults is 60% to 97%.[10] In such countries, community-wide epidemics account for a significant proportion of disease. Propagation of HAV infection occurs until all susceptible persons have been infected. The most common vehicle for source outbreaks has been raw or partially cooked shellfish; shellfish filter large volumes of water and thus concentrate both bacteria and viruses, including HAV. Outbreaks from a single contaminated source may become an increasingly important source of infection as the number of susceptible adults increases. In low-endemic areas (Northern and Western Europe, United States, Canada, Australia), peak infection rates occur among adolescents and young adults, with outbreaks occasionally occurring in daycare centers and residential institutions and in situations where water or food is contaminated.[10] In low-endemic countries, the seroprevalence rates in adults vary from 13% in Sweden to 62% in Australia.[10] In these areas, groups at high risk of acquiring HAV have been identified: travelers to high-endemic areas, health care personnel (mainly pediatric nurses), cleaning personnel in hospitals, military and prison populations, staff in daycare centers, and sewage workers.[12]

Table 68–3 | **Patterns of HAV Prevalence**

CHARACTERISTIC	LOW	INTERMEDIATE	HIGH
Age at infection	Adolescents and adults	Older children and adolescents	Early childhood
Clinical course	Frequently symptomatic, high risk of fulminant cases	Frequently symptomatic	Frequently asymptomatic
Immunity in the adult population (seroprevalence rates)	15%–60%	60%–90%	99%–100%
Geographic areas	Northern and western Europe, US, Canada, Australia	Southern and Eastern Europe, republics of former Soviet Union, parts of the Americas and Asia	Africa, Asia, Central and South America

In the United States, the reported incidence of hepatitis A is 9.1 per 100,000. Rates in men are consistently higher than in women by about 20%.[12] Between 1983 and 1990, the overall seroprevalence was 38%, with rates increasing from 11% in children under the age of 5 years to 74% in adults of 50 years or older. This increase in prevalence with age was seen for all ethnic and racial groups and for both genders.[12] In 1990, Native Americans had the highest incidence of hepatitis A, which is consistent with the known prevalence of HAV in this ethnic group.[12]

In the Viral Hepatitis Surveillance Study, the most common risk factor for HAV acquisition was personal contact with a person infected with HAV (26% of patients). Other risk factors included employment or attendance at a daycare facility (14%), injection drug use (11%), a history of recent travel (4%), and association with a suspected food or waterborne outbreak (3%). In 42% of cases, no known source of infection was reported.[12] International travel to developing countries is a well-recognized risk factor for HAV. HAV is the most common potentially preventable infection that occurs in travelers. The risk is higher for those who travel to highly endemic areas with poor hygiene conditions (e.g., backpackers). Both travelers[13] and those at occupational risk[14] are obvious candidates for vaccination.

Pathogenesis

Most evidence indicates that hepatocyte injury is secondary to a host immune response. HLA-restricted, virus-specific, cytotoxic $CD8^+$ T cells have been isolated from the livers of patients with acute HAV infection, and $CD8^+$ clones react specifically against HAV-infected fibroblasts.[15] Nonspecific immune mechanisms involving natural killer (NK) and lymphokine-activated killer cells may also play a central role in hepatocyte injury in acute HAV prior to the initiation of damage due to cytotoxic T lymphocytes (CTLs). Although circulating immune complexes composed of immunoglobulin (Ig)M and HAV capsid polypeptides and RNA have been found in the sera of infected chimpanzees, they are present before the onset of histological disease and likely reflect the viremic phase of the infection.[16] Immunohistochemical analysis has revealed IgM in the sinusoidal cells and HAVAg in Kupffer cells. Viral antigen has been postulated to cause functional impairment of Kupffer cells and the histologic manifestations of disease.[17]

Clinical Manifestations and Diagnosis

HAV results in acute infection only (see Table 68–2). The clinical spectrum of disease ranges from silent asymptomatic infection to fulminant hepatitis. Atypical manifestations include cholestasis, relapse after recovery, extrahepatic symptoms, and the possible triggering of autoimmune diseases.

Acute Infection

The incubation period is 15 to 49 days (average, 25 days). Serial changes in symptoms, serum alanine aminotransferase (ALT) levels, and tests for HAV that occur during acute infection are shown in Figure 68–2.

Clinical Symptoms

Prodromal symptoms include fatigue and weakness, anorexia, nausea and vomiting, and abdominal pain.[18] Less common symptoms include fever, headache, arthralgia, myalgia, and diarrhea. In more than 90% of patients, the development of jaundice and dark urine occurs within 1 to 2 weeks of the onset of prodromal symptoms.[18] Anicteric infections are 3.5 times more likely than icteric infections, with the vast majority of anicteric infections occurring in children.[19] Although more than 90% of children under the age of 5 are asymptomatic, 70% to 80% of adults are symptomatic.[18, 19] With the appearance of jaundice, pruritus may become prominent, and extrahepatic manifestations may be seen (see later section). In general, with the exception of anorexia, prodromal symptoms tend to abate with the onset of jaundice. Tenderness and mild enlargement of the liver are present in 85% of patients, splenomegaly in 15%, and posterior cervical lymphadenopathy in 15%.[18] The duration of jaundice is less than 2 weeks in the majority of patients; complete clinical and biochemical recovery is seen in 60% of patients within a period of 2 months and in nearly 100% of patients by 6 months. Persistent elevation of serum aminotransferase and serum bilirubin levels beyond 12 months has been reported but is rare. Overall, the prognosis in acute HAV infection is excellent, and chronic hepatitis does not occur.

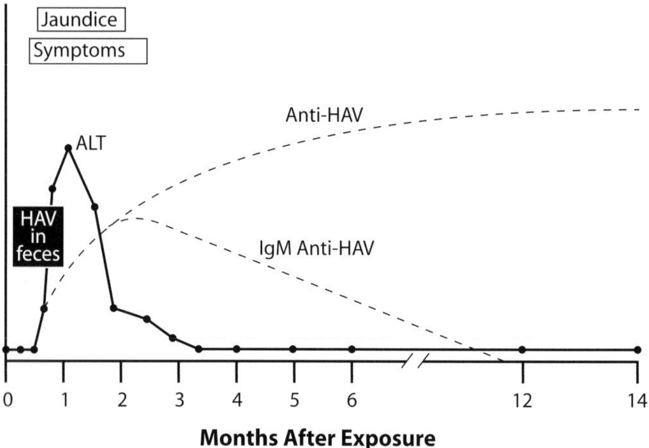

Figure 68–2. Typical course of a case of acute hepatitis A. ALT, alanine aminotransferase; HAV, hepatitis A virus; anti-HAV, antibody to HAV. (Reproduced from Hoofnagle JH, DiBisceglie AM: Serologic diagnosis of acute and chronic viral hepatitis. Semin Liver Dis 11:73, 1991.)

Biochemical Abnormalities

Levels of serum aminotransferases increase during the prodromal phase, and the peak is typically heralded by intense nausea, anorexia, and vomiting, which precede the onset of jaundice. Peak aminotransferase levels are commonly above 500 U/L and decrease at a rate of 75% per week initially, then decline more slowly. Serum bilirubin levels peak after aminotransferase activity and are usually less than 10 mg/dL. The bilirubin levels fall more slowly than the aminotransferase levels but return to normal in 85% of patients by 3 months.

The severity of illness is age dependent. Patients over 50 years of age have the most severe disease, whereas infection in children is usually asymptomatic or, if symptomatic, nonicteric.[19] Pregnancy is not associated with an increased severity of disease, and there is no increase in fetal loss or fetal abnormalities.[20] Severe HAV infection and the development of fulminant hepatitis are associated with underlying chronic hepatitis B virus (HBV) or hepatitis C virus (HCV) infection, especially when chronic hepatitis or cirrhosis is present.[20–24] Overall, fulminant hepatitis (acute liver failure) is rare, and case-fatality rates for hepatitis A are only 0.14% in hospitalized patients. Fatality rates, however, vary with age: infants and children have a fatality rate of 0.1%; adolescents and young adults (ages 15–39) have a fatality rate of 0.4%; and patients 40 years of age or older have a fatality rate of 1.1%.[20, 24]

Atypical Courses

Two atypical courses of acute infection are well described: 1) prolonged cholestasis and 2) relapsing hepatitis.[25] In patients with prolonged cholestasis, the duration of jaundice exceeds 12 weeks and is associated with symptoms of pruritus, fatigue, loose stools, and weight loss. Aminotransferase levels during the period of cholestasis are typically less than 500 U/L. Spontaneous recovery occurs, although glucocorticoids have been recommended by some authorities to hasten resolution of the cholestatic phase.[25] An abdominal ultrasound is appropriate to exclude biliary disease, but invasive testing (liver biopsy and cholangiography) is rarely necessary. Relapsing or polyphasic hepatitis A occurs in 6% to 12% of cases, has been described in both children and adults, and is typified by an initial phase of acute infection followed by a period of remission (lasting 4–15 weeks) with subsequent relapse.[26] Aminotransferase levels often return to normal during remission but increase to greater than 1000 U/L during relapse. HAV is frequently recovered from the stools during relapse, and HAV RNA is detectable in the serum. The pathogenesis of relapsing hepatitis is unknown.

Diagnosis

There are a range of diagnostic methods available for detection of HAV antigen and anti-HAV. HAV may be detected directly in stool and body fluids by electron microscopy, but this technique is impractical. Viral RNA may be detected in body fluids and serum using polymerase chain reaction (PCR) amplification, but such methods, although sensitive, are expensive, not readily available, and used primarily for research purposes.

Most patients present when virus is no longer detectable in stool. Thus, detection of anti-HAV in serum by radioimmunoassay (RIA) or enzyme-linked immunoassay (EIA) is the gold standard for diagnosis. Detection of IgM anti-HAV in a patient who presents with clinical features of hepatitis or in an asymptomatic person with elevated serum aminotransferase levels is confirmatory of acute HAV infection (see Fig. 68–2). IgG anti-HAV indicates previous exposure and immunity to HAV; a rising titer of IgG anti-HAV is indicative of recent exposure. Occasionally, serologic evidence of acute HAV infection is documented in the absence of serum aminotransferase elevations. Serum IgM anti-HAV levels peak during the acute or early convalescent phases of infection and decline to undetectable levels by 3 to 4 months in the majority of patients. In 25% of patients, IgM anti-HAV persists for 6 months or more. IgG anti-HAV typically appears in the early convalescent phase and remains detectable for decades after acute infection, with slowly declining titers. Both the EIA and RIA methods of antibody detection are sensitive, specific, and sufficiently reliable to allow diagnosis of acute infection from a single serum sample.

An experimental antibody assay has been developed recently that detects antibodies to the 3C proteinase of HAV. Such antibodies develop regularly in persons who are infected with the virus but not in those who are immunized with HAV vaccine.[27]

Extrahepatic Manifestations

Extrahepatic manifestations are less frequent in acute HAV infection than in acute HBV infection and consist most commonly of an evanescent rash (14%) and arthalgias (11%) and less commonly of leukocytoclastic vasculitis, glomerulonephritis, and arthritis, in which immune-complex disease is believed to play an etiologic role.[25] Cutaneous vasculitis is typically seen on the legs and buttocks; skin biopsies reveal the presence of IgM anti-HAV and complement in the blood vessel walls. The arthritis also appears to have a predilection for the lower extremities. Both vasculitis and arthritis have been associated with cryoglobulinemia, although cryoglobulinemia, in general, is more frequently associated with HCV infection (see later section). The cryoglobulin has been shown to contain IgM anti-HAV. Other rare extrahepatic manifestations that may be immune-complex related include toxic epidermal necrolysis, fatal myocarditis, renal failure in the absence of liver failure, optic neuritis, transverse myelitis, and polyneuritis. Hematologic complications include thrombocytopenia, aplastic anemia, and red-cell aplasia. Patients with more protracted illness appear to have a higher frequency of extrahepatic manifestations.[25]

Complications

A post-hepatitis syndrome is characterized by prolonged malaise, elevated serum aminotransferase levels, and persistence of IgM anti-HAV in serum.[28] Acute HAV infection has been linked with the development of type 1 autoimmune hepatitis.[29] Acute liver failure is a rare complication that occurs more frequently in patients who are either over the age of 40 or under the age of 11[20, 24] or in those with underlying chronic liver disease[20–24] (see Chapter 80).

Pathology

Histologic assessment of the liver is rarely needed in a patient with acute hepatitis A. As with other forms of acute viral hepatitis, hepatocyte ballooning, degeneration, and acidophilic body formation are present. These changes are most prominent near the terminal hepatic venule, and in mild cases the injury is confined to this area. The lobular architecture remains intact, but collapse of the reticulin network in the region of the terminal hepatic venule (Rappaport zone 3) may be seen. Portal tracts are variably expanded by a mixed inflammatory infiltrate of mainly mononuclear and lymphocytic cells but may also contain plasma cells, neutrophils, and eosinophils. Kupffer cell proliferation is prominent, particularly in areas of hepatocytolysis. Regenerative activity begins within 48 hours of hepatocyte injury, frequently coexists with hepatocyte destruction, and is manifested by variability in the size of hepatocytes, a cobblestone pattern of hydropic hepatocytes, hepatocytes with more than one nucleus, and small foci of twinning of cell plates. Cholestasis is more pronounced in patients with acute hepatitis A, particularly in those with the cholestatic variant of HAV infection, than in those with acute HBV or HCV infection; the associated pathologic appearance includes bile thrombi, cholestatic liver cell rosettes, and ductular transformation of hepatocytes.[30] The acute changes resolve completely, and no chronic sequelae occur.

Natural History

Hepatitis A is typically a benign, self-limited infection, with the majority of patients exhibiting complete recovery within 2 months of the onset of disease. The severity of the disease is age dependent, with increased fatality rates in patients aged 40 years or greater.[20, 24] Underlying chronic liver disease is also associated with increase severity and an increased risk of acute liver failure.[20–24] A small subset of patients experience symptoms for more prolonged periods of time or have the relapsing variant.[25, 26] Fulminant HAV infection is rare. Chronic HAV infection does not occur.

Prevention

General Measures

Prevention requires attention to public and personal health measures. The virus is inactivated by boiling for 20 minutes, chlorination (concentration-dependent), ultraviolet light, and a 1:4000 formalin mixture. Strict adherence to handwashing in the hospital, daycare, and institutional setting is important in preventing person-to-person spread. Travelers to endemic areas should be advised to avoid drinking water or beverages with ice from sources of unknown purity, eating uncooked shellfish, or eating uncooked and unpeeled fruits and vegetables.[13]

Passive Immunoprophylaxis with Immune Globulin

Pooled human immune globulin (IG) has been used since 1945 to provide passive protection against HAV infection (Table 68-4). Administration of IG before exposure will prevent infection in 85% to 95% of exposed persons, administration within 1 to 2 weeks of exposure will prevent or attenuate infection, and administration beyond 2 weeks is ineffective.[31] The dose that has been shown to be consistently protective is 0.02 mL/kg. The duration of protection appears to be dose related, with the 0.02 mL/kg dose providing protection for approximately 3 months and a 0.05 mL/kg dose providing protection for 4 to 6 months.[31] Patients in whom attenuated infection develops (so-called passive-active immunization) excrete virus at some stage of their illness and theoretically may be at risk for HAV transmission, although this risk appears to be minimal. Lifelong immunity may develop in patients who undergo passive-active immunization. IG has a good safety record, the main side effect being local discomfort.

Passive immunization is recommended for several "at-risk" groups, including travelers to endemic areas and household contacts of index cases with HAV infection, unless there is a well-documented history of HAV infection. Although the secondary attack rates are highest among children, adults are at greatest risk of symptomatic disease, and therefore contacts of all ages should be given IG. Contacts outside the home (i.e., at work or school) do not require passive immunoprophylaxis unless repeated cases are occurring, suggesting the presence of a common-source outbreak. For containment of HAV outbreaks in nursing homes or other institutions, administration of IG may be required in addition to strict adherence to preventive measures.

Reports of hepatitis A that develops despite apparently adequate passive immunoprophylaxis have raised concerns about the potency of the current IG product. IG anti-HAV titers have declined, consistent with the changing prevalence of anti-HAV in the donor population.[32] It is unclear whether the somewhat lower titers of anti-HAV are associated with a significant reduction in efficacy of IG; HAV vaccination of plasma donors may be one method to produce IG with high titers of anti-HAV.

Table 68–4 | **Basic Characteristics and Comparisons of Immune Globulin and HAV-Inactivated Vaccine**

CHARACTERISTIC	IMMUNE GLOBULIN	VACCINE
Anti-HAV production	No	Yes
Time to anti-HAV detection	Immediate	1–2 wk
Peak anti-HAV titer	150 IU/L	4000 IU/L
Preexposure protective efficacy	90%–95%	95%–100%
Duration of protection	4–6 mo	>20 yr
Side effects	Mild and rare	Mild and rare

Active Immunoprophylaxis

Three different strategies have been utilized in vaccine development: a live attenuated virus vaccine, an inactivated virus vaccine, and a recombinant polypeptide vaccine (see Table 68–4).

Live Attenuated Vaccines

The live attenuated vaccine, produced by serial passage of HAV in cell culture to create a virus with reduced infectivity but with retained antigenicity, was the first available HAV vaccine.[33] The vaccine induces the development of anti-HAV in 100% of vaccinees, with persistence of neutralizing antibody for 3 to 6 months. Adverse effects are minimal.

Inactivated Vaccines

Because of the potential risk of reversion of a live vaccine to a virulent strain, inactivated virus vaccines have been developed. For inactivated vaccines, the virus is grown in cell culture and then inactivated by exposure to formalin. Two commercially available and licensed HAV vaccines (Havrix, Glaxo Smith Kline; and VAQTA, Merck Sharp and Dohme) have been studied extensively and found to be safe and efficacious.[34–36] These vaccines are highly immunogenic, with 90% to 98% seroconversion rates after a single 25-U dose and a 100% seroconversion rate after three doses.[34, 35] Lower rates of seroconversion after a single dose may occur with increasing age and a body weight greater than 77 kg, and in these persons, two 25-U doses given 2, 4, or 8 weeks apart are necessary to obtain early seroconversion.[34, 35] It is anticipated that protective antibody levels will last for more than 20 years.[37] In vaccinees in whom titers of anti-HAV have fallen to borderline levels, an anamnestic response is seen when a booster dose is given and antibody persists for at least 12 months.[34, 35] Administration of IG in combination with HAV vaccine results in lower titers of anti-HAV, and a booster dose of vaccine is recommended in persons who receive this combination.[38] Seroconversion results in protection against HAV infection. Postvaccination testing for a serologic response is not indicated because of the high rate of vaccine response in normal subjects.[37]

The association between severe HAV infection and underlying chronic liver disease has led to the recommendation that patients with chronic liver disease be vaccinated against HAV.[37, 39] Recent data have provided evidence that supports the efficacy and immunogenicity of the HAV vaccine in patients with mild-to-moderate chronic liver disease.[40] Postvaccination testing is not recommended in these patients. However, HAV vaccination has uncertain efficacy in patients with advanced liver disease[41] and in liver transplant recipients.[42] In these groups, postvaccination testing is recommended. Although scarce, available data suggest that testing for anti-HAV in patients with chronic liver disease before vaccination is cost-effective in light of the high prevalence of anti-HAV in this patient population (approximately 50%–75%).[43]

Recombinant Polypeptide Vaccines

The development of immunogenic recombinant polypeptides offers the potential advantage of large-scale production of a highly purified, safe, and potentially less expensive product. Sequences from the VP0, VP1, and VP3 proteins have been inserted into expression vectors to generate the corresponding polypeptides, and further progress with both attenuated and recombinant polypeptide vaccines can be anticipated.

Treatment

Supportive measures are the only treatment necessary in most cases of acute HAV infection. Sedatives and narcotics should be avoided. There are no mandatory dietary modifications. Hospitalization is advised in patients with severe or persistent anorexia or vomiting and in those with indices of developing acute liver failure (see Chapter 80). In patients with severe cholestasis, a short course of prednisolone (30 mg/day with a taper over 1–2 weeks) may reduce the severity of symptoms, such as pruritus and malaise, and the serum bilirubin level. Prolonged administration of glucocorticoids is not recommended. Cholestyramine is the drug of choice for pruritus. Acute liver failure should prompt early consideration of liver transplantation.

Cost

As the incidence of hepatitis A declines in the United States, there is an increasing number of susceptible adolescents and adults. Severe HAV infection, which is associated with greater morbidity and mortality, is more likely to develop in such persons than in younger persons infected with HAV. The economic burden of hepatitis A was recently evaluated in order to assess the potential economic benefit of vaccination programs. Under base-case assumptions, annual hepatitis A costs were estimated to be $488.8 million in 1997.[44] These costs could be reduced by universal vaccination of children, which has been shown to be cost-effective if the cost of the two-dose vaccine is reduced to less than $75.[45]

Current recommendations of the Advisory Committee on Immunization Practices for use of HAV vaccine target high-risk persons (Table 68–5) and those with underlying chronic liver disease. This strategy will likely not achieve a sustained reduction of disease incidence, which will probably require universal infant vaccination with catch-up immunization of adolescents. Furthermore, the recommendation to vaccinate patients with underlying chronic liver disease was recently questioned in a study that showed a lack of cost-effectiveness for this approach, with a current annual incidence of hepatitis A of only 0.01%.[46]

Table 68–5 | **Persons at Increased Risk of Hepatitis A in Whom Hepatitis A Vaccine Is Recommended**

Travelers to countries with high or intermediate HAV endemism
Men who have sex with men
Illicit drug users
Persons who work with HAV-infected primates or with HAV in a research laboratory
Persons with clotting factor disorders
Persons who live in communities with high or intermediate rates of hepatitis A
Children living in areas where rates of hepatitis A are at least twice the national average (eg, ≥20 cases per 100,000 population)

HEPATITIS B VIRUS

The first recognition of a form of hepatitis that was transmissible through blood or blood products was reported by Lurman in Germany in 1883.[47] He reported on a large group of persons who received a smallpox vaccine that had been prepared from human sera. Jaundice developed in 15% of that group over the next several weeks to months, but in none of their coworkers who had not undergone immunization. A vaccine derived from human serum was again implicated in the transmission of hepatitis during World War II. In this case, there was a high incidence of jaundice among a specific group of soldiers who received a yellow fever vaccine that was made from human serum.[48] In the late 1960s, a unique antigen was identified in the serum of an Australian aborigine patient with acute leukemia, and subsequently this antigen was found to occur most commonly in patients who had received multiple blood transfusions.[49–51] The antigen was called the Australia antigen, and further studies established a relationship between the Australia antigen and the development of hepatitis B. This association eventually led to the development of the first specific diagnostic tests for HBV infection.[50] Ultimately, it was recognized that the Australia antigen was the hepatitis B surface antigen (HBsAg) protein. Confirmation of the hypothesis that hepatitis B is a viral infection and that it is associated with the Australia antigen was achieved through the recognition by electron microscopy of specific virions that reacted with serum directed against the Australia antigen.[51] These virions were termed "Dane particles," and they were subsequently shown in fact to be the etiologic agent responsible for HBV infection.

Virology

Hepadnaviruses

HBV is a member of a family of distinct viruses, known as the Hepadnaviridae, which infect humans and a few animal species (duck, ground squirrel, and woodchuck) (see Table 68–1). Characteristics of these viruses include the presence of partially double-stranded DNA that is surrounded by an outer lipoprotein envelope and an inner core composed of nucleocapsid proteins (see Table 68–1). The virus encodes a polymerase that catalyzes by reverse transcription both the generation of DNA complementary to the viral RNA template and the synthesis of positive-strand viral DNA from the negative-strand DNA template of the virus (Fig. 68–3).[52, 53] In contrast to most other viruses, hepadnaviruses massively overproduce viral envelope proteins (e.g., HBsAg). The reason for this overproduction is poorly understood. Finally, these viruses are all predominantly hepatotropic, although other organs can be infected.

Animal models of HBV have been extremely useful in

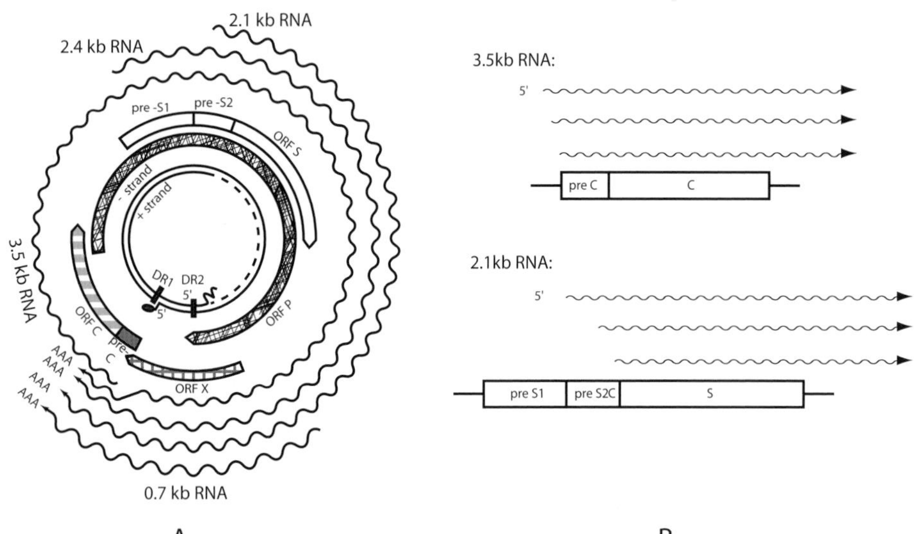

Figure 68–3. Genomic organization of HBV. *A,* The partially double-stranded DNA *(complete minus strand and partial plus strand);* the major viral mRNA coded by these regions *(wavy lines on the outer circle);* and resultant proteins (S, P, C, and X) from the four open reading frames (ORF). The filled circle at the 5′ end of the minus-strand DNA represents the terminal protein; the wavy line at the 5′ end of the plus strand denotes the terminal RNA. DR1 and DR2 are the direct repeats, which are important for the initiation of viral DNA synthesis. *B,* Details of the viral transcripts of the preC/C regions *(top)* and preS/S regions *(bottom)* (see text for greater detail). (From Ganem D: Hepadnaviridae: The viruses and their replication. In Fields BN, Knipe DM, Hawley, PM: [eds]: Fundamental Virology, 3rd ed. Philadelphia, Lippincott-Raven, 1996, pp 1199–1234.)

elucidating the biology of hepadnaviruses. Differences among these animal models make them more or less applicable to human disease. The ground squirrel (GSHV) and woodchuck hepatitis virus (WHV) are similar to HBV morphologically and share approximately 60% homology in nucleotide sequence with HBV. As with HBV, GSHV and WHV exhibit strong hepatotropism and are associated with acute and chronic liver disease as well as with the development of hepatocellular carcinoma (HCC). Chronic WHV infection is associated with minimal hepatitis yet a strong propensity for the development of HCC, thereby implicating mechanisms other than cell turnover in the pathogenesis of HCC. In vivo studies of viral kinetics have shown that the plasma half-life of HBV is 24 hours, with a daily turnover of 50% and a daily production of 10^{11} virions.[54]

Duck hepatitis B virus (DHBV) is more genetically distinct from HBV than are the other hepadnaviruses, and hence many biologic and immunologic features of this virus differ from those of HBV. DHBV is much less hepatotropic than HBV, is associated with mild or no hepatitis, and has not been strongly implicated in HCC. Nevertheless, DHBV has been a useful model for investigating the hepadnavirus life cycle and for screening potential antiviral drugs. Woodchucks infected with WHV also have been useful for the testing of safety and efficacy of antiviral agents.

Structure

HBV is a remarkably compact virus with four open reading frames (ORF) (S, P, C, and X) that encode four major proteins (surface, polymerase, core, and X protein, respectively) (see Fig. 68–3). Intact HBV virions are 42 nm in diameter and are readily visualized by electron microscopy. HBsAg, or S protein, which is 24 kD in size, is the major envelope protein of the virus. Two other proteins, L and M, which are 39 kD and 31 kD, respectively, are also present in the viral envelope. Both of these proteins include the S protein fused to peptides of variable length at the amino terminal end. The L protein, which is synthesized from an AUG initiation codon upstream from the S gene in the pre-S1 region, is believed to play a role in binding virus to a receptor on the hepatocyte surface. The function of the M protein, which is synthesized from an AUG initiation site between the pre-S1 and S gene in the pre-S2 region, is unknown. These three envelope proteins can be either glycosylated or nonglycosylated.

Within the envelope is a 27-nm structure known as the nucleocapsid core, which consists of 180 copies of the viral core protein, or hepatitis B core antigen (HBcAg), surrounding the viral DNA and the virally encoded polymerase. This icosahedral structure protects the viral DNA from degradation by exogenous nucleases. The nucleic acid itself is a relaxed circular molecule that consists of a 3.2-kB minus strand and a smaller, complementary DNA plus strand of variable length (see Figs. 68–3 and 68–4). The circular structure of HBV is maintained by hydrogen bonds between 250 bp at the two 5′ ends of the plus and minus strands. The 5′ ends of the DNA strands are each linked covalently to additional structures that are essential for the initiation of DNA synthesis: the polymerase, which is bound to the 5′ end of the minus strand; and an oligo RNA, which is linked to the 5′ end of the plus strand. Two short repeat sequences known as DR1 and DR2, which are present at the 5′ ends of the plus and minus strands, are important for the initiation of DNA synthesis (see later section).

The viral polymerase is bound to the 5′ end of the minus strand, where it functions as both a reverse transcriptase for synthesis of the negative DNA strand from genomic RNA and an endogenous DNA polymerase. Its function as a polymerase includes synthesis of completely double-stranded, relaxed, circular DNA by using the 3′ end of the plus strand as a primer and the 5′ end of the minus strand as a template. The HBV polymerase, which is encoded by the P gene of the virus, is distantly related to reverse transcriptase (RT) enzymes of retroviruses such as human immunodeficiency virus (HIV). This similarity to retroviral RT has been exploited in the development of drugs, such as lamivudine, that inhibit the activities of both enzymes (see later section).

The function of the X protein has not been fully elucidated, but the X protein appears to be essential for replica-

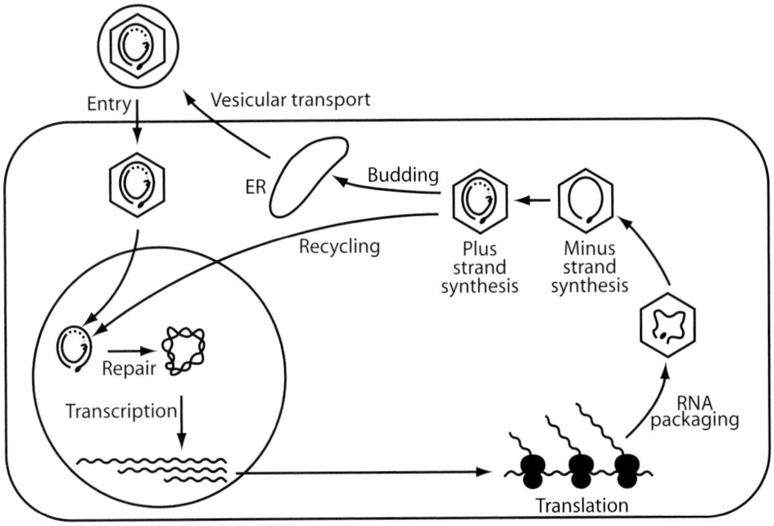

Figure 68–4. Life cycle of hepatitis B virus. See text for details. ER, endoplasmic reticulum. (From Ganem D: Hepadnaviridae: The viruses and their replication. In Fields BN, Knipe DM, Hawley PM [eds]: Fundamental Virology, 3rd ed. Philadelphia, Lippincott-Raven, 1996, pp 1199–1234.)

tion because viral genomes with mutations in the X ORF fail to produce active infection in culture. X protein appears to function as a transcriptional activator that influences the transcription of HBV genes as well as those of other viruses (e.g., HIV) by regulating the activity of transcriptional promoters.[55] The clinical relevance of these in vitro observations remains to be determined.

In addition to intact virions, serum and HBV-infected hepatocytes of infected persons contain subviral particles, which are produced in great excess. These 20-nm spheres and long filamentous structures consist predominantly of S protein, with a lesser contribution from L and M proteins. These subviral particles are not infectious because they contain no viral DNA. They are, however, strongly immunogenic and stimulate the production of neutralizing antibodies in the host. This property was exploited in the development of the first HBV vaccines. The function of these subviral particles in the life cycle of the virus is unknown.

Genomic Organization

Despite its small size (3.2 kb), HBV encodes four major proteins: the surface, core, and X proteins and the polymerase. This compactness is achieved by the use of overlapping ORFs, so that more than one half of the nucleotides are used in a different frame for the transcription of different viral messenger RNAs (mRNAs). These mRNAs are in turn translated into more than one viral protein. For example, the S gene, which encodes HBsAg, is used in its entirety in another frame to encode part of the polymerase (see Fig. 68–3). Multiple related proteins are also produced by differential translation at multiple AUG translation initiation codons within the same ORF. For example, three proteins, S, pre-S1 or L, and pre-S2 or M, are synthesized from the pre-S/S gene (see previous discussion). Two related proteins are produced by a similar mechanism from translation of mRNAs encoded by the core gene. One of these, the core peptide, is a 21-kD protein that forms the nucleocapsid core of the virus; the translation of the second protein, the hepatitis B e antigen (HBeAg), is initiated at a start codon upstream from the core AUG codon and consists of the core peptide plus a 30-amino-acid residue encoded by the precore region. The precore region contains a signal sequence that directs the protein to the endoplasmic reticulum, where host proteases cleave much of the C-terminus of the protein to form HBeAg, which is subsequently excreted from the cell. The function of this 16kD protein is unknown, but it is clearly not necessary for viral replication because replication-competent mutant viruses in which translation of the precore sequence is inhibited have been well described both in vitro and in vivo. These so-called "precore mutants" in humans are associated with active viral replication (readily detectable HBV DNA in serum), lack of HBeAg production, and progressive liver disease (see later section). In light of the cross-immunoreactivity between HBcAg and HBeAg, a possible function of HBeAg is to divert the immune response of the host away from virally infected hepatocytes that express HBcAg on their surfaces. In this model, the absence of HBeAg production would be associated with a vigorous and, for the virus, potentially lethal immune response against the hepatocyte. However, direct evidence that HBeAg is an immunologic "smoke screen" is lacking.

HBeAg is also a marker of active viral replication. HBeAg is translated from genomic-length mRNA transcripts that are similar to those used for synthesis of viral DNA by RT. Thus, production of high levels of HBeAg is indicative of synthesis of large amounts of full-length genomic mRNA, which in turn reflects active viral replication.

During transcription, viral mRNAs specific for each related protein are transcribed from separate sites within the ORF of each gene (see Fig. 68–3). Thus, the translation initiation start codon, which is positioned near the 5′ end of the mRNA, can be efficiently recognized by the host ribosomes and the viral protein that is translated. There are distinct mRNAs encoding the three envelope proteins, the X protein, and the two precore proteins. However, the largest mRNA transcript, which is 3.5 kb in length, is translated into two proteins, the polymerase and core protein, that is, it is bicistronic. The 5′ end of this mRNA is used for the translation of the core protein, and the translation initiation codon for the polymerase is 500 nucleotides downstream. It is unclear how the ribosome initiates translation of the polymerase at this second internal entry site.

Replication

Much of our understanding of the mechanism of HBV replication is derived from experiments performed in ducks, woodchucks, and ground squirrels. Although extremely useful, extrapolation of these results to human disease must be made with caution. For example, activation of host oncogenes by WHV has been clearly described in hepatic oncogenesis in WHV, yet comparable activation has not been demonstrated in HBV-associated HCC in man.

The duck model has been particularly useful because these animals are available commercially, and primary duck hepatocytes in culture support efficient DHBV replication. In contrast, normal human hepatocytes are limited in their availability, have limited longevity in culture, and can only be infected with HBV with low efficiency. Certain transformed cell lines, such as HepG2 cells, can be transfected with cloned HBV DNA and produce infectious virions. This human system has been used extensively to examine the effects of mutations in different viral genes on the replication competence of these viruses.

The life cycle of HBV includes the following steps (see Fig. 68–4):

1. Viral binding and entry: Early events in viral binding and entry are poorly understood. However, these first steps likely determine the host range and relative hepatotropism of HBV, because other cell lines can support HBV replication if viral DNA is introduced by transfection (which bypasses viral binding and cell entry). In DHBV, there is convincing evidence that sequences in the pre-S region determine viral binding. Supportive, although less convincing, data suggest that the same is true for human HBV infection.
2. Viral uncoating in the cytoplasm: After viral entry, which likely occurs by direct membrane fusion rather than receptor-mediated endocytosis, the virus is uncoated, and the nucleocapsid core is transported to the nucleus, perhaps by passive diffusion or microtubule-dependent transport. Uncertainty exists as to how the viral DNA enters the nucleus, because the nucleocapsid is too large to traverse the nuclear pores. The viral genome may be uncoated in the cytoplasm, with transport of the naked DNA into the nucleus.
3. Synthesis of complete double-stranded DNA in the nucleus: Once in the nucleus, the viral genome is repaired (i.e., the gap in the positive-strand genome is filled in), and covalently closed circular DNA (cccDNA), which is completely double stranded, is formed. Synthesis of cccDNA is catalyzed by the viral DNA polymerase.
4. Synthesis of genomic or pregenomic RNA and viral transcripts necessary for viral protein production: The cccDNA is the template for synthesis of genomic and subgenomic transcripts, catalyzed by host RNA polymerase II (see Fig. 68–4). Each of the four major viral transcripts is expressed by its own promoter. The core promoter is central to replication because it controls the production of the genomic RNA, which is the template for future DNA minus-strand synthesis.[56]
5. Translation of viral transcripts: Viral RNA transcripts are transported into the cytoplasm, where translation yields the viral envelope, core, precore, and X proteins and the viral DNA polymerase.
6. Encapsidation: Viral packaging, or encapsidation, occurs in the cytoplasm, a reaction that is initiated by the binding of viral polymerase to a unique stem-loop structure at the 5′ end of the genomic RNA. This stem-loop structure serves as an encapsidation signal for assembly of the viral core (consisting of 180 molecules of core protein), which occurs simultaneously with DNA synthesis. The encapsidation sequence (or ϵ) is found at the 5′ end of pregenomic RNA and at the 3′ end of subgenomic RNA, but is not present in cellular mRNA. Because this sequence is only recognized when present at the 5′ end of the molecule, only pregenomic RNA is incorporated into the viral core; subgenomic and cellular RNA are excluded.
7. Reverse transcription and synthesis of DNA strands: Central to the replication of HBV is the production of an RNA intermediate followed by the synthesis of viral DNA by RT, mostly within the viral core in the cytoplasm. The two DNA strands of HBV are made sequentially rather than simultaneously as occurs in conventional DNA replication. The template for the minus strand is pregenomic mRNA, and the template for synthesis of the plus strand is minus-strand DNA. Minus-strand DNA synthesis is initiated by the viral polymerase, which uses the bulge of the ϵ stem-loop as the initial template.[57] With synthesis of the plus strand, the RNA template is degraded by specific RNAaseH activity, which resides in the viral polymerase.[58] Once minus-strand synthesis is complete, plus-strand synthesis is initiated with use of an RNA primer at the 5′ end of pregenomic RNA.[59]
8. Envelopment: After replication is complete, the viral core can either be transported into the nucleus or, as occurs more frequently, pass through the endoplasmic reticulum or Golgi apparatus, where the core acquires the envelope proteins (surface, L, and M) before exportation from the cell by vesicular transport. The envelope proteins of HBV are directed to the endoplasmic reticulum by specific sequences in the S gene, where they span the membrane. During the passage of the viral cores through the endoplasmic reticulum, these proteins, in conjunction with lipid from the endoplasmic reticulum, surround the core, which is then budded off from the Golgi.[60] Surface and pre-S1 (L) proteins are essential for envelopment; pre-S2 (M) protein is not. The pre-S1 protein contains the putative receptor-binding region of HBV that facilitates cell-surface binding to hepatocytes and is likely arranged on the outside of the envelope. Early in infection, nucleocapsid cores are preferentially transported back to the nucleus, where synthesis of the plus strand is completed and stable cccDNA molecules are formed. The cccDNA molecules form a reservoir of transcriptional templates so that after cell division of the infected hepatocyte, infection will be propagated to daughter hepatocytes. When infection is well established, nucleocapsid cores are preferentially exported from the hepatocyte, thereby facilitating horizontal spread of infection throughout the liver.

In contrast to classical retroviruses such as HIV, integration of HBV DNA into the host genome is not necessary for viral RNA synthesis, and HBV transcripts are synthesized entirely from episomal DNA. Integration of HBV DNA (either intact or, more frequently, in fragments) does occur in chronic infection. Although integrants may be important for hepatic carcinogenesis, they are not required for viral replication. Indeed, because integration of virus requires disruption of the integrity of the DNA strand and every nucleotide of HBV encodes a viral protein, integration of viral DNA will reduce and most often abolish the replication potential of the integrant.

The unique life cycle of this family of viruses affords special opportunities for the development of antiviral agents (see later section). The similarities between sequences of the viral polymerases of HBV and HIV made it apparent that some inhibitors of HIV polymerase/RT might have activity against the HBV polymerase (see later section).

Epidemiology

Incidence and Prevalence

Chronic hepatitis B is a common disease with an estimated global prevalence of over 300 million carriers, or approximately 5% of the world's population. In the United States, approximately 1 to 1.25 million people are chronically infected with HBV, as indicated by HBsAg positivity.[61] There are wide ranges in the prevalence of HBV infection in different parts of the world. In the Far East (Southeast Asia, China, the Philippines, Indonesia), the Middle East, Africa, and parts of South America, the prevalence is high, with HBsAg positivity rates ranging from 8% to 15%.[62] The only region in the United States of high prevalence is Alaska, where the prevalence rate in the native population is 6.4%.[63] In regions of high seroprevalence, serologic evidence of prior HBV infection (antibody to HBcAg [anti-HBc] or antibody to HBsAg [anti-HBs] positivity) is almost universal in persons without active infection. Regions of intermediate prevalence (2%–7%) include Japan, parts of South America, Eastern and Southern Europe, and parts of central Asia. Prevalence is lowest (<2%) in the United States and Canada, Northern Europe, Australia, and the southern part of South America.

The prevalence of HBV infection in a particular community is influenced by local factors, including the ethnic mix of the population, frequency of injection drug use, and proportion of the population that engages in high-risk sexual activity. In the United States, the estimated incidence of acute HBV infection has been falling from a peak in 1985 of 70 cases per 10,000 population to 40 cases per 100,000 in 1991.[64] This falling incidence is believed to be the result of changes in behavior (e.g., an increase in safe sexual practices related to HIV education efforts) that have led to decreased transmission of infection, rather than the result of the introduction of effective vaccination programs.[64] Reliable information regarding the incidence of acute HBV infection in developing countries is not available. In the United States, the greatest prevalence of HBV is in certain ethnic groups (Alaskan natives, Pacific Islanders) and in first-generation immigrants from regions of high prevalence (Southeast Asia). Rates of HBsAg positivity range from 5% to 15% in these immigrant groups; rates of other serologic markers of HBV infection range from 43% to 65%. Other high-prevalence groups include injection drug users and men who have sex with men. African-Americans are at greater risk of HBV infection than are Caucasians (14% and 3%, respectively).[64] HBV infection is more common in men than in women, with the peak prevalence in men occurring between the ages of 10 and 29. Other patient groups at risk include household contacts and sexual partners of HBV-infected carriers, patients with multiple sexual contacts, health-care workers, and patients on hemodialysis.

In the United States, spread of infection is predominantly by horizontal routes, and adults and adolescents are at greatest risk of acquiring HBV infection.[64] However, children of certain ethnic groups are at substantial risk for infection, probably from both vertical transmission and horizontal spread in early childhood from mothers and other family members. Because the vast majority of these infections are subclinical, the true epidemiology of subclinical infection in the United States is not known.

It is well established that the risk of persistent infection is much greater in infants than in adults. Although only 1% to 3% of all reported cases of HBV infection in the United States are thought to occur in children, 20% to 30% of all chronic HBV infections in the United States occur in children under the age of 5 years.[62] The incidence of infection in different age groups in the United States is difficult to determine accurately because of current methods of reporting. The Sentinel Counties study, which was established by the Centers for Disease Control (CDC) a number of years ago to assess the epidemiology of viral hepatitis in the United States, relies largely on clinical presentation of patients with symptoms of viral hepatitis. Because children are less likely than adults to have symptoms associated with acute HBV infection, the incidence of infection in children is likely to be underestimated by the current reporting mechanisms. Nevertheless, adolescents and young adults appear to be at greatest risk of infection in the United States, presumably because of acquisition from sexual activity and, to a lesser extent, injection drug use. The epidemiology of infection is much different in the Far East and developing countries, where neonates and young children are at high risk of infection because of perinatal or early childhood transmission.

Transmission

HBV is parenterally transmitted via blood or blood products or by sexual or perinatal exposure, the same routes as for HIV; hence, there are many similarities in the epidemiology of these two viruses. Viral particles, which are capable of transmitting infection to chimpanzees, are detectable in body secretions, including semen and saliva. Thus, contact with mucous membranes and their secretions is likely to be a mode of transmission of HBV.[61]

Perinatal and Early Childhood Transmission

HBV is most prevalent in people born in regions of high HBV endemism and their descendants. High levels of virus in serum (signified by HBV DNA and HBeAg positivity) have been associated with an increased risk of transmission by needlestick exposure and by vertical routes.[61] Infants born to HBeAg-positive mothers who have high levels of viral replication (HBV DNA level >80 pg/mL) have a 70% to 90% risk of perinatal acquisition in the absence of interventions. In contrast, the risk of mother-to-infant transmission from HBeAg-negative mothers is substantially lower (10%–

40%). Infection occurs through occult inoculation of the infant at the time of birth or shortly thereafter. IgM anti-HBc is not detectable in cord blood, so that intrauterine infection is unlikely to have occurred. Even with active and passive immunization, 5% to 10% of babies may acquire HBV infection at birth.

Children of HBsAg-positive mothers who are not infected at birth remain at high risk of early childhood infection; 60% become infected by the age of 5 years.[65] The mechanism of this later infection, which is neither perinatal nor sexual, is unknown. Although HBsAg can be detected in breast milk, breast-feeding is not believed to be an important mode of transmission. Children living in areas of high endemism may acquire infection outside the family.

Sexual Transmission

Sexual activity is probably the single most important mode of HBV transmission in areas of the world such as North America, where the prevalence of infection is low. From 1980 to 1985, men who had sex with men were at particularly high risk of HBV infection and accounted for 20% of all reported cases of HBV infection.[64] Factors associated with a high risk of viral acquisition in this patient population included multiple sexual partners, anal-receptive intercourse, and duration of sexual activity.[64] The risk has fallen markedly in recent reports (to 8% of all cases), probably because of modifications of sexual behavior in response to the acquired immunodeficiency syndrome (AIDS) epidemic.[62] Unfortunately, advanced liver disease from HBV infection is emerging as an important medical problem for patients infected with HIV (see later).

Heterosexual sex now accounts for the majority of cases of HBV infection (26%) with an identifiable risk factor in the United States.[62] In heterosexuals, factors associated with an increased risk of HBV infection include duration of sexual activity, number of sexual partners, a history of sexually transmitted diseases, and positive serologic results for syphilis.[64] Sexual partners of injection drug users, prostitutes, and clients of prostitutes are at particularly high risk of HBV infection.[64]

Sexual partners of persons infected with HBV are at risk for infection, even in the absence of high-risk behavior. Studies of sexual and household contacts of HBV carriers have shown that 0% to 3% of the spouses or sexual partners and 4% to 9% of the children are HBsAg positive. Moreover, there is a high prevalence of markers of prior HBV infection in these two groups (29%–59% of spouses or sexual contacts and 9%–12% of children).[53] Because many patients with chronic HBV infection are unaware of their infection and are "silent carriers," sexual transmission is likely to be an important mode of transmission worldwide. As with perinatal transmission, sexual transmission is facilitated by active viral replication in the infected person.[53] The risk of heterosexual transmission is greater when the infected person is female than when the infected person is male.[53] The use of condoms appears to reduce the risk of sexual transmission. Sexual transmission may also account for some of the approximately 30% to 40% of all cases in the United States in which no known risk factor can be identified.[64]

Injection Drug Use

In the United States and Western Europe, injection drug use remains a very important mode of HBV transmission (23% of all cases).[62] The risk of HBV infection increases with duration of drug use, so that serologic markers of ongoing or prior HBV infection are almost universal after 5 years of drug use.

Other Modes of Transmission

Other risk factors for HBV infection include working in a health-care setting (3% of cases in the United States), transfusions and dialysis (1% each), acupuncture, tattooing, travel abroad, and residence in an institution.[62] Although the risk of transfusion-associated HBV infection has been greatly reduced with the screening of blood (with tests to detect HBsAg and anti-HBc) as well as exclusion of donors who engage in high-risk activities, it is estimated that 1 in 50,000 transfused units transmits HBV infection. Acupuncture has been associated with outbreaks of HBV infection. In World War II, contaminated plasma-stabilized yellow-fever vaccine was associated with one of the largest epidemics of HBV infection, in which icteric hepatitis developed in 50,000 U.S. army personnel.[48] Nosocomial spread of HBV infection in hospitals, particularly in dialysis units as well as in dental units, has been well described, even when current infection control practices are followed.[62] HBV infection has been linked to multiple-use heparin vials. As with other modes of transmission, high viral titers in serum have been related to an increased risk of transmission. HBV remains infectious in the environment for 7 days or longer, so that contaminated surfaces may account for transmission in the absence of a known exposure.

Epidemiology of Subtypes and Genotypes

Although there are a variety of serotypes and genotypes of HBV, there is remarkably little genomic variability in this virus. Geographic differences in the distribution of HBV subtypes have facilitated epidemiologic tracking of infection to the country of origin. There are four major serologic types of HBV (adw, ayw, adr, and ayr), which have different geographic distributions but unclear clinical differences. Classification of HBV into subtypes is dependent on serologic responses to minor differences in the proteins encoded by the nucleotide sequence of the surface gene. Common to all these subtypes is an immunodominant epitope, the "a" determinant, which is the target of neutralizing antibody in HBV infection (anti-HBs). Because of the commonality of sequence encoding the "a" determinant among subtypes of HBV, infection with one subtype is cross-protective against infection with other subtypes. Thus, coinfection with more than one subtype of HBV is rare. Mutations in the "a" determinant have been shown to arise in association with virologic "escape" from neutralizing antibodies (see later section).

There has been increasing interest in the clinical significance of HBV genotypes. As for HCV infection, there are geographic differences in the distribution of genotypes (Table 68–6). The clinical significance of these differences is under investigation but appears to be related in part to the stability of the stem-loop structure of the HBV genome and the association with precore variants of HBV (see later section).

Pathogenesis

Immune Pathogenesis

Clinical observations suggest that the immune response of the host is more important than viral factors in the pathogenesis of liver injury caused by HBV. Chronic HBV carriers who have normal liver enzyme levels and normal or near-normal liver histologic studies, despite high levels of viral replication, have been well described; significant liver injury would be predicted if the virus were directly cytopathic. Similarly, HBV can be grown in hepatocyte culture with no adverse effect on cell viability. Other clinical observations point to the importance of an intact immune response in mediating liver injury. Infants with immature immune systems who acquire HBV infection at birth have a high rate of chronic infection and replication yet typically have only mild liver injury. Conversely, HBV-induced fulminant hepatic failure is associated with a vigorous immune response, low serum levels of virus, and massive hepatocellular necrosis.

There has been extensive investigation in both humans and experimental animals of specific immune responses associated with HBV clearance (or conversely persistence) and liver injury. In acute infection, a specific immune response to multiple viral antigens can be demonstrated in both major histocompatibility complex (MHC) class II–restricted and MHC class I–restricted T cells ($CD4^+$ and $CD8^+$, respectively, the latter making up the majority of CTLs).[66] T helper cell responses to core and polymerase proteins are particularly strong, with lesser responses to the envelope proteins. In patients with chronic HBV infection who fail to clear the virus, the number of both $CD4^+$ and $CD8^+$ T cells is markedly reduced. In contrast, the humoral immune response is preserved in both acute and chronic HBV infection, although anti-HBs usually cannot be detected in the latter because of antigen excess.

There are few animals models with which to investigate the pathogenesis of liver injury and the mechanisms of viral clearance in hepadnaviral infections. Transgenic mouse models have been used to examine specific mechanisms by which CTLs clear virus and cause hepatocyte necrosis. These mice are naturally tolerant to the "transgene," that is, to different components of the HBV genome, yet their immune response can be reconstituted with infusion of CTLs from non-transgenic mice immunized with different HBV proteins.[67] Acute liver injury associated with CTL infiltration of the liver develops in a dose-dependent manner in recipients of these cells.

It has been widely accepted that CTLs are responsible for destruction of virally infected hepatocytes and for viral clearance. However, the number of CTLs involved is generally much fewer than the number (10^{11}) of virally infected hepatocytes. Thus, secondary non–antigen-specific immune responses, such as those mediated by inflammatory cytokines, may be more important for viral clearance than the CTL-mediated mechanism. Recent data point to the importance of tumor necrosis factor-α (TNF-α) and gamma-interferon as prime mediators of this non–antigen-specific clearance of HBV.[68] These cytokines activate two independent pathways that result in elimination of HBV nucleocapsid cores and destabilization of viral RNA.[69] These cytokines may also be important in the clearance of HBV in chronically infected patients who become superinfected with other hepatotropic viruses.[69, 70]

Table 68–6 | **Hepatitis B Virus Genotypes: Geographic Distribution**

SUBTYPES	GENOTYPE	GEOGRAPHIC DISTRIBUTION
ayw1 adw2	A*	Northern Europe, U.S.
ayw1 adw	B†	Eastern Asia, Far East
ayr adr adrq-	C†	Eastern Asia, Far East
ayw2 ayw3	D†	Worldwide; prevalent in Mediterranean area, Near and Middle East, South Asia
ayw4	E†	Western Sub-Saharan areas
adw4q-	F*	America, Africa
adw2	G	Recently isolated in France and U.S.

*Stable stem-loop base pairing.
†Stem-loop base pairing predisposes to development of HBV precore variants.

Viral Pathogenesis

Variant Viruses

Although there are a variety of serotypes and genotypes of HBV, there is remarkably little genomic variability in this virus. Nevertheless, mutant forms of HBV with mutations in the precore, surface, and X genes, as well as the core promoter region, have been implicated in a number of clinical syndromes. Polymerase variants that are selected by exposure to nucleoside analogues have recently been described. These polymerase variants may be less replication-competent and even less pathogenic than the wild-type virus[71] and are discussed in greater detail in the section on treatment. Several recent review articles describe the clinical significance of HBV variants and suggest changes in the nomenclature of the mutations associated with these variants.[71, 72]

Precore/Core Variants

Although the majority of Northern European and American patients with chronic HBV infection and active viral replication are HBeAg positive, many Southern European and Asian patients have severe liver disease and active viremia in the absence of HBeAg.[73] Sequence analysis of the precore region of HBV isolated from such patients has revealed a point mutation (G to A) at nucleotide position 1896 that results in the production of a translational stop codon predicted to stop translation of HBeAg.[73] In contrast, production of core peptide continues because translation of this protein is initiated at a start codon downstream from the site of mutation. Such variant viruses have also been described in association with fulminant liver failure and severe chronic liver disease.[74, 75] Whether these precore mutants are etiologically important in these syndromes or whether they merely emerge in association with severe disease remains controversial. Moreover, if the precore mutants are etiologically associated with these syndromes, the mechanism by which the virus causes these syndromes is unknown. Several hypotheses have been put forward, including 1) a heightened immune response against core peptide expressed on hepatocytes in the absence of "immune deflection" by HBeAg in serum (see previous section); 2) direct cytopathicity of the truncated HBeAg fragment that is synthesized as a result of early termination of translation of precore/core mRNA; 3) enhanced replication of mutant virus over wild-type virus because of increased stability of the hairpin stem-loop of the HBV genome, which encodes the encapsidation signal for viral packaging.[76] In the United States, only a small proportion of all cases of HBsAg-positive fulminant liver failure is associated with variant viruses.[77]

Mutations in the core promoter region have also been proposed to result in failure of HBeAg production.[78] These mutant viruses, which involve nucleotide substitutions at positions 1762 and 1764, may decrease transcription of mRNA that encodes HBeAg. Core promoter variants have been described in association with 10% of cases of fulminant HBV infection, 10% of cases of acute self-limited hepatitis, and 27% of cases of progressive chronic hepatitis.[78]

Although there has been a great deal of interest generated by the discovery of HBV variants, the clinical significance of these mutant viruses, particularly those described in association with severe liver disease, remains controversial. The presence of precore variants is also associated with the distribution of HBV genotypes. In patients with genotype A HBV infection (the predominant genotype in North America and Europe), nucleotide (nt) 1858 is a C. In this genotype, both a mutation at nt 1896 (G to A) and nt 1858 (C to T) would be required to stabilize the stem-loop structure of the HBV genome. Without a compensatory mutation at nt 1858 in genotype A, impaired base pairing results when C-1858 tries to pair with A-1896, thereby destabilizing the stem-loop structure of the packaging signal and leading to a decrease in encapsidation and in viral replication. Thus, precore stop codon mutations may be less frequent in genotype A because of the need for two mutational events. By contrast, in countries where precore mutants are common, genotypes B, C, D, and E are predominant (see Table 68–6).[79] In these patients only one mutation at nt 1896 is required to yield a precore mutant with stable stem-loop pairing of the genome.

Surface Gene Mutants

Immune escape from neutralizing antibodies occurs in a region of HBV known as the "a" determinant.[80] This hydrophilic region from amino acids 124 to 147 is highly conserved between subtypes of HBV and is believed to be important in eliciting protection against infection. The glycine at amino acid 145 in particular is highly conserved among HBV subtypes, and a G-to-A nucleotide substitution produces amino acid changes at this position that result in major antigenic changes in the virus. Escape mutants have been described in babies who have received immunoprophylaxis with polyclonal hepatitis B immune globulin (HBIG).[80] Despite protective levels of antibody, these babies became HBsAg positive and developed chronic liver disease. Virus from such a baby demonstrated a G-to-A substitution at amino acid 145 compared with the viral isolate from the mother, and the mutant virus bound HBIG with lower affinity than did the "wild-type" virus. Emergence of surface gene mutants in liver transplant recipients receiving monoclonal HBIG therapy has also been described.[81] As with the "vaccine-escape" mutants, these viruses fail to bind anti-HBs with high affinity.[82] Because of the very compact nature of the genomic organization of HBV, changes in the "a" determinant have the potential to alter the function of the HBV polymerase, an enzyme essential for viral replication. The G-to-A mutation in the "a" determinant may give rise to a stop codon (TAG) (if the nucleotide before this mutation is a T), which would have profound effects on viral replication and the pathogenesis of disease.

Low-Level HBV Infection

The existence of HBsAg-negative HBV infection has long been debated.[71, 83] Low-level HBV infection is implicated or has been documented in the following clinical situations: a) HBV infection has been transmitted by transfusion of a unit of blood from an HBsAg-negative, anti-HBc-positive blood donor; b) HBV DNA has been detected in serum and liver from persons lacking all serologic markers of HBV infection. Serum from serologically negative, HBV DNA–positive persons can transmit HBV infection to chimpanzees; c) occult HBV infection has been reported in association with apparent fulminant hepatic failure in patients who lack all serologic markers of HBV or HAV infection (so-called non-A, non-B fulminant hepatic failure), although these results are controversial[53, 85]; d) low-level HBV infection has been detected in patients with a variety of causes of chronic liver disease and in association with primary hepatocellular carcinoma.[86] Even in regions of low endemism for HBV, such as France, 11 of 22 HBsAg-negative patients with hepatocellular carcinoma had detectable HBV DNA in serum.[86] Molecular studies have demonstrated selective accumulation of RNA encoded by the X gene in association with HBsAg-negative hepatocellular carcinoma;[87] e) HBsAg-negative patients may become HBsAg positive and develop overt hepatitis with cancer chemotherapy or immunosuppression following kidney transplantation. Presumably low-level HBV infection is the source of viral reactivation that is unmasked by immunosuppression.

Whether viral or host immune factors enable persistence of HBV infection in the absence of HBsAg is unclear. Two hypotheses have been proposed to explain the atypical serologic profiles in these patients. The first hypothesis suggests that mutations in the viral genome result in impaired antigen production by the virus. Numerous mutations in HBV, particularly in the region of the gene for HBsAg, have been reported and may facilitate viral persistence.[88] The second hypothesis suggests that the host immune system keeps the virus in a quiescent or latent state until immunosuppressive therapy results in viral reactivation.

Clinical Manifestations and Diagnosis

Acute Infection

The incubation period from acute exposure to clinical symptoms ranges from 60 to 180 days (see Table 68–2). Clinical presentation varies from asymptomatic infection to cholestatic hepatitis with jaundice, and rarely liver failure. In acute infection (Fig. 68–5*A*), HBsAg and markers of active viral replication (HBeAg and HBV DNA by hybridization assays) become detectable approximately 6 weeks after inoculation, before the onset of clinical symptoms or biochemical abnormalities. These tests remain positive throughout the prodromal phase and during the early clinical phase of the illness. Biochemical abnormalities usually coincide with the prodromal phase of the acute illness and may persist for several months. With the onset of symptoms, IgM anti-HBc becomes detectable. IgM anti-HBc may persist for many months, and IgG anti-HBc may persist for many years, if not a lifetime. Anti-HBs is the last serologic test to become positive and is a marker of resolving infection (as HBsAg titers fall). Much has been made of the serologic window period when neither HBsAg nor anti-HBs is detectable and IgM anti-HBc is the only marker of acute infection. However, with currently available serologic assays, this window period is rare.

The biochemical diagnosis of acute hepatitis depends largely on measurements of serum bilirubin and aminotransferase levels. The serum alanine aminotransferase (ALT) level is typically higher than the serum aspartate aminotransferase (AST) level, and levels of both aminotransferases are usually 500 U/L or greater. Bilirubin elevations are usually modest (5–10 mg/dL), although they may be higher in the setting of hemolysis or renal failure.

The most profound complication of acute HBV infection is fulminant hepatic failure, defined as the onset of hepatic encephalopathy within 8 weeks of the onset of symptoms. Although this complication is infrequent (occurring in less than 1% of cases), the prognosis is poor once encephalopathy has developed. When patients present with acute hepatitis, it is essential to obtain tests of hepatic synthetic function (prothrombin time, serum albumin). Evidence of a prolonged prothrombin time (International Normalized Ratio [INR] of 1.5 or greater or prothrombin time of 17 seconds or longer) should raise concern regarding the potential development of fulminant hepatic failure. If clinical symptoms of hepatic failure develop, patients should be referred for consideration of liver transplantation.

Current serologic assays for the diagnosis of acute and chronic HBV infection (HBsAg and HBeAg) are both sensitive and specific. HBsAg, HBeAg, anti-HBc, and anti-HBe are detected by standardized enzyme-linked immunoassays (EIAs). The detection of HBsAg indicates active HBV infection, and the detection of HBeAg indicates active viral replication and increased infectivity. Characteristic serologic changes develop in relation to clinical symptoms and biochemical abnormalities in acute resolving infection and in acute followed by chronic infection (see Figs. 68–5*A* and *B*).

Chronic Infection

In acute HBV infection that progresses to chronicity (see Fig. 68–5*B*), early events are similar to those in acute HBV infection that resolves. However, with chronic infection, HBsAg, HBeAg, and HBV DNA remain positive for 6 months or longer. After the acute phase of infection, serum ALT levels fall but often remain persistently abnormal (from 50 to 200 U/L). IgM anti-HBc titers typically fall to undetectable levels after 6 months but may become detectable again during reactivation of infection. IgG anti-HBc persists indefinitely. HBV DNA is detectable by hybridization assays during the acute and chronic phases of disease. With time, there may be a spontaneous loss of HBV DNA and HBeAg, frequently in association with a flare of serum ALT levels and seroconversion to anti-HBe positivity. Spontaneous loss of HBsAg is rare. Anti-HBs may be detected simultaneously with HBsAg in serum in fewer than 10% of cases. In some cases of chronic infection, active viral replication (HBV DNA positivity) occurs in the absence of HBeAg (see previous section).

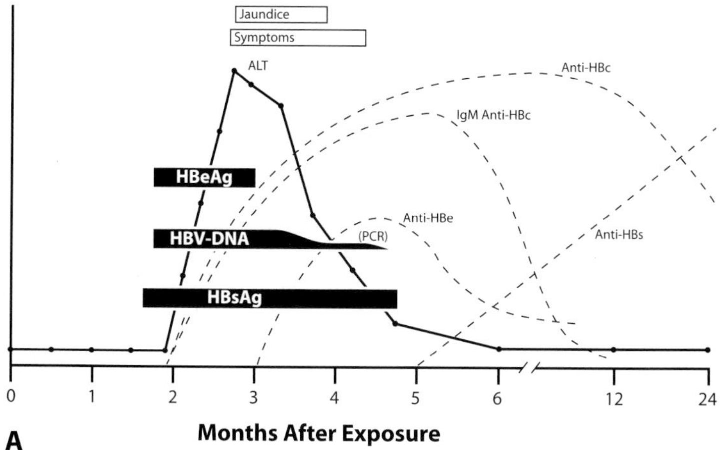

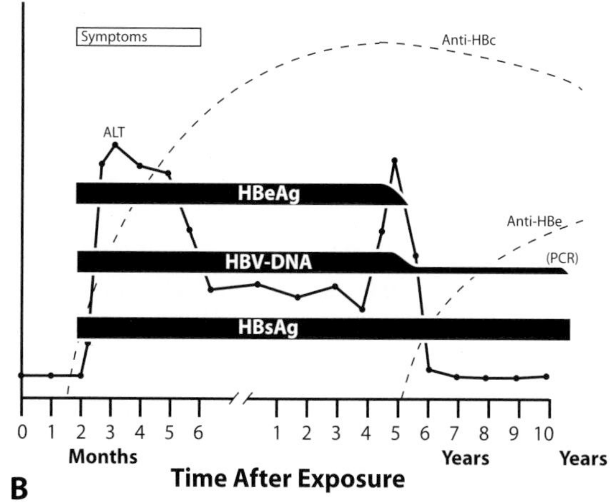

Figure 68–5. Sequence of events after acute hepatitis B virus (HBV) infection. *A*, Acute HBV infection with resolution (for explanation of these events, see text). *B*, Acute HBV infection going to chronicity (for explanation of these events, see text). (From Hoofnagle JH, DiBisceglie AM: Serologic diagnosis of acute and chronic viral hepatitis. Semin Liver Dis 11:73, 1991.)

The presence of anti-HBs is associated with immunity to HBV infection. Isolated anti-HBs is more likely to be acquired by vaccination than by natural infection, in which both anti-HBs and IgG anti-HBc are typically present. Much confusion surrounds the interpretation of isolated anti-HBc positivity. The significance of this finding depends on the patient population in which it is observed. Fifty percent of patients with chronic HCV infection are anti-HBc positive, and in these patients, who have had frequent parenteral exposure, the anti-HBc positivity likely represents resolved HBV infection or low-level HBV infection of minor clinical significance. In Alaskan natives, a group with a high prevalence of HBV infection, vaccination against HBV has been used to determine whether isolated anti-HBc signifies prior exposure; those with a primary immune anti-HBs response were deemed to have a false-positive anti-HBc, whereas those with an anamnestic response were deemed to have a true-positive anti-HBc, indicative of prior or ongoing low-level HBV infection. In blood donors who have been prescreened for parenteral risk factors, an isolated anti-HBc, particularly if it is of low optical density on EIA, likely represents a false-positive result. Because there is no readily available "gold standard" for the diagnosis of resolved or ongoing low-level HBV infection, the interpretation of an isolated positive anti-HBc remains problematic.

Diagnosis

Serologic assays for the diagnosis of acute and chronic infection are described in Figures 68–5*A* and *B*. Assays for the quantitation of HBV DNA are in development, and none are yet approved by the Food and Drug Administration (FDA). HBV DNA quantification is generally performed by signal or target amplification tests; the liquid hybridization test (Genostics assay [Abbott Laboratories, Abbott Park, Chicago. IL]) uses a liquid phase to hybridize ^{125}I-HBV DNA after the sample HBV DNA has been denatured. The lower detection limit of the assay is 1–2 pg/mL or 6×10^5 copies/mL. The RNA-DNA hybrid assay (Digene Hybrid Capture II HBV DNA Test) uses an HBV-RNA probe to capture serum HBV DNA and has a sensitivity of 0.018 pg/mL or 5×10^5 copies/mL. The branched DNA assay (Bayer, Emeryville, CA) is a compound nucleic hybridization assay that uses a synthetic oligonucleotide to bind single-stranded HBV DNA to a solid phase. Different oligonucleotides bind to other areas of HBV DNA (throughout the genome) and also bind amplifier oligonucleotides (branched DNA) that enhance the chemiluminescent signal by having multiple branches of the same sequence that bind alkaline phosphatase–labeled probes. The sensitivity limit is 7×10^5 DNA equivalents/mL. The polymerase chain reaction (PCR) assay is based on the amplification of viral DNA, together with an internal standard, using HBV-specific complementary primers usually to the precore/core region. The PCR method can now be performed automatically in the Cobas analyzer after the manual extraction of viral DNA (Cobas Amplicor HBV Monitor or Cobas-AM)[89] or using real-time fluorescent-probe PCR (TaqMan).[90] The sensitivity of the Cobas-Amplicor assay is between 100 and 400 copies/mL, and that for the Taqman method is as low as 10 copies/mL; both assays are more sensitive than the branched DNA and Genostics assays. These last tests are especially less sensitive in the detection of HBV DNA in HBsAg-positive, HBeAg-negative patients (13% and 25%, respectively) but have a high specificity (100% for each assay).[91]

In summary, convenient methods for detection of HBV DNA are now available but are expensive and are not yet standardized across different commercial assays. In the future these new, very sensitive methods will be necessary to evaluate viral replication especially in patients with precore mutant forms of HBV and in those patients undergoing therapy with antiviral nucleoside analogues.

Extrahepatic Manifestations

Extrahepatic findings are common in patients with acute HBV infection. Arthralgias and rashes occur in 25% of cases. A severe serum sickness–like syndrome with immune complex deposition occurs more rarely and can result in angioneurotic edema. Polyarteritis nodosa with a systemic vasculitis can occur with either acute or chronic HBV infection. This syndrome typically presents with abdominal pain resulting from arteritis of the medium-sized arteries with ischemia to the intestine or gallbladder. Other manifestations of HBV-associated vasculitis include neuropathy (mononeuritis), renal disease, cutaneous vasculitis, arthritis, and Raynaud's phenomenon.[92] Chronic, and to a lesser extent acute, HBV infection has also been associated with membranoproliferative glomerulonephritis resulting from deposition of immune complexes in the basement membrane of the glomerulus. The syndrome of type II mixed essential cryoglobulinemia was previously believed to be caused largely by HBV infection but has been shown to be associated more frequently with chronic HCV infection (see later section).[93] Neurologic manifestations of HBV infection include Guillain-Barré syndrome and a polyneuropathy (usually related to polyarteritis). HBV infection is rarely associated with pericarditis and pancreatitis.

Complications

Patients with chronic HBV infection are at risk of developing long-term complications of portal hypertension and hepatic decompensation, such as variceal bleeding, ascites, and hepatorenal syndrome, as well as HCC, which may ultimately result in death. When complications occur, referral for liver transplantation should be considered. Evolving antiviral therapies, discussed later, have greatly improved the outcome of patients with HBV infection after liver transplantation.

Patients with chronic liver disease, particularly those with established cirrhosis, are at increased risk of developing HCC (see Chapter 81). The risk of developing HCC is increased 10- to 390-fold in patients with chronic HBV infection compared with those who are HBsAg negative and is greater in those who acquired HBV infection perinatally than in those who acquired the infection as adults. In regions where HBV is endemic, HCC is the leading cause of cancer-related deaths.[94]

Despite this strong epidemiologic link between HBV infection and HCC, and despite active research in this area for more than a decade, the mechanism by which HBV causes malignant transformation has not been elucidated. Comparison of HBV DNA sequences with those of known oncogenes has failed to identify a specific viral oncogene. Activation of an adjacent host cellular oncogene may occur during the process of HBV genome integration, but the viral genome does not integrate into the host genome in any consistent pattern. Cirrhosis of the liver is present in more than 90% of patients with HCC related to HBV, suggesting that the presence of cirrhosis is a risk factor for HCC development. Chronic inflammation associated with active viral replication, together with ongoing cellular proliferation and regeneration associated with cirrhosis, is likely a predisposing factor that leads to cellular transformation and frank malignancy.

Coinfection with Other Viruses

Risk factors for acquisition of HBV infection are similar to those for acquisition of HIV infection. Both viruses have an increased prevalence in persons with multiple sexual partners and in injection drug users.[53] In contrast, sexual transmission of HDV and HCV is relatively inefficient, so that coinfection with HBV and these two viruses is seen primarily in patients with injection drug use as their risk factor for infection.[53] Patients with vertically acquired HBV infection rarely have coexisting infection with other viruses.

Markers of prior or active HBV infection are present in more than 80% of patients with HIV infection, approximately 10% of whom are HBsAg positive.[95] Conversely, HIV infection can be prevalent in patients with chronic HBV infection. In one study of 260 patients with chronic HBV infection, HIV coexisted in 13%.[96] After acute infection with HBV, patients with HIV infection are at greater risk of developing chronic HBV infection than are those without HIV infection. Compared with patients with HBV infection alone, HBV/HIV coinfected patients have higher levels of viral replication, lower serum ALT values, and milder histologic disease. Historically, HBV infection has not adversely affected survival in HIV-positive patients,[95] although with improving survival of HIV-infected patients, liver disease is emerging as an important clinical problem. Coinfected patients have reduced rates of response to alpha-interferon. Treatment of HBV infection is made more problematic in persons with coinfection, because the majority of infected persons have been exposed to lamivudine as part of their HIV regimen and are infected with lamivudine-resistant variants of HBV. In patients coinfected with HBV and HCV, preliminary data suggest that viral interactions result in lower serum HBV DNA levels than in those with HBV infection alone.[70] The significance of such viral interactions remains to be determined.

Pathology

As with other chronic viral hepatitides, HBV infection is associated with a predominantly lymphocytic infiltrate that may or may not be confined to the portal tracts. Prior classification of liver injury into chronic persistent, chronic lobular, and chronic active hepatitis, with or without cirrhosis, has been largely replaced with a histologic scoring system that quantifies the degree of inflammation and fibrosis on a scale of 0 to 4 (see Chapter 75). Characteristic of chronic HBV infection is the presence of ground-glass hepatocytes, in which the cytoplasm is stained pink with hematoxyline and eosin, reflecting the massive overproduction of HBsAg in these chronically infected cells. A specific histologic entity known as *fibrosing cholestatic hepatitis* has been described in liver transplant recipients with severe recurrent HBV infection in the allograft.[53] The pathology is characterized by massive hepatocellular necrosis in the absence of a strong inflammatory response, with striking overexpression of viral proteins. Immunohistochemical and molecular methods have been developed to detect viral antigens and viral DNA, respectively, in liver tissue. The role of these methods in the clinical management of patients with chronic HBV infection remains to be defined.

Natural History

Chronic HBV infection is usually defined as detectable hepatitis B surface antigenemia for a period of six months or more.[97] The risk of chronic infection is related to two major factors: the age at which infection is acquired and the immune state of the host. Detection of HBV DNA by sensitive molecular techniques has brought the standard definition of chronic HBV infection into question, because viral DNA and infectious virions can clearly be detected in patients who are HBsAg negative.[83, 84]

The risk of chronicity after acute HBV infection is low in immunocompetent adults.[48, 97] The reported risk of chronic infection after acute exposure in adults ranges from less than 1% to 12%, but the consensus is that the risk of chronicity is less than 5%.[48] Follow-up studies conducted on 597 World War II veterans who had been infected in 1942 as a result of immunization with a contaminated lot of yellow fever vaccine found that the rate of chronicity after acute infection was less than 1%.[48] The epidemic affected approximately 330,000 army personnel, 50,000 of whom became jaundiced and 1% of whom died of fulminant liver failure. Of the 597 who were tested 40 years later, only one was HBsAg positive. This result may be an underestimate of the true proportion in whom chronic infection developed, because some patients who initially had chronic infection may have subsequently seroconverted spontaneously.

The risk of chronic infection is greatly increased in patients who have a reduced ability to recognize and clear viral infection (e.g., patients on chronic hemodialysis, those on exogenous immunosuppression following solid organ transplantation, and those receiving cancer chemotherapy). Patients with concomitant HIV infection are also at significant risk of developing chronic infection (20%–30% remain HBsAg positive after acute infection). The risk of chronicity after neonatally acquired infection is extremely high (up to 90%), presumably because neonates have an immature immune system. One possible mechanism is that the fetus is tolerized in utero to HBV following transplacental passage of viral proteins. Children below the age of 6 years have a lower yet nevertheless significant risk of chronic infection (approximately 30%).

The prognosis of chronic HBV infection is determined predominantly by the presence or absence of active viral replication and by the degree of histologic liver damage.[98]

Approximately one half of all chronic HBV carriers have evidence of active viral replication, particularly if serum aminotransferase levels are elevated.[99] Chronic HBV carriers with evidence of active viral replication are at highest risk for the development of progressive disease; cirrhosis develops in 15% to 20% of them within 5 years, even if histologic liver damage is initially mild.[53] Longitudinal follow-up of such patients has shown that the spontaneous loss of HBeAg is 7% to 20% per year; therefore, the prevalence of HBeAg declines with age.[100] HBeAg loss, which may occur spontaneously or in association with the use of antiviral therapy, is often accompanied by an exacerbation of liver disease. HBsAg loss occurs much less frequently, at a rate of 1% to 2% per year, and thus most carriers remain infected for their entire lifetime. In a prospective study of 379 HBV carriers in the United States, the 5-year survival rate was 97% in patients with early histologic changes, including chronic persistent hepatitis (in which inflammation is limited to the portal areas), compared with 86% in patients with chronic active hepatitis (in which liver cell necrosis and inflammation extend to the hepatic parenchyma) and 55% in patients with established cirrhosis.[99]

Many patients with chronic HBV infection have normal serum aminotransferase levels, normal or near-normal liver histologic findings, and no symptoms.[101] These "healthy carriers" appear to be immunologically tolerant of the virus, and their prognosis is excellent.[102] Liver biopsies obtained from 92 asymptomatic HBsAg-positive carriers who were identified during blood donation showed no or minimal changes in the majority.[102] Only 5% of patients had evidence of significant histologic liver damage (chronic active hepatitis), and none had histologic evidence of cirrhosis. The majority of patients included in the study were HBeAg and HBV DNA negative. When followed prospectively for a mean of 130 months (range, 70 to 170 months), 12% had sustained elevations of serum aminotransferase levels, and only 2% developed histologic progression of disease.[102] In a minority of patients, spontaneous flares of serum aminotransferase levels were noted in association with evidence of active viral replication. With 7 to 11 years of follow-up, spontaneous loss of HBsAg was seen in 15% of patients.[102] In summary, HBV infection in asymptomatic carriers tends to be a mild disease, and few complications develop even after prolonged periods of follow-up.

Prevention

Three main strategies exist for the prevention of HBV infection: 1) behavior modification to prevent disease transmission, 2) passive immunoprophylaxis, and 3) active immunization.

Behavior Modification

Changes in sexual practices in response to HIV infection have probably contributed to the falling incidence of HBV infection in the United States, and improved screening measures of blood products in blood banks have reduced the risk of transfusion-associated hepatitis B. Other primary preventive measures, such as needle exchange programs in injection drug users, are more difficult to implement. Behavior modification is unlikely to be beneficial in developing countries, where neonates and young children are at greatest risk of acquiring infection. In these groups, immunoprophylaxis, both passive and active, will be most effective.

Passive Immunoprophylaxis

Passive immunoprophylaxis is used in four situations: 1) neonates born to HBsAg-positive mothers; 2) after needlestick exposure; 3) after sexual exposure; and 4) after liver transplantation in patients who are HBsAg positive pretransplantation. The mechanism by which hepatitis B immune globulin (HBIG) prevents HBV infection is uncertain. Immunoprophylaxis is currently recommended for all infants born to HBsAg-positive mothers and should ideally be performed in combination with universal screening of all pregnant women for HBsAg, as recommended by the CDC. Current dosing recommendations are 0.13 mL/kg of HBIG immediately after delivery, or within 12 hours after birth, in combination with the first dose of the recombinant vaccine, followed by the remainder of the vaccine series (see later). This combination results in a greater than 90% level of protection against perinatal acquisition of HBV.[103] Between 3% and 15% of infants still acquire HBV infection perinatally from HBV-infected mothers.[104] Failure of passive and active immunoprophylaxis in this setting may be the result of 1) in utero transmission of HBV infection, 2) perinatal transmission related to a high inoculum, or 3) the presence of surface gene escape mutants (see later section).

After sexual or needlestick exposure, current recommendations are to administer HBIG in a dose of 0.05 to 0.07 mL/kg as soon after exposure as possible, preferably within 48 hours of exposure and no more than 7 days after exposure. A second dose 30 days later may decrease the risk of transmission of HBV.[53] Active immunization should be administered concurrently.

Active Immunization

Preventing primary infection by vaccination is an important strategy to decrease the risk of chronic HBV infection and its subsequent complications. Effective vaccines have been available since the early to mid-1980s. Vaccination programs targeted at high-risk groups (e.g., health care workers, parenteral drug users, and infants of infected mothers) have failed. In 1988, the CDC recommended screening of all pregnant women in the United States for HBV infection. Subsequently, in 1991, universal childhood vaccination against HBV infection was recommended. In 1994, the CDC expanded its recommendations to include all 11- and 12-year-old children who had not previously been vaccinated and all children less than 11 years of age who belonged to ethnic groups at high risk for HBV infection (Alaskan Natives and Pacific Islanders). In areas of the world with high endemism of HBV infection, current recommendations are for universal vaccination. The major difficulty in implementing these recommendations is the high cost to developing countries of vaccinating large populations. In many states in the United States, immunization of infants is now routine.

Plasma-derived vaccines were the first available HBV vaccines, but concerns about transmission of other infectious agents led to the development of recombinant vaccines. The early plasma-derived vaccines are no longer routinely available. Recombinant vaccines are made by incorporating the surface gene of HBV into different expression vectors (yeast, *Escherichia coli*, or mammalian cell lines). The yeast-derived recombinant vaccines are most widely available. Two licensed HBV vaccines are available in the United States: Engerix-B, which is manufactured by Glaxo SmithKline, and Recombivax HB, which is made by Merck Sharp and Dohme. The standard regimen is 10 to 20 μg in adults, with the same dosing intervals (generally 0, 1, and 6 months) as used for the plasma-derived vaccine. With this schedule, the rate of induction of protective immunity is comparable to that for the plasma-derived vaccine. Current recommendations are to administer the vaccine by intramuscular injection in the deltoid muscle for adults and in the lateral aspect of the thigh in children. The dose administered to infants of HBV-infected mothers differs with the two recombinant vaccines and is 5 μg and 10 μg for Recombivax HB and Engerix-B, respectively. The dose for infants of HBsAg-negative mothers and other children under the age of 11 years is 2.5 μg and 10 μg of Recombivax HB and Engerix-B, respectively. Doses for each vaccine in children aged 11 to 19 years are 5 μg and 20 μg, respectively, and for adults more than 20 years of age, the vaccine dose is 10 μg for Recombivax HB and 20 μg for Engerix-B. Prevaccination testing of patients is not usually cost-effective in areas where the prevalence of markers for HBV infection is less than 20%.

HBV vaccine is highly effective. Anti-HBs develops in over 95% of vaccine recipients, and the attack rate of all HBV infections is only 3.2% in vaccine recipients compared with 25.6% in recipients of placebo. In Alaska, broad-based vaccination programs have markedly reduced the incidence of HBV infection.[63, 105] If patients fail to develop protective antibodies in response to the standard vaccine regimen, an additional dose of either the plasma-derived or recombinant vaccine will result in an adequate response in only a small proportion of patients.[53] Because of the high seroconversion rates in immunocompetent individuals, postvaccination testing is usually not necessary. Protective levels of antibody persist in the majority of responders (68% at 4 years).[53] Even if antibody levels decline to the point that anti-HBs is no longer detectable, protection is not necessarily lost. Hence, routine testing of vaccinated persons and routine booster vaccination are not recommended. In select circumstances, particularly when persons at high risk of acquiring HBV infection are vaccinated (such as children of HBV-infected mothers), documentation of seroconversion may be prudent. Moreover, revaccination of such high-risk persons after 5 to 10 years may be appropriate if anti-HBs titers have declined below 10 IU/L.

Immunocompromised patients, including those on hemodialysis, have a reduced chance of mounting a protective immune response after vaccination.[53] Additional doses of the vaccine appear to increase the response rate.[53] Patients over the age of 40 years also exhibit a decreased response rate. There is evidence that vaccine response is genetically determined. A dominant immune-response gene in the MHC determines vaccine response.[53] Immunocompetent patients who are homozygous for this gene have a low response rate.

Treatment

Treatment of acute HBV infection is largely supportive, and antiviral therapy is not indicated (Table 68–7). Attention should be paid to indices of hepatic synthetic function (prothrombin time, serum bilirubin level, and serum albumin level), and evidence of significant impairment should prompt close monitoring, preferably in a hospital setting, and, if hepatic failure is progressive, prompt referral for liver transplantation.

Treatment of chronic HBV infection requires knowledge of the natural history of untreated HBV infection as well as the potential benefits of intervention. Knowledge of HBV virology has been essential for the development of drugs such as lamivudine, which inhibit viral replication. Equally important is an understanding of the host immune response to infection. The primary goal of treatment is the prevention of the complications of liver disease. A secondary goal is to decrease the number of chronic carriers who serve as a reservoir for HBV transmission. Because complications may take many years to develop, most treatment trials of patients with chronic HBV infection have used intermediate endpoints, such as inhibition of viral replication and improvement in liver histologic appearance, to evaluate efficacy. Loss of HBV DNA and seroconversion from HBeAg to anti-HBe are usually associated with normalization of liver enzymes and a decrease in inflammation on liver biopsy specimens.

Interferon

Alpha-interferon has been studied most extensively. In the largest trial in the United States, 169 patients were randomized to treatment with interferon-α-2b 5 million units (mU) daily, 1 mU daily, 6 weeks of oral prednisone followed by 5 mU daily, or observation for a period of 16 weeks.[106] Disappearance of HBV DNA and loss of HBeAg occurred in 37% of patients who received 5 mU daily, a significantly higher rate than that observed in patients who received 1 mU daily (17%), or patients who received no therapy (7%). A decrease in inflammation was evident on the liver biopsies of patients who responded. Loss of HBV DNA was typically preceded by an increase in serum ALT activity, which was believed to result from interferon-induced, immune-mediated hepatocyte necrosis. This flare, defined as a greater than twofold rise in the serum ALT level, occurred more commonly in responders (63%) than in nonresponders (27%). Ten percent of all treated patients lost HBsAg. The majority of patients experienced minor side effects during interferon treatment, but these side effects rarely led to cessation of therapy. In patients who have not lost HBV DNA after 16 weeks but in whom serum HBV DNA levels are falling, extending the duration of interferon therapy may improve response.

Long-term follow-up of patients treated with interferon indicates that remission is maintained in the majority of those who initially respond to therapy and that additional

Table 68–7 | **Therapeutic Options for the Treatment of Chronic Hepatitis B Infection**

TREATMENT	STATUS OF DEVELOPMENT*	REASON
Drugs Acting Predominantly As Antivirals		
Adenine arabinoside (ara-A)		Promising efficacy but neurotoxicity
Adenine arabinoside 5′-monophosphate (ara-AMP)		
Acyclovir and related compounds		
Ganciclovir		Limited efficacy, nephrotoxicity at high doses
Famciclovir (prodrug for penciclovir)		Limited efficacy, good safety profile, mutations
Lamivudine (2′-deoxy, 3′-thiacytidine)	FDA-approved	Significant efficacy, good safety profile, YMDD mutations
Clevudine (fluorothiocytidine)	Phase II–III trial	HBV antiviral activity, safety, and resistance profile under evaluation
Adefovir dipivoxil	Phase III trial	Significant efficacy, no reported resistance
Entecavir	Phase II–III trial	Potent HBV antiviral activity; full safety and resistance profile unknown
Other Dideoxynucleosides		
Azidothymidine (AZT)		Limited efficacy
2′,3′-dideoxyinosine (ddI)		Limited efficacy
2′,3′-dideoxycytosine (ddC)		Limited efficacy
Cis-5-fluoro-1-(2-(hydromethyl)-1,3-oxythiolane-5-yl) cytidine (FTC)		Significant in vitro efficacy, unknown in vivo efficacy
D-carbocyclic-2′-deoxyguanosine (CDG)		Significant in vitro efficacy, unknown in vivo efficacy
β-L-2′-dideoxynucleosides		
β-L-2′-deoxycytidine (L-dC)		Significant in vitro efficacy
β-L-2′-deoxyadenosine (L-dA)		Significant in vitro efficacy
β-L-thymidine (L-dT)	Phase II trial	Significant in vitro efficacy
Drugs Acting Predominantly As Immunomodulators		
Interferon: IFN-α-2b and -2a	FDA-approved	Significant efficacy but typical interferon side effects
Lymphoblastoid interferon		Limited U.S. data
Consensus-IFN, IFN-β, IFN-γ		
Pegylated interferon α-2a	Phase II trial	Safety and efficacy data not available
Glucocorticoids		Limited efficacy in combination with interferon in patients with low serum alanine aminotransferase levels
Thymosin alpha 1		Good safety profile but limited efficacy
Interleukin-2		Limited efficacy and significant toxicity
Interleukin-12		Limited efficacy
Ribavirin		Limited efficacy
Granulocyte-macrophage colony stimulation factor		Limited efficacy
Therapeutic HBV vaccine		Limited efficacy
Gene-based approaches		Safety and efficacy data not available

*Unless otherwise indicated, drug development is on hold.
FDA, U.S. Food and Drug Administration; YMDD, tyrosine-methionine-aspartate-aspartate.

instances of seroconversion occur after treatment is complete.[107] HBV DNA is absent in the serum of the majority of patients who clear HBeAg, and loss of HBeAg and HBV DNA in serum is usually associated with disappearance of replicative forms of HBV DNA in the liver.[108] Thus, patients with chronic HBV appear to derive long-term benefit from interferon.[109, 110]

The patients included in most clinical trials of interferon-α represent a highly select group of chronic HBV carriers.[111] In particular, patients with decompensated liver disease have been excluded. These patients frequently have leukopenia and thrombocytopenia because of hypersplenism, which limits the dose of interferon that can be administered. Because of the availability of other therapies for patients with decompensated HBV disease, interferon is rarely administered to and is not advised in this group.

Pretreatment variables associated with a sustained loss of HBeAg and HBV DNA are high serum AST and ALT levels, low serum HBV DNA levels, short duration of infection, and a histologic picture of active hepatitis.[112] Patients with serum HBV DNA levels less than 200 pg/mL are more likely to respond than are those with higher levels. The age at the time of infection as well as the duration of infection are likely important in determining the rate of response. Patients who acquire the infection in the perinatal period typically have low serum aminotransferase levels and are less likely to respond to interferon than are older persons. Patients coinfected with HIV have lower rates of response than do immunocompetent patients.[113] In summary, interferon is one of the few FDA-approved treatments for chronic HBV infection, and it is the only approved therapy that has not been associated with viral resistance. Interferon has also been approved by the FDA for treatment of children with chronic hepatitis B. Moreover, there are subsets of patients (those with mild liver disease and high pretreatment levels of serum ALT and low levels of HBV DNA) in whom sustained viral clearance and improved survival can be achieved in a cost-effective manner with treatment.[114]

Nucleoside Analogues

Lamivudine

Lamivudine, or 3TC (the [−] enantiomer of 2′-deoxy-3′-thiacytadine), belongs to the family of nucleoside inhibitors that possess the negative "unnatural" L-enantiomeric structure (see Table 68–7). This orally administered compound is an inactive prodrug that gains potency once it is converted intracellularly into its triphosphorylated form. It has been shown in multiple in vitro studies that the activated drug is a potent inhibitor of the HBV reverse transcriptase.[18, 119] Lamivudine 5′-triphosphate is a competitive inhibitor of deoxycytadine (dCTP) incorporation into viral DNA, and its incorporation results in chain termination of the elongating nucleic acid strand. Fortunately, it also has been shown that lamivudine 5′-triphosphate is a poor substrate for both nuclear and mitochondrial DNA polymerases, which in turn accounts for its good safety profile. Early clinical trials showed that orally administered lamivudine given for 4 to 12 weeks was well tolerated and resulted in a rapid and pronounced inhibition of HBV replication. However, these studies also showed that the response was transient and that almost all patients had recurrence of detectable serum HBV DNA after cessation of treatment. Fewer than 10% of treated patients underwent HBeAg seroconversion.

Studies of the kinetics of HBV clearance during treatment with lamivudine predicted that prolonged treatment of 1 to 5 years' duration is required to clear HBV infection reliably.[117] However, it is known from in vivo experience with HIV, as well as with HBV, that prolonged use of lamivudine can lead to the development of viral mutations that confer resistance to this agent.[115] HBV has a high rate of viral turnover, and its polymerase is quite error prone, particularly the reverse transcriptase component. The most common mutation leading to lamivudine resistance is a specific point mutation in the conserved tyrosine-methionine-aspartate-aspartate (YMDD) motif of the HBV polymerase in which a methionine residue is changed to a valine or isoleucine.[119] The identical mutation has also been identified in the YMDD motif of the HIV reverse transcriptase enzyme and confers lamivudine resistance to that virus as well. The emergence of YMDD mutants in the context of lamivudine therapy results in diminished therapeutic antiviral activity.[120] However serum HBV DNA and aminotransferase levels are typically lower in the presence of the mutant virus when compared with wild-type infection. Hence, the YMDD variant appears to have diminished replicative competence and is potentially less injurious to hepatocytes than is the wild-type virus.[121]

A number of trials have examined extended-duration lamivudine therapy. Two placebo-controlled trials of continuous lamivudine administration for 1 year to patients with chronic HBV infection demonstrated substantial benefit.[122, 123] One study was conducted in Asia, and the other study was conducted in the United States. Lamivudine was well tolerated, and the antiviral response, defined as HBeAg seroconversion and undetectable serum HBV DNA using a solution hybridization assay, was observed in 16% and 17% of patients in the Asian and American studies, respectively, who received active drug, compared with 4% and 6% of those who received placebo. These studies also demonstrated a rate of HBeAg loss of approximately 32%, which was similar to that observed with interferon treatment. Loss of HBsAg was detected in only 1 (2%) patient treated with lamivudine in the United States study. Histologic improvement, defined as a decrease in the Knodell necroinflammatory score by at least 2 points, was noted in 56% and 52% of treated patients and in 25% and 23% of controls. Similar results have been reported in an international study. Extended therapy may improve response.[124] A limitation of these studies was the use of solution hybridization assays, which have a lower limit of detection of 10^6–10^7 genomes/mL. Many of the patients with apparent loss of HBV DNA have detectable virus by more sensitive tests. These trials demonstrated similar effects of lamivudine treatment in both United States and Asian populations, in contrast to interferon, in which the beneficial effects seemed to be confined largely to non-Asian patients.[125] The only independent predictive factor of HBeAg seroconversion is the pretreatment aminotransferase level. HBeAg seroconversion occurred in 64%, 26%, and 5% of patients with pretreatment serum ALT levels greater than five times, two to five times, and less than two times the upper limit of normal, respectively.[126] These data suggest that, as with interferon-α, a successful antiviral response to lamivudine therapy is dependent on an endogenous immune response to HBV. Furthermore, lamivudine may lack efficacy on the covalently closed-circular DNA (cccDNA), the template for transcription of pregenomic RNA.

The beneficial results demonstrated in these studies came at the expense of induction of a resistant mutant virus. The most common mutation affects the YMDD motif in the catalytic domain of the HBV polymerase and results in substitution of methionine to valine (M552V) or isoleucine (M552I). The M552V mutation is frequently found in association with another mutation in an upstream region that results in substitution of leucine to methionine (528M). Lamivudine-resistant mutants were detected in 14% and 32% of patients at the end of a 1-year course of treatment in the Asian and United States studies, respectively. Lamivudine resistance is usually manifested as breakthrough infection, defined as reappearance of HBV DNA in serum after its initial disappearance. Most patients continue to have lower serum HBV DNA and ALT levels compared with pretreatment values, a finding attributed to the decreased fitness of the mutants.

On the basis of available data, it is clear that a 1-year course of treatment with lamivudine is insufficient to achieve a sustained antiviral response in most patients. Recently, the second-year results of the multicenter Asian study were reported.[127] Patients who had received 25 or 100 mg lamivudine in the first year were randomized to continue original therapy or to receive placebo in a ratio of 3:1. Of the 93 patients who received 100 mg daily for 2 years, HBeAg seroconversion increased from 18% at the end of the first year to 25% at the end of the second year.

Unfortunately, of the 154 patients who received lamivudine continuously for 2 years, resistant mutants were detected in a total of 62 (40%) patients. For patients who received continuous lamivudine, results from the first 4 years have been analyzed. There was an increase in the HBeAg seroconversion rate in each of the 4 years as follows: 22%, 29%, 40%, and 47%, respectively. However YMDD variants emerged over time with a cumulative rate of 17%, 40%, 55%, and 67% at the end of each of the 4 years. Short-term follow-up showed that most patients with resistant mutants continued to have lower HBV DNA and serum ALT levels compared with pretreatment values. Indeed, 23% of patients who remained on lamivudine achieved HBeAg seroconversion after the emergence of the mutants. Thus, longer follow-up is needed to determine the long-term clinical significance of the lamivudine-resistant variants. Current recommendations are to treat with lamivudine until loss of HBeAg, with or without acquisition of anti-HBe. It is hoped that loss of HBeAg will occur before the development of resistance, although in many persons, this unfortunately is not the case. Because the risk of developing lamivudine resistance is substantial in patients who receive prolonged treatment, caution is advised before instituting treatment in patients with mild histologic liver disease even in the presence of active viral replication. It is unclear whether lamivudine should be continued in patients in whom evidence of resistance develops. New therapies in development appear to be effective against the resistant variants. However, it is still controversial as to whether these drugs will be used sequentially (i.e., lamivudine, another nucleoside, or interferon first, followed by an alternative drug when the first drug is unsuccessful) or whether more than one drug will be given in combination from the start.

Lamivudine therapy also has been tested in patients with precore variants of HBV. As in patients with wild-type infection, lamivudine produces a complete response in approximately two thirds of patients, as shown by the normalization of the serum ALT and loss of serum HBV DNA associated with a greater than 2-point reduction in the Knodell necroinflammatory score.[128] However, the frequency of a sustained response is unknown. Preliminary data suggest that most patients relapse and that a longer duration of treatment will be necessary to achieve a sustained response. In patients with decompensated cirrhosis, treatment with lamivudine produces clinical improvement with a reduction in serum ALT and HBV DNA levels and improvement in the Child-Turcotte-Pugh score.[129] However, on stopping lamivudine, most patients experience an increase in serum HBV DNA levels, and there is concern that relapse of disease may be associated with a flare of liver disease and worsening hepatic decompensation. For this reason, it seems advisable to continue lamivudine therapy indefinitely in a patient with advanced HBV-related liver disease.

Famciclovir

Another potential source of candidate therapies for HBV infections was identified in the group of acyclic deoxyguanosine analogues that were originally developed to treat herpesvirus infections. These drugs include acyclovir, ganciclovir, and penciclovir (the oral form of which is famciclovir), and they are known to have activity against the DNA-dependent DNA polymerases of the herpesviruses. The most clinical experience in HBV infection is with famciclovir. Famciclovir can effectively reduce serum HBV DNA levels in patients with chronic hepatitis B and in those who have had a liver transplant,[130] although the overall clinical efficacy of this agent is less than that of lamivudine. There are a number of mutations associated with resistance to famciclovir. Most of them are clustered in the B domain region of the HBV polymerase (as opposed to the C domain that contains the YMDD motif associated with lamivudine resistance),[131] but there are other resistance mutations scattered throughout the polymerase/reverse transcriptase domain of the viral genome. In addition, there are some famciclovir-associated variants that demonstrate mutations in the C domain and that confer cross-resistance to both famciclovir and lamivudine, but these are not the most commonly observed variants. Because of the relatively weak potency of famciclovir (approximately one log drop in viral DNA with treatment as compared with a two to three log drop seen with lamivudine) and the cost associated with daily administration of 1.5 g of drug, it is unlikely that famciclovir will ever be first-line therapy for HBV infection.

Adefovir Dipivoxil

Adefovir dipivoxil is the oral prodrug of an acyclic nucleotide monophosphate analogue (9-(2-phosphonylmethoxyethyl)-adenine [PMEA]). The active drug is a selective inhibitor of numerous species of viral nucleic acid polymerases and reverse transcriptases and has been shown to have broad-spectrum antiviral activity against retroviruses, hepadnaviruses, and herpesviruses. Orally administered adefovir dipivoxil exhibits an inhibitory effect on both the HIV and HBV reverse transcriptases. Importantly, adefovir appears to be capable of inhibiting the enzymatic activity of both wild-type and YMDD-mutant variants of both of these viruses.[132]

Studies of adefovir in the treatment of HIV infection demonstrated a toxicity profile that was deemed unacceptable by reviewers at the FDA. Toxicities included renal insufficiency and frequent development of hypophosphatemia. However, doses used for HIV are significantly higher than those used for HBV infection. Phase II clinical trials of adefovir (at 5 mg, 30 mg, and 60 mg daily) in hepatitis B demonstrated a dose-dependent antiviral effect associated with an increased rate of HBeAg seroconversion when compared with placebo controls.[133] In one study of 15 HBV-infected patients, 12 weeks of treatment with 30 mg of adefovir daily was associated with a 4.1 log reduction in serum HBV DNA.[134] In vitro studies have demonstrated synergistic inhibitory activity of adefovir and lamivudine or famciclovir against duck HBV, and it has further been shown that adefovir retains activity against various HBV strains that have acquired both lamivudine or famciclovir resistance.[135]

Further large-scale clinical trials are underway to evaluate the safety and efficacy of adefovir. However, adefovir appears to be a promising therapeutic agent with novel, nonoverlapping resistance characteristics when compared with agents already in use against HBV infection. In an initial case series of patients who had undergone liver transplantation, adefovir was shown to be active against lamivudine-resistant variants.[136] Adefovir has also been shown to be viral suppressive in patients with HBV/HIV coinfection, many of whom have lamivudine resistance. Trials of both adefovir monotherapy and lamivudine/adefovir combination therapy are currently underway in previously untreated and lamivudine-resistant patients.

Entecavir

Entecavir [1S-(1α,3α,4β]-2-amino-1,9-dihydro-9[4-hydroxy-3-(hydroxymethyl)-2-methylenecyclopentyl]-6H-purin-6-one]) (BMS-200475) is a carbocyclic deoxyguanosine analogue with potent antiherpes and antihepadnaviral activity. In woodchucks infected with WHV, treatment with entecavir produced 2 to 3 log reductions in viral load with undetectable serum HBV DNA in all treated woodchucks. However, relapse occurred shortly after discontinuation of brief periods of treatment. Adefovir and entecavir are effective against all common lamivudine-resistant variants, although higher doses of these compounds are necessary to inhibit variants with multiple rather than single mutations.[137] Phase II and III clinical studies have been initiated. Adverse events associated with entecavir include headache, dizziness, and photophobia.

Other Antiviral Agents

Adenine arabinoside (ara-A) and the monophosphate form (ara-AMP), which is more soluble, are synthetic purine nucleosides that suppress HBV DNA replication, but long-term toxicity, including peripheral neuropathy, has limited their use. Many dideoxynucleosides demonstrate significant activity against HBV in vitro and in vivo. In cell culture systems, azidothymidine (AZT), ddI (2′,3′-dideoxyinosine), ddC (ZT-dideoxycytosine), FTC (cis-5-fluoro-l-[2-[hydroxymethyl]-l,3-oxythiolane-5-yl] cytidine), and CDG (D-carbocyclic-Z′-deoxyguanosine) demonstrate potent anti-HBV activity. It has also been shown recently in animal models that the 3′-OH group of the β-L-2′-deoxyribose of the β-L-2′-deoxynucleoside series confers specific anti-HBV activity. In this chemical series, the unsubstituted nucleosides β-L-2′deoxycytidine (L-dC), β-L-thymidine (L-dT), and β-L-2′deoxyadenosine (L-dA) had an important selective and specific antiviral activity against HBV replication. The current status of clinical development of these compounds is summarized in Table 68–7. The new anti-HBV drugs that have been tested in humans are capable of reducing viral loads very rapidly, but the initial response is invariably followed by slower elimination of residual virus. Long-term treatment that is required to eliminate residual virus carries an increased risk of cumulative toxicity and drug resistance.

Fialuridine, or FIAU, is a nucleoside analogue with antiviral activity against several DNA viruses. Analogues of FIAU inhibit HBV replication in WHV and DHBV models. FIAU is phosphorylated by viral and cellular enzymes, and this triphosphate analogue is a potent inhibitor of HBV DNA polymerase activity. Because FIAU was readily bioavailable by the oral route and had potent inhibitory effects on HBV DNA levels in vivo and in vitro, it appeared to be an ideal agent for treating chronic HBV infection. Initial phase I and II studies in immunocompetent patients with chronic HBV infection showed a rapid and significant fall in DNA polymerase activity with FIAU. In these early studies, FIAU was well tolerated for the 1-month treatment period. However, the clinical trial of more prolonged therapy was terminated prematurely when severe toxicity, including lactic acidosis, pancreatitis, and renal failure, developed.[138] The clinical, biochemical, and histologic picture associated with this delayed toxicity suggested that the underlying mechanism was at least in part related to inhibition of mitochondrial function.

Therapeutic Vaccines

Theradigm-HBV™ (Cytel, San Diego, CA) is a therapeutic vaccine that consists of three components: the viral protein (HBV core antigen peptide); a T helper peptide (tetanus toxoid peptide), which enhances immunogenicity; and two palmitic acid molecules. The vaccine is capable of inducing an HBV-specific MHC class I–restricted CTL response in healthy volunteers, but results of phase I/II studies in patients with chronic HBV infection showed only modest benefits, if any.[139]

Other Immunomodulators

Thymosin derivatives have been shown to regulate multiple aspects of T-cell function (see Table 68–7). Thymosin has been chemically synthesized. Despite apparent antiviral activity in animal models (WHV) and in pilot studies of patients with chronic HBV infection, large randomized trials have failed to show any clear evidence of a sustained clinical or virologic effect. Interferons-β and -γ have been used as monotherapy and as combination therapy. Because of the limited sample size and uncontrolled nature of most published studies, there is insufficient information to determine efficacy of interferon-β and interferon-γ, either alone or in combination. Glucocorticoids have been studied as monotherapy and in combination therapy with interferon-α. Increased viral replication occurs in association with glucocorticoid administration, and prolonged therapy can delay seroconversion from HBeAg to anti-HBe. Withdrawal of glucocorticoids is associated with an enhancement of the immune response with subsequent fall in HBV DNA levels, but with deleterious effects in some patients. Glucocorticoids in combination with interferon-α (concurrent or sequential administration) offer no advantage over interferon therapy alone, although a subgroup of patients with serum ALT levels less than 100 U/L at baseline may benefit.[106]

Combination Therapy

Regimens combining interferon-α with another agent have shown no clear advantage over interferon-α alone. Specifically, the combination of lamivudine and interferon did not show superiority over lamivudine monotherapy in patients who had previously failed to respond to interferon alone. Although one trial of lamivudine plus interferon in the treatment of previously untreated patients suggested a benefit of the combination over either drug alone,[140] further investigation is required to determine the optimal timing and duration of combination therapy. To date, the efficacy of combination therapy with nucleoside analogues has not been fully evaluated. However, in vitro study and a preliminary in vivo study showed that the combination of famciclovir and lamivudine may be more efficacious than therapy with either agent alone.[141] Further studies will be required to determine whether use of combinations of nucleotide analogues will not only improve the therapeutic efficacy of regimens to treat chronic hepatitis B but also delay or possibly even prevent the development of resistance to single agents.

Liver Transplantation

HBV infection accounts for less than 10% of all liver transplantations performed in the United States. Because the causative viral agent is not eradicated, infection of the allograft is certain if no interventions are undertaken.[142] However, because of many improvements in the treatment of hepatitis B after transplantation, orthotopic liver transplantation is now the standard of care for patients with decompensated HBV-induced liver disease.[143] The risk of HBV reinfection is at least 80% without prophylaxis, and HBV-associated graft failure is the leading cause of death in patients with recurrent HBV infection. Because of these poor outcomes, many transplant centers have specifically excluded HBsAg-positive patients, particularly those with active pretransplantation viral replication. However, because of successful therapies, 2-year survival rates have improved from 70% to 80% in the most recent cohort of patients with HBV-related cirrhosis and from 56% to 80% in those with fulminant hepatitis B, and HBV infection is now considered an appropriate indication for liver transplantation, with the expectation that the outcome will be successful.[144, 145]

Long-term passive immunization with HBIG has become an effective way to prevent or delay hepatitis B recurrence.[142] The mechanism of action of HBIG is not known but likely involves binding to HBsAg with neutralization of circulating virions, thereby preventing entry of the virus into the hepatocyte. HBIG immunoprophylaxis given at the time of liver transplantation and in the post-transplantation period reduces the rate of HBV recurrence from 90% to approximately 20%.[143] Because HBIG therapy is expensive and associated with side effects during the infusion, alternatives to indefinite post-transplantation therapy are being sought. However, limiting HBIG to short-term treatment (6 months or less) frequently results in viral recurrence, and until nucleoside analogues became available, long-term post-transplantation HBIG, administered monthly intravenously at high doses, was considered the standard of care in the United States.

The next major intervention was the nucleoside analogue lamivudine, 100 mg orally per day. Both North American and European multicenter trials of lamivudine monotherapy have shown that pre-emptive therapy results in a post-transplant recurrence rate that is similar to that associated with HBIG monotherapy but that lamivudine is substantially less expensive and potentially less toxic.[146] However, recurrence rates with monotherapy are unacceptably high. Case series of patients treated with a combination of lamivudine and high doses of HBIG have demonstrated very low rates of recurrence (5%–10%),[144] although the optimal approach remains controversial.

Both HBIG and lamivudine administered as monotherapeutic agents are associated with the development of resistance mutations. With lamivudine, these mutations are in the polymerase gene, whereas with HBIG, mutations are in the "a" determinant of the surface gene.[147] The risk of developing lamivudine resistance in a patient awaiting liver transplantation is dependent on the duration of therapy with lamivudine (in one large series, this risk was 15%–20%).[146] There is also concern that polymerase mutations can result in decreased efficacy of HBIG (see later section). Against these risks is the potential benefit of improving hepatic synthetic function with lamivudine in patients with decompensated liver disease. Although there are no controlled studies, there are several reports of improvement in the patient's Child-Turcotte-Pugh status and even abrogation of liver transplantation.[129, 148] Thus, lamivudine appears to be appropriate for patients with decompensated HBV cirrhosis awaiting liver transplantation. Lamivudine is also likely to be beneficial in patients with advanced HBV-related disease who, because of contraindications, are not candidates for liver transplantation.

Nevertheless, there is some risk in treating a patient who is awaiting liver transplantation with lamivudine monotherapy, because the development of active viral replication associated with resistance before transplantation could reduce the chance of a successful outcome after transplantation. Because of the overlapping nature of polymerase and surface genes of HBV, there is at least a theoretical risk that lamivudine-associated polymerase mutations could result in alteration of the surface gene such that HBIG would no longer be neutralizing. However, there are case reports of patients with pretransplantation lamivudine resistance who received HBIG at transplantation without evidence of post-transplantation recurrence.[149] Moreover, as other HBV therapies are developed, particularly those with demonstrated activity against lamivudine-resistant variants, the risk associated with pretransplantation lamivudine therapy will be greatly outweighed by the potential benefit to the patient in terms of stabilization and even improvement in decompensated liver disease. Thus, a combination of lamivudine and HBIG is currently the standard of care in patients with decompensated HBV who undergo liver transplantation. The controversies surrounding the administration of combination therapy relate to the timing, dosing, and duration of each therapy. In many transplant centers, HBIG therapy is given perioperatively and at regular intervals intravenously postoperatively for 6 to 12 months. Because of the cost and side effects associated with high-dose intravenous HBIG, some centers give lower doses of HBIG intramuscularly. Adefovir has been used successfully to suppress HBV replication in a small case series that included patients with lamivudine-resistant variants present both before and after liver transplantation.[136]

Despite effective prevention of HBV infection of the graft with current interventions, there remain a number of patients with HBV infection after liver transplantation who are at risk for graft failure. These include patients who either underwent liver transplantation in the pre-HBIG, pre-lamivudine era or who appear to have acquired HBV infection in the peritransplantation period (de novo HBV infection). Sources of apparently de novo HBV infection include occult HBV infection in the organ donor as well as reactivation under immune suppression of low-level HBV infection present in the recipient before liver transplantation.[150, 151] In these patients, lamivudine given after transplantation suppresses viral replication and improves liver histology,[152] but the likelihood that resistance to lamivudine will develop is high (up to 50%).

There is one more treatment intervention available for lamivudine resistance, namely, other nucleoside or nucleotide analogues. Two drugs under study are adefovir and entecavir.[136] Both have activity against lamivudine-resistant variants, but both are potentially more toxic than lamivudine. Currently, these agents may be used as "salvage" therapy either for patients awaiting liver transplantation or for those with lamivudine-resistant HBV infection after liver transplantation.

HEPATITIS C VIRUS

Hepatitis C virus (HCV) is an important public health problem because it is a major cause of chronic hepatitis, cirrhosis, and HCC and a major indication for liver transplantation worldwide. The most striking feature of this virus is its ability to induce persistent infection in at least 85% of infected persons despite a vigorous humoral and cellular host immune response.

Virology

Structure

Knowledge of the structure and mechanism of replication of HCV is incomplete, largely because of the lack of an in vitro system to study viral replication and of suitable animal models. HCV is an enveloped virus approximately 50 nm in diameter that is visualized on electron microscopy within cytoplasmic vesicles of lymphoblastoid cells in culture (see Table 68–1).[153] Immune electron microscopy has demonstrated both HCV core and envelope proteins in these particulate structures. HCV appears to be associated with immunoglobulins and low-density lipoproteins in vivo.[154] HCV consists of a positive-strand RNA surrounded by the core (nucleocapsid), which is surrounded by two envelope proteins (E1 and E2).[155] The negative strand of HCV RNA is produced as a replicative intermediate during replication and is acknowledged to be a marker of ongoing viral replication.[156] On entry into a susceptible cell, the genomic RNA is released from the particle, binds ribosomes, and is translated.

Genomic Organization

HCV is a single-stranded positive-sense RNA virus that belongs to the Flaviviridae family (Fig. 68–6).[1, 157] All members of the Flaviviridae family are positive-strand RNA viruses that encode a single long polypeptide, which is cleaved post-translationally. The genome of HCV has approximately 9600 nucleotides and contains a single open reading frame (ORF) capable of encoding a large viral polypeptide precursor of 3010 to 3033 amino acids (the length of which varies slightly among HCV isolates), with regions at the 5′ and 3′ ends that are not translated. The cleavage of the protein by cellular and viral proteases results in a series of structural (nucleocapsid [C, p21], envelope 1 [E1, gp31], and envelope 2 [E2, gp70]) and nonstructural (NS2, NS3, NS4a, NS4b, NS5a, and NS5b) proteins. The amino terminal region of NS3 encodes a viral serine protease that is important in post-translational cleavage of viral peptides.[158] The carboxy end of NS3 functions as a helicase, which is essential for unwinding of viral RNA during replication.[159] By analogy with other positive-strand RNA viruses, the NS5b protein functions as an RNA-dependent RNA polymerase. The function of the NS5A protein is unknown, but recent observations linking mutations in this region with sensitivity to interferon therapy and low levels of virus suggest that the NS5A protein may play a role in the viral regulation of replication.[160] The noncoding 5′ terminal region (5′NTR) and portions of the 3′ noncoding region (3′NTR) are the most conserved parts of the HCV genome and contain signals for replication and translation. The 5′NTR of 349 to 352 base pairs has a highly complex secondary RNA structure with four stem root structures and contains an internal ribosomal entry site.[161] This region is essential for viral protein synthesis and probably also for replication. The reported 3′NTR of HCV consists of a hypervariable segment of 416 nucleotides, a poly-U element that is variable in size, and a recently discovered additional, highly conserved region of approximately 100 nucleotides.[162] Unlike the 5′NTR, the 3′NTR has a very stable secondary structure. Like the 5′NTR, this region appears to be essential for translation and replication.

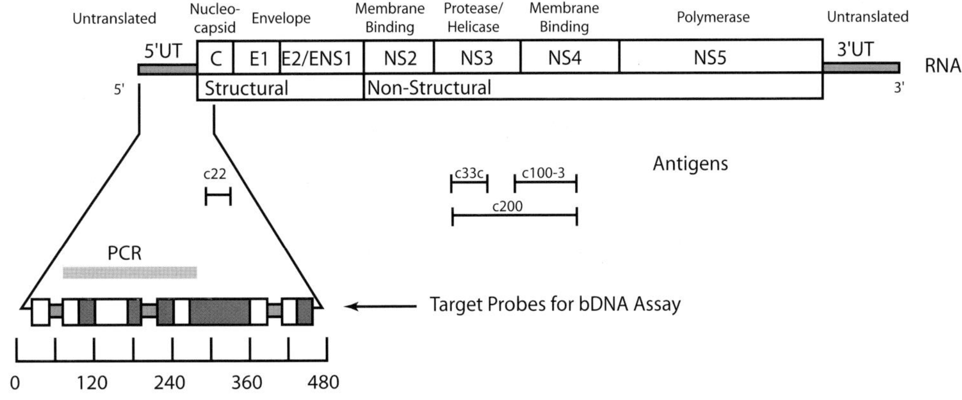

Figure 68–6. Putative functional regions of the hepatitis C virus (HCV) genome and regions used for diagnostic assays. Major structural (core and two envelope) and nonstructural proteins (NS2, NS3, NS4, and NS5) are shown, as well as the regions of HCV most commonly used for PCR (5′ UTR), serologic assays (recombinant antigens c22, c33c, c100-3, and c200), and branched DNA (bDNA) assay (5′ UTR and core). (From Wilber J, Polito A: Serological and virological diagnostic tests for hepatitis C virus infection. Semin Gastrointest Dis 6:13, 1995.)

The positive-strand RNA of HCV has three potential functions: 1) as a template for synthesis of negative-strand RNA during replication, 2) as a template for translation of viral proteins, and 3) as genomic RNA to be packaged into new virions. In contrast to HBV, HCV has no DNA intermediate and therefore cannot integrate into the host genome.

Replication

Early events in viral binding to the hepatocyte surface are still poorly understood. Two different putative cellular receptors for HCV have been proposed: low-density lipoproteins[154] and, more recently, CD81.[163] CD81 is a cell surface protein called tetraspanin that has four loops (two of which are extracellular and two intracellular) and that is expressed on most human cells, except red blood cells and platelets. The HCV envelope protein E2 has been shown to bind specifically to CD81, suggesting that CD81 may be the receptor for HCV.[163]

Knowledge of the mechanism of replication comes in part from studies in chimpanzees and in part from extrapolation of the mechanisms used by other flaviviruses. HCV RNA is detectable within 3 days of infection in chimpanzees and persists in serum during the peak serum ALT elevation. This period is associated with the appearance of viral antigens in hepatocytes, the major site of HCV replication. The importance of extrahepatic reservoirs of HCV replication (such as peripheral blood mononuclear cells) is uncertain, and current studies are clouded by technical issues related to the specificity of methods used to detect minus-strand RNA.[164] Studies of the kinetics of HCV in patients have shown that the turnover of virus is rapid, with high production of virus in vivo in the order of 10^{10}–10^{12} virions per day.[165] These high turnover rates may explain the rapid emergence of viral diversity in patients with chronic infection and the frequent persistence of infection, through immune escape, after acute exposure. The actual mechanism of formation of minus-strand RNA from the plus-strand template is also poorly understood, again in large part because of the lack of an effective in vitro system. By analogy to other RNA viruses, the NS5b region of the genome encodes an RNA-dependent RNA polymerase that catalyzes formation of the minus strand.[164]

The 5′ UTR contains several stem-loop structures that function as an internal ribosomal entry site (IRES), allowing efficient translation at the first AUG of the long open reading frame.[161] Some investigators have suggested that the IRES may downregulate translation and induce a low rate of viral protein synthesis. This low rate of protein synthesis may play a role in long-term viral persistence by making it difficult for the immune system to recognize infected cells.[166] The cleavage of the viral polyprotein is achieved by a host signal peptidase and two viral proteinases that cleave the polypeptide at the NS2–3 and NS3–4A regions. The function of the viral serine protease, which is located at the amino terminal region of NS3, is enhanced by its cofactor NS4A (see Fig. 68–6).[158, 159, 167] Mechanisms of viral packaging and release from the hepatocyte are poorly understood. By analogy with Pestiviruses, HCV packaging and release may be inefficient because much of the virus remains cell associated. Host secretory mechanisms may be utilized by HCV for packaging and release of virions via budding from the Golgi. After being released, the viral particles may either infect adjacent hepatocytes or enter the circulation, where they are available for infection of a new host.

Genotypes and Quasispecies

Like many RNA viruses, HCV has an inherently high mutation rate that results in considerable heterogeneity throughout the genome.[168] As with other positive-strand RNA viruses, the RNA-dependent RNA polymerase of HCV lacks 3′ to 5′ exonuclease proofreading ability to remove mismatched nucleotides incorporated during replication. This lack of proofreading ability results in increasing viral diversity with each cycle of replication. The first designation used to describe genetic heterogeneity is the *genotype*, which refers to genetically distinct groups of HCV isolates that have arisen during the evolution of the virus.[168] Nucleotide sequencing has shown that differences of up to 34% exist between different HCV variants.[168] The most conserved region (5′ UTR) has a maximum of 9% nucleotide sequence divergence among genotypes, whereas the highly variable regions that encode the putative envelope proteins (E1 and E2) exhibit 35% to 44% nucleotide sequence divergence among genotypes.[168] The existence of different classification systems has led to confusion when results from different studies are compared. A group of investigators has proposed a system of nomenclature based on phylogenetic analysis of nucleotide sequences of complete genome or subgenomic regions.[169] There is evidence for a clustering of sequences into six major "types" (designated by Arabic numbers), with sequence similarities of 66% to 69%, and more than 50 different "subtypes" (designated by a lower case letter) within these types, with sequence similarities of 77% to 80%. In this scheme, the first variant cloned by Choo and associates is designated type 1a.[170] Different genotypes are associated with differences in geography, the mode of acquisition, and responsiveness to antiviral therapy.[168, 171] The association between genotype and disease severity is still unclear, and although some studies have reported an association between genotype 1b and more severe liver disease, other studies have failed to find such an association.[171] Several confounding factors may explain these discrepancies, one of which is that patients infected with genotype 1b are older than those infected with other genotypes, thus suggesting that a cohort effect, with a longer duration of infection among genotype 1b infected patients, is the likely explanation for the association between this genotype and more severe liver disease. Indeed, all genotypes have been found to be both hepatotropic and pathogenic, and similar levels of viremia exist among patients infected with different genotypes. In the United States, genotype 1 is most prevalent (approximately 75%), with an equal distribution of subtypes 1a and 1b.[168, 171] Genotypes 2 (2.2% 2a, 8.6% 2b) and 3 (5.8%) are less common.

The second component of genetic heterogeneity is known as *quasispecies*.[168, 171] Quasispecies are closely related yet heterogeneous sequences of the HCV genome within a single infected person that result from mutations during viral replication. The rate of nucleotide changes varies significantly among the different genomic regions, with an overall mutation rate of 0.144% to 0.192% nucleotide changes per year.[168, 171] The highest proportion of mutations has been found in the E1 and E2 regions at both the nucleotide (1.2%–3.4%) and the amino acid (1.4%–2.7%) levels, particularly in the hypervariable region (HVR) at the amino terminal end of E2.[168, 171] Even though this region represents only a minor part of the E2/NS1 region, it accounts for approximately 50% of the nucleotide changes and 60% of the amino acid substitutions within the envelope region. Recent studies have shown that the rate of mutations within the HVR may be accelerated by interferon therapy.[172] Antibodies reactive to the HVR of a particular isolate of HCV are specific to that particular epitope and do not cross-react with epitopes of different isolates.[173, 174] The quasispecies nature of HCV may be one of the mechanisms by which the virus escapes immune responses.[171] Furthermore, strain-specific viral factors, not distinguishable on the basis of genotype, may play a significant role in disease severity, thereby potentially explaining different courses of disease. Other clinical implications of HCV genotypes and quasispecies are summarized in Table 68–8. The clinical significance of genotypes and quasispecies continues to be an area of active investigation.

Chimeras, Replicons, and Infectious Cloned Transcripts

Although an efficient cell culture system has not been devised so far, both replicons (capable of RNA amplification but not production of mature viruses)[175] and chimeric viruses are available to enhance our understanding of HCV replication and gene expression. These experimental systems may also be used to develop antiviral drugs.[175] Finally, infectious cloned transcripts provide a novel source for studying HCV replication and pathogenesis. Recently, plasmids containing full-length copies of HCV RNA have been developed[176, 177] and will likely open new doors to the understanding of the interactions between the host and the virus in producing persistent infection and liver damage[178] and into the development of improved antiviral therapies.

Table 68–8 | **Clinical Implications of HCV Genotypes and Quasispecies**

PARAMETER	TYPE OF ASSOCIATION	STRENGTH OF ASSOCIATION
Genotypes		
Disease severity	Genotype 1b→more severe liver disease	Conflicting data
Response to antiviral therapy	Genotypes 1 and 4→poor response to therapy	Consistent data
Viral transmission	Genotype 3a→intravenous drug use Genotype 1b→blood transfusion	Consistent data
Quasispecies		
HCV persistence	HVR1 variability→immune system escape	Consistent data*
Outcome following acute hepatitis	Emergence of a homogeneous viral population with relative evolutionary stasis→acute resolving hepatitis Genetic evolution early after infection→chronicity	Few studies
Disease severity	Higher viral heterogeneity→progressive liver disease	Conflicting data
Response to antiviral therapy	Higher viral heterogeneity→lower response to therapy	Conflicting data
Viral transmission	Presence of antibodies to HVR1→selective transmission of viral variants	Few studies

*Additional mechanisms have been suggested since experimental studies in chimpanzees with infectious molecular clones have recently shown persistent infection despite the lack of a viral quasispecies in the inoculum and of mutations in the HVR1.

HVR, hypervariable region.

Epidemiology

Incidence and Prevalence

The worldwide seroprevalence of HCV infection, based on antibody to HCV (anti-HCV), is estimated to be 3%. However, marked geographic variation exists, from 0.4% to 1.1% in North America to 9.6% to 13.6% in North Africa.[179] Currently, there are approximately 3 to 4 million persons infected with HCV in the United States, with an estimated prevalence of HCV antibody of approximately 1.8% in the general population and 0.6% in volunteer blood donors. The prevalence is higher in persons between the ages of 30 and 49 years than in older or younger age groups, higher in males than females (2.5% vs. 1.2%), and higher among certain ethnic groups, such as African Americans and Mexican Americans, than whites.[180] Worldwide, three different epidemiologic patterns of HCV infection can be identified: 1) In countries like the United States and Australia, most HCV infections are found among persons between 30 and 49 years of age, indicating that most HCV transmission occurred in the relatively recent past, primarily among young adults infected through intravenous drug use; 2) in areas like Japan or Southern Europe, the prevalence of HCV infection is highest in older persons, suggesting that the risk of HCV transmission was greatest in the distant past (>30 years ago). In these countries, health care–related procedures, particularly unsafe injection practices with reuse of contaminated glass syringes, and folk medicine practices may have played a major role in viral spread; and 3) in countries like Egypt, high rates of infection are observed in all age groups, suggesting that an ongoing high risk of acquiring HCV exists (see later sections).

In the United States, the incidence of acute hepatitis C is falling. The incidence was estimated to be 180,000 cases per year in the mid-1980s (peak incidence) but declined to approximately 30,000 new cases per year in 1995.[180] Persons at highest risk of infection are those who were born between

1940 and 1965.[181] The major factor contributing to the falling incidence of acute hepatitis C has been risk reduction as a result of changes in medical practices, including widespread blood donor screening in the early 1990s, and educational and syringe-exchange programs.[182]

Transmission

The modes of transmission of HCV infection can be divided into percutaneous (blood transfusion and needlestick inoculation) and nonpercutaneous (sexual contact, perinatal exposure). The latter group may represent occult percutaneous exposure. Overall, blood transfusion from unscreened donors and injection drug use are the two best documented risk factors. Indeed, in initial studies, HCV was shown to be the etiologic agent in more than 85% of cases of post-transfusional non-A, non-B hepatitis. After the introduction of anti-HCV screening of blood donors in 1991, transfusion-related cases of HCV infection declined significantly, and non–transfusion-related cases became more important.[183] Currently, among patients presenting with acute and chronic HCV infection, injection drug use is the most common risk factor identified and is present in 40% or more of patients.[179]

Percutaneous Transmission

With the introduction of donor screening by first-generation anti-HCV testing, the risk of transfusion-related hepatitis declined to approximately 0.6% per patient and 0.03% per unit transfused.[183] Since the introduction of more sensitive second-generation assays for anti-HCV, the risk of HCV-related transfusion hepatitis is estimated to be only 0.01% to 0.001% per unit of blood transfused, accounting for only 4% of all acute HCV infections.[184]

The prevalence of HCV infection in injection drug users is 48% to 90%. The risk of anti-HCV positivity correlates with the prevalence of HBV and HIV infection but is markedly higher for HCV than for these other viruses. Unlike transfusion-associated hepatitis, the prevalence of HCV infection associated with injection drug use has not declined, and this population remains an important reservoir of HCV infection.[179] The majority of injection drug users become positive for anti-HCV within 6 months of initiating injection.[185] Those engaging in injection drug use should refrain from sharing syringes, cotton, and cooking equipment.

Chronic hemodialysis is associated with both endemic cases and, more rarely, sporadic outbreaks of HCV infection. The prevalence of anti-HCV in hemodialysis patients has been noted to be as high as 45%, although studies have more commonly found a prevalence of 10% to 20%.[179] Serologic assays (anti-HCV) may underestimate the prevalence of HCV infection in this relatively immunocompromised population, and virologic assays (for HCV RNA by PCR amplification) may be necessary for accurate diagnosis in dialysis patients (Fig. 68–7).[179] A correlation has been found between increasing years on dialysis and anti-HCV positivity, independent of a history of blood transfusion. These data suggest that HCV might be transmitted among these patients because of incorrect implementation of infection-control procedures.

Anti-HCV seroconversion rates have been 0% to 4% in

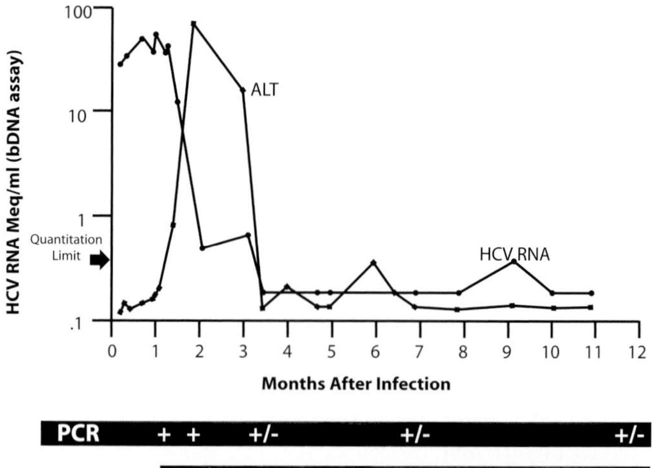

Figure 68–7. Typical course of a case of acute hepatitis C infection. Changes in HCV RNA and serum ALT levels after acute post-transfusion hepatitis C. Note that viral RNA is detectable for several weeks before anti-HCV seroconversion. (Courtesy of Chiron Corporation, Emeryville, CA). EIA, enzyme immunoassay; PCR, polymerase chain reaction.

longitudinal studies of health care workers with documented needlestick exposures to anti-HCV–positive patients.[179, 186] If PCR is used to detect infection, the risk of HCV acquisition after percutaneous exposure is as high as 10%.[187] However, health care professionals, including those with a high likelihood of percutaneous exposure to blood, have prevalence rates of anti-HCV similar to those described in the general population.[179]

Transmission may also occur from health care worker to patient.[188] Because acute HCV infection is often subclinical, nosocomial transmission may occur with greater frequency than has previously been recognized. Strict adherence to universal precautions to protect the health care worker and the patient are critically important.

Nonpercutaneous Transmission

The nonpercutaneous modes of transmission of HCV include transmission between sexual partners and perinatal transmission. Available evidence indicates that, in contrast to the percutaneous modes of transmission, transmission by nonpercutaneous routes is inefficient; this is particularly true for sexual transmission of HCV, which, although infrequent, clearly occurs. Although 10% of patients with sporadic acute HCV have a history of sexual exposure, most seroepidemiologic studies have demonstrated anti-HCV in only a small number of sexual contacts of infected persons.[179] Even in female sexual partners of male hemophiliacs, the overwhelming majority of whom are infected with HCV, anti-HCV is detected in no more than 3%.[179] If the index sexual partner is also infected with HIV, the transmissibility may be somewhat increased, probably because of the high level of HCV viremia present in coinfected persons.[179]

Overall, sexual partners of index patients with anti-HCV have prevalences rates of infection ranging from 0% to 27%.[179, 189] Sexual partners of low-risk index subjects without liver disease and without high-risk behavior (injection drug use or promiscuity) have anti-HCV prevalence rates ranging from 0% to 7%.[179] In contrast, sexual partners of subjects with liver disease or with high-risk behavior (the partners may themselves participate in high-risk behavior) have anti-HCV prevalence rates between 11% and 27%.[179] Several serologic surveys of the sexual partners of homosexual men and promiscuous heterosexuals with HCV infection have shown an increase in prevalence of anti-HCV. More data are needed to determine the risk for, and factors related to, transmission of HCV between long-term steady partners as well as among persons with high-risk sexual practices and to determine whether other sexually transmitted diseases promote transmission of HCV by influencing the level of viremia or modifying mucosal barriers.[190] Although the efficiency of sexual transmission of HCV remains controversial, safe sexual practices should be encouraged and barrier precautions recommended, particularly in nonmonogamous relationships.[190]

In contrast to the high efficiency of perinatal transmission of HBV from mothers to infants, the efficiency of perinatal transmission of HCV is low,[179] with a risk estimated to range from 0% to 10%. The prevalence of anti-HCV positivity in pregnant women ranges from 0.7% to 4.4%,[192] with a rate of HCV RNA detectability in anti-HCV–positive women of 65% to 72%.[192] Because anti-HCV can be acquired passively by the infant, recent studies have utilized HCV RNA by PCR to detect HCV infection in the infant.[179] Testing of the infant for anti-HCV before 18 months is not recommended. Perinatal transmission occurs exclusively from mothers who are HCV RNA positive at the time of delivery. As with sexual transmission, high titers of circulating HCV RNA in the mother may place the infant at greater risk of acquiring HCV infection, although the required levels of HCV RNA differ among studies.[191–193] There is considerable controversy as to whether the rate of vertical transmission is higher when the mother is coinfected with HIV, as suggested in early studies. However, in a recent large study of 370 anti-HCV–positive women, 4% were coinfected with HIV but did not transmit HCV to their infants. Interestingly, all women were on antiretroviral therapy during pregnancy, and such therapy was believed to reduce HIV-related immunosuppression.[192] Data regarding the risk associated with vaginal delivery as opposed to caesarean delivery are controversial.[192, 194] The risk posed to the infant from breast-feeding is believed to be negligible.[190] Further studies are needed, however, to delineate the time of infection (in utero or at the time of delivery), the importance of breast-feeding in neonatal transmission, and the natural history of HCV infection in children.

Sporadic HCV Infection

In earlier epidemiologic reports, approximately 40% of patients with HCV infection were reported to have no identifiable risk factors.[179] More recent data, however, suggest that the source of transmission is now considered to be unknown for fewer than 10% of new cases.[195] The high rate of unknown risk factors in prior reports may have been related to patients' denial of high-risk behavior.[196] "Sporadic" HCV infection may result from a prevalent nonpercutaneous or percutaneous route yet to be identified. For example, alternative routes of illicit drug use, such as intranasal cocaine use, may be associated with transmission,[196] although data regarding the potential risk associated with this practice are conflicting.[197] Likewise, tattoing and body piercing are potential routes of transmission when performed with contaminated equipment.[197] In some countries, such as Egypt, the use of reusable syringes for treatment of other diseases may have been a major route of transmission of HCV.[198]

Pathogenesis

Mechanisms of viral persistence and hepatocellular injury in patients with chronic HCV infection are poorly understood and may be distinct. The primary determinant of viral persistence appears to be the quasispecies nature of HCV[171–173] (see previous section), although other potential mechanisms may include 1) an inadequate innate immune response; 2) insufficient induction or maintainence of the adaptive response; 3) viral evasion from efficient immune responses through several mechanisms, such as infection of immunologically privileged sites, viral interference with antigen processing or other immune responses, or viral suppression of the effectiveness of antiviral cytokines; and 4) induction of immunologic tolerance. Independent of the mechanisms used to induce persistence, it is clear that the net result of the host-virus interplay is that despite the development of antibodies against several viral proteins, the majority of infected patients are unable to eradicate the virus. Furthermore, the immune responses are highly strain specific, so that animals that recover from HCV are susceptible to reinfection.[199, 200] Whether this is also true for humans who clear HCV infection remains to be determined.

In general, viral infection can produce cellular injury by direct cytopathicity and indirect immune-mediated injury.

Viral Mechanisms

Viral factors may be important in the pathogenesis of disease either directly, through cell injury associated with accumulation of the intact virus or viral proteins, or indirectly, through a differential immune response associated with one viral strain but not with another. If HCV were directly cytopathic, one would predict a positive correlation between the level of virus and the degree of cellular injury. Using the branched DNA assay to quantitate levels of HCV RNA, such a correlation has been demonstrated, with higher serum HCV RNA levels seen in patients with greater lobular inflammatory activity than in those with minimal inflammation. However, not all studies have demonstrated such a correlation.[201] A lack of correlation does not exclude the possibility of a direct cytopathic mechanism, because liver cell injury may require a certain critical level of intracellular HCV antigen accumulation. Support for this occurrence comes from a report of severe liver dysfunction in an immunocompromised transplant recipient who, despite exhibiting subfulminant liver failure, had only moderate inflammation on biopsy yet high serum levels of HCV RNA.[202]

In studies from Europe, infection with genotype 1 HCV has been associated with higher levels of viral replication, and infection with HCV subtype 1b has been associated with more advanced liver disease than has infection with other genotypes.[203] Studies from the United States have been unable to confirm these findings but have, in contrast, shown a positive correlation between HCV genotype 2 infection and severe disease.[204] In the latter study, levels of virus were lower in patients with genotype 2 infection than in patients infected with other genotypes, adding further confusion to the relationship between genotype, level of virus, and severity of liver injury.[204] Duration of infection is a factor that has not been included in many of these studies but that would be expected to influence disease severity. Unfortunately, duration of infection is often difficult to estimate because the initial infection is frequently subclinical and the time of acquisition is unknown. A recent study found that the prevalence of different genotypes has changed with time (with genotype 1b being more common before 1977 than after 1985).[203] Thus, there may be a cohort effect, with genotype 1b being over-represented in patients with severe liver disease simply because this subtype was more prevalent than other subtypes 20 or more years ago.[205]

Immune-Mediated Mechanisms

HCV infection elicits a specific antibody response, both circulating and liver-infiltrating virus-specific $CD8^+$ and $CD4^+$ T-cells, and NK cell activity. Although the cellular immune response may play a pivotal role in the pathogenesis of HCV infection, the importance of the antibody response in generating liver damage is less clear.

The HCV-specific $CD8^+$ T-cell response is polyclonal and directed against different epitopes of both structural and nonstructural regions of the viral polyprotein (core, envelope, NS3, NS4, and NS5) in the context of different MHC alleles.[206] Recent studies using MHC tetramers estimated the frequency of HCV-specific $CD8^+$ T cells to range from 0.01% to 1.2% of total $CD8^+$ T cells.[206, 207] Data from the chimpanzee model and from studies in patients with acute infection suggest that HCV-specific $CD8^+$ T cells, and particularly the number of interferon-γ–producing $CD8^+$ T cells, early in infection are involved in viral clearance.[208–210] HCV-specific $CD8^+$ T-cell responses to HCV antigens are detectable for up to 20 years after infection in persons in whom hepatitis C resolves, but not in those with persistent HCV infection,[210] suggesting that the maintenance of HCV-specific $CD8^+$ T cells determines a benign course of the disease.

Helper/inducer ($CD4^+$) T cells also may be important in modifying hepatocellular damage in chronic HCV infection. The ultimate expression of HCV depends on the balance between type 1 (Th1) and type 2 (Th2) $CD4^+$ responses. The Th1 cells secrete interleukin-2 (IL-2) and interferon-γ, which are important stimuli for the host antiviral immune response, including CTL generation and NK-cell activation. The Th2 cells produce IL-4 and IL-10, which enhance antibody production and downregulate the Th1 response. The $CD4^+$ T-cell response against HCV is also multispecific and frequently found in patients with chronic hepatitis C.[206] However, this $CD4^+$ T-cell response is probably impaired, because the proportion of chronic carriers able to mount an effective $CD4^+$ T-cell response to HCV is small.[211] In turn, an early and multispecific $CD4^+$ T-cell proliferative response seems more frequent and stronger in patients in whom acute infection resolves with clearance of HCV viremia. In these cases, there is a predominance of Th1 $CD4^+$ T cells in the peripheral blood,[206] most of which produce interferon-γ. This "protective" HCV-specific $CD4^+$ T-cell response is detected 18 to 20 years after infection in the majority of asymptomatic recovered patients, but in only a minority of patients in whom chronic HCV infection develops,[212] and loss of virus-specific $CD4^+$ T cells is associated with HCV reactivation after acute infection.[213] The primary causes of these different early immune responses in acute HCV infection are unknown.

Liver-infiltrating $CD8^+$ and $CD4^+$ lymphocytes are detected in portal, periportal, and lobular areas of the liver in patients with chronic HCV infection. $CD8^+$ lymphocytes predominate, suggesting that CTLs are the main perpetrators of hepatocellular injury. Direct cytotoxicity against HCV antigens was noted with intrahepatic $CD8^+$ T lymphocytes cloned from HCV-infected chimpanzees with active HCV infection.[208] Intrahepatic $CD8^+$ lymphocytes that recognize multiple epitopes of the putative HCV core, E1, E2/NS1, and NS3 genomic regions have been cloned from chronically infected patients[206] and may represent a high proportion of the intrahepatic T-cell infiltrate.[207] HCV-specific $CD4^+$ T cells are also enriched in the liver, and the majority of these intrahepatic $CD4^+$ T cells secrete cytokines typical of Th1 cells but not IL-4 or IL-5, probably favoring HCV $CD8^+$ T-cell activity in the liver. Patients with detectable intrahepatic CTL activity show lower levels of viremia, higher ALT values, and more active liver disease than those without HCV-specific CTLs, suggesting a correlation between the $CD8^+$ T-cell response and the degree of hepatocellular injury. Most of the intrahepatic HCV-specific $CD8^+$ T cells express the activation molecule CD69, which shows very low expression in circulating virus-specific $CD8^+$ T cells,[207] probably indicating that these cells become activated in the liver after contact with specific HCV antigens. Hepatic expression of other markers of lymphocyte activation vary. Although there is low expression of IL-2 and transferrin receptors, a large proportion of intrahepatic $CD8^+$ lymphocytes express T11/3, an activation-inducer molecule. These findings suggest that some hepatic $CD8^+$ lymphocytes are activated by an alternative antigen-independent pathway.

Molecular mechanisms for hepatic injury in chronic hepatitis C are currently under investigation. As mentioned previously, it seems clear that HCV-specific T cells are enriched at the site of viral replication compared with the peripheral blood.[206, 207] An upregulated expression of adhesion molecules in the portal tracts probably reflects active recruitment and priming of T cells in the inflamed liver.[214] The T-cell immune reponse in the liver may result in direct cytolysis of the infected cells and also in the inhibition of viral replication by secreted antiviral cytokines.[215] Programmed cell-death pathways are probably involved in HCV-related liver damage, and Fas antigen (FasAg) mRNA transcription seems to be upregulated by intrahepatic HCV replication. Taken together, these data support an important role for T-cell–mediated cytotoxicity in the pathogenesis of hepatocyte injury. The role of T cells in the pathogenesis of HCV infection has been further substantiated by the establishment of a human $CD3^+$ (pan T-cell marker), $CD8^+$, and $CD56^+$ lymphocyte clone capable of lysing autologous and allogeneic hepatocytes. Because $CD56^+$ is a marker of NK cells, the observed cytotoxicity is not HLA class I restricted. Non-

HLA class I–restricted $CD3^+$, $CD16^+$, and $CD56^+$ peripheral blood lymphocytes are found more commonly in patients with chronic HCV infection than in uninfected controls.

The humoral response against HCV is targeted against epitopes within all viral proteins. The role of circulating anti-HCV antibodies in the pathogenesis of hepatocyte injury is unknown. In contrast to the cellular immune response, the antibody response to HCV antigens continues to be evident with time in patients with a chronic outcome but is lost in most recovered patients, suggesting that T cells and not antibodies effect the resolution of acute hepatitis C.[210] Indeed, several studies have shown that neutralizing antibodies are produced during natural HCV infection despite the high rate of viral persistence, suggesting that this humoral immune response is inadequate for viral clearance. Neutralizing antibodies are usually detected between 7 and 31 weeks after infection. The most likely explanation for the ineffectiveness of the antibody response against HCV is that rapid occurrence of viral mutations within the epitopes recognized by neutralizing antibodies abrogates antibody recognition of the new variant. The quasispecies nature of HCV with high viral turnover is likely to play a major role in viral persistence, with rapid generation of viral variants that are capable of evading the host immune response. These hypotheses need further evaluation. Indeed, although several studies have suggested that an early antibody response to the hypervariable region (HVR1) is associated with a self-limited course of HCV infection and that increased heterogeneity of the quasispecies is associated with viral persistence,[171] other recent studies have shown clearance of HCV in chimpanzees in the absence of any antibody against the envelope region and HCV persistence in the absence of mutations in the HVR1 or in the absence of the whole HVR1.[216] In summary, although the humoral response may play some role in viral clearance, it is likely that other mechanisms predominate.

Other immunologic factors such as HLA class I and class II alleles likely contribute to HCV-related disease severity and viral persistence. Indeed, some HLA-DR and HLA-DQ alleles have been associated with HCV clearance.[217]

Clinical Manifestations and Diagnosis

Acute and Chronic Infection

HCV accounts for approximately 20% of cases of acute hepatitis. Acute infection is, however, rarely seen in clinical practice, because the vast majority of patients experience no clinical symptoms[218] (see Table 68–2). Jaundice may develop in 25% of these patients, whereas 10% to 20% may present with nonspecific symptoms such as fatigue, nausea, and vomiting indistinguishable from symptoms of other types of acute viral hepatitis. HCV RNA appears in the blood within 2 weeks of exposure and is followed by an increase in serum aminotransferase levels several weeks later. Serum aminotransferase levels may exceed 1000 U/L in 20% of cases and generally follow a fluctuating pattern during the first months. In patients in whom jaundice develops, peak serum bilirubin levels are usually less than 12 mg/dL, and elevations typically resolve in 1 month. Fulminant hepatitis is rare. HCV infection is self-limiting in only 15% of patients in whom HCV RNA in serum becomes undetectable and ALT levels return to normal. A person who initially tests negative for HCV RNA in serum may eventually test positive, suggesting that in clinical practice, virologic outcome should be assessed by long-term follow-up.

Approximately 85% of infected patients do not clear the virus by 6 months, and chronic hepatitis develops. Of these, the majority will have elevated or fluctuating serum ALT levels, whereas one third have persistently normal ALT values, despite continued liver injury and detectable viremia (see later section). The most common complaint of patients with chronic HCV infection is fatigue, the severity of which is not necessarily related to the severity of the underlying liver disease. Other nonspecific symptoms include depression, nausea, anorexia, abdominal discomfort, and difficulty with concentration. Once cirrhosis of the liver develops, patients are at risk for complications of portal hypertension (ascites, gastrointestinal bleeding, encephalopathy, etc.). Jaundice is rarely seen in chronic HCV infection until hepatic decompensation has occurred. Once complications of portal hypertension or evidence of hepatic synthetic failure (reduction in serum albumin, rise in serum bilirubin, or prolongation of the prothrombin time) develop, referral for liver transplantation should be considered.

Extrahepatic Manifestations

HCV has been recognized increasingly as a cause of significant extrahepatic disease. Reported extrahepatic manifestations of HCV infection include membranoproliferative glomerulonephritis, essential mixed cryoglobulinemia, porphyria cutanea tarda, leukocytoclastic vasculitis, focal lymphocytic sialadenitis, Mooren corneal ulcers, lichen planus, rheumatoid arthritis, non-Hodgkin's lymphoma, and diabetes mellitus.[219] Some of these associations are more convincing than others. Extrahepatic manifestations will develop in approximately 1% to 2% of HCV-infected patients. Furthermore, nonorgan-specific autoantibodies are frequently expressed in patients with HCV infection (antinuclear antibodies with a titer >1 : 40 in 21%, antismooth muscle antibody with a titer >1 : 40 in 21%, and anti-liver kidney microsomal antibodies in 5%).

HCV infection is strongly implicated in the pathogenesis of essential mixed cryoglobulinemia and membranoproliferative glomerulonephritis, presumably by immune complex deposition. Anti-HCV antibodies are found in serum in 50% to 90% of patients with essential mixed cryoglobulinemia. Furthermore, cryoglobulins are found in approximately one half of patients infected with HCV. Many studies have found HCV RNA concentrated in cryoprecipitate. Clinical symptoms develop in only 25% to 30% of HCV-infected patients with cryoglobulinemia, with symptoms ranging from fatigue, arthralgias, or arthritis to purpura, Raynaud's phenomenon, vasculitis, peripheral neuropathies, and glomerulonephritis. Treatment with immunosuppressive agents is ineffective. Therapy with interferon-α has resulted in improvement in symptoms and reduction in serum HCV RNA levels in patients with HCV-related essential mixed cryoglobulinemia, although the effect appears to be transient.[220] The addition of ribavirin may reduce the rate of relapse but requires further study. Glomerular disease, gener-

Table 68–9 | **Diagnostic Tests for Hepatitis C**

I. Serologic assays
  1. Screening assays
    EIA-1
    EIA-2
    EIA-3
  2. Confirmatory assays (RIBA)
II. Virologic assays
  1. HCV RNA detection
    Qualitative
    Quantitative
      PCR-based methods
      bDNA assays
  2. Genotyping
    Sequencing and phylogenetic analysis
    PCR with genotype-specific primers
    Restriction fragment length polymorphism
    Line-probe or reverse dot-blot hybridization assay
    Serotyping with genotype-specific antibodies
  3. Analysis of HCV quasispecies
    Molecular cloning of RT-PCR amplicons and sequencing
    Single-stranded conformation polymorphism
    Temperature-gradient gel electrophoresis
    Heteroduplex mobility assay

bDNA, branched DNA; EIA, enzyme immunoassay; PCR, polymerase chain reaction; RIBA, recombinant immunoblot assay; RT-PCR, reverse transcription PCR.

ally in the form of membranoproliferative glomerulonephritis, is another frequent extrahepatic disease in patients with HCV infection. Most affected patients also have essential mixed cryoglobulinemia. Clinically, patients may present with nephrotic syndrome, non–nephrotic-range proteinuria, or renal insufficiency. Hypocomplementemia is frequent, as is positivity for rheumatoid factor. Interferon therapy in patients with membranoproliferative glomerulonephritis has been associated with a reduction in proteinuria (65%) but typically no significant changes in renal function.[221] Approximately 10% of affected patients will progress to end-stage renal failure and require dialysis. Use of pulse methylprednisolone therapy may result in some benefit in patients with severe progressive disease.

Diagnosis

There are several immunologic and molecular assays for the detection and assessment of hepatitis C (Table 68–9). The immunologic or serologic tests identify the presence of anti-HCV, which indicates exposure to the virus without differentiating among acute, chronic, and resolved infection.[222] In contrast, the molecular or virologic assays detect specific viral nucleic acid sequences (HCV RNA), which indicate persistence of the virus.[222] Whereas serologic assays are typically used for screening and first-line diagnosis, virologic assays are needed to confirm active infection or to monitor the effects of therapy (see Table 68–9).

Serologic Tests

There are two types of anti-HCV assay, the enzyme immunoassay (EIA) and the recombinant immunoblot assay (RIBA). Both detect antibodies to different HCV antigens from the core and nonstructural proteins and were developed using recombinant antigens derived from cloned HCV transcripts (see Fig. 68–6). The time course of symptoms and the detection of anti-HCV and HCV RNA after acute infection are shown in Fig. 68–7. Serologic assays are typically used for screening and first-line diagnosis. The actual use of the serologic assays is being questioned with the advent of the more sensitive and specific molecular techniques. Three successive generations of EIAs have resulted in increasing sensitivity and a progressive decrease in the duration of the window period (Table 68–10). Because first-generation EIAs lacked sensitivity and specificity, confirmatory RIBAs were systematically used in samples positive by EIA. With the newer EIAs and the increased use of molecular assays, confirmatory RIBAs are needed less frequently. A proposed algorithm for the evaluation of a serologically positive patient is outlined in Figure 68–8.

Screening Assays

The c100-3 antigen was the antigen used to develop the first-generation antibody assays, which were approved by the FDA in 1990. These assays were reactive in 80% to 90% of patients with post-transfusional non-A, non-B hepatitis, but antibody was not detectable during the earliest stages of acute infection. As with other immunoassays, screening of low-risk populations yielded a large number of false-positive results. Second-generation assays incorporated the recombinant antigens c22-3 from the nucleocapsid (core) region and c33c from the nonstructural region NS3. c33c was combined with c100-3 to form a single-expression protein called c200 from the NS3 and NS4 regions. The second-generation EIA-2, approved by the FDA in 1992, resulted in earlier detection of HCV antibody and identification of a greater number of cases of acute and chronic non-A, non-B hepatitis (10%–30% more than first-generation assays).[222] The latest EIA-3 assay has incorporated a recombinant antigen from the NS5 region that confers a slightly increased sensitivity and shorter time to seroconversion (see Table 68–10). Although second-generation EIAs are the most widely used assays, several blood banks and clinical laboratories have switched to the EIA-3. Despite the high sensitivity of these recent EIA assays, the specificity differs according to the popula-

Table 68–10 | **Enzyme Immunoassays for the Diagnosis of HCV Infection**

ASSAY	SENSITIVITY (%)*	POSITIVE PREDICTIVE VALUE IN LOW-RISK GROUPS (%)†	POSITIVE PREDICTIVE VALUE IN HIGH-RISK GROUPS (%)†	WINDOW PERIOD (WK)‡
EIA-1	70–80	30–50	70–85	15
EIA-2	90–95	50–60	90–95	9–10
EIA-3	95–98	25	–	7–8

*Compared with HCV RNA testing.
†High-risk patients are considered those with a definitive risk factor for HCV acquisition and elevated serum aminotransferase levels. Low-risk patients include blood donors, patients with normal aminotransferase levels, and those with no risk factor for HCV acquisition.
‡Window period: time between acquisition of infection and first positive result.

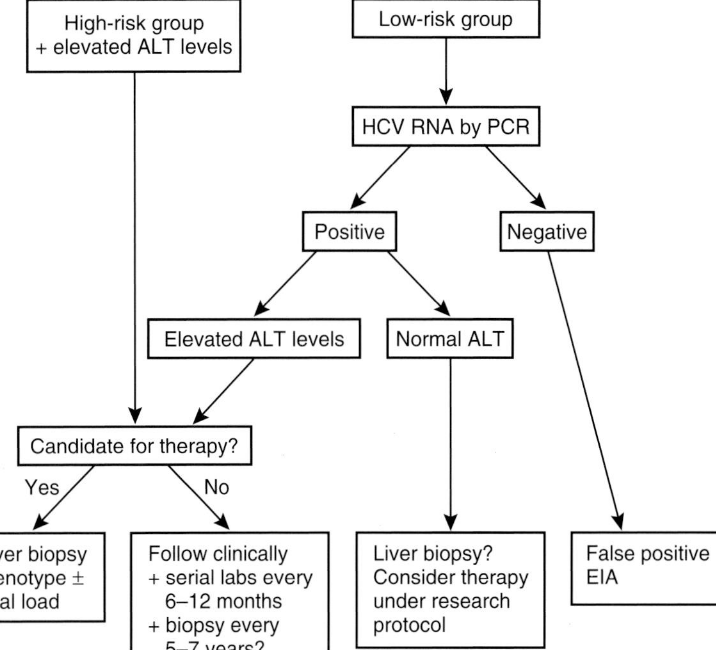

Figure 68–8. A proposed algorithm for the evaluation of a serologically positive patient. ALT, alanine aminotransferase; EIA, enzyme immunoassay; PCR, polymerase chain reaction.

tion tested (see Table 68–10). In low-risk populations, confirmatory tests are still generally helpful.

Confirmatory Assays

The RIBA tests use the same antigens as the corresponding EIA tests but in a strip immunoblot assay format. Their sensitivity is generally lower than that of EIAs, but their specificity is superior. The 4-antigen RIBA-2 (RIBA HCV 2.0 Strip Immunoassay, Chiron Corporation, Emeryville, CA) was approved by the FDA in June 1993. This assay incorporated antigens 5-1-1, c100-3, c22-3, c33c, and superoxide dismutase (SOD). With this assay, a specimen is considered positive if two or more bands, representing at least two different HCV gene products, are detectable. If a specimen reacts with bands from only one region, such as 5-1-1- and c100-3 (both from the NS4 region), the result is considered indeterminate. If a specimen reacts with the SOD band in addition to two or more HCV antigen bands, the result is also considered indeterminate. In a patient with a positive RIBA-2 result, HCV RNA is detectable with PCR methods in 72% to 100% of cases.[222] Most patients and blood donors who are RIBA-2 negative are also PCR negative.[222] Absence of detectable HCV RNA in a sample that is serologically positive by RIBA-2 may result from one or more of the following: 1) mishandling of specimens with resulting degradation of viral RNA; 2) intermittent viremia with levels intermittently below detection by standard assays; 3) viral heterogeneity that results in failure to detect true infection by routine assays; or 4) false-positive serologic results.[222] Therefore, seropositivity (EIA and RIBA positive), even in the absence of detectable viral RNA, likely represents true infection. A RIBA-2 indeterminate result in low-risk groups rarely yields a positive HCV RNA result, but in high-risk groups, it is associated with positive viremia in 20% to 50% of cases. The third-generation RIBA-3 assay (RIBA HCV 3.0 Strip Immunoassay, Chiron Corporation, Emeryville, CA) includes two recombinant antigens (c33c and NS5) and synthetic peptides from the nucleocapsid (c22) and the NS4 (c100-3) regions. RIBA-3 has been approved for use by blood banks as a supplemental test for EIA-3–positive test results. This new RIBA format is able to identify correctly HCV-negative and HCV-positive results in samples that are RIBA-2 indeterminate. RIBA assays are more difficult to perform and more expensive than EIA tests, and despite their high reproducibility and potential for distinguishing false- from true-positive results in low-risk populations, their clinical use has been limited by the availability of molecular assays.[223]

Virologic Tests

Because no methods for culturing HCV are available, detection of viral RNA in serum is used as a marker of the virus itself. Viral detection is accomplished by amplification methods such a PCR or quantitative assays such as the branched DNA (bDNA) signal amplification assay (Quantiplex HCV RNA, Chiron Corporation) or the PCR-based Amplicor assay (Roche Diagnostics).[222]

Qualitative PCR testing for HCV RNA is very sensitive and may detect as few as 100 viral copies/mL, usually within 1 week of exposure. To achieve these results, specifc procedures should be followed carefully, including separation of serum or plasma from whole blood within 4 hours of venipuncture and rapid storage of specimens at −70°C. Qualitative PCR testing should be used in the evaluation of seronegative acute or chronic hepatitis of unknown cause; chronic liver disease with several possible causes, including the presence of HCV antibodies; chronic hepatitis C with repeatedly normal serum aminotransferase levels; babies born to HCV-infected mothers; and immunosuppressed patients with possible hepatitis C and to monitor antiviral therapy.

The quantitative tests allow measurement of serum HCV RNA levels (viral load) and may be useful in assessing the effectiveness of antiviral therapy and in evaluating the likelihood of a treatment response.[222] Their use is limited, however, by expense and lack of standardization. The bDNA assay uses capture and target probes from the conserved 5′ UTR and core regions. Captured HCV RNA is amplified with synthetic branched DNA oligonucleotides (signal amplification) and labeled with alkaline phosphatase probes, and the entire complex is incubated with a chemiluminescent substance. The light emitted corresponds to an exact level of RNA, determined from a standardized curve. The lower limit of detection with the second-generation bDNA assay is approximately 250,000 viral equivalents per milliliter. The third-generation bDNA assay can detect 600 IU/mL. The more recently developed Amplicor assay provides a semiquantitative measurement of viral RNA. HCV target RNA is reverse transcribed and amplified using primers from the most conserved region of the HCV genome. Internal quantitative standards are coamplified with the target to monitor the efficacy of this step. A microwell plate detection system with chemiluminescent label is used. The amount of viral RNA present in the amplified sample is estimated from a standardized dilutional series. The lower limit of detection with the Amplicor assay is approximately 1000 viral copies per milliliter or 600 IU/mL.

Several recent large trials have shown a relationship between pretreatment viral load and the response to antiviral therapy. In these trials, the Superquant assay (National Genetics Institute, Los Angeles, CA), an "in-house" competitive PCR-based technique using multiple cycles, was used to measure viral load. Unfortunately, the recommendations issued from these trials have been difficult to apply universally because most laboratories use one of the two commercial assays described above. Indeed, there are few data comparing the results of HCV quantitation using different methods.[224, 225] Furthermore, a value obtained by one method does not necessarily correlate with a specific result obtained by another method. To permit universal standardization of HCV RNA quantitation units, a recent collaborative study established the World Health Organization (WHO) International Standard for HCV RNA quantitation. A lyophilized sample of HCV RNA, genotype 1, was accepted as the candidate standard and was assigned a titer of 10^5 IU/mL. This standard has been used to calibrate HCV RNA concentration panels and to express HCV RNA load in IU/mL in the commercial assays.[226] Roche Molecular Systems recently released the first semiautomated HCV RNA quantitation assay with results expressed in IU/mL, the Cobas Amplicor HCV Monitor assay version 2.0 (Cobas v2.0). More data are needed regarding these standardized assays. In the meantime, data from a recent study have suggested that commercially available quantitation tests are roughly equivalent to the noncommercial NGI Superquant and thus, despite their limitations, may be used in clinical laboratories.[227] Some important guidelines have been provided regarding the use of the commercial assays: 1) high-end quantification using quantitative PCR tests (Monitor and SuperQuant) is often inaccurate without a previous 100-fold dilution; 2) a perfect linear range extending from low to high viral load is often unachievable with these assays, and the bDNA 2.0 test performs better at high viral loads than either the Monitor or SuperQuant assays; and 3) the newer assays (bDNA v2.0 and Cobas v2.0) perform equally well with regard to HCV genotypes.[224–227] In summary, although the tests cannot be used interchangeably, changes in viral load that occur over time in a single patient can be measured consistently with a single assay.

Genotypes

The high spontaneous mutational rate that is characteristic of many RNA viruses results in considerable heterogeneity throughout the HCV genome.[171] The most highly conserved regions of the genome are the 5′ and 3′ UTRs; the most variable are the envelope regions (E1 and E2). Genetic heterogeneity has been classified under two headings: genotype and quasispecies. As discussed previously, quasispecies represent the genetic heterogeneity of the HCV population within an individual patient, and genotype represents the genetic heterogeneity of the virus between patients.[171]

Differentiation of these genotypes is accomplished by direct sequencing, differential PCR using type-specific primers, detection of PCR products with type-specific probes (the Line Probe Assay), restriction fragment length polymorphism (RFLP) analysis, and serotyping with type-specific antibody. These techniques have been used in the 5′ untranslated, NS4, NS5, and core regions. Of the many methods available for genotyping, direct sequencing is regarded as the most accurate. However, sequencing methods are technically demanding and time-consuming. A recent study comparing sequencing, type-specific primers, serotyping, and RFLP demonstrated over 90% concordance among the various methods.[228]

Selection of Serologic and Virologic Tests

A proposed algorithm for the evaluation of an anti-HCV–seropositive person is shown in Figure 68–8. Initial diagnostic testing of HCV infection is currently made by detecting specific antibody by second- or third-generation EIA tests (see Table 68–9). For low-risk patients, a negative EIA test result is sufficient to exclude HCV infection. In contrast, for high-risk, recently exposed, or immunocompromised patients (including HIV-infected, chronic hemodialysis, and transplant patients), further confirmatory testing is required. For years, confirmation was performed using RIBA testing. More recently, PCR testing has supplanted the RIBA test as the confirmatory test of choice. RIBA tests still may be used for distinguishing resolved infection from a false-positive EIA test (for example, a high-risk patient with positive EIA but negative PCR results).

Screening in Blood Banks

The risk of acquiring HCV infection from blood products has declined substantially since the advent of donor screening with specific serologic tests for HCV and is now estimated to be extremely low (0.01%–0.001% per unit transfused).[184] With the most recent EIA and RIBA-3 assays, the number of false or indeterminate test results is very low. One major limitation of these assays, however, is the existence of a window period in which the patient may transmit the virus before anti-HCV is detectable. With recent assays, the average delay until anti-HCV appears is approximately 80 days. For this reason, many blood banks are exploring the feasibility of testing all donors with qualitative PCR assays.

Diagnosis in Hemodialysis Units

Because of the high rate of HCV infection in hemodialysis units, routine testing for HCV is recommended in hemodialyzed patients. Although the EIA-1 tests had poor sensitivity and specificity in this setting, EIA-2 tests perform with a high efficiency, and over 90% of EIA-2–positive patients have detectable HCV RNA, whereas false-positive results are uncommon.

Diagnosis in Immunocompromised Patients

Antibody tests underestimate the prevalence of HCV infection in immunocompromised populations, and detection of viral RNA is frequently required for diagnosis. In a study comparing RNA assays to standard antibody tests (EIA-2 and RIBA-2) for the diagnosis of HCV infection after liver transplantation, EIA-2 failed to detect HCV infection in 12% of patients with HCV RNA detectable by PCR and bDNA assays. RIBA-2 produced indeterminate samples in 24% and negative samples in 17% of patients in whom HCV RNA was detectable. Thus, antibody assays lack sensitivity in the transplant setting. A decrease in antibody titer to specific viral antigens (c100-3 and c33c) or complete loss of reactivity has been demonstrated in kidney and bone marrow transplant recipients.[229] Other antigens, such as c25, Ne1, and e2, are less affected.

In HIV-infected patients with HCV coinfection, a fall in seroreactivity to certain viral antigens in the RIBA-2 assay can produce an increase in the frequency of indeterminate results. Most HIV/HCV coinfected patients with indeterminate RIBA-2 results are HCV RNA positive, independent of whether the serum ALT level is abnormal or not.[230] In contrast, a minority of HIV-negative patients with indeterminate RIBA-2 results and normal serum ALT levels have detectable HCV RNA in serum. HCV infection in the absence of seropositivity can occur in immunocompromised HIV-infected patients but is less common than in other immuncompromised hosts.

Pathology

The pathology of HCV infection has been summarized in an excellent review.[231] The range of histologic findings in patients with chronic HCV infection is broad, from minimal periportal lymphocytic inflammation to active hepatitis with bridging fibrosis, hepatocyte necrosis, and frank cirrhosis. Steatosis, lymphoid aggregates, and bile duct damage are frequent in the liver biopsy specimens from patients with HCV infection, but there is considerable overlap with the histologic findings in patients with chronic HBV infection and autoimmune hepatitis.[231] Grading and staging systems for liver biopsy specimens from these patients are in evolution. The Histologic Activity Index (HAI) developed by Knodell and associates is still used to quantify the degree of liver damage in many trials of antiviral therapy, but it is cumbersome to use. A simplified system in which inflammation is graded from 0 to 4 and fibrosis is staged from 0 to 4 has been developed by Scheuer and colleagues and is gaining widespread use in clinical practice. Although the prognostic implications of specific histologic findings are not clear,[231] mild inflammation and negligible fibrosis are associated with a low risk of progression to cirrhosis, whereas patients with severe necroinflammatory activity and advanced fibrosis will likely evolve to cirrhosis with time.

The role of a liver biopsy in the management of HCV-infected patients is not settled to date. The potential risks associated with a biopsy contrast with the importance of the information generated, especially in the absence of appropriate surrogate markers of hepatic fibrosis. Recent consensus conferences have stated that a liver biopsy is mandatory in patients with chronic hepatitis C and elevated serum aminotransferase levels so that correct grading and staging can be performed. This information is particularly relevant when considering antiviral therapy or when other causes of liver disease may be present. A post-treatment liver biopsy is not necessary because most trials have demonstrated that a sustained virologic response is generally associated with stable or improved histologic findings (see later section). In contrast, in patients with normal serum aminotransferase levels, the role of a liver biopsy is less clear. Although the frequency of progression of fibrosis appears to be low in these patients, only 20% have absolutely normal liver histologic findings, and a small percentage (<15%) have significant liver damage.[232] Because no surrogate markers allow the identification of this subset of patients, many authors recommend a liver biopsy in them. In patients in whom the diagnosis of cirrhosis is suggested by clinical or ultrasound findings (ascites, splenomegaly, spider angioma, low platelet count, prolonged prothrombin time, reduced portal flow, nodularity of the liver), histologic confirmation is usually not needed.

Natural History

An understanding of the natural history of HCV infection is essential for guiding physicians when counseling patients about their prognosis and the need for therapeutic intervention. Infection with HCV, once established, persists in the vast majority of patients. Disease progression is largely silent, and patients often are identified only on routine biochemical screening or blood donation. Several strategies have been used to assess the natural history of chronic HCV infection: 1) cross-sectional studies in which patients with end-stage disease are evaluated and assessed concurrently for markers of HCV infection; 2) retrospective/prospective studies in which patients with established liver disease are assessed by estimating the time of initial infection and then measuring the natural history of infection from that time forward; 3) prospective studies in which patients are evaluated at the onset of disease and are followed longitudinally for a defined period; and 4) long-term cohort studies of subjects with a defined parenteral exposure, in which the HCV status of the person at the time of initial exposure was known and outcome was assessed after more than 15 years of follow-up. Each approach has its limitations. As would be predicted, the most severe outcomes have been described in cross-sectional and retrospective studies.

Studies of Patients with End-Stage Disease (Cross-Sectional Studies)

Evaluation of patients with established chronic hepatitis, cirrhosis, or non-HBV HCC with use of antibody assays provides evidence for an association between HCV infection and liver disease. Anti-HCV is detectable in 8% to 69% of patients with cryptogenic cirrhosis, with most studies finding rates of approximately 50%.[218] Anti-HCV is also detectable in 6% to 76% of persons with HCC.[218] As impressive as these findings are, they have limitations. Cross-sectional studies fail to establish cause and effect; specifically, the presence of HCV infection before the development of liver complications cannot be shown conclusively. Furthermore, these studies fail to determine the proportion of HCV-infected persons who do not achieve these serious end points and, in doing so, tend to exaggerate the proportion of patients in whom end-stage cirrhosis and HCC develop.

Retrospective/Prospective Studies

These studies have been conducted by referral centers and include patients in whom complications of HCV infection have developed. In particular, two sets of investigators have used this approach to evaluate the natural history of HCV infection resulting from blood transfusion. Patients with HCV-related liver disease were observed prospectively for 1 to 27 years, and the rate of disease progression was calculated from the time of presumed infection (based on the history of transfusion).[233, 234] Despite disparate geographic backgrounds (Japan and the United States), the studies yielded similar results. In the Japanese study, chronic hepatitis was identified 10 ± 11.3 years after transfusion, cirrhosis 21.2 ± 9.6 years after transfusion, and HCC 29 ± 13.2 years after transfusion.[233] The longest interval from transfusion to HCC was 62 years, and the shortest was 16 years, demonstrating the variability in rate of progression. In the United States study, the mean interval between transfusion and chronic hepatitis was 13.7 ± 10.9 years, cirrhosis 20.6 ±10.1 years, and HCC 28.3 ± 11.5 years.[234] Although these studies demonstrate unequivocally the potential of HCV infection to induce severe liver disease, they cannot address the frequency of serious disease among all HCV-infected persons. For such an estimate, population-based studies are required.

Prospective Studies

Because non-A, non-B hepatitis and hepatitis C have been recognized only since 1974, prospective studies are typically less than 20 years in duration. Table 68–11 summarizes eight representative studies with follow-up ranging from 7 to 15 years.[218] These studies provide unequivocal evidence of the progressive nature of chronic HCV infection. Infection often can be subclinical, and in symptomatic patients, fatigue is the most frequent complaint. Cirrhosis, defined histologically or clinically, is present in 8% to 42% of patients. In some cases, cirrhosis was identified as early as 15 months after the episode of acute hepatitis. In approximately 10% of cases, decompensated disease was present, with splenomegaly, ascites, coagulopathy, and esophageal varices. HCC is rare in European and North American series but is described more frequently in studies from Japan. Although the duration of follow-up was limited and a control group to assess disease-associated risk was frequently lacking, available prospective studies indicate that at least two decades of infection is required for clinically significant disease. Death from end-stage liver disease is uncommon, but clearly liver failure and HCC occur. The higher rate of HCC in Japan compared with that in Western countries is unexplained but may relate to differences in HCV genotypes or concomitant exposure to other hepatotoxic agents.

Table 68–11 | **Consequences of Chronic Non-A, Non-B Hepatitis in Follow-up Studies of Less Than 15 Years**

AUTHOR	COUNTRY	NUMBER OF PATIENTS	DISEASE ONSET	MEAN FOLLOW-UP (YRS)	SYMPTOMS (%)	CIRRHOSIS (%)	HCC (%)	DEATH FROM LIVER DISEASE (%)
Tremolada	Italy	135	Acute	7.6	3.7	15.6	0.7	3.6
Mason	Sweden	66	Acute	13.0	11.5	8–11	N.R.	1.6
DiBisceglie	U.S.	39	Acute	9.7	12.8	20.0	0	6.0
Koretz	U.S.	80	Acute	14.0	10.0	18–20	1.3	2.5
Hopf	Germany	86	Acute/Chronic	8.0	4.7	24.0	N.R.	N.R.
Roberts	Australia	57	Chronic	15.0	50.0*	8.0	N.R.	N.R.
Takashi	Japan	100	Chronic	11.0	N.R.	42.0	19.0	N.R.
Yano	Japan	155	Chronic	8.7	N.R.	30.0	15.0	N.R.

*All symptomatic patients had vague symptoms.
HCC, hepatocellular carcinoma; N.R., not reported.
From Seeff L: Natural history of viral hepatitis type C. Semin Gastrointest Dis 6:20, 1995.

Cohort Studies with Prolonged Follow-up after a Defined Parenteral Exposure

Cohort studies allow assessment of not only patients in whom persistent infection and significant liver disease developed but also those with mild disease and those who cleared the infection. In the study of Seeff and colleagues, 568 patients with post-transfusional non-A, non-B hepatitis were compared with 984 matched controls who received transfusions but did not develop hepatitis.[235] After an average follow-up of 18 years, all-cause mortality rates (determined from death certificates) did not differ between the cases and controls (50.5% and 50.9%, respectively). The death rate attributable to liver disease was quite low but was higher in the cases than controls (3.3% and 1.5%, respectively). Reanalysis of this study group after a follow-up of 20 years again showed no difference in all-cause mortality rates between cases and controls.[218] Seventy-two percent of tested patients were anti-HCV positive. Mortality in the anti-HCV–positive cases was not significantly different from that of the anti-HCV–negative controls (51% versus 54%, respectively). Of the 205 cases available for re-evaluation, 75% had either biochemical or serologic evidence of HCV infection, compared with 19% of the 335 controls. Liver biopsy specimens were obtained in one half of the patients with biochemical abnormalities, the majority of whom were anti-HCV positive, and almost 90% had evidence of chronic hepatitis or cirrhosis. Although none of the patients with chronic hepatitis had clinical signs of liver disease, one half of those with cirrhosis had overt signs of chronic liver disease (splenomegaly, ascites, hypoalbuminemia). From this large multicenter study with a mean follow-up of 20 years, the natural history of post-transfusional HCV infection could be defined as follows: 1) 25% of patients had spontaneous recovery with loss of HCV RNA in serum (10% also had concomitant loss of serologic markers of prior HCV infection); and 2) of the 75% with persistent infection, severe progressive liver disease occured in only 15% to 20%, whereas in the remainder, a benign evolution was observed. It remains to be seen if this benign evolution will continue with prolonged follow-up.

An iatrogenic outbreak has given us insight into the natural history of HCV. In 1977, young Irish women were accidentally infected with HCV when a contaminated lot of anti-D serum was administered to them. In a surveillance program, 438 who were viremic with HCV were identified. All were infected with HCV genotype 1b. However, on prolonged follow-up (more than 18 years) few had developed cirrhosis (2%) and none had developed complications of liver disease.[236] A similar study was recently reported in Germany and involved 152 women also infected through contaminated Rh immune globulin.[237] After 15 years of infection, none of the women had evidence of chronic hepatitis or cirrhosis. These are two of the few studies that assessed the natural history in people infected at a young age and, as such, probably have important implications for people infected through injection drug use, the majority of whom are infected in their teens and twenties. However, compared with other studies, these studies appear to document a slower progressive course of HCV infection. The slower progression may be the result of several factors, such as 1) gender (disease progression is slower in women compared with men),[238] 2) infection at a young age, which is thought to be predictive of slow disease progression, and 3) the specific route of infection, with a probable small inoculum of virus compared with that acquired through blood transfusions.

A 45-year natural history study of 8568 military recruits, 0.2% of whom tested positive for anti-HCV on second- and third-generation assays, has had the longest follow-up to date. In this study, mortality from liver disease in the HCV-positive group was very low, with small differences when compared with the control group. These data suggest that HCV is a less progressive disease than previously believed and that only 15% to 20% of HCV-infected persons eventually progress to potentially serious end-stage liver disease, while the remainder will die of causes other than liver disease.[239]

Finally, studies performed in children infected at an early age also suggest that the natural history of HCV may be more benign than previously thought. In a study performed in Germany, 458 children infected with HCV through cardiac surgery before the implementation of blood donor screening were observed for a mean of 17 years.[240] After this time, almost one half of the infected children had spontaneously cleared the infection, and of the remainder, only one had persistently abnormal serum ALT levels. Of the 17 patients who underwent a liver biopsy, only 2 had portal fibrosis, and both of them had chronic congestive heart failure, which could have accounted for the more aggressive histologic picture.[240]

If the data from all these studies are combined, we can conclude that when the entire population of HCV-infected persons is observed, only a small percentage have severe outcomes during the first two decades of infection.

Factors Associated with Disease Progression

The factors that contribute to the histologic progression of liver disease and development of HCC are under investigation but will be important to identify in order to focus therapy on those patients who are at greatest risk for progressive liver disease. Age (older than 40 years), male gender, and increased alcohol intake (>50 g daily) have been documented as variables associated with disease progression.[238] Immunosuppression is clearly linked with more aggressive disease. Indeed, studies from patients with humoral immunodeficiency (hypogammaglobulinemic patients)[241] or cellular immune impairment (liver or kidney transplant recipients, HIV-infected patients with a low $CD4^+$ count)[242, 243] have all shown rates of progression to cirrhosis significantly higher than those observed in immunocompetent patients (see later). Other less consistently documented prognostic factors include mode of transmission (higher disease progression when infection is through blood transfusion than through injection drug use)[244, 245] and coinfection with HBV. In contrast, viral-related factors such as genotype and viral load do not appear to affect the clinical course of HCV-infected individuals. Conflicting results have been reported regarding the role played by genotypes or quasispecies in disease severity (see previous section).

Natural History of Clinically Compensated HCV-Related Cirrhosis

Complications may develop once a patient has cirrhosis. Interestingly, even after the development of cirrhosis, the short- and medium-term natural history is fair. Actuarial survival rates are 91% at 5 years and 79% at 10 years in the absence of clinical decompensation. The survival drops to 50% at 5 years among those in whom clinical decompensation develops. The cumulative probability of an episode of decompensation is only 5% at 1 year, increasing to 30% at 10 years from the diagnosis of cirrhosis.[246–248] The risk of HCC is 1% to 4% per year once cirrhosis is established. In some, but not all, studies, interferon therapy has been shown to reduce the risk of hepatic decompensation and HCC.[246–249]

Disease in Patients with Persistently Normal Aminotransferase Levels

Approximately one third of anti-HCV–positive patients have normal serum ALT levels. Most of these patients have some degree of histologically proven chronic liver damage, ranging from mild chronic hepatitis to cirrhosis.[250] The wide range in disease severity in previous studies may be related to the absence of a well-defined definition of these patients. Indeed, different types of patients typically have been included in these studies, with differences in 1) duration of ALT normalization, 2) requirement that the ALT level be normal or that both the AST and ALT be normal, and 3) presence of detectable viremia. Strictly speaking, patients considered as "HCV carriers" should be those with persistently normal serum ALT levels over a period of at least 12 months, with measurement of ALT levels on several occasions at least 1 month apart and with detectable HCV RNA in serum. Disease progression appears to be slower in these patients than in those with elevated ALT levels, and progression to cirrhosis is considered a rare event.[232]

Disease in Immunocompromised Patients

Dialysis and Renal Transplant Recipients

Dialysis and renal transplant recipients have a higher prevalence of HCV infection than the general population, in part because of the frequent risk factors in these patients (prior blood transfusion and prior injection drug use), and in part because of nosocomial spread within dialysis units. Using anti-HCV tests, the prevalence of HCV is 6% to 22%, and the incidence rate is 4.9% per year.[251]

De novo acquisition of HCV from infected organs or blood products has been well documented. A large study of 3078 cadaveric organ donors from eight organ procurement agencies in the United States found a frequency of HCV (by EIA-2) and of HCV RNA (by PCR) of 4.2% and 2.4%, respectively.[252] Recipients of organs from seropositive donors with detectable viremia were more likely to be viremic after transplantation and to develop post-transplantation liver disease than were recipients of organs from donors lacking these markers. This finding strongly suggests that the presence of HCV RNA in the donor is associated with transmission of HCV. After renal transplantation, elevated serum aminotransferase levels are more common in anti-HCV–positive than in anti-HCV–negative patients (median, 48% and 14%, respectively). Several studies have shown that over the long term, there are differences in patient and graft survival rates between anti-HCV–positive and anti-HCV–negative kidney transplant recipients and that the increased mortality rate is related to liver dysfunction.[253]

Transmission of HCV to heart transplant recipients has also been described, particularly in patients who underwent transplantation before 1992. The outcome of de novo hepatitis C in these patients appears to be milder than in liver transplant recipients. Although the majority of patients develop histologic and biochemical signs of chronic hepatitis, long-term survival is similar to that in uninfected controls. However, a small subset of infected heart transplant recipients will develop severe HCV-related hepatitis, typically in the form of cholestatic hepatitis, which is associated with a poor outcome.[254, 255]

Bone marrow transplant recipients have multiple risk factors for chronic liver disease, including hepatitis virus infections. The cumulative frequency of cirrhosis has been estimated to be 0.6% after 10 years and 3.8% after 20 years. HCV infection is a major cause of cirrhosis and liver-related mortality in this population.[256]

Liver Transplant Recipients

HCV infection is an important issue in liver transplantation for several reasons. First, chronic HCV infection is the most common indication for liver transplantation in the United States. HCV infection alone or in association with alcoholic liver disease is present in approximately 40% of patients who undergo liver transplantation in the United States.[257] Second, recurrence of HCV infection after liver transplantation is nearly universal because most patients are viremic at the time of transplantation and have a 15-fold increase in serum levels of HCV RNA after transplantation.[258] Third, the progression of HCV-related liver disease is signficantly faster than that observed in immunocompetent patients, and the time to develop cirrhosis is short in this population.[242] Although histologic evidence of liver injury will develop in approximately one half of the patients within the first year post-transplantation, severe graft dysfunction in the short term is infrequent. With longer follow-up (5–7 years), HCV-related graft cirrhosis will develop in a substantial proportion of patients, ranging from 8% to 30%. Furthermore, in 5% of patients, an accelerated course of liver injury, leading to rapid development of liver failure reminiscent of that previously described in HBV-infected recipients with fibrosing cholestatic hepatitis, has been observed.[202]

The accelerated natural history of recurrent hepatitis C, as compared with that described in immunocompetent patients, is present not only before the development of cirrhosis[242] but also afterward.[261] Once the patient has reached the stage of clinically compensated cirrhosis, the risk of decompensation is approximately 40% at 1 year,[261] a much higher percentage than the 4% to 6% described in immunocompetent patients.[246–248] Disease progression is highly variable, however, and likely depends on the interaction among several host, viral, and external factors.[257] Viral factors include the viral load at the time of transplantation and the infecting genotype; host-related factors include the type of immune response mounted toward the virus and the genetic background (e.g., race, HLA type); and external factors include the type and amount of immunosuppression. Other variables include the grade of activity and stage of fibrosis early after transplantation and the age of the donor. Of these variables, serum HCV RNA levels before and early after transplantation,[262] severe early acute hepatitis,[260] and strong immunosuppression[242, 260] appear to be the three variables most consistently associated with a poor outcome, but further studies are needed to confirm these conclusions. Preliminary data suggest that disease progression after transplantation for HCV-related cirrhosis has increased in recent years.[242] The reasons for this worsening outcome are under evaluation and include the increasing age of donors and the use of more potent immunosuppressive drugs with "abrupt reconstitution" of the immune response. Short-term survival is not affected by HCV recurrence. However, with continued follow-up, survival is decreased as compared with nonviral indications for transplantation.

HIV/HCV Coinfection

Because of shared transmission routes, coinfection with HCV and HIV is common. However, the efficiency of the transmission of hepatitis viruses and HIV by the parenteral or sexual route appears to differ, thus explaining the wide variability of HCV seropositivity among HIV-infected subjects. Indeed, rates of HCV seropositivity ranging from 4% to 100% have been reported, depending on the transmission category, with higher rates among injection drug users and recipients of blood transfusions than among men who have sex with men and heterosexual contacts.[263]

There is increasing evidence that the effects of HCV infection can be modified at the molecular and clinical level by coinfection with HIV. Critical to these interplays are changes in the natural history of HIV infection. Indeed, a decline in mortality has been reported in the late 1990s and early 2000s in HIV-infected patients, probably as a result of increased availability of effective antiretroviral therapy as well as the use of prophylactic therapy to prevent opportunistic infections. As a consequence, chronic hepatitis C is a growing cause of morbidity and mortality in patients who are HIV positive. Indeed, several studies have shown that HIV/HCV–coinfected patients have more severe liver injury and a worse prognosis than do patients with HCV infection alone.[263] The reasons why hepatic decompensation develops more rapidly in coinfected patients than in those with HCV infection alone are unknown. Several hypotheses have been raised: 1) HIV does not seem to be cytopathic to hepatocytes, but it can be demonstrated in Kupffer cells in patients with AIDS and could have pathologic effects on the liver by stimulating abnormal production of fibrogenic cytokines; 2) hepatic decompensation could be precipitated by AIDS-related opportunistic infections in patients who have already developed cirrhosis as a result of chronic HCV infection; 3) HIV immunosuppression enhances serum HCV RNA levels, which have been shown in some studies to be associated with more severe liver damage; and 4) distribution of HCV genotypes and HCV diversity may be different in coinfected patients compared with those infected with HCV alone.

Additional specific features of HCV infection have been proposed to occur more frequently in coinfected patients as compared with patients infected with HCV alone. These include 1) lack of sensitivity of serologic assays in diagnosing HCV infection, 2) enhancement of HCV replication, and 3) higher risk of heterosexual and perinatal transmission of HCV infection. Data to support some of these observations are stronger than others.

Data regarding the impact of HCV infection on HIV disease progression and HIV transmission are only now emerging but are conflicting. Early reports in longitudinal cohorts failed to demonstrate a detrimental effect of HCV infection on HIV disease progression. In contrast, studies that have included HIV-infected persons treated with new antiretroviral drugs have suggested that HIV-infected patients coinfected with HCV genotype 1 experience more rapid progression to AIDS and death than those infected with other genotypes.[264] Further longitudinal studies are required to confirm or refute the association between HCV infection or HCV genotype and HIV disease progression.

Common Variable Immunodeficiency

An "iatrogenic accident" has provided an opportunity to examine the natural history of infection in patients with impaired humoral immunity. Immune globulin contaminated with HCV was infused into patients with varying types of hypogammaglobulinemia.[241] The rate of transmission of HCV (as determined by detection of HCV RNA in serum) was high (85% of the recipients of the contaminated batch), and the natural history was aggressive. During a follow-up period of approximately 10 years, two patients died of liver failure, and one required liver transplantation. Liver histologic studies were abnormal in all 15 patients who underwent biopsy, with cirrhosis in six. In addition, there is anecdotal evidence that patients with common variable immunodeficiency who undergo liver transplantation for HCV infection have severe recurrent disease post-transplantation.[265] The unusually severe recurrence may be related to the combined effects of both humoral and cellular immunodeficiency. These preliminary findings suggest a central role for the humoral immune response in the pathogenesis of HCV-related liver damage.

Prevention

General Measures

Because there is no effective vaccine and no effective post-exposure prophylaxis against HCV, a major effort should be placed on counseling both HCV-infected patients and those at risk of infection.[182, 190] In addition, adequate sterilization of medical and surgical equipment is mandatory. Efforts should also be made to modify injection practices among persons involved in folk medicine, rituals, and cosmetic procedures. Persons at high risk of HCV infection, such as recipients of blood and blood product transfusions before 1990 and drug users, should be tested for anti-HCV, as should sexual partners of persons infected with HCV. HCV-infected patients should be instructed to avoid sharing razors and toothbrushes and to cover any open wounds. In addition, safe sexual practices, such as the use of latex condoms, should be encouraged in patients with multiple sexual partners. No change in sexual practices among persons involved in long-term monogamous relationships is recommended. Information regarding the risk associated with sexual transmission should be provided to these patients. Because of the low rate of vertical transmission, pregnancy is not contraindicated in HCV-infected women. No recommendations have been issued regarding the mode of delivery. Breast-feeding is not contraindicated. Finally, it is recommended that HCV-infected patients be vaccinated against HAV and HBV because of the high risk of severe liver disease if superinfection with these viruses occurs.[21–23]

Passive Immunoprophylaxis

Immune globulin (IG) has not been studied in the prevention of HCV infection since this virus was isolated in 1989. Nevertheless, there are several lines of evidence which would suggest that such measures are unlikely to be effective. First, studies from the 1970s of IG as a means of prophylaxis against post-transfusional non-A, non-B hepatitis failed to demonstrate clear benefit.[266] Second, the neutralizing immune response to HCV infection, even in healthy adults, appears to be weak, and it would seem unlikely that IG would contain sufficient neutralizing antibody to be effective. Finally, HCV has an inherently high mutational rate that would be predicted to facilitate rapid escape from immune recognition with consequent establishment of persistent infection even if the antibodies in IG were initially neutralizing. Polyclonal immunoglobulins containing anti-HCV have been shown to decrease the incidence of recurrent HCV viremia measured 1 year after liver transplantation.[267] The development of hyperimmune serum containing polyclonal immunoglobulin may be possible through the immunization of healthy adults with HCV proteins. Whether such sera will be protective in the setting of exposure to HCV remains to be determined.

Active Immunoprophylaxis

Development of a vaccine for HCV appears to be encountering the same difficulties encountered in the development of a vaccine against HIV infection. Vaccination of chimpanzees with composite proteins from the envelope regions of the virus (El/E2 fusion protein) has been demonstrated to be protective against challenge with viruses that contain homologous but not heterologous sequences.[268] The absence of natural protective immunity in chimpanzees to challenge with heterologous, and even homologous, strains of virus bodes poorly for rapid vaccine development.[175] Nevertheless, neutralizing antibodies to HCV can be elicited during natural infection and have been demonstrated to be effective at preventing viral transmission to experimental animals when used to neutralize virus in vitro.[176] Currently, there is active investigation into the development of HCV vaccines.[269]

Treatment

Goals of Therapy

The primary goal of therapy for HCV infection is to eradicate the infection early in the course of the disease to prevent progression to end-stage liver disease and eventually to HCC. However, these end points are difficult to achieve because of the long natural history of hepatitis C. Intermediate end points that have been used to assess successful therapy include normalization of serum aminotransferase levels, loss of serum HCV RNA measured by a variety of methods, and improvement in histologic findings. It is likely, although unproven, that the achievement of these end points will translate into long-term benefit from therapy, as measured by reductions in the rate of disease progression, need for liver transplantation, and rate of development of HCC and by improvement in survival. A lesser goal of therapy is to reduce the secondary spread of infection by eradicating viremia.

End Points

Normalization of serum ALT levels was the end point of therapy in early clinical trials. After the discovery of HCV, both loss of HCV RNA and normalization of serum ALT levels have been used as treatment end points. These responses are usually evaluated at the end of treatment (*end of treatment response*) and 6 months after discontinuation of treatment (*sustained response*). Sustained biochemical and virologic responses, which are often accompanied by histologic improvement, are the current standard therapeutic end points. Indeed, several studies have shown that, in patients with sustained biochemical and virologic responses, the durability of the response is greater than 95% for up to 10 years.[270] Although the effect on clinical end points is more difficult to prove, data from some studies suggest that the risk of hepatic decompensation and HCC may be reduced in patients with cirrhosis who have been treated with interferon.[248, 249] These data need confimation.

Available Drugs

Interferon-α–based regimens constitute the cornerstone of current antiviral therapies (Table 68–12). There are several types of alpha interferon available, including recombinant forms (interferon-α-2a and -α-2b and Consensus interferon) and naturally occurring forms (lymphoblastoid interferon) (see Table 68–12). Interferons are naturally occurring proteins that exert a wide array of antiviral, antiproliferative, and immunomodulatory effects. For years, interferon given as monotherapy was the standard treatment in patients with chronic hepatitis C, with modest results at best.[271] New formulations of interferon, *pegylated interferons*, have been developed recently.[272, 273] They consist of interferon bound to a molecule of polyethylene glycol of varying length, which increases the half-life of the molecule and reduces the volume of distribution, thereby allowing once-weekly dosing. These new interferons are able to sustain more uniform

Table 68–12 | **Treatments for HCV Infection**

FDA-Approved for Treatment of Previously Untreated Patients
Interferon α-2a (3 MU tiw for up to 12 mo)
Interferon α-2b (3–6 MU tiw for up to 12 mo)
Consensus interferon (9 μg tiw for 6 mo)
Lymphoblastoid interferon (3 MU tiw for 6 mo)
Interferon α-2b (3 MU tiw) plus ribavirin (1000/1200 mg/d)
Pegylated interferon α-2b (12 kD) (1.0 μg/kg per week)
Pegylated interferon α-2b (12 kD) (1.5 μg/kg per week) plus ribavirin (800 mg/d)
Experimental for Treatment of Previously Untreated Patients
Pegylated interferon α-2a (40 kD) (180 μg per week)
Pegylated interferon α-2a (40 kD) (180 μg per week) plus ribavirin (1000/1200 mg/d)
VX 497 (inosine monophosphate dehydrogenase inhibitor)
Levorin (ribavirin analogue)
Heptazyme (HCV ribozyme)

tiw, three times a week.

plasma levels, as opposed to the fluctuations observed with every-other-day dosing, and consequently enhance viral suppression. Comparison of the pharmacokinetic properties of the two pegylated interferons is shown in Table 68–13.

Ribavirin is an antiviral agent with activity against DNA and RNA viruses. It is given orally, making it an attractive alternative to interferon, which must be given by injection. In immunocompetent patients with chronic HCV infection, ribavirin improves serum ALT levels, but the effect is transient and no direct antiviral activity is observed.[274, 275] Ribavirin is generally well tolerated, although significant hemolysis is seen.[275] Because of the potential to cause a sudden fall in hemoglobin, ribavirin is contraindicated in patients with a history of myocardial infarction or cardiac arrhythmia. Because ribavirin is teratogenic, patients and partners are required to avoid pregnancy during therapy and for 6 months after cessation of treatment. Ribavirin has a long cumulative half-life and is excreted by the kidney, so that severe side effects, particularly hemolysis, can occur in patients with renal failure. Therefore, ribavirin cannot be removed by hemodialysis. Hence, ribavirin should not be administered to patients with a serum creatinine level greater than 1.5 mg/dL. Overall, in 10% to 15% of patients who receive ribavirin, there is a need for a dose reduction or even discontinuation. This percentage increases significantly when the drug is combined with interferon and continued for 12 months.

Efficacy

Several recent, large, randomized controlled trials have shown that treatment with a combination of interferon-α (3 MU three times weekly) plus ribavirin (1000–1200 mg/day) results in a higher frequency of sustained biochemical and virologic response than does treatment with interferon alone (Table 68–14),[276, 277] so that in the absence of contraindications to ribavirin, combination therapy is currently the standard. Overall, the success rate with combination therapy in previously untreated ("naive") patients is 38% to 42% and is largely dependent on genotype and pretreatment viral load (see Table 68–14). Likewise, patients who relapse after discontinuation of interferon monotherapy show a significantly higher sustained response rate if retreated with combination

Table 68–13 | **Pegylated Interferons: Pharmacokinetic Comparison with Interferon-α**

PHARMACOKINETIC PARAMETER	INTERFERON-α	PEGINTERFERON-α-2b (12 kD)	PEGINTERFERON-α-2a (40 kD)
Absorption	Rapid	Rapid	Sustained
Distribution	Wide	Wide	Blood, organs
Clearance	—	10-fold decrease (renal and hepatic)	100-fold decrease (hepatic)
Terminal elimination half-life	3–5 h	30–50 h	50–80 h
Weight-based interferon dosing	No	Yes	No
Increased levels with multiple dosing	No	Yes	Yes
Protected from degradation	No	Likely	Yes

Table 68–14 | **Results of Combination Treatment Trials for HCV Infection: Interferon α-2b Alone Versus Interferon α-2b Plus Ribavirin**

	COMBINATION THERAPY FOR 24 WK	COMBINATION THERAPY FOR 48 WK	INTERFERON THERAPY ALONE FOR 48 WK
Previously Untreated Patients			
Overall efficacy (%)	33	41	16
Genotype 1			
$> 2 \times 10^6$ copies/mL	10	27	4
$< 2 \times 10^6$ copies/mL	32	33	29
Genotypes 2 and 3			
$> 2 \times 10^6$ copies/mL	60	64	33
$< 2 \times 10^6$ copies/mL	67	64	34
Relapsers after Interferon Alone			
Overall efficacy (%)	47	–	5
Genotype 1			
$> 2 \times 10^6$ copies/mL	25	–	0
$< 2 \times 10^6$ copies/mL	40		12
Genotypes 2 and 3			
$> 2 \times 10^6$ copies/mL	65	–	3
$< 2 \times 10^6$ copies/mL	100		18

From references 276–278.

therapy than with interferon monotherapy.[278] In contrast, the efficacy in patients who are nonresponders to interferon monotherapy is low, either when using combination therapy or a second course of interferon monotherapy in higher doses for longer durations. These patients should be included in therapeutic trials whenever possible.

Factors Predictive of a Sustained Response

Factors associated with a better outcome include low serum HCV RNA levels, viral genotype other than 1, absence of cirrhosis, female gender, and age less than 40 years.[276–279] Some specifics need to be addressed regarding factors predictive of treatment response. African Americans have been shown to respond poorly to interferon monotherapy as well as to combination therapy. The negative predictive value of cirrhosis needs to be re-evaluated with the advent of the new therapies, although in general, patients with advanced fibrosis have lower response rates to all current therapies than do patients with milder liver disease.[273, 280, 281] However, the presence of clinically compensated cirrhosis should not exclude patients from antiviral therapy. In terms of pretreatment viral load, although a value of 2 million copies/mL (800,000 IU/mL) was initially considered the boundary separating patients with a low response rate from those with a high response rate, recent reanalysis has established an upper limit of 3.5 million copies/mL as more predictive of a response.[279] With interferon monotherapy, absence of a virologic response at 12 weeks was a strong predictor of end-of-treatment nonresponse, and further treatment was abandoned. This statement may not be true for combination therapy, because approximately 10% of patients with detectable HCV RNA at 12 weeks of therapy will become sustained responders if combined treatment is continued. Recent studies suggest that response to treatment can be predicted by the degree to which the serum HCV RNA level decreases or by the quasispecies genetic divergence within the first weeks of treatment.[171]

Indications and Contraindications

Theoretically, all patients with ongoing HCV infection with persistently elevated serum aminotransferase levels are potential candidates for antiviral therapy.[282] However, because 1) therapy is still imperfect in terms of efficacy and is associated with significant side effects[275, 283] and 2) the natural history of hepatitis C is benign in the majority of patients, both physicians and patients need to evaluate carefully the chances of benefit, costs, and risks before initiating therapy. Ironically, patients with the lowest likelihood of progression are precisely the ones who are most likely to respond to treatment. In contrast, those with the least likelihood of responding or with the least tolerance to side effects are often the ones with the greatest need for treatment. Nevertheless, in patients with a low chance of disease progression (immunocompetent setting, infection at age less than 40 years, female gender, no alcohol consumption, minimal histologic inflammation and fibrosis), there are as many arguments in favor of starting treatment as there are for waiting until safer and more effective treatments are available.

For some situations, there are no established guidelines regarding treatment. In particular, treatment is not recommended outside clinical trials in patients with persistently normal serum ALT levels,[284] in patients with minimal histologic abnormalities, or in those with decompensated cirrhosis.[285] Regarding the last group, interferon is particularly poorly tolerated. The rationale for initiating therapy in patients with cirrhosis is to reduce the risk of development of HCC,[248, 249] to stabilize the liver disease as a bridge to liver transplantation, and to reduce the levels of viremia because high serum levels of HCV RNA pretransplantation have been associated with a worse outcome post-transplantation.[242, 262] However, clinical data to support these reasons to treat such patients are lacking.

The decision to treat a patient younger than age 18 or older than age 60 years must also be evaluated by carefully weighing risks and benefits. Patients with HIV coinfection should be treated with combination therapy, with particular attention to the development of anemia. Preliminary data suggest that the rate of sustained response does not differ from that observed in HIV-negative patients as long as the patient is immunocompetent.[286, 287] Interferon has produced short-term improvement in the symptoms and signs of cryoglobulinemia in patients who demonstrate a virologic response, although recurrence of viremia and cryoglobulinemia is the rule when treatment is discontinued.[220] Interferon has been used successfully to treat HCV-associated membranoproliferative glomerulonephritis. There is a strong theoretical rationale for treating patients with acute HCV infection, because the majority develop persistent infection and chronic liver disease. The few studies that have addressed this issue suggest that higher rates of disease remission (39%–98%) are observed in patients treated with interferon at an early stage as compared with untreated controls (0%).[288] However, these studies have included relatively few patients and have used different doses and lengths of treatment. Even if early intervention is effective, identification of acute cases in the nontransfusion setting is difficult, and early treatment will be limited to a small number of patients. Nevertheless, early treatment of acute HCV infection appears to be warranted. Interferon is not approved for use in children with chronic hepatitis C in the United States, but response rates appear to be similar to that in adults.[289]

Treatment Choices

In previously untreated patients with documented HCV infection, persistently elevated serum aminotransferase levels, and moderate-to-severe necroinflammatory activity with portal or bridging fibrosis, the current standard treatment is either standard or pegylated interferon-α given subcutaneously combined with ribavirin orally. Long-acting (pegylated) interferons as monotherapy are less effective than interferon/ribavirin combination therapy. Pegylated interferons will likely become the standard of care in combination with ribavirin. The optimal dose of ribavirin in combination with pegylated interferon is under investigation. The results of two large prospective randomized trials of pegylated interferon plus ribavirin compared with standard interferon plus ribavirin are shown in Table 68–15.

In patients who have relapsed after a course of interferon

Table 68–15 | **Results of Combination Treatment Trials for Hepatitis C Virus (HCV) Infection with Pegylated Interferon**

PEGYLATED (12 KD) INTERFERON-α-2b PLUS RIBAVIRIN VERSUS INTERFERON-α-2b PLUS RIBAVIRIN FOR CHRONIC HCV INFECTION			
Sustained Virologic Response	**PEG 1.5 μg/kg/wk Plus Ribavirin 800 mg/d**	**PEG 0.5 μg/kg/wk Plus Ribavirin 1000/1200 mg/d**	**Interferon 3 mU Three Times a Week Plus Ribavirin 1000/1200 mg/d**
Overall	54%	47%	47%
Genotype 1	42%	34%	33%
Genotype non-1	82%	80%	79%

PEGYLATED (40 KD) INTERFERON-α-2a PLUS RIBAVIRIN VERSUS INTERFERON-α2b PLUS RIBAVIRIN VERSUS PEGYLATED (40 KD) INTERFERON-α2a PLUS PLACEBO FOR CHRONIC HCV INFECTION			
Sustained Virologic Response	**PEG 180 μg/wk Plus Ribavirin 1000/1200 mg/d**	**PEG 180 μg/wk Plus Placebo**	**Interferon 3 mU Three Times a Week Plus Ribavirin 1000/1200 mg/d**
Overall	57%	30%	45%
Genotype 1	46%	Not available	37%
Genotype non-1	76%	Not available	60%

From Manns MP, McHutchison JP, Gordon S, et al: Peginterferon alfa-2b plus ribavirin compared to interferon alfa-2b plus ribavirin for the treatment of chronic hepatitis C: 24-week treatment analysing of a multicenter multinational phase III randomized controlled trial (Abstract). Hepatology 2000;32:297A.

From Fried MW, Shiffman ML, Reddy RK, et al: Pegylated (40 kDa) interferon alfa-2a (Pegasys) in combination with ribavirin: Efficacy and safety results from a phase III, randomized, actively controlled, multicenter study (Abstract). Gastroenterology 2001;120(suppl 1):A-55.

PEG, pegylated interferon.

monotherapy, combination therapy is the treatment of choice. Alternatively, these patients can be retreated with a 12-month course of higher doses of interferon-α. The treatment of choice for patients who have relapsed after an initial course of combination therapy has yet to be established.

There are no proven treatments for nonresponders to prior treatment with interferon alone. Combination therapy administered during 12 months with either interferon-α or pegylated interferon may achieve a response in a minority.[285] Nonresponders to combination therapy should enter trials evaluating new alternative treatments.

Monitoring of Therapy

Before starting therapy, blood tests should be conducted to establish the patient's baseline status, including liver biochemical tests, complete blood cell count (CBC count), and thyroid-stimulating hormone (TSH). A pregnancy test is needed before initiating ribavirin therapy in women. Genotyping and quantitation of the serum viral level will help in selecting the best strategy. During the first month of therapy, a CBC should be done weekly because most side effects, particularly hemolytic anemia due to ribavirin, occur within this period. Approximately 10% of patients will have a fall in hemoglobin to below 10 g/dL with a mean decrease of approximately 3 g/dL. After the first month, serum ALT values and a CBC count should be obtained monthly and a TSH level obtained every 3 months. Doses of drugs should be modified according to the severity of side effects. At 3 months of treatment, a qualitative HCV RNA test is useful to determine whether treatment should be continued when interferon is used in monotherapy (see previous section). At the end of treatment and at 6 months after discontinuation of treatment, HCV RNA testing should be repeated to assess the patient's response. If a sustained response is achieved, it is recommended that HCV RNA testing be performed annually for at least 2 years after completion of therapy. A repeat liver biopsy after treatment is rarely necessary. In nonresponders or relapsers in whom no additional treatment is considered, the follow-up should be similar to that for untreated patients, with yearly check-ups and repeated liver biopsy every 3 to 5 years to assess disease progression.

The rate of withdrawal from treatment is known only from clinical trials in which an unusually high level of commitment is typical. In these settings, the withdrawal rate increases with both the duration of treatment and the use of combination therapy.[276–278] For example, therapy was stopped in 13% to 14% of patients treated with interferon monotherapy for 48 weeks compared with 19% to 21% of patients receiving combination therapy for the same duration. The withdrawal rate for combination therapy was lower when therapy was administered for only 24 weeks (8%).

Cost-Effectiveness of Hepatitis C Treatment

In a cost-effectiveness analysis of interferon in a hypothetical cohort of 25- to 35-year-old patients with HCV infection, interferon treatment (3 MU tiw for 6 months) was associated with savings in health care costs and years of life.[96] However, the underlying assumptions of this cost-effectiveness analysis have been criticized. In a second analysis, the benefit of a 6-month course of interferon in treating histologically mild disease was examined,[290] the rationale being that patients with mild disease are more likely to have a sustained benefit from treatment than are patients with advanced disease. In this model, early rather than delayed treatment with interferon led to a greater likelihood of viral eradication, improved survival, and overall reduction in health care costs.[290] However, the rate of disease progression in patients with mild disease is likely to be slow, so that it could be argued that these are the patients who are least in need of therapy. Unfortunately, our knowledge of the natural history of HCV infection, particularly in those who acquire HCV at a young age, is incomplete, making the assumptions involved in these analyses problematic. Economic analysis of combination therapy has also been reported.[291] Retreatment with standard interferon-α for 12 months was compared with combination therapy given for the same duration, and ribavirin was found to add significant cost to the treatment. The cost-effectiveness of combination therapy diminished significantly if the difference in efficacy between the combination and interferon monotherapy was less than 30%.

Algorithm for the Treatment of Patients with Chronic Hepatitis C

The National Institutes of Diabetes and Digestive and Kidney Disease (NIDDK) has proposed new treatment guidelines for the use of combination therapy in patients with chronic hepatitis C (Fig. 68–9).[292] In the algorithm proposed, the decision to treat and the duration of therapy are based mainly on HCV genotype, which should be determined before discussing side effects and possible outcomes of treatment with the patient. However, Poynard and colleagues have criticized this "simplistic approach" based on only one predictive factor and proposed an alternative approach. In an analysis of 1774 patients from the two large multicenter interferon/ribavirin studies, five independent variables were found to be associated with a sustained response: genotype 2 or 3, baseline serum HCV RNA level less than 3.5 million copies/mL, no or minimal portal fibrosis, female gender, and age of less than 40 years. After 24 weeks of combined treatment, the authors recommend discontinuation of therapy if HCV RNA remains detectable in serum. If HCV RNA is undetectable, the treatment should be continued until week 48 if the patient has fewer than four favorable variables. In contrast, treatment can be discontinued if four or more favorable variables are present.[279] The choice of standard interferon versus pegylated interferon, in combination with ribavirin, depends on review of the efficacy and side effect profiles as well as cost.

Liver Transplant Recipients

Preemptive therapy with interferon either alone or in combination with ribavirin in the early post-transplantation period has been attempted to reduce the frequency and severity of recurrent hepatitis C.[293, 294] In one study, 86 recipients were randomized within 2 weeks of liver transplantation to receive either interferon alone (n=38) or placebo (n=48) for one year.[293] Although patient and graft survival rates at 2 years did not differ between the groups and the rate of viral persistence was not affected by treatment, histologic disease recurrence was observed less frequently in interferon-treated patients (8 of 30 evaluable at 1 year) than in those who were not treated (22 of 41; P=0.01). In a second controlled trial, 24 recipients were randomized at 2 weeks post-transplantation to receive interferon or placebo for 6 months.[294] No differences in graft or patient survival rates were observed. Although neither the frequency of histologic recurrence nor its severity differed between the groups, a delay in the development of HCV hepatitis was observed among treated patients (408 days vs 193 days, P=0.05). However, the lack of effect of interferon on serum HCV RNA levels suggests that if treatment is beneficial, it is through a mechanism other than the antiviral effect of the drug. Although side effects were common in these studies, with leukopenia being the most frequently observed, the frequency of rejection was not increased by interferon therapy. Interferon in combination with ribavirin has also been evaluated in the early post-transplant period in case series, with interesting results that need confirmation in additional studies.[295]

Treatment of recurrent HCV disease with interferon or ribavirin as single agents has thus far been disappointing.[295–298] Interferon alone has failed to clear serum HCV

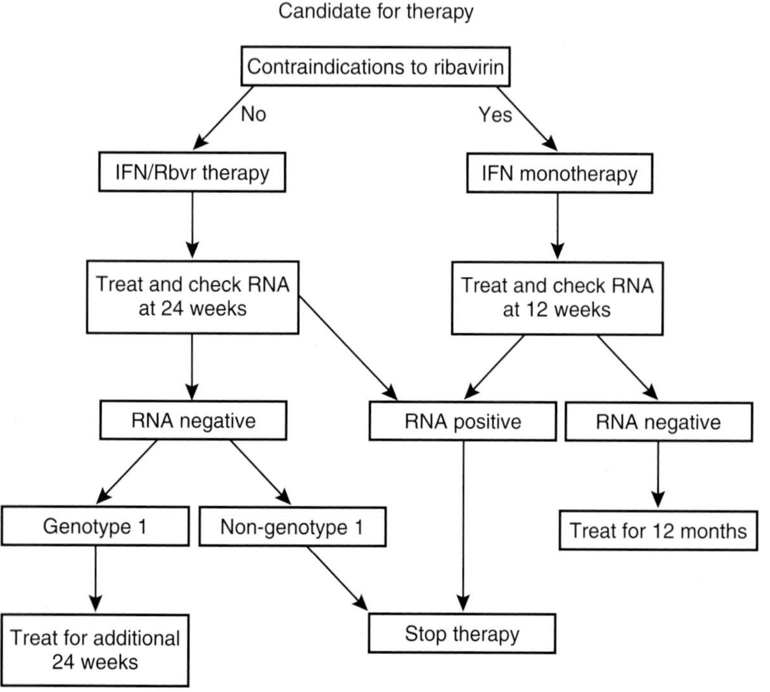

Figure 68–9. Proposed algorithm for the treatment of HCV infection. IFN, interferon; Rbvr, ribavirin; RNA, serum hepatitis C RNA level.

RNA, despite transient normalization of serum ALT values in a subset of patients treated (0%–28%), with minor or no histologic improvement. Furthermore, there has been concern about using interferon in the transplant setting, because interferon can upregulate the expression of HLA class I and II antigens and, theoretically, may increase the risk of allograft rejection. In contrast to the renal transplant experience, interferon-induced rejection appears to be rare in the setting of liver transplantation. Ribavirin monotherapy has been evaluated in liver transplant recipients, with biochemical improvement observed in many but virologic clearance seen in none.[295, 298] Initial results of combination therapy with interferon and ribavirin are encouraging.[299] In one pilot study, viral clearance was achieved in 50% of patients treated with both drugs, with reappearance of viremia in one half of these when interferon was discontinued and ribavirin was maintained as monotherapy. Despite reappearance of viremia, serum aminotransferase levels normalized and liver histologic characteristics improved in most of the patients who tolerated the treatment. Safety and tolerability were satisfactory, with reversible hemolytic anemia being the most common side effect. This pilot study of combination therapy is encouraging. Recent data from a U.S. multicenter study were less enthusiastic[300] for several reasons, including 1) low tolerability of the treatment with a significant percentage of patients requiring reduction in the dose or interruption of ribavirin because of significant side effects and 2) lower virologic response rates, with only 25% of patients clearing HCV RNA at the end of the combination treatment phase. Reasons for the somewhat discrepant results are unknown but may include differences in the timing of treatment, infecting strain, or antiviral regimens. In summary, although results with combination therapy appear promising, when used prophylactically or therapeutically, follow-up data have not been provided so far. Duration and doses are as yet unclear. The need for ribavirin maintenance following discontinuation of interferon is also unknown. Finally, whether early preemptive treatment reduces the likelihood of post-transplant HCV-related disease or just delays its occurrence is still under evaluation.

HEPATITIS D VIRUS

Virology

Classification

The *delta agent* was discovered by Rizzetto and colleagues in 1977, when liver tissue specimens from patients with chronic hepatitis B infection were found to stain for hepatitis B core antigen by immunofluorescence in nuclei even though no hepatitis B core particles were present by electron microscopy.[301] This new antigen, designated hepatitis D virus (HDV), was found only in the nuclei of hepatocytes and was present in some but not all patients with hepatitis B. HDV is a small animal virus that shares several properties with defective RNA plant viruses, including viroids, satellite viruses, and satellite RNAs (see Table 68–1). Like viroids and satellite RNAs, HDV replicates by a "rolling circle" mechanism, in which extensive intramolecular base pairing occurs and leads to the formation of an unbranched rod-like genome. Like satellite viruses, HDV encodes a protein that is required for encapsidation, and it requires the helper function of another virus (HBV).

Structure

On electron microscopy, HDV is a 36-nm particle that contains RNA and delta antigen (HDVAg). Delta antigen exists in two forms, large delta antigen (LHDAg) of 27 kDa and small delta antigen (SHDAg) of 24 kDa, which differ in length by 19 amino acids at the carboxy terminus. SHDAg supports replication, whereas LHDAg acts predominantly to suppress replication. LHDAg, together with HBsAg, is necessary for assembly of HDV. HDV RNA and HDVAg are encapsidated by envelope proteins derived from the pre-S and S antigens of HBV.

Genomic Organization

The HDV genome is a single-stranded positive-sense RNA molecule. Because of extensive intramolecular base pairing, the circular RNA of 1679 to 1683 bases collapses into an unbranched rod-like conformation under denaturing conditions. There are two highly conserved regions, each approximately 265 nucleotides in length, which are believed to be important for viral replication as well as autocleavage and ligation. Comparison of full-length RNA sequences reveals significant heterogeneity among isolates with up to 39% sequence variability.[302] A genotypic classification has been proposed.[303] Type 1 predominates in most areas of the world. Type 2 was originally discovered in Taiwan, where it is the predominant genotype and where an association with less severe disease has been proposed. Type 3 is found in South America and is associated with a more severe form of hepatitis. The relationship between genotype and clinical characteristics is under investigation.

Replication Cycle

Replication of HDV is restricted to the liver. Although replication of HDV can occur within hepatocytes in the absence of HBV, HBV is necessary for coating the HDV virions and allowing their spread from cell to cell.

The HDV genome replicates via an RNA intermediate, the anti-genome. Both genomic and anti-genomic RNA can be folded into highly base-paired, rod-shaped structures. An essential enzyme in the replication process is the host's RNA-dependent RNA polymerase. During replication, genomic strands (+), which exist predominantly as single strands, are present in excess compared with anti-genomic strands (−), which are found in double-stranded molecules hybridized to genomic RNA. During replication, the genomic, positive-strand, circular HDV RNA becomes the template for successive rounds of minus-strand synthesis. The multimeric but linear minus strand then serves as the template for plus-strand synthesis. Following autocleaving and ligation, unit-length circular genomes are produced from the multimeric precursor. The process of autocleavage is a critical part of the replication process and involves a highly conserved region within the genome. HDVAg is translated from a cytoplasmic, polyadenylated anti-genomic mRNA that is 800 base pairs in length. The mRNA for HDVAg is much less abundant than the genomic RNA, and the significance of this finding has not been fully elucidated. HDVAg appears to be essential for viral replication. Mutations in the HDVAg open reading frame that result in frameshift mutations have a significant effect (40-fold decrease) on the level of replication in transfected hepatoma cell lines. HDVAg has RNA-binding capabilities that are specific for HDV RNA.

During the replication cycle, RNA editing occurs at position 1012 of the RNA anti-genome. The editing changes A to G and results in the formation of a UAG codon, tryptophan, which allows the translation of LHDAg with the additional 19–amino-acid extension at the carboxy end. The production of LHDAg leads to suppression of RNA replication and initiates viral particle assembly. In the absence of this editing, the UAG stop codon results in the production of SHDAg. The precise mechanisms of RNA editing are under investigation.

HDV particles consist of HBsAg, HDVAg (both LHDAg and SHDAg), and HDV RNA. Assembly thus can only occur in the presence of the helper virus HBV. Cotransfection experiments indicate that HBsAg and LHDAg are essential and sufficient for the assembly of particles, whereas HDV RNA and SHDAg are not required. The precise mechanism by which HBsAg, which resides in the cytoplasm of the hepatocyte, and LHDAg, which is in the nucleus, interact to initiate viral assembly is unknown. Although HDV RNA is not required for assembly of viral particles, it is incorporated into the particles when present, probably via an interaction with LHDAg. LHDAg can interact with both genomic and anti-genomic RNA, but only genomic RNA is incorporated into viral particles. Only the major form of HBsAg is needed for particle formation, but for the HDV particles to be infectious, the large form of HBsAg (L protein, see earlier section) must be present, probably because of the necessity of L protein of HBV to interact with cell surface receptors. The M protein of HBV is not needed for infectivity of HDV.

Epidemiology

Incidence and Prevalence

There are 15 million persons infected with HDV worldwide. Areas of high prevalence include Italy, certain parts of Eastern Europe, the Amazon basin, Colombia, Venezuela, Western Asia, and some Pacific Islands. In the United States, an estimated 7500 HDV infections occur annually.[24] The prevalence of HDV infection in patients with HBV infection is low in the general population, as represented by blood donors, and highest among persons with percutaneous exposures, such as injection drug users (20%–53%) and hemophiliacs (48%–80%).[24] Intermediate rates of HDV infection are found in HBsAg-positive persons with less apparent parenteral risk factors, such as residents of institutions (0%–30%). Although HBV is required for replication of HDV, the geographic distribution of HDV does not match that of HBV precisely, suggesting that other factors, such as age of infection, may determine the prevalence of HDV within a population of HBV-infected persons. For example, infection with HDV is infrequent in populations such as the Alaskan Natives, in which HBV acquisition occurs during infancy and childhood.[24] A changing pattern of chronic hepatitis D has recently been shown in Southern Europe, with a substantial reduction in the number of new cases and severe forms of hepatitis D. Most patients currently infected with HDV represent cohorts infected years ago who have survived the immediate medical impact of hepatitis D.[304]

Transmission

The modes of transmission of HDV are similar to those of HBV infection, and percutaneous exposures are the most efficient. Intravenous drug use is among the commonest modes of HDV transmission in areas of low prevalence, such as North America. In a severe outbreak of HDV among injection drug users in New York, approximately 50% were found to be coinfected with HBV and HDV.[305] The reported frequency of HDV infection among HBsAg-positive injection drug users varies from 31% in Ireland to 91% in Taiwan. Drug abusers with HBV infection have higher histologic activity on liver biopsy and a greater likelihood of cirrhosis than HBV-infected patients with other risks for exposure (such as sexual activity), presumably because of the common occurrence of HDV coinfection in HBsAg-positive drug abusers. Injection drug users are also at risk for HIV infection. In a study of 88 HBV-infected drug users in New York, HDV and HIV infections were present in 67% and 58%, respectively.[306] Although HDV was associated with more severe liver disease, the severity of liver disease was not further aggravated by concomitant HIV infection.[306] Some HDV-infected HBV carriers, particularly those in southern Italy, where the incidence of HDV infection is high, appear to have a more benign clinical course. Hemophiliacs and other persons who receive large amounts of pooled blood products are at increased risk of acquiring HDV infection. Studies from the 1980s, before the introduction of more modern methods of viral inactivation and donor screening, indicate that the prevalence of HBV infection in hemophiliacs was 50%.[307] Routine testing of blood donors for HBsAg and anti-HBc has likely contributed to the decreased risk of HDV infection among hemophiliacs. Screening of blood donors for HDV is considered unnecessary because the frequency of HDV replication in the absence of HBsAg is very low.

Sexual transmission of HDV is less efficient than that of HBV.[24] In a prospective study of the sexual partners of drug users with HDV infection, 33% were infected with HDV, suggesting that HDV also can be transmitted sexually.[308] Stronger evidence of sexual transmission of HDV is provided by sequence analysis of three HBsAg-positive couples who were infected with HDV.[309] High sequence homology between sexual partners provided strong support for a common source of infection. However, the very low prevalence of HDV infection among HBsAg-positive homosexual men argues against sexual transmission as an important risk factor for HDV infection. Perinatal transmission of HDV is rare, and, to our knowledge, there are no documented cases of vertical transmission of HDV in the United States.[24]

Pathogenesis

There is some evidence that HDVAg and HDV RNA may be directly cytotoxic to hepatocytes. SHDAg, but not LHDAg, is directly cytotoxic to hepatocytes when expressed in large quantities.[310] However, several stably transformed cell lines that express SHDAg and LHDAg do not exhibit direct cytotoxic effects. Additionally, transgenic mice that overexpress SHDAg or LHDAg at a level similar to that seen in humans with HDV infection do not show any hepatopathicity.[310] Likewise, transgenic mice that express HDV RNA with active RNA replication show no evidence of cytopathicity. Alternatively, HDV RNA may cause cytopathicity indirectly by interfering with protein processing. There is an extensive degree of sequence homology between antigenomic HDV RNA and a structure involved in the translocation of secretory and membrane-associated proteins called 7SL RNA. The replicative intermediate of HDV may injure cells by annealing to host RNA and thereby interfere with cellular protein sorting.

The other mechanism of cell injury is immune mediated, and the presence of inflammatory cells around hepatocytes that contain HDVAg suggests that the immune response may be important in pathogenesis.[310] Several autoantibodies have been described in association with chronic HDV infection.[311, 312] The asialoglycoprotein receptor antibody, a liver-specific autoantigen, is associated with the severity of liver disease but not with the presence or absence of HDV.[312] Nonorgan-specific autoantibodies, including basal cell layer antibodies, thymic stellate epithelial cell antibodies, thymic reticular antibodies, nuclear lamin C antibodies, perithymocytic cell antibodies, and liver-kidney microsomal antibodies, also have been identified in patients with HDV infection, but the specificity of these autoantibodies for infection is controversial.[311, 312] Much attention has been focused on the relationship between HDV and liver-kidney microsomal antibody (LKM) type 3. The major LKM-3 antigen appears to be a family of uridine diphosphate-glucuronosyltransferases (UGTs), which are hepatic enzymes involved in phase II drug metabolism.[311] One study found LKM-3 antibodies in 18% of HDV-infected patients. Whether LKM-3 or the other autoantibodies described have a role in the pathogenesis of liver disease in HDV infection or merely represent secondary phenomena is not known. Autoimmunity may be one mechanism by which liver disease is propagated and may explain, in part, the differences in disease severity seen in patients with HDV and HBV coinfection compared with those with HBV infection alone.

Clinical Manifestations and Diagnosis

Acute Infection

Acute HDV infection can occur in a patient with established HBV infection (*superinfection*) or concurrently with HBV infection (*coinfection*) (see Table 68–2). The liver transplant setting has also highlighted a third pattern of infection, termed *latent HDV infection*, in which HDV infection is identified in the liver allograft before overt reinfection of the graft with HBV.[313]

Coinfection with HDV and HBV is characterized by a biphasic increase in serum aminotransferase activity, a finding that is rare in acute HBV infection alone. The time course of symptoms, biochemical changes, and detection of HBV and HDV in acute HBV/HDV coinfection are shown in Figure 68–10. In coinfection, the synthesis of HBV is transient, and expression of HDV is short-lived. Thus, the HDV infection has little impact on the natural history of HBV infection in coinfected persons, and complete clinical recovery with no chronic sequelae is the rule. Coinfected persons are more likely to have a fulminant presentation than are patients with HBV infection alone, for unclear reasons.

In superinfection with HDV, the presence of established HBV infection provides the ideal substrate for HDV, and, as a consequence, chronic progressive liver disease develops in over 90% of patients.[314] Uncommonly, HDV superinfection produces a self-limited infection followed by subsequent clearance of HDV and HBV. Fulminant hepatitis may result from HDV superinfection and is characterized by the presence of HDV markers and the absence of IgM anti-HBc in serum (see Chapter 80).

Patients who undergo liver transplantation for HDV- and HBV-related liver disease may have latent asymptomatic recurrence of HDV infection in the allograft, which only becomes clinically manifest when the graft becomes reinfected with HBV.[313]

Chronic Infection

The clinical features of chronic HDV infection are not specific and, in general, cannot be distinguished from chronic hepatitis of other causes on clinical grounds alone. However, there are certain patients in whom infection with HDV should be considered: 1) anti-HBe–positive patients with chronic hepatitis, 2) HBsAg-positive patients who experience a "flare" or unexpected rise in serum aminotransferase activity, and 3) HBsAg-positive patients with rapidly progressive disease or presentation with cirrhosis early after infection. In

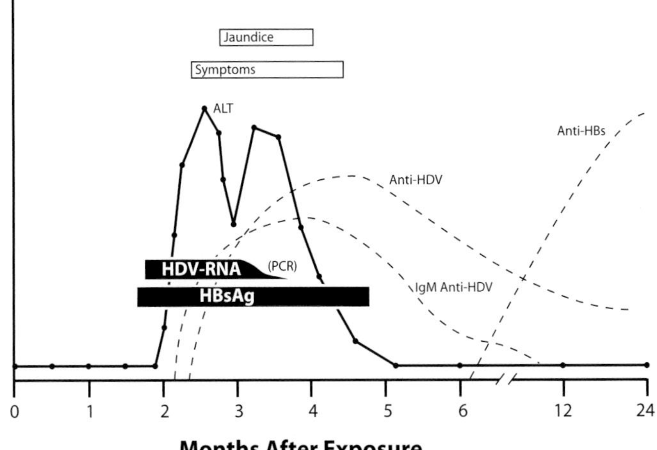

Figure 68–10. Time course of symptoms, biochemical changes, and detection of HBV and HDV in acute HBV/HDV coinfection. (ALT, alanine aminotransferase; Anti-HBs, antibody to hepatitis B surface antigen; Anti-HDV, antibody to hepatitis D virus; HBsAg, hepatitis B surface antigen; HDV, hepatitis D virus; PCR, polymerase chain reaction.)

chronic HDV infection, IgG anti-HDV and IgM anti-HDV are present in the serum, and HDVAg is demonstrable with immunohistochemical staining or in situ hybridization of the liver tissue (see later section).

Diagnosis

Both EIA and RIA for the detection of total and IgM anti-HDV are commercially available. Detection of HDV RNA is only available on a research basis but has utility in distinguishing ongoing from prior infection (see later section).[303] Measurement of total anti-HDV is not helpful for diagnosing acute HDV infection because the antibody typically becomes positive only late in the clinical course of infection. However, in the chronic setting, an IgG anti-HDV titer greater than 1 : 1000 correlates well with the presence of ongoing viral replication. IgM anti-HDV is detectable during the early phase of acute infection and therefore serves as a useful marker of acute disease. In patients with acute but self-limiting HDV infection, the IgM anti-HDV response is short-lived. In patients with chronic HDV infection, IgM anti-HDV is present early and persists in a variable titer for long periods. IgM anti-HDV is not useful in distinguishing coinfection (HBV and HDV acquired simultaneously) and superinfection (HDV acquired in a chronic HBV carrier). Rather, this distinction is made by the presence or absence of IgM anti-HBc. In acute coinfection with HDV and HBV, IgM anti-HDV and HDV RNA are present in the serum together with IgM anti-HBc, whereas in patients with superinfection, the HDV markers are present in the absence of IgM anti-HBc. Anti-HDV remains detectable if the infection is persistent, and the titer of antibody correlates with the severity of clinical disease.

Delta antigen (HDVAg) is present in serum in the late incubation period of acute infection and persists into the symptomatic phase in approximately 20% of cases. Because HDVAg is often present transiently, repeat testing may be necessary for detection. Detection of HDVAg by EIA and RIA is limited by the need to collect serum at the right time and by the availability of the assay only as a research test. In immunodeficient patients, the former limitation is less important because HDVAg is detectable at low titers for longer periods of time. During persistent infection, HDVAg may not be detectable because it is complexed with anti-HDV.

HDV RNA is an early marker of acute infection and a useful marker of HDV replication in patients with chronic infection. Using conventional hybridization techniques and either cloned DNA or strand-specific cloned RNA probes, the sensitivity is in the range of 10^4 to 10^6 molecules. In acute HDV infection, serum HDV RNA is detectable in up to 90% of cases during the symptomatic phase of the illness and becomes undetectable after clinical resolution. In chronic HDV infection, serum HDV RNA is detectable in 60% to 75% of patients.[315] There is a good correlation between detection of HDV RNA by dot hybridization, positive results for IgM anti-HDV in serum, and positive immunohistochemistry for HDVAg in liver biopsy specimens.[315] RT-PCR–based assays are more sensitive and have a lower limit of detection, as few as 10 genomic copies. Because only a few regions of the HDV genome are highly conserved among different genotypes of HDV, the efficiency of RT-PCR is dependent on the choice of primers for amplification. Sequence analysis of HDV from genetically divergent isolates is needed to determine the optimal primers for PCR-based assays.

Detection of HDVAg by immunohistochemical analysis of liver tissue is considered the gold standard for diagnosis of persistent HDV infection; however, HDVAg staining is available only in research laboratories. Moreover, this test becomes less accurate with time because HDVAg staining decreases, so that only 50% of biopsies are positive in patients with chronic HDV infection of 10 years or more.[303] Detection of HDV RNA by in situ hybridization is more sensitive than HDVAg staining.

Complications

Patients with chronic HDV infection are at risk of developing cirrhosis with portal hypertension and hepatic decompensation. When these complications occur, referral for liver transplantation is necessary. Compared with patients with HBV infection alone, the risk of reinfection of the allograft with HBV after transplantation is lower in patients with HDV coinfection (see later section).

Although HBV infection is a well-established risk factor for the development of HCC, there is a negative association between HDV infection and HCC.[316] The reason for the low frequency of HCC in patients with HDV infection is unknown. Possible explanations are that 1) HDV directly interferes with the development of HCC (tumor protective effect); 2) HDV markers in patients with HCC disappear because the time between infection and detection of cancer is longer than that for patients with HCC from other causes; or 3) HDV results in a more severe chronic hepatitis that leads to death from end-stage liver disease before HCC can develop. An understanding of the relationship between HDV infection and HCC may provide insights into the mechanisms of carcinogenesis in HBV infection.

Pathology

The histologic features of viral hepatitis caused by HDV are similar to those of hepatitis B, and in the absence of immunohistologic staining, the two diseases are indistinguishable. However, HDV infection is usually associated with significant pathology and may be more commonly associated with large numbers of acidophilic bodies or hepatocytes with acidophilic cytoplasmic degeneration, often in the absence of inflammatory cells (suggesting that the virus is directly cytopathic). A unique pathologic variant of HDV has been described in the Amazon basin in which intense microvesicular fatty change is seen with acidophilic degeneration of hepatocytes.[317]

By immunohistochemistry, HDVAg can be identified in the nuclei of hepatocytes in small amounts in the cytoplasm. In acute HDV infection superimposed on chronic HBV infection, variable degrees of nuclear HDVAg staining are seen with an approximately even distribution from one lobule to another and with suppression of HBsAg and HBcAg staining. In chronic HDV infection, HDVAg exhibits greater nuclear staining among lobules; HBcAg staining may be absent, but HBsAg is typically present.

Natural History

Acute hepatitis caused by coinfection with HDV and HBV is associated with a higher risk of severe or fulminant liver disease than is hepatitis caused by HBV alone. In one study, 34% of patients with fulminant HBV infection were anti-HDV positive, whereas only 4% of patients with nonfulminant acute HBV infection were anti-HDV positive.[306] The rate of chronicity following coinfection with HBV and HDV is equal to that of HBV infection alone. As indicated previously, superinfection with HDV is associated with a high rate of chronicity. Although HDV has been thought to hasten progression to cirrhosis and liver failure, recent studies indicate that the course may be more variable.[314] Approximately 15% of patients who are superinfected with HDV will have disease that is rapidly progressive, with cirrhosis developing within 12 months of infection. A further 15% of patients have a benign course with spontaneous remission of the histologic disease. The remaining 70% have a slowly progressive course leading to cirrhosis. The more aggressive disease is typically seen in adults with intravenous drug use as their risk factor for acquisition of infection. The slowly progressive disease course is typical of patients without overt percutaneous risk factors who reside in areas where HDV is endemic. The rate of disease progression has been positively correlated with the level of viral replication.[306] HBeAg status has been linked to the risk of developing fulminant disease. HBsAg-positive patients with anti-HBe who are superinfected with HDV usually develop chronic disease, whereas HBsAg-positive patients with HBeAg who become superinfected with HDV develop fulminant disease.[306] However, because superinfection with HDV is associated with increased conversion from HBeAg to anti-HBe, the relationship between HBeAg status and risk of fulminant disease is complex.

Prevention

HDV replication is dependent on HBV replication, and thus HBV/HDV coinfection can be prevented by either preexposure or postexposure prophylaxis for HBV (see previous section). However, HBIG and HBV vaccine are of no value in preventing superinfection, because HBV infection is already established. Prevention of HDV superinfection depends primarily on behavior modification, such as use of condoms to prevent sexual transmission and needle exchange programs to prevent transmission by intravenous drug use. The introduction of measures to prevent the spread of AIDS, the large-scale application of HBV vaccination programs, and improvements in social and hygienic conditions in endemic areas all play a role in preventing HDV transmission.

Treatment

General Approach

The management of acute HDV infection is supportive. There have been no studies of antiviral therapy in this context. The frequency of fulminant hepatic failure is greater with HDV infection than with HBV infection alone, and patients should be monitored closely for evidence of encephalopathy, coagulopathy, and other signs of liver failure. Liver transplantation is the treatment of choice for patients with fulminant or end-stage liver disease secondary to HDV. In patients with chronic HDV infection, antiviral therapy must be considered in the context of the natural history of the disease, which is severe and rapidly progressive in some patients. The only drug that has been examined in randomized controlled trials is interferon-α.[314]

Antiviral Therapy

Pilot studies suggested that patients with chronic HDV infection who receive interferon-α therapy for periods of 3 to 4 months derive some benefit, with improvement in serum aminotransferase activity and a decrease in inflammatory activity on histologic evaluation. Markers of active HDV replication (HDV RNA in serum and HDVAg in liver) decrease or disappear. Unfortunately, the beneficial effects are transitory, with return of biochemical and histologic abnormalities in association with the presence of HDV replicative activity. As a consequence, trials utilizing interferon-α for longer periods and at higher doses have been pursued with the hope of enhancing the durability of response. A total of five controlled trials have been completed, with doses of interferon varying from 3 to 9 MU three times weekly and four of five trials using treatment periods of 12 months.[215] Patients who received 9 MU three times weekly had a higher rate of response (normalization of ALT levels and loss of HDV RNA from serum) than patients treated with 3 MU three times weekly (50% vs 21%, respectively), and both treated groups had a higher rate of response than control patients (0%).[219] Treatment with 9 MU three times weekly was associated with an improvement in histologic disease, and a decrease in HDVAg in the liver was seen in responders.[318] A biochemical response was maintained in 50% of the patients, but virologic relapse occurred in all patients after interferon was discontinued.[318] Tapering the dose of interferon does not appear to prevent relapse; lowering of interferon dose from 5 MU to 3 MU three times weekly is typically associated with a breakthrough of aminotransferase activity (rise in ALT after initial normalization).[314] Interferon therapy may lead to clearance of HBV DNA and seroconversion from HBeAg to anti-HBe, but without improvement in aminotransferase activity. Whether eradication of HBV replication with persistence of HDV replication alters the rate of disease progression remains to be determined. Side effects are dose related.

Because response to treatment is associated with histologic and biochemical improvement, patients with compensated chronic HDV infection should be counseled regarding treatment. The available data indicate that treatment for 12 months is beneficial, but it is unknown whether treatment for longer periods of time would prove beneficial, particularly with regard to viral eradication. The appropriate end points of therapy remain to be determined. If HBsAg is lost, treatment can be safely stopped without risk of relapse. Loss of HDV RNA from serum and HDVAg from the liver at the end of treatment is not always predictive of a sustained response. However, if the loss of these markers of viral replication occurs in conjunction with improvement in histologic and biochemical indices, then interferon should be stopped and the patient monitored for relapse. The long-term clinical benefits of retreatment are unknown. Also unknown is when to stop therapy in patients who are not responding. With HBV and HCV, failure to respond within the first 2 to 4 months of interferon treatment is generally predictive of a lack of response by the end of treatment. With HDV, the response can take up to 10 months. Thus, to determine the response status with HDV, administration of interferon for a period of 1 year is recommended.

Predictors of response to interferon have been sought. There are no clinical, serologic, or virologic factors that are associated consistently with response or lack of response.[314] The duration of disease may be important, because impressive results have been obtained in patients who have acquired their infection via intravenous drug use (response rates of 66%–71%) and in whom the duration of infection is presumably shorter than that of patients in endemic areas in whom the infection is acquired early in life.[314] Because these studies were uncontrolled and involved small numbers of patients, verification of the association between disease duration and response is needed.

Alternative Therapeutic Agents

More efficacious therapies for HDV infection are needed. Suramin and ribavirin have been shown to have anti-HDV efficacy in primary woodchuck hepatocytes.[319] However, suramin is excessively toxic in humans. Ribavirin has been examined in two small studies, with no apparent benefit.[314] Nucleoside analogues that have been evaluated for the treatment of chronic HBV infection, such as lamivudine, may provide benefit in the management of chronic HDV infection, but data are limited. Eradication of HBV may render the HDV latent and perhaps result in eradication, if HBsAg remains undetectable in serum. This approach is analogous to administering HBIG to HDV-positive liver transplant recipients (see later section).[320]

Liver Transplantation

For patients with decompensated cirrhosis, liver transplantation is the appropriate therapy. Interferon should not be used in these patients, because further decompensation of the liver disease may be precipitated by therapy. The most important predictor of outcome after transplantation for chronic HBV infection is the pretransplant level of HBV replication. Patients who undergo liver transplantation for chronic HDV infection have lower rates of HBV infection post-transplantation than do patients with HBV infection alone, and it has been suggested that HDV has an inhibitory effect on HBV replication. After liver transplantation, the rate of HBV reinfection was 67% in patients with chronic HBV infection compared with 32% in patients with chronic HDV infection.[142] Three-year survival rates were also significantly higher in patients transplanted for HDV cirrhosis than in those transplanted for HBV cirrhosis alone, 88% versus 44%, respectively.[142] Survival in patients who undergo liver transplantation for acute HDV infection is intermediate between the survival for those with chronic HBV and chronic HDV infection (approximately 65% at 3 years).

HBIG administered perioperatively and postoperatively effectively reduces the rate of HBV reinfection after liver transplantation (see earlier section). Thus, the outcome of patients who undergo liver transplantation for end-stage HDV infection is comparable to that of patients transplanted for other indications. Liver transplantation, therefore, is the recommended therapy for patients with liver failure caused by HDV. In a longitudinal study of patients who underwent transplantation for chronic HDV infection and received long-term HBIG therapy, the rate of HBV recurrence was 10%.[320] Four virologic and clinical patterns of HBV and HDV recurrence were observed in this study: 1) HBV and HDV replication occurred together with clinical evidence of hepatitis; 2) HBV and HDV replication were evident but without substantial clinical, biochemical, or histologic effects; 3) HDVAg was present in the liver or HDV RNA was present in the serum, but patients were HBsAg negative; this pattern was generally seen during the first year post-transplantation, and in subsequent follow-up, the HDV markers were lost; and 4) HBV and HDV markers were absent in serum and liver. Administration of long-term HBIG decreases the rate of HBV reinfection and improves survival. Although data on the use of lamivudine for HBV/HDV infection in the setting of liver transplantation are limited, it seems prudent to give combination therapy with lamivudine plus HBIG, as for patients with HBV infection alone.

HEPATITIS E VIRUS

Virology

Classification

Clarification of the taxonomy of hepatitis E virus (HEV) remains unsettled to date (see Table 68–1). Based on early studies of physicochemical properties, HEV was initially grouped into the Calicivirus family. With DNA cloning of prototypic HEV and calicivirus, comparative analysis of the genomic organization revealed no significant similarities in the two genomic sequences. In fact, subsequent amino acid sequence analysis has indicated that HEV is most similar to viruses of the alpha-like supergroup of positive-strand RNA viruses, which include rubella virus and some plant furoviruses.[321]

Structure

HEV is an icosahedral, nonenveloped virus approximately 27 to 34 nm in diameter. Initial identification of the virus was made by immune electron microscopy in stool samples from infected persons.[322] Subsequent establishment of infection in cynomolgus macaques led to the cloning and sequencing of the virus.[323]

Genomic Organization

The HEV genome is a single-stranded polyadenylated RNA that is approximately 7.5 kilobases in length and consists of three ORFs (Fig. 68–11). Unlike HAV, the other enterically transmitted hepatitis virus, HEV has an RNA genome that encodes structural and nonstructural proteins through the use of discontinuous and partially overlapping ORFs. HEV ORF1 encodes nonstructural proteins, ORF2 encodes structural protein(s), and the ORF3-derived protein is of undetermined function. The HEV ORF1 polyprotein has several consensus sequences that are present in other positive-stranded RNA viruses, including an RNA-dependent RNA polymerase (located at the extreme carboxy end of the ORF1 polyprotein), an RNA helicase, a methyltransferase (at the extreme amino terminal end of the ORF1 polyprotein), and a virally encoded cysteine protease.[321, 324]

Geographically distinct isolates of HEV have been identified and are classified roughly into four distinct genotypes. Isolates from North America (genotype 3) show substantial divergence from Asian isolates (genotype 1) (Burma, China, Pakistan, and the former Soviet Union) with only 77% homology at the nucleotide level and 87% to 90% homology at the amino acid level,[324] in contrast to 94% homology at the nucleotide level and 95% homology at the amino acid levels between Asian isolates (Burma and the Soviet Union). Genotype 2 comprises a single isolate from Mexico, whereas genotype 4 comprises isolates from some parts of China and Taiwan. Individual isolates from several European countries have recently been described, but their classification remains unsettled.[325] Such analyses are useful in the investigation of evolutionary changes of HEV. Despite the presence of genetically different isolates of HEV, there appears to be only one serotype. The presence of one major cross-reactive epitope has facilitated the development of serologic assays for HEV.[324]

Epidemiology

Incidence and Prevalence

A large epidemic of waterborne viral hepatitis was reported from India in 1955 and 1956, when raw sewage from the flooding Yamuna river resulted in 30,000 cases of jaundice.[326] Although initially presumed to be caused by HAV, subsequent analysis of stored serum samples indicated that this epidemic was caused by HEV. It is now recognized that HEV is the most common cause of epidemic enterically transmitted hepatitis, and HEV is viewed as a significant health problem by the World Health Organization.

Worldwide, two geographic patterns can be differentiated: areas of HEV prevalence, in which major outbreaks and a substantial number of sporadic cases occur, and nonendemic regions, in which HEV accounts for a few cases of acute viral hepatitis, mainly among travelers to endemic regions.

Endemic disease is geographically distributed around the equatorial belt, including Central America, Africa and the Middle East, subcontinental India, Asia, and the Southeast

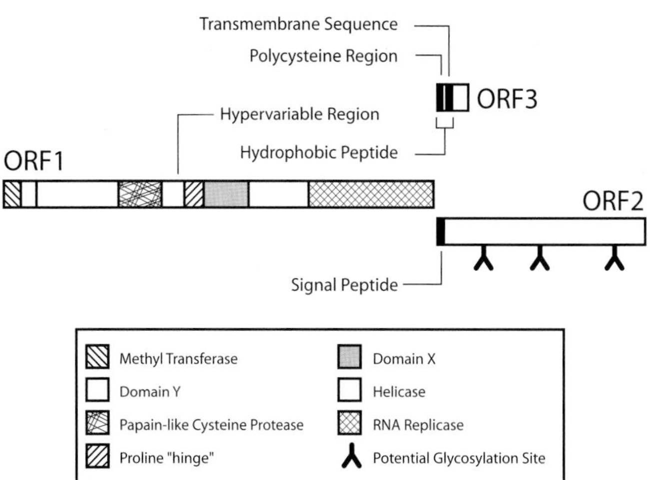

Figure 68–11. Genomic organization of HEV. ORF, open reading frame.

Pacific. In these areas, which are generally characterized by inadequate environmental sanitation, major outbreaks of HEV infection involving thousands of cases have been reported. The largest reported outbreak occurred in the Xinjiang region of China between 1986 and 1988 and involved 120,000 cases.[327] Studies of this and other large outbreaks of HEV infection have provided important information on the clinical and epidemiologic features of HEV infection. Classic features of these outbreaks[328] included a high fatality rate (0.5%–4%), mainly among pregnant women (20%), and high rate of clinically evident disease among persons 15 to 40 years of age, a pattern that contrasts with HAV infection, in which children have the highest attack rates.[328, 329] In fact, significant differences exist between the two enterically transmitted human hepatitis viruses A and E (see Table 68–2).

In endemic areas, outbreaks have a periodicity of 5 to 10 years, which in part reflects the patterns of heavy rainfall. The reservoir for HEV during interepidemic periods is unknown. Sporadic HEV infection in endemic areas may be sufficient to maintain the virus within the community during the interepidemic periods. Indeed, HEV accounts for up to 50% of the cases of acute sporadic hepatitis in adults and children in some endemic areas.[328] Another possibility is that a nonhuman HEV reservoir exists. HEV has been isolated from swine,[330] and antibodies to HEV have been detected in a number of animal species, including swine, sheep, cattle, chickens, rats, and captive monkeys.[331] Moreover, viruses recovered from swine have been identified as variants related to human HEV strains found in the same geographic regions.[332]

In nonendemic countries, cases of acute HEV infection are uncommon and occur primarily in travelers returning from endemic areas. Secondary transmission has not been reported in these cases. Acute hepatitis E without a history of travel has also been described, and the source of HEV infection in such cases has not yet been determined. Indeed, the seroprevalence of HEV antibodies (anti-HEV) in blood donors in the United States is 1% to 2%,[333, 334] a frequency that is much higher than that of acute HEV infection. The reasons for the high frequency of anti-HEV in industrialized countries, where the disease is rarely reported, are currently unknown. Potential explanations have been proposed, including serologic cross-reactivity with other agents (related but nonpathogenic human viruses or an HEV variant that causes subclinical disease), false-positive test results, or subclinical HEV infection.

Transmission

HEV is transmitted by the fecal-oral route, and the most common vehicle of transmission during epidemics is the ingestion of fecally contaminated water. Outbreaks in endemic areas occur most frequently during the rainy season, after floods and monsoons, or following recession of flood waters. These climatic conditions in conjunction with inadequate sanitation and poor personal hygiene lead to epidemics of HEV infection, primarily when the water supply becomes contaminated.

There is a low rate of clinical illness among household contacts of infected patients, an unexpected finding because the virus is transmitted by the fecal-oral route. Reported secondary attack rates in households of HEV-infected persons range from 0.7% to 2.2%, in contrast to secondary attack rates of 50% to 75% in households of HAV-infected persons.[334] The reasons for this difference may be related to instability of HEV in the environment, differences in infectious dose needed to produce infection, or a higher frequency of subclinical disease among persons secondarily infected with HEV. Available evidence suggests that nosocomial transmission of HEV occurs but is relatively inefficient.[335]

Pathogenesis

Cynomolgus macaques have provided a model to study the events surrounding hepatocyte injury in acute HEV infection. In these models, infection with HEV results in hepatitis that is very similar to that observed in humans. The earliest findings after intravenous inoculation with HEV consist of a rise in the serum ALT level (days 10–19), the appearance of HEV antigen (HEVAg) in the liver (days 14–22), and the appearance of virus in the bile,[336] indicating that the virus is replicating in the liver. Mild histologic changes in the liver are present during this time (days 12–14), but the most prominent histologic changes are seen on days 18 to 25. Serum anti-HEV becomes detectable on days 27 to 39 just before or coinciding with the ALT peak. By day 39, hepatic HEVAg is no longer detectable, but the pathologic abnormalities persist.

HEV replication in the liver is the initial event that allows early detection of HEVAg in the liver and bile. A rise in serum ALT level and presence of mild histologic injury at this time would be consistent with a direct cytopathic effect of the virus or an early immune-mediated effect. Later, hepatic HEVAg becomes undetectable, indicating that viral replication has stopped, and during this time the histologic changes are more pronounced, suggesting that the injury at this time is primarily immune mediated. The delayed appearance of anti-HEV (if true and not the result of insensitivity of antibody testing) suggests that antibody is not essential for initiating hepatocyte injury but may be important in perpetuating it. It is also possible that development of an antibody response occurs independent of hepatocyte injury. The loss of HEVAg from the liver coincident with the rise in antibody production suggests a pathogenic link between antibody production or some other immune mechanism and viral clearance.

In summary, the mechanism of cell death is not known, but early in the course of infection the mechanism may be predominantly direct cytopathicity and later predominantly immune mediated.

Clinical Manifestations and Diagnosis

Acute Infection

HEV infection is self-limited and not different from other causes of viral hepatitis. The incubation period after exposure to HEV is 15 to 60 days (average, 40 days) (see Table 68–2). Two phases of illness have been described, a *prodromal and preicteric phase* characterized by fever and malaise and an *icteric phase* characterized by jaundice, dark urine, clay-colored stools, anorexia, nausea, vomiting, and abdominal pain. Overall, malaise is present in 95% to 100% of patients, anorexia in 66% to 100%, nausea and vomiting in 20% to 100%, abdominal pain in 37% to 82%, fever in 23% to 97%, and hepatomegaly in 10% to 85%.[329] Less common symptoms include diarrhea, pruritus, arthalgias, and urticarial rash. Generally, acute HEV infection is mild and self-limited, with no chronic sequelae. Symptoms generally resolve within 6 weeks.

Fulminant hepatitis has been described in association with HEV infection (see Chapter 80). Pregnant women are at increased risk of a fulminant course. The maternal case-fatality rate increases with the term of pregnancy.[330] In the south Xinjiang epidemic, the maternal mortality rate was 1.5% for infections in the first trimester of pregnancy, 8.5% for those in the second trimester, and 21% for those in the third trimester.[327] The frequency of fetal death in utero and immediately after birth is also increased above that seen with acute viral hepatitis of other etiologies.[337, 338]

Peak serum aminotransferase levels coincide with the onset of the icteric phase and generally return to normal within 1 to 6 weeks.[339] The stools become positive for HEV RNA at the onset of the icteric phase, and HEV RNA typically persists for approximately 10 days beyond the period of icterus. Viral shedding for up to 52 days after the onset of icterus has been described.[340] HEV RNA can be detected in the serum during the preicteric phase and before the detection of virus in stool but becomes undetectable after the peak in serum aminotransferase activity.[339] The detection of HEV RNA in serum during the preicteric phase suggests that sporadic transmission of the virus may occur via the parenteral route. Because HEV RNA is not detectable in the serum during the symptomatic phase of the illness, diagnostic tests based on HEV RNA detection in serum have limited application. Additionally, the correlation between detection of HEV RNA by sensitive techniques, such as PCR, and infectivity is yet to be demonstrated. Protracted periods of viremia have been described and may be one of the mechanisms that allows the virus to survive in an endemic area between epidemics.[340]

The IgM antibody to HEV becomes detectable just before the peak ALT activity; peak antibody titers occur at approximately the same time as peak ALT levels and decline rapidly thereafter. In the majority of patients, IgM anti-HEV is undetectable 5 to 6 months after the onset of illness. IgG anti-HEV is detectable shortly after IgM anti-HEV becomes detectable, increases in titer throughout the acute and convalescent phases of infection, and remains detectable in most patients one year after acute infection.[329] The duration of the IgG anti-HEV response is unknown, but high titers have been measured up to 14 years after acute infection.[341] The duration of protective immunity is not known. However, in the short term, there appears to be protection from reinfection.[342] Acute infection diagnosed by the presence of HEV RNA in serum and stool, in the absence of a detectable antibody response, is well described[340] and may be related to the timing of the blood samples in relation to symptomatic infection, as the IgM anti-HEV response may be short lived or biphasic.[340] Alternatively, lack of an antibody response may represent a defective immune response by the host.

Diagnosis

The first assays for detection of anti-HEV used immune electron microscopy to detect HEVAg on the surface of HEV particles in stool or serum and immunohistochemistry to detect HEVAg in liver tissue.[343] Subsequently, a fluorescent antibody blocking assay was developed to identify anti-HEV reacting to HEVAg in serum, and although highly specific, this assay had a sensitivity rate of only 50% to 70% in patients with acute hepatitis during outbreaks of HEV.[344] Successful cloning and sequencing of the HEV genome led to the development of Western blot assays and EIAs that detect anti-HEV by using recombinant-expressed proteins or synthetic peptides from the immunodominant epitopes of the putative structural regions of HEV (ORF2 and ORF3).[329] Limited data are available on the comparability of the different methods of antibody detection. The serologic assays utilize different target antigens from different HEV strains and different expression systems for the production of the recombinant proteins, factors that may affect the performance characteristics of the assay. ORF2-derived antigens expressed from baculovirus in insect cells and, to a lesser extent, antigens expressed in *E. coli* have yielded the best serologic tests, whereas synthetic peptides have yielded tests that have been relatively insensitive.[345] The assays that use recombinant proteins have greater sensitivity than the fluorescent blocking assays and detect 80% to 100% of cases during outbreaks of acute hepatitis E. Assays for detecting IgG anti-HEV and IgM anti-HEV are available for distinguishing acute from past infection.

HEVAg also can be detected in liver tissue and stool using an immunofluorescent probe prepared from convalescent-phase serum aggregating HEV particles.[329]

Finally, although amplification and detection of HEV RNA from serum, liver, or stool using RT-PCR can be used to diagnose HEV infection, this methodology has been used primarily for research purposes. Quantitative assays for HEV RNA are not available.

In clinical practice, the diagnosis of acute HEV infection is usually made by exclusion. Most clinical laboratories do not have diagnostic tests for HEV. In a patient with symptoms and biochemical evidence of acute hepatitis, serologic tests for excluding acute hepatitis A (IgM anti-HAV), B (HBsAg, IgM anti-HBc), C (anti-HCV), cytomegalovirus, and Epstein-Barr virus are obtained. In nonendemic areas, suspicion of acute HEV should be heightened by a history of travel to areas endemic for HEV. In endemic areas, an outbreak may be associated with a common contaminated water source, and such information should be sought. In endemic areas, infection with HEV may be seen in association with other hepatotropic viruses (A, B, and C), and in the absence of specific anti-HEV testing, the diagnosis of acute HEV coinfection or superinfection may be missed.

Pathology

Much of the what is known about the pathology of acute HEV infection has been obtained from studies of enterically transmitted non-A, non-B hepatitis epidemics occurring in developing countries before the discovery of HEV.[329] The morphologic findings are of two main types: 1) a typical acute hepatitis picture and 2) a cholestatic variant. In the latter, prominent features include bile stasis in canaliculi, gland-like transformation of hepatocytes, and extensive proliferation of small bile ductules. There is also prominent cholestasis in the centroacinar zone. Degenerative changes in hepatocytes and focal areas of necrosis are less frequent than in the noncholestatic type. Kupffer cells that contain lipofuscin granules are prominent. Portal tracts are expanded; polymorphonuclear leukocytes are conspicuous in the portal tract infiltrates, but lymphocytes predominate. Phlebitis of portal and central veins may be seen. Intralobular infiltrates consist mainly of polymorphonuclear leukocytes and macrophages. With the noncholestatic type of HEV infection, focal hepatocyte necrosis, ballooned hepatocytes, acidophilic degeneration of hepatocytes, and acidophilic body formation are frequent. An important morphologic feature is the focal intralobular areas of hepatocyte necrosis with prominent accumulations of mononuclear macrophages and activated Kupffer cells in the presence of lymphocytes. The histologic severity of the hepatitis is variable, but in one well-documented epidemic, 78% of biopsy specimens were graded as at least moderately severe. In fatal cases, severe acute hepatitis with submassive or massive hepatocyte necrosis is observed. No chronic histologic manifestations have been described.

In acute but nonfulminant cases of HEV infection, electron microscopy reveals considerable hepatocyte polymorphism. Some hepatocytes show ballooning degeneration and vesiculation of the perinuclear envelope and rough endoplasmic reticulum, whereas other hepatocytes show shrinking and condensation of cytoplasm and cell organelles to form a web-like pattern. The bile canaliculi are dilated, and intracanalicular and intracytoplasmic bile stasis is seen. In fulminant cases of HEV infection, hepatocytes show extensive organelle damage.

Natural History

In nonfatal cases, acute hepatitis is followed by complete recovery without chronic sequelae. There appears to be protection from reinfection for a time, but the duration of this protection is unknown. Long-term serologic studies will be needed to determine the duration of protective immunity and the nature of the anamnestic response.

Prevention

General Measures

Effective prevention relies primarily on improved sanitation, because immunoprophylaxis is not currently available. Provision of a clean water source is one of the principal preventive maneuvers during an epidemic, because contaminated drinking water is the most common source of infection. Although limited studies are available, boiling water appears to inactivate HEV effectively. Travelers to endemic areas should be advised to avoid drinking water or beverages with ice from sources of unknown purity, eating uncooked shellfish, or eating uncooked and unpeeled fruits and vegetables.

Passive Immunoprophylaxis

In cynomolgus macaques, passive immunization with anti-HEV–titered convalescent-phase plasma from a previously infected animal ameliorated the clinical disease after intravenous challenge but did not prevent infection.[346]

Limited studies have evaluated the efficacy of pre- and postexposure IG prophylaxis in the prevention of acute HEV infection in humans. Administration of IG during an outbreak in India produced no statistically significant difference in disease rates.[347, 348] Titers of IgG anti-HEV in IG preparations derived from persons living in endemic areas may have been insufficient to be protective. The geometric mean titer of anti-HEV in IG from endemic areas such as India is <1 : 1000 in the general population. In contrast, the titer of anti-HEV used for passive immunization in studies with cynomolgus monkeys was 1 : 10,000.[346] Immune globulin prepared in nonendemic countries would be expected to have even lower levels of anti-HEV and hence would be of little benefit as pre-exposure prophylaxis for travelers to endemic areas.

Active Immunoprophylaxis

In cynomolgus monkeys, immunization with a 55-kDA recombinant HEV fusion protein from the second ORF of HEV provided protection against cross-challenge with live HEV.[346] Immunized animals developed IgM anti-HEV and IgG anti-HEV responses after HEV challenge, and no HEV RNA was detectable in the serum or feces in animals given two doses of vaccine. Animals that received a single dose had fecal shedding of virus, but virus was not detected in the blood. Serum ALT levels remained normal, and there was no histologic evidence of hepatitis in immunized animals.

Several recombinant HEV proteins are being evaluated as candidate vaccines in humans,[349] including trpE-C2 fusion protein (derived from ORF2) expressed in *E. coli* and baculovirus-expressed C2 protein. Further studies are needed to determine the optimal recombinant immunogen, most efficient adjuvant, and best immunization schedule. Potential applications of the vaccine include control of outbreaks and sporadic infection in endemic areas and prophylaxis of travelers in nonendemic areas.

Treatment

Supportive care is the cornerstone of therapy. Infection is usually self-limited, and no specific interventions are required. Uncommonly, fulminant hepatitis occurs and should prompt consideration of liver transplantation.

HEPATITIS G VIRUS AND THE GB AGENTS

There has long been evidence that infectious agents in addition to those discussed previously are associated with liver disease. The evidence can be briefly summarized as follows: 1) Multiple bouts of aminotransferase elevations have been observed in patients with non-A, non-B hepatitis who have been observed longitudinally. Although these bouts may be caused by fluctuations of disease in patients infected with a single agent, an alternative interpretation is that these patients are serially infected with different parenterally transmitted viruses; 2) short and long incubation periods have been observed in prospective studies of patients in whom hepatitis developed after blood transfusion, suggesting that two or more transfusion-transmitted agents are involved in this disease; 3) chronic liver disease, as well as acute liver failure, that is not explained by all known infectious, metabolic, or toxic etiologies continues to occur; and 4) cross-challenge studies in chimpanzees have failed to demonstrate cross-protection between two agents with different physicochemical properties. A chloroform-sensitive agent was subsequently demonstrated to be HCV; a chloroform-resistant agent remains to be identified.

Virology

Hepatitis G Virus

Hepatitis G virus (HGV) was identified from the plasma of a patient with community-acquired non-A, non-B hepatitis who was initially believed to have clinically significant hepatitis unrelated to HCV.[350] A cloned DNA library was constructed, the corresponding proteins were synthesized, and the clones were used to screen plasma from the original patient with immunologic methods. Immunoreactive clones were identified, and a consensus sequence was constructed from these clones as well as from clones from two other patients with non-A through E hepatitis. The original cloning source, determined to have non-A, non-B hepatitis through the Sentinel Counties Study of Viral Hepatitis, was believed to lack HCV infection (because anti-HCV was negative by EIA-1). However, subsequently, testing by EIA-2 confirmed HCV infection, making an association with clinical hepatitis problematic.

GB Agents

At approximately the same time, another parenterally acquired agent was identified by investigators at Abbott Laboratories. Infectious serum from a 35-year-old surgeon with acute hepatitis was inoculated into marmosets and passed serially through marmosets and tamarins. Representational difference analysis was used to identify and characterize further the sequence of three flaviviridae, GBV-A, GBV-B, and GBV-C. GBV-C and HGV were subsequently shown to be minor variants of the same positive-strand virus, with a length of approximately 9400 nucleotides that encode approximately 2900 amino acids.[351, 352] The deduced organization is similar to that of HCV, with structural proteins at the 5′ end and nonstructural proteins at the 3′ end of the virus. One major difference between HCV and the GB agents is that the capsid region of the latter is defective, so that a core protein does not appear to be encoded. How this defect influences the replicative capacity of this virus is unknown. In contrast to HCV, the region of the genome encoding the envelope gene or genes appears to be relatively conserved, with only minor differences among viral species. The nonstructural proteins encoded by the 3′ end of the virus include a metalloproteinase, which is likely important for processing the polyprotein; a helicase, which is important for unwinding of viral RNA during replication; and an RNA-dependent RNA polymerase, which is essential for viral replication.

Comparisons of the nucleotide sequences of HGV, the GB agents, and HCV have demonstrated that HGV and GBV-C are minor variants of the same virus (86% nucleotide and >95% amino acid sequence homology between the two). There is 44% and 28% nucleotide homology between HGV and GBV-A and GBV-B, respectively. HGV/GBV-C is clearly distinct from HCV because there is only 27% nucleotide homology between HGV/GBV-C and HCV.[353]

Human Studies

The transmissibility of HGV has been clearly demonstrated both in humans and in experimental animals. HGV viremia has persisted in three prospectively observed transfusion recipients from the National Institutes of Health.[350, 354]

Epidemiology

HGV infection is present in a substantial proportion of volunteer blood donors[350–354] and more frequently in patient groups with parenteral risk factors.[350, 354–357] Of interest, HGV viremia is no more common in volunteer blood donors with a normal aminotransferase level than in rejected blood donors with an elevated ALT level.[350, 355] This finding has two major implications. First, HGV infection is common in blood donors and is not eliminated by the exclusion of blood donors with an elevated ALT level. Second, HGV infection is equally frequent in blood donors with and without an elevated ALT level, bringing into question the association between HGV infection and clinical liver disease.

Clinical Manifestations and Diagnosis

A substantial number of clinical studies have shown that although the virus 1) is transmitted through blood transfusions,[350, 354–356] 2) is found in cases of non-A to C acute and chronic hepatitis,[350, 354–356] and 3) may persist for many years,[350, 354–356] it does not cause liver disease.[357] Further, no relationship has been found between the level of viremia and the degree of liver damage assessed both biochemically and histologically. Finally the virus has not been proven to replicate in the liver.[358] Thus, HGV does not appear to be a hepatotropic virus.

TT VIRUS

TT virus (TTV) is a new virus that was identified by representational difference analysis in the serum of a patient with non–A-G post-transfusional hepatitis in Japan in 1997.[359]

Virology

Structure and Classification

TTV is a nonenveloped, single-stranded, and circular DNA virus of negative polarity closely related to a family of animal viruses, the circoviridae, not previously associated with human disease.[360] The taxonomic place of TTV remains controversial, and it may represent a novel virus group. Neither the size nor the morphology of the virion have been determined, but some of its characteristics have been revealed through biophysical studies[361]: 1) a buoyant density ranging from 1.26 to 1.36 g/mL that does not change with detergent treatment, implying lack of a viral envelope, and 2) a genome sensitive to DNase I and Mung Bean Nuclease, implying that it is a single-stranded DNA.

Genomic Organization

The full sequence consists of approximately 3.9 kb that contain at least three overlapping ORFs. The larger ORF1 extends from nt 589 to 2898, whereas the smaller ORF2 extends from nt 107 to 712. Considerable diversity exists among several geographic isolates, and a genotyping classification has been proposed from phylogenetic analysis of different strains.[362] There are at least 16 genotypes separated by a sequence difference of greater than 30% from one another, with the highest divergence between members exceeding 50%.[363]

Epidemiology

Incidence and Prevalence

TTV has been found in 1% to 40% of healthy blood donors in different countries.[364–370] As more inclusive primers are used that encompass a broader spectrum of the heterogeneous TTV family, the prevalence of infection in healthy blood donors rises dramatically, reaching rates close to 100%.[362]

Transmission

Epidemiologic studies have demonstrated that TTV is a parenterally transmitted agent with a high prevalence of infection among hemophiliacs, intravenous drug users, and transplant recipients. Furthermore, donor-recipient linkage has been confirmed in transfused patients.[359, 365–367] In addition, TTV has been shown to be transmitted enterically, with high titers of TTV DNA recovered from feces of viremic patients.[367] In fact, the high prevalence of TTV in healthy blood donors in different countries[364, 365, 368, 369] may result from viral circulation in the community because of fecal-oral transmission.

Clinical Manifestations and Diagnosis

Clinical Manifestations

In the original study from Japan, viremia was first detected at 6 to 8 weeks postexposure and 2 weeks before the rise in serum ALT levels. Loss of viral DNA documented by PCR was associated with normalization of serum ALT levels.[359] Subsequently, several studies found high "carrier rates" in patients with various kinds of chronic liver disease and in healthy blood donors.[364–370] Clinical manifestations of TTV infection are, however, currently unknown. The virus can clearly persist for many years. As with HGV, the studies published to date do not support a causal association between TTV infection and liver disease.

Diagnosis

To date, no serologic tests have been developed for the diagnosis of TTV infection, which is based on DNA detection by virologic methods. The high diversity of the genome may have significant implications for viral detection. Indeed, PCR protocols based on different regions of the genome have yielded very different results.[363, 364]

Disease Association

TTV may persist for many years and is present in patients with different types of liver disease[364–370] but has yet to be demonstrated to cause liver disease. Thus, the clinical manifestations, natural history, and pathogenesis of disease have yet to be defined. Although TTV has been claimed to be a hepatotropic virus on the basis of the higher titers of virus detected in liver compared to serum[363] and detection of TTV in liver cells by in situ hybridization, no morphologic changes in the liver cells with a positive hybridization signal have been visualized, and the majority of TTV-infected patients do not show biochemical or histologic evidence of liver damage.

Treatment

No formal treatment studies of this virus have been performed.

SANBAN, YONBAN, TLMV, AND SEN VIRUSES

Since the discovery of TTV in Japan in 1997, several new TTV-like viruses with a relatively small DNA genome (approximately 3.5–4 kb) have been isolated in Japan and denominated Sanban, Yonban, and TLMV. These viruses are linked by common biophysical characteristics to TTV.[371, 372] They are readily transmitted by parenteral routes but also appear to be transmitted by enteric routes. The association of these agents with liver disease is uncertain. They may be responsible for clinical manifestations not restricted to the liver. Alternatively, they may be viruses, like cytomegalovirus or Epstein-barr virus, that occasionally cause mild liver disease.

At the same time, a new virus was recently discovered by Diasorin Corporation from the serum of a patient infected with HIV. Using highly degenerative primers from the prototype TTV, a new viral sequence with little homology to previously known viruses was discovered and named SEN virus for the initials of the patients in whom it was found.[373] Nucleotide sequencing has shown homology of only 50% with the prototype TTV, whereas amino acid homology is only 30%. Like TTV, SEN virus is a small, nonenveloped, single-stranded DNA virus, but unlike TTV, the SEN genome is linear.

Subsequent sequencing studies have shown that there are several variants, each differing by 15% to 50% from the others. Although these variants differ by as much as 40% to 60% from the prototype TTV strain, they are closely related to the new family of circoviridae viruses.[374] Preliminary data suggest that, as with TTV strains, this family of viruses is parenterally transmitted but rarely, if at all, causally associated with liver disease. It is possible that there are certain populations, such as persons who are immunocompromised, in which this virus does cause liver disease.

REFERENCES

1. Francki RIB, Fauquet CM, Knudson DL, Brown F: Classification of nomenclature of viruses. Fifth report of the International Committee on Taxonomy of viruses. Arch Virol Suppl 2:320, 1991.
2. Lemon S, Jansen R, Brown E: Genetic, antigenic and biological differences between strains of hepatitis A virus. Vaccine 10 Suppl 1:S40, 1992.
3. Feinstone S, Kapikian A, Purcell R: Hepatitis A: Detection by immune electron microscopy of a virus-like antigen associated with acute illness. Science 182:1026, 1973.
4. Schultheiss T, Kusov Y, Gauss-Muller V: Proteinase 3C of hepatitis A virus (HAV) cleaves the HAV polyprotein P2–P3 at all sites including VP1/2A and 2A/2B. Virology 198:275, 1994.
5. Ping L, Jansen R, Stapleton J, et al: Identification of an immunodominant antigenic site involving the capsid protein VP3 of hepatitis A virus. Proc N Acad Sci USA 85:8281, 1988.
6. Stapleton J, Lemon S: Neutralization escape mutants define a dominant immunogenic neutralization site on hepatitis A virus. J Virol 61: 491, 1987.
7. Balayan M. Natural hosts of hepatitis A virus. Vaccine 10 Suppl 1: S27, 1992.
8. Provost P, Hilleman M: Propagation of human hepatitis A virus in cell culture in vitro. Proc Soc Exp Biol Med 160:213, 1997.
9. Blank CA, Anderson DA, Beard M, Lemon SM: Infection of polarized cultures of human intestinal epithelial cells with hepatitis A virus: Vectorial release of progeny virions through apical cellular membranes. J Virol 74:6476, 2000.
10. Melnick J. History and epidemiology of hepatitis A virus. J Infect Dis 171(suppl 1):S2, 1995.
11. Manucci PM, Gdovin S, Gringeri A, et al: Transmission of hepatitis A to patients with hemophilia by factor VIII concentrates treated with organic solvent and detergent to inactivate viruses. Ann Intern Med 20:1, 1993.
12. Shapiro C, Coleman P, McQuillan G, Alter M, Margolis H: Epidemi-

ology of hepatitis A: Seroepidemiology and risk groups in the USA. Vaccine 10(suppl 1):S59, 1992.
13. Steffen R, Kane M, Shapiro C, Billo N, Schoellhorn J, van Damme P: Epidemiology and prevention of hepatitis A in travelers. JAMA 272(11):885, 1994.
14. Hofman F, Wehrle G, Berthold H, Koster D: Hepatitis A as an occupational hazard. Vaccine 10(suppl 1):S82, 1992.
15. Vallbracht A, Maier K, Stierhof Y, et al: Liver-derived cytotoxic T cells in hepatitis A virus infection. J Infect Dis 160:209, 1989.
16. Margolis H, Nainan O: Identification of virus components in circulating immune complexes isolated during hepatitis A virus infection. Hepatology 11:31, 1990.
17. Sciot R, De Vos R, De Wolf-Peeters C, Desmet V: Hepatitis A: A Kupffer cell disease? J Clin Pathol 39:1160, 1986.
18. Lednar W, Lemon S, Kirkpatrick J, Redfield R, Fields M, Kelly P: Frequency of illness associated with epidemic hepatitis A virus infections in adults. Am J Epidemiol 122:226, 1985.
19. Romero R, Lavine J: Viral hepatitis in children. Sem Liv Dis 14(3): 289, 1994.
20. Hu M, Kang L, Yao G: An outbreak of hepatitis A in Shanghai. In Bianchi L, Gerok W, Maier K, Deinhardt F (eds): Infectious Diseases of the Liver. London, Kluwer, 1990, pp 361–72.
21. Keefe EB: Is hepatitis A more severe in patients with chronic hepatitis B and other chronic liver diseases? Am J Gastroenterol 90:201, 1995.
22. Vento S, Garofano T, Renzini C, et al: Fulminant hepatitis associated with hepatitis A superinfection in patients with chronic hepatitis C. N Engl J Med 338:286, 1998.
23. Berenguer M, Wright TL: Are HCV-infected individuals candidates for hepatitis A vaccine? Lancet 351(9107):924, 1998.
24. Centers for Disease Control: Hepatitis Surveillance Report. MMWR 53:23, 1990.
25. Schiff E: Atypical clinical manifestations of hepatitis A. Vaccine 10 suppl 1:S18, 1992.
26. Glikson M, Galun E, Oren R, Tur-Kaspa R, Shouval D: Relapsing hepatitis A: Review of 14 cases and literature survey. Medicine 71:14, 1992.
27. Stewart DR, Morris TS, Purcell RH, Emerson SU: Detection of antibodies to the nonstructural 3C proteinase of hepatitis A virus. J Infect Dis 176:593, 1997.
28. Cook D, Riddell R, Chernesky M, Salena B: Relapsing hepatitis A infection with immuological sequelae. Can J Gastroenterol 3:145, 1989.
29. Vento S, Garofano T, Di Perri G, Dolci L, Concia E, Bassetti D: Identification of hepatitis A virus as a trigger for autoimmune chronic hepatitis type 1 in susceptible individuals. Lancet 337:1183, 1991.
30. Sciot R, Vandamme B, Desmet V: Cholestatic features in hepatitis A. J Hepatol 3:172, 1986.
31. Stapleton J: Passive immunization against hepatitis A. Vaccine 10(suppl 1), 1992.
32. Thorpe R, Minor P, Wood D: Hepatitits A concentration in immunoglobulin preparation. Lancet 337:497, 1991.
33. Provost P, Conti P, Giesa P, et al: Studies in chimpanzees of live attenuated hepatitis A vaccine candidates. Proc Soc Exp Biol Med 172:357, 1983.
34. Werzberger A, Mensch B, Ketter R, et al: A controlled trial of formalin-inactivated hapatitis A vaccine in healthy children N Engl J Med 327:453, 1992.
35. Innis BL, Snitbhan R, Kunasol P, et al: Protection against hepatitis A by an inactivated vaccine. JAMA 271:1328, 1994.
36. Braconier JH, Wennerholm S, Norrby SR: Comparative immunogenicity and tolerance of Vaqta and Havrix. Vaccine 17:2182, 1999.
37. Centers for Disease Control and Prevention: Prevention of hepatitis A through active of passive immunization: Recommendations of the Advisory Committee on Immunization Practices (ACIP). MMWR 48:137, 1999.
38. Green M, Cohen D, Lerman Y, et al: Depression of the immune response to an inactivated hepatitis A vaccine adminstered concomitantly with immune globulin. J Infect Dis 168:740, 1993.
39. Consensus Development Conference Panel Statement: Management of hepatitis C. Hepatology 26(suppl 1):2S, 1997.
40. Keeffe EB, Iwarson S, McMahon BJ, et al: Safety and immunogenicity of hepatitis A vaccine in patients with chronic liver disease. Hepatology 27:881, 1998.
41. Dumont JA, Barnes DS, Younossi Z, et al: Immunogenicity of hepatitis A vaccine in decompensated liver disease. Am J Gastroenterol 94: 1601, 1999.
42. Stark K, Gunther M, Neuhaus R, et al: Immunogenicity and safety of hepatitis A vaccine in liver and renaltransplant recipients. J Infect Dis 180:2014, 1999.
43. Sjogren MH: Preventing acute liver disease in patients with chronic liver disease (editorial). Hepatology 27:887, 1998.
44. Berge JJ, Drennan DP, Jacobs RJ, et al: The cost of hepatitis A infections in American adolescents and adults in 1997. Hepatology 31: 469, 2000.
45. Ananya DAS: An economic analysis of different strategies of immunization against hepatitis A virus in developed countries. Hepatology 29: 548, 1999.
46. Myers RP, Gregor JC, Marotta PJ: The cost-effectiveness of hepatitis A vaccination in patients with chronic hepatitis C. Hepatology 31:834, 2000.
47. Lurman A: Eine icterus Epidemic. Wochenschr 22:20, 1855.
48. Seeff LB, Beebe GW, Hoofnagle JH, et al: A serological follow-up of the 1942 epidemic of post-vaccination hepatitis in the United States Army. N Engl J Med 316:965, 1987.
49. Blumberg BS, Alter HJ, Visnich S: A "new" antigen in leukemia serum. JAMA 191:541, 1965.
50. Blumberg BS: Australia antigen and the biology of hepatitis B. Science 197:17, 1977.
51. Dane DS, Cameron CH, Briggs M: Virus-like particles in serum of patients with Australia antigen associated hepatitis. Lancet i:695, 1970.
52. Summers J, Mason WS: Replication of the genome of a hepatitis B-like virus by reverse transcription of an RNA intermediate. Cell 29: 403, 1982.
53. Zarski JP, Ganem D, Wright TL, Terrault NA: Hepatitis B virus. Clin Virol (in press).
54. Nowak, Thomas H: HBV kinetics. Proc Natl Acad Sci 93:4398, 1996.
55. Rossner M: Hepatitis B virus X gene product: A promiscous transcriptional activator. J Med Virol 36:101, 1992.
56. Seeger C, Baldwin B, Tennant BC: Expression of infectious woodchuck hepatitis virus in murine and avian fibroblasts. J Virol 63:4665, 1989.
57. Wang GH, Seeger C: The reverse transcriptase of hepatitis B virus acts as a protein primer for viral DNA synthesis. Cell 71:663, 1992.
58. Chang LJ, Hirsch R, Ganem D, Varmus H: Effects of insertional and point mutations on the functions of the duck hepatitis B virus polymerase. J Virol 64:5553, 1990.
59. Seeger C, Ganem D, Varmus HE: Genetic and biochemical evidence for the hepatitis B virus replication strategy. Science 232:477, 1986.
60. Simon K, Lingappa V, Ganem D: Secreted hepatitis B surface antigen polypeptides are derived from a transmembrane transporter. J Cell Biol 10:2163, 1988.
61. Alter M, Mast E: The epidemiology of viral hepatitis in the United States. Gastroenterol Clin North Am 23:437, 1994.
62. Margolis H, Alter M, Hadler S: Hepatitis B: Evolving epidemiology and implications for control. Semin Liver Dis 11:84, 1991.
63. McMahon B, Rhoades E, Heyward W, et al: A comprehensive programme to reduce the incidence of hepatitis B virus infection and its sequelae in Alaskan natives. Lancet 2:1134, 1987.
64. Alter M, Hadler S, Margolis H, et al: The changing epidemiology of hepatitis B in the United States. Need for alternative vaccination strategies. JAMA 263:1218, 1990.
65. Beasley R, Huang L: Postnatal infectivity of hepatitis B surface antigen-carrier mothers. J Infect Dis 147:185, 1983.
66. Chisari FV, Ferrari C: Hepatitis B virus immunopathogenesis. Ann Rev Imm 13:29, 1995.
67. Moriyama T, Guilhot S, Klopchin K, et al: Immunobiology and pathogenesis of hepatocellular injury in hepatitis B virus transgenic mice. Science 248:361, 1990.
68. Guidotti LG, Ishikawa T, Hobbs MV, Matzke B, Schreiber R, Chisari FV: Intracellular inactivation of the hepatitis B virus by cytotoxic T lymphocytes. Immunity 4:25, 1996.
69. Guidotti LG, Borrow P, Hobbs MV, et al: Viral cross talk: Intracellular inactivation of the hepatitis B virus during an unrelated viral infection of the liver. Proc Natl Acad Sci USA 93:4589, 1996.
70. Huang E, Wright TL, Lake JR, Combs C, Ferrell LD: Hepatitis B and C coinfections and persistent heaptitis B infections: Clinical outcome and liver pathology after transplantation. Hepatology 23:396, 1996.
71. Hunt CM, McGill JM, Allen MI, Condreay LD: Clinical relevance of hepatitis B mutations. Hepatology 31:1037, 2000.
72. Stuyver LJ, Locarnini SA, Lok A, Richman DD, Carmen WF, Dienstag JL, Schinazi RF: Nomenclature for anti-viral resistant human hepatitis B mutations in the polymerase region. Hepatology 32:751, 2001.

73. Thomas HC, Carman WF: Envelope and precore/core variants of hepatitis B virus. Gastroenterol Clin North Am 23:499, 1994.
74. Liang T, Hasegawa K, Rimon N, Wands J, Ben-Porath E: A hepatitis B virus mutant associated with an epidemic of fulminant hepatitis. N Engl J Med 324:1705, 1991.
75. Omata M, Ehata T, Yokosuka O, Hosoda K, Ohto M: Mutations in the precore region of hepatitis B virus DNA in patients with fulminant and severe hepatitis. N Engl J Med 324:1705, 1991.
76. Tong S, Liang T, Vitvitski L, Kay A, Trepo C: Evidence for a base-paired region of the hepatitis B virus pregenome encapsidation signal which influences the pattern of precore mutant abolishing HBe protein expression. J Virol 67:5651, 1993.
77. Liang T, Hasegawa K, Munoz S, et al: Hepatitis B virus precore mutation and fulminant hepatitis in the United States. A polymerase chain reaction-based assay for the detection of specific mutation. J Clin Invest 93:550, 1994.
78. Laskus T, Rakela J, Nowicki MJ, Persing DH: Hepatitis B core promotor sequence analysis in fulminant and chronic hepatitis B. Gastroenterology 109:1618, 1995.
79. Kao JH, Chen PJ, Lai MY, Chen DS: Hepatitis B genotypes correlate with clinical outcomes in patients with chronic hepatitis B. Gasteroenterology 118:554, 2000.
80. Zanetti A, Tanzi E, Manzillo G, et al: Hepatitis B variants in Europe. Lancet 2:1132, 1988.
81. McMahon G, Ehrlich P, Moustafa Z, et al: Genetic alterations in the gene encoding the major HBsAg: DNA and immunological analysis of recurrent HBsAg derived from monoclonal antibody-treated liver transplant patients. Hepatology 15:757, 1992.
82. Waters JA, Kennedy M, Voet P, et al: Loss of the common "a" determinant of hepatitis B surface antigen by a vaccine induced escape mutant. J Clin Invest 90:2543, 1992.
83. Brechot C, Thiers V, Kremsdorf D, et al: Persistent hepatitis B virus infection in subjects without hepatitis B surface antigen: Clinically significant or purely "occult"? Hepatology 34:194, 2001.
84. Cacciola I, Pollicino T, Cerenzia G, Orlando ME, Raimondo G: Occult hepatitis B virus infection in patients with chronic hepatitis C liver disease. N Engl J Med 341:22, 1999.
85. Teo EK, Ostapowicz G, Hussain M, et al: Hepatitis B infection in patients with acute liver failure in the United States. Hepatology 33: 972, 2001.
86. Paterlini P, Driss F, Nalpas B, et al: Persistence of hepatitis B and hepatitis C viral genomes in primary liver cancers from HBsAg-negative patients: A study of a low-endemic area. Hepatology 17:20, 1993.
87. Paterlini P, Poussin K, Kew M, Franco D, Brechot C: Selective accumulation of the X transcript of hepatitis B virus in patients negative for hepatitis B surface antigen with hepatocellular carcinoma. Hepatology 21:313, 1995.
88. Liang T, Blum H, Wands J: Characterization and biologic properties of a hepatitis B virus isolated from a patient without hepatitis B virus serologic markers. Hepatology 12:204, 1990.
89. Noborg U, Gusdal A, Pisa EK, Hedrum A, Lindh M: Automated quantitative analysis of hepatitis B virus DNA by using the Cobas Amplicor HBV monitor test. J Clin Microbiol 37:2793, 1999.
90. Loeb, K, Jerome K, Goddard J, Huang M, Cent A, Corey L: High throughput quantitative analysis of hepatitis B virus DNA in serum using the TaqMan fluorogenic detection system. Hepatology 32:626, 2000.
91. Chan HL, Leung NW, Lau TC, Wong ML, Sung JJ: Comparison of three different sensitive assays for hepatitis B virus DNA in monitoring of responses to antiviral therapy. J Clin Microbiol 38:3205, 2000.
92. McMahon BJ, Rhoades E, Heyward W, et al: Hepatitis B-associated polyarteritis nodosa in Alaskan eskimos: Clinical and epidemiological features and long-term follow-up. Hepatology 9:97, 1989.
93. Agnello V, Chung R, Kaplan L: A role for hepatitis C virus infection in type II cryoglobulinemia. N Engl J Med 327:1490, 1992.
94. Beasley R: Hepatitis B. The major etiology of hepatocellular carcinoma. Cancer 61:1942, 1988.
95. Scharschmidt B, Held M, Hollander H, et al: Hepatitis B in patients with HIV infection: Relationship to AIDS and patient survival. Ann Intern Med 117:837, 1992.
96. Housset C, Pol S, Carnot F, et al: Interactions between human immunodeficiency virus 1, hepatitis delta virus and hepatitis B virus infections in 260 chronic carriers of hepatitis B virus. Hepatology 15:578, 1992.
97. Hyams KC: Risks of chronicity following acute hepatitis B virus infection: A review. Clin Infect Dis 20:992, 1995.
98. Fattovich G, Brollo L, Giustina G, et al: Natural history and prognostic factors for chronic hepatitis type B. Gut 32:294, 1991.
99. Weissberg J, Andres L, Smith C, et al: Survival in chronic hepatitis B: An analysis of 379 patients. Ann Intern Med 101:613, 1984.
100. Lok A, Lai C, Wu P, Leung E, Lam T: Spontaneous hepatitis B e antigen to antibody seroconversion and reversion in Chinese patients with chronic hepatitis B virus infection. Gastroenterology 92:1839, 1987.
101. Hoofnagle J, DiBisceglie A, Waggoner J, Park Y: Interferon alfa for patients with clinically apparent cirrhosis due to chronic hepatitis B. Gastroenterology 104:1116, 1993.
102. de Franchis R, Meucci G, Vecchi M, et al: The natural history of asymptomatic hepatitis B surface antigen carriers. Ann Intern Med 118:191, 1993.
103. Stevens CE, Taylor PE, Tong MJ, et al: Yeast-recombinant hepatitis B vaccine: Efficacy with hepatitis B immune globulin in prevention of perinatal hepatitis B virus transmission. JAMA 257:2612, 1987.
104. Tong MJ, Hwang S-J: Hepatitis B virus infection in Asian Americans. Gastroenterol Clin North Am 23:569, 1994.
105. Harpaz R, McMahon BJ, Margolis HS, Shapiro CN, Havron D, Carpenter G, Bulkow LR, Wainwright RB: Elimination of new chronic hepatitis B infections: Results of the Alaska immunization program. J Infect Dis 181;413, 2000.
106. Perrillo R, Schiff E, Davis G, et al: A randomized, controlled trial of interferon alfa-2b alone and after prednisone withdrawal for the treatment of chronic hepatitis B. N Engl J Med 323:295, 1990.
107. Korenman J, Baker B, Waggoner J, Everhart J, DiBisceglie A, Hoofnagle J: Long-term remission of chronic hepatitis B after alpha-interferon therapy. Ann Intern Med 114:629, 1991.
108. Lok A, Lai C, Lau J: Interferon alfa therapy in patients with chronic hepatitis B virus infection. Effects on hepatitis B virus DNA in the liver. Gastroenterology 100:756, 1991.
109. Niederau C, Heinges T, Lange S, et al: Long-term follow-up of the HBeAg-positive patients treated with interferon alfa for chronic hepatitis B. N Engl J Med 334:1422, 1996.
110. Fattovich G, Giustina G, Realdi G, Corrocher R, Schalm SW: Long-term outcome of hepatitis B e antigen-positive patients with compensated cirrhosis treated with interferon alfa. European concerted action on Viral Hepatitis (EUROHEP). Hepatology 26:1338, 1997.
111. Malik AH, Lee WM: Chronic hepatitis B virus infection: Treatment strategies for millennium. Ann Intern Med 132:723, 2000.
112. Perrillo R, Brunt E: Hepatic histologic and immunohistochemical changes in chronic hepatitis B after prolonged clearance of hepatitis B e antigen and hepatitis B surface antigen. Ann Intern Med 115:113, 1991.
113. Wong D, Cheung A, O'Rourke K, Naylor C, Detsky A, Heathcote J: Effect of alpha-interferon treatment in patients with hepatitis B e antigen-positive chronic hepatitis B. A meta-analysis. Ann Intern Med 119:312, 1993.
114. Wong JB, Koff RS, Tine F, Pauker SG: Cost-effectiveness of interferon-alpha 2b treatment for hepatitis B e antigen-positive hepatitis B. Ann Intern Med 122:664, 1995.
115. Zoulim F, Dannaoui E, Borel C, et al: 2',3'-dideoxy-b-L-5-fluorocytidine inhibits duck hepatitis B virus reverse transcription and suppresses viral DNA synthesis in hepatocytes, both in vitro and in vivo. Antimicrob Agents Chemother 40:448, 1996.
116. Doong S, Tsai CH, Schinazi RF, Liotta DC, Cheng YC: Inhibition of the replication of hepatitis B virus in vitro by 2',3'-dideoxy-3'thiacytidine and related analogues. Proc Natl Acad Sci USA 88:8495, 1991.
117. Nowak M, Bonhoeffer S, Hill A, Boehme R, et al: Viral dynamics in hepatitis B virus infection. Proc Natl Acad Sci USA 93:4398, 1996.
118. Zoulim F, Trepo C: Drug therapy for chronic hepatitis B: Antiviral efficacy and the influence of hepatitis B virus polymerase mutations on the outcome of therapy. J Hepatol 29:151, 1998.
119. Ling R, Mutimer D, Ahmed M, et al: Selection of mutations in the hepatitis B virus polymerase during therapy of transplant recipients with lamivudine. Hepatology 24:711, 1996.
120. Chayama K, Suzuki Y, Kobayashi M, et al: Emergence and takeover of YMDD motif mutant hepatitis B virus during long-term lamivudine therapy and re-takeover by wild type after cessation of therapy. Hepatology 27:1711, 1998.
121. Allen M, Deslauriers, M, Andrews CW, et al: Identification and characterization of mutations in hepatitis B virus resistant to lamivudine. Hepatology 27:1670, 1998.
122. Dienstag JL, Schiff ER, Wright TL, et al: Lamivudine as initial treat-

ment for chronic hepatitis B infection in the United States. N Engl J Med 341:1256, 1999.
123. Lai C-L, Chien R-N, Leung NWY, et al: A one year trial of lamivudine for chronic hepatitis B. N Engl J Med 339:61, 1998.
124. Dienstag J, Schiff ER, Mitchell M, Casey DE, Gitlin N, et al: Extended lamivudine retreatment for chronic hepatitis B: Maintenance of viral suppression after discontinuation of therapy. Hepatology 30:1082, 1999.
125. Perrillo R: Factors influencing response to interferon in chronic hepatitis B: Implications for Asian and western populations. Hepatology 12: 1433, 1990.
126. Chien RN, Liaw YF, Atkins M: Pretherapy alanine transaminase level as a determinant for hepatitis B e antigen seroconversion during lamivudine therapy in patients with chronic hepatitis B. Asian Hepatitis Lamivudine Trial Group. Hepatology 30:770, 1999.
127. Liaw YF, Leung NW, Chang TT, et al: Effects of extended lamivudine therapy in Asian patients with chronic hepatitis B. Asia Hepatitis Lamivudine Study Group. Gastroenterology 119:172, 2000.
128. Tassopoulos NC, Volpes R, Pastore G, et al: Efficacy of lamivudine in patients with hepatitis B e antigen-negative hepatitis B virus DNA-positive (precore mutant) chronic hepatitis B. Lamivudine Precore Mutant Study Group. Hepatology 29:88996, 1999.
129. Villeneuve J, Condreay LD, Willems B, et al: Lamivudine treatment for decompensated cirrhosis resulting from chronic hepatitis B. Hepatology 31:207, 2000.
130. De Man, RA, Marcellin P, Habal F, et al: A randomized, placebo-controlled study to evaluate the efficacy of 12-month famciclovir treatment in patients with chronic hepatitis B e antigen-positive hepatitis B. Hepatology 32:413, 2000.
131. Tillmann H, Trautwein C, Bock T, et al: Mutational pattern of hepatitis B virus on sequential therapy with famciclovir and lamivudine in patients with hepatitis B virus reinfection occurring under HBIG immunoglobulin after liver transplantation. Hepatology 30:244, 1999.
132. Xiong X, Flores C, Yang H, et al: Mutations in hepatitis B DNA polymerase associated with resistance to lamivudine do not confer resistance to adefovir in vitro. Hepatology 28:1669, 1998.
133. Heathcote E, Jeffers L, Wright T, et al: Loss of serum HBV DNA and HBeAg and seroconversion following short-term (12 week) adefovir dipivoxil therapy in chronic hepatitis B: Two placebo controlled phase II studies [abstract]. Hepatology 38:317A, 1998.
134. Jeffers L, Heathcote E, Wright T, et al: A phase II dose-ranging, placebo-controlled trial of adefovir dipivoxil for the treatment of chronic hepatitis B virus infection [abstract]. Antiviral Res 37:A197, 1998.
135. Shaw T, Colledge D, Locarnini SA: Synergistic inhibition of in vitro hepadnaviral replication by PMEA and penciclovir or lamivudine [abstract]. Antiviral Res 34:A33, 1997.
136. Perrillo R, Schiff E, Yoshida E, et al: Adefovir dipivoxil for the treatment of lamivudine-resistant hepatitis B mutants Hepatology 32: 129, 2000.
137. Ono SK, Kato N, Shiratori Y, et al: The polymerase L528M mutation cooperates with nucleotide binding-site mutations, increasing hepatitis B virus replication and drug resistance. J Clin Invest 107:449, 2001.
138. McKenzie R, Fried M, Sallie R, et al: Hepatic failure and lactic acidosis due to fialuridine (FIAU), an investigational nucleoside analogue for chronic hepatitis B. N Engl J Med 333:1099, 1995.
139. Heathcote J, Lee S, McHutchison J, et al: A pilot study of the CY-1899 T-cell vaccine in subjects chronically infected with hepatitis B virus. Hepatology 30:531, 1999.
140. Schalm SW, Heathcote J, Cianciara J, et al: Lamivudine and alpha interferon combination treatment of patients with chronic hepatitis B infection: A randomised trial Gut 46:562, 2000.
141. Lau GK, Tsiang M, Hou J, et al: Combination therapy with lamivudine and famciclovir for chronic hepatitis B-infected Chinese patients: a viral dynamics study. Hepatology 32:394, 2000.
142. Samuel D, Muller R, Alexander G, et al: Liver transplantation in European patients with the hepatitis B surface antigen. N Engl J Med 329:1842, 1993.
143. Terrault NA, Zhou S, Combs C, et al: Prophylaxis in liver transplant recipients using a fixed dosing schedule of hepatitis B immunoglobulin. Hepatology 24:1327, 1996.
144. Markowitz JS, Martin P, Conrad AJ, et al: Prophylaxis against hepatitis B recurrence following liver transplantation using combination lamivudine and hepatitis immune globulin. Hepatology 28:585, 1998.
145. Shouval D, Samuel D: Hepatitis B immune globulin to prevent hepatitis B virus graft reinfection following liver transplantation: A concise review. Hepatology 32:1189, 2000.
146. Perrillo R, Wright T, Rakela J, et al and the lamivudine transplant group. A multi-center U.S.-Canadian trial to assess lamivudine monotherapy before and after liver transplantation for chronic hepatitis B. Hepatology 33:424, 2001.
147. Terrault NA, Zhou S, McGory RW, et al: Incidence and clinical consequences of surface and polymerase gene mutations in liver transplant recipients on hepatitis B immune globulin. Hepatology 28:555, 1998.
148. Yao FY, Bass NM: Lamivudine treatment in patients with severely decompensated cirrhosis due to replicating hepatitis B infection. J Hepatol 33:301, 2000.
149. Saab S, Kim M, Wright TL, Han SN, Busuttil RW: Successful orthotopic liver transplantation for lamivudine-resistant YMDD mutant virus. Gastroenterology 119:1382, 2000.
150. Dickson RC, Everhart JE, Lake JR, et al: Transmission of hepatitis B by transplantation of livers from donors positive for antibody to hepatitis B core antigen. Gastroenterology 113:1668, 1997.
151. Chazouilleres O, Mamish D, Kim M, et al: "Occult" hepatitis B viral infection: An important source of transmission to the liver transplant recipient. Lancet 343:142, 1994.
152. Perrillo R, Rakela J, Dienstag J, et al and the Lamivudine Transplant Group: Multicenter study of lamivudine therapy for recurrent hepatitis B after liver transplantation. Hepatology 29:1581, 1999.
153. Shimizu YK, Feinstone SM, Kohara M, Purcell RH, Yoshikura H: Hepatitis C virus: Detection of intracellular virus particles by electron microscopy. Hepatology 23:205, 1996.
154. Agnello V, Abel G, Elfahal M, Knight GB, Zhang QX: Hepatitis C virus and other flaviviridae viruses enter cells via low density lipoprotein receptor. Proc Natl Acad Sci USA 96:12766, 1999.
155. Choo Q, Richman K, Han J, et al: Genetic organization and diversity of the hepatitis C virus. Proc Natl Acad Sci USA 88:2451, 1991.
156. Agnello V, Abel G, Knight GB, Muchmore E: Detection of widespread hepatocyte infection in chronic hepatitis C. Hepatology 28:573, 1998.
157. Houghton M, Weiner A, Han J, Kuo G, Choo Q: Molecular biology of the hepatitis C viruses: Implications for diagnosis, development and control of viral disease. Hepatology 14:381, 1991.
158. Grakoui A, McCourt DW, Wychowski C, Feinstone SM: Characterization of the hepatitis C virus-encoded serine proteinase: Determination of proteinase-dependent polyprotein cleavage sites. J Virol 67:2832, 1993.
159. Kim JL, Morgenstern KA, Griffith JP, et al: Hepatitis C virus NS3 RNA helicase domain with a bound oligonucleotide: The crystal structure provides insights into the modes of unwinding. Structure 6:89, 1998.
160. Enomoto N, Sakuma I, Asahina Y, et al: Mutations in the nonstructural protein 5A gene and response to interferon in patients with chronic hepatitis C virus 1b infection. N Engl J Med 334:77, 1996.
161. Tsukiyama-Kohara K, Kohara I, Nomoto A: Internal ribosome entry site within hepatitis C virus RNA. J Virol 66:1476, 1992.
162. Tanaka T, Kato N, Cho M, Shimotohno K: A novel sequence found at the 3' terminus of hepatitis C virus genome. Biochem Biophys Res Commum 215:744, 1995.
163. Pileri P, Uematsu Y, Campagnoli S, et al: Binding of hepatitis C virus to CD81. Science 282:938, 1998.
164. Gowans EJ: Distribution of markers of hepatitis C virus infection throughout the body. Semin Liv Dis 20:85, 2000.
165. Zeuzem S, Schmidt JM, Lee JH, Ruster B, Roth WK: Effect of interferon alfa of the dynamics of hepatitis C virus turnover in vivo. Hepatology 23:366, 1996.
166. Honda M, Brown EA, Lemon SM: Stability of a stem-loop involving the initiator AUG controls the efficiency of internal initiation of translation on hepatitis C virus RNA. RNA 2:955, 1992.
167. Shimotohno K, Tanji Y, Hirowatari Y, Komoda Y, Kato N, Hijikata M: Processing of the hepatitis C virus precursor protein. J Hepatol 22: 87, 1995.
168. Bukh J, Miller R, Purcell R: Genetic heterogeneity of hepatitis C virus: Quasispecies and genotypes. Semin Liver Dis 15:41, 1995.
169. Simmonds P, Alberti A, Alter H, et al: A proposed system for the nomenclature of hepatitis C virus genotypes. Hepatology 19:1321, 1994.
170. Choo Q, Kuo G, Weiner A, Overby L, Bradley D, Houghton M: Isolation of a cDNA derived from a blood-borne non-A, non-B viral hepatitis genome. Science 244:359, 1989.

171. Farci P, Purcell RH: Clinical significance of hepatitis C virus genotypes and quasispecies. Semin Liver Dis 20:103, 2000.
172. Enomoto N, Sato C, Kurosaki M, Marumo F: Hepatitis C virus after interferon treatment has the variation in the hypervarible region of the envelope 2 gene. J Hepatol 20:252, 1994.
173. Weiner AJ, Geysen HM, Christopherson C, et al: Evidence for immune selection of hepatitis C virus (HCV) putative envelope glycoprotein variants: Potential role in chronic HCV infection. Proc Natl Acad Sci USA 89:3468, 1992.
174. Kato N, Ostsuyuma Y, Sekiya H, et al: Genetic drift in hypervariable region 1 of the viral genome in persistent hepatitis C virus infection. J Virol 68:4776, 1994.
175. Branch AD: Hepatitis C virus RNA codes for proteins and replicates: Does it also trigger the interferon response. Semin Liver Dis 20:57, 2000.
176. Yanagi M, Purcell RH, Emerson SU, Bukh J: Transcripts from a single full-length cDNA clone of hepatitis C virus are infectious when directly transfected into the liver of a chimpanzee. Proc Natl Acad Sci USA 94:8738, 1997.
177. Kolykhalov AA, Agapov EV, Blight K, et al: Transmission of hepatitis C by intrahepatic inoculation with transcribed RNA. Science 277: 570, 1997.
178. Major ME, Mihalik K, Fernandez J, et al: Long-term follow-up of chimpanzees inoculated with the first infectious clone for hepatitis C virus. J Virol 73:3317, 1999.
179. Wasley A, Alter MJ: Epidemiology of hepatitis C: Geographic differences and temporal trends. Semin Liver Dis 20:1, 2000.
180. Alter MJ, Kruszon-Moran D, Nainan OV, et al: Prevalence of hepatitis C virus infection in the United States, 1988–1994. N Engl J Med 341:556, 1999.
181. Armstrong GL, Alter MJ, McQuillan GM, Margolis HS: The past incidence of hepatitis C virus infection: Implications for the future burden of chronic liver disease in the United States. Hepatology 31: 777, 2000.
182. Anonymous: Recommendations for the prevention and control of hepatitis C virus (HCV) infection and HCV-related chronic liver disease. MMWR 47:1, 1998.
183. Donahue J, Munoz A, Ness P, et al: The declining risk of post-transfusion hepatitis C virus infection. N Engl J Med 327:369, 1992.
184. Schreiber GB, Busch MP, Kleinman SH, et al: The risk of transfusion-transmitted viral infection. N Engl J Med 334:1685, 1996.
185. Garfein RS, Vlahov D, Galai N, et al: Viral infections in short-term injection drug users: The prevalence of hepatitis C, hepatitis B, human immunodeficiency and human T-lymphotropic viruses. Am J Pub Health 86:655, 1996.
186. Kiyosawa K, Sodeyama T, Tanaka E, et al: Hepatitis C in hospital employees with needlestick injuries. Ann Intern Med 115:367, 1991.
187. Mitsui T, Iwano K, Masuko K, et al: Hepatitis C virus infection in medical personel after needlestick accident. Hepatology 166:1109, 1992.
188. Esteban JI, Gomez J, Martell M, et al: Transmission of hepatitis C by a cardiac surgeon. N Engl J Med 334:555, 1996.
189. Akahane Y, Aikawa T, Sugai Y, Tsuda F, Okamoto H, Mishiro S: Transmission of HCV between spouses. Lancet 339:10591060, 1992.
190. Lavanchy D: Hepatitis C: Public strategies. J Hepatol 31(suppl 1):146, 1999.
191. Ohto H, Terazawa S, Sasaki N, et al: Transmission of hepatitis C virus from mothers to infants. N Engl J Med 330:744, 1994.
192. Conte D, Fraquella M, Prati D, et al: Prevalence and clinical course of chronic hepatitis C virus (HCV) infection and rate of HCV vertical transmission in a cohort of 15,250 pregnant women. Hepatology 31: 751, 2000.
193. Zanetti AR, Tanzi E, Paccagnini S, et al: Mother-to-infant transmission of hepatitis C virus. Lancet 345:289, 1995.
194. Granovsky MO, Minkoff HL, Tess BH, et al: Hepatitis C virus infection in the mothers and infants cohort study. Pediatrics 102:355, 1998.
195. National Institutes of Health: Consensus development conference panel statement: Management of hepatitis C. Hepatology 26(suppl 1): 2S, 1997.
196. Conry-Contilena C, Vanraden M, Gibble J, et al: Routes of infection, viremia, and liver disease in blood donors found to have hepatitis C virus infection. N Engl J Med 334:1691, 1996.
197. Murphy EL, Bryzman SM, Glynn SA, et al: Risk factors for hepatitis C virus infection in the United States blood donors. Hepatology 31: 756, 2000.
198. Frank C, Mohamed MK, Strickland GT, et al: The role of parenteral antischistosomal therapy in the spread of hepatitis C in Egypt. Lancet 355:887, 2000.
199. Farci P, Alter HJ, Govindarajan S, et al: Lack of protective immunity against reinfection with hepatitis C virus. Science 258:135, 1992.
200. Lai ME, Mazzoleni AP, Argiolu F, et al: Hepatitis C virus in multiple episodes of acute hepatitis in polytransfused thalassemic children. Lancet 343:388, 1994.
201. Nousbaum J, Pol S, Nalpas B, et al: Hepatitis C virus type 1b (II) infection in France and Italy. Ann Intern Med 122:161, 1995.
202. Schluger L, Sheiner P, Thung S, et al: Severe recurrent cholestatic hepatitis C following orthotopic liver transplantation. Hepatology 23: 971, 1996.
203. Pol S, Thiers V, Nousbaum J, et al: The changing relative prevalence of hepatitis C virus genotypes: Evidence in hemodialyzed patients and kidney recipients. Gastroenterology 108:581, 1995.
204. Mahaney K, Tedeschi V, Maertens G, et al: Genotypic analysis of hepatitis C virus in American patients. Hepatology 20:1405, 1994.
205. Lopez-Labrador FX, Ampurdanes S, Forns X, et al: Hepatitis C virus (HCV) genotypes in Spanish patients with chronic HCV infection: Relationship between HCV genotype 1b, cirrhosis and hepatocellular carcinoma. J Hepatol 27:959, 1997.
206. Rehermann B: Interactions between the hepatitis C virus and the immune system. Semin Liver Dis 20:127, 2000.
207. He XS, Rehermann B, López-Labrador FX, et al: Quantitative analysis of hepatitis C virus-specific CD8(+) T cells in peripheral blood and liver using peptide-MHC tetramers. Proc Natl Acad Sci USA 96:5692, 1999.
208. Cooper S, Erickson AL, Adams EJ, et al: Analysis of a successful immune response against hepatitis C virus. Immunity 10:439, 1999.
209. Lechner F, Wong DK, Dunbar PR, et al: Analysis of successful immune responses in persons infected with hepatitis C virus. J Exp Med 191:1499, 2000.
210. Gruner NH, Gerlach TJ, Jung MC, et al: Association of hepatitis C virus-specific CD8+ T cells with viral clearance in acute hepatitis C. J Infect Dis 181:1528, 2000.
211. Cramp ME, Carucci P, Rossol S, et al: Hepatitis C virus (HCV) specific immune responses in anti-HCV positive patients without hepatitis C viraemia. Gut 44:424, 1999.
212. Takaki A, Wiese M, Maertens G, et al: Cellular immune responses persist and humoral responses decrease two decades after recovery from a single-source outbreak of hepatitis C. Nat Med 6:578, 2000.
213. Gerlach JT, Diepolder HM, Jung MC, et al: Recurrence of hepatitis C virus after loss of virus-specific CD4(+) T-cell response in acute hepatitis C. Gastroenterology 117:933, 1999.
214. García-Monzón C, Sánchez-Madrid F, García-Buey L, García-Arroyo A, García-Sánchez A, Moreno-Otero R: Vascular adhesion molecule expression in viral chronic hepatitis: Evidence of neoangiogenesis in portal tracts. Gastroenterology 108:231, 1999.
215. Guidotti LG, Rochford R, Chung J, Shapiro M, Purcell R, Chisari FV: Viral clearance without destruction of infected cells during acute HBV infection. Science 284:825, 1999.
216. Forns X, Thimme R, Govindarajan S, et al: Hepatitis C virus lacking the hypervariable region 1 of the second envelope protein is infectious and causes acute resolving or persistent infection in chimpanzees. Proc Natl Acad Sci USA 97:13318, 2000.
217. Asti M, Martinetti M, Zavaglia C, Cuccia MC, Gusberti L, Tinelli C, et al: Human leukocyte antigen class II and III alleles and severity of hepatitis C virus-related chronic liver disease. Hepatology 29:1271, 1999.
218. Alter HJ, Seeff LB: Recovery, persistence and sequelae in hepatitis C virus infection: A perspective on long-term outcome. Sem Liver Dis 20:17, 2001.
219. Zignego AL, Brechot C: Extrahepatic manifestations of HCV infection: Facts and controversies. J Hepatol 31:369, 1999.
220. Misiani R, Bellavita P, Fenili D, et al: Interferon alfa-2a therapy in cryoglobulinemia associated with hepatitis C virus. N Engl J Med 330:751, 1994.
221. Johnson RJ, Gretch GR, Yamabe H, et al: Membranoproliferative glomerulonephritis associated with hepatitis C virus infection. N Engl J Med 328:465, 1993.
222. Morishima C, Gretch DR: Clinical use of hepatitis C virus tests for diagnosis and monitoring during therapy. Clin Liver Dis 3:717, 1999.
223. Pawlotsky JM, Lonjon I, Hezode C, et al: What strategy should be used for diagnosis of hepatitis C virus infection in clinical laboratories. Hepatology 27:1700, 1999.

224. Lunel F, Cresta P, Vitour D, et al: Comparative evaluation of hepatitis C virus RNA quantitation by branched DNA, NASBA and Monitor assays. Hepatology 29:528, 1999.
225. Pawlotsky JM, Bouvier-Alias M, Hezode C, et al: Standardization of hepatitis C virus RNA quantification. Hepatology 32:654, 2000.
226. Saldanha J, Lelie N, Heath A: Establishment of the first international standard for nucleic acid amplification technology (NAT) assays for HCV RNA. Vox Sang 76:149, 1999.
227. Martinot-Peignoux M, Boyer N, Le Breton V, et al: A new step toward standardization of serum hepatitis C virus-RNA quantification in patients with chronic hepatitis C. Hepatology 31:726, 1999.
228. Lau J, Mizokami M, Kolberg J, et al: Application of six hepatitis C virus genotyping systems to sera from chronic hepatitis C patients in the United States. J Infect Dis 171:281, 1995.
229. Lok A, Chien D, Choo Q, et al: Antibody response to core, envelope and nonstructural hepattitis C virus antigens: Comparison of immunocompetent and immunosuppressed patients. Hepatology 18:497, 1993.
230. Marcellin P, Martinot-Peignoux M, Elias A, et al: Hepatitis C virus (HCV) viremia in human immunodeficiency virus-seronegative and seropositive patients with indeterminate HCV recombinant immunoblot assay. J Infect Dis 170:433, 1994.
231. Goodman ZD, Ishak KG: Histopathology of hepatitis C virus infection. Semin Liver Dis 15:70, 1995.
232. Mathurin P, Moussalli J, Cadranel JF, et al: Slow progression rate of fibrosis in hepatitis C virus patients with persistently normal alanine aminotransferase activity. Hepatology 27:868, 1998.
233. Kiyosawa K, Sodeyama T, Tanaka E, et al: Interrelationship of blood transfusion, non-A, non-B hepatitis and hepatocellular carcinoma: Analysis by detection of antibody to hepatitis C virus. Hepatology 12: 671, 1990.
234. Tong MJ, El-Farra NS, Reikes AR, Co RL: Clinical outcomes after transfusion-associated hepatitis C infection. N Engl J Med 332:1463, 1995.
235. Seeff L, Buskell-Bales, Wright EC, et al: Long-term mortality after transfusion-associated non-A, non-B (NANB) hepatitis. N Engl J Med 327:1906, 1992.
236. Kenny-Walsh E for the Irish Hepatology Research Group: Clinical outcomes after hepatitis infection from contaminated antiglobulin. N Engl J Med 340:1228, 1999.
237. Muller R: The natural history of hepatitis C: Clinical experiences. J Hepatol 24(suppl):52, 1996.
238. Poynard T, Bedossa P, Opolon P, for the OBSVIRC, METAVIR, CLINIVIR and DOSVIRC groups: Natural history of liver fibrosis progression in patients with chronic hepatitis C. Lancet 349:825, 1997.
239. Seef LB, Miller RN, Rabkin CS, et al: 45-year follow-up of hepatitis C virus infection in healthy young adults. Ann Intern Med 132:105, 2000.
240. Vogt M, Lang T, Frosner G, et al: Prevalence and clinical outcomes of hepatitis C infection in children who underwent cardiac surgery before the implementation of blood-donor screening. N Engl J Med 341:866, 1999.
241. Bjoro K, Froland SS, Yun Z, et al: Hepatitis C infection in patients with primary hypogammaglobulinemia after treatment with contaminated immune globulin. N Engl J Med 331:1607, 1994.
242. Berenguer M, Ferrell L, Watson J, et al: HCV-related fibrosis progression following liver transplantation: Increase in recent years. J Hepatol 32:673, 2000.
243. Benhamou Y, Bochet M, Di Martino V, et al: Liver fibrosis progression in human immunodeficiency virus and hepatitis C virus coinfected patients. The Multivirc Group. Hepatology 30:1054, 1999.
244. Gordon SC, Eloway RS, Long JC, et al: The pathology of hepatitis C as a function of mode of transmission. Blood transfusion vs intravenous drug use. Hepatology 18:1338, 1993.
245. Roudot-Thoraval F, Bastie A, Pawlotsky JM, et al: Epidemiological factors affecting the severity of hepatitis C-virus related liver disease: A French survey of 6,664 patients. Hepatology 26:485, 1997.
246. Hu K-Q, Tong MJ: The long-term outcomes of patients with compensated hepatitis C virus related cirrhosis and history of parenteral exposure in the United States. Hepatology 29:1311, 1999.
247. Fattovitch G, Giustina G, Degos F, et al: Morbidity and mortality in compensated cirrhosis type C: A retrospective follow-up study of 384 patients. Gastroenterology 112:463, 1997.
248. Serfarty L, Aumaître H, Chazouillères O, et al: Determinants of outcome of compensated hepatitis C virus-related cirrhosis. Hepatology 27:1435, 1998.
249. International Interferon-α Hepatocellular Carcinoma Study Group: Effect of interferon-α on progression of cirrhosis to hepatocellular carcinoma: A retrospective cohort study. Lancet 351:1535, 1998.
250. Marcellin P: Hepatitis C: The clinical spectrum of the disease. J Hepatol 31(suppl.1):9, 1999.
251. Chan T, Lok A, Cheng I, Chan R: Prevalence of hepatitis C virus infection in hemodialysis patients: A longitudinal study comparing the results of RNA and antibody assays. Hepatology 17:5, 1993.
252. Pereira B, Wright T, Schmid C, et al: Screening and confirmatory testing of cadaver organ donors for hepatitis C virus infection: A US national collaborative study. Kidney Int 46:886, 1994.
253. Hanafusa T, Ichikawa Y, Kishikawa H, et al: Retrospective study on the impact of hepatitis C virus infection on kidney transplant patients over 20 years. Transplantation 66:471, 1998.
254. Lunel F, Cadranel JF, Rosenheim M, et al: Hepatitis virus infections in heart transplant recipients: Epidemiology, natural history, characteristics, and impact on survival. Gastroenterology 119:1064, 2000.
255. Ong JP, Barnes DS, Younossi ZM, et al: Outcome of the novo hepatitis C virus infection in heart transplant recipients. Hepatology 30:1293, 1999.
256. Strasser SI, Sullivan KM, Myerson D, et al: Cirrhosis of the liver in long-term marrow transplant survivors. Blood 93:3259, 1999.
257. Berenguer M, Wright TL: Hepatitis C and liver transplantation. Gut 45:159, 1999.
258. Chazouilleres O, Kim M, Combs C, et al: Quantitation of hepatitis C virus RNA in liver transplant recipients. Gastroenterology 106:994, 1994.
259. Gane EJ, Portmann BC, Naoumov N, et al: Long-term outcome of hepatitis C infection after liver transplantation. N Engl J Med 334:815, 1996.
260. Prieto M, Berenguer M, Rayón M, et al: High incidence of allograft cirrhosis in hepatitis C virus genotype 1b infection following transplantation: Relationship with rejection episodes. Hepatology 29:250, 1999.
261. Berenguer M, Lopez-Labrador FX, Wright TL: Hepatitis C and liver transplantation. J Hepatol 35:666, 2001.
262. Charlton M, Seaberg E, Wiesner R, et al: Predictors of patient and graft survival following liver transplantation for hepatitis C. Hepatology 28:823, 1998.
263. Berenguer M, Wright TL: Hepatitis C infection. In Sande M, Volberding P (eds): Medical Management of AIDS. Philadelphia, WB Saunders, 2000.
264. Sabin C, Telfer P, Philips AN, et al: The association between hepatitis C virus genotype and human immunodeficiency virus disease progression in a cohort of hemophilic men. J Infect Dis 175:164, 1997.
265. Smith M, Webster D, Dhillon A, et al: Orthotopic liver transplantation for chronic hepatitis in two patients with common variable immunodeficiency. Gastroenterology 108:879, 1995.
266. Seeff LB, Zimmerman HJ, Wright EC, et al: A randomized, double-blind controlled trial of the efficacy of immune serum globulin for the prevention of post-transfusion hepatitis: A Veterans Administration Cooperative Study. Gastroenterology 72:111, 1977.
267. Feray C, Gigou M, Samuel D, et al: Incidence of hepatitis C in patients receiving different preparations of hepatitis B immunoglobulins after liver transplantation. Ann Intern Med 128:810, 1998.
268. Choo Q, Quo G, Ralston R: Vaccination of chimpanzees against infection by the hepatitis C virus. Proc Natl Acad Sci U S A 91:1294, 1994.
269. Lechmann M, Liang TJ: Vaccine development for hepatitis C. Semin Liver Dis 20:211, 2000.
270. Marcellin P, Boyer N, Gervais A, et al: Long-term histologic improvement and loss of detectable intrahepatic HCV RNA in patients with chronic hepatitis C and sustained response to interferon-alfa therapy. Ann Intern Med 127:875, 1997.
271. Poynard T, Bedossa P, Chevallier M, et al: A comparison of three α-2b interferon regimes for long term treatment of chronic non-A non-B hepatitis. N Engl J Med 332:1457, 1995.
272. Zeuzem S, Feinman V, Rasenack J, et al: Peginterferon alfa-2a in patients with chronic hepatitis C. N Engl J Med 343:1666, 2000.
273. Heathcote J, Shiffman M, Cooksley G, et al: Peginterferon alfa-2a in patients with chronic hepatitis C and cirrhosis. N Engl J Med 343: 1673, 2000.
274. DiBisceglie A, Conjeevaram H, Fried M, et al: Ribavirin as therapy for chronic hepatitis C. Ann Intern Med 123:897, 1995.
275. Bodenheimer HC Jr, Lindsay KL, Davis GL, et al: Tolerance and

efficacy of oral ribavirin treatment for chronic hepatitis C: A multicenter trial. Hepatology 26:473, 1997.
276. McHutchinson JG, Gordon SC, Schiff ER, et al: Interferon alfa-2b alone or in combination with ribavirin as initial treatment for chronic hepatitis C. N Engl J Med 339:1485, 1998.
277. Poynard T, Marcellin P, Lee SS, et al: Randomized trial of interferon alfa-2b plus ribavirin for 48 weeks or for 24 weeks verus interferon alfa-2b plus placebo for 48 weeks for treatment of chronic infection with hepatitis C virus. Lancet 352:1426, 1998.
278. Davis GL, Esteban-Mur R, Rustgi V, et al: Interferon alfa-2b alone or in combination with ribavirin for the treatment of relapse of chronic hepatitis C. N Engl J Med 339:1493, 1998.
279. Poynard T, McHutchinson J, Goodman Z, Ling M, Albrecht J: Is an "a la carte" combination interferon alfa-2b plus ribavirin regimen possible for the first line treatment in patietns with chronic hepatitis C? Hepatology 31:211, 2000.
280. Valla DC, Chevallier M, Marcelin P, et al: Treatment of hepatitis C virus-related cirrhosis: A randomized controlled trial of interferon alfa-2b versus no treatment. Hepatology 29:1870, 1999.
281. Everson G, Jensen DM, Craig JR, et al: Efficacy of interferon treatment for patients with chronic hepatitis C: Comparison of response in cirrhotics, fibrotics or nonfibrotics. Hepatology 30:271, 1999.
282. Consensus statement: EASL international consensus conference on hepatitis C. Paris, 26–28 February 1999. J Hepatol 30:956, 1999.
283. Duscheiko G: Side-effects of alpha-interferon in chronic hepatitis C. Hepatology 26(suppl.1):112S, 1997.
284. Marcellin P, Martinot M, Boyer N, Levy S: Treatment of hepatitis C patients with normal aminotransferase levels. Clin Liver Dis 3:843, 1999.
285. Heathcote J: Antiviral therapy for patients with chronic hepatitis C. Semin Liver Dis 20:185, 2000.
286. Pérez-Olmeda M, González J, García-Samaniego J, Arribas J, Peña J, Soriano V: Interferon plus ribavirin in HIV-infected patients with chronic hepatitis C. J Acquir Immune Defic Syndr 22:308, 1999.
287. Landau A, Batisse D, Duong J, et al: Efficacy and safety of combination therapy with interferon-alpha 2b and ribavirin for severe chronic hepatitis C in HIV-infected patients. AIDS 14:839, 2000.
288. Orland JR, Wright TL, Cooper S: Acute hepatitis C. Hepatology 32: 321, 2001.
289. Ruiz-Moreno M, Rua M, Castillo I, et al: Treatment of children with chronic hepatitis C with recombinant interferon alfa: a pilot study. Hepatology 16:882, 1992.
290. Bennet WG, Inoue Y, Beck JR, et al: Estimates of the cost-effectiveness of a single course of interferon-alfa-2b in patients with histologically mild chronic hepatitis C. Ann Intern Med 127:855, 1997.
291. Kim WR, Poterucha JJ, Dickson ER, et al: Economics analysis of interferon/ribavirin treatment in patients with chronic hepatitis C who relapse following initial interferon therapy. Gastroenterology 114: 1274A, 1998.
292. National Institute of Diabetes and Digestive and Kidney Disease: Chronic hepatitis C: current disease management. www.niddk.nih.gov/health/digest/pubs/chrnhepc/chrnhepc.htm Accessed 2000.
293. Sheiner P, Boros P, Klion FM, et al: The efficacy of prophylactic interferon alfa-2b in preventing recurrent hepatitis C after liver transplantation. Hepatology 28:831, 1998.
294. Singh N, Gayowski T, Wannstedt C, et al: Interferon-α for prophylaxis of recurrent viral hepatitis C in liver transplant recipients. Transplantation 65:82, 1998.
295. Berenguer M, Wright T: Treatment strategies for recurrent hepatitis C after liver transplantation. Clin Liver Dis 3:883, 1999.
296. Wright T, Combs C, Kim M, et al: Interferon-alpha therapy for hepatitis C virus infection after liver transplantation. Hepatology 20:773, 1994.
297. Feray C, Samuel D, Gigou M,, et al: An open trial of interferon alfa recombinant for hepatitis C after liver transplantation: Antiviral effects and risk of rejection. Hepatology 22:1084, 1995.
298. Gane EJ, Lo SK, Riordan SM, et al: A randomized study comparing ribavirin and interferon alfa monotherapy for hepatitis C recurrence after liver transplantation. Hepatology 27:1403, 1998.
299. Bizollon T, Palazzo U, Ducerf C, et al: Pilot study of the combination of interferon alfa and ribavirin as therapy of recurrent hepatitis C after liver transplantation. Hepatology 26:500, 1997.
300. Shakil AO, McGuire B, Crippin JS, et al: Interferon-alfa 2b and ribavirin combination therapy in liver transplant recipients with recurrent hepatitis C [abstract]. Hepatology 32:221, 2000.
301. Rizzetto M, Verme G, Recchia S, et al: Immunoflorescence detection of a new antigen-antibody system (delta-antidelta) associated to the hepatitis virus in the liver and the serum of HBsAg carriers. Gut 18: 996, 1977.
302. Negro F, Rizzetto M: Diagnosis of hepatitis delta virus infection. J Hepatol 22(Suppl 1):136, 1995.
303. Casey J, Brown T, Colan E, Wignall F, Gerin J: A genotype of hepatitis D virus RNA that occurs in northern South America. Proc Natl Acad Sci U S A 90:9016, 1993.
304. Rosina F, Conoscitore P, Cuppone R, et al: Changing pattern of chronic hepatitis D in Southern Europe. Gastroenterology 117:161, 1999.
305. Lettau L, McCarthy J, Smith M, et al: Outbreak of severe hepatitis due to delta and hepatitis B viruses in parenteral drug abusers and their contacts. N Engl J Med 317:1256, 1987.
306. Govindarajan S, Chin KP, Redeker AG, Peters RL:: Fulminant B viral hepatitis: Role of delta agent. Gastroenterology 86:1417, 1984.
307. Rizzetto M, Morello C, Mannucci P, et al: Delta infection and liver disease in haemophiliac carriers of the hepatitis B surface antigen. J Infect Dis 145:18, 1982.
308. Leon A, Lopez J, Contreras G, Echevarria J: Antibodies to hepatitis delta virus in intravenous drug addicts and male homosexuals in Spain. Eur J Clin Microbiol Infect Dis 7:533, 1988.
309. Wu J, Chen C, Sheen I, Lee S, Tzeng H, Choo K: Evidence of transmission of hepatitis D virus to spouses from sequence analysis of the viral genome. Hepatology 22:1656, 1995.
310. Lai M: The molecular biology of hepatitis delta virus. Annu Rev Biochem 64:259, 1995.
311. Philipp T, Straub P, Durazzo M, Tukey R, Manns M: Molecular analysis of autoantigens in hepatitis D. J Hepatol 22(Suppl 1):132, 1995.
312. McFarlane B, Bridger C, Smith H, et al: Autoimmune mechanism in chronic hepatitis B and delta virus infections. Eur J Gastroenterol Hepatol 7:615, 1995.
313. Ottobrelli A, Marzano A, Smedile A, et al: Patterns of hepatitis delta virus reinfection and disease in liver transplantation. Gastroenterology 101:1649, 1991.
314. Rosino F, Cozzolongo R: Interferon for HDV infection. Antiviral Res 24:165, 1994.
315. Smedile A, Rizzetto M, Denniston K, et al: The clinical signficance of hepatitis D RNA in serum as detected by a hybridzation-based assay. Hepatology 6:1297, 1986.
316. Raimondo G, Craxi A, Longo G, et al: Delta infection in hepatocellular carcinoma positive for hepatitis B surface antigen. Ann Intern Med 101:343, 1984.
317. Popper H, Buitrago B, Hadler S, et al: Pathology of hepatitis delta infection in the Amazon Basin. Prog Clin Biol Res 234:121, 1987.
318. Farci P, Mandas A, Coiana A, et al: Treatment of chronic hepatitis D with interferon alfa-2a. N Engl J Med 330:88, 1994.
319. Rasshofer R, Choi S, Wolfi P: Interference of antiviral substances with replication of hepatitis delta virus RNA in primary woodchuck hepatocytes. In Gerin J, Purcell R, Rizzetto M, (eds): The Delta Hepatitis Virus. New York, Wiley Liss, 1992, pp 223–34.
320. Samuel D, Zignego A, Reynes M, et al: Long-term clinical and virological outcome after liver transplantation for cirrhosis caused by chronic delta hepatitis. Hepatolgy 21:333, 1995.
321. Koonin E, Gorbalenya A, Purdy M, Rozanov M, Reyes G, Bradley D: Computer-assisted assignment of functional domains in the nonstructural polyprotein of hepatitis E virus: Delineation of an additional group of positive-strand RNA plant and animal viruses. Proc Natl Acad Sci USA 89:8259, 1992.
322. Kane M, Bradley D Shrestha S, et al: Epidemic non-A, non-B hepatitis in Nepal: Recovery of a possible etiologic agent and transmission studies in marmosets. Am J Med 87:11S, 1984.
323. Reyes G, Purdy M, Kim J, et al: Isolation of a cDNA from the virus responsible for enterically transmitted non-A, non-B hepatitis. Science 247:1335, 1990.
324. Bradley D, Purdy M, Reyes G: Hepatitis E virus genome. J Hepatology 13(suppl 4):S152, 1991.
325. Schlauder GG, Desai SM, Zanetti AR, et al: Novel hepatitis E virus (HEV) isolates from Europe: Evidence for additional genotypes of HEV. J Med Virol 57:243, 1999.
326. Washwanathan R: Infectious hepatitis in Delhi (1955–1956): a critical study: Epidemiology. Indian J Med Res 45(suppl):1, 1957.
327. Cao XY, Ma XZ, Liu YZ, et al: Epidemiological and etiological studies on enterically transmitted non-A, non-B hepatitis in the south part of Xinjiang. In Shikata T, Purcell R, Uchida T (eds): Viral Hepatitis C, D and E. Amsterdam, Excerpta Medica, 1991, pp 297–312.

328. Khuroo M, Rustagi V, Dawson G, et al: Spectrum of hepatitis E virus infection in India. J Med Virol 43:281, 1994.
329. Mast E, Krawczynski K: Hepatitis E: An overview. Ann Rev Med 47: 257, 1996.
330. Balayan M, Usamov R, Zamyatina N, et al: Experimental hepatitis E infection in domestic pigs. J Med Virol 132:58, 1990.
331. Labrique AB, Thomas DL, Stoszek SK, et al: Hepatitis E: An emerging infectious disease. Epidemiol Rev 21:162, 1999.
332. Hsieh SY, Meng XJ, Wu YH, et al: Identity of a novel swine hepatitis E in Taiwan forming a monophyletic group with Taiwan isolates of human hepatitis E virus. J Clin Microbiol 37:3828, 1999.
333. Paul DA, Knigge MF, Ritter A, et al: Determination of hepatitis E virus seroprevalence by using recombinant fusion proteins and synthetic peptides. J Infect Dis 169:801, 1994.
334. Lok ASF, Soldevilla-Pico C: Epidemiology and serologic diagnosis of hepatitis E. J Hepatol 20:567, 1994.
335. Robson S, Adams S, Brink N, et al: Hospital outbreak of hepatits E. Lancet 339:1424, 1992.
336. Longer C, Denny S, Caudill J, et al: Experimental hepatitis E: pathogenesis in cynomolgus macaques (Macaca fascicularis). J Infect Dis 168:602, 1993.
337. Tsega E, Hansson B, Krawszynski K, Nordenfeldt E: Acute sporadic viral hepatitis in Ethiopia: Causes, risk factors and effects on pregnancy. Clin Infect Dis 14:961, 1992.
338. Khuroo MS, Kamill S, Jameel S: Vertical transmission of hepatitis E virus. Lancet 315:1025, 1995.
339. Chauhan A, Jameel S, Dilawari J, Chawla Y, Kaur U, Ganguly N: Hepatitis E virus transmission to a volunteer. Lancet 341:149, 1993.
340. Nanda S, Ansari I, Acharya S, Jameel S, Panda S: Protracted viremia during acute sporadic hepatitis E virus infection. Gastroenterology 108:225, 1995.
341. Khuroo M, Kamili S, Dar M: Hepatitis E and long-term antibody status. Lancet 341:1355, 1993.
342. Bryan J, Tsarev S, Iqbal M, et al: Epidemic hepatitis E in Pakistan: patterns of serologic response and evidence that antibody to hepatitis E protects against disease. J Infect Dis 170:517, 1994.
343. Balayan M, Andjaparidze A, Savinskaya S, et al: Evidence for a virus in non-A, non-B hepatitis transmitted via the fecal-oral route. Intervirology 20:23, 1983.
344. Purdy M, Carson D, McCaustland K, et al: Viral specificity of hepatitis E virus antigens identified by flourescent antibody assay using recombinant HEV proteins. J Med Virol 44:212, 1994.
345. Dawson G, Chau K, Cabal C, Yarbough P, Reyes G, Mushahwar I: Solid-phase enzymes-linked immunosorbent assay for hepatitis E virus IgG and IgM antibodies utilizing recombinant antigens and synthetic peptides. J Virol Meth 38:175, 1992.
346. Tsarev S, Tsareva T, Emerson S, et al: Successful passive and active immunization of cynomolgus monkeys against hepatitis E. Proc Natl Acad Sci USA 91:10198, 1994.
347. Khuroo M, Dar M: Hepatitis E: Evidence for person-to-person transmission and inability of low dose immune serum globulin from an Indian source to prevent it. Indian J Gastroenterol 11:113, 1992.
348. Joshi Y, Babu S, Sarin S, et al: Immunoprophylaxis of epidemic non-A, non-B hepatitis. Indian J Med Res 81:18, 1985.
349. Tsarev SA, Tsareva TS, Emerson SU, et al: Recombinant vaccine against hepatitis E: dose and protection against heterologous challenge. Vaccine 15:1834, 1997.
350. Linnen J, Wages J, Zhang-Keck ZY, et al: Molecular cloning and disease association of hepatitis G virus: A transfusion-transmissible agent. Science 271:505, 1996.
351. Simons J, Leary T, Dawson G, et al: Isolation of novel virus-like sequences associated with human hepatitis. Nature Med 1:564, 1995.
352. Simons J, Pilot-Matias T, Leary T, et al: Identification of two flavivirus-like genomes in the GB hepatitis agent. Proc Natl Acad Sci U S A 92:3401, 1995.
353. Muerhoff A, Leary T, Simons J, et al: Genomic organization of GB viruses A and B: two new members of the Flaviviridae associated with GB agent hepatitis. J Virol 69:5621, 1995.
354. Alter HJ, Nakatsuji Y, Melpolder J, et al: The incidence of transfusion-associated hepatitis G virus infection and its relationship to liver disease. N Engl J Med 336:747, 1997.
355. Sauleda JM, Hernandez JM, Tussell J, et al: Prevalence of hepatitis G virus among blood donors and blood product recipients in Barcelona, Spain. Hepatology 24:415, 1996.
356. Alter MJ, Gallagher M, Morris TT, et al: Acute non A–E hepatitis in the United States and the role of hepatitis G virus infection. N Engl J Med 336:741, 1997.
357. Kiyosawa K, Tanaka E: GB virus C/hepatitis G virus. Intervirology 42:185, 1999.
358. Pessoa MG, Terrault NA, Detmer J, et al: Quantitation of hepatitis G and C viruses in the liver: Evidence that hepatitis G is not hepatotropic. Hepatology 27:877, 1998.
359. Nishizawa T, Okamoto H, Konishi K, et al: A novel DNA virus (TTV) associated with elevated transaminase levels in posttransfusion hepatitis of unknown etiology. Biochem Biophys Res Comm 241:92, 1997.
360. Okamoto H, Nishizawa T, Kato N, et al: Molecular cloning and characterization of a novel DNA virus (TTV) associated with posttransfusion hepatitis of unknown etiology. Hepatol Res 10:1, 1998.
361. Mushahwar IK, Erker JC, Muerhoff AS, et al: Molecular and biophysical characterization of TT virus: Evidence for a new virus family infecting humans. Proc Natl Acad Sci U S A 96:3177, 1999.
362. Okamoto H, Takahashi N, Nishizawa T, et al: Marked genomic heterogeneity and frequent mixed infection of TT virus demonstrated by PCR with primers from coding and noncoding regions. Virology 259: 428, 1999.
363. Khudyakov YE, Cong ME, Nichols B, et al: Sequence heterogeneity of TT virus and closely related viruses. J Virol 74:2990, 2000.
364. Berg T, Schreier E, Heuft HG, et al: Occurrence of a novel DNA virus (TTV) in patients with liver disease and its frequency in blood donors. J Med Virol 59:117,1999.
365. Desai SM, Muerhoff AS, Leary TP, et al: Prevalence of TT virus infection in US blood donors and populations at risk for acquiring parenterally transmitted viruses. J Infect Dis 179:1242, 1999.
366. Charlton M, Adjei P, Poterucha J, et al: TT virus infection in North American blood donors, patients with fulminant hepatic failure, and cryptogenic cirrhosis. Hepatology 28:839, 1998.
367. Kato T, Mizokami M, Orito E, et al: High prevalence of TT virus infection in Japanese patients with liver diseases and in blood donors. J Hepatol 31:221, 1999.
368. Simmonds P, Davidson F, Lycett C, et al: Detection of a novel DNA virus (TTV) in blood donors and blood products. Lancet 352:191, 1998.
369. Gimenez-Barcons M, Forns X, Ampurdanes S, et al: Infection with a novel human DNA virus (TTV) has no pathogenic significance in patients with liver diseases. J Hepatol 30:1028, 1999.
370. Naoumov NV, Petrova EP, Thomas MG, Williams R: Presence of a newly described human DNA virus (TTV) in patients with liver disease. Lancet 352:195, 1998.
371. Takahashi K, Hijikata M, Samokhvalov EI, Mishiro S: Full or near full length nucleotide sequences of TT virus variants (types SANBAN and YONBAN) and the TT virus-like mini virus. Intervirology 43:119, 2000.
372. Hijikata M, Takahashi K, Mishiro S: Complete circular DNA genome of a TT virus variant (isolate name SANBAN) and 44 partial ORF2 sequences implicating a great degree of diveristy beyond genotypes. Virology 260:17, 1999.
373. Primi D, Fiordalisi G, Mantero GL, et al: Identification of SENV genotypes. International publication: WO 00/28039; 2000 (International application published under the patent cooperation treaty).
374. Tanaka Y, Primi D, Wang RYH, et al: Genomic and molecular evolutionary analysis of a newly identified infectious agent (SEN virus) and its relationship to the TT virus family. J Infec Dis 183:359, 2001.

Chapter 69

Liver Abscess and Bacterial, Parasitic, Fungal, and Granulomatous Liver Disease

Raymond T. Chung and Lawrence S. Friedman

The liver serves as the initial site of filtration of absorbed luminal contents and is particularly susceptible to contact with microbial antigens of all varieties. Other than hepatotropic viruses, the liver can be affected by: 1) spread of bacterial or parasitic infection from outside the liver; 2) primary infection by spirochetal, protozoal, helminthic, or fungal organisms; or 3) systemic effects of bacterial or granulomatous infections. This chapter describes pyogenic and amebic liver abscesses; other bacterial and spirochetal infections that affect the liver; parasitic diseases, including protozoal and helminthic diseases; fungal infections with prominent hepatic manifestations; and infectious and other causes of granulomatous liver disease.

LIVER ABSCESS

Pyogenic Liver Abscess

Until recently, most cases of pyogenic liver abscess were a consequence of appendicitis complicated by pylephlebitis in a young patient.[1] This presentation is less common today as a result of earlier diagnosis and effective antibiotic therapy. Most cases now are cryptogenic or occur in older men with underlying biliary tract disease.[2]

Pathogenesis

Infections of the biliary tract (e.g., cholangitis, cholecystitis) are the most common identifiable source of liver abscess. Infection of the liver may occur via the bile duct, along a penetrating vessel, or from an adjacent septic focus. Pyogenic liver abscess may arise as a late complication of endoscopic sphincterotomy for bile duct stones or within 3 to 6 weeks of a surgical biliary-intestinal anastomosis.[2] Pyogenic liver abscesses may complicate recurrent pyogenic cholangitis, which is found predominantly in east and southeast Asia and characterized by recurring episodes of cholangitis, intrahepatic stone formation and, in many cases, biliary parasitic infections (see Chapter 59). Less commonly, liver abscess is a complication of bacteremia arising from underlying abdominal disease, such as diverticulitis, perforated or penetrating peptic ulcer, gastrointestinal malignancy, inflammatory bowel disease, or peritonitis, or rarely from bacterial endocarditis. Occasionally, a pyogenic liver abscess may be the presentation of a hepatocellular or gallbladder carcinoma or a complication of chemoembolization of a hepatic neoplasm.[3]

In approximately 40% of cases of pyogenic liver abscess, no obvious source of infection can be identified. Oral flora have been proposed to be a potential source in such cases, particularly in patients with severe periodontal disease.[4]

Microbiologic Evaluation

Most pyogenic liver abscesses are polymicrobial.[5] The bacterial organisms that have been cultured from liver abscesses are listed in Table 69–1. The most frequently isolated organisms are *Escherichia coli* and *Klebsiella*, *Proteus*, *Pseudo-*

Table 69–1 | **Organisms That May Be Isolated From Abscess and Blood in Pyogenic Liver Abscess**

AEROBES			
Gram-Negative	**Gram-Positive**	**ANAEROBES**	**OTHERS**
Escherichia coli	Enterococci	*Bacteroides* spp.	*Candida albicans*
Klebsiella pneumoniae	*Streptococcus pyogenes*	*Fusobacterium* spp.	Tuberculosis
Enterobacter spp.	*Staphylococcus aureus*	Streptococci	
Pseudomonas spp.	*Listeria monocytogenes* (rare)	*Peptostreptococcus* spp.	
Citrobacter spp.	*Streptococcus milleri* (microaerophilic)	*Peptococcus* spp.	
Morganella spp.		*Prevotella* spp. (rare)	
Proteus spp.		*Clostridium* spp. (rare)	
Salmonella spp.		*Actinomyces* spp. (rare)	
Serratia marcescens (rare)			
Yersinia spp. (rare)			
Burkholderia pseudomallei (rare)			
Capnocytophaga canimorsus (rare, capnophilic)			
Pasteurella multocida (rare)			

monas, and *Streptococcus* species, particularly *Streptococcus milleri*. With improved cultivation methods and earlier diagnosis, the number of cases identified as being caused by anaerobic organisms has increased. The most commonly identified anaerobic species are *Bacteroides fragilis*, *Fusobacterium necrophorum*, and anaerobic streptococci. Pyogenic abscess associated with recurrent pyogenic cholangitis may be caused by *Salmonella typhi*. *Clostridium* and *Actinomyces* species are uncommon causes of liver abscess, and rare cases are caused by *Yersinia enterocolitica*, septic melioidosis, *Pasteurella multocida*, *Haemophilus parainfluenzae*, and *Listeria* species. Liver abscesses caused by *Staphylococcus aureus* infection are most common in children and patients with septicemia or impaired host resistance. Fungal abscesses of the liver may occur in immunocompromised hosts, particularly in those with a hematologic malignancy.[6]

Diagnosis

In the past, patients with a pyogenic liver abscess typically presented with acutely spiking fevers, pain in the right upper quadrant, and, in many cases, shock. Since the introduction of antibiotics, the presentation of pyogenic liver abscess has become less acute, often insidious, and characterized by malaise, low-grade fever, weight loss, and dull abdominal pain that may increase with movement. Symptoms may be present for 1 month or more before a diagnosis is made. Multiple abscesses are typical when biliary disease is the source and are associated with a more acute systemic presentation, often with sepsis and shock, than is the case with solitary abscesses. When an abscess is situated near the dome of the liver, pain may be referred to the right shoulder, or a cough resulting from diaphragmatic irritation or atelectasis may be present.

A physical examination usually discloses hepatomegaly and liver tenderness, which is accentuated by movement or percussion. Splenomegaly is unusual, except with a chronic abscess. Ascites is rare, and, in the absence of cholangitis, jaundice is present only late in the course of the illness. Portal hypertension may follow recovery if there has been thrombosis of the portal vein.

Laboratory findings include anemia, leukocytosis, an elevated erythrocyte sedimentation rate, and abnormal liver biochemical tests, especially an elevated serum alkaline phosphatase level. Blood culture specimens may identify the causative organism in 50% of cases.[7]

Ultrasonography is the initial imaging modality of choice and may help to distinguish solid from fluid-filled lesions.[1, 2] Abscesses as small as 1 cm can be detected. Ultrasonography is inexpensive and accurate and can guide needle aspiration of the abscess. Culture specimens of aspirated material yield positive results in 90% of cases (although the yield is probably lower if the patient has been receiving antibiotics).[7] Computed tomography (CT) is also accurate, with a sensitivity approaching 100%, but is more expensive than ultrasonography. Hepatic abscesses are usually hypodense on a CT scan and may display a "rim" of contrast enhancement in 20% of cases. CT is the procedure of choice when it is critical to determine the precise location of an abscess and its relationship to adjacent structures. Endoscopic retrograde cholangiopancreatography is indicated in patients with imaging evidence of biliary stones or prominent cholestasis.[8] Magnetic resonance imaging and arteriography may each be of value in selected clinical situations.

Prevention and Treatment

Pyogenic liver abscesses are best prevented by prompt treatment of acute biliary and abdominal infections and by adequate drainage of infected intra-abdominal collections under appropriate antibiotic coverage. Treatment of a hepatic abscess requires antibiotic therapy directed at the causative organism(s) and, in most cases, drainage of the abscess, usually percutaneously with radiologic guidance. Placement of an indwelling drainage catheter in the abscess may be necessary until the cavity has resolved. With multiple abscesses, only the largest abscess may need to be aspirated; smaller lesions often resolve with antibiotic treatment alone, but rarely, each lesion may need drainage. For a small abscess, antibiotic therapy without drainage may suffice. Biliary decompression is essential when a hepatic abscess is associated with biliary obstruction and may be accomplished through the endoscopic or transhepatic route (see Chapter 61). Surgical drainage of a hepatic abscess may be necessary in patients with incomplete percutaneous drainage, unresolved jaundice, renal impairment, a multiloculated abscess, or a ruptured abscess.[9] A laparoscopic approach may be feasible in selected cases.

Initial antibiotic coverage, pending culture results, should be broad spectrum and include ampicillin and an aminoglycoside (suspected biliary source) or a third-generation cephalosporin (suspected colonic source), plus, in either case, metronidazole, to cover anaerobic organisms. If amebiasis is suspected, metronidazole therapy should be started before aspiration is performed. After culture results and sensitivity profiles have been obtained, antibiotic therapy directed at the specific organism(s) should be administered intravenously for 2 weeks and then orally for 6 weeks. For streptococcal infections, the use of high-dose oral antibiotics for 6 months may be preferable.

The mortality rate for patients with hepatic abscesses treated with antibiotics and percutaneous drainage has improved over the past two decades but remains about 8%.[9] A worse prognosis is associated with a delay in diagnosis, multiple organisms cultured from blood, a fungal cause, jaundice, hypoalbuminemia, a pleural effusion, an underlying biliary malignancy, severe multiorgan dysfunction, or other associated medical diseases.[2] Complications of pyogenic liver abscess include empyema, pleuropericardial effusion, portal or splenic vein thrombosis, rupture into the pericardium, thoracic and abdominal fistula formation, and sepsis.

Amebic Liver Abscess

Pathogenesis

Amebiasis occurs in 10% of the world's population and is most common in tropical and subtropical regions. In the United States, it is a disease of young, often Hispanic, adults. Endemic areas include Africa, Southeast Asia, Mexico, Venezuela, and Colombia. Amebic liver abscess is the most common extraintestinal manifestation of amebiasis. Compared to affected persons who reside in an endemic area, persons in whom an amebic liver abscess develops after travel to an endemic area are older and more likely to be male, have marked hepatomegaly, and have a large abscess or multiple abscesses. The occurrence of an amebic liver abscess in a person who has not traveled to or resided in an endemic area should raise the suspicion of underlying immunosuppression, particularly the acquired immunodeficiency syndrome (AIDS).[10]

During its life cycle, *Entamoeba histolytica* exists as trophozoite or cyst forms (Fig. 69–1). After infection, amebic cysts pass through the gastrointestinal tract and become trophozoites in the colon, where they invade the mucosa and produce typical "flask-shaped" ulcers. The organism is carried by the portal circulation to the liver, where an abscess may develop. Occasionally, organisms travel beyond the liver and can establish abscesses in the lung or brain. Rupture of an amebic liver abscess into the pleural, pericardial, and peritoneal spaces can also occur.

Clinical Features

An amebic liver abscess is more likely than a pyogenic liver abscess to have an acute presentation.[7] Symptoms are present on average for 2 weeks by the time a diagnosis is made. There may be a latency period between intestinal and liver infection of up to many years, and fewer than 10% of patients report an antecedent history of bloody diarrhea with amebic dysentery.

Abdominal pain is typically well localized to the right upper quadrant. Fever is nearly universal but may be intermittent. Malaise, myalgias, and arthralgias are common. Jaundice occurs more frequently than in patients with a pyogenic liver abscess, and pulmonary symptoms may be present. Laboratory features resemble those found in pyogenic abscess.

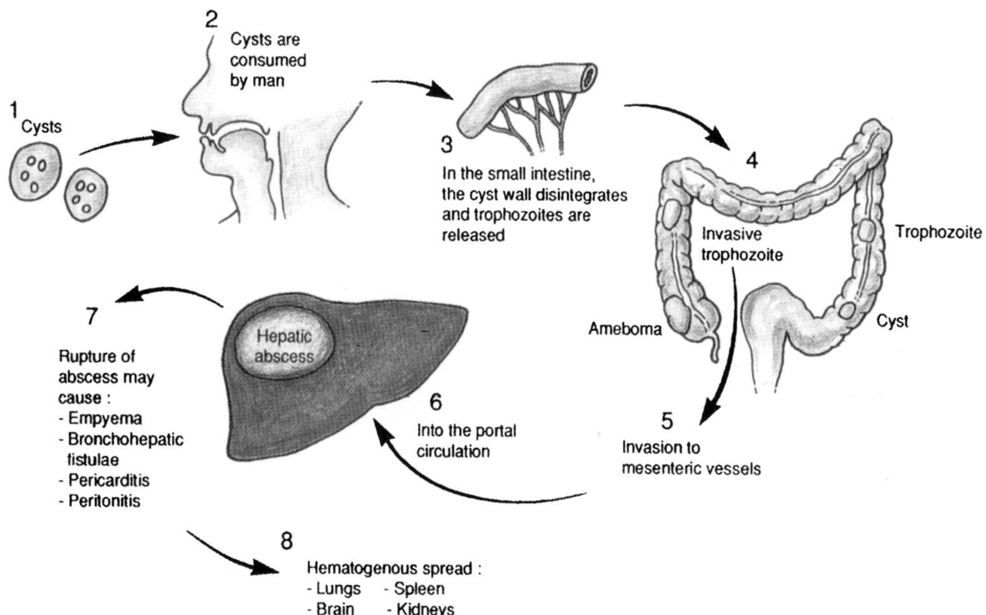
1 Cysts
2 Cysts are consumed by man
3 In the small intestine, the cyst wall disintegrates and trophozoites are released
4
Invasive trophozoite
Trophozoite
Ameboma
Cyst
5 Invasion to mesenteric vessels
6 Into the portal circulation
Hepatic abscess
7 Rupture of abscess may cause :
- Empyema
- Bronchohepatic fistulae
- Pericarditis
- Peritonitis
8 Hematogenous spread :
- Lungs - Spleen
- Brain - Kidneys

Figure 69–1. The life cycle of *Entamoeba histolytica* in amebiasis. (From Gitlin N, Strauss R: Atlas of Clinical Hepatology. Philadelphia, WB Saunders, 1995, p 64.)

Diagnosis

The diagnosis of amebic liver abscess is based on clinical suspicion, hepatic imaging, and serologic testing. Hepatic imaging studies cannot distinguish a pyogenic from an amebic liver abscess (Fig. 69–2). An amebic abscess is commonly localized to the right hepatic lobe, close to the diaphragm, and is usually single (Table 69–2). Available serologic tests include enzyme-linked immunosorbent assay (ELISA), indirect hemagglutination, countercurrent immunoelectrophoresis, latex fixation, indirect fluorescent antibody, complement fixation, and immunodiffusion. Serologic test results must be interpreted in the clinical context, because serum antibody levels may remain elevated for years after recovery or cure. The sensitivity of these tests approaches 95%, and a negative result makes an amebic abscess an unlikely diagnosis. Polymerase chain reaction–based tests to detect amebic DNA are available in the research setting.[2]

Aspiration of an amebic abscess should be performed only if the diagnosis remains uncertain. The presence of a reddish-brown pasty aspirate ("anchovy paste" or "chocolate sauce") is typical; trophozoites are rarely identified. Aspiration may also be considered in rare cases resistant to antibiotic therapy or when an abscess in the left lobe of the liver is close to the pericardium.

Treatment

Standard therapy consists of metronidazole, 750 mg three times daily, by mouth or, if necessary, intravenously for 5 to 10 days. Chloroquine may be substituted for metronidazole. The response to treatment is usually rapid. Following a course of metronidazole, most authorities recommend the addition of an oral luminal amebicide such as iodoquinol, 650 mg three times daily for 20 days, diloxanide furoate, 500 mg three times daily for 10 days, or paromomycin 25 to 35 mg/kg daily in three divided doses for 7 days, to eradicate residual amebae in the gut. The rate of pyogenic superinfection of an amebic liver abscess is low once treatment is begun. Rare complications of amebic abscesses can include intraperitoneal and intrathoracic rupture and multiorgan failure.

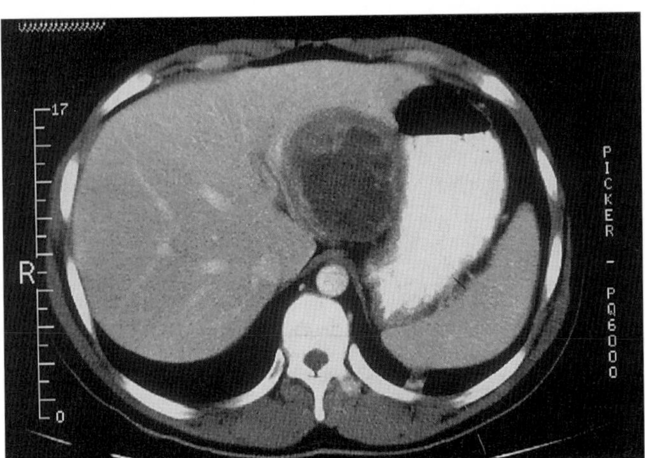

Figure 69–2. Computed tomographic scan showing a large amebic abscess in the left lobe of the liver. (Courtesy of Mark Feldman, MD, Dallas VA Hospital, Dallas, TX.)

Table 69–2 | **Pyogenic and Amebic Liver Abscess: Clinical Distinctions**

PARAMETER	PYOGENIC LIVER ABSCESS	AMEBIC LIVER ABSCESS
Number	Often multiple	Usually single
Location	Either lobe	Usually right hepatic lobe, near the diaphragm
Presentation	Subacute	Acute
Jaundice	Mild, if present	Moderate, if present
Diagnosis	US or CT ± aspiration	US or CT and serology
Treatment	IV antibiotics ± drainage	Metronidazole, 750 mg tid for 5 d orally or IV followed by iodoquinol, 650 mg orally tid for 20 d; diloxanide furoate, 500 mg orally tid for 10 d; or paromomycin 25–35 mg/kg orally in three divided doses for 7 d

CT, computed tomography; IV, intravenous; US, ultrasonography.

BACTERIAL AND SPIROCHETAL INFECTIONS OF THE LIVER

Manifestations of Extrahepatic Bacterial Infections

A number of extrahepatic infections can lead to derangements of hepatic function, ranging from mild abnormalities on liver biochemical testing to frank jaundice and, rarely, hepatic failure.

Legionellosis

Legionella pneumophila, a fastidious gram-negative bacterium, is the cause of Legionnaire's disease. While pneumonia is the predominant clinical manifestation, abnormalities of liver biochemical tests occur frequently, with elevations in serum aminotransferase levels in 50%, alkaline phosphatase levels in 45%, and bilirubin levels in 20% of cases (but usually without jaundice). Involvement of the liver does not influence clinical outcome. Liver histologic characteristics include microvesicular steatosis and focal necrosis; organisms can be seen occasionally. The diagnosis is confirmed by direct fluorescence of antibody in the serum or sputum or of antigen in the urine.[11]

Staphylococcus aureus *Infection (Toxic Shock Syndrome)*

Toxic shock syndrome is a multisystem disease caused by the staphylococcal toxic shock syndrome toxin. Originally described in association with tampon use, this syndrome is now more frequently a complication of *S. aureus* infections in surgical wounds. Typical findings include a scarlatiniform rash, mucosal hyperemia, hypotension, vomiting, and diarrhea. Hepatic involvement is almost always present, can be extensive, and is marked by deep jaundice and high serum aminotransferase levels.[12] Histologic findings in the liver include microabscesses and granulomas. The diagnosis is confirmed by culture of toxigenic *S. aureus* from the wound, blood, or other body sites.

Clostridial Infection

Clostridial myonecrosis involving *Clostridium perfringens* is usually a mixed anaerobic infection that results in the rapid development of local wound pain, abdominal pain, and diarrhea. The skin lesions become discolored and even bullous, and gas gangrene spreads rapidly, leading to a high mortality rate. Jaundice may develop in up to 20% of patients with gas gangrene and is predominantly a consequence of massive intravascular hemolysis caused by the exotoxin elaborated by the bacterium.[13] Liver involvement may include abscess formation and gas in the portal vein. Hepatic involvement does not appear to affect mortality.

Listeriosis

Hepatic invasion in adult human *Listeria monocytogenes* infection is uncommon. One report described three cases of disseminated listeriosis associated with hepatitis.[14] In almost all cases with overt hepatic involvement, underlying liver disease was present, including cirrhosis, hemochromatosis, or chronic hepatitis. Hepatic histologic findings include multiple abscesses and granulomas. The diagnosis of disseminated listerial infection is based on a positive result on blood cultures.[15]

Gonococcal Infection

In approximately 50% of patients with disseminated gonococcal infection, serum alkaline phosphatase levels are elevated, and in 30% to 40% of patients, aspartate aminotransferase levels are elevated.[16] Jaundice is uncommon.

The most common hepatic complication of gonococcal infection is the Fitz-Hugh-Curtis syndrome, a perihepatitis that is believed to result from the direct spread of infection from the pelvis.[16] Clinically, patients describe a sudden, sharp pain in the right upper quadrant. This pain may be confused with acute cholecystitis or pleurisy. Most patients have a history of pelvic inflammatory disease. The syndrome is distinguished from gonococcal bacteremia by a characteristic friction rub over the liver and negative results of blood cultures. The diagnosis is made by vaginal cultures for gonococcus. The overall prognosis of gonococcal infection appears to be unaffected by the presence of perihepatitis.[17]

Burkholderia pseudomallei *Infection (Melioidosis)*

Burkholderia pseudomallei is a soil-borne and water-borne gram-negative bacterium that is found predominantly in southeast Asia. The clinical spectrum of melioidosis ranges from asymptomatic infection to fulminant septicemia with involvement of the lungs, gastrointestinal tract, and liver.[18] Histologic changes in the liver include inflammatory infiltrates, multiple microabscesses, and focal necrosis. Organisms can be visualized with a Giemsa stain of liver biopsy specimens.[18] With chronic disease, granulomas may be seen.

Shigellosis and Salmonellosis

Several case reports have described cholestatic hepatitis attributable to enteric infection with *Shigella*.[19, 20] Histologic findings in the liver have included portal and periportal polymorphonuclear infiltration, hepatocyte necrosis, and cholestasis.

Typhoid fever, caused by *Salmonella typhi*, is a systemic infection that frequently involves the liver. Some patients may present with an acute hepatitis-like picture, characterized by fever and tender hepatomegaly. Mild elevations of serum bilirubin levels (in up to 16% of cases) and aminotransferase levels (in 50%) are common.[21] Cholecystitis and liver abscess may complicate hepatic involvement with *S. typhi*.

Hepatic damage by *S. typhi* appears to be mediated by bacterial endotoxin, although organisms can be visualized within the liver tissue. Circulating endotoxin may produce focal necrosis, a periportal mononuclear infiltrate, and Kupffer cell hyperplasia. These changes resemble those seen in gram-negative sepsis. Characteristic typhoid nodules scattered throughout the liver are the result of profound hypertrophy and proliferation of Kupffer cells. The clinical course can be severe, with a mortality rate approaching 20%, particularly with delayed treatment or in patients with other complications of *Salmonella* infection.[21]

S. paratyphi A and B are the predominant causes of paratyphoid fever. As in typhoid fever, abnormalities in liver biochemical tests, with or without hepatomegaly, are common. Serum aminotransferase elevations are frequent (82%); less commonly, elevations in alkaline phosphatase (39%) and bilirubin (19%) levels are seen.[21]

Yersiniosis

Infection with *Yersinia enterocolitica* presents as ileocolitis in children and terminal ileitis and mesenteric adenitis in adults. Arthritis, cellulitis, erythema nodosum, and septicemia may complicate *Yersinia* infection. Most patients with complicated disease have underlying comorbidity, such as diabetes mellitus, cirrhosis, or hemochromatosis. Excess tissue iron, in particular, may be a predisposing factor, because growth of the *Yersinia* bacterium is enhanced by iron.

The subacute septicemic form of the disease resembles typhoid fever or malaria. Multiple abscesses are diffusely distributed in the liver and spleen.[22] In some cases, the occurrence of *Y. enterocolitica* liver abscesses may lead to the detection of underlying hemochromatosis.[23, 24] The mortality rate is approximately 50%.

Coxiella burnetii *Infection (Q Fever)*

Infection by *Coxiella burnetii*, typically acquired by inhalation of animal dusts, causes the clinical syndrome of Q fever, which is characterized by relapsing fevers, headache, myalgias, malaise, pneumonitis, and culture-negative endocarditis. The liver is commonly affected.[25] The predominant abnormality is an elevated serum alkaline phosphatase level, with minimal elevations of aspartate aminotransferase or bilirubin. The histologic hallmark in the liver is the presence of characteristic fibrin-ring granulomas. The diagnosis is confirmed by serologic testing for complement-fixing antibodies.[25]

Rocky Mountain Spotted Fever

In recent decades, mortality caused by this systemic tick-borne rickettsial illness has decreased considerably as a result of prompt recognition of the classic maculopapular rash in association with fever and an exposure history. However, a small subset of patients exists who present with multiorgan manifestations and in whom the mortality rate has remained high.[26] A characteristic severe vasculitis develops in these patients that is thought to be the result of a microbe-induced coagulopathy. Hepatic involvement is frequent in multiorgan Rocky Mountain spotted fever (RMSF). In one postmortem study, rickettsiae were identified in the portal triads of eight of nine fatal cases.[27] Portal inflammation, portal vasculitis, and sinusoidal erythrophagocytosis were consistent findings, but hepatic necrosis was negligible. The predominant clinical manifestation was jaundice; elevations of serum aminotransferase and alkaline phosphatase levels were variable. Jaundice is likely due to a combination of inflammatory bile ductular obstruction and hemolysis.[27]

Actinomycosis

Actinomycosis is caused most commonly by *Actinomyces israelii*, a gram-positive anaerobic bacterium. While cervicofacial infection is the most frequent manifestation of infection, gastrointestinal involvement occurs in 13% to 60% of cases.[28, 29] Hepatic involvement is present in 15% of cases of abdominal actinomycosis and is thought to result from metastatic spread from other abdominal sites. Common presenting symptoms of actinomycotic liver abscess include fever, abdominal pain, and anorexia with weight loss.[30] The course is more indolent than that seen with the usual causes of pyogenic hepatic abscess. Anemia, leukocytosis, an elevated erythrocyte sedimentation rate, and an elevated serum alkaline phosphatase level are nearly universal.[30] Radiographic findings are nonspecific; multiple abscesses may be seen in both lobes of the liver.

The diagnosis is based on aspiration of an abscess cavity and either visualization of characteristic sulfur granules or positive results on an anaerobic culture. Most abscesses resolve with prolonged courses of intravenous penicillin or oral tetracycline. Large abscesses can be drained percutaneously.[30]

Bartonellosis

Endemic to Colombia, Ecuador, and Peru, *Bartonella bacilliformis* is a gram-negative coccobacillus that causes an acute febrile illness accompanied by jaundice, hemolysis, hepatosplenomegaly, and lymphadenopathy.[31] Centrilobular necrosis of the liver and splenic infarction may occur. As many as 40% of patients die of sepsis or hemolysis. Prompt treatment with chloramphenicol or tetracycline prevents fatal complications.

Brucellosis

Brucellosis may be acquired from infected pigs, cattle, goats, and sheep (*Brucella suis*, *B. abortus*, *B. melitensis*, and *B. ovis*, respectively) and typically presents as an acute febrile illness. Hepatic abnormalities are seen in the majority of infected persons, and jaundice may be present in severe cases. Typically, multiple noncaseating hepatic granulomas are found on liver biopsy specimens; less often, there is focal mononuclear infiltration of the portal tracts or lobules.[32] The diagnosis can be made by isolation of the organism from a culture specimen of liver tissue and is confirmed by serologic testing with use of counterimmunoelectrophoresis in combination with a history of exposure to animals.

Bacterial Sepsis and Jaundice

Jaundice may complicate systemic sepsis caused by gram-negative or gram-positive organisms. Exotoxins and endotoxin liberated in overwhelming infection can directly or indirectly, through cytokines such as tumor necrosis factor-alpha (TNF-α), inhibit the transport of bile acids and other organic anions across the hepatic sinusoidal and bile canalicular membranes, thereby leading to intrahepatic cholestasis.[33, 34] Serum bilirubin levels can reach 15 mg/dL or higher. The magnitude of the jaundice does not correlate with mortality. Results of culture of liver biopsy specimens are usually negative.

Spirochetal Infections of the Liver

Leptospirosis

Leptospirosis is one of the most common zoonoses in the world and has a wide range of domestic and wild animal reservoirs. Humans acquire the spirochete by contact with infected urine or contaminated soil or water. In humans, disease can occur as anicteric leptospirosis or Weil's syndrome.

Anicteric leptospirosis accounts for more than 90% of cases and is characterized by a biphasic illness. The first phase begins, often abruptly, with viral illness–like symptoms associated with fever, leptospiremia, and conjunctival suffusion, which serves as an important diagnostic clue. Following a brief period of improvement, the second phase in 95% of cases is characterized by myalgias, nausea, vomiting, abdominal tenderness, and, in some cases, aseptic meningitis.[35] During this phase, a few patients have elevated serum aminotransferase and bilirubin levels with hepatomegaly.

Weil's syndrome is a severe icteric form of leptospirosis and constitutes 5% to 10% of all cases. The first phase of this illness is often marked by jaundice, which may last for weeks. During the second phase, fever may be high, and hepatic and renal manifestations predominate. Jaundice may be marked, with serum bilirubin levels approaching 30 mg/dL (predominantly conjugated). Serum aminotransferase levels usually do not exceed five times the upper limit of normal.[36] Acute tubular necrosis often develops and can lead to renal failure, which may be fatal. Hemorrhagic complications are frequent and are the result of capillary injury due to immune complexes.[35] Spirochetes are seen in renal tubules in the majority of autopsy specimens but are rarely found in the liver. Hepatic histologic findings are generally nonspecific and without necrosis. Altered mitochondria and disrupted membranes in hepatocytes on electron microscopy suggest the possibility of a toxin-mediated injury.

The diagnosis of leptospirosis is made on clinical grounds in conjunction with a positive result of a blood or urine culture specimen in the first or second phase, respectively. Serologic testing confirms the diagnosis when culture results are unrevealing. Doxycycline is effective if given within the first several days of illness. Most patients recover without residual organ impairment.

Syphilis

Syphilis may involve the liver in congenital, secondary, and tertiary, or late, infection.

Secondary Syphilis

Liver involvement is characteristic of secondary syphilis.[37] The frequency of hepatitis in secondary syphilis ranges from 1% to 50%.[31, 37, 38] Symptoms are usually nonspecific, including anorexia, weight loss, fever, malaise, and sore throat. A characteristic pruritic maculopapular rash involves the palms and soles.[31] Jaundice, hepatomegaly, and tenderness in the right upper quadrant are less common. Almost all patients exhibit generalized lymphadenopathy.[31] Biochemical testing generally reveals low-grade elevations of serum aminotransferase and bilirubin levels, with a disproportionate elevation of the serum alkaline phosphatase; isolated elevation of the alkaline phosphatase is common. Proteinuria may be present.

A histologic examination of the liver in syphilitic hepatitis generally discloses focal necrosis in the periportal and centrilobular regions. The inflammatory infiltrate typically includes polymorphonuclear cells, plasma cells, lymphocytes, eosinophils, and mast cells.[31, 37, 38] Kupffer cell hyperplasia may be seen, but bile ductular injury is rare. Spirochetes may be demonstrated by silver staining in up to one half of patients. Resolution of these findings without sequelae follows treatment with penicillin.

Tertiary (Late) Syphilis

Tertiary syphilis is now rare. Although hepatic lesions are common in late syphilis, most patients are asymptomatic. Some patients describe anorexia, weight loss, fatigue, fever, or abdominal pain.[31]

The characteristic lesion in tertiary syphilis is the gumma, which can be single or multiple. It is necrotic centrally with surrounding granulation tissue consisting of a lymphoplasmacytic infiltrate and endarteritis and can lead to exuberant deposition of scar tissue, giving the liver a lobulated appearance (hepar lobatum). If hepatic involvement is unrecognized, hepatocellular dysfunction and portal hypertension with jaundice, ascites, and gastroesophageal varices can ensue.[39] Hepatic gummas may resolve after therapy with penicillin.

Lyme Disease

Lyme disease is a multisystem disease caused by the tick-borne spirochete *Borrelia burgdorferi*. Predominant manifestations are dermatologic, cardiac, neurologic, and musculoskeletal. Hepatic involvement has been described. Among 314 patients, abnormalities in liver biochemical tests and generally increased serum aminotransferase and lactate dehydrogenase levels were seen in 19%.[40] Clinical findings included anorexia, nausea and vomiting, weight loss, right upper quadrant pain, and hepatomegaly, usually within days to weeks of the onset of illness and often accompanied by the sentinel rash, erythema chronicum migrans.[40]

In early stages of the illness, the spirochetes are thought to disseminate hematogenously from the skin to other organs, including the liver.[41] One report has suggested that the Lyme spirochete can also cause acute hepatitis as a manifestation of reactivation,[42] although the possibility of reinfection cannot be fully excluded. Histologic examination of the liver in Lyme hepatitis reveals hepatocyte ballooning, marked mitotic activity, microvesicular fat, Kupffer cell hyperplasia, a mixed sinusoidal infiltrate, and intraparenchymal and sinusoidal spirochetes.[41]

The diagnosis of Lyme disease is confirmed with serologic studies in patients with a typical clinical history. Hepatic involvement does not appear to affect overall outcome,

Table 69–3 | **Parasitic Infections of the Hepatobiliary Tree: Classification by Pathologic Process**

PATHOLOGIC PROCESS	DISEASES
Hepatocellular	
Granulomatous hepatitis	Schistosomiasis Fascioliasis Toxocariasis Hepatic capillariasis Strongyloidiasis
Portal fibrosis	Schistosomiasis
Hepatic abscesses or necrosis	Amebic liver disease Toxoplasmosis
Cystic liver disease	Echinococcosis
Peliosis hepatis	Bacillary angiomatosis
Reticuloendothelial Disease	
Kupffer cell infection or hyperplasia	Visceral leishmaniasis Malaria Babesiosis Toxoplasmosis
Biliary Disease	
Cholangitis	Fascioliasis Clonorchiasis/opisthorchiasis
Biliary hyperplasia	Ascariasis Cryptosporidiosis (see Chapter 28) Fascioliasis Clonorchiasis
Cholangiocarcinoma	Clonorchiasis/opisthorchiasis

Table 69–4 | **Parasitic Diseases of the Liver and Biliary Tract**

DISEASE (CAUSE)	ENDEMIC AREAS	PRE-DISPOSITION	PATHO-PHYSIOLOGY	MANIFESTATIONS	DIAGNOSIS	TREATMENT
Protozoans						
Amebiasis *(Entamoeba histolytica)*	Worldwide, especially Africa, Asia, Mexico, South America	Poor sanitation, sexual transmission	Hematogenous spread and tissue invasion, abscess formation	Fever, RUQ pain, peritonitis, elevated right hemidiaphragm	Cysts in the stool, serology (CIE, IHA), hepatic imaging	Metronidazole 750 mg po or IV tid × 5–10 d followed by diloxanide furoate 500 mg po tid × 10 d; or iodoquinol 650 mg po tid × 20 d
Malaria *(Plasmodium falciparum, P. malariae, P. vivax, P. ovale)*	Africa, Asia, South America	Blood transfusion, intravenous drug use	Sporozoite clearance by hepatocytes; exoerythrocytic replication in liver	Tender hepatomegaly; splenomegaly, rarely hepatic failure *(P. falciparum)*	Identification of the parasite on a blood smear	1. *P. falciparum*: (chloroquine-sensitive) mefloquine or quinine and either doxycycline or clindamycin or pyrimethamine-sulfadoxine (Fansidar) or atavaquone/proguanil (chloroquine-resistant) 2. *P. malariae*: Chloroquine 3. *P. vivax, ovale*: Chloroquine and primaquine (chloroquine-sensitive) or mefloquine and primaquine (chloroquine-resistant) (eliminate exoerythrocytic forms)
Visceral leishmaniasis *(Leishmania donovani)*	Old World, Central America, South America	Immunosuppression (AIDS, organ transplant)	Infection of RE cells	Fever, weight loss, hepatosplenomegaly, secondary bacterial infection, hyperpigmentation (kala-azar)	Amastigotes seen in the spleen, liver, marrow biopsy	1. Pentavalent antimorix (pertostain) 2. Gamma interferon and allopurinol (refractory cases) 3. Liposomal amphotericin B, (IV) aminosidine 4. Miltefosine po × 4 wk (investigational)
Toxoplasmosis *(Toxoplasma gondii)*	Worldwide	Intrauterine infection, immunosuppression (AIDS, organ transplant)	Replication in the liver leading to inflammation, necrosis	Fever, lymphadenopathy, occasionally hepatosplenomegaly, atypical lymphocytosis	Serology (IF, ELISA), isolation of the organism in the tissue	Pyrimethamine × 4 wk Sulfadiazine × 4–6 wk Leucovorin
Nematodes						
Ascariasis *(Ascaris lumbricoides)*	Tropical climates	Ingestion of raw vegetables	Larval migration to the liver, adult invasion of the bile ducts	Abdominal pain, fever, jaundice, biliary obstruction, perioval granulomas	Ova or adult in stool or contrast study	Albendazole 400 mg × 1 dose; or Mebendazole 500 mg × 1 dose; or Mebendazole 100 mg bid × 3 d; or Pyrantel pamoate 11 mg/kg up to 1g
Toxocariasis *(Toxocara canis, T. cati)*	Worldwide	Exposure to dogs or cats, especially children younger than five years of age	Larval migration in liver (visceral larva migrans)	Granuloma formation with eosinophilia	Larvae in tissue serology (ELISA)	Diethylcarbamazine 3 mg/kg tid × 21 d; or Thiabendazole 50 g/kg/d × 5 d; or Albendazole 5–10 mg/kg/d × 5 d
Hepatic capillariasis *(Capillaria hepatica)*	Worldwide	Exposure to rodents	Larval migration to the liver; inflammatory reaction to eggs	Acute, subacute hepatitis, tender hepatomegaly, occasionally splenomegaly, eosinophilia	Adult worms or eggs in a liver biopsy	Supportive, possibly dithiazine iodide, sodium stibogluconate, thiabendazole
Strongyloidiasis *(Strongyloides stercoralis)*	Asia, Africa, South America, Southern Europe, United States	Immunosuppression (AIDS, chemotherapy, organ transplant)	Larval penetration from the intestine to the liver	Hepatomegaly, occasionally jaundice, larvae in the portal tract or lobule	Larvae in the stool or duodenal aspirate	Ivermectin 200 μg/kg/d × 2 d; or albendazole 400 mg/d × 3 d
Trichinosis *(Trichinella spiralis)*	Temperate climates	Ingestion of undercooked meat	Hematogenous dissemination to the liver	Occasionally jaundice, biliary obstruction, larvae in hepatic sinusoids	History, eosinophilia, fever, muscle biopsy	1. Glucocorticoids for allergic symptoms 2. Albendazole 400 mg/d × 3 d or mebendazole 200 mg/d × 5 d

Table 69–4 | **Parasitic Diseases of the Liver and Biliary Tract** *Continued*

DISEASE (CAUSE)	ENDEMIC AREAS	PRE-DISPOSITION	PATHO-PHYSIOLOGY	MANIFESTATIONS	DIAGNOSIS	TREATMENT
Trematodes						
Schistosomiasis (*Schistosoma mansoni, S. japonicum*)	Asia, Africa, South America, Caribbean	Travelers exposed to fresh water	Fibrogenic host immune response to eggs in portal vein	*Acute*: eosinophilic infiltrate; *chronic*: hepatosplenomegaly, presinusoidal portal hypertension, perioval granuloma formation	Ova in the stool, rectal or liver biopsy	Praziquantel 60 mg/kg × 1 d; or Oxamniquine 15–60 mg/kg/d × 1–2 d. Acute toxemic schistosomiasis: Praziquantal 75 mg/kg in three divided doses × 1 d
Fascioliasis (*Fasciola hepatica*) (watercress)	Worldwide	Cattle or sheep raising, stone formation	Larvae migrate through the liver Penetration of the bile ducts or surgery	*Acute*: fever, abdominal pain, jaundice, hemobilia; *chronic*: hepatomegaly	Ova in the stool, flukes in the bile ducts at ERCP	Bithionol 50 mg/kg/d × 10 d (CDC); or Dehydroemetine 1 mg/kg/d × 14 d (CDC)
Clonorchiasis/opisthorchiasis (*Clonorchis sinensis, Opisthorchis viverrini, O. felineus*)	Southeast Asia, China, Japan, Korea, Eastern Europe, Southeast Asian immigrants	Ingestion of raw freshwater fish	Migration through the ampulla; egg deposition in the bile ducts	Biliary hyperplasia, obstruction, sclerosing cholangitis, stone formation, cholangiocarcinoma	Ova in the stool, flukes in the bile ducts at ERCP or surgery	Praziquantel 75 mg/kg in three divided doses × 1 d
Cestodes						
Echinococcosis (*Echinococcus granulosus, E. multilocularis*)	Worldwide	Sheep and cattle raising (*E. granulosa*)	Larval migration to the liver, encystment (hydatid)	Tender hepatomegaly, fever, eosinophilia, cyst rupture, biliary obstruction	Serology (IHA, ELISA), hepatic imaging	1. Surgical resection or percutaneous drainage 2. Perioperative albendazole 400 mg bid × 8 wk

AIDS, acquired immunodeficiency syndrome; CDC, Centers for Disease Control; CIE, counterimmunoelectrophoresis; ELISA, enzyme-linked immunosorbent assay; ERCP, endoscopic retrograde cholangiopancreatography; IF, immunofluorescence; IHA, indirect hemagglutination assay; RE, reticuloendothelial; RUQ, right upper quadrant

which is excellent in primary disease after institution of treatment with oral doxycycline, amoxicillin, clarithromycin, or azithromycin. Ceftriaxone is the drug of choice for late disease.[41]

PARASITIC DISEASES THAT INVOLVE THE LIVER (see Tables 69–3 and 69–4)

Protozoal Infections

Malaria

It is estimated that 300 to 500 million persons in more than 100 countries are infected with malaria each year. The liver is affected during two stages of the malarial life cycle: first in the pre-erythrocytic phase; then in the erythrocytic phase, which coincides with clinical illness. The life cycle of the prototypical malarial parasite is illustrated in Figure 69–3.

Pathobiology of the Malaria Life Cycle

Malarial sporozoites injected by an infected mosquito circulate to the liver and enter hepatocytes. Maturation to a schizont ensues. When the schizont ruptures, merozoites are released into the bloodstream, where they enter erythrocytes. The four major species of *Plasmodium* responsible for malaria differ with respect to the number of merozoites released and the maturation times. Infection by *P. falciparum* and *P. malariae* is not associated with a residual liver stage after the release of merozoites, whereas infection by *P. vivax* and *P. ovale* is associated with a persistent exoerythrocytic stage, the hypnozoite, which persists in the liver and, when activated, can divide and mature into schizont forms.

The extent of hepatic injury varies with the malarial species (most severe with *P. falciparum*) and the severity of infection. Unconjugated hyperbilirubinemia is most commonly seen as a result of hemolysis, but hepatocyte dysfunction can also be seen, leading to conjugated hyperbilirubinemia. There may be moderate elevations of serum aminotransferase and 5′-nucleotidase levels.[43] Synthetic dysfunction (e.g., prolongation of the prothrombin time, hypoalbuminemia) may be seen as well. In severe falciparum malaria, hypoglycemia and lactic acidosis are late and life-threatening complications.[44] Reversible reductions in portal venous blood flow have been described during the acute phase of falciparum malaria, presumably as a consequence of micro-occlusion of portal venous branches by parasitized erythrocytes.[44]

Histopathology

In acute falciparum malaria in a previously unexposed person, hepatic macrophages hypertrophy, and large quantities of malarial pigment (the result of hemoglobin degradation by

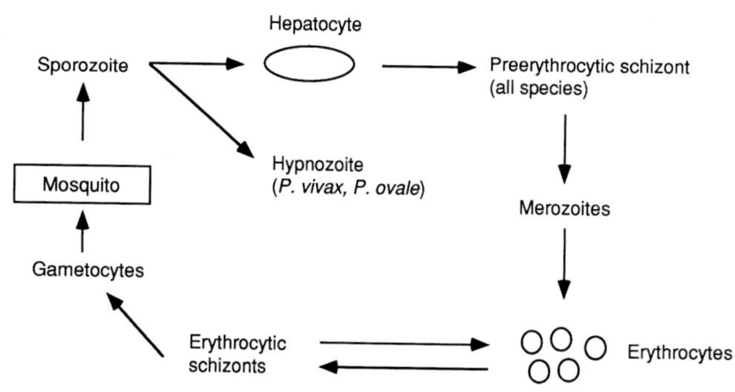

Figure 69–3. The life cycle of *Plasmodium*.

the parasite) accumulate in Kupffer cells, which phagocytose parasitized and unparasitized erythrocytes.[45] Histopathologic findings include Kupffer cell hyperplasia with pigment deposition and a mononuclear infiltrate. Hepatocyte swelling and centrizonal necrosis may be seen. All abnormalities are reversible with treatment.

Clinical Presentation

Only the erythrocytic stage of malaria is associated with clinical illness. Symptoms of acute infection develop 30 to 60 days following exposure and include fever, often hectic; malaise; anorexia; nausea; vomiting; diarrhea; and myalgias. Jaundice due to hemolysis is common in adults, especially in heavy infection with *P. falciparum*. In general, hepatic failure is seen only in association with concomitant viral hepatitis or with severe *P. falciparum* infection.[43] Tender hepatomegaly with splenomegaly is common.[45] Cytopenias are common in acute infection. The differential diagnosis includes viral hepatitis, gastroenteritis, amebic liver abscess, yellow fever, typhoid, tuberculosis, and brucellosis.

Diagnosis

The diagnosis of acute malaria rests on the clinical history, physical examination, and identification of parasites on peripheral thick blood smears. Because the number of parasites in the blood may be small, repeated smear examinations should be performed when the index of suspicion is high. Serologic assays are more useful for chronic than for acute infection.[43, 46]

Treatment

The treatment of acute malaria depends on the species of parasite, and, for falciparum infection, the pattern of chloroquine resistance. Chloroquine is generally effective for *P. malariae*, *P. vivax*, *P. ovale*, and *P. falciparum* in areas endemic for chloroquine-sensitive species. Resistant falciparum infections can be treated with mefloquine alone; quinine and either doxycycline or clindamycin; pyrimethamine-sulfadoxine (Fansidar); or a combination of atovaquone and proguanil. For *P. vivax* and *P. ovale* infections, the addition of primaquine (in persons without glucose-6-phosphate dehydrogenase deficiency) to chloroquine or mefloquine is indicated to eliminate the exoerythrocytic hypnozoites in the liver.[47]

Hyperreactive Malarial Splenomegaly (Tropical Splenomegaly Syndrome)

In endemic areas, with repeated exposure to malaria, an aberrant immunologic response may lead to overproduction of B lymphocytes, malarial antibody, and increased levels of circulating immune complexes, resulting in dense hepatic sinusoidal lymphocytosis and stimulation of the reticuloendothelial cell system. This can lead to massive splenomegaly, markedly elevated antimalarial antibody levels, and high serum IgM levels. Severe debilitating anemia due to hypersplenism, especially in women of childbearing age, can result. Variceal bleeding may occur but is uncommon.[48] Treatment consists of lifelong antimalarial therapy and blood transfusions.

Babesiosis

Babesiosis, caused by *Babesia* species, is a malaria-like illness transmitted by the tick *Ixodes dammini*. The disease is endemic to coastal areas of the Northeast and areas of the Midwest in the United States. Clinical features include fever, anemia, mild hepatosplenomegaly, abnormal liver biochemical tests, hemoglobinuria, and hemophagocytosis on bone marrow biopsy specimen. The disease is especially severe in asplenic and immunocompromised patients. In rare cases, marked pancytopenia occurs. Hepatic involvement reflects the severity of the systemic illness but generally is not severe. Uncomplicated cases are treated with oral clindamycin 600 mg three times daily and quinine 650 mg three times daily for 7 days. In severe cases, the clindamycin may be given intravenously.

Leishmaniasis

Visceral leishmaniasis is caused by *Leishmania donovani* and is endemic in the Mediterranean, central Asia, the former Soviet Union, the Middle East, China, India, Pakistan, Bangladesh, Africa, Central America, and South America.[49] Amastigotes are ingested by the sandfly (*Lutzomyia* in the New World, *Phlebotomus* in the Old World) and become flagellated promastigotes. Following injection into the human host, the promastigotes are phagocytosed by macrophages in the reticuloendothelial system, where they multiply.

Histopathology

Visceral leishmaniasis can usually be found in mononuclear phagocytes of the liver, spleen, bone marrow, and lymph nodes. Proliferation of Kupffer cells is often seen, and amastigotes can be detected within these cells.[50] Occasionally, parasite-bearing cells aggregate within noncaseating granulomas.[51] Hepatocyte necrosis is mild compared with that seen in cutaneous leishmaniasis. Healing is accompanied by fibrous deposition, and occasionally the liver takes on a cirrhotic appearance. However, complications of chronic liver disease are rare.

Clinical Presentation

Visceral infection caused by *L. donovani* begins with a papular or ulcerative skin lesion at the site of the sandfly bite. Following an incubation period of 2 to 6 months (sometimes years), intermittent fevers, weight loss, diarrhea (of bacillary, amebic, or leishmanial origin), and progressive painful hepatosplenomegaly develop, often accompanied by pancytopenia and a polyclonal hypergammaglobulinemia. Secondary bacterial infections resulting from suppression of reticuloendothelial cell function are important causes of mortality and include pneumonia, pneumococcal infection, and tuberculosis.

Physical findings include hepatomegaly, massive splenomegaly, jaundice or ascites in severe disease, generalized lymphadenopathy, and muscle wasting. Cutaneous gray hyperpigmentation, which prompted the name *kala-azar* (black fever), is characteristically seen in patients in India. Oral and nasopharyngeal nodules due to granuloma formation may also be seen.

Diagnosis

The diagnosis is based on the history, physical examination, and microscopic demonstration of amastigotes in affected tissue samples. The highest yield (90%) comes from aspiration of the spleen. The yield of liver biopsy is almost as great and less risky. The yield of bone marrow aspiration is 80% and that of lymph node aspirates is 60%.[47] Serologic testing (ELISA, immunofluorescence, direct agglutination) can be used to support a presumptive diagnosis of visceral leishmaniasis. The leishmanin skin test (Montenegro test) is not helpful in acute visceral disease.

Treatment

Pentavalent antimonial compounds are the drugs of choice for all forms of leishmaniasis. Parenteral sodium stibogluconate (Pentostam) is available through the Centers for Disease Control and Prevention for treatment of infections in the United States. Gamma-interferon and allopurinol have been used in combination with antimonials in cases refractory to antimonials alone. Alternative parenteral agents include liposomal amphotericin B and aminosidine.[47] Treatment with antimonials should be administered for at least 4 weeks. However, patients with AIDS and leishmaniasis often fail to respond to or relapse following treatment with conventional regimens.[45] Miltefosine, a phosphocholine analog administered orally, has recently shown promise in visceral leishmaniasis, with a reported cure rate of 97% in phase 2 trials.[52]

Toxoplasmosis

Toxoplasmosis caused by *Toxoplasma gondii* is found worldwide. In the United States, serologic surveys suggest that 20% to 40% of the population has been exposed to *T. gondii*.[53] The infection may be congenitally transmitted or may be an opportunistic infection causing cerebral mass lesions in patients with AIDS (see Chapter 28). Oocysts of *T. gondii* in soil, water, or contaminated meat are ingested and mature in the intestinal tract of humans to become sporozoites, which penetrate the intestinal mucosa, become tachyzoites, and circulate systemically, invading a wide array of cell types.[54] Hepatic involvement has been observed in severe, disseminated infection.

Clinical Presentation

Acquired toxoplasmosis can present as a mononucleosis-like illness with fever, chills, headache, and regional lymphadenopathy. Hepatomegaly, splenomegaly, and minimal elevations of serum aminotransferase levels are uncommon.[55] Infections of immunocompromised hosts can result in pneumonia, myocarditis, encephalitis, and, rarely, hepatitis.[56] Toxoplasmosis can produce atypical lymphocytosis, an otherwise unusual feature of parasitic disease.

Diagnosis

The diagnosis is best made by detecting specific IgM or IgG antibody using highly specific indirect immunofluorescence or an enzyme immunoassay.[57, 58] Specialized histologic staining techniques and tissue culture systems can provide adjunctive diagnostic support.

Treatment

Antibiotic therapy should be administered to all persons with severe symptomatic infection and immunocompromised or pregnant patients with acute uncomplicated infection. Treatment consists of a combination of pyrimethamine for 4 weeks and sulfadiazine for 4 to 6 weeks, plus leucovorin to minimize hematologic toxicity.[57]

Helminthic Infections

Nematodes (Roundworms)

Nematodes are nonsegmented roundworms that have a thick cuticle covering the body. Toxocariasis and capillariasis present with major hepatobiliary manifestations, whereas ascariasis, strongyloidiasis, and trichinosis affect the liver less frequently or less severely.

Ascariasis

Ascaris lumbricoides infects at least one billion persons, particularly in areas of lower socioeconomic standing.[59] Humans are infected by ingesting embryonated eggs, usually in raw vegetables. The eggs hatch in the small intestine, and the larvae penetrate the mucosa, enter the portal circulation, and reach the liver, pulmonary artery, and lungs, where they grow in the alveolar spaces, are regurgitated and swallowed, and become mature adults in the intestine 2 to 3 months after ingestion, whereupon the cycle repeats itself.

Clinical Presentation

Symptoms are generally proportionate to the worm burden; most infected persons are asymptomatic. Cough, fever, dyspnea, wheezing, substernal chest discomfort, and hepatomegaly may occur in the first 2 weeks. Chronic infection is more frequently characterized by episodic epigastric or periumbilical pain. If the worm burden is particularly heavy, small bowel complications such as obstruction, intussusception, volvulus, perforation, and appendicitis may occur.[60] Fragments of disintegrating worms within the biliary tree can serve as a nidus for the development of biliary calculi.[61] Preexisting disease of the biliary tree or pancreatic duct can predispose to worm migration into the bile ducts, with development of obstructive jaundice, cholangitis, or intrahepatic abscesses.[62] Chest radiography may show an infiltrate, and eosinophilia may be present.

Diagnosis

A history of regurgitating a worm or passing a large worm (15 to 40 cm) in the stool suggests ascariasis. In the absence of such a history, the diagnosis is made by identification of characteristic eggs in stool specimens. Larvae may also be identified in sputum and gastric washings and in liver and lung biopsy specimens. In patients with biliary or pancreatic symptoms, ultrasonography or endoscopic retrograde cholangiopancreatography (ERCP) is performed. ERCP offers the additional potential of extracting the worm.[63]

Treatment

One of the following regimens may be used: 1) a single dose of albendazole 400 mg; 2) a single dose of mebendazole, 500 mg; 3) mebendazole, 100 mg twice daily for 3 days; or 4) pyrantel pamoate, 11 mg/kg up to a maximum of 1 g.[63, 64] Intestinal or biliary obstruction may require endoscopic or surgical intervention.

Toxocariasis

Toxocara canis and *T. cati* infect dogs and cats, respectively. Infection occurs worldwide, especially in children, and is acquired when embryonated eggs are ingested from soil or contaminated food. The eggs hatch in the small intestine and release larvae that penetrate the intestinal wall, enter the portal circulation, and reach the liver and systemic circulation. Blocked by narrowing vascular channels, the immature worms bore through vessel walls and migrate through the tissues, leading to hemorrhagic, necrotic, and secondary inflammatory responses. When larvae become trapped in tissue, they provoke granuloma formation with a predominance of eosinophils. Tissue larvae may remain within inflammatory capsules or granulomas for months to years.[57] The liver, brain, and eye are most frequently affected.

Clinical Presentation

Most infected persons are asymptomatic. Two clinical syndromes are recognized: visceral larva migrans; and occult infections associated with nonspecific symptoms, including abdominal pain, anorexia, fever, and wheezing.[65]

Visceral larva migrans is seen most commonly in children with a history of pica. Findings include fever, hepatomegaly, urticaria, leukocytosis with persistent eosinophilia, hypergammaglobulinemia, and elevated blood group isohemagglutinins.[66] Pulmonary manifestations include asthma and pneumonitis. Neurologic involvement can result in focal or generalized seizures, encephalopathy, and abnormal behavior.[66] Ocular larva migrans is often associated with visual loss and strabismus and can present as a unilateral raised retinal lesion that resembles an ocular tumor.

Diagnosis

The diagnosis should be considered in persons with a history of pica, exposure to dogs or cats, and persistent eosinophilia. Stool studies are not useful for toxocariasis, because these organisms do not produce eggs in humans nor do they remain in the gastrointestinal tract. A definitive diagnosis is made by identification of the larvae in affected tissues, although blind biopsies are not routinely recommended.[67] A liver biopsy may be necessary to differentiate visceral larva migrans from hepatic capillariasis (see later section). A strongly positive result on the ELISA using larval antigens provides support for the diagnosis.

Treatment

Treatment is primarily supportive. Diethylcarbamazine, 3 mg/kg three times daily for 21 days; or thiabendazole, 50 mg/kg/day for 5 days, can be given to kill larvae and prevent migration. Alternatively albendazole, 5 to 10 mg/kg/day for 5 days, is better tolerated.[68, 69] Significant pulmonary, cardiac, ophthalmologic, or neurologic manifestations may warrant use of systemic glucocorticoids.[68]

Hepatic Capillariasis

Human infection with *Capillaria hepatica* is rare. Infection with *C. hepatica* is acquired by ingesting soil, food, or water contaminated with embryonated eggs. Larvae released in the cecum penetrate the intestinal mucosa, enter the portal venous circulation, and lodge in the liver. Four weeks after infection, adult worms disintegrate, releasing eggs into the hepatic parenchyma and producing an intense inflammatory reaction with macrophages, eosinophils, and giant cells. Resolution is accompanied by marked peri-egg fibrosis.

Clinical Presentation

Hepatic capillariasis typically presents as acute or subacute hepatitis. Findings include fever, nausea, vomiting, diarrhea or constipation, anorexia, myalgias, arthralgias, tender hepatomegaly, and occasionally splenomegaly. Laboratory investigation may reveal leukocytosis with eosinophilia; mild elevations of serum aspartate aminotransferase, alkaline phosphatase, and bilirubin levels; anemia; and an increased erythrocyte sedimentation rate. A chest radiograph may show pneumonitis.[70]

Diagnosis

The diagnosis is established by detection of adult worms or eggs in the liver (Fig. 69–4). Histologic findings in the liver include necrosis, fibrosis, and granuloma formation.[70] A finding of *C. hepatica* eggs in stool is not indicative of acute infection and likely reflects passage of undercooked liver from an infected animal.

Treatment

Treatment of hepatic capillariasis has, in general, been unsuccessful. Anecdotal benefit has been reported with dithiazanine iodide, sodium stibogluconate, and thiabendazole.[71]

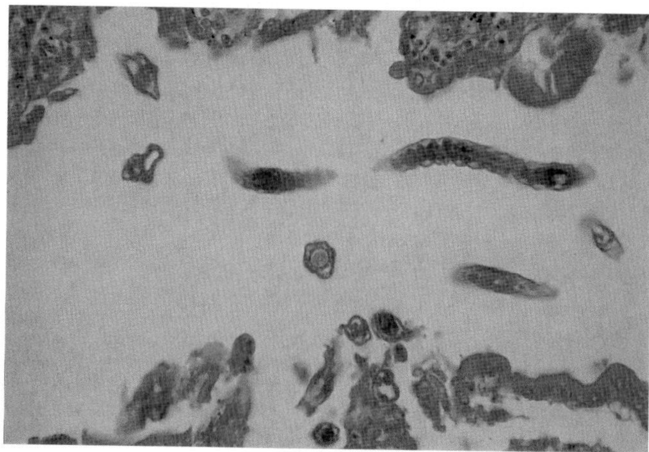

Figure 69–4. A liver biopsy specimen demonstrating *Capillaria hepatica* organisms (80×, hematoxyline-eosin stain). (Courtesy of Dr. Fiona Graeme-Cook, Massachusetts General Hospital, Boston.)

Strongyloidiasis

Strongyloides stercoralis is prevalent in the tropics and subtropics, southern and eastern Europe, and the United States. Infection is usually asymptomatic (see also Chapter 99). Humans are infected by the filariform larvae, which penetrate intact skin, are carried to the lungs, migrate through the alveoli, and are swallowed to reach the intestine, where maturation ensues. Autoinfection can occur if the rhabditiform larvae transform into infective filariform larvae in the intestine; reinfection occurs by penetration of the bowel wall or perianal skin. Symptomatic infection results from a heavy infectious burden or infection in an immunocompromised patient. In the latter case, a hyperinfection syndrome may result from dissemination of filariform larvae into tissues not usually infected.[72]

Clinical Presentation

Acute infection can lead to a pruritic eruption followed by fever, cough, wheezing, abdominal pain, diarrhea, and eosinophilia. In immunocompromised patients, the hyperinfection syndrome may be characterized by invasion of any organ, including the liver, lung, and brain. When the liver is affected, jaundice and cholestatic liver function test abnormalities can be seen. A liver biopsy specimen may show periportal inflammation, eosinophilic granulomatous hepatitis, or both. Larvae may be observed in intrahepatic bile canaliculi, lymphatic vessels, and small branches of the portal vein.[72]

Diagnosis

Serologic tests include counterimmunoelectrophoresis and ELISA, but the diagnosis rests on the identification of larvae in the stool or intestinal biopsy specimens. An obstructive hepatobiliary picture in a person with known strongyloidiasis should alert the clinician to the possibility of dissemination.

Treatment

For acute infection, the drug of choice is ivermectin 200 μg/kg/day for 2 days. Clearance rates are high. An alternative is albendazole 400 mg/day for 3 days for adults and children older than 2 years of age, but re-treatment may be necessary, and this drug is less effective for disseminated disease. The hyperinfection syndrome requires longer courses of treatment than does the primary acute infection.[72]

Trichinosis

Humans may be infected with *Trichinella spiralis* by eating raw or undercooked pork bearing larvae, which are released in the small intestine, penetrate the mucosa, and disseminate through the systemic circulation (see also Chapter 99). Larvae can be found in the myocardium, cerebrospinal fluid, brain, and, less commonly, liver and gallbladder. The larvae then re-enter the circulation and reach striated muscle, where they become encapsulated.

Clinical Presentation

Clinical manifestations occur when the worm burden is high and include diarrhea, fever, myalgias, periorbital edema, and leukocytosis with marked eosinophilia. Rarely, larvae can be seen invading hepatic sinusoids on a liver biopsy specimen. Jaundice due to biliary obstruction may occur.

Diagnosis

The diagnosis is suggested by a characteristic history in a patient with fever and eosinophilia. Serologic studies for antibody to *Trichinella* may not be helpful in the acute phase of infection but can be useful after 2 weeks.[73] Muscle biopsy may help to confirm the diagnosis. DNA-based tests are investigational.

Treatment

Treatment consists of corticosteroids to relieve allergic symptoms followed by antihelminthic treatment with albendazole 400 mg/day for 3 days or mebendazole 200 mg/day for 5 days.[73]

Trematodes (Flukes)

Blood Flukes: Schistosomiasis (Bilharziasis)

About 200 million persons are infected with trematodes of the genus *Schistosoma* worldwide (see also Chapter 99). *S. mansoni* is found in the western hemisphere, Africa, and the Middle East; *S. haematobium* is found in Africa and the Middle East; *S. japonicum* and *S. mekongi* are found in the Far East; and *S. intercalatum* is found in parts of central Africa. The last two species are much less common than the other three and cause liver disease and colonic disease, respectively.[47]

The infectious cycle is initiated by penetration of the skin

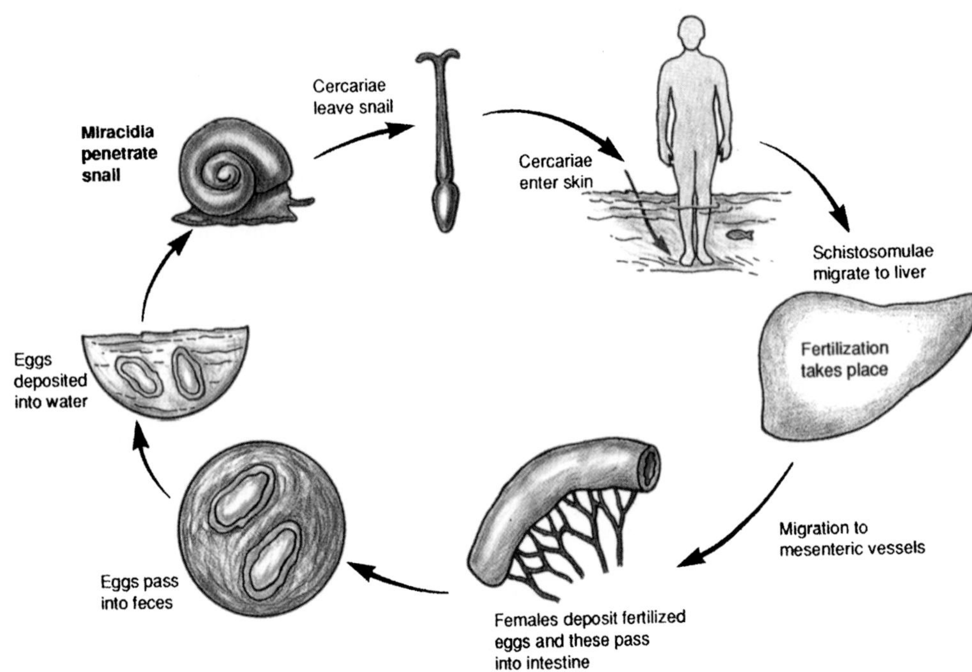

Figure 69–5. The life cycle of *Schistosoma* species (From Gitlin N, Strauss R: Atlas of Clinical Hepatology. Philadelphia, WB Saunders, 1995, p 72.)

by free cercariae in fresh water (Fig. 69–5). The cercariae reach the pulmonary vessels within 24 hours, pass through the lungs, and reach the liver, where they lodge, develop into adults, and mate. Adult worms then migrate to their ultimate destinations in the inferior mesenteric venules (*S. mansoni*), superior mesenteric venules (*S. japonicum*), or the veins around the bladder (*S. haematobium*). These locations correlate with the clinical complications associated with each species. Each female fluke can lay 300 to 3000 eggs daily. The eggs are deposited in the terminal venules and eventually migrate into the lumen of the involved organ, after which they are expelled in the stool or urine. Eggs remaining in the organ provoke a robust granulomatous response. Excreted eggs hatch immediately in fresh water, liberating early intermediate miracidia, which infect their snail hosts. The miracidia transform into cercariae within the snails and are then released into the water from which they may again infect humans.[74]

CLINICAL PRESENTATION. Acute toxemic schistosomiasis (Katayama syndrome), presumably a consequence of the host immunologic response to mature worms and eggs, occurs about 4 to 6 weeks after exposure. Manifestations include headache, fever, chills, cough, diarrhea, myalgias, arthralgias, tender hepatomegaly, and eosinophilia.

Untreated acute schistosomiasis invariably progresses to chronic disease. Mesenteric infection leads to hepatic complications, including periportal fibrosis, presinusoidal occlusion, and, ultimately, portal hypertension, as a result of the inflammatory reaction to eggs deposited in the liver. The lungs and central nervous system may be affected when eggs or adult worms pass via the liver into the systemic circulation, especially in *S. japonicum* infection; pulmonary hypertension and cor pulmonale may result.[45] With severe schistosomal infection, portal hypertension becomes progressive, leading to gastroesophageal varices, splenomegaly, and rarely ascites.

Chronic schistosomal infection may be complicated by increased susceptibility to *Salmonella* infections.[45] Hepatitis B viral coinfection is also common in persons living in endemic areas and may accelerate the progression of liver disease and the development of hepatocellular carcinoma.[45] In African intestinal schistosomiasis, pseudopolyps of the colon may develop, leading in some cases to protein-losing enteropathy and an inflammatory mass in the descending colon.

Laboratory findings of chronic schistosomiasis include anemia from recurrent luminal gastrointestinal bleeding or hypersplenism, leukocytosis with eosinophilia, an elevated erythrocyte sedimentation rate, and increased serum IgE levels. Liver biochemical tests are generally normal until the disease is at an advanced stage.

DIAGNOSIS. The diagnosis of acute schistosomiasis should be considered in a patient with a history of exposure, abdominal pain, diarrhea, and fever. Multiple stool examinations for ova may be required to confirm the diagnosis, because results are frequently negative in the early phase of disease. Serologic testing using counterimmunoelectrophoresis or ELISA has proved useful for early diagnosis.[75] Sigmoidoscopy or colonoscopy may reveal rectosigmoid or transverse colonic involvement and may be useful in chronic disease when few eggs pass in the feces. Ultrasonography and liver biopsy are useful for demonstrating periportal (or "pipestem") fibrosis (Fig. 69–6) but not for diagnosing acute infection, due to their insensitivity for visualizing schistosomal eggs.

TREATMENT. Praziquantel, 60 mg/kg given in 1 day in three divided doses 4 hours apart, is the treatment of choice. Oxamniquine, 15 to 60 mg/kg for 1 to 2 days, is an effec-

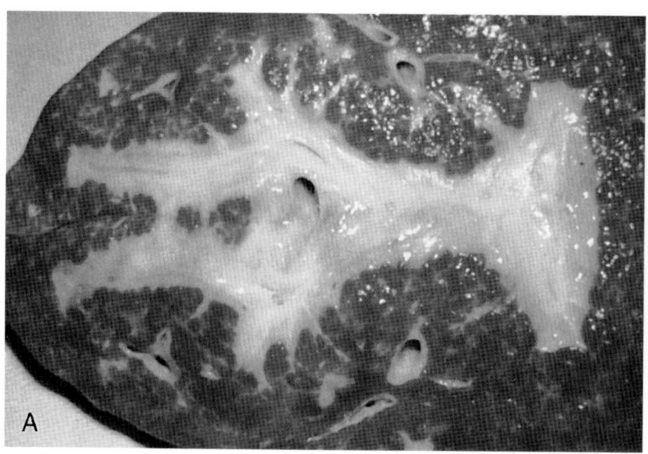

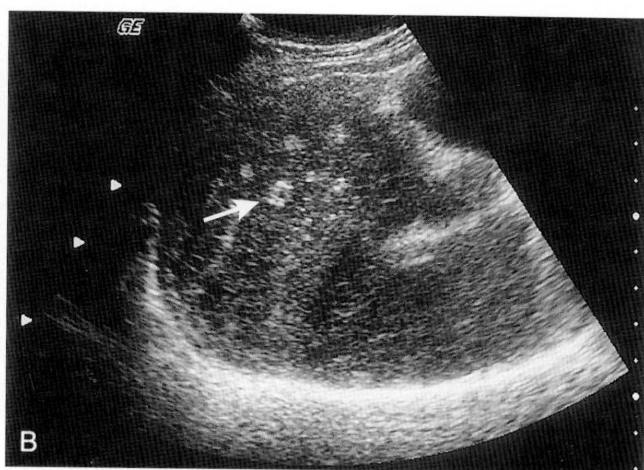

Figure 69–6. *A,* Gross liver resection specimen demonstrating characteristic pipestem fibrosis due to long-term infection with *Schistosoma mansoni.* (Courtesy of Dr. Fiona Graeme-Cook, Massachusetts General Hospital, Boston.) *B,* Ultrasound scan of liver from a patient with schistosomiasis demonstrating the pipestem fibrosis as echodense circles surrounding vessels (*arrow*). (Courtesy of Mark Feldman, Dallas VA Medical Center, Dallas, TX.)

tive alternative regimen in patients who cannot tolerate praziquantel. Treatment of acute toxemic schistosomiasis requires praziquantel, 75 mg/kg in 1 day in three divided doses, in some cases with prednisone for the prior 2 to 3 days to suppress immune-mediated helminthicidal or drug reactions.[47]

Band ligation and injection sclerotherapy of varices is effective in controlling variceal bleeding. Management of advanced chronic schistosomal liver disease may require a distal splenorenal shunt with or without splenopancreatic disconnection or esophagogastric devascularization with splenectomy. Fortunately, since the advent of praziquantel, complicated schistosomal liver disease has become uncommon.

Liver Flukes: Fascioliasis

Fascioliasis is endemic in parts of Europe and Latin America, North Africa, Asia, the Western Pacific, and some parts of the United States (see also Chapter 99). Fascioliasis is caused by the sheep liver fluke *Fasciola hepatica*. Eggs passed in the feces of infected mammals into fresh water give rise to miracidia that penetrate snails and eventually emerge as mobile cercariae, which attach to aquatic plants such as watercress. Hosts become infected when they consume plants containing encysted metacercariae, which then bore into the intestinal wall, enter the abdominal cavity, penetrate the hepatic capsule, and eventually settle in the bile ducts, where they attain maturity. Mature flukes release eggs that are passed in the host's feces to complete the life cycle.[76]

CLINICAL PRESENTATION. Three syndromes are recognized: acute or invasive, chronic latent, and chronic obstructive.[45] The acute phase corresponds to the migration of young flukes through the liver and is marked by fever, pain in the right upper quadrant, and eosinophilia. Urticaria with dermatographia and nonspecific gastrointestinal symptoms are common. A physical examination often reveals fever and a tender, enlarged liver. Splenomegaly is seen in up to 25% of cases, but jaundice is rare and liver biochemical test abnormalities are mild. Eosinophilia can be profound, sometimes exceeding 80% of the differential leukocyte count.[76]

The latent phase corresponds with the settling of the flukes into the bile ducts and can last for months to years. Affected patients may experience vague gastrointestinal symptoms. Eosinophilia persists, and fever can occur.

The chronic obstructive phase is a consequence of intrahepatic and extrahepatic bile ductal inflammation and hyperplasia evoked by adult flukes. Recurrent biliary colic, cholangitis, cholelithiasis, and biliary obstruction may result. Blood loss from epithelial injury occurs, but overt hemobilia is rare. Liver biochemical testing commonly demonstrates a pattern suggestive of biliary obstruction.[76] Long-term infection may lead to biliary cirrhosis and secondary sclerosing cholangitis, but there is no convincing association with biliary tract or hepatic malignancy.[77, 78]

DIAGNOSIS. The diagnosis should be considered in patients with prolonged fever, abdominal pain, diarrhea, tender hepatomegaly, and eosinophilia. Because eggs are not passed during the acute phase, diagnosis depends on the detection of antibody by counterimmunoelectrophoresis or ELISA. In the latent and chronic phases, a definitive diagnosis is based on the detection of eggs in stool, duodenal aspirate specimens, or bile. On occasion, ultrasonography or ERCP will demonstrate flukes in the gallbladder and common bile duct.[78, 79, 80]

Hepatic histologic findings include necrosis and granuloma formation with eosinophilic infiltrates and Charcot-Leyden crystals. Eosinophilic abscesses, epithelial hyperplasia of the bile ducts, and periportal fibrosis may be seen.[76]

TREATMENT. The drug of choice is bithionol, a halogenated phenol derivative, 50 mg/kg/day for ten doses. Intramuscular dehydroemetine, 1 mg/kg/day for 14 doses, is also effective but is more toxic (associated with cardiac, gastrointestinal, and hepatic reactions). Both drugs are available only through the Centers for Disease Control and Prevention. Encouraging preliminary reports support the eventual use of a single dose of the benzimidazole derivative triclabendazole.[81] Praziquantel is not effective for fascioliasis.

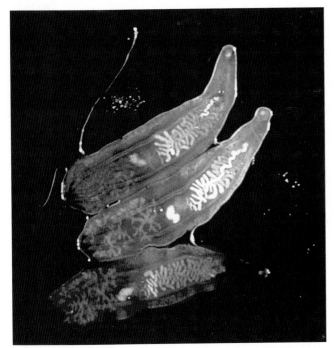

Figure 69–7. The fluke of *Clonorchis sinensis.* (Courtesy of Dr. Fiona Graeme-Cook, Massachusetts General Hospital, Boston.)

Liver Flukes: Clonorchiasis and Opisthorchiasis

Clonorchis sinensis, *Opisthorchis viverrini*, and *O. felineus* are trematodes of the family Opisthorchioideae (see also Chapter 99). Infection by *C. sinensis* and *O. viverrini* is widespread in East and Southeast Asia and is linked to lower socioeconomic status. *O. felineus* infects humans and domestic animals in eastern Europe. All three have similar life cycles and result in similar clinical manifestations. Eggs are passed in the feces into fresh water, consumed by snails, and hatch as free-swimming cercariae, which seek and penetrate fish or crayfish, encysting in skin or muscle as metacercariae. The mammalian host is infected when it consumes raw or undercooked fish. The metacercariae excyst in the small bowel and migrate into the ampulla of Vater and into the bile ducts, where they mature into adult flukes. Infection can be maintained for two decades or longer.[82]

CLINICAL PRESENTATION. In general, acute infection is clinically silent. Occasional symptoms include fever, abdominal pain, and diarrhea. Chronic manifestations correlate with the fluke burden and are dominated by hepatobiliary features: fever, pain in the right upper quadrant, tender hepatomegaly, and eosinophilia. If the worm burden in the bile ducts is heavy, chronic or intermittent biliary obstruction can ensue, with frequent cholelithiasis, cholecystitis, jaundice, and, ultimately, recurrent cholangitis (recurrent pyogenic cholangitis is described in Chapter 59). Liver biochemical tests, especially serum alkaline phosphatase and bilirubin levels, are elevated. Long-standing infection leads to exuberant inflammation, resulting in periportal fibrosis, marked biliary epithelial hyperplasia and dysplasia, and, ultimately, a substantially increased risk of cholangiocarcinoma.[78] Cholangiocarcinoma resulting from clonorchiasis or opisthorchiasis tends to be multicentric and arises in the secondary biliary radicles of the hilum of the liver.[78] Cholangiocarcinoma should be suspected in infected persons with weight loss, jaundice, epigastric pain, or an abdominal mass.

DIAGNOSIS. The diagnosis of clonorchiasis or opisthorchiasis is made by detection of characteristic fluke eggs in the stool, except late in the disease, when biliary obstruction has supervened. In these cases, the diagnosis is made by identifying flukes in the bile ducts or gallbladder at surgery or in bile obtained by postoperative drainage or percutaneous aspiration (Fig. 69–7). Endoscopic or intraoperative cholangiography reveals slender, uniform filling defects within intrahepatic ducts that are alternately dilated and strictured, mimicking sclerosing cholangitis. Serologic methods of diagnosis are generally not helpful.[77, 83]

TREATMENT. All patients with clonorchiasis or opisthorchiasis should be treated with praziquantel, which is uniformly effective in a dose of 75 mg/kg in three divided doses over 1 day. Side effects are uncommon and include headache, dizziness, and nausea. After treatment, dead flukes may be seen in the stool or biliary drainage. When the burden of infecting organisms is high, the dead flukes and surrounding debris or stones may cause biliary obstruction, necessitating endoscopic or surgical drainage.[77]

Cestodes (Tapeworms)

Echinococcus

Infections with *Echinococcus granulosus* can be found worldwide in areas where dogs are used to help raise livestock (see also Chapter 81). *E. multilocularis* is distributed in northern North America and Eurasia, whereas *E. vogeli* is found in scattered areas of Central and Latin America. Infection occurs when humans eat vegetables contaminated by dog feces containing embryonated eggs. The eggs hatch in the small intestine and liberate oncospheres that penetrate the mucosa and migrate via vessels or lymphatics to distant sites. The liver is the most common destination (70%), followed by the lungs (20%), kidney, spleen, brain, and bone. In these organs, the hydatid cyst develops by vesiculation, resulting in the production of thousands of protoscolices. The cyst wall contains three layers: an outer adventitial layer, which is host-derived and can calcify, and an intermediate acellular layer and an inner germinal layer, which are worm-derived. A protoscolex is produced asexually within small secondary cysts that develop from the inner layer. Rupture of the hydatid cyst releases the viable protoscolices, which set up daughter cysts in secondary sites. Dogs acquire the infection by consuming organs of sheep, cattle, or other livestock bearing the hydatid cyst.

CLINICAL PRESENTATION. As the cysts of *E. granulosus* grow within the liver (Fig. 69–8), they begin to cause low-grade fever, tender hepatomegaly (usually the right hepatic lobe), and eosinophilia. If the cysts grow large enough, they may rupture into the lungs, leading to dyspnea and hemoptysis. More extensive rupture into the peritoneum or lungs may lead to a life-threatening anaphylactic reaction to the cyst contents. Rupture into the biliary tract can cause cholangitis and obstruction. Superinfection of the hepatic cysts

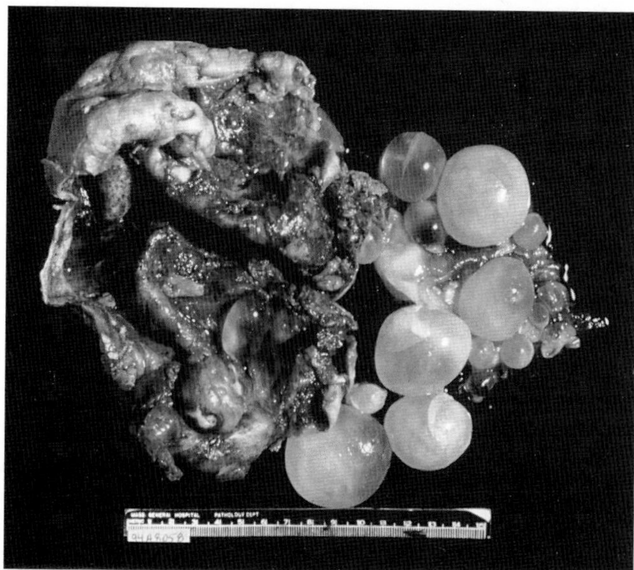

Figure 69–8. Gross liver resection specimen of a hydatid cyst due to *Echinococcus granulosus.* Multiple daughter cysts can be readily appreciated. (Courtesy of Dr. Fiona Graeme-Cook, Massachusetts General Hospital, Boston.)

can lead to pyogenic liver abscesses in up to 20% of patients with hepatic disease. In fact, echinococcal disease is the most common cause of pyogenic hepatic abscess in Greece and Spain.[84, 85]

E. multilocularis is highly invasive and leads to solid masses in the liver that are easily confused with cirrhosis or carcinoma. Alveolar hydatid disease is the term applied to hepatic nodules that appear on microscopy as alveolus-like microvesicles.[86] Unfortunately, infection is generally not diagnosed until the lesions are inoperable due to extensive invasion or distant metastatic disease,[86] and mortality rates are high, approaching 90%.[86]

Infection with *E. vogeli* has clinical features intermediate between those of the other two species and is characterized by multiple fluid-filled cysts containing daughter cysts and protoscolices. Although not as aggressive as *E. multilocularis*, *E. vogeli* can spread to contiguous sites.

DIAGNOSIS. A history of exposure in a patient with hepatomegaly and an abdominal mass is highly suggestive of hepatic echinococcosis, but the most important diagnostic tools are radiography and serology. Ring-like calcifications in up to one fourth of hepatic cysts are visible on plain abdominal radiographs in patients infected with *E. granulosus*. The sensitivity and specificity of both ultrasonography and CT in confirming the diagnosis are high.[85, 87] Both modalities can demonstrate intracystic septations and daughter cyst formation in about one half of the cysts.[88, 89] Contrast-enhanced CT may display avascular cysts with ring enhancement. Percutaneous aspiration of the cyst has traditionally been discouraged because of concern about anaphylactic reactions. However, encouraging reports suggest that under carefully controlled conditions with use of thin needles and concomitant antihelminthic therapy, percutaneous aspiration for diagnosis and therapy may be safe. The detection of protoscolices or acid-fast hooklets in the cyst fluid confirms the diagnosis.[90] Both an ELISA and an indirect hemagglutination assay may also be used for diagnosis, with a sensitivity of 90%.[45] Assays for detecting circulating antigen are likely to provide additional diagnostic benefit in the future. The Casoni skin test, used in the past, is nonspecific and no longer recommended.

E. multilocularis infection can be diagnosed with a combination of ELISA and CT, which often shows scattered areas of calcified necrotic tissue. In *E. vogeli* infection, CT demonstrates polycystic lesions in the liver or peritoneal space.

TREATMENT. Until recently, accessible cysts in younger persons have been treated surgically. The goal has been removal of the cestode without disruption of cyst contents. Successful approaches have included cystectomy, endocystectomy, omentoplasty, and marsupialization. In complicated cases, hepatic lobectomy or hemihepatectomy may be necessary. Promising data indicate that careful percutaneous drainage is a safe and effective alternative to surgery for the treatment of complicated cysts.[91] In addition to surgery or drainage, administration of an antihelminthic, such as albendazole, 10 mg/kg/day for 8 weeks, is recommended.[91, 92] A recent report from Italy has demonstrated that *p*uncture, *a*spiration, *i*njection (of a scolicidal agent), and *r*e-aspiration (PAIR) can be performed safely with long-term control of echinococcal cysts.[93]

Surgical resection is curative in up to one third of cases of *E. multilocularis* infection. In most cases the disease is advanced when the diagnosis is made. In such cases, palliative drainage procedures or long-term treatment with albendazole may increase the chance of survival.[86] Surgery appears to be the most effective approach for *E. vogeli* infection.

FUNGAL LIVER DISEASE

Candidiasis

Candida species may cause invasive systemic infection with hepatic involvement in severely immunocompromised persons. The liver can become infected by *C. albicans* in the setting of disseminated, multiorgan disease. Most disseminated infections occur in leukemic patients undergoing high-dose chemotherapy and become manifest during the period of recovery from severe neutropenia. In several series of predominantly leukemic patients, hepatic candidiasis was present in 51% to 91% of patients.[6, 94] Disease is often overwhelming, with high mortality rates.[94]

Other less frequent presentations in the compromised host are isolated or focal hepatic candidiasis or hepatosplenic candidiasis.[95] Focal candidiasis is thought to result from colonization of the gastrointestinal tract by *Candida*, which disseminates locally following the onset of neutropenia and mucosal injury caused by high-dose chemotherapy.[95] Resultant fungemia of the portal vein seeds the liver and leads to hepatic microabscesses and macroabscesses.

In either focal or disseminated candidiasis involving the liver, clinical features include fever, abdominal pain and distention, nausea, vomiting, diarrhea, and tender hepatomegaly. The serum alkaline phosphatase level is almost invariably elevated, with variable elevations in serum aminotransferase and bilirubin levels. CT of the abdomen is the most sensitive test to detect hepatic or splenic abscesses, which are often multicentric.[96] In cases diagnosed ante-mortem, liver biopsy or laparoscopy reveals macroscopic nodules, necrosis with microabscess formation, and characteristic yeast or hyphal forms of *Candida*.[96, 97] The results of cultures of biopsy material are negative in most cases.

Response rates to therapy with intravenous amphotericin B 0.8 to 1.0 mg/kg/d IV are better (almost 60%) for focal hepatic candidiasis than for disseminated disease. However, the success of treatment is currently far from optimal. Alternatives to amphotericin B are fluconazole 800 mg/d IV and liposomal amphotericin 5 mg/kg/d IV.

Histoplasmosis

Infection with *Histoplasma capsulatum* is acquired through the respiratory tract and, in most cases, confined to the lungs. However, severely immunocompromised persons (e.g., those with AIDS) are predisposed to disseminated histoplasmosis. The liver can be invaded in both acute and chronic progressive disseminated histoplasmosis. Fever, oropharyngeal ulcers, hepatomegaly, and splenomegaly may be present in chronic disease.[98] In children with acute hepatic disease, which appears to be an extension of primary pulmonary infection, marked hepatosplenomegaly is universal and is associated with high fever and lymphadenopathy. Serum alanine aminotransferase and alkaline phosphatase levels are often elevated. Hepatosplenomegaly is present in approximately 30% of adults with acute disease (often the AIDS-defining illness).

Yeast forms can be identified in sections of liver biopsy specimens with standard hematoxylin and eosin staining. The silver methenamine method is superior for detecting yeast forms in areas of caseating necrosis or granuloma formation. The organism is difficult to culture and almost never grows from biopsy specimens. Serologic testing for complement-fixing antibodies is therefore helpful in confirming the diagnosis. In immunocompromised persons who may not be capable of mounting an antibody response, detection of *H. capsulatum* antigens in urine and serum can be useful.[98]

GRANULOMATOUS LIVER DISEASE

Hepatic granulomas represent a complex interplay between the presenting antigen and the host immune response. They are found in a wide variety of disorders and in 2% to 10% of all liver biopsy specimens[99] (Table 69–5). Poorly degraded antigens or drugs provide the nidus for granuloma formation. The center consists of epithelioid and giant cells and $CD4^+$ helper T cells. The periphery consists of antigen-presenting macrophages associated with $CD8^+$ cytotoxic T lymphocytes. Eventually, the granuloma becomes infiltrated by fibroblasts with deposition of a fibrous capsule. There may or may not be central caseation and necrosis. Granulomas caused by some entities have distinctive histologic characteristics, such as lipogranulomas caused by ingestion of mineral oil and fibrin-ring granulomas caused by Q fever.[100]

The liver is a common site for granuloma formation, because of its rich blood supply and large number of reticuloendothelial cells. Although granulomas can be found anywhere in the liver, they are usually located near portal tracts. There is usually little perturbation of hepatic function, and most patients are minimally symptomatic or asymptomatic.

A suggested workup for granulomatous liver disease in-

Table 69–5 | **Causes of Hepatic Granulomas**

INFECTIOUS	NEOPLASTIC	MEDICATIONS	MISCELLANEOUS
Bacteria			
Tuberculosis	Hodgkin's disease	Allopurinol	Sarcoidosis
Mycobacterium avium complex	Non-Hodkin's lymphoma	Carbamazepine	Primary biliary cirrhosis
Brucellosis	Renal cell carcinoma	Chlorpropamide	Berylliosis
Tularemia		Diltiazem	Talc
Listeriosis		Gold	Whipple's disease
Lepromatous leprosy		Halothane	Inflammatory bowel disease
BCG		Hydralazine	Wegener's granulomatosis
Syphilis (secondary)		Methyldopa	Lymphomatoid granulomatosis
Viruses		Nitrofurantoin	Idiopathic
Cytomegalovirus		Penicillin	
Epstein-Barr virus		Phenylbutazone	
Fungi		Phenytoin	
Histoplasmosis		Procainamide	
Coccidioidomycosis		Quinidine	
Cryptococcosis		Quinine	
Parasites		Sulfonamides	
Toxoplasmosis			
Schistosomiasis			
Visceral larva migrans			
Fascioliasis			
Hepatic capillariasis			
Ascariasis			
Rickettsioses			
Coxiella burnetii (Q fever)			

BCG, bacille Calmette-Guérin.

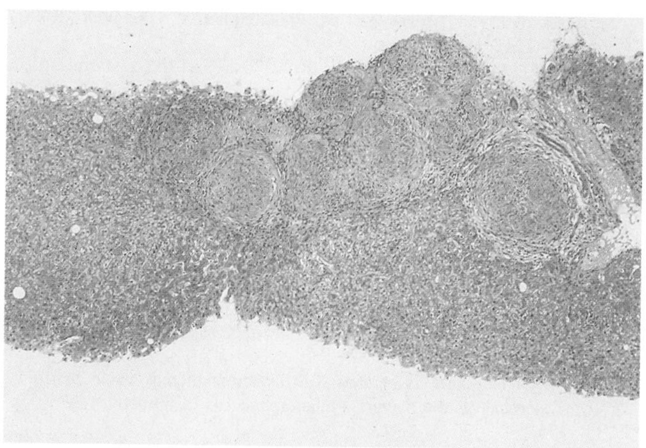

Figure 69–9. A liver biopsy specimen demonstrating multiple granulomas in a patient with sarcoidosis (80×, trichrome stain). (Courtesy of Edward Lee, MD, Dallas VA Hospital, Dallas, TX.)

cludes chest radiography; cultures for bacteria (including *Brucella* and mycobacteria) and fungi; serologic testing for Q fever, *Brucella*, syphilis, and viral hepatitis; a tuberculin skin test; and an antimitochondrial antibody test.

Sarcoidosis

Sarcoidosis and tuberculosis account for up to 50% to 60% of cases of hepatic granulomatous disease worldwide[99] (see also Chapter 82). Noncaseating hepatic granulomas occur in 60% to 95% of patients with sarcoidosis (Fig. 69–9). Cirrhosis is uncommon. Portal hypertension may develop as a result of granulomatous phlebitis of the portal and hepatic veins,[101, 102] but variceal bleeding is rare. Occasionally, granulomatous cholangitis can lead to loss of intrahepatic bile ducts and chronic cholestasis.[102] Rare complications are hepatic vein thrombosis and biliary tract obstruction due to hilar adenopathy or bile duct strictures.[102] Serum levels of angiotensin-converting enzyme are often elevated in patients with hepatic sarcoidosis. Glucocorticoids do not appear to improve histologic findings or prevent complications. Symptomatic and biochemical improvement has been reported with ursodeoxycholic acid[103] and with methotrexate.[104] Chloroquine and azathioprine have been used as glucocorticoid-sparing agents. Rarely, liver transplantation is required.

A subset of patients, usually young black men, presents with an acute picture of fever, weight loss, jaundice, and hepatosplenomegaly. Patients with this form of sarcoid involvement of the liver have a poor prognosis.

Tuberculosis

Granulomas are found in liver biopsy specimens in about 25% of persons with pulmonary tuberculosis and 80% of those with extrapulmonary tuberculosis.[99] Tuberculous granulomas can be distinguished from sarcoid granulomas by central caseation, acid-fast bacilli, and the presence of fewer granulomas with a tendency to coalesce.[105] Multiple granulomas in the liver may also be seen following vaccination with bacille Calmette-Guérin, especially in persons with an impaired immune response. Patients with multiple granulomas due to tuberculosis rarely have clinically significant liver disease. Occasionally, tender hepatomegaly is found. Jaundice with elevated serum alkaline phosphatase levels may occur in miliary infection. The treatment of tuberculous granulomatous disease of the liver is the same as that for active pulmonary tuberculosis, namely, four-drug therapy.[105]

Granulomatous Hepatitis

The designation of granulomatous hepatitis is applied when a specific underlying cause for hepatic granulomas cannot be identified. Patients are typically middle-aged to elderly men with prolonged fever and mild elevations of liver biochemical tests. The condition often resolves spontaneously, but in prolonged cases, a short trial of glucocorticoids or low-dose oral pulse methotrexate may be warranted.[106]

Acquired Immunodeficiency Syndrome

Numerous infectious agents may cause hepatic granulomas in persons with AIDS. The most common of these is *Mycobacterium avium* complex (MAC), which typically causes fatigue, malaise, low-grade fever, night sweats, elevated serum alkaline phosphatase levels, and, less frequently, hepatomegaly. Treatment of MAC infection is of unproven value but is generally attempted in patients with systemic symptoms and positive blood culture results. Other causes of hepatic granulomas in AIDS include *M. tuberculosis*, cytomegalovirus infection (see Chapter 28), histoplasmosis (see previous section), toxoplasmosis (see previous section), and cryptococcosis, as well as lymphoma and drug reactions.[100]

BACILLARY ANGIOMATOSIS AND ACQUIRED IMMUNODEFICIENCY SYNDROME

Bacillary angiomatosis is an infectious disorder that primarily affects persons with AIDS or other immunodeficiency states. The causative agents have been identified as the gram-negative bacilli *Bartonella henselae* and, in some cases, *B. quintana*.[107] Infection is frequently associated with exposure to cats.

Bacillary angiomatosis is characterized most commonly by multiple blood-red papular skin lesions, but disseminated infection with or without skin involvement has also been described.[108] The causative bacilli can infect liver, lymph nodes, pleura, bronchi, bones, brain, bone marrow, and spleen. Additional manifestations include persistent fever, bacteremia, and sepsis. Hepatic infection should be suspected when serum aminotransferase levels are elevated in the absence of other explanations.

Hepatic infection in persons with bacillary angiomatosis may present as peliosis hepatis, or blood-filled cysts. Histologically, peliosis in patients with AIDS is characterized by an inflammatory myxoid stroma containing clumps of bacilli surrounding the blood-filled peliotic cysts. Diagnosis of *Bartonella* infection by polymerase chain reaction–based methods is being used more often.[109]

Bacillary angiomatosis responds uniformly to therapy

with erythromycin. For visceral infection, at least 6 weeks of treatment with erythromycin, 500 mg four times daily, or doxycycline should be administered.

REFERENCES

1. Srivasta ED, Mayberry JF: Pyogenic liver abscess: A review of etiology, diagnosis, an intervention. Dig Dis 8:287, 1990.
2. Rockey DC: Hepatobiliary infections. Curr Opin Gastroenterol 17:257, 2001.
3. Yeh TS, Jan YY, Leng LB: Hepatocellular carcinoma presenting as pyogenic liver abscess: Characteristics, diagnosis, and management. Clin Infect Dis 26:1224, 1998.
4. Crippin JS, Wang KK: An unrecognized etiology for pyogenic hepatic abscesses in normal hosts: Dental disease. Am J Gastroenterol 7:1740, 1992.
5. Brook I, Frazier EH: Microbiology of liver and spleen abscesses. J Med Microbiol 47:1075, 1998.
6. Lipsett PA, Huang C-J, Lillemoe KD, et al: Fungal hepatic abscesses: Characterization and management. J Gastrointest Surg 1:78, 1997.
7. Barnes PF, DeCock KM, Reynolds TN, et al: A comparison of amebic and pyogenic abscesses of the liver. Medicine 66:472, 1987.
8. Lam YH, Wong SK, Lee DW, et al: ERCP and pyogenic liver abscess. Gastrointest Endosc 50:340, 1999.
9. Barakate MS, Stephen MS, Waugh RC: Pyogenic liver abscess: A review of 10 years' experience. Aust NZ J Surg 69:205, 1999.
10. Hung CC, Chen PJ, Hsieh SM, et al: Invasive amoebiasis: An emerging parasitic disease in patients with HIV in an area endemic for amoebic infection. AIDS 13:2421, 1999.
11. Cunha BA: Clinical features of legionnaires' disease. Semin Respir Infect 13:116, 1998.
12. Stevens DL: The toxic shock syndromes. Infect Dis Clin North Am 10:727, 1996.
13. Meer RR, Songer JG, Park DL: Human disease associated with Clostridium perfringens enterotoxin. Rev Environ Contam Toxicol 150:75, 1997.
14. Yu VL, Miller WP, Wing EJ, et al: Disseminated listeriosis presenting as acute hepatitis. Am J Med 73:773, 1982.
15. Hof H, Nichterlein T, Kretschmar M: Management of listeriosis. Clin Microbiol Rev 10:345, 1997.
16. Holmes KK, Counts GW, Beaty HN: Disseminated gonococcal infection. Ann Intern Med 74:979, 1971.
17. Ross JD: Systemic gonococcal infection. Genitourin Med 72:404, 1996.
18. Leelarasamee A: Melioidosis in southeast Asia. Acta Trop 74:129, 2000.
19. Stern MS, Gitnick GL: Shigella hepatitis. JAMA 235:2628, 1976.
20. Nasrallah SM, Nassar VH: Enteric fever: A clinicopathologic study of 104 cases. Am J Gastroenterol 69:63, 1978.
21. Pramoolsinsap C, Viranuvatti V: Salmonella hepatitis. J Gastroenterol Hepatol 13:745, 1998.
22. Strungs I, Farrell DH, Matar LD, et al: Multiple hepatic abscesses due to Yersinia enterocolitica. Pathology 27:374, 1995.
23. Vadilla M, Corbella X, Pac V, et al: Multiple liver abscesses due to Yersinia enterocolitica discloses primary hemochromatosis: Three case reports and review. Clin Infect Dis 18:938, 1994.
24. Santoro MJ, Chen YK, Seid NS, et al: Yersinia enterocolitica liver abscesses unmasking idiopathic hemochromatosis. J Clin Gastroenterol 18:253, 1994.
25. Rice PS, Kudesia G, McKendrick MW, et al: Coxiella burnetii serology in granulomatous hepatitis. J Infect 27:63, 1993.
26. Lee SMK: Viscerotropic Rocky Mountain spotted fever in Southeastern Texas. South Med J 82:640, 1989.
27. Adams JS, Walker DH: The liver in Rocky Mountain spotted fever. Am J Clin Pathol 75:156, 1981.
28. Jonas RB, Brasitus TA, Chowdhury L: Actinomycotic liver abscess. Dig Dis Sci 32:1435, 1987.
29. Weese WC, Smith IM: A study of 57 cases of actinomycosis over a 36-year period. Arch Intern Med 135:1562, 1975.
30. Miyamoto MI, Fang FC: Pyogenic liver abscess involving actinomyces: Case report and review. Clin Infect Dis 16:303, 1993.
31. Goldman IS, Farber BF, Brandborg LL: Bacterial and miscellaneous infections of the liver. In Zakim DS, Boyer TD (eds): Hepatology: A Textbook of Liver Disease, 3rd ed. Philadelphia, WB Saunders, 1996, pp 1232–1242.
32. Ablin J, Mevorach D, Eliakim R: Brucellosis and the gastrointestinal tract. The odd couple. J Clin Gastroenterol 24:25, 1997.
33. Roelofsen H, Schoemaker B, Bakker C, et al: Impaired hepatocanalicular organic anion transport in endotoxemic rats. Am J Physiol 269: G427, 1995.
34. Moseley RH: Sepsis-associated jaundice. Hepatology 24:969, 1996.
35. Sperber SJ, Schleupner CJ: Leptospirosis. South Med J 82:1285, 1989.
36. Feigin RD, Anderson DC: Human leptospirosis. CRC Crit Rev Clin Lab Sci 5:413, 1975.
37. Baker A, Kaplan M, Wolfe H, et al: Liver disease associated with early syphilis. N Engl J Med 284:1422, 1971.
38. Feher J, Somogyi T, Timmer M, et al: Early syphilitic hepatitis. Lancet 2:896, 1978.
39. Klatskin G: Hepatitis associated with systemic infections. In Schiff L (ed): Diseases of the Liver. Philadelphia, JB Lippincott, 1975, pp 711–754.
40. Steere AC, Bartenhagen NH, Craft JE, et al: The early clinical manifestations of Lyme disease. Ann Intern Med 99:76, 1983.
41. Nadelman RB, Wormser GP: Lyme borreliosis. Lancet 352:557, 1998.
42. Goellner MH, Agger WA, Burgess JJ, Duray PH: Hepatitis due to recurrent Lyme disease. Ann Intern Med 108:707, 1988.
43. World Health Organization: WHO expert committee on malaria: 18th report. World Health Organization, 1986.
44. Molyneux ME, Looareesuwan S, Menzies IS, et al: Reduced hepatic flow and intestinal malabsorption in severe falciparum malaria. Am J Trop Med Hyg 40:470, 1989.
45. Dunn MA: Parasitic diseases. In Schiff ER, Sorrell MF, Maddrey WC (eds): Diseases of the Liver, 8th ed. Philadelphia, Lippincott-Raven, 1999, pp 1533–1548.
46. Strickland GT: Malaria. In Strickland GT (ed): Hunter's Tropical Medicine. Philadelphia, WB Saunders, 1991, pp 586–617.
47. Murray HW, Pépin J, Nutman TB, et al: Tropical medicine. BMJ 320: 490, 2000.
48. Bates I: Hyperreactive tropical splenomegaly in pregnancy. Trop Doct 21:101, 1991.
49. Smith DH: Visceral leishmaniasis: Human aspects. In Gilles HM (ed): Recent Advances in Tropical Medicine. Edinburgh, Churchill Livingstone, 1984, pp 79–87.
50. Sen Gupta PC: The liver in kala-azar. Ann Trop Med Parasitol 50: 252, 1956.
51. Moreno A, Marazuela M, Yebra M, et al: Hepatic fibrin-ring granulomas in visceral leishmaniasis. Gastroenterology 95:1123, 1988.
52. Jha TK, Sundar S, Thakur CP, et al: Miltefosine, an oral agent, for the treatment of Indian visceral leishmaniasis. N Engl J Med 341: 1795, 1999.
53. Sever JL, Ellenberg JH, Ley AC, et al: Toxoplasmosis: Maternal and pediatric findings in 23,000 pregnancies. Pediatrics 82:181, 1988.
54. Frenkel JK: Pathophysiology of toxoplasmosis. Parasitol Today 4:273, 1988.
55. Beneson MW, Takafuji ET, Lemon SM, et al: Oocyst-transmitted toxoplasmosis associated with ingestion of contaminated water. N Engl J Med 307:666, 1982.
56. Ruskin J, Remington JS: Toxoplasmosis in the compromised host. Ann Intern Med 84:193, 1976.
57. Bryan RT, Michelson MK: Parasitic infections of the liver and biliary tree. In Surawicz C, Owen RL (eds): Gastrointestinal and Hepatic Infections. Philadelphia, WB Saunders, 1995, pp 405–454.
58. Vischer TL, Bernheim C, Engelbrecht E: Two cases of hepatitis due to Toxoplasma gondii. Lancet 2:919, 1967.
59. World Health Organization: Prevention and control of intestinal parasitic infections: Report of a WHO expert committee. World Health Organization, 1987.
60. Hlaing T: A profile of ascariasis morbidity in Rangoon Children's Hospital, Burma. J Trop Med Hyg 90:165, 1987.
61. Schulman A: Non-western patterns of biliary stones and the role of ascariasis. Radiology 162:425, 1987.
62. Uflacker R, Duarte D, Silva P: Association of congenital cystic dilatation of the common bile duct and congenital diverticulum of the hepatic duct with concomitant ascariasis. Gastrointest Radiol 3:407, 1978.
63. Khuroo MS: Ascariasis. Gastroenterol Clin North Am 3:553, 1996.
64. Cline BL: Current drug regimens for the treatment of intestinal helminth infections. Med Clin North Am 66:721, 1982.

65. Taylor MRH, Keane CT, O'Connor P, et al: The expanded spectrum of toxocaral disease. Lancet 1:692, 1988.
66. Huntley CC, Costas MC, Lyerly A: Visceral larva migrans syndrome: Clinical characteristics and immunologic studies in 51 patients. Pediatrics 36:523, 1965.
67. Nichols RL: The etiology of visceral larva migrans: I. Diagnostic morphology of infective second-stage Toxocara larvae. J Parasitol 42: 349, 1956.
68. World Health Organization: WHO model prescription information: Drugs used in parasitic diseases. World Health Organization, 1990.
69. Overgaauw PA: Aspects of Toxocara epidemiology: Human toxocarosis. Crit Rev Microbiol 23:215, 1997.
70. Grencis RK, Cooper ES: Enterobius, Trichuris, capillaria, and hookworm, including Ancylostoma caninum. Gastroenterol Clin North Am 25:579, 1996.
71. Berger T, Degremont A, Gebbers JO, et al: Hepatic capillariasis in a 1-year-old child. Eur J Pediatr 149:333, 1990.
72. Mahmoud AA: Strongyloidiasis. Clin Infect Dis 23:949, 1996.
73. Capó V, Despommier DD: Clinical aspects of infection with trichinella spp. Clin Microbiol Rev 9:47, 1996.
74. World Health Organization: The control of schistosomiasis. World Health Organization, 1985.
75. Hancock K, Tsang VCW: Development and optimization of the FAST-ELISA for detecting antibodies to Schistosoma mansoni. J Immunol 92:167, 1986.
76. Bunnag D, Thanongsak B, Goldsmith R: Fascioliasis. In Strickland GT (ed): Hunter's Tropical Medicine. Philadelphia, WB Saunders, 1991, pp 823–826.
77. Chan CW, Lam SK: Diseases caused by liver flukes and cholangiocarcinoma. In: Bailliere's Clinical Gastroenterology, vol. 1. London, Bailliere Tindall, 1987, pp 297–318.
78. Osman M, Lausten SB, El-Sefi T, et al: Biliary parasites. Dig Surg 15:287, 1998.
79. Takeyama N, Nobuyoshi O, Sakai Y, et al: Computed tomography findings of hepatic lesions in human fascioliasis: Report of two cases. Am J Gastroenterol 81:1078, 1986.
80. Beers B, Pringot J, Geubel A, et al: Hepatobiliary fascioliasis: Noninvasive imaging findings. Radiology 174:809, 1990.
81. Loutan L, Bouvier M, Rojanawisut B, et al: Single treatment of invasive fascioliasis with triclabendazole. Lancet 2:383, 1989.
82. Bunnag D, Thanongsak B, Goldsmith R: Clonorchiasis. In Strickland GT (ed): Hunter's Tropical Medicine. Philadelphia, WB Saunders, 1991, pp 822–823.
83. Dennis MJS, Dennison AR, Morris DL: Parasitic causes of obstructive jaundice. Ann Trop Med Parasitol 83:159, 1989.
84. Schantz PM, Okelo GBA: Echinococcosis (hydatidosis). In Warren KS, Mahmoud AAF (eds): Tropical and Geographical Medicine. New York, McGraw-Hill, 1990, pp 505–518.
85. Schaefer JW, Khan MY: Echinococcosis (hydatid disease): Lessons from experience with 59 patients. Rev Infect Dis 13:243, 1991.
86. Akingolu A, Demiyurek H, Guzel C: Alveolar hydatid disease of the liver: A report on thirty-nine surgical cases in eastern Anatolia, Turkey. Am J Trop Med Hyg 45:182, 1991.
87. Kalovidouris A, Pissiotis C, Pontifex C, et al: CT characterization of multivesicular hydatid cysts. J Comput Assist Tomogr 10:428, 1986.
88. Filice C, Di Perri G, Strosselli M, et al: Parasitologic findings in percutaneous drainage of human hydatid liver cysts. J Infect Dis 161: 1290, 1990.
89. Mathisen GE, Sokolov RT, Meyer RD: Fever, abdominal pain and headache in an Iranian woman. Rev Infect Dis 12:529, 1990.
90. Hira PR, Lindberg LG, Francis I, et al: Diagnosis of cystic hydatid disease: Role of aspiration cytology. Lancet 1:655, 1988.
91. Khuroo MS, Wani NA, Javid G, et al: Percutaneous drainage compared with surgery for hepatic hydatid cysts. N Engl J Med 337: 881, 1997.
92. Horton RJ: Chemotherapy of Echinococcus infection in man with albendazole. Trans R Soc Trop Med Hyg 83:97, 1989.
93. Crippa FG, Bruno R, Brunetti E, Filice C: Echinococcal liver cysts: Treatment with echo-guided percutaneous puncture PAIR for echinococcal liver cysts. Ital J Gastroenterol Hepatol 31:884, 1999.
94. Myerowitz RL, Pazin GJ, Allen CM: Disseminated candidiasis: Changes in incidence, underlying diseases, and pathology. Am J Clin Pathol 68:29, 1977.
95. Tashjian LS, Abramson JS, Peacock JE: Focal hepatic candidiasis: A distinct clinical variant of candidiasis in immunocompromised patients. Rev Infect Dis 6:689, 1984.
96. Semelka RC, Shoenut JP, Greenberg HM, et al: Detection of acute and treated lesions of hepatosplenic candidiasis: Comparison of dynamic contrast-enhanced CT and MR imaging. J Magn Reson Imaging 2:341, 1992.
97. Phillips EH, Carroll BJ, Chandra M, et al: Laparoscopic-guided biopsy for diagnosis of hepatic candidiasis. J Laparoendosc Surg 2:33, 1992.
98. Bullock WE: Histoplasma capsulatum. In Mandell GL, Bennett JE, Dolin R (eds): Principles and Practice of Infectious Diseases. New York, Churchill Livingstone, 1995, pp 2340–2353.
99. Reynolds TB, Campra JL, Peters RL: Granulomatous liver disease. In Zakim D, Boyer TD (eds): Hepatology: A Textbook of Liver Diseases, 3rd ed. Philadelphia, WB Saunders, 1996, pp 1472–1489.
100. Lefkowitch JH: Hepatic granulomas. J Hepatol 30:40, 1999.
101. Moreno-Merlo F, Wanless IR, Shimamatsu K, et al: The role of granulomatous phlebitis and thrombosis n the pathogenesis of cirrhosis and portal hypertension in sarcoidosis. Hepatology 26:554, 1997.
102. Ishak KG: Sarcoidosis of the liver and bile ducts. Mayo Clin Proc 73: 467, 1998.
103. Bécheur H, Dall'osto H, Chatellier G: Effect of ursodeoxycholic acid on chronic intrahepatic cholestasis due to sarcoidosis. Dig Dis Sci 42: 789, 1997.
104. Baughman RP: Methotrexate for sarcoidosis. Sarcoidosis Vasc Diffuse Lung Dis 15:147, 1998.
105. Alvarez SZ: Hepatobiliary tuberculosis. J Gastroenterol Hepatol 13: 833, 1998.
106. Knox TA, Kaplan MM, Gelfand JA, Wolff SM: Methotrexate treatment of idiopathic granulomatous hepatitis. Ann Intern Med 122:592, 1995.
107. Tompkins DC, Steigbigel RT: Rochalimaea's role in cat scratch disease and bacillary angiomatosis. Ann Intern Med 118:388, 1993.
108. Cotell SL, Noskin GA: Bacillary angiomatosis: Clinical and histologic features, diagnosis, and treatment. Arch Intern Med 154:524, 1994.
109. Gasquet S, Maurin M, Brouqui P, et al: Bacillary angiomatosis in immunocompromised patients. AIDS 12:1793, 1998.

Chapter 70

VASCULAR DISEASES OF THE LIVER

Daniel F. Schafer and Michael F. Sorrell

Whether counting spider angiomas, noting the caput medusae, or injecting esophageal varices, the physician caring for the patient with liver disease is involved with blood vessels. Most often vascular problems are a complication of liver disease. The adaptive (or maladaptive) response of the portal venous system to increased hepatic resistance is responsible for much morbidity and mortality (see Chapter 77). This chapter deals with those less common cases in which the cardiovascular system is involved in the initiation or perpetuation of liver disease. Discussed are a potpourri of syndromes of varied causes and pathophysiologic characteristics, recognition of which is important in the management of patients with liver disease.

BUDD-CHIARI SYNDROME

Rare in occurrence, varied in cause, inconsistent in presentation, unpredictable in progression, and challenging in therapy, the Budd-Chiari syndrome (BCS) tests the insight and judgment of the most experienced clinician. With the advent of more effective treatment, simply making the diagnosis is insufficient. Optimal patient outcomes require careful assessment of the cause, pace, severity, and reversibility of the injury suffered.

BCS is a collection of anatomic and physiologic changes brought about by reduction of hepatic venous outflow. The reduction can be caused by impediments to flow anywhere from the right atrium to small radicles of the hepatic veins, in which it shares features with veno-occlusive disease (VOD). In its classic form, BCS is a nearly complete obstruction to flow caused by the acute formation of blood clot at the opening of the hepatic veins into the inferior vena cava. This sudden event is followed by the onset of hepatomegaly, pain, ascites, and liver failure. The early mortality rate in untreated patients with this classic form of the syndrome is very high. Improved methods of imaging the hepatic vasculature have resulted in recognition of more subtle forms of BCS. Innovative and sophisticated therapies also have played a role in reducing morbidity and mortality rates. The widening spectrum of causes, presentations, diagnostic studies, and therapies has transferred BCS from a pathologist's curiosity to a clinician's challenge.

The literature on BCS is extensive. Two major reviews of the world literature collected data on cases reported before 1980.[1, 2] Reviews of over 100 cases each have appeared from Japan, India, China, and South Africa.[3–6] The review from India is especially helpful in understanding the geographic diversity of this syndrome.

Etiology

The major causes of BCS are outlined in Table 70–1. In Western countries, the leading cause is idiopathic, accounting for 40% of collected cases. Newly recognized causes will reduce this number. Examples include antiphospholipid syndrome,[7] occult myeloproliferative disease,[8] and coagulation factor mutations.[9] One fourth of cases of BCS are caused by hematologic conditions, primarily polycythemia rubra vera. Tumors, infections, and pregnancy each cause about 10% of cases. When intensively studied, many patients with BCS are found to have multiple contributory conditions.[10]

In series from Asia, membranous obstruction of the inferior vena cava (MOVC) represents about 40% of cases of BCS; the remainder are distributed in much the same ratios as those of Western cases (Fig. 70–1). The pathophysiologic characteristics of MOVC are poorly understood. Because of the occurrence of MOVC in childhood and the developmental complexity of the inferior vena cava, some authors argue for a congenital origin of the lesion. Others point to the peak incidence in the fourth decade and the anatomic variability of lesions as arguments for an acquired origin. Some histologic studies have pointed out that the membrane itself may develop from a thrombus. Also unexplained is the pre-

Table 70–1 | **Causes of Budd-Chiari Syndrome**

Hypercoagulable States	Cancer
Antiphospholipid syndrome	Adrenal carcinoma
Antithrombin III deficiency	Bronchogenic carcinoma
Essential thrombocytosis	Hepatocellular carcinoma (including fibrolamellar variant)
Factor V Leiden mutation	Leiomyosarcoma
Lupus anticoagulant	Leukemia
Myeloproliferative disorder	Renal cell carcinoma
Paroxysmal nocturnal hemoglobinuria	Rhabdomyosarcoma
Polycythemia rubra vera	**Miscellaneous**
Postpartum thrombocytopenic purpura	Behçet's syndrome
Protein C deficiency	Celiac sprue
Protein S deficiency	Crohn's disease
Prothrombin mutation G20210A	Laparoscopic cholecystectomy
Sickle cell disease	Membranous obstruction of vena cava
Infections	Oral contraceptives
Amebic liver abscess	Polycystic disease
Aspergillosis	Pregnancy
Filariasis	Sarcoidosis
Pyogenic liver abscess	Trauma
Hydatid cysts	
Pelvic cellulitis	
Schistosomiasis	
Syphilis	
Tuberculosis	

dilection of MOVC for persons living in Asia and Africa. Western cases are reported but are rare. The distinctiveness of BCS with MOVC has led some authors to refer to it as a separate clinical entity, obliterative hepatocavopathy. The propensity of this variant to be complicated by hepatocellular carcinoma is another distinctive feature.[11]

Among the tumors associated with BCS, hepatocellular carcinoma represents a special case because it can be both a cause and a complication of the syndrome. In some cases, it may be impossible to determine the causative sequence of pathologic events.

Of the hematologic causes of BCS, some are lifelong (antithrombin III deficiency), some are chronic (polycythemia rubra vera, which may be occult), and others are transient (protein S or C deficiency due to liver disease). In most cases it is extremely difficult to identify the proximate causes of BCS in these at-risk patients.

Clinical Features

The epidemiologic characteristics of BCS (except in those cases associated with MOVC) parallel those of its underlying conditions. BCS is exceedingly rare in infants and young children; the largest number of pediatric cases are reported in South African children with MOVC.

The presentation of BCS can be fulminant, acute, or chronic. Fulminant BCS is seen most often in women who have pregnancy-related BCS. Severe pain, hepatomegaly, jaundice, ascites, and rapid deterioration of hepatic function are characteristic. Because many of these patients also have encephalopathy, this type of BCS may be considered a form of fulminant hepatic failure. Few of these patients survive without prompt intervention.

Acute nonfulminant BCS is characterized by ascites, tender hepatomegaly, and abdominal pain but not hepatic coma. The duration of illness is usually measured in weeks. Some of these patients may have a remitting course. A wide range of laboratory result abnormalities have been reported; hepatocellular damage is more prominent than is cholestatic features. The clinical findings depend on the location of the thrombus, the stage of evolution, and the percentage of liver tissue deprived of venous drainage. In the past, in such patients the thrombus has usually progressed to include features of chronic disease. With current diagnostic modalities, the patients affected are now candidates for therapies directed at removing or dissolving the thrombus, whereas urgent portocaval shunt may be used to preserve threatened liver. Acute BCS represents one fourth to one third of cases.

Chronic BCS accounts for most cases in all large series. Such patients have many features of chronic, decompensated cirrhosis. Many of them, in fact, have cirrhosis. The liver is large and firm. Ascites is variably present, but evidence of collateral circulation can almost always be found. Some patients experience variceal hemorrhage. The patient's history reveals evidence of liver disease that extends back months to years. Such patients have obviously survived the acute interruption of hepatic venous outflow and have had what has been called *hepatic parenchymal extinction.* Prognosis depends on the underlying disease, severity of liver failure, and success of treatment.

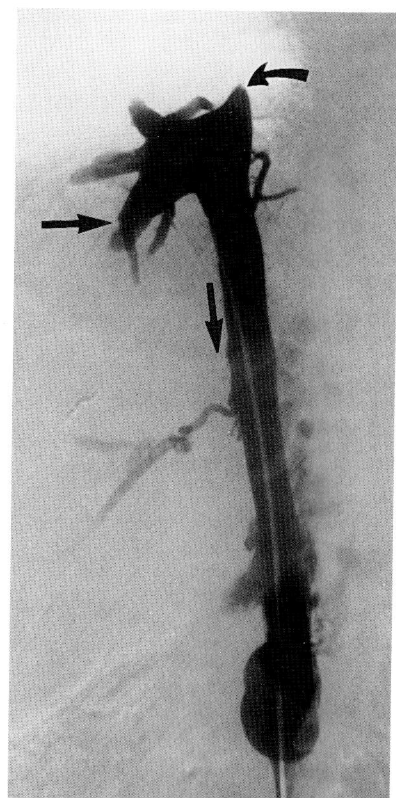

Figure 70–1. Membranous obstruction of the vena cava. Injection of contrast medium into the inferior vena cava demonstrates retrograde flow toward the legs *(downward arrow)* and into the hepatic veins *(horizontal arrow)*, rather than antegrade flow toward the right atrium. The membranous obstruction is nearly complete; only a tiny opening is visible as a small protrusion *(curved arrow)*. (Courtesy of Drs. Jeanne LaBerge, Roy Gordon, Robert Kerlin, and Ernest Ring of the University of California, San Francisco.)

Although the progress of BCS may be indolent, few cases have been known to regress. Some form of intervention is needed in most patients.

Pathologic Features

Acutely, the features of centrizonal congestion, cell necrosis, and hemorrhage predominate (Fig. 70–2). This lesion evolves into cirrhosis in chronic cases. Occasionally, patients who have chronic disease do not have cirrhosis. Whether these patients have zonal disease or have had sufficient drainage to prevent cell death must be determined by other diagnostic methods.

Radiology

Traditionally, catheterization of the inferior vena cava or percutaneous transhepatic hepatovenography has been needed to establish the diagnosis of BCS. These studies may still be necessary in planning of surgery or in unusually difficult cases, but Doppler ultrasonography is now the diagnostic procedure of choice. The typical ultrasonographic features of BCS include inability to visualize normal hepatic venous connections to the vena cava, comma-shaped intrahepatic collateral vessels, and absence of waveform in the hepatic veins. Magnetic resonance imaging and computed tomography may also demonstrate characteristic findings but do not add much to the findings of an adequate ultrasonographic examination.[12]

Treatment

Decisions about the therapy for BCS depend on the cause, anatomic characteristics, and pace of disease (Fig. 70–3). Because most patients require some form of surgery, early consultation of an experienced hepatobiliary surgeon is recommended.

If a patient has the fulminant form of BCS with encephalopathy and laboratory evidence of hepatocellular failure (vi-

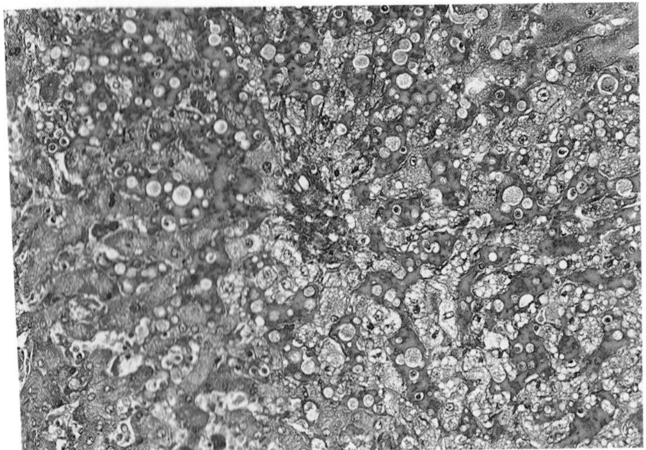

Figure 70–2. Histology of Budd-Chiari syndrome. This low-power view shows the centrizonal congestion, hemorrhage, and hepatocyte necrosis typical of the acute type of Budd-Chiari syndrome. (Courtesy of Edward Lee, MD, Dallas, TX.)

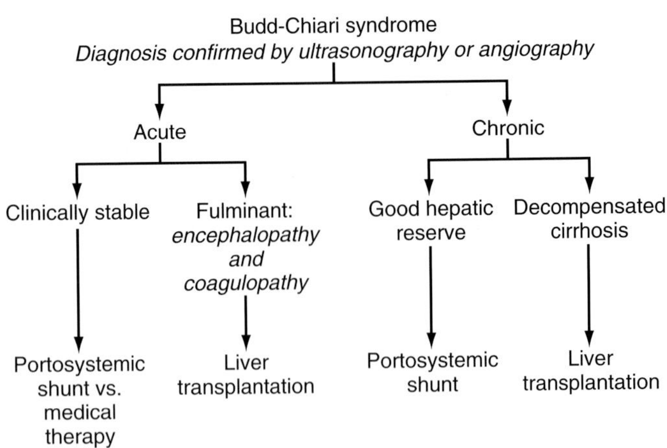

Figure 70–3. Approach to patients with the Budd-Chiari syndrome. Although each case must be considered individually, this algorithm shows typical treatment options for the various forms of Budd-Chiari syndrome. Patients with either fulminant disease or decompensated cirrhosis are unlikely to benefit from any therapy other than transplantation. Patients with clinically stable, acute disease have the widest number of options open to them. Special efforts should be made to determine local or transient causes of the syndrome that might yield to less invasive therapies.

tamin K–resistant coagulopathy, factor V level less than 20% of normal, hypoalbuminemia), orthotopic liver transplantation should be considered.[13] Similarly, a case of chronic disease with evidence of decompensated cirrhosis and encephalopathy would rarely benefit from portacaval shunt surgery.[14] If technically feasible, transplantation may be the only therapeutic option. A third clear indication for liver transplantation is continued deterioration after a portosystemic shunt procedure.[15]

Evidence of hepatic reserve and recent onset of disease present a more varied and challenging range of options. Consideration should be given to the potential cause of the syndrome. Several causes of BCS are either local (hepatic abscesses, tumors, webs), transient (pregnancy, acquired hypercoagulable state), or treatable (Crohn's disease). In such cases, the use of thrombolytic agents with or without surgery has been attempted. Operations include resection of a tumor[16] and transcardiac membranotomy.[17] Nonsurgical approaches to localized disease include balloon angioplasty[18] and placement of metallic stents in the inferior vena cava.[19] Treatment with thrombolytics alone most often has been used when paroxysmal nocturnal hemoglobinuria is the underlying cause of BCS.[20] Portocaval shunting provides a method of saving liver threatened by continued congestion and ischemia. The treatment of selected patients with anticoagulation alone has received some support. In a historical study of more than 100 patients treated at three hospitals in France, patients with favorable prognostic features were as likely to survive when treated with anticoagulation as they were when treated with a surgical shunt.[21]

For the patient with chronic BCS of any cause and evidence of adequate hepatic reserve, the most common therapy employs some sort of surgical shunt, the type of which depends on the extent of thrombosis[22] and the extent to which the hypertrophied caudate lobe obstructs the inferior vena cava. The only acceptable shunts are those that decompress the portal circulation (e.g., side-to-side shunts). The shunt with the highest patency rate is the direct side-to-side anastomosis between the portal vein and the intrahepatic inferior vena cava.[23, 24] Placing a mesocaval interposition graft of venous material or synthetic polyester textile fiber (Dacron) is a much simpler operation, which eliminates the need for hilar dissection. Unfortunately, shunt thrombosis occurs in one fourth to one half of patients.[25] Regardless of the design of the shunt, the pressure difference between the splanchnic vein used for the shunt and the receiving vessel must be at least 10 mm Hg to prevent shunt thrombosis. Alternatively, splanchnic blood can be returned directly to the heart by means of a mesoatrial shunt. This operation is continuing to evolve, and several variants have been described.

An even more ambitious approach has been described by Senning.[26] In this operation, the diseased portion of the inferior vena cava and outflow tracts of the liver are resected and the liver is anastomosed directly to the right atrium, allowing hepatic blood to enter directly. The 5-year survival rate has been reported to be 76%, and in some patients with extensive thrombosis and hepatic reserve this surgery may be the only alternative to transplantation.[27]

Transjugular intrahepatic portosystemic shunts (TIPS) have gained popularity in the emergency treatment of complications of portal hypertension and as a "bridge" to liver transplantation (see Chapter 77). Although the use of these devices would seem to be precluded by hepatic vein occlusion, several reports have described creative attempts to place a TIPS in patients with BCS. Access to the liver substance can be obtained by cannulation of the caudate vein, piercing of the inferior vena cava, or puncture of a vein stump.[28] No long-term studies of use of TIPS as definitive therapy for BCS have been published, but encouraging results of treatment of patients with fulminant and subfulminant disease who might not otherwise survive long enough to undergo transplantation have been published.[29]

Liver transplantation as a therapy for BCS carries the burden of lifelong immunosuppression and its attendant complications. In rare circumstances (e.g., protein C deficiency), transplantation corrects an underlying hypercoagulable state,[30] but most patients will require anticoagulation as well. Despite these perils, transplantation has achieved 5-year survival rates ranging from 45% to 80%. The determination of which patients to treat by shunt and which to treat by transplantation has become clearer as centers that perform both operations report their experiences.[31] Patients with acute or chronic liver failure probably fare best with transplantation, whereas those with only portal hypertension may do best with a shunt. Obtaining a liver biopsy specimen can be crucial in making this judgment.[32] Whether a shunt is placed or transplantation is performed, recurrent thrombosis remains a major threat to any patient treated for BCS. The challenge of establishing and maintaining anticoagulation in the survivors of BCS is as great as that of determining an initial course of therapy.

VENO-OCCLUSIVE DISEASE

Occlusion of the terminal hepatic venules and hepatic sinusoids has been classified as a subset of the Budd-Chiari syndrome, which it resembles clinically; however, the causes, epidemiologic and pathophysiologic characteristics and prognosis are sufficiently distinct to identify this syndrome as a separate entity.

Etiology

VOD was first recognized in Jamaica and related to the ingestion of pyrrolizidine alkaloids contained in plants of the genera *Senecio, Crotalaria*, and *Heliotropium*.[33] Epidemics have been described in India, Afghanistan, South Africa, the Middle East, and the United States. Rare familial clusters have been reported in association with immunodeficiency states.[34] Hepatic irradiation and a variety of antineoplastic drugs also have been implicated as causes of VOD, but the most common setting for VOD in the United States is early after bone marrow transplantation.[35, 36]

Clinical Features and Course

The insidious onset of portal hypertension is characteristic of VOD. In bone marrow transplantation recipients, VOD occurs within 2 weeks of transplantation. Weight gain and jaundice (reaching a peak at day 17 after marrow transplantation) are followed by hepatomegaly, abdominal pain, ascites, and encephalopathy. Predisposing factors include older age and pretransplantation elevations in serum aminotransferase levels. The differential diagnosis of VOD is complicated by the many types of liver injury to which marrow transplantation recipients are vulnerable. Graft-versus-host disease rarely occurs before day 15. Drug toxicities and bacteremia rarely cause hepatomegaly and ascites. Post-transfusion hepatitis also tends to occur later in the course of transplantation and causes signs of portal hypertension only if fulminant hepatic failure results. If there is any question about the diagnosis, liver biopsy can be performed if the platelet count is above 60,000/mm^3. Probably safer is the measurement of a wedged hepatic venous pressure gradient, in which a gradient of more than 10 mm Hg has been found to be quite specific for VOD. Ultrasonography may reveal signs of portal hypertension and a thickened gallbladder wall; results of Doppler flow studies are usually normal. Increased lung uptake of ^{99m}Tc-sulfur colloid during hepatic scintigraphy has been found to be useful both to predict the occurrence of VOD before it has been manifested clinically and to stage the severity of the disease.[37] Standard laboratory tests are not specific for VOD. Serum procollagen type III levels have been found to be increased in children and adults with VOD,[38, 39] whereas levels of von Willebrand factor are unaltered.

The outcome of transplantation-related VOD varies from a fulminant course with early death to complete recovery within 3 weeks. As more sophisticated and sensitive diagnostic tests are used to identify cases and as clinical suspicion of this syndrome has increased, a greater number of transient cases has been reported. In a large series of affected patients treated with supportive care, VOD was believed to contribute to death in 32% of cases, the course was prolonged in 13%, and the disease resolved in 55%.[40]

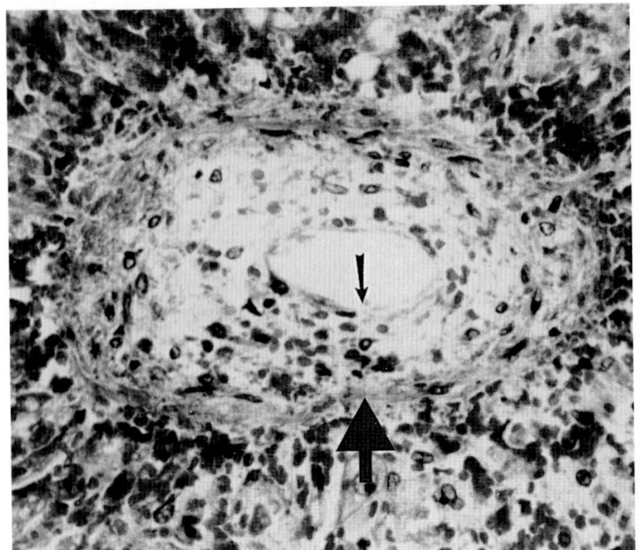

Figure 70–4. Pathology of veno-occlusive disease. This medium-power view of a terminal hepatic venule (central vein) shows the extensive intimal hyperplasia characteristic of the endothelial injury of veno-occlusive disease. The small arrow is inside what remains of the venular lumen. The large arrow is at the outer extent of the hyperplasia. The supporting collagenous ring just inside the large arrow suggests the normal size of the venule. Red blood cells (stained dark) surround the venule. They are congesting the sinusoids and have hemorrhaged into the surrounding liver. Higher power views would confirm that the hepatocytes are necrotic.

Pathologic Features

The primary lesion of VOD is endothelial toxicity with progressive occlusion of the terminal hepatic venules and sinusoids with cellular debris, exfoliated hepatocytes, activated coagulation factors, and stagnant red blood cells. Intimal change results in phlebosclerosis and narrowing (Figs. 70–4 and 70–5). Fibrosis extends from the terminal hepatic venules into the sinusoids. Intrahepatic hemorrhage and centrizonal (acinar zone 3) necrosis complete the histologic findings. Later, abnormal architecture with recanalization of veins and centrilobular cholestasis are prominent features. One study, which attempted to relate the symptoms and signs of VOD to histologic changes, found that the total severity of the histologic change had a higher correlation with clinical outcome than any single histologic feature.[41]

Treatment

Aggressive diuresis and pulmonary support are mandatory in severely ill patients. Prevention has been attempted by adjusting busulfan doses and pharmacokinetic monitoring of conditioning regimens. Prophylactic use of heparin has been found to reduce the frequency of VOD in at least one randomized, prospective trial.[42] A similar trial using prophylactic ursodeoxycholic acid reduced the frequency of VOD after bone marrow transplantation by more than 50%.[43] Treatment of the established syndrome with almost every agent known to influence hemostasis has been reported; these agents include recombinant tissue plasminogen activator, urokinase, gabexate mesylate, and prostaglandins, alone and in various combinations.[44] *N*-acetylcysteine has been reported to have a beneficial effect on established VOD in a small trial.[45]

The severity of portal hypertensive symptoms in VOD has led several investigators to attempt to place a TIPS in these patients. In 10 such cases, it was found that the shunts could be placed safely and effectively to lower portal pressures, but the outcomes were not good: 5 patients died within 10 days and 4 more died within months. Only one patient recovered. The authors suggest that earlier placement of a TIPS might improve survival rate.[46]

As a last resort, liver transplantation has been used. Although strict guidelines cannot be given for the management of bone marrow transplantation–related VOD at the present time, the combination of primary prevention, improved surveillance, more accurate diagnosis, and earlier intervention should reduce the morbidity and mortality rates of this syndrome.

PORTAL VEIN THROMBOSIS

The formation of thrombus in the portal vein results in a predictable sequence of events. Pressure rises in the portal vein remnant and is transmitted into the splenic vein. The spleen enlarges in response to the pressure. Alternatively, collateral channels begin to open to carry portal blood to the systemic circulation. Increased flow in these small potential veins dilates them to form esophageal, gastric, duodenal, and jejunal varices. Varices proliferate in the porta hepatis and may include venous channels in the gallbladder bed. Meanwhile, normal evolution of the clot occurs. Fibroblasts transform the clot into a firm, collagenous plug in which tortuous venous channels develop. This "cavernous transformation" occurs over 5 weeks to 12 months (Fig. 70–6). The bowels, meanwhile, are engorged with venous blood. The stomach

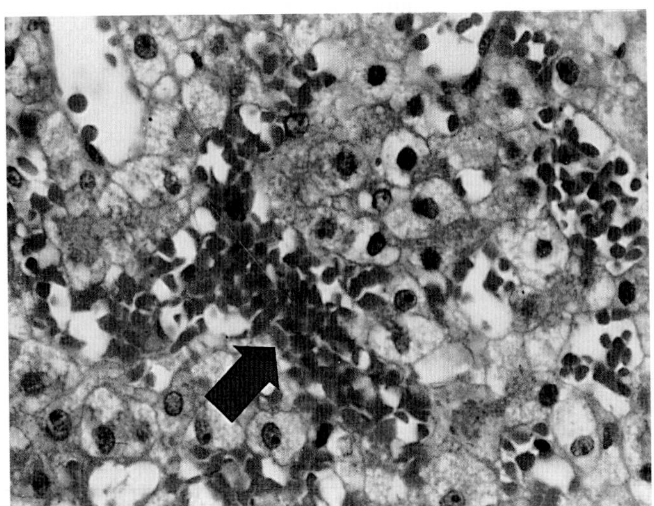

Figure 70–5. Pathology of veno-occlusive disease. This higher power view of the hepatic lobule shows liver cell plates between expanded, red blood cell–filled sinusoids. The arrow points to a collection of dark red blood cells in an expanded sinusoid. This view could be seen in any of the vascular liver diseases causing hepatic outflow obstruction, including Budd-Chiari syndrome and congestive hepatopathy.

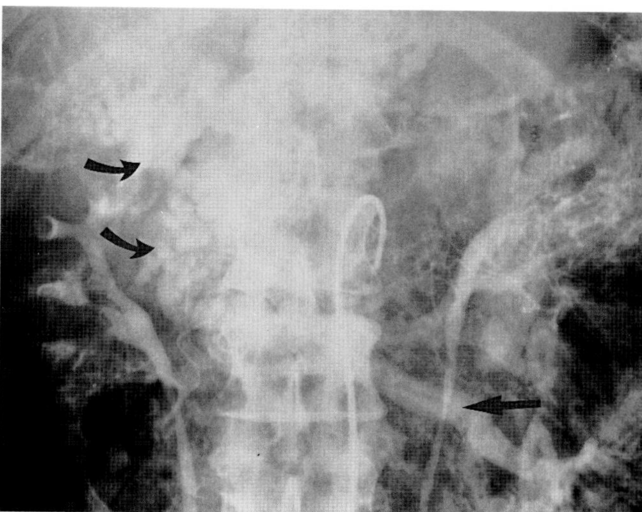

Figure 70–6. Cavernous transformation of the portal vein. The venous phase of this splanchnic arteriogram demonstrates the splenic vein *(straight arrow)* but no clearly delineated portal vein. Rather, the normal portal vein is replaced by a tangle of smaller tortuous vessels *(curved arrows).*

takes on the endoscopic appearance of portal hypertensive gastropathy. The liver, deprived of portal flow, scavenges whatever blood it can from perihepatic varices and, sustained by hepatic arterial flow, usually maintains its synthetic and excretory functions. An equilibrium is reached. Ascites, which may have formed during the initial stages of portal hypertension, recedes. In outward appearance, the child or adult in whom the portal vein has clotted seems unaffected. Careful examination discloses the enlarged spleen. Years later hemorrhage occurs; a varix ruptures, and large amounts of blood are vomited or passed per rectum. The person with portal vein thrombosis now becomes a patient and, with supportive care, survives hemorrhage.

Etiology

The chief cause of portal vein thrombosis (PVT) in children is infection, most often umbilical sepsis. The frequency with which umbilical sepsis leads to PVT is unknown, but it must not be high. This complication developed in none of the 86 children with umbilical infections observed prospectively for PVT.[47] Table 70–2 lists other causes of PVT. New procoagulant mutations continue to be described and are increasingly recognized as causes of portal vein thrombosis. Among these is a mutation of the 3′-untranslated region of the prothrombin gene: factor II G20210A.[48] This mutation is related to familial venous thrombosis and has been found in 4 of 10 patients who had idiopathic PVT. Better understanding of the multiple causes of hypercoagulability has led to the recognition of patients in whom multiple coexisting risk factors have resulted in PVT. PVT in adults is strongly related to cirrhosis or a history of splenectomy. Most often, the thrombosis results from sluggish blood flow in the portal vein. Approximately 16% of patients evaluated for liver transplantation have ultrasonographic findings of PVT. In adults with PVT and normal liver function, hypercoagulable states, often secondary to neoplasm, are usually responsible.

Clinical Features and Course

Portal vein thrombosis is found with equal frequency in adults (peak, age 40) and children (peak, age 6). The presenting symptom is almost always variceal hemorrhage with melena. A report of abdominal pain should alert the clinician to the possibility of more extensive mesenteric thrombosis with intestinal ischemia. Doppler ultrasonography reveals an echogenic thrombus in the portal vein, extensive collateral circulation near the porta hepatis, and an enlarged spleen. Flow in the remainder of the portal vein is usually hepatofugal and without respiratory variation. At times the portal vein is not visualized. In practice, the ultrasonographer can be greatly assisted by an indication of the possibility of this diagnosis before the examination is performed. If, because of bowel gas or body habitus, diagnostic ultrasonography cannot be performed, magnetic resonance angiography is probably the procedure of choice. The limitation of computed tomography is its inability to provide important axial images. Many surgeons request angiography before performing a shunt.

The endoscopic evaluation of PVT is usually done in conjunction with therapeutic efforts to control variceal hemorrhage. Variceal banding or sclerotherapy[49] should be considered as first-line therapy in PVT. Multiple sessions are needed to control varices. Varices may form in unusual sites in patients with PVT. Gallbladder varices were found in 30% of 74 patients studied by Doppler ultrasonography.[50] All 16 patients with PVT who were studied with endoscopic retrograde cholangiopancreatography had evidence of varices in the common bile duct that mimicked cholangiocarcinoma.[51] Such varices can cause obstructive jaundice.[52] Colonic varices also occur. Occasionally, PVT with esophageal varices is encountered before bleeding has occurred. Such

Table 70–2 | **Causes of Portal Vein Thrombosis**

Hypercoagulable States	**Complications of Medical Intervention**
Antiphospholipid syndrome	Alcohol injection
Factor V Leiden mutations	Ambulatory dialysis
Paroxysmal nocturnal hemoglobinuria	Chemoembolization
Prothrombin mutation G20210A	Islet cell injection
Myeloproliferative diseases	Liver transplantation
Oral contraceptives	Partial hepatectomy
Polycythemia rubra vera	Sclerotherapy
Pregnancy	Splenectomy
Protein S deficiency	Transjugular intrahepatic portosystemic shunt
Methylenetetrahydrofolate reductase mutation TT677	Umbilical catheterization
Sickle cell disease	**Infections**
Inflammatory Diseases	Actinomycosis
Behçet's syndrome	Appendicitis
Crohn's disease	*Candida albicans* infection
Pancreatitis	Diverticulitis
Ulcerative colitis	**Miscellaneous**
	Cirrhosis
	Bladder cancer
	Nodular regenerative hyperplasia

patients experience no bleeding for an average of 4 years, and in up to 10% bleeding may never occur.[53] In such cases, reversibility of cause, risk of therapy, constitutional ability to survive hemorrhage, and access to medical emergency care must all be factored into the treatment recommendation.

Rebleeding after endoscopic therapy and bleeding from varices distal to the esophagus are indications for surgical shunts. Both mesocaval and splenorenal shunts have been performed with low mortality rates and long survival.[54] Radical esophagogastric devascularization (Sugiura) procedures have been attempted in small numbers of patients outside Asia.[55] Results seem promising if the procedure can be accomplished electively in good-risk patients. Emergency surgery of this type cannot be recommended.

The usefulness of beta blockade to prevent recurrent variceal bleeding caused by PVT has not been studied in controlled trials. However, we believe that such treatment can be justified by analogy to treatment of cirrhotic portal hypertension.

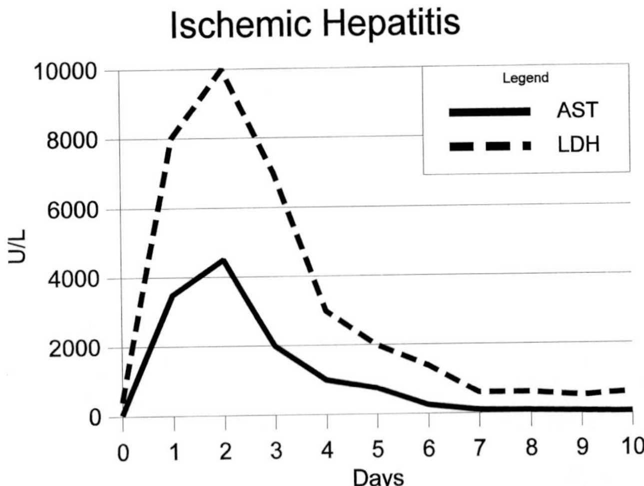

Figure 70–7. The dramatic rise and fall of serum aspartate aminotransferase (AST) and lactate dehydrogenase (LDH) levels in ischemic hepatitis are shown in this graph. (Adapted from Gitlin NG, Serio KM: Ischemic hepatitis: Widening horizons. Am J Gastroenterol 7:831, 1992.)

ISCHEMIC HEPATITIS

If *hepatitis* implies inflammation of the liver, the term *ischemic hepatitis* is a misnomer. *Hepatic infarction, centrilobular necrosis, shock liver,* and other terms have been used as synonyms. Convenience and usage, however, have settled on *ischemic hepatitis* for the syndrome described here. Acute circulatory failure of the liver may be the most underappreciated and underdiagnosed form of vascular liver disease. The practice of frequent biochemical monitoring in severely ill patients has drawn more cases to the attention of consultants.

Etiology

Ischemic hepatitis is typically preceded by hypotension, hypoxemia, or both. As one would expect, the most common cause of sustained systemic hypotension is cardiovascular disease. In one study, the causes of all serum aspartate aminotransferase (AST) levels more than 100 times the upper limit of normal were investigated over the period of 1 year.[56] At least 90% of cases were caused by liver disease. One half of the cases related to hypotension were seen in patients who had acute myocardial infarction or were undergoing cardiac surgery. Hypotension caused by sepsis was the next leading cause. Other studies have shown that ischemic hepatitis can be detected biochemically in 0.3% to 2.6% of all patients admitted to a hospital for cardiac events. Trauma, dehydration, hemorrhage, heat stroke, burns, and obstructive sleep apnea all have caused transient ischemic injury to the liver.

Diagnosis

The diagnosis of ischemic hepatitis is typically first recognized by the laboratory finding of extraordinarily high aminotransferase values on a screening panel. Most often, the patient is in the hospital for problems not primarily associated with the liver, so the report is often greeted with raised eyebrows, followed by a bedside visit and request for a battery of hepatitis serologic tests. Drug lists are scrutinized for the names of known hepatotoxins. Findings of physical examination are not revealing, although altered mental status has been described in a few patients. Results of laboratory tests may be abnormal at the time of presentation. The lactate dehydrogenase (LDH) level is profoundly elevated. The ratio of alanine aminotransferase (ALT) to LDH is much higher in acute viral hepatitis than it is in ischemic hepatitis.[57] The prothrombin time may be prolonged by 2 or 3 seconds. Tests of kidney function (blood urea nitrogen and creatinine levels) are likely to yield abnormal results caused by coincident acute tubular necrosis generated by the hypotensive episode. In many cases, a secure diagnosis cannot be made until the characteristic normalization of liver function test results occurs within a few days (Fig. 70–7). Liver biopsy, which is usually not necessary, reveals bland, centrizonal necrosis with preservation of hepatic architecture (Fig. 70–8).

Clinical Course

In the most severely affected patients, ischemic hepatitis is one manifestation of multiorgan failure and has a poor prognosis. Likewise, in the few patients whose liver injury is so severe that the syndrome of fulminant hepatic failure develops, ischemic hepatitis may be lethal. Fortunately, most cases are transient and subclinical.[58]

CONGESTIVE HEPATOPATHY

Right-sided heart failure results in transmission of increased central venous pressure directly to the liver through the inferior vena cava and the hepatic veins. In the days before the use of potent diuretics, pathologists regularly interpreted the findings of increased liver weight and hepatic fibrosis as signs of prolonged cardiac disease. Clinicians took advantage of the elastic storage properties of the liver to demonstrate that compression of the liver raises the central venous pres-

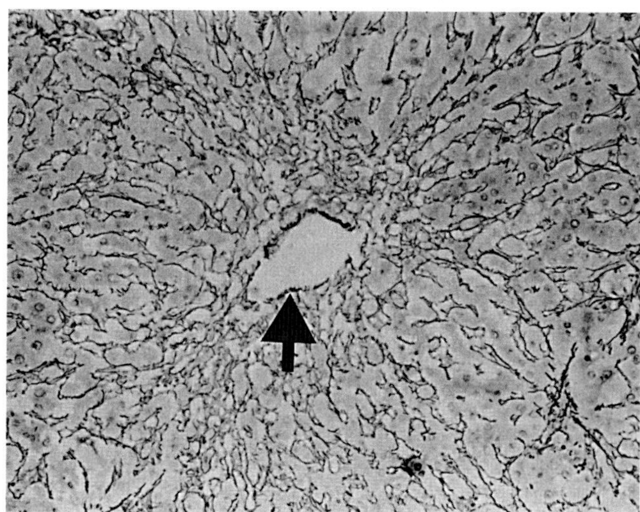

Figure 70–8. Pathology of ischemic hepatitis. This is a medium-power view of a reticulin stain demonstrating the loss of hepatocytes surrounding a terminal hepatic venule (central vein). The arrow points to the venule. Note that the thin dark lines are uniformly seperated by plates of hepatocytes on the periphery of the image. Toward the center of the image, radiating lines have collapsed owing to the necrosis and dropout of ischemic liver cells. The architecture is intact, and if oxygenated blood flow is restored, the liver will regenerate to complete normality.

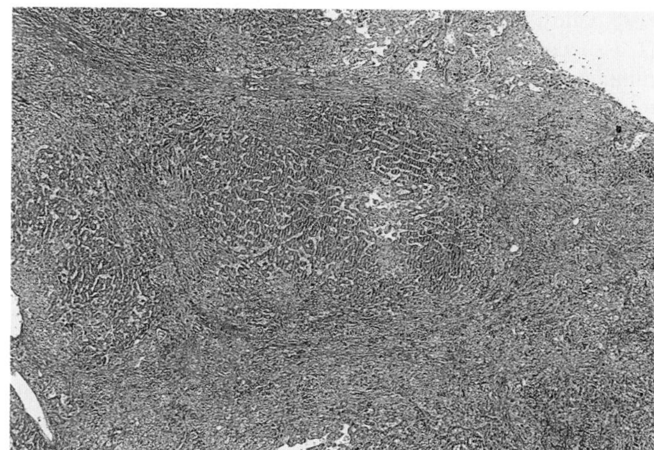

Figure 70–9. Pathology of cardiac cirrhosis. This low-power view shows a portal tract in the center of a regenerative nodule and fibrotic bands bridging central veins. The size of the scar and the presence of the ducts attest to the long-term development of the fibrotic process. Even at low power, one can see the bland nature of the cirrhosis. No inflammatory cells are evident. The sinusoids are dilated and congested. (Courtesy of Edward Lee, MD, Dallas, TX.)

sure (i.e., the hepatojugular reflux). Most often, the effects of heart failure on the liver were prolonged and insidious, but occasionally they were acute and severe, especially in cases of constrictive pericarditis and acute cardiomyopathy. The clinical presentation of congestive hepatopathy is generally masked by the customary symptoms and signs of right-sided heart failure. Dull aching in the right upper quadrant in association with hepatomegaly is common. Jaundice is seen in less than 10% of patients. Laboratory studies are not helpful in making this diagnosis. In a study of 175 patients with severe right-sided heart failure, no results of standard laboratory tests (ALT, AST, alkaline phosphatase, bilirubin, albumin levels) were abnormal in most patients who had either acute or chronic disease.[59] The prothrombin time was abnormal in three fourths of both groups and returned to normal very slowly with improvement in the heart failure. There is no evidence that the presence of congestive liver disease worsens the prognosis of patients with heart failure, whose mortality rate is dominated by the severity of the cardiac disease.

The histologic manifestations of chronic passive congestion include atrophy of hepatocytes, distention of sinusoids, and centrilobular fibrosis. The fibrosis can become extensive with bridging to adjacent lobules and the replacement of normal architecture with regenerative nodules, so-called cardiac cirrhosis (Fig. 70–9). Centrilobular necrosis is often associated with passive congestion. To define the clinical events that correlate with these histologic findings better, Arcidi and coworkers reviewed findings of 1000 autopsies in adults and compared the hepatic histologic lesions with clinical and histologic cardiac findings.[60] They observed that passive congestion frequently coexists with centrilobular necrosis but that the lesions differ in pathophysiologic characteristics. The congestive lesion is associated with high venous pressure, whereas the centrilobular necrosis is related to shock.

The straightforward sequence of increased pressure leading to fibrosis evolving into cirrhosis has been challenged. Wanless and coworkers have noted that the distribution of fibrosis is irregular in cardiac cirrhosis (see Fig. 70–9).[61] Careful study of the vascular lesions seen in the distribution of fibrotic areas suggests that cardiac failure leads to sinusoidal thrombosis that propagates to both central veins and branches of the portal vein. The thrombosis leads to local ischemia, parenchymal extinction, and fibrosis.

PELIOSIS HEPATIS

Peliosis hepatis is the occurrence of multiple blood-filled cysts in the liver. The cysts can range from a few millimeters to 3 cm and are usually seen in association with dilated hepatic sinusoids (Fig. 70–10). Fibrosis, regenerative nodules, and tumors also may be seen with the peliosis. In the

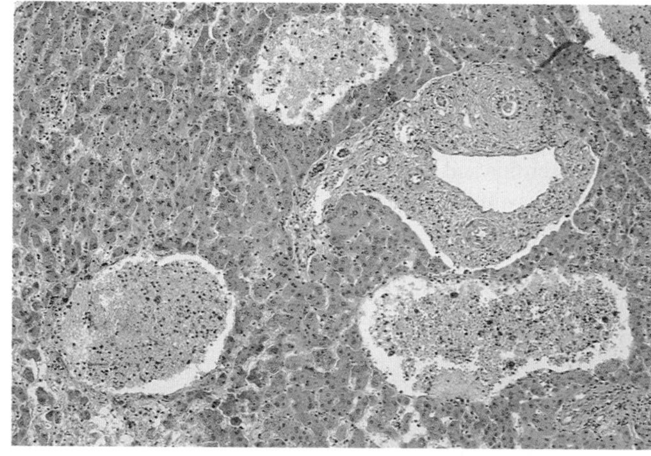

Figure 70–10. Pathology of peliosis hepatis. Note three blood-filled cysts without lining cells and an adjacent portal tract. Sinusoidal dilation is also present. (Courtesy of Edward Lee, MD, Dallas, TX.)

past, peliosis hepatis was largely a histologic curiosity, but its associations with renal transplantation and the acquired immunodeficiency syndrome have increased clinical awareness of this syndrome.

Peliosis was often noted in the liver of persons who died of wasting diseases, particularly tuberculosis and carcinomatosis.[62] At times the cysts are lined with endothelial cells and are contiguous with dilated sinusoids. At other times the cysts are not lined but are surrounded by hepatic parenchymal cells. Both types of cysts may be present in the same liver. Although the pathogenesis of the syndrome is not established, most investigators presume that the inciting lesion is damage to sinusoidal lining cells. Etiologic associations have been made with use of anabolic steroids, oral contraceptives, urethane, vitamin A, vinyl chloride, thorium dioxide, tamoxifen, glucocorticoids, and thioguanine (6-TG). Similar histologic lesions can be seen in myeloproliferative diseases such as agnogenic myeloid metaplasia[63] and malignant histiocytosis.[64]

Although fatal hemorrhage, liver failure, hepatomegaly, and jaundice have all been caused by peliosis, more often peliosis is indicated by abnormal results of liver tests. If they are large enough, the cysts can be identified by radiologic tests, including ultrasonography, computed tomography, and magnetic resonance imaging.[65]

Bacillary peliosis hepatis is caused by *Bartonella henselae*, the organism responsible for cat-scratch disease in both immunocompetent[66] and immunodeficient[67] persons. The identification of this organism capped the search for the cause of a pseudoneoplastic vascular proliferative disease of skin and viscera in human immunodeficiency virus–positive persons. The lesions in both skin and liver respond to antibiotic therapy (see Chapter 69).

Vascular diseases of the liver, including peliosis hepatis, occur with increased frequency in kidney transplant recipients. The cause has been assumed to be prolonged exposure to azathioprine.[68] Two studies have helped to define the natural history and inciting agents involved in the pathogenesis of this syndrome. Serial laparoscopies were performed in patients with renal failure.[69] Nodular transformation and peliosis appeared after transplantation and persisted despite modification of immunosuppression. The authors believed that cyclosporine as well as azathioprine may contribute to the liver abnormalities. Another group retrospectively reviewed 32 histologically identified cases of peliosis hepatis in renal transplant recipients.[70] Twenty patients had mild findings, whereas 12 had major abnormalities. Two patients died as a complication of the peliotic lesions. These authors thought that vascular liver disease was an important source of the morbidity and mortality rates in their patients and that azathioprine withdrawal did not clearly modify the course of the disease.

HEPATIC ARTERY ANEURYSM

The majority of hepatic artery aneurysms are saccular, extrahepatic defects caused by atherosclerosis, amyloidosis, infection, trauma, surgery, invasive radiologic procedures, or arteritis.[71] The older literature stresses presentations of advanced disease, including jaundice, abdominal mass, and hemorrhage into the duodenum, peritoneum, or pancreas. More recent literature stresses the ability to diagnose earlier and smaller aneurysms by using advanced imaging techniques. Earlier diagnosis has led to improved elective surgical methods. When grafting is performed, inclusion of flow from the gastroduodenal artery appears to be important to maintaining graft patency.

One of the unusual presentations of a hepatic artery aneurysm is fistula formation with a branch of the portal vein to cause portal hypertension.[72] This type of fistula has become more common as a result of the increased number of transhepatic invasive procedures performed. Its presence should be sought in any case of development of portal hypertension after such a procedure. Typically, such patients may bleed from varices, but ascites is unlikely to form in the absence of coexisting liver disease. Often, one can hear a murmur over the liver and the presence of the fistula can be confirmed by Doppler ultrasonography.

ATHEROSCLEROSIS

Despite its frequency in the general population, atherosclerosis is rarely a cause of liver disease. There are scattered reports of hepatic arterial aneurysms[73] and hepatic infarctions attributed to atherosclerotic vascular disease. Dr. Hans Popper, in a discussion of the aging liver, explained this rarity as follows:

> The ample supply of blood to the liver . . . far exceeds the organ's needs and serves the action of the liver on the circulating blood. Liver function is thus greatly protected from the effects of vascular diseases like arteriosclerosis, which cause senescent alterations in such organs as the kidney, with similar proliferative potential.[74]

This is not to say that atherosclerosis does not occur in the liver. The presence of atherosclerosis limits the utilization of livers from older donors for liver transplantation. Not only are arterial anastomoses more difficult to secure in these livers, but also there is a feeling that the lack of regulatory control in the stiffened hepatic arteries renders the organs more susceptible to transport and reperfusion injuries. If these acute problems can be overcome, the livers function well, just as they do in most cases of diffuse vascular disease.

POLYARTERITIS NODOSA

Polyarteritis nodosa involves small- and medium-sized arteries throughout the body in an unpredictable distribution. The segmental, inflammatory lesions result in aneurysms, dissection, rupture, occlusion, and fibrosis of the arteries. Ischemic infarction of kidneys, heart, neural tissue, adrenals, lung, and skin is common. Hepatic arterial involvement can be found in one half of cases at autopsy.[75] Histologically, such lesions show inflammatory destruction of hepatic arterial intima and media with primarily lymphocytic infiltration and fibrinoid necrosis. Thrombotic occlusion may be seen. Healing occurs with scarring and thickening. Presence of any of these lesions is unusual on a percutaneous biopsy specimen. Because one half of the cases of polyarteritis nodosa are associated with hepatitis B virus infection, the biopsy specimen more often reveals the changes of the viral infection. The benign nature of the liver lesions of polyarteritis nodosa has been illustrated by a study of prognostic factors in this syndrome.[76] Cardiac and renal involvement greatly increased the mortality risk, but elevated serum aminotransferase levels were strongly predictive of a reduced mortality rate.

In the rare cases in which hepatic disease is important, hepatic arterial aneurysms may rupture, with hemoperitoneum. Also, involvement of the gallbladder may mimic acute cholecystitis.

POLYMYALGIA RHEUMATICA

Polymyalgia rheumatica, temporal arteritis, and giant cell arteritis are systemic diseases of unknown cause that attack large and small arteries. Up to one third of patients may have abnormal liver test results. A liver biopsy specimen may show the characteristic findings of numerous giant cells in the arterial walls. Other inflammatory cells and lipocytes may be seen.[77] In a study of 74 patients who had polymyalgia rheumatica and giant cell arteritis, 27 had abnormal serum levels of alkaline phosphatase that fell to normal with treatment, usually within 3 weeks. Seven of these patients had persistently abnormal nuclear medicine liver scan findings. Measurements of arterial hepatic blood flow were also abnormal but improved with treatment. All of these findings were more common in patients with giant cell arteritis than in those with polymyalgia rheumatica alone.[78] Liver biochemical test result abnormalities in a person with one of these syndromes should be considered a marker for widespread arterial disease.

REFERENCES

1. Parker RGF: Occlusion of the hepatic veins in man. Medicine 38:369, 1959.
2. Mitchell MC, Boitnott JK, Kaufman S, et al: Budd-Chiari syndrome: Etiology, diagnosis and management. Medicine 61:199, 1982.
3. Okuda H, Yamagata H, Obata H, et al: Epidemiological and clinical features of Budd-Chiari syndrome in Japan. J Hepatol 22:1, 1995.
4. Dilawari JB, Bambery P, Chawla Y, et al: Hepatic outflow obstruction (Budd-Chiari syndrome). Medicine 73:21, 1994.
5. Wang Z, Zhu Y, Wang S, et al: Recognition and management of Budd-Chiari syndrome: Report of one hundred cases. J Vasc Surg 10: 149,1989.
6. Simson IW: Membranous obstruction of the inferior vena cava and hepatocellular carcinoma in South Africa. Gastroenterology 88:576, 1985.
7. Pelletier S, Landi B, Piette JC, et al: Antiphospholipid syndrome as the second cause of non-tumorous Budd-Chiari syndrome. J Hepatol 21:76, 1994.
8. Valla D, Dhumeaux D, Babany C, et al: Primary myeloproliferative disorder and hepatic vein thrombosis. Ann Intern Med 103:329, 1985.
9. Denninger M-H, Beldjord K, Durand F, et al: Budd-Chiari syndrome and factor V Leiden mutation. Lancet 345:525, 1995.
10. Denninger M-H, Chait Y, Casadevall N, et al: Cause of portal or hepatic venous thrombosis in adults: The role of multiple concurrent factors. Hepatology 31:587, 2000.
11. Okuda K, Kage M, Shrestha SM: Proposal of new nomenclature for Budd-Chiari syndromes: Hepatic vein thrombosis versus thrombosis of the inferior vena cava at its hepatic portion. Hepatology 28:1191, 1998.
12. Kane R, Eustace S: Diagnosis of Budd-Chiari syndrome: Comparison between sonography and MR angiography. Radiology 195:117, 1995.
13. Halff G, Todo S, Tzakis AG, et al: Liver transplantation for the Budd-Chiari syndrome. Ann Surg 211:43, 1990.
14. Knoop M, Lemmers HP, Bechstein WO, et al: Treatment of the Budd-Chiari syndrome with orthotopic liver transplantation and long-term anticoagulation. Clin Transplant 8:67, 1994.
15. Thompson NP, Miller AD, Hamilton G, et al: Emergency rescue hepatic transplantation following shunt surgery for Budd-Chiari syndrome. Eur J Gastroenterol Hepatol 6:835, 1994.
16. Fabre JM, Domergue J, Fagot H, et al: Leiomyosarcoma of the inferior vena cava presenting as Budd-Chiari syndrome. Eur J Surg Oncol 1:86, 1995.
17. Kimura L, Matsuda S, Koie H, et al: Membranous obstruction of the hepatic portion of the inferior vena cava. Surgery 72:551, 1972.
18. Puri SK, Goel M, Kumar N, et al: Percutaneous transluminal balloon angioplasty in suprahepatic IVC obstruction–Budd-Chiari syndrome. Trop Gastroenterol 16:39, 1995.
19. Venbrux AC, Mitchell SE, Savander SJ, et al: Long-term results with the use of metallic stents in the inferior vena cava for treatment of Budd-Chiari syndrome. J Vasc Interv Radiol 5:411, 1994.
20. McMullin MF, Hillmen P, Jackson J, et al: Tissue plasminogen activator for hepatic vein thrombosis in paroxysmal hemoglobinuria. J Intern Med 1:85, 1994.
21. Zeitoun G, Escolano S, Hadengue A, et al: Outcome of Budd-Chiari syndrome: A multivariate analysis of factors related to survival including portosystemic shunting. Hepatology 30:84, 1999.
22. Tilanus HW: Budd-Chiari syndrome. Br J Surg 82:1023, 1995.
23. Orloff MJ, Orloff MS, Daily PO: Long-term results of treatment of Budd-Chiari syndrome with portal decompression. Arch Surg 127:1182, 1992.
24. Klein AS, Cameron JL: Diagnosis and management of the Budd-Chiari syndrome. Am J Surg 160:128, 1990.
25. Terpstra OT, Ausema B, Bruining HA, et al: Late results of mesocaval interposition shunting for bleeding esophageal varices. Br J Surg 74: 787, 1987.
26. Senning A: Transcaval posterocranial resection of the liver as treatment of the Budd-Chiari syndrome. World J Surg 7:632, 1983.
27. Pasic M, Senning A, von Segesser L, et al: Transcaval liver resection with hepatoatrial anastomosis for treatment of patients with Budd-Chiari syndrome: Late results. J Thorac Cardiovasc Surg 106:275, 1993.
28. Dolmatch BL, Cooper BS, Chang PP, et al: Percutaneous hepatic venous reanastomosis in a patient with Budd-Chiari syndrome. Cardiovasc Intervent Radiol 18:46, 1995.
29. Ochs A, Sellinger M, Haag K, et al: Transjugular intrahepatic portosystemic stent-shunt (TIPS) in the treatment of Budd-Chiari syndrome. J Hepatol 18:217, 1993.
30. Lang H, Oldhafer KJ, Kupsch E, et al: Liver transplantation for Budd-Chiari syndrome—palliation or cure? Transpl Int 7:115, 1994.
31. Ringe B, Lang H, Oldhafer KJ, et al: Which is the best surgery for Budd-Chiari syndrome: Venous decompression or liver transplantation? A single center experience with 50 patients. Hepatology 21:1337, 1995.
32. Panis Y, Belghiti J, Valla D, et al: Portosystemic shunt in Budd-Chiari syndrome: Long-term survival factors affecting shunt patency in 25 patients in Western countries. Surgery 115:276, 1994.
33. Bras G, Jelliffe DB, Stuart KL: Veno-occlusive disease of the liver with non-portal type of cirrhosis, occurring in Jamaica. Arch Pathol 57: 285, 1954.
34. Mellis C, Bale PM: Familial veno-occlusive disease with probable immune deficiency. J Pediatr 88:236, 1976.
35. Shulman HM, Fisher LB, Schoch HG, et al: Veno-occlusive disease of the liver after marrow transplantation: Histological correlates of clinical signs and symptoms. Hepatology 19:1171, 1994.
36. Shulman HM, Gooley T, Dudley MD, et al: Utility of transvenous liver biopsies and wedged hepatic venous pressure measurements in sixty marrow transplant recipients. Transplantation 59:1015, 1995.
37. Jacobson AF, Teefey SA, Higano CA, et al: Increased lung uptake of ^{99m}Tc-sulphur colloid as an early indicator of the development of hepatic veno-occlusive disease in bone marrow transplant patients. Nucl Med Commun 14:706, 1993.
38. Heikinheimo M, Halila R, Fasth A: Serum procollagen type III is an early and sensitive marker for veno-occlusive disease of the liver in children undergoing bone marrow transplantation. Blood 83:3036, 1994.
39. Rio B, Bauduer F, Arrago JP, et al: N-terminal peptide of type III procollagen: A marker for the development of hepatic veno-occlusive disease after BMT and a basis for determining the timing of prophylactic heparin. Bone Marrow Transplant 11:471, 1993.
40. McDonald GB, Sharma P, Matthews DE, et al: The clinical course of 53 patients with veno-occlusive disease of the liver after marrow transplantation. Transplantation 36:603, 1985.

41. Shulman HM, Fisher LB, Schoch HG, et al: Veno-occlusive disease of the liver after marrow transplantation: Histological correlates of signs and symptoms. Hepatology 19:1171, 1994.
42. Attal M, Huguet F, Rubie H, et al: Prevention of hepatic veno-occlusive disease after bone marrow transplantation by continuous infusion of low-dose heparin: A prospective, randomized trial. Blood 79:2834, 1992.
43. Essell JH, Schroeder MT, Harman GS, et al: Ursodiol prophylaxis against hepatic complications of allogenic bone marrow transplantation: A randomized, double-blind, placebo-controlled trial. Ann Intern Med 128:975, 1998.
44. Bearman SI: The syndrome of hepatic veno-occlusive disease after marrow transplantation. Blood 85:3005, 1995.
45. Ringden O, Remberger M, Lehmann S, et al: *N*-acetylcysteine for veno-occlusive disease after allogenic stem cell transplantation. Bone Marrow Transplant 25:993, 2000.
46. Azoulay D, Castaing D, Lemoine A, et al: Transjugular intrahepatic portosystemic shunt (TIPS) for severe veno-occlusive disease of the liver following bone marrow transplantation. Bone Marrow Transplant 25:987, 2000.
47. Thompson EN, Sherlock S: The aetiology of portal vein thrombosis with particular reference to the role of infection and exchange transfusion. Q J Med 132:465, 1964.
48. Chamouard P, Pencreach E, Maloisel F, et al: Frequent factor II G20210A mutation in idiopathic portal vein thrombosis. Gastroenterology 118:144, 1999.
49. Karrer FM, Holland RM, Allshouse MJ, et al: Portal vein thrombosis: Treatment of variceal hemorrhage by endoscopic variceal ligation. J Pediatr Surg 29:1149, 1994.
50. Chawla Y, Dilawari JB, Katariya S: Gallbladder varices in portal vein thrombosis. AJR Am J Roentgenol 162:643, 1994.
51. Bayraktar Y, Balkanci F, Kayhan B, et al: Bile duct varices or "pseudo-cholangiocarcinoma sign" due to cavernous transformation of the portal vein. Am J Gastroenterol 87:1801, 1992.
52. Lohr JM, Kuchenreuter S, Grebmeier H, et al: Compression of the common bile duct due to portal-vein thrombosis in polycythemia vera. Hepatology 17:586, 1993.
53. Webb IJ, Sherlock S: The aetiology, presentation and natural history of extrahepatic portal venous obstruction. Q J Med 192:627, 1979.
54. Boles ET, Wise WE, Birken G: Extrahepatic portal hypertension in children: Long term evaluation. Am J Surg 151:734, 1986.
55. Dagenais M, Langer B, Taylor ER, et al: Experience with radical esophagogastric devascularization procedures (Suguira) for variceal bleeding outside Japan. World J Surg 18:222, 1994.
56. Johnson RD, O'Connor ML, Kerr RM: Extreme serum elevations of aspartate aminotransferase. Am J Gastroenterol 90:1244, 1995.
57. Cassidy WM, Reynolds TB: Serum lactic dehydrogenase in the differential diagnosis of acute hepatocellular injury. J Clin Gastroenterol 19: 118, 1994.
58. Gitlin NG, Serio KM: Ischemic hepatitis: Widening horizons. Am J Gastroenterol 7:831, 1992.
59. Richman SM, Delman AJ, Grob D: Alterations in indices of liver function in congestive heart failure with particular reference to serum enzymes. Am J Med 30:211, 1961.
60. Arcidi JM, Moore GW, Hutchins GM: Hepatic morphology in cardiac dysfunction: A clinicopathologic study of 1000 subjects at autopsy. Am J Pathol 104:159, 1981.
61. Wanless IR, Liu JJ, Butany J: Role of thrombosis in the pathogenesis of congestive hepatic fibrosis (cardiac cirrhosis). Hepatology 21:1232, 1995.
62. Yanoff M, Rawson AJ: Peliosis hepatis: An anatomic study with demonstration of two varieties. Arch Pathol Lab Med 77:159, 1964.
63. Makdisi WJ, Cherian R, Vanvelddhuizen PJ, et al: Fatal peliosis of the liver and spleen in a patient with agnogenic myeloid metaplasia treated with danazol. Am J Gastroenterol 90:317, 1995.
64. Fine KD, Solano M, Polter DE, et al: Malignant histiocytosis in a patient presenting with hepatic dysfunction and peliosis hepatis. Am J Gastroenterol 90:485, 1995.
65. Jamadar DA, D'Souza SP, Thomas EA, et al: Case report: Radiological appearances in peliosis hepatis. Br J Radiol 67:102, 1994.
66. Dolan MJ, Wong MT, Regnery RL, et al: Syndrome of *Rochalimaea henselae* adenitis suggesting cat-scratch disease. Ann Intern Med 118: 331, 1993.
67. Tappero JW, Mohle-Boetani J, Koehler JE, et al: The epidemiology of bacillary angiomatosis and bacillary peliosis. JAMA 269:770, 1993.
68. Gerlag PGG, Lobatto S, Driessen WMM: Hepatic sinusoidal dilation with portal hypertension during azathioprine treatment after kidney transplantation. J Hepatol 1:339, 1985.
69. Izumi S, Nishiuchi M, Kameda Y, et al: Laparoscopic study of peliosis hepatis and nodular transformation of the liver before and after renal transplantation: Natural history and aetiology in follow-up cases. J Hepatol 20:129, 1994.
70. Cavalcanti R, Pol S, Carnot F, et al: Impact and evolution of peliosis hepatis in renal transplant recipients. Transplantation 58:315, 1994.
71. Dougherty MJ, Gloviczki P, Cherry KJ, et al: Hepatic artery aneurysms: Evaluation and current management. Int Angiol 12:178, 1993.
72. Lumsden AB, Allen RC, Sreeram S, et al: Hepatic arterioportal fistula. Am Surg 59:722, 1993.
73. Dougherty MJ, Gloviczki P, Cherry KJ, et al: Hepatic artery aneurysms: Evaluation and treatment. Int Angiol 2:178, 1993.
74. Popper H: Aging and the liver. Prog Liver Dis 8:659, 1986.
75. Weinblatt ME, Teser JRP, Gilliam JH: The liver in rheumatic diseases. Semin Arthritis Rheum 11:399, 1982.
76. Fortin PR, Larson MG, Watters AK, et al: Prognostic factors in systemic necrotizing vasculitis of the polyarteritis nodosa group—a review of 45 cases. J Rheumatol 22:78, 1995.
77. Leong AS-Y, Alp MH: Hepatocellular disease in the giant-cell arteritis polymyalgia rheumatica syndrome. Ann Rheum Dis 40:92, 1981.
78. Kyle V, Wraight EP, Hazleman BL: Liver scan abnormalities in polymyalgia rheumatica/giant cell arteritis. Clin Rheumatol 10:294, 1991.

Chapter 71

ALCOHOLIC LIVER DISEASE

Jacquelyn J. Maher

EPIDEMIOLOGY

Alcohol is one of the most openly available and generally consumed mood-altering substances. Despite the accessibility of alcohol to all populations, patterns of intake vary among different geographic regions. On average, persons in northern Europe drink more than 10 L/year of pure ethanol. By contrast, persons in Southeast Asia consume approximately one fourth this amount. Americans fall between these two groups, drinking 8.4 L/year of pure ethanol.[1] Longitudinal data indicate that drinking trends have changed dramatically during the 1990s. Between 1990 and 1998, per capita alcohol consumption in northern Europe and the United States declined by as much as 6% to 12%. In Latin America and Asia and in other countries, alcohol use increased, leaving worldwide totals relatively flat.

Epidemiologic studies from around the world have documented a direct correlation between per capita ethanol consumption and liver-related mortality rates.[2–4] Figure 71–1 shows that in the United States, deaths from cirrhosis dropped sharply during Prohibition (1916–1932) and then rose in the post–World War II era as ethanol consumption increased. Cirrhosis-related mortality rates began to decline again in the mid-1970s for unclear reasons, as per capita alcohol consumption rose progressively in the United States from 1960 to 1980. Alcohol consumption started to decline in 1980 (Fig. 71–2) and continued to drop through 1998, along with the cirrhosis-related mortality rate. The liver-related mortality rate in the United States is now at its lowest level in a century, and alcohol consumption is remaining steady at levels similar to those reported in 1965 (see Fig. 71–2).[1]

Although alcohol consumption in the United States is declining, 13.8 million persons still meet diagnostic criteria for alcoholism.*[5] Among this group, more than 2 million are suspected of having liver disease, and 14,000 people die of cirrhosis each year. The number of deaths that are alcohol-related is difficult to determine, because of the inaccurate reporting of ethanol use.[6] Men who drink more than 80 g of ethanol (eight 12-ounce beers, 1 L of wine, or 1/2 pint of distilled spirits) per day are at substantial risk for development of clinical liver disease.[7–10] Liver disease in women who drink excessively is two to four times more likely to develop than in men who drink excessively.[8–10] In 1997, investigators examined the relationship between ethanol intake and alcoholic liver disease in entire populations rather than individuals. The results indicate that the risk of liver disease begins at relatively low levels of alcohol consumption (30 g/day).[2] This finding has led to a general recommendation that the maximal safe level of ethanol consumption is 20 g/day of ethanol, or two "drinks" per day.

It should be noted that although the relative risk of alcoholic liver disease begins to rise in individuals who consume more than 30 g/day of ethanol, the absolute risk remains small. Indeed, even among those who ingest large amounts of alcohol (more than 60 g/day), serious liver disease develops in only approximately 1 in 10.[2] When disease occurs, it can take many forms, ranging from steatosis, to alcoholic hepatitis, to hepatic fibrosis or cirrhosis. The severity of liver disease is not readily predicted by the amount of ethanol consumed.[9] Because alcohol does not cause liver disease in all individuals, and because disease severity does not correspond to classic dose dependency, other factors are likely to play an important role in pathogenesis. These factors may be hereditary, environmental, or both (discussed later).

ETHANOL METABOLISM

Hepatic Metabolism

The liver is the primary site of ethanol metabolism. Within the liver, ethanol can be oxidized by three enzyme systems: the alcohol dehydrogenases (ADHs), cytochrome P-4502E1 (CYP2E1), and catalase. The enzyme system of catalase, which is present in peroxisomes and mitochondria, is the least important of the three pathways. The remaining two

*Diagnostic criteria for alcohol abuse, alcohol dependence, or both are defined in the *Diagnostic and Statistical Manual of Mental Disorders*, 4th edition (DSM-IV).

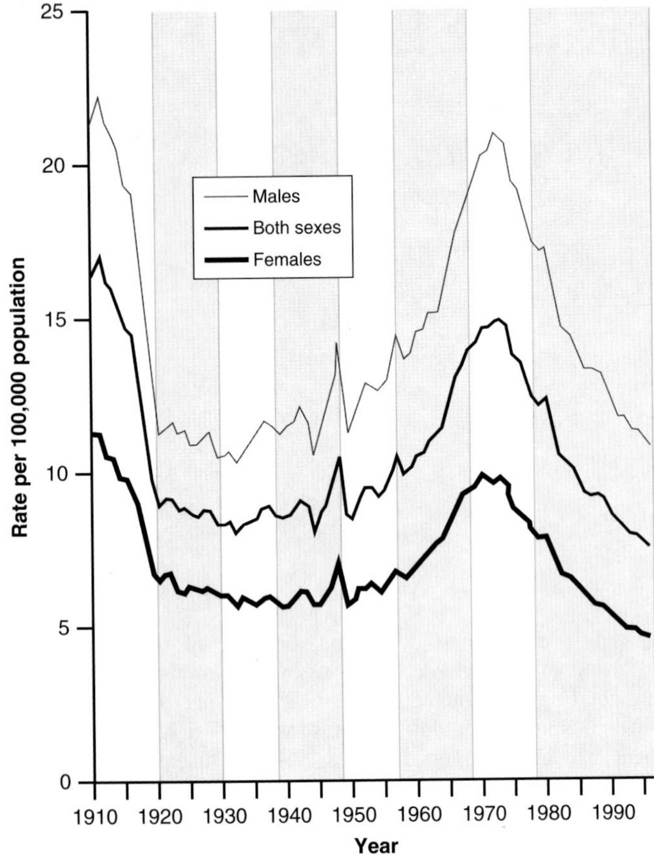

Figure 71–1. Age-adjusted death rates from liver cirrhosis: Death Registration States, 1910–1932, and United States, 1933–1996. (From Saadatmand F, Stinson FS, Grant BF, et al: NIAAA Surveillance Report No. 52, Washington, D.C., CSR, Inc., 2000.)

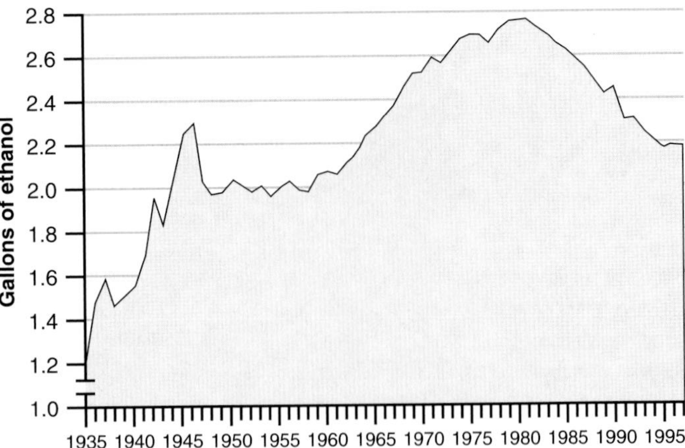

Figure 71–2. Total per capita ethanol consumption, United States, 1935–97. (From Nephew TM, Williams GD, Stinson FS, et al: NIAAA Surveillance Report No. 51, Washington, D.C., CSR, Inc., 1999.)

enzyme systems oxidize most of the ethanol that reaches the liver.

The ADHs are cytoplasmic enzymes with numerous isoforms in human liver.[11] The class I enzymes, which have the lowest K_m values and highest substrate specificity for ethanol, are encoded by three separate genes, ADH1, ADH2, and ADH3. The genes are translated into α, β, and γ peptide subunits, respectively (Table 71–1). For ADH2 and ADH3, polymorphisms have been identified, leading to further subdivision of the β and γ subunits into β_1, β_2, and γ_1, γ_2, and γ_3. Typically, the active enzymes are formed by homodimerization of individual subunits ($\alpha\alpha$, $\beta\beta$, $\gamma\gamma$). However, heterodimers can sometimes form. Variations in ADH isoforms can account for significant differences in ethanol elimination rates among ethnic groups. For example, individuals of Asian descent, who typically have the β_2 ADH subunit, metabolize ethanol 20% faster than northern Europeans, who possess the β_1 subunit.[12]

ADH is the enzyme responsible for alcohol metabolism when blood and tissue ethanol concentrations are low. However, when tissue levels exceed 10 mM (approximately 50 mg/dL), CYP2E1 can also contribute. Chronic ethanol consumption induces the activity of CYP2E1 in the liver by as much as 5- to 10-fold. Ethanol can up-regulate both CYP2E1 messenger ribonucleic acid (mRNA) and protein. Ethanol-related induction of CYP2E1 is likely to account for the more rapid elimination of ethanol observed in chronic alcoholics.

Both ADH and CYP2E1 convert ethanol to acetaldehyde (Fig. 71–3). Acetaldehyde is then oxidized to acetate, primarily by a low-K_m aldehyde dehydrogenase in hepatocyte mitochondria designated *ALDH2*. Rarely, acetaldehyde can be oxidized by alternative pathways involving aldehyde oxidase or xanthine oxidase. Acetaldehyde is a highly reactive and potentially toxic metabolite of ethanol. Fortunately, equilibrium conditions in the liver strongly favor elimination of this compound. If the ability of the liver to remove acetaldehyde is decreased, acetaldehyde can accumulate in the liver and in the circulation. Acetaldehyde produces symptoms of flushing and tachycardia and can provoke circulatory collapse. Approximately one half of Japanese and Chinese individuals are susceptible to these symptoms after alcohol consumption.[13] The problem results from inheritance of the *ALDH2*2* allele, which encodes a completely inactive form of ALDH2. Persons who are homozygous for the mutant enzyme experience severe side effects from acetaldehyde and thus rarely consume ethanol.

Gastric Metabolism

Although the liver is the primary site of alcohol metabolism, ethanol can also be oxidized in the gastrointestinal tract. ADH isoenzymes with subunits different from those described previously have been identified in the stomach and intestine. Gastric ADH has been implicated in a so-called

Table 71–1 | **Class I ADH Genes and Their Encoded Enzyme Subunits***

ADH1-α	ADH2-β		ADH3-γ	
α	ADH2*1	β_1	ADH3*1	γ_1
	ADH2*2	β_2	ADH3*2	γ_2
			ADH3*3	γ_3

*Subunits can form homodimers (e.g., $\alpha\alpha$, $\beta_1\beta_1$, $\gamma_2\gamma_2$) or heterodimers (e.g., $\alpha\beta_1$, $\beta_2\gamma_1$, $\alpha\gamma_3$).
ADH, alcohol dehydrogenase.

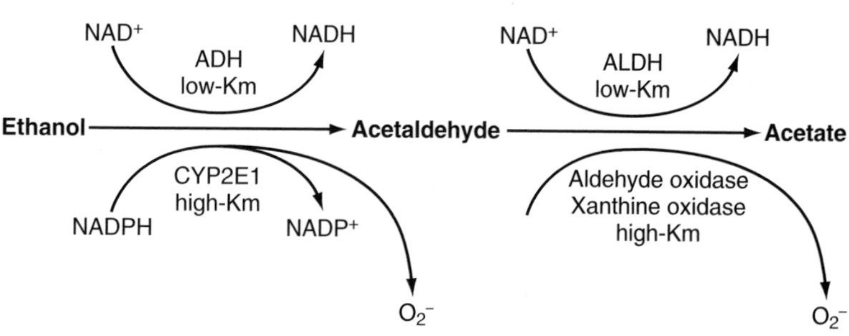

Figure 71–3. Ethanol metabolism in the liver is catalyzed primarily by ADH and CYP2E1. ADH predominates at low ethanol concentrations; at concentrations above 10 mM, CYP2E1 also contributes. Both enzymes convert ethanol to acetaldehyde. ADH-mediated ethanol oxidation is coupled to the conversion of NAD^+ to NADH. CYP2E1 utilizes NADPH and forms oxyradicals as a byproduct. Acetaldehyde is oxidized to acetate primarily by ALDH. Aldehyde oxidase and xanthine oxidase, which produce oxyradicals, are used only rarely. (ADH, alcohol dehydrogenase; CYP2E1, cytochrome P4502E1; NAD, nicotinamide-adenine dinucleotide; ALDH, aldehyde dehydrogenase; NADPH, nicotinamide-adenine dinucleotide phosphate.)

gastric first-pass metabolism of ethanol; by oxidizing ethanol directly in the stomach, this enzyme may limit the amount of ingested ethanol that is delivered to the portal circulation.

Gastric ADH activity is lower in women than in men[14] and can also be inhibited by certain drugs, such as aspirin and histamine H_2 receptor blockers.[15, 16] When gastric ADH activity is reduced, blood ethanol levels after ethanol ingestion are increased. Some investigators have argued that individuals with reduced gastric ADH activity are more susceptible to liver disease, because of increased delivery of ethanol to the liver; however, in light of the many factors involved in ethanol absorption and elimination, this hypothesis has not been proved. Overall, the importance of gastric ADH and gastric first-pass metabolism to the pathophysiologic mechanisms of alcoholic liver disease is unsettled.[17]

PATHOGENESIS OF ALCOHOLIC LIVER INJURY

Toxic and Metabolic Mechanisms

REDOX ALTERATION. ADH-mediated ethanol oxidation is accompanied by the reduction of oxidized nicotinamide-adenine dinucleotide (NAD^+) to reduced NAD (NADH) (see Fig. 71–3). Excess NADH shifts the redox state of hepatocytes, which in turn affects other NAD^+-dependent processes, including lipid and carbohydrate metabolism. One consequence of the redox shift is hepatic steatosis. Excess reducing equivalents provoke steatosis by stimulating fatty acid synthesis and inhibiting mitochondrial beta oxidation. Fatty acids accumulate in the hepatocyte cytoplasm, where they are esterified and stored as triglyceride. NADH also interferes with gluconeogenesis, by limiting the availability of the substrates oxaloacetate, pyruvate, and dihydroxyacetone phosphate and by inhibiting the activity of gluconeogenic enzymes. In patients who have underlying carbohydrate malnutrition, disturbances in this pathway can lead to profound hypoglycemia (see Chapter 63).

The redox shift and the resulting metabolic disturbances are acute consequences of ethanol oxidation. Consequently, they are reversible with abstinence. Chronic ethanol consumption, however, can prolong the redox shift by damaging hepatocyte mitochondria and preventing reoxidation of NADH to NAD^+ (discussed later).

OXIDANT STRESS. Ethanol oxidation leads to formation of several free radical species in the liver, including the hydroxyethyl radical, the superoxide anion (O_2^-), and the hydroxyl radical (OH·). These free radicals can inflict oxidative damage on a wide range of intracellular compounds.[18] Radical formation has classically been considered a consequence of ethanol oxidation by CYP2E1 (see Fig. 71–3),[19] but studies of experimental animals suggest that ethanol-induced radicals also derive importantly, if not primarily, from Kupffer cells. The role of CYP2E1 in the formation of ethanol-derived free radicals was called into question after a study of CYP2E1-knockout mice in 1999.[20] When these mice were fed ethanol, they showed evidence of free radical formation in the liver despite a complete lack of CYP2E1 activity. This study and others[21] indicate that ethanol can induce radical formation in the liver by more than one mechanism and in more than one type of cell. Although CYP2E1 has not been dismissed as a contributor to alcohol-induced oxidant stress, it is important to note that other factors can contribute to free radical formation. Even within hepatocytes, the excess NADH generated by ethanol metabolism promotes mobilization of iron from ferritin. In the reduced state, ferritin can interact with hydrogen peroxide to form hydroxyl radical. Recruited leukocytes can also contribute to alcohol-induced oxidant stress. Neutrophils, which figure prominently in alcoholic hepatitis (discussed later), are stimulated by ethanol to produce superoxide radical.

When free radicals attack unsaturated lipids, a chain reaction of lipid peroxidation is initiated. Chronic ethanol consumption leads to lipid peroxidation in the liver,[22] an event that is associated with both acute tissue damage and fibrosis.[23–25] Free radicals can also attack cellular deoxyribonucleic acid (DNA); mitochondrial DNA is more susceptible to oxidative damage than nuclear DNA, because of reduced protection by histone and nonhistone proteins and because of a decreased capacity for repair. Oxidants can cause both deletions and mutations in mitochondrial DNA, thereby leading to mitochondrial dysfunction. Although in rats chronic ethanol feeding does not produce significant abnormalities in mitochondrial DNA content and transcription, studies in humans have identified mitochondrial DNA deletions in alcoholics with microvesicular steatosis.[26, 27]

The effects of radicals on the liver may be amplified if ethanol also reduces antioxidant defenses. Chronic alcohol consumption causes depletion of several antioxidants in the liver, including vitamins A and E and glutathione. Ethanol-induced vitamin E deficiency enhances hepatic lipid peroxidation; vitamin A depletion causes lysosomal damage. Ethanol-induced glutathione depletion, which occurs selectively in hepatic mitochondria, impairs mitochondrial function and sensitizes cells to apoptosis (see Chapter 63).[28] Ethanol depletes mitochondrial glutathione preferentially by inhibiting transport of glutathione from the hepatocyte cytoplasm.

S-adenosyl-methionine (SAMe), a glutathione precursor, can replete mitochondrial glutathione stores and correct some of the functional alterations.[29, 30] Interestingly, the beneficial effect of SAMe does not appear to be related to its conversion to glutathione. SAMe may act instead by preventing or reversing the glutathione transport defect.[30]

HYPOXIA. Another means by which ethanol may preferentially damage pericentral hepatocytes is through tissue hypoxia. There is evidence that chronic ethanol consumption induces a hypermetabolic state in the liver with increased oxygen consumption by liver cells. The hypermetabolic state has been postulated to enhance the portal-to-central oxygen gradient, leaving pericentral hepatocytes in a state of relative hypoxia. Pericentral hypoxia has been documented in human alcoholics[31]; however, hypoxia may occur only during periods of abstinence or withdrawal. When ethanol is present in the bloodstream, hepatic oxygen consumption increases but is believed to be offset by a concomitant increase in splanchnic blood flow. Studies in experimental animals have indicated that cellular hypoxia can be induced in the liver by both acute and chronic ethanol exposure,[32, 33] thereby leading to adenosine triphosphate (ATP) depletion and liver injury.

EFFECTS OF ACETALDEHYDE. Although acetaldehyde is usually metabolized rapidly in the liver to acetate, in alcoholics the metabolism of acetaldehyde is slowed and can result in acetaldehyde accumulation. If acetaldehyde reaches a high enough concentration, it can become a substrate for the enzymes aldehyde oxidase and xanthine oxidase, which produce free radicals (see Fig. 71–3). Acetaldehyde impairs mitochondrial beta oxidation of fatty acids (discussed later) and can also react with specific amino acid residues on cellular proteins to form acetaldehyde-protein adducts. Acetaldehyde-protein adducts, as well as hybrid adducts formed by acetaldehyde and malondialdehyde, are demonstrable in the liver of alcoholics[34–36] and of alcohol-fed animals.[37, 38] In most instances, the adducts localize preferentially to the pericentral zone, where liver injury is most pronounced. Aldehyde-protein adducts may contribute to alcoholic liver disease by forming neoantigens that stimulate immune responses or by promoting hepatic collagen synthesis (discussed later). If acetaldehyde forms adducts with cytoskeletal proteins such as tubulin, microtubule assembly can be impaired and in turn disturb critical transport processes in hepatocytes, including receptor- and non-receptor-mediated endocytosis as well as protein secretion. Acetaldehyde-induced impairment of protein secretion has been implicated as the major event underlying hepatocellular swelling ("ballooning") in alcoholic liver disease.[39]

Immune and Inflammatory Mechanisms of Liver Injury

KUPFFER CELL ACTIVATION AND CYTOKINE PRODUCTION. Kupffer cells, which are the resident macrophages of the liver, produce oxidants and cytokines for the purpose of host defense. Chronic ethanol consumption, however, causes abnormal activation of Kupffer cells. In this setting, the cytokines and oxidants elaborated by these cells can inflict damage on the liver itself. The central role of Kupffer cells in the pathogenesis of alcoholic liver disease has been demonstrated by eliminating these cells from the livers of experimental animals. When ethanol is fed to rats that lack functional Kupffer cells, liver injury is abrogated.[40] Ethanol is postulated to activate Kupffer cells by promoting leakage of bacterial endotoxin from the intestine into the portal circulation. Indeed, when endotoxin is removed from the gut by treatment with nonabsorbable antibiotics,[41] or when gut flora are altered by administration of *Lactobacillus* species,[42] experimental alcoholic liver injury is reduced.

Among the many compounds produced by activated Kupffer cells, tumor necrosis factor (TNF), transforming growth factor-β (TGF-β), and superoxide appear to be the most pertinent to alcoholic liver injury. In chronic ethanol exposure, TNF promotes hepatocyte apoptosis.[28] TNF also induces hepatic expression of many other cytokines and cell adhesion molecules that cause leukocyte recruitment to the liver. Among these cytokines and molecules are interleukin-1 (IL-1), IL-6, IL-8, monocyte chemoattractant protein-1 (MCP-1), macrophage inflammatory protein-1α and -1β (MIP-1α and MIP-1β), and growth-related oncogene-α (GRO-α).[43, 44] These proinflammatory cytokines contribute importantly to the syndrome of alcoholic hepatitis. TNF and IL-8 are of particular interest because their circulating levels correlate with disease severity.

Superoxide produced by Kupffer cells can have many of the same adverse effects as TNF. Superoxide activates the transcription factor nuclear NF-κB, which directly regulates the transcription of genes encoding cytokines and cell adhesion molecules. Indeed, NF-κB controls transcription of TNF itself, and data from 2000 suggest that oxidants begin the process of alcoholic liver injury by providing a mechanism for the induction of TNF and other inflammatory compounds.[21] Kupffer cell–derived TGF-β does not appear to play a critical role in alcoholic hepatitis but has been implicated in hepatic fibrogenesis (discussed later).

IMMUNE RESPONSES TO ALTERED HEPATOCELLULAR PROTEINS. If hepatocellular proteins form adducts with either aldehyde or hydroxyethyl radicals, they can be altered sufficiently to provoke immune responses. Antibodies directed against these protein adducts are detectable in the blood of alcoholic patients.[36, 45, 46] The role of autoantibodies in the pathogenesis of alcoholic liver injury is uncertain, because many of the target antigens are either retained within cells or released into the circulation. Neither of these processes lends itself to hepatic targeting of the immune response. Some neoantigens, however, are present on the hepatocyte surface and in the hepatic extracellular space. Some animal experiments support the notion that autoantibodies are pathogenic in alcoholic liver disease. In two reports, ethanol was fed to guinea pigs that had been immunized previously with acetaldehyde-protein adducts. Within 90 days, signs of hepatic injury and even fibrosis developed in the guinea pigs, with circulating autoantibodies against the adducts.[47, 48]

Mechanisms of Fibrosis

Liver fibrosis is a serious and potentially irreversible consequence of chronic ethanol use. Fibrosis occurs in only 10% to 15% of alcoholics but can be found in almost 50% of alcoholics who have evidence of liver disease.[49, 50] Central to the pathophysiologic mechanisms of alcoholic liver fibrosis is activation of hepatic stellate cells. Stellate cells reside in Disse's space between hepatocytes and sinusoidal endothelia. In normal liver, stellate cells exhibit a quiescent phenotype and play an important role in hepatic vitamin A storage. In liver injury, however, whether caused by alcohol abuse or by other toxic or infectious insults, stellate cells alter their phenotype to become proliferative, myofibroblast-like cells.[51] Activated stellate cells are the principal collagen producing cells of the liver. They are responsible for the perisinusoidal fibrosis that is characteristic of alcoholic liver disease.

The precise stimulus that initiates stellate cell activation in vivo is unknown. However, a number of compounds present in the alcoholic liver can perpetuate or enhance stellate cell activation and collagen synthesis. Acetaldehyde and aldehyde-protein adducts increase stellate cell collagen synthesis in culture.[52] Oxidants and products of lipid peroxidation also can stimulate collagen synthesis.[53] Yet another stimulus to liver fibrosis is TGF-β, which is a potent inducer of stellate cell collagen synthesis in culture.[54] Stellate cells from alcohol fed rats appear to have increased sensitivity to the fibrogenic effects of TGF-β. In rats, chronic ethanol feeding stimulates Kupffer cells to produce TGF-β. Stellate cells also secrete TGF-β; this autocrine pathway of cytokine production may amplify and perpetuate the fibrogenic process.

COFACTORS IN THE DEVELOPMENT OF ALCOHOLIC LIVER DISEASE

Heritable Factors

Because liver disease develops in only a small proportion of alcoholics, factors other than ethanol itself must play a role in the pathogenesis of alcoholic liver disease. The 1980s witnessed the beginning of an intense search for a hereditary predisposition to alcoholic liver disease. Initially, histocompatibility (human leukocyte antigen [HLA]) antigens were investigated as potential predictors of liver injury; although the frequencies of HLA-A1, -A9, -A28, -B13, -B15, -BW35, and -B40 were noted to be increased in patients with alcoholic cirrhosis,[55–58] none of these associations was confirmed on repeat testing.[59–62]

Hereditary variations in ethanol metabolism have also been explored as risk factors for alcoholic liver disease. Studies have focused on polymorphisms in ADH, CYP2E1, and ALDH, which together cause a wide range of ethanol elimination rates. Among the ADH alleles, the *ADH2*2* allele encodes an enzyme that metabolizes ethanol rapidly. Because this allele is more common in nonalcoholics than in alcoholics, some researchers suggest that rapid metabolism leads to ethanol avoidance.[63, 64] Asians who inherit the slower allele, *ADH2*1,* tend to consume more alcohol[65] and experience more liver disease than those with *ADH2*2*.[66, 67] Unlike ADH, the *CYP2E1* allele associated with liver disease is the one that encodes the more active enzyme.[68] Researchers suggest that the *c2* allele of *CYP2E1,* which is more active than its counterpart *c1,* leads to liver disease by shifting more ethanol metabolism through *CYP2E1,* particularly when *c2* is inherited with a slow-metabolizing allele of ADH such as *ADH3*2*.[69] Reports from Japan, where the *c2* allele is more common than elsewhere, suggest that *c2* is a risk factor for alcoholic liver disease.[65, 68] Confirmation of this association is lacking, however, in other series from both Japan and China.[66, 70, 71] The contribution of *c2* to alcoholic liver disease in whites is also controversial.[69, 72–74]

For ALDH, the mutant allele *ALDH2*2* has been implicated in the development of alcoholic liver disease. As mentioned earlier, *ALDH2*2* homozygotes have a strong aversion to ethanol caused by acetaldehyde toxicity. *ALDH2*1/*2* heterozygotes, however, do occasionally abuse ethanol and experience liver injury. One study from Japan suggests that liver injury develops in *ALDH2*1/*2* heterozygotes with a higher frequency and at a lower dose than in *ALDH2*1/*1* homozygotes.[75] Similar findings have not been reported from China, despite a larger study population.[76]

Hereditary factors other than the rate of ethanol metabolism may play a role in the development of alcoholic liver disease. Researchers have identified two polymorphisms in the promoter region of the *TNF* gene that modify production of this proinflammatory cytokine. One of the polymorphisms, *TNFA-A,* is associated with increased TNF production. In a case control study of patients who had alcoholic liver disease, inheritance of the *TNFA-A* allele did not differ in the alcoholic group from that in the healthy control population. However, among patients who have alcoholic liver disease, those with *TNFA-A* had twice the frequency of steatohepatitis of those without *TNFA-A*.[77] Overall, the absolute number of patients who inherited the abnormal allele was small, and the frequency of more advanced liver disease (i.e., cirrhosis) did not differ in individuals with *TNFA-A* and those with the normal allele.[77] Further study is required to determine the significance of *TNFA-A* in the pathogenesis of alcoholic liver disease.

Gender

Women are more susceptible to serious alcoholic liver injury than men.[8–10] Not only are women at increased risk of alcoholic liver injury, but they also exhibit a tendency toward disease progression even with abstinence.[78, 79] This gender-specific difference in the risk of alcoholic liver disease is unexplained. One theory implicates the reduced levels of gastric ADH in women as a causative factor (discussed earlier). Accelerated alcoholic liver injury in women also may be related to gender-specific differences in fatty acid metabolism. If the fatty acids that accumulate in liver cells as a result of impaired beta oxidation are not converted to triglyceride, they can induce liver injury. This problem may be circumvented by diversion of the fatty acids to alternative routes of metabolism, such as cytochrome P-4504A1–mediated omega hydroxylation. This compensatory pathway is efficiently up-regulated in male rats but not in female rats. Fatty acid binding capacity is also reduced in female rats after long-term ethanol feeding. This reduced binding capacity may contribute to fatty acid toxicity.

Diet and Nutrition

Studies in baboons indicate that ethanol can induce liver injury despite adequate protein-calorie and vitamin nutrition. In human beings, however, alcoholic liver injury appears to be influenced strongly by nutritional status. Interestingly,

Table 71–2 | **Prevalence of Malnutrition in Alcoholic Patients with and without Alcoholic Liver Disease of Varying Severity**

NUTRITIONAL ASSESSMENT	NO DISEASE, % (*n* = 21)	MILD DISEASE, % (*n* = 129)	MODERATE DISEASE, % (*n* = 83)	SEVERE DISEASE, % (*n* = 72)
Normal	38.1	0	0	0
Abnormal but not diagnostic	61.9	50.4	25.3	13.9
Kwashiorkor	0	2.3	13.3	8.3
Marasmus	0	42.6	14.5	5.6
Kwashiorkor and marasmus	0	4.6	47.0	72.2

Data from Mendenhall CL, Anderson S, Weesner RE, et al: Protein-calorie malnutrition associated with alcoholic hepatitis: Veterans Administration Cooperative Study Group on Alcoholic Hepatitis. Am J Med 76:211, 1984.

both undernutrition and overnutrition have been implicated as risk factors in the development of alcoholic liver disease. Patient based studies, such as the Veterans Administration (VA) Cooperative Study on Alcoholic Hepatitis, have shown that alcoholics with liver disease are much more poorly nourished than alcoholics without liver disease (Table 71–2).[80] Mendenhall and coworkers have demonstrated that in patients who have established alcoholic liver disease, a low caloric intake coincides with a high 6-month mortality rate.[81] By contrast, population based studies suggest that the dietary abnormality that places individuals at risk for alcoholic liver disease is excess intake. Nanji and French reported that alcoholic liver disease is most prevalent in populations who consume large amounts of polyunsaturated fat.[82] Other investigators have documented that drinkers who are obese have a two- to threefold higher risk of alcoholic liver disease than those with normal body mass.[83] Obesity is now well recognized as an independent risk factor for hepatic steatosis and steatohepatitis[84–86]: when alcohol consumption is superimposed on obesity, the risk of liver disease rises almost sixfold.[87]

In addition to fat and calories, dietary iron can influence the development of liver disease in alcoholics. Chronic ethanol ingestion promotes absorption of iron from the intestine, and over time hepatic iron stores increase; because iron is an important catalyst of free radical production, it can contribute to liver disease by enhancing the oxidant stress that accompanies hepatic ethanol metabolism.

Coexistent Viral Hepatitis

Roughly 18% to 25% of alcoholics are infected with the hepatitis C virus (HCV).[88–91] In alcoholics with liver disease, the frequency of HCV infection is even higher: some studies report seropositivity rates of 40% or more.[88, 89, 92, 93] The combination of alcohol and HCV infection significantly accelerates the progression of liver disease over that seen with either insult alone.[90, 91, 94] One study indicates that HCV infection in alcoholics increases the probability of development of cirrhosis 8- to 10-fold.[94] This association may be related to the effects of alcohol on HCV replication or on the host immune response to the virus.[95–97]

Like HCV, hepatitis B virus (HBV) accelerates the progression of alcoholic liver disease. Limited experimental studies suggest that ethanol enhances expression of hepatitis B surface antigen and other viral envelope proteins in vitro.[98] Epidemiologic surveys indicate that HBV infection hastens mortality in alcoholics.[90, 99]

DIAGNOSIS

Alcohol should be strongly suspected as a cause of liver disease in any patient who consumes more than 80 g/day of ethanol. Although the risk may be lower in persons who drink less, confounding factors such as gender or HCV infection warrant consideration of alcoholic liver disease even in individuals who consume two drinks of ethanol daily. One must also take into account that patients often underreport ethanol intake. Corroboration of the drinking history by an objective outsider is a helpful adjunct to diagnosis.

Physical Findings

The most extensive demographic information on alcoholic liver disease in the United States is that from studies of hospitalized patients who were assigned a diagnosis based on clinical and histologic parameters.[49, 50] Although these studies did not include a potentially large number of patients who were asymptomatic,[100, 101] they provide a useful guide to diagnosis. The most common physical finding in individuals with alcoholic liver disease is hepatomegaly. Liver enlargement is detectable in more than 75% of patients, regardless of disease severity.[49, 50] Jaundice and ascites are also found in approximately 60% of patients but are more frequent in those with severe disease (Table 71–3).[49, 50] Among the patients who have mild, moderate, and severe disease illustrated in Table 71–3, the high frequency of jaundice in the moderate and severe groups results from use of hyperbilirubinemia (level >5 mg/dL) as a diagnostic criterion. However, even when patients are stratified solely by histologic criteria, the frequency of jaundice increases as the disease progresses.[49]

Other clinical features are noteworthy in patients with alcoholic liver disease. First, an unusually large proportion of patients exhibit hepatic encephalopathy (44.6%), even with mild disease (27.3%). Chedid and colleagues[49] have confirmed this finding: they reported a 19% frequency of encephalopathy and a 28% frequency of portal hypertension in patients whose liver biopsy results indicated only fatty liver. Portal hypertension has been reported in patients with hepatic steatosis[102] and may be related to compression of the

Table 71–3 | **Symptoms and Signs in Hospitalized Patients with Alcoholic Liver Disease**

Symptom or sign	GROUP I (n = 89) Mild (%)	GROUP II (n = 58) Moderate (%)	GROUP III (n = 37) Severe (%)	OVERALL (%)
Hepatomegaly	84.3	94.7	79.4	86.7
Jaundice	17.4	100	100	60.1
Ascites	30.3	79.3	86.5	57.1
Anorexia	39.3	56.9	59.5	48.9
Hepatic encephalopathy	27.3	55.2	70.3	44.6
Alcohol withdrawal	35.9	30.0	14.6	29.0
Weight loss	37.1	27.6	8.1	28.3
Splenomegaly	18.0	30.9	39.4	26.0
Fever	18.0	31.0	21.6	22.8
Infection	3.4	12.1	18.7	9.2

Data from Mendenhall CL: Alcoholic hepatitis. Clin Gastroenterol 10:420, 1981.

hepatic sinusoids by enlarged hepatocytes.[103] Also worth mentioning is that whereas in approximately 25% of patients with alcoholic hepatitis fever is present, demonstrable infection is found in only 9.2%. This discrepancy suggests a possible contribution by ethanol-induced cytokines.[104]

Laboratory Findings

At least 75% of patients with alcoholic liver disease have a macrocytic anemia (Table 71–4). Leukocytosis is also common, with a mean white blood cell count of 12,400/mm^3. Serum aspartate aminotransferase (AST) and alanine aminotransferase (ALT) levels are only modestly elevated; AST and ALT levels rarely exceed 300 U/L and do not correlate well with disease severity.[49, 50]

The AST/ALT ratio often exceeds 2 in patients who have alcoholic liver disease (Figure 71–4).[49, 105] This finding together with the relatively low values of AST and ALT helps to distinguish alcoholism from other types of liver diseases. Although an AST/ALT ratio greater than 1 is used by some investigators to predict alcoholic liver disease, Figure 71–4 demonstrates that, in the range between 1 and 2, there is substantial overlap with viral hepatitis and postnecrotic cirrhosis. A ratio greater than or equal to 3 strongly suggests alcoholic liver disease.

The high AST/ALT ratio in alcoholics with liver disease has been attributed to pyridoxine deficiency, which causes a reduction in the AST and ALT content of hepatocytes, and a disproportionate reduction in ALT content. The changes in intracellular AST and ALT content are more reflective of alcohol consumption than of alcoholic liver injury; consequently, in the setting of pyridoxine deficiency, any insult

Table 71–4 | **Laboratory Values in Hospitalized Patients with Alcoholic Liver Disease***

	GROUP I (n = 89) Mild	GROUP II (n = 58) Moderate	GROUP III (n = 37) Severe
Hematocrit (%)	38	36	33
MCV (μm^3)	100	102	105
WBC count (per mm^3)	8,000	11,000	12,000
Serum AST level (U/L)	84	124	99
Serum ALT level (U/L)	56	56	57
Serum alkaline phosphatase level (IU/mL)	166	276	225
Serum bilirubin level (mg/dL)	1.6	13.5	8.7
Prothrombin time (sec prolonged)	0.9	2.4	6.4
Serum albumin level	3.7	2.7	2.4

*Moderate disease was defined by bilirubin level >5 mg/dL and severe disease by bilirubin level >5 mg/dL and prothrombin time >4 seconds prolonged. ALT, alanine aminotransferase; AST, aspartate aminotransferase; MCV, mean corpuscular volume; WBC, white blood cell.

Data from Mendenhall CL: Alcoholic hepatitis. Clin Gastroenterol 10:422, 1981.

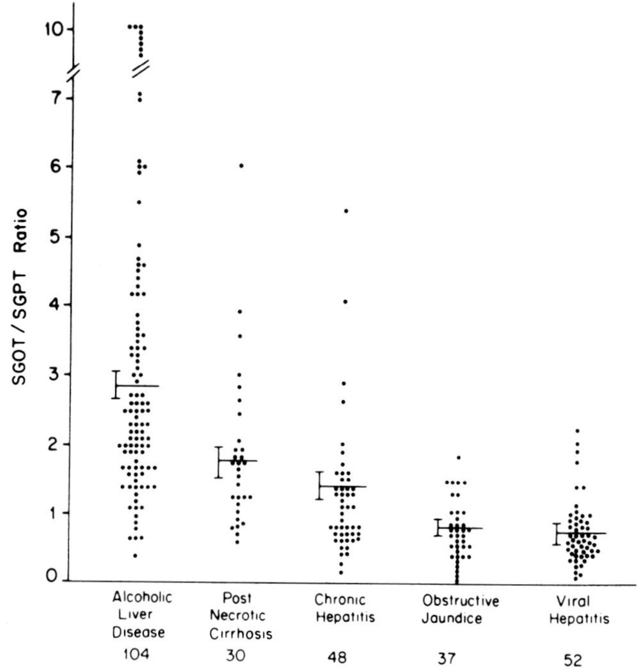

Figure 71–4. SGOT/SGPT (AST/ALT) ratios in patients with biopsy-proven liver disease. (From Cohen JA, Kaplan, MM: The SGOT/SGPT ratio—an indicator of alcoholic liver disease. Dig Dis Sci 24:835, 1979.)

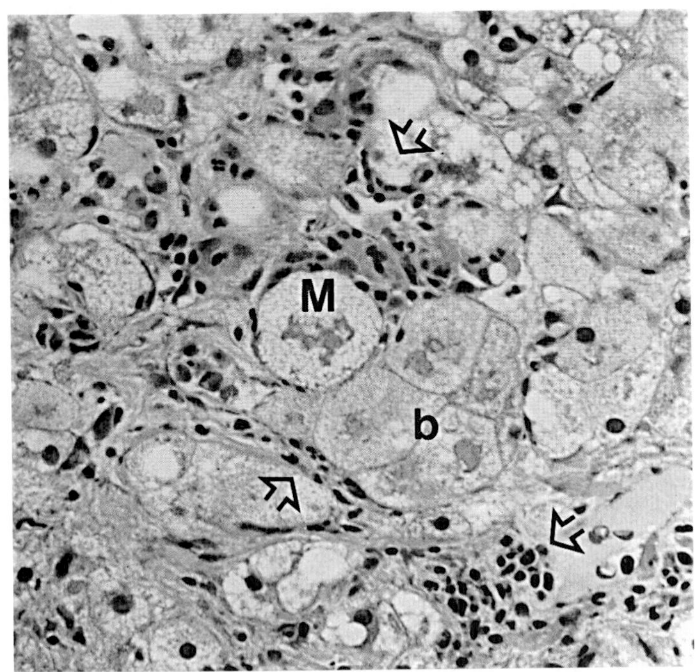

Figure 71–5. Light photomicrograph illustrating acute alcoholic liver injury. Note ballooning degeneration (b); Mallory's bodies (M); neutrophilic inflammatory infiltrate *(arrows)*.

that causes hepatocellular necrosis provokes an increase in aminotransferase levels with a predominance of AST level. This phenomenon is likely to explain the high AST/ALT ratio in alcoholics who have acetaminophen toxicity. Even in therapeutic doses, acetaminophen can cause severe hepatic necrosis in actively drinking patients (see Chapter 73). In active drinkers, acetaminophen hepatotoxicity is characterized by dramatic elevations in serum aminotransferase levels with a high AST/ALT ratio.[106] That severe nonalcoholic liver injury can occur in alcoholics and can be associated with the typical AST/ALT ratio of alcohol-induced disease underscores the importance of considering the absolute aminotransferase values before making a diagnosis. A marked aminotransferase level elevation (>300 U/L) in an alcoholic, even with an AST/ALT ratio greater than 2, should raise concern about acute nonalcoholic liver injury.

The serum bilirubin level and prothrombin time (PT) are useful predictors of the severity of liver disease in alcoholics. The two parameters have been used to stratify patients with alcoholic liver disease into mild, moderate, and severe categories (Tables 71–3 and 71–4).[50] Maddrey and associates[107] also used the bilirubin level and PT to generate a "discriminant function" that identifies patients who have a significant short-term mortality rate:

$$\text{Discriminant function} = 4.6 \times (\text{PT in seconds} - \text{control in seconds}) + \text{bilirubin (mg/dL)}$$

A discriminant function greater than 32 predicts a 1-month mortality rate of approximately 50%. Some researchers believe that calculation of the discriminant function is unnecessary for patients who have encephalopathy, because of evidence from North American studies that encephalopathy alone predicts a high short-term mortality rate.[108]

Several blood tests have been evaluated as markers of recent alcohol consumption. These tests include mitochondrial AST,[109] carbohydrate deficient transferrin,[110] and antibodies against acetaldehyde-protein adducts.[111] Collagen propeptides also have been studied, not only as markers of alcohol consumption, but as noninvasive markers of liver fibrosis. Interestingly, in some studies collagen propeptides have been better predictors of hepatic inflammation than of fibrosis.[112–115] None of these tests has proved sufficiently accurate or reliable for routine clinical use.

Histology

Liver biopsy is viewed by many authorities as the standard for diagnosing alcoholic liver injury. Indeed, in one study as many as 20% of cases of alcoholic liver disease were misdiagnosed by clinical criteria alone.[116] Although the true error rate in diagnosis is probably closer to 10%, liver biopsy is still quite useful for diagnosis and for prediction of prognosis. Among the most common histologic features of alcoholic liver disease are (1) steatosis, (2) ballooning degeneration of hepatocytes, (3) presence of Mallory's bodies, (4) neutrophilic inflammation, and (5) pericellular fibrosis (Fig. 71–5).

Steatosis is present in 60% to 95% of alcoholic liver disease patients.[49, 50, 117] Fat is most prominent pericentrally, although in severe cases it exhibits a panlobular distribution. Macrovesicular steatosis is the rule; large fat droplets in hepatocytes displace the nucleus to an eccentric position. Microvesicular steatosis, or "foamy degeneration,"[118] also can occur in the livers of alcoholics (Fig. 71–6). Although once considered rare, microvesicular steatosis in alcoholics[119] has been shown by close review of biopsy findings to be a common accompaniment to ballooning degeneration.[49]

Ballooning degeneration of hepatocytes is characterized by marked cell swelling with a pale appearance of the cytoplasm. Ballooning is a nonspecific marker of hepatocyte in-

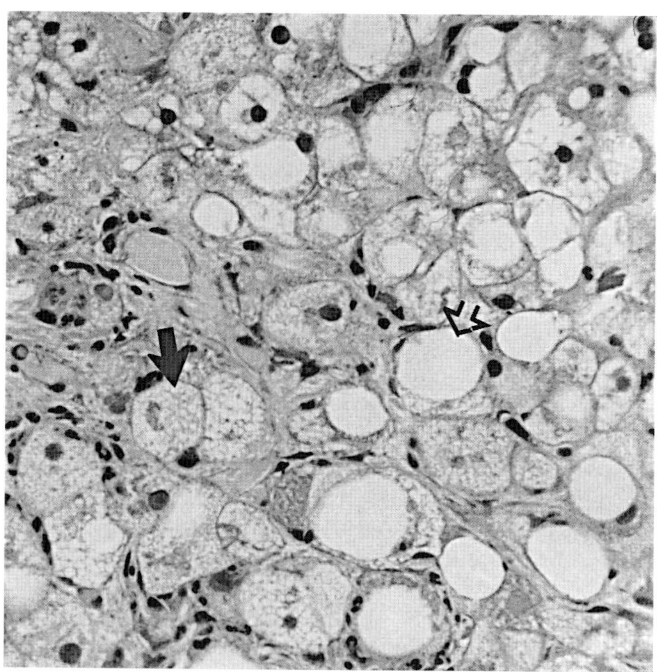

Figure 71–6. Light photomicrograph of alcoholic liver injury illustrating macrovesicular *(open arrow)* and microvesicular *(solid arrow)* steatosis.

jury and is often accompanied by acidophil (apoptotic) bodies. Both features are found in 60% to 90% of patients with alcoholic liver disease.[49, 117] Also common in alcoholic liver disease are Mallory's bodies, crescent shaped eosinophilic structures that represent intermediate filaments that have undergone condensation. Mallory's bodies are found in 70% to 75% of patients who undergo biopsy examination for alcoholic liver disease[49, 50] and are classically found to be wrapped around the nucleus of hepatocytes (see Fig. 71–5). Despite their prevalence in alcoholics, Mallory's bodies are not pathognomonic of alcoholic liver disease. They also appear in patients who have primary biliary cirrhosis and Wilson disease and in those who are prescribed griseofulvin or amiodarone.

Hepatic inflammation is present in 50% to 85% of patients with alcoholic liver disease.[49, 50] Polymorphonuclear leukocytes (neutrophils) are prominent components of the inflammatory infiltrate, and their presence helps to distinguish alcohol-induced inflammation from other forms of hepatitis. Neutrophils are typically found beside ballooned hepatocytes or cells containing Mallory's bodies. Mononuclear cells also can be seen. Some degree of periportal inflammation is observed in 75% of patients who have alcoholic liver injury; that finding suggests that this lesion may be caused by ethanol as well.[49] However, the detection of classic interface hepatitis suggests coexistent viral infection.

Fibrosis, which occurs in 50% to 75% of patients who have alcoholic liver injury, begins with deposition of connective tissue around the terminal hepatic venule and then extends into the hepatic parenchyma in a pericellular fashion ("chicken-wire" fibrosis). As fibrosis advances, broader septa are formed, with central-central and central-portal bridging. The cirrhosis that evolves is micronodular.

In 1991, Chedid and colleagues[49] defined four histologic categories of alcoholic liver disease for the purpose of predicting survival: (1) fatty liver (FL), (2) alcoholic hepatitis (AH), (3) cirrhosis (C), and (4) cirrhosis with alcoholic hepatitis (C+AH). The two main criteria used to stratify patients into the four categories were hepatic inflammation (absent in FL and present in AH) and cirrhosis (present in C and C+AH but not in FL or AH). Using these criteria they found statistically significant differences in 4-year survival rates among the 4 groups (70% FL; 58% AH; 49% C; 35% C+AH). These results parallel data published in 1987 by Orrego and colleagues.[120]

Differential Diagnosis

Distinguishing alcoholic liver disease from nonalcoholic steatohepatitis (NASH) can present a major challenge (see Chapter 72). Both syndromes have strikingly similar clinical and histologic features. One parameter that may be helpful in the differential diagnosis is the AST/ALT ratio. Whereas in alcoholics, the AST/ALT ratio typically exceeds 2, in NASH the ratio averages about 1.0.[86, 121] As NASH progresses toward fibrosis, the AST/ALT ratio rises. However, even in advanced disease, the ratio remains below 1.5.[122] Thus, an AST/ALT ratio above 1.5 suggests alcoholic liver disease.

Alcoholic liver disease also can be difficult to distinguish from hereditary hemochromatosis, in the event of findings of a high serum iron saturation and siderosis on liver biopsy. In this situation, genetic testing for hemochromatosis may be useful (see Chapter 66). Hepatic iron quantitation also can be performed on biopsy material for the purpose of calculating a hepatic iron index.

COMPLICATIONS

The complications of alcoholic liver disease are similar to those encountered in other types of chronic liver injury. Among these are ascites, gastrointestinal hemorrhage, and encephalopathy, as well as hypoalbuminemia and hypoprothrombinemia arising from hepatocellular dysfunction. These complications and others are discussed in detail in Chapters 77 to 79.

When alcoholic liver disease progresses to cirrhosis, hepatocellular carcinoma (HCC) may develop. Alcohol alone appears to be an independent risk factor for HCC, albeit a weaker one than viral hepatitis.[123, 124] One Japanese study reported 10-year frequency rates for HCC to be 18.5% in patients with liver disease caused by alcohol alone, 56.5% in those with liver disease caused by HCV infections alone, and 80.7% in those with liver disease caused by both alcohol and HCV.[123] Data from a study in 2000 show that alcohol increases the risk of HCC in patients with HCV infection 1.5- to 2.5-fold.[125] Not all studies have found alcohol to be an independent risk factor for HCC, but studies with negative results have tended to have the shortest follow-up periods.[126, 127] Most investigators in the field are in agreement that alcohol consumption, when combined with viral hepatitis, poses a high risk of HCC.[128] Among alcoholics, men older than 50 years of age appear to be most vulnerable to development of HCC.[92, 129]

TREATMENT

Abstinence

The mainstay of treatment for alcoholic liver disease is abstinence, which in itself can improve survival rates substantially in persons with alcoholic liver disease even if cirrhosis and portal hypertension are present at the time of diagnosis (discussed later). In severe alcoholic liver disease, however, abstinence and supportive medical care may not be sufficient to improve the patient's clinical status, and pharmacologic therapy may provide an important adjunct. Several agents have been used in the treatment of alcoholic hepatitis and alcoholic fibrosis. The rationales for their use and a general assessment of their efficacy are discussed in the sections that follow.

Nutritional Supplements

The VA Cooperative Study Group reported that malnutrition worsens the prognosis of alcoholic hepatitis. The study found that patients who had severe protein-calorie malnutrition had a 6-month mortality rate of 20% to 50%, in contrast to mildly malnourished patients in whom the mortality rate was 0% to 9%.[80] The outcome of severely malnourished patients improved if the nutritional status was partially corrected during 30-day hospitalization.[80] The concept that nutritional support could improve the outcome of patients with alcoholic hepatitis led to several controlled trials of enteral and parenteral supplements in hospitalized patients. Although individual studies employed different nutritional formulas and different routes of administration, the chosen end points were similar, and the results were remarkably consistent. Contrary to expectations, nutritional supplements produced little or no improvement in nutritional status, laboratory parameters of liver injury, or survival rate (Table 71–5).[130–135]

Despite these negative results, enteral supplements may still be of general value in hospitalized patients with alcoholic hepatitis, particularly in anorexic patients who consume less than 75% of their calculated energy and protein requirements per day.[136] Branched-chain amino acid formulas (e.g., Hepatic-Aid II Instant Drink) need not be used rather than conventional amino acid preparations. Branched-chain amino acid formulas are expensive, and conventional preparations have not been proved to cause hepatic encephalopathy, even in patients who have cirrhosis and portal hypertension.[130, 132]

Anti-inflammatory Drugs

GLUCOCORTICOIDS. Because of their broad anti-inflammatory and immunosuppressive properties, glucocorticoids have been viewed as a logical treatment for alcoholic hepatitis. Between 1971 and 1989, at least 11 published placebo controlled trials examined the effects of glucocorticoids on patients who had acute alcoholic liver disease.[107, 137–146] Although the studies involved a total of 562 patients, they yielded widely disparate results. Only 4 of the 11 trials demonstrated a reduction in short-term mortality by glucocorticoids. The variable outcomes were attributed to numerous factors, including differences in gender, liver disease severity, renal function, nutritional status, and even location. In an effort to settle the controversy regarding the efficacy of glucocorticoids, Imperiale and McCullough performed a meta-analysis of the 11 clinical trials.[108] On combining all the data, they found that the relative risk of short-term mortality was 0.63 in patients who were treated with glucocorticoids. When they restricted their analysis to include only the highest-quality studies, glucocorticoids demonstrated even more impressive benefit, with a relative mortality risk of 0.41.[108] Glucocorticoids were effective whether administered orally or intravenously (as prednisolone 40 mg/day or methylprednisolone 32 mg/day). In the trials demonstrating efficacy, full-dose treatment was continued for 28 to 30 days, followed in most instances by a 2- to 4-week taper. Serious infections sometimes occurred in glucocorticoid treated patients,[140, 143] but they were rare and apparently no more frequent than in patients who received placebo.[143]

The meta-analysis confirmed a suspicion raised in several of the individual trials that glucocorticoids are effective only in the subgroup of alcoholics who have the most severe liver disease. One means of identifying these patients is the discriminant function of Maddrey and coworkers.[107] Encephalopathy also identifies patients with a high short-term mortality rate; in fact, in the meta-analysis, encephalopathy was the strongest predictor of a response to glucocorticoids. The concept that encephalopathy is required for a response to glucocorticoids has been challenged by Ramond and col-

Table 71–5 | **Studies Evaluating the Effect of Supplemental Enteral or Parenteral Nutrition on Short-Term Survival Rate in Alcoholic Hepatitis**

REFERENCE	YEAR	*n*	ROUTE	FORMULA	MORTALITY RATE
130	1980	35	Enteral	Amino acids	78% Control 100% Amino acids
131	1985	57	Enteral	BCAA	20.6% Control 16.7% BCAA
132	1985	64	Enteral/Parenteral	BCAA/conventional	32% Control 33% BCAA 43% Conventional
134	1987	28	Parenteral	Amino acids	21% Control 7% Amino acids
135	1991	54	Parenteral	Amino acids	19% Control 21% Amino acids

BCAA, branched-chain amino acids

leagues,[147] who studied 61 patients with a discriminant function greater than 32 and showed that glucocorticoids improved survival rate significantly whether or not encephalopathy was present.[147] In a subsequent study, Mathurin and associates reported that peripheral neutrophilia (greater than 5500/mm^3) could also be used to predict a favorable response to glucocorticoids.[148] Of note, the study by Mathurin and colleagues was the first to report long-term follow-up data for patients treated with glucocorticoids for alcoholic hepatitis. Their results indicated that the survival benefit of a 4-week course of prednisolone lasted for at least 1 year.[148]

In the meta-analysis of Imperiale and McCullough,[108] only when patients who had gastrointestinal hemorrhage were excluded from consideration did treatment improve survival rate. Glucocorticoids did not enhance the risk of gastointestinal hemorrhage, but bleeding had such a high independent mortality risk that it dampened the effect of glucocorticoids. Poor renal function at randomization can also limit the benefit of glucocorticoids. Patients with alcoholic hepatitis who exhibited a serum creatinine level greater than 2.5 mg/dL had a high risk of progression to renal failure and a short-term mortality rate of 75%, with or without glucocorticoid therapy.[143] When evaluating patients for glucocorticoid therapy, certain confounding illnesses should be excluded, including active infection, pancreatitis, and possibly insulin-dependent diabetes mellitus.

A second meta-analysis that examined the benefit of glucocorticoids for alcoholic hepatitis was published in 1995.[149] The authors of this study drew the opposite conclusion, namely, that glucocorticoids do not improve patient survival rates. In their analysis, they employed statistical adjustment to correct for imbalances of confounding variables. This methodology differed from that of the first study, in which outlying data were excluded. At present, therefore, there remains some controversy over the use of glucocorticoids for alcoholic hepatitis, not only because efficacy is uncertain but also because many potential candidates for therapy exhibit one or more exclusion criteria. Despite their limited target population, glucocorticoids are considered sufficiently beneficial to be recommended by the American College of Gastroenterology for treatment of alcoholic hepatitis.[150]

PENTOXIFYLLINE. Pentoxifylline can reduce inflammation by inhibiting the synthesis of TNF. This drug was studied in 2000 as a treatment for alcoholic hepatitis in a randomized controlled trial involving 101 patients.[151] All patients had severe alcoholic hepatitis as judged by a discriminant function greater than 32; 49 were treated with pentoxifylline (400 mg orally three times a day) for 4 weeks, and 52 received placebo. Pentoxifylline did not cause a significant decrease in plasma TNF levels in treated patients. It did, however, afford a survival benefit and significant protection against the hepatorenal syndrome. The 4-week mortality rate in the placebo group was 46.1%, as would be predicted by the discriminant function. In the pentoxifylline group, the mortality rate over the same interval was 24.5%. In addition, pentoxifylline reduced the frequency of hepatorenal syndrome from 34.6% to 8.2%. The mechanism of action of pentoxifylline may be related to beneficial effects of the drug on the microcirculation, particularly within the kidney. Results with pentoxifylline appear promising but require confirmation.

Antioxidants

POLYENYLPHOSPHATIDYLCHOLINE. Alterations in mitochondrial phospholipids have been noted in the liver of alcohol-fed animals and are implicated in alcohol-induced hepatic mitochondrial dysfunction. One proposed means of ameliorating ethanol-induced mitochondrial dysfunction is to provide supplemental phospholipids. A soybean extract containing polyunsaturated lecithin (PUL) has putative membrane stabilizing effects; this compound was first tested by Lieber and colleagues[152] in the treatment of alcohol-fed baboons. In a study lasting 10 years, PUL did not prevent ethanol-induced mitochondrial abnormalities in liver cells.[152] The compound did, however, significantly attenuate hepatic fibrosis (75% versus 0% fibrosis in control versus treated groups, $n = 8$).

The active phospholipid species in PUL is polyenylphosphatidylcholine (PPC).[153] In cell culture, PPC is capable of inhibiting hepatic stellate cell activation,[154, 155] also decreases CYP2E1 induction, and may reduce ethanol-related apoptosis in vivo.[156, 157] In intact animals, PPC decreases ethanol-induced lipid peroxidation and restores hepatic glutathione.[156] A controlled trial of PPC is currently under way in humans with alcoholic liver disease.

***S*-ADENOSYL-METHIONINE.** *S*-adenosyl-methionine (SAMe) preserves mitochondrial glutathione stores in alcohol treated hepatocytes[30] and may protect them against alcohol-induced injury. A study in baboons showed SAMe to be a promising treatment for alcoholic liver disease[29] and was followed by a randomized controlled trial in humans.[158] In the study, 123 patients with alcoholic cirrhosis (84% biopsy-proven) received either SAMe 400 mg orally three times a day or placebo for 2 years. The primary end point was death or liver transplantation. Over 90% of patients had Child-Turcotte-Pugh class A or B cirrhosis; one half of them continued to drink alcohol during the study. SAMe improved the overall 2-year survival rate from 70% to 84%, but the difference was not statistically significant. When Child-Turcotte-Pugh class C patients were excluded, the gap widened just enough to achieve statistical significance ($P = 0.046$). Deaths in both groups were primarily liver-related. Like PPC, SAMe may have a role in the long-term treatment of alcoholic liver disease. However, because the effects of this single study were quite modest, additional patients must be treated to determine whether the drug has true benefit. Whether SAMe can ameliorate acute alcoholic hepatitis, rather than chronic alcoholic liver disease, has not been investigated.

SILYMARIN. Silymarin, an antioxidant compound derived from the milk thistle plant, has been examined as a long-term treatment for alcoholic liver disease. In one study, 91 patients with alcoholic cirrhosis were randomized to receive either silymarin, 140 mg orally three times a day, or placebo for 2 years.[159] Silymarin improved the 4-year survival rate in treated patients, but the effect was restricted to individuals who had Child-Turcotte-Pugh class A cirrhosis. That alcohol consumption was not strictly controlled in this population possibly accounts for the relatively low 4-year survival rates of 50% and 80% in the control and silymarin groups, respectively. A second study of silymarin was conducted on

200 patients with alcoholic cirrhosis, about one half of whom were designated Child's class B.[160] These patients also received silymarin, 150 mg orally three times a day, or placebo for 2 years. In contrast to the first study, this trial showed no survival benefit of silymarin treatment. The overall 5-year survival rate in the second study was good for patients in Child-Turcotte-Pugh class B (71% in the silymarin group, 76% in the placebo group). The authors attributed the favorable outcome to their rigorous attempts to enforce abstinence. Together, these studies suggest that silymarin provides no greater benefit than abstinence alone does in promoting survival in patients who have alcoholic liver disease. Silymarin may be of benefit in patients who continue to drink, but only those with Child's A cirrhosis.

ANTIOXIDANT VITAMINS. Although vitamins A and E have been used in animals and humans as a potential treatment for alcoholic liver disease, results have been disappointing.[161–165] Vitamin A has a very narrow toxic-to-therapeutic ratio[162, 163] and is not likely to be useful as a single agent.

Drugs with Unconfirmed Benefit

COLCHICINE. Colchicine inhibits leukocyte migration and function and has been reported to attenuate toxin-induced liver injury in experimental animals. Colchicine was evaluated in a randomized controlled trial involving 72 patients with a serum bilirubin level greater than 5 mg/dL; it was administered at a dose of 1 mg/day for 30 days. At the end of the study interval, no differences were observed in either survival rate or liver biochemical test results.[166] Colchicine also has reported antifibrotic effects and has been evaluated as a treatment for cirrhosis. Kershenobich and colleagues[167] studied the efficacy of colchicine therapy in 100 cirrhotic patients, 45% of whom had alcohol-induced liver disease. Colchicine, 1 mg/day, or placebo was administered for up to 14 years (mean 4.7 years). Life table analysis indicated a significant survival benefit in patients receiving colchicine, with 75% and 34% 5-year survival rates in the treatment and control groups, respectively.[167] In some colchicine treated patients, serial liver biopsies demonstrated resolution of fibrosis. Although the long-term results with colchicine seemed impressive, careful scrutiny revealed problems with the study. Almost three fourths of the patients who had Child-Turcotte-Pugh class A cirrhosis at the time of enrollment would have been predicted to have a 5-year survival rate much greater than 34% (see later discussion). The poor survival rate in the control group largely resulted from problems other than liver disease; when non–liver disease deaths were excluded from analysis, the survival rate for the placebo group rose to equivalence with that for the colchicine group. In light of these findings, there is no clear benefit to the use of colchicine for either acute or chronic alcoholic liver disease.

PROPYLTHIOURACIL. The hypermetabolic state induced by ethanol (discussed earlier) is similar to that encountered in hyperthyroidism. This observation prompted several trials of propylthiouracil (PTU) as treatment for alcoholic hepatitis. In the first study, PTU, 300 mg/day, was administered to 103 patients with varying degrees of alcoholic liver disease. Over a treatment period of 42 days, PTU accelerated the clinical improvement of the most severely ill patients but did not affect survival rate.[168] An independent group conducted a second trial of PTU in 67 alcoholic hepatitis patients. This study, which included only patients who had severe liver disease, showed no benefit of PTU despite an identical dose and duration of therapy.[169] In both trials PTU exhibited a demonstrable antithyroid effect, reflected by a rise in serum thyroid-stimulating hormone levels.

A third long-term study examined outpatients who had alcoholic liver disease. In this 2-year trial, patients in the treatment group received PTU, 300 mg/day, in a 3-months-on/1-month-off regimen. PTU reduced the mortality rate significantly, from 25% to 13%.[170] As with the original short-term trial, patients who had the most severe liver disease were afforded the greatest benefit (55% versus 25% mortality rates in the placebo and PTU groups, respectively). Patients who had mild alcoholic liver injury did not derive any survival benefit from PTU, as their underlying mortality rate was quite low (3%).[170]

Despite the encouraging results of the long-term study, PTU has not gained acceptance as a treatment for alcoholic liver disease, in part because of concerns that PTU might provoke hypothyroidism and in part because of uncertainties about the patient populations in which PTU is effective. The issue of hypothyroidism has been addressed in a follow-up study that demonstrated almost no side effects in patients who received PTU for up to 4 years.[171] However, concerns over efficacy remain. Studies have shown that the ethanol-induced hypermetabolic state is transient, disappearing within 30 days of abstinence. Thus, if PTU is exerting its effect by diminishing the hypermetabolic state, the effect should be greatest in patients who continue to drink. This was not the finding in the clinical trials; indeed, in order to derive benefit from PTU, patients had to remain abstinent or drink only modestly.[170, 171] Why PTU is most effective in abstainers remains unexplained.

Liver Transplantation

Advanced alcoholic liver disease patients may be candidates for liver transplantation (see Chapter 83). For patients in Child-Turcotte-Pugh class C, transplantation can improve 5-year survival rate significantly.[172] Patients who have transplantation for alcohol-induced liver disease have survival rates comparable to those of patients who have transplantation for nonalcoholic liver disease.[173–175] Some investigators have argued that transplantation is successful even in the setting of acute alcoholic hepatitis.[176] Others warn that active alcoholic liver disease in the explanted liver portends a poor prognosis.[177] For patients who survive transplantation surgery, recidivism occurs in 20% to 50% of patients postoperatively.[175, 178]

Identifying alcoholic patients with a potential for recidivism is a major challenge for transplantation professionals. Although 6 months of pretransplantation abstinence has been used as a criterion to reduce the risk of post-transplant recidivism, other investigators favor a risk scale that considers a number of factors independent of the duration of sobriety.[179, 180] Efforts are ongoing to refine risk scores and incorporate them as standard transplantation selection criteria for alcoholics.

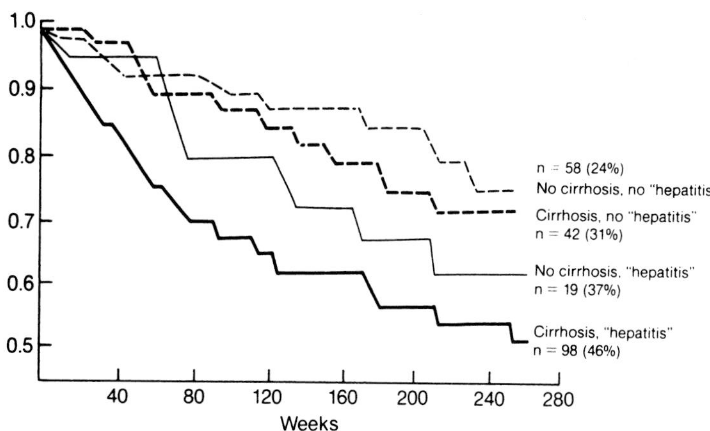

Figure 71–7. Five-year survival of patients with alcoholic liver disease stratified by histologic disease severity. (From Orrego H, Blake JE, Blendis LM, et al: Prognosis of alcoholic cirrhosis in the presence and absence of alcoholic hepatitis. Gastroenterology; 92: 208, 1987.)

PROGNOSIS

Alcoholic steatosis has been viewed as a benign lesion. Although fat can cause acute morbidity as a result of portal hypertension, such consequences typically reverse with abstinence. In 1996, however, activated stellate cells were identified in the liver of alcoholics whose routine histologic evaluation results demonstrated only steatosis.[181] This finding suggests that fat alone may be sufficient to stimulate hepatic fibrogenesis. Longitudinal studies of alcoholics in which serial liver biopsy results were obtained support the suggestion that steatosis carries a risk of disease progression. For example, Marbet and colleagues[9] reported progression from steatosis to liver fibrosis in 5 of 16 patients over an interval of 8 years. Similarly over 10 years, Sorensen and colleagues[182] and Teli and colleagues[183] reported progression from steatosis to fibrosis or cirrhosis in 13% to 18% of 336 patients. On an initial liver biopsy evaluation disease progression may be heralded by the presence of perivenular fibrosis.[184]

In patients who exhibit clinical evidence of alcoholic liver injury, the natural history of the disease is dependent largely on severity. Even patients with mild disease have a significant mortality risk; patients who are sick enough to be hospitalized, even if they do not have jaundice or hypoprothrombinemia, have a 1-month mortality rate close to 20%.[50] Patients who have severe disease have a short-term mortality rate of approximately 50%.[50, 107] When disease severity is assessed by histologic rather than clinical criteria, survival rate is somewhat better (1-year survival rate of 60% to 70% for patients who have severe disease).[49, 120]

Table 71–6 | **Five-Year Survival Rates in Patients with Alcoholic Cirrhosis as a Function of Drinking Behavior**

	FIVE-YEAR SURVIVAL RATES	
	Abstinent, %	**Drinking, %**
All patients	63.0	40.5
No complications	88.9	68.2
Complications	60.1	34.1

Data from Powell WJ Jr, Klatskin G: Duration of survival in patients with Laennec's cirrhosis: Influence of alcohol withdrawal, and possible effects of recent changes in general management of the disease. Am J Med 44:406, 1968.

Interestingly, hepatic inflammation and cirrhosis appear to be equally ominous histologic lesions in predicting prognosis. Cirrhosis alone is an indicator of poor prognosis; indeed, Goldberg and colleagues,[185] who assessed the outcome of 34 patients with biopsy-proven alcoholic cirrhosis but clinical signs of only mild disease, found the 30-month mortality rate to be 29% (compared with 18% for the group without cirrhosis). However, alcoholic hepatitis also carries a high independent risk of mortality and in some series has proved to be more deadly than inactive cirrhosis (Fig. 71–7).[120] In studies that have examined the natural history of alcoholic liver disease on the basis of histologic characteristics at diagnosis, patients with fatty liver or the equivalent have had the best outcome (70% to 80% survival rate at 4 to 5 years); those with alcoholic hepatitis or cirrhosis, an intermediate outcome (50% to 75% survival rate at 4 to 5 years); and those with cirrhosis combined with alcoholic hepatitis, the worst outcome (30% to 50% survival rate at 4 to 5 years). Considering all patients with alcoholic liver disease as a single group, the average 1-year and 5-year survival rates are approximately 80% and 50%, respectively.[49, 50, 186]

Continued drinking is another factor that impacts the survival rate significantly in alcoholic liver disease.[187, 188] Powell and Klatskin[187] showed that abstinence can improve patient outcome regardless of disease severity at diagnosis (Table 71–6). Abstinence is not a guarantee of improvement, however, and some studies have reported progression of liver injury despite cessation of ethanol intake.[78, 79] The latter finding may be particularly true for women.[78, 79]

The natural history of alcoholic liver disease may be modified by specific nutritional or pharmacologic therapy (discussed earlier). The greatest impact of such therapies to date has been on short-term survival rate and on improvements in laboratory indices. The long-term impact of drug therapy on outcomes other than survival, such as progression to cirrhosis, is not yet known.

REFERENCES

1. Nephew TM, Williams GD, Stinson FS, et al: Apparent Per Capita Alcohol Consumption: National, State, and Regional Trends, 1977–97 (NIAAA Surveillance Report No. 5), Washington, D.C., CSR, Inc., 1999.
2. Bellantani S, Saccoccio G, Costa G, et al: Drinking habits as cofactors of risk for alcohol induced liver damage. Gut 41:845, 1997.

3. Kerr WC, Fillmore KM, Marvy P: Beverage-specific alcohol consumption and cirrhosis mortality in a group of English-speaking beer-drinking countries [see comments]. Addiction 95:339, 2000.
4. Ramstedt M: Per capita alcohol consumption and liver cirrhosis mortality in 14 European countries. Addiction 96:S19, 2001.
5. Drinking in the United States: Main Findings from the 1992 National Longitudinal Alcohol Epidemiologic Survey (NLAES) (NIH Publication No. 99-3519). 1998.
6. Saadatmand F, Stinson FS, Grant BF, et al: Liver Cirrhosis Mortality in the United States, 1970–97 (NIAAA Surveillance Report No. 52). Washington, D.C., CSR, Inc., 2000.
7. Lelbach WK: Cirrhosis in the alcoholic and its relation to the volume of alcohol abuse. Ann N Y Acad Sci 252:85, 1975.
8. Tuyns AJ, Pequignot G: Greater risk of ascitic cirrhosis in females in relation to alcohol consumption. Int J Epidemiol 13:53, 1984.
9. Marbet UA, Bianchi L, Meury U, et al: Long-term histological evaluation of the natural history and prognostic factors of alcoholic liver disease. J Hepatol 4:364, 1987.
10. Mezey E, Kolman CJ, Diehl AM, et al: Alcohol and dietary intake in the development of chronic pancreatitis and liver disease in alcoholism. Am J Clin Nutr 48:148, 1988.
11. Bosron WF, Ehrig T, Li TK: Genetic factors in alcohol metabolism and alcoholism. Semin Liver Dis 13:126, 1993.
12. Hanna JM: Metabolic responses of Chinese, Japanese and Europeans to alcohol. Alcohol Clin Exp Res 2:89, 1978.
13. Goedde HW, Agarwal DP, Harada S, et al: Population genetic studies on aldehyde dehydrogenase isozyme deficiency and alcohol sensitivity. Am J Hum Genet 35:769, 1983.
14. Frezza M, di Padova C, Pozzato G, et al: High blood alcohol levels in women: The role of decreased gastric alcohol dehydrogenase activity and first-pass metabolism. N Engl J Med 322:95, 1990.
15. Roine R, Gentry RT, Hernandez-Munoz R, et al: Aspirin increases blood alcohol concentrations in humans after ingestion of ethanol. JAMA 264:2406, 1990.
16. Caballeria J, Baraona E, Deulofeu R, et al: Effects of H_2-receptor antagonists on gastric alcohol dehydrogenase activity. Dig Dis Sci 36: 1673, 1991.
17. Smith T, DeMaster EG, Furne JK, et al: First-pass gastric mucosal metabolism of ethanol is negligible in the rat. J Clin Invest 89:1801, 1992.
18. Nordmann R, Ribiere C, Rouach H: Implication of free radical mechanisms in ethanol-induced cellular injury. Free Radic Biol Med 12:219, 1992.
19. Albano E, Clot P, Morimoto M, et al: Role of cytochrome P4502E1–dependent formation of hydroxyethyl free radical in the development of liver damage in rats intragastrically fed with ethanol. Hepatology 23:155, 1996.
20. Kono H, Bradford BU, Yin M, et al: CYP2E1 is not involved in early alcohol-induced liver injury. Am J Physiol 277:G1259, 1999.
21. Kono H, Rusyn I, Yin M, et al: NADPH oxidase–derived free radicals are key oxidants in alcohol-induced liver disease. J Clin Invest 106:867, 2000.
22. Niemela O, Parkkila S, Britton RS, et al: Hepatic lipid peroxidation in hereditary hemochromatosis and alcoholic liver injury. J Lab Clin Med 133:451, 1999.
23. Nanji AA, Zhao S, Lamb RG, et al: Changes in cytochromes P-450, 2E1, 2B1, and 4A, and phospholipases A and C in the intragastric feeding rat model for alcoholic liver disease: Relationship to dietary fats and pathologic liver injury. Alcohol Clin Exp Res 18:902, 1994.
24. Tsukamoto H, Horne W, Kamimura S, et al: Experimental liver cirrhosis induced by alcohol and iron. J Clin Invest 96:620, 1995.
25. Niemela O, Parkkila S, Yla-Herttuala S, et al: Sequential acetaldehyde production, lipid peroxidation, and fibrogenesis in micropig model of alcohol-induced liver disease. Hepatology 22:1208, 1995.
26. Fromenty B, Grimbert S, Mansouri A, et al: Hepatic mitochondrial DNA deletion in alcoholics: Association with microvesicular steatosis. Gastroenterology 108:193, 1995.
27. Mansouri A, Fromenty B, Berson A, et al: Multiple hepatic mitochondrial DNA deletions suggest premature oxidative aging in alcoholic patients. J Hepatol 27:96, 1997.
28. Colell A, Garcia-Ruiz C, Miranda M, et al: Selective glutathione depletion of mitochondria by ethanol sensitizes hepatocytes to tumor necrosis factor. Gastroenterology 115:1541, 1998.
29. Lieber CS, Casini A, DeCarli LM, et al: *S*-adenosyl-L-methionine attenuates alcohol-induced liver injury in the baboon. Hepatology 11: 165, 1990.
30. Garcia-Ruiz C, Morales A, Colell A, et al: Feeding *S*-adenosyl-L-methionine attenuates both ethanol-induced depletion of mitochondrial glutathione and mitochondrial dysfunction in periportal and perivenous rat hepatocytes. Hepatology 21:207, 1995.
31. Hayashi N, Kasahara A, Kurosawa K, et al: Oxygen supply to the liver in patients with alcoholic liver disease assessed by organ-reflectance spectrophotometry. Gastroenterology 88:881, 1985.
32. Arteel GE, Raleigh JA, Bradford BU, et al: Acute alcohol produces hypoxia directly in rat liver tissue in vivo: Role of Kupffer cells. Am J Physiol 271:G494, 1996.
33. Arteel GE, Iimuro Y, Yin M, et al: Chronic enteral ethanol treatment causes hypoxia in rat liver tissue in vivo. Hepatology 25:920, 1997.
34. Niemela O, Juvonen T, Parkkila S: Immunohistochemical demonstration of acetaldehyde-modified epitopes in human liver after alcohol consumption. J Clin Invest 87:1367, 1991.
35. Holstege A, Bedossa P, Poynard T, et al: Acetaldehyde-modified epitopes in liver biopsy specimens of alcoholic and nonalcoholic patients: Localization and association with progression of liver fibrosis. Hepatology 19:367, 1994.
36. Rolla R, Vay D, Mottaran E, et al: Detection of circulating antibodies against malondialdehyde-acetaldehyde adducts in patients with alcohol-induced liver disease. Hepatology 31:878, 2000.
37. Lin RC, Zhou FC, Fillenwarth MJ, et al: Zonal distribution of protein-acetaldehyde adducts in the liver of rats fed alcohol for long periods. Hepatology 18:864, 1993.
38. Tuma DJ, Thiele GM, Xu D, et al: Acetaldehyde and malondialdehyde react together to generate distinct protein adducts in the liver during long-term ethanol administration. Hepatology 23:872, 1996.
39. Tuma DJ, Sorrell MF: Effects of ethanol on protein trafficking in the liver. Semin Liver Dis 8:69, 1988.
40. Adachi Y, Bradford BU, Gao W, et al: Inactivation of Kupffer cells prevents early alcohol-induced liver injury. Hepatology 20:453, 1994.
41. Adachi Y, Moore LE, Bradford BU, et al: Antibiotics prevent liver injury in rats following long-term exposure to ethanol. Gastroenterology 108:218, 1995.
42. Nanji AA, Khettry U, Sadrzadeh SM: Lactobacillus feeding reduces endotoxemia and severity of experimental alcoholic liver (disease). Proc Soc Exp Biol Med 205:243, 1994.
43. Maltby J, Wright S, Bird G, et al: Chemokine levels in human liver homogenates: Associations between GRO alpha and histopathological evidence of alcoholic hepatitis. Hepatology 24:1156, 1996.
44. Afford SC, Fisher NC, Neil DA, et al: Distinct patterns of chemokine expression are associated with leukocyte recruitment in alcoholic hepatitis and alcoholic cirrhosis. J Pathol 186:82, 1998.
45. Niemela O, Klajner F, Orrego H, et al: Antibodies against acetaldehyde-modified protein epitopes in human alcoholics. Hepatology 7: 1210, 1987.
46. Clot P, Bellomo G, Tabone M, et al: Detection of antibodies against proteins modified by hydroxyethyl free radicals in patients with alcoholic cirrhosis. Gastroenterology 108:201, 1995.
47. Yokoyama H, Ishii H, Nagata S, et al: Experimental hepatitis induced by ethanol after immunization with acetaldehyde adducts. Hepatology 17:14, 1993.
48. Yokoyama H, Nagata S, Moriya S, et al: Hepatic fibrosis produced in guinea pigs by chronic ethanol administration and immunization with acetaldehyde adducts. Hepatology 21:1438, 1995.
49. Chedid A, Mendenhall CL, Gartside P, et al: Prognostic factors in alcoholic liver disease: VA Cooperative Study Group. Am J Gastroenterol 86:210, 1991.
50. Mendenhall CL: Alcoholic hepatitis. Clin Gastroenterol 10:417, 1981.
51. Friedman SL: The cellular basis of hepatic fibrosis. N Engl J Med 328:1828, 1993.
52. Lee KS, Buck M, Houglum K, et al: Activation of hepatic stellate cells by TGF alpha and collagen type I is mediated by oxidative stress through c-myb expression. J Clin Invest 96:2461, 1995.
53. Nieto N, Greenwel P, Friedman SL, et al: Ethanol and arachidonic acid increase alpha 2(I) collagen expression in rat hepatic stellate cells overexpressing cytochrome P450 2E1: Role of H_2O_2 and cyclooxygenase-2. J Biol Chem 275:20136, 2000.
54. Casini A, Pinzani M, Milani S, et al: Regulation of extracellular matrix synthesis by transforming growth factor beta 1 in human fat-storing cells. Gastroenterology 105:245, 1993.
55. Melendez M, Vargas-Tank L, Fuentes C, et al: Distribution of HLA histocompatibility antigens, ABO blood groups and Rh antigens in alcoholic liver disease. Gut 20:288, 1979.

56. Bell H, Nordhagen R: HLA antigens in alcoholics, with special reference to alcoholic cirrhosis. Scand J Gastroenterol 15:453, 1980.
57. Doffoel M, Tongio MM, Gut JP, et al: Relationships between 34 HLA-A, HLA-B and HLA-DR antigens and three serological markers of viral infections in alcoholic cirrhosis. Hepatology 6:457, 1986.
58. Monteiro E, Alves MP, Santos ML, et al: Histocompatibility antigens: Markers of susceptibility to and protection from alcoholic liver disease in a Portuguese population. Hepatology 8:455, 1988.
59. Scott BB, Rajah SM, Losowsky MS: Histocompatibility antigens in chronic liver disease. Gastroenterology 72:122, 1977.
60. Faizallah R, Woodrow JC, Krasner NK, et al: Are HLA antigens important in the development of alcohol-induced liver disease? BMJ (Clin Res Ed) 285:533, 1982.
61. Mills PR, MacSween RN, Dick HM, et al: Histocompatibility antigens in patients with alcoholic liver disease in Scotland and northeastern England: Failure to show an association. Gut 29:146, 1988.
62. List S, Gluud C: A meta-analysis of HLA-antigen prevalences in alcoholics and alcoholic liver disease. Alcohol Alcohol 29:757, 1994.
63. Chao YC, Liou SR, Chung YY, et al: Polymorphism of alcohol and aldehyde dehydrogenase genes and alcoholic cirrhosis in Chinese patients. Hepatology 19:360, 1994.
64. Whitfield JB: Meta-analysis of the effects of alcohol dehydrogenase genotype on alcohol dependence and alcoholic liver disease. Alcohol Alcohol 32:613, 1997.
65. Tanaka F, Shiratori Y, Yokosuka O, et al: Polymorphism of alcohol-metabolizing genes affects drinking behavior and alcoholic liver disease in Japanese men. Alcohol Clin Exp Res 21:596, 1997.
66. Yamauchi M, Maezawa Y, Mizuhara Y, et al: Polymorphisms in alcohol metabolizing enzyme genes and alcoholic cirrhosis in Japanese patients: A multivariate analysis. Hepatology 22:1136, 1995.
67. Tanaka F, Shiratori Y, Yokosuka O, et al: High incidence of ADH2*1/ALDH2*1 genes among Japanese alcohol dependents and patients with alcoholic liver disease. Hepatology 23:234, 1996.
68. Tsutsumi M, Takada A, Wang JS: Genetic polymorphisms of cytochrome P4502E1 related to the development of alcoholic liver disease. Gastroenterology 107:1430, 1994.
69. Grove J, Brown AS, Daly AK, et al: The RsaI polymorphism of CYP2E1 and susceptibility to alcoholic liver disease in Caucasians: Effect on age of presentation and dependence on alcohol dehydrogenase genotype. Pharmacogenetics 8:335, 1998.
70. Carr LG, Yi IS, Li TK, et al: Cytochrome P4502E1 genotypes, alcoholism, and alcoholic cirrhosis in Han Chinese and Atayal natives of Taiwan. Alcohol Clin Exp Res 20:43, 1996.
71. Chao YC, Young TH, Tang HS, et al: Alcoholism and alcoholic organ damage and genetic polymorphisms of alcohol metabolizing enzymes in Chinese patients. Hepatology 25:112, 1997.
72. Pirmohamed M, Kitteringham NR, Quest LJ, et al: Genetic polymorphism of cytochrome P4502E1 and risk of alcoholic liver disease in Caucasians. Pharmacogenetics 5:351, 1995.
73. Carr LG, Hartleroad JY, Liang Y, et al: Polymorphism at the P450IIE1 locus is not associated with alcoholic liver disease in Caucasian men. Alcohol Clin Exp Res 19:182, 1995.
74. Wong NA, Rae F, Simpson KJ, et al: Genetic polymorphisms of cytochrome p4502E1 and susceptibility to alcoholic liver disease and hepatocellular carcinoma in a white population: A study and literature review, including meta-analysis. Mol Pathol 53:88, 2000.
75. Enomoto N, Takase S, Takada N, et al: Alcoholic liver disease in heterozygotes of mutant and normal aldehyde dehydrogenase-2 genes. Hepatology 13:1071, 1991.
76. Chao YC, Wang MF, Tang HS, et al: Genotyping of alcohol dehydrogenase at the ADH2 and ADH3 loci by using a polymerase chain reaction and restriction-fragment-length polymorphism in Chinese alcoholic cirrhotics and non-alcoholics. Proc Natl Sci Counc Repub China B 18:101, 1994.
77. Grove J, Daly AK, Bassendine MF, et al: Association of a tumor necrosis factor promoter polymorphism with susceptibility to alcoholic steatohepatitis. Hepatology 26:143, 1997.
78. Galambos JT: Natural history of alcoholic hepatitis. 3. Histological changes. Gastroenterology 63:1026, 1972.
79. Pares A, Caballeria J, Bruguera M, et al: Histological course of alcoholic hepatitis: Influence of abstinence, sex and extent of hepatic damage. J Hepatol 2:33, 1986.
80. Mendenhall CL, Tosch T, Weesner RE, et al: VA Cooperative Study on Alcoholic Hepatitis. II. Prognostic significance of protein-calorie malnutrition. Am J Clin Nutr 43:213, 1986.
81. Mendenhall C, Roselle GA, Gartside P, et al: Relationship of protein calorie malnutrition to alcoholic liver disease: A reexamination of data from two Veterans Administration Cooperative Studies. Alcohol Clin Exp Res 19:635, 1995.
82. Nanji AA, French SW: Dietary factors and alcoholic cirrhosis. Alcohol Clin Exp Res 10:271, 1986.
83. Naveau S, Emilie D, Borotto E, et al: Interleukin-1 receptor antagonist plasma concentration is specifically increased by alpha-2A-interferon treatment. J Hepatol 27:272, 1997.
84. Diehl AM: Nonalcoholic steatohepatitis. Semin Liver Dis 19:221, 1999.
85. Sheth SG, Gordon FD, Chopra S: Nonalcoholic steatohepatitis. Ann Intern Med 126:137, 1997.
86. Neuschwander-Tetri BA, Bacon BR: Nonalcoholic steatohepatitis. Med Clin North Am 80:1147, 1996.
87. Bellantani S, Saccoccio G, Masutti F, et al: Prevalence of and risk factors for hepatic steatosis in northern Italy. Ann Intern Med 132: 112, 2000.
88. Pares A, Barrera JM, Caballeria J, et al: Hepatitis C virus antibodies in chronic alcoholic patients: Association with severity of liver injury [see comments]. Hepatology 12:1295, 1990.
89. Nalpas B, Driss F, Pol S, et al: Association between HCV and HBV infection in hepatocellular carcinoma and alcoholic liver disease. J Hepatol 12:70, 1991.
90. Mendenhall CL, Seeff L, Diehl AM, et al: Antibodies to hepatitis B virus and hepatitis C virus in alcoholic hepatitis and cirrhosis: Their prevalence and clinical relevance: The VA Cooperative Study Group (No. 119). Hepatology 14:581, 1991.
91. Caldwell SH, Li X, Rourk RM, et al: Hepatitis C infection by polymerase chain reaction in alcoholics: False-positive ELISA results and the influence of infection on a clinical prognostic score. Am J Gastroenterol 88:1016, 1993.
92. Poynard T, Aubert A, Lazizi Y, et al: Independent risk factors for hepatocellular carcinoma in French drinkers. Hepatology 13:896, 1991.
93. Shimizu S, Kiyosawa K, Sodeyama T, et al: High prevalence of antibody to hepatitis C virus in heavy drinkers with chronic liver diseases in Japan. J Gastroenterol Hepatol 7:30, 1992.
94. Corrao G, Arico S: Independent and combined action of hepatitis C virus infection and alcohol consumption on the risk of symptomatic liver cirrhosis. Hepatology 27:914, 1998.
95. Sawada M, Takada A, Takase S, et al: Effects of alcohol on the replication of hepatitis C virus. Alcohol Alcohol Suppl 1B:85, 1993.
96. Oshita M, Hayashi N, Kasahara A, et al: Increased serum hepatitis C virus RNA levels among alcoholic patients with chronic hepatitis C. Hepatology 20:1115, 1994.
97. Pessione F, Degos F, Marcellin P, et al: Effect of alcohol consumption on serum hepatitis C virus RNA and histological lesions in chronic hepatitis C. Hepatology 27:1717, 1998.
98. Ganne-Carrie N, Kremsdorf D, Garreau F, et al: Effects of ethanol on hepatitis B virus Pre-S/S gene expression in the human hepatocellular carcinoma derived HEP G2 hepatitis B DNA positive cell line. J Hepatol 23:153, 1995.
99. Shiomi S, Kuroki T, Minamitani S, et al: Effect of drinking on the outcome of cirrhosis in patients with hepatitis B or C. J Gastroenterol Hepatol 7:274, 1992.
100. Levi AJ, Chalmers DM: Recognition of alcoholic liver disease in a district general hospital. Gut 19:521, 1978.
101. Bruguera M, Bordas JM, Rodes J: Asymptomatic liver disease in alcoholics. Arch Pathol Lab Med 101:644, 1977.
102. Leevy C: Fatty liver: A study of 270 patients with biopsy-proven fatty liver and a review of the literature. Medicine 41:249, 1962.
103. Israel Y, Orrego H, Colman JC, et al: Alcohol-induced hepatomegaly: Pathogenesis and role in the production of portal hypertension. Fed Proc 41:2472, 1982.
104. McClain C, Hill D, Schmidt J, et al: Cytokines and alcoholic liver disease. Semin Liver Dis 13:170, 1993.
105. Cohen JA, Kaplan MM: The SGOT/SGPT ratio—an indicator of alcoholic liver disease. Dig Dis Sci 24:835, 1979.
106. Seeff LB, Cuccherini BA, Zimmerman HJ, et al: Acetaminophen hepatotoxicity in alcoholics: A therapeutic misadventure. Ann Intern Med 104:399, 1986.
107. Maddrey WC, Boitnott JK, Bedine MS, et al: Corticosteroid therapy of alcoholic hepatitis. Gastroenterology 75:193, 1978.
108. Imperiale TF, McCullough AJ: Do corticosteroids reduce mortality from alcoholic hepatitis? A meta-analysis of the randomized trials. Ann Intern Med 113:299, 1990.

109. Fletcher LM, Kwoh-Gain I, Powell EE, et al: Markers of chronic alcohol ingestion in patients with nonalcoholic steatohepatitis: An aid to diagnosis. Hepatology 13:455, 1991.
110. Rosman AS, Basu P, Galvin K, et al: Utility of carbohydrate-deficient transferrin as a marker of relapse in alcoholic patients. Alcohol Clin Exp Res 19:611, 1995.
111. Lin RC, Shahidi S, Kelly TJ, et al: Measurement of hemoglobin-acetaldehyde adduct in alcoholic patients. Alcohol Clin Exp Res 17: 669, 1993.
112. Annoni G, Colombo M, Cantaluppi MC, et al: Serum type III procollagen peptide and laminin (Lam-P1) detect alcoholic hepatitis in chronic alcohol abusers. Hepatology 9:693, 1989.
113. Niemela O, Risteli L, Sotaniemi EA, et al: Aminoterminal propeptide of type III procollagen in serum in alcoholic liver disease. Gastroenterology 85:254, 1983.
114. Torres-Salinas M, Pares A, Caballeria J, et al: Serum procollagen type III peptide as a marker of hepatic fibrogenesis in alcoholic hepatitis. Gastroenterology 90:1241, 1986.
115. Niemela O, Risteli J, Blake JE, et al: Markers of fibrogenesis and basement membrane formation in alcoholic liver disease: Relation to severity, presence of hepatitis, and alcohol intake. Gastroenterology 98:1612, 1990.
116. Levin DM, Baker AL, Riddell RH, et al: Nonalcoholic liver disease: Overlooked causes of liver injury in patients with heavy alcohol consumption. Am J Med 66:429, 1979.
117. French SW, Nash J, Shitabata P, et al: Pathology of alcoholic liver disease: VA Cooperative Study Group 119. Semin Liver Dis 13:154, 1993.
118. Uchida T, Kao H, Quispe-Sjogren M, et al: Alcoholic foamy degeneration—a pattern of acute alcoholic injury of the liver. Gastroenterology 84:683, 1983.
119. Montull S, Pares A, Bruguera M, et al: Alcoholic foamy degeneration in Spain: Prevalence and clinico-pathological features. Liver 9:79, 1989.
120. Orrego H, Blake JE, Blendis LM, et al: Prognosis of alcoholic cirrhosis in the presence and absence of alcoholic hepatitis. Gastroenterology 92:208, 1987.
121. Matteoni CA, Younossi ZM, Gramlich T, et al: Nonalcoholic fatty liver disease: A spectrum of clinical and pathological severity. Gastroenterology 116:1413, 1999.
122. Sorbi D, Boynton J, Lindor KD: The ratio of aspartate aminotransferase to alanine aminotransferase: Potential value in differentiating nonalcoholic steatohepatitis from alcoholic liver disease. Am J Gastroenterol 94:1018, 1999.
123. Yamauchi M, Nakahara M, Maezawa Y, et al: Prevalence of hepatocellular carcinoma in patients with alcoholic cirrhosis and prior exposure to hepatitis C. Am J Gastroenterol 88:39, 1993.
124. Miyakawa H, Sato C, Tazawa J, et al: A prospective study on hepatocellular carcinoma in liver cirrhosis: Respective roles of alcohol and hepatitis C virus infection. Alcohol Alcohol 29:75, 1994.
125. Khan KN, Yatsuhashi H: Effect of alcohol consumption on the progression of hepatitis C virus infection and risk of hepatocellular carcinoma in Japanese patients. Alcohol Alcohol 35:286, 2000.
126. Tsukuma H, Hiyama T, Tanaka S, et al: Risk factors for hepatocellular carcinoma among patients with chronic liver disease. N Engl J Med 328:1797, 1993.
127. Miyakawa H, Izumi N, Marumo F, et al: Roles of alcohol, hepatitis virus infection, and gender in the development of hepatocellular carcinoma in patients with liver cirrhosis. Alcohol Clin Exp Res 20:91A, 1996.
128. Bosch FX, Ribes J, Borras J: Epidemiology of primary liver cancer. Semin Liver Dis 19:271, 1999.
129. Aizawa Y, Shibamoto Y, Takagi I, et al: Analysis of factors affecting the appearance of hepatocellular carcinoma in patients with chronic hepatitis C: A long term follow-up study after histologic diagnosis. Cancer 89:53, 2000.
130. Nasrallah SM, Galambos JT: Aminoacid therapy of alcoholic hepatitis. Lancet 2:1276, 1980.
131. Mendenhall C, Bongiovanni G, Goldberg S, et al: VA Cooperative Study on Alcoholic Hepatitis. III. Changes in protein-calorie malnutrition associated with 30 days of hospitalization with and without enteral nutritional therapy. JPEN J Parenter Enteral Nutr 9:590, 1985.
132. Calvey H, Davis M, Williams R: Controlled trial of nutritional supplementation, with and without branched chain amino acid enrichment, in treatment of acute alcoholic hepatitis. J Hepatol 1:141, 1985.
133. Diehl AM, Boitnott JK, Herlong HF, et al: Effect of parenteral amino acid supplementation in alcoholic hepatitis. Hepatology 5:57, 1985.
134. Achord JL: Malnutrition and the role of nutritional support in alcoholic liver disease. Am J Gastroenterol 82:1, 1987.
135. Mezey E, Caballeria J, Mitchell MC, et al: Effect of parenteral amino acid supplementation on short-term and long-term outcomes in severe alcoholic hepatitis: A randomized controlled trial. Hepatology 14: 1090, 1991.
136. Soberon S, Pauley MP, Duplantier R, et al: Metabolic effects of enteral formula feeding in alcoholic hepatitis. Hepatology 7:1204, 1987.
137. Helman RA, Temko MH, Nye SW, et al: Alcoholic hepatitis: Natural history and evaluation of prednisolone therapy. Ann Intern Med 74: 311, 1971.
138. Porter HP, Simon FR, Pope CE 2nd, et al: Corticosteroid therapy in severe alcoholic hepatitis: A double-blind drug trial. N Engl J Med 284:1350, 1971.
139. Campra JL, Hamlin EM Jr, Kirshbaum RJ, et al: Prednisone therapy of acute alcoholic hepatitis: Report of a controlled trial. Ann Intern Med 79:625, 1973.
140. Blitzer BL, Mutchnick MG, Joshi PH, et al: Adrenocorticosteroid therapy in alcoholic hepatitis: A prospective, double-blind randomized study. Am J Dig Dis 22:477, 1977.
141. Lesesne HR, Bozymski EM, Fallon HJ: Treatment of alcoholic hepatitis with encephalopathy: Comparison of prednisolone with caloric supplements. Gastroenterology 74:169, 1978.
142. Shumaker JB, Resnick RH, Galambos JT, et al: A controlled trial of 6-methylprednisolone in acute alcoholic hepatitis: With a note on published results in encephalopathic patients. Am J Gastroenterol 69: 443, 1978.
143. Depew W, Boyer T, Omata M, et al: Double-blind controlled trial of prednisolone therapy in patients with severe acute alcoholic hepatitis and spontaneous encephalopathy. Gastroenterology 78:524, 1980.
144. Theodossi A, Eddleston AL, Williams R: Controlled trial of methylprednisolone therapy in severe acute alcoholic hepatitis. Gut 23:75, 1982.
145. Carithers RL Jr, Herlong HF, Diehl AM, et al: Methylprednisolone therapy in patients with severe alcoholic hepatitis: A randomized multicenter trial. Ann Intern Med 110:685, 1989.
146. Mendenhall CL, Anderson S, Garcia-Pont P, et al: Short-term and long-term survival in patients with alcoholic hepatitis treated with oxandrolone and prednisolone. N Engl J Med 311:1464, 1984.
147. Ramond MJ, Poynard T, Rueff B, et al: A randomized trial of prednisolone in patients with severe alcoholic hepatitis. N Engl J Med 326:507, 1992.
148. Mathurin P, Duchatelle V, Ramond MJ, et al: Survival and prognostic factors in patients with severe alcoholic hepatitis treated with prednisolone. Gastroenterology 110:1847, 1996.
149. Christensen E, Gluud C: Glucocorticoids are ineffective in alcoholic hepatitis: A meta-analysis adjusting for confounding variables. Gut 37: 113, 1995.
150. McCullough AJ, O'Connor JF: Alcoholic liver disease: Proposed recommendations for the American College of Gastroenterology. Am J Gastroenterol 93:2022, 1998.
151. Akriviadis E, Botla R, Briggs W, et al: Pentoxifylline improves short-term survival in severe acute alcoholic hepatitis: A double-blind, placebo-controlled trial. Gastroenterology 119:1637, 2000.
152. Lieber CS, DeCarli LM, Mak KM, et al: Attenuation of alcohol-induced hepatic fibrosis by polyunsaturated lecithin. Hepatology 12: 1390, 1990.
153. Lieber CS, Robins SJ, Li J, et al: Phosphatidylcholine protects against fibrosis and cirrhosis in the baboon. Gastroenterology 106:152, 1994.
154. Brady LM, Fox ES, Fimmel CJ: Polyenylphosphatidylcholine inhibits PDGF-induced proliferation in rat hepatic stellate cells. Biochem Biophys Res Commun 248:174, 1998.
155. Poniachik J, Baraona E, Zhao J, et al: Dilinoleoylphosphatidylcholine decreases hepatic stellate cell activation. J Lab Clin Med 133:342, 1999.
156. Aleynik MK, Leo MA, Aleynik SI, et al: Polyenylphosphatidylcholine opposes the increase of cytochrome P-4502E1 by ethanol and corrects its iron-induced decrease. Alcohol Clin Exp Res 23:96, 1999.
157. Mi LJ, Mak KM, Lieber CS: Attenuation of alcohol-induced apoptosis of hepatocytes in rat livers by polyenylphosphatidylcholine. Alcohol Clin Exp Res 24:207, 2000.
158. Mato JM, Camara J, Fernandez de Paz J, et al: *S*-adenosylmethionine

in alcoholic liver cirrhosis: A randomized, placebo-controlled, double-blind, multicenter clinical trial. J Hepatol 30:1081, 1999.
159. Ferenci P, Dragosics B, Dittrich H, et al: Randomized controlled trial of silymarin treatment in patients with cirrhosis of the liver. J Hepatol 9:105, 1989.
160. Pares A, Planas R, Torres M, et al: Effects of silymarin in alcoholic patients with cirrhosis of the liver: Results of a controlled, double-blind, randomized and multicenter trial. J Hepatol 28:615, 1998.
161. Sadrzadeh SM, Meydani M, Khettry U, et al: High-dose vitamin E supplementation has no effect on ethanol-induced pathological liver injury. J Pharmacol Exp Ther 273:455, 1995.
162. Leo MA, Kim C, Lowe N, et al: Interaction of ethanol with beta-carotene: Delayed blood clearance and enhanced hepatotoxicity. Hepatology 15:883, 1992.
163. Ahmed S, Leo MA, Lieber CS: Interactions between alcohol and beta-carotene in patients with alcoholic liver disease. Am J Clin Nutr 60: 430, 1994.
164. Butcher GP, Rhodes JM, Walker R, et al: The effect of antioxidant supplementation on a serum marker of free radical activity and abnormal serum biochemistry in alcoholic patients admitted for detoxification. J Hepatol 19:105, 1993.
165. de la Maza MP, Petermann M, Bunout D, et al: Effects of long-term vitamin E supplementation in alcoholic cirrhotics. J Am Coll Nutr 14: 192, 1995.
166. Akriviadis EA, Steindel H, Pinto PC, et al: Failure of colchicine to improve short-term survival in patients with alcoholic hepatitis. Gastroenterology 99:811, 1990.
167. Kershenobich D, Vargas F, Garcia-Tsao G, et al: Colchicine in the treatment of cirrhosis of the liver. N Engl J Med 318:1709, 1988.
168. Orrego H, Kalant H, Israel Y, et al: Effect of short-term therapy with propylthiouracil in patients with alcoholic liver disease. Gastroenterology 76:105, 1979.
169. Halle P, Pare P, Kaptein E, et al: Double-blind, controlled trial of propylthiouracil in patients with severe acute alcoholic hepatitis. Gastroenterology 82:925, 1982.
170. Orrego H, Blake JE, Blendis LM, et al: Long-term treatment of alcoholic liver disease with propylthiouracil. N Engl J Med 317:1421, 1987.
171. Orrego H, Blake JE, Blendis LM, et al: Long-term treatment of alcoholic liver disease with propylthiouracil. Part 2. Influence of drop-out rates and of continued alcohol consumption in a clinical trial. J Hepatol 20:343, 1994.
172. Poynard T, Naveau S, Doffoel M, et al: Evaluation of efficacy of liver transplantation in alcoholic cirrhosis using matched and simulated controls: 5-year survival. Multi-centre group. J Hepatol 30:1130, 1999.
173. Wiesner RH, Lombardero M, Lake JR, et al: Liver transplantation for end-stage alcoholic liver disease: An assessment of outcomes. Liver Transpl Surg 3:231, 1997.
174. Stefanini GF, Biselli M, Grazi GL, et al: Orthotopic liver transplantation for alcoholic liver disease: Rates of survival, complications and relapse. Hepatogastroenterology 44:1356, 1997.
175. Jain A, DiMartini A, Kashyap R, et al: Long-term follow-up after liver transplantation for alcoholic liver disease under tacrolimus. Transplantation 70:1335, 2000.
176. Shakil AO, Pinna A, Demetris J, et al: Survival and quality of life after liver transplantation for acute alcoholic hepatitis. Liver Transpl Surg 3:240, 1997.
177. Conjeevaram HS, Hart J, Lissoos TW, et al: Rapidly progressive liver injury and fatal alcoholic hepatitis occurring after liver transplantation in alcoholic patients. Transplantation 67:1562, 1999.
178. Pereira SP, Howard LM, Muiesan P, et al: Quality of life after liver transplantation for alcoholic liver disease. Liver Transpl 6:762, 2000.
179. Anand AC, Ferraz-Neto BH, Nightingale P, et al: Liver transplantation for alcoholic liver disease: Evaluation of a selection protocol. Hepatology 25:1478, 1997.
180. Yates WR, Martin M, LaBrecque D, et al: A model to examine the validity of the 6-month abstinence criterion for liver transplantation. Alcohol Clin Exp Res 22:513, 1998.
181. Reeves HL, Burt AD, Wood S, et al: Hepatic stellate cell activation occurs in the absence of hepatitis in alcoholic liver disease and correlates with the severity of steatosis. J Hepatol 25:677, 1996.
182. Sorensen TI, Orholm M, Bentsen KD, et al: Prospective evaluation of alcohol abuse and alcoholic liver injury in men as predictors of development of cirrhosis. Lancet 2:241, 1984.
183. Teli MR, Day CP, Burt AD, et al: Determinants of progression to cirrhosis or fibrosis in pure alcoholic fatty liver. Lancet 346:987, 1995.
184. Worner TM, Lieber CS: Perivenular fibrosis as precursor lesion of cirrhosis. JAMA 254:627, 1985.
185. Goldberg S, Mendenhall C, Anderson S, et al: VA Cooperative Study on Alcoholic Hepatitis. IV. The significance of clinically mild alcoholic hepatitis—describing the population with minimal hyperbilirubinemia. Am J Gastroenterol 81:1029, 1986.
186. Orrego H, Israel Y, Blake JE, et al: Assessment of prognostic factors in alcoholic liver disease: Toward a global quantitative expression of severity. Hepatology 3:896, 1983.
187. Powell WJ Jr, Klatskin G: Duration of survival in patients with Laennec's cirrhosis: Influence of alcohol withdrawal, and possible effects of recent changes in general management of the disease. Am J Med 44:406, 1968.
188. Borowsky SA, Strome S, Lott E: Continued heavy drinking and survival in alcoholic cirrhotics. Gastroenterology 80:1405, 1981.

Chapter 72

Nonalcoholic Fatty Liver Disease

Anna Mae Diehl and Fred Poordad

Nonalcoholic steatohepatitis (NASH) is a form of chronic hepatitis with histologic features of alcohol-induced liver disease that occurs in persons who do not consume a significant amount of alcohol. Several other terms have been used to refer to this entity, including *pseudoalcoholic liver disease, alcohol-like hepatitis, fatty liver hepatitis, diabetic hepatitis, nonalcoholic Laënnec's disease, steatonecrosis*,[1, 1a] and, most recently, *nonalcoholic fatty liver disease* (NAFLD).[2] The last term is increasingly preferred. In this chapter, NASH is considered to be part of the spectrum of NAFLD. A number of retrospective studies have suggested that NAFLD is an uncommon disorder that occurs most often in middle-aged obese women. Obesity, hyperglycemia, and hyperlipidemia are commonly associated with NAFLD and are thought to be predisposing conditions. Other identified risk factors include total parenteral nutrition, protein-calorie malnutrition, jejunoileal (J-I) bypass, and use of certain drugs.[1]

A 1994 report suggested that NAFLD may be more common than originally suspected and that many affected persons lack typical risk factors for the disorder.[3] In fact, ultrasonographic surveys of the general population demonstrate fatty liver in about 25% of adults in the United States.[4] Furthermore, NAFLD is the most common explanation for an elevated serum alanine aminotransferase (ALT) level in blood donors.[5] The prevalence of NAFLD in the general population parallels the prevalence of obesity and insulin resistance, the two most common risk factors for this type of liver disease.[2, 6] At present, the clinical implications of NAFLD have not been clearly defined. Progression to cirrhosis does occur. Indeed, studies in 1999 and 2000 from the United States and France documented advanced fibrosis or cirrhosis on liver biopsy specimens in up to two thirds of patients with NAFLD who were older than age 45 years and had type 2 diabetes, obesity, or hypertriglyceridemia.[6, 7] Clinical manifestations of portal hypertension, hepatic failure, and hepatocellular carcinoma may develop in patients with NAFLD and significant hepatic fibrosis.[3, 8] In a 1999 series, liver disease was the second leading cause of death in patients with NAFLD; the liver-related mortality rate was 11% in those with evidence of fibrosis or cirrhosis on liver biopsy specimens.[2] On the other hand, many other patients with NAFLD appear to have an indolent course.[9]

The prevalence of NAFLD and lack of information about its natural history have generated controversy about the wisdom of recommending invasive diagnostic tests or attempting to develop specific therapies for patients with this disease. Efforts to prevent or improve NAFLD also have been limited by our poor understanding of its pathogenesis. Careful epidemiologic studies and basic investigation are needed to provide new data to guide the management of patients with NAFLD.

ETIOLOGY

Many different agents and conditions have been associated with NAFLD. These may be divided into two broad categories: (1) drugs and toxins and (2) metabolic abnormalities—either acquired or congenital. Potential causes of NAFLD are listed in Table 72–1. Although some or all of the histologic features of NAFLD have been documented in a wide variety of settings, most published series of patients with NAFLD emphasize a predisposition to steatohepatitis in middle-aged women who are obese or who have non-insulin-dependent diabetes mellitus or hyperlipidemia.[1]

PATHOGENESIS

In light of the variety of conditions that have been associated with NAFLD, it is not surprising that no common mechanism has been identified to explain the pathogenesis of this condition. The lack of a common pathogenesis has prompted speculation that NASH may be the result of several diverse insults, that is, that the pathogenesis is multifactorial. Several mechanisms have been proposed as causes of NASH, including amino acid imbalance, hyperglycemia (caused by diabetes mellitus or excessive administration of glucose), excessive circulating levels of anabolic (e.g., insulin) relative to catabolic (e.g., leptin) hormones, and endotoxemia (caused by sepsis or starvation-associated bacterial translocation).[10] Clearly, each of these processes can shift metabolism to favor net lipogenesis rather than lipolysis, and the mechanisms are not mutually exclusive. Although some evidence supports a role for one or more of these mechanisms in steatosis associated with starvation, diabetes, total parenteral nutrition, and J-I bypass surgery, the possibility

Table 72–1 | **Potential Causes of Nonalcoholic Fatty Liver Disease**

Toxins and Drugs

Metals
- Antimony
- Barium salts
- Borates
- Carbon disulfide
- Chromates
- Phosphorus
- Rare earths of low atomic numbers
- Thallium compounds
- Uranium compounds

Cytotoxic/cytostatic drugs
- L-Asparaginase
- Azacitidine
- Azauridine
- Methotrexate

Antibiotics
- Azaserine
- Bleomycin
- Puromycin
- Tetracycline

Other drugs
- Amiodarone
- Coumadin
- Dichloroethylene
- Ethionine
- Ethyl bromide
- Estrogens
- Flectol H
- Glucocorticoids
- Hydrazine
- Hypoglycin
- Orotate
- Perhexilene maleate
- Safrole

Inborn Errors of Metabolism
- Abetalipoproteinemia
- Familial hepatosteatosis
- Galactosemia
- Glycogen storage disease
- Hereditary fructose intolerance
- Homocystinuria
- Systemic carnitine deficiency
- Tyrosinemia
- Refsum's syndrome
- Schwachman syndrome
- Weber-Christian syndrome
- Wilson disease

Acquired Metabolic Disorders
- Diabetes mellitus
- Inflammatory bowel disease
- Jejunoileal bypass
- Kwashiorkor and marasmus
- Obesity
- Serum lipid abnormalities
- Starvation and cachexia
- Severe anemia
- Total parenteral nutrition

that some of them may be sequelae (rather than causes) of NAFLD has not been excluded. Furthermore, because hepatitis and cirrhosis are much less frequent than steatosis, it is conceivable that only a few causes of steatosis can provoke histologic progression to cirrhosis or that an additional insult is necessary to produce this outcome.

Similarities in the histologic features and natural histories of alcoholic liver disease and NAFLD suggest that common mechanisms may be involved in the pathogenesis of these two disorders (Table 72–2). Chronic oxidative stress is thought to be important in the genesis of alcohol-related liver damage. Processes that increase oxidant production in the liver during chronic alcohol exposure include the metabolism of ethanol to its reactive intermediate, acetaldehyde; induction of microsomal ethanol oxidizing enzymes, such as cytochrome P-450IIE1; inhibition of mitochondrial electron transport chain activity; and depletion of mitochondrial glutathione.[11] The observations that mice with obesity-related fatty livers have increases in the endogenous production of ethanol,[12] activation of microsomal enzymes,[13] and mitochondrial production of reactive oxygen species[14] suggest that chronic oxidative stress also may be involved in the pathogenesis of NAFLD.

Studies in animal models of NAFLD have raised the intriguing possibility that endogenously produced ethanol may play a role in the pathogenesis of NAFLD. Increased production of ethanol by gastrointestinal flora has been demonstrated in aging ob/ob mice, in which fatty livers develop as the mice become progressively more obese during adulthood.[12] In the 1970s, Mezey and colleagues noted that blood ethanol levels were elevated in some morbidly obese patients who had undergone J-I bypass surgery to facilitate weight reduction; this finding prompted speculation that intestinally derived ethanol might account for the rapid progression of NAFLD that follows J-I bypass surgery. However, at the time, investigators concluded that increased intestinal ethanol production probably did not cause post–J-I bypass-related steatohepatitis, because the correlation between the severity of liver disease and blood ethanol levels was weak.[15] However, data from patients with a range of NAFLD (from simple steatosis to cirrhosis) complement the findings in NAFLD animal models and suggest that the original theory merits reevaluation. These preliminary studies show that, in patients with NAFLD, the content of ethanol in the breath increases progressively with body mass index and is independent of serum liver enzyme levels or histologic evidence of fibrosis.[16] These findings suggest that endogenous ethanol might promote the earliest stage of obesity-related NAFLD (i.e., steatosis). If confirmed, these results have exciting diagnostic and therapeutic implications. At the very least, they provide a potential explanation for the poor diagnostic specificity of tests that attempt to differentiate alcoholic from nonalcoholic fatty liver disease.

Endotoxin and endotoxin-inducible cytokines, particularly tumor necrosis factor-α (TNF-α), are required for the patho-

Table 72–2 | **Pathogenesis of Steatosis and Steatohepatitis**

CONTRIBUTING FACTOR	ALCOHOLIC LIVER DISEASE	NAFLD
Microsomal enzyme activation	+	+
Endotoxin	+	+
Macrophage activation/TNF-α	+	+
Mitochondrial abnormalities	+	+
Decreased hepatocyte ATP	+	+

ATP, adenosine triphosphate; NAFLD, nonalcoholic fatty liver disease; TNF-α, tumor necrosis factor-α.

genesis of alcohol-induced liver disease in experimental animals, as supported by the finding in mice that alcoholic liver damage is prevented by disruption of the gene that encodes type 1 TNF receptors.[17] Serum and adipose tissue levels of TNF-α are increased in obesity,[18, 19] and leptin, a satiety factor that is produced by adipose tissue,[20] modulates the toxic actions of TNF-α.[21] Obese, leptin-deficient mice have defects in macrophages and lymphocytes that promote TNF-α–mediated liver damage,[22, 23] and these animals are unusually susceptible to endotoxin-induced liver injury.[21, 24] Analogously, steatohepatitis occurs commonly in obese patients who have undergone J-I bypass surgery and in patients receiving long-term total parenteral nutrition (TPN); both conditions promote intestinal bacterial overgrowth, portal endotoxemia, and hepatic TNF-α production.[25, 26] Also supportive of the importance of endotoxin-induced cytokines in the progression of NAFLD is the observation that treatment with metronidazole improves the liver disease that is related to J-I bypass and TPN.[27, 28]

How TNF-α and oxidative stress promote the progression of alcohol-related fatty liver disease or NAFLD remains poorly understood. Studies in obese mice suggest that hepatocytes in fatty livers experience chronic apoptotic and oxidative stress and survive by accumulating various mitochondrial adaptations that make the cell more vulnerable to necrosis.[14, 29] Consistent with this concept is the observation that hepatic recovery from depletion of adenosine triphosphate (ATP) is impaired in obese mice[30] and humans[31] with NAFLD. Moreover, structural abnormalities[32] of liver mitochondria, including deletions of mitochondrial deoxyribonucleic acid (DNA),[33] have been documented in patients with NAFLD.

Studies in the 1990s of lean mice with experimentally induced or naturally occurring mutations in genes that regulate fatty acid beta oxidation by peroxisomes or mitochondria suggest that polymorphisms in these enzymes may modulate both lipid accumulation and hepatic oxidative stress.[34–36] For example, steatosis, steatohepatitis, and hepatocellular carcinoma develop spontaneously in mice that are genetically deficient in peroxisome proliferator-activated receptor-α (PPARα) (which activates the transcription of the genes for mitochondrial and peroxisomal fatty acid oxidizing enzymes) as they age.[36] Unlike patients with NASH, who are at increased risk for cirrhosis,[2, 7] mice that have fatty acid oxidation defects do not develop cirrhosis, even though such mice have severe NASH.[34–36] Nevertheless, these studies suggest that inherited or acquired defects in one or more of the fatty acid beta-oxidizing enzymes may promote the progression from steatosis to steatohepatitis in some patients with NAFLD. Insulin itself inhibits mitochondrial beta oxidation,[37] and this observation may explain the correlation between hyperinsulinemia and NASH.[6, 38] Metformin, an antihyperglycemic agent that reduces hyperinsulinemia in patients with type 2 diabetes,[39] reverses NASH in obese, leptin-deficient mice,[40] an observation that supports the possibility that hyperinsulinemia promotes the progression from steatosis to steatohepatitis.

Evidence from studies since 1998 suggests that leptin may promote hepatic fibrogenesis. Activated hepatic stellate cells can produce leptin,[41] and carbon tetrachloride–induced cirrhosis is inhibited in leptin deficient mice.[42]

CLINICAL FEATURES

Symptoms and Signs

The clinical features of NAFLD are summarized in Table 72–3. Like patients who have other types of chronic liver disease, most patients with NAFLD are asymptomatic. Hence, NAFLD is often diagnosed after serum liver biochemical abnormalities are noted during routine laboratory testing.[1] Some patients may come to medical attention because of fatigue, malaise, and vague right upper quadrant abdominal discomfort. In a study by Bacon and associates these symptoms antedated the histologic diagnosis of steatohepatitis in about one third of patients.[3] Although many patients deny symptoms of liver disease, hepatomegaly has been noted in up to three fourths of patients in several studies.[1, 3, 8] Stigmata of portal hypertension appear to occur less frequently, although splenomegaly was noted at the time of diagnosis in about 25% of the patients in one series.[3]

In contrast with most patients with steatohepatitis related to obesity and type 2 diabetes, some patients with certain types of drug-induced fatty liver (steatosis) experience rapid evolution of hepatic failure. Fulminant liver failure and death have been reported in patients treated with certain nucleoside analogs, antimitotic agents, and tetracycline.[10] In other patients with inborn errors of metabolism, such as tyrosinemia, steatosis appears to progress rapidly to cirrhosis and commonly leads to death from various liver-related complications, including hepatocellular carcinoma.

Laboratory Findings

The suspicion of NAFLD is usually prompted by abnormal serum liver biochemical findings. Typically, these laboratory test result abnormalities are noted when persons have routine testing or seek attention for other illnesses. Increased serum alanine aminotransferase (ALT) and aspartate aminotransferase (AST) activity is the predominant laboratory abnormality reported in patients with NAFLD.[1, 2, 3, 8] Usually the levels of ALT, AST, or both, are mildly to moderately increased,

Table 72–3 | **Clinical Features of Nonalcoholic Fatty Liver Disease**

Symptoms
Often asymptomatic
Fatigue, malaise, right upper quadrant discomfort
Signs
Hepatomegaly (common)
Splenomegaly (in some)
Portal hypertension (unusual)
Laboratory Findings
Increased serum aminotransferase levels (typical)
Increased alkaline phosphatase, gamma-glutamyl transpeptidase levels (occasional)
Increased serum cholesterol and triglyceride levels (common)
Increased glucose level (common)
Viral markers absent
Autoantibodies absent
Abnormal iron study results (sometimes)
Imaging Findings
Fatty liver
Stigmata of portal hypertension (unusual)

and the serum levels of these enzymes cannot be used to predict the histologic severity of hepatic inflammation or fibrosis. As many as 25% to 30% of patients with minimally elevated serum liver enzyme levels caused by NAFLD have significant fibrosis or cirrhosis detected on liver biopsy specimens.[2, 6, 7] Unlike hospitalized patients with alcohol-induced steatohepatitis, who typically manifest disproportionate increases in the AST level relative to the ALT level, patients with NAFLD usually have an AST/ALT ratio of less than 1,[1, 2] although the AST/ALT ratio tends to increase as cirrhosis develops.[6] Increases in serum alkaline phosphatase and gamma-glutamyl transpeptidase (GGTP) levels are not uncommon in patients with NAFLD. In fact, there is some evidence that an elevated serum GGTP level is a sensitive marker for insulin resistance.[38] Hence, increases in GGTP levels may be among the earliest biochemical findings in NAFLD.[7, 38] However, hyperbilirubinemia, prolongation of the prothrombin time, and hypoalbuminemia are noted infrequently in most series.[1–3, 8]

Abnormal serum lipid profiles (e.g., hypercholesterolemia, hypertriglyceridemia) and elevated serum glucose concentrations are also common in patients with NAFLD and have been reported in 25% to 75% of cases.[1] The pathophysiologic significance of hyperlipidemia remains uncertain, because some,[7] but not other,[6] series have demonstrated a positive correlation between hypertrigylceridemia and histologically advanced NAFLD. On the other hand, a growing body of evidence links insulin resistance, intermittent hyperglycemia, and overt diabetes with histologically advanced forms of NAFLD.[2, 6, 7, 38] Because most of these reports are derived from retrospective data analyses, whether insulin resistance is a cause or a consequence of the liver disease remains uncertain.

In an Australian report, elevated serum ferritin or iron levels or an increased transferrin saturation occurred commonly in patients with NASH, and about one third of patients were hetero- or homozygous for hemochromatosis gene *(HFE)* mutations.[43] The authors noted a trend toward more severe hepatic fibrosis in patients with NASH and a genetic basis for hepatic iron overload. However, other series from the United States[2, 7] and Europe[7] have been unable to document an association between hepatic iron overload or the hemochromatosis mutations and NASH.

Another report demonstrated an association between cryptogenic chronic hepatitis and celiac sprue and sparked interest in the possibility that subclinical gluten sensitivity may be a cause of NAFLD.[44] However, there are no published data to support this association conclusively.

A diagnosis of NAFLD can be established only in patients who do not consume significant amounts of alcohol. There is reasonably good evidence that the incidence of alcohol-induced liver disease begins to increase only after certain "threshold" levels of alcohol consumption (i.e., 20 g/day of ethanol in women and 80 g/day of ethanol in men) are exceeded habitually.[10] Thus, alcohol is not incriminated as the cause of liver disease in persons who report an alcohol intake that falls consistently below these threshold doses. However, it is conceivable that alcohol may contribute to liver disease in some obese persons with NAFLD who appear to be unusually sensitive to alcohol-mediated hepatotoxicity.[45] In addition, there has long been skepticism about the validity of self-reporting as a measure of alcohol consumption. Some physicians even doubt that the histologic features of alcoholic liver disease can ever occur in the absence of alcohol consumption.

There is no perfect test to identify alcohol use, particularly in the context of underlying liver disease. Indeed, results of some commonly used tests to identify habitual alcohol use (e.g., abnormally elevated serum aminotransferase levels, GGTP levels, or mean corpuscular volume [MCV]) are increased by liver disease per se and may overestimate alcohol use in patients with liver disease. For this reason, the diagnostic utility of these markers in differentiating NAFLD from alcohol-induced liver disease is limited. Other biochemical markers, specifically partially desialylated transferrin (dTf) and the mitochondrial isozyme of AST (mAST), have been advocated as tests for active alcohol use in patients with liver disease. The ratio of dTf to total Tf appears to be the best single marker of chronic excessive alcohol consumption in such patients.[10] In one study, which included patients with liver disease, a dTf/Tf ratio of 1.3% or greater was a reliable indicator of excessive chronic alcohol consumption, with a sensitivity of 81% and a specificity of 98%. In contrast, the ratio of serum mAST to total AST was not useful in distinguishing patients with NAFLD from alcoholic subjects.[10] Despite early promising results with dTf testing, it is premature to conclude that the test is required to exclude alcohol abuse in order to establish the diagnosis of NAFLD.

Testing to exclude viral hepatitis has become a prerequisite for the diagnosis of NAFLD. A study published in 1992 suggested that hepatitis C virus (HCV) is not involved in the pathogenesis of NAFLD, because markers of HCV infection are negative in the great majority of NAFLD patients.[46] Similarly, there is no evidence that the prevalence of hepatitis G viral infection is increased in patients with NAFLD. An increasing number of reports suggest that, although HCV infection does not cause NAFLD,[46] NAFLD may increase the severity of HCV-related liver damage. In particular, regression analysis has identified hepatic steatosis as an independent predictor of cirrhosis in patients with chronic hepatitis C.[47, 48] A large French study has demonstrated that obesity-related steatosis has the same ominous prognostic implications as alcohol-induced steatosis in patients infected with HCV.[48]

Several noninvasive imaging techniques, including ultrasonography, computed tomography, and magnetic resonance imaging (MRI), can identify hepatic steatosis and have been advocated as diagnostic tests for NAFLD.[1] Of these, phase contrast MRI appears to be the most promising, because its results correlate well with the degree of histologic steatosis. Ultrasonography is a reasonable, relatively inexpensive, noninvasive screening test to detect hepatic steatosis.[4] However, none of these imaging techniques is sufficiently sensitive to detect hepatic inflammation, fibrosis, or cirrhosis. Overall, currently available imaging modalities are relatively insensitive and nonspecific and can neither definitively establish a diagnosis of NAFLD nor grade its severity. Therefore, liver biopsy remains the best diagnostic test for confirming the clinical suspicion of NAFLD and staging the severity of liver injury and fibrosis.

A 1999 study from the Mayo Clinic suggested that older age, obesity, diabetes mellitus, and a serum AST/ALT ratio greater than 1 can help identify a subset of patients with

NAFLD who are most likely to have severe fibrosis indicated on liver biopsy.[6] A French group reached the same conclusion but suggested that hypertriglyceridemia may be more important than diabetes in their patient population.[7] The presence or absence of these risk factors may help clinicians select patients with suspected NAFLD for liver biopsy.

HISTOLOGIC FEATURES

The major histologic features of NAFLD resemble those of alcohol-induced liver disease and include steatosis (fatty liver), steatohepatitis (fatty liver plus parenchymal inflammation with or without accompanying focal necrosis), and variable degrees of fibrosis (including cirrhosis) (Fig. 72–1).[49] As in alcoholic liver disease, steatosis in NAFLD is predominantly macrovesicular and generally distributed diffusely throughout the liver lobule, although prominent microvesicular steatosis or zone 3 (perivenular) steatosis has been reported occasionally. In NASH, lobular infiltration, with both acute and chronic inflammatory cells, and Mallory's bodies resemble the findings noted in some patients with alcoholic liver disease. Patients with NASH can also have perivenular and sinusoidal fibrosis, reminiscent of that observed in alcohol-induced liver disease. As in patients with alcohol-induced liver disease, fibrosis can progress to cirrhosis in NAFLD.[2, 50] In light of the similarities between the histologic features of NAFLD and alcohol-induced liver disease, it is likely that the two diseases have a similar natural history. In both, steatosis is the principal early finding, but episodes of steatohepatitis can punctuate the course, and eventually cirrhosis develops in some affected persons. Failure to appreciate time-dependent variations in the histologic features of NAFLD may explain some of the confusion about its prognosis. Uncertainty about the prognosis is compounded by the dearth of long-term epidemiologic studies in patients with NAFLD.

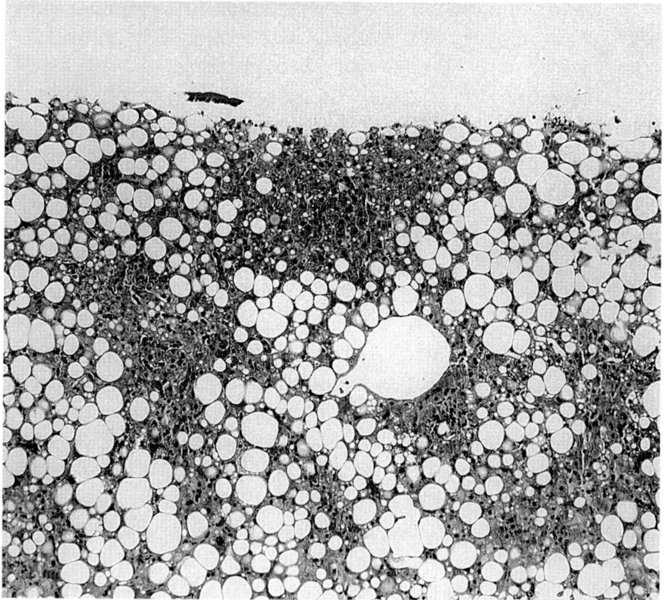

Figure 72–1. Low-power liver biopsy specimen showing typical histologic features of NAFLD, in particular diffuse macrovesicular steatosis and focal necroinflammation.

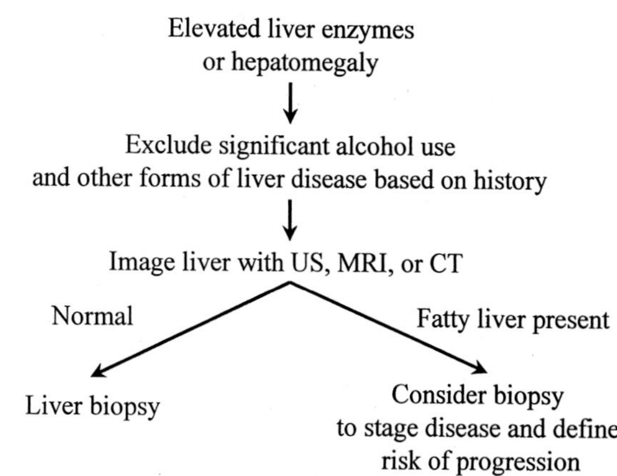

Figure 72–2. Diagnostic approach to NAFLD. Histologic and clinical outcomes are similar to those reported in alcoholic liver disease. US, ultrasound; MRI, magnetic resonance imaging; CT, computed tomography.

Role of Liver Biopsy in Diagnosis

The combination of the history, physical examination, noninvasive blood tests, and imaging studies is useful for excluding other diseases as an explanation for abnormal liver enzyme levels. Liver biopsy is seldom necessary simply to diagnose NAFLD, which is currently a diagnosis that is made by excluding other causes of chronic hepatitis in patients with fatty liver (Fig. 72–2). On the other hand, liver biopsy is the only diagnostic test that can reliably identify and quantify hepatic necrosis, inflammation, and fibrosis. Liver biopsy is the most sensitive and specific means to stage patients with NAFLD. As discussed later, histologic features provide important prognostic information about NAFLD and may guide recommendations concerning the advisability of other diagnostic testing (e.g., endoscopy to screen for gastroesophageal varices or serum α-fetoprotein testing with or without ultrasonography to screen for hepatocellular carcinoma in patients with cirrhosis) and may provide a justification for aggressive treatment strategies and frequent follow-up visits. However, because so little is known about the natural history of untreated or treated NAFLD, the clinical prognosis is difficult to predict unless advanced fibrosis is present.

PROGNOSIS

Major controversy concerning the prognosis of NAFLD persists. Specifically, it is not known whether information gathered from studies of large numbers of patients with alcohol-induced liver disease (Fig. 72–3) can be used to predict the outcome of patients with liver disease that is histologically similar to but is not caused by alcohol (see Chapter 71). In this regard, it is instructive to recall that, although even modest alcohol intake reliably leads to steatosis, cirrhosis is a relatively infrequent complication of alcohol abuse and occurs in only 15% to 20% of persons who have consumed as much as 180 g/day of ethanol for more than a decade.[10]

Episodes of alcoholic steatohepatitis are generally believed to increase the likelihood of eventual cirrhosis. However, several studies indicate that cirrhosis is not an inevitable sequela of alcoholic hepatitis but develops in only approximately one half of patients followed for 3 to 5 years after an index episode of alcoholic hepatitis.[51] Even after alcohol-induced cirrhosis is established, the clinical prognosis is extremely variable[52, 53] (Fig. 72–4). Thus, experience has shown that histologic progression and clinical outcome are highly variable in patients with alcohol-induced steatosis, steatohepatitis, or cirrhosis.

In light of this information, it is curious that there is reluctance to consider that NAFLD may portend an ominous prognosis. However, many small series include a sizable fraction of patients with histologically advanced disease. Severe fibrosis has been noted in 15% to 50% of patients, whereas well-established cirrhosis has been documented in 7% to 16% of patients.[1–3, 6–8, 54] Relatively few patients with NAFLD have been followed prospectively to delineate the natural history of the disease. The few follow-up studies that have been reported include small numbers of patients with various stages of NAFLD at the time of initial diagnosis. In general, studies that predominantly include patients with simple steatosis suggest that NAFLD has a benign long-term prognosis,[9] whereas those that are enriched with cases of steatohepatitis suggest a less favorable outcome.[2, 6–8] Therefore, patient heterogeneity coupled with relatively short durations of follow-up confounds the interpretation of these divergent results. Nevertheless, it is clear that progressive liver disease develops within a decade of the diagnosis of NAFLD in at least some patients.[2, 3, 8]

Even less certain is how often NAFLD evolves to a stage at which clinical complications are likely. The apparent discrepancy between the frequency of steatosis and that of life-threatening cryptogenic cirrhosis remains poorly understood. For example, steatosis has been documented in at least 40% of obese patients who have elective surgery to induce weight loss,[55] yet autopsy series suggest that only about 2% of obese persons become cirrhotic; these same autopsy series, however, also demonstrate that obesity is the only identifiable cause of liver disease in 12% of cirrhotic patients and that cirrhosis is approximately six times as prevalent in obese persons as in the general population.[56] The latter observations prompt speculation that steatosis is a risk factor for more progressive liver disease but requires the superimposition of other, ill-defined insults before cirrhosis can develop. This theory is consistent with evidence that both cirrhosis and liver-related mortality occur commonly after patients with obesity-related steatosis undergo J-I bypass surgery,[55] consume excessive alcohol,[45] or are exposed to other hepatotoxins.[57]

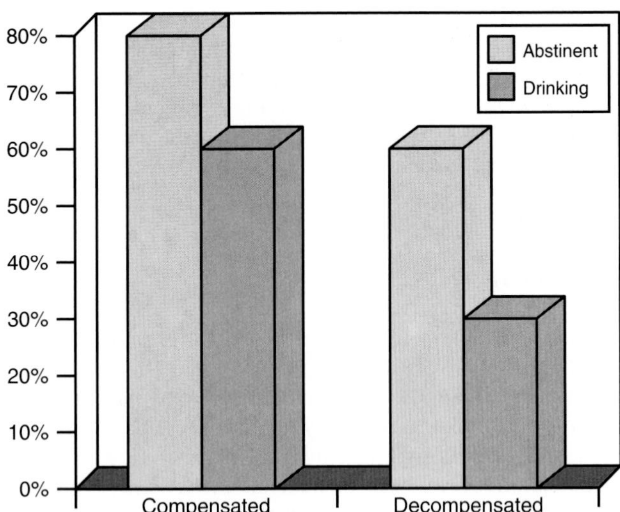
80%
70%
60%
50%
40%
30%
20%
10%
0%
Abstinent
Drinking
Compensated
Decompensated

Figure 72–4. Alcoholic cirrhosis: 5-year survival.

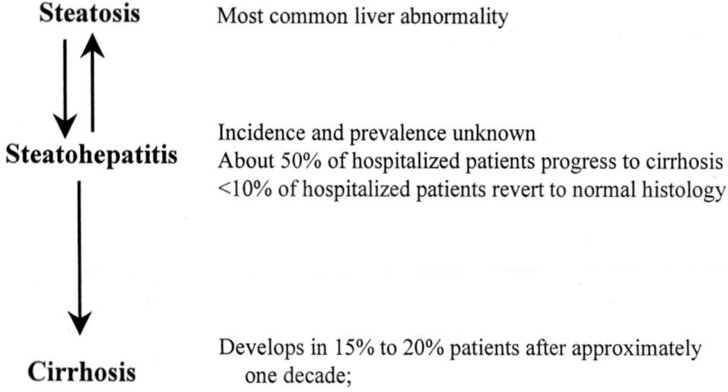
Steatosis
Most common liver abnormality
Steatohepatitis
Incidence and prevalence unknown
About 50% of hospitalized patients progress to cirrhosis
<10% of hospitalized patients revert to normal histology
Cirrhosis
Develops in 15% to 20% patients after approximately one decade;
The ultimate consequence of antecedent steatohepatitis

Figure 72–3. Natural history of alcoholic liver disease. Compensated patients have normal serum bilirubin and albumin levels at the time of diagnosis. Decompensated patients have jaundice, ascites, gastrointestinal bleeding, or encephalopathy.

Emerging evidence suggests that clinically significant liver disease is probably no more rare in NAFLD than in chronic hepatitis C or other types of chronic hepatitis.[2] Indeed, evidence from Caldwell and colleagues in 1999 suggests that NAFLD is likely to have been the underlying liver disease for most patients with cryptogenic cirrhosis[50]; it follows that NAFLD may be as important a cause of cirrhosis in the United States as alcohol or hepatitis C infection. Unfortunately, comorbidity resulting from associated medical conditions, such as obesity or diabetes, limits the use of liver transplantation in the management of patients with NAFLD. Moreover, NAFLD may recur after liver transplantation, particularly in patients with an intact J-I bypass.[58] Final resolution of existing controversies about the clinical implications of NAFLD will require large epidemiologic studies that track affected persons for several decades as well as a better understanding of the pathogenesis of NAFLD.

TREATMENT: CURRENT AND FUTURE

The current therapy of NAFLD emphasizes the elimination or modification of the factors that are commonly associated with NAFLD (Fig. 72–5). The mainstays of therapy are weight loss, treatment of hyperlipidemia and hyperglycemia, and discontinuation of use of potentially toxic drugs.[1] Unfortunately, efforts to modify a patient's life-style are often unsuccessful, and these approaches cure only a minority of affected persons.[1] Moreover, rapid weight reduction may even accelerate the progression of NAFLD.[59] Encouraging results have been reported in a few, highly selected patients who were treated with various agents, such as ursodeoxycholic acid, metronidazole, supplemental amino acids, glutamine, glucagon, or lipid-lowering drugs.[10] However, it is not

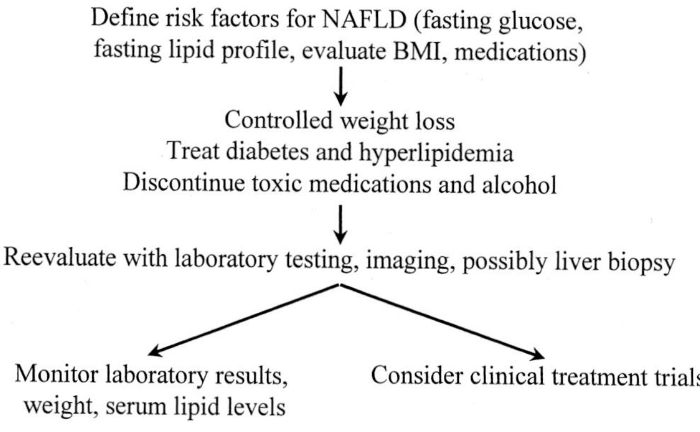
Define risk factors for NAFLD (fasting glucose, fasting lipid profile, evaluate BMI, medications)
Controlled weight loss
Treat diabetes and hyperlipidemia
Discontinue toxic medications and alcohol
Reevaluate with laboratory testing, imaging, possibly liver biopsy
Monitor laboratory results, weight, serum lipid levels
Consider clinical treatment trials
BMI = body mass index

Figure 72–5. Current therapy of NAFLD.

known whether these treatments are generally beneficial. Furthermore, many NAFLD patients lack known risk factors for the disease[3] and are not candidates for any of the management recommendations mentioned previously.

New therapeutic methods should capitalize on our improved understanding of the pathogenesis of NAFLD (Fig. 72–6). Potential future therapies for NAFLD are summarized in Table 72–4. For example, because hormonal imbalances (e.g., those between insulin and leptin discussed previously) promote NAFLD in experimental animals,[40, 60] it is reasonable to evaluate hormonal supplements, such as leptin, and pharmacologic agents, such as metformin or thiazolidinediones, that reduce hyperinsulinemia as potential therapies for NAFLD. However, caution is necessary because thiazolidinediones have caused acute liver disease in some patients,[61] and leptin may promote hepatic fibrogenesis.[42] In light of these concerns, anti-inflammatory agents may be more prudent choices as therapeutic agents for NAFLD. Soluble cytokine receptors, neutralizing anticytokine antibodies, and selective cyclooxygenase inhibitors have excellent safety profiles. Moreover, there is strong evidence that proinflammatory cytokines are necessary for experimental alcoholic liver disease[17] and that hepatic inflammation is a major risk factor for progressive NAFLD in humans.[2, 7] However, use of the newer anti-inflammatory agents for such a chronic disease as NAFLD will be limited by their expense.

The increased hepatic production of oxidants is also a logical therapeutic target in alcoholic and nonalcoholic fatty liver disease. Certain antioxidants, such as vitamin E (α-tocopherol), are safe and relatively inexpensive. Data from the 1960s demonstrate that α-tocopherol inhibits alcohol- and carbon tetrachloride–induced steatosis,[62] and in 2000 vitamin E was reported to improve serum ALT level elevations in some pediatric patients with NASH.[63] Other antioxidants, such as *S*-adenosyl methionine (SAMe), have also shown some benefit in patients with alcohol-induced steatohepatitis,[64] but SAMe is more expensive and less available than vitamin E. As in alcoholic liver disease, in NAFLD, chronic oxidative stress probably results from activation of microsomal enzymes and hepatic mitochondrial dysfunction. Excessive oxidants also can injure mitochondria (causing further mitochondrial dysfunction) and damage nuclear DNA, promoting the activation of DNA repair enzymes, such as poly (adenosine diphosphate-ribose) (poly [ADP-ribose]) polymerase (PARP). In extreme cases, the resulting disruption of normal redox balance causes hepatocyte ATP depletion, energy failure, and necrosis. Fatty livers are extremely vulnerable to injury from ischemia and reperfusion and from other insults that deplete liver ATP stores.[30] Therefore, treatments that prevent activation of PARP or that provide alternative energy sources for the liver may prove

Table 72–4 | **Potential Future Therapies for Nonalcoholic Fatty Liver Disease**

Agents That May Correct Hormonal Imbalances
Leptin
Pharmacologic agents that reduce hyperinsulinemia (Metformin, thiazolidinediones)
Agents That May Prevent Inflammation
By limiting macrophage activation
Intestinal decontamination with oral antibiotics or *Lactobacillus* species
Antiendotoxin antibodies
COX-2 inhibitors
By neutralizing inflammatory mediators
Anticytokines (TNF-α antibodies and soluble receptors)
Agents That May Constrain Hepatocyte Reactive Oxygen Species Production
Antioxidants
Vitamin E, glutathione prodrugs
Agents That May Protect Hepatocyte ATP Stores
Poly (ADP-ribose) polymerase inhibitors
Alternative energy substrates

ADP, adenosine diphosphate; ATP, adenosine triphosphate; COX-2, cyclooxygenase-2; TNF-α, tumor necrosis factor-α.

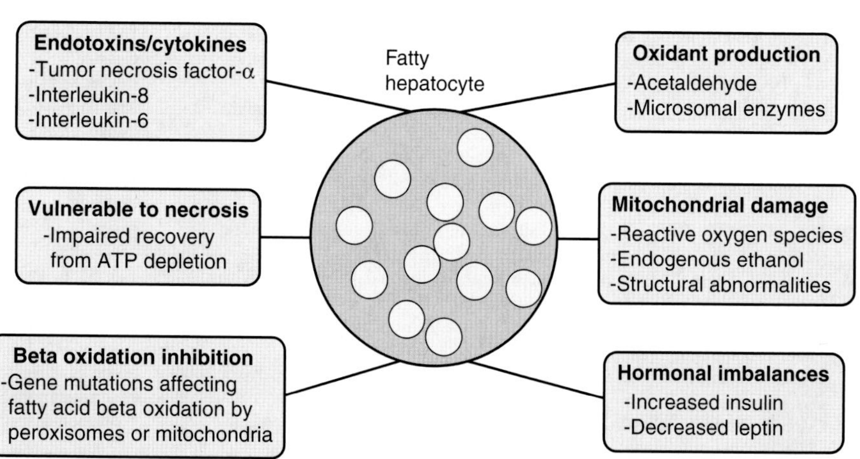
Endotoxins/cytokines
-Tumor necrosis factor-α
-Interleukin-8
-Interleukin-6
Fatty hepatocyte
Oxidant production
-Acetaldehyde
-Microsomal enzymes
Vulnerable to necrosis
-Impaired recovery from ATP depletion
Mitochondrial damage
-Reactive oxygen species
-Endogenous ethanol
-Structural abnormalities
Beta oxidation inhibition
-Gene mutations affecting fatty acid beta oxidation by peroxisomes or mitochondria
Hormonal imbalances
-Increased insulin
-Decreased leptin

Figure 72–6. NAFLD—pathogenic mechanisms.

useful in selected patients with NAFLD. Carefully controlled trials will be required to determine whether any of these strategies is beneficial in patients with NAFLD.

FOCAL FATTY LIVER

In contrast to NAFLD, which is a diffuse parenchymal process, focal fatty liver is a localized or patchy process that simulates a space-occupying lesion in the liver. Since it was first described by Brawer and colleagues[65] in 1980, this condition has become increasingly recognized, as a result of the improved sensitivity of abdominal imaging by ultrasonography, computed tomography (CT) and MRI. Focal fatty liver has characteristic patterns on CT: usually a nonspherical shape, absence of mass effect, and CT attenuation values consistent with those of soft tissue.[66] The density of focal fatty liver is close to that of water, unlike that of liver metastases, which have a density that is closer to that of hepatocytes.[66] Ultrasonography and MRI can be helpful to confirm the diagnosis of focal fatty liver.[67, 68] The presence of mass effect, areas of mixed hypo- and hyperechogenicity, an irregular shape, or a history of prior malignancy makes the diagnosis of focal fatty liver by noninvasive means difficult. In such patients, ultrasonographically guided fine-needle biopsy is helpful in distinguishing focal fatty liver from other mass lesions.[69] There is no evidence that the pathogenesis of focal fatty liver is similar to that of NAFLD. Furthermore, in the absence of accompanying or background liver disease, this lesion often regresses. Thus, no specific treatment is justified.

REFERENCES

1. Sheth SG, Gordon FD, Chopar S: Nonalcoholic steatohepatitis. Ann Intern Med 126:137–145, 1997.

1a. Reid AE. Nonalcoholic steatohepatitis. Gastroenterology 121:710, 2001.

2. Matteoni C, Younossi ZM, Gramlich T, et al: Nonalcoholic fatty liver disease: A spectrum of clinical pathological severity. Gastroenterology 116:1413–1419, 1999.
3. Bacon B, Faravash MJ, Janney CG, et al: Nonalcoholic steatohepatitis: An expanded clinical entity. Gastroenterology 107:1103–1106, 1994.
4. el-Hassan AY, Ibrahim EM, al-Mulhim FA, et al: Fatty infiltration of the liver: Analysis of prevalence, radiological and clinical features and influence on patient management. Br J Radiol 65:774–778, 1992.
5. Bizzaro N, Tremolada F, Casarin C, et al: Serum alanine aminotransferase levels among volunteer blood donors: Effect of sex, alcohol intake and obesity. Ital J Gastroenterol Hepatol 24:237–241, 1992.
6. Angulo P, Deach JC, Batts KP, Lindor Kc: Independent predictors of liver fibrosis in patients with nonalcoholic steatohepatitis. Hepatology 30:1356–1362, 1999.
7. Ratziu V, Giral P, Charlotte F, et al: Liver fibrosis in overweight patients. Gastroenterology 118:1117–1123, 2000.
8. Powell EE, Cooksley GE, Hanson R, et al: The natural history of nonalcoholic steatohepatitis: A follow-up study of 42 patients for up to 21 years. Hepatology 11:74–80, 1990.
9. Teli M, James OF, Burt AD, et al: A natural history of nonalcoholic fatty liver: A follow-up study. Hepatology 22:1714–1717, 1995.
10. Okolo PI, Diehl AM: Nonalcoholic steatohepatitis and focal fatty liver. In Feldman M, Scharschmidt BF, Sleisenger MH (eds.): Sleisenger and Fordtran's Gastrointestinal and Liver Disease, 6th ed. Philadelphia: WB Saunders, 1998, pp 1215–1220.
11. Lieber CS: Biochemical factors in alcoholic liver disease. Semin Liver Dis 13:136–147, 1993.
12. Cope K, Risby T, Diehl AM: Increased gastrointestinal ethanol production in obese mice: Implications for fatty liver disease pathogenesis. Gastroenterology 119:1340–1347, 2000.
13. Leclercq IA, Farrell GC, Field J, et al: Cyp2E1 and Cyp4A as microsomal catalysts of lipid peroxides in murine nonalcoholic steatohepatitis. J Clin Invest 105:1067–1075, 2000.
14. Yang SQ, Zhu H, Li Y, et al: Mitochondrial adaptations to obesity-related oxidant stress. Arch Biochem Biophys 378:259–268, 2000.
15. Mezey E, Imbembo AL, Potter JJ, et al: Endogenous ethanol production and hepatic disease following jejunoileal bypass for morbid obesity. Am J Clin Nutr 28:1277–1283, 1975.
16. Nair S, Cope K, Risby T, Diehl AM: Obesity and female gender increase breath ethanol concentration: Potential implications for the pathogenesis of nonalcoholic steatohepatitis. Am J Gastroenterol 96: 1200–1204, 2001.
17. Yin M, Wheeler MD, Kono H, et al: Essential role of tumor necrosis factor alpha in alcohol-induced liver injury in mice. Gastroenterology 117:942–952, 1999.
18. Hotamisligil GS, Peraldi SP, Budavari A, et al: IRS-1-mediated inhibition of insulin receptor tyrosine kinase activity in TNF-alpha- and obesity-induced insulin resistance. Science 271:665–668, 1996.
19. Kern PA, Saghizaheh M, Ong JM, et al: The expression of tumor necrosis factor in human adipose tissue: Regulation by obesity, weight loss, and relationship to lipoprotein lipase. J Clin Invest 95:2111–2119, 1995.
20. Friedman JM, Leibel R, Siegel DS, et al: Molecular mapping of the mouse ob mutation. Genetics 11:1054–1062, 1991.
21. Faggioni R, Fantuzzi G, Gabay C, et al: Leptin deficiency enhances sensitivity to endotoxin-induced lethality. Am J Physiol 276:R136–R142, 1999.
22. Lee F-Y, Li Y, Yang EK, et al: Phenotypic abnormalities in macrophages from leptin-deficient, obese mice. Am J Physiol Cell Physiol 276:C386–C394, 1999.
23. Guebre-Xabier M, Yang SQ, Lin HZ, et al: Altered hepatic lymphocyte subpopulations in obesity-related fatty livers. Hepatology 31:633–640, 1999.
24. Yang SQ, Lin HZ, Lane MD, et al: Obesity increases sensitivity to endotoxin liver injury: Implications for pathogenesis of steatohepatitis. Proc Natl Acad Sci U S A 94:2557–2562, 1997.
25. Leung FW, Drenick EJ, Stanley TM: Intestinal bypass complications involving the excluded small bowel segment. Am J Gastroenterol 77: 67–72, 1982.
26. Jorizzo JL, Apisarnthanarax P, Subrt P, et al: Bowel-bypass syndrome without bowel bypass: Bowel-associated dermatosis-arthritis syndrom. Arch Intern Med 143:457–461, 1983.
27. Moxley RT, Posefsky T, Lockwood DH: Protein nutrition and liver disease after jejunoileal bypass for morbid obesity. N Engl J Med 290: 921–925, 1974.
28. Capron JP, Herve MA, Ginestron JL, et al: Metronidazole in prevention of cholestasis associated with total parenteral nutrition. Lancet 1:446–449, 1983.
29. Rashid A, Wu T-C, Huang CC, et al: Mitochondrial proteins that regulate apoptosis and necrosis are induced in mouse fatty liver. Hepatology 29:1131–1138, 1999.
30. Chavin K, Yang SQ, Lin HZ, et al: Obesity induces expression of uncoupling protein-2 in hepatocytes and promotes liver ATP depletion. J Biol Chem 274:5692–5700, 1999.
31. Cortez-Pinto H, Chatham J, Chacko VP, et al: Alterations in liver ATP homeostasis in human nonalcoholic steatohepatitis: A pilot study. JAMA 282:1659–1664, 1999.
32. Caldwell SH, Swerdlow RH, Khan EM, et al: Mitochondrial abnormalities in nonalcoholic steatohepatitis. J Hepatol 31:430–434, 1999.
33. Mansouri A, Gaou I, Fromenty B, et al: Premature oxidative aging of hepatic mitochondiral DNA in Wilson's disease. Gastroenterology 113: 599–605, 1997.
34. Kuwajima M, Kono N, Horiuchi M, et al: Animal model of systemic carnitine deficiency: Analysis in C3H-2 strain of mouse associated with juvenile visceral steatosis. Biochem Biophys Res Commun 174:1090–1094, 1991.
35. Fan C-Y, Pan J, Usuda N, et al: Steatohepatitis, spontaneous peroxisome proliferation and tumors in mice lacking peroxisomal and fatty acyl-CoA oxidase. J Biol Chem 273:15639–15645, 1998.
36. Leone TC, Weinheimer CJ, Kelly DP: A critical role for the peroxisome proliferator-activated receptor alpha (PPAR alpha) in the cellular fasting response: The PPAR alpha–null mouse as a model of fatty acid oxidation disorders. Proc Natl Acad Sci U S A 96:7473–7478, 1999.

37. Moller DE, Flier JS: Insulin resistance: Mechanisms, syndromes, and implications. N Engl J Med 325:938–948, 1991.
38. Marchesini G, Brizi M, Morselli-Labate AM, et al: Association of nonalcoholic fatty liver disease with insulin resistance. Am J Med 107: 450–455, 1999.
39. Stumvoll M, Nurjhan N, Perriello G, et al: Metabolic effects of metformin in non-insulin-dependent diabetes mellitus. N Engl J Med 333: 550–554, 1995.
40. Lin HZ, Yang SQ, Kujhada F, et al: Metformin reverses nonalcoholic fatty liver disease in obese leptin-deficient mice. Nat Med 6:998–1003, 2000.
41. Potter JJ, Womack L, Mezey E, Anania FA: Transdifferentiation of rat hepatic stellate cells results in leptin expression. Biochem Biophys Res Commun 244:178–182, 1998.
42. Leclerq IA, Farrell GC: Leptin is required for the development of hepatic fibrosis. Hepatology 32:302A, 2000.
43. George DK, Goldwurm S, MacDonald GA, et al: Increased hepatic iron concentration in nonalcoholic steatohepatitis is associated with increased fibrosis. Gastroenterology 114:311–318, 1998.
44. Volta U, De Franceshi L, Lari F, et al: Coeliac disease hidden by cryptogenic hypertransaminasemia. Lancet 352:26–29, 1998.
45. Giraud NS, Borotto E, Aubert A, et al: Excess weight risk factor for alcoholic liver disease. Hepatology 25:108–111, 1997.
46. Rogers DW, Lee CH, Pound DC, et al: Hepatitis C virus does not cause nonalcoholic steatohepatitis. Dig Dis Sci 37:1644–1649, 1992.
47. Czaja AJ, Carpenter HA, Santrach PJ, Moore SB: Host- and disease-specific factors affecting steatosis in chronic hepatitis C. J Hepatol 29: 198–206, 1998.
48. Poupon RY, Serfaty LD, Amorim M, et al: Combination of steatosis and alcohol intake is the main determinant of fibrosis progression in patients with hepatitis C. Hepatology 30:406A, 1999.
49. Ludwig J, Viggiano RT, McGill DB: Nonalcoholic steatohepatitis: Mayo Clinic experiences with a hitherto unnamed disease. Mayo Clin Proc 55:342–348, 1980.
50. Caldwell SH, Oelsner DH, Iezzoni JC, et al: Cryptogenic cirrhosis: Clinical characterization and risk factors for underlying disease. Hepatology 29:664–669, 1999.
51. Pares A, Caballeria J, Brugera M: Histologic course of alcoholic hepatitis: Influence of abstinence, sex, and extent of hepatic damage. J Hepatol 2:33–38, 1986.
52. Galambos J: Natural history of alcoholic hepatitis III: Histologic changes. Gastroenterology 56:515–522, 1972.
53. Lelbach WK: Epidemiology of alcoholic liver disease. Prog Liver Dis 5:494–513, 1976.
54. Diehl AM, Goodman Z, Ishak KG: Alcohol-like liver disease in nonalcoholics: A clinical and histopathological comparison with alcohol-induced liver injury. Gastroenterology 95:1056–1060, 1989.
55. Vyberg M, Ravn V, Andersen B: Patterns of progression of liver injury following jejunoileal bypass for morbid obesity. Liver 7:271–276, 1987.
56. Wanless IR, Lentz JS: Fatty liver hepatitis (steatohepatitis) and obesity: An autospy study with analysis of risk factors. Hepatology 12:1106–1110, 1990.
57. Hodgson M, Van Thiel DH, Goodman-Klein B: Obesity and hepatotoxin risk factors for fatty liver disease. Br J Ind Med 48:690–695, 1991.
58. D'Souze-Gburek S, Batta KP, Nikias GA, et al: Liver transplantation for jejunoileal bypass–associated cirrhosis: Allograft histology in the setting of an intact bypassed limb. Liver Transpl Surg 3:23–27, 1997.
59. Capron JP, Delamarre M, Dupas JL, et al: Fasting in obesity: Another cause of liver injury with alcoholic hyaline? Dig Dis Sci 54:374–377, 1982.
60. Shimomura I, Hammer RE, Ikemoto S, et al: Leptin reverses insulin resistance and diabetes mellitus in mice with congenital lipodystrophy. Nature 401:73–76, 1999.
61. Kohlroser J, Mathai J, Reichheld J, et al: Hepatotoxicity due to troglitazone: Report of two cases and review of adverse events reported to the United States Food and Drug Administration. Am J Gastroenterol 95: 272–276, 2000.
62. DiLuzio N, Costales F: Inhibition of ethanol and carbon tetrachloride induced fatty liver by antioxidants. Exp Mol Pathol 4:141–145, 1965.
63. Lavine JE: Vitamin E treatment of non-alcoholic steatohepatitis in children: A pilot study. J Pediatr 136:734–738, 2000.
64. Friedel HA, Goa KL, Benfield P: *S*-adenosylmethionine: A review of its pharmacological properties and therapeutic potential in liver dysfunction and affective disorders in relation to its physiological role in cell metabolism. Drugs 38:389–416, 1989.
65. Brawer MK, Austin GE, Lewin KJ: Focal fatty change of the liver, a hitherto poorly recognized entity. Gastroenterology 78:247, 1980.
66. Halvorsen RA, Korobkin M, Ram PC, et al: CT appearance of focal fatty infiltration of the liver. AJR Am J Roentgenol 139:277, 1982.
67. Wang SS, Chiang JH, Tsai YT, et al: Focal hepatic liver infiltration as a cause of pseudotumors: Ultrasonographic patterns and clinical differentiation. J Clin Ultrasound 18:401, 1990.
68. Kane AG, Redwine MD, Cossi AF: Characterization of focal fatty change in the liver with a fat-enhanced inversion-recovery sequence. J Abdom Imaging 3:581, 1993.
69. Caturelli E, Rapaccini GL, Sabelli C, et al: Ultrasonography and echo-guided fine-needle biopsy in the diagnosis of focal fatty liver change. Hepatogastroenterology 34:137, 1987.

Chapter 73

Liver Disease Caused by Drugs, Anesthetics, and Toxins

Geoffrey C. Farrell

DEFINITIONS AND GENERAL IMPORTANCE OF DRUGS AND TOXINS AS CAUSES OF LIVER DISEASE

Hepatotoxicity is liver injury caused by drugs and other chemicals. *Adverse drug reactions* are noxious, unintentional effects that occur at doses used for prophylaxis and therapy. Adverse drug reactions that affect the liver are more difficult to define because the biochemical tests used to detect liver injury may also be elevated as an *adaptive response* to drugs. In general, however, *liver injury* is present when abnormalities of liver tests include an increase, to more than twice the upper limit of normal, of serum alanine aminotransferase (ALT), alkaline phosphatase (AP), or bilirubin levels. The severity of drug-induced liver injury varies from minor nonspecific changes in hepatic structure and function to fulminant hepatic failure, cirrhosis, and liver cancer. The term *drug-induced liver disease* should be confined to cases in which the nature of liver injury has been characterized histologically.

Hepatotoxicity accounts for less than 5% of cases of jaundice or acute hepatitis in the community and for even fewer cases of chronic liver disease.[1–3] However, drugs are an important cause of more severe types of liver disease and of liver disease in older people; for instance, they accounted for 10% of cases of severe hepatitis requiring hospitalization in France,[4] 20% to 75% of cases of acute liver failure in Western countries (approximately one third of cases in the United States),[5, 6] and 43% of cases of hepatitis among patients aged 50 years and older.[7] The incidence of most types of drug-induced liver disease is in the order of 1 per 10,000 to 1 per 100,000 persons exposed. However, hepatic drug reactions produce an array of clinical syndromes and liver pathologies that mimic all known hepatobiliary diseases, and one agent can produce several clinicopathologic syndromes. In complex medical situations, drug toxicity can interact with other causes of liver injury. Noteworthy examples include bone marrow transplantation, cancer chemotherapy, highly active antiretroviral therapy (HAART) for human immunodeficiency virus (HIV) and acquired immunodeficiency syndrome (AIDS), chronic viral hepatitis, and nonalcoholic steatohepatitis (NASH) in patients with the metabolic syndrome. For all these reasons, drug-induced liver disease poses a diagnostic challenge to physicians and pathologists.

The hepatotoxic nature of many drugs and industrial toxins was recognized during the first 6 decades of the past century,[2, 3] and many such agents have been removed from use. Since the 1960s, a common feature of hepatic adverse drug reactions has been delayed recognition until many years after release and widespread use of individual agents. Initial reports of hepatotoxicity are then followed by clusters of case reports that evoke the appearance of "mini-epidemics." Examples include isoniazid, α-methyldopa (methyldopa), halothane, chlorpromazine, erythromycin, amoxicillin/clavulanate, oxypenicillins, various nonsteroidal anti-inflammatory drugs (NSAIDs), and troglitazone. As drugs become known as potential hepatotoxic agents, they have usually been replaced by more acceptable alternatives. However, the burgeoning number of therapeutic agents now includes hundreds that can be cited as rare causes of drug-induced liver disease. The increasing number of agents implicated as potential causes of liver disease poses several challenges to clinicians.[2, 3, 8–12] These challenges include concern about what constitutes an adequate level of patient information at the time a drug is prescribed and the reliability of evidence linking individual agents to particular types of liver injury.[2, 11–15]

This chapter reviews contemporary issues in drug-induced liver disease, including epidemiology, etiopathogenesis, clinicopathologic spectrum, and practical approaches to diagnosis, prevention, and management. Particular reference is made to more recently described examples of drug-induced liver disease and drugs of continuing importance. Industrial and environmental hepatotoxicity is less important now than in the past but remains a topic of medicolegal interest; it is discussed briefly. On the other hand, complementary and alternative therapies, including traditional herbal medicines and vitamins, are implicated increasingly as causes of liver injury, and they are considered in more detail.

EPIDEMIOLOGY

Epidemiologic studies confirm the rarity of drug-induced liver disease with currently used agents. For example, for NSAIDs, the risk of liver injury lies between 1 and 10 per 100,000 exposed persons;[16, 17] amoxicillin/clavulanic acid has been associated with cholestatic hepatitis in 1 to 2 per 100,000 exposed persons;[18–20] and low-dose tetracyclines have caused hepatotoxicity in less than one case per million exposed persons.[21] The frequency may be higher for agents that exert a metabolic type of hepatotoxicity. For instance, isoniazid causes liver injury in up to 2% of those exposed, with the risk depending on age, gender, concomitant exposure to other agents, and, possibly, the presence of chronic hepatitis B.

In most types of drug-related liver injury, drugs are the sole cause of hepatic damage. In other cases, drugs increase the *relative risk* for types of liver disease that may occur in the absence of drug exposure. Examples include salicylates in Reye's syndrome,[22] oral contraceptive steroids in hepatic venous thrombosis (Budd-Chiari syndrome),[23] methotrexate in hepatic fibrosis associated with alcoholic and diabetic types of fatty liver disease, and tamoxifen in NASH.

The best term for expressing how common drug reactions are is *frequency* or *risk*—that is, the number of adverse reactions for a given number of persons exposed. The time-dependent terms *incidence* and *prevalence* are not appropriate for drug reactions because the frequency is not linearly related to the duration of exposure. Instead, the onset of most reactions occurs within a relatively short exposure time, although some types of chronic liver disease occur after a *latent period* of many months or years.

The reported rate of drug reactions is a crude indicator of risk because of the inherent inaccuracies of case definition (see section on Diagnosis),[2, 11, 15] and because case recognition and reporting depend on the skill and motivation of observers. More appropriate epidemiologic methods can be applied to hepatotoxicity, such as prescription event monitoring, record linkage, and case-control studies. The first two methods have been used to estimate the frequency of liver injury with some antimicrobial agents (erythromycins, sulfonamides, tetracyclines, flucloxacillin, amoxicillin/clavulanate) and NSAIDs,[16, 17, 24] whereas the case-control studies have been used to define attributable risk for industrial toxins, aspirin and Reye's syndrome,[22] and oral contraceptives and liver tumors[25, 26] or hepatic vein thrombosis.[23]

Individual Risk Factors

Many factors influence the risk of drug-induced liver disease (Table 73–1). These factors include the dose, blood level, and duration of intake for dose-dependent hepatotoxins like acetaminophen and methotrexate. Some idiosyncratic reactions also are partly dependent on these factors; examples include tetracyclines, dantrolene, tacrine, and the oxypenicillins. For these drugs, however, other host determinants such as age, gender, genetic factors, exposure to other substances, and concomitant diseases are more relevant.

AGE. Most hepatic drug reactions are more common in adults than in children. Exceptions include valproic acid hepatotoxicity, which is most common in children less than 3 years of age and rare in adults,[27, 28] and Reye's syndrome, in which salicylates play a key role.[22, 29, 30] As discussed later, both drugs may cause mitochondrial toxicity. In adults, the risk of isoniazid-associated hepatotoxicity is greater in persons more than 40 years of age. Similar observations have been made for nitrofurantoin, halothane, etretinate, diclofenac, and troglitazone. However, the overall increased frequency of adverse drug reactions in older subjects is largely the result of increased exposure, use of multiple agents, and altered drug disposition. Clinical severity increases strikingly with age, as exemplified by reactions to isoniazid and halothane.

GENDER. Women are particularly predisposed to drug-induced hepatitis, a difference that cannot be attributed simply to increased exposure. Examples include halothane, nitrofurantoin, sulfonamides, flucloxacillin, minocycline, and troglitazone. Drug-induced chronic hepatitis caused by nitrofurantoin, diclofenac, or minocycline has an even more pronounced female preponderance. Conversely, equal gender frequency or even male preponderance is common for some drug reactions characterized by cholestasis; an example is amoxicillin/clavulanic acid, which is more common in men than in women (see later). Male renal transplant recipients are also more likely than female recipients to develop aza-

Table 73–1 | **Factors Influencing Risk of Liver Diseases Caused by Drugs**

FACTOR	EXAMPLES OF DRUGS AFFECTED	INFLUENCE
Age	Isoniazid, nitrofurantoin, halothane, troglitazone	Age >60 yr: increased frequency, increased severity
	Valproic acid, salicylates	More common in children
Gender	Halothane, minocycline, nitrofurantoin	More common in women, especially chronic hepatitis
	Amoxicillin/clavulanic acid, azathioprine	More common in men
Dose	Acetaminophen, aspirin; some herbal medicines (see text)	Blood levels directly related to risk of hepatotoxicity
	Tetracycline, tacrine, oxypenicillins	Idiosyncratic reactions, but partial relationship to dose
	Methotrexate, vitamin A	Total dose, dose frequency, and duration of exposure related to risk of hepatic fibrosis
Genetic factors	Halothane, phenytoin, sulfonamides	Multiple cases in families, in vitro test results
	Amoxicillin/clavulanic acid	Strong HLA association (see text)
	Valproic acid	Familial cases, association with mitochondrial enzyme deficiencies
History of other drug reactions	Isoflurane, halothane, enflurane Erythromycins Diclofenac, ibuprofen, tiaprofenic acid Sulfonamides, COX-2 inhibitors (see text)	Instances of cross-sensitivity have been reported among members of each class of drugs but are rare
Other drugs	Acetaminophen	Isoniazid, zidovudine, phenytoin lower dose threshold and increase severity of hepatotoxicity
	Valproic acid	Other antiepileptics increase risk of hepatotoxicity
	Anticancer drugs	Interactive vascular toxicity
Excessive alcohol use	Acetaminophen hepatotoxicity	Lowered dose threshold, poorer outcome
	Isoniazid, methotrexate	Increased risk of liver injury, hepatic fibrosis
Nutritional status:		
Obesity	Halothane, troglitazone, tamoxifen, methotrexate	Increased risk of liver injury; hepatic fibrosis
Fasting	Acetaminophen	Increased risk of hepatotoxicity
Preexisting liver disease	Hycanthone, pemoline	Increased risk of liver injury
	Antituberculosis drugs, ibuprofen	Increased risk of liver injury with chronic hepatitis B and C
Other Diseases		
Diabetes mellitus	Methotrexate	Increased risk of hepatic fibrosis
HIV/AIDS	Sulfonamides (cotrimoxazole)	Increased risk of hypersensitivity
Renal failure	Tetracycline; methotrexate	Increased risk of liver injury; hepatic fibrosis
Organ transplantation	Azathioprine, thioguanine, busulfan	Increased risk of vascular toxicity

AIDS, acquired immunodeficiency syndrome; COX, cyclooxygenase; HIV, human immunodeficiency virus; HLA, human leukocyte antigens.

thioprine-induced liver disease (see section on Vascular Toxicity).

GENETIC FACTORS. Genetic determinants predispose to drug-induced liver disease,[31] as they do to other drug reactions like penicillin allergy. It has been stated that atopic patients have an increased risk of some types of drug hepatitis, but this association has not been proved. Genetic factors determine the activity of drug-activating and antioxidant pathways, encode pathways of canalicular bile secretion, and modulate the immune response and cell death pathways. Documented examples of familial predisposed adverse hepatic drug reactions are few and include valproic acid[32] and phenytoin.[33] Inherited mitochondrial diseases are a risk factor for valproic acid–induced hepatotoxicity.[27, 34] There are strong associations between some forms of drug-induced liver disease and human leukocyte antigens (HLA), as illustrated by cholestatic reactions to amoxicillin/clavulanic acid[19, 35] and tiopronin (see later).[36]

PAST HISTORY. A previous history of adverse drug reactions generally increases the risk of adverse reactions to the same drug and to other agents. However, instances of cross-sensitivity to related agents in cases of drug-induced liver disease are surprisingly uncommon. Examples of agents discussed later include anesthetics (halothane, isoflurane, enflurane); erythromycins; phenothiazines and tricyclic antidepressants; isoniazid and pyrazinamide; sulfonamides and other sulfur-containing compounds (e.g., some cyclooxygenase-2 [COX-2] inhibitors); and some NSAIDs. *A previous reaction to the same drug* is the major factor predisposing to the severity of drug-induced liver injury (see Acute Drug Hepatitis; Chronic Liver Disease).[37]

CONCOMITANT EXPOSURE TO OTHER AGENTS. Patients taking multiple drugs are more likely to experience an adverse reaction than are those taking single agents.[2, 14, 38–41] The mechanisms include enhanced cytochrome P450 (CYP)–mediated metabolism of the second drug to a toxic intermediate. Examples of agents discussed later include acetaminophen, isoniazid, valproic acid, and anticancer drugs.[42] Alternatively, drugs may alter the disposition of other agents by reducing bile flow or competing with canalicular pathways for biliary excretion; this mechanism may account for apparent interactions between oral contraceptive steroids (OCS) and other drugs to produce cholestasis.[43] Drugs or their metabolites may also interact via toxic mechanisms involving mitochondrial injury, cell signaling, and regulation of key hepatic genes, such as those involved with controling the response to stress and injury and triggering cell death processes.[44]

ALCOHOL. Chronic excessive alcohol ingestion decreases the dose threshold and enhances the severity of acetaminophen-induced hepatotoxicity, increases the risk and severity of isoniazid hepatitis and the risk of niacin (nicotinamide) hepatotoxicity, and predisposes to methotrexate-induced hepatic fibrosis.

NUTRITIONAL STATUS. Obesity is strongly associated with the risk of halothane hepatitis and appears to be an independent risk factor for NASH and hepatic fibrosis in patients taking methotrexate or tamoxifen (see later). Conversely, fasting predisposes to acetaminophen hepatotoxicity.[45] A role for nutritional factors in isoniazid hepatotoxicity also has been proposed.[46]

PREEXISTING LIVER DISEASE. In general, liver diseases such as alcoholic cirrhosis and cholestasis do not predispose to adverse hepatic reactions. Exceptions include some anticancer drugs,[47] niacin (nicotinamide),[14, 48] pemoline,[49, 50] and hycanthone.[51] Preexisting liver disease is also a critical determinant of risk for methotrexate-induced hepatic fibrosis. More recently, patients with chronic viral hepatitis and possibly those with HIV infection or AIDS have been found to have a heightened risk of liver injury during antituberculosis[52] or HAART chemotherapy,[53] after exposure to ibuprofen and possibly other NSAIDs,[54] and possibly after taking antiandrogens, such as flutamide and cyproterone acetate.[55]

OTHER DISEASES. Rheumatoid arthritis appears to increase the risk of salicylate hepatotoxicity.[56] Diabetes, obesity, and renal failure predispose to methotrexate-induced hepatic fibrosis (see later), whereas HIV infection and AIDS carry a high risk of sulfonamide hypersensitivity.[57] Renal transplantation is a risk factor for azathioprine-associated vascular injury,[2] and renal failure predisposes to tetracycline-induced fatty liver.[3] A curious, unexplained observation is that hepatitis associated with sulfasalazine appears to be more common in patients with rheumatoid arthritis than in those with inflammatory bowel disease.[1] Finally, veno-occlusive disease induced by anticancer drugs is apparently more common after bone marrow transplantation.[47]

PATHOPHYSIOLOGY

Role of the Liver in Drug Elimination

By virtue of the portal circulation, the liver is highly exposed to drugs and other toxins absorbed from the gastrointestinal tract. Most drugs tend to be lipophilic compounds that are readily taken up by the liver and that are not readily excreted in bile or urine. However, the liver is well equipped to handle high concentrations of drugs and toxins by an adjustable series of metabolic pathways. These pathways include those that alter the parent molecule (phase 1 drug metabolism), those that synthesize a conjugate of the drug or its metabolite with a more water-soluble moiety, such as a sugar, amino acid, or sulfate molecule (phase 2 metabolism), and energy-dependent pathways of excretion for either the parent molecule or the drug/drug metabolite conjugate from the hepatocyte (phase 3 elimination). For any given compound, one, two, or three of these steps may participate in drug elimination.

Pathways of Drug Metabolism

Drugs can be rendered more hydrophilic, and thus excretable in water, by enzyme-dependent processes termed *biotransformation;* the liver is the main site of drug metabolism. Phase 1 pathways include oxidation, reduction, and hydrolytic reactions. The products can be readily conjugated or excreted without further modification. Drug metabolism is reviewed elsewhere,[58, 59] and only issues salient to drug-induced liver disease are summarized here.

Cytochrome P450 (CYP)

Most type 1 reactions are catalyzed by microsomal drug oxidases, the key component of which is a hemoprotein of the CYP gene superfamily. The apparent promiscuity of drug oxidases toward drugs, environmental toxins, steroid hormones, lipids, and bile acids results from the existence of multiple, closely related CYP proteins. Members of the same CYP subfamily are structurally similar but catalyze the same reactions at vastly different rates. There are more than 20 CYP enzymes in the human liver.[59]

The reaction cycle has been described fully elsewhere.[58, 59] In brief, iron in the heme prosthetic group binds oxygen, which is then reduced by accepting an electron from nicotinamide-adenine dinucleotide phosphate (NADPH)-CYP reductase, a flavoprotein reductase. The resulting "activated oxygen" is incorporated into lipophilic substrates, such as drugs, toxins, fatty acids, or steroid hormones. Reduction of oxygen and insertion into a substrate for "mixed function oxidation" can result in formation of chemically reactive intermediates, including free radicals, electrophilic "oxy-intermediates" (e.g., unstable epoxides, quinone imines), and reduced (and therefore reactive) oxygen species (ROS). A typical example is the CYP2E1-catalyzed metabolite of acetaminophen, *N*-acetyl-*p*-benzoquinone imine (NAPQI), an oxidizing and arylating metabolite that is responsible for liver injury during acetaminophen hepatotoxicity. Other quinone metabolites are potential reactive metabolites of such agents as troglitazone,[60] quinine, and methyldopa,[58] whereas epoxide metabolites of diterpenoids may be hepatotoxic metabolites of some plant toxins.[61, 62] ROS appear to have broad significance in the production of tissue injury, particularly by contributing to the production of oxidative stress (see later).[63]

CYP proteins are distributed selectively in the hepatic acinus (or lobule). In particular, there is a higher content in zone 3, and localization of CYP2E1 is confined to a narrow rim of hepatocytes 1 to 2 cells thick around the terminal hepatic venule. Following exposure to inducing agents, enzyme protein extends peripherally through the lobule. The localization of CYP proteins explains in part the zonality of hepatic lesions produced by drugs and toxins that are converted to reactive metabolites, such as acetaminophen and carbon tetrachloride.

Genetic and Environmental Determinants of CYP Enzymes

PHARMACOGENETICS AND POLYMORPHISMS OF CYP EXPRESSION. The hepatic expression of each CYP enzyme is genetically determined. This observation largely explains the fourfold or greater differences in rates of drug metabolism in healthy subjects. Some CYPs, particularly minor forms, are also subject to polymorphic inheritance; occasional persons completely lack the encoded protein.[59] One example is CYP2D6, which codes the enzyme responsible for metabolism of debrisoquine and perhexiline. Poor metabolizers lack CYP2D6 protein and accumulate perhexiline when treated with usual doses of the drug; absence of CYP2D6 is the critical determinant of serious adverse effects of perhexiline, including chronic hepatitis and cirrhosis.[64] Other examples include CYP2C9 which affects *S*-warfarin, tolbutamide, and phenytoin metabolism, and 2C19, which affects *S*-mephenytoin metabolism;[59] 3% of white populations and 15% of Asians are poor metabolizers of *S*-mephenytoin.

DEVELOPMENTAL REGULATION AND CONSTITUTIVE EXPRESSION. Expression of several CYPs is developmentally regulated. During adult life, there may be a slight (up to 10%) decline in some CYPs with advancing age,[65] but this change is trivial compared with genetic variation and environmental influences. Gender differences in expression of CYPs 3A4 and 2E1 may explain the slightly enhanced metabolism of certain drugs (erythromycin, chlordiazepoxide, midazolam) in women,[66] but it remains unclear whether this difference contributes to the increased risk of hepatic drug reactions in women.

NUTRITION AND DISEASE-RELATED CHANGES. Nutritional status influences the expression of certain CYPs, both in health and in the presence of liver disease.[67] It is particularly noteworthy that CYP2E1 activity is increased by obesity and fasting.[14, 58, 59] Certain diseases can also alter expression of hepatic CYPs; these include diabetes mellitus (increased CYP2E1), hypothyroidism (decreased CYP1A), and hypopituitarism (decreased CYP3A4).[59] Severe liver disease is associated with decreased levels of total CYP and with reduced hepatic perfusion; the result is a decrease in the clearance of drugs that are rapidly metabolized by the liver.[59]

ADAPTIVE RESPONSE AND ENZYME INDUCTION. Exposure to lipophilic substances results in an adaptive response by the CYP system that usually involves synthesis of new enzyme protein, a process termed *enzyme induction*. The molecular basis for genetic regulation of constitutive and inducible expression of the major human hepatic P450, CYP3A4, has recently been determined.[68] Agents like rifampicin, a powerful inducer of CYP3A4, interact with the pregnane X-receptor (PXR), a member of the orphan nuclear receptor family of transcriptional regulators.[69] The activated PXR and the analogous constitutive androstane receptor (CAR) in turn bind to cognate nucleotide sequences upstream to the CYP3A4 structural gene within a "xenobiotic responsive enhancer module" (XREM).[68, 70] This interaction regulates the CYP3A4 promoter downstream and ultimately the transcription of CYP3A4 protein. Similar control mechanisms apply to several other CYP pathways, particularly those involved with bile acid synthesis, in which the nuclear receptors implicated include the farnesyl X-receptor (FXR).[68, 70]

Common examples of induction of microsomal enzymes by environmental compounds include the effect of smoking cigarettes and cannabis on CYP1A2[71] and of alcohol on CYP2E1 and possibly CYP3A4.[14, 72] Several drugs are potent inducers of CYP enzymes. Isoniazid induces CYP2E1, whereas phenobarbital and phenytoin increase the expression of multiple CYPs.[59] Rifampicin is a potent inducer of CYP3A4. So too is hypericum,[73] the active ingredient of St. John's wort, a herbal medication commonly used in Europe and elsewhere; rifampicin and hypericum exert the effect on CYP3A4 transcription by binding to and activating RXR.[73] Further descriptions of the regulation of hepatic drug-metabolizing enzymes have been published elsewhere.[58, 59] The implications for drug-induced liver disease are twofold. First, enzyme induction often involves more than the CYP system, possibly because of activation of the nuclear orphan receptor transcriptional regulators; such activation accounts for increases in serum alkaline phosphatase and gamma-glutamyl transpeptidase (GGTP) levels, which are part of "hepatic adaptation" to chronic drug ingestion. Second, the influence of one drug on expression and activity of drug-metabolizing enzymes can alter the metabolism of other agents. Such drug-drug interactions are important pharmacologically and may also be relevant to mechanisms of hepatotoxicity in drug-induced liver disease.

INHIBITION OF DRUG METABOLISM. Alternatively, some chemicals inhibit drug metabolism, as reviewed elsewhere.[58, 59] The contribution of this phenomenon to drug-induced liver disease is less clear, although it could be relevant to persons taking more than one medication. For example, competition for phase 2 pathways, such as glucuronidation and sulfation, may allow more unconjugated drugs to be presented to the CYP system; this mechanism appears to explain in part why agents like zidovudine and phenytoin lower the dose threshold for acetaminophen-induced hepatotoxicity.

Other Pathways of Drug Oxidation

In addition to the role of CYP enzymes of the smooth endoplasmic reticulum, electron transport systems of mitochondria may lead to the generation of tissue-damaging reactive intermediates during the metabolism of some drugs. These intermediates may include nitroradicals from nitrofuran derivatives (nitrofurantoin, cocaine),[44, 58] which in turn can lead to electron transfer by flavoprotein reductases into molecular oxygen to form superoxide and other ROS. Other compounds, including some anticancer drugs like doxorubicin (Adriamycin), and the imidazole antimicrobial agents also can participate in redox cycling reactions that generate ROS.

Phase 2 (Conjugation) Reactions

Phase 2 reactions involve formation of ester links to the parent compound or a drug metabolite. The responsible enzymes include glucuronosyl transferases, sulfatases, glutathione S-transferases, and acetyl and amino acid *N*-transferases. The resulting conjugates are highly water soluble and can be excreted readily in bile or urine. Conjugation reactions are impaired by depletion of cofactors (glucuronic acid, inorganic sulfate), and their relatively low capacity can restrict the rate of drug elimination when substrate concentrations exceed enzyme saturation. Reviews on phase 2 reactions are published elsewhere.[58, 74] In general, drug conjugates are nontoxic, and phase 2 reactions are considered to be detoxification reactions, but there are exceptions. For example, some glutathione conjugates can undergo cysteine S-conjugate β-lyase-mediated activation to highly reactive intermediates.[58] Little is known about the regulation of such enzymes and their potential significance for drug-induced liver disease.

Phase 3 Pathways of Drug Elimination from the Liver

The general importance of energy-dependent pathways by which drugs, drug metabolities, or their conjugates are excreted from the liver has only recently been appreciated. These pathways, now often referred to as phase 3 of hepatic drug elimination, involve the ATP-binding cassette (ABC) transport proteins, which derive the energy for their transport functions from the hydrolysis of ATP. ABC transport proteins are distributed widely in nature and include the cystic fibrosis transmembrane conductance regulator (CFTR) and the canalicular and intestinal copper transporters (see Chapters 52 and 67). The role of ABC transport proteins in secretion of bile is discussed in Chapter 54 and has been reviewed.[75, 76] Multidrug resistance protein (MDR, or mdr-1 in humans, formerly termed p-glycoprotein) is highly expressed on the apical (canalicular) membrane of hepatocytes, where it transports cationic drugs, particularly anticancer agents, into bile. Another family of ABC transporters, the multidrug resistance-related proteins (MRP), is also expressed in liver. At least two members of this family serve to excrete drug (and other) conjugates from hepatocytes; MRP-1 (and probably MRP-5) on the lateral surface facilitates passage of drug conjugate into the sinusoidal circulation, whereas MRP-2 is expressed on the canalicular membrane. Formerly known as the canalicular multipurpose organic anion transporter (cMOAT), this protein stimulates the energy-dependent pumping of endogenous conjugates (e.g., bilirubin diglucuronide, leukotriene-glutathionyl conjugates) and drug conjugates into bile. Regulation of the membrane expression and activity of these drug elimination pathways is complex and currently under intense study. The possibility that altered expression or impaired activity could predispose to drug accumulation, impairment of bile flow, or cholestatic liver injury has already been demonstrated for estrogens[77, 78] and may have much wider mechanistic importance for drug-induced liver disease.

Toxic Mechanisms of Liver Injury

Direct Hepatotoxins and Reactive Metabolites

Highly hepatotoxic chemicals directly produce irreversible lesions of key subcellular structures, particularly mitochondria and the plasma membrane. The damage arrests energy generation, dissipates ionic gradients, and disrupts the physical integrity of the cell. This type of lethal "king hit" does not apply to currently relevant hepatotoxins, most of which require *metabolic activation* to mediate damage to liver cells.

The types of chemically reactive species that can be formed by CYP-mediated drug oxidation include carbon-based radicals, nitroradicals, electrophilic oxymetabolites, and ROS. Much less commonly, secondary reactions to drug conjugates can produce chemically reactive intermediates. These *reactive metabolites* can interact with critical cellular target molecules, particularly those with nucleophilic substituents such as thiol-rich proteins and nucleic acids. They also can act as oxidizing species within the hepatocyte to establish a state of *oxidative stress,* an imbalance between pro-oxidants and antioxidants, with the former predominating.[63] Alternatively, reactive metabolites bind irreversibly to macromolecules, particularly proteins and lipids. Such *covalent binding* may produce injury by inactivating key enzymes or by forming protein-drug adducts that are potential targets for immune-mediated liver injury.

Oxidative Stress and the Glutathione System

The liver is exposed to oxidative stress by the propensity of hepatocytes to activate oxygen, both in mitochondrial and microsomal electron transport systems, and by NADPH-oxidase–catalyzed formation of ROS and nitroradicals in Kupffer cells, endothelial cells, and stimulated polymorphonuclear leukocytes and macrophages. To combat oxidative stress, the liver is well-endowed with antioxidant mechanisms. These mechanisms include micronutrients, such as vitamin E and vitamin C, thiol-rich proteins, metal-sequestering proteins (e.g., ferritin), and enzymes that metabolize reactive metabolites (e.g., epoxide hydrolases), ROS (e.g., catalase, superoxide dismutase), and lipid peroxides (e.g., glutathione peroxidases). By far the most important antioxidant in the mammalian liver is the *glutathione* (L-gamma-glutamyl-L-cysteine-glycine) *system,* as reviewed elsewhere.[44, 79, 80]

Glutathione is found in high concentrations (5 to 10 mmol/L) in hepatocytes, the exclusive site of glutathione synthesis. Hepatic levels of glutathione can be increased by enhancing its synthesis through the supply of cysteine; this mechanism is the cornerstone of thiol antidote therapy for acetaminophen poisoning (see later). Glutathione is a critical cofactor for several antioxidant pathways, including thiol/disulfide exchange reactions and a cofactor for *glutathione peroxidase*. Glutathione peroxidase has a higher affinity for hydrogen peroxide than does catalase and disposes of organic peroxides, free radicals, and electrophilic drug metabolites. Reduced glutathione is a cofactor for conjugation reactions catalyzed by the *glutathione S-transferases*. Other reactions proceed nonenzymatically; the products include glutathione/protein mixed disulfides and oxidized glutathione. The latter can be converted back to reduced glutathione by proton donation catalyzed by *glutathione reductase*.

Normally, most glutathione within the hepatocyte is in the reduced state, indicating the importance of this pathway for maintenance of the redox capacity of the cell. Formation of NADPH, an essential cofactor for glutathione reductase, requires ATP, thereby illustrating an *essential link between the energy-generating capacity of the liver and its ability to withstand oxidative stress*.[80] There is also compartmentalization of glutathione within the hepatocyte, with highest concentrations in the cytosol. It is essential that levels of glutathione are adequate within mitochondria, where ROS are constantly being formed as a minor by-product of oxidative respiration. Mitochondrial glutathione is maintained by active uptake from the cytosol; this transport system is altered by chronic ethanol exposure and is therefore another potential target of drug toxicity.[44]

Biochemical Mechanisms of Cellular Injury

Mechanisms once thought to be central to hepatotoxicity, such as covalent binding to cellular enzymes and peroxidation of membrane lipids, are no longer regarded as exclusive pathways of cellular damage. Oxidation of proteins, phospholipid fatty acyl side chains, and nucleosides appears to be common. Secondary reactions also may play a role; these reactions include post-translational modification of proteins via mono (ADP)-ribosylation or protease activation, cleavage of DNA by activation of endogenous endonucleases, and disruption of lipid membranes by activated phospholipases. Some of these catabolic reactions could be set in motion by a rise in cytosolic ionic calcium concentration $[Ca^{2+}]_i$, as a result of increased Ca^{2+} entry or release from internal stores like the endoplasmic reticulum and mitochondria (these processes have been reviewed elsewhere).[2, 14] However, the concept that hepatotoxic chemicals cause hepatocyte cell death by a *biochemical final common pathway* (e.g., activation of catalytic enzymes by a rise in $[Ca^{2+}]_i$) has proved inadequate to explain the diverse processes that can result in lethal hepatocellular injury. Rather, a variety of processes can damage key organelles, thereby initiating either programmed cell death (apoptosis), necrosis, or both.

Types of Cell Death

APOPTOSIS. Apoptosis is an energy dependent, genetically programmed form of cell death that typically results in controlled deletion of individual cells. In addition to its major roles in developmental biology, tissue regulation, and carcinogenesis, apoptosis is important in toxic, viral, and immune-mediated liver injury.[81, 82] The ultrastructural features of apoptosis are cell and nuclear shrinkage, condensation and margination of nuclear chromatin, plasma membrane blebbing, and ultimately fragmentation of the cell into membrane-bound bodies that contain intact mitochondria and other organelles. Engulfment of these *apoptotic bodies* by surrounding epithelial and mesenchymal cells conserves cell fragments that contain nucleic acid and intact mitochondria. These fragments can then be digested by lysosomes and recycled without release of bioactive substances. As a consequence, apoptosis in its purest form does not incite an inflammatory tissue reaction.

The role of apoptosis in toxic liver injury has been reviewed elsewhere.[44, 81, 82] Hepatocytes undergo apoptosis when pro-apoptotic intracellular signaling pathways are activated, either because of toxic biochemical processes within the cell or because cell surface receptors are activated to transduce cell death signals. Such pro-apoptotic receptors include Fas, tumor necrosis factor receptor (TNFR), and other members of the TNFR superfamily. The toxic processes that can trigger intracellular pro-apoptotic pathways include oxidative stress and mitochondrial injury.[44, 80, 82] In addition to model hepatotoxins, like menadione (a redox cycling quinone), and hydrogen peroxide, drugs known to be converted into pro-oxidant reactive metabolites (e.g., acetaminophen, plant diterpenoids) have now been shown to set in motion the following sequence: CYP-mediated metabolism to form reactive metabolites; glutathione depletion; mitochondrial injury with release of cytochrome c and operation of the mitochondrial membrane permeability transition; caspase activation; apoptosis.[61, 62, 83]

The operation of intracellular processes and activation of pro-apoptotic receptors are not mutually exclusive pathways of cell death in toxic liver injury.[44] In fact, there are several reasons why drug toxicity could predispose the injured hepatocyte to apoptosis mediated by TNFR or Fas-operated pathways. Further details of apoptosis-initiating pathways, the role of caspases in executing cell death, and the targets of cell execution are of broad relevance in several areas of hepatology and are well discussed elsewhere.[81–83]

NECROSIS. In contrast to apoptosis, necrosis is a relatively uncontrolled process. It can result from extensive damage to the plasma membrane with disturbance of ion transport, dissolution of membrane potential, cell swelling, and eventually rupture of the cell. Drug-induced injury to the mitochondrion can impair energy generation, whereas membrane permeability transition can release stored Ca^{2+} into the cytosol and perturb other ionic gradients. Mitochondrial enzymes appear to be a particular target of NAPQI, the reactive metabolite of acetaminophen. Reye's syndrome–like drug toxicity also may result from injury to the mitochondrion (e.g., caused by tetracycline, aspirin [in febrile children], valproic acid, and some nucleoside analogues—fialuridine, didanosine, zidovudine, zalcitabine).[84] Mitochondrial injury can result in cell death by either apoptosis or necrosis;[44] determination of the type of cell death pathway may depend primarily on the energy state of the cell as well as the rapidity and severity of the injury process. In the presence of ATP, cell death can proceed by apoptosis, but when mitochondria are de-energized, the mechanism of cell death is necrosis. This apparent dichotomy between cell death processes is probably artificial, and apoptosis and necrosis more likely represent the ends of a spectrum of overlapping morphologic and mechanistic cell death processes.[44, 85]

One important way in which necrosis differs from apoptosis is that uncontrolled dissolution of the cell liberates macromolecular breakdown products, including lipid peroxides, aldehydes, and eicosanoids. These products act as *chemoattractants for circulating leukocytes,* which enjoin an inflammatory response in the hepatic parenchyma. Even before cell death occurs, oxidative stress produced during drug toxicity can up-regulate *adhesion molecules and chemokines* that are expressed or secreted by endothelial cells.[83] These processes contribute to recruitment of cells to the hepatic inflammatory response, which is prominent in some types of drug-induced liver disease. Lymphocytes and macrophages also may be attracted to the liver as part of a cell-mediated hypersensitivity reaction.

ROLE OF HEPATIC NONPARENCHYMAL CELLS. In addition to migratory cells, activation of nonparenchymal liver cell types plays an important role in drug- and toxin-induced liver injury.[86]

Kupffer cells function as resident macrophages and antigen-presenting cells. They may be activated to release ROS, nitroradicals, leukotrienes, and proteases. Some of the toxic effects of activated Kupffer cells, as well as of recruited leukocytes, may be mediated by *release of cytokines,* such as TNF, which under some circumstances that are present during toxic liver injury can induce cell death in hepatocytes by apoptosis or necrosis.[85]

Endothelial cells of the hepatic sinusoid or terminal hepatic veins are vulnerable to injury by some hepatotoxins because of their low glutathione content. One example is the pyrrolizidine alkaloids, which are an important cause of hepatic veno-occlusive disease.[87] Other types of drug-induced vascular injury also may be caused primarily by involvement of the sinusoidal endothelial cells.

Hepatic *stellate cells* (formerly termed fat-storing or Ito cells) are the principal liver cell type involved in matrix deposition and hepatic fibrosis. Stellate cells are activated in methotrexate-induced hepatic fibrosis, and the possibility that vitamin A, drugs, or drug metabolites can transform stellate cells into collagen-synthesizing myofibroblasts is of considerable interest.

Immunologic Mechanisms

In addition to the activation of inflammatory processes in the liver by toxic mechanisms, as just described, immunologic mechanisms could account for certain aspects of idiosyncratic adverse drug reactions. The most convincing evidence for a drug allergy includes: (1) delayed onset after initial exposure and accelerated onset after rechallenge, (2) hepatic inflammatory infiltrates with eosinophilia, and (3) fever, rash, lymphadenopathy, and involvement of other organs. In some types of drug hepatitis, the liver is clearly implicated as part of a systemic hypersensitivity reaction; sulfonamides, phenytoin, nitrofurantoin, and minocycline are examples of causative agents. It is unclear why the liver is a predominant site of injury in some persons, whereas different organs are involved in others. In many other idiosyncratic drug reactions, the liver is the only organ implicated (e.g., halothane, diclofenac, isoniazid).

One possible immunopathogenic mechanism for drug-induced liver disease is the *altered antigen concept,* in which an initial interaction between drug metabolites and cellular proteins results in the formation of *neoantigens or drug/protein adducts.* This mechanism is typified by the formation of trifluoroacetylated (TFA) adducts after exposure to halothane or other haloalkane anesthetics. For these adducts to initiate tissue-damaging immune responses, (1) they should be presented in an immunogenic form (e.g., by Kupffer cells, in association with mixed histocompatibility (MHC) molecules), (2) appropriately responsive $CD4^+$ T cells must be present to provide help to induce an immune response, and (3) the drug-derived antigen, together with a class II MHC molecule, must be expressed on the target cells in order to attract $CD8^+$ (cytotoxic) T cells. That bile duct epithelial cells are more likely than hepatocytes to express class II MHC antigens may explain why these cells are possible targets in drug-induced cholestatic hepatitis.

Although antibodies directed against TFA-protein adducts circulate in the majority of patients after recovery from halothane-induced liver injury,[88] the specificity and pathogenicity of these antibodies remain in doubt. Another way in which circulating drug-induced antibodies could result in immune-mediated lysis of hepatocytes is through molecular mimicry with host enzymes.[89] There is also experimental evidence, in the case of diclofenac, for antibody-dependent cell-mediated immunity as a potential mechanism for drug-induced liver disease.[90]

A second type of immunopathogenic mechanism that could operate in some types of drug-induced liver disease is dysregulation of the immune system, termed *drug-induced autoimmunity.* This mechanism can lead to formation of drug-induced autoantibodies (e.g., liver-kidney microsomal [LKM] antibodies) directed against microsomal enzymes. For tienilic acid, CYP2C9 is the target of LKM, whereas the autoantibodies that circulate after halothane hepatitis are directed at CYP2E1. Nontissue-specific autoantibodies, such as antinuclear and smooth muscle antibodies, may be present in nitrofurantoin, methyldopa, or minocycline hepatitis. Like spontaneous autoimmunity, drug-induced autoimmunity may involve genetic predisposition through anomalies of immune tolerance. Additional information on immune-mediated drug injury is provided in an authoritative review.[91]

CLINICOPATHOLOGIC FEATURES OF DRUG-INDUCED LIVER DISEASE

Classification

Hepatic drug reactions mimic all known liver diseases, but classification is often difficult because of overlap among categories. Some drugs may be associated with more than one syndrome, and there may be discordance between the clinical and laboratory features of liver disease and the hepatic histology. Thus, although recognition of specific patterns or syndromes is a clue to the diagnosis of drug-induced liver disease, the chronologic relationship between drug administration and liver injury is a more important clue.

Drugs are often divided into *dose-dependent,* or *predictable, hepatotoxins* and *dose-independent,* or *unpredictable (idiosyncratic), hepatotoxins.* Dose-dependent hepatotoxins generally require metabolic activation to toxic metabolites

Table 73–2 | **Clinicopathologic Classification of Drug-Induced Liver Disease**

CATEGORY	DESCRIPTION	EXAMPLES
Hepatic adaptation	No symptoms; raised GGTP and AP (occasionally ALT)	Phenytoin, warfarin
	Hyperbilirubinemia	Rifampicin, flavaspidic acid
Dose-dependent hepatotoxicity	Symptoms of hepatitis; zonal, bridging, and massive necrosis; ALT > fivefold increased, often >2000 U/L	Acetaminophen, nicotinic acid, amodiaquine, hycanthone
Other cytopathic, acute steatosis	Microvesicular steatosis, diffuse or zonal; partially dose-dependent, severe liver injury, features of mitochondrial toxicity (lactic acidosis)	Valproic acid, didanosine, HAART, fialuridine, L-asparaginase, some herbal medicines
Acute hepatitis	Symptoms of hepatitis; focal, bridging, and massive necrosis; ALT > fivefold increased; extrahepatic features of drug allergy in some cases	Isoniazid, dantrolene, nitrofurantoin, halothane, sulfonamides, phenytoin, disulfiram, acebutolol, etretinate, ketoconazole, terbinafine, troglitazone
Chronic hepatitis	Duration >3 mo; interface hepatitis, bridging necrosis, fibrosis, cirrhosis; clinical and laboratory features of chronic liver disease; autoantibodies in some types of reaction (see Table 73–6)	Nitrofurantoin, etretinate, diclofenac, minocycline, trazadone (see also Table 73–6)
Granulomatous hepatitis	Hepatic granulomas with varying hepatitis and cholestasis; raised ALT, AP, GGTP	Allopurinol, carbamazepine, hydralazine, quinidine, quinine (see also Table 73–5)
Cholestasis without hepatitis	Cholestasis, no inflammation; AP > twofold normal	Oral contraceptives, androgens
Cholestatic hepatitis	Cholestasis with inflammation; symptoms of hepatitis; raised ALT and AP.	Chlorpromazine, tricyclic antidepressants, erythromycins, amoxicillin/clavulanic acid
Cholestasis with bile duct injury	Bile duct lesions and cholestatic hepatitis; clinical features of cholangitis	Chlorpromazine, flucloxacillin, dextropropoxyphene
Chronic cholestasis	Cholestasis present >3 mo	Chlorpromazine, flucloxacillin, trimethoprim-sulfamethoxazole
Vanishing bile duct syndrome	Paucity of small bile ducts; resembles primary biliary cirrhosis but AMA negative	
Sclerosing cholangitis	Strictures of large bile ducts	Intra-arterial floxuridine, intralesional scolicidals
Steatohepatitis	Steatosis, focal necrosis, Mallory's hyaline, pericellular fibrosis, cirrhosis; chronic liver disease, portal hypertension	Perhexiline, amiodarone
Vascular disorders	Many—see Table 73–9	See Table 73–9
Tumors	Many—see Table 73–10	See Table 73–10

ALT, alanine aminotransferase; AMA, antimitochondrial antibody; AP, alkaline phosphatase; GGTP, gamma-glutamyl transpeptidase; HAART, highly active antiretroviral therapy.

and interfere with subcellular organelles and processes like mitochondria or canalicular bile secretion.[76, 77] Liver injury produced by dose-dependent hepatotoxins usually occurs after a short latent period (hours), is characterized by zonal necrosis or microvesicular steatosis, and can be reproduced in other species. In contrast, idiosyncratic hepatotoxins cause a wide range of histologic changes, do not reliably cause injury in other species, and exhibit a variable latent period to onset of injury. The distinction between dose-dependent and idiosyncratic hepatotoxins is blurred by agents like dantrolene, tacrine, perhexiline, flucloxacillin, cyclophosphamide, nucleoside analogues, anticancer drugs, and cyclosporine. Liver injury caused by each of these drugs is partly dose dependent, but reactions occur in only a small proportion of exposed persons.

Two general types of mechanisms have been proposed to account for idiosyncratic hepatotoxicity—metabolic idiosyncrasy and immunoallergy. *Metabolic idiosyncrasy* refers to the susceptibility of rare individuals to hepatotoxicity from a drug that, in conventional doses, is usually safe. Such susceptibility may be the result of genetic or acquired differences in drug metabolism, canalicular secretion, mitochondrial defects, or cell death receptor signaling. *Immunoallergy* indicates operation of the immune system in mediating the response to a drug. These two mechanisms may be interrelated; the resulting patterns of liver disease are discussed in more detail later.

To the clinician, a more useful classification of drug toxicity is one based on clinical, laboratory, and histologic features, as summarized in Table 73–2. This classification provides a framework for discussing drug-related conditions in relation to other hepatobiliary disorders but is imperfect because the clinical and pathologic features are not always congruent. There is also much overlap among categories, particularly in the spectrum from severe necrosis (which may result from dose-dependent or idiosyncratic hepatotoxicity) to focal necrosis with lobular inflammation (*hepatitis*) to cholestasis. Some researchers include a further category of *mixed cholestatic/hepatocellular reactions,* but many drugs produce a spectrum of syndromes from hepatitis to cholestasis, whereas granulomatous hepatitis also is associated with liver test abnormalities that suggest hepatitis, cholestasis, or both.

Drugs can alter liver biochemical tests without causing

significant liver injury. Such *adaptive responses* include hyperbilirubinemia associated with drugs like rifampicin and flavaspidic acid (male fern extract), and raised serum GGTP and alkaline phosphatase levels associated with agents like phenytoin and warfarin.[2, 3] The latter effect is probably attributable to microsomal enzyme induction. Conversely, liver tumors or hepatic fibrosis may develop insidiously without significant abnormalities of liver tests, the former in association with sex steroids or vinyl chloride monomer and the latter with methotrexate, arsenic, and hypervitaminosis A.

The duration of the disorder is another dimension that must be considered in classifying drug-induced liver diseases. In general, chronic liver disease is less commonly attributable to drugs and toxins, although not to consider this possibility can lead to missed diagnosis.[15, 37] An important exception is vascular disorders, for which drugs and toxins are the most important cause (see later). Drugs also have been associated with chronic cholestasis, chronic hepatitis, NASH, hepatic fibrosis, cirrhosis, and benign and malignant liver tumors.

Histopathology

Although there are no pathognomic features of drug-induced liver disease, certain patterns suggest a drug etiology. These features include zonal necrosis or microvesicular steatosis (which accompanies mitochondrial injury) and mixed histologic features of hepatocellular necrosis and cholestasis. Necrotic lesions that are disproportionately severe compared with the clinical picture indicate a possible drug cause. Destructive bile duct lesions, prominent neutrophils, and eosinophils may be suggestive of drug-induced cholestatic hepatitis. Hepatic granulomas are another common type of hepatic drug reaction. In cases of hepatic fibrosis or liver tumors, there are no specific clues to a drug cause, although sex steroids increase the vascularity of hepatic tumors and are frequently associated with sinusoidal dilatation or peliosis hepatis. Some drugs implicated as causing steatohepatitis are associated with more severe forms that closely resemble alcoholic hepatitis, whereas with other drugs the lesions appear identical to those found in NASH attributable to the insulin resistance syndrome. Hall,[92] Lee,[8] and Zimmerman[3] provide detailed discussions of this topic in well-illustrated reviews. Indications for liver biopsy are summarized in the section "A Practical Approach to Diagnosis."

Clinical Features

The history and physical examination can provide important clues to the diagnosis of hepatic drug reactions. The most important is the *temporal pattern of disease evolution* in relation to exposure to drugs or toxins. The identification of *specific risk factors for hepatotoxicity* (e.g., chronic excessive alcohol intake in a person taking acetaminophen) and the presence of *systemic features of drug hypersensitivity* may indicate the correct diagnosis. Such features include fever, rash, mucositis, eosinophilia, lymphadenopathy, mononucleosis-like syndrome, bone marrow suppression, vasculitis, renal failure, pneumonitis, and pancreatitis.

For idiosyncratic reactions, there is a *latent period* between the commencement of drug intake and onset of clinical and laboratory abnormalities. This period is commonly 2 to 8 weeks for immunoallergic types of drug hepatitis but often 6 to 20 weeks or longer for agents like isoniazid and dantrolene. Occasionally, liver injury may become evident after discontinuation of the causative agent; for oxypenicillins and amoxicillin/clavulanate, the delay may be as long as 2 weeks after the end of therapy. In other cases, hepatotoxicity is rare after the first exposure but increasingly frequent and more severe after subsequent courses. Typical examples include halothane, nitrofurantoin, and dacarbazine. A history of previous reaction to the drug in question *(inadvertent rechallenge)* may therefore be the key to diagnosis of drug-induced liver disease.

Another aspect of the temporal relationship between drug ingestion and hepatotoxicity is the response to discontinuation of the drug, or *dechallenge*. Dechallenge should be accompanied by discernible and progressive improvement within days or weeks of stopping the incriminated agent. Exceptions include ketoconazole, troglitazone, coumarol, etretinate, and amiodarone; with these agents, reactions may be severe, and clinical recovery may be delayed for months. However, although some types of drug-induced cholestasis also can be prolonged, failure of jaundice to resolve in suspected drug reactions is most often indicative of an alternative diagnosis. Rarely (see later), *deliberate rechallenge* may be used to confirm the diagnosis of drug-induced liver disease or to prove the involvement of one particular agent when the patient has been exposed to several drugs.

A Practical Approach to Diagnosis

Because there are no specific diagnostic tests, diagnosis requires clinical suspicion, a careful drug history, consideration of the temporal relationships between drug ingestion and liver disease, and exclusion of other disorders. The objective weighing of evidence for and against individual agents, *causality assessment,* is a probabilistic form of diagnosis. Several clinical scales have been described to incorporate and give weight to various features,[93, 94] and although the performance of these scales is modest, they serve as a framework for aspects to be addressed in cases of suspected hepatic adverse drug reactions in order to improve consistency of diagnosis.[15, 95] In some cases, a liver biopsy may be indicated to exclude other diseases and to provide further clues to a drug etiology. In the future, in vitro tests may provide confirmatory evidence for particular drugs,[88, 94] but rechallenge remains the gold standard test for drug-induced liver disease.

PHYSICIAN AWARENESS. Physician awareness is crucial for the diagnosis of drug-induced liver disease. The sources of potential hepatotoxins include not only prescribed medications, but also over-the-counter drugs, complementary and alternative medicines (CAM) (discussed later), substances taken for recreational use (e.g., ecstasy) or self-poisoning, and environmental contaminants in food and water supplies and in the home, workplace, and community. Unfortunately, patients and physicians do not always heed early nonspecific symptoms associated with reactions to hepatotoxic drugs. Isoniazid is a classic example; preventable deaths from liver failure still occur more than 30 years after the recognition that isoniziad can cause drug hepatitis. Continuing education and availability of information about potentially hepatotoxic drugs are important issues, and there is a professional and legal obligation for physicians to inform patients carefully about possible adverse drug reactions.

Particularly in cases of obscure or poorly explained liver disease, possible drug toxicity should be considered. Relevant circumstances include mixed or atypical patterns of cholestasis and hepatitis; cases of cholestasis in which common causes have been excluded, particularly in elderly patients; and histologic features that suggest a drug etiology. It is then mandatory to *address the drug history as a special investigation,* with attention paid to separate sources of information (household members, primary care providers), examination of household drug cupboard contents, and consideration of nonprescribed medications or environment toxins.

EXCLUSION OF OTHER DISEASES. Exclusion of other diseases is essential before ascribing a form of hepatobiliary disease to a drug. For acute and chronic hepatocellular reactions, viral and autoimmune causes of hepatitis and vascular and metabolic disorders must be considered.[2, 8] In one study,[96] 60% of cases reported as drug-related syndromes were found later to be associated with hepatitis C. On the other hand, some types of drug-induced chronic hepatitis are associated with autoantibodies, thereby superficially resembling autoimmune hepatitis. An approach to the correct diagnosis is described later (see "Nitrofurantoin"). Drug-induced cholestasis should be considered when dilation of the common bile duct has been excluded by imaging. The potential interactions between drugs and NASH are more complex, as detailed in a later section.

EXTRAHEPATIC FEATURES. Extrahepatic features such as skin rash, eosinophilia, and involvement of other organs are relatively specific for adverse drug reactions. However, their *absence* is not helpful because they are present in only a minority of cases. *Specific diagnostic tests* for individual drug-induced liver diseases have been described[88, 97] but are not yet generally accepted or widely available. In the case of dose-dependent hepatotoxins, *blood levels* may be helpful; acetaminophen and aspirin are examples.

CHRONOLOGIC RELATIONSHIPS. For most drugs, the chronologic relationships among drug ingestion, onset, and resolution of liver injury remain the most important consideration in diagnosis.[15, 93, 98, 99] The criteria for *temporal eligibility* include relationship to onset, course of the reaction after discontinuation of the drug, and response to readministration of the drug.[98] *Deliberate rechallenge* is rarely indicated for logistic and ethical reasons because it can be hazardous, but inadvertent rechallenge may have occurred. It is regarded as positive if the serum alaninine aminotransferase (ALT) or alkaline phosphatase level is increased at least twofold.[98] Deliberate rechallenge may be considered when there is a need to ascertain whether a drug that is important for an individual patient is responsible for hepatotoxicity (e.g., amiodarone for refractory ventricular tachycardia). In other cases, it may be desirable to document the propensity of newer agents, hitherto unrecognized as hepatotoxins, to cause liver injury. Written informed consent is required for such deliberate rechallenge.

WHICH DRUG? New and nonproprietary compounds should arouse particular suspicion. For patients taking multiple drugs, the agent most likely responsible is the one started most recently before the onset of liver injury. If that agent is unlikely to be the culprit and another well-known hepatotoxin is being taken, the latter is more likely. When possible, the most likely hepatotoxin or all therapeutic agents should be discontinued. If the patient improves, the drugs that are unlikely to be responsible can be carefully reintroduced.

Drug-Induced Liver Injury in Patients with Viral Hepatitis

Patients with chronic hepatitis B or C may be at higher risk of liver injury from antituberculosis chemotherapy, ibuprofen, and possibly other NSAIDs.[52, 54, 55] A more common clinical problem is the patient who at a routine clinic visit has a serum ALT value of greater than 300 U/L, with previous values of less than 150 U/L. Particularly with hepatitis C, this rise in ALT is more likely to be the result of drug toxicity than a spontaneous change in the activity of the disease, and with ALT values of greater 1000 U/L, drugs are almost always the cause. The most commonly implicated agents are acetaminophen taken in moderate doses under conditions of increased risk (fasting, alcohol excess, other medication; see later), or CAM, typically Chinese herbal medicines. Clinical suspicion is essential for recognizing the drug cause of liver injury so that appropriate advice can be given; blood levels of acetaminophen also may be useful in difficult cases, but values can be difficult to interpret in the context of regular ingestion, as opposed to a single episode of self-poisoning (see later).

PREVENTION AND MANAGEMENT

With the exception of acetaminophen hepatotoxicity (discussed later), there is little effective treatment for drug-induced liver disease. Special emphasis is therefore placed on *prevention* and *early detection* of liver injury, as well as on *prompt withdrawal* of the offending agent. Safe use of self-medication with agents like acetaminophen and CAM is an important issue that will be discussed in more detail in later sections. Clear and open communication between physicians and their patients and appropriate recommendations about dose limitations would prevent many instances of liver injury from these agents.

The majority of drugs associated with drug-induced liver disease are idiosyncratic hepatotoxins. Thus, liver injury occurs rarely. The overall frequency of adverse hepatic reactions can be minimized only through avoidance of overuse of these drugs; antibiotics such as amoxicillin/clavulanic acid and flucloxacillin are pertinent examples. Similarly, polypharmacy should be avoided where possible. The rarity of adverse drug reactions also means that the hepatotoxic potential of new agents may not be recognized until after their introduction.[100] Thus, all physicians share the responsibility to report suspected adverse effects to monitoring agencies during postmarketing surveillance of new drugs.

For dose-dependent hepatotoxins, prevention depends on adherence to dosage guidelines or use of blood levels. This approach has virtually abolished some forms of drug-induced liver injury, like tetracycline-induced fatty liver, aspirin hepatitis, and methotrexate-induced hepatic fibrosis. In cases with specific risk factors, strategies to avoid toxicity are essential (e.g., avoidance of the use of valproic acid with other drugs in the very young, avoidance of the use of methotrexate in persons who consume alcohol to excess). Likewise, moderate acetaminophen dosing is contraindicated in heavy drinkers and after fasting,[45] and administration of halothane should not be repeated within 28 days or in persons suspected of previous sensitivity to haloalkane anesthetics.

Early detection is also critical. Patients should be warned to report any untoward symptoms, particularly unexplained nausea, malaise, right upper quadrant abdominal pain, lethargy, or fever. These nonspecific features may represent the prodrome of drug-induced hepatitis. They are an indication to perform liver tests and, if the results suggest liver injury, to stop treatment.

A more difficult issue is protocol screening with liver tests.[100–102] Although often recommended by investigators and drug manufacturers, the efficiency and cost-effectiveness are unknown. It has been shown that the onset of liver injury is often rapid, rendering monthly or even second weekly screening futile; moreover, 7.5% of persons receiving placebo in clinical trials have persistently raised serum ALT levels.[102] If liver tests are monitored, the level of abnormality at which drugs should be discontinued is uncertain.[100] A classic example is isoniazid, which causes some liver test abnormality in 30% of exposed subjects. Generally, it is recommended that the drug be stopped if serum ALT values exceed 250 U/L or more than five times the upper limit of normal, but the presence of abnormalities in serum bilirubin or albumin concentrations or prothrombin time provides a clearer indication to stop therapy. Conversely, a rise in GGTP levels or minor elevation in alkaline phosphatase does not usually indicate liver injury. I do not routinely recommend protocol screening, but it could be useful for agents such as valproic acid, isoniazid, pyrazinamide, ketoconazole, dantrolene, tacrine, thioridazone antidiabetics, and synthetic retinoids, either because the onset of liver injury may be delayed and gradual in some cases or to underscore the hepatotoxic potential of particular drugs in the minds of patients and physicians. Liver biopsy has a special place in the assessment of methotrexate and hepatic fibrosis (see later).

Occupational exposure to hepatotoxic chemicals raises special issues of prevention. These issues include the avoidance of highly toxic solvents, most of which have been abandoned; adequate ventilation; and use of masks and protective clothing. In some cases, liver tests are performed routinely, but abnormalities are more likely to reflect diseases such as chronic hepatitis C, alcoholism, and NASH than toxic liver injury. In the case of vinyl chloride exposure, periodic physical examination (for hepatomegaly) and hepatic imaging with ultrasonography may be useful.

Active management might include removal of the drug and the administration of antidotes and anti-inflammatory and cytoprotective agents. In practice, management is usually confined to *discontinuation of hepatotoxic drugs*. Failure to discontinue a drug that is the cause of liver injury is the single most important factor leading to poor outcomes, such as acute liver failure and chronic liver disease.[37] For ingested toxins like metals, poisonous mushrooms, and acetaminophen, *removal of unabsorbed drug* through the aspiration of stomach contents may be appropriate. Methods to remove absorbed hepatotoxins, such as hemodialysis through charcoal columns and forced diuresis, are not effective for hepatotoxins. For chlordecone, an organochlorine insecticide that is lipid soluble and excreted in bile, cholestyramine enhances bodily removal by interrupting the enterohepatic cycle.[103] Thiol replacement therapy, usually *N*-acetylcysteine (NAC), is indicated as an antidote for acetaminophen poisoning. Whether NAC or other antioxidants have a role in other types of acute hepatotoxicity is unclear, but the flavonoid silybin is traditionally used for *Amanita phalloides* toxicity,[104] and tocopherol analogues show promise in experimental hepatotoxicity.

Beyond discontinuation of the offending agent, the management of drug hepatitis and cholestasis is symptomatic and supportive. In cases of acute liver failure, hepatic transplantation should be considered[6] (See Chapters 80 and 83). Ursodeoxycholic acid has some promise for chronic cholestasis and pruritus, as discussed later.[14] Glucocorticoids have little role in the management of drug-induced cholestasis or hepatitis and are ineffective in chlorpromazine-, methyldopa-, and isoniazid-induced hepatitis and in drug-induced fulminant hepatic failure. Case reports attest to their occasional effectiveness in protracted cases of hepatitis caused by etretinate, allopurinol, diclofenac, or ketoconazole.[2] Glucocorticoids should be reserved for atypical and refractory cases, particularly those with vasculitis. There is no clinical evidence of the effectiveness of putative hepatoprotective agents, such as prostaglandin analogues.

DOSE-DEPENDENT HEPATOTOXICITY

The number of clinically important dose-dependent hepatotoxins has diminished; examples include acetaminophen, some herbal medicines, plant and fungal toxins, amodiaquine, hycanthone, vitamin A, methotrexate, cyclophosphamide, anticancer drugs, carbon tetrachloride, phosphorus, and metals (especially iron, copper, and mercury). Acetaminophen is by far the most important of these agents; herbal medicines (as part of CAM), vitamin A, and methotrexate are discussed in later sections.

Acetaminophen

General Nature, Frequency, and Predisposing Factors

Acetaminophen (paracetamol) is a widely used analgesic that is available without prescription. It is very safe when taken in the recommended therapeutic dose of 1 to 4 g daily, but hepatotoxicity produced by *self-poisoning with acetaminophen* has been recognized since the 1960s. Despite the effectiveness of thiol-based antidotes, acetaminophen remains the most common cause of drug-induced liver injury in most countries and an important cause of acute liver failure.[5, 104–111] Parasuicide and suicide are the usual reasons for overdose;[105, 110, 111] but many cases of poisoning arise through what Zimmerman and Maddrey termed *therapeutic misadventure*.[109] This occurrence is especially common in persons who habitually drink alcohol to excess[109, 112] and has also been recognized after daily ingestion of *moderate therapeutic doses (10 to 20 g over 3 days) of acetaminophen in subjects who are fasting*[45] or taking drugs that interact with the metabolism of acetaminophen.[109, 113]

Single ingestions of acetaminophen exceeding 7 to 10 g (150 mg/kg body weight in children) may cause liver injury, although this outcome is not inevitable. Severe liver injury (serum ALT > 1000 U/L) or fatal cases usually involve doses of at least 15 to 25 g, but interindividual variability is such that survival is possible even after ingestion of massive doses (>50 g).[114] Indeed, among untreated subjects with acetaminophen overdose, severe liver injury occurred in only 20%, and among those with severe liver injury the mortality was 20%.[114] Conversely, among heavy drinkers, daily doses of 2 to 6 g have been associated with fatal hepatotoxicity.[109, 112]

The risk factors for acetaminophen-induced hepatotoxicity are summarized in Table 73–3. Children are relatively resistant to acetaminophen-induced hepatotoxicity,[115] but therapeutic misadventure after multiple dosing, especially exceeding weight-based recommendations, has a high mortality.[116] Relative resistance in children may result from a tendency to ingest smaller doses, vomiting, or biologic resistance. Conversely, the presence of underlying liver disease does not predispose to acetaminophen hepatotoxicity.[56] Self-poisoning with acetaminophen is more common in young women, but fatalities are more frequent in men, possibly because of alcoholism and late presentation.[105, 107, 109] Late presentation is a critical factor in mortality because thiol therapy given within 12 hours of acetaminophen poisoning virtually abolishes significant liver injury[105–111]; therapeutic misadventure is also associated with a worse outcome.[110, 111] Concomitant use of agents such as phenobarbital, phenytoin, isoniazid,[113, 117] and zidovudine is another risk factor for acetaminophen hepatotoxicity. These drugs may promote the oxidative metabolism of acetaminophen to NAPQI by inducing CYP2E1 (for isoniazid) or CYP3A4 (for phenytoin) or by competing with glucuronidation pathways (for zidovudine).[14] Alcohol and fasting have dual effects by enhancing expression of CYP2E1 and depleting hepatic glutathione. Fasting also may impair acetaminophen conjugation through both the glucuronidation and sulfation pathways.[45]

Table 73–3 | **Risk Factors for Acetaminophen-Induced Hepatotoxicity**

FACTOR	RELEVANCE
Age	Children may be more resistant than adults
Dose	Minimal hepatotoxic dose 7.5 g in adults; >150 mg/kg body weight in children Severe toxicity possible if dose is >15 g
Blood level	Influenced by dose, time after ingestion, gastric emptying Best indicator of risk of hepatotoxicity (see text and Fig. 73–1)
Chronic excessive alcohol ingestion	Toxic dose threshold lowered; worsens prognosis (also related to late presentation); nephrotoxicity common
Fasting	Toxic dose threshold lowered—therapeutic misadventure (see text)
Concomitant medication	Toxic dose threshold lowered—therapeutic misadventure; worsens prognosis—e.g., isoniazid, phenytoin, zidovudine
Time of presentation	Late presentation or treatment (>16 hr) predicates worse outcome

Acetaminophen hepatotoxicity produces zone 3 necrosis, with extension into bridging (submassive) or panacinar (massive) necrosis in severe cases.[92] Inflammation is minimal, and recovery is associated with complete resolution without fibrosis. The zonal pattern of acetaminophen-induced necrosis is related to the mechanism of hepatotoxicity, particularly the role of CYP2E1, which is expressed in this part of the hepatic lobule, and to glutathione levels, which are lower in zone 3 than elsewhere in the liver.

Clinical Course, Outcomes, and Prognostic Indicators

There are no features of liver injury in the first 2 days after acetaminophen self-poisoning; nausea, vomiting, and drowsiness are often caused by concomitant ingestion of alcohol and other drugs. After 48 to 72 hours, serum ALT levels may be elevated, and anorexia, nausea and vomiting, fatigue, and malaise may occur. Pain over the liver may be pronounced. In severe cases, the course is characterized by repeated vomiting, jaundice, hypoglycemia, and other features of acute liver failure, particularly coagulopathy and hepatic encephalopathy. The liver may shrink as a result of severe necrosis. Levels of ALT are often between 2000 and 10,000 U/L. These high levels (and those of other intracellular proteins like ferritin and glutathione S-transferases) may provide the clue to the diagnosis in complex settings, including alcoholic subjects, and distinguish acute drug toxicity from viral hepatitis.[109, 112]

The following are indicators of a poor outcome:[107, 108] grade IV hepatic coma, acidosis, severe and sustained impairment of coagulation factor synthesis, renal failure, and the pattern of falling ALT in conjunction with a worsening prothrombin time (see Chapter 80). Renal failure reflects acute tubular necrosis or the hepatorenal syndrome. Myocardial injury also has been attributable to acetaminophen toxicity.[114] Death occurs between 4 and 18 days, usually from cerebral edema and sepsis complicating hepatic and multiorgan failure. However, in the majority of cases recovery occurs and is usually complete. Cases of apparent chronic hepatotoxicity have rarely been attributed to continued ingestion of acetaminophen (2 to 6 g/day), usually in a susceptible host, such as a heavy drinker, or in a person with preexisting, unrecognized liver disease.[2, 3]

Management

In patients who present within 4 hours of acetaminophen ingestion, the stomach should be emptied with a wide-bore gastric tube. There is little place for osmotic cathartics or binding agents. Charcoal hemoperfusion has no established role. Management centers around the identification of patients who should receive thiol-based antidote therapy, and, in established severe liver injury, assessment of candidacy for liver transplantation.

Acetaminophen blood levels should be determined at the time of presentation. However, because of delayed gastric

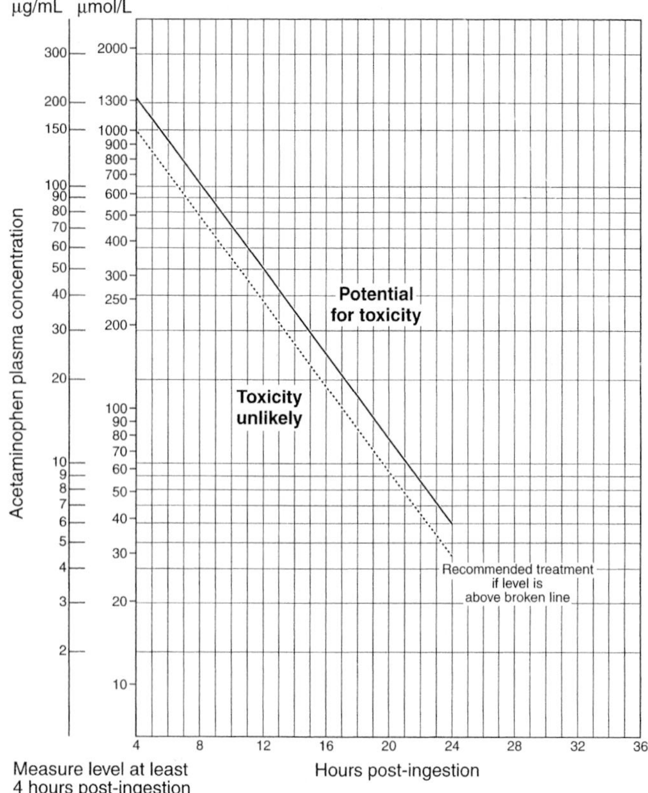

Figure 73–1. Acetaminophen toxicity nomogram. The risk of hepatotoxicity correlates with the plasma acetaminophen level and the time after ingestion.[106]

emptying, blood levels within 4 hours of ingestion may not be a reliable estimate of the extent of exposure. After 4 hours, *acetaminophen blood levels give a reliable indicator of the risk of liver injury*, which is estimated by reference to a nomogram (Fig. 73–1).[106, 114] Indications for antidote therapy include a reliable history of major poisoning (more than 10 g), and blood acetaminophen levels in the moderate or high-risk bands.[106, 114] At-risk cases should be admitted to the hospital for monitoring.

Hepatic necrosis occurs only when concentrations of reduced glutathione fall below a critical level, thereby allowing the CYP-generated metabolite of acetaminophen, NAPQI, to produce liver injury. Administration of cysteine donors stimulates hepatic synthesis of reduced glutathione, thereby protecting the liver. Many cysteine precursors or thiol-donors could be used, but NAC has become the agent of choice. Oral administration is preferred in the United States,[8, 106] with a loading dose of 140 mg/kg followed by administration of half this dose every 4 hours for 72 hours. Despite the theoretical disadvantage that delayed gastric emptying and vomiting may reduce absorption, oral administration of NAC is highly effective.[118] In Europe and Australia, NAC is administered by slow bolus intravenous injection followed by infusion.[105, 114] This route could be associated with a higher rate of hypersensitivity reactions because of the much higher systemic blood levels achieved.[2] Adverse reactions to NAC may be severe, with rash, angioedema and occasionally fatal shock. Therefore, NAC should be administered under close supervision and only for appropriate indications. In patients known to be sensitized to NAC, methionine is probably just as effective but is not available in a commercial preparation; it must be made up fresh, and it often causes vomiting.[114]

Cases of severe liver injury are virtually abolished if NAC is administered within 12 hours and possibly within 16 hours of acetaminophen ingestion.[105, 106] After 16 hours, thiol donation is unlikely to affect the development of liver injury, because oxidation of acetaminophen to NAPQI and consequent oxidation of thiol groups is complete and mitochondrial injury and activation of cell death pathways are likely to be established. Nevertheless, NAC decreased the mortality of acetaminophen-induced hepatotoxicity when administered 16 to 36 hours after self-poisoning,[107] possibly because NAC stabilizes vascular reactivity in liver failure. Therefore, it is recommended that NAC be administered to late presenters after acetaminophen overdose. Other strategies to protect the liver against acetaminophen poisoning, such as inhibition of CYP-dependent metabolism through the use of cimetidine or prostaglandin analogues (which are efficacious in rats),[119] have not been established as clinically useful.

Hepatic transplantation has been advocated as a therapeutic option for selected patients who develop liver failure after acetaminophen poisoning.[107, 108] The selection of cases is based on the aforementioned prognostic indicators and is strongly influenced by the prospects for successful psychological rehabilitation, as reviewed elsewhere.[107, 110, 108, 120] In several series, about 60% of listed patients have been transplanted, and survival rates have exceeded 70%.[120]

Prevention

Safe use of acetaminophen involves not only adherence to the recommended maximum dose for healthy subjects, but also education about the risk factors that lower the toxic dose threshold. Moderate acetaminophen dosing (more than 2 g each day) is contraindicated in heavy drinkers, in persons taking other medications (particularly phenytoin, zidovudine, and isoniazid), and during fasting, and care should also be taken with prolonged use of acetaminophen in patients with severe cardiorespiratory disease or advanced cirrhosis. Use of acetaminophen for self-poisoning continues despite attempts at public education about the risks involved. Attempts to limit harm from what are usually suicide gestures include smaller package size and tighter individual unit packaging (e.g., blister packs) that hampers ready access to tablets or capsules.[121, 122]

Niacin (Nicotinic Acid)

Hepatotoxicity associated with use of nicotinic acid (3-pyridinecarboxylic acid, niacin) has been noted since the 1960s. When used to treat hypercholesterolemia, niacin has been an important cause of liver injury.[14, 48, 123] The clinicopathologic spectrum encompasses mild and transient increases in aminotransferase levels, jaundice, cholestasis, and rare cases of acute liver failure. Hepatotoxicity is dose dependent; toxic doses usually exceed 2 g/day. The risk is much greater with sustained release niacin than with unmodified crystalline (immediate release) forms. Other predisposing factors are alcohol use, preexisting liver disease, and concurrent therapy with sulfonylureas.[14, 123] There is no association with age, diet, or insulin-managed diabetes. The onset of liver injury is usually within 6 months but may be as late as 4 years. Product substitution without dose adjustment should be avoided; switching from immediate- to sustained-release preparations requires a 50% to 70% reduction in dose.

Other Types of Cytopathic Liver Injury

Some hepatotoxins are not as clearly dose-dependent as acetaminophen but cause cytopathic or cytotoxic changes, such as extensive hydropic change, diffuse or zonal microvesicular steatosis, and zonal necrosis, or combinations of these lesions.[2, 3] Injury likely represents *metabolic idiosyncrasy* in which the drug or one of its metabolites accumulates and interferes with protein synthesis or intermediary metabolism. The mitochondrion often appears to be the main subcellular target, and other metabolically active tissues can be involved. Thus, pancreatitis and renal tubular injury may accompany severe liver injury caused by tetracycline, valproic acid, and HAART, and metabolic acidosis with a shocklike state is common. The first agent recognized to cause this clinicopathologic syndrome was tetracycline administered in high doses (>2 g/day for more than 4 days, usually intravenously) during pregnancy, in men receiving estrogens, or in the presence of renal failure;[3] with appropriate dose limitations, this reaction no longer occurs.

Valproic Acid (Sodium Valproate)

This effective antiepileptic has been associated with severe hepatotoxicity.[2, 124] Children are most at risk, particularly those less than 3 years old.[27] Cases in adults have been described rarely.[28] Concomitant administration of other antiepileptics is another predisposing factor, with the frequency of liver injury increasing in proportion to the number of agents ingested. The frequency of valproic acid hepatotoxicity varies from 1 per 500 high-risk persons exposed to 1 per 37,000 low-risk persons.[27] Another risk factor is a family history of mitochondrial enzyme deficiencies (particularly of the urea cycle or long-chain fatty acid transport), Reye's syndrome, or a sibling affected by valproate hepatotoxicity.[34, 125]

There is no relationship to dose, but blood levels tend to be high in one half of affected persons. It is of interest that 4-en-valproic acid, a desaturated metabolite produced by CYP-catalyzed metabolism of valproic acid, is a dose-dependent hepatotoxin in animals and in vitro. Thus the concept has emerged that valproic acid is an occult dose-dependent toxin in which accumulation of a hepatotoxic metabolite (favored by coexposure to CYP-inducing antiepileptics) produces mitochondrial injury in a susceptible host (e.g., young children, especially those with partial deficiencies of mitochondrial enzymes).[2, 34, 125]

The clinicopathologic features resemble idiopathic Reye's syndrome or tetracycline-induced fatty liver. The onset occurs after 4 to 12 weeks of valproic acid treatment and is characterized by nonspecific clinical features such as lethargy, muscle weakness, worsening seizures, drowsiness, facial swelling, and malaise. In typical cases, features of hepatotoxicity follow, including anorexia, nausea, vomiting, abdominal discomfort over the liver, and weight loss.[2, 3, 124] Jaundice ensues, coagulopathy and encephalopathy are often profound, and ascites may be present.

In some cases, a neurologic syndrome characterized by ataxia, mental confusion, and coma predominates, with little evidence of hepatic involvement.[125] In others, fever and tender hepatomegaly suggestive of Reye's syndrome may be present; such cases tend to have a better prognosis. Other features may include alopecia, hypofibrinogenemia, thrombocytopenia, and pancreatitis. The terminal phase is often indicated by renal failure, hypoglycemia, metabolic acidosis, and severe bacterial infection.

Laboratory features include modest elevation of serum bilirubin and ALT levels; the aspartate aminotransferase (AST) is usually higher than ALT. Profound impairment of clotting factor levels, hypoalbuminemia, and raised serum ammonia levels are common. Hepatic imaging shows a small liver with increased echogenicity suggesting steatosis or extensive necrosis. Liver histology shows zonal or panlobular necrotic lesions in two thirds of cases, often with centrilobular congestion; microvesicular steatosis, either zonal or generalized, predominates in the remainder. Both steatosis and necrotic lesions may be present. Ultrastructural studies indicate conspicuous abnormalities of the mitochondria.

Treatment is supportive. There have been at least 60 reported fatalities, and the mortality rate remains high. Thus prevention is crucial. It has been shown that 90% of cases can be avoided by careful adherence to prescribing guidelines, particularly avoiding valproic acid in combination with other agents in the first 3 years of life or in children with possible mitochondrial enzyme defects.[27] Liver test abnormalities develop in at least 40% of patients taking valproic acid; therefore, these tests are unreliable predictors of severe hepatotoxicity. It is more important to warn patients and parents about the need to report any adverse symptoms during the first 6 months of valproic acid therapy.

Fialuridine

Fialuridine (FIAU; 1-[2′-deoxy-2′-fluoro-b-D-arabinofuranosyl]-5-idoouracil), a nucleoside analogue that acts as a chain terminator for DNA synthesis, is a potent inhibitor of hepatitis B virus replication that showed promise in short-term trials. A study to examine efficacy and safety of a 6-month course was stopped as soon as toxicity was recognized.[126] The onset of toxicity was delayed. Hepatic and renal dysfunction, often with peripheral and autonomic neuropathy, myopathy, and pancreatitis, developed in 14 of 15 patients; severe complications occurred in 7 of the 10 patients who received the drug for more than 8 weeks, and 5 died.[126]

The constellation of metabolic acidosis with hepatic and renal failure is best explained as a form of mitochondrial toxicity, as supported by ultrastructural changes.[127] Further work is required to explain completely the delayed onset of hepatic toxicity; phosphorylation of FIAU and inhibition of mitochondrial DNA synthesis are likely to be involved.[128, 129]

Antiretroviral Treatment

Abnormal liver tests and clinical evidence of liver disease are common in patients with HIV infection and AIDS. There are many reasons, including chronic hepatitis B or C, other hepatobiliary infections, lymphoma and other tumors, and possibly effects of HIV infection itself. However, the commonest cause of liver injury is hepatotoxicity from drugs used to treat HIV infection and AIDS; the possibility that concurrent chronic hepatitis C may increase this risk is unproved. In the earlier years of HIV monotherapy, individual nucleoside analogues were associated with uncommon episodes of severe cytopathic liver injury, as illustrated later by didanosine, and because of the experience with fialuridine, there was concern about a general mitochondrial toxicity from nucleoside analogues.

The frequency of hepatic injury with three- to four-agent HAART is at least 10%.[53, 130] Nucleosides and nucleotides that block HIV reverse transcriptase are also weak inhibitors of mitochondrial DNA polymerase gamma in vitro; the order of potency is zalcitabine > didanosine > stavudine > lamivudine > zidovudine > abacavir.[131] In clinical studies, zidovudine and didanosine have been implicated most often in hepatotoxicity, but no particular nucleoside or nucleotide analogue appears to be more hepatotoxic than the others[84, 132–134]; it is possible that drug combinations are more toxic than individual agents.[135] However, lamivudine seems free of this adverse effect, as now shown with the extensive experience of its use against hepatitis B (see Chapter 68).

All the protease inhibitors have been part of combinations associated with liver injury; rotinavir[53, 136, 137] and indinavir[138, 139] seem most often incriminated. The pattern of liver injury is often mixed, with prominent steatosis, focal liver injury, and cholestasis. Myopathy or neuromyopathic changes are often associated, and it seems likely though unproven that the toxicity may be a form of mitochondrial injury. Mitochondrial lesions have been found in more severe syndromes associated with lactic acidosis and liver failure, usually after at least 6 months of nucleoside-based anti-HIV therapy.[135] Protease inhibitors are associated with various types of lipodystrophy and with insulin resistance, the hallmark of metabolic predisposition to NASH. Possibly because the hepatic lesions are more closely related to NASH than to other types of cytopathic change, recovery is usually slow after discontinuation of HAART.

DIDANOSINE. Didanosine (2′,3′-dideoxyinosine) is a nucleoside analogue that inhibits the reverse transcriptase of HIV. Adverse reactions include peripheral neuropathy and pancreatitis. Several cases of didanosine-induced fulminant hepatic failure have been reported.[14, 140] The livers show microvesicular fatty change with cholestasis but no inflammation; hepatic necrosis is variable. Onset occurs at 13 to 15 weeks after the start of therapy with didanosine, with vomiting, diarrhea, and dyspnea and with biochemical tests that indicate lactic acidosis and hepatic and renal failure.

The clinical course is characterized by severe metabolic acidosis and fulminant liver and multiorgan failure, with death occurring within 3 to 8 days despite the discontinuation of didanosine. There is evidence for partial dose dependence, but individual susceptibility must also be involved. Incorporation of the phosphorylated cytoplasmic form of didanosine (2′,3′-dideoxy-ATP) into mitochondrial DNA might lead to mitochondrial dysfunction and resulting hepatotoxicity. Patients receiving didanosine should be monitored regularly with serum AST, prothrombin time, and serum bicarbonate testing during the first 4 months of therapy and should be counseled to report the onset of nausea, vomiting, diarrhea, or dyspnea.

STAVUDINE. Stavudine has been shown by rechallenge to cause a similar albeit less severe form of hepatic steatosis with lactic acidosis.[141, 142]

Aspirin

Aspirin has occasionally been associated with major increases in serum ALT levels suggestive of drug hepatitis, but hepatotoxicity occurs only when blood salicylate concentrations exceed 25 mg/100 mL.[2, 56, 143] Patients with juvenile rheumatoid arthritis, Still's disease, or systemic lupus erythematosus appear to be at particular risk. Patients do not develop clinical or laboratory features of chronic liver disease, and there are no features of drug allergy. Management requires suspecting the correct diagnosis and reducing the dose of (or stopping) aspirin. Recovery is usually rapid. Aspirin can be used again in lower doses, but other NSAIDs have displaced the use of high-dose aspirin for most conditions. Aspirin increases the risk of Reye's syndrome in febrile children,[22] and the incidence of Reye's syndrome in the United States, Britain, and elsewhere has fallen dramatically since avoidance of aspirin use in children with a viral illness was introduced as a public health measure.[29, 30] Misdiagnosis of earlier cases which have subsequently been shown to be inborn errors of metabolism that mimic Reye's syndrome may be part of the reason for the decline in the reported incidence of Reye's syndrome.[144]

Other Drugs

L-Asparaginase is an antileukemic drug that often causes hepatotoxicity. Toxicity is usually reversible but can result in liver failure associated with diffuse microvesicular steatosis.[145]

Phosphorus is one of the few truly direct hepatotoxins, but hepatotoxicity is rarely seen because phosphorus is no longer a component of rat poisons and matches. The clinical picture is one of vomiting and acute hepatorenal failure.[3]

Cocaine, phencyclidine, and 5-methoxy-3,4-methylenedioxymethamphetamine (MDMA, ecstasy) are recreational drugs that can cause liver failure, with some evidence of dose dependency. However, the direct relationship of the drug to liver injury is somewhat controversial.[43] *Cocaine* is a hepatotoxin in mice but not in several other species. In humans severely intoxicated with cocaine, liver injury is usually secondary to other factors, such as hypoxia, hypotension, and hyperthermia.[43]

Phencyclidine (angel dust) has been associated with liver injury in cases of severe toxicity with hyperthermia, rhabdomyolysis, and respiratory and renal failure.[2]

Ecstasy has been associated with several cases of severe liver failure; some have been fatal and some have been treated by liver transplantation.[2, 146, 147] Hepatomegaly, jaundice, pruritus, severe hyperbilirubinemia, and a disproportionate increase in serum AST compared with ALT have been noted, and liver biopsy has shown acute hepatitis of variable severity.[148] Liver injury has not always been related to the dose; an underlying abnormality of muscle metabo-

Table 73–4 | **Types of Drug-Induced Acute Hepatitis: Comparison of Immunoallergic Reactions with Those Possibly Caused by Metabolic Idiosyncrasy**

CHARACTERISTIC	IMMUNOALLERGIC TYPE	METABOLIC IDIOSYNCRASY
Frequency	<1 case per 10,000 persons exposed	0.01%–2% of persons exposed
Gender predilection	Females, often ≥2:1	Variable, slightly more common in females
Latent period to onset	Fairly constant, 2 to 10 weeks	More variable, 2 to 24 weeks, occasionally longer than 1 year
Relationship to dose	None	Usually none (occasional exceptions)
Interactions with other agents	None	Alcohol; occasionally other drugs (e.g., isoniazid/rifampicin)
Course after stopping drug	Prompt improvement (rare exceptions, e.g., minocycline)	Variable; occasionally slow improvement or deterioration (e.g., troglitazone)
Positive rechallenge	Always, often fever within 3 days	Usual (two thirds), abnormal liver tests in 2 to 21 days
Fever	Usual, often initial symptom, part of prodrome	Infrequent, less prominent
Extrahepatic features (rash, lymphadenopathy)	Common	Rare
Eosinophilia:		
Blood	33% to 67% of cases	<10% of cases
Tissue	Usual, a major cell type	Common but minor
Autoantibodies	Often positive	Rarely positive
Examples	Nitrofurantoin (see text), phenytoin, methyldopa, sulfonamides, etretinate, minocycline	Isoniazid (see text), pyrazinamide, ketoconazole, dantrolene, troglitazone

lism similar to that associated with the malignant hyperthermia syndrome has been suggested. CYP2D6 is the major hepatic drug oxidation pathway for ecstasy and related designer drugs,[149] but whether persons lacking this enzyme (and therefore exhibiting a debrisoquine slow metabolizer phenotype) are at risk of liver injury from ecstasy has not been studied. Unexplained liver test abnormalities and hepatomegaly in young people should prompt inquiry into illicit drug use.[146–148]

Amodiaquine, a 4-aminoquinolone antimalarial, has been associated with fatal hepatotoxicity as well as with agranulocytosis.[150] A possible relationship to total dose has been noted. Amodiaquine should be reserved for active treatment of chloroquine-resistant falciparum malaria, and dose recommendations should be strictly observed.

Hycanthone is an antischistosomal agent for which risk factors for hepatotoxicity include concomitant administration of phenothiazines or estrogens and preexisting liver injury and bacterial infection. The most important risk factor, however, is dose.[51]

DRUG-INDUCED ACUTE HEPATITIS

The term *acute hepatitis* is used for lesions characterized by the presence of hepatic inflammation with conspicuous hepatocyte cell death or degeneration. More severe lesions include zonal and bridging necrosis or massive (panlobular) hepatic necrosis; these lesions may be associated with *fulminant* or *subfulminant hepatic failure*.[4] Acute hepatitis accounts for nearly one half of reported adverse drug reactions involving the liver,[1] and there are many causative agents.[1–3, 7, 8, 13, 151]

Two broad types of drug hepatitis are those with clinical and laboratory features consistent with drug allergy (immunoallergic reactions) and those without such features. The latter could be the result of metabolic idiosyncrasy; partial dose dependence, relationship to metabolism of the drug, and histologic or ultrastructural features consistent with chemical toxicity are often found. The clinical and laboratory features that suggest one of these processes are summarized in Table 73–4. Nitrofurantoin is discussed next as an example of immunoallergy, whereas isoniazid will be used to illustrate metabolic idiosyncrasy. Other relatively frequent examples of drug hepatitis are described briefly, as are granulomatous reactions and chronic hepatitis.

Immunoallergic Reactions

Nitrofurantoin

Nitrofurantoin, a synthetic furan-based compound, is a urinary antiseptic with a range of uncommon adverse effects. Abnormal liver tests are commonly noted during the first few weeks of administration but are of doubtful importance. The range of liver disease associated with nitrofurantoin includes acute hepatitis, sometime with features of cholestasis, hepatic granulomas, chronic hepatitis with autoimmune phenomena, acute liver failure, and cirrhosis.[2, 152, 153] Causality has been proven by rechallenge. There is no relationship to dose; cases have even been described after ingestion of milk from a nitrofurantoin-treated cow. The frequency of nitrofurantoin hepatic injury ranges from 0.3 to 3 cases per 100,000 exposed persons,[2, 152] and it increases with age, particularly after age 64 years. Two thirds of acute cases occur in women, and the gender ratio is 8:1 for chronic hepatitis.[152, 153]

There has been debate about the relative frequencies of hepatocellular versus cholestatic or mixed reactions[152, 153] and acute versus chronic hepatitis.[2] The first issue occurs because reactions cover a spectrum of biochemical and histologic features, but these have no apparent relevance to clinical outcome. Chronicity depends mostly on the duration of drug ingestion and has been less than 6 weeks in acute cases but more than 6 months in 90% of chronic cases.[152, 153] Patients with chronic hepatitis often have continued taking nitrofurantoin despite symptoms attributable to adverse drug effects, or they have been exposed to another course after previous adverse effects. The mortality rate of chronic nitrofurantoin hepatitis is 20%, compared with 5% to 10% for acute hepatitis.[152]

The latent period to onset is from a few days to 6 weeks after the start of drug ingestion. Early symptoms may be nonspecific (e.g., fever, myalgia, arthralgia, fatigue, malaise, anorexia, and weight loss) and are followed by more specific features of hepatitis, such as nausea and vomiting, hepatic pain or discomfort, dark urine, jaundice, and occasionally pruritus. Rash occurs in 20%, and lymphadenopathy may be present. Pneumonitis coexists with hepatitis in 20% of cases and is suggested by cough and dyspnea. Rarely, liver failure develops, with ascites, coagulopathy, and encephalopathy. In cases of chronic hepatitis, there also may be clinical findings to suggest chronic liver disease, such as spider angiomata, hepatosplenomegaly, muscle wasting, and ascites.

Liver tests may show pronounced elevation of serum ALT levels, but more often there is a mixed picture with some increase in the serum alkaline phosphatose level as well or relatively nonspecific changes in liver tests. In other cases, the results suggest cholestasis. Serum bilirubin levels tend to be increased in proportion to the severity of the reaction. Unlike most types of acute drug hepatitis, serum albumin concentrations are often low. An increase in serum globulins is more likely with chronic hepatitis.[152] Eosinophilia occurs in 33% of cases. Antinuclear antibodies are present in some cases of acute hepatitis but in 80% of chronic cases. Smooth muscle antibodies are also present in most patients with nitrofurantoin-induced chronic hepatitis. In contrast to spontaneous autoimmune hepatitis, there is no association with an increased frequency of the histocompatibility antigens HLA-B8 and DRw3.[152, 153]

There is no specific treatment. Glucocorticoids have no role, even in chronic hepatitis with autoimmune features. Recovery is rapid after discontinuation of nitrofurantoin. Adverse outcomes are usually related to continued intake of the drug after the onset of symptoms of drug reaction or to inadvertent re-exposure in a sensitized individual. Monitoring liver tests in users of nitrofurantoin is unlikely to be useful or cost-effective.

Other Agents

Methyldopa was one of the first drugs described to cause immunoallergic drug hepatitis. Cases now rarely occur, because better antihypertensive agents are available. Hepatic reactions to methyldopa vary from abnormal liver tests, severe acute hepatitis, granulomas, and cholestasis to chronic hepatitis with bridging necrosis and cirrhosis. The female predilection, clinical and laboratory changes, course, and extrahepatic features of drug allergy are similar to those for nitrofurantoin.[2, 3]

Phenytoin causes severe acute drug hepatitis in fewer than one per 10,000 persons exposed.[33] There is an equal gender incidence, and cases can occur in childhood. Blacks may be affected more often than whites. Rash, fever, eosinophilia, lymphadenopathy, a pseudomononucleosis syndrome, and other allergic features are common. Although these findings suggest immunoallergy, a familial enzymatic defect in disposal of phenytoin arene oxide also has been detected among patients with phenytoin reactions,[33] thereby implicating a possible metabolic factor in predisposition to phenytoin reactions.

The mortality rate is 10% to 40%. Some deaths result from liver failure; others are the result of severe systemic hypersensitivity, bone marrow suppression, exfoliative dermatitis, or vasculitis involving skin and kidney. Rarer hepatic associations with phenytoin reactions include cholestatic hepatitis and bile duct injury.[2] The most common association with phenytoin therapy is an adaptive response of the liver with microsomal enzyme induction; at least two thirds of patients have raised serum GGTP levels, and one third exhibit raised alkaline phosphatase levels. Ground-glass cytoplasm, which represents hypertrophied smooth endoplasmic reticulum, is usually present in hepatocytes.

Barbiturates, including *phenobarbital,* are also rarely associated with acute hepatitis. Described cases have been similar to phenytoin reactions; fever and rash are usual and the mortality rate as a result of liver failure is high.[154] Among newer antiepileptic drugs, felbamate[155] and topiramate[156] have been associated with acute liver failure.

Sulfonamides are a cause of drug hepatitis that is relatively common with combination drugs such as co-trimoxazole (sulfamethoxazole and trimethoprim).[1, 157] Trimethoprim alone has been associated with some cases of cholestatic hepatitis; the estimated risk is 1.4 cases per 100,000 exposed persons.[157] Reactions to co-trimoxazole resemble those of trimethoprim more closely than those of sulfonamides; cholestasis is more common. Patients with HIV infection and AIDS are predisposed to sulfonamide hypersensitivity.[57] Some other drugs have a sulfa moiety that differs from that of sulfonamides but may increase the risk of cross-sensitivity reactions; thus, COX-2 inhibitor celecoxib has recently been observed to cause severe hepatitis in two women with a past history of sulfonamide sensitivity.[158] Likewise, sulfonylureas, such as *gliclazide,* have rarely been associated with drug hepatitis showing features of immunoallergy.[159]

The latent period to onset of sulfonamide hepatitis is 5 to 14 days, and clinical features often include fever, rash, mucositis (Stevens-Johnson syndrome), lymphadenopathy, and vasculitis.[2, 3] Reactions may be severe, and deaths have occurred. The serum ALT level is usually more increased than the alkaline phosphatase, but mixed or cholestatic reactions occur. A few cases of hepatic granulomas and of chronic hepatitis also have been associated with sulfonamides.[42]

Sulfasalazine (salicylazosulfapyrine, salazopyrine) also has been associated with rare cases of acute hepatitis, often severe.[1, 160] Although it has been assumed that the sulfonamide moiety is responsible, this notion has been challenged by the observation of one patient in whom hepatitis recurred after exposure to *mesalamine* (mesalazine, 5-aminosalicylic acid).[161] This observation implicates the salicylate moiety, and like salicylate hepatitis (discussed earlier), sulfasalazine hepatotoxicity appears to be more common in patients with rheumatoid arthritis than in those with inflammatory bowel disease.[1] Another case of mesalamine hepatitis with autoimmune features and chronic hepatitis was diagnosed after 21 months of mesalamine treatment.[162]

Minocycline and other tetracyclines used in conventional low doses are a rare but important cause of drug hepatitis,[21, 163, 164] including cases that have resulted in acute liver failure requiring liver transplantation.[165] Minocycline is one of the few agents in current use that can lead to drug-induced autoimmune hepatitis, as discussed later.

Disulfiram (Antabuse) has rarely been associated with acute hepatitis, occasionally leading to liver failure.[1, 166, 167] Hepatotoxicity from disulfuram is usually easy to distinguish from alcoholic hepatitis by the tenfold or greater elevation of serum ALT levels.

β-Adrenergic blocking agents have rarely been incriminated in hepatotoxicity. *Acebutolol,*[168] *labetalol,*[169] and *metoprolol*[170] have each been associated with cases of acute hepatitis; some cases were proved by rechallenge. Reactions were hepatocellular and severe. There are insufficient data to indicate whether or not immunoallergy is likely.

The *calcium channel blockers nifedipine,*[171] *verapamil,*[172] and *diltiazem*[173] have a good safety record, but rare cases of acute hepatitis with a short incubation period (5 days to 6 weeks) and other features of immunoallergy have been reported.

Etretinate, a synthetic retinoid, is useful for treating several skin diseases. Unlike vitamin A (see later), synthetic retinoids are not predictable hepatotoxins, but etretinate has been associated with abnormal liver tests in 10% to 25% of treated patients.[2, 174] Tests may normalize with a reduction in dose, suggesting partial dose dependency. Approximately ten cases of severe hepatitis have been attributed to etretinate; some have been proved by rechallenge.[2, 174] Most patients were women over the age of 50 years. Two were associated with chronicity, and one patient appeared to respond to glucocorticoids.

Etretinate has a half-life of 100 days; it is therefore recommended that serum ALT levels be monitored. Progressive increases in ALT levels above twice the upper limit of normal are an indication to stop the drug or perform a liver biopsy to assess the significance of the changes.[174] *Acitretin* is another synthetic retinoid that has been associated with a single case of severe acute hepatitis.[1]

Gastric acid suppression drugs have an excellent safety record, although rare adverse hepatic reactions have been reported.[2, 7, 8, 151] The histamine H_2 receptor blocker *oxmetidine* was removed from clinical trials because of hepatotoxicity, and more recently *ebrotidine* was withdrawn because of many cases of liver injury.[175] *Cimetidine,*[176] *ranitidine,*[177] and *famotidine*[178] have all been associated with cases of acute hepatitis, mostly mild and often with cholestatic features. Some cases have been proved by rechallenge. Features of immunoallergy have been present in some of the cimetidine reactions. Cases of hepatotoxicity attributed to the proton pump blocker *omeprazole* are few, and causality has not been proved.[179, 180]

Zafirlukast, a leukotriene receptor antagonist effective against asthma, has been reported to cause severe liver injury, with acute liver failure in two of three cases.[181] *Ticlopidine* is an antiplatelet agent that has been incriminated in at least one case of microvesicular steatosis.[182]

Metabolic Idiosyncrasy

Isoniazid

Isoniazid-induced liver injury has been characterized since the 1970s, but deaths still occur.[183–186] Hepatitis develops in approximately 21 per 1000 persons exposed to isoniazid; 5% to 10% of cases are fatal. The risk and severity increase with age; the risk is 0.3% in the third decade of life and increases to 2% or higher after age 50 years.[183, 184] The overall frequency is the same in men and women, but 70% of fatal cases are in women; black and Hispanic women may be at particular risk.[183, 184] There is no relationship to dose or blood level. The importance of genetic factors has been controversial. Slow acetylators of isoniazid may be at increased risk, but the data are conflicting.[2] Chronic excessive alcohol intake increases the frequency and severity of hepatotoxicity,[183, 184] as may rifampicin and pyrazinamide.[185] Pyrazinamide and acetaminophen have been associated with several cases that were fatal or led to hepatic transplantation.[14, 185] Some studies have found that the risk of liver injury from isoniazid and other anti-tuberculous drugs is increased among persons with chronic hepatitis B,[52] but conflicting findings have been reported.[187] Malnutrition may play a role in some countries.[46] Likewise, in patients with chronic hepatitis C or HIV infection (or both) the risk of significant ALT elevation during anti-tuberculous treatment may be increased several-fold;[188] successful antiviral treatment of hepatitis C allowed antituberculous drugs to be reintroduced safely in four patients.

In 10% to 36% of persons, ALT levels rise in the first 10 weeks of taking isoniazid. Abnormalities are typically minor and resolve spontaneously. In persons in whom hepatitis develops, the latent period is from 1 week to more than 6 months, with a median of approximately 8 weeks, or 12 weeks for severe cases.[183, 184] Re-exposure may be associated with an accelerated onset, although the experience in India is that gradual reintroduction of isoniazid and rifampicin therapy can be achieved in the majority of cases after resolution of drug hepatitis.[46] Prodromal symptoms occur in one third of patients and include malaise, fatigue, and early symptoms of hepatitis such as anorexia, nausea, and vomiting. Jaundice appears several days later and is the only feature in approximately 10% of cases. Fever, rash, arthralgia, and eosinophilia are uncommon.

Liver tests indicate hepatocellular injury; AST exceeds ALT in one half of patients. The serum bilirubin level is usually elevated; values that are increased more than tenfold indicate a poor prognosis. In one study,[183] one third of patients had a prolonged prothrombin time, and 60% of these cases were fatal. Most liver biopsy samples show hepatocellular injury, which is focal in approximately one half of cases, often with marked hydropic change in residual hepatocytes. The remaining are cases of zonal, submassive, or massive necrosis in which inflammation is confined to the portal tracts. Cholestasis and lobular regeneration suggestive of early cirrhosis are rare.

Cases with a fatal outcome have been associated with a longer duration of therapy or continued ingestion of isoniazid after the onset of symptoms.[183–186] Thus, most deaths from isoniazid hepatitis could be prevented if patients report early symptoms and isoniazid is discontinued.[186, 189] In New York, isoniazid hepatitis has become the most common hepatic drug reaction requiring liver transplantation.[189]

Recovery is rapid if isoniazid is discontinued before severe liver injury is established. Management of liver failure is supportive; transplantation is indicated in the most severe cases.[14] Prevention is the most appropriate way to deal with this problem, and it is critical to determine whether the risks of preventive therapy with isoniazid outweigh those of latent tuberculosis.[189] The optimal approach to monitoring for isoniazid toxicity is uncertain; second-weekly or monthly monitoring of serum ALT levels will not always prevent the rapid onset of severe hepatotoxicity. Effective prevention depends on awareness of early symptoms, no matter how nonspecific, that could indicate drug toxicity.

Other Agents

OTHER ANTI-TUBERCULOUS DRUGS. Most cases in which *rifampicin* has been implicated with liver injury have occurred in patients taking isoniazid,[190] but a few cases have been observed when rifampicin was given alone to patients with underlying liver disease.[191] *Pyrazinamide* (and the related *ethionamide*) was known as a dose-dependent hepatotoxin in earlier years.[2, 3] It is used in lower doses (1.5 to 2 g/day) because of the emergence of resistant strains of mycobacteria. Hepatotoxicity in patients taking combinations that include isoniazid and pyrazinamide may be particularly severe.[185] Monitoring ALT levels throughout therapy is recommended. There may be cross-sensitivity between isoniazid, pyrazinamide, and ethionamide.[2, 3]

ANTIFUNGAL AGENTS. *Ketoconazole* is associated with raised liver enzymes in 5% to 17% of treated patients.[2, 192–194] Symptomatic hepatitis occurs in 7 to 9 per 100,000 exposed individuals; increasing age and female gender are risk factors. Reactions are usually mild but can be severe, including rare cases of acute liver failure[195]; the mortality rate is 3% to 7%.[192, 193] The onset is 6 to 12 weeks after starting ketoconazole, and rarely after stopping the drug. There is no relation to dose. Continued drug ingestion after the onset of symptoms leads to an adverse outcome. Patients present with jaundice or symptoms of hepatitis; features of drug allergy are rare. Liver tests are mostly hepatocellular or mixed, but cholestatic hepatitis or bland cholestasis may occur.[192] Resolution of jaundice is usual within 12 weeks but may take months.[192, 193] The role of glucocorticoids in cases that are slow to resolve is unclear.

Terbinafine is an allylamine antifungal agent effective against onychomycosis. Several cases of cholestatic hepatitis have been reported[14, 196–198]; the frequency has been estimated at 2 to 3 cases per 100,000 persons exposed.[197] The onset is usually after 30 to 40 days. Recovery may be slow, and some cases have resulted in chronic cholestasis.[199] Monitoring of ALT levels may be indicated.

Fluconazole and *itraconazole* appear to be less hepatotoxic than ketoconazole and terbinafine; elevations of liver tests occur in fewer than 5% of patients. Rare cases of severe hepatic necrosis have been ascribed to fluconazole, but other causes were not excluded.[14]

ANTIDIABETIC DRUGS. *Troglitazone (Rezulin)* is a thiazolidinedione, the first of a new class of agents that improve glycemic control and hypertriglyceridemia in type 2 diabetes mellitus by reducing insulin resistance, particularly in extrahepatic tissues. These agents are peroxisome proliferator activator-γ [PPARγ] agonists. Troglitazone appeared to be free of serious hepatotoxicity during clinical trials, but during the early marketing phase several cases of acute liver failure were reported, and the drug was withdrawn in Britain in 1997, and in the United States in 1999. At least 20 fatal cases of troglitazone hepatotoxicity have been reported in the literature, and many more to the U.S. Food and Drug Administration (FDA).[200–205] The frequency may be as high as 1.9%.[204] Extrahepatic features of drug allergy are inconspicuous with troglitazone hepatotoxicity. The pathogenic mechanism remains unclear but appears to be a form of metabolic idiosyncrasy. Whether toxicity could be related to formation of a quinone type of metabolite by CYPs 2C8 and 3A4 is unclear.[60]

Among other thiazolidinediones, *rosiglitazone* appears safer on the basis of early data[206] but has been associated with two reports of hepatotoxicity[207, 208]; in both cases, the onset was much earlier than in cases associated with troglitazone use, and both patients survived.

There is no clear relationship between the dose of troglitazone and hepatotoxicity. Reported cases were generally in older women and in obese persons, but there are no relevant epidemiologic studies, and these associations may only reflect the characteristics of patients with type 2 diabetes. There is no evidence that preexisting liver disease or other medications predispose to troglitazone hepatotoxicity.[209] A notable feature of hepatic injury attributable to troglitazone is the delayed onset, which is commonly as long as 9 months and, in two reported cases, was more than 12 months after commencement of therapy[210]; rare cases have had a much earlier onset.[211] Screening with serum ALT testing has several potential problems. First, abnormal liver tests are common in persons with type 2 diabetes but are rarely caused by antidiabetic agents.[212] Second, monitoring ALT on a monthly basis may not always detect significant cases of troglitazone-induced liver disease because the clinical onset appears to be abrupt; however, the efficacy of screening has not been studied.

Patients present with nausea, fatigue, jaundice, vomiting, and symptoms of liver failure. Progression to acute liver failure is often rapid and may occur despite discontinuation of troglitazone ingestion. There is a high mortality, particularly in older patients,[209] and several cases have been treated by liver transplantation. Biopsy, explant, and autopsy studies have shown submassive or massive hepatic necrosis, with postcollapse scarring, bile duct proliferation, and some eosinophils.

DRUGS USED IN NEUROLOGIC DISORDERS. Several neuroleptic agents have been associated with drug hepatitis, as reviewed elsewhere.[213] In keeping with their varying structures, some agents have been associated with immunoallergic types of drug hepatitis, whereas others conform to the pattern of apparent metabolic idiosyncrasy. There have been reactions to commonly used antidepressants, such as *fluoxetine,*[214, 215] *paroxetine,*[216] *venlafaxine,* [217, 218] *trazodone,* [41, 219] *tolcapone,*[220] and *nefazodone*[221–223]; the reactions to nefazodone and tolcapone have included several cases of acute liver failure. Hypnotics, such as *alpidem,*[224] *zolpidem,*[225] and *bentazepam,*[226] also have been implicated in hepatotoxicity; in three reported cases with bentazepam, the clinicopathologic pattern resembled chronic hepatitis but without autoantibodies or other immunologic features.[226]

Tacrine is a reversible choline esterase inhibitor that improves cognition in Alzheimer's disease. A survey of tacrine-related adverse effects in 2446 patients with Alzheimer's disease showed that serum ALT levels more than three times the upper limit of normal occurred in 25%, more often in women than men, and were elevated more than 20-fold in 2%.[227] There was no dose effect. ALT elevations occurred abruptly, not after a gradual rise, and discontinuation of tacrine led to resolution of abnormalities. Symptoms were rare; only nausea and vomiting correlated with major ALT elevations. In liver biopsies from three patients, steatosis and mild lobular hepatitis were observed. Thus, minor degrees of hepatocellular injury occur in one half of the recipients of tacrine, but tolerance to this minor form of liver injury eventually develops. Isolated reports of jaundice indicate a rare potential for tacrine to cause more significant hepatotoxicity.[2, 42] Weekly monitoring of ALT during the first 3 months of therapy with tacrine and discontinuation of the drug if values reach three times normal should prevent significant hepatotoxicity.[227]

Dantrolene, a direct-acting muscle relaxant that is valuable against spasticity, causes hepatitis in approximately 1% of patients; the case fatality rate has been approximately 28%.[228] Cases have been severe, and hepatitis continued in some cases when the drug was not discontinued. Most patients have been more than 30 years old, suggesting that susceptibility increases with age. One third of cases are asymptomatic; the remainder of patients present with jaundice and symptoms of hepatitis. Hepatic lesions are hepatocellular, often with submassive or massive necrosis.[2, 228] Dantrolene should initially be used on a trial basis with second-weekly liver test monitoring. If there is clinical benefit at 45 days and liver tests are normal, continuation is recommended, whereas the presence of abnormal liver enzymes is an indication to stop dantrolene.

Other neurotropic drugs and muscle relaxants implicated as idiosyncratic hepatotoxins include *riluzole* (used for amyotrophic lateral sclerosis),[229, 230] *tizanidine* (a centrally acting muscle relaxant),[231] and *alverine* (a smooth muscle relaxant).[232]

Nonsteroidal anti-inflammatory drugs can rarely cause drug-induced liver disease, with or without immunoallergic features and with varying degrees of hepatocellular injury and cholestasis.[2, 151] Bromfenac is a phenylacetic acid derivative that was withdrawn recently because of several cases of severe hepatotoxic reactions resulting in acute liver failure, which led to liver transplantation or death.[233–236] Most patients had received therapeutic doses of bromfenac for longer than 90 days before experiencing a prodrome of malaise and fatigue that was followed by symptoms of severe hepatitis and progressive liver failure over 5 to 37 days. There were no features to suggest immunoallergy. Hepatic lesions were characterized by confluent necrosis with a predominantly lymphocytic infiltrate. Bromfenac was withdrawn in the United States in 1998.

COX-2 inhibitors appear to be relatively free of hepatic drug reactions, but their release is too recent to allow definitive statements to be made about the risks and nature of hepatotoxicity. A small number of cases of hepatotoxicity have been reported in association with nimesulide and celecoxib.[158, 237, 238]

Leflunomide (Arava) is a novel agent against rheumatoid arthritis. A statement from the European Medicines Evaluation Agency (EMEA) in March 2001 indicated that 296 liver reactions had been reported in association with the use of this agent, including 129 serious cases, 15 cases of liver failure, and two cases of cirrhosis. Monitoring ALT levels before and during therapy is now recommended.

Ritodrine is a beta-sympathicomimetic agent used as a tocolytic agent for treatment of premature labor; a small number of cases of hepatotoxicity have been described.[239]

Cyproterone acetate is an antiandrogenic compound rarely associated with drug-induced liver disease; two cases of fatal acute liver failure have been reported.[240]

DRUG-INDUCED GRANULOMATOUS HEPATITIS

Granulomatous reactions are a common type of drug-induced liver disease,[2, 241] and drugs account for 2% to 29% of cases of *granulomatous hepatitis* (see Chapter 69). The number of drugs and foreign compounds associated with hepatic granulomas exceeds 40; some are summarized in Table 73–5.[242–250] Not all are associated with systemic inflammation or with persuasive evidence of causality. Many are associated more commonly with other patterns of liver injury (e.g., halothane, methyldopa, nitrofurantoin, troglitazone, amiodarone, amoxicillin/clavulanic acid[251]). Some of these associations may be fortuitous.

The clinical picture is heralded by fever and systemic symptoms (e.g., malaise, headache, myalgia) between 10 days and 4 months after the start of treatment. Hepatomegaly and hepatic tenderness are common; splenomegaly is present in 25% of cases. Extrahepatic features of drug hypersensitivity are common, as is eosinophilia (30%). Liver tests are typically mixed because of the infiltrative nature of hepatic granulomas and the frequent presence of some hepatocellular necrosis or cholestasis. For several drugs that cause granulomatous hepatitis, continued exposure leads to more severe types of liver disease, such as cholestatic hepatitis, with or without bile duct injury, or hepatic necrosis. Small vessel vasculitis is another adverse syndrome and may involve the kidneys, bone marrow, skin, and lungs; the mortality rate is high.[2]

DRUG-INDUCED CHRONIC HEPATITIS

Chronic hepatitis is defined as hepatitis continuing for more than 6 months, but for drug reactions, the definition has often been based inappropriately on histologic features alone.[252, 253] These features include periportal (piecemeal) necrosis, bridging necrosis, and hepatic fibrosis; such features may be present as early as 6 weeks after the onset of severe

Table 73–5 | **Drug-Induced Granulomatous Hepatitis: Major Causative Agents, Frequency, Clinicopathologic Characteristics, and Outcomes**

CAUSATIVE AGENTS*	KEY REFERENCE	FREQUENCY, RISK FACTORS	CLINICOPATHOLOGIC CHARACTERISTICS, OUTCOME
Allopurinol	242	Very rare (<40 cases) Older men, black race, renal failure, use of thiazides	Acute hepatitis, cholestatic hepatitis, bile duct injury also frequent; rash (exfoliative dermatitis), nephritis, vasculitis usual; mortality rate 15%, especially with vasculitis
Carbamazepine	243	16:100,000 treatment years Age >40 yr, no gender predilection	Two thirds of cases show granulomatous hepatitis; remainder show acute hepatitis, cholangitis; no features of drug allergy; no reported mortality, rapid recovery
Phenylbutazone	244	2:10,000 exposed No age/gender predilection	Severe acute hepatitis, cholestasis, and bile duct injury also reported; features of drug allergy common; occasional vasculitis; mortality rate 25%, particularly in cases with hepatocellular necrosis
Hydralazine	245	Rare; older patients, possibly slow acetylators	Other types of reaction also common: acute hepatitis, cholestatic hepatitis, cholangitis; features of drug allergy uncommon; vasculitis not described; reactions severe but no mortality reported
Quinine	246	Very rare; no recognized risk factors	Acute hepatitis in two thirds of cases; rash, interstitial pneumonitis, positive Coombs' test, thrombocytopenia; vasculitis not described; good prognosis

*Other drugs that have been reliably reported to cause granulomatous hepatitis include quinidine[247], phenytoin (usually with vasculitis),[248] sulfonamides,[42] (usually with vasculitis), nitrofurantoin, aspirin, papaverine, procainamide, sulfasalazine, mesalamine,[249] and glyburide.[250] Single case reports have implicated many other agents, as referred to briefly in the text and detailed in reviews.[2, 241]

reactions and do not confirm chronicity. The diagnosis of chronic hepatitis is more convincing when clinical or biochemical evidence of hepatitis has been present for more than 3 months and when there are clinical and laboratory features of chronic liver disease or histologic evidence of established hepatic fibrosis.

As defined earlier, drugs are an uncommon cause of chronic hepatitis (Table 73–6). Implicated agents, like *oxyphenisatin*[2, 252, 253] and *methyldopa*, are now rarely used, and with the increasing importance of chronic viral hepatitis (see Chapter 68), only a small proportion (2% to 6%, depending on location) of cases of chronic hepatitis are drug related.[2, 37] Indeed, several cases reported in the past were subsequently found to be cases of chronic hepatitis C.[96] However, recognition of a drug cause remains important because a poor outcome is usually attributable to continued drug ingestion after clinical onset of the disorder.[37]

Women are approximately four times more prone to drug-

Table 73–6 | **Drug-Induced Chronic Hepatitis: Causative Agents, Risk Factors, Clinicopathologic Characteristics, and Outcomes**

CAUSATIVE AGENT*	RISK FACTORS	CLINICOPATHOLOGIC CHARACTERISTICS, OUTCOME
Nitrofurantoin	Age >40 yr; 90% of cases in women; continued ingestion after onset	Clinical features of chronic hepatitis, liver failure; some cases have features of cholestasis; 20% pneumonitis; hyperglobulinemia usual, ANA, SMA positive; mortality rate 10%
Methyldopa	Age >50 yr; 80% of cases in women; repeated courses, continued ingestion in sensitized patient	Jaundice, systemic features, diarrhea, liver failure; hyperglobulinemia, ANA, SMA positive; protracted course, high mortality rate
Diclofenac	Age >65 yr; most cases in women	Clinical features of chronic hepatitis, liver failure; ANA, SMA, hyperglobulinemia; response to glucocorticords in a few cases
Minocycline	Young women; prolonged ingestion of minocycline	Often part of drug-induced systemic lupus erythematosus syndrome (arthritis, rash, nephritis); ANA positive; hyperglobulinemia; cases may be severe with fatal outcome or need for liver transplantation; glucocorticoid treatment may be indicated
Isoniazid	Age >50 yr; continued drug ingestion after onset; duration of therapy	Not well documented clinically; severe and fatal cases with cirrhosis histologically; immune phenomena not apparent; high mortality rate or need for liver transplantation
Dantrolene	Age >30 yr; dose, duration of therapy	Jaundice, liver failure; no immune phenomena; high mortality rate
Etretinate	Age >50 yr; two thirds in women	Jaundice, weight loss, liver failure; deterioration after stopping drug; response to glucocorticoids in two cases
Acetaminophen	Regular intake at moderate doses (2 to 6 g/day); alcohol, fasting, other drugs	No features of chronic liver disease, no autoimmune phenomena; these are cases of chronic toxicity; rapid normalization of liver tests after stopping drug

*Other drugs include oxyphenisatin and tienilic acid, which are now of historic interest,[2, 3] and clometacin, for which many affected patients have now been shown to have had hepatitis C.[96] Several other agents, including sulfonamides, aspirin, halothane, cimetidine, methotrexate, trazadone, fluoxetine, fenfibrate, and germander have been mentioned as associated with chronic hepatitis, but details are not always convincing.[2]

ANA, antinuclear antibody; SMA, smooth muscle antibody.

induced chronic hepatitis than are men.[252, 253] Older patients appear to be at greater risk, and the reaction is virtually unknown in children. Drugs associated with chronic hepatitis more commonly cause acute hepatitis, and the latent period to recognition tends to be longer in cases of chronic hepatitis; thus, duration of drug ingestion may be a risk factor.

There are two syndromes. In the first, cases appear to be identical to acute hepatitis but are more severe, more prolonged, or later in onset, perhaps as a result of failure of recognition. These cases may more appropriately be termed *chronic toxicity*. Clinical and laboratory features of chronic liver disease are rare, and there are no hallmarks of autoimmunity. Management consists of drug withdrawal and treatment of liver failure (for examples, see Table 73–6).

The second syndrome more closely resembles autoimmune hepatitis by the presence of spider angiomata, firm liver edge, and splenomegaly and the development of liver failure. Ascites, bruising, bleeding esophageal varices, and hepatic encephalopathy are common. In addition to raised serum ALT and bilirubin levels, hypoalbuminemia and hyperglobulinemia are usual. The prothrombin time is prolonged in severe cases. Autoantibodies, particularly antinuclear and smooth muscle antibodies, are frequent. In contrast to idiopathic autoimmune hepatitis, other hallmarks of autoimmunity, such as a history of other autoimmune diseases and genetic predisposition indicated by HLA-B8 and DRw3, are not found. Immunosuppressive treatment is not usually indicated; the clinical condition improves spontaneously after withdrawal of the causative drug. However, in individual cases (see later discussion), glucocorticoids occasionally appear to hasten recovery.

Diclofenac

Diclofenac is one of the world's most prescribed NSAIDs and appears to be at least as safe as comparable agents. Significant hepatotoxicity occurs in 1 to 5 per 100,000 persons exposed, or 0.4 per 1 million defined daily doses; the latter rate is minimally greater than that for phenylbutazone (0.2 per 1 million) and piroxicam (0.3 per 1 million) but less than that for benoxaprofen (12.6 per 1 million)[16] and bromfenac,[233–236] which was recently withdrawn (discussed earlier). There have now been at least 30 cases of diclofenac hepatitis reported,[2, 254, 255] including several proved by inadvertent rechallenge. Four fatalities and five cases have been reasonably regarded as chronic hepatitis. The risk is increased in women and with aging.

Affected persons are seen between 1 and 11 months (usually less than 3 months) after the start of diclofenac. A prodromal illness or symptoms of hepatitis are followed by jaundice and liver failure in severe cases. Fever and rash occur in 25% of cases. In some patients, features suggest chronic liver disease, such as ascites, hypoalbuminemia, and hyperglobulinemia. Liver tests and histology usually reflect acute hepatitis, but some features of cholestasis may be present, and other cases show bridging necrosis, fibrous expansion of portal tracts, and periportal necrosis. Recovery has often,[254] but not always,[255] followed cessation of diclofenac. In a few cases, recovery was not evident by 3 months, and glucocorticoids were administered with apparent benefit.[2, 255]

Cross-sensitivity among NSAIDs seems to be rare, but one patient with diclofenac hepatitis also had an adverse reaction to ibuprofen, and another had an adverse reaction to tiaprofenic acid.[2, 254] The rarity of severe diclofenac-induced hepatotoxicity makes biochemical monitoring unrealistic. Patients need to be advised to report adverse effects, and clinicians must be aware that diclofenac can cause both acute and chronic hepatitis.

Minocycline

Minocycline has been associated with rare cases of drug-induced systemic lupus erythematosus syndrome (rash, polyarthritis, hyperglobulinemia, antinuclear antibodies), chronic hepatitis with autoimmune features, or both syndromes in the same patient.[163, 164, 256, 257] The onset is often after treatment with minocycline for more than 6 months, and young women appear to be particularly affected. The reactions are severe; some patients have died or required liver transplantation, and the course may be prolonged after discontinuing the drug; several cases have been treated with glucocorticoids.[257]

DRUG-INDUCED CHOLESTASIS

Importance, Types of Reaction, and Diagnosis

Drugs are an important cause of acute cholestasis, with or without hepatitis. The full spectrum of drug-related disorders includes *cholestatic hepatitis with cholangitis* and *chronic cholestasis,* with either a *vanishing bile duct syndrome* resembling primary biliary cirrhosis or *biliary strictures* reminiscent of sclerosing cholangitis.[2, 258, 259] The clinical and biochemical features of drug-induced cholestasis resemble those of several hepatobiliary disorders, and it is therefore critical that clinicians take a thorough drug history from all patients with cholestasis. The prompt discontinuation of exposure to a causative agent prevents an adverse outcome and avoids unnecessary invasive investigations or surgery.

The clinical syndrome of cholestasis is indicated by pruritus, dark urine, pale stools, and, often, jaundice. It is typically reflected by liver tests that show a predominant elevation of serum alkaline phosphatase levels with lesser increases in ALT levels, elevation of other "biliary" enzymes such as GGTP and 5′-nucleotidase, raised serum bile acid levels, and conjugated hyperbilirubinemia. However, ALT may be elevated up to eightfold, either because of the toxic effects of acute bile retention on hepatocellular integrity or because of concomitant "hepatitis." In such cases, the ratio of the ALT to alkaline phosphatase level is important; it is typically less than 2:1 in cholestasis.[99, 258] Cases of *mixed cholestasis and hepatitis* are highly suggestive of a drug reaction.

Hepatobiliary imaging is essential to exclude dilation of large bile ducts produced by biliary obstruction and to exclude hepatic and pancreatic mass lesions. In the absence of such findings, drug-induced cholestasis is more likely, and a liver biopsy is often advisable. Certain histologic features suggest a hepatic drug reaction, whereas others (e.g., edema of the portal tracts) suggest biliary obstruction. When the temporal relationship to drug ingestion indicates a high probability of a drug reaction, particularly when the agent is known to be potentially hepatotoxic, it is appropriate to discontinue the incriminated drug and observe whether improvement occurs.

Management is confined to symptom relief, with particular attention to pruritus.[2, 258–260] Glucocorticoids have no role. Pruritus is often ameliorated with cholestyramine. Phenobarbital and antihistamines are usually ineffective or cause oversedation. In intractable cases, ursodeoxycholic acid has shown promise.[14, 260, 261] Rifampicin can be tried; phototherapy, plasmapheresis, and morphine receptor antagonists (e.g., nalorphine) have been used as third-line therapy.[260]

Cholestasis without Hepatitis

Reactions associated with cholestasis without hepatitis are characterized by the retention of bile in canaliculi, Kupffer cells, and hepatocytes, with minimal inflammation or hepatocellular necrosis. Synonyms are *pure, canalicular,* or *bland cholestasis*. Cholestasis without hepatitis reflects a primary disturbance in bile flow. Sex steroids are the typical causative agent. Some drugs more often associated with cholestatic hepatitis occasionally produce bland cholestasis (e.g., amoxicillin/clavulanic acid, sulfonamides, griseofulvin, ketoconazole, tamoxifen, warfarin, ibuprofen).[2, 258, 259] *Cyclosporine* is associated with liver test abnormalities; the features partly resemble cholestasis, but hyperbilirubinemia is usually predominant.[2] The reaction is mild and reverses rapidly with a reduction in dose.

Estrogen-Induced Cholestasis

Combination oral contraceptive steroids are associated with cholestasis that resembles cholestasis of pregnancy. In Western Europe, the frequency is approximately 1 per 10,000 exposed, whereas in Chile and Scandinavia, approximately 1 in 4000 women are affected.[262] The estrogenic component is most likely responsible; pure estrogens also may cause cholestasis. Estrogen-induced cholestasis can occur in women with a history of cholestasis of pregnancy and also has been observed in sisters, suggesting that there is a genetic predisposition. Studies in rats indicate that canalicular bile transporters may be implicated,[75–78] particularly MRP-2.[77] The reaction is partially dose-dependent and is less common with low-dose estrogen preparations. The onset is usually between 2 and 3 months after initial exposure but may occur up to 9 months after the start of estrogens. There may be a mild transient prodrome of nausea and malaise, followed by pruritus and jaundice. In the early stages, serum ALT levels may be elevated, but eventually the biochemical profile is typical of cholestasis. Liver biopsy is rarely required; it shows normal bile ducts and cholestasis but no portal or lobular inflammation. Recovery is usually prompt, but symptoms may occasionally take 4 to 10 weeks to resolve, and a few cases of chronic cholestasis have followed the use of estrogens, especially in combination with other drugs that cause cholestasis.[42]

Cholestasis with Hepatitis

Cholestasis with hepatitis is a common type of hepatic drug reaction characterized by conspicuous cholestasis and hepatocellular necrosis. Histologic lesions include lobular and portal tract inflammation, often with neutrophils and eosinophils as well as mononuclear cells. This type of reaction overlaps with drug-induced acute hepatitis (occasionally resulting in acute liver failure), cholestasis without hepatitis, and cholestasis with bile duct injury. Causative agents include chlorpromazine (see later), antidepressants and other psychotropic agents, erythromycins and other macrolide antibiotics,[263] sulfonamides,[2, 3] oxypenicillins,[2, 10, 259, 264–266] ketoconazole (discussed earlier),[192, 193] sulfonylureas,[2] sulindac,[267] ibuprofen,[151, 268] phenylbutazone,[244] piroxicam,[269] captopril,[270] flutamide,[271, 272] enalapril,[2] pravastatin,[273] atorvastatin,[274] ticlopidine,[275] ciprofloxacin,[276] norfloxacin,[277, 278] and metformin.[279]

Chlorpromazine

Chlorpromazine hepatitis, the prototypic drug-induced cholestatic hepatitis,[2, 258, 280] has been recognized since the 1950s, but cases still occur.[261] The full spectrum of hepatic reactions to chlorpromazine includes asymptomatic liver test abnormalities in 20% to 50% of those exposed and rare cases of fulminant hepatic failure. The frequency of cholestatic hepatitis varies from 0.2% to 2.0% depending on the study; the lower value is probably more representative of the risk in the general population.[2] There is no relationship to dose or underlying liver disease. Female predominance is evident. Reactions do not appear to be more common with increasing age but are rare in children.

The onset is 1 to 6 weeks after the start, or occasionally 5 to 14 days after discontinuation, of chlorpromazine. Accelerated onset occurs with rechallenge. A prodromal illness of fever and nonspecific symptoms is usual, followed by the development of gastrointestinal symptoms and jaundice. Pruritus is common, occurring later than in cholestasis without hepatitis. In a small proportion of patients, right upper quadrant abdominal pain is significant. Rash is infrequent. Liver tests show elevation of both ALT and alkaline phosphatase levels and hyperbilirubinemia. Eosinophilia is present in 10% to 40%. Most patients with chlorpromazine hepatitis recover completely, one third within 4 weeks, another third between 4 and 8 weeks, and the remainder after that time.[258, 280] In approximately 7%, full recovery has not occurred by 6 months (see later).

Amoxicillin/Clavulanic Acid (Augmentin)

More than 150 cases of cholestatic hepatitis have been reported in association with the use of amoxicillin/clavulanic acid, a commonly prescribed antibiotic. The overall frequency is 1 to 2 cases per 100,000 persons exposed[20]; men, those older than age 55 years, and possibly those taking the antibiotic for a prolonged period are at increased risk.[18, 281] It seems likely that the clavulanic acid component is responsible because amoxicillin rarely causes liver disease, whereas similar lesions have been noted with ticarcillin-clavulanic acid.[282, 283] The onset is from 1 to 6 weeks after starting the drug (mean, 18 days) to as long as 6 weeks after completing a course of amoxicillin/clavulanic acid. The illness is either a cholestatic hepatitis or drug-induced cholestasis with minimal hepatic inflammation. Granulomatous hepatitis has rarely been observed,[251] and one case of prolonged cholestasis with vanishing bile duct syndrome has been reported.[284] Liver biopsy shows cholestasis with mild portal inflammation and focal injury to interlobular bile ducts.[19, 285] The main clinical features are nausea, pruritus, jaundice, fever, and abdominal pain. Most patients recover completely in 4 to 16 weeks, but rare cases have had a fatal outcome[286] or led to vanishing bile duct syndrome, cirrhosis, and liver transplantation.[287] There is a strong association with the DRB1*1501-DRB5*0101-DQB1*062 haplotype, supporting the view that an immunologic idiosyncrasy mediated through HLA class II antigens could play a pathogenetic role in this form of drug-induced cholestatic hepatitis.[19, 35] However, the presence of this haplotype has no influence on the clinical characteristics, severity, and outcome of the disease.

Cholestatic Hepatitis with Bile Duct Injury

Bile duct (cholangiolytic) injury is observed with several drugs that cause cholestatic hepatitis, such as chlorpromazine[258, 280] and flucloxacillin.[14, 274] The severity of bile duct injury may be a determinant of the vanishing bile duct syndrome (see later).[288, 289] The clinical features may resemble those of bacterial cholangitis, with upper abdominal pain, fever, rigors, tender hepatomegaly, jaundice, and cholestasis. Liver tests are typical of cholestasis. Compounds associated with this syndrome include arsphenamine,[3] carbamazepine,[290] dextropropoxyphene,[291] and methylenediamine, an industrial toxin responsible for the Epping jaundice, which was an outbreak of jaundice associated with the ingestion of bread made from contaminated flour.[292]

Dextropropoxyphene

Dextropropoxyphene, an opioid analgesic used alone or in compound analgesics, caused cholestasis with bile duct injury in at least 25 reported cases,[14, 291] some proved by inadvertent rechallenge. There is a female predominance. The onset is usually less than 2 weeks after the start of dextropropoxyphene. It is often heralded by abdominal pain, which may be severe and simulate other causes of cholangitis. Jaundice is usual. The bile ducts are normal on cholangiography. Liver biopsy demonstrates cholestasis with expansion of the portal tracts by inflammation and mild fibrosis; portal tract edema also may be present. There is irregularity and necrosis of the biliary epithelium, together with close application of neutrophils and eosinophils to the outer surface of bile ducts. Bile ductular proliferation is universal. Recovery has occurred in all reported cases.[291] Liver tests normalize between 1 to 3 months of discontinuation of the drug. It is important to distinguish this type of hepatic drug reaction from bile duct obstruction and bacterial cholangitis.

CHRONIC CHOLESTASIS

Chronicity of drug-induced liver disease is considered to be present when typical biochemical changes last longer than 3 months[98, 99]; earlier definitions required the presence of jaundice for more than 6 months or anicteric cholestasis (raised serum alkaline phosphatase and GGTP levels) for more than 12 months after stopping the implicated agent.[258] Drug-induced chronic cholestasis is uncommon but has now been ascribed to more than 45 compounds.[2, 42, 258–260, 280, 289, 293, 294] Chronicity complicates approximately 7% of cases of chlorpromazine hepatitis[258, 261, 280] and is a feature in 10% to 30% of cases of flucloxacillin hepatitis.[2, 14, 259, 264] Chronicity has been reported in less than 5% of cases of erythromycin hepatitis,[260, 280, 293] and in only isolated instances for other agents, such as tetracycline,[294] amoxicillin/clavulanic acid,[284] ibuprofen,[268, 295] and trimethoprim-sulfamethoxazole.[296]

Chronic cholestasis is always preceded by an episode of acute cholestatic hepatitis. The episode tends to be severe, occasionally associated with the Stevens-Johnson syndrome,[2, 295] and one study indicated that the severity of bile duct lesions at the time of the initial hepatic reaction is a critical determinant of a chronic course.[288] Other possible mechanisms include continuing toxic or immunologic destruction of the biliary epithelium.[289] The histologic lesion is paucity of smaller (septal, interlobular) bile ducts and ductules, often with residual cholestasis, and portal tract inflammation focused on injured bile ducts. These changes may lead to an irreversible loss of biliary patency and the vanishing bile duct syndrome.[297]

The clinical features are those of chronic cholestasis. Pruritus is the dominant symptom; it is often severe. There may be continuing jaundice, dark urine, and pale stools, but these symptoms are not invariable and may resolve despite continuing biochemical abnormalities. In severe cases, malabsorption, weight loss, and bruising caused by vitamin K deficiency may occur; xanthelasma, tuberous xanthomas, and other complications of severe hypercholesterolemia also have been noted. Firm hepatomegaly may remain, but splenomegaly is unusual unless portal hypertension develops. Antimitochondrial antibodies are not a feature of drug-induced chronic cholestasis. Cases usually have a favorable outcome, with resolution of jaundice in most instances. Progression to biliary cirrhosis is rare[258, 259] and is associated with a severe reduction in the number of bile ducts.[92]

Flucloxacillin

Flucloxacillin is one of the most important causes of drug-induced cholestatic hepatitis in Europe, Scandinavia, and Australia.[2, 10, 14, 259, 264, 265] Flucloxacillin hepatotoxicity is usually severe, and several fatalities have resulted from the systemic features and associated cholestatic hepatitis. The course is prolonged, with a high proportion of cases progressing to chronic cholestasis and the vanishing bile duct syndrome.[10, 264] Other oxypenicillins appear less prone to cause this complication, but it has been reported with dicloxacillin and cloxacillin.[265, 266]

Fibrotic Bile Duct Strictures

Another type of drug-induced chronic cholestasis results from *fibrotic strictures of the larger bile ducts*. This complication has been associated with *intralesional therapy of hepatic hydatids* with formalin[298] and *intra-arterial infusion of floxuridine* for metastatic colorectal carcinoma.[289, 299] After several months of floxuridine infusion, the frequency of toxic hepatitis, bile duct injury, or both, is 25% to 55%. Acalculous cholecystitis is another complication.[2] Cholangiography shows strictures, typically in the common hepatic duct and the left and right hepatic ducts. Unlike idiopathic sclerosing cholangitis, there is sparing of the common bile duct and the smaller intrahepatic bile ducts. Ischemia has been a suspected pathogenetic factor,[2, 268] but toxicity to biliary epithelial cells is another possibility. Recovery may occur after discontinuation of infusion therapy. Other cases require dilation or stenting of biliary strictures.

LIVER DISEASE CAUSED BY ANESTHETIC AGENTS AND JAUNDICE IN THE POSTOPERATIVE PERIOD

Postoperative jaundice has become uncommon with modern techniques of anesthesia and resuscitation and more accurate preoperative diagnosis of hepatobiliary disease. It may be caused by an underlying hepatobiliary disorder or by abnormalities resulting from tissue hypoxia or systemic infection (see also Chapters 14 and 64). The topic is considered here because adverse reactions to an anesthetic agent or other drugs are possible causes of liver disease in the postoperative period. Most interest has centered around halothane, a highly effective, safe, pleasant, and convenient anesthetic that is rarely associated with severe liver injury. This section describes halothane-induced liver injury and its nature and preventability and discusses whether other haloalkane anesthetics are hepatotoxic.

Halothane-Induced Liver Injury

Halothane was introduced in the 1950s. Its initial safety and efficacy records were so impressive that early reports of possible hepatotoxicity were treated with skepticism. Indeed, the National Halothane Study confirmed that halothane was at least as safe as other anesthetic agents, even when used for patients with underlying hepatobiliary disease.[300] Most cases of postoperative massive liver necrosis were readily attributable to nonanesthetic causes, such as shock and hypoxia, but cases of *unexplained massive hepatic necrosis after anesthesia* appeared to be more common after halothane than after the use of other agents.[300] The reproducible clinical syndrome, characteristic temporal relationships, and, in particular, observations from deliberate or inadvertent rechallenge led eventually to the acceptance that *halothane hepatitis* is a real entity.[2] Rare cases of halothane-induced liver injury also have occurred after workplace exposure among anesthetists, surgeons, nurses, and laboratory staff, and after halothane sniffing for "recreational" use. Despite its rarity, the severity of cases of halothane hepatitis has led to the virtual abandonment of halothane in many centers, perhaps prematurely in light of its other advantages (especially in children) and lower cost. Mechanistic studies continue to be of interest, as halothane is a model idiosyncratic hepatotoxin.

General Nature, Frequency, and Predisposing Factors

Two types of postoperative liver injury are associated with use of halothane. Minor elevations in the serum ALT level occur between the first and tenth postoperative day in 10% to 20% of patients; the risk is higher after a second use of halothane than with subsequent use of agents like enflurane, isoflurane, and desflurane.[2, 301, 302] There are no symptoms, and the change in liver tests is rapidly reversible. The explanation is unclear, as is the relationship to the more severe lesions of halothane hepatitis. Severe halothane-induced hepatotoxicity (halothane hepatitis) is a rare, dose-independent hepatic drug reaction. After one exposure to halothane anesthetic, the frequency is low (0.3 to 1.5 per 10,000 exposed persons), but after two or more exposures within a 28-day period, the frequency increases to 15 per 10,000 exposed persons.[2, 126, 127] There is often zonal, bridging, or panlobular necrosis, and the mortality rate is between 10% and 50%.[2, 303, 304] The reaction is unrelated to the type of surgery, duration of anesthesia, or preexisting liver disease.

RISK FACTORS. Several risk factors have been identified.[2] The reaction is extremely rare in childhood and more severe in persons over age 40 years. Two thirds of cases are in women. Repeated exposure to halothane, especially within a relatively short period of time, is a feature in 80% of cases, and many patients give a history of previous *unexplained, delayed-onset fever, nausea, or jaundice in the postoperative period.* After repeat exposure, the onset is earlier, and the severity typically increases with each exposure. Obesity is another risk factor, possibly related to increased storage of halothane or induction of hepatic CYP2E1, an enzyme involved in halothane metabolism. The induction of CYP enzymes has been implicated experimentally in the pathogenesis of halothane-induced liver injury, and one study indicated that coadministration of antiepileptics predisposes patients to halothane hepatitis.[305] A genetic predisposition to halothane-induced liver injury is evident in guinea pigs, and there are data in humans to invoke familial predisposition, such as instances of several closely related family members who experience halothane hepatitis.[32] Likewise, with the use of an in vitro test to detect injury to peripheral blood mononuclear cells after exposure to phenytoin epoxide, increased susceptibility was noted among the relatives of patients with halothane hepatitis, as well as in the patients themselves.[306]

Clinical and Laboratory Features

Fever is common in the first 48 hours after any major surgery, but fever associated with an adverse reaction to halothane is typically delayed in onset (5 to 14 days). It may be associated with chills and rigors; occasionally a rash is noted. Jaundice occurs within 21 days of halothane exposure; the median time to onset is 9 days after a single anesthetic exposure and 5 days after multiple exposures. Jaundice is usually preceded or accompanied by symptoms of hepatitis. The liver may be swollen and tender, but in severe cases it decreases in size as a result of extensive hepatic necrosis. Liver failure is then present, with bruising, bleeding, and clouding of consciousness.

Liver tests indicate severe hepatocellular necrosis; serum ALT levels typically exceed 1000 U/L and may be much higher. The serum bilirubin level is increased according to severity, and the prothrombin time is prolonged in severe cases. In liver failure, hypoglycemia and metabolic acidosis occur, and in the terminal phase, the serum ALT level decreases as a result of impaired hepatic protein synthesis and loss of hepatic parenchyma. Leukocytosis is a nonspecific feature of severe hepatic necrosis that is present in some patients; eosinophilia has been reported in 10% to 30%. Bone marrow suppression is rare. Renal failure may develop as part of the hepatorenal syndrome, but acute tubular necrosis may result from a nephrotoxic effect of halothane, as has been better documented for methoxyflurane.

Liver Histology

In nonfatal cases, focal necrosis and a portal tract infiltrate are present. Bridging or zonal necrosis is common in severe cases, and confluent (massive) necrosis is noted at autopsy. Hepatocellular regeneration may also be present. Hepatic granulomas, steatosis, cholestasis, and predominant eosinophils are seen occasionally, but features of chronic hepatitis with hepatic fibrosis are rare.[307, 308] It is unclear whether these are cases of repeated halothane exposure with continuing or intermittent liver injury[307] or cases of chronic hepatitis attributable to other etiologies and exacerbated by surgery and anesthesia.

Course and Outcome

In milder cases, symptoms may not be attributed to a halothane reaction. Thus, it is crucial to take a full history of earlier anesthetic exposures to prevent fatal cases of halothane-induced liver injury. In more severe cases, hepatic failure may follow a fulminant course, and in many countries halothane was the leading cause of drug-induced liver failure other than acetaminophen poisoning until the mid-1980s.

The reported mortality rate is 10% to 80%, but the higher rates reflect referral to specialized centers.[304, 306] When recovery occurs, symptoms usually resolve within 5 to 14 days, and recovery is usually complete. Rare cases in which halothane was implicated as the cause of chronic liver disease have been reported, as discussed earlier.[2, 307, 308]

Prevention and Management

There is no specific treatment. Although an immunologic mechanism has been invoked,[88, 89, 91] immunosuppressive agents do not alter the outcome. Management centers around intensive medical support. Liver transplantation must be considered in cases with a poor prognosis, as presaged by previous episodes, early onset, a serum bilirubin level of more than 200 μmol/L (10 mg/dL), and prolongation of the prothrombin time.

In many countries, anesthesiologists have virtually abandoned halothane in favor of the equally well-tolerated (for induction of anesthesia) sevoflurane and desflurane or isoflurane, but halothane is occasionally used in children. In adults, halothane-induced liver disease could have been prevented in 90% of reported cases by attention to the previous history and adherence to safety guidelines. As many as two thirds of cases occur in persons with a history of previous reactions to halothane, and the majority of cases are associated with repeated use of halothane within 28 days, especially in obese, middle-aged women. Because halothane may leach out of the tubing of anesthetic devices, prevention of recurrence in sensitized patients requires that the equipment used for anesthesia should never have been exposed to halothane. Cross-sensitivity between halothane and other haloalkane anesthetics is best documented for methoxyflurane, an agent that is no longer in use. Cross-sensitivity with enflurane and possibly isoflurane is possible, as described later, but has not been reported for desflurane and sevoflurane.

Differential Diagnosis of Jaundice in the Postoperative Period

Although much interest has surrounded use of an antibody test that is claimed to be 80% sensitive,[88] there is no readily available diagnostic test for halothane hepatitis. The diagnosis of halothane hepatitis therefore requires a careful consideration of the present and past relationships of liver injury to halothane exposure and rests on the exclusion of other causes of liver disease in the postoperative period, as summarized in Table 73–7 (see also Chapters 14 and 64). Besides drug-induced liver injury, postoperative liver disease may be caused by unrecognized underlying liver disease, mechanical obstruction of the bile ducts, hepatic dysfunction related indirectly to surgery and anesthesia (e.g., reduction in hepatic blood flow causing ischemic hepatitis or ischemia/reperfusion injury),[309] and the syndrome of *benign postoperative cholestasis*.[2, 310] The latter is likely to be identical to jaundice observed in critically ill patients. Predisposing factors include severe sepsis, multiple trauma, hypoxia, blood transfusion, and repeated and prolonged operations, particularly abdominal, trauma, or cardiac surgery. Jaundice is noted 2 to 4 days after surgery and peaks at 3 to 10 days. The remarkable feature of the liver tests is hyperbilirubinemia. Values may be extremely high, even exceeding 500 μmol/L (25 mg/dL) if renal failure is also present. In contrast, other liver tests such as the ALT and alkaline phosphatase are minimally abnormal, tests of synthetic function are normal, and there are no clinical features of liver failure, such as ascites, coagulopathy, and encephalopathy.

Other Agents

Methoxyflurane caused hepatotoxicity similar to halothane hepatitis, with cross-sensitivity to halothane and a high frequency of nephrotoxicity that led to its withdrawal.[2, 3] General anesthetic agents in use other than halothane have rarely been associated with postoperative liver failure and massive hepatic necrosis. However, the evidence that such agents cause idiosyncratic hepatic drug reactions is strong only for *enflurane*.[2, 311, 312] The likelihood that individual haloalkane anesthetics can cause liver injury appears to be related to the extent to which they are metabolized by hepatic CYP enzymes: 20% for halothane, 2% for enflurane, 1% for sevoflurane, and 0.2% or less for isoflurane and desflurane. Likewise, the extent of acylation of hepatic proteins in rats exposed to anesthetic concentrations of these agents for 8 hours was greatest for halothane, followed by enflurane, isoflurane, desflurane, and oxygen (which did not differ from each other).[313] Accordingly, the estimated frequency of enflurane-related hepatitis is much less than that for halothane.

Table 73–7 | **Causes of Jaundice in the Postoperative Period**

CAUSE	DIAGNOSTIC CLUES
Unrecognized preexisting liver disease: Hepatitis B or C Autoimmune hepatitis Cirrhosis: alcoholic, primary biliary, NASH, and others	History, features of chronic liver disease, liver tests; specific diagnostic tests, hepatitis serology, autoantibodies, serum lipids, blood glucose, hepatic imaging (see Chapters 68 and 75)
Post-transfusion hepatitis	Appropriate incubation period (usually >3 wk), now rare; use of hepatitis serology and viral studies (e.g., HCV RNA)
Ischemic hepatitis (ischemia-reperfusion injury)	Documentation of profound and prolonged hypoxemia or shock; type of surgery (hepatic resections, cardiac, trauma); short latent period; very high ALT levels (>2000 U/L)
Drug-induced liver disease: Anesthetics: halothane, enflurane, isoflurane, others? Others (e.g., antibiotics, acetaminophen, dextropropoxyphene, neuroleptic agents, herbal medicines)	History, risk factors; onset 2 to 20 days; clinicopathologic syndrome relevant to individual agents
Extrahepatic biliary obstruction	Type of surgery; later onset, presence of cholestasis; dilated biliary tree on biliary imaging (e.g., ultrasonography, MRCP, or ERCP)
Benign postoperative cholestasis (jaundice in critically ill patients)	Clinical setting: critically ill patient, sepsis, multiple trauma, blood transfusion; onset 2–4 days; liver tests: very high bilirubin levels, other tests normal or minimally elevated; no biliary obstruction, no liver failure

ALT, alanine aminotransferase; ERCP, endoscopic retrograde cholangiopancreatography; HCV, hepatitis C virus; MRCP, magnetic resonance cholangiopancreatography; NASH, nonalcoholic steatohepatitis; RNA, ribonucleic acid.

The clinical syndrome is similar to that for halothane, with onset of fever within 3 days and jaundice in 3 to 19 days; at least one case has been proved by positive rechallenge.[311] Two thirds of patients had previously been exposed to either enflurane or halothane.

ISOFLURANE. The possibility that *isoflurane* could be responsible for drug-induced liver injury is more contentious. More than 50 suspected cases had been reported to the FDA by 1986, but in two thirds of these cases another potential cause of liver injury was more likely.[314] In the remainder, isoflurane was only one of several possible factors that could have caused hepatic damage. During the 1990s, there were a small number of case reports in which isoflurane seemed to be the likely cause of fatal hepatotoxicity, because of repeated exposure to isoflurane in the absence of other potential causes of liver injury[315–320] or because isoflurane had been administered after possible previous sensitization to halothane[321] or enflurane.[322] Isoflurane should be regarded as a possible but rare cause of hepatotoxicity; the pathogenic mechanism remains unclear.

The newer haloalkane anesthetics sevoflurane and desflurane appear to be essentially free of adverse hepatic events, although rare isolated reports have noted an association between liver injury and desflurane anesthesia, none of which have been proven by rechallenge.[323, 324]

DRUG-INDUCED STEATOHEPATITIS, HEPATIC FIBROSIS, AND CIRRHOSIS

Drug-induced liver disease can produce cirrhosis by a variety of processes; chronic hepatitis and chronic cholestasis with the vanishing bile duct syndrome have already been discussed. *Steatohepatitis* is a form of chronic liver disease in which fatty change is associated with focal liver cell injury, Mallory's hyaline, focal inflammation of mixed cellularity, including polymorphonuclear leukocytes, and progressive hepatic fibrosis in a pericentral and pericellular distribution[325] (see Chapters 71 and 72). Alcohol is a common etiology. NASH can be associated with diabetes, obesity, and several drugs (e.g., perhexiline maleate[64] and amiodarone; see later).[326] In addition to steatohepatitis or chronic injury to liver cells or bile ducts, some foreign compounds appear to promote hepatic fibrogenesis directly, most likely through effects on hepatic nonparenchymal cells. Stellate (fat-storing or Ito) cells are central to this process (see Chapter 71). Compounds that stimulate hepatic fibrosis include arsenic, vitamin A, and methotrexate (discussed later).

Amiodarone-Induced Liver Disease

Amiodarone is an iodinated benzofuran derivative used for therapy-resistant ventricular tachyarrhythmias. Adverse effects lead to discontinuation of therapy in 25% of patients and include pulmonary infiltrates, worsening cardiac failure, hypothyroidism, peripheral neuropathy, nephrotoxicity, and corneal deposits, but liver disease is one of the most serious. The spectrum of abnormalities includes abnormal liver tests in 15% to 80% of patients and clinically significant liver disease in 0.6%, including rare cases of acute liver failure.[327–330, 331] The most typical lesion is steatohepatitis; cirrhosis is present in 15% to 50% of persons with steatohepatitis.[327, 328]

A feature that differs from most other types of drug-induced liver disease is that progression of the disease may occur despite discontinuation of amiodarone.[2, 328, 332] Amiodarone is highly concentrated in the liver, and after a few weeks of treatment, the drug accounts for as much as 1% of the wet weight of the liver. The iodine content absorbs radiation, so that the liver appears opaque on computed tomography.[331] Although odd, this appearance is not clinically significant. Hepatic storage of amiodarone also produces phospholipidosis, a storage disorder characterized by enlarged lysosomes stuffed with whorled membranous material *(myeloid bodies)*.[92] In animals fed amiodarone, development of phospholipidosis is time- and dose-dependent.[329] It may result from the direct inhibition of phospholipase or from the formation of nondegradable drug-phospholipid complexes but appears to have no relationship to NASH and hepatocyte injury. Other occasional hepatic abnormalities include granulomas and acute liver failure, apparently caused by severe acute hepatitis or a Reye's syndrome–like illness.[2, 333] Amiodarone is concentrated in mitochondria by virtue of its physicochemical properties and may interrupt mitochondrial electron transport.[334] Thus, in rats and mice, treatment with amiodarone has produced microvesicular steatosis, augmented mitochondrial production of ROS, and caused lipid peroxidation.[335, 336]

Chronic liver disease may be detected 1 year or more after starting amiodarone (median, 21 months). There is a relationship between the occurrence of chronic liver disease and the duration of amiodarone therapy and possibly the total dose,[333, 337] but there is no clear relationship to the incremental dose. However, the frequency of other toxic effects of amiodarone (most are thought to be dose dependent) is increased in patients with liver disease.[337] Patients may complain of fatigue, nausea and vomiting, malaise, weight loss, or abdominal swelling as a result of ascites. Hepatomegaly, jaundice, bruising, and other features of chronic liver disease may be present. Liver test abnormalities include increased serum aminotransferase levels, most often to at least fivefold the upper limit of normal, and minor increases in the serum alkaline phosphatase. The ratio of AST to ALT is close to unity, a finding that differs from that of alcoholic hepatitis. In severe cases, hyperbilirubinemia, low serum albumin levels, and prolongation of the prothrombin time are evident. It is often difficult to determine the cause of abnormal liver tests and hepatomegaly in patients taking amiodarone, and a liver biopsy is then indicated. The histologic changes include phospholipidosis, steatosis, focal necrosis with Mallory's hyaline, infiltration with polymorphonuclear leukocytes, and pericellular fibrosis.[92, 328] Cirrhosis is often present.

Prevention and management of amiodarone-induced liver disease are problematic because liver test abnormalities are common in patients taking amiodarone, particularly in patients with cardiac failure. In asymptomatic or less severe cases, features resolve in 2 weeks to 4 months. In cases of severe liver disease, the mortality rate is high.[328, 337] Cessation of amiodarone therapy does not always result in clinical improvement, presumably because of prolonged hepatic storage of amiodarone, and in one study, the outcome was worse (usually from fatal arrhythmias) in those who stopped therapy.[328] Thus, although serial liver tests are recommended in those taking amiodarone,[337] it is not known whether testing will prevent significant hepatotoxicity.

Tamoxifen and Other Causes of Drug-Induced Steatohepatitis

Perhexiline maleate and *coralgil (4,4′-diethylaminoethoxyhexestrol)* are definite toxic causes of steatohepatitis but have been withdrawn.[2, 3, 326] Among agents associated with steatosis and steatohepatitis during the 1990s, causality is harder to prove,[326] particularly because steatosis is a common disorder among patients with insulin resistance or metabolic syndrome (syndrome X) (see Chapter 72). Thus, calcium channel blockers used for arterial hypertension or cardiac arrhythmias have rarely been associated with steatohepatitis[338, 339]; and methyldopa has been reported in association with NASH and cirrhosis in obese middle-aged women,[340] but this association may have been fortuitous. Other drugs, including estrogens[341] and glucocorticoids,[342] may precipitate fatty liver or NASH in persons predisposed because of their effects on the risk factors: insulin resistance, type 2 diabetes, obesity, and hypertriglyceridemia. The association between NASH and *tamoxifen* appears to be much stronger.

Tamoxifen is an estrogen receptor ligand with both agonist and antagonist actions and is widely used in the prevention and treatment of breast cancer. Several forms of liver injury have been attributed to tamoxifen[343]: cholestasis,[344] hepatocellular carcinoma,[345] peliosis hepatis,[346] acute hepatitis, massive hepatic necrosis,[343] steatosis, and NASH, occasionally with cirrhosis.[326, 347–353] In one series of 66 women with breast cancer who had received tamoxifen for 3 to 5 years, 24 showed radiologic evidence of hepatic steatosis.[350] Seven others were diagnosed with NASH after taking tamoxifen for 7 to 33 months.[348, 349, 351]

The metabolic profile of women in whom radiologic evidence of hepatic steatosis (or histologic proof of NASH) develops while taking tamoxifen appears similar to those of most patients with NASH; one half are obese, and raised body mass index (BMI) correlates with hepatic steatosis among women taking tamoxifen.[354] Tamoxifen also can induce hypertriglyceridemia, another risk factor for NASH, and in two women, treatment with bezafibrate, a PPARα stimulator, led to a marked decrease in steatosis as assessed radiologically.[354] It therefore seems possible that tamoxifen may play a synergistic role with other factors like hyperlipidemia, obesity, and insulin resistance to cause fatty liver or NASH. Physicians need to be aware of the apparent high frequency (approximately 30%) of hepatic steatosis, as determined by hepatic imaging, or NASH in women treated with tamoxifen. Monitoring patients for this adverse effect should include physical examination for hepatomegaly and liver tests, and some researchers have recommended that hepatic imaging (ultrasonography or computed tomography) be performed on an annual basis.[355] Liver biopsy may be required to establish the severity of the disorder, particularly if liver test abnormalities fail to resolve after discontinuation of tamoxifen, or to exclude metastatic breast cancer in difficult cases. Many cases seem to improve after discontinuation of tamoxifen, but it is not yet clear whether treatment should always be withdrawn permanently.

Toremifene, an analogue of tamoxifen, has also been reported to cause steatosis or steatohepatitis. However, the frequency is lower (less than 10%) than with tamoxifen.[355]

Methotrexate-Induced Hepatic Fibrosis

Methotrexate is a dose-dependent toxin. In higher doses, it produces bone marrow suppression, mucocutaneous reactions, pneumonitis, and hepatotoxicity. In the 1950s, it became apparent that previous methotrexate treatment of leukemia caused severe hepatic fibrosis and cirrhosis[2, 3]; a few cases were complicated by hepatocellular carcinoma.[356] In the 1960s, the use of methotrexate for psoriasis was associated with development of hepatic fibrosis and cirrhosis in as many as 25% of cases.[357] A clearer picture of methotrexate as a dose-dependent promoter of hepatic fibrosis emerged, particularly in persons who drank alcohol to excess or had preexisting liver disease. Strict guidelines were instituted for scheduled pretreatment and interval liver biopsies to monitor the safety of methotrexate therapy. The problem of methotrexate-induced cirrhosis has now been overcome in large part by the avoidance of daily dosing with methotrexate and the reduction in weekly treatment regimens to doses of 5 to 15 mg.[358–360]

Risk Factors

Risk factors for methotrexate-induced hepatic fibrosis are listed in Table 73–8. Dose, alcohol intake, and preexisting liver disease are the most significant.[359, 360] Total dose, incremental dose, dose interval, and duration of methotrexate therapy each influence the risk of hepatic fibrosis. After cumulative ingestion of 3 g, there is a 20% chance of histologic progression, but only 3% of patients have advanced histologic abnormalities.[360] Obesity and diabetes mellitus may be important because they predispose to NASH and are associated with induction of CYP2E1. Increasing age, impaired renal function, and other drugs decrease the elimination of methotrexate or facilitate tissue uptake by displacing methotrexate from plasma protein binding sites. Psoriasis and rheumatoid arthritis are associated with hepatic abnormalities that vary from abnormal liver tests (in 25% to 50% of cases) and minor histologic changes (50% to 70%) to fibrosis (11% of patients with psoriasis) and cirrhosis (1% in patients with psoriasis). In psoriasis, alcoholism is often a complicating factor. In a meta-analysis,[360] alcohol was the most important determinant of significant hepatic fibrosis in patients treated with methotrexate; the risk of progressive hepatic fibrosis was 73% in patients who drank more than 15 g of alcohol daily, compared with 26% in those who did not.

The possibility that low-dose (5 to 15 mg) methotrexate given as a single weekly dose can cause hepatic fibrosis has been debated.[10, 358–360] The available data are limited by a lack of controlled studies with pretreatment liver histology; the latter is a particularly serious deficiency given the high frequency of liver abnormalities among patients with rheumatoid arthritis. It appears that regimens that are currently in use can promote hepatic fibrosis, at least at the ultrastructural level, but cases of clinically significant liver disease are now virtually unknown. Indeed, repeat biopsies in some series have shown a reduction in fibrosis despite continuation of methotrexate in lower doses.[361] Thus, although methotrexate remains a potential cause of liver disease, significant hepatic fibrosis is in large part preventable.

Clinicopathologic Features

Abnormal liver tests are common among patients taking methotrexate, but significant hepatic fibrosis occasionally can develop without such abnormalities. Likewise, nausea, fatigue, and abdominal pain are common adverse effects of methothrexate, but patients with hepatic fibrosis are typically asymptomatic unless complications of liver failure or portal hypertension, such as bleeding esophageal varices, develop. A firm liver edge, hepatomegaly, splenomegaly, or ascites may be noted. Liver tests are either normal or show nonspe-

Table 73–8 | **Risk Factors for Methotrexate-Induced Hepatic Fibrosis**

RISK FACTOR	IMPORTANCE	IMPLICATIONS FOR PREVENTION
Age	Increased risk >60 yr; possibly related to renal clearance and/or biologic effect on fibrogenesis	Greater care in use of methotrexate in older people
Dose	Incremental dose Dose frequency Duration of therapy Cumulative (total) dose	5–15 mg/wk very safe Weekly bolus (pulse) safer than daily schedules Consider review of hepatic status each 2–3 yr Review hepatic status after each 2 g of methotrexate
Alcohol consumption	Increased risk with daily levels of >15 g (1 to 2 drinks)	Avoid methotrexate use if intake not curbed Consider pretreatment liver biopsy with relevant history
Obesity	Increased risk	Consider pretreatment and interval liver biopsies
Diabetes mellitus	Increased risk if obese (type 2 diabetes)	Consider pretreatment and interval liver biopsies
Preexisting liver disease	Greatly increased risk Particularly related to alcohol, obesity, and diabetes (NASH)	Pretreatment liver biopsy mandatory Avoid methotrexate, or schedule interval biopsies according to severity of hepatic fibrosis, total dose, and duration of methotrexate therapy Conduct monitoring liver tests during therapy (see text)
Systemic disease	Possibly risk greater with psoriasis than rheumatoid arthritis (may depend on preexisting liver disease, alcohol)	None
Impaired renal function	Increased risk because of reduced clearance of methotrexate	Reduce dose; greater caution with use
Other drugs	Possibly NSAIDs increase risk; vitamin A, arsenic may increase risk	Greater caution with use; liver test monitoring

NASH, nonalcoholic steatohepatitis; NSAIDs, nonsteroidal anti-inflammatory drugs.

cific changes, including minor elevations of the ALT and GGTP. In more advanced cases, hypoalbuminemia is present, but elevation of serum bilirubin levels and coagulation disturbances are rare. Thrombocytopenia may be present in cases with cirrhosis.

Liver histology is often graded according to the system of Roenigk, which has been useful in analyzing the published literature.[92, 360] The features vary from minor hepatocellular abnormalities of steatosis, nuclear pleomorphism, and focal degeneration and inflammation to Kupffer cell proliferation, stellate cell enlargement, and varying degrees of portal, periportal, pericellular, and bridging fibrosis (Roenigk grade 3b) and cirrhosis (Roenigk grade 4). Most pathologists have interpreted the hepatic fibrosis as developing in the absence of conspicuous portal and periportal inflammation, but rare cases have been ascribed to the histologic lesion of "chronic active hepatitis," whereas other observers have considered the lesions to resemble steatohepatitis.[362]

Outcome and Prevention

Serious clinical sequelae (portal hypertension, liver failure, hepatocellular carcinoma) caused by methotrexate-induced liver disease are now rarely seen. Cases that have come to liver transplantation generally have been associated with suboptimal supervision of methotrexate therapy.[363] Cases of severe hepatic fibrosis (Roenigk grades 3b and 4) are often associated with lack of progression and even improvement after discontinuation of methotrexate or a reduction in the dose.[361] In less severe cases, a balanced judgment must be made about the appropriateness of continuing or discontinuing methotrexate. A scheduled liver biopsy after an additional 2 years or 2 g of methotrexate may be judicious in a patient who is found to have minor fibrosis. Recommendations for preventing methotrexate-induced hepatic fibrosis have been made.[359, 364] If at all possible, methotrexate should be avoided when the risk of liver injury is high. Persons should abstain from alcohol use during treatment, and those who drink more than 100 g of ethanol per week should not be given methotrexate.[359, 360, 364] Pretreatment liver biopsy is indicated only if the liver tests are abnormal or if the history (e.g., of alcoholism) and clinical features (e.g., hepatomegaly) indicate possible underlying liver disease.[10]

The use of liver tests to monitor progress is recommended but is problematic because of their lack of specificity and sensitivity; 4 to 6 sets of liver tests each year are often performed in patients taking methotrexate. Persistent or recurrent elevations in serum AST or ALT levels, any decrease in the serum albumin level, and development of hepatomegaly each warrant investigation by liver biopsy.[10] It is recommended that scheduled liver biopsies be performed after 4 g of methotrexate or 2 years of treatment,[360] but whether a biopsy is necessary in patients with normal liver tests and without major risk factors remains unclear.[361, 364] Biochemical tests that indicate progressive hepatic fibrosis, such as procollagen peptide-3, have not proved sufficiently accurate for monitoring use of methotrexate.[2]

VASCULAR TOXICITY

Vascular injury gives rise to several unusual types of liver disease, including hepatic venous outflow obstruction, dilation and destruction of hepatic sinusoids (peliosis hepatis), noncirrhotic portal hypertension, and nodular regenerative hyperplasia. Drugs and chemical toxins are the most common cause of hepatic vascular injury.[23, 343, 365] The mechanism is primarily dose-dependent toxicity to sinusoidal and other vascular endothelial cells, but additional risk factors include interactions between drugs used in combination and concurrent radiotherapy. Activation of inflammatory cells, such as those of the immune system, also may be important. Individual drugs have been associated with more than one vascular syndrome (e.g., azathioprine, described later). There is overlap among individual disorders, which may evolve from one type to another, and vascular injury may give rise to a continuum of disorders, each resulting from injury in different components of the hepatic vasculature. The essential features of these disorders are summarized in Table 73–9, and the more important conditions are described later.

Table 73–9 | **Types of Drug-Induced Hepatic Vascular Disorders: Clinicopathologic Features and Major Etiologic Agents**

DISORDER	CLINICOPATHOLOGIC FEATURES AND OUTCOME	IMPLICATED ETIOLOGIC AGENTS
Veno-occlusive disease	Abdominal pain, tender hepatomegaly, ascites, liver failure; occasionally chronic liver disease, portal hypertension, ascites; high mortality, possibly some cases evolve into nodular regenerative hyperplasia	Especially in bone marrow transplantation: 6-thioguanine, busulfan; dactinomycin, azathioprine, mitomycin; pyrrolizidine alkaloids (e.g., in comfrey)
Nodular regenerative hyperplasia	Portal hypertension, encephalopathy, especially after variceal bleeding; diagnosed by histology; relatively good prognosis	Anticancer drugs: busulfan, dactinomycin; azathioprine
Noncirrhotic portal hypertension	Splenomegaly, hypersplenism, varices; ascites if associated hepatocellular disease; prognosis depends on cause and associated liver injury	Vitamin A, methotrexate, azathioprine, arsenic, vinyl chloride, anticancer drugs
Peliosis hepatis	Incidental finding, hepatomegaly, hepatic rupture, liver failure; diagnosed from appearances at surgery, vascular imaging; prognosis depends on cause and complications	Anabolic steroids, azathioprine, 6-thioguanine
Sinusoidal dilatation	Hepatomegaly, abdominal pain; may regress after stopping oral contraceptives	Oral contraceptive steroids

Hepatic imaging and measurement of portal venous pressure play a role in the diagnosis of these conditions, some of which are difficult to confirm in needle biopsy specimens.

Veno-occlusive Disease

Veno-occlusive disease is a form of hepatic venous outflow obstruction that results from nonthrombotic occlusion of the terminal hepatic venules and small intrahepatic veins (see also Chapters 27 and 70). It results from endothelial damage, with intimal edema and thickening and fragmentation of the venular wall. Hepatic veno-occlusive disease is the commonest type of drug-induced vascular injury and is often fatal. More than 20 drugs and toxic alkaloids have been identified as causative agents; all contain a strong alkylating agent that can destroy the vascular endothelium as well as surrounding hepatocytes. Hepatotoxicity is, at least in part, dose dependent.[366] Veno-occlusive disease complicates at least 1% of cases during use of anticancer drugs, and risks as high as 54% have been reported after bone marrow transplantation, depending on the regimen used.[47, 145, 366, 367] Pyrrolizidine alkaloids are another important cause.[368, 369]

The onset is 2 to 10 weeks after starting therapy. Patients usually present with abdominal pain and hepatomegaly, and their condition is rapidly complicated by acute liver failure, jaundice, ascites, and severe coagulopathy. Other cases may resemble the acute Budd-Chiari syndrome, with tender hepatomegaly and ascites caused by acute portal hypertension (see Chapter 70). Liver tests reflect acute hepatocellular necrosis, secondary to hepatic ischemia and congestion, and liver failure. The results of hepatic imaging may be similar to those for the Budd-Chiari syndrome,[2] except that patency of the large hepatic veins can be demonstrated (e.g., by Doppler ultrasonography or magnetic resonance imaging). Most cases are not confirmed histologically because of the severe coagulation disturbance. There is no specific treatment. The prognosis has generally been regarded as poor, with death occurring within a few weeks in most patients with liver failure. Recovery is possible, however, particularly in less severe cases. It has been suggested that some cases diagnosed as veno-occlusive disease on clinical grounds may actually be instances of nodular regenerative hyperplasia (see later). Alternatively, nodular regenerative hyperplasia may evolve during recovery from veno-occlusive disease. Veno-occlusive disease can sometimes give rise to a chronic form of hepatic venous outflow obstruction complicated by portal hypertension and cirrhosis, as originally documented for pyrrolizidine alkaloids consumed in Jamaican bush teas[2, 3] and later in comfrey.[368, 369]

Nodular Regenerative Hyperplasia

Nodular regenerative hyperplasia is characterized by the presence of regenerative nodules in the absence of hepatic fibrosis (see also Chapter 82). The critical lesion is obliterative portal venopathy (i.e., obstruction to terminal radicals of hepatic arterioles and portal venules, possibly secondary to endothelial cell damage). The resulting hepatic ischemia may be responsible for induction of the nodular regenerative change. Nodular regenerative hyperplasia is associated with myeloproliferative and immunologic disorders (see Chapter 82), but cases attributed to the use of anticancer drugs and azathioprine are well documented (see Table 73–9).[343] Nodular regenerative hyperplasia appears to be the cause of portal hypertension among patients with chronic myeloid leukemia who received both busulfan and thioguanine.[370] Among 103 patients undergoing bone marrow transplantation, nodular regenerative hyperplasia was found in 23%, and veno-occlusive disease was found in 9% (see Chapter 27).[371]

The clinical features are those of portal hypertension, often complicated by bleeding esophageal varices. After an episode of severe upper gastrointestinal hemorrhage, hepatic encephalopathy may occur. Liver tests may be normal or show minor nonspecific changes. The diagnosis is made histologically, although a wedge biopsy may be required. In general, the prognosis for nodular regenerative hyperplasia is good; complete reversibility may occur in some drug-induced cases.[371]

Noncirrhotic Portal Hypertension

Noncirrhotic portal hypertension induced by drugs is usually the result of obstruction of the portal vein or its terminal branches (see "Nodular Regenerative Hyperplasia"), hepatic venous outflow obstruction (see "Veno-occlusive Disease"), or compression, damage, and distortion of the hepatic sinusoids (see also Chapter 77). Such distortion may result from processes other than cirrhosis, including compression from swollen hepatocytes and perisinusoidal cells. A variable extent of perisinusoidal fibrosis is usual. Cases with more extensive hepatic fibrosis that apparently arises from the portal tracts *(hepatoportal sclerosis)* may be a variant of this type of injury. Agents associated with noncirrhotic portal hypertension include vitamin A (see later), azathioprine,[343] methotrexate, cytotoxic agents,[145] arsenic,[372] and vinyl chloride monomer.[373] The clinical features include splenomegaly, hypersplenism, bleeding esophageal varices, and portal hypertensive gastropathy, a common cause of iron deficiency anemia. The liver may be enlarged because of associated disorders.

Peliosis Hepatis

Peliosis hepatis refers to blood-filled cavities that do not have an endothelial lining.[23, 92] At laparoscopy, peliosis appears as bluish-black cystic lesions on the surface of the liver, with varying diameters ranging from 1 mm to several centimeters. The lesions correspond to dilation and disruption of the sinusoidal architecture caused by disintegration of the reticulin framework with resulting atrophy of surrounding hepatocytes. Peliosis hepatis may occur in association with androgens,[2] azathioprine,[343] estrogens,[365] tamoxifen,[374] 6-thioguanine,[375] and possibly vitamin A.[376] It is also a common finding in association with sex steroid-induced liver tumors (see later). In some cases, regression of peliosis has been recorded after discontinuation of a causative drug.[375] The diagnosis is rarely suspected before surgery or liver biopsy; the latter is contraindicated if peliosis is suspected. The diagnostic clue is unexplained hepatomegaly in a patient taking a drug known to cause this lesion. However, cases often present with shock and abdominal pain as a result of hemorrhage or spontaneous rupture of the liver. Hepatic imaging by ultrasonography may fail to demonstrate the lesions, but dual-phase helical computed tomography, angiocomputed tomography, and magnetic resonance imaging are more sensitive. Hepatic arteriography demonstrates typical changes, in particular pooling of contrast in the late venous phase.

Azathioprine

Liver disease is a rare but important complication of azathioprine. The overall frequency is less than 0.1%, but many cases occur in complex medical situations, particularly after organ transplantation, in which activation of the immune system, viral infections, and other agents may increase the risk of hepatotoxicity. The central role of azathioprine has been confirmed in some cases that resolved after discontinuation of the drug and others in which a positive rechallenge was documented.[343, 377] Azathioprine is associated with an extraordinary range of hepatic disorders, including liver test abnormalities in asymptomatic patients, bland cholestasis, cholestatic hepatitis, bile duct injury, and vascular injury. Cholestatic hepatitis is probably the most common; several cases have been associated with zone 3 necrosis and congestion, suggesting acute vascular injury,[378] and azathioprine shares the vascular toxicity of other thiopurines (see Table 73–9). All the hepatic syndromes that result from vascular injury have been associated with azathioprine, particularly after organ transplantation. Cases of azathioprine-induced nodular regenerative hyperplasia and veno-occlusive disease have also been reported with other medical conditions, including inflammatory bowel disease.[379]

There is no relation to dose or duration of azathioprine therapy, but men are almost exclusively involved in cases of hepatic vascular injury following renal transplantation.[2, 23, 343] The onset of cholestatic reactions is 2 weeks to 22 months after the start of azathioprine, but vascular toxicity is recognized later; 3 months to 3 years is usual after transplantation,[14, 379] and cases have been described after 9 years.[380] The presentation and clinical features depend on the type of reaction. Cases of later onset are the result of delayed recognition and tend to be associated with complications of portal hypertension, ascites, and liver failure. Recovery can occur in such cases,[379] but the overall mortality rate is high.

LIVER TUMORS

Several associations between pharmacologic and environmental agents and liver tumors have been described, but causality has been difficult to prove because of the rarity of these associations. However, for some sex steroid–related tumors, as well as vinyl chloride–induced angiosarcoma, the relative risk attributable to the causative agent has been determined. Prevention and early detection are crucial to improve outcomes. The most important associations between drugs or toxins and hepatic tumors are summarized in Table 73–10, along with the evidence for causality and the principal clinicopathologic features. The major tumors of interest

Table 73–10 | **Associations between Drugs or Toxins and Hepatic Tumors**

TUMOR	IMPLICATED AGENTS, EVIDENCE FOR CAUSALITY	CLINICAL SIGNIFICANCE
Focal nodular hyperplasia	OCS: *weak evidence*—clinical observations, no case-control studies, no overall increased incidence	Benign lesions; possibly reactive hepatic changes in response to vascular lesion or possibly hamartomas OCS increase vascularity, size, risk of complications
Hepatic adenoma	OCS: *conclusive evidence*—case-control studies, biologic dependence Anabolic steroids: *persuasive evidence*—clinical observations, biologic dependence	Prevention: avoid prolonged, uninterrupted exposure to OCS and high-dose estrogens Diagnosis by vascular imaging Need to resect for diagnosis or to prevent rupture and malignant transformation if large Avoid further use of OCS, estrogens, pregnancy
Cavernous hemangioma	OCS: *rare association*—causative role unlikely or minor	Possible trophic effect of OCS on vasculature Note possible association with focal nodular hyperplasia
Hepatocellular carcinoma	OCS: *persuasive, but weak role/not discernible in high-incidence areas*—case-control studies, biologic dependence Anabolic steroids: *controversial*—biologic dependence	Same as for hepatic adenoma Regression has been reported, but resection always required Cases associated with anabolic steroids difficult to separate from adenomas Prognosis guarded, late recurrence common
Angiosarcoma	Arsenic, vinyl chloride monomer, thorium dioxide: *strong associations* Sex steroids: very rare and possibly fortuitous association	Prevention by avoiding industrial and environmental contamination; poor prognosis
Mixed cholangiocarcinoma, hepatoblastoma, epithelioid hemangioendothelioma	Rare clinical observations in individual cases; estrogens implicated, but significance dubious	Unclear; very rare malignant hepatic tumors with poor prognosis

OCS, oral contraceptive steroids.

are discussed briefly, have been reviewed elsewhere,[381, 382] and are described in more detail in Chapter 81.

Focal Nodular Hyperplasia

The significance of any association between oral contraceptive steroids (OCS) and focal nodular hyperplasia has been difficult to assess. Case reports in the early 1970s emphasized focal nodular hyperplasia among cases of oral contraceptive pill–related liver tumors that were large and vascular and occasionally ruptured.[2, 381, 382] On the other hand, focal nodular hyperplasia has always been more common in young women than others and does not appear to have increased in frequency since the introduction of OCS.[383] Some observations have supported an etiologic role of estrogens; thus, 86% of affected patients in two major centers had been exposed to exogenous estrogens.[384] Estrogens also have been reported to have a trophic effect on established lesions, thereby enhancing their size and vascularity, and have been associated with rare cases of hemorrhage.[2, 381] Thus, patients with large focal nodular hyperplasias should be counseled, and consideration should be given to discontinuation of OCS. Lesions greater than 5 cm in diameter should be resected if they are associated with pain or if the diagnosis is not clear.

Hepatic Adenoma

In contrast to focal nodular hyperplasia, there is a clear relationship between hepatic adenomas and the use of OCS. The results of two large case-control studies indicate that the annual risk is approximately 3 to 4 per 100,000 exposed persons,[25, 385] corresponding to a relative risk (compared with nonusers) of approximately 20-fold among those taking OCS for less than 10 years and more than 100-fold in those exposed for more than 10 years. The risk is increased with age and estrogen dose and is likely much lower with agents used since the 1980s.

Rare cases also have been associated with androgens, usually C17-alkylated anabolic steroids. There has been debate about whether some of these cases involved adenomas or well-differentiated hepatocellular carcinomas, because the histology is similar.[382, 386] Many of the androgen-associated cases have been in patients with Fanconi's familial hypoplastic anemia, a condition associated with chromosomal breaks, leukemia, and other malignancies, but some cases have occurred in female transsexuals taking androgens as conditioning agents, weight lifters, and patients with impotence or hypoplastic anemia.[2, 387] Danazol, a synthetic steroid that is a weak androgen, has been associated with a small number of liver tumors, both adenomas and hepatocellular carcinomas.[388] Danazol is the most effective agent for preventing hereditary angioedema, but among 11 patients taking the steroid for this indication for more than 10 years, hepatic adenomas developed in three.[389]

Although regression of sex steroid–related hepatic adenomas has been well documented after the withdrawal of steroids,[2, 381, 387] resection is indicated in large or symptomatic lesions and may be needed to make a firm diagnosis. Transition to hepatocellular carcinoma, as well as association with hepatocellular carcinoma in the same liver, has been documented.[390] The continued use of sex steroids and pregnancy are contraindicated in a patient who has had a hepatic adenoma, because of the risk of recurrence;[2] the recurrence rate was 12.5% in one series.[25] To prevent hepatic adenomas, OCS preparations with low estrogenic potency are favored, and long uninterrupted periods of oral contraceptive use should be avoided. During long-term treatment with danazol, ultrasonographic surveillance of the liver is indicated at least once a year.[389]

Hepatocellular Carcinoma

The risk of hepatocellular carcinoma is increased approximately twofold in women who have ever taken OCS, and the relative risk in long-term users (>8 years) is increased more than sevenfold compared with age-matched controls.[26, 391, 392] However, estrogen-related hepatocellular carcinoma is rare,[393] accounting for less than 10% of all OCS-related liver tumors and less than 2% of primary liver cancers in Western countries.[381] In areas endemic for hepatitis B virus, there is no statistical relationship between hepatocellular carcinoma and sex steroids because of the overwhelmingly greater etiologic role of chronic viral hepatitis.[26] The median age of presentation for estrogen-related tumors is 30 years. Patients have typically been taking combination OCS for more than 5 years. The tumors are well differentiated and include some instances of the fibrolamellar variant. The surrounding liver is normal or exibits other estrogen-related effects, particularly sinusoidal dilation.

Approximately 30 cases of hepatocellular carcinoma have been reported in association with use of androgenic anabolic steroids,[2, 382, 386, 387] but there have been no case-control studies, and in many cases there have been possible confounding variables (e.g., multiple blood transfusions before 1989). Instances of hepatic adenomas and hepatocellular carcinoma in the same patient, cases among weight lifters and female transsexuals without other liver disease, and regression of tumors after discontinuation of androgens all indicate a possible biologic role for androgens in some hepatocellular carcinomas. In androgen-associated tumors, peliosis hepatis is common.

Although regression is well documented for both estrogen and anabolic steroid–related hepatocellular carcinomas,[381, 382] subsequent recurrence[387, 393] or transmogrification to a more malignant tumor[390] has been recorded. Thus, appropriate treatment is resection or an alternative method of physical ablation. The 3-year survival rate is substantially better than that for more common types of hepatocellular carcinoma in cirrhotic livers (see Chapter 81), but many patients eventually succumb to recurrence with massive liver replacement or metastases.

Angiosarcoma

Angiosarcoma is a rare liver tumor attributable, in approximately one third of cases, to toxic agents: arsenic,[394] copper salts, thorium dioxide,[3, 365] and vinyl chloride monomer (see later). Rare cases have been associated with androgens and estrogens.[2] All the agents implicated in hepatic angiosarcoma are sometimes associated with noncirrhotic portal hypertension, a disorder associated with injury to the hepatic microvasculature (see earlier), and with precursor lesions consisting of hypertrophied sinusoidal lining cells.

VINYL CHLORIDE. Vinyl chloride has been associated with an epidemic of angiosarcoma.[395, 396] Cases occurred in plastics factory workers who were responsible for cleaning the heating vats used for polymerization of vinyl chloride monomer in the manufacture of polyvinyl chloride (PVC). Intake was mainly through inhalation. Lack of ventilation and failure to use protective clothing and ventilators were characteristic of working conditions before this hazard was recognized in 1974.[395] Levels of exposure to vinyl chloride monomer were commonly 100 parts per million, compared with the recommended limit of 1 part per million per 8 hours of time-weighted exposure. No cases have been attributable to initial exposure to vinyl chloride after 1974. The risk of angiosarcoma among at-risk workers exposed before that time is between five- and 300-fold, depending on cumulative exposure levels and time after exposure.[395, 396] Contamination with vinyl chloride monomer is insignificant after exposure to PVC, even though small amounts may leach out of new water piping and during burning of PVC. However, there have been cases of angiosarcoma among persons exposed as a result of contaminated industrial sites or toxic waste dumps before 1970.[395]

Cases of angiosarcoma are diagnosed 15 to 40 years (median, 22 years) after exposure to vinyl chloride monomer. In persons previously exposed to vinyl chloride, regular clinical examination is recommended for early detection of liver tumors.[395] Hepatic imaging is also indicated in patients with known chronic liver disease or high levels of exposure. In persons working in PVC plants, regular biochemical monitoring of liver tests is conducted, and those with persistent abnormalities are removed from workplace exposure.

Other Liver Tumors

Estrogens probably do not increase the incidence of *cavernous hemangiomas,* the most common benign tumor of the liver. However, they have been suspected of increasing the size of these lesions and thus the frequency with which they cause symptoms.[365] *Hepatoblastoma, cholangiocarcinoma, mixed carcinosarcoma,* and *epithelioid hemangioendothelioma* have rarely been reported in association with various therapeutic agents, particularly sex steroids.[2] Such sporadic cases are vanishingly rare, and there is no plausible biologic explanation for their etiology to suggest a causal role.

COMPLEMENTARY AND ALTERNATIVE MEDICINES AND ENVIRONMENTAL AGENTS

In addition to prescribed drugs, hepatotoxicity can be caused by other medicinal compounds, such as vitamins, dietary supplements, food additives, and the herbal and nonproprietary remedies collectively termed *complementary and alternative medicines (CAM).* In addition, toxic substances consumed in the diet and in drinking water or inhaled in the work environment can lead to liver disease.[2, 397] Arsenic, vinyl chloride, and nicotinic acid have already been referred to in this chapter, and other hepatotoxins that cause liver injury are summarized in Table 73–11. Plant toxins include the pyrrolizidine alkaloids, an important cause of veno-occlusive disease (see earlier), and constituents of Chinese traditional remedies (see later). Hypervitaminosis A (discussed later) is an example of an unusual type of chronic liver disease resulting from nonprescription medication. Other dietary toxins include poisonous mushrooms, particularly *Amanita phalloides,* a potent cause of severe hepatocellular necrosis,[398] and aflatoxin, a fungal toxin that is a potent hepatic carcinogen.

Amanita phylloides toxicity is more common in Western Europe, where mushroom hunting is popular, than in the United States. Consumption of a single mushroom can lead to fulminant hepatic failure and death. Amatoxins (mainly amanitine) are largely responsible for the toxicity by interfering with mRNA synthesis and causing hepatocyte necrosis. Three clinical phases are typical: (1) crampy abdominal pain, nausea, vomiting, and profuse diarrhea mimicking gastroenteritis 6 to 24 hours after ingestion; (2) a latent period of 12 to 24 hours during which symptoms improve but liver biochemical test results become abnormal; and (3) rapid progression to fulminant hepatic failure. In addition to supportive treatment, administration of high doses of penicillin may be beneficial. Liver transplantation may be life-saving. The overall mortality rate is now less than 20%.

For a more complete discussion of this topic, several relevant reviews are available.[2, 343, 368, 399, 400] Significant hepatotoxicity from industrial exposure (see Table 73–11) is uncommon with modern standards of workplace hygiene and abandonment of highly hepatotoxic chemicals; the topic has been reviewed elsewhere.[2, 395, 397]

Herbal Medicines

Many herbal remedies regarded as harmless for hundreds of years eventually have been shown to be hepatotoxic (Table 73–12)[368, 399, 400]; these remedies include germander,[401] pennyroyal oil,[402] pyrrolizidine alkaloids in comfrey,[369] mistletoe, motherwort, valerian, asafetida, hops, gentian, skullcap, chaparral leaf,[368, 403, 404] and senna fruit extract.[405] Use of alternative medicine in Western society is extensive and increasing.[406–412] In Australia, just over one half of the population use complementary medicines (excluding calcium, iron, and prescribed vitamins) each year,[411, 413] and in the United States, use of alternative medicine rose from 34% of the population in 1990 to 42% in 1997[407–409]; nearly 20% of the population took complementary medicines at the same time as conventional prescriptions. Use of herbal products is even more popular among patients with chronic hepatitis.[414, 415] Such agents are occasionally associated with toxic effects, particularly, but not exclusively, when recommended toxic dose thresholds are exceeded. Thus, public education is required to counter the assumption that "natural" or herbal products are invariably safe.[406, 409, 410]

Until 1997, the Australian Adverse Drug Reactions Advisory Committee (ADRAC) had received only 154 reports related to use of CAM in 25 years[410]; however, even though the safety of CAM seems good compared with that of conventional pharmaceuticals,[411, 416] the small number of cases is probably the result of underreporting. The safety record of Chinese proprietary medicines is good,[416] but serious poison-

Table 73–11 | **Environmental Agents That Cause Toxic Liver Injury**

AGENT	TYPE OF EXPOSURE	NATURE OF LIVER INJURY
Pyrrolizidine alkaloids (also Table 73–12)	Herbal and bush teas; contaminated crops	Veno-occlusive disease, cirrhosis
Vitamin A (see text)	Health tonic; skin disorders (no longer appropriate); massive ingestion of liver	Noncirrhotic portal hypertension, hepatic fibrosis, liver failure with or without cirrhosis, peliosis hepatis
Amanita phalloides, other toxic mushrooms	Accidental ingestion, as little as one mushroom	Fulminant hepatic failure
Aflatoxin	Contaminated crops, foodstuffs	Hepatocellular carcinoma (p53 deletions)
Arsenic	Nonproprietary medications; contaminated water supply; industrial exposure (pesticides, herbicides)	Hepatic fibrosis, cirrhosis, noncirrhotic portal hypertension, angiosarcoma
Bordeaux mixture (copper salts, lime)	Vineyard sprayers	Hepatic granulomas, noncirrhotic portal hypertension, angiosarcoma
Vinyl chloride monomer	Industrial exposure; contaminated sites	Acute hepatocellular injury; hepatic fibrosis, noncirrhotic portal hypertension, angiosarcoma
Carbon tetrachloride	Solvent, fumigant, refrigerant (historical)	Acute cytopathic injury (zonal steatosis, necrosis); ?cirrhosis, HCC
Beryllium	Industrial exposure, contaminated clothes	Hepatic granulomas
Dimethylformamide	Industrial exposure	Hepatocellular injury (minor); possibly steatohepatitis[326]
Dimethylnitrosamine	Industrial, laboratory exposure	Acute hepatic necrosis, HCC
Methylenedianiline	Epoxyresin hardener: industrial, domestic exposure; contaminated food (the Epping jaundice)[292]	Acute cholestasis with bile duct injury
Phosphorus	Industrial exposure; domestic exposure in matches, rodenticides (historical)	Acute cytopathic injury: zonal necrosis and steatosis
Chlordecone (Kepone)	Industrial exposure (insecticides)	Hepatocellular injury (minor); hepatic adaptation
2,3,7,8-Tetrachloro-dibenzo *p*-dioxin (TCDD)	Industrial and environmental contaminant (e.g., in polychlorinated biphenyls)	Hepatic adaptation (induction of cytochrome P450), porphyria cutanea tarda
Tetrachloroethane	Industrial solvent, dry cleaning	Acute, subacute hepatocellular necrosis
Tetrachloroethylene	Industrial solvent, degreasing agent	Hepatocellular necrosis
2,4,5-Trinitrotoluene	Explosive, industrial exposure	Acute hepatocellular necrosis (severe), cirrhosis, HCC
1,1,1-Trichloroethane	Domestic and industrial solvent	Steatosis, minor hepatocellular injury
Toluene and xylene	Paint solvent and thinners, glues	*Only with massive and prolonged exposure;* steatosis, possibly minor hepatocellular injury, NASH[326]

See reviews 2, 14, 397, 398.
HCC, hepatocellular carcinoma; NASH, nonalcoholic steatohepatitis.

ing may result from some components, and preparations often contain small amounts of Western medicines, arsenic, or cadmium. These herbal products are available through mail order or the Internet and in some countries do not conform to the high standards of manufacturing required for pharmaceutical products, nor do they undergo tests of purity. It is important for clinicians to inquire about ingestion of herbal remedies as a routine part of the drug history and particularly to consider self-prescribing with herbal medicines when investigating unusual cases of liver injury.

Jin Bu Huan

Jin Bu Huan Anodyne tablets (*Lycopodium serratum*) are a traditional herbal remedy that has been used as a sedative and an analgesic for more than 1000 years; it has been available in the United States for approximately 15 years. Symptoms of acute hepatitis developed in 7 adults at a mean of 20 weeks (range, 7 to 52 weeks) after the start of Jin Bu Huan ingestion.[417] In two patients, rechallenge showed Jin Bu Huan to be the cause of liver injury. In another, there was evidence of dose dependency. All patients were taking doses within the recommended range. Other than female predominance, no predisposing factors were evident. Fever, fatigue, nausea, pruritus, abdominal pain, jaundice, and hepatomegaly were common features. Liver tests showed 20- to 50-fold increases in serum ALT levels with minor increases in the alkaline phosphatase, except for one patient with cholestasis. Hyperbilirubinemia was prominent in the more severe cases. Liver biopsy showed lobular hepatitis with prominent eosinophils among the inflammatory infiltrate and, in a patient who had taken the herbal remedy for 12 months, mild hepatitis with microvesicular steatosis and fibrotic expansion of the portal tracts. Others have reported chronic hepatitis induced by Jin Bu Huan.[418, 419] Resolution of liver injury occurs within 8 weeks.[417]

Other Examples of Herbal Toxicity

Hepatic injury and fatal liver failure (each in one patient) have been attributed to use of *Chinese herbal teas* for eczema and psoriasis.[420] The latent period to onset in the first case was 8 weeks before the first episode and 3 days after resuming the Chinese herbs, whereas the second patient had taken the preparation for 6 months. Other reports of herbal hepatotoxicity have described cases of acute and chronic hepatitis,[418–425] cholestatic hepatitis,[426] hepatic fibrosis,[417] zonal or diffuse hepatic necrosis, bile duct injury,[427] veno-occlusive disease, acute liver failure resulting in death or requiring liver transplantation,[428–430] and carcinogenesis.[368, 399, 400] The toxic ingredients of Chinese herbal medicines are not known, although *Scutellaria* (also found in skullcap), *Paeonia, Dictomanus dasycarpus*, and glycyrrhizin have been implicated in some reports.[420, 427] Skullcap, germander, and other *Teucrium* species contain diterpenoids, which are hepatotoxic in experimental systems.[61, 62, 83]

CHAPARRAL. Chaparral *(Larrea tridentata)* is marketed as a dietary and "energy" supplement; hepatic, skin, and renal

Table 73–12 | **Herbal Remedies Implicated as Causes of Toxic Liver Injury**

HERBAL REMEDY	USE	TOXIC CONSTITUENT	NATURE OF LIVER INJURY
African remedy	Multiple uses	*Atractylis gummifera*	Diffuse hepatic necrosis
Chaparral leaf	Multiple uses	*Larrea tridentata*	Zone 3 necrosis; chronic hepatitis
Chinese herbal medicines (see text)	Multiple; skin diseases; health tonic; hepatitis B and C	Many (see text)	Liver injury (no histologic studies); veno-occlusive disease; chronic cholestasis with vanishing bile duct syndrome
Comfrey; gordolobo yerba maté tea; Chinese medicinal tea	Health tonic	Pyrrolizidine alkaloids; Compositae	Veno-occlusive disease
Dai-saiko-to (TJ-9)*	Liver disease, especially chronic viral hepatitis	*Scutellaria;* glycyrrhiza	Acute and chronic hepatitis
European remedy	Gallstones	*Chelidonium majus*	Hepatitis; fibrosis
Germander (tea, capsules)	Weight reduction; health tonic	Neoclerodane diterpenes (*Teucrium chamaedrys L.*)	Acute and chronic hepatitis; zone 3 necrosis; fibrosis, cirrhosis
Jin Bu Huan Anodyne tablets (see text)	Sedation; analgesic	*Lycopodium serratum*	Acute and chronic hepatitis; steatosis; fibrosis
Kombucha "mushroom"	Health tonic	Yeast-bacteria aggregate	Liver injury (no histologic studies)
Ma-huang	Weight reduction	Ephedrine	Acute hepatitis
Margosa oil	Health tonic	*Melia azedarach indica*	Reye's syndrome
Mediterranean traditional remedy	Anti-inflammatory	*Teucrium polium*	Zone 3 necrosis; acute liver failure; fibrosis
Mixed preparations: mistletoe, skullcap, valearian	Herbal tonics	Not identified; ?*Scutellaria*	Liver injury (no histologic studies)
"Natural laxatives"	Cathartic	Senna, podophyllin, aloin	Liver injury (no histologic studies)
Oil of cloves	Dental pain	Eugenol	Dose-dependent hepatotoxin; zonal necrosis
Pennyroyal oil (squaw mint)	Abortifacient; herbal remedy	*Labitae*	Liver injury (no histologic studies)
Prostata (saw palmetto)	Prostatism	*Serenoa repens; S. serrulata*	Hepatitis; fibrosis
Sho-saiko-to (TJ-9)*	Health tonic; viral hepatitis	*Scutellaria;* glycyrrhiza; others	Zonal and bridging necrosis; fibrosis; microvesicular steatosis
Zulu remedy	Health tonic	*Callilepsis laureola*	Hepatic necrosis

*TJ-9 is a herbal preparation used in Japan and China; there are several alternative spellings, including Sho-saiko-to and Dai-saiko-to. See reviews 2, 14, 343, 368, 399, 400.

toxicity have been reported. Among 18 reports of chaparral-associated illness between 1992 and 1994 evaluated by the FDA, liver injury was present in 13 reports, 11 in women.[404] The onset of illness was between 3 and 24 weeks of starting chaparral ingestion. The predominant pattern was cholestatic hepatitis, but severe cases of hepatic necrosis have been associated with chaparral,[368] including two patients who had been taking chaparral for longer than 1 year and in whom end-stage liver disease requiring hepatic transplantation developed.[404]

Hypervitaminosis A

Vitamin A is a dose-dependent hepatotoxin, and severe liver disease may result from hypervitaminosis A.[2, 376, 431–434] Earlier cases resulted from the use of large doses of vitamin A for keratinizing dermatoses, such as congenital ichthyosis,[436] but most cases now arise from self-medication.[431–433] Despite the adequacy of a dietary supply of vitamin A, it has been estimated that 35% of the U.S. population take vitamin supplements containing vitamin A, with as many as 3% of supplements providing a daily dose of 25,000 IU or more.[432] Doses of more than 10,000 IU/day may be toxic.[434] This observation highlights the need to inquire about exposure to vitamins and other dietary supplements in cases of unexplained liver injury.

The average daily dose of vitamin A in reported cases of liver disease has been 96,000 IU, and the average duration of ingestion has been 7.2 years, for a mean cumulative dose of 229 million units.[2, 433] Liver injury has been described with daily doses of 15,000 to 45,000 IU,[431, 432] and cirrhosis has occurred after a daily intake of 25,000 IU for 6 years or longer.[433] The severity of liver disease depends on duration as well as dose; the half-life of vitamin A in the liver varies between 50 days and 1 year.[434] Individual susceptibility may be an additional factor.[436] Rare cases of hypervitaminosis A have been described in persons who consumed enormous amounts of liver.[437]

The clinicopathologic spectrum of hypervitaminosis A–related liver disease includes minor changes with abnormal liver tests and stellate cell hyperplasia, noncirrhotic portal hypertension with perisinusoidal fibrosis, cirrhosis, or fatal chronic liver disease with hepatocellular failure in the absence of cirrhosis.[431–437] Rare cases of peliosis hepatitis also have been attributed to hypervitaminosis A.[376] Liver biopsy specimens show increased storage of vitamin A as characteristic greenish autofluorescence after irradiation with ultraviolet light. The excess vitamin A is stored initially in stellate cells that lie in the space of Disse; these cells are both swollen and hyperplastic in hypervitaminosis A. Under light microscopy, the enlarged clear stellate cells compress the hepatic sinusoids and give rise to a "Swiss cheese," or honeycombed, appearance. Hepatocellular injury is usually minor, with microvesicular steatosis and focal degeneration but minimal necrosis or inflammation. Hepatic fibrosis is the other striking histologic feature. It begins in a perisinusoidal distribution and most likely arises from activated stellate cells that transform into myofibroblasts.[431]

Other clinical features of hypervitaminosis A are usually present (e.g., fatigue, muscle and bone pain, dry skin, alopecia, gingivitis, xanthosis [yellowish discoloration of the skin], headache and neurologic or psychiatric disturbances, hypercalcemia, and growth retardation).[437] Hepatomegaly is common, and in severe cases, splenomegaly and ascites may be evident. Cases with portal hypertension can present with bleeding esophageal varices. Liver tests are abnormal in two thirds of cases, but the changes are nonspecific. In advanced cases, low serum albumin concentrations, hyperglobulinemia (especially IgM), hyperbilirubinemia, and prolongation of prothrombin time may be present. The diagnosis rests on obtaining the relevant dietary and medication history and on clinical suspicion informed by the diverse manifestations of hypervitaminosis A (vitamin ingestion is occasionally denied). Plasma vitamin A levels may be normal, and it is more reliable to demonstrate increased hepatic storage of vitamin A and characteristic histology. The average duration of vitamin A intake before diagnosis is 18 months, but in some cases diagnosis has been delayed for several years because of failure to suspect the cause of liver injury.[433]

Gradual improvement occurs after discontinuation of vitamin A ingestion, but deterioration may continue in cases of severe intoxication, particularly when cirrhosis is present.[433, 435] Features of liver failure and established cirrhosis at diagnosis indicate a poor prognosis; most patients die or require liver transplantation.[433, 435] There is a need for better public education to prevent hypervitaminosis A, as well as restriction on the sale of high-dose vitamin A preparations (this is in force in some countries). Clinicians need to make a prompt diagnosis to avoid possible adverse sequelae. Alcohol should be avoided because of possible interactive hepatotoxicity, and vitamin A supplements generally should be avoided in other types of liver disease because of possible accentuation of hepatic injury and fibrosis.[434]

REFERENCES

1. Friis H, Andreasen PB: Drug-induced hepatic injury: An analysis of 1100 case reports to The Danish Committee on Adverse Drug Reactions between 1978 and 1987. J Intern Med 232:133, 1992.
2. Farrell GC: Drug-Induced Liver Disease. Edinburgh, Churchill Livingstone, 1994.
3. Zimmerman HJ: Hepatotoxicity. The Adverse Effects of Drugs and Other Chemicals on the Liver, 2nd ed. Philadelphia, Lippincott, Williams and Wilkins, 1999.
4. Bernuau J, Rueff B, Benhamou JP: Fulminant and subfulminant liver failure: Definitions and causes. Semin Liver Dis 6:97, 1986.
5. Ostapowicz G, Lee WM: Acute hepatic failure: A western perspective. J Gastroenterol Hepatol 15:480, 2000.
6. Schiodt FV, Atillasoy E, Shakil AO, et al: Etiology and outcome for 295 patients with acute liver failure in the United States. Liver Transpl Surg 5:29, 1999.
7. Pessayre D, Larrey D: Acute and chronic drug-induced hepatitis. Bailliére's Clin Gastroenterol 2:385, 1988.
8. Lee WM: Drug-induced hepatotoxicity. N Engl J Med 333:1118, 1995.
9. Biour M, Poupon R, Grange J-D, et al: Drug-induced liver injury. Twelfth updated edition of the bibliographic database of liver injuries related to drugs. Gastroenterol Clin Biol 23:310, 1999.
10. Farrell GC: Drug-induced hepatic injury. J Gastroenterol Hepatol 12 (Suppl):S242, 1997.
11. Larrey D: Drug-induced liver diseases. J Hepatol 32 (suppl 1):77, 2000.
12. Lewis JH: Drug-induced liver disease. Med Clin North Am 84:1275, 2000.
13. Stricker BHCh: Drug-induced hepatic injury. In Dukes MNG (ed): Drug-induced Disorders, Vol 5; 2nd ed. Amsterdam, Elsevier, 1992.
14. Farrell GC, Weltman D: Drug-induced liver disease. In Gitnick G (ed): Current Hepatology, Vol 16. Chicago, Mosby–Year Book, 1996, p 143.
15. Kaplowitz N: Causality assessment versus guilt-by-association in drug hepatotoxicity. Hepatology 33:308, 2001.
16. Kromann-Andersen H, Pedersen A: Reported adverse reactions to and consumption of nonsteroidal anti-inflammatory drugs in Denmark over a 17-year period. Dan Med Bull 35:187, 1988.
17. García Rodríguez LA, Gutthann SP, Walker AM, et al: The role of non-steroidal anti-inflammatory drugs in acute liver injury. Br Med J 305:865, 1992.
18. Larrey D, Vital T, Babany G, et al: Hepatitis associated with amoxicillin-clavulanic acid combination. Report of 15 cases. Gut 33:368, 1992.
19. O'Donohue J, Oien KA, Donaldson P, et al: Co-amoxiclav jaundice: Clinical and histological features and HLA class II association. Gut 47:717, 2000.
20. García Rodríguez LA, Stricker BH, Zimmerman HJ: Risk of acute liver injury associated with the combination of amoxicillin and clavulanic acid. Arch Intern Med 156:1327, 1996.
21. Bjornsson E, Lindberg J, Olsson R: Liver reactions to oral low-dose tetracyclines. Scand J Gastroenterol 32:390, 1997.
22. Hurwitz ES, Barrett MJ, Bregman D, et al: Public Health Service study of Reye's syndrome and medications. JAMA 257:1905, 1987.
23. Valla D, Benhamou J-P: Drug-induced vascular and sinusoidal lesions of the liver. Baillière's Clin Gastroenterol 2:481, 1988.
24. Carson JL, Strom BL, Duff A, et al: Acute liver disease associated with erythromycins, sulfonamides, and tetracyclines. Ann Intern Med 119:576, 1993.
25. Rooks JB, Ory HW, Ishak KG, et al: Epidemiology of hepatocellar adenoma. The role of oral contraceptive use. JAMA 242:644, 1979.
26. Prentice RL: Epidemiologic data on exogenous hormones and hepatocellular carcinoma and selected other cancers. Prevent Med 20:38, 1991.
27. Bryant AE, Dreifuss FE: Valproic acid hepatic fatalities. III. US experience since 1986. Neurology 46:465, 1996.
28. Konig SA, Schenk M, Sick C, et al: Fatal liver failure associated with valproate therapy in a patient with Friedreich's disease: Review of valproate hepatotoxicity in adults. Epilepsia 40:1036, 1999.
29. Belay ED, Bresee JS, Holman RC, et al: Reye's syndrome in the United States from 1981 through 1997. N Engl J Med 340:1377, 1999.
30. Hardie RM, Newton LH, Bruce JC, et al: The changing clinical pattern of Reye's syndrome 1982–1990. Arch Dis Child 74:400, 1996.
31. Larrey D, Pageaux GP: Genetic predisposition to drug-induced hepatotoxicity. J Hepatol 26(suppl2):12, 1997.
32. Hoft RH, Bunker JP, Goodman HI, et al: Halothane hepatitis in three pairs of closely related women. N Engl J Med 304:1023, 1981.
33. Gennis MA, Vemuri R, Burns EA, et al: Familial occurrence of hypersensitivity to phenytoin. Am J Med 91:631, 1991.
34. Krähenbühl S, Bandner S, Kleinle S, et al: Mitochondrial diseases represent a risk factor for valproate-induced fulminant hepatic failure. Liver 20:346, 2000.
35. Hautekeete ML, Horsmans Y, Van Waeyenberge C, et al: HLA association of amoxicillin-clavulanate–induced hepatitis. Gastroenterology 117:1181, 1999.
36. Kurosaki M, Takagi H, Mori M: HLA-A33/B44/DR6 is highly related to intrahepatic cholestasis induced by tiopronin. Dig Dis Sci 45:1103, 2000.
37. Aithal PG, Day C: The natural history of histologically proved drug induced liver disease. Gut 44:731, 1999.
38. Hokkanen OT, Sotaniemi EA: Liver injury and multiple drug therapy. Arch Toxicol (Suppl):173, 1978.
39. Smith DW, Cullity GJ, Silberstein EP: Fatal hepatic necrosis associated with multiple anticonvulsant therapy. Aust NZ J Med 18:575, 1988.
40. Perez Gutthann S, Garcia Rodriguez LA: The increased risk of hospitalizations for acute liver injury in a population with exposure to multiple drugs. Epidemiology 4:496, 1993.
41. Hull M, Jones R, Bendall M: Fatal hepatic necrosis associated with trazodone and neuroleptic drugs [letter]. Br Med J 309:378, 1994.
42. Moertel CG, Fleming TR, Macdonald JS, et al: Hepatic toxicity associated with fluorouracil plus levamisole adjuvant therapy. J Clin Oncol 11:2386, 1993.
43. George J, Farrell GC: Drug-induced liver disease. In Gitnick G (ed):

Current Hepatology, Vol 12. St. Louis, Mosby–Year Book, 1992, p 131.
44. Kaplowitz N: Mechanisms of liver cell injury. J Hepatol 32 (suppl 1): 39, 2000.
45. Whitcomb DC, Block GD: Association of acetaminophen hepatotoxicity with fasting and ethanol use. JAMA 272:1845, 1994.
46. Singh J, Garg PK, Tandon RK: Hepatotoxicity due to antituberculosis therapy. Clinical profile and reintroduction of therapy. J Clin Gastroenterol 22:211, 1996.
47. McDonald GB, Sharma P, Matthews DE, et al: Venoocclusive disease of the liver after bone marrow transplantation: Diagnosis, incidence, and predisposing factors. Hepatology 4:116, 1984.
48. Gray DR, Morgan T, Chretien SD, et al: Efficacy and safety of controlled-release niacin in dyslipoproteinemic veterans. Ann Intern Med 121:252, 1994.
49. Nehra A, Mullick F, Ishak KG, et al: Pemoline-associated hepatic injury. Gastroenterology 99:1517, 1990.
50. Marotta PJ, Roberts EA: Pemoline hepatotoxicity in children. J Pediatr 132:894, 1998.
51. Dennis EW: Fatal hepatic necrosis in association with the use of hycanthone. South Afr Med J 54:137, 1978.
52. Wong WM, Wu PC, Yuen MF, et al: Antituberculosis drug-related liver dysfunction in chronic hepatitis B infection. Hepatology 31:201, 2000.
53. Sulkowski MS, Thomas DL, Chaisson RE, et al: Hepatotoxicity associated with antiretroviral therapy in adults infected with human immunodeficiency virus and the role of hepatitis C or B virus. JAMA 283: 74, 2000.
54. Riley TR 3rd, Smith JP: Ibuprofen-induced hepatotoxicity in patients with chronic hepatitis C: A case series. Am J Gastroenterol 93: 1563, 1998.
55. Pu YS, Liu CM, Kao JH, et al: Antiandrogen hepatotoxicity in patients with chronic viral hepatitis. Eur Urol 36:293, 1999.
56. Benson GB: Hepatotoxicity following the therapeutic use of antipyretic analgesics. Am J Med 75(Suppl):85, 1983.
57. Gordin FM, Simon GL, Wofsy CB, et al: Adverse reactions to trimethoprim-sulfamethoxazole in patients with acquired immunodeficiency syndrome. Ann Intern Med 100:495, 1984.
58. Murray M: Role of the liver in drug metabolism. In Farrell GC (ed), Drug-induced Liver Disease. Edinburgh, Churchill Livingstone, 1994, p 3.
59. Hasler JA, Estrabrook R, Murray M, et al: Human cytochromes P450. Molec Aspects Med 20:1, 1999.
60. Yamazaki H, Shibata A, Suzuki M, et al: Oxidation of troglitazone to a quinone-type metabolite catalyzed by cytochrome P-450 2C8 and P-450 3A4 in human liver microsomes. Drug Metab Dispos 27:1260, 1999.
61. Fau D, Lekehal M, Farrell G, et al: Diterpenoids from germander, an herbal medicine, induce apoptosis in isolated rat hepatocytes. Gastroenterology 113:1334, 1997.
62. Haouzi D, Lekehal M, Moreau A, et al: Cytochrome P450–generated reactive metabolites cause mitochondrial permeability transition, caspase activation, and apoptosis in rat hepatocytes. Hepatology 32:303, 2000.
63. Sies H: Oxidative stress: From basic research to clinical application. Am J Med 91:31S, 1991.
64. Morgan MY, Reshef R, Shah RR, et al: Impaired oxidation of debrisoquine in patients with perhexiline liver injury. Gut 25:1057, 1984.
65. George J, Byth K, Farrell GC: Age but not gender selectively affects expression of individual cytochrome P450 proteins in human liver. Biochem Pharmacol 50:727, 1995.
66. Hunt CM, Westerkam WR, Stave GM: Effect of age and gender on the activity of human hepatic CYP3A. Biochem Pharmacol 44:275, 1992.
67. George J, Byth K, Farrell GC: Influence of clinicopathological variables on CYP protein expression in human liver. J Gastroenterol Hepatol 11:33, 1996.
68. Goodwin B, Hodgson E, Liddle C: Orphan human pregnane X receptor mediates the transcriptional activation of CYP3A4 by rifampicin through a distal enhancer module. Mol Pharmacol 56:1329, 1999.
69. Moore LB, Parks DJ, Jones SA, et al: Orphan nuclear receptors constitutive androstane receptor and pregnane X receptor share xenobiotic and steroid ligands. J Biol Chem 275:15122, 2000.
70. Del Castillo-Olivares A, Gil G: Role of FXR and FTF in bile acid–mediated suppression of cholesterol 7-alpha-hydroxylase transcription. Nucleic Acids Res 28:3587, 2000.
71. Sesardic D, Boobis AR, Edwards RJ, et al: A form of cytochrome P450 in man, orthologous to form d in the rat, catalyses the O-deethylation of phenacetin and is inducible by cigarette smoking. Br J Clin Pharmacol 26:363, 1988.
72. Sinclair JF, Szakacs JG, Wood SG, et al: Acetaminophen hepatotoxicity precipitated by short-term treatment of rats with ethanol and isopentanol: Protection by triacetyloleandomycin. Biochem Pharmacol 59: 445, 2000.
73. Moore LB, Goodwin B, Jones SA, et al: St. John's wort induces hepatic drug metabolism through activation of the pregnane X receptor. Proc Natl Acad Sci USA 97:7500, 2000.
74. Meech R, Mackenzie PI: Structure and function of uridine diphosphate glucuronosyltransferases. Clin Exp Pharmacol Physiol 24:907, 1997.
75. Lee J, Boyer JL: Molecular alterations in hepatocyte transport mechanisms in acquired cholestatic liver disorders. Semin Liver Dis 20:373, 2000.
76. Trauner M, Meier PJ, Boyer JL: Molecular pathogenesis of cholestasis. N Engl J Med 339:1217, 1998.
77. Huang L, Smit JW, Meijer DK, et al: Mrp2 is essential for estradiol-17beta(beta-D-glucuronide)-induced cholestasis in rats. Hepatology 32: 66, 2000.
78. Steiger B, Fattiger K, Madon J, et al: Drug- and estrogen-induced cholestasis through inhibition of the hepatocellular bile salt export pump (Bsep) of rat liver. Gastroenterology 118:422, 2000.
79. Meister A: Glutathione. In Arias IM, Jakoby WB, Popper H, et al (eds): The Liver. Biology and Pathobiology, 2nd ed. New York, Raven Press, 1988, p 401.
80. Kaplowitz N, Tsukamoto H: Oxidative stress and liver disease. Prog Liver Dis 14:131, 1996.
81. Galle PR: Apoptosis in liver disease. J Hepatol 27:405, 1997.
82. Patel T, Steer CJ, Gores GJ: Apoptosis and the liver: A mechanism of disease, growth regulation, and carcinogenesis. Hepatology 30:811, 1999.
83. Kaplowitz N: Hepatotoxicity of herbal remedies: Insights into the intricacies of plant-animal warfare and cell death. Gastroenterology 113:1408, 1997.
84. Lewis W, Dalakas MC: Mitochondrial toxicity of antiviral drugs. Nat Med 1:417, 1995.
85. Lemasters J: Mechanisms of hepatic toxicity V. Necrapoptosis and the mitochondrial permeability transition: Shared pathways to necrosis and apoptosis. Am J Physiol 276:G1, 1999.
86. Laskin DL: Nonparenchymal cells and hepatotoxicity. Semin Liver Dis 10:293, 1990.
87. DeLeve LD, McCuskey RS, Wang X, et al: Characterization of a reproducible rat model of hepatic veno-occlusive disease. Hepatology 29:1779, 1999.
88. Smith GCM, Kenna JG, Harrison DJ, et al: Autoantibodies to hepatic microsomal carboxylesterase in halothane hepatitis. Lancet 342:963, 1993.
89. Gut J, Christen U, Huwyler J, et al: Molecular mimicry of trifluoroacetylated human liver protein adducts by constitutive proteins and immunochemical evidence for its impairment in halothane hepatitis. Eur J Biochem 210:569, 1992.
90. Kretz-Rommel A, Boelsterli UA: Cytotoxic activity of T cells and non-T cells from diclofenac-immunized mice against cultured syngeneic hepatocytes exposed to diclofenac. Hepatology 22:213, 1995.
91. Mackay IR: The immunological mediation of drug reactions affecting the liver. In Farrell GC (ed): Drug-induced Liver Disease. Edinburgh, Churchill Livingstone, 1994, p 61.
92. Hall P de la M: Histopathology of drug-induced liver disease. In Farrell GC (ed): Drug-induced Liver Disease. Edinburgh, Churchill Livingstone, 1994, p 115.
93. Danan G, Benichou C: Causality assessment of adverse reactions to drugs. I. A novel method based on the conclusions of international consensus meetings: Application to drug-induced liver injuries. J Clin Epidemiol 46:1323, 1993.
94. Maria VA, Victorino RM: Development and validation of a clinical scale for the diagnosis of drug-induced hepatitis. Hepatology 26:664, 1997.
95. Lucena MI, Camargo R, Andrade RJ, et al: Comparison of two clinical scales for causality assessment in hepatotoxicity. Hepatology 33: 123, 2001.
96. Laurent-Puig P, Dussaix E, de Paillette L, et al: Prevalence of hepatitis C RNA in suspected drug-induced liver diseases [letter]. J Hepatol 19:487, 1993.

97. Maria VA, Victorino RM: Diagnostic value of specific T cell reactivity to drugs in 95 cases of drug induced liver injury. Gut 41:534, 1997.
98. Benichou C: Criteria for drug-induced liver disorders. Report of an International Consensus Meeting. J Hepatol 11:272, 1990.
99. Benichou C, Danan G, Flahault A: Causality assessment of adverse reactions to drugs. II. An original model for validation of drug causality assessment methods: Case reports with positive rechallenge. J Clin Epidemiol 46:1331, 1993.
100. Kaplowitz N: Avoiding hepatic injury from drugs. Gastroenterology 117:759, 1999.
101. Amacher DE: Serum transaminase elevations as indicators of hepatic injury following the administration of drugs. Regul Toxicol Pharmacol 27:119, 1998.
102. Rosenzweig P, Miget N, Brohier S: Transaminase elevation on placebo during phase I trials. Br J Clin Pharmacol 48:19, 1999.
103. Cohn WJ, Boylan JJ, Blanke RV, et al: Treatment of chlordecone (Kepone) toxicity with cholestyramine. Results of a controlled clinical trial. N Engl J Med 298:243, 1978.
104. Pond SM, Olson KR, Woo OF, et al: Amatoxin poisoning in Northern California, 1982–1983. West J Med 145:204, 1986.
105. Brotodihardjo A, Batey RG, Farrell GC, et al: Hepatotoxicity from paracetamol self-poisoning in western Sydney: A continuing challenge. Med J Aust 157:382, 1992.
106. Smilkstein MJ, Knapp GL, Kulig KW, et al: Efficacy of oral *N*-acetylcysteine in the treatment of acetaminophen overdose. Analysis of the National Multicentre Study (1976–1985). N Engl J Med 319: 1557, 1988.
107. Makin AJ, Wendon J, Williams R: A 7-year experience of severe acetaminophen-induced hepatotoxicity (1987–1993). Gastroenterology 109:1907, 1995.
108. Mutimer DJ, Ayres RCS, Neuberger JM, et al: Serious paracetamol poisoning and the results of liver transplantation. Gut 35:809, 1994.
109. Zimmerman HJ, Maddrey WC: Acetaminophen (paracetamol) hepatotoxicity with regular intake of alcohol: Analysis of instance of therapeutic misadventure. Hepatology 22:767, 1995.
110. Broughan TA, Soloway RD: Acetaminophen hepatotoxicity. Dig Dis Sci 45:1553, 2000.
111. Schiødt FV, Rochling FA, Casey DL, Lee WM: Acetaminophen toxicity in an urban county hospital. N Engl J Med 337:1112, 1997.
112. Denison H, Kaczynski J, Wallerstedt S: Paracetamol medication and alcohol abuse: A dangerous combination for the liver and kidney. Scand J Gastroenterol 22:701, 1987.
113. Crippin JS: Acetaminophen hepatotoxicity: Potentiation by isoniazid. Am J Gastroenterol 88:590, 1993.
114. Prescott LF, Critchley JAJH: The treatment of acetaminophen poisoning. Annu Rev Pharmacol Toxicol 23:87, 1983.
115. Penna A, Buchanan N: Paracetamol poisoning in children and hepatotoxicity. Br J Clin Pharmacol 32:143, 1991.
116. Heubi JE, Barbacci MB, Zimmerman HJ: Therapeutic misadventures with acetaminophen: Hepatotoxicity after multiple doses in children. J Pediatr 132:22, 1998.
117. Nolan CM, Sandblom RE, Thummel KE, et al: Hepatotoxicity associated with acetaminophen usage in patients receiving multiple drug therapy for tuberculosis. Chest 105:408, 1994.
118. Buckley NA, Whyte IM, O'Connell DL, Dawson AH: Oral or intravenous *N*-acetylcysteine: Which is the treatment of choice for acetaminophen (paracetamol) poisoning? J Toxicol Clin Toxicol 37:759, 1999.
119. Lim SP, Andrews FJ, O'Brien PE: Misoprostil protection against acetaminophen-induced hepatotoxicity in the rat. Dig Dis Sci 39:1249, 1994.
120. Bernal W, Wendon J, Rela M, et al: Use and outcome of liver transplantation in acetaminophen-induced acute liver failure. Hepatology 27:1050, 1998.
121. Robinson D, Smith AM, Johnston GS: Severity of overdose after restriction of paracetamol availability: Retrospective study. Br Med J 321:926, 2000.
122. Turvill JL, Burroughs AK, Moore KP: Change in occurrence of paracetamol overdose in UK after introduction of blister packs. Lancet 355:2048, 2000.
123. McKenny JM, Proctor JD, Harris S, et al: A comparison of the efficacy and toxic effects of sustained- vs immediate-release niacin in hypercholesterolemic patients. JAMA 271:672, 1994.
124. Powell-Jackson PR, Tredger JM, Williams R: Hepatotoxicity to sodium valproate: A review. Gut 25:673, 1984.
125. Appleton RE, Farrell K, Applegarth DA, et al: The high incidence of valproate hepatotoxicity in infants may relate to familial metabolic defects. Can J Neurol Sci 17:145, 1990.
126. McKenzie R, Fried MW, Sallie R, et al: Hepatic failure and lactic acidosis due to fialuridine (FIAU), an investigational nucleoside analogue for chronic hepatitis B. N Engl J Med 333:1099, 1995.
127. Kleiner DE, Gaffey MJ, Sallie R, et al: Histopathologic changes associated with fialuridine hepatotoxicity. Mod Pathol 10:192, 1997.
128. Klecker RW, Katki AG, Collins JM: Toxicity, metabolism, DNA incorporation with lack of repair, and lactate production for 1-(2′-fluoro-2′-deoxy-b-D-arabinofuranoxyl)-5-iodouracil in U-937 and MOLT-4 cells. Mol Pharmacol 46:1204, 1994.
129. Horn DM, Neeb LA, Colacino JM, et al: Fialuridine is phosphorylated and inhibits DNA synthesis in isolated rat hepatic mitochondria. Antiviral Res 34:71, 1997.
130. Dove LM, Alonzo J, Wright TL: Clinicopathological conference: Hepatitis C in a patient with human immunodeficiency virus infection. Hepatology 32:147, 2000.
131. Kakuda TN: Pharmacology of nucleoside and nucleotide reverse transcriptase inhibitor–induced mitochondrial toxicity. Clin Ther 22:685, 2000.
132. Stein D: A new syndrome of hepatomegaly with severe steatosis in HIV seropositive patients. AIDS Clinical Care 6:17, 1994.
133. Sundar K, Suarez M, Banogon PE, Shapiro JM: Zidovudine-induced fatal lactic acidosis and hepatic failure in patients with acquired immunodeficiency syndrome: Report of two patients and review of the literature. Crit Care Med 25:1425, 1997.
134. Chariot P, Drogou I, de Lacroix-Szmania I, et al: Zidovudine-induced mitochondrial disorder with massive liver steatosis, myopathy, lactic acidosis, and mitochondrial DNA depletion. J Hepatol 30:156, 1999.
135. ter Hofstede HJ, de Marie S, Foudraine NA, et al: Clinical features and risk factors of lactic acidosis following long-term antiretroviral therapy: 4 fatal cases. Int J STD AIDS 11:611, 2000.
136. Picard O, Rosmorduc O, Cabane J: Hepatotoxicity associated with ritonavir [letter]. Ann Intern Med 129:670, 1998.
137. Benveniste O, Longuet P, Duval X, et al: Two episodes of acute renal failure, rhabdomyolysis, and severe hepatitis in an AIDS patient successfully treated with ritonavir and indinavir. Clin Infect Dis 28:1180, 1999.
138. Bräu N, Leaf HL, Wieczorek RL, Margolis DM: Severe hepatitis in three AIDS patients treated with indinavir [letter]. Lancet 349:924, 1997.
139. Matsuda J, Gohchi K, Yamanaka M: Severe hepatitis in patients with AIDS and haemophilia B treated with indinavir [letter]. Lancet 350: 364, 1997.
140. Lai KK, Gang DL, Zawacki JK, et al: Fulminant hepatic failure associated with 2′,3′-dideoxyinosine (ddI). Ann Intern Med 115:283, 1991.
141. Bleeker-Rovers CP, Kadir SW, van Leusen R, Richter C: Hepatic steatosis and lactic acidosis caused by stavudine in an HIV-infected patient. Neth J Med 57:190, 2000.
142. Miller KD, Cameron M, Wood LV, et al: Lactic acidosis and hepatic steatosis associated with use of stavudine: Report of four cases. Ann Intern Med 133:192, 2000.
143. O'Gorman T, Koff RS: Salicylate hepatitis. Gastroenterology 72:726, 1977.
144. Orlowski JP: Whatever happened to Reye's syndrome? Did it ever exist? Crit Care Med 27:1582, 1999.
145. Zimmerman HJ: Hepatotoxic effects of oncotherapeutic agents. In Popper H, Schaffner F (eds): Progress in Liver Disease, Vol 8. New York, Grune & Stratton, 1986, p 621.
146. Dykhuizen RS, Brunt PW, Atkinson P, et al: Ecstasy induced hepatitis mimicking viral hepatitis. Gut 36:939, 1995.
147. Jones AL, Simpson KJ: Mechanisms and management of hepatotoxicity in ecstasy (MDMA) and amphetamine intoxications. Alim Pharmacol Ther 13:129, 1999.
148. Fidler H, Dhillon A, Gertner D, Burroughs A: Chronic ecstasy (3,4-methylenedioxymetamphetamine) abuse: A recurrent and unpredictable cause of severe acute hepatitis. J Hepatol 25:563, 1996.
149. Kreth K-P, Kovar K-A, Schwab M, Zanger UM: Identification of the human cytochromes P450 involved in the oxidative metabolism of "ecstasy"-related designer drugs. Biochem Pharmacol 59:1563, 2000.
150. Bernuau J, Larrey D, Campillo B, et al: Amodiaquine-induced fulminant hepatitis. J Hepatol 6:109, 1988.
151. Zimmerman HJ: Update of hepatotoxicity due to classes of drugs in

common clinical use: Non-steroidal, anti-inflammatory drugs, antibiotics, antihypertensives, and cardiac and psychotropic agents. Semin Liver Dis 10:322, 1990.
152. Stricker BCCh, Blok APR, Claas FHJ, et al: Hepatic injury associated with the use of nitrofurans: A clinicopathological study of 52 reported cases. Hepatology 8:599, 1988.
153. Sharp JR, Ishak KG, Zimmerman HJ: Chronic active hepatitis and severe hepatic necrosis associated with nitrofurantoin. Ann Intern Med 92:14, 1980.
154. Mockli G, Crowley M, Stern R, et al: Massive hepatic necrosis in a child after administration of phenobarbital. Am J Gastroenterol 84: 820, 1989.
155. Pellock JM, Brodie MJ: Felbamate: 1997 update. Epilepsia 38:1261, 1997.
156. Bjøro K, Gjerstad L, Bentdal Ø, et al: Topiramate and fulminant liver failure. Lancet 352:1119, 1998.
157. Lindgren A, Olsson R: Liver reactions from trimethoprim. J Intern Med 236:281, 1994.
158. Jones B: Untitled letter. Med J Aust 174:368, 2001.
159. Dourakis SP, Tzemanakis E, Sinani C, et al: Gliclazide-induced acute hepatitis. Eur J Gastroenterol Hepatol 12:119, 2000.
160. Besnard M, Debray D, Durand P, et al: Fulminant hepatitis in two children treated with sulfasalazine for Crohn's disease. Arch Pediatr 6: 643, 1999.
161. Hautekeete ML, Bougeois N, Potvin P, et al: Hypersensitivity with hepatotoxicity to mesalazine after hypersensitivity to sulfasalazine. Gastroenterology 103:1925, 1992.
162. Deltenre P, Berson A, Marcellin P, et al: Mesalazine (5-aminosalicylic acid)-induced chronic hepatitis. Gut 44:886, 1999.
163. Malcolm A, Heap TR, Eckstein RP, et al: Minocycline-induced liver injury. Am J Gastroenterol 91:1641, 1996.
164. Goldstein PE, Deviere J, Cremer M: Acute hepatitis and drug-related lupus induced by minocycline treatment. Am J Gastroenterol 92:143, 1997.
165. Pohle T, Menzel J, Domschke W: Minocycline and fulminant hepatic failure necessitating liver transplantation. Am J Gastroenterol 95:560, 2000.
166. Bartle WR, Fisher MM, Kerenyi N: Disulfiram-induced hepatitis. Report of two cases and review of the literature. Dig Dis Sci 30:834, 1985.
167. Rabkin JM, Corless CL, Orloff SL, et al: Liver transplantation for disulfiram-induced hepatic failure. Am J Gastroenterol 93:830, 1998.
168. Tanner LA, Bosco LA, Zimmerman HJ: Hepatic toxicity after acebutolol therapy. Ann Intern Med 111:533, 1989.
169. Clark JA, Zimmerman HJ, Tanner LA: Labetalol hepatotoxicity. Ann Intern Med 113:210, 1990.
170. Larrey D, Henrion J, Heller F, et al: Metoprolol-induced hepatitis: Rechallenge and drug oxidation phenotyping. Ann Intern Med 108:67, 1988.
171. Shaw DR, Misan GMH, Johnson RD: Nifedipine hepatitis. Aust NZ J Med 17:447, 1987.
172. Hare DL, Horowitz JD: Verapamil hepatotoxicity: A hypersensitivity reaction. Am Heart J 11:610, 1986.
173. Shallcross H, Padley SPG, Glynn MJ, et al: Fatal renal and hepatic toxicity after treatment with diltiazem. Br Med J 295:1236, 1987.
174. Roenigk HH Jr: Liver toxicity of retinoid therapy. J Am Acad Dermatol 19:199, 1988.
175. Andrade RJ, Lucena MI, Martin-vivaldi R, et al: Acute liver injury associated with the use of ebrotidine, a new H_2-receptor antagonist. J Hepatol 31:641, 1999.
176. Kimura H, Akamatsu K, Sakaue H, et al: Fulminant hepatitis induced by cimetidine. J Gastroenterol Hepatol 3:223, 1988.
177. Black M, Scott WE Jr, Kanter R: Possible ranitidine hepatotoxicity. Ann Intern Med 101:208, 1984.
178. Hashimoto F, Davis RL, Egli D: Hepatitis following treatments with famotidine and then cimetidine. Ann Pharmacother 28:37, 1994.
179. Jochem V, Kirkpatrick R, Greenson J, et al: Fulminant hepatic failure related to omeprazole. Am J Gastroenterol 87:523, 1992.
180. Koury SI, Stone CK, La Charite DD: Omeprazole and the development of acute hepatitis. Eur J Emerg Med 5:467, 1998.
181. Reinus JF, Persky S, Burkiewicz JS, et al: Severe liver injury after treatment with the leukotriene receptor antagonist zafirlukast. Ann Intern Med 133:964, 2000.
182. Remy AJ, Heran B, Galindo G, et al: A new drug responsible for microvesicular steatosis: Ticlopidine. Gastroenterol Clin Biol 23:151, 1999.
183. Mitchell JR, Zimmerman HJ, Ishak KG, et al: Isoniazid liver injury: Clinical spectrum, pathology and probable pathogenesis. Ann Intern Med 84:181, 1976.
184. Maddrey WC: Isoniazid-induced liver disease. Semin Liver Dis 1:129, 1981.
185. Durand F, Bernuau J, Pessayre D, et al: Deleterious influence of pyrazinamide on the outcome of patients with fulminant or subfulminant liver failure during antituberculous treatment, including isoniazid. Hepatology 21:929, 1995.
186. Moulding TS, Redeker AG, Kanel GC: Twenty isoniazid-associated deaths in one state [letter]. Ann Intern Med 114:431, 1991.
187. Hwang SJ, Wu JC, Lee CN, et al: A prospective clinical study of isoniazid-rifampicin-pyrazinamide–induced liver injury in an area endemic for hepatitis B. J Gastroenterol Hepatol 12:87, 1997.
188. Ungo JR, Jones D, Ashkin D, et al: Antituberculosis drug-induced hepatotoxicity. The role of hepatitis C virus and the human immunodeficiency virus. Am J Respir Crit Care Med 157:1871, 1998.
189. Halpern M, Meyers B, Miller C, et al: Severe isoniazid-associated hepatitis—New York, 1991–1993. JAMA 270:809, 1993.
190. Pessayre D, Bentata M, Deggott C, et al: Isoniazid-rifampicin fulminant hepatitis: A possible consequence of enhancement of isoniazid hepatotoxicity by enzyme induction. Gastroenterology 72:284, 1977.
191. Bachs L, Parés A, Elena M, et al: Effects of long-term rifampicin administration in primary biliary cirrhosis. Gastroenterology 102:2077, 1992.
192. Lewis JH, Zimmerman HJ, Benson GD, et al: Hepatic injury associated with ketoconazole therapy. Analysis of 33 cases. Gastroenterology 86:503, 1984.
193. Lake-Bakaar G, Scheuer PJ, Sherlock S: Hepatic reactions associated with ketoconazole in the United Kingdom. Br Med J 294:419, 1987.
194. Chien RN, Yang LJ, Lin PY, et al: Hepatic injury during ketoconazole therapy in patients with onychomycosis: A controlled cohort study. Hepatology 25:103, 1997.
195. Findor JA, Sorda JA, Igartua EB, Avagnina A: Ketoconazole-induced liver damage. Medicina (B Aires) 58:277, 1998.
196. van't Wout JW, Herrmann WA, de Vries RA, et al: Terbinafine-associated hepatic injury. J Hepatol 21:115, 1994.
197. Gupta AK, del Rosso JQ, Lynde CW, et al: Hepatitis associated with terbinafine therapy: Three case reports and a review of the literature. Clin Exp Dermatol 23:64, 1998.
198. Fernandes NF, Geller SA, Fong TL: Terbinafine hepatotoxicity: Case report and review of the literature. Am J Gastroenterol 93:459, 1998.
199. Mallat A, Zafrani ES, Metreau JM, et al: Terbinafine-induced prolonged cholestasis with reduction of interlobular bile ducts. Dig Dis Sci 42:1486, 1997.
200. Gitlin N, Julie NL, Spurr CL, et al: Two cases of severe clinical and histologic hepatotoxicity associated with troglitazone. Ann Intern Med 129:36, 1998.
201. Neuschwander-Tetri BA, Isley WL, Oki JC, et al: Troglitazone-induced hepatic failure leading to liver transplantation. Ann Intern Med 129:38, 1998.
202. Vella A, de Groen PC, Dinneen SF: Fatal hepatotoxicity associated with troglitazone [letter]. Ann Intern Med 129:1080, 1998.
203. Murphy EJ, Davern TJ, Shakil O, et al: Troglitazone-induced fulminant hepatic failure. Dig Dis Sci 45:549, 2000.
204. Kohlroser J, Mathai J, Reichheld J, et al: Hepatotoxicity due to troglitazone: Report of two cases and review of adverse events reported to the United States Food and Drug Administration. Am J Gastroenterol 95:272, 2000.
205. Schiano T, Dolehide K, Hart J, Baker AL: Severe but reversible hepatitis induced by troglitazone. Dig Dis Sci 45:1039, 2000.
206. Balfour JA, Plosker GL: Rosiglitazone. Drugs 57:921, 1999.
207. Forman LM, Simmons DA, Diamond RH: Hepatic failure in a patient taking rosiglitazone. Ann Intern Med 132:118, 2000.
208. Al-Salman J, Arjomand H, Kemp DG, Mittal M: Hepatocellular injury in a patient receiving rosiglitazone. A case report. Ann Intern Med 132:121, 2000.
209. Malik AH, Prasad P, Saboorian MH, et al: Hepatic injury due to troglitazone. Dig Dis Sci 45:210, 2000.
210. Bell DSH, Ovalle F: Late-onset troglitazone-induced hepatic dysfunction [letter]. Diabetes Care 23:128, 2000.
211. Jagannath S, Rai R: Rapid-onset subfulminant liver failure associated with troglitazone [letter]. Ann Intern Med 132:677, 2000.
212. Jick SS, Stender M, Myers MW: Frequency of liver disease in type 2 diabetic patients treated with oral antidiabetic agents. Diabetes Care 22:2067, 2000.

213. Selim K, Kaplowitz N: Hepatotoxicity of psychotropic drugs. Hepatology 29:1347, 1999.
214. Cai Q, Benson MA, Talbot TJ, et al: Acute hepatitis due to fluoxetine therapy. Mayo Clin Proc 74:692, 1999.
215. Johnston DE, Wheeler DE: Chronic hepatitis related to use of fluoxetine. Am J Gastroenterol 92:1225, 1997.
216. Benbow SJ, Gill G: Paroxetine and hepatotoxicity [letter]. Br Med J 314:1387, 1997.
217. Cardona X, Avila A, Castellanos P: Venlafaxine-associated hepatitis [letter]. Ann Intern Med 132:417, 2000.
218. Horsmans Y, De Clercq M, Sempoux C: Venlaxafine-associated hepatitis [letter]. Ann Intern Med 130:944, 1999.
219. Fernandes NF, Martin RR, Schenker S: Trazodone-induced hepatotoxicity: A case report with comments on drug-induced hepatotoxicity. Am J Gastroenterol 95:532, 2000.
220. Spahr L, Rubbia-Brandt L, Burkhard PR, et al: Tolcapone-related fulminant hepatitis. Electron microscopy shows mitochrondrial alterations. Dig Dis Sci 45:1881, 2000.
221. Aranda-Michel J, Koehler A, Bejarano PA, et al: Nefazodone-induced liver failure: Report of three cases. Ann Intern Med 130:285, 1999.
222. Lucena MI, Andrade RJ, Gomez-Outes A, et al: Acute liver failure after treatment with nefazodone. Dig Dis Sci 44:2577, 1999.
223. Schrader GD, Roberts-Thompson IC: Adverse effect of nefazodone: Hepatitis. Med J Aust 170:452, 1999.
224. Ausset P, Malavialle P, Vallet A, et al: Subfulminant hepatitis due to alpiderm, treated by hepatic transplantation. Gastroenterol Clin Biol 19:222, 1995.
225. Karsenti D, Blanc P, Bacq Y, et al: Hepatotoxicity associated with zolpidem treatment. Br Med J 318:1179, 1999.
226. Andrade RJ, Lucena MI, Aguilar J, et al: Chronic liver injury related to use of bentazepam. An unusual instance of benzodiazepine hepatotoxicity. Dig Dis Sci 45:1400, 2000.
227. Watkins PB, Zimmerman HJ, Knapp MJ, et al: Hepatotoxic effects of tacrine administration in patients with Alzheimer's disease. JAMA 271:992, 1994.
228. Wilkinson SP, Portmann B, Williams R: Hepatitis from dantrolene sodium. Gut 20:33, 1979.
229. Remy AJ, Camu W, Ramos J, et al: Acute hepatitis after riluzole administration. J Hepatol 30:527, 1999.
230. Castells LI, Gámex J, Cervera C, Guardia J: Icteric toxic hepatitis associated with riluzole [letter]. Lancet 351:648, 1998.
231. de Graaf EM, Oosterveld M, Tjabbes T, Stricker BH: A case of tizanidine-induced hepatic injury. J Hepatol 25:772, 1996.
232. Malka D, Pham BN, Courvalin JC, et al: Acute hepatitis caused by alverine associated with antilamin A and C autoantibodies. J Hepatol 27:399, 1997.
233. Fontana RJ, McCashland TM, Benner KG, et al: Acute liver failure associated with prolonged use of bromfenac leading to liver transplantation. The Acute Liver Failure Study Group. Liver Transpl Surg 5: 480, 1999.
234. Hunter EB, Johnston PE, Tanner G, et al: Bromfenac (Duract)–associated hepatic failure requiring liver transplantation. Am J Gastroenterol 94:2299, 1999.
235. Moses PL, Schroeder B, Alkhatib O, et al: Severe hepatotoxicity associated with bromfenac sodium. Am J Gastroenterol 94:1393, 1999.
236. Rabkin JM, Smith MJ, Orloff SL, et al: Fatal fulminant hepatitis associated with bromfenac use. Ann Pharmacother 33:945, 1999.
237. Romero-Gomez M, Nevado Santos M, Fobelo MJ, et al: Nimesulide acute hepatitis: Description of 3 cases. Med Clin (Barc) 113:357, 1999.
238. McCormick PA, Kennedy F, Curry M, Traynor O: COX-2 inhibitor and fulminant failure [letter]. Lancet 353:40, 1999.
239. Ceriani R, Borroni G, Bissoli F: Ritodrine-related liver injury. Case reports and review of the literature. Ital J Gastroenterol Hepatol 30: 315, 1998.
240. Friedman G, Lamoureux E, Sherker AH: Fatal fulminant hepatic failure due to cyproterone acetate. Dig Dis Sci 44:1362, 1999.
241. McMaster KR, Hennigar GR: Drug-induced granulomatous hepatitis. Lab Invest 44:61, 1981.
242. Al-Kawas FH, Seeff LB, Berendson RA, et al: Allopurinol hepatotoxicity. Report of two cases and review of the literature. Ann Intern Med 95:588, 1981.
243. Williams SJ, Ruppin DC, Grierson JM, et al: Carbamazepine hepatitis: The clinicopathological spectrum. J Gastroenterol Hepatol 1:159, 1986.
244. Benjamin SE, Ishak KG, Zimmerman HJ, et al: Phenylbutazone liver injury: A clinico-pathological survey of 23 cases and review of the literature. Hepatology 1:255, 1981.
245. Myers JL, Augur NA: Hydralazine-induced cholangitis. Gastroenterology 87:1185, 1984.
246. Mathur S, Dooley J, Scheuer PJ: Quinine-induced granulomatous hepatitis and vasculitis [letter]. Br Med J 300:613, 1990.
247. Knobler H, Levij IS, Gavish D, et al: Quinidine-induced hepatitis. A common and reversible hypersensitivity reaction. Arch Intern Med 146:526, 1986.
248. Mullick FG, Ishak KG: Hepatic injury associated with diphenylhydantoin therapy. A clinicopathological study of 20 cases. Am J Clin Pathol 74:442, 1980.
249. Braun M, Fraser GM, Kunin M, et al: Mesalamine-induced granulomatous hepatitis. Am J Gastroenterol 94:1973, 1999.
250. Saw D, Pitman E, Maung M, et al: Granulomatous hepatitis associated with glyburide. Dig Dis Sci 41:322, 1996.
251. Sylvain C, Fort E, Levillain P: Granulomatous hepatitis due to combination of amoxicillin and clavulanic acid. Dig Dis Sci 37:150, 1992.
252. Maddrey WC, Boitnott JK: Drug-induced chronic liver disease. Gastroenterology 72:1348, 1977.
253. Seeff LB: Drug-induced chronic liver disease, with emphasis on chronic active hepatitis. Semin Liver Dis 1:104, 1981.
254. Scully LJ, Clarke D, Bar J: Diclofenac-induced hepatitis. 3 cases with features of autoimmune chronic active hepatitis. Dig Dis Sci 38:744, 1993.
255. Iveson TJ, Ryley NG, Kelly PMA, et al: Diclofenac-associated hepatitis. J Hepatol 10:85, 1990.
256. Gough A, Chapman S, Wagstaff K, et al: Minocycline-induced autoimmune hepatitis and systemic lupus erythematosus-like syndrome. Br Med J 312:169, 1996.
257. Teitelbaum JE, Perez-Atayde AR, Cohen M, et al: Minocycline-related autoimmune hepatitis: Case series and literature review. Arch Pediatr Adolesc Med 152:1132, 1998.
258. Larrey D, Erlinger S: Drug-induced cholestasis. Bailliére's Clin Gastroenterol 2:423, 1988.
259. Chitturi S, Farrell GC: Drug-induced cholestasis. Semin Gastroenterol 12:113, 2001.
260. Chitturi S, Farrell GC: Drug-induced liver disease. Curr Treat Options Gastroenterol 3:457, 2000.
261. Moradpour D, Altorfer J, Flury R, et al: Chlorpromazine-induced vanishing bile duct syndrome leading to cirrhosis. Hepatology 20: 1437, 1994.
262. Kreek MJ: Female sex steroids and cholestasis. Semin Liver Dis 7:8, 1987.
263. Pessayre D, Larrey D, Funck-Bretano C, et al: Drug interactions and hepatitis produced by some macrolide antibiotics. J Antimicrob Chemother 16(suppl A):181, 1985.
264. Koek GH, Sticker BHCh, Blok APR, et al: Flucloxacillin-associated hepatic injury. Liver 14:225, 1994.
265. Olsson R, Wiholm BE, Sand C, et al: Liver damage from flucloxacillin, cloxacillin and dicloxacillin. J Hepatol 15:154, 1992.
266. Gosbell IB, Turnidge JD, Tapsall JW, et al: Toxicities of flucloxacillin and dicloxacillin—is there really a diference? Med J Aust 173:500, 2000.
267. Tarazi EM, Harter JG, Zimmerman HJ, et al: Sulindac-associated hepatic injury: Analysis of 91 cases reported to the Food and Drug Administration. Gastroenterology 104:569, 1993.
268. Alam I, Ferrell LD, Bass NM: Vanishing bile duct syndrome temporally associated with ibuprofen use. Am J Gastroenterol 91:1626, 1996.
269. Hepps KS, Maliha GH, Estrada R, Goodgame RW: Severe cholestatic jaundice associated with piroxicam. Gastroenterology 101:1737, 1991.
270. Crantock L, Prentice R, Powell L: Cholestatic jaundice associated with captopril therapy. J Gastroenterol Hepatol 6:528, 1991.
271. Cetin M, Demirci D, Unal A, et al: Frequency of flutamide-induced hepatotoxicity in patients with prostate carcinoma. Hum Exp Toxicol 18:137, 1999.
272. Andrade RJ, Lucena MI, Fernandez MC, et al: Fulminant liver failure associated with flutamide therapy for hirsuitism [letter]. Lancet 33: 983, 1999.
273. Hartleb M, Rymarczyk G, Januszewski K: Acute cholestatic hepatitis associated with pravastatin. Am J Gastroenterol 94:1388, 1999.
274. Jimenez-Alonso J, Osorio JM, Gutierrez-Cabello F, et al: Atorvastatin-induced cholestatic hepatitis in a young woman with systemic lupus

erythematosus. Grupo Lupus Virgen de las Nieves. Arch Intern Med 159:1811, 1999.
275. Iqbal M, Goenka P, Young MF, et al: Ticlopidine-induced cholestatic hepatitis: Report of three cases and review of the literature. Dig Dis Sci 43:2223, 1998.
276. Labowitz JK, Silverman WB: Cholestatic jaundice induced by ciprofloxacin. Dig Dis Sci 42:192, 1997.
277. Hautekeete ML, Kockx MM, Naegels S, et al: Cholestatic hepatitis related to quinolones: A report of two cases. J Hepatol 23:759, 1995.
278. Lucena MI, Andrade RJ, Sanchez-Martinez H, et al: Norfloxacin-induced cholestatic jaundice. Am J Gastroenterol 93:2309, 1998.
279. Babich MM, Pike I, Shiffman ML: Metformin-induced acute hepatitis. Am J Med 104:490, 1998.
280. Ishak KG, Irey NS: Hepatic injury associated with the phenothiazines. Clinicopathologic and follow-up study of 36 patients. Arch Pathol 93: 283, 1972.
281. Thompson JA, Fairley CK, Ugoni AM, et al: Risk factors for the development of amoxycillin-clavulanic acid associated jaundice. Med J Aust 162:638, 1995.
282. Ryan J, Dudley F: Cholestasis with ticarcillin-potassium clavulanate (Timentin). Med J Aust 156:291, 1992.
283. Sweet JM, Jones MP: Intrahepatic cholestasis due to ticarcillin-clavulanic acid [letter]. Am J Gastroenterol 90:675, 1995.
284. Richardet J-P, Mallat A, Zafrani ES, et al: Prolonged cholestasis with ductopenia after administration of amoxicillin/clavulanic acid. Dig Dis Sci 44:1997, 1999.
285. Hautekeete ML, Brenard R, Horsmans Y, et al: Liver injury related to amoxycillin-clavulanic acid: Interlobular bile-duct lesions and extrahepatic manifestations. J Hepatol 22:71, 1995.
286. Hebbard GS, Smith KG, Gibson PR, et al: Augmentin-induced jaundice with a fatal outcome. Med J Aust 156:285, 1992.
287. Chawla A, Kahn E, Yunis EJ, Daum F: Rapidly progressive cholestasis: An unusual reaction to amoxicillin/clavulanic acid therapy in a child. J Pediatr 136:121, 2000.
288. Degott C, Feldmann G, Larrey D, et al: Drug-induced prolonged cholestasis in adults: A histological semiquantitative study demonstrating progressive ductopenia. Hepatology 15:244, 1992.
289. Geubel AP, Sempoux SL: Drug and toxin-induced bile duct disorders. J Gastroenterol Hepatol 15:1232, 2000.
290. Forbes GM, Jeffrey GP, Shilkin KB, et al: Carbamazepine hepatotoxicity: Another cause of the vanishing bile duct syndrome. Gastroenterology 102: 1385, 1992.
291. Rosenberg WMC, Ryley NG, Trowell JM, et al: Dextropropoxyphene-induced hepatotoxicity: A report of nine cases. J Hepatol 19:470, 1993.
292. Kopelman H, Scheuer PJ, Williams R: The liver lesion of the Epping jaundice. Q J Med 35:553, 1966.
293. Lazarczyk DA, Duffy M: Erythromycin-induced primary biliary cirrhosis. Dig Dis Sci 45:1115, 2000.
294. Hunt CM, Washington K: Tetracycline-induced bile duct paucity and prolonged cholestasis. Gastroenterology 107:1844, 1994.
295. Srivastava M, Perez-Atayde A, Jonas MM: Drug-associated acute-onset vanishing bile duct and Stevens-Johnson syndromes in a child. Gastroenterology 115:743, 1998.
296. Yao F, Behling CA, Saab S, et al: Trimethoprim-sulfamethoxazone–induced vanishing bile duct syndrome. Am J Gastroenterol 92:167, 1997.
297. Desmet VJ. Cholangiopathies: Past, present and future. Semin Liver Dis 7:67, 1987.
298. Belghiti J, Benhamou J-P, Houry H, et al: Caustic sclerosing cholangitis. A complication of the surgical treatment of hydatid disease of the liver. Arch Surg 121:1162, 1986.
299. Anderson SD, Holley HC, Berland LL, et al: Causes of jaundice during hepatic artery infusion chemotherapy. Radiology 161:439, 1986.
300. National Halothane Study: Summary of the National Halothane Study: Possible association between halothane anesthesia and postoperative hepatic necrosis. JAMA 197:123, 1966.
301. Wright R, Eade OE, Chisholm M, et al: Controlled prospective study of the effect on liver function of multiple exposures to halothane. Lancet 1:817, 1975.
302. Schmidt CC, Suttner SW, Piper SN, et al: Comparison of the effects of desflurane and isoflurane anaesthesia on hepatocellular function assessed by alpha-glutathione S-transferase. Anaesthesia 54:1207, 1999.
303. Inman HW, Mushkin WW: Jaundice after repeated exposure to halothane: An analysis of reports to the Committee on Safety of Medicines. Br Med J 1:5, 1974.
304. Böttiger LE, Dalén E, Hallén B: Halothane-induced liver damage: An analysis of the material reported to the Swedish Adverse Drug Reaction Committee, 1966–1973. Acta Anaesthesiol Scand 20:40, 1976.
305. Nomura F, Hatano H, Ohnishi K, et al: Effects of anticonvulsant agents on halothane-induced liver injury in human subjects and experimental animals. Hepatology 6:952, 1986.
306. Farrell GC, Prendergast D, Murray M: Halothane hepatitis. Detection of a constitutional susceptibility factor. N Engl J Med 313:1300, 1985.
307. Klatskin G, Kimberg DV: Recurrent hepatitis attributable to halothane sensitization in an anesthetist. N Engl J Med 280:515, 1969.
308. Moore DH, Benson GD: Prolonged halothane hepatitis. Prompt resolution of severe lesion with corticosteroid therapy. Dig Dis Sci 31:1269, 1986.
309. Gelman S: General anesthesia and hepatic circulation. Can J Physiol Pharmacol 65:1762, 1987.
310. LaMont JT: Postoperative jaundice. Surg Clin North Am 54:637, 1974.
311. Lewis JH, Zimmerman HJ, Ishak KG, et al: Enflurane hepatotoxicity. A clinicopathologic study of 234 cases. Ann Intern Med 98:984, 1983.
312. Egar EI II, Smuckler EA, Ferrell LD, et al: Is enflurane hepatotoxic? Anesth Analg 65:21, 1986.
313. Njoku D, Laster MJ, Gong DH, et al: Biotransformation of halothane, enflurane, isoflurane, and desflurane to trifluoroacetylated liver proteins: Association between protein acylation and hepatic injury. Anesth Analg 84:173, 1997.
314. Stoelting RK, Blitt CD, Cohen PJ, et al: Hepatic dysfunction after isoflurane anesthesia. Anesth Analg 66:147, 1987.
315. Brunt EM, White H, Marsh JW, et al: Fulminant hepatic failure after repeated exposure to isoflurane anesthesia: A case report. Hepatology 13:1017, 1991.
316. Zimmerman HJ: Even isoflurane. Hepatology 13:1251, 1991.
317. Scheider DM, Klygis LM, Tsang TK, Caughron MC: Hepatic dysfunction after repeated isoflurane administration. J Clin Gastroenterol 17:168, 1993.
318. Sinha A, Clatch RJ, Stuck G, et al: Isoflurane hepatotoxicity: A case report and review of the literature. Am J Gastroenterol 91:2406, 1996.
319. Gelven PL, Cina SJ, Lee JD, Nichols CA: Massive hepatic necrosis and death following repeated isoflurane exposure: Case report and review of the literature. Am J Forensic Med Pathol 17:61, 1996.
320. Turner GB, O'Rourke D, Scott GO, Beringer TR: Fatal hepatotoxicity after re-exposure to isoflurane: A case report and review of the literature. Eur J Gastroenterol Hepatol 12:955, 2000.
321. Hasan F: Isoflurane hepatotoxicity in a patient with a previous history of halothane-induced hepatitis. Hepatogastroenterology 45:518, 1998.
322. Weitz J, Kienle P, Bohrer H, et al: Fatal hepatic necrosis after isoflurane anaesthesia. Anaesthesia 52:892, 1997.
323. Martin JL, Plevak DJ, Flannery KD, et al: Hepatotoxicity after desflurane anesthesia. Anesthesiology 83:1125, 1995.
324. Berghaus TM, Baron A, Geier A, et al: Hepatotoxicity following desflurane anesthesia. Hepatology 29:613, 1999.
325. Brunt EM, Janney CG, Di Bisceglie AM, et al: Nonalcoholic steatohepatitis: A proposal for grading and staging the histological lesions. Am J Gastroenterol 94:2467, 1999.
326. Farrell GC: Drugs and non-alcoholic steatohepatitis. In Falk 121: Steatohepatitis (NASH and ASH). Kluwer Academic 121:132, 2000.
327. Rigas B: The evolving spectrum of amiodarone hepatotoxicity. Hepatology 10:116, 1989.
328. Lewis JH, Ranard RC, Caruso A, et al: Amiodarone hepatotoxicity: Prevalence and clinicopathologic correlations among 104 patients. Hepatology 9:679, 1989.
329. Pirovino M, Müller O, Zysset T, et al: Amiodarone-induced hepatic phospholipidosis: Correlation of morphological and biochemical findings in an animal model. Hepatology 8:591, 1988.
330. Breuer HW, Bossek W, Haferland C, et al: Amiodarone-induced severe hepatitis mediated by immunological mechanisms. Int J Clin Pharmacol Ther 36:350, 1998.
331. Beuers U, Heuck A: Images in hepatology. Iodine accumulation in the liver during long-term treatment with amiodarone. J Hepatol 26:439, 1997.
332. Chang CC, Petrelli M, Tomashefski JF, McCullough AJ: Severe intrahepatic cholestasis caused by amiodarone toxicity after withdrawal of the drug: A case report and review of the literature. Arch Pathol Lab Med 123:251, 1999.

333. Richer M, Roberts S: Fatal hepatotoxicity following oral administration of amiodarone. Ann Pharmacother 29:582, 1995.
334. Fromenty B, Fisch C, Labbe G, et al: Amiodarone inhibits the mitochondrial β-oxidation of fatty acids and produces microvesicular steatosis of the liver in mice. J Pharmacol Exp Ther 255:1371, 1990.
335. Letteron P, Fromenty B, Terris B, et al: Acute and chronic hepatic steatosis lead to in vivo lipid peroxidation in mice. J Hepatol 24:200, 1996.
336. Berson A, De Beco V, Letteron P, et al: Steatohepatitis-inducing drugs cause mitochondrial dysfunction and lipid peroxidation in rat hepatocytes. Gastroenterology 114:764, 1998.
337. Hilleman D, Miller MA, Parker R, et al: Optimal management of amiodarone therapy: Efficacy and side effects. Pharmacotherapy 18: 138S, 1998.
338. Babany G, Uzzan F, Larrey D, et al: Alcoholic-like liver lesions induced by nifedipine. J Hepatol 9:252, 1989.
339. Beaugrand M, Denis J, Callard P: Tous les inhibiteurs calciques peuvent-ils entrainer des lesions d'hepatite alcoolique? Gastroenterol Clin Biol 1:76, 1987.
340. Sotaniemi EA, Hokkanen OT, Ohakas JT, et al: Hepatic injury and drug metabolism in patients with alpha-methyldopa–induced liver damage. Eur J Clin Pharmacol 12:429, 1977.
341. Seki K, Minami Y, Nishikawa M, et al: Nonalcoholic steatohepatitis induced by massive doses of synthetic estrogen. Gastroenteral Jpn 18: 197, 1983.
342. Itoh S, Igarashi M, Tsukada Y, Ichinoe A: Nonalcoholic fatty liver with alcoholic hyaline after long-term glucocorticoid therapy. Acta Hepato-Gastroenterol 24:415, 1977.
343. Lee AU, Farrell GC: Drug-induced liver disease. Curr Opin Gastroenterol 13:199, 1997.
344. Agrawal BL, Zelkowitz L: Bone "flare" hypercalcemia and jaundice after tamoxifen therapy [letter]. Arch Intern Med 141:2140, 1981.
345. Moffat DF, Oien KA, Dickson J, et al: Hepatocellular carcinoma after long-term tamoxifen therapy. Ann Oncol 11:1195, 2000.
346. Blackburn WR, Amiel SA, Millis RR, Rubens RD: Tamoxifen and liver damage. Br Med J 289:288, 1984.
347. Cai Q, Bensen M, Greene R, Kirchner J: Tamoxifen-induced transient multifocal hepatic fatty infiltration. Am J Gastroenterol 95:277, 2000.
348. Pratt DS, Knox TA, Erban J: Tamoxifen-induced steatohepatitis [letter]. Ann Intern Med 123:236, 1995.
349. Cortez-Pinto H, Baptista A, Camilo ME, et al: Tamoxifen-associated steatohepatitis—report of three cases. J Hepatol 23:95, 1995.
350. Ogawa Y, Murata Y, Nishioka A, et al: Tamoxifen-induced fatty liver in patients with breast cancer [letter]. Lancet 351:725, 1998.
351. Van Hoof M, Rahier J, Horsmans Y: Tamoxifen-induced steatohepatitis [letter]. Ann Intern Med 124:855, 1996.
352. Oien KA, Moffat D, Curry GW, et al: Cirrhosis with steatohepatitis after adjuvant tamoxifen [letter]. Lancet 353:36, 1999.
353. Dray X, Tainturier MH, De La Lande P, et al: Cirrhosis with nonalcoholic steatohepatitis: Role of tamoxifen. Gastroenterol Clin Biol 24: 1122, 2000.
354. Saibara T, Ogawa Y, Takahashi M, et al: Tamoxifen-induced nonalcoholic steatohepatitis and bezafibrate [abstract]. J Gastroenterol Hepatol 15 (Suppl):F96, 2000.
355. Hamada N, Ogawa Y, Saibara T, et al: Toremifene-induced fatty liver and NASH in breast cancer patients with breast-conservation treatment. Int J Oncol 17:1119, 2000.
356. Ruymann FB, Mosijczuk AD, Sayers RJ: Hepatoma in a child with methotrexate-induced hepatic fibrosis. JAMA 238:2631, 1977.
357. Zachariae H, Kragbelle K, Søgaard H: Methotrexate-induced liver cirrhosis: Studies including serial liver biopsies during continued treatment. Br J Dermatol 102:407, 1980.
358. Shergy WJ, Polisson RP, Caldwell DS, et al: Methotrexate-associated hepatotoxicity: Retrospective analysis of 210 patients with rheumatoid arthritis. Am J Med 85:771, 1988.
359. Lewis JH, Schiff ER: Methotrexate-induced chronic liver injury: Guidelines for detection and prevention. Am J Gastroenterol 88:1337, 1988.
360. Whiting-O'Keefe QE, Fyfe KH, Sack KD: Methotrexate and histologic hepatic abnormalities: A meta-analysis. Am J Med 90:711, 1991.
361. Zachariae H, Søgaard H: Methotrexate-induced liver cirrhosis: A follow up. Dermatologica 175:178, 1987.
362. Langman G, Hall P de la M: Personal communication, 2000.
363. Gilbert SC, Klintmalm G, Menter A, et al: Methotrexate-induced cirrhosis requiring liver transplantation in three patients with psoriasis. Arch Intern Med 150:889, 1990.
364. Kremer JM, Alarcon GS, Lightfoot RW Jr, et al: Methotrexate for rheumatoid arthritis. Suggested guidelines for monitoring liver toxicity. Arthritis Rheum 37:316, 1994.
365. Zafrani ES, Pinaudeau Y, Dhumeaux D: Drug-induced vascular lesions of the liver. Arch Intern Med 143:495, 1983.
366. Doll DC, Ringenberg QS, Yarbro JW: Vascular toxicity associated with antineoplastic agents. J Clin Oncol 4:1405, 1986.
367. McDonald GB, Hinds MS, Fisher LD, et al: Veno-occlusive disease of the liver and multiorgan failure after bone marrow transplantation: A cohort study of 355 patients. Ann Intern Med 118:255, 1993.
368. Chitturi S, Farrell GC: Herbal hepatotoxicity: An expanding but poorly defined problem. J Gastroenterol Hepatol 15:1093, 2000.
369. Ridker PM, Ohkuma S, McDermott WV, et al: Hepatic venoocclusive disease associated with the consumption of pyrrolizidine-containing dietary supplements. Gastroenterology 88:1050, 1985.
370. Key NS, Kelly PMA, Emerson PM, et al: Oesophageal varices associated with busulphan-thioguanine combination therapy for chronic myeloid leukaemia. Lancet 2:1050, 1987.
371. Snover DC, Weisdorf S, Bloomer J, et al: Nodular regenerative hyperplasia of the liver following bone marrow transplantation. Hepatology 9:443, 1989.
372. Nevens F, Fevery J, Van Steegbergen W, et al: Arsenic and non-cirrhotic portal hypertension. A report of eight cases. J Hepatol 11:80, 1990.
373. Thomas LB, Popper H, Berk PD, et al: Vinyl-chloride–induced liver disease. From idiopathic portal hypertension (Banti's syndrome) to angiosarcomas. N Engl J Med 292:17, 1975.
374. Loomus GN, Aneja P, Bota RA: A case of peliosis hepatis in association with tamoxifen therapy. Am J Clin Pathol 80:881, 1983.
375. Larrey D, Fréneaux E, Berson A, et al: Peliosis hepatis induced by 6-thioguanine administration. Gut 29:1265, 1988.
376. Zafrani ES, Bernuau D, Feldmann G: Peliosis-like ultrastructural changes of the hepatic sinusoids in human chronic hypervitaminosis A: Report of three cases. Hum Pathol 15:1166, 1984.
377. Sterneck M, Weisner R, Ascher N, et al: Azathioprine hepatotoxicity after liver transplantation. Hepatology 14:806, 1991.
378. Duvoux C, Kracht M, Lang P, et al: Nodular regenerative hyperplasia of the liver associated with azathioprine therapy. Gastroenterol Clin Biol 15:968, 1991.
379. Gane E, Portmann B, Saxena R, et al: Nodular regenerative hyperplasia of the liver graft after liver transplantation. Hepatology 20:88, 1994.
380. Liaño F, Moreno A, Matesanz R, et al: Veno-occlusive hepatic disease of the liver in renal transplantation: Is azathioprine the cause? Nephron 51:509, 1989.
381. Ishak KG: Hepatic lesions caused by anabolic and contraceptive steroids. Semin Liver Dis 1:116, 1981.
382. Anthony PP: Liver tumours. Bailliére's Clin Gastroenterol 2:501, 1988.
383. Kerlin P, Davis GL, McGill DB, et al: Hepatic adenoma and focal nodular hyperplasia: Clinical, pathologic and radiologic features. Gastroenterology 84:994, 1983.
384. Pain JA, Gimson AES, Williams R, et al: Focal nodular hyperplasia of the liver: Results of treatment and options in management. Gut 32: 524, 1991.
385. Edmondson HA, Henderson B, Benton B: Liver-cell adenomas associated with use of oral contraceptives. N Engl J Med 294:470, 1976.
386. Farrell GC, Joshua DE, Uren R, et al: Androgen-induced hepatoma. Lancet 1:430, 1975.
387. Westaby D, Portmann B, Williams R: Androgen-related primary hepatic tumors in non-Fanconi patients. Cancer 51:1947, 1983.
388. Kahn H, Manzarbeita C, Theise N, et al: Danazol-induced hepatocellular adenoma. A case report and review of the literature. Arch Pathol Lab Med 115:1054, 1991.
389. Bork K, Pitton M, Harten P, Koch P: Hepatocellular adenomas in patients taking danazol for hereditary angio-edema [letter]. Lancet 353:1066, 1999.
390. Tesluk H, Lawrie J: Hepatocellular adenoma. Its transformation to carcinoma in a user of oral contraceptives. Arch Pathol Lab Med 105: 296, 1981.
391. La Vecchia C, Negri E, Parazzini F: Oral contraceptives and primary liver cancer. Br J Cancer 59:460, 1989.
392. La Vecchia C, Tavani A, Franceschi S, Parazzini F: Oral contraceptives and cancer. A review of the evidence. Drug Saf 14:260, 1996.
393. Gleeson D, Newbould MJ, Taylor P, et al: Androgen-associated hepatocellular carcinoma with an aggressive course. Gut 32:1084, 1991.

394. Falk H, Herbert JT, Edmonds L, et al: Review of four cases of childhood hepatic angiosarcoma — elevated environmental arsenic exposure in one case. Cancer 47:382, 1981.
395. Harrison R, Hathaway G, Welch L, et al: Case studies in environmental medicine. Vinyl chloride toxicity. Clin Toxicol 28:267, 1990.
396. Simonato L, L'Abbe KA, Andersen A, et al: A collaborative study of cancer incidence and mortality among vinyl chloride workers. Scand J Work Environ Health 17:159, 1991.
397. Pond SM: Effects on the liver of chemicals encountered in the workplace. West J Med 137:506, 1982.
398. Pond SM, Olson KR, Woo OF, et al: Amatoxin poisoning in Northern California, 1982–1983. West J Med 145:204, 1986.
399. Larrey D. Hepatotoxicity of herbal remedies. J Hepatol 26 (Suppl 1): 47, 1997.
400. Stickel F, Egerer G, Seitz HK: Hepatotoxicity of botanicals. Public Health Nutr 3:113, 2000.
401. Larrey D, Vial T, Pauwels A, et al: Hepatitis after germander *(Teucrium chamaedrys)* administration: Another instance of herbal medicine hepatotoxicity. Ann Intern Med 117:129, 1992.
402. Sullivan JB Jr, Rumack BH, Thomas H Jr, et al: Pennyroyal oil poisoning and hepatotoxicity. JAMA 242:2873, 1979.
403. Katz M, Saibil F: Herbal hepatitis: Subacute hepatic necrosis secondary to chaparral leaf. J Clin Gastroenterol 12:203, 1990.
404. Sheikh NM, Philen RM, Love LA: Chaparral-associated hepatotoxicity. Arch Intern Med 157:913, 1997.
405. Beuers U, Spengler U, Pape GR: Hepatitis after chronic abuse of senna [letter]. Lancet 337:372, 1991.
406. Delbanco TL: Bitter herbs: Mainstream, magic, and menace. Ann Intern Med 121:803, 1994.
407. Eisenberg DM, Davis RB, Ettner SL, et al: Trends in alternative medicine use in the United States, 1990–1997. JAMA 280:1569, 1998.
408. Winslow LC, Kroll DJ: Herbs as medicines. Arch Intern Med 158: 2192, 1998.
409. Angell M, Kassirer JP: Alternative medicine—the risks of untested and unregulated remedies. N Engl J Med 339:839, 1998.
410. Drew AK, Myers SP: Safety issues in herbal medicine: Implications for the health professions. Med J Aust 166:538, 1997.
411. Bensoussan A: Complementary medicine—where lies its appeal? Med J Aust 170:247, 1999.
412. Lewith GT: Complementary and alternative medicine: An educational, attitudinal and research challenge. Med J Aust 2000;172:102.
413. MacLennan AH, Wilson DH, Taylor AW: Prevalence and cost of alternative medicine in Australia. Lancet 347:569, 1996.
414. Berk BS, Chaya C, Benner KC, et al: Comparison of herbal therapy for liver disease: 1996 versus 1999 [abstract]. Hepatology 30:A478, 1999.
415. Peyton BG, Spears TL, Lindsey A, et al: A survey of the use of herbal medicine in patients with hepatitis C [abstract]. Hepatology 30: A191, 1999.
416. Chan TYK, Chan JCN, Tomlinson B, et al: Chinese herbal medicines revisited: A Hong Kong perspective. Lancet 342:1532, 1993.
417. Woolf GM, Petrovic LM, Roijter SE, et al: Acute hepatitis associated with the Chinese herbal product Jin Bu Huan. Ann Intern Med 121: 729, 1994.
418. Picciotti A, Campo N, Brizzolara R, et al: Chronic hepatitis induced by Jin Bu Huan. J Hepatol 28:165, 1998.
419. Horowitz RS, Feldhaus K, Dart RC, et al: The clinical spectrum of Jin Bu Huan toxicity. Arch Intern Med 156:899, 1996.
420. Kane JA, Kane SP, Jain S: Hepatitis induced by traditional Chinese herbs: Possible toxic components. Gut 36:146, 1995.
421. Nadir A, Agarwal S, King PD, et al: Acute hepatitis associated with the use of a Chinese herbal product, Ma-huang. Am J Gastroenterol 91:1436, 1996.
422. Melchart D, Linde K, Weidenhammer W, et al: Liver enzyme elevation in patients treated with traditional Chinese medicine. JAMA 282: 28, 1999.
423. Benninger J, Schneider HT, Schuppan D, et al: Acute hepatitis induced by Greater Celandine *(Chelidonium majus)*. Gastroenterology 117:1234, 1999.
424. Kamiyama T, Nouchi T, Kojima S, et al: Autoimmune hepatitis triggered by administration of a herbal medicine. Am J Gastroenterol 92: 703, 1997.
425. Park GJ-H, Mann SP, Ngu MC: Acute hepatitis induced by Shou-Wu-Pian, a herbal product derived from *Polygonum multiflorum*. J Gastroenterol Hepatol 16:115, 2001.
426. Hamid S, Rojter S, Vierling J: Protracted cholestatic hepatitis after the use of Prostata [letter]. Ann Intern Med 127:169, 1997.
427. Itoh S, Marutani K, Nishijima T, et al: Liver injuries induced by herbal medicine, syo-saiko-to (xiao-chai-hu-tang). Dig Dis Sci 40: 1845, 1995.
428. Mattei A, Rucay P, Samuel D, et al: Liver transplantation for acute liver failure after herbal medicine *(Teucrium polium)* administration [letter]. J Hepatol 22:597, 1995.
429. Yoshida EM, McLean CA, Cheng ES, et al: Chinese herbal medicine, fulminant hepatitis and liver transplantation [letter]. Am J Gastroenterol 91:2647, 1996.
430. Hullar TE, Sapers BL, Ridker PM, et al: Herbal hepatotoxicity and fatal hepatic failure. Am J Med 106:267, 1999.
431. Farrell GC, Bhathal PS, Powell LW: Abnormal liver function in chronic hypervitaminosis A. Am J Dig Dis 22:724, 1977.
432. Kowalski TE, Falestiny M, Furth E, et al: Vitamin A hepatotoxicity: A cautionary note regarding 25,000 IU supplements. Am J Med 97: 523, 1994.
433. Geubel AP, De Galocsy C, Alves N, et al: Liver damage caused by therapeutic vitamin A administration: Estimation of dose-related toxicity in 41 cases. Gastroenterology 100:1701, 1991.
434. Leo MA, Lieber CS: Hypervitaminosis A: A liver lover's lament. Hepatology 8:412, 1988.
435. Russell RM, Boyer JL, Bagheri SA, et al: Hepatic injury from chronic hypervitaminosis A resulting in portal hypertension and ascites. N Engl J Med 291:435, 1974.
436. Sarles J, Scheiner C, Sarran M, et al: Hepatic hypervitaminosis A: A familial observation. J Pediatr Gastroenterol Nutr 10:71, 1990.
437. Inkeles SB, Conner WE, Illingworth DR: Hepatic and dermatologic manifestations of chronic hypervitaminosis A in adults. Report of two cases. Am J Med 80:491, 1986.

Chapter 74

Pregnancy-Related Hepatic and Gastrointestinal Disorders

Caroline A. Riely and Rene Davila

Pregnancy is a state of altered, but normal, physiologic processes. Gastroenterologists and internists often are not well versed in the physiologic characteristics of pregnancy and may be uneasy when confronted with a pregnant patient who has a gastrointestinal or liver disorder. Because some disorders affect pregnant women uniquely, physicians may be unsure as to which diagnostic tools are safe to use and which medications are safe to prescribe in this setting. Patients who have chronic gastrointestinal or hepatic disorders may have pressing questions about the effects of their underlying condition on a possible pregnancy. In many instances, the answers are unclear because of the lack of prospective studies and an incomplete understanding of the pathogenesis of these conditions. Nevertheless, the care of the pregnant woman who has gastrointestinal or liver disease is usually extremely gratifying, because most such persons are basically healthy and involved in a joyful event.

LIVER PROBLEMS UNIQUE TO PREGNANCY

Cholestasis of Pregnancy

Cholestasis of pregnancy is a form of intrahepatic cholestasis that is associated with itching, elevation of serum bile acid levels, and bland cholestasis on a liver biopsy specimen during pregnancy.[1, 2] The condition is not rare and may have a variable course, making diagnosis difficult.[3] The diagnosis has serious implications for fetal well-being and must be addressed promptly.[4]

CLINICAL FEATURES. Cholestasis of pregnancy usually occurs in the third trimester of gestation but can begin earlier. The initial, and the most characteristic, symptom is pruritus, and patients may be referred initially to a dermatologist. As with all forms of cholestasis, pruritus is most severe at night and on the palms and soles. In this condition, the pruritus is often intractable and can be difficult to tolerate, leading in rare patients to threats of suicide. Jaundice develops in only a minority of patients during the course of the disease. Laboratory testing confirms the presence of cholestasis, with elevations in serum levels of bile acids and, in some patients, with bilirubinuria or even an elevation in the serum bilirubin level.[5] The level of alkaline phosphatase is modestly elevated, but the gamma glutamyl transpeptidase (GGTP) level is normal or only minimally elevated, an unexpected finding that is atypical of cholestasis in adults.[5] The phenomenon of cholestasis with a normal GGTP level is similar to that of cholestasis in pediatric patients who have progressive familial intrahepatic cholestasis caused by an inherited defect, as in Byler's syndrome.[6] The levels of serum aminotransferases are also elevated, occasionally to values of 1000 U/L or higher; therefore, distinguishing cholestasis of pregnancy from hepatitis is difficult.[7] When monitored serially, the laboratory test results, and even the symptoms, may vary. The intense cholestasis is associated with steatorrhea, which is usually subclinical but may lead to fat-soluble vitamin deficiencies, most notably a deficiency in vitamin K.

Amelioration in the symptoms and improvement in the laboratory test results begin with delivery and are usually, although not invariably, prompt and complete. Rare patients experience prolonged cholestasis; this occurrence should suggest an alternate diagnosis, such as primary biliary cirrhosis or primary sclerosing cholangitis.[8, 9] Women who have cholestasis of pregnancy have no hepatic sequelae but are at increased risk for the development of gallstones. The disorder may recur with subsequent gestations, and 60% to 70% of patients affected in their initial pregnancy have a recurrence, although not necessarily as severe as the first episode. Patients who have experienced a previous episode and who have had cholecystectomy are at greater risk for cholestasis of pregnancy on subsequent gestations than those who have not had cholecystectomy.[10]

The fetus fares less well than the mother, and there are many reports of an increased frequency of fetal distress, unexplained stillbirth, and need for premature delivery and neonatal care.[4, 11] These risks may be minimized by heightened surveillance through close monitoring of an affected mother.[12] Not all studies, however, have reached the same conclusion, and stillbirth may occur even after a monitoring session.[13] Electively planned early delivery shortly after the fetal lungs have matured has been recommended.[4, 14]

PATHOGENESIS. The pathogenesis of cholestasis of pregnancy is unclear. The condition is most common in certain ethnic groups, especially in Chile and Scandinavia.[1] The condition may have some relation to the season of the year, and it is seen more commonly in the colder months in both Chile and Scandinavia. Other environmental factors may play a significant role, and, of interest, the prevalence in Chile has fallen in the past several years, perhaps in response to increases in mean serum selenium levels in the population.[15] In some patients, there is a clear family history,[16, 17] and a heightened sensitivity to the cholestatic effects of exogenous estrogen has been demonstrated in family members (including male relatives) of affected women.[18] There has been much recent interest in the unfolding discovery of gene defects that result in cholestatic syndromes in children, and two groups have described women with cholestasis of pregnancy and elevated GGTP levels who have a defect in the multidrug resistance type 3 (MDR-3) gene.[19, 20] There is no relationship to human leukocyte antigen (HLA) types.[21] Administration of estrogen to susceptible women can precipitate cholestasis,[22] and in the experimental setting, estrogen clearly causes cholestasis.[23] Progesterone use during pregnancy is associated with cholestasis of pregnancy.[24] The finding that ursodeoxycholic acid therapy alters the metabolism of progesterone[25] perhaps explains its mode of action (discussed later). It is possible that affected persons have an inherited enhanced sensitivity to estrogen or alteration in the metabolism of progesterone and that clinical cholestasis develops in response to a variety of stimuli, including medications and dietary factors.

DIFFERENTIAL DIAGNOSIS. The differential diagnosis of cholestasis of pregnancy is broad and includes other cholestatic states such as primary biliary cirrhosis, primary sclerosing cholangitis, benign recurrent intrahepatic cholestasis, viral hepatitis, and biliary obstruction. Liver biopsy in patients who have cholestasis of pregnancy reveals a bland cholestasis but is usually not warranted. A family of sisters with progressive liver disease associated with recurrent severe cholestasis in pregnancy, atypical of the usual cholestasis of pregnancy, was described in 1997.[8] The clinician should remember that pregnancy can exacerbate underlying cholestasis related to a preexisting disease (which may be subclinical), such as primary biliary cirrhosis or familial intrahepatic cholestasis.

MANAGEMENT. Management of this cholestatic syndrome is difficult and is primarily symptomatic. Ursodeoxycholic acid has been shown to be helpful and is well tolerated by the patient and fetus.[4, 26] Its mechanism of action is uncertain; studies have demonstrated improvement in the bile acid profile in both the mother's serum and amniotic fluid,[27, 28] as well as improved transport of bile acids across the placenta.[29] Most investigators have used a conventional dose (15 mg/kg/day), although a 2001 report suggests that a higher dose (20 to 25 mg/kg/day) is more beneficial.[28] The use of bile acid binders such as cholestyramine or guar gum[30] may help, but the treating physician should bear in mind that this therapy worsens steatorrhea and fat-soluble vitamin deficiency.[31] Therapy with *S*-adenosylmethionine (SAMe) was reported to be successful in one study but not in others.[4, 32, 33] Therapy with a combination of both ursodeoxycholic acid and SAMe may have some utility.[34, 35] A short course of oral dexamethasone has been reported to reduce itching and serum levels of bile acids[16] but was associated with clinical deterioration in one case.[36] Central sedatives, such as phenobarbital, may produce some symptomatic relief but have implications for the fetus. Ultraviolet B light treatment has been suggested. As with other cholestatic syndromes, no therapy is always or completely efficacious, and the only sure therapy is delivery, which affected patients may urge.

Liver Disease of Preeclampsia

Preeclampsia/eclampsia, the disorder previously known as "toxemia of pregnancy," is a disease of unclear cause that is difficult to define and, on occasion, to diagnose.[37] The disorder is not rare and complicates 3% to 10% of all pregnancies. It occurs more commonly in women who are primiparas or have a multiple gestation than in other pregnant women.[38] It is a multisystemic disease that begins in the second half of gestation, in which the manifestations may be lacking in any one system.[39] The usual criteria for making the diagnosis include sustained hypertension after the 20th week of pregnancy, with a blood pressure of 140/90 mm Hg or higher, in a woman known previously to be normotensive, with proteinuria of 500 mg/L or greater indicated on 24-hour urine testing.[40] Many patients are hyper-reflexic, and many are edematous. Liver disease is now recognized as a common, and ominous, complication of preeclampsia. The liver disease usually takes the form of the hemolysis, elevated liver enzymes, and low platelets (HELLP) syndrome. Since it was named by Weinstein in 1982,[41] HELLP syndrome has been recognized increasingly. It is presumed to underlie the even more ominous complications of hepatic hematoma and rupture in pregnancy[42, 43] and infarct of the liver (discussed later).[44] Preeclampsia is commonly present in patients who have acute fatty liver of pregnancy and may play an important role in the pathogenesis of this disorder, although acute fatty liver of pregnancy is not usually classified as one of the preeclamptic liver diseases.[45]

Hemolysis, Elevated Liver Enzymes, and Low Platelets Syndrome

CLINICAL FEATURES. HELLP syndrome is common, complicating the course of pregnancy in almost 20% of women who have severe preeclampsia.[46] Patients may exhibit HELLP syndrome as their major problem. They may report epigastric or right upper quadrant abdominal and chest pain, nausea and vomiting, and symptoms typical of preeclampsia (thirst, headache, and blurred vision) (Table 74–1). In such patients, the diagnosis is usually arrived at with ease. Other patients may have an asymptomatic fall in the platelet count during observation prompted by preeclampsia. Some patients have no hypertension or proteinuria at the initial medical consultation.[47] Some patients complain of malaise that suggests "flu."[48] Most patients seek treatment after the 27th week of gestation, but up to 11% may do so earlier. Presentation of the disorder after delivery, with no signs of preeclampsia at delivery, occurs in up to 30% of cases.[49, 46]

DIAGNOSIS. The diagnosis rests on clinical grounds (see Table 74–1). The hemolysis is modest and associated with fragmented cells on blood smear and with an elevated serum lactate dehydrogenase (LDH) level. The serum aminotransferase levels are elevated, ranging from modest elevations to levels of several thousand without substantial elevations in levels of cholestatic enzymes.[46, 50] The serum bilirubin level is often elevated but usually to a low levels. Serum levels of glutathione *S*-transferase alpha may be a more sensitive indicator of liver involvement than aspartate aminotransferase (AST).[51] Elevations in serum levels of D-dimer,[52] tissue polypeptide antigen (TPA),[53] and fibronectin[54] have been described in patients with HELLP syndrome, and these tests may have some utility in predicting severe disease. Imaging of the abdomen may be useful and should be performed for any patient who has severe abdominal pain, neck or shoulder pain, or hypotension. One report has documented abnormalities in 45% of such patients; computed tomography (CT) and magnetic resonance imaging (MRI) were the most useful imaging techniques.[42]

Table 74–1 | **Clinical Characteristics of Hemolysis, Elevated Liver Enzymes, and Low Platelets (HELLP) Syndrome**

Presenting Symptom	Percentage Affected	
Pain, right upper quadrant or epigastric	65	
Nausea or vomiting	36	
Headache	31	
Bleeding	9	
Jaundice	5	
Laboratory Findings (Normal Range)	**Median**	**Range**
AST level (<40 U/L)	249	70–663
Total bilirubin (<1 mg/dL)	1.5	0.5–25
Platelet count (>125 × 10^3/mm^3)	57	7–99
Outcome, Maternal Complications	**Percentage**	
Disseminated intravascular coagulation	21	
Abruptio placentae	16	
Acute renal failure	8	
Subcapsular hematoma of liver	1	
Death	1	

AST, aspartate aminotransferase.

Adapted from Sibai BH, Ramadan MK, Usta I, et al: Maternal morbidity and mortality in 442 pregnancies with hemolysis, elevated liver enzymes, and low platelets (HELLP syndrome). Am J Obstet Gynecol 169:100–106, 1993.

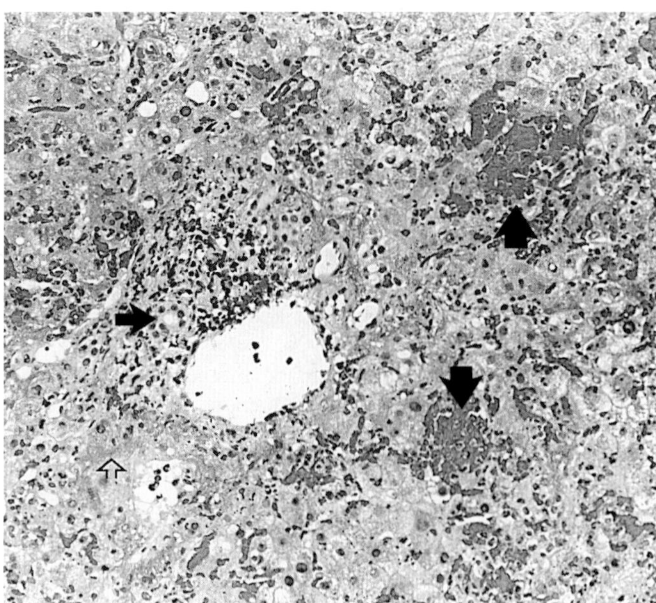

Figure 74–1. Histology of HELLP syndrome. The portal triad, on the left of the figure (the *horizontal arrow* points to an interlobular bile duct in the portal triad), is surrounded by pockets of hemorrhage *(vertical arrows)* and by an area of fibrin deposition (to the left of the portal triad).

Liver biopsy specimens demonstrate periportal hemorrhage and fibrin deposition with periportal hepatic necrosis typical of preeclampsia (Fig. 74–1). Both macrovesicular and microvesicular fat are present,[55, 56] but steatosis is usually modest and is unlike the pericentral microvesicular fat seen in acute fatty liver of pregnancy. There is little if any correlation between the severity of the histologic lesion on liver biopsy and the abnormalities in laboratory testing results (primarily platelet count and serum aminotransferase levels); modest laboratory result abnormalities should not be interpreted to indicate only modest hepatic involvement.[57] Liver biopsy is rarely warranted and should be approached with caution, because of the possibility of hepatic hematoma or contained rupture.

Although most women with thrombocytopenia in association with preeclampsia have HELLP syndrome, the differential diagnosis is not limited to this disorder.[58, 59] Also to be considered are other diseases that cause thrombocytopenia, including idiopathic thrombocytopenic purpura, thrombotic thrombocytopenic purpura,[60] and the antiphospholipid antibody syndrome.[61] The liver involvement of HELLP syndrome is most frequently misdiagnosed as viral hepatitis,[62] although thrombocytopenia is unexpected in hepatitis. Acute fatty liver of pregnancy should be considered but is usually associated with more severe liver failure (although often with lower serum aminotransferase levels) and is not necessarily associated with thrombocytopenia.

PATHOGENESIS. The pathogenesis of preeclampsia remains elusive, a surprising fact in light of the frequency of the syndrome.[37] Any hypothesis must include the known characteristics of the disorder: it is more common in primiparas, and patients have inappropriately high systemic vascular resistance with an inappropriately low plasma volume. Preeclampsia follows, and is presumably a consequence of, a problem with placentation: there is a failure of trophoblast invasion of the uterine lining, which leads to a failure of dilation of the spiral arteries and an inability to increase uteroplacental perfusion appropriately as gestation proceeds.[63] There is often a family history of preeclampsia or eclampsia in the patient's mother, and, in some populations, evidence exists to support inheritance as either an autosomal recessive trait or an autosomal dominant trait with variable penetrance.[64, 65] Preeclampsia is less common the longer the parents of the fetus have been cohabiting sexually and also is less common when there has been a previous miscarriage or delivery of a fetus of the same father.[66] In contrast, the disorder is more common in multiparous women who have had a change in sexual partner and a change in paternity of the fetus; in these circumstances, the risk for preeclampsia approaches that for primiparous women.[67] These data suggest that immune mechanisms play a role; for example, natural immune tolerance may develop over time with exposure to the father's sperm.[68, 69] There is an increased risk of early and severe preeclampsia in women who have an underlying procoagulant such as factor V Leiden mutation or an anticardiolipin antibody.[70, 71] Preeclampsia also occurs with greater frequency in women who have polycystic ovary syndrome.[72]

Preeclampsia is common, although not invariable, in women who have acute fatty liver of pregnancy, and these two disorders may share a common pathogenesis. Women who have long-chain 3-hydroxyacyl-CoA dehydrogenase (LCHAD) deficiency, an underlying defect in intramitochondrial beta oxidation of fatty acids, have been reported to have preeclampsia and HELLP syndrome while pregnant with an affected fetus.[73] Other studies have not demonstrated LCHAD deficiency in women with HELLP syndrome.[74] Other hypotheses include ongoing lipid peroxidation and oxidative stress in response to an unknown primary insult, dysfunction of the endothelium,[54, 75] abnormal fluidity of the endothelial cell membrane, abnormal permeability of the cells to calcium, or inheritance of a molecular variant of angiotensin known to be associated with hypertension.[76] Interestingly, there is no animal model for the human syndrome of preeclampsia, and the histologic characteristics of this condition are unique and are not similar to those of any other known liver disease in humans or animals.

OUTCOME AND MANAGEMENT. In most affected patients, the clinical course of HELLP syndrome is marked by prompt return to normal of all abnormalities after delivery, which is the treatment of choice.[77] Transient diabetes insipidus has been reported.[78] In rare patients the condition worsens progressively before delivery, with further diminution of the platelet count to dangerously low levels and development of sepsis, multisystem organ failure, or hepatic failure with disseminated intravascular coagulation. Death of the mother can occur but is rare.[79] Untreated, or undiagnosed, patients may experience progression to renal failure, hepatic hematoma, hepatic rupture, and death. Neither the serum aminotransferase levels nor platelet count is predictive of the outcome.[80] Patients are at risk for obstetric complications including preeclampsia during subsequent pregnancies but are at low risk for recurrent HELLP syndrome,[81] although it can recur.[82] The offspring of affected pregnancies may experience the consequences of intrauterine growth retardation or prematurity but are not at risk of thrombocytopenia.[83, 84]

Management is primarily supportive; once the diagnosis is made the patient should be observed and supported in an intensive care unit, until the baby can be delivered safely. The delivery should be accomplished by the safest route, which may be vaginal. Some patients may be "tided over," that is, carried with close inpatient observation without delivery, and may show improvement in the platelet count and serum aminotransferase levels.[85] This temporizing management is tried if the woman is at an early stage of gestation and may result in delaying delivery and prolonging gestation,[85] but it may not be successful, because the fetus usually fails to grow in the setting of preeclampsia. Patients may require platelet transfusion or even dialysis. Full recovery with no sequelae is anticipated, and every effort should be made to support the patient. Plasmapheresis after delivery has been advocated by some authorities but is expensive and has not been proved to alter the course.[49, 86] Glucocorticoid therapy also has been advocated, and many affected women receive glucocorticoids before delivery not as a result of the disease, but as a method of speeding fetal lung maturity.[87] Glucocorticoids have been used with success but have not been tested in controlled trials.[88–90] Liver transplantation has been used in the treatment of HELLP syndrome but with early diagnosis and prompt delivery should not be needed.[91]

Hepatic Rupture, Hematoma, and Infarct

Spontaneous rupture of the liver can be a complication of preeclampsia and of the HELLP syndrome. Patients with this feared and often fatal disorder seek medical attention in the third trimester, usually close to term, or in the early postpartum period with abdominal pain and distention and cardiovascular collapse.[92–96] In contrast with most preeclampsia patients, patients who experience spontaneous hepatic rupture tend to be older and to have had multiple previous pregnancies. If the condition is undiagnosed or untreated, death results for both mother and fetus. Diagnosis depends on identification of hemoperitoneum, which can be detected by paracentesis, and demonstration on CT, ultrasonography, or MRI of the ruptured liver, often with a partially contained subcapsular hematoma (Fig. 74–2).[42, 97, 98] Laparoscopy demonstrates the subcapsular hemorrhages.[99] Management should be aggressive, with rapid delivery of the fetus and repair of the liver, which is best carried out by surgeons who have expertise in trauma surgery. Affected patients have a protracted course that can include disseminated intravascular coagulation and hepatic failure. Rare patients have been treated with liver transplantation, with removal of the fractured liver followed by interval portosystemic shunting while a donor organ is urgently sought.[92, 100] In rare instances, a patient who has a hepatic rupture and is in a hemodynamically stable condition can be successfully treated expectantly without surgery.[101] Patients who survive may have uneventful subsequent pregnancies[101] or recurrence of the hematoma with rupture.[102]

Some patients may have a contained subcapsular hematoma without frank rupture into the peritoneum. In such patients, pain is the usual symptom. Management in these

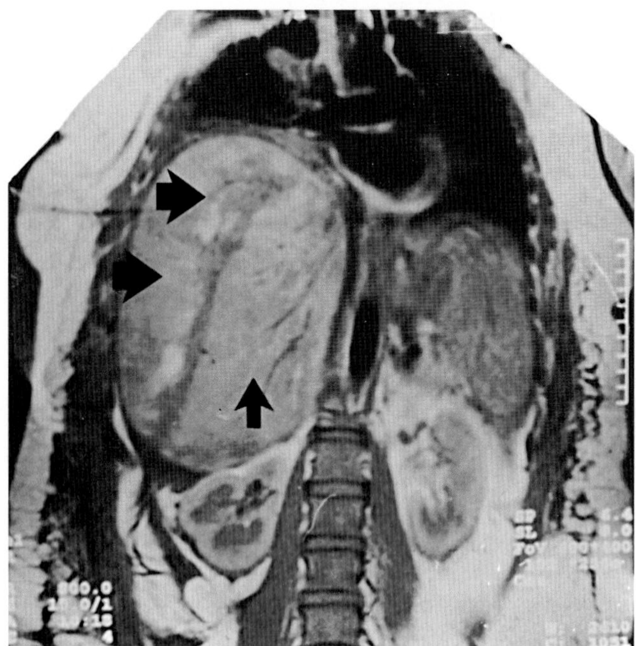

Figure 74–2. Subcapsular hepatic hematoma in preeclampsia. This coronal section of a T1-weighted MRI scan demonstrates the subcapsular clot or hemorrhage *(horizontal arrows)* adjacent to the liver *(vertical arrow).* (From Barton JR, Sibai BM: Hepatic imaging in HELLP syndrome [hemolysis, elevated liver enzymes, and low platelet count]. Am J Obstet Gynecol 174:1820–1825, 1996.)

cases can be expectant, with serial imaging by CT scanning and careful prevention of pressure to the liver.[42, 102] Some experts have recommended angiographic embolization of the hepatic artery in such cases.

Hepatic rupture complicating preeclampsia results from extravasation of blood, presumably from one or several microscopic areas of periportal hemorrhage under Glisson's capsule, as is typical of HELLP syndrome.[96] The capsule is then torn off the surface of the liver by the expanding hematoma, leaving behind multiple bleeding sites on the denuded surface of the liver. When the pressure under the capsule becomes excessive, the capsule ruptures, with resulting hemoperitoneum.

Necrotic infarcts of the liver also occur as a complication of preeclampsia. Patients have unexpected anemia with fever, leukocytosis, and marked elevation in the serum aminotransferase levels.[42, 44, 103] There may be accompanying hepatic failure. With time, the disorder may resolve completely, or may lead to death from multiorgan failure. Confluent infarcts can best be seen on CT scanning. Needle aspiration of the abnormal areas yields blood or necrotic tissue. The immediately adjacent liver tissue shows the periportal hemorrhage and fibrin deposition typical of preeclampsia. Hepatic infarction has been associated with the presence of an underlying procoagulant state such as factor V Leiden mutation or an antiphospholipid antibody.[104]

Acute Fatty Liver of Pregnancy

Acute fatty liver of pregnancy (AFLP), a fascinating disorder unique to human gestation, is widely feared, and justifiably so.[105, 106] It is a form of true hepatic failure, with coagulopathy and often encephalopathy, in contrast to HELLP syndrome, which is only exceptionally associated with true hepatic dysfunction. Criteria needed for a diagnosis of AFLP include prolongation of elevation in the prothrombin time with a low serum fibrinogen level in a woman who is in the second half of gestation. The characteristic abnormality is microvesicular fatty infiltration. The condition is rare; a 1999 report indicated a frequency of 1/6659 deliveries for clinically diagnosed cases.[107] Subclinical cases exist[45]; published series in 1994 and 1997 included up to 32 patients.[108, 109] The pathogenesis of this disorder is unclear, although at least some affected patients have an inherited LCHAD deficiency, which also affects their offspring.[110]

CLINICAL FEATURES. Patients are affected late in pregnancy at 34 to 37 weeks of gestation, although cases that began as early as 19 to 20 weeks have been recorded. Rarely, the onset may occur after delivery. The initial symptoms reported are variable but usually include nausea and vomiting. Abdominal pain and confusion are common, and many patients have pregnancy-related conditions, such as premature labor, vaginal bleeding, or a decrease in fetal movement. The disorder is more common in patients who are primipara or carrying a multiple gestation.[111] There is a higher than normal number of male infants (2.7 : 1) among the babies born in pregnancies complicated by AFLP.[112] Preeclampsia is common (21%[107] to 64%[109]) but not invariable in AFLP patients and is similarly more common in primiparas, women who have twin pregnancies, and women who have male infants. Pruritus may be an initial symptom, and overlap with cholestasis of pregnancy may occur rarely.[113]

Laboratory testing of affected women demonstrates prolongation of the prothrombin time and a decrease in serum fibrinogen levels. Moderate elevations in serum aminotransferase levels (≤750 U/L) are usual, but rare patients may have very high or normal levels. Jaundice is common but not invariable. Initial laboratory findings usually indicate renal dysfunction with elevations in serum uric acid, creatinine, and blood urea nitrogen levels. Leukocytosis is common.

The course of AFLP is also quite variable. Hypoglycemia and hyperammonemia occur and should be suspected when patients exhibit an altered mental state. Other complications of liver failure, including ascites, pleural effusions, acute pancreatitis, respiratory failure, renal failure, and infection, may occur. Bleeding, often from the vagina or from a cesarean section wound, is common. Transient diabetes insipidus is not uncommon.[114] Rare complications include coronary artery dissection leading to myocardial infarction[115] and pulmonary fat emboli.[116]

DIAGNOSIS. The diagnosis of AFLP usually is based on a typical clinical evaluation of a patient who is at the expected stage in gestation with compatible laboratory features. The histologic features are strongly suggestive and, in the applicable circumstances, are pathognomonic. The hallmark is microvesicular fatty infiltration, most prominent in the central zone, with sparing of the periportal hepatocytes (Fig. 74–3). This microvesicular change can be inconspicuous; affected cells may appear ballooned and vacuolated, without obvious fat droplets. Thus, to confirm the diagnosis, special stains for fat must be used, either oil red O stain on frozen

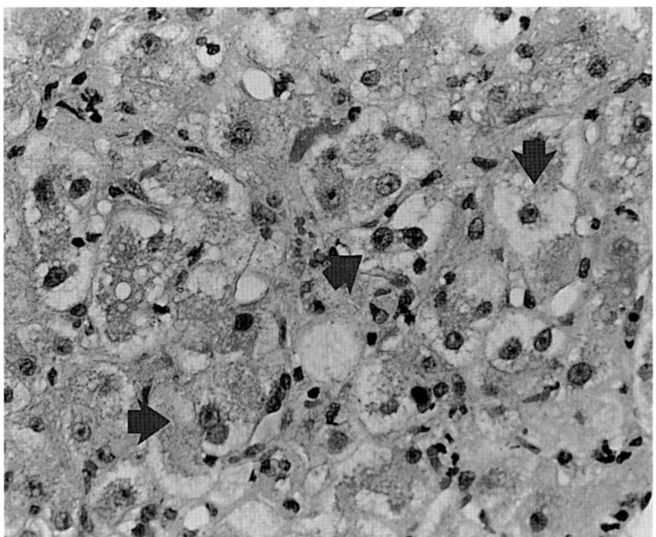

Figure 74–3. Histology of acute fatty liver of pregnancy. The perivenular hepatocytes (selected hepatocytes are designated with *arrows*) are pleomorphic and vacuolated, with lobular disarray. Large fat droplets are not seen.

tissue or electron microscopy on glutaraldehyde fixed tissue. To accomplish either, plans must be made before the biopsy is performed. Other histologic findings may be misleading; they may include lobular disarray suggestive of viral hepatitis and biliary ductular proliferation and inflammation suggestive of cholangitis.[45, 117] The periportal hemorrhage and fibrin deposition typical of preeclampsia are not found in patients with AFLP, and specialized staining of biopsy specimens differs in these two conditions.[118] Despite initial enthusiasm, imaging techniques, including ultrasonography, CT, and MRI, have not been consistently useful in confirming the diagnosis of AFLP.[119]

The differential diagnosis in patients with AFLP includes forms of acute hepatic failure not associated with pregnancy, including viral hepatitis and drug-induced injury. Uncommon forms of viral hepatitis may be more severe in pregnant than in nonpregnant women, and hepatitis E and herpes simplex hepatitis should be considered.[120, 121] These possibilities can be excluded by history taking, physical examination (identifying rashes on the skin and genitalia), and appropriate serologic studies. More difficult is distinguishing AFLP from other forms of liver disease associated with pregnancy, particularly preeclamptic liver disease, including severe HELLP syndrome and hepatic infarct or rupture. For example, patients with AFLP may have complicating disseminated intravascular coagulation with attendant thrombocytopenia, thus fulfilling the diagnostic criteria for HELLP syndrome. The distinction is usually not clinically relevant, however, because both conditions are treated by delivery.

Although the liver biopsy findings can be diagnostic in AFLP, biopsy is often contraindicated by the attendant coagulopathy as well as the possibility of hepatic rupture. Thus, as in Reye's syndrome, the diagnosis usually rests on clinical grounds. The biopsy can be useful, however, when the obstetrician has reservations about delivery. In such a case, the finding of microvesicular fat would mandate delivery; a biopsy can be obtained either percutaneously or via the transjugular route once the possibility of hepatic hematoma or rupture has been ruled out by CT or MRI.

PATHOGENESIS. An understanding of the pathogenesis of AFLP, like that of preeclampsia, has been elusive. Initially, AFLP was thought to be associated with exposure to a toxin such as chloroform anesthesia or intravenous tetracycline. These agents are either no longer in use or no longer given to pregnant women, yet AFLP continues to occur. Because of the concurrence of preeclampsia in many affected patients, AFLP has been considered to be the severe end of the spectrum of preeclamptic liver disease.[45, 55, 56] Against this supposition is the absence of liver biopsy evidence of the histologic hallmarks of preeclampsia in women affected with AFLP. Further complicating this issue is the continued inability to define the pathogenic mechanisms leading to preeclampsia.

The association between inherited defects in beta oxidation of fatty acids and AFLP is now well established and is easy to comprehend in light of the similarity in histologic characteristics and clinical course of AFLP and Jamaican vomiting sickness, which is caused by a toxin present in unripe akee fruit that disables intramitochondrial beta oxidation of fatty acids. Work in 1999 showed that AFLP may occur regardless of the mother's genotype if her fetus is deficient in LCHAD and carries at least one allele for the G1528C mutation.[110] In affected families, prenatal diagnosis based on chorionic villus sampling has proved to be both feasible and accurate.[122] Another defect in beta oxidation, carnitine palmitoyltransferase I deficiency, also has been associated with AFLP,[123] and deoxyribonucleic acid (DNA) analysis for this deficiency is also available.[124] Not all investigators have been able to confirm the association between AFLP and beta oxidation defects,[125] and other pathogenic mechanisms, as yet not elucidated, may exist.

MANAGEMENT. Management in a medical or obstetric intensive care unit is appropriate; most patients require maximal monitoring and supportive care administered by a multidisciplinary team. The cornerstone of treatment is early diagnosis with prompt delivery by the most expeditious route, followed by maximal supportive care as the liver recovers. This support may include infusion of blood products, surgical exploration of the abdomen or uterus, mechanical ventilation, dialysis, and administration of antibiotics. Hepatic encephalopathy is treated in the usual fashion with lactulose and catharsis. Infusions of concentrated glucose may be required to support the blood sugar level. Although many patients have disseminated intravascular coagulation and depression of antithrombin III levels, treatment with heparin or antithrombin III is not recommended.[126] Diabetes insipidus can be managed with 1-deamino-8-D-vasopressin (DDAVP).[114] Liver transplantation, either orthotopic or auxiliary, has been reported for patients with AFLP[127, 128] but should be reserved for severely ill women whose diagnosis and prompt delivery are not carried out. Most affected women recover completely, some after a long and complicated course requiring maximal support. Recovery begins with delivery, shortly after which the prothrombin time begins to improve. Persistent or increasing hyperbilirubinemia and multiple complications should not be interpreted as indicating the need for liver transplantation rather than the need for continued supportive care. There is one report of resolution without delivery and with a subsequent normal outcome of the gestation in a patient whose liver biopsy findings and course were compatible with AFLP.[129]

OUTCOME. With prompt diagnosis and maximal supportive care, maternal outcome in the present era should be excellent, and a 100% survival rate of affected mothers has been reported.[107, 109, 130] Survival rates for infants of affected mothers also have improved: perinatal mortality rates have been reported to be 6% to 7% or less. The surviving baby may have LCHAD deficiency, and the pediatrician should be alert to signs of nonketotic hypoglycemia with associated coma. Recurrence of AFLP is rare but clearly documented.[131–133] Mother, infant, and father should be tested for the G1528C mutation in LCHAD.[110]

LIVER DISORDERS COMPLICATING PREGNANCY

The pregnant woman is not protected from routine diseases, and liver diseases that occur in the nonpregnant population also occur in pregnancy and may necessitate special consideration related to the pregnant state. Some disorders of the general population run a more severe course if they occur during pregnancy. Also, although rare during pregnancy, chronic liver disease requires special consideration when it occurs.

Viral Hepatitis

Viral hepatitis is the most prevalent liver disease worldwide and commonly affects women of childbearing age. Viral hepatitis in pregnancy may be manifested as acute viral hepatitis during a previously normal gestation or may occur during the pregnancy of a woman who has chronic hepatitis.

In most cases, acute hepatitis A or B does not appear to affect the natural course of pregnancy, and pregnancy does not appear to affect the natural course of the acute infection. For hepatitis E and herpes simplex, however, acute infection during pregnancy, particularly during the third trimester of gestation, may lead to acute liver failure.

Hepatitis E is widely distributed in the underdeveloped world but is rare in the United States (see Chapter 68). It is common during monsoon conditions of flooding in Pakistan, India, and the Middle East. Rare cases have been reported in the United States in travelers from endemic areas, particularly Mexico. Acute infection during the third trimester of pregnancy has a high risk of acute liver failure and a maternal mortality rate of up to 20%.[120] Hepatitis E also has been associated with reported cases of intrauterine deaths,[134, 135] but whether such deaths are related to maternal factors or to direct effects of the virus is not clear. The risk of abortion and of intrauterine death is higher in women with hepatitis E in any trimester of gestation than in their nonaffected counterparts. Maternal-fetal transmission of hepatitis E that resulted in neonatal symptomatic hepatitis has been reported.[136] There are no therapeutic agents currently available to prevent vertical transmission of the virus.

Hepatitis caused by herpes simplex virus is common and subclinical during primary infection but becomes clinically evident during pregnancy or conditions of immunosuppression. Infection during pregnancy, particularly during the third trimester, may result in fulminant hepatitis accompanied by encephalopathy.[121] Clinical examination indicates anicteric hepatic failure. The encephalopathy may be worsened by the development of encephalitis. Pregnant women may show subtle vesicular lesions of the oropharynx and genital areas as well as elevated serum aminotransferase levels and prolongation of the prothrombin time. Serologic tests may be useful for diagnosis if the clinician suspects the infection. Liver biopsy specimens usually reveal characteristic inclusion bodies and punched-out hemorrhagic lesions. Acyclovir is an effective treatment, which appears to prevent transmission of the virus to the fetus.[121]

Most cases of chronic viral hepatitis are caused by hepatitis B, C, and D viruses. The presence of chronic viral hepatitis in pregnancy must be recognized early in order to initiate measures to prevent maternal-fetal transmission of infection related to prenatal, peripartum, and postpartum events.

Most young women who have hepatitis B are healthy carriers. Most of these hepatitis B carriers have a low risk of development of liver failure or decompensated liver disease during pregnancy or delivery. Chronic hepatitis B infection has little effect on the course of pregnancy. Pregnancy has no adverse effects on the course of hepatitis B infection and does not result in significant changes in serum aminotransferase levels. Maternal-fetal transmission of hepatitis B virus is responsible for most cases of the chronic carrier state worldwide, particularly in endemic areas such as Southeast Asia and Africa.[137] Mothers who have hepatitis B e antigen in serum have higher viremia levels and higher rates of vertical transmission of the hepatitis B virus.[138] Mothers who have hepatitis B e antibody in serum may also transmit the virus to their neonates but at a much lower rate.[139] If untreated, 90% of infants born to hepatitis B e antigen–positive mothers are infected by the virus, compared with 10% of infants born to hepatitis B e antigen–negative mothers. Infants born to mothers who have hepatitis B surface antigen in serum should receive hepatitis B immunoglobulin at birth as well as hepatitis B vaccine on day 1 and at month 1 and month 6 after birth.[140] Interferon therapy is not used during pregnancy for the chronic carrier state. The use of lamivudine, a nucleoside analog, for treatment of hepatitis B during pregnancy cannot be recommended until further data are obtained.

Chronic hepatitis C does not appear to affect the outcome of pregnancy.[141] One report has suggested that pregnancy may worsen the histopathologic liver injury associated with hepatitis C.[142] Currently available data suggest that most mothers who have hepatitis C antibody in serum maintain normal serum aminotransferase levels during pregnancy. In the absence of human immunodeficiency virus (HIV) coinfection, perinatal transmission of hepatitis C is uncommon.[143] The increased risk of transmission in hepatitis C virus–HIV coinfected women is most likely the result of increased levels of hepatitis C viremia found in immunosuppressed patients. Available data also suggest that the rate of perinatal transmission of hepatitis C is not related to the route of infant delivery, that is, vaginal delivery or cesarean section. Reports to date show that infants who are breast-fed by infected mothers who have high levels of hepatitis C viral ribonucleic acid (RNA) in blood appear to be free of infection 1 year postpartum. Isolated cases of hepatitis C transmission via transplacental amniocentesis have been reported.[144] Factors associated with an increased risk of perinatal transmission of hepatitis C are prolonged duration of membrane rupture, use of internal fetal monitoring devices, and meconium staining of amniotic fluid.[145] The use of immunoglobulin has been ineffective in preventing maternal-fetal transmission of hepatitis C, and multiple attempts to develop vaccines against this virus have been unsuccessful. Current treatment regimens for hepatitis C infection are not used during pregnancy.

Hepatitis D viral infection requires the presence of hepatitis B viral infection. There is no evidence that pregnancy has any impact on the natural course of acute or chronic hepatitis D. Current data reveal no adverse effects of hepatitis D during pregnancy. Prevention of maternal-fetal transmission of hepatitis D is accomplished by vaccination against maternal hepatitis B or treatment of hepatitis B virus with interferon or lamivudine before pregnancy. No data related to the use of immunoglobulin to prevent vertical transmission of the hepatitis D virus have been published.

Portal Hypertension Caused by Chronic Liver Disease

Chronic liver disease may result in cirrhosis and hepatic decompensation (see Chapters 77, 78, and 79). As a result of hormonal changes, anovulatory cycles, and amenorrhea, affected women are unlikely to become pregnant. Portal hypertension can develop in noncirrhotic fertile women, as in patients who have portal or splenic vein thrombosis, congenital hepatic fibrosis, or hepatoportal sclerosis. Portal hypertension may lead to development of varices (esophageal or gastric) and ascites. Because pregnancy is associated with increased blood volume as well as increased azygous venous flow caused by the pressure of the gravid uterus on the inferior vena cava, portal venous pressure, and variceal size increase during gestation.

The risk of variceal bleeding during pregnancy in women who have portal hypertension remains unclear. The treatment of variceal bleeding during pregnancy also remains controversial. The use of vasopressin or octreotide is not indicated because of the potential of these drugs to cause uterine ischemia and to induce premature labor. Emergency sclerotherapy of bleeding varices with sodium tetradecyl sulfate or ethanolamine oleate has been reported. Some authors have suggested prophylactic band ligation or sclerotherapy, portocaval shunting, and delivery by cesarean section to decrease the risk of bleeding. The possible role of beta blockers to reduce portal hypertension and prevent variceal bleeding during pregnancy remains to be determined.

Ascites and hepatic encephalopathy are not more common in pregnant women who have chronic liver disease than in nonpregnant women who have liver disease. The use of spironolactone for management of ascites appears to be acceptable during pregnancy.

Wilson Disease

Wilson disease is associated with amenorrhea and infertility in women of childbearing age (see Chapter 67). Successful treatment of Wilson disease with copper chelation therapy may result in resumption of ovulatory cycles and subsequent pregnancy. Both D-penicillamine and trientine have proved safe in pregnancy. Chelation therapy should continue during pregnancy because discontinuation can lead to sudden copper release, acute liver failure, and death.[146] The use of zinc sulfate for pregnant patients with Wilson disease remains controversial.[147]

Autoimmune Liver Disease

Autoimmune diseases are more common in women than in men. Consequently, clinicians may encounter autoimmune hepatitis in pregnant women. Immunosuppression for autoimmune hepatitis should be continued during pregnancy (see Chapter 75). The low doses of azathioprine used in standard treatment regimens are not known to be teratogenic. Occasionally autoimmune hepatitis may flare after delivery when the relative immunosuppression of pregnancy resolves. Therefore, patients with autoimmune hepatitis should have frequent measurements of serum aminotransferase levels for up to 6 months after delivery.

Primary biliary cirrhosis is more common in women past childbearing age than in younger women (see Chapter 76). Pregnant women who have primary biliary cirrhosis may experience an exacerbation in pruritus.[148] Ursodeoxycholic acid has been used successfully to treat pruritus during pregnancy,[149] but its safety during pregnancy remains to be proven.

Hepatic Neoplasia

A liver mass may be discovered during pregnancy, usually as an incidental finding on ultrasonography. Benign neoplasms of the liver include adenomas, focal nodular hyperplasias, and hemangiomas (see Chapter 81). Hepatic adenoma is associated with the use of oral contraceptives. Adenomas may enlarge during pregnancy, with subsequent hemorrhage into the adenoma and possible rupture into the abdominal cavity. Focal nodular hyperplasias and hemangiomas also have been reported to hemorrhage during pregnancy.[150] Women known to have a benign hepatic neoplasm should seek medical advice about whether to become pregnant. If pregnancy occurs, serial ultrasonography to measure the size of the tumor or to detect evidence of hemorrhage is indicated. Hepatocellular carcinoma during pregnancy may be suggested by the detection of high α-fetoprotein levels during screening (higher than the modest elevations usually associated with pregnancy).[151] Other causes of an elevated (α-fetoprotein level during pregnancy include Down's syndrome, neural tube defects, and hydatidiform mole.

Budd-Chiari Syndrome

Pregnancy is a relatively hypercoagulable state, particularly at delivery, and thrombosis of the hepatic veins, Budd-Chiari syndrome, can complicate it. Budd-Chiari syndrome has been associated with HELLP syndrome[152] and with preeclampsia in women who have an antiphospholipid antibody (see Chapter 70).[153] In patients who have Budd-Chiari syndrome and are not pregnant, an underlying procoagulant state, such as factor V Leiden mutation, should be sought.[154, 155]

Liver Transplant Recipients

In women of childbearing age successful liver transplantation may result in relatively uneventful pregnancies and infant deliveries. Women who become pregnant after liver transplantation should continue immunosuppressive therapy with close monitoring of the gestation (see Chapter 83). Although teratogenicity has not been reported in this group of patients, common adverse effects of immunosuppressive therapy such as hypertension and hyperglycemia may result in increased fetal distress or preeclampsia. In rare instances, the pregnancy may be complicated by organ rejection.

GASTROINTESTINAL DISORDERS COMPLICATING PREGNANCY

Nausea and Vomiting of Pregnancy and Hyperemesis Gravidarum

Nausea and vomiting are common during the first trimester of pregnancy and occur in 60% to 70% of pregnancies (see Chapter 8). Most pregnant women who experience nausea and vomiting are able to obtain sufficient oral nutrition and hydration to preclude the need for further medical intervention.

Hyperemesis gravidarum is characterized by severe, persistent vomiting that affects 0.5 to 10/1000 pregnancies.[156] Hyperemesis usually requires hospitalization of the pregnant patient for intravenous hydration, electrolyte replacement, and nutritional supplementation. Factors associated with an increased risk of hyperemesis gravidarum are nulliparity, high body weight,[157] multiple gestations, and hydatidiform mole.

In affected women, nausea, vomiting, and ptyalism develop between the sixth and eighth weeks of pregnancy. Hospitalization is indicated when patients have hypotension and tachycardia, ketosis, weight loss, or muscle wasting. Hyperemesis may require multiple hospitalizations and is likely to recur in subsequent pregnancies. Laboratory abnormalities include hypokalemia, hyponatremia, and ketonuria. In approximately 60% of patients with hyperemesis, free thyroxine levels increase, consistent with clinical hyperthyroidism.[158] The abnormal thyroid function does not require treatment, because it does not appear to affect the course of pregnancy. Clinical hyperthyroidism resolves with resolution of hyperemesis but is known to recur with subsequent pregnancies. Mild increases in serum aminotransferase and bilirubin levels have been detected in 25% to 40% of patients with hyperemesis.[159]

The pathogenesis of hyperemesis gravidarum remains unclear. Factors associated with the severity of hyperemesis are elevated thyroxine, estriol, and human chorionic gonadotropin levels. Other factors that may be associated with the development of hyperemesis include autonomic dysfunction, abnormal gastric emptying, and psychological factors.

The management of hyperemesis gravidarum is directed to the replacement of intravenous fluids and electrolytes. Studies suggest that thiamine and pyridoxine supplements are useful in the treatment of hyperemesis. The use of antiemetics remains controversial and requires further studies in the United States. Metoclopramide and prochlorperazine are widely prescribed during pregnancy on the basis of studies showing that they are not teratogenic and do not cause adverse outcomes, although they may cause extrapyramidal side effects in up to 30% of patients. The limited number of studies of the use of glucocorticoids in the treatment of hyperemesis gravidarum are inconclusive. The role of psychological therapy in the management of hyperemesis remains to be determined. Total parenteral nutrition is indicated in cases of severe, prolonged hyperemesis gravidarum.

Gastroesophageal Reflux Disease

Heartburn occurs in 30% to 50% of all pregnant women (see Chapter 33). During gestation, the lower esophageal sphincter is affected by extrinsic pressures and intrinsic factors. The enlarging gravid uterus increases intra-abdominal and intragastric pressures and may displace the lower esophageal sphincter. Resting lower esophageal sphincter pressure decreases during the second trimester of pregnancy but normalizes after delivery. Esophageal clearance may be decreased during pregnancy as a result of an increase in the frequency of low-amplitude contractions.

The clinical characteristics of gastroesophageal reflux in pregnant women are similar to those in the general population. In addition to heartburn, women may experience regurgitation, nausea, dysphagia, and emesis. Atypical symptoms of gastroesophageal reflux include persistent cough, wheezing, and chest pain. The symptoms are usually present by the end of the second trimester of gestation and worsen during the third trimester. Careful medical history taking is necessary for diagnosis and exclusion of other causes of atypical symptoms. Esophagogastroduodenoscopy is seldom necessary for diagnosis but is safe during pregnancy.[160] The role of 24-hour ambulatory esophageal pH monitoring in the diagnosis of gastroesophageal reflux during pregnancy remains to be determined, because no data are available regarding esophageal exposure to gastric acid during the different stages of pregnancy. Complications of gastroesophageal reflux such as severe erosive or ulcerated esophagitis or esophageal stricture formation are rarely seen in pregnancy unless the patient was symptomatic before gestation.

The first line of management of gastroesophageal reflux during pregnancy includes dietary and life-style changes. A diet low in fatty foods should be accompanied by avoidance of substances that decrease the lower esophageal sphincter pressure, such as coffee and chocolate, as well as substances with a high acidic content. Elevation of the head of the bed and cessation of smoking are two of the life-style changes that should be strongly recommended for symptom relief. The use of non-calcium-based antacids appears to be safe in pregnancy.

Severe gastroesophageal reflux may require the use of drugs to suppress gastric acid secretion. Data regarding the use of histamine H_2 receptor antagonists reveal that cimetidine should be avoided because it has antiandrogenic effects and may affect normal male fetal development. The short-term use of ranitidine during pregnancy appears to be safe. Animal studies of proton pump inhibitors reveal that omeprazole and pantoprazole may be toxic to the fetus. Lansoprazole does not seem to cause fetal toxicity in animals. No data are available on the use of prokinetic agents for the treatment of gastroesophageal reflux in pregnancy.

Constipation and Diarrhea

Constipation is common in pregnancy, with a frequency of 11% to 40% (see Chapter 12). The pathogenesis of constipation during pregnancy has not been firmly established, but one study showed a potential association between increased serum progesterone levels during the third trimester and decreased colonic smooth muscle activity.[161] Extrinsic compression of the sigmoid colon by the gravid uterus also has been implicated in the pathogenesis of constipation during pregnancy. Other factors that have been postulated to contribute to constipation in pregnant women include oral iron supplementation and increased absorption of electrolytes and water. A complete medical history should be obtained in order to exclude other causes of constipation such as hypothyroidism and other causes of mechanical intestinal obstruction.

The management of constipation in pregnancy includes increased intake of dietary fiber and fluid and use of bulk forming agents such as psyllium. The use of laxatives containing anthraquinone or cascara derivatives is contraindicated during pregnancy because of the potential to cause congenital malformations. Castor oil has been found to induce premature uterine contractions and should be avoided. Phenolphthalein laxatives should not be used during breastfeeding. The use of stool softeners during pregnancy requires further study. Common complications of constipation include exacerbation of hemorrhoids, fecal impaction, and worsening back pain.

Evaluation of diarrhea during pregnancy is the same as that for diarrhea in the nonpregnant population (see Chapter 9). Inflammatory bowel disease may occur initially during pregnancy, particularly because the onset of the disease often takes place in young adulthood.

Hemorrhoidal Disease

Hemorrhoidal disease may occur initially during pregnancy (see Chapter 117). Pregnant women commonly experience anorectal discomfort or pain, bleeding, or anal pruritus, particularly during the third trimester of gestation. Factors associated with the development of hemorrhoids during pregnancy include mechanical compression of veins by the enlarging uterus, worsening constipation accompanied by straining during defecation, and hormone-induced vascular changes. Initial therapy should be instituted with conservative measures such as sitz baths and suppositories. Injection sclerotherapy has been used safely during pregnancy. Intractable cases can be referred safely for surgical hemorrhoidectomy.[162] The efficacy of rubber band ligation of hemorrhoids during pregnancy deserves further study.

Gallstone Disease

The incidence of cholelithiasis appears to increase in pregnancy (see Chapter 55). The prevalence of gallstones in asymptomatic pregnant women is 2.5% to 12%. The prevalence of cholelithiasis appears to be directly related to increased parity and older age.[163]

Abnormalities in gallbladder motility during pregnancy lead to increased residual gallbladder volume in both the fasting and fed states. Pregnancy also results in changes in the composition of bile, including cholesterol supersaturation, decreased concentrations of chenodeoxycholic acid, increased concentrations of cholic acid, and increased bile acid pool size.[164, 165]

Pregnant women are at increased risk of gallstone formation because of the increase in gallbladder volume and changes in bile composition. Potential complications of cholelithiasis include biliary colic, cholecystitis, and gallstone pancreatitis.

The clinical characteristics of gallstone disease in pregnancy are similar to those in nonpregnant women. Acute cholecystitis is probably more common in the postpartum period than during gestation.[166] Abdominal ultrasonography is a safe diagnostic tool during pregnancy. Conservative management with antibiotics and intravenous fluid replacement is preferable until the postpartum period.[166] Endoscopic retrograde cholangiopancreatography with stone removal has been performed in a limited number of cases with adequate lead shielding and minimal use of fluoroscopy or direct radiography.[167] Cholecystectomy during pregnancy is indicated for patients who do not respond to conservative therapy or who have sepsis. Laparoscopic cholecystectomy is usually not recommended because of high risk of damage to the gravid uterus. Open cholecystectomy during the first trimester may contribute to a risk of abortion, whereas surgery during the third trimester may induce labor.

Pancreatitis

Acute pancreatitis is rare during pregnancy, with an incidence of 0.009% (see Chapter 48). Gallstones are responsible for approximately 90% of cases of pancreatitis among pregnant women. Other causes of pancreatitis during pregnancy include alcohol use, hypertriglyceridemia, hypercalcemia, and trauma. The clinical characteristics of acute pancreatitis in pregnancy are similar to those in nonpregnant women. Abdominal ultrasonography is helpful as a diagnostic tool for pancreatitis in pregnancy.

Pregnant women who have acute pancreatitis should be admitted to an intensive care unit or high-risk obstetric unit for supportive management. Bowel rest, intravenous fluids, and nasogastric suction are usually instituted. The role of endoscopic retrograde cholangiopancreatography in the management of gallstone pancreatitis in pregnancy has not been clearly established. Surgery for management of complications such as pseudocysts, fistulas, abscesses, and necrotizing pancreatitis should be reserved for patients who have life-threatening conditions.

Inflammatory Bowel Disease

Women with ulcerative colitis have fertility rates similar to those of unaffected women (see Chapters 103 and 104). In women who have Crohn's disease fertility can be affected by altered ovulation, scarring of fallopian tubes, dyspareunia associated with perianal involvement of disease, decreased libido, and malnutrition.[168]

Ulcerative colitis may have its onset in the first two trimesters of gestation. Exacerbation of ulcerative colitis during pregnancy is uncommon in women whose disease is asymptomatic before pregnancy. Women who have active ulcerative colitis at the time of conception may experience worsening of symptoms during the first trimester and marked improvement of symptoms during the second trimester, when amelioration has been associated with increased serum cortisol levels. Most pregnant women who have ulcerative colitis deliver normal full-term babies. The incidences of congenital malformations, stillbirths, and spontaneous abortions in patients with ulcerative colitis are comparable to those of unaffected women.

Crohn's disease is rarely diagnosed initially during pregnancy. Two thirds of women who have inactive disease at the time of conception do not experience relapse of disease during pregnancy. Women are advised to attempt to conceive when they are symptom-free, because active disease has been associated with an increased risk of premature birth. There is no increased risk, however, of congenital malformations, stillbirths, or spontaneous abortions.[169]

Sulfasalazine is well tolerated during pregnancy and does not pose any risk for fetal abnormalities. Folate supplementation is necessary because sulfasalazine causes folate malabsorption. Oral 5-aminosalicylic acid preparations and glucocorticoids also can be used safely during pregnancy.[170, 171] The use of metronidazole for treatment of perianal Crohn's disease during pregnancy requires further study.[172] Initiation of immunosuppressive therapy with azathioprine or 6-mercaptopurine should generally be avoided during pregnancy.

The data regarding potential congenital abnormalities that result from immunosuppressive therapy remain controversial. The experience of pregnant women who received immunosuppressive therapy after renal transplantation seems to suggest that there is no increased risk of adverse effects to the fetus. The use of immunosuppressive therapy is not an absolute contraindication to pregnancy nor an absolute indication for termination of pregnancy.

REFERENCES

1. Lammert F, Marschall H, Glantz A, Matern S: Intrahepatic cholestasis of pregnancy: Molecular pathogenesis, diagnosis and management. J Hepatol 33:1012–1021, 2000.
2. Reyes H, Simon F: Intrahepatic cholestasis of pregnancy: An estrogen-related disease. Semin Liver Dis 13:289–301, 1993.
3. Reyes H: The enigma of intrahepatic cholestasis of pregnancy: Lessons from Chile. Hepatology 2:87–96, 1982.
4. Davies M, da Silva C, Jones S, et al: Fetal mortality associated with cholestasis of pregnancy and the potential benefit of therapy with ursodeoxycholic acid. Gut 37:580–584, 1995.
5. Bacq Y, Myara A, Brechot M-C, et al: Serum conjugated bile acid profile during intrahepatic cholestasis of pregnancy. J Hepatol 22:66–70, 1995.
6. Schneider J: Genetic cholestasis syndromes. J Pediatr Gastroenterol Nutr 28:124–131, 1999.
7. Wilson JAP: Intrahepatic cholestasis of pregnancy with marked elevation of transaminases in a black American. Dig Dis Sci 32:665–668, 1987.
8. Leevy C, Koneru B, Klein K: Recurrent familial prolonged intrahepatic cholestasis of pregnancy associated with chronic liver disease. Gastroenterology 113:966–972, 1997.
9. Olsson R, Tysk C, Aldenborg F, Holm B: Prolonged postpartum course of intrahepatic cholestasis of pregnancy. Gastroenterology 105: 267–271, 1993.
10. Glasinovic J, Marinovic I, Mege R, et al: Intrahepatic cholestasis of pregnancy in cholecystectomized women: An epidemiological study. In Reyes H, Leuschner U, Arias I (eds): Pregnancy, Sex Hormones, and the Liver: Proceedings of the 89th Falk Symposium, Nov 10–11, 1995, Santiago, Chile. Hingham, MA: Kluwer Academic, 1995, pp 248–249.
11. Heinonen S, Kirkinen P: Pregnancy outcome with intrahepatic cholestasis. Obstet Gynecol 94:189–193, 1999.
12. Rioseco A, Ivankovic M, Manzur A, et al: Intrahepatic cholestasis of pregnancy: A retrospective case-control study of perinatal outcome. Am J Obstet Gynecol 170:890–895, 1994.
13. Alsulyman O, Ouzounian J, Ames-Castro M, Goodwin T: Intrahepatic cholestasis of pregnancy: Perinatal outcome associated with expectant management. Am J Obstet Gynecol 175:957–960, 1996.
14. Fagan E: Intrahepatic cholestasis of pregnancy. BMJ 309:1243–1244, 1994.
15. Reyes H, Baez M, Gonzalez M, et al: Selenium, zinc and copper plasma levels in intrahepatic cholestasis of pregnancy, in normal pregnancies and in healthy individuals, in Chile. J Hepatol 32:542–549, 2000.
16. Hirvioja M, Kivinen S: Inheritance of intrahepatic cholestasis of pregnancy in one kindred. Clin Genet 43:315–317, 1993.
17. Holzbach R, Sivak D, Braun W: Familial recurrent intrahepatic cholestasis of pregnancy: A genetic study providing evidence for transmission of a sex-limited, dominant trait. Gastroenterology 85:175–185, 1983.
18. Reyes H, Ribalta J, Gonzalez M, et al: Sulfobromophthalein clearance tests before and after ethinyl estradiol administration, in women and men with familial history of intrahepatic cholestasis of pregnancy. Gastroenterology 81:226–231, 1981.
19. Dixon P, Weerasekera N, Linton K, et al: Heterozygous MDR3 missense mutation associated with intrahepatic cholestasis of pregnancy: Evidence for a defect in protein trafficking. Hum Mol Genet 9:1209–1217, 2000.
20. Jacquemin E, Cresteil D, Manouvrier S, et al: Heterozygous non-sense mutation of the MDR3 gene in familial intrahepatic cholestasis of pregnancy. Lancet 353:210–211, 1999.
21. Mella J, Roschmann E, Glasinovic J, et al: Exploring the genetic role of the HLA-DPB1 locus in Chileans with intrahepatic cholestasis of pregnancy. J Hepatol 24:320–323, 1996.
22. Kreek M, Weser E, Sleisenger M, Jeffries G: Idiopathic cholestasis of pregnancy: The response to challenge with the synthetic estrogen, ethinyl estradiol. N Engl J Med 277:1391–1395, 1967.
23. Vore M: Estrogen cholestasis—membranes, metabolites, or receptors? Gastroenterology 93:641–650, 1987.
24. Bacq Y, Sapey T, Brechot M-C, et al: Intrahepatic cholestasis of pregnancy: A French prospective study. Hepatology 26:358–364, 1997.
25. Meng L, Reyes H, Axelson M, et al: Progesterone metabolites and bile acids in serum of patients with intrahepatic cholestasis of pregnancy: Effect of ursodeoxycholic acid therapy. Hepatology 26:1573–1579, 1997.
26. Palma J, Reyes H, Ribalta J, et al: Ursodeoxycholic acid in the treatment of cholestasis of pregnancy: A randomized, double-blind study controlled with placebo. J Hepatol 27:1022–1028, 1997.
27. Brites D, Rodrigues C, Oliveira N, et al: Correction of maternal serum bile acid profile during ursodeoxycholic acid therapy in cholestasis of pregnancy. J Hepatol 28:91–98, 1998.
28. Mazzella G, Nicola R, Francesco A, et al: Ursodeoxycholic acid administration in patients with cholestasis of pregnancy: Effects on primary bile acids in babies and mothers. Hepatology 33:504–508, 2001.
29. Serrano M, Brites D, Larena M, et al: Beneficial effect of ursodeoxycholic acid on alterations induced by cholestasis of pregnancy in bile acid transport across the human placenta. J Hepatol 28:829–839, 1998.
30. Riikonen S, Savonius H, Gylling H, et al: Oral guar gum, a gel-forming dietary fiber, relieves pruritus in intrahepatic cholestasis of pregnancy. Acta Obstet Gynecol Scand 79:260–264, 2000.
31. Sadler L, Lane M, North R: Severe fetal intracranial haemorrhage during treatment with cholestyramine for intrahepatic cholestasis of pregnancy. Br J Obstet Gynaecol 102:169–170, 1995.
32. Frezza M, Centini G, Cammareri G, et al: *S*-adenosylmethionine for the treatment of intrahepatic cholestasis of pregnancy: Results of a controlled clinical trial. Hepatogastroenterology 37:122–125, 1990.
33. Ribalta J, Reyes H, Gonzalez M, et al: *S*-adenosy-L-methionine in the treatment of patients with intrahepatic cholestasis of pregnancy: A randomized, double-blind, placebo-controlled study with negative results. Hepatology 13:1084–1089, 1991.

34. Floreani A, Paternoster D, Melis A, Grella P: *S*-adenosylmethionine versus ursodeoxycholic acid in the treatment of intrahepatic cholestasis of pregnancy: Preliminary results of a controlled trial. Eur J Obstet Gynecol Reprod Biol 67:109–113, 1996.
35. Nicastri P, Diaferia A, Tartagni M, et al: A randomized placebo-controlled trial of ursodeoxycholic acid and *S*-adenosylmethionine in the treatment of intrahepatic cholestasis of pregnancy. Br J Obstet Gynaecol 105:1205–1207, 1998.
36. Kretowicz E, McIntyre H: Intrahepatic cholestasis of pregnancy, worsening after dexamethasone. Aust N Z J Obstet Gynaecol 34:211–213, 1994.
37. Broughton Pipkin F, Rubin P: Pre-eclampsia—the "disease of theories." Br Med Bull 50:381–396, 1994.
38. Sibai B, Hauth J, Caritis S, et al: Hypertensive disorders in twin versus singleton gestations: National Institute of Child Health and Human Development Network of Maternal-Fetal Medicine Units. Am J Obstet Gynecol 182:938–942, 2000.
39. Roberts JM, Redman CW: Pre-eclampsia: More than pregnancy-induced hypertension. Lancet 341:1447, 1993.
40. Broughton Pipkin F: The hypertensive disorders of pregnancy. BMJ 311:609–613, 1995.
41. Weinstein L: Syndrome of hemolysis, elevated liver enzymes, and low platelet count: A severe consequence of hypertension in pregnancy. Am J Obstet Gynecol 142:159–167, 1982.
42. Barton J, Sibai B: Hepatic imaging in HELLP syndrome (hemolysis, elevated liver enzymes, and low platelet count). Am J Obstet Gynecol 174:1820–1825, 1996.
43. Manas K, Welsh J, Rankin R, Miller D: Hepatic hemorrhage without rupture in preeclampsia. N Engl J Med 312:424–426, 1985.
44. Krueger K, Hoffman B, Lee W: Hepatic infarction associated with eclampsia. Am J Gastroenterol 85:588–592, 1990.
45. Riely C, Latham P, Romero R, Duffy T: Acute fatty liver of pregnancy: A reassessment based on observations in nine patients. Ann Intern Med 106:703–706, 1987.
46. Sibai B, Ramadan M, Usta I, et al: Maternal morbidity and mortality in 442 pregnancies with hemolysis, elevated liver enzymes, and low platelets (HELLP syndrome). Am J Obstet Gynecol 169:1000–1006, 1993.
47. Aarnoudse J, Houthoff H, Weits J, et al: A syndrome of liver damage and intravascular coagulation in the last trimester of normotensive pregnancy: A clinical and histopathological study. Br J Obstet Gynecol 93:145–155, 1986.
48. Tomsen T: HELLP syndrome (hemolysis, elevated liver enzymes, and low platelets) presenting as generalized malaise. Am J Obstet Gynecol 172:1876–1880, 1995.
49. Julius C, Dunn Z, Blazina J: HELLP syndrome: Laboratory parameters and clinical course in four patients treated with plasma exchange. J Clin Apheresis 9:228–235, 1994.
50. Catanzarite V, Steinberg S, Mosley C, et al: Severe preeclampsia and fulminant and extreme elevation of aspartate aminotransferase and lactate dehydrogenase levels: High risk for maternal death. Am J Perinatol 12:310–313, 1995.
51. Steegers E, Mulder T, Bisseling J, et al: Glutathione *S*-transferase alpha as marker for hepatocellular damage in pre-eclampsia and HELLP syndrome. Lancet 345:1571–1572, 1995.
52. Neiger R, Trofatter M, Trofatter KJ: D-Dimer test for early detection of HELLP syndrome. South Med J 88:416–419, 1995.
53. Schrocksnadel H, Daxenbichler G, Artner E, et al: Tumor markers in hypertensive disorders of pregnancy. Gynecol Obstet Invest 35:204–208, 1993.
54. Paternoster D, Stella A, Simioni P, et al: Coagulation and plasma fibronectin parameters in HELLP syndrome. Int J Gynaecol Obstet 50:263–268, 1995.
55. Dani R, Mendes G, Medeiros JD, et al: Study of the liver changes occurring in preeclampsia and their possible pathogenetic connection with acute fatty liver of pregnancy. Am J Gastroenterol 91:292–294, 1996.
56. Minakami H, Oka N, Sato T, et al: Preeclampsia: A microvesicular fat disease of the liver. Am J Obstet Gynecol 159:1043–1047, 1988.
57. Barton J, Riely C, Adamec T, et al: Hepatic histopathologic condition does not correlate with laboratory abnormalities in HELLP syndrome (hemolysis, elevated liver enzymes, and low platelet count). Am J Obstet Gynecol 167:1538–1543, 1992.
58. Goodlin RC: Preeclampsia as the great imposter. Am J Obstet Gynecol 164:1577–1581, 1991.
59. Martin J, Stedman C: Imitators of preeclampsia and HELLP syndrome. Obstet Gynecol Clin North Am 18:181–198, 1991.
60. Hsu H, Belfort M, Vernino S, et al: Postpartum thrombotic thrombocytopenic purpura complicated by Budd-Chiari syndrome. Obstet Gynecol 85:839–843, 1995.
61. Ibery M, Jones A, Sampson J: Lupus anticoagulant and HELLP syndrome complicated by placental abruption, hepatic, dermal and adrenal infarction. Aust N Z J Obstet Gynaecol 35:215–217, 1995.
62. Mizutani S, Nomura S, Hirose R, et al: Intra-uterine fetal death due to pre-eclampsia which was misdiagnosed to be complicating with hepatitis. Horm Metab Res 25:187–189, 1993.
63. Pijnenborg R, Anthony J, Davey D, et al: Placental bed spiral arteries in the hypertensive disorders of pregnancy. Br J Obstet Gynaecol 98: 648–655, 1991.
64. Arngrimsson R, Bjornsson S, Geirsson R, et al: Genetic and familial predisposition to eclampsia and pre-eclampsia in a defined population. Br J Obstet Gynaecol 97:762–769, 1990.
65. Chesley L, Cooper D: Genetics of hypertension in pregnancy: Possible single gene control of pre-eclampsia and eclampsia in the descendants of eclamptic women. Br J Obstet Gynaecol 93:898–908, 1986.
66. Robillard P-Y, Hulsey T, Perianin J, et al: Association of pregnancy-induced hypertension with duration of sexual cohabitation before conception. Lancet 344:973–975, 1994.
67. Tubbergen P, Lachmeijer A, Althuisius S, et al: Change in paternity: A risk factor for preeclampsia in multiparous women? J Reprod Immunol 45:81–98, 1999.
68. Dekker G, Sibai B: The immunology of preeclampsia. Semin Perinatol 23:24–33, 1999.
69. Koelman C, Coumans A, Nijman H, et al: Correlation between oral sex and a low incidence of preeclampsia: A role for soluble HLA in seminal fluid? J Reprod Immunol 46:155–166, 2000.
70. Dizon-Townson D, Nelson L, Easton K, Ward K: The factor V Leiden mutation may predispose women to severe preeclampsia. Am J Obstet Gynecol 175:902–905, 1996.
71. van Pampus M, Dekker G, Wolf H, et al: High prevalence of hemostatic abnormalities in women with a history of severe preeclampsia. Am J Obstet Gynecol 180:1146–1150, 1999.
72. de Vries M, Dekker G, Schoemaker J: Higher risk of preeclampsia in the polycystic ovary syndrome: A case control study. Eur J Obstet Gynecol Reprod Biol 76:91–95, 1998.
73. Tyni T, Ekholm E, Pihko H: Pregnancy complications are frequent in long-chain 3-hydroxyacyl–coenzyme A dehydrogenase deficiency. Am J Obstet Gynecol 178:603–608, 1998.
74. den Boer M, Ijlst L, Wijburg F, et al: Heterozygosity for the common LCHAD mutation (1528G>C) is not a major cause of HELLP syndrome and the prevalence of the mutation in the Dutch population is low. Pediatr Res 48:151–154, 2000.
75. Friedman S, Lubarsky S, Ahokas R, et al: Preeclampsia and related disorders: Clinical aspects and relevance of endothelin and nitric oxide. Clin Perinatol 22:343–355, 1995.
76. Ward K, Hata A, Jeunemaitre X, et al: A molecular variant of angiotensinogen associated with preeclampsia. Nat Genet 4:59–61, 1993.
77. Makkonen N, Harju M, Kirkinen P: Postpartum recovery after severe pre-eclampsia and HELLP-syndrome. J Perinat Med 24:641–649, 1996.
78. Ferrara J, Malatesta R, Kemmann E: Transient nephrogenic diabetes insipidus during toxemia in pregnancy. Diagn Gynecol Obstet 2:227–230, 1980.
79. Isler C, Rinehart B, Terrone D, et al: Maternal mortality associated with HELLP (hemolysis, elevated liver enzymes, and low platelets) syndrome. Am J Obstet Gynecol 181:924–928, 1999.
80. Haddad B, Barton J, Livingston J, et al: Risk factors for adverse maternal outcomes among women with HELLP (hemolysis, elevated liver enzymes, and low platelet count) syndrome. Am J Obstet Gynecol 183:444–448, 2000.
81. Sibai B, Ramadan M, Chari R, Friedman S: Pregnancies complicated by HELLP syndrome (hemolysis, elevated liver enzymes, and low platelets): Subsequent pregnancy outcome and long-term prognosis. Am J Obstet Gynecol 172:125–129, 1995.
82. Sullivan C, Magaan E, Perry KJ, et al: The recurrence risk of the syndrome of hemolysis, elevated liver enzymes, and low platelets (HELLP) in subsequent gestations. Am J Obstet Gynecol 171:940–943, 1994.
83. Harms K, Rath W, Herting E, Kuhn W: Maternal hemolysis, elevated liver enzymes, low platelet count, and neonatal outcome. Am J Perinatol 12:1–6, 1995.

84. Kandler C, Kevekordes B, Zenker M, et al: Prognosis of children born to mothers with HELLP-syndrome. J Perinat Med 26:486–490, 1998.
85. Visser W, Wallenburg H: Maternal and perinatal outcome of temporizing management in 254 consecutive patients with severe preeclampsia remote from term. Eur J Obstet Gynecol Reprod Biol 63: 147–154, 1995.
86. Martin JJ, Files J, Blake P, et al: Postpartum plasma exchange for atypical preeclampsia-eclampsia as HELLP (hemolysis, elevated liver enzymes, and low platelets) syndrome. Am J Obstet Gynecol 175: 506–507, 1995.
87. Magann E, Bass D, Chauhan S, et al: Antepartum corticosteroids: Disease stabilization in patients with the syndrome of hemolysis, elevated liver enzymes, and low platelets (HELLP). Am J Obstet Gynecol 171:1148–1153, 1994.
88. Martin JJ, Perry KJ, Blake P, et al: Better maternal outcomes are achieved with dexamethasone therapy for postpartum HELLP (hemolysis, elevated liver enzymes, and thrombocytopenia) syndrome. Am J Obstet Gynecol 177:1011–1017, 1997.
89. O'Brien J, Milligan D, Barton J: Impact of high-dose corticosteroid therapy for patients with HELLP (hemolysis, elevated liver enzymes, and low platelet count) syndrome. Am J Obstet Gynecol 183:921–924, 2000.
90. Tompkins M, Thiagarajah S: HELLP (hemolysis, elevated liver enzymes, and low platelet count) syndrome: The benefit of corticosteroids. Am J Obstet Gynecol 181:304–309, 1999.
91. Strate T, Broering D, Bloechle C, et al: Orthotopic liver transplantation for complicated HELLP syndrome: Case report and review of the literature. Arch Gynecol Obstet 264:108–111, 2000.
92. Erhard J, Lange R, Niebel W, et al: Acute liver necrosis in the HELLP syndrome: Successful outcome after orthotopic liver transplantation: A case report. Transpl Int 6:179–181, 1993.
93. Risseeuw J, de Vries J, van Eyck J, Arabin B: Liver rupture post partum associated with preeclampsia and HELLP syndrome. J Matern Fetal Med 8:32–35, 1999.
94. Sheikh R, Yasmeen S, Pauly M, Riegler J: Spontaneous intrahepatic hemorrhage and hepatic rupture in the HELLP syndrome. J Clin Gastroenterol 28:323–328, 1999.
95. Stevenson J, Graham D: Hepatic hemorrhage and the HELLP syndrome: A surgeon's perspective. Am Surg 61:756–760, 1995.
96. Wilson R, Marshall B: Postpartum rupture of a subcapsular hematoma of the liver. Acta Obstet Gynecol Scand 71:394–397, 1992.
97. Chan A, Gerscovich E: Imaging of subcapsular hepatic and renal hematomas in pregnancy complicated by preeclampsia and the HELLP syndrome. J Clin Ultrasound 27:35–40, 1999.
98. Zissin R, Yaffe D, Fejgin M, et al: Hepatic infarction in preeclampsia as part of the HELLP syndrome: CT appearance. Abdom Imaging 24: 594–596, 1999.
99. Gordon S, Meyer R, Rosenberg B: Laparoscopic diagnosis of subcapsular hepatic hemorrhage in pre-eclamptic liver disease. Gastrointest Endosc 38:718–720, 1992.
100. Hunter S, Martin M, Benda J, Zlatnik F: Liver transplant after massive spontaneous hepatic rupture in pregnancy complicated by preeclampsia. Liver Transpl 85:819–822, 1995.
101. Alleman J, Delarue M, Hasaart T: Successful delivery after hepatic rupture in previous pre-eclamptic pregnancy. Eur J Obstet Gynecol Reprod Biol 47:76–79, 1992.
102. Greenstein D, Henderson J, Boyer T: Liver hemorrhage: Recurrent episodes during pregnancy complicated by preeclampsia. Gastroenterology 106:1668–1671, 1994.
103. Chiang K, Athey P, Lamki N: Massive hepatic necrosis in the HELLP syndrome: CT correlation. J Comput Assist Tomogr 15:845–847, 1991.
104. Seige M, Schweigart U, Moessmer G, et al: Extensive hepatic infarction caused by thrombosis of right portal vein branches and arterial vasospasm in HELLP syndrome associated with homozygous factor V Leiden. Am J Gastroenterol 93:473–474, 1998.
105. Bacq Y: Acute fatty liver of pregnancy. Semin Perinatol 22:134–140, 1998.
106. Riely C: Acute fatty liver of pregnancy. Semin Liver Dis 7:47–54, 1987.
107. Castro M, Fassett M, Reynolds T, et al: Reversible peripartum liver failure: A new perspective on the diagnosis, treatment, and cause of acute fatty liver of pregnancy, based on 28 consecutive cases. Am J Obstet Gynecol 181:389–395, 1999.
108. Pereira S, O'Donohue J, Wendon J, Williams R: Maternal and perinatal outcome in severe pregnancy-related liver disease. Hepatology 26: 1258–1262, 1997.
109. Usta I, Barton J, Amon E, et al: Acute fatty liver of pregnancy: An experience in the diagnosis and management of fourteen cases. Am J Obstet Gynecol 171:1342–1347, 1994.
110. Ibdah J, Bennett M, Rinaldo P, et al: A fetal fatty-acid oxidation disorder as a cause of liver disease in pregnant women. N Engl J Med 340:1723–1731, 1999.
111. Malone F, Kaufman G, Chelmow D, et al: Maternal morbidity associated with triplet pregnancy. Am J Perinatol 15:73–77, 1998.
112. James W: Sex ratios of offspring and the causes of placental pathology. Hum Reprod 10:1403–1406, 1995.
113. Vanjak D, Moreau R, Roche-Sicot J, et al: Intrahepatic cholestasis of pregnancy and acute fatty liver of pregnancy. Gastroenterology 100: 1123–1125, 1991.
114. Kennedy S, Hall P, Seymour A, Hague W: Transient diabetes insipidus and acute fatty liver of pregnancy. Br J Obstet Gynaecol 101: 387–391, 1994.
115. Coulson C, Kuller J, Bowes W: Myocardial infarction and coronary artery dissection in pregnancy. Am J Perinatol 12:382, 1995.
116. Jones M: Pulmonary fat emboli associated with acute fatty liver of pregnancy [letter to the editor]. Am J Gastroenterol 88:791–792, 1993.
117. Rolfes D, Ishak K: Acute fatty liver of pregnancy: A clinicopathologic study of 35 cases. Hepatology 5:1149, 1985.
118. Halim A, Kanayama N, El Maradny E, et al: Immunohistological study in cases of HELLP syndrome (hemolysis, elevated liver enzymes and low platelets) and acute fatty liver of pregnancy. Gynecol Obstet Invest 41:106–112, 1996.
119. Castro M, Ouzounian J, Colletti P, et al: Radiologic studies in acute fatty liver of pregnancy: A review of the literature and 19 new cases. J Reprod Med 41:839–843, 1996.
120. Hamid S, Jafri S, Khan H, et al: Fulminant hepatic failure in pregnant women: Acute fatty liver or acute viral hepatitis. J Hepatology 25:20–27, 1996.
121. Klein N, Mabie W, Shaver D, et al: Herpes simplex virus hepatitis in pregnancy. Gastroenterology 100:239–244, 1991.
122. Ibdah J, Zhao Y, Viola J, et al: Molecular prenatal diagnosis in families with fetal mitochondrial trifunctional protein mutations. J Pediatr 138:396–399, 2001.
123. Innes A, Seargeant L, Balachandra K, et al: Hepatitic carnitine palmitoyltransferase I deficiency presenting as maternal illness in pregnancy. Pediatr Res 47:43–45, 2000.
124. Ijlst L, Mandel H, Oostheim W, et al: Molecular basis of hepatic carnitine palmitoyltransferase I deficiency. J Clin Invest 102:527–531, 1998.
125. Mansouri A, Fromenty B, Durand F, et al: Assessment of the prevalence of genetic metabolic defects in acute fatty liver of pregnancy. J Hepatol 25:781, 1996.
126. Castro M, Goodwin T, Shaw K, et al: Disseminated intravascular coagulation and antithrombin III depression in acute fatty liver of pregnancy. Am J Obstet Gynecol 174:211–216, 1996.
127. Franco J, Newcomer J, Adams M, Saeian K: Auxiliary liver transplant in acute fatty liver of pregnancy. Obstet Gynecol 95:1042, 2000.
128. Ockner SA, Brunt EM, Cohn SM, Krul ES: Fulminant hepatic failure caused by acute fatty liver of pregnancy treated by orthotopic liver transplantation. Hepatology 11:59–64, 1990.
129. Miguil M, Sadraoui S, Moutaouakkil B: La steatose hepatique aigue gravidique peut guerir malgre la poursuite de la grossesse. J Gynecol Obstet Biol Reprod 23:308, 1994.
130. Reyes H, Sandoval L, Wainstein A, et al: Acute fatty liver of pregnancy: A clinical study of 12 episodes in 11 patients. Gut 35:101–106, 1994.
131. MacLean M, Cameron A, Cumming G, et al: Recurrence of acute fatty liver of pregnancy. Br J Obstet Gynaecol 101:453–454, 1994.
132. Meicler P, Bernuau J, Darai E, et al: Steatose aigue hepatique gravidique recidivante. Rev Fr Gynecol Obstet 89:44–48, 1994.
133. Wilcken B, Leung K-C, Hammond J, et al: Pregnancy and fetal long-chain 3-hydroxyacyl coenzyme A hydrogenase deficiency. Lancet 341: 407–408, 1993.
134. Khuroo M, Kamili S, Jameel S: Vertical transmission of hepatitis E virus. Lancet 345:1025–1026, 1995.
135. Nanda S, Ansari I, Acharya S, et al: Protracted viremia during acute sporadic hepatitis E virus infection. Gastroenterology 108:225–230, 1995.
136. Rab M, Bile M, Mubarik M, et al: Water-borne hepatitis E virus epidemic in Islamabad, Pakistan: A common source outbreak traced to the malfunction of a modern water treatment plant. Am J Trop Med Hyg 57:151–157, 1997.

137. Lok A: Natural history and control of perinatally acquired hepatitis B virus infection. Dig Dis 10:46–52, 1992.
138. Beasley R, Trepo C, Stevens C, Szmuness W: The e antigen and vertical transmission of hepatitis B surface antigen. Am J Epidemiol 102:94–98, 1977.
139. Beath S, Boxall E, Watson R, et al: Fulminant hepatitis B in infants born to anti-HBe hepatitis B carrier mothers. BMJ 304:1169–1170, 1992.
140. American Academy of Pediatrics Committee on Infectious Diseases: Universal hepatitis B immunization. Pediatrics 89:795–800, 1989.
141. Silverman N, Jenkin B, Wu C, et al: Hepatitis C virus in pregnancy: Seroprevalence and risk factors for infection. Am J Obstet Gynecol 169:583–587, 1993.
142. Fontaine H, Nalpas B, Carnot F, et al: Effect of pregnancy on chronic hepatitis C: A case-control study. Lancet 356:1328–1329, 2000.
143. La Torre A, Biadaioli R, Capobianco T, et al: Vertical transmission of HCV. Acta Obstet Gynecol Scand 77:889–892, 1998.
144. Delamare C, Carbonne B, Heim N, et al: Detection of hepatitis C virus RNA (HCV RNA) in amniotic fluid: A prospective study. J Hepatol 31:416–420, 1999.
145. Mast E, Hwang L, Seto D: Perinatal hepatitis C virus transmission: Maternal risk factors and optimal timing of diagnosis. Hepatology 30: 499A, 1999.
146. Walshe J: The management of pregnancy in Wilson's disease treated with trientine. QJM 58:81–87, 1986.
147. Brewer G, Johnson V, Dick R, et al: Treatment of Wilson's disease with zinc. XVII. Treatment during pregnancy. Hepatology 31:531–532, 2000.
148. Olsson R, Loof L, Wallerstedt S: Pregnancy in patients with primary biliary cirrhosis—a case for dissuasion? The Swedish Internal Medicine Liver Club. Liver 13:316–318, 1993.
149. Rudi J, Schonig T, Stremmel W: Therapy with ursodeoxycholic acid in primary biliary cirrhosis in pregnancy. Z Gastroenterol 34:188–191, 1996.
150. Athanassiou A, Craigo S: Liver masses in pregnancy. Semin Perinatol 22:166–177, 1998.
151. Lau W, Leung W, Ho S, et al: Hepatocellular carcinoma during pregnancy and its comparison with other pregnancy-associated malignancies. Cancer 75:2669–2676, 1995.
152. Gordon S, Polson D, Shirkhoda A: Budd-Chiari syndrome complicating pre-eclampsia: Diagnosis by magnetic resonance imaging. J Clin Gastroenterol 13:460–462, 1991.
153. Segal S, Shenhav S, Segal O, et al: Budd-Chiari syndrome complicating severe preeclampsia in a parturient with primary antiphospholipid syndrome. Eur J Obstet Gynecol Reprod Biol 68:227–229, 1996.
154. Deltenre P, Denninger M, Hillaire S, et al: Factor V Leiden related Budd-Chiari syndrome. Gut 48:264–268, 2001.
155. Fickert P, Ramschak H, Kenner L, et al: Acute Budd-Chiari syndrome with fulminant hepatic failure in a pregnant woman with factor V Leiden mutation. Gastroenterology 111:1670–1673, 1996.
156. Hod M, Orvieto R, Kaplan B, et al: Hyperemesis gravidarum: A review. J Reprod Med 39:605–612, 1994.
157. Abell T, Riely C: Hyperemesis gravidarum. Gastroenterol Clin North Am 21:835–849, 1992.
158. Goodwin T, Montoro M, Mestman J: Transient hyperthyroidism and hyperemesis gravidarum: Clinical aspects. Am J Obstet Gynecol 167(3):648–652, 1992.
159. Rotman P, Hassin D, Mouallem M, et al: Wernicke's encephalopathy in hyperemesis gravidarum: Association with abnormal liver function. Isr J Med Sci 30:225–228, 1994.
160. Cappell M: The safety and efficacy of gastrointestinal endoscopy during pregnancy. Gastroenterol Clin North Am 27:37–71, 1998.
161. Wald A, Van Thiel D, Hoechstetter L, et al: Effect of pregnancy on gastrointestinal transit. Dig Dis Sci 27:1015–1018, 1982.
162. Saleeby R, Rosen L, Stasik J, et al: Hemorrhoidectomy during pregnancy: Risk or relief? Dis Colon Rectum 34:260–261, 1991.
163. Basso L, McCollum P, Darling M, et al: A study of cholelithiasis during pregnancy and its relationship with age, parity, menarche, breast-feeding, dysmenorrhea, oral contraception and a maternal history of cholelithiasis. Surg Gynecol Obstet 175:41–46, 1992.
164. Scott L: Gallstone disease and pancreatitis in pregnancy. Gastroenterol Clin North Am 21:803–815, 1992.
165. Valdivieso V, Covarrubias C, Siegel F, Cruz F: Pregnancy and cholelithiasis: Pathogenesis and natural course of gallstones diagnosed in early puerperium. Hepatology 17:1–4, 1993.
166. Dixon N, Faddis D, Silberman H: Aggressive management of cholecystitis during pregnancy. Am J Surg 154:292–294, 1987.
167. Jamidar P, Beck G, Hoffman B, et al: Endoscopic retrograde cholangiopancreatography in pregnancy. Am J Gastroenterol 90:1263–1267, 1995.
168. Korelitz B: Inflammatory bowel disease and pregnancy. Gastroenterol Clin North Am 27:213–214, 1998.
169. Woolfson K, Cohen Z, McLeod R: Crohn's disease and pregnancy. Dis Colon Rectum 33:869–873, 1990.
170. Diav-Citrin O, Park Y, Veerasuntharam G, et al: The safety of mesalamine in human pregnancy: A prospective controlled cohort study. Gastroenterology 114:23–28, 1998.
171. Habal F, Hui G, Greenberg G: Oral 5-aminosalicylic acid for inflammatory bowel disease in pregnancy: Safety and clinical course. Gastroenterology 105:1057–1060, 1993.
172. Diav-Citrin O, Shechtman S, Gotteiner T, et al: Pregnancy outcome after gestational exposure to metronidazole: A prospective controlled cohort study. Teratology 63:186–192, 2001.

Chapter

75 AUTOIMMUNE HEPATITIS

Albert J. Czaja

Autoimmune hepatitis (AIH) is a self-perpetuating hepatocellular inflammation of unknown cause. It is characterized by the presence of interface hepatitis on histologic examination (Fig. 75–1), hypergammaglobulinemia, and autoantibodies in serum.[1] Diagnosis requires the exclusion of other chronic liver diseases that have similar features, including Wilson disease, chronic viral hepatitis, α_1-antitrypsin deficiency, genetic hemochromatosis, drug-induced liver disease, nonalcoholic steatohepatitis, and the immune cholangiopathies of primary biliary cirrhosis (PBC), primary sclerosing cholangitis (PSC), and autoimmune cholangitis.

DIAGNOSTIC CRITERIA

An international panel codified the diagnostic criteria of AIH in 1992, and an expanded panel updated them in 1999.[2] The propensity for an acute, and rarely fulminant, presentation has been recognized; the requirement for 6 months of disease activity to establish chronicity has been waived; and lobular hepatitis is now part of the histologic spectrum (Fig. 75–2).[2] Cholestatic histologic changes, including bile duct injury and ductopenia, are incompatible features, and the nonviral nature of AIH has been reaffirmed.

The immunoserologic tests essential for diagnosis are assays for antinuclear antibodies (ANA), smooth muscle antibodies (SMA), and antibodies to liver/kidney microsome type 1 (anti-LKM1).[3] These assays are based on the indirect immunofluorescence of rodent tissues or Hep-2 cell lines or on enzyme immunoassays using microtiter plates with adsorbed recombinant or highly purified antigens. Perinuclear anti-neutrophil cytoplasmic antibodies (pANCAs) are common in type 1 AIH, and they are routinely available in most clinical laboratories. These antibodies have been useful in evaluating patients who lack the conventional autoantibodies.

Clinical Criteria

The *definite* diagnosis of AIH requires the exclusion of other similar diseases; laboratory findings that indicate substantial immunoreactivity; and histologic features of interface hepatitis (Fig. 75–3).[2] A *probable* diagnosis is justified when findings are compatible with AIH but insufficient for a definite diagnosis (see Fig. 75–3).[2] Patients who lack conventional autoantibodies but who are seropositive for investigational markers, such as antibodies to the asialoglycoprotein receptor (anti-ASGPR), soluble liver antigen/liver-pancreas (anti-SLA/LP), actin (antiactin), or liver cytosol type 1 (anti-LC1), are classified as having *probable* disease.

Scoring Criteria

A scoring system proposed by the International Autoimmune Hepatitis Group accommodates the diverse manifestations of AIH and renders an aggregate score that reflects the net strength of the diagnosis before and after glucocorticoid treatment (Table 75–1).[2] By weighing each component of the syndrome, discrepant features can be accommodated and biases associated with isolated inconsistencies prevented. The scoring system is rarely necessary in clinical practice. However, it does have investigational value as a means to ensure compatible study populations in clinical trials and to assess objectively the resemblance of various chronic liver diseases to definite AIH.[4]

PATHOGENESIS

The pathogenic mechanisms of AIH are unknown. The most popular hypotheses evoke a constellation of interactive factors that include a triggering agent, a genetic predisposition, and various determinants of autoantigen display, immunocyte activation, and effector cell expansion.[5] Multiple triggering factors have been proposed, and they include infectious

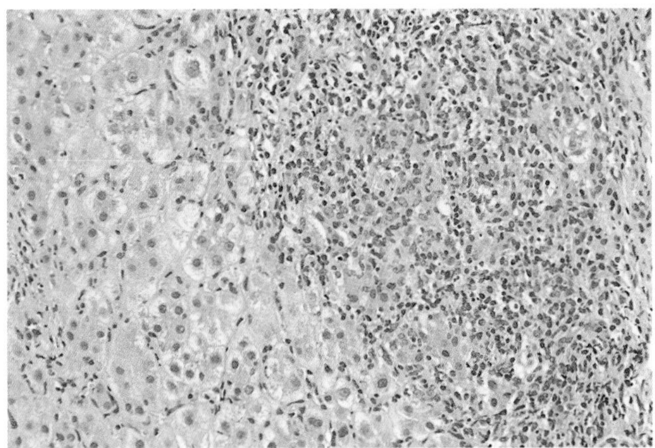

Figure 75–1. Interface hepatitis. The limiting plate of the portal tract is disrupted by a lymphoplasmacytic infiltrate. This histologic pattern is the hallmark of autoimmune hepatitis, but it is not disease specific. Hematoxylin and eosin, ×200.

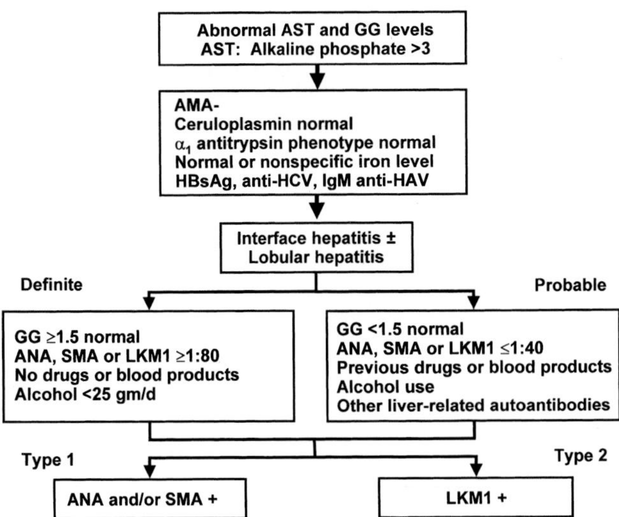

Figure 75–3. Diagnostic algorithm for autoimmune hepatitis. Diagnosis requires predominant elevation of the serum aminotransferase levels, exclusion of other similar disorders (especially Wilson disease, drug-induced hepatitis, and viral hepatitis), interface hepatitis on histologic examination, and manifestations of immunoreactivity, including serum gamma globulin (GG) elevation and seropositivity for antinuclear antibodies (ANA), smooth muscle antibodies (SMA), or antibodies to liver/kidney microsome type 1 (LKM1). The degree of immunoreactivity and the presence of confounding etiologic factors, such as alcohol or drug exposure, distinguish definite from probable autoimmune hepatitis. Classification into the descriptive categories of type 1 or type 2 autoimmune hepatitis is based on the nature of the autoantibodies. (AST, aspartate aminotransferase; HBsAg, hepatitis B surface antigen; anti-HCV, antibody to hepatitis C virus; IgM, immunoglobulin M; anti-HAV, antibody to hepatitis A virus.)

agents, drugs, and toxins. There can be a long lag time between exposure to the trigger and onset of the disease, and the triggering factor may not be needed for perpetuation of the disorder.

Molecular mimicry of a foreign antigen and a self-antigen is the most common explanation for the loss of self-tolerance, but there have been no autoimmune diseases in which this mechanism has been established.[5] Genetic factors influence autoantigen presentation and CD4+ helper T cell recognition. The antigen binding groove of the class II molecule of the major histocompatibility complex (MHC) is encoded by alleles that determine its configuration and its ability to activate immunocytes. The susceptibility alleles of AIH reside on the *DRB1* gene, and among white northern European and North American patients, they are *DRB1*0301* and *DRB1*0401*.[6]

Different ethnic groups have different susceptibility alleles, and these findings support a shared motif hypothesis of pathogenesis.[7] According to this hypothesis, risk of disease relates to amino acid sequences in the antigen binding groove of the class II MHC molecule, and multiple alleles encode the same or a similar sequence (shared motif). The critical shared motif in AIH in white northern Europeans and North Americans is represented by the six-amino-acid code LLEQKR, where lysine (K) is in position 71 of the DRβ polypeptide chain of the class II MHC molecule.[7] *DRB1*0301* and *DRB1*0401* encode identical sequences in this region. *DRB1*0404* and *DRB1*0405*, which are the susceptibility alleles in Mexican, Japanese, and Argentine adults, encode a similar sequence except for an arginine (R) for lysine (K) at the DRβ71 position.[7]

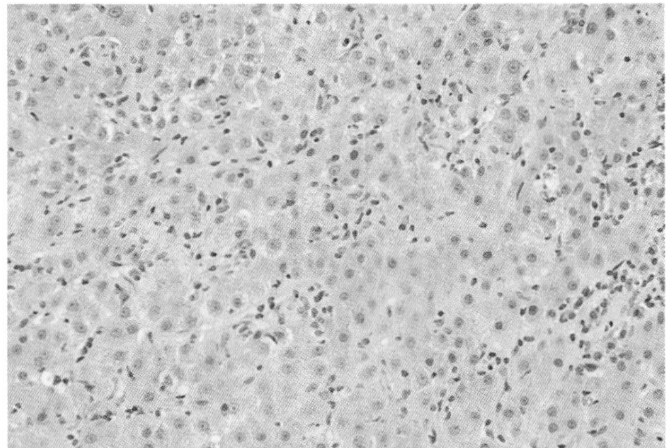

Figure 75–2. Lobular hepatitis. Mononuclear inflammatory cells line the sinusoidal spaces. Typically, lobular hepatitis coexists with interface hepatitis, but it may be pronounced during acute onset or during relapse after treatment withdrawal. Hematoxylin and eosin, ×200.

Antigenic peptides are selected for display by the nature of the amino acids that interact with residues within the antigen binding groove.[7] The critical six-amino-acid motif in AIH restricts the range of peptides that can be accommodated. Multiple self-antigens or foreign antigens may satisfy the minimal structural requirements and serve as immunogenic peptides. Only the cytochrome monooxygenase P-450 IID6 (CYP2D6) has been recognized as a target autoantigen in AIH.[8]

Liver cell destruction is accomplished by either cell-mediated cytotoxicity, antibody-dependent cell-mediated cytotoxicity, or a combination of both mechanisms.[1, 5] Cell-mediated cytotoxicity depends on the clonal expansion of CD8+ cytotoxic T cells that accomplish liver cell injury through the release of lymphokines. This mechanism is regulated by type 1 cytokines, and a genetic polymorphism that affects tumor necrosis factor-α (TNF-α) production may facilitate this pathway.[9] Antibody-dependent cell-mediated cytotoxicity is regulated by type 2 cytokines, and the natural killer cell

Table 75–1 | **Scoring System for Diagnosis of Autoimmune Hepatitis**

CATEGORY	FACTOR	SCORE	CATEGORY	FACTOR	SCORE
Gender	Female	+2	Immune disease	Thyroiditis, colitis, synovitis, others	+2
AP/AST (or AP/ALT) ratio	>3	−2	Other liver defined autoantibodies	Anti-SLA/LP, antiactin, anti-LC1, pANCA	+2
	<1.5	+2			
Gamma globulin or IgG levels above normal	>2.0	+3	Histologic features	Interface hepatitis	+3
	1.5–2.0	+2		Plasmacytic	+1
	1.0–1.5	+1		Rosettes	+1
	<1.0	0		None of above	−5
				Biliary changes	−3
				Other features	−3
ANA, SMA, or anti-LKM1 titers	>1:80	+3	Treatment response	Complete	+2
	1:80	+2		Relapse	+3
	1:40	+1			
	<1:40	0			
AMA	Positive	−4			
Viral markers	Positive	−3			
	Negative	+3			
Drugs	Yes	−4	**Pretreatment Score**		
	No	+1	Definite diagnosis		>15
			Probable diagnosis		10–15
Alcohol	<25 g/day	+2	**Post-treatment Score**		
	>60 g/day	−2	Definite diagnosis		>17
			Probable diagnosis		12–17
HLA	DR3 or DR4	+1			

AMA, antimitochondrial antibodies; ANA, antinuclear antibodies; anti-LC1, antibodies to liver cytosol type 1; anti-LKM1, antibodies to liver/kidney type 1; anti-SLA/LP, antibodies to soluble liver antigen/liver pancreas; AP/AST (or AP/ALT) ratio, ratio of serum alkaline phosphatase level to serum aspartate aminotransferase (or serum alanine aminotransferase) level; HLA, human leukocyte antigen; IgG, serum immunoglobulin G level; pANCA, perinuclear antineutrophil cytoplasmic antibodies; SMA, smooth muscle antibodies.

accomplishes liver cell destruction by the binding of its Fc receptor with an antigen–antibody complex on the hepatocyte surface. The predominant mechanism depends on the phenotypic differentiation of the CD4+ helper T cell, which in turn reflects the cytokine milieu. The cytokine milieu may reflect polymorphisms of the cytokine genes that favor excessive production of some modulators, such as TNF-α, or deficient production of others.[10]

SUBCLASSIFICATIONS

Three types of AIH have been proposed on the basis of immunoserologic markers.[1] Only two types have almost mutually exclusive autoantibodies, and none has been ascribed a unique cause, distinctive clinical phenotype, individual management strategy, or special type of behavior.[11] The International Autoimmune Hepatitis Group has not endorsed subclassification of AIH, and subtyping by autoantibody profile has mainly been of descriptive value (see Fig. 75–3).

Type 1 Autoimmune Hepatitis

Type 1 AIH is characterized by the presence of SMA and/or ANA in serum (Table 75–2).[1, 11] Antibodies to actin have greater specificity for the diagnosis than SMA, but they have less sensitivity, and the assay for antiactin is not generally available.[12] Perinuclear antineutrophil cytoplasmic antibodies (pANCAs), which occur in patients who have PSC and chronic ulcerative colitis, are found in up to 90% of patients who have type 1 AIH and may be surrogate markers for the disease.[13]

Type 1 AIH has a bimodal age distribution (see Table 75–2).[1] Seventy-eight percent of patients are women (female-to-male ratio, 3.6 : 1), and 41% have concurrent extrahepatic immunologic diseases. Autoimmune thyroiditis (12%), Graves' disease (6%), and chronic ulcerative colitis (6%) are the most common associated immune disorders. Rheumatoid arthritis, pernicious anemia, systemic sclerosis, Coombs' test–positive hemolytic anemia, idiopathic thrombocytopenic purpura, symptomatic cryoglobulinemia, leukocytoclastic vasculitis, nephritis, erythema nodosum, systemic lupus erythematosus, and fibrosing alveolitis may also occur (less than 1% each). Cholangiography is warranted in all patients who have concurrent chronic ulcerative colitis to exclude PSC.[14]

In 40% of patients who have type 1 AIH, the onset of symptoms is acute and the disease may appear in a fulminant fashion.[15] Typically, patients who have an acute presentation have clinical (ascites, esophageal varices, or spider angiomas), laboratory (thrombocytopenia, hypoalbuminemia, or hypergammaglobulinemia), and histologic changes (cirrhosis) that suggest chronic liver disease. The acute presentation frequently reflects preexisting subclinical disease that is

Table 75–2 | **Subclassifications of Autoimmune Hepatitis Based on Autoantibodies***

CLINICAL FEATURES	TYPE 1	TYPE 2	TYPE 3
Conventional autoantibodies	Smooth muscle Nuclear	Liver/kidney microsome type 1	None
Novel autoantibodies	pANCA *Actin* *Asialoglycoprotein receptor*	*Liver cytosol type 1*	*Soluble liver antigen/liver-pancreas*
Putative autoantigen	Unknown *Asialoglycoprotein receptor* possible	CYP2D6	Transfer ribonucleoprotein (tRNP) involved in selenocysteine metabolism
Age (years)	Bimodal (10–20 and 45–70)	Pediatric (2–14)	Adults (30–50)
Women (%)	78	89	90
Concurrent immune diseases (%)	41	34	58
Organ-specific antibodies (%)	4	30	Uncertain
Gamma globulin elevation	Marked	Mild	Moderate
Low IgA	No	Occasional	No
HLA associations	-B8, -DR3, -DR4	-B14, -DR3, *-C4A-Q0*, -DR7	Uncertain
Allelic risk factors	*DRB1*0301* and **0401* (White North Americans and northern Europeans)	*DRB1*07* (Germans and Brazilians)	Uncertain
Glucocorticoid responsive	+++	+++	+++

*Autoantibodies in italics are investigational only and are not available for routine clinical use.

HLA, human leukocyte antigen; IgA, immunoglobulin A; pANCA, perinuclear antineutrophil cytoplasmic antibody; +++, very responsive; ++, moderately responsive; +, mildly responsive.

unmasked by progression or a spontaneous exacerbation of disease. Eight percent of patients have no features of chronicity, and the presentation of the disorder is indistinguishable from that of acute viral or toxic hepatitis.

The target autoantigen of type 1 AIH is unknown, but the asialoglycoprotein receptor (ASGPR) is a candidate.[16] The ASGPR is expressed on the hepatocyte surface and is associated a with high titer of autoantibody (anti-ASGPR) and sensitized liver infiltrating lymphocytes. Antibodies to ASGPR, especially those directed against human-derived antigen, are specific for AIH; titers correlate with the laboratory and histologic indices of inflammatory activity; and persistence of seropositivity during therapy identifies patients who commonly relapse after withdrawal of therapy.[17]

Human leukocyte antigen (HLA)-DR3 *(DRB1*0301)* and -DR4 *(DRB1*0401)* are independent risk factors for type 1 AIH.[6] *DRB1*0301* is associated most closely with the disease in white patients of northern European extraction, and *DRB1*0401* has a secondary association. Over 80% of white patients in Great Britain and the United States possess either *DRB1*0301* or *DRB1*0401*, compared with 42% of a normal white population. These findings indicate that type 1 AIH is a polygenic disorder.

Type 2 Autoimmune Hepatitis

Type 2 AIH is characterized by the presence of anti-LKM1 in serum (see Table 75–2).[18] Mainly children are affected (ages 2 to 14 years), but adults can also be afflicted. In Europe, especially in Germany and France, 20% of patients are adults,[18] whereas in the United States, only 4% of patients are older than 18 years.[19] The regional differences in prevalence may relate to genetic polymorphisms in the expression of cytochrome monooxygenase P-450 IID6 (CYP2D6), which is the target autoantigen.

Type 2 AIH patients are younger than type 1 patients, and they may have different clinical and laboratory features (see Table 75–2).[18] An acute or fulminant presentation is possible, and it is essential to screen all patients who have an acute decompensation for type-specific autoantibodies. Earlier perceptions that type 2 AIH had a worse outcome than type 1 disease have not been corroborated, and both types respond well to glucocorticoids.[20] Type 2 AIH is associated with HLA-B14, -DR3, and *-C4A-Q0*. *DRB1*07* has also been implicated as a susceptibility factor in German and Brazilian patients.[21, 22] These findings suggest that type 2 AIH has a distinctive genetic predisposition.

The target antigen of type 2 AIH is CYP2D6.[8] This protein is a 50-kd microsomal drug metabolizing enzyme, and its expression on the hepatocyte surface can be modulated by interleukins and TNF-α. Antibodies to LKM1 inhibit the activity of CYP2D6 in vitro but not in vivo, and lymphocytes extracted from the liver tissue of patients who have the disease exhibit immunoreactivity specific to the antigen.

Recombinant CYP2D6 has been used to define the epitopes of anti-LKM1, and reactivity is restricted mainly to a short linear 33-amino-acid sequence.[8] Of the sera reactive to this sequence, 50% are reactive to an even shorter eight-amino-acid sequence. Sera from type 2 AIH patients bind mainly to the peptide sequence 254–271 of recombinant CYP2D6, and this region has been designated as its core motif. Antibodies to LKM1 are present in some patients with chronic hepatitis C, but their reactivities are usually to epitopes outside the core motif.[23]

A distinct form of anti–LKM-positive AIH occurs in association with the autoimmune polyendocrinopathy disorder (APECED),[24] which is marked by the presence of numerous organ- and non-organ-specific autoantibodies and multiple concurrent autoimmune diseases. Autoimmune polyendocrine syndrome type 1 (APS1) is caused by a single-gene mutation located on chromosome 21q22.3.[25] The APS1 gene encodes a transcription factor, called the *autoimmune regulator* (AIRE), which is expressed in epithelial and dendritic cells within the thymus, where it may regulate clonal deletion of autoreactive T cells and affect self-tolerance. Features of the disease are ectodermal dystrophy, mucocutaneous candidiasis, multiple endocrine gland failure (parathyroids, adrenals, ovaries), autoantibody production, and AIH in various combinations.[26] Unlike other autoimmune diseases, APS1 has a mendelian pattern of inheritance, complete penetrance of the gene, no HLA-DR associations, and no female predominance. Patients who have APS1 and AIH have a particularly aggressive liver disease that does not respond well to standard immunosuppressive regimens.[26] Earlier reports of type 2 AIH that described a poor outcome and high frequency of other autoimmune disorders may have included these patients.

Type 3 Autoimmune Hepatitis

Type 3 AIH is characterized by the presence of anti-SLA/LP in serum (see Table 75–2).[27, 28] Antibody to soluble liver antigen (anti-SLA) and antibody to liver/pancreas (anti-LP) were originally proposed as independent markers of type 3 AIH, but they are now recognized to have identical reactivities. Glutathione S-transferases have been nominated as the target autoantigens,[29] but a 50-kd protein was described in 2000 as the more likely target.[30] The candidate antigen is a transfer ribonucleoprotein ($tRNP^{(Ser)Sec}$) involved in the incorporation of selenocysteine into peptide chains. Patients who have anti-SLA/LP have clinical and laboratory features that are indistinguishable from those of type 1 AIH patients, and they respond well to glucocorticoids.[31, 32] For these reasons, anti-SLA/LP does not define a valid subgroup of AIH. Testing for anti-SLA/LP may be useful in reclassifying patients with cryptogenic chronic hepatitis,[31] and a standardized enzyme immunoassay based on recombinant antigen is available in Europe as a commercial kit.[32]

VARIANT FORMS

Patients who have atypical features of AIH currently lack an established identity, official designation, and confident treatment strategy.[33] They have autoimmune features but do not satisfy the criteria for a definite or probable diagnosis of AIH. Such patients typically have manifestations of AIH and another type of chronic liver disease (overlap syndrome), or they have findings that are incompatible with the diagnosis of AIH by current diagnostic criteria (outlier syndrome) (Table 75–3).

Overlap with Primary Biliary Cirrhosis

Patients with AIH who also have antimitochondrial antibodies (AMAs) and histologic findings of cholangitis constitute an overlap syndrome with patients who have PBC (see Table 75–3).[33, 34] Typically, these patients have low titers of AMA and concurrent features of bile duct injury or loss. Antibodies against the PBC-specific M2 mitochondrial antigens may be present; histologic features of cholangitis, including destructive cholangitis, may be seen, and copper staining of hepatic tissue indicative of cholestasis may yield positive findings.[34] The occurrence varies from 5% of patients originally diagnosed as having AIH to 19% of patients originally diagnosed as having PBC.[34]

The behavior of the disease and response to treatment depend mainly on the component of the disease that predominates. Patients who have high serum aspartate aminotransferase levels, serum alkaline phosphatase concentrations less than twice normal, moderate to severe interface hepatitis on histologic examination, and high diagnostic scores for AIH commonly respond to glucocorticoid therapy.[34] In contrast, patients who have serum alkaline phosphatase levels greater than twice normal, serum gamma glutamyl transpeptidase concentrations at least five times normal, and florid bile duct lesions on histologic examination mainly have PBC. These patients commonly respond to ursodeoxycholic acid in combination with glucocorticoids.[35]

Overlap with Primary Sclerosing Cholangitis

Histologic changes of lymphocytic, pleomorphic, or fibrous cholangitis; cholestatic laboratory findings; concurrent inflammatory bowel disease; and failure to respond to glucocorticoids are justifications for cholangiography in patients who have AIH.[14, 34] As many as 41% of these individuals

Table 75–3 | **Variant Forms of Autoimmune Hepatitis**

DISTINCTIVE FEATURES	AIH + PBC	AIH + PSC	AUTOIMMUNE CHOLANGITIS	CRYPTOGENIC CHRONIC HEPATITIS
Clinical	AIH features AMA present	AIH features CUC AMA absent Abnormal cholangiogram	ANA and/or SMA present AMA absent No CUC Normal cholangiogram	AIH features No autoantibodies HLA-B8 or -DR3
Histologic	Cholangitis Cholestasis	Cholangitis Cholestasis	Cholangitis Cholestasis	Interface hepatitis
Treatment	Empirical prednisone if AP ≤ twice normal; prednisone and ursodeoxycholic acid if AP > twice normal and/or florid duct lesions	Empirical prednisone and ursodeoxycholic acid	Empirical prednisone and/or ursodeoxycholic acid	Empirical conventional regimens for AIH

AIH, autoimmune hepatitis; AMA, antimitochondrial antibodies; ANA, antinuclear antibodies; AP, serum alkaline phosphatase level; CUC, chronic ulcerative colitis; HLA, human leukocyte antigen; PBC, primary biliary cirrhosis; PSC, primary sclerosing cholangitis; SMA, smooth muscle antibodies.

have cholangiographic changes of PSC and are classifiable as having overlap variants (see Table 75–3). Furthermore, 54% of patients who have PSC have aggregate scores that support a probable or definite diagnosis of AIH and also have an overlap syndrome.[34, 36] The absence of characteristic cholangiographic changes does not preclude the diagnosis of PSC, because small duct disease may be present (see Table 75–3).[14]

Diagnostic difficulties occur mainly in children. Autoimmune sclerosing cholangitis is a disorder described in children who have the clinical phenotype of AIH but abnormal cholangiographic results.[20, 37] Because these children have features of AIH and PSC, they satisfy the criteria for an overlap syndrome. Inflammatory bowel disease, however, is frequently absent, and these children respond as well to glucocorticoid therapy as do their counterparts who have classic AIH. Consequently, they are distinct from the adults who have the overlap syndrome and are best categorized separately.

Treatment is empirical. Glucocorticoids have been effective only in those adults whose serum alkaline phosphatase levels are less than twice normal.[34] Ursodeoxycholic acid can be considered for patients who have dominant cholestatic features, but it has generally not been useful in PSC. The combination of glucocorticoids and ursodeoxycholic acid is rational but of uncertain value.

Autoimmune Cholangitis

Autoimmune cholangitis is a chronic hepatocellular inflammation that has features of AIH and AMA-negative PBC or small-duct PSC (see Table 75–3).[38] Antinuclear antibodies or SMA (or both) are typically present in conjunction with cholestatic biochemical changes and histologic findings of bile duct injury, and the cholangiographic result is normal (see Table 75–3).

Persons who have autoimmune cholangitis are variably responsive to glucocorticoids and ursodeoxycholic acid. Preliminary experience suggests that these therapies can improve the clinical and laboratory findings but not the histologic changes. This recalcitrance to therapy with glucocorticoids is another feature that favors separate classification of the disorder.

Cryptogenic Chronic Hepatitis

Thirteen percent of adults who have nonviral chronic hepatitis satisfy consensus criteria for the diagnosis of AIH, but because they lack characteristic autoantibodies, they are considered to have an outlier syndrome (see Table 75–3). These patients are commonly designated as having cryptogenic chronic hepatitis, and they may be excluded inappropriately from therapies of potential benefit.

Autoantibody-negative patients who have severe inflammatory activity are similar in age, female predominance, frequency of concurrent immunologic diseases, histologic features, and laboratory findings to patients with classical AIH.[39] Furthermore, they have similar frequencies of HLA-B8, -DR3, and A1-B8-DR3, and they respond as well to glucocorticoid treatment as do their autoantibody-positive counterparts. These patients probably have a form of AIH that has escaped detection by conventional immunoserologic assays, and they are candidates for a closely monitored treatment trial of glucocorticoids. Investigational assays for anti-SLA/LP occasionally yield positive findings in these patients, and successive testing for conventional autoantibodies may demonstrate the late appearance of typical autoimmune markers in some (see Table 75–3).[40]

PREVALENCE

The incidence of AIH among white northern Europeans is 1.9 cases per 100,000 persons per year, and its point prevalence is 16.9 cases per 100,000 persons per year.[41] In the United States, AIH affects 100,000 to 200,000 persons,[42] and it accounts for 2.6% of the transplantations in the European Liver Transplant Registry and 5.9% in the National Institutes of Health Liver Transplantation Database.[43] The frequency of AIH among patients with chronic liver disease in North America is between 11% and 23%.

The impact of genetic risk factors must be considered when assessing the occurrence of disease in different regions. The prevalence of AIH is greatest among northern European white groups who have a high frequency of HLA-DR3 and -DR4, and it is found with similar frequency in the derivative populations of North America and Australia.[44] The Japanese have a low frequency of HLA-DR3, and their AIH reflects an association with HLA-DR4.[45] All populations are susceptible to the disease, and it has been described in African Americans, Brazilians, Argentines, Arabs, Japanese, and Indians.

PROGNOSTIC INDICES

The prognosis of AIH relates mainly to the severity of liver inflammation at the initial medical consultation, as reflected in the laboratory indices and the histologic findings. HLA status influences treatment outcome (Table 75–4).[46]

Laboratory Indices

The serum aspartate aminotransferase (AST) and gamma globulin levels reflect severity of disease and immediate prognosis. Sustained severe derangements indicate a poor outcome unless therapy is started. Less severe laboratory abnormalities are associated with a better prognosis (see Table 75–4).[46]

Spontaneous resolution is possible in 13% to 20% of patients regardless of disease activity.[46] There are no features that predict this outcome, and patients should not be managed with this expectation. Of the individuals who survive the early, most active stage of the disease, inactive cirrhosis develops in 41%. Untreated patients who have initial severe disease and survive the first 2 years of illness typically survive long term. These observations suggest that a critical determinant of survival in the untreated patient is early tolerance to the disease.

Histologic Findings

The histologic findings at presentation are also indices of disease severity, and each pattern of liver cell injury has its

Table 75–4 | **Prognostic Indices of Autoimmune Hepatitis**

PROGNOSTIC INDICES BEFORE TREATMENT*	OUTCOME	PROGNOSTIC INDICES AFTER TREATMENT	COMMENTS
AST ≥ 10-fold normal *or* AST ≥ 5-fold normal + gamma globulin ≥ 2-fold normal	50% 3-Year mortality 90% 10-Year mortality	HLA-B8, -DR3 or *DRB1*0301*	Onset at young age Severe inflammation at presentation Relapse propensity Treatment failure common Liver transplantation frequent
AST < 10-fold normal + gamma globulin < 2-fold normal	49% Cirrhosis at 15 years 10% 10-Year mortality	HLA-DR4 or *DRB1*0401*	Onset in old age Women Concurrent immunologic diseases Good response to glucocorticoids
Interface hepatitis	17% Cirrhosis at 5 years Normal 5-year survival	C4A gene deletions	Low serum complement level Early-onset disease Associated with HLA-DR3
Bridging necrosis *or* multilobular necrosis	82% Cirrhosis at 5 years 45% 5-Year mortality	Multilobular necrosis and failure to improve on treatment; hyperbilirubinemia after 2 weeks	High mortality rate
Cirrhosis	58% 5-Year mortality	Failure to enter remission within 4 years and first sign of decompensation (ascites)	High mortality rate

AST, serum aspartate aminotransferase level; HLA, human leukocyte antigen.

own prognostic implication (see Table 75–3).[47] Esophageal varices develop in 54% of patients with cirrhosis, and death from hemorrhage occurs in 20% of those with varices if treatment is not instituted. Hepatocellular carcinoma can also occur in patients with cirrhosis, but the risk is small.[48]

Human Leukocyte Antigen Status

Patients who have HLA-B8, which is in tight linkage dysequilibrium with HLA-DR3, typically are younger and have more active disease than patients who have other HLA types (see Table 75–4).[49] Individuals with HLA-DR3 respond less well to glucocorticoids; those with HLA-DR4 have different clinical features and better outcomes than those with HLA-DR3.[50, 51] These findings indicate that there are important associations between the genetic predisposition of the host and the outcome of the disease.

Patients who have *DRB1*0401* have less severe disease initially, relapse less frequently after drug withdrawal, and have the disease later in life than do their counterparts with *DRB1*0301*.[50] Null allotypes at the C4A and C4B locus occur in 90% of patients with early-onset disease,[52] and a 21-hydroxylase A pseudogene in adults has been associated with increased mortality rates and frequency of relapse.[53] The HLA alleles determine the ability of each class II molecule of the MHC to bind and present antigens to CD4+ helper T cells. Consequently, they directly influence the immune response and, in turn, the clinical manifestations and behavior of AIH. At present, the clinical applications of HLA testing in AIH are uncertain, and determinations are not routinely made.

CLINICAL MANIFESTATIONS

The clinical manifestations of AIH reflect chronic hepatocellular inflammation (Table 75–5). Cholestatic features may

Table 75–5 | **Clinical Manifestations of Autoimmune Hepatitis**

FINDINGS	OCCURRENCE (%)
Symptoms	
Fatigue	85
Jaundice	77
Upper abdominal discomfort	48
Pruritus (mild)	36
Anorexia	30
Polymyalgias	30
Diarrhea	28
Cushingoid features	19
Fever (≤40°C)	18
Physical Findings	
Hepatomegaly	78
Jaundice	69
Splenomegaly	≥32
Spider angiomas	58
Ascites	20
Encephalopathy	14
Concurrent immune diseases	≤48
Laboratory Features	
Aspartate aminotransferase level elevation	100
Hypergammaglobulinemia	92
Increased immunoglobulin G level	91
Hyperbilirubinemia	83
Alkaline phosphatase level ≥2-fold normal	33
Immunoserologic Markers*	
SMA, ANA, or anti-LKM1	100
Perinuclear antineutrophil cytoplasm	92 (Type 1 only)
Antiasialoglycoprotein receptor	82
Antiactin	74
Anti-liver cytosol 1	32 (Type 2 only)
Anti-soluble liver antigen/liver-pancreas	11–17

*Autoantibodies in italics are investigational and are not available for routine clinical use.

ANA, antinuclear antibody; anti-LKM1, antibody to liver/kidney type 1; SMA, smooth muscle antibody.

Table 75–6 | **Treatment Indications**

FINDINGS	INDICATIONS		
	Absolute	Relative	None
Clinical	Incapacitating symptoms	Mild or no symptoms	Asymptomatic with mild laboratory changes
	Relentless clinical progression		Previous intolerance to prednisone and/or azathioprine
Laboratory	AST ≥ 10-fold normal	AST 3- to 9-fold normal	AST < 3-fold normal
	AST ≥ 5-fold normal and gamma globulin ≥ 2-fold normal	AST < 5-fold normal and gamma globulin < 2-fold normal	Severe cytopenia
Histologic	Bridging necrosis	Interface hepatitis	Inactive cirrhosis
	Multilobular necrosis		Portal hepatitis
			Decompensated cirrhosis with variceal bleeding

AST, serum aspartate aminotransferase level.

be present, but they do not dominate the clinical picture. Similarly, manifestations of liver decompensation, such as ascites, hepatic encephalopathy, and variceal bleeding, are uncommon findings at the initial medical consultation.[54, 55]

Ready fatigability is the most common symptom (85%) (see Table 75–5).[54] Weight loss is uncommon and intense pruritus argues against the diagnosis. Hepatomegaly is the most common physical finding (78%), and jaundice is found in 69%. Splenomegaly can be present in patients with and without cirrhosis (56% and 32%, respectively), as can spider angiomas.

Hyperbilirubinemia is present in 83% of patients, but the serum level is greater than threefold normal in only 46%.[54] Similarly, the serum alkaline phosphatase level is commonly increased (81%), but elevations of more than two times (33%) or four times (10%) normal are uncommon (see Table 75–5).

The hypergammaglobulinemia of AIH is polyclonal; the immunoglobulin G fraction predominates.[54] Paraproteins with immunoreactivity are common, and patients may have diverse, nonspecific immunoserologic findings, including antibodies to bacteria (*Escherichia coli*, bacteroides, and *Salmonella* species) and viruses (measles, rubella, and cytomegalovirus). Cryoglobulinemia may be present, but symptomatic disease is rare.

Concurrent immunologic diseases are common and involve diverse organ systems, most frequently the thyroid.[56] Smooth muscle antibodies, ANA, and anti-LKM1 are required for the diagnosis, but other autoantibodies may be present, as shown in Table 75–5. These autoantibodies do not have routine clinical applications, and their use is investigational.

TREATMENT

Indications

The indications for treatment are shown in Table 75–6.[1, 57] They are based on manifestations of inflammation rather than measures of hepatic dysfunction.

Treatment Regimens

Prednisone alone or at a lower dose in combination with azathioprine is effective (Table 75–7).[1, 57] No findings at presentation preclude a satisfactory response to therapy. The presence of ascites or hepatic encephalopathy identifies patients with a poor prognosis. These individuals, however, can still respond to glucocorticoid therapy and should be treated before a decision regarding liver transplantation is made.[58] When decompensated patients with multilobular necrosis have at least one laboratory parameter that fails to normalize or hyperbilirubinemia that does not improve during a 2-week treatment period, the immediate mortality rate is high and evaluation for liver transplantation is warranted (see Table 75–4). In contrast, when these parameters improve, patients have an excellent immediate survival rate, and their drug treatment should be continued.

Drug-Related Side Effects

Cosmetic changes, such as facial rounding, dorsal hump formation, obesity, acne, or hirsutism, occur in 80% of patients after 2 years of treatment regardless of regimen.[57] Severe side effects, including osteopenia with vertebral compression, diabetes, cataracts, emotional lability, and hypertension, usually develop only after protracted therapy (more than 18 months) and on the higher dose prednisone schedule (20 mg/day). Azathioprine with prednisone is preferred to prednisone alone because the combination produces fewer glucocorticoid-related side effects during comparable periods of treatment (10% versus 44%). Premature discontinuation of treatment is justified in 13% of patients, mainly because of intolerable obesity, cosmetic changes, or osteoporosis.[57, 59]

Postmenopausal patients are at risk for vertebral compression and must be carefully selected for therapy before institution of a glucocorticoid regimen.[60] A regular program of exercise, calcium and vitamin D supplementation, and hormonal replacement therapy may help preserve bone density. Bisphosphonates, such as alendronate (10 mg/day) or etidronate (400 mg/day for 2 weeks every 3 months), should be

Table 75–7 | **Preferred Treatment Regimens**

COMBINATION THERAPY		SINGLE-DRUG THERAPY
Prednisone (mg/day)	Azathioprine (mg/day)	Prednisone (mg/day)
30 mg × 1 Week 20 mg × 1 Week 15 mg × 2 Weeks 10 mg Until end point	50 mg Until end point	60 mg × 1 Week 40 mg × 1 Week 30 mg × 2 Weeks 20 mg Until end point

considered for patients with osteopenia.[61] Carefully selected postmenopausal patients respond as well as others to initial therapy; protracted therapy, however, especially retreatment after relapse, is associated with an increased risk of complications.

Treatment with azathioprine can be complicated by cholestatic hepatotoxicity, nausea, emesis, rash, and cytopenia.[57] These side effects occur in fewer than 10% of patients treated with 50 mg/day and reverse with a reduction in dose or termination of therapy. Teratogenicity and oncogenicity are theoretical complications, and the risk of nonhepatic malignancy in patients on long-term immunosuppressive therapy is 1.4-fold greater than that in an age- and sex-matched normal population.[62] This low but increased risk of malignancy does not contraindicate therapy, but it does emphasize the importance of maintaining strict indications for treatment. In women who are pregnant or contemplating pregnancy, it is appropriate to avoid azathioprine.

Treatment End Points

Glucocorticoid therapy is continued until remission, treatment failure, incomplete response, or drug toxicity occurs (Fig. 75–4).[46, 57] *Remission* implies the absence of symptoms; resolution of inflammatory indices (except for a serum AST level no greater than twice normal); and histologic improvement to normal or minimal activity. Histologic resolution lags behind clinical and laboratory resolution by 3 to 6 months, and therapy must be extended accordingly. Liver biopsy examination before drug withdrawal ensures an optimal end point. Improvement of the liver tissue to normal is associated with a frequency of relapse of only 20% after cessation of treatment. In contrast, improvement to portal hepatitis is associated with a 50% frequency of relapse. Progression to cirrhosis or persistence of interface hepatitis is associated with a 100% frequency of relapse.

Treatment failure connotes deterioration during therapy.[46, 57] It is made evident by worsening of the serum AST or bilirubin levels by at least 67% of previous values, progressive histologic activity, or onset of ascites or encephalopathy. Conventional glucocorticoid therapy should be stopped, and a high-dose regimen should be instituted.

Incomplete response connotes improvement that is insufficient to satisfy remission criteria.[46, 57] Failure to achieve remission within 3 years indicates that remission is unlikely and warrants discontinuation of conventional treatment.

Drug toxicity justifies premature withdrawal of medication or reduction in dose.[46, 57] Many side effects are reversible, and some consequences such as cataracts and osteopenia with vertebral compression have effective therapies. Weight gain, acne, edema, and diabetes may be consequences of the disease rather than of the drugs.

TREATMENT RESULTS

Prednisone alone or in combination with azathioprine induces a clinical, biochemical, and histologic remission in 65% of patients within 3 years.[46, 57] The average treatment interval until remission is 22 months. Most importantly, therapy improves the survival rate: the 10-year life expectancies for treated patients with and without cirrhosis at the time of the initial medical consultation are 89% and 90%, respectively.[55] The overall 10-year survival rate is 93% and is comparable to that of an age- and sex-matched cohort from the population at large (94%).[55] Patients who have histologic cirrhosis respond as well as noncirrhotic patients and should be treated similarly, with the same expectation of success.

Relapse

Patients who enter remission commonly experience an exacerbation after drug withdrawal.[46, 57] Relapse occurs in 50% within 6 months, and most (70% to 86%) experience exacer-

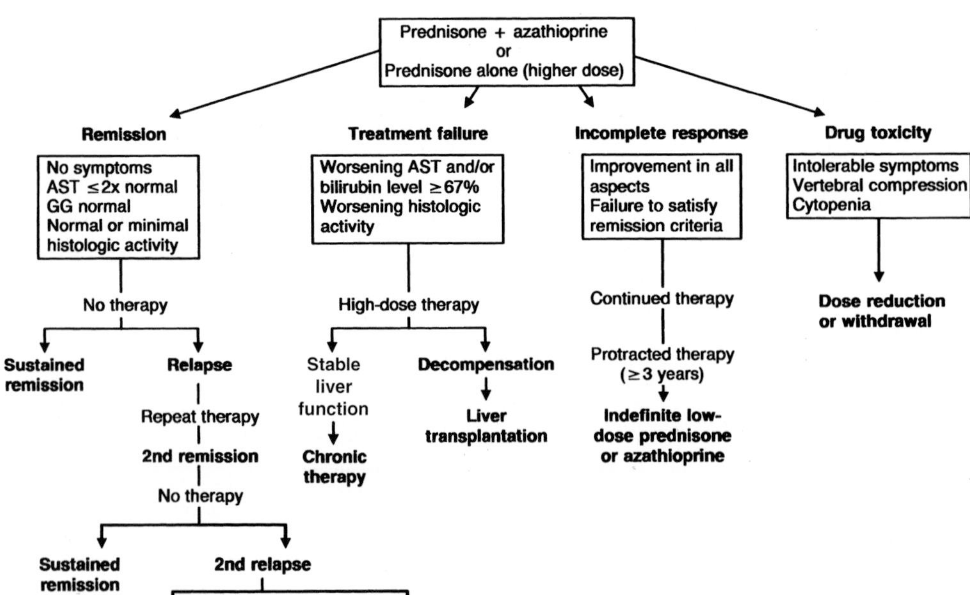

Figure 75–4. Treatment algorithm for autoimmune hepatitis. Patients who satisfy absolute or relative indications for glucocorticoid therapy are treated with prednisone in combination with azathioprine or a higher dose of prednisone alone. Treatment is continued until the criteria for a treatment end point are met. Possible end points are remission, treatment failure, incomplete response, and drug toxicity. Therapy can then be discontinued, increased in dose, or reduced in dose. Responses to the dose adjustments determine the need for other actions. The principal indices of inflammatory activity are serum aspartate aminotransferase (AST) and gamma globulin (GG) levels.

bation within 3 years. Reinstitution of the original treatment induces another remission, but relapse commonly recurs after termination of therapy. The major consequence of relapse and retreatment is the development of drug-related complications, which occur in 70% of those who have multiple relapses and retreatments.[59]

Patients who have had at least two relapses require indefinite therapy with either prednisone or azathioprine (see Fig. 75–4). Eighty-seven percent of patients can be managed long term on prednisone at less than 10 mg/day (median dose, 7.5 mg/day).[63] The dose is titrated to the lowest level needed to prevent symptoms and maintain serum aminotransferase levels below fivefold normal. Side effects attributable to previous glucocorticoid therapy resolve in 85%; the immediate survival rate is comparable to that of conventionally treated individuals (91% versus 90%); and new complications do not occur.

Continuous azathioprine therapy (2 mg/kg/day) is an alternative strategy and can be used in patients who are not severely cytopenic or pregnant.[64] Eighty-three percent of individuals remain in remission for up to 10 years. Symptoms of glucocorticoid withdrawal (arthralgias and myalgias) occur in 56% but are self-limited. Myelosuppression (6%) and nonhepatic malignancies (7%) are infrequent. The prednisone and azathioprine regimens have not been compared directly, and there is no objective basis for prefering one to the other. The teratogenic and oncogenic risks of indefinite azathioprine therapy remain uncertain, and concerns about these risks may influence the selection of treatment. In 2000, mycophenolate mofetil was reported to maintain remission in patients resistant to or intolerant of azathioprine.[65] Future studies are needed to determine whether this inhibitor of de novo purine nucleotide synthesis can replace azathioprine in the management of relapse.

Treatment Failure

The condition of 9% of patients deteriorates during glucocorticoid therapy (treatment failure) (see Fig. 75–4).[46, 57] High doses of prednisone alone (60 mg/day) or prednisone (30 mg/day) in conjunction with azathioprine (150 mg/day) are the standard treatments in this group. Each schedule induces clinical and biochemical improvement in 70% of patients within 2 years. Histologic resolution, however, occurs in only 20%, and long-term therapy is frequently necessary. These patients are at risk for liver failure and serious drug toxicity. Liver transplantation must be considered at the first sign of hepatic decompensation, which usually appears with ascites (see Table 75–4).[66]

Liver transplantation is effective in the decompensated patient for whom glucocorticoid therapy has failed[66] (see Chapter 83). After transplantation, the autoantibodies and hypergammaglobulinemia disappear within 2 years, and the 5-year survival rate is 96%. Recurrent disease after transplantation is common but has been described mainly in patients who have inadequate immunosuppression.[67] Progression to cirrhosis and graft failure are possible, but usually adjustments in the immunosuppressive regimen are sufficient to suppress the manifestations.

Alternative management strategies for treatment failure have included the administration of cyclosporine, ursodeoxycholic acid, budesonide, 6-mercaptopurine, methotrexate, and cyclophosphamide.[68–70] In each instance, experience has been limited, and in most reports the preliminary results have been encouraging but uncorroborated. Among the new drugs used in treatment failure, only ursodeoxycholic acid has been evaluated by a randomized controlled clinical trial, which yielded the one negative report.[68]

Incomplete Response

Thirteen percent of patients improve during therapy but do not satisfy remission criteria (see Fig. 75–4).[46, 57] The diminishing benefit-to-risk ratio of protracted therapy justifies an alternative strategy. A low-dose prednisone regimen similar to that used after relapse is reasonable. The goal of treatment is to control disease activity on the lowest possible dose of medication. A similar strategy can be applied to patients who have emerging drug-related side effects.

Drug Toxicity

Treatment can usually be continued with the single tolerated drug (prednisone or azathioprine) in an adjusted dose (see Fig. 75–4). Cyclosporine, 6-mercaptopurine, and cyclophosphamide have also been used successfully after drug toxicity in isolated cases.

FUTURE DIRECTIONS

Future investigations must focus on the clarification of pathogenic mechanisms, characterization of target autoantigens, identification of host susceptibility factors, and assessment of alternative treatment strategies. Future drug trials must include more powerful immunosuppressive agents, novel cytoprotective drugs, and combinations of both. Site-specific interventions are possible when the pathogenic mechanisms are clarified. These therapies may include peptides to block autoantigen display within the class II major histocompatibility complex (MHC) molecules, agents such as cytotoxic T lymphocyte antigen 4 to temper immunocyte response, T cell vaccination, oral tolerance regimens, and cytokine manipulations.[70] A logical strategy by which to evaluate the interactions between the class II MHC molecules and the immune response is to develop animal models based on the transgenic expression of the immunoreactive unit. Similar models already exist for multiple sclerosis, rheumatoid arthritis, and autoimmune diabetes, and one is sorely needed for AIH.

REFERENCES

1. Czaja A: Autoimmune hepatitis: Evolving concepts and treatment strategies. Dig Dis Sci 40:435, 1995.
2. Alvarez F, Berg P, Bianchi F, et al: International Autoimmune Hepatitis Group report: Review of criteria for diagnosis of autoimmune hepatitis. J Hepatol 31:929, 1999.
3. Czaja A, Homburger H: Antibodies in liver disease. Gastroenterology 120:239, 2001.
4. Czaja A, Carpenter H: Validation of a scoring system for the diagnosis of autoimmune hepatitis. Dig Dis Sci 41:305, 1996.
5. Czaja A: Immunopathogenesis of autoimmune-mediated liver damage.

In Moreno-Otero R, Clemente-Ricote G, Garcia-Monzon C (eds): Immunology and the Liver: Autoimmunity. Madrid, Aran Ediciones, 2000, p. 73.
6. Strettell M, Donaldson P, Thomson L, et al: Allelic basis for HLA-encoded susceptibility to type 1 autoimmune hepatitis. Gastroenterology 112:2028,1997.
7. Czaja A, Donaldson P: Genetic susceptibilities for immune expression and liver cell injury in autoimmune hepatitis. Immunol Rev 174:250, 2000.
8. Manns M, Griffin K, Sullivan K, et al: LKM-1 autoantibodies recognize a short linear sequence in P450IID6, a cytochrome P-450 monooxygenase. J Clin Invest 88:1370, 1991.
9. Czaja A, Cookson S, Constantini P, et al: Cytokine polymorphisms associated with clinical features and treatment outcome in type 1 autoimmune hepatitis. Gastroenterology 117:645, 1999.
10. Czaja A, Sievers C, Zein N: Nature and behavior of serum cytokines in type 1 autoimmune hepatitis. Dig Dis Sci 45:1028, 2000.
11. Czaja A, Manns M: The validity and importance of subtypes of autoimmune hepatitis: A point of view. Am J Gastroenterol 90:1206, 1995.
12. Czaja A, Cassani F, Cataleta M, et al: Frequency and significance of antibodies to actin in type 1 autoimmune hepatitis. Hepatology 24:1068, 1996.
13. Targan S, Landers C, Vidrich A, et al: High-titer antineutrophil cytoplasmic antibodies in type 1 autoimmune hepatitis. Gastroenterology 108:1159, 1995.
14. Perdigoto R, Carpenter H, Czaja A: Frequency and significance of chronic ulcerative colitis in severe corticosteroid-treated autoimmune hepatitis. J Hepatol 14:325, 1992.
15. Nikias G, Batts K, Czaja A: The nature and prognostic implications of autoimmune hepatitis with an acute presentation. J Hepatol 21:866, 1994.
16. Poralla T, Treichel U, Lohr H, et al: The asialoglycoprotein receptor as target structure in autoimmune liver diseases. Semin Liver Dis 11:215, 1991.
17. Czaja A, Pfeifer K, Decker R, et al: Frequency and significance of antibodies to asialoglycoprotein receptor in type 1 autoimmune hepatitis. Dig Dis Sci 41:1733, 1996.
18. Homberg J, Abuaf N, Bernard O, et al: Chronic active hepatitis associated with anti–liver-kidney microsome antibody type 1: A second type of "autoimmune" hepatitis. Hepatology 7:1333, 1987.
19. Czaja A, Manns M, Homburger H: Frequency and significance of antibodies to liver/kidney microsome type 1 in adults with chronic active hepatitis. Gastroenterology 103:1290, 1992.
20. Gregorio G, Portmann B, Reid F, et al: Autoimmune hepatitis in childhood: A 20 year survey. Hepatology 25:541, 1997.
21. Czaja A, Kruger M, Santrach P, et al: Genetic distinctions between types 1 and 2 autoimmune hepatitis. Am J Gastroenterol 92:2197, 1997.
22. Bittencourt P, Goldberg A, Cancado E, et al: Genetic heterogeneity in susceptibility to autoimmune hepatitis types 1 and 2. Am J Gastroenterol 94:1906, 1999.
23. Yamamoto A, Cresteil D, Homberg J, et al: Characterization of the anti–liver-kidney microsome antibody (anti-LKM1) from hepatitis C virus–positive and–negative sera. Gastroenterology 104:1762, 1993.
24. The Finnish-German APECED Consortium: An autoimmune disease, APECED, caused by mutations in a novel gene featuring two PHD-type zinc finger domains. Nat Genet 17:399, 1997.
25. Nagamine K, Peterson P, Scott H, et al: Positional cloning of the APECED gene. Nat Genet 17:393, 1997.
26. Clemente M, Obermayer-Straub P, Meloni A, et al: Cytochrome P450 1A2 is a hepatic autoantigen in autoimmune polyglandular syndrome type 1. J Clin Endocrinol Metab 82:1353, 1997.
27. Manns M, Gerken G, Kyriatsoulis A, et al: Characterization of a new subgroup of autoimmune chronic active hepatitis by autoantibodies against a soluble liver antigen. Lancet 1:292, 1987.
28. Stechemesser E, Klein R, Berg P: Characterization and clinical relevance of liver-pancreas antibodies in autoimmune hepatitis. Hepatology 18:1, 1993.
29. Wesierska-Gadek J, Grimm R, Hitchman E, et al: Members of the glutathione *S*-transferase gene family are antigens in autoimmune hepatitis. Gastroenterology 114:329, 1998.
30. Wies I, Brunner S, Henninger J, et al: Identification of target antigen for SLA/LP autoantibodies in autoimmune hepatitis. Lancet 355:1510, 2000.
31. Czaja A, Carpenter H, Manns M: Antibodies to soluble liver antigen, P450IID6, and mitochondrial complexes in chronic hepatitis. Gastroenterology 105:1522, 1993.
32. Kanzler S, Weidemann C, Gerken G, et al: Clinical significance of autoantibodies to soluble liver antigen in autoimmune hepatitis. J Hepatol 31:635, 1999.
33. Czaja A: The variant forms of autoimmune hepatitis. Ann Intern Med 125:588, 1996.
34. Czaja A: Frequency and nature of the variant syndromes of autoimmune liver disease. Hepatology 28:360, 1998.
35. Chazouilleres O, Wendum D, Serfaty L, et al: Primary biliary cirrhosis–autoimmune hepatitis overlap syndrome: Clinical features and response to therapy. Hepatology 28:296, 1998.
36. Boberg K, Fausa O, Haaland T, et al: Features of autoimmune hepatitis in primary sclerosing cholangitis: An evaluation of 114 primary sclerosing cholangitis patients according to a scoring system for the diagnosis of autoimmune hepatitis. Hepatology 23:1369, 1996.
37. Mieli-Vergani G, Vergani D: Immunological liver diseases in children. Semin Liver Dis 18:271, 1998.
38. Czaja A, Carpenter H, Santrach P, et al: Autoimmune cholangitis within the spectrum of autoimmune liver disease. Hepatology 31:1231, 2000.
39. Czaja A, Carpenter H, Santrach P, et al: The nature and prognosis of severe cryptogenic chronic active hepatitis. Gastroenterology 104:1755, 1993.
40. Czaja A: Behavior and significance of autoantibodies in type 1 autoimmune hepatitis. J Hepatol 30:394, 1999.
41. Boberg K, Aadland E, Jahnsen J, et al: Incidence and prevalence of primary biliary cirrhosis, primary sclerosing cholangitis, and autoimmune hepatitis in a Norwegian population. Scand J Gastroenterol 33:99, 1998.
42. Jacobson D, Gange S, Rose N, et al: Epidemiology and estimated population burden of selected autoimmune diseases in the United States. Clin Immunol Immunopathol 84:223, 1997.
43. Wiesner R, Demetris A, Belle S, et al: Acute allograft rejection: Incidence, risk factors, and impact on outcome. Hepatology 28:638, 1998.
44. Mackay I: Autoimmune diseases of the liver: Chronic active hepatitis and primary biliary cirrhosis. In Rose N, Mackay I (eds): The Autoimmune Diseases. Orlando, Fla, Academic Press, 1985, p 291.
45. Seki T, Ota M, Furuta S, et al: HLA class II molecules and autoimmune hepatitis susceptibility in Japanese patients. Gastroenterology 103: 1041, 1992.
46. Czaja A: Diagnosis, prognosis, and treatment of classical autoimmune chronic active hepatitis. In Krawitt E, Wiesner R (eds): Autoimmune Liver Disease. New York, Raven Press, 1991, p 143.
47. Schalm S, Korman M, Summerskill W, et al: Severe chronic active liver disease: Prognostic significance of initial morphologic patterns. Am J Dig Dis 22:973, 1977.
48. Park S, Nagorney D, Czaja A: Hepatocellular carcinoma in autoimmune hepatitis. Dig Dis Sci 45:1944, 2000.
49. Czaja A, Rakela J, Hay J, et al: Clinical and prognostic implications of human leukocyte antigen B8 in corticosteroid-treated severe autoimmune chronic active hepatitis. Gastroenterology 98:1587, 1990.
50. Czaja A, Strettell M, Thomson L, et al: Associations between alleles of the major histocompatibility complex and type 1 autoimmune hepatitis. Hepatology 25:317, 1997.
51. Czaja A, Carpenter H, Santrach P, et al: Significance of HLA DR4 in type 1 autoimmune hepatitis. Gastroenterology 105:1502, 1993.
52. Scully L, Toze C, Sengar D, et al: Early-onset autoimmune hepatitis is associated with a C4A gene deletion. Gastroenterology 104:1478, 1993.
53. Doherty D, Underhill J, Donaldson P, et al: Polymorphisms in the human complement C4 genes and genetic susceptibility to autoimmune hepatitis. Autoimmunity 18:243, 1994.
54. Czaja A: Natural history, clinical features, and treatment of autoimmune hepatitis. Semin Liver Dis 4:1, 1984.
55. Roberts S, Therneau T, Czaja A: Prognosis of histologic cirrhosis in type 1 autoimmune hepatitis. Gastroenterology 110:848, 1996.
56. Czaja A, Carpenter H, Santrach P, et al: Genetic predispositions for the immunological features of chronic active hepatitis. Hepatology 18:816, 1993.
57. Czaja A: Drug therapy in the management of type 1 autoimmune hepatitis. Drugs 57:49, 1999.
58. Czaja A, Rakela J, Ludwig J: Features reflective of early prognosis in corticosteroid-treated severe autoimmune chronic active hepatitis. Gastroenterology 95:448, 1988.
59. Czaja A, Beaver S, Shiels M: Sustained remission following corticosteroid therapy of severe HBsAg-negative chronic active hepatitis. Gastroenterology 92:215, 1987.

60. Wang K, Czaja A: Prognosis of corticosteroid-treated hepatitis B surface antigen–negative chronic active hepatitis in postmenopausal women: A retrospective analysis. Gastroenterology 97:1288, 1989.
61. Guanabens N, Pares A, Monegal A, et al: Etidronate versus fluoride for treatment of osteopenia in primary biliary cirrhosis: Preliminary results after 2 years. Gastroenterology 113:219, 1997.
62. Wang K, Czaja A, Beaver S, et al: Extrahepatic malignancy following long-term immunosuppressive therapy of severe hepatitis B surface antigen–negative chronic active hepatitis. Hepatology 10:39, 1989.
63. Czaja A: Low dose corticosteroid therapy after multiple relapses of severe HBsAg–negative chronic active hepatitis. Hepatology 11:1044, 1990.
64. Johnson P, McFarlane I, Williams R: Azathioprine for long-term maintenance of remission in autoimmune hepatitis. N Engl J Med 333:958, 1995.
65. Richardson P, James P, Ryder S: Mycophenolate mofetil for maintenance of remission in autoimmune hepatitis patients resistant to or intolerant of azathioprine. J Hepatol 33:371, 2000.
66. Sanchez-Urdazpal L, Czaja A, van Hoek B, et al: Prognostic features and role of liver transplantation in severe corticosteroid-treated autoimmune chronic active hepatitis. Hepatology 15:215, 1992.
67. Ratziu V, Samuel D, Sebagh M, et al: Long-term follow-up after liver transplantation for autoimmune hepatitis: Evidence of recurrence of primary disease. J Hepatol 30:131, 1999.
68. Czaja A, Carpenter H, Lindor K: Ursodeoxycholic acid as adjunctive therapy for problematic type 1 autoimmune hepatitis: A randomized placebo-controlled treatment trial. Hepatology 30:1381, 1999.
69. Czaja A, Lindor K: Failure of budesonide in a pilot study of treatment-dependent autoimmune hepatitis. Gastroenterology 119:1312, 2000.
70. Czaja A, Manns M, McFarlane I, et al: Autoimmune hepatitis: The investigational and clinical challenges. Hepatology 31:1194, 2000.

Chapter 76

PRIMARY BILIARY CIRRHOSIS

Paul Angulo and Keith D. Lindor

Primary biliary cirrhosis (PBC) is an autoimmune liver disease that generally affects middle-aged women and is the most common chronic cholestatic liver disease in adults in the United States. PBC is characterized by ongoing inflammatory destruction of the interlobular and septal bile ducts that leads to chronic cholestasis and biliary cirrhosis, with consequent complications such as portal hypertension and liver failure. Although the designation *primary biliary cirrhosis* has been used for several decades, the term is potentially misleading because in most affected patients cirrhosis is not found on liver biopsy at the time of diagnosis. Evidence for an immunologic cause of PBC includes immunohistochemical data showing the presence of activated T cells in areas of bile duct destruction, the presence of highly specific autoantibodies reactive with antigens on the surface of biliary epithelial cells, and the association of PBC with other disorders thought to be autoimmune in nature. PBC may be discovered incidentally on routine blood testing but also can present with pruritus or fatigue. The diagnosis should be considered in the setting of elevated serum alkaline phosphatase, cholesterol, and immunoglobulin M (IgM) levels. The presence of antimitochondrial antibody in serum is highly characteristic of the disease. Ursodeoxycholic acid (UDCA) is the only medication of proven benefit for patients with PBC; liver transplantation represents a life extending alternative for patients who have end-stage PBC. It also is important to recognize and treat the complications of chronic cholestasis, such as osteopenic bone disease, fat-soluble vitamin deficiency, hypercholesterolemia, and steatorrhea. Survival models are used in determining the prognosis of the disease as well as the timing of liver transplantation.

EPIDEMIOLOGY

PBC occurs worldwide and predominantly in women with a female-to-male ratio of 9:1. The median age of onset is approximately 50 years, with a range of 21 to 91 years. PBC has not been documented in children or adolescents. The true prevalence and incidence of PBC are unclear. Until the early 1970s, PBC was considered to be rare and thought to present with persistent jaundice, with almost inevitable progression to end-stage liver disease. A better understanding of the pathogenesis of PBC since the 1980s along with recent clinical and epidemiologic studies have modified our concepts about this condition. As a result of increasing awareness of the disease and identification of asymptomatic patients through the widespread use of screening tests, such as serum cholesterol levels and liver biochemical tests, PBC now appears to be more common than was previously believed.

The highest incidence and prevalence of PBC have been reported in northern Europe.[1] Prevalence rates reported from various countries are quite variable, ranging from 19 cases per million in Australia[2] to 240 cases per million in northeastern England.[1] Inconsistency in case definition and case finding methods as well as imprecision in defining the study area, the populations evaluated, and the dates of diagnosis, make comparisons of studies difficult. Estimates of annual incidence range from 2 to 22 per million.[1, 3] The prevalence of PBC seems to have increased over time: 18 cases per million were reported in 1976[4] and 240 cases per million in 1994.[1] Without a clear increase in the incidence rate, however, the increase in prevalence may reflect an increase in survival in PBC patients.

Only one study has reported age adjusted incidence and prevalence rate of PBC in the United States:[5] 45 and 654 per million, respectively, for women and 7 and 121, respectively, for men (27 and 402, respectively, overall).

The occurrence of PBC in relatives and the detection of abnormalities of cell-mediated immunity in first-degree relatives of affected patients suggest a genetic association. Although no significant link between PBC and human leukocyte antigen (HLA) class I phenotypes has been found, class

II HLA phenotypes may contribute to the development of PBC. An association with HLA-DR8 is most frequently observed; however, that association is found in only about one third of cases.[6] Conversely, the DQA1*0102 haplotype seems to be strongly associated with resistance to the disease.[7] HLA class III antigens whose genes code for complement components C2 and C4 and factor B have been studied less extensively; an increased frequency of haplotype C4B2 has been reported. An excess frequency of haplotype C4A*Q0 also has been found to be associated with PBC with a significant relative risk (*RR* = 184).[8]

PATHOGENESIS

Although the cause of PBC is unknown, available evidence suggests that an autoimmune process underlies the pathogenesis of this condition. Autoimmunity is suggested by the presence of highly specific antimitochondrial antibodies (AMA), a frequent association with other autoimmune diseases, involvement of T cells in the destruction of the bile ducts, and numerous defects in immunologic regulation. The disease seems to be triggered by an immune-mediated response to allo- or autoantigen(s), which leads to progressive destruction of bile ducts, chronic cholestasis, and eventual development of biliary cirrhosis. Immunohistochemical phenotyping of inflammatory cells surrounding the bile ducts of patients with PBC shows a combination of CD4+ and CD8+ T cells. There is abundant evidence that bile duct destruction is induced directly by the cytotoxicity of CD4+ and CD8+ T cells in contact with biliary epithelium. B lymphocytes are relatively uncommon in the inflammatory reaction, although they are sometimes present in clusters. Intracellular adhesion molecules (ICAMs) (e.g., ICAM-1) are strongly expressed on many biliary epithelial cells, particularly in areas of lymphocyte damage[9]; these molecules may facilitate the interaction of destructive lymphocytes and their targets.

Autoantibodies in Primary Biliary Cirrhosis

Much attention has been devoted recently to the humoral immune system, in particular the identification of the antigens recognized by AMAs.[10–12] These autoantibodies have been shown to be directed against the E2 component of the pyruvate dehydrogenase complex (PDC-E2), the E2 unit of the branched-chain 2-oxo-acid dehydrogenase complex (BCOADC-E2), and the E2 subunit of the 2-oxo-glutarate dehydrogenase complex (OGDC-E2), as well as the E1 subunit of PDC and protein X. These enzymes all are located on the inner mitochondrial membranes. At least one of these components usually reacts with AMA in patients with PBC. The most frequent antigen against which AMAs are directed is PDC-E2; PDC-E2 reacting antibodies are present in more than 90% of PBC patients. The mechanisms by which AMAs develop against proteins located on the inner surface of mitochondrial membranes are unknown. In patients with PBC PDC-E2 or a cross-reacting molecule is overexpressed on biliary epithelial cells, predominantly in the luminal domain, and PDC-E2–specific CD4+ T cells are present in portal inflammatory infiltrates.[10] Although AMAs are predominantly of the IgG1 and IgG3 classes, a characteristic feature of PBC is an elevation in serum levels of IgM, perhaps caused by faulty switching from IgM to IgG synthesis after exposure to an unknown antigen or defective suppressor T cell activity. It is uncertain, however, why the lesions in PBC are confined to the small intrahepatic bile ducts, whereas the antigens on the inner mitochondrial membrane are found in all tissues of the body. These antigens appear to share a common epitope with antigens in the cytoplasmic region of bile duct epithelial cells in patients with PBC.[13, 14] AMA-negative PBC patients have immunoreactive material on the damaged bile ducts similar to that in AMA-positive PBC patients.[15] The main targets of the immune reactions in PBC are the epithelial cells of the interlobular bile ducts. Although most patients with PBC have AMAs, these autoantibodies do not appear to be cytotoxic: the AMAs persist after liver transplantation without evidence of disease recurrence; disease severity is unrelated to the titer of AMA; AMAs do not always occur in PBC; and AMAs develop in animal models after the injection of recombinant PDC-E2 protein but are not accompanied by bile duct destruction or inflammation.

AMAs are not the only PBC-specific autoantibodies. Antibodies against the nuclear pore protein gp210, a transmembrane glycoprotein, are found in 25% of patients who have AMA-positive PBC and in up to 50% of those who have AMA-negative PBC. Their specificity for PBC when detected by immunoblotting is above 99%,[16] and they seem to have prognostic importance.[17] Antibodies against p62, a nuclear pore glycoprotein, are found in about 25% of patients with PBC[18] and are highly specific for PBC. Anti-p62 antibodies and anti-gp210 antibodies appear to be mutually exclusive in PBC patients.

Complement System in Primary Biliary Cirrhosis

The complement system is chronically activated in patients with PBC. Serum concentrations of several complement components are increased. Some patients have circulating immune complexes that result from either increased production or defective clearance by the reticuloendothelial system. These immune complexes may contain antigens that are partially identical to or cross-reacting with epithelial antigens of bile ducts or mitochondria.[19] A C4 abnormality found in patients with PBC[8, 20] may contribute to deposition of immune complexes or to defective viral clearance, thereby leading to chronic infection and possibly triggering autoimmunity. Suppressor T cell activity is abnormal in patients with PBC,[21] and in a substantial proportion of their healthy first-degree relatives. This abnormality may be responsible for the increased number of circulating B cells capable of producing AMA spontaneously in vitro.[21, 22]

Other Incriminated Agents

Infectious agents, such as bacteria, yeast antigens, and viruses, have been incriminated in triggering the immune response in PBC. Defective sulfoxidation of certain compounds, such as bile acids, estrogen, or drugs, and selenium deficiency have also been proposed as underlying mechanisms leading to the development of PBC. However, all these hypotheses are far from established.[23]

CLINICAL FEATURES

Asymptomatic Disease

Widespread use of screening laboratory tests has led to an increase in the frequency of diagnosing PBC at an asymptomatic stage. In up to 25% of patients, a diagnosis of PBC is made when an asymptomatic person is found to have an elevated serum alkaline phosphatase level and AMA during routine health evaluations or investigation of an unrelated symptom, including autoimmune diseases known to be associated with PBC. Most asymptomatic individuals who have AMA but normal liver biochemical findings have features consistent with PBC on liver biopsy and eventually have typical symptoms and cholestasis.[24, 25]

Symptomatic Disease

The patient with PBC is usually a middle-aged woman who reports fatigue or pruritus. Other symptoms include right upper quadrant abdominal pain, anorexia, and jaundice (Table 76–1). Fatigue, although relatively nonspecific in PBC, is the most common symptom and is found in about two thirds of patients; it generally becomes worse as PBC progresses. Pruritus may occur at any point in the course of the disease. Generally, pruritus is intermittent during the day and most troublesome in the evening and at night. Often, pruritus resolves as the disease progresses, but in some patients severe intractable pruritus develops in earlier stages of the disease and may be an indication for liver transplantation. Most patients with PBC do not have jaundice at the time of diagnosis. Jaundice occurs later in the course of the disease and is usually persistent and associated with a poor prognosis. Symptoms also may be related to fat-soluble vitamin deficiency, bone pain with or without spontaneous fractures, or an associated autoimmune disease (Table 76–2). Symptoms of advanced liver disease, such as ascites, bleeding from gastroesophageal varices, and encephalopathy, usually occur late in the course of PBC. On physical examination the most common findings are hyperpigmentation, hepatosplenomegaly, xanthelasma, and, in more advanced disease, jaundice and signs of portal hypertension.

A minority of patients are men. Symptoms and autoimmune manifestations, especially Sjögren's syndrome, appear to be less frequent in men than in women. Otherwise, the disease is clinically identical in men and women.

Table 76–1 | **Symptoms and Signs of Primary Biliary Cirrhosis at Presentation**

FINDING	FREQUENCY, %
Fatigue	70
Pruritus	55
Jaundice	10
Hyperpigmentation	25
Hepatomegaly	25
Splenomegaly	15
Xanthelasma	10
None	25

Table 76–2 | **Diseases Associated with Primary Biliary Cirrhosis**

DISEASE	FREQUENCY, %
Keratoconjunctivitis sicca	72–100
Arthritis/arthropathy	4–42
Scleroderma and variants	15–20
Scleroderma	3–4
CREST or any of its components	7
Raynaud's disease	8
Autoimmune thyroiditis	15–20
Cutaneous disorders (lichen planus, discoid lupus, pemphigoid)	11
Renal tubular acidosis (proximal or distal)	50–60
Gallstones	33
Hepatocellular cancer	1–2
Pulmonary fibrosis	Rare
Celiac sprue	Rare

CREST, calcinosis, Raynaud's phenomenon, esophageal dysmotility, sclerodactyly, telangiectases.

Associated Diseases

Many of the diseases found frequently in patients with PBC are thought to be related to disturbances in immune mechanisms (see Table 2). These include Sjögren's syndrome, characterized by dry eyes (keratoconjunctivitis sicca) and dry mouth; scleroderma and its variants; rheumatoid arthritis; some cutaneous disorders; renal tubular acidosis; and thyroiditis. The cause of renal tubular acidosis is unclear, but it may relate to excess copper deposition within the kidney, as in Wilson disease, or to an undefined autoimmune process.

There is an increase in the incidence of malignancy in patients with PBC. An increased risk of breast cancer in women with PBC was found in studies from 1984 and 1985[26, 27] but was not confirmed by larger studies in 1994 and 1999.[28, 29] Although hepatocellular carcinoma is uncommon, occurring in 1% to 2% of patients, patients with PBC have a substantially higher risk of hepatocellular carcinoma than the general population.[28] Gallstones can be found in up to one third of patients with PBC, but other associated disorders, such as inflammatory bowel disease and interstitial pulmonary fibrosis, are rare.

DIAGNOSIS

The diagnosis of PBC is established by biochemical test results that are consistent with cholestasis, presence of serum AMA by indirect immunofluorescence or immunoblotting techniques, and compatible or diagnostic histologic features.

Biochemical Changes

Liver biochemical tests show a cholestatic picture. Almost all patients have increased serum levels of alkaline phosphatase (three to four times normal) and gamma-glutamyl transpeptidase. Serum aspartate aminotransferase (AST) and alanine aminotransferase (ALT) levels are mildly elevated

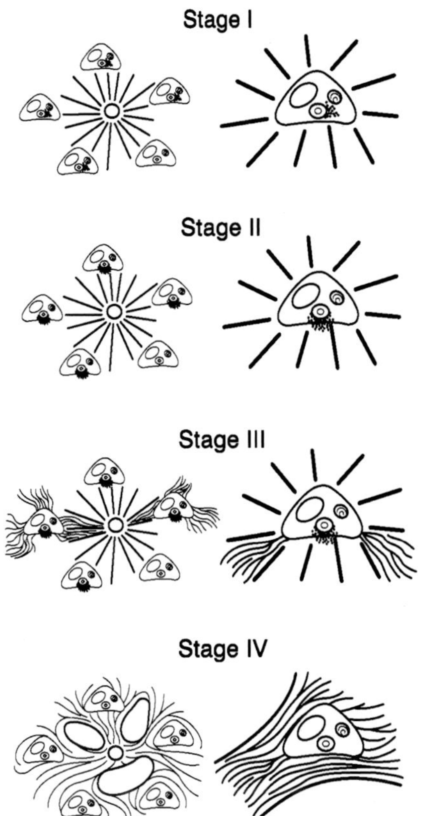

Figure 76–1. Schematic representation of the staging system of primary biliary cirrhosis (Ludwig's classification). Stage I is inflammation within the portal space, focused on the bile duct. Stage II is inflammation extending into the hepatic parenchyma (interface hepatitis or piecemeal necrosis). Stage III is fibrosis, and stage IV is cirrhosis with regenerative nodules.

(usually less than three times normal); marked elevations (more than five times normal) are distinctly unusual and may suggest a PBC–autoimmune hepatitis overlap syndrome or coexisting viral hepatitis.[30] Serum bilirubin levels are usually normal in the early stages of PBC, increase slowly over the course of the disease, and may reach levels exceeding 20 mg/dL. A high serum bilirubin level, low serum albumin level, and prolonged prothrombin time all suggest a poor prognosis for advanced disease. Levels of serum immunoglobulins, especially IgM levels, serum bile acid levels, in particular cholic and chenodeoxycholic acid levels, and serum cholesterol levels are all increased.

Serologic Diagnosis

AMAs are present in serum in approximately 90% to 95% of patients with PBC. The M2 antibody, which is directed against the pyruvate dehydrogenase complex of the inner mitochondrial membrane, has a sensitivity rate of 98% and specificity rate of 96% for the diagnosis of PBC. Other autoantibodies found in patients with PBC are rheumatoid factor (70%), anti–smooth muscle antibody (66%), antithyroid (antimicrosomal, antithyroglobulin) antibody (41%), and antinuclear antibody (35%).

Liver Histologic Features

Liver biopsy has been considered necessary for the final diagnosis of PBC and exclusion of other liver diseases. The initial lesion on liver biopsy specimens is damage to epithelial cells of the small bile ducts (Fig. 76–1). The most important and only diagnostic clue in many cases is *ductopenia,* defined as the absence of interlobular bile ducts in more than 50% of portal tracts. The florid duct lesion, in which the epithelium of the interlobular and segmental bile ducts degenerates segmentally, with the formation of poorly defined, noncaseating epithelioid granulomas, is nearly diagnostic of PBC but is found in a relatively small number of cases, mainly in the early stages. The two most popular histologic staging systems are those of Ludwig and associates[31] and of Scheuer,[32] which classify PBC into four stages. Both systems describe progressive pathologic changes, initially in the portal areas surrounding the bile ducts, with eventual progression to cirrhosis.

In stage 1 of Ludwig's classification, there is inflammatory destruction of the intrahepatic septal and interlobular bile ducts that have a diameter of up to 100 μm. Often these lesions are focal and are described as florid duct lesions characterized by marked inflammation and necrosis around the bile ducts. The portal tracts usually are expanded by lymphocytes and only sparse neutrophils or eosinophils are seen. In stage 2 disease, the inflammation extends from the portal tract into the hepatic parenchyma, a lesion called *interface hepatitis* or *piecemeal hepatitis* (formerly *piecemeal necrosis*). Destruction of bile ducts with proliferation of bile ductules can be seen. In stage 3 disease lymphocytic involvement of the portal and periportal areas as well as the hepatic parenchyma can be seen; this stage is characterized by extensive fibrosis without regenerative nodules. Stage 4 disease is marked by cirrhosis with fibrous septa and regenerative nodules.

The rate of histologic progression in PBC has been described, using the data from 916 liver biopsy procedures performed in 222 PBC patients over 779 patient-years of follow-up.[33] In this series, most patients had histologic progression; only a few had prolonged histologic stability; and sustained regression was rare. A time course Markov model was used to describe the rate of histologic progression over time (Table 76–3).

Imaging Studies

Cross-sectional imaging with ultrasonography, computed tomography, or, less frequently, magnetic resonance imaging is

Table 76–3 | **Time Course of Histologic Progression in Precirrhotic Patients with Primary Biliary Cirrhosis**

	INITIAL HISTOLOGIC STAGE		
RATE OF PROGRESSION	1	2	3
1 Year	41%	43%	35%
2 Years	62%	62%	50%

From Locke RG III, Therneau TM, Ludwig J, et al: Time course of histological progression in primary biliary cirrhosis. Hepatology 23:52, 1996.

useful to exclude biliary obstruction. Other than indicating increased liver echogenicity and signs consistent with parenchymal liver disease or portal hypertension, findings of cross-sectional imaging are usually unremarkable. A number of patients may have adenopathy in the hilar area.[34] Adenopathy, noted in about 24% of PBC patients, is not progressive; it is important that adenopathy be recognized to prevent confusion or undue concern about the presence of an underlying malignancy. Large, bulky adenopathy, however, should raise the question of associated malignancy, such as lymphoma or, less often, metastatic adenocarcinoma.

NATURAL HISTORY

The natural history of PBC has been described in patients who have symptoms attributable to PBC and in asymptomatic patients who have normal or abnormal liver biochemical test results.[35] Prognostic models useful in predicting survival in individual patients have been developed.

Asymptomatic Primary Biliary Cirrhosis

In 1986, Mitchison and colleagues[36] reported on 29 patients who had AMA in serum (titer ≥1 : 40), normal liver biochemical findings, and no symptoms of liver disease. Liver histologic features were compatible with or diagnostic of PBC in 24 patients (83%) and normal in only 2 patients. The entire cohort of patients was followed for a median of 17.8 years (range 11 to 24 years).[36] Persistently abnormal liver biochemical test results developed in 24 patients (83%), and in 22 patients (76%) persistent symptoms attributable to PBC, including fatigue, pruritus, and right upper abdominal discomfort, developed. Five patients died, none as a result of liver disease, after a median of 11.7 years (range 6.4 to 16.8 years) after the first positive AMA result. The median time from first positive AMA test result to persistently abnormal liver biochemical findings was 5.6 years (range 0.9 to 19 years). Four of ten patients who had a second liver biopsy during a median follow-up of 11.4 years (range 1.3 to 14.3 years) showed progression of histologic stage, but in none of the patients in this cohort did cirrhosis or portal hypertension develop during the follow-up period. This study shows clearly that asymptomatic patients who have AMA but normal liver biochemical test results have very early PBC, which may over time develop into clinically obvious PBC. These patients may represent a subgroup of patients with PBC in whom the natural history may be different from that of the general PBC patient population.

Several reports have described the natural history of asymptomatic patients who are AMA-positive and have abnormal liver biochemical findings consistent with cholestasis and liver histologic findings diagnostic of or compatible with PBC. The patients who are asymptomatic at their initial medical consultation survive longer than those with symptoms, but most eventually have progressive disease. Patients who remain asymptomatic for several years may have a significantly longer survival rate than symptomatic patients, but their life expectancy is still less than that of age- and gender-matched healthy control subjects. Symptoms of PBC develop in approximately 40% of initially asymptomatic patients in 5 to 7 years of follow-up. Once symptoms develop, life expectancy falls significantly and is the same as that for other symptomatic patients, with a median survival time of approximately 10 years.[35–37] Unfortunately, there is no way to predict in which asymptomatic patients symptoms of PBC will develop; nevertheless, patients who have normal serum bilirubin levels and histologic stage 1 disease may have a better long-term prognosis than patients who have more severe liver disease at the time of diagnosis.

Symptomatic Primary Biliary Cirrhosis

Compared with asymptomatic patients, patients who have symptoms of chronic cholestasis progress more rapidly to end-stage liver disease and associated complications and a worse prognosis. The several independent predictors of a poor prognosis identified in this group include advanced age, high serum bilirubin level, poor synthetic function, hepatomegaly, fluid retention (edema, ascites), variceal bleeding, and advanced histologic stage (Table 76–4).[37–42]

Most patients who have PBC and portal hypertension have cirrhosis on liver biopsy. However, portal hypertension can be found in some patients who have findings of moderate to severe inflammation without cirrhosis on liver biopsy. The development of esophageal varices is an ominous sign that occurs in about one third of patients with PBC during extended follow-up. About 40% of these patients experience one or more episodes of variceal bleeding within 3 years of development of varices; variceal bleeding may be associated with a decreased survival rate.[43]

Prediction of Survival in Patients with Primary Biliary Cirrhosis

When untreated, PBC may follow a course that extends over a 15- to 20-year period. However, in patients who have

Table 76–4 | **Independent Predictors of Survival in Patients with Primary Biliary Cirrhosis in Six Studies**

YALE (38)*	EUROPEAN (42)	MAYO (37)	OSLO (39)	GLASGOW (40)	AUSTRALIA (41)
Age Bilirubin level Hepatomegaly Fibrosis Cirrhosis	Age Bilirubin level Albumin level Cirrhosis Cholestasis	Age Bilirubin level Albumin level Prothrombin time Edema	Variceal bleeding Bilirubin level	Age Bilirubin level Ascites Variceal bleeding Fibrosis Cholestasis Mallory's bodies	Age Bilirubin level Albumin level

*Reference number.

Table 76–5 | **Prognostic Models in Primary Biliary Cirrhosis**

AUTHOR (REFERENCE)	PREDICTIVE VARIABLE	FORMULA (IF USED)	EXTRAMURAL VALIDATION
Dickson et al. (37)	Age Total bilirubin level Serum albumin level Prothrombin time Edema score	$R = 0.871 \log_e$ (bilirubin, mg/dL) − $2.53 \log_e$ (albumin, g/dL) +0.039 (age in years) + $2.38 \log_e$ (prothrombin time, sec) +0.859 edema	Yes
Rydning et al. (39)	Bleeding varices Bilirubin level	$\log_e R = 1.68$ (bleeding − 0.25) + $2.03 \log_e$ (bilirubin − 30.3)	No
Christensen et al. (42)	Bilirubin level Ascites Albumin level Age Gastrointestinal bleeding Central cholestasis Cirrhosis IgM level	Calculated from pocket chart and tables in reference 42	Yes

IgM, immunoglobulin M.

serum bilirubin levels greater than 10 mg/dL, the average life expectancy is reduced to 2 years. In order to predict survival in patients with PBC, prognostic models, some of which rely on Cox's proportional hazard analysis, have been reported[37, 39, 42] (Table 76–5). Of these models, the Mayo risk score,[34, 44] based on the patient's age, serum bilirubin level, serum albumin level, prothrombin time, and presence of edema, has been cross-validated and widely used in predicting survival and guiding physicians in referring patients for liver transplantation. These prognostic models also can be used to monitor the effect of experimental drugs in clinical trials. Although the models undoubtedly assist in the clinical decision-making process, they should not replace the clinician's judgment in determining the optimal time for liver transplantation for an individual patient.

MEDICAL TREATMENT

A large number of controlled and uncontrolled trials evaluating drugs with different properties in the treatment of PBC have been published. These drugs can be separated according to their mechanisms of action as immunosuppressive, anti-inflammatory, cupruretic, or antifibrotic or as bile acids.[45]

GLUCOCORTICOIDS. Although reports in the early 1950s described the beneficial clinical and biochemical effects of glucocorticoids, only one placebo controlled trial has been conducted.[46] For 36 patients who received prednisolone, after one year of treatment clinical and biochemical test result improvement as well as a reduction in inflammation on liver biopsy specimens were noted. The study was continued in a single-blind manner for a further 2 years, and the mortality rate was similar in both groups. Worsening osteopenic bone disease is the main concern in using glucocorticoids in the treatment of PBC, and these drugs cannot be recommended currently outside the context of prospective trials.

BUDESONIDE. Budesonide is a new glucocorticoid that is structurally related to 16-α hydroxyprednisolone. Budesonide undergoes extensive first-past hepatic metabolism and has minimal systemic availability; in theory, it shoud be devoid of glucocorticoid-associated systemic effects. Budesonide was evaluated in combination with UDCA in studies in 1999 and 2000.[47, 48] In previously untreated patients with PBC, treatment with a combination of budesonide and UDCA led to a greater improvement of serum alkaline phosphatase, AST, and Ig levels as well as greater improvement in the degree of inflammation and fibrosis on liver biopsy specimens than UDCA alone.[47] Unfortunately, the effect of such a combination on serum bilirubin levels and the Mayo risk score was not reported, and the effect of budesonide on these important prognostic markers remains uncertain. In the second study,[48] the combination of budesonide and UDCA did not benefit patients who had responded incompletely to UDCA alone administered for a number of years. In that study[48] the combination of UDCA and budesonide did not improve serum bilirubin levels or the Mayo risk score but led to significant worsening of osteoporosis and cosmetic side effects, particularly in patients who had more advanced liver disease.

D-PENICILLAMINE. Increased hepatic copper concentrations in patients with PBC prompted assessment of the potential benefit of D-penicillamine. Eight controlled trials of more than 700 patients have been reported.[45] D-Penicillamine was associated with a modest and transitory improvement in liver biochemical findings in some studies, but had no effect on survival. Furthermore, serious side effects developed in approximately one fifth of patients. Therefore, D-penicillamine is not used in the treatment of PBC.

COLCHICINE. Colchicine has anti-inflammatory and antifibrotic effects. Three placebo controlled trials involving a total of 181 patients have been reported.[45] Colchicine was associated with some improvement in liver biochemical findings, but had no effects on symptoms related to cholestasis, histologic progression to cirrhosis, or the overall survival rate.[49] The minimal toxicity of colchicine has led some physicians to recommend its use in PBC; however, on the basis of an analysis of these studies, colchicine does not seem to benefit patients with PBC.

AZATHIOPRINE. Azathioprine, which is currently used to prevent allograft rejection, was evaluated in a large international study involving 248 patients with PBC.[50] After the first 18 months of follow-up, no significant benefit was noted on the clinical course, liver biochemical test results, liver histologic findings, or survival rate.[50] With extended follow-up, and after adjustment for a slight imbalance in mean serum bilirubin levels between the two study groups, a statistical improvement in the survival rate was shown with azathioprine.[42] Because of uncertainty about the conclusions of this trial, in light of the large number of withdrawals, missing data, and initially reported negative results, azathioprine is rarely used in patients with PBC.

CHLORAMBUCIL. Chlorambucil was evaluated in a small controlled trial involving 24 patients with a mean follow-up period of 4.1 years.[51] Although liver biochemical test results and inflammation on liver biopsy specimens improved, no effect on the histologic stage of disease was noted, and the study was too small to allow evaluation of any benefit in survival. One third of patients experienced bone marrow toxicity, necessitating discontinuation of the drug and making chlorambucil an unattractive drug for further evaluation; therefore, chlorambucil cannot be recommended for routine use in PBC.

CYCLOSPORINE. Cyclosporine has proved effective in preventing immune-mediated rejection of transplanted human allografts. A large European study of 349 PBC patients with a follow-up of up to 6 years (mean 2.5), with death or liver transplantation as the main end points, showed biochemical test improvement but no effect on histologic progression or survival.[52] A multivariate analysis suggested a reduction in the mortality rate for patients treated with cyclosporine. However, the use of this drug is associated with a high incidence of side effects, such as hypertension and renal dysfunction, which largely preclude long-term use of cyclosporine in PBC.

METHOTREXATE. Anecdotal reports of clinical, biochemical, and histologic improvement in patients with PBC treated with methotrexate have been reported.[53] However, only one placebo-controlled trial of methotrexate had been conducted up to 1999.[54] In this study, methotrexate in a dose of 7.5 mg/week given for up to 6 years was not only not beneficial, but also associated with more unfavorable outcomes than placebo.

URSODEOXYCHOLIC ACID. UDCA, the 7-ß epimer of chenodeoxycholic acid, is the drug that has been most widely evaluated in the treatment of PBC. UDCA occurs naturally in small quantities in human bile (less than 4% of total bile acids). Introduced for the dissolution of radiolucent gallstones in the 1970s, UDCA is the only medication approved by the United States Food and Drug Administration for the treatment of PBC. Several mechanisms for the protective actions of UDCA have been proposed, including inhibition of the intestinal absorption of toxic, hydrophobic, endogenous bile salts; stabilization of hepatocyte membranes against toxic bile salts; replacement of endogenous bile acids, some of which may be hepatotoxic, by UDCA, which is not hepatotoxic; and reduction of the expression of major histocompatibility (MHC) class I and class II antigens on the biliary epithelium. During therapy with UDCA, there is a variable increase in total serum bile acids levels. The proportion of UDCA in serum and bile increases to about 30% to 60% of the total bile acids,[55–58] and the proportion of endogenous bile acids, such as cholic, chenodeoxycholic, deoxycholic, and lithocholic acids, decline consequently. The degree of enrichment of the bile acid pool with UDCA is similar in all histologic stages of PBC,[59] and there is a correlation between the degree of enrichment and improvement in both liver biochemical test results and the Mayo risk score.[59, 60]

Because of its safety and a high rate of patient compliance, UDCA is the drug that has received most attention for treatment of PBC. Treatment of patients with UDCA leads to a rapid improvement in results of liver biochemical tests.[55–59, 61] Improvement in several histologic features, such as interface hepatitis, inflammation, cholestasis, bile duct paucity, and bile duct proliferation, occurs after 2 years of therapy with UDCA.[56–58, 61, 62] The drug also decreases the risk of gastroesophageal varices[63] and delays progression to cirrhosis.[64] The therapeutic benefit of UDCA in PBC was questioned in 1999 in a meta-analysis of therapeutic trials of UDCA in PBC.[65] However, the meta-analysis suffered from serious methodologic flaws, primarily mixing of different patient populations, some of whom had been treated with suboptimal doses of UDCA for too short a period to demonstrate an effect.[66] When an effective dose of UDCA (13 to 15 mg/kg/day) has been used and an appropriate number of patients treated for an appropriate period, UDCA has clearly been shown to improve the duration of survival free of liver transplantation,[67–69] as shown in Figure 76–2.

During UDCA therapy, there is a significant decrease in the Mayo risk score, a cross-validated index of survival in PBC[55–58]; with UDCA therapy, the Mayo risk score retains its validity in predicting survival, as it does when applied to untreated patients.[70] The most cost-effective dose of UDCA in PBC is 13 to 15 mg/kg/day,[59] which can be divided into three or four doses given with meals. In patients who are also prescribed cholestyramine, UDCA should be taken at least 2 hours before or after the cholestyramine to ensure optimal intestinal absorption.

COMBINATION THERAPY. The use of combinations of drugs with different properties and some efficacy in PBC has been evaluated in open and controlled trials.[45] These combinations include UDCA and methotrexate, UDCA and colchicine, cyclosporine and prednisone, chlorambucil and prednisolone, UDCA and glucocorticoid, UDCA and budesonide, UDCA and sulindac, and UDCA, prednisone, and azathioprine. Although some short-term improvement in liver biochemical test results has been reported for several of these combinations, the small number of patients enrolled, the short period of follow-up, and the potential for drug-related side effects do not allow recommendation of any of these combinations for the treatment of PBC. Furthermore, no combination of drugs seems to be more effective than UDCA alone.

COMPLICATIONS OF CHRONIC CHOLESTASIS AND THEIR MANAGEMENT

Bone Disease

Osteopenic bone disease, with its predisposition to spontaneous fractures, is a common complication of chronic chole-

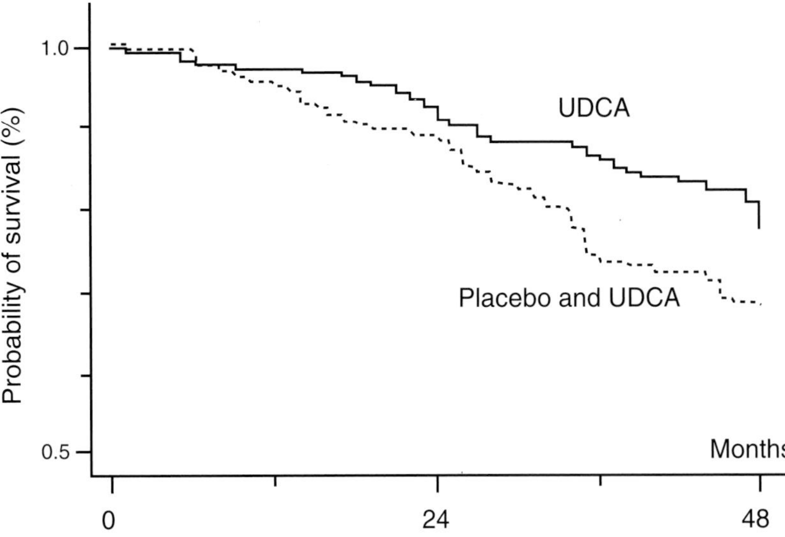

Figure 76–2. Survival in 548 patients with PBC. The probability of survival free of liver transplantation was significantly greater in patients treated for 4 years with ursodeoxycholic acid (UDCA) than in those who first received placebo and then UDCA ($P < 0.001$; relative risk, 1.92; 95% confidence interval, 1.30–2.82). (Adapted from Poupon R, Lindor KD, Cauch-Dudek K, et al: Combined analysis of French, American and Canadian randomized controlled trials of ursodeoxycholic acid therapy in primary biliary cirrhosis. Gastroenterology 113:884–890, 1997.)

static liver disease.[71] In North America, most patients who have osteopenia as a result of cholestasis have underlying osteoporosis rather than osteomalacia. *Osteoporosis* is defined as defective bone formation, whereas *osteomalacia* is defective bone mineralization caused by vitamin D deficiency. The cause of osteoporosis associated with PBC is poorly understood but seems to be related to the cholestasis itself. Women who have PBC lose bone mass at a rate approximately twice that of age-matched controls,[72] and this accelerated bone loss is the result of decreased formation rather than increased resorption of bone.[73] The severity and progression of bone disease can be assessed by measurement of bone mineral density in different sites, in particular the lumbar spine and femur. Dual-energy radiographic absorptiometry and dual-photon absorptiometry are noninvasive techniques that provide excellent quantification of bone mass. Approximately 20% of patients with PBC have osteoporosis, as defined by a T-score below −2.5 for either the lumbar spine or the femoral neck, at the time of referral for or diagnosis of the liver disease; approximately 10% of patients have severe bone disease as defined by a Z-score below −2.[74, 75] The risk of osteoporosis (T-score below −2.5) in patients with PBC is more than eight times that of a healthy gender-matched population, whereas the risk of severe bone disease (Z-score below −2) is more than four times that of a healthy gender- and age-matched population.[75] In patients with PBC, as in the general population, older age, postmenopausal status, and a lower body mass index are independent risk factors for the development of osteoporosis. In patients with PBC, however, the severity of osteoporosis increases as liver disease advances; in patients who have stage 1 or 2 PBC, bone mass is similar to that of a normal age- and gender-matched population, whereas bone mass is significantly lower in patients who have stage 3 or 4 PBC. Fifty percent of patients with PBC who undergo liver transplantation have severe bone disease, and pathologic fractures occur in one half of patients with PBC during the first months after liver transplantation, almost exclusively in those who already are osteopenic at the time of transplantation.[76] Higher serum bilirubin levels contribute significantly to a higher rate of bone loss.[75]

Treatment of bone disease in patients with PBC usually includes adequate exercise and supplemental calcium and vitamin D (25,000 to 50,000 IU orally once or twice per week). Estrogens are useful for postmenopausal osteoporosis; in two small series, estrogens were suggested to benefit PBC patients.[77, 78] However, estrogens should be used cautiously by patients with PBC because of their potential to cause cholestasis, induce menstruation, and possibly cause cancer. Raloxifene, a selective estrogen receptor modulator, is a promising alternative to estrogen replacement therapy for postmenopausal osteoporosis and is currently under evaluation in patients with PBC. Bisphosphonates also may hold promise for the treatment of osteoporosis in patients with PBC; conflicting results have been reported for etidronate,[79, 80] but further studies of residronate, alendronate, and palmidronate are warranted.

Fat-Soluble Vitamin Deficiency

Most patients with PBC who have fat-soluble vitamin deficiency have advanced liver disease with jaundice. Fat-soluble vitamin deficiency is almost always caused by malabsorption that results from a decreased amount of bile salts in the intestinal lumen. Vitamin D deficiency should be excluded in patients with PBC. When deficiency is encountered, 25,000 to 50,000 IU of oral vitamin D given once or twice per week usually is sufficient to achieve a normal serum vitamin D level. Because 25-hydroxylation of vitamin D is reported in patients with PBC, vitamin D, rather than the more expensive 25-hydroxy vitamin D or 1,25-hydroxy vitamin D, can be used.

Vitamin A deficiency, which may cause blindness, may occur in patients with PBC. When blood levels of vitamin A are low, replacement therapy with 25,000 to 50,000 IU orally two to three times per week should be instituted, usually beginning at lower levels and assessing the adequacy of replacement by repeated serum assays and evaluation of dark adaptation if indicated.

Vitamin K deficiency also occurs in patients who have severe cholestasis and is manifested by an increased prothrombin time. A trial of vitamin K (5 to 10 mg orally) should be given to determine whether the prothrombin time improves. If the prothrombin time improves, patients should be maintained on oral water-soluble vitamin K 5 mg/day.

Deficiency of vitamin E has been reported in a few patients with PBC. Typically, vitamin E deficiency causes a neurologic abnormality that primarily affects the posterior columns and is characterized by areflexia or loss of proprioception and ataxia. Despite the disappointing response to vitamin E replacement, patients who have chronic cholestasis and low levels of serum vitamin E should have replacement therapy, usually 50 to 200 U orally per day for 2 weeks.

Hypercholesterolemia and Hyperlipidemia

Lipid abnormalities are found in up to 85% of patients with PBC. High-density lipoprotein cholesterol levels usually are most prominently elevated in the early stages of PBC; however, as the disease progresses, the high-density lipoprotein cholesterol levels decrease, and low-density lipoprotein levels increase. There appears to be no increased risk of atherosclerosis in patients who have hyperlipidemia.[81] In some patients who have hyperlipidemia, xanthelasmas may develop and may be troublesome. Treatment with UDCA has been shown to lower the low-density lipoprotein cholesterol levels in patients with PBC and has been useful in some patients who have xanthelasma[82]; surgical removal of these cholesterol deposits is seldom successful and should not be performed.

Pruritus

The cause of pruritus in PBC remains an enigma. The bile acid–binding resin cholestyramine was the first medication described to alleviate this symptom. Cholestyramine therapy is successful in most patients who can tolerate the unpleasant side effects of bad taste, bloating, and occasional constipation. The recommended dose of 4 to 16 g/day orally is most effective when given before and after breakfast to allow maximal bile acid binding as the gallbladder empties. All drugs that potentially can be bound to this anion exchange resin (e.g., thyroxine, digoxin, and contraceptive pills) as well as UDCA should be taken several hours before or after cholestyramine. Not all patients with pruritus are helped by cholestyramine. The antibiotic rifampin is effective in reducing the pruritus of PBC. Most patients respond within a 1 week of starting therapy. The starting dose is 150 mg twice a day, but occasionally higher doses are needed. Rifampin induces drug metabolizing enzymes, and caution is required when prescribing other drugs. Rifampin has been associated with liver injury in up to 15% of patients (see Chapter 73). In some patients, treatment with UDCA alleviates pruritus, although on occasion pruritus may worsen on initiation of UDCA.

In warm countries, exposure to ultraviolet light without sun block can alleviate pruritus, and not surprisingly the pruritus of PBC often improves during the summer months. Some researchers have hypothesized that pruritus may be related to the release of endogenous opioids.[83] Intravenous infusion of naloxone has shown a clear benefit in a double-blind trial.[84] In other trials, oral opiate receptor antagonists such as nalmefene[85] and naltrexone[86] led to impressive amelioration of pruritus in patients with PBC, although further trials are needed to evaluate their safety.

Antihistamines are helpful only as sedatives to combat the insomnia associated with pruritus, which is always more troublesome at night. Phenobarbital may have a similar effect. Finally, the pruritus of PBC is almost always cured by liver transplantation, which is a viable option for patients who have severe intractable pruritus.

Steatorrhea

Steatorrhea can occur in patients who have advanced PBC. Several causes have been described, the most important of which is decreased delivery of bile acid to the small intestine with insufficient micellar concentrations. Occasionally, exocrine pancreatic insufficiency can occur as part of the more widespread glandular dysfunction seen in some patients with PBC. Coexisting celiac sprue has been reported in a small number of patients with PBC, and intestinal bacterial overgrowth may be the cause of steatorrhea in some patients with PBC and scleroderma. Because the treatment of each of these conditions is specific, determining the exact cause of steatorrhea in patients with PBC is important. Patients who have a decreased intestinal bile acid concentration usually benefit from dietary substitution of medium-chain triglycerides for long-chain triglycerides and a decrease in total fat intake. Patients who have exocrine pancreatic insufficiency benefit from pancreatic replacement therapy; patients who have celiac sprue, from gluten withdrawal from the diet; and patients who have bacterial overgrowth, from intermittent oral antibiotic therapy.

LIVER TRANSPLANTATION

The best therapeutic alternative for patients who have end-stage PBC is liver transplantation (see Chapter 83). Although many factors should be considered in determining the optimal timing of liver transplantation, the survival rate improves when transplantation is performed earlier in the course of the disease than after the patient has experienced a life-threatening complication or is on life support.[87] As for other chronic liver diseases, liver transplantation should be considered in patients with PBC who have major complications related to portal hypertension, including bleeding from gastroesophageal varices, diuretic resistant ascites, hepatorenal syndrome, and hepatic encephalopathy. In addition, liver transplantation for PBC may be considered in the absence of cirrhosis on liver biopsy when patients have complications associated with chronic cholestasis that make quality of life poor, such as disabling fatigue, intractable pruritus, and severe muscle wasting, as well as persistent increases in serum bilirubin levels in the absence of hepatic malignancy. Data from 1998 suggest that optimal survival and resource utilization can be achieved by liver transplantation for patients with PBC who have a Mayo risk score that does not exceed 7.8.[88] Liver transplantation clearly improves the survival rate as well as quality of life; 1-year survival rates after liver transplantation are currently higher than 90%; 5-year survival rates are higher than 80% in most transplantation centers.

PBC-specific autoantibodies against mitochondria and gp210 protein generally persist after liver transplantation. PBC may recur in the allograft, and the rate of recurrence increases with time; by 10 years, histologic recurrence may be found in 30% to 50% of patients. Although no risk factors that predict recurrent PBC have been identified, the pattern and degree of immunosuppression may be relevant. Recurrent PBC after liver transplantation seems to follow a benign course, at least in the medium term, and cirrhosis has been reported only rarely.[89]

AUTOIMMUNE CHOLANGITIS OR ANTIMITOCHONDRIAL ANTIBODY–NEGATIVE PRIMARY BILIARY CIRRHOSIS

Autoimmune cholangitis, or AMA-negative PBC, is characterized by classic clinical, biochemical, and histologic features of PBC, but without serum AMA by indirect immunofluorescence or immunoblotting techniques. Most patients have antinuclear or anti–smooth muscle antibodies, or both, and tend to have a clinical course and therapeutic response to UDCA similar to those of AMA-positive PBC patients.[90–93] Furthermore, it has been demonstrated that although these patients may be distinguished by the lack of AMA in serum, the specific AMA antigen PDC-E2 is expressed on the apical region of the biliary epithelium, as occurs in AMA-positive patients, suggesting that both conditions may have the same pathogenesis.[21] Interestingly, this staining reaction, which is found before HLA class II expression is detected, may be the earliest specific lesion of PBC. Whether there is different genetic susceptibility for the development of AMA-positive and AMA-negative PBC is still uncertain. Patients who have AMA-negative PBC or autoimmune cholangitis should be treated with UDCA (13 to 15 mg/kg/day)[93]; however, when features in the liver biopsy suggest superimposed autoimmune hepatitis,[94, 95] the combination of glucocorticoids and UDCA should be considered.

REFERENCES

1. Metcalf JV, Bhopal RS, Gray J, et al: Incidence and prevalence of primary biliary cirrhosis in the city of Newcastle upon Tyne, England. Int J Epidemiol 26:830, 1997.
2. Watson RG, Angus PW, Dewar M, et al: Low prevalence of primary biliary cirrhosis in Victoria, Australia: Melbourne Liver Group. Gut 36:927, 1995.
3. Remmel T, Remmel H, Uibo R, et al: Primary biliary cirrhosis in Estonia: With especial reference to incidence, prevalence, clinical features and outcome. Scand J Gastroenterol 30:367, 1995.
4. Myszor M, James OFW: The epidemiology of primary biliary cirrhosis in the northeast of England: An increasingly common disease? QJM 75:377, 1990.
5. Kim WR, Lindor KD, Locke GR III, et al: Epidemiology and natural history of primary biliary cirrhosis in a US community. Gastroenterology 119:1631, 2000.
6. Underhill J, Donaldson P, Bray G, et al: Susceptibility to primary biliary cirrhosis is associated with HLA-DR8–DQB1*0402 haplotype. Hepatology 16:1404, 1992.
7. Begovich AB, Klitz W, Moosamy PV, et al: Genes within the HLA class II region confer both predisposition and resistance to primary biliary cirrhosis. Tissue Antigens 43:71, 1994.
8. Manns MP, Bremm A, Schneider PM, et al: HLA DRw8 and complement C4 deficiency as risk factor in primary biliary cirrhosis. Gastroenterology 101:1367, 1991.
9. Lim AG, Jazrawi RP, Ahmed HA, et al: Soluble intercellular adhesion molecule-1 in primary biliary cirrhosis: Relationship with disease stage, immune activity, and cholestasis. Hepatology 20:882, 1994.
10. Van de Water J, Ansari AA, Surh CD, et al: Evidence for the targeting by 2-oxo-dehydrogenase enzymes in the T cell response of primary biliary cirrhosis. J Immunol 146:89, 1991.
11. Leung PSC, Chuang DT, Wynn RM, et al: Autoantibodies to BCOADC-E2 in patients with primary biliary cirrhosis recognize a conformational epitope. Hepatology 22:505, 1995.
12. Maeda T, Loveland BE, Rowley MJ, et al: Autoantibody against dihydrolipoamide dehydrogenase, the E3 subunit of the 2-oxoacid dehydrogenase complex: Significance for primary biliary cirrhosis. Hepatology 14:994, 1991.
13. Tsuneyuma K, Van De Water J, Leung PSC, et al: Abnormal expression of the E2 component of the pyruvate dehydrogenase complex on the luminal surface of biliary epithelium occurs before major histocompatibility complex class II and BBI-B7 expression. Hepatology 21:1031, 1995.
14. Joplin RE, Johnson GD, Matthews JB, et al: Distribution of pyruvate dehydrogenase dihydrolipoamide acetyltransferase (PDC-E2) and another mitochondrial marker in salivary glands and biliary epithelium from patients with primary biliary cirrhosis. Hepatology 19:1375, 1994.
15. Tsuneyama K, Van De Water J, Van Thiel D, et al: Abnormal expression of PDC-E2 on the apical surface of biliary epithelial cells in patients with antimitochondrial antibody negative primary biliary cirrhosis. Hepatology 22:1440, 1995.
16. Bandin O, Courvalin J, Poupon R, et al: Specificity and sensitivity of gp210 autoantibodies detected using an enzyme-linked immunosorbent assay and a synthetic polypeptide in the diagnosis of primary biliary cirrhosis. Hepatology 23:1020, 1996.
17. Itoh S, Ichida T, Yoshida T, et al: Autoantibodies against a 210 kDa glycoprotein of the nuclear pore complex as a prognostic marker in patients with primary biliary cirrhosis. J Gastroenterol Hepatol 13:257, 1998.
18. Wasleska-Gadek J, Honenauer H, Hitchman E, et al: Autoantibodies against nucleoporin p62 constitute a novel marker of primary biliary cirrhosis. Gastroenterology 110:840, 1996.
19. Penner EH, Goldenberg H, Albini B, et al: Immune complexes in primary biliary cirrhosis contain mitochondrial antigens. Clin Immunol Immunopathol 22:394, 1982.
20. Potter EJ, Elias E, Thomas HC, et al: Complement metabolism in chronic liver disease: Catabolism of C1q in chronic liver disease and primary biliary cirrhosis. Gastroenterology 78:1034, 1980.
21. James SP, Elson CO, Jones EA, et al: Abnormal regulation of immunoglobulin synthesis in vitro in primary biliary cirrhosis. Gastroenterology 79:242, 1980.
22. Lohse AW, Reckmann A, Kyriatsoulis A, et al: In vitro secretion of specific antimitochondrial antibodies in primary biliary cirrhosis. J Hepatol 16:165, 1992.
23. Kaplan MM: Primary biliary cirrhosis. N Engl J Med 335:1570, 1996.
24. Mitchison HC, Bassendine MF, Hendrick A, et al: Positive antimitochondrial antibody but normal alkaline phosphatase: Is this primary biliary cirrhosis? Hepatology 6:1279, 1986.
25. Metcalf JV, Mitchison HC, Palmer JM, et al: Natural history of early primary biliary cirrhosis. Lancet 348:1399, 1996.
26. Wolke AM, Schaffner F, Kapleman B, et al: Malignancy in primary biliary cirrhosis: High incidence of breast cancer in affected women. Am J Med 76:1075, 1984.
27. Goudie BM, Burt AD, Boyle P, et al: Breast cancer in women with primary biliary cirrhosis. BMJ 291:1597, 1985.
28. Nijhawan PK, Therneau TM, Dickson ER, et al: Incidence of cancer in primary biliary cirrhosis: The Mayo experience. Hepatology 29:1396, 1999.
29. Loof L, Adami HO, Sparen P, et al: Cancer risk in primary biliary cirrhosis: A population-based study from Sweden. Hepatology 20:101, 1994.
30. Czaja AJ: Frequency and nature of the variant syndrome of autoimmune liver disease. Hepatology 28:360, 1998.
31. Ludwig J, Dickson ER, McDonald GSA: Staging of chronic non-suppurative destructive cholangitis (syndrome of primary biliary cirrhosis). Virchows Arch 379:103, 1978.
32. Scheuer PJ: Primary biliary cirrhosis: Chronic non-suppurative destructive cholangitis. Am J Pathol 46:387, 1965.
33. Locke RG III, Therneau TM, Ludwig J, et al: Time course of histological progression in primary biliary cirrhosis. Hepatology 23:52, 1996.

34. Lazaridis K, Angulo P, Keach JC, et al: Lymphadenopathy in patients with cholestatic liver disease. Hepatology 32:512A, 2000.
35. Balasubramaniam K, Grambsch PM, Wiesner RH, et al: Diminished survival in asymptomatic primary biliary cirrhosis: A prospective study. Gastroenterology 98:1567, 1990.
36. Mitchison HC, Lucey MR, Kelly, et al: Symptom development and prognosis in primary biliary cirrhosis: A study of two centers. Gastroenterology 99:778, 1990.
37. Dickson ER, Grambsch PM, Flemming TR, et al: Prognosis in primary biliary cirrhosis: Model for decision making. Hepatology 10:1, 1989.
38. Roll J, Boyer JL, Barry D, et al: The prognostic importance of clinical and histologic features in asymptomatic and symptomatic primary biliary cirrhosis. N Engl J Med 308:1, 1983.
39. Rydning A, Schrumpf E, Abdelnoor M, et al: Factors of prognostic importance in primary biliary cirrhosis. Scand J Gastroenterol 25:119, 1990.
40. Goudie BM, Burt AD, Macfarlane GJ, et al: Risk factors and prognosis in primary biliary cirrhosis [published erratum appears in Am J Gastroenterol 84:1474, 1989]. Am J Gastroenterol 84:713, 1989.
41. Jeffrey GP, Reed WD, Shilkin KB: Natural history and prognostic variables in primary biliary cirrhosis (PBC) [abstract]. Hepatology 12: 955, 1990.
42. Christensen E, Neuberger J, Crowe J, et al: Beneficial effect of azathioprine and prediction of progression in primary biliary cirrhosis: Final results of an international trial. Gastroenterology 89:1084, 1985.
43. Gores GJ, Wiesner RH, Dickson ER, et al: A prospective evaluation of esophageal varices in primary biliary cirrhosis: Development, natural history and influence on survival. Gastroenterology 96:1552, 1989.
44. Murtaugh PA, Dickson ER, van Dam GM, et al: Primary biliary cirrhosis: Prediction of short-term survival based on repeated patient visits. Hepatology 20:126, 1994.
45. Angulo P, Lindor KD: Management of primary biliary cirrhosis and autoimmune cholangitis. Clin Liver Dis 2:333, 1998.
46. Mitchison HC, Bassendine MF, Malcolm AJ, et al: A pilot double-blind controlled 1-year trial of prednisolone treatment in primary biliary cirrhosis: Hepatic improvement but greater bone loss. Hepatology 10:420, 1989.
47. Leuschner M, Maier KP, Schlichting J, et al: Oral budesonide and ursodeoxycholic acid for treatment of primary biliary cirrhosis: Results of a prospective double-blind trial. Gastroenterology 117:918, 1999.
48. Angulo P, Jorgensen RA, Keach JC, et al: Oral budesonide in the treatment of patients with primary biliary cirrhosis with a suboptimal response to ursodeoxycholic acid. Hepatology 31:318, 2000.
49. Zifroni A, Schaffner F: Long-term follow-up of patients with primary biliary cirrhosis on colchicine therapy. Hepatology 14:990, 1991.
50. Crowe J, Christensen E, Smith M, et al: Azathioprine in primary biliary cirrhosis: A preliminary report on an international trial. Gastroenterology 78:1005, 1980.
51. Hoofnagle JH, Davis GL, Schafer DF, et al: Randomized trial of chlorambucil for primary biliary cirrhosis. Gastroenterology 91:1327, 1986.
52. Lombard M, Portmann B, Neuberger J, et al: Cyclosporine A treatment in primary biliary cirrhosis: Results of a long-term placebo controlled trial. Gastroenterology 104:519, 1993.
53. Angulo P, Dickson ER: Methotrexate in the treatment of primary biliary cirrhosis: The hype and the hope. Gastroenterology 117:492, 1999.
54. Hendrickse MT, Rigney E, Giaffer MH, et al: Low-dose methotrexate is ineffective in primary biliary cirrhosis: Long-term results of a placebo-controlled trial. Gastroenterology 117:400, 1999.
55. Lindor KD, Dickson ER, Baldus WP, et al: Ursodeoxycholic acid in the treatment of primary biliary cirrhosis. Gastroenterology 106:1284, 1994.
56. Heathcote EJ, Cauch-Dudek K, Walker V, et al: The Canadian multicenter double-blind randomized controlled trial of ursodeoxycholic acid in primary biliary cirrhosis. Hepatology 19:1149, 1994.
57. Combes B, Carithers RL, Maddrey WC, et al: A randomized, double-blind, placebo-controlled trial of ursodeoxycholic acid in primary biliary cirrhosis. Hepatology 22:759, 1995.
58. Poupon RE, Balkau B, Eschwege E, et al: A multicenter, controlled trial of ursodiol for the treatment of primary biliary cirrhosis. N Engl J Med 324:1548, 1991.
59. Angulo P, Dickson ER, Therneau TM et al: Comparison of three doses of ursodeoxycholic acid in the treatment of primary biliary cirrhosis: A randomized trial. J Hepatol 30:830, 1999.
60. Lindor KD, Lacerda MA, Jorgensen RA, et al: Relationship between biliary and serum bile acids and response to ursodeoxycholic acid in patients with primary biliary cirrhosis. Am J Gastroenterol 93:1498, 1998.
61. Pares A, Caballeria L, Rodes J, et al: Long-term effects of ursodeoxycholic acid in primary biliary cirrhosis: Results of a double-blind controlled multicentric trial. J Hepatol 32:561, 2000.
62. Batts KP, Jorgensen RA, Dickson ER, et al: Effects of ursodeoxycholic acid on hepatic inflammation and histological stage in patients with primary biliary cirrhosis. Am J Gastroenterol 91:2314, 1996.
63. Lindor KD, Jorgensen RA, Dickson ER, et al: Ursodeoxycholic acid delays the onset of esophageal varices in primary biliary cirrhosis. Mayo Clin Proc 72:1137, 1997.
64. Angulo P, Batts KP, Therneau TM, et al: Long-term ursodeoxycholic acid delays histologic progression in primary biliary cirrhosis. Hepatology 29:644, 1999.
65. Goulis J, Leandro G, Burroughs AK: Randomized controlled trials of ursodeoxycholic acid therapy for primary biliary cirrhosis: A meta-analysis. Lancet 354:1053, 1999.
66. Lindor KD, Poupon R, Poupon RE, et al: Ursodeoxycholic acid for primary biliary cirrhosis. Lancet 355:657, 2000.
67. Poupon RE, Poupon R, Balkau B, et al: Ursodiol for the long-term treatment of primary biliary cirrhosis. N Engl J Med 330:1342, 1994.
68. Lindor KD, Therneau TM, Jorgensen RA, et al: Effects of ursodeoxycholic acid on survival in patients with primary biliary cirrhosis. Gastroenterology 110:1515, 1996.
69. Poupon R, Lindor KD, Cauch-Dudek K, et al: Combined analysis of French, American and Canadian randomized controlled trials of ursodeoxycholic acid therapy in primary biliary cirrhosis. Gastroenterology 113:884, 1997.
70. Angulo P, Lindor KD, Therneau TM, et al: Utilization of the Mayo risk score in patients with primary biliary cirrhosis receiving ursodeoxycholic acid. Liver 19:115, 1999.
71. Hay JE: Bone disease in cholestatic liver disease. Gastroenterology 108:276, 1995.
72. Eastell R, Dickson ER, Hodgson SF, et al: Rate of vertebral bone loss before and after liver transplantation in women with primary biliary cirrhosis. Hepatology 14:296, 1991.
73. Janes CH, Dickson ER, Okazaki R, et al: Role of hyperbilirubinemia in the impairment of osteoblast proliferation associated with cholestatic jaundice. J Clin Invest 95:2581, 1995.
74. Springer JE, Cole DE, Rubin LA, et al: Vitamin D–receptor genotypes as independent genetic predictors of decreased bone mineral density in primary biliary cirrhosis. Gastroenterology 118:145, 2000.
75. Menon N, Angulo P, Weston S, et al: Predictors and rate of progression of bone disease in patients with primary biliary cirrhosis [abstract]. Gastroenterology 116:A1239, 1999.
76. Porayko M, Wiesner RH, Hay JE, et al: Bone disease in liver transplant recipients: Incidence, timing and risk factors. Transplant Proc 23: 1462, 1991.
77. Crippin JS, Jorgensen RA, Dickson ER, et al: Hepatic osteodystrophy in primary biliary cirrhosis: Effects of medical treatment. Am J Gastroenterol 89:47, 1994.
78. Olsson R, Mattsson LA, Obrant K, Mellstrom D: Estrogen-progestogen therapy for low bone mineral density in primary biliary cirrhosis. Liver 19:188, 1999.
79. Guanabens N, Pares A, Monegal A, et al: Etidronate versus fluoride for treatment of osteopenia in primary biliary cirrhosis: Preliminary results after 2 years. Gastroenterology 113:219, 1997.
80. Lindor KD, Jorgensen RA, Tiegs RD, et al: Etidronate for osteoporosis in primary biliary cirrhosis: A randomized trial. J Hepatol 33:878, 2000.
81. Crippin JS, Lindor KD, Jorgensen RA, et al: Hypercholesterolemia and atherosclerosis in primary biliary cirrhosis: What is the risk? Hepatology 15:858, 1992.
82. Balan V, Dickson ER, Jorgensen RA, et al: Effect of ursodeoxycholic acid on serum lipids of patients with primary biliary cirrhosis. Mayo Clin Proc 69:923, 1994.
83. Jones EA, Bergasa NV: The pruritus of cholestasis. Hepatology 29: 1003, 1999.
84. Bergasa NV, Alling DW, Talbot TL, et al: Effect of naloxone infusion in pâtients with the pruritus of cholestasis: A double-blind, randomized, controlled trial. Ann Intern Med 123:161, 1995.
85. Bergasa NV, Schmidt JM, Talbot TL, et al: Open-label trial of oral nalmefene therapy for the pruritus of cholestasis. Hepatology 27:679, 1998.
86. Wolfhagen FHJ, Sternieri E, Hop WCJ, et al: Oral naltrexone treatment

for cholestatic pruritus: A double-blind, placebo-controlled study. Gastroenterology 113:1264, 1997.

87. Angulo P, Dickson ER: The timing of liver transplantation in primary biliary cirrhosis. Bailieres Best Pract Res Clin Gastroenterol 14:657, 2000.
88. Kim WR, Wiesner RH, Therneau TM, et al: Optimal timing for liver transplantation for primary biliary cirrhosis. Hepatology 28:33, 1998.
89. Neuberger J: Recurrent primary biliary cirrhosis. Bailieres Best Pract Res Clin Gastroenterol 14:669, 2000.
90. Mitchieletti P, Wanless IR, Katz A, et al: Antimitochondrial antibody negative primary biliary cirrhosis: A distinct syndrome of autoimmune cholangitis. Gut 35:260, 1994.
91. Lacerda MA, Ludwig J, Dickson ER, et al: Antimitochondrial antibody–negative primary biliary cirrhosis. Am J Gastroenterol 90:247, 1995.
92. Invernizzi P, Crogsinani A, Battezzati PM, et al: Comparison of the clinical features and clinical course of antimitochondrial antibody–positive and –negative primary biliary cirrhosis. Hepatology 25:1090, 1997.
93. Kim WR, Poterucha JJ, Jorgensen RA, et al: Does antimitochondrial antibody status affect response to treatment in patients with primary biliary cirrhosis? Outcomes of ursodeoxycholic acid therapy and liver transplantation. Hepatology 26:22, 1997.
94. Ben-Ari Z, Dhillon AP, Sherlock S: Autoimmune cholangiopathy: Part of the spectrum of autoimmune chronic active hepatitis. Hepatology 18: 10, 1993.
95. Chazouilleres O, Wendum D, Serfaty L, et al: Primary biliary cirrhosis–autoimmune hepatitis overlap syndrome: Clinical features and response to therapy. Hepatology 28:296, 1998.

Chapter 77

PORTAL HYPERTENSION AND VARICEAL BLEEDING

Nathan M. Bass and Francis Y. Yao

The problem of therapy for hemorrhage in cirrhosis will continue to be a serious one.

ALLEN O. WHIPPLE, 1945

That gastrointestinal bleeding could occur as a consequence of derangement of the portal circulation was certainly appreciated by physicians in the 17th century. The concept that esophageal varices develop as a result of obstruction to portal flow in liver cirrhosis was well established by the end of the 19th century, and the term *portal hypertension* was introduced by Gilbert and Carnot in 1902.[1] Whipple made his dour comment in 1945,[2] at a time of considerable innovation in the surgical therapy of portal hypertension, yet it remains applicable today. There have been considerable advances since the late 1970s, but the complications of portal hypertension—gastrointestinal hemorrhage, ascites, and portosystemic encephalopathy—continue to pose difficult challenges to the physician managing patients with end-stage liver disease and remain the cause of substantial morbidity and mortality rates. Liver transplantation is a highly successful cure for end-stage liver disease, but donor livers are in short supply, and there remains the need for managing portal hypertension in patients who are awaiting transplantation or who are not considered transplantation candidates. Substantial progress has been achieved in the management of portal hypertension, particularly in the understanding of its pathophysiologic characteristics.[3–12] Translation from research into therapeutic applications has been rapid and has fostered the growth of pharmacologic therapies.[10, 13] Other important therapeutic options that are now used widely include endoscopic therapies, a variety of surgical shunt and nonshunt procedures, and the transjugular intrahepatic portosystemic shunt (TIPS), an interventional technique that since the 1990s has established its place among therapeutic options.[14] Many questions remain regarding the optimal use and timing of these therapies, but continued progress in our understanding of the natural history, pathophysiologic features, and hemodynamic derangements that attend portal hypertension holds promise for the development of new treatments and management strategies that will prove more effective and minimize iatrogenic morbidity and cost.

ETIOLOGY AND PATHOPHYSIOLOGY OF PORTAL HYPERTENSION

Normal Liver Blood Flow

The normal anatomic characteristics of the portal and hepatic arterial circulation are described in Chapter 62 (see Fig. 62–3). Hepatic blood flow is normally about 1500 mL/minute, representing 15% to 20% of cardiac output. One third of this flow and 30% to 60% of the oxygen consumed by the liver are provided by the hepatic artery. Approximately two thirds of the hepatic blood supply is provided by portal venous blood.[7, 11] The high-pressure, well-oxygenated arterial blood mixes completely with the low-pressure, low-oxygen-containing, nutrient-rich portal venous blood within the hepatic sinusoids. After perfusing the sinusoids, blood flows, sequentially, into the hepatic venules, hepatic veins, and inferior vena cava. A fraction of the plasma entering the space of Disse is drained into lymphatic vessels.

A unique feature of the normal hepatic sinusoidal microcirculation is its low perfusion pressure. This low pressure is attributed to the unusually high precapillary to postcapillary resistance in the liver.[11] It appears that the sinusoids are normally protected from upstream portal perfusion pressure and fluctuations in that pressure by a presinusoidal site of high resistance, probably within the terminal portal venous radicals.[15] Because the sinusoids are lined by an endothelium that lacks a continuous basement membrane and contains a multitude of large (50 to 200 nm), highly permeable fenestrae, maintenance of a low pressure in the hepatic sinusoids is critical to the maintenance of normal rates of transudation of sinusoidal fluid into the space of Disse.

Another feature that is unique to the hepatic circulation is the close interrelationship between blood flow in the portal vein and that in the hepatic artery. When portal blood flow increases, hepatic arterial flow decreases; when portal flow decreases, hepatic arterial flow increases. This phenomenon has been termed the *hepatic arterial buffer response* and is an adenosine-mediated vascular reflex that ensures the maintenance of a relatively constant state of sinusoidal perfusion in the face of changes in portal inflow that occur, for example, with meals.[7, 11]

Hemodynamic Alterations in Portal Hypertension

General Principles

The pathogenesis of portal hypertension involves the relationship between portal venous blood flow and the resistance offered to this blood flow within the liver (the portohepatic resistance) and within portosystemic collateral blood vessels (the portocollateral resistance) that form during the evolution of portal hypertension (Fig. 77–1).

The movement of blood within the portal vascular system is driven by a pressure difference or gradient that exists along the length of the system. The portal pressure gradient (ΔP), that is, the difference in pressure between the portal and systemic venous systems, is the resultant product of portal venous blood flow (Q) and the vascular resistance to this flow (R), as expressed by Ohm's law

$$\Delta P = Q \times R.$$

R, in turn, is derived by Poiseuille's law from the relationship

$$R = 8\eta l/\pi r^4$$

where η is the coefficient of viscosity, l is the length of the vessel, and r is the radius. It is clear from this relationship that small changes in vessel radius lead to disproportionate increases in resistance, and hence pressure. Also the incremental influence on resistance of an increase in the hematocrit value, and hence viscosity, as a result of blood transfusions administered to a patient who has recently bled from varices can be appreciated.[11] Normal, uncorrected pressure in the portal vein ranges from 5 to 10 mm Hg and is influenced by intra-abdominal pressure. Hepatic venous pressure is similarly affected by intra-abdominal pressure and also reflects central venous filling pressure. In order to eliminate the contribution of intra-abdominal pressure and central venous pressure and thus express portal pressure as the intrinsic pressure difference between the portal and systemic venous compartments, portal pressure is usually expressed as a portal pressure gradient (ΔP). In practical terms, this is most often determined in patients with cirrhosis as the hepatic venous pressure gradient (HVPG), a technique similar in principle to the measurement of the pulmonary capillary wedge pressure[3, 4] (Fig. 77–2). In brief, the technique is as follows: A pressure measurement is made via a catheter wedged into a hepatic vein via either a femoral or a transjugular approach. This measurement is termed the *wedged hepatic venous pressure* (WHVP). After withdrawal of the catheter tip into the hepatic vein, a free hepatic vein pressure (FHVP) is obtained. The HVPG is obtained by subtracting the value of the WHVP from the FHVP. Normally, the HVPG does not exceed 5 mm Hg. Portal hypertension exists if the HVPG exceeds this value.

From the foregoing discussion, it is apparent that a rise in portal pressure could, in theory, result from an increase in either portal flow or vascular resistance. Increased flow into the portal system from a massively enlarged spleen was initially believed to be the cause of elevated portal pressure in patients with cirrhosis (Banti's hypothesis). This view was subsequently abandoned when the crucial role of increased resistance to portal flow at various sites became evident. Since the 1980s, the pendulum has swung back once more,

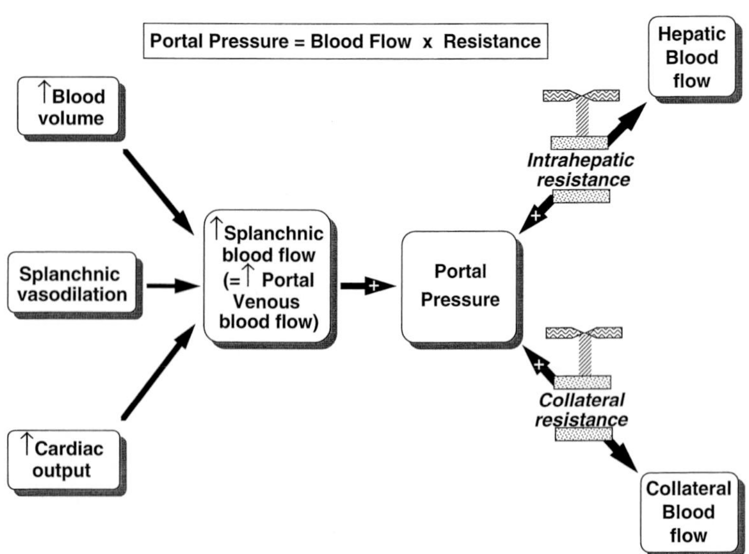

Figure 77–1. Hemodynamic principles in portal hypertension. The schematic summarizes the contribution and interplay of the major hemodynamic forces underlying the pathogenesis of portal hypertension. (See also Fig. 77–2 and Table 77–2.)

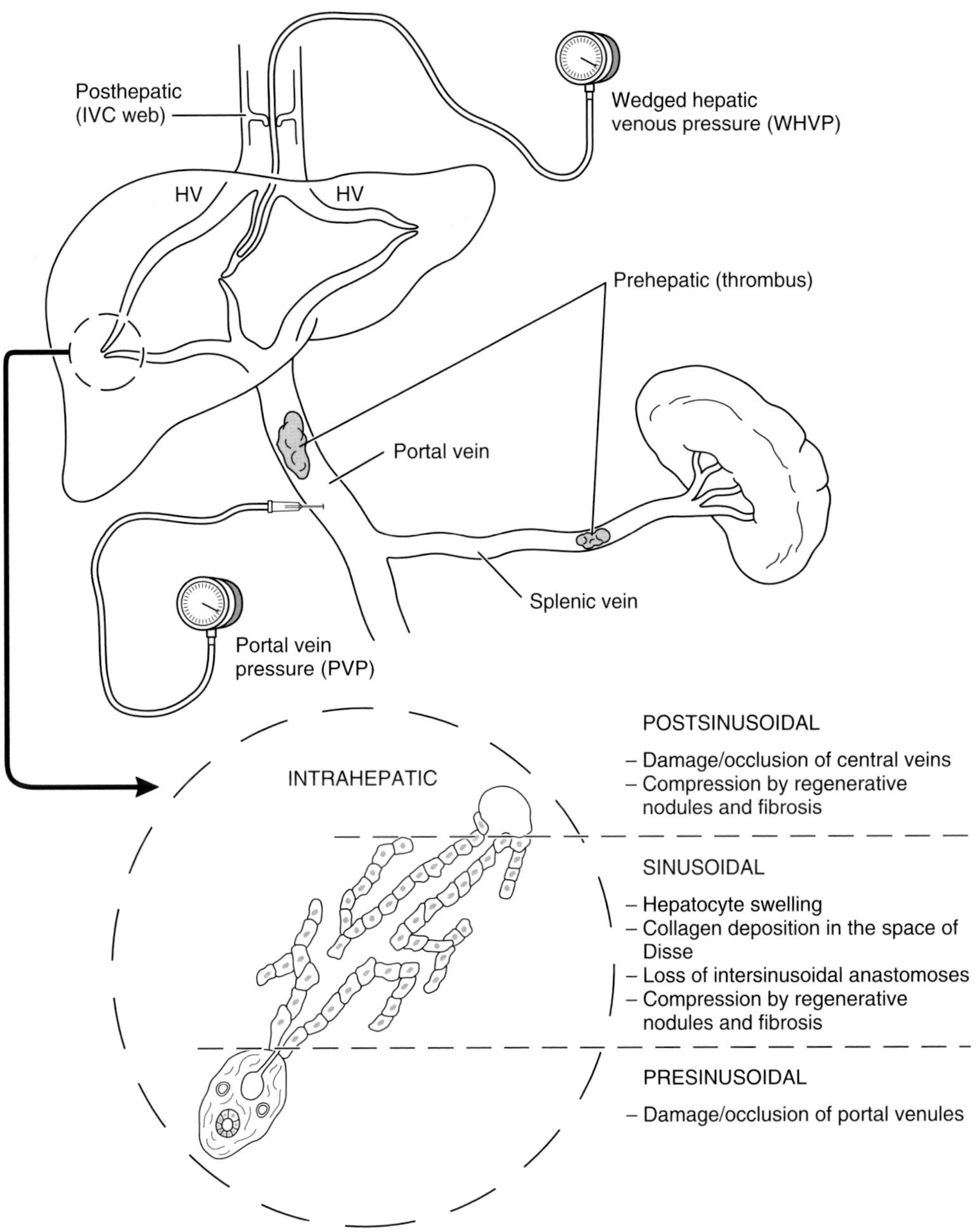

Figure 77–2. Sites of obstruction (resistance) to portal venous flow and measurement of portal pressure. The schematic illustrates the major locations of extrahepatic (prehepatic and posthepatic) and intrahepatic (presinusoidal, sinusoidal, and postsinusoidal) obstruction. A catheter tip is also shown wedged into a small hepatic vein for the measurement of the WHVP. When the catheter tip is withdrawn into the hepatic vein, the FHVP is obtained. HVPG = WHV − FHVP. Direct measurement of the PVP is accomplished intraoperatively either by catheterization of the umbilical vein or by catheterization of the portal vein via the transjugular or transhepatic approach. HVPG, hepatic venous pressure gradient; WHVP, wedged hepatic venous pressure; FHVP, free hepatic vein pressure; PVP, portal venous pressure.

on the basis of a plethora of elegant experimental and clinical studies that have demonstrated the presence of a hyperdynamic circulatory state in portal hypertension, with increased splanchnic blood flow contributing to the increase in portal pressure. The relative extent to which increased splanchnic portal inflow—the so-called forward force—as opposed to vascular resistance (backward force) is responsible for the increase in portal pressure in any given clinical situation is of considerable practical importance in the understanding of the fundamental pathophysiologic characteristics of portal hypertension as well as the development of rational pharmacologic therapy.

The Role of Increased Resistance

Cirrhosis, mainly from alcohol and chronic viral hepatitis, is the most important cause of portal hypertension in the Western world, but there are many other causes, most of which are noncirrhotic; for example schistosomiasis is a particularly prevalent cause in the developing world. Improved understanding of the pathologic mechanisms of these conditions has confirmed the existence of resistance to portal flow at a variety of different anatomic levels in portal hypertension of various causes. Thus, the causes of portal hypertension are conventionally classified according to the localization of the site of maximal resistance to portal flow (see Fig. 77–2 and Table 77–1). The three major categories of portal hypertension are prehepatic, intrahepatic, and posthepatic, for which the site of increased resistance is usually obvious. Thus, portal vein thrombosis exemplifies prehepatic portal hypertension, whereas an inferior vena caval web typifies posthepatic portal hypertension. In the case of intrahepatic causes, the site of resistance is conventionally subdivided further into presinusoidal, sinusoidal, and postsinusoidal. Precise

Table 77–1 | **Causes of Portal Hypertension**

Primary increased flow
Arterial-portal venous fistula
Intrahepatic
Intrasplenic
Splanchnic
Splenic capillary hemangiomatosis
Primary increased resistance
Prehepatic
Thrombosis/cavernous transformation of the portal vein
Splenic vein thrombosis
Intrahepatic
Presinusoidal
Schistosomiasis*
Sarcoidosis*
Myeloproliferative diseases and myelofibrosis*
Congenital hepatic fibrosis
Idiopathic portal hypertension (hepatoportal sclerosis)
Chronic arsenic hepatotoxicity
Azathioprine hepatotoxicity
Vinyl chloride hepatotoxicity
Early primary biliary cirrhosis*
Early primary sclerosing cholangitis*
Partial nodular transformation
Sinusoidal/mixed
Cirrhosis secondary to chronic hepatitis
Alcoholic cirrhosis
Cryptogenic cirrhosis
Methotrexate
Alcoholic hepatitis
Hypervitaminosis A
Incomplete septal fibrosis
Nodular regenerative hyperplasia
Postsinusoidal
Veno-occlusive disease
Hepatic vein thrombosis (Budd-Chiari syndrome)
Posthepatic
Inferior vena caval web
Constrictive pericarditis
Tricuspid regurgitation
Severe right-sided heart failure

*Usually presinusoidal early in the course, often progressing to a sinusoidal or mixed type of portal hypertension when more advanced.

classification of portal hypertension according to the intrahepatic site of maximal resistance has been limited by the lack of technical means to measure pressure directly within the hepatic sinusoids. Most of the relevant information has been provided by direct measurement of pressure in the portal system and indirect estimation of the intrasinusoidal pressure from the WHVP in conjunction with details of the morbid anatomic features.[3, 11] For example, in both prehepatic and intrahepatic presinusoidal portal hypertension, the directly measured portal venous pressure (PVP) is always elevated in the presence of a normal WHVP and HVPG. In sinusoidal and intrahepatic postsinusoidal portal hypertension, the WHVP tends to approximate or equal the directly measured PVP, and the HVPG is increased proportionately. In posthepatic portal hypertension, the WHVP equals the increased PVP. Because the FHVP is also abnormally high in this scenario, the HVPG is usually normal.

As a rule, the intrahepatic localization of maximal resistance tends to be more clearly established in noncirrhotic disease than in cirrhosis.[16] Thus, veno-occlusive disease, resulting from either pyrrolizidine alkaloids or chemotherapeutic agents (see Chapters 70 and 73), is readily apparent as a cause of postsinusoidal intrahepatic portal hypertension, whereas the portal-based granulomatous inflammation and fibrosis of early hepatic schistosomiasis is a well-studied example of presinusoidal intrahepatic portal hypertension. However, even such widely accepted examples of presinusoidal portal hypertension as schistosomiasis[16, 17] and idiopathic portal hypertension[18] are more complicated when one considers that over the course of time, hepatic pathologic processes usually progress and may generate a more complex or mixed pattern of vascular resistance.

The main site of intrahepatic vascular resistance in cirrhosis has been difficult to establish. Most measurements in nonalcoholic cirrhosis show a higher PVP than WHVP. Because the WHVP is an estimate of the intrasinusoidal pressure, this finding has been variously interpreted to indicate either the presence of a presinusoidal component of resistance, probably related to inflammatory activity or fibrotic changes in the portal tracts, or the presence of intersinusoidal anastomoses that partially decompress the sinusoids during wedged pressure measurement.[3] In patients who have alcoholic liver disease, the WHVP is usually equal to the PVP, suggesting that the site of the increase in resistance in alcoholic cirrhosis includes the entire sinusoid and that there are fewer decompressive intersinusoidal anastomoses in this disease, possible because of greater intrasinusoidal fibrosis.[15]

The pathogenesis of the increased sinusoidal resistance in alcoholic cirrhosis is not fully understood. Architectural derangement produced by the development of fibrotic septa and regenerative nodules are important, as are pathologic changes within the sinusoids. These changes include hepatocyte enlargement, resulting from alcohol-induced accumulation of fat and protein, with compression of the liver sinusoids and obstruction of flow, and collagen deposition in the space of Disse[15] (see Fig. 77–2). From the standpoint of the location of maximal resistance, alcoholic cirrhosis is by no means a homogeneous entity. The site of predominant resistance may vary according to the stage, activity, and predominant pathologic morphologic features. Thus, hepatocyte swelling may be an important contributor to the partially reversible sinusoidal portal hypertension in acute alcoholic hepatitis.[16] On the other hand, the lesions of perivenular fibrosis and central hyaline sclerosis that characterize some cases of alcoholic liver disease could account for a substantial component of postsinusoidal resistance.[3] In addition, thrombus formation in the medium- to large-caliber portal and hepatic veins appears to be common in advanced alcoholic cirrhosis.[19] This portal and hepatic venopathy may contribute further to the pre- and postsinusoidal mix of resistance elements.

The morphologic derangements that occur in chronic liver disease are undoubtedly the most important factor in the increased intrahepatic resistance. However, substantial data also suggest a role for dynamic, contractile factors that can lead to increased vascular tone. Present in fibrous scars and perisinusoidal areas of cirrhotic, but not normal, livers are contractile cells, the myofibroblasts.[20] These cells appear to develop from activated hepatic stellate cells and exhibit a contractile response to vasoconstrictors such as endothelin (ET),[8, 20] levels of which are increased in the blood and liver tissue of patients with cirrhosis.[20–22] The emergence of myofibroblasts in the cirrhotic liver may account for the observation that infusion of vasodilators into a normal liver is not associated with a change in vascular tone, whereas in the cirrhotic liver, a similar infusion causes a decrease in pressure.[20] Therefore, in cirrhosis portal pressure may change in an active manner, depending on intrahepatic contractile elements and the action of vasoactive compounds in the blood. Although the hepatic stellate cell is regarded as a key cellular element in the pathogenesis of fibrosis in the cirrhotic liver, the contribution of this cell to dynamic intrahepatic resistance in cirrhosis remains unsettled.[8, 15]

With the development of portosystemic collaterals during the evolution of portal hypertension, the overall resistance encountered by total portal venous flow (R_P) is determined by the parallel resistances offered by the portohepatic vascular resistance (R_H) and the portocollateral resistance (R_C) according to the following relationship

$$1/R_P = 1/R_H + 1/R_C$$

The portosystemic collateral vessels have a substantial amount of smooth muscle and thus may show active changes in diameter in response to vasoactive substances. Therefore, perhaps to an even greater extent than R_H, R_C is subject to modulation resulting from changes in the diameter of the collateral vessels, rendering this source of resistance dynamic and amenable to pharmacologic manipulation, as discussed more fully later in this chapter.

Portal Blood Flow

The contribution of increased portal venous blood flow to the pathogenesis of portal hypertension is supported by several distinct clinical and experimental observations.

PRIMARY HIGH PORTAL FLOW STATES. Although uncommon, conditions leading to high-flow states in the portal system (arterioportal fistulas, splenomegaly resulting from myelofibrosis or myeloid metaplasia) are well-recognized causes of portal hypertension. In fact, the development of portal hypertension in patients who have these conditions invariably reflects the combined effect of increased flow and increased resistance in the liver.[3, 11, 16] For example, idiopathic portal hypertension, an entity that is common in Asia but rare in the United States, was long believed to be a primary disorder of the spleen (hence the older term *tropical splenomegaly*) with a marked increase in splenic arterial and hence splenoportal venous blood flow. In reality, idiopathic portal hypertension is a disease of the preterminal branches of the portal vein (hepatoportal sclerosis),[18] and portal hypertension in idiopathic portal hypertension is not abrogated by splenectomy.[23] Nevertheless, the importance of the contribution of high portal flow in certain instances is amply illustrated by the observation that clinical evidence of portal hypertension, including ascites and esophageal varices, may regress dramatically after the normalization of portal flow that follows closure of an arterioportal fistula.[24]

THE PORTOSYSTEMIC COLLATERAL PARADOX. When portal pressure reaches a critical value, portosystemic collaterals begin to develop. In alcoholic cirrhosis, a portal pressure gradient of 10 to 12 mm Hg appears to be necessary for the development of esophageal varices.[3, 9] Collateral veins are believed to develop as a result of dilatation of embryonic channels or redirection of flow within existing veins, rather than as a result of the formation of new blood vessels. As collaterals form, they would be expected to decompress the portal system and lower portal pressure. Paradoxically, the extent of collaterals often correlates with the degree of portal pressure,[11] and therefore either a compensatory increase in portal inflow occurs as collaterals form or the resistance within the collateral bed must be unusually high. The latter does not apply, because the vascular resistance of the collateral bed, although higher than normal portohepatic resistance, is still lower than the resistance of the obstructed portal system.[6, 11] Hence, portal hypertension is maintained during collateral formation by increased portal inflow, and, as a consequence, portal hypertension persists even when all portal flow escapes through collaterals.

In portal hypertension, therefore, splanchnic arterial blood flow into the portal venous system (portal venous inflow) equals flow of portal blood through the liver *plus* portocollateral blood flow. Under normal physiologic conditions, the flow of portal blood through the liver essentially equals all the blood entering the splanchnic system (portal venous inflow). In portal hypertension, perfusion of the liver by portal blood is decreased and may be negligible. In approximately 10% of patients, flow within the portal vein may even be reversed (retrograde or hepatofugal portal flow).[25, 26] This situation develops when hepatic arterial blood flow encounters greater resistance to flow in its usual anterograde course through the sinusoids than via the path offered by the portal venous radicals backward to the portal venous circulation. This loss of hepatic arterial blood flow, or hepatic arterial steal, via collaterals is associated with a high risk of impaired hepatic function and hepatic encephalopathy.[25, 26] This principle, as discussed later, also applies to therapeutic side-to-side portosystemic shunts.[14]

Although increased portal venous inflow has been well characterized in animal models of portal hypertension,[3, 4, 6, 27] and, albeit to a lesser extent, in portal hypertensive patients,[3, 4] its precise contribution to the maintenance of elevated portal pressure in patients who have portal hypertension has been less clear.[6, 11] Reduction in flow from one part of the splanchnic circulation is rapidly compensated by an increase from other parts. For example, patients who have portal hypertension and in whom splenic arterial flow is temporarily interrupted by balloon occlusion show a fall in portal flow and pressure. These reductions, however, are less than expected from the loss of splenic blood flow as a result of a marked compensatory increase in mesenteric venous blood flow.[28] The current view, therefore, considers increased resistance as the major and driving force in cirrhotic portal hypertension and supports a role for increased splanchnic arterial flow in contributing to the maintenance of elevated portal pressure.[11]

HYPERDYNAMIC CIRCULATION OF PORTAL HYPERTENSION. The increase in splanchnic blood flow in portal hypertension occurs as a result of a more generalized hyperdynamic circulatory disturbance.[29, 30] An association between portal hypertension and a hyperdynamic circulatory state was first described by Kowalski and Abelmann in 1953,[31] and its hallmarks are increased cardiac output and reduced arterial blood pressure. Increased cardiac output results from an increase in heart rate and possibly an increase in stroke volume and total blood volume; decreased blood pressure results from a reduction in systemic vascular resistance secondary to peripheral arterial vasodilation. The severity of the hyperkinetic circulatory abnormalities that accompany cirrhosis correlates with clinical indices of hepatic dysfunction,[32] although the same abnormalities are also present in patients who have noncirrhotic portal hypertension.[29] Nevertheless, patients who have noncirrhotic portal hypertension have an extensive portosystemic collateral circulation, suggesting that portosystemic shunting rather than decompensation of hepatic function is the main factor in the development of the hyperdynamic circulatory state. The systemic consequences of the hyperdynamic circulation in end-stage liver disease are complex and represent a form of multisystem organ dysfunction.[30] Significant effects on the circulation of the kidneys, brain, and lungs have all been described. In the case of the lungs, pulmonary vasodilation leads to arterial hypoxemia, which is observed in approximately one third of cirrhotic patients in the absence of detectable cardiorespiratory diseases, the hepatopulmonary syndrome (see Chapter 79). In this syndrome, reduced vascular tone of the pulmonary circulation is believed to result in a perfusion-diffusion mismatch, which is responsible for the arterial hypoxemia.[33]

The mechanisms of the systemic hemodynamic changes observed in portal hypertension are currently explained via two opposing, although not mutually exclusive, theories. The essential difference between these two theories relates to whether the primary event is viewed as a reduction in vascular resistance with a compensatory increase in cardiac output or as an increase in cardiac output with a compensatory reduction in systemic vascular resistance.

The peripheral vasodilation theory[34] (see Chapter 78) proposes that a factor or factors associated with cirrhosis or portosystemic shunting cause arterial vasodilation, primarily in the splanchnic circulation. A necessary consequence of the peripheral vasodilation would then be an increase in cardiac output due to afterload reduction, thereby producing a hyperdynamic circulatory state. An alternative theory proposes that there is a primary stimulus (hepatorenal reflex) to sodium and water retention that is a direct consequence of the presence of portal hypertension.[29, 30, 35] As a result of this primary increase in salt and water retention in portal hypertension, blood volume increases and causes an increase in cardiac output. According to this theory, peripheral vasodilation occurs as an adaptation to these earlier events.

At present, neither theory explains completely all the systemic hemodynamic changes described in patients who have portal hypertension.[30] Rather, there appears to be a continuum of changes that progress as the liver disease progresses and portal hypertension supervenes. Most important are the collective data from hemodynamic studies in patients who have portal hypertension who are treated with selective and nonselective beta-blockers that point to a role for both increased cardiac output (β_1 receptor–mediated) and splanchnic arteriolar vasodilation (β_2 receptor–mediated) in generating the increase in portal venous inflow that contributes to the maintenance of portal hypertension.

Vasoactive Mediators in the Pathogenesis of Portal Hypertension

Vasoactive humoral and autocrine factors play a key role in the pathogenesis of portal hypertension. Both vasodilator and vasoconstrictor substances have been implicated and may act by either mediating systemic and splanchnic vasodilation and hence portocollateral blood flow or promoting an increase in vascular resistance within the intrahepatic and portal-collateral beds (Table 77–2).

Table 77–2 | **Vasoactive Mediators in Portal Hypertension**

VASODILATORS	VASOCONSTRICTORS
Glucagon	Norepinephrine
Prostacyclin	Serotonin
Substance P	Endothelins
Adenosine	Angiotensin II
Atrial natriuretic factor	Vasopressin
Bile acids	
Histamine	
Vasoactive intestinal peptide	
γ-Aminobutyric acid	
Leu and met enkephalins	
Endotoxin	
Tumor necrosis factor-α	
Nitric oxide (NO)	

Vasoactive Mediators and Splanchnic Vasodilation

There is abundant evidence for increased sympathetic nervous system tone in patients with cirrhosis. Serum norepinephrine levels are increased. However, considerable data point to the attenuation of sympathetic neurotransmitter effects in portal hypertension, in part as a result of down-regulation of adrenergic receptor density and in part as a result of postreceptor antagonism by opposing vasodilator influences.[10, 36]

Earlier studies showed that cross-perfusion between portal hypertensive and normal animals produces arteriolar vasodilation in the latter, lending support to the hypothesis that a transferable humoral vasodilator is present in the blood in portal hypertension.[6] Much attention has since focused on putative vasoactive mediators responsible for the arteriolar vasodilation in splanchnic organs that underlies the increase in portal venous inflow.[36, 37] Investigators have postulated that endogenous vasodilators normally present in portal blood and cleared by the liver may escape hepatic removal either as a result of portosystemic shunting via portosystemic collaterals or as a result of impaired hepatocellular metabolism. A further possibility is that liver disease and portal hypertension lead to an increase in the production of certain vasodilators within either the hepatic or the splanchnic vascular beds. These vasodilators then reach high concentrations in the systemic circulation, thereby leading to systemic and splanchnic arterial vasodilation.

Several gut peptide hormones have been proposed as vasodilator mediators in portal hypertension. Glucagon has been a prime candidate.[6] Serum glucagon levels are increased in experimental models of portal hypertension and in patients with cirrhosis.[6, 38, 39] Glucagon impairs systemic vascular sensitivity to norepinephrine.[39] A role for glucagon in portal hypertension is also supported by the finding of a significant reduction in splanchnic blood flow after infusion of a glucagon-specific antiserum.[40] However, this reduction in splanchnic blood flow was not accompanied by a reduction in systemic vasodilation. In addition, other investigators have found no correlation between the magnitude of arterial vasodilation and circulating levels of glucagon.[41] On the other hand, infusion of pharmacologic doses of somatostatin or its synthetic analog octreotide, which decreases glucagon release, produces vasoconstriction of both the splanchnic and the systemic circulation.[42] Because somatostatin also inhibits the release of several other peptide vasodilators, such as substance P, vasoactive intestinal peptide (VIP), and calcitonin gene-related peptide (CGRP), it is conceivable that the effects of somatostatin on the circulation in portal hypertension may be mediated by other peptides in addition to, or apart from, glucagon. Also, somatostatin may exert a direct vasoconstrictive effect on vascular smooth muscle.[10] Therefore, understanding of the role of glucagon as a mediator of systemic vasodilation in portal hypertension remains inconclusive, but on the basis of available data, hyperglucagonemia may account for approximately 30% to 40% of the splanchnic vasodilation of chronic portal hypertension.[36]

Vasoactive factors produced by the vascular endothelium have attracted considerable attention with respect to a potential role in the pathogenesis of portal hypertension. There is increasing evidence for the involvement of nitric oxide (NO) and prostacyclin in the pathogenesis of the circulatory abnormalities in portal hypertension.

NO is a powerful endogenous vasodilator that is generated in several tissues by a constitutive vascular endothelial NO synthase (eNOS) and an inducible NO synthase (iNOS) from the amino acid L-arginine.[37] NO is produced constitutively by eNOS and by liver parenchymal and nonparenchymal cells after induction of iNOS by cytokines and endotoxin. An increasing body of evidence suggests that excessive NO biosynthesis by eNOS may be involved in the pathogenesis of the low systemic and splanchnic vascular resistance and hence increased splanchnic arterial flow associated with portal hypertension.[37, 43, 44]

Tumor necrosis factor-α (TNF-α) mediates the effects of endotoxin, a potent stimulant of NOS. A dramatic amelioration in the hyperdynamic circulation and the increased portal pressure has been described in portal hypertensive rats treated with antibody to TNF-α.[45]

Administration of specific NO antagonists to animals with portal hypertension induces splanchnic and systemic vasoconstriction, thereby attenuating the hyperdynamic circulation.[43, 44] In addition, inhibition of NO synthesis, at least partially, corrects the blunted vascular responsiveness to vasoconstrictors that is characteristic of portal hypertension.[37] The finding that patients with cirrhosis have increased serum and urinary concentrations of nitrite and nitrate (end-products of NO oxidation) also supports a role for NO in the genesis of the circulatory disturbances of portal hypertension.[46] However, NO inhibition attenuates but does not normalize the hyperkinetic state of portal hypertension.[43, 44] Also, in one study chronic NO inhibition delayed but did not prevent the development of splanchnic vasodilation in experimental animals.[47] These and other data suggest that other factors in addition to NO are involved in the vasodilatory phenomena associated with the hyperdynamic circulation of portal hypertension.

Several studies have supported a role for prostaglandins in the hyperdynamic circulation of portal hypertension.[48, 49] Prostacyclin levels have also been found to be increased in the portal vein of portal hypertensive rats,[48] whereas patients with cirrhosis have increased systemic and portal levels of prostacyclin.[48, 49] Portal levels of prostacyclin correlate with the degree of portal pressure elevation in these patients. In one study inhibition of prostaglandin biosynthesis by indomethacin reduced the hyperdynamic circulation and portal pressure in patients who had cirrhosis and portal hypertension.[36]

A variety of other circulating vasodilators have been evaluated, including bile acids, histamine, adenosine, and substance P (see Table 77–2), without convincing evidence to date that they contribute to the systemic hyperdynamic state of portal hypertension.

Vasoactive Mediators and Vascular Resistance

INTRAHEPATIC VASCULAR RESISTANCE. As discussed earlier, there is evidence, albeit controversial, that hepatic stellate cell contraction may contribute to a dynamic component of increased intrahepatic resistance in portal hypertension.[8, 15, 20] Vasoactive mediators, both vasoconstrictors and vasodilators, may modulate intrahepatic vascular resistance through contraction or relaxation of these cells or other contractile elements, such as vascular sphincters, in the liver.[15, 50, 51]

The endothelins, a family of at least three homologous 21-amino-acid peptides (ET-1, ET-2, and ET-3),[52] are active contractile agonists of stellate cells.[20, 50] ET-1 release from vascular endothelial cells is stimulated by epinephrine and angiotensin II.[52] ET-1, in turn, increases the release of these same pressor factors, which, with vasopressin, increase intrahepatic vascular resistance.[53] Infusion of ET-1 increases portal pressure, and ET has also been shown to promote the closing of endothelial fenestrae in normal rat liver,[37, 54] thus contributing to the process of sinusoidal "capillarization" and increased resistance in portal hypertension. Plasma and hepatic levels of ET are increased in patients with cirrhosis, particularly in those with ascites.[21, 22] The mechanisms responsible for increased ET production in cirrhosis are not known, but stimulation of ET production by transforming growth factor-β, TNF, or fluid-mechanical stress has been suggested.[21]

Although mainly studied with respect to a potential role in arterial vasodilation in portal hypertension, NO also has been implicated in the modulation of dynamic intrahepatic resistance elements and may have a major function in the regulation of the intrahepatic portal circulation in health and disease. Available evidence points strongly to a state of relative NO deficiency within the cirrhotic liver, as a result of sinusoidal endothelial cell dysfunction.[20, 37, 43] NO deficiency in cirrhotic liver may have important consequences, resulting not only in impaired relaxation of contractile resistance elements, but also in loss of other important protective effects of NO, including antifibrogenic and antithrombotic effects.[37] Hepatic NO deficiency in cirrhosis may therefore serve to promote the variety of mechanisms responsible for increased hepatic resistance (Fig. 77–3).

PORTOCOLLATERAL RESISTANCE. In advanced portal hypertension, the collateral circulation may carry over 90% of the

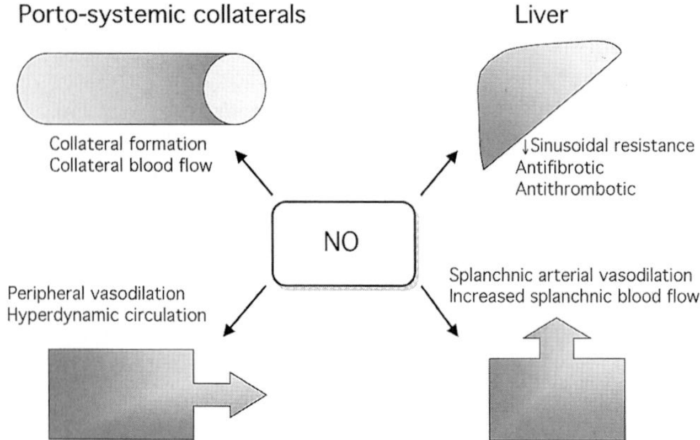

Figure 77–3. The central role of nitric oxide (NO) in the circulatory disorder of portal hypertension. A relative deficiency of NO in the cirrhotic liver leads to increased microcirculatory (sinusoidal) resistance to blood flow. Loss of the antithrombotic and antifibrogenic effects of NO also contributes to increased intrahepatic vascular resistance. In the systemic and splanchnic arterial beds, NO overproduction leads to vasodilation, increased arterial blood flow, a hyperdynamic circulation, and increased portal venous inflow. Finally, NO appears to be involved in the development of portosystemic collateral vessels and the modulation of collateral vessel tone and resistance.

blood entering the portal system. Under these circumstances, it is obvious that the vascular resistance of collateral vessels may markedly influence the overall resistance to portal blood flow and therefore portal pressure.[37] The factors that modulate collateral resistance are not well characterized. Studies to date suggest that NO is also important in the formation of portosystemic collaterals and in reduction of the vascular tone of these vessels and hence their resistance to blood flow.[36, 37] Figure 77–3 summarizes the current view of the central hemodynamic role played by NO in portal hypertension.

An important vasoconstrictor role for serotonin, mediated by 5-hydroxytryptamine (5-HT_2) receptors in the splanchnic venous circulation, has also been demonstrated. In portal hypertensive animals and humans, the administration of the selective 5-HT_2 receptor blockers ketanserin and ritanserin has been shown to cause a significant decrease in portal pressure without modifying systemic hemodynamics or portal inflow, thereby suggesting that a dynamic element of portocollateral resistance is responsible in part for the elevated portal pressure.[10, 36]

ANATOMIC SITES OF COLLATERAL FORMATION AND BLEEDING

Varices

Spontaneous portosystemic collaterals develop in patients who have portal hypertension in a number of anatomic sites. The following are the major sites of collateral formation:

1. *The squamocolumnar epithelial junctions of the gastrointestinal tract.* It is at these sites that gastroesophageal varices (gastroesophageal junction) and hemorrhoids (anorectal junction) form in patients who have portal hypertension. Esophageal varices are the most important site of bleeding in portal hypertension and are supplied mainly by an enlarged coronary (left gastric) vein and by the short gastric veins arising from the splenic bed. Esophageal varices drain cephalad into the azygous vein, which is enlarged as a consequence with a considerable increase in blood flow.
2. *The recanalized umbilical vein that communicates with the paraumbilical plexus in the abdominal wall.* This occurrence gives rise to the physical signs of a caput medusae and a Cruveilhier-Baumgarten venous hum in the epigastrium.
3. *The retroperitoneum.* The veins of abdominal viscera are commonly in contact with the abdominal wall. Retroperitoneal collaterals frequently communicate with the left renal vein.
4. *Sites of previous abdominal surgery or intra-abdominal trauma.* Stomal varices surrounding a colostomy or ileostomy are an example of the latter.
5. *Various other sites in the gastrointestinal tract.* Sites include the duodenum, ileum, cecum, and rectum especially in patients who have had previous abdominal surgery.[55] Hemoperitoneum in patients who have portal hypertension rarely may result from spontaneous rupture of intraperitoneal varices[56] but is encountered more commonly as a complication of paracentesis.

Esophageal varices appear as serpentine venous channels that course through several levels from the lamina propria to the deep submucosa of the esophagus. They communicate via perforating veins with an extensive paraesophageal collateral circulation[57] (Fig. 77–4), achieve their greatest prominence, as a rule, 2 to 3 cm above the gastroesophageal junction, and in time may extend cephalad to the midesophagus. Factors invoked in this specific localization of esophageal varices include normal and abnormal pressure gradients in the vicinity of the lower esophageal sphincter.[4]

The next most common site for the formation of clinically significant varices is the stomach, either in obvious continuity with esophageal varices, that is, true gastroesophageal varices, or as free-standing gastric varices. Various classifications for the different locations of gastric varices have been proposed. The most simple, and practical, classifies type I gastric varices as those that appear as an inferior extension of esophageal varices; type II, as varices in the gastric fundus in continuity with esophageal varices; and type III, as isolated gastric varices in the fundus or body and antrum of the stomach without esophageal varices.[58] The appearances of gastric varices varies from a relatively subtle, bluish discoloration of otherwise normal appearing gastric mucosal folds to more obvious, classic cerebriform clusters of veins. There is considerable interobserver variation in the identification of gastric varices, and estimates of their prevalence in patients who have portal hypertension vary greatly. The largest study to date found gastric varices in 20% of patients who had portal hypertension from a variety of causes.[59] Factors that promote the formation of gastric varices are poorly understood. The notion that they arise more frequently in patients who have had endoscopic obliteration of esophageal varices has been noted by some, but not all, observers. Gastric fundal varices in the absence of esophageal varices should raise the suspicion of splenic vein throm-

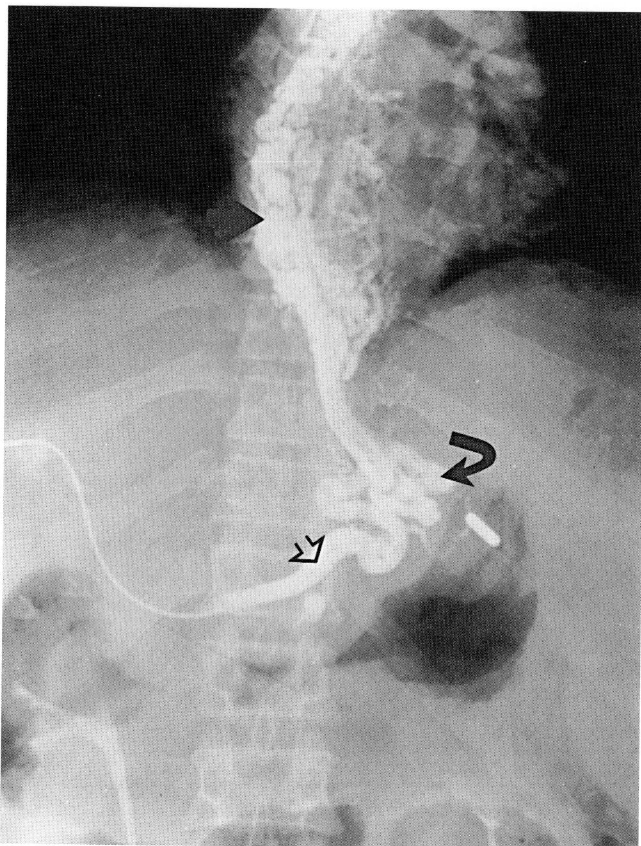

Figure 77–4. Transhepatic portal venogram illustrating esophageal and paraesophageal portosystemic collaterals. The right branch of the portal vein has been entered percutaneously and the catheter advanced into the coronary vein *(open arrow)*. Contrast injection illuminates the coronary vein and the extensive leash of esophageal varices in the area of the gastric fundus *(curved arrow)* and paraesophageal collateral veins draining cephalad toward the azygous vein *(solid straight arrow)*. This approach was used for the percutaneous transhepatic embolization of varices, an interventional therapy popular two decades ago that was abandoned because of its high failure rate and high frequency of portal vein thrombosis.

bosis, although in most cases fundal varices are simply a manifestation of portal hypertension caused by cirrhosis.[60]

Nonvariceal Mucosal Lesions

Portal hypertension is associated with a widespread abnormality in gastrointestinal mucosal microcirculatory integrity. Characterized as venous and capillary ectasia in the mucosa and submucosa with little associated inflammatory activity, this mucosal manifestation of portal hypertension has been studied most extensively in the stomach, where ectasia is manifested as portal hypertensive gastropathy.[61–64] Venous and capillary ectasia has been described to a lesser extent in the colon and other areas of the gastrointestinal tract.[65, 66] Portal hypertensive gastropathy is a common finding in patients who have portal hypertension.[62, 63] There is evidence for increased gastric mucosal blood flow,[64, 65, 67] but the importance of "passive" congestion from portal back pressure remains unclear. The primacy of portal hypertension in the pathogenesis of the gastropathy is demonstrated unequivocally by the cessation of bleeding from gastropathy after relief of portal hypertension by either surgical decompression[68] or beta-blockade.[69] Many abnormalities in gastric mucosal function in portal hypertensive gastropathy have been reported, but it is unclear whether these are secondary disturbances or whether they play an important primary role in the development of the condition. Relative hypochlorhydria with hypergastrinemia has been reported by some investigators. Although previous sclerotherapy has been noted by some authors to increase the risk of gastropathy,[62] there is little agreement on this point.[61]

Portal hypertensive gastropathy is often graded by endoscopic appearance from mild to severe, with mild gastropathy characterized by a mosaic or "snakeskin" pattern of erythema and severe gastropathy by a variety of morphologic characteristics including bright red punctate erythema, diffuse hemorrhagic lesions, and black or brown spots indicating submucosal hemorrhages.[58, 63, 64] The natural history of portal hypertensive gastropathy is highly variable; gastropathy may progress or remit spontaneously but is more often slowly progressive.[62, 63] Portal hypertensive gastropathy accounts for 8% to 20% of acute bleeding in patients who have portal hypertension and also has been identified as an important source of chronic blood loss.[61, 63]

Gastric antral vascular ectasia (GAVE), or "watermelon stomach," may occur with increased frequency in cirrhosis. The lesion may be confused with portal hypertensive gastropathy but shows little relation to portal hypertension and is not ameliorated by portal decompressive procedures.[70]

NATURAL HISTORY AND PROGNOSIS OF VARICEAL HEMORRHAGE

Determinants of Variceal Bleeding

The mechanisms by which varices rupture have not been fully elucidated. The "corrosion" hypothesis postulated that reflux of gastric acid injures the mucosa of the lower part of the esophagus with subsequent erosion into the submucosal varices. This theory has fallen out of favor in view of a lack of evidence to support increased gastroesophageal reflux in patients who have bleeding esophageal varices, acid-peptic damage to the lower esophageal mucosa after acute variceal hemorrhage, or any benefit of long-term H_2 receptor antagonist therapy in preventing variceal bleeding.

Attention has shifted to the "explosion" theory, in which the key event is an increase in variceal elastic wall tension to a critical level at which explosive rupture occurs.[4, 11, 71] Wall tension *(T)* in a varix varies as a function of the transmural pressure *(TP)*, vessel radius *(r)*, and wall thickness *(w)* as represented by LaPlace's law:

$$T = TP \cdot r/w$$

The wall tension T resists the expanding force $TP \cdot r/w$, and when the latter exceeds the former, rupture occurs. Esophageal varices rupture most commonly at or near the gastroesophageal junction, the area of the esophagus where the veins are most superficial and, therefore, least surrounded by supportive tissues. These properties encourage the progressive widening and wall thinning of varices at this site.

The explosion theory places considerable emphasis on

variceal size, wall thickness, and transmural pressure as risk factors for bleeding (Table 77–3).[72, 73] This emphasis appears justified. Several groups have confirmed that variceal size is an important risk factor for variceal bleeding,[4, 11, 72] and several systems for grading varices according to their size and the presence of so-called red signs have been proposed (Fig. 77–5). Red signs, including cherry red spots and red wale markings (longitudinal, raised, red streaks) are usually associated with the most advanced grade of varices and are thought to represent focal weaknesses, or "blowouts," in the variceal wall ("varices-on-varices"). They also clearly carry additional weight as risk factors for bleeding.[72]

The relationship between portal pressure and the risk of variceal rupture is more subtle. Although all patients who have variceal bleeding have increased portal pressure, there is no clear correlation between portal pressure and the risk of bleeding. However, several groups have confirmed that there is an important threshold phenomenon with respect to the portal pressure gradient (HVPG) and the risk of bleeding.[4, 11, 71] Thus, it is well recognized that varices rarely bleed below an HVPG of 12 mm Hg, but there is no direct correlation between the risk of bleeding and the HVPG above this threshold value. There may be a more quantitative relationship between pressure and risk of bleeding from varices that depends on where the pressure is measured (i.e., HVPG versus intravariceal pressure)[74, 75] and when it is measured in relation to an episode of acute variceal hemorrhage.[76] Furthermore, a reduction in HVPG of at least 20% by pharmacologic intervention appears to be as reliably predictive of a significant reduction in the risk of bleeding as is a reduction of the absolute HVPG below the 12–mm Hg threshold.[75]

Inasmuch as they contribute to portal and intravariceal pressure, total blood volume and variceal collateral blood flow are two factors that also may contribute to the risk of variceal rupture. Variceal blood flow measured as total azygous vein blood flow has not shown a clear correlation with the risk of variceal bleeding. On the other hand, reduction of plasma volume with diuretics in patients who have portal hypertension lowers portal and variceal pressure,[77, 78] whereas expansion of intravascular volume may be a significant determinant of variceal hemorrhage and, in particular, ongoing acute bleeding. Intra-abdominal pressure clearly influences several hemodynamic variables in portal hypertension, but there is no convincing evidence that tense ascites per se, as opposed to decompensated liver disease, increases the risk of variceal bleeding.[79, 80]

Patients who have decompensated liver disease bleed more often and have a worse prognosis than patients who have compensated liver disease.[81, 82] The severity of the underlying liver disease (as assessed by the Child-Turcotte-Pugh class) correlates with variceal size[83] (see Table 77–3), appears to be an important independent predictor of variceal hemorrhage, and may influence bleeding risk via several other factors, including poor nutritional state and worsening coagulopathy.[84, 85] The North Italian Endoscopic Club[72] studied 321 patients with cirrhosis who had esophageal varices that had not yet bled and calculated an index using three variables: Child's class, size of varices, and presence of "red

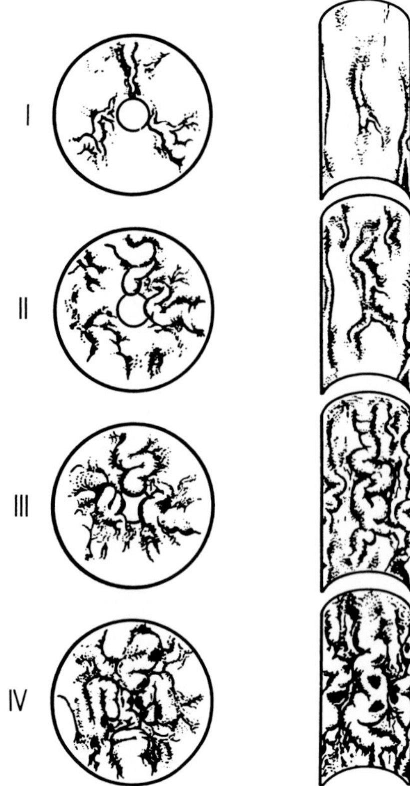

Figure 77–5. Endoscopic grading of esophageal varices according to Paqet.[73] Grade I: small varices without luminal prolapse; grade II: moderate-sized varices showing luminal prolapse with minimal obscuring of the gastroesophageal junction; grade III: large varices showing luminal prolapse substantially obscuring the gastroesophageal junction; grade IV: very large varices completely obscuring the gastroesophageal junction. The presence of red signs *(black spots)* is noted separately. (From Paquet, KJ: Prophylactic endoscopic sclerosing treatment of the esophageal wall in varices: A prospective controlled trial. Endoscopy 14:4, 1982.)

Table 77–3 | **Determinants of Variceal Bleeding**

Local Factors			
Variceal size, vessel radius			
Variceal wall thickness, red signs			
Hemodynamic Factors			
Portal (intravariceal) pressure: threshold HVPG of 12 mm Hg			
Blood volume			
Collateral blood flow (?)			
Intra-abdominal pressure (?)			
Severity of Liver Disease (Child-Turcotte-Pugh Class)			
	Numerical score		
Parameter	1	2	3
Ascites	None	Slight	Moderate/severe
Encephalopathy	None	Slight/moderate	Moderate/severe
Bilirubin (mg/dL)	<2.0	2–3	>3.0
Albumin (mg/L)	>3.5	2.8–3.5	<2.8
Prothrombin time (seconds increased)	1–3	4–6	>6.0
Total numerical score		***Child-Turcotte-Pugh class***	
5–6		A	
7–9		B	
10–15		C	
Other			
Continued alcohol abuse (?)			
Use of salicylates and nonsteroidal anti-inflammatory agents			
Bacterial infection			

HVPG, hepatic venous pressure gradient.

wale" markings. Over a 2-year follow-up period, patients with the lowest score (mild hepatic dysfunction, small varices, no red markings) had a 6% risk of variceal bleeding, whereas those with the highest scores (poor liver function, large varices, and many red signs) had a risk of bleeding of 76%.

Spontaneous regression of varices may occur in alcoholic patients who are strictly abstinent from alcohol,[86] and continued alcohol abuse has long been held to play a role in promoting the risk of variceal bleeding in patients with alcoholic cirrhosis. Oddly, this relationship has been surprisingly difficult to prove.[79, 87] On the other hand, suspicions relating to a role for aspirin and nonsteroidal anti-inflammatory drugs in the precipitation of portal hypertensive bleeding have been substantiated,[88] and patients who have portal hypertension are best advised to avoid these agents.

An interesting hypothesis by Goulis and colleagues[89] postulates that bacterial infections in patients who have variceal hemorrhage may be a critical factor that triggers bleeding. They suggest that the release of endotoxin into the systemic circulation during episodes of bacterial infection results in a further increase in portal pressure through the induction of ET and possibly vasoconstrictive cyclooxygenase products. Furthermore, endotoxin-induced NO and prostacyclin could inhibit platelet aggregation, thereby possibly leading to a further deterioration of primary hemostasis at the level of the varix.

Risk of Bleeding from Other Sites

Gastric varices located in the fundus, whether isolated or in continuity with esophageal varices, carry a particularly high risk of bleeding.[58, 59] In patients who have portal hypertensive gastropathy, bleeding occurs more commonly with more severe grades of gastropathy; mild or chronic bleeding occurs in one third of patients who have mild gastropathy and 90% of patients who have severe gastropathy. Overt bleeding occurs in 30% of those who have mild gastropathy and 60% of those who have severe gastropathy.[64]

Natural History of Variceal Bleeding

Gastroesophageal varices develop in 50% to 60% of cirrhotic patients, and approximately 30% of them experience an episode of variceal hemorrhage within 2 years of the diagnosis of varices.[71, 82] Variceal bleeding accounts for 2% to 20% of all upper gastrointestinal hemorrhage in Western series but for a much higher proportion of patients (50%) who have severe, persistent bleeding.[90, 91]

The greatest risk of initial variceal bleeding is within a 6- to 12-month period after their discovery. Beyond this time, the risk of bleeding tends to diminish in those who have not already bled.[11, 92] A diurnal periodicity of variceal bleeding has been noted by several groups; bleeding episodes tend to occur in the early morning and late evening.[92] After a variceal bleed, the risk of rebleeding is particularly high, approximately 60% to 70% over a 24-month period. The risk of rebleeding is greatest, however, within hours or days after an acute bleed.[81, 91, 92] Once bleeding has occurred, a number of factors that increase the risk of early rebleeding have been identified. These factors include bleeding from gastric varices, thrombocytopenia, encephalopathy, a diagnosis of alcoholic cirrhosis, large varices, active bleeding at the time of diagnostic endoscopy, and a high HVPG.[59, 76, 81, 92]

McCormick and colleagues[92] have suggested that secondary hemodynamic changes in the splanchnic circulation after a bleed may contribute to the risk of further bleeding. These changes include an increase in portocollateral resistance after hypotension, increased splanchnic blood flow stimulated by blood in the gut, and an increase in PVP as a result of overzealous volume expansion during resuscitation. The net effect of these changes is to "overshoot" the portal pressure and blood flow during resuscitation, thereby encouraging continued variceal bleeding.

Prognosis

Variceal hemorrhage is the most serious complication of portal hypertension and accounts for approximately one fifth to one third of all deaths in cirrhotic patients.[12, 79, 90, 91] The mortality rate after a variceal bleed ranges from 40% to 70% in various series, with an average of approximately 50% within 6 weeks.[79] As noted by several authors, this high early mortality rate may have a profound effect on survival in therapeutic trials depending on the interval between the patient's presentation with bleeding and inclusion in the study.[79, 82] The high early mortality rate also has been the prime motivation for the development of prophylactic therapy. The most important determinant of survival is the patient's level of hepatic function. The prognosis associated with variceal bleeding is generally much better in patients without significant liver impairment, such as those with noncirrhotic portal vein thrombosis or idiopathic portal hypertension.[18, 93] In cirrhotic patients, the prognosis is also worse in the presence of concomitant alcoholic hepatitis, hepatocellular carcinoma, or portal vein thrombosis.[94–96]

DIAGNOSIS

The initial presentation of portal hypertension may be accompanied by gastrointestinal hemorrhage or by other signs of liver disease. Congestive gastropathy may appear with iron deficiency anemia. An initial presentation with acute bleeding in an otherwise healthy appearing person is typical in patients who have prehepatic portal hypertension, as from portal vein thrombosis[93] or schistosomiasis[16]; patients who have cirrhosis or postsinusoidal portal hypertension (e.g., Budd-Chiari syndrome) more often exhibit other signs of advanced liver disease, including ascites, hepatic encephalopathy, jaundice, spider angiomas, and coagulopathy.[91]

Clinical or laboratory evidence of liver disease in a patient who has gastrointestinal bleeding should raise the possibility of portal hypertension as the cause. In nonbleeding, hemodynamically stable patients who have portal hypertension, the skin may be warm, the pulse rapid, and systemic blood pressure low, often in the range of 100 to 110 mm Hg systolic. The presence of splenomegaly, dilated abdominal wall veins, or the rarely encountered epigastric Cruveilhier-Baumgarten venous hum or caput medusae is a useful clue. The presence of hepatomegaly is variable and depends on the cause and stage of the underlying liver disease. Splenomegaly secondary to portal hypertension usually is associated with hypersplenism; a low platelet count is the earliest manifestation. Distinguishing portal hypertensive splenomegaly and hypersplenism caused by a primary hematologic disorder is usually straightforward when the clinical, laboratory, and radiologic evidence of liver disease and portal hypertension is unequivocal. Portal vein thrombosis occurs most frequently as a complication of portal hypertension but also may occur as a complication of myeloproliferative disorders and inherited or acquired hypercoagulable states.[93]

Endoscopy

Bleeding from esophageal varices usually occurs with hematemesis and melena; less frequently melena or hematochezia alone occurs. The standard diagnostic approach to patients who have acute gastrointestinal bleeding is discussed in Chapter 13. Endoscopy is undertaken after initial hemodynamic resuscitation and is essential for the precise diagnosis of the type of bleeding as well as initiation of endoscopic therapy. Although patients with cirrhosis can and do bleed as a result of sources other than portal hypertension, at least 60% to 80% of bleeding episodes in these patients are from esophageal varices. Approximately 7% of episodes are from gastric varices, and 5% to 20% are from congestive gastropathy. Peptic ulcer, Mallory-Weiss tears, and other sources account for the remaining cases.[61, 63, 91, 97]

Endoscopy often requires endotracheal intubation when patients have severe hepatic decompensation and altered mental status. At endoscopy, bleeding may be attributed to varices if any of the following is seen: a nonpulsatile venous spurt of active bleeding, venous ooze, or clot adherent to a varix. In the absence of these signs, varices are implicated as the source of recent bleeding only in the reliable absence of other lesions to account for bleeding.[97]

Imaging Studies

Imaging studies are useful in patients who have portal hypertension for elective diagnosis and for the more precise definition of portal venous anatomic features before surgical or interventional procedures. Duplex-Doppler ultrasonography is the initial procedure of choice because of its low cost and ability to provide sophisticated information. Pertinent findings in portal hypertension may include increased hepatic echogeneity, splenomegaly, a dilated portal vein, thrombotic occlusion or cavernous transformation of the portal vein, collaterals, and gallbladder wall thickening.[12, 98] In addition, information on the direction and velocity of portal flow is obtained.[26] The venous phase of visceral angiography is quite valuable for the more precise definition of portal anatomic characteristics, particularly if portal vein occlusion is diagnosed by the less invasive ultrasonographic approach. Computed tomography (CT) and magnetic resonance imaging (MRI) are rarely useful in the primary investigation of portal hypertension, but MR angiography[99] is used increasingly for the noninvasive investigation of portal venous system patency, particularly in patients with renal compromise in whom it is desirable to avoid radiographic contrast medium.

Pressure Measurement

Measurement of portal pressure is rarely indicated in the everyday clinical diagnosis of portal hypertension, which most often rests on the identification of varices or other collaterals and a compatible cause. Portal pressure measurement is most often used in hemodynamic and therapeutic research studies and has a role in clinical practice that is confined largely to the assessment of the adequacy of portal pressure reduction by pharmacologic agents or shunt procedures.[13, 14, 75, 100] Many approaches to portal pressure measurement have been described.[3, 4, 74] With the exception of newer techniques for endoscopic measurement of intravariceal pressure,[74] most approaches are relatively invasive, and their use is rarely justified. Both HVPG measurement[75] and noninvasive measurement of variceal pressure with a surface transducer[74] have been reported to aid in predicting the risk of bleeding and guiding therapeutic decisions in patients who have varices. These techniques require specialized equipment and considerable expertise, and more data on cost-effectiveness are needed before they can be adopted for more routine use in clinical practice. HVPG remains a useful tool for the investigation of the occasional patient in whom the diagnosis or cause of portal hypertension remains uncertain.

MANAGEMENT

Principles and Goals of Management

Acute bleeding from varices or nonvariceal sites in a patient who has portal hypertension often poses a life-threatening medical emergency. Prompt and appropriate hemodynamic resuscitation should be followed by implementation of measures aimed at arresting and preventing the recurrence of bleeding. The main goals of therapy for portal hypertensive bleeding are (1) prevention of the initial bleeding episode, (2) control of acute hemorrhage, and (3) prevention of recurrent variceal bleeding, while minimizing morbidity and not limiting the performance of future liver transplantation in potential candidates. The major therapies available for the achievement of these goals rely on one of two fundamental approaches: lowering of portal pressure or local obliteration

Table 77–4 | **Goals and Principles of Managing Variceal Hemorrhage**

Goals of Management
Prevent first bleed
Control acute bleeding
Prevent recurrent bleeding
Principles of Management
Reduce portal pressure
Pharmacologic therapy
Surgical or interventional (TIPS) shunts
Local control, obliteration of varices
Balloon tamponade
Endoscopic sclerotherapy
Endoscopic ligation (banding)
Surgical devascularization (transection, Sugiura procedure)

TIPS, transjugular intrahepatic portosystemic shunt.

of the varices (Table 77–4). The goal of preventing or delaying the initial bleed from portal hypertension arises from an appreciation of the considerable mortality rate associated with this bleed.[79] Realization of this goal has been difficult to achieve because it requires not only safe and effective treatment, but also an aggressive approach to the diagnosis of portal hypertension and esophageal varices in patients with liver disease who have never bled and who may be asymptomatic.

The following section considers the techniques, clinical outcomes, and complications of endoscopic therapy, pharmacologic treatment, balloon tamponade, surgical therapy, and TIPS, with emphasis on recent advances. Finally, a general approach to the management of bleeding in portal hypertension is outlined.

Overview of the Principles and Techniques of the Major Treatment Modalities

Endoscopic Therapy

Endoscopy is the cornerstone of the management of gastrointestinal hemorrhage both as a diagnostic and as a therapeutic modality. Once esophageal varices are identified as the source or likely source of bleeding, endoscopic options for treatment include injection sclerotherapy and variceal band ligation. Although these techniques do not treat the underlying portal hypertension, they have been shown to be effective in controlling variceal hemorrhage.[101, 102] The rates of success and complications of these endoscopic techniques depend in part on the experience of the operator and the technique employed.

ENDOSCOPIC SCLEROTHERAPY. A variety of techniques have been employed in performing endoscopic sclerotherapy (EST) with the goal of arresting acute bleeding and preventing recurrent bleeding through the obliteration of varices by repeated injections. Injections may be directed into the veins (intravariceal injection) or into the esophageal wall adjacent to the variceal channels (paravariceal injection). Both techniques are effective, but intravariceal injection is more widely employed.[101, 103] Additionally, several different sclerosants are available, including 5% sodium morrhuate, 1% to 3% sodium tetradecyl sulfate (used in the United States), 5% ethanolamine oleate, 0.5% to 1% polidocanol (used in Europe), and absolute alcohol. Adhesives such as *N*-butyl-2-cyanoacrylate (tissue glue) have been used successfully.[104] An optimal sclerosant for EST has not emerged; however, there are potentially important differences among these agents. For example, 1.5% sodium tetradecyl sulfate may be associated with more local ulceration and stricturing than polidocanol or ethanolamine oleate.[105] The optimal volume of sclerosant to inject during a single session of EST is controversial. Typically 1 to 2 mL of sclerosant is used per injection and total volumes in the range of 10 to 15 mL seem to be optimal with regard to efficacy and safety.

The appropriate interval for performing follow-up EST after control of the initial hemorrhage also remains somewhat arbitrary. After the initial injection to control bleeding, a follow-up session 2 to 3 days later is common practice, usually followed by weekly or biweekly procedures until variceal obliteration is achieved. Thereafter, surveillance for reappearance of varices is usually conducted at intervals that extend from 1 month to 3 months and then 6 months. However, EST may be performed according to a variety of schedules, depending on patient tolerance, response to EST, and the development of sclerotherapy ulcers or other complications.

ENDOSCOPIC VARICEAL LIGATION. The relatively high frequency of complications after EST (discussed later) led to the development of an alternative endoscopic therapy, endoscopic variceal ligation (EVL), also referred to as *variceal banding*.[101, 102] This technique was developed on the basis of principles established for the banding of hemorrhoids and involves the placement of elastic O ring ligatures on the varices, thereby causing strangulation of the veins (Fig. 77–6). The original EVL device allowed only one band placement at a time, and the endoscope had to be removed to reload a new band after each ligation. Consequently, a plastic overtube was required to facilitate repeated esophageal intubation. Newer multiple-band devices have now replaced the original single-band device, thereby allowing the deployment of 6 to 10 rubber bands with a single esophageal

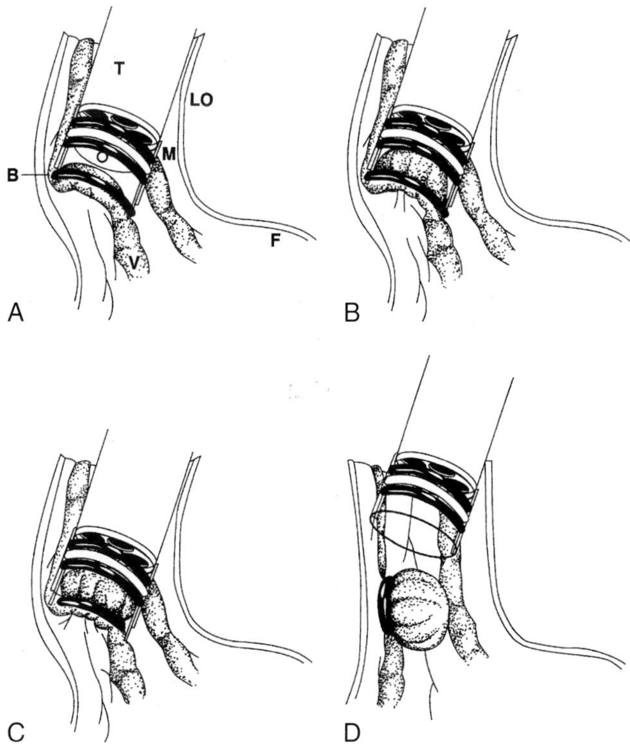

Figure 77–6. Band ligation of esophageal varices using the multishot band technique. *A,* Approximation of the endoscope tip mounted with the multiband ligator until there is full contact with the varix. *B,* Suction of the esophageal mucosa, submucosa, and the varix. *C,* Displacement of the rubber band by pulling the trip wire. *D,* Strangulation of the varix with the rubber band. The endoscope is now ready to band other varices. (From Helmy A, Hayes PC: Review article: Current endoscopic therapeutic options in the management of variceal bleeding. Aliment. Pharmacol Ther 15:575, 2001.) B, a rubber band; F, fundus of stomach; LO, lower esophagus; M, esophageal mucosa; T, tip of the endoscope; V, varix.

intubation. Despite the improved technology, the use of EVL in the actively bleeding patient is still challenging because the plastic cylinder that carries the bands at the tip of the endoscope limits the operator's field of vision. EVL is typically begun at the level of the gastroesophageal junction with additional bands deployed proximally. An endoscopic technique for EVL reported in 1999 that preserves the operator's field of vision and employs detachable snares awaits further evaluation.[106]

Complications of Endoscopic Therapy

ENDOSCOPIC SCLEROTHERAPY. Although sclerotherapy provides effective treatment for variceal hemorrhage, EST is associated with a variety of complications, some of which can be disastrous. These risks must be borne in mind when the decision to utilize sclerotherapy is taken. Minor complications, including chest pain, temporary dysphagia, fever, and small pleural effusions, are common and usually not serious. Although esophageal ulcers are seen in most treated patients, most such ulcers are uncomplicated. However, recurrent bleeding from mucosal ulceration occurs in up to 20% of patients. Esophageal strictures leading to dysphagia are seen in approximately 15% of patients, although the frequency and severity of this complication vary widely. Proton pump inhibitors are probably the most effective treatment for esophageal ulcer, and also are recommended for prophylactic use to prevent both ulcers and strictures after EST.[107]

Uncommon but serious complications of EST include bacterial peritonitis, esophageal perforation, mediastinitis, brain abscess, spinal cord paralysis, and pericarditis. Rarely, portal vein thrombosis has followed EST and has compromised subsequent liver transplantation. Whether or not obliteration of esophageal varices increases the risk of bleeding from portal hypertensive gastropathy remains controversial.[62, 64] Actively bleeding patients are at increased risk of aspiration pneumonia during EST, which can potentially be prevented by endotracheal intubation of patients whose ability to protect their airway is impaired.

ENDOSCOPIC VARICEAL LIGATION. Although EVL requires the same sedation and analgesia required for EST, it was hoped that this new technique would produce fewer systemic and local complications. Indeed, esophageal strictures, bleeding from treatment-induced ulcers, pulmonary infection, bacterial peritonitis, and death have all been reported less commonly with EVL than with EST, although in one meta-analysis, only the reduced frequency of esophageal stricture reached statistical significance.[103] Currently, the use of multiple-band ligators has prevented the complications induced by an overtube, such as esophageal tears resulting from trapping of mucosa between the overtube and the endoscope.[108]

Pharmacologic Therapy

A variety of pharmacologic agents are available for the treatment of acute hemorrhage as well as for prophylactic therapy.[10, 13, 109] Theoretically ideal, pharmacologic therapy is relatively inexpensive, is not operator-dependent, and can be administered at any time of the day. The combination of different pharmacologic agents, as well as their adjunctive use with endoscopic therapy, remains an important area of ongoing investigation. Drugs that are currently in common use include beta-blockers, long-acting nitrates, vasopressin with or without nitroglycerin, terlipressin, and somatostatin or octreotide. Several other drugs also have been studied, but their efficacy in the clinical setting is unproved or their use is still confined to experimental studies (Table 77–5).

Table 77–5 | **Principles of Pharmacologic Therapy for Portal Hypertension**

HEMODYNAMIC DISTURBANCE	PHARMACOLOGIC PRINCIPLE	EXAMPLES
Increased blood volume	Diuretic	Spironolactone* Furosemide*
Increased cardiac output	Sympatholytic	Beta-blockers (β_1 blocking effects)
Splanchnic arteriolar vasodilation	Vasoconstrictor	Vasopressin Somatostatin and octreotide Beta-blockers (β_2-blocking effects)
Increased hepatic and collateral resistance (venoconstriction)	Vasodilator (increased NO production)	Short-acting nitrates (nitroglycerin) Long-acting nitrates (isosorbide-5-mononitrate) Prazosin* Clonidine* Molsidomine* Serotonin 5-HT_2 receptor antagonists*
Increased variceal blood flow	Increase in lower esophageal sphincter tone by prokinetic agents	Metoclopramide* Domperidone*

*Data on clinical efficacy are limited.
5-HT, 5-hydroxytryptamine; NO, nitric oxide.

Drugs used in the treatment of portal hypertension exert their effect by reducing portal inflow or reducing intrahepatic or collateral resistance. Other less validated but readily available drugs may reduce collateral blood flow by increasing lower esophageal sphincter tone or reducing circulating plasma volume (see Table 77–5). As discussed earlier, varices rarely bleed when the portosystemic pressure gradient, or HVPG, is less than 12 mm Hg.[4] Although this degree of reduction of portal pressure cannot always be achieved by pharmacologic means, it has been demonstrated that a 20% decrease in the pressure gradient from its baseline value reduces the risk of variceal rebleeding significantly.[10, 75, 100]

Transjugular Intrahepatic Portosystemic Shunt

Attempts to devise a less invasive approach to portal decompression led to the development of a nonsurgical shunt, the TIPS.[14] The potential advantages of this technique include avoidance of general anesthesia, decreased procedural morbidity and mortality rates, and avoidance of surgery in the region of the hepatic hilum, which may be important in potential liver transplantation candidates.

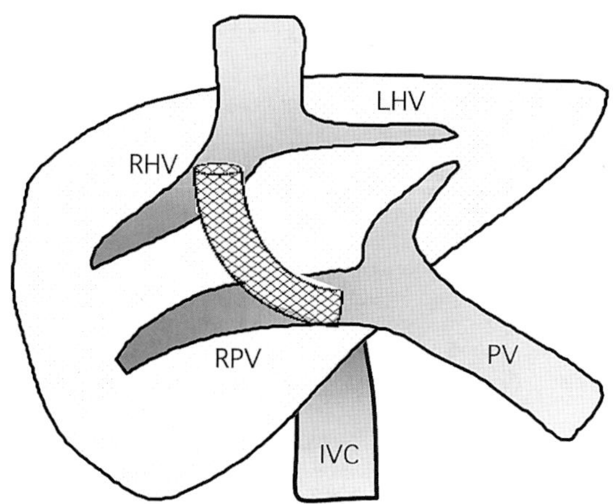

Figure 77–7. Schematic representation of a TIPS shunt in situ. See text for description of technique. A metal mesh stent is shown placed within a parenchymal tract joining the right hepatic vein with the right portal vein. (IVC, inferior vena cava; LHV, left hepatic vein; PV, portal vein; RHV, right hepatic vein; RPV, right portal vein.)

A percutaneous method of creating a portosystemic shunt was first conceived in the late 1960s. Although technically successful, the shunts were short-lived, and all thrombosed within a few days. The development of expandable, implantable metallic stents provided a means, albeit imperfect, for maintaining shunt patency and allowed the widespread clinical implementation of this technique. The use of the flexible Wallstent endoprosthesis (Schneider, Minneapolis, MN) and several technical modifications have reduced procedure times to the range of 1 to 3 hours.[110, 111] Although a TIPS can be created successfully in over 95% of patients, considerable operator skill and experience in vascular and hepatobiliary interventional procedures are required.

A schematic representation of the TIPS principle is shown in Figure 77–7. There are minor variations in the technique among centers, and a variety of stents are in use. In brief, the technique employed at the University of California, San Francisco, is as follows: with the patient under sedation and analgesia, the right internal jugular vein is punctured percutaneously, and a vascular sheath is advanced into the inferior vena cava and then into a hepatic vein. Next, a Colapinto transjugular needle is advanced through the sheath caudally and anteriorly into the liver parenchyma. Portal vein puncture is detected by aspiration of blood and confirmed by injection of contrast medium. The portal pressure is measured after a branch of the portal venous system is entered. Subsequently, a guidewire is introduced and manipulated into the main portal vein. The needle is removed, an angioplasty balloon catheter is advanced over the guidewire, and the tract between the hepatic and portal veins is dilated. An 8- or 10-mm-diameter expandable metallic Wallstent is then deployed across the tract, with care taken to prevent intrusion of the stent into the portal vein or inferior vena cava in a manner that might compromise subsequent liver transplantation surgery. Portal venography is then repeated, and postshunt portal and vena caval pressures are determined. A representative venogram before and after TIPS is shown in Figure 77–8.

Ideally, the portal vein–inferior vena cava gradient is decreased to less than 12 mm Hg, the threshold below which varices rarely bleed. However, achieving this hemodynamic goal is not always possible with the relatively small stents used in the TIPS procedure. Typically, portal decompression is judged adequate if the gradient falls to 15 mm Hg or lower and varices can no longer be demonstrated radiographically after injection of contrast medium into the splenic vein. When the gradient remains greater than 15 mm Hg or variceal flow persists, the stent is expanded to 10 or 12 mm in diameter, and, if necessary, a second parallel shunt is placed and the varices embolized with coils or alcohol. Patients are then monitored closely for bleeding for 12 to 24 hours. A Doppler ultrasonographic examination is performed the day after TIPS to assess patency of the shunt.

The indication and contraindications to TIPS are shown in Table 77–6. TIPS should not be performed in patients who have polycystic liver disease or cholangiohepatitis with intrahepatic bile duct dilation because of the high risk of traversing a cyst or bile duct, respectively. Like all portosystemic shunts, TIPS acutely increases right-sided cardiac pressure and therefore should not be performed in patients who have right-sided heart failure or primary pulmonary hypertension. Relative contraindications to TIPS include biliary obstruction, active intrahepatic or systemic infection, severe hepatic encephalopathy, and portal vein thrombosis.

Complications of Transjugular Intrahepatic Portosystemic Shunt

Procedural complications are generally seen in 10% or fewer patients after TIPS.[112] Severe life-threatening bleeding has been reported in 1% to 2% of cases because of either puncture of the liver capsule with resulting hemoperitoneum or inadvertent puncture of the biliary tree with resulting hemobilia. Other major complications include contrast medium–induced renal failure, heart failure, stent migration, fever, infection, transient arrhythmias, and inadvertent puncture of the gallbladder or other organs adjacent to the liver. Hemolysis, which is typically self-limited and mild, is not uncommon after TIPS.[14]

Although procedural complications are relatively infrequent, hepatic encephalopathy is a common complication after TIPS, with a frequency in the range of 20% to 30%.[113–115] This figure is not unexpected: TIPS represents a side-to-side portosystemic shunt that often results in complete diversion of portal flow, as well as a proportion of hepatic arterial blood flow, into the shunt (hepatofugal flow).

Related to post-TIPS encephalopathy, but much more ominous, is the development of accelerated liver failure after TIPS as a result of a critical loss of hepatic perfusion. A retrospective study at the University of California, San Francisco, noted clinically significant increases in serum bilirubin or alanine aminotransferase levels or prolongation of the prothrombin time in over one fourth of patients after TIPS.[116] This deterioration in liver function is typically transient, but in a minority (about 5%) of patients progressive liver failure develops leading to expedited liver transplantation or death. Determining the natural history of liver function after TIPS will be an important challenge in the years to come and will be important for the understanding of the long-term utility of TIPS as well as for optimal patient selection.

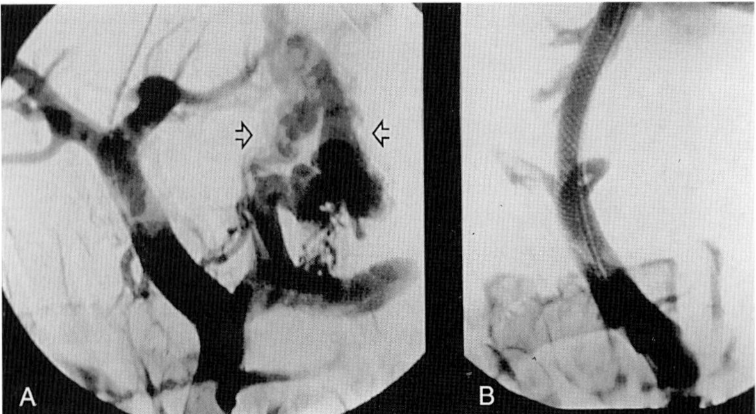

Figure 77–8. Total portal diversion after TIPS. *A*, Portal venogram before TIPS shows filling of large esophageal varices *(arrows)*. *B*, After insertion of an 8-mm TIPS, flow to varices is eliminated. Intrahepatic portal vein flow is now reversed, and the direction of intrahepatic flow is toward the TIPS. (From LaBerge JM, Ring EJ, Lake JR, et al: Transjugular intrahepatic portosystemic shunts: preliminary results in 25 patients. J Vasc Surg 16:258, 1992.)

The 30-day mortality rate after TIPS varies from 3% to 44% but is typically in the range of 10% to 15%.[110, 111, 115–123] Appropriate patient selection is the key to reducing the mortality rate after TIPS. Death after TIPS is usually related to decompensated hepatic function and is caused by liver failure, infection, renal insufficiency, or multisystem organ failure. The paradox is that patients in whom TIPS is most clearly indicated for refractory bleeding or ascites often have advanced liver disease and are at greatest risk of dying after the procedure. Identification of specific prognostic factors that will help identify patients at greatest risk of death after TIPS has therefore been undertaken in a number of studies,[116–122] as summarized in Table 77–7. Independent prognostic variables identified in these studies have been used to formulate models and nomograms that can be used to calculate risk scores and the probability of short-term mortality after TIPS.[120–122] Although this approach is clearly valuable, none of the predictive models published to date has been

Table 77–6 | **Transjugular Intrahepatic Portosystemic Shunt: Indications and Contraindications**

Indications
- Accepted indications
  - Control of refractory* acute variceal bleeding
  - Prevention of refractory* recurrent variceal bleeding in Child class B and C patients
  - Refractory† hepatic hydrothorax
  - Budd-Chiari syndrome
  - Refractory† ascites
- Promising but unproven
  - Hepatorenal syndrome
  - Veno-occlusive disease
- Unproven
  - Prevention of refractory* recurrent variceal bleeding in Child class A patients
  - Initial therapy of acute variceal hemorrhage
  - Initial therapy to prevent recurrent variceal hemorrhage
  - Prevention of initial variceal hemorrhage
  - Reduction in intraoperative morbidity rate during liver transplantation or other major surgery in patients with portal hypertension
  - Hepatopulmonary syndrome

Contraindications
- Absolute contraindications
  - Right-sided heart failure
  - Primary pulmonary hypertension
  - Polycystic liver disease
  - Severe hepatic failure
  - Portal vein thrombosis with cavernous transformation
- Relative contraindications
  - Biliary obstruction
  - Active intrahepatic or systemic infection
  - Severe hepatic encephalopathy poorly controlled by medical therapy
  - Portal vein thrombosis without cavernous transformation

*Refractory acute or recurrent variceal bleeding implies failure of medical treatment, including pharmacologic and endoscopic therapy, to control bleeding, or limitation of these therapies as a result of adverse effects, complications, or patient intolerance.

†Refractory ascites or hepatic hydrothorax implies the failure to control fluid retention by dietary salt restriction and high doses of diuretics, the need for frequent large-volume abdominal paracentesis or thoracentesis, or the limitation of these therapies by complications, most commonly compromised renal function or serum electrolyte disturbances.

Adapted from Bass NM: Role of TIPS in portal hypertension: Variceal bleeding and ascites. Technol Vasc Intervent Radiol 1:44, 1998.

Table 77–7 | **Predictors of Liver Failure and Mortality after Transjugular Intrahepatic Portosystemic Shunt**

REFERENCE	PROGNOSTIC VARIABLES IDENTIFIED
117†	Child-Turcotte-Pugh class C Hyponatremia
118†	Child-Turcotte-Pugh class C Urgent TIPS
116	Serum bilirubin level >10 mg/dL within the first month post TIPS PT ≥ 17 sec before TIPS Nonalcoholic cause of liver disease
119†	Child-Turcotte-Pugh class C Older age
122*	Moderate or severe ascites Need for ventilation Elevated WBC count Low platelet count Elevated PTT Elevated serum creatinine level
120†	TIPS performed as an emergency Serum bilirubin level >3 mg/dL
121‡	Elevated serum bilirubin level Elevated serum creatinine level Increased INR Nonalcoholic or noncholestatic cause of liver disease

*Included only patients treated for acute variceal bleeding.
†Predictors of 30-day mortality.
‡Components of the Model for End-Stage Liver Disease (MELD) (see Chapter 83).
INR, international normalized ratio; PT, prothrombin time; PTT, partial thromboplastin time; TIPS, transjugular portosystemic shunt; WBC, white blood cell.

validated independently and prospectively. They are best used currently to complement clinical judgment and to counsel patients and their families accordingly.

Another major problem that has limited the utility of TIPS is occlusion or stenosis of the shunt. Narrowing or occlusion of TIPS stents may occur as an early event secondary to thrombosis or more chronically over a period of weeks or months as a result of pseudointimal hyperplasia. The latter occurrence is the much more common cause of significant shunt insufficiency after TIPS. From 30% to 50% of cases of shunt insufficiency present with recurrent variceal hemorrhage or ascites; the remainder are discovered during routine monitoring, a practice necessitated by the high frequency of shunt dysfunction.[115, 124] The actuarial frequency of shunt insufficiency ranges from 30% to 50% at 12 months and 47% to 68% at 24 months.[115, 125–127] The higher frequencies of shunt insufficiency reported by some centers reflect, in part, a more aggressive approach to monitoring of TIPS patency with frequent venography, as well as classification of any narrowing as an abnormality. A more conservative and practical approach is to monitor shunt patency every 3 to 4 months by Doppler ultrasound, with venography performed when a suggestive ultrasonographic abnormality is found.[128] Such abnormalities include a reduction in mean peak flow velocity in the TIPS below 0.5 m/second, reversal of previous hepatofugal flow to hepatopetal flow, and reversal of flow in the stented hepatic vein. Useful venographic criteria for shunt insufficiency include narrowing of the lumen by 75% or more or a pressure gradient across the shunt of 15 mm Hg or higher.[124, 129]

The development of strategies to prevent shunt stenosis is the focus of active research. Potential strategies include pharmacologic approaches to reduce shunt intimal hyperplasia, the primary cause of stenosis, and engineering and testing of stents covered by selectively permeable materials like polytetrafluoroethylene.[14]

Surgical Treatments

SHUNT OPERATIONS. A variety of surgical shunts have been devised for control of variceal bleeding.[130, 131] Shunt operations traditionally have been classified as total, partial, or selective, on the basis of their intended impact on portal blood flow. Total shunts divert all portal blood flow into the inferior vena cava. The end-to-side portacaval shunt, which is the best example, involves transection of the portal vein at its bifurcation and creation of an anastomosis between the end of the portal vein and the side of the inferior vena cava, thereby diverting all portal flow. The side-to-side portacaval shunt differs in that the portal vein is not transected; rather a side-to-side anastomosis is created between the portal vein and inferior vena cava. This operation was designed to divert only part of the portal stream into the vena cava; the remainder, it was hoped, would continue to perfuse the liver. In reality, not only does the side-to-side portacaval shunt usually allow total diversion of portal blood flow into the lower pressure inferior vena cava, but it also may encourage reversal of portal venous flow with diversion of part of the hepatic arterial blood flow into the vena cava as well. This hepatic arterial steal has been recognized increasingly as a potential complication of all shunts that employ a side-to-side principle, including TIPS, and is believed to underlie the higher frequency of encephalopathy and hepatic decompensation seen with these types of shunt. Other surgical approaches to the side-to-side shunt have used large diameter interposition prosthetic H grafts.[132] An interposition shunt also can be performed by creating an anastomosis between the superior mesenteric vein and the inferior vena cava (mesocaval shunt). This operation has the advantage of avoiding the hepatic hilum and preserving the portal vein, which may be important in potential liver transplantation candidates. Nonselective and partial shunt operations are generally faster and easier to perform than selective shunt procedures and are often preferred to selective shunts in the emergency setting.

Another surgical alternative is the partial shunt. As noted earlier, variceal hemorrhage does not occur with a portal pressure gradient below 12 mm Hg. Therefore, partial decompression of the portal system below this threshold may prevent rebleeding while maintaining prograde or hepatopetal portal flow. This goal is typically achieved with the use of a small-diameter H graft between the portal vein or superior mesenteric vein and the inferior vena cava. One study showed that decreasing the diameter of the portacaval H graft from 16 to 20 mm to 8 mm led to maintenance of portal perfusion in most patients with a fall in the frequency of encephalopathy from 39% to 9%.[132] These observations were extended to a randomized trial that compared small-diameter partial shunts to large-diameter total shunts.[133] Both shunts were 100% effective in controlling hemorrhage. However, the partial shunts preserved hepatopetal flow in 90% of patients and were associated with a significantly lower frequency of encephalopathy.

The term *selective shunt* is used to describe a shunt that selectively decompresses variceal flow, while preserving portal blood flow. The distal splenorenal shunt (DSRS) was designed as a selective shunt to avoid the high rate of encephalopathy seen with total shunts. In this operation, the varices are decompressed by anastomosis of the splenic vein, which drains the varices via the short gastric veins, to the distal left renal vein. Meticulous ligation of the coronary vein and other collaterals is also performed to disconnect the main portal watershed from the azygous watershed. This procedure maintains prograde portal flow into the liver, although with time the shunt tends to reconnect with the portal vein, thereby losing its selective nature and becoming a partial or even a total shunt.[134] Indeed, studies comparing the DSRS with total shunts have yielded inconsistent results: three trials demonstrated a lower frequency of encephalopathy with the DSRS, and three trials showed no difference in the frequency of encephalopathy.[130, 135]

ESOPHAGEAL DEVASCULARIZATION. Direct surgical devascularization of the lower esophagus and stomach offers the potential for control of bleeding without the shunt-related complication of encephalopathy. Simple surgical variceal ligation with esophageal transection is an effective means of controlling acute variceal bleeding, but bleeding frequently recurs as additional varices develop. Improved long-term control of bleeding has been reported with the Sugiura operation, a more extensive procedure consisting of transthoracic paraesophageal devascularization, esophageal transection, splenectomy, esophagogastric devascularization, pyloroplasty, and vagotomy.[136, 137] Although excellent results have been achieved with this procedure in Europe and Asia, experience with this procedure in the United States is limited.

COMPLICATIONS OF SURGICAL TREATMENT FOR VARICEAL HEMORRHAGE. Encephalopathy is a major concern after portosystemic shunt surgery. Large-diameter shunts typically have been associated with a 20% to 50% rate of encephalopathy.[132] Although the risk of encephalopathy is probably lower with DSRS and partial shunts, all risk is not eliminated. In addition, DSRS is technically quite demanding and often associated with worsening ascites postoperatively. Diversion of portal blood flow is associated with accelerated progression of liver failure in some patients. These problems, combined with the perioperative morbidity rates associated with major surgery in patients with cirrhosis, mandate careful patient selection for these operations and avoidance of such procedures for patients who have advanced liver disease.[131]

Prophylaxis of Initial Variceal Hemorrhage

Pharmacologic Therapy

Nonselective beta-blockers (propranolol and nadolol) and long-acting nitrates have been studied extensively in attempts to prevent a first variceal hemorrhage.[10, 13, 109] These agents lower portal pressure by decreasing cardiac output via β_1 receptor blockade. In addition, β_2 receptor blockade leads to unopposed α-adrenergic activity, which results in splanchnic vasoconstriction and reduced portal pressure and variceal flow. The optimal end point of therapy remains controversial. Measurement of the HVPG is not done commonly in clinical practice. With beta-blocker therapy, a 25% decrease in the resting pulse rate from baseline is often used as a surrogate marker of efficacy; however, the validity of this end point as an indicator of portal pressure reduction has been questioned.[10]

Data are available from 11 trials that compared beta-blockers with placebo in a prevention of the first variceal hemorrhage.[109] Eight of these studies used propranolol, and three used nadolol. There was relative homogeneity among the studies, as all but one small trial showed a reduction in the frequency of a first bleed. This trial was atypical in that the bleeding rate for control subjects was only 8%. The rate of first variceal bleeds in patients taking beta-blockers (15%) was significantly less than that for patients taking placebo (25%). There was a smaller reduction in the mortality rate in the beta-blocker treated patients, but the difference was not statistically significant.[109] However, an earlier study in which the data of individual patients from four beta-blocker trials were pooled and analyzed found that death from bleeding was reduced significantly by beta-blocker therapy.[138] The authors found that 90% of patients in the beta-blocker group had not had a fatal hemorrhage at 2 years as compared with 82% of the control patients (p = .01). This study also demonstrated that, although beta-blockers were most effective in patients who had well-preserved liver function, they also had a protective effect in subjects who had ascites and advanced liver disease.

Several issues regarding the use of prophylactic drug therapy in portal hypertension need to be clarified. These issues include patient and drug selection as well as optimal drug dosing. Some, but not all, studies have suggested that patients with alcoholic liver disease and large varices are especially likely to benefit from this type of prophylactic therapy.[138, 139] A cost-effectiveness analysis in 1997, on the other hand, supports the use of propanolol as the most cost-effective therapy for primary prophylaxis of variceal bleeding in cirrhotic patients who have esophageal varices regardless of their Child's class and the risks of bleeding.[140] It is uncertain whether propranolol or nadolol is more effective than the other. Nadolol has become popular largely on the basis of its convenient once-a-day dosage regimen and lack of extensive hepatic metabolism.

On the basis of the available data, it is appropriate clinical practice to perform screening endoscopy in patients with cirrhosis to look for moderate to large varices and to treat these patients prophylactically with beta-blockers.[101] Whether to limit prophylactic therapy to a subset of cirrhotic patients (e.g., those who have a platelet count less than 88,000/mm^3) likely to have large varices is the subject of controversy and ongoing study.

Long-acting nitrates such as isosorbide-5-mononitrate also appear to be effective in preventing a first variceal bleed and may prove to be useful in patients intolerant of beta-blockers.[141] These agents produce venodilation by forming NO. They are believed to lower portal pressure through a combination of reducing splanchnic flow via venous pooling and reducing transhepatic sinusoidal resistance.[10] The potential benefit of isosorbide mononitrate used in combination with nadolol in the primary prophylaxis of variceal bleeding also has been evaluated in an Italian multicenter study, with a follow-up analysis of long-term treatment for up to 7 years.[142] Combination therapy was associated with a risk of first variceal bleeding less than one half that associated with nadolol alone (12% versus 29%), without causing deleterious side effects, de novo ascites, or a significant impact on survival.

Endoscopic Treatment

The utility of sclerotherapy for the primary prophylaxis of variceal hemorrhage has been investigated in a sizable number of studies but remains controversial.[101, 102] An early trial reported a lower frequency of variceal hemorrhage and higher survival rate with prophylactic EST than with conservative management.[73] However, meta-analyses have since identified marked heterogeneity among the large number of trials that followed this initial report, not only of study design and patient characteristics, but also in the impact of EST on bleeding and mortality rates.[101, 102] Although the pooled estimates show a benefit of EST in reducing the frequencies of bleeding and death, considerable study heterogeneity renders these data suspect. Indeed, the largest of these studies, the Veterans Administration Cooperative trial, showed an almost twofold increase in mortality rate in the patients who had prophylactic EST, a finding that led to early termination of the trial.[143] Although there was no clear explanation for the excess deaths in the EST group, the deaths appeared to have been associated with the use of EST. The lack of compelling evidence to support prophylactic EST, combined with the risk of procedure-related complications, make it an inappropriate therapeutic undertaking at this time.

The lower rate of associated complications makes EVL a potentially attractive option for prophylactic therapy. Although a few clinical trials have suggested a potential benefit of EVL over no treatment in reducing the risk of a first variceal bleed,[144, 145] it is the general consensus that beta-blocker therapy should be considered the standard of care for the prophylaxis of first variceal bleeding and that other therapeutic interventions should be compared with beta-blockers.[146] The efficacy of EVL relative to propanolol in the primary prophylaxis of first variceal bleeding was reported in 1999 by investigators in India.[147] The rate of first variceal bleeding at 18 months was significantly lower in the EVL group (15%) than in the propanolol group (43%). However, the rate of bleeding in the propanolol group was higher than the expected rate of approximately 20% according to pooled data from previous studies of propanolol for primary prophalaxis,[138] and the dose of propanolol used in this study was relatively low. Moreover, the preliminary results of a 1998 trial suggest that EVL confers no advantage over propanolol.[148] Until more conclusive data are available, a nonselective beta-blocker should remain the treatment of choice for the primary prevention of variceal hemorrhage among patients at high risk for variceal bleeding.

Shunt Surgery

Shunt surgery was compared with nonsurgical treatment in four trials in the 1960s and 1970s.[130, 131] Not surprisingly, bleeding was less common in patients randomized to surgical prophylaxis. However, rates of both encephalopathy and mortality were worse, and this approach was abandoned. A series in Japan found a reduced mortality rate with prophylactic devascularization or selective shunt surgery,[149] but these results have not been confirmed and must be questioned, because a variety of surgical procedures were employed and the mortality rate was unexpectedly high in the control group.

Transjugular Intrahepatic Portosystemic Shunt

There are no data to support the use of TIPS for the primary prophylaxis of variceal hemorrhage. Because TIPS requires technical expertise, can have serious adverse effects, and is expensive, at present TIPS should not be used for this indication.

Management of Acute Variceal Hemorrhage

Resuscitation

There is often great temptation to perform endoscopy immediately when a patient has massive bleeding. However, the need for adequate and careful resuscitation cannot be overemphasized. The principles of resuscitation in gastrointestinal hemorrhage are reviewed in Chapter 13. Several special issues pertain to the resuscitation of patients who have portal hypertension. These patients often have altered mental status as a result of hepatic encephalopathy, and airway protection with endotracheal intubation must be considered. Transfusion of platelets and fresh frozen plasma is often required to correct coagulopathy, in addition to transfusion of packed red blood cells to correct the volume deficit. Although resuscitation should be prompt and vigorous, volume overload should be avoided so as not to "overfill" the venous circulation and precipitate further bleeding.[92] It is currently widely recommended that all patients with cirrhosis who have acute gastrointestinal bleeding receive a short course of prophylactic antibiotics to lower the high risk of associated infection.[150] Typically, once the patient has a good urine output, stable blood pressure, improvement in tachycardia, adequate peripheral perfusion, and a hematocrit value of 25% to 30%, fluid administration can be reduced to maintenance levels.

Pharmacologic Therapy

Pharmacotherapy of acute variceal bleeding theoretically is an ideal approach to the treatment of acute variceal bleeding, because it is noninvasive, is immediately available, and does not require special technical expertise. The major agents used in this setting have been intravenous vasopressin and its analogs, with or without nitroglycerin, and somatostatin or its analog, octreotide (see Table 77–5).

VASOPRESSIN AND TERLIPRESSIN. Vasopressin is a potent but nonselective vasoconstrictor that has been used for many years in the treatment of variceal bleeding. Vasopressin lowers portal pressure by causing splanchnic arterial vasoconstriction and decreasing splanchnic blood flow. Vasopressin is typically given as a bolus, followed by a continuous intravenous infusion. However, this agent controls acute variceal hemorrhage in only about 50% of patients.[109] In addition, vasospastic side effects are seen in approximately 25% of patients on vasopressin, and the risk of myocardial infarction raises greatest concern. To reduce this risk and potentially to lower portal pressure further, nitroglycerin has been used in combination with vasopressin. The pharmacologic rationale for using nitroglycerin is that nitrates are believed to reduce collateral and possibly portohepatic resistance by increasing local concentrations of NO and causing vascular smooth muscle relaxation. Three trials have compared vasopressin alone with vasopressin plus a nitroglycerin preparation, and in each study there was a trend toward improved control of hemorrhage with combination therapy, as well as fewer side effects, thereby rendering monotherapy with vasopressin obsolete.[109] Another approach has been to use a vasopressin analog, triglycyl-lysine vasopressin (terlipressin [Glypressin]), which undergoes cleavage of the glycyl residues to allow a slow release of lysine-vasopressin. Although terlipressin has not been proved more efficacious than vasopressin, terlipressin has been associated with fewer side effects. This agent is unavailable in the United States at present.

SOMATOSTATIN AND OCTREOTIDE. Somatostatin and its longer-acting analog octreotide have generated a great deal of interest as pharmacologic treatments for variceal hemorrhage. These agents have a variety of physiologic actions, including inhibition of the release of several vasodilatory hormones such as glucagon and direct effects on vascular smooth muscle.[10] The net pharmacologic action of somatostatin is to induce splanchnic vasoconstriction selectively. The true impact of somatostatin and octreotide on portal hemodynamics remains controversial, and variable changes in portal pressure and intravariceal pressure in response to these drugs have been reported in different studies.[10, 109] However, both agents have been shown consistently to decrease azygous blood flow, a measure of blood flow through the varices. The optimal methods of administering these drugs remains to be determined; most authorities favor an initial intravenous bolus (somatostatin, 250 μg; octreotide, 50 μg) followed by a continuous infusion (somatostatin, 250 μg/hour; octreotide, 50 to 100 μg/hour).[151]

Three randomized, controlled trials have compared somatostatin with placebo.[152–154] One trial showed failure to control bleeding in 35% of patients treated with somatostatin compared with 59% of those treated with placebo.[152] By contrast, another trial showed no benefit to the use of somatostatin.[153] However, this study was quite atypical in having an 83% response rate to placebo. None of these trials showed any beneficial effect on survival.

Somatostatin has been compared with vasopressin in seven trials, with a trend toward a lower rate of failure to control bleeding with somatostatin (pooled odds ratio, 0.68; 95% CI, 0.45 to 1.04).[109, 135] In addition, there were significantly fewer complications with somatostatin. Three trials that compared somatostatin or octreotide with terlipressin showed no significant differences in either control of bleeding or mortality rate.[109]

An active area of investigation has been the comparison of these vasoconstrictor agents with endoscopic therapy. Several trials have suggested that somatostatin and octreotide are as effective as EST in controlling acute variceal hemorrhage.[109, 155, 156] For example, one trial that compared octreotide infusion with EST showed no differences in rates of mortality, control of hemorrhage, or transfusion.[155]

Another important use of somatostatin and octreotide is as an adjunct to endoscopic therapy of an actively bleeding patient to assist in the control of acute bleeding and the prevention of early rebleeding.[156, 157] The results of studies to date support a role for combination pharmacologic and endoscopic therapy, and it appears that these drugs may be safely used for longer periods (up to 5 or 7 days) than has traditionally been regarded as appropriate.[152, 157, 158] Long-term subcutaneous administration of octreotide for 15 days after an acute bleed also was shown to reduce rebleeding significantly at 42 days in a 1998 study.[159] Further studies are needed to confirm these results. On the other hand, long-acting octreotide has shown no benefit in preventing recurrent variceal bleeding to date.

In summary, vasopressin plus nitroglycerin, terlipressin, and somatostatin or octreotide all appear to be useful in the treatment of acute variceal hemorrhage. A beneficial side effect profile favors the use of somatostatin or octreotide. However, these agents are not universally available. Current opinion favors endoscopic therapy as first-line therapy for acute variceal hemorrhage, with pharmacologic therapy of particular value in patients who are too unstable for endoscopy or who have bleeding that is not immediately controlled by endoscopy and as a valuable adjunct to endoscopic therapy to prevent early rebleeding.

Balloon Tamponade

Balloon tamponade has been used for many years to diminish variceal flow and control bleeding by compressing the varices.[102, 160] Several different tubes are available for this purpose; tubes have a gastric balloon or both gastric and esophageal balloons. Balloon tamponade can control active bleeding in more than 90% of cases. However, on deflation of the balloons rebleeding occurs in a high proportion of patients. In addition, balloon tamponade may result in serious complications, including esophageal perforation, aspiration pneumonia, and rarely asphyxiation.

Because of the high rate of rebleeding when the balloon is deflated, as well as the high rate of complications, we view balloon tamponade as a temporizing measure in patients who have active, life-threatening hemorrhage that is refractory to endoscopic and pharmacologic therapy. If the patient remains hemodynamically unstable, it is appropriate to place a balloon to allow adequate resuscitation before more definitive therapy, such as surgery or TIPS, is undertaken. The quadruple-lumen Minnesota tube is regarded by many authorities as the safest type because the tube allows continuous aspiration of secretions above the esophageal balloon via a separate port. Patients should be intubated for airway protection before insertion of the tube, and the position of a partly inflated gastric balloon should be confirmed radiographically before full inflation. Of greatest importance, the tube should be placed by an experienced physician, the patient should be monitored continuously, and the tube should be removed at the earliest possible time, with continuous inflation for no more than 24 hours.

Endoscopic Therapy

It is difficult to compare trials of EST for acute variceal hemorrhage because the definition of acute hemorrhage is highly variable. However, several studies have shown that EST can achieve control of acute hemorrhage in 60% to 100% of patients, and most trials have demonstrated an effectiveness rate of approximately 90%.[101, 102] In addition, endoscopic therapy affords the opportunity to visualize the outcome of treatment immediately and to assess the need for adjunctive pharmacologic therapy. When compared with EST to alternative treatments, EST is generally more effective than balloon tamponade or vasopressin, but it may not be significantly better than infusion of either somatostatin[109] or octreotide[155] in the control of bleeding or in improving survival. Surgical shunts are more effective than EST in controlling active hemorrhage, but their use is associated with high morbidity and mortality rates, especially in advanced liver disease patients.[131] On the basis of diagnostic and therapeutic value and efficacy in stopping hemorrhage, EST is considered to be the treatment of choice for the management of active variceal hemorrhage. The major drawback to the use of EST in this setting is the potential for complications. A promising approach is the combined use of EST and drug therapy. In two 1995 trials in which a total of

299 patients were randomized to a 5-day infusion of octreotide in combination with either EST or EVL or to endoscopic therapy alone,[157, 158] the survival rate did not differ between the two groups, but octreotide was associated with a lower rate of early rebleeding in both trials. Combined endoscopic-pharmacologic therapy thus holds promise for reducing the high frequency of variceal rebleeding during the days immediately after an index bleed and should become the standard of practice if these results are confirmed.

As mentioned earlier, EVL is quite challenging in the setting of active hemorrhage, because the banding device significantly narrows the field of view. Nevertheless, randomized trials to date have found EVL to be equivalent to EST in controlling active hemorrhage (pooled odds ratio 1.14 [95% CI, 0.44 to 2.90]).[102]

Transjugular Intrahepatic Portosystemic Shunt

Approximately 10% of patients who exhibit an acute variceal hemorrhage require a TIPS when two sessions of endoscopic therapy within 24 hours fail to control the acute hemorrhage.[161] Several large series that have included patients who have active variceal hemorrhage, as well as series that specifically addressed this indication, have documented the efficacy of TIPS for acute variceal hemorrhage.[110, 111, 162, 163] Placement of a TIPS was successful in over 90% of patients. Common causes of failure to place the TIPS included preexisting portal vein thrombosis and anomalous hepatic vein anatomic features. The gradient between the portal vein and hepatic vein pressures was typically reduced below 12 to 15 mm Hg. However, available data suggest that a decrease in the portosystemic gradient of approximately 50%, rather than a decrease to 12 to 15 mm Hg, is usually sufficient to achieve a significant reduction in the risk of bleeding[164] with an acceptable risk of hepatic encephalopathy. In as many as 10% of cases, adequate portal decompression requires creation of a shunt lumen greater than 10 mm in diameter. Acute variceal bleeding is controlled in almost all patients after a technically successful TIPS. Continued bleeding after placement of a TIPS should prompt a repeat endoscopy to look for an alternative source of hemorrhage. One such source that has been noted commonly is bleeding from sclerotherapy-induced ulcers that overlie varices. If the site of ongoing hemorrhage is variceal, Doppler ultrasonography or TIPS venography should be performed to look for an early occlusion of the shunt.

Surgical Shunts

Surgical shunts and esophageal transection are highly effective in controlling acute variceal hemorrhage and produce more effective control of bleeding than can be achieved with endoscopic therapy.[130, 131] However, this improvement in the control of bleeding is offset by an increase in the rate's procedural morbidity and mortality, as well as shunt-related complications such as encephalopathy. Meticulous perioperative and postoperative care can improve the results of emergency shunt surgery.[165] Today most centers avoid the use of emergency shunt surgery, especially when TIPS is available and for potential liver transplantation candidates. If bleeding cannot be controlled medically and surgery is planned, a mesocaval shunt is effective, avoids the hepatic hilum, and is relatively simple to construct.

Prevention of Recurrent Hemorrhage

Pharmacologic Therapy

Studies of the prevention of subsequent hemorrhage (secondary prophylaxis) have focused on beta-blockers, long-acting nitrates, and combined drug therapy.[10, 13, 109] Concerns have been raised regarding the difficulty in hemodynamically resuscitating patients on beta-blocker therapy, but in practice this problem is uncommon and has not been identified as a cause of morbidity or mortality. Beta-blockers have the additional benefit of reducing the risk of bleeding from portal hypertensive gastropathy.[166]

Twelve randomized, controlled trials published in the English language literature have compared nonselective beta-blockers with no active treatment in the prevention of recurrent variceal hemorrage.[13, 109] Propranolol was used in 10 studies, nadolol in 1 study, and both propranolol and atenolol, in addition to placebo, in one study. There was a lower rate of variceal rebleeding with beta-blocker therapy in each trial. Eight meta-analyses concluded that beta-blockers significantly reduce the risk of variceal rebleeding. However, only one meta-analysis[167] found a significant improvement in survival rate with the use of beta-blockers.

Only one published trial has compared the efficacy of combination therapy with isosorbide mononitrate and beta-blocker with therapy with a beta-blocker alone.[168] Although a lower rate of rebleeding was associated with the use of isosorbide mononitrate and propanolol than with propanolol alone, the difference was not statistically significant (40.4% versus 57.4%, $p = .09$). Approximately 15% of patients in the combination group had to discontinue one of the two drugs because of adverse events.

Beta-blockers also have been compared directly with EST in 10 randomized studies. EST was associated with a lower rate of rebleeding but no survival advantage. A 1993 trial in which these two modalities were compared highlighted some of the issues that are critical to choosing the most appropriate form of secondary prophylaxis.[169] In this study, initial treatment of active variceal bleeding was conservative, thereby avoiding the impact of acute EST on long-term rebleeding risk. The actuarial probability of rebleeding at 1 year was 33% in the EST group and 53% in the propranolol group, and almost all of the difference between the groups occurred in the first 2 months. As expected, the rate of complications was higher with EST. The authors suggested that the benefits of EST in preventing rebleeding may be balanced by an increased rate of complications.

Another interesting study compared nadolol plus isosorbide mononitrate with EST in the prevention of variceal rebleeding.[170] In this study of 86 patients who were followed for a median of 18 months, the actuarial probability of remaining free of variceal rebleeding at 2 years was 75% in the group receiving drug therapy and 45% in the group having EST (p = .002). There was also a trend toward improved survival in the group that received combination medical therapy.

Endoscopic Therapy

Variceal rebleeding rates reported in different trials vary significantly, as do the timing of randomization and initiation of therapy.[82] However, with expectant management alone, the risk of recurrent variceal bleeding is in the range of 47% to 84%.[79] Therefore, after an initial variceal hemorrhage is controlled, patients are typically scheduled for a course of repeated EST or EVL to reduce the risk of recurrent hemorrhage. Ten studies have compared EST with conservative management for the prevention of rebleeding.[101, 102] The rebleeding rate was lower with EST, with a pooled odds ratio of 0.57 (95% CI 0.45 to 0.71). Moreover, the use of EST was associated with a lower mortality rate (pooled odds ratio 0.72 [95% CI 0.57 to 0.90]). However, one study suggested that most of the benefit of EST was due to its effectiveness as emergency treatment and that use of EST only on an emergency basis might be as effective as use in an elective, serial manner.[171] Trials comparing EST with beta-blockers also have tended to favor EST in terms of lower rebleeding rates (pooled odds ratio 0.64 [95% CI 0.48 to 0.85]), but the heterogeneity among these trials has been substantial, and no difference in mortality rates with these two treatments has been demonstrated.[102]

EVL has proved to be a major advance in the treatment of patients who have variceal hemorrhage. Although originally designed to reduce the frequency of complications associated with EST by reducing the depth of injury to the esophageal wall, EVL has also been shown to be more effective therapeutically than EST. EST has been compared with EVL for the secondary prophylaxis of variceal bleeding in 13 trials to date.[101, 102] EVL was found to be better than EST in preventing rebleeding in all studies (significantly in five; pooled odds ratio 0.46 [95% CI 0.30 to 0.60]).[102] However, meta-analysis revealed no difference in mortality rates between the two treatment modalities. The mean number of treatment sessions needed to achieve variceal eradication was also lower with EVL. In light of the finding of lower rates of complications, rebleeding, and time to eradication for EVL, EVL has emerged as the endoscopic treatment of choice for the prevention of variceal rebleeding. Attempts to hasten variceal eradication by combining EVL with EST have not shown additional benefit when compared with EVL alone.[172] A 1998 study, however, supports the use of low-volume EST to achieve complete eradication of residual small esophageal varices after a course of EVL with a substantially lower rate of variceal rebleeding.[173] More data are needed to confirm the efficacy of this combined approach.

Although endoscopic therapy reduces the risk of recurrent variceal hemorrhage, rebleeding still occurs in 30% to 50% of patients during a course of endoscopic treatment for variceal obliteration.[102] Attempts have been made to reduce the rebleeding rate further by combining beta-blocker therapy with repeated therapy. Only one such randomized trial has emerged, in which EVL alone was compared with EVL in combination with nadolol and sucralfate for the prevention of variceal rebleeding.[174] The combination of EVL, sucralfate, and nadolol was found to be significantly more effective than EVL alone in the prevention of rebleeding from all causes, including esophageal varices. A trend toward a lower mortality rate in the combination group was also noted, but the difference did not achieve statistical significance. Although used commonly in clinical practice and unlikely to do harm, the efficacy of combination therapy will be unproven until its benefits are confirmed by further studies.

At present, both pharmacologic and endoscopic options are effective in reducing the risk of rebleeding. Which modality is best as first-line therapy remains an unsettled issue and may vary with local experience and expertise. Moreover, EVL has largely replaced EST as a safer, more effective procedure of first choice for the prevention of recurrent variceal hemorrhage.

Transjugular Intrahepatic Portosystemic Shunt

TIPS has been compared with endoscopic therapy for the prevention of recurrent variceal bleeding in 11 randomized controlled studies.[175–185] A total of 811 patients were included in these studies. TIPS was compared with EST alone in five studies,[175–178, 183] with EST or EVL combined with beta-blocker therapy in three studies,[178, 182, 185] and with EVL alone in three studies.[179, 181, 184] Despite the heterogeneity in study design, the outcomes have been remarkably consistent, as evaluated in 1999 by meta-analysis.[186, 187] The results are shown in Figure 77–9. The overall variceal rebleeding rate with TIPS was 19% compared with 47% with endoscopic therapy. The number of hospital admissions for variceal rebleeding was lowered after TIPS, but the overall number of days of hospitalization after treatment was not clearly lower with TIPS than with endoscopic therapy.[186] The reason is that although TIPS reduces the number of hospitalizations for rebleeding, the additional days that patients spend in the hospital after TIPS for treatment of hepatic encephalopathy or shunt insufficiency negate this advantage. TIPS yields rates of survival similar to that for endoscopic therapy. Although eight of the randomized studies showed fewer deaths in the endoscopically treated patients and three showed fewer deaths in the TIPS treated group, no single trial showed a significant difference in mortality rates, and the overall mortality rate did not differ significantly for the two treatments (see Fig. 77–9). With its greater effectiveness in controlling bleeding and lower rate of local complications when compared with EST, EVL might be anticipated to narrow the advantages of TIPS. Surprisingly, the results of three studies to date have been quite similar to those for TIPS and EVS in that TIPS resulted in a lower rate of rebleeding than EVL and no significant difference in survival rate was detected.[179, 181, 184]

These results are indeed quite favorable with respect to TIPS, especially because most, if not all, the trials to date have really compared TIPS with endoscopic therapy plus TIPS "salvage." In the absence of TIPS salvage, the results may have been even more favorable for TIPS as a primary option for preventing variceal rebleeding. A careful comparison of the quality of life of patients treated with TIPS and

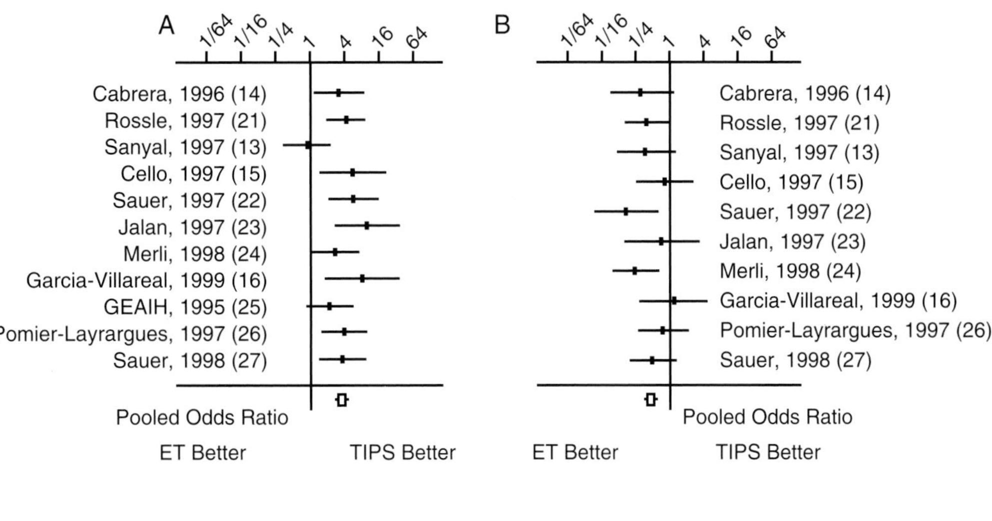

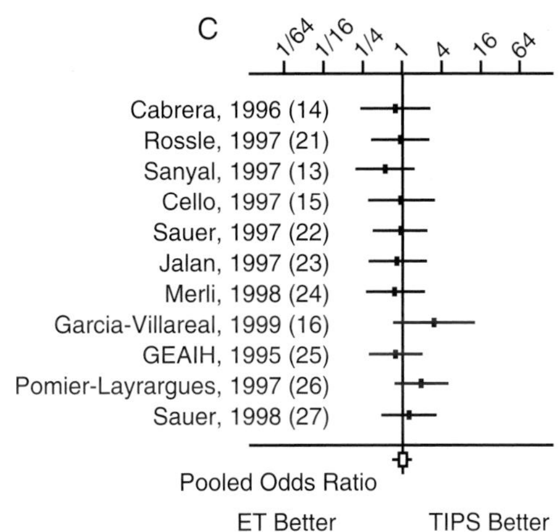

Figure 77–9. Meta-analysis of randomized, controlled trials comparing TIPS with endoscopic therapy for variceal bleeding. The panels show the results for pooled odds ratio and 95% confidence intervals for (*A*) recurrent bleeding, (*B*) hepatic encephalopathy, and (*C*) survival. ET, endoscopic therapy; TIPS, transjugular intrahepatic portosystemic shunt. (From Papatheodoridis GV, Goulis J, Leandro G, et al: Transjugular intrahepatic portosystemic shunt compared with endoscopic treatment for prevention of variceal rebleeding: A meta-analysis. Hepatology 80:612, 1999.)

those treated with endoscopic therapy has not yet been undertaken. Although the frequency of hepatic encephalopathy is higher in patients who have had TIPS, the encephalopathy is usually readily controlled with medical treatment. On the other hand, the frequency of symptomatic esophageal ulceration and ascites is higher in the endoscopically treated patients.[182–184] Comparisons of costs of TIPS and EST or EVL in the randomized studies found either no difference,[176] a lower cost for TIPS,[179] or a higher cost for TIPS.[188] Results of a decision analysis[189] in 2000 may explain this discrepancy by revealing that TIPS is more cost-effective in the short term by preventing recurrent esophageal variceal bleeding, but this advantage narrows in the long term because of the accumulating costs of managing TIPS stenosis.

Reduction in the frequency of TIPS stenosis is clearly identified by the aforementioned studies as essential for improving the cost-effectiveness of this therapy. Until compelling data to the contrary become available, EVL is currently regarded as the first-line treatment for the elective, secondary prophylaxis of variceal bleeding. In the future, the choice between TIPS and endoscopic therapy as the initial approach to secondary prophylaxis of variceal bleeding will likely incorporate considerations of cost, quality of life, and the expectations and circumstances of the individual patient.

Surgical Shunts

EST has been compared with shunt surgery for the secondary prophylaxis of variceal hemorrhage in seven trials, four with a DSRS and three with a portacaval shunt.[130, 131, 135] Patients were randomized more than 1 week after the bleeding episode in all but one study. It is not unexpected that the pooled data of these studies demonstrate a lower rate of rebleeding (pooled odds ratio 0.18 [95% CI 0.12 to 0.28]) but a higher rate of encephalopathy with shunt surgery. It is rather surprising, however, that the mortality rate did not differ for surgery and EST. A meta-analysis of the trials that compared DSRS with EST revealed a trend toward an increased frequency of encephalopathy after surgery.[190] The results of one study suggested that EST should be considered the treatment of first choice, with surgical "rescue" for patients for whom EST fails.[191] However, this study was not designed specifically to test this hypothesis. Moreover, EVL has now emerged as a superior endoscopic option.

The role of surgical therapy or TIPS in the prevention of rebleeding from varices is primarily of importance for patients for whom pharmacologic and endoscopic therapy has failed or is unfeasible (see Table 77–6). One prospective, randomized, controlled study[192] compared the complex end point of treatment failure (defined as technical failures, shunt occlusion, major rebleeds, liver failure, or death) in patients for whom conventional therapy failed and who were randomized to either a TIPS or a small-diameter portacaval prosthetic H graft. Although no single outcome differed for the surgical and TIPS groups, there was a significant difference in the total failure rate (TIPS 57%, surgical shunt 26%; $p < .02$). Pairwise randomization in this study may have been a source of bias, and as a result, the patients in the TIPS group may have been sicker than those in the shunt group at the start of the trial.

Although patients who are liver transplantation candidates or who have Child-Turcotte-Pugh class C cirrhosis are more suitable candidates for TIPS than for a surgical shunt because of the risks attendant with the latter, patients who have Child-Turcotte-Pugh class A cirrhosis may not need transplantation for many years and may lead productive lives of excellent quality as long as bleeding is held in check. This group may be better served, once they are fully stable from a bleeding perspective, by a selective surgical shunt (DSRS, mesocaval shunt, or small-diameter H-graft portacaval shunt), which offers the advantages of a considerably lower frequency of shunt stenosis and hence recurrent variceal bleeding. Because shunt insufficiency is a rare complication of these surgical shunts, there is also no need for frequent Doppler ultrasonography to assess shunt patency. With the DSRS there is also the advantage, albeit less well substantiated, of a lower risk of hepatic encephalopathy.[193] On the basis of the available data, a decision analysis comparing TIPS with DSRS in patients who have Child's class A cirrhosis found TIPS to be prohibitively less cost-effective than the surgical shunt.[194]

Management of Other Sources of Hemorrhage Resulting from Portal Hypertension

Gastric Varices

Bleeding from gastric varices can arise from varices that appear as extensions of esophageal varices or from distinct fundal varices. Pharmacologic therapy to reduce variceal flow can lead to cessation of active hemorrhage, as can endoscopic therapy or balloon tamponade. However, EST may produce extensive gastric ulceration and does not lead to effective variceal obliteration. Beta-blockers may reduce the risk of recurrent hemorrhage.[13] However, in patients who have massive or recurrent hemorrhage or in those who are considered to have a high risk of mortality, more definitive therapy, such as TIPS or a surgical shunt, should be considered.

Isolated gastric varices may occur in splenic vein thrombosis resulting from pancreatitis, trauma, or other causes. Splenectomy is the treatment of choice in this setting and is typically curative.[195] Bleeding also may occur as a result of rupture of ectopic varices (e.g., small bowel, stomal, rectal), and recurrent bleeding from hemorrhoids may be troublesome and occasionally severe.[196] These lesions may require portal decompression, and TIPS is usually effective in these situations.[197]

Portal Hypertensive Gastropathy

Bleeding from portal hypertensive gastropathy may be occult or may occur as acute hemorrhage. In one study of patients who had portal hypertensive gastropathy, the actuarial percentage of patients bleeding from portal hypertensive gastropathy at 1 year was 35% in patients who were taking propranolol compared with 62% in those on placebo ($p < .05$).[198]

In cases of severe acute or recurrent hemorrhage from gastropathy, portal decompression may be necessary. Portacaval shunt surgery has been shown to prevent recurrent hemorrhage,[87] and preliminary studies indicate that TIPS is also highly effective.[70, 186]

Management Decisions and Liver Transplantation

Orthotopic liver transplantation has emerged as a highly successful treatment for patients with end-stage liver disease (see Chapter 83). Transplantation cures portal hypertension but is expensive, requires lifelong immunosuppression, and is limited by a significant donor shortage. Therefore, liver transplantation should not be viewed as a primary treatment for variceal hemorrhage, particularly for patients who have well-preserved hepatic function.

Patients who have variceal hemorrhage should be stabilized and their risk of recurrent hemorrhage minimized without potentially interfering with future liver transplantation surgery. For example, although shunt surgery does not preclude transplantation, prior shunt surgery is associated with longer operative times and increased use of blood products during liver transplantation.[199] Nonrandomized studies of patients who have liver transplantation with either a surgical shunt or a TIPS in place have suggested that patients who have a surgical shunt have a longer duration of transplantation surgery when compared with those who have TIPS, although the mortality rate is unaffected.[200] Although TIPS is emerging as the preferred portal decompressive procedure for liver transplantation candidates, misplacement of the stent too far into the vena cava or main portal vein may complicate a subsequent transplantation operation.[201] In addition, TIPS has not been shown to have any significant impact on liver transplantation in terms of total operative time, blood product requirements, survival rate, or length of hospital stay.[202] Consequently, preoperative portal decompression solely to facilitate liver transplantation is not an acceptable indication for TIPS.

Summary of Treatment Strategies

Individual treatment decisions must consider a patient's desires, local expertise, comorbid illnesses, severity of underlying liver disease, and candidacy for liver transplantation. Moreover, newer techniques such as EVL and TIPS require further study to define their role in management. However, numerous studies have provided a framework with which to approach patients who have variceal hemorrhage (Fig. 77–10).

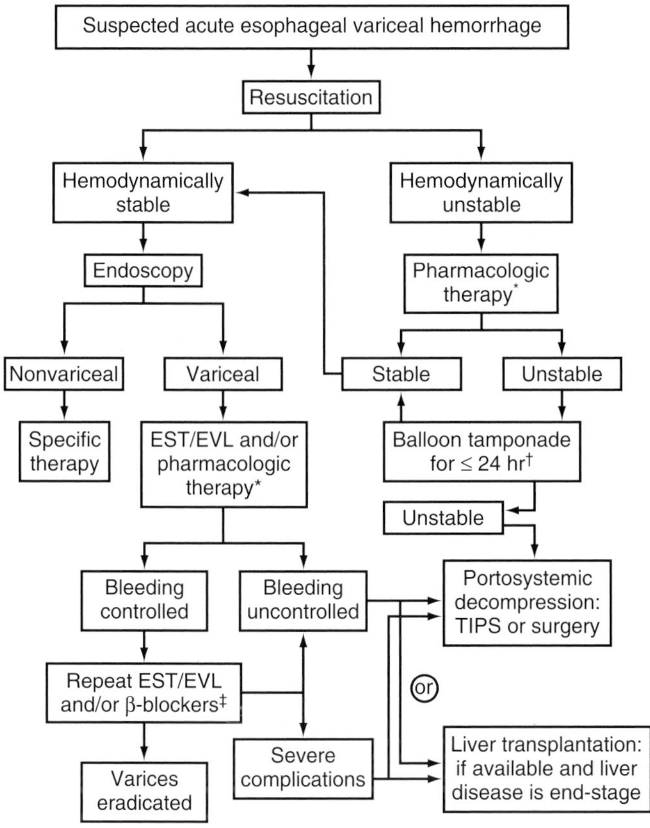

Figure 77–10. Algorithm for the management of hemorrhage from esophageal varices. *Pharmacologic agents for acute hemorrhage include vasopressin plus nitroglycerin, terlipressin, somatostatin, and octreotide. †If at all possible, endoscopy should be performed before TIPS or surgery to confirm the site of bleeding. ‡Long-term treatment with β-blockers may be a reasonable alternative in selected patients (see text for details). EST, endoscopic sclerotherapy; EVL, endoscopic variceal ligation; TIPS, transjugular intrahepatic portosystemic shunt.

Initial therapeutic efforts (after hemodynamic resuscitation) should be aimed at the control of acute hemorrhage by endoscopic and pharmacologic means. If the bleeding cannot be controlled, balloon tamponade provides a temporizing measure before more definitive therapy is undertaken. In liver transplantation candidates and patients with advanced liver disease, TIPS now appears to be the best option for portal decompression. In patients who have well-preserved hepatic function who are not expected to require transplantation for many years, emergency shunt surgery should be considered.

If initial attempts to control active hemorrhage are successful, patients should have obliterative endoscopic therapy, preferably with EVL, to reduce the risk of recurrent bleeding. Long-term treatment with beta-blockers may be a reasonable alternative for selected patients, particularly those in whom complications of endoscopic therapy have developed or in whom bleeding from sites other than or in addition to esophageal varices is not amenable to endoscopic control. Treatment with beta-blockers may also be used in combination with endoscopic therapy with added benefit. Failure to control bleeding with endoscopic or pharmacologic measures on a long-term basis can be managed with TIPS in liver transplantation candidates, although transplantation is preferable if advanced liver disease is present. TIPS is also the procedure of choice for patients in whom endoscopic and pharmacologic therapy fail and who are judged to be poor surgical candidates. Shunt surgery should be reserved for patients who have well-preserved hepatic function.

Finally, in patients known to have cirrhosis or portal hypertension, it is important to establish by endoscopic examination whether varices or gastropathy are present and to institute appropriate pharmacotherapy in patients who have these lesions, particularly if the varices are large in size (larger than grade II; see Fig. 77–5). Therapeutic options include nadolol or propranolol at doses sufficient to reduce the resting pulse by 25%. Although unproven therapeutically in preventing portal hypertensive bleeding, diuretic therapy with dietary salt restriction may benefit even patients who do not have overt fluid retention by reducing portal pressure.[14, 78] The use of diuretics for patients with hepatic disease is not, however, without risk and may produce renal impairment or encephalopathy; therefore, their role in the management of the bleeding complications of portal hypertension needs further study.[109]

REFERENCES

1. Sandblom P: The history of portal hypertension. J R Soc Med 86:544, 1993.
2. Whipple AO: The problem of portal hypertension in relation to the hepatosplenopathies. Ann Surg 1223:449, 1945.
3. Groszmann RJ, Atterbury CE: The pathophysiology of portal hypertension. Semin Liver Dis 2:177, 1982.
4. Polio J, Groszmann RJ: Hemodynamic factors involved in the development and rupture of esophageal varices: A pathophysiologic approach to treatment. Semin Liver Dis 6:318, 1986.
5. Bosch J, Mastai R, Kravetz D, et al: Hemodynamic evaluation of the patient with portal hypertension. Semin Liver Dis 6:309, 1986.
6. Benoit JN, Granger DN: Splanchnic hemodynamics in chronic portal hypertension. Semin Liver Dis 6:287, 1986.
7. Huet P-M, Pomier-Layrargues G, Villeneuve J-P, et al: Intrahepatic circulation in liver disease. Semin Liver Dis 6:277, 1986.
8. Pinzani M, Gentilini P: Biology of hepatic stellate cells and their possible relevance in the pathogenesis of portal hypertension in cirrhosis. Semin Liver Dis 19:397, 1999.
9. Roberts LR, Kamath PS: Pathophysiology of variceal bleeding. Gastrointest Endosc Clin N Am 9:167, 1999.
10. Garcia-Pagan JC, Escorsell A, Moitinho E, et al: Influence of pharmacological agents on portal hemodynamics: Basis for its use in the treatment of portal hypertension. Semin Liver Dis 19:427, 1999.
11. Boyer TD: Portal hypertensive hemorrhage: Pathogenesis and risk factors. Semin Gastrointest Dis 6:125, 1995.
12. Fevery J, Nevens F: Oesophageal varices: Assessment of the risk of bleeding and mortality. J Gastroenterol Hepatol 15:842, 2000.
13. Tripathi D, Hayes PC: Review article: A drug therapy for the prevention of variceal haemorrhage. Aliment Pharmacol Ther 15:291, 2001.
14. Bass NM, Yao FY: The role of the interventional radiologist: Transjugular procedures. Gastrointest Endosc Clin N Am 11:131, 2001.
15. Ekataksin W, Kaneda K: Liver microvascular architecture: An insight into the pathophysiology of portal hypertension. Semin Liver Dis 19: 359, 1999.
16. Lebrec D, Benhamou JP: Noncirrhotic intrahepatic portal hypertension. Semin Liver Dis 6:332, 1986.
17. Da Silva LC, Carrilho FJ: Hepatosplenic schistosomiasis: Pathophysiology and treatment. Gastroenterol Clin North Am 21:163, 1992.
18. Ludwig J, Hashimoto E, Obata H, et al: Idiopathic portal hypertension. Hepatology 17:1157, 1993.
19. Wanless IR, Wong F, Blendis LM, et al: Hepatic and portal vein thrombosis in cirrhosis: Possible role in development of parenchymal extinction and portal hypertension. Hepatology 21:1238, 1995.

20. Rockey D: The cellular pathogenesis of portal hypertension: Stellate cell contractility, endothelin, and nitric oxide. Hepatology 25:2, 1997.
21. Moller S, Henriksen JH: Endothelins in chronic liver disease. Scand J Clin Lab Invest 56:481, 1996.
22. Alam I, Bass NM, Gee L, et al: Hepatic tissue levels of endothelin-1 correlate with severity of chronic liver disease and ascites. Am J Gastroenterol 95:199, 2000.
23. Matsubara S, Ouchi K, Matsuno S: Portal venous pressure following splenectomy in patients with portal hypertension of differing etiology. Eur Surg Res 24:372, 1992.
24. Vauthey JN, Tomczak RJ, Helmberger T, et al: The arterioportal fistula syndrome: Clinicopathologic features, diagnosis, and therapy. Gastroenterology 113:1390, 1997.
25. Rector WG Jr, Hoefs JC, Hossack KF, et al: Hepatofugal portal flow in cirrhosis: Observations on hepatic hemodynamics and the nature of the arterioportal communications. Hepatology 8:16, 1988.
26. Gaiani S, Bolondi L, Li Bassi S, et al: Prevalence of spontaneous hepatofugal portal flow in liver cirrhosis: Clinical and endoscopic correlation in 228 patients. Gastroenterology 100:160, 1991.
27. Sugita S, Ohnishi K, Saito M, et al: Splanchnic hemodynamics in portal hypertensive dogs with portal fibrosis. Am J Physiol 252:G748, 1987.
28. Nishida O, Moriyasu F, Nakamura T, et al: Interrelationship between splenic and superior mesenteric venous circulation manifested by transient splenic arterial occlusion using a balloon catheter. Hepatology 7: 442, 1987.
29. Ready J, Rector WG: Systemic hemodynamic changes in portal hypertension. Semin Gastrointest Dis 6:134, 1995.
30. Groszmann RJ: Hyperdynamic circulation of liver disease 40 years later: Pathophysiology and clinical consequences. Hepatology 20:1359, 1994.
31. Abelmann WH: Hyperdynamic circulation in cirrhosis: A historical perspective. Hepatology 20:1356, 1994.
32. Meng H, Lin H, Tsai Y, et al: Relationships between the severity of cirrhosis and hemodynamic values in patients with cirrhosis. J Gastroenterol Hepatol 9:148, 1994.
33. Lange PA, Stoller JK: The hepatopulmonary syndrome. Ann Intern Med 122:521, 1995.
34. Schrier RW, Arroyo V, Bernardi M, et al: Peripheral arterial vasodilation hypothesis: A proposal for the initiation of renal sodium and water retention in cirrhosis. Hepatology 8:1151, 1988.
35. Rector WG Jr, Robertson AD, Lewis FW, et al: Arterial underfilling does not cause sodium retention in cirrhosis. Am J Med 95:286, 1993.
36. García-Pagán JC, Bosch J, Rodés J: The role of vasoactive mediators in portal hypertension. Semin Gastrointest Dis 6:140, 1995.
37. Wiest R, Groszmann RJ: Nitric oxide and portal hypertension: Its role in the regulation of intrahepatic and splanchnic vascular resistance. Semin Liver Dis 19:411, 1999.
38. Silva G, Navasa M, Bosch J, et al: Hemodynamic effects of glucagon in portal hypertension. Hepatology 11:668, 1990.
39. Pizcueta MP, Casamitjana R, Bosch J, et al: Decreased systemic vascular sensitivity to norepinephrine in portal hypertensive rats: Role of hyperglucagonism. Am J Physiol 258:G191, 1990.
40. Benoit JN, Zimmermann B, Preman AJ, et al: Role of glucagon in splanchnic hyperemia of chronic portal hypertension. Am J Physiol 251:G674, 1986.
41. Sikuler E, Groszmann RJ: Hemodynamic studies in long and short term portal hypertensive rats: The relation to systemic glucagon levels. Hepatology 6:414, 1986.
42. Albillos A, Colombato LA, Lee FY: Chronic octreotide treatment ameliorates peripheral vasodilation and prevents sodium retention in portal hypertensive rats. Gastroenterology 104:568, 1993.
43. Bomzon A, Blendis LM: The nitric oxide hypothesis and the hyperdynamic circulation in cirrhosis. Hepatology 20:1343, 1994.
44. Sogni P, Moreau R, Gadano A, et al: The role of nitric oxide in the hyperdynamic circulatory syndrome associated with portal hypertension. J Hepatol 23:218, 1995.
45. Lopez-Talavera JC, Merrill WW, Groszmann RJ: Tumor necrosis factor alpha: A major contributor to the hyperdynamic circulation in prehepatic portal–hypertensive rats. Gastroenterology 108:761, 1995.
46. Guarner C, Soriano G, Tomas A, et al: Increased serum nitrite and nitrate levels in patients with cirrhosis: Relationship to endotoxemia. Hepatology 18:1139, 1993.
47. García-Pagan JC, Fernández M, Bernadich C, et al: Effects of continued nitric oxide inhibition on the portal hypertensive syndrome after portal vein stenosis in the rat. Am J Physiol 30:984, 1994.
48. Guarner C, Soriano G: Prostaglandin and portal hypertension. Prostaglandins Leukot Essent Fatty Acids 48:203, 1993.
49. Guarner C, Soriano G, Such J, et al: Systemic prostacyclin in cirrhotic patients: Relationship with portal hypertension and changes after intestinal decontamination. Gastroenterology 102:303, 1992.
50. Kawada N, Tran-Thi TA, Klein H, et al: The contraction of hepatic stellate cells stimulated with vasoactive substances: Possible involvement of endothelin-1 and nitric oxide in the regulation of sinusoidal tonus. Eur J Biochem 213:815, 1993.
51. Zhang JX, Pegoli W, Clemens MG: Endothelin-1 induces direct constriction of hepatic sinusoids. Am J Physiol 266:G624, 1994.
52. Levin ER: Mechanisms of disease: Endothelins. N Engl J Med 333: 356, 1995.
53. Ballet F, Chretien Y, Rey C, et al: Differential response of normal and cirrhotic liver to vasoactive agents: A study in the isolated perfused rat liver. J Pharmacol Exp Ther 244:233, 1988.
54. Reichen J, Gerbes AL, Steiner MJ, et al: The effect of endothelin and its antagonist Bosentan on hemodynamics and microvascular exchange in cirrhotic rat liver. J Hepatol 28:1020, 1998.
55. Cappell MS, Price JB: Characterization of the syndrome of small and large intestinal variceal bleeding. Dig Dis Sci 32:422, 1987.
56. Ben-Ari Z, McCormick AP, Jain S, et al: Spontaneous haemoperitoneum caused by ruptured varices in a patient with non-cirrhotic portal hypertension. Eur J Gastroenterol Hepatol 7:87, 1995.
57. Hashizume M, Kitano S, Sugimachi K, et al: Three-dimensional view of the vascular structure of the lower esophagus in clinical portal hypertension. Hepatology 8:1482, 1988.
58. Hashizume M, Sugimachi K: Classification of gastric lesions associated with portal hypertension. J Gastroenterol Hepatol 10:339, 1995.
59. Sarin SK, Lahoti D, Saxena S, et al: Prevalence, classification and natural history of gastric varices: A long-term follow-up study in 568 portal hypertension patients. Hepatology 16:1343, 1992.
60. Levine MS, Kieu K, Rubesin SE, et al: Isolated gastric varices: Splenic vein obstruction or portal hypertension? Gastrointest Radiol 15:188, 1990.
61. Gostout CJ, Viggiano TR, Balm RK: Acute gastrointestinal bleeding from portal hypertensive gastropathy: Prevalence and clinical features. Am J Gastroenterol 88:2030, 1993.
62. Sarin SK, Shahi HM, Jain M, et al: The natural history of portal hypertensive gastropathy: Influence of variceal eradication. Am J Gastroenterol 95:2888, 2000.
63. Primignani M, Carpinelli L, Preatoni P, et al: Natural history of portal hypertensive gastropathy in patients with liver cirrhosis: The New Italian Endoscopic Club for the Study and Treatment of Esophageal Varices (NIEC). Gastroenterology 119:181, 2000.
64. Toyonaga A, Iwao T: Portal-hypertensive gastropathy. J Gastroenterol Hepatol 13:865, 1998.
65. Bini EJ, Lascarides CE, Micale PL, et al: Mucosal abnormalities of the colon in patients with portal hypertension: An endoscopic study. Gastrointest Endosc 52:511, 2000.
66. Nagral AS, Joshi AS, Bhatia SJ, et al: Congestive jejunopathy in portal hypertension. Gut 34:694, 1993.
67. Ohta M, Hashizume M, Higashi H, et al: Portal and gastric mucosal hemodynamics in cirrhotic patients with portal-hypertensive gastropathy. Hepatology 20:1432, 1994.
68. Orloff MJ, Orloff MS, Orloff SL, et al: Treatment of bleeding from portal hypertensive gastropathy by portacaval shunt. Hepatology 21: 1011, 1995.
69. Munoz SJ: Propranolol for portal hypertensive gastropathy: Another virtue of beta-blockade? Hepatology 15:554, 1992
70. Kamath PS, Lacerda M, Ahlquist DA, et al: Gastric mucosal responses to intrahepatic portosystemic shunting in patients with cirrhosis. Gastroenterology 118:905, 2000.
71. Navarro VJ, Garcia-Tsao G: Variceal hemorrhage. Crit Care Clin 11: 391, 1995.
72. North Italian Endoscopic Club for the Study and Treatment of Esophageal Varices: Prediction of the first variceal hemorrhage in patients with cirrhosis of the liver and esophageal varices. N Engl J Med 319: 983, 1988.
73. Paquet KJ: Prophylactic endoscopic sclerosing treatment of the esophageal wall in varices: A prospective controlled trial. Endoscopy 14:4, 1982.
74. Nevens F, Bustami R, Scheys I, et al: Variceal pressure is a factor predicting the risk of a first variceal bleeding: A prospective cohort study in cirrhotic patients. Hepatology 27:15, 1998.

75. Merkel C, Bolognesi M, Sacerdoti D, et al: The hemodynamic response to medical treatment of portal hypertension as a predictor of clinical effectiveness in the primary prophylaxis of variceal bleeding in cirrhosis. Hepatology 32:930, 2000.
76. Ready JB, Robertson AD, Goff JS, et al: Assessment of the risk of bleeding from esophageal varices by continuous monitoring of portal pressure. Gastroenterology 100:1403, 1991.
77. Katsuta Y, Aramaki T, Sekiyama T, et al: Plasma volume contraction in portal hypertension. J Hepatol 17(suppl 2):S19, 1993.
78. Nevens F, Lijnen P, VanBilloen H, et al: The effect of long-term treatment with spironolactone on variceal pressure in patients with portal hypertension without ascites. Hepatology 23:1047, 1996.
79. Burroughs AK: The natural history of varices. J Hepatol 17(suppl 2): S10 1993.
80. Luca A, Cirera I, García-Pagan JC, et al: Hemodynamic effects of acute changes in intra-abdominal pressure in patients with cirrhosis. Gastroenterology 104:222, 1993.
81. De Franchis R, Primignani M: Why do varices bleed? Gastroenterol Clin North Am 21:85, 1992.
82. Burroughs AK, Mezzanotte G, Phillips A, et al: Cirrhotics with variceal hemorrhage: The importance of the time interval between admission and the start of analysis for survival and rebleeding rates. Hepatology 9:801, 1989.
83. Cales P, Zabotto B, Meskens C, et al: Gastroesophageal endoscopic features in cirrhosis: Observer variability, interassociations, and relationship to hepatic dysfunction. Gastroenterology 98:156, 1990.
84. Violi F, Ferro D, Basili S, et al: Hyperfibrinolysis increases the risk of gastrointestinal hemorrhage in patients with advanced cirrhosis. Hepatology 15:672, 1992.
85. Møller S, Bendtsen F, Christensen E, et al: Prognostic variables in patients with cirrhosis and oesophageal varices without prior bleeding. J Hepatol 21:940, 1994.
86. Muting D, Kalk JF, Fischer R, et al: Spontaneous regression of oesophageal varices after long-term conservative treatment: Retrospective study in 20 patients with alcoholic liver cirrhosis, posthepatitic cirrhosis and haemochromatosis with cirrhosis. J Hepatol 10:158, 1990.
87. McCormick PA, Morgan MY, Phillips A, et al: The effects of alcohol use on rebleeding and mortality in patients with alcoholic cirrhosis following variceal haemorrhage. J Hepatol 14:99, 1992.
88. De Lèdinghen V, Heresbach D, Fourdan O, et al: Anti-inflammatory drugs and variceal bleeding: A case-control study. Gut 44:270, 1999.
89. Goulis J, Patch D, Burroughs AK: Bacterial infection in the pathogenesis of variceal bleeding. Lancet 353:139, 1999.
90. Brewer TG: Treatment of acute gastroesophageal variceal hemorrhage. Med Clin North Am 77:993, 1993.
91. Pagliaro L, D'Amico G, Luca A, et al: Portal hypertension: Diagnosis and treatment. J Hepatol 23:36, 1995.
92. McCormick PA, Jenkins SA, McIntyre N, et al: Why portal hypertensive varices bleed and bleed: A hypothesis. Gut 36:100, 1995.
93. Valla DC, Condat B: Portal vein thrombosis in adults: Pathophysiology, pathogenesis and management. J Hepatol 32:865, 2000.
94. Orrego H, Blake JE, Blendis LM, et al: Prognosis of alcoholic cirrhosis in the presence and absence of alcoholic hepatitis. Gastroenterology 92: 208, 1987.
95. Lo GH, Lin CY, Lai KH, et al: Endoscopic injection sclerotherapy versus conservative treatment for patients with unresectable hepatocellular carcinoma and bleeding esophageal varices. Gastrointest Endosc 37:161, 1991.
96. Sarfeh IJ: Portal vein thrombosis associated with cirrhosis. Arch Surg 114:902 1989.
97. Burroughs AK: The management of bleeding due to portal hypertension. 1. The management of acute bleeding episodes. QJM 67:447, 1988.
98. Shapiro RS, Stancato-Pasik A, Glajchen N, et al: Color Doppler applications in hepatic imaging. Clin Imaging 22:272, 1998.
99. Stafford-Johnson DB, Chenevert TL, Cho KJ, et al: Portal venous magnetic resonance angiography: A review. Invest Radiol 33:628, 1998.
100. Sanyal AJ: Hepatic venous pressure gradient: To measure or not to measure, that is the question. Hepatology 32:1175, 2000.
101. Helmy A, Hayes PC: Review article: Current endoscopic therapeutic options in the management of variceal bleeding. Aliment Pharmacol Ther 15:575, 2001.
102. de Franchis R, Primignani M: Endoscopic treatments for portal hypertension. Semin Liver Dis 19:439, 1999.
103. Laine L, Cook D: Endoscopic ligation compared with sclerotherapy for treatment of esophageal variceal bleeding: A meta-analysis. Ann Intern Med 123:280, 1995.
104. Binmoeller KF, Soehendra N: "Superglue": The answer to variceal bleeding and fundal varices? Endoscopy 27:392, 1995
105. Bhargava DK, Singh B, Dogra R, et al: Prospective randomized comparison of sodium tetradecyl sulfate and polidocanol as variceal sclerosing agents. Am J Gastroenterol 87:182, 1992.
106. Shim CS, Cho JY, Park YJ, et al: Mini-detachable snare ligation for the treatment of esophageal varices. Gastrointest Endosc 50:673, 1999.
107. Gimson A, Polson R, Westaby D, et al: Omeprazole in the management of intractable esophageal ulceration following injection sclerotherapy. Gastroenterology 99:1829, 1990.
108. Holderman WH, Etzkorn KP, Patel SA, et al: Endoscopic findings and overtube-related complications associated with esophageal variceal ligation. J Clin Gastroenterol 21:91, 1995.
109. D'Amico G, Pagliaro L, Bosch J: Pharmacological treatment of portal hypertension: An evidence-based approach. Semin Liver Dis 19:475, 1999.
110. Rössle M, Haag K, Ochs A, et al: The transjugular intrahepatic portosystemic stent-shunt procedure for variceal bleeding. N Engl J Med 330:165, 1994.
111. LaBerge JM, Ring EJ, Gordon RL, et al: Creation of transjugular intrahepatic portosystemic shunts with the Wallstent endoprosthesis: Results in 100 patients. Radiology 187:413, 1993.
112. Freedman AM, Sanyal AJ, Tisnado J, et al: Complications of transjugular intrahepatic portosystemic shunt: A comprehensive review. Radiographics 13:1185, 1993.
113. Sanyal AJ, Freedman AM, Shiffman ML, et al: Portosystemic encephalopathy after transjugular intrahepatic portosystemic shunt: Results of a prospective controlled study. Hepatology 20:46, 1994.
114. Somberg KA, Riegler JL, Doherty MM, et al: Hepatic encephalopathy following transjugular intrahepatic portosystemic shunts (TIPS): Incidence and risk factors. Am J Gastroenterol 90:549, 1995.
115. LaBerge JM, Somberg KA, Lake JR, et al: Two-year outcome following transjugular intrahepatic portosystemic shunts for variceal bleeding: Results in 90 patients. Gastroenterology 108:1143, 1995.
116. Rouillard SS, Bass NM, Roberts JP, et al: Severe hyperbilirubinemia after creation of transjugular intrahepatic portosystemic shunts: Natural history and predictors of outcome. Ann Intern Med 128:374, 1998.
117. Jalan R, Elton RA, Redhead DN, et al: Analysis of prognostic variables in the prediction of mortality, shunt failure, variceal rebleeding and encephalopathy following the transjugular intrahepatic portosystemic stent-shunt for variceal haemorrhage. J Hepatol 23:123, 1995.
118. Jabbour N, Zajko AB, Orons PD, et al: Transjugular intrahepatic portosystemic shunt in patients with end-stage liver disease: Results in 85 patients. Liver Transpl Surg 2:139, 1996.
119. Williams D, Waugh R, Gallagher N, et al: Mortality and rebleeding following transjugular intrahepatic portosystemic stent shunt for variceal haemorrhage. J Gastroenterol Hepatol 13:163, 1998.
120. Chalasani N, Clark WS, Martin LG, et al: Determinants of mortality in patients with advanced cirrhosis after transjugular intrahepatic portosystemic shunting. Gastroenterology 118:138, 2000.
121. Malinchoc M, Kamath PS, Gordon FD, et al: A model to predict poor survival in patients undergoing transjugular intrahepatic portosystemic shunts. Hepatology 31:864, 2000
122. Patch D, Nikolopoulou V, McCormick A, et al: Factors related to early mortality after transjugular intrahepatic portosystemic shunt for failed endoscopic therapy in acute variceal bleeding. J Hepatol 28:454, 1998
123. Bass NM: Role of TIPS in portal hypertension: Variceal bleeding and ascites. Technol Vasc Intervent Radiol 1:44, 1998.
124. LaBerge J, Feldstein VA: Ultrasound surveillance of TIPS—why bother? Hepatology 28:1433, 1998
125. Haskal ZJ, Pentecost MJ, Soulen MC, et al: Transjugular intrahepatic portosystemic shunt stenosis and revision: Early and midterm results. AJR Am J Roentgenol 163:439, 1994.
126. Lind CD, Malisch TW, Chong WK, et al: Incidence of shunt occlusion or stenosis following transjugular intrahepatic portosystemic shunt placement. Gastroenterology 106:1277, 1994
127. Saxon RS, Ross PL, Mendel-Hartvig J, et al: Transjugular intrahepatic portosystemic shunt patency and the importance of stenosis location in the development of recurrent symptoms. Radiology 207:683, 1998.
128. Pasha TM, Kamath PS: Shunt stenosis post TIPS: Ultrasonography is the most cost-effective detection strategy. Gastroenterology 110: A1306, 1996.

129. Feldstein VA, Patel MD, LaBerge JM: Transjugular intrahepatic portosystemic shunts: Accuracy of Doppler US in determination of patency and detection of stenoses. Radiology 201:141, 1996.
130. Henderson JM: Surgical treatment of portal hypertension. Baillieres Best Pract Res Clin Gastroenterol 14:911, 2000.
131. Collins JC, Sarfeh IJ: Surgical management of portal hypertension. West J Med 162:527, 1995.
132. Sarfeh IJ, Rypins EB, Mason GR: A systematic appraisal of portacaval H-graft diameters: Clinical and hemodynamic perspectives. Ann Surg 204:356, 1986.
133. Sarfeh IJ, Rypins EB: Partial versus total portacaval shunt in alcoholic cirrhosis—results of a prospective, randomized clinical trial. Ann Surg 219:353, 1994.
134. Henderson JM, Millikan WJ Jr, Wright-Bacon L, et al: Hemodynamic differences between alcoholic and nonalcoholic cirrhotics following distal splenorenal shunt—effect on survival? Ann Surg 198:325, 1983.
135. D'Amico G, Pagliaro L, Bosch J: The treatment of portal hypertension: A meta-analytic review. Hepatology 22:332, 1995.
136. Mathur SK, Shah SR, Soonawala ZF, et al: Transabdominal extensive oesophagogastric devascularization with gastro-oesophageal stapling in the management of acute variceal bleeding. Br J Surg 84:413, 1997.
137. Shah SR, Nagral SS, Mathur SK: Results of a modified Sugiura's devascularisation in the management of "unshuntable" portal hypertension. HPB Surg 11:235, 1999.
138. Poynard T, Calès P, Pasta L, et al: Beta-adrenergic-antagonist drugs in the prevention of gastrointestinal bleeding in patients with cirrhosis and esophageal varices: An analysis of data and prognostic factors in 589 patients from four randomized clinical trials. N Engl J Med 324: 1532, 1991.
139. Conn HO, Grace ND, Bosch J, et al: Propranolol in the prevention of the first hemorrhage from esophagogastric varices: A multicenter, randomized clinical trial. Hepatology 13:902, 1991.
140. Teran JC, Imperiale TF, Mullen KD, et al: Primary prophylaxis of variceal bleeding in cirrhosis: A cost-effectiveness analysis. Gastroenterology 112:473, 1997.
141. Angelico M, Carli L, Piat C, et al: Effects of isosorbide-5-mononitrate compared with propanolol on first bleeding and long-term survival in cirrhosis. Gastroenterology 113:1632 1997.
142. Merkel C, Marin R, Sacerdoti D, et al: Long-term results of a clinical trial of nadolol with or without isosorbide mononitrate for primary prophylaxis of variceal bleeding in cirrhosis. Hepatology 31:324, 2000
143. The Veterans Affairs Cooperative Variceal Sclerotherapy Group: Prophylactic sclerotherapy for esophageal varices in men with alcoholic liver disease: A randomized, single-blind, multicenter clinical trial. N Engl J Med 324:1779, 1991.
144. Lay CS, Tsai YT, Teg CY, et al: Endoscopic variceal ligation in prophylaxis of first variceal bleeding in cirrhotic patients with high-risk esophageal varices. Hepatology 25:134, 1997.
145. Lo GH, Lai KH, Cheng TS, et al: Prophylactic banding ligation of high-risk esophageal varices in patients with cirrhosis: A prospective, randomized trial. J Hepatol 31:451, 1999.
146. Grace ND, Groszmann RJ, Garcia-Tsao G, et al: Portal hypertension and variceal bleeding: An AASLD single topic symposium. Hepatology 28:868, 1998.
147. Sarin SK, Lamba GS, Kumar M, et al: Comparison of endoscopic ligation and propanolol for the primary prevention of variceal bleeding. N Engl J Med 340:998, 1999.
148. Stanley AJ, Forrest EH, Lui HF, et al: Banding ligation versus propanolol or isosorbide mononitrate in the primary prophylaxis of variceal haemorrhage: Preliminary results of a randomized controlled trial. Gut 42(suppl 1):A19, 1998.
149. Inokuchi K: Cooperative Study Group of Portal Hypertension of Japan: Improved survival after prophylactic portal nondecompression surgery for esophageal varices, a randomized clinical trial. Hepatology 12:1, 1990.
150. Bernard B, Grange JD, Khac EN, et al: Antibiotic prophylaxis for the prevention of bacterial infections in cirrhotic patients with gastrointestinal bleeding: A meta-analysis. Hepatology 29:1655, 1999.
151. Cirera I, Feu F, Luca A, et al: Effect of bolus injections and continuous infusions of somatostatin and placebo in patients with cirrhosis: A double blind hemodynamic investigation. Hepatology 22:106, 1995.
152. Burroughs AK, McCormick PA, Hughes MD, et al: Randomized, double-blind, placebo-controlled trial of somatostatin for variceal bleeding: Emergency control and prevention of early variceal rebleeding. Gastroenterology 99:1388, 1990.
153. Valenzuela JE, Schubert T, Fogel MR, et al: A multicenter, randomized, double-blind trial of somatostatin in the management of acute hemorrhage from esophageal varices. Hepatology 10:958, 1989.
154. Gotzsche PC, Gjorup I, Bonnen H, et al: Somatostatin v placebo in bleeding oesophageal varices: Randomised trial and meta-analysis. BMJ 310:1495, 1995.
155. Sung JJ, Y, Chung SCS, Lai C-W, et al: Octreotide infusion or emergency sclerotherapy for variceal haemorrhage. Lancet 342:637, 1993.
156. Jenkins SA, Shields R, Davies M, et al: A multicentre randomized trial comparing octreotide and injection sclerotherapy in the management and outcome of acute variceal haemorrhage. Gut 41:526, 1997.
157. Besson I, Ingrand P, Person B, et al: Sclerotherapy with or without octreotide for acute variceal bleeding. N Engl J Med 333:555, 1995.
158. Sung JJ, Chung SC, Yung MY, et al: Prospective randomised study of effect of octreotide on rebleeding from oesophageal varices after endoscopic ligation. Lancet 346:1666, 1995.
159. D'Amico G, Politi F, Morabito A, et al: Octreotide compared with placebo in a treatment strategy for early rebleeding in cirrhosis: A double blind, randomized pragmatic trial. Hepatology 28:120, 1998.
160. Panés J, Terés J, Bosch J, et al: Efficacy of balloon tamponade in treatment of bleeding gastric and esophageal varices, results in 151 consecutive episodes. Dig Dis Sci 33:454, 1988.
161. Kamath PS, McKusick MA: Transvenous intrahepatic portosystemic shunts. Gastroenterology 111:1700, 1996.
162. McCormick PA, Dick R, Panagou EB, et al: Emergency transjugular intrahepatic portosystemic stent shunting as salvage treatment for uncontrolled variceal bleeding. Br J Surg 81:1324, 1994.
163. Sanyal AJ, Freedman AM, Luketic VA, et al: Transjugular intrahepatic portosystemic shunts for patients with active variceal hemorrhage unresponsive to sclerotherapy. Gastroenterology 111:138, 1996.
164. Rössle M, Haag K, Berger E, et al: How much reduction in the portosystemic pressure gradient is essential to prevent rebleeding? Hepatology 26:139A, 1997
165. Orloff MJ, Orloff MS, Orloff SL, et al: Three decades of experience with emergency portacaval shunt for acutely bleeding esophageal varices in 400 unselected patients with cirrhosis of the liver. J Am Coll Surg 180:257, 1995.
166. Pérez-Ayuso RM, Piqué J, Bosch J, et al: Propranolol in prevention of recurrent bleeding from severe portal hypertensive gastropathy in cirrhosis. Lancet 337:1431, 1991.
167. Bernard B, Lebrec D, Mathurin P, et al: Beta-adrenergic antagonists in the prevention of gastrointestinal rebleeding in patients with cirrhosis: A meta-analysis. Hepatology 25:63, 1997.
168. Gournay J, Masliah C, Martin T, et al: Isosorbide mononitrate and propanolol compared with propanolol alone for the prevention of variceal rebleeding. Hepatology 31:1239, 2000.
169. Terés J, Bosch J, Bordas JM, et al: Propranolol versus sclerotherapy in preventing variceal rebleeding: A randomized controlled trial. Gastroenterology 105:1508, 1993.
170. Villanueva C, Balanzó J, Novella MT, et al: Nadolol plus isosorbide mononitrate compared with sclerotherapy for the prevention of variceal rebleeding. N Engl J Med 334:1624, 1996.
171. Burroughs AK, McCormick PA, Siringo S, et al: Prospective randomized trial of long term sclerotherapy for variceal bleeding using the same protocol to treat rebleeding in all patients: Final report. J Hepatol 9(suppl 1):S12, 1989.
172. Laine L, Stein C, Sharma V: Randomized comparison of ligation versus ligation plus sclerotherapy in patients with bleeding esophageal varices. Gastroenterology 110:529, 1996.
173. Lo GH, Lai KH, Cheng JS, et al: The additive effect of sclerotherapy to patients receiving repeated endoscopic variceal ligation: A prospective, randomized trial. Hepatology 28:391, 1998.
174. Lo GH, Lai KH, Cheng JS, et al: Endoscopic variceal ligation plus nadolol and sucralfate compared with ligation alone for the prevention of variceal rebleeding: A prospective, randomized trial. Hepatology 32:461, 2000.
175. Cabrera J, Maynar M, Granados R, et al: Transjugular intrahepatic portosystemic shunt versus sclerotherapy in the elective treatment of variceal hemorrhage. Gastroenterology 110:832, 1996.
176. Cello JP, Ring EJ, Olcott EW, et al: Endoscopic sclerotherapy compared with percutaneous transjugular intrahepatic portosystemic shunt after initial sclerotherapy in patients with acute variceal hemorrhage—a randomized, controlled trial. Ann Intern Med 126:858, 1997.
177. Garcia-Villarreal L, Martinez-Lagares F, Sierra A, et al: Transjugular

intrahepatic portosystemic shunt versus endoscopic sclerotherapy for the prevention of variceal rebleeding after recent variceal hemorrhage. Hepatology 29:27, 1999.

178. Groupe d'Etude des Anastomoses Intra-Hépatiques: TIPS versus sclerotherapy and propranolol in the prevention of variceal rebleeding: Preliminary results of a multicenter randomized trial. Hepatology 22: 297A, 1995.
179. Jalan R, Forrest EH, Stanley AJ, et al: A randomized trial comparing transjugular intrahepatic portosystemic stent-shunt with variceal band ligation in the prevention of rebleeding from oesophageal varices. Hepatology 26:1115, 1997.
180. Merli M, Salerno F, Riggio O, et al: Transjugular intrahepatic portosystemic shunt versus endoscopic sclerotherapy for the prevention of variceal bleeding in cirrhosis: A randomized multicenter trial. Gruppo Italiano Studio TIPS (GIST). Hepatology 27:48, 1998.
181. Pomier-Layrargues G, Dufresne MP, et al: TIPS versus endoscopic variceal ligation in the prevention of variceal rebleeding in cirrhotic patients: A comparative randomized clinical trial (interim analysis). Hepatology 26:137A, 1997.
182. Rössle M, Deibert P, Haag K, et al: Randomised trial of transjugular-intrahepatic-portosystemic shunt versus endoscopy plus propranolol for prevention of variceal rebleeding. Lancet 349:1043, 1997
183. Sanyal AJ, Freedman AM, Luketic VA, et al: Transjugular intrahepatic portosystemic shunts compared with endoscopic sclerotherapy for the prevention of recurrent variceal hemorrhage—a randomized, controlled trial. Ann Intern Med 126:849, 1997.
184. Sauer P, Benz C, Theilmann L, et al: Transjugular intrahepatic portosystemic stent shunt (TIPS) versus endoscopic banding in the prevention of variceal rebleeding: Final results of a randomized study. Gastroenterology 114:A1334, 1998.
185. Sauer P, Thielmann L, Stremmel W, et al: Transjugular intrahepatic portosystemic stent shunt versus sclerotherapy plus propranolol for variceal bleeding. Gastroenterology 113:1623, 1997.
186. Burroughs AK, Patch D: Transjugular intrahepatic portosystemic shunt. Semin Liver Dis 19:457, 1999.
187. Papatheodoridis GV, Goulis J, Leandro G, et al: Transjugular intrahepatic portosystemic shunt compared with endoscopic treatment for prevention of variceal rebleeding: A meta-analysis. Hepatology 30: 612, 1999.
188. Meddi P, Merli M, Lionetti R, et al: Cost analysis for the prevention of variceal rebleeding: A comparison between transjugular intrahepatic portosystemic shunt and endoscopic sclerotherapy in a selected group of Italian cirrhotic patients. Hepatology 29:1074, 1999.
189. Russo MW, Zacks SL, Sandler RS, et al: Cost-effectiveness analysis of transjugular intrahepatic portosystemic shunt (TIPS) versus endoscopic therapy for the prevention of recurrent esophageal variceal bleeding. Hepatology 31:358, 2000.
190. Spina GP, Henderson JM, Rikkers LF, et al: Distal spleno-renal shunt versus endoscopic sclerotherapy in the prevention of variceal rebleeding: A meta-analysis of 4 randomized clinical trials. J Hepatol 16:338, 1992.
191. Henderson JM, Kutner MH, Millikan WJ Jr: Endoscopic variceal sclerosis compared with distal splenorenal shunt to prevent recurrent variceal bleeding in cirrhosis. Ann Intern Med 112:262, 1990.
192. Rosemurgy AS, Goode SE, Zwiebel BR, et al: A prospective trial of transjugular intrahepatic portosystemic stent shunts versus small-diameter prosthetic H-graft portacaval shunts in the treatment of bleeding varices. Ann Surg 224:378, 1996.
193. Rikkers LF, Jin G, Langnas AN, et al: Shunt surgery during the era of liver transplantation. Ann Surg 226:51, 1997.
194. Zacks SL, Sandler RS, Biddle AK, et al: Decision-analysis of transjugular intrahepatic portosystemic shunt versus distal splenorenal shunt for portal hypertension. Hepatology 29:1399, 1999.
195. Moossa AR, Gadd MA: Isolated splenic vein thrombosis. World J Surg 9:384, 1985.
196. Norton ID, Andrews JC, Kamath PS: Management of ectopic varices. Hepatology 28:1154, 1998.
197. Shibata D, Brophy DP, Gordon FD, et al: Transjugular intrahepatic portosystemic shunt for treatment of bleeding ectopic varices. Dis Colon Rectum 42:1581, 1999.
198. Perez-Ayuso R, Pique J, Bosch J, et al: Propranolol in prevention of recurrent bleeding from severe portal hypertensive gastropathy in cirrhosis. Lancet 337:1431, 1991.
199. Langnas AN, Marujo WC, Stratta RJ, et al: Influence of a prior portosystemic shunt on outcome after liver transplantation. Am J Gastroenterol 87:714, 1992.
200. Abouljoud MS, Levy MF, Rees CR, et al: A comparison of treatment with transjugular intrahepatic portosystemic shunt or distal splenorenal shunt in the management of variceal bleeding prior to liver transplantation. Transplantation 59:226, 1995.
201. Millis JM, Martin P, Gomes A, et al: Transjugular intrahepatic portosystemic shunts: Impact on liver transplantation. Liver Transplant Surg 4:229, 1995.
202. Somberg KA, Lombardero MS, Lawlor SM, et al: A controlled analysis of the transjular intrahepatic portosystemic shunt in liver transplant recipients: The National Institute of Diabetes and Digestive and Kidney Diseases (NIDDK) Liver Tranplantation Database. Transplantation 63:1074, 1997.

Chapter 78

ASCITES AND SPONTANEOUS BACTERIAL PERITONITIS

Bruce A. Runyon

Ascites is of Greek derivation ("askos") and refers to a bag or sack. The word is a noun and describes pathologic fluid accumulation within the peritoneal cavity. The adjective *ascitic* is used in conjunction with the word *fluid* to describe the liquid per se.

PATHOGENESIS OF ASCITES FORMATION

Liver Disease

Ascites forms in the setting of cirrhosis as a result of the sequence of events detailed in Figure 78–1. The most recent theory of ascites formation, the "peripheral arterial vasodilation hypothesis," proposes that both older hypotheses, the underfill and overflow theories, are correct, but that each is operative at a different stage.[1] The first abnormality that develops appears to be portal hypertension. Portal pressure increases above a critical threshold, and nitric oxide levels increase. Nitric oxide leads to vasodilation. As the state of vasodilation worsens, plasma levels of vasoconstrictor, sodium-retentive hormones increase, and renal function deteriorates; ascites develops, that is, decompensation occurs.

The explanation for the neurohumoral excitation, which is characteristic of volume depletion, in the setting of volume overload in a patient with cirrhosis and ascites may have to do with volume sensors. Animals have sophisticated systems for detecting and preserving vascular perfusion pressures and intravascular osmolality. However, an organism's ability to detect changes in intravascular volume (especially volume overload) is limited and is linked to pressure receptors. This may explain in part the paradox of dramatic volume overload in the face of sympathetic nervous traffic and hormone levels that are indicative of intravascular volume depletion.

Noncirrhotic Ascites

The mechanism of fluid retention in patients with malignancy-related ascites depends on the location of the tumor. Peritoneal carcinomatosis appears to cause ascites through the production of proteinaceous fluid by tumor cells lining the peritoneum. Extracellular fluid enters the peritoneal cavity to reestablish oncotic balance.[2] Fluid accumulates in patients with massive liver metastases because of portal hypertension caused by stenosis or occlusion of portal veins by tumor nodules or tumor emboli.[3] In patients with hepatocellular carcinoma, ascites forms because of the underlying cirrhosis-related portal hypertension, tumor-induced portal vein thrombosis, or both. Chylous ascites in patients with malignant lymphoma appears to be caused by lymph node obstruction by tumor and rupture of chyle-containing lymphatics.

Ascites can complicate high-output or low-output heart failure or nephrotic syndrome. As in cirrhosis, effective arterial blood volume appears to be decreased, and the vasopressin, renin-aldosterone, and sympathetic nervous systems are activated.[4] These changes lead to renal vasoconstriction and sodium and water retention. Fluid then weeps from the congested hepatic sinusoids as lymph, as in cirrhotic ascites. Tuberculosis, *Chlamydia* infection, and coccidioidomycosis probably cause ascites through the production of proteinaceous fluid, as in peritoneal carcinomatosis. Spontaneous bacterial peritonitis (SBP) does not appear to cause fluid to accumulate; infection develops only in preexisting ascites.

In patients with pancreatic or biliary ascites, fluid forms by leakage of pancreatic juice or bile into the peritoneal cavity or by a "chemical burn" of the peritoneum. After abdominal surgery, especially extensive retroperitoneal dissection, lymphatics may be transected and may leak lymph for variable amounts of time.[5] The mechanism of formation of ascites in this condition is similar to that for malignant chylous ascites, namely, lymphatic leak.

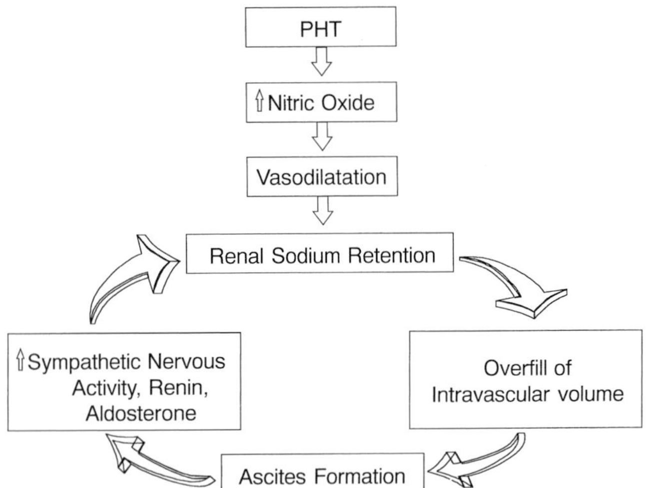

Figure 78–1. Pathogenesis of ascites formation in the setting of cirrhosis. (PHT, portal hypertension.)

CLINICAL FEATURES OF ASCITES

History

Most patients (~80%) with ascites in the United States have cirrhosis. The three most common causes of cirrhosis at the present time are alcohol, chronic hepatitis C, and nonalcoholic steatohepatitis (NASH) related to obesity. Many patients have two of these conditions, and some have all three.[6, 7] In about 20% of patients with ascites, there is a nonhepatic cause of fluid retention (Table 78–1). Ascites frequently develops as part of the patient's first decompensation of alcoholic liver disease. Ascites can develop early in alcoholic liver disease in the precirrhotic, alcoholic hepatitis stage. At this stage, portal hypertension and the resulting predisposition to sodium retention are reversible with abstinence from alcohol.[8] Patients with precirrhotic alcoholic liver disease may lose their predisposition to fluid retention when they reduce or cease consumption of alcohol. In contrast, patients in whom ascites develops in the setting of nonalcoholic liver disease tend to have persistent fluid retention thereafter, probably because of the late stage at which ascites forms in nonalcoholic liver disease and the lack of effective therapy other than liver transplantation.

Patients with ascites should also be questioned about risk factors for liver disease other than alcohol, such as intravenous drug use, blood transfusions, sex with a member of the same sex, acupuncture, tattoos, ear piercing, and country of origin. Quite commonly, the cause of ascites in a middle-aged or elderly woman is viral hepatitis–induced cirrhosis resulting from a remote, often forgotten blood transfusion. Another cause of "cryptogenic" cirrhosis and ascites is NASH from long-standing obesity.[9] Many patients who have been obese will spontaneously lose 50 or even 100 pounds after their liver disease decompensates. Unless the physician asks about lifetime maximum body weight and usual adult body weight, the possibility of NASH-related cirrhosis may not be considered. With a careful history and appropriate laboratory testing, the percentage of patients with cirrhosis who are now labeled cryptogenic has approached zero.[10]

Table 78–1 | **Causes of Ascites**

CAUSE	% OF TOTAL NUMBER OF PATIENTS
Cirrhosis (with or without infection)	85
Miscellaneous portal hypertension-related (including 5% with two causes, including portal hypertension)	8
Cardiac ascites	3
Peritoneal carcinomatosis	2
Miscellaneous nonportal hypertension-related	2

Data from Runyon BA, Montano AA, Akriviadis EA, et al: The serum-ascites albumin gradient is superior to the exudate-transudate concept in the differential diagnosis of ascites. Ann Intern Med 117:215, 1992.

Patients with a long history of stable cirrhosis and the sudden development of ascites should be suspected of harboring a hepatocellular carcinoma that has precipitated the decompensation.

Patients with ascites who have a history of cancer should be suspected of having malignancy-related ascites. However, cancer in the past does not guarantee a malignant cause of ascites. For example, patients with tobacco-related lung cancer and alcohol abuse may have cirrhotic ascites. Breast, lung, colon, and pancreatic cancers are regularly complicated by ascites.[3] Abdominal pain is a helpful distinguishing feature. Malignancy-related ascites frequently is painful, whereas cirrhotic ascites usually is not, unless there is superimposed bacterial peritonitis or alcoholic hepatitis.

A history of heart failure may raise the possibility of cardiac ascites. Alcoholics in whom ascites develops may have alcoholic cardiomyopathy or alcoholic liver disease, but usually not both.

Tuberculous peritonitis is usually manifested by fever and abdominal pain. Many affected patients are recent immigrants from an endemic area. In the United States, more than half the patients with tuberculous peritonitis have underlying alcoholic cirrhosis, which may contribute to the formation of ascites.

Ascites may develop in patients with acute hemorrhagic pancreatitis or a ruptured pancreatic duct from chronic pancreatitis or trauma. Often, troublesome ascites also may develop in a small percentage of patients on hemodialysis. Fitz-Hugh–Curtis syndrome caused by *Chlamydia* may cause inflammatory ascites in a sexually active woman.[11] Patients in whom ascites and anasarca develop in the setting of diabetes should be suspected of having nephrotic ascites. Ascites in a patient with symptoms and signs of myxedema should prompt measurement of thyroid function. Serositis in connective tissue disease may be complicated by ascites.[12]

Physical Examination

On the basis of the history and the appearance of the abdomen, the diagnosis of ascites is readily suspected and usually easily confirmed on physical examination. The presence of a full, bulging abdomen should lead to percussion of the flanks. If the amount of flank dullness is greater than usual (i.e., if the percussed air-fluid level is higher than that normally found on the lateral aspect of the abdomen with the patient supine), then the examiner should check for "shifting." If there is no flank dullness, there is no reason to check for shifting. Approximately 1500 mL of fluid must be present before dullness is detected.[13] If flank dullness is not present, the chance that the patient has ascites is less than 10%.[13] A fluid wave is not worth testing for.[13]

Gaseous distention of the bowel, a thick panniculus, and an ovarian mass can mimic ascites. Gaseous distention should be readily apparent on percussion. Ovarian masses usually cause tympanic flanks with central dullness. An obese abdomen may be diffusely dull to percussion, and abdominal ultrasonography may be required to determine if fluid is present. As the percentage of patients with ascites and obesity increases, the use of ultrasound to detect the presence or absence of fluid will also increase. Ultrasonographic scans can detect as little as 100 mL of fluid in the abdomen.[14]

The presence of palmar erythema, large pulsatile spider angiomata, large abdominal wall collateral veins, or fetor hepaticus is suggestive of parenchymal liver disease and portal hypertension. The presence of large veins on the patient's back suggests inferior vena cava blockage. An immobile mass in the umbilicus, the Sister Mary Joseph nodule, is suggestive of peritoneal carcinomatosis.

The neck veins of patients with ascites should always be examined. Constrictive pericarditis is one of the few curable causes of ascites. Most patients with cardiac ascites have impressive jugular venous distention. Some have no visible jugular venous distention but such high central venous pressures that their bulging forehead veins rise to the tops of their skulls. When present, peripheral edema in patients with liver disease is usually found in the lower extremities and occasionally may involve the abdominal wall. Patients with nephrotic syndrome or cardiac failure may have total body edema (anasarca).

DIAGNOSIS

Although the diagnosis of ascites may be suspected on the basis of the history and physical examination, final confirmation is based on successful abdominal paracentesis. Determination of the cause of ascites is based on the results of the history, physical examination, and ascitic fluid analysis. In general, few other tests are required.

Abdominal Paracentesis

Indications

Abdominal paracentesis with appropriate ascitic fluid analysis is probably the most rapid and cost-effective method of diagnosing the cause of ascites. Also, because of the possibility of ascitic fluid infection in a cirrhotic patient admitted to the hospital, a surveillance paracentesis performed on admission may detect unexpected infection.[15] Not all patients with ascitic fluid infection are symptomatic; many have subtle symptoms, such as mild hepatic confusion noticed only by the family. Detection of infection at an early asymptomatic stage may reduce mortality. Therefore, ascitic fluid should be sampled in all inpatients and outpatients with the new onset of ascites and in all patients with ascites who are admitted to the hospital. Paracentesis should be repeated in patients (whether in the hospital or not) in whom symptoms, signs, or laboratory abnormalities suggestive of infection develop (e.g., abdominal pain or tenderness, fever, encephalopathy, hypotension, renal failure, acidosis, or peripheral leukocytosis).

Contraindications

There are few contraindications to paracentesis. Coagulopathy is a potential contraindication; however, most patients with cirrhotic ascites have coagulopathy, and if mild coagulopathy were viewed as a contraindication to paracentesis, few cirrhotics would undergo this procedure.[16] In the author's opinion, coagulopathy should preclude paracentesis only when there is clinically evident fibrinolysis or clinically evident disseminated intravascular coagulation.[16] These conditions occur in less than 1 per 1000 taps. There are no data to support a cut-off for coagulation parameters beyond which paracentesis should be avoided. Even after multiple paracenteses, bloody ascites usually does not develop in patients with severe prolongation of prothrombin time. Cirrhotic patients without clinically obvious coagulopathy simply do not bleed excessively from needlesticks unless a blood vessel is entered.[16]

Studies regarding complications of paracentesis in patients with ascites have documented no deaths or infections caused by the paracentesis.[16, 17] There have been no episodes of hemoperitoneum or entry of the paracentesis needle into the bowel. Complications have included only abdominal wall hematomas in approximately 2% of cases, even though 71% of the patients had an abnormal prothrombin time and 21% had a prothrombin time prolonged by longer than 5 seconds.[16] Complication rates may be higher when paracentesis is performed by an inexperienced operator.

Some physicians give blood products (fresh-frozen plasma or platelets) routinely before paracentesis in cirrhotic patients with coagulopathy, presumably to prevent hemorrhagic complications. This policy is not supported by data. Because a hematoma that requires blood transfusion develops in only approximately 1% of patients who undergo paracentesis without prophylactic transfusion of plasma or platelets, approximately 100 to 200 units of fresh-frozen plasma or platelets would have to be given to prevent the transfusion of approximately 2 units of red blood cells.

On the basis of the complications (reported in the older literature) of paracentesis performed with large-bore trocars, many physicians had avoided diagnostic paracentesis in the evaluation of the patient with ascites. However, in view of the documented safety of this procedure and the frequency of ascitic fluid infection, paracentesis is now performed more frequently.[16]

Patient Position, Choice of Needle Entry Site, and Needle

The volume of fluid in the abdomen and the thickness of the abdominal wall determine in part how the patient should be positioned in preparation for the procedure. Patients with a large volume of ascites and thin abdominal walls can be "tapped" successfully in the supine position with the head of the bed or examining table elevated slightly. Patients with less fluid can be placed in the lateral decubitus position and tapped in the midline or in the right or left lower quadrant while supine (see later). Patients with small amounts of fluid may be tapped successfully only in the face-down position or with ultrasound guidance.[16]

The choice of the site for inserting the needle has changed in recent years because of the increasing prevalence of obesity and the increasing frequency of therapeutic paracentesis. Obese patients pose special problems. Using ultrasound guidance, the author has found that in obese patients, the abdominal wall is usually substantially thicker in the midline than in the lower quadrants. The abdominal wall may even be thicker than the length of a 3.5-inch paracentesis needle. Also, on physical examination, it is frequently difficult to determine whether ascites is present or absent in the obese patient. Ultrasound is helpful in confirming the presence of fluid and in guiding the paracentesis needle to obtain a fluid sample. It is preferable to insert the needle through the left lower quadrant than the right lower quadrant because the cecum may be distended with gas from lactulose therapy. Also the right lower quadrant is more likely to have a surgical scar (e.g., from appendectomy) than the left. When therapeutic paracentesis is performed, more fluid can be obtained via a lower quadrant needle insertion site than a midline site.

Surgical scars also must be considered when one is selecting a site for needle insertion. The bowel may be adherent to the peritoneal surface of the abdomen near a scar, and a needle inserted there may enter the bowel.[16] The needle must be placed several centimeters from the scar. A long midline scar precludes midline paracentesis. An appendectomy scar precludes a right lower quadrant site, in general.

The author usually chooses a site in the left lower quadrant two fingerbreadths cephalad and two fingerbreadths medial to the anterior superior iliac spine. In a patient with multiple abdominal scars, ultrasound guidance may be required.

In the patient who is not overweight, the author prefers to use a standard metal 1.5-inch 22-gauge needle. Obese patients require a longer needle, for example, a 3.5-inch 22-gauge variety. Steel needles are preferable to plastic-sheathed cannulas because of the risk that the plastic sheath will shear off into the peritoneal cavity and the tendency of the plastic sheath to kink and obstruct the flow of fluid after the cannula is removed. Metal needles do not puncture bowel unless the bowel is adherent to a scar or there is severe gaseous distention.

Technique of Diagnostic Paracentesis

Drapes, gown, hat, and mask are optional, but sterile gloves should be used when paracentesis is performed. The skin is disinfected with an iodine solution. The skin and subcutaneous tissue should be infiltrated with a local anesthetic. The sterile package insert enclosing the gloves can be used as a sterile field on which to place syringes, needles, gauze, and other supplies. When sterile gloves are not used, ascitic fluid cultures frequently grow skin contaminants. Only one viable organism will grow to detectable levels in blood culture bottles.

To prevent leakage of ascites after the needle is withdrawn, the needle is inserted using a "Z tract." This is accomplished by displacing (with one gloved hand) the skin approximately 2 cm downward and then slowly inserting the paracentesis needle mounted on the syringe held in the other hand. The skin is not released until the needle has penetrated the peritoneum and fluid flows. This technique requires that the hand holding the syringe stabilize it and retract its plunger simultaneously. A steady hand and experience are needed. When the Z tract is used and the needle is finally removed, the skin resumes its original position and seals the needle pathway. If the needle is not inserted by this technique, the fluid will leak out more easily because the pathway is straight. The needle should be advanced slowly in about 5-mm increments. Slow insertion allows the operator to see blood if a vessel is entered, so that the needle can be withdrawn immediately before further damage is done. Slow insertion also allows the bowel to move away from the needle, thereby avoiding bowel puncture. The syringe that is attached to the needle should be aspirated intermittently during insertion. If continuous suction is applied, bowel or omentum may be drawn to the end of the needle as soon as the needle enters the peritoneal cavity, thereby occluding flow and resulting in an apparently unsuccessful tap. Slow insertion also allows time for the elastic peritoneum to "tent" over the end of the needle and be pierced by it. The most common causes for an unsuccessful paracentesis are continuous aspiration during insertion of the needle and rapid insertion and withdrawal of the needle before the peritoneum is pierced. If the operator is certain that the needle tip is inserted far enough but no fluid is apparent, the syringe and needle can be twisted 90 degrees to pierce the peritoneum and permit flow of fluid.

Approximately 30 mL of fluid is obtained using one or more syringes. The author prefers to use a 5- or 10-mL syringe for the initial portion of a diagnostic tap and then twist this syringe off of the needle and replace it with a 30-mL syringe to obtain the remainder of the sample. The initial use of a small syringe allows the operator to have better control and to see fluid more easily as it enters the hub of the syringe. The syringe and attached needle are then pulled out of the abdomen, and the needle is removed and discarded. A sterile needle is then placed on the larger syringe, and an appropriate amount of fluid is inoculated into each of a pair of prepared blood culture bottles (see later). Usually, 5 to 10 mL is inoculated into 50-mL bottles, and 10 to 20 mL into 100-mL bottles. The next aliquot is placed into a "purple-top" ethylenediaminetetraacetic acid tube for a cell count, and the final aliquot is placed into a "red-top" tube for chemistries. Inoculating the culture bottles first with a sterile needle minimizes contamination. The fluid then must be placed promptly into the anticoagulant-containing tube to avoid clotting; clotted fluid cannot be analyzed for cell count.

Technique of Therapeutic Paracentesis

Therapeutic paracentesis is similar to diagnostic paracentesis except that a larger bore needle is used and additional equipment is required. In the patient who is not overweight, the author prefers to use a standard metal 1.5-in 16- to 18-gauge needle. Obese patients may require a longer needle, for example, a 3.5-inch 18-gauge needle. Recently, 15-gauge 5-

hole needles have been produced specifically for therapeutic abdominal paracentesis; these needles may replace the spinal needles used currently for paracentesis in obese patients. The new needles have a removable sharp inner component and a blunt outer cannula; they range in length from 3.25 to 5.9 in.

An old method of using a 60-mL syringe, stopcock, and collection bag is tedious. Use of vacuum bottles (1 or 2 L) connected to the needle with noncollapsible tubing is much faster. Use of a peristaltic pump is even faster than vacuum bottles.[18] Unless the needle is allowed to drift subcutaneously, the needle (or blunt steel cannula) can be left in the abdomen during a therapeutic paracentesis without injury. Larger bore needles or cannulas permit more rapid removal of fluid, but leave larger defects if they enter vessels or the bowel inadvertently.

Once fluid is flowing, the needle should be stabilized to ensure steady flow. It is not unusual for flow to cease intermittently. With respiratory movement, the needle may gradually work its way out of the peritoneal cavity and into the soft tissue, and some serosanguineous fluid may appear in the needle hub or tubing. When this happens, the pump should be turned off or a clamp placed on the tubing connected to the vacuum bottle. The tubing is removed from the needle, and the needle is twisted a few degrees. If flow does not resume, the needle is twisted a bit more. If flow still does not resume, the needle is inserted in 1- to 2-mm increments until there is brisk dripping of fluid from the needle hub. The tubing is then reattached, and more fluid is removed. Occasionally, fluid cannot be aspirated but drips from the needle hub. In this situation, fluid is allowed to drip into a sterile container for collection, as in a lumbar puncture.

As the fluid is removed, the bowel and omentum draw closer to the needle and eventually block the flow of ascites. The patient then must be repositioned so gravity causes the fluid to pool near the needle. It is useful to reposition the patient a few times during a total paracentesis to maximize the amount of fluid removed. Excessive manipulation of the needle is avoided to minimize the risk of trauma to the bowel or blood vessels.

After samples of fluid are obtained for testing, 2 to 4 L of fluid is removed to relieve the pressure of tense ascites in patients with new or diuretic-sensitive ascites. A sodium-restricted diet and diuretics are prescribed to further reduce the fluid (see later). If a patient is known to be diuretic-resistant, a "total tap" is performed, that is, all the fluid that is accessible is removed. If less is removed, the tap will need to be repeated soon (see later section, "Refractory Ascites").

Ascitic Fluid Analysis

Gross Appearance

Non-neutrocytic (i.e., ascitic fluid neutrophil count <250/mm^3 [0.25 × 10^9/L]) ascitic fluid is transparent and usually slightly yellow (Fig. 78–2). Ascitic fluid with a very low protein concentration may have no pigment and look like water. The opacity of many cloudy ascitic fluid specimens is caused by neutrophils. The presence of neutrophils leads to a shimmering effect when a glass tube containing the fluid is rocked back and forth in front of a light. Fluid with an absolute neutrophil count under 1000/mm^3 (1.0 × 10^9/L) may be nearly clear. Fluid with a count over 5000/mm^3 (5.0 × 10^9/L) is quite cloudy, and fluid with a count over 50,000/mm^3 (50.0 × 10^9/L) resembles mayonnaise.

Ascitic fluid specimens are frequently blood-tinged or frankly bloody. A red blood cell count of 10,000/mm^3 (10.0 × 10^9/L) is the threshold for a pink appearance; smaller concentrations result in clear or turbid fluid. Ascitic fluid with a red blood cell count greater than 20,000/mm^3 (20.0 × 10^9/L) is distinctly red. Many ascitic fluid specimens are bloody because of a traumatic tap; these specimens are blood-streaked and frequently clot unless the fluid is immediately transferred to the anticoagulant tube (for the cell count). In contrast, nontraumatic or remotely traumatic blood-tinged ascitic fluid is homogenous and does not clot because it has already clotted and the clot has lysed. Some patients with portal hypertension have bloody hepatic lymph leading to bloody ascitic fluid, perhaps because of rupture of lymphatics that are under high pressure. Samples from patients with hepatocellular carcinoma are regularly bloody, but only about 10% of samples from patients with peritoneal carcinomatosis are red.[3] Although many physicians have the impression that tuberculosis results in bloody ascites, less than 5% of tuberculous samples are hemorrhagic in the author's experience.

Ascitic fluid is frequently lipid-laden. Lipid opacifies the fluid. The degree of opalescence of ascitic fluid ranges from slightly cloudy to completely opaque and chylous. Most opaque milky fluid has a triglyceride concentration greater than 200 mg/dL (2.26 mmol/L), usually greater than 1000 mg/dL (11.30 mmol/L). Fluid that has the appearance of dilute skim milk has a triglyceride concentration between 100 mg/dL (1.13 mmol/L) and 200 mg/dL (2.26 mmol/L). A substantial minority of cirrhotic ascitic fluid samples are neither transparent nor frankly milky. These opalescent samples have slightly elevated triglyceride concentrations ranging from 50 mg/dL (0.56 mmol/L) to 200 mg/dL (2.26 mmol/L).[19] The opacity of these fluids does not have the shimmering characteristics of ascitic fluid with an elevated white blood cell count. The lipid usually layers out when a tube of ascitic fluid is placed in the refrigerator for 48 to 72 hours. In contrast to older published reports, most patients with chylous or opalescent ascites have cirrhosis.[19, 20]

Dark-brown fluid with a bilirubin concentration greater than that of serum usually indicates biliary perforation.[21] Deeply jaundiced patients have bile-stained ascitic fluid, but the bilirubin level and the degree of pigmentation are visually less than those of the corresponding serum. Pancreatic ascites may be pigmented because of the effect of pancreatic enzymes on red blood cells. The red blood cells may have to be centrifuged before the discolored supernatant is revealed. The degree of pigmentation ranges from tea-colored to jet black, as in hemorrhagic pancreatitis. Black ascites may also be found in patients with malignant melanoma.

Ascitic Fluid Tests

The practice of ordering every conceivable body fluid test on every ascitic fluid specimen is expensive and can be more confusing than helpful, especially when unexpectedly abnormal results are encountered. An algorithm for the anal-

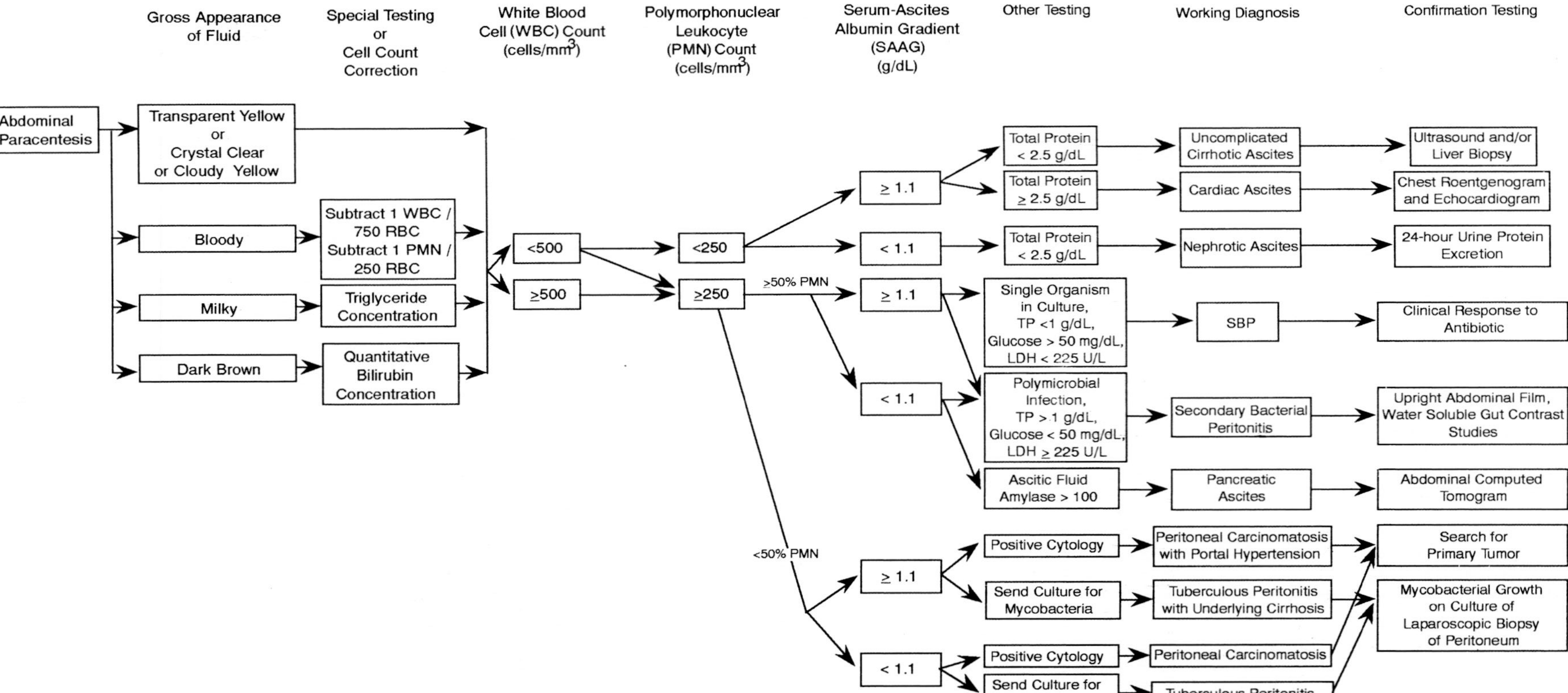

Figure 78–2. Approach to the differential diagnosis of ascites. (RBC, red blood cells; TP, total protein; LDH, lactate dehydrogenase; SBP, spontaneous bacterial peritonitis.)

Table 78–2 | **Ascitic Fluid Laboratory Data**

ROUTINE	OPTIONAL	UNUSUAL	UNHELPFUL
Cell count	Culture in blood culture bottles	TB smear and culture	pH
Albumin	Glucose	Cytology	Lactate
Total protein	LDH	Triglyceride	Cholesterol
	Amylase	Bilirubin	Fibronectin
	Gram's stain		α_1-Antitrypsin
			Glycosaminoglycans

LDH, lactate dehydrogenase; TB, tuberculosis.

ysis of ascitic fluid, shown in Figure 78–2, works quite well in the author's experience. The basic concept is that screening tests are performed on the initial specimen. Additional testing is performed only when necessary based on the results of the screening tests. Further testing usually requires another paracentesis. However, because most specimens consist of uncomplicated cirrhotic ascites, no further testing is usually needed in the majority of specimens.

Based on cost analysis, tests can be classified as routine, optional, unusual, and unhelpful (Table 78–2).[22] Each test is discussed subsequently in detail in order of decreasing importance. The cell count is the single most helpful ascitic fluid test. Only about 10 μL of fluid is required for a standard manual hemocytometer count. Therefore, if only one drop of fluid can be obtained, it should be sent for cell count. However, more fluid is almost always obtainable. The fluid should be submitted in an anticoagulant tube (i.e., ethylenediaminetetraacetic acid) to prevent clotting. Because the decision to begin empiric antibiotic treatment of suspected ascitic fluid infection is based largely on the absolute neutrophil count (which should have a turnaround time of a few minutes) rather than the culture (which takes 12 to 48 hours to demonstrate growth), the cell count is more important than the culture in the early detection and treatment of ascitic fluid infection.

CELL COUNT. Surprisingly, ascitic fluid cell counts have not been standardized. Some laboratories count mesothelial cells in addition to white blood cells (WBCs) and label the sum as "nucleated cells." The usefulness of mesothelial cell counts is not clear. The WBC count in uncomplicated cirrhotic ascites is usually less than 500 cells/mm^3 (0.5 × 10^9/ see Fig. 78–2).[22–24] During diuresis in patients with cirrhotic ascites, the WBC count can concentrate to more than 1000 cells/mm^3 (1.0 × 10^9/L).[23] However, a diagnosis of diuresis-related elevation of the ascitic fluid WBC count requires that a prediuresis count is available and normal, that there is a predominance of lymphocytes in the fluid, and that there are no unexplained clinical symptoms or signs (e.g., fever or abdominal pain).

The upper limit of normal for the absolute polymorphonuclear leukocyte (PMN) count in uncomplicated cirrhotic ascitic fluid is usually stated to be lower than 250/mm^3 (0.25 × 10^9/L).[22–24] The short survival of PMNs results in relative stability of the absolute PMN count during diuresis.[23] Therefore, the 250-cell/mm^3 (0.25 × 10^9/L) "cut-off" remains reliable even after diuresis.

Any inflammatory process can result in an elevated ascitic fluid WBC count. Spontaneous bacterial peritonitis (SBP) is the most common cause of inflammation of ascitic fluid and the most common cause of an elevated ascitic WBC count. The total WBC count, as well as the absolute PMN count, is elevated in SBP, and PMNs usually account for more than 70% of the total WBC count. Also, in tuberculous peritonitis and peritoneal carcinomatosis, there frequently is an elevated total ascitic WBC count but usually with a predominance of lymphocytes.[3]

Most bloody ascites is the result of a slightly traumatic tap. Leakage of blood into the peritoneal cavity leads to an elevated ascitic fluid WBC count. Because neutrophils predominate in blood, the ascitic fluid differential count may be altered by contamination of ascitic fluid with blood. To correct for this, 1 PMN is subtracted from the absolute ascitic fluid PMN count for every 250 red blood cells (see Fig. 78–2).[23] If the leakage of blood occurred at a remote time, the PMNs will have lysed, and the corrected PMN count will be a negative number. If the corrected PMN count in a bloody specimen is greater than 250 cells/mm^3 (0.25 × 10^9/L), the patient must be assumed to be infected.

EXUDATE/TRANSUDATE. Before the 1980s, the ascitic fluid total protein concentration was used to classify ascites into exudates (>2.5 g/dL [25 g/L]) and transudates (<2.5 g/dL [25 g/L]). Unfortunately, this classification does not work well in ascitic fluid, and these terms, as applied to ascitic fluid, were never carefully defined or validated. Attempts at using combinations of lactate dehydrogenase (LDH) and serum-to-ascitic fluid ratios of LDH and protein also have not been shown to classify ascitic fluid accurately into exudates and transudates.[24]

SERUM-ASCITES ALBUMIN GRADIENT. The *serum-ascites albumin gradient (SAAG)* has been proved in multiple studies to categorize ascites better than either the total protein concentration or other parameters do (Table 78–3).[25–27] The SAAG is based on oncotic-hydrostatic balance.[25] Portal hypertension results in an abnormally high hydrostatic pressure gradient between the portal bed and ascitic fluid. There must be a similarly large difference between ascitic fluid and intravascular oncotic forces.[25] Albumin exerts greater oncotic force per gram than do other proteins. Therefore, the difference between the serum and ascitic fluid albumin concentrations correlates directly with portal pressure.[25]

Calculating the SAAG involves measuring the albumin concentration of serum and ascitic fluid specimens and sim-

Table 78–3 | **Classification of Ascites by Serum-Ascites Albumin Gradient**

HIGH GRADIENT ≥1.1 G/DL (11 G/L)	LOW GRADIENT <1.1 G/DL (11 G/L)
Cirrhosis	Peritoneal carcinomatosis
Alcoholic hepatitis	Tuberculous peritonitis
Cardiac ascites	Pancreatic ascites
"Mixed" ascites	Bowel obstruction or infarction
Massive liver metastases	Biliary ascites
Fulminant hepatic failure	Nephrotic syndrome
Budd-Chiari syndrome	Postoperative lymphatic leak
Portal vein thrombosis	Serositis in connective tissue diseases
Veno-occlusive disease	
Myxedema	
Fatty liver of pregnancy	

ply *subtracting* the ascitic fluid value from the serum value. Unless there is a laboratory error, the serum albumin concentration is always the larger value. *The gradient is calculated by subtraction and is not a ratio.* If the *SAAG is greater than or equal to 1.1 g/dL (11 g/L), the patient can be diagnosed with portal hypertension with an accuracy of approximately 97%.*[26] Also, if the serum albumin–ascitic fluid *total protein* gradient is greater than or equal to 1.1 g/dL (11 g/L), the patient has portal hypertension, because the ascitic fluid albumin concentration cannot be greater than the ascitic fluid total protein concentration. Conversely, *if the SAAG is less than 1.1 g/dL (11 g/L), the patient does not have portal hypertension with an accuracy of approximately 97%.* The SAAG does not explain the pathogenesis of ascites formation, nor does it explain where the albumin came from, that is, liver or bowel. It simply gives the physician an indirect but accurate index of portal pressure. The accuracy of the test is about 97%, even with ascitic fluid infection, diuresis, therapeutic paracentesis, intravenous infusions of albumin, and varying causes of liver disease.[26]

Measurement of the ascitic fluid albumin concentration has been routine in some laboratories for almost 20 years. However, before sending ascitic fluid for the first time to a laboratory to measure the albumin concentration, a physician should discuss the test with the laboratory chemist. Ensuring accuracy of the albumin assay at low albumin concentrations (e.g., <1 g/dL [10 g/L]) is important because many patients with ascites have a serum albumin concentration in the range of 2.0 g/dL (20 g/L) and an ascitic fluid albumin concentration in the range of 0 to 1.0 g/dL (0 to 10 g/L). If the assay for albumin is not accurate at low levels, errors will occur. Also, if a cirrhotic patient has a serum albumin level less than 1.1 g/dL (11 g/L; as occurs in less than 1% of patients with cirrhotic ascites), the gradient will be falsely low.

There are other situations in which the accuracy of the SAAG is reduced, as when specimens of serum and ascites are not obtained nearly simultanously. The specimens should be obtained on the same day, preferably within the same hour. Both serum and ascitic fluid albumin concentrations change over time; however, these values change in parallel such that the difference is stable. Arterial hypotension may result in a decrease in the portal pressure and a narrowing of the SAAG. Lipid interferes with the assay for albumin, and chylous ascites may result in a falsely high SAAG.

Serum hyperglobulinemia (>5 g/dL [50 g/L]) leads to a high ascitic fluid globulin concentration and can narrow the albumin gradient by contributing to the oncotic forces. A narrowed gradient caused by high serum globulin levels occurs in only approximately 1% of ascitic fluid specimens. To correct the SAAG in the setting of a high serum globulin level, the uncorrected SAAG is multiplied by (0.16) × (serum globulin [in g/dL] + 2.5).[27]

A problem with the exudate/transudate system of classification is that it has no provision for patients with two causes of ascites, that is, "mixed" ascites. Most of these patients have portal hypertension from cirrhosis plus another cause of ascites, such as tuberculosis or peritoneal carcinomatosis.[26] Approximately 5% of patients with ascites have mixed ascites (see Table 78–1). The albumin gradient is high (≥1.1 g/dL [11 g/L]) in mixed ascites, as a reflection of the underlying portal hypertension.[26]

The presence of a high SAAG does not confirm a diagnosis of cirrhosis; it simply indicates the presence of portal hypertension. There are many causes of portal hypertension other than cirrhosis (see Tables 78–1 and 78–3). A low SAAG does not confirm a diagnosis of peritoneal carcinomatosis. Although peritoneal carcinomatosis is the most common cause of a low SAAG, there are other causes (see Table 78–3). The SAAG needs only to be determined on the first paracentesis in a given patient; it does not need to be repeated in subsequent specimens, if the first value is definitive. If the first result is borderline (e.g., 1.0 or 1.1 g/dL [10 or 11 g/L]), repeating the paracentesis and analysis usually provides a definitive result.

"High albumin gradient" and "low albumin gradient" should replace the terms "transudative" and "exudative" in the classification of ascites.[25–27]

CULTURE. The technique of ascitic fluid culture has undergone a dramatic change based on recently published data.[15, 28, 29] The older method of culture assumed that most episodes of ascitic fluid infection were polymicrobial with high colony counts, as in surgical peritonitis. However, the most common bacterial infection of ascitic fluid, SBP, is monomicrobial with a low bacterial concentration (median colony count of only 1 organism/mL).[28] The older method of culture was designed to detect bacteria in the setting of polymicrobial infections with high colony counts and consisted of inoculation (in the microbiology laboratory) of each of three agar plates and some broth with a few drops of fluid. This method of culturing ascitic fluid as if it were urine or stool is predictably insensitive in detecting monomicrobial infections with low colony counts. SBP is more like bacteremia, in terms of numbers of bacteria present. Predictably, culturing ascitic fluid as if it were blood has a high yield.

In fact, the sensitivity of culture in detecting bacterial growth in neutrocytic ascites (i.e., ascitic fluid with a PMN count greater than or equal to 250 cells/mm^3 [0.25 × 10^9/L]) varies widely depending on the method of culture used. In published studies, the older method of culture has been found to detect bacterial growth in approximately 50% of neutrocytic samples, whereas bedside inoculation of blood culture bottles with ascitic fluid detects growth in approximately 80%.[15] Multiple prospective studies have demonstrated the superiority of the blood-culture-bottle method.[15] Also, bedside inoculation is superior to delayed laboratory inoculation of blood culture bottles in the laboratory.[29] Gene probes are now commercially available for the detection of bacteremia; hopefully, they will also lead to rapid (30-minute) and accurate detection of organisms in ascitic fluid.[30] However, culture will continue to be required for assessment of the susceptibility of the organism to antibiotics.

TOTAL PROTEIN. The antiquated exudate/transudate system of ascitic fluid classification, which is based on ascitic fluid total protein concentration, is problematic. The protein concentration in cirrhotic ascites is determined almost entirely by the serum protein concentration and portal pressure.[25] A cirrhotic patient with a relatively high serum protein concentration will have a relatively high ascitic fluid protein concentration. Because of this relationship, almost 20% of uncomplicated cirrhotic ascites samples have a protein concentration of greater than 2.5 g/dL (25 g/L). The ascitic fluid total protein concentration does not increase during SBP; it remains stable before, during, and after infection.[31] In fact, patients with the lowest ascitic protein concentrations are the most susceptible to spontaneous peritonitis.[32] During a 10-kg diuresis, the ascitic fluid total protein concentration doubles, and 67% of such patients with cirrhotic ascites have a protein greater than 2.5 g/dL (25 g/L) by the end of diuresis.[23] In almost one third of patients with malignant ascites, the ascites is caused by massive liver metastases or hepatocellular carcinoma; the ascitic fluid in these patients has a low protein concentration.[3] In cardiac ascites, the ascitic fluid protein concentration is greater than 2.5 g/dL (25 g/L).[33]

Therefore, the exudate/transudate method of classification of ascites places many patients with cirrhotic ascites and all patients with cardiac ascites in the exudate category, and many patients with malignant ascites and essentially all patients with spontaneously infected ascites in the transudate category. Clearly, this method of classification is not useful. In contrast, the SAAG classifies fluid by the presence or absence of portal hypertension and is much more physiologic and intuitive.[25, 26] The albumin gradient classifies cardiac ascites in the high SAAG category, similar to cirrhotic ascites. The high SAAG of cardiac ascites is presumably the result of high right-sided cardiac pressures.

Measurement of the combination of ascitic fluid total protein, glucose, and LDH is of value in distinguishing SBP from gut perforation into ascites (Fig. 78–3).[34] Patients who have neutrocytic ascitic fluid, in whom there is clinical suspicion of bacterial peritonitis (rather than peritoneal carcinomatosis or tuberculous peritonitis) and who meet two of the following three criteria, are likely to have surgical peritonitis and warrant immediate radiologic evaluation to determine if gut perforation into ascites has occurred: Total protein greater than 1 g/dL (10 g/L), glucose less than 50 mg/dL (2.8 mmol/L), and LDH greater than the upper limit of normal for serum.[34]

GLUCOSE. The glucose molecule is small enough to diffuse readily into body fluid cavities. Therefore, the concentration of glucose in ascitic fluid is similar to that in serum unless glucose is being consumed by ascitic fluid WBCs or bacteria.[34] In early SBP, the ascitic fluid glucose is similar to that of sterile fluid.[34] However, in late SBP and in the setting of gut perforation into ascitic fluid, the ascitic glucose concentration usually drops to 0 mg/dL (0 mmol/L) because of large numbers of stimulated neutrophils and bacteria.[34]

LACTATE DEHYDROGENASE. LDH enters ascitic fluid by diffusion from blood and by release from disintegrating ascitic fluid WBCs. The LDH molecule is too large to enter ascitic fluid readily from blood.[34] The ascitic fluid concentration of LDH is usually less than half of the serum level in uncomplicated cirrhotic ascites. In SBP, the ascitic fluid LDH level rises because of the release of LDH from neutrophils, and the ascitic fluid concentration is greater than that of serum. In secondary peritonitis, the LDH level is even higher than that seen in SBP and may be several-fold higher than the serum LDH level.[34]

AMYLASE. In uncomplicated cirrhotic ascites, the ascitic fluid amylase concentration is usually half that of the serum value, approximately 50 U/L.[35] In patients with acute pancreatitis or gut perforation (with release of luminal amylase into the fluid), the ascitic fluid amylase concentration is elevated markedly, usually greater than 2000 U/L and approximately five-fold greater than simultaneous serum values.[34, 35]

GRAM'S STAIN. Gram's stains of body fluids demonstrate bacteria only when there are more than 10,000 bacteria/mL. The median ascitic concentration of bacteria in SBP is only 1 organism/mL, similar to the colony count in bacteremia.[28] Requesting an ascitic fluid Gram's stain to detect bacteria in SBP is analagous to requesting Gram's stain of blood to detect bacteremia. Bacteria are present only when there is an overwhelming infection, as in advanced SBP or asplenic pneumococcal sepsis. Gram's stain of ascitic fluid is most helpful in the diagnosis of free perforation of the gut into ascites. In this setting, sheets of multiple different bacteria are found. Gram's stain of the centrifuged sediment of 50

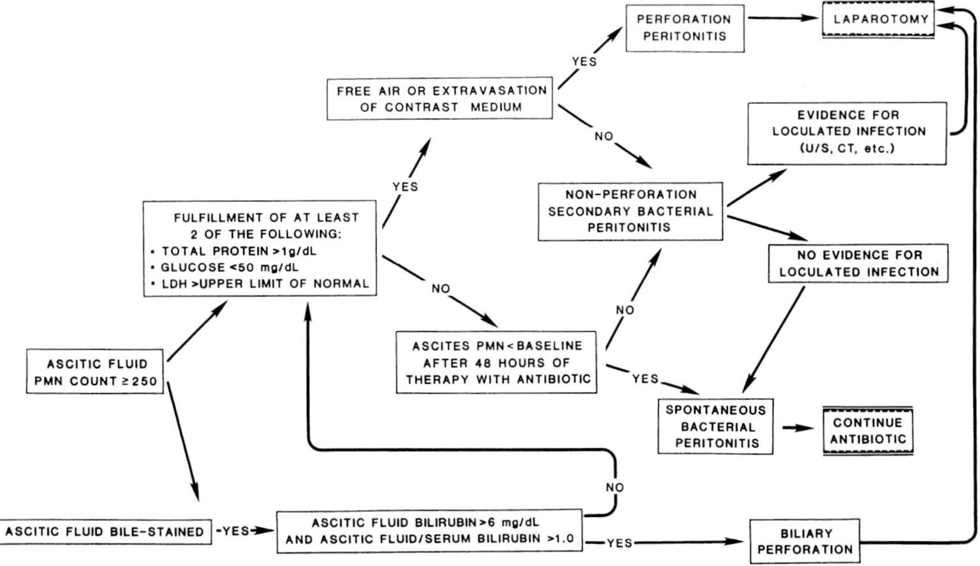

Figure 78–3. Algorithm for differentiating spontaneous from secondary bacterial peritonitis in patients with neutrocytic ascites (i.e., neutrophil count ≥ 250 cells/mm^3 [0.25×10^9/L]) in the absence of hemorrhage into ascites, tuberculosis, peritoneal carcinomatosis, or pancreatitis. U/S, ultrasound, LDH, lactate dehydrogenase; CT, computed tomography. (Reproduced with permission from Akriviadis EA, Runyon BA. The value of an algorithm in differentiating spontaneous from secondary bacterial peritonitis. Gastroenterology 98:127, 1990. Copyright 1990 by the American Gastroenterological Association.)

mL of ascites has a sensitivity rate of only 10% for visualizing bacteria in SBP.[28]

SMEAR AND CULTURE FOR TUBERCULOSIS. The direct smear of ascitic fluid to detect mycobacteria is almost never positive because of the rarity of tuberculous peritonitis and the low concentration of mycobacteria in ascitic fluid in tuberculous peritonitis.[36, 37] The older literature suggests that 1 L of fluid should be cultured. However, the largest centrifuge tube found in most laboratories has a capacity of 50 mL. In general, only one 50-mL aliquot of fluid is centrifuged, and the pellet is cultured. In contrast to a sensitivity rate of approximately 50% for ascitic fluid mycobacterial culture with optimal processing, laparoscopy with histology and culture of peritoneal biopsies has a sensitivity rate of approximately 100% in detecting tuberculous peritonitis.[36] Tuberculous peritonitis easily can be confused with SBP because both conditions are associated with abdominal pain and fever, and one half of the patients with tuberculous peritonitis have cirrhosis. However, a negative bacterial culture and predominance of mononuclear cells in the differential count provide clues to the diagnosis of tuberculous peritonitis. DNA probes are now available to detect mycobacteria and will probably replace older methods of detection.[38] However, cultures will be required to determine susceptibility to antimicrobial agents.

CYTOLOGY. In the past, it was assumed that malignant ascites was caused only by peritoneal carcinomatosis. Massive liver metastases and hepatocellular carcinoma superimposed on cirrhosis were not recognized as causes of "malignant ascites." Also, the results of cytology were not compared with a "gold standard" diagnostic test, such as autopsy, laparotomy, or laparoscopy. Cytology was reported to have a sensitivity rate of only about 60% in detecting "malignant ascites."[39] However, cytology can be expected to detect malignancy only when tumor cells line the peritoneal cavity and exfoliate into the ascitic fluid, that is, in peritoneal carcinomatosis. Cytology should not be expected to detect tumor when the peritoneum is uninvolved, as in hepatocellular carcinoma or massive liver metastases causing ascites because of portal hypertension, or malignant lymphoma causing ascites by lymph node obstruction.[3] In one study in which the location and type of tumor causing ascites were confirmed by a gold standard test, only approximately two thirds of patients with malignancy-related ascites were found to have peritoneal carcinomatosis.[3] Essentially 100% of patients with peritoneal carcinomatosis were reported to have a positive fluid cytology.[3] The remaining one third of patients with massive liver metastases, chylous ascites caused by lymphoma, or hepatocellular carcinoma had a negative cytology.[3] Therefore, the sensitivity rate for cytology is approximately 100% for detecting peritoneal carcinomatosis but lower for detecting malignancy-related ascites caused by conditions other than peritoneal carcinomatosis. Cytology should not be falsely positive if performed carefully; the author has never encountered a false-positive result. Because hepatocellular carcinoma rarely metastasizes to the peritoneum, a positive cytology in a patient with hepatocellular carcinoma is unusual enough to be the subject of a case report.[40] Measurement of the serum alpha-fetoprotein concentration (which is always higher in serum than in ascitic fluid) may be of value in detecting hepatocellular carcinoma; alpha-fetoprotein is much more sensitive than ascitic cytology for this purpose.[3] Malignancy-related ascites may have an elevated PMN count, presumably because dying tumor cells attract neutrophils into the fluid.[3, 41] The elevated PMN count may cause confusion with SBP; however, there usually is a predominance of lymphocytes in malignancy-related ascites. Flow cytometry of ascitic fluid as an adjunct to cytology may further increase diagnostic accuracy.

TRIGLYCERIDE. A triglyceride level should be measured on opalescent or frankly milky ascitic fluid (see Fig. 78–2). By definition, chylous ascites has a triglyceride concentration greater than 200 mg/dL (2.26 mmol/L) and greater than the serum level; usually the level is greater than 1000 mg/dL (11.30 mmol/L).[42] In sterile cirrhotic ascitic fluid specimens that are slightly cloudy without an elevated cell count (i.e., opalescent), the triglyceride concentration is elevated—64 $\pm$ 40 mg/dL (0.72 $\pm$ 0.45 mmol/L), compared with 18 $\pm$ 9 mg/dL (0.20 $\pm$ 0.10 mmol/L) for clear cirrhotic ascites.[19]

BILIRUBIN. The bilirubin concentration should be measured in ascitic fluid that is dark brown. An ascitic fluid bilirubin level greater than 6 mg/dL (102 μmol/L) and greater than the serum level of bilirubin suggests biliary or upper gut perforation into ascites.[21, 34]

TESTS THAT ARE SELDOM HELPFUL. Tests that have been proposed to be helpful in the analysis of ascitic fluid but shown subsequently to be unhelpful include pH, lactate, fibronectin, and cholesterol. The studies that attempted to validate the value of pH and lactate included small numbers of patients and used suboptimal culture techniques. In the two largest and most recent studies, which did not have some of the deficiencies of the earlier studies, the ascitic fluid pH and lactate were found not to be helpful.[43, 44] The pH was found to have no impact on decision-making regarding the use of empiric antibiotics.[43]

Fibronectin and cholesterol have been proposed to be useful in detecting malignant ascites. The basic premise of studies of these markers was that ascitic fluid cytology is insensitive. Unfortunately, the design of the studies was problematic, several subgroups of malignancy-related ascites (e.g., massive liver metastases, hepatocellular carcinoma with cirrhosis) were not acknowledged, and appropriate control groups (e.g., patients with ascites caused by conditions other than cirrhosis or peritoneal carcinomatosis) were not included. Other studies have demonstrated that in patients with massive liver metastases, ascitic fluid fibronectin and cholesterol concentrations are not abnormally elevated.[45, 46] Therefore, in patients with malignancy-related ascites and a negative cytology, these "humoral tests of malignancy" usually are negative. Additionally, patients with high-protein noncirrhotic ascites nearly always have false-positive ascitic fibronectin and cholesterol elevations.[3, 45, 46]

Carcinoembryonic antigen (CEA) in ascitic fluid has been proposed as a helpful test for detecting malignant ascites.[47] However, the study that attempted to validate this test was flawed, and more studies, with various subgroups of patients, are required before ascitic fluid CEA can be considered validated.

Adenosine deaminase has been proposed as a useful test in detecting peritoneal tuberculosis. However, in the United

States, where more than 50% of patients with tuberculous peritonitis have underlying cirrhosis, adenosine deaminase has been found to be too insensitive to be helpful.[37]

DIFFERENTIAL DIAGNOSIS

Although cirrhosis is the cause of ascites in most patients evaluated by internists, a cause other than liver disease is found in approximately 20% of patients (see Table 78–1). Approximately 5% of patients have two causes of ascites, that is, "mixed" ascites.[26] Usually, these patients have cirrhosis plus one other cause, such as peritoneal carcinomatosis or peritoneal tuberculosis (see Table 78–1). Because tuberculosis is potentially fatal but curable and frequently occurs in cirrhotic patients with preexisting ascites, the physician must not assume that liver disease is the only cause of ascites in a febrile alcoholic patient if the ascitic fluid analysis is atypical. For example, if the ascitic fluid lymphocyte count is unusually high, peritoneal tuberculosis may be present. Interpretation of ascitic fluid analysis is difficult in patients with mixed ascites but crucial to accurate diagnosis and treatment. Additionally, liver diseases other than cirrhosis (e.g., fulminant hepatic failure) may cause ascites (see Table 78–1).

An algorithm for the differential diagnosis of ascites is shown in Figure 78–2. This proposed strategy is applicable to the majority of patients with ascites, including many with the causes listed in Table 78–1. However, not every patient (including patients with rare causes of ascites) can be categorized readily with such an algorithm. Many patients with enigmatic ascites eventually are found to have two or even three causes of ascites (e.g., heart failure, cirrhosis caused by nonalcoholic steatohepatitis, and diabetic nephropathy). In these cases, the sum of predisposing factors leads to sodium and water retention even though each individual factor may not be severe enough by itself to cause fluid overload.

In most patients with ascites, cirrhosis is the cause. Cirrhotic ascites, especially low-protein cirrhotic ascites, is complicated frequently by SBP (see later). Other forms of ascites are complicated by spontaneous peritonitis so rarely that they are the subjects of case reports or small series.[48–50]

The gut can perforate into ascites of any cause, cirrhosis or otherwise. The ascitic fluid analysis in gut perforation is dramatically different from that in SBP (see Fig. 78–3).[34] Distinguishing SBP from surgical peritonitis in a patient with cirrhosis is critical to the patient's survival; SBP is treated with antibiotics alone, whereas surgical peritonitis is treated with antibiotics and emergent surgical intervention.

Cancer accounts for less than 10% of cases of ascites (see Table 78–1). Not all malignancy-related ascites is caused by peritoneal carcinomatosis; the characteristics of the ascitic fluid and the treatments vary depending on the pathophysiology of ascites formation, for example, peritoneal carcinomatosis versus massive liver metastases (Table 78–4; see also section, "Ascitic Fluid Analysis").[3]

Heart failure accounts for less than 5% of cases. Cardiac ascites is characterized by a high albumin gradient, high ascitic protein concentration, and normal blood hematocrit value.[33] Patients with cardiac ascites usually have alcoholic cardiomyopathy, with cardiomegaly on chest x-ray and four-chamber enlargement of the heart on echocardiogram. Clinically, heart failure may mimic cirrhosis, including the presence of small nonbleeding esophageal varices and hepatic encephalopathy.[51] Cirrhotic ascites has a high albumin gradient like cardiac ascites but a low protein concentration, and patients with cirrhosis and ascites have a lower mean blood hematocrit value of 32%.[33]

Table 78–4 | **Classification of Malignancy-Related Ascites**

Peritoneal carcinomatosis
Massive liver metastases
Peritoneal carcinomatosis with massive liver metastases
Hepatocellular carcinoma
Malignant lymph node obstruction
Malignant Budd-Chiari syndrome (tumor emboli in hepatic veins)

In the United States, tuberculous peritonitis is generally a disease of Asian and Latin American immigrants to the West Coast, poor blacks, and the elderly. Tuberculous peritonitis was a rare disease between 1955 and 1985, but it has increased in prevalence because of the acquired immunodeficiency syndrome (AIDS). Fifty percent of patients with tuberculous peritonitis have underlying cirrhosis (i.e., "mixed" ascites). Although most patients with liver disease are not unusually predisposed to the hepatotoxicity of antituberculous drugs, they tolerate drug toxicity less well than do patients with normal livers.[52] Therefore, a diagnosis of mixed tuberculous and cirrhotic ascites is important. Underdiagnosis can lead to unnecessary deaths from untreated tuberculosis, whereas overdiagnosis and overtreatment of suspected but unproven tuberculous peritonitis may lead to unnecessary deaths from the hepatotoxicity of isoniazid. If the clinical circumstances (e.g., a febrile immigrant from an area endemic for tuberculosis) and initial ascitic fluid analysis (high lymphocyte count) suggest tuberculosis, strong consideration should be given to an urgent laparoscopy with histology and culture of peritoneal biopies. If the peritoneum has the typical "millet-seed" and "violin-string" appearance, antituberculous therapy can be started immediately. Blind peritoneal biopsy may be performed in the patient without cirrhosis, but in a cirrhotic patient, the predictable presence of peritoneal collateral veins makes blind biopsy potentially hazardous. Laparoscopically guided biopsy is preferable. Suspected tuberculous peritonitis is one of the few principal indications for diagnostic laparoscopy.[53] Peritoneal coccidioidomycosis can mimic tuberculous peritonitis, including its appearance at laparoscopy, and can occur in patients without AIDS.[54] There has been a resurgence of tuberculous peritonitis coincident with the AIDS epidemic.[55]

The high sensitivity rates of cytology for peritoneal carcinomatosis and ultrasound-guided biopsy for focal liver lesions have obviated the need for laparoscopy in detecting tumor, for all practical purposes.[3]

Pancreatic ascites, an uncommon condition, occurs in patients with clinically obvious severe acute pancreatitis or a history of chronic pancreatitis. It is not necessary to order an ascitic fluid amylase level on all ascitic fluid samples, only for patients in whom pancreatitis is suspected or the initial ascitic fluid is nondiagnostic (see Table 78–2). Patients with alcohol-related pancreatic ascites also may have underlying alcoholic cirrhosis. Pancreatic ascites is frequently neutrocytic and also may be complicated by bacterial infection. Patients with an ascitic fluid neutrophil count greater than or equal to 250 cells/mm^3 (0.25 × 10^9/L) warrant empirical antibiotic coverage, at least until the cause of the elevated neutrophil count is explained.

Nephrogenous ascites is a poorly understood form of ascites that develops in patients undergoing hemodialysis.[56] On careful evaluation, most of these patients are found to have another cause of ascites, usually cirrhosis from alcohol abuse or hepatitis C. The presence of a second cause for fluid overload explains why these patients have ascites, whereas the majority of patients on dialysis do not.

Chlamydia peritonitis should be suspected in sexually active, young women with fever and neutrocytic, high-protein, low-gradient ascites and no evidence of liver disease.[11] This infection responds rapidly to oral doxycycline and is one of the few curable causes of ascites.

Although the nephrotic syndrome used to be a common cause of ascites in children, it is rare in adults.[57] When it occurs in adults, there is usually a second cause of ascites, just as in nephrogenous ascites.[57] The ascitic fluid usually is characterized by a low protein concentration and low albumin gradient and can be complicated by SBP.

In some patients, pathologic accumulations of fluid develop in the peritoneal cavity as a result of leakage from a ruptured viscus (e.g., "bile ascites" from a ruptured gallbladder).[21] The ascitic fluid analysis is critical to the preoperative diagnosis of this condition (see earlier section, "Ascitic Fluid Analysis" and Fig. 78–3).

Chylous ascites develops when intra-abdominal lymphatics containing chyle are ruptured. The older literature suggests that this form of ascites is caused by a malignancy in almost 90% of patients.[42] In contrast, cirrhosis is the cause of chylous ascites in more than 90% of the patients that the author has encountered (see Table 78–1).[20, 26] The high lymphatic flow and pressure must be the cause of lymphatic rupture in patients with cirrhosis. Retroperitoneal surgery and radical pelvic surgery in patients with cancer can transect lymphatics and lead to chylous ascites as well.

Causes of ascites excluded from or not encountered in the list in Table 78–1 include ambulatory peritoneal dialysis fluid, Budd-Chiari syndrome, myxedema, connective tissue disease, postoperative ascites, and rare causes. The iatrogenic form of ascites associated with peritoneal dialysis usually is not under the care of gastroenterologists. Although the Budd-Chiari syndrome is regularly complicated by ascites, hepatic vein thrombosis itself is rare enough that it accounts for less than 0.1% of cases of ascites. Ascites in patients with myxedema appears to be of cardiac origin, related to heart failure.[58] Treatment of the hypothyroidism cures the fluid retention. Serositis with ascites formation may complicate systemic lupus erythematosus.[12]

The development of ascites after abdominal surgery (in particular, after inappropriate cholecystectomy in the setting of asymptomatic gallstones and abnormal liver tests) is a common mode of presentation of previously undiagnosed cirrhosis.[5] Resection of hepatocellular carcinoma in the setting of cirrhosis regularly leads to hepatic decompensation, which all too often starts a downward spiral ending in fatality.[59]

Aggressive hormone administration to induce ovulation can lead to ascites from "ovarian hyperstimulation syndrome."[60] Other rare causes of ascites include the POEMS syndrome (polyneuropathy, organomegaly, endocrinopathy, M component, and skin changes) and chemotherapy with 5-fluorouracil for colon cancer.[61, 62]

COMPLICATIONS OF ASCITES

Infection

Ascitic fluid infection can be classified into five categories based on ascitic culture results, PMN count, and presence or absence of a surgical source of infection (Table 78–5). An abdominal paracentesis must be performed and ascitic fluid must be analyzed before a confident diagnosis of ascitic fluid infection can be made. A "clinical diagnosis" of infected ascitic fluid without a paracentesis is not adequate.

Subtypes

Of the three subtypes of spontaneous ascitic fluid infection, the prototype is SBP. The diagnosis of SBP is made when there is a positive ascitic fluid culture and an elevated ascitic fluid absolute PMN count (i.e., at least 250 cells/mm^3 [0.25 × 10^9/L]) without evidence of an intra-abdominal surgically treatable source of infection.[15] When Conn coined the term *spontaneous bacterial peritonitis* in 1975, his goal was to distinguish this form of infection from surgical peritonitis,[63] a very important distinction. Therefore, although many patients with SBP have a focus of infection (e.g., urinary tract infection or pneumonia), they are labeled SBP unless the focus requires surgical intervention (e.g., a ruptured viscus). The author has not encountered a convincing case of polymicrobial SBP. All the patients presumed to have SBP in whom ascitic fluid cultures initially grew more than one organism eventually were found to have surgical peritonitis or an erroneous culture result (e.g., a pathogen plus a contaminant or two colony morphologies of one species of bacteria).

The criteria for a diagnosis of monomicrobial non-neutrocytic bacterascites (MNB) include (1) a positive ascitic fluid culture for a single organism, (2) an ascitic fluid PMN count lower than 250 cells/mm^3 (0.25 × 10^9/L), and (3) no evidence of an intra-abdominal surgically treatable source of infection.[64] In the older literature, MNB was either grouped with SBP or labeled "asymptomatic bacterascites." Because many patients with bacterascites have symptoms, the modifier "asymptomatic" seems inappropriate.

Culture-negative neutrocytic ascites (CNNA) is diagnosed when (1) the ascitic fluid culture grows no bacteria, (2) the ascitic fluid PMN count is equal to or higher than 250 cells/mm^3 (0.25 × 10^9/L), (3) no antibiotics have been given (not even a single dose), and (4) there is no other explanation for an elevated ascitic PMN count (e.g., hemorrhage into ascites, peritoneal carcinomatosis, tuberculosis, or pancreatitis).[65]

Table 78–5 | **Classification of Ascitic Fluid Infection**

Spontaneous ascitic fluid infection
Spontaneous bacterial peritonitis
Monomicrobial non-neutrocytic bacterascites
Culture-negative neutrocytic ascites
Secondary bacterial peritonitis
Polymicrobial bacterascites (needle perforation of the bowel)

This variant of ascitic fluid infection is seldom diagnosed when sensitive culture methods are used.[28, 29]

Secondary bacterial peritonitis is diagnosed when (1) the ascitic fluid culture is positive (usually for multiple organisms), (2) the PMN count is equal to or greater than 250 cells/mm^3 (0.25 × 10^9/L), and (3) there is an identified intra-abdominal surgically treatable primary source of infection (e.g., perforated gut, perinephric abscess).[34] The importance of distinguishing this variant from SBP is that secondary peritonitis usually requires emergency surgical intervention.

Polymicrobial bacterascites is diagnosed when (1) multiple organisms are seen on Gram stain or cultured from the ascitic fluid and (2) the PMN count is lower than 250 cells/mm^3 (0.25 × 10^9/L).[66] This diagnosis should be suspected when the paracentesis is traumatic or unusually difficult because of ileus, or when stool or air is aspirated into the paracentesis syringe. Polymicrobial bacterascites is essentially diagnostic of gut perforation by the paracentesis needle.

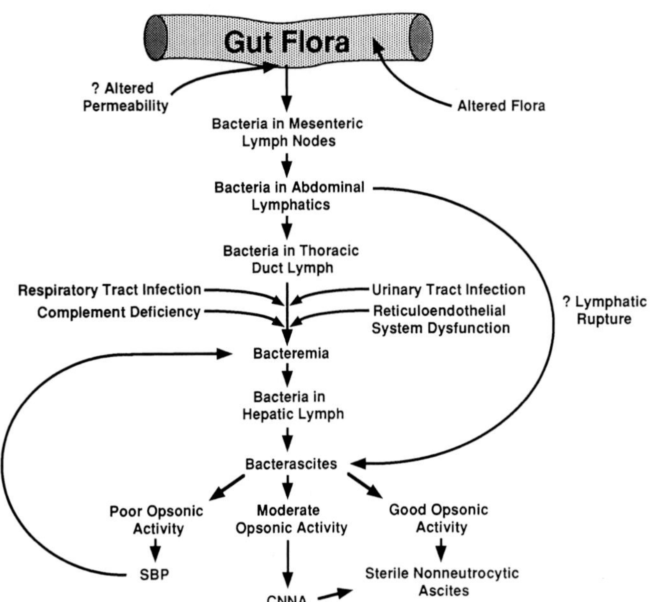

Figure 78–4. Proposed pathogenesis of spontaneous ascitic fluid infection. (SBP, spontaneous bacterial peritonitis; CNNA, culture-negative neutrocytic ascites.)

Clinical Setting

The spontaneous variants of ascitic fluid infection (SBP, CNNA, and MNB) occur only in the setting of severe liver disease. The liver disease is usually chronic (cirrhosis), but may be acute (fulminant hepatic failure) or subacute (alcoholic hepatitis). Cirrhosis of all causes can be complicated by spontaneous ascitic fluid infection. Spontaneous infection of noncirrhotic ascites is rare enough to be the subject of case reports.[48–50]

Essentially all patients with SBP have an elevated serum bilirubin level and abnormal prothrombin time, and they usually have Child-Pugh class B or C cirrhosis.[15] Ascites appears to be a prerequisite to the development of SBP. It is unlikely that SBP precedes the development of ascites. Usually, the infection develops when the volume of ascites is at its maximum.

Secondary bacterial peritonitis and polymicrobial bacterascites can develop in ascites of any type. The only prerequisite, in addition to the presence of ascites, for the development of secondary bacterial peritonitis is an intra-abdominal surgical source of infection.[34] Such an infection can result from penetration of a needle into the bowel during attempted paracentesis.[66]

Pathogenesis

Over the past several years, the elusive source of SBP has become clearer, and the pathogenesis of spontaneous forms of ascitic fluid infection has been partially elucidated (Fig. 78–4). The body of currently available evidence suggests that the spontaneous forms of ascitic fluid infection are the result of overgrowth of a specific organism in the gut, "translocation" of that microbe from the gut to mesenteric lymph nodes, and resulting spontaneous bacteremia and subsequent colonization of susceptible ascitic fluid (see Fig. 78–4).[67–69]

Once bacteria enter the fluid in the abdomen, by whatever route, a battle ensues between the virulence factors of the organism and the immune defenses of the host.[70] The ascitic fluid protein concentration does not change with development of spontaneous infection.[31] Low-protein ascitic fluid (e.g., <1 g/dL [10 g/L]) is particularly susceptible to SBP.[32] The endogenous antimicrobial activity (opsonic activity) of human ascitic fluid correlates directly with the protein concentration of the fluid.[70] Patients with deficient ascitic fluid opsonic activity are predisposed to SBP.[71] Patients with detectable ascitic fluid opsonic activity appear to be protected from SBP unless they are exposed to a particularly virulent organism (e.g., *Salmonella*).[50, 70, 71]

Recent studies in both patients and animals with cirrhosis demonstrate that MNB is common.[64, 72] In both humans and rats, most episodes of bacterascites resolve without antibiotic treatment.[64, 72] The fluid frequently becomes sterile without a rise in ascitic PMN. Apparently, the host's defense mechanisms are able to eradicate the invading bacteria on most occasions. It is probable that uncontrolled infection develops only when the defenses are weak or the organism is virulent (see Fig. 78–4). Bacterascites is probably more common than SBP. It is conceivable that cirrhotic ascites is regularly colonized by bacteria, and almost just as regularly, the colonization resolves. The entry of PMNs into the fluid probably signals failure of the peritoneal macrophages to control the infection.[73] The majority of episodes of MNB appear to resolve in cirrhotic rats and humans, whereas untreated SBP frequently is fatal. In summary, MNB probably represents an early stage of ascitic fluid infection, which can resolve to CNNA or progress to SBP.

Most episodes of CNNA are diagnosed by insensitive culture methods for which there are insufficient numbers of bacteria to reach the threshold of detectability.[28] Inoculation of ascitic fluid into blood culture bottles can lead to detection of a single organism in the cultured aliquot of fluid, whereas the older method of culture probably requires at least 100 organisms/mL.[28] However, even when optimal culture methods are used, a small percentage of patients grow no bacteria from their neutrocytic ascitic fluid. A study of

Table 78–6 | **Symptoms and Signs of Ascitic Fluid Infection***

	SBP	BACTERASCITES	CNNA	SECONDARY PERITONITIS	POLYMICROBIAL BACTERASCITES
Fever	68	57	50	33	10
Abdominal pain	49	32	72	67	10
Tender abdomen	39	32	44	50	10
Rebound	10	5	0	17	0
Altered mental status	54	50	61	33	0

*Data presented as % of the total number of patients in that group. CNNA, culture-negative neutrocytic ascites; SBP, spontaneous bacterial peritonitis. Data from references 34, 64–66.

rapid sequential paracenteses (before the initiation of antibiotic treatment) in patients with CNNA demonstrated that in most cases, the PMN count dropped spontaneously and the culture remained negative in the second specimen.[74] When sensitive culture techniques are used, CNNA probably represents spontaneously resolving SBP in which the paracentesis is performed after all bacteria have been killed by host defenses, but before the PMN count has normalized.

The pathogenesis of secondary bacterial peritonitis is more straightforward than that of SBP. When the gut perforates, billions of bacteria flood into the ascites. In the absence of a frank perforation, bacteria may cross inflamed tissue planes and enter the ascites. The pathogenesis of polymicrobial bacterascites is also apparent.[66] The paracentesis needle enters the bowel, and the bowel contents are released into the ascites.

Symptoms and Signs

Although 87% of patients with SBP are symptomatic at the time the infection is diagnosed, the symptoms and signs of infection are often subtle, such as a slight change in mental status.[64] Without prompt paracentesis, the diagnosis and treatment of infected ascites may be delayed, often resulting in the death of the patient. The symptoms and signs manifested in all five variants of ascitic fluid infection are listed in Table 78–6.

Prevalence

Before the 1980s, abdominal paracentesis was not performed routinely because of fear that complications of the procedure would occur and because the utility of ascitic fluid analysis in the differential diagnosis of ascites was not fully recognized. Now, paracentesis is performed routinely at the time of admission to the hospital in many patients with ascites. Routine admission paracenteses have provided data regarding the prevalence of ascitic fluid infection. In the 1980s, about 10% of patients with ascites were infected at the time of hospital admission; of the subgroup of patients with cirrhotic ascites, about 27% were infected.[15, 32] At the present time, because of measures to prevent SBP, this prevalence has dropped significantly (see later). Of patients with culture-positive ascitic fluid, about two thirds have neutrocytic ascitic fluid (SBP), and one third have MNB.[64] The frequency of CNNA depends largely on the culture technique (see earlier). Polymicrobial bacterascites occurs in only 1 in 1000 paracenteses. Secondary bacterial peritonitis occurs in only 0% to 2% of patients with ascites at the time of admission to the hospital.[15, 34]

Bacteriology

Escherichia coli, streptococci (mostly pneumococci), and *Klebsiella* cause most episodes of SBP and MNB in patients who are not receiving selective intestinal decontamination (Table 78–7; see later). CNNA is by definition culture-negative. Polymicrobial bacterascites is by definition polymicrobial. The most apparent difference between the spontaneous forms of ascitic fluid infection and the secondary forms (secondary peritonitis and polymicrobial bacterascites) is that the former are always monomicrobial and the latter are usually polymicrobial. Although older papers reported that anaerobic bacteria were present in approximately 6% of cases of SBP, the detection of anaerobes probably reflected unrec-

Table 78–7 | **Pathogens in Ascitic Fluid Infection***

ORGANISM	SBP	MONOMICROBIAL NON-NEUTROCYTIC BACTERASCITES	SECONDARY BACTERIAL PERITONITIS	SBP WITH SID
Monomicrobial				
Escherichia coli	37	27	20	0
Klebsiella pneumoniae	17	11	7	7
Pneumococcus	12	9	0	29
Streptococcus viridans	9	2	0	0
Staphylococcus aureus	0	7	13	0
Misc gram-negative	10	14	7	7
Misc gram-positive	14	30	0	50
Polymicrobial	1	0	53	7

*Data reported as % of total in that group. SBP, spontaneous bacterial peritonitis; SID, selective intestinal decontamination. Data from references 37, 64, 75.

ognized cases of secondary bacterial peritonitis. In recent series, anaerobes have been found in approximately 1% of cases of SBP and MNB.[28, 64]

Selective intestinal decontamination causes a change in the bacteria isolated from patients who develop an ascitic infection. Gram-positive organisms usually are cultured from the ascitic fluid of these patients (see Table 78–7).[75]

Risk Factors

Patients with cirrhosis are unusually predisposed to bacterial infection because of multiple defects in immune defense. The concept that cirrhosis is a form of acquired immunodeficiency (in the generic sense) is rather new. In a recently published prospective study, a bacterial infection occurred in more than 40% of consecutive cirrhotic patients at the time of admission to the hospital or during the hospitalization.[76] Low ascitic fluid total protein concentrations, as well as the phagocytic (both motile and stationary) dysfunction associated with cirrhosis, are risk factors for bacterial infection.

Paracentesis itself has been proposed as a risk factor for ascitic fluid infection. This theoretical risk has not been substantiated in prospective studies of paracentesis-related complications.[16] SBP is statistically more likely to be diagnosed on the first paracentesis than on subsequent taps.[16] Needle-induced ascitic fluid infections do not occur unless the bowel is penetrated by the paracentesis needle.[16, 66] Fortunately, this occurs in only one in 1000 taps. One would expect skin flora such as *Staphylococcus aureus* to be isolated more frequently if poor paracentesis technique were the cause of many cases of SBP; yet skin flora are very seldom isolated from ascites.[28] Iatrogenic peritonitis is most likely to occur when the paracentesis needle enters the bowel during a difficult paracentesis.

Gastrointestinal hemorrhage is an under-recognized risk factor for the development of spontaneous bacteremia and SBP. The cumulative probability of infection during a single hospitalization for bleeding is approximately 40%.[77] The risk appears to peak 48 hours after the onset of hemorrhage. The high risk of infection is probably mediated by a shock-induced increase in the translocation of bacteria from the gut to extraintestinal sites.[78] Urinary tract infections are also an under-recognized risk factor for SBP.[79]

Diagnosis

Timely diagnosis of ascitic fluid infection requires a high index of suspicion and a low threshold for performing a paracentesis. Clinical deterioration, especially fever or abdominal pain, in a patient with ascites should raise the suspicion of infection and prompt a paracentesis. If the ascitic fluid PMN count is elevated, the working diagnosis is ascitic fluid infection until proven otherwise. Although peritoneal carcinomatosis, pancreatitis, hemorrhage into ascites, and tuberculosis can lead to an elevated ascitic fluid PMN count, most cases of neutrocytic ascites are caused by infection. A predominance of PMNs in the WBC differential count lends further credence to the diagnosis of infection. In patients with peritoneal carcinomatosis, pancreatitis, and tuberculosis, there usually is not a predominance of PMNs in the ascites. An elevated absolute ascitic fluid PMN count with a predominance of neutrophils in a clinical setting compatible with infection should prompt empirical antibiotic therapy (Table 78–8; also, see details later in text).

Table 78–8 | **Indications for Empirical Antibiotic Therapy of Suspected Spontaneous Ascitic Fluid Infection**

Ascitic fluid neutrophil count ≥ 250/mm³ (0.25 × 10⁹/L)
Convincing symptoms or signs of infection

Although SBP is approximately six times as common as surgical peritonitis in a patient with ascites, secondary peritonitis should be considered in any patient with neutrocytic ascites. Clinical symptoms and signs do not distinguish patients with secondary peritonitis from those with SBP (see Fig. 78–3).[34] Even with free perforation of the colon into ascitic fluid, a classic surgical abdomen does not develop. Peritoneal signs require contact of inflamed visceral and parietal peritoneal surfaces. Such contact does not occur when there is a large volume of fluid separating these surfaces. Gut perforation can be suspected and pursued if a specimen of ascites is neutrocytic and meets two of the following three criteria (see Fig. 78–3): Total protein greater than 1 g/dL (10 g/L), glucose less than 50 mg/dL (2.8 mmol/L), and LDH greater than the upper limit of normal for serum.[34] In the setting of a perforated viscus, cultures of ascitic fluid nearly always disclose multiple organisms, except gallbladder rupture, which is usually monomicrobial.[21] Brown ascitic fluid with a bilirubin concentration that is greater than 6 mg/dL (102 μmol/L) and greater than the serum level is indicative of biliary or upper gut perforation into ascites.[21] An ascitic fluid amylase level that is greater than five-fold that of the serum level also may be indicative of gut rupture (except gallbladder rupture) and the release of luminal amylase.[34, 35]

The initial ascitic fluid analysis is helpful in delineating which patients are likely to have a ruptured viscus (see Fig. 78–3). Within minutes of the detection of neutrocytic ascitic fluid, these patients should undergo a radiologic evaluation to confirm and localize the site of rupture. Plain and upright abdominal films and water-soluble contrast studies of the upper and lower gut should be obtained. If perforation is documented, emergency surgical intervention is the next step. Timing is crucial; after septic shock occurs, death is nearly certain. Antibiotic therapy without surgical intervention in the treatment of a ruptured viscus is predictably unsuccessful.

In contrast to patients with peritonitis resulting from perforation of a viscus, patients with secondary peritonitis unrelated to perforation tend not to have a diagnostic initial ascitic fluid analysis.[34] It is less urgent to make the diagnosis of secondary peritonitis in patients without free perforation, and there may be time to evaluate the response of the ascitic PMN count and fluid culture to treatment with antibiotics. The best time to repeat the paracentesis to assess the response to treatment is after 48 hours of therapy; by 48 hours in essentially every patient with SBP who has been treated with an appropriate antibiotic, the ascitic PMN count will be lower than the pretreatment value, and the ascitic culture will be negative.[34] Before 48 hours of treatment, the ascitic PMN count may rise to a value higher than baseline in either SBP or secondary peritonitis.[34] The culture remains positive in secondary peritonitis and becomes rapidly negative in SBP (see Fig. 78–3).[34] Antibiotics alone cannot control secondary peritonitis, but medical therapy rapidly cures SBP.[34]

Treatment

Patients with an ascitic fluid PMN count greater than or equal to 250 cells/mm^3 (0.25 × 10^9/L) and a clinical picture compatible with ascitic fluid infection should receive empirical antibiotic treatment (Table 78–9; see also Table 78–8).[15] Patients with hemorrhage into ascites, peritoneal carcinomatosis, pancreatic ascites, or tuberculous peritonitis may have an elevated PMN count that is unrelated to SBP and usually do not require empirical antibiotic treatment. If they do receive antibiotics, the ascitic PMN count usually fluctuates randomly, in contrast to the dramatic reduction in PMN count typical of SBP. If the clinical picture initially is unclear, the physician should err on the side of antibiotic treatment (with a non-nephrotoxic antibiotic). Usually in patients with uninfected neutrocytic ascitic fluid (except those with hemorrhage), lymphocytes predominate in the ascitic fluid differential count, in contrast to SBP, in which PMNs predominate. In patients with bloody ascites, a "corrected" PMN count should be calculated (as discussed earlier). Antibiotic therapy is not necessary for patients with bloody ascites unless the corrected ascitic PMN count is greater than or equal to 250 cells/mm^3 (0.25 × 10^9/L).

The decision to begin empirical antibiotic treatment in patients with bacterascites must be individualized. Many episodes resolve without treatment.[64] However, the hospital mortality rate of 22% to 43% in patients with MNB is due at least in part to infection.[64, 80] Therefore, treatment appears to be warranted in many patients. By definition, the ascitic PMN count is lower than 250 cells/mm^3 (0.25 × 10^9/L) in this variant of ascitic fluid infection, and the PMN count cannot be the only parameter on which to base the decision about empirical therapy. Most patients with MNB in whom the colonization does not resolve progress to SBP and have symptoms or signs of infection at the time of the paracentesis that documents bacterascites.[64] Therefore, patients with cirrhotic ascites who have convincing symptoms or signs of infection should receive treatment regardless of the ascitic PMN count. Empirical treatment can be discontinued after only 2 to 3 days if the culture demonstrates no growth. Asymptomatic patients may not need treatment.[64, 80] The paracentesis should be repeated for cell count and culture in patients without clinical evidence of infection, once it is known that the initial culture is positive. If the PMN count has risen to at least 250/mm^3 (0.25 × 10^9/L) or if symptoms or signs of infection have developed, treatment should be started. Culture results usually are negative in patients without a rise in the ascitic PMN count on repeat paracentesis and without clinical evidence of infection, and these persons do not require treatment.[64] In these patients, colonization has been eradicated by host immune defenses.

The physician will not know initially that the ascitic culture is destined to be negative in a patient with CNNA; therefore, empirical antibiotic treatment should be started. When the preliminary culture demonstrates no growth, it is helpful to repeat the paracentesis after 48 hours of therapy to assess the response of the PMN count to antibiotics. A dramatic decline in PMN count (always below the baseline pretreatment value and frequently a greater than 80% reduction) confirms a response to treatment. In such cases, a few more days of therapy probably is warranted.[81] A stable ascitic PMN count, especially if there is a predominance of lymphocytes and monocytes, suggests a nonbacterial (or mycobacterial) cause of ascitic neutrocytosis, and sending fluid for cytology and mycobacterial culture is appropriate. Because a negative culture may be the result of insensitive culture techniques, the prevalence of CNNA in a hospital that still uses conventional methods of culture can be reduced by convincing the microbiology laboratory to accept and process ascitic fluid submitted in blood culture bottles.[28]

Gram stain of the ascitic fluid is most helpful in detecting secondary peritonitis, in which multiple different bacterial forms are seen. Gram stain is of little value in guiding the choice of empirical antibiotic treatment for spontaneous ascitic infections. The author has found that Gram stain did not help narrow the antibiotic coverage in even 1 patient of approximately 500 with SBP. Only approximately 10% of Gram stains demonstrate organisms in SBP.[28] If Gram stain indicates secondary peritonitis, coverage of anaerobic flora, in addition to coverage of aerobic and facultative anaerobic flora, is required, as is an emergency search for the source of the infection (see Fig. 78–3 and Table 78–9).[34] Therefore, a positive Gram stain may lead to broader antibiotic coverage rather than narrower coverage. Choosing narrow coverage (e.g., penicillin alone) based on a misinterpretation of the significance of the results of Gram stain may lead to the patient's death from uncontrolled infection before it be-

Table 78–9 | **Treatment of Subtypes of Ascitic Fluid Infection**

DIAGNOSIS	TREATMENT
Spontaneous bacterial peritonitis	Five days of intravenous antibiotic to which the organism is highly susceptible (e.g., cefotaxime 2 g every 8 hours empirically followed by more narrow spectrum therapy after susceptibility results are available)
Monomicrobial non-neutrocytic bacterascites	Five days of intravenous antibiotic to which the organism is highly susceptible, if the patient is symptomatic or persistently culture-positive. Not all patients with bacterascites require treatment
Culture-negative neutrocytic ascites	Five days of intravenous third-generation cephalosporin (e.g., cefotaxime 2 g q8h)
Secondary bacterial peritonitis	Surgical intervention plus approximately 2 weeks of intravenous cephalosporin (e.g., cefotaxime 2 g q8h) plus an antianaerobic drug such as metronidazole
Polymicrobial bacterascites	Intravenous third-generation cephalosporin (e.g., cefotaxime 2 g q8h) plus an antianaerobic drug such as metronidazole. Duration is determined by clinical response and serial ascitic fluid PMN counts and cultures

PMN, polymorphonuclear neutrophil.

comes apparent that the isolated organism is resistant to the chosen antibiotic.

Until the results of susceptibility testing are available, relatively broad-spectrum antibiotic therapy is warranted in patients with suspected ascitic fluid infection. After sensitivities are known, the spectrum of coverage usually can be narrowed. The antibiotics that have been recommended for empirical treatment have changed over the past several years. In 1978, the combination of ampicillin and gentamicin was promoted, but this recommendation was not based on susceptibility testing or efficacy data. In recent years, it has become apparent that gentamicin has an unpredictable volume of distribution in patients with ascites and that the serum creatinine level (and even the creatinine clearance) is a poor index of the glomerular filtration rate in patients with ascites.[82, 83] Therefore, it is difficult to determine appropriate loading and maintenence doses of gentamicin for this patient population. Use of aminoglycosides without reaching toxic serum levels requires that frequent "stat" serum and ascitic fluid levels of the drug be obtained. There are no evidence-based guidelines to follow. In the author's experience, even if high serum levels are avoided, nephrotoxicity still develops in most patients treated with aminoglycosides.[84, 85] There is no evidence that newer aminoglycosides are less problematic than gentamicin.

Several nonaminoglycoside antibiotics are now available for the treatment of ascitic fluid infection. Aztreonam is a monobactam that has been used in SBP, but it has little gram-positive coverage and is associated with an unacceptable superinfection rate of 19%.[86] If aztreonam is used as empirical therapy, a second drug that covers gram-positive bacteria also must be used. The first- and second-generation cephalosporins cover less than 80% of the organisms that cause SBP.[87] Infection with organisms that are resistant to the empirical antibiotic may cause the patient's death before susceptibility testing results are available. Cefotaxime, a third-generation cephalosporin, has been shown in a controlled trial to be superior to ampicillin plus tobramycin for the treatment of SBP.[88] Fully 98% of causative organisms were susceptible to cefotaxime, which did not result in superinfection or nephrotoxicity.[88] Cefotaxime or a similar third-generation cephalosporin appears to be the treatment of choice for suspected SBP.[15] Anaerobic coverage is not needed, nor is coverage for *Pseudomonas* or *Staphylococcus*.[28] Cefotaxime 2 g intravenously every 8 hours has been shown to result in excellent ascitic fluid levels (20-fold killing power after one dose).[89] In patients with a serum creatinine level greater than 3 mg/dL, the dosing interval may be extended to 12 hours.[89] Neither a loading dose nor an intraperitoneal dose appears to be necessary or appropriate.

Intravenous Albumin Plus Antibiotic

Intravenous albumin (1.5 g/kg body weight at the time the infection is detected and 1.0 g/kg on day 3) in combination with cefotaxime has been shown in a large randomized trial to reduce the risk of renal failure and improve survival.[90] A confirmatory trial is needed. However, because of the survival advantage, the use of intravenous albumin as an adjunct to antibiotic treatment has been recommended by other authors.[91]

Other Intravenous Antibiotics

Amoxicillin-clavulanic acid has been shown to be as effective as cefotaxime in the treatment of SBP.[92] However, a parenteral formulation is not available in the United States. Other antibiotics have been recommended as well but have been less well studied than cefotaxime.

Oral Antibiotic Treatment

Oral ofloxacin has been reported in a controlled trial to be as effective as parenteral cefotaxime in the treatment of SBP in patients who are not vomiting, in shock, bleeding, or in renal failure.[93] The dose studied was 400 mg twice daily.[93] Another study has demonstrated the efficacy of intravenous ciprofloxacin 200 mg every 12 hours for 2 days followed by oral ciprofloxacin 500 mg every 12 hours for 5 days.[94] However, because of the possibility of quinolone resistance in patients receiving quinolones to prevent SBP (see later), it is best to avoid the empirical use of a quinolone to treat suspected SBP.[95] Fortunately, bacterial isolates from patients with SBP who were receiving quinolones to prevent SBP remain susceptible to cefotaxime.[75]

Narrowing the Spectrum of Coverage

After the results of susceptibility testing are available, an antibiotic with a narrower spectrum of activity usually can be substituted for the broad-spectrum drug (e.g., pneumococci usually will be sensitive to penicillin, and most *E. coli* species usually will be sensitive to ampicillin).

Duration of Treatment

Most infectious disease subspecialists recommend 10 to 14 days of antibiotic therapy for life-threatening infections. However, there are no data to support this duration of treatment in spontaneous ascitic fluid infections. The ascitic fluid culture becomes sterile after one dose of cefotaxime in 86% of patients.[34] After 48 hours of therapy, the ascitic fluid PMN count is always less than the pretreatment value in patients with a spontaneous ascitic fluid infection treated with appropriate antibiotics; frequently, there is an 80% reduction at 48 hours.[34] A randomized controlled trial involving 100 patients has demonstrated that 5 days of treatment is as efficacious as 10 days in the treatment of SBP and CNNA.[96] The author has been treating SBP and CNNA for 5 days for longer than 10 years, with excellent results.

The average duration of oral ofloxacin treatment was 8 days in the only published trial.[93]

Follow-Up Paracentesis in Spontaneous Bacterial Peritonitis

The question often arises, "Should a paracentesis be repeated to assess the response to the treatment of SBP?" On the basis of a large database of repeat paracenteses during and after the treatment of SBP,[34, 96] it appears that a follow-up paracentesis is not needed if the setting (advanced cirrhosis with symptoms and signs of infection), bacterial isolate (monomicrobial with a typical organism), and response to treatment (dramatic reduction in symptoms and signs of infection) are typical.[97] Paracentesis should be repeated after 48 hours of treatment if the course is atypical.[34, 97]

Treatment of Ascitic Fluid Infection Other Than Spontaneous Bacterial Peritonitis

Because of the predictable presence of anaerobes, patients with suspected secondary peritonitis require empirical antibiotic coverage that is broader in spectrum than that needed by those with SBP, in addition to an emergency evaluation to assess the need for surgical intervention (see earlier discussion, and Table 78–8 and Fig. 78–3). Cefotaxime plus metronidazole appears to provide excellent initial empirical therapy of suspected secondary peritonitis.[34]

Polymicrobial bacterascites (needle perforation of the bowel) is relatively well tolerated. Peritonitis developed in only 1 in 10 patients with a needle perforation of the gut into ascitic fluid in the one relevant study.[66] The single episode of paracentesis-related peritonitis was not fatal. It appears that patients with low-protein ascitic fluid are at most risk of developing a PMN response and clinical peritonitis related to needle perforation of the gut.[66] Most of the patients with a higher protein concentration in the ascites (e.g., >1 g/dL [10 g/L]) did not receive antibiotics and yet did well. However, many physicians would probably feel uncomfortable withholding antibiotic treatment if needle perforation is suspected. If a decision to treat is made, anaerobic coverage should be included (e.g., cefotaxime and metronidazole; see Table 78–9). Whether or not treatment is begun, a follow-up paracentesis is helpful (if it can be performed safely) to follow the ascitic PMN count and culture. If a decision is made not to treat and the number of organisms does not decrease or a rise in the PMN count occurs in the second specimen, antibiotic treatment should be initiated (see Table 78–9).

Prognosis

In the past, 48% to 95% of patients with a spontaneous ascitic fluid infection died during the hospitalization in which the diagnosis was made, despite antibiotic treatment.[90–96] The most recent series report the lowest mortality rate, probably because of earlier detection and treatment of infection in the 1990s, as well as the avoidance of nephrotoxic antibiotics. In the older series, about 50% of the patients with SBP died of the infection despite antibiotic treatment; now less than 5% of patients die of infection if appropriate antibiotics are administered in a timely fashion.[96] However, even now, many patients are cured of their infection and yet die of liver or renal failure or gastrointestinal bleeding, because of the severity of the underlying liver disease. In fact, spontaneous ascitic fluid infection is a good marker of end-stage liver disease and has been proposed as an indication for liver transplantation in a patient who is otherwise a candidate.

In order to maximize survival, it is important that paracentesis be performed in all patients with ascites at the time of hospital admission so that infection can be detected and treated promptly. The ascitic cell count should be reviewed as soon as the results are available (~60 min), and appropriate treatment instituted when indicated.

Paracentesis should be repeated during the hospitalization if any clinical deterioration occurs, including pain, fever, a change in mental status, renal failure, acidosis, peripheral leukocytosis, or gastrointestinal bleeding. In the past, a delay in diagnosis was responsible, at least in part, for the excessive mortality rate. If the physician waits until convincing symptoms and signs of infection have developed in a patient before performing a paracentesis, the infection is likely to be advanced by the time the diagnosis is made. There have been no reported survivors of SBP when the diagnosis is made after the serum creatinine level has risen above 4 mg/dL (350 μmol/L), or after shock has developed.

Without surgical intervention, the mortality rate for secondary peritonitis in hospitalized patients with ascites approaches 100%. When secondary peritonitis is diagnosed early and treated with emergency laparotomy, the mortality rate is in the same range as that for SBP, approximately 50%.[34]

Prevention

The identification of risk factors for SBP (including an ascitic fluid protein concentration <1.0 g/dL, variceal hemorrhage, and prior episode of SBP) has led to controlled trials of prophylactic antibiotics.[32, 98–100] Norfloxacin 400 mg/day orally has been reported to reduce the risk of SBP in inpatients with low-protein ascites and patients with prior SBP.[98, 99] Norfloxacin 400 mg orally twice daily for 7 days helps prevent infection in patients with variceal hemorrhage.[100] However, oral antibiotics do not prolong survival and do select for resistant organisms in the gut flora, which can subsequently cause spontaneous ascitic infection.[75, 98–101] For the primary prevention of ascitic infection in patients with low-protein ascites, it is appropriate to restrict the use of prophylactic antibiotics to inpatients only, with discontinuation of the drug at the time the patient is discharged from the hospital.[102] According to a randomized trial, this strategy may be the best compromise for preventing ascitic infection without selecting resistant organisms.[102]

Trimethoprim-sulfamethoxazole also has been shown to be effective in preventing SBP in an animal model and in patients.[103, 104]

Parenteral antibiotics to prevent endoscopic sclerotherapy or banding-related infections do not appear to be warranted, based on a controlled trial.[105] Active bleeding, not the endoscopic treatment, appears to be the risk factor for ascitic infection.

Tense Ascites

Some patients with ascites do not seek medical attention until they can no longer breathe or eat comfortably because of the pressure that the intra-abdominal fluid exerts on their diaphragms. Tense ascites requires urgent therapeutic paracentesis. Contrary to folklore, tense ascites can be drained without untoward hemodynamic effects.[106–108] "Total paracentesis," even more than 20 L, has recently been demonstrated to be safe.[108] In the setting of tense ascites, therapeutic paracentesis improves venous return and hemodynamics.[107] The myth of paracentesis-related hemodynamic disasters was based on observations in small numbers of patients.

Pleural Effusions

"Sympathetic" pleural effusions are common in patients with cirrhotic ascites. They are usually unilateral and right-sided but occasionally may be bilateral and larger on the right side than the left. A unilateral left-sided effusion suggests tuberculosis.[109] A large effusion in a patient with cirrhotic ascites is referred to as *hepatic hydrothorax*.[110] Most carefully studied patients with hepatic hydrothorax have been shown to have a small defect in the right hemidiaphragm. Occasionally, the effusion develops acutely with sudden shortness of breath as the abdomen decompresses. With large diaphragmatic defects, ascites may be undetectable on clinical examination despite a large pleural effusion.

The most common symptom associated with hepatic hydrothorax is shortness of breath. Infection of the fluid can occur, usually as a result of SBP and transmission of bacteria across the diaphragm.[111] The analysis of uncomplicated hepatic hydrothorax fluid is similar, but not identical, to that of ascites because the pleural fluid is subject to hydrostatic pressures different from those that affect the portal bed. The total protein concentration is higher (by approximately 1.0 g/dL [10 g/L]) in the pleural fluid than in ascites.

The treatment of hepatic hydrothorax has been difficult until the availability of transjugular intrahepatic portosystemic stent shunts (TIPS; see later).[110] The effusions tend to occur in patients who are the least compliant with or most refractory to therapy. Some authors have recommended chest tube insertion and sclerosis of the pleurae with tetracycline. However, chest tubes inserted to treat hepatic hydrothorax usually are difficult to remove.[112] Shortness of breath may recur when the tube is clamped, and fluid may leak around the insertion site of the tube. Direct surgical repair of the diaphragmatic defect can be considered, but these patients typically are poor operative candidates. A peritoneovenous shunt (see later) can be considered when the patient with hepatic hydrothorax has a large volume of ascites, but the shunt usually clots after a short time. Sodium restriction and use of diuretics constitute the safest and most effective first-line therapy of hepatic hydrothorax. TIPS has been reported to be successful and is reasonable second-line treatment.[110] If the patient is a candidate for liver transplantation, proceeding with a transplant evaluation may be the best approach.

Abdominal Wall Hernias

Abdominal wall hernias are common in patients with ascites. They are usually umbilical or incisional but occasionally inguinal. There is little published information about these hernias. In one study, almost 20% of cirrhotic patients with ascites were found to have umbilical hernias at the time of admission to the hospital.[113] Many of these hernias incarcerate or perforate. Because of these potential complications, elective surgical treatment should be considered in all patients with hernias and ascites. However, the ascites should be medically removed preoperatively because the hernia recurs in 73% of patients who have ascites at the time of hernia repair but only 14% of those who have no ascites at the time of repair.[114] Hernia repair is not without hazard. Many transplant surgeons prefer to postpone repair of the hernia until the time of liver transplantation.

Surgery should be performed semiemergently for skin ulceration, crusting, or black discoloration. Emergency surgery should be performed for refractory incarceration or rupture. Rupture is the most feared complication of umbilical hernias.

TREATMENT OF ASCITES

Appropriate treatment of the patient with ascites depends on the cause of fluid retention. Accurate determination of the etiology of ascites is crucial. The SAAG is helpful diagnostically, as well as in therapeutic decision-making. Patients with a low SAAG usually do not have portal hypertension and do not respond to salt restriction and diuretics (except nephrotic syndrome). Conversely, patients with a high SAAG have portal hypertension and usually are responsive to these measures.[2]

Low Albumin-Gradient Ascites

Peritoneal carcinomatosis is the most common cause of low albumin-gradient ascites.[3] Peripheral edema in these patients responds to diuretics. Patients without peripheral edema who are treated with diuretics lose only intravascular volume without loss of ascites.[2] The mainstay of treatment of nonovarian peritoneal carcinomatosis is outpatient therapeutic paracentesis.[2] Patients with peritoneal carcinomatosis usually live only a few months. Patients with ovarian malignancy are an exception to this rule; these patients may have a good response to surgical debulking and chemotherapy.

Ascites caused by tuberculous peritonitis (without cirrhosis) is cured by antituberculous therapy. Diuretics do not speed weight loss unless the patient has underlying portal hypertension from cirrhosis. More than 50% of patients with tuberculous peritonitis in the United States have underlying cirrhosis.[37] Pancreatic ascites may resolve spontaneously, require endoscopic stent placement in the pancreatic duct or operative intervention, or respond to treatment with somatostatin.[115] A postoperative lymphatic leak from a distal splenorenal shunt or radical lymphadenectomy also may resolve spontaneously but on occasion may require surgical intervention or peritoneovenous shunting. *Chlamydia* peritonitis is cured by tetracycline.[11] Ascites caused by lupus serositis may respond to glucocorticoids.[12] Dialysis-related ascites may respond to aggressive dialysis.[56]

High Albumin-Gradient Ascites

Cirrhosis is the most common cause of liver disease that leads to high albumin-gradient ascites (see Table 78–1). Many patients with cirrhosis have multiple insults to the liver, including excessive alcohol use, NASH, and chronic hepatitis C.[6, 7] One of the most important steps in treating high albumin-gradient ascites is to treat the underlying liver disease by convincing the patient to stop drinking alcohol. In a period of months, abstinence from alcohol can result in healing of the reversible component of alcoholic liver disease.[8] Ascites may resolve or become more responsive to medical therapy during this time. Patients with other forms of treatable liver disease (e.g., autoimmune hepatitis, hemochromatosis, or Wilson disease) should receive specific therapy for these diseases. Specific therapy may improve their liver function and ease the overall management of their ascites. However, these diseases are less reversible than alcoholic liver disease, and by the time ascites is present, these patients may be candidates for liver transplantation rather than protracted medical therapy.

HOSPITALIZATION. Outpatient treatment of patients with small-volume ascites can be attempted initially. However, patients with large-volume ascites and those who are resistant to outpatient treatment usually require hospitalization for definitive diagnosis and management of the fluid overload, as well as the underlying liver disease.[22, 116] Many of these patients also have gastrointestinal hemorrhage, encephalopathy, infection, or hepatocellular carcinoma. An intensive period of inpatient education and treatment may be required to convince the patient that the diet and diuretics actually are effective and worth the effort that it will take to follow the regimen at home.

PRECIPITATING CAUSE. It may be of value to determine the precipitating cause of ascites formation (e.g., dietary indiscretion or noncompliance with diuretics). Further education about diet may help prevent future hospitalizations for ascites. Ascites may be precipitated by saline infusions given perioperatively or to treat variceal hemorrhage, in which case the ascites may resolve without the need for long-term treatment.

DIET EDUCATION. Fluid loss and weight change are related directly to sodium balance in patients with portal hypertension–related ascites. In the presence of avid renal retention of sodium, dietary sodium restriction is essential. The patient and the food preparer should be educated by a dietitian about a sodium-restricted diet. Severely sodium-restricted diets (e.g., 500 mg, or 22 mmol, sodium/day) are feasible (but not palatable) in an inpatient setting but unrealistic for outpatients. The dietary sodium restriction that the author recommends for inpatients and outpatients is 2 grams (88 mmol) per day.

FLUID RESTRICTION. Indiscriminate restriction of fluid in treating the patient with cirrhotic ascites is inappropriate; hypernatremia may result.[117] Sodium restriction, not fluid restriction, results in weight loss; fluid follows sodium passively. The chronic hyponatremia usually seen in patients with cirrhotic ascites is seldom morbid. Attempts to correct hyponatremia rapidly in this setting can lead to more complications than the hyponatremia itself. Severe hyponatremia (e.g., serum sodium concentration <120 mmol/L) does warrant fluid restriction in the patient with cirrhotic ascites.[116, 118] Symptoms from hyponatremia usually do not develop in cirrhotic patients until the serum sodium concentration is below 110 mmol/L, unless the decline in sodium concentration is rapid. Indiscriminate fluid restriction serves only to alienate patients, nurses, and dietitians.

NO BED REST. Although it is traditional to order bed rest, there are no controlled trials to support this practice.[119] An upright posture may aggravate the plasma renin elevation found in most cirrhotic patients with ascites and, theoretically, increase renal sodium retention. However, in all likelihood, strict bed rest is unnecessary and may lead to decubitus ulcers in these emaciated patients.

URINE SODIUM EXCRETION. The 24-hour urinary sodium excretion is a helpful parameter to follow in patients with portal hypertension–related ascites. The completeness of the urine collection can be assessed by measuring the urinary creatinine excretion. Cirrhotic men should excrete 15 to 20 mg/kg/day of creatinine, and women should excrete 10 to 15 mg/kg/day.[116, 119] Excretion of less creatinine indicates an incomplete collection. Only the 10% to 15% of patients who have significant spontaneous natriuresis can be considered for dietary sodium restriction as sole therapy of ascites (i.e., without diuretics).[22] However, when given a choice, most patients would prefer to take some diuretics with a more liberal intake of sodium than to take no pills with severe restriction of sodium intake. Contrary to popular belief, compliant patients, including outpatients, can collect complete 24-hour specimens.[121]

Because urine is the most important route of excretion of sodium in the absence of diarrhea or hyperthermia, and because dietary intake is the only source of nonparenteral sodium, dietary intake and urinary excretion of sodium should be roughly equivalent if the patient's weight is stable. Nonurinary sodium losses are less than 10 mmol per day in these patients.[120] A suboptimal decline in body weight may be the result of inadequate natriuresis, failure to restrict sodium intake, or both. Monitoring 24-hour urinary sodium excretion and daily weight will clarify the issue. Patients who are compliant with an 88-mmol/day sodium diet and who excrete more than 78 mmol/day of sodium in the urine should lose weight. If the weight is increasing despite urinary losses in excess of 78 mmol/day, one can assume that the patient is eating more sodium than is prescribed in the diet.

URINE SODIUM/POTASSIUM RATIO. Although 24-hour specimens are the gold standard, one study has demonstrated that when a random urine specimen has a sodium concentration that is greater than the potassium concentration, a 24-hour specimen will reveal sodium excretion greater than 78 mmol/day in 95% of cases.[121] Therefore, a random urine sodium/potassium concentration ratio greater than 1 predicts that the patient should lose weight if the sodium-restricted diet is followed. Patients who do not lose weight despite a Grandom urine sodium/potassium ratio greater than 1 are probably not compliant with the diet.

AVOID USE OF URINARY BLADDER CATHETERS. Many physicians promptly insert a bladder catheter in inpatients with cirrhosis in order to monitor urine output more accurately. Unfortunately, these immunocompromised patients regularly have urinary tract infections at the time of admission to the hospital.[79] Urethral trauma from insertion of the catheter in the setting of cystitis can lead to bacteremia. Prolonged catheterization predictably leads to cystitis and possibly to urosepsis in these patients. The author inserts urinary catheters only in the intensive care unit setting; these portals of entry for bacteria should be removed as soon as possible. Twenty-four-hour urine specimens can be collected completely without catheters.

DIURETICS. Spironolactone is the mainstay of treatment for cirrhotic ascites but is slow to increase natriuresis. Single-agent diuretic therapy with spironolactone requires several days to induce weight loss. Although spironolactone alone has been shown to be superior to furosemide alone in the treatment of cirrhotic ascites,[122] the author prefers to start spironolactone and furosemide together on the first hospital day in initial doses of 100 mg and 40 mg, respectively, each taken once in the morning.[116] Amiloride 10 mg per day can be substituted for spironolactone; amiloride is less widely available and more expensive than spironolactone but more rapidly effective, and it does not cause gynecomastia. The half-life of spironolactone is approximately 24 hours in normal control subjects but markedly prolonged in patients with cirrhosis; almost 1 month is required to reach a steady state.[123] There is no reason to dose the drug multiple times per day in view of its long half-life. A loading dose may be appropriate but has not been studied. Single daily doses are most appropriate and enhance compliance; 25-, 50-, and 100-mg spironolactone tablets are available. Furosemide is also recommended to be given once a day.[124]

If the combination of spironolactone 100 mg/day (or 10 mg/day of amiloride) and furosemide 40 mg/day orally is ineffective in increasing urinary sodium or decreasing body weight, the doses of both drugs should be increased simultaneously as needed (e.g., spironolactone 200 mg plus furosemide 80 mg, then 300 mg plus 120 mg, and finally 400 mg plus 160 mg). Starting both drugs at once speeds the onset of diuresis, in the author's experience. Slowly increasing the dose of spironolactone to 400 to 600 mg/day before adding furosemide delays diuresis and results in hyperkalemia.

The 100:40 ratio of the daily doses of spironolactone and furosemide usually maintains normokalemia. The ratio of spironolactone and furosemide can be adjusted to correct abnormal serum potassium levels. Occasionally, an alcoholic patient who has had no recent food intake will have hypokalemia at the time of admission and for a variable interval thereafter. Such a patient should receive spironolactone alone until the serum potassium normalizes; then furosemide can be added. When combined with a sodium-restricted diet in a study of almost 4000 patients, the regimen of spironolactone and furosemide has been demonstrated to achieve successful diuresis in more than 90% of cirrhotic patients.[125]

Intravenous diuretics cause acute decreases in the glomerular filtration rate in cirrhotic patients with ascites and should be avoided.[126] If rapid weight loss is desired, therapeutic paracentesis should be performed (see later). There is no limit to the acceptable daily weight loss of patients who have massive edema. Once the edema has resolved, a reasonable maximum weight loss is probably 0.5 kg/day.[127] Encephalopathy, a serum sodium concentration less than 120 mmol/L despite fluid restriction, or a serum creatinine level greater than 2.0 mg/dL (180 μmol/L) should result in cessation of diuretics and reassessment of the situation. Abnormalities in potassium levels almost never prohibit diuretic use because the ratio of the two diuretics can be readjusted. Patients with parenchymal renal disease (e.g., diabetic nephropathy) usually require higher doses of furosemide and lower doses of spironolactone than those mentioned earlier. Patients in whom complications develop despite a careful attempt at diuretic treatment usually require second-line therapy. Prostaglandin inhibitors (e.g., nonsteroidal anti-inflammatory drugs) should be avoided in patients with cirrhotic ascites because they inhibit diuresis, may promote renal failure, and cause gastrointestinal bleeding.[128]

Reducing the quantity of fluid in the abdomen can improve the patient's comfort and prevent hepatic hydrothorax and hernias. Also, by concentrating the ascitic fluid, diuresis increases the opsonic activity of fluid 10-fold, and theoretically, may be of value in preventing spontaneous ascitic fluid infection.[129]

In the past, patients with ascites frequently occupied hospital beds for prolonged periods because of uncertainty regarding the diagnosis and optimal treatment and because of iatrogenic complications. Although a "dry" abdomen is a reasonable ultimate goal, complete resolution of ascites should not be a prerequisite for discharge from the hospital. Patients who are stable, with ascites as their major problem, can be discharged after it has been determined that they are responding to the medical regimen. Following early discharge from the hospital, a patient must be seen in the outpatient setting promptly, preferably in 7 to 14 days.

NO SODIUM BICARBONATE. Mild renal tubular acidosis develops in a substantial minority of patients with cirrhosis and ascites. Many nephrologists recommend oral sodium bicarbonate administration in this setting. Clearly, such treatment increases sodium intake dramatically and cannot be advocated in the absence of evidence to support its use.

AQUARETICS. A new class of drugs, the aquaretics, have been used in animals and preliminarily in patients with cirrhosis.[130] Whether these drugs will improve severe hyponatremia without causing hypotension awaits randomized trials.

OUTPATIENT MANAGEMENT. After discharge from the hospital, the patient's body weight, orthostatic symptoms, serum electrolytes, urea, and creatinine should be monitored. Twenty-four-hour urine specimens or random urine sodium/potassium ratios can be collected to assist with treatment decisions. It is the author's experience that compliant outpatients can collect complete specimens successfully, when adequate written instructions are provided. The subsequent frequency of follow-up is determined by the response to treatment and the stability of the patient. The author usually evaluates these patients every 2 to 4 weeks until it is clear that they are responding to treatment and are not experiencing problems. Intensive outpatient follow-up helps prevent subsequent hospitalizations.

Diuretic doses and dietary sodium intake are adjusted to achieve weight loss and negative sodium balance. Patients who are gaining fluid weight despite diuretics should not be labeled as diuretic-resistant until they are demonstrated to be compliant with the diet. Monitoring the urine sodium concentration provides insight into compliance. Patients who excrete more than 78 mmol/day of sodium in the urine or have a random urine sodium/potassium ratio greater than 1 should be losing weight if they are consuming less than 88 mmol/day of sodium. The author has encountered patients who were labeled as diuretic-resistant despite dramatic noncompliance with the diet and weight gain with urinary sodium excretion of more than 500 mmol/day. Most patients who are thought initially to be diuretic-resistant are eventually found to be noncompliant with the diet in the author's experience. Diet education is crucial to the successful treatment of such patients. Truly diuretic-resistant patients excrete nearly sodium-free urine despite maximum doses of diuretics.

During long-term follow-up, abstinent alcoholic patients may become more sensitive to diuretics, which may be tapered and even discontinued.

Refractory Ascites

Refractory ascites is defined as ascites unresponsive to a sodium-restricted diet and high-dose diuretic treatment. Refractoriness may be manifested by minimal or no weight loss despite diuretics or the development of complications of diuretics.[131] Several studies have shown that *less than 10% of patients with cirrhotic ascites are refractory to standard medical therapy*.[122, 125]

In the 1960s, portacaval shunts were used to treat refractory ascites, but operative hemorrhagic complications and portosystemic encephalopathy led to the abandonment of this approach.[119] In Europe in the 1970s, the Paris pump was used to ultrafilter ascitic fluid and reinfuse it intravenously.[119] Unfortunately, this approach was complicated by disseminated intravascular coagulation and was abandoned.

Viable options for patients refractory to routine medical therapy include liver transplantation, serial therapeutic paracenteses, TIPS, and peritoneovenous shunts (Fig. 78–5).[116]

LIVER TRANSPLANTATION. Orthotopic liver transplantation should be considered among the treatment options of patients with cirrhosis and ascites (see also Chapter 83). In areas where there are long waiting times for liver transplantation, the patient should be evaluated early after the first evidence of hepatic decompensation. Once ascites becomes refractory to routine medical therapy, the patient should be prioritized for transplant. In many areas of the United States, patients are not offered transplantation until hepatorenal syndrome has developed. The 12-month survival rate for patients with ascites refractory to medical therapy is only 25%.[132] The survival rate for liver transplantation is far superior to this value.

In patients who are transplant candidates, procedures that would make transplantation difficult should be avoided. Surgery in the right upper quadrant causes adhesions that become vascularized and difficult to remove during transplant surgery. Even peritoneovenous shunting can lead to the formation of a "cocoon" in the right upper quadrant that can involve the bowel and liver.[133]

SERIAL PARACENTESES. Therapeutic abdominal paracentesis is one of the oldest medical procedures. In the 1980s, after 2000 years of use, scientific data regarding large-volume paracentesis were reported, and patients were documented to tolerate large-volume paracentesis very well, just as the patients had in the 1940s and earlier.[134–137] In one large randomized controlled trial, therapeutic paracentesis plus intravenous infusion of colloid led to fewer minor (asymptomatic) changes in serum electrolyte and creatinine levels than did diuretic therapy.[137] However, no differences in morbidity or mortality rates could be demonstrated.[137] Therapeutic paracentesis now appears to be first-line therapy for patients with tense ascites and second-line therapy for cirrhotic patients who are refractory to diuretics (see Fig. 78–5).[116]

COLLOID REPLACEMENT. One controversial issue regarding therapeutic paracentesis is that of colloid replacement. In one study, patients with tense ascites were randomized to receive albumin (10 g/L of fluid removed) versus no albumin after therapeutic paracentesis.[137] In the group that did not receive albumin, statistically significantly more (asymptomatic) changes in electrolytes, plasma renin, and serum creatinine developed than in the group that received albumin, but there was no more clinical morbidity or mortality. Although an-

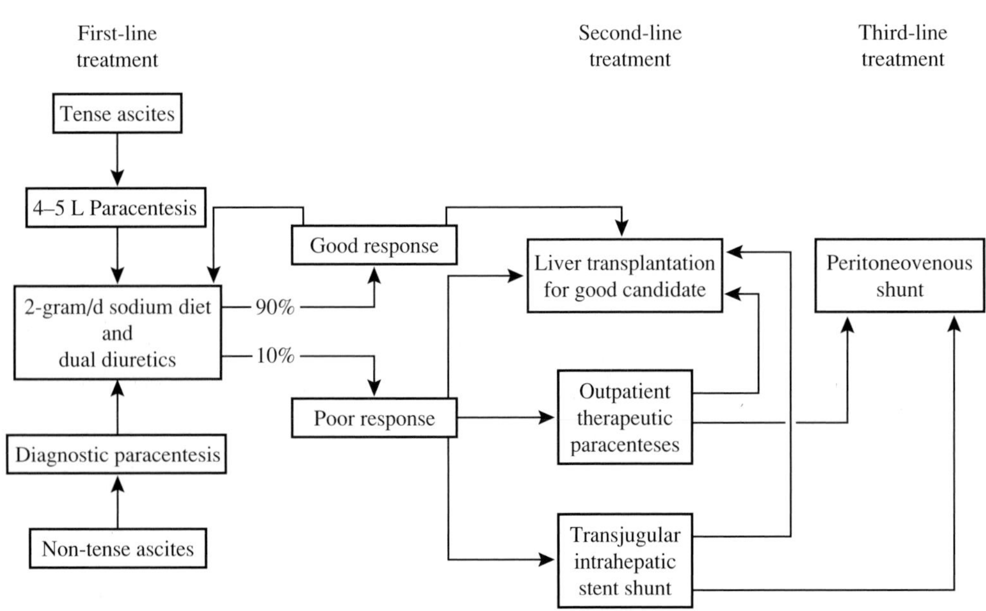

Figure 78–5. Overview of the treatment of patients with cirrhotic ascites.

other study has documented that the patients with a postparacentesis rise in plasma renin levels have a decreased life expectancy compared with those with stable renin levels, no study has demonstrated a decreased survival in patients not given plasma expander compared with patients given albumin after paracentesis.[138] A new phrase, "paracentesis-induced circulatory dysfunction," has been coined to describe the rise in plasma rennin levels after paracentesis.[139] Despite the lack of a direct effect of albumin infusion on survival, the authors of the two studies cited previously recommend routine infusion of albumin after therapeutic paracentesis.[137, 138] However, albumin infusions markedly increase the degradation of albumin, and albumin is expensive.[140, 141] In a study performed more than 30 years ago, 58% of infused albumin was offset by increased degradation, and a 15% increase in the serum albumin level led to a 39% increase in degradation.[140] Increasing the concentration of albumin in cell culture media has been shown to decrease albumin synthesis.[142] In view of the cost ($2 to $25/g or $100 to $1250/tap), it is difficult to justify the expense of routine infusions of albumin based on the available data.

The confusion regarding albumin infusion relates in part to the design of the relevant studies. In the studies from Barcelona, patients with "tense" ascites could be entered into the trial of albumin versus no albumin, and 31% of these patients were not even receiving diuretics.[137] It seems more appropriate to study the population that really needs chronic paracenteses, specifically, the diuretic-resistant group, rather than all patients with tense ascites.[143] Another group has shown that patients with cirrhosis and diuretic-resistant ascites tolerate a 5-L paracentesis without a change in plasma renin levels.[144] This author's approach to patients with tense ascites is to take off enough fluid (4 to 5 L) to relieve intra-abdominal pressure and then to rely on diuretics to eliminate the remainder. To remove all the fluid by paracentesis when most of it can be removed with diuretics seems inappropriate, in part because paracentesis removes opsonins, whereas diuresis concentrates opsonins.[129] In addition, patients with early cirrhosis seem to be more sensitive than patients with advanced cirrhosis to changes in volume; this finding may also help explain the differences between the studies.[145] Patients with early cirrhosis and diuretic-sensitive ascites should be treated with diuretics, not large-volume paracentesis; these patients may be sensitive to paracentesis-related volume depletion.[145] Chronic therapeutic paracenteses should be reserved for the 10% of patients who fail diuretic treatment.

Other studies have compared less expensive plasma expanders with albumin. However, there were no differences in electrolyte imbalance or clinically relevant complications between the groups.[146] In addition, the most recent studies advocate giving one half of the plasma expander immediately after the paracentesis and the other half 6 hours later.[138, 146] This approach converts an otherwise simple outpatient procedure into an all-day clinic visit or even a brief hospitalization. This approach seems unwarranted.

Recent consensus statements and systematic reviews have pointed out some of the hazards of albumin infusion and have recommended against its liberal use.[147, 148] Until there are more convincing data involving appropriate groups of patients, it seems reasonable to (1) avoid serial large-volume paracenteses in patients with diuretic-sensitive ascites; (2) withhold albumin after taps of 5 L or less; and (3) consider albumin infusion optional after taps of larger volume in patients with diuretic-resistant ascites.[91, 116]

TERLIPRESSIN. A recent uncontrolled study has advocated the use of parenteral terlipressin for the short-term treatment of refractory ascites and hepatorenal syndrome.[149] However, this drug is not available in the United States. A randomized trial and availability of this drug are required before its use can be recommended.

TRANSJUGULAR INTRAHEPATIC PORTOSYSTEMIC STENT SHUNT (TIPS). TIPS is a side-to-side portacaval shunt that is placed by an interventional radiologist, usually under local anesthesia. It was first used for the treatment of refractory variceal bleeding, but it has also been advocated for diuretic-resistant ascites.[150] TIPS was received with great enthusiasm in the 1990s, similar to the enthusiasm for the peritoneovenous shunt in the 1970s. Just as with peritoneovenous shunting, TIPS was overused until serious complications and suboptimal efficacy were reported. A randomized trial in diuretic-resistant patients has demonstrated a survival advantage following placement of a TIPS compared with serial paracenteses.[151] Although TIPS dysfunction is common and must be managed with repeated manipulation of the stent, maintaining a TIPS is logistically less challenging than large-volume paracenteses performed every 2 weeks. (See also Chapter 77.)

PERITONEOVENOUS SHUNT. In the mid-1970s, the peritoneovenous shunt was promoted as a new "physiologic" treatment for the management of ascites. Reports of shunt failure, fatal complications following shunt insertion, and randomized trials demonstrating no survival advantage have led to the relegation of this procedure to third-line therapy in patients with cirrhosis and ascites (see Fig. 78–5).[125] Patients who are not candidates for liver transplantation and who have a scarred abdomen that is not amenable to repeated paracenteses or who have failed an attempt at TIPS make up this small subset of patients.

SUMMARY OF TREATMENT OF PATIENTS WITH CIRRHOSIS AND ASCITES

The mainstay of therapy for patients with cirrhotic ascites is dietary sodium restriction and diuretics (see Fig. 78–5). Standard medical therapy is effective in 90% of patients. Evaluation for liver transplantation should be considered at the time of first decompensation. However, psychosocial issues frequently preclude transplantation. A therapeutic paracentesis should be performed promptly in patients with tense ascites and as second-line long-term treatment in the 10% of patients who are refractory to medical therapy. Therapeutic paracenteses can be repeated indefinitely or until a more definitive treatment is provided. TIPS is a second-line treatment that should be reserved for (1) diuretic-resistant patients who are not candidates for transplantation, as well as those who are awaiting transplantation, or (2) patients with hepatic hydrothorax. Peritoneovenous shunting is a third-line therapy and should be reserved for special and unusual circumstances. For patients with no psychosocial contraindications, evaluation for liver transplantation is even more urgent once ascites has become diuretic-resistant.

PROGNOSIS

Cirrhosis complicated by ascites is associated with significant morbidity and mortality, related in part to the severe underlying liver disease and in part to the ascites per se. In half of the patients in whom cirrhosis is detected before "decompensation" (i.e., ascites, jaundice, encephalopathy, or gastrointestinal hemorrhage), ascites develops within 10 years.[152] Once ascites appears, the expected mortality rate is approximately 50% in just 2 years.[153] With liver transplantation, survival is improved dramatically.

REFERENCES

1. Martin P-Y, Gines P, Schrier RW: Nitric oxide as a mediator of hemodynamic abnormalities and sodium and water retention in cirrhosis. N Engl J Med 339:533, 1998.
2. Pockros PJ, Esrason KT, Nguyen C, et al: Mobilization of malignant ascites with diuretics is dependent on ascitic fluid characteristics. Gastroenterology 103:1302, 1992.
3. Runyon BA, Hoefs JC, Morgan TR: Ascitic fluid analysis in malignancy-related ascites. Hepatology 8:1104, 1988.
4. Schrier RW: Pathogenesis of sodium and water retention in high-output and low-output cardiac failure, nephrotic syndrome, cirrhosis, and pregnancy. N Engl J Med 319:1065, 1988.
5. Brown MW, Burk RF: Development of intractable ascites following upper abdominal surgery in patients with cirrhosis. Am J Med 80:879, 1986.
6. Naveau S, Giraud V, Borotto E, et al: Excess weight risk factor for alcoholic liver disease. Hepatology 25:108, 1997.
7. Hourigan LF, MacDonald GA, Purdie D, et al: Fibrosis in chronic hepatitis C correlates significantly with body mass index. Hepatology 29:1215, 1999.
8. Reynolds TB, Geller HM, Kuzma OT, et al. Spontaneous decrease in portal pressure with clinical improvement in cirrhosis. N Engl J Med 263;734, 1960.
9. Powell EE, Cooksley WGE, Hanson R, et al: The natural history of nonalcoholic steatohepatitis: A follow-up study of 42 patients for up to 21 years. Hepatology 11:74, 1990.
10. Caldwell SH, Oelsner DH, Iezzoni JC, et al: Cryptogenic cirrhosis: Clinical characterization and risk factors for underlying disease. Hepatology 29:664, 1999.
11. Muller-Schoop JW, Wang SP, Munzinger J, et al: *Chlamydia trachomatis* as possible cause of peritonitis and perihepatitis in young women. Br Med J 1:1022, 1978.
12. Wilkins KW, Hoffman GS: Massive ascites in systemic lupus erythematosus. J Rheumatol 12:571, 1985.
13. Cattau EI, Benjamin SB, Knuff TE, et al: The accuracy of the physical exam in the diagnosis of suspected ascites. JAMA 247:1164, 1982.
14. Goldberg BB, Goodman GA, Clearfield HR: Evaluation of ascites by ultrasound. Radiology 96:15, 1970.
15. Such J, Runyon BA: Spontaneous bacterial peritonitis. Clin Infect Dis 27:669, 1998.
16. Runyon BA: Paracentesis of ascitic fluid: A safe procedure. Arch Intern Med 146:2259, 1986.
17. McVay PA, Toy PTCY: Lack of increased bleeding after paracentesis and thoracentesis in patients with mild coagulation abnormalities. Transfusion 13:164, 1991.
18. Runyon BA, Sheikh MY, Heck M: A peristaltic pump with multi-hole needle removes ascitic fluid safely and more rapidly than conventional equipment. Gastroenterology 112:A1368, 1997.
19. Runyon BA, Akriviadis EA, Keyser AJ: The opacity of portal hypertension–related ascites correlates with the fluid's triglyceride concentration. Am J Clin Pathol 96:142, 1991.
20. Rector WG: Spontaneous chylous ascites of cirrhosis. J Clin Gastroenterol 6:369, 1984.
21. Runyon BA: Ascitic fluid bilirubin concentration as a key to the diagnosis of choleperitoneum. J Clin Gastroenterol 9:543, 1987.
22. Runyon BA: Care of patients with ascites. N Engl J Med 330:337, 1994.
23. Hoefs JC: Increase in ascites WBC and protein concentrations during diuresis in patients with chronic liver disease. Hepatology 1:249, 1981.
24. Runyon BA: Ascites. In Yamada T, Alpers D, Owyang C, et al (eds): Textbook of Gastroenterology, 2nd ed. Philadelphia, JB Lippincott, 1995, p 927.
25. Hoefs JC: Serum protein concentration and portal pressure determine the ascitic fluid protein concentration in patients with chronic liver disease. J Lab Clin Med 102:260, 1983.
26. Runyon BA, Montano AA, Akriviadis EA, et al: The serum-ascites albumin gradient is superior to the exudate-transudate concept in the differential diagnosis of ascites. Ann Intern Med 117:215, 1992.
27. Hoefs JC: Globulin correction of the albumin gradient: Correlation with measured serum to ascites colloid osmotic gradient. Hepatology 16:396, 1992.
28. Runyon BA, Canawati HN, Akriviadis EA: Optimization of ascitic fluid culture technique. Gastroenterology 95:1351, 1988.
29. Runyon BA, Antillon MR, Akriviadis EA, et al: Bedside inoculation of blood culture bottles with ascitic fluid is superior to delayed inoculation in the detection of spontaneous bacterial peritonitis. J Clin Microbiol 28:2811, 1990.
30. Davis TE, Fuller DD: Direct identification of bacterial isolates in blood cultures using a DNA probe. J Clin Microbiol 29:2193, 1991.
31. Runyon BA, Hoefs JC: Ascitic fluid analysis before, during, and after spontaneous bacterial peritonitis. Hepatology 5:257, 1985.
32. Runyon BA: Low-protein-concentration ascitic fluid is predisposed to spontaneous bacterial peritonitis. Gastroenterology 91:1343, 1986.
33. Runyon BA: Cardiac ascites: A characterization. J Clin Gastroenterol 10:410, 1988.
34. Akriviadis EA, Runyon BA: The value of an algorithm in differentiating spontaneous from secondary bacterial peritonitis. Gastroenterology 98:127, 1990.
35. Runyon BA: Amylase levels in ascitic fluid. J Clin Gastroenterol 9: 172, 1987.
36. Manohar A, Simjee AA, Pettengill KE: Symptoms and investigative findings in 145 patients with tuberculous peritonitis diagnosed by peritoneoscopy and biopsy over a five year period. Gut 31:1130, 1990.
37. Hillebrand DJ, Runyon BA, Yasmineh W, et al: Ascitic fluid adenosine deaminase insensitivity in detecting tuberculous peritonitis. Hepatology 19:731, 1994.
38. Altamirano M, Kelly MT, Wong A, et al: Characterization of a DNA probe for detection of *Mycobacterium tuberculosis* complex in clinical samples by polymerase chain reaction. J Clin Microbiol 30:2173, 1992.
39. Cardozo PL: A critical evaluation of 3000 cytologic analyses of pleural fluid, ascitic fluid, and pericardial fluid. Acta Cytol 10:455, 1966.
40. Chetty R, Learmonth GM, Taylor DA: Giant cell hepatocellular carcinoma. Cytopathology 1:233, 1990.
41. Wang S-S, Lu C-W, Chao Y, et al: Malignancy-related ascites: A diagnostic pitfall of spontaneous bacterial peritonitis by ascitic fluid polymorphonuclear cell count. J Hepatol 20:79, 1994.
42. Press OW, Press NO, Kaufman SD: Evaluation and management of chylous ascites. Ann Intern Med 96:358, 1982.
43. Runyon BA, Antillon MR: Ascitic fluid pH and lactate: Insensitive and nonspecific tests in detecting ascitic fluid infection. Hepatology 13:929, 1991.
44. Albillos A, Cuervas-Mons V, Millan I, et al: Ascitic fluid polymorphonuclear cell count and serum to ascites albumin gradient in the diagnosis of bacterial peritonitis. Gastroenterology 98:134, 1990.
45. Runyon BA: Elevated ascitic fluid fibronectin: A non-specific finding. J Hepatol 3:219, 1986.
46. Runyon BA: Editorial: Malignancy-related ascites and ascitic fluid "humoral tests of malignancy." J Clin Gastroenterol 18:94, 1994.
47. Loewenstein MS, Rittgers RA, Feinerman AE, et al: CEA assay of ascites and detection of malignancy. Ann Intern Med 88:635, 1978.
48. Runyon BA: Spontaneous bacterial peritonitis associated with cardiac ascites. Am J Gastroenterol 79:796, 1984.
49. Kurtz RC, Bronzo RL: Does spontaneous bacterial peritonitis occur in malignant ascites? Am J Gastroenterol 77:146, 1982.
50. Wolfe GM, Runyon BA: Spontaneous *Salmonella* infection of high protein non-cirrhotic ascites. J Clin Gastroenterol 12:430, 1990.

51. Arora A, Seth S, Acharya SK, et al: Hepatic coma as a presenting feature of constrictive pericarditis. Am J Gastroenterol 88:430, 1993.
52. Wong W-M, Wu P-C, Yuen M-F, et al: Antituberculosis drug-related liver dysfunction in chronic hepatitis B infection. Hepatology 31:201, 2000.
53. De Groen PC, Rakela J, Moore C, et al: Diagnostic laparoscopy in gastroenterology: A 14-year experience. Dig Dis Sci 32:677, 1987.
54. Weisman IM, Moreno AJ, Parker AL, et al: Gastrointestinal dissemination of coccidioidomycosis. Am J Gastroenterol 81:589, 1986.
55. Cappell MS, Shetty V: A multicenter, case-controlled study of the clinical presentation and etiology of ascites and of the safety and clinical efficacy of diagnostic abdominal paracentesis in HIV seropositive patients. Am J Gastroenterol 89:2172, 1994.
56. Han S-HB, Reynolds TB, Fong T-L: Nephrogenic ascites: Analysis of 16 cases and review of the literature. Medicine 77:233, 1998.
57. Ackerman Z: Ascites in nephrotic syndrome: Incidence, patients' characteristics and complications. J Clin Gastroenterol 22:31, 1996.
58. Mauer K, Manzione NC: Usefulness of the serum-ascites albumin gradient in separating transudative from exudative ascites: Another look. Dig Dis Sci 33:1208, 1988.
59. Ikeda Y, Kanematsu T, Matsumata T, et al: Liver resection and intractable postoperative ascites. Hepato-Gastroenterol 40:14, 1993.
60. Schenker JG, Weinstein D: Ovarian hyperstimulation syndrome: A current survey. Fertil Steril 30:255, 1978.
61. Case Record. N Engl J Med 327:1014, 1992.
62. Kemeny N, Seiter K, Martin D, et al: A new syndrome: Ascites, hyperbilirubinemia, and hypoalbuminemia after biochemical modulation of fluorouracil with N-phosphonacetyl-L-aspartate (PALA). Ann Intern Med 115:946, 1991.
63. Correia JP, Conn HO: Spontaneous bacterial peritonitis in cirrhosis: Endemic or epidemic. Med Clin North Am 59:963, 1975.
64. Runyon BA: Monomicrobial nonneutrocytic bacterascites: A variant of spontaneous bacterial peritonitis. Hepatology 12:710, 1990.
65. Runyon BA, Hoefs JC: Culture-negative neutrocytic ascites: A variant of spontaneous bacterial peritonitis. Hepatology 4:1209, 1984.
66. Runyon BA, Canawati HN, Hoefs JC: Polymicrobial bacterascites: A unique entity in the spectrum of infected ascitic fluid. Arch Intern Med 146:2173, 1986.
67. Berg RD, Garlington AW: Translocation of certain indigenous bacteria from the gastrointestinal tract to the mesenteric lymph nodes and other organs in a gnotobiotic mouse model. Infect Immun 23:403, 1979.
68. Guarner C, Runyon BA, Young S, et al: Intestinal bacterial overgrowth and bacterial translocation in an experimental model of cirrhosis in rats. J Hepatol 26:1372, 1997.
69. Runyon BA, Squier SU, Borzio M: Translocation of gut bacteria in rats with cirrhosis to mesenteric lymph nodes partially explains the pathogenesis of spontaneous bacterial peritonitis. J Hepatol 21:792, 1994.
70. Runyon BA, Morrissey R, Hoefs JC, et al: Opsonic activity of human ascitic fluid: A potentially important protective mechanism against spontaneous bacterial peritonitis. Hepatology 5:634, 1985.
71. Runyon BA: Patients with deficient ascitic fluid opsonic activity are predisposed to spontaneous bacterial peritonitis. Hepatology 8:632, 1988.
72. Runyon BA, Sugano S, Kanel G, et al: A rodent model of cirrhosis and spontaneous bacterial peritonitis. Gastroenterology 100:1737, 1991.
73. Dunn DL, Barke RA, Knight NB, et al: Role of resident macrophages, peripheral neutrophils, and translymphatic absorption in bacterial clearance from the peritoneal cavity. Infec Immun 49:257, 1985.
74. McHutchison JG, Runyon BA: Spontaneous bacterial peritonitis. In Surawicz CM, Owen RL (eds): Gastrointestinal and Hepatic Infections. Philadelphia, WB Saunders, 1994, p 455.
75. Llovet J, Rodriguez-Iglesias P, Moitinho E, et al: Spontaneous bacterial peritonitis in patients with cirrhosis undergoing selective intestinal decontamination. J Hepatol 26:88, 1997.
76. Caly WR, Strauss E: A prospective study of bacterial infections in patients with cirrhosis. J Hepatol 18:353, 1993.
77. Bernard B, Cadranel J-F, Valla D, et al: Prognostic significance of bacterial infection in bleeding cirrhotic patients: A prospective study. Gastroenterology 108:1828, 1995.
78. Sorell WT, Quigley EMM, Jin G, et al: Bacterial translocation in the portal-hypertensive rat: Studies in basal conditions and on exposure to hemorrhagic shock. Gastroenterology 104:1722, 1993.
79. Cadranel J-P, Denis J, Pauwels A, et al: Prevalence and risk factors of bacteriuria in cirrhotic patients: A prospective case-control multicenter study in 244 patients. J Hepatol 31:464, 1999.
80. Pelletier G, Lesur G, Ink O, et al: Asymptomatic bacterascites: Is it spontaneous bacterial peritonitis? Hepatology 14:112, 1991.
81. Runyon BA: Four days of antibiotics can be effective therapy of culture-negative neutrocytic ascites or of delayed growth culture-positive spontaneous peritonitis. Hepatology 6:1139, 1986.
82. Gill MA, Kern JW: Altered gentamicin distribution in ascitic patients. Am J Hosp Pharm 36:1704, 1979.
83. Papadakis MA, Arieff AI: Unpredictability of clinical evaluation of renal function in cirrhosis: Prospective study. Am J Med 82:945, 1987.
84. Cabrera J, Arroyo V, Ballesta AM, et al: Aminoglycoside nephrotoxicity in cirrhosis. Gastroenterology 82:97, 1982.
85. Moore RD, Smith CR, Lietman PS: Increased risk of renal dysfunction due to interaction of liver disease and aminoglycosides. Am J Med 80:1093, 1986.
86. Ariza J, Gudiol F, Dolz C, et al: Evaluation of aztreonam in the treatment of spontaneous bacterial peritonitis in patients with cirrhosis. Hepatology 6:906, 1986.
87. Sader HS, Runyon BA, Erwin ME, et al: Antimicrobial activity of eleven newer and investigational drugs tested against isolates from spontaneous bacterial peritonitis. Diag Micro Infect Dis 21:105, 1995.
88. Felisart J, Rimola A, Arroyo V, et al: Randomized comparative study of efficacy and nephrotoxicity of ampicillin plus tobramycin versus cefotaxime in cirrhotics with severe infections. Hepatology 5:457, 1985.
89. Runyon BA, Akriviadis EA, Sattler FR, et al: Ascitic fluid and serum cefotaxime and desacetylcefotaxime levels in patients treated for bacterial peritonitis. Dig Dis Sci 36:1782, 1991.
90. Sort P, Navasa M, Arroyo V, et al: Effect of intravenous albumin on renal impairment and mortality in patients with cirrhosis and spontaneous bacterial peritonitis. N Engl J Med 341:403, 1999.
91. Runyon BA: Albumin infusion for spontaneous bacterial peritonitis. Lancet 354:1838, 1999.
92. Ricart E, Soriano G, Novella MT, et al: Amoxicillin-clavulanic acid versus cefotaxime in the therapy of bacterial infections in cirrhotic patients. J Hepatol 32:596, 2000.
93. Navasa M, Follo A, Llovet JM, et al: Randomized, comparative study of oral ofloxacin versus intravenous cefotaxime in spontaneous bacterial peritonitis. Gastroenterology 111:1011, 1996.
94. Terg R, Cobas S, Fassio E, et al: Oral ciprofloxacin after a short course of intravenous ciprofloxacin in the treatment of spontaneous bacterial peritonitis: Results of a multicenter, randomized study. J Hepatol 33:564, 2000.
95. Aparicio JR, Such J, Pascual S, et al: Development of quinolone-resistant strains of *Escherichia coli* in stools of patients with cirrhosis undergoing norfloxacin prophylaxis: Clinical consequences. J Hepatol 31:277, 1999.
96. Runyon BA, McHutchison JG, Antillon MR, et al: Short-course vs long-course antibiotic treatment of spontaneous bacterial peritonitis: A randomized controlled trial of 100 patients. Gastroenterology 100: 1737, 1991.
97. Akriviadis EA, McHutchison JG, Runyon BA: Follow-up paracentesis is usually not necessary in patients with typical spontaneous bacterial peritonitis. Hepatology 26:288A, 1997.
98. Soriano G, Teixedo M, Guarner C, et al: Selective intestinal decontamination prevents spontaneous bacterial peritonitis. Gastroenterology 100:477, 1991.
99. Gines P, Rimola A, Planas R, et al: Norfloxacin prevents spontaneous bacterial peritonitis recurrence in cirrhosis: Results of a double-blind, placebo-controlled trial. Hepatology 12:716, 1990.
100. Soriano G, Guarner C, Tomas A, et al: Norfloxacin prevents bacterial infection in cirrhotics with gastrointestinal hemorrhage. Gastroenterology 103:1267, 1992.
101. Runyon BA, Borzio M, Young S, et al: Effect of selective bowel decontamination with norfloxacin on spontaneous bacterial peritonitis, translocation, and survival in an animal model of cirrhosis. Hepatology 21:1719, 1995.
102. Novella M, Sola R, Soriano G, et al: Continuous versus inpatient prophylaxis of the first episode of spontaneous bacterial peritonitis with norfloxacin. Hepatology 25:532, 1997.
103. Guarner C, Runyon BA, Heck M, et al: Effect of long-term trimethoprim-sulfamethoxazole prophylaxis on ascites formation, bacterial translocation, spontaneous bacterial peritonitis and survival in cirrhotic rats. Dig Dis Sci 44:1957, 1999.

104. Singh N, Gayowski T, Yu VL, et al: Trimethoprim-sulfamethoxazole for the prevention of spontaneous bacterial peritonitis in cirrhosis: A randomized trial. Ann Intern Med 122:595, 1995.
105. Rolando N, Gimson A, Philpott-Howard J, et al: Infectious sequelae after endoscopic sclerotherapy of oesophageal varices: Role of antibiotic prophylaxis. J Hepatol 18:290, 1993.
106. Reynolds TB: Therapeutic paracentesis: Have we come full circle? Gastroenterology 93:386, 1987.
107. Guazzi M, Polese A, Magrini F, et al: Negative influences of ascites on the cardiac function of cirrhotic patients. Am J Med 59:165, 1975.
108. Tito L, Gines P, Arroyo V, et al: Total paracentesis associated with intravenous albumin management of patients with cirrhosis and ascites. Gastroenterology 98:146, 1990.
109. Mirouze D, Juttner HU, Reynolds TB: Left pleural effusion in patients with chronic liver disease and ascites: Prospective study of 22 cases. Dig Dis Sci 26:984, 1981.
110. Strauss RM, Boyer TD: Hepatic hydrothorax. Semin Liver Dis 17:227, 1997.
111. Xiol X, Castellote J, Baliellas C, et al: Spontaneous bacterial empyema in cirrhotic patients: Analysis of eleven cases. Hepatology 11: 365, 1990.
112. Runyon BA, Greenblatt M, Ming RHC: Hepatic hydrothorax is a relative contraindication to chest tube insertion. Am J Gastroenterol 81:566, 1986.
113. Belghiti J, Durand F: Abdominal wall hernias in the setting of cirrhosis. Semin Liver Dis 17:219, 1997.
114. Runyon BA, Juler GL: Natural history of umbilical hernias in patients with and without ascites. Am J Gastroenterol 80:38, 1985.
115. Oktedalen O, Nygaard K, Osnes M: Somatostatin in the treatment of pancreatic ascites. Gastroenterology 99:1520, 1990.
116. Runyon BA: Management of adult patients with ascites caused by cirrhosis. Hepatology 27:264, 1998.
117. Adrogue HJ, Madias NE: Hypernatremia. N Engl J Med 342:1493, 2000.
118. Adrogue HJ, Madias NE: Hyponatremia. N Engl J Med 342:1581, 2000.
119. Runyon BA: Historical aspects of treatment of patients with cirrhosis and ascites. Semin Liver Dis 17:163, 1997.
120. Eisenmenger WJ, Blondheim SH, Bongiovanni AM, et al: Electrolyte studies on patients with cirrhosis of the liver. J Clin Invest 29:1491, 1950.
121. Runyon BA, Heck M: Utility of 24-hr urine sodium collections and urine Na/K ratios in the management of patients with cirrhosis and ascites. Hepatology 24:571A, 1996.
122. Perez-Ayuso RM, Arroyo V, Planas R, et al: Randomized comparative study of efficacy of furosemide vs. spironolactone in nonazotemic cirrhosis with ascites. Gastroenterology 84:961, 1983.
123. Sungaila I, Bartle WR, Walker SE, et al: Spironolactone pharmacokinetics and pharmacodynamics in patients with cirrhotic ascites. Gastroenterology 102:1680, 1992.
124. Cohn JN: The management of chronic heart failure. N Engl J Med 335:490, 1996.
125. Stanley MM, Ochi S, Lee KK, et al: Peritoneovenous shunting as compared with medical treatment in patients with alcoholic cirrhosis and massive ascites. N Engl J Med 321:1632, 1989.
126. Daskalopoulos G, Laffi G, Morgan T, et al: Immediate effects of furosemide on renal hemodynamics in chronic liver disease with ascites. Gastroenterology 92:1859, 1987.
127. Pockros PJ, Reynolds TB: Rapid diuresis in patients with ascites from chronic liver disease: The importance of peripheral edema. Gastroenterology 90:1827, 1986.
128. Mirouze D, Zipser RD, Reynolds TB: Effect of inhibitors of prostaglandin synthesis on induced diuresis in cirrhosis. Hepatology 3:50, 1983.
129. Runyon BA, Antillon MR, Montano AA: Effect of diuresis versus therapeutic paracentesis on ascitic fluid opsonic activity and serum complement. Gastroenterology 97:158, 1989.
130. Gadano A, Moreau R, Pessione F, et al: Aquaretic effects of niravoline, a kappa-opioid agonist, in patients with cirrhosis. J Hepatol 32: 38, 2000.
131. Arroyo V, Gines P, Gerbes AL, et al: Definition and diagnostic criteria of refractory ascites and hepatorenal syndrome in cirrhosis. Heptology 23:164, 1996.
132. Bories P, Garcia-Compean D, Michel H, et al: The treatment of refractory ascites by the LeVeen shunt: A multi-center controlled trial (57 patients). J Hepatol 3:212, 1986.
133. Stanley MM, Reyes CV, Greenlee HB, et al: Peritoneal fibrosis in cirrhotics treated with peritoneovenous shunting for ascites. Dig Dis Sci 41:571, 1996.
134. Gines P, Arroyo V, Quintero E, et al: Comparison of paracentesis and diuretics in the treatment of cirrhotics with tense ascites: Results of a randomized study. Gastroenterology 93:234, 1987.
135. Kao HW, Rakov NE, Savage E, et al: The effect of large volume paracentesis on plasma volume—a cause of hypovolemia? Hepatology 5:403, 1985.
136. Pinto PC, Amerian J, Reynolds TB: Large-volume paracentesis in nonedematous patients with tense ascites: Its effect on intravascular volume. Hepatology 8:207, 1988.
137. Gines P, Tito L, Arroyo V, et al: Randomized comparative study of therapeutic paracentesis with and without intravenous albumin in cirrhosis. Gastroenterology 94:1493, 1988.
138. Gines A, Fernandez-Esparrach G, Monescillo A, et al: Randomized trial comparing albumin, dextran 70 and polygeline in cirrhotic patients with ascites treated by paracentesis. Hepatology 111:1002, 1996.
139. Ruiz-del-Arbol L, Monescillo A, Jimenez W, et al: Paracentesis-induced circulatory dysfunction: Mechanism and effect on hepatic hemodynamics in cirrhosis. Gastroenterology 113:579, 1997.
140. Rothschild M, Oratz M, Evans C, et al: Alterations in albumin metabolism after serum and albumin infusions. J Clin Invest 43:1874, 1964.
141. Wilkinson P, Sherlock S: The effect of repeated albumin infusions in patients with cirrhosis. Lancet ii:1125, 1962.
142. Pietrangelo A, Panduro A, Chowdhury JR, et al: Albumin gene expression is down-regulated by albumin or macromolecule infusion in the rat. J Clin Invest 89:1755, 1992.
143. Runyon BA: Patient selection is important in studying the impact of large-volume paracentesis on intravascular volume. Am J Gastroenterol 92:371, 1996.
144. Peltekian KM, Wong F, Liu PP, et al: Cardiovascular, renal, and neurohumoral responses to single large-volume paracentesis in patients with cirrhosis and diuretic-resistant ascites. Am J Gastroenterol 92: 394, 1997.
145. Moller S, Bendtsen F, Henriksen JH: Effect of volume expansion on systemic hemodynamics and central and arterial blood volume in cirrhosis. Gastroenterology 109:1917, 1995.
146. Planas R, Gines P, Arroyo V, et al: Dextran-70 versus albumin as plasma expanders in cirrhotic patients with tense ascites treated with total paracentesis. Gastroenterology 99:1736, 1990.
147. Vermeulen LC, Ratko TA, Erstad BL, et al: The University Hospital Consortium guidelines for the use of albumin, nonprotein colloids, and crystalloid solutions. Arch Intern Med 155:373, 1995.
148. Cochrane Injuries Group Albumin Reviewers: Human albumin administration in critically ill patients: Systematic review of randomized trials. BMJ 317:235, 1998.
149. Uriz J, Gines P, Cardenas A, et al: Terlipressin plus albumin infusion: An effective and safe therapy of hepatorenal syndrome. J Hepatol 33: 43, 2000.
150. Ochs A, Rossle M, Haag K, et al: The transjugular intrahepatic portosystemic stent-shunt procedure for refractory ascites. N Engl J Med 332:1192, 1995.
151. Rossle M, Ochs A, Gulberg V, et al: A comparison of paracentesis and transjugular intrahepatic portosystemic shunting in patients with ascites. N Engl J Med 342:1701, 2000.
152. Gines P, Quintero E, Arroyo V, et al: Compensated cirrhosis: Natural history and prognostic factors. Hepatology 7:12, 1987.
153. D'Amico G, Morabito A, Pagliaro L, Marubini E: Survival and prognostic indicators in compensated and decompensated cirrhosis. Dig Dis Sci 31:468, 1986.

Chapter 79

Hepatic Encephalopathy, Hepatopulmonary Syndromes, Hepatorenal Syndrome, Coagulopathy, and Endocrine Complications of Liver Disease

J. Gregory Fitz

The liver plays a central role in the regulation of other organ systems by virtue of its functions in nutrition, metabolism, and secretion of xenobiotics and endobiotics. Consequently, chronic liver disease can lead to a broad range of systemic manifestations that may dominate the clinical course and represent principal indications for liver transplantation. Some of these complications result from a decreased number of functioning hepatocytes and concomitant loss of synthetic and metabolic capacity. Others reflect the increased pressure in the portal circulation, leading to opening of vascular collaterals and shunting of blood away from hepatic lobules. These manifestations of cirrhosis—decreased synthetic reserve and altered perfusion—are functionally interrelated and can change over time in response to varying physiologic demands. Consequently, the systemic effects of cirrhosis on other organ systems are also dynamic, with symptoms frequently developing in the absence of obvious deterioration of the standard biochemical tests of liver function.

Despite the diversity of the organ systems affected by cirrhosis, the complications affecting these organs in the early stages share a common mechanistic bond in that they are largely functional in nature, representing a secondary effect of cirrhosis and not a primary abnormality of the target organs. Thus, replacement of a failing liver by transplantation can lead to full restoration of associated renal, neurologic, and other abnormalities. Moreover, specific diagnostic features are not always present, and patients with liver disease are also susceptible to other disease processes. In certain systemic diseases such as cystic fibrosis (pulmonary) or Wilson disease (brain), multiple organ systems are targeted by the same pathophysiologic mechanisms. This chapter provides an overview of the pathophysiology of the most common systemic manifestations of chronic liver disease and focuses particularly on their diagnosis and management.

HEPATIC ENCEPHALOPATHY

Definition

Hepatic encephalopathy, or portosystemic encephalopathy, represents a reversible decrease in neurologic function caused by liver disease.[1] It occurs most notably in patients with portal hypertension and shunting of blood away from the liver. In the setting of chronic liver disease, the onset is often insidious and is characterized by subtle and sometimes intermittent changes in memory, personality, concentration, and reaction times.[2, 3] Typically, early changes are subclinical and are recognized only in retrospect, but latent encephalopathy can be clinically significant. For example, early studies of patients with compensated cirrhosis and no clinical evidence of hepatic encephalopathy indicated that more than one half were unfit to drive an automobile, as assessed by a battery of psychometric tests.[3] Although these results cannot be extended to all patients with cirrhosis,[4] the implications for patients and for society are important in view of the prevalence of cirrhosis.

With progression of encephalopathy, the neurologic abnormalities become more apparent and are commonly graded on a numeric scale that reflects increasing degrees of neurologic dysfunction, as described in Table 79–1.[1] The manifestations of stage 1 encephalopathy reflect involvement of higher cortical functions, with decreases in attention span, changes in personality, irritability, and impaired computational and construction skills. A change in sleep pattern with wakefulness at night and drowsiness during the day is observed. The electroencephalogram (EEG), if measured, is usually normal but may show subtle slowing of the dominant frequency. Progression to stage 2 is characterized by an exaggeration of these cortical manifestations, with more drowsiness and lethargy, and by the appearance of movement disorders that reflect increasing involvement of the descending reticular system or other neurologic structures. These movement disturbances include tremors, incoordination, and asterixis.[5, 6] In cooperative patients, asterixis is commonly evaluated by asking the patient to hold the arms extended with the wrists dorsiflexed. Asterixis is characterized by an abrupt loss of flexor tone with a characteristic wristdrop that occurs in a periodic manner every 2 to 3 seconds. Alternatively, the periodic relaxations become apparent if the examiner grips the patient's hand and lightly holds the wrist in a dorsiflexed position. In a patient with mental confusion, drowsiness, and personality changes, the presence of asterixis is suggestive of underlying hepatic encephalopathy. An EEG performed in stage 2 usually shows slower rhythms with triphasic waves in the frontal regions.

Progression to stage 3, defined as increasing obtundation in a still arousable patient, or to stage 4, in which the patient is comatose, reflects either severe bilateral cortical dysfunction or involvement of the brainstem and reticular activating system. Asterixis may be lost, and hyperreflexia and muscle rigidity become apparent.[1] The EEG shows severe slowing with frequencies in the theta and delta ranges. Even though the clinical features may be fully reversible with treatment (see later), encephalopathy of this degree is generally a manifestation of advanced liver disease and is associated with a poor long-term prognosis.

The clinical features of hepatic encephalopathy are nonspecific. Similar manifestations can accompany hypoxia, acidosis, drug toxicity, and other metabolic and toxic insults. Consequently, it is important to consider and exclude these possibilities by the use of appropriate drug screens and diagnostic testing. The neurologic manifestations of hepatic encephalopathy are generally (but not always) symmetrical. The appearance of focal neurologic motor or sensory abnormalities, such as cranial nerve dysfunction or paresis, should always prompt investigation for other causes of structural neurologic disease, such as intracranial hemorrhage.

Histologic examination of the brains of patients with chronic liver disease who have had recurrent or chronic encephalopathy has identified several abnormalities, the most notable of which is a decrease in the number of astrocytes, which may contribute to the neuropathologic abnormality found in hepatic encephalopathy.[7, 8] However, it is difficult to assess whether these changes represent a cause or an effect of encephalopathy. Evidence for and against increased signals on T1-weighted magnetic resonance images of the globus pallidus has also been presented.[9] However, most early cases of encephalopathy are fully reversible with treatment, arguing against a structural basis for encephalopathy and for a toxic or neurohumoral cause.

Table 79–1 | **Clinical Stages of Hepatic Encephalopathy**

CLINICAL STAGE	INTELLECTUAL FUNCTION	NEUROMUSCULAR FUNCTION
Subclinical	Normal examination, but work or driving may be impaired	Subtle changes on psychometric or number connection tests
Stage 1	Impaired attention, irritability, depression, or personality change	Tremor, incoordination, apraxia
Stage 2	Drowsiness, behavioral changes, poor memory and computation, sleep disorders	Asterixis, slowed or slurred speech, ataxia
Stage 3	Confusion and disorientation, somnolence, amnesia	Hypoactive reflexes, nystagmus, clonus, and muscular rigidity
Stage 4	Stupor and coma	Dilated pupils and decerebrate posturing; oculocephalic reflex; absence of response to stimuli in advanced stages

Pathophysiology

Despite the frequency and characteristic clinical features of hepatic encephalopathy, the precise mechanisms involved are not fully defined. However, decades of experience with animal models, including dogs with a surgically created Eck fistula (end-to-side portacaval shunt),[10] have resulted in identification of the essential elements. In the setting of portosystemic shunting where portal blood is diverted away from the liver and into the vena cava, ingestion of a protein meal is associated with the onset of encephalopathy and progression to coma and death. Although the precise mechanisms are still not established, these findings point toward a key role for nitrogenous by-products of proteins absorbed from the colon into the portal circulation.

This model is in some ways simplistic and does not account for other potentially important parameters, such as changes in central neurotransmitters and the blood–brain barrier.[11, 12] However, the model fits well with clinical experience and makes no assumptions about the precise identity of the toxins involved. For example, although creation of a portacaval anastomosis is highly effective for treating the bleeding associated with portal hypertension, the clinical consequences include increased shunting and an increase in the frequency and severity of encephalopathy.[13] Thus, recognition of these key features—portosystemic shunting and defective hepatic clearance of nitrogenous metabolites—continues to form the basis for the standard treatments of hepatic encephalopathy.

Is ammonia the toxin responsible for hepatic encephalopathy? Yes, but not the only one, and the mechanisms whereby ammonia produces neuropsychiatric abnormalities are not fully defined. In most clinical series, elevated blood ammonia levels are detected in 60% to 80% of patients with cirrhosis and encephalopathy, and therapy aimed at decreasing the concentration of ammonia results in resolution of encephalopathy.[2, 6, 14] It is clear, however, that multiple metabolic abnormalities coexist, including changes in the profile of circulating amino acids, mercaptans, and central nervous system levels of dopamine and other neurotransmitters.[12, 15, 16] These alterations, which are summarized in Table 79–2, are present to a varying extent in different clinical scenarios and probably work in a complementary manner to modify neurologic function in patients with cirrhosis.[12] Even if ammonia is not the only cause, or even the predominant cause, of hepatic encephalopathy, it is a clinically useful marker for the production of enteric toxins from nitrogenous substrates.

Detailed reviews of the pathogenesis of hepatic encephalopathy have been published.[1, 2] In the following sections, emphasis is placed on a brief review of the role of ammonia and on the potential role of inhibitory neurotransmission through γ-aminobutyric acid (GABA) receptors in the central nervous system. This focus is based on the importance of ammonia as a guide to therapy and on emerging support for the GABA receptor complex as a target for newer therapies. Other mechanisms involving changes in central neurotransmitters and circulating amino acids are also relevant, but their therapeutic implications are not as well defined.

Table 79–2 | **Pathogenesis of Hepatic Encephalopathy**

MECHANISM	HYPOTHESIS
Toxins (ammonia, mercaptans)	Ammonia and mercaptans produced by the action of intestinal bacteria on urea and protein are elevated in blood and brain as a result of defective hepatic clearance and lead to impaired neural function through cytotoxicity, cell swelling, and depletion of glutamate
GABAergic neurotransmission	Defective hepatic clearance of GABA produced by intestinal bacteria, increased neuronal GABA synthesis, and increased production of benzodiazepine receptor agonists leads to neuronal inhibition through stimulation of the GABA receptor complex in postsynaptic membranes
False neurotransmitters	Increases in the ratio of plasma aromatic amino acids to branched-chain amino acids increase brain levels of aromatic amino acid precursors of false neurotransmitters

GABA, γ-aminobutyric acid.

Ammonia Hypothesis

Ammonia is a key intermediate in nitrogen and protein metabolism, and the dynamics of ammonia handling in man are well defined.[17, 18] The gastrointestinal tract is the primary site of ammonia production. Nitrogenous compounds in the colon, which include ingested proteins and secreted urea, are degraded by bacteria with liberation of ammonia, which is then absorbed into the portal circulation, where concentrations are 5- to 10-fold greater than in mixed venous blood.[18] The first-pass extraction of ammonia by the liver is high,[17] resulting in clearance of ammonia from the portal system and prevention of its entry into the systemic circulation. Within hepatocytes, ammonia is converted rapidly by a series of enzymatic reactions to nontoxic glutamine and, in separate reactions, synthesized into urea for secretion by the kidneys. Although abnormalities in urea cycle enzymes occur in congenital syndromes, enzyme deficiencies are not the major concern in most patients with cirrhosis, in whom ammonia bypasses the liver through portosystemic shunting.

In addition to a role in urea transport, the kidneys are a site of ammonia generation and actively secrete ammonia into the urine.[17] Indeed, there is a net increase in the concentration of ammonia in renal veins as compared with renal arteries; in addition, the concentration of ammonia in the renal veins is increased by hypokalemia and the use of diuretics.[18, 19] Clinical studies support a role for hypokalemia in precipitating hepatic encephalopathy through effects on renal ammoniagenesis.[20]

Following bolus injection of radiolabeled ammonia, the liver, bladder, and brain show appreciable uptake of ammonia.[17] In hepatic encephalopathy, arterial ammonia levels increase, and the rate of brain ammonia accumulation also increases from 32 ± 3 μmol/min to 53 ± 7 μmol/min.[17] Because muscle is an important site of ammonia clearance, the muscle atrophy seen in advanced cirrhosis may contribute to the increase in brain uptake of ammonia.[17]

Although the implications of these observations regarding ammonia metabolism, portosystemic shunting, and the pathogenesis of hepatic encephalopathy are not fully defined, collectively they indicate a clear relationship between hepatic encephalopathy and abnormal ammonia handling. Difficulties in the measurement and interpretation of blood ammonia levels include (1) substantial variations in venous as compared with arterial levels, (2) exercise-induced release of ammonia from skeletal muscle, (3) a poor correlation between the absolute value of the plasma ammonia level and the degree of encephalopathy, and (4) differences in time course between the rise in plasma ammonia levels and the onset of symptoms.[21] Despite these limitations, measures to lower arterial ammonia levels remain a cornerstone of the management of hepatic coma.[14, 22, 23]

Patients with cirrhosis are subject to changes in systemic fluid and electrolyte balance by virtue of the sodium and water retention that accompanies cirrhosis and because of the frequent use of potent diuretics. Because encephalopathy is commonly precipitated by metabolic events,[24] it is instructive to consider how abnormalities in acid-base and electrolyte balance influence ammonia metabolism, with the assumption that increases in ammonia levels increase the severity of encephalopathy. The effects of uremia are predictable because urea diffuses into the colon, where it is metabolized to liberate ammonia after bacterial degradation. The effects of hypokalemia and alkalosis are more subtle, although hypokalemia frequently develops in cirrhotic patients as a consequence of diuretic-induced urinary losses, diarrhea, vomiting, and nutritional deficiencies. First, hypokalemia increases ammonia production by the kidney.[19, 20] Second, hypokalemia and alkalosis favor cellular uptake of ammonia.[21] Because most of the body's potassium stores are found in the intracellular space, lowering potassium concentrations in the extracellular fluid stimulates efflux of potassium out of cells to restore extracellular concentrations. Cells compensate for the loss of potassium by a net uptake of sodium and hydrogen ions to maintain electroneutrality, leading to relative alkalinization of the extracellular space and acidification of the intracellular space.[21] Because ammonia (NH_3) and ammonium ion (NH_4^+) exist in equilibrium, the extracellular alkalosis increases the portion of membrane-permeable ammonia, whereas the intracellular acidosis serves to trap ammonium ion within the cell. Thus, the net effect of hypokalemia is a shift of ammonia into neurons or other cells, where it exerts its toxic effects. Consequently, normalization of hypokalemia has therapeutic importance.[25]

Despite the strong evidence that implicates ammonia as an important contributor to hepatic encephalopathy, the precise cellular mechanisms involved remain elusive. Several potential mechanisms of ammonia-induced neuronal dysfunction have been described. Ammonia has been reported to decrease the concentration of glycogen in cultured astrocytes,[7] impair glial-neuronal communication,[8] and interfere with synaptic transmission.[15] Over longer periods, sustained elevation of plasma ammonia levels induces pathologic changes in perineural astrocytes.[15] Because glycogen stores in astrocytes represent an important energy reserve for the brain, disruption of glial-neuronal signaling may play a role in the pathogenesis of hepatic encephalopathy.[7, 26] Observations in animal models of hepatic encephalopathy and hyperammonemia support these general conclusions,[22] although the multiple effects of ammonia and its metabolites have not been fully resolved.

γ-Aminobutyric Acid (GABA) Hypothesis

Ammonia causes some of the symptoms and signs of hepatic encephalopathy only after it is metabolized by glutamine synthetase in the brain. In an animal model of hepatic encephalopathy, portacaval shunting leads to increases in plasma and brain ammonia concentrations, as well as increases in brain glutamine and tryptophan concentrations, as a result of the action of glutamine synthetase.[27] Inhibition of glutamine synthetase results in normalization of brain glutamine concentrations and normalization of brain glucose consumption (and other parameters), supporting a role for glutamine synthesis in the development of cerebral metabolic abnormalities in hyperammonemic states.[27] Thus, ammonia alone does not explain the central nervous system abnormalities associated with hepatic encephalopathy.

Recent studies in humans and in animal models have implicated the GABA receptor complex as a key contributor to neuronal inhibition in hepatic encephalopathy.[16, 28] The GABA receptor complex (Fig. 79–1) is localized to postsyn-

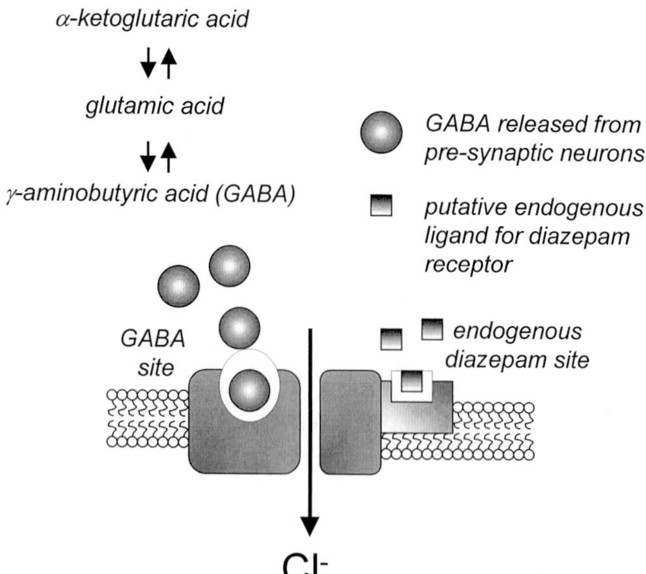

Figure 79–1. γ-Aminobutyric acid (GABA) receptor-chloride channel complex in the postsynaptic membrane.

aptic membranes and constitutes the principal inhibitory network within the central nervous system. The complex consists of (1) a GABA-binding site facing the extracellular surface, (2) a chloride-selective pore that opens in response to GABA binding to permit influx of chloride and produce membrane hyperpolarization, and (3) closely associated barbiturate and benzodiazepine receptor sites that potentiate the effects of GABA. The endogenous ligands for the benzodiazepine receptor are not known.

Theoretically, increases in GABAergic transmission could result from increased availability of extracellular GABA or benzodiazepine receptor ligands. The liver contains high concentrations of GABA and GABA transaminase.[29] Liver injury disrupts GABA homeostatic mechanisms and may contribute to the pathogenesis of hepatic encephalopathy. In addition, ammonia combines with α-ketoglutarate in the central nervous system to form glutamate, which, in turn, is amidated to produce GABA. Thus, increased production of GABA would be expected to correlate with ammonia levels.[1, 22] However, there is better evidence for the role of endogenous benzodiazepine receptor ligands.[16, 28, 30]

In the absence of known ligands, putative benzodiazepine receptor agonists are identified by their competitive inhibition of flumazenil binding.[16, 31] In both animal[32] and human models,[31] hepatic encephalopathy is associated with an increase in benzodiazepine receptor ligands. Similarly, there is increased benzodiazepine-like activity in cerebrospinal fluid, blood, and urine in human hepatic encephalopathy.[2] Several additional points merit emphasis. First, gut bacteria lead to production of precursors of benzodiazepine receptor ligands just as well as to ammonia production.[33] Impairment of hepatic clearance of such ligands in cirrhosis parallels the effects on ammonia, and treatment to lower ammonia would be expected to have similar effects on benzodiazepine receptor ligands. Second, the concentration of benzodiazepine ligands in plasma correlates roughly with the stage of hepatic encephalopathy.[31] Finally, hepatic encephalopathy is ameliorated in some patients by the benzodiazepine receptor antagonist flumazenil[30] and its structurally related analogs Ro 15-3505 and Ro 15-4513.[28]

Evaluation of the efficacy of flumazenil in the treatment of hepatic encephalopathy has been the subject of several clinical trials. In general, infusion of flumazenil (0.4 to 1 mg) results in modest but rapid improvement in the EEG and a more delayed improvement in mental status.[34, 35] In published trials, some responders had received pharmaceutical benzodiazepines. Other studies, including blinded crossover trials, have failed to identify a beneficial effect of flumazenil.[36] The reasons for these different results are not clear. However, even beneficial responses are usually incomplete, without full recovery to normal mental status, and are short-lived, possibly because flumazenil-like drugs are incomplete blockers, or, more likely, because other factors such as ammonia, mercaptans, and amino acids contribute to hepatic encephalopathy as well.[1]

Nevertheless, these studies support a role for benzodiazepine receptor ligands in the pathogenesis of hepatic encephalopathy and suggest that flumazenil or other benzodiazepine receptor antagonists may be useful in the treatment of the disorder. Clearly, benzodiazepine receptor antagonists are of benefit in reversing the effects of exogenous benzodiazepines and also may aid in the differential diagnosis of coma.[28] Although findings in animal models are not necessarily generalizable to all forms of liver injury, the implications are intriguing and imply that encephalopathy is caused in part by increased inhibitory neurotransmitter tone within the central nervous system.

Diagnosis

Hepatic encephalopathy presents as a spectrum of neurologic abnormalities, but the principal clinical features are all nonspecific. Subtle impairments of memory, consciousness, and personality are easily overlooked if the underlying liver disease is not recognized. Alternatively, even if there have been well-defined periods of encephalopathy, it may be difficult to assess whether recovery has been complete. In contrast, the clinical features of advanced encephalopathy with asterixis in a patient with known cirrhosis and portal hypertension are quite characteristic, and the combination of asterixis, hyperammonemia, and other clinical features permits confident recognition of hepatic encephalopathy.

The recognition of latent encephalopathy is of particular importance because of the high prevalence of associated cirrhosis. In the absence of characteristic features, subtle abnormalities of neuropsychiatric function are generally assessed by more specialized neuropsychiatric testing, such as the Reitan trail test, block design and digit symbol tests, and visual reaction times.[4] In addition, there is evidence to support the use of brainstem auditory evoked responses and somatosensory evoked responses[37]; however, these are specialized tests that are not readily available in the clinical setting. Consequently, a high index of suspicion in patients at risk, such as those with a recent surgical or transjugular portosystemic shunt,[13, 38, 39] and a beneficial response to a therapeutic trial are more clinically useful approaches to diagnosis outside of research settings.

Special attention has been paid to deficits in cerebral function in patients with latent or subclinical hepatic encephalopathy with regard to fitness to drive an automobile and quality of life. Driving requires complex response and spatial recognition skills; in an early series of cirrhotic patients without clinical signs of portosystemic encephalopathy, psychometric testing indicated that 60% were unfit to drive, and an additional 25% had questionable driving skills.[3] Some, but not all, recent studies have confirmed a reasonably high frequency of subclinical encephalopathy in persons with cirrhosis, but there is no consensus on whether the ability to drive is impaired in the absence of major abnormalities on neuropsychiatric testing.[4, 40–43] Thus, decisions regarding driving should be made on a case-by-case basis, with no clear support for the strict prohibition of driving in persons with compensated cirrhosis but without overt encephalopathy. Still, administration of lactulose seems to improve psychometric performance in these persons.[40]

With progression to clinically apparent hepatic encephalopathy, two modes of presentation are common. These include an acute onset of encephalopathy with rapid deterioration of mental function and coma in the absence of prior symptomatology and a chronic, relapsing clinical course that usually occurs in patients with more pronounced portal hypertension. In either case, it is important to emphasize that hepatic encephalopathy in chronic cirrhosis is usually reversible and that a precipitating cause for the deterioration can usually be identified and corrected, as is summarized in Table 79–3. The relative contributions of these precipitants were analyzed in 100 hospital admissions by Fessel and Conn[24] and are illustrated in Figure 79–2. Many of these precipitants are readily understood on the basis of their effects on ammonia. An increase in nitrogenous substances from azotemia and gastrointestinal hemorrhage together accounted for almost one half of the admissions. Iatrogenic causes from medications also figured prominently. These cases included precipitation of coma directly from increased sensitivity to tranquilizers and sedatives and indirectly through hypokalemia, dehydration, and alkalosis associated with diuretic use. The important lessons are that identification and correction of these causes is the cornerstone of effective therapy and that few patients with chronic cirrhosis develop encephalopathy because of an irreversible loss of hepatocyte mass and synthetic capacity.

Arterial ammonia levels should be measured whenever hepatic encephalopathy is suspected, both for diagnostic purposes and as a general guide to treatment. However, normal values do not exclude the diagnosis of encephalopathy and

Table 79–3 | **Common Clinical Factors that May Precipitate Hepatic Encephalopathy in Patients with Cirrhosis**

NITROGENOUS ENCEPHALOPATHY	NON-NITROGENOUS ENCEPHALOPATHY
Uremia/azotemia	Sedatives, benzodiazepines
Gastrointestinal bleeding	Barbiturates
Dehydration	Hypoxia, hypoglycemia
Metabolic alkalosis	Hypothyroidism
Hypokalemia	Anemia
Constipation	
Excessive dietary protein	
Infection	

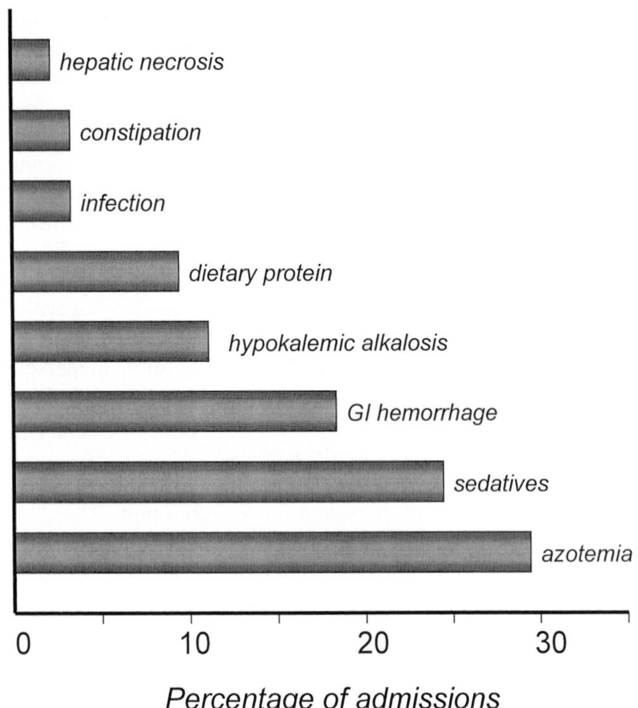

Figure 79–2. Clinical causes of portal-systemic encephalopathy. GI, gastrointestinal. (Fessel JM, Conn HO: An analysis of the causes and prevention of hepatic coma. Gastroenterology 62:191, 1972.)

should not delay initiation of ammonia-lowering therapy. Approximately one fourth of patients will have non-nitrogenous causes of encephalopathy, such as adverse reactions to sedatives or fluid and electrolyte imbalances. In light of the potential involvement of the GABA receptor complex in encephalopathy, it is not surprising that these patients respond to treatment in a manner similar to those with elevated ammonia levels. Other diagnostic tests, including measurement of glutamine levels in the spinal fluid and EEG, can provide important confirmation of the clinical impression but alone are not sensitive or specific enough to establish the diagnosis of encephalopathy.

The clinical stages of hepatic encephalopathy provide a general index of severity in the acute setting but are not sufficiently quantitative to assess subtle changes in clinical performance. Consequently, there is a need for reliable, reproducible tests that can be easily administered. The trailmaking test provides a semiquantitative measure of the degree of encephalopathy that has proven useful. In this test, the subject connects 25 consecutively numbered circles, and the number of seconds required to complete the task is recorded.[6] An alternative figure-making test has also been introduced for patients who cannot recognize numbers and has been validated, with detection of subclinical encephalopathy in 48% of subjects.[44] None of these measures alone is entirely satisfactory, and these semiquantitative tests are best used when administered serially to assess changes over time. The Portosystemic Encephalopathy Index, introduced by Conn and colleagues nearly 20 years ago, is based on an arbitrary measure of the degree of abnormality of five factors—clinical assessment of mental state, trailmaking time, EEG, asterixis, and arterial ammonia—and is still not surpassed as a clinical research tool.[6] Although complex, the index emphasizes the need for taking multiple parameters into account in the overall assessment and diagnosis of hepatic encephalopathy.

In the near future, the diagnosis of hepatic encephalopathy is likely to include cerebral imaging studies. Currently, computed tomography (CT) and magnetic resonance imaging (MRI) are used to exclude structural causes of altered mental status, such as intracerebral bleeding. However, MRI imaging and ^{1}H spectroscopy of the brains of patients with cirrhosis detect abnormalities in brain metabolites that correlate with encephalopathy and are restored to normal 3 to 7 months after liver transplantation.[45] The overall sensitivity of these techniques is not yet established, but they offer the possibility of real-time imaging of encephalopathy-specific brain metabolite changes.

Management

The principles involved in the management of hepatic encephalopathy are straightforward: Identify and correct the precipitating causes, initiate ammonia-lowering therapy, and minimize the potential medical complications of cirrhosis and depressed consciousness (Table 79–4). Among these, careful scrutiny for and correction of the underlying cause of the deterioration, such as bleeding, tranquilizers, electrolyte abnormalities, or azotemia, are most important. These basic steps are relatively easy and effective, with excellent recovery to basal function in most patients when comorbid factors are absent.

Correction of the underlying cause of encephalopathy depends on a careful review of potential contributors. Many of these, such as gastrointestinal bleeding, dehydration, hypokalemia, and azotemia, are readily apparent from the initial physical examination and basic laboratory studies. Particular attention should be paid to the possibility of gastrointestinal bleeding because of the high risk of bleeding in the setting of portal hypertension and because of the need for specific therapeutic intervention. Catabolism of blood in the intestine, with liberation of ammonia, presumably benzodiazepine re-

Table 79–4 | **Treatment of Hepatic Encephalopathy**

1. *Identify and correct the precipitating cause(s)*
   a. Assess volume status, vital signs
   b. Evaluate for gastrointestinal bleeding
   c. Eliminate sedatives, tranquilizers, or similar drugs
   d. Perform screening tests for hypoxia, hypoglycemia, anemia, hypokalemia, and other potential metabolic or endocrine factors and correct as indicated
2. *Initiate ammonia-lowering therapy*
   a. Nasogastric lavage, lactulose ± other cathartics or enemas to remove the source of ammonia from the colon
   b. Minimize or eliminate dietary protein
   c. Initiate treatment with lactulose or lactitol to produce 2 to 4 bowel movements per day
   d. Consider oral nonabsorbable antibiotics to reduce intestinal bacterial counts
   e. Consider flumazenil and other benzodiazepine receptor antagonists (see text)
3. *Minimize the potential complications of cirrhosis and depressed consciousness*
   a. Provide supportive care with attention to airway, hemodynamic, and metabolic status

ceptor ligands, and other mediators, is a classic cause of nitrogenous encephalopathy.

It is essential that action be taken as soon as potential precipitating factors are identified. If azotemia is the cause of encephalopathy, rehydration and attention to other prerenal factors are indicated. If bleeding is the cause, then the bleeding must be controlled. Medications should be reviewed in detail, with specific attention to tranquilizers and sedatives and to the adverse effects of diuretics. When any doubt exists, all potential contributing medicines should be discontinued. Moreover, general measures to correct and maintain the glucose level, oxygenation, and acid-base balance are essential.

The second step in treatment is directed toward lowering elevated ammonia levels by removing the source of the ammonia from the intestinal tract, trapping ammonia in the colon to prevent systemic absorption, and, in some patients, providing specific therapy to decrease the number of ammonia-producing bacteria in the colon. In patients with gastrointestinal bleeding, removing the source of ammonia involves elimination of blood from the gastrointestinal tract. For hemorrhage in the upper gastrointestinal tract, nasogastric lavage to remove blood and initiation of lactulose or other cathartics to speed the transit of blood through the colon are appropriate. For chronic encephalopathy not associated with bleeding, excessive protein ingestion or constipation may elevate ammonia levels sufficiently to cause encephalopathy[24]; the same treatment principles apply, including a decrease in dietary protein to approximately 60 g/day and initiation of lactulose or other laxatives to eliminate protein from the colon (see later). In addition, there appears to be some advantage to substituting vegetable protein for other protein sources because of a lower rate of ammonia production.[46] In severe encephalopathy, dietary protein should be eliminated until there is sufficient improvement to allow institution of a stable therapeutic regimen.

The synthetic disaccharides lactulose (1,4-galactosidofructose)[6] and lactitol (beta-galactosidosorbitol)[47] represent the mainstays of medical therapy for nitrogenous hepatic encephalopathy. These agents target the production and absorption of ammonia and benzodiazepine receptor ligands in the gut. Lactulose was introduced approximately 30 years ago as a therapy for hepatic encephalopathy based on the concept that the drug acidifies the contents of the colon and favors both trapping of ammonium ion in the lumen and prevention of absorption. In the colon, lactulose is metabolized by bacteria to release lactic, acetic, and other organic acids, thereby decreasing stool pH to approximately 5.5.[6] Lactulose is clinically effective in more than 80% of patients, in whom serum ammonia levels decrease and encephalopathy improves.[6, 14, 47] The benefit extends to persons with subclinical encephalopathy revealed by psychometric testing.[40] Treatment is well tolerated, and the principal toxicity is abdominal cramping, diarrhea, and flatulence. When administered orally to normal adults in amounts up to 160 g/day, lactulose decreases fecal ammonia production and increases fecal nitrogen excretion approximately four-fold owing to an increase in stool volume.[23] Thus, an increase in the number of bowel movements to 2 to 4 soft stools per day is an important therapeutic goal.

Several clinical trials have evaluated the relative efficacies of lactulose and lactitol in the treatment of hepatic encephalopathy. In general, these drugs are equally effective, but there is a trend toward better palatability and fewer adverse effects with lactitol.[47]

Antibiotics of several types, including neomycin, ampicillin, and rifaximin, are also effective in lowering blood ammonia levels.[6, 14, 48] This effect on ammonia results in large part from a decreased number of colonic bacteria and a concomitant decrease in bacterial urease and protease activity, the main enzymes responsible for ammonia generation.[48] In addition, decreasing colonic bacteria appears to decrease the production of benzodiazepine receptor ligands.[33] In most patients, the response to antibiotics is equivalent to that for lactulose, and, in small series, use of antibiotics has been associated with improved patient compliance.[6, 14] However, nonspecific use of antibiotics in the absence of an established or suspected infection raises certain concerns. Neomycin, for example, can be absorbed systemically in concentrations sufficient to induce ototoxicity and nephrotoxicity, particularly when given over longer periods; also, the alterations in gut flora associated with antibiotic use can contribute to diarrhea, malabsorption, and staphylococcal and other overgrowth syndromes. Thus, long-term therapy with antibiotics should be reserved for patients who cannot tolerate oral lactulose or lactitol therapy, and neomycin should be avoided.

Treatment of hepatic encephalopathy in the absence of elevated ammonia levels follows the same principles, including a careful review of the use of sedatives or analgesics. Prolonged recovery from sedatives administered during endoscopy or other procedures is characteristic. In addition, ammonia-lowering steps may be effective because of their effects on GABAergic transmission[1, 33] or on other agents derived from the colon that contribute to hepatic encephalopathy.

The role of flumazenil and other benzodiazepine receptor antagonists in the treatment of hepatic encephalopathy is not yet defined.[28] In clinical trials, evidence for[34, 35] and against[36] clinical benefit has been presented. Even when the response was favorable, however, recovery was rarely complete and was short-lived because of the pharmacokinetic properties of the drug. Thus, much remains to be learned regarding the origin, overall contribution, and therapy of increased GABAergic transmission in hepatic encephalopathy. At present, according to the guidelines of Jones and others, therapy with flumazenil should be limited to the following situations: (1) reversing the effects of exogenous benzodiazepines, (2) aiding in the establishment of a diagnosis of encephalopathy, and (3) providing information about prognosis and optimizing brain function in hepatic encephalopathy.[1, 28, 30] These indications are likely to evolve with additional clinical experience and the development of more selective and effective analogs.

There is a long history of clinical trials involving other experimental approaches to the treatment of hepatic encephalopathy. These approaches include, but are not limited to, use of levodopa, branched-chain amino acids, and charcoal hemoperfusion.[1, 2] Although anecdotal reports have been encouraging, the benefit of these approaches has not been established sufficiently to allow recommendation of their widespread application.

HEPATOPULMONARY SYNDROMES

Definition

Patients with cirrhosis are at increased risk for specific abnormalities of pulmonary mechanics, hemodynamics, and ventilation-perfusion matching that can adversely affect both quality of life and longevity (Table 79–5). In the early stages, subtle symptoms such as exertional dyspnea and tachypnea are commonly attributed to poor conditioning and nonspecific effects of chronic disease. With progression, dyspnea may occur at rest and may be associated with clubbing of the digits, cyanosis, and cutaneous arteriovenous malformations. The degree of liver dysfunction does not predict the magnitude of the pulmonary process.[49] However, hypoxemia or intrapulmonary shunting is common in patients with cirrhosis, affecting 20% to 40% of those tested, and the hypoxemia may be severe, with a PaO_2 less than 60 mm Hg in selected patients.[49–51] Thus, the development of hypoxia as a complication of cirrhosis indicates a high-risk patient with a poor long-term prognosis unless definitive therapy is administered.

Two of the most common pulmonary manifestations of cirrhosis are alterations in lung mechanics caused by the presence of ascites and intrapulmonary shunting and abnormal gas exchange, which together constitute the *hepatopulmonary syndrome*. There are other significant causes of pulmonary dysfunction in patients with cirrhosis. Some of these causes reflect involvement of both lung and liver in specific disease processes, such as primary biliary cirrhosis, cystic fibrosis, and sarcoidosis.[18] Others result from the adverse effects of therapy. For example, sclerotherapy of bleeding esophageal varices has been reported to decrease PaO_2 and vital capacity in some patients, possibly because of the development of a restrictive defect caused by sclerosant embolization to the lung.[52] Finally, there is increasing evidence that elevation of pulmonary artery pressure (to >40 mm Hg), a condition referred to as portopulmonary hypertension, occurs with increased frequency in patients with cirrhosis and carries a poor prognosis.

Table 79–5 | **Pulmonary Syndromes Associated with Cirrhosis**

PULMONARY MANIFESTATION	DIAGNOSTIC FEATURES
Systemic diseases affecting both lung and liver	
Cystic fibrosis	Sweat test, obstructive airway disease, juvenile onset
α_1-Antitrypsin deficiency	Emphysematous changes, phenotype
Sarcoidosis	Granulomatous inflammation, hilar adenopathy, black race
Drug toxicity	Exposure history, restrictive airway disease, chest radiograph
Mechanical effects of ascites	Tense ascites ± pleural effusion Decreased lung volumes Therapeutic response to large-volume paracentesis
Hepatopulmonary syndrome[49]	Presence of liver disease Absence of primary cardiopulmonary disease Normal chest radiograph except for basilar shadowing Pulmonary gas exchange defects, including an increased $D(A\text{-}a)O_2$, with or without hypoxemia Evidence of intrapulmonary vascular shunting
Pulmonary hypertension	Loud pulmonic component of second heart sound Right ventricular heave Right ventricular dilation or hypertrophy on echocardiography Elevated pulmonary artery pressure (>40 mm Hg) by echocardiography

$D(A\text{-}a)O_2$, alveolar-arterial oxygen content difference.

Pathophysiology

Mechanical Effects of Ascites

Accumulation of ascites can lead to significant abnormalities of pulmonary mechanics through effects on intra-abdominal and intrathoracic pressures and accompanying alterations of thoracic volumes. Generally, the clinical findings are not subtle; typically, the onset of respiratory symptoms and hypoxia is associated with worsening ascites and fluid accumulation. In some patients, the ascitic fluid may cross the diaphragm through dilated lymphatics and accumulate in the intrapleural space. Thus, the pleural fluid can represent an "ascites equivalent," requiring treatment aimed at controlling portal hypertension, and is not the result of a specific pulmonary process.

With compression of the diaphragm, standard pulmonary function tests are characterized by a decrease in mean lung volumes, including functional residual capacity and total lung capacity.[53, 54] In many patients, the diffusion capacity also is decreased.[53, 55] Air flow dynamics such as forced expiratory volumes (FEV_1 or FEV_{25-75}) generally are not affected unless there is coexisting airway disease.[53, 54] With a large amount of ascites, dyspnea is attributable in large part to an increase in the work of breathing. Indeed, many patients improve symptomatically after large-volume paracentesis even without appreciable changes in PaO_2.[54] However, the progressive loss of lung volumes and functional alveolar surface area can result in overt hypoxemia.

Hepatopulmonary Syndrome

The hepatopulmonary syndrome is more complex than the mechanical effects of ascites from a pathophysiologic perspective and frequently is not as obvious clinically.[56] In individual patients, the hepatopulmonary syndrome may coexist with mechanical pulmonary dysfunction from ascites. However, intrapulmonary shunting resulting from pulmonary vascular dilation is the main determinant of impaired gas exchange and can develop in the absence of ascites or other signs of advanced liver disease.[56] Indeed, the pulmonary symptoms may be sufficiently severe to warrant orthotopic liver transplantation even when the other clinical manifestations of cirrhosis are stable and well compensated. Impaired hypoxic vasoconstriction and ventilation-perfusion mismatching also contribute in varying degrees to the hypoxia of the hepatopulmonary syndrome.[51]

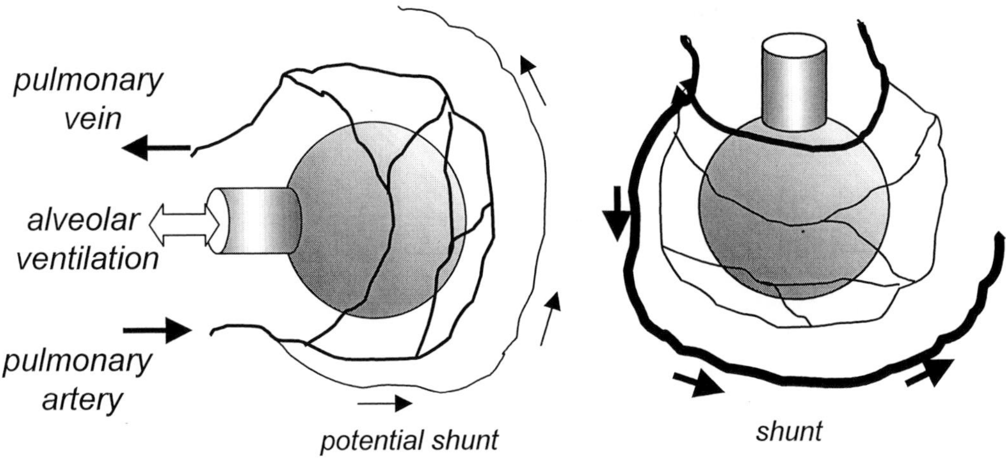

Figure 79–3. Intrapulmonary shunting of blood from pulmonary artery to pulmonary vein. Moving from a supine to an upright position can result in preferential perfusion of basilar regions and increased shunting and hypoxia (orthodeoxia). The drawing represents the level of a single acinus, but preferential perfusion of lung bases where shunts are most prominent contributes importantly to the decrease in PaO_2.

The hepatopulmonary syndrome is generally associated with a hyperdynamic circulatory state and elevations in cardiac output, cardiac index, oxygen delivery, and oxygen consumption. Both pulmonary vascular resistance and systemic vascular resistance are low.[51, 57] Clinically, the low-resistance vascular channels in the pulmonary circuit reflect shunt pathways, where blood from the pulmonary arteries bypasses functional alveoli and returns to the systemic circulation without full oxygenation, leading to desaturation of arterial blood[55] (Fig. 79–3). The effects of intrapulmonary shunting may be severe. In a series of nine cirrhotic patients with an average PaO_2 of 64 mm Hg, the shunt fraction determined during pure oxygen breathing averaged 20%.[51] This measurement indicates that 20% or more of the cardiac output bypassed functioning alveoli. The shunt fraction can increase with exercise, and there frequently are postural changes in oxygen saturation that are referred to as orthodeoxia.[51, 58] When an affected patient assumes an upright position, blood shifts to the dilated precapillary beds in the basal zones because of the effects of gravity, thereby resulting in increased shunting and exacerbation of hypoxemia[58] (see Fig. 79–3). The underlying pathophysiology is the focus of a recent review.[56]

Several theories have been proposed to account for the circulatory changes associated with hepatopulmonary syndrome. In human studies, elevated plasma catecholamine (epinephrine) levels correlate with the hyperkinetic circulation, suggesting a causal role.[59] In animal studies, glucagon also has been shown to have potent vasodilatory actions.[60] Plasma glucagon levels increase in chronic bile duct–ligated rats, and the degree of elevation correlates positively with the cardiac index and negatively with systemic vascular resistance.[60] These animals also show impaired hypoxic pulmonary vasoconstriction, consistent with a role for glucagon in hepatopulmonary syndrome.[60] More recently, elevated endothelin-1 levels have been detected in some models of cirrhosis and have been associated with vasodilation.[61] Studies of other potential mediators, including nitric oxide, somatostatin, and thromboxane A2, suggest that ultimately more than one factor will be implicated in the pathogenesis.[55, 62]

Pulmonary Hypertension

The underlying pathophysiology of the pulmonary hypertension is distinct and characterized by elevation of pulmonary artery pressures, as opposed to the pulmonary vascular dilation and intrapulmonary shunting described previously. Little is known about the pathogenesis of this process. Primary pulmonary hypertension is quite rare, but there is a general consensus among transplant centers that the frequency of pulmonary hypertension is increased in patients with cirrhosis. Unfortunately, there are few studies to assess the prevalence of pulmonary hypertension in this population. It is attractive to speculate that pulmonary hypertension develops in some patients when vasoactive molecules bypass the cirrhotic liver because of portal hypertension and portosystemic shunting and then mediate vasoconstriction when they reach the pulmonary circulation. Unfortunately, neither this nor other theories have withstood critical appraisal. Although much additional study is needed, it is important to emphasize that portopulmonary hypertension is probably underdiagnosed, and case studies suggest that, when diagnosed early, it can be cured by liver transplantation with restoration of normal portal dynamics.

Diagnosis

The increase in morbidity and mortality associated with the hepatopulmonary syndrome means that a high index of suspicion and a systematic approach to diagnosis and management are required. In patients with known cirrhosis, worsening fatigue or dyspnea should not be ascribed to chronic liver disease without further evaluation. Initially, oxygen saturation should be measured noninvasively at rest and after exercise to identify patients at risk. Arterial blood gases provide a more definitive measure of oxygen delivery and help to categorize the defect in oxygenation as mild (PaO_2 > 80 mm Hg), moderate (PaO_2 60 to 80 mm Hg), or severe (PaO_2 < 60 mm Hg). Exercise-induced desaturation is common, and the severity of pulmonary compromise may be underestimated if gas exchange is assessed under basal conditions only. Spirometry provides further documentation of changes in pulmonary volume and diffusion capacity and helps to exclude other causes of hypoxia, such as restrictive or obstructive airway disease. These alternative diagnoses are particularly relevant in disorders such as primary biliary cirrhosis in which the lungs may be a primary target of injury.[63]

The finding of tense ascites or pleural effusion on physical examination suggests the possibility of decreased lung volumes and increased work of breathing. After measurement of oxygen saturation and assessment of the possibility of coexisting pleural effusions or pulmonary parenchymal disease, the best diagnostic information often is provided by the therapeutic response to a large-volume paracentesis (see later). Prompt resolution of symptoms within several hours of fluid removal is characteristic.[53]

Digital clubbing, cyanosis, and spider angiomata are more suggestive of hepatopulmonary syndrome than of ascites-induced pulmonary compromise. Four diagnostic criteria that emphasize the functional nature of this disorder have been proposed[49] (see Table 79–5): (1) presence of chronic liver disease; (2) absence of intrinsic cardiopulmonary disease with a normal chest radiograph, or findings attributable to vascular redistribution, such as nodular shadowing in the bases; (3) pulmonary gas exchange abnormalities, including an increased alveolar-arteriolar oxygen gradient with or without hypoxemia; and (4) evidence of intrapulmonary vascular shunting. These criteria make no assumptions about the severity of the underlying liver disease.

There are several options for assessing the degree of shunting in suspected hepatopulmonary syndrome. Inert gas elimination techniques to assess ventilation-perfusion ratios, arterial blood gas measurements, and measurement of shunt fraction and alveolar-arterial oxygen content difference [$D(A\text{-}a)O_2$] represent standard approaches and are available through most hospital-based pulmonary function laboratories.[51, 55, 57] The presence of a large intrapulmonary shunt fraction in the setting of cirrhosis and hypoxemia is suggestive of hepatopulmonary syndrome. The effect of postural changes on shunt fraction, oxygenation, and $D(A\text{-}a)O_2$ can be used to demonstrate the basis of orthodeoxia and provide further support for the presence of intrapulmonary shunts in a basilar distribution.[51, 58] Right-sided heart catheterization and measurement of pulmonary artery pressures and hemodynamics provides an important adjunct in many patients.[57] Moreover, in patients with severe hypoxia, a pulmonary angiogram should be considered to rule out the possibility of large, dominant shunts. Some medical centers have developed expertise in embolization or other therapeutic approaches to close dominant shunts and improve oxygenation.

More recently, noninvasive measures, such as whole-body nucleotide scanning with technetium-99m (^{99m}Tc) macroaggregated albumin and contrast echocardiography, have proved to be useful in the detection of shunting.[49, 64, 65] Under normal conditions, ^{99m}Tc macroaggregated albumin spheres are approximately 20 μm in diameter, are trapped in pulmonary capillaries, and provide a reliable measure of lung perfusion. In cirrhosis and other conditions associated with intrapulmonary shunting, the opening of low-resistance vascular pathways allows the albumin spheres to bypass the capillary beds and appear in the systemic circulation, where they can be detected by whole-body imaging. Enhanced uptake of isotope by extrapulmonary organs indicates the presence of a shunt.[64] Using an entirely different approach, contrast echocardiography also can detect dilation of intrapulmonary vascular beds. When compared directly in a recent study, contrast echocardiography proved to be a more useful screening test because of its increased sensitivity.[50] In that study, 38% of cirrhotic patients had positive contrast echocardiography results, and 18% had both positive echocardiography results and gas exchange abnormalities. None of the patients had positive lung scans with negative echocardiography results.[50] Even in normoxemic patients with cirrhosis, contrast echocardiography detects pulmonary vasodilation in up to 10% of cases.[66]

Although these tests focus primarily on the detection of shunting, it is important to emphasize that shunting is not the sole cause of hypoxemia in the hepatopulmonary syndrome. Ventilation-perfusion mismatching, impaired oxygen diffusion, changes in cardiac output, and systemic hemodynamics each can play a role.[49] In addition, it is important to consider the possibility that symptoms are caused by pulmonary hypertension associated with the hepatopulmonary syndrome and not with shunting. Although rare, the index of suspicion for pulmonary hypertension should be increased when a loud pulmonic component of the second heart sound and a right ventricular heave are found on physical examination. Additional evaluation by echocardiography is usually sufficient to confirm the diagnosis in the presence of a dilated right ventricle, right ventricular hypertrophy, and pulmonary artery pressure greater than 40 mm Hg. When pulmonary hypertension is suspected, patients should be referred to a transplant center for definitive management.

Management

The clinical management of mechanical abnormalities of ventilatory function focuses on control of ascites and of fluid retention. In the short term, supplemental oxygen administered via nasal prongs or face mask provides symptomatic relief, and a careful clinical assessment should be conducted to assure adequate intravascular volume and the absence of pneumonia or other contributing factors. Blood is obviously the best treatment for a low intravascular volume when the hemoglobin level is less than 10 mg/dL. In addition, careful consideration of hepatopulmonary shunting is warranted in most patients.

Large-volume paracentesis of 3 L or more has proved to be safe and effective in the management of dyspnea associated with tense ascites.[53] Following paracentesis, lung volumes increase significantly, with the greatest increase in expiratory reserve volume (105%), and significant increases in vital capacity, functional residual capacity, and total lung capacity.[53, 54] Air flow generally is not affected, and there are variable effects on oxygenation.[53, 54, 67] Nevertheless, the improved work of breathing and increase in lung volumes provide marked symptomatic improvement that is detectable within hours in most patients and is sustained as long as the ascites does not reaccumulate.[54] The response to paracentesis is so reliable that the absence of significant improvement should prompt a more rigorous search for other contributing causes of dyspnea.

When pleural effusions coexist with ascites, there is no specific requirement for a therapeutic thoracentesis unless either the effusion is unusually large or there is diagnostic uncertainty. The majority of these effusions improve over several days or weeks with control of the ascites. In troublesome cases in which the size of the pleural effusion seems to be out of proportion to the amount of ascites, free communication between the intrathoracic and intra-abdominal spaces can be documented by injection of a marker such as methylene blue or a radioisotope label into the ascites. Rapid appearence in the pleural space indicates the presence of low-resistance pathways between the pleural and peritoneal cavities. Isotopes have the advantage of being detectable by nuclear imaging without the need for thoracentesis.

Although paracentesis is effective in the short term and can be repeated when needed, long-term management requires control of ascites formation through sodium restriction, diuretics to promote natriuresis and diuresis, and lowering of portal venous pressure. Several medical regimens have been demonstrated to be effective[68] (see Chapter 78). In the absence of renal impairment, sodium restriction and bed rest are successful in only approximately 10% of patients. The addition of spironolactone in doses up to 400 mg/day to antagonize the effects of aldosterone increases the proportion of responding patients to approximately 65%, and addition of furosemide or other loop diuretics allows effective control of ascites in up to 85% of patients.[68, 69] The goal of medical therapy is to minimize fluid accumulation and prevent pulmonary symptoms from developing. In patients with ascites refractory to medical management, early consideration of liver transplantation is warranted. In the interim, placement of a transjugular intrahepatic portosystemic shunt (TIPS) to lower portal pressure may improve fluid balance in approximately two thirds of patients and aid in control of recurrent pleural and abdominal fluid.[70] However, several weeks may be required before the improvement in ascites is appreciated. It should be noted that the risks of increased encephalopathy and shunt stenosis detract from the feasibility of this approach as a long-term management strategy.[13, 71]

Because the pathophysiology underlying the hepatopulmonary syndrome is complex, involving intrapulmonary shunting, ventilation-perfusion mismatching, and impaired oxygen diffusion, clinical management can be challenging.[49, 56] However, the therapeutic approach is largely supportive and often disappointing (Table 79–6). Supplemental oxygen is required to overcome any contribution of ventilation-perfusion mismatching and impaired hypoxic vasoconstriction and to improve tissue oxygen delivery. In addition, control of ascites and optimization of systemic and pulmonary hemodynamics can be important adjuncts.[49] Small series have reported beneficial responses to pharmacologic agents such as almitrine, which increases pulmonary vascular resistance and pulmonary artery pressures.[57] However, there is no standard pharmacologic approach that has proved to be effective over longer periods.[51, 55, 58] Occasional patients may benefit from right-sided heart catheterization and measurement of pulmonary pressures to optimize filling pressures and oxygen delivery. This approach may be particularly relevant to patients anticipating surgery. A pulmonary angiogram may also be considered in patients with severe hypoxemia to detect and correct dominant shunts. Similarly, measurement of right-sided heart pressures by echocardiography or right-sided heart catheterization is essential when pulmonary hypertension is being considered.

With supportive therapy, the prognosis of patients with the hepatopulmonary syndrome is poor, with an overall mortality rate of 41% after 2.5 years in a representative series.[58] However, orthotopic liver transplantation can effectively reverse pulmonary shunting or pulmonary hypertension and correct the associated hypoxia.[49, 61, 64, 72, 73] Undoubtedly, the risk of transplantation is increased by coexisting hypoxia,[51, 64] but transplantation of selected patients remains the only effective therapeutic option. Consequently, patients with suspected hepatopulmonary syndrome should be referred to a liver transplant center early in their clinical courses. This recommendation applies especially to children with biliary atresia, in whom the risk of pulmonary arteriovenous shunting is increased.[64] In general, patients with a

Table 79–6 | **Guide to the Management of Hypoxemia in Cirrhosis**

Supplemental oxygen to maintain $PaO_2 > 60$ mm Hg
Large-volume paracentesis and medical therapy of ascites; consider diagnostic or therapeutic thoracentesis
Spirometry and radiographic evaluation to identify intrinsic cardiopulmonary disease
Quantitate gas exchange abnormalities, including alveolar-arteriolar oxygen gradient
Echocardiography to evaluate right ventricular function and to estimate pulmonary artery pressure
Assess evidence for intrapulmonary vascular shunting through inert gas elimination, arterial blood gas measurements, and measurement of shunt fraction using pulmonary scanning, contrast echocardiography, or other approaches
Consider right-sided heart catheterization, pulmonary angiography
Liver transplantation

PaO_2 greater than 60 mm Hg should undergo liver transplantation as soon as possible before the shunting becomes more severe. Those with advanced disease marked by a PaO_2 of 60 mm Hg or less require careful evaluation by the transplant team with respect to operative candidacy and risk (see Chapter 83).[56, 72]

HEPATORENAL SYNDROME

Definition

There is a spectrum of hyperkinetic changes in the circulatory system in patients with cirrhosis and portal hypertension. At the extreme lies the hepatorenal syndrome, which is defined as functional renal failure in the setting of cirrhosis and in the absence of intrinsic renal disease.[74, 75] The hepatorenal syndrome is characterized by intense constriction of renal cortical vasculature with resulting oliguria and avid sodium retention.[71, 76, 77] Histologically, the kidneys are normal,[71, 78] and function is restored when the kidneys are removed and transplanted into a noncirrhotic recipient[78, 79] or following correction of portal hypertension by liver transplantation.[80]

Unfortunately, the probability that hepatorenal syndrome will develop in a patient with cirrhosis and portal hypertension is relatively high. In a recent series of 234 nonazotemic patients with cirrhosis and ascites, functional renal failure developed within 1 year in 18% and within 5 years in 39%.[81] Typically, hepatorenal syndrome occurs in the setting of portal hypertension and ascites and is characterized by a rise in the serum creatinine level and oliguria with urine outputs of 400 to 800 mL/day. The course is generally progressive, and laboratory studies demonstrate (1) relatively hyperosmolar urine, (2) a high ratio (typically >30) of urinary creatinine to plasma creatinine concentrations, and (3) a low urine sodium concentration, usually <10 mEq/L, even in the presence of diuretics.[78] Importantly, central filling pressures must be normal. In a retrospective evaluation of nonazotemic patients with cirrhosis and ascites, multivariate analysis revealed only three factors that were independent predictors of the future development of hepatorenal syndrome: a low serum sodium concentration, high plasma renin activity, and absence of hepatomegaly.[81] Other risk factors identified on univariate analysis included ascites, poor nutritional status, and esophageal varices.[81]

Patients with cirrhosis also are at increased risk for other causes of renal insufficiency. This risk is related in part to the frequent involvement of both the liver and kidney in the same disease process. Primary biliary cirrhosis, for example, is associated with lymphocytic infiltration of the renal parenchyma and interstitial nephritis, and tubular damage in Wilson disease frequently leads to renal tubular acidosis and impaired renal potassium secretion. Indeed, renal tubular acidosis and impaired acid secretion are relatively common in cirrhosis of many causes. A greater clinical concern is hypovolemia associated with diuretic use, lactulose therapy, or bleeding. The clinical features of hypovolemia may be difficult to assess with confidence in the setting of low systemic vascular resistance, and the laboratory features of prerenal azotemia are indistinguishable from those of hepatorenal syndrome. A beneficial response to volume expansion is suggestive of prerenal azotemia.

Pathophysiology

The liver plays an important role in the regulation of renal function under normal conditions.[82] In the absence of cirrhosis, uptake of amino acids by the liver stimulates an increase in renal blood flow, glomerular filtration rate, and urine volume.[82, 83] The mechanisms that have been proposed to link liver and kidney function include release both of glucagon, nitric oxide, and angiotensin II from the liver and of intrarenal prostaglandins, but the respective roles of these mediators remain controversial. There is speculation that other factors, referred to collectively as liver-borne diuretic factors or glomerulopressin, are released by the liver and target the kidney.[82] Although these substances have not been isolated and identified, the presence of such factors is an attractive hypothesis because they might account for the effect of protein loading on glomerular filtration rate and because their absence in liver failure could contribute to impaired renal function.[82]

Functional renal failure in cirrhosis is characterized by sodium retention, water retention, and renal vasoconstriction[74, 75]; it is associated with decreases in renal blood flow, glomerular filtration rate, and urinary output that contribute to the azotemia.[74, 77] However, the pathophysiologic mechanisms responsible for these functional changes are not fully defined. Hepatorenal syndrome appears to represent a final stage of the complex hemodynamic derangements associated with portal hypertension and ascites that include systemic vasodilation, effective hypovolemia, and a hyperkinetic circulation.[75, 76]

Three main hypotheses for ascites formation have been proposed: vascular underfilling, vascular overflow, and peripheral arterial vasodilation[75, 78] (see Chapter 78). These hypotheses are not mutually exclusive, and each likely accounts for part of the process.[74] The traditional underfilling hypothesis focuses on the intrahepatic blockade of hepatic blood flow as an initial event, leading to an increase in hydrostatic pressure within the hepatic and splanchnic circulation. Ascites develops when hepatic lymph production exceeds the capacity for lymphatic return, and contraction of the blood volume with underfilling leads to secondary renal dysfunction. The vascular overflow model is based on the observation that renal sodium retention often precedes the onset of ascites and can lead to an increase in blood volume. The increased volume, in turn, leads to ascites formation and reflex vasodilation to compensate for the increased volume.[74]

More recently, the peripheral arterial vasodilation model, illustrated in Figure 79–4, has been proposed because many of the features of ascites and renal dysfunction could not be explained fully by the underfilling and overflow hypotheses.[74, 85, 86] Arterial hypotension is nearly universal in advanced liver disease because of peripheral vasodilation. According to this model, peripheral and splanchnic arterial vasodilation related to portal hypertension is the initial abnormality. This vasodilation initiates adaptive reponses that stimulate both renal vasoconstriction and renal sodium and water retention, including stimulation of the sympathetic nervous system and renin-angiotensin-aldosterone system, as well as nonosmotic release of arginine vasopressin. Initially, intrarenal responses, including release of prostaglandins and atrial natriuretic factor, counteract these effects by stimulating renal vasodilation. Ultimately, the balance between the

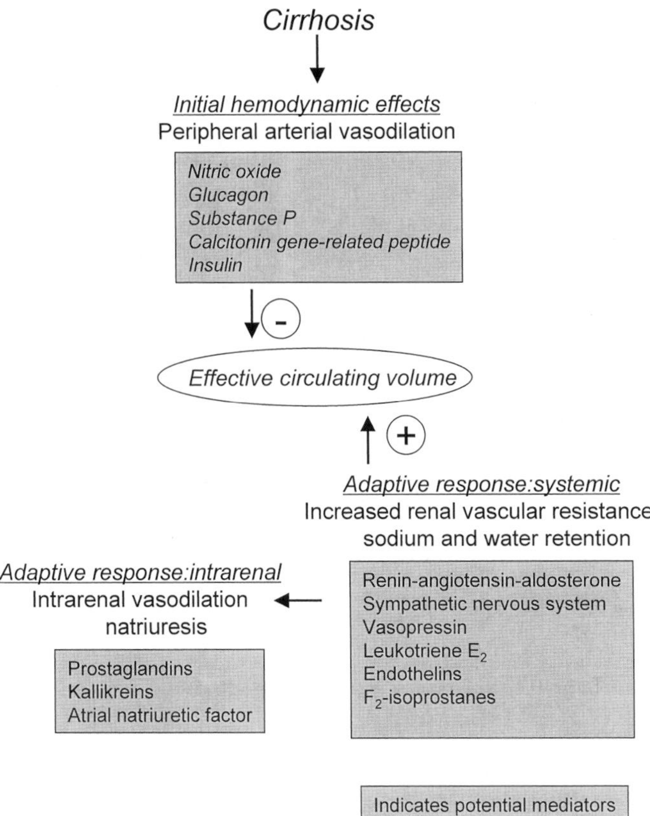

Figure 79–4. Pathogenesis of hepatorenal syndrome. Peripheral arterial vasodilation appears to be an early event in the pathogenesis of fluid retention and the hepatorenal syndrome. Following initial vasodilation, maintenance of normal renal perfusion depends on a balance between vasodilatory and vasoconstricting factors. Hepatorenal syndrome represents the clinical manifestation of markedly increased renal vascular resistance with a decreased glomerular filtration rate and avid sodium and water retention.

vasoconstrictive and vasodilatory effects is lost, leading to striking increases in renal vascular resistance and functional renal failure (see Fig. 79–4). The vasoconstrictor-mediated increase in proximal sodium resorption in the kidney accounts in part for diminished delivery of sodium to the distal tubule, the site of action of aldosterone and atrial natriuretic peptide.[85–87]

The precise factors involved in the initiation of peripheral arterial vasodilation remain obscure.[88] A role for chronic increases in levels of nitric oxide, a highly reactive diffusible gas,[77, 89] has been proposed as a cause of both the hyperdynamic circulatory changes[90] and the renal failure.[78] Similarly, plasma levels of glucagon,[89] substance P,[77] and calcitonin gene-related peptide are elevated. Calcitonin gene-related peptide is a potent vasodilator, and circulating levels are increased in patients with alcoholic cirrhosis with ascites but not in controls or cirrhotic patients without ascites.[91]

Regardless of the etiology, peripheral arterial vasodilation and underfilling of the arterial compartment initiate a sequence of responses aimed at restoring arterial filling pressure.[76, 85] Activation of the sympathetic nervous system,[92, 93] renin-angiotensin-aldosterone system,[81, 94] vasopressin,[95, 96] and other factors collectively increases renal vascular resistance[76] and renal sodium and water retention.[85, 97]

Nonosmotic stimulation of arginine vasopressin release appears to account for the impaired ability to excrete a water load that is characteristic of advanced cirrhosis.[95] In humans and in animal models, serum levels of arginine vasopressin are elevated in cirrhosis, and vasopressin metabolic clearance rates are reduced, with an increase in the half life of vasopressin in serum. In addition, there is evidence for increased gene expression of the vasopressin-regulated water channels.[98] The combination of increased vasopressin levels and an increase in the number of water channels would be expected to increase reabsorption of water in the distal nephron. In fact, both mRNA and protein levels for water channels are increased in the kidneys of cirrhotic rats and correlate with the amount of ascites, a finding consistent with the proposed formulation[98] and with the role of vasopressin in the fluid retention and dilutional hyponatremia of cirrhosis.

In addition, there are elevated plasma levels of the vasoconstrictor endothelin-1 in several pathologic conditions characterized by sodium retention.[99, 100] In heathy subjects, infusion of low doses of endothelin-1 decreases sodium excretion by 36%; infusion of high doses decreases sodium excretion further and increases renal vascular resistance by 37%.[99] These effects are partially blocked by the calcium channel blocker nifedipine.[99] Arterial and hepatic venous levels of endothelin-1 and endothelin-3 are increased in patients with cirrhosis[100]; values are higher in the presence than in the absence of ascites.[101] In addition, plasma levels of endothelin-1 and endothelin-3 correlate with significantly elevated serum creatinine levels[100–102] and negatively with central and arterial blood volume, diastolic blood pressure, and serum sodium levels.[100, 102]

Recently, F2-isoprostanes, including 8-epi-prostaglandin F2a, also have been implicated in renal vasoconstriction through effects on endothelin release.[103, 104] 8-Epi-prostaglandin F2a is an extremely potent renal vasoconstrictor, and plasma levels are markedly elevated in the hepatorenal syndrome but not in compensated cirrhosis, normal control subjects, or patients with other forms of renal disease.[104] The F2-isoprostanes are generated in response to oxidative stress by a free radical–catalyzed lipid peroxidation mechanism that does not require cyclooxygenase.[103] In cultured endothelial cells, they bind to specific receptors that are closely related to thromboxane receptors and stimulate the release of endothelin-1.[103] The stimulation of the production of F2-isoprostanes in response to hypoxia is intriguing and suggests a potential relationship between prostanoids and hepatopulmonary syndromes, alcohol, and other forms of oxidative stress.

Both local and systemic factors counterbalance renal vasoconstriction to promote natriuresis. For example, intravascular volume expansion causes release of atrial natriuretic factor.[87, 93] Initially, this response may be sufficient to counteract antinatriuretic influences at the expense of an expanded intravascular volume. As fluid retention progresses, elevated atrial natriuretic factor levels are inadequate, and diminished distal tubule delivery of sodium appears to account for the failure of some patients to escape from the sodium-retaining effects of aldosterone and resistance to atrial natriuretic factor.[85] Epstein and associates have concluded that the role of atrial natriuretic factor in cirrhosis is primarily beneficial in compensating for antinatriuretic forces in the compensated stage but that renal resistance to atrial natriuretic factor develops in later stages.[79, 87] Thus, abnormalities of atrial natriuretic factor are not likely to represent a primary cause of hepatorenal syndrome.

Renal vasoconstriction also leads to intrarenal production of vasodilating prostaglandins and kallikreins.[76] Ultimately, when the balance between renal vasoconstriction and vasodilation is lost, renal vascular resistance increases dramatically (and renal blood flow decreases), with development of hepatorenal syndrome and uremia (see Figure 79–4).

Diagnosis

Diagnostic Criteria for Hepatorenal Syndrome

Hepatorenal syndrome should be suspected in any patient with acute or chronic liver disease and portal hypertension when there is a rise in serum creatinine to above 1.5 mg/dL. In general, hepatorenal syndrome occurs in the setting of relatively advanced liver disease, and the risk of hepatorenal syndrome is increased in patients with hyponatremia, high plasma renin activity, and small liver size.[105] However, neither the etiology of the liver disease nor the Child-Turcotte-Pugh score has significant predictive value.[105]

Criteria for the diagnosis of hepatorenal syndrome have been summarized in a thoughtful review by the International Ascites Club and are summarized in Table 79–7.[74] The criteria are divided into major criteria, which must be present for the diagnosis, and minor criteria, which provide support for the diagnosis. The major criteria include (1) the presence of chronic or acute liver disease with advanced hepatic failure and portal hypertension; (2) low glomerular filtration rate as indicated by a serum creatinine greater than 1.5 mg/dL or a creatinine clearance less than 40 mL/min; (3) absence of nephrotoxic drugs, shock, infection, recent fluid losses, or other potential causes of nephrotoxicity; (4) lack of sustained improvement in renal function following diuretic withdrawal and volume expansion with 1.5 L of isotonic saline; and (5) no evidence of significant proteinuria, renal obstruction, or parenchymal renal disease.[74]

The minor criteria are based largely on functional evidence of low glomerular filtration rate and avid sodium retention and include (1) a urine volume less than 500 mL/day; (2) urine sodium concentration less than 10 mEq/L; (3) urine osmolality greater than plasma osmolality; (4) absence of significant hematuria; and (5) serum sodium concentration less than 130 mEq/L. Although not required for the diagnosis, these associated features are sufficiently common that their absence should raise doubts about the diagnosis and prompt further investigation.

These diagnostic features require that patients with suspected hepatorenal syndrome be scrutinized for other causes of renal insufficiency, undergo a careful physical examination to evaluate volume status, and have a careful urinalysis to exclude other causes of renal insufficiency. In addition, a renal ultrasound should be obtained to exclude renal parenchymal disease and obstruction, and postvoid residual bladder volumes should be assessed if there is a question of bladder outlet obstruction.

Table 79–7 | **Criteria for the Diagnosis of Hepatorenal Syndrome**[74]

MAJOR CRITERIA

1. Chronic or acute liver disease with advanced hepatic failure and portal hypertension
2. Low glomerular filtration rate, indicated by serum creatinine level > 1.5 mg/dL or creatinine clearance < 40 mL/min
3. Absence of treatment with nephrotoxic drugs, shock, infection, or significant recent fluid losses
4. No sustained improvement in renal function following diuretic withdrawal and volume expansion with 1.5 L isotonic saline
5. Proteinuria < 500 mg/dL and no ultrasonographic evidence of obstruction or parenchymal renal disease

ADDITIONAL CRITERIA

1. Urine volume < 500 mL/day
2. Urine sodium < 10 mEq/L
3. Urine osmolality greater than plasma osmolality
4. Urine red blood cells < 50 per high-power field
5. Serum sodium concentration < 130 mEq/L

From Arroyo V, Gines P, Gerbes AL, et al: Definition and diagnostic criteria of refractory ascites and hepatorenal syndrome in cirrhosis. Hepatology 23:164, 1996.

Limitations of Creatinine Measurements

One difficult issue in the early detection of hepatorenal syndrome is that there are significant limitations in the use of serum creatinine as a marker of renal function in patients with cirrhosis. In general, estimates of the glomerular filtration rate based on serum creatinine levels and creatinine clearance tend to overestimate the actual glomerular filtration rate in the presence of cirrhosis.[106] For example, when compared with inulin clearance in 56 cirrhotic patients, the sensitivity of the serum creatinine (18%) and creatinine clearance (74%) for detecting renal insufficiency was marginal; these tests overestimated the actual glomerular filtration rate by approximately 50% in persons with reduced inulin clearance.[106] The overestimation appears to result from increased tubular secretion of creatinine.[106]

Serum creatinine and creatinine clearance may be inadequate markers of renal function even in patients with well-compensated cirrhosis.[107] In 68 nonazotemic cirrhotic patients with uncomplicated cirrhosis, evidence for renal dysfunction was detected in nearly two thirds,[108] including 21 patients with a creatinine clearance of 50 to 80 mL/min and 25 patients with a creatinine clearance of less than 50 mL/min. Detection of renal insufficiency is clinically important because there is an associated substantial increase in mortality. With a mean follow-up of 180 days, the mortality rate was 24% in patients with a creatinine clearance of 50 to 80 mL/min and 36% in those with a creatinine clearance of less than 50 mL/min, as compared with 9% in those with normal renal function.[108]

Alternative Methods for Early Detection of Hepatorenal Syndrome

Ideally, the glomerular filtration rate should be measured in cirrhotic patients with the use of sensitive techniques such as iothalamate clearance, but this is not feasible in most clinical settings.[74] Because hepatorenal syndrome is characterized by renal vasoconstriction that appears before clinically recognized disease, several studies have evaluated alternative diagnostic approaches. One of the most promising is the use of Doppler ultrasonography to assess the resistive index of the renal vasculature, a measure of vascular flow resistance.[105] In 180 patients with liver disease in the absence of azotemia, renal vascular waveform analysis indicated an increase in resistive index in 42%; kidney dysfunction subsequently developed in 55%, as compared with only 6% of those with a normal resistive index. Hepatorenal syndrome occurred in 26% of those with an elevated resistive index, as compared with only 1% of those with normal values.[105] In cirrhotic patients with kidney failure, the resistive index correlates with the glomerular filtration rate, arterial pressure, plasma renin activity, and free water clearance[109] and has a sensitivity rate and specificity rate for the detection of kidney failure of 71% and 80%, respectively.[109]

Can measurement of the resistive index identify high-risk patients when standard renal function tests are still normal? The resistive index increases progressively from normal values in control patients (0.53 ± 0.03) to higher values in nonascitic cirrhotic patients (0.67 ± 0.06) and those with ascites. Values are also higher in Child-Turcotte-Pugh class B and C cirrhotic patients as compared with those with class A cirrhosis.[110] Although abnormal values may allow identification of high-risk patients,[105] operator experience is important, and considerably more information is required before this method can be recommended as a standard technique.

Management

In general, hepatorenal syndrome emerges in the setting of diuretic treatment of portal hypertension and ascites. Such treatment generally involves bed rest, sodium restriction, and intensive diuretic use with spironolactone in doses up to 400 mg/day and, in some patients, supplemental furosemide in doses up to 160 mg/day.[68, 69] These measures led to control of ascites in up to 85% of patients, but at some risk of prerenal azotemia, hypokalemia, and encephalopathy.[68, 69] Treated patients who fail to respond with natriuresis and diuresis after 1 week of intensive therapy can be considered to have refractory ascites, a frequent prelude to hepatorenal syndrome.[74]

A rise in the serum creatinine to values greater than 1.5 mg/dL in this setting represents a demanding clinical challenge. Initially, all potential nephrotoxic agents, including nonsteroidal anti-inflammatory drugs, aminoglycosides, and other antibiotics, must be discontinued. In addition, prerenal azotemia can mimic the clinical and laboratory features of hepatorenal syndrome, including oliguria, low urine sodium concentration, and high urine osmolality. Because cirrhotic patients are at risk for prerenal azotemia caused by diuretics, bleeding, and other volume losses, an intravascular volume challenge is required in most patients. This is one of the major diagnostic criteria of the International Ascites Club, which advocates diuretic withdrawal and a volume challenge of 1.5 L isotonic saline.[74] Ultimately, the diagnosis of hepatorenal syndrome is one of exclusion. When in doubt, central filling pressures should be assessed by right-sided heart catheterization.

The emergence of diuretic resistance, related perhaps to impaired mineralocorticoid escape,[86] represents a major limitation of current treatments. Moreover, diuretic use in the setting of an elevated serum creatinine level is problematic because it increases the risk of deterioration of the glomerular filtration rate through effects on plasma volume. Consequently, alternative therapies are often considered. Large-volume paracentesis causes a significant increase in cardiac output and a rapid fall in portal pressure, as well as a fall in plasma renin and aldosterone levels, and has been reported to improve serum creatinine and blood urea nitrogen levels.[111] However, the creatinine clearance may decrease following large-volume paracentesis, even when the blood urea nitrogen and serum creatinine remain unchanged, presumably because of effects on intravascular volume.[108] There is also limited evidence to support extracorporeal albumin dialysis[112] and pharmacologic treatment with low-dose dopamine, the combination of norepinephrine and dopamine,[113] terlipressin,[114] or the vasopressin analog ornipressin.[68, 76, 115] Studies of these agents are not sufficiently compelling to warrant their widespread application in clinical practice.

Several case reports have proposed a role for transjugular intrahepatic portosystemic shunts (TIPS) in the reversal of hepatorenal syndrome.[71, 116] In a series of patients with refractory ascites, TIPS increased mean urinary sodium excretion and improved serum creatinine and glomerular filtration rate.[98] This response was associated with a decrease in plasma aldosterone levels and renin activity. Clinical improvement in ascites was detected in 74% of treated patients, and the mean use of diuretics was decreased by one half.[98] The majority of patients, however, did not have overt hepatorenal syndrome. Therefore, the use of TIPS may be appropriate for some patients with diuretic-resistance ascites, but its role in hepatorenal syndrome remains to be established.

Head-out water immersion has proved to be a valuable model for studying the pathogenesis and treatment of resistant ascites.[79, 93] In patients with ascites, head-out water immersion increases central blood volume and promotes marked natriuresis and diuresis, with two- to three-fold increases in urine volume and urine sodium excretion.[93, 117] Plasma levels and urinary excretion of norepinephrine decrease, and there generally is a prompt increase in immunoreactive atrial natriuretic factor level.[93] Thus, if facilities are available, the hemodynamic response to immersion is favorable.

The onset of renal failure in patients with cirrhosis carries a poor prognosis. Plasma renin activity, plasma concentration of antidiuretic hormone, and serum sodium concentration have some value as predictors of survival,[109] but in the absence of clearly reversible causes, treatment is largely supportive. The traditional view is that dialysis is futile in hepatorenal syndrome except when used as a bridge to liver transplantation.[118] In patients with preexisting liver disease and acute renal failure (including, but not limited to, hepatorenal syndrome) that requires dialysis, the relative risk of dying is increased substantially in those with thrombocytopenia (platelet count < 100,000 mm^3), hepatic encephalopathy, or an elevated prothrombin time. In the absence of these features, the 1-year survival is 38%.[118] Renal failure alone in the absence of other contraindications may not exclude dialysis, but the risks are significant.

Orthotopic liver transplantation remains the ultimate treatment for hepatorenal syndrome. When successful, full recovery from functional renal failure can be expected. However, delaying transplantation until the onset of renal failure imposes great risks. Transplant recipients with hepatorenal syndrome have a significantly decreased survival rate at 5 years compared with those without hepatorenal syndrome.[80] In addition, longer stays in the intensive care unit, longer hospitalizations, and more dialysis sessions are required.[80] Thus, early transplantation remains the best course whenever possible.

ENDOCRINE DYSFUNCTION

Definition

The presence of advanced cirrhosis invariably leads to abnormal regulation and function of multiple endocrine systems.[119] However, the effects are complex, as anticipated from the diverse roles of the liver (1) as a target organ with functions that are regulated by circulating hormones, and (2) as a site for hormone uptake and metabolism and for production of serum hormone–binding globulins.[120–122] The prevalence and severity of endocrine dysfunction are increased in diseases in which both liver and endocrine organs are damaged by a common pathophysiologic process. For example, iron accumulation in the testes, hypothalamus, and pancreatic beta cells leads to an increased frequency of hypogonadism and diabetes in hemochromatosis,[123] and autoimmune damage to the thyroid gland frequently accompanies primary biliary cirrhosis (Table 79–8). However, cirrhosis per se is sufficient to alter regulation along the hypothalamic-pituitary-endocrine gland axis,[124] and the clinical manifestations of feminization and hypogonadism, which include gynecomastia, spider angiomata, and palmer erythema, are so common that they are considered to be characteristic of advanced liver disease.

Table 79–8 | **Endocrine Syndromes Associated with Cirrhosis**

ENDOCRINE MANIFESTATION	DIAGNOSTIC FEATURES
Systemic diseases affecting both endocrine organ(s) and liver	
Hemochromatosis	Gonadal insufficiency Hypothalamic dysfunction Diabetes
PBC	Autoimmune thyroid disease Metabolic bone disease
Alcoholic cirrhosis	Gonadal insufficiency Hypothalamic dysfunction
Feminization and hypogonadism	Elevated estrone Decreased total and free testosterone levels Loss of diurnal variation Elevated sex hormone–binding globulin Hypothalamic dysfunction Testicular atrophy
Hypothyroidism	Decreased triiodothyronine Normal or increased thyroxine-binding globulin
Diabetes	Elevated fasting glucose Insulin resistance

PBC, primary biliary cirrhosis.

In this section, emphasis is placed on the effects of cirrhosis on sex and thyroid hormone functions because of their frequency and clinical impact.[119, 122, 125, 126] These endocrine abnormalities are frequently overlooked, but approximately 60% of cirrhotic patients have a history of diminished libido, loss of well-being, and impotence.[123, 127, 128] Diabetes also merits special mention because of its prevalence in patients with cirrhosis. However, the detection and management of insulin resistance[129] is similar to that of patients without cirrhosis, except for a higher risk of complications from oral hypoglycemic medications because of prolonged drug half-life and secondary hypoglycemia.

Pathophysiology

Normal regulation of both thyroid and sex hormone levels depends on an intact hypothalamic-pituitary axis and on peripheral factors, including the level of hormone-binding globulins, that influence the availability and distribution of free (not protein-bound) hormone.

Feminization and Hypogonadism

Feminization and hypogonadism in men with cirrhosis result from a decrease in serum testosterone levels and a relative increase in circulating estrogen levels. The degree of abnormality can be striking in advanced cirrhosis, as was illustrated in a recent study in which serum free testosterone levels were lower (0.11 ± 0.02 vs 0.22 ± 0.03 nmol/L) and the serum estrogen/free testosterone ratio was significantly higher (10.3 ± 2.5 vs 2.6 ± 0.5) in cirrhotic men than in healthy control subjects.[130] The decrease in serum testosterone levels results in part from diminished testicular synthesis, and the increase in serum estrone or estradiol levels appears to be related to increased peripheral conversion of weak androgens to estrogens.[131]

The clinical features of feminization include loss of libido, decreased sperm counts,[124] decreased muscle mass, testicular atrophy, appearance of spider angiomata, and changes in hair distribution; these features presumably reflect the effects of the increased estrogen/free testosterone ratio on target organs that express androgen and estrogen receptors. An exception may be gynecomastia, for which the prevalence among cirrhotic patients of 44% does not appear to be different from that in nonobese controls without cirrhosis.[130] Moreover, estradiol levels are not different in cirrhotic patients with and without gynecomastia.[130] Thus, factors other than estrogen excess may contribute to the development of gynecomastia and perhaps other features of feminization as well.

Interpretation of the significance of sex hormone levels depends in large part on parallel measurements of sex hormone–binding globulin (SHBG), a glycoprotein with high-affinity binding for 17 β-hydroxysteroid hormones, including testosterone and estradiol.[121] SHBG is produced in the liver, and plasma concentrations are regulated by androgen/estrogen balance, thyroid hormones, and insulin.[121] Thus, the amount of free (biologically active) hormone is a function of the amount of SHBG present in the circulation. Levels of SHBG are increased significantly in patients with compensated cirrhosis.[126, 132] Thus, total testosterone levels may be normal or only slightly decreased when free testosterone levels are low because of increased SHBG levels. With progression of cirrhosis, serum free testosterone and the testosterone/SHBG ratio decrease, and serum estradiol, free estradiol, and the estradiol/testosterone ratio increase.[126] The net effect is estrogen excess and loss of androgen stimulation.

Several other factors contribute to the alterations in estrogen/testosterone balance. First, there is loss of the normal circadian rhythm of testosterone release.[131] Second, there are alterations in hepatic uptake of sex steroids, which accounts for 20% to 50% of their metabolic clearance, consistent with an important role in their bioavailability.[120] Finally, there is decreased production of testosterone as a result of impaired hypothalamic regulation. Typically, leuteinizing hormone (LH) and follicle-stimulating hormone (FSH) levels are normal or slightly increased in patients with cirrhosis, but not to the degree expected for the low testosterone levels.[127] Stimulation of pituitary gonadotropin release with clomiphene[131] or gonadotropin-releasing hormone (GnRH) increases LH and FSH release.[127] Thus, pituitary and gonadal function are relatively preserved in compensated cirrhosis, and defective hypothalamic sensing of low hormone levels or defective release of GnRH appears to contribute importantly to gonadal insufficiency. This interpretation is consistent with the elevated prolactin levels seen in some patients with cirrhosis. Pituitary secretion of prolactin is under tonic inhibitory regulation by the hypothalamus by way of the prolactin inhibitory factor dopamine. Loss of hypothalamic dopamine regulation leads to prolactin release.[133]

Similar effects occur in women with cirrhosis, but they have not been as well studied because feminization is not a great clinical concern in women in the early stages of cirrhosis. In postmenopausal women, in whom the effects of menstrual cycle variations are minimized, both estradiol levels and the estradiol/testosterone ratio are increased as compared with control subjects.[134] Testosterone, LH, and FSH levels are typically decreased.[134] In younger women, these endocrine abnormalities can lead to amenorrhea.[135] It is notable that injection of GnRH stimulates an increase in LH and FSH levels, indicating preservation of pituitary responsiveness.[135] Moreover, the findings in women are consistent with those in men, in whom the hypothalamus rather than the pituitary represents a primary site of disturbance in gonadotropin secretion.[135]

The complicating effects of alcohol merit special mention. Alcohol, even in moderate amounts, can have substantial effects on estradiol, testosterone, and estrogen-responsive pituitary hormone levels in normal postmenopausal women.[136] However, these effects are exaggerated in the presence of cirrhosis.[136] In addition, SHBG levels are elevated in most cases of cirrhosis, but the increase is greater in alcohol-related disease.[131] However, these abnormalities of sex hormone regulation are not limited to alcohol-related disease. They clearly occur in cirrhosis of other causes, and the degree of endocrine regulatory dysfunction tends to correlate with the severity of liver disease[134] and portal hypertension[124, 125, 136, 137] rather than the cause of the liver disease.

Hypothyroidism

Changes in free thyroxine levels parallel those associated with sex hormones in that the levels are influenced by thyroxine-binding globulins (TBGs), which frequently are increased in patients with cirrhosis.[138] Although this increase complicates the interpretation of standard thyroid tests, hypothyroidism is thought to be relatively common in patients with cirrhosis. However, there are few studies of the prevalence and mechanisms involved early in the disease process; the clinical features of advanced liver disease and hypothyroidism are similar and include loss of energy and appetite and depressed affect, in part because of the development of the sick-euthyroid state in advanced cirrhosis.

In patients with nonalcoholic cirrhosis and hepatic encephalopathy, serum triiodothyronine (T_3) and free T_4 levels are typically decreased,[139] and there are elevated levels of TBG and total T_4.[138] Clinical interpretation of these findings requires measurement of thyroid-stimulating hormone (TSH), which is usually normal in compensated patients and elevated in those with true hypothyroidism.[138] In 73 men with alcohol-related cirrhosis, the decrease in serum T_3 concentrations and increase in serum TSH levels correlated with the degree of liver dysfunction and testosterone levels, respectively, suggesting that there might be a relationship between testosterone and thyroid function.[140] There is evidence for both central and peripheral defects in thyroid secretion in cirrhosis. Alcohol in particular appears to have direct toxic effects on the thyroid gland.[141] In addition, in patients with cirrhosis and low total T_3 and T_4 levels, the TSH response to injected thyrotropin-releasing hormone (TRH) is frequently subnormal or delayed.[142]

Is hypothyroidism good or bad for the patient with cirrhosis? Paradoxically, an intriguing clinical study suggests that relative hypothyroidism may have beneficial effects on the outcome of cirrhosis.[122] In a retrospective analysis, there was a significant negative correlation between TSH levels and tests of liver function. Because many of the synthetic and metabolic functions of the liver are regulated by thyroid hormones, subtle hypothyroidism may minimize the rate of progression of liver disease and decrease the frequency of bleeding, ascites, and encephalopathy.[122] These findings are interesting but highly theoretical and require additional investigation.

Diagnosis

Feminization and hypogonadism are typically suspected on the basis of clinical findings of estrogen excess, including palmar erythema, spider angiomata, and an altered secondary hair pattern. In men, decreased libido and a history of impotence are common, and physical examination shows testicular atrophy and a loss of muscle mass. In women, decreased libido and amenorrhea or menstrual irregularity are frequently present.

The laboratory evaluation begins with measurement of total and free testosterone and estrogen levels to assess gonadal release and of LH and FSH levels to evaluate the pituitary response. In the early stages of compensated cirrhosis, the only findings are increases in the mean serum concentrations of estrone and SHBG.[137] With progression, low levels of free and total testosterone may become apparent, and the estrone levels increase markedly.[137] Large increases in LH and FSH are uncommon and, when present, suggest primary gonadal failure. In contrast, suppression of LH and FSH in the setting of low testosterone levels implies a central regulatory defect. When the diagnosis is uncertain, the effects of GnRH on LH, FSH, and testosterone can be assessed, and the hypothalamic-pituitary axis can be imaged by computed tomography, although these tests are rarely indicated.

The clinical features of hypothyroidism are nonspecific and are easily attributable to the systemic manifestations of cirrhosis. Consequently, every patient with cirrhosis, regardless of the etiology, should have screening studies to assess serum thyroid hormone and TSH levels. The risk of hypothyroidism is widely recognized to be increased in diseases such as primary biliary cirrhosis, but the risk is also increased in the large pool of patients with chronic viral hepatitis C, as well as those with cryoglobulinemia and those treated with interferon. Low levels of free T_3 are suggestive of hypothyroidism, but clinically significant hypothyroidism may be difficult to distinguish from sick-euthyroid states. Typically, the TSH level is normal or slightly decreased in sick-euthyroid disease and increased in hypothyroidism. When the diagnosis is uncertain, pituitary responsiveness can be assessed with a TRH stimulation test, or a clinical trial of thyroid hormone replacement can be undertaken. Clinical improvement and normalization of thyroid hormone levels and TSH would support continuation of therapy.

Management

The endocrine abnormalities associated with cirrhosis become more frequent and more severe with progression of liver disease and portal hypertension.[124] Persons with advanced liver disease (Child-Turcotte-Pugh class C) are more likely to have severe feminization, hypogonadism, or hypothyroidism. In light of the poor prognosis of advanced liver disease, it is understandable that there is little definitive information regarding the effects of hormone replacement on survival, quality of life, or disease progression. Consequently, treatment decisions must be individualized according to the patient's response and are often based on criteria developed for other diseases.

The aim of treatment for hypothyroidism with synthetic T_4 is to improve the fatigue, metabolic abnormalities, and other systemic manifestations resulting from diminished thyroid hormone levels. Therapy is initiated in conventional doses of 50 to 100 μg/day, and the dose is adjusted gradually to achieve the desired clinical effect and to maintain serum thyroid hormone and TSH levels in the normal range. There are no large controlled clinical series evaluating the efficacy of prolonged therapy. It is apparent that early detection and initiation of therapy before progression to advanced cirrhosis is likely to improve the outcomes in affected patients.

Several clinical trials have evaluated the role of testosterone replacement therapy in cirrhotic men with feminization and hypogonadism. In some studies, testosterone enanthate 250 mg intramuscularly every 4 weeks has been shown to be safe and apparently to improve libido, well-being, and sexual potency.[123] However, in larger series, testosterone in different forms has shown no consistent benefit with respect to liver function, hemodynamics, general well-being, sexual function, or survival.[132, 143] Oral testosterone therapy (200 mg three times daily) appears to decrease the prevalence of gynecomastia.[143] It is likely that early recognition before the development of advanced liver disease may identify selected patients who would benefit from testosterone replacement therapy. Short-term treatment with clomiphene increases serum LH and FSH levels and increases testicular androstenedione release[131]; there are no long-term trials of its safety or efficacy.

The long-term effects of liver transplantation on recovery of endocrine function are not fully defined. In one series, liver transplantation resulted in a trend toward normalization of total and free testosterone levels and SHBG levels.[127] The beneficial effects appear be greater in patients with alcohol-related disease than in those with other causes of liver disease.[144] However, recovery is incomplete, suggesting that there may be residual damage to the hypothalamic-pituitary-gonadal axis that persists despite liver replacement.[127, 144] Thus continued clinical and laboratory monitoring of endocrine status is required after transplantation until the etiology and natural history of these important disorders are better defined.

COAGULATION DISORDERS

Definition

The risk of bleeding in patients with cirrhosis is increased by the development of specific disorders of coagulation. The pathogenesis of coagulopathy is complex and involves abnormalities of platelets, intrinsic and extrinsic coagulation cascades, and fibrinolysis.[40] When acute bleeding occurs, correction of these abnormalities represents one of the main goals of therapy. In the absence of bleeding, coagulation disorders cause no specific symptoms and are detected by screening laboratory studies. In general, the severity of the hemostatic defects tends to increase with advancing liver disease, and their detection identifies a subset of cirrhotic patients with a high risk for a poor outcome. For example, decreases in factor VII levels, decreases in platelet counts, and increases in fibrinolysis have each been shown to increase the probability of bleeding and to affect survival adversely in different clinical scenarios.[145–147] Consequently, standard measures of hemostasis, including the platelet count, prothrombin time (PT), and partial thromboplastin time (PTT), are important for monitoring cirrhotic patients, managing bleeding, and evaluating patients before biopsies or other invasive procedures. Moreover, the prothrombin time serves as a key element of most of the grading systems designed to quantitate the severity of disease in order to determine organ allocation priorities.[148]

Pathophysiology

The parenchymal cells of the liver produce most of the factors involved in coagulation and fibrinolysis, and the reticuloendothelial cells of the liver play an active role in clearance of endotoxins, fibrin degradation products, and other factors that contribute to the balance between thrombin deposition and removal. Therefore, a variety of hemostatic disorders have been described in cirrhotic patients. In general, these disorders can be categorized into abnormalities of platelet number or function, increased fibrinolysis, or deficient synthesis of clotting factors (Table 79–9). Because

Table 79–9 | **Coagulation Abnormalities in Cirrhosis**

ABNORMALITY	LABORATORY FEATURES
Thrombocytopenia and thrombopathy	Platelet count < 80,000 mm^3 Bleeding time > 9 min Impaired aggregation
Altered synthesis of vitamin K–dependent coagulation factors	Prolonged prothrombin time Decreased factor VII levels Normal factor VIII levels
Dysfibrinoginemia	Fibrinogen normal or low Increase in fibrin degradation products, D-dimer Prolonged thrombin time Prolonged reptilase time

these abnormalities frequently coexist in individual patients, a systematic approach to their evaluation is warranted.

Cirrhosis is associated with both quantitative and qualitative platelet abnormalities. Approximately 40% of cirrhotic patients have prolongation of the bleeding time to values of more than 10 minutes and a decrease in the platelet count to less than 100,000/mL.[149] The severity of the thrombocytopenia increases with the Child-Turcotte-Pugh score, and platelet counts of less than 50,000/mL are common.[150] This decrease in the number of circulating platelets is related in part to pooling of platelets in the spleen caused by portal hypertension and splenomegaly and in part to immunologic destruction of platelets. In a representative study of 31 cirrhotic patients with an average platelet count of 46,000/mL, splenic uptake of the radiolabeled platelet pool ranged from 43% to 54%, and platelet survival decreased to 6.5 days from control values of 9.3 days.[151] Several studies have confirmed the presence of platelet-associated immunoglobulin G (IgG) in cirrhosis, and immunoglobulin levels increase in proportion to the severity of liver disease.[150–152] This phenomenon is a particular concern in patients with hepatitis C, in whom platelet-associated IgG is increased and thrombocytopenia is observed in 41% of patients (as compared with 19% of patients with hepatitis B).[153] In addition, hepatitis C may have direct effects on platelets, because viral RNA can be detected in circulating platelets.[153] The relative contributions of splenic sequestration and immune-mediated destruction are difficult to assess in individual patients. In addition, there is no consensus on the role of thrombopoietin, with evidence for both decreased production of thrombopoietin and decreased sensitivity of the bone marrow to thrombopoietin. Defining the precise role of thrombopoietin is of great interest because thrombopoietin could represent an alternative treatment in some cirrhotic patients with thrombocytopenia. The key point is that lower platelet counts, regardless of the cause, generally predict a poorer clinical outcome in patients with cirrhosis.

Cirrhosis is also associated with functional abnormalities whereby circulating platelets are not activated in a normal manner, resulting in defective clot formation.[154, 155] The decrease in platelet aggregation, as measured by the ristocetin test, may be related to decreases in glycoprotein Ib levels in the platelet membrane[156] or to defective signal transduction within the platelets.[157] Patients with bleeding times longer than 7 min or a clinical history of bleeding have the lowest glycoprotein Ib levels.[156] Other abnormalities are likely to play a role in platelet dysfunction as well.[158]

Dysfibrinogenemia represents an activation of fibrinolysis and is detected by increased blood levels of fibrin degradation products, D-dimer, and tissue plasminogen activator in the presence of cirrhosis. Fibrinogen levels may be normal, but the thrombin time and reptilase time generally are prolonged. Enhanced fibrinolysis increases the risk of gastrointestinal hemorrhage[147] and presumably other causes of bleeding as well. Increased levels of both tissue plasminogen activator and plasminogen activator inhibitors are frequently detected and appear to contribute to the underlying disorder.[159–162] However, the causative mechanisms are not clear. It has been proposed that there is an exchange between plasma and ascitic fibrinolytic proteins that regulates plasma fibrinolytic potential[161] and that endotoxin derived from intestinal bacteria enters the blood to activate the fibrinolytic cascade.[163] The relative contribution of these and other factors appears to vary from patient to patient. In more severe cases, dysfibrinogenemia may progress to disseminated intravascular coagulation. The plasma concentration of antithrombin III appears to be important in this regard.[164] Thrombin formation is increased in cirrhosis but is controlled if sufficient antithrombin III is present. At low levels of antithrombin III (<0.3 U/mL), thrombin is not inactivated, which may lead to sustained interactions with fibrin and an increase in the risk of disseminated intravascular coagulation.[164]

With loss of functioning liver parenchymal cells, clotting factor deficiencies develop and may become quite severe.[165] Vitamin K–dependent factors, including II, VII, IX, and X, and proteins S and C are affected early.[165] Factor VII, with a half-life of only 4 to 7 hours, is particularly important clinically.[67] After synthesis, vitamin K serves as a cofactor for a hepatic carboxylase that modifies these factors to provide a site for calcium binding, an essential step in their function. As factor VII levels decrease, there is a progressive increase in the prothrombin time, reflecting decreased function of the extrinsic coagulation cascade (see Chapter 63). Prolongation of the prothrombin time occurs with sufficient frequency that the prothrombin time is a standard component of the Child-Turcotte-Pugh score used to assess the severity of cirrhosis (see Chapter 77).

Diagnosis

Acquired hemostatic abnormalities in patients with cirrhosis have important clinical implications, but because there are no associated specific clinical findings, a laboratory-based approach to their evaluation is required. Generally, the diagnosis of coagulopathy is straightforward using standard laboratory tests that are readily available. Surveillance studies include the platelet count, prothrombin time, and partial thromboplastin time and should be performed at regular intervals or whenever hemorrhage is suspected. Low platelet counts are commonly detected in patients with physical manifestations of portal hypertension, including ascites and splenomegaly. Generally, platelet counts above 70,00/mL are well tolerated and do not cause prolongation of the bleeding time unless there are associated qualitative platelet abnormalities. Other causes of thrombocytopenia, including bone marrow suppression from alcohol, interferon, or other medications, must be excluded by history and bone marrow examination when necessary. Splenic sequestration is most often a diagnosis of exclusion, but increased platelet trapping can be visualized directly using ^{111}indium tropolone–labeled platelets when uncertainty exists.[152] Platelet-associated IgG levels (antiplatelet antibodies) should be measured, especially in patients with hepatitis C and autoimmune hepatitis, to assess the possible contribution of immune-mediated platelet destruction.[152] Prolongation of the bleeding also can reflect impaired platelet function in vivo.[149] When necessary, formal studies of platelet aggregation induced by ristocetin can be performed.[156]

Dysfibrinogenemia involves activation of fibrinolysis and is detected by increased levels of fibrin degradation products and D-dimer. Fibrinogen levels may be normal, but the thrombin time and reptilase time are generally prolonged. In patients with compensated cirrhosis, levels of thrombin-antithrombin III complexes are increased.[164] The presence of overt disseminated intravascular coagulation should prompt a rigorous evaluation for endotoxemia and other reversible causes.

Deficiencies in vitamin K–dependent clotting factors are detected by prolongation of the prothrombin time.[165] Direct measurement of factor VII levels is more sensitive because factor VII has a comparatively short half-life and levels must decrease to less than 60% of control values before the prothrombin time becomes abnormal. Decreases in levels of other vitamin K–dependent factors and in protein S and protein C can also contribute to prolongation of the prothrombin time. A therapeutic trial of vitamin K is important in distinguishing the potential contribution of vitamin K deficiency from diminished parenchymal synthetic capacity.

Management

Management strategies differ according to the urgency of the clinical situation. In patients with acute bleeding or undergoing invasive procedures, the goal is to improve hemostasis for the short term. The detection of coagulopathy in patients with cirrhosis identifies a high-risk subset of patients who should be evaluated for liver transplantation early in the clinical course.

In urgent settings, prolongation of the bleeding time caused by thrombocytopenia and thrombopathies generally can be managed by platelet transfusions. In addition, administration of desmopressin may improve the bleeding time[166] shorten the activated partial thromboplastin time, and increase factor VIII, XI, and XII levels.[166] The prothrombin time generally is not affected.

In patients with thrombocytopenia related to portal hypertension and splenic sequestration, there has been some clinical experience with splenic embolization with the aim of achieving a 40% to 60% reduction in splenic blood flow. Although the procedure is associated with some short-term morbidity, it effectively prolongs platelet survival time and decreases the spleen/liver ratio of platelet uptake.[152] In addition, splenic embolization decreases platelet-associated IgG levels, suggesting that the improvement in platelet count is caused not only by effects on splenic pooling but also by immunologic mechanisms.[150, 152, 167] The clinical experience with splenic embolization is decreasing with the increasing availability of liver transplantation.

From a theoretical perspective, transjugular intrahepatic portosystemic shunts (TIPS) represent an attractive approach to the treatment of splenic platelet sequestration by lowering portal venous pressures. However, clinical series are limited in number and do not yet allow definitive conclusions about the efficacy of TIPS. In a retrospective analysis of 21 patients, there was a significant rise in platelet counts following TIPS placement in patients with a postshunt portal pressure gradient of less than 12 mm Hg.[168] In a larger prospective series, however, TIPS had no beneficial effect on thrombocytopenia.[169] Thus, TIPS cannot be advocated as a definitive treatment for thrombocytopenia in the absence of further investigation.

The treatment of dysfibrinogenemia is clinically challenging. Generally, when the underlying cirrhosis is of sufficient severity to cause dysfibrinogenemia, other hematologic abnormalities are present as well. Consequently, therapy is largely supportive, with the aim of minimizing any effects of endotoxemia through surveillance cultures and antibiotics and of correcting associated platelet and factor deficiencies. Despite the poor prognosis associated with enhanced fibrinolysis,[146] the syndrome has multiple causes, and there are no clinical studies of antifibrinolytic drugs that are sufficiently compelling to recommend the use of these agents except in specific situations, such as liver transplantation or management of operative bleeding.[165]

Factor deficiencies related to decreased hepatic synthesis are detected by prolongation of the prothrombin time and quantitation of factor levels, particularly factor VII. In the urgent setting, factor deficiencies can be corrected by administration of fresh frozen plasma in amounts sufficient to lower the prothrombin time and control bleeding. Use of fresh frozen plasma is generally preferable to specific replacement of factor VII (or use of other factor concentrates) because the synthetic defects associated with cirrhosis cause multiple abnormalities in the coagulation cascade, and other important factors such as protein S and protein C are not readily quantitated. In addition, vitamin K should be administered to optimize hepatic carboxylation of vitamin K–dependent factors even when malabsorption or malnutrition is not suspected on clinical grounds.[165]

REFERENCES

1. Basile AS, Jones EA, Skolnick P: The pathogenesis and treatment of hepatic encephalopathy: Evidence for the involvement of benzodiazepine receptor ligands. Pharm Rev 43:27–62, 1991.
2. Rodes J: Clinical manifestations and therapy of hepatic encephalopathy. Adv Expt Med Biol 341:39–44, 1993.
3. Schomerus H, Hamster W, Blunck H, et al: Latent portosystemic encephalopathy. I. Nature of cerebral functional defects and their effect on fitness to drive. Dig Dis Sci 26:622–630, 1981.
4. Srivastava A, Mehta R, Rothke SP, et al: Fitness to drive in patients with cirrhosis and portal-systemic shunting: A pilot study evaluating driving performance. J Hepatol 21:1023–1028, 1994.
5. Conn HO: Asterixis in non-hepatic disorders. Am J Med 29:647–661, 1960.
6. Conn HO, Leevy CM, Vlachevic ZR, et al: Comparison of lactulose and neomycin in the treatment of chronic portal-systemic encephalopathy. Gastroenterology 72:573–583, 1977.
7. Dombro RS, Hutson DG, Norenberg MD: The action of ammonia on astrocyte glycogen and glycogenolysis. Mol Chem Neuropathol 19: 259–268, 1993.
8. Norenberg MD, Neary JT, Bender AS, Dombro RS: Hepatic encephalopathy: A disorder in glial-neuronal communication. Prog Brain Res 94:261–269, 1992.

9. Thuluvath PJ, Edwin D, Yue NC, et al: Increased signals seen in globus pallidus in T1-weighted magnetic resonance imaging in cirrhotics are not suggestive of chronic hepatic encephalopathy. Hepatology 21:440–442, 1995.
10. Fischer JE, Funovics JM, Aquirre A: The role of plasma amino acids in hepatic encephalopathy. Surgery 78:276–288, 1975.
11. Mousseau DD, Perney P, Latrargues GP, Butterworth RF: Selective loss of pallidal dopamine D2 receptor density in hepatic encephalopathy. Neurosci Lett 162:192–196, 1993.
12. Zieve L, Doizaki WM, Zieve FJ: Synergism between mercaptans and ammonia or fatty acids in the production of coma: A possible role in the pathogenesis of hepatic coma. J Lab Clin Med 83:16–28, 1974.
13. Somberg KA, Riegler JL, LaBerge JM, et al: Hepatic encephalopathy after transjugular intrahepatic portosystemic shunts: Incidence and risk factors. Am J Gastroenterol 90:531–533, 1995.
14. Bucci L, Palmieri GC: Double blind, double dummy comparison between treatment with rifaximin and lactulose in patients with medium to severe degree hepatic encephalopathy. Curr Med Res Opin 13:109–118, 1993.
15. Szerb JC, Butterworth RF: Effect of ammonium ions on synaptic transmission in the mammalian central nervous system. Prog Neurobiol 39:135–153, 1992.
16. Basile AS, Hughes RD, Harrison PM, et al: Elevated brain concentrations of 1,4-benzodiazepines in fulminant hepatic failure. N Engl J Med 325:473–478, 1991.
17. Lockwood AH, McDonald JM, Reiman RE, et al: The dynamics of ammonia metabolism in man. J Clin Invest 63:449–460, 1979.
18. McDermott WV: Metabolism and toxicity of ammonia. N Engl J Med 257:1076–1081, 1957.
19. Conn HO: Effects of high-normal and low-normal serum potassium levels on hepatic encephalopathy: Facts, half-facts or artifacts. Hepatology 20:1637–1640, 1994.
20. Gabuzda GJ, Hall PW: Relation of potassium depletion to renal ammonium metabolism and hepatic coma. Medicine 45:481–490, 1966.
21. Conn HO: Hepatic encephalopathy. In Schiff L, Schiff ER (eds): Diseases of the Liver. Philadelphia, JB Lippincott, 1993, pp 1036–1060.
22. Mullen KD, Birgisson S, Gacad RC, Conjeevaram H: Animal models of hepatic encephalopathy and hyperammonemia. Adv Exp Med Biol 368:1–10, 1994.
23. Mortensen PB: The effect of oral-administered lactulose on colonic nitrogen metabolism and excretion. Hepatology 16:1350–1356, 1992.
24. Fessel JM, Conn HO: An analysis of the causes and prevention of hepatic coma. Gastroenterology 62:191, 1972.
25. Zavagli G, Ricci G, Bader G, et al: The importance of the highest normokalemia in the treatment of early hepatic encephalopathy. Miner Electrolyte Metab 19:362–367, 1993.
26. Albrecht J, Faff L: Astrocyte-neuron interactions in hyperammonemia and hepatic coma. Adv Exp Med Biol 368:45–54, 1994.
27. Hawkins RA, Jessy J, Mans AM, De Joseph MR: Effect of reducing brain glutamine synthesis on metabolic symptoms of hepatic encephalopathy. J Neurochem 60:1000–1006, 1993.
28. Jones EA, Basile AS, Yurdaydin C, Skolnich P: Do benzodiazepine ligands contribute to hepatic encephalopathy? Adv Exp Med Biol 341:57–69, 1993.
29. Minuk GY: Gamma-aminobutyric acid and the liver. Dig Dis 11:45–54, 1993.
30. Hoffman EJ, Warren EW: Flumazenil: A benzodiazepine antagonist. Clin Pharm 12:641–656, 1993.
31. Basile AS, Harrison PM, Hughes RD, et al: Relationship between plasma benzodiazepine receptor ligand concentrations and severity of hepatic encephalopathy. Hepatology 19:112–121, 1994.
32. Yurdaydin C, Gu ZQ, Nowak G, et al: Benzodiazepine receptor ligands are elevated in an animal model of hepatic encephalopathy: Relationship between brain concentration and severity of encephalopathy. J Pharm Exp Ther 265:565–571, 1993.
33. Yurdaydin C, Walsh TJ, Engler HD, et al: Gut bacteria provide precursors of benzodiazepine receptor ligands in a rat model of hepatic encephalopathy. Brain Res 679:42–48, 1995.
34. Cadrenal JF, el Younsi M, Pidoux B, et al: Flumazenil therapy for hepatic encephalopathy in cirrhotic patients: A double-blind pragmatic randomized, placebo study. Eur J Gastroenterol Hepatol 7:325–329, 1995.
35. Pomier-Layrargues G, Giguere JF, Lavoie J, et al: Flumazenil in cirrhotic patients in hepatic coma: A randomized double-blind placebo-controlled crossover trial. Hepatology 19:32–37, 1994.
36. Van der Rijt CC, Schalm SW, Meulstee J, Stijnen T: Flumazenil therapy for hepatic encephalopathy. A double-blind crossover study. Gastroenterol Clin Biol 19:572–580, 1995.
37. Kullmann F, Hollerbac S, Holstege A, Scholmerich J: Subclinical hepatic encephalopathy: The diagnostic value of evoked potentials. J Hepatol 22:101–110, 1995.
38. Chalasani N, Clark WS, Martin LG, et al: Determinants of mortality in patients with advanced cirrhosis after transjugular intrahepatic portosystemic shunting. Gastroenterology 118:138–144, 2000.
39. Pomier-Layrargues G: TIPS and hepatic encephalopathy. Semin Liver Dis 16:315–320, 1996.
40. Dhiman RK, Sawhney MS, Chawla YK, et al: Efficacy of lactulose in cirrhotic patients with subclinical hepatic encephalopathy. Dig Dis Sci 45:1549–1552, 2000.
41. Hartmann IJ, Groeneweg M, Quero JC, et al: The prognostic significance of subclinical hepatic encephalopathy. Am J Gastroenterol 95: 2029–2034, 2000.
42. Groeneweg M, Moerland W, Quero JC, et al: Screening of subclinical hepatic encephalopathy. J Hepatol 32:748–753, 2000.
43. Groeneweg M, Quero JC, De Bruijn I, et al: Subclinical hepatic encephalopathy impairs daily functioning. Hepatology 28:45–49, 1998.
44. Dhiman RK, Saraswat VA, Verma M, Naik SR: Figure connection test: A universal test for assessment of mental state. J Gastroenterol Hepatol 10:14–23, 1995.
45. Naegele T, Grodd W, Viebahn R, et al: MR imaging and (1)H spectroscopy of brain metabolites in hepatic encephalopathy: Time-course of renormalization after liver transplantation. Radiology 216:683–691, 2000.
46. Conn HO: Animal versus vegetable protein diet in hepatic encephalopathy. J Intern Med 233:369–371, 1993.
47. Camma C, Fiorello F, Tine F, et al: Lactitol in treatment of chronic hepatic encephalopathy. A metaanalysis. Dig Dis Sci 38:916–922, 1993.
48. Alexander T, Thomas K, Cherian AM, Kanakasabapathy A: Effect of three antibacterial drugs in lowering blood and stool ammonia production in hepatic encephalopathy. Indian J Med Res 96:292–296, 1992.
49. Rodriguez-Roisin R, Agusti AG, Roca J: The hepatopulmonary syndrome: New name, old complexities. Thorax 47:897–902, 1992.
50. Abrams GA, Jaffe CC, Hoffer PB, et al: Diagnostic utility of contrast echocardiography and lung perfusion scan in patients with hepatopulmonary syndrome. Gastroenterology 109:1283–1288, 1995.
51. Andrivet P, Cadranel J, Housset B, et al: Mechanisms of impaired arterial oxygenation in patients with liver cirrhosis and severe respiratory insufficiency. Chest 103:500–507, 1993.
52. Samuels T, Lovett MC, Campbell IT, et al: Respiratory function after injection sclerotherapy of oesophageal varices. Gut 35:1459–1463, 1994.
53. Berkowitz KA, Butensky MS, Smith RI: Pulmonary function changes after large volume paracentesis. Am J Gastroenterol 88:905–907, 1993.
54. Angeuira CE, Kadakia SC: Effects of large volume paracentesis on pulmonary function in patients with tense cirrhotic ascites. Hepatology 20:825–828, 1994.
55. Soderman C, Juhlin-Dannfelt A, Lagerstrand L, Eriksson LS: Ventilation-perfusion relationships and central hemodynamics in patients with cirrhosis. Effects of a somatostatin analogue. J Hepatol 21:52–57, 1994.
56. Fallon MB, Abrams GA: Hepatopulmonary syndrome. Curr Gastroenterol Rep 2:40–45, 2000.
57. Nakos G, Evrenoglou D, Vassilakis N, Lampropoulos S: Haemodynamics and gas exchange in liver cirrhosis: The effect of orally administered almitrine bismesylate. Respir Med 87:93–98, 1993.
58. Krowka MJ, Dickson ER, Cortese DA: Hepatopulmonary syndrome. Clinical observations and lack of response to somatostatin analogue. Chest 104:515–521, 1993.
59. Braillon A, Gaudin C, Poo JL, et al: Plasma catecholamine concentrations are a reliable index of sympathetic vascular tone in patients with cirrhosis. Hepatology 15:58–62, 1992.
60. Ohara N, Jaspan J, Chang SW: Hyperglucagonemia and hyperdynamic circulation in rats with biliary cirrhosis. J Lab Clin Med 121:142–147, 1993.
61. Luo B, Abrams GA, Fallon MB: Endothelin-1 in the rat bile duct ligation model of hepatopulmonary syndrome: Correlation with pulmonary dysfunction. J Hepatol 29:571–578, 1998.
62. Chang SW, Ohara N: Increased pulmonary vascular permeability in

rats with biliary cirrhosis: Role of thromboxane A2. Am J Physiol 264:L245–L252, 1993.
63. Costa C, Sambataro A, Baldi S, et al: Primary biliary cirrhosis: Lung involvement. Liver 15:196–201, 1995.
64. Barbe T, Losay J, Gromin G, et al: Pulmonary arteriovenous shunting in children with liver disease. J Pediatr 126:571–579, 1995.
65. Aller R, Moya JL, Moreira V, et al: Diagnosis and grading of intrapulmonary vascular dilatation in cirrhotic patients with contrast transesophageal echocardiography. J Hepatol 31:1044–1052, 1999.
66. Mimidis KP, Karatza C, Spiropoulos KV, et al: Prevalence of intrapulmonary vascular dilatations in normoxaemic patients with early liver cirrhosis. Scand J Gastroenterol 33:988–992, 1998.
67. Chang SC, Chang HI, Chen FJ, et al: Effects of ascites and body position on gas exchange in patients with cirrhosis. Proc Nat Sci Counc Repub China B 19:143–150, 1995.
68. Gerbes AL. Medical treatment of ascites. J Hepatol 17:S4–S9, 1993.
69. Arroyo V, Gines P, Planas R: Treatment of ascites in cirrhosis. Diuretics, peritovenous shunt, and large-volume paracentesis. Gastroenterol Clin North Am 21:237–256, 1992.
70. Somberg KA, Lake JR, Tomlanovich SJ, et al: Transjugular intrahepatic portosystemic shunts for refractory ascites: Assessment of clinical and hormonal response and renal function. Hepatology 21:709–716, 1995.
71. Spahr L, Fenyves D, N'Guyen VV, et al: Improvement of hepatorenal syndrome by transjugular intrahepatic portosystemic shunt. Am J Gastroenterol 90:1169–1171, 1995.
72. Hobeika J, Houssin D, Bernard O, et al: Orthotopic liver transplantation in children with chronic liver disease and severe hypoxemia. Transplantation 57:224–228, 1994.
73. Koneru B, Admed S, Weisse AB, et al: Resolution of pulmonary hypertension of cirrhosis after liver transplantation. Transplantation 58: 1133–1135, 1994.
74. Arroyo V, Gines P, Gerbes AL, et al: Definition and diagnostic criteria of refractory ascites and hepatorenal syndrome in cirrhosis. Hepatology 23:164–176, 1996.
75. Gines P: Diagnosis and treatment of hepatorenal syndrome. Baillieres Best Pract Res Clin Gastroenterol 14:945–957, 2000.
76. Badalamenti S, Graziani G, Salerno F, Ponticelli C: Hepatorenal syndrome. New perspectives in pathogenesis and treatment. Arch Intern Med 153:1957–1967, 1993.
77. Lang F, Gerok W, Haussinger D: New clues to the pathophysiology of hepatorenal failure. Clin Invest Med 71:93–97, 1993.
78. Epstein M: Hepatorenal syndrome: Emerging perspectives of pathophysiology and therapy. J Am Soc Nephrol 4:1735–1753, 1994.
79. Epstein M: Renal sodium retention in liver disease. Hosp Pract 30:33–37, 1995.
80. Gonwa TA, Klintmalm GB, Levy M, et al: Impact of pretransplant renal function on survival after liver transplantation. Transplantation 59:361–365, 1995.
81. Gines A, Escorsell A, Gines P, et al: Incidence, predictive factors, and prognosis of the hepatorenal syndrome. Gastroenterology 105:229–236, 1993.
82. Lang F, Tschernko E, Haussinger D: Hepatic regulation of renal function. Exp Physiol 77:663–673, 1992.
83. Lang F, Ottl I, Haussinger D, et al: Renal hemodynamic response to intravenous and oral amino acids in animals. Semin Nephrol 15:415–418, 1995.
84. DeSanto NG, Cirillo M, Anastasio P, et al: Renal response to an acute oral protein load in healthy humans and in patients with renal disease or liver disease. Semin Nephrol 15:433–448, 1995.
85. Abraham WT, Schrier RW: Body fluid volume regulation in health and disease. Adv Intern Med 39:23–47, 1994.
86. Schrier RW: Peripheral arterial vasodilation in cirrhosis and impaired mineralocorticoid escape. Gastroenterology 102:2165–2168, 1992.
87. Warner L, Skorecki K, Blendis LM, Epstein M: Atrial natriuretic factor and liver disease. Hepatology 17:500–513, 1993.
88. Castro M, Krowka MJ, Schroeder DR, et al: Frequency and clinical implications of increased pulmonary artery pressures in liver transplant patients. Mayo Clin Proc 71:543–551, 1996.
89. Michielsen PP, Pelckmans PA: Haemodynamic changes in portal hypertension. Acta Gastroenterol Belg 57:194–205, 1994.
90. Abrams GA, Nathanson MH: Nitric oxide and liver disease. Gastroenterologist 3:220–233, 1995.
91. Gupta S, Morgan TR, Gordan GS: Calcitonin gene-related peptide in hepatorenal syndrome. A possible mediator of peripheral vasodilation? J Clin Gastroenterol 14:122–126, 1992.
92. Henriksen JH, Ring-Larsen H: Hepatorenal disorders: Role of the sympathetic nervous system. Semin Liver Dis 14:35–43, 1994.
93. Grossman E, Goldstein DS, Hoffman A, et al: Effects of water immersion on sympathoadrenal and dopa-dopamine systems in humans. Am J Physiol 262:R993–R999, 1992.
94. Bernardi M, Trevisani F, Gasbarrini A, Gasbarrini G: Hepatorenal disorders: Role of the renin-angiotensin-aldosterone system. Semin Liver Dis 14:23–34, 1994.
95. Kim JK, Sumner SN, Schrier RW: Vasopressin gene expression in rats with experimental cirrhosis. Hepatology 17:143–147, 1993.
96. Solis-Herruzo JA, Gonzalez-Gamarra A, Castellano G, Munoz-Yague MT: Metabolic clearance rate of arginine vasopressin in patients with cirrhosis. Hepatology 16:974–979, 1992.
97. Gines P, Arroyo V, Rodes J: Ascites and hepatorenal syndrome: Pathogenesis and treatment strategies. Adv Intern Med 43:99–142, 1998.
98. Asahina Y, Izumi N, Enomoto N, et al: Increased gene expression of water channel in cirrhotic rat kidneys. Hepatology 21:169–173, 1995.
99. Rabelink TJ, Kaasjager KA, Boer P, et al: Effects of endothelin-1 on renal function in humans: Implications for physiology and pathophysiology. Kidney Int 46:376–381, 1994.
100. Moller S, Gulberg V, Henriksen JH, Gerbes AL: Endothelin-1 and endothelin-3 in cirrhosis: Relations to systemic and splanchnic haemodynamics. J Hepatol 23:135–144, 1995.
101. Ucihara M, Izumi N, Sato C, Marumo F: Clinical significance of elevated plasma endothelin concentrations in patients with cirrhosis. Hepatology 16:95–99, 1992.
102. Moller S, Emmeluth C, Henriksen JH: Elevated circulating plasma endothelin-1 concentrations in cirrhosis. J Hepatol 19:285–290, 1993.
103. Fukunaga M, Yura T, Badr KF: Stimulatory effect of 8-epi-PGF2 alpha, an F2-isoprostane, on endothelin-1 release. J Cardiovasc Pharmacol 26:S51–S52, 1995.
104. Morrow JD, Moore KP, Awad JA, et al: Marked overproduction of non-cyclooxygenase derived prostanoids (F2-isoprostanes) in the hepatorenal syndrome. J Lipid Mediat Cell Signal 6:417–420, 1993.
105. Platt JF, Elis JH, Rubin JM, et al: Renal duplex Doppler ultrasonography: A noninvasive predictor of kidney dysfunction and hepatorenal failure in liver disease. Hepatology 20:362–369, 1994.
106. Caregaro L, Menon F, Angeli P, et al: Limitations of serum creatinine level and creatinine clearance as filtration markers in cirrhosis. Arch Intern Med 154:201–205, 1994.
107. DeSanto NG, Anastasio P, Loguercio C, et al: Creatinine clearance: An inadequate marker of renal filtration in patients with early posthepatic cirrhosis (Child A) without fluid retention and muscle wasting. Nephron 70:421–424, 1995.
108. Amarapurkar DN, Dhawan P, Kalro RH: Role of routine estimation of creatinine clearance in patients with liver cirrhosis. Indian J Gastroenterol 13:79–82, 1994.
109. Maroto A, Gines A, Salo J, et al: Diagnosis of functional kidney failure or cirrhosis with Doppler sonography: Prognostic value of resistive index. Hepatology 20:839–844, 1994.
110. Sacerdoti D, Bolognesi M, Merkel C, et al: Renal vasoconstriction in cirrhosis evaluated by duplex Doppler ultrasonography. Hepatology 17:219–224, 1993.
111. Luca A, Feu F, Garcia-Pagan JC, et al: Favorable effects of total paracentesis on splanchnic hemodynamics in cirrhotic patients with tense ascites. Hepatology 20:30–33, 1994.
112. Mitzner SR, Stange J, Klammt S, et al: Improvement of hepatorenal syndrome with extracorporeal albumin dialysis MARS: Results of a prospective, randomized, controlled clinical trial. Liver Transpl Surg 6:277–286, 2000.
113. Durkin RJ, Winter SM: Reversal of hepatorenal syndrome with the combination of norepinephrine and dopamine. Crit Care Med 23:202–204, 1995.
114. Hadengue A, Gadano A, Moreau R, et al: Beneficial effects of the 2-day administration of terlipressin in patients with cirrhosis and hepatorenal syndrome. J Hepatol 29:565–570, 1998.
115. Guevara M, Gines P, Fernandez-Esparrach G, et al: Reversibility of hepatorenal syndrome by prolonged administration of ornipressin and plasma volume expansion. Hepatology 27:35–41, 1998.
116. Sturgis TM: Hepatorenal syndrome: Resolution after transjugular intrahepatic portosystemic shunt. J Clin Gastroenterol 20:241–243, 1995.
117. Yersin B, Burnier M, Magnenat P: Improvement of renal failure with repeated head-out water immersions in patients with hepatorenal syndrome associated with alcoholic hepatitis. Am J Nephrol 15:260–265, 1995.

118. Keller F, Heinze H, Jochimsen F, et al: Risk factors and outcome of 107 patients with decompensated liver disease and acute renal failure: The role of hemodialysis. Ren Fail 17:135–146, 1995.
119. Madersbacher S, Ludvik G, Stulnig T, et al: The impact of liver transplantation on endocrine status in men. Clin Endocrinol 44:461–466, 1996.
120. Guechot J, Vaubourdolle M, Ballet F, et al: Hepatic uptake of sex steroids in men with alcoholic cirrhosis. Gastroenterology 92:203–207, 1987.
121. Selby O: Sex hormone binding globulin: Origin, function and clinical significance. Ann Clin Biochem 27:532–541, 1990.
122. Oren R, Brill S, Dotan I, Halpern Z: Liver function in cirrhotic patients in the euthyroid versus the hypothyroid state. J Clin Gastroenterol 27(4):339–341, 1998.
123. Kley HK, Stremmel W, Kley JB, Schlaghecke R: Testosterone treatment of men with idiopathic hemochromatosis. Clin Invest Med 70: 566–572, 1992.
124. Kaymakoglu S, Okten A, Cakaloglu Y, et al: Hypogonadism is not related to the etiology of liver cirrhosis. J Gastroenterol 30:745–750, 1995.
125. Wang YJ, Lee SD, Lin HC, et al: Changes in sex hormone levels in patients with hepatitis B vius–related postnecrotic cirrhosis: Relationship to the severity of portal hypertension. J Hepatol 18:101–105, 1993.
126. Maruyama Y, Adachi Y, Aoki N, et al: Mechanism of feminization in male patients with non-alcoholic liver cirrhosis: Role of sex hormone binding globulin. Gastroenterol Jpn 26:435–439, 1991.
127. Handelsman DJ, Strasser S, McDonald JA, et al: Hypothalamic-pituitary-testicular function in end-stage non-alcoholic liver disease before and after liver transplantation. Clin Endocrinol 43:331–337, 1995.
128. Wang YJ, Wu JC, Lee SD, et al: Gonadal dysfunction and changes in sex hormones in postnecrotic cirrhotic men: A matched study with alcoholic cirrhotic men. Hepatogastroenterology 38:531–534, 1991.
129. Vidal J, Ferrer JP, Esmatjes E, et al: Diabetes mellitus in patients with liver cirrhosis. Diabetes Res Clin Pract 25:19–25, 1994.
130. Cavanaugh J, Niewoeher CB, Nuttall FQ: Gynecomastia and cirrhosis of the liver. Arch Intern Med 150:563–565, 1990.
131. Martinex-Riera A, Santolaria-Fernandez F, Gonzalez Riemers E, et al: Alcoholic hypogonadism: Response to clomiphene. Alcohol 12:581–587, 1995.
132. Gluud C: Testosterone and alcoholic cirrhosis. Epidemiologic, pathophysiologic and therapeutic studies in men. Dan Med Bull 35:564–575, 1988.
133. Molitich ME: Pathologic hyperprolactinemia. Endocrinol Metab Clin North Am 21:877–901, 1992.
134. Gavaler JS, Van Thiel DH: Hormonal status of postmenopausal women with alcohol-induced cirrhosis: Further findings and review of the literature. Hepatology 16:312–319, 1992.
135. Bell H, Rakerud N, Falch JA, Haug E: Inappropriately low levels of gonadotrophins in amenorrheic women with alcoholic and non-alcoholic cirrhosis. Eur J Endocrinol 132:444–449, 1995.
136. Gavaler JS: Alcohol effects on hormone levels in normal postmenopausal women and in postmenopausal women with alcohol-induced cirhosis. Recent Dev Alcohol 12:199–208, 1995.
137. De Besi L, Zucchetta P, Zotti S, Mastrogiacomo I: Sex hormones and sex hormone binding globulin in males with compensated and decompensated cirrhosis of the liver. Acta Endocrinol 120:271–276, 1989.
138. Huang MJ, Liaw YF: Clinical associations between thyroid and liver disease. J Gastroenterol Hepatol 10:344–350, 1995.
139. Guven K, Kelestimur F, Yucesoy M: Thyroid function tests in non-alcoholic patients with hepatic encephalopathy. Eur J Med 2:83–85, 1993.
140. Becker U, Gluud C, Bennett P: Thyroid hormones and thyroxine-binding globulin in relation to liver function and serum testosterone in men with alcoholic cirrhosis. Acta Med Scand 224:367–373, 1988.
141. Hegedus L, Rasmussen N, Ravn V, et al: Independent effects of liver disease and chronic alcoholism on thyroid function and size: The possibility of a toxic effect of alcohol on the thyroid gland. Metabolism 37:229–233, 1988.
142. Huang TS, Wu HP, Huang LS, et al: A study of thyroidal response to thyrotropin (TSH) in decompensated liver cirrhosis. Thyroidology 1: 119–125, 1989.
143. Anonymous: Testosterone treatment of men with alcoholic cirrhosis: A double-blind study. The Copenhagen Study Group for Liver Diseases. Hepatology 6:807–813, 1986.
144. Van Thiel DH, Kumar S, Gavaler JS, Tarter RE: Effect of liver transplantation on the hypothalamic-pituitary-gonadal axis of chronic alcoholic men with advanced liver disease. Alcohol Clin Exp Res 14: 478–481, 1990.
145. Plevris JN, Dhariwal A, Elton RA, et al: The platelet count as a predictor of variceal hemorrhage in primary biliary cirrhosis. Am J Gastroenterol 90:959–961, 1995.
146. Violi F, Ferro D, Basili S, et al: Prognostic value of clotting and fibrinolytic systems in a follow-up of 165 liver cirrhotic patients. CALC Group. Hepatology 22:96–100, 1995.
147. Violi F, Ferro D, Basili S, et al: Hyperfibrinolysis increases the risk of gastrointestinal hemorrhage in patients with advanced cirrhosis. Hepatology 15:672–676, 1992.
148. Kamath PS, Wiesner RH, Malinchoc M, et al: A model to predict survival in patients with end-stage liver disease. Hepatology 33:464–470, 2001.
149. Violi F, Leo R, Vezza E, et al: Bleeding time in patients with cirrhosis: Relation with degree of liver failure and clotting abnormalities. C.A.L.C. Group. J Hepatol 20:531–536, 1994.
150. Kajiwara E, Akagi K, Azuma K, et al: Evidence for an immunological basis of thrombocytopenia in chronic liver disease. Am J Gastroenterol 90:962–966, 1995.
151. Aoki Y, Hirai K, Tanikawa K: Mechanism of thrombocytopenia in liver cirrhosis: Kinetics of indium-111 tropolone labelled platelets. Eur J Nucl Med 20:123–129, 1993.
152. Noguchi H, Hirai K, Aoki Y, et al: Changes in platelet kinetics after a partial splenic arterial embolization in cirrhotic patients with hypersplenism. Hepatology 22:1682–1688, 1995.
153. Nagamine T, Ohtuka T, Takehara K, et al: Thrombocytopenia associated with hepatitis C viral infection. J Hepatol 24:135–140, 1996.
154. Laffi G, Marra F, Gresele P, et al: Evidence for a storage pool defect in platelets from cirrhotic patients with defective aggregation. Gastroenterology 103:641–646, 1992.
155. Laffi G, Cinotti S, Filimberti E, et al: Defective aggregation in cirrhosis is independent of in vivo platelet aggregation. J Hepatol 24:436–443, 1996.
156. Sanchez-Roig MJ, Rivera J, Moraleda JM, Garcia VV: Quantitative defect of glycoprotein Ib in severe cirrhotic patients. Am J Hematol 45:10–15, 1994.
157. Laffi G, Marra F, Failli P, et al: Defective signal transduction in platelets from cirrhotics is associated with increased cyclic nucleotides. Gastroenterology 105:148–156, 1993.
158. Beer JH, Clerici N, Baillod P, et al: Quantitative and qualitative analysis of platelet GPIb and von Willebrand factor in liver cirrhosis. Thromb Haemost 73:601–609, 1995.
159. Leiper K, Croll A, Moore NR, et al: Tissue plasminogen activator, plasminogen activator inhibitors, and activator-inhibitor complex in liver disease. J Clin Pathol 47:214–217, 1994.
160. Cimminiello C, Soncini M, Gerosa MC, et al: Lipoprotein a and fibrinolytic system in liver cirrhosis. Coagulation Abnormalities in Liver Cirrhosis (CALC) Study Group. Biomed Pharmacother 49:364–368, 1995.
161. Toschi V, Rocchini GM, Motta A, et al: The hyperfibrinolytic state of liver cirrhosis: Possible pathogenetic role of ascites. Biomed Pharmacother 47:345–352, 1993.
162. Violi F, Ferro D, Basili S, et al: Hyperfibrinolysis resulting from clotting activation in patients with different degrees of cirrhosis. The CALC Group. Hepatology 17:78–83, 1993.
163. Violi F, Ferro D, Basili S, et al: Association between low grade disseminated intravascular coagulation and endotoxemia in patients with liver cirrhosis. Gastroenterology 109:531–539, 1995.
164. Bakker CM, Knot EA, Stibbe J, Wilson JH: Disseminated intravascular coagulation in liver cirrhosis. J Hepatol 15:330–335, 1992.
165. Mammen EF: Coagulation defects in liver disease. Med Clin North Am 78:545–554, 1994.
166. Agnelli G, Parise P, Levi M, et al: Effects of desmopressin on hemostasis in patients with liver cirrhosis. Haemostasis 25:241–247, 1995.
167. Sangro B, Bilbao I, Herrero I, et al: Partial splenic embolization for the treatment of hypersplenism in cirrhosis. Hepatology 18:309–314, 1993.
168. Lawrence SP, Lezotte DC, Durham JD, et al: Course of thrombocytopenia after transjugular intrahepatic portosystemic shunts (TIPS). A retrospective analysis. Dig Dis Sci 40:1575–1580, 1995.
169. Sanyal AJ, Freedman AM, Purdum PP, et al: The hematological consequences of transjugular intrahepatic portosystemic shunts. Hepatology 23:32–39, 1996.

Chapter 80

ACUTE LIVER FAILURE

Hal F. Yee Jr. and Steven D. Lidofsky

Acute liver failure (ALF), also known as fulminant hepatic failure, is a rare manifestation of liver disease and constitutes a medical emergency. The syndrome arises from loss of hepatic parenchyma that may result from a variety of insults to the liver. Despite advances in medical management and the availability of liver transplantation, mortality rates in patients with ALF remain substantial. It has been estimated that in the United States, 2000 deaths a year are attributable to ALF.[1] This chapter reviews the (1) definition, (2) causes, (3) clinical presentation, (4) differential diagnosis, (5) predictors of outcome, and (6) management of ALF.

DEFINITION

ALF has been defined by three criteria: (1) rapid development of hepatocellular dysfunction (e.g., jaundice, coagulopathy), (2) encephalopathy, and (3) absence of a prior history of liver disease. Thus, ALF is a clinical syndrome that represents a final common pathway for a wide variety of diseases that rapidly produce severe liver injury. Such injury is caused most often by hepatocellular necrosis, as with acetaminophen toxicity or viral hepatitis, but it can be the result of massive hepatocellular replacement, as with malignant infiltration. ALF originally was defined by an interval between the onset of illness and appearance of encephalopathy of 8 weeks or less,[2] but there is marked heterogeneity among affected patients with respect to the temporal progression of disease.

The time course of ALF has etiologic, biologic, and prognostic significance. For example, an illness of 1 week or less before the development of encephalopathy is characteristic of ALF caused by hepatic ischemia or acetaminophen toxicity. In contrast, an interval longer than 4 weeks is more likely to be caused by viral hepatitis or ALF of unknown etiology.[3] Patients with a duration of illness longer than 2 weeks before the onset of encephalopathy have a higher likelihood of developing manifestations of portal hypertension, such as ascites or renal failure,[4] whereas patients with a duration of illness of less than 4 weeks have an increased likelihood of developing cerebral edema.[5] Finally, the presence of jaundice for at least 1 week before the onset of encephalopathy is associated with a poor prognosis.[6]

The relationship between the time course of symptoms and the spectrum of complications has led to proposals for more restrictive definitions of ALF. Some investigators have suggested that the term *fulminant hepatic failure* be reserved for cases in which encephalopathy develops within 2 weeks of the onset of jaundice and that the term *subfulminant hepatic failure* be applied to cases in which encephalopathy develops between 2 weeks and 3 months of the onset of jaundice.[7] Others have proposed that ALF be redefined to comprise three distinct syndromes: hyperacute liver failure (onset of encephalopathy within 1 week of jaundice), acute liver failure (development of encephalopathy between 1 and 4 weeks of jaundice), and subacute liver failure (development of encephalopathy within 5 to 12 weeks of jaundice).[3] Unfortunately, there is great overlap in prognosis among patients with varying presentations, regardless of which nomenclature is used. Moreover, no universally accepted nomenclature has yet been adopted. The original definition of ALF (encephalopathy within 8 weeks of the onset of illness) will be used here, because it has been used in most published clinical studies.[2]

CAUSES

The most common causes of ALF are drugs (notably acetaminophen) and hepatotropic viruses (Table 80–1). However, many other conditions can lead to ALF, albeit uncommonly (Table 80–2). Despite serologic and molecular advances in the diagnosis of viral infections, ALF of unknown etiology continues to represent a substantial proportion of the patients affected by this syndrome (see Table 80–1).

Drugs

Most cases of drug-related ALF result from acetaminophen overdose. In fact, acetaminophen is the most common single cause of ALF in many locations (see Table 80–1). Acetaminophen is directly hepatotoxic and predictably produces hepatocellular necrosis with an overdose (>12 g). Because of its easy availability, acetaminophen is a common mode of suicide and, occasionally, a cause of unintentional overdose. Even recommended therapeutic dosages of acetaminophen

Table 80–1 | **Frequencies (%) of Causes of Acute Liver Failure Reported by Several Centers**

CENTER	ETIOLOGY					
	Hepatitis A Virus	Hepatitis B Virus	Acetaminophen Toxicity	Other Drug/Toxin	Other	Cryptogenic*
London (n = 941)[19]	9	9	53	7	5	17
Clichy (n = 330)[7]	4	47	2	15	10	22
Birmingham (n = 73)[78]	0	3	45	5	14	33
Barcelona (n = 62)[33]	2	40	0	8	6	44
San Francisco (n = 60)[52]	8	15	18	15	5	39
Camperdown (n = 22)[79]	0	36	9	14	14	27
Multicenter (USA) (n = 295)[80]	7	10	20	12	36	15
OVERALL (n = 1783)	7	18	34	10	12	19

*Etiology unknown and seronegative for acute infection from hepatitis A or B virus (non-A, non-B hepatitis).

(as low as 4 g) can sometimes result in ALF in patients who are fasting or who chronically use alcohol or drugs that induce cytochrome oxidases.[8, 9] Such "therapeutic misadventures" are a particular problem with over-the-counter remedies that contain acetaminophen as an active ingredient.

Numerous other drugs, including halothane, isoniazid, valproate, sulfonamides, phenytoin, thiazolidinediones, and certain herbal remedies, have been implicated in ALF. In most cases, drug-related ALF is rare and idiosyncratic. Hepatotoxic drugs are discussed further in Chapter 73.

Hepatotropic Viruses

Hepatitis A and hepatitis B viruses are major causes of ALF (see Table 80–1). These viruses are discussed in greater detail in Chapter 68. Infection with hepatitis A virus (HAV) rarely leads to ALF, and when it does, the prognosis is relatively good. Although hepatitis B virus (HBV) is the most common viral cause of ALF (see Table 80–1), ALF is an uncommon manifestation of HBV infection. Infection with hepatitis D virus (HDV) requires coinfection with HBV. In certain geographic regions, HDV can account for almost 5% of the cases of ALF in patients who are positive for hepatitis B surface antigen and approximately 4% of the cases of ALF in patients who are positive for IgM antibody to hepatitis B core antigen.[10]

Table 80–2 | **Uncommon Causes of Acute Liver Failure**

Wilson disease (initial presentation)
Other infections (e.g., Epstein-Barr and herpesviruses, tuberculosis)
Vascular abnormalities (e.g., Budd-Chiari syndrome, hepatic veno-occlusive disease)
Toxins (e.g., *Amanita phalloides* ingestion, sea anenome sting, CCl_4)
Fatty liver of pregnancy
Autoimmune hepatitis (initial presentation)
Malignant infiltration (e.g., lymphoma, melanoma, breast cancer)
Ischemia (e.g., hypotension, heat stroke)
Reye's syndrome
Primary graft nonfunction following liver transplantation

CCl_4, carbon tetrachloride.

Acute Liver Failure of Unknown Etiology

ALF of unknown etiology, defined by negative serologic testing for hepatitis A and B and the absence of other known causes, constitutes 15% to 44% of the total cases of ALF (see Table 80–1). It had been anticipated that new sensitive molecular methods such as the polymerase chain reaction (PCR) would identify a viral etiology for ALF of unknown cause, but most cases remain cryptogenic. For example, occult HBV infection has been identified in the sera or livers of some patients with ALF of unknown etiology by PCR-based assays by some,[11, 12] but not all, investigators.[13, 14] Although hepatitis C virus (HCV) has been implicated as a cause of ALF in a few patients,[15, 16] it appears that HCV is an exceedingly rare cause of ALF in Western countries.[11, 13, 14, 17–19] In Japan, however, HCV may be a more common cause of ALF.[20] Hepatitis E virus (HEV), an acknowledged cause of ALF in central Asia and other parts of the developing world, has not been found to cause ALF in the United States or the European continent.[11–13, 18] Despite the identification of hepatitis G virus (HGV) in patients with ALF of unknown etiology, HGV does not appear to cause ALF.[21]

Several other viruses merit comment. Togavirus-like particles have been identified by electron microscopy in 7 of 18 liver explants from patients who underwent transplantation for ALF[22] but are unlikely to be responsible for a substantial portion of these cryptogenic cases. The TT virus has been found in patients with ALF in the United States and Japan, but it is uncertain whether this virus can cause ALF.[23] Finally, parvovirus B19 has been postulated to be an important cause of ALF, but this postulate remains to be verified.[24] Although these viruses warrant further investigation as causes of ALF, it is doubtful that any of these viral causes will explain the etiology of a significant portion of the cases of cryptogenic ALF.

Historically, ALF of unknown etiology has been attributed to non-A, non-B hepatitis. However, hepatitis C and E must now be ruled out as well. Moreover, despite the expectation that one or more viruses may be discovered to be responsible for most cases of ALF of unknown etiology, it is not clear that cryptogenic ALF necessarily has a viral pathogenesis.

CLINICAL PRESENTATION

The clinical features of ALF may result directly from loss of critical hepatocellular functions (e.g., protein synthesis, intermediary metabolism, and detoxification) and from effects on distant organs. The major complications of ALF, as well as their pathogenesis and medical management, are outlined in Table 80–3. The initial presentation of ALF may include nonspecific complaints such as nausea, vomiting, fatigue, and malaise, but jaundice develops soon after.

Hepatocellular Dysfunction

Hepatocellular injury or loss leads to impaired elimination of bilirubin; depressed synthesis of coagulation factors I, II, V, VII, IX, and X; diminished glucose synthesis; and decreased lactate uptake or increased generation of intracellular lactate as a result of anaerobic glycolysis. These derangements manifest clinically as jaundice, coagulopathy, hypoglycemia, and metabolic acidosis, respectively. Besides portending liver failure, coagulopathy increases the risk of gastrointestinal and intracranial hemorrhage, hypoglycemia can contribute to brain injury, and acidosis can produce cardiovascular dysfunction.

Hepatic Encephalopathy and Cerebral Edema

Encephalopathy is a defining criterion for ALF. The severity of encephalopathy can range from subtle changes in affect, insomnia, and difficulties with concentration (stage 1); to drowsiness, disorientation, and confusion (stage 2); to marked somnolence and incoherence (stage 3); to frank coma (stage 4). The pathophysiologic mechanisms underlying ALF-associated encephalopathy are multifactorial. Many features of ALF, including hypoglycemia, sepsis, hypoxemia, occult seizures, and cerebral edema, can contribute to neurologic abnormalities. Notably, neurologic conditions account for approximately 25% of patients with ALF who are excluded from liver transplantation and for more than 20% of postoperative deaths after liver transplantation.[25]

Continuous monitoring of cerebral activity by electroencephalogram (EEG) identifies subclinical seizures in almost 33% of ALF patients with at least stage 3 encephalopathy who are mechanically ventilated and paralyzed.[26] Cerebral edema is found in up to 80% of patients who die in the setting of ALF and is virtually universal among patients with coma.[27]

Progressive cerebral edema will produce intracranial hy-

Table 80–3 | **Pathogenesis and Medical Management of the Major Complications of ALF**

MAJOR COMPLICATIONS	PATHOGENESIS	MANAGEMENT
Hypoglycemia	Diminished glucose synthesis	Blood glucose monitoring Intravenous glucose administration
Encephalopathy	Cerebral edema	CT scan (if advanced encephalopathy) ICP monitoring (if patient is in coma) Careful positioning of patient Consider osmotherapy (mannitol) or barbiturates
	Other common reversible factors (e.g., hypoglycemia, hypoxemia)	Standard therapy; avoid benzodiazepines and other sedative medications
Sepsis, pneumonia, other organ system infections	Bacterial or fungal infection	Aseptic medical/nursing care Surveillance cultures Antimicrobial agents
Hemorrhage (e.g., gastrointestinal, intracerebral)	Stress ulceration	H_2 receptor antagonists, proton pump inhibitors, nasogastric aspiration
	Coagulopathy	Vitamin K Platelet or fresh-frozen plasma infusions
Hypotension	Hypovolemia	Hemodynamic monitoring of central pressures Volume repletion with blood or colloid
	Decreased vascular resistance	α-Adrenergic agents
Respiratory failure	ARDS	Hemodynamic monitoring of central pressures Mechanical ventilation
Renal failure	Hypovolemia	Hemodynamic monitoring of central pressures Volume repletion with blood or colloid
	Hepatorenal syndrome or acute tubular necrosis	Avoid nephrotoxic agents (e.g., aminoglycosides, aspirin, contrast dye) Hemofiltration/dialysis

ALF, acute liver failure; ARDS, acute respiratory distress syndrome; CT, computed tomography; ICP, intracranial pressure.

pertension, which results in cerebral hypoperfusion and irreversible neurologic damage. The pathogenesis of cerebral edema in ALF is poorly understood. It has been proposed to result from the actions of gut-derived neurotoxins that escape hepatic clearance and are released into the systemic circulation.[27, 28] Two principal mechanisms appear to contribute to the development of cerebral edema in this setting: brain cell swelling (cytotoxic edema) and disruption of the blood-brain barrier (vasogenic edema). In the cerebral tissue of patients who die of ALF, there is swelling in endothelial and astroglial cells, a phenomenon indicative of cytotoxic edema, as well as vacuolization in the basement membranes of capillaries, consistent with disruption of the blood-brain barrier and suggestive of vasogenic edema. Progressive cerebral edema can impair cerebral perfusion, which may lead to irreversible neurologic damage or even result in uncal herniation and death.

Infection

Infections develop in as many as 80% of patients with ALF, and bacteremia is present in 20% to 25%.[29, 30] Uncontrolled infection accounts for approximately 25% of patients with ALF who are excluded from liver transplantation and approximately 40% of postoperative deaths.[25] At least three factors place patients with ALF at increased risk for infection. First, gut-derived microorganisms may enter the systemic circulation from portal venous blood as a result of damage to hepatic macrophages (Kupffer cells). Second, impaired neutrophil function may result from reduced hepatocellular synthesis of acute-phase reactants, such as components of the complement cascade. Third, patients with ALF are often subjected to invasive procedures (e.g., intravascular and urethral catheterization, endotracheal intubation), and physical barriers to infection, including skin and airway, are thus breached. Indeed, the major sites of infection are the respiratory and urinary tracts.[29] It is not surprising therefore that the most common bacteria isolated are staphylococcal and streptococcal species and gram-negative rods.

Fungal infections develop in up to one third of patients with ALF.[31] The majority of these infections are caused by *Candida albicans*. Although *Aspergillus* infections have been thought to be uncommon in the setting of ALF,[31] they may be more prevalent than appreciated previously. Aspergillosis may account for up to one half of fatal infections in the period immediately following liver transplantation for ALF.[32, 33] These infections probably are acquired preoperatively. Risk factors for fungal infections are renal failure and prolonged antibiotic therapy for bacterial infections. Characteristically, fungal infection is associated with fever or leukocytosis refractory to broad-spectrum antibiotics.[31] It is unknown whether the high prevalence of fungal infections among patients with ALF is a result of disturbances in immune function or prolonged antibiotic administration.

Gastrointestinal Bleeding

Patients with ALF have an increased risk of hemorrhage because of deficiencies in coagulation factors and thrombocytopenia. Such critically ill patients thus have a propensity for gastrointestinal stress ulceration and consequent bleeding.[34] In contrast to patients with chronic liver failure, those with ALF rarely exhibit bleeding from varices.

Multiple Organ Failure Syndrome

A potential consequence of ALF is the syndrome of multiple organ failure. This syndrome manifests clinically as peripheral vasodilation with hypotension, pulmonary edema, acute tubular necrosis, and disseminated intravascular coagulation. Liver failure may trigger the microcirculatory derangements that underlie this syndrome by two mechanisms. First, polymerization of actin (released from dying hepatocytes) within the capillary lumen and platelet activation may produce endothelial injury.[35] Second, impaired hepatic clearance may lead to the accumulation of vasoactive substances in the systemic circulation.[36] Multiple organ failure is a significant contributor to patient mortality and a major contraindication to liver transplantation. For example, acute tubular necrosis is associated with a 50% decrease in survival among patients with acetaminophen-induced ALF,[37] and the mortality rate is more than doubled in patients with multiple organ failure.[38]

Hypotension is observed frequently in patients with ALF and can result from decreases in vascular resistance, which often accompany ALF, or intravascular volume depletion related to extravascular third spacing or frank blood loss.

Respiratory failure commonly is associated with ALF. In one series, 37% of patients with ALF had pulmonary edema.[39] In another study, acute respiratory distress syndrome (ARDS) was present in 33% of patients with acetaminophen-associated ALF.[40] Furthermore, ARDS was associated with intracranial hypertension, the requirement for vasopressive agents, and, most important, a higher rate of mortality.

The cause of renal failure in ALF (seen in more than one third of patients in one series)[36] is multifactorial. Hepatorenal syndrome is often difficult to differentiate from intravascular volume depletion, which is also a common finding in ALF. Acute renal tubular acidosis is a prominent component of multiple organ failure syndrome.

DIFFERENTIAL DIAGNOSIS

The diagnosis of ALF is made clinically on the basis of the physical examination (jaundice, altered mental status) and laboratory findings (hyperbilirubinemia, prolonged prothrombin time) that are consistent with hepatic dysfunction, in the absence of a history of liver disease. Infrequently, ALF may be confused with other clinical entities that manifest as jaundice, coagulopathy, and encephalopathy. The differential diagnosis includes sepsis, preeclampsia/eclampsia, and an acute decompensation of chronic liver disease.

In particular, both sepsis and ALF have similar hemodynamic pictures, with decreases in peripheral vascular resistance accompanied by high cardiac output. Encephalopathy, a hallmark of ALF, also may be a manifestation of the sepsis syndrome. If the hepatic manifestations of sepsis are severe, the clinical picture can be mistaken for ALF. In this situation, jaundice and coagulopathy may result from the cholestasis of sepsis and disseminated intravascular coagulation, respectively. Measurement of levels of factor VIII, which is not synthesized by the liver, may be helpful in differentiating sepsis (low factor VIII level) from ALF (factor VIII level generally not suppressed). This differential diagnosis has practical importance in patient management.

In the pregnant patient, preeclampsia/eclampsia also can be difficult to differentiate from ALF, particularly ALF resulting from fatty liver of pregnancy. Differentiating between these two syndromes is of little practical concern, however, because delivery of the fetus is the management of choice in either situation and, if performed early enough, is almost always curative. Moreover, it has been suggested that overlap may exist between preeclampsia/eclampsia syndrome and fatty liver of pregnancy.[41] (See Chapter 74.)

Finally, an acute exacerbation of liver dysfunction in patients with underlying chronic liver disease is occasionally confused with ALF. Examples include alcoholic hepatitis in patients with alcoholic cirrhosis and flares of chronic viral hepatitis.

PREDICTORS OF OUTCOME

Patients with ALF fall into two broad categories: (1) those in whom intensive medical care enables recovery of hepatic function and (2) those who require liver transplantation to survive. Thus, it is critical to determine rapidly the group into which a particular patient may belong. It is also critical to avoid the following two scenarios: (1) death of the patient despite intensive medical care without consideration of transplantation and (2) unnecessary liver transplantation when recovery would have occurred spontaneously. Clinical decision making has been aided by the identification of prognostic markers.

The etiology of disease and clinical presentation have predictive relevance. For example, patients with ALF caused by hepatitis A have a better prognosis than those with ALF of unknown etiology.[37] Patients who reach stage 3 or stage 4 encephalopathy tend to do worse than those who reach only stage 1 or stage 2.[2] However, these indicators do not allow accurate prediction of the need for transplantation.

A number of liver transplantation centers have examined the utility of a variety of predictive criteria to identify high-risk patients for consideration of liver transplantation. The most extensive analysis has been performed by investigators at King's College in London. These investigators performed a multivariate analysis of clinical and biochemical variables and their relation to mortality in 588 patients with ALF.[37] In the analysis, a major distinction was made between patients with acetaminophen toxicity and those with other causes of ALF. The following characteristics were associated with a poor outcome: negative serology for hepatitis A or B, younger (<10 years) or older (>40 years) age, prolonged duration of jaundice, markedly elevated serum bilirubin level, marked prolongation of the prothrombin time, and in patients with acetaminophen toxicity, arterial acidosis, and an elevated serum creatinine level. The significance of these adverse prognostic characteristics was validated prospectively.[37] Among patients with a cause of ALF other than acetaminophen toxicity, the presence of any single adverse prognostic characteristic was associated with a mortality rate of 80%, and the presence of three adverse characteristics was associated with a mortality rate of more than 95%. For patients with acetaminophen-induced liver failure, the presence of any one adverse characteristic was associated with a mortality rate of at least 55%, and severe acidosis was associated with a mortality rate of 95%. These mortality rates vastly exceed those associated with liver transplantation. Thus, the presence of any single indicator of a poor prognosis should prompt serious consideration of placing the patient immediate on a waiting list for liver transplantation. These selection criteria are simple, and acquisition of the necessary data requires only history taking, routine laboratory studies, and serologic testing for hepatitis A and B, all of which can be obtained within 24 hours of hospital admission. Moreover, the utility of these criteria has been confirmed, albeit with slightly lower predictive accuracy, at another center.[42]

A severity scoring system with a comparable predictive value has been devised, but it demands cumbersome arithmetic and has not been validated prospectively.[43] Serum Gc-globulin levels also have been shown to have comparable predictive value to the King's College criteria, but the assay for this protein is technically difficult and not generally available.[44, 45] Liver histology does not predict outcome.[46] Other investigators have examined the prognostic utility of measuring plasma factor V levels[47] and hepatic volumetry,[48] but these parameters do not appear to add significantly to the assessment of outcome.

MANAGEMENT

Historically, the mortality rate associated with ALF was very high, and management consisted of hopeful supportive care. The advent of intensive medical care heralded modest improvements in survival. Although intensive medical care enabled some patients with ALF to survive long enough to allow the liver to regenerate, the majority of patients still died. A wide variety of therapies have been proposed and utilized for the specific treatment of ALF, including glucocorticoids, prostaglandins, and exchange transfusions, but none of these have proved efficacious. Only liver transplantation has permitted salvage of patients with irreversible liver failure. Unfortunately, many patients with irreversible ALF do not undergo transplantation because of contraindications or the unavailability of donor livers. Patients with ALF should be evaluated for liver transplantation as soon as possible and, if no contraindications are found, placed on a liver transplant waiting list. If and when a donor organ becomes available, patients listed for transplantation should be reassessed for the continued need and for contraindications to transplantation. An algorithm depicting the management of ALF is shown in Figure 80–1.

Issues in Medical Management

Initial Evaluation and Management

The initial management of ALF should include an attempt to identify the cause of ALF. A small number of causes of ALF can be treated specifically. For example, acetaminophen toxicity can be treated with *N*-acetylcysteine,[49] and herpes-induced fulminant hepatitis has been reported to respond to intravenous acyclovir.[50] Therapy of ALF caused by fatty liver of pregnancy is emergency delivery. Especially critical

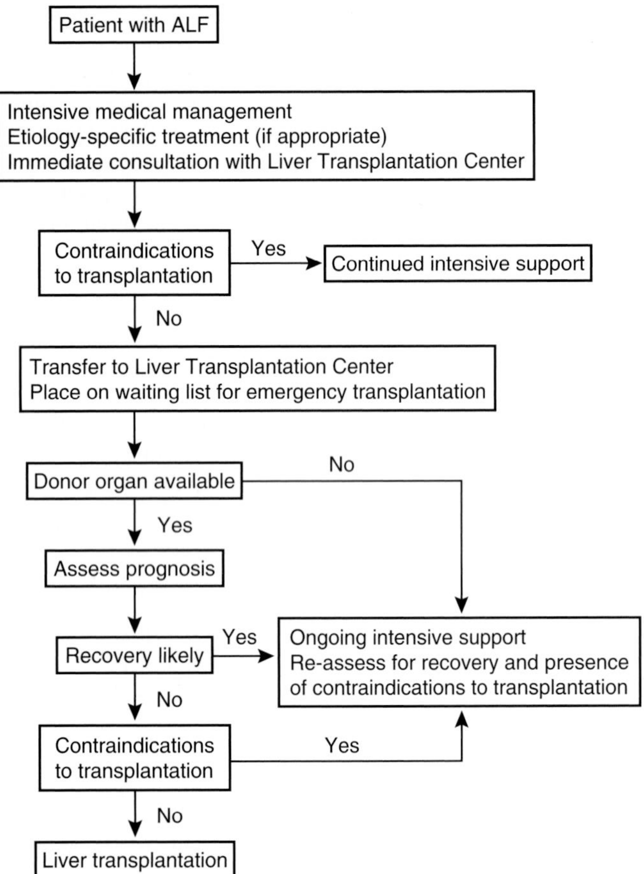

Figure 80–1. Algorithm for the management of acute liver failure (ALF). The initial approach to patient management includes intensive care support and prompt contact with a liver transplantation center. Even if contraindications to liver transplantation are present at the time of admission, urgent patient transfer to a transplantation center may be beneficial in selected circumstances.

in the early evaluation of patients with ALF is the decision regarding the patient's candidacy for liver transplantation. Urgent transfer to a liver transplantation center is advisable for all potential liver transplantation candidates. Rapid clinical deterioration is common in patients with ALF, and transporting the patient may be dangerous later in the course.

Intensive medical care is warranted in all patients with ALF. Initial laboratory studies should include tests to determine the cause (e.g., viral serologic profiles, toxicology screening for acetaminophen and other drugs) and assess the severity of liver failure (e.g., liver biochemical and renal function tests, arterial blood gas measurements).

Coagulopathy

The management of coagulopathy in patients with ALF requires careful consideration. The risk of upper gastrointestinal hemorrhage can be reduced by agents such as intravenous H_2 receptor antagonists.[51] It is likely that proton pump inhibitors have similar effects. Placement of a nasogastric tube to monitor bleeding and gastric pH has been recommended in intubated patients. It is also reasonable to administer a trial of subcutaneous vitamin K to treat coagulopathy possibly related to vitamin K deficiency. The decision to replace clotting factors in nonbleeding patients should be tempered by two issues: first, infusion of agents such as fresh-frozen plasma may normalize the prothrombin time and thereby reduce its accuracy with respect to assessing the patient's prognosis, and second, infusion of plasma can present a significant volume challenge. In patients with renal insufficiency, infusion of plasma can lead to volume overload and respiratory failure. Unless the patient is bleeding or an invasive procedure will be performed, the potential drawbacks of plasma infusions outweigh the potential benefits. Empiric administration of fresh-frozen plasma has not been shown to improve the clinical outcome of patients with ALF.

Hypoglycemia

Hypoglycemia commonly occurs in patients with ALF. It is thus critical to monitor blood glucose levels frequently. Hypoglycemia generally responds to parenteral administration of glucose (e.g., an intravenous bolus of 50% dextrose followed by continuous intravenous infusion of a dextrose solution).

Encephalopathy and Cerebral Edema

Unlike chronic hepatic encephalopathy, the encephalopathy associated with ALF tends to be progressive unless liver failure is reversed. Sedative-hypnotic drugs, which may exacerbate encephalopathy, should be avoided. Lactulose is of no proven benefit. Reversible conditions associated with ALF that could contribute to altered mental status (e.g., hypoglycemia, hypoxemia) must be treated immediately. More difficult to diagnose and treat are subclinical seizures, cerebral edema, and intracranial hypertension.

Patients with profound encephalopathy (i.e., stage 3 and stage 4) should undergo endotracheal intubation and mechanical ventilation for airway protection, particularly before being transported to a liver transplantation center. However, many mechanically ventilated patients are also deeply sedated or paralyzed, and evidence of generalized seizure activity may be concealed. Such seizure activity may worsen encephalopathy. Thus, it may be valuable to monitor deeply sedated or paralyzed patients for subclinical seizures by EEG. Treatment of subclinical seizures with phenytoin or other antiepileptic medications is appropriate, but the efficacy of prophylactic therapy to prevent seizure activity has not been proved.[26]

Intracranial hypertension can be suspected noninvasively or detected directly. Noninvasive modalities such as physical examination and radiologic imaging have important limitations. Impaired pupillary responses, posturing, or seizures, which may suggest the presence of intracranial hypertension, are not sensitive, particularly when sedatives or neuromuscular blocking agents are used in mechanically ventilated patients. Computed tomographic (CT) scanning of the head is valuable for identifying mass lesions, intracranial hemorrhage, and evidence of brainstem herniation. Because these diagnoses may affect clinical decision making, a CT scan of the head should be obtained in all patients with advanced encephalopathy. Nevertheless, the correlation between CT evidence of cerebral edema and measured intracranial pressure (ICP) is imperfect, ranging from 60% to 75%.[52, 53]

ICP monitoring represents the most accurate way to detect intracranial hypertension. However, there are several potential limitations of ICP monitoring. First, placement of an ICP transducer requires correction of underlying coagulopathy (discussed earlier). Second, the ICP transducer represents a potential portal of entry for infectious organisms. Third, placement of the transducer can precipitate intracranial hemorrhage, which can be fatal. The frequency of significant complications ranges from 4% to 20%.[54] If ICP monitoring is contemplated, the transducer should be inserted at an experienced transplantation center.

Elevation of the head of the bed (and avoidance of the head-down position) is a simple measure to reduce ICP. If this maneuver fails, specific treatment is required. Osmotherapy and barbiturates are two options for treating intracranial hypertension. Osmotherapy with mannitol requires preserved renal function (or hemofiltration) and is effective in controlling intracranial hypertension in approximately 60% of cases.[55] Uncontrolled data support the intravenous use of the barbiturate thiopental; its efficacy is similar to that of mannitol.[56] Thiopental has two relative advantages: its onset of action is rapid, and its use does not require preserved renal function. Potential drawbacks of thiopental are hypotension and, more importantly, masking of clinical indicators of neurologic recovery or deterioration. In general, it is reasonable to use mannitol as first-line therapy and to reserve barbiturates for patients with renal insufficiency or refractory intracranial hypertension. Glucocorticoids are of no benefit.[55]

Infection

Clinical recognition of infection may be difficult, because signs such as hypothermia, hypotension, leukocytosis, and acidosis may reflect the underlying liver failure. For these reasons, surveillance cultures in patients with ALF are extremely helpful. The advisability of prophylactic antibiotics in the setting of ALF is debatable. On one hand, prophylactic antibiotics may offset the development of infections that limit the applicability of liver transplantation. On the other hand, they may increase the risk of superinfection with resistant bacteria or fungi. This issue has been addressed in a small randomized trial.[57] Patients treated with prophylactic intravenous cefuroxime had a significant reduction in the rate of documented infections (from 61% to 32%) compared with those treated conservatively, and a modest (but statistically insignificant) increase in the rate of survival (from 45% to 67%). Enteral decontamination does not appear to alter the clinical outcome of patients with ALF who receive systemic prophylactic antimicrobials.[58] The utility of systemic prophylactic antibiotics warrants further investigation. In the interim, a high level of suspicion for infection should be maintained in patients with ALF, as should a low threshold for administering antibiotics. If infection is suspected, the choice of antibiotics should be based on the spectrum of likely bacterial pathogens (e.g., *Staphylococcus*, gram-negative aerobes) and local hospital microbial sensitivities. A reasonable empiric regimen is vancomycin and a third-generation cephalosporin.

Multiple Organ Failure Syndrome

The fundamental goals of management of multiple organ failure syndrome in patients with liver failure are similar to those in patients with other causes of multiple organ failure: to optimize arterial pressure and tissue oxygenation. Ideally, the mean arterial pressure (MAP) should be maintained above 60 mm Hg. If the MAP falls below this value, cerebral perfusion can drop precipitously.[59] Hemodynamic monitoring with a central venous or pulmonary arterial catheter may be useful for deducing the patient's intravascular volume status. Hypotension resulting from intravascular volume depletion should be corrected with blood or colloids. If hypotension is caused by reduced vascular resistance, administration of α-adrenergic agonists may be useful. Although pressors can be used to maintain MAP within a physiologic range, they have the potential to further impair tissue oxygenation.[60] In small, short-term studies, *N*-acetylcysteine and prostacyclin, which have been proposed to reverse microcirculatory derangements, have been shown to improve tissue oxygenation without adverse effects on hemodynamics.[60, 61] The impact of these agents on overall patient outcome has not yet been investigated.

Endotracheal intubation and mechanical ventilation frequently are necessary for patients with ALF. Hypoxemia can result from respiratory depression caused by coma or impaired gas exchange caused by ARDS or superimposed pneumonia. Endotracheal surveillance cultures are thus useful (see previous section).

If renal failure is present, a major practical issue in management is whether the renal failure is caused by intravascular volume depletion (and is readily reversible) or other causes, such as acute tubular necrosis or hepatorenal syndrome. Nephrotoxic drugs, especially aminoglycosides and nonsteroidal anti-inflammatory agents, must be avoided, and care must be taken when contrast dye is used. Measurement of central venous (or pulmonary capillary wedge) pressure provides a direct guide to fluid therapy. Patients with ALF tolerate volume overload poorly, in light of their propensity to develop ARDS. Early measurement of central venous or pulmonary arterial pressure in oliguric patients is preferable to empiric administration of fluid boluses. If oliguria persists in the face of adequate central filling pressures, continuous arteriovenous hemofiltration should be initiated. Continuous arteriovenous hemofiltration has been shown to be superior to intermittent machine hemofiltration with regard to hemodynamic stability and tissue oxygen delivery in oliguric patients with ALF.[62]

Liver Transplantation

Liver transplantation has transformed the management of patients with ALF and is discussed in greater detail in Chapter 83. Before the era of liver transplantation, fewer than one half of patients with ALF survived. In contrast, survival rates for patients with ALF who undergo liver transplantation have been substantially higher, with an overall rate of 63% for all transplants performed for ALF in the United States between 1987 and 1991,[63] and greater than 70% when the results of several major transplantation centers are considered (Table 80–4). The decision to transplant a patient with ALF must balance the likelihood of spontaneous recovery with the risks of surgery and long-term immunosuppression. Furthermore, contraindications to transplantation, particularly irreversible brain damage, active extrahepatic infection, or multiple organ failure syndrome, must be considered. In some countries, where cadaveric livers are not

Table 80–4 | **Results of Liver Transplantation for Acute Liver Failure**

CENTER	NUMBER OF PATIENTS	STUDY PERIOD	SURVIVAL (%)
Pittsburgh[81]	42	1980–1987	59
Cambridge[6]	33	1982–1988	70
San Francisco[52]	28	1988–1991	89
Barcelona[33]	28	1988–1992	69
Berlin[82]	26	1988–1994	89
Omaha[83]	24	1986–1988	58
Chicago[84]	19	1984–1988	58
Toronto[85]	18	1986–1988	72
Philadelphia[86]	18	1985–1990	65
Villejuif[87]	17	1986–1987	71
Birmingham[78]	16	1984–1987	55
USA (multicenter)[80]	121	1994–1996	76
OVERALL	390		71

readily available for transplantation, living-related liver transplantation is performed with success.[64, 65] Although recent changes in the rules governing donor liver allocation have shortened waiting times for patients with ALF in the United States, the decision to place a patient on the waiting list for transplantation must still be made promptly, because a delay increases the likelihood that complications such as infection, multiple organ failure, and intracranial hypertension will develop. These complications can preclude liver transplantation, thereby virtually assuring death of the patient.

Experimental Therapy

Recent advances in the therapy of ALF have been limited. Treatment strategies, such as charcoal hemoperfusion and administration of prostaglandin E_1, which showed early promise, have not been shown to be superior to standard care when analyzed in randomized studies.[66, 67] Plasmapheresis and hepatectomy have been suggested as possible "bridging" mechanisms to liver transplantation, but prospective trials have yet to be performed.[68, 69] Four additional forms of therapy may provide a bridge to liver transplantation or to regeneration of the native liver with spontaneous recovery: auxiliary liver transplantation, bioartificial liver devices, nonhuman liver transplantation, and hepatocyte transplantation.

Auxiliary liver transplantation as a temporary bridge to spontaneous recovery from ALF has been investigated by a number of centers.[70, 71] In this procedure, the donor graft is implanted orthotopically beside the native liver (after it has been surgically reduced) or heterotopically inferior to the native liver. The advantage of this procedure is that if spontaneous recovery of the native liver occurs, then immunosuppression can be stopped. The allograft can then be removed or permitted to atrophy. However, the utility of this operation is limited by the difficulty of predicting which patients with ALF are likely to recover spontaneously. Although early results are promising, the benefits of this procedure remain to be shown.

Extracorporeal liver support devices fall into two broad categories: hemodiadsorption systems and bioartificial livers.[72] Hemodiadsorption systems employ hemodialysis in combination with perfusion of the patient's plasma through a series of hollow fiber filters impregnated with charcoal, resins, and albumin, respectively. Although these devices may remove circulating toxins, they do not replace other liver functions. At this time, published information about the efficacy of these systems in ALF is quite limited.

Bioartificial liver devices contain liver cells grown within specialized hollow fiber cartridges through which the patient's plasma is perfused. The success of such devices depends largely on the mass of cells they contain, the extent to which these cells maintain liver-specific functions, and the duration that these functions are maintained. Because the devices under current clinical investigation contain only hepatocytes, derangements attributable to hepatocyte injury are corrected, but those originating from injured nonparenchymal cells, such as Kupffer cells and biliary epithelia, are not. The published experience with such devices in patients with ALF is limited. Although case reports and small series suggest that bioartificial liver systems may improve encephalopathy and coagulopathy in patients with ALF,[73] a survival benefit has not yet been demonstrated objectively. Determination of the ultimate utility of these devices awaits the results of controlled clinical trials.

Transplantation of nonhuman livers (i.e., xenotransplantation) has been proposed as a solution to the shortage of human donor livers. If major problems with trans-species rejection can be solved, xenotransplantation, particularly utilizing porcine or nonhuman primate livers, offers the potential for developing a renewable source of donor livers. In the meantime, xenotransplantation has been suggested as a means to support patients with ALF until a human donor liver becomes available. In some case reports, porcine livers were used for extracorporeal perfusion or heterotopic transplantation to treat patients with ALF until human livers became available for transplantation.[74, 75] Controlled studies remain to be conducted.

Hepatocyte transplantation represents an alternative approach. Its utility is likely to be similar to that of the bioartificial liver devices just described, that is, as a bridge to liver transplantation or regeneration. Preliminary reports suggest that hepatocyte transplantation may be useful in patients with ALF.[76, 77] However, further study is necessary.

REFERENCES

1. Hoofnagle JH, Carithers RL Jr, Shapiro C, et al: Fulminant hepatic failure: Summary of a workshop. Hepatology 21:240, 1995.
2. Trey C, Davidson C: The management of fulminant hepatic failure. Prog Liver Dis 3:292, 1970.
3. O'Grady JG, Schalm SW, Williams R: Acute liver failure: Redefining the syndromes. Lancet 342:273, 1993.
4. Dhiman RK, Makharia GK, Jain S, et al: Ascites and spontaneous bacterial peritonitis in fulminant hepatic failure. Am J Gastroenterol 95: 233, 2000.
5. Gimson AE, O'Grady J, Ede RJ, et al: Late-onset hepatic failure: Clinical, serological and histological features. Hepatology 6:288, 1986.
6. O'Grady JG, Alexander GJ, Thick M, et al: Outcome of orthotopic liver transplantation in the aetiological and clinical variants of acute liver failure. Q J Med 68:817, 1988.
7. Bernuau J, Rueff B, Benhamou JP: Fulminant and subfulminant liver failure: Definitions and causes. Semin Liver Dis 6:97, 1986.
8. Makin AJ, Wendon J, Williams R: A 7-year experience of severe acetaminophen-induced hepatotoxicity (1987–1993). Gastroenterology 109:1907, 1995.
9. Whitcomb DC, Block GD: Association of acetaminophen hepatotoxicity with fasting and ethanol use. JAMA 272:1845, 1994.

10. Feray C, Chitnis DS, Artwani KK, et al: Prevalence of anti-delta antibodies in central India. Trop Gastroenterol 20:29, 1999.
11. Feray C, Gigou M, Samuel D, et al: Hepatitis C virus RNA and hepatitis B virus DNA in serum and liver of patients with fulminant hepatitis. Gastroenterology 104:549, 1993.
12. Wright TL, Mamish D, Combs C, et al: Hepatitis B virus and apparent fulminant non-A, non-B hepatitis. Lancet 339:952, 1992.
13. Kuwada SK, Patel VM, Hollinger FB, et al: Non-A, non-B fulminant hepatitis is also non-E and non-C. Am J Gastroenterol 89:57, 1994.
14. Theilmann L, Solbach C, Toex U, et al: Role of hepatitis C virus infection in German patients with fulminant and subacute hepatic failure. Eur J Clin Invest 22:569, 1992.
15. Farci P, Alter HJ, Shimoda A, et al: Hepatitis C virus–associated fulminant hepatic failure. N Engl J Med 335:631, 1996.
16. Villamil FG, Hu KQ, Yu CH, et al: Detection of hepatitis C virus with RNA polymerase chain reaction in fulminant hepatic failure. Hepatology 22:1379, 1995.
17. Wright TL, Hsu H, Donegan E, et al: Hepatitis C virus not found in fulminant non-A, non-B hepatitis. Ann Intern Med 115:111, 1991.
18. Liang TJ, Jeffers L, Reddy RK, et al: Fulminant or subfulminant non-A, non-B viral hepatitis: The role of hepatitis C and E viruses. Gastroenterology 104:556, 1993.
19. Sallie R, Silva AE, Purdy M, et al: Hepatitis C and E in non-A non-B fulminant hepatic failure: A polymerase chain reaction and serological study. J Hepatol 20:580, 1994.
20. Yoshiba M, Dehara K, Inoue K, et al: Contribution of hepatitis C virus to non-A, non-B fulminant hepatitis in Japan. Hepatology 19:829, 1994.
21. Hadziyannis SJ: Fulminant hepatitis and the new G/GBV-C flavivirus. J Viral Hepat 5:15, 1998.
22. Fagan EA, Ellis DS, Tovey GM, et al: Toga virus–like particles in acute liver failure attributed to sporadic non-A, non-B hepatitis and recurrence after liver transplantation. J Med Virol 38:71, 1992.
23. Charlton M, Adjei P, Poterucha J, et al: TT-virus infection in North American blood donors, patients with fulminant hepatic failure, and cryptogenic cirrhosis. Hepatology 28:839, 1998.
24. Karetnyi YV, Beck PR, Markin RS, et al: Human parvovirus B19 infection in acute fulminant liver failure. Arch Virol 144:1713, 1999.
25. Lidofsky SD: Fulminant hepatic failure. Crit Care Clin 11:415, 1995.
26. Ellis AJ, Wendon JA, Williams R: Subclinical seizure activity and prophylactic phenytoin infusion in acute liver failure: A controlled clinical trial. Hepatology 32:536, 2000.
27. Ede RJ, Williams RW: Hepatic encephalopathy and cerebral edema. Semin Liver Dis 6:107, 1986.
28. Blei AT, Larsen FS: Pathophysiology of cerebral edema in fulminant hepatic failure. J Hepatol 31:771, 1999.
29. Rolando N, Harvey F, Brahm J, et al: Prospective study of bacterial infection in acute liver failure: An analysis of fifty patients. Hepatology 11:49, 1990.
30. Wyke RJ, Canalese JC, Gimson AE, et al: Bacteraemia in patients with fulminant hepatic failure. Liver 2:45, 1982.
31. Rolando N, Harvey F, Brahm J, et al: Fungal infection: A common, unrecognised complication of acute liver failure. J Hepatol 12:1, 1991.
32. Rakela J, Perkins JD, Gross JB Jr, et al: Acute hepatic failure: The emerging role of orthotopic liver transplantation. Mayo Clin Proc 64: 424, 1989.
33. Castells A, Salmeron JM, Navasa M, et al: Liver transplantation for acute liver failure: Analysis of applicability. Gastroenterology 105:532, 1993.
34. Cook DJ, Fuller HD, Guyatt GH, et al: Risk factors for gastrointestinal bleeding in critically ill patients. Canadian Critical Care Trials Group. N Engl J Med 330:377, 1994.
35. Lee WM, Galbraith RM: The extracellular actin-scavenger system and actin toxicity. N Engl J Med 326:1335, 1992.
36. Bihari DJ, Gimson AE, Williams R: Cardiovascular, pulmonary and renal complications of fulminant hepatic failure. Semin Liver Dis 6: 119, 1986.
37. O'Grady JG, Alexander GJ, Hayllar KM, et al: Early indicators of prognosis in fulminant hepatic failure. Gastroenterology 97:439, 1989.
38. Pitre J, Soubrane O, Dousset B, et al: How valid is emergency liver transplantation for acute liver necrosis in patients with multiple-organ failure? Liver Transpl Surg 2:1, 1996.
39. Trewby PN, Warren R, Contini S, et al: Incidence and pathophysiology of pulmonary edema in fulminant hepatic failure. Gastroenterology 74: 859, 1978.
40. Baudouin SV, Howdle P, O'Grady JG, et al: Acute lung injury in fulminant hepatic failure following paracetamol poisoning. Thorax 50: 399, 1995.
41. Sibai BM, Kustermann L, Velasco J: Current understanding of severe preeclampsia, pregnancy-associated hemolytic uremic syndrome, thrombotic thrombocytopenic purpura, hemolysis, elevated liver enzymes, and low platelet syndrome, and postpartum acute renal failure: Different clinical syndromes or just different names? Curr Opin Nephrol Hypertens 3:436, 1994.
42. Anand AC, Nightingale P, Neuberger JM: Early indicators of prognosis in fulminant hepatic failure: An assessment of the King's criteria. J Hepatol 26:62, 1997.
43. Takahashi Y, Kumada H, Shimizu M, et al: A multicenter study on the prognosis of fulminant viral hepatitis: Early prediction for liver transplantation. Hepatology 19:1065, 1994.
44. Lee WM, Galbraith RM, Watt GH, et al: Predicting survival in fulminant hepatic failure using serum Gc protein concentrations. Hepatology 21:101, 1995.
45. Schiodt FV, Bondesen S, Petersen I, et al: Admission levels of serum Gc-globulin: Predictive value in fulminant hepatic failure. Hepatology 23:713, 1996.
46. Hanau C, Munoz SJ, Rubin R: Histopathological heterogeneity in fulminant hepatic failure. Hepatology 21:345, 1995.
47. Pauwels A, Mostefa-Kara N, Florent C, et al: Emergency liver transplantation for acute liver failure. Evaluation of London and Clichy criteria. J Hepatol 17:124, 1993.
48. Sekiyama K, Yoshiba M, Inoue K, et al: Prognostic value of hepatic volumetry in fulminant hepatic failure. Dig Dis Sci 39:240, 1994.
49. Harrison PM, Keays R, Bray GP, et al: Improved outcome of paracetamol-induced fulminant hepatic failure by late administration of acetylcysteine. Lancet 335:1572, 1990.
50. Klein NA, Mabie WC, Shaver DC, et al: Herpes simplex virus hepatitis in pregnancy. Two patients successfully treated with acyclovir. Gastroenterology 100:239, 1991.
51. Martin LF, Booth FV, Karlstadt RG, et al: Continuous intravenous cimetidine decreases stress-related upper gastrointestinal hemorrhage without promoting pneumonia. Crit Care Med 21:19, 1993.
52. Lidofsky SD, Bass NM, Prager MC, et al: Intracranial pressure monitoring and liver transplantation for fulminant hepatic failure. Hepatology 16:1, 1992.
53. Muñoz SJ, Robinson M, Northrup B, et al: Elevated intracranial pressure and computed tomography of the brain in fulminant hepatocellular failure. Hepatology 13:209, 1991.
54. Blei AT, Olafsson S, Webster S, et al: Complications of intracranial pressure monitoring in fulminant hepatic failure. Lancet 341:157, 1993.
55. Canalese J, Gimson AE, Davis C, et al: Controlled trial of dexamethasone and mannitol for the cerebral oedema of fulminant hepatic failure. Gut 23:625, 1982.
56. Forbes A, Alexander GJ, O'Grady JG, et al: Thiopental infusion in the treatment of intracranial hypertension complicating fulminant hepatic failure. Hepatology 10:306, 1989.
57. Rolando N, Gimson A, Wade J, et al: Prospective controlled trial of selective parenteral and enteral antimicrobial regimen in fulminant liver failure. Hepatology 17:196, 1993.
58. Rolando N, Wade JJ, Stangou A, et al: Prospective study comparing the efficacy of prophylactic parenteral antimicrobials, with or without enteral decontamination, in patients with acute liver failure. Liver Transpl Surg 2:8, 1996.
59. Muñoz SJ, Moritz MJ, Martin P, et al: Relationship between cerebral perfusion pressure and systemic hemodynamics in fulminant hepatic failure. Transplant Proc 25:1776, 1993.
60. Wendon JA, Harrison PM, Keays R, et al: Effects of vasopressor agents and epoprostenol on systemic hemodynamics and oxygen transport in fulminant hepatic failure. Hepatology 15:1067, 1992.
61. Harrison PM, Wendon JA, Gimson AE, et al: Improvement by acetylcysteine of hemodynamics and oxygen transport in fulminant hepatic failure. N Engl J Med 324:1852, 1991.
62. Davenport A, Will EJ, Davidson AM: Improved cardiovascular stability during continuous modes of renal replacement therapy in critically ill patients with acute hepatic and renal failure. Crit Care Med 21:328, 1993.
63. Detre K, Belle S, Beringer K, et al: Liver transplantation for fulminant hepatic failure in the United States: October 1987 through December 1991. Clin Transplant 8:274, 1994.
64. Uemoto S, Inomata Y, Sakurai T, et al: Living donor liver transplantation for fulminant hepatic failure. Transplantation 70:152, 2000.
65. Miwa S, Hashikura Y, Mita A, et al: Living-related liver transplantation for patients with fulminant and subfulminant hepatic failure. Hepatology 30:1521, 1999.
66. O'Grady JG, Gimson AE, O'Brien CJ, et al: Controlled trials of char-

coal hemoperfusion and prognostic factors in fulminant hepatic failure. Gastroenterology 94:1186, 1988.
67. Sterling RK, Luketic VA, Sanyal AJ, et al: Treatment of fulminant hepatic failure with intravenous prostaglandin E_1. Liver Transpl Surg 4: 424, 1998.
68. Larsen FS, Hansen BA, Jorgensen LG, et al: High-volume plasmapheresis and acute liver transplantation in fulminant hepatic failure. Transplant Proc 26:1788, 1994.
69. Ejlersen E, Larsen FS, Pott F, et al: Hepatectomy corrects cerebral hyperperfusion in fulminant hepatic failure. Transplant Proc 26:1794, 1994.
70. Sudan DL, Shaw BW Jr, Fox IJ, et al: Long-term follow-up of auxiliary orthotopic liver transplantation for the treatment of fulminant hepatic failure. Surgery 122:771, 1997.
71. van Hoek B, de Boer J, Boudjema K, et al: Auxiliary versus orthotopic liver transplantation for acute liver failure. EURALT Study Group. European Auxiliary Liver Transplant Registry. J Hepatol 30:699, 1999.
72. Stockmann HB, Hiemstra CA, Marquet RL, et al: Extracorporeal perfusion for the treatment of acute liver failure. Ann Surg 231:460, 2000.
73. Watanabe FD, Shackleton CR, Cohen SM, et al: Treatment of acetaminophen-induced fulminant hepatic failure with a bioartificial liver. Transplant Proc 29:487, 1997.
74. Makowka L, Cramer DV, Hoffman A, et al: The use of a pig liver xenograft for temporary support of a patient with fulminant hepatic failure. Transplantation 59:1654, 1995.
75. Chari RS, Collins BH, Magee JC, et al: Brief report: Treatment of hepatic failure with ex vivo pig-liver perfusion followed by liver transplantation. N Engl J Med 331:234, 1994.
76. Habibullah CM, Syed IH, Qamar A, et al: Human fetal hepatocyte transplantation in patients with fulminant hepatic failure. Transplantation 58:951, 1994.
77. Mito M, Kusano M, Kawaura Y: Hepatocyte transplantation in man. Transplant Proc 24:3052, 1992.
78. Vickers C, Neuberger J, Buckels J, et al: Transplantation of the liver in adults and children with fulminant hepatic failure. J Hepatol 7:143, 1988.
79. Sheil AG, McCaughan GW, Isai HI, et al: Acute and subacute fulminant hepatic failure: The role of liver transplantation. Med J Aust 154: 724, 1991.
80. Schiodt F, Atillasoy E, Shakil A, et al: Etiology and outcome for 295 patients with acute liver failure in the United States. Liver Transpl Surg 5:29, 1999.
81. Iwatsuki S, Stieber AC, Marsh JW, et al: Liver transplantation for fulminant hepatic failure. Transplant Proc 21:2431, 1989.
82. Raakow R, Blumhardt G, Bechstein WO, et al: Liver transplantation for fulminant hepatic failure caused by viral infections. Transplant Proc 26: 3606, 1994.
83. Schafer DF, Shaw BW Jr: Fulminant hepatic failure and orthotopic liver transplantation. Semin Liver Dis 9:189, 1989.
84. Emond JC, Aran PP, Whitington PF, et al: Liver transplantation in the management of fulminant hepatic failure. Gastroenterology 96:1583, 1989.
85. Gallinger S, Greig PD, Levy G, et al: Liver transplantation for acute and subacute fulminant hepatic failure. Transplant Proc 21:2435, 1989.
86. Muñoz SJ, Moritz MJ, Martin P, et al: Liver transplantation for fulminant hepatocellular failure. Transplant Proc 25:1773, 1993.
87. Bismuth H, Samuel D, Gugenheim J, et al: Emergency liver transplantation for fulminant hepatitis. Ann Intern Med 107:337, 1987.

HEPATIC TUMORS AND CYSTS

Chapter 81

Michael C. Kew

Mass lesions of the liver occur sufficiently often that clinicians interested in liver disease should have a thorough understanding of their presentations, diagnosis, and treatment. Hepatic mass lesions include tumors, tumor-like lesions, abscesses, cysts, hematomas, and confluent granulomas. The frequency with which each is seen varies appreciably in different geographic regions and different population groups. The more common hepatic tumors and cysts and those important for other reasons are reviewed in this chapter.

HEPATIC TUMORS

Hepatic tumors may either originate in the liver—from hepatocytes, bile duct epithelium, or mesenchymal tissue—or spread to the liver from primary lesions in remote or adjacent organs.

In adults in most parts of the world, hepatic metastases are more common than primary malignant tumors of the liver, although the converse is true in sub-Saharan Africa and parts of the Far East. In children, primary malignant tumors outnumber both metastases and benign tumors of the liver. Except for cavernous hemangiomas, benign hepatic tumors are rare in all geographic regions and in all age groups.

Primary Malignant Tumors

Hepatocellular Carcinoma

Incidence and Geographic Distribution

Hepatocellular carcinoma is the most common primary malignant tumor of the liver. It is the fifth most common cancer in men and the eighth in women.[1, 2] Information on incidence derived from a limited number of cancer registries makes it possible to classify countries into broad risk categories only. Moreover, in developing countries, especially in Africa, hepatocellular carcinoma is likely to be underdiagnosed and underreported, in some instances by as much as 50%. Despite these sources of inaccuracy, it is evident that hepatocellular carcinoma has an unusual geographic distribution (Fig. 81–1).[1, 2] The tumor is not necessarily uniformly common throughout countries with a high incidence, such as China[3] and Mozambique.[4] The incidence of hepatocellular carcinoma has increased considerably in Japan during the past 3 decades,[5] and lesser increases have been recorded in a number of European countries, parts of North America, and Israel, India, and Puerto Rico.[1, 2] Some of the lesser increases may be apparent rather than real, because of changes in the composition of the population over time or an increase in the reliability of diagnosis.

Migrants from countries with a low incidence of hepatocellular carcinoma to those with a high incidence usually retain the low risk of their country of origin, even after several generations in the new environment.[2] The consequences for migrants from countries with a high incidence to those with a low incidence differ, depending on the major risk factors for the tumor in their country of origin and on whether chronic hepatitis B virus infection, if this is the major risk factor, is acquired predominantly by the perinatal or horizontal route.[2, 6, 7]

Sex Distribution

Men are generally more susceptible than women to hepatocellular carcinoma. Male predominance is, however, more obvious in populations at high risk of the tumor (mean ratio 3.7 : 1.0) than in those at low or intermediate risk (2.4 : 1.0).[1, 2] In industrialized countries, patients with hepatocellular carcinoma in the absence of cirrhosis have an approximately equal sex distribution.

Age Distribution

The incidence of hepatocellular carcinoma increases progressively with advancing age in all populations, although it tends to level off in the oldest age groups.[1, 2] However, in ethnic Chinese and even more in black African populations, the mean age is definitely younger. This phenomenon is most striking in Mozambique, where more than 50% of Shangaan men with hepatocellular carcinoma are younger than 30 years of age, and their mean age is 33 years.[8] Hepatocellular carcinoma is rare in children.[9]

Clinical Presentation

When far advanced, hepatocellular carcinoma generally presents with typical symptoms and physical signs, and diagnosis is easy. Before this late stage is reached, however, clinical recognition is often difficult for a number of reasons.

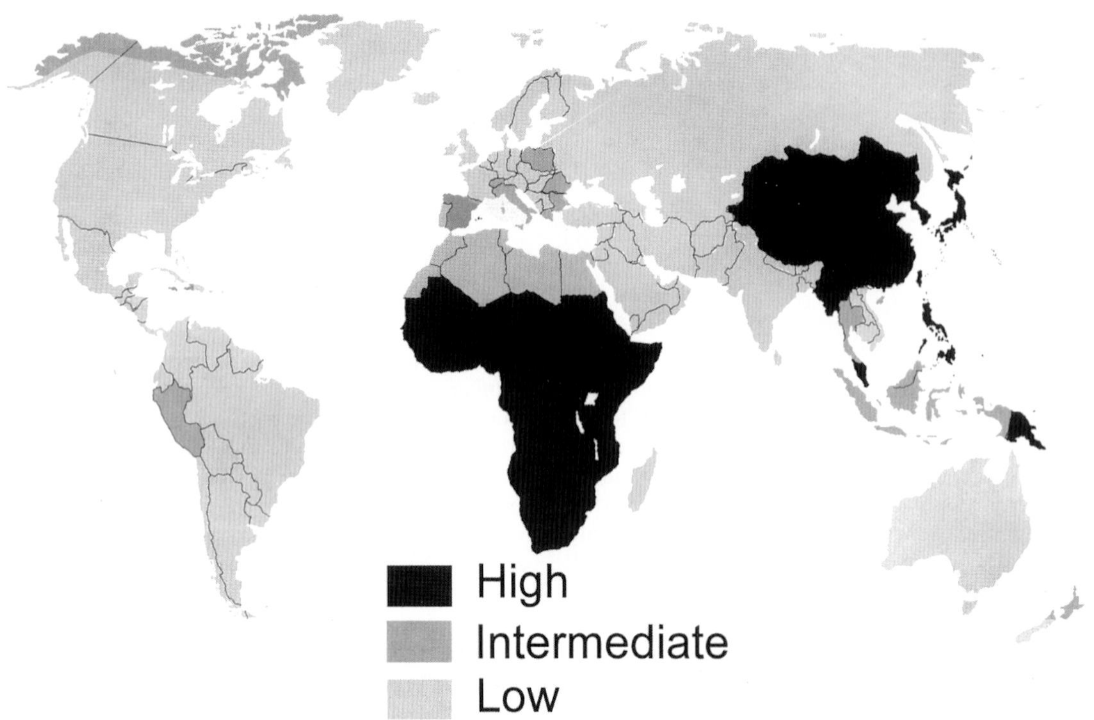

Figure 81–1. Incidence of hepatocellular carcinoma in different parts of the world. Key: High, age-adjusted rate of more than 15 per 100,000 of the population per annum; intermediate, age-adjusted rate of 5–15 per 100,000 of the population per annum; low, age-adjusted rate of fewer than 5 per 100,000 of the population per annum.

The liver is relatively inaccessible to the examining hand, and its large size dictates that the tumor must reach a substantial size before it can be felt or before it invades adjacent structures. The functional reserve of the liver is such that jaundice and other evidence of hepatic dysfunction do not appear until a large part of the organ has been replaced by tumor. The ease of recognizing hepatocellular carcinoma clinically also differs among geographic regions. In countries where the tumor is common, clinicians are especially mindful of hepatocellular carcinoma and its many and diverse presentations. Consequently, they recognize the tumor more readily than do clinicians in countries where hepatocellular carcinoma is rare. Moreover, hepatocellular carcinoma often coexists with cirrhosis,[10] and this association influences diagnosis differently in regions with a high or a low (or an intermediate) incidence of the tumor. In regions of low incidence (but also in Japan, a country of high incidence), hepatocellular carcinoma commonly develops as a complication of long-standing *symptomatic* cirrhosis, and the patient has few, if any, symptoms attributable to the tumor.[10] If, in addition, the tumor is small (as it often is in a cirrhotic liver), it may not be obvious in the presence of advanced cirrhosis. One circumstance that should alert the clinician to the possibility that hepatocellular carcinoma has supervened in a cirrhotic liver is a sudden unexplained change in the patient's condition: he or she may complain of abdominal pain or weight loss; ascites may worsen or become more difficult to treat or blood-stained; the liver may enlarge rapidly or develop a bruit; or hepatic failure may ensue. In contrast, in populations at high risk of hepatocellular carcinoma, the symptoms, if any, of the coexisting cirrhosis are overshadowed by those of the tumor. Hepatocellular carcinomas are generally considerably larger in these populations, and their symptoms and signs are, accordingly, more florid, thereby facilitating diagnosis.[11]

SYMPTOMS. Patients with hepatocellular carcinoma are often unaware of its presence until the tumor has reached an advanced stage. Black Africans, in particular, seek treatment late in the illness.[11, 12] The most common—and frequently the first—symptom is right hypochondrial or epigastric pain (Table 81–1). Although sometimes severe, the pain is usually a dull continuous ache that becomes more intense in the

Table 81–1 | **Frequency of Clinical Features of Hepatocellular Carcinoma**

SYMPTOMS	(%)	PHYSICAL SIGNS	(%)
Abdominal pain	59–95	Hepatomegaly	54–98
Weight loss	34–71	Hepatic bruit	6–25
Weakness	22–53	Ascites	35–61
Abdominal swelling	28–43	Splenomegaly	27–42
Nonspecific gastrointestinal symptoms	25–28	Jaundice	4–35
		Wasting	25–41
		Fever	11–54
Jaundice	5–26		

later stages of the illness. It may be accompanied by weakness and weight loss. Less common complaints are an awareness of a lump in the upper abdomen, poor appetite, early satiety or discomfort after eating, generalized abdominal swelling, diarrhea, and constipation. Jaundice is an infrequent initial complaint; when present, it may be obstructive.[13] Rarely, hepatocellular carcinoma presents with an "acute abdomen" when the tumor ruptures, causing hemoperitoneum. Other rare presentations are bone pain resulting from skeletal metastases, sudden paraplegia secondary to vertebral destruction, and cough or dyspnea caused by multiple pulmonary metastases or a markedly raised right hemidiaphragm.[14]

These symptoms may be surprisingly short-lived when the extent of the tumor burden is first appreciated. This rapid course occurs especially in black African and in Chinese patients, who often admit to symptoms of only 4 or 6 weeks' duration.

PHYSICAL FINDINGS. Physical findings vary according to the stage of the disease at which the patient is first seen. Early on, there may either be evidence of cirrhosis alone or no abnormal findings (see Table 81–1). More often, the tumor is advanced at the time of the first visit. The liver is then almost always enlarged, sometimes massively, particularly in black African and ethnic Chinese patients. Hepatic tenderness is common and may be severe, especially in the latter stages of the illness. The surface of the enlarged liver is smooth, irregular, or frankly nodular. Although the consistency is characteristically stony hard, it may be merely firm. An arterial bruit may be heard over the tumor.[12, 15, 16] The bruit occurs in systole and is rough in character and not affected by changing the position of the patient. Although not pathognomonic, the bruit is a useful clue to the diagnosis of hepatocellular carcinoma. Less often, a friction rub is heard over the tumor, although this sign is more typical of hepatic metastases or abscesses.

Ascites may be present when the patient is first seen. The majority of patients with ascites have had long-standing cirrhosis, and ascites is the result of portal hypertension, but in some it is caused by invasion of the peritoneum by the primary tumor or by metastases (in which case the ascites is likely to be blood-stained). Ascites may appear or increase with progression of the tumor. In a proportion of patients, hepatocellular carcinoma invades the hepatic veins and tense ascites results.[14] Splenomegaly may be evident, reflecting coexisting cirrhosis and portal hypertension.

The patient may be slightly or moderately wasted when first seen. Thereafter, progressive muscle wasting is the rule, and patients are typically emaciated in the final stages of the illness. Jaundice is unusual at first presentation and, when present, is mild. It commonly appears or deepens with progression of the disease. A low to moderate intermittent or remittent fever may be present, and in rare instances the tumor may masquerade as a fever of unknown origin.

Physical evidence of cirrhosis is common in patients in industrialized countries but unusual in black African and ethnic Chinese patients. Severe pitting edema extending up to the groins occurs when hepatocellular carcinoma that has invaded the hepatic veins propagates into the inferior vena cava and obstructs the lumen.[14] A Virchow-Trosier node is rarely present, as is a Sister Mary Joseph's nodule.

PARANEOPLASTIC MANIFESTATIONS. Some of the deleterious effects of hepatocellular carcinoma are not caused by either local effects of the tumor or metastases (Table 81–2). These systemic or remote sequelae result, directly or indirectly, from synthesis and secretion of biologically active substances by the tumor. Most often, clinically recognizable effects are caused by the secretion of hormones or hormone-like substances. Paraneoplastic phenomena may antedate the local effects of the tumor and direct attention to its presence. In addition, some effects, such as hypoglycemia and hypercalcemia, have implications for treatment.

The majority of paraneoplastic syndromes in hepatocellular carcinoma are rare. One of the more important is type B hypoglycemia, which occurs in fewer than 5% of patients and manifests as severe hypoglycemia early in the course of the disease.[14] Characteristically, the hypoglycemia is the reason that the patient seeks medical attention. Affected patients present with confusion, delirium, acute neuropsychiatric disturbances, convulsions, stupor, or coma. Not surprisingly, the presence of the underlying tumor is easily overlooked. Type B hypoglycemia is believed to result from the defective processing by malignant hepatocytes of the precursor to insulin-like growth factor II (pro-IGF-II).[17] The resulting *big* IGF-II circulates in 60-kd complexes that are appreciably smaller than the normal complexes. They transfer more readily across capillary membranes and increase access of IGF-II to IGF-I, IGF-II, and insulin receptors. The effect is to increase glucose uptake by tissues greatly and thereby cause severe hypoglycemia. In contrast, type A hypoglycemia is a milder form of glycopenia that occurs in the terminal stages of hepatocellular carcinoma (and other malignant tumors of the liver). It results from the inability of a liver extensively infiltrated by tumor and often cirrhotic to satisfy the demands for glucose by both a large, often rapidly growing tumor and other tissues of the body.

Another important paraneoplastic syndrome is polycythemia (erythrocytosis), which occurs in fewer than 10% of patients with hepatocellular carcinoma.[18] If polycythemia develops in a patient known to have cirrhosis, hepatocellular carcinoma is highly likely. This syndrome is probably caused by the synthesis of erythropoietin by malignant hepatocytes.[18]

A patient with hepatocellular carcinoma, especially the sclerosing variety, may present with hypercalcemia in the absence of osteolytic metastases. When hypercalcemia is se-

Table 81–2 | **Paraneoplastic Syndromes Associated with Hepatocellular Carcinoma**

Hypoglycemia
Polycythemia (erythrocytosis)
Hypercalcemia
Sexual changes: isosexual precocity, gynecomastia, feminization
Systemic arterial hypertension
Watery diarrhea syndrome
Porphyria
Carcinoid syndrome
Osteoporosis
Hypertrophic osteoarthropathy
Thyrotoxicosis
Thrombophlebitis migrans
Polymyositis
Neuropathy

vere, the patient is drowsy and lethargic and may be stuporous. The probable cause is secretion of parathyroid hormone-related protein (PTHrP) by the tumor.[19]

Cutaneous manifestations of hepatocellular carcinoma are rare except for *pityriasis rotunda*, which may be a useful cutaneous marker of the tumor in black Africans. The disorder is characterized by single or multiple, round or oval, hyperpigmented scaly lesions on the trunk and thighs that range in size from 0.5 to 25 cm.[20]

Diagnosis

Conventional tests of hepatic function do not distinguish hepatocellular carcinoma from other hepatic masses or from cirrhosis. Accordingly, they contribute little to the diagnosis of this tumor. Although not sufficiently useful to be measured routinely, the serum cholesterol concentration may sometimes help in making a diagnosis. Hypercholesterolemia occurs in 11% to 38% of patients with hepatocellular carcinoma,[21] and its presence in a patient with noncholestatic liver disease should raise suspicion of hepatocellular carcinoma. The increased de novo cholesterol biosynthesis by malignant hepatocytes results from the absence in these cells of the normal feedback inhibition of the rate-limiting enzyme, β-methyl glutaryl coenzyme A reductase.[21]

SERUM TUMOR MARKERS

Many of the substances synthesized and secreted by hepatocellular carcinoma are not biologically active. Nevertheless, a few are produced by a sufficiently large proportion of tumors to warrant use as serum markers of the tumor (Table 81–3). The most helpful of these is α-fetoprotein.

α-Fetoprotein. α-Fetoprotein is an α_1-globulin normally present in high concentration in fetal serum but in only minute amounts thereafter. Reappearance of high serum levels of α-fetoprotein strongly suggests the diagnosis of hepatocellular carcinoma (and hepatoblastoma).[22, 23] This finding is especially true in populations in which hepatocellular carcinoma is most prevalent: the great majority of ethnic Chinese and black African patients have a raised serum concentration (more than 20 ng/mL [20μg/L]), and about 75% have a diagnostic level (more than 500 ng/mL [500μg/L]). These percentages are lower in populations at low or intermediate risk of the tumor, and consequently, α-fetoprotein is a less useful tumor marker in these groups. The mean serum value of α-fetoprotein in affected patients in high incidence regions of hepatocellular carcinoma is 60,000 to 80,000 ng/mL, compared with about 3000 ng/mL in regions with a low or intermediate incidence of the tumor. Raised serum values range over six orders of magnitude, although concentrations of greater than 1 million are rare. The reason 500 ng/mL (500μg/L) is used as a diagnostic level is that serum concentrations below this value may be found in patients with a variety of acute and chronic benign liver diseases, such as acute and chronic hepatitis and cirrhosis.[22, 23] False-positive results may also occur in patients with tumors of endodermal origin and undifferentiated teratocarcinomas or embryonal cell carcinomas of the ovaries or testis.[22, 23] A progressively rising serum α-fetoprotein concentration, even if below the diagnostic level, is highly suggestive of hepatocellular carcinoma.

Because not all hepatocellular carcinomas produce α-fetoprotein, its presence is not essential to hepatocellular carcinogenesis, and there is no evidence that tumors that do not produce α-fetoprotein are biologically different from the majority of hepatocellular carcinomas. Synthesis of α-fetoprotein by a tumor is permanent and age-related: the younger the patient, the more likely the serum value is to be raised and the higher the level attained. Provided that patients are age-matched, there is no sex difference in α-fetoprotein production. No obvious correlation exists between the serum concentration of α-fetoprotein and any of the clinical or biochemical features of the tumor or the survival time after diagnosis. However, small presymptomatic tumors are associated with an appreciably lower serum level of α-fetoprotein than are symptomatic tumors.[24] Attempts to correlate the degree of differentiation of hepatocellular carcinoma with production of α-fetoprotein have produced conflicting results.

Because both false-positive and false-negative results are obtained when α-fetoprotein is used as a serum marker for hepatocellular carcinoma, the search for an ideal marker continues. A number of alternative markers have been suggested, although none has proved to be more useful than α-fetoprotein.

Fucosylated α-Fetoprotein. α-Fetoprotein is heterogeneous in structure. Its microheterogeneity results from differences in the oligosaccharide side chain and accounts for the differential affinity of the glycoprotein for lectins. The α-fetoprotein secreted by malignant hepatocytes contains unusual and complex sugar chains that are not found in the α-fetoprotein present in the nontransformed hepatocytes. The sugar chains have the same core structure, but the number of the outer chain trisaccharides differ. The asparagine-linked sugar chains all contain two outer chains, and no tri- or tetraantenerary chains are found. Several reports have attested to

Table 81–3 | **Tumor Markers of Hepatocellular Carcinoma***

	SENSITIVITY (%)	SPECIFICITY (%)	ADVANTAGES	DISADVANTAGES
α-Fetoprotein	In high-incidence populations, 80–90; in low-incidence populations, 50–70	90	Relatively quick and easy to measure, most extensively studied	Relatively expensive
Des-γ-carboxy-prothrombin	58–91	84	Quick and easy to measure	Much more expensive than α-fetoprotein
α-L-Fucosidase	75	70–90	Quick and easy to measure; relatively inexpensive	

*Note that sensitivity and specificity rates vary both with the population under study and the absolute level of the marker. Thus, the specificity of a markedly elevated α-fetoprotein level in high-risk patients greatly exceeds the sensitivity of mildly elevated levels in persons without cirrhosis.

the usefulness of the reactivity of α-fetoprotein with *lens culinaris* agglutinin A in differentiating hepatocellular carcinoma from benign hepatic parenchymal disease and, to a lesser extent, the reactivity with concanavalin A in distinguishing hepatocellular carcinoma from other tumors that produce this protein.[25] This refinement is particularly useful in the differential diagnosis of hepatocellular carcinoma when the serum α-fetoprotein concentration is less than 500 ng/mL [500 μg/L],[26] and it may improve the diagnostic yield of α-fetoprotein in presymptomatic tumors. Unfortunately, the method now used to measure fucosylated α-fetoprotein is rather complex and costly.

Des-γ-carboxy Prothrombin. Serum concentrations of des-γ-carboxy prothrombin (also known as prothrombin produced by vitamin K absence or antagonism II [PIVKA II]) are raised in the majority of patients with hepatocellular carcinoma.[27] In populations in which the incidence of hepatocellular carcinoma is low, the abnormal prothrombin may prove to be a better marker than α-fetoprotein, and it could be used as a first-line tumor marker. In black Africans, however, des-γ-carboxy prothrombin is less sensitive and less specific than α-fetoprotein.[28] Moreover, when the diagnostic cut-off level is increased in an attempt to eliminate false-positive results seen in benign hepatic parenchymal diseases, hepatic metastases, and hepatic abscesses, the sensitivity for hepatocellular carcinoma declines from 91% to 67%.[28]

α-L-Fucosidase. A number of isomers of α-L-fucosidase have been identified in human tissue, including two hepatic forms. α-L-Fucosidase was first reported to have a sensitivity of 75% and a specificity of 90% for the diagnosis of hepatocellular carcinoma.[29] In a subsequent study, however, the marker failed to distinguish cirrhosis from hepatocellular carcinoma.[30] Moreover, in black Africans this marker is less sensitive and less specific and has a lower predictive value than α-fetoprotein.[31] When the specificity of each of these markers was increased to 95% by raising the diagnostic cut-off level, the sensitivity of α-L-fucosidase decreased to 21%, whereas that of α-fetoprotein remained at 78%.[31]

None of a number of other substances claimed to be serum markers of hepatocellular carcinoma has sufficient sensitivity or specificity to warrant routine use in the diagnosis of this tumor.[23] CA 125, tissue polypeptide antigen, and tumor-associated isoenzymes of 5′-nucleotide phosphodiesterase have high sensitivity but poor specificity. Tumor-associated isoenzymes of γ-glutamyl transpeptidase and variant alkaline phosphatase have high specificity but low sensitivity, and both sensitivity and specificity are low for ferritin, carcinoembryonic antigen, CA 19-9, and calcitonin. Two tumor markers—abnormal vitamin B_{12}-binding protein and neurotensin—have been linked specifically to the fibrolamellar variant of hepatocellular carcinoma. When present, they provide useful confirmatory evidence of this variant, but both markers have low sensitivity.

HEMATOLOGIC CHANGES

More than half of ethnic Chinese and black African patients with hepatocellular carcinoma are anemic when they are first seen, although anemia is less common in other populations. Severe anemia is rare, however, and should suggest the possibility of intraperitoneal bleeding. Slight or moderate leukocytosis may be present. As discussed earlier, polycythemia rarely may occur as a paraneoplastic complication of hepatocellular carcinoma.

RADIOLOGIC INVESTIGATIONS

Plain chest radiography may help in the diagnosis of hepatocellular carcinoma. Pulmonary metastases may be seen on plain chest radiography, particularly often in black African and ethnic Chinese patients.[32] They are almost always multiple and may enlarge rapidly. The right hemidiaphragm may be raised.[32] Skeletal metastases are seen occasionally.

HEPATIC IMAGING

The imaging modalities used most often for the diagnosis of symptomatic hepatocellular carcinoma are ultrasonography and computed tomography (CT). Magnetic resonance imaging (MRI) also may be useful.

Ultrasonography. Ultrasonography detects the majority of hepatocellular carcinomas but does not distinguish this tumor from other solid lesions in the liver. Its advantages include safety, availability, and cost effectiveness, although it has the drawbacks of being nonstandardized and examiner-dependent. Approximately two thirds of symptomatic hepatocellular carcinomas are uniformly hyperechoic, whereas the remainder are partly hyperechoic and partly hypoechoic (Fig. 81–2).[33] Tumors located immediately under the right hemidiaphragm may be difficult to detect. In Japanese patients in particular, hepatocellular carcinoma may have a well-defined—even a thick—capsule, which can be seen on ultrasonography. Ultrasonography with Doppler is useful for assessing the patency of the inferior vena cava, portal vein and its larger branches, hepatic veins, and biliary tree.[33]

Ultrasonographic evaluation of intranodular blood flow is important because the pattern is closely related to pathologic findings and the grade of malignancy. Dynamic contrast-enhanced Doppler ultrasonography with intra-arterial infusion of CO_2 microbubbles and intravenous enhanced color Doppler ultrasonography are recent refinements that, by characterizing hepatic arterial and portal venous flow in tumorous nodules, facilitate the diagnosis of malignant and benign hepatic nodules.[34]

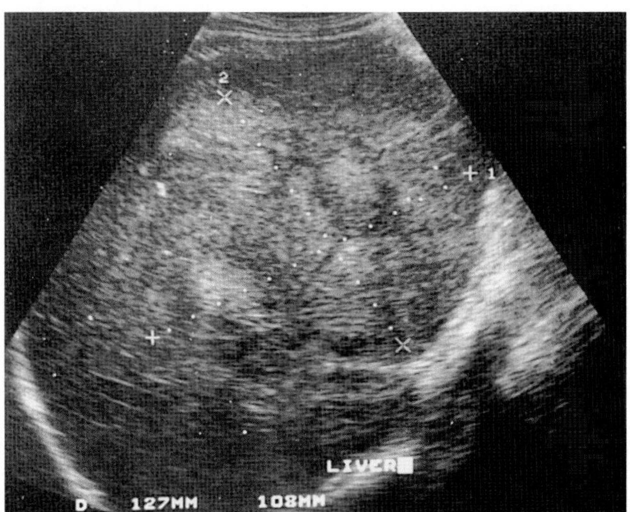

Figure 81–2. Ultrasonographic picture of hepatocellular carcinoma showing a nodular hyperechoic pattern with scattered hypoechoic areas. The edges of the tumor are ill-defined.

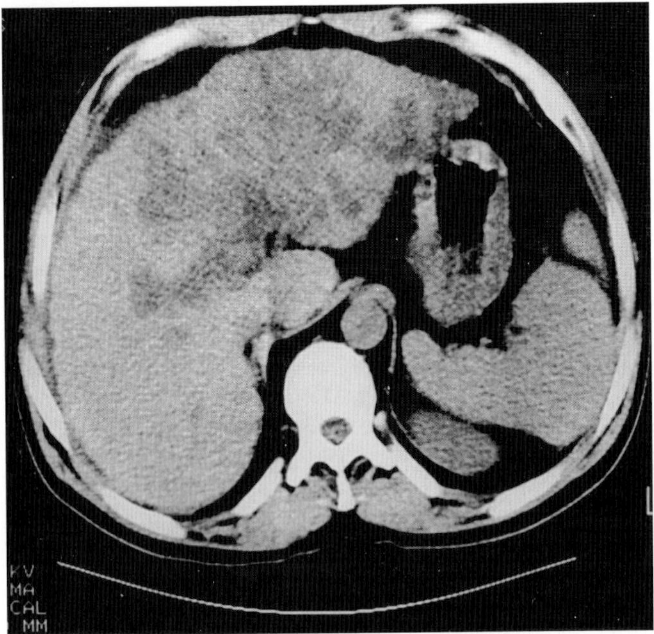

Figure 81–3. Computed tomographic image of hepatocellular carcinoma involving much of the left lobe and the adjacent part of the right lobe of the liver.

Computed Tomography. Spiral (helical) CT and CT during arterial portography have greatly improved the diagnosis of hepatocellular carcinoma by CT.[34] The images of hepatocellular carcinoma obtained with CT are, however, not specific.[34–36] Nevertheless, CT is especially useful in defining the extent of the tumor within and beyond the liver (Fig. 81–3) and showing the course, caliber, and patency of blood vessels. Because iodized poppy seed oil (Lipiodol) is concentrated and retained in hepatocellular carcinoma tissue, injection of this material at the end of hepatic arteriography can be used in conjunction with CT, performed after a suitable delay, to detect small tumors.

Magnetic Resonance Imaging. MRI provides another way of distinguishing hepatocellular carcinoma from normal liver tissue. Most tumors have a low signal intensity on T_1-weighted images and a high signal intensity on T_2-weighted images.[34, 36, 37] Gradient-echo sequences and turbo spin-echo sequences have greatly reduced the time needed for MRI. Furthermore, the use of a contrast agent, such as gadopentetate dimeglumine and superparamagnetic iron oxide, increases the accuracy of MRI, especially in detecting small hepatocellular carcinomas in cirrhotic livers and distinguishing small hepatocellular carcinomas from hemangiomas or dysplastic nodules discovered in surveillance programs.[34]

HEPATIC ANGIOGRAPHY

Hepatic digital subtraction angiography is helpful in recognizing small hypervascular hepatocellular carcinomas but may miss early, well-differentiated hypovascular tumors. Dynamic contrast-enhanced ultrasonography with intra-arterial infusion of CO_2 microbubbles can be used to detect these hypovascular tumors and also to differentiate hepatocellular carcinoma from other hepatic nodules.[34] Angiography is also essential in delineating the hepatic arterial anatomy when planning surgical resection, transplantation, bland or chemoembolization of the tumor, or infusion of cytotoxic drugs directly into the hepatic artery or its branches. Angiography will also confirm patency of the portal vein. Hepatocellular carcinomas are often densely vascular, although multinodular tumors may be relatively avascular.[38] The arteries in the tumor are irregular in caliber and do not taper in the usual way, and the smaller branches may show a bizarre pattern (Fig. 81–4).[38] The hepatic veins fill early, and retrograde filling of the portal veins results from the presence of arteriovenous anastomoses within the tumor. In addition, there is a delay in capillary emptying, which is seen as a blush. The center of some large tumors may be avascular as a result of necrosis or, less often, hemorrhage.

Examination of the portal venous circulation during recirculation after celiac axis arteriography or during portal venography may show tumor invasion.[38] Less often, invasion of the hepatic veins can be demonstrated, and the tumor may be seen to propagate into the lumen of the inferior vena cava.

LAPAROSCOPY

Laparoscopy can be used to detect peritoneal and other extrahepatic spread, ascertain whether the nontumorous part of the liver is cirrhotic and obtain a biopsy under direct vision.

Pathology

Definitive diagnosis of hepatocellular carcinoma depends on demonstrating typical histologic features. Suitable tissue

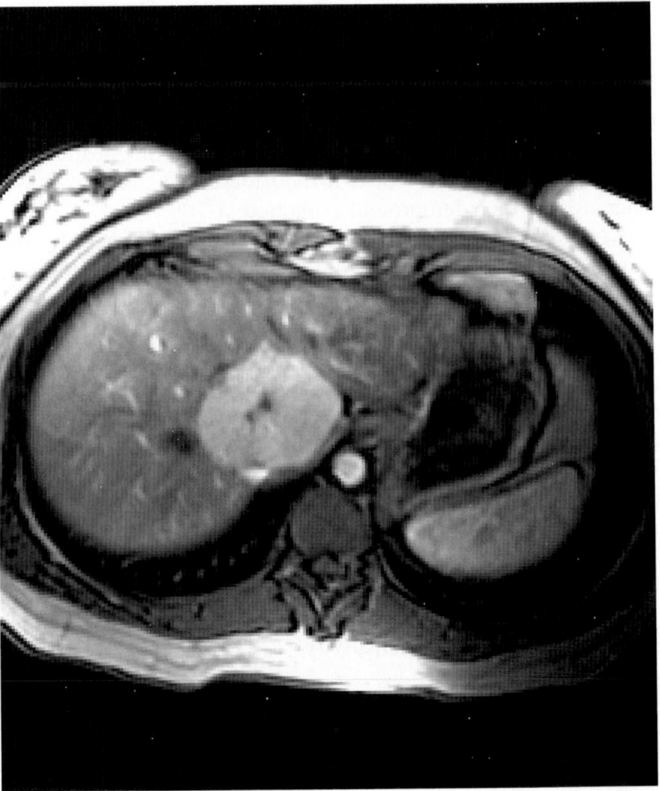

Figure 81–4. Hepatic arteriogram showing the typical features of a highly vascular hepatocellular carcinoma.

samples generally can be obtained by percutaneous biopsy or fine-needle aspiration. The yield and safety of the procedure can be increased by aiming the needle under ultrasonographic guidance. Laparoscopically directed biopsy is an alternative approach. Because there is a risk of local, regional, or systemic dissemination of hepatocellular carcinoma by needle biopsy or aspiration of the tumor, many clinicians believe that these procedures should be avoided if the tumor is thought to be operable.

GROSS APPEARANCE

Hepatocellular carcinoma may take three forms—nodular, massive, or diffuse.[39–41] The nodular variety accounts for about 75% of hepatocellular carcinomas and usually coexists with cirrhosis. It is characterized by numerous round or irregular nodules of various sizes scattered throughout the liver, some of which are confluent. The massive type is more common in younger patients with a noncirrhotic liver. It is characterized by a large circumscribed mass, often with small satellite nodules. This type of tumor is most prone to rupture. The diffusely infiltrating variety is rare. In this type, a large part of the liver is infiltrated homogeneously by indistinct minute tumor nodules, which may be difficult to distinguish from the regenerating nodules of cirrhosis that are almost invariably present. Hepatocellular carcinoma rarely, if ever, umbilicates. The tumor may be monoclonal (with intrahepatic metastases accounting for other tumor deposits) or polyclonal.

In the nodular and massive varieties, the tumor tissue is usually soft and bulges above the surrounding cut surface of the liver. Areas of necrosis and hemorrhage are common. Well-differentiated tumors are light brown, whereas anaplastic tumors are yellowish white or gray. Bile production may cause greenish brown discoloration of the tumor. The portal vein and its branches are infiltrated by tumor in up to 70% of cases seen at necropsy; the hepatic veins and bile ducts are invaded less often.

MICROSCOPIC APPEARANCE

Hepatocellular carcinoma is classified histologically into well-differentiated, moderately differentiated, and undifferentiated (pleomorphic) forms.[39–41]

Well-differentiated Appearance. Despite the aggressive nature and poor prognosis of hepatocellular carcinoma, most tumors are well differentiated. Trabecular and acinar (pseudoglandular) varieties occur, sometimes in a single tumor. In the trabecular variety the malignant hepatocytes grow in irregular anastomosing plates separated by sinusoids lined by flat cells resembling Kupffer cells. The sinusoids may be inconspicuous, however. The trabeculae resemble those of normal adult liver, although they are often thicker and may be composed of several layers of cells. Scanty collagen fibers may be seen adjacent to the sinusoid walls. The malignant hepatocytes are polygonal, with abundant, slightly granular cytoplasm that is less eosinophilic than that of normal hepatocytes. The nuclei are large and hyperchromatic with prominent nucleoli. Bile production is the hallmark of hepatocellular carcinoma, regardless of the pattern.

A variety of glandlike structures are present in the acinar variety. They are composed of layers of malignant hepatocytes surrounding the lumen of a bile canaliculus, which may contain inspissated bile. A tubular or pseudopapillary appearance may be produced by degeneration and loss of cells, or cystic spaces may form in otherwise solid trabeculae. The individual cells may be more elongated and cylindrical than in the trabecular variety.

Moderately Differentiated Appearance. Solid, scirrhous, and clear cell varieties are described. In the solid variety, the cells are usually small, although they vary considerably in shape. Pleomorphic multinucleated giant cells are occasionally present. The tumor grows in solid masses or cell nests. Evidence of bile secretion is rare, and connective tissue is inconspicuous. Central ischemic necrosis is common in larger tumors. In the scirrhous variety, the malignant hepatocytes grow in narrow bundles separated by abundant fibrous stroma. Ductlike structures are occasionally present. In most tumors the cells resemble hepatocytes. In an occasional tumor, the malignant hepatocytes are predominantly or exclusively clear cells. More often, tumors contain areas of clear cells. The appearance of these cells usually results from a high glycogen content, although in some cases fat is the cause.

Undifferentiated Appearance. The cells are pleomorphic, varying greatly in size and shape. The nuclei are also extremely variable. Large numbers of bizarre-looking giant cells are present. The cells may be spindle-shaped, resembling those of sarcomas.

Globular hyaline structures may be seen in all types of hepatocellular carcinoma. These reflect the presence of α-fetoprotein, α_1-antitrypsin, or other proteins. Mallory's hyaline is occasionally present.

Extrahepatic metastases are present at necropsy in 40% to 57% of patients with hepatocellular carcinomas.[42] They are more common (~70%) in patients without coexisting cirrhosis than in those with cirrhosis (~30%). The most common sites are the lungs (up to 50% in some populations) and regional lymph nodes (~20%).

Fibrolamellar Hepatocellular Carcinoma. This variant of hepatocellular carcinoma typically occurs in young patients, has an approximately equal sex distribution, does not secrete α-fetoprotein, is not caused by chronic hepatitis B (HBV) or C (HCV) virus infection, and almost always arises in a noncirrhotic liver.[40] Fibrolamellar hepatocellular carcinoma is more often amenable to surgical treatment and, therefore, generally has a better prognosis than conventional hepatocellular carcinoma. It does not, however, respond to chemotherapy any better than other forms of hepatocellular carcinoma. The hepatocytes are characteristically plump and deeply eosinophilic and are encompassed by abundant fibrous stroma composed of thin, parallel fibrous bands that separate the cells into trabeculae or nodules. The cytoplasm is packed with swollen mitochondria and, in approximately half the tumors, contains pale or hyaline bodies. Nuclei are prominent, and mitoses are rare.

Etiology and Pathogenesis

Hepatocellular carcinoma is multifactorial in etiology and complex in pathogenesis. Four major and several minor causal associations with the tumor have been identified (Table 81–4). The blend of risk factors differs in different parts of the world, and this may explain in part the diverse biologic characteristics of hepatocellular carcinoma in different populations.[43]

HEPATITIS B VIRUS

There are 387 million carriers of HBV in the world today, and hepatocellular carcinoma will develop in as many as 25% of them. HBV accounts for as much as 80% of the cases of hepatocellular carcinoma that occur with such high frequency in ethnic Chinese and black African populations.[43, 44] Persistent HBV infection antedates the development of hepatocellular carcinoma by several to many years, an interval commensurate with a cause-and-effect relationship between the virus and the tumor. Indeed, in ethnic Chinese and black Africans the carrier state is established in early childhood.[45, 46] The carrier state acquired early in life carries a lifetime relative risk for developing hepatocellular carcinoma of over 100.[47] An effective vaccine against HBV has been available for several years, and in countries in which this vaccine has been included in the Expanded Program of Immunization for a sufficient length of time, there has been a decrease in the carrier rate among children by as much as 10-fold. A recent report from Taiwan, where universal immunization was started in 1984, and where the rate of HBV carriage among children has decreased considerably, has shown that there has already been a 50% reduction in the mortality rate from hepatocellular carcinoma among children.[48] This finding gives promise for the ultimate eradication of HBV-induced hepatocellular carcinoma and provides further evidence for the oncogenic potential of HBV.

HBV DNA is integrated into cellular DNA in about 95% of HBV-related hepatocellular carcinomas.[43, 44] The sites of chromosomal insertion appear to be random, and it is not yet certain whether integration is essential for hepatocarcinogenesis. The virus appears to be both directly and indirectly carcinogenic.[49] Possible direct carcinogenic effects include *cis*-activation of cellular genes as a result of viral integration, transcriptional activation of cellular genes by HBV-encoded proteins, particularly the X protein, and effects resulting from viral mutations. The transcriptional activity of the HBV X protein may be mediated by interaction with specific transcription factors, activation of the MAP kinase and JAK/STAT pathways, an effect on apoptosis, and modulation of DNA repair.[49] Indirect carcinogenic effects are the result of the chronic necroinflammatory hepatic disease induced by the virus. The increased hepatocyte turnover rate resulting from continuous or recurring cycles of cell necrosis and regeneration acts as a potent tumor promoter.[49] In addition, the distorted architecture characteristic of cirrhosis contributes to the loss of control of hepatocyte growth, and hepatic inflammation generates mutagenic reactive oxygen species. The transgenic mouse model of Chisari and coworkers has provided indirect support for the role of prolonged hepatocyte injury in hepatocarcinogenesis.[50]

Table 81–4 | **Risk Factors for Hepatocellular Carcinoma in Humans**

MAJOR RISK FACTORS
Chronic hepatitis B virus infection
Chronic hepatitis C virus infection
Cirrhosis
Repeated dietary exposure to aflatoxin B_1
MINOR RISK FACTORS
Oral contraceptive steroids
Cigarette smoking
Dietary iron overload in Africans
Hereditary hemochromatosis
Wilson disease
α_1-Antitrypsin deficiency
Type 1 hereditary tyrosinemia
Types 1 and 2 glycogen storage disease
Hypercitrullinemia
Ataxia telangiectasia
Membranous obstruction of the inferior vena cava

HEPATITIS C VIRUS

There are approximately 170 million people in the world today who are chronically infected with HCV and are at increased risk for the development of hepatocellular carcinoma.[44] In Japan, Italy, and Spain, HCV is the cause of as much as 83% of cases of hepatocellular carcinoma, and in other industrialized countries this virus is emerging as a major causal association with the tumor, often in combination with alcohol abuse.[44] Patients with HCV-induced hepatocellular carcinoma are generally older than those with HBV-related tumors, and it is likely that the HCV infection is acquired mainly in adult life.

Almost all HCV-induced hepatocellular carcinomas arise in cirrhotic livers, and most of the exceptions are associated with chronic hepatitis. This observation strongly suggests that chronic hepatic parenchymal disease plays a key role in the genesis of HCV-related tumors.[49] Evidence is emerging, however, that HCV also may be directly oncogenic.[49] Because the HCV genome does not integrate into host DNA, the virus would have to exert its carcinogenic effect from an extra-chromosomal position, and a number of possible ways in which such an effect may be achieved are under investigation.

CIRRHOSIS

In all parts of the world, hepatocellular carcinoma frequently coexists with cirrhosis.[10] In ethnic Chinese and black African populations, the cirrhosis is typically of the macronodular variety and is attributed to chronic HBV infection, whereas in other populations it is commonly of the mixed macronodular/micronodular or micronodular variety and results from chronic HCV infection, alcohol abuse, or both. All etiologic forms of cirrhosis may be complicated by tumor formation.[10] Male sex, age, and duration of cirrhosis are the major risk factors for hepatocellular carcinoma in cirrhotic patients. Cirrhosis contributes to hepatocarcinogenesis in a number of ways, but mainly by acting as a potent tumor promoter.[49]

AFLATOXIN B_1

Aflatoxin B_1, derived from *Aspergillus flavus* and *Aspergillus parasiticus*, is an important risk factor for hepatocellular carcinoma in parts of Africa and Asia. *A. flavus* is ubiquitous in nature and contaminates a number of staple foodstuffs in tropical and subtropical regions. Epidemiologic studies have shown a strong positive correlation between the dietary intake of aflatoxin B_1 and the incidence of hepatocellular carcinoma.[51] Aflatoxin B_1 and HBV may interact in the pathogenesis of hepatocellular carcinoma. One possible way in which aflatoxin B_1 may contribute to hepatocarcinogenesis is suggested by the correlation between heavy dietary exposure to this mycotoxin and an inactivating mutation of the third base of codon 249 of the p53 tumor suppressor gene.[52, 53]

MINOR RISK FACTORS

Hepatocellular carcinoma develops in as many as 45% of patients with hereditary hemochromatosis.[54] Malignant transformation was thought to occur only in the presence of cirrhosis (and is certainly more likely to do so), but in recent years this complication has been reported in a few patients without cirrhosis.[55] This observation suggests that excessive free iron in tissue per se may be carcinogenic, perhaps by generating mutagenic reactive oxygen species,[56] a possibility that has gained further support from the observation that black Africans with dietary iron overload are at greatly increased risk of hepatocellular carcinoma.[57] Hepatocellular carcinoma develops occasionally in patients with Wilson disease, but only in the presence of cirrhosis.[58] Malignant transformation has been attributed to the cirrhosis but also may result from oxidant stress secondary to the accumulation of copper in the liver.[59] Hepatocellular carcinoma also may develop in patients with other inherited metabolic disorders that are complicated by cirrhosis, such as α_1-antitrypsin deficiency and type 1 hereditary tyrosinemia, whereas in patients with other diseases, for example type 1 glycogen storage disease, tumors develop in the absence of cirrhosis.

A statistically significant correlation between the use of oral contraceptive steroids and the occurrence of hepatocellular carcinoma has been demonstrated in countries in which the incidence of the tumor is low and there is no overriding risk factor for the tumor.[60] This group of patients, however, constitutes a small proportion of all patients with hepatocellular carcinoma. The patients are usually relatively young. The increased risk persists for more than 10 years after the agents are discontinued.[61] Epidemiologic evidence of a link between cigarette smoking and the occurrence of hepatocellular carcinoma is conflicting, although most of the evidence suggests that smoking is a minor risk factor.[62] Heavy smokers have an approximately 50% higher risk than nonsmokers. The cytochrome P450 system, which is responsible for the metabolic activation of a number of chemical carcinogens, is highly inducible by smoking.

Hepatocellular carcinoma develops in about 40% of patients with membranous obstruction of the inferior vena cava, a rare congenital or acquired anomaly. Continuous cycles of hepatocyte necrosis followed by regeneration resulting from the severe and unremitting hepatic venous congestion render the cells susceptible to environmental mutagens and spontaneous mutations.[63, 64]

Natural History and Prognosis

Symptomatic hepatocellular carcinoma carries a grave prognosis; in fact, the annual incidence and mortality rates for the tumor are virtually the same. The main reasons for the poor outcome are the extent of tumor burden when the patient is first seen and the presence of coexisting cirrhosis. The natural history of hepatocellular carcinoma in its florid form is one of rapid progression with increasing hepatomegaly, pain, wasting, and deepening jaundice. In black African and ethnic Chinese populations, death often ensues within 4 months,[11, 12] although in industrialized countries the tumor generally runs a somewhat more indolent course with longer survival times.[16] Rare instances of spontaneous tumor regression have been reported.

Treatment

No form of treatment for hepatocellular carcinoma has been shown conclusively or consistently to be better than no treatment, or superior, in terms of survival, to any other form of treatment.[65] The treatment of hepatocellular carcinoma depends on the extent of the disease, presence or absence of cirrhosis, and degree of hepatic dysfunction. The many patients who show evidence of liver failure are seldom suitable for any active treatment.

SURGICAL RESECTION

Resection or liver transplantation offers the best chance of cure for hepatocellular carcinoma (Table 81–5). For resection to be considered, the tumor must be confined to one lobe of the liver and be favorably located, and ideally, the nontumorous liver tissue should not be cirrhotic. Resection can, however, be considered if the tumor is limited to the left lobe and the cirrhosis of the right lobe is not severe, or if the tumor is favorably located in either lobe, allowing the surgeon to perform a segmentectomy or limited nonanatomic resection. Unfortunately, the proportion of symptomatic patients with resectable tumors is small in countries where hepatocellular carcinoma is most common,[66, 67] although the situation is less bleak in industrialized countries.[68] Overall, resection is feasible in only about 15% of patients. Resection carries an operative mortality rate of around 5% in noncirrhotic and 10% to 15% in cirrhotic livers. One of the most disappointing aspects of resecting hepatocellular carcinoma is the very high recurrence rate.[69, 70]

LIVER TRANSPLANTATION

Liver transplantation is performed in patients in whom the tumor is not resectable but is confined to the liver or in whom advanced cirrhosis and poor liver function preclude resection.[71] Even patients with well-compensated cirrhosis may be served better by transplantation than by resection.[71]

Table 81–5 | **Treatment Options for Hepatocellular Carcinoma**

Surgical resection: Offers best chance for cure, but is seldom possible when the tumor is symptomatic. May be technically difficult. High rate of recurrence after resection.

Liver transplantation: May be successful in selected patients. Requires transfer to a transplant center and, postoperatively, lifelong immunosuppression. High recurrence rate. Expensive.

Alcohol injection or radiofrequency ablation: Palliative for small (usually multiple) tumors that cannot be resected. May be difficult to confirm that all the malignant cells have been destroyed.

Chemoembolization: May shrink selected tumors to the point that they may become resectable. Effect is palliative for localized but unresectable tumors.

Chemotherapy: Palliative only; can be used as an adjunct to surgical resection or transplantation. Drug toxicity is common.

The early experience with transplantation was disappointing, with unacceptably high recurrence rates and short survival times after recurrence.[72] With more careful selection of patients, particular attention to tumor size and vascular invasion, improved surgical techniques, and perhaps adjunctive anticancer treatment, better results have been obtained.[71, 73, 74] However, because of undetected spread of the tumor before transplantation, the rate of tumor recurrence remains high, particularly in patients with an unresectable tumor in a noncirrhotic liver.

OTHER TREATMENTS

Small tumors not amenable to resection, because they are multiple or inaccessible or because of severe hepatic dysfunction, have been treated with a variety of intralesional techniques.[75] The first of these was ethanol injection, a relatively effective and safe technique that is still widely used.[76] Following ethanol injection it may be difficult to establish that necrosis of tumor tissue is complete. There is also a risk of disseminating the tumor by facilitating the passage of malignant cells into the blood stream. More recently, radiofrequency ablation of the tumor has been introduced, but its efficacy and safety, as compared to ethanol ablation, remain to be determined.

Arterial embolization and chemoembolization are additional palliative methods in selected patients.[77–80] They also are used to reduce the size of the tumor in an attempt to make resection possible or to allow a more conservative resection.

CHEMOTHERAPY

A large number of anticancer drugs, including alkylating agents, antitumor antibiotics, antimetabolites, plant alkyloids, platinum derivatives, and procarbazine, have been tried alone and in various combinations, and by different routes of administration, in the treatment of hepatocellular carcinoma, but response rates have invariably been less than 20%.[81] Because single agents have limited value in treating hepatocellular carcinoma, it is not surprising that combinations of these agents are also disappointing. Multidrug resistance is an important factor in the poor outcomes, and the development and testing of drugs that reverse this resistance is in progress. Biologic response modifiers tested to date have not proved to be of value.

Screening for Small Presymptomatic Hepatocellular Carcinoma

Because symptomatic hepatocellular carcinoma is seldom amenable to surgical cure and responds poorly to conservative modalities of treatment, there is a pressing need either to prevent the tumor or to diagnose it at a presymptomatic stage, when surgical intervention is still possible. Programs for detecting subclinical hepatocellular carcinomas are of two kinds: (1) screening whole populations that have a high incidence of the tumor and (2) long-term surveillance of persons known to be at high risk for developing hepatocellular carcinoma.[24] Mass population screening has been attempted in a number of ethnic Chinese and black African populations at high risk of hepatocellular carcinoma. The serum α-fetoprotein concentration was the sole screening method used. Because only 45% of presymptomatic hepatocellular carcinomas produce a diagnostic level of this marker,[24] an appreciable number of small tumors are missed in programs of this sort. Nonetheless, subclinical tumors have been detected in this way. For example, 147 instances of a raised serum α-fetoprotein concentration were detected among 344,000 unselected subjects in China, 88% of whom were proved to have hepatocellular carcinoma.[82] Clearly, this type of mass screening can be contemplated only in countries with the highest incidence rates of hepatocellular carcinoma, and even then, the enormity of the task is daunting.

Long-term surveillance of persons at high risk for the development of hepatocellular carcinoma is more feasible,[24] and such programs have been shown to be cost effective. Surveillance involves periodic ultrasonographic examination of the liver and testing of serum for α-fetoprotein, but difficulties are encountered. In addition to the limited sensitivity of serum α-fetoprotein levels in detecting presymptomatic hepatocellular carcinoma, slightly raised serum levels are difficult to interpret because benign hepatic diseases known to be complicated by tumor formation also produce such slight elevations.[24]

Ultrasonography is used for initial screening because it is noninvasive, carries no radiation hazard, and can be done quickly, cheaply, and repeatedly. With experienced operators and sophisticated equipment, tumors smaller than 1 cm in diameter can be visualized. Hepatocellular carcinomas uncovered in this way are frequently hypoechoic, although the pattern changes as the tumor grows.[83] For persons at high risk (Table 81–6), ultrasonography and serum α-fetoprotein measurement should be performed at 4- or 6-month intervals, and for those at moderate risk, α-fetoprotein levels should be measured every 6 months, and ultrasonography should be performed annually. Other imaging modalities, which have similar sensitivities to ultrasonography, are used in doubtful cases or special circumstances. One problem encountered in monitoring programs is differentiating small hepatocellular carcinomas from benign hepatic lesions, especially regenerating nodules in cirrhotic livers and hemangiomas.[24]

Persons at risk for hepatocellular carcinoma should be counseled about (1) their chances of developing hepatocellular carcinoma, (2) the limited treatment options should a

Table 81–6 | **Factors Influencing Screening for Hepatocellular Carcinomas**

FACTORS	RISK			SCREENING	
	High	Moderate	Low	Yes	No
HBV carriage					
Early onset	+			+	
Later onset		+		+	
Chronic HCV infection	+			+	
Hereditary hemochromatosis	+			+	
Membranous obstruction of the inferior vena cava (in black Africans)	+			+	
Cirrhosis of most other causes			+		+

HBV = hepatitis B virus; HCV = hepatitis C virus.

tumor develop, (3) the natural history and prognosis of hepatocellular carcinoma, (4), the availability, advantages, and shortcomings of monitoring programs, and (5) the results of treating subclinical tumors discovered in a surveillance program. Persons who agree to surveillance should be enrolled in such a program. Surveillance is not recommended for patients with a type of cirrhosis at low risk for tumor formation.

If the tumor detected during monitoring is small and accessible to surgery, and if hepatic function is adequate, surgical resection offers the best chance of cure.[24] Five-year survival rates of up to 68% have been achieved, although tumor recurrence, both intrahepatic and extrahepatic, is disturbingly frequent.

Cholangiocarcinoma

Cholangiocarcinomas may originate from small intrahepatic bile ducts (peripheral cholangiocarcinoma), large intrahepatic bile ducts (hilar cholangiocarcinoma or Klatskin tumor), or extrahepatic ducts (bile duct carcinoma) (see Chapter 60).

Epidemiology and Pathogenesis

The occurrence of peripheral cholangiocarcinoma shows geographic variation,[84, 85] although not to the same extent as hepatocellular carcinoma. Frequency rates relative to those for hepatocellular carcinoma range from 5% to 30%. The higher ratios are found in parts of the Far East, such as Hong Kong and Canton, but most notably in northeastern Thailand, where chronic infestation of the biliary tree with the liver flukes *Clonorchis sinensis* and *Opistorchis viverrini* is causally related to this tumor.[86] Occasionally, cholangiocarcinoma also occurs years after a patient has received the radiographic contrast medium thorium dioxide (Thorotrast)[87] or in a patient with α_1-antitrypsin deficiency.[88] Hilar cholangiocarcinoma may complicate long-standing sclerosing cholangitis,[89] biliary atresia,[90] von Meyenburg complexes,[91] or intrahepatic cholelithiasis.[92]

Intrahepatic cholangiocarcinomas are more common in older than younger persons; the average age at presentation is between 50 and 60 years.[84, 85] The sex distribution is approximately equal.[84, 85]

Clinical Presentation

A peripheral cholangiocarcinoma seldom produces symptoms until the tumor is advanced. The clinical features are then similar to those of hepatocellular carcinoma, except that jaundice may be more frequent, earlier, and prominent.[84, 85] In addition, the liver tends not to be as enlarged, a bruit is not heard, ascites is much less common, and fever and extrahepatic metastases are less frequent. The clinical presentation of hilar cholangiocarcinoma is one of progressive obstructive jaundice, with or without weight loss.[93]

Diagnosis

Apart from higher serum concentrations of bilirubin, alkaline phosphatase, and γ-glutamyl transpeptidase in peripheral cholangiocarcinoma, the results of liver biochemical testing are similar to those of hepatocellular carcinoma.[84, 85] These tumors occasionally produce hypercalcemia in the absence of osteolytic metastases. In one patient, hypercalcemia resulted from ectopic production of immunoreactive parathormone by the tumor.[94] In hilar cholangiocarcinoma, the biochemical picture is that of obstructive jaundice.[93] Only occasionally is α-fetoprotein produced by cholangiocarcinoma.[84, 85, 93] The appearances of peripheral cholangiocarcinoma on ultrasonography and CT are similar to those of hepatocellular carcinoma.[84, 85] Larger hilar tumors and the resulting ductal dilatation can be seen with these imaging techniques. Endoscopic retrograde or transhepatic cholangiography localizes the site of these tumors. In peripheral cholangiocarcinomas, a characteristic picture is evident on hepatic arteriography[95]; the marked desmoplastic reaction that characteristically occurs with this tumor causes the branches of the hepatic artery to appear scanty, stretched, and attenuated.

Pathology

Peripheral cholangiocarcinomas usually are large and solitary tumors, but they may be multinodular.[40, 41, 96] They are grayish white, firm, and occasionally umbilicated. The tumor is poorly vascularized and rarely bleeds internally or ruptures. Vascular invasion and tumor necrosis also are less common than in hepatocellular carcinoma. Peripheral cholangiocarcinoma arises in a noncirrhotic liver. Hilar cholangiocarcinoma may take the form of a firm, intramural tumor encircling the bile duct, a bulky mass centered on the duct or hilar region that radiates into the hepatic tissue, or a spongy friable mass within the lumen of the duct.[40, 41, 96] Metastatic nodules may be distributed irregularly throughout the liver. The bile ducts peripheral to the tumor may be dilated, and in long-standing cases biliary cirrhosis may be present.

Microscopically, cholangiocarcinomas have acinar or tubular structures resembling those of other adenocarcinomas.[40, 41, 96] Most tumors are well differentiated. Secretion of mucus may be demonstrable, but bile production is not seen. The tumor cells provoke a variable desmoplastic reaction, and in many tumors the collagenized stroma may be the most prominent feature.

A peripheral cholangiocarcinoma is often complicated by intrahepatic metastases and tumor growth along the biliary tracts.[96] Metastases in regional lymph nodes occur in about 50% of cases.[96]

Treatment and Prognosis

Early diagnosis of a peripheral cholangiocarcinoma is unusual, and the tumor carries the same poor prognosis as hepatocellular carcinoma.[84, 85] Resection is rarely possible, and the results of radiation therapy and chemotherapy are disappointing. Liver transplantation has, however, been performed successfully in some patients. Resection of a hilar cholangiocarcinoma may be feasible, depending on its position and size and whether it has spread. Inoperable hilar cholangiocarcinomas tend to progress more slowly than peripheral tumors.[93] For inoperable cases, biliary drainage must be established, usually be an endoscopic or radiologic approach.

Hepatoblastoma

Epidemiology

Hepatoblastoma is the most common malignant hepatic tumor in children. It occurs almost exclusively in the first 3 years of life; boys are affected twice as often as girls.[40, 41, 98]

Clinical Presentation

The great majority of children with hepatoblastoma come to medical attention because of abdominal swelling.[40, 41, 98] Other reasons include failure to thrive, weight loss, poor appetite, abdominal pain, irritability, and intermittent vomiting and diarrhea. The tumorous liver is almost always enlarged, firm, and possibly tender, and the surface is smooth or nodular. Pallor is common, but the patient seldom has jaundice. Hepatoblastomas rarely rupture. This tumor occasionally causes isosexual precocity in boys, as a result of the ectopic production of human chorionic gonadotrophin.[99]

Diagnosis

α-Fetoprotein is present in high concentration in the serum of 80% to 90% of patients with hepatoblastoma and is a useful clue to diagnosis.[97, 98, 100] Anemia is common, and occasionally the platelet count may be either high or low.[97, 98] Pulmonary metastases and, rarely, mottled calcification in the tumor, may be seen on plain radiography. The tumor is visualized as an echogenic mass on ultrasonography and an avascular mass on hepatic arteriography. In neither instance is the picture specific.[97, 98]

Pathology

Hepatoblastomas are the malignant derivatives of incompletely differentiated hepatocyte precursors. Their constituents are diverse, reflecting both the multipotentiality of their mesodermal origin and the progressive stages of embryonic and fetal development. Hepatoblastomas are classified morphologically into an *epithelial type*, composed predominantly of epithelial cells of varying maturity, and a *mixed epithelial and mesenchymal type,* which contains, in addition, tissues of mesenchymal derivation.[40, 41, 97, 98] The tumors are usually solitary, ranging in size from 5 to 25 cm, and always well circumscribed (about half are encapsulated). They vary in color from tan to grayish white and contain foci of hemorrhage, necrosis, and calcification. Vascular channels may be prominent on the capsular surface. *Epithelial* hepatoblastomas are solid, whereas the *mixed variety* are often separated into lobules by white bands of collagen tissue.

Two types of epithelial cells are present in the tumor.[40, 41, 97, 98] The first resemble *fetal* hepatocytes and are arranged in irregular plates, usually two cells thick, with bile canaliculi between individual cells and sinusoids between plates. The cytoplasm of the cells is eosinophilic and appears granular or vacuolated. Few mitotic figures are seen. Extramedullary hematopoiesis is generally present. The *embryonal* type of epithelial cells are less differentiated. They show weak cohesiveness and are usually arranged in sheets or ribbons. Individual cells are small, fusiform, and dark-staining, with irregular, ill-defined outlines. The cytoplasm of these cells is scanty and amphophilic. Nuclei contain abundant chromatin and large nucleoli.

Mixed hepatoblastomas contain mesenchymal tissue consisting of areas of a highly cellular primitive type of mesenchyme intimately admixed with epithelial elements. The cells are elongated and spindle-shaped, with delicate processes arising from the tapering ends. The cytoplasm is scanty, and the nuclei are elongated but plump. These tumors also contain areas in which the cells are intermediate between primitive mesenchyme and the acellular collagen of fibrous septa. The cells in these areas show parallel orientation, and collagen fibers are present between the cells. Cartilage may be present, as may striated muscle. Hepatoblastomas may show foci of squamous cells, with or without keratinization, and giant cells of the foreign-body type may occur in these foci. Vascular invasion may be evident. Metastases most commonly involve lung, abdominal lymph nodes, and brain.

Treatment and Prognosis

Hepatoblastoma is a rapidly progressive tumor.[97, 98] The *fetal* variety carries the least favorable prognosis; the *embryonal* and *mixed* types have a slightly better outlook. If the lesion is solitary and sufficiently localized to be resectable, surgery may be curative.[97, 98] In some patients in whom the tumor is thought to be inoperable, chemotherapy, with or without radiotherapy, may reduce the size of the tumor sufficiently that resection becomes feasible.[101] Encouraging results also have been obtained with liver transplantation.[102] If surgery is not an option, the prognosis is poor, because hepatoblastomas do not respond consistently to radiotherapy or to currently used cancer chemotherapeutic agents.

Angiosarcoma

Epidemiology

Although rare, angiosarcoma (also known as malignant hemangioendothelioma, hemangioendothelial sarcoma, or Kupffer cell sarcoma) is the most common malignant mesenchymal tumor of the liver.[40, 41, 103–105] It occurs almost exclusively in adults and is most prevalent in the sixth and seventh decades of life.[40, 41, 103–105] Men are affected four times more often than women.[40, 41, 103–105]

Pathogenesis

Despite its rarity, hepatic angiosarcoma is of special interest because specific risk factors have been identified, although no cause is discerned in the majority of tumors. In early reports, the tumor became evident about 20 years after the patient had been exposed to thorium dioxide (Thorotrast).[106] Angiosarcoma has also occurred in German vintners who used arsenic-containing insecticides and drank wine adulterated with arsenic.[107] A few patients with angiosarcoma had taken potassium arsenite (Fowler's solution) for many years to treat psoriasis.[108] Hepatic angiosarcoma in workers exposed to vinyl chloride monomers was first reported in 1974.[103, 105, 109] Vinyl chloride monomers are converted by enzymes of the endoplasmic reticulum to reactive metabolites that bind covalently to DNA.[100, 102, 108] Angiosarcomas have occurred after exposures of 11 to 37 years (or sooner with a heavy initial exposure).[103, 105, 109] The mean age of patients at diagnosis is 48 years.

Clinical Presentation

The most common presenting symptom is upper abdominal pain, but other frequent complaints are abdominal swelling, rapidly progressing liver failure, malaise, weight loss, poor appetite, and nausea.[103–105, 109] Vomiting occasionally occurs. The duration of symptoms is generally between 1 week and 6 months, but a few patients have had symptoms for as long as 2 years. The liver is almost always enlarged and usually tender. Its surface may be irregular, or a definite mass may be felt.[103–105, 109] An arterial bruit occasionally is heard over the enlarged liver. Splenomegaly may be present and is attributed to the hepatic fibrosis and consequent portal hypertension that are also complications of exposure to vinyl chloride monomers. Ascites is not infrequent, and the fluid may be blood-stained. The patient often has jaundice. Fever and dependent edema are less common. Approximately 15% of patients present with acute hemperitoneum following tumor rupture. Rarely, pulmonary or skeletal metastases are present.

Diagnosis

There may be a rising serum bilirubin concentration and other evidence of progressive hepatic dysfunction, especially in the later stages of the tumor.[103–105, 109] Plain radiography may show pulmonary metastases, a raised right hemidiaphragm, or rarely, skeletal metastases. In patients who received thorium dioxide, radiopaque deposits of the material may be evident in the liver and spleen.[103–105, 109] One or more mass lesions may be demonstrated on ultrasonography, but diffusely infiltrating tumor may not be visualized. Hepatic arteriography reveals a characteristic appearance.[110] The hepatic arteries are displaced by the tumor, which shows a blush and puddling during the middle of the arterial phase that persist for many seconds, except in the central area, which may be hypovascular.[110]

Complications and Prognosis

Hepatic angiosarcomas grow rapidly, and the prognosis is poor; death ensues within 6 months.[103–105, 109] Patients may have thrombocytopenia resulting from entrapment of platelets within the tumor (Kasabach-Merritt syndrome),[104] disseminated intravascular coagulation with secondary fibrinolysis,[111] or microangiopathic hemolytic anemia as a result of fragmentation of erythrocytes within the tumor circulation.[112]

Pathology

Angiosarcomas are usually multicentric.[40, 41, 113] Their hallmark is blood-filled cysts, although solid growth is also evident. The lesions are fairly well circumscribed but not encapsulated. Larger masses are spongy and bulge beneath Glisson's capsule.

The earliest microscopic change is the presence of hypertrophic sinusoidal lining cells with hyperchromatic nuclei in ill-defined loci throughout the liver.[40, 41, 113] With progression of the lesion, sinusoidal dilatation and disruption of hepatic plates occurs, and the malignant cells become supported by collagen tissue. Enlarging vascular spaces lined by malignant cells cause the tumor to become cavernous. The malignant endothelial cells are usually multilayered and may project into the cavity in intricate fronds and tufts supported by fibrous tissue. They are commonly elongated with ill-defined borders.[40, 41, 113] The cytoplasm is clear and faintly eosinophilic. Nuclei are hyperchromatic and vary greatly in size and shape, and some cells are multinucleate. Evidence of phagocytosis may be seen. Foci of extramedullary hematopoiesis are common and invasion of the portal and central veins occurs in most cases. Distant metastases occur in 50% of tumors.

Treatment

Operative treatment is usually precluded by the advanced stage of the tumor.[103, 105] Even when surgery is undertaken, the patient commonly survives only 1 to 3 years.[103, 105] The results of irradiation and chemotherapy are poor.

Hepatic Metastases

The liver is the most frequent target for metastatic spread of tumors. Hepatic metastases occur in 40% to 50% of adult patients with extrahepatic primary malignancies.[40, 114] Foremost among the reasons for the high frequency of hepatic metastases are the double blood supply of the liver and the presence of fenestrations in the sinusoidal endothelium that facilitate penetration of malignant cells into the hepatic parenchyma.[115] Hepatic metastases commonly originate from primary sites in the distribution of the portal venous system. Outside this system, the lung and the breast are the most common organs of origin of hepatic metastases.[40, 114]

Clinical Presentation

Often, hepatic metastases are clinically silent, or their symptoms are overshadowed by those of the primary tumor. Occasionally, the symptoms and signs attributable to metastases are the presenting manifestations of an asymptomatic primary tumor. In such cases, the likely symptoms are malaise, weight loss, and upper abdominal pain. Jaundice, when present, is generally a complication of the primary tumor and seldom attributable to replacement of hepatic tissue by metastases. Depending on the extent of the metastatic disease, the liver may be enlarged, sometimes markedly. Its surface may be irregular, and umbilicated nodules may be felt. A friction rub may be heard over hepatic metastases.

Macroscopic Appearance

Hepatic metastases are almost always multiple.[40, 114] Their pathologic features vary depending on their site of origin. They are expansive, when they are discrete, or infiltrative. Individual metastases may reach a large size, and with multiple metastases, the liver may be large. Metastases are commonly gray-white and may show scattered hemorrhages or central necrosis. Individual metastases may be surrounded by a zone of venous stasis. Subcapsular lesions are often umbilicated. The old teaching that cirrhotic livers are less likely than noncirrhotic livers to harbor metastatic deposits remains to be verified.

Microscopic Appearance

The microscopic features, including the degree of stromal growth, of most hepatic metastases duplicate those of the tumor of origin. Metastatic deposits are usually delineated easily from the surrounding liver tissue. Invasion of portal or hepatic veins may be seen, although less often than with hepatocellular carcinoma.[40, 114]

Diagnosis

Ultrasonography is generally used for initial screening, although CT is the most useful imaging technique.[116] CT portography, contrast-enhanced CT, and spiral CT are more sensitive than conventional CT. Dynamic contrast-enhanced Doppler ultrasonography with intra-arterial infusion of CO_2 microbubbles also has a place in the diagnosis of hepatic metastases.[34] T_1-weighted MRI may also be useful, and iron-oxide enhanced MRI is even better. Hepatic arteriography shows most hepatic metastases to have a poor blood supply.

Treatment and Prognosis

The extent of the replacement of liver tissue by metastases generally determines the patient's prognosis. The greater the tumor burden, the worse the outlook, and only about 50% of patients survive for 3 months after the onset of symptoms; fewer than 10% survive beyond 1 year.[117] Improved imaging modalities, advances in surgical techniques for resection and transplantation, and new chemotherapeutic agents and regional therapies have, however, made it possible to achieve long-term survival in individual patients.[117] Long-term survival has been accomplished most often by resection of hepatic metastases in patients with colorectal cancer, for which a substantial number of patients have been cured or have obtained up to 20 years of disease-free survival.[117–119] If the primary tumor has been removed completely and metastases are confined to the liver, resection of hepatic metastases is worth considering, if feasible. Liver transplantation, with or without chemotherapy, has been performed in a few patients. Less invasive methods of destroying metastases, such as ethanol injection, radiofrequency ablation, freezing with cryoprobes, and laser vaporization, warrant further study. Radiation therapy and intra-arterial infusion of cytotoxic drugs have limited roles.

Benign Liver Tumors

Hepatocellular Adenoma

Epidemiology and Pathogenesis

Hepatocellular adenomas were extremely rare before the use of oral contraceptive steroids became widespread. They are still rare in men, but the number of women in whom this tumor develops while or after they take contraceptive steroids strongly implies a cause-and-effect relationship.[120–123] Nevertheless, in light of the large number of women who use this form of contraception, the risk of hepatic adenoma is small, and its occurrence implies some form of genetic predisposition to this complication.[123] The association is particularly strong with prolonged use; the estimated risk for women who use oral contraceptive agents continuously for 5 to 7 years is five times the normal rate, and this figure increases to 25 times with use longer than 9 years. Treatment with preparations that have a high potency of hormone further increases the risk. Contraceptive pill–associated hepatocellular adenomas are more likely to develop in older than younger women.[120–123]

Hepatocellular adenomas have been linked to both types of synthetic estrogen and all forms of progestogen contained in oral contraceptive preparations.[120–123] Current evidence favors estrogens as the culprit, although progestogens may contribute through their enzyme-inducing properties. The growth of hepatocellular adenomas appears to be hormone dependent,[120–123] as evidenced by occasional instances of the slow regression of the tumor after cessation of oral contraceptive use and an increase in size during pregnancy.

Hepatocellular adenomas also may occur in persons receiving long-term anabolic androgenic steroids[40] and in those with a number of inherited metabolic disturbances, especially type 1 glycogen storage disease, in which one or more hepatocellular adenomas occur in about 60% of patients.[122]

Clinical Presentation

Hepatocellular adenomas present in a number of ways.[120–123] They may produce no symptoms and, if large, may be discovered during routine physical examination or, if small, during imaging of the upper abdomen for other reasons. About one fourth of patients experience pain in the right hypochondrium or epigastrium. The pain is usually mild and ill-defined but may be severe as a result of bleeding into or infarction of the tumor. If enlarged, the surface of the liver is usually smooth and may be slightly tender. The most alarming presentation is with an acute hemoperitoneum following rupture of the adenoma. This complication is not uncommon, especially with tumors linked to oral contraceptive use, and carries an appreciable mortality rate.[120–123] Tumors that rupture are generally large and solitary, although the most important determinant of rupture is a superficial location. Often, the affected woman is menstruating at the time.

Diagnosis

Serum α-fetoprotein concentrations are normal. Ultrasonography is used for initial imaging. Tissue harmonic imaging, which is obtained by receiving the second harmonic frequency signals, is capable of increased spatial and contrast resolution and less acoustic artifact than standard ultrasound and has facilitated the detection of these (and other) tumors in obese subjects.[34] Hepatic angiography is the most useful aid to diagnosis.[123] Approximately 50% of hepatocellular adenomas are avascular, with draping of the hepatic arteries around the lesion; the remainder are hypervascular. The tumor has a clearly defined margin and, often, nearly parallel vessels entering it from the periphery ("spoke-wheel appearance"). Alternatively, the lesion contains tortuous vessels coursing irregularly through it. When hypervascular, the adenoma may have focal avascular areas as a result of hemorrhage or necrosis. MRI may prove to be a useful alternative to hepatic angiography in the diagnosis of hepatocellular adenomas. Because adenomas mimic normal liver tissue microscopically, needle biopsy and fine-needle aspiration may be of limited value.

Pathology

A hepatocellular adenoma generally occurs as a solitary, relatively soft, light brown to yellow tumor. It is sharply circumscribed but does not have a true capsule, although a pseudocapsule is formed by compression of the surrounding liver tissue[40, 41, 123, 124] (Fig. 81–5*A*). Hepatocellular adenomas arise in an otherwise normal liver. Occasionally, two or more tumors are present. Adenomas range in size from 1 to 30 cm, but are commonly 8 to 15 cm in diameter. They are larger in women taking contraceptive steroids and usually occupy a subcapsular position and project slightly from the surface of the liver. A pedunculated variety is seen occasionally. The cut surface of the tumor may show ill-defined lobulation but is never nodular or fibrotic. Foci of hemorrhage or necrosis are frequent, and bile staining may be evident.

Microscopically, a hepatocellular adenoma may mimic normal liver tissue to an astonishing degree[40, 41, 123, 124] (Fig. 81–5*B*). It is composed of sheets or cords of normal-looking or slightly atypical hepatocytes that show no features of malignancy. The cells occasionally have an acinar arrangement. The hepatocytes are usually slightly larger and may be paler than normal, with cytoplasm that is finely vacuolated or granular, and may be loaded with glycogen. Eosinophilic inclusions containing α_1-antitrypsin are often present. The nuclei show minimal variation in structure or size. Sinusoids are focally dilated, and Kupffer cells are either markedly reduced in number or absent. There are few or no portal tracts or central veins, and bile ducts are conspicuously absent. Only an infrequent fibrous or vascular septum traverses the lesion. An essentially normal reticulin pattern is demonstrable throughout the adenoma. The walls of arteries and veins are thickened. Some areas with vascular abnormalities are infarcted, and thromboses may be seen. Peliosis hepatis may be found in relation to the tumor.

Treatment and Prognosis

Because of the danger that a hepatocellular adenoma will rupture, surgical treatment is recommended.[124] Resection is

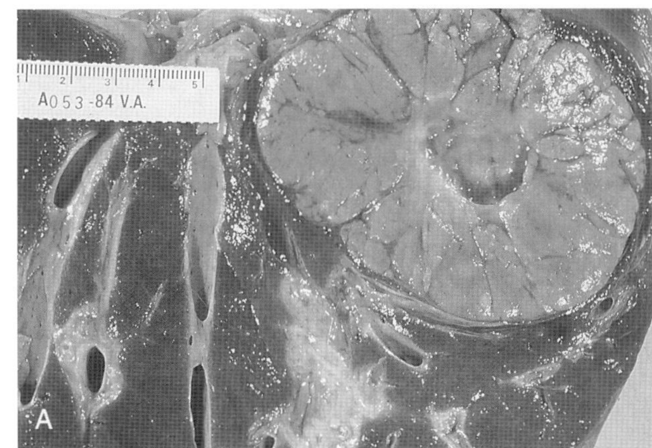

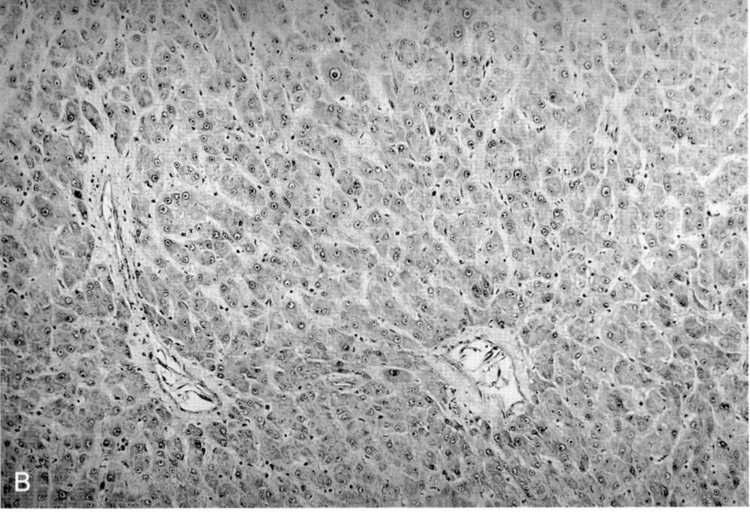

Figure 81–5. (*A*) Gross specimen of a large hepatocellular adenoma. The tumor is yellowish and slightly lobular with a central cavitation and a pseudocapsule. (Courtesy of Edward Lee, MD, Dallas VA Medical Center, Dallas, TX.) (B) Photomicrograph of a hepatocellular adenoma showing the resemblance to normal liver tissue, with cords of normal-looking, although generally slightly larger, hepatocytes and Kupffer cells (although fewer in number than normal) lining the sinusoids. Bile ducts and central veins are not seen, but the presence of abnormal vascular structures is evident. (Courtesy of Professor A. C. Paterson.)

usually feasible in an uncomplicated case. When rupture has occurred, emergency resection should be performed if possible. (It may be necessary to clamp the hepatic artery first to stop the bleeding.) If resection cannot be accomplished, the hepatic artery should be ligated. The patient must refrain from taking oral contraceptive steroids, whether or not the tumor is removed. If the adenoma is not resected, pregnancy should be avoided.

Hepatocellular carcinoma occurs in a small number of women taking oral contraceptive steroids,[60, 125] and there is speculation that hepatocellular adenomas might undergo malignant transformation. Indeed, this sequence has been documented in a few instances.[126] Therefore, there is a risk to managing hepatocellular adenomas merely by discontinuing the use of contraceptive steroids.

Cavernous Hemangioma

Epidemiology

Cavernous hemangioma is the most common benign tumor of the liver and is present in as many as 7% of necropsies.[40, 124] The lesion is thought to be a congenital malformation or hamartoma that increases in size initially with growth of the liver and thereafter by ectasia. Cavernous hemangiomas present at all ages, although most often in the third, fourth, and fifth decades. Women are predominantly affected (4 : 1 to 6 : 1) and often present at a younger age and with larger tumors than men.[40, 124] Cavernous hemangiomas increase in size with pregnancy or the administration of estrogens and are more common in multiparous than nulliparous women.[40, 124]

Clinical Presentation

The great majority of cavernous hemangiomas are small and asymptomatic and are discovered incidentally when the liver is imaged for another reason, at necropsy, or at laparotomy.[40, 124] Larger or multiple lesions produce symptoms. Those larger than 4 cm are called giant cavernous hemangiomas, which may be as large as 27 cm. Upper abdominal pain is the most common complaint and results from partial infarction of the lesion or pressure on adjacent tissues. Early satiety, nausea, and vomiting also may occur. Cavernous hemangiomas occasionally rupture. The only physical finding may be an enlarged liver. Occasionally, an arterial bruit is heard over the tumor.

Diagnosis

The ultrasonographic appearance is variable and nonspecific, although the lesion is usually echogenic.[127] Provided that the cavernous hemangioma is larger than 3 cm, single-photon emission computed tomography (SPECT) with colloid 99^{m}Tc-labeled red blood cells shows the tumor to be highly vascular and has a sensitivity and accuracy similar to that of MRI.[128] Almost all cavernous hemangiomas can be diagnosed by bolus-enhanced CT with sequential scans.[127] The center of the lesion remains hypodense, whereas the peripheral zone, which varies in thickness and may have a corrugated inner margin, enhances. MRI has a high degree of specificity and a central role in the diagnosis of small hemangiomas (Fig. 81–6).[129] Another useful investigation is hepatic arteriography.[127] The branches of the hepatic artery may be displaced and crowded together or stretched around the lesion. They do, however, taper normally. There is early opacification of irregular areas or lakes, and the contrast material persists in these lakes long after arterial emptying. With small hemangiomas, the contrast material may appear as ring-shaped or C-shaped, with an avascular center resulting from fibrous obliteration; this appearance is pathognomonic. Thrombocytopenia resulting from sequestration and destruction of platelets in large hemangiomas (Kasabach-Merritt syndrome) is seen occasionally in children but rarely in adults.[130] Hypofibrinogenemia, attributed to fibrin deposition in the tumor with secondary fibrinolysis, is also described.[131] Malignant transformation has not been reported.

Because of the risk of severe bleeding, percutaneous needle biopsy should not be performed if a cavernous heman-

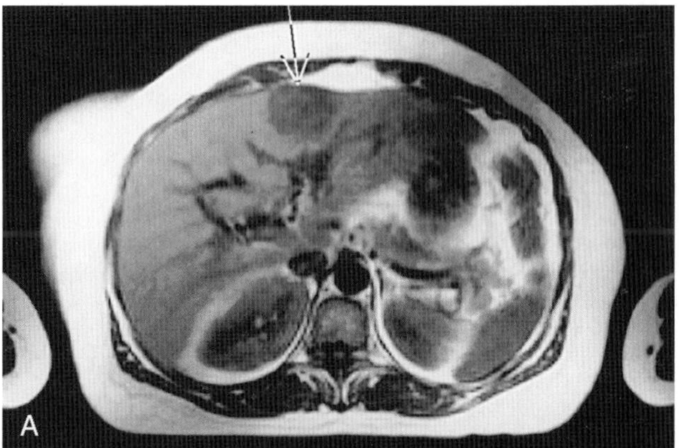

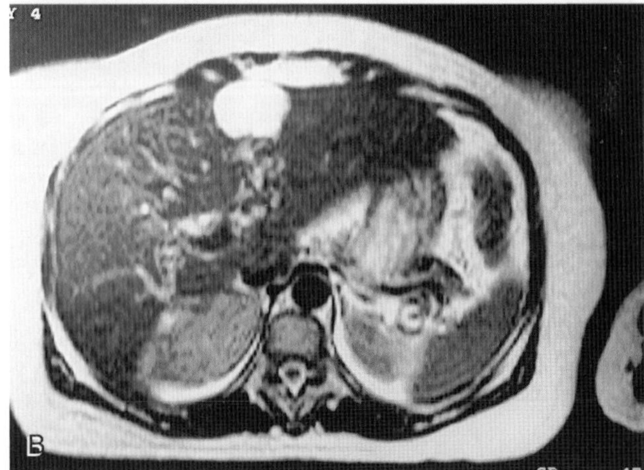

Figure 81–6. Magnetic resonance image of a small cavernous hemangioma in the liver (arrow). *A*, T1-weighted image shows a rounded mass with a uniform raised T1 signal (low signal). *B*, Heavily T2-weighted image shows a mass with a uniform raised T2 signal (bright signal compared with the water signal of cerebrospinal fluid). (Courtesy of Dr. P. Sneider.)

gioma is suspected. Moreover, a needle biopsy is of limited diagnostic value.

Pathology

Cavernous hemangiomas are usually solitary, although multiple tumors occur in 10% of patients.[40, 41, 124] Reddish purple or bluish masses are seen under Glisson's capsule or deep in the substance of the liver. The larger lesions may be pedunculated. Cavernous hemangiomas are well circumscribed but seldom encapsulated. They may show central necrosis, and in some instances, the whole tumor has a firm grayish white appearance. Microscopically, hemangiomas are composed of multiple vascular channels of varying sizes, lined by a single layer of flat epithelium and supported by fibrous septa.[40, 41, 124] The vascular spaces may contain thrombi.

Occasionally, cavernous hemangiomas are associated with hemangiomas in other organs. They also may coexist with cysts in the liver or pancreas.[132] von Meyenburg complexes,[133] or focal nodular hyperplasia.[134]

Treatment

The great majority of cavernous hemangiomas can be left alone safely. A cavernous hemangioma that is large, but localized, and the cause of incapacitating symptoms, should be resected.[135] If resection is not feasible, reduction in the size of the tumor with relief of symptoms is rarely achieved with irradiation, arterial ligation, arteriographic embolization, or systemic glucocorticoids.[136, 137] If a cavernous hemangioma has ruptured, it may be necessary to embolize or clamp the hepatic artery to stop bleeding before proceeding to resection.

Infantile Hemangioendothelioma

Epidemiology and Clinical Presentation

Benign infantile hemangioendothelioma (also known as multinodular hepatic hemangiomatosis) is a rare but important tumor of the liver. Its importance stems from the high incidence of congestive cardiac failure in infants with this tumor and the resulting 70% mortality rate. The tumor almost invariably presents in the first 6 months of life and is twice as common in girls as boys.[40, 122, 138, 139] Hepatic hemangioendothelioma often coexists with hemangiomas in other organs, especially the skin (in about 50% of patients). When benign hemangiomas are present in three or more organs, the condition is referred to as diffuse neonatal hemangiomatosis.

Small hemangioendotheliomas are asymptomatic.[122, 138, 139] The presence of a large lesion is recognized clinically by the diagnostic triad of an enlarged liver, high-output cardiac failure, and multiple cutaneous hemangiomas.[122, 138, 139] The size of the liver is disproportionate to the severity of the cardiac failure, and hepatomegaly persists after the latter has been treated successfully. When hemangioendotheliomas occur diffusely throughout the liver, as they usually do, their combined effect is to act as a large peripheral arteriovenous shunt. Shunts of this size are responsible for the cardiac failure.[122, 138, 139] About one third of patients have jaundice. They may be anemic, owing in part to the dilutional effect of the increased circulating plasma volume that develops with large peripheral arteriovenous fistulas. A microangiopathic hemolytic anemia may contribute.[139] In addition, thrombocytopenia may be present (Kasabach-Merritt syndrome).[139] Malignant change is a rare complication.[40]

Diagnosis

Ultrasonography may show one or more echogenic masses in the liver. Hepatic angiography is particularly helpful in diagnosis and shows stretching, but not displacement, of the intrahepatic arteries.[140] Abnormal vessels arise from the hepatic arteries and promptly opacify the liver, thereby giving rise to the characteristic blush of an arteriovenous shunt. The circulation time through the liver is short. Focal avascular areas may be evident when hemorrhage into, or necrosis of, the tumor has occurred. CT with enhancement or MRI are as specific as hepatic arteriography for the diagnosis of hemangioendotheliomas. Percutaneous biopsy is contraindicated because of the danger of bleeding.

Pathology

Infantile hemangioendotheliomas are typically multifocal and produce a nodular deformity of the whole liver.[40, 41, 124, 138, 139] The nodules range in size from a few millimeters to many centimeters and are well demarcated but not encapsulated. At laparotomy, the nodules can be seen to pulsate. They are reddish purple, although large tumors are gray to tan. They may show hemorrhages, fibrosis, or calcification. Microscopically, infantile hemangioendothelioma is composed of layers of plump endothelial cells.[40, 41, 124, 138, 139] A single layer characterizes a *type I pattern*, whereas several layers characterize a *type II pattern*. In some areas of the tumor, solid masses of mesoblastic primordial cells that differentiate early into vascular structures are observed. Fibrous septa may be prominent, and extramedullary hematopoiesis occurs frequently. Thrombosis may be followed by scarring and calcification.

Treatment and Prognosis

The course of infantile hemangioendothelioma is characterized by growth during the early months of life, followed by gradual involution.[139] If the child survives, the tumor involutes completely. Life-threatening aspects of the disorder are intractable congestive cardiac failure and, to a lesser extent, rupture of the tumor. Cardiac failure should be treated by conventional means initially, but, if these measures fail, more aggressive forms of treatment, such as embolization, ligation of the hepatic artery, or surgical resection, should be tried.[138, 139, 141] Gucocorticoids have been successful in many (but not all) patients,[142] whereas irradiation has seldom been beneficial. When the tumor is confined to one lobe, surgical resection is curative, even in the presence of cardiac failure.[139, 140]

TUMOR-LIKE LESIONS

Focal Nodular Hyperplasia

Focal nodular hyperplasia is a circumscribed, usually solitary, lesion composed of nodules of benign hyperplastic hepatocytes surrounding a central stellate fibrous scar.[39, 40]

Epidemiology and Pathogenesis

Although rare, focal nodular hyperplasia is more common than hepatocellular adenoma. The lesion is seen more often in women than men, although the sex difference is less striking than that of hepatocellular adenoma.[120–122] Focal nodular hyperplasia occurs at all ages, but the great majority of patients present in the third and fourth decades,[120–122] an age distribution similar to that of hepatocellular adenomas.

The cause of focal nodular hyperplasia is unknown. Abnormalities in arteries in small and medium-sized portal tracts have been described, and an ischemic origin, related to vascular malformation, is possible. A role for oral contraceptive steroids in the development of the lesion was suggested, but there is no unequivocal evidence in support of such an association.[120–122] There is, nevertheless, some evidence that focal nodular hyperplasia is hormone dependent.[120–122, 143] Contraceptive steroids may accentuate the vascular abnormalities in focal nodular hyperplasia and cause the lesion to enlarge, become more symptomatic, and, rarely, rupture.

Clinical Presentation

Most of these lesions do not produce symptoms and are discovered during upper abdominal imaging for other reasons, during abdominal surgery or necropsy, or because the clinician detects an enlarged liver on routine examination.[120–122] Mild pain may be felt, particularly with bleeding into or necrosis of the lesion. This presentation is more common in patients taking contraceptive steroids.[120–122] Focal nodular hyperplasia seldom ruptures, even in patients taking oral contraceptive steroids.

Diagnosis

Serum α-fetoprotein levels are normal. The mass lesion seen on ultrasonography and CT is not specific for focal nodular hyperplasia,[123] although the central scar may be seen (Fig. 81–7). The picture obtained with dynamic contrast-enhanced Doppler ultrasonography with intra-arterial infusion of CO_2 microbubbles is, however, characteristic.[34] Selective hepatic arteriography shows one or more highly vascular lesions.[123, 144] The vessels within the lesion are tortuous. In about 50% of cases, septation of the mass is visible during the capillary phase, which is also characterized by irregular granularity. However, it is often impossible to distinguish focal nodular hyperplasia from hepatocellular adenoma on the basis of the arteriographic findings.

Pathology

Focal nodular hyperplasia presents as a firm, coarsely nodular light brown or yellowish gray mass of variable size with

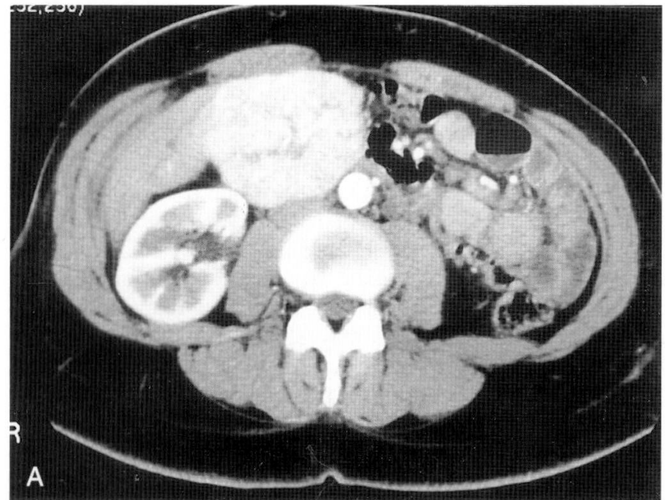

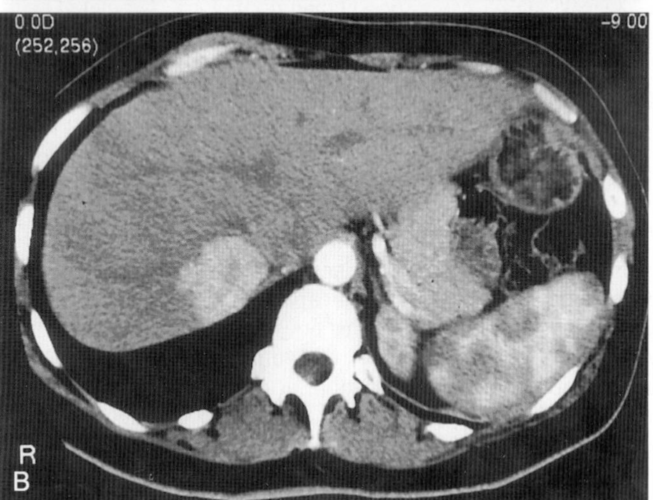

Figure 81–7. Contrast-enhanced computed tomogram in a 41-year-old woman with two lesions of focal nodular hyperplasia, one in the left hepatic lobe (*A*), the other in the right (*B*). The central stellate scar with radiating bands of fibrosis can be seen in each of the lesions.

a dense, central stellate scar and radiating fibrous septa that divide the lesion into lobules.[40, 41, 120–122, 144] The nodule may be small, resembling a cirrhotic nodule, or extremely large. Focal nodular hyperplasia usually occupies a subcapsular position and may be pedunculated. It is generally solitary, but there may be multiple lesions. Larger lesions may show foci of hemorrhage or necrosis, although these are seen less frequently than in hepatocellular adenomas. The fibrous septa are sometimes poorly developed, and the central scar may be absent. The lesion is sharply demarcated from the surrounding liver tissue, which is normal, but there is no true capsule. Focal nodular hyperplasia is associated with hepatic hemangiomas in 5% to 10% of patients.

Microscopically, focal nodular hyperplasia closely resembles inactive cirrhosis.[40, 41, 120–122, 144] Individual hepatocytes are indistinguishable from those of normal liver, but they lack the normal cord arrangement in relation to sinusoids, central veins, and portal tracts. The cytoplasm is finely granular but may be vacuolated. Kupffer cells are present. Characteristically, the fibrous septa contain numerous bile ductules and vessels. In addition, there are heavy infiltrations of lymphocytes and, to a lesser extent, plasma cells and histiocytes. Bile duct proliferation in portal tracts also may be evident. Branches of the hepatic artery and portal vein show various combinations of intimal and smooth muscle hyperplasia, subintimal fibrosis, thickening of the wall, occlusive luminal lesions, and, at times, occluding thrombosis. Whether these vascular changes are primary or secondary is not known. Peliosis hepatis may be an associated lesion. The histologic features almost always make it possible to distinguish focal nodular hyperplasia from hepatocellular adenoma, although the distinction may be extremely difficult in a few instances.

Treatment

Large symptomatic or complicated lesions should be resected, usually by segmental resection or enucleation. Recurrence after resection is rare. Otherwise, focal nodular hyperplasia should be left alone. If the lesion is not resected, any contraceptive steroids should be discontinued. Pregnancy should also be avoided. Periodic ultrasonography should be performed if a firm diagnosis of focal nodular hyperplasia has not been made, and a lesion seen to increase substantially in size should be resected. There is no convincing evidence that focal nodular hyperplasia is a premalignant condition.

Other Nodular Disorders

Nodular regenerative hyperplasia is characterized by nodularity of the liver without fibrosis[40] (see also Chapters 62 and 82). This rare condition may be associated with a number of diseases, such as rheumatoid arthritis and Felty syndrome. Although generally diffuse, the nodularity is occasionally focal, in which case it may be mistaken for a tumor. Patients with nodular regenerative hyperplasia typically present clinically with portal hypertension. Partial nodular transformation is characterized by nodules that are limited to the perihilar region of the liver. These patients also present with portal hypertension.[40, 41]

Macroregenerative nodules may occur in advanced cirrhosis or after massive hepatic necrosis. They are believed to be premalignant conditions and may, in addition, be mistaken for hepatic tumors during hepatic imaging. Inflammatory pseudotumor is a rare entity resulting from focal infection and that may be mistaken for a hepatic tumor.[41] It occurs particularly in young men, who present with intermittent fever, abdominal pain, jaundice, vomiting, and diarrhea. Leukocytosis, an elevated erythrocyte sedimentation rate, and polyclonal hyperglobulinemia are present in about 50% of the patients. The lesion may be solitary or multiple and shows a mixture of chronic inflammatory cells, with plasma cells predominating. Focal fatty infiltration, or focal fatty sparing in the presence of diffuse fatty infiltration, may also be mistaken for a hepatic tumor.[145]

HEPATIC CYSTS

Hepatic cysts are of three main types—hydatid cysts, a group of conditions collectively known as fibrocystic diseases of the liver, and solitary congenital cysts.

Hydatid Cysts

Hydatid cysts (echinococcosis) of the liver are caused by small tapeworms of the genus *Echinococcus* (see also Chapter 69). The disease in humans results from infestation by *Echinococcus granulosis*, less often *Echinococcus multilocularis*, or rarely, *Echinococcus vogeli*.

Echinococcus granulosis

E. granulosis has a worldwide distribution but is most prevalent in sheep- and cattle-raising regions. The adult tapeworm lives in the upper small bowel of the definitive host, usually a domestic dog. Other definitive hosts include wolves, jackals, hyenas, dingoes, kangaroos, pumas, reindeer, and domestic cats. Sheep, cattle, pigs, and humans are the intermediate hosts of the larval stage of the infestation.

The adult tapeworm consists of a scolex, which contains a rostellum with 20 to 50 hooklets and 4 suckers, a neck, and an immature, mature, and gravid proglottid. The gravid proglottid ruptures, either in the bowel or after passage in the feces, and the eggs are ingested as a contaminant by the intermediate host. The external shell of the egg is digested by gastric juice or pancreatic enzymes, freeing the larvae (embryos), which penetrate the bowel mucosa, enter portal venous blood, and are carried to the liver. About 70% of the larvae are trapped in the liver, and approximately 20% in the lungs. The remainder are carried through the circulation to organs such as the spleen, kidney, and brain. The embryos that survive the host's defense mechanisms become encysted and grow at a rate of about 1 cm per year. The hydatid cyst is composed of a fibrous and inflammatory outer layer of host origin, a laminated cuticle, and a germinal membrane. The germinal membrane forms daughter cysts. The life cycle is completed when the definitive host ingests infected viscera of the intermediate host, the scolices are freed, and the cysts become attached to the bowel mucosa and grow into adult worms.

Most patients with a hydatid cyst in the liver have no symptoms,[146, 147] and the presence of a cyst becomes evident when the liver is found to be enlarged or a cystic lesion is noted when the liver is imaged for other reasons. Large cysts (usually more than 10 cm in diameter) may cause pain, but otherwise symptoms are the result of complications of the cyst.[146–148] The cyst may rupture into the biliary system, either spontaneously or more usually after blunt abdominal trauma.[148] The patient then presents with cholangitis, with or without obstructive jaundice, accompanied by marked eosinophilia. Pancreatitis may develop as a complication. Cysts also may become infected, obstruct major intrahepatic bile ducts, or, rarely, cause portal hypertension.[146, 147] Subcapsular cysts may become pedunculated or may rupture into the peritoneal cavity (when the patient may present with anaphylactic shock) or into the bowel. Subdiaphragmatic cysts may perforate the diaphragm and enter the pleural cavity, lung, or pericardial sac.[146, 147]

Apart from eosinophilia, which is present in about 40% of patients, routine laboratory investigations are of little help in diagnosis.[149] Serologic tests for hydatidosis are positive in up to 90% of patients.[149] The Casoni test is no longer used. Plain abdominal radiography may show show calcification of the cyst lining.[150] Ultrasound examination and CT are useful in diagnosis, especially when daughter cysts are visualized.[150]

The treatment of hydatid cysts in the liver is primarily surgical.[149] A small superficial cyst can be excised with a rim of liver tissue. With larger cysts, great care must be taken to avoid spillage of the cyst contents into the peritoneal cavity. The area around the cyst should be isolated using lotion cloths soaked in 20% saline, and a small-bore needle should be used to aspirate the contents of the cyst. Twenty percent saline, cetrimide, or silver nitrate should then be injected into the cyst and allowed to remain for at least 10 minutes, to kill the daughter cysts, before being aspirated from the cavity. The cyst can then be removed. Calcified cysts need not be removed, and small cysts located deep within the liver are better treated nonoperatively.

Cysts that cannot be removed surgically should be treated with albendazole, preferably, or mebendazole.[149, 151] Large doses are required, and they need to be given over a prolonged period. In general, the results of nonoperative treatment of hydatid cysts are disappointing, although long-term control has been described using a technique of cyst aspiration, injection of a scolicidal agent, and reaspiration (see Chapter 69.)

Echinococcus Multilocularis

The definitive hosts of *E. multilocularis* are foxes, dogs, wolves, and domestic cats, and the intermediate hosts are small rodents (such as tundra mice) and humans. The cysts have a wide geographic distribution; the main endemic areas are central Europe, Russia, Turkey, Japan, Kurile islands, China, Alaska, and northern Canada.[152] *E. multilocularis* occurs less frequently than *E. granulosis*. *E. multilocularis* has the same basic structure as *E. granulosis* but with some internal differences. The liver is the primary site of the infestation in 90% of patients. Daughter cysts arise from the germinal membrane by budding on the outside of the original cyst in an uncontrolled manner. This results in "invasion" of the surrounding parenchyma by the scolices, a pattern of growth reminiscent of that in malignant neoplasms.[152] There is no cyst wall. Invasion of bile ducts and vessels and necrosis of the central parts of the parasitic tissue may result in cholangitis, liver abscess formation, septicemia, portal hypertension, hepatic vein occlusion, or biliary cirrhosis.[152, 153] The daughter hydatids may "metastasize" to distant organs, especially the lungs, which are involved in 20% of patients. Unless the lesion can be resected entirely or liver transplantation performed, the prognosis is poor.[152, 153] Long-term progression of the disease may be slowed by the administration of benzimadazole carbamates.[152, 153]

Fibrocystic Diseases of the Liver

This group of conditions originates from abnormal persistence or defects in the progressive remodeling of the ductal plate. The result is ductal plate malformation, with variations that give rise to a spectrum of congenital diseases of the intrahepatic bile ducts[154, 155] (see also Chapter 52). The cystic disorders of the liver included are polycystic liver disease, solitary congenital cysts, Caroli's disease (type V choledochal cyst), and von Meyenburg complexes. (The other diseases are congenital hepatic fibrosis and type IV choledochal cyst.)

Polycystic Liver Disease

Polycystic liver disease may present in childhood, when it has an autosomal recessive inheritance and is usually rapidly fatal as a consequence of the associated (autosomal recessive) polycystic kidney disease.[156–158] The liver cysts are microscopic rather than macroscopic and present a picture indistinguishable from congenital hepatic fibrosis. Complications of portal hypertension are the usual hepatic manifestations of the disease.[156–158]

More commonly, multiple cysts of the liver are diagnosed in adulthood. They present either in association with autosomal dominant polycystic kidney disease (ADPKD)[156] or as isolated polycystic liver disease.[159, 160] The gene affected in ADPKD1 is located on the short arm of chromosome 16 (q13–q23) and expresses a ubiquitous protein, polycystin-1.[161] The gene responsible for ADPKD2 is located on chromosome 4 and expresses polycystin-2.[162] The two polycystins are believed to work in concert to regulate calcium flux and cell signaling. The genetic defect underlying isolated polycystic liver disease has not yet been identified.[160]

Autosomal dominant polycystic kidney disease carries a better prognosis than the recessive variety.[156–158] Polycystic kidney disease has a more deleterious effect on kidney function than does the polycystic liver disease on hepatic function and largely determines the outcome. Hepatic cysts, which manifest later in life than the renal cysts, are usually diagnosed in the fourth or fifth decades.[156–158] The size and number of cysts correlate with the patient's age, severity of the renal disease, and worsening renal function. Women tend to have larger and more numerous cysts, and there is a correlation with the number of pregnancies. The use of exogenous female sex hormones may accelerate the rate of growth and size of the cysts. In the autosomal dominant variety, there also may be cysts in the pancreas and spleen and less often in other organs. In addition, autosomal dominant polycystic liver disease may coexist with the other fibropolycystic liver diseases, such as congenital hepatic fibrosis (in which the patient is likely to present with portal hypertension), Caroli's disease, or von Meyenburg complexes,[156–158] as well as other conditions such as berry aneurysms, mitral valve prolapse, diverticular disease, and inguinal hernias.

The hepatic cysts in polycystic liver disease, whether or not they occur in association with renal cysts, rarely cause morbidity, and many affected patients are asymptomatic.[156–159] These patients possess only a few cysts or cysts smaller than 2 cm in diameter. With the more widespread use of hepatic imaging, asymptomatic cysts are being discovered more often now than in the past. Symptoms occur in patients with more and larger cysts (10% to 15% of patients, almost always women), usually as abdominal discomfort or pain, postprandial fullness, an awareness of an upper abdominal mass, a protuberant abdomen, and shortness of breath. Severe pain may be felt with rupture or infection of a cyst, bleeding into a cyst, or torsion of a pedunculated cyst. The liver is enlarged in approximately 80% of patients. The associated polycystic kidneys are also often palpable. Jaundice is

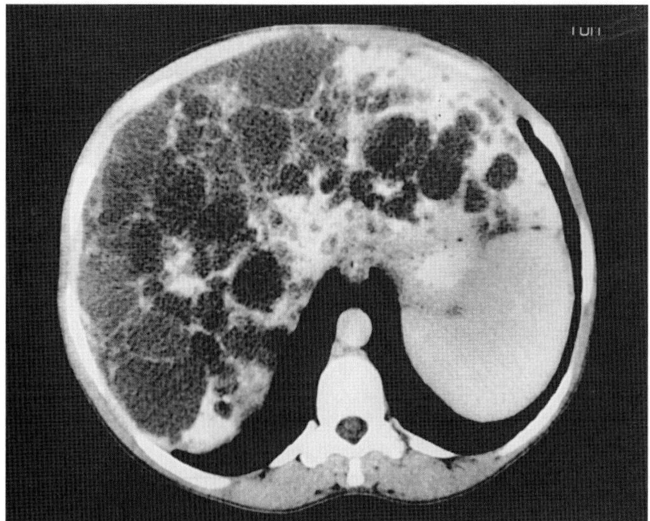

Figure 81–8. CT of liver in a patient with severe autosomal-dominant (adult) polycystic liver disease.

evident in about 5% of patients and is caused by compression of the major intrahepatic or extrahepatic bile ducts. Ascites, if present, is the result of portal hypertension, which is generally caused by the associated congenital hepatic fibrosis but occasionally by compression of the hepatic veins by the cysts.

Liver biochemical tests are generally not abnormal, although the alkaline phosphatase and γ-glutamyl transpeptidase levels may be increased. A raised right hemidiaphragm may be evident on a plain radiography of the chest in severe polycystic liver disease. The diagnosis of polycystic liver disease is confirmed by ultrasound examination or CT (Fig. 81–8).[163] Hepatic arteriography shows multiple avascular lesions with displacement of the vessels.

The cysts range in size from a few millimeters to 10 cm or more. They contain clear, colorless, or straw-colored fluid. The cysts are lined by a single layer of cuboidal or columnar epithelium, resembling that of bile ducts.[156–159] Rarely, the cysts may be lined by squamous epithelium, and these cysts may be complicated by the development of squamous carcinoma. In addition to the nature of their lining epithelium, evidence for a biliary origin is suggested by the composition of the cystic fluid, which has a low glucose content and contains secretory immunoglobulin A and γ-glutamyl transpeptidase. The cysts are thought to arise as a result of ductal plate malformation. This process gives rise to von Meyenburg complexes, which become disconnected from the biliary tree during development and growth and dilate progressively to form the cysts.[156–158]

On the rare occasions when a cyst requires treatment, fenestration should be performed.[156, 164] Cyst fenestration was originally done at laparotomy but is now performed laparoscopically. Cysts also have been treated by percutaneous injection of sclerosing substances such as alcohol or doxycycline, but most patients have too many cysts of insufficient size to warrant this approach. Patients who fail to respond to cyst fenestration may be considered for partial hepatic resection or liver transplantation (sometimes combined with renal transplantation).

Solitary Hepatic Cysts

Solitary hepatic cysts are relatively common, occurring in up to 3.6% of the population, and are typically asymptomatic.[165] They are discovered incidentally during upper abdominal imaging and are commonly less than 5 cm in diameter (Fig. 81–9). Solitary cysts occur more often in women than men, and their prevalence increases with age. Larger cysts or those complicated by intracystic bleeding or infection may produce discomfort or pain.

Asymptomatic solitary hepatic cysts should be left alone. If intervention is required, percutaneous aspiration and sclerosis with alcohol or doxycycline will almost always ablate the cyst, and recurrences are rare.[165] An alternative and equally successful approach is laparoscopic (or, less often, open surgical) fenestration.

Other Cystic Diseases of the Liver

von Meyenburg Complexes

von Meyenburg complexes (also known as biliary microhamartomas) are common and do not produce symptoms. von Meyenburg complexes are small and usually multiple. Each complex is composed of cystically dilated intra- and inter-lobular bile ducts embedded in a fibrous stroma.[41, 65] The cysts are lined by cuboidal or flat epithelium. They occur in almost all patients with congenital hepatic fibrosis and may coexist with Caroli's disease or autosomal dominant polycystic kidney disease. von Meyenburg complexes are found in or adjacent to portal tracts and are believed to arise as a result of malformation of the ductal plate. They may be complicated by the development of peripheral cholangiocarcinoma.[91]

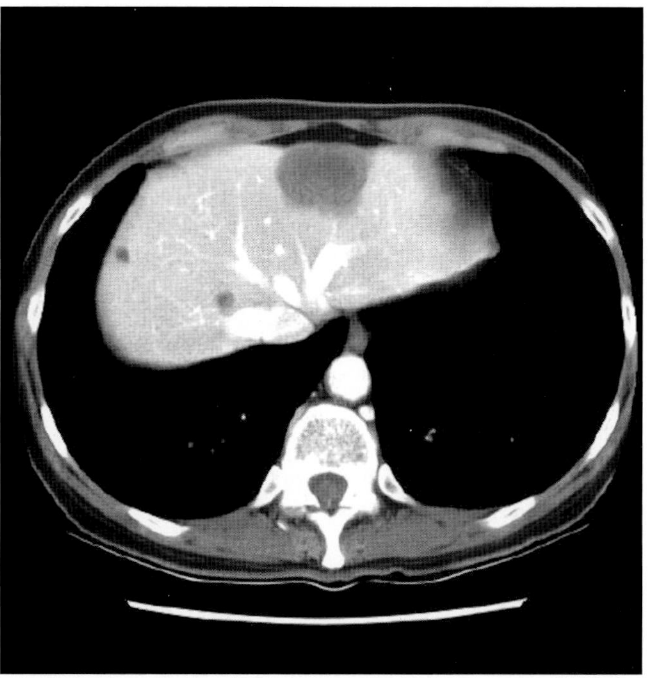

Figure 81–9. Computed tomogram showing a large solitary congenital cyst in the liver.

Caroli's Disease

Caroli's disease is characterized by gross segmental dilation of the intrahepatic bile ducts.[40, 165–167] The disease has been included in the classification of choledochal cysts (type V)[156, 165] and may occur in association with either medullary sponge kidney (in 60% to 80% of patients) or congenital hepatic fibrosis.[40] Caroli's disease is believed to be caused by an intrauterine event that arrests ductal plate remodeling at the level of the larger intrahepatic bile ducts.[155] The resulting bile duct ectasia may be diffuse or localized. Both autosomal recessive and dominant modes of inheritance have been proposed. Caroli's disease affects men and women equally and usually becomes symptomatic in early adulthood (more than 80% of patients present with symptoms before the age of 30 years).

Patients typically present with recurrent episodes of fever and abdominal pain caused by cholangitis. The liver may be enlarged. Ductal ectasia predisposes to bile stagnation, which in turn may lead to cholangitis, abscess formation, and septicemia.[166, 167] Gallstones form in the ectatic ducts in one third of patients.[166, 167] The result of these complications may be cholangiocarcinoma, which develops in 7% of patients.

Caroli's disease is usually discovered when the liver is imaged during investigation of suspected cholangitis. Irregular dilatations of the larger intrahepatic bile ducts are seen.

Attacks of cholangitis require treatment with antibiotics. Endoscopic retrograde cholangiography may be used to remove sludge or stones from the accessible part of the biliary system, and percutaneous transhepatic cholangiography may be used to drain the cysts. Localized forms of the disease may be treated by surgical resection.[168] Liver transplantation has been performed in patients with recurrent bouts of cholangitis unresponsive to endoscopic or radiologic intervention or with complications of the associated congenital hepatic fibrosis.

Peliosis Hepatis

Peliosis hepatis is characterized by blood-filled cavities in the liver of varying sizes that may or may not be lined by epithelium.[41, 169] The lesions may be diffuse or focal. They occur in a variety of chronic diseases, such as malnutrition, tuberculosis, aquired immunodeficiency syndrome, and a number of malignant diseases and also are associated with long-term administration of anabolic androgenic steroids.

Mild forms of the disease produce no symptoms or signs, but severe peliosis hepatis presents with hepatomegaly, hepatic failure, ascites, and esophageal varices and is associated with a poor prognosis.

APPROACH TO THE PATIENT WITH HEPATIC MASS LESIONS

The approach to the diagnosis of a liver harboring a mass will be influenced by the age and sex of the patient and whether or not the lesion is symptomatic (Fig. 81–10). It is seldom possible to make a specific diagnosis of a mass lesion in the liver solely on clinical grounds. Nevertheless, a detailed history should provide important clues to the probable benign or malignant nature of the lesion. In addition, clues to the diagnosis may be obtained from various risk factors, as in the patient known to be chronically infected with hepatitis B or C virus, to have taken oral contraceptive steroids or anabolic androgenic steroids for a long time, or to have been exposed to vinyl chloride monomers. Likewise, certain diagnoses are more readily excluded in the absence of a particular risk factor, as for hydatid cysts when there has been no contact with the definitive hosts for this worm. Patients known to have chronic hepatic parenchymal disease who present with a solid liver mass should be presumed to have hepatocellular carcinoma until proved otherwise. Neoplastic and non-neoplastic masses may mimic each other in their clinical presentations. For example, patients with an amebic (or pyogenic) liver abscess or hepatocellular carcinoma may present with a short history of upper abdominal pain, fever, and an enlarged tender liver. Although a liver enlarged by a mass lesion may show features that favor a particular pathologic condition, such as umbilication with hepatic metastases, an arterial bruit with hepatocellular carcinoma, or a friction rub with metastases or abscesses, these findings usually are insufficient to support a firm diagnosis. Severe muscle wasting obviously favors a malignant tumor but does not specify its nature. Moreover, some benign hepatic diseases, such as tuberculous hepatitis and chronic amebic abscess, also can cause wasting. Evidence of extrahepatic metastases makes it likely that the hepatic mass is malignant, although the primary tumor may not necessarily be in the liver. The presence of cutaneous hemangiomas in a child with mass lesions in the liver points strongly to a diagnosis of infantile hemangioendothelioma.

The circumstances in which the mass lesion became evident must be considered. With the increasing use of sophisticated imaging modalities, more asymptomatic hepatic lesions are being discovered. Although these lesions sometimes prove to be malignant, the great majority are benign. Subclinical malignant lesions must not be missed because they are the ones most amenable to cure. Likewise, subclinical benign lesions should be found because some have life-threatening complications, such as the propensity of hepatocellular adenomas to rupture.

Because it is difficult to make a specific diagnosis at the bedside, available investigations must be used rationally to arrive at the correct diagnosis with the least delay and without undue cost. The approach must take into consideration the likely diagnosis and the expected treatment and prognosis. Plain radiographic films of the chest should always be obtained because they may show a raised right hemidiaphragm (especially with hepatocellular carcinoma and amebic liver abscess), pulmonary metastases, hydatid cysts, or calcification in the liver. Conventional biochemical tests of liver function are of limited use in the differential diagnosis. However, raised serum alkaline phosphatase and γ-glutamyltranspeptidase concentrations in the presence of normal or slightly elevated serum bilirubin and aminotransferase levels suggest the presence of a space-occupying or infiltrative lesion in the liver.

Ultrasonography determines if the lesion is cystic or solid and if the intrahepatic bile ducts are dilated. It is the cheapest and most widely available of the several hepatic imaging modalities now in use but is operator dependent. Congenital cysts are completely anechoic and have a clearly defined

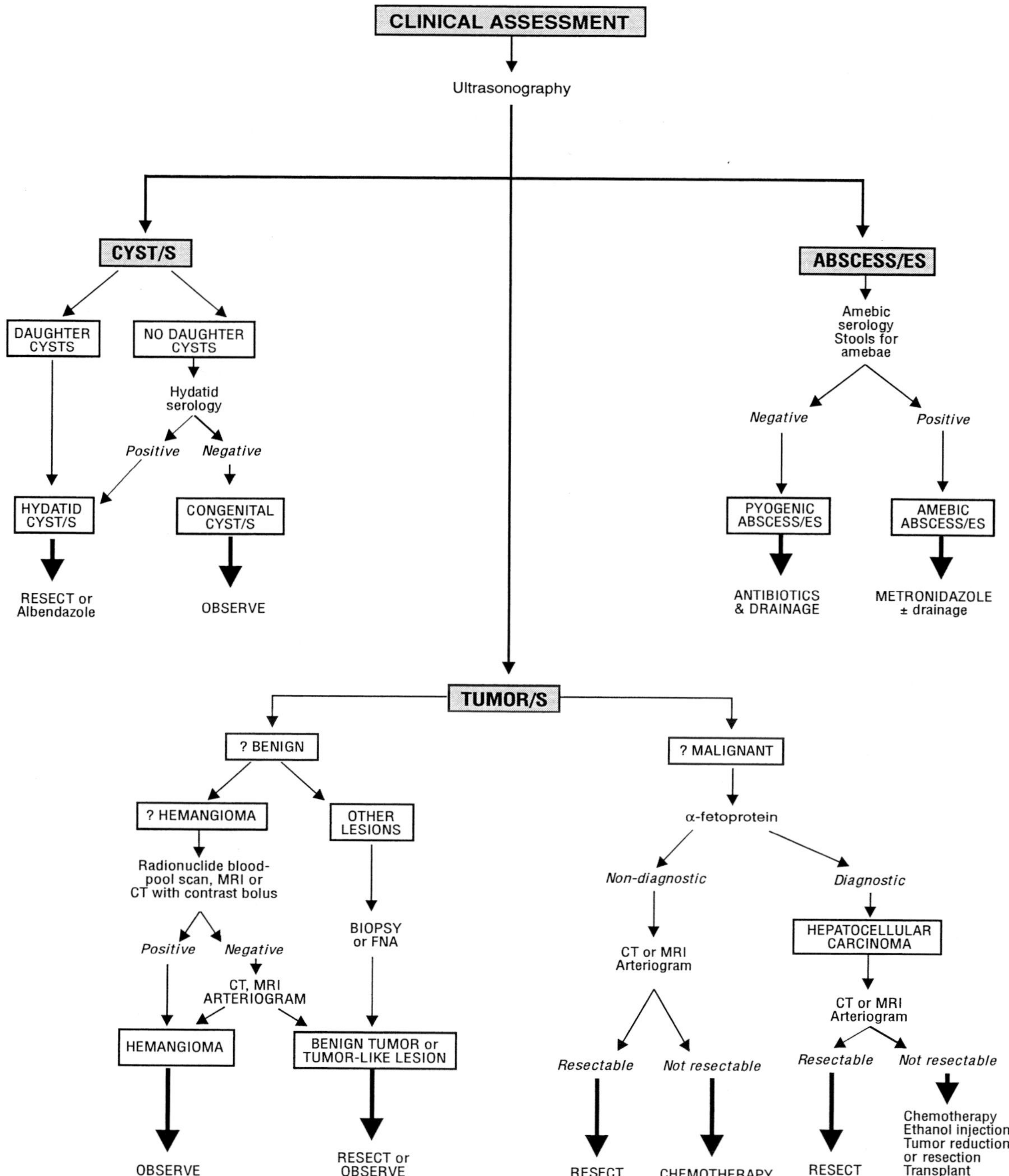

Figure 81–10. Algorithm depicting the approach to the patient with a hepatic mass (CT, computed tomography; MRI, magnetic resonance imaging; FNA, fine-needle aspiration).

thin wall; no further investigations are needed to establish this diagnosis. Ultrasonography is also an effective way to demonstrate the presence of daughter cysts within hydatid cysts. If daughter cysts are not seen, serologic tests may help distinguish hydatid from congenital cysts. Although abscesses are hypoechoic and have a thick irregular wall, early amebic abscesses may be hyperechoic and may be mistaken for a solid hepatic mass. If an abscess is suspected on clinical grounds, treatment should be commenced and the ultrasonography repeated after 3 or 4 days, by which time an abscess will have become hypoechoic. Some tumors may be partly cystic, e.g., biliary cystadenoma and cystadenocarcinoma. In addition, solid tumors may show hypoechoic areas interspersed with the expected hyerechoic picture. The hypoechoic areas result from the histologic characteristics of the tumor or from necrosis or hemorrhage in the tumor. Focal fatty change produces focal hypoechoic areas that are also hypodense on CT. Hemangiomas are typically hyperechoic. Ultrasonography does not enable a specific diagnosis of hepatic tumors to be made, and additional information needs to be obtained by dynamic contrast-enhanced ultrasonography with intra-arterial infusion of CO_2 microbubbles, CT, or MRI. Each of these techniques has limitations, however, and at present, there is no ideal method for imaging the liver.

Cavernous hemangiomas larger than 3 cm in diameter may be recognized on scintigraphy following the injection of radiolabeled red blood cells. Hepatic arteriography may show the typical features of vascular malignant tumors but is not always helpful. If hepatocellular carcinoma or hepatoblastoma is suspected, the serum α-fetoprotein concentration should be measured. Laparoscopy may demonstrate unsuspected tumor seeding or the presence of cirrhosis.

Definitive diagnosis of solid hepatic lesions depends on demonstrating the typical histologic features of the tumor. Histologic confirmation can usually be achieved by percutaneous needle biopsy or fine-needle aspiration.

REFERENCES

1. Parkin DM, Muir CS, Whelan SL, et al: Cancer Incidence in Five Continents, Vol. 5. IARC Publication No. 120. Lyon, International Agency for Research on Cancer, 1997.
2. Bosch FX, Ribes J, Borras J: Epidemiology of primary liver cancer. Semin Liver Dis 13:271, 1999.
3. Terry WD: Primary cancer of the liver. In Kaplan HS, Tsuchtani PJ (eds): Cancer in China. New York, Alan R. Liss, 1978, p 101.
4. Harington JS, McGlashan ND, Bradshaw E, et al: A spatial and temporal analysis of four cancers in African goldminers from southern Africa. Br J Cancer 31:665, 1976.
5. Okuda K, Fugimoto J, Hanai A, et al: Changing incidence of hepatocellular carcinoma in Japan. Cancer Res 7:4976, 1987.
6. Kew MC, Kassianides C, Hodkinson J, et al: Hepatocellular carcinoma in urban-born blacks: Frequency and relation to hepatitis B virus infection. Br Med J 293:1339, 1986.
7. Kew MC, Kassianides C, Berger EL, et al: Prevalence of chronic hepatitis B virus infection in pregnant black women living in Soweto. J Med Virol 22:263, 1987.
8. Prates MD, Torres EO: A cancer survey in Lourenco Marques. Portugese East Africa. J Natl Cancer Inst 35:729, 1965.
9. Shorter RG, Baggenstoss AH, Logan GB, et al: Primary carcinoma of the liver in infancy and childhood. Pediatrics 25:191, 1960.
10. Kew MC: The role of cirrhosis in hepatocarcinogenesis. In Bannasch P, Keppler D, Weber G (eds): Liver Cell Carcinoma. Dordrecht, Kluwer Academic, 1989, p 37.
11. Bagshawe A, Cameron HM: The clinical problem of liver cell cancer in a high incidence area. In Cameron HM, Linsell DA, Warwick GP (eds): Liver Cell Cancer. Amsterdam, Elsevier, 1976, 45.
12. Kew MC, Geddes EW: Hepatocellular carcinoma in rural southern African blacks. Medicine (Balt) 61:98, 1982.
13. Lau WY, Leung WY, Ho S, et al: Obstructive jaundice secondary to hepatocellular carcinoma. Surg Oncol 4:308, 1995.
14. Kew MC, Paterson AC: Unusual clinical presentations of hepatocellular carcinoma. J Trop Gastroenterol 6:10, 1985.
15. Clain D, Wartnaby K, Sherlock S: Abdominal arterial bruits in liver disease. Lancet 2:516, 1966.
16. Kew MC, Dos Santos HA, Sherlock S: Diagnosis of primary cancer of the liver. Br Med J 4:408, 1971.
17. Zapf J, Futo E, Martina P, et al: Can *big* insulin-like growth factor-II in the serum of a tumor patient account for the development of extrapancreatic tumor hypoglycemia? J Clin Invest 90:2574, 1990.
18. Kew MC, Fisher JW: Serum erythropoietin concentrations in patients with hepatocellular carcinoma. Cancer 58:2485, 1986.
19. Yen T-C, Hwang S-J, Lee S-D, et al: Hypercalcemia and parathyroid hormone-related protein in hepatocellular carcinoma. Liver 13:311, 1993.
20. DiBisceglie AM, Hodkinson HJ, Berkowitz I, et al: *Pityriasis rotunda*—A cutaneous sign of hepatocellular carcinoma in southern African blacks. Arch Dermatol 122:802, 1986.
21. Danilewitz MD, Herrera G, Kew MC, et al: Autonomous cholesterol biosynthesis in murine hepatoma: A receptor defect with normal coated pits. Cancer 54:1562, 1984.
22. Alpert E: Human α_1-fetoprotein. In Okuda K, Peters RL (eds): Hepatocellular Carcinoma. New York, Wiley, 1976, p 353.
23. Kew MC: Tumor markers in hepatocellular carcinoma. J Gastroenterol Hepatol 4:373, 1989.
24. Kew MC: The detection and treatment of small hepatocellular carcinoma. In Hollinger FB, Lemon SM, Margolis H (eds): Viral Hepatitis and Liver Disease. Baltimore, Williams & Wilkins, 1991, p 515.
25. Taketa A, Sekiya C, Namiki M, et al: Lectin-reactive profiles of α-fetoprotein characterizing hepatocellular carcinoma and related conditions. Gastroenterology 99:508, 1990.
26. Du M-Q, Hutchinson WL, Johnson PJ, et al: Differential α-fetoprotein lectin binding in hepatocellular carcinoma; Diagnostic utility at low levels. Cancer 67:476, 1991.
27. Liebman HA, Furie B, Tong MJ, et al: Des-γ-carboxy (abnormal) prothrombin as a serum marker of primary hepatocellular carcinoma. N Engl J Med 310:427, 1984.
28. King MA, Kew MC, Kuyl JM, et al: A comparison between des-γ-carboxy prothrombin and α-fetoprotein as markers of hepatocellular carcinoma in southern African blacks. J Gastroenterol Hepatol 4:17, 1989.
29. Deugnier Y, David V, Brissot P, et al: Serum α-L-fucosidase: A new marker for the diagnosis of primary liver cancer? Hepatology 4:889, 1984.
30. Di Coccio RA, Barlow JJ, Motta KL: Evaluation of α-L-fucosidase as a marker of primary liver cancer. IRCS Med Sci 23:849, 1985.
31. Bukofzer S, Stass PM, Kew MC, et al: α-L-Fucosidase as a serum marker of hepatocellular carcinoma in southern African blacks. Br J Cancer 59:417, 1989.
32. Levy JI, Geddes EW, Kew MC: The chest radiograph in primary liver cancer. S Afr Med J 15:1323, 1976.
33. Kudo M: Ultrasound. In Okuda K, Tabor E (eds): Liver Cancer. New York, Churchill Livingstone, 1997, p 331.
34. Kudo M: Imaging diagnosis of hepatocellular carcinoma and premalignant/borderline lesions. Semin Liver Dis 19:291, 1999.
35. Choi BI: CT diagnosis of liver cancer. In Okuda K, Tabor E (eds): Liver Cancer. New York, Churchill Livingstone, 1997, p 516.
36. Moss AM, Goldberg HI, Stark DB, et al: Hepatic tumors. Magnetic resonance and computed tomography. Radiology 150:142, 1984.
37. Ebara M: MRI diagnosis of hepatocellular carcinoma. In Okuda K, Tabor E (eds): Liver Cancer. New York, Churchill Livingstone, 1997, p 361.
38. Takayasu K: Hepatic angiography. In Okuda K, Tabor E (eds): Liver Cancer. New York, Churchill Livingstone, 1997, p 347.
39. Kojiro M: Pathology of hepatocellular carcinoma. In Okuda K, Tabor E (eds): Liver Cancer. New York, Churchill Livingstone, 1997, p 165.
40. Craig JR, Peters RL, Edmondson HA, et al: Fibrolamellar carcinoma of the liver: A tumor of adolescents and young adults with distinctive clinicopathologic features. Cancer 46:372, 1980.
41. Anthony PP: Tumors and tumor-like lesions of the liver and biliary tract. In MacSween RNM, Anthony PP, Scheuer PJ, et al (eds): Pathology of the Liver, Edinburgh, Churchill Livingstone, 1994, p 635
42. Yuki K, Hirohashi S, Sakamoto M, et al: Growth and spread of hepatocellular carcinoma. A review of 240 autopsy cases. Cancer 66: 2174, 1990.
43. Kew MC: Clinical, pathologic, and etiologic heterogeneity in hepatocellular carcinoma: Evidence from southern Africa. Hepatology 1:366, 1981.
44. Hepatitis Viruses. IARC Monographs on the Evaluation of Carcinogenic Risks to Humans, Vol. 59. Lyon, International Agency for research on Cancer, 1994, p 202.
45. Stevens CE, Szmuness W: Vertical transmission of hepatitis B and neonatal hepatitis B. In Bianchi LO, Gerock W, Sickinger K, et al (eds): Virus and the Liver. Lancaster, MTP Press, 1980, p 285.
46. Botha JA, Ritchie MJJ, Dusheiko GM, et al: Hepatitis B virus carrier state in black children in Ovamboland: Role of perinatal and horizontal infection. Lancet 2:1209, 1984.
47. Beasley RP, Hwang L-Y: Hepatocellular carcinoma and hepatitis B virus. Semin Liver Dis 4:113, 1984.
48. Chang M-H, Chen C-J, Lai M-S, et al: Universal hepatitis B virus vaccination in Taiwan and the incidence of hepatocellular carcinoma in children. N Engl J Med 336:1855, 1997.
49. Arbuthnot P, Kew MC: Hepatitis B virus and hepatocellular carcinoma. Int J Exp Pathol 82:77,2001.
50. Chisari FV, Filippe P, Buras J, et al: Structural and pathological effects of synthesis of hepatitis B virus large envelope polypeptide in transgenic mice. Proc Natl Acad Sci USA 84:6909, 1987.
51. Wogan GN: Aflatoxin exposure as a risk factor in the etiology of hepatocellular carcinoma. In Okuda K, Tabor E (eds): Liver Cancer. New York, Churchill Livingstone, 1997, p 51.
52. Hsu IC, Metcalf RA, Sun T, et al: Mutational hotspot in the p53 gene in human hepatocellular carcinomas. Nature 350:427, 1991.
53. Bressac B, Kew MC, Wands JR, et al: Selective G to T mutation in

the p53 gene in hepatocellular carcinoma from southern Africa. Nature 350:429, 1991.

54. Deugnier YM, Guyader D, Crantock L, et al: Primary liver cancer in genetic hemochromatosis: A clinical, pathological, and pathogenetic study of 54 cases. Gastroenterology 104:228, 1993.
55. Kew MC: Pathogenesis of hepatocellular carcinoma in hereditary hemochromatosis: Occurrence in non-cirrhotic patients. Hepatology 11: 806, 1990.
56. Loeb LA, James EA, Waltersdorff AM, et al: Mutagenesis by the auto-oxidation of iron with isolated DNA. Proc Natl Acnd Sci USA 85:3918, 1988.
57. Mandishona E, McPhail AP, Gordeuk VR, et al: Dietary iron overload as a risk factor for hepatocellular carcinoma in black Africans. Hepatology 27:1563, 1998.
58. Polio J, Enriquez RE, Chow A, et al: Hepatocellular carcinoma in Wilson's disease: Case report and review of the literature. J Clin Gastroenterol 11:220, 1989.
59. Tokol RJ, Twedt T, McKim JM, et al: Oxidant injury to mitochondria in patients with liver disease and Bedlington terriers with copper toxicosis. Gastroenterology 107:1788, 1994.
60. Collaborative MILTS project team: Oral contraceptives and liver cancer. Results of a multicenter international liver tumor study (MILTS). Contraception 56:275, 1997.
61. Thomas DB: Exogenous steroid hormones and hepatocellular carcinoma. In Tabor E, DiBisceglie AM, Purcell RH (eds): Etiology, Pathology, and Treatment of Hepatocellular Carcinoma in North America. Houston, Gulf Publishing Co., 1991, p 77.
62. Austin A: The role of tobacco use and alcohol consumption in the etiology of hepatocellular carcinoma. In Tabor E, DiBisceglie AM, Purcell RH (eds): Etiology, Pathology, and Treatment of Hepatocellular Carcinoma in North America. Houston, Gulf Publishing Co, 1991, p 57.
63. Simson IM: Membranous obstruction of the inferior vena cava and hepatocellular carcinoma in South Africa. Gastroenterology 82:171, 1982.
64. Kew MC, McKnight A, Hodkinson HJ, et al: The role of membranous obstruction of the inferior vena cava in the etiology of hepatocellular carcinoma in southern African blacks. Hepatology 9:121, 1989.
65. Johnson PJ: Benign and malignant tumors of the liver. In Bacon BR, DiBisceglie AM (eds): Liver Disease: Diagnosis and Management. New York, Churchill Livingstone, 2000, p 310.
66. Balasegaram M: Management of primary liver cancer. Am J Surg 130: 33, 1975.
67. Maraj J, Kew MC, Hyslop RJ: Resectability rate of hepatocellular carcinoma in rural southern African blacks. Br J Surg 75:335, 1988.
68. Foster JA, Berman MM: Solid Liver Tumors. Philadelphia, WB Saunders, 1977.
69. Bathe OF, Scudamore CH, Caron NR, et al: Resection of hepatocellular carcinoma. In Okuda K, Tabor E (eds): Liver Cancer. New York, Churchill Livingstone, 1997, p 511.
70. Tang Z-Y: Surgery of hepatocellular carcinoma—Current status and future prospects. J Gastroenterol Hepatol 15 (Suppl):11, 2000.
71. Bismuth H, Majno PE, Adam R: Liver transplantation for hepatocellular carcinoma. Semin Liver Dis 19:311, 1999.
72. Yokoyama Y, Carr B, Saitsu H, et al: Accelerated growth rates of hepatocellular carcinoma after liver transplantation. Cancer 68:2095, 1991.
73. Ringe BR, Wittekind C, Bechstein WO, et al: The role of liver of recurrent transplantation in hepatobiliary malignancy: A retrospective study of 95 patients with particular regard to tumor stage and recurrences. Am Surg 209:88, 1989.
74. Rolles K: Transplantation for liver cancer. In Okuda K, Tabor E (eds): Liver Cancer. New York, Churchill Livingstone, 1997, p 531.
75. Okada S: Local ablation of hepatocellular carcinoma. Semin Liver Dis 19:323, 1999.
76. Livraghi T: Ethanol injection for the treatment of hepatocellular carcinoma. In Okuda K, Tabor E (eds): Liver Cancer. New York, Churchill Livingstone, 1997, p 497.
77. Wu C-C, Ho Y-Z, Ho WL, et al: Preoperative transcatheter arterial chemoembolization for resectable large hepatocellular carcinoma: A reappraisal. Br J Surg 82:122. 1985.
78. Stephanini GF, Amorati P, Bisseli M, et al: Efficacy of transarterial targeted treatments on survival in patients with hepatocellular carcinoma. Cancer 75:2927, 1995.
79. Nakamura H, Murakami T: Arterial embolization. In Okuda K, Tabor E (eds): Liver Cancer. New York, Churchill Livingstone, 1997, p 449.
80. Bronowicki J-P, Vetter D, Doffoel M: Chemoembolization of hepatocellular carcinoma. In Okuda K, Tabor E (eds): Liver Cancer. New York, Churchill Livingstone, 1997, p 463.
81. Falkson G, Falkson CI: Current approaches in the management of patients with hepatocellular carcinoma. Oncol Res 4:87, 1992.
82. Tang Z-Y: Sub-clinical Hepatocellular Carcinoma. Historical Aspects and General Considerations. Beijing, China Academic Publishers, 1985, p 1.
83. Ebara M, Ohto M, Shinagawa T, et al: Natural history of minute hepatocellular carcinoma smaller than 3 cm complicating cirrhosis. Gastroenterology 90:289, 1986.
84. Okuda K, Kubo Y, Ozaki N, et al: Clinical aspects of intrahepatic bile duct carcinoma, including hilar carcinoma. Cancer 19:232, 1977.
85. Nakanuma Y, Hoso M, Terada T: Clinical and pathologic features of cholangiocarcinoma. In Okuda K, Tabor E (eds): Liver Cancer. New York, Churchill Livingstone, 1997, p 279.
86. Srivatanakul P, Parkin DM, Yiang Y-Z, et al: The role of infection by *Opistorchis viverrini*, hepatitis B virus, and aflatoxin exposure in liver cancer in Thailand. Cancer 68:2411, 1991.
87. Wogan AM: The induction of liver cancer by chemicals. In Cameron H, Linsell CA, Warwick GP (eds): Liver Cell Cancer. New York, Wiley, 1976, p 6.
88. Eriksson S, Hagerstrand I: Cirrhosis and malignant hepatoma in α_1-antitrypsin dfeciency. Acta Med Scand 195:451, 1974.
89. Stauffer MH, Sauer WG, Dearing WH, et al: The spectrum of cholestatic liver disease. JAMA 191:829, 1965.
90. Kulkarny PB, Beatty EC: Cholangiocarcinoma associated with biliary atresia. Am J Dis Child 31:442, 1977.
91. Dekker A, Ten Kate FJW, Terpstra OT: Cholangiocarcinoma associated with multiple bile duct hamartomas of the liver. Dig Dis Sci 34: 592, 1989.
92. Sane S, MacCallum JD: Primary carcinoma of the liver: Cholangiocarcinoma in hepatolithiasis. Am J Pathol 18:675, 1942.
93. Klatskin G: Adenocarcinoma of the hepatic duct at its bifurcation within the porta hepatis. Am J Med 38:241, 1965.
94. Knill-Jones RP, Buckle RM, Parsons V, et al: Hypercalcemia and parathyroid activity in primary hepatoma. N Engl J Med 282:704, 1970.
95. Kaude J, Rian R: Cholangiocarcinoma. Radiology 100:573, 1971.
96. Sugihara S, Kojiro M: Pathology of cholangiocarcinoma. In Okuda K, and Ishak KG (eds): Neoplasms of the Liver. Tokyo, Springer Verlag, 1987, p 143.
97. Stocker JT, Iskak KG: Hepatoblastoma. In Okuda K, Ishak KG (eds): Neoplasms of the Liver. Tokyo, Springer Verlag, 1987, p 127.
98. Exelby PR, Filler RM, Groshield JM: Liver tumors in children with particular reference to hepatoblastoma and hepatocellular carcinoma. J Pediat Surg 10:329, 1975.
99. McArthur JW, Toll GD, Russfield AB, et al: Sexual precocity attributed to ectopic gonadotropin secretion by hepatoblastoma. Am J Med 54:390, 1973.
100. Hasegawa H, Mukojima T, Hattori N, et al: Embryonal carcinoma and α-fetoprotein. Cancer Res 14:129, 1973.
101. Reynolds M, Douglass EC, Finegold M, et al: Chemotherapy can convert unresectable hepatoblastoma. J Pediat Surg 27:1080, 1992.
102. Koneru B, Flye MW, Busitill RW, et al: Liver transplantation for hepatoblastoma: The American experience. Ann Surg 213:118, 1991.
103. Tamburro CH: Relationship of vinyl chloride to liver cancers: angiosarcoma and hepatocellular carcinoma. Semin Liver Dis 4:158, 1984.
104. Locker GY, Duroshaw JH, Zwelling IA, et al: The clinical features of hepatic angiosarcoma: A report of four cases and a review of the literature. Medicine (Balt) 58:48, 1979.
105. Makk L, Delmore F, Creech JI, et al: Clinical and morphological features of hepatic angiosarcoma in vinyl chloride workers. Cancer 37: 149, 1976.
106. Visfeldt J, Polse H: Of the histopathology of the liver and liver tumors in thorium dioxide patients. Acta Pathol Microbiol Scand 80A: 97, 1972.
107. Roth F: Arsen-leber-tumoren hemangioendotheliom. Arch Pathol 60: 493, 1955.
108. Regelson W, Kim U, Ospina J, et al: Hemangioendothelial sarcoma of the liver from chronic arsenic intoxication by Fowler's solution. Cancer 21:514, 1968.
109. Creech JL, Johnson MN: Angiosarcoma of the liver in the manufacture of polyvinyl chloride. J Occup Med 16:150, 1974.
110. Whelan JG, Creech JL, Tamburro CH: Angiographic and radionuclide characteristics of hepatic angiosarcoma found in vinyl chloride workers. Radiology 118:549, 1976.
111. Truell JE, Peck SD, Reiguam CW: Hemangiosarcoma of the liver

complicated by disseminated intravascular coagulation. Gastroenterology 65:936, 1973.
112. Alpert LI, Benisch B: Hemangioepithelioma of the liver associated with microangiopathic hemolytic anemia. Am J Med 48:624, 1970.
113. Ishak KG: Malignant mesenchymal tumors of the liver. In Okuda K, Ishak KG (eds): Neoplasms of the Liver. Tokyo, Springer Verlag, 1987, p 159.
114. Pickren JW, Tsukada Y, Lane WW: Liver metastasis: Analysis of autopsy data. In Weiss L, Gilbert HA (eds): Liver Metastases. Boston, CK Hall, 1982, p 2.
115. Dingemans KP, Roos E: Ultrastructural aspects of the invasion of the liver by cancer cells. In Weiss L, Gilbert HA (eds): Liver Metastases, Boston, CK Hall, 1982, p 51.
116. Ward BA, Miller DL, Frank JA, et al: prospective evaluation of hepatic imaging studies in the detection of colorectal metastases: Correlation with surgical findings. Surgery 105:180, 1989.
117. Sheiner PA, Brower ST: Treatment of metastatic cancer. Semin Liver Dis 14:169, 1994.
118. Hughes K, Scheele J: Surgery for colorectal cancer metastatic to the liver. Surg Clin North Am 69:339, 1989.
119. Barr LC, Skene AI, Thomas JN: Metastectomy. Br J Surg 79:1268, 1992.
120. Prentice RL, Thomas DB: On the epidemiology of oral contraceptives and disease. Adv Cancer Res 49:285, 1987.
121. Vessey MP, Kay CR, Baldwin JA, et al: Oral contraceptives and benign liver tumors. 1:164, 1977.
122. Nagorney DM: Benign hepatic tumors, focal nodular hyperplasia, and hepatocellular adenoma. World J Surg 19:13, 1995.
123. Knowles DM, Casarella WJ, Johnson PM, et al: The clinical, radiologic, and pathologic characterization of benign hepatic adenomas. Alleged association with oral contraceptives. Medicine (Balt) 57:223, 1978.
124. Goodman ZD: Benign tumors of the liver. In Okuda K, Ishak KG (eds): Neoplasms of the Liver. Toyko, Springer Verlag, 1987, p 105.
125. Tavani A, Negri E, Parazinni F, et al: Female hormone utilization and risk of hepatocellular carcinoma. Br J Cancer 67:635, 1993.
126. Gyoffy E, Bredfeldt JE, Black WC: Transformation of hepatic cell adenoma to hepatocellular carcinoma due to oral contraceptive use. Ann Intern Med 110:489, 1989.
127. Freeny PC, Vimant TR, Barnett TC: Cavernous hemangioma of the liver: Ultrasonography, arteriography, and computed tomography. Radiology 132:143, 1979.
128. Krause T, Hauenstein K, Studier-Fischer B, et al: Improved evaluation of technetium 99m red blood cell SPECT in hemangioma of the liver. J Nucl Med 34:375, 1993.
129. Yamauchi T, Minami M, Yshiro N: Non-invasive diagnosis of small hemangioma of the liver: Advantage of magnetic resonance imaging. Radiology 145:1195, 1985.
130. Cooper WH, Martin JF: Hemangioma of the liver with thrombocytopenia. Am J Radiol 88:751, 1962.
131. Martinez J, Shapiro SS, Halbrun RR, et al: Hypofibrinogenemia associated with hemangioma of the liver. Am J Clin Pathol 29:160, 1958.
132. Feldman M: Hemangioma of the liver. Special reference to its association with cysts of the liver and pancreas. Am J Clin Pathol 29:160, 1958.
133. Chung EB: Multiple bile duct hamartomas. Cancer 26:287, 1970.
134. Banz EJ, Baggenstoss AH: Focal cirrhosis of the liver: Its relation to the so-called hamartoma (adenoma, benign hepatoma). Cancer 6:743, 1953.
135. Hanson SW, Gray HK, Dockerty MB: Benign tumors of the liver. II. Hemangiomas. Surg Gynecol Obstet 103:327, 1956.
136. Park WC, Phillips R: The role of radiation therapy in the management of hemangiomas of the liver. JAMA 21:1496, 1970.
137. Schwartz S, Husser WC: Cavernous hemangioma of the liver. Ann Surg 2905:456, 1987.
138. McLean RH, Moller JH, Warwick J, et al: Multinodular hemangiomatosis of the liver in infancy. Pediatrics 49:563, 1972.
139. Holcomb GW, O'Neill JA, Mahboubi S, et al: Experience with hepatic hemangioendothelioma in infancy and childhood. J Pediat Surg 23:661, 1988.
140. Mortensen W, Petersonn H: Infantile hemangioendothelioma. Angiographic considerations. Acta Radiol (Diagn) (Stockh) 20:161, 1979.
141. Rake MO, Liberman MM, Dawson JL: Ligation of the hepatic artery in the treatment of heart failure due to hepatic hemangiomatosis. Gut 11:512, 1970.
142. Frost NC, Esterley NB: Successful treatment of juvenile hemangiomas with prednisone. J Pediat 72:351, 1968.
143. Ross D, Pinna J, Mirza M, et al: Regression of focal nodular hyperplasia after discontinuation of oral contraceptives. Ann Intern Med 85: 203, 1976.
144. Knowles DM, Wolff M, Johnson PM: Focal nodular hyperplasia and liver cell adenoma: Radiologic and pathologic differentiation. Am J, Radiol 131:393, 1978.
145. Wang SS, Chiang J, Tsai Y, et al: Focal hepatic fatty infiltration as a cause of pseudotumors: Ultrasonographic patterns and clinical differentiation. J Clin Ultrasound 18:401, 1990.
146. Barros JL: Hydatid disease of the liver. Am J Surg 135:597, 1978.
147. Lewis JW, Koss N, Kerstein MD: A review of echinococcal disease. Ann Surg 181:390, 1975.
148. Lygidakis NJ: Diagnosis and treatment of intrabiliary rupture of hydatid cyst of the liver. Arch Surg 118:1186, 1983.
149. Kuhn GA, Jones T, Sali A: Hydatid disease in Australia: Prevention, clinical presentation, and treatment. Med J Aust 3:385, 1983.
150. Beggs I: The radiological appearances of hydatid disease of the liver. Clin Radiol 34:555, 1983.
151. Saimot AG, Meulemains A, Cremieux AC, et al: Albendazole as a potential treatment for human hydatidosis. Lancet 2:652, 1983.
152. Wilson JF, Rausch RL: Alveolar hydatid disease: A review of clinical features of 33 indigenous cases of Echinococcus multilocularis infection in Alaskan Eskimos. Am J Trop Med Hyg 29:1340, 1980.
153. Bresson-Hani S, Koch S, Beuerton I, et al: Primary disease recurrence after liver transplantation for alveolar echinococcosis.: Long-term evaluation in 15 patients. Hepatology 30:857, 1999.
154. Jorgensen MJ: The ductal plate malformation. Acta Pathol Microbiol Scand Suppl A 257:1, 1977.
155. Desmet VJ: Congenital diseases of intrahepatic bile ducts; variations on the theme "ductal plate malformation." Hepatology 16:1069, 1992.
156. D'Agata ID, Jonas MM, Perez-Atayde AR, et al: Combined cystic disease of the liver and kidney. Semin Liver Dis 14:215, 1994.
157. Lai ECS, Wong J: Symptomatic non-parasitic cysts of the liver. World J Surg 14:452, 1990.
158. Summerfield JA, Nagafuchi Y, Sherlock S, et al: Hepatobiliary fibropolycystic diseases: A clinical and histologic review. J Hepatol 2:141, 1986.
159. Karhunen PJ, Tenhu M: Adult polycystic liver and kidney diseases are separate entities. Clin Genet 30:29, 1985.
160. Pirson Y, Lannoy N, Peters D, et al: Isolated polycystic liver disease as a distinct genetic disease, unlinked to polycystic kidney disease 1 and polycystic kidney disease 2. Hepatology 23:249, 1996.
161. Reeders ST, Breuning MH, Davies KE, et al: A highly polymorphic DNA marker linked to adult polycystic kidney disease on chromosome 16. Nature 317:542, 1985.
162. Everson GT: Hepatic cysts in autosomal dominant polycystic kidney disease. Am J Kidney Dis 22:520, 1993.
163. Barnes PA, Thomas JL, Bernadino ME: Pitfalls in the diagnosis of hepatic cysts by computed tomography. Radiology 141:1209, 1981.
164. Que F, Nagorney DM, Gross TB, et al: Liver resection and cyst fenestration in the treatment of severe polycystic liver disease. Gastroenterology 108:407, 1995.
165. Everson GT, Shrestha R: Cystic disorders of the liver and biliary tree. In Bacon BR, DiBisceglie AM (eds): Liver Disease: Diagnosis and Management. New York, Churchill Livingstone, 2000, p 321.
166. Caroli S: Diseases of the intrahepatic biliary tree. Clin Gastroenterol 2:147, 1973.
167. Mathias K, Waldmann D, Daikeler G, et al: Intrahepatic cystic duct dilatations and stone formation: A new case of Caroli's disease. Acta Hepatogastroenterol 25:30, 1978.
168. Ramond JM, Huequet C, Danan G, et al: Partial hepatectomy in the treatment of Caroli's disease. Dig Dis Sci 29:67, 1984.
169. Valla D, Benhamou JP: Disorders of the hepatic venous system, peliosis, and sinusoidal dilatation. In Bacon BR, DiBisceglie AM (eds): Liver Disease: Diagnosis and Management. New York, Churchill Livingstone, 2000, p 331.

Chapter 82

HEPATIC MANIFESTATIONS OF SYSTEMIC DISEASE AND OTHER DISORDERS OF THE LIVER

Dwain L. Thiele

HEMATOLOGIC MALIGNANCIES

Liver involvement in hematologic malignancies is only rarely life-threatening or a source of great morbidity. Nevertheless, the liver is a major component of the reticuloendothelial system, and it is not surprising that malignant infiltration of the liver commonly occurs in such diseases. As is detailed in Table 82–1, the frequency of malignant infiltration varies from less than 10% to nearly 100% depending on the nature of the underlying hematologic malignancy. In addition to histologic and biochemical abnormalities related to malignant infiltration, a variety of other hepatic abnormalities are observed in a substantial portion of such patients. Many of these abnormalities are related to the toxicity of pharmacologic or radiation therapies or to the secondary opportunistic or transfusion-related infections that commonly occur in such patients. In addition, a variety of nonspecific histologic abnormalities of uncertain etiology, such as steatosis, fibrosis, hemosiderosis, and nonspecific portal lymphocytic infiltrates, are observed in both treated and untreated patients. Other hepatic manifestations that are associated with specific malignancies also may occur. Such notable paraneoplastic manifestations include granuloma formation and pronounced intrahepatic cholestasis in patients with Hodgkin's disease and deposition of amyloid in patients with multiple myeloma.

Hodgkin's Disease

As shown in Table 82–1, malignant infiltration of the liver is observed in only a minority of patients with untreated Hodgkin's disease.[1, 2] However, autopsy series have noted hepatic involvement in as many as 55% of patients,[3] suggesting that hepatic involvement increases with progression of the disease. Although Reed-Sternberg cells have been reported in only 8% of liver biopsies at the time of initial evaluation, fully one third of specimens exhibit nonspecific mononuclear cell infiltrates in portal tracts, and approximately 10% to 25% have noncaseating hepatic granulomas that are not associated with malignant histiocytes or infectious etiologies.[1, 4, 5] Moderate elevations in serum alkaline phosphatase levels often are observed, especially in febrile patients or patients with advanced disease.[6] Although such elevations are almost invariably derived from the hepatic fraction of alkaline phosphatase,[6] not all patients with elevated alkaline phosphatase levels have tumor infiltration of the liver.[1, 6] All patients with hepatic involvement of Hodgkin's disease have been reported to have splenic involvement,[1, 4] but splenic infiltration does not invariably imply liver involvement.[4]

Although Hodgkin's disease may involve the extrahepatic bile ducts or lymph nodes in the porta hepatis and cause extrahepatic obstruction,[7] multiple reports describe an addi-

Table 82–1 | **Involvement of the Liver in Patients with Hematologic Malignancies**

	FREQUENCY OF LIVER INFILTRATION		OTHER NOTABLE HISTOLOGIC ABNORMALITIES (FREQUENCY)
	Clinical Evaluation	Post Mortem	
Hodgkin's disease	8–14%	55%	Portal lymphocytic infiltrates (32%), granulomas (9–25%), steatosis (11%), hemosiderosis (9%), idiopathic cholestasis (<5%)
Non-Hodgkin's lymphoma	16–57%	52%	Portal lymphocytic infiltrates (20–25%), steatosis (7%)
Multiple myeloma	30–40%	40–50%	Amyloidosis (10%), light chain deposition, extramedullary hematopoiesis
Leukemias			
ALL	—	>95%	
AML	—	~75%	
CCL	—	98%	
HCL	100%	100%	Angiomatous lesions (64%)
LGLL	75–100%	—	

ALL, acute lymphocytic leukemia; AML, acute myelogenous leukemia; CLL, chronic lymphocytic leukemia; HCL, hairy cell leukemia; LGLL, large granular lymphocyte leukemia.

Data abstracted from references 1–5, 8, 9, 12–15, 22–27, and 31.

tional syndrome of idiopathic intrahepatic cholestasis unrelated to hepatic infiltration, extrahepatic obstruction, or other identifiable causes.[8–10] The degree of cholestasis is often disproportionate to the apparent tumor load.[8, 10] Cholestasis has been reported to resolve with response to systemic therapy,[8] but in some cases this syndrome has been associated with intractable, fatal liver damage.[10] Recently, progressive loss of small intrahepatic bile ducts has been documented in some affected patients,[10] suggesting that this syndrome may be caused by destruction of bile duct epithelial cells either by the direct effects of tumor cells that invade the intrahepatic bile ducts or by the indirect effects of cytokines that are released from lymphoma cells.

Because liver involvement in a patient with Hodgkin's disease signifies stage IIIE or IV disease,[11] identification of the cause of abnormal liver biochemistries in a patient with the disease is important in determining prognosis and therapy. Numerous studies have noted the superiority of laparotomy or laparoscopy over blind percutaneous liver biopsy in detecting hepatic involvement with Hodgkin's disease, presumably because of the relatively small volume of tissue obtained by percutaneous liver biopsy and the difficulty in finding diagnostic Reed-Sternberg cells in the liver. With improved noninvasive imaging techniques and increased understanding of the adverse immunologic consequences of splenectomy, staging laparotomies are performed less often now than in the past.[11] However, laparoscopy appears to provide a diagnostic yield equivalent to that obtained at laparotomy[2, 12] and appears to be a satisfactory method for assessing hepatic involvement by Hodgkin's disease.

Non-Hodgkin's Lymphoma

As is noted in Table 82–1, the frequency of liver involvement on initial clinical staging is significantly higher in patients with non-Hodgkin's lymphoma than in those with Hodgkin's disease. When evaluated by percutaneous liver biopsy, 16% to 26% of patients with non-Hodgkin's lymphoma are found to have liver infiltration[13, 14]; higher percentages of patients are found to have hepatic involvement when evaluated at staging laparotomy (56%)[12] or at autopsy (52%).[4] In both Hodgkin's and non-Hodgkin's lymphomas, the majority of infiltrative lesions are located in the portal tracts.[4, 15] Although the overall frequency of hepatic involvement appears to be similar in patients with different histologic types of lymphoma,[13] primary hepatic lymphoma is an unusual variant that occurs more often in diffuse large cell lymphomas of B cell origin than in T cell or non-B, non-T cell lymphomas.[16, 17] In contrast to secondary lymphomatous involvement of the liver, which is often detected only by histologic evaluation, patients with primary lymphoma commonly have evidence of mass lesions on computed tomography, magnetic resonance imaging, or other hepatic imaging procedures; these mass lesions may mimic primary or metastatic carcinoma.[16–18] Some reports have suggested an association between primary hepatic lymphomas and immunosuppression or chronic viral hepatitis in a minority of cases.[16, 17]

Recently, hepatosplenic $\gamma\delta$ T cell lymphoma has been recognized as a distinct type of lymphoma.[19] This extremely rare form of lymphoma typically occurs in young men who present with hepatosplenomegaly secondary to diffuse hepatic sinusoidal and splenic sinus infiltration with clonal populations of $\gamma\delta$ T cell receptor (TCR) expressing cells. Lymphadenopathy is absent, but bone marrow involvement is common on presentation. Cytogenetic analysis commonly reveals an isochromosome 7q and trisomy 8.[19]

The most common liver test abnormality reported in patients with non-Hodgkin's lymphoma is a moderately elevated serum alkaline phosphatase level. However, liver test abnormalities are poorly predictive of the presence or absence of lymphomatous infiltration of the liver,[12, 14] in part because the histologic abnormalities often are nonspecific[4, 13, 15] and include portal lymphocytic infiltrates, hemosiderosis, and steatosis. Patients with lymphomatous liver infiltrates may have normal liver tests.[14] Noncaseating granulomas also have been found in the portal tracts of patients with non-Hodgkin's lymphoma, although the frequency is lower than that observed in Hodgkin's disease.[4, 20] Extrahepatic biliary obstruction secondary to nodal involvement in the porta hepatis also may occur.[12]

Percutaneous liver biopsy has been found to be of value in detecting hepatic involvement with lymphoma.[14, 21] If biopsy specimens are processed properly, immunotyping can be performed to characterize the phenotype of the malignant cells.[21] However, a sufficient quantity of tissue is needed, and biopsy at laparotomy is superior to either blind percutaneous or laparoscopic biopsy for the diagnosis of hepatic infiltration by non-Hodgkin's lymphoma.[12]

Multiple Myeloma

Hepatomegaly and abnormalities of liver biochemical tests are commonly observed in patients with multiple myeloma.[22] In up to one half of patients who undergo a hepatic histologic evaluation, either diffuse sinusoidal or portal infiltration or, less commonly, nodule formation by malignant plasma cells has been observed.[15, 22, 23] The frequency of jaundice has ranged from 0% to 30% in series of patients with hepatic infiltration by multiple myeloma.[22, 23] Ascites has been reported to complicate the course of disease in 10% to 35% of patients with massive hepatic infiltration[21, 22]; esophageal varices occur more rarely. Portal hypertension secondary to tumor infiltration appears to be the cause of ascites in most affected patients; other potential causes include congestive heart failure, dissemination of myeloma cells into the peritoneal cavity, and tuberculous peritonitis. In addition to direct malignant infiltration of the liver, hemosiderosis, or portal lymphocytic infiltrates, multiple myeloma is complicated in approximately 10% of patients by deposition of amyloid or nonamyloid containing immunoglobulin light chains in the space of Disse.[21–25] Extramedullary hematopoiesis also may contribute to hepatomegaly or liver test abnormalities in these patients.[22] Clinical staging and follow-up of patients with multiple myeloma are based largely on the assessment of marrow, osseous, serum, and urinary abnormalities, and thus histologic evaluation of the liver is considered only occasionally. As is discussed later in the section dealing with amyloidosis, the potential diagnostic benefits of liver biopsy must be weighed against concerns regarding bleeding complications.

Leukemias

At the time of initial presentation, hepatomegaly is present in the majority of patients with acute lymphocytic leukemia (ALL) and in a substantial minority of patients with acute myelogenous leukemia (AML). In autopsy series of patients dying in advanced stages of these acute leukemias, liver involvement has been reported in more than 95% of patients with ALL and in three fourths of those with AML.[26] The hemorrhagic complications of these acute leukemias rarely permit histologic evaluation of the liver in patients with early, active disease. Therefore, it is difficult to discern the relative contributions of leukemic infiltration, extramedullary hematopoiesis, and infectious or toxic complications of the underlying leukemia (or the therapies employed) to the development of hepatomegaly and liver test abnormalities.

In patients with a leukemia that runs a more chronic course, hepatic involvement is much more commonly detected on histologic evaluation than is indicated initially by clinical or laboratory assessment.[25–31] In an autopsy series, 98% of patients with chronic lymphocytic leukemia (CLL) were found to have leukemic infiltration, which consisted predominantly of portal infiltrates that usually left the hepatic limiting plates intact.[27] However, in some cases, leukemic infiltrates were observed to bridge adjacent portal tracts and to be associated with hepatocellular necrosis, bridging necrosis, and occasionally pseudolobule formation. In contrast to the predominantly portal pattern of hepatic infiltration in CLL, liver involvement in hairy cell leukemia (HCL), large granular lymphocytic leukemia (LGLL), and the adult T cell leukemia/lymphoma syndrome associated with human T lymphotropic virus type I (HTLV-1) infection is usually characterized by diffuse sinusoidal infiltration or a mixed pattern of portal and sinusoidal involvement.[28–31]

As in the case of CLL, nearly all patients with HCL, including some without hepatomegaly or liver test abnormalities, demonstrate hepatic infiltration on histologic evaluation.[29, 30] Although liver infiltration by HCL occasionally may be missed on conventional histologic evaluation, use of tartrate-resistant acid phosphatase staining[29] and immunotyping by staining with monoclonal antibodies against lymphocyte cell surface markers[21] has been reported to enhance diagnostic sensitivity and specificity. HCL also has been associated with angiomatous lesions in the liver that are created by disruption of the sinusoidal wall, with resulting wide areas of communication between the sinusoidal lumen and the space of Disse and replacement of the sinusoidal cell lining by tumor cells that are in direct contact with hepatocytes.[30]

Other Myeloproliferative Syndromes

Because the liver is a major site of extramedullary hematopoiesis, hepatomegaly or mild liver biochemical test abnormalities secondary to extramedullary hematopoiesis may occur in a variety of myeloproliferative disorders or marrow-infiltrating malignancies.[24] Benign or malignant proliferations of histiocytes (macrophages) or dendritic cells may be complicated by hepatomegaly or jaundice resulting from the diffuse infiltration of hepatic sinusoids by erythrophagocytic histiocytes, peliosis hepatis, or intrahepatic or extrahepatic invasion of bile ducts and portal tracts by histiocytes or Langerhans (dendritic) cells.[32–35] Erythrophagocytosis may be a manifestation of malignant histiocytosis or may represent a reactive benign histiocyte proliferation in patients with advanced T cell lymphomas.[32] Thus, assessment of involved tissues for malignant cells of T cell or, more rarely, B cell origin should be included in the diagnostic evaluation of myeloproliferative disorders of uncertain origin. Liver biopsies are commonly abnormal in patients with Langerhans cell histiocytosis (formerly termed histiocytosis X). The most common abnormality in this disorder is mild mononuclear cell infiltration of the portal tracts.[35] However, portal triaditis associated with periportal fibrosis, cirrhosis, or extrahepatic cholangiographic evidence of sclerosing cholangitis also may be seen and in some patients may lead to severe cholestatic liver disease.[34, 35]

HEPATIC SARCOIDOSIS

Sarcoidosis is a systemic disease of uncertain etiology that is characterized by the presence of granulomas in multiple organs. Hepatic involvement is not a source of significant morbidity in most patients with sarcoidosis, but in some reports as many as 80% to 95% of North or South American

Table 82–2 | **Hepatic Involvement in Sarcoidosis**

Most common
- Incidental hepatic granulomas in active pulmonary, skin, or ocular disease

Common
- Hepatic granulomas, fever, and weight loss with or without extrahepatic disease

Rare
- Severe intrahepatic cholestasis
- Portal hypertension secondary to cirrhosis, extensive granulomas, or nodular hyperplasia

patients with sarcoidosis have hepatic granulomas on liver biopsy[36, 37] (see also Chapter 69). As is summarized in Table 82–2, hepatic involvement in sarcoidosis may be associated with a number of disparate clinical syndromes. In most affected patients, hepatic granulomas appear incidental to a disease primarily involving the lung or other organs. However, because of the highly variable clinical picture of sarcoidosis, liver test abnormalities, the presence of noncaseating epithelioid granulomas on liver biopsy specimens, and symptoms apparently related to the presence of hepatic involvement may be among the earliest manifestations of the disease.[38, 39] Additionally, liver biopsy results may prove helpful in confirming the diagnosis of sarcoidosis in patients with suspected sarcoid involvement of other organs.

Pathologic Findings

Sarcoid granulomas are scattered diffusely throughout the hepatic lobule with increased frequency in the portal tracts or periportal areas.[24, 37, 39] They consist of epithelioid cells, sometimes with multinucleated giant cells, surrounded by lymphocytes or macrophages. Rarely, hepatic granulomas contain laminated concretions (Schaumann's bodies), asteroid bodies, or calcium oxalate crystals. Although frank caseation is not seen, central granular necrosis of granulomas may occur. Sarcoid granulomas typically are small and not detected on radiographic studies. However, sarcoid granulomas may cluster to form large aggregates and may be surrounded by significant fibrosis or inflammation,[24, 39] leading occasionally to the appearance on ultrasound, computed tomographic, or magnetic resonance images of multiple, 0.1- to 3.0-cm nodules.[40]

In addition to granulomas, patients with hepatic sarcoidosis commonly have varying degrees of Kupffer cell hyperplasia and mononuclear cell infiltration in both the portal tracts and hepatic lobules.[37, 39] In patients with clinical manifestations of portal hypertension or liver disease, additional vascular and cholestatic lesions also have been observed. Granulomatous phlebitis of portal and hepatic veins has been observed in association with multiple foci of parenchymal fibrosis or with diffuse nodular regenerative hyperplasia.[41, 42] In patients with cholestasis, ductopenia (loss of intrahepatic bile ducts), bile duct lesions similar to those seen in primary biliary cirrhosis, and periductal fibrosis reminiscent of primary sclerosing cholangitis have been observed.[42] Finally, among patients with clinical evidence of liver disease, cirrhosis has been noted in 6% and lesser degrees of fibrosis in an additional 15% of cases.[42]

Clinical Manifestations and Treatment

In approximately one third of patients with sarcoidosis, liver biochemical test abnormalities are characterized by elevated serum alkaline phosphate levels with or without less prominent elevations in serum aminotransferase levels.[38, 43] Most patients with sarcoidosis and liver biochemical test abnormalities have no symptoms or signs of liver disease, and on follow-up, the liver enzyme abnormalities improve initially in one half or more of patients, irrespective of the use of immunosuppressive therapy.[43] Small subsets of patients with hepatic sarcoidosis present with jaundice or pruritus resulting from chronic intrahepatic cholestasis[39, 44, 45] or with complications of portal hypertension.[39, 46, 47] In patients with prominent intrahepatic cholestasis, the histologic evolution of the disease is characterized by progressive destruction of bile ducts by granulomas, leading in turn to progressive depletion of interlobular bile ducts, periportal fibrosis, and the development of "biliary" cirrhosis reminiscent of the late stages of primary biliary cirrhosis.[44, 45] Most patients with cholestatic liver disease in the setting of systemic sarcoidosis lack antimitochondrial antibodies.[44] However, rare patients with multiorgan granulomas and antimitochondrial antibodies appear to fulfill common diagnostic criteria for both sarcoidosis and primary biliary cirrhosis.[46, 48] Recent reports have described improvement in symptoms and liver biochemical tests in patients with sarcoidosis and intrahepatic cholestasis following treatment with ursodeoxycholic acid, but this therapy has not yet been studied in controlled trials.[48a, 48b]

Patients with sarcoidosis who present with complications of portal hypertension may have histologic evidence of cirrhosis, extensive granulomas, or nodular regenerative hyperplasia. In some patients with nodular regenerative hyperplasia, measurement of wedged hepatic vein pressure has been normal, suggesting that the cause of portal hypertension is granulomatous infiltration[47] or granulomatous phlebitis, either of which leads to obliteration of portal vein branches and presinusoidal portal hypertension.[41] Portal hypertension has been observed to develop in patients on glucocorticoid therapy. Moreover, in patients presenting with jaundice caused by severe intrahepatic cholestasis or with complications of portal hypertension, improvement on glucocorticoids has not been observed consistently.[39, 44–47] Indeed, many authors have reported that the severity of glucocorticoid-induced adverse effects tends to exceed the therapeutic benefit achieved in this group of patients.[39, 44, 46] Liver transplantation has been performed successfully in such patients with advanced hepatic disease.[49]

Another group of patients with hepatic sarcoidosis has been reported to present with systemic symptoms, including fever and weight loss, with markedly elevated serum alkaline phosphatase levels but without jaundice or other complications of chronic liver disease. Such patients tend not to have prominent symptomatic or radiographic evidence of pulmonary sarcoidosis. Evidence of multiorgan granulomatous disease is usually confirmed by biopsy of skin, lymph nodes, or conjunctiva.[38, 50] Such patients with symptomatic, predominantly extrapulmonary sarcoidosis are indistinguishable clinically from a group of patients characterized as having idiopathic granulomatous hepatitis without evidence of extrahepatic involvement.[36, 51–54] The relative proportion of patients with hepatic granulomas who are classified as having systemic sarcoidosis versus idiopathic granulomatous hepatitis varies greatly from series to series[36, 38, 50, 54] and may depend on referral patterns, length of follow-up, or persistence in the pursuit of evidence of extrahepatic involvement. In evaluating such patients, it is important to exclude infectious or other causes of granulomas (see Chapter 69) and to observe patients for the possibility of spontaneous remission.[38, 51] However, in patients with a prolonged symptomatic course and no defined etiology of hepatic granulomatous disease except for sarcoidosis or idiopathic granulomatous hepatitis, the symptomatic response to glucocorticoid therapy has been reported to be gratifying.[38, 51–54] Improvement in symptoms, liver biochemical tests, or both, also has been reported following low-dose methotrexate therapy in patients with idiopathic granulomatous hepatitis[54a] and systemic sarcoidosis with hepatic involvement.[54b] Although relapses are common in patients who are treated for only brief periods with glucocorticoids, most such patients experience remission of systemic symptoms again and exhibit some improvement in liver enzyme on retreatment with glucocorticoids or other immunosuppressive agents.[38, 51–54] Such patients rarely have significant fibrosis on initial or follow-up liver biopsies and lack manifestations of portal hypertension.[38, 53] It is unclear whether the relatively benign course is a characteristic of this variant of sarcoidosis or an effect of immunosuppressive therapy.

HEPATIC AMYLOIDOSIS

Amyloidosis is a disorder of protein metabolism that leads to extracellular deposition of insoluble proteinaceous material, which consists of three components: (1) a nonfibrillar glycoprotein, serum amyloid P (SAP), that is present as a minor component in every form of amyloid deposit; (2) a fibrillar protein that varies in different forms of the disease (Table 82–3); and (3) glycosoaminoglycans, predominantly of the heparan sulfate and dermatan sulfate type, that are noncovalently associated with the fibrillar proteins. Amyloid deposits appear homogeneous and amorphous under the light microscope and, when stained with Congo red, produce a green birefringence when viewed with a polarizing microscope. Despite these relatively uniform and specific staining characteristics, amyloid deposits are produced by a variety of diseases of diverse etiology and may be present in single or multiple organs.

Classification

The original attempts to classify amyloidosis were based on apparent etiology and perceived differences in organ involvement. The most popular such classification[55–57] subdivided amyloidosis into *primary amyloidosis*, a syndrome having no apparent preceding or coexisting disease; *secondary amyloidosis*, a syndrome associated with a variety of chronic inflammatory diseases; *localized* or *tumor-forming amyloidosis*; *familial amyloidosis*; and *amyloidosis associated with multiple myeloma*. Early descriptions emphasized apparent differences in organ involvement among the various syndromes, with primary amyloidosis found to involve principally the tongue, heart, gastrointestinal tract, muscle, nerves, and skin and secondary amyloidosis reported to involve predominantly the liver, spleen, kidneys, and adrenal glands. Differences in histologic characteristics also were noted, with primary amyloidosis having variable staining patterns and more nodular deposits and secondary amyloidosis having more uniform staining properties.[55, 58] However, a significant overlap between these syndromes became apparent, serum M-paraproteins were found to be associated with a high percentage of cases classified as either primary or secondary, and the liver was found to be involved commonly in all forms of systemic amyloidosis.[57, 58]

As the basic biochemical and molecular properties of amyloid deposits have become better understood, classification systems based on the nature of the fibrillar protein component, underlying disease pathogenesis, and extent of organ involvement have become more useful.[59–60] Table 82–3 details the nature of fibrillar protein found in amyloid deposits that are present in the liver and other organs involved in various forms of systemic amyloidosis. In the classification system used in Table 82–3, the letter A designates amyloid fibril protein and is modified by a second letter (or letters) to indicate the specific fibrillar protein. Thus, the amino terminal fragment of immunoglobulin light chains found in the majority of amyloid deposits in both primary amyloidosis and amyloidosis associated with multiple myeloma is designated AL, and the amyloid A component found in secondary

Table 82–3 | **Nomenclature and Classification of Systemic Amyloidosis Syndromes**

AMYLOID PROTEIN	PRECURSOR OF FIBRIL PROTEIN	CLINICAL SYNDROME
AA	Serum amyloid A protein (SAA)	Reactive (secondary) amyloidosis associated with chronic disease, familial Mediterranean fever, Muckle-Wells syndrome
AL	Immunoglobulin light chains, $\kappa\lambda$	Amyloidosis associated with multiple myeloma, macroglobulinemia, monoclonal gammopathy, or occult immunocyte dyscrasia
AH	Heavy chain of IgG_1	Same as above
$A\beta_2M$	Plasma β_2-microglobulin	Hemodialysis-associated amyloidosis
ATTR	Normal plasma transthyretin or genetic variants Thr45, Ala60, Ser80, Met111, Ile122	Senile systemic amyloidosis, autosomal dominant familial amyloid polyneuropathy
ACys	Genetic variant Glu68 of cystatin A	Hereditary cerebral hemorrhage with amyloidosis, Icelandic type
AGel	Genetic variant Asn187 or Tyr187 of gelsolin	Familial amyloid polyneuropathy (Finland)
AApoAI	Genetic variant Arg26 or Arg60 of apolipoprotein AI	Non-neuropathic systemic amyloidosis (Ostertag type)
ALys	Genetic variants Thr56 or His67 of lysozyme	Non-neuropathic systemic amyloidosis (Ostertag type)
AFib	Genetic variant Leu554 of fibrinogen α chain	Non-neuropathic systemic amyloidosis (Ostertag type)

Data from references 59 and 60.

amyloidosis is designated AA. Not included in Table 82–3 are additional amyloid proteins not known to be deposited in the liver, such as Aβ, the amyloid β-protein found in brain deposits in Alzheimer's disease, or AIAPP, the islet amyloid polypeptide deposited in islets of Langerhans in type II diabetes mellitus.

Pathologic Findings

Despite the apparent diversity of proteins that may serve as precursors for amyloid fibrils, the fibrils in all forms of amyloidosis share a similar ultrastructural morphology. They are rigid, twisting, nonbranching fibrils that are 7 to 15 nm in diameter and that take up Congo red dye from alkaline alcoholic salt-saturated solutions and display strong apple green uniaxial positive birefringence when viewed in polarized light. This common staining pattern is thought to reflect either a common intermolecular packing motif shared by all amyloid fibrils[61, 62] or a common secondary structure that gives rise to antiparallel β-pleated sheets arranged with their long axes perpendicular to the long axis of the fibril.[63] Other proteins with repeating β-sheet motifs are also insoluble and highly resistant to proteinase; thus, the common structural motif of the amyloid proteins may explain similarities in patterns of both histologic staining and pathologic involvement in amyloidosis caused by highly disparate precursor protein abnormalities.

In the liver, as in other organs, amyloidosis gives rise to amorphous, hyaline extracellular deposits in the walls of arteries and arterioles, with less involvement of portal or hepatic veins. In the liver, the space of Disse also is a major site of amyloid involvement. Three patterns of hepatic amyloid deposits have been described: (1) extensive space of Disse and sinusoidal intralobular or parenchymal involvement (Fig. 82–1), (2) vascular and periportal involvement, and (3) a mixture of parenchymal and periportal involvement.[64, 65] An additional unusual histologic presentation of amyloid deposition in the liver is the presence of oval globular deposits, 5 to 40 μm in diameter, in the space of Disse or portal triads of patients without typical nonglobular parenchymal or vascular involvement[66] (Fig. 82–2). Patients with predominantly sinusoidal or parenchymal involvement may present with massive hepatomegaly occasionally associated with ascites; on light microscopy, they are found to have amyloid deposits that distort and compress the normal hepatocyte plates, often leaving little of the hepatic parenchyma normal. Other patients may present only with infiltration of the portal blood vessel walls with amyloid deposits that spare the hepatic parenchyma. Such patients typically have less prominent or no hepatomegaly.

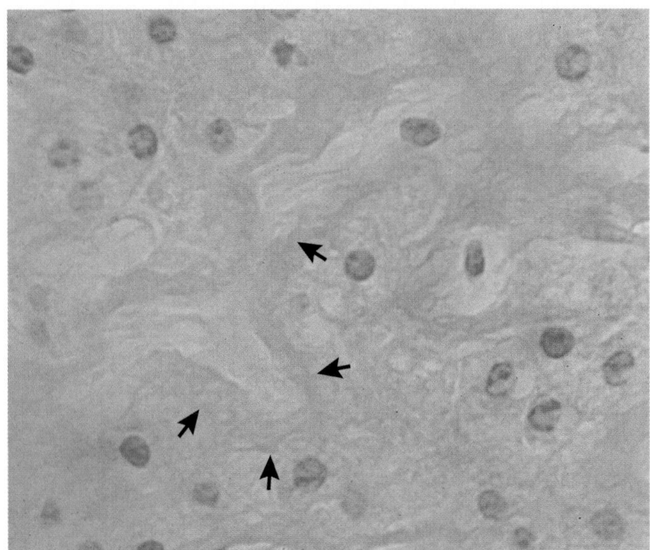

Figure 82–1. Liver biopsy showing extracellular amyloid diffusely present in space of Disse *(arrows)*. Congo red stain, 200×.

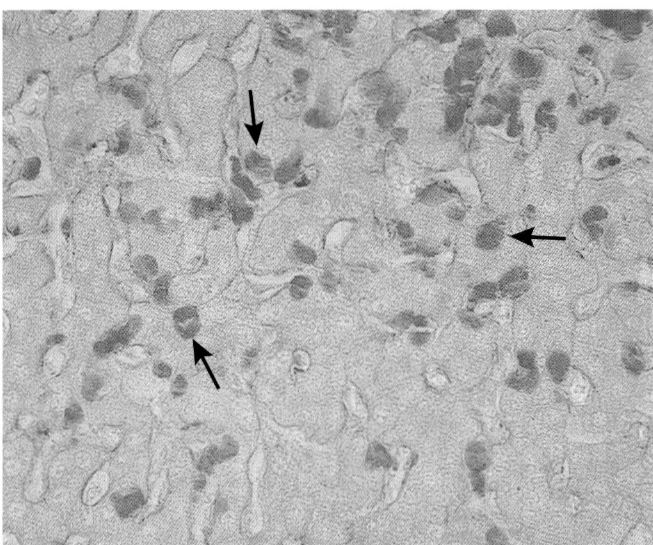

Figure 82–2. Liver biopsy showing globular deposition of amyloid in numerous Kupffer cells *(arrows)* in hepatic sinusoids occasionally indenting adjacent hepatocytes. Congo red stain, 100×.

Although previous reports suggested that primary AL forms of amyloidosis were more likely to be associated with vascular involvement in the liver and that secondary AA amyloidosis was more commonly associated with parenchymal infiltration, more recent reports have found frequent vascular involvement in AA forms of amyloidosis, as well as nearly universal parenchymal infiltration in AL amyloidosis.[64, 65] The differences in patterns of amyloid deposition between AL and AA amyloidosis may be statistically significant, but the degree of overlap is so great that histologic characterization would seem to have little value in ascribing an etiology to individual cases of hepatic amyloidosis.[64, 65] Instead, current diagnostic efforts tend to focus on specific immunohistochemical techniques that attempt to identify the nature of the amyloid fibril proteins in combination with clinical evaluation of the patient for potential underlying diseases or amyloid fibril protein precursor abnormalities. Commercially available antibodies to serum amyloid A and β_2-microglobulin have been reported to be almost universally successful in staining AA and Aβ_2M amyloid deposits, respectively[59]; antibodies against other known amyloid fibril proteins are also available.[67] AL fibril proteins most commonly derive from the amino terminal variable region of immunoglobulin light chains, with λ light chains more frequently the source than κ light chains. Perhaps for these reasons, commercially available antisera stain AL deposits in only approximately one half of cases[59] because they react predominantly with invariant epitopes on κ and λ chains and less often with variable regions. However, in AL amyloidosis, careful investigation of serum and urine samples usually reveals the source of the monoclonal light chain fibril protein.

Clinical and Laboratory Findings

Systemic amyloidosis usually presents after age 40 and is slightly more common in men than women.[57] The most common symptoms are fatigue, weight loss, and edema, each of which is reported by 40% to 70% of patients.[57] Weight loss is noted by more than one half of patients and often is severe.[57] Edema is usually associated with congestive heart failure but rarely with ascites or other stigmata of portal hypertension.[57] In addition to such nonspecific systemic complaints, approximately 25% of patients with systemic amyloidosis report paresthesias, which are even more common in certain familial forms of amyloidosis.[57, 59, 60] Other complaints may include cough or dyspnea secondary to pulmonary involvement, purpuric or papular lesions of the skin, carpal tunnel syndrome, orthostatic hypotension secondary to autonomic neuropathy, and gastrointestinal bleeding, diarrhea, or malabsorption secondary to gastrointestinal involvement.[57] Presenting complaints referable to hepatic involvement are uncommon and may include right upper quadrant discomfort related to hepatomegaly or, rarely, severe cholestasis,[68, 69] hepatic encephalopathy, or intractable ascites. Severe cholestatic presentations appear to be limited largely to patients with advanced AL amyloidosis.[69]

Hepatomegaly is noted on physical examination in 40% to 50% of patients with the more common forms of systemic amyloidosis (AL and AA). Modest elevations of serum alkaline phosphatase levels and hypoalbuminemia are common, whereas elevated serum aminotransferase levels are less common and elevated serum bilirubin levels rare.[57] The prothrombin time also may be abnormal.[70] However, there is a poor correlation between the degree of liver biochemical test abnormalities and the extent of hepatic amyloid deposition. In addition, patients without hepatomegaly or abnormal liver biochemical tests may prove to have histologic evidence of hepatic involvement.

Diagnosis of Systemic Amyloidosis with Hepatic Involvement

In patients with hepatomegaly and mild liver test abnormalities that develop in the setting of a known monoclonal gammopathy, a chronic inflammatory disease, or a constellation of systemic symptoms or signs typical of systemic amyloidosis, hepatic amyloid deposition should be suspected. Because there is no laboratory test capable of making a specific diagnosis of amyloidosis, a histologic diagnosis is required for confirmation. Liver biopsy has a high diagnostic yield in systemic amyloidosis. However, previous reports of serious hemorrhagic complications following needle biopsy of the liver or of other organs with amyloid deposits[70] suggest that, when possible, diagnostic biopsies should be limited to sites accessible to local control of bleeding. Patients with hepatic amyloidosis almost invariably have involvement of other organ sites that are as or more amenable to diagnostic biopsies. Needle aspiration of abdominal subcutaneous fat and rectal biopsy are two alternative approaches that have been recommended and have a high diagnostic yield with lower rates of life-threatening hemorrhage.[60, 70] Hepatic dysfunction is rarely a source of great morbidity in systemic amyloidosis, and the degree or type of hepatic involvement has little direct bearing on therapeutic decisions. Moreover, scintigraphy using radiolabeled serum amyloid P (SAP) has proved to have high sensitivity and specificity in demonstrating liver involvement in systemic amyloidosis.[67] Thus, liver biopsy is rarely necessary to confirm infiltration of the liver in patients with amyloid involvement that can be demonstrated in other organs.

However, in many cases of hepatic amyloidosis, patients present initially with hepatomegaly or liver test abnormalities and lack other clinical findings suggestive of systemic amyloidosis. In such cases, the differential diagnosis usually includes disorders that are unlikely to be demonstrated on histologic evaluation of subcutaneous or rectal tissues. Moreover, in some cases of systemic amyloidosis, attempts to obtain a histologic diagnosis from extrahepatic sites may prove to be unproductive. In such situations, liver biopsy may be appropriate if coagulation test results are acceptable and patients have not had prior evidence of a bleeding dyscrasia. One review of bleeding manifestations in 100 patients with amyloidosis noted that all patients with hemorrhagic complications of diagnostic procedures had a prior history of a bleeding disorder.[70] In this study, 41 of 100 patients had hemorrhagic manifestations at some point in their course, and 45 had abnormalities of one or more coagulation tests. Only the presence of a prolonged prothrombin time correlated with the risk of bleeding complications, but many patients with hemorrhagic complications had normal coagulation tests. Among eight patients who had episodes of bleeding induced by diagnostic or therapeutic procedures, no coagulation test was found to be predictive of bleeding, but all eight patients had other bleeding problems such as intracutaneous hemorrhage (ecchymoses), gastrointestinal bleeding, hematuria, or hemoptysis[70] preceding the diagnostic procedure. These findings suggest that although coagulation abnormalities may complicate amyloidosis, other factors such as amyloid infiltration of blood vessel walls also play a role in the propensity to hemorrhagic complications.

Treatment and Prognosis

Systemic amyloidosis is often an incurable and inevitably progressive disease. The majority of deaths are related to cardiac or renal complications or, in the case of multiple myeloma, to progression of the underlying malignancy.[57, 59] Morbidity and mortality is rarely determined by the extent of hepatic involvement. Nevertheless, patients who present with initial hepatic manifestations may survive for prolonged intervals. Thus, careful thought must be given to additional therapeutic approaches that may improve the prognosis in these patients.

In general, therapy of amyloidosis is directed at management of renal, cardiac, or other organ complications and, when possible, reduction of the amount of amyloid precursor protein to prevent or slow the rate of further amyloid deposition. In selected patients, renal or cardiac transplantation has been performed with an apparent increase in survival and improvement in the quality of life.[59, 71] Traditional chemotherapy regimens directed at reducing the level of monoclonal immunoglobulin light chains in patients with AL amyloidosis have proven only marginally beneficial,[72] although apparent regression of amyloidosis with reduction in organomegaly and improvement in organ function has been reported in rare individual cases in which the abnormal B or plasma cell clone has responded well to cytoreductive therapy.[73] More recently, scintigraphy using ^{123}I-labeled SAP has been used to monitor progression or regression of amyloid deposits during therapy[74, 75] and has led to a greater appreciation of the frequency with which diminution and even disappearance of visceral amyloid deposits occur in patients treated with agents designed to block production of the precursor of the offending amyloid fibril protein.[59, 67, 74–76] Indeed, in small studies, one half of patients treated with high-dose melphalan in combination with stem cell rescue have been observed to enter complete remission of the underlying plasma cell dyscrasia and to show improvement in amyloid-related organ dysfunction.[67, 76]

In contrast to the generally poor response of AL amyloidosis to therapeutic maneuvers, AA amyloidosis has been noted more frequently to improve with therapies designed to prevent initial amyloid deposition or disease progression. Treatment with colchicine therapy decreases symptoms and prevents amyloid deposition in patients with familial Mediterranean fever and appears also to benefit patients who have already developed amyloidosis.[77] In other cases of AA amyloidosis secondary to Crohn's disease, juvenile rheumatoid arthritis, or chronic infections such as tuberculosis or leprosy, progression of the disease appears to cease following initiation of specific therapy for the underlying disorder.[59, 78, 79] Finally, liver transplantation has proven effective in halting progression and inducing modest improvement in neurologic symptoms and regression of systemic amyloid deposits in patients with amyloid transthyretin (ATTR) (type I familial amyloid neuropathy) amyloidosis.[80, 81] Liver transplantation has also been employed successfully in other forms of genetic amyloidosis, including AApoAI, Alys, and AFib amyloidosis.[67] The salutary effects of liver transplantation in ATTR (and potentially in AapoAI and AFib) amyloidosis appear to relate to the rapid disappearance of variant transthyretin (formerly prealbumin) from the circulation following replacement of the liver, the predominant site of synthesis of this serum protein.[82] Because ATTR amyloidosis rarely involves the liver, has never been associated with liver failure, and usually does not manifest extrahepatic complications until the third decade of life or later, ATTR liver explants are considered suitable for sequential ("domino") transplantation into older recipients or into recipients with primary hepatic malignancies.[67, 80, 81]

SICKLE CELL DISEASE INVOLVING THE LIVER

Sickle cell anemia and its variants are inherited disorders of hemoglobin structure that are characterized by chronic hemolytic anemia and recurrent episodes of vascular occlusion leading to ischemia and distal tissue infarction in multiple organs. As in other cases of chronic hemolytic anemia, there is a high frequency of black pigment (calcium bilirubinate) gallstones.[83, 84] Blood transfusions are frequently employed in the therapy of sickle cell anemia, and such patients are at increased risk of hepatitis C and other forms of post-transfusion hepatitis.[85] Multitransfused teenage and adult patients with sickle cell anemia also may have varying degrees of excess hepatic iron stores that are comparable with those noted in thalassemia major.[86] In addition to liver dysfunction related to extrahepatic obstruction, viral hepatitis, or pathologic iron overload, patients with sickle cell disease often have evidence of acute or chronic ischemic damage to the liver that appears to be related to intrasinusoidal sickling, impaired intrahepatic blood flow, and reduced delivery of oxygen to hepatocytes.[87, 88]

Hepatic Pathology

When histologic evaluation of the liver has been performed in patients with sickle cell anemia at autopsy, cholecystectomy, or diagnostic percutaneous liver biopsy, dilated sinusoids, erythrophagocytosis by Kupffer cells (Fig. 82–3), and varying degrees of parenchymal atrophy in the central zones of the liver have been observed frequently.[87–93] In association with hepatic sinusoids engorged by phagocytosed, sickled red blood cells, adjacent areas of ischemic necrosis have been reported in patients with acute episodes of jaundice, right upper quadrant pain, fever, and leukocytosis thought to be secondary to intrahepatic sickle cell crises.[87–89, 93, 94] Accumulation of collagen or thin basement membranes within the space of Disse,[89] perisinusoidal fibrosis,[93] and an apparently high frequency of cirrhosis in patients with sickle cell anemia[87] have suggested that recurrent ischemic injury secondary to intrahepatic sickling may also be a cause of chronic liver disease.

Although early reports suggested that viral hepatitis was an unusual cause of acute or chronic liver disease in such patients,[89, 90] studies conducted in the 1980s suggested that both hepatitis B[91, 92] and hepatitis C[85] are common infections in patients with sickle cell anemia and may account for

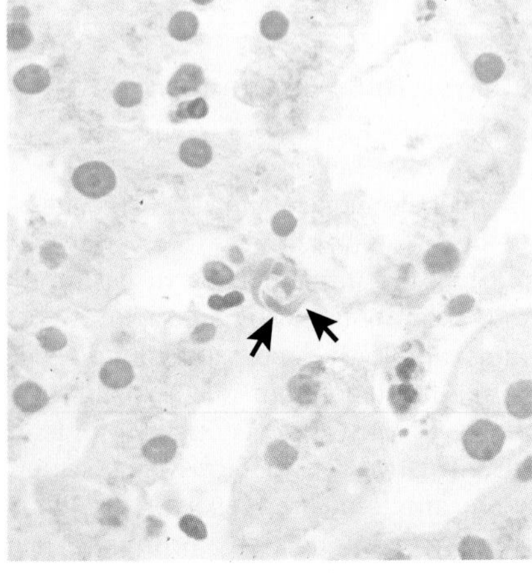

Figure 82–3. Liver biopsy showing sickled red blood cells in Kupffer cell (erythrophagocytosis) *(arrows)* in hepatic sinusoid of a patient with sickle cell disease. Hematoxylin and eosin stain, 200×.

many episodes of acute or chronic liver disease previously attributed to sickle cell hepatopathy. In a recent study, more than 20% of patients with sickle cell anemia were found to have antibody to hepatitis C virus (HCV).[85] The prevalence of antibody to hepatitis C was highest in recipients of multiple units of blood products. There also was a significant correlation between the presence of antibody to hepatitis C and the presence of persistent serum alanine aminotransferase (ALT) elevations in this patient population; 9 of 11 patients with persistently elevated serum ALT levels were anti-HCV seropositive compared with only 14% of patients with normal ALT values.[85] In studies performed in Los Angeles, acute and chronic hepatitis B infections were found to be the most common causes of liver disease in a group of patients with hemoglobin SS or SC disease.[91, 92]

In these studies, intrasinusoidal sickling and Kupffer cell erythrophagocytosis (see Fig. 82–3) were found almost invariably in all patients with sickle cell anemia irrespective of the apparent cause of liver disease or degree of serum ALT elevation. Intrasinusoidal sickling also was found in two liver biopsies performed after recovery from acute viral hepatitis. To some extent, the presence of nonphagocytosed sickled red blood cells in hepatic sinusoids could be attributed to the observation that formalin fixation was noted to induce irreversible sickling of red blood cells in patients with hemoglobin SS or SC disease.[92] In addition, Omata and colleagues[92] have suggested that Kupffer cell erythrophagocytosis may reflect the role of Kupffer cells in the clearance of sickled red cells in functionally asplenic patients with sickle cell anemia. Thus, the degree of intrasinusoidal sickling or even Kupffer cell erythrophagocytosis is a poor indicator of possible ischemic liver injury in patients with sickle cell anemia. In contrast, other features of vascular insufficiency such as acute ischemic necrosis, sinusoidal dilatation, and perisinusoidal fibrosis appear to be more specific markers of vascular injury in patients with symptomatic liver dysfunction in the absence of viral hepatitis or other causes of hepatocellular injury.[93]

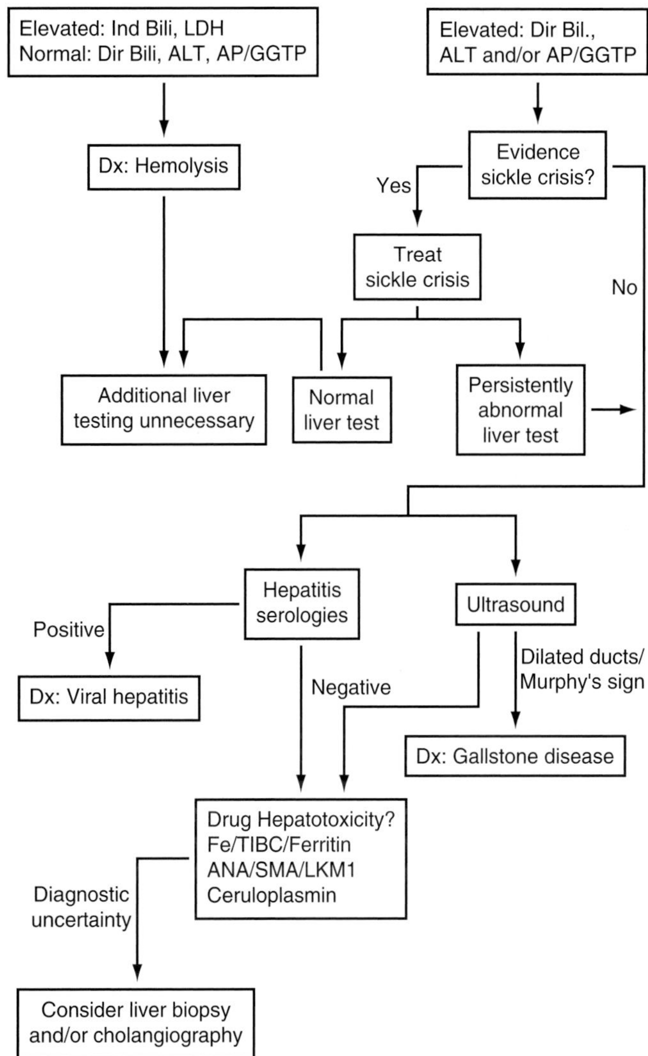

Figure 82–4. Algorithm for the evaluation of abnormal liver tests in patients with sickle cell anemia. (ALT, alanine aminotransferase; ANA, antinuclear antibody; AP, alkaline phosphatase; Dir Bili, direct bilirubin; Dx, diagnosis; Fe, iron; GGTP, gamma glutamyl transpeptidase; Ind Bili, indirect bilirubin; LDH, lactate dehydrogenase; LKM1, liver kidney microsomal antibodies type 1; SMA, smooth muscle antibodies; TIBC, total iron-binding capacity.)

Diagnosis and Management of Liver Disease in Patients with Sickle Cell Anemia

Diggs[88] reported in 1965 that 10% of patients presenting with acute sickle crises were jaundiced. A more recent assessment of the prevalence of liver disease in patients with sickle cell anemia has found persistent elevations in one or more serum liver enzymes in 24% of patients with sickle cell anemia.[91] In addition, 48 of 72 (67%) patients without other biochemical evidence of liver disease had a total serum bilirubin level of greater than 2 mg/dL (>34 μmol/L). Thus, laboratory abnormalities suggesting possible liver disease are common in patients with sickle cell anemia and frequently lead to diagnostic evaluations, as detailed in Figure 82–4.

In patients with sickle cell anemia without liver disease, hyperbilirubinemia is exclusively unconjugated, or indirect, and only uncommonly exceeds levels of 4.5 mg/dL (77 μmol/L). In more severely jaundiced patients, higher serum lactate dehydrogenase levels are also seen and suggest higher rates of hemolysis.[91] However, in the setting of acute viral hepatitis or other causes of liver dysfunction, extreme levels of hyperbilirubinemia consisting of relatively equal amounts of direct and indirect bilirubin are observed.[91, 95] Although early reports suggested that a total serum bilirubin level of greater than 25 mg/dL (>428 μmol/L) was a grave prognostic sign,[88, 96] patients with extreme degrees of hyperbilirubinemia have been noted to have relatively benign courses of acute viral hepatitis or presumed intrahepatic sickle cell crises.[91, 95, 97] The degree of serum ALT or aspartate aminotransferase (AST) elevation in patients with sickle cell anemia and acute viral hepatitis is similar to that observed in other patients with acute viral hepatitis, with most symptomatic patients having elevations more than 10-fold the upper limit of normal.[90, 95] However, among patients with jaundice and other symptoms such as fever, leukocytosis, and intense right upper quadrant pain attributed to intrahepatic sickling, serum AST and ALT values have often been found to be only modestly elevated,[90, 96, 97] although in some cases, elevations in excess of 15 times the upper limit of normal have been noted.[89] Thus, in patients with jaundice and prominent ALT elevations, both acute viral hepatitis and ischemic injury related to sickle cell anemia itself must be considered as possible etiologies. In addition, coincidental causes of liver disease such as autoimmune hepatitis[98, 99] have been reported in patients with sickle cell anemia and clinically apparent liver disease that was initially ascribed incorrectly to complications of sickle cell anemia. Thus, when evaluating liver disease in these patients, one must take care to consider the full spectrum of possible etiologies.

Although the majority of patients with acute hepatocellular dysfunction thought to be secondary to either viral hepatitis or intrahepatic sickle cell crises recover after receiving supportive care, a number of cases of acute hepatic failure have been reported.[87, 90, 94, 100] Most such patients have presented with right upper quadrant pain, jaundice, modest serum aminotransferase elevations (<10-fold elevated), and progressive coagulopathy; at post-mortem examination, they have had histologic findings that suggest that the initiating cause of liver failure was centrilobular necrosis secondary to vascular complications of sickle cell disease.[94] Recovery from severe cholestasis and coagulopathy has been reported after exchange transfusions.[101] It also has been suggested that sickle cell anemia may be a predisposing factor to the development of acute hepatic failure in children with acute viral hepatitis.[100] Thus, even in cases of liver failure with an apparent viral etiology, aggressive measures directed at reversal or prevention of intrahepatic sickling may be warranted.

In all patients with sickle cell anemia and direct hyperbilirubinemia, and especially those with right upper quadrant pain, fever, and leukocytosis, acute cholecystitis with or without choledocholithiasis must be investigated as a possible primary or contributing cause. A number of reports indicate that common bile duct stones are found in a substantial proportion of patients with sickle cell anemia who undergo cholecystectomy for symptomatic biliary tract disease.[102, 103] However, other studies have noted no evidence of choledocholithiasis or acute or chronic cholecystitis in many patients with sickle cell anemia who undergo cholecystectomy for presumed symptomatic biliary tract disease. These observations have led to speculation that intrahepatic ischemia may better explain the symptoms and signs of liver disease in many of these patients.[93]

A significant rate of operative and anesthetic complications has been reported in patients with sickle cell anemia.[102–104] Therefore, cholecystectomy is not recommended in asymptomatic patients with cholelithiasis. However, several reports have noted that in patients with sickle cell anemia and recurrent bouts of right upper quadrant pain and jaundice, a marked decrease in such symptomatic episodes is noted after cholecystectomy.[93, 103, 104] Thus, cholecystectomy is recommended in recurrently symptomatic patients with gallstones in whom there is difficulty in distinguishing cholecystitis from intrahepatic crisis.[104] However, in such patients, special attention should be directed toward minimizing the risk of anoxic injury during surgery by preoperative transfusion of red blood cells and expansion of intravascular volume and by intraoperative and postoperative oxygen therapy.

HEPATIC DYSFUNCTION DURING SYSTEMIC INFECTION

Structural and functional hepatic abnormalities occur commonly during systemic infections. In many spirochetal, rickettsial, viral, and mycobacterial infections, hepatic abnormalities can be attributed to direct involvement of the liver by a multiorgan or systemic infection[105] (see Chapter 69). However, in a variety of bacterial infections, intrahepatic cholestasis is observed in the absence of evidence of direct invasion of the liver by the infectious agent. Jaundice is a well-recognized complication of severe bacterial infection in neonates[106–108] but is less frequent in adults with bacteremia. In one survey of bacteremia in adult patients, only 7 of 1150 patients (0.6%) were noted to develop jaundice in the absence of evidence of primary hepatic or biliary disease.[109] However, the frequency of subclinical liver dysfunction detected by laboratory testing alone is likely to be much higher.[105, 110–112] Moreover, in some diseases such as lobular pneumonia attributed to *Streptococcus pneumoniae* infection, the frequency of hepatic dysfunction has been noted to be much higher, with clinically apparent jaundice in 3% to 68% of patients and biochemical abnormalities in nearly all.[105, 110]

Although most early reports of cholestasis and serum liver enzyme abnormalities in patients with lobular pneumonia involved illness attributed to pneumococcal infection, similar clinical, biochemical, and histologic hepatic abnormalities have been reported in patients with pneumonia attributed to infection by *Klebsiella pneumoniae* and other bacterial agents. Similarly, cholestasis has been noted in bacteremic patients infected with a wide variety of gram-positive and gram-negative organisms.[105–113] The primary site of bacterial infection in such patients is also quite variable, with jaundice and other markers of hepatic dysfunction reported in patients not only with pneumonia, but also with pyelonephritis, diverticulitis, appendicitis, endocarditis, and pulmonary, soft tissue, abdominal, or pelvic abscesses.[105, 109, 111–113]

In some series, 40% to 90% mortality rates have been observed in patients in whom jaundice developed in the setting of extrahepatic bacterial infection,[109, 113] although hepatic failure appeared to play little or no direct role in such deaths. Such observations seem to indicate that hepatic dysfunction is related to the severity of the underlying disease and that the development of jaundice may be a sign of poor prognosis. However, among the subset of patients who become clinically jaundiced in the course of extrahepatic bacterial infection, the level of serum bilirubin does not appear to differ between survivors and nonsurvivors.[113] Moreover, in patients with pneumococcal pneumonia, the development of jaundice does not seem to correlate with a poor prognosis.[105, 110]

Laboratory and Histologic Features

Patients with jaundice in the setting of generalized sepsis usually exhibit a cholestatic pattern of biochemical and histologic abnormalities. In the majority of patients, serum alkaline phosphatase levels rise to only 1 to 3 times the upper limit of normal. In rare patients, 5- to 10-fold elevations in serum alkaline phosphatase levels, with similar elevations in serum gamma glutamyl transpeptidase levels, have been noted.[111, 112] Serum aminotransferase elevations tend to be modest.[111–113] Peak serum bilirubin levels typically range from 5 to 10 mg/dL (86 to 171 μmol/L), invariably with a significant component of conjugated hyperbilirubinemia[105, 110–113] However, serum bilirubin levels of 10 to 20 mg/dL (171 to 342 μmol/L) have been reported in 30% of patients with cholestasis ascribed to extrahepatic infection,[113] and levels as high as 30 to 50 mg/dL (513 to 855 μmol/L) have occasionally been noted.[105] The levels of serum enzymes and bilirubin may appear to be discrepant, with deeply jaundiced patients often having normal or nearly normal alkaline phosphatase levels, and some anicteric patients having prominent elevations of the serum alkaline phosphatase and γ-glutamyl transpeptidase levels.[111–113] Jaundice and liver enzyme abnormalities usually develop within several days of the onset of bacteremia and resolve following adequate treatment of the underlying infection. Coagulopathy related to hepatic dysfunction is not a feature of this syndrome, although hypoalbuminemia and hyperglobulinemia are common in both icteric and anicteric patients.[111, 113] Pruritus is usually absent, even in deeply jaundiced persons, but mild hepatomegaly is frequently noted on physical examination.[113]

In patients with cholestasis related to extrahepatic infection, liver histology usually reveals minimal or no histologic evidence of hepatocyte necrosis. Central and midzonal bile stasis is apparent in the majority of liver biopsies obtained from jaundiced patients. In some cases, a more striking picture of acute cholangiolitis, called "cholangitis lenta" (Fig. 82–5), is noted.[114] In these cases, portal tracts are surrounded by dilated cholangioles containing deeply stained bile thrombi. Neutrophils are usually present within and around these dilated cholangioles but do not involve ducts within the portal tracts, thus presenting a picture distinct from that seen with extrahepatic obstruction. However, in the majority of cases, histologic findings are less distinctive and may include a variety of nonspecific findings such as mild portal mononuclear cell infiltrates, either mild or occasionally extensive fatty change, parenchymal foci of cell dropout, Kupffer cell hyperplasia, and inflammatory infiltrates.[109, 111–113]

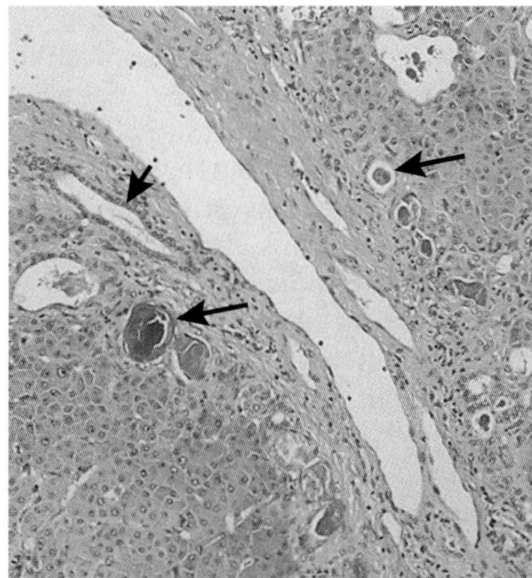

Figure 82–5. Liver biopsy specimen from a septic patient with marked hyperbilirubinemia and normal serum alkaline phosphatase levels with histologic picture of *cholangitis lenta.* Bile is inspissated in proliferated periportal bile ductules *(long arrows).* The interlobular bile ducts in the portal tract are normal in appearance without bile stasis or injury *(short arrows).* Hematoxylin and eosin stain, 25×.

Pathogenesis

The diversity of bacteria and extrahepatic sites of infection that have been implicated in cases of cholestasis suggests that the factors that initiate hepatic dysfunction are humoral and common to most if not all forms of bacterial infection. Circulating endotoxin has been observed to impair both basolateral and canalicular bile acid and organic anion transport.[115] Endotoxin also impairs bile acid–independent bile flow by impairing glutathione and bicarbonate excretion, while also blocking the choleretic effect of endotoxin-induced nitric oxide.[116] This profound cholestatic effect of endotoxin is mediated in part by a reduction in mRNA and protein levels of the ATP-dependent canalicular multispecific organic anion transporter.[117] Endotoxin stimulates the release of proinflammatory cytokines such as tumor necrosis factor, interleukin-1 (IL-1), and interleukin-6 (IL-6) that have been implicated as mediators of the cholestatic effects of endotoxin.[118–121] Administration of tumor necrosis factor in humans also causes frequently mild and occasionally severe hepatotoxicity[122] and has been implicated in the evolution of hepatic dysfunction in other diseases such as acute alcoholic hepatitis.[123] Finally, elevated levels of IL-6 have been observed in close association with paraneoplastic cholestasis syndromes in patients with renal cell carcinoma (Stauffer's syndrome) or other malignancies such as Hodgkin's disease that are known to secrete cytokines such as IL-6, IL-1, and tumor necrosis factor.[10, 124] Thus, these cytokines appear to be the final common mediators of cholestasis associated with a variety of inflammatory diseases.

A number of observations suggest that other factors also play a contributing role in the development of jaundice in patients with cholestasis associated with severe extrahepatic infection. In patients with lobar pneumonia, jaundice occurs more frequently in patients with a history of alcoholism and appears to be especially common among black men.[105, 125] These observations suggest that preexisting liver disease and hemolysis associated with glucose-6-phosphate deficiency may play a role in the development of jaundice in many of these patients.[105, 125] Because many patients with jaundice associated with severe bacterial infection have life-threatening illnesses and prerenal azotemia,[113] it is likely that both decreased hepatic perfusion resulting from septic shock and decreased urinary excretion of conjugated bilirubin play a significant role in determining the degree of hyperbilirubinemia in such patients.

Diagnosis and Management

Cholestasis induced by systemic or severe extrahepatic infection rarely contributes to morbidity or mortality. The major impact of cholestasis relates to potential errors in diagnosis or to inappropriate treatment directed at suspected primary hepatic or biliary diseases. In patients who present with fever and jaundice in the absence of prominent serum aminotransferase elevations or symptoms suggestive of primary hepatic or biliary tract disease, it is important to consider bacterial sepsis and other extrahepatic bacterial infections such as lobar pneumonia, pyelonephritis, appendicitis, and diverticulitis. Because the biochemical features of cholestasis associated with systemic infection cannot be readily distinguished from those found in patients with extrahepatic obstruction or hepatic abscess,[111] ultrasonographic evaluation of the liver and biliary tree is almost always indicated. However, a careful evaluation for bacteremia and for extrahepatic sites of bacterial infection should also be undertaken. When the presence of an extrahepatic or systemic infection has been established in a patient with a biochemical, clinical, and ultrasonographic picture consistent with intrahepatic cholestasis, additional radiologic and endoscopic procedures to exclude intrahepatic or biliary tract disease are often best deferred until the initial response to appropriate antimicrobial therapy can be assessed. In patients with mild jaundice and liver enzyme abnormalities, significant improvement in these abnormalities is usually apparent within the first week of therapy.[105, 111]

Table 82–4 | **Factors Contributing to Postoperative Jaundice**

Increased bilirubin production
Destruction of transfused erythrocytes
Hemolysis secondary to preexisting conditions (glucose-6-phosphate dehydrogenase deficiency, hemoglobinopathies, etc.)
Hemolysis secondary to mechanical prostheses
Resorption of hematomas
Hepatocellular injury
Ischemic hepatitis
Drug- or anesthetic-induced hepatotoxicity
Viral hepatitis
Extrahepatic biliary obstruction
Bile duct ligation
Choledocholithiasis
Postoperative pancreatitis
Extrinsic mass compression of bile duct
Intrahepatic cholestasis
Sepsis, bacterial abscess
Drug-induced cholestasis
Total parenteral nutrition
Preexisting abnormalities in bilirubin metabolism or secretion
Chronic liver disease
Gilbert's syndrome

POSTOPERATIVE CHOLESTASIS

Mild abnormalities of liver function are common after surgery[126] and likely relate to multiple factors that influence hepatic function in the perioperative setting (Table 82–4). Frank jaundice is much less common in the postoperative setting,[126] but severe cholestasis occasionally develops in the absence of extrahepatic obstruction or obvious hepatic parenchymal injury.[127, 128]

Clinical, Laboratory, and Pathologic Features

The syndrome of postoperative cholestasis is characterized by the development of jaundice 2 to 10 days after a prolonged, complicated operation. Serum bilirubin levels may rise to 10 to 40 mg/dL (171 to 684 μmol/L) in association with mild to occasionally prominent alkaline phosphatase elevations and generally less pronounced rises in serum aminotransferase levels.[126–128] Although early reports of this syndrome described a 50% or greater mortality rate because of the severity of the underlying disease,[127, 128] the course of the liver disease appeared to be benign, encephalopathy and other evidence of hepatic insufficiency did not develop, and jaundice resolved within 2 to 3 weeks of onset in surviving patients.[126–128] Histologic evaluation of the liver on biopsy or post-mortem examination in such patients usually shows only features of intrahepatic cholestasis, although Kupffer cell erythrophagocytosis and centrilobular congestion also have been noted.[127, 128] Episodes of benign postoperative cholestasis have almost invariably been preceded by long, complicated operative procedures associated with periods of hypotension and multiple blood transfusions. Thus, it is likely that increased bilirubin loads related to premature destruction of transfused erythrocytes or resorption of hematomas and the effects of transient ischemia and passive hepatic congestion play major roles in the pathogenesis of this syndrome.[126–128] In addition, many reported cases of postoperative cholestasis have been noted to be associated with peritonitis or other infectious complications during the postoperative period, suggesting that cholestatic responses to severe bacterial infection also play a role.[127]

Diagnosis and Management

Because of the multitude of factors that may influence liver function in the perioperative period (see Table 82–4), determination of the etiology of postoperative jaundice is rarely straightforward. Ischemic injury to the liver and hepatotoxicity caused by drugs or anesthetics such as halothane and related agents are generally readily distinguishable from other causes of cholestasis by the presence of more dramatic elevations of the serum aminotransferases.[127, 129–131] However, in patients with cholestatic biochemical abnormalities, exclusion of sepsis, bacterial abscess, extrahepatic biliary obstruction, and acalculous cholecystitis,[132] all of which require specific therapeutic intervention, necessitates additional bacteriologic and radiologic investigation. Preexisting liver disease or Gilbert's syndrome also may contribute significantly to postoperative jaundice.[126] In patients with delayed onset of postoperative jaundice or liver enzyme abnormalities, hepatic abnormalities associated with parenteral nutrition,[133] wound infection, drug toxicity, or the multiple organ failure syndrome[134, 135] should be considered in the differential diagnosis.

LIVER ABNORMALITIES IN RHEUMATOID ARTHRITIS

Abnormal liver biochemical tests, especially elevated serum alkaline phosphatase levels of hepatobiliary origin,[136–138] are observed commonly in patients with rheumatoid arthritis. In one large series,[137] 18% of patients with rheumatoid arthritis had elevated levels of serum alkaline phosphatase, and 11% had hepatomegaly. Fluctuations in serum alkaline phosphatase levels also have been reported to correlate with the activity of rheumatoid arthritis.[136–138] However, the degree of alkaline phosphatase elevation usually is modest, with the mean level being less than two-fold the upper limit of normal.[137] Furthermore, other clinical signs of liver disease are usually absent, and liver biopsy and autopsy studies have not revealed consistent or specific findings. The most common histologic abnormalities are fatty change, Kupffer cell hyperplasia, and mild mononuclear cell infiltration of the portal tracts or rare parenchymal foci of hepatocyte necrosis.[137, 139–142] Periportal fibrosis is also present in a few cases.[142] Determination of the etiology of hepatic dysfunction in patients with active rheumatoid arthritis is complicated by the observation that many drugs used currently or in the past to treat the disease have a known potential for liver injury.[141–145]

Primary Hepatic Disease in Patients with Rheumatoid Arthritis

In a small subset of patients with rheumatoid arthritis or Sjögren's syndrome, serum antimitochondrial antibodies are detectable, as are the biochemical and histologic features of primary biliary cirrhosis.[146–148] The incidence of primary biliary cirrhosis and autoimmune hepatitis appears to be much higher in patients with Sjögren's syndrome alone than in those with Sjögren's syndrome and rheumatoid arthritis or rheumatoid arthritis alone.[146–148] Hepatic amyloidosis also may rarely complicate long-standing rheumatoid arthritis.[59, 78] Because chronic hepatitis C and rheumatoid arthritis are both relatively common diseases of adults, it is not surprising that these two entities are found concurrently in some patients. However, it also has been noted that 75% of persons with chronic hepatitis C infection develop a rheumatoid factor,[149, 150] and a subset of these rheumatoid factor–positive persons develop essential mixed cryoglobulinemia, which may manifest in part by the development of arthralgias.[151, 152] Liver disease in such persons is often asymptomatic, and biochemical abnormalities are modest or even absent.[152] Thus, some persons with essential mixed cryoglobulinemia associated with chronic hepatitis C may be labeled erroneously as having rheumatoid arthritis. Alternatively, in some genetically susceptible persons, hepatitis C infection may precede and play a role in triggering the development of rheumatoid arthritis.[153]

Liver Abnormalities in Felty's Syndrome

Perhaps the most distinctive association between rheumatoid arthritis and hepatic abnormalities is seen in the subset of patients with rheumatoid arthritis in whom splenomegaly and neutropenia develop *(Felty's syndrome)*. Felty's syndrome is associated with an even higher frequency of hepatomegaly and liver biochemical test abnormalities than is seen in uncomplicated rheumatoid arthritis.[154, 155] However, there is little correlation between the level of serum hepatic enzyme abnormalities and hepatic histopathologic findings.[154, 155] Nevertheless, more than one half of patients with Felty's syndrome have hepatic histologic abnormalities that range from sinusoidal lymphocytosis and portal fibrosis to a more distinctive picture of nodular regenerative hyperplasia,[154–157] which, in one small prospective series, was found to be present in 5 of 18 (28%) patients. Hepatic encephalopathy and other manifestations of liver failure have not been reported in patients with Felty's syndrome and nodular regenerative hyperplasia, but portal hypertension and esophageal variceal hemorrhage may occur.[155–157]

Liver Abnormalities in Adult Still's Disease

In contrast to the lack of significant hepatic dysfunction in classic rheumatoid arthritis, adults with the systemic form of juvenile rheumatoid arthritis known as adult Still's disease present with features of mild hepatitis in the majority of cases and rarely with life-threatening acute liver failure.[158–162] Variable degrees of serum aminotransferase and alkaline phosphatase elevations are typically observed in such patients during symptomatic flares of the disease. Liver biopsy usually reveals moderate portal mononuclear cell infiltration with occasional focal hepatocyte necrosis.[159] Biopsies obtained in patients with jaundice and biochemical evidence of severe hepatitis have been found to have interface and lobular hepatitis with lymphoplasmacytic inflammation reminiscent of autoimmune hepatitis.[162] Most cases of severe hepatitis have been observed in patients treated previously with salicylates or other nonsteroidal anti-inflammatory drugs,[159, 162] but liver enzyme abnormalities are also commonly noted before such therapy is provided. Some patients with severe hepatitis have been reported to respond to immunosuppressive therapy,[162] whereas others have required liver transplantation or have died of liver failure.[158, 160–162] Although severe hepatitis is a rare complication of adult Still's disease, liver failure appears to be the most common cause of death related to this disease.[158]

NODULAR DISORDERS OF THE LIVER

Nodular hepatocellular lesions have been classified broadly into nodules composed of regenerative hepatocytes or those containing dysplastic cells.[163] Dysplastic or neoplastic lesions are discussed in Chapter 81. Nodular lesions in the liver created by regenerative changes include focal nodular hyperplasia (also discussed in Chapter 81), lobular or segmental hyperplasia, and regenerative nodules either associated or not associated with fibrous septa or cirrhosis.

Lobar or segmental hyperplasia represents diffuse enlargement of a lobe or portion of a lobe and is usually associated with developmental anomalies (see Chapter 62) or with atrophy, necrosis, or fibrosis of other lobes. For example, in the Budd-Chiari syndrome, the caudate lobe is often hyperplastic because its hepatic drainage may be preserved when the main hepatic veins are occluded.[163, 164] In addition, in patients with cirrhosis, the mean percentage of liver volume occupied by both the caudate lobe and the lateral segment of the left lobe tends to increase.[165] Developmental abnormalities of the liver include anomalous lobulations or projections from the right (Riedel's lobe) or left lobe of the liver, accessory lobes or ectopic tissue with or without pedicles connecting to the liver, and hypoplasia or absence of a hepatic lobe.[166] Uncommon liver lobulations may be perceived as abdominal or perigastric masses and raise concerns about neoplastic disease. Liver imaging studies often clarify the benign nature of these malformations.

Regenerative nodules have been classified by histologic criteria as either monoacinar nodules, which contain only a single portal tract, or multiacinar nodules, which contain two or more portal tracts.[163] In cirrhotic livers, these nodules are surrounded by fibrous septa and are usually referred to as *cirrhotic nodules*. In contrast, *nodular regenerative hyperplasia* is a distinct regenerative abnormality of the liver that occurs in the absence of cirrhosis. The unifying characteristic of all cases of nodular regenerative hyperplasia appears to be the presence of obliterative lesions in small portal veins, or more rarely, hepatic veins.[163, 164, 167, 168] Obstruction of the portal venous blood supply is associated with ischemia and atrophy followed by hyperplasia of acini with preserved arterial blood flow.[163, 168] In autopsy series, a strong association between nodular regenerative hyperplasia and increasing age has been noted,[163] and it has been proposed that this pattern of regeneration represents a secondary, nonspecific adaptation to altered blood flow to the liver, rather than a single, specific entity.[163] Nodular regenerative hyperplasia is composed of multiple monoacinar nodules, without fibrous septa, that usually involve most of the liver. Nevertheless, this diagnosis may be difficult to establish based on findings in small needle biopsies.[156, 163] As is illustrated in Figure 82–6, reticulin stains are especially useful in identifying the unique structural features of nodular regenerative hyperplasia.

Nodular regenerative hyperplasia was originally described as a rare lesion in Felty's syndrome (see previous section)[156, 157] and in patients with various hematologic disorders associated with portal or hepatic vein thrombosis.[169] Many such cases were discovered during the evaluation of patients with complications of portal hypertension. However,

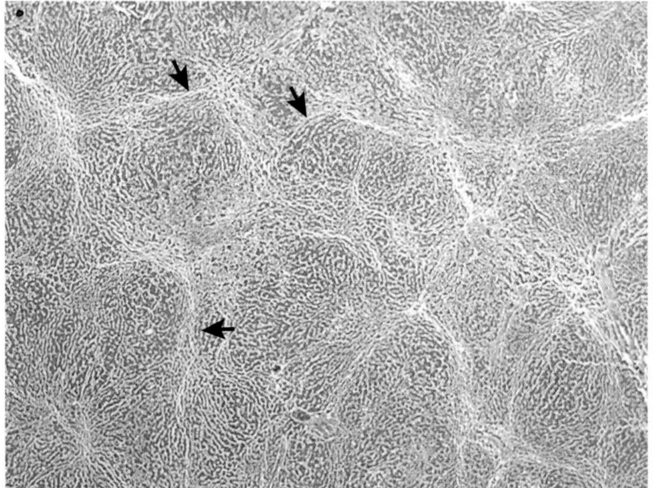

Figure 82–6. Liver biopsy specimen from a patient with polycythemia vera and portal hypertension from nodular regenerative hyperplasia. The liver is finely nodular because of nodular proliferation of hepatocytes that compress the liver plates at the periphery of nodules *(arrows)* without an increase in fibrosis. Trichrome stain, 5×.

nodular regenerative hyperplasia has been found in 0.7% to 2.6% of autopsies,[170–172] with only a minority of cases having evidence of portal hypertension.[170–172] Thus, it appears that this lesion occurs more frequently than would be suspected by clinical manifestations. Although mild-to-moderate elevation of the serum alkaline phosphatase level is often noted in patients with nodular regenerative hyperplasia, radiologic evaluation often suggests an apparently normal liver. In some cases, well-defined nodules appear hypodense on computed tomography or display abnormal echogenicity on ultrasonography.[173–175] This pseudotumoral appearance on ultrasonographic and computed tomographic images can be clarified by magnetic resonance imaging, which usually reveals subtle focal lesions with dynamic behavior similar to that of normal liver parenchyma.[175] Rarely, monoacinar nodules form confluent masses in the perihilar area that may be many centimeters in diameter. This syndrome was formerly known as partial nodular transformation and is often associated with high-grade obstruction of medium-sized or large portal veins.[163]

Nodular regenerative hyperplasia has been described in association with Felty's syndrome and other immunologically mediated diseases such as systemic lupus erythematosus, progressive systemic sclerosis, sarcoidosis, and polymyalgia rheumatica and has been reported in patients with polycythemia vera, agnogenic myeloid hyperplasia, and a variety of other hematologic disorders.[41, 171] An association with use of azathioprine,[176] thioguanine,[177] and other chemotherapeutic agents[178] also has been reported. Finally, a histologically identical lesion has been found to occur in the early stages of primary biliary cirrhosis.[178] In these patients, nodular transformation is reported to be focal rather than diffuse in the majority of cases. However, this lesion may be associated with evidence of portal hypertension in patients with primary biliary cirrhosis in whom cirrhosis has not yet developed.[178]

Although hepatic function remains normal in patients with nodular regenerative hyperplasia, complications of portal hypertension such as variceal hemorrhage, hypersplenism, or, rarely, ascites develop in some patients.[170–173] When the diagnosis of nodular regenerative hyperplasia is made, implicated medications should be discontinued, and associated conditions should be treated. Variceal hemorrhage should be managed initially with endoscopic band ligation or sclerotherapy with selective portosystemic shunt surgery or a transjugular intrahepatic portosystemic shunt in refractory cases, as in other cases of portal hypertension in which hepatic function is preserved (see Chapter 77).

REFERENCES

1. Abt AB, Kirschner RH, Belliveau RE, et al: Hepatic pathology associated with Hodgkin's disease. Cancer 33:1564, 1974.
2. Coleman M, Lightdale CJ, Vinciguerra VP, et al: Peritoneoscopy in Hodgkin disease. Confirmation of results by laparotomy. JAMA 236: 2634, 1976.
3. Trotter MC, Cloud GA, Davis M, et al: Predicting the risk of abdominal disease in Hodgkin's lymphoma. A multifactorial analysis of staging laparotomy results in 255 patients. Ann Surg 201:465, 1985.
4. Kim H, Dorfman RF, Rosenberg SA: Pathology of malignant lymphomas in the liver: Application in staging. In Popper H, Schaffner F (eds): Progress in Liver Diseases, vol V. New York, Grune & Stratton, 1976, p 683.

5. Kadin ME, Donaldson SS, Dorfman RF: Isolated granulomas in Hodgkin's disease. N Engl J Med 283:859, 1970.
6. Aisenberg AC, Kaplan MM, Rieder SV, et al: Serum alkaline phosphatase at the onset of Hodgkin's disease. Cancer 26:318, 1970.
7. Davey FR, Doyle WF: Hepatic alterations in Hodgkin's disease. N Y State J Med 73:1981, 1973.
8. Perera DR, Greene ML, Fenster LF: Cholestasis associated with extrabiliary Hodgkin's disease. Report of three cases and report of four others. Gastroenterology 67:680, 1974.
9. Meinders LE, Werre JM, Brandt KH, et al: Intrahepatic cholestasis in Hodgkin's disease. Neth J Med 19:287, 1976.
10. Hubscher SG, Lumley MA, Elias E: Vanishing bile duct syndrome: A possible mechanism for intrahepatic cholestasis in Hodgkin's lymphoma. Hepatology 17:70, 1993.
11. Burke JS: Hodgkin's disease: Histopathology and differential diagnosis. In Knowles DM (ed): Neoplastic Hematopathology. Baltimore, Williams & Wilkins, 1992, p 497.
12. Bagley CJ Jr, Thomas LB, Johnson RE, et al: Diagnosis of liver involvement by lymphoma: Results in 96 consecutive peritoneoscopies. Cancer 31:840, 1973.
13. Roth A, Kolaric K, Dominis M: Histologic and cytologic liver changes in 120 patients with malignant lymphomas. Tumori 64:45, 1978.
14. Kolaric K, Roth A, Dominis M, et al: The diagnostic value of percutaneous liver biopsy in patients with non-Hodgkin's lymphoma—a preliminary report. Acta Hepato-Gastroenterol 24:440, 1977.
15. Scheimberg IB, Pollock DJ, Collins PW, et al: Pathology of the liver in leukaemia and lymphoma. A study of 110 autopsies. Histopathology 26:311, 1995.
16. Lei KIK: Primary non-Hodgkin's lymphoma of the liver. Leuk Lymphoma 29:293, 1998.
17. Avlonitis VS, Linos C: Primary hepatic lymphoma: A review. Eur J Surg 165:725, 1999.
18. Fukuya T, Honda H, Murata S, et al: MRI of primary lymphoma of the liver. J Comput Assist Tomogr 17:596, 1993.
19. Weidmann E: Hepatosplenic T cell lymphoma. A review on 45 cases since the first report describing the disease as a distinct entity in 1990. Leukemia 14:991, 2000.
20. Kim H, Dorfman RF: Morphological studies of 84 untreated patients subjected to laparotomy for the staging of non-Hodgkin's lymphomas. Cancer 33:657, 1974.
21. Verdi CJ, Grogan TM, Protell R, et al: Liver biopsy immunotyping to characterize lymphoid malignancies. Hepatology 6:6, 1986.
22. Thomas FB, Clausen KP, Greenberger NJ: Liver disease in multiple myeloma. Arch Intern Med 132:195, 1973.
23. Perez-Soler R, Esteban R, Allende E, et al: Liver involvement in multiple myeloma. Am J Hematol 20:25, 1985.
24. MacSween RNM: Liver pathology associated with diseases of other organs. In MacSween RNM, Anthony PP, Scheuer PJ (eds): Pathology of the Liver. Edinburgh, Churchill Livingstone, 1987, p 646.
25. Randall RE, Williamson WC, Mullinax F, et al: Manifestations of systemic light chain deposition. Am J Med 60:293, 1976.
26. Goldberg GM, Rubenstone I, Saphir O: A study of malignant lymphomas and leukemias. III. Stem cell, blast cell, and monocytic leukemias (with reference to their lymphogenous or myelogenous origin). Cancer 19:21, 1961.
27. Schwartz JB, Shamsuddin AM: The effects of leukemic infiltrates in various organs in chronic lymphocytic leukemia. Hum Pathol 12:432, 1981.
28. Foucar K, Carroll TJ Jr, Tammous R, et al: Nonendemic adult T-cell leukemia/lymphoma in the United States: Report of two cases and review of the literature. Am J Clin Pathol 83:18, 1985.
29. Grouls V, Stiens R: Hepatic involvement in hairy cell leukemia: Diagnosis by tartrate-resistant acid phosphatase enzyme histochemistry on formalin fixed and paraffin-embedded liver biopsy specimens. Pathol Res Pract 174:332, 1984.
30. Zafrani ES, Degos F, Guigui B, et al: The hepatic sinusoid in hairy cell leukemia: An ultrastructural study of 12 cases. Hum Pathol 18: 801, 1987.
31. Agnarsson BA, Loughran TP Jr, Starkebaum G, et al: The pathology of large granular lymphocyte leukemia. Hum Pathol 20:643, 1989.
32. Weiss LM: Histiocytic and dendritic cell proliferations. In Knowles DM (ed): Neoplastic Hematopathology. Baltimore, Williams & Wilkins, 1992, p 1459.
33. Fine KD, Solano M, Polter DE, et al: Malignant histiocytosis in a patient presenting with hepatic dysfunction and peliosis hepatis. Am J Gastroenterol 90:485, 1995.
34. Rand EB, Whitington PF: Successful orthotopic liver transplantation in two patients with liver failure due to sclerosing cholangitis with Langerhans cell histiocytosis. J Pediatr Gastroenterol Nutr 15:202, 1992.
35. Heyn RM, Hamoudi A, Newton WA Jr: Pretreatment liver biopsy in 20 children with histiocytosis X: A clinicopathologic correlation. Med Pediatr Oncol 18:110, 1990.
36. Klatskin G: Hepatic granulomata: Problems in interpretation. Ann N Y Acad Sci 278:427, 1976.
37. de Carvalho Hercules H, Bethlem NM: Value of liver biopsy in sarcoidosis. Arch Pathol Lab Med 108:831, 1984.
38. Israel HL, Margolis ML, Rose LJ: Hepatic granulomatosis and sarcoidosis. Further observations. Dig Dis Sci 29:353, 1984.
39. Maddrey WC, Johns CJ, Boitnott JK, et al: Sarcoidosis and chronic hepatic disease: A clinical and pathologic study of 20 patients. Medicine 49:375, 1970.
40. Scott GC, Berman JM, Higgins JL: CT patterns of nodular hepatic and splenic sarcoidosis: A review of the literature. J Comput Assist Tomogr 21:369, 1997.
41. Moreno-Merlo F, Wanless IR, Shimamatsu K, et al: The role of granulomatous phlebitis and thrombosis in the pathogenesis of cirrhosis and portal hypertension in sarcoidosis. Hepatology 26:554, 1997.
42. Devaney K, Goodman ZD, Epstein MS, et al: Hepatic sarcoidosis. Clinicopathologic features in 100 patients. Am J Surg Pathol 17:1272, 1993.
43. Vatti R, Sharma OP: Course of asymptomatic liver involvement in sarcoidosis: Role of therapy in selected cases. Sarcoidosis Vasc Diffuse Lung Dis 14:73, 1997.
44. Rudzki C, Ishak KG, Zimmerman HJ: Chronic intrahepatic cholestasis of sarcoidosis. Am J Med 59:373, 1975.
45. Murphy JR, Sjogren MH, Kikendall JW, et al: Small bile duct abnormalities in sarcoidosis. J Clin Gastroenterol 12:555, 1990.
46. Valla D, Pessegueiro-Miranda H, Degott C, et al: Hepatic sarcoidosis with portal hypertension. A report of seven cases with a review of the literature. Q J Med 63:531, 1987.
47. Tekeste H, Latour F, Levitt RE: Portal hypertension complicating sarcoid liver disease: Case report and review of the literature. Am J Gastroenterol 79:389, 1984.
48. Fagan EA, Moore-Gillon JC, Turner-Warwick M: Multiorgan granulomas and mitochondrial antibodies. N Engl J Med 308:572, 1983.
48a. Bécheur H, Dall'osto H, Chatellier G, et al: Effect of ursodeoxycholic acid on chronic intrahepatic cholestasis due to sarcoidosis. Dig Dis Sci 42:789, 1997.
48b. Baratta L, Cascino A, Delfino M, et al: Ursodeoxycholic acid treatment in abdominal sarcoidosis. Dig Dis Sci 45:1559, 2000.
49. Casavilla FA, Gordon R, Wright HI, et al: Clinical course after liver transplantation in patients with sarcoidosis. Ann Intern Med 18:865, 1993.
50. Israel HL, Goldstein RA: Hepatic granulomatosis and sarcoidosis. Ann Intern Med 79:669, 1973.
51. Eliakim M, Eisenberg S, Levij IS, et al: Granulomatous hepatitis accompanying a self-limited febrile disease. Lancet i:1348, 1968.
52. Simon HB, Wolff SM: Granulomatous hepatitis and prolonged fever of unknown origin: A study of 13 patients. Medicine 52:1, 1973.
53. Zoutman DE, Ralph ED, Frei JV: Granulomatous hepatitis and fever of unknown origin. An 11-year experience of 23 cases with three years' follow-up. J Clin Gastroenterol 13:69, 1991.
54. Sartin JS, Walker RC: Granulomatous hepatitis: A retrospective review of 88 cases at the Mayo Clinic. Mayo Clin Proc 66:914, 1991.
54a. Knox TA, Kaplan MM, Gelfand JA, et al: Methotrexate treatment of idiopathic granulomatous hepatitis. Ann Intern Med 122:592, 1995.
54b. Lower EE, Bauchman RP: The use of low dose methotrexate in refractory sarcoidosis. Am J Med Sci 299:153, 1990.
55. Reimann HA, Koucky RF, Eklerd CM, et al: Primary amyloidosis limited to tissue of mesenchymal origin. Am J Pathol 11:977, 1935.
56. Dahlin DC: Primary amyloidosis, with report of 6 cases. Am J Pathol 25:105, 1949.
57. Kyle RA, Bayrd EC: Amyloidosis: Review of 236 cases. Medicine 54: 271, 1975.
58. Isobe T, Osserman EF: Patterns of amyloidosis and their association with plasma-cell dyscrasia, monoclonal immunoglobulins and Bence-Jones Proteins. N Engl J Med 290:473, 1974.
59. Pepys MB: Amyloidosis. In Frank MM, Austen KF, Claman HN, Unanue ER (eds): Samter's Immunologic Diseases. Boston, Little, Brown, 1994, p 637.

60. Buxbaum JN, Tagoe CE: The genetics of the amyloidoses. Annu Rev Med 51:543, 2000.
61. Lansbury PT: In pursuit of the molecular structure of amyloid plaque: New technology provides unexpected and critical information. Biochemistry 31:6865, 1992.
62. Turnell WG, Finch JT: Binding of the dye Congo red to the amyloid protein pig insulin reveals a novel homology amongst amyloid-forming peptide sequences. J Mol Biol 227:1205, 1992.
63. Glenner GG: Amyloid deposits and amyloidosis—the β-fibrilloses. II. N Engl J Med 302:1333, 1980.
64. Chopra S, Rubinow A, Koff RS, et al: Hepatic amyloidosis. A histopathologic analysis of primary (AL) and secondary (AA) forms. Am J Pathol 115:186, 1984.
65. Looi LM, Smithran E: Morphologic differences in the pattern of liver infiltration between systemic AL and AA amyloidosis. Hum Pathol 19: 732, 1988.
66. Kanel GC, Uchida T, Peters RL: Globular hepatic amyloid—an unusual morphologic presentation. Hepatology 1:647, 1981.
67. Gillmore JD, Lovat LB, Hawkins PN: Amyloidosis and the liver. J Hepatol 30:17, 1999.
68. Levy M, Fryd CH, Eliakim M: Intrahepatic obstructive jaundice due to amyloidosis of the liver. Gastroenterology 61:234, 1971.
69. Rockey DC: Striking cholestatic liver disease: A distinct manifestation of advanced primary amyloidosis. South Med J 92:236, 1999.
70. Yood RA, Skinner M, Rubinow A, et al: Bleeding manifestations in 100 patients with amyloidosis. JAMA 249:1322, 1983.
71. Stone MJ: Amyloidosis: A final common pathway for protein deposition in tissues. Blood 75:531, 1990.
72. Kyle RA, et al: Primary systemic amyloidosis. Comparison of melphalan/prednisone versus colchicine. Am J Med 79:708, 1985.
73. Kyle RA, Wagoner RD, Holley KE: Primary systemic amyloidosis. Resolution of the nephrotic syndrome with melphalan and prednisolone. Arch Intern Med 142:1445, 1982.
74. Hawkins PN, Lavender JP, Pepys MB: Evaluation of systemic amyloidosis by scintigraphy with ^{123}I-labeled serum amyloid P component. N Engl J Med 323:508, 1990.
75. Hawkins PN, Richardson S, MacSweeney JE, et al: Scintigraphic quantification and serial monitoring of human visceral amyloid deposits provide evidence for turnover and regression. Q J Med 86:365, 1993.
76. Comenzo RL, Vosburgh E, Falk RH, et al: Dose-intensive melphalan with blood stem-cell support for the treatment of AL (amyloid light-chain) amyloidosis: Survival and responses in 25 patients. Blood 91: 3662, 1998.
77. Zemer D, et al: Colchicine in the prevention and treatment of amyloidosis of familial Mediterranean fever. N Engl J Med 314:1001, 1986.
78. David J: Amyloidosis in juvenile chronic arthritis. Clin Exp Rheumatol 9:73, 1991.
79. Fausa O, Nygaard K, Elgjo K: Amyloidosis and Crohn's disease. Scand J Gastroenterol 12:657, 1977.
80. Azoulay D, Samuel D, Castaing D, et al: Domino liver transplants for metabolic disorders: Experience with familial amyloidotic polyneuropathy. J Am Coll Surg 189:584, 1999.
81. Suhr OB, Herlenius G, Friman S, et al: Liver transplantation for hereditary transthyretin amyloidosis. Liver Transplantation 6:263, 2000.
82. Holmgren G, Steen L, Ekstedt J, et al: Biochemical effect of liver transplantation in two Swedish patients with familial amyloidotic polyneuropathy (FAP-met30). Clin Genet 40:242, 1991.
83. Barrett-Connor E: Cholelithiasis in sickle cell anemia. Am J Med 45: 889, 1968.
84. Cameron JL, Maddrey WC, Zuidema GC: Biliary tract disease in sickle cell anemia: Surgical considerations. Ann Surg 174:702, 1971.
85. DeVault KR, Friedman LS, Westerberg S, et al: Hepatitis C in sickle cell anemia. J Clin Gastroenterol 18:206, 1994.
86. Brittenham GM, Cohen AR, McLaren CE, et al: Hepatic iron stores and plasma ferritin concentration in patients with sickle cell anemia and thalassemia major. Am J Hematol 42:81, 1993.
87. Green TW, Conley CL, Berthrong M: The liver in sickle cell anemia. Bull J Hopkins Hosp 92:99, 1953.
88. Diggs LW: Sickle cell crises. Am J Clin Pathol 44:1, 1965.
89. Rosenblate HJ, Eisenstein R, Holmes AW: The liver in sickle cell anemia. A clinical-pathologic study. Arch Pathol 90:235, 1970.
90. Sheehy TW: Sickle cell hepatopathy. South Med J 70:533, 1977.
91. Johnson CS, Omata M, Tong MJ, et al: Liver involvement in sickle cell disease. Medicine 64:349, 1985.
92. Omata M, Johnson CS, Tong M, et al: Pathological spectrum of liver diseases in sickle cell disease. Dig Dis Sci 31:247, 1986.
93. Charlotte F, Bachir D, Nenert M, et al: Vascular lesions of the liver in sickle cell disease. A clinicopathological study in 26 living patients. Arch Pathol Lab Med 119:46, 1995.
94. Owen DM, Aldridge JE, Thompson RB: An unusual hepatic sequela of sickle cell anemia: A report of five cases. Am J Med Sci XX:175, 1965.
95. Barrett-Connor E: Sickle cell disease and viral hepatitis. Ann Intern Med 69:517, 1968.
96. Klion FM, Weiner MJ, Schaffner F: Cholestasis in sickle cell anemia. Am J Med 37:829, 1964.
97. Buchanan GR, Glader BE: Benign course of extreme hyperbilirubinemia in sickle cell anemia: Analysis of six cases. J Pediatr 91:21, 1977.
98. El Younis CM, Min AD, Fiel MI, et al: Autoimmune hepatitis in a patient with sickle cell disease. Am J Gastroenterol 91:1016, 1996.
99. Chuang E, Ruchelli E, Mulberg AE: Autoimmune liver disease and sickle cell anemia in children: A report of three cases. J Pediatr Hematol Oncol 19:159, 1997.
100. Yohannan MD, Arif M, Ramia S: Aetiology of icteric hepatitis and fulminant hepatic failure in children and the possible predisposition to hepatic failure by sickle cell disease. Acta Paediatrica Scand 79:201, 1990.
101. Sheehy TW, Law DE, Wade BH: Exchange transfusion for sickle cell intrahepatic cholestasis. Arch Intern Med 140:136, 1980.
102. Flye MW, Silver C: Biliary tract disease and sickle cell disease. Surgery 72:361, 1972.
103. Solanki D, McCurdy PR: Cholelithiasis in sickle cell anemia: A case for elective cholecystectomy. Am J Med Sci 277:319, 1979.
104. Schubert TT: Hepatobiliary system in sickle cell disease. Gastroenterology 90:2013, 1986.
105. Zimmerman HJ, Fang M, Utili R, et al: Jaundice due to bacterial infection. Gastroenterology 77:362, 1979.
106. Bernstein J, Brown AK: Sepsis and jaundice in early infancy. Pediatrics 29:873, 1962.
107. Hamilton JR, Sass-Kortsak A: Jaundice associated with severe bacterial infections in young infants. J Pediatr 63:121, 1963.
108. Escobedo MB, Barton LL, Marshall RE: The frequency of jaundice in neonatal bacterial infections. Clin Pediatr 13:656, 1974.
109. Vermillion SE, Gregg JA, Baggenstoss AH, et al: Jaundice associated with bacteremia. Arch Intern Med 124:611, 1969.
110. Zimmerman HJ, Thomas LJ: The liver in pneumococcal pneumonia: Observations in 94 cases on liver function and jaundice in pneumonia. J Lab Clin Med 35:556, 1950.
111. Neale G, Caughey DE, Mollin DL, et al: Effects of intrahepatic and extrahepatic infection on liver function. Br Med J 1:382, 1966.
112. Fang MH, Ginsberg AL, Dobbins WO III: Marked elevation in serum alkaline phosphatase activity as a manifestation of systemic infection. Gastroenterology 78:592, 1980.
113. Miller DJ, Keeton GR, Webber BL, et al: Jaundice in severe bacterial infection. Gastroenterology 71:94, 1976.
114. Lefkowitch JH: Bile ductular cholestasis: An ominous histopathologic sign related to sepsis and "cholangitis lenta." Hum Pathol 13:19, 1982.
115. Bolder U, Ton-Nu H-T, Schteingart CD, et al: Hepatocyte transport of bile acids and organic anions in endotoxemic rats: Impaired uptake and secretion. Gastroenterology 112:214, 1997.
116. Trauner M, Nathanson MH, Rydberg SA, et al: Endotoxin impairs biliary glutathione and HCO_3^- excretion and blocks the choleretic effect of nitric oxide in rat liver. Hepatology 25:1184, 1997.
117. Trauner M, Arrese M, Soroka CJ, et al: The rat canalicular conjugate export pump (Mrp2) is down-regulated in intrahepatic and obstructive cholestasis. Gastroenterology 113:255, 1997.
118. Whiting JF, Green RM, Rosenbluth AB, et al: Tumor necrosis factor-alpha decreases hepatocyte bile salt uptake and mediates endotoxin-induced cholestasis. Hepatology 22:1273, 1995.
119. Green RM, Beier D, Gollan JL: Regulation of hepatocyte bile salt transporters by endotoxin and inflammatory cytokines in rodents. Gastroenterology 111:193, 1996.
120. Moseley RH, Wang W, Takeda H, et al: Effect of endotoxin on bile acid transport in rat liver—a potential model for sepsis-associated cholestasis. Am J Physiol 271:G137, 1996.
121. Green RM, Whiting JF, Rosenbluth AB, et al: Interleukin-6 inhibits hepatocyte taurocholate uptake and sodium potassium-adenosine triphosphatase activity. Am J Physiol 267:G1094, 1994.
122. Schilling PJ, Murray JL, Markowitz AB: Novel tumor necrosis factor toxic effects. Pulmonary hemorrhage and severe hepatic dysfunction. Cancer 69:256, 1992.

123. Thiele DL: Tumor necrosis factor, the acute phase response and the pathogenesis of alcoholic liver disease. Hepatology 9:497, 1989.
124. Blay J-Y, Rossi J-F, Wijdenes J, et al: Role of interleukin-6 in the paraneoplastic inflammatory syndrome associated with renal-cell carcinoma. Int J Cancer 72:424, 1997.
125. Tugswell P, Williams O: Jaundice associated with lobar pneumonia. Q J Med 66:97, 1977.
126. LaMont JT, Isselbacher KJ: Current concepts of postoperative hepatic dysfunction. Conn Med 39:461, 1975.
127. Schmid M, Hefti ML, Gattiker R, et al: Benign postoperative intrahepatic cholestasis. N Engl J Med 272:545, 1965.
128. Kantrowitz PA, Jones WA, Greenberger NJ, et al: Severe postoperative hyperbilirubinemia simulating obstructive jaundice. N Engl J Med 276:591, 1967.
129. Gibson PR, Dudley FJ: Ischemic hepatitis: Clinical features, diagnosis and prognosis. Aust N Z J Med 14:822, 1984.
130. Touloukian J, Kaplowitz N: Halothane-induced hepatic disease. Semin Liver Dis 1:134, 1981.
131. Lewis JH, Zimmerman HJ, Ishak KG, et al: Enflurane hepatotoxicity. Ann Intern Med 98:984, 1983.
132. Orlando R III, Gleason E, Drezner AC: Acute acalculous cholecystitis in the critically ill patient. Am J Surg 145:472, 1983.
133. Baker AL, Rosenberg IH: Hepatic complications of total parenteral nutrition. Am J Med 82:489, 1987.
134. Carrico JC, Meakins JL, Marshall JC, et al: Multiple organ-failure syndrome. Arch Surg 121:196, 1986.
135. Te Boeckhorst T, Urlus M, Doesburg W, et al: Etiologic factors of jaundice in severely ill patients: A retrospective study in patients admitted to an intensive care unit with severe trauma or with septic intra-abdominal complications following surgery and without evidence of bile duct obstruction. J Hepatol 77:111, 1988.
136. Kendall MJ, Cockel R, Becker J, et al: Raised serum alkaline phosphatase in rheumatoid disease: An index of liver dysfunction. Ann Rheum Dis 29:537, 1970.
137. Whaley K, Webb J: Liver and kidney disease in rheumatoid arthritis. Clin Rheum Dis 3:527, 1977.
138. Aida S: Alkaline phosphatase isoenzyme activities in rheumatoid arthritis: Hepatobiliary enzyme dissociation and relation to disease activity. Ann Rheum Dis 52:511, 1993.
139. Rau R, Pfenninger K, Boni A: Liver function tests and liver biopsies in patients with rheumatoid arthritis. Ann Rheum Dis 34:198, 1975.
140. Dietrichson O, From A, Christoffersen P, et al: Morphological changes in liver biopsies from patients with rheumatoid arthritis. Scand J Rheumatol 5:65, 1976.
141. Mills PR, Sturrock RC: Clinical associations between arthritis and liver disease. Ann Rheum Dis 41:295, 1982.
142. Ruderman EM, Crawford JM, Maier A, et al: Histologic liver abnormalities in an autopsy series of patients with rheumatoid arthritis. Br J Rheumatol 36:210, 1997.
143. Rich RR, Johnson JS: Salicylate hepatotoxicity in patients with juvenile rheumatoid arthritis. Arthritis Rheum 16:1, 1973.
144. Shergy WJ, Polisson RP, Caldwell DS, et al: Methotrexate-associated hepatotoxicity: Retrospective analysis of 210 patients with rheumatoid arthritis. Am J Med 85:771, 1988.
145. Kremer JM, Alarcon GS, Lightfood RW Jr, et al: Methotrexate for rheumatoid arthritis. Suggested guidelines for monitoring liver toxicity. Arthritis Rheum 37:316, 1994.
146. Whaley K, Goudie RB, Williamson J, et al: Liver disease in Sjogren's syndrome and rheumatoid arthritis. Lancet i:861, 1970.
147. Lindgren S, Manthorpe R, Eriksson S: Autoimmune liver disease in patients with primary Sjogren's syndrome. J Hepatol 20:354, 1994.
148. Skopouli FN, Barbatis C, Moutsopoulos HM: Liver involvement in primary Sjogren's syndrome. Br J Rheumatol 33:745, 1994.
149. Pawlotsky JM, Roudot-Thoraval F, Simmonds P, et al: Extrahepatic immunologic manifestations in chronic hepatitis C and hepatitis C virus serotypes. Ann Intern Med 122:169, 1995.
150. Clifford BD, Donahue D, Smith L, et al: High prevalence of serologic markers of autoimmunity in patients with chronic hepatitis C. Hepatology 21:613, 1995.
151. Gumber SC, Chopra S: Hepatitis C: A multifaceted disease. Review of extrahepatic manifestations. Ann Intern Med 123:615, 1995.
152. Misiani R, Bellavita P, Fenili D, et al: Hepatitis C virus infection in patients with essential mixed cryoglobulinemia. Ann Intern Med 117: 573, 1992.
153. Hirohata S, Inoue T, Ito K: Development of rheumatoid arthritis after chronic hepatitis caused by hepatitis C virus infection. Intern Med 31: 493, 1992.
154. Rosenstein ED, Kramer N: Felty's and pseudo-Felty's syndromes. Semin Arthritis Rheum 21:129, 1991.
155. Thorne C, Urowitz MB, Wanless I, et al: Liver disease in Felty's syndrome. Am J Med 73:35, 1982.
156. Blendis LM, Parkinson MC, Shilkin KB, et al: Nodular regenerative hyperplasia of the liver in Felty's syndrome. Q J Med XLIII:25, 1974.
157. Ruiz FP, Orte Martinez FJ, Zea Mendoza AC, et al: Nodular regenerative hyperplasia of the liver in rheumatic diseases: Report of seven cases and review of the literature. Semin Arthritis Rheum 21:47, 1991.
158. Reginato AJ, Schumacher HR, Baker DG, et al: Adult onset Still's disease: Experience in 23 patients and literature review with emphasis on organ failure. Semin Arthritis Rheum 1117:39, 1987.
159. Pouchot J, Sampalis JS, Beudet F, et al: Adult Still's disease: Manifestations, disease course, and outcome in 62 patients. Medicine 70: 118, 1991.
160. Dino O, Provenzano G, Giannuoli G, et al: Fulminant hepatic failure in adult onset Still's disease. J Rheumatol 23:784, 1996.
161. McFarlane M, Harth M, Wall WJ: Liver transplant in adult Still's disease. J Rheumatol 24:2038, 1997.
162. Janssen HLA, Van Laar JM, Van Hoek BV, et al: Severe hepatitis and pure red cell aplasia in adult Still's disease: Good response to immunosuppressive therapy. Dig Dis Sci 44:1639, 1999.
163. International Working Party: Terminology of nodular hepatocellular lesions. Hepatology 22:983, 1995.
164. Tavill AS, Wood EJ, Kreel L, et al: The Budd-Chiari syndrome: Correlation between hepatic scintigraphy and the clinical, radiological, and pathological findings in nineteen cases of hepatic venous outflow obstruction. Gastroenterology 68:509, 1975.
165. Torres WE, Whitmire LF, Gedgaudas-McClees K, et al: Computed tomography of hepatic morphologic changes in cirrhosis of the liver. J Comput Asst Tomogr 10:47, 1986.
166. Battle WM, Laufer I, Moldofsky PJ, et al: Anomalous liver lobulation as a cause of perigastric masses. Dig Dis Sci 24:65, 1979.
167. De Sousa JMM, Portmann B, Williams R: Nodular regenerative hyperplasia of the liver and the Budd-Chiari syndrome. J Hepatol 12:28, 1991.
168. Shimamatsu K, Wanless IR: Role of ischemia in causing apoptosis, atrophy, and nodular hyperplasia in human liver. Hepatology 26:343, 1997.
169. Wanless IR, Godwin TA, Allen F, et al: Nodular regenerative hyperplasia of the liver in hematologic disorders: A possible response to obliterative portal venopathy. A morphometric study of nine cases with a hypothesis on the pathogenesis. Medicine 59:367, 1980.
170. Colina F, Alberti N, Solis JA, et al: Diffuse nodular regenerative hyperplasia of the liver (DNRH). A clinicopathologic study of 24 cases. Liver 9:253, 1989.
171. Wanless IR: Micronodular transformation (nodular regenerative hyperplasia) of the liver: A report of 64 cases among 2,500 autopsies and a new classification of benign hepatocellular nodules. Hepatology 11: 787, 1990.
172. Nakanuma Y: Nodular regenerative hyperplasia of the liver: Retrospective survey in autopsy series. J Clin Gastroenterol 12:460, 1990.
173. Dachman AH, Ros PR, Goodman ZD, et al: Nodular regenerative hyperplasia of the liver: Clinical and radiologic observations. Am J Roentgenol 148:717, 1987.
174. Pelletier G, Roche A, Boccaccio F, et al: Imagerie de l'hyperplasie nodulaire regenerative du foie. Etude de 9 cas. Gastroenterol Clin Biol 12:687, 1988.
175. Casillas C, Marti-Bonmati L, Galant J: Pseudotumoral presentation of nodular regenerative hyperplasia of the liver: Imaging in five patients including MR imaging. Eur Radiol 7:654, 1997.
176. Duvoux C, Kracht M, Lang P, et al: Hyperplasie nodulaire regenerative du foie associee a la prise d'azathioprine. Gastroenterol Clin Biol 15:968, 1991.
177. Shepherd PC, Fooks J, Gray R, et al: Thioguanine used in maintenance therapy of chronic myeloid leukaemia causes non-cirrhotic portal hypertension. Results from MRC CML. II. Trial comparing busulphan with busulphan and thoguanine. Br J Haematol 79:185, 1991.
178. Colina F, Pinedo F, Solis JA, et al: Nodular regenerative hyperplasia of the liver in early histological stages of primary biliary cirrhosis. Gastroenterology 102:1319, 1992.

Chapter 83

LIVER TRANSPLANTATION

Paul Martin and Hugo R. Rosen

Orthotopic liver transplantation (OLT) has evolved rapidly since its initial widespread application nearly two decades ago. The focus of management of the OLT recipient has shifted increasingly from the prevention of rejection to the threat of disease recurrence, with potentially serious consequences for the allograft and patient. Although the propensity of hepatitis B virus (HBV) to recur had become a major concern by the late 1980s, it has now been overshadowed by recurrent hepatitis C, because of the frequency of the latter as an indication for OLT, high rate of graft reinfection, and lack of effective prophylaxis.[1] Recurrence of nonviral liver diseases also has become apparent and has led to recognition that immunosuppressive regimens may need to be tailored to the specific indication for OLT, with more intensive immunosuppression maintained in disorders of putative autoimmune etiology (primary biliary cirrhosis, primary sclerosing cholangitis, and autoimmune hepatitis) and more rapid tapering of immunosuppressive doses in patients transplanted for chronic viral hepatitis.[2] The apparently intractable shortage of cadaveric donors has led to an increasing number of fatalities among patients listed for OLT. Although innovations such as the splitting of cadaveric grafts and use of living-related organ donors as well as the use of so-called marginal grafts, including those from older and nonheart-beating donors, have provided alternative access to OLT in individual cases, it is likely that the cadaveric donor shortage will continue to be the rate-limiting step that prevents a further substantial increment in the number of patients transplanted.[3]

The number of persons listed for OLT in the United States and elsewhere has continued to increase exponentially despite the relatively static cadaveric donor supply. The resulting discrepancy is reflected in the increasing number of patients who succumb to complications of liver disease, as waiting times for OLT become even more protracted (Fig. 83–1).[4] For example, between 1988 and 1997, the number of patients awaiting transplantation increased almost 16-fold, and the number of waiting-list deaths increased almost six-fold.[3] However, for the individual patient who undergoes OLT, the chances for long-term survival are excellent despite concerns about recurrent disease. Thus, the likely 1-year survival rate for patients with decompensated cirrhosis is less than 10% without OLT but approximately 85% to 90% at 1 year and 75% at 5 years after transplantation for most indications.[3]

A major influence on patient survival post-OLT is the severity of hepatic decompensation and associated debility at the time of surgery; in some candidates OLT may no longer be feasible by the time a suitable donor is identified. Although access to OLT has transformed the management of advanced liver disease, the increase in waiting times has resulted in an expanding cohort of increasingly decompensated patients who require frequent medical attention. Because the best outcomes following OLT are obtained in patients who have not already experienced multiple complications of liver disease, it is appropriate to initiate referral for transplant evaluation when a cirrhotic patient has had an index complication, such as the onset of ascites.

The field of transplant hepatology has emerged as a distinct subspecialty, that, despite encompassing aspects of gastroenterology, multidisciplinary internal medicine, and intensive care, represents a unique discipline requiring unique skills and training.[5]

INDICATIONS

The major indications for OLT in adults mirror the most common forms of liver disease, notably chronic hepatitis C and to a lesser extent chronic hepatitis B, alcoholic liver disease, primary biliary cirrhosis, primary sclerosing cholangitis, and autoimmune hepatitis (Table 83–1). Other indications include fulminant hepatic failure and cirrhosis of other causes, such as nonalcoholic fatty liver disease and hemochromatosis. The role of OLT in patients with hepatic malignancy has become more circumscribed in recent years, although there is clearly a subset of patients with hepatocellular carcinoma who can be cured. The major indication for

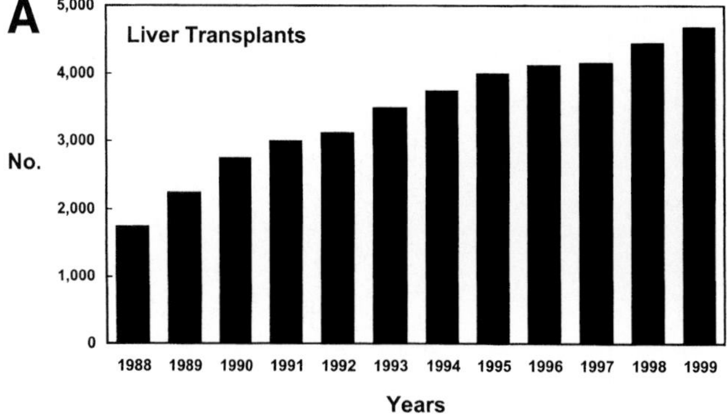

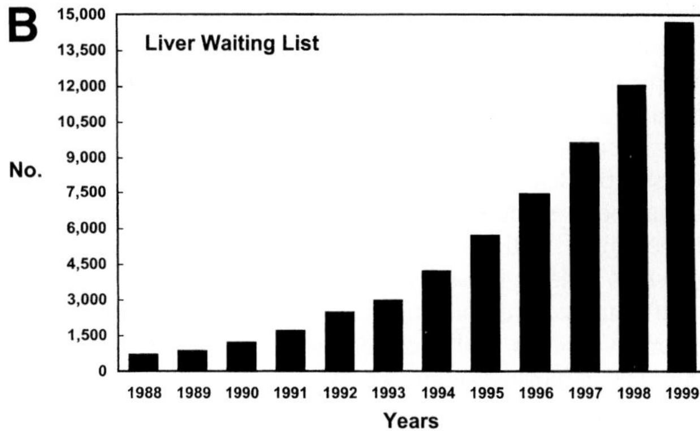

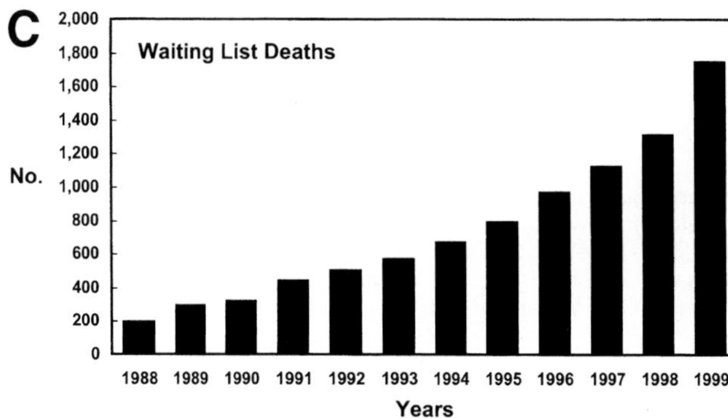

Figure 83–1. UNOS liver transplant data showing differential increases from 1988 to 1999 in *(A)* number of liver transplants (from 1713 to 4700); *(B)* number of patients on liver transplant waiting list (from 616 to 14,709); and *(C)* number of pretransplant waiting list deaths (from 195 to 1753). (From Keeffe EB: Liver transplantation: Current status and novel approaches to liver replacement. Gastroenterology 120:749–762, 2001.)

pediatric OLT is biliary atresia following a failed Kasai procedure (portoenterostomy) or delayed recognition of the diagnosis. Other major pediatric indications include α_1-antitrypsin deficiency and other metabolic disorders.[6]

One of the key issues in assessing severe liver disease is the appropriate timing of transplantation, which should be performed before advancing hepatic decompensation and associated morbidity diminish the likelihood of a successful outcome but not before medical options have been exhausted. For example, in a patient with decompensated cirrhosis caused by HBV, effective suppression of viral replication by the antiviral agent lamivudine may result in clinical improvement, allowing OLT to be deferred safely.[7] However, the course of chronic liver disease is unpredictable, and it is sobering to observe how an apparently well-compensated patient can deteriorate dramatically because of an intercurrent complication such as variceal bleeding. Anticipation of complications of cirrhosis may permit prophylactic intervention. Notable examples include identification of esophageal varices with endoscopic features such as large size or a red wale sign indicative of a high likelihood of bleeding, followed by administration of beta blockers to reduce the risk of hemorrhage, and antibiotic prophylaxis to prevent spontaneous bacterial peritonitis.[8] Although the utility of surveillance for hepatocellular carcinoma remains unproved as measured in terms of improved outcome, the recognition of hepatocellular carcinoma in an OLT candidate may enhance the patient's priority for OLT under current United Network for Organ Sharing (UNOS) rules, if the tumor burden is low enough that there is a high likelihood of cure by OLT.

Although a diagnosis of cirrhosis carries the potential for major complications, the prognosis of cirrhosis in the absence of complications is actually quite good. For example, Fattovich and colleagues observed that in well-compensated cirrhosis related to hepatitis C virus (HCV) infection, the rate of development of decompensated liver disease, e.g., ascites and variceal hemorrhage, was lower than 30% at 10 years (Fig. 83–2).[9] However, the likelihood of survival of a cirrhotic patient diminishes significantly with the onset of hepatic decompensation, and once the limits of medical therapy are reached, survival is measured in months; for example, after the development of ascites refractory to diuretics, only 25% of patients will survive beyond 1 year.

The development of predictive models based on the natural history of primary biliary cirrhosis (PBC) (see Chapter 76) and primary sclerosing cholangitis (PSC) (see Chapter

Table 83–1 | **Liver Diseases of Adult Transplant Recipients in the United States**

PRIMARY LIVER DISEASE	NUMBER	%
Chronic hepatitis C	5155	20.7
Alcoholic liver disease	4258	17.1
Alcoholic liver disease and hepatitis C	1106	4.4
Chronic hepatitis B	1368	5.5
Cryptogenic cirrhosis	2719	10.9
Primary biliary cirrhosis	2317	9.3
Primary sclerosing cholangitis	2178	8.7
Autoimmune hepatitis	1194	4.8
Acute liver failure	1555	6.2
Hepatic malignancy	951	3.8
Metabolic diseases	923	3.7
Other	1050	4.2
Unknown	126	0.5

NOTE: United Network for Organ Sharing Database 1987–1998; n = 24,900 patients. Adapted and reprinted with permission from Keeffe EB: Liver transplantation: Current status and novel approaches to liver replacement. Gastroenterology 120:749–762, 2001.

59) has helped in clinical decision making in patients with these cholestatic disorders, which tend to progress in a fairly stereotypical fashion.[10] Until recently, similar models have not been available for the noncholestatic forms of cirrhosis, and the decision to refer a patient for OLT generally has been based on disease severity, although the patient's quality of life has been an additional important factor.[11]

The cardinal indications for OLT are based on disease severity that reflects hepatocellular failure, such as coagulopathy and jaundice; complications of portal hypertension, such as refractory ascites and recurrent variceal bleeding; or the combination of portosystemic shunting and diminished hepatocellular function, as in hepatic encephalopathy. With validation of predictive models for the natural history of PBC and PSC, it is possible to predict an individual patient's course based on simple clinical parameters, the most ominous of which is a rising serum bilirubin level. Although the patient's quality of life is not included in assigning the UNOS status for transplantation, the presence of potentially disabling symptoms such as pruritus and osteopenia in patients with cholestatic and other forms of cirrhosis, as well as recurrent bacterial cholangitis in those with PSC, are important considerations in deciding when to refer a patient for OLT. Ideally, OLT should occur before a protracted period of disability, because subsequent post-transplantation rehabilitation to full employment and social functioning is more likely. Unfortunately, with increasing waiting times, many patients may have to cope with the consequences and hardship of unemployment for medical reasons; therefore, once liver disease starts to have an impact on the patient's ability to function normally, referral to a transplant program should be considered.

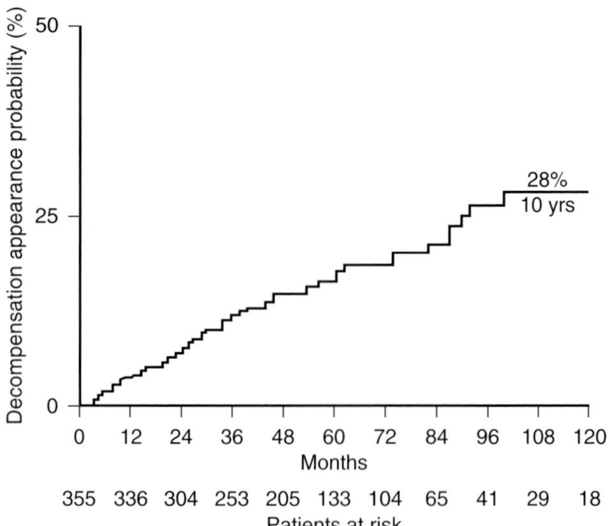

Figure 83–2. Low rate of development of major complications (decompensation) in well-compensated cirrhosis due to hepatitis C. (From Fattovich G, Giustina G, Degos F, et al: Morbidity and mortality in compensated cirrhosis type C: A retrospective follow-up study of 384 patients. Gastroenterology 112:463–472, 1999.)

LISTING CRITERIA AND POLICIES OF THE UNITED NETWORK FOR ORGAN SHARING

Organ allocation within the United States is administered by UNOS, which considers only disease severity in determining a patient's priority for OLT. Innovations such as transjugular intrahepatic portosystemic shunts (TIPS) to manage complications of cirrhosis like variceal hemorrhage or tense ascites may make it possible to delay OLT in some patients but do not treat the underlying liver disease.[12]

In an effort to achieve a consensus about eligibility for OLT in the United States and to ensure equitable and uniform practices by individual transplant programs, the concept of *minimal listing criteria* was developed in 1997.[13] A Child-Turcotte-Pugh (CTP) score of at least 7 (Table 83–2), based on an anticipated 1-year survival rate of less than 90%, was proposed as the minimal disease severity for placing a patient on a transplant waiting list. Disease-specific criteria also were developed for conditions in which survival and outcome may be inadequately reflected by the CTP score, including primary hepatic malignancy (e.g., hepatocellular carcinoma [HCC]) and cholestatic liver diseases (i.e., PBC and PSC). For PBC and PSC, the Mayo mathematical model and the Mayo risk score, respectively, predict survival more reliably than the CTP score. It was recommended that patients with PBC and PSC be listed for OLT if the risk score predicts a 1-year survival rate of less than 95%. Other suggested minimal criteria included a minimum period of abstinence of 6 months if alcohol is implicated in the pathogenesis of liver disease. For patients with HCC, generally accepted criteria for OLT include a solitary tumor less than 5 cm in diameter or three or fewer tumor nodules with the largest lesion measuring less than 3 cm in diameter, without metastases. The UNOS status, which determines a candidate's priority for organ allocation, is based on disease severity, as noted in Table 83–3.

More recently, the Model for End-Stage Liver Disease (MELD) has been proposed as a more objective and accurate way to stratify OLT candidates for organ allocation and to eliminate time waiting for a donor organ as a determining factor (see also Chapter 77).[14] This new scale overcomes some of the inherent limitations of the CTP system, including limited discriminatory ability and subjective interpretation of parameters such as presence or absence of ascites based on physical examination. Inclusion of the serum creatinine level reflects the major prognostic importance of renal dysfunction in advanced liver disease.

ABSOLUTE AND RELATIVE CONTRAINDICATIONS

As experience with OLT has expanded, contraindications to OLT also have evolved and changed. An absolute contraindication (Table 83–4) to OLT is a clinical circumstance in which the likelihood of a successful outcome is so remote that OLT should not be offered; alternatively, transplantation is contraindicated if the patient has compensated cirrhosis without complications, i.e., a CTP score of less than 7. A relative contraindication implies a reduced chance of a good outcome, although OLT may still be considered in some patients.

An example of a contraindication to OLT in evolution is human immunodeficiency virus (HIV) infection, which was

Table 83–2 | **Nondisease-Specific Minimal Listing Criteria**

Immediate need for liver transplantation
Estimated 1-yr survival ≤ 90%
Child-Turcotte-Pugh score ≥ 7 (Child-Turcotte-Pugh class B or C)
Portal hypertensive bleeding or a single episode of spontaneous bacterial peritonitis, irrespective of Child-Turcotte-Pugh score

Adapted from Lucey MR, Brown KA, Everson GT, et al: Minimal criteria for placement of adults on the liver transplant waiting list: A report of a national conference organized by the American Society of Transplant Physicians and the American Association for the Study of Liver Diseases. Liver Transpl Surg 3:628–637, 1997.

an absolute contraindication until recently because of earlier experience that HIV-infected patients succumbed rapidly following OLT. However, with the advent of effective antiretroviral therapy, this issue is being readdressed by some transplant programs, and in the future HIV infection in the absence of the acquired immunodeficiency syndrome (AIDS) may be regarded as a relative rather than absolute contraindication to OLT. As discussed later, OLT for chronic HBV infection was regarded as a contraindication in the late 1980s, because of the likelihood of graft reinfection, and the United States Medicare program excluded HBV-associated OLT from reimbursement.[15] This policy has now been reversed, based on data showing that in patients transplanted for HBV who are treated indefinitely with high-dose hepatitis B immune globulin (HBIG), the survival rate and quality of life are excellent and may exceed those of patients transplanted for hepatitis C–related liver failure.[16]

The role of OLT in the management of hepatic malignancies, in contrast, has become more limited with the recognition that a large tumor burden in patients with primary HCC is associated with a high probability of metastatic spread within a short time of OLT and that some tumors such as cholangiocarcinoma almost inevitably recur. However, even this dogma has been challenged recently by the success of a Mayo Clinic protocol involving external beam irradiation and chemotherapy in a selected subset of patients with cholangiocarcinoma.[17] The results of OLT have been so poor for angiosarcoma that its diagnosis remains an absolute contraindication, whereas patients with epithelioid hemangioendothelioma have been transplanted successfully, despite an extensive tumor burden, with documented regression of extrahepatic metatases.

For a transplant candidate with a prior extrahepatic malignancy, curative therapy needs to have been performed, and the pathologic specimen must indicate a low likelihood of metastatic spread. A 2-year period without recurrence after definitive resection is sufficient for most nonhepatic malignancies before OLT can be considered, although for breast cancer, colon cancer, and malignant melanoma, longer periods of recurrence-free survival are desirable. Myeloproliferative disorders are not infrequent in patients presenting with Budd-Chiari syndrome, but fortunately, the rate of evolution to acute leukemia is not accelerated following OLT.

Ongoing alcohol or recreational drug use is an absolute contraindication to OLT. If there is concern about continued abuse, random toxicology screens are appropriate.[18] Although medicinal marijuana use is sanctioned for palliation, it is contraindicated in the setting of OLT because of concerns about the overall compliance of users as well as possible pulmonary side effects. A history of prescription narcotic abuse is also a cause for concern because it may contribute to difficulties with pain management post-OLT, and nonnarcotic alternatives should be attempted for chronic pain. However, other analgesics such as the nonsteroidal anti-inflammatory drugs (NSAIDs) also are contraindicated in persons with end-stage liver disease because of potential renal and gastrointestinal complications.

Table 83–3 | **UNOS Liver Status for Patients 18 Years of Age and Older According to Disease Severity**

Status 1	Fulminant liver failure with life expectancy < 7 days Fulminant hepatic failure as traditionally defined Primary graft nonfunction < 7 days after transplantation Hepatic artery thrombosis < 7 days after transplantation Acute decompensated Wilson disease
Status 2A	Hospitalized in ICU for chronic liver failure with life expectancy < 7 days
Status 2B	Continuously hospitalized in acute care bed for at least 5 days or ICU-bound
Status 3	Requires continuous medical care—in hospital < 5 days or at home
Status 7	Temporarily inactive

United Network for Organ Sharing (http://www.ew3.att.net/unos). Implemented on July 30, 1997.
ICU, intensive care unit.

During the course of evaluating a patient for OLT, other medical conditions may come to light, including cardiac and pulmonary disease. The frequency of coronary artery disease in adult patients presenting for an evaluation for OLT has been estimated to range from 5% to 10%. In one study of patients with coronary artery disease who underwent OLT, including a subset of patients who had undergone coronary artery bypass grafting 6 months to 12 years before OLT, mortality and morbidity rates were found to be 50% and 81%, respectively.[19] Discrete coronary artery stenoses can be managed by angioplasty. Although surgical bypass grafting may be contraindicated because of significant perioperative risk of excessive bleeding in a patient with decompensated cirrhosis, such surgery, if successful, may render a patient an acceptable candidate for OLT.[19] Pre-OLT cardiac evaluation may overestimate cardiac performance, and impaired cardiac function may become apparent only after the protective ef-

Table 83–4 | **Contraindications to Liver Transplantation**

Acquired immunodeficiency syndrome (AIDS)
Extrahepatic malignancy
Cholangiocarcinoma
Hemangiosarcoma
Uncontrolled sepsis
Active alcoholism or substance abuse
Fulminant hepatic failure with sustained ICP > 50 mm Hg or CPP < 40 mm Hg*
Advanced cardiac or pulmonary disease
Child-Turcotte-Pugh score < 7
Anatomic abnormality precluding liver transplantation
Persistent noncompliance

*ICP is intracranial pressure; CPP is cerebral perfusion pressure and equals the mean arterial pressure minus ICP.

fect of the decreased systemic vascular resistance that characterizes cirrhosis is lost after OLT, when afterload increases because of the hypertensive effects of the primary immunosuppressive agents and when overvigorous volume repletion may occur. Emerging data suggest that dobutamine stress echocardiography is the screening test of choice, in terms of sensitivity, specificity, and cost, to assess cardiac function pre-OLT.[19] Specific forms of cirrhosis may have extrahepatic manifestations that diminish long-term survival. For example, lethal cardiac arrythmias may result in poorer survival for patients who undergo liver transplantation for decompensated cirrhosis caused by hemochromatosis.[20]

Pulmonary evaluation in the OLT candidate also may reveal abnormal arterial oxygenation (see Chapter 79). Although severe chronic obstructive pulmonary disease or pulmonary fibrosis precludes liver transplantation, respiratory restriction caused by ascites or diminished respiratory muscle strength caused by chronic illness is reversible and should not preclude OLT. Even patients who undergo OLT for alpha$_1$-antitrypsin deficiency may show improvement in pulmonary function tests postoperatively. The hepatopulmonary syndrome is characterized by the triad of chronic liver disease, pulmonary vascular dilation (with right-to-left shunting), and hypoxemia and was formerly an absolute contraindication to OLT.[21] The diagnosis is suggested by the finding of a PaO_2 value of less than 70 mm Hg on arterial blood gas obtained from the patient in the supine position. Definitive diagnosis is made by the demonstration of intrapulmonary vascular dilation by perfusion lung scanning with technetium 99m-labeled macroaggregated albumin, pulmonary arteriography, or contrast-enhanced echocardiography, which is the most sensitive technique.[21, 22] Detection of contrast in the left side of the heart within several beats after its appearance in the right atrium indicates intrapulmonary shunting. Predictors of reversibility of the hepatopulmonary syndrome post-OLT include younger age, a lesser degree of preoperative hypoxemia, and adequate correction of hypoxemia with an inspiration of 100% oxygen (PaO_2 > 200 mm Hg). In the majority of patients with hepatopulmonary syndrome, hypoxemia resolves within several months of OLT, although they may require a protracted period of ventilatory support in the immediate postoperative period. In the candidate for OLT, it is crucial to recognize portopulmonary hypertension, which is distinct from hepatopulmonary syndrome and is associated with high perioperative mortality and frequently unchanged pulmonary hemodynamics despite OLT.[21] Specifically, documentation of a mean pulmonary arterial pressure greater than 35 mm Hg, pulmonary vascular resistance greater than 300 dynes/s/cm^{-5}, and cardiac output less than 8 L/min are indicative of a high perioperative risk.

Active uncontrolled extrahepatic infection is an absolute contraindication to OLT. Because OLT may be the only option for a patient with recurrent bacterial cholangitis in the setting of PSC or repeated episodes of spontaneous bacterial peritonitis (SBP), it should be attempted only after infection has been controlled by antibiotic therapy. A particularly ominous finding is fungemia, which can be impossible to eradicate in a debilitated cirrhotic patient and may be a harbinger of mortality in this setting.

With increased surgical experience, vascular abnormalities, most notably portal vein thrombosis, have declined in significance as technical obstacles to OLT. However, more extensive vascular thrombosis with involvement of the superior mesenteric vein may still prevent OLT because of lack of a suitable venous anastomosis for the graft. The presence of a prior portosystemic shunt, particularly a nonselective shunt such as a side-to-side or end-to-side portocaval shunt, increases the technical complexity of OLT but is no longer regarded as a contraindication. However, pretransplant studies of the vascular anatomy may be required. Initially, it had been suggested that insertion of a TIPS decreases intraoperative blood loss during OLT, but more extensive experience has not confirmed this observation.[23] Still, besides controlling bleeding resulting from portal hypertension that is not amenable to endoscopic intervention in the OLT candidate, TIPS can provide an important temporizing option for relief of intractable ascites and hydrothorax (see Chapters 77 and 78).

Although age restrictions for recipients and donors have been relaxed, in the evaluation of the older OLT candidate close attention must be paid to comorbid conditions and the likelihood that after OLT the candidate will be able to return to an active lifestyle, particularly because severe liver disease may cause more debility in older than in younger patients. However, because a subset of older recipients have good outcomes after OLT, candidates in their late 60s who are otherwise in good health should be considered for OLT.

The differential diagnosis of renal insufficiency in patients with advanced liver disease includes hepatorenal syndrome, which is potentially reversible, but renal failure remains an important predictor of a poor outcome post-OLT. In OLT recipients with decompensated cirrhosis, renal insufficiency severe enough to require dialysis or combined liver-kidney transplantation has been associated consistently with poorer patient and graft outcomes. Inclusion of the serum creatinine level in the new MELD score reflects the major prognostic importance of renal insufficiency in advanced liver disease.[14]

One of the major systemic manifestations of decompensated cirrhosis is malnutrition, and many OLT candidates have experienced substantial loss of muscle mass, which in turn increases the likelihood of perioperative morbidity, the need for more prolonged ventilator support, and poorer patient survival.[24] Nutritional assessment may be difficult because peripheral edema and ascites make changes in body weight or anthropometric measurements unreliable. Deficiency of fat-soluble vitamins, reflecting intestinal malabsorption, can occur in patients with cholestatic liver disease, and appropriate supplementation should be prescribed. Consultation with a dietitian is an integral part of the evaluation of the OLT candidate. Attempts to improve the nutritional status of OLT candidates have included enteral and parenteral feeding, which may result in a modest improvement in some patients. In contrast, obesity has not been a major source of morbidity in OLT recipients except for an increased frequency of wound infections. Still, weight reduction is advisable in the obese OLT candidate, particularly because further weight gain is typical after OLT.[25]

TRANSPLANT EVALUATION AND LISTING

The formal transplant evaluation provides the opportunity for the patient and his or her family to become acquainted with the details of OLT as well as to complete a rigorous medical assessment to confirm that OLT is the best option for managing the patient's liver disease and that no absolute contraindications exist. The patient typically is seen by a transplant surgeon, hepatologist, psychiatrist, and social worker, with additional consultations if clinically indicated. As increasingly older candidates are evaluated, it is imperative to identify potential causes of perioperative morbidity, such as carotid artery stenosis. More detailed abdominal imaging studies may be required if there is concern about the patency of the portal vasculature or if hepatocellular carcinoma is suspected. As discussed later, there are disease-specific issues that may need to be addressed, such as the likelihood of recidivism in the alcoholic patient or of cure in the patient with hepatocellular carcinoma, and that impact on acceptance for OLT. The need and appropriateness of OLT for the individual candidate is then discussed formally by the members of the transplant team. Following acceptance, the candidate is placed on the transplant list for an OLT with matching by the blood type and weight of potential cadaveric donors. The patient's priority for OLT is based on disease severity and the time spent waiting.

With the critical and seemingly intractable shortage of cadaveric donor organs, a major challenge for UNOS and similar organ allocation agencies elsewhere in the world has been to develop an equitable system of allocation in an effort to ensure that hepatic allografts are not used for patients whose prognosis without OLT remains good. Disease severity increasingly has been the basis for assigning priority for OLT, although the other major consideration has been time already spent on the waiting list for OLT. UNOS stages have been defined and redefined in an attempt to ensure uniform and equitable access to donor organs (see Table 83–3). Until now, the CTP score has been used to stratify cirrhotic patients, in addition to a consideration of complications such as hepatorenal syndrome and SBP. However, because the clinical components of the CTP score, specifically ascites and encephalopathy, rely on subjective clinical evaluation, and because normal ranges for the biochemical values (albumin, bilirubin, prothrombin time) vary depending on the local laboratory, there has been interest in developing a more objective assessment of disease severity for OLT candidates. Furthermore, the CTP score may not adequately reflect the severity of liver disease in certain patient groups, such as those with cholestatic disorders, because no greater weight is given to a serum bilirubin level of 30 mg/dL than to a level of 3 mg/dL, even though a patient with the markedly higher bilirubin level clearly has more advanced liver disease. The recently described MELD incorporates the serum creatinine level, serum bilirubin level, and International Normalized Ratio (INR) into a mathematical formula that predicted survival accurately in four different groups of cirrhotic patients. The MELD system ultimately may replace the CTP score in stratifying patients with regard to the need for OLT. Additional methods will need to be devised to accommodate special circumstances not well served by any prognostic scoring system, such as persons with metabolic disorders like hyperoxaluria, cancer, or intractable pruritus.[26]

Once the evaluation process is complete and if the patient is accepted for OLT, financial clearance is sought from the patient's private, state, or federal payor to fund the procedure. The criteria for coverage for OLT vary among payors, and the transplant center must have expertise in funding issues.

DISEASE-SPECIFIC INDICATIONS

Alcoholic Liver Disease

Despite the prominence of chronic HCV as an indication for OLT, alcoholic liver disease (ALD) remains the most frequent cause of decompensated chronic liver disease (see Chapter 71). The application of OLT for ALD has continued to be controversial, albeit less so than the early 1990s. Major concerns in the past included possible recidivism following OLT as well as potentially poor compliance in this population. In addition, it was feared that the sheer number of patients with ALD would easily outstrip the cadaveric donor supply. In fact, patients with acute alcoholic hepatitis generally have had poor outcomes following OLT, with a high rate of recidivism. However, with increased clinical experience, ALD is now universally accepted as a worthwhile indication for OLT because well-selected candidates have excellent survival rates, with a low likelihood of returning to abusive alcohol consumption. Excellent graft and patient survival rates are typical following OLT for ALD, and rehabilitation of these patients is generally successful. However, only a rigorously selected subset of patients with ALD have had access to OLT. Key factors in determining the alcoholic patient's suitability for OLT include acceptance by the patient of the role alcohol has played in the pathogenesis of the person's liver disease, participation in some form of alcohol rehabilitation, such as attendance at Alcoholics Anonymous, stable social support, and a defined period of abstinence from alcohol, usually 6 months.

Nevertheless, despite rigorous efforts to preclude patients likely to resume alcohol use after OLT, a substantial proportion of the recipients resume drinking after OLT, although graft loss or death attributable to alcohol abuse remains uncommon. A higher rate of return to alcohol use is elicited by use of anonymous questionnaires or toxicology screening than by direct questioning of patients, and at least 10% to 15% of alcoholic OLT recipients are found to consume alcohol. A particularly difficult dilemma arises in the alcoholic patient with severely decompensated liver disease and recent use of alcohol and little likelihood of surviving without prompt OLT. Clearly enunciated criteria, including a contractual commitment by the patient to sobriety and active involvement in some form of alcohol rehabilitation such as participation in Alcoholics Anonymous, ensure that the selection process is equitable under these circumstances. One report from the University of Pittsburgh of 23 recipients who resumed consumption of alcohol demonstrated that Mallory's hyaline developed in all 23, central sclerosis in 22, and cirrhosis in 4 of the allografts.[27] Although earlier reports had suggested that even alcoholics who return to abusive drinking continue to take their medications regularly and that death post-transplantation is rarely attributable to alcohol abuse alone, a recent study by Lucey and colleagues[28] showed that recidivisim may indeed be associated with failure to adhere to the immunosuppressant protocol. Moreover, patients who return to pathologic drinking after OLT appear to have a higher rate of medical problems, including pneumonia, cellulitis, and pancreatitis, that require hospital admissions and occasionally lead to graft loss and death. In addition, alcoholic OLT recipients are prone to develop de novo oropharyngeal and lung tumors, likely reflecting other aspects of an alcoholic lifestyle, most notably cigarette consumption.

Hepatitis B

Graft reinfection by HBV clearly was shown to result in reduced patient and graft survival rates by the late 1980s.[29] Subsequently, the recognition of the key role of active viral replication pre-OLT with detection in serum of hepatitis B e antigen or HBV DNA by molecular hybridization as a predictor of recurrent hepatitis B in the graft and of the protective effect of long-term high-dose hepatitis B immunoglobulin (HBIG) led to markedly improved outcomes for patients transplanted for HBV-related cirrhosis. The OLT candidate with chronic HBV infection is now readily accepted for OLT, albeit with the requirement for inconvenient and expensive immunoprophylaxis. In a seminal European study, Samuel and colleagues[30] observed that patients with a fulminant presentation of acute HBV infection or hepatitis D (delta) virus coinfection had a reduced risk of recurrent hepatitis B post-OLT in the absence of immunoprophylaxis, because of the lower level of HBV replication in these persons. The widespread use of chronic high-dose HBIG administered intravenously has resulted in markedly reduced rates of recurrence of hepatitis B post-OLT but has a number of limitations, including high expense and a high frequency of side effects. The optimal dosing regimen for HBIG has been difficult to establish in the absence of controlled clinical data. Some groups have titrated HBIG doses according to trough serum levels of antibody to hepatitis B surface antigen (anti-HBs). Recent interest has focused on intramuscular administration of HBIG, which is less expensive. HBV infection that recurs despite use of HBIG may reflect inadequate dosing or a genomic mutation at the "a" moiety of the hepatitis B surface antigen (HBsAg) that results in less avid binding of the virus to HBIG.

Lamivudine, a nucleoside analog that effectively suppresses HBV replication, also has been used to prevent recurrent HBV infection post-OLT, but the efficacy of lamivudine monotherapy has been limited by frequent (~40%) mutations in the YMDD sequence of the HBV polymerase gene, leading in turn to graft reinfection. However, the combination of lamivudine and HBIG has been highly effective in protecting against graft reinfection with an apparently low rate of selecting HBV mutants (Fig. 83–3).[16] Patients in whom viral resistance to lamivudine develops with combined therapy may still respond to a new antiviral agent, adefovir dipivoxil[31] (see also Chapter 68).

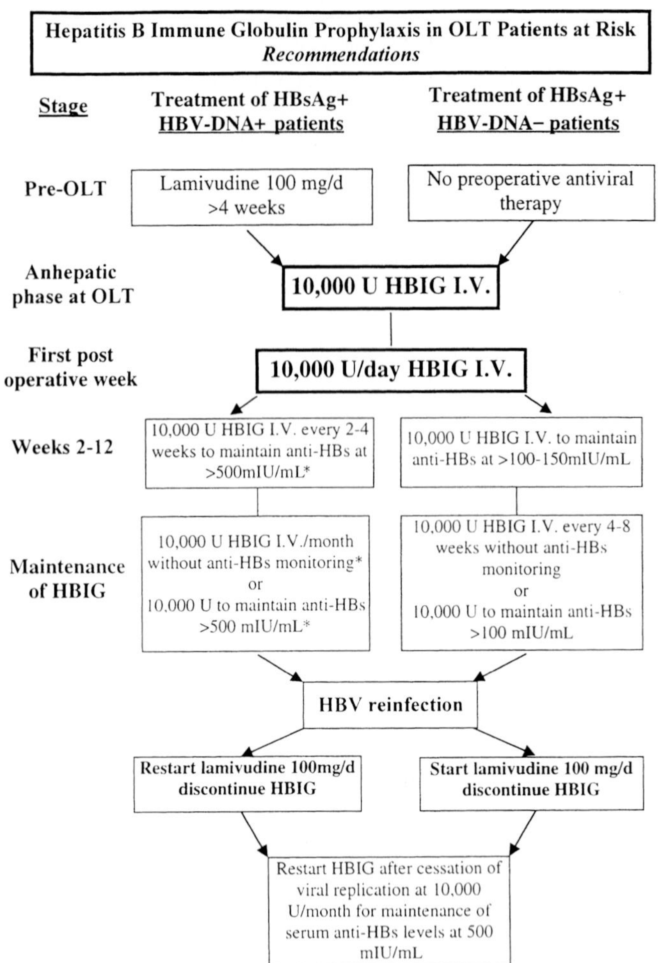

Figure 83–3. Flow chart guidelines for administration of HBIG for prevention of HBV graft reinfection following liver transplantation. HBIG, hepatitis B immune globulin; IV, intravenous; OLT, orthotopic liver transplantation. (From Shouval D, Samuel D: Hepatitis B immune globulin to prevent hepatitis B virus graft reinfection following liver transplantation: A concise review. Hepatology 32:1189–1195, 2000.)

Hepatitis C

An increasing concern about OLT for HCV-related liver disease is the burden of recurrent HCV infection post-OLT. After HCV was identified, early reports suggested that recurrent HCV infection post-OLT, based on detection of viremia, was frequent but did not have an adverse impact on overall patient or graft survival in the first several years after OLT. However, with more extensive clinical experience, it has become clear that in a subset of HCV-infected recipients, severe graft injury and failure develop as a result of recurrent hepatitis C. Analysis of serial liver biopsies from OLT recipients with recurrent hepatitis C has indicated accelerated fibrosis and progression to cirrhosis when compared with immunocompetent patients with hepatitis C. In a seminal report from King's College in London, approximately 20% of the HCV-infected patients had evidence of allograft cirrhosis on 5-year protocol biopsies.[32] Although studies with longer follow-up are required to determine the proportion of patients who will ultimately develop allograft cirrhosis related to recurrent hepatitis C, it appears that fewer than 10% of patients with mild hepatitis at 1 year progress to allograft cirrhosis at 5 years. In contrast, two thirds of the patients with at least moderate hepatitis at 1 year progress to cirrhosis by 5 years.[32] The majority of patients generally have indolent progression of recurrent hepatitis clinically. However, in some cases, an ominous finding is prominent biochemical and histologic cholestasis that not infrequently is the precursor to rapid allograft failure.[33]

Reliable predictors of severe recurrent hepatitis C have

Table 83–5 | **Factors Associated with More Severe HCV Recurrence Following Liver Transplantation**[34–38]

VIRAL
High hepatitis C viral RNA levels pre-OLT and within 2 wk post-OLT
Viral genotype 1b
Absence of pretransplant hepatitis B viral coinfection
Cytomegalovirus coinfection
IMMUNOSUPPRESSION
Multiple episodes of rejection (indicating a high cumulative prednisone dose)
Use of OKT3 for rejection
OTHER
High tumor necrosis factor-α production in the graft
Impaired HCV-specific CD4+ T-cell responses
Nonwhite recipients
Ischemic-preservation injury

HCV, hepatitis C virus; OLT, orthotopic liver transplantation.

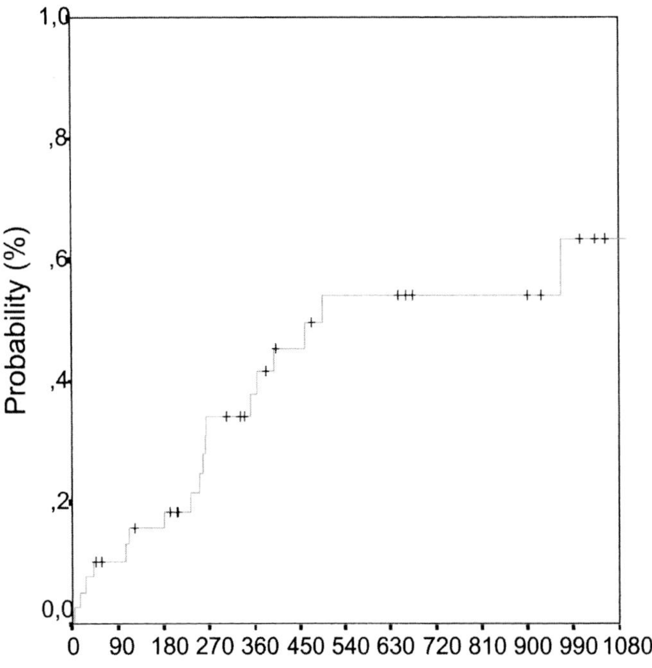

Figure 83–4. High rate of hepatic decompensation in cirrhosis due to recurrent hepatitis C following liver transplantation. (From Berenguer M, Prieto M, Rayon JM, et al: Natural history of clinically compensated hepatitis C virus–related graft cirrhosis after liver transplantation. Hepatology 32:852–858, 2000.)

been difficult to identify, although a number of viral and nonviral factors have been implicated (Table 83–5). Infection with viral genotype 1b has been suggested as one such predictor, but this observation has not been universal. Higher serum viral levels pre-OLT and immediately post-OLT and possibly more rapid HCV quasispecies evolution have been described in patients with more aggressive recurrent hepatitis C. Episodes of acute cellular rejection, particularly if multiple, lead to a greater likelihood of severe recurrent hepatitis C.[36] A major challenge is to distinguish recurrent hepatitis C from graft rejection, particularly because many of the histologic hallmarks of acute rejection, including bile duct injury, are also consistent with recurrent hepatitis C (Table 83–6). Serial liver biopsies may help clarify this issue. The use of OKT3 to treat glucocorticoid-resistant rejection also has been recognized to increase the severity of recurrent hepatitis C.[39, 40] After the introduction of the immunosuppressant tacrolimus, there was concern that its use led to more severe recurrent hepatitis C when compared with cyclosporine-based immunosuppression, although recent experience has not borne this difference out.[41]

A study by Berenguer and associates evaluated the natural history of HCV-related graft cirrhosis to define the rate of clinical decompensation and mortality.[42] Thirty-nine patients with clinically compensated allograft cirrhosis were studied; at least one episode of decompensation developed in eighteen (46%) at a mean follow-up of approximately 8 months (Fig. 83–4). This rate of decompensation was considerably higher than that reported by Fattovich and colleagues[9] in immunocompetent cirrhotic patients. Moreover, patient survival rates after development of allograft decompensation were abysmal: 93%, 61%, and 41% at 1, 6, and 12 months, respectively. Variables associated with decompensation and death included a short interval between OLT and development of allograft cirrhosis and a high CTP score (>A). The study concluded that retransplantation, if considered, should be performed promptly once decompensation develops.

In contrast to recurrent HBV infection, it has not been

Table 83–6 | **Histologic Features of Recurrent Hepatitis C Virus (HCV) Versus Acute Cellular Rejection**

	RECURRENT HCV	REJECTION
Time post-OLT	Anytime; onset usually within first yr	Usually in first 2 months
Portal inflammation	Most cases	Always
Lymphocytes	Bland, uniform	Activated
Aggregates	Usually	Occasionally
Follicles	50% of cases	Very rarely
Eosinophils	Inconspicuous	Almost always
Steatosis	Often	Never
Acidophilic bodies	Common	Uncommon
Duct damage	About 50% of cases	Very common
Atypical features	Cholestasis, ballooning degeneration without significant inflammation, marked ductular proliferation mimicking obstruction, granulomas	Prominent periportal and lobular necroinflammatory activity without subendothelial venular inflammation

OLT, orthotopic liver transplantation.
From Rosen HR, Martin P: Liver transplantation. In Schiff ER, Sorrell MF, Maddrey WC (eds): Schiff's Diseases of the Liver, 3rd ed. Philadelphia, Lippincott- Raven, 1999, pp 1589–1615.

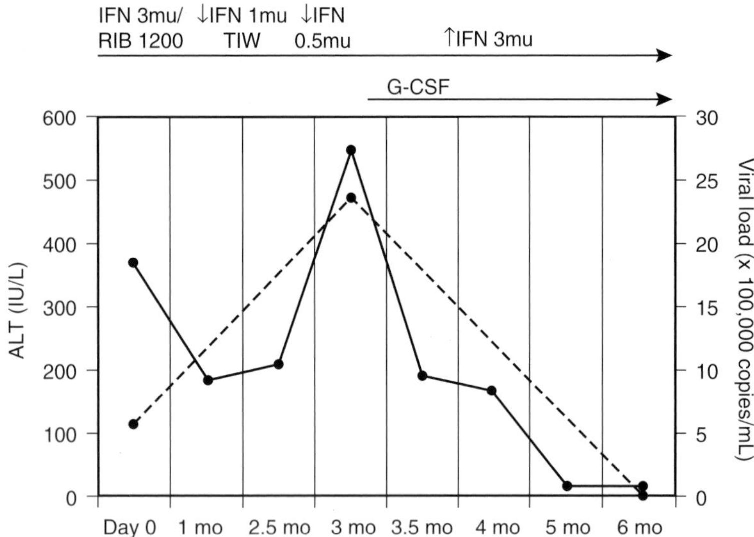

Figure 83–5. Response to therapy with interferon-α (IFN) and ribavirin (RIB) in a patient with early, severe recurrent hepatitis C. A reduction in the dose of IFN was required because of marked leukopenia at 5 weeks into therapy. A rise in serum levels of viremia *(dashed line)* and alanine aminotransferase (ALT) *(solid line)* occurred at 3 months into IFN/RIB therapy. Initiation of therapy with granulocyte colony stimulating factor (G-CSF) 300 μg SQ daily allowed reinstitution of IFN/RIB and subsequent clearance of hepatitis C virus (reflected in an undetectable serum viral RNA level) 6 months after completion of therapy. Serum total bilirubin levels on the day therapy was initiated and 3 and 6 months later were 7.1 mg/dL, 10.2 mg/dL, and 0.9 mg/dL, respectively. (From Gopal DV, Rabkin JM, Berk BS, et al: Treatment of progressive hepatitis C recurrence following liver transplantation with combination interferon plus ribivirin. Liver Transplantation 2001; 7:181–190.)

possible to develop effective prophylaxis against recurrent HCV infection.[43] Interferon alfa monotherapy generally has been ineffective in treating established recurrent hepatitis C. When interferon is used with ribavirin, the rate of virologic response is increased, but at the cost of frequent and potentially severe side effects. Leukopenia is a particularly vexing problem in patients undergoing such treatment, and adjunctive granulocyte colony-stimulating factor (G-CSF) may be beneficial in permitting continuation of standard doses of interferon (Fig. 83–5).[44] A more promising approach is preemptive antiviral therapy started shortly after OLT but before histologic recurrence is established; in particular, the use of long-acting pegylated interferons is currently the focus of ongoing clinical trials. Based on earlier reports of rejection and graft loss in renal transplant recipients treated with interferon as well as preliminary experience in OLT recipients, there had been concern that interferon therapy would increase the risk of graft rejection, but the risk appears to be less significant than initially thought. Increasingly, recurrent hepatitis C is recognized as the cause of graft failure in OLT recipients, and the dilemma arises as to whether repeat OLT is justified. As discussed later, a subset of patients retransplanted for graft loss caused by recurrent hepatitis C have reasonable survival rates, if they do not have deep jaundice or renal failure (see also Chapter 68).

Acute Liver Failure

Acute liver failure is an important but infrequent indication for OLT. The outcome of OLT for acute liver failure is often excellent unless irreversible complications have occurred. In the past, OLT for acute liver failure was associated with poorer patient survival rates than those for other indications, such as PBC. However, more recent experience has shown that excellent patient survival rates are possible if liver failure is recognized promptly and the patient is referred for OLT before irreversible complications, especially neurologic, have supervened and made full recovery unlikely, despite a technically satisfactory transplant. The clinical syndrome of fulminant hepatic failure is defined as the onset of hepatic encephalopathy within 8 weeks of the initial symptoms of liver disease and has a variety of etiologies (see Chapter 80). On clinical grounds and even by computed tomographic (CT) scanning of the head, it may be impossible to exclude cerebral edema that complicates worsening encephalopathy; therefore, direct intracranial pressure monitoring may be required to detect and manage this frequently lethal complication of fulminant hepatic failure. Specific criteria to identify patients with fulminant hepatic failure who are unlikely to recover spontaneously without OLT are shown in Table 83–7. Ongoing trials will clarify whether full recovery without OLT may be possible in patients with fulminant hepatic failure and adverse prognostic characteristics who are treated with liver support systems and whether these systems can provide a "bridge to transplantation" in the face of clinical deterioration.

Cholestatic Liver Disease

Although less common than other major causes of cirrhosis, PBC and PSC have been major indications for OLT in many transplant centers and have facilitated the development of the Mayo disease models to predict the course of these disorders and to aid in decision making regarding the timing of referral for OLT. Patient and graft survival rates after OLT for PBC have been regarded as benchmarks for results of OLT for other types of cirrhosis and generally have been excellent. Patients with PBC and PSC should be referred for OLT evaluation if their Mayo risk scores predict a one-year survival rate of less than 95%. The Mayo model for PBC uses bilirubin, albumin, age, prothrombin time, and the presence of edema, whereas the model for PSC includes bilirubin, age, splenomegaly, and edema to predict survival. However, these models do not take into account prominent and frequently disabling complications of cholestatic liver disease, such as pruritus, osteopenia, or recurrent bouts of bacterial cholangitis in PSC. Despite the generally excellent results of OLT for these disorders, there is increasing concern that they may recur in the graft. A recent series of over 700 patients transplanted for these diseases demonstrated the risk of histologic recurrence to increase from 1% to 4% in the first year to 21% to 25% in the tenth year post-OLT.[45]

Table 83–7 | **Criteria for Liver Transplantation in Fulminant Hepatic Failure**

CRITERIA OF KING'S COLLEGE, LONDON:
Acetaminophen patients
  Arterial pH < 7.3, or
  INR > 6.5 and serum creatinine > 3.4 mg/dL
Nonacetaminophen patients
  INR > 6.5, or
  Any three of the following variables:
    Age < 10 yr or > 40 yr
    Etiology: non-A, non-B hepatitis; halothane hepatitis; idiosyncratic drug reaction
    Duration of jaundice before encephalopathy > 7 days
    INR > 3.5
    Serum bilirubin > 17.6 mg/dL
CRITERIA OF HOPITAL PAUL-BROUSSE, VILLEJUIF:
Hepatic encephalopathy, and
Factor V level < 20% in patients < age 30 yr, or
Factor V level < 30% in patients ≥ age 30 yr

INR, International Normalized Ratio. Reprinted with permission from Keeffe EB: Liver transplantation: Current status and novel approaches to liver replacement. Gastroenterology 120:749–762, 2001.

Biliary stricturing similar to that in the native diseased liver can be identified in a minority of patients following OLT for PSC and may represent recurrent disease. Differentiation of recurrent disease from other important causes of graft injury such as chronic rejection or ischemia may be difficult. Graft loss caused by recurrent PBC and PSC has been recognized but is uncommon, at least in patients followed for less than 5 years after OLT. Management at present consists of excluding other causes of hepatic dysfunction and intensifying immunosuppression, which may arrest disease recurrence in at least some recipients.

Hepatic Malignancy

Hepatocellular carcinoma (HCC) is the most common primary hepatic malignancy and usually occurs with cirrhosis as a precursor (see Chapter 81). Tumors discovered incidentally in the explanted liver with diameters of less than 2 cm typically do not have an adverse impact on patient survival.[46] However, the likelihood of tumor recurrence increases markedly with tumor burden, vascular invasion, and multiple lesions. Based on a large European experience reported by Mazzaferro and colleagues, generally accepted criteria for OLT in patients with HCC include a tumor diameter of less than 5 cm if the tumor is solitary or, if multiple, three lesions or less with the diameter of the largest lesion being no greater than 3 cm.[47] Survival rates comparable to those for transplantation for decompensated cirrhosis in the absence of complicating HCC (75% at 4 years) have been reported. The preoperative metastatic work-up should include a bone scan and chest CT in addition to abdominal imaging. Portal vein occlusion in a patient with HCC is regarded as evidence of metastatic spread and precludes OLT.

Use of a variety of adjuvant interventions has been reported in patients transplanted for HCC. Recurrent tumor occurs frequently in the graft, and the rationale for adjuvant therapy has been to eliminate micrometastatic disease, which is typically disseminated via the vascular system. Systemic chemotherapy given perioperatively as well as for varying durations before and after OLT and usually incorporating doxorubicin has been reported by a number of a transplant centers, although the benefit of this approach has been difficult to establish in the absence of controlled data. More recently, transarterial chemoembolization (TACE) administered directly into the tumor arterial supply has found favor with the aim of reducing tumor burden during the often protracted wait for OLT. This intervention can be hazardous in patients with decompensated cirrhosis, and its benefit in patients with favorable tumor characteristics remains to be determined. Confounding the management of the OLT candidate with HCC is the frequent observation that the tumor burden in the explant is significantly underestimated by preoperative imaging studies and that, in retrospect, withholding interventions such as TACE may not have been appropriate. Despite these caveats, there is clearly a subset of patients with HCC who can be cured by OLT and who would not have tolerated surgical resection of the tumor because of associated cirrhosis.

The fibrolamellar variant of HCC presents in younger adults without underlying cirrhosis and often comes to medical attention when the tumor burden is already large.[46] Extensive resection is tolerated because cirrhosis is absent. OLT may still be performed in patients who have recurrent tumor after resectional surgery. Post-OLT tumor recurrence may be delayed, and survival rates are acceptable. Hepatoblastoma is a rare pediatric tumor that also occurs in the absence of underlying parenchymal liver disease. Initial management consists of surgical resection; adjuvant chemotherapy is indicated for metastatic disease. OLT is an option when the tumor cannot be resected.

Cholangiocarcinoma remains the only major tumor of primarily hepatic origin for which a convincing role for OLT has been difficult to establish. The results of OLT for cholangiocarcinoma diagnosed preoperatively have been so poor that its presence has been regarded as a contraindication to OLT. Recurrence is almost invariable and prompt in OLT recipients. Only a subset of patients with a hilar location of the tumor and absence of nodal involvement have been reported to have good 5-year survivals. The extent of cholangiocarcinoma frequently is more extensive than suspected on pre-OLT imaging; often there is local, lymphatic, and perineural spread. The addition of en bloc pancreaticoduodenectomy has not resulted in improved survival post-OLT. Other approaches to treatment include preoperative irradiation and chemotherapy, with careful intraoperative tumor staging followed by OLT, with encouraging results in a preliminary report from the Mayo Clinic.[17, 48] The occasional patient with cholangiocarcinoma discovered incidentally in the explant can have a good long-term survival.[49]

Metabolic Disorders

Patients with congenital hepatic enzyme deficiencies and other inborn errors of metabolism can be cured by implantation of a normal liver (see Chapters 65, 66, and 67). Metabolic disorders considered for hepatic transplantation fall into two broad categories: diseases dominated clinically by obvious hepatocyte injury (e.g., Wilson disease, hemochromatosis) and those without any evidence of clinical or histologic hepatic injury (e.g., primary hyperoxaluria, familial hypercholesterolemia).[50] Although metabolic disorders are most prominent as indications for OLT in the pediatric population, important adult diseases managed by OLT include Wilson disease and hemochromatosis. Substantial neurologic improvement can occur following OLT for Wilson disease presenting with decompensated cirrhosis and neurologic involvement. Wilsonian crisis with severe hemolysis is an indication for urgent OLT. Hemochromatosis has been associated with poorer outcomes following OLT than other forms of cirrhosis, mainly because of an increased risk of cardiac deaths resulting from arrthymias. Ongoing studies will clarify whether iron depletion pre-OLT will improve post-OLT survival. Iron reaccumulation occurs in the grafts of patients with hemochromatosis after OLT, and continued iron depletion therapy may be required.

OLT also has been performed for a variety of systemic disorders, including adult polycystic disease with extensive and symptomatic hepatic cysts and as a curative procedure in combination with renal transplantation for primary hyperoxaluria in which end-organ damage is confined to the kidney but the metabolic defect is hepatic. The biliary type of cirrhosis associated with cystic fibrosis has been managed by OLT. Nonalcoholic steatohepatitis has been recognized increasingly as a frequent cause of hepatic dysfunction that progresses to decompensated cirrhosis in some patients. Graft injury apparently resulting from recurrent steatohepatitis has been observed following OLT.

Vascular Disorders

Budd-Chiari syndrome is characterized by hepatic venous outflow obstruction of the liver (see Chapter 70). Important associations are myeloproliferative disorders, hypercoagulable states, and vena caval webs. Medical approaches to management often are disappointing and fail to retard the often progressive natural history to liver failure and death. Liver biopsy may be helpful in determining whether the therapeutic approach should be decompression with a portosystemic shunt or liver transplantation. Good long-term results have been described in patients who undergo prompt shunt surgery, but patients with advanced fibrosis on liver biopsy should undergo liver transplantation.[51]

Veno-occlusive disease (VOD) is a similar disorder manifested by necrosis of zone 3 hepatocytes and fibrous obliteration of the central venule lumen. Most commonly seen after bone marrow transplantation (BMT), VOD may lead to hepatic failure and death in up to 25% of patients despite an otherwise successful BMT. Although the experience with liver transplantation for hepatic complications of BMT is limited, liver transplantation appears to be the only intervention that consistently alters the course of advanced VOD. Similarly, liver transplantation has been shown to be effective in the management of severe post-BMT graft-versus-host disease with predominantly hepatic involvement (see also Chapters 27 and 70).[52] Both hypocoagulable (e.g., hemophilias A and B) and hypercoagulable (e.g., protein C and S deficiencies) hematologic disorders have been cured with liver transplantation.[50]

Autoimmune Hepatitis

Failure of immunosuppressive therapy to arrest progression of severe autoimmune hepatitis with the development of hepatic decompensation is an indication to consider OLT. Human leukocyte antigen (HLA)-DR3 is associated with a lower likelihood of a therapeutic response to immunosuppression in autoimmune hepatitis. Excellent long-term survival is usual after OLT. However, the autoimmune diathesis may result in higher rates of acute cellular rejection. In addition, recurrent autoimmune hepatitis has been recognized increasingly in recent years and may require higher maintenance doses of immunosuppression. Graft survival is generally not diminished by recurrent autoimmune hepatitis.

Other Indications

Data compiled by UNOS reveal that benign tumors were the indication for OLT in approximately 0.5% of 9347 adult patients, with 0.1% transplanted for a hepatocellular adenoma.[4] OLT also is indicated in cases of multiple adenomas associated with glycogen storage disease and not only eliminates the risk for progression to HCC but also corrects the underlying metabolic disease. Multiorgan diseases for which OLT has been performed include Alagille's syndrome, amyloidosis, sarcoidosis, and adult polycystic disease.

SURGICAL ASPECTS OF LIVER TRANSPLANTATION

Once a potential organ donor is identified, the local organ procurement organization coordinates harvesting and supplies pertinent donor medical information to centers with suitable potential recipients listed with UNOS. In contrast to other types of organ transplants, including kidney and bone marrow, absence of HLA incompatibility does not appear to reduce liver graft survival, and donor-recipient matching is based only on ABO blood compatibility and physical characteristics. In critically ill recipients, an ABO-incompatible organ may be implanted, with the recognition that graft survival may be diminished and hemolytic anemia can develop. In addition to screening serologic studies and routine liver biochemical testing, particular attention is paid to the donor's medical history, including cardiovascular instability and need for pressor support before the determination of brain death.[53] With the critical shortage of cadaveric organ donors, expansion of the donor pool has included acceptance of older donors age 70 years and greater. The typical donor has had a catastrophic head injury or an intracerebral bleed with brain death but without multisystem failure. Electrolyte imbalance and hepatic steatosis are particular concerns as predictors of subsequent graft nonfunction.

The harvesting team makes a visual and if necessary histologic assessment of the donor organ, which is preserved in University of Wisconsin solution to maintain its viability during transport to the transplant center and allow organ preservation for up to 24 hours. Particular note is made during the harvesting procedure of anatomic variants in the hepatic arterial supply that need to be preserved to ensure graft viability. Once the circulation is interrupted, the organ is rapidly infused with cold University of Wisconsin solution to help preserve it before hepatectomy. Donor iliac arteries and veins also are retrieved in case vascular grafting is required. After its arrival at the recipient institution, further vascular dissection, with arterial reconstruction if necessary, is performed before implantation.

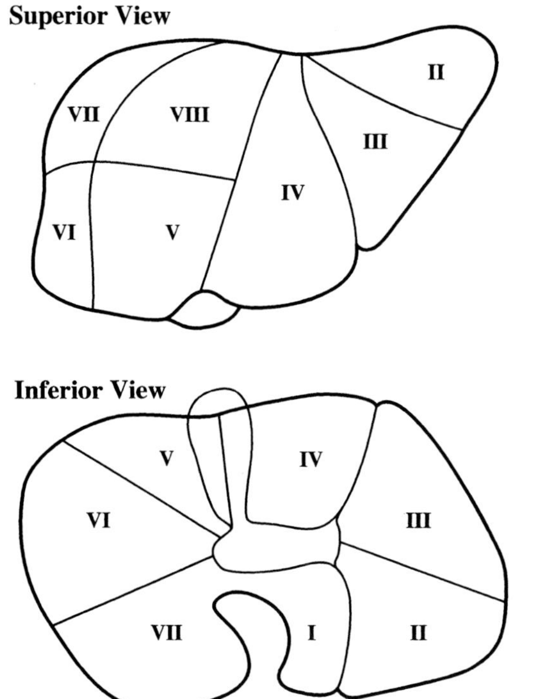

Figure 83–6. Segmental anatomy of the liver in the superior and inferior view. Segment VIII is visible only on the superior view, and segment I (caudate lobe) is visible only on the inferior view. (From Keeffe EB: Liver transplantation: Current status and novel approaches to liver replacement. Gastroenterology 120:749–762, 2001.)

Splitting cadaveric donor livers either in situ during harvesting or ex vivo on return to the transplant center allows two recipients to receive portions of the same hepatic allograft, if the volume and quality are sufficient. An adult cadaveric liver is divided into two functioning grafts. The left lateral segment (segments 2 and 3) is used for a pediatric recipient, and the right trisegment (segments 4 to 8) is used for an adult recipient. Acceptable graft and patient survival rates can be obtained with split grafts, although high-risk unstable recipients may have poorer outcomes with this technique. Figure 83–6 shows the segmental anatomy of the liver, which forms the basis of dissection for both split and living donor liver transplantation. Combined data suggest that in vivo split liver transplantation may yield superior survival rates and lower complication rates than the ex vivo technique. A recent series from the University of California at Los Angeles of 102 pediatric and adult patients who received in vivo split grafts demonstrated graft and patient survival rates comparable to those for standard OLT.[54]

Native Hepatectomy

Removal of the native liver is a technically challenging part of OLT. Previous abdominal surgery, especially a portosystemic shunt, and severe portal hypertension add to the complexity of the hepatectomy. However, hepatectomy is easier after placement of a TIPS than after a surgical portosystemic shunt, and TIPS is now regarded as a better choice for treatment of intractable variceal bleeding in a patient who ultimately will require OLT. Hilar dissection is performed to access the major hepatic vessels and devascularize the liver. Clamping of the portal vein during hepatectomy and liver implantation results in increased bleeding during dissection, mesenteric congestion, and production of lactate, whereas clamping of the inferior vena cava aggravates venous stasis and causes renal hypertension,[53] with diminished venous return to the heart. To circumvent these problems, venovenous bypass is achieved by cannulation of the portal vein and inferior vena cava via the femoral vein and return of blood via the axillary vein to the right side of the heart. This technique is routine in adult OLT and older pediatric recipients. In some recipients, only a suprahepatic anastomosis to the vena cava is performed, and the inferior vena cava is ligated below the graft. This is called the "piggyback" technique, in contrast to the more usual circumstance in which anastomosis to the vena cava is performed above and below the graft. The piggyback technique may be applicable if uninterrupted caval flow during OLT is particularly beneficial, as in a recipient with cardiac instability, if a prior portosystemic shunt obviates the need for portal bypass, or if the recipient is a pediatric patient in whom venovenous bypass may not be possible. The portal venous anastomosis is performed after portal bypass is terminated and is followed by the hepatic arterial anastomosis. The bile duct anastomosis is then fashioned either directly, duct-to-duct with or without a T-tube, or with a hepaticojejunostomy. The latter is favored if there is intrinsic bile duct disease such as primary sclerosing cholangitis or a major discrepancy in donor and recipient bile duct diameters. Microscopic surgical techniques facilitate the donor-recipient biliary and vascular anastomoses. Vascular anatomic anomalies increase the complexity of surgery further. Until recently, direct duct-to-duct anastomosis was typically facilitated by placement of a T-tube, with the added advantage of easy assessment of bile flow and access for cholangiography postoperatively. However, the risk of a bile leak during subsequent removal of the T-tube has led many transplant programs to abandon routine placement of a T-tube.

The use of a live donor involves implantation of a portion of the liver and is even more technically challenging than use of a whole cadaveric organ. Auxiliary cadaveric OLT is the placement of a graft without removal of the native liver. This technique usually has been performed in critically ill patients such as those with fulminant hepatic failure who are too unstable to tolerate native hepactectomy.

Irrespective of the type of graft used, after the anastomoses are complete, the newly implanted graft is reperfused with restoration of normal blood flow. The resulting release of vasoactive agents from pooled blood in the lower half of the body can lead to potentially lethal cardiovascular instability and tachyarrhythmias. Prompt bile production should occur if graft function is adequate. Hyperacute rejection is rare but devastating in OLT and leads to rapid graft necrosis within hours, with the need for urgent retransplantation.

Living Donor Liver Transplantation

Living donor liver transplantation (LDLT) in adults has expanded in recent years after becoming the standard of care for children in many transplant centers. The donor (generally a relative of the recipient) should be a healthy person and undergo careful evaluation by the transplant team; in most centers, a hepatologist not involved in the care of the recipi-

Table 83–8 | **Protocol for Evaluation of Potential Living-Related Donors**

Stage 1	Complete history and physical examination
	Laboratory blood tests: Liver biochemical tests, blood chemistry, hematology, coagulation profile, urinalysis, alpha-fetoprotein, carcinoembryonic antigen, and serologies for hepatitis A, B, and C, cytomegalovirus, Epstein-Barr virus, and human immunodeficiency virus
	Imaging studies: abdominal ultrasound and chest radiograph
Stage 2	Complete psychiatric and social evaluation
	Imaging studies: Computed tomographic scan of the abdomen
	Other studies: pulmonary function tests, echocardiography
Stage 3	Histology: liver biopsy
	Imaging studies: celiac and superior mesenteric angiography with portal phase
Stage 4	Imaging studies: Magnetic resonance cholangiogram
	Informed consent obtained

From Ghobrial RM, Amersi F, Busuttil RW: Surgical advances in liver transplantation. Clin Liver Dis 4:553–565, 2000.

ent performs an assessment of the donor. Morbidity and mortality rates in donors undergoing hepatic resection are 10% and 0.5%, respectively, and carefully obtained informed consent is essential.[3] Preoperative evaluation of the donor at a typical center is performed in four stages over a period of 1 to 3 months (Table 83–8). After undergoing complete evaluation, only a relatively small proportion of potential donors are deemed satisfactory candidates.

Right lobes (segments 5 to 8), extended right grafts (segments 4 to 8), or left hepatic grafts (segments 2 to 4) have been used successfully in adult-to-adult LDLT.[55] Adult LDLT provides obvious advantages to the recipient, including reduction in the mortality rate of patients awaiting OLT and a theoretical (but as yet unproved) reduction in the risk of rejection, because the donor usually is a relative. Table 83–9 outlines comparisons between in vivo split liver transplantation and adult LDLT.[55]

IMMUNOSUPPRESSION

Immunosuppressive strategies have by convention been classified into induction (initial immunosuppression), maintenance immunosuppression, and treatment of acute cellular rejection. A wide array of immunosuppressive agents are currently in use. The primary goal of immunosuppression is to prevent graft rejection and loss; a secondary goal is to avoid the adverse consequences of the antirejection therapy.

A list of the commonly used immununosuppressive agents, routes of administration, methods of monitoring, and common adverse effects is shown in Table 83–10. Common drug-drug interactions are shown in Table 83–11. The calcineurin inhibitors cyclosporine and tacrolimus are the basis for the majority of induction and maintenance immunosuppressive regimens, and both agents have substantial toxicity. Tacrolimus is now frequently used for primary immunosuppression instead of cyclosporine. In addition, patients may be converted from cyclosporine to tacrolimus following glucocorticoid- or OKT3-refractory rejection, late rejection (> 6

Table 83–9 | **Split Liver Versus Adult Living-Related Transplantation**

	SPLIT LIVER TRANSPLANTATION	ADULT LIVING-RELATED TRANSPLANTATION
Advantages	Increases pediatric and adult donor pools	Increases donor pool
	Dissection distant from hilar structures	Allows elective intervention
	Organs can be shared by different centers	Quality of graft can be assessed in living donor
	Applicable in urgent recipients	Allows early transplantation of recipients
		Provides the recipient with an optional allograft
		Decreases cold ischemia time
Disadvantages	Longer duration of procurement	Dissection at hilum is technically difficult
	Technically demanding	Complications in donor
	Splitting is restricted to perfect donor organs	Applicability to urgent recipient questionable

From Ghobrial RM, Amersi F, Busuttil RW: Surgical advances in liver transplantation. Clin Liver Dis 4:553–565, 2000.

Table 83–10 | **Major Immunosuppressive Agents**

	MODE OF ACTION	MONITORING	TOXICITIES
Cyclosporine	Calcineurin inhibitor: suppresses IL-2 dependent T-cell proliferation	Blood level	Renal, neurologic, hyperlipidemia, hypertension, hirsutism
Tacrolimus	Same as cyclosporine	Blood level	Renal, neurologic, diabetes mellitus
Prednisone	Cytokine inhibitor (IL-1, IL-2, IL-6, TNF, and IFN gamma)	None	Hypertension, diabetes mellitus, obesity, osteoporosis, infection
Azathioprine	Inhibits T- and B-cell proliferation by interfering with purine synthesis	White blood cell count	Bone marrow depression, hepatotoxicity
Mycophenolate mofetil	Selective inhibition of T- and B-cell proliferation by interfering with de novo purine synthesis	White blood cell count	Diarrhea, bone marrow depression
Sirolimus	Inhibits late T-cell functions	Blood level	Neutropenia, thrombocytopenia, hyperlipidemia
OKT3	Blocks T-cell CD3 receptor, preventing stimulation by antigen	CD3 count	Cytokine release syndrome, pulmonary edema, increased risk of infections
IL-2 receptor blocker	Competitive inhibition of IL-2 receptor on activated lymphocytes	None	Hypersensitivity reactions with basiliximab

IFN, interferon, IL, interleukin; TNF, tumor necrosis factor. Adapted from Everson GT, Karn I: Immediate postoperative care. In Maddrey WC, Schiff ER, Sorrell MF (eds): Transplantation of the Liver, 3rd ed. Philadelphia, Lippincott Williams & Wilkins, 2001, pp 131–162.

Table 83–11 | **Clinically Relevant Drug Interactions with Immunosuppressive Drugs**

Drugs that increase blood levels of cyclosporine and tacrolimus:
- Antifungals: fluconazole, ketoconazole, itraconazole
- Antibiotics: erythromycin, clarithromycin
- Calcium channel blockers: diltiazem, verapamil
- Others: bromocriptine, metoclopramide, allopurinol

Drugs that decrease levels of cyclosporine and tacrolimus:
- Anticonvulsants: phenytoin, phenobarbitone
- Antibiotics: rifampin, nafcillin

Drugs that increase nephrotoxicity of cyclosporine and tacrolimus:
- Gentamicin, ketoconazole, nonsteroidal anti-inflammatory drugs

Drugs that interact with mycophenolate mofetil:
- Acyclovir, ganciclovir
- Antacids
- Cholestyramine (inhibits absorption)

Drugs that interact with azathioprine:
- Allopurinol, angiotensin-converting enzyme (ACE) inhibitors, warfarin

months post-OLT), histologically diagnosed chronic rejection, severe cholestasis, intestinal malabsorption of cyclosporine, or cyclosporine toxicity (e.g., hirsutism, gingivitis, severe hypertension).[56] Tacrolimus used as rescue therapy for chronic rejection is less effective in the subgroup of patients with a serum total bilirubin level above 10 mg/dL, underscoring that its early recognition is imperative for a favorable outcome.

There are considerable differences from transplant center to transplant center in the rate at which the level of immunosuppression is reduced. For example, one center may withdraw prednisone as early as 2 weeks post-OLT, whereas another may keep patients on low-dose prednisone (5 mg/d) indefinitely.[57] A protocol recently adapted at the University of Colorado involves rapid, 14-day glucocorticoid withdrawal in the immediate postoperative period, with the patient taking either cyclosporine or tacrolimus, with or without mycophenolate mofetil. This protocol has led to marked reductions in the frequency of post-OLT diabetes mellitus, hypertension, hypercholesterolemia, and opportunistic infections, without an increase in the risk of graft loss or mortality.[57]

POSTOPERATIVE COURSE

Initial Phase to Discharge from Hospital

Because of the complexity of OLT and the often markedly decompensated state of OLT recipients, invasive monitoring with arterial and pulmonary venous lines is necessary in the first few postoperative days. If a T tube has been placed, hepatocellular recovery can be monitored at the bedside, with dark copious bile providing reassuring evidence of good graft function. The patient's overall status, including neurologic recovery from anesthesia, urinary output, and cardiovascular stability, also reflect graft function. Routine antimicrobial prophylaxis includes bowel decontamination with oral nonabsorbable antibiotics, perioperative systemic broad-spectrum antibiotics, antifungal agents, and ganciclovir to prevent cytomegalovirus infection. Markedly abnormal liver biochemistries are typical during the initial 48 to 72 postoperative hours and reflect a number of insults to the graft, including ischemia following harvesting, preservation, and subsequent reperfusion.[58] However, the overall trend in serum aminotransferase levels should be downward, with a corresponding improvement in coagulopathy and a falling serum bilirubin level.

Clinical features that are worrisome include scanty, pale bile, metabolic acidosis, depressed mentation, and continued need for pressor support with worsening liver biochemistries. Hepatic artery thrombosis needs to be excluded promptly by Doppler ultrasound, because it usually requires urgent retransplantation. Hepatic artery thrombosis is more common in pediatric recipients because of the smaller size of the vessels. Primary nonfunction of the graft is also an indication for urgent retransplantation and is suggested by the absence of bile production in the first several hours after transplantation, as well as an unstable overall clinical status. Donor characteristics that are associated with an increased likelihood of primary nonfunction include marked hepatic steatosis and profound hyponatremia. However, if graft function is adequate, pressor support can be tapered and weaning parameters can be obtained to facilitate extubation, although the recipient who is markedly debilitated from advanced cirrhosis may require several days of ventilatory support. Poor graft function and renal insufficiency also can impede weaning from the ventilator.

Within the first week post-OLT, liver biochemistries should steadily improve as ischemia and reperfusion injury resolve. Acute cellular rejection (ACR) becomes an important and frequent cause of graft dysfunction at 1 week and beyond. ACR is suggested by a rise in serum aminotransferase, alkaline phosphatase, and bilirubin levels. Because the biochemical features are nonspecific, there is a low threshold for performing a liver biopsy to evaluate other diagnostic possibilities, which include slowly resolving reperfusion injury, biliary tract obstruction, and cholestasis related to sepsis. Histologic findings characteristic of ACR are bile duct injury, portal inflammation with eosinophils, and, with more severe injury, endothelitis (Fig. 83–7). High doses of glucocorticoids (1000 mg of methylprednisolone or the equivalent) followed by a taper (200 to 20 mg/d) extending over several days are the first line of therapy. A response is suggested by a return of liver biochemistries toward normal values.

For the occasional patient with presumed ACR who fails to have a biochemical response to glucocorticoids, enhancement of immunosuppression may be necessary with the monoclonal antibody OKT3, although successful treatment also has been described with the substitution of tacrolimus for cyclosporine.[56] Liver biopsy should be repeated to confirm a lack of histologic response before more intensive therapy is initiated and to exclude other important causes of graft dysfunction such as ischemia.

The ability of recurrent HCV infection to mimic virtually all the histologic features of ACR has led to a re-evaluation of the need to treat apparent ACR aggressively under all circumstances.[59] Routine (protocol) liver biopsies also have fallen out of favor because histologic evidence of ACR can be noted in the absence of worsening graft function with no apparent clinical significance. A routine cholangiogram is obtained prior to clamping the T tube, if one is present. A nonsustained rise in liver biochemistries can be anticipated as a result. The timing of various infectious complications following liver transplantation is shown in Figure 83–8.

A number of other important medical issues are common in the first weeks following OLT and may require evaluation

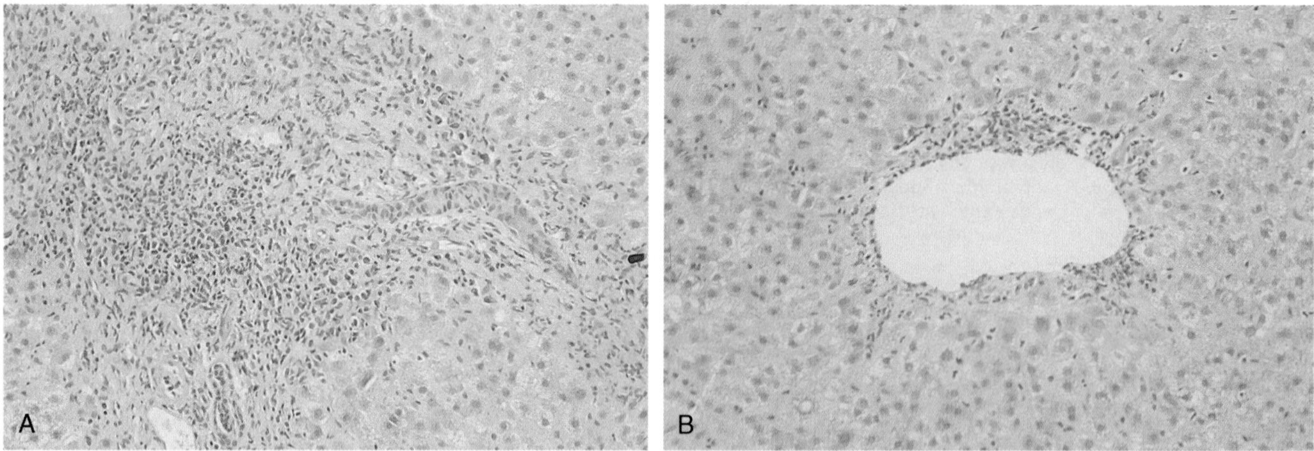

Figure 83–7. Acute cellular rejection of a liver graft. *A*, The portal tract shows a lymphocytic and plasma cell infiltrate that spills over into the periportal hepatocytes and bile duct. An atypical bile duct is also present. *B*, The central vein shows attachment of lymphocytes to the endothelium (endotheliitis). (From Cotran RS, Kumar V, Collins T (eds). Robbins' Pathologic Basis of Disease, 6th edition, CD-ROM. Philadelphia, WB Saunders.)

(Table 83–12). Neurologic dysfunction can present as an acute confusional state or seizures, and the differential diagnosis may include the lingering effects of hepatic encephalopathy, electrolyte imbalance, poor graft function, sepsis, uremia, and side effects of medications. A particular concern is the development of neurologic toxicity caused by the major immunosuppressive agents, the most dramatic presentation of which is central pontine myelinolysis. Overly rapid correction of hyponatremia perioperatively has been implicated in the genesis of central pontine myelinolysis, with evidence of demyelination demonstratable on magnetic resonance imaging. Management includes correcting the electrolyte imbalance if present and reducing baseline immunosuppression with the calcineurin inhibitors, which has been facilitated in recent years by the availability of mycophenolate mofetil. Diabetes mellitus, which is common in persons with cirrhosis, can occur for the first time in the postoperative period and usually requires insulin for control. Recent data demonstrate that HCV infection further increases the risk of post-OLT diabetes.[60] Renal impairment post-OLT may reflect a number of factors, including pre-OLT hepatorenal syndrome or renal failure of other etiologies, intraoperative hypotension resulting in acute tubular necrosis, and, importantly, the nephrotoxic effects of cyclosporine and tacrolimus, which cause renal afferent arteriolar vasoconstriction and a corresponding fall in the glomerular filtration rate. Adjunctive therapy with mycophenolate mofetil allows a reduction in the doses of cyclosporine and tacrolimus while

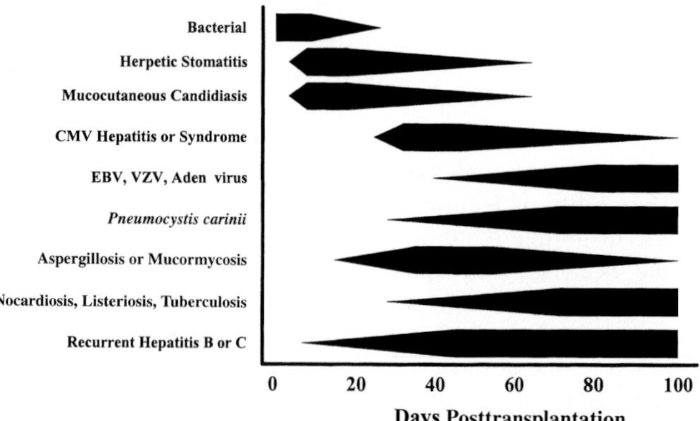

Figure 83–8. The time course of various infectious complications in liver transplant recipients. (From Everson GT, Kam I: Immediate postoperative care. In Maddrey WC, Schiff ER, Sorrell MF (eds): Transplantation of the Liver, 3rd ed., Philadelphia, Lippincott Williams & Wilkins, 2001, pp 131–162.)

Table 83–12 | **Medical Complications Occurring in the Immediate Postoperative Period**

Infections
Bacterial
Viral
Cytomegalovirus
Epstein-Barr virus
Fungal
Candidiasis, torulopsosis
Pneumocystis carinii pneumonia
Aspergillosis, mucormycosis
Respiratory complications
Pneumonia
Pulmonary edema
Acute respiratory distress syndrome
Portopulmonary hypertension
Hepatopulmonary syndrome
Renal failure
Cardiovascular disease
Hypertension
Myocardial ischemia
Valvular heart disease
Cardiomyopathy
Idiopathic hypertrophic subaortic stenosis
Hemochromatosis
Neurologic complications
Central pontine myelinolysis
Seizures
Central nervous system hemorrhage
Ischemic events
Coagulopathy
Thrombocytopenia
Disseminated intravascular coagulation
Diabetes mellitus

From Everson GT, Karn I: Immediate postoperative care. In Maddrey WC, Schiff ER, Sorrell MF (eds): Transplantation of the Liver, 3rd ed. Philadelphia, Lippincott Williams & Wilkins, 2001.

providing adequate immunosuppression. However, short-term hemodialysis may be necessary until renal function improves. In the first 3 to 4 weeks post-OLT, infections are typically bacterial and related to surgical complications such as intra-abdominal bleeding, bile leak, or wound infection.

Following Discharge from Hospital

If the postoperative course is smooth, planning for discharge may be possible by the second week after OLT. However, recovery often is more protracted, particularly in debilitated recipients. Once discharged, patients are seen at frequent intervals during the first postoperative month. The liver biochemistries should reach normal levels within a few weeks of OLT. Further graft dysfunction is an indication for prompt liver biopsy, because ACR remains a concern during this time; in addition, cytomegalovirus (CMV) becomes an important consideration three or more weeks post-OLT. Histologic features suggestive of CMV hepatitis include "owl's eye" inclusion bodies in the hepatocytes as well as neutrophilic abscesses with focal necrosis of the parenchyma.[61] Recipients who have had no prior exposure to CMV are at particularly high risk of CMV infection, particularly if they receive a graft from a CMV-seropositive donor, and are candidates for more intensive prophylaxis. Early recurrence of HCV infection also may become apparent, and, as noted earlier, it is crucial to recognize that many of the histologic features of ACR, such as bile duct inflammation and endotheliitis, are mimicked by HCV infection (see Table 83–6).

In addition to graft hepatitis, other important manifestations of de novo CMV infection include pneumonitis and diarrhea. Reactivation of CMV in a previously infected recipient tends to be less clinically severe than de novo infection. The diagnosis of CMV infection is confirmed by culture of tissue or blood, but not isolation from urine. Many transplant centers now have access to rapid tissue culture techniques with indirect immunofluorescence that allow prompt diagnosis. High-dose intravenous ganciclovir is highly effective in the treatment of CMV infection, but viral resistance has been described. Other therapies include a CMV hyperimmune globulin and foscarnet. Not only is CMV infection an important cause of morbidity and mortality in OLT recipients, but it also has been implicated in other complications, notably chronic graft rejection and recurrent HCV infection.[35, 62]

If the liver biopsy shows features to suggest biliary obstruction or if graft dysfunction is associated with clinical features of cholangitis such as fever and abdominal pain, a cholangiogram is obtained via the T tube, if present, by endoscopic retrograde cholangiopancreatography (ERCP) if a T tube is not present and the anastomosis is duct-to-duct, or by percutaneous transhepatic cholangiography if choledochojejunostomy has been performed. A stricture in a choledochocholedochostomy at the site of anastomosis is usually managed initially by balloon dilation at the time of diagnosis by cholangiography, followed by placement of a temporary internal stent. Surgical intervention is reserved for patients who do not respond to this approach, in which case the anastomosis is converted to a Roux-en-Y anastomosis. Anastomotic stricturing also can occur at the site of a choledochojejunostomy and requires access, usually by a percutaneous approach, to dilate the stenotic area.

A crucial point in management is to distinguish anastomotic stricturing from stricturing caused by ischemia. The bile duct in the OLT recipient is prone to ischemia because of its relatively tenuous arterial blood supply, and the development of a biliary stricture (unless it is obviously anastomotic) may reflect hepatic artery thrombosis. Ischemic stricturing is generally diffuse but can be predominantly hilar. Although temporizing measures such as balloon dilation may have some utility, if hepatic artery thrombosis is present or stricturing is widespread, such efforts are generally futile, and retransplantation will be required. Other etiologies of nonanastomotic stricturing include the use of an ABO-incompatible graft and protracted cold ischemia after harvesting. Biliary stricturing also can be a feature of recurrent primary sclerosing cholangitis. A T tube, if present, is removed by the sixth postoperative month, and removal is best performed at the transplant center, because bile leaks are common. When a bile leak occurs, prompt ERCP with nasobiliary drainage or stenting usually allows the tear in the bile duct to heal uneventfully.

In addition to prophylaxis against CMV infection in the early postoperative months, long-term antibiotics, most frequently sulfamethoxazole-trimethoprim, are prescribed to prevent infection with *Pneumocystis carinii* (PCP). In patients intolerant of sulfa drugs alternative options are dapsone tablets or inhaled pentamidine. Because PCP infection occurs most commonly in the first postoperative year, prophylaxis needs to be continued for at least this period of time.

Fungal infections pose a major threat to the OLT recipient, particularly in the setting of marked debilitation, intensive immunosuppression for rejection, or retransplantation. Major sites of infection are mucocutaneous (oral and esophageal), pulmonary, and intracerebral. Despite prolonged therapy with amphotericin or more recently with itraconazole, a fatal outcome is usual. A diagnosis of a brain abscess in a patient with invasive *Aspergillus* infection implies a dismal prognosis. It is important to distinguish superficial skin infections and simple colonization from invasive fungal infection, because topical antifungal agents such as nystatin or clotrimazole can eradicate the former. Similarly, bladder irrigation with amphotericin can cure candidal cystitis without the need for systemic antifungal therapy.

Opportunistic infections remains a concern in the OLT recipient during long-term follow-up. Patients need prompt assessment of symptoms of infection. Standard antibiotic therapy is appropriate for community-acquired respiratory infections, but a more extensive work-up is indicated for unusually severe symptoms or failure of an infection to resolve rapidly with treatment. Enteric bacteremia may be an initial clue to hepatic artery thrombosis in an otherwise stable recipient. Reactivation of tuberculosis may present in an atypical fashion post-OLT. Bronchoscopy to obtain cultures or lumbar puncture may be necessary, as clinically indicated.

LONG-TERM MANAGEMENT

General Preventive Medicine

Long-term management of the OLT recipient requires continued cooperation and communication between the primary care physician and the transplant center. Many of the disorders related to long-term survival after OLT are common diseases, including systemic hypertension, hyperlipidemia, and diabetes. Regular determination of a complete blood count, electrolytes, liver biochemical tests, and immunosuppressive drug levels should be arranged and the results forwarded to the transplant center.

Systemic hypertension is a frequent complication of OLT and is related to calcineurin inhibitor–induced renal vasoconstriction, as well as other drugs such as glucocorticoids.[63] Reduction in the level of immunosuppression unfortunately is generally ineffective in ameliorating hypertension. Other contributing factors include mild renal insufficiency, which is frequent post-OLT even when absent preoperatively. Initial antihypertensive therapy usually consists of a calcium channel blocker; angiotensin-converting enzyme inhibitors, as well as potassium-sparing diuretics, are relatively contraindicated because of their propensity to accentuate hyperkalemia, which is frequent in OLT recipients because of renal tubular acidosis caused by the calcineurin inhibitors. Cyclosporine and tacrolimus levels are increased by verapamil and diltiazem, and nifedipine is the agent of choice. Beta-blockers are the second-line antihypertensive agents used; diuretics are generally avoided because of concern about exacerbating renal insufficiency and electrolyte imbalances in the OLT recipient. Furosemide is the diuretic of choice if fluid overload is present. In the minority of patients in whom hypertension is not controlled, a centrally acting agent such as clonidine is introduced. For the occasional patient with intractable hypertension on cyclosporine-based immunosuppression, substitution of tacrolimus for cyclosporine may aid blood pressure control. However, both cyclosporine and tacrolimus are nephrotoxic and accentuate the renal impairment that exists perioperatively. Although acute nephrotoxicity may respond to interruption of or a reduction in the dose of these drugs, chronic renal impairment is usually irreversible, and drastic dose reductions should be avoided for fear of precipitating graft rejection. Cofactors implicated in the progression to chronic dialysis include recurrent HCV infection with associated glomerulonephritis as well as diabetes and systemic hypertension. Renal transplantation may be performed successfully in OLT recipients who become dialysis-dependent after otherwise successful liver transplantation.

Osteopenia is a frequent cause of morbidity in OLT recipients. Although hepatic osteodystrophy is typically associated with the cholestatic liver diseases, it is also prevalent in other forms of cirrhosis. Factors implicated in the pathogenesis include poor nutritional status, immobility, the calciuric effect of many diuretics, hypogonadism, and glucocorticoid use in patients with autoimmune hepatitis. In the initial several months post-OLT, osteopenia is accelerated further by high-dose glucocorticoid therapy as well as the other major immunosuppressive agents.[64] Atraumatic fractures may occur in trabecular bone such as vertebrae or ribs. However, patients begin to rebuild bone mass after immunosuppressive doses are reduced and the patient's mobility increases. Supplemental calcium and vitamin D are frequently prescribed for patients with symptomatic osteopenia; the role of the bisphosphonates is currently an area of active investigation.

De novo malignancies are increased in frequency following OLT. Post-transplant lymphoproliferative disorder (PTLD) varies from a low-grade indolent process to an aggressive neoplasm. Uncontrolled proliferation of B cells post-OLT, typically in response to primary Epstein-Barr virus infection, can be polyclonal or monoclonal. Pediatric recipients are at particular risk because of absence of prior Epstein-Barr viral infection. Intensive immunosuppression with OKT3 for severe rejection increases the risk of PTLD, which can present as a mononucleosis-like syndrome, lymphoproliferation, or malignant lymphoma. Clinical features suggestive of the diagnosis of PTLD include lymphadenopathy, unexplained fever, and systemic symptoms such as weight loss. After the diagnosis is made histologically by biopsy of involved areas (which can include the liver graft and gastrointestinal tract as well as lymph nodes), therapy includes a reduction in the level of immunosuppression and antiviral therapy with acyclovir or, more recently, ganciclovir directed against Epstein-Barr virus. Systemic chemotherapy may be required in patients who present with a malignant lymphoma. The higher frequency of PTLD in pediatric recipients has led to surveillance by polymerase chain reaction methodology for Epstein-Barr viremia and reduction of immunosuppression in those who are positive, before clinical features of PTLD occur. In addition, antiviral prophylaxis is used in high-risk recipients, including those who are seronegative for Epstein-Barr virus and receive a liver from a seropositive donor. Chronic rejection is increased in frequency in survivors of PTLD because of the deliberate reduction in the level of immunosuppression, which may be cautiously increased after PTLD is contained.

Screening for prostatic carcinoma should be performed by yearly digital rectal examination in male OLT recipients over age 40 years, in conjunction with serum prostate specific antigen (PSA) testing.[63] Screening for colorectal cancer should also be performed by colonoscopy every 3 to 5 years after age 50 in asymptomatic recipients; and in patients with a history of PSC and ulcerative colitis, yearly colonoscopy with surveillance mucosal biopsies should be considered.[63] In the setting of chronic immunosuppression, it seems appropriate to screen female transplant recipients over age 40 years for breast cancer by yearly mammography, although the cost-effectiveness of this approach is undefined. Other malignancies that are increased in frequency in organ transplant recipients include skin, female genital tract, and perineal cancers; alcoholic patients may be particularly prone to malignancies of the oropharynx. Patients should be encouraged to wear sunscreen and undergo appropriate surveillance for these malignancies.

Hyperlipidemia is observed in up to one half of OLT recipients and reflects a number of factors, including diabetes mellitus, obesity, renal dysfunction, and immunosuppressive agents, especially cyclosporine.[65] Pharmacologic therapy is indicated if hypercholesterolemia fails to respond to weight reduction and tight diabetic control. Pravastatin, a 3-hydroxy-3-methylglutaryl coenzyme A (HMG-CoA) reductase inhibitor, is well tolerated and efficacious in OLT recipients. Diabetes mellitus is common in OLT recipients and occurs in approximately one third of patients for the first time postoperatively. The pathogenesis is multifactorial; immunosuppressive therapy is a major factor because of the hyperglycemic effects of prednisone, cyclosporine, tacrolimus, azathioprine, and mycophenolate mofetil. In most dia-

Table 83–13 | **Multivariate Models Developed to Predict Survival Following Liver Retransplantation**

AUTHORS, YEAR	NO. OF PATIENTS	PROGNOSTIC PREDICTIVE FACTORS	COMMENTS
Rosen,[73] 1999	1356	Recipient age, bilirubin, creatinine, UNOS status, and cause of graft failure	UNOS database; HCV positivity, donor age significant by univariate analysis
Wong,[69] 1997	70	Age, UNOS status, inpatient status, creatinine, and bilirubin	Single site: King's College
Doyle,[70] 1996	418	Recipient age, mechanical ventilatory status, creatinine, and bilirubin	Single site: University of Pittsburgh
Markman,[71] 1999	150	Age group (pediatric vs. adult), mechanical ventilatory status, organ ischemia time >12 hr, creatinine, bilirubin	Single site: UCLA
Kim,[72] 1999	447	Interval to retransplantation (better prognosis if within 30 days)	Single site: Mayo Clinic; limited to patients with PBC or PSC
Rosen,[74] 1999	207	Creatinine (>2.0 mg / dL); bilirubin (>10 mg / dL)	UNOS database; limited to HCV-positive patients retransplanted for causes other than primary nonfunction

From Rosen HR: Disease recurrence following liver transplantation. Clin Liver Dis 4:675–689, 2000.
HCV, hepatitis C virus; PBC, primary biliary cirrhosis; PSC, primary sclerosing cholangitis; UNOS, United Network for Organ Sharing.

betic recipients, therapy with insulin is required. The high frequency of diabetes following OLT has led to the development of glucocorticoid-sparing immunosuppressive regimens.

A related problem is obesity, which is frequent even in OLT recipients who were profoundly malnourished preoperatively. Factors responsible for weight gain post-OLT include glucocorticoid use, increased caloric intake, and decreased physical activity during recuperation from surgery. Immunosuppression with tacrolimus has been reported to result in less weight gain than cyclosporine, which to a large extent may reflect the lower glucocorticoid doses employed with tacrolimus. Management of obesity in this population includes a reduction in the dose of glucocorticoid and even complete withdrawal if possible. The advent of mycophenolate mofetil may permit effective immunosuppression without glucocorticoids.

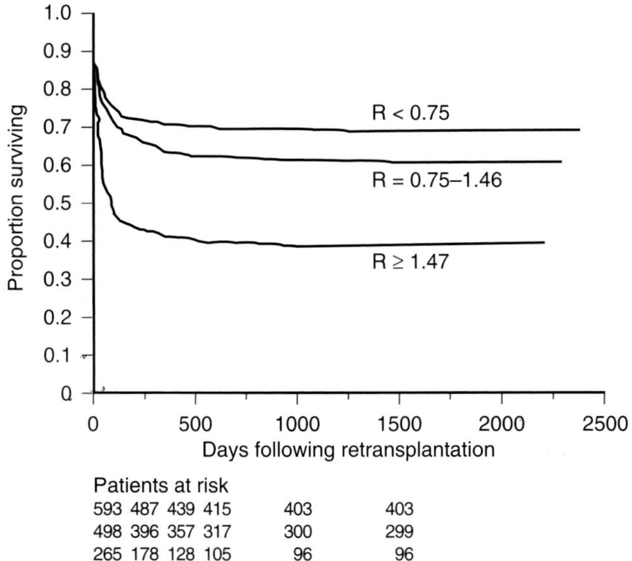

Figure 83–9. Kaplan-Meier analysis of survival for patients undergoing hepatic retransplantation stratified into low (R < 0.75), medium (R = 0.75–1.46), and high-risk groups (R ≥ 1.47) using prognostic predictive factors listed in Table 83–13 ($P < .00001$ by Wilcoxon rank sum). The number or patients in each group at various time points is also indicated. (From Rosen HR, Madden JP, Martin P: A model to predict survival following hepatic retransplantation. Hepatology 29:365–369, 1999.)

Immunizations and Bacterial Prophylaxis

Immunization against hepatitis A and B, influenza, pneumoccocus, tetanus, and diphtheria is part of the standard pretransplantation evaluation. A substantial proportion of patients may be unable to mount adequate antibody responses. Indeed, a number of recent studies point to a high rate of primary nonresponse to HAV or HBV vaccines in chronically HCV-infected patients.[66] Vaccines based on live or attenuated microorganisms (e.g., measles, mumps, rubella, oral polio, bacille Calmette-Guérin [BCG], vaccinia) are contraindicated because of the risk of reactivation. It is recommended that prophylactic antibiotics be taken for any dental procedure, even basic cleaning.

When to Call the Transplant Center

A number of common symptoms, signs, and laboratory abnormalities warrant a call by the local physician to the transplant center. These problems include fever, abdominal pain, neurologic symptoms, anticipated surgery, and a possible change in the patient's immunosuppressive regimen. When an unexplained abnormality of liver biochemical tests occurs, a complete work-up for possible causes is imperative. Although liver biopsy can be obtained by the patient's local physician, a local pathologist may be inexperienced in allograft interpretation, and it is critical that the specimen be reviewed at the transplant center so that appropriate decisions regarding management can be obtained. Additionally, many transplant programs prefer to perform indicated interventional biliary tract studies, because therapeutic intervention often is required, and immediate access to the transplant team permits more rapid decision making. Any evidence of graft failure needs to be attended to immediately by referral to the transplant center.

Hepatic Retransplantation

Although improved immunosuppressive regimens have led to a lower rate of graft loss because of chronic rejection, recurrence of the underlying liver disease has been recognized increasingly as a cause of graft failure. The rates and severity of recurrent disease are highly variable and probably related to a complex interplay of host factors (including the underlying liver disease), therapeutic decisions (e.g., immunosuppression, antiviral treatment), and possibly genetic variability of the allograft (perhaps through effects on the nature and magnitude of the inflammatory response within the graft).[45] Understanding the full impact of recurrent disease, especially non-viral disease, on patient and graft survival will require long-term follow-up studies. For example, although the rate of histologic recurrence of viral hepatitis is greatest in the first year post-OLT, recurrent PBC or PSC develops in less than 5% of patients by the first year, whereas more than 20% demonstrate histologic recurrence 10 years post-OLT. As patients enter their second and third decades post-OLT, it is possible that the number of patients needing retransplantation will further strain the donor pool.[67] This issue is compounded by the observation that patients undergoing retransplantation experience an approximately 20% overall reduction in survival but consume increased resources when compared with primary OLT recipients.[68] Based on these considerations, a number of investigators have developed models to predict survival following retransplantation.[69–74] Preoperative serum bilirubin and serum creatinine levels consistently provide prognostic information (Table 83–13; Fig. 83–9).[73, 75] Although these models only estimate the probability of survival for the individual patient and do not take into account the patient's quality of life, they can be used as adjuncts to clinical judgment. Application of retransplantation to low-risk patients is associated with survival comparable to that for primary liver transplantation; whether retransplantation is justified in patients with high-risk scores will require prospective studies.

REFERENCES

1. Rosen HR, Martin P: Hepatitis B and C in the liver transplant recipient. Semin Liver Dis 20:465–480, 2000.
2. Reding R: Steroid withdrawal in liver transplantation. Benefits, risks and unanswered questions. Transplantation 70:405–410, 2000.
3. Keeffe EB: Liver transplantation: Current status and novel approaches to liver replacement. Gastroenterology 120:749–762, 2001.
4. United Network for Organ Sharing. http: 2000; //www.unos.org.
5. Rosen HR, Bass N, Brown RS, et al: Curricular guidelines for training in transplant hepatology training. Liver Transplant 8:85–87, 2002.
6. Abramson O, Rosenthal P: Current status of pediatric liver transplantation. Clin Liver Dis 4:533–552, 2000.
7. Yao FY, Bass N: Lamivudine treatment in patients with severely decompensated cirrhosis due to replicating hepatitis B infection. J Hepatol 33:301–307, 2000.
8. Donovan JP: Endoscopic management of the liver transplant recipient. Clin Liver Dis 4:607–618, 2000.
9. Fattovich G, Giustina G, Degos F, et al: Morbidity and mortality in compensated cirrhosis type C: A retrospective follow-up study of 384 patients. Gastroenterology 112:463–472, 1999.
10. Wiesner RH, Porayko MK, Dickson ER, et al: Selection and timing of liver transplantation in primary biliary cirrhosis and primary sclerosing cholangitis. Hepatology 16:1290, 1999.
11. Gralnek IM, Hays RD, Rosen HR, et al: Development and evaluation of the liver disease quality of life instrument, LDQOL 1.0. Am J Gastroenterol 95:3552–3565, 2000.
12. Jenkins RL: Defining the role of transjugular intrahepatic portosystemic shunts in the management of portal hypertension. Liver Transpl Surg 1: 225, 1999.
13. Lucey MR, Brown KA, Everson GT: Minimal criteria for placement of adults on the liver transplant waiting list: A report of a national conference organized by the American Society of Transplant Physicians and the American Association for the Study of Liver Diseases. Liver Transpl Surg 3:628–637, 1997.
14. Kamath P, Wiesner RH, Malinchoc M, et al: A model to predict survival in patients with endstage liver disease. Hepatology 33:464–470, 2001.
15. Rosen HR, Martin P: Viral hepatitis following liver transplantation. Infect Dis Clin North Am 14:761–784, 2000.
16. Shouval D, Samuel D: Hepatitis B immune globulin to prevent hepatitis B virus graft reinfection following liver transplantation: A concise review. Hepatology 32:1189–1195, 2000.
17. DeVreede I, Steers JL, Ruch PA: Prolonged disease-free survival after orthotopic liver transplantation plus adjuvant chemoirradiation for cholangiocarcinoma. Liver Transplant 6:309–316, 2000.
18. Lucey MR, Merion RM, Henley KS, et al: Selection for and outcome of liver transplantation in alcoholic liver disease. Gastroenterology 102: 1736, 1999.
19. Plotkin JS, Johnson LB, Rustgi V, Kuo PC: Coronary artery disease and liver transplantation: The state of the art. Liver Transplant 6:S53–S56, 2000.
20. Farrell FJ, Nguyen M, Woodley S, et al: Outcome of liver transplantation in patients with hemochromatosis. Hepatology 20:404, 1999.
21. Krowka MJ: Hepatopulmonary syndrome versus portopulmonary hypertension: Distinctions and dilemmas. Hepatology 25:1282–1284, 1999.
22. Krowka MJ: What are we learning from interventional radiology, liver transplantation, and other disorders? Hepatopulmonary syndrome. Gastroenterology 109:1009, 1999.
23. Somberg KA, Lombardero MS, Lawlor SM, et al: A controlled analysis of the transjugular intrahepatic portosystemic shunt in liver transplant recipients. Transplantation 63:1074–1079, 1999.
24. Selberg O, Bottcher J, Tusch G, et al: Identification of high- and low-risk patients before liver transplantation: A prospective cohort study of nutritional and metabolic parameters in 150 patients. Hepatology 25: 652–657, 1999.
25. Keeffe EB, Gettys C, Esquivel CO: Liver transplantation in patients with severe obesity. Transplantation 57:309, 1999.
26. Forman L, Lucey MR: Predicting the prognosis of chronic liver disease: An evolution from Child to MELD. Hepatology 33:473–475, 2001.
27. Baddour N, Demetris AJ, Shah G, et al: The prevalence, rate of onset and spectrum of histologic liver disease in alcohol-abusing liver allograft recipients [abstract]. Gastroenterology 102:A779, 1992.
28. Lucey MR, Carr K, Beresford TP: Alcohol use after liver transplantation in alcoholics: A clinical cohort follow-up study. Hepatology 25: 1223–1227, 1997.
29. Todo S, Demetris A, Van Thiel D: Orthotopic liver transplantation for patients with hepatitis B virus-related liver disease. Hepatology 13:619, 1991.
30. Samuel D: Liver transplantation in European patients with the hepatitis B surface antigen. N Engl J Med 329:1842–1846, 1999.
31. Perrillo R, Schiff ER, Yoshida E, et al: Adefovir dipivoxil for the treatment of lamivudine-resistant hepatitis B mutants. Hepatology 32: 129–134, 2000.
32. Gane EJ, Portmann BC, Naoumouv NV, et al: Long-term outcome of hepatitis C infection after liver transplantation. N Engl J Med 334:821–827, 1999.
33. Rosen HR, Gretch DR, Oehlke M, et al: Timing and severity of hepatitis C Recurrence following liver transplantation as predictors of long-term allograft injury. Transplantation 65:1178–1182, 1999.
34. Rosen HR, Hinrichs DJ, Gretch DR, et al: Association of multispecific CD4(+) response to hepatitis C and severity of recurrence after liver transplantation. Gastroenterology 117:1012–1014, 1999.
35. Rosen HR, Chou S, Gretch DR, et al: Cytomegalovirus viremia: Risk factor for allograft cirrhosis following liver transplantation for hepatitis C. Transplantation 64:721–726, 1999.

36. Sheiner PA, Schwartz ME, Mor E, et al: Severe or multiple rejection episodes are associated with early recurrence of hepatitis C after orthotopic liver transplantation. Hepatology 21:30–34, 1995.
37. Rosen HR, Lentz JJ, Rose SL: Donor polymorphism of tumor necrosis factor gene associated with variable severity of hepatitis C recurrence following liver transplantation. Transplantation 68:1898–1902, 1999.
38. Feray C, Caccamo L: European Collaborative Study on factors influencing outcome after liver transplantation for hepatitis C. Gastroenterology 117:619–625, 1999.
39. Rosen HR, Martin P: OKT3 and hepatitis C: Defining the risks. Transplantation 63:171–172, 1999.
40. Rosen HR, Shackleton CR, Higa L, et al: Use of OKT3 associated with early and severe hepatitis C recurrence following liver transplantation. Am J Gastroenterol 92:1453–1456, 1999.
41. Wiesner RH, United States FK506 Study Group: A long-term comparison of tacrolimus (FK506) versus cyclosporine in liver transplantation. Transplantation 66:493–499, 1999.
42. Berenguer M, Prieto M, Rayon JM, et al: Natural history of clinically compensated hepatitis C virus-related graft cirrhosis after liver transplantation. Hepatology 32:852–858, 2000.
43. Sheiner P: The efficacy of prophylactic interferon alfa-2b in preventing recurrent hepatitis C after liver transplantation. Hepatology 28:831–838, 1999.
44. Gopal DV, Rabkin JM, Berk BS, et al: Treatment of progressive hepatitis recurrence after liver transplantation with combination interferon plus ribavirin. Liver Transplantation 7:181–190, 2001.
45. Rosen HR: Disease recurrence following liver transplantation. Clin Liver Dis 4:675–689, 2000.
46. Penn I: Hepatic transplantation for primary and metastatic cancers of the liver. Surgery 110:726, 1999.
47. Mazzaferro V, Regalia E, Doci R, et al: Liver transplantation for the treatment of small hepatocellular carcinomas in patients with cirrhosis. N Engl J Med 11:693–699, 1996.
48. Bismuth H: Revisiting liver transplantation for patients with hilar cholangiocarcinoma: The Mayo Clinic Proposal. Liver Transplant 6:317–319, 2000.
49. Goss JA, Shackleton CR, Farmer DG, et al: Orthotopic liver transplantation for primary sclerosing cholangitis: A twelve-year single-center experience. Ann Surg 225:472–481, 1997.
50. Rosen HR, Martin P: Liver transplantation. In Schiff ER, Maddrey WC, Sorrel MF (eds): Schiff's Diseases of the Liver. Philadelphia, Lippincott-Raven, pp 1589–1615, 1999.
51. Bismuth H, Sherlock S: Portosystemic shunting versus liver transplantation for the Budd-Chiari syndrome. Ann Surg 214:581–586, 1991.
52. Rosen HR, Martin P, Schiller GJ, et al: Orthotopic liver transplantation for bone-marrow-transplant–associated veno-occlusive disease and graft-versus-host disease of the liver. Liver Transpl Surg 2:225–230, 1996.
53. Balan V, Marsh JW, Rakela J: Liver transplantation. In Bircher J, Benhamou JP, McIntyre N, et al (eds): eds. Oxford Textbook of Clinical Hepatology, 2nd ed. London, Oxford University Press, pp 2039–2061, 1999.
54. Ghobrial RM, Yersiz H, Farmer DG, et al: Predictors of survival after in vivo split liver transplantation: Analysis of 110 consecutive patients. Ann Surg 232:312–323, 2000.
55. Ghobrial RM, Amersi F, Busuttil RW: Surgical advances in liver transplantation. Clin Liver Dis 4:553–565, 2000.
56. Cronin II, Faust TW, Brady L, et al: Modern immunosuppression. Clin Liv Dis 4:619–655, 2000.
57. Everson GT, Kam I: Immediate postoperative care. In Maddrey WC, Schiff ER, Sovell MF (eds): Transplantation of the Liver, 3rd ed. Philadelphia, Lippincott Williams & Wilkins, 131–162, 1999.
58. Rosen HR, Martin P, Goss J, et al: The significance of early aminotransferase elevation following liver transplantation. Transplantation 65: 68–72, 1999.
59. Prieto M, Berenguer M, Rayon JM, et al: High incidence of allograft cirrhosis in hepatitis C virus genotype 1b infection following transplantation: Relationship with rejection episodes. Hepatology 29:250–256, 1999.
60. Zein NN, Abdulkarim AS, Wiesner RH, et al: Prevalence of diabetes mellitus in patients with end-stage liver cirrhosis due to hepatitis C, alcohol, or cholestatic disease. J Hepatol 32:209–217, 2000.
61. Rubin RH: Infectious disease problems. In Maddrey WC, Schiff ER, Sorrell MF (eds): Transplantation of the Liver, 3rd ed. Philadelphia, Lippincott Williams & Wilkins, pp. 279–295, 1999.
62. Rosen HR, Corless CL, Rabkin J, Chou S: Association of cytomegalovirus genotype and graft rejection after liver transplantation. Transplantation 66:1627–1631, 1998.
63. Munoz SJ, Rothstein KD, Reich D, Manzarbeitia C: Long-term care of the liver transplant recipient. Clin Liver Dis 4:691–710, 2000.
64. Hay JE: Bone disease after liver transplantation. Liver Transpl Surg, 1: 55–61, 1995.
65. Munoz SJ: Hyperlipidemia and other coronary risk factors after orthotopic liver transplantation: Pathogenesis, diagnosis and treatment. Liver Transpl Surg 1:29–35, 1995.
66. Keeffe EB, Iwarson S, McMahon BLK, et al: Safety and immunogenicity of hepatitis A vaccine in patients with chronic liver disease. Hepatology 27:881–886, 2001.
67. Wall WJ: Recurrent disease after liver transplantation: Implications for the future. Liver Transpl Surg 3:S62–S67, 1997.
68. Evans RW, Manninen DL, Dong FB, McLynne DA: Is retransplantation cost effective? Transplant Proc, 25:1694–1697, 1999.
69. Wong T, Devlin J, Rolando N, et al: Clinical characteristics affecting the outcome of liver retransplantation. Transplantation 27:878–882, 1997.
70. Doyle HR: Hepatic retransplantation: An analysis of risk factors associated with outcome. Transplantation 61:1499–1505, 1999.
71. Markmann JF, Gornbein J, Markowitz JS: A simple model to estimate survival after retransplantation of the liver. Transplantation 67:422–430, 1999.
72. Kim WR, Wiesner RH, Poterucha JJ: Hepatic retransplantation in cholestatic liver disease: Impact of the interval to retransplantation on survival and resource utilization. Hepatology 30:395–400, 2001.
73. Rosen HR, Madden JP, Martin P: A model to predict survival following hepatic retransplantation. Hepatology 29:365–369, 1999.
74. Rosen HR, Martin P: Hepatitis C infection in patients undergoing liver retransplantation. Transplantation 66:1612–1616, 1998.
75. Rosen HR: Disease recurrence following liver transplantation. Clin Liver Dis 4:675–690, 2001.

Section Ten

SMALL AND LARGE INTESTINE

Chapter 84

Anatomy, Histology, Embryology, and Developmental Anomalies of the Small and Large Intestine

David J. Keljo and Cheryl E. Gariepy

INTESTINAL ANATOMY

Gross Morphology of the Small Intestine

The small intestine is a specialized tubular structure within the abdominal cavity that is continuous proximally with the stomach and distally with the colon. It is responsible for the absorption of nutrients, salt, and water. The small bowel increases 20-fold in length, from 200 cm in the newborn to almost 6 m in the adult. The average length of the small intestine is nearly approximated by three times the length of the infant or standing height of the child or adult.[1]

The duodenum is the most proximal portion of the small intestine and begins at the duodenal bulb, travels in the retroperitoneal space around the head of the pancreas, and ends on its return to the peritoneal cavity at the ligament of Treitz. The remainder of the small intestine is suspended within the peritoneal cavity by a thin, broad-based mesentery attached to the posterior peritoneal wall. This arrangement allows free movement of the small bowel within the abdominal cavity. The proximal 40% of the mobile small intestine is called the *jejunum* and the remaining 60% is called the *ileum*. There is no clear delineation between the jejunum and the ileum on external examination, although the jejunum feels thicker to the surgeon.

Visual examination of the luminal surface of the small intestine reveals a concentration of mucosal folds, the *plicae circulares*, in the proximal jejunum that decrease in number in the distal small bowel and are absent in the terminal ileum. Lymphoid follicles are scattered throughout the small intestine but are found in highest concentrations in the distal ileum. They are more prominent during infancy and childhood and in certain disease states such as giardiasis and immunodeficiency.[2] Aggregates of lymphoid follicles, which can measure up to 3 cm in length within the ileum, are designated *Peyer's patches*.

The small bowel connects to the colon at the ileocecal valve, which is composed of upper and lower lips that protrude into the cecum. The valve is frequently more prominent in children because of additional lymphoid tissue. The ileocecal valve opposes reflux of colonic contents and gas into the small bowel. This appears to be a function of the angulation between the ileum and cecum maintained by superior and inferior ileocecal ligaments.[3] There does not appear to be a tonic, sphincter-type pressure in this region.

Gross Morphology of the Colon

The colon is a tubular structure of approximately 30 to 40 cm in length at birth that reaches 1.5 m in length in the adult. It is continuous proximally at the ileocecal valve with the small intestine and ends distally at the anal verge (Fig. 84–1).[4] The external appearance of the colon differs from that of the small bowel because of differences in their musculature. Although both organs have inner circular and outer longitudinal muscle layers, the colonic longitudinal muscle fibers coalesce into three discrete bands *(teniae)* located at 120-degree intervals about the colonic circumference. The teniae start at the base of the appendix and run continuously to the proximal rectum. (In surgery they are frequently followed to locate the appendix.) Outpouchings of the colon *(haustra)* separate the teniae. The folds between the haustra have a semilunar appearance when viewed from within the colon. On the outside of the colon are fatty-filled sacs of peritoneum called *appendices epiploicae* or *omental appendices*.

The first portion of the colon, the cecum, lies in the right iliac fossa, and is slightly dilated compared with the rest of the colon. Because of its large diameter (approximately 8 cm), it is the part of the bowel most subject to rupture with distal obstruction, and tumors of the cecum can grow to be quite large while remaining asymptomatic. The cecum may also have some degree of mobility, predisposing it to volvulus (see Chapter 20). The vermiform appendix is a blind outpouching of the cecum that begins inferior to the ileocecal valve. Clinically relevant features of appendiceal anatomy are discussed in Chapter 107.

The *ascending colon* extends cranially from the cecum for 12 to 20 cm along the right side of the peritoneal cavity to the undersurface of the liver. In most individuals, the mesentery of the ascending colon has fused with the parietal peritoneum such that this segment of the colon is a retroperitoneal structure.

At the hepatic flexure the colon turns medially and anteriorly to emerge into the peritoneal cavity as the *transverse colon*. This segment of the colon is about 45 cm in length and supports the greater omentum. The transverse colon can be quite mobile on its mesentery, even dipping down below the pelvic brim before reaching its attachment to the diaphragm at the splenic flexure.

The *descending colon* travels posteriorly and then inferiorly in the retroperitoneal compartment to the pelvic brim. There it emerges into the peritoneal cavity as the *sigmoid colon*. This is an S-shaped redundant segment of variable length. Its mobility and tortuosity challenge the endoscopist and radiologist and also cause it to be susceptible to volvulus (see Chapter 20). The narrowest portion of the colon (approximately 2.5-cm diameter) is in the sigmoid, explaining why tumors in this region may be symptomatic early.

The *rectum* begins at the peritoneal reflection and follows

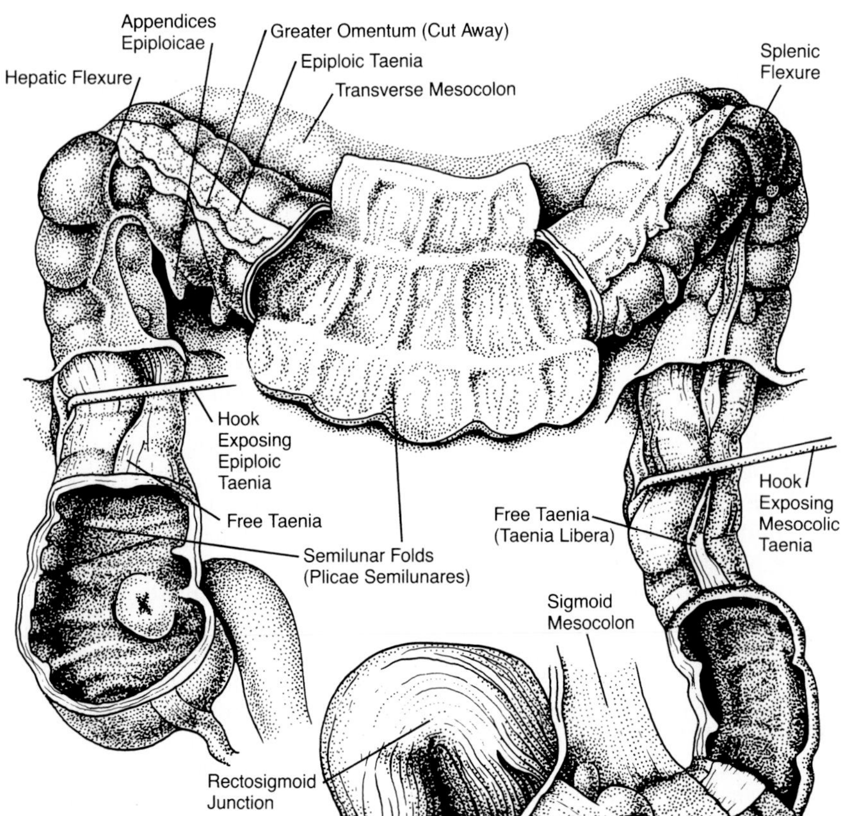

Figure 84–1. Contour and gross anatomy of the colon. Note the ileocecal junction, which is not labeled. (Courtesy of the CIBA Collection of Medical Illustrations by Frank H. Netter, M.D.)

the curve of the sacrum, ending at the anal canal. The anal canal begins at the mucocutaneous junction, where the lining of the canal changes from columnar epithelium to the stratified squamous epithelium of skin. The distal 3 cm of rectum and anal canal is marked by longitudinal folds called the *columns of Morgagni,* which terminate in the anal papillae.

In the proximal rectum, fibers of the teniae fan out to envelop the rectum. The circular inner smooth muscle layer becomes the *internal sphincter* at the upper anal canal. The anal canal passes through the muscular pelvic diaphragm where it is surrounded by the *external sphincter,* which is separated from the internal sphincter by a thin layer of elastic fibers and the longitudinal muscle coat of the rectum. The fibers of the external sphincter blend with those of the levator ani and are attached posteriorly to the coccyx and anteriorly to the perineal body. The function of these muscles is described in more detail in Chapter 11.

Intestinal Vascular Supply

(see also Chapter 119)

The superior mesenteric artery delivers oxygenated blood to the distal duodenum, the entire jejunum and ileum, the ascending colon, and portions of the transverse colon. The remainder of the colon is supplied primarily from branches of the inferior mesenteric artery. The anal canal is supplied from branches of the internal iliac arteries. Veins follow the arterial supply, with the superior and inferior mesenteric veins emptying into the portal vein.

Intestinal Lymphatic Drainage

The lymphatic drainage of both the small bowel and colon follows their respective blood supplies to lymph nodes in the celiac, superior, and inferior preaortic regions. Lymphatic drainage proceeds to the cisterna chyli and then through the thoracic duct into the left subclavian vein. The perianal region drains to the inguinal lymph nodes.

Intestinal Extrinsic Innervation

The vagus nerve supplies parasympathetic innervation to the small bowel and proximal colon. Pelvic parasympathetic fibers supply the distal colon and rectum. Upper thoracic sympathetic fibers supply the small bowel, and the lower thoracic sympathetic fibers supply the proximal colon. The distal colon and rectum are innervated by lumbar sympathetic fibers. Neurons within the gut project out of the bowel and innervate prevertebral sympathetic ganglia, as well as ganglia in the gallbladder and pancreas.

INTESTINAL HISTOLOGY

Layers of the Intestinal Wall

The four layers of the intestinal wall are the serosa, the muscularis, the submucosa, and the mucosa (Fig. 84–2). The *serosa* consists of a single layer of mesothelial cells that

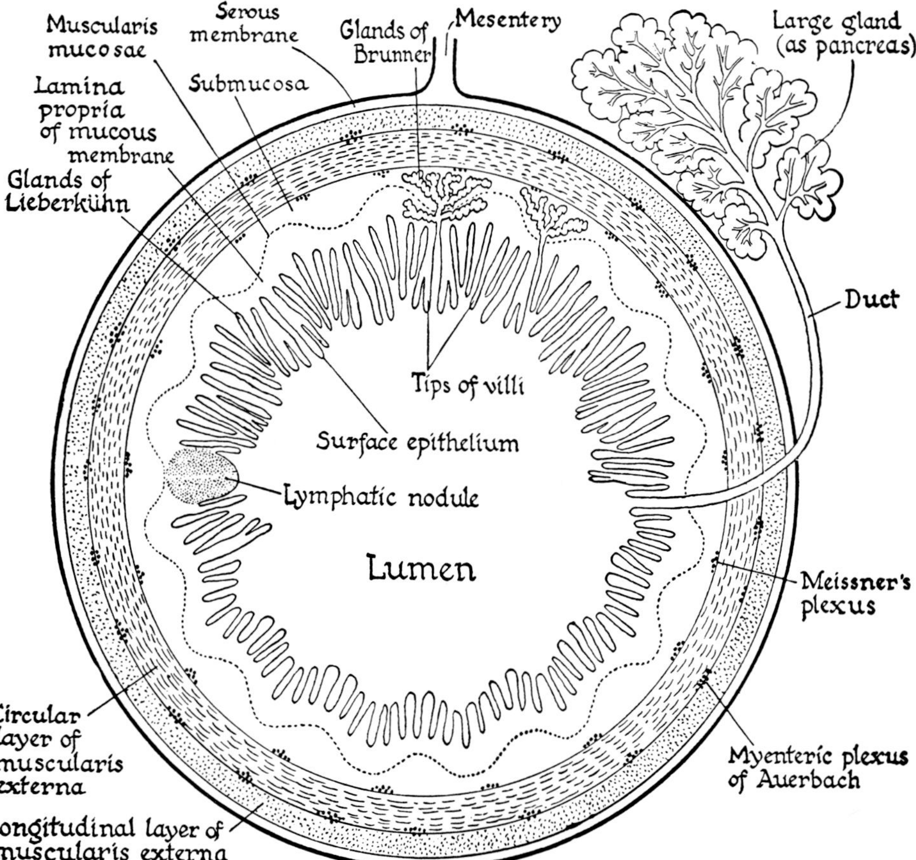

Figure 84–2. Schematic diagram of a cross section of the intestinal tract. (From Bloom W-N, Fawcett DW: A Textbook of Histology. Philadelphia, WB Saunders, 1968.)

extend from the peritoneum and encase the intestine to form its outermost layer. The *muscularis* contains both the outer longitudinal and inner circular layers of smooth muscle fibers. Between these muscular layers are found ganglion cells of the myenteric (Auerbach's) plexus. Within the *submucosa* is a heterogeneous population of cells, including lymphocytes, plasma cells, macrophages, eosinophils, fibroblasts, and mast cells embedded within a dense connective tissue. The nature and admixture of these cells vary in disease states.[5] In addition, an intricate network of nerve fibers, ganglion cells (Meissner's plexus), vascular, and lymphatic elements can be found. The *mucosa* is separated into three layers: the muscularis mucosae, the lamina propria, and the intestinal epithelium (see Fig. 84–2). The muscularis mucosae is a thin sheet of smooth muscle cells, three to ten cells thick, that separates the mucosa from the submucosa. The lamina propria is a continuous connective tissue space bounded by the muscularis mucosae below and intestinal epithelium above. It contains a variety of cell types similar to those found within the submucosa. The intestinal epithelium is a layer of highly specialized cells that absorb and secrete products essential to sustain life.

The mucosa of both the small and large intestine contains crypts, which are small cylindrical structures containing epithelial stem cells, as well as Paneth cells, enteroendocrine cells, goblet cells, and undifferentiated cells.

Small Bowel Epithelium

The small intestinal epithelium is fashioned into crypts and villi (Figs. 84–3 and 84–4).[6] The villi are delicate, fingerlike structures that extend out into the intestinal lumen. They are 0.5 to 1 mm in height, tallest in the jejunum and progressively shorter in the ileum. Those villi that are in proximity to a lymphoid follicle, Peyer's patch, or Brunner's gland appear flattened or stubby. The villi are covered primarily by absorptive cells with an elaborate microvillous apical membrane. Present also on the villi are some goblet cells and intraepithelial lymphocytes (IELs). Each villus receives cells from six to ten different crypts. As undifferentiated crypt cells migrate up the villus, they differentiate and acquire the properties of absorptive cells. Epithelial cells are extruded from the villus tips. Turnover time of cells in the small intestinal epithelium appears to be about 4 to 6 days.[5]

Colonic Epithelium

The colonic epithelium, unlike that of the small intestine, lacks villi (Fig. 84–5). Colonic mucosa consists of tightly packed crypts lined primarily by goblet cells with intervening flat epithelial surfaces covered by absorptive cells.[7] Cells are generated in the crypts and extruded from the flat intercrypt region on the surface. The average lifespan of a colonocyte appears to be 3 to 5 days.[5]

Vascular Anatomy of the Intestinal Mucosa

The vascular anatomy of the small intestinal villus is complex.[8] One or two arterioles originating within the submucosa proceed unbranched to the tip of the villus where the vessels then branch into a dense network of subepithelial vessels that subsequently collect into venules at different levels within the villus (see Fig. 84–3). This vascular anatomy may allow a countercurrent multiplier mechanism to function during absorption by the intestinal villus. Blood vessels supplying the colonic mucosa are located in the submucosa.

Lymphatic vessels in the lamina propria of the small intestinal villus participate in fat absorption and drain to mesenteric lymph nodes. Lymphatics are lacking in the colonic mucosa but run in a circular direction in the submucosa before draining into epicolic and pericolic lymph nodes on the outer and inner margins of the bowel, respectively.

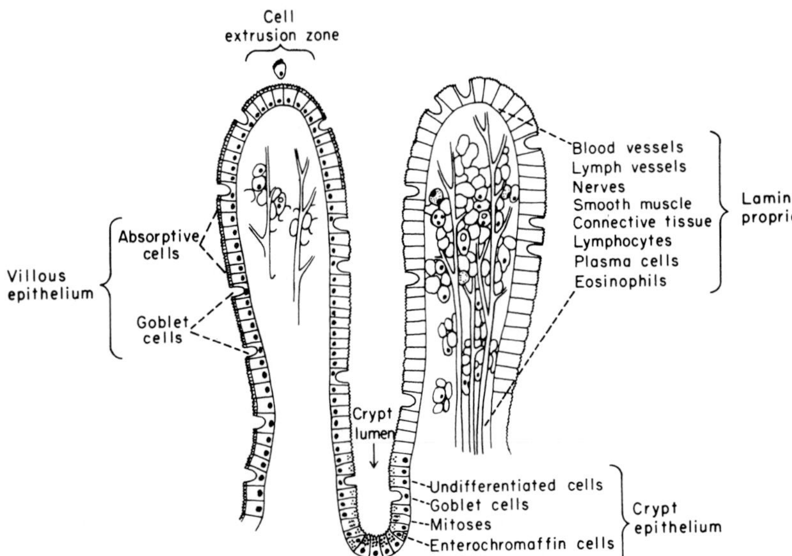

Figure 84–3. Schematic diagram of two sectioned villi and a crypt to illustrate the histologic organization of the small intestinal mucosa.

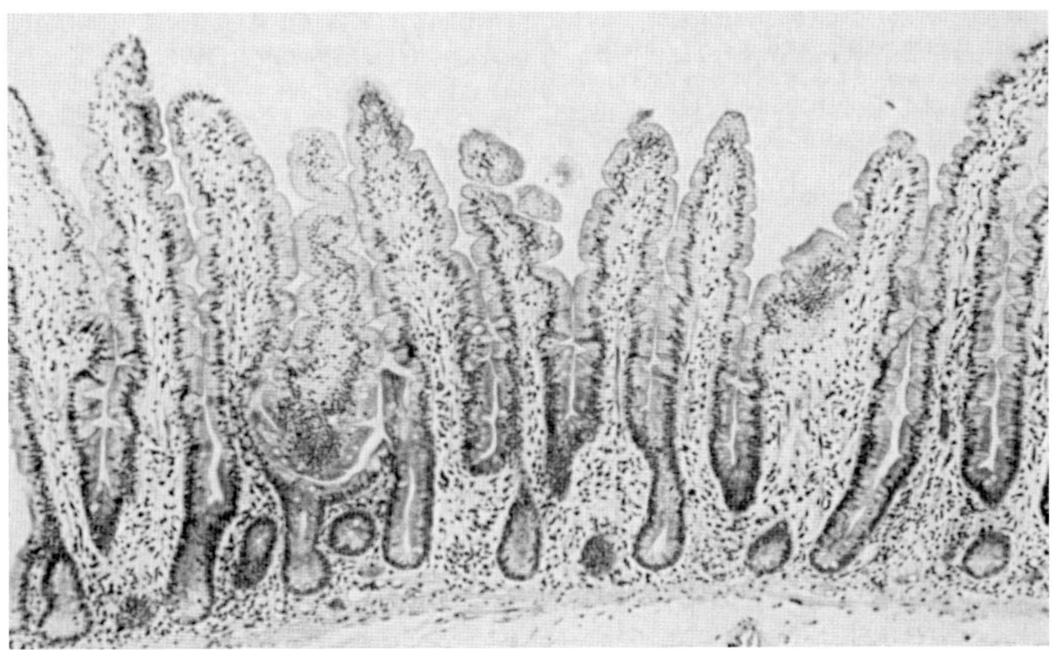

Figure 84–4. Light micrograph of a section of mucosa obtained by peroral biopsy from the proximal jejunum of a normal man. Hematoxylin-eosin stain. Magnification, approximately ×93.

Intestinal Nervous System and Pacemaker Cells

The *enteric nervous system* (ENS) is an independent branch of the peripheral nervous system. It consists of ganglia arranged throughout the gut wall in two concentric rings. The myenteric plexus forms the outer ring, between the longitudinal and circular smooth muscle layers. The inner ring is the submucosal plexus. The ENS rivals the central nervous system (CNS) in neuronal phenotype diversity and contains as many neurons as the spinal cord.[9]

The ENS contains intrinsic sensory neurons and interneurons that produce reflex activity in the absence of CNS input. It also contains motor neurons that excite or inhibit enteric smooth muscle, glands, and blood vessels. The role of the ENS in gut motility is discussed in Chapters 85 and 86.

Interstitial cells of Cajal (ICC) form a distinct layer just internal to the circular smooth muscle layer of the small intestine and are closely associated with myenteric neurons. Pacemaker activity in intestinal smooth muscle is generated by the spontaneous excitability of ICC. ICC propagate slow waves and are electrically coupled to smooth muscle cells. An apparently distinct population of ICC are also found in the deep muscular plexus, closely associated with enteric motor neurons.[10]

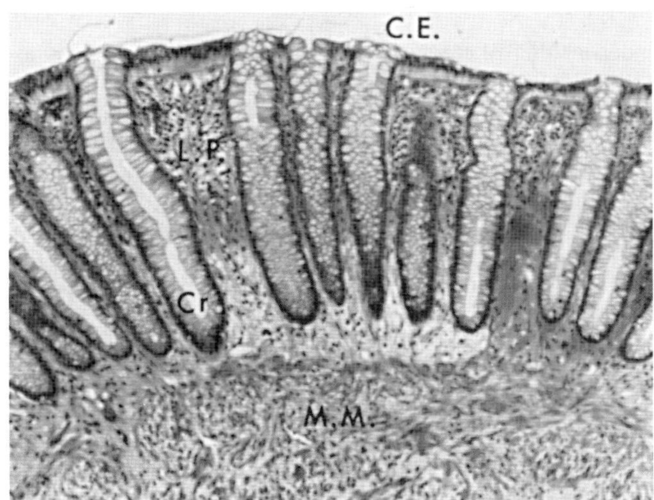

Figure 84–5. Biopsy of normal adult human rectum, showing rectal mucosa. CE, columnar epithelium; LP, lamina propria; Cr, crypt; MM, muscularis mucosae. Magnification ×100.

Cell Types in the Intestinal Epithelium

Stem cells are nonmigratory, pluripotential cells located within the first seven cell positions at the base of the crypt. They are capable of proliferation and self-maintenance.[11] Stem cells cannot be distinguished from other undifferentiated cells within the crypt.[6]

Undifferentiated crypt cells, the most common cell type within the small intestinal crypt, secrete water and chloride into the intestinal lumen. As might be expected, they have fewer, less well-developed intracellular organelles and microvilli than do enterocytes.[12] Mitotic figures are common within this cell population, likely reflecting rapid proliferation.

Paneth cells are located at the base of the crypt and can be identified by their basophilic cytoplasm and trapezoid appearance. Apical eosinophilic secretory granules contain growth factors, digestive enzymes, and antimicrobial peptides that can be discharged into the intestinal lumen.[13] Only the proximal third of the colon normally contains Paneth cells. Like stem cells, Paneth cells remain in the crypts.[11]

Goblet cells are the most common cell type in the colonic crypt. They are also found throughout the gastrointestinal tract.[5] They share a common lineage with other gastrointestinal columnar epithelial cells. Mucin release by goblet cells, an integral part of the host immune system, is influenced by dietary and immune factors.[14]

Enteroendocrine cells may not be readily identified with a hematoxylin or eosin stain. Transmission electron microscopy highlights their distinctive features: a narrow apex, broad base, and spare and irregular microvilli. Their secretory granules are generally located at the base of the cell and are thought to influence epithelial function via receptors located in the basal lateral membrane of the enterocytes (see Chapter 1).

Enterocytes (absorptive cells) are members of the family of polarized epithelial cells. They are connected to one another by a junctional complex that separates their apical from their basal-lateral domains (Fig. 84–6).[6] The apical domain faces the intestinal lumen and contains microvilli (Fig. 84–7). These are much more numerous in small intestinal absorptive cells than they are in colonic absorptive cells. Small bowel enterocyte microvilli are estimated to increase the luminal surface area of the cell 14- to 40-fold. This apical membrane contains a variety of digestive enzymes and a complement of transporters and ion channels. The transporters and ion channels on the apical membrane are different from those found on the basal-lateral membrane. The polarized distribution of transport proteins allows for vectorial transport of ions and other solutes. The nature of the vectorial transport varies from region to region of the intestine, depending on the structure of the local epithelium. Fluid and electrolyte transport is discussed in Chapter 87, and nutrient absorption is discussed in Chapter 88.

Located also on the basal-lateral surface of the epithelial cell are receptors for growth factors, hormones, and neurotransmitters. The basal surface of the enterocyte is applied closely to the basement membrane that is interposed between the epithelium and the lamina propria. Epithelial permeability, solute transport and cell replication, migration, and differentiation are regulated by a variety of factors: cell-cell interactions at junctional complexes; cell interactions with the basement membrane; nutrient effects on cell function; and modulation of cellular activity by hormones, neurotransmitters, and other peptides.[15–17]

Two components of the intestinal immune system, *M cells* and *IELs*, are found in the normal intestinal mucosa. M cells are specialized epithelial cells overlying lymphoid follicles in both small bowel and colon. They selectively bind, process, and deliver pathogens directly to lymphocytes, macrophages, or other components of the mucosal lymphoid system.[5, 18] IELs are a specialized subpopulation of memory T cells that migrate from the peripheral circulation to intercalate between the basal lateral membranes of mucosal epithelial cells.[19] IELs appear to play an important role in mucosal immune defense, as increased numbers are identified in small intestinal diseases such as giardiasis and celiac disease. Gut immunology is discussed in more detail in Chapter 2.

EMBRYOLOGY OF THE INTESTINE AND PATHOGENESIS OF BOWEL MALFORMATIONS

The major malformations and constellations of malformations affecting the midgut and hindgut can best be understood in terms of the embryology of the organism. A number of processes take place during development that have major impact on the structure of the gastrointestinal tract.[20–22]

Separation of Endoderm, Ectoderm, and Mesoderm

The embryo begins the 3rd week of development as a bilaminar germ disk. During the 3rd week of development, in a process known as *gastrulation,* this disk becomes a trilaminar disk. The surface facing the yolk sac then becomes the definitive endoderm (precursor of epithelial linings). The surface facing the amniotic sac becomes the ectoderm (the source of skin, nerves, and other structures). The middle layer or mesoderm is the source of muscle, bone, connective tissue, vessels, and septae of various organs.

The long axis and left-right axis of the embryo are also established at this time. The position for the oral opening is marked by the buccopharyngeal membrane. The location of the future opening of the urogenital and digestive tracts becomes identifiable as the cloacal membrane.[23]

The effects of defects in mesodermal migration can be protean and are probably represented in the VACTERL syndrome (see later). Improper formation of the cloacal membrane leads to a variety of anal and urogenital anomalies. Defective separation of neural, vertebral, and primordial precursors from gut endoderm caudally gives rise to the Curarino triad (see later) as well as mesenteric and neurenteric cysts.[24]

Genetic Control of Intestinal Morphogenesis

Understanding of the genetic control of morphogenesis is as yet incomplete. A full discussion of the current state of knowledge is beyond the scope of this chapter, but certain principles are important.[1] Hox genes, a family of genes encoding homeodomain-containing transcription factors, play a regulatory role in mesoderm to endoderm signaling. Hox genes are expressed in an organ/region-specific pattern in the mesoderm of the gut tube. Alterations in the expression of these genes cause relatively localized abnormalities in gut development. Hox genes have been shown to play a role in, for example, patterning of the sphincters of the gastrointestinal tract.[25]

Developmental defects can result from a complex combination of genetic abnormalities affecting cell migration, proliferation, and differentiation. Recent advances in our understanding of ENS development and Hirschsprung's disease illustrate the complexity of these developmental processes. For example, the endothelin-B receptor is normally expressed by ENS precursors, whereas its ligand (endothelin-3)

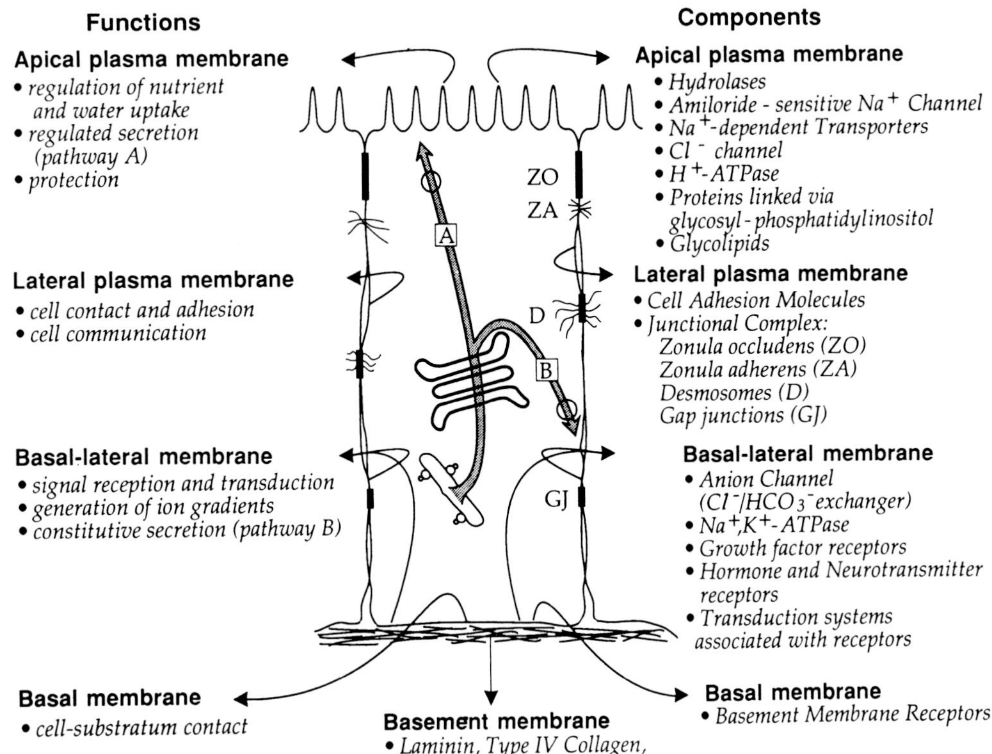

Figure 84–6. Functional diagram of an epithelial cell. (From Rodriguez-Boulan E, Nelson WJ: Morphogenesis of the polarized epithelial cell phenotype. Science 245:719, 1989).

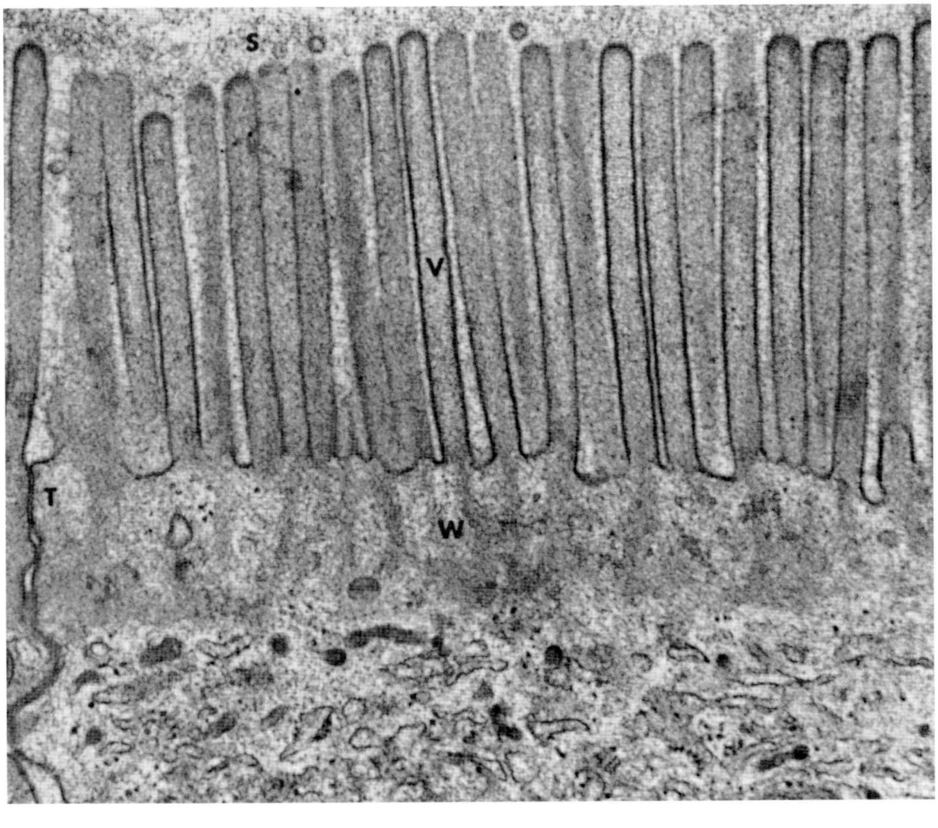

Figure 84–7. Apical cytoplasm of an absorptive cell from a jejunal villus from a normal adult man. The well-developed filamentous surface coat (S) lining the microvilli (V) is apparent. A tight junction (T) between adjacent cells is seen to the left at the level of the terminal web (W). Magnification approximately ×27,200.

is expressed by the mesenchyme of the developing gut. Activation of the endothelin-B receptor on ENS precursor cells can apparently be communicated to surrounding ENS precursor cells.[26] It is not yet clear whether this communication occurs by direct cell-cell contact, secretion of a soluble factor, or altered matrix secretion. Activation of the endothelin-B receptor is proposed to delay differentiation of ENS precursors, thereby allowing them to complete aboral colonization of the embryonic gut. The complexity of molecular events in ENS development is reflected in the genetics of Hirschsprung's disease. Mutations in six genes are implicated in the pathogenesis of Hirschsprung's disease. These include the transcription factor SOX10, the receptor tyrosine kinase RET and its ligand (the glial cell line–derived neurotrophic factor), the endothelin-B receptor and its ligand (endothelin-3), and the activating enzyme of endothelin-3 (endothelin-converting enzyme-1). Mutations causing Hirschsprung's disease are generally heterozygous with incomplete penetrance. No mutation in any of these genes can be identified in more than 50% of individuals with Hirschsprung's disease. This means that individuals carrying one of these mutations can be considered only to be at increased risk of having Hirschsprung's disease. The extent of the increased risk is difficult to define without extensive family study.[27]

Children with gross chromosomal defects also commonly have gastrointestinal malformations. Gastrointestinal defects are common in Down's syndrome and other trisomies, as well as 2p, 13q, and 5p (cri-du-chat) chromosomal defects.[28]

Folding of the Embryo and Formation of the Gut Tube and the Fetal Abdominal Cavity

During the 4th week of development, the embryo grows rapidly, the yolk sac remains static, and the embryonic disc assumes a convex shape that folds over to enclose the yolk sac. The endodermal, mesodermal, and ectodermal layers fuse in zipper fashion. The endoderm forms the gut tube, which communicates only with the yolk sac. The ectoderm then becomes the entire outer surface of the embryo, except where the yolk sac and connecting stalk (future umbilical cord) protrude. That yolk sac communication narrows by the 6th week to form the vitelline duct. Expansion of the amnion brought about by increasing amniotic fluid volume over the next 4 weeks causes envelopment of the yolk sac and connecting stalk by amnion, forming the umbilical cord. Generally, by the end of gestation the yolk sac and vitelline duct are obliterated. Persistence of the vitelline duct results in the spectrum of defects seen in Meckel's diverticulum (see later) (Fig. 84–8).

With folding of the embryo during the 4th week of devel-

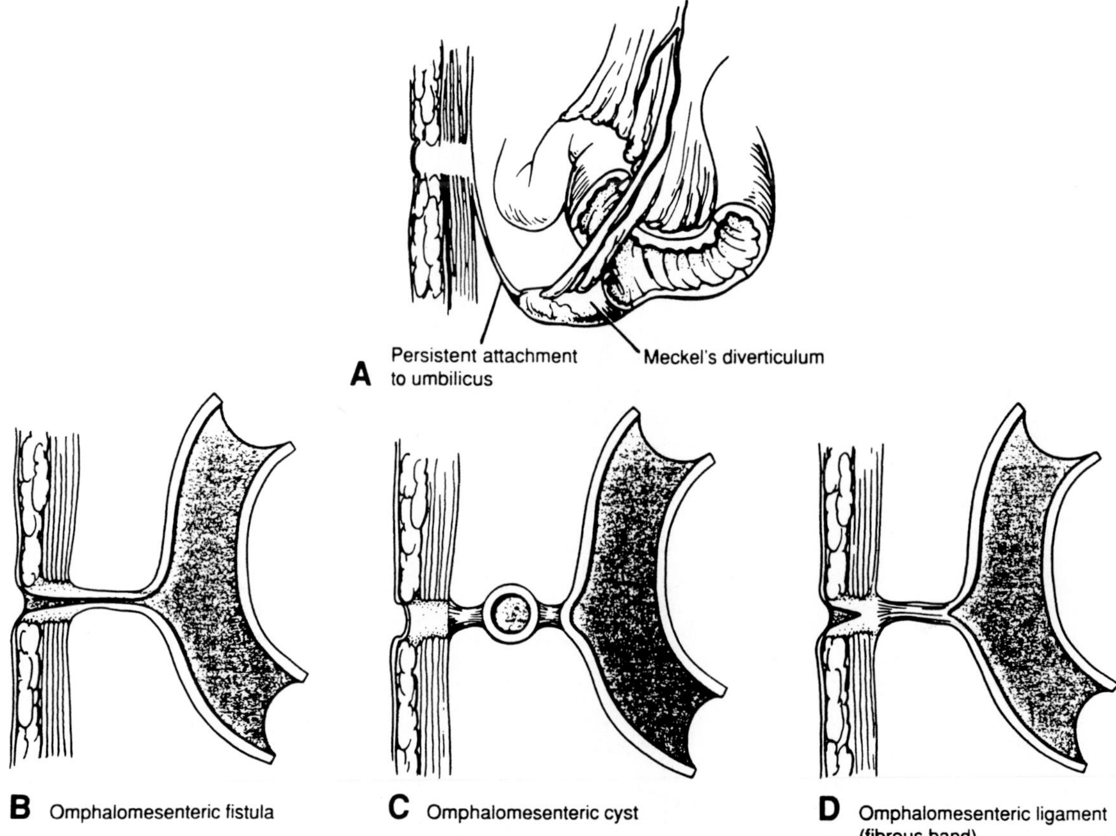

Figure 84–8. Meckel's diverticulum. A typical Meckel's diverticulum *(A)* is a finger-like projection of the ileum located approximately 100 cm proximal to the cecum. A Meckel's diverticulum may form *(B)* a patent fistula connecting the umbilicus with the ileum, *(C)* an isolated cyst suspended by ligaments, or *(D)* a fibrous band connecting the ileum and anterior body wall at the level of the umbilicus. (Photograph courtesy of Children's Hospital Medical Center, Cincinnati, Ohio.)

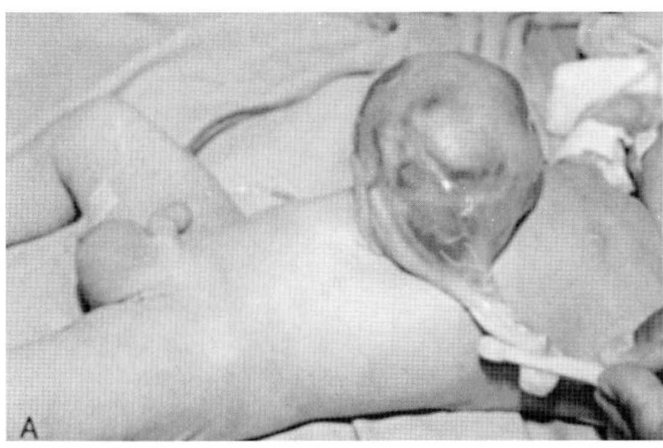

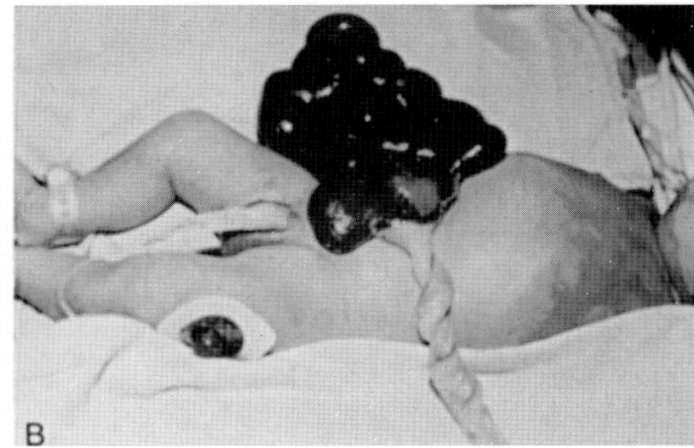

Figure 84–9. *A,* Infant with an omphalocele. Note how abdominal wall contents are enclosed in a saclike structure that is related to the umbilical cord. *B,* Infant with gastroschisis. Note the thickened abdominal viscera and the position of the umbilical cord. (Courtesy of Robert Shamberger.)

opment, the mesodermal layer splits, and that which adheres to endoderm forms the visceral peritoneum while that which adheres to ectoderm forms the parietal peritoneum. The space between layers forms the coelom, which disperses to form the embryonic and, subsequently, the peritoneal cavity. Incomplete closure of the mesodermal and ectodermal layers in the region of the umbilical cord leads to one form of omphalocele where the prolapsed organs are only covered by a layer of amnion (see later) (Fig. 84–9*A*). Omphaloceles are frequently associated with other anomalies. Several genetically defined lines of mice exhibit complex syndromes including omphalocele.[29, 30–32]

Gastroschisis, an abdominal wall defect adjacent to (but not involving) the umbilicus, may be secondary to vascular accidents involving the right umbilical vein. Bowel protruding through such a defect is not covered by amnion or peritoneum (Fig. 84–9*B*). Accompanying anomalies other than bowel atresias are uncommon in gastroschisis.

Defects in septation of the abdominal from chest cavities result in diaphragmatic hernia, discussed in Chapter 20.

Lengthening of the Gut Tube, Intestinal Herniation into the Umbilicus, Rotation, and Return to the Abdomen

Starting at about the 5th week of gestation, the ileum begins to lengthen more rapidly than can be accommodated by the abdominal cavity and the bowel herniates into the umbilical cord (Fig. 84–10). It forms a loop with the vitelline duct at the apex and the superior mesenteric artery, forming the long axis of the loop. Between weeks 5 and 9, the intestine grows in length, and during the 10th week, the bowel is retracted into the abdomen. In the process of extrusion and retraction the bowel rotates 270 degrees relative to the posterior abdominal wall. As a result, the cecum is located in the right lower quadrant and the duodenojejunal junction is located to the left of the spine. Return of the intestine to the abdomen is completed by 11 weeks. Subsequently, the mesenteries of the ascending and descending colons shorten and fold, and these portions of the colon become retroperitoneal. The duodenum is similarly pushed against the posterior abdominal wall and becomes retroperitoneal, possibly as a result of pressure from the transverse colon. There is variation in the extent of resorption of these mesenteries. Errors in rotation and fixation can predispose to torsion of the bowel about the mesenteric artery with bowel obstruction and vascular compromise (see later).

Because molecular functions controlling sidedness are involved, the incidence of gut malrotation is increased in children with congenital cardiac malformations. Many genes are reported to play important roles in left-right asymmetry and intestinal rotation in mice. These genes encode microtubule proteins, signaling molecules and receptors, and transcription factors.[33]

Development of the Vasculature and Lymphatics

During the 3rd week of development, blood vessel formation begins in the splanchnopleuric mesoderm of both the yolk sac and the embryonic disc. The yolk sac is completely vascularized by the end of the 3rd week. These arteries and veins become the vitelline system that, through remodeling and reanastomosis, supplies the thoracic arteries to the esophagus and abdominal arteries (celiac axis, superior and inferior mesenteric arteries) by 7 weeks.

The molecular mechanisms controlling vascular development are being revealed. Vascular endothelial growth factor (VEGF)-A and its receptors, VEGFR-1 and VEGFR-2, are important for endothelial cell proliferation, migration, and sprouting.[34, 35] Angiopoietins and their receptors, Tie1 and Tie2, appear to play a role in remodeling and maturation of the developing vasculature.[35] Activating mutations in Tie2 cause inherited vascular malformations in humans.[36] Vascular malformations are discussed in Chapter 120.

Lymphatic channels begin to appear at about 5 weeks in the head and neck and 6 weeks in the trunk and lower body. The thoracic duct is identifiable by 16 weeks. The origin of lymphatic vessels has been controversial. Recent evidence supports the theory of lymphatic development originally proposed by Sabin in 1902. Isolated primitive lymph sacs originate in endothelial budding from the veins. From primary lymph sacs, the peripheral lymphatic system spreads by endothelial sprouting into the surrounding tissues and organs. Flt4 (also known as VEGFR-3), a receptor for VEGF, plays a role in development of both the vascular and lymphatic systems.[37] Overexpression of VEGF-C, a ligand of Flt4, results in hyperplasia of lymphatic vessels in transgenic

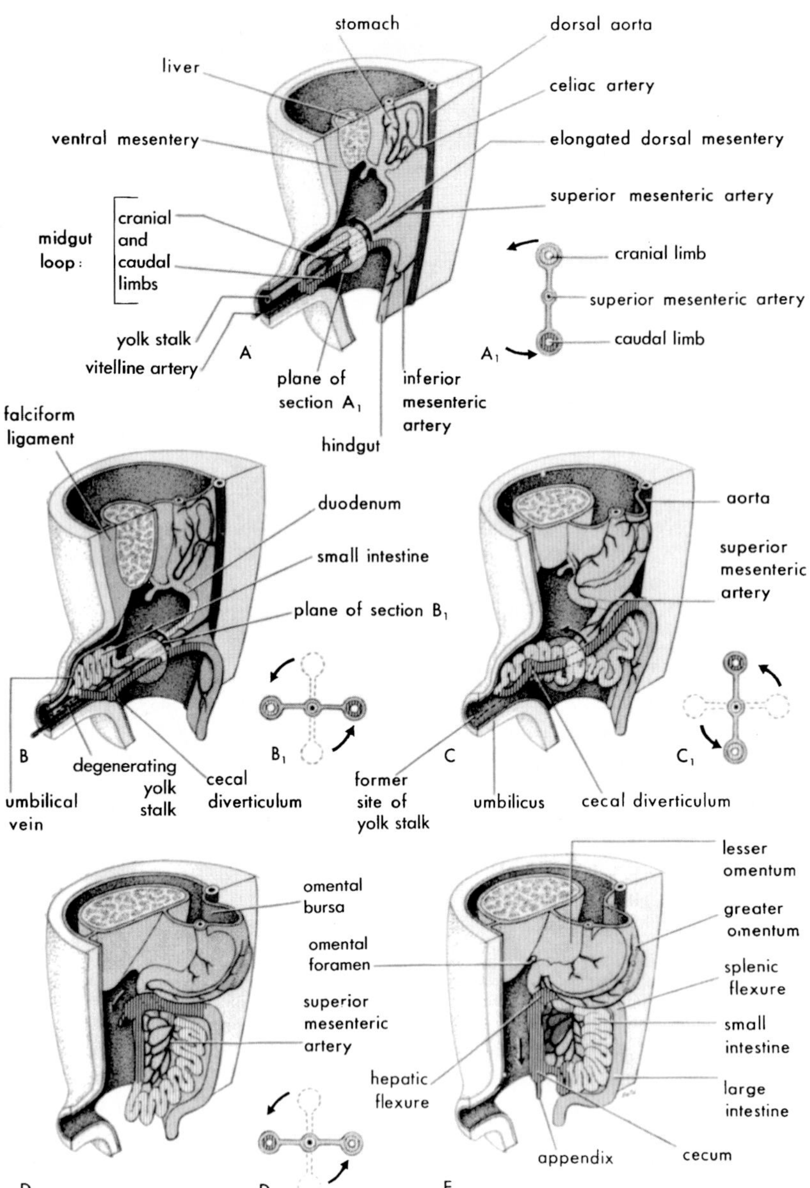

Figure 84–10. Stages of intestinal rotation during development. See text for details. (From Moore KL, Persaud TVN. The Developing Human: Clinically Oriented Embryology, 5th ed., Philadelphia, WB Saunders, 1993.)

mice.[38] The homeobox gene Prox1 is essential for normal development of the lymphatic system. Mice heterozygous for targeted disruption of the Prox1 gene die shortly after birth with chyle-filled intestine, suggesting an important role for Prox1 in the normal development of the enteric lymphatic system. Abnormalities in enteric lymphatic development in humans can result in intestinal lymphangiectasia, which is discussed in Chapter 25.

Development of the Enteric Nervous System

During the 3rd week of development, neural crest cells begin to migrate away from the neural tube. Enteric neural precursors from the vagal region of the neural crest proceed along the course of the vagus nerves, enter the foregut mesenchyme, and colonize the developing gut in a rostral-to-caudal progression. Whereas neural crest cells from the sacral region enter the caudal hindgut before the arrival of the vagal crest cells have arrived, the distribution of vagal crest–derived cells correlates with the ultimate distribution of neurons in the gut. Defects in migration or penetration of the gut by neural crest cells results in Hirschsprung's disease. The genetics of Hirschsprung's disease were discussed earlier.

Study of gene mutations producing intestinal dysganglionosis in rodents has led to the discovery of lineages within the ENS. For example, development of the ENS of the esophagus and gastric cardia is dependent on different transcription factors/signaling molecules than the more distal ENS. Further, the genetic/signaling requirements for ENS development in the colon appear to be distinct from the genetic/signaling requirements for colonization of the small intestine.

Ncx, a homeobox transcription factor (also known as Enx and Hox11L.1) may play a role in proper neuronal identity and pattern formation after colonization. Mice with targeted disruption of the Ncx gene develop intestinal obstruction and die in the first weeks of life. Histologic examination reveals an increase in both excitatory and inhibitory neurons in the colons of these mice after 2 weeks of age. Ncx "knock-out" mice may be an animal model of intestinal neuronal dysplasia (IND).

Proliferation of Epithelium with Obliteration of the Lumen Followed by Recanalization

During the 6th week of embryonic development, exuberant epithelial proliferation obliterates the lumen of the bowel. Vacuoles then form in this tissue over the next couple of weeks until recanalization has occurred by about 9 weeks. Errors in recanalization are thought to contribute to formation of a variety of duplications, webs, and stenoses of the gastrointestinal tract (Fig. 84–11).

During the 9th week, the epithelium begins to differentiate from the endothelial lining with villus formation and elaboration of a variety of types of epithelial cells. Organogenesis is complete by about 12 weeks.

Bowel Atresias Occurring Postorganogenesis

Vascular accidents can cause segmental atresias of the small intestine. Obliteration of the superior mesenteric artery results in an "apple-peel" atresia in which the distal small bowel is supplied retrograde from the inferior mesenteric artery via the ileocolic artery, and the remaining small bowel is coiled like an apple peel around the ileocolic artery (Fig. 84–12). Cystic fibrosis most commonly causes bowel obstruction in the newborn secondary to thick meconium but also appears to be responsible for a significant fraction of ileal atresias. Intrauterine volvulus of a malrotated bowel can cause atresia of the entire midgut. Bowel that has prolapsed through an abdominal wall defect (particularly gastroschisis) can twist with subsequent necrosis and involution or it can be damaged in the birth canal during a vaginal delivery.

CLINICAL PRESENTATIONS OF ANOMALIES OF THE GASTROINTESTINAL TRACT

Abnormalities in the anatomy of the gastrointestinal tract may present in many ways (Table 84–1). Some anomalies will be obvious on inspection of the infant. Abdominal wall defects will be grossly apparent at birth. Most anorectal malformations will be apparent on the initial physical examination. If the anal opening is large enough to allow stools to pass, the problem may not be appreciated until the child is older and presents with constipation. Management of abdominal wall defects and imperforate anus is discussed later.

A variety of anomalies can present as intestinal obstruction in the newborn (see Table 84–1). Symptoms of intestinal obstruction in the neonate include polyhydramnios, bilious emesis, abdominal distention, failure to pass meconium, and jaundice. Passage of meconium does not rule out proximal obstruction. History of bilious emesis in a child must always be investigated because of the possibility of intermit-

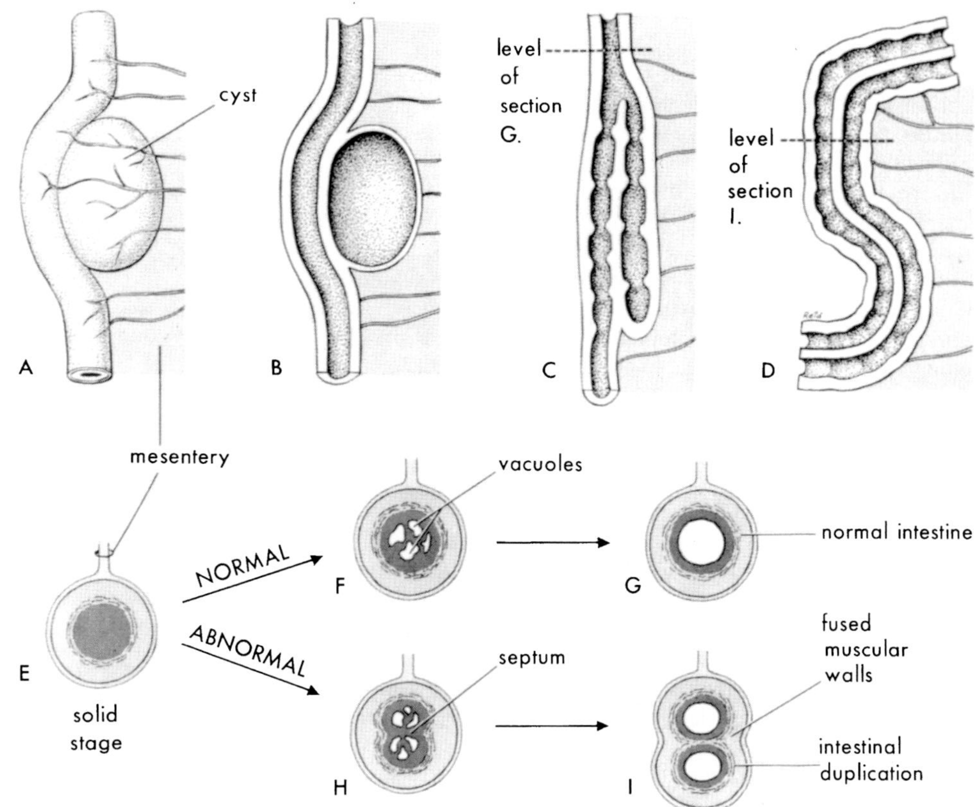

Figure 84–11. *A,* Cystic duplication of the small intestine. Note that it is on the mesenteric side and receives branches from the arteries supplying the intestine. *B,* Longitudinal section of the duplication shown in A. It does not communicate with the intestine, but its musculature is continuous with the gut wall. *C,* A short tubular duplication of the small intestine. *D,* A long duplication of the small intestine showing a partition consisting of the fused muscular walls. *E,* Transverse section of the intestine during the solid stage. *F,* Normal vacuole formation. *G,* Coalescence of the vacuoles and reformation of the lumen. *H,* Two groups of vacuoles have formed. *I,* Coalescence of the vacuoles illustrated in *H* results in intestinal duplication. (From Moore KI, Persaud TVN: The Developing Human: Clinically Oriented Embryology, 5th ed., Philadelphia, WB Saunders, 1993.)

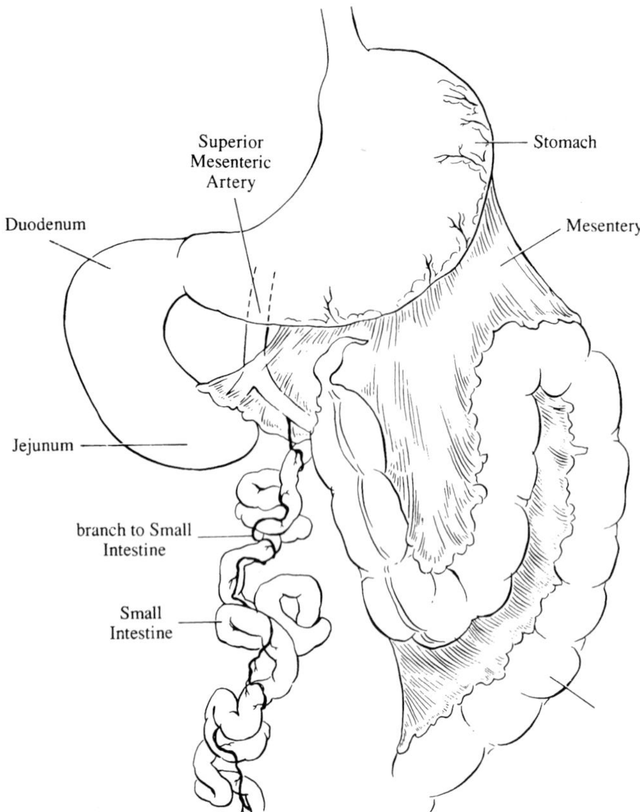

Figure 84–12. Schematic drawing of typical "apple peel" atresia. Superior mesenteric artery gives a branch to proximal jejunum and a branch to right colon and then ends abruptly (vessels are drawn larger than scale for the purpose of illustration). Small branch of right colic artery courses retrograde through a thin remnant of mesentery to supply remaining distal small bowel. (From Seashore JH, Collins FS, Markowitz RI, Seashore MR: Familial apple peel jejunal atresia: Surgical, genetic, and radiographic aspects. Pediatrics 80:541, 1987.)

tent obstruction from a self-limited volvulus. Nonhemolytic, indirect hyperbilirubinemia, when it occurs, is seen more frequently in patients with proximal than distal obstruction. The mechanism is thought to be related to either increased enterohepatic circulation of bilirubin or altered glucuronyl transferase activity.

The evaluation and management of infants with evidence of small bowel obstruction must occur simultaneously. Aggressive, supportive care is initiated to maintain the infant's temperature and fluid needs. Orogastric suction relieves abdominal distention. Plain radiographs of the abdomen (prone and upright) identify the bowel gas pattern, peritoneal calcifications, or impacted meconium. A contrast study of the colon, performed by a radiologist experienced in the techniques required for ill neonates, can determine if the obstruction is in the large or small bowel and evaluate intestinal rotation (Fig. 84–13). Water-soluble contrast agents have replaced barium if a potential intestinal perforation exists. A hyperosmolar contrast enema can be both diagnostic and therapeutic for patients with meconium plug or meconium ileus. If malrotation remains a concern, a contrast study of the upper intestine can determine the location of the ligament of Treitz.

Painless rectal bleeding (usually hemodynamically significant in quantity) can be an indication of a Meckel's diverticulum or of a duplication. *Abdominal masses* can reflect intestinal duplications, mesenteric cysts, or omphalomesenteric cysts. *Protein-losing enteropathy* can be the result of malrotation with partial volvulus or of intestinal lymphangiectasia. *Abdominal pain* can result from torsion of malrotated bowel, bowel tethered by vitelline duct remnants, from intussusception of Meckel's diverticuli or duplications, or mass effect of duplications. *Severe secretory diarrhea* beginning in the newborn period can indicate an epithelial cell defect.

ASSOCIATED MALFORMATIONS

It is important to recognize that many malformations are frequently associated with other malformations. Some of the common mechanisms were discussed earlier in the embryology section. Table 84–2 lists some particularly common associations that are unlikely to be obvious on physical examination.

DEVELOPMENTAL ANOMALIES OF THE INTESTINE

Abdominal Wall Defects (Omphalocele and Gastroschisis)

Omphalocele and gastroschisis are distinct clinical entities.[39] Both are present at birth. The incidence of omphalocele is about 2.5 in 10,000 births. The incidence of gastroschisis is approximately 1 in 10,000 births overall, but approaches 7 in 10,000 for mothers younger than 20 years of age and may be increasing for reasons that are poorly understood.

An *omphalocele* is a herniation of the abdominal viscera

Table 84–1 | **Presentations of Congenital Anomalies of the Midgut and Hindgut**

Abnormal physical examination
- Abdominal wall defects
- Anorectal malformations, including imperforate anum

Bowel obstruction
- Malrotation with or without midgut volvulus
- Intestinal duplication
- Intestinal atresia
- Meconium ileus
- Meconium plug syndrome
- Hirschsprung's disease
- Absence of the musculature of the distal ileum

Painless rectal bleeding
- Meckel's diverticulum
- Intestinal duplication

Abdominal mass
- Intestinal duplication
- Mesenteric cyst
- Omphalomesenteric cyst

Intractable diarrhea
- Ion transport defect

Abdominal pain
- Torsion
- Intussusceptions
- Duplications

Protein-losing enteropathy
- Malrotation with partial volvulus
- Intestinal lymphangiectasia

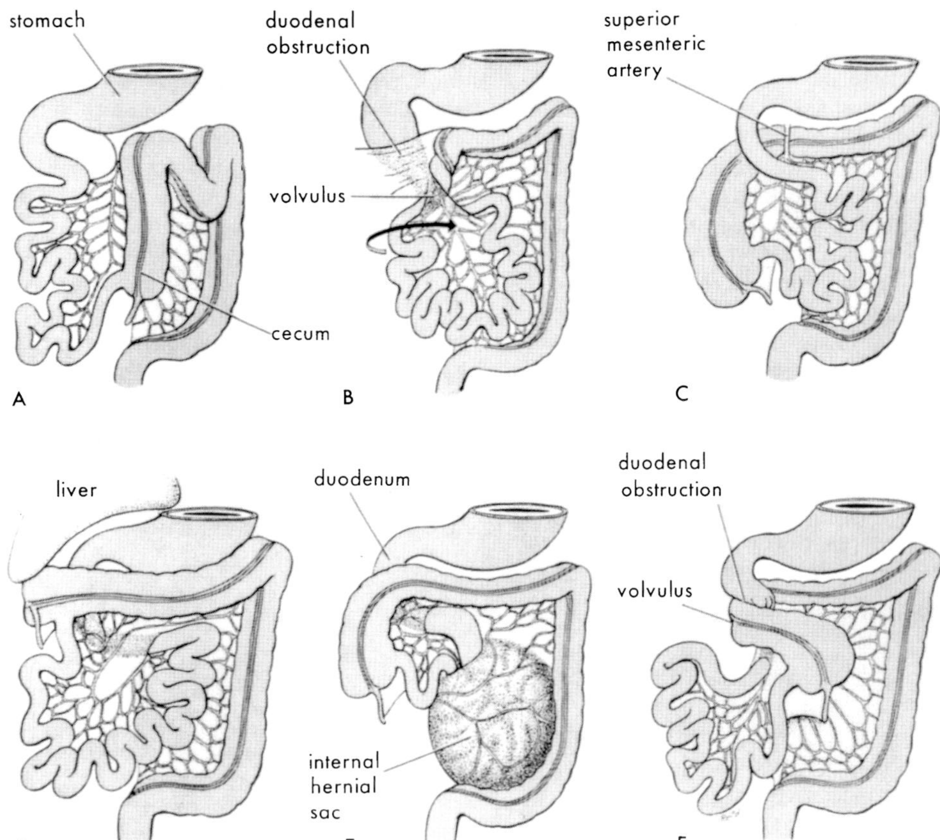

Figure 84–13. Drawings illustrating various abnormalities of midgut rotation. *A,* Nonrotation. *B,* Mixed rotation and volvulus. *C,* Reversed rotation. *D,* Subhepatic cecum and appendix. *E,* Internal hernia. *F,* Midgut volvulus. (From Moore KL, Persaud TVN: The Developing Human: Clinically Oriented Embryology, 5th ed., Philadelphia, WB Saunders, 1993.)

and, on occasion, the liver, into the base of the umbilical cord. The defect is usually less than 4 cm (see Fig. 84–9*A*). The abdominal contents appear normal and are contained within a membranous sac into which the umbilical cord inserts. On occasion, only remnants of the sac are present. Three of four patients with omphalocele have extraintestinal birth defects, most commonly trisomy 13 or 18 and Beckwith-Wiedemann syndrome (also known as exomphalos-macroglossia-gigantism syndrome).[40]

Gastroschisis results from an abdominal wall defect lateral to the umbilicus. The bowel, unprotected by a sac or remnant, appears abnormal and is matted and thickened owing to its extended exposure to amniotic fluid (see Fig. 84–9*B*). Other abdominal organs, including the urinary bladder, kidneys, ovaries, and uterus, may be contained within the eviscerated mass. The umbilical cord has a normal insertion. Fewer than one in four patients with gastroschisis has additional birth defects, which include gallbladder and renal agenesis.

Table 84–2 | **Common Malformation Associations***

Anorectal malformation	Occult spinal anomalies Renal anomalies Cardiac anomalies Tracheoesophageal fistula
Anal stenosis	Abnormal sacrum Presacral mass
Dextrocardia/polysplenia	Malrotation
Trisomy 21	Hirschsprung's disease

*When a disorder in the left column is encountered, an associated condition in the right column should be thought of.

Surgical repair of these defects is initiated on the first day of life. Expert clinical judgment and experience are needed to assess whether the abdominal cavity can accept the exposed viscera. Primary closure is accomplished in half of the cases, whereas a staged reduction is needed for the other half.[41] Postoperative complication rates are not significantly different between the two procedures. Immediate postoperative morbidity and mortality are higher in patients with omphalocele and are likely related to more frequent associated congenital anomalies. For patients with gastroschisis, long-term morbidity and mortality are higher due to necrotizing enterocolitis, bowel perforation or necrosis, and complications related to prolonged parenteral alimentation.[42]

Anomalies of Rotation and Fixation

As already discussed, between the 6th and 10th weeks of gestation, the bowel herniates into the umbilical cord and rotates on return to the abdominal cavity, ideally fixing the base of the mesentery in a stable fashion (see Fig. 84–10). Anomalies of intestinal rotation and fixation include nonrotation, incomplete rotation, reversed rotation, and anomalous fixation of the mesentery (see Fig. 84–13).[43] Nonrotation results from an arrest of stage I of normal intestinal rotation. As a consequence, the bowel is suspended by a narrow dorsal mesentery (see Fig. 84–13*A*). Although obstructing bands are not present, the bowel is susceptible to torsion about its long axis. This abnormality is often associated with other anomalies such as omphalocele, gastroschisis, duodenal atresia and stenosis, Meckel's diverticulum, biliary atresia, annular pancreas, and imperforate anus.[44] An arrest in stage II of intestinal rotation is manifested by three clinical conditions. The cecal loop rotates and fixates, but the duodenal loop does not. This entraps the duodenum with abnormal bands (Ladd's bands) (see Fig. 84–13*B*). Less commonly, both duodenal and cecal loops rotate in the reverse direction causing colonic obstruction due to external compression by the superior mesenteric vessels (see Fig. 84–13*C*) or the duodenal loop can rotate in a reverse fashion with normal rotation of the cecal loop, thus encasing the small bowel in its mesentery (see Fig. 84–13*E*). With disturbances of stage III, the duodenal loop is properly rotated and fixed but the cecum is not and results in a nonfixed midgut loop on a narrow pedicle. A poorly fixed cecum that sits high in the right upper quadrant with or without abnormal bands is part of the spectrum of an interruption of stage III of intestinal rotation (see Fig. 84–13*D*).

Clinical Features

Up to 90% of patients with abnormalities of intestinal rotation will present in the first 2 months of life with symptoms of intestinal obstruction. Bilious emesis and abdominal distention in addition to symptoms that suggest an abdominal catastrophe such as hypotension, shock, and bloody stools are seen in some patients. Others can have more subtle, chronic symptoms such as abdominal pain, poor weight gain, diarrhea with malabsorption, constipation, irritability, lethargy, hematochezia, and intermittent vomiting.[45] Rarely, intestinal malrotation occurs in multiple family members to suggest a genetic predisposition.[46] Presentation may be delayed in mild cases in to the 2nd, 3rd, or 4th decade of life. Those who present acutely require aggressive fluid resuscitation and immediate surgical exploration. If the patient's condition allows, and malrotation is considered in the differential diagnosis, both an upper gastrointestinal series and a barium enema may be necessary to secure the diagnosis preoperatively.

Management is surgical with the procedure described by Ladd preferred for all patients. With improved perioperative management, nutritional support, and a heightened index of suspicion, mortality has fallen from 23% in 1937 to 2.9% in 1987.[44] Significant morbidity may result if surgical resection leaves the patient with an inadequate length of small intestine to sustain life without parenteral nutrition (see also Chapters 16 and 92). Also, an ill-defined disorder of intestinal dysmotility may contribute to persistent symptoms following surgical correction of malrotation.[47]

Duplications

An enteric duplication is a rare congenital malformation of unclear pathogenesis. One autopsy study noted an incidence of 2 in 9000 children.[48] Duplications are cystic, tubular, or diverticular structures located on the mesenteric border of the intestine and likely result from disordered recanalization of the fetal intestine (see Fig. 84–11). Although the jejunum and ileum are the most common sites, they may occur anywhere along the intestinal tract.[49] The lumen of the duplication is usually not in continuity with the normal intestine, but the two structures share a portion of the muscular coat and vascular supply. Gastric mucosa, in various stages of maturation, may line the wall of duplications. This feature allows some lesions to be detected by a technetium-99m radioisotope (Meckel's) scan (see later).[50] Malignant transformation can occur in adults.

Intestinal duplications are usually symptomatic and present within the first year of life with intestinal obstruction or a palpable mass. Adults may experience similar symptoms with acute presentations attributed to recent hemorrhage or malignant transformation within the duplication. The diagnosis is made with ultrasonogram, Meckel's scan, or computed tomography of the abdomen.[51] Treatment involves surgical resection of the duplication and adjacent bowel with end-to-end anastomosis. If this approach involves the removal of a large amount of normal small bowel, surgical alternatives are available.[52]

Meckel's Diverticulum

Meckel's diverticulum, based on autopsy studies, occurs in 1% to 3% of the population and is the most common congenital anomaly of the gastrointestinal tract.[53] The omphalomesenteric duct, a structure that bridges the yolk sac with the developing gut, is normally obliterated by the 8th week of gestation. Failure to do so results in either an omphalomesenteric fistula, an enterocyst, a fibrous band connecting the small bowel to the umbilicus, or, most commonly, a Meckel's diverticulum (see Fig. 84–8).[54] In contrast with intestinal duplications, a Meckel's diverticulum arises from the antimesenteric border, contains all layers of the intestinal wall, has its own mesentery, and derives its blood supply from a terminal branch of the superior mesenteric artery. Diverticula that do not contain normal ileal mucosa will commonly harbor gastric mucosa. Pancreatic acinar tissue, Brunner's glands, colonic mucosa, hepatobiliary tissue or a combination of these tissues is noted on occasion. Although Meckel's diverticula have been described as proximal as the ligament of Treitz, most are within 100 cm of the ileocecal valve. Congenital anomalies such as cleft palate, bicornate uterus, and annular pancreas have been noted in association with Meckel's diverticulum. Meckel's may be found more frequently in patients with Crohn's disease than in the general population.

Painless, often hemodynamically significant (though not life-threatening) lower intestinal bleeding is a common presentation.[55] Bleeding is more common in children and occurs at a mean age of 5 years. Stools are most often maroon but can be tarry or bright red, depending on intestinal transit. Hemorrhage typically results from ulceration within the diverticulum or adjacent intestinal mucosa as a consequence of acid secretion from ectopic gastric mucosa. A prior history of intestinal bleeding can be elicited in some patients. Intestinal obstruction is more common in older patients and can be caused by intussusception, volvulus, herniation, or entrapment of a loop of bowel through a defect in the diverticular mesentery. Symptoms reminiscent of acute appendicitis can occur as a result of Meckel's diverticulitis, *Helicobacter pylori* infection of the ectopic gastric mucosa, or a foreign body in the diverticular lumen. Neoplastic transformation has

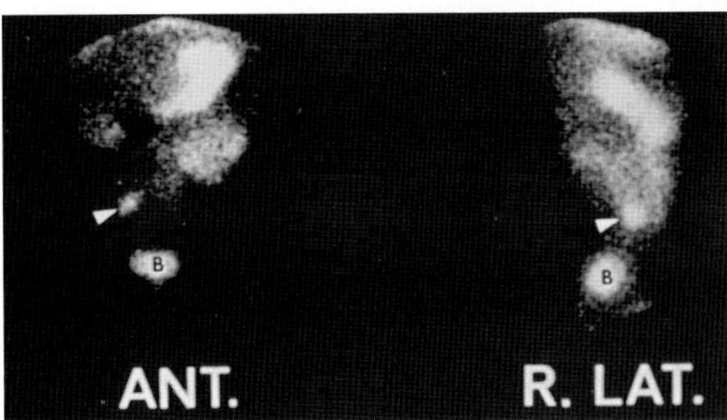

Figure 84–14. ^{99m}Tc scan of Meckel's diverticulum demonstrating ectopic uptake *(arrowheads)* in an area superior to the bladder *(B)* in the anterior projection and in the right lateral projection.

been reported, with carcinoid tumors, sarcomas, benign mesenchymal tumors, and adenocarcinomas being the most common.[56]

Diagnosis is made by a technetium-99m pertechnetate scintigraphic study (Fig. 84–14). A high index of suspicion is required to include Meckel's diverticulum in the preoperative differential diagnosis. Although a Meckel's diverticulum can rarely be visualized with a small bowel series or barium enema, the nuclear scan should precede a barium study to avoid interference with the scintigraphic counter. The likelihood of obtaining a false-negative Meckel's scan is minimized by pretreatment of the patient with pentagastrin or a histamine$_2$ receptor antagonist. Causes of a false-positive scan include intussusception, Crohn's disease, ureteral obstruction, intestinal hemangioma, or an aortic aneurysm.[57] Selective superior mesenteric artery angiography, when performed to evaluate or treat significant intestinal hemorrhage of unclear etiology, may detect a Meckel's diverticulum as the source.

Surgical resection is the treatment of choice for all symptomatic Meckel's diverticula. However, the morbidity associated with diverticulectomy precludes routine surgical resection of a Meckel's diverticulum found incidentally at surgery. However, if it is suspected to contain ectopic mucosa on palpation, if fibrous bands extend to the umbilicus, if mesodiverticular bands are present, or if there is surrounding inflammation, the Meckel's diverticulum should be removed.[55]

Intestinal Atresia

Intestinal atresia refers to a congenitally acquired complete obstruction of the lumen of the bowel. Stenosis indicates an incomplete or partial obstruction. In the small intestine, 50% of atresias occur in the duodenum, 36% in the jejunum, and 14% in the ileum.[58] Colonic atresias are far less common and represent only 10% of all bowel atresias.[59]

The reported incidence for small bowel atresia ranges from 1 in 330 to 1 in 1500 live births. Although there are no gender differences, the prevalence of isolated jejunal atresia is higher among black infants, low-birth-weight infants, and twins.[58] Apple-peel jejunal atresia, a rare variant that accounts for less than 5% of all atresias, is more common in families with another affected sibling, which suggests a genetic predisposition for this anomaly (see Fig. 84–12).[60] Multiple unrelated defects are more common in patients with isolated duodenal and jejunal atresias than in those with ileal atresia (Table 84–3). Approximately 10% of white infants with jejunoileal atresias will have cystic fibrosis.[61] Familial intestinal atresias, possibly due to defective canalization, have been described.[62] Isolated reports of jejunal atresia occurring with maternal use of Cafergot for migraine headaches or cocaine use during pregnancy, congenital rubella, and immunodeficiency have been documented.[63–65]

Treatment involves resection of the atretic portion with primary end-to-end anastomosis. The dilated proximal segment may need to be surgically tapered. The entire bowel is searched for additional atretic segments prior to closing the abdomen. Postoperative recovery depends on the length and function of the remaining bowel. Altered intestinal motility, involving the dilated proximal segment, can lead to long-term complications such as feeding intolerance, bacterial overgrowth, and malabsorption.[66] Hirschsprung's disease has been described in colon distal to a colonic atresia, presumably because the lesion occurred early enough to prevent neuronal migration. Some patients require prolonged intravenous or enteral nutritional support (see Chapter 16).[67] Aggressive nutritional and surgical care has improved morbidity and mortality, with many survivors able to achieve normal growth without chronic intestinal problems.

Anorectal Malformations

Incidence, Associated Malformations, and Etiology

Anorectal malformations are relatively common, with an incidence of approximately 1 in 2000 to 1 in 5000 live births.[68, 69] They are also noted with some frequency in stillbirths and spontaneously aborted fetuses. The high forms of anorectal malformations are somewhat more common in male than in female infants. About half occur as isolated defects, and half are associated with a wide variety of other defects. The most common group of defects has been designated the VATER or VACTERL association (acronym for *v*ertebral, *a*nal, *c*ardiac, *t*racheo*e*sophageal, *r*enal and *l*imb anomalies).[70] Table 84–4 summarizes the vast array of other anomalies encountered in patients with anorectal malformations.

Table 84–3 | **Anomalies Associated with Intestinal Atresia**

Annular pancreas
Malrotation
Ectopic anus
Gastroschisis
Omphalocele
VATER sequence*
Congenital heart disease
Ileal duplication
Genetic defects (more common with duodenal atresia)
Trisomy 21 (Down's syndrome)
2p- chromosomal defect
13q- chromosomal defect
5p- chromosomal defect (cri-du-chat)

**V*ertebral, *a*nal, *t*racheo*e*sophageal, and *r*enal anomalies.

Table 84–4 | **Anomalies Associated with Anorectal Malformations**

Neurologic
Hydrocephalus
Spinal cord—lipoma, tethered cord, syrinx, meningomyelocele
Cardiac
Ventral and atrial septal defects, tetralogy of Fallot, and many others
Urinary
Renal—dysplasia, hypoplasia, malposition, hydronephrosis
Ureteral—absent, blocked
Genital
Male—hypospadias, undescended testes
Female—septate vagina, vaginal atresia, duplicated uterus, hydrometrocolpos
Ambiguous genitalia
Other gastrointestinal
Tracheoesophageal atresia, fistula
Small bowel atresia, stenosis
Gastroschisis, omphalocele
Meckel's diverticulum
Malrotation
Skeletal
Vertebral asymmetry, agenesis, spina bifida
Polydactyly
Clubfoot
Radial aplasia, hypoplasia
Sensory
Sensorineural deafness
Ocular malformations
Chromosomal
Down syndrome, trisomy 8 mosaicism, fragile X syndrome, others

Data from references 70, 73, 75, and 90.

The etiology of these defects is uncertain. The embryology is summarized earlier. Vascular accidents are postulated to cause more localized defects.[71] Mesodermal abnormalities are invoked to explain several patterns of associated malformations.[72] Consanguinity is not statistically linked to the VACTERL association.[73] Diabetes and drug ingestion (including thalidomide, phenytoin, and tridione) are more common in mothers of infants with anorectal malformations.[64, 74, 75] Occupational exposures are more common in fathers of children with anorectal malformations. A variety of rare syndromes, some clearly hereditary, include anorectal malformations.[28]

Classification

Anorectal malformations are categorized by the location of the terminal bowel relative to the levator muscles that form the pelvic diaphragm. Infants in whom the terminal portion of the colon passes through the levator muscles are said to have a "low malformation" and can generally be treated with a relatively localized surgery with a good outcome. When the colon ends in or above the levator muscles (a "high malformation"), it usually communicates with the urinary tract (males) or genital tract (females) and the surgical repair becomes more complex. Diagrams of the most common lesions are provided in Figures 84–15 for males and 84–16 for females. From a practical standpoint, the key issue is whether or not a diverting ostomy is needed prior to definitive repair. This distinction is summarized in Table 84–5.

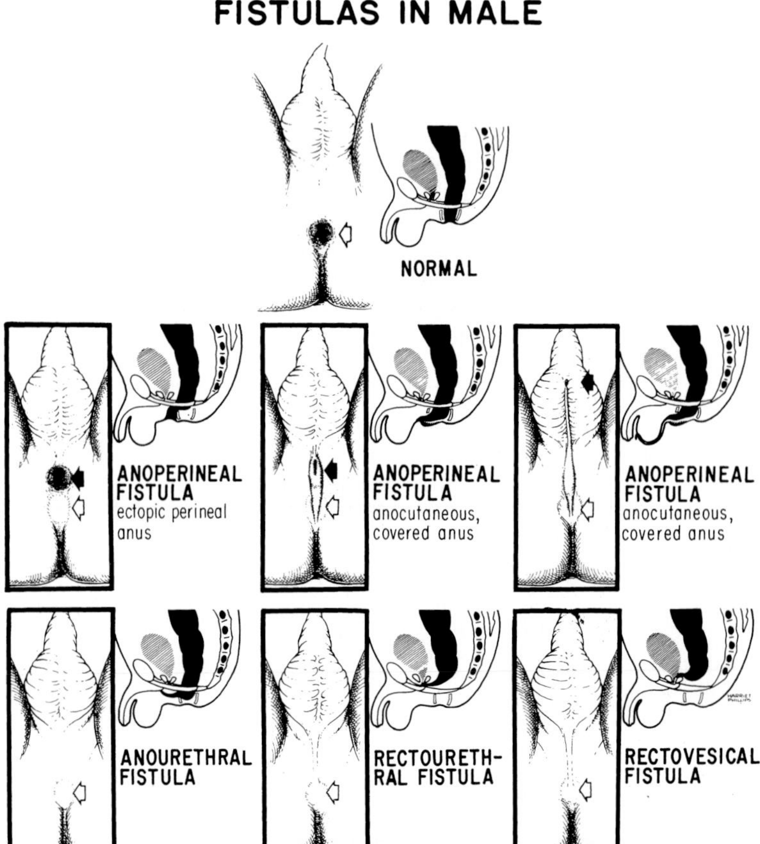

Figure 84–15. Anorectal anomalies in the male with fistula formation. Note relationship of the rectum to the puborectalis sling of the levator ani muscle. Anoperineal fistulas may be located anywhere between the perineoscrotal junction and the anal dimple. In the ectopic perineal anus, the opening resembles a normal anus. In the anocutaneous fistula or covered anus, the orifice is usually small and is anterior to a thickened median band. Anourethral fistulas are rare and open into the bulbar or membranous urethra. The common rectourethral and the rare rectovesical fistulas represent high anomalies in which the bowel has not traversed the sling. (From Santulli TV, Kiesewetter WB, Bill AH Jr: Anorectal anomalies: A suggested international classification. J Pediatr Surg 5:281, 1970.)

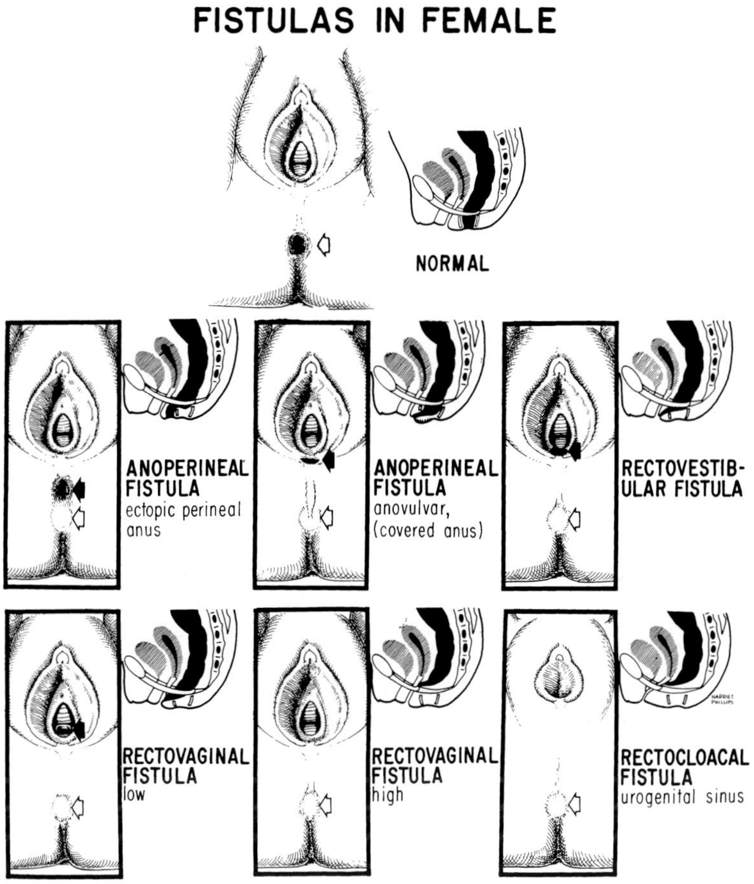

FISTULAS IN FEMALE

NORMAL

ANOPERINEAL FISTULA
ectopic perineal anus

ANOPERINEAL FISTULA
anovulvar, (covered anus)

RECTOVESTIBULAR FISTULA

RECTOVAGINAL FISTULA
low

RECTOVAGINAL FISTULA
high

RECTOCLOACAL FISTULA
urogenital sinus

Figure 84–16. Anorectal anomalies in the female with anoperineal fistulas, which may be either an ectopic perineal anus or an anovulvar fistula, which is in the fourchette. The rectovestibular fistula lies within the vestibule of the vagina and courses cephalad, paralleling the posterior vaginal wall. The anovulvar fistula is directed posteriorly and is relatively superficial to the skin. Rectovaginal fistulas are usually low but may be located high in the posterior vaginal wall. The rectocloacal fistula occurs as a high communication in a urogenital sinus. The bowel traverses the sling in all except the last two malformations. (From Santulli TV, Kiesewetter WB, Bill AH Jr: Anorectal anomalies: A suggested international classification. J Pediatr Surg 5:281, 1970.)

Nomenclature in the literature is greatly influenced by associated malformations. Hence, patients may be lumped in artificial groupings as "VATER syndrome," or "caudal regression syndrome," or "sacral agenesis syndrome." It is not clear that these are distinctly different syndromes. It is most important to identify the other anomalies that may be present. Infant mortality increases with the number of malformations. Cardiac and renal disease are the major causes of death in these infants, so early identification and therapy of lesions in these systems is critical.[68] Continence following surgery is strongly dependent on innervation. This in turn may be affected by sacral vertebral, spinal cord, and CNS anomalies. Identification and treatment of a tethered spinal cord or hydrocephalus are particularly important. In female infants with anorectal malformations, genital malformations are common. Careful evaluation and treatment of this area are essential to successful reproductive function later.[76]

Table 84–5 | **Classification of Anorectal Malformations by Need for Ostomy Either to Protect the Urinary Tract or to Protect Repair**

	MALES	FEMALES
Colostomy not required	Perineal (cutaneous) fistula	Perineal (cutaneous) fistula
Colostomy required	Rectourethral fistula (bulbar or prostatic)	Vestibular fistula
	Rectovesical fistula	Persistent cloaca
	Imperforate anus without fistula	Imperforate anus without fistula
	Rectal atresia	Rectal atresia

Adapted from Pena A, Spitz L, Coran AG. (eds): Rob and Smith's Operative Surgery: Pediatric Surgery, 5th ed. New York, Chapman & Hall, 1995.

Diagnosis and Management

Although a few patients with anorectal malformations are diagnosed antenatally by sonography, most are identified by careful examination of the perineum at birth. If the anal opening is large enough to allow stooling, the problem may not be appreciated until the child is older and presents with constipation.

The key features of the initial management of an infant with imperforate anus are to decompress the gut by orogastric or nasogastric suction, to rule out an obstructive uropathy by ultrasonography, and to wait 24 hours to allow fistulas to fill to establish if there is a perineal membrane or fistula that can be approached directly.[77] Patients with anal stenosis frequently have also sacral agenesis and a presacral mass (lipoma, teratoma, or meningocele), and surgical intervention should be planned accordingly.[78] If no anal opening or perineal membrane or fistula is seen, efforts are then made to determine the location of the bowel and any fistula.

In both males and females, evaluation for vertebral anomalies, spinal cord anomalies, cardiac anomalies, and other gastrointestinal anomalies (i.e., malrotation, tracheoesophageal fistula) is also important.

In patients for whom the location of the fistula is not

Table 84–6 | **Types of Anorectal Defects, Frequency, and Functional Outcome**

	NO. OF PATIENTS STUDIED	NORMAL SACRUM	VOLUNTARY STOOLS	SOILING
Males				
Bulbourethral fistula	22	17	12	12/17
Prostatic fistula	29	19	16	10/19
Vesical fistula	9	6	2	3/6
Females				
Vestibular fistula	11	10	10	2/10
Vaginal fistula	2	1	1	1/1
Cloacal fistula	11	4	4	3/4
Both sexes				
No fistula	12	9	8	3/9
Rectal atresia/stenosis	4	4	4	1/4
Low malformation (perineal fistula)	4	4	4	0/4
Patients missing more than 3 sacral vertebrae	10	–	2	6/10

Adapted from Pena A: Posterior sagittal anorectoplasty: Results in the management of 332 cases of anorectal malformations. Pediatr Surg Int 3:94–104, 1988.

obvious, once the diverting loop ostomy has been formed, the distal limb is injected with water-soluble contrast agent under pressure (distal colostography) to fill and thereby visualize fistulas as well as to identify the height of the rectum.[79] This is then used to guide the surgical approach.[77] If the fistula from the rectum enters the genitourinary tract, reconstruction of genitourinary structures is also done at the time of bowel repair, and adequate planning is crucial to success here as well.[76] The anorectal surgery attempts to preserve normal muscle anatomy and innervation, most commonly by using a posterior sagittal approach. Here the surgeon operates in the midline, minimizing potential damage to perineal nerves and using a muscle stimulator to facilitate identification both of the muscles and of the midline. Great efforts are taken to preserve both the levator sling and the superficial and deep portions of the external anal sphincter. Because sensation in the lower anal canal is also important for continence, every attempt is made to preserve this portion of bowel. In some cases of high lesions, a transabdominal approach may also be necessary to identify and correct the anomaly. These patients generally have a single opportunity for successful repair, and it needs to be performed by an experienced and meticulous surgeon.

Outcome

The goals of surgical repair are fecal continence and adequate sexual and reproductive function. Continence appears to depend on proper rectal location within intact perineal muscles, normal innervation, and adequate anal sensation. Table 84–6 summarizes the outcomes in one series.[80] Although most patients achieve socially adequate continence (60% to 90%), only a few achieve complete continence, making some sort of bowel program generally necessary. A few require an ostomy for continence purposes. Limited follow-up suggests the posterior sagittal approach may have better anatomic and continence results than transabdominal approaches.[81, 82] Bladder dysfunction is rare in patients treated with the posterior sagittal approach, if the sacrum is normal.[83] Urinary incontinence and sexual dysfunction are common when the pelvic nerve routes are disrupted or are congenitally absent.[84] Vesicoureteral reflux with potential for obstructive uropathy can develop with or without neurogenic bladder.

Anal dilations to prevent stricture formation are a routine part of the management program following posterior sagittal anoplasty. Fecal impaction is common and needs to be treated aggressively to avoid permanent sigmoid dysfunction as well as to protect the urinary tract. Fecal soiling is dependent on stool consistency as well as the quality of the perineal muscles and their innervation. Careful evaluation is important to distinguish between impaction with overflow incontinence and simple leakage of soft stool. Loperamide has helped some patients; biofeedback training has been helpful for others, but a few may require continence enemas or even a permanent ostomy.[85]

Anomalies of Intrinsic Innervation and Motility

Hirschsprung's disease, or congenital distal intestinal aganglionosis, is a developmental defect characterized by the complete absence of the ENS in a portion of the intestinal tract. Hirschsprung's disease is a relatively common condition, affecting approximately 1 in 5000 live births worldwide. More than 80% of cases of Hirschsprung's disease involve aganglionosis restricted to the distal colon and rectum. In the remaining patients, aganglionosis begins in the more proximal colon or small bowel and extends to the rectum. In the aganglionic gut, the residual extrinsic nerves are often hypertrophic. Lack of submucosal ganglion cells, particularly when accompanied by hypertrophic submucosal nerves and/or an abnormal acetylcholinesterase (AchE)-staining pattern, is sufficient to establish the diagnosis of Hirschsprung's disease. Genetics of this condition were discussed earlier. Diagnostic and clinical aspects are discussed in Chapter 110.

Intestinal neuronal dysplasia (IND) is a controversial entity. Two types of IND are defined: IND-A and IND-B. IND-A is defined as a rare form of enteric dysganglionosis, and little has been published on the subject. The term *IND* has become almost synonymous with IND-B.

Most of the features of IND-B are nonspecific. Disagreement exists among groups that recognize the existence of

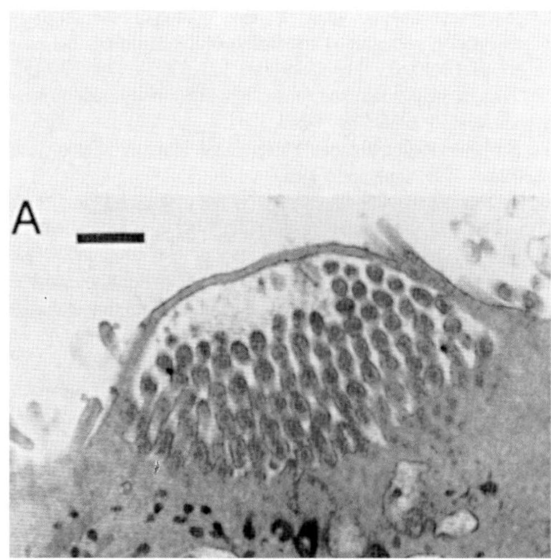

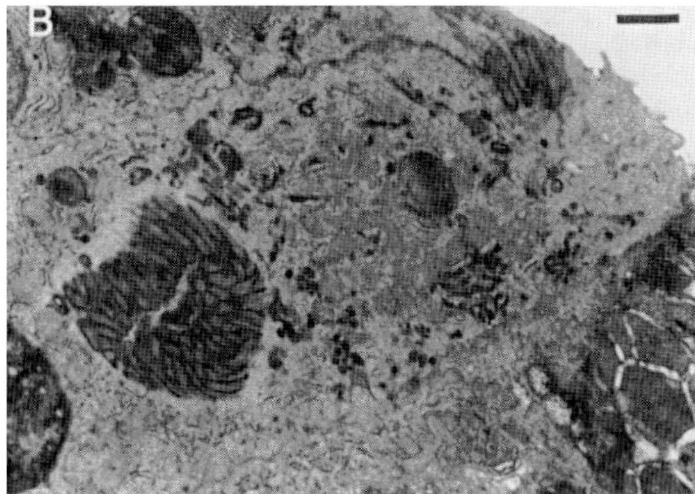

Figure 18–17. Ultrastructural appearance of microvillous inclusion disease. *A,* Microvillous inclusion with microvilli on lower inner face of vesicle (magnification, ×17,640; bar = 480 nm). *B,* Microvillous inclusion within cytoplasm (magnification, ×9660; bar = 870 nm). (From Phillips AD, Schmitz J: Familial microvillus atrophy: A clinicopathological survey of 23 cases. J Pediatr Gastroenterol Nutr 14:387, 1992.)

IND-B as to the significance of the histopathologic findings. They have been interpreted as signs of immaturity in the submucosal plexus that spontaneously resolve in most patients, as secondary phenomena to other intestinal disorders, or as a primary developmental defect responsible for intestinal dysmotility.[27]

Microvillous Membrane and Epithelial Defects

A number of rare, congenital, likely autosomal recessive disorders of the enterocyte are described. *Microvillous inclusion disease* or *familial microvillous atrophy* describes two similar disorders of the intestinal microvillus (Fig. 84–17).[86, 87] All patients present in infancy, usually within the first 3 weeks, with intractable, high-output, nonbloody diarrhea that persists despite withdrawal of oral feedings. Occasionally, symptoms are delayed until 6 to 8 weeks of life. Light microscopy of the small intestine reveals severe villous atrophy without significant crypt lengthening. Periodic acid–Schiff-positive material is demonstrated in the apical cytoplasm of the epithelial cell. On transmission electron microscopy, the apical surface is almost devoid of microvilli, whereas vesicles filled with microvilli are contained under the apical membrane. As many as 75% of patients succumb to their disease, and those who survive are dependent on parenteral nutrition.

Tufting enteropathy is clinically similar both in presentation and outcome to microvillous inclusion disease but is histologically different (Fig. 84–18).[88] The surface epithelium shows focal epithelial "tufts" composed of tightly packed enterocytes, while transmission electron microscopy reveals relatively normal enterocyte microvilli and no inclu-

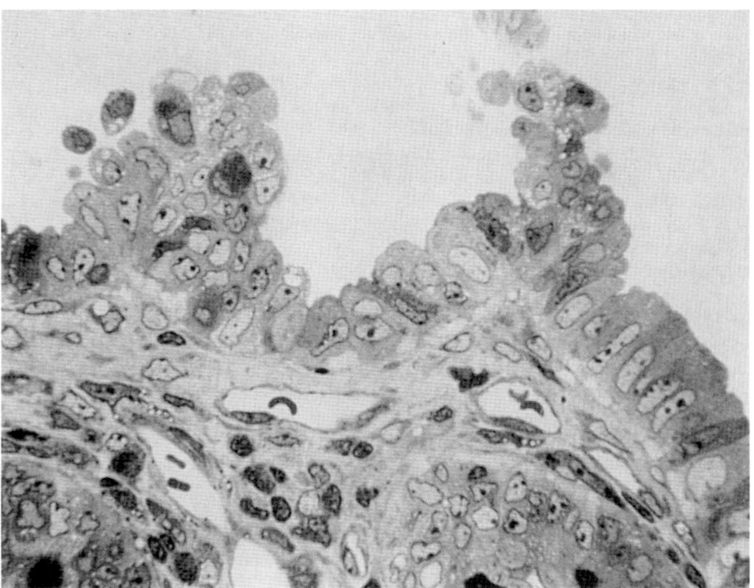

Figure 18–18. Tufting enteropathy. Villous surface epithelium shows disorganization with crowding and focal tufting. (From Goulet O, Kedinger M, Brousse N, et al: Intractable diarrhea of infancy with epithelial and basement membrane abnormalities. J Pediatr 127:214, 1995.)

sions. An abnormality in epithelial-mesenchymal cell interaction is proposed as a possible mechanism for the disease.[89]

REFERENCES

1. Montgomery RK, Grand RJ: Development of the human gastrointestinal system. In The Undergraduate Teaching Project in Gastroenterology and Liver Disease. Timonium, MD, American Gastroenterological Association/Milner-Fenwick, 1999, pp 1–35.
2. Ward H, Jalan KN, Maitra TK, et al: Small intestinal nodular lymphoid hyperplasia in patients with giardiasis and normal serum immunoglobulins. Gut 24:120–126, 1983.
3. Kumar D, Phillips SF: The contribution of external ligamentous attachments to function of the ileocecal junction. Dis Colon Rectum 6:410–416, 1987.
4. Moore KL: Clinically Oriented Anatomy, 3rd ed. Baltimore, Williams & Wilkins, 1992.
5. Lewin KJ, Riddell RH, Weinstein WM (eds): Small and large bowel structure, developmental, and mechanical disorders. In Gastrointestinal Pathology and Its Clinical Implications. New York, Igaku-Shoin, 1992, pp 703–749.
6. Madara JL, Trier JS. Johnson LR (eds): The functional morphology of the mucosa of the small intestine. In Physiology of the Gastrointestinal Tract, 3rd ed. New York, Raven Press, 1994, pp 1577–1622.
7. Goldman H, Antonioli DA: Mucosal biopsy of the rectum, colon, and distal ileum. Hum Pathol 13:981–1012, 1982.
8. Jodal M, Lundgren O: Countercurrent mechanisms in the mamalian gastrointestinal tract. Gastroenterology 91:225–241, 1986.
9. Gershon MD: Genes and lineages in the formation of the enteric nervous system. Curr Opin Neurobiol 7:101–109, 1997.
10. Sanders KM, Ordog T, Koh SD, et al: Development and plasticity of interstitial cells of Cajal. Neurogastroenterol Motil 11:311–338, 1999.
11. Potten CS, Loeffler M: Stem cells: Attributes, cycles, spirals, pitfalls, and uncertainties: Lessons for and from the crypt. Development 110: 1001–1020, 1990.
12. Madara JL, Trier JS, Neutra MR: Structural changes in the plasma membrane acompanying differentiation of epithelial cells in human and monkey small intestine. Gastroenterology 78:963–975, 1980.
13. Ouellette A, Hsieh MM, Nosek MT, et al: Mouse paneth cell defensins: Primary structures and antibacterial activities of numerous cryptdin isoforms. Infect Immunol 62:5040–5047, 1994.
14. Ishikawa N, Horii Y, Suganuma T, Nawa Y: Goblet cell mucins as the selective barrier for the intestinal helminths: T-cell–independent alteration of goblet cell mucins by immunologically "damaged" *Nippostrongylus brasiliensis* worms and its significance on the challenge infection with homologous and heterologous parasites. Immunology 81:480–486, 1994.
15. Geiger B, Ayalon O: Cadherins. Annu Rev Cell Biol 8:307–332, 1992.
16. Dignass AU, Podolsky DK: Cytokine modulation of intestinal epithelial cell restitution: Central role of transforming growth factor-beta. Gastroenterology 105:1323–1332, 1993.
17. Nsi-Emvo E, Foltzer-Jourdainne C, Raul F, et al: Precocious and reversible expression of sucrase-isomaltase unrelated to intestinal cell turnover. Am J Physiol 266:G568–G575, 1994.
18. Neutra MR, Kraehenbuhl JP: The role of transepithelial transport by M cells in microbial invasion and host defense. J Cell Sci 17(Suppl):209–215, 1993.
19. Cerf-Bensussan N, Guy-Grand D: Intestinal intraepithelial lymphocytes. Gastroenterol Clin North Am 20:549–576, 1991.
20. Moore KL, Persaud TVN: The Developing Human, 5th ed. Philadelphia, WB Saunders, 1993.
21. Larsen WJ: Human Embryology, 2nd ed. New York, Churchill Livingstone, 1997.
22. Montgomery RK, Mulberg AE, Grand RJ: Development of the human gastrointestinal tract: Twenty years of progress. Gastroenterology 116: 702–731, 1999.
23. Kluth D, Lambrecht W: Current concepts in the embryology of anorectal malformations. Semin Pediatr Surg 6:180–186, 1997.
24. Dias MS, Azizkhan RG: A novel embryogenetic mechanism for Currarino's triad: Inadequate dorsoventral separation of the caudal eminence from hindgut endoderm. Pediatr Neurosurg 28:223–229, 1998.
25. Zakany J, Duboule D: Hox genes and the making of sphincters. Nature 401:761–762, 1999.
26. Kapur RP, Sweetser DA, Doggett B, et al: Intercellular signals downstream of endothelin receptor-B mediate colonization of the large intestine by enteric neuroblasts. Development 121:3787–3795, 1995.
27. Kapur RP: Hirschsprung disease and other enteric dysganglionoses. Crit Rev Clin Lab Sci 36:225–273, 1999.
28. Jones KL: Smith's Recognizable Patterns of Human Malformation, 5th ed. Philadelphia, WB Saunders, 1997.
29. Klootwijk R, Franke B, van der Zee CE, et al: A deletion encompassing Zic3 in bent tail, a mouse model for X-linked neural tube defects. Hum Mol Genet 9:1615–1622, 2000.
30. Eggenschwiler J, Ludwig T, Fisher P, et al: Mouse mutant embryos overexpressing IGF-II exhibit phenotypic features of the Beckwith-Wiedemann and Simpson-Golabi-Behmel syndromes. Genes Dev 11:3128–3142, 1997.
31. Rauch F, Prud AA, Dedhar S, St-Arnaud R: Heart, brain, and body wall defects in mice lacking calreticulin. Exp Cell Res 256:105–111, 2000.
32. Carter MG, Johns MA, Zeng X, et al: Mice deficient in the candidate tumor suppressor gene Hic1 exhibit developmental defects of structures affected in the Miller-Dieker syndrome. Hum Mol Genet 9:413–419, 2000.
33. Kioussi C, Rosenfeld MG: Body's left side. Cell Mol Biol 1999:517–522, 1999.
34. Flamme I, Frolich T, Risau W: Molecular mechanisms of vasculogenesis and embryonic angiogenesis. J Cell Physiol 173:206–210, 1997.
35. Gale NW, Yancopoulos GD: Growth factors acting via endothelial cell–specific receptor tyrosine kinases: VEGFs, angiopoietins, and ephrins in vascular development. Gene Dev 13:1055–1066, 1999.
36. Vikkula M, Boon LM, Carraway KL, et al: Vascular dysmorphogenesis caused by an activating mutation in the receptor tyrosine kinase TIE2. Cell 87:1181–1190, 1996.
37. Kukk E, Lymboussaki A, Taira S, et al: VEGF-C receptor binding and pattern of expression with VEGFR-3 suggests a role in lymphatic vascular development. Development 122:3829–3837, 1996.
38. Jeltsch M, Kaipainen A, Joukov V, et al: Hyperplasia of lymphatic vessels in VEGF-C transgenic mice [erratum in Science 277(5325):463, 1997]. Science 276:1423–1425, 1997.
39. Torfs C, Cruuy C, Roeper P: Gastroschisis. J Pediatr 116:1–6, 1990.
40. Weng EY, Moeschler JB, Graham JM: Longitudinal observations on 15 children with Wiedemann-Beckwith syndrome. Am J Med Genet 56: 366, 1995.
41. Caniano DA, Brokaw B, Ginn-Pease ME: An individualized approach to the management of gastroschisis. J Pediatr Surg 25:297–300, 1990.
42. Oldham KT, Coran AG, Drongowski RA, et al: The development of necrotizing enterocolitis following repair of gastroschisis: A surprisingly high incidence. J Pediatr Surg 23:945–949, 1988.
43. Rees JR, Redo SF: Anomalies of intestinal rotation and fixation. Am J Surg 116:834–841, 1968.
44. Ford EG, Senac MO, Srikanth MS, Weitzman JJ: Malrotation of the intestine in children. Ann Surg 215:172–178, 1992.
45. Powell DM, Othersen HB, Smith CD: Malrotation of the intestines in children: The effect of age on presentation and therapy. J Pediatr Surg 24:777–780, 1989.
46. Stalker HJ, Chitayat D: Familial intestinal malrotation with midgut volvulus and facial anomalies: A disorder involving a gene controlling the normal gut rotation? Am J Med Genet 44:46–47, 1992.
47. Coombs RC, Buick RG, Gornall PG, et al: Intestinal malrotation: The role of small intestinal dysmotility in the cause of persistent symptoms. J Pediatr Surg 26:553–556, 1991.
48. Potter EL (ed): Pathology of the Fetus and Infant. Chicago, Year Book, 1961.
49. Bissler JJ, Klein RL: Alimentary tract duplications in children. Clin Pediatr 27:152–157, 1988.
50. Mathur M, Gupta SD, Bajpai M, Rohatagi M: Histochemical pattern in alimentary tract duplications of children. Am J Gastroenterol 86:1419–1423, 1991.
51. Geller A, Wang KK, DiMagno EP: Diagnosis of foregut duplication cysts by endoscopic ultrasonography. Gastroenterology 109:838–842, 1995.
52. Balen EM, Hernandez-Lizoain JL, Pardo F, et al: Giant jejunoileal duplication: Prenatal diagnosis and complete excision without intestinal resection. J Pediatr Surg 28:1586–1588, 1993.
53. Turgeon DK, Barnett JL: Meckel's diverticulum. Am J Gastroenterol 85:777–781, 1990.
54. Vane DW, West KW, Grosfeld JL: Vitelline duct anomalies: Experience with 217 childhood cases. Arch Surg 122:542–547, 1987.

55. St-Vil D, Brandy ML, Panic S, et al: Meckel's diverticulum in children: A 20-year review. J Pediatr Surg 26:1289–1292, 1991.
56. Dixon AY, McAnaw M, McGregor DH: Dual carcinoid tumors of Meckel's diverticulum presenting as metastasis in an inguinal hernia sac: Case report with literature review. Am J Gastroenterol 83:1283–1288, 1988.
57. Rodgers BM, Youssef S: "False positive" scan for Meckel diverticulum. J Pediatr 87:239–240, 1975.
58. Cragan JD, Martin ML, Moore CA, Khoury MJ: Descriptive epidemiology of small intestinal atresia, Atlanta, Georgia. Teratology 48:441–450, 1993.
59. Dalla VL, Grosfeld JL, West KW, et al: Intestinal atresia and stenosis: A 25-year experience with 277 cases. Arch Surg 133:490–496, 1998.
60. Imaizumi K, Kimura J, Masuno M, et al: Apple-peel intestinal atresia associated with balanced reciprocal translocation t(2;3)(q31.3 4.2) mat. Am J Med Genet 87:434–435, 1999.
61. Roberts HE, Cragan JD, Cono J, et al: Increased frequency of cystic fibrosis among infants with jejunoileal atresia. Am J Med Genet 78:446–449, 1998.
62. Puri P, Fujimoto T: New observations on the pathogenesis of multiple intestinal atresias. J Pediatr Surg 23:221–225, 1988.
63. Graham JM, Marin-Padilla M, Hoefnagel D: Jejunal atresia associated with Cafergot ingestion during pregnancy. Clin Pediatr 22:226, 1983.
64. Hoyme HE, Jones KL, Dixon SD, et al: Prenatal cocaine exposure and fetal vascular disruption. Pediatrics 85:743, 1990.
65. Moreno LA, Gottrand F, Turk D, et al: Severe combined immunodeficiency syndrome associated with autosomal recessive familial multiple gastrointestinal atresias: Study of a family. Am J Med Genet 37:143, 1990.
66. Masumoto K, Suita S, Nada O, et al: Abnormalities of enteric neurons, intestinal pacemaker cells, and smooth muscle in human intestinal atresia. J Pediatr Surg 34:1463–1468, 1999.
67. Ward HC, Leake J, Milia PJ, Spitz L: Brown bowel syndrome: A late complication of intestinal atresia. J Pediatr Surg 27:1593–1595, 1992.
68. Shaul DB, Harrison EA: Classification of anorectal malformations—initial approach, diagnostic tests, and colostomy. Semin Pediatr Surg 6:187–195, 1997.
69. Stoll C, Alembik Y, Roth MP, Dott B: Risk factors in congenital anal atresias. Ann Genet 40:197–204, 1997.
70. Weaver DD, Mapstone CL, Yu PL: The VATER association: Analysis of 46 patients. Am J Dis Child 140:225–229, 1986.
71. Chadha R, Bagga D, Malhotra CJ, et al: The embryology and management of congenital pouch colon associated with anorectal agenesis. J Pediatr Surg 29:439–446, 1994.
72. Duncan PA, Shapiro LR, Klein RM: Sacrococcygeal dysgenesis association. Am J Med Genet 41:153–161, 1991.
73. Schuler L, Salzano FM: Patterns in multimalformed babies and the question of the relationship between sirenomelia and VACTERL. Am J Med Genet 49:29–35, 1994.
74. Ives EJ: Thalidomide and anal anomalies. Can Med Assoc J 87:670–675, 1962.
75. Boocock GR, Donnai D: Anorectal malformations: Familial aspects and associated anomalies. Arch Dis Child 62:576–579, 1987.
76. Sheldon CA, Gilbert A, Lewis AG, et al: Surgical implications of genitourinary tract anomalies in patients with imperforate anus. J Urol 152:196–199, 1994.
77. Pena A, Spitz L, Coran AG (eds): Anorectal anomalies. In Rob and Smith's Operative Surgery: Pediatric Surgery, 5th ed. New York, Chapman & Hall Medical, 1995, pp 423–451.
78. Currarino G, Votteler TP, Kirks DR: Anal agenesis with rectobulbar fistula. Radiology 126:457–461, 1978.
79. Gross GW, Wolfson PJ, Pena A: Augmented-pressure colostogram in imperforate anus with fistula. Pediatr Radiol 21:560–562, 1991.
80. Pena A: Posterior sagittal anorectoplasty: Results in the management of 332 cases of anorectal malformations. Pediatr Surg Int 3:94–104, 1988.
81. Hedlund H, Pena A, Rodriguez G, Maza J: Long-term anorectal function in imperforate anus treated by a posterior sagittal anorectoplasty: Manometric investigation. J Pediatr Surg 27:906–909, 1992.
82. Holschneider AM, Pfrommer W, Gerresheim B: Results in the treatment of anorectal malformations with special regard to the histology of the rectal pouch. Eur J Pediatr Surg 4:303–309, 1994.
83. Boemers TM, Bax KM, Rovekamp MH, van Gool JD: The effect of posterior sagittal anorectoplasty and its variants on lower urinary tract function in children with anorectal malformations. J Urol 153:191–193, 1995.
84. Rintala R, Lindahl H, Marttinen E, Sariola H: Constipation is a major functional complication after internal sphincter–saving posterior sagittal anorectoplasty for high and intermediate anorectal malformations. J Pediatr Surg 28:1054–1058, 1993.
85. Pena A, Guardino K, Tovilla JM, et al: Bowel management for fecal incontinence in patients with anorectal malformations. J Pediatr Surg 33:133–137, 1998.
86. Rhoads JM, Vogler RC, Lacey SR, et al: Microvillus inclusion disease. Gastroenterology 100:811–817, 1991.
87. Phillips AD, Schmitz J: Familial microvillous atrophy: A clinicopathological survey of 23 cases. J Pediatr Gastroenterol Nutr 14:380–396, 1992.
88. Reifen RM, Cutz E, Griffiths AM, et al: Tufting enteropathy: A newly recognized clinicopathological entity associated with refractory diarrhea in infants. J Pediatr Gastroenterol Nutr 18:379–385, 1994.
89. Goulet O, Kedinger M, Brousse N, et al: Intractable diarrhea of infancy with epithelial and basement membrane abnormalities. J Pediatr 127:212–219, 1995.
90. Spouge D, Baird PA: Imperforate anus in 700,000 consecutive liveborn infants. Am J Med Genet 2(Suppl):151–161, 1986.

Chapter 85

SMALL INTESTINAL MOTOR PHYSIOLOGY

Jane M. Andrews and John Dent

The two most important goals of small intestinal (SI) motor function are the efficient absorption of nutrients and the maintenance of orderly aborad movement of chyme and indigestible residues along the small intestine. SI motility is also critically important in keeping bacterial concentrations down to their normally low levels.

Net movement of contents along the small intestine is antegrade, but retrograde flows also occur. Most often, retrograde flows occur over short distances and are likely to be important in mixing digested food with gut secretions and bringing contents into contact with the epithelium; such contact is important for both the absorption and "sensing" of nutrients within the lumen. Both absorption and mucosal sensing of nutrients exert significant feedback control on gastric and SI motor function. This interplay is thought to optimize the rate at which additional nutrient is presented to the absorptive epithelium and to minimize the amount of nutrient lost to the colon. Preceding emesis, and in association with nausea, retrograde movement of SI contents also occurs over longer distances, when a unique pattern characterized by a strong zone of phasic SI contractions travels in an orad direction over a large proportion of the small intestine. These contractions deliver luminal contents back to the stomach for ejection into the esophagus during the straining efforts of emesis. This coordinated motor pattern underscores the versatile modulation of SI motility according to physiologic need.

The motor function of the small intestine depends directly on smooth muscle in the gut wall, which contains the basic control mechanisms that initiate contractions and control their frequency. Overlying these basic control mechanisms are the enteric nervous system (ENS), the motor autonomic nervous system (ANS), and the spinal and vagal extrinsic sensory neurons, along with the central nervous system (CNS). In addition, a number of hormones modulate the frequency and patterning of SI contractions. Each of these factors plays a role in the motility of the small intestine in health, and specific damage of each component in some diseases has helped significantly to define their discrete roles.

In recent years there have been major advances in the definition of the anatomy of the sensory and motor control systems of the small intestine at the microscopic level. New techniques have allowed direct correlation of structure and function for some aspects of these systems. Moreover, identification of neural and other structures that have specific roles in the control of SI motor function is now allowing researchers to define the cellular mechanisms that underlie the functioning of these elements. Because of the close linkage of structure to function, the anatomy of the sensory and motor control systems is presented here in some detail.

This chapter concentrates on the physiology of normal SI motility. Basic definitions and concepts, including measurement techniques, that are relevant to an understanding of the field are discussed first. Subsequently, SI anatomy and neurophysiology are reviewed. This is followed by commentary on specialized tests used to assess SI motility clinically and a brief discussion of disease states in which SI motor function is affected. Finally, a general approach to the patient with suspected SI motor dysfunction is presented.

MAJOR CONCEPTS IN THE EVALUATION OF SMALL INTESTINAL MOTILITY: INSIGHTS AND LIMITATIONS OF MEASUREMENTS

General Considerations

The outcomes of SI motor activity basically depend on the patterning of SI contractions in both space and time; that is, *where and when do the contractions occur with respect to each other*? Measurement methods for assessing SI motor physiology must address substantial technical challenges to gather functionally relevant information on the temporospatial organization of SI motility, especially in humans. These challenges arise from the great length of the organ, the spatial and temporal complexity of motor events, and the time frame of several hours over which SI motor activity determines the successful absorption and movement of nutrients.

In the healthy small intestine, the occurrence and patterning of a large number of individual motor events determine the outcomes of absorption and transit, so that "whole animal" measures of transit and absorption yield a gross, or summary, report of motor function. More detailed descriptions of SI motility report great variability in the patterning of individual contractile events, depending, in part, on the technique used to assess motility and the time frame over which it is observed and on the temporal and spatial resolution of the measurements.

If one seeks to understand the relationship between individual motor events and transport in the small intestine, the temporal resolution of the measurement technique must be greater than the duration of each discrete motor event. Based on similar principles, the spatial resolution of the measurement technique is also an important parameter to consider if relationships between motor events and intraluminal flow are to be defined adequately. The importance of temporospatial resolution can be appreciated more clearly by considering Figure 85–1. Direct evaluation of SI motility requires methods of measurement with a time resolution of at least 2 seconds, because in humans the intrinsic frequency of SI contractions in the duodenum is up to 12 per minute. Although the optimal spatial resolution for studies of SI motor function has not been determined, the spatial patterning of pressures is known to vary over relatively small distances,[1] with most pressure wave sequences traveling less than 6 cm. Spatial resolution is also complicated by the fact that one ideally seeks high spatial resolution between measurement points and a long span over which measurements are made.

Evaluation of Single Cell Functions

At a cellular level, a number of techniques can be used to yield insights into SI motor physiology. Intracellular recordings of electrical potential can be obtained from a number of cell types within the small intestine and its neural control system. These recordings give detailed information about the signals received and transmitted by individual cells, with excellent temporal resolution, but cannot generally be applied concurrently over a significant length of gut and therefore have limited real-time spatial resolution with regard to motor events.

Recently, novel approaches that combine retrograde labeling of specific neurons from which recordings have been made have allowed important correlations between structure and function to be described.[2] Immunohistochemistry, in combination with high-resolution microscopy, has also made a significant contribution to the understanding of the neurophysiology of SI motility.[2–5] Although neurophysiologic methods provide information on structure, neurotransmitters used, and proximity to other elements, they cannot describe the actual resulting motility and its temporospatial organization. Although these single cell techniques generally have been applied to animal tissues, the results are probably also applicable to humans, because a similar structural organization of the control elements is found in human tissue.

Recording of Muscle Contractions

Direct recording of increased muscle tension is generally done with strain gauges. These can be used in muscle strips, isolated loops of intestine, and whole-organ preparations or even chronically implanted in animals. Strain gauges are capable of excellent temporal resolution of motor events, but the spatial resolution is limited by the size and number of strain gauges that are used concurrently in the selected preparation. Over short lengths of intestine, a spatial resolution of approximately 1 cm is possible. Unfortunately, strain gauges are not suitable for use in human subjects, but they have provided much valuable information on the organization of motor events in animals.[6] Muscle contractions can also be recorded by surrogate measurement techniques that record phenomena associated with contractions. One such approach is the fluorescent measurement of "calcium transients" (rapid increases in free intracellular calcium) in smooth muscle.[7] Over short sections of gut tissue (1 to 2 mm), such measurements provide excellent temporospatial resolution but are likely to be more helpful in elucidating neurophysiologic control than in describing whole-organ function. Other measurement techniques that record phenomena resulting from contractions of the smooth muscle include luminal manometry, fluoroscopy, and transit studies performed by a number of approaches.

Luminal manometry measures the change in intraluminal pressure that results mainly from lumen-occlusive or near-lumen–occlusive contractions. Fortunately, because the small intestine is tubular, with a relatively small diameter, a large proportion of motor events are recognized as pressure rises. Moreover, it has been suggested that contractions that do not result in a detectable change in intraluminal pressure are less important in determining the movement of intraluminal contents; thus, little mechanical information is lost by the failure to detect such events with manometry. Manometry can be applied in several settings, ranging from short isolated intestinal segments to clinical use in humans. Appropriately designed manometric assemblies can access any part of the human small intestine and are moderately well tolerated. Modern computer-based recording systems give excellent temporal resolution (10 Hz is routinely achieved), and spatial resolution can be tailored to give either close

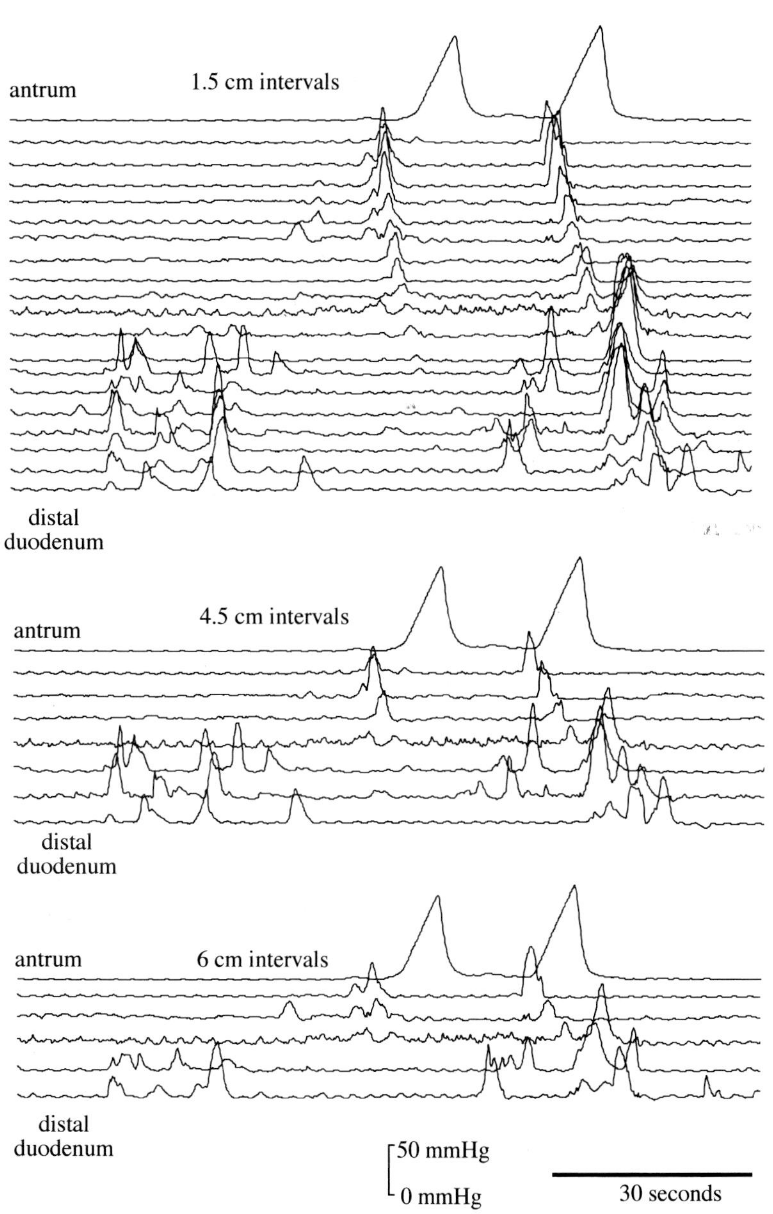

Figure 85–1. Multichannel manometric recording from the human duodenum, with recording points at varying intervals: 1.5 cm (*upper panel*), 4.5 cm (*middle panel*), and 6 cm (*lower panel*). These data exemplify some of the limitations of varying the interval between recording points: As a phasic contraction travels along a section of gut, the associated rise in pressure is detected only at each measurement point. If the interval between recording points is too wide, unrelated pressures may be judged to be related, or a propagated pressure wave sequence may be judged to be a limited phasic event. One can see the oversimplification of pressure patterning that may arise as spatial detail is lost by broadening of the recording intervals.

resolution (1- to 2-cm intervals) over a 20- to 40-cm length or wider spatial resolution to cover a longer segment of the small intestine. Perfused side-hole manometric assemblies are now capable of routinely recording at up to 22 sites.

Wall Motion and Transit Studies

Contrast fluoroscopy yields detailed information on the time and space patterning of motor events and useful insights into associated movements of luminal contents. When used in combination with other techniques, such as manometry or strain gauges, useful correlations can be made between contractions or luminal pressures and transit of contents, particularly in animals. These insights are likely to lead to improved understanding of pressure patterns, which may in turn enable us to better interpret manometry in humans. Improving the interpretation of manometry is important, because radiation exposure severely restricts the usefulness of fluoroscopy in humans, and many other measures of motility are too invasive for use in humans.

Other imaging methods that can view SI wall motion and associated movement of intraluminal contents include magnetic resonance imaging (MRI) and ultrasonography. Both approaches have been used in research studies, and although suitable for human use and capable of good temporal resolution, they have significant practical limitations when applied to the small intestine. By contrast with fluoroscopy, MRI allows prolonged observation but currently has inadequate spatial resolution of the small intestine and is prohibitively expensive. Further development may at least partly overcome these limitations, but currently MRI is restricted to research use for the study of SI motility. Ultrasonography also allows prolonged observation but only of short segments of the intestine and has relatively poor spatial resolution. It is limited in many instances by subject factors such as body habitus and intestinal gas and is operator dependent.

Transit and absorption measurements demonstrate whether

or not mass transit occurs and give no information on the mechanical pattern by which the transport of contents is achieved. Methodology for transit studies includes breath tests and scintigraphy. Breath tests are based on the exhalation of gases such as H_2 or CO_2 labeled with C^{13} or C^{14}, which are generated when a test meal reaches the colon. Scintigraphic tests visually assess the arrival of a labeled meal into the cecum. These transit techniques yield the lowest temporospatial resolution in assessing SI motility but nonetheless are sometimes clinically useful and are further discussed later in the chapter.

STRUCTURAL ELEMENTS THAT DETERMINE SMALL INTESTINAL MOTILITY

General Anatomy (see also Chapter 84)

The small intestine is approximately 3 to 7 m long, extending from the duodenal side of the pylorus to the ileocecal valve. It is divided into three regions—duodenum, jejunum, and ileum—based on structural and functional considerations. Although some structural and functional differences among these three regions exist, the regions exhibit largely similar motor characteristics. At each end of the small intestine, however, the pylorus and the ileocecal region have distinctly different motor patterns that give them the ability to act as controllers of flow between the antrum and duodenum and the ileum and colon, respectively. The motor function of the pylorus is discussed in Chapter 37, and the ileocecal region is discussed in Chapter 86. The duodenum is a fixed, largely retroperitoneal structure located in the upper abdomen, and the distal ileum is generally anchored in the right iliac fossa by its attachment to the cecum. Except for these regions, the small intestine is mobile within the peritoneal cavity.

Small Intestinal Smooth Muscle

The wall of the small intestine comprises the mucosa (consisting of the epithelium and lamina propria), submucosa, muscular layer, and serosa (Fig. 85–2). The muscularis is composed of inner circular and outer longitudinal layers of smooth muscle that are present in continuity along the length of the small intestine. Contractions within these layers are responsible for gross SI motility. A much smaller additional muscular layer, the muscularis mucosae, presents between the mucosa and submucosa and plays a role in mucosal or villus motility,[8] but it does not contribute to gross motility and is not considered further in this chapter.

The smooth muscle cells within each muscle layer form a syncytium. Myocytes communicate electrically with each other via physically specialized areas of cell-to-cell contact, *gap junctions*, which are visible on electron microscopy. This intimate contact between adjacent myocytes gives low-resistance electrical contact or coupling among them, thereby enabling them to be excited as a unit. Mechanical connections among myocytes in each layer enable them to function as a contractile unit. At a cellular level, the mechanical connections are provided by *intermediate junctions*, and at a tissue level, mechanical connections are provided by the dense extracellular stroma of collagen filaments between bundles of smooth muscle cells.[9] Within each layer the smooth muscle cell bodies are arranged in parallel, so that the circular muscle layer encircles the lumen, and the longitudinal layer extends axially along the small intestine. Hence, SI muscle contractions can reduce luminal diameter and shorten SI length.[10]

The myocytes themselves are spindle-shaped cells that derive their contractile properties from specialized cytoplasmic filaments and from the attachment of these filaments to cytoskeletal elements (Fig. 85–3). On electron microscopy, condensations of electron-dense, amorphous material are noted around the inner aspect of the cell membrane (dense bands) and throughout the cytoplasm (dense bodies). The contractile filaments—actin and myosin—are arranged in a fashion similar to that in skeletal muscle and insert onto the dense bands and bodies approximately in parallel with the long axis of the cell. Thus, when the contractile filaments are activated to slide over each other, shortening of the cell results. Activation of the contractile filaments is triggered by an increase in free intracellular calcium, which results from both release of calcium from intracellular stores and entry of extracellular calcium.

Interstitial Cells of Cajal

The *interstitial cell of Cajal* (ICC) is another specialized type of cell within the smooth muscle layer that in recent

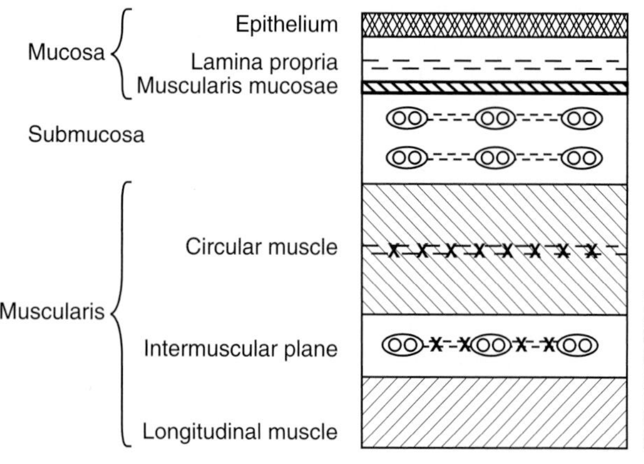

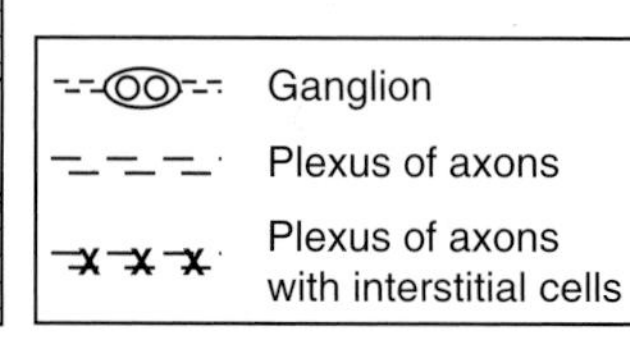

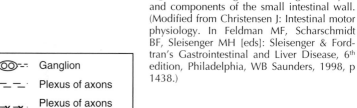

Figure 85–2. Diagram showing the layers and components of the small intestinal wall. (Modified from Christensen J: Intestinal motor physiology. In Feldman MF, Scharschmidt BF, Sleisenger MH [eds]: Sleisenger & Fordtran's Gastrointestinal and Liver Disease, 6th edition, Philadelphia, WB Saunders, 1998, p 1438.)

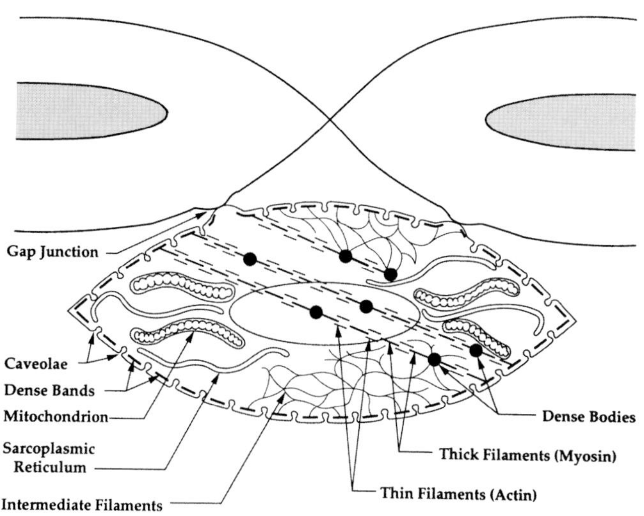

Figure 85–3. Diagram of a smooth muscle cell to show ultrastructural features discussed in the text. (From Christensen J: Gastrointestinal motility. In West JB [ed]: Best and Taylor's Physiologic Basis for Medical Practice. Baltimore, Williams & Wilkins, 1990, p 614.)

years has been recognized as vital for normal SI motor function.[11] ICCs generate the electrical slow wave that plays an important pacemaker role in determining the basic rhythmicity of SI contractions.[11] They are pleomorphic mesenchymal cells that form an interconnecting network via long, tapering cytoplasmic processes. ICCs lie in close proximity to axons and myocytes with which they form gap junctions. Recent studies[12, 13] have implicated ICCs in amplifying both inhibitory and excitatory neural signals to the myocytes, and they have the power to vary the myocyte membrane potential and thus, contractile activity. The exact mechanisms by which these effects are achieved remain to be defined. SI ICCs are located in the intramural neural plexi and are most numerous in the myenteric plexus but also present in the deep muscular plexus within the circular muscle layer. Absence or inactivity of ICCs has been implicated in a number of clinical disorders that manifest as disturbed gut motility.

Neural Control System

The small intestine is richly innervated with both extrinsic and intrinsic neurons. Intrinsic neurons have their cell bodies within the wall of the small intestine and comprise the ENS. Extrinsic neurons have their cell bodies outside the gut wall but have projections that end within the gut wall. Extrinsic neurons can be classified anatomically according to the location of their cell bodies and the route along which their projections travel. Extrinsic motor neurons belong to the ANS and connect the CNS with the ENS intrinsic motor neurons or directly with the SI smooth muscle. Extrinsic sensory neurons from the small intestine do not belong to the ANS and are classified as spinal or vagal, depending on the route they follow to the CNS (Fig. 85–4).

SI ENS elements can be subdivided into three functional groups: primary sensory neurons, motor neurons, and interneurons. There are other categories of neurons, including secretomotor and vasomotor neurons and motor neurons to endocrine cells, but these are not considered further in this chapter. Many distinct groups of enteric neurons are now well characterized both structurally and functionally and are reviewed elsewhere.[3]

The cell bodies of ENS neurons are grouped together in ganglia (clusters of cell bodies) of the two main intramural plexuses. These plexuses lie in the submucosa (submucosal plexus) and between the two muscle layers (myenteric plexus). A deep muscular plexus exists within the circular muscle, but it does not contain ganglia. The ganglia are connected by interganglionic fascicles, which are comprised predominantly of the axons of motor and interneurons, because sensory nerve processes (dendrites) do not often extend for any distance outside the ganglia. The myenteric plexus consists of ganglia spaced at regular intervals connected by a network of interganglionic fascicles. This major

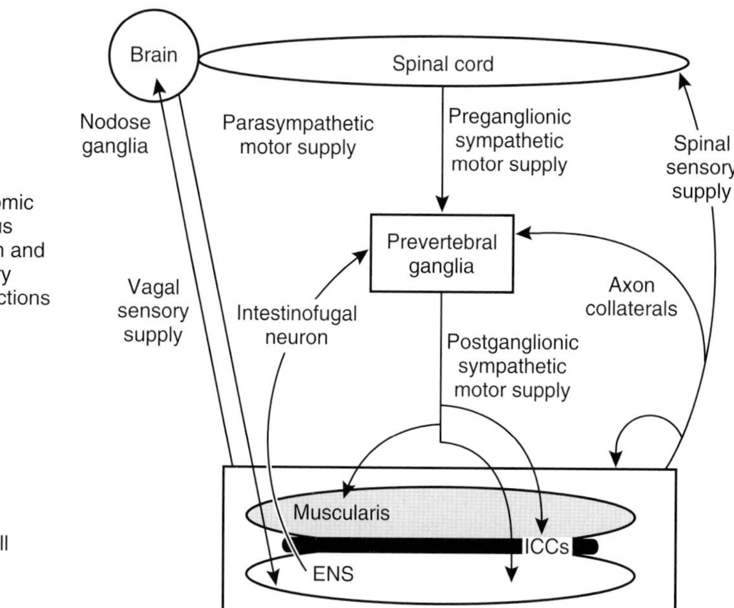

Figure 85–4. A schematic representation of the relationship between the component elements of the small intestinal motor control system. ICCs, interstitial cells of Cajal; ENS, enteric nervous system; CNS, central nervous system. For further details, see text.

network is known as the *primary plexus*. Within this main structure, smaller branches of nerve bundles arise from the primary plexus and form the *secondary plexus*, and still smaller branches form the *tertiary plexus*. The submucosal plexus has two layers, one close to the mucosa and another nearer to the circular muscle layer, which are connected by interganglionic fascicles. The submucosal plexus does not have a hierarchy of subordinate plexuses.

Because most "sensation" from the small intestine is not perceived at a conscious level, the term *afferent* neural supply is often used, in contrast to the motor, or *efferent*, supply. This terminology, however, is somewhat cumbersome, and in this chapter the afferent supply is referred to as the *sensory component* and the efferent supply as the *motor component*. Although the importance of motor innervation for motility is self-evident, the importance of sensory function has been less well appreciated. The importance of the sensory innervation is emphasized by the observation that at least 80% of vagal fibers are afferent.[14]

The rapidly increasing knowledge in the area of gastrointestinal neurophysiology has raised several contentious issues. These issues include the relative importance of sensory input from intrinsic sensory neurons as compared to axon collaterals from extrinsic sensory neurons in subserving local reflexes; the presence of specialized tension receptors in the gut wall; and the precise role of the ICC in neuromuscular coupling. Each of these issues is discussed briefly.

Sensory Pathways

EXTRINSIC SENSORY SUPPLY. The pathway of vagal sensory innervation is relatively straightforward. The vagal sensory neurons have endings in the intestinal wall and cell bodies within the nodose and jugular ganglia, which deliver input directly to the brainstem. The spinal sensory input is via perivascular nerves to the prevertebral ganglia (where neurons do not end but may give off an axon collateral that synapses on postganglionic sympathetic motor neurons), then into the thoracic spinal cord via the splanchnic nerves. The spinal sensory neurons enter the spinal cord via the dorsal roots and have their cell bodies in the dorsal root ganglia. Spinal sensory neurons may also give off axon collaterals closer to the gut wall, which synapse on components of the ENS, blood vessels, smooth muscle, or secretory elements (see Fig. 85–4).

Previously, it was believed that extrinsic sensory endings in the gut did not show ultrastructural specialization, except for pacinian corpuscles (pressure receptors) in the mesentery. Therefore, extrinsic sensory neurons were classified according to their response to chemical or mechanical stimuli. Regardless of morphology, the response patterns of sensory nerve endings are thought to be primarily determined by their location within the gut wall; mucosal nerve endings are well placed to sense the luminal environment, release of local hormones, and mucosal deformation, whereas receptors within the muscle layer are better placed to sense stretch and motor activity.

Recently, specialized SI tension receptors have been described. Vagal sensory endings have now been well studied morphologically with a fluorescent dye (1,1′-diotadecyl-3,3,3′,3′-tetramethyl-indo-carbocyanine perchlorate [DiI]), which is injected into the nodose ganglia, taken up by the cell bodies of the sensory neurons, and transported distally along their axons, thereby labeling their nerve endings. Berthoud and Powley[5] have used this approach to describe two specialized vagal receptors: *intramuscular arrays* (IMAs) and *intraganglionic laminar endings* (IGLEs). IMAs consist of multiple fine, branching nerve endings that aborize within the muscularis and are aligned with the long axis of the myocytes. Although structure and function have not yet been correlated for IMAs, they are hypothesized to be tension receptors. Moreover, IMAs have been confirmed to be sensory rather than motor endings by concurrent labeling of extrinsic primary motor neurons with a second dye (4-4-dihexadecylaminostyryl-*N*-methyl-pyridium [DiA]). Berthoud and associates[4] have also demonstrated fine vagal terminal branches with multiple arborizations within the villi of the rat duodenum. These vagal endings, although in close proximity to the basal lamina, did not appear to be in direct contact with the epithelium but may be the vagal means whereby intraluminal nutrients are sensed, giving rise to reflexes that delay gastric emptying, stimulate pancreatic secretion, and lead to satiation.

IGLEs have been further investigated using this retrograde labeling technique in combination with focused electrophysiology recordings.[2] This approach has enabled elegant concurrent observations of structure and function. After locating and recording from nerve fibers that responded to stretch, the specific nerve fibers from which the recordings had been made were labeled with DiI. Because each neuron has a characteristic electrophysiologic response pattern, the investigators were able to further define each field receptive to mechanical stimulation (to tens of microns in size) and then to examine this specific, small area microscopically for neural structures. In this fashion, IGLEs that specifically respond to stretch have been demonstrated in the myenteric plexus (Fig. 85–5).

INTRINSIC SENSORY SUPPLY. The primary sensory neurons of the ENS are morphologically Dogiel type II neurons (neurons with a single process and smooth cell body). The cell bodies of mucosal chemosensitive neurons are in the myenteric plexus, although their endings have not yet been defined anatomically.[3] The myenteric plexus also contains the cell bodies of intrinsic sensory neurons that fire in response to muscle activity or stretch.[3] Intrinsic sensory neurons that respond to mucosal mechanical stimulation are also thought to exist, based on enteric reflexes seen in extrinsically denervated preparations. The cell bodies and processes of these neurons have not yet been definitively identified, but available evidence is consistent with the presence of their cell bodies in the submucosal ganglia.[3] Intrinsic sensory neurons synapse in the intramural plexuses with intrinsic motor and interneurons.

Motor Pathways

EXTRINSIC MOTOR SUPPLY. The extrinsic motor pathways to the small intestine are supplied by the sympathetic and parasympathetic divisions of the ANS. The SI parasympathetic supply is cranial and cholinergic, whereas the sympathetic supply is spinal (thoracic) and adrenergic. These two motor pathways are not entirely separate, however, because

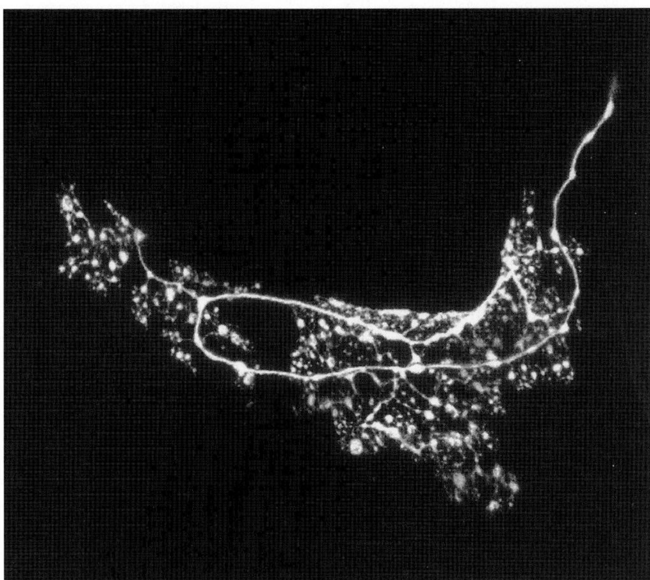

Figure 85–5. An intraganglionic laminar ending (IGLE) of a primary vagal sensory neuron, retrogradely labeled with DiI, a fluorescent dye, in the myenteric plexus of a guinea pig esophagus. Note the extensive branching and multiple varicosities. These endings are intimately related to other cells in the myenteric plexus. (From Zagorodruk VP, Brookes SJU: Transduction sites of vagal mechanoreceptor in the guinea-pig oesophagus. J Neuroscience 20:6249–6255, 2000.)

postganglionic sympathetic fibers arising from cervical ganglia are sometimes found within the vagus nerve.

The SI parasympathetic motor neurons have cell bodies within the dorsal motor nuclei of the vagi in the CNS. Their axons extend via the vagi to the intestinal intramural plexuses, where they synapse with motor cells of the ENS. The sympathetic motor supply is more complex; a primary motor neuron within the intermediolateral horn of the thoracic spinal cord synapses with a second-order neuron in the prevertebral ganglia. These second-order neurons then synapse either with ENS motor neurons within the intestinal intramural plexuses, directly with smooth muscle, or possibly even with ICCs.

There is both excitatory and inhibitory extrinsic motor output to the small intestine. Excitatory outputs depolarize, and inhibitory outputs hyperpolarize the smooth muscle, thereby facilitating or impeding the development of contractions, respectively. In general, the sympathetic motor supply is inhibitory to the ENS, and this ENS inhibition leads to decreased smooth muscle activity, with the opposite effect seen in sphincter regions. Direct sympathetic inhibitory and excitatory outputs onto smooth muscle also exist. The parasympathetic motor output to the ENS is more diffuse, with each primary motor neuron supplying a large area. There is parasympathetic motor output onto both inhibitory and excitatory ENS motor neurons.

INTRINSIC MOTOR SUPPLY. The axons of the intrinsic motor neurons that supply SI smooth muscle exit the intramural ganglia and enter either the circular or longitudinal muscle layer, where they pass in close proximity to both the myocytes and ICCs. There are no specific neuromuscular junctions as in skeletal muscle, although the multiple varicosities along the motor axons are likely to represent specialized areas of neurotransmission. The motor axons discharge along their length, potentially activating large numbers of myocytes and ICCs. The lack of exclusive, specific neuromuscular junctions, the gap junctions among myocytes, and the overlap of innervation of myocytes from more than one motor axon means that functionally discrete motor units in the gut smooth muscle do not appear to exist, in contrast to skeletal muscle. The ENS motor supply itself is both inhibitory and excitatory, and intrinsic motor neurons generally contain both a fast and a slow neurotransmitter. The predominant excitatory transmitters are acetylcholine and substance P, and the inhibitory ones are nitric oxide, vasoactive intestinal peptide, and adenosine triphosphate.

Interneurons

Interneurons connect ENS neurons of the same or different class with one another. They permit local communication within limited lengths of gut wall (measured in millimeters or centimeters) and are implicated in simple local responses. There also is some evidence for connections within the gut wall along greater distances, but these neural pathways are not well defined. These connections may be provided anatomically by the ENS or via connections between the ENS and ANS.

A special type of interneuron, *the intestinofugal neuron,* may be important for local reflex control, has its cell body within the myenteric plexus, and projects to the prevertebral ganglia, where it synapses with sympathetic motor neurons (see Fig. 85–4).

Central Connections of Neural Control Elements

Centrally, the sensory and motor supplies to the gut are closely interrelated; the vagal sensory input and the parasympathetic motor output are closely located, as are the spinal sensory input and the sympathetic motor output. Both the vagal/parasympathetic and the spinal/sympathetic supplies have widespread connections to many other areas throughout the CNS that are implicated in feeding, arousal, mood, and other "reflex" behaviors. The proximity of these CNS areas involved in SI regulation and their interconnections make it likely that the vagal/parasympathetic and the spinal/sympathetic control mechanisms are interconnected and may function less independently than previously thought.

The parasympathetic primary motor neurons originate from the ipsilateral dorsal motor nucleus of the vagus in the brainstem. The dorsal motor nucleus of the vagus lies close to, and receives a substantial input from, the nucleus tractus solitarius, which receives the vagal sensory (afferent) fibers via the nodose ganglia and the tractus solitarius. The nucleus tractus solitarius also has extensive connections to other CNS regions, and several of these same regions have input to the dorsal motor nucleus of the vagus, thereby influencing vagal motor output to the gut.

The central connections of the spinal and sympathetic supply to the gut are less well described. The spinal sensory neurons enter the spinal cord, where they synapse ipsilaterally on a second-order sensory neuron and also feedback directly onto sympathetic primary motor neurons (via axon collaterals). The second-order sensory neurons then cross the spinal cord to ascend contralaterally, where they terminate in numerous areas,[16] including the raphe nuclei and periaqueductal gray in the brainstem and the thalamus. The thalamus has extensive ramifications throughout the CNS. The central influence on sympathetic motor output is complex and not well understood, but stress and arousal level play a role. These influences have their output via the brainstem and descending tracts to the sympathetic primary motor neurons in the intermediolateral horn of the spinal cord, which send their axons to the prevertebral ganglia.

CONTROL OF MOTOR ACTIVITY

Integrative Control Mechanisms

As described earlier, sensory and motor aspects of SI motility are closely interwoven and do not function independently. As detailed earlier, basic circuits capable of driving motility exist within the ENS. At their simplest, these circuits comprise a sensory and a motor neuron that synapse either directly or via an interneuron. These local circuits can be excitatory or inhibitory. Their function also may be modulated by ANS efferent output, which in turn may be influenced by locally or centrally processed information gathered from primary sensory neurons or spinal or vagal afferents. Synapses outside the CNS in the spinal sensory and sympathetic motor arms of the extrinsic neural supply to the intestine are capable of subserving intestino-intestinal reflexes,[15] which are potentially important in the minute-to-minute regulatory control of motility. SI neuromuscular function is also influenced by a number of hormones acting in either endocrine or paracrine fashions. Most of this integration of function occurs beneath consciousness but is sometimes perceived.[15, 16]

There is little direct information on the precise contribution of each control element on SI motor function in humans. Vagal sensory input is generally thought to be important for integration of major SI functions, such as motility, secretion, and the control of food and water intake.[4, 15, 16] The SI spinal sensory innervation is not so well studied because spinal afferent nerve recordings present an extraordinary technical challenge. Moreover, recordings from mesenteric nerves are likely to include both vagal and spinal afferents. Previously, spinal sensory nerves were thought to be primarily concerned with the perception of noxious stimuli[16] and to respond to mechanical and chemical stimulation, particularly of the serosa, rather than to modulate normal SI functions. However, these concepts are now being challenged, as investigators examine spinal sensory input from the gut in more detail.

Control of Contractions at a Fixed Point

The increased smooth muscle tension arising from contractions can result in increased intraluminal pressure, decreased intraluminal diameter, SI shortening, or a combination of these effects. Smooth muscle contractions can be tonic or phasic, but common usage has labeled tonic contractions as *tone* and phasic motor events as *contractions*. Human SI phasic contractions generally last 0.8 to 6.0 seconds.

SI electrical recordings reveal the presence of a continuous cyclical oscillation in electrical potential, the *slow wave*, *basic electrical rhythm*, or *pacesetter potential*. This slow wave is generated by the ICCs in the myenteric and deep muscular plexuses at a frequency that varies with the region of intestine. In humans, the slow-wave frequency decreases from a peak of 12 per minute in the duodenum to approximately 7 per minute in the distal ileum. A SI contraction arises when an electrical action potential, or spike burst, is superimposed on the slow wave (Fig. 85–6). Spike bursts may be caused by the intrinsic motor output from the ENS to the ICCs and are likely to also be modulated by the extrinsic motor supply. Except during phase III of the interdigestive motor cycle (IDMC) (or migrating motor complex) (see later), not every slow wave leads to a phasic contraction. The region-specific frequency of the slow wave thus controls SI rhythmicity by determining the timing and maximal frequency of contractions.

Smooth muscle contraction results from a rapid increase in free intracellular calcium that activates actin and myosin filaments to move over each other and shorten. These calcium transients can be visualized with fluorescent techniques. They appear to spread in a coordinated fashion over an area of smooth muscle and extend over variable distances of the gut wall. These calcium transients are extinguished by collision with each other or by encountering locally refractory regions.[7]

Control of Contractions That Travel Along the Small Intestine

The electrical slow wave migrates along the SI in an aborad direction so that each subsequent site along the gut is depo-

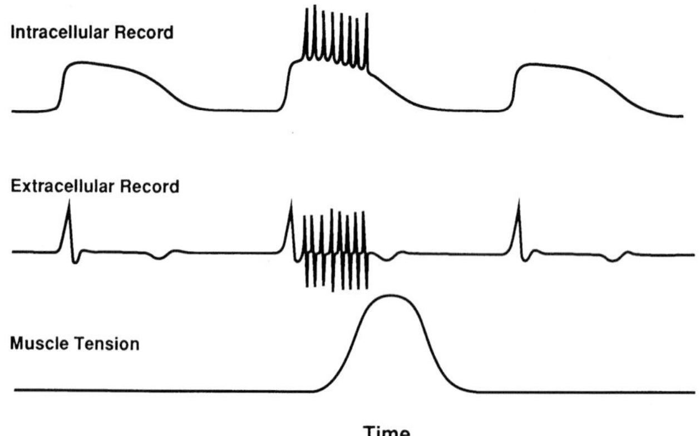

Figure 85–6. A schematic demonstrating the relationship among slow waves, spike bursts, and muscle contraction. The top tracing is from an intracellular electrode in the muscle, the middle tracing from an extracellular electrode, and the bottom tracing shows muscle tension. The cyclic fluctuation in membrane potential in the top tracing is the slow wave. When spike bursts are superimposed on the slow wave, the muscle is depolarized and contraction occurs. (From Christensen J: Gastrointestinal motility. In West JB [ed]: Best and Taylor's Physiologic Basis for Medical Practice. Baltimore, Williams & Wilkins, 1990; p 614.)

larized sequentially. In this manner, the slow wave determines the maximal rate of travel of contractions. When a slow wave results in contraction, the propagation of the slow wave along the SI will also lead to the propagation of the contraction along the gut. The propagation velocity of the slow wave thus determines the maximal rate at which contractions can travel along the gut. However, because not every slow wave leads to a contraction, manifest contractions will not always travel at this maximal rate. Additionally, the distance over which muscular excitation or inhibition spreads appears also to be determined by ENS influences via local inhibitory and excitatory circuits.[7]

Contraction sequences may travel in an antegrade (aborad) or retrograde (orad) direction. There has been little accurate information on the length and direction of travel of SI contractions in humans because of the low spatial resolution of most motility recordings. However, from animal data and some recent high spatial resolution human studies, we know that a large proportion of contractions travel along the SI, rather than remain static, but most contractions are limited to only a few centimeters in extent.[1, 6] Further data are needed to determine the contribution that these short contraction sequences make to overall transit as compared with the less frequent, longer sequences.

Currently Recognized Motility Patterns

From experiments on isolated SI segments, *ascending excitation* and *descending inhibition* are the simplest well-recognized patterns of motility. *Ascending excitation* refers to the contraction that occurs orad to a stimulus, and *descending inhibition* refers to the inhibition of motor activity that occurs distal to a stimulus. These simple reflexes can be demonstrated in the absence of any extrinsic innervation and are thus subserved entirely by the ENS, although extrinsic influences may modulate their occurrence. These two patterns are thought to be responsible for peristalsis and retroperistalsis when they travel in a coordinated fashion along the gut.

Recordings of human SI motility show isolated (stationary) phasic contractions, but frequently spatial patterns are more complex. The limited spatial resolution of many recording techniques may lead to over-reporting of the proportion of stationary contractions. Frequently, phasic motor activity consists of a recognizable group of contractions associated both in space, along the small intestine, and time. Phase III activity of the IDMC (see later), is a good example. Several other types of grouped SI contractions have been described and include those associated with emesis[17] and discrete clustered contractions, which are said to be common in irritable bowel syndrome (IBS)[18] (see Chapter 91). However, the most commonly observed motor patterns in the healthy small intestine are described simply as the postprandial, or fed, pattern and the fasting pattern, or IDMC, as described later.

CLINICAL MEASUREMENT OF SMALL INTESTINAL MOTILITY

The major outcome of SI motor activity is the transit of gastric effluent to the terminal ileum in a way that optimizes nutrient absorption and prevents debris from accumulating in the small intestine. Prevention of SI bacterial overgrowth is an important indirect outcome that is achieved by net aborad flow of luminal contents during both the fed and fasting states, probably with the assistance of the "gatekeeper" function of the ileocecal junction, which prevents backflow of cecal contents.

The broader issues of measurement of SI motor function have been considered earlier, and the discussion that follows is limited to the clinical techniques used to assess SI motor function. Additional techniques, available in specialized centers (such as MRI), are not considered here.

Small Intestinal Transit Studies

SI transit time can be measured with breath tests or scintigraphic observation of the movement of intraluminal contents. Unless the test substance is delivered past the pylorus by tube, these techniques also include gastric emptying (and thus gastric function) in the measurement. They are therefore imprecise about actual SI transit time and are more accurately termed tests of orocecal transit time. Because each technique measures a different aspect of motility, the results obtained from different techniques are not directly comparable.

The lactulose breath test is perhaps the best known and most widely used of these techniques. Lactulose is nonabsorbable and is fermented on reaching the bacteria-laden environment of the colon. The H_2 that is formed is rapidly absorbed and exhaled from the lungs. Samples of exhaled gases are taken at baseline and at regular intervals after the ingestion of lactulose. The orocecal transit time is taken as the time at which a sustained rise in exhaled H_2 is seen. An early rise, or a high baseline level, may be evidence of small bowel bacterial overgrowth, but this measure is said to be relatively insensitive for bacterial overgrowth. Similar principles are used in recently developed C^{13} or C^{14} breath tests that measure gastric emptying in combination with the completeness of SI absorption of specific nutrients. Acetate, octanoic acid, and triolein have been used. Acetate appears to be a good liquid marker, octanoic acid is better suited for solids, and triolein is useful in suspected cases of malabsorption. This nutrient-focused assessment of SI function can be combined with the H_2 breath test to measure orocecal transit time as well. These methods are still being refined and are confined to laboratories with a special interest in human SI function.

The more familiar visual/anatomic scintigraphic measurement of SI transit is also technically challenging but more widely available. The major difficulty with these studies is the lack of a reliable anatomic landmark for the cecum. The cecum is either defined arbitrarily as the right iliac fossa and a skin marker is used or is considered retrospectively as the area in which radioisotope accumulates. Two approaches are used to report the scintigraphic orocecal transit time. In the simplest approach, the time of first appearance of isotope in the cecum is given; in the other, the initial activity of the radiolabeled meal is quantified in the stomach, and the orocecal transit time is reported as the time taken for 50% of this initial gastric activity to reach the cecum. Values obtained vary depending on which of these methods is used, and each laboratory should ideally set its own normal range.

Fluoroscopy

Contrast fluoroscopy is useful for detecting mucosal disease and fixed narrowings of the lumen that may induce secondary changes in motility, transit, and absorption. However, fluoroscopy is insensitive for detection of abnormal nutrient absorption and measurement of transit time. Clinical fluoroscopy is limited by short observation times because of radiation exposure and, therefore, may only detect gross disturbances of motor activity. Once a substantial amount of contrast has entered the small intestine, the usefulness of fluoroscopy is further reduced, because overlying loops of bowel hinder the interpretation of the movement of contrast.

Manometry

SI manometry gives the most direct measurement of the forces that are applied to luminal contents as a result of motor function in humans. Manometry can be performed over hours or even days and over either long or short segments and is capable of excellent spatial resolution, but it also has major practical limitations. Placement of a manometric assembly along the small intestine is demanding even in healthy subjects but is especially challenging in patients who have major abnormalities of motor function. Manometry allows recognition of some abnormal patterns of pressure over time at individual recording points, but there is a lack of critical evaluation of the best spacing of pressure recording points and of diagnostic criteria for abnormal pressure patterns that make a clear distinction between health and disease. This lack of criteria reflects the current, limited understanding of the relationship between SI intraluminal time-space pressure patterning and the achievement of mixing and propulsion within the small intestine. Because of practical limitations on the number of recording points that can be included on an assembly, the choice must be made between high spatial resolution over a short segment or lower spatial resolution over a longer segment of intestine. Both approaches are likely to be necessary in achieving an accurate understanding of SI motor physiology, perhaps in conjunction with a technique to assess wall motion or intraluminal flow.

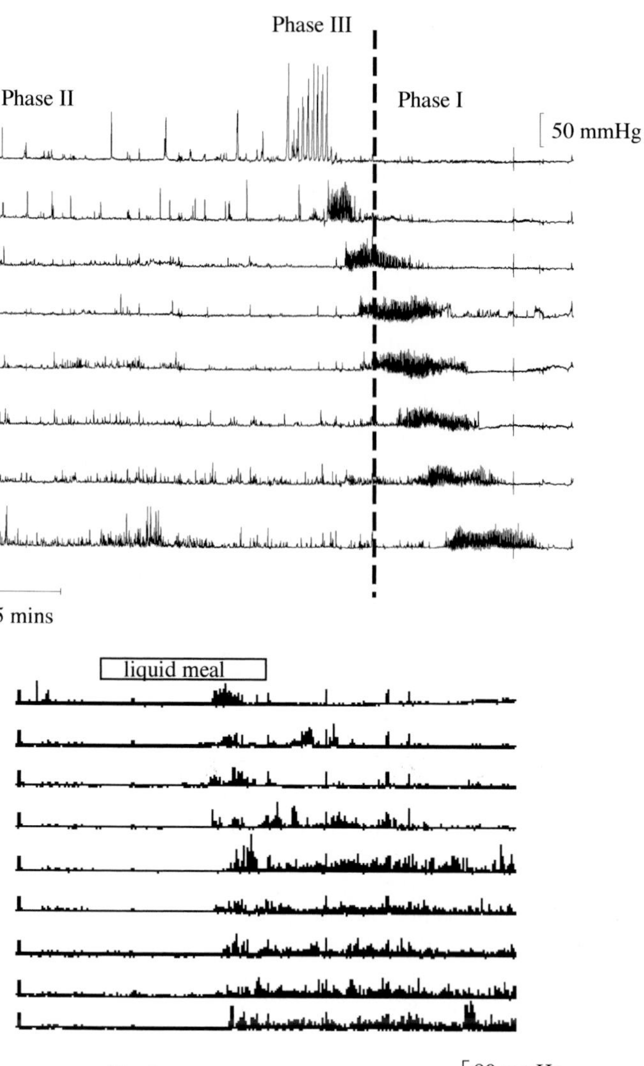

Figure 85–7. Fasting small intestine motility, showing the three phases of the IDMC (unpublished data: JM Andrews), and the conversion to a fed motor pattern by the presence of SI nutrients (data by kind permission from Dr RJ Fraser). In the top figure, at a given time-point (*dashed vertical line*), all three phases of the IDMC can be encountered at different points along the small intestine. The similarity of phase II and the fed motor pattern can be appreciated by comparing the top and bottom figures.

NORMAL SMALL INTESTINAL MOTOR FUNCTION IN HUMANS

The small intestine exhibits two predominant motor patterns: the fed (postprandial) pattern and the fasting (interdigestive) pattern (Fig. 85–7). The pattern at a given time is determined by the presence or absence of a significant amount of nutrient within the small intestine. Despite a large number of studies on fasting motility, there is a paucity of studies of human postprandial SI motility, probably because of the difficulty in knowing which aspects of postprandial motility to study, in contrast to fasting motility, which has an easily recognized cyclical patterning and thus easily studied parameters. The fed motor pattern ensures transit of SI contents at a rate consistent with normal digestion and absorption. The fasting motor pattern is less concerned with orderly luminal transport and is thought to serve important roles in clearing the upper gut of solid residues, which otherwise may accumulate and form bezoars, maintaining relative sterility of the SI by keeping it empty, and preventing net orad migration of colonic bacteria.

Within 10 to 20 minutes of the consumption of a meal, the interdigestive motor cycle (IDMC) in progress at the time of eating is interrupted.[19] The presence of intraluminal nutrients is "sensed" by mucosal nutrient contact; portal or intravenous nutrients do not have the same effects as those consumed orally.[20] Several neural and humoral signals result from mucosal nutrient contact, including vagal afferent signals, cholecystokinin, and glucagon-like peptide-1 (GLP-1), and are implicated in the induction of the fed motor pattern.

Moreover, the sensing of intraluminal nutrients is relatively complex, because different types of nutrient, or varying amounts of the same nutrient, generate recognizably different motor responses.[1, 6, 21, 22] In general, the presence of unabsorbed SI nutrients slows SI transit by decreasing the frequency and length of travel of phasic contractions, so that the rate at which a substance is absorbed limits its transit rate. In the absence of sufficient proximal SI nutrient stimulation, the fasting motor pattern re-emerges 4 to 6 hours after a meal. In the absence of interruption by intraluminal nutrients, the IDMC repeats continuously.

Distention, intraluminal pH changes, and hyperosmolar contents are capable of stimulating SI motor activity. Hyperosmolar contents and pH changes are probably sensed by mucosal receptors, whereas distention is signaled by IGLEs and probably IMAs, as well as mucosal deformation. In the normal course of events, these stimuli occur concurrently with the presence of nutrients, and the significance of their isolated effects in healthy subjects is unclear.

The small intestine also exerts negative feedback control on the rate of gastric emptying via neural and humoral means. This negative feedback is achieved by the release of neural signals and gut hormones that suppress phasic gastric motor activity, relax the gastric fundus, and increase tonic and phasic pyloric pressures subsequent to mucosal sensing of SI nutrients.[23] This process indirectly also prolongs "whole-meal" SI transit time, by slowing the input of SI chyme. The small intestine, in particular the duodenum, is also thought to offer direct mechanical resistance to gastric emptying by acting as a capacitance resistor[24] and by reaugmenting gastric contents as a result of duodenogastric reflux.[25]

Fed Motor Patterns

Radiologic Observations

Early radiologic observations of the small intestine in animals described several different patterns of wall motion and transit of intestinal contents. Cannon[17, 26] observed both localized contractions over short segments of intestine in association with to-and-fro movement of contents and intermittent episodes of propulsion of contents over greater distances caused by aborally traveling waves of peristalsis. In the fed state, the most common pattern of wall motion observed in a number of species was termed *rhythmic segmentation*, whereby short columns of chyme were recurrently divided and united into new aliquots by localized circular contractions that caused temporary local occlusion of the lumen over distances of less than 1 to 2 cm.[17, 26] These contractions did not travel along the small intestine and did not result in much, if any, net orad movement of contents.[17, 26] Peristalsis was also commonly observed, often in combination with segmentation. During SI nutrient loading, peristalsis was noted to have two forms: a slow advance of chyme over short distances in association with segmentation, and rapid transit of chyme over longer distances, sometimes several loops, of the SI. This "fast peristalsis" was frequently seen in the cat duodenum.[26] Similar observations have been made in other animal species[6, 17] and correlate with some of the motor patterns seen during clinical radiologic studies in humans (although these studies are usually performed when the subject is fasting and show the rapid peristaltic pattern more than the segmenting postprandial activity).

Transit Time Observations

The SI transit time for a meal varies greatly according to the amount and nature of what is consumed, because the caloric content and physical form of a meal determine both the gastric emptying rate and the rate of transport along the intestine.[27–30] Depending on the test and parameter used, postprandial orocecal transit time is usually less than 6 hours. However, as assessed by lactulose breath testing, orocecal transit time can be as rapid as approximately 70 minutes with low nutrient loads. There is a need for a systematic evaluation of the optimal conditions for nutrient loading to reveal abnormal SI motor function using transit studies.

Manometric Observations

Postprandial SI motility is characterized by irregular phasic pressure waves without a discernible cyclical pattern. Most SI motility data are quite limited in spatial resolution (interval between sensors and length of small intestine spanned by sensors) because of the length of the small intestine. Despite this, it is thought that most phasic pressures (pressure wave sequences) travel only a short distance[1, 6] and represent the mixing contractions noted in earlier radiologic studies.[17, 26] In animal studies, postprandial SI motility is more "segmenting" than is fasting phase II activity, with phasic pressures occurring less frequently and traveling shorter distances along the bowel, thereby resulting in slower transit of the contents.[6] A similar suppression in the frequency of pressure wave sequences has now been found as well in human duodenum.[1] This segmenting motor pattern is thought to assist in mixing food with digestive enzymes and maximizing the exposure of food to the mucosa to optimize absorption.

Fasting Motor Patterns

During fasting, SI motor activity adopts a repetitive cyclic motor pattern—the IDMC. The IDMC is absent in a number of disease states associated clinically with stasis of SI contents, malabsorption, and small bowel bacterial overgrowth, presumably because of a primary neuropathic process. For more detailed reviews see References 18 and 19.

Radiologic Observations

Radiologic contrast agents may stimulate SI mucosal receptors sensitive to pH, caloric content, and osmolarity changes. It is possible, therefore, that radiologic studies of "fasting" motility are not truly representative of the fasting state. Nonetheless, in general, contrast agent appears to move more swiftly through the small intestine during fasting than during the postprandial state and to be associated with more episodes of peristalsis over one or more loops and fewer segmenting contractions. When the phase of the IDMC is assessed concurrently (see later), little net movement of SI contents is seen during phase I, but residual luminal contents are swept through the small intestine and into the terminal ileum during late phase II and phase III of the IDMC. This finding is not surprising, because by definition, phase I is the absence of measurable phasic pressure waves, which are likely to be necessary to generate a sufficient intraluminal pressure gradient to cause intraluminal flow.

Transit Time Observations

Studies of SI transit time also probably do not represent a true assessment of fasting motor function, because most of the substrates used to measure transit also interact with SI mucosal receptors. The lower the caloric content, the more closely fasting motility will be assessed (see earlier).

Manometric Observations

The IDMC is defined manometrically and comprises three main phases. Phase I is defined as motor quiescence ($<$ 3 pressure waves per 10 minutes at any one site); phase II is characterized by random pressure waves at less than the maximal rate; and phase III is characterized by pressure waves at the maximal rate (for the region) for longer than 2 minutes (and, ideally, extending over $>$ 40 cm). Some authors also include a fourth phase (phase IV) as a transitional period between phases III and I, although this approach is not universal. Phases I and III are quite distinctive and easily recognized, whereas phase II can be recognized reliably only when sandwiched between phases I and III, because it superficially resembles the fed pattern. The phases of the IDMC start proximally and migrate distally over varying distances, with few phase IIIs reaching the ileum.[31] Moreover, phase III of each IDMC may start at a variable location; approximately one third of IDMCs have a gastroduodenal component, and most onsets of phase III occur by the proximal jejunum.[31] The length of the SI and the velocity of travel of the IDMC mean that one part of the SI can be in phase I, while other parts are in phase II or III (see Fig. 85–7). The normal periodicity of the IDMC varies greatly both within and between subjects; however, its median duration is 90 to 120 minutes.

CLINICAL CONSEQUENCES OF DISORDERED SMALL INTESTINAL MOTOR FUNCTION

Most of the time, the overall outcome of SI motility is achieved without conscious awareness; however, a range of symptoms may arise when an optimal outcome is not attained. Fortunately, like other organs, the small intestine has a substantial reserve capacity and copes with many insults,

Table 85–1 | **Diseases and Clinical Settings Associated with Abnormal Small Intestinal Motility**

CLINICAL SETTING	SMOOTH MUSCLE	NEURAL EFFECTS	SENSORY EFFECTS	MOTOR OUTCOME
Irritable bowel syndrome			Increased visceral sensitivity	Alterations in fasting phase III, increased "clustered contractions"
Acute illness	Decreased strength of contractions	Altered neurotransmission		Ileus
Pregnancy	Decreased strength of contractions			Slowed transit
Diabetes		Altered neurotransmission	Enhanced perception of gastrointestinal stimuli	Abnormal patterning of contractions, slow or rapid transit
Metabolic disturbances	Possible decreased strength of contractions	Altered neurotransmission	Nausea, altered sensory perception	Variable outcome: ileus, rapid transit
Drugs	Possible decreased strength of contractions	Altered neurotransmission		Ileus, slow or rapid transit, disordered contractions
Obstruction	Hypertrophy if chronic			High-amplitude forceful contractions
Pseudo-obstructive syndromes		Multiple neural abnormalities, neuron loss, plexus abnormalities, altered distribution of neurotransmitters		Feeble contractions, absent phase III IDMC, eventually leads to failure of transit
Scleroderma and other connective tissue diseases	Ischemia and fibrosis	Nerve loss in gut wall; may also lose extrinsic neural supply due to vasculitis		Feeble contractions, thickening of bowel wall, transit failure
Neurologic syndromes		Neural absence or loss	Afferent information for reflex control lost	Disorganized IDMC, failure to convert to "fed" pattern, transit failure
Rare myopathies	Myocyte and mitochondrial abnormalities; inadequate contractile force			Insufficient force for transit and mixing

IDMC, interdigestive motor cycle.

including infection, resection, inflammation, and denervation, before clinical problems become manifest. In the most common clinical syndrome in which altered motility is implicated, IBS, the sufferer's physical well-being is rarely threatened even when symptoms are considerable. Rarely, the motor disturbances are sufficiently severe to disrupt a person's ability to maintain oral nutrition.

The most important diseases and clinical settings associated with abnormal SI motility are listed in Table 85–1. Because these disorders are covered elsewhere, they are mentioned here only with regard to the associated SI motor disturbances.

In IBS a number of abnormalities of visceral sensation have been documented. It is likely that these sensory abnormalities also lead to disordered motility. However, whereas some investigators have documented motor abnormalities in patients with IBS, others have not (see Chapter 91). Because it appears increasingly likely that IBS is an as yet undefined generalized enteric neuropathy, it is possible that failure to define motor abnormalities results from a poor understanding of normal SI motor physiology and the relatively gross measures by which motility in IBS patients has been assessed.

SI motility is severely disrupted in acutely ill persons and is increasingly recognized as an important factor to consider in patients in the intensive care unit. The disturbances are likely to result from several factors, including sepsis and drugs, which disrupt the slow wave rhythm; abdominal trauma or surgery, which stimulate reflex motor responses; and inflammatory mediators, which affect neurotransmission within the CNS, ANS, and ENS. For a more detailed review see Reference 32.

Pregnancy is known to alter lower esophageal sphincter function, delay gastric emptying, and disturb the frequency of gastric slow waves. It is also associated frequently with constipation. In view of these widespread complaints and findings related to altered gut motility, it is likely that SI motor function also is altered. Recently, in guinea pigs, the strength of the contraction of intestinal circular smooth muscle has been shown to be impaired during pregnancy by down-regulation of G proteins (which mediate contraction) and up-regulation of $G_s$alpha protein (which mediates relaxation).[33]

Diabetes has widespread effects on the motility of the gastrointestinal tract. Acute effects are the result of changes in blood glucose levels but also may result from the autonomic neuropathy that develops in patients with long-standing diabetes. Based predominantly on studies of the stomach, hyperglycemia may alter the rhythm of the slow wave, modulate sensory signaling, lead to changes in the temporospatial pattern of phasic contractions, and even stimulate inappropriate phase III–like IDMC activity in the small intestine.

Metabolic disturbances of potassium, magnesium, and calcium homeostasis are likely to impair SI motor function because these chemicals are vital for normal neuromuscular function. The effects of abnormal levels of these electrolytes on normal human SI function have not been studied specifically, but in organ bath experiments, alterations of these electrolytes have caused gross disturbances in neural and muscular function. Renal and hepatic failure also are likely to alter SI motility because of the multiple homeostatic inputs of the affected organs. However, altered SI motility is usually not a prominent feature of these clinical conditions.

Many drugs affect SI motility, especially those that alter ion transport, such as antidepressants (of several classes), calcium channel blockers, and beta blockers. Sedatives and narcotic analgesics also alter motility but usually do not cause clinically important SI motor dysfunction, except in critically ill patients or those with acute severe pain.

Pseudo-obstruction, scleroderma and other connective tissue diseases, dysautonomia, visceral myopathies, and other rare diseases in which abnormal SI motor function occurs are discussed in detail in Chapters 29 and 111. These diseases may be the most uncommon causes of disordered SI motility, but they have increased our understanding of normal motility because, in some cases, the neural and myopathic processes are impaired separately.

APPROACH TO PATIENTS WITH POSSIBLY DISORDERED SMALL INTESTINAL MOTOR FUNCTION

Taking a thorough history is a vital first step in approaching a patient who may have abnormal SI motility. A review of exposures to drugs and toxins, family history, and, in the younger patient, milestones of growth and development are especially important. The physical examination in this setting is often unremarkable. First-line investigations are generally suggested by the history, physical examination, and age of the patient and may include a plain abdominal radiograph (to look for dilated SI loops, thickened wall, air-fluid levels), complete blood count with red blood cell indices (to look for evidence of malabsorption), serum albumin and electrolyte levels, and a random blood glucose or glycosylated hemoglobin level. How much further one proceeds with investigation depends on these results and the severity of the patient's condition.

Special investigations may be indicated to answer particular questions. There is no standard approach, however, and local interest and expertise often determine which investigations are available. Fluoroscopy is widely available and may help exclude medically or surgically treatable problems. Endoscopy with small bowel biopsy or aspiration is useful if celiac sprue, SI bacterial overgrowth, or intestinal infection is considered likely. Analysis of the stool may be necessary to exclude malabsorptive or secretory causes of SI diarrhea. SI manometry, if available, may help distinguish neuropathic from myopathic forms of disordered motility, although in many settings the abnormalities associated with these two forms overlap (see Table 85–1). Manometry also may show features typical of intestinal obstruction, although radiology is a better tool to identify an obstruction. In selected cases, a full-thickness biopsy of the SI will be necessary, but for a full-thickness biopsy to be of value, it should be performed only in centers with expertise in immunohistochemistry of gut neurons, because standard histologic approaches often yield little useful information.

FUTURE OUTLOOK

SI motor physiology is much better understood now than 10 years ago, but progress is still needed. Although traditionally regarded as a limited, circumscribed area of clinical gastroenterology, motility probably has a large impact on many common clinical conditions encountered in the practice of gastroenterology. A better understanding of normal SI motility will clarify the pathophysiology of disordered motility, which in turn will assist in the development of specific, targeted interventions. Treatments that improve disordered SI motility have the potential to improve the quality of life of a substantial proportion of the population and to facilitate the maintenance of enteral nutrition in selected groups of patients.

Acknowledgments
We gratefully acknowledge the invaluable advice and assistance in interpretation of a complex neurophysiology literature provided by Dr. L. Ashley Blackshaw (BSc, PhD, Sheffield).

REFERENCES

1. Andrews JM, Doran SD, Hebbard GS, et al: Nutrient-induced spatial patterning of human duodenal motor function. Am J Physiol Gastrointest Liver Physiol 280:G501–G509, 2001.
2. Zagorodruk UP, Brookes SJH: Transduction sites of vagal mechanoreceptors in the guinea pig oesophagus. J Neurosci 20:6249–6255, 2000.
3. Furness JB: Types of neurons in the enteric nervous system. J Auton Nerv Syst 81:87–96, 2000.
4. Berthoud HR, Kressel M, Raybould HE, Neuhuber WL: Vagal sensors in the rat duodenal mucosa: Distribution and structure as revealed by in vivo DiI-tracing. Anat Embryol 191:203–212, 1995.
5. Berthoud HR, Powley TL: Vagal afferent innervation of the rat fundic stomach: Morphological characterisation of the gastric tension receptor. J Comp Neurol 319:261–276, 1992.
6. Huge A, Weber E, Ehrlein HJ: Effects of enteral feedback inhibition on motility, luminal flow, and absorption of nutrients in proximal gut of minipigs. Dig Dis Sci 40:1024–1034, 1995.
7. Stevens RJ, Publicover NG, Smith TK: Induction and organisation of Ca^{2+} waves by enteric neural reflexes. Nature 399:62–66, 1999.
8. Lee JS: Relationship between intestinal motility, tone, water absorption, and lymph flow in the rat. J Physiol (Lond) 345:489–499, 1983.
9. Christensen J: Intestinal motor physiology. In Feldman M, Friedman LS, Sleisenger MH (eds): Sleisenger and Fordtran's Gastrointestinal and Liver Disease, 6th ed. Philadelphia, WB Saunders, 1997, pp 1437–1450.
10. Sarna SK: Gastrointestinal longitudinal muscle contractions. Am J Physiol 265:G156–G164, 1993.
11. Sanders KM: A case for interstitial cells of Cajal as pacemakers and mediators of neurotransmission in the gastrointestinal tract. Gastroenterology 111:492–515, 1996.
12. Ward SM, Morris G, Reese L, et al: Interstitial cells of Cajal mediate enteric inhibitory neurotransmission in the lower esophageal and pyloric sphincters. Gastroenterology 115:314–329, 1998.
13. Ward SM, Beckett EA, Wang X, et al: Interstitial cells of Cajal mediate cholinergic neurotransmission from enteric motor neurons. J Neurosci 20:1393–1403, 2000.
14. Agostini E, Chinnok JE, Daly MD, Murray JG: Functional and histological studies of the vagus nerve and its branches to the heart, lungs and abdominal viscera. J Physiol (Lond) 135:182–205, 1957.
15. Grundy D, Scratcherd T: Sensory afferents from the gastrointestinal tract. In American Physiological Society (eds): Handbook of Physiology: The Gastrointestinal System. Washington DC, Raven Press, 1989, pp 593–620.
16. Cervero F: Sensory innervation of the viscera: Peripheral basis of visceral pain. Physiol Rev 74:95–138, 1994.
17. Cannon WB: The mechanical factors of digestion. London, Edward Arnold, 1911, pp 131–147.
18. Husebye E: The patterns of small bowel motility: Physiology and implications in organic diseases and functional disorders. Neurogastroenterol Motil 11:141–161, 1999.
19. Sarna SK: Cyclic motor activity: Migrating motor complex. Gastroenterology 89:894–913, 1985.
20. Gielkins HAJ, van den Biggelaar A, Vetch J, et al: Effect of intravenous amino acids on interdigestive antroduodenal motility and small bowel transit time. Gut 44:240–245, 1999.
21. Rao SSC, Safadi R, Lu C, Schulze-Delrieu K: Manometric responses of human duodenum during infusion of Hcl, hyperosmolar saline, bile, and oleic acid. Neurogastroenterol Motil 8:35–43, 1996.
22. Rao SSC, Lu C, Schulze-Delrieu K: Duodenum as an immediate brake to gastric outflow: A videofluoroscopic and manometric assessment. Gastroenterology 110:740–747, 1996.
23. Horowitz M, Dent J: The study of gastric mechanics: A Mad Hatter's Tea Party starting to make sense [editorial]. Gastroenterology 107:37–46, 1994.
24. Shirazi S, Schulze-Delrieu K, Brown CK: Duodenal resistance to the emptying of various solutions from the isolated cat stomach. J Lab Clin Med 111:654–660, 1988.
25. Hausken T, Odegaars S, Matre K, Berstad A: Antroduodenal motility and movements of luminal contents studied by duplex sonography. Gastroenterology 102:1583–1590, 1992.
26. Cannon WB: The movements of the intestines studied by means of the rontgen rays. Am J Physiol 6:251–277, 1902.
27. Hunt JN, Smith JL, Jiang CL: Effect of meal volume and energy density on the gastric emptying of carbohydrates. Gastroenterology 89: 1326–1330, 1985.
28. Benini L, Castellani G, Brighenti F, et al: Gastric emptying of a solid meal is accelerated by the removal of dietary fibre naturally present in food. Gut 36:825–830, 1995.
29. Lin HC, Doty JE, Reedy TJ, Meyer JH: Inhibition of gastric emptying by sodium oleate depends on length of intestine exposed to nutrient. Am J Physiol 259:G1031–G1036, 1990.
30. Lin HC, Zhao XT, Wang L: Jejunal brake: Inhibition of intestinal transit by fat in the proximal small intestine. Dig Dis Sci 41:326–329, 1996.
31. Kellow J, Borody TJ, Phillips SF, et al: Human interdigestive motility: Variations in patterns from oesophagus to colon. Gastroenterology 91: 386–395, 1986.
32. Ritz MA, Fraser R, Tam W, et al: Impacts and patterns of disturbed gastrointestinal function in critically ill patients. Am J Gastroenterol 95: 3044–3052, 2000.
33. Chen Q, Xiao ZL, Biancani P, Behar J: Downregulation of Galphaq-11 protein expression in guinea pig antral and colonic circular muscle during pregnancy. Am J Physiol 276:G895–G900, 1999.

Chapter 86

MOTILITY OF THE LARGE INTESTINE

Ian J. Cook and Simon J. Brookes

Each day, from 1200 to 1500 mL of ileal effluent enters the colon, and 200 to 400 mL is excreted as stool. The colon stores excreta for extended periods and mixes the contents to facilitate the transmural exchange of water, electrolytes, and short-chain fatty acids. This process involves rhythmic to-and-fro motions, together with short step-wise movements of contents, resulting in an overall net aborad flow rate that averages approximately 1 cm per hour. When dehydration threatens survival, such as water deprivation or severe diarrhea, the ability of the colon to reabsorb fluid is of major physiologic significance. Appropriate motility patterns are important in achieving this function. For example, the colon has the capacity to increase its fluid absorption fivefold, when required, but this ability is greatly impaired when transit is accelerated. Under normal circumstances, viscous contents are occasionally propelled aborally at a rapid rate and, if circumstances are appropriate, stool is evacuated under voluntary control. Thus, the colon is capable of showing a diverse range of motor patterns that are suited for particular physiologic functions. The generic term *motility* describes the range of motor patterns and the mechanisms that control them.

STUDYING COLONIC MOTILITY

Common sensorimotor symptoms, such as constipation, diarrhea, bloating, abdominal pain, or rectal urgency, can arise from disturbances of ileocolonic delivery, colonic propulsion, or stool expulsion. Clearly, these symptoms and dysmotility must be linked, although our current understanding of these links is limited, due largely to the technical difficulties involved in studying the human colon. Interspecies differences require care in extrapolating from animal studies to humans. For many years, intraluminal motility recordings in humans were obtained mainly from the rectum and sigmoid. It is now clear that the motor activity of these distal regions is not representative of the colon as a whole. The contents of the colon become increasingly viscous distally, and their mobility is affected. This alteration complicates the relationship between propulsion and the contractile activity of the smooth muscle. Colonic movements are much less frequent and transit is considerably slower than in other regions of the gut. The highly propulsive, stereotypic motor patterns that are associated with stool expulsion generally occur only once or twice daily. Hence, in vivo study of the motor patterns in the human cannot be achieved using contrast radiography. Prolonged recording techniques must be used to capture such infrequent motor patterns. Recording of intraluminal pressure, via manometric catheters inserted per rectum, requires prior bowel cleansing, which may modify colonic motility. Interpretation of intraluminal pressure measurements is complicated, because many contractions of the wall of the colon do not occlude the lumen and are, therefore, undetectable by manometry. Smooth muscle electromyography gives good insight into the patterning of muscle activity but generally requires access to the muscular wall of the colon, which is ethically difficult in humans. Scintigraphy, with suitably high frame rates (15 to 30 seconds per frame) can resolve discrete movements of the contents but is suboptimal for measuring actual wall motion. Study of the cellular basis of motility in vitro, usually using isolated specimens of colon, faces fewer technical and ethical limitations. However, data obtained at the cellular level, often under highly nonphysiologic conditions, can be difficult to relate to the more complex situation in vivo. Nonetheless, although each of these approaches has intrinsic limitations, in combination they have provided important insights into the relationships among muscle activity, wall motion, intraluminal pressure, and flow.

ANATOMY, INNERVATION, AND BASIC CONTROL MECHANISMS

Macroscopic Structure of the Colon

(See also Chapter 84)

The human colon is just over one meter long and is divided anatomically into the cecum; the ascending, transverse, descending, sigmoid colon; and the rectum, which lies between the rectosigmoid junction and the anal canal. The outer longitudinal smooth muscle layer forms three thick, cord-like structures called the taenia coli, which are spaced evenly around the circumference. Between the taenia, the longitudinal smooth muscle is much thinner, allowing the wall to bulge noticeably. In addition, irregularly spaced circumferential constrictions pinch the gut into a series of pockets, called haustra, which give the colon a sacculated appearance for most of its length. The haustra are not fixed structures, but move, disappear, and re-form during the propulsion of the contents and appear to be caused by sustained contractions of the circular muscle. The taenia fuse to form a continuous outer longitudinal smooth muscle layer at the rectosigmoid junction; this layer is continuous down to the distal margin of the anal canal. Throughout the length of the colon, the circular smooth muscle layer consists of thick bundles of cells, which are separated by connective tissue. The internal anal sphincter consists of a thickening of the circular muscle layer over the last 2 to 4 cm of the anal canal.

Structure and Activity of Colonic Smooth Muscle

Smooth muscle cells in the human colon are spindle-shaped, nucleolated cells with tapered ends. The surface area of the cell membrane is greatly increased by numerous caveolae, or small pits. Individual smooth muscle cells are connected to neighboring cells by gap junctions, which allow ions and small molecules (with a molecular weight of up to about 1000) to diffuse between the cells, thus ensuring that the cells are electrically coupled to one another. Therefore, the smooth muscle cells do not contract as individual cells. Rather, they contract together in large, coordinated assemblies. Like smooth muscle cells throughout the gastrointestinal tract, colonic smooth muscle typically shows spontaneous, oscillatory electrical activity, even when all neural activity is blocked. Two types of rhythmic myoelectrical activity occur.[1] Small amplitude, rapid oscillations, with a frequency of 12 to 20 per minute, originate from the plane of the myenteric plexus. These small oscillations spread, via gap junctions, into both the longitudinal and circular smooth muscle layers. They have been termed *myenteric potential oscillations* (MPOs) and often reach the threshold potential for generating smooth muscle action potentials. In the circular muscle layer, MPOs, with superimposed action potentials, generate small phasic contractions of the circular muscle layer. When the muscle is strongly excited by neurotransmitters released by enteric excitatory motor neurons, each MPO evokes an action potential, and the phasic contractions summate into powerful contractions, which last several seconds.

A second pacemaker region is located at the submucosal border of the circular muscle. This region produces larger amplitude, slower myogenic oscillations in membrane potential called *slow waves,* which also spread through the circular smooth muscle via gap junctions. These slow waves also often reach the threshold for triggering smooth muscle action potentials and can evoke strong contractions. Slow waves occur throughout the colon at a frequency of approximately 2 to 4 per minute. The currents produced by pacemaker cells at the myenteric and submucosal borders decay as they spread through the thickness of the circular muscle layer. Thus, in the middle of the circular smooth muscle layer, there is complex spontaneous electrical activity consisting of a mixture of MPOs and slow waves, with superimposed smooth muscle action potentials. There is some indication that under normal circumstances the slow waves tend to determine the contractile activity of the smooth muscle and favor nonpropulsive mixing movements. During times of strong enteric neuronal activity, however, MPO-derived contractions can summate, giving rise to powerful contractions of much longer duration than the slow waves. Action potentials in the smooth muscle can be readily recorded in vivo with electrodes attached to the serosal surface, thereby giving a high-resolution measurement of "myoelectric activity" or "spike bursts."

Ion Channels in Colonic Smooth Muscle

The membrane of colonic smooth muscle cells contains a variety of ion channels, including potassium channels, calcium channels, chloride channels, and nonselective cation channels.[2] Although the physiologic role of many of these ion channels is currently uncertain, the high-threshold, voltage-operated calcium channels (L-type calcium channels) play a crucial role in colonic muscle contractility. They open when the membrane potential of smooth muscle cells is depolarized beyond a voltage threshold and are responsible for the rapid upstroke of smooth muscle action potentials. The influx of calcium through L-type calcium channels during action potentials is a major trigger for activation of the contractile apparatus. It is not surprising that pharmacologic blockade of L-type calcium channels by dihydropyridine drugs such as nifedipine can reduce the contractility of colonic smooth muscle substantially. However, release of calcium from intracellular stores, which is triggered by excitatory neurotransmitters, also may play a role in muscle contraction.

Interstitial Cells of Cajal: Smooth Muscle Pacemakers

Since 1991, the interstitial cells of Cajal (ICCs) have been shown to play at least two important roles in the control of gastrointestinal motility. They are non-neuronal in origin but

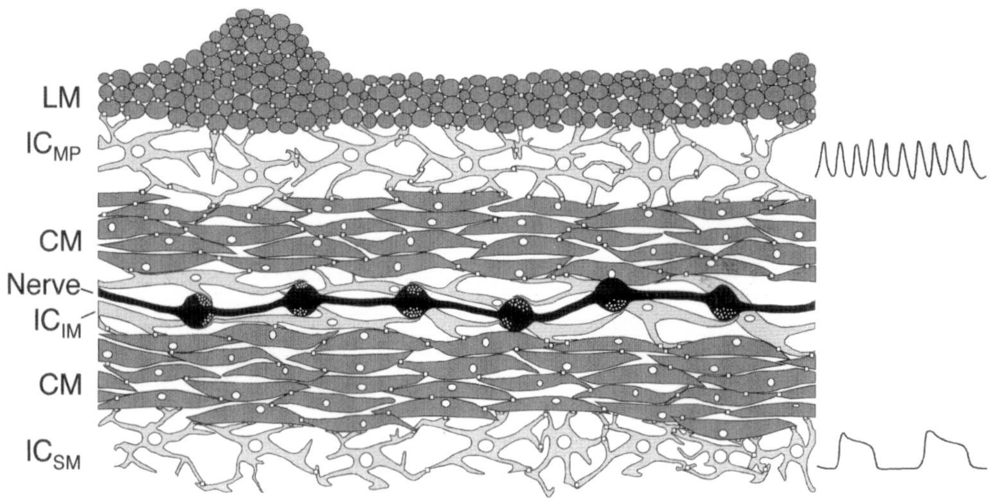

Figure 86–1. Schematic cross section of the muscularis externa of the human colon. The outer longitudinal smooth muscle layer (LM) is thickened at the taenia. In the plane of the myenteric plexus (not shown) is a network of interstitial cells of Cajal (ICCs), which generate a rapid myenteric potential oscillation (IC_{MP}, see wave form on the right). The circular muscle layer (CM) is innervated by axons of enteric motor neurons with transmitter release sites (clusters of clear vesicles) that are associated with specialized intramuscular ICCs (IC_{IM}). At the outer border of the circular muscle is another network of submucosal ICCs, which generate slow waves (IC_{SM}, see wave form on the right). There are also axons of motor neurons in the longitudinal muscles and IC_{IM} (not shown in this cross section). The tiny white squares represent gap junctions.

are derived from common progenitors of smooth muscle. Mutant mice and rats that are deficient in ICCs have profoundly disturbed intestinal motility, an observation that provides insight into the roles of ICCs in the human gastrointestinal tract. In the human colon, there are three types of ICCs, which are named according to their location. There are ICCs in the plane of the myenteric plexus (IC_{MP}), ICCs near the submucosal plexus (IC_{SM}), and intramuscular ICCs located between the circular and longitudinal muscle layers (IC_{IM}). IC_{MP} and IC_{SM} form extensive networks along the colon and are electrically coupled to one another and to the smooth muscle layers by gap junctions (Figs. 86–1 and 86–2). IC_{MP} are probably the pacemakers for the small, rapid (12 to 20/min) oscillations in membrane potential (MPOs) of longitudinal and circular smooth muscle layers. IC_{SM} are the pacemakers for the large amplitude, slow waves (2 to 4/min) originating in the plane of the submucosal plexus; these slow waves have a powerful influence on the patterning of circular muscle contraction. Exactly how IC_{MP} and IC_{SM} give rise to MPOs and slow waves in gastrointestinal smooth muscle is not entirely clear; however, oscillations in membrane potential are an intrinsic property of IC_{MP} and IC_{SM}. Intramuscular ICCs (IC_{IM}) probably play a different role: they are a major target of neurotransmitters released from the axons of excitatory and inhibitory enteric motor neurons. Acetylcholine and nitric oxide (and probably several other motor neuron transmitters) evoke changes in the membrane potential of IC_{IM}, which then spread through the smooth muscle via gap junctions. Some IC_{IM} have been shown to contain nitric oxide synthase and other transmitter-related enzymes and probably amplify the effects of nitric oxide released from motor neurons.

The discovery that cellular mechanisms that were long considered to be the properties of smooth muscle cells are actually mediated by ICCs may have important clinical implications. For example, in the distal bowel, reduced num-

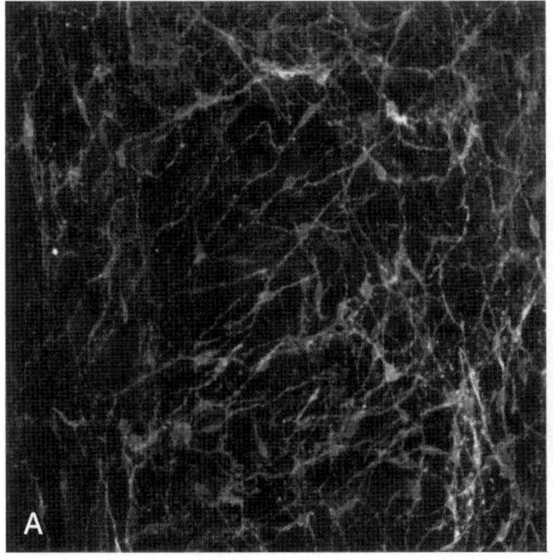

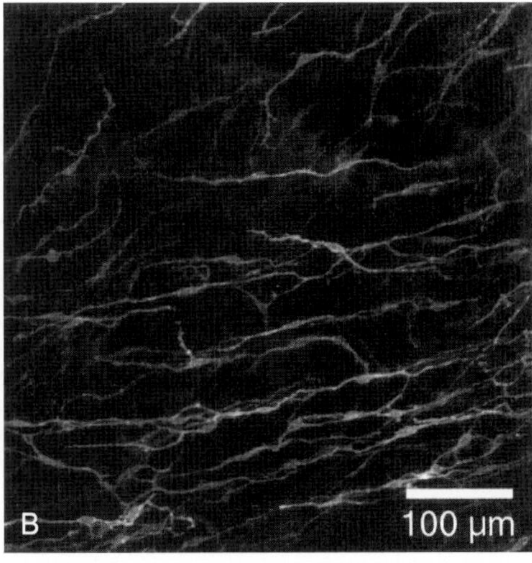

Figure 86–2. Micrographs of interstitial cells of Cajal, labeled by c-kit immunohistochemistry in the human colon. *A,* ICCs in the plane of the myenteric plexus (IC_{IM}) have an irregular shape, form a dense network of cells, and probably function as pacemakers. *B,* A different plane of focus of the same region shows spindle-shaped intramuscular ICCs (IC_{IM}) in the overlying circular muscle layer. These are probably involved in neuromuscular transmission to the smooth muscle. (Images courtesy of Liz Murphy and David Wattchow.)

bers of ICCs, or a reduction in the total volume of ICCs, has been associated with anorectal malformations, colonic manifestations of Chagas' disease, and possibly some cases of slow transit constipation.[3] There have been reports that the density of ICCs may be affected in the aganglionic segments of colon in Hirschsprung's disease, but this finding has not been consistent.[3]

Innervation of the Colon: The Enteric Nervous System

Direct neuronal control of colonic motility is mediated mostly by the enteric nervous system. Although the enteric nervous system is capable of expressing a diverse repertoire of motor patterns, its functions are modulated by sympathetic, parasympathetic, and extrinsic afferent pathways (Fig. 86–3). In terms of numbers of nerve cells, the enteric nervous system is by far the largest component of the autonomic nervous system, with considerably more neurons than the parasympathetic and sympathetic divisions combined. The nerve cell bodies of the enteric nervous system are located in plexuses of myenteric ganglia (Auerbach's plexus), which are located between the longitudinal and circular muscle layers of the muscularis externa, or in the submucosal ganglia, which lie between the circular muscle and mucosa (Fig. 86–4). The submucosal plexus is divisible into at least two networks: Meissner's plexus, which lies closer to the mucosa, and Schabadasch's plexus, which lies adjacent to the circular muscle. Internodal strands that contain hundreds of axons run within and between the different plexuses. Finer nerve trunks innervate the various target tissues of the gut wall, including the longitudinal muscle layer, circular muscle, muscularis mucosa, mucosal crypts, and mucosal epithelium. Within the ganglia of each plexus, different functional classes of enteric nerve cell bodies are randomly mixed. However, there are differences in the proportions of cell types among the plexuses. It has recently become clear that there is an exquisite degree of organization in the enteric nervous system, with each class of nerve cell making highly specific and precise projections to its particular target.

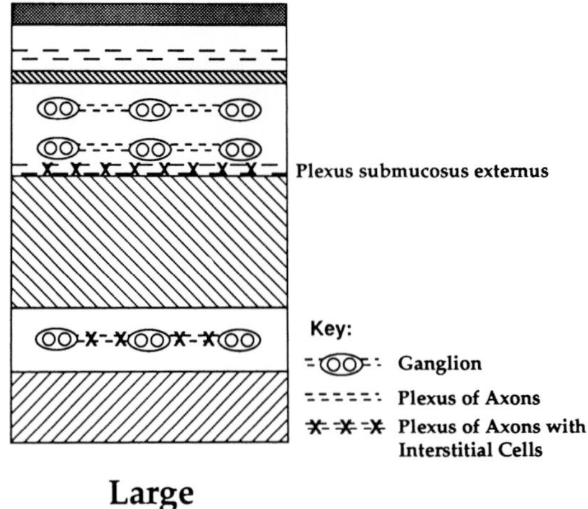

Figure 86–4. Block diagram shows the layers and components of the intestinal wall. The lumen is at the top and the longitudinal muscle layer is at the bottom. The terms at the right identify the plexuses that may be related to the origin of rhythmic activity. The plexus submucosus externus (Stach's plexus) is prominent in the colon. These plexuses contain the interstitial cells of Cajal, the electrical pacemaking system of the gut.

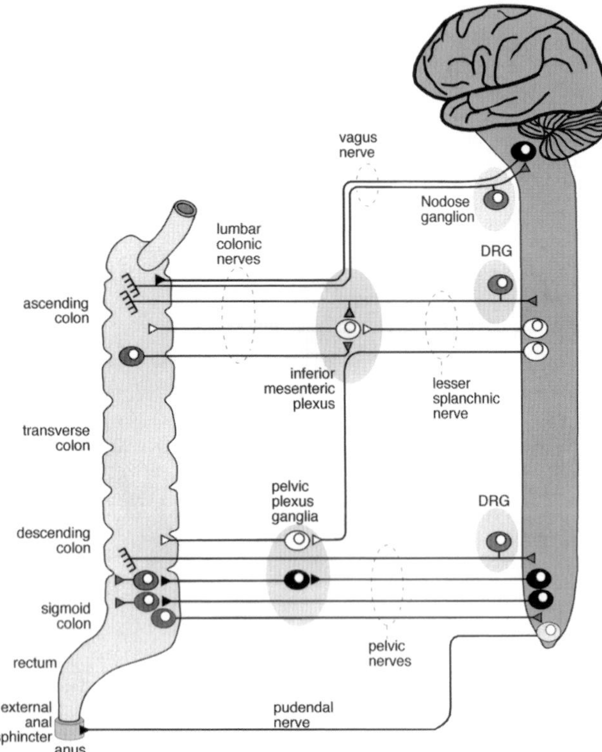

Figure 86–3. The extrinsic innervation of the human colon. Parasympathetic efferent pathways (black cell bodies) arise from the dorsal motor nucleus of the vagus in the brainstem and pass through the vagus nerve and prevertebral sympathetic ganglia to the colon, through the lumbar colonic nerves. There are also parasympathetic pathways from nuclei in the sacral spinal cord that run through the pelvic nerves and either synapse in the pelvic plexus ganglia or run directly into the gut wall. Sympathetic pathways (white cell bodies) consist of preganglionic neurons in the thoracic spinal cord that synapse onto sympathetic postganglionic neurons in either the inferior mesenteric plexus or the pelvic plexus. Enteric nerve cell bodies (located within the colon) receive input from both parasympathetic and sympathetic pathways. Viscerofugal enteric neurons project out of the gut to the prevertebral ganglia. A rectospinal pathway has been described in animal studies, with enteric neurons that project directly to the spinal cord. Afferent pathways consist of vagal afferent neurons from the proximal colon with cell bodies in the nodose ganglion. In addition, spinal afferents with cell bodies in dorsal root ganglia (DRG) run through both the lesser splanchnic and lumbar colonic nerve pathway and via the pelvic nerves. Lastly, the striated muscles of the pelvic floor (including the external anal sphincter) are supplied by motor neurons with cell bodies in the spinal cord and axons that run in the pudendal nerves. Triangles represent transmitter release sites; "combs" represent sensory transduction sites.

Enteric Primary Afferent Neurons

Much of the motor and secretory activity of the gut can be conceptualized as a series of reflexes evoked by mechanical or chemical stimuli. These reflexes involve activation of enteric primary afferent neurons, integration by interneurons, and execution of appropriate responses by motor neurons. The first neurons in these reflex circuits are primary afferent neurons (sometimes called "sensory" neurons, although they do not give rise to conscious sensation). These neurons are located in both myenteric and submucosal plexuses and characteristically have several long axonal processes. Some primary afferents fire action potentials in response to stretch or tension in the gut wall. Others are activated by chemical or mechanical stimuli to the mucosa. These mucosal stimuli probably work, at least in part, by activating specialized entero-endocrine cells in the mucosal epithelium, such as the serotonin-containing enterochromaffin cells. The primary afferent neurons then release synaptic transmitters (acetylcholine or tachykinins or both) to excite other classes of enteric neurons in nearby ganglia. Enteric primary afferent neurons also make excitatory synaptic contacts onto other neurons of their own class, so that they fire in coordinated assemblies.

Enteric Motor Neurons

Enteric motor neurons typically have a smaller cell body than afferent neurons, with a few short dendrites and a single long axon. Separate populations of motor neurons innervate the circular and longitudinal muscle layers. *Excitatory motor neurons* synthesize acetylcholine, which they release from their varicose endings in the smooth muscle layers. In addition, some of them also release the tachykinin peptides, substance P and neurokinin A, which excite smooth muscle. Typically, the axons of excitatory motor neurons project either directly to the smooth muscle close to their cell bodies or orad for up to 10 mm.[4] Once in the smooth muscle layers, the axons turn and run parallel to the smooth muscle fibers for several millimeters; they branch extensively and form many small varicosities, or transmitter release sites, which are associated with intramuscular ICCs (IC_{IM}).

Inhibitory motor neurons are typically slightly larger than excitatory motor neurons but fewer in number. They also have short dendrites and a single axon, but, unlike excitatory motor neurons, they project aborally to the smooth muscle layer for distances of 1 to 15 mm in the human colon.[4] Once the axon reaches the smooth muscle, it branches extensively and forms multiple varicose release sites. Inhibitory motor neurons release a cocktail of transmitters that inhibit smooth muscle cells, including nitric oxide, adenosine triphosphate (ATP), and peptides, such as vasoactive intestinal polypeptide (VIP) and pituitary adenyl cyclase-activating peptide (PACAP). The varicose transmitter release sites of inhibitory motor neurons are also associated with IC_{IM}. There is evidence that inhibitory motor neurons may be tonically active, modulating the ongoing contractile activity of the colonic circular smooth muscle. Inhibitory motor neurons are particularly important in relaxing sphincteric muscles in the ileocecal junction and internal anal sphincter.

Enteric Interneurons

When a region of colon is stimulated, for example by a bolus that distends it, primary afferent neurons are activated. These neurons then activate excitatory and inhibitory motor neurons, which, because of their polarized projections, cause contraction of the muscle orad to the bolus and relaxation aborally. These effects tend to propel the contents aborally. From the new position of the bolus, another set of polarized reflexes is triggered, and peristaltic propulsion results. The *ascending excitatory reflex* and the *descending inhibitory reflex* are sometimes called "the law of the intestine." These reflexes spread farther than predicted by the projections of the excitatory and inhibitory motor neurons, because interneurons are also involved in these reflex pathways. Orally directed, cholinergic interneurons in the human colon run for up to 40 mm and extend the spread of ascending excitatory reflex pathways. There are also several classes of descending interneurons in the human colon that project up to 70 mm anally. Some of these interneurons are involved in spreading descending inhibition along the colon, but others are likely to be involved in the propagation of migratory contractions. In addition to the sensory, inter-, and motor neurons, viscerofugal nerve cells project to the sympathetic prevertebral ganglia, vasomotor neurons innervate blood vessels, and secretomotor neurons stimulate secretion from the colonic epithelium.

Sympathetic Innervation of the Colon

The major sympathetic innervation of the proximal colon arises from the inferior mesenteric ganglion and projects via the lumbar colonic nerves to the ascending and transverse colon (see Fig. 86–3). A small number of sympathetic neurons in the celiac and superior mesenteric ganglia, in the paravertebral chain ganglia, and in the pelvic plexus ganglia also project to the colon (see Fig. 86–3). These neurons receive a powerful cholinergic input from preganglionic nerve cell bodies in the intermedio-lateral column of the spinal cord (segments L2 to L5), which is a major pathway by which the central nervous system modifies gut activity, for example during exercise. They also receive input from the enteric viscerofugal neurons and from extrinsic, spinal sensory neurons with cell bodies in the dorsal root ganglia.

Sympathetic nerve fibers from prevertebral ganglia cause vasoconstriction of the blood vessels in the submucosa and mucosa. Other cells project to the enteric ganglia, where they cause presynaptic inhibition of synaptic activity in the enteric nervous system and thus down-regulate motility. Another target for sympathetic axons is the circuitry of the submucosal plexus involved in controlling epithelial secretion. Hence, these pathways markedly inhibit colonic motor activity, reduce blood flow, and inhibit secretion to limit water loss from the body during times of sympathetic activation. In addition, some sympathetic axons innervate the smooth muscle directly, particularly the ileocecal junction and internal anal sphincter, where they cause contraction. These effects also are consistent with a shutting-down of enteric motor activity during sympathetic arousal.

Parasympathetic Innervation of the Colon

The colon receives parasympathetic innervation from both the vagus nerve and pathways in the sacral spinal cord. Branches of the vagus nerve reach the prevertebral ganglia and then run with sympathetic axons to the ceco-ascending and transverse colon. The distal colon is supplied largely by sacral parasympathetic axons via the pelvic nerves. Some of these axons synapse first onto nerve cell bodies in the pelvic plexus, whereas others project directly to the colon. From their point of entry into the colon, many of the axons run in an orad direction and form thick trunks called *shunt fascicles*. Parasympathetic axons project to the enteric ganglia in the colon where they make excitatory cholinergic synapses onto enteric nerve cell bodies. Sacral parasympathetic pathways play an important role in increasing the propulsive activity of the distal colon prior to defecation.

Extrinsic Afferent Pathways from the Colon

Sensation from the colon is mediated by primary afferent neurons with cell bodies outside the gut wall. Vagal afferent neurons, with nerve cell bodies located in the nodose and jugular ganglia, project to the proximal colon and run with the vagal efferent parasympathetic pathways. Their exact role in reflex control and sensation is not understood, but they are unlikely to be involved in the transmission of pain sensation from the colon.

The entire colon is also innervated by spinal primary afferent neurons with nerve cell bodies in the dorsal root ganglia. Many spinal afferents project via the lumbar splanchnic nerves through the prevertebral ganglia and via the lumbar colonic nerves to the colon, where they terminate in sensory endings in the mesentery, serosa, muscular layers, and mucosa. There also is a population of sacral afferents, with cell bodies in the sacral dorsal root ganglia, that project via the pelvic nerves to the colon and traverse the pelvic plexus en route. Spinal afferents respond to distention of the gut wall, traction of the mesenteric membranes, powerful colonic contractions, or chemical stimulation of the mucosa by bile acids, high osmolarity, and other stimuli. It is well established that the sensitivity of many spinal afferents is increased greatly by inflammation in the gut wall. It is not clear whether there are true, specialized nociceptors, because many spinal afferents have a wide dynamic range and respond in a graded fashion to a spectrum that spans small, nonpainful stimuli to strong aversive stimuli. Hence, it is likely that these neurons give rise to graded sensations ranging from fullness, to urgency, to pain, with increasing distention of the colon or rectum. In addition to their role in sensation, spinal afferents also have axon branches (collaterals) in enteric ganglia and prevertebral sympathetic ganglia and on mucosal blood vessels, where they may play a role in generating peripheral reflex responses to noxious stimuli. However, some spinal afferents do appear to have high thresholds and may function mainly in pain pathways.

RELATIONSHIPS AMONG CELLULAR EVENTS, PRESSURE, AND FLOW

Smooth muscle activation is often divided into two components. The first component is the tonic, ongoing activation that gives smooth muscle its basal resistance to stretch (i.e., its "tone"). Second, there are the dynamic, phasic contractions that mix and propel contents. *Compliance* is a term used to describe the extent to which the gut wall will stretch to accommodate contents. A muscle that is very distensible (for example, because of powerful inhibitory motor neuron activity) has a high compliance. During phasic contractions there is a transient increase in the resistance of the gut wall to stretch (in other words, a decrease in its compliance). If the contents are fluid and there is no downstream resistance to impede flow, the smooth muscle will shorten rapidly. The contents will then be propelled, with a minimal increase in intraluminal pressure. If, on the other hand, there is resistance to forward flow of contents, for example by a lumen-occluding contraction distally, the smooth muscle will not shorten significantly but its tension will increase. This increase in tension will increase intraluminal pressure but will not cause propulsion. In most situations in vivo, smooth muscle contraction causes a mixture of shortening and increased tension.

In light of the complex, dynamic relationship among smooth muscle length and tension, intraluminal pressure, tone, and compliance, it can be difficult to relate complex motility patterns to the cellular events. However, a few features appear to be explicable. The frequency of nonpropagating, mixing, or segmenting contractions of the colon in vivo is often 2 to 4 cycles per minute, similar to the frequency of the spontaneous myogenic slow waves generated by IC_{SM} at the submucosal border of the circular muscle.[1, 5] The timing of these nonpropagating contractions is probably affected relatively little by enteric motor neural activity but is very dependent on the degree of wall distention. In contrast, when excitatory motor neurons are active, contractions evoked by MPOs summate, giving rise to powerful, lumen-occlusive contractions that can last much longer than slow waves and that may propagate along the colon. The process of propagation is controlled both by pathways intrinsic to the enteric neural circuitry and by triggering sequences of polarized reflexes that cause peristaltic propulsion.

REGULATION OF COLONIC FILLING, TRANSPORT, AND DEFECATION

The Colon as a Storage Organ

The region of preferential storage of colonic content is not entirely settled. In 1902, Cannon proposed on the basis of radiologic observations that the proximal colon is the site of storage and mixing, whereas the distal colon acts as a conduit during expulsion. Subsequent studies, however, found no difference in the dwell time for radiopaque markers in the middle, proximal, and distal colon (roughly 11 hours in each). Dietary composition influences regional transit and probably accounts for some discrepancies among studies. On a liquid diet, the right colon empties rapidly (1 to 2 hours), whereas the transverse colon retains isotope for 20 to 40 hours. A solid diet retards transit through the cecum and ascending colon. With a mixed diet, particulate matter and liquids are stored in both the ascending and transverse colon, as suggested by Cannon's earlier radiologic observations.[6]

Regulation of Colonic Filling: The Contribution of the Ileocecal Junction

In humans, the ileocolonic junction (ICJ) regulates colonic filling and prevents colo-ileal reflux in order to avoid contamination of the small bowel by colonic bacteria. In the fasted state, cecal filling is slow and erratic, and ileal chyme is retained in the distal ileum for prolonged periods.[7] The close physical link between the terminal ileum and cecum by the ileocecal ligaments behaves functionally as a valve and is responsible in part for continence of the ICJ. A specialized band of muscle forms a low-pressure tonic sphincter.[8] Prominent 6 cycles-per-minute (cpm) phasic contractions contribute to the regulatory function of the ICJ. Phasic and tonic activity are inhibited concurrently with episodic terminal ileal flow or distention of the ileum, and the tone of the ICJ increases in response to cecal distention.[8] Phase III of the interdigestive motor cycle (IDMC) [or migrating myoelectric complex (MMC)], a motor pattern that occurs every 90 to 120 minutes in the upper gut during fasting (see Chapter 85), does not contribute to ileocecal transit because it rarely reaches the terminal ileum in the human. Most ileal chyme, driven by ileal propagating contractions in synchrony with inhibition of phasic contractions of the ICJ, enters the cecum in a pulsatile fashion within 90 minutes of a meal. Around 30% of the propagating contractions in the ileum are followed closely by propagating pressure waves in the cecum, a finding which suggests that cecal filling is one trigger for colonic propagating pressure waves.

Regulation of Emptying of the Proximal Colon

Emptying of the proximal colon occurs more rapidly when wall tone is increased, for example, by fatty acids, than when the tone is low. The volume and consistency of the contents also affect the rate of emptying and correlate with both stool frequency and weight.[9] Isotonic fluid infused into the proximal colon stimulates proximal colonic emptying, a finding which suggests that distention per se can activate propulsive motor patterns. However, chemical stimulation in the proximal colon triggers propagating contractions much more reliably than does distention alone.[10] Hence, proximal colonic emptying is influenced by a combination of increased wall tone and the initiation of propagating contractions, probably under the influence of both chemical and mechanical factors.

It has been suggested, from animal studies, that "antiperistaltic" waves of contraction occur in the proximal colon and may contribute to the retention of content. Retrograde movement of contents was first demonstrated in the feline proximal colon, and later retrogradely migrating myoelectrical activity was shown to be present. Manometric and electromyographic methods have demonstrated motor patterns in the proximal colon that are propagated in an orad direction, either spontaneously or in response to stimuli. Scintigraphy and time-lapse barium contrast cineradiography suggest that such retrograde movements are infrequent in humans. In addition, retrograde movements probably traverse only short segments and may be prompted by voluntary suppression of defecation.

Regional Variation in Pressure Patterns and Flow

Mass movements, recorded using radiographic techniques, are associated with the movement of stool over long distances. High-amplitude propagating pressure waves are associated with defecation.[11] However, mass movements and defecation are relatively infrequent events. In contrast, movements of colonic contents occur episodically throughout the day; most happen in a step-wise fashion over short distances.[6, 12]

Recently, using a combination of pan-colonic manometry and high-frame-rate scintigraphy, it has become possible to record intraluminal pressure and colonic flow with high temporal resolution. This methodology has identified some of the motor patterns that give rise to propulsion. It has also demonstrated significant differences in motor patterns among the various regions of the colon in terms of prevalence, amplitude, velocity, distance covered, and ability to propel contents (Fig. 86–5).[12] For example, propagating pressure waves originate nearly four times as frequently in the proximal colon as in the distal colon (Fig. 86–5). The mean distance covered by antegrade pressure waves starting in the cecum is 50 cm, compared with only 20 cm for sequences originating in the descending and sigmoid colon. Still, pressure waves arising proximally do not generally propagate beyond the midcolon (Fig. 86–5). It is now clear that slower propagation rates favor the effective propulsion of contents. The conduction velocity of pressure waves increases as the waves migrate caudally (Fig. 86–6). Indeed, such events frequently accelerate to the point of synchronicity, which arrests the progress of contents. In addition, nonpropagating (segmenting) pressure waves make up a higher proportion of activity in the distal colon than in more proximal regions. Thus, most motor activity in the distal colon functions to retard forward flow, perhaps to minimize challenges to continence.

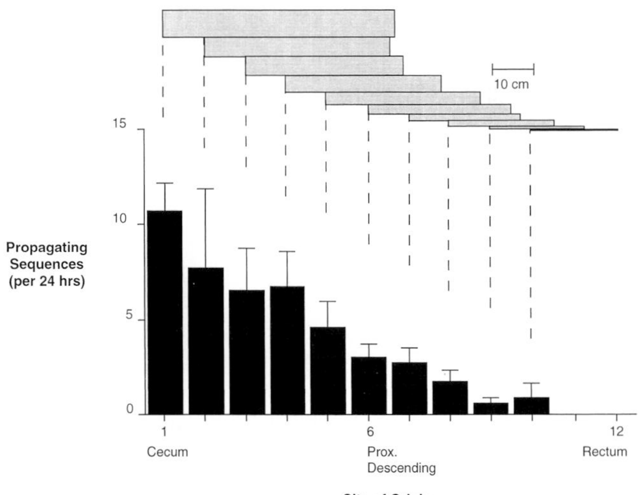

Figure 86–5. Regional variation in the frequency of initiation and extent of propagation of propagating sequences. The histogram at the bottom shows the distribution of antegrade propagating sequences grouped according to the site of origin. The horizontal bars at the top show the mean extent of propagation by sequences originating at the same site. Note that propagating sequences originate significantly more frequently in the proximal colon than more distally. The extent of propagation is much greater for sequences originating in the proximal than the distal colon. The vertical thickness of each horizontal bar at the top is proportional to the propagating sequence frequency shown at the bottom and indicates that the "density" of component pressure waves is highest in the midcolon and lowest in the distal colon. (From Cook IJ, Furukawa Y, Panagopoulos V, et al: Relationships between spatial patterns of colonic pressure and individual movements of content. Am J Physiol 278:G329–G341, 2000.)

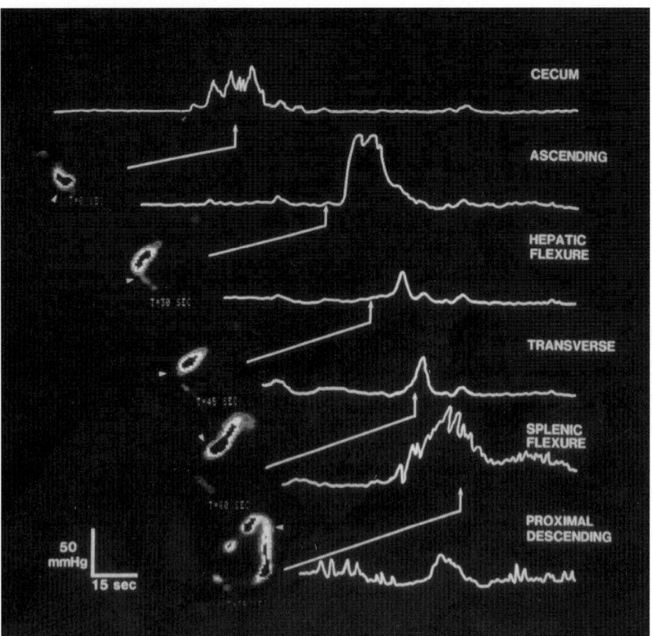

Figure 86–6. Intracolonic pressures and corresponding scintiscans showing a clear correlation between a propagating pressure wave sequence and discrete movement of colonic content from the cecum to the sigmoid colon. This particular movement was associated with neither defecation nor sensation. The vertical arrows (scintiscan images) correspond to the time (horizontal axis) of acquisition of each 15-second scintigraphic frame. Small arrowheads indicate the location of the manometric sidehole from which the corresponding pressure tracing was recorded. In the proximal and midcolon (channels 2 3, and 4 from the top), there is a close temporal relationship between movement of the isotope and the onset of the propagating pressure wave upstroke. When the pressure wave reaches the splenic flexure, however, the entire descending colon is seen to expand to accommodate the isotope, consistent with loss of lumen occlusion at this region. The pressure waves in channels 5 and 6 do not appear to correspond to lumen occluding contractions. Note also that propagating pressure wave amplitudes in channels 3 and 4 are only 30 and 39 mm Hg, respectively, yet the motor pattern is clearly propulsive. (From Cook IJ, Furukawa Y, Panagopoulos V, et al: Relationships between spatial patterns of colonic pressure and individual movements of content. Am J Physiol 278: G329–G341, 2000.)

What Determines Whether a Pressure Wave Is Propulsive?

Approximately one third of episodic movements of colonic content are related to repetitive, nonpropagating pressure waves that move content only short distances in either direction. Another one third of movements of content are attributable to pressure wave sequences that propagate over longer distances (see Fig. 86–6).[12] The remaining one third of episodic movements of content cannot be associated with any measurable changes in intraluminal pressure, according to currently available recording techniques. This finding may reflect the occurrence of contractions at points remote from the recording sites. Alternatively, propulsion may sometimes be caused by motor events that do not affect intraluminal pressure significantly, such as longitudinal muscle shortening, nonlumen-occluding circular muscle contractions, or alterations in regional wall tone.

When propagating pressure wave sequences are detectable, only approximately 40% of them throughout the day actually propel colonic contents. This relative propulsive "inefficiency" may be desirable, by minimizing challenges to continence and retaining content for appropriate times to allow optimal fluid and electrolyte absorption. The question remains as to why some propagating sequences are propulsive and others are not. It appears that a higher pressure wave amplitude and slower conduction velocity favor propulsion (see Fig. 86–6). Sequences recorded proximally have these characteristics, and more than 80% of all propagating sequences originating in the ceco-ascending colon are propulsive. In contrast, only 30% of sequences originating distal to the hepatic flexure propel significant quantities of material.[12]

In summary, the distal colon displays a combination of fewer propagating sequences, shorter extent of propagation, higher conduction velocity, and lower probability of propulsion of content than the proximal colon. In addition, there are more nonpropagating (segmenting) pressure waves in the distal colon than proximally. Considered together, these features would be expected to retard flow into the distal sigmoid and rectum, thus minimizing challenges to continence while maximizing the mixing of content more proximally.

Colonic Function Relating to Defecation

Variations in propagating motor activity along the colon, as just described, would limit or even prevent content from ever reaching the rectum and being expelled. Clearly, additional mechanisms must operate in the colon to facilitate the process of defecation. Traditionally, defecation was conceptualized as an exclusively recto-anal function. However, evidence for the integration of motor activity in the colon with defecation has come from several sources. Radiopaque marker and scintigraphic recordings confirm that the great proportion of the entire colonic content may be evacuated in some cases.[6, 13] Furthermore, pancolonic manometric studies recently have demonstrated that the preparatory phase of defecation not only involves the greater part of the colon, but also commences up to 1 hour before stool expulsion. In this predefecatory phase, there is a characteristic progressive increase in the frequency of propagating pressure wave sequences. These sequences start first in the proximal colon, with each successive sequence originating slightly more distal to the preceding one. These "priming" sequences do not evoke conscious sensation. In contrast, in the 15 minutes leading up to defecation, there is a dramatic increase in the frequency of these propagating sequences, which lead to a strong defecatory urge. In the last 15 minutes of the predefecatory phase, propagating pressure waves begin to originate in the distal colon. However, in this late phase, each successive propagating sequence originates from a site *proximal* to the site of origin of the preceding one. Each sequence also tends to run for a slightly longer distance and has a higher amplitude than the preceding propagating sequence (Fig. 86–7). These final sequences provide potent forces to fill and distend the rectum, thus further heightening the defecatory urge and prompting the expulsive phase in which the anorectum comes into play.

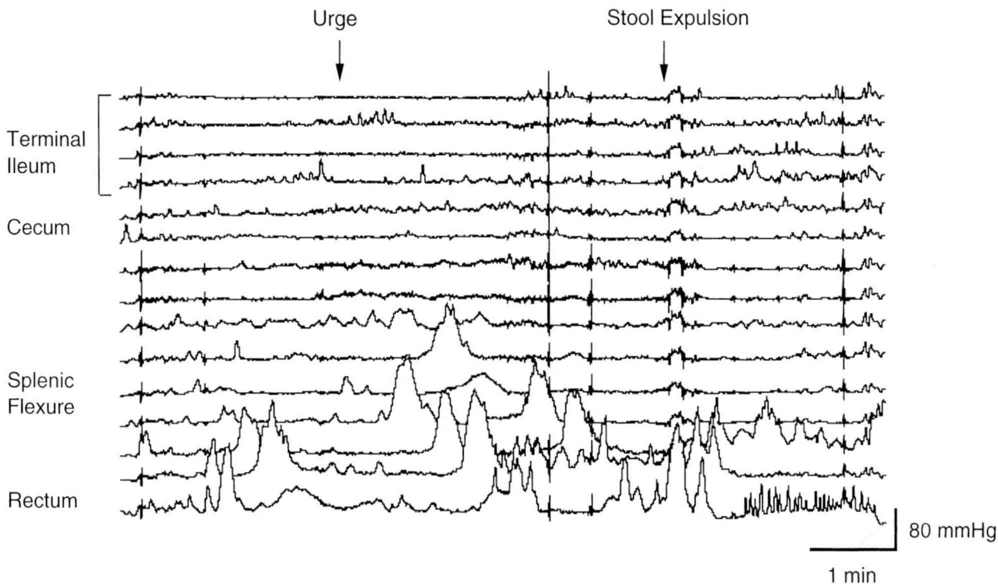

Figure 86–7. Intracolonic pressures leading up to spontaneous defecation by the healthy, unprepared human colon. Recordings were made with a Silastic perfused catheter passed transnasally so that 15 recording sites at 7.5-cm intervals extended from the distal ileum (*top*) to the rectum (*bottom*). There are four propagating pressure wave sequences leading up to actual stool expulsion. Each propagating sequence originates from a site more proximal than the preceding sequence. Note also the increase in amplitude and slowing of propagation velocity with successive sequences leading to stool expulsion, which in this example, is achieved by a combination of voluntary strain and colonic propulsion. (From Bampton PA, Dinning PG, Kennedy ML, et al: Spatial and temporal organization of pressure patterns throughout the unprepared colon during spontaneous defecation. Am J Gastroenterol 95:1027–1035, 2000.)

ANORECTAL MOTILITY

Anorectal Anatomy and Innervation

Before considering anorectal function during defecation, it is necessary to understand the gross morphology of the anorectum. Although the rectum is in direct continuity with the colon, the longitudinal muscle layer is not concentrated in the taenia. Rather, it forms a continuous outer longitudinal muscle layer, uniformly encircling the rectum, insinuating distally between the internal and external anal sphincters, and extending to the distal end of the 3- to 4-cm-long anal canal. The narrowed distal rectum, or anorectal junction, is formed by the sling fibers of the puborectalis muscle, attachments of the levator ani muscles, and proximal margins of the internal and external anal sphincters. The puborectalis and levator ani muscles have important roles in maintaining continence and during defecation. These striated muscles form part of the pelvic floor and are in a state of constant tone that serves to pull the rectum anteriorly and elevate it, thereby reducing the anorectal angle. This mechanical effect tends to prevent entry of stool into the upper anal canal. The internal anal sphincter (IAS) is a thickened band of smooth muscle, with relatively high spontaneous tone, which is in continuity with the circular smooth muscle of the rectum. On the other hand, the external anal sphincter (EAS) is a striated muscle and is located distal to, but partly overlying, the IAS. The EAS also has a high resting tone but, unlike the IAS, can be influenced by voluntary efforts, to help maintain continence.

As expected, the sources of innervation of the internal and external anal sphincters are different. The IAS is innervated extrinsically, via the pelvic plexus, by lumbar sympathetic and sacral parasympathetic nerves and receives a powerful inhibitory innervation from enteric inhibitory motor neurons with cell bodies in the enteric ganglia. The EAS and other pelvic floor muscles are innervated, via the pudendal nerve (S3–S4), by motor neurons with cell bodies in the spinal cord. The rectum and proximal anal canal are richly supplied with sensory receptors that respond to rectal stretch and detect the composition of the contents. These receptors are important for detecting rectal filling, triggering sensations of urgency, facilitating rectal accommodation, and differentiating the composition (stool or gas) of rectal content.

Rectal Filling, Capacitance, and Accommodation and Motility of Anal Sphincters

If stool or gas enters the rectum, the rectal wall is stretched, thereby activating an enteric descending inhibitory reflex that causes relaxation of the IAS. Simultaneously, an extrinsic reflex pathway that leads to contraction of the EAS is also triggered. The rectoanal inhibitory reflex can be tested formally in the laboratory by balloon distention of the rectum. Because the reflex is mediated by intramural enteric neural circuits, its presence reflects the integrity of enteric neural pathways. For example, the rectoanal inhibitory reflex is absent in Hirschsprung's disease, in which there is loss of enteric ganglia in the rectal myenteric plexus. In health, this reflex permits entry of a small amount of content into the upper anal canal, while continence is maintained by the reflexive EAS contraction. This "sampling" of the content by the sensory receptors in the proximal anal canal permits the distinction between solid or liquid stool and gas. "Sampling reflexes" of this kind occur many times each day in response to low-volume rectal distentions, are not registered consciously, and do not cause an urge to defecate. A large-volume rectal distention causes an IAS relaxation of longer duration, which is registered consciously and which necessitates extra voluntary contraction of the EAS to maintain continence, while the person decides how the content (stool or gas) may best be dealt with. Suppression of the defecation urge at this time, together with receptive accommodation of the rectum (see later), results in delayed temporary storage of stool or gas in the rectum or retrograde transport of the stool or gas back to the sigmoid colon.

Although the rectum is generally empty, it has the capacity to temporarily store feces until convenient evacuation can be arranged. More prolonged rectal storage is made possible by the ability of the rectum to accommodate an increasing volume without a corresponding increase in intrarectal pressure, in a manner similar to gastric fundic relaxation.[14] This adaptive increase in rectal compliance, mediated by inhibitory nerves, is important for maintaining continence by permitting prolonged fecal storage without a constant urge to defecate. Such rectal distention also has negative feedback effects on the proximal gut and inhibits gastric emptying, slows small bowel transit, reduces the frequency of proximal colonic propagating pressure waves, and delays colonic transit. Typically, rectal tone is increased following a meal. A pathologic loss of rectal compliance, as seen, for example, after pelvic radiotherapy, causes rectal urgency. Conversely, excessive compliance, as in megarectum, attenuates the urge to defecate.

Anorectal Motility During Defecation

If the processes just described give rise to the urge to defecate and the social circumstances are appropriate, the full defecation process is activated. This process involves a combination of pelvic reflexes coordinated in the medulla and pons. Rectal distention by a large volume of stool in the rectum stimulates reflex relaxation of the IAS, and the stool moves into the upper anal canal and heightens the sense of urge. Postural changes and straining facilitate this process in several ways: sitting or squatting causes descent of the anorectal junction, and straining causes further rectal descent. Both activities serve to increase the anorectal angle and reduce resistance to outflow. At this point, if the person

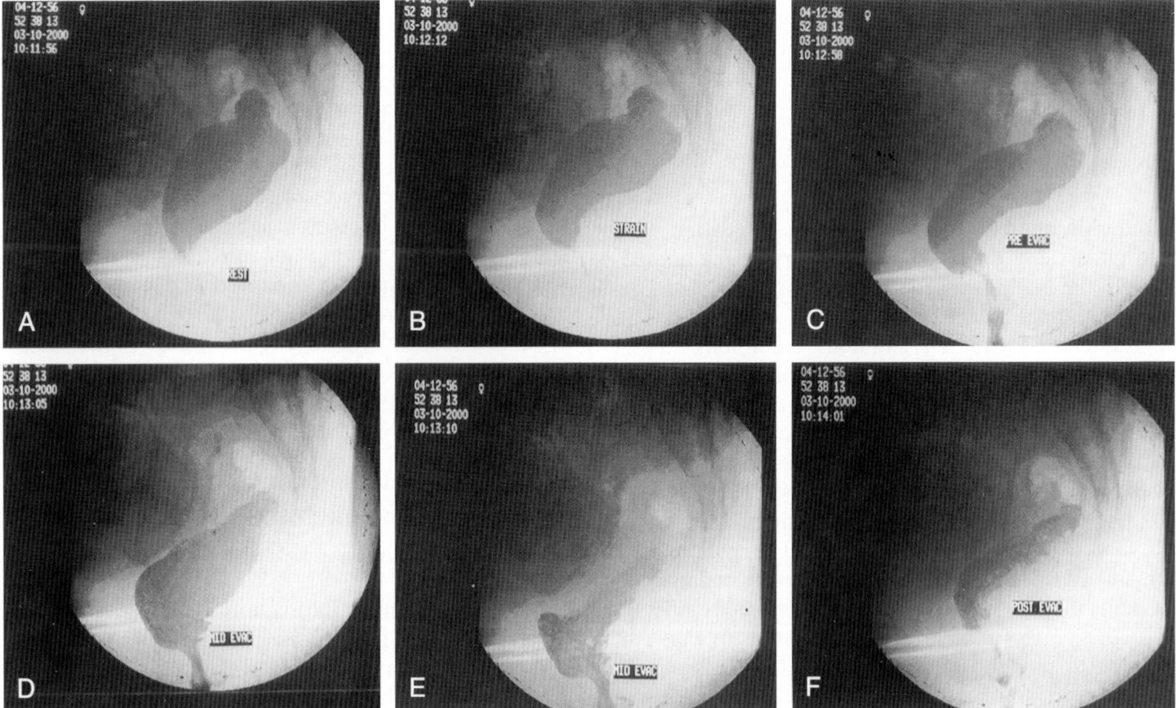

Figure 86–8. Sequential radiographs of simulated defecation of thickened barium during defecation proctography illustrating some of the mechanical processes that facilitate stool expulsion. *A,* The rectum at rest with a normal resting angle of around 90 degrees and the anal canal is closed. *B,* On straining, as the anterior rectal wall begins to flatten, the proximal anal canal begins to funnel as contrast is forced into it. *C,* As more pressure is exerted, the anterior rectal wall is seen to flatten further, contrast fills the anal canal, and evacuation begins. At this time, the puborectalis muscle and external anal sphincter are relaxing, resulting in the onset of descent of the rectoanal junction. At the same time, the levator ani muscles are activated and help control the descent of the rectoanal junction (e.g., note posterior indentation due to pubococcygeus muscle contraction). *D,* The puborectalis is fully relaxed and, in combination with vigorous straining, descent of the rectoanal junction is nearly complete. Note the position of the rectoanal junction, which in this frame is well below the horizontal pale artifact (due to the water-filled toilet seat) compared with the previous frame, in which the junction was level with this artifact. Note that this descent has now opened up the anorectal angle, thereby reducing further the resistance outflow through the anal canal. *E,* Rectal emptying continues and anterior rectal compression is more obvious. *F,* Postevacuation, note the anorectal junction has now ascended to its original position and the anorectal angle returns to its more acute resting angle. (Images courtesy of Dr D. Z. Lubowski.)

wishes to proceed to expel stool, the EAS is relaxed voluntarily. At the same time, the puborectalis muscle is relaxed (further increasing the anorectal angle); the levator ani muscles contract; the perineum descends further; and stool is funneled into the anal canal and expelled by increasing strain-induced, intrarectal pressure (Fig. 86–8). Once the expulsion phase has commenced, evacuation of stool can proceed in some cases without further straining, as a consequence of the anally propagating colonic contractions (see Fig. 86–7).[15] However, expulsion of stool is possible in response to strain alone without rectosigmoid contractions, although a contribution from increased rectal wall tone cannot be excluded.

MODULATORS OF COLONIC MOTILITY

Physiologic Modulators: Food, Sleep, and Stress

Twenty-four hour recordings of myoelectrical activity or intraluminal pressure show that colonic phasic and tonic activity is predictably increased 1 to 2 hours after a meal (the "gastrocolonic" response) and markedly suppressed at night.[11, 16, 17] It is interesting that a minimum caloric load of around 300 kcal is required to generate the colonic response to a meal,[16] and the response also is highly dependent on the fat content of the caloric load. For example, 600 kcal of fat induces the response, whereas equicaloric loads of protein or carbohydrate do not. The entire colon responds to the meal, and there is an increase in colonic wall tone, migratory long spike bursts, and propagating and segmenting contractile patterns. The mechanism of the response to the meal remains unclear. Non-nutrient gastric distention, by balloon or water, can stimulate rectosigmoid motility.[18] However, neither the stomach nor the spinal cord need to be intact to display the response. Moreover, infusion of lipid into the duodenum will also induce the response.[18] It has been suggested that hormones released during the meal may be involved. Cholecystokinin (CCK), which is released by fats and fatty acids in the duodenum, can reproduce the gastrocolonic response but only at doses exceeding those occurring postprandially. In addition, the CCK-A antagonist loxiglumide blocks the effects of CCK on the colon but does not abolish the gastrocolonic response, thus making CCK an unlikely mediator of the response.

Colonic myoelectrical and pressure activity is profoundly suppressed at night.[11, 16, 17] During stable sleep, propagating pressure waves virtually cease, thereby reducing the challenges to continence at a time when anal sphincter tone and awareness of colorectal sensations are minimal. If the subject moves to a lighter level of sleep, even without actually waking up, there is an immediate increase in propagating and nonpropagating pressure waves (Fig. 86–9). Forced waking at night and spontaneous early morning waking both stimulate an immediate increase in colonic propagating pressure waves.[11, 17] This phenomenon is clearly linked with the readily identifiable habit of defecation soon after awakening in the morning and demonstrates the potential for profound modulation of colonic motor activity by the central nervous system. Stress and emotional factors have long been assumed to influence colonic motility, but currently evidence for this influence is conflicting, possibly because of reliance on distal colonic recording sites. In light of the profound waking response, it is likely, but unproven, that stress induces propagating pressure waves.

Pharmacologic Modulators

Laxatives exert their diarrheal action by increasing mucosal secretion or stimulating colonic propulsive activity. For ex-

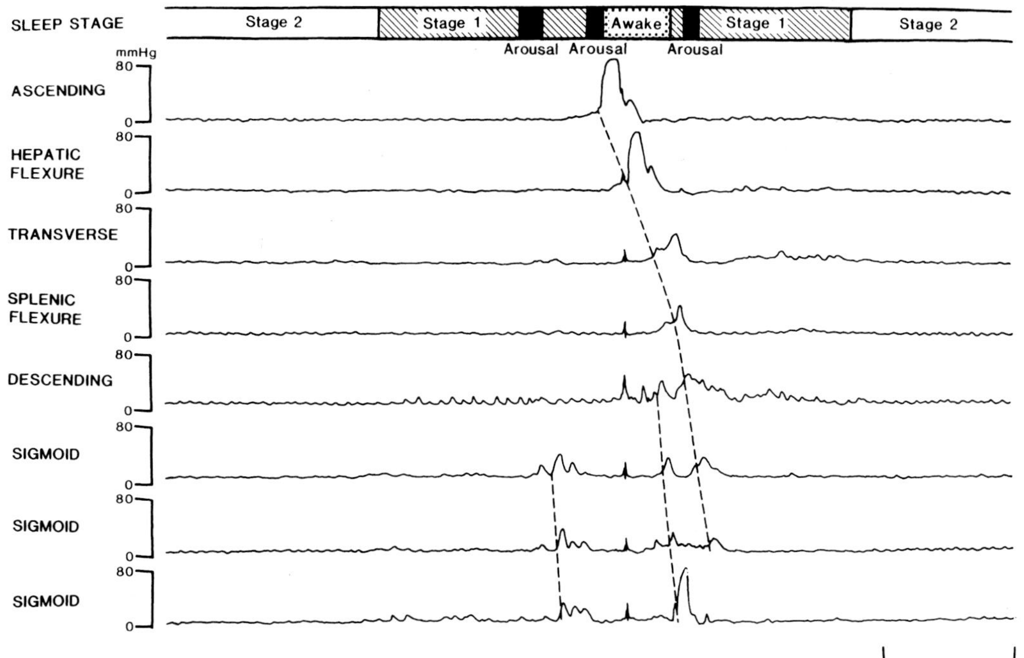

Figure 86–9. Relationship of propagating pressure wave sequences to nocturnal arousals. An arousal represents a lightening of the level of sleep, which need not necessarily culminate in waking. This example demonstrates an arousal-induced event propagating from the proximal to distal sigmoid colon followed by another arousal-induced event propagating from the ascending colon to the sigmoid. Only the second arousal culminated in a brief period of wakefulness. Repetitive propagating sequences of this type are seen also on early morning waking. (From Furukawa Y, Cook IJ, Panagopoulos V, McEvoy RD, Sharp DJ, Simula M. Relationship between sleep patterns and human colonic motor patterns. Gastroenterology 107: 1372–1381, 1994.)

ample, the irritant laxative bisacodyl and the bile acid chenodeoxycholic acid both stimulate colonic propagating sequences, thereby leading to mass movements. Bisacodyl exerts its motor effect via afferent nerve fibers in the mucosa, because the response can be blocked by topical application of lidocaine to the mucosa. In addition to the local response, these agents, when administered rectally, also can induce an increase in motor activity in the proximal colon, a finding that indicates the existence of long reflex pathways between the rectum and proximal colon. A newer class of colonic prokinetic agonists at 5-hydroxytryptamine$_4$ ($5HT_4$) receptors have shown promise in the treatment of constipation. The $5HT_4$ agonists accelerate colonic transit by inducing propagating contractions.[19]

Opiates are well known to have an antidiarrheal effect, but their mechanism of action is less clear. In the human colon in vivo, morphine increases phasic segmenting activity, which is likely to retard flow, and may promote mixing and enhance absorption. Barostat studies have shown that morphine also reduces colonic tone and attenuates the response to a meal.[20] Opiates are known to cause both presynaptic and postsynaptic inhibition of enteric neural circuitry. Therefore, it seems likely that these drugs reduce neurally dependent propagating contractions and favor myogenic mixing movements; both effects contribute to the constipating effect.

DISORDERS OF COLONIC MOTILITY

Disorders attributable to disturbed colonic motor function are discussed elsewhere in this textbook. It is useful, however, to consider how disturbances in the mechanisms of colonic motility described in this chapter may relate to symptoms or pathophysiologic phenomena.

Constipation (See Chapter 12)

Intuitively, one would expect that constipation and diarrhea should be manifestations of hypomotility and hypermotility, respectively. Sometimes this is true, but in the distal colon, at least, the converse may be true. A paradoxical increase in nonpropagating (segmenting) contractions and myoelectrical short spike bursts has been reported in the rectosigmoid region of constipated patients. Conversely, patients with diarrhea have hypomotility in this region.[21] It is likely that segmenting activity retards forward flow, whereas suppression of such activity permits unrestricted access of stool to the rectum, where a defecatory urge is initiated. Thus, constipation may be a consequence either of infrequent or ineffective propagating pressure waves or of an increase in segmenting distal colonic pressure waves, or perhaps both. Prolonged manometric studies of the mid- and distal colon of patients with severe constipation have confirmed a reduction in the overall number of high-amplitude propagating pressure waves. The underlying pathogenesis of severe slow transit constipation is unclear, but changes in the populations of enteric excitatory motor neurons to the smooth muscle in patients with severe slow transit constipation have been described.[22]

Diarrhea (See Chapter 9)

Detailed scintigraphic studies in patients with diarrhea have shown the dominant feature to be early and rapid transit through the ascending and transverse colon.[23] Normally, propagating sequences are more frequent in these proximal regions than elsewhere. There is a surprising lack of manometric data from the entire colon in patients with diarrhea to help explain these observations. A relative lack of distal colonic segmenting activity, perhaps in combination with increased proximal colonic propagating pressure waves, may explain this preferential acceleration of proximal colonic transit, but proof of this hypothesis is awaited.

Irritable Bowel Syndrome (See Chapter 91)

Although colonic transit is generally slower in constipation-predominant irritable bowel syndrome (IBS) and faster in diarrhea-predominant IBS, no colonic motor pattern is specific for IBS. Exaggerated responses to stimuli such as meals, CCK, and mechanical stimuli have been reported, but a consistent disturbance has not emerged, probably because of the heterogeneity of the disease and the methodologies used. In addition, there has been remarkably little study to date of the proximal colon in IBS. At present, compelling evidence suggests a major contribution by afferent hypersensitivity, in addition to a variable alteration in colonic motor function, in the pathophysiology of IBS.

Colonic Motility Disturbances Secondary to Nonmotor Disorders

Altered motility secondary to underlying inflammation or a hormonal disturbance can contribute to the colonic symptoms of an underlying disease. The diarrhea of idiopathic inflammatory bowel disease, for example, results from a combination of enhanced secretion, reduced absorption, and altered colonic motor function. In ulcerative colitis, rectosigmoid-segmenting, nonpropagating pressure waves are diminished, whereas postprandial propagating pressure waves are increased.[6] Rectal compliance is also reduced, and together, these effects may exacerbate diarrhea, as suggested by rapid rectosigmoid transit in ulcerative colitis. The motility of the healthy colon also can be perturbed by ileal diseases. For example, exposure of the healthy proximal colon to supranormal concentrations of bile salts (resulting, for example, from terminal ileal disease or resection) not only stimulates net colonic secretion but also initiates high-amplitude propagating pressure waves, thus accelerating colonic transit.

REFERENCES

1. Rae MG, Fleming N, McGregor DB, et al: Control of motility patterns in the human colonic circular muscle layer by pacemaker activity. J Physiol 510(Pt 1):309–320, 1998.
2. Farrugia G: Ionic conductances in gastrointestinal smooth muscles and interstitial cells of Cajal. Annu Rev Physiol 61:45–84, 1999.
3. Sanders KM, Ordog T, Torihashi S, Ward SM: Development and plasticity of interstitial cells of Cajal. Neurogastroenterol Motil 11:311–338, 1999.

4. Porter AJ, Wattchow DA, Brookes SJ, Costa M: The neurochemical coding and projections of circular muscle motor neurons in the human colon. Gastroenterology 113:1916–1923, 1997.
5. Sarna SK: Physiology and pathophysiology of colonic motor activity: Part 1. Dig Dis Sci 36:827–862, 1991.
6. O'Brien MD, Phillips SF: Colonic motility in health and disease. Gastroenterol Clin North Am 25:147–162, 1996.
7. Spiller RC, Brown ML, Phillips SF: Emptying of the terminal ileum in intact humans. Influence of meal residue and ileal motility. Gastroenterology 92:724–729, 1987.
8. Dinning PG, Bampton PA, Kennedy ML, et al: Basal pressure patterns and reflexive motor responses in the human ileocolonic junction. Am J Physiol 276:G331–G340, 1999.
9. Hammer J, Phillips SF: Fluid loading of the human colon: Effects on segmental transit and stool composition. Gastroenterology 105:988–998, 1993.
10. Hardcastle JD, Mann CV: Physical factors in the stimulation of colonic peristalsis. Gut 11:41–46, 1970.
11. Bassotti G, Crowell MD, Whitehead WE: Contractile activity of the human colon: Lessons from 24-hour studies. Gut 34:129–133, 1993.
12. Cook IJ, Furukawa Y, Panagopoulos V, et al: Relationships between spatial patterns of colonic pressure and individual movements of content. Am J Physiol 278:G329–G341, 2000.
13. Lubowski DZ, Meagher AP, Smart RC, Butler SP: Scintigraphic assessment of colonic function during defecation. Int J Colorect Dis 10:91–93, 1995.
14. Bell AM, Pemberton JH, Hanson RB, Zinsmeister AR: Variations in muscle tone of the human rectum: Recordings with an electromechanical barostat. Am J Physiol 260:G17–G25, 1991.
15. Bampton PA, Dinning PG, Kennedy ML, et al: Spatial and temporal organization of pressure patterns throughout the unprepared colon during spontaneous defecation. Am J Gastroenterol 95:1027–1035, 2000.
16. Frexinos J, Bueno L, Fioramonti J: Diurnal changes in myoelectric spiking activity of the human colon. Gastroenterology 88:1104–1110, 1985.
17. Furukawa Y, Cook IJ, Panagopoulos V, et al: Relationship between sleep patterns and human colonic motor patterns. Gastroenterology 107: 1372–1381, 1994.
18. Wiley J, Tatum D, Keinath R, Owyang C: Participation of gastric mechanoreceptors and intestinal chemoreceptors in the gastrocolonic response. Gastroenterology 94:1144–1149, 1988.
19. Grider JR, Foxx-Orenstein AE, Jin J-G: 5-Hydroxytryptamine$_4$ receptor agonists initiate the peristaltic reflex in human, rat and guinea pig intestine. Gastroenterology 115:370–380, 1998.
20. Kamath PS, Phillips SF, O'Connor MK, et al: Colonic capacitance and transit in man: Modulation by luminal contents and drugs. Gut 31:443–449, 1990.
21. Connell AM: The motility of the pelvic colon. II. Paradoxical motility in diarrhoea and constipation. Gut 3:342–348, 1962.
22. Porter AJ, Wattchow DA, Hunter A, Costa M: Abnormalities of nerve fibres in the circular muscle of patients with slow transit constipation. Int J Colorect Dis 13:208–216, 1998.
23. Vassallo MJ, Camilleri M, Phillips SF, et al: Transit through the proximal colon influences stool weight in the irritable bowel syndrome. Gastroenterology 102:102–108, 1992.

Chapter 87

Intestinal Electrolyte Absorption and Secretion

Joseph H. Sellin, MD

The gut is challenged on a daily basis to transform an intake highly variable in volume and composition into a manageable pool of fluid from which it extracts nutrients, minerals, and water; excludes bacteria and potentially harmful antigens; and excretes waste. It predictably reduces an input of 8 to 9 L, primarily of endogenous origins, by 98% to 100 to 200 mL/day. This is accomplished through an elaborate array of pathways that the small intestine and colon have developed (Fig. 87–1). These transport pathways represent the traffic routes that ions and nutrients necessarily follow. The traffic is regulated by several different agonists, including neurotransmitters, hormones, inflammatory mediators, and intraluminal contents. Normally this traffic runs smoothly, but occasionally the regulation goes awry, as may occur with an enteric infection, and diarrhea results.

In this chapter we review the cellular mechanisms involved in the intestinal trafficking of ions and solutes, the regional differences in transport, the intracellular and extracellular regulators of transport, and the events involved in aberrant transport leading to diarrhea. An understanding of these processes is critical to an appreciation of normal intestinal function, the pathophysiology of a host of intestinal abnormalities, and the development of diagnostic and therapeutic strategies for specific diseases.

OVERVIEW OF INTESTINAL ELECTROLYTE TRAFFIC

The intestines are one of several transport epithelia that are capable of bulk transport of fluid across a membrane. These transport epithelia share common properties: a polarity of membranes with distinct apical (luminal) and basolateral (serosal) membranes demarcated by tight junctions joining one cell to the next; a sodium (Na) pump (ouabain-inhibitable Na, K-ATPase) located on the basolateral membrane, exchanging intracellular Na for extracellular potassium (K); and a characteristic electrochemical potential profile, in which the intracellular potential difference is negative and the intracellular Na concentration is low compared with the extracellular environment (Fig. 87–2). These common properties provide an initial framework for understanding the basic mechanisms of ion and water transport that apply to all epithelia. The distinct characteristics of a particular segment of intestine are determined by what additional factors may be added to the apical or basolateral membrane or to the tight junctions (e.g., pumps, channels, carriers, etc.).

Molecular Biology and Intestinal Transport

Much of the recent focus of research in gastrointestinal transport has involved use of molecular biology to identify specific genes and gene products involved in ion transport. With this level of identification, characterization of transport involves localization and measurement of changes in specific molecules in addition to the classic descriptions of the underlying biophysical characteristics of the specific transporter. However, identification of a gene or molecule does not, in and of itself, necessarily answer the relevant physiologic and clinical questions. Thus, molecular biology has sometimes advanced our understanding but at other times has raised new issues, or sharpened the questions that still need to be asked.

Molecular approaches can provide insight into rare genetic diseases such as glucose-galactose malabsorption in which mutations of a specific carrier protein, SGLT1, can now be identified. However, even in cystic fibrosis, identifi-

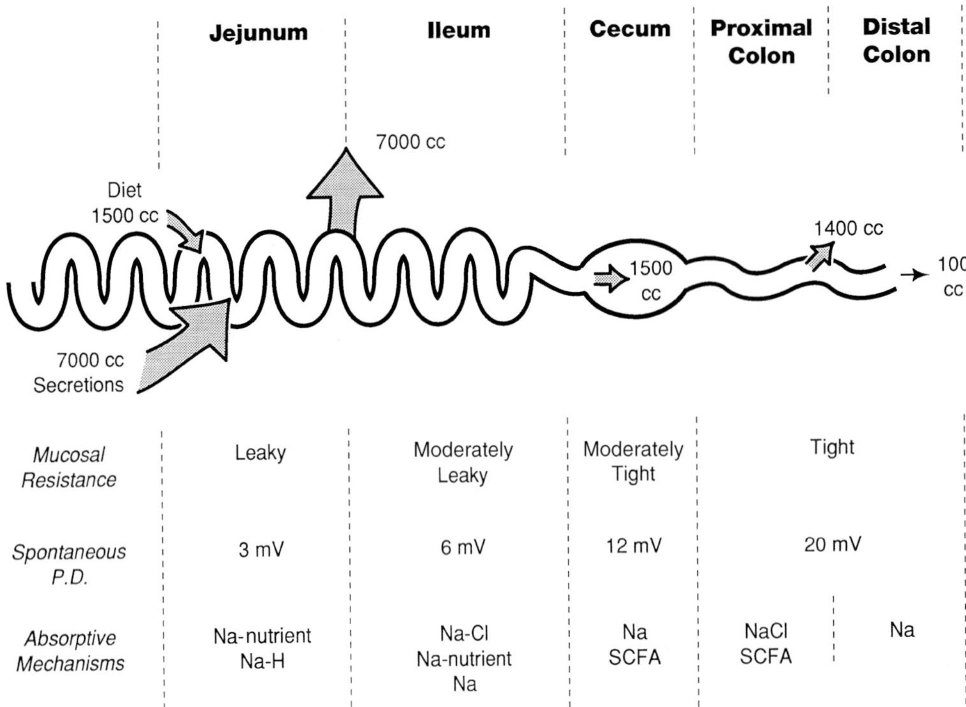

Figure 87–1. Overview of intestinal fluid balance. Eight to nine liters of fluid flow into the intestine. Salivary, gastric, biliary, pancreatic, and intestinal secretions make up the bulk of this amount. Most intestinal fluid is absorbed in the small bowel, with approximately 1500 mL of fluid crossing the ileocecal valve. The colon extracts most of this fluid, leaving 100 to 200 mL of still water daily. As one progresses down the intestine, it becomes progressively "tighter." Spontaneous potential difference measured in vitro demonstrates a corresponding rise. Absorptive mechanisms in each segment of the gut differ, whereas chloride secretion is found throughout the intestine.

cation and characterization of the abnormal gene (*CFTR*) and gene product have not necessarily answered how chloride (Cl) channels work but rather have opened up new questions concerning intracellular trafficking and regulation. Cloning and structural analysis can identify similarities between seemingly disparate biologic activities, such as has occurred with Na channels. Occasionally, molecular techniques leapfrog physiology, and investigators find themselves with transport molecules in search of a clear biologic function. Identification of specific transport molecules necessarily leads to more physiologic issues of function and regulation.

Segmental Heterogeneity of Transport

Different regions of the gut exhibit a different array of transporters (see Fig. 87–1). Some of these have long been recognized, such as the difference between jejunum and distal colon, whereas others have only been appreciated more recently. It is now apparent that the cecum, proximal colon, and distal colon exhibit distinctly different transporters.[1–4] The difference in transport characteristics is indicative of diverse physiologic function and, perhaps, pathophysiologic response. For example, the glucose and amino acid–coupled transporters in the jejunum are well suited for absorption of large volumes of nutrients and water. Electrogenic Na absorption in the distal colon accomplishes the necessary fluid extraction in preparation of feces. In other instances, although we may recognize the differences in transport pathways, the differences in function are not as clear (e.g., variations in intestinal bicarbonate transport or mechanisms of colonic Na absorption).

Segmental differences have also been noted along the crypt-villus axis in the small intestine and the crypt-surface axis in the colon. As epithelial cells migrate away from the proliferative zone, several important changes occur. The complexity of the tight junctions increases. There are changes in cytoskeletal-associated proteins and protein kinase C isozymes.[5, 6] The levels of some transport-associated proteins remain relatively constant (e.g., Na pump), but there is increased expression of several additional transporters associated with absorption. Na-nutrient–coupled transporters and apical Na-H exchangers are present primarily in mature villus cells but absent from crypt cells.[7, 8] One exception is the cyclic AMP-associated Cl channel, cystic fibrosis transmembrane regulator (CFTR), which tends to decrease in more mature cells. The same agonist may elicit different responses from similar transporters, depending on their position along the crypt-villus axis.[9]

This spatial distribution of these transporters (Fig. 87–3) is consistent with a model in which secretory function resides primarily in the crypts and absorption occurs in villus or surface cells. However, this dichotomy between absorptive surface cells and secretory crypt cells is far from absolute.[10] Colonic crypts absorb Na and fluid and surface cells secrete Cl.[11–13] Changes in the rates of maturation and migration may alter the distribution of transporters along the crypt-villus axis and account for some of the changes in transport function seen in various clinical settings.

Basic Epithelial Cell Model

A fundamental characteristic of epithelial cells is distinct apical and basolateral membranes separated by intercellular junctions. Although there are differences in the lipid composition, the most important feature distinguishing these membrane domains is the sorting of proteins specifically to either the apical or basolateral pole of the cell. The factors controlling the traffic of membrane proteins within the cell are only partially understood. In some cases, a particular structural component of the protein determines its destination; proteins with a glycerophosphoinosital anchor (e.g., alkaline phosphatase or carcinoembryonic antigen) are directed toward the

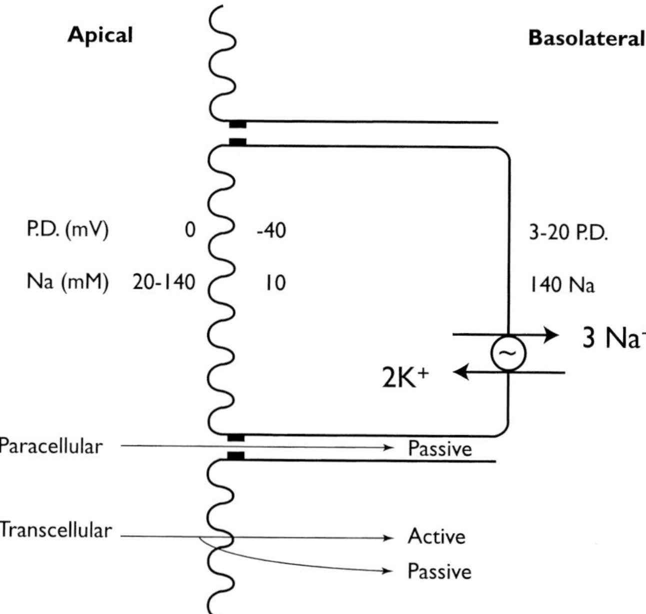

Figure 87–2. Basic cell model. Intestinal epithelial cells have several design characteristics that make them particularly adept at vectorial transport. (1) The cell membrane is divided into distinct apical and basolateral zones by the tight junctions; the asymmetric distribution of transporters in these two membranes promotes vectorial transport; (2) there is a characteristic electrochemical profile across the epithelium that permits "downhill" entry of sodium into the cell from either the apical or basolateral side (not shown); (3) the sodium pump on the basolateral membrane is integral to maintaining the electrochemical profile, exchanging 3 intracellular Na^+ for 2 extracellular K^+; (4) water and solutes can cross the epithelium either around the cell (paracellular) or through the cell (transcellular).

apical membrane. In other instances, proteins may at first randomly insert into either apical or basolateral domains but then may be retained in the basolateral pole by specific membrane components such as ankyrin.[14] Cytoskeletal elements may serve as tracks directing membrane proteins to their eventual destination. Regulation of intracellular trafficking to ensure delivery of the right protein to the right membrane is obviously critical for establishing polarized epithelia and vectorial transport.

The cell interior maintains a low intracellular concentration of Na due to the activity of the Na pump on the basolateral membrane (see Fig. 87–2). The interior of the cell is characteristically electronegative compared with both the mucosal and serosal borders because the Na pump is electrogenic, extruding three Na ions in exchange for two K ions; there is a greater membrane permeability for K over Na that favors diffusional potassium exit from the cell over Na entry; and there are a large number of intracellular proteins with fixed negative charges.

These two basic features of the epithelial cell interior (low [Na] and electronegativity) establish a favorable electrochemical gradient for passive Na entry into the cell. This "downhill" movement of Na into the cell is pivotal for most absorptive and secretory processes. This obviously relates to mechanisms for Na transport, but, more generally, it applies to other ions and solutes that harness the energy of the Na gradient to enter the cell either across the apical or basolateral membrane.

Movement across the Epithelium

Ions and solute may cross the epithelium by either active or passive transport. Passive transport of uncharged solutes may occur through diffusion or convection (solvent drag); diffusion of an uncharged particle is determined solely by differences in concentration across a membrane. Passive movement of ions is determined by concentration gradients and additionally by the electrical potential difference across a membrane. Thus, ions move passively in response to an *electrochemical gradient* rather than a simple concentration gradient. Because epithelial cells exhibit a negative intracellular voltage compared with either the apical or basolateral bathing solutions, this favors the entry of cations into the cell and the exit of anions from the cell. This negative membrane potential may lead to the curious situation in which ions move passively against their concentration gradient.

Gradients are established across the epithelium in two ways. Quite obviously, the characteristics of ingested food and liquid are different from plasma; thus, the upper reaches of the gut are exposed to large concentration differences between lumen and plasma. Second, active transport may establish chemical and electrical gradients across the epithelium. Active transport is the net movement of a solute or ion in the absence of or against an electrochemical gradient. Active transport necessarily requires the expenditure of energy that in the gut is linked to the hydrolysis of ATP. In both the small bowel and the colon, the serosa is electropositive compared with the mucosal border. In general, this can be ascribed either to the absorption of cations (Na, K) or to the secretion of anions (Cl, HCO_3).

Active transport is always through cells (transcellular) because it requires the expenditure of energy. Passive transport may either be transcellular or occur around cells, through their tight junctions (paracellular). The presence of a gradient by itself does not ensure effective movement of a solute or ion because the cell membrane and tight junction both present barriers to diffusion. The lipid bilayer of the cell membrane precludes simple passive diffusion of ions and

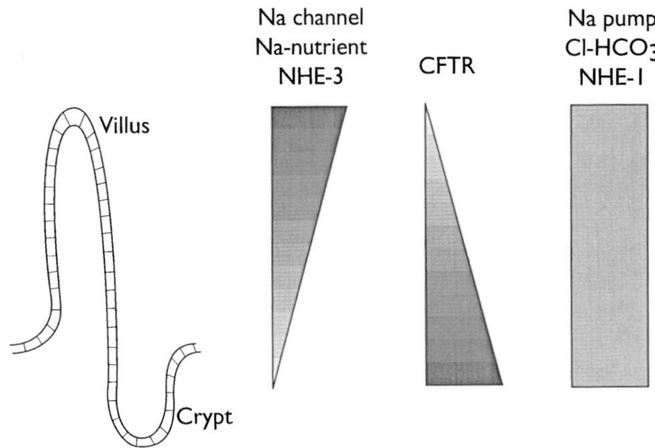

Figure 87–3. Gradients from crypt to villus. There is a significant spatial geometry of transport proteins along the crypt-villus (crypt-surface) axis. Some transport molecules are found at relatively constant concentrations along the axis, some exhibit a greater density in the base of the crypt, and others exhibit a greater density toward the villus or surface.

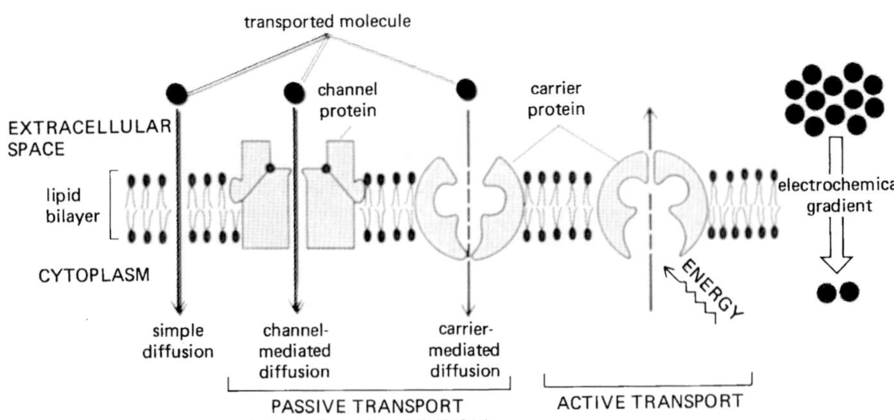

Figure 87–4. Channels, carriers, and pumps. Because only nonpolar molecules freely cross the lipid domain of the membrane by simple diffusion, transfer of ions and charged molecules necessitates specific transmembrane proteins to modulate entry and exit. Ion specific channels mediate membrane transport through passive electrodiffusion. Carriers permit facilitated diffusion. Active transport occurs against an electrochemical gradient and requires input of metabolic energy. (From Pedley KC, Naftalin RJ: Evidence from fluorescence microscopy and comparative studies that rat, ovine and bovine colonic crypts are absorptive. J Physiol [Lond] 460:525–547, 1993; originally published in Alberts B, Bray D, Lewis J, et al. [eds]: Molecular Biology of the Cell, 2nd ed. New York and London, Garland Publishing, 1983, p. 303.)

large molecules into the cell. The movement of ions and solutes into the cell is controlled by specialized membrane proteins, termed channels, carriers, and pumps. The specific characteristics of the tight junctions within a segment of the gut will, in large part, determine the relative contribution of paracellular fluxes to overall transport (see following discussion).

Water moves across epithelia passively. How exactly water gets across the gut has not been definitively answered. Mechanisms operative in other transport epithelia, such as water channels (aquaporins), seem to have only a minor role in the intestine. Linkage of water to ion or solute transporters across apical membranes is an attractive hypothesis, but only limited evidence supports this theory. The most widely accepted mechanism is that of a response to osmotic gradients created by the movement of ions. An increase in osmolarity in the intercellular and subcellular spaces, created by active transcellular transport of ions and solutes, causes movement of water across the epithelium, through either the cell or the paracellular pathways. Recent theoretical approaches have implicated the cellular pathway as the principal route for water absorption.[15–17] Solvent drag refers to the entraining of solutes and fluid nonspecifically in movement across the paracellular pathway.

There is two-way traffic of ions and solutes across the epithelium. Part of this bidirectional movement represents diffusion, primarily through the paracellular pathways. In relatively leaky epithelia, this may be the major component of both absorptive and secretory fluxes. But, in addition, there are separate transcellular routes for absorption and secretion. Both processes may occur simultaneously. A net change in transport can occur through a change in either (or both) an absorptive or secretory flux of a particular ion.

Although a huge panoply of factors determines fluid and electrolyte transport, experiments to investigate the mechanisms are necessarily reductionist and focus on specific aspects of transport. Thus, an in vitro approach using Ussing chambers is particularly appropriate for assessing active transport but could not easily measure solvent drag; in contrast, an in vivo triple-lumen perfusion technique in humans may be ideal for characterizing solvent drag but could not determine changes in intracellular potential differences. In comparing results of different studies, one must be aware of the limitations of the techniques used, which in part may explain some of the apparently conflicting results in different studies.

Channels, Carriers, and Pumps

Channels, carriers, and pumps are all integral membrane proteins involved in transport of ions and solutes into and out of the cell (Fig. 87–4). They provide the means for controlled passage through the lipid barrier of the cell membrane. However, there are important structural and functional differences among these proteins that are critical to understanding the nature of transport mechanisms.[18]

Channels are protein pores within a cell membrane that are generally specific for a particular ion. The precise mechanisms for this ionic specificity are unknown, but specificity is not based solely on either charge or size. For example, Na channels exclude K despite similar charge and a smaller size. Our understanding of the "molecular physiology" of channel behavior has expanded rapidly with the advent of the patch-clamp technique, in which a "patch of membrane" is isolated in a microelectrode, permitting study of the electrical behavior of single channels.

Channels open and close rapidly. In the open state, more than a million ions per second can pass through a channel, but when closed they effectively exclude passage of any charge. Channels are characterized by their density within the membrane, the proportion of time they remain open, and the rate of ionic passage through a single open channel. The opening and closing of channels are regulated ("gated") by several different signals. Channels may be regulated by voltage, relative ionic concentrations, and intracellular mediators. Ions pass through channels by electrodiffusion.

Carriers are also integral proteins that may carry either solutes or multiple ions across a membrane. The transport rate through a carrier is several orders of magnitude lower than through channels. Carriers exhibit a high degree of structural specificity, for example, transporting D-glucose but not L-glucose. Carrier-mediated transport can be modeled in a manner similar to that of enzyme kinetics, with saturation and competitive inhibition. Although it is now considered unlikely that carrier proteins actually shuttle or flip-flop across the membrane, the precise mechanisms for transporting solutes into and out of the cell remain unclear.

Carriers may be involved in either facilitated diffusion or secondary active transport. Like simple diffusion, facilitated diffusion involves movement from regions of higher to lower concentrations. The carrier mechanisms permit the downhill movement of a solute across an otherwise impermeable barrier (i.e., the cell membrane). In contrast, secondary active transport reverses the diffusional flow of a specific solute or ion, similar to primary active transport. However, instead of a direct link to energy expenditure, secondary active transport harnesses the electrochemical energy established by the downhill movement of a second ion, usually Na. Na-coupled solute absorption and Cl secretion (see following discussion) are paradigms of secondary active transport.

Pumps are carriers responsible for movement of a solute against an electrochemical gradient, directly linked to the expenditure of energy. Pumps mediate primary active transport. The most important intestinal epithelial pump is the Na pump, a.k.a. Na, K-ATPase, which directly uses energy from the metabolism of ATP to move Na across the basolateral membrane against both electrical and chemical gradients. Other pumps that may be important in intestinal epithelial transport include a K, H-ATPase and a Ca-ATPase.

The Na pump extrudes three Na ions in exchange for two inward moving K ions, associated with the hydrolysis of one molecule of ATP. Thus, the Na pump is responsible for maintaining the characteristic intracellular ionic environment of high K and low Na. The unbalanced movement of charge (3:2) contributes to the electronegativity of the cell interior. The pump is a major source of cellular energy consumption and, in addition to its transport function, is integral in maintaining cell volume and osmotic balance.

Tight and Leaky Epithelia

Epithelia in a variety of organs are generally classified as "tight" or "leaky." The images conjured up of an impermeable or, alternatively, porous membrane, although not physiologically exact, are quite useful. Leaky epithelia, in general, transfer large amounts of fluid of approximately similar composition (i.e., isotonic absorption). The jejunum is a classic leaky epithelium. In contrast, tight epithelia usually effect net solute transfer against a gradient. The rectum and distal colon are examples of a tight epithelium.

The "tightness" of an epithelium is determined by the paracellular (shunt) pathway rather than by the apical or basolateral membranes. The in vitro electrical parameters predict the tightness of an epithelium. Tight epithelia exhibit both a high transepithelial voltage and resistance, whereas leaky epithelia have a low voltage and low resistance (see Fig. 87–1). The paracellular shunt conductance provides a mechanism for maintaining or dissipating the transcellular potential difference; thus, in a leaky epithelium, the relatively high shunt conductance tends to short circuit the potential difference generated by transcellular transport.

The lateral borders of adjacent cells are linked by several complex structures (Fig. 87–5); the two major ones are the zona adherens (ZA) and the zona occludens (ZO), the tight junction. The ZA is primarily responsible for cell to cell adhesion and cell polarity. Cadherins are transmembrane glycoproteins in the ZA that establish the link from one cell to another by binding across the intercellular space. Cadherins, in turn, bind to a family of adhesion molecules called catenins. Alterations in cadherin/catenin distribution and/or function have been implicated in carcinogenesis.[19, 20] The tight junction, or ZO, is the most apical complex and is thought to control permeability across the paracellular pathway through a series of strands and grooves. As with the ZA, molecular definition of the specific components of the tight junction (e.g., ZO-1, ZO-2, occludin, cingulin) may permit a clearer understanding of how the ZO functions as a barrier for ions and macromolecules.[21]

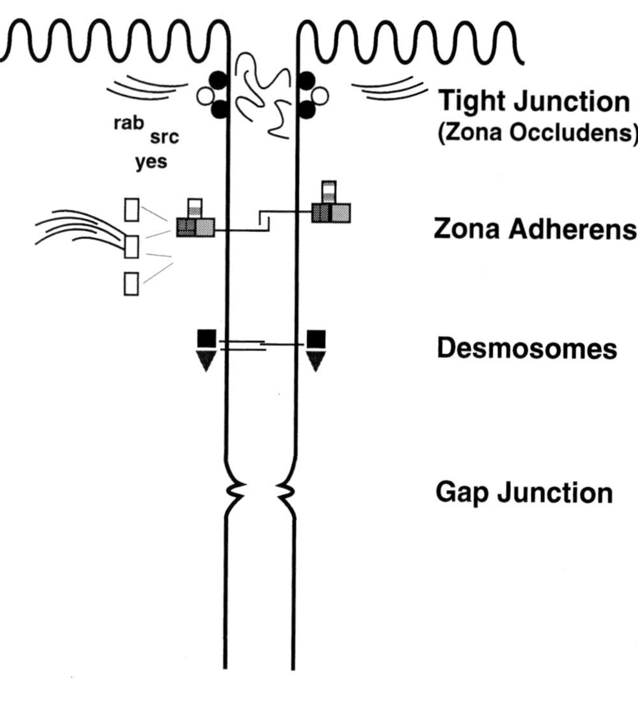

Figure 87–5. Paracellular structures in intestinal epithelial cells. The paracellular pathway is characterized by a series of structures, originally defined microscopically but now by specific molecular distributions. The tight junction is made up of a network of strands and grooves (occludins) attached to a group of membrane proteins, which are then linked to the cytoskeleton. Cadherins span the paracellular pathway across the zona adherens (ZA) and are responsible for cell-cell attachment and maintenance of cell polarity. Cadherins bind to catenins, which are linked to the actin cytoskeleton through an additional family of molecules, including radixim, vinculin, and α actinin. Catenins and other molecules associated with the ZA, including rab, src, and yes, are involved with intracellular signaling through second messengers. Desmosomes are another point of cell attachment in which cadherin-like molecules are linked to intermediate filaments.

Original models of the paracellular pathway as a static barrier are being replaced by a more dynamic model in which the junctional complexes are involved in signaling and regulation, most likely through protein phosphorylation or dephosphorylation.[22] There may be significant interaction between the ZO and the ZA. Both are intricately associated with the cytoskeleton and hence to more distant parts of the cell. Several transport proteins are also directly linked to the cytoskeleton,[23–25] raising the possibility of a complex regulatory web. In this new paradigm, paracellular permeability may be altered by extracellular agonists, tyrosine kinases, and changes in transport and cell volume.

Unstirred Layers

The gut constantly mixes the luminal contents by its peristaltic activity and reduces the distance that an individual molecule must diffuse to reach the apical membrane. The depth of that unstirred layer may be a major factor in determining the rate of absorption of a solute independent of the mechanisms of cellular transport. The relative permeability barriers posed by the unstirred water layers and the apical membrane determine their importance in the absorption of a specific solute. The unstirred layer is a more important factor for larger lipid-soluble molecules such as long-chain fatty acids and solutes rapidly transported across the apical membrane. Estimates of the thickness of the unstirred layer can vary greatly depending on the experimental techniques used; the thickness of the layer may be <40 μm, much less than previously estimated.[26] The kinetics of nutrient absorption are significantly altered without consideration of unstirred layers; even this reduced layer may be the rate-limiting step for compounds rapidly transported across the apical membrane. Unstirred water layers in the subcellular space may also be an important factor in modulating absorption and secretion.

ION TRANSPORTERS

Apical Sodium Channel

Ion-specific Na channels in the apical membrane permit the entry of Na into the cell down its electrochemical gradient with subsequent exit across the basolateral membrane via the Na pump (Fig. 87–6). Because this transport is not linked to the movement of other ions and involves the net transfer of charge across the epithelium, it is electrogenic. Colonic epithelia demonstrate electrogenic Na absorption blocked by amiloride and stimulated by mineralocorticoids. The Na channel from aldosterone-treated rat distal colon has been cloned and its structure analyzed.[27–30] The Na channel is composed of three discrete subunits. The specific biologic roles of the subunits remain to be clarified. Because of structural similarities with genes involved in neuronal degeneration, investigators have recognized an Na channel/degenerin gene family that has expanded to include a variety of channels in the brain, nervous system, tongue, and lymphocytes.[30, 31] Immunohistochemistry and in situ hybridization studies have demonstrated, as expected, the presence of the channel in surface cells of the distal colon.[29] Electrogenic Na absorption is also present in cecum and ileum but is not readily inhibited by amiloride; this raises the possibility of a different class of channels or other proteins that modulate electrogenic Na absorption in the more proximal reaches of the bowel.[32]

Nutrient-Coupled Na Transport

Nutrient absorption is generally linked to sodium transport.[7] Although the fetal colon transiently exhibits nutrient-coupled Na absorption,[33] this rapidly disappears at birth. Thus, nutrient-coupled Na transport (glucose, amino acids, vitamins) is restricted to the small intestine. This transport system consists of a family of apical membrane carriers that, after binding both Na and a nutrient, transport both into the cell (see Fig 87–6). The electrochemical gradient for Na provides the driving force for accumulation of the nutrient intracellularly against its own concentration gradient. Nutrient exit across the basolateral membrane is diffusional.

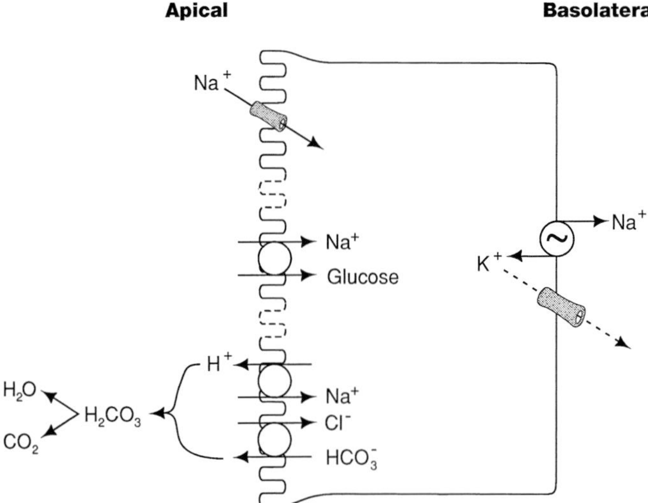

Figure 87–6. Apical sodium transporters. Sodium crosses the apical membrane of the epithelial cell, down an electrochemical gradient. The mechanisms for this may be (1) an ion-specific channel that can be blocked by amiloride, (2) a carrier that couples the movement of sodium and nutrients, such as glucose, e.g., SGLT1, or (3) a carrier that allows electroneutral entry of sodium in exchange for intracellular hydrogen (antiport carrier), e.g., NHE-3. The common exit pathway across the basolateral membrane is the sodium pump.

Molecular approaches in the study of glucose transport have led to the identification of two families of proteins: sodium glucose transporters (SGLTs), which mediate Na-coupled transport, and glucose transporters (GLTs), which mediate facilitated diffusion.[34, 35] SGLT1 is localized to the apical surface of epithelial cells in the upper villus. It binds two Na for a single glucose molecule and transports them into the cell. Because there is a net transfer of charge (two cations), this transport is electrogenic. Glucose accumulates in the epithelial cell at concentrations higher than in the surrounding intercellular fluid. It therefore diffuses across the basolateral membrane via a specific membrane protein, GLT2.[34, 35]

Despite the elegant molecular details provided by studies of SGLT1, it is still surprisingly unclear how Na-coupled glucose absorption alters the mechanisms of epithelial water and solute absorption. Glucose exiting across the basolateral membrane creates a hypertonic compartment in the intercellular space, causing water to move from the lumen, through the tight junction (or cell), into the intercellular space to maintain osmotic equilibrium. Several investigators,[36–39] but not all[40] found that a significant amount of glucose, along with other inert solutes such as D-xylose, is absorbed paracellularly. Because glucose stimulates water absorption, this would be an expected consequence of solvent drag (see earlier discussion). However, although some studies have found that glucose-induced changes in the cytoskeleton lead to significant alterations in the permeability of the tight junctions,[36, 37] others found no such changes.[39] Clarifying these mechanisms will be important to understand basic aspects of intestinal function and designing optimal strategies for enteral nutrition and fluid replacement.

Na-H Exchangers

Na-H exchange activity can be demonstrated in essentially every cell type. Exchange of extracellular Na for intracellular H is driven by both the electrochemical gradient for Na and a pH gradient that results from a moderately acidic intracellular environment. Five isoforms of Na-H exchangers (NHE) have been cloned.[41–44] NHE-1 is found in both epithelial and nonepithelial cells. It most likely represents the ubiquitous "housekeeper" involved in regulation of intracellular pH, cell volume, and growth.[45] In polarized epithelia, NHE-1 is localized to the basolateral membrane, consistent with its housekeeping role. NHE-2 and NHE-3 are localized to the apical membrane of surface/villus cells. Although both isoforms are presumably involved in Na absorption, they are subject to different hormonal, pharmacologic, and dietary influences.[46–54] Making sense of the different roles of NHE-2 and NHE-3 is complicated by different experimental models. Nevertheless, it appears that NHE-3 is the isoform responsible for the bulk of apical Na-H exchange, but NHE-2 may account for some of the variability in physiologic and pathophysiologic response. Interdigestive salt and water absorption probably occurs via NHE-3. Knockout mice lacking NHE-3 exhibit a severe absorptive defect in Na absorption, but little diarrhea, suggesting compensatory mechanisms. In contrast, NHE-2 knockouts did not have marked transport abnormalities but did exhibit an unexpected and somewhat inexplicable decrease in gastric parietal cells.[51, 52] The apical NHE appears to be linked to tyrosine kinase and growth factor receptors, providing another potential level of regulation.[55]

Electroneutral NaCl Absorption

A considerable portion of Na absorption in the intestine is linked (or coupled) to chloride through synchronous functions of NHE and a Cl-HCO_3 anion exchanger.[56–59] Because the rates of cation and anion transport are similar, this process does not involve the net transfer of charge and is therefore electroneutral.

One of the fundamentals underlying the dual antiporter model is that the movement of Na and Cl is linked by an intracellular signal, most probably cell pH and/or HCO_3. Downhill Na entry drives H exit across the apical membrane, alkalinizing the cell; this creates a favorable gradient for HCO_3 exit that, in turn, permits Cl entry into the cell. Cl accumulates in the cell above its electrochemical equilibrium. If these two exchangers operate at roughly the same rate, the net result is cellular uptake of NaCl, maintenance of a constant intracellular pH, and luminal secretion of water and CO_2. Inhibition of apical membrane Na influx and NHE is associated with a decrease in intracellular pH, supporting this model.[60, 61] Cellular acidification decreases intracellular HCO_3, thus inhibiting Cl-HCO_3 exchange. Although this model would predict tight coupling between Na-H and Cl-HCO_3 exchangers, there is considerable variability ranging from NHEs operating solo (jejunum) to unaccompanied Cl-HCO_3 exchangers (distal colon).[62] How this happens is unclear but may be due to different molecular isoforms or varying regulatory factors.

Chloride Absorption

In vivo, most Cl absorption probably occurs through diffusion, generated by the orientation of the potential difference across the epithelium.[63] Electrogenic Na absorption creates an electrical potential profile that favors movement of anions from the lumen through the paracellular pathway. Cellular transport of Cl occurs linked to Na through the dual antiporter system noted earlier. There also is a family of anion exchangers with differing affinities for Cl, HCO_3, hydroxyl ions, sulfate, and other anions.[64] These transporters may provide the gut with the flexibility to handle a variety of luminal anions.

Chloride Secretion

Whereas Na flux provides the principal driving force for intestinal absorption of fluid, Cl fulfills the analogous role for fluid secretion (Fig. 87–7). The intestinal epithelium exhibits a basal rate of Cl secretion, which can be augmented by a variety of hormonal, paracrine, neural, luminal, and inflammatory mediators. This basal rate of Cl secretion hydrates and lubricates intestinal contents to ensure smooth passage through the gastrointestinal tract. Increased rates of intestinal Cl secretion are the underlying basis of secretory diarrheas, with water and other electrolytes moving in response to osmotic gradients. Increased Cl secretion probably

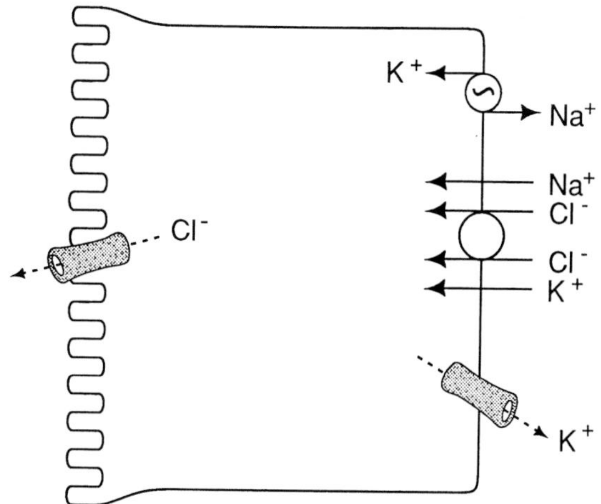

Figure 87–7. Chloride secretion. Discrete basolateral entry steps and apical exit steps are integral to chloride secretion. A carrier couples the movement of sodium, potassium, and chloride in a 1:1:2 stoichiometry and permits chloride to accumulate in the cell above its electrochemical equilibrium. Chloride exits the cell across the apical membrane via a chloride channel, e.g., CFTR. The sodium and potassium that entered with the chloride are recycled by, respectively, the sodium pump and a basolateral potassium channel.

serves a protective function, flushing toxins out of the intestine and colon.

A common mechanism of electrogenic Cl secretion exists in several epithelia, including the small intestine and colon. This consensus model of secretion entails both discrete basolateral entry steps into the cell and an exit step across the apical membrane. The basolateral Cl entry step couples the uphill movement of Cl to Na entry and is electroneutral. In contrast to electroneutral NaCl absorption, mediated by dual ion exchangers, this pathway is mediated by a single carrier that binds three ionic species in the ratio 1 Na 1K 2Cl and is inhibited by the loop diuretics bumetanide and furosemide.[65] Na then exits across the basolateral membrane via the Na pump, resulting in no net transcellular Na movement. Potassium entering through the Na K 2Cl carrier is recycled through K channels in both the basolateral and apical membranes. Although recycling of K may seem inefficient, the linkage of K to NaCl influx serves several purposes. Basolateral K exit electrically balances the large Cl flux across the apical membrane. The rate of K exit through these channels modulates the electrochemical driving force for apical Cl transport and provides an additional regulatory point for controlling Cl secretion (see Intracellular Mediators, following discussion).[66]

Cl accumulates in the cell above its electrochemical equilibrium and then exits the cell through specific Cl channels into the intestinal lumen. Electrophysiologic fingerprints detected by patch clamping exist for several different types of Cl channels in secretory epithelia, including the intestine. These may respond uniquely or in combination to different agonists, including cyclic AMP, Ca^{2+}, and volume. A relatively small Cl channel, activated by cyclic AMP, has evoked particular interest because it has been identified as the defective gene product in cystic fibrosis. This channel has been termed CFTR (cystic fibrosis transmembrane regulator) and is the Cl channel activated by several agonists implicated in secretory diarrhea.[67, 68] The physiologic significance of Ca-activated channels in the intestine remains controversial.[69, 70]

Determination of CFTR mRNA by in situ hybridization showed a remarkable segmental heterogeneity with decreasing gradients of expression along the crypt-villus axis (see Fig. 87–3) and along a proximal-distal gut axis.[71] The distribution of CFTR along the crypt-villus axis is consistent with the generalized model localizing secretion to the crypts; however, the implications of finding decreasing CFTR message as one moves down the gut are less clear. Although the gene and the gene product associated with CF have been identified, the pathophysiology of the defect has not been clarified; the abnormality in CF may be in the trafficking of CFTR from the endoplasmic reticulum through the Golgi apparatus to specific docking targets on the apical membrane.[72–76]

Potassium Transport

There are specific absorptive and secretory pathways for potassium in the gut; in general, secretion tends to predominate, but in the appropriate clinical and experimental settings, K absorption is significant. In the small intestine, most K secretion is passive, secondary to the lumen negative potential difference developed across the epithelium. The colon actively secretes K. This pathway is mediated by uptake of potassium across the basolateral membrane by the Na,K-ATPase and/or the Na-K-2Cl carrier and exit across the apical membrane via a K channel. Several secretory stimuli enhance both Cl and K secretion, suggesting that the two transport functions are linked.[77] However, they can clearly be separated during development and with appropriate pharmacologic manipulations.

K absorption occurs in the distal colon, via apical uptake of K by a primary active transport process mediated by K-ATPase pumps. Apparently, at least two K-ATPases can be delineated by molecular and pharmacologic techniques; one may be localized to surface cells and the other to crypts.[78, 79] These transporters are similar to the K, H-ATPase found in gastric parietal cells.

Bicarbonate Transport

Bicarbonate secretion is a major function of intestinal epithelia, occurring in duodenum, ileum, and colon. In contrast to the elegant descriptions of the molecular basis for Cl secretion or NHE, the mechanisms of bicarbonate transport remain more problematic. To a certain extent, bicarbonate secretion is a chameleon. In clinically significant secretory diarrheas, the principal anion lost in the stool is bicarbonate. However, cholera toxin or its surrogates stimulate Cl secretion in vitro. The reason for this remains elusive, but Cl and bicarbonate secretion may be intertwined in a yet-to-be-determined mechanism. Bicarbonate is a transported species, a metabolic product, and a regulator of intracellular processes. Recent studies using measurements of intracellular pH suggest that intracellular bicarbonate may modulate Cl secretion and that P_{CO_2} and pH may regulate NHE.[80, 81]

Bicarbonate secretion has both electrogenic and electroneutral components. As with other transepithelial ion fluxes, there are discrete apical and basolateral transporters. Bicarbonate may enter across the basolateral membrane either by diffusion of CO_2 or by a specific ion transport mechanism, perhaps Na-HCO_3 cotransport,[82, 83] or alternatively may originate from intracellular metabolic processes.[84, 85]

The apical exit step(s) for bicarbonate secretion has not been fully delineated, but it is clear that CFTR is pivotal to duodenal bicarbonate secretion.[86, 87] Drawing from models in the pancreas and the bladder, bicarbonate secretion may involve the synchronized function of an apical Cl channel (CFTR) and an anion (Cl-HCO_3) exchanger. In this model, electrogenic Cl secretion provides luminal Cl that is then recycled across the apical membrane in exchange for intracellular HCO_3. Alternatively, HCO_3 may exit across the apical membrane through an anion-specific channel, either CFTR or an HCO_3 specific channel.[85, 88] Cyclic AMP activation of CFTR appears to be the major pathway for bicarbonate secretion; however, in the absence of CFTR other pathways may become operative.[83, 87]

HCO_3 secretion may depend on the geographic separation of antiporter systems along the crypt-villus axis in the ileum. Although villus cells possess both apical and basolateral NHEs, crypt cells apparently exhibit only a basolateral NHE. In contrast, Cl-HCO_3 exchangers are found on apical but not basolateral membranes of both crypt and villus cells. This separation provides a mechanism for villus cells to absorb NaCl but for crypt cells to secrete HCO_3. Inhibition of bicarbonate secretion by adrenergic agonists may depend on a differential effect on crypt and villus NHEs.[9] Additionally, there may be adrenergic-sensitive bicarbonate absorption.[84]

Short-Chain Fatty Acid Transport

Short-chain fatty acids (SCFAs), not Cl or bicarbonate, are the principal luminal anions in the colon. They are two to four carbon compounds (acetate, propionate, butyrate) that originate from bacterial metabolism of carbohydrates and protein passing through the ileocecal valve. The magnitude of the daily colonic load and absorption of SCFAs is comparable with that of colonic Na. SCFAs are the preferred metabolic substrate for colonocytes, have important effects of epithelial growth and differentiation, and have been implicated in the pathogenesis and/or therapy of several colonic diseases.

SCFAs are rapidly cleared from the colon and enhance Na absorption.[89, 90] Like other weak electrolytes, SCFAs may be either protonated or ionized. Although it has generally been assumed that protonated (un-ionized) SCFAs can readily diffuse across membranes, there may be a unique apical diffusion barrier in the colon. At normal colonic luminal pH, most SCFAs are ionized. In vitro studies have demonstrated several mechanisms for SCFA transport. Propionate absorption in rabbit proximal colon is linked to the activity of Na-H exchange, suggesting that H^+ secretion may create a low pH microclimate at the apical surface that promotes diffusion of the protonated SCFA into the cell.[91] Other studies in ileum and colon have suggested specific anion exchangers that operate with SCFAs and bicarbonate.[92, 93] The large concentration gradient for SCFAs across the colonic epithelium (>50 mM) may be important in stimulating Na absorption, but the specific mechanism(s) linking SCFAs to Na transport remains to be determined.[94] The presence of active transcellular SCFA transport implies that it may be subject to physiologic regulation and pathophysiologic alteration.[95–97] SCFAs may have ancillary benefits in reversing toxin-induced secretion in cholera and other diarrheas.[98]

PARACRINE IMMUNONEURO-ENDOCRINE SYSTEMS

Multiple extracellular factors regulate epithelial ion transport. In a reductionist approach, it is possible to delineate the paracrine, immunologic, neural, and endocrine inputs into the enterocyte; however, the borders separating these systems have become increasingly blurred, because there is so much overlap and interplay among them. For example, Verner-Morrison syndrome (pancreatic cholera) is mediated by pancreatic islet cell tumors producing large amounts of vasoactive intestinal peptide (VIP). VIPomas are often cited as the classic example of a hormonally mediated secretory diarrhea, because, under these conditions, VIP is a circulating mediator that fits the classic definition of a hormone. However, VIP is not normally found in the adult pancreas; its physiologic role in the gut is as a peptidergic neurotransmitter in the enteric nervous system, affecting both epithelial cells and smooth muscle. A similar dilemma of classification applies to serotonin and other mediators. A single agonist such as prostaglandins or cholera toxin may simultaneously stimulate neural, paracrine, and immune responses, in addition to exerting a direct effect on epithelial cells. Neurotransmitters may stimulate the release of immune modulators, and inflammatory mediators may alter neural regulation of the epithelium.

Within the subepithelium, structural elements of the neural, immune, and paracrine system lie in close proximity to each other. For example, mucosal mast cells are strategically located adjacent to enteric neurons, blood vessels, and epithelial cells. Release of mast cell mediators may easily target neurons or vice versa. Therefore, although it is possible to dissect out the specific effects of an individual component in vitro, clinically they are inextricably intertwined.

Thus, it makes more sense, heuristically, scientifically, and clinically, to lump, rather than split, these multiple components into a single, complex, superregulatory system for which the acronym PINES (*p*aracrine *i*mmuno*n*euro*e*ndocrine *s*ystem) can be used. PINES emphasizes the inherent interplay among these factors in providing the extracellular messages necessary for the epithelial cell to set its transport machinery appropriately. Fluid secretion is the major component of diarrhea, an organism's defense response to intestinal challenge; however, other mechanisms, including motility, mucus secretion, and blood flow, all regulated by PINES, are important adjuncts. The recognition that elements of PINES frequently are potent regulators of intestinal motility helps resolve the dichotomy between epithelial and muscle elements in the etiology of diarrhea. Clinically, intestinal motility is a critical factor in diarrhea; patients with rapid intestinal transit (e.g., after gastrectomy), altered anorectal motility (e.g., small volume diarrhea), or decreased motility (e.g., bacterial overgrowth) may have significant diarrhea with a primary muscle component. However, more commonly, inflammatory mediators such as prostaglandins or bacterial enterotoxins may target both the epithelium and the muscle to elicit a coordinated secretory response. Similarly, absorptive stimuli such as opiates/enkephalins may have a complementary effect on motility to further enhance their absorptive effect. Thus, PINES provides the opportunity for a coordinated and integrated response to multiple, varied, extracellular signals.

EXTRACELLULAR REGULATION

Extracellular signals may be divided into those that stimulate Na and water absorption (absorbagogues) (Table 87–1) and those that either inhibit Na absorption or stimulate Cl and water secretion (secretagogues) (Tables 87–2 and 87–3). Quite obviously, if the secretory signals predominate, an individual is subject to diarrhea. Whether there is a clinical corollary for a predominant absorptive pattern is unclear.

Neural Regulation

Neural input is critical in the regulation of fluid and electrolyte transport (Fig. 87–8). Three divisions of the autonomic nervous system are involved in regulation of epithelial transport: parasympathetic, sympathetic, and enteric. The basic

Table 87–1 | **Intestinal Absorbagogues**

Endogenous absorbagogues
Aldosterone
Glucocorticoids
α-Adrenergic agonists
Enkephalins
Somatostatin
Angiotensin
Peptide YY
Neuropeptide Y
Prolactin
Growth hormone
Short-chain fatty acids
Growth factors (EGF,FGF)?
Pharmacologic agents
Mineralocorticoids
Glucocorticoids
Octreotide (somatostatin analog)
Cyclo-oxygenase inhibitors (NSAIDs)
Lithium
Clonidine (α_2-agonist)
Propranolol
Opiates
Berberine
Phenothiazines

EGF, epidermal growth factor; FGF, fibroblastic-derived growth factor; NSAIDs, nonsteroidal anti-inflammatory drugs.

Table 87–2 | **Endogenous Secretagogues**

AGONIST	INTRACELLULAR MEDIATOR	SOURCE(S)
Prostaglandins	Cyclic AMP	Immune, mesenchymal
Bradykinin	Cyclic AMP	Immune
Arachidonic acid	Cyclic AMP	Immune, cell membranes
VIP	Cyclic AMP	ENS/VIPoma
Secretin	Cyclic AMP	Paracrine
Peptide histadine isoleucine	Cyclic AMP	ENS
Platelet-activating factor	Cyclic AMP	Immune
Reactive oxygen metabolites	Cyclic AMP	Immune
Adenosine	Cyclic AMP	Immune
Leukotrienes	??	Immune
Acetylcholine	Calcium	ENS
Serotonin	Calcium	ENS, carcinoid
Histamine	Calcium	Immune
Substance P	Calcium	ENS, carcinoid
Neurotensin	Calcium	ENS
Atrial natriuretic peptide	Cyclic GMP	
Guanylin	Cyclic GMP	Goblet, epithelial cells
Nitric oxide	Cyclic GMP(?)	Immune, mesenchymal
Calcitonin/cGRP	??	ENS, MCT
Gastrin	??	Paracrine
GIP	??	??
Motilin	??	??
Bombesin/gastrin-releasing peptide	??	ENS

cGRP, calcitonin gene-related peptide; MCT, medullary carcinoma of the thyroid; GIP, gastrointestinal inhibitory peptide; ENS, enteric nervous system; VIP, vasoactive intestinal peptide.

framework of extrinsic innervation mediated by cholinergic stimulation of secretion, predominantly through vagal input, and adrenergic stimulation of absorption via prevertebral and sympathetic ganglia have long been recognized as fundamental neural factors affecting the intestinal epithelium. However, a fuller appreciation of the labyrinthine innervation of the gut has added several additional layers of complexity to our understanding of neural regulation.[99, 100]

The enteric nervous system (ENS) independently integrates and coordinates the neural effects on the epithelia, muscles, and blood vessels of the gut, with input and modification from the central nervous system.[101] The hubs of the ENS are two ganglionated plexuses of Meissner (submucosal) and Auerbach (myenteric).[102] The ENS has reflex arcs that may have important clinical implications. As in any neural circuit, there are sensory neurons, interneurons, and motor neurons. Sensory input into the ENS would logically come from changes in the luminal environment or luminal volume. Relatively little is known about the sensory input into the ENS; endocrine and paracrine cells may function as auxiliary sensors for the ENS with subsequent input into the system further upstream. Capsaicin-sensitive nerves may elicit secretion[103] and may be important in the response to bacterial toxins.[104] ENS reflexes may regulate colonic epithelial responses to distant small bowel challenges.[105] Interneurons are primarily cholinergic. Two broad categories of motor neurons innervate epithelial and submucosal cells: cholinergic and VIPergic, with each having additional neuroactive substances. Target cells for neurons include other components of PINES, vascular and smooth muscle cells, and, of course, epithelial cells.

Tonic sympathetic and parasympathetic tone modulates ion transport. A good deal of evidence suggests a basal cholinergic secretory drive.[106, 107] Loss of sympathetic neural regulatory mechanisms in diabetic autonomic neuropathy is associated with the development of "diabetic diarrhea" and may be corrected by α_2-adrenergic agonists.[108]

Several examples emphasize the intricacies of neural control. The number of potential neuroactive agents has been steadily increasing. Peptidergic neurons may release specific combinations of mediators (VIP, cholecystokinin, gastrin-releasing peptide, etc.) rather than a single substance.[99] Sorting

Table 87–3 | **Luminal Secretagogues**

BACTERIAL ENTEROTOXINS	INTRACELLULAR MEDIATOR
V. cholera	Cyclic AMP
V. cholera enterotoxin	Cyclic AMP
Zona occludens toxin	??
Accessory cholera enterotoxin	??
Escherichia coli (heat labile)	Cyclic AMP
Salmonella	Cyclic AMP
Campylobacter jejuni	Cyclic AMP
Aeromonas	Cyclic AMP
E. coli (heat stable)	Cyclic GMP
Y. enterocolitica	Cyclic GMP
C. perfringens	??
C. difficile (A)	??
MISCELLANEOUS	**INTRACELLULAR MEDIATOR**
Bile salts	Cyclic AMP/calcium
Long-chain fatty acids	Cyclic AMP/calcium
Laxatives	??

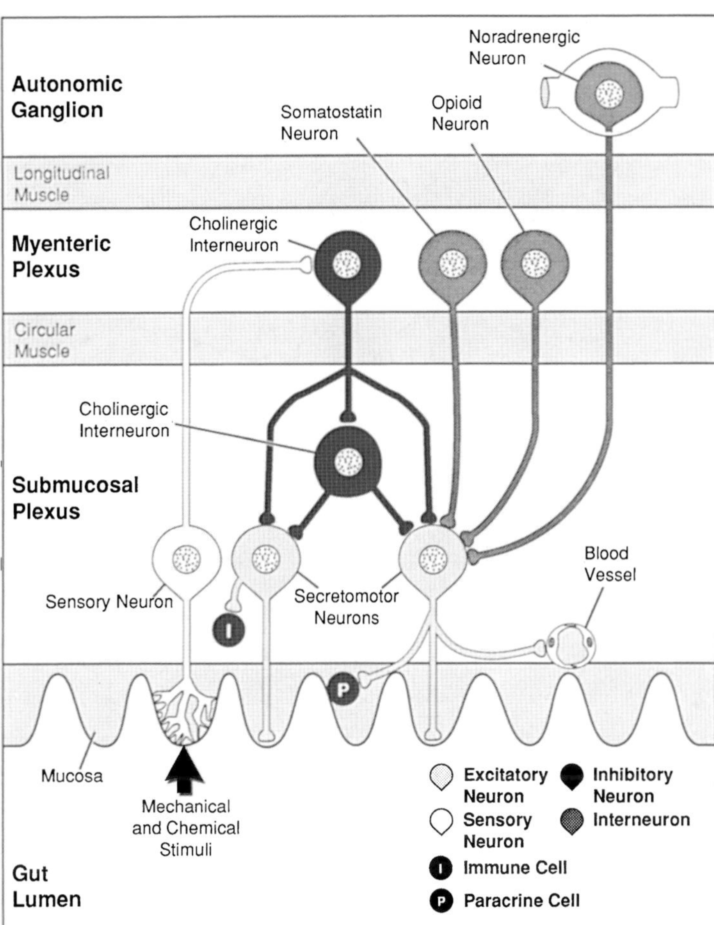

Figure 87–8. Neural regulation of ion transport. This model depicts the integral components of the enteric nervous system, including (1) sensory neurons responsive to intraluminal mechanical/chemical stimuli, (2) interneurons in either the myenteric or submucosal plexi, (3) secretory neurons releasing the vasoactive intestinal peptide and acetylcholine that act on epithelial cells, (4) additional neural input from somatostatin, opiate, and noradrenergic neurons that modulate the function of the secretory neurons, and (5) interaction between secretory neurons and blood vessels, immune cells, and paracrine cells. (Adapted from Castro GA: Gut immunophysiology: regulatory pathways within a common mucosal immune system. NIPS 4:59–64, 1989.)

out the physiologic effects of the release of a mix of agonists may be exponentially more difficult than tracing the effects of a single agonist. Agents may act as either classic neurotransmitters or neuromodulators, fine tuning the neuronal circuits of presynaptic sites of source neuron or other neurons. Individual neurotransmitters may have biphasic effects varying with concentrations. The ability to map the neuronal circuitry of the gut has, to a certain extent, outstripped our understanding of the biologic significance of specific neuroactive agents.

Immunologic Regulation

The clinical correlation between inflammation in the intestine and diarrhea is obvious. Ulcerations, exudation of protein, changes in motility, and loss of absorptive surface area have been frequently implicated as etiologies for the fluid loss in inflammatory diarrheas. Recent investigation has focused on the effect of immune cells in the lamina propria on regulation of salt and water transport. Immunocytes and their vast array of soluble products play an integral role in fluid regulation and are intimately intertwined with the ENS and the paracrine-endocrine network.

The lamina propria is home for a family of immunocompetent cells. Most of these, under normal (noninflamed) conditions, are T lymphocytes (60%) with smaller numbers of B lymphocytes and plasma cells (25% to 30%), macrophages (8% to 10%), and mast cells and polymorphonuclear cells (2% to 5%), usually eosinophils.[109] Inflammation elicits an increase in the number of immunocytes within the intestine. However, the etiology of the inflammation may determine the increase in a particular cell population. Acute bacterial infections result in an increase in polymorphonuclear leukocytes; lymphocytes characteristically increase in celiac sprue. In a rat model of parasitic infections, the intestinal mast cell population is dramatically enlarged.[110] In inflammatory bowel disease, there is activation of all components of the immune system with an increase in IgG-secreting cells.[111] Thus, the etiology of the inflammatory reaction may determine the type of inflammatory cells recruited and the range of cytokines released.

Cytokines, eicosanoids, and other soluble peptide mediators may interact with other immunocytes, neurons, or epithelial cells directly to alter rates of ion transport or the barrier function of the intestine (Fig. 87–9). Mucosal mast cells and their secretory products are central to several inflammatory reactions.[112] These mast cells are strategically located in close proximity to enteric neurons, blood vessels, and epithelial cells[113]; this intimate relation suggests that mast cell mediators have important localized effects. Histamine, serotonin, and adenosine are potent secretagogues in vivo and in vitro. These mediators elicit secretion both by direct effects on the epithelial cells and by indirect neural stimulation and prostaglandin release.[112, 114]

The mechanisms of how polymorphonuclear infiltration of

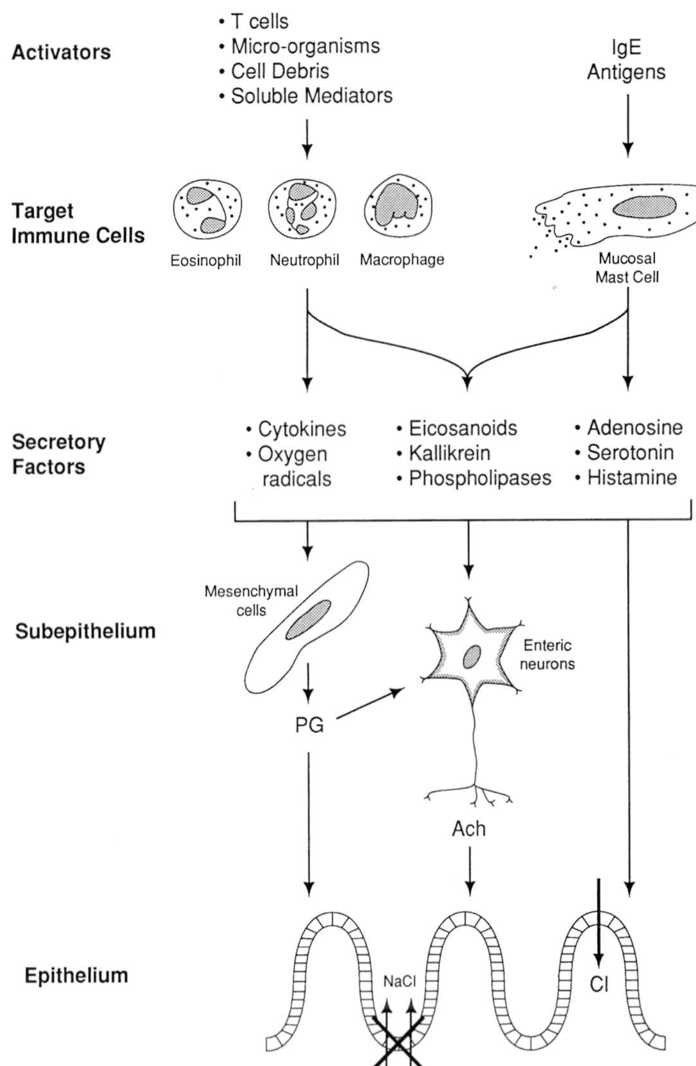

Figure 87–9. Immune responses. Multiple activators can stimulate target immune cells. These intestinal cells can release an array of secretory factors, which may act either directly on the epithelium or indirectly by stimulating the mesenchymal cells or enteric neurons to release prostaglandins or acetylcholine.

the mucosa stimulates secretion have become clearer. Polymorphonuclear leukocytes, responding to a variety of chemoattractants, interact with epithelial cells. White cells burrow through the intercellular space of colonic cell lines in a complex integrin-dependent process.[115] Migrating leukocytes release 5′AMP, which is converted to the more potent secretagogue, adenosine, by apical membrane enzymes. This adenosine-stimulated secretion may serve as a mechanism to cleanse the crypt lumen.[116] In a model of enterohemorrhagic *Escherichia coli* diarrhea in rabbits, treatment with anti-integrin antibodies prevented both inflammation and changes in electrolyte transport.[117] Thus, complex specific immunocyte–epithelial cell interactions are important in alterations of electrolyte secretion associated with mucosal inflammation.

Other novel secretagogues associated with inflammation have been identified. Oxidants such as superoxides, hydrogen peroxide, and hydroxyl radicals released from neutrophils stimulate Cl secretion.[118] Cytokines such as interleukins -1 and -3 stimulate intestinal secretion.[119] Arachidonic acid, platelet-activating factor, substance P, kallikreins, and bradykinin may be important factors in the secretory response associated with inflammation. Inflammatory mediators such as interferon-γ may also alter intestinal permeability and barrier function.[120, 121]

Eicosanoids (leukotrienes and, particularly, prostaglandins) are central to the secretory response associated with inflammation. Studies using cyclooxygenase inhibitors to block prostaglandin production demonstrate that the secretory response of most inflammatory mediators is linked to prostaglandins. Bradykinin and other inflammatory mediators liberate arachidonic acid and stimulate prostaglandin production. Prostaglandins also affect other components of the PINES, particularly enteric neurons.[122]

In assessing the role of inflammatory mediators in ion transport, the common strategy has been to identify potential mediators that are increased in inflamed tissue and then test their effects in normal model systems. However, this approach ignores the likelihood that cells damaged by the inflammatory process simply cannot perform their normal function. Studies examining transport parameters in colonic specimens from patients with inflammatory bowel disease suggest that it is a loss of the normal absorptive capacity rather than a stimulation of secretion that predominates in this clinical entity.[123]

Systemic Regulation

Acid-base balance modulates intestinal electrolyte transport both in vivo and in vitro. Metabolic acidosis stimulates electroneutral NaCl absorption, whereas metabolic alkalosis inhibits this transport process.[124–126] Measurements of intracellular pH suggest that intracellular bicarbonate concentrations may modulate basal Cl secretion. Intracellular pH and PCO_2 may alter Na-H exchange.

Volume status and intestinal blood flow may alter ion transport. Both active absorption and secretion have been associated with increased intestinal blood flow.[127, 128] A decrease in intravascular volume, such as may be associated with hemorrhage, elicits a series of responses that increase fluid absorption. Cardiopulmonary mechanoreceptors and carotid baroreceptors increase sympathetic input into the ENS, resulting in decreased secretion. Angiotensin II, antidiuretic hormone, and atrial natriuretic peptide may also contribute to regulation of intestinal fluid transport in these conditions.[129–131]

The metabolic status of the gut has an impact on its transport capability. A well-fed gut transports more effectively.[132] There are segmental preferences for metabolic fuels. Although the entire intestinal tract uses glucose, the small bowel effectively uses glutamine and the colon SCFAs, particularly butyrate.[133, 134]

Osmotic Effects

Unlike the kidney, there is no evidence to suggest that the intestinal epithelium can maintain an osmotic gradient. In normal physiology, the duodenum and upper jejunum are subject to major fluid shifts as they adjust to dietary intake of hypertonic foods and liquids. Rapid equilibration is usually accomplished by movement of water into the intestinal lumen. Absorptive processes along the remainder of the gut steadily decrease the luminal volume. However, the continued presence of a nonabsorbable solute within the intestinal lumen may negate functioning absorptive pathways in the distal gut. This is the basis for osmotic diarrhea (see Chapter 9).

Carbohydrates, usually disaccharides, are a frequent source of a nonabsorbable solute. Because disaccharides must be converted to simple sugars before they can cross the apical membrane of the small intestine, the absence of a specific brush border disaccharidase will prevent absorption (see Chapter 90). The most frequent clinical example of this is lactose intolerance, in which the glucose-galactose disaccharide cannot be broken down because of a lactase deficiency. Because the human gut does not naturally possess a lactulase, the disaccharide lactulose will reliably cause an increase in small bowel fluid.

The physiology of carbohydrate-induced osmotic diarrhea is complicated by the fact that what may be a nonabsorbable solute in the small bowel can be converted into an absorbable solute by colonic bacteria. Almost all classes of carbohydrates malabsorbed by the small bowel are rapidly converted to SCFAs once they cross the ileocecal valve and encounter the bacterial flora of the colon; these SCFAs are then absorbed across the colonic mucosa. Thus, depending on the rate of conversion to SCFAs and the colonic capacity for SCFA absorption, small bowel fluid loss may be compensated by colonic fluid absorption. However, the degree of carbohydrate malabsorption may be sufficient to either overproduce SCFA to the extent that the SCFA absorptive capacity of the colon is exceeded or allow unmetabolized carbohydrate to pass through the colon and continue its osmotic effect as a nonabsorbable solute.[135]

Cations such as magnesium or anions like sulfate are absorbed poorly by the normal gut. Thus, increased ingestion of these ions can easily lead to an osmotic diarrhea.[136] This either can be an intended therapeutic effect, as with laxatives, or may be the etiology of an iatrogenic diarrhea, as may occur with magnesium-containing antacids.

In clinical situations in which there is malabsorption or a generalized destruction of the epithelium, solutes normally absorbed readily may remain in the intestinal lumen and thereby contribute an osmotic component to an inflammatory diarrhea or a malabsorptive state. Osmolality is an important factor in enteral nutrition. For example, complex carbohydrates provide a significant amount of calories with minimal osmolality compared with simple sugars. Absorption of di- and tripeptides instead of amino acids reduces intestinal osmolality. This balance between calories and osmolality becomes clinically relevant in effectively designing appropriate tube-feeding regimens. It has also become apparent that variations in osmolarity alter the effectiveness or oral rehydration therapies. Hypotonic solutions may stimulate water absorption. Rice-based or glucose polymer solutions appear to deliver similar absorptive stimuli at lower osmolar cost to the intestine.

Specific Regulatory Factors

Absorptive Stimuli

Mineralocorticoids increase Na absorption. Aldosterone and its analogs affect primarily those segments of the gut that exhibit electrogenic Na absorption, such as the distal colon.[137, 138] In epithelia that do not spontaneously exhibit electrogenic Na absorption, aldosterone may have no effect (ileum) or may induce new electrogenic Na transport (rat colon).[139, 140] Aldosterone increases the number of Na channels in the apical membrane, thereby increasing the rate of Na entry in the cell. This may occur either by synthesis of new channels or by insertion of channels from a preexisting cellular pool. There is a secondary increase in the activity of the Na pump. Aldosterone also increases K absorption and K secretion.[141, 142] Clinically, the role of aldosterone can be seen in the increased colonic absorption after Na depletion or in the diarrhea associated with Addison's disease. Neonates exhibit a correlation between high circulating levels of aldosterone and enhanced colonic Na absorption.[143, 144]

Glucocorticoids also are potent stimulators of Na absorption. Glucocorticoids are a more "global" absorbagogue, enhancing Na absorption independent of the presence of amiloride-sensitive Na conductance. Thus, glucocorticoids increase Na absorption in the small intestine and in the colon.[145, 146] The action of glucocorticoids may be directed more to the stimulation of the Na pump rather than an alteration in specific apical entry mechanisms.[147] Although there have been some lingering doubts about whether glucocorticoids have an effect on ion transport independent of aldosterone, the weight of recent studies suggests a specific glucocorticoid effect.[148, 149] Thus, in addition to their anti-inflammatory effect, glucocorticoids directly stimulate intestinal Na and water absorption. This may account, in part, for their potent antidiarrheal action in a wide variety of clinical settings.

Catecholamines, opioids, and *somatostatin* all are absorbagogues with a similar pattern of action: stimulation of electroneutral Na absorption. Acting as an α_2-adrenergic agonist, epinephrine stimulates NaCl absorption in ileum and colon and decreases bicarbonate secretion in the ileum.[2, 150, 151] The effects on NaCl absorption and bicarbonate transport are not necessarily linked.[2] Another catecholamine found in the intestine, dopamine, has similar absorptive properties.[152] The theoretical basis for the use of clonidine as an antidiarrheal, particularly in diabetic diarrhea, is rooted in this adrenergic absorptive pathway.[153]

Historically, opioids have been the most effective class of antidiarrheals. Characterization of the role of enkephalins and endorphins in the gut has provided a physiologic understanding of their therapeutic effect. There are multiple opiate receptor subtypes. In the intestine, the μ, κ, and δ receptors all regulate smooth muscle tone; activation of the δ receptor also stimulates electrolyte absorption.[154] Given the relative affinities of the currently available opioid drugs (loperamide, codeine) for specific receptor subtypes, the effect on smooth muscle may be more important than the proabsorptive effect.[155]

The development of long-acting analogs of somatostatin has transformed this hormone from a physiologically fascinating regulator to a clinically relevant pharmacologic agent. Somatostatin and its receptors are found throughout the body. In the gut, endocrine-like D cells produce somatostatin. Somatostatin stimulates salt and water absorption in ileum and colon and also blocks the effects of several secretory agents.[156, 157] Somatostatin analogs are effective in treating several types of diarrheal diseases, particularly endocrine-related secretory diarrheas.[158] Their therapeutic effect is due to a combination of actions, including inhibition of hormone release by tumors, slowing of intestinal transit, and a direct effect on epithelial cells. On a cellular level, somatostatin appears to activate the inhibitory subunit of the guanine nucleotide protein of adenylate cyclase, reducing cellular cyclic AMP. Paradoxically, increasing somatostatin levels, as encountered in somatostatinomas or with large pharmacologic doses of somatostatin analog, may precipitate diarrhea, due in large part to steatorrhea.

SECRETORY FACTORS

Eicosanoids are a family of 20-carbon oxygenated metabolites of arachidonic acid. There is a complex metabolism of eicosanoids originating from the conversion of membrane phospholipids to arachidonic acid and the subsequent metabolism into cyclooxygenase products (prostaglandins) and lipoxygenase products (leukotrienes). Intestinal eicosanoids are produced primarily in the subepithelium. More than 95% of gut prostaglandins arise from inflammatory cells in the submucosa.[159, 160] However, there is a preferential metabolism of eicosanoids by the epithelial cells. Prostaglandin effects are, in part, modulated by the enteric nerves and, to a major extent, by a direct effect on epithelial cells. Prostaglandins also have significant extraepithelial effects on intestinal motility and blood flow.

There are subtle differences in the biologic actions within the families of prostaglandins and leukotrienes, but in general they inhibit electroneutral NaCl absorption and stimulate electrogenic Cl secretion. The principal intracellular second messenger for prostaglandins is cyclic AMP,[161] although there is some evidence to suggest a role for intracellular calcium.[162] Prostaglandins may contribute to the basal secretory tone of the epithelium.[163]

The role of prostaglandins in the diarrhea of inflammatory bowel disease is enigmatic. Clearly, there is increased intestinal production of eicosanoids. Given the role of steroids in decreasing prostaglandin synthesis and the therapeutic effect of mesalamine and sulfasalazine, one might expect cyclooxygenase inhibitors to have a beneficial effect. They do not.[164, 165] This has led to a reassessment of the pharmacology of the salicylate derivatives used in inflammatory bowel disease.[166, 167] Leukotrienes and other inflammatory mediators may be pivotal in the etiology of the diarrhea associated with inflammatory bowel disease (see Chapters 103 and 104).

Acetylcholine, Vasoactive Intestinal Peptide, Serotonin, and Additional Secretagogues

A host of hormones and neurotransmitters has been implicated as modulators of intestinal ion transport. Although a few are clearly clinically relevant (VIP and serotonin), the specific physiologic or pathophysiologic role of many others remains to be determined. Acetylcholine and muscarinic cholinergic agonists act directly on epithelial cells to increase cell calcium (Ca) and cause secretion.[168] VIP increases intracellular cyclic AMP, inhibits electroneutral NaCl absorption, and stimulates Cl secretion. Peptides structurally related to VIP, such as secretin, peptide histidine isoleucine, and peptide histidine methionine, have similar effects.

Serotonin (5-hydroxytryptamine) is normally found in enterochromaffin cells and enteric neurons. Increased amounts of serotonin (and other peptides) cause the diarrhea associated with carcinoid tumors (see Chapter 112). Serotonin increases intracellular Ca in enterocytes and, like VIP, inhibits electroneutral NaCl absorption and stimulates Cl secretion.[169] Adenosine, a potent secretagogue in vitro, may have a unique role interacting with the colonic epithelium to stimulate secretion in vivo. Reductionist models of crypt abscesses have demonstrated that after leukocytes traverse the tight junctions into the luminal space, they release a weak secretagogue (5′ AMP) that is converted by specific apical membrane enzymes into a more powerful secretagogue, adenosine.[116, 170] Thus, it appears that, in the right setting, epithelial and inflammatory cells provide an intricate coordinated series of actions to stimulate secretion.

Recently recognized, clinically relevant secretagogues include *guanylin, reactive oxygen metabolites*, and, perhaps, *nitric oxide* (NO). The search for an endogenous activator of the *E. coli* stable enterotoxin receptor led to the discovery of guanylin, a small peptide synthesized in goblet and columnar cells, which increases intracellular cyclic GMP and elicits

Cl secretion.[171, 172] Guanylin may represent a mechanism through which the gut can calibrate its rate of secretion.

Leukocytes release multiple reactive oxygen metabolites, including oxygen free radicals, hydrogen peroxide, and chloramines, which cause Cl secretion in vitro.[173] These may provide a direct link between inflammation and diarrhea. Multiple additional agonists stimulate secretion (see Table 87–2). Interestingly, most of these agents also affect intestinal motility.

Enterotoxins and Infectious Diarrheas

Worldwide, infectious diarrhea is a major cause of morbidity and mortality; it certainly has a far greater clinical significance than the relatively rare hormonally mediated secretory diarrheas. With the re-emergence of cholera in the Americas, toxin-induced diarrhea may no longer be a traveler's nuisance or an exotic curiosity.

Bacterial toxins may cause diarrhea by different mechanisms. Cytotoxins kill mammalian cells, usually by inhibition of protein synthesis. The archetypical cytotoxin is produced by *Shigella* and is responsible for the dysentery-like symptoms associated with impaired absorption and damage to the mucosa.[138] In contrast, enterotoxins produced a diarrhea by capturing and turning on the secretory machinery of the epithelium. The paradigm for enterotoxin-medicated diarrhea is cholera. The toxin binds to the brush border membrane of the small intestine before localizing to the adenylate cyclase system on the basolateral membrane; there, through a specific ADP-ribosylation of the stimulating Gs protein (see subsequent text), the toxin produces an unregulated increase in cyclic AMP and thus secretion.

Our understanding of how cholera affects the gut has undergone continuous revision. It is now apparent that *Vibrio cholera* produces multiple toxins, including one directed at the tight junction (ZO).[174] Cholera affects the epithelium directly but also recruits multiple components of the PINES, including enteric neurons and enterochromaffin cells, and multiple mediators such as prostaglandins and serotonin to produce a complex secretory response.[175, 176] There also may be effects beyond the small intestine, with a reflex secretory response in the colon.[105]

Cholera toxin blocks electroneutral NaCl absorption and stimulates electrogenic chloride secretion in the small bowel. The volume of secretion can be staggering and life-threatening (see Chapter 96). However, despite the degree of secretion, specific intestinal absorptive pathways remain fully intact and operational. Na-coupled nutrient pathways (Na-glucose, Na-amino acids) are unaltered by the toxin. This forms the physiologic basis for the oral rehydration therapy in which nutrient-driven Na absorption permits water absorption to continue in the face of massive diarrhea.[177]

Multiple additional enterotoxins and cytotoxins have been identified (see Table 87–3). Many act in a manner similar to that of cholera toxin, elevating intracellular cyclic AMP, but others, such as the heat stable enterotoxins produced by *E. coli* and *Yersinia enterocolitica*, stimulate Cl secretion by increasing cycle GMP. Other enterotoxins may have relatively selective effects on intestinal permeability by altering tight junction properties.[178] Nonbacterial pathogens may also elicit secretory diarrheas. The mechanism of diarrhea in cryptosporidiosis is complex and may vary according to the patient's immune status; however, there is evidence that the massive watery diarrhea sometimes encountered in cryptosporidiosis is due to an enterotoxin.[179, 180] In addition to its effect on epithelial integrity, *Entamoeba histolytica* may elicit a Ca-mediated secretory diarrhea, perhaps related to release of serotonin from the organism itself.[181] Although it has been assumed that rotavirus elicits diarrhea by damaging mature absorptive cells, there is now emerging evidence that a rotavirus protein (NSP4) can elicit Ca-mediated Cl secretion.[182] NSP4-induced Cl secretion does not depend on CFTR but probably involves a novel Ca-dependent Cl channel. There is an age dependency of NSP4-induced diarrhea that parallels the clinical pattern of rotavirus-induced diarrhea.[183]

Thus, the spectrum of toxin-induced mechanisms of secretion is expanding. Delineating the mechanisms of toxin-induced secretion is obviously important for understanding the pathophysiology of infectious diarrheas; additionally, characterizing these effects can lead to insights about intrinsic regulation of the epithelium. Infectious agents frequently use molecular mimicry as a subterfuge to take control of the transport mechanisms of the cell. Identifying the bacterial mechanism (e.g., *E. coli* heat stable toxin) can lead to the discovery of endogenous regulators (e.g., guanylin).

Bile Salts and Other Luminal Factors

Small bowel malabsorption of bile acids or oral intake of pharmacologic amounts of certain bile acids causes diarrhea. Only dihydroxy bile acids with the hydroxyl groups in the alpha, but not beta, position cause diarrhea. This seemingly obscure detail of bile acid biochemistry indicates why chenodeoxycholic acid ($3\alpha7\alpha$) but not ursodeoxycholate ($3\alpha7\beta$) is associated with diarrhea. Bile acids have multiple effects on the colonic epithelium. At high concentrations they act as a detergent on the epithelial membrane, increasing intestinal permeability. At more physiologic concentrations, bile salts stimulate Cl secretion, both by directly acting on epithelial cells with increases in cyclic AMP and Ca or indirectly through activation of mast cells.[184, 185]

Long-chain fatty acids within the colonic lumen arise when triglycerides are digested by lipase but are malabsorbed within the small bowel in clinical conditions such as sprue. These long-chain fatty acids have similar mechanisms of action as bile acids. Hydroxylated fatty acids (e.g., ricinoleic acid) are more potent secretagogues than the corresponding long-chain fatty acid. They originate from colonic bacterial metabolism or may be given as the active ingredient of castor oil.

INTRACELLULAR MEDIATORS

The intestinal epithelial cell is exposed to a barrage of potential stimuli. These external messages need to be translated into an intracellular "language" that allows the cell to regulate its transport machinery. The second messengers of the cell that perform this regulatory function are the adenylate cyclase and guanylate cyclase systems, intracellular Ca, and the inositol phosphate-diacyl glycerol cascade. These systems are common to several epithelia and other organ systems. Gastric acid secretion, pancreatic enzyme secretion, and hormonal effects all depend on basically similar systems. More detailed descriptions of second messenger systems can be found in Chapter 1 and elsewhere.[186, 187]

In general, an increase in any of these systems inhibits absorption or stimulates secretion. They elicit an increase in apical chloride and basolateral K conductances associated with electrogenic Cl secretion. They can inhibit Na-H exchange in intestinal epithelia, which is in contrast to the regulatory response in other tissues. The second messengers appear to have little effect on Na conductances in the colon, again in contrast to other epithelia.

Protein kinases execute second messages rapidly. The kinases are both mediator and target specific. They phosphorylate either a membrane transport protein or a modulator of transport. Kinases takes the terminal phosphate from ATP and put it on the hydroxyl group of a serine, threoninine, or tyrosine of a target protein, leading to a conformational change and a change in function. Specifically, characterization of phosphorylated targets of protein kinases involving NHEs and Cl channels will be critical to understanding the regulation of the transport pathways involving these proteins.[188]

The complexities of the adenylate cyclase system have been well characterized (Fig. 87–10). Located on the basolateral membrane of epithelial cells, adenylate cyclase has two distinct receptors, one stimulatory and the other inhibitory. Each receptor is linked to a corresponding guaninine-nucleotide binding protein, either stimulatory (Gs) or inhibitory (Gi), which when activated modifies the activity of catalytic subunit. The catalytic subunit converts ATP to cyclic AMP, which then goes on to activate a protein kinase. Specific agonists are known to have either stimulatory or inhibitory effects on the system.

Intracellular Ca is tightly regulated at relatively low levels, maintaining a 100-fold gradient with the extracellular environment (Fig. 87–11). Transient elevations in intracellular Ca elicit a series of events that may alter ion transport and a host of other cellular events. Increased membrane permeability, presumably through ion-specific Ca channels, can increase intracellular Ca. This mechanism, activated by substance P, depends on extracellular Ca and may be blocked by Ca-channel blockers. An alternative mechanism depends on the release of Ca from intracellular stores. In this system, receptor-mediated events cause the release of phosphoinositol metabolites and diacylglycerol from the cell membrane. Inositol triphosphate triggers the release of calcium from poorly defined nonmitochondrial sources.

Ca-related intracellular events occur through activation of Ca-calmodulin complex, which subsequently activates multiple kinases; diacyl glycerol activation of a specific kinase, protein kinase C; and direct activation of Ca-sensitive channels.[189, 190] Low cell Ca can be restored by Ca-ATPases or Na-Ca exchangers, which promote Ca exit from the cell. Diacylglycerol may have a negative effect on inositol triphosphate–stimulated release of intracellular Ca. Pharmacologic agents may affect intracellular Ca metabolism. Phenothiazines and loperamide may exert some of their effects through interference in Ca metabolism.

The guanylate cyclase system in the intestine forms a parallel secretory apparatus, with a distinct set of agonists (guanylin, atrial natriuretic peptide, nitric oxide, heat stable enterotoxins) and a specific protein kinase.[191] Both cyclic AMP and cyclic GMP target CFTR as a regulator of Cl secretion. Although representing three distinct regulatory systems, there is probably considerable interaction among the cyclic nucleotides and Ca in eliciting their physiologic effects. Cyclic AMP and Ca-related agonists exhibit synergistic actions on Cl secretion. This potentiation may be related to different target sites (Cl channels or K channels) or may be due to modulation of the intracellular signaling process.[192] Studies have suggested that cyclic nucleotides may have broader effects than previously realized, perhaps altering Na-glucose cotransport.[193]

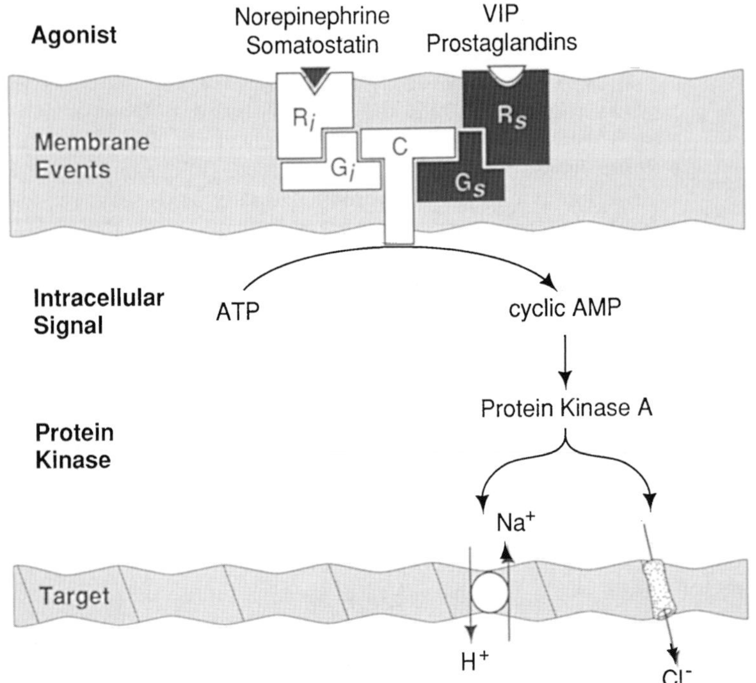

Figure 87–10. Second messengers: cyclic AMP. Five steps are involved in the transduction of an external signal into a change in cellular function: (1) Binding of either a stimulatory or an inhibitory agonist to appropriate receptor of the membrane bound adenylate cyclase system; (2) binding activates the corresponding G protein, which modulates the catalytic subunit (c); (3) an intracellular signal results from production of cyclic AMP from ATP; (4) increased intracellular cyclic AMP results in activation of protein kinases such as protein kinase A; (5) protein kinases mediated phosphylation of specific target proteins results in change in the activity of chloride channel or the sodium hydrogen exchanger.

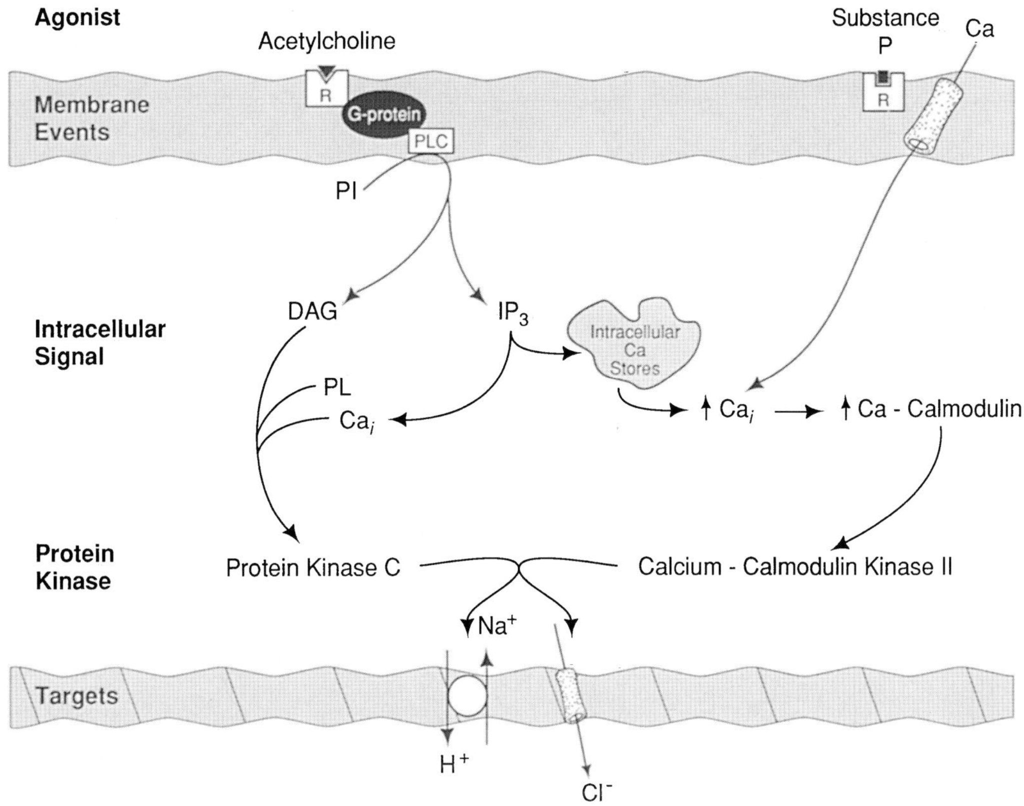

Figure 87–11. Second Messengers: intracellular calcium. The signal transduction by intracellular calcium can be modeled into five steps. (1) Agonist binding to a specific membrane protein, e.g. acetylcholine, (2) resulting in activation of a G protein, which stimulates phospholipase C (PLC), (3) converting phospholinositols (PI) to diacylglycerol and inositol trisphosphate (DAG and IP3). (4) Elevated diacylglycerol in combination with phospholipids and intracellular calcium functions as an intracellular signal that activates protein kinase C, which (5) then acts on its specific target protein, modulating the activity of sodium hydrogen exchanger and chloride channel.

Inositol trisphosphate will (3) increase intracellular calcium, by release from intracellular stores, which then functions as an intracellular signal, binding calmodulin, which will activate its protein kinases, such as calcium calmodulin kinase 2, and then (5) subsequently act on membrane target proteins.

A different pathway for calcium modulation exists in which agonists such as substance P (1) bind to specific membrane receptors leading to (2) activation of a calcium channel, (3) thereby increasing intracellular calcium, which (4) activates the particular protein kinases, and (5) ending with action on the target protein.

ADDITIONAL REGULATORY MECHANISMS

On one level, regulation of transport is like throwing a switch. The intact machinery is simply waiting for the right input. This can occur with nutrient-coupled transport as in oral rehydration therapy. On another level, obviously, altering the abundance of specific transporter will alter function of the gut. This occurs in several different circumstances: as part of the maturation process as cells migrate along the crypt-villus axis, in response to hormonal input, or as part of genetic programming (e.g., lactase deficiency). Specific disease states may selectively alter individual transport molecule abundance; this occurs in the diabetic intestine, which exhibits up-regulation of the sodium-glucose cotransporter.[194] However, given the complexities of the intestinal epithelium, we are only beginning to appreciate several additional levels of regulation.

The epithelium takes cues and clues from the luminal environment above and beyond the immediate stimulation of a specific transport pathway. Nutrient–gene interactions occur in the gut both in a feed-forward and feedback mechanism. There may be more generalized types of regulation. Butyrate in vitro and fiber (pectin) in vivo increase colonic NHE-3, suggesting that dietary factors may alter global parameters of transport.[50]

Changes in epithelial turnover may alter the transport function of the intestine. The balance between immature "secretory" crypt cells and mature "absorptive" villus cells may have an impact on the overall fluid balance of the gut. In experimental models of rapidly proliferating colon, there is a dramatic increase in both CFTR and secretory capacity concomitant with an increase in crypt cells.[195] There may be clinical correlates such as celiac sprue.

How molecules move around in cells may have a profound impact on their function.[196] Three different types of intracellular trafficking may regulate transport function.

1. Establishment of vectorial transport requires directed cellular trafficking of specific molecules to either the apical or basolateral membrane. This is critical to a polarized epithelium (see previous section, Basic Epithelial Cell Model).

2. The rate of transport may be controlled by rapid recycling of molecules between the apical membrane and a subapical compartment. NHE-3, SGLT1, and CFTR, for example, cycle between the plasma membrane and endocytic vesicles. At times of increased demand for transport, the vesicles

are rapidly directed to the cell surface, fuse with the plasma membrane, and increase the number of transport molecules and thus the maximal transport velocity. This endosomal recycling is regulated by growth factors and second messengers.[75, 197, 198]

3. There is now emerging evidence that transporters and their regulating factors may be brought together in localized membrane domains by scaffolding proteins that bind them together. This proximity increase the effectiveness of the regulatory process.[199–201]

Finally, there is the concept of homocellular regulation. Simply put, what goes in must come out. Apical and basolateral entry and exit activity must be coordinated to maintain cell volume within an acceptable range. If not, the cell will either shrink or explode owing to a rapid change in ionic content and osmolality. Given the vicissitudes in luminal content, intestinal epithelial cells must be prepared for large and rapid changes in the rates of ion and nutrient transport. Exactly how the cell fine tunes discrete events at its opposite borders is still not well understood.

FLUID AND ELECTROLYTE TRANSPORT IN CONTEXT

Intestinal regulation of solute and water absorption has multiple levels of intricate control. The specific transport pathways within each segment of the intestine in large part define their physiologic function. Characterization of these transport pathways is therefore important in assessing the role of different regions of the gut in normal physiology and pathologic responses. Control of transport function is both intracellular and extracellular. Subepithelial components, including neural, hormonal, and immunologic, are a dominant factor in determining the balance between absorption and secretion. Recognition of the importance of these factors in ion transport has led to increasing investigation of their alterations in various disease states such as inflammatory bowel disease or infectious diarrhea. Additionally, it is now apparent that the dichotomy between epithelial function and motility that has plagued research in diarrheal disease may be an artifact of the investigational technique; in fact, epithelial transport and intestinal motility may be subject to common regulatory factors in the subepithelium.

These multiple levels of control generally serve the gut well. However, the intestine may be challenged by poorly absorbable luminal contents, diminished absorptive capacity, or the stimulation of secretion. The presence of a nonabsorbable solute may precipitate an osmotic diarrhea. Decreased absorptive function, occurring through resection, selective villous damage (sprue, viral enteritides), or rare congenital absence of a transporter (congenital chloridorrhea) may lead to diarrhea. Both exogenous and endogenous factors may stimulate a secretory diarrhea.

The intestine can adapt to increased intestinal fluid losses. The colon can increase its absorptive capacity two- to threefold in the face of increased small bowel losses. Carbohydrate malabsorption by the small bowel may be minimized through colonic salvage of SCFAs. The intestinal epithelium clearly can adapt after resection (see Chapter 92).

Transferral of the physiology of intestinal transport to clinical application is integral to the treatment of diarrhea. This is readily apparent in the use of oral rehydration therapy in the management of cholera. Drugs that interfere with stimulus-secretion coupling, such as somatostatin, may be particularly suitable for therapy in diarrhea. As our understanding of the molecular physiology and biology of ion transport increases, it provides the opportunity for more precise therapeutic interventions in the treatment of intestinal disorders.

REFERENCES

1. Sellin JH, Oyarzabal H, Cragoe EJ: Electrogenic sodium absorption in rabbit cecum in vitro. J Clin Invest 81:1275–1283, 1988.
2. Sellin JH, DeSoignie R: Rabbit proximal colon: a distinct transport epithelium. Am J Physiol 246:G603–G610, 1984.
3. Foster ES, Budinger ME, Hayslett JP, et al: Ion transport in proximal colon of the rat. J Clin Invest 77:228–235, 1986.
4. Hatch M, Freel RW: Electrolyte transport across the rabbit caecum in vitro. Pflugers Arch 411:333–338, 1988.
5. Cartwright CA, Mamajiwalla S, Skolnick SA, et al: Intestinal crypt cells contain higher levels of cytoskeletal-associated pp60c-src protein tyrosine kinase activity than do differentiated enterocytes. Oncogene 8:1033–1039, 1993.
6. Saxon ML, Zhao X, Black JD: Activation of protein kinase C isozymes is associated with post-mitotic events in intestinal epithelial cells in situ. J Cell Biol 126:747–763, 1994.
7. Hopfer U: Membrane transport mechanisms for hexoses and amino acids in the small intestine. In Johnson LR (ed): Physiology of the Gastrointestinal Tract. New York, Raven, 1987, pp 1499–1526.
8. Bookstein C, DePaoli AM, Xie Y, et al: Na/H exchangers, NHE-1 and NHE-3, of rat intestine: expression and localization. J Clin Invest 93:106–113, 1994.
9. Sundaram U: Mechanism of intestinal absorption effect of clonidine on rabbit ileal villus and crypt cells. J Clin Invest 95:2187–2194, 1995.
10. Powell DW: Dogma destroyed: colonic crypts absorb. J Clin Invest 96:2102–2103, 1995.
11. Diener M, Rummel W, Mestres P, et al: Single chloride channels in colon mucosa and isolated colonic enterocytes of the rat. J Memb Biol 108:21–30, 1989.
12. Singh SK, Binder HJ, Boron WF, et al: Fluid absorption in isolated perfused colonic crypts. J Clin Invest 96:2373–2379, 1995.
13. Pedley KC, Naftalin RJ: Evidence from fluorescence microscopy and comparative studies that rat, ovine and bovine colonic crypts are absorptive. J Physiol (Lond) 460:525–547, 1993.
14. Nelson WJ: Regulation of cell surface polarity from bacteria to mammals. Science 258:948, 1992.
15. Persson B, Spring K: Gallbladder epithelial cell hydraulic water permeability and volume regulation. J Gen Physiol 79:481–505, 1982.
16. Spring KR: Routes and mechanisms of fluid transport by epithelia. Annu Rev Physiol 60:105–119, 1998.
17. Spring KR: Epithelial fluid transport—a century of investigation. News Physiol Sci 14:92–98, 1999.
18. Alberts B, Bray D, Lewis J, et al: Molecular Biology of the Cell. New York, Garland, 1991:300.
19. Nathke IS, Hinck LE, Nelson WJ: Epithelial cell adhesion and development of cell surface polarity: possible mechanisms for modulation of cadherin function, organization and distribution. J Cell Sci 106(Suppl 17):139–145, 1993.
20. Fish EM, Molitoris BA: Alterations in epithelial polarity and the pathogenesis of disease states. N Engl J Med 330:1580–1588, 1994.
21. Anderson JM, Van Itallie CM: Tight junctions and the molecular basis for regulation of paracellular permeability. Am J Physiol Gastrointest Liver Physiol 269:G467–G476, 1995.
22. Staddon JM, Herrenknecht K, Smales C, et al: Evidence that tyrosine phosphorylation may increase tight junction permeability. J Cell Sci 108:609–619, 1995.
23. Matthews JB, Awtrey CS, Thompson R, et al: Na^+-K-$2Cl^-$ cotransport and Cl- secretion evoked by heat-stable enterotoxin is microfilament dependent in T84 cells. Am J Physiol Gastrointest Liver Physiol 265:G370–G378, 1993.
24. Rotin D, Bar-Sagi D, O'Bradovich H, et al: An SH3 binding region in

the epithelial Na channel (alpha rENaC) mediates its localization at the apical membrane. EMBO J 13:4440–4450, 1994.

25. Watson AJM, Levine S, Donowitz M, et al: Serum regulates Na+/H+ exchange in Caco-2 cells by a mechanism which is dependent on F-actin. J Biol Chem 267:956–962, 1992.
26. Levitt MD, Furne JK, Strocchi A, et al: Physiological measurement of luminal stirring in the dog and human small bowel. J Clin Invest 86: 1540, 1990.
27. Horisberger J-D, Canessa C, Rossier BC: The epithelial sodium channel: recent developments. Cell Physiol Biochem 3:283–294, 1993.
28. Canessa CM, Schild L, Buell G, et al: Amiloride-sensitive epithelial Na+ channel is made of three homologous subunits. Nature 367:463–467, 1994.
29. Duc C, Rarman N, Canessa CM, et al: Cell specific expression of epithelial sodium channel alpha, beta and gamma subunits in aldosterone responsive epithelia from the rat: localization by in situ hybridization and immunohistochemistry. J Cell Biol 127:1907–1921, 1994.
30. Palmer LG: Epithelial Na channels and their kin. News in Physiol Sci 10:61–67, 1995.
31. Canessa CM, Horisberger JD, Rossier BC: Epithelial sodium channel related to proteins involved in neurodegeneration. Nature 361:467–470, 1993.
32. Goldner AM, Schultz SG, Curran PF: Sodium and sugar fluxes across the mucosal border of rabbit ileum. J Gen Physiol 53:362, 1969.
33. Potter GD, Schmidt KL, Lester R: Glucose absorption by in vitro perfused colon of the fetal rat. Am J Physiol 245:G424–G430, 1983.
34. Hediger MA, Coady MJ, Ikeda TS, et al: Expression cloning and cDNA sequencing of the Na+/glucose co-transporter. Nature 330: 379–380, 1988.
35. Hediger MA, Kanai Y, You G, et al: Mammalian ion-coupled solute transporters. J Physiol 482.P:7S–17S, 1995.
36. Pappenheimer JR, Reiss KZ: Contribution of solvent drag through intercellular junctions to absorption of nutrients by the small intestine of the rat. J Memb Biol 100:123–135, 1987.
37. Madara JL: Loosening tight junctions. Lessons from the intestine. J Clin Invest 183:1089–1094, 1989.
38. Turner JR, Madara JL: Physiological regulation of intestinal epithelial tight junctions as a consequence of Na+-/coupled nutrient transport. Gastroenterology 109:1391–1396, 1995.
39. Fine KD, Santa Ana CA, Porter JL, et al: Effect of D-glucose on intestinal permeability and its passive absorption in human small intestine in vivo. Gastroenterology 105:1117–1125, 1993.
40. Schwartz RM, Furne JK, Levitt MD: Paracellular intestinal transport of six-carbon sugars is negligible in the rat. Gastroenterology 109: 1206–1213, 1995.
41. Sardet C, Franchi A, Pouyssegur J: Molecular cloning, primary structure and expression of the human growth factor activatable Na/H antiporter. Cell 56:271–280, 1989.
42. Orlowski J, Kandasamy RA, Shull GE: Molecular cloning of putative members of the NHE exchanger gene family. cDNA cloning, deduced amino acid sequence, and mRNA tissue expression of the rat NHE exchanger NHE-1 and two structurally related proteins. J Biol Chem 267:9331–9339, 1992.
43. Tse CM, Ma AI, Yang VW, et al: Molecular cloning and expression of a cDNA encoding the rabbit ileal villus cell basolateral membrane Na-H exchanger. EMBO J 10:1957–1967, 1991.
44. Tse C-M, Brant SR, Walker MS, et al: Cloning and sequencing of a rabbit cDNA encoding an intestinal and kidney-specific Na^+/H^+ exchanger isoform (NHE-3). J Biol Chem 267:9340–9346, 1992.
45. Rothstein A: The Na/H exchange system in cell pH and volume control. Rev Physiol Biochem Pharmacol 112:235–257, 1989.
46. Knickelbein RG, Aronson PS, Dobbins JW: Characterization of Na/H exchangers on villus cells in rabbit ileum. Am J Physiol Gastrointest Liver Physiol 259:G802–G806, 1990.
47. Ikuma M, Kashgarian M, Binder JH, et al: Differential regulation of NHE isoforms by sodium depletion in proximal and distal segments of rat colon. Am J Physiol Gastrointest Liver Physiol 39:G539–G549, 1999.
48. Cho JH, Musch MW, Bookstein CM, et al: Aldosterone stimulates intestinal Na^+ absorption in rats by increasing NHE3 expression of the proximal colon. Am J Physiol 274:C586–C594, 1998.
49. McSwine RL, Musch MW, Bookstein C, et al: Regulation of apical membrane Na+/H+ exchangers NHE2 and NHE3 in intestinal epithelial cell line C2/bbe. Am J Physiol 275:C693–C701, 1998.
50. Musch MW, Bookstein C, Xie Y, et al: Short chain fatty acids regulate intestinal Na absorption: region- and isoform-specific regulation of luminal membrane Na-H exchangers in vivo and in human intestinal C2/BBE cells. Am J Physiol 280:G687–G693, 2001.
51. Schultheis PJ, Clarke LL, Meneton P, et al: Renal and intestinal absorptive defects in mice lacking the NHE-3 Na+/H+ Exchanger. Nat Genet 19:282–285, 1998.
52. Schultheis PJ, Clarke LL, Meneton P, et al: Targeted disruption of the murine Na/H exchanger isoform 2 gene causes reduced viability of gastric parietal cells and loss of net acid secretion. J Clin Invest 101: 1243–1253, 1998.
53. Yun CHC, Gurubhagavatula S, Levine SA, et al: Glucocorticoid stimulation of ileal Na^+ absorptive cell brush border Na^+/H^+ exchange and association with an increase in message for NHE-3, an epithelial Na^+/H^+ exchanger isoform. J Biol Chem 268:206–211, 1993.
54. Tse M, Levine S, Yun C, et al: Structure/function studies of the epithelial isoforms of the mammalian Na^+/H^+ exchanger gene family. J Membr Biol 135:93–108, 1993.
55. Donowitz M, Montgomery JLM, Walker MS, et al: Brush border tyrosine phosphorylation stimulates ileal neutral NaCl absorption and brush border Na+-H+ exchange. Am J Physiol Gastrointest Liver Physiol 266:G647–G656, 1994.
56. Nellans HN, Frizzell RA, Schultz SG: Coupled sodium-chloride influx across the brush border of rabbit ileum. Am J Physiol 225:467–475, 1973.
57. Liedtke CM, Hopfer U: Mechanism of Cl translocation across small intestinal brush border membrane. I. Absence of NaCl contransport. Am J Physiol 242:G263–G271, 1982.
58. Kleinman JG, Harig JM, Barry JA, et al: Na and H transport in human jejunal brush-border membrane vesicles. Am J Physiol 255: G206–G211, 1988.
59. Gunther RD, Wright EM: Na, Li, and Cl transport by brush border membranes from rabbit jejunum. J Memb Biol 74:85–94, 1983.
60. Semrad CE, Chang EB: Calcium mediated cyclic AMP inhibition of Na-H exchange in small intestine. Am J Physiol 252:C315–C322, 1987.
61. Ahn J, Chang EB, Field M: Phorbol ester inhibition of Na-H exchange in rabbit proximal colon. Am J Physiol 249:C527–C530, 1985.
62. Schultz SG: Cellular models of sodium and chloride absorption by mammalian small and large intestine. In Field M, Fordtran JS, Schultz SG (eds): Secretory Diarrhea. Bethesda, Md., American Physiology Society, 1980, pp 1–9.
63. Sellin JH, Duffey ME: Mechanisms of intestinal chloride absorption. In Duffey M, Lebenthal E (eds): Textbook of Secretory Diarrhea. New York, Raven, 1990, pp 81–94.
64. Knickelbein R, Aronson PS, Dobbins JW: Substrate and inhibitor specificity of anion exchangers on the brush border membrane of rabbit ileum. JMB 88:199–204, 1985.
65. O'Grady SM, Palfry HC, Field M: Characteristics and functions of Na-K-Cl cotransport in epithelial tissues. Am J Physiol 253:C177–C192, 1987.
66. Mandel KG, McRoberts JA, Beuerlein G, et al: Ba inhibition of VIP- and A23187-stimulated Cl secretion by T-84 cell monolayers. Am J Physiol 250:C486, 1986.
67. Kartner NJ, Hanrahan W, Jensen TJ, et al: Expression of the cystic fibrosis gene in nonepithelial invertebrate cells produces a regulated anion conductance. Cell 64:681–691, 1991.
68. Bear CE, Duguay F, Naismith AL, et al: Cl channel activity in *Xenopus* occytes expressing the cystic fibrosis gene. J Biol Chem 266: 19142–19145, 1991.
69. Rao MC: Absorption and secretion of water and electrolytes. In Ratnaike RRN (ed): Small Bowel Disorders. London, Arnold, 2000, pp 116–134.
70. Barrett KE, Keely SJ: Chloride secretion by the intestinal epithelium: molecular basis and regulatory aspects. Annu Rev Physiol 62:535–572, 2000.
71. Strong TV, Boehm K, Collins FS: Localization of cystic fibrosis transmembrane conductance regulator mRNA in the human gastrointestinal tract by in situ hybridization. J Clin Invest 93:347–354, 1994.
72. Cohn JA, Nairn AC, Marino CR, et al: Characterization of the cystic fibrosis transmembrane conductance regulator in a colonocyte cell line. Proc Natl Acad Sci USA 89:2340–2344, 1992.
73. Demming GM, Anderson MP, Amara JF, et al: Processing of mutant cystic fibrosis transmembrane conductance regulator is temperature-sensitive. Nature 358:761–764, 1992.

74. Morris AP, Cunningham SA, Tousson A, et al: Polarization-dependent apical membrane CFTR targeting underlies cAMP-stimulated Cl^- secretion in epithelial cells. Am J Physiol Cell Physiol 266:C254–C268, 1994.
75. Peters KW, Qi J, Watkins S, et al: Mechanisms underlying regulated CFTR trafficking. Med Clin North Am 84:633–640, 2000.
76. Peters KW, Qi J, Watkins SC, et al: Synthaxin 1A inhibits regulated CFTR trafficking in xenopus oocytes. Am J Phyiol 277:C174–C180, 1999.
77. Smith PL, Sullivan SK, McCabe RD: Potassium absorption and secretion by intestinal epithelium. In Lebenthal E, Duffey M (eds): Textbook of Secretory Diarrhea. New York, Raven, 1990, pp 109–118.
78. Abrahamse SL, Vis A, Bindels RJM, et al: Regulation of intracellular pH in crypt cells from rabbit distal colon. Am J Physiol Gastrointest Liver Physiol 267:G409–G415, 1994.
79. Lee J, Rajendran VM, Mann AS, et al: Functional expression and segmental localization of rat colonic K-adenosine triphosphatase. J Clin Invest 96:2002–2008, 1995.
80. Dagher PC, Egnor RW, Charney AN: Effect of intracellular acidification on colonic NaCl absorption. Am J Physiol Gastrointest Liver Physiol 264:G569–G575, 1993.
81. Dagher PC, Morton TZ, Joo CS, et al: Modulation of secretagogue-induced chloride secretion by intracellular bicarbonate. Am J Physiol Gastrointest Liver Physiol 266:G929–G934, 1994.
82. Shumaker H, Amlal H, Frizzell R, et al: CFTR drives Na^+-$nHCO_3$ cotransport in pancreatic duct cells: a basis for detective HCO_3 secretion in CF. Am J Physiol 776:C6–C25, 1999.
83. Janecki A: Why should a clinician care about the molecular biology of transport? Curr Gastroenterol Rep 2:378–386, 2000.
84. Sellin JH, DeSoignie R: Regulation of bicarbonate transport by rabbit ileum. pH stat studies. Am J Physiol 257:G607–G615, 1989.
85. Minhas BS, Sullivan SK, Field M: Bicarbonate secretion in rabbit ileum: electrogenicity, ion dependence, and effects of cyclic nucleotides. Gastroenterology 105:1617–1629, 1993.
86. Hogan DL, Crombie DL, Isesnberg JI, et al: CFTR mediates camp- and Ca^{2+}-activated duodenal epithelial HCO3-secretion. Am J Physiol 272:G872–G878, 1997.
87. Pratha VS, Hogan DL, Martensson BA, et al: Identification of transport abnormalities in duodenal mucosa and duodenal enterocytes from patients with cystic fibrosis. Gastroenterology 118:1051–1060, 2000.
88. Smith JJ, Welsh MJ, Baccam DN: cAMP stimulates bicarbonate secretion across normal, but not cystic fibrosis airway epithelia. J Clin Invest 89:1148–1153, 1992.
89. Argenzio RA, Southworth M, Lowe JE, et al: Interrelationship of Na, HCO_3 and volatile fatty acid transport by equine large intestine. Am J Physiol 233:E469–E478, 1977.
90. Ruppin H, Bar-Meir S, Soergel KH, et al: Absorption of short-chain fatty acids by the colon. Gastroenterology 78:1500–1507, 1980.
91. Sellin JH, DeSoignie R: Short-chain fatty acid absorption in rabbit colon in vitro. Gastroenterology 99:676–683, 1990.
92. Mascolo N, Rajendran VM, Binder HJ: Mechanisms of short-chain fatty acid uptake by apical membrane vesicles of rat distal colon. Gastroenterology 101:331–338, 1991.
93. Harig JM, Soergel KH, Barry JA, et al: Transport of propionate by human ileal brush border membrane vesicles. Am J Physiol 260: G776–G782, 1991.
94. Sellin JH, DeSoignie R: Short-chain fatty acids have polarized effects on sodium transport and intracellular pH in rabbit proximal colon. Gastroenterology 114:734–747, 1998.
95. Harig JM, Soergel KH, Komorowski RA, et al: Treatment of diversion colitis with short-chain fatty acid irrigation. N Engl J Med 320:23–28, 1989.
96. Breuer RI, Buto SK, Christ ML, et al: Rectal irrigation with short-chain fatty acids for distal ulcerative colitis: preliminary report. Dig Dis Sci 36:185–187, 1991.
97. Roediger WEW: The colonic epithelium in ulcerative colitis—an energy deficient disease. Lancet 2:712–715, 1980.
98. Ramakrishna BS, Venkataraman S, Srinivasan P, et al: Amylase-resistant starch plus oral rehydration solution for cholera. N Engl J Med 342:308–313, 2000.
99. Cooke HJ: Hormones and neurotransmitters regulating intestinal ion transport. In Field M (ed): Diarrheal Diseases. New York, Elsevier, 1991, pp 23–48.
100. Makhlouf GM: Neural and hormonal regulation of function in the gut. Hosp Pract 25:59–78, 1990.
101. Fogel R, Michelson G, Senler T, et al: Central administration of benzodiazepines alters water absorption by the rat ileum in vivo. Gastroenterology 93:330–334, 1987.
102. Jodal M, Holmgren S, Lundgren O, et al: Involvement of the myenteric plexus in the cholera toxin-induced net fluid secretion in the rat small intestine. Gastroenterology 105:1286–1293, 1993.
103. Vanner S, MacNaughton WK: Capsaicin-sensitive afferent nerves activate submucosal secretomotor neurons in guinea pig ileum. Am J Physiol Gastrointest Liver Physiol 269:G203–G209, 1995.
104. Moore BA, Sharkey KA, Mantle M: Neural mediation of cholera toxin-induced mucin secretion in the rat small intestine. Am J Physiol Gastrointest Liver Physiol 265:G1050–G1056, 1993.
105. Nocerino A, Iafusco M, Guandalini S: Cholera toxin-induced small intestinal secretion has a secretory effect on the colon of the rat. Gastroenterology 108:34–39, 1995.
106. Hubel KA: Intestinal ion transport. Effect of norephinephrine, pilocarpine and atropine. Am J Physiol 231:252–257, 1976.
107. Morris AI, Turnberg LA: The influence of a parasympathetic agonist and antagonist on human intestinal transport in vivo. Gastroenterology 79:861–866, 1980.
108. Chang EB, Bergenstal EM, Field M: Diarrhea of streptocozin-treated rats. Loss of adrenergic regulation of intestinal fluid and electrolyte transport. J Clin Invest 75:1666–1670, 1985.
109. Sartor RB, Powell DW: Mechanisms of diarrhea in intestinal inflammation and hypersensitivity. In Field M (ed): Diarrheal Diseases. New York, Elsevier, 1991, pp 75–114.
110. Castro GA: Gut immunophysiology: regulatory pathways within a common mucosal immune system. NIPS 4:59–64, 1989.
111. MacDermott RP: Alterations in the mucosal immune system in ulcerative colitis and Crohn's disease. Med Clin North Am 78:1207–1231, 1994.
112. Perdue MH, Masson S, Wershil BK, et al: Role of mast cells in ion transport abnormalities associated with intestinal anaphylaxis. Collection of the diminished secretory response in genetically mast cell-deficient W/W mice by bone marrow transplantation. J Clin Invest 87: 687–693, 1991.
113. Stead RH, Tomioka M, Quinonez G, et al: Intestinal mucosal mast cells in normal and nematode-infected rat intestines are in intimate contact with peptidergic nerves. Proc Natl Acad Sci USA 84:2975–2979, 1987.
114. Castro GA, Harari Y, Russell D: Mediators of anaphylaxis-induced ion transport changes in small intestine. Am J Physiol 253:G540–G548, 1987.
115. Parkos CA, Delp C, Arnaout MA, et al: Neutrophil migration across a cultured intestinal epithelium. J Clin Invest 88:1605–1612, 1991.
116. Madara JL, Patapoff TW, Gillece-Castro B, et al: 5′ Adenosine monophosphate is the neutrophil derived paracrine factor that elicits Cl secretion from T84 intestinal epithelial monolayers. Clin Invest 91: 2320–2325, 1993.
117. Elliott E, Li A, Bell C, et al: Modulation of host response to *Escherichia coli* 0157:H7 infection by anti-CD18 antibody in rabbits. Gastroenterology 106:1554–1561, 1994.
118. Karayalcin SS, Sturbaum CW, Wachsman JT, et al: Hydrogen peroxide stimulates rat colonic prostaglandin production and alters electrolyte transport. J Clin Invest 86:60–68, 1990.
119. Chang EB, Musch MW, Mayer L: Interleukins 1 and 3 stimulate anion secretion in chicken intestine. Gastroenterology 98:1518–1524, 1990.
120. Grisham MB, Gaginella TS, Von Ritter C, et al: Effects of neutrophil-derived oxidants on intestinal permeability, electrolyte transport and epithelial cell viability. Inflammation 14:531–542, 1990.
121. Madara JL, Stafford J: Interferon-gamma directly affects barrier function of cultured intestinal epithelial monolayers. J Clin Invest 83:724–727, 1989.
122. Bern MJ, Sturbaum CW, Karayalcin SS, et al: Immune system control of rat and rabbit colonic electrolyte transport. J Clin Invest 83:1810–1820, 1989.
123. Sandle GI, Higgs N, Crowe P, et al: Cellular basis for defective electrolyte transport in inflamed human colon. Gastroenterology 99: 97–105, 1990.
124. Charney AN, Feldman GM: Systemic acid-base disorders and intestinal electrolyte transport. Am J Physiol 247:G1–G12, 1984.
125. DeSoignie R, Sellin JH: Acid-base regulation of ion transport in rabbit ileum in vitro. Gastroenterology 99:132–141, 1990.
126. Charney AN, Egnor RW: NaCl absorption in the rabbit ileum. Effect of acid-base variables. Gastroenterology 100:403–409, 1991.

127. Mialman D: Blood flow and intestinal absorption. Fed Proc 41:2096–2100, 1982.
128. Granger DN, Richardson PDI, Kvietys PR, et al: Intestinal blood flow. Gastroenterology 78:837–863, 1980.
129. Levens NR: Control of intestinal absorption by the renin-angiotensin system. Am J Physiol 249:G3–G15, 1985.
130. Soergel KH, Whalen GE, Harris JA, et al: Effect of ADH on human small intestinal water and solute transport. J Clin Invest 47:1071–1082, 1968.
131. Moriarty KJ, Higgs NB, Leese M, et al: Influence of atrial natriuretic peptide on mammalian large intestine. Gastroenterology 98:647–653, 1990.
132. Penn D, Lebenthal E: Intestinal mucosal energy metabolism—a new approach to therapy of gastrointestinal disease. J Pediatr Gastro Nutr 10:1–4, 1990.
133. Rhoads JM, Keku EO, Quinn J, et al: L-Glutamine stimulates jejunal sodium and chloride absorption in pig rotavirus enteritis. Gastroenterology 100:683–691, 1991.
134. Bugaut M, Bentejac M: Biological effects of short-chain fatty acids in nonruminant mammals. Annu Rev Nutr 13:217–241, 1993.
135. Eherer AJ, Fordtran JS: Fecal osmotic gap and pH in experimental diarrhea of various causes. Gastroenterology 103:545–551, 1992.
136. Fine KD, Santa Ana CA, Fordtran JS: Diagnosis of magnesium-induced diarrhea. N Engl J Med 324:1012–1017, 1991.
137. Frizzell RA, Schultz SG: Effect of aldosterone on ion transport by rabbit colon in vitro. JMB 39:233–256, 1978.
138. Fromm M, Schulzke JD, Hegel U: Control of electrogenic Na^+ absorption in rat late distal colon by nanomolar aldosterone added in vitro. Am J Physiol Endocrinol Metab 264:E68–E73, 1993.
139. Will PC, DeLisle RC, Cortwright RN, et al: Induction of amiloride-sensitive sodium transport in the intestines by adrenal steroids. Ann N Y Acad Sci 81:64–78, 1981.
140. Turnamian SG, Binder HJ: Regulation of active sodium and potassium transport in the distal colon of the rat. J Clin Invest 84:1924–1929, 1989.
141. Sweiry JH, Binder HJ: Characterization of aldosterone-induced potassium secretion in rat distal colon. J Clin Invest 83:844–851, 1989.
142. Pandiyan V, Rajendran VM, Binder HJ: Mucosal ouabain and Na^+ inhibit active Rb^+ (K^+) absorption in normal and sodium-depleted rat distal colon. Gastroenterology 102:1846–1853, 1992.
143. O'Loughlin EV, Hunt DM, Kreutzmann D: Postnatal development of colonic electrolyte transport in rabbits. Am J Physiol 258:G447–G453, 1990.
144. Jenkins HR, Fenton TR, McIntosh N, et al: Development of colonic sodium transport in early childhood and its regulation by aldosterone. Gut 31:194–197, 1990.
145. Charney AN, Kinsey MD, Myers L, et al: Na-K-activated adenosine triphosphatase and intestinal electrolyte transport. J Clin Invest 56:653–660, 1975.
146. Sellin JH, Field M: Physiologic and pharmacologic effects of glucocorticoids on ion transport across rabbit ileal mucosa in vitro. J Clin Invest 67:770–778, 1981.
147. Sellin JH, DeSoignie RC: Methylprednisolone increases absorptive capacity of rabbit ileum in vitro. Am J Physiol 245:G562–G567, 1983.
148. Maurusic ET, Hayslett JP, Binder HJ: Corticosteroid-binding studies in cytosol of colonic mucosa of the rat. Am J Physiol 240:G417–G423, 1981.
149. Sellin JH, Field M: Physiologic and pharmacologic effects of glucocorticoids on ion transport across rabbit ileal mucosa in vitro. J Clin Invest 67:770–778, 1981.
150. Chang EB, Field M, Miller RJ: Alpha 2-adrenergic receptor regulation of ion transport in rabbit ileum. Am J Physiol 242:G237–G242, 1982.
151. Sellin JH, DeSoignie R: Regulation of Na-Cl absorption in rabbit proximal colon in vitro. Am J Physiol 252:G445–G551, 1987.
152. Donowitz M, Cusolito S, Battisti L, et al: Dopamine stimulation of active Na and Cl absorption in rabbit ileum. J Clin Invest 69:1008–1016, 1982.
153. Fedorak RN, Field M, Chang EB: Treatment of diabetic diarrhea with clonidine. Ann Intern Med 102:197–199, 1985.
154. Dobbins JW, Racusen L, Binder HJ: Effect of D-alanine methionine enkephalin amide on ion transport in rabbit ileum. J Clin Invest 66:19–28, 1980.
155. Kachur JF, Miller RJ, Field M: Control of guinea pig intestinal electrolyte secretion by a delta-opiate receptor. Proc Natl Acad Sci USA 77:2753–2756, 1980.
156. Guandalini S, Kachur JF, Smith PL, et al: In vitro effects of somatostatin on ion transport in rabbit intestine. Am J Physiol 238:G67–G74, 1980.
157. Dharmsathaphorn K, Racusen L, Dobbins JW: Effects of somatostatin on ion transport in the rat colon. J Clin Invest 66:813–820, 1980.
158. Kvols LK, Moertel CG, O'Connel MJ, et al: Treatment of the malignant carcinoid syndrome. Evaluation of a long-acting somatostatin analogue. N Engl J Med 315:663–666, 1986.
159. Craven PA, DeRubertis FR: Patterns of prostaglandin synthesis and degradation in isolated superficial and proliferative colonic epithelial cells compared to residual colon. Prostaglandins 225:583–604, 1983.
160. Lawson LD, Powell DW: Bradykinin-stimulated eicosanoid synthesis and secretion by rabbit ileal components. Am J Physiol 252:G783–G790, 1987.
161. Gaginella TS: Eicosanoid-mediated intestinal secretion. In Duffey M, Lebenthal E (eds): Textbook of Secretory Diarrhea. New York, Raven, 1990, pp 15–30.
162. Beubler E, Bukhave K, Rask-Madsen J: Significance of calcium for the prostaglandin E2-mediated secretory response to 5-hydroxytryptamine in the small intestine of the rat in vivo. Gastroenterology 90:1972–1977, 1986.
163. Clarke LL, Argenzio RA: NaCl transport across equine proximal colon and the effect of endogenous prostanoids. Am J Physiol 259:G62–G69, 1990.
164. Kaufmann HJ, Taubin HL: Nonsteroidal anti-inflammatory drugs activate quiescent inflammatory bowel disease. Ann Intern Med 107:513–516, 1987.
165. Bjarnason I, Guiseppe Z, Smith T, et al: Nonsteroidal antiinflammatory drug-induced inflammation in humans. Gastroenterology 93:480–489, 1987.
166. Smith PL, Montzka DP, McCafferty GP, et al: Effect of sulfidopeptide leukotrienes D4 and E4 on ileal ion transport in vitro in the rat and rabbit. Am J Physiol 255:G175–G183, 1988.
167. Musch MW, Miller RJ, Field M, et al: Stimulation of colonic secretion by lipoxygenase metabolites of arachidonic acid. Science 217:1255–1256, 1982.
168. Tapper EJ: Local modulation of intestinal ion transport by enteric neurons. Am J Physiol 244:G457–G468, 1983.
169. Donowitz M, Tai Y-H, Asarkof N: Effect of serotonin on active electrolyte transport in rabbit ileum, gallbladder and colon. Am J Physiol 239:G463–G472, 1980.
170. Madara JL, Parkos C, Colgan S, et al: Cl^- secretion in a model intestinal epithelium induced by a neutrophil-derived secretagogue. J Clin Invest 89:1938–1944, 1992.
171. Cohen MB: Wherefore art thou guanylin? Gastroenterology 109:2039–2042, 1995.
172. Li Z, Taylor-Blake B, Light AR, et al: Guanylin, an endogenous ligand for C-type guanylate cyclase, is produced by goblet cells in the rat intestine. Gastroenterology 109:1863–1875, 1995.
173. Gaginella TS, Kachur JF, Tamai H, et al: Reactive oxygen and nitrogen metabolites as mediators of secretory diarrhea. Gastroenterology 109:2019–2028, 1995.
174. Fasano A, Trucksis M, Comstock L, et al: Cholera toxin (CT), zona occludens toxin (ZOT), and accessory cholera toxin (ACE): three distinct toxins elaborated by the same pathogen. Gastroenterology 104:A247, 1993.
175. Kandel G, Donohue-Rolfe A, Donowitz M, et al: Pathogenesis of *Shigella* diarrhea. J Clin Invest 84:1509–1517, 1989.
176. Beubler E, Kollar G, Saria A, et al: Involvement of 5-hydroxytryptamine, prostaglandin E2, and cyclic adenosine monophosphate in cholera toxin-induced fluid secretion in the small intestine of the rat in vivo. Gastroenterology 96:368–376, 1989.
177. Field M, Fromm D, al Awqati Q, et al: Effect of cholera enterotoxin on ion transport across isolated ileal mucosa. J Clin Invest 51:796–804, 1972.
178. Fasano A, Fiorentini C, Donnelli G, et al: Zonula ocludens toxin modulates tight junctions through protein kinase C-dependent actin reorganization in vitro. J Clin Invest 96:710–720, 1995.
179. Argenzio RA, Liacos JA, Levy ML, et al: Villous atrophy, crypt hyperplasia, cellular infiltration and impaired glucose-Na absorption in enteric cryptosporidiosis of pigs. Gastroenterology 98:1129–1140, 1990.
180. Guarino A, Canani RB, Pozio E, et al: Enterotoxic effect of supernatant of cryptosporidium-infected calves on human jejunum. Gastroenterology 106:28–34, 1994.

181. McGowan K, Piver G, Stoff JS, et al: Role of prostaglandins and calcium in the effects of *Entamoeba histolytica* on colonic electrolyte transport. Gastroenterology 98:873–880, 1990.
182. Ball JM, Tian P, Zeng C, et al: Age-dependent diarrhea is induced by a rotaviral nonstructural glycoprotein. Science 272:101–104, 1996.
183. Morris AP, Scott JR, Ball JM, et al: NSP4 elicits age-dependent diarrhea and Ca^{++} mediated I-influx into intestinal crypts of CF mice. Am J Physiol 277:G431–G444, 1999.
184. Dharmsathaphorn K, Huott PA, Vongkovit P, et al: Chloride secretion induced by bile salts. J Clin Invest 84:945–953, 1989.
185. Gelbmann CM, Schteingart CD, Thompson SM, et al: Mast cells and histamine contribute to bile acid-stimulated secretion in the mouse colon. J Clin Invest 95:2831–2839, 1995.
186. DeJonge HR, Rao MC: Cyclic nucleotide-dependent kinases. In Duffey M, Lebenthal E (eds): Textbook of Secretory Diarrhea. New York, Raven, 1990, pp 191–208.
187. Rao MC, DeJonge HR: Ca and phospholipid-dependent protein kinases. In Duffey M, Lebenthal E (eds): Textbook of Secretory Diarrhea. New York, Raven 1990, pp 209–233.
188. Moe OW, Amemiya M, Yamaji Y: Activation of protein kinase A acutely inhibits and phosphorylates Na/H exchanger NHE-3. J Clin Invest 96:2187–2194, 1995.
189. Donowitz M, Cohen ME, Gould M, et al: Elevated intracellular Ca^{2+} acts through protein kinase C to regulate rabbit ileal NaCl absorption. Evidence for sequential control by Ca^{2+}/calmodulin and protein kinase. J Clin Invest 83:1953–1962, 1989.
190. Emmer E, Rood RP, Wesolek HJ, et al: Role of calcium and calmodulin in the regulation of the rabbit ileal brush-border membrane Na+-H+ antiporter. J Memb Biol 108:207–215, 1989.
191. Markert T, Vaandrager AB, Gambaryan S, et al: Endogenous expression of type II cGMP-dependent protein kinase mRNA and protein in rat intestine. J Clin Invest 96:822–830, 1995.
192. Vajanaphanich M, Schultz C, Tsien RY, et al: Cross-talk between calcium and cAMP-dependent intracellular signaling pathways. J Clin Invest 96:386–393, 1995.
193. Grubb BR: Ion transport across the jejunum in normal and cystic fibrosis mice. Am J Physiol Gastrointest Liver Physiol 268:G505–G513, 1995.
194. Burant CF, Flink S, DePaoli AM, et al: Small intestine hexose transport in experimental diabetes. Increased transporter mRNA and protein expression in enterocytes. J Clin Invest 93:578–585, 1994.
195. Umar S, Scott J, Sellin J, et al: Murine colonic mucosa hyperproliferation. 1. Elevated CFTR expression and enhanced cAMP-dependent Cl secretion. Am J Physiol 278:G753–G764, 2000.
196. Forte JG: Regulation of secretion and absorption by recruitment and recycling of primary transport proteins. Gastroenterology 109:1706–1710, 1995.
197. Janecki AJ, Janecki M, Akhter S, et al: Basic fibroblast growth factor stimulates surface expression and activity of the Na^+/H^+ exchanger NHE via mechanisms involving phosphatidylinositol 3-kinase. J Biol Chem 275:8133–8142, 2000.
198. Janecki AJ, Montrose MH, Zimniak P, et al: Subcellular redistribution is involved in acute regulation of the brush border Na+/H+ exchanger isoform 3 in human colon adenocarcinoma cell line Caco-2: protein kinase C-mediated inhibition of the exchanger. J Biol Chem 273:8790–8798, 1998.
199. Weinman EJ, Steplock D, Donowitz M, et al: NHERF associations with sodium-hydrogen exchanger isoform 3 (NHE3) and ezrin are essential for cAMP-mediated phosphorylation and inhibition of NHE3. Biochemistry 39:6123–6129, 2000.
200. Sun F, Hug MJ, Lelwarchik CM, et al: E3KARP mediates the association of ezrin and protein kinase A with the cystic fibrosis transmembrane conductance regulator in airway cells. J Biol Chem 275:29539–29546, 2000.
201. Yun CH, Oh S, Zizak M, et al: cAMP-mediated inhibition of the epithelial brush border Na+/H+ exchanger, NHE3, requires an associated regulatory protein. Proc Natl Acad Sci USA 94:3010–3015, 1997.

Chapter 88

Digestion and Absorption of Nutrients and Vitamins

James J. Farrell

Most nutrients are absorbed with remarkable efficiency: less than 5% of ingested carbohydrate, fat, and protein is excreted in the stool of adults taking their normal diet.[1] Even much indigestible dietary fiber is absorbed from the colon as short-chain fatty acids that are liberated by bacterial breakdown of fiber.[2] The intestinal tract of neonates is less efficient, as a glance at a baby's stool confirms. Infants fail to absorb 10% to 15% of their dietary fat, and in prematurity as much as 25% to 35% may be lost in the stool.[3, 4] In old age, however, nutrient absorption remains highly efficient unless the intestine becomes diseased.

Despite considerable variations in types of food and nutritional intake across national and racial groups, absorption remains efficient. There is good evidence that absorptive mechanisms adapt to the nature and amount of various nutrients presented to the intestinal tract. Such changes occur not only during early development[5] but also throughout life and at times of specific need, as during pregnancy.[6] In achieving the overall objective of nutrient absorption, the different parts of the gastrointestinal (GI) tract act in a closely integrated and coordinated manner under the control of neural and humoral regulatory mechanisms.

In this chapter, integration of intestinal function with the dietary intake, digestion, and absorption of major nutrients (fat, carbohydrate, and protein) and essential micronutrients (vitamins and trace elements) is discussed.

This chapter is a revision of the chapter on the same topic from the 6th edition of this text, written by M. N. Marsh and S. A. Riley. The author and editors acknowledge the valuable contribution of Marsh and Riley.

DIGESTION AND ABSORPTION OF NUTRIENTS

An Overview of Gastrointestinal Integration

The cerebral phase of digestion, whether triggered by the sight, smell, or thought of food, initiates the digestive process. Salivary and gastric secretory responses to this type of stimulus are mediated via the autonomic nervous system, and there is modest stimulation of pancreaticobiliary secretion via the vagus nerve.[7] The further stimulus of nutrients in the mouth and upper GI tract markedly potentiates secretion by both humoral and local neural mechanisms (see Chapter 1).[8]

The speed at which food is normally chewed and swallowed affords little time for significant oral digestion of nutrients; however, good mastication and mixing with saliva initiate digestion of starch by salivary amylase and, particularly in infants, of fat by gastric lipase in the stomach. Gastric acid would soon switch off these enzymes were it not for the buffering capacity of food that allows some digestion to continue. The optimal pH of gastric lipases is 4.5 to 6.0, and it has been suggested that a considerable proportion of dietary triglyceride may be digested by these lipases.[9, 10] Protein digestion begins in the stomach with secretion of gastric pepsinogens and their rapid conversion to pepsins by gastric acid. Pepsins become increasingly active as luminal pH falls.

During ingestion of food the stomach is distended, but intragastric pressure rises little because of neurally mediated receptive relaxation. The mechanisms by which subjects perceive satiety and, therefore, cease eating are complex and are due only partly to a sensation of fullness. Cholecystokinin (CCK), gastrin-releasing peptide, and apolipoprotein A-IV have all been implicated as messengers that transmit the satiety signal to the central nervous system (CNS).[11–13] They potentiate each other's actions, and a combination of these agents may participate in the satiety signal.

The major digestive processes occur in the duodenum. The delivery of chyme from the stomach is delicately adjusted so that it enters the duodenum at a controlled rate, thus allowing efficient mixing with pancreaticobiliary secretions. Control of gastric emptying is thus critical to ensuring optimal digestion. The characteristics of gastric contents that determine this rate of emptying include their consistency, pH, osmolality, and lipid and calorie content (Fig. 88–1).[14]

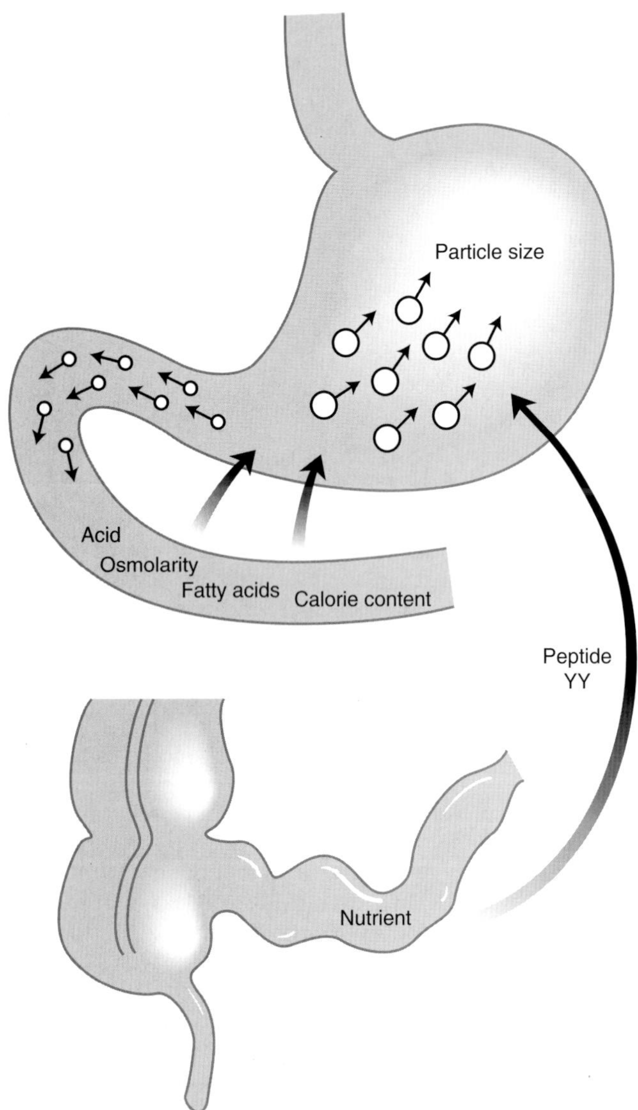

Figure 88–1. Some factors that delay gastric emptying. Receptors for osmolarity, acid (pH), fatty acids, and other nutrients in the duodenum signal gastric delay via neurohumoral mechanisms. Food particles larger than 2 mm in diameter are rejected by the antrum. Nutrients in the ileum and colon also influence gastric emptying by the so-called ileal brake mechanism, which may involve release of peptide YY.

The pylorus is selective in that it allows rapid passage of liquids but retains solid particles with diameters of 2 mm or larger.[15] Thus, large particles are retained and progressively reduced in size by the gastric "mill" until they are small enough to ensure reasonably close apposition to digestive enzymes once the nutrient is allowed to enter the duodenum. Meals of high viscosity empty more slowly than those of low viscosity.

Duodenal mucosal receptors for pH and osmolality trigger a delay in gastric emptying when gastric effluent is acidic or hyper- or hypotonic.[16, 17] When duodenal luminal contents are neutralized by pancreaticobiliary bicarbonate and osmolality is adjusted by water fluxes, gastric emptying is encouraged once more. This careful titration in the duodenal lumen ensures that the nutrient is presented optimally to the pancreatic enzymes, which function best at neutral pH.

The total calorie content of meals also controls gastric emptying rates; on average, the human stomach delivers about 150 kcal/hr to the duodenum.[18] An increase in the size or energy density of a meal leads to a corresponding increase in the rate of delivery. Receptors for fatty acids, amino acids, and carbohydrates in duodenal mucosa are involved in this response, which is probably mediated by both neural and humoral feedback mechanisms.[19]

Gastric emptying is additionally controlled by a mechanism involving the ileum and colon. If much nutrient escapes digestion and absorption in the jejunum, its presence in the ileum and colon delays GI transit, and this again provides more time for digestion and absorption.[20, 21] This "brake" is probably mediated by a neurohumoral mechanism, and various neurotransmitters and hormones have been implicated. Peptide YY appears to play a key role (see Chapter 1).[22]

The gallbladder is stimulated to contract and the pancreas to secrete simultaneously in response to the presence of nutrient in the duodenal lumen. A range of nutrient receptors stimulates the release of CCK and secretin from mucosal endocrine cells into the portal circulation, and these receptors are largely responsible for this release. The simultaneous release of bile salts, pancreatic enzymes, and bicarbonate provides optimal conditions for further nutrient digestion. Critically important to the activation of pancreatic proteolytic enzymes is the simultaneous release of enteropeptidase (enterokinase) from duodenal mucosa. This releases trypsin from trypsinogen, thus encouraging proteolysis within the duodenal lumen rather than the pancreatic duct. That these three factors—bile, pancreatic enzymes, and enteropeptidase—remain separate until they are mixed in the intestinal lumen ensures that they become operative at the site of nutrient delivery.

Adequate lipid digestion depends critically on the presence of bile salts and pancreatic lipase and colipase at nearly neutral pH.[23] On the other hand, digestion of carbohydrate and protein depends on the combined effects of secreted enzymes in the lumen and, for the final stages, of enzymes sited on the brush border membrane and within the intestinal mucosa. The close physical relationship, at the brush border, between the sites for terminal digestion of protein and carbohydrate and the active absorption of digestive products provides a very efficient mechanism for dealing with these nutrients.

Two other simultaneous phenomena encourage efficient

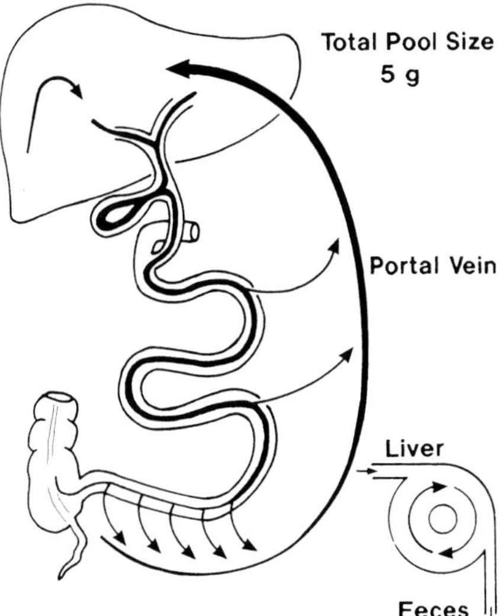

Figure 88–2. Enterohepatic circulation of bile salts. Active transport in the ileum retrieves most bile salts, and the small fraction lost into the colon is made up by fresh hepatic synthesis.

digestion and absorption. Ingestion of a meal stimulates salt and water secretion by the jejunal mucosa, and this maintains luminal contents in a sufficiently fluid state for proper mixing and digestion (see Chapter 87).[24] The other phenomenon is the motor response of the gut. After feeding, the characteristic repetitive pattern of motility that occurs during fasting is disrupted. Instead, an apparently disordered pattern is seen, which presumably ensures that the nutrient is well mixed and brought into close contact with intestinal mucosa (see Chapter 85). There is close integration of the neurohumoral control mechanisms involving the motor and secretory responses of the intestine.[25] For rapidly absorbed molecules, intestinal blood flow may be the rate-limiting step.[26]

Efficient conservation and recycling mechanisms ensure that GI secretions are not entirely lost. Gastric acid secretion is balanced to a large extent by pancreaticobiliary bicarbonate secretion, so that the overall acid-base balance is not disturbed. Although intact digestive enzymes are reabsorbed only in trace amounts, the nitrogen they contain is reabsorbed after their digestion. Finally, efficient enterohepatic circulation recycles bile salts several times a day so that they may be utilized about twice for each meal.[27] Although bile salts are passively reabsorbed throughout the small intestine, most reach the terminal ileum, where they are reabsorbed via specific active absorptive mechanisms. Thus, bile salts remain in the lumen, where they are needed for lipid digestion, but are largely reabsorbed at the last moment to avoid being lost by the colon (Fig. 88–2; see Chapter 54).

Once intestinal chyme leaves the ileum and enters the colon, most nutrients have been digested and absorbed and colonic function largely resolves itself into dehydration of luminal contents through absorption of salt and water and storage of the residuum. Dietary fiber may be digested by bacteria, with release of short-chain fatty acids, which are avidly absorbed; however, short-chain fatty acids do not usually have much nutritional significance, except in areas of the world where the major source of energy is a high-fiber diet.

DIGESTION AND ABSORPTION OF FAT

Dietary Intake

About 40% of adult energy requirements is supplied by lipids, of which triglycerides form the majority.[28] The average daily intake in the United States in the 1960s was about 150 g/day, two thirds of which was derived from animal fat and one third from vegetable fat.[29] There is evidence that average fat intake is falling—in the United Kingdom it has now reached 90 g/day, compared with 120 g/day in 1969.[28] Similar trends have been observed in the United States. The proportion of fat contributed by saturated fatty acids also appears to be declining (from 45% in 1980 to 41% in 1990 in the United Kingdom), and the proportion of polyunsaturates has increased from 10% to 15%.[28]

The majority of fatty acids present in dietary triglyceride are oleate and palmitate (C18:1 and C16:0, respectively).[30] In animal triglyceride, most fatty acids are long-chain saturated ones (i.e., longer than C14 chain length; Fig. 88–3). Polyunsaturated fatty acids such as linoleic and linolenic acid are derived from phospholipid of vegetable origin and, since they cannot be synthesized de novo, are considered essential fatty acids (Table 88–1).

The average range of phospholipid ingestion lies between 2 and 8 g/day. The commonest ingested phospholipid is phosphatidylcholine (lecithin), and the predominant fatty acids in phospholipid are linoleate and arachidonate (see Fig. 88–3). Rather more phospholipid is found in the duodenal lumen (10 to 22 g/day), but the majority is derived from endogenous sources, particularly bile.

Cholesterol intake varies widely but averages about 200 to 250 mg/day.[30] Some people consume as much as 500 mg/

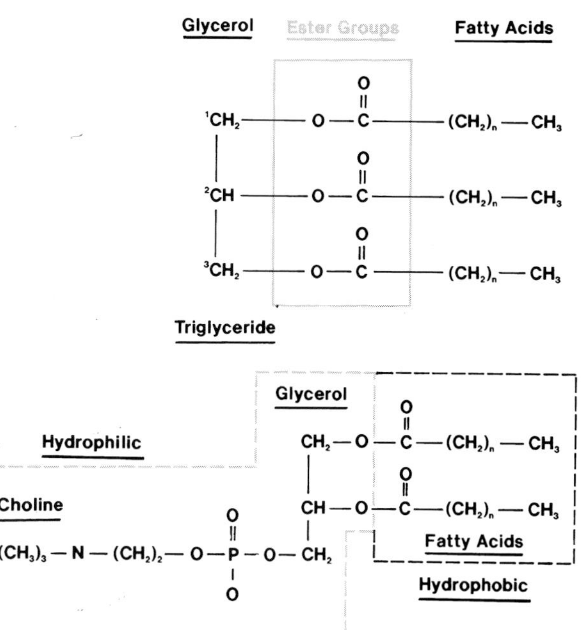

Figure 88–3. General molecular structure of triglycerides and a phospholipid (phosphatidylcholine and lecithin).

Table 88–1 | **Common Dietary Fatty Acids***

SATURATED FATTY ACIDS	
Butyric	C4:0
Caproic	C6:0
Lauric	C12:0
Myristic	C14:0
Palmitic	C16:0
Stearic	C18:0
MONOUNSATURATED FATTY ACIDS	
Oleic	C18:1
Palmitoleic	C16:1
POLYUNSATURATED FATTY ACIDS	
Linoleic	C18:2
Linolenic	C18:3
Arachidonic	C20:4

*By convention, the number of carbon atoms in the chain is given by the first figure and the number of double bonds in the chain by the second.

day, and one unusual patient has been described who for many years ate 25 eggs per day (almost 500 mg of cholesterol) without apparent harm.[31]

Commercial hydrogenation of unsaturated bonds in the fatty acids of natural oils raises their melting points, thus allowing production of margarines and spreads of variable consistency. Hydrogenation, in addition to saturation, results in isomerization of *cis* to *trans* double bonds.[32] Although many commercial products contain partially hydrogenated fats, the content of *trans* fatty acids in some margarines exceeds 60%, thus raising anxious concerns about their relationship to cancer induction.[33]

Digestion

Most dietary lipid is absorbed by the upper two thirds of the jejunum, although the rate and extent of absorption by the jejunum are influenced by the presence of other foods, particularly dietary fiber, which reduces the rate of absorption.[34] The types of ingested fat also appear to influence the absorptive process both by modifying the morphologic structure of the intestinal mucosa and by influencing its absorptive function for other nutrients such as carbohydrate.[35]

The problem of the insolubility of fat in water dominates the mechanisms that have been developed to digest and absorb lipid. Within the lumen, ingested fat has to be physically released and broken down into emulsion droplets. Following digestion, the products have to be transported across the bulk (lumen) water phase to the lipoid epithelial cell membrane. Transfer across the lipid membrane is followed, within the epithelium, by reconstitution into larger lipid molecules, predominantly triglyceride, which then require specialized processing to permit export from the cell. Thus, lipid goes through three phases: water in the lumen, lipid in the epithelial membrane, and water in the lymphatics and blood stream. Despite these potential barriers, more than 95% of ingested fat is absorbed by adults.

Triglyceride

Liberation of fatty acids from the glycerol backbone of triglycerides (lipolysis) is achieved by lipases acting at the surface of emulsified droplets. This occurs initially in the stomach (also see Chapter 38) and then in the small intestine. Studies suggest that normal intragastric lipolysis may account for 20% to 30% of total intraluminal lipid digestion[36]; gastric lipase, which is of fundic origin, has been demonstrated in the gastric contents of premature neonates and in mucosal biopsy specimens from adults up to 80 years of age. For either gastric or small intestinal lipolysis to occur, two conditions are critical. First, a stable emulsion is required of fat droplets of such a size that they present a large surface area to the digestive enzyme; second, a mechanism for bringing enzyme and triglyceride into close apposition within the emulsion is needed.

Emulsification

A number of factors assist in optimal production of an emulsion. Physical release of fat by mastication and gastric "milling" of food produce a relatively unstable emulsion that is delivered into the duodenum. To permit its stabilization, the droplets in this emulsion have to be coated, and *phospholipid* in the diet provides one such coat. The ratio of ingested phospholipid to triglyceride is approximately 1:30; this is sufficient for the purpose, and more phospholipid is added in the duodenum from bile.[37] In breast milk (Table 88–2), emulsion droplets are smaller, and proteins as well as phospholipid are incorporated into their surface trilayer.[38] Emulsification is also enhanced by the fatty acids liberated by intragastric lipolysis and, within the duodenum, by bile salts (Fig. 88–4). The final product in the duodenum is an emulsion consisting predominantly of triglyceride, together with cholesterol esters and some diglyceride, and coated by phospholipid, partially ionized fatty acids, monoglyceride, and bile salts.

Lipase

This stable emulsion is then presented to pancreatic lipase. Unlike other soluble enzymes, which can act in a three-dimensional solution, lipase has to act at the two-dimensional surface of the emulsion droplet, and this poses particular problems.[39] Certain characteristics of the enzyme itself are important. Thus, the lipolytic "zone" of the molecule is hydrophobic and lies deep within it, shielded from the aqueous phase. It is revealed to the lipid only on close apposition to its surface. The presence of a coat on the lipid droplet

Table 88–2 | **Characteristics of Lipase Activity in Infancy**

MILK-DERIVED LIPASE
Stimulated by bile salts
Optimal pH is 7.0 (inactivation by acid is reversible)
Active against 1, 2, and 3 ester bonds*
GASTRIC LIPASE
Optimal pH is 4.0–6.0
Inhibited by pancreatic proteolysis
Preference for 1 ester bond*
PANCREATIC LIPASE
Optimal pH is 7.0
Active against 1 and 3 ester bonds*

*See Figure 88–3.

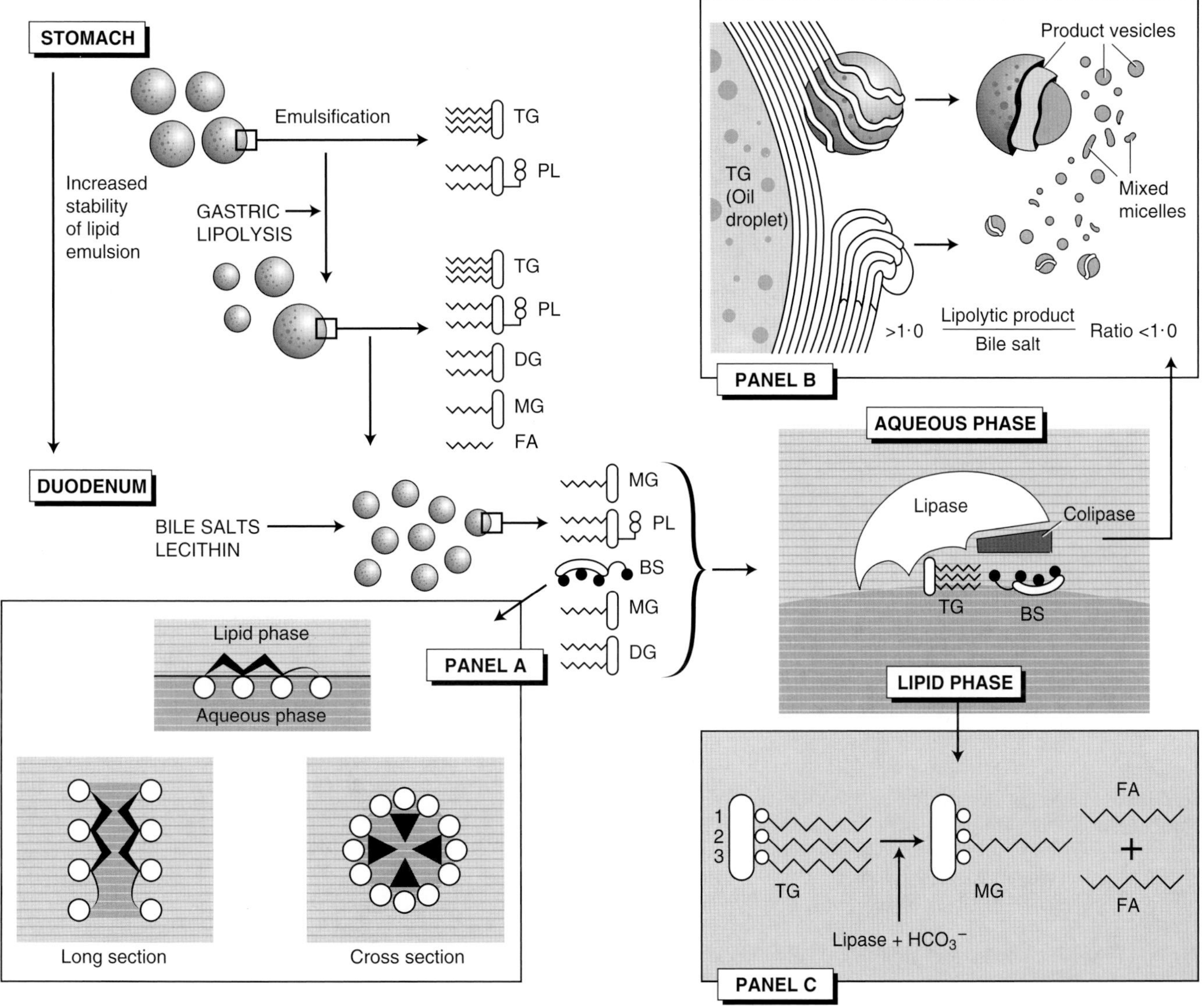

Figure 88–4. The initial step in lipolysis is to increase the stability of the fatty emulsion. Gastric lipase acts to yield fatty acids and diglyceride (the latter enhancing emulsification). This step is further enhanced in the duodenum by bile salts and phospholipid, which enable lipase, in the presence of colipase, to act at the surface of the emulsion droplet to bring it close to the triglyceride molecule, whence monoglyceride and fatty acids are released. Lipolysis in the duodenum, yielding fatty acids (from the α_1 and α_3 positions) and monoglyceride, occurs in a rapid and efficient manner at nearly neutral pH. In panel *A* are bile salt molecules (*top*), oriented at an oil-water interface with hydrophobic sterolic backbone in oil phase and their hydrophylic hydroxyl and either taurine or glycine conjugates in aqueous phase. At concentrations above the critical micellar concentration, bile salts aggregate as simple micelles in water with their hydrophylic groups facing into the water. In this diagram, three hydroxyl groups (cholate) are shown as open circles and an additional polar group represents either taurine or glycine. In panel *B* is a diagrammatic sketch of the dispersion of the products of lipolysis into lamellae at the surface of the oil phase, each about 4 to 5 nm thick with water spacings up to 8 nm, and thence into vesicles of about 20 to 130 nm in diameter. Fatty acids and monoglyceride within the vesicles pass on into mixed micelles (panel *C*).

thus poses a barrier to the action of lipase, and assistance is required to bring it into close contact with the triglyceride. The presence of colipase, secreted by the pancreas with lipase (molar ratio 1:1), is critical in approximating lipase to triglyceride (see Fig. 88–4). Colipase attaches to the ester bond region of the triglyceride, lipase then binding strongly to colipase by electrostatic interactions.[37] Phospholipase A_2 digestion of the phospholipid on the surface of the lipid emulsion allows exposure of the triglyceride core to the colipase–lipase complex, further enhancing colipase-dependent anchoring of lipase to the lipid emulsion. Phospholipase A_2 digestion requires bile salts and Ca^{2+} for activation, which may further assist colipase–lipase-mediated triglyceride lipolysis by providing a mechanism for removal of lipolytic products. In the absence of colipase, bile salts on the surface of the emulsion droplet inhibit lipase activity.

The colipase gene is located in chromosome 6, and the amino acid sequence of the lipid-binding domain, the lipase-binding domain, and the activation peptide appear to be highly conserved.[40] Colipase is secreted by the pancreas as pro-colipase,[41] which is activated by cleavage by trypsin of a pentapeptide from the *N*-terminus after entering the small intestinal lumen. It is interesting that the pentapeptide cleaved from the pro-colipase by trypsin, called enterostatin, seems to be a specific satiety signal for the ingestion of fat.[42]

Since pancreatic lipase is most active at nearly neutral pH, secretion of bicarbonate by the pancreas and biliary tree is critically important and provides the necessary neutralization of gastric acid; however, luminal pH falls to about 6 in the jejunum, and here the fact that bile salts lower the pH optimal for lipase activity from 8 to 6 may be significant. In the presence of colipase and optimal pH, lipase activity releases fatty acids and monoglyceride extremely rapidly and efficiently (see Fig. 88–4). Pancreatic lipase also binds strongly to the mucosal brush border membrane,[43] where it may participate in lipolysis of cholesteryl esters or triglyceride-releasing fatty acids, monoglyceride, and free cholesterol in proximity to the brush border membrane, where fatty acids, monoglyceride and free cholesterol undergo rapid uptake.

Micelles and Other Lipid-Containing Particles

The products of lipolysis are distributed among the aqueous, oil, and intermediate (aqueous/oil) phases in a number of forms prepared for transfer across the lumen to the mucosal brush border membrane. The shuttling of these products depends, in part, on the formation of micelles with bile salts. The concentration of bile salts secreted in bile is about 35 mmol, and this is further decreased by dilution to 10 to 20 mmol in the duodenum. This concentration lies well above the critical concentration for micelle formation. Mixed micelle production depends on a number of other factors, including pH, presence or absence of lipids, and types of bile salts that are secreted (see Chapter 54).[23]

Bile salts are capable of forming micelles because they are amphipathic (having in their molecules both water-soluble and lipid-soluble parts), and they have a particular three-dimensional structure (see Fig. 88–4). They orient themselves at an oil-water interface and thus are ideal emulsifying agents. In addition, micelles are formed when bile salt levels fall above critical concentrations and, thus, are able to aggregate in disklike particles with their hydrophobic, sterolic backbones oriented toward each other and their hydrophilic, polar groups facing outward into the aqueous phase. Bile salt micelles have the capacity to "dissolve" fatty acids, monoglycerides, and cholesterol, but not triglyceride.[44] The mixed micelles thus formed are arranged so that the insoluble lipid is surrounded by the bile salts oriented with their hydrophilic groups facing outward. Mixed micelles are about 50 to 80 nm in diameter and, unlike emulsion droplets, are too small to scatter light. Thus, micellar solutions are clear. The presence of phospholipid secreted in bile enlarges mixed micelles and makes them more efficient in the dissolution of fat.

Other lipid-containing particles participate in their transfer to the mucosa. As the emulsion droplet shrinks during lipolysis, liquid crystalline structures are formed at its surface.[45, 46] These vesicular structures with multilamellar and unilamellar forms can be seen under the electron microscope, budding off the surface of emulsion droplets and, occasionally, close to the brush border membrane of the intestinal mucosa.[47] This physical phase of lipid within the lumen may provide a significant mechanism for transfer of lipid to the mucosa, over and above that provided by bile salt micelles. Its presence could explain the observation that, in the absence of bile salts, some 50% or more of dietary triglyceride may be absorbed. In the presence of adequate concentrations of bile salts, however, these vesicles undergo rapid spontaneous dissolution and release their lipid into micelles, which are likely to be the major route for lipid traffic (see Fig. 88–4). Numerically, micelles are much more common than lipid vesicles.

Importance of Intraluminal pH

Lipid digestion and absorption depend critically on intraluminal pH at several steps in the chain. Pancreatic lipase operates best in the presence of bile salts and at least pH 6. It therefore functions well at the pH of the luminal duodenum, where the majority of lipid digestion occurs. Glycine-conjugated bile salts precipitate below pH 5; furthermore, fatty acids are in their protonated form below approximately pH 6 and have limited solubility in bile salt micelles. Thus, in conditions in which intraluminal pH becomes more acid, as for example in the Zollinger-Ellison syndrome, pancreatic lipase is inactive, bile acids precipitate out of solution, and fatty acid partitioning is reduced. It is not surprising, therefore, that steatorrhea (without any other nutrient or hematologic disturbances) is a feature of this syndrome. Biologic characteristics of lipases, including effect of pH on activities, are detailed in Table 88–2.

Unstirred Water Layer

There is an unstirred water layer on the surface of the epithelium that in humans previously was thought to be some 100 to 700 μm deep, although recent reappraisal indicates a more realistic value of about 40 μm.[48] This layer may be rate limiting for uptake of long-chain fatty acids but not for short- or medium-chain fatty acids, whose limiting step occurs at the brush border membrane.[37] The provision of a high concentration of fatty acid in the microenvironment adjacent to the epithelium depends on the diffusion of micelles into this region. The microclimate here is slightly acidic, owing to activity of a sodium-hydrogen (Na^+/H^+) exchanger at the brush border membrane, and at pH between 5 and 6 the solubility of fatty acids in micelles decreases, thus encouraging liberation of fatty acids close to the mucosa. The high concentration of fatty acids necessary for diffusion across the mucosal membrane is thus achieved, and evidence for this model is increasingly persuasive.[49] The low-microclimate pH also encourages the fatty acids to be presented in an undissociated, protonated form. Thus, the pH partition hypothesis would predict that fatty acids could diffuse passively into the cell as protonated species and, at the near-neutral intracellular pH, become trapped in the ionized form.

A surfactant-like material has been discovered close to the brush border membrane, although its role in absorption, if any, is uncertain.[50] It is secreted by enterocytes, contains phosphatidylcholine and alkaline phosphatase, and appears as flat lamellae or vesicles adjacent to the brush border membrane.

Transfer Across the Brush Border Membrane

Much of the current understanding of the micellar solubilization and uptake of dietary lipids comes from the work of Hofmann and Borgstrom, who described the uptake of lipid digestion products by enterocytes.[51] Further work by Carey and associates discovered the coexistence of unilamellar liposomes with bile salt–lipid mixed micelles in the small intestine.[52] Although the uptake of lipid digestion products by enterocytes has been accepted as a passive process, recent work has raised the possibility that some lipids may be taken up by enterocytes via carrier-mediated processes that are energy dependent.[53]

Studies with brush border membrane vesicles suggest that linoleic acid uptake occurs by facilitated diffusion.[54] Absorption of oleic and arachidonic acid also appears to occur by a saturable process, suggesting the possibility of active transport. The brush border membrane–fatty acid–binding protein, which is likely to be concerned with transfer of fatty acids into the cell, could provide one explanation for facilitated diffusion and the observed saturability of absorption.[55] Using a purified rat jejunal microvillus membrane, an affinity-purified ligand specific for long-chain fatty acids has been identified. This ligand co-elutes exclusively with long-chain fatty acids, whereas incubation with phospholipid or cholesteryl ester fails to produce a co-elution pattern. Although no specific membrane carrier has been identified for monoglyceride or cholesterol, this microvillus membrane fatty acid–binding protein (MVM-FABP) may be involved in mediating uptake of these lipids. The evidence for this is based on substrate competition and MVM-FABP antibody inhibition of lipid uptake in vitro.[55]

Cholesterol, unlike beta-sitosterol (plant sterol), is well absorbed by the small intestine,[56] although both are present in the human diet, suggesting that intestinal cholesterol absorption is an active process possibly mediated by a transporter at the brush border membrane. Thurnhofer and Hauser first described the presence of a possible binding protein in the small intestinal brush border that facilitates the uptake of cholesterol by the small intestine.[57] However, this 14 kd protein was later identified as sterol carrier protein-2 (SCP-2), which is an intracellular protein.[58] Evidence favoring a cholesterol membrane transporter is seen in individuals with beta-sitosterolemia, a condition in which the intestine fails to discriminate between cholesterol and beta-sitosterol. The genetic defect of beta-sitosterolemia is linked to chromosome 2p21.[59] Seven different mutations in two adjacent genes have been described that are responsible for encoding new members of the ABC transporter (ABCG5 and ABCG8) in sitosterolemia patients. Feeding cholesterol to mice upregulated these genes, thus suggesting that ABCG5 and ABCG8 work together to limit intestinal cholesterol absorption by cholesterol efflux from small intestinal epithelial cells.[60]

A number of other proteins have also been demonstrated to bind lipids, but their precise role in facilitated lipid absorption remains unclear. These include GP 330 (also called megalin),[61–63] CD 36,[64] and caveolin.[65]

Digestion of Other Lipids

Phosphatidylcholine, the major dietary phospholipid, is hydrolyzed by pancreatic phospholipase A_2 (PLA_2) to yield fatty acid and lysophosphatidylcholine. Pancreatic PLA_2 is secreted as an anionic zymogen, which is activated in the small intestine by tryptic cleavage of an *N*-terminal heptapeptide, has a molecular weight of approximately 14,000, and requires calcium for activation and the presence of bile salts for its activity. It has multiple isoforms and apparently requires a 2:1 bile salt–to-phosphatidylcholine molar ratio for optimal activity. Although the bulk of intestinal PLA_2 activity is derived from pancreatic juice, there is some contribution from the intestinal mucosa, where the enzyme is concentrated in the brush border.[66]

Cholesterol esters, in the presence of bile salts and calcium, are hydrolyzed by pancreatic cholesterol esterase to release the free sterol, in which form it is absorbed. Pancreatic esterase is well conserved and shares 78% homology in the rat and human.[67] Using site-directed mutagenesis, the serine at position 194, the histidine at position 435, and the aspartic acid at position 320 are important for catalytic activity.[68–70]

Both hydrolytic enzymes act on the emulsion phase at the surface of droplets, and the products of digestion are released into multilamellar and unilamellar vesicles and, thence, to mixed micelles. Fatty acids and monoglycerides increase the solubility of cholesterol in micelles, thus encouraging its absorption. The products of phospholipid and cholesterol hydrolysis thus pursue the same route to the brush border membrane as the fatty acids and monoglyceride, which originate from dietary triglyceride.

Unabsorbed long-chain fatty acids that enter the colon are not absorbed by the colon, and they undergo a series of bacterial modifications, principally hydroxylation. In healthy persons, undigested triglyceride is not found in the stool, and the standard fecal fat estimate of approximately 7 g/day reflects the cumulative total excretion of saponification products (i.e., fatty acids) that arise principally from membrane phospholipid and bacteria.

Intracellular Processing

Once within the enterocyte, fatty acids bind to specific fatty acid–binding proteins (FABPs), which are found predominantly in the jejunum and more in villous cells than in crypt cells. There are at least two FABPs in enterocytes; the I-FABP and the L-FABP (I for intestine, and L for liver, where they were first isolated). They have greater affinity for unsaturated fatty acids than for saturated ones, and very little affinity, if any, for short-chain or medium-chain fatty acids.[23] Based on nuclear magnetic resonance (NMR) binding studies, it is suggested that the binding of I-FABP is involved in the intracellular transport of fatty acids, whereas the L-FABP is involved in the intracellular transport of monoglycerides and lysophosphatidylcholine.[71] I-FABP and L-FABP may as-

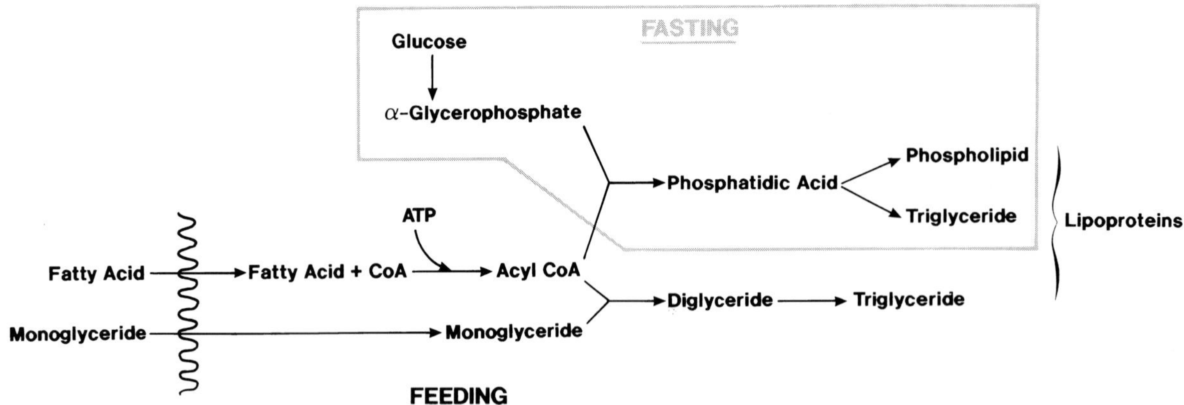

Figure 88–5. Metabolic fate of absorbed fatty acid and monoglyceride in enterocytes. During feeding, triglyceride is resynthesized largely from absorbed fatty acid and monoglyceride. During fasting, triglyceride and phospholipid are synthesized from α-glycerophosphate, derived from glucose entering across the basolateral membrane, and from fatty acids. Unsaturated fatty acids tend to form the phospholipid.

sist transfer across the cytoplasm to the endoplasmic reticulum for triglyceride resynthesis.

In addition, two sterol carrier proteins, SCP-1 and SCP-2, have been isolated and characterized. SCP-1 is important in the microsomal conversion of squalene to lanosterol,[72] whereas SCP-2 participates in the microsomal conversion of lanosterol to cholesterol, as well as the intracellular transport of cholesterol from cytoplasmic lipid droplets to mitochondria.[73]

In the endoplasmic reticulum, triglyceride is resynthesized by two processes (Fig. 88–5).[74] (1) In the first process, monoglyceride is re-esterified with absorbed fatty acid after it has been activated to form acyl coenzyme A (CoA) (the monoglyceride pathway). Microsomal acyl CoA-ligase is necessary to synthesize acyl CoA from the fatty acid before esterification. Diglyceride and then triglyceride are formed sequentially in reactions that favor long-chain fatty acid absorption from the lumen. This route, involving monoglyceride esterification, accounts for the majority of the triglyceride synthesized during the absorptive phase, no more than 4% being formed by acylation of absorbed glycerol. It is thought that the synthesis of triglyceride from diglyceride is catalyzed by the enzyme acyl CoA:diglyceride acyl transferase.[75] The gene for this enzyme has been isolated, and a knockout mouse model of this gene synthesized triglyceride in the intestinal mucosa, suggesting that another enzyme may be involved in the formation of triglyceride from diglyceride.[76, 77]

(2) During fasting, triglyceride (and phospholipid) is synthesized via the second route, which involves acylation of α-glycerophosphate with the formation of phosphatidic acid and, then, triglyceride or phospholipid (see Fig. 88–5). The α-glycerophosphate is synthesized largely in the cytoplasm from glucose. The relative importance of the monoglyceride pathway and the α-glycerophosphate pathway depends on the availability of 2-monoacylglycerol and fatty acid. During normal lipid absorption, when 2-monoacylglycerol is sufficiently present, the monoglyceride pathway facilitates the conversion of 2-monoacylglycerol and fatty acid to form triglyceride and aids in inhibiting the α-glycerophosphate pathway. Conversely, when the supply of 2-monoacylglycerol is lacking or insufficient, the α-glycerophosphate pathway becomes the major pathway for formation of triglyceride.

Some absorbed lysophosphatidylcholine is reacylated to form phosphatidylcholine. The remaining absorbed lysophosphatidylcholine is hydrolyzed to form glycero-3-phosphorylcholine. The liberated fatty acid is used for triglyceride synthesis, whereas the glycero-3-phosphorylcholine is readily transported via the portal blood for use in the liver.

Absorbed dietary cholesterol enters a free cholesterol pool within enterocytes that also contain cholesterol from endogenous sites (nondietary absorbed sources [e.g., biliary cholesterol], cholesterol derived from plasma lipoproteins, and cholesterol synthesized de novo). Cholesterol is transported mainly as esterified cholesterol and almost exclusively by the lymphatic system. Cholesterol esterase and acyl-CoA cholesterol acyltransferase (ACAT) are thought to be predominantly responsible for cholesterol esterification. ACAT is stimulated by the feeding of a high-cholesterol diet and appears to play a more important role in mucosal cholesterol esterification than does cholesterol esterase.[78] Two ACAT proteins have been identified: ACAT-1 and ACAT-2.[79, 80] The role of ACAT-2 in intestinal cholesterol absorption is supported by resistance to diet-induced hypercholesterolemia due to defective cholesterol esterification and absorption by the small intestine in the ACAT-2 knockout mouse model.[81]

Once synthesized, triglyceride, cholesterol and its esters, and phospholipids are packaged for export in the form of chylomicrons and very-low-density lipoproteins (VLDL). During fasting, VLDL are the major triglyceride-rich lipoproteins that emerge from the epithelium; after feeding, chylomicrons predominate. VLDL triglycerides have a different fatty acid composition from those in chylomicrons, because different pathways are involved in their formation. Furthermore, the fatty acids derived from dietary triglyceride go predominantly into the formation of chylomicrons, whereas those derived from phospholipid appear to be utilized in the formation of VLDL.[37]

The diameter of chylomicrons ranges between 750 and 6000 nm; their cores comprise triglycerides, whereas cholesterol ester and phospholipid form more than 80% of the surface coat. Forming a smaller proportion of the surface of chylomicrons is the essential component, apolipoprotein (apo). Apo A is an important apoprotein for all lipoproteins, including chylomicrons, VLDL, and high-density lipoproteins (HDL). Apo A is synthesized in the small intestine and is found in bile.[82] Apo B probably is synthesized in the Golgi cisternae and is found in the rough endoplasmic reticulum. After feeding, it is found in association with the chylomicrons in the smooth endoplasmic reticulum. The absence of apo B prevents synthesis and secretion of chylomicrons. However, data suggest that the supply of apo B is not the rate-limiting step for forming chylomicrons. For example, the apo B output in lymph does not change after intraduodenal infusion of lipid, despite the fact that lymphatic triglyceride output increases sevenfold to eightfold.[83, 84]

Abetalipoproteinemia is a rare genetic disorder resulting in complete failure of the liver and intestine to make triglyceride-rich lipoproteins.[85] It was previously thought that abetalipoproteinemic patients have a problem synthesizing apo B. However, apo B synthesis is reduced, but not abolished, suggesting that failure to synthesize apo B by the gut and liver may not be the reason abetalipoproteinemic patients do not produce chylomicrons and VLDL.[86] This has been confirmed by the finding that the abetalipoproteinemia results from mutations of the microsomal triglyceride transfer protein gene.[84, 87]

Anderson's disease (also known as chylomicron retention disorder) is another disorder in the formation or secretion of chylomicrons by the small intestine. There is no defect in genes that carry known apoproteins or microsomal triglyceride transfer protein.[88] This fact suggests that this disease is caused by an unknown factor central to secretion of chylomicrons.

Once the chylomicrons have formed in the smooth endoplasmic reticulum, they are transferred to the Golgi apparatus. Golgi-derived chylomicron vesicles are then incorporated into the basolateral membrane and secreted by exocytosis into the lymphatic circulation (Fig. 88–6). During absorption, lacteals distend and endothelial cells, which overlap each other in the fasting state, move apart and open gaps through which chylomicrons can readily pass.[89]

Medium-chain fatty acids are absorbed by way of the portal vein, but as the chain length of saturated fatty acids increases they are increasingly absorbed via the lymphatics. Polyunsaturated fatty acids may pass directly across the basolateral membrane and into the portal circulation.

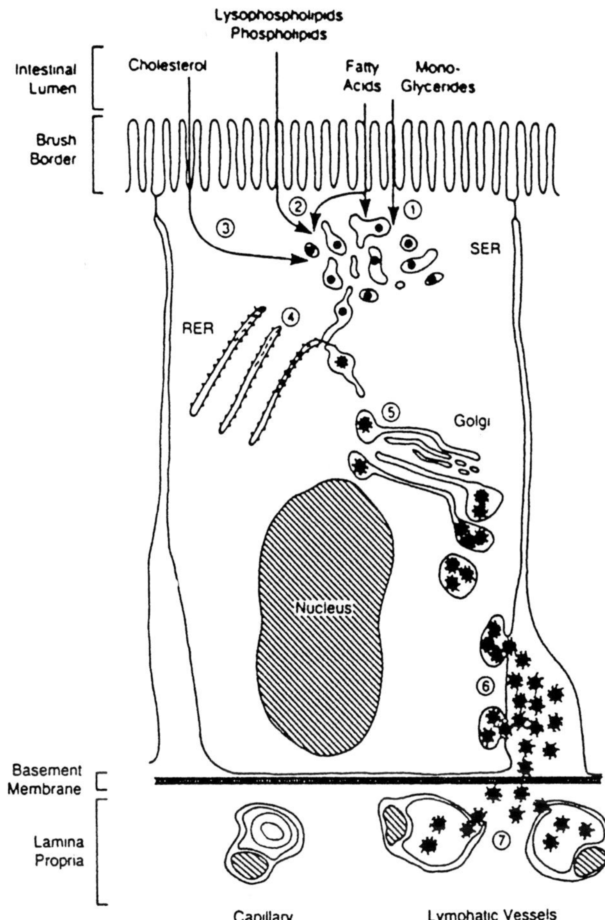

Figure 88–6. Pathway taken by lipids during passage across the enterocyte. Triglyceride and phospholipid are synthesized in the smooth endoplasmic reticulum (SER) and accumulate there as dense droplets. Apolipoproteins, synthesized in the rough endoplasmic reticulum (RER), assist in the formation of chylomicrons and very low-density lipoproteins in the tubular endoplasmic reticulum and Golgi apparatus, and these particles are finally released across the basolateral membrane by exocytosis, where the particles enter lymphatic vessels.

CARBOHYDRATE

Dietary Intake

In Western civilization, about 45% of a body's total energy requirement is provided by carbohydrate.[90] The volume of carbohydrate ingestion appears to be declining, owing in part to a reduction in the intake of purified sugar.[28, 89] Overall, total calorie intake is on the decline because of reductions in dietary fat and carbohydrate by affluent, but diet-conscious, Western societies. The proportion of carbohydrate ingested as fruit and vegetables is rising as the intake of raw fiber increases.

About half the digestible carbohydrate in an average Western diet is starch derived from cereals and plants, in which it is the major storage form. Starch (as either amylose or amylopectin) is made up of long chains of glucose molecules. Amylose, a linear polymer in which each glucose molecule is coupled to its neighbor by α-1,4 linkage, has a molecular weight of 10^6. Amylopectin, on the other hand, is a branched-chain polymer in which α-1,6 links provide the angulations between adjacent chains of α-1,4–linked glucose molecules (Fig. 88–7): it has a molecular weight greater than 10^9. Although the ratio varies widely, most starches usually contain more amylopectin than amylose. Starches are relatively easily digested, but food preparation can influence their biologic utilization. Utilization may also be determined by protein associated with the starch, particularly gluten.[1]

Other major sources of dietary carbohydrate include sugars derived from milk (lactose), contained within the cells of fruit and vegetables (fructose, glucose, sucrose), or purified from cane or beet sources (sucrose). Processed foods form a major source of dietary sugars, particularly fructose and corn syrup, which contains not only fructose but oligosaccharides and polysaccharides. The sugar alcohol sorbitol is often used in the manufacture of "diabetic" sweets and

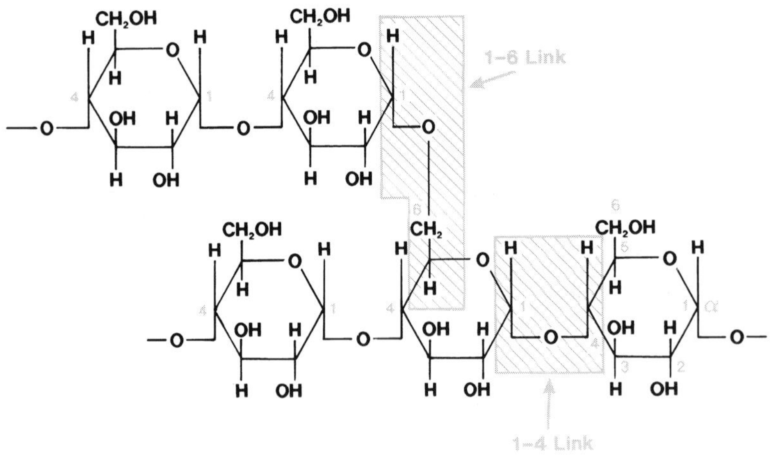

Figure 88–7. Part of an amylopectin molecule indicating the disposition of α-1,4 and α-1,6 linkages between glucose molecules.

preserves. The aldehyde group of glucose is hydrogenated to an alcohol group during manufacture, which slows its rate of absorption and thus diminishes its effect on blood sugar concentrations.[30]

Glycogen is the major storage form of polysaccharide in animals, but the amounts ingested in a normal diet are small. The structure of glycogen is similar to that of amylose, comprising straight chains of α-1,4–linked glucose monomers. "Nonstarch polysaccharides" form the majority of the "unavailable" carbohydrate. The dietary fiber component of unavailable carbohydrate is found most abundantly in cereals, peas, beans, carrots, and peanuts, and in the United Kingdom some 10 to 15 g of dietary fiber, consisting predominantly of celluloses and hemicelluloses, are consumed by each person every day.[28] Cellulose is made up of β-1,4–linked glucose molecules in straight chains, and hemicelluloses are pentose and hexose polymers with both straight and branched chains. Both forms are resistant to digestion in the small bowel because the β-1,4 bond, unlike the α-bond in starch, is resistant to amylases. However, both forms are broken down to some extent by colonic bacteria to yield short-chain fatty acids, which are avidly absorbed by colonic mucosa.[91] The quantity of cellulose and hemicellulose in vegetables and fruit varies markedly and depends on their age and "ripeness."

Other "unavailable carbohydrates" include pectins, gums, and alginates, which are only partially metabolized in the colon. Lignins, elaborated by plants in the process of becoming woody, are completely indigestible.[30]

It is well recognized that increased intake of dietary fiber eases constipation by increasing fecal bulk, with the increase in the mass of fecal flora being largely responsible. However, dietary fiber has other roles, since it has important effects on the absorption of other nutrients. It delays absorption of sugars and fats and curtails the insulin response to a carbohydrate meal. Some, such as lignins, may lower serum cholesterol by binding bile salts. Perhaps these effects have led to the widespread recommendation of a high-fiber diet for management or prevention of such diseases as diabetes mellitus and atherosclerosis. Satiety is achieved more rapidly from a diet rich in fiber than from a low-fiber diet, and it takes longer to ingest a high-fiber meal. Advantage of this is taken in the management of obesity.

Intraluminal Digestion

Salivary and Pancreatic Amylase

Salivary and pancreatic amylases are endoenzymes; that is, they cleave the α-1,4 links internal to, or at the second or third bond from, the end of the polysaccharide chain. The products of amylase digestion therefore comprise short, linear oligosaccharides with maltotriose and maltose (Fig. 88–8). Since α-1,6 links, and the adjacent α-1,4 bonds in the branched chains of amilopectin are not hydrolyzed by amylase, the products of amylopectin digestion include short, branched oligosaccharides, termed α-limit dextrins. Amylase proteins are encoded by a clustered gene family located on human chromosome 1 and mouse chromosome 3.[92] In humans, the *AMY1* gene is expressed in the parotid gland, and the *AMY2* gene is expressed in the pancreas.[93] The sequences of the pancreatic and salivary cDNAs are 94% similar, encoding for polypeptides with the same number of amino acids.[94]

Salivary amylase depends for its effect on its proximity to the ingested starches and the time spent within the mouth. Thus, careful, slow chewing affords a good start to diges-

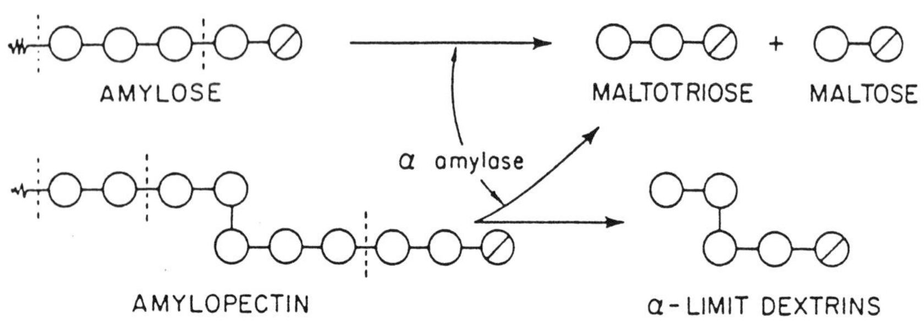

Figure 88–8. Action of pancreatic α-amylase on amylose and amylopectin molecules. Because the α-1,6 link in the latter is resistant to amylase, the products include α-limit dextrin. O, glucose units; ⊘, reducing glucose units. (From Gray GM: Carbohydrate absorption and malabsorption. In Johnson LR [ed]: Physiology of the Gastrointestinal Tract. New York, Raven Press, 1981, p 1064.)

tion, whereas rapid swallowing of poorly chewed foods—often a problem for edentulous persons—may cause suboptimal salivary amylase action.

Salivary amylase is rapidly inactivated by gastric acid, but some activity may persist within the food bolus, while short-chain oligosaccharides offer further protection for the enzyme against inactivation at acid pH. Despite these factors, it is uncertain what proportion of dietary starch is digested before it reaches the duodenum.

Pancreatic amylase is the major enzyme of starch digestion and, as with salivary amylase, produces short oligosaccharides, maltotriose, maltose, and α-limit dextrins; glucose monomer is not produced. Most of this hydrolysis occurs within the lumen, but because amylase also attaches itself to the brush border membrane of enterocytes, some digestion may occur at this site. Amylase concentration becomes limiting for starch hydrolysis only in severe cases of pancreatic insufficiency, in which luminal amylase activity levels are reduced to below 10% of normal.[95] Human milk contains amylase activity, which may be important for carbohydrate digestion in infants.[96]

Brush Border Membrane Hydrolases

The terminal products of luminal starch digestion, together with the major disaccharides in the diet (sucrose and lactose), cannot be absorbed intact and are hydrolyzed by specific brush border membrane hydrolases that are maximally expressed in the villi of duodenum and jejunum. Several types have been identified (Table 88–3).[97]

Lactase hydrolyzes lactose to produce 1 molecule of glucose and 1 of galactose.

Sucrase-isomaltase (SI, sucrase-α-dextrinase) possesses 2 subunits of the same molecule, each with distinct enzyme activity. Sucrase hydrolyzes sucrose to yield 1 molecule of glucose and 1 of fructose. Both enzymes remove glucose molecules from the nonreducing end of α-limit dextrins. Critically important is the ability of isomaltase ("debrancher" enzyme) in hydrolyzing the 1,6 glycosidic linkage in α-limit dextrins. The concerted action of sucrase and isomaltase thus yields monomeric glucose molecules from sucrose and α-limit dextrins (Fig. 88–9).

In addition, two other carbohydrases participate in terminal hydrolysis of starch products. Maltase (glucoamylase) acts on 1,4–linked oligosaccharides containing as many as 9 glucose residues, liberating glucose monomers. It has been suggested that, whereas isomaltase hydrolyzes the smallest α-limit dextrin, another enzyme, α-limit dextrinase, is responsible for rapid hydrolysis of penta- and hexa-α–limit dextrins.[98]

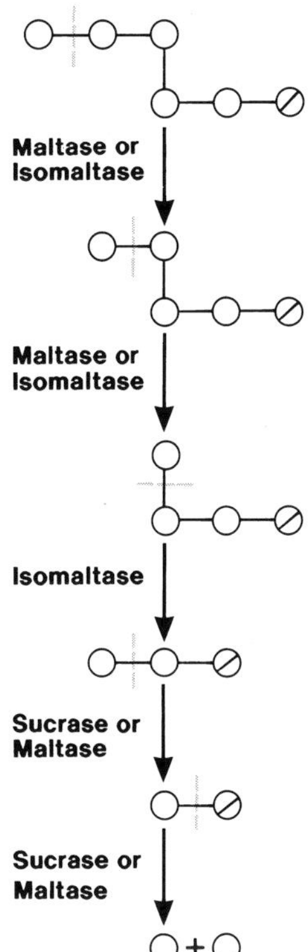

Figure 88–9. Actions of brush border membrane hydrolases. The combined actions of maltase, isomaltase, and sucrase yield glucose molecules from α-limit dextrins. Isomaltase is necessary to split the α-1,6 link. O, glucose unit; ⊘, reducing unit.

Table 88–3 | **Characteristics of Brush Border Membrane Carbohydrases**

ENZYME	SUBSTRATE	PRODUCT
Lactase	Lactose	Glucose Galactose
Maltase (glucoamylase)	α-1,4–linked oligosaccharides up to 9 residues	Glucose
Sucrase-isomaltase (sucrose-α-dextrinase)		
Sucrase	Sucrose	Glucose Fructose
Isomaltase	α-limit dextrin α-1,6 link	Glucose
Both enzymes	α-limit dextrin α-1,4 link at nonreducing end	Glucose
Trehalase	Trehalose	Glucose

The combination of sucrase-isomaltase, maltase, and α-limit dextrinase serves to liberate glucose monomers very rapidly and close to hexose carriers, thus encouraging efficient absorption. Since free hexoses are found in the intestinal lumen, it is likely that the transport process is the rate-limiting step for uptake of monomers into the epithelium rather than the actions of the carbohydrases. Trehalose is a disaccharide found predominantly in mushrooms. It is therefore an insignificant element of the normal diet, but nevertheless there is a specific brush border enzyme, trehalase, for its hydrolysis.

Disaccharidase Biosynthesis and Regulation

Much has been learned of the gene regulation, biosynthesis, and processing of the disaccharidases.[99–102] Sucrase-isomaltase is encoded by a single gene in humans,[103] which is located on the human chromosome 3 at locus 3q-25-26.[104] The 5′-flanking region of the sucrase-isomaltase gene has a number of DNA regulatory regions that control initiation of gene transcription.[105, 106] Using mouse genetics, all four epithelial cell types in the small intestinal mucosa have the transcriptional machinery to express the SI gene.[107] The elements necessary to direct intestinal epithelial cell-specific expression are embodied in a 201-nucleotide, evolutionary-conserved, 5′-flanking region of the gene.[108] At least two types of transcriptional proteins are involved in sucrase-isomaltase promoter transcription, including hepatocyte nuclear factor 1 (HNF1)[109] and caudal-related homeodomain proteins (Cdx).[110] The interaction of tissue-specific and tissue-restricted transcription factors facilitates the transcription of genes in a single cell type.

Changes in diet have a marked effect on the expression of sucrase-isomaltase. Starvation leads to a decline in brush border proteins and sucrase-isomaltase activity. This decline in sucrase-isomaltase activity is restored rapidly after refeeding. The type of carbohydrate ingested is important for regulation of sucrase-isomaltase expression. Although starch and sucrose induce sucrase-isomaltase activity, sucrose is a more potent inducer.[111] Study of the intestinal cell line Caco-2 has shown that a promoter region of the human sucrase gene (nucleotides −370 to +30) can down-regulate sucrase-isomaltase transcription in the presence of glucose.[112]

The human lactase gene is approximately 55 kb long, with 17 exons, and is located on the long arm of chromosome 2.[113, 114] Studies in intestinal cell lines have identified functional DNA elements in the lactase gene promoter that interact with nuclear transcription factors.[115] Cdx proteins and GATA6, a member of the GATA-type zinc-finger transcription factor family, have been shown to interact with the human lactase gene promoter and activate transcription.

Disaccharidase synthesis occurs within the endoplasmic reticulum, and the proenzymes then follow the path for secretory proteins through the Golgi complex before being inserted into the brush border membrane. All are glycoproteins, and all undergo extensive intracellular processing, with removal of redundant segments of the molecule. In the case of sucrase-isomaltase, final processing occurs on insertion into the brush border membrane after exposure to luminal pancreatic proteases (Fig. 88–10). At this point, it is cleaved into its two active subunits. Lactase, on the other hand, is already completely processed before its insertion.

In their final active form, the carbohydrases project into the lumen, forming part of the glycocalyx, and they are attached to the membrane by a hydrophobic anchor that represents about 10% of the total mass of the molecule.

Disaccharidases are synthesized by both crypt and villous cells but are expressed only on villous cells. The expression of these genes in the intestine exhibits a complex spatial pattern along the vertical (crypt-to-villus) and horizontal (proximal-to-distal) axes.[116] There is little sucrase-isomaltase activity in the crypts and villous tip cells, with maximal activity in lower and midvillus.[117] The major mechanism for regulating the expression of the SI protein along the crypt-villus axis is the steady-state level of sucrase-isomaltase mRNA. However, post-transcriptional and post-translational regulation likely play a role in the expression of the functional SI protein along the intestinal crypt-villus axis.[118]

A functional difference also exists between the jejunum and distal ileum that reflects differences in the expression of different genes, or gradients of gene expression, along the proximal-distal axis of the intestine. For example, sucrase-isomaltase activity is fourfold to fivefold greater in the jejunum than in the ileum[119]; however, sucrase-isomaltase mRNA appears to be similar in the two areas. Although there are minor differences in the pattern of glycosylation in the Golgi apparatus, the major difference in regulation between the jejunum and ileum appears to be at the level of mRNA translation.[120]

There are also developmental changes in the expression of disaccharidases. For example, in humans, lactase is expressed in fetal small intestine at a time in gestation just after the onset of expression of sucrase-isomaltase. This expression is maintained throughout development and during childhood, although at some time during childhood, lactase activity declines to 5% to 10% of early childhood levels in the majority of worldwide populations. This decline occurs at the same time that sucrase-isomaltase activity in the intestine is increasing. Ingestion of milk or milk products by persons with diminished lactase activity leads to flatulence, abdominal cramping, and diarrhea. In selected populations, such as in Northern Europe, where dairy cattle have been

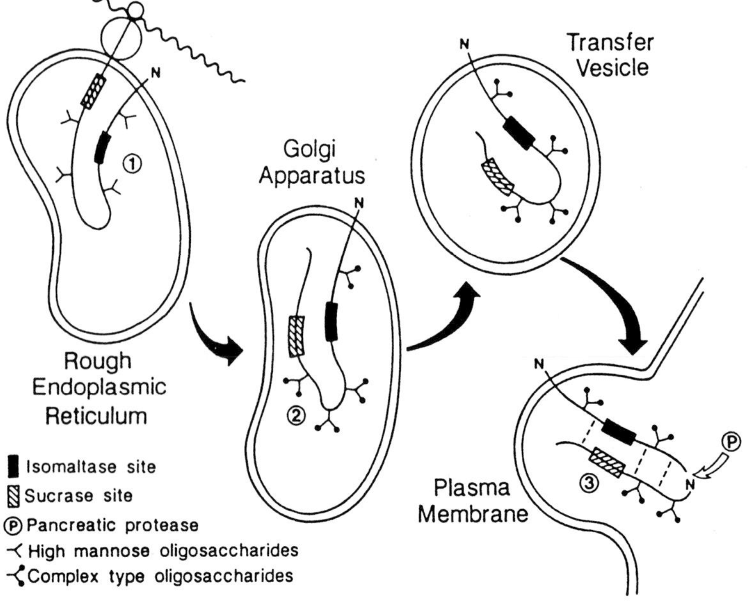

Figure 88–10. Biosynthesis of sucrase isomaltase. The nascent polypeptide is translocated across the endoplasmic reticulum membrane after ribosomal mRNA translation. Oligosaccharide side chains join the polypeptide to be transferred to the Golgi for further processing. After incorporation in the plasma membrane, luminal proteases cleave the molecule into its active subunits. (From Lloyd ML, Olsen WA: Intestinal carbohydrases. Viewpoints Dig Dis 3:13–18, 1991.)

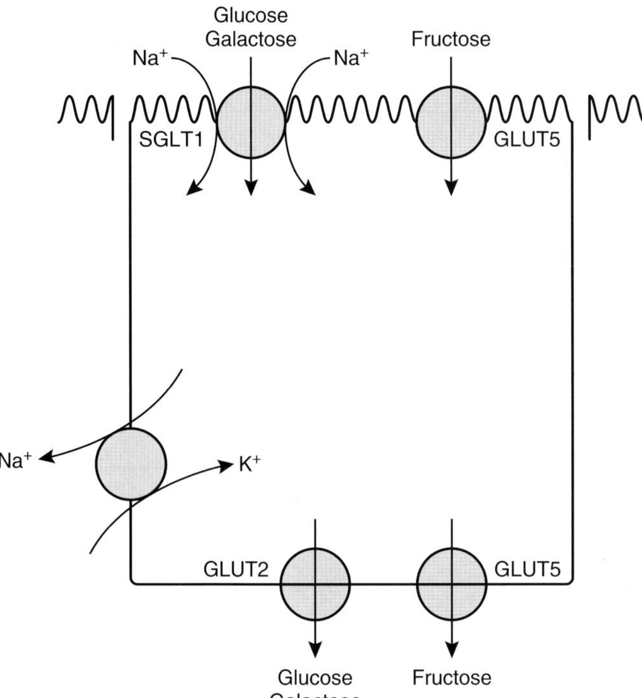

Figure 88–11. Monosaccharide transport across the intestinal epithelium. The sodium pump (sodium-potassium-ATPase) at the basolateral membrane generates a low intracellular sodium concentration. Sodium passes down the concentration gradient so created across the apical membrane coupled to glucose on a common carrier (SGLT1). The sodium pump thus generates the energy for this system. Glucose leaves the cell through facilitated diffusion (GLUT2) across the basolateral membrane. Fructose employs the facilitative transporter GLUT5 for transport across the apical and basolateral membrane.

developed as a source of milk, intestinal lactase activity persists throughout adulthood.

Pancreatic proteolytic enzymes shorten the half-life of the carbohydrases.[121] Sucrase isomaltase half-life may drop as low as 4.5 hours after meals, compared with more than 20 hours during fasting. Presumably, proteolysis, as largely determined by meals, is responsible for the diurnal variation in carbohydrase activity.[30]

The levels of sucrase-isomaltase and other saccharidases may also decrease with infection and inflammation. In some cases a decline in enzyme activity leads to malabsorption of carbohydrates and symptoms of diarrhea, flatulence, and weight loss. In most disease processes, however, the diminished levels of SI are associated with global dysfunction of the mucosa of the small intestine.

Transport Across the Mucosa

The three major diet-derived monosaccharides, glucose, galactose, and fructose, are absorbed by saturable carrier-mediated transport systems located in the brush border membrane of enterocytes.[122] The active transport of glucose and galactose is achieved by the same transport protein that acts as a sodium cotransporter[123]: active glucose transport is driven by the sodium gradient across the apical cell membrane (Fig. 88–11). A low intracellular sodium concentration is generated by the sodium pump sodium-potassium-adenosine triphosphatase (Na^+,K^+-ATPase) located in the basolateral membrane, which transports $3Na^+$ out of the cell and $2K^+$ into the cell. Sodium then enters the cell across the apical membrane and moves down its concentration gradient, bringing with it glucose or galactose in a one-to-one molar ratio. Fructose absorption occurs by facilitated diffusion; that is, transport occurs not against a concentration gradient but with a carrier protein to achieve transport rates greater than one would expect from simple diffusion.

Values for the K_m (that concentration of substrate at which half-maximal absorptive rates are achieved) for glucose have been estimated to be in the range of 2 to 20 mmol, a value that matches well with the concentrations of glucose found in the intestinal lumen under normal conditions (0.4 to 24 mmol; maximum, 48 mmol under experimental conditions).[124] These recent figures, being much lower than previous estimates of luminal glucose concentration (greater than 250 mmol), help remove the paradox that was posed by such high concentrations associated with low K_m and maximal transport rates for the glucose transporter.

The sodium-glucose cotransporter (SGLT1) has been extensively characterized.[125–128] Activity of the cotransporter in the intestinal brush border membrane rests on the presence of four independent, identical subunits arranged in a homotetramer. Having cloned and sequenced the sodium-glucose cotransporter and demonstrated that the gene for this resides on chromosome 22, investigators have demonstrated that a single missense mutation resulting in a change of amino acid residue 28 from an aspartate to an asparaginase is responsible for the defective sodium-glucose cotransporter in familial glucose/galactose malabsorption.[129] The cloned cDNA encodes for transport activity with the same relative specificity as the previously characterized native transport system: D-glucose > alpha-methyl-D-glucose > D-galactose > 3-O-methyl-D-glucopyranose >>> L-glucose.[128] The cDNA encodes a 662-amino acid protein with a predicted molecular weight that correlates well with the biochemically defined size. SGLT1 is predicted to have 14 membrane-spanning domains, with one asparagine-linked carbohydrate group on the third extracytoplasmic loop.[129]

The expression and activity of glucose transport in the intestinal brush border are regulated by both short-term and longer-term processes. In the short term, activity of glucose transport is increased by both protein kinase A– and C–dependent processes.[130] The mechanism of this enhanced activity is an increase in the number of membrane transporters, mediated by changes in exocytosis and endocytosis of membrane vesicles that contain the transport protein. Longer-term regulation of glucose transport is mediated by changes in the expression of SGLT, which is controlled by changes in the nutrient environment.[131]

Studies in humans have shown that there is a saturable, facilitative transport system for fructose in the intestinal epithelium that has a lower activity than the system for transport of glucose and galactose. The protein responsible for most apical membrane fructose transport is a member of the facilitative monosaccharide transporter family called GLUT5. This 501-amino acid protein in humans has 12 membrane-spanning domains, as do other GLUT (glucose transporter) molecules, and transports fructose exclusively.[132] Little fructose is metabolized in the enterocytes; fructose is transported across the basolateral membrane and is taken up and metabolized rapidly by the liver, resulting in low postabsorptive blood levels of fructose. There may be more than one type of fructose transport system. Malabsorption of fructose in humans can be prevented by the administration of glucose together with fructose, suggesting that there maybe another, glucose-responsive system present in the enterocytes.

Debate has developed over the mechanism of the passive or "diffusive" component of intestinal glucose absorption and, indeed, whether it even exists.[133] Pappenheimer and Reiss proposed that paracellular solvent drag contributes a passive component, which, at high concentrations of sugars similar to those in the jejunal lumen immediately after a meal, is severalfold greater than the active component mediated by the Na^+-glucose cotransporter SGLT1.[134] Others have argued that the kinetics of glucose absorption can be explained solely in terms of SGLT1 and that a passive or paracellular component plays little, if any, part.[135] More recent data suggest that the passive component of glucose absorption exists but is in fact facilitated by the rapid, glucose-dependent activation and recruitment of the facilitative glucose transporter GLUT2 to the brush border membrane. This is regulated through a protein kinase C–dependent pathway activated by glucose transport through SGLT1 and also involves mitogen-activated protein kinase (MAP kinase) signalling pathways.[136]

Exit from the Epithelium

Most hexoses are exported from the epithelial cell by way of the basolateral membrane, although small amounts are utilized for intracellular metabolism. Exit across the basolateral membrane depends on facilitated diffusion (not requiring energy) via a specific carrier. Two genes that are expressed in the small intestine, GLUT2, which is the basolateral membrane-associated glucose transporter, and GLUT5, which is an apical membrane fructose transporter, encode these facilitative sugar transport proteins.[137] GLUT2 has molecular structural characteristics similar to those of the other members of this family of genes. The protein has 500 amino acids, with many hydrophobic residues that predict a total of 12 membrane-spanning domains. One long extracellular loop between membrane-spanning domains 1 and 2 contains an asparagine that is *N*-glycosylated and there is another long cytoplasmic loop between membrane-spanning domains 6 and 7. Once the hexoses have entered the interstitial space, they pass onward by diffusion into the portal circulation.

Not all potentially digestible carbohydrate is absorbed in the small intestine. As much as 20% of dietary starch may escape into the colon, particularly that derived from cereals and potatoes.[2] Most of this, however, is metabolized by colonic bacteria, and the short-chain fatty acids thus derived are readily absorbed. Hydrogen and methane are also generated, and they contribute to flatus.

PROTEINS

Dietary Intake

Dietary proteins are the major source of amino acids and, in the average Western diet, provide about 10% to 15% of energy intake. Affluent populations ingest more protein than needed to maintain a normal balance. An average adult in a Western country consumes at least 70 g of protein per day, whereas poor people in Asia and Africa consume 50 g or less per day.[30] Recommended dietary requirements vary from 0.75 to 1 g/kg of body weight per day, but deficiency states are rare even with intakes of 0.5 g/kg per day or less. In the United Kingdom, protein intake has remained fairly steady since the mid-1970s, but with the marked decline in fat and carbohydrate ingestion the ratio of protein to nonprotein energy intake has risen.[30] Little harm appears to occur in the unusual subgroups of society who consume very large amounts of protein, although renal function can be impaired. The Masai tribes of Africa and the gauchos of South America, who consume 250 to 300 g (largely of animal origin) per day, suffer no obvious untoward effects.[30]

The variety of types of animal and plant proteins is enormous. Generally, plant proteins are less digestible than those derived from animals, but some fibrous animal proteins, such as keratin and collagen, are also relatively indigestible. High-proline proteins such as the glutenins are less thoroughly digested than others. The "quality" of proteins depends largely on their amino acid composition; those proteins rich in essential amino acids are regarded as being "high quality."

Food processing, by heat for example, may cause inter- and intramolecular bonding in the proteins to produce polymeric forms that are relatively resistant to hydrolysis.[1] Other constituents of the diet may also interfere with protein digestion—for example, starch and reducing sugars have the potential to impair digestion.[30] Despite this, digestion and absorption of proteins is remarkably complete, and only about 3% to 5% of ingested nitrogen is lost in the stool, probably because of the resistance of some peptide bonds to hydrolysis.[1] A few selected proteins are resistant to proteolysis in the small bowel, including secretory IgA and intrinsic factor. Among the 20 common amino acids that form animal and plant proteins, 8 cannot be synthesized by animals. These eight "essential" amino acids have to be ingested, usually in plant-derived foods. They are leucine, isoleucine, lysine, methionine, phenylalanine, threonine, tryptophan, and valine. Histidine is also required for growth in infants.

Proteins of Endogenous Source

Almost half of all protein that enters the intestine is derived from endogenous sources. Of this, about 20 to 30 g/day is derived from secretions of salivary, gastric, biliary, pancreatic, and mucosal origin. Another 30 g/day of protein is provided by epithelial cells desquamated from the villous tips, and 2 g of plasma proteins are delivered into the intestinal lumen each day.

Intraluminal Digestion

Pepsins

Digestion of proteins begins in the stomach with the action of pepsins secreted by gastric mucosa. They are released from their precursor pepsinogens by autoactivation in an acid pH with the loss of a small basic peptide. Pepsinogen release from chief cells is stimulated by gastrin, histamine, and acetylcholine and closely mirrors acid secretion.[138]

The pepsins are a family of proteolytic enzymes that can

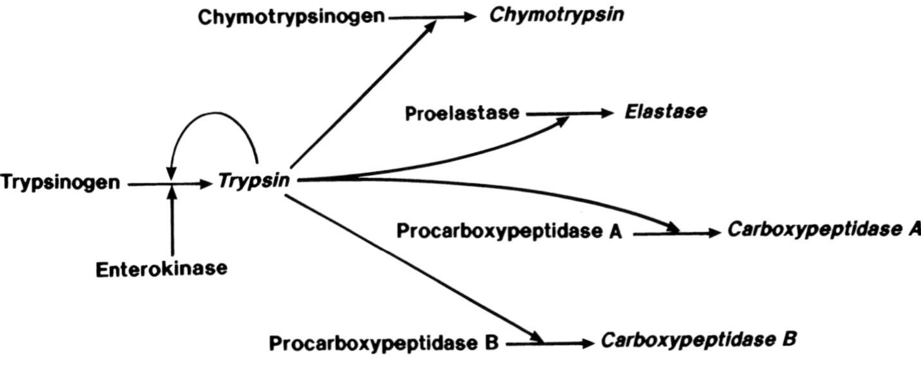

Figure 88–12. Activation of pancreatic proteolytic enzymes. Enterokinase (enteropeptidase) plays a critical role in activating trypsinogen to form trypsin. Trypsin in turn activates not only more trypsinogen but also the other proteolytic enzyme precursors.

be distinguished electrophoretically and immunologically. There are two immunologically distinct groups (groups 1 and 2), whereas electrophoresis reveals eight fractions. Both immunologically separated species are secreted by chief cells, but group 2 isoforms are present in mucous cells in the oxyntic and pyloric areas of the stomach and in Brunner's glands of the duodenum. Their substrate specificities vary little, but their pH optima differ slightly (between 1.8 and 3.5); all are irreversibly inactivated in alkali.

Pepsins remain active at the acid pH of gastric contents to produce a mixture of peptides with a small portion of amino acids. The completeness of gastric proteolysis depends, in part, on the rate of gastric emptying, the pH of intragastric contents, and the types of protein ingested. Subjects who are achlorhydric or who have lost control of gastric emptying as a result of pyloroplasty or partial gastrectomy do not appear to have a problem with assimilation of protein, which suggests that gastric proteolysis is not an essential component of digestion.

Pancreatic Proteases

Each of the pancreatic proteases is secreted as a proenzyme and, thus, must be activated within the lumen, in contradistinction to amylase and lipase, which are secreted in their active forms. Enterokinase (enteropeptidase) plays a key role. It is liberated from its superficial position in the brush border membrane by the action of bile acids,[139] its action being to convert trypsinogen to trypsin by removing its NH_2 terminus, the hexapeptide. Trypsin in turn activates the other proteases and continues to split more trypsin from trypsinogen (Fig. 88–12).

The proteases are classified into endo- and exopeptidases, according to the sites of the peptide bonds against which they are most active. Endopeptidases include trypsin, chymotrypsin, and elastase, and exopeptidases include carboxypeptidase A and B (Table 88–4).

Trypsin, chymotrypsin, and elastase have specificity for peptide bonds adjacent to certain specific amino acids. They split peptide bonds in the protein molecule, whereas exopeptidases remove a single amino acid from the carboxyl terminal end of the peptide. Trypsin produces short-chain oligopeptides, which are further hydrolyzed by the exopeptidases: carboxypeptidase A acting on aromatic and aliphatic carboxyl terminals, and carboxypeptidase B acting on peptides containing basic carboxyl terminals. The final products of intraluminal digestion are thus produced by cooperative activity of endo- and exopeptidases and consist of a number of neutral and basic amino acids, together with peptides of 2 to 6 amino acids in length. About 30% of luminal amino nitrogen is found in amino acids and about 70% in oligopeptides.[140]

In addition to nutrient protein hydrolysis, pancreatic proteases have other functions. They split vitamin B_{12} from the R protein to which it is linked so that it then can bind intrinsic factor. They increase the turnover of brush border membrane hydrolytic enzymes, and, as discussed earlier, they initiate the final steps in the processing of the sucrase-isomaltase complex. Finally, they may have a role in the inactivation of some organisms.[1]

Digestion at the Brush Border Membrane and in the Cytoplasm

In contrast to the absorption of carbohydrate, which is largely restricted to uptake of hexose monomers across the brush border membrane, amino acids can be absorbed either as monomers or as di- or tripeptides. Indeed, amino acid

Table 88–4 | **Pancreatic Proteolytic Enzymes and Some of Their Characteristics**

ENZYME	ACTION	PRODUCTS
Trypsin	Endopeptidase; cleaves internal bonds at lysine or arginine residues; cleaves other pancreatic proenzymes	Oligopeptides
Chymotrypsin	Endopeptidase; cleaves bonds at aromatic or neutral amino acid residues	Oligopeptides
Elastase	Endopeptidase; cleaves bonds at aliphatic amino acid residues	Oligopeptides
Carboxypeptidase A	Exopeptidase; cleaves aromatic amino acids from carboxyl terminal end of protein and peptides	Aromatic amino acids and peptides
Carboxypeptidase B	Exopeptidase; cleaves arginine or lysine from carboxyl terminal end of proteins and peptides	Arginine, lysine, and peptides

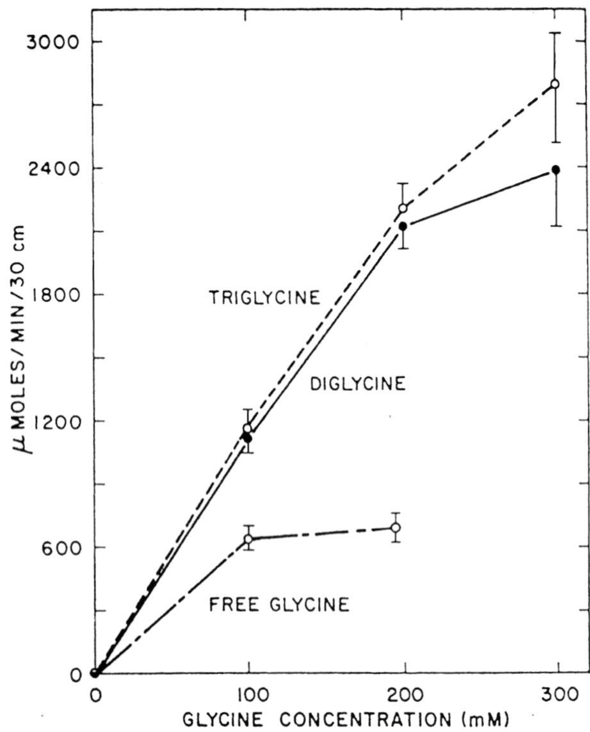

Figure 88–13. Rates of glycine absorption (mean ± standard error of mean) from perfusion solutions containing equivalent amounts of glycine in free or peptide form. Results are from studies in the jejunum of four normal humans. (From Adibi SA, et al: Evidence for two different modes of tripeptide disappearance in human intestine. Uptake by peptide carrier systems and hydrolysis by peptide hydrolases. J Clin Invest 56:1355–1363, 1975.)

absorption is achieved more efficiently with amino acids in the form of peptides than as single amino acids (Fig. 88–13).[141] However, the fact that the great majority of the end-products of protein digestion that reach the portal circulation are amino acids speaks strongly in favor of the presence of peptidases in the epithelium.

Patients with cystinuria and Hartnup's disease, who have specific defects in the absorption of basic and neutral amino acids, respectively, do not develop protein deficiency states because the absorption of peptides in these patients is normal.[142] The discovery that di- and tripeptides are actively transported by the brush border membrane of enterocytes has been valuable in explaining this observation, and it emphasizes the need for critical evaluation of the supposed nutritional advantage provided by elemental diets that consist only of free amino acids.

A range of peptidases is present in the brush border membrane and in the cytoplasm for the hydrolysis of oligopeptides up to about 8 amino acid residues in length (Table 88–5).[143–145] The peptidases on the brush border membrane differ in several important respects from those within the cytoplasm (Table 88–6). About 90% of the dipeptidases are found in the cytoplasm and only about 10% in the brush border, whereas the distribution of hydrolases for tetrapeptides is the reverse of this. Peptidases for pentapeptides and larger molecules are confined almost entirely to the brush border membrane. Cytoplasmic enzymes are much more heat labile than those in the brush border, and there are differences in the electrophoretic mobility patterns for the two sets of enzymes.[75]

Most oligopeptidases appear to be aminopeptidases; that is, they act by removing residues from the amino terminus. The chain length of the peptides is an important factor that determines not only whether the site at which hydrolysis occurs is at the brush border or within the cell but also its rate. Thus, rates of brush border membrane hydrolysis for tripeptides are most rapid, for dipeptides least rapid, whereas tetra- and pentapeptide hydrolysis rates occupy an intermediate position.[141]

Distinct from the amino oligopeptidases are at least three other peptidases. Aminopeptidase A has specificity for peptides with acidic amino acids at their amino termini. Aminopeptidases 1 and 3 (distinguished on electrophoretic mobility) have specificities for different substrates with different amino acid peptide bonds.[1]

Proline-containing oligopeptides are not readily hydrolyzed by most proteases, despite the fact that many proteins—including collagen, gliadin, and casein—are rich in proline. However, two proline-specific carboxypeptidases have been demonstrated in the brush border membrane and have slightly different substrate specificities.[146] Together with a cytoplasmic proline dipeptidase, these are likely to be responsible for hydrolysis of proline-rich peptides.

Table 88–5 | **Peptidases Found on the Brush Border Membrane and in the Cytoplasm of Villous Epithelial Cells**

PEPTIDASE	ACTION	PRODUCT(S)
Brush Border Membrane Peptidases		
Amino-oligopeptidases (at least two types)	Cleave amino acids from carboxy terminus of 3–8 amino acid peptides	Amino acids and dipeptides
Aminopeptidase A	Cleaves dipeptides with acidic amino acids at amino terminus	Amino acids
Dipeptidase I	Cleaves dipeptides containing methionine	Amino acids
Dipeptidase III	Cleaves glycine-containing dipeptides	Amino acids
Dipeptidyl aminopeptidase IV	Cleaves proline-containing peptides with free α-amino groups	Peptides and amino acids
Carboxypeptidase P	Cleaves proline-containing peptides with free carboxy terminus	Peptides and amino acids
γ-Glutamyl transpeptidase	Cleaves γ-glutamyl bonds and transfers glutamine to amino acid or peptide acceptors	γ-Glutamyl amino acid or peptide
Folate conjugase	Cleaves pteroyl polyglutamates	Monoglutamate
Cytoplasmic Peptidases		
Dipeptidases (several types)	Cleave most dipeptides	Amino acids
Aminotripeptidase	Cleaves tripeptides	Amino acids
Proline dipeptidase	Cleaves proline-containing dipeptides	Proline and amino acids

Table 88–6 | **Distribution of Peptidase Activity in Enterocytes**

SUBSTRATE	BRUSH BORDER MEMBRANE (%)	CYTOPLASM (%)
Dipeptides	5–10	80–95
Tripeptides	10–60	30–60
Tetrapeptides	90	1–10
Higher peptides	98	Nil

A number of other brush border membrane peptidases should be mentioned. Gamma-glutamyl transpeptidase hydrolyzes gamma-glutamyl peptide bonds, with the transfer of the gamma-glutamyl group to another amino acid to form a gamma-glutamyl amino acid or peptide derivative.[1] The role of this brush border membrane in the intestine is not yet clear. Folate conjugase, an enzyme concerned with hydrolysis of dietary folate, will be considered later. The recent demonstration of angiotensin I–converting enzyme (AICE) in intestinal mucosa suggests that it, too, may hydrolyze dietary peptides.[147] Indirect evidence suggests that endopeptidases also may be present on the brush border membrane, since protein digestion occurs, even in the complete absence of pancreatic function; these enzymes have yet to be isolated.

As with other proteins, synthesis of each specific peptidase occurs in the rough endoplasmic reticulum (RER), and, following transfer to the Golgi apparatus, the proteins are transported to the brush border membrane, where they are inserted by exocytic fusion.[148, 149] They are attached to this membrane by short anchoring pieces in a manner analogous to the attachment of disaccharidases[150]; however, unlike the latter enzymes, there is little post-translational processing, either within the cytoplasm or by pancreatic enzymes on the brush border.

Of the dipeptidases in the cytoplasm, the most abundant appears to be one with broad specificity for neutral amino acid–containing dipeptides. The tripeptidase isolated has broad specificity for amino terminal residues. It also has high specificity toward tripeptides containing proline as the amino terminal residue, which distinguishes it from the brush border membrane amino oligopeptidase. Other characteristics of the tripeptide that are required for rapid hydrolysis include a free α-amino group, an α-carboxyl group, and an L configuration for the two amino acid residues.[151]

Absorption

Peptides

Substrate inhibition studies indicate that tri- and dipeptides inhibit intestinal uptake of either dipeptides or tripeptides, respectively, from the lumen, but intestinal uptake of dipeptides and tripeptides is not affected by single amino acids. Such evidence suggests that small peptides utilize a transporter system separate from those utilized by single amino acids. On the other hand, tetrapeptide absorption is inhibited by single amino acids but not by di- and tripeptides, suggesting that tetrapeptides are split before absorption.

The advantage of dipeptide absorption over single amino acid absorption has been demonstrated experimentally largely with single peptides containing a single amino acid, usually glycine.[141] However, several studies have demonstrated the kinetic advantage of peptides over amino acids, even in complex mixtures of partial digests of proteins.[152, 153] Absorption was greater from tryptic hydrolysates of proteins than from a mixture of amino acids. Furthermore, the wide variation in rates of absorption seen with different individual amino acids was reduced when they were presented as a tryptic hydrolysate.

A number of other factors influence digestion and absorption. The presence of amino acids in the lumen inhibits peptide hydrolysis (product inhibition), whereas luminal glucose and luminal acidification each inhibit amino acid and peptide absorption.[141] There is good evidence to suggest that di- and tripeptides are taken up by a single type of transporter and that there is some stereospecificity, because the length of the amino acid side chains on the di- or tripeptides is important; the longer the side chain, the more preferred the substrate for the absorption site (Table 88–7).[154] The L isomers of the amino acids in dipeptides are much preferred to the D isomers, whereas the presence of acidic and basic amino acid residues in dipeptides reduces affinity for the transport system, compared with neutral amino acid residues. Affinity is also greater for dipeptides than for tripeptides, at least in the example of peptides containing glycine. The transporter for peptides is not dependent on sodium, but cotransport with protons may occur instead.[155]

The peptide transporter for human small intestine has been cloned[156, 157] and is a member of a superfamily of H^+-coupled peptide transporters. The human protein consists of 708 amino acids, with a predicted core molecular size of 79 kd, which contains 12 transmembrane domains. The gene is located on chromosome 13. In humans, it is expressed in the small intestine (duodenum, jejunum, and ileum) but not in the esophagus, stomach or colon. In the small intestine it is expressed only on absorptive epithelium. It recognizes a variety of neutral, anionic, and cationic dipetides as substrates.[158, 159] This explains the broad substrate specificity of the intestinal peptide transport system.

The most interesting feature of this transport process is that it uses a transmembrane electrochemical H^+-gradient rather than a transmembrane electrochemical Na^+-gradient as the driving force.[160] An acid pH microclimate on the luminal surface of the intestinal brush border membrane creates an H^+-gradient across the brush border membrane in vivo. This acid pH microclimate is generated and maintained by the combined action of the Na^+-H^+ exchanger in the brush border membrane and Na^+,K^+-ATPase in the basolateral membrane of the enterocyte. As shown in Figure 88–14, the mechanism of the transport process is a simultaneous translocation of H^+ and peptide substrate involving a single H^+ binding site on the protein.[161, 162]

Table 88–7 | **Relative Specificities of Intestinal Peptide Transporters for Various Peptides**

Dipeptides	> Tripeptides
L-Form of amino acids in peptide	> D-Form
Neutral amino acids in peptide	> Acidic or basic amino acids
Long side chain amino acids in peptides	> Short side chains

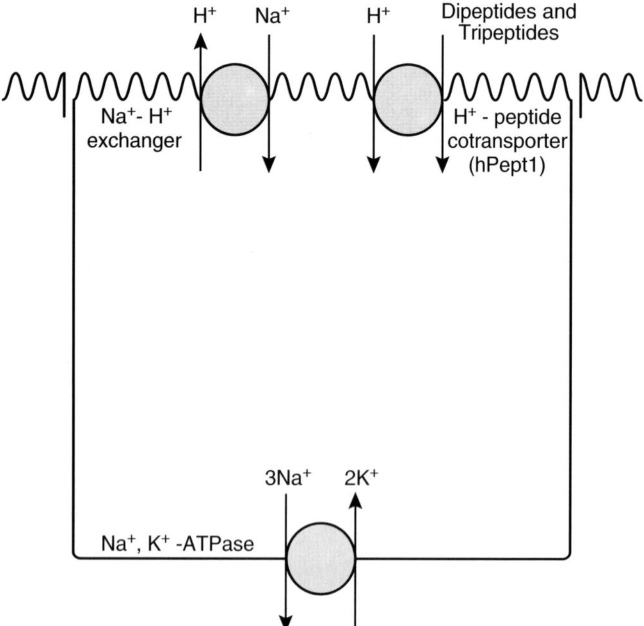

Figure 88–14. Peptide transport across the intestinal epithelium. This transport process uses a transmembrane H^+-gradient rather than a transmembrane electrochemical Na^+-gradient as the driving force. The acid pH microclimate on the luminal surface of the intestinal brush border membrane is generated and maintained by the combined action of the Na^+-H^+ exchanger in the brush border membrane and Na^+,K^+-ATPase in the basolateral membrane of the enterocyte. The mechanism of the transport process is a simultaneous translocation of H^+ and peptide substrate involving a single H^+ binding site on the protein.

Amino Acids

Although there appears to be only one type of dipeptide transporter in the brush border membrane for the 400 different possible dipeptides, a multiplicity of transport mechanisms exists for the 20 amino acids. In adults, these are sited on villous enterocytes and involve carrier-mediated active transport or facilitated diffusion processes; a small proportion may be absorbed by simple diffusion. There has been some difficulty in defining the number and types of transporters because of their overlapping specificities; several amino acids utilize a number of different transport systems (Table 88–8). On the basis of kinetic studies, at least four active processes for transport of *neutral* amino acids across the apical cell membrane have been identified. Each is electrogenic and sodium dependent. One has broad specificity for a number of neutral amino acids (NBB system); a second provides another route for phenylalanine and methionine (PHE system); a third provides a mechanism for imino acid absorption (IMINO system); and the fourth transports beta-amino acids.

The molecular nature of several of the amino acid transport systems has been elucidated.[163–165] For example, the neutral amino acid transport system is a 541-amino acid protein that contains 10 transmembrane domains.[163] The gene coding for the protein is located on chromosome 19, and even though this transport system preferentially recognizes neutral amino acids as substrates at neutral pH, anionic amino acids are recognized as substrates to a significant extent at acid pH. This suggests that, under the acid pH microclimate that exists in vivo in the intestine, this system may mediate the absorption of both neutral and anionic amino acids.

Separate sodium-dependent, active transport processes for *basic* and *acidic* amino acids also have been demonstrated, and there is some evidence to suggest that facilitated diffusion of these types of amino acids also occurs, although this is likely to be a minor pathway. The fact that there are a number of different congenital disorders of amino acid transport that affect the intestine, each with a characteristic and specific defect, speaks for the presence of multiple different transporters; however, until these transporters have been more clearly defined at the molecular level, their individuality will remain uncertain.

Several hormones have been shown to alter the amino acid and peptide transport process in the intestine. Somatostatin and vasoactive intestinal polypeptide decrease these transport processes. In contrast, epidermal growth factor, neurotensin, cholecystokinin, and secretin enhance transport. Human Pept1 appears to be inhibited by protein kinase C[166] and cyclic adenosine monophosphate (cAMP).[167] The expression of the intestinal peptide transporter is also modulated by diet protein content.[168] Even though the peptide transporter is expressed along the entire small intestine, the diet-induced changes in the expression of the transporter are specific to certain regions. A high-protein diet increases the steady-state levels of the transporter specific messenger RNA in the middle and distal regions of the small intestine. The expression of the brush border peptidases dipeptidylcarboxypeptidase and dipeptidylaminopeptidase IV, which release dipeptides from oligopeptides, is also enhanced by a high-protein diet.

Exit from the Epithelium

Exit through the basolateral membrane operates through a number of different mechanisms that involve active transport and diffusion of both facilitated types.[169] Active, sodium-dependent processes exist at this membrane for the uptake of neutral amino acids, which presumably supplies nutrients for crypt cells and for villous enterocytes during fasting when a luminal source is unavailable (see Table 88–8). Villous enterocytes normally receive the amino acids necessary for production of their own protein from luminal nutrients; crypt

Table 88–8 | **Major Amino Acid Transport Systems Detected in Intestinal Epithelial Cells**

TRANSPORT SYSTEM	SUBSTRATES
Brush Border Membrane	
Neutral amino acids:	
NBB system	Broad specificity for neutral amino acids
PHE system	Phenylalanine and methionine
IMINO system	Imino acids: proline, hydroxyproline
Basic amino acids	Lysine, cysteine, basic amino acids
Acidic amino acids	Glutamate, aspartate
Basolateral Membrane	
L	Broad selectivity
A	Broad selectivity
ASC	Neutral amino acids: alanine, serine, cysteine
N	Glutamine, histidine, asparagine

cells obtain their supply from the portal circulation. Of all the amino acids, glutamine appears to be a unique, major source of energy for enterocytes, ammonia being an important metabolic by-product. Active uptake of glutamine at the basolateral membrane, as well as via apical membrane processes, is thus of particular importance.

It has been estimated that about 10% of amino acids are utilized in the production of enterocyte protein. Some of these proteins are secreted across the basolateral membrane specifically by villous enterocytes, including the apolipoproteins A1 and A1v, secretion of which increases manyfold after a fatty meal.[30]

The intestinal basolateral membrane possesses a set of amino acid transport systems that is different from those in the brush border membrane. The amino acid transport systems in the basolateral membrane function to export amino acids from the enterocytes into the portal circulation during feeding. They also participate in the import of amino acids from the splanchnic circulation into the enterocyte for cellular metabolism when amino acids are not available from the intestinal lumen, such as between meals. The intestinal basolateral membrane also possesses a peptide transporter system probably identical to that in the brush border membrane. This transport system facilitates the exit of hydrolysis-resistant small peptides from the enterocyte into the portal circulation.

Although very small amounts of dipeptides have been detected in the portal circulation after a meal, the great majority of absorbed products of protein digestion that reach the circulation are in the form of single amino acids. It is somewhat surprising that digestion of protein continues into the ileum, with approximately 40% of ingested protein undergoing transport in this segment of small intestine.[170]

VITAMINS

Water-Soluble Vitamins

Although in the past it has been thought that the absorption of water-soluble vitamins depended simply on passive diffusion across the intestinal mucosa, the improvement of specific carrier-mediated processes has been recognized increasingly (Table 88–9). Furthermore, several of these vitamins are present in the diet as conjugates or coenzymes that require hydrolysis before or during their absorption.

Table 88–9 | **Water-Soluble Vitamins**

VITAMIN	REFERENCE NUTRIENT INTAKE*	TRANSPORT MECHANISM
Ascorbic acid	40 mg/day	Active; Na-dependent process at BBM
Folic acid	200 μg/day	Hydrolysis of dietary polyglutamates by folate conjugase at BBM; Na-dependent active transport or facilitated diffusion of monoglutamate at BBM
Cobalamin (B_{12})	1.5 μg/day	Intrinsic factor binding; uptake of intrinsic factor/B_{12} complex at BBM by way of specific receptor
Thiamine	1 mg/day	Na-dependent active transport
Riboflavin	1.3 mg/day	Thiamine and riboflavin absorption includes hydrolytic and phosphorylation steps
Pantothenic acid	3–7 mg/day†	
Biotin	10–200 μg/day†	
Pyridoxine	1.5 mg/day	Simple diffusion
Niacin	18 mg/day	?

*Reference nutrient intakes quoted are calculated as 2 SD above the estimated average intake for normal adult men. These figures provide an adequate intake for nonpregnant adults.

†Nutrient intakes for pantothenic acid and biotin are given as "safe intakes" because insufficient data are available on human needs. These values provide a range over which there is no risk of deficiency or toxicity.

BBM, brush border membrane.

Ascorbic Acid (Vitamin C)

Although most species synthesize all their vitamin C requirements, primates, guinea pigs, and some birds have lost this capacity and thus depend on diet for their needs. Vitamin C is found in a wide range of foods, but the most abundant sources are fresh fruits and fruit juices. Black currants are particularly rich (200 mg/100 g), and apples and pears less so (5 mg/100 g). Of animal sources, raw liver contains about 20 mg/100 g, milk about 2 mg/100 g, but fresh meat traces only. The ingestion of as little ascorbic acid as 10 mg/day prevents scurvy, and the recommended daily intake of 40 mg thus seems reasonable.[90]

Cooking destroys some of the ascorbic acid, but this can be minimized by shortening cooking times and not keeping foods hot for prolonged periods before they are eaten. Prolonged storage of foods also depletes vitamin C content.

With the loss of the capacity for hepatic synthesis, a specific absorptive mechanism has developed in humans (and guinea pigs). Transport across the apical membrane of small intestinal enterocytes occurs by an active, sodium-dependent process.[171] Electrically neutral, uphill transport of vitamin C probably occurs in the form of sodium ascorbate. A variable proportion of luminal vitamin C is present in the oxidized form as dehydroascorbic acid, which is also actively absorbed.

Folic Acid

Folic (pteroyl monoglutamic) acid consists of the complex pterin molecule conjugated to para-aminobenzoic acid and glutamic acid. Although much dietary folate is in the form of polyglutamates comprising at least six glutamic acid residues, much is present as formyl- and methylhydrofolate. The folates are widely distributed in the diet, particularly rich sources being spinach (200 mg/100 g), liver (140 mg/100 g), and peanuts and beans (100 mg/100 g). Meat, chicken, potatoes, and fruit (except orange juice) are poor sources (less than 15 mg/100 g). Food preparation, especially prolonged cooking, destroys its value. Recommended dietary intakes are on the order of 200 mg/day in adults and 400 mg/day during pregnancy.[90]

Absorption of dietary polyglutamates depends on hydrolysis at the brush border membrane, followed by transport into the cytoplasm.[172, 173] The apical membrane hydrolase in human intestine is a carboxypeptidase, cleaving a single glu-

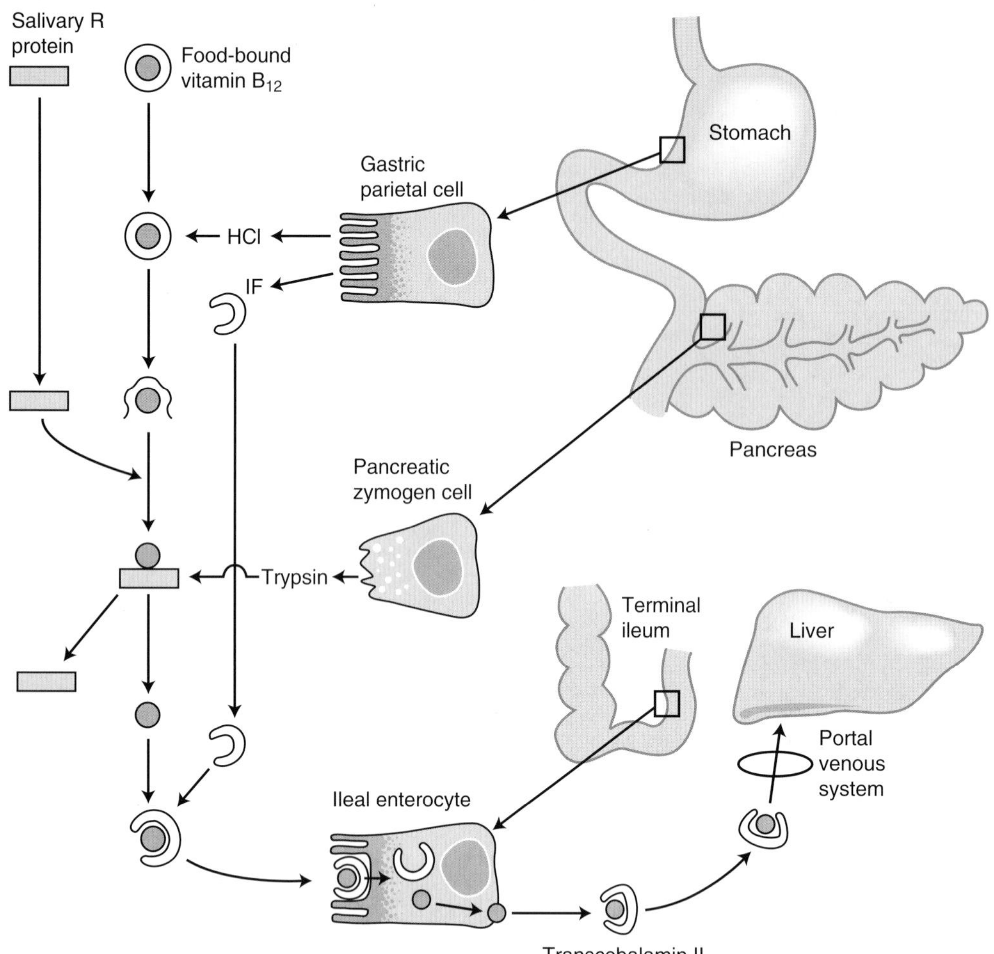

Figure 88–15. Steps in the chain leading to the binding of vitamin B_{12} to intrinsic factor (IF). Food-bound B_{12} is released by gastric acid-peptic activity and picked up preferentially by salivary R protein in the stomach. Proteolysis of R protein by duodenal trypsin from the pancreas releases B_{12} for binding to intrinsic factor. The subsequent binding and uptake of the intrinsic factor–B_{12} complex occurs through a specific receptor-mediated process on the brush border membrane of ileal enterocytes. Vitamin B_{12} is released at an intracellular site, transported across the basolateral membrane, and there taken up by transcobalamin II for transport into the portal circulation.

tamic acid residue at a time. There is also a cytoplasmic folate hydrolase, an endopeptidase prominent in several species and present in humans; its role in the latter is uncertain.

Uptake is achieved by a specific carrier-mediated, sodium-dependent, pH-sensitive process that is active at acid pH. It is not absolutely clear whether this transport mechanism is an active process against a concentration gradient or by facilitated diffusion. It is inhibited by diphenylhydantoin and sulfasalazine, which also depresses hydrolysis. Prolonged exposure to ethanol inhibits hydrolysis (but not uptake), and this may be relevant to the folate deficiency sometimes found in alcoholic patients.

Vitamin B_{12} (Cobalamin)

Cobalamin exists largely as hydroxycobalamin, methylcobalamin, and adenosylcobalamin, and these are found almost entirely in animal sources. Liver, kidney, beef, fish, eggs, and milk provide most cobalamin in a normal diet.[30] Vegetables are almost entirely lacking the vitamin, and strict vegans' intake may be inadequate. About 10 to 20 μg is ingested per day in an average diet, and of this about 1 to 2 μg/day is required to provide for normal needs.[174]

Three types of binding proteins are concerned with the absorption of cobalamin—one in saliva, one in gastric juice, and one in the circulation.[174] The vitamin is released by gastric acid from the various dietary proteins with which it is associated (Fig. 88–15). Here the first specific binding protein secreted in saliva, the R protein, takes up the free cobalamin and binds it with strong affinity. At intragastric pH values below 3, intrinsic factor has much weaker affinity for the vitamin than has R protein.[175] Only in the duodenum, where the R protein is hydrolyzed by pancreatic enzymes, is intrinsic factor able to bind the cobalamin that has been released.[176]

In humans, intrinsic factor is secreted from parietal cells; rats and mice secrete it from chief cells. Its release is stimulated in response to the same agonists that stimulate acid secretion—histamine, gastrin, and cholinergic agonists. Unlike R proteins, of which there are several that can bind a wide variety of cobalamin analogs, intrinsic factor is much more selective and specific for cobalamin. It has been suggested that the nonspecificity of binding to the R protein that exists in plasma may offer an advantage in binding potentially harmful compounds.[177] Intrinsic factor has a very strong affinity for cobalamin and binds it tightly by enclosing the vitamin in its cuplike interior. This complex resists pancreatic proteolysis, passes down the intestine to the terminal ileum, and there binds to specific receptors on ileal enterocytes. These are patchily distributed in the ileal mucosa.[178] Estimates suggest that there are about 300 to 400 receptors per enterocyte, or 1 per microvillus, located deeply between the microvilli.[179] The number of receptors available determines how much vitamin can be absorbed; absorption doubles during pregnancy by a doubling of the number of available receptors.[180]

After binding to the receptor, the intrinsic factor–cobalamin complex probably enters the cell intact by translocation (see Fig. 88–15). Intracellular events have not been fully elucidated, but B_{12} accumulates in the mitochondria, and the complex is split at some point within the enterocyte. Free cobalamin leaves the base of the cell, where it is immediately bound to an ileal pool of transcobalamin II, which transports it into the portal circulation.

It is clear that this complicated series of events can be prevented at a number of different points in the pathway. Lack of pancreatic proteolysis would lead to a defect in the release of the vitamin from the R protein for intrinsic factor binding; lack of intrinsic factor would fail to provide the complex necessary for binding and absorption at the ileal mucosa; loss of ileal receptors would prevent absorption; and defects within ileal enterocytes may prevent release of the vitamin into the circulation.

Other Water-Soluble Vitamins[30, 181]

Thiamine (vitamin B_1) is widely distributed, but the only important dietary sources are seeds of plants. Germs of cereals, nuts, peas, beans, and pulses (legumes) are major sources, whereas green vegetables and fruit are relatively poor ones. White flour or bread and purified rice have virtually no thiamine. It is very water soluble and is readily lost in the cooking water.

Niacin (nicotinic acid) and nicotinamide are widely distributed in foods, but the availability of the vitamins in these foods varies. About half of the dietary intake of North Americans and Europeans is supplied in meat and fish. The niacin content of legumes, however, is largely bound and unavailable. It can be released by treatment with alkali, but unfortunately the food preparation methods widely employed in Asia and Africa for maize, for example, do not render the niacin available. Nicotinic acid can be synthesized in humans from tryptophan, 60 mg of the latter being required for the synthesis of 1 mg of niacin. The concept of the "nicotinic acid equivalent" has thus arisen, and foods lacking in niacin may remain valuable in preventing pellagra because of high tryptophan content. Such is the case with milk and eggs, for example.

Riboflavin is linked with phosphoric acid in most animal and plant tissues to form flavin mononucleotide, and with adenosine monophosphate (AMP) to form flavinadenine dinucleotide. The richest dietary sources are liver, eggs, milk, green vegetables, and beer. It is also synthesized by colonic bacteria, but its availability from this site is uncertain. Cooking does not destroy much riboflavin, but exposure to sunlight may.

Pantothenic acid is usually found as its calcium salt and is derived largely from animal tissues, especially liver and kidney, and egg yolk, wheat germ, and peanuts. It is almost completely lacking in many processed foods but is not lost in normal cooking.

Biotin is so very widely available that spontaneous deficiency states in humans have rarely been described. Many yeasts and bacteria contain biotin and may provide a sufficient supply in normal foods. Liver, legumes, nuts, and vegetables are reasonable sources.

Pyridoxine occurs in the diet in one of three forms: pyridoxamine phosphate, pyridoxal phosphate, and pyridoxine phosphate. Its presence is widespread in plant and animal tissues; cereals, peanuts, bananas, and liver are good sources.

Absorptive Mechanisms

A specific sodium-dependent active transport process has been demonstrated for each of these vitamins: thiamine, riboflavin, pantothenic acid, and biotin.[30, 181, 182] Pyridoxine appears to be absorbed by simple diffusion, whereas the mechanism for niacin uptake awaits further study.

Riboflavin is presented to the mucosa in the form of coenzymes, so it is necessary for these to be hydrolyzed at the brush border membrane before active transport occurs into the cell. Once within the cell, rephosphorylation occurs. Thiamine is also phosphorylated in the enterocyte after absorption and is transported out of the cell, possibly by the basal membrane sodium-potassium-ATPase. This exit step is inhibited by ethanol. Dietary deficiency of thiamine, ascorbic acid, and biotin appears to enhance specific mechanisms for their uptake, although evidence of a similar adaptive mechanism for other vitamins is lacking.[30]

Fat-Soluble Vitamins

Vitamins A, D, E, and K are structurally different from each other, but all can be classified as polar, nonswelling, insoluble lipids. Although their chemical structures are known, the retention of a letter to signify their individuality is valuable because each consists of a number of closely related compounds with similar properties (Table 88–10).[30]

Vitamin A (retinol) is found in the diet in milk and milk products, egg yolk, and fish oils. Beta-carotene is a precursor that consists of 2 conjoined molecules of retinol (Fig.

Table 88–10 | **Absorptive Mechanisms of Fat-Soluble Vitamins**

VITAMIN	REFERENCE NUTRIENT INTAKE*	MECHANISM OF ABSORPTION
Vitamin A (retinol)	700 μg/day	Passive diffusion
Vitamin D (cholecalciferol)	10 μg/day†	Passive diffusion
Vitamin E (α-tocopherol)	>4 mg/day‡	Passive diffusion
Vitamin K (phytomenadione [K_1] and menaquinones [K_2])	1 μg/kg/day‡	K_1, carrier-mediated uptake K_2, passive diffusion

*Reference nutrient intakes quoted are calculated as 2 SD above the average intake of normal male adults.

†Normal adults with normal exposure to sunlight do not require any dietary intake of vitamin D.

‡Figures for vitamin E and K are "safe intake" values that provide safe and adequate amounts for normal nutrition. Excessive intake of vitamins A and D produces toxic effects, and the figures quoted in the table are safe in normal men, but not necessarily in infants.

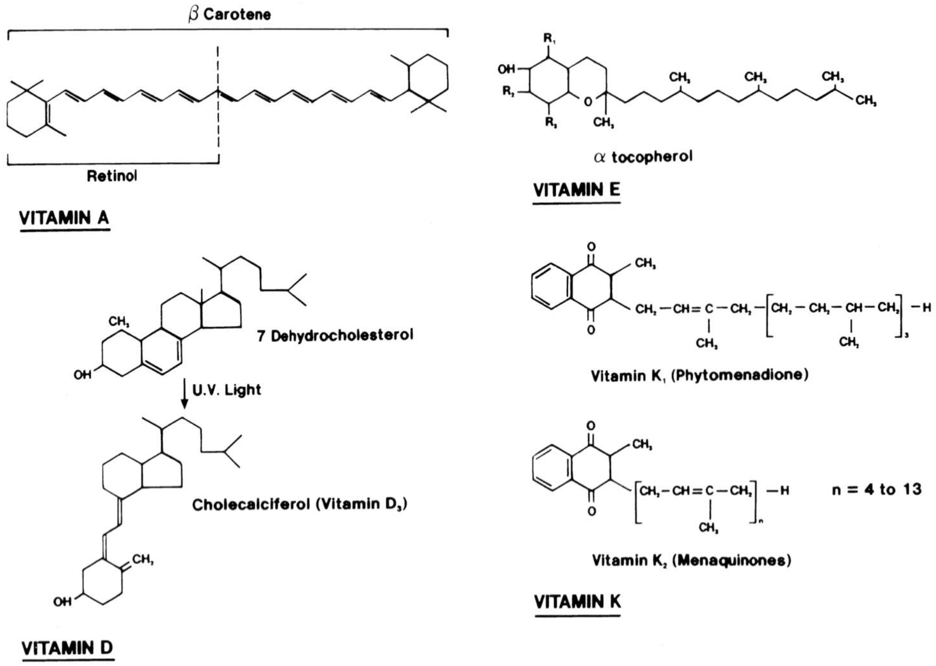

Figure 88–16. Structural formulae of the fat-soluble vitamins A, D, E, and K.

88–16). There are many other carotenoids in the diet, but these contain only 1 retinol molecule. The carotenoids are found predominantly in green vegetables and carrots, and in the United States and Europe these sources account for about half the dietary intake. Retinol and the carotenes are stable to normal cooking.

Both retinol and carotene are absorbed in the small bowel, carotene less readily than retinol.[183, 184] Beta-carotene is split by an oxygenase in the brush border membrane, yielding two molecules of retinol, but it is unclear whether this is a prerequisite for absorption. Transport across the apical membrane appears to occur by passive diffusion, but facilitated diffusion cannot be excluded. Vitamin A leaves the mucosa largely in chylomicrons as retinyl palmitate.

Vitamin D is a group of sterols that have antirachitic properties, but the only two nutritionally important members are vitamins D_2 (ergocalciferol) and D_3 (cholecalciferol). Both are produced by ultraviolet irradiation of their precursor sterols, ergosterol and 7-dehydrocholesterol, respectively (see Fig. 88–16). Ergosterol, found in fungi and yeasts, is an unusual constituent of the normal diet, whereas vitamin D_3 is the major dietary form. It is found in a restricted range of foods, predominantly the oils of fatty fish, which themselves ingest it in plankton found near the surface of the sea.[30] Human breast milk contains sufficient vitamin D to prevent rickets, but cow's milk is a poor source. Most of a person's requirement for vitamin D, however, is supplied by endogenous synthesis in the skin during exposure to sunlight, and dietary intake becomes critical only when such exposure is inadequate (see Table 88–10).

Like absorption of vitamin A, vitamin D absorption occurs by simple passive diffusion in the small intestine.[185] Bile salts are unnecessary, but luminal pH influences absorption. Absorption is reduced at neutral pH and increased in acid.[186] Most absorbed vitamin D passes into the lymphatics unchanged.

Vitamin E is still seeking a role in humans. It comprises a group of eight or so tocopherols, the most potent of which in animals is α-tocopherol (Fig. 88–16).[106] It is very widely distributed in the diet: vegetable oils, cereals, eggs, and fruit are good sources. Margarines are particularly rich in vitamin E, and breast milk contains much more vitamin E than does cow's milk. Although a variety of diseases can result from deficiency of vitamin E in a variety of animals, it has proved difficult to ascribe a human disease to vitamin E deficiency.

Vitamin E is absorbed passively across the intestinal mucosa.[187] The ester form, in which many vitamin preparations are presented, is hydrolyzed prior to absorption, but the ester can be absorbed intact.[188] Vitamin E is transported into the lymphatics largely unchanged.

Vitamin K is found in two forms: K_1, derived largely from plants, is phytomenadione; K_2 comprises a group of bacteria-produced compounds, the multiprenyl menaquinones. K_1, the major dietary form, is found in green vegetables, but beef liver is another good source. K_2 is produced by colonic bacteria, and, although some may be absorbed from the colon, this alone is an inadequate source if K_1 absorption is impaired. Absorption of K_1 from the small intestine depends on luminal bile salts, and uptake is achieved by a carrier-mediated process,[189] whereas K_2 absorption is entirely passive.[190]

MINERALS AND TRACE ELEMENTS

Various divalent ions are essential nutrients; some are absorbed in milligram amounts and are major constituents of the body; others are necessary only in trace amounts. Iron, calcium, magnesium, phosphorus, and sulfur are in the former category, and specialized absorptive mechanisms are concerned with their assimilation.

Calcium

Milk and cheese are the most valuable sources of calcium, although cereals, legumes, and other vegetables contribute. Phytic acid or oxalate in vegetables binds strongly to calcium, thus reducing its availability. Dietary fiber also binds calcium and may interfere with its absorption. On the other hand, dietary lactose enhances absorption.[191] Fractional, or true, absorption is only about 20% to 30% of total dietary calcium, the remainder being excreted in stool.

Absorption across the intestinal mucosa is achieved by two parallel processes—an active, transcellular transport process and a passive, paracellular diffusive process.[192–194] Under normal dietary conditions, the duodenum is the major site for active transport, whereas passive, paracellular transfer occurs throughout the small intestine. Despite this localization of the active transport site, quantitatively more calcium may be absorbed in the jejunum and ileum than in the duodenum because of the relative amounts of time luminal contents spend in these regions of the intestine. The human jejunum absorbs calcium faster than the ileum, and absorption rates in both are increased by treatment with vitamin D.[195]

The paracellular route, via the tight junctions, may be capable of modifying calcium transport because passive transport increases in response to treatment with vitamin D.[196] Furthermore, recent evidence suggests that tight junctional permeability increases during sugar transport, and this may provide another mechanism for control of paracellular transport.[197]

The transcellular route involves transport across the apical membrane, transfer across the cytoplasm, and exit across the basolateral membrane (Fig. 88–17). Entry probably occurs via specific calcium channels in the apical membrane and down the prevailing electrochemical gradient. Within the cytoplasm, a key step is binding to a calcium-binding protein, calbindin.[198] Maximal transport rates correlate closely with calbindin concentrations. This protein, present in concentrations of 0.1 to 0.2 mM, must rapidly take up the calcium entering the cell because intracellular free calcium concentrations are carefully maintained at very low values (about 10^{-7} M). Transient rises in intracellular calcium act as key second messenger signals for secretory responses in enterocytes. Absorbed calcium is thus presumably segregated from that concerned with cell signalling, and calbindin plays a vital role here by bringing calcium to the transporter at the basolateral membrane.[199] An active mechanism is then necessary to drive calcium uphill against the electrochemical gradient, for which a calcium-dependent ATPase is responsible.[198] Calcium arrives at the basolateral pole bound to a site at the cytoplasmic aspect of the calcium-dependent ATPase that spans the basolateral membrane. A phosphorylation-induced change in the conformation of the calcium-dependent ATPase follows, and the calcium ion is extruded through the channel formed by the enzyme transmembrane elements.[200]

The rate-limiting step in the absorption process is the intracellular calbindin concentration, which is regulated by a metabolite of vitamin D, 1,25-dihydroxyvitamin D (1,25-$[OH]_2D$), produced in the kidneys from 25-hydroxyvitamin D (25-[OH]D) converted by the liver from absorbed vitamin D.[193] The vitamin also has a modest effect on the calcium entry step and enhances activity of the basolateral calcium ATPase. Up-regulation of the calbindin gene in response to vitamin D occurs largely in villous cells.[201]

There is evidence, too, of colonic absorption of calcium, which can be enhanced in response to vitamin D.[202] The presence of the colon has advantages for calcium absorption in patients with short bowel syndrome.[203]

Active duodenal calcium absorption is increased in calcium deficiency states and reduced in calcium repletion states. Increased production of the active 1,25-$(OH)_2$ vitamin D metabolite in response to a small drop in plasma calcium concentration is responsible for increasing calcium absorption, and this change occurs within a day of changing from a high-calcium to a low-calcium diet.[204] It is also likely to be the cause of the enhanced calcium absorption seen during late pregnancy and lactation.

At birth, the active vitamin D–dependent, absorptive

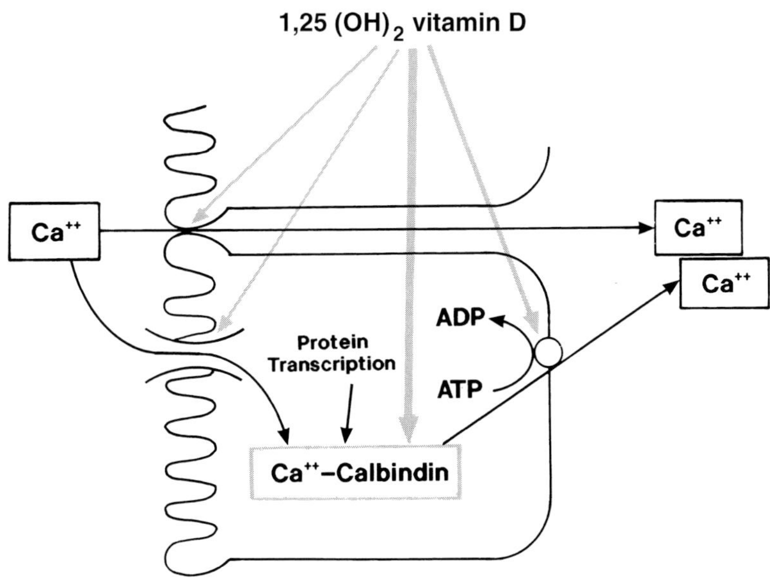

Figure 88–17. Mechanisms of calcium transport across the intestinal epithelium. A paracellular route allows bidirectional flux. Transport into the epithelial cell occurs through specific channels down an electrochemical gradient. A critical step is the binding to calbindin, which then presents calcium for export through a calcium-dependent ATPase on the basolateral membrane. Each of these processes appears to be influenced by 1,25-$(OH)_2$ vitamin D, although the maximal effect is on synthesis of fresh calbindin.

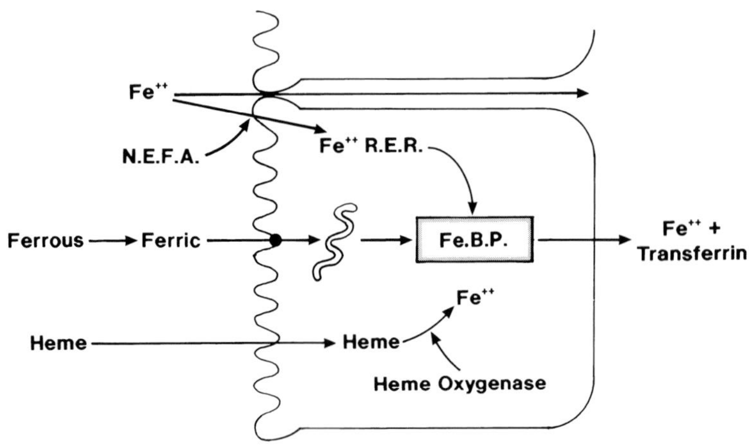

Figure 88–18. Mechanisms of iron transport in the intestine. A small amount of inorganic iron may pass through the paracellular route. Inorganic iron is converted into its ferric form at the brush border membrane before transport into the cell. Another route appears to be stimulated by nonessential fatty acids. Heme iron is transported into the cell by a separate mechanism. Within the cell, one or more iron-binding proteins take up iron and transfer it to the basolateral membrane for delivery across the membrane and subsequent binding to transferrin. R.E.R., rough endoplasmic reticulum.

mechanisms are present in the human duodenum. Ingestion of large amounts of calcium, together with lactose, in breast milk ensures adequate intake at this critical stage of life. Calcium absorption declines with age, but this may be due in part to a lack of vitamin D.[191]

Magnesium

An average diet provides about 300 to 500 mg of magnesium per day in a wide range of vegetables. Its absorption has been less thoroughly investigated than that of calcium, but it seems likely that the mechanisms involved are different. In contrast to calcium, absorption in the basal state is greater in the human ileum than in the jejunum.[195] Jejunal absorption is increased by vitamin D, whereas ileal absorption is not. Ileal transport involves both a paracellular, diffusive pathway and a transcellular, carrier-mediated, saturable process.[205] There is some competition from calcium for the diffusive pathway but not for the saturable, presumably carrier-mediated process.[205] Quantitatively, magnesium fluxes across ileal mucosa are severalfold greater than those for calcium.

Iron

Meat-eating affluent societies ingest about 20 to 30 mg of iron per day, largely as myoglobin or hemoglobin. Vegetarian societies in poor countries ingest much less than this in wheat and vegetables, and iron in these foods is less readily available for absorption. A careful balance of absorption and loss is maintained in normal adults: both inputs and losses are about 1 mg/day. Developing children and adolescents need to absorb about 0.5 mg/day more, to build up total body iron to adult values. Iron is present in breast milk in the form of lactoferrin, for which a specific brush border membrane receptor has been demonstrated.[206, 207] This facilitates absorption in neonates. During reproductive life, normal women need to compensate for menstrual losses, which are of the order of 5 to 50 mg/month, and for each pregnancy, about 500 mg.

Since dietary intake often markedly exceeds the body's need for iron, it is clearly necessary to absorb only a small portion of that ingested. Overall, there is a positive and linear relationship between the *amount* ingested and that absorbed, but the *proportion* absorbed decreases as more is taken in.[208]

Most absorption occurs in the proximal small intestine, and the ferrous (Fe^{2+}) form is absorbed better than the ferric (Fe^{3+}) form. The latter is insoluble at pH values above 3, and gastric acid and some sugars and amino acids render it more available for absorption. The presence of some anions, such as oxalate, phosphate, and phytate, precipitates iron out of solution and reduces its absorption. The presence of bile enhances absorption, but the mechanism is unclear.

The iron in hemoglobin and myoglobin is well absorbed, and although these apparently compete with inorganic iron for absorption, the organic molecules are absorbed intact by a separate process.[209] The presence of the globin nucleus enhances absorption even though this part is split off before absorption. The iron is released by mucosal heme oxygenase in the epithelium.[210]

A small proportion of the iron crossing the mucosa utilizes a paracellular route by simple diffusion. Another component, utilizing a transcellular route, is encouraged by nonessential fatty acids. A third component is one that is regulated and dependent on metabolic energy (Fig. 88–18).[211]

Dietary iron is predominantly found in the ferric form, but Fe^{3+} is highly insoluble under physiologic conditions. During intestinal uptake, ferrous iron is converted to the ferric form at the apical membrane before it attaches to an acceptor protein in the membrane. The ability of intestinal mucosa to reduce Fe^{3+} to Fe^{2+} has been documented,[212] and a ferrireductase activity has been characterized for intestinal cell lines.[212, 213] A functional role for Fe^{3+} reduction in iron transport across the brush border is inferred by the fact that inhibition of ferrireductase activity reduces apical iron uptake. Furthermore, increased ferrireductase activity correlates with enhanced iron uptake induced by iron deficiency and hypoxia.[213, 214]

A number of brush border iron-binding proteins have been described, including a 520-kd membrane complex called paraferritin. This complex contains integrin, mobilferrin (a calreticulin homolog), and flavin mono-oxygenase, and it is theorized that the complex participates in uptake of dietary iron bound in the gut lumen by mucin. How these various iron-binding moieties mediate uptake and what their relative contributions are to the dietary absorptive process remain unclear.[213, 215]

An iron transport protein called divalent metal ion transporter 1 (DMT-1, also called DCT-1 or Nramp2) that is responsible for dietary iron absorption in the villous cells of the small intestine has been identified.[216] The symport activity of DMT-1 is proton-coupled, with a stoichiometry of $1Fe^{2+}:H^{+}$. In order of substrate preference, DMT-1 can mediate import of Fe^{2+}, Zn^{2+}, Mn^{2+}, Co^{2+}, Cd^{2+}, Cu^{2+}, Ni^{2+}, and Pb^{2+}. The idea that the transporter responsible for dietary iron absorption recognizes other divalent cations agrees well with observations that Zn^{2+}, Mn^{2+}, Cd^{2+}, and Cu^{2+} all can inhibit this process. DMT-1 mRNA is found in many different tissues, but the protein and its mRNA are most abundant in the proximal duodenum, with decreasing absorption along the distal axis, consistent with a function in intestinal iron absorption.[217] Furthermore, iron depletion results in increased DMT-1 mRNA levels in the intestine, which suggests that iron-responsive elements (IREs) in the gene's 3′-untranslated region bind and stabilize the DMT-1 mRNA.[217] Although the major route for dietary iron absorption is likely to be mediated by DMT-1, this transporter is found only in the apical surface of enterocytes. Thus, other factors must be involved in the transfer across the intestinal epithelium.

DMT-1 may be involved in the pathogenesis of hereditary hemochromatosis (HH). *HFE* is the gene responsible for HH. HFE protein is found in the crypt cells of the duodenum associated with β_2-microgobulin and transferrin receptor. It is hypothesized that HFE protein may facilitate transferring receptor-dependent iron uptake into crypt cells and that mutant HFE protein may lose this ability, leading to a "relative" iron deficiency in duodenal crypt cells. In turn, this may lead to an increase in the expression of DMT-1, resulting in increased iron absorption in HH. Up-regulation of DMT-1 expression has been confirmed in the HFE-knockout mouse and in humans with HH (see Chapter 66).[218]

Once in the intestinal cell, iron is transferred to the RER for onward transmission to the basolateral membrane. A number of nonferritin iron-binding proteins have been demonstrated in enterocyte cytoplasm, and it has been proposed that one or more of these controls the rate of iron absorption.[208] When these proteins are replete with iron, derived from both the lumen and plasma, they are less available to accept more absorbed iron. Shedding of enterocytes at the villous tips also sheds their iron content. In iron depletion, free iron-binding protein is available for more uptake from the lumen, and this is passed on across the basolateral membrane. Some of these iron-binding proteins also have an affinity for other divalent cations; this could explain the observation of reciprocal regulation of absorption of one by the other. Although the mechanism by which iron is released from the intestinal enterocyte remains ambiguous, it may involve hephaestin, a ceruloplasmin homolog, which is abundant in the small intestine and colon and is anchored to the cell surface via a single transmembrane-spanning domain.[219]

The stimuli for increased iron absorption include iron deficiency, hypoxia, increased erythropoiesis, and pregnancy,[220] but the circulating signal to the intestine is unknown. It is not the hemoglobin or serum iron concentration, nor does it appear to be erythropoietin. Transferrin may be involved.[221] In any event, absorption of both inorganic iron and hemoglobin iron is increased, and both iron uptake and exit are enhanced.[222] This is achieved by an increase in maximum absorptive capacity rather than in the "affinity" of the system.[223]

Trace Elements

The importance of zinc, copper, and iodine in human nutrition has long been recognized, and they have received increasing attention in recent years as their roles in defined enteral and parenteral forms of nutrition have been demonstrated. The value of selenium also has been emphasized, and the need for manganese and chromium is receiving attention. Despite this interest, surprisingly few systematic studies of their absorption have been undertaken.

Zinc is present in the body in about half the amount of iron (about 2 g), largely in a wide variety of enzymes. It also plays important roles in maintaining configuration of gene transcription proteins and the integrity of membranes. It is found particularly in meat, shellfish, cereals, and legumes. Daily requirements are approximately 12 to 15 mg in adults. Persons who consume a low-energy diet may take in marginal amounts of zinc, and requirements are increased during pregnancy and lactation. Absorption is impaired by phytic acid phytates and oxalates in the diet, and food processing may render it less available for absorption.[30, 224]

There is enterohepatic circulation of zinc, and reabsorption appears to be maximal in the distal small intestine.[225] Studies with vesicles of jejunal brush border membranes of pigs have identified two uptake processes: a saturable, carrier-mediated process and a "nonsaturable," diffusive process.[226] The relative importance of each is not known. The recently characterized zinc transporters (ZnT) have significantly increased understanding of the interrelationships of cellular zinc uptake and efflux but do not yet account for observations at the whole body level.[227, 228] ZnT-1 is a ubiquitously expressed protein that has been found in the villi of the proximal small bowel. In response to manipulation of dietary zinc, however, expression in rats was increased in response to zinc supplementation but not to zinc restriction.[229] These and other observations have led to the current consensus that ZnT-1 functions mainly as a zinc exporter and may play a role in zinc homeostasis as a mechanism for zinc acquisition and elimination under conditions of excess zinc.[227]

The role of metallothionen (MT), an intracellular metal-binding protein, in the regulation of zinc absorption, particularly in conjunction with the zinc transporters, also remains unclear. This binding protein may be concerned with zinc absorption because changing dietary loads of zinc rapidly affect protein synthesis with changes in binding capacity.[230] Subjects on a low-zinc diet respond by decreasing their urinary excretion rate and by increasing absorption rates.[225, 231] Absorption increases in pregnancy and during lactation.[232] In experiments with knockout and transgenic mice, the rise in serum zinc after a single dose of zinc was much greater than in the control animals. In contrast, the serum zinc response of the MT transgenic animals was blunted compared with that of the control animals. The expression of ZnT-1 was also measured and found to be directly related to serum zinc levels but unaffected by MT levels.[233] Thus, MT may function in cellular responses to limit free zinc concentrations within narrow ranges and function as a zinc pool.[227, 233] Another transporter potentially involved in zinc and other metal uptake is DCT-1, a transmembrane polypeptide that is found in the duodenum in the crypts and lower villi and may be available for the uptake of several metal ions.[228]

Copper is found in green vegetables and fish, and the average Western diet provides 1 to 3 mg/day, which is adequate for a daily need of about 1 mg/day. Dietary copper is absorbed from the stomach and small intestine. Although the precise mechanisms involved in copper absorption remain incomplete, within physiologic ranges of intake absorption is probably by active transport. Competition between copper and zinc for absorption may be demonstrable with large doses but not with normal dietary intakes.[234] Its uptake may increase in pregnancy.[235] In mammals, one candidate protein has been identified. A human complementary DNA (cDNA) encoding a putative high-affinity Cu transport protein, denoted hCtrl, has been identified by functional complementation of the respiratory defect in yeast cells defective in Cu transport due to an inactivation of both the CTR1 and CTR3 genes.[236] Human CTR1 is a 190-amino acid protein with three transmembrane domains, with significant homology to yeast CTR1 and CTR3, suggesting that mammalian high-affinity Cu transporters may have evolved from both CTR1 and CTR3. RNA blotting analysis has demonstrated that hCTR1 is expressed in all organs and tissues examined, with liver, heart, and pancreas exhibiting the highest levels of expression and intermediate levels of expression in the intestine, while expression in the brain and muscle is low. Whether hCTR1 plays an important role in Cu uptake into intestinal mucosal cells has yet to be firmly established.[237]

Two putative low-affinity mammalian Cu transporters, hCTR12 and Nramp2, also have been identified. It is unclear what role hCTR2 plays in Cu homeostasis, as its mRNA levels are highest in the placenta and very low in liver, intestine, and colon.[236, 237] The Nramp2 protein also has been identified as a proton-coupled metal ion transporter of a broad range of metal ions.[217] Once transported into intestinal mucosal cells, MNK is required for Cu transport into the portal circulation. MNK is a P-type ATPase defective in Menkes disease patients in whom Cu has accumulated in intestinal cells.[238] Once entering the plasma, Cu is bound with albumin and histidine in the portal blood and rapidly deposited in the liver, where hCTR1 may play a role in this process. Ceruloplasmin, a major Cu-containing protein in plasma, is synthesized in the liver with incorporation of Cu by the Wilson disease protein, which has a high homology with MNK and is defective in Wilson disease patients who suffer from copper accumulation in the liver (see Chapter 67).

Iodine is present in varying amounts in a wide range of foods, depending on the soil content in the region where animals have been reared and vegetation has grown. Seafoods are particularly rich in iodine. It is absorbed largely as inorganic iodide, but some iodine is also transported as amino acid complexes.[239]

Selenium is found predominantly in association with amino acids, and about 60% of dietary selenium is absorbed. Selenium deficiency states have been reported in China (Keshan disease), where there is very little selenium in soil and water,[240] but not in New Zealand, where intake is equally sparse.[241] Absorption of selenium occurs rapidly when it is associated with amino acids, as in selenomethionine, probably by active transport mechanisms operative for the amino acid.[242] Inorganic selenium is absorbed more slowly, possibly by simple diffusion.

The mechanisms underlying the absorption of other trace elements, including manganese and chromium, are largely unknown.[239] Trace element deficiencies are rare in normal people, even in those with poor protein and calorie intake. Exceptions occur when local geographic availability is suboptimal, as may occur with iodine, and possibly with selenium.

ADAPTATION TO CHANGES IN NEED OR LOAD

One of the most fascinating aspects of intestinal function, observed for more than 30 years, is the phenomenon of adaptation. Two specific forms of intestinal adaptation have been identified in the intestine: (1) mucosal hypertrophy[6] leading to a global increase in absorption of all nutrients, and (2) an increase in specific transport mechanisms induced in response to specific dietary needs or availability.[243]

Mucosal Hypertrophy

Resection of more than 50% of the human intestine results in increased fecal nitrogen losses, which slowly return toward normal, thus implying that mucosal adaptation has occurred. This is due largely to hypertrophy of intestinal mucosa, which is manifested in increases in the number of villous enterocytes and in villous height without obvious increase in the absorption rate per individual cell.[153] Absorption increases for all nutrients, and absorptive capacity, may be enhanced up to fivefold in response to intestinal resection. Jejunal adaptation following ileal resection appears to be less efficient than ileal adaptation in response to jejunal resection.

Although hypertrophy in response to resection is the best-characterized example, other causes also have been discerned, at least in experimental animals. Thus, during lactation and pregnancy,[244] in diabetes,[245] and in the physiologic response to extreme cold,[246] hypertrophy is evident, but this may be due, at least in part, to the hyperphagia that accompanies these conditions.

The mechanisms by which hypertrophy occurs have been the subject of much study (Fig. 88–19). The presence of luminal nutrition appears to be a major stimulus to growth,[6] in addition to pancreaticobiliary secretions in the lumen.[247] Certain peptide hormones also have been implicated, particularly enteroglucagon and glucagon-like peptides.[248] Gastrin and CCK display trophic effects on the GI tract,[249] and more recently other trophic factors such as epidermal growth factor and insulin-like growth factors have been implicated.[250, 251] It is uncertain whether they act as local paracrine mediators or as circulating hormones.

Polyamines are other important local mediators of mucosal hypertrophy[252] since epithelial production of polyamines

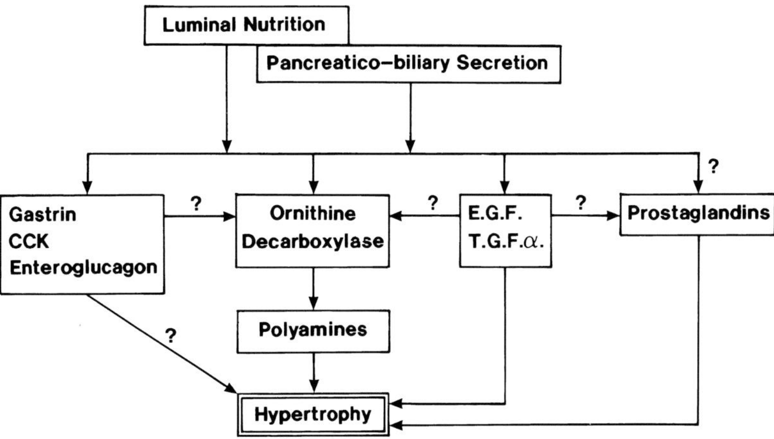

Figure 88–19. Intestinal adaptation. Interrelationships between the major factors concerned with inducing mucosal hypertrophy, such as may follow intestinal resection.

follows intestinal resection, whereas inhibiting their synthesis prevents the hypertrophy usually associated with resection. Polyamines also may play a role in the maintenance of normal mucosal structure, since their mucosal level in the intestines of experimental animals decreases rapidly in response to a 24-hr fast and increases within a few hours of refeeding.[253] Although certain prostaglandins have been shown to enhance cell proliferation in the stomach and intestine, their role in adaptation is uncertain.[254]

Specific Reversible Adaptation

Pancreatic Enzyme Secretion

It has long been known that the digestive capacity of pancreatic juice can be altered by changes in nutritional intake, but it is now clear that specific responses occur after different types of dietary manipulation.[255] A high-protein diet enhances proteolytic enzyme production, a high-carbohydrate diet enhances amylase secretion, and a high-fat diet stimulates lipase secretion (Fig. 88–20). In part, these changes appear to depend on specific polypeptide hormone release. Prolonged administration of caerulein (an analog of CCK) stimulates trypsinogen and inhibits amylase secretion,[255] whereas secretin stimulates lipase secretion (Fig. 88–21).[256] Insulin released from pancreatic beta cells, in response to carbohydrate ingestion, appears to be involved indirectly in enhancing amylase secretion.[255] A high-fat diet also induces increased capacity to secrete gastric lipase, but the mechanisms involved are not known.[257]

The underlying molecular biologic events that lead to pancreatic adaptation have been studied, and, as might be expected, responses depend on the period over which a dietary stimulus is applied. Responses to short-term stimulation, as after a single meal, appear to depend on enhanced translation of mRNAs for enzymes.[255] Protein synthesis increases within the first 2 hours of hormonal stimulation and appears to be due entirely to translational events; however, more prolonged stimulation—over several days—increases mRNA production by increased transcription, leading to enhanced biochemical commitment to enzyme secretion.[258] A single stimulus after a prolonged period of high protein intake, therefore, results in much greater proteolytic enzyme output than it does in persons whose protein intake is low.

It is clear, therefore, that the polypeptide hormones secretin, CCK, and possibly insulin, liberated in response to a meal, not only cause immediate release of pancreatic enzymes but also stimulate gene expression over the longer term and thus increase secretory capacity.

Mucosal Responses

Adaptive responses to changes in dietary intake influence mucosal digestive and absorptive processes. Activity of the disaccharidase enzymes sucrase and maltase increases in response to high carbohydrate intake over several days but

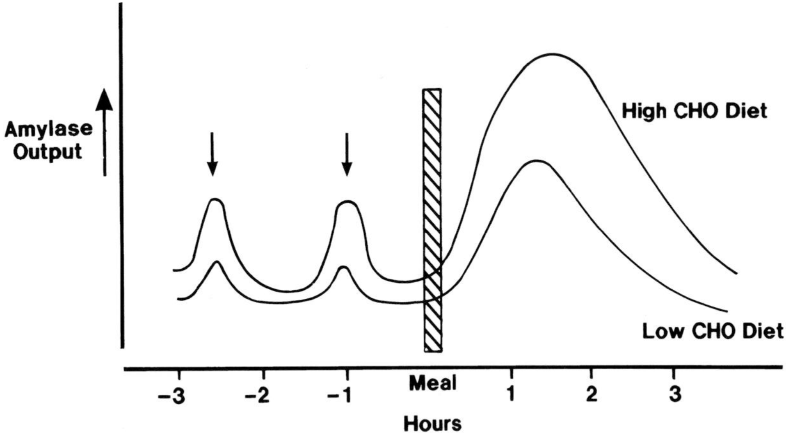

Figure 88–20. Pancreatic enzyme adaptation to dietary manipulation. Diagram of typical pancreatic amylase outputs in normal subjects fed either a high- or a low-carbohydrate diet for 2 weeks. Greater amylase secretion rates occur, both during the interdigestive phasic periods (↓) and in response to a standard meal, in subjects given a high-carbohydrate diet.

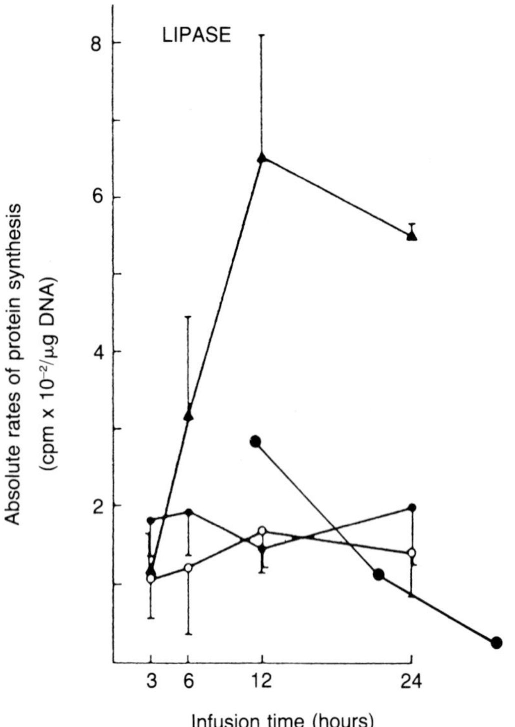

Figure 88–21. Pancreatic enzyme responses to prolonged hormone stimulation in rats. The lipase synthesis rate rose in response to secretin (16 units/kg/h) (*triangles*), but not to caerulein (0.25 µg/kg/h) (*closed circles*), or saline (*open circles*), infused for up to 24 h. (From Rausch U: Synthesis of lipase in the rat pancreas is regulated by secretin. Pancreas 1:522–528, 1986.)

not to manipulation of protein intake.[259] Sucrase levels increase first in crypt cells, about 24 hours after refeeding sucrose following a period of starvation. Thus, synthesis of the disaccharidases is stimulated but their breakdown is also diminished. On the other hand, lactase is an enzyme that appears not to respond to manipulation of dietary intake of lactose.[260]

Absorptive function also adapts to dietary manipulation.[135] It has been widely assumed that there is a considerable reserve of absorptive function in normal circumstances, but Diamond and colleagues argued eloquently that it would be inefficiently costly in biosynthetic energy for the intestine to have a large spare capacity.[135, 261] Furthermore, it has been subsequently shown that there is a fairly close match between absorptive capacity for many nutrients and dietary load. There is a clear need, therefore, for adaptation to occur in response to changes in load, and there is good evidence to suggest that most nutrients regulate their specific mucosal transporter. Two major adaptive responses are discernible in the mucosa (Fig. 88–22).[135]

In the first, as exemplified by sugars, peptides, and nonessential amino acids, transport activity rises in response to increased dietary loads. Experimental animals fed diets high and low in glucose increase or decrease their maximum capacity for glucose transport, respectively, over a twofold range, probably by changing the number of transporters. An analogous response to increased dietary load is seen with protein ingestion, in which peptide transporters and some amino acid transporters are increased.

In the second type of mucosal response, as exemplified by a number of vitamins and trace elements, absorptive mechanisms are switched on by low dietary loads and switched off by a large load. Here absorption is enhanced in nutrient deficiency but inhibited with nutrient excess, when potentially toxic effects may result.

A mixed pattern is seen with other types of nutrients, as with essential, predominantly basic, and neutral amino acids, when absorption is enhanced at very low dietary levels; presumably in an effort to ensure adequate intake. Absorptive mechanisms are at their minimum with average dietary intake but rise as dietary ingestion increases above that range.[135]

The signal for up-regulation of brush border membrane glucose absorption is glucose itself, although an actively transported but unmetabolized sugar stimulates glucose uptake too.[261] Fructose stimulates its own absorption by a separate mechanism from that which stimulates glucose transport.[262] Regulation of mucosal transport of acidic amino acids and imino acids follows the same pattern as that for sugars; that is, an increase in dietary load up-regulates transport. There is an interesting cross-induction of transport mechanisms by one type of amino acid with another. Thus, the basic amino acid arginine up-regulates acidic as well as basic amino acid transport, and the acidic amino acid aspartate induces maximal transport of basic amino acids as well as acidic ones.[263] This cross-stimulation occurs between amino acids and peptides, each of which stimulates the absorption of the other.

Enhanced absorption could result from increased numbers of transporters or from increased activity of each transporter.[135] There is evidence in favor of both mechanisms, although the former probably predominates. It is uncertain whether an increase in transporter number is caused by increased synthesis, secondary to either transcription or translation; decreased degradation; or an increase in the insertion of preformed transporters into the brush border membrane. Because dietary regulation of glucose and amino acid transporters takes 2 to 3 days, it is likely that regulation occurs at the level of crypt cells.

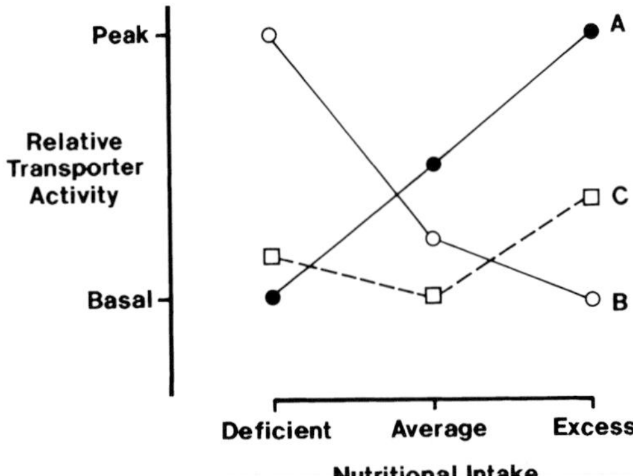

Figure 88–22. Three types of adaptive responses of intestinal transporters to variation in nutritional intake. Type A (*filled circles*) characterizes hexose and nonessential amino acid transport; type B (*open circles*), elements such as iron and calcium and some vitamins; and type C (*open squares*) is a mixed pattern seen with some essential amino acids. (Adapted from Ferraris RP, Diamond JM: Specific regulation of intestinal nutrient transporters by their dietary substrates. Annu Rev Physiol 51: 125–141, 1989, with permission.)

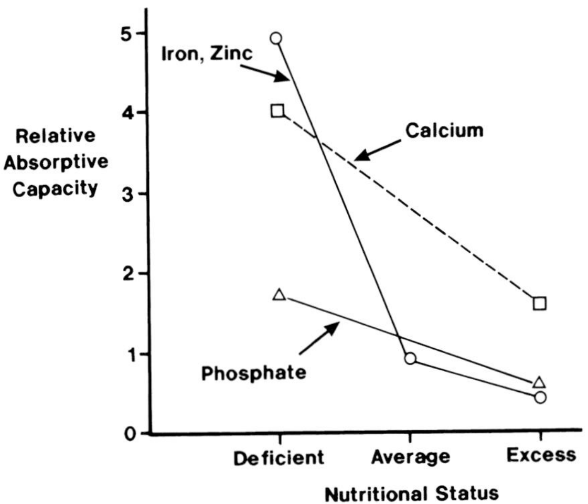

Figure 88–23. Changes in absorptive capacity for some nutrients in response to nutritional requirements. (Adapted from Ferraris RP, Diamond JM: Specific regulation of intestinal nutrient transporters by their dietary substrates. Annu Rev Physiol 51:125–141, 1989, with permission.)

In diabetes mellitus, the persistent hyperglycemia stimulates both basolateral and apical membrane glucose transport, which can be inhibited by protein synthesis inhibitors such as cyclohexamide, suggesting a role for increased synthesis of new glucose transporters.[264]

Vitamins and Trace Elements

Deficiencies of vitamins and trace elements are associated with up-regulation of their absorptive mechanisms. This is seen, for example, with biotin, thiamine, and ascorbic acid and with iron, calcium, zinc, and phosphate (Fig. 88–23).[135] Because some of these are potentially toxic, most down-regulate their transport mechanisms when present in higher concentrations. Furthermore, low body stores of iron, zinc, calcium, and phosphate signal enhanced absorptive mechanisms. Zinc deficiency enhances zinc absorption approximately fivefold by increasing transport capacity. Dietary calcium deficiency stimulates calcium uptake in the proximal intestine by a vitamin D–dependent mechanism involving increases in a cytosolic calcium-binding protein and by stimulating transport across the brush border membrane and at the basolateral membrane. These changes occur within a few hours, suggesting that mature enterocytes on the villi are capable of being regulated. This contrasts with the effects of dietary regulation of glucose and amino acids, which takes 2 to 3 days.

The difference in time scales over which GI responses to stimulation by various nutrients occur provides fascinating insights into the molecular and biologic events underlying these phenomena. Immediate responses seen within seconds to a few minutes after exposure are likely to involve release, or activation, of preformed proteins. Adaptive responses found within 2 to 3 hours of stimulation are probably due to increased translation; responses that take several hours or days are likely to be due to increased transcription and production of more mRNA.[265]

THE NEONATAL INTESTINE

Development and Adaptation of Nutrient Digestion and Absorption

Nutrient requirements vary markedly during early postnatal development, and this is mirrored by alterations in digestive and absorptive capacity. Some of these changes are genetically determined and programmed and do not appear to be greatly influenced by changes in dietary load.[5] Thus, for most of the world's population, excluding white persons, the decline in activity of the disaccharidase lactase, which occurs after infancy, cannot be prevented by maintaining a high milk intake.[135]

Some early postnatal responses and most responses in adult life, however, appear to be purposive and reversible in parallel with changes in dietary intake, in terms of both digestive enzyme production and absorptive capacity. Such adaptations may occur in response to changes in dietary load or altered body needs.[135, 255]

Developmental Changes

Some 50% of the total calorie requirement of infants is provided by the fat in milk. Breast milk contains 3.5% to 4% of lipid, of which 95% is in the form of triglyceride.[176] The fatty acid composition is a mixture of medium- and long-chain fatty acids.

In neonates, pancreatic lipase secretion is low, and the digestion of triglyceride in milk relies on the other lipases present in milk or secreted by the tongue or gastric mucosa. Pancreatic lipase secretion rises after weaning, as milk-derived lipase is no longer available (Fig. 88–24).[265]

Protein digestion is incomplete in infancy, and many proteins, such as human milk protein (whey), may partially escape digestion.[266] This relative immaturity also may have advantages for the infant because some biologically important peptides and immunoglobulins are preserved.

Proteolytic enzymes are derived from a variety of sources, which are also changing during early neonatal life. Thus, there are several specific proteases, including trypsin and elastase, in breast milk.[266] Gastric acid and pepsin are secreted at birth and increase toward adult values over the

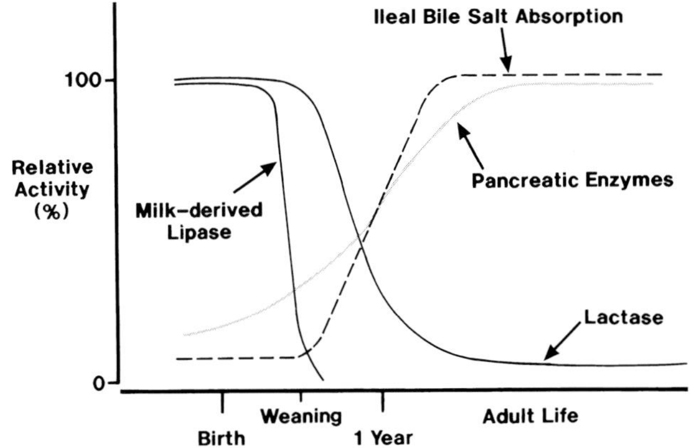

Figure 88–24. Diagram of the major changes in digestive function in neonates.

following 3 to 4 months. Despite this, little protein digestion appears to occur in the stomach during the first couple of weeks of life, possibly owing to the presence of protease inhibitors in milk. Likewise, luminal proteolytic machinery in the small intestine is not fully developed at birth, although enterokinase and pancreatic proteolytic enzymes are easily detectable. Rates of chymotrypsin and trypsin secretion are slower in infancy than in adult life, and responses to stimulation with CCK are depressed.[267]

Low rates of pancreatic enzyme secretion at birth may be attributable in part to the retarded display of polypeptide hormone receptors on the basolateral membrane of acinar cells. Digestive enzymes appear at different times after birth, suggesting that the genes that code for these enzymes may be activated at different times during development.[267]

One of the most characteristic changes in the postnatal period is the decline in lactase activity seen in most of the world's populations, apart from Western white persons.[268] After weaning, lactase activity greatly diminishes in most species, as milk is normally expected to be withdrawn from the diet. This change is genetically determined and not prevented or reversed by continued lactose ingestion. Recent observations suggest that a novel mechanism may underlie the decline in enzyme levels. Continued synthesis of substantial amounts of lactase proteins appeared to occur in adult rat enterocytes, but the further processing necessary for the active enzyme to be produced was impaired.[32]

Changes in epithelial membrane transport of nutrients take place when the intestine is suddenly and rapidly expected to assume the role of the placenta in providing nutrients at the moment of birth and immediately thereafter. Brush border membrane glucose and most amino acid transporters are present in the human fetal intestine well before birth,[5] when, in contrast to adult intestine, they are found throughout the crypt-villus axis. Fructose absorptive capacity rises rapidly after weaning when this sugar is presented in the diet. Transporters for bile salts are not programmed to appear on ileal enterocytes until weaning.[243]

Triglyceride Digestion in Neonates and Infants

There are some differences, compared with adults, in the way infants digest triglyceride, which they receive in milk. In contradistinction to other dietary sources, the triglyceride in milk is packaged in smaller emulsion droplets, each surrounded by a trilaminar membrane that includes both phospholipid and proteins (albumin and beta-lactoglobulin).[265] At a time in life when the newborn infant relies for over half its energy requirements on milk-derived triglyceride, pancreatic lipase secretion rates are only about half that of adults when expressed in terms of body surface area. Only at weaning does pancreatic lipase secretion begin to rise to adult levels.[269]

Two other lipases are important at this stage in life (see Table 88–2). The first is secreted by the mammary gland but is inactive in milk and requires the presence of bile salts to activate it. It begins to function, therefore, on entering the duodenum.[265] The second lipase is secreted either from serous glands at the base of the tongue or from gastric mucosa (or both), depending on the species. In humans, this "preduodenal" lipase is largely, if not entirely, derived from chief cells in the mucosa of the body of the stomach.[270] In the rat it is derived from the tongue. This lipase has an optimal pH of 4 to 6, which is lower than that of pancreatic lipase. It preferentially cleaves the 1α-position on triglyceride and releases fatty acid and diacylglycerol, as opposed to the monoglyceride produced by pancreatic lipase. It is not stimulated by bile salts and is released during feeding by autonomic nervous stimulation. Gastric lipase appears to be particularly active at the surface membrane of droplets derived from milk; pancreatic lipase is less so. Although the amount of lipolysis that occurs within the stomach is relatively small, the release of even modest amounts of fatty acids, particularly from the shorter- and medium-chain triglycerides, may be important in the emulsification of fat in the duodenum and in enhancing pancreatic lipase activity. Gastric lipase is rapidly inactivated in the duodenum by proteolytic enzymes. However, there is conflicting evidence about the importance of intragastric lipolysis, and some researchers have suggested that as much as 30% of fat may be digested here.[38] However, the rapid "product" inhibition of gastric lipase activity by released fatty acids makes this unlikely.

Each of the three lipases has a different specificity for the ester bonds in triglyceride. Gastric lipase preferentially cleaves the bond in the 1α-position, and pancreatic lipase the bonds in the 1 and 3 α-positions; milk-derived, bile salt–stimulated lipase is nonselective and splits the bonds at the 1, 2, and 3 α-positions. Thus, newborns' luminal contents contain more fatty acids and less monoglyceride and diglyceride than do adults' luminal contents, and this is probably advantageous for absorption. Smaller amounts of bile salts are available in neonates than in adults, in part at least because active ileal reabsorption is immature.[265] Under these conditions, fatty acids are likely to be absorbed more readily than monoglyceride. In addition, the low bile salt availability makes it likely that transfer of fat to the brush border membrane depends more on unilamellar liquid crystalline vesicles.

Gastric lipase persists into adult life, and the amounts found in biopsies of adult gastric mucosa are similar to those found in infant gastric mucosa. Recent studies suggest it may hydrolyze as many as one in four triglyceride acyl chains during digestion of a meal.[10]

Carbohydrate Digestion and Absorption in the Neonate

Lactose is the major carbohydrate in breast milk, and the need for an amylase before weaning is therefore minimal. An α-amylase is present in milk, however, and an amylase is also secreted in saliva at birth.[268] Both these amylases are inactivated by acid in the stomach but may resume their activity at nearly neutral pH on reaching the duodenum. It has been estimated that 15% to 40% of amylase activity in the duodenum of infants is of salivary origin.[269] Pancreatic amylase secretion is low, and stimulation with exogenous agonists produces little response, indicating the prematurity of the pancreas at this stage. In any event, the need for any amylase in neonates is slender unless starch is introduced early. Most infant formula feeds do not contain starches, but some contain glucose polymers.

Digestion of any starch ingested during the first 2 or 3

months of life relies on salivary amylase and mucosal α-glucosidases, as well as colonic "salvage" by fermentation of undigested carbohydrate by bacteria.

Mucosal lactase is present at birth in high concentration, as are the other glucosidases.[271] Despite this fact, lactose absorption may be incomplete in neonates, particularly in premature ones. Estimates of the amount of lactose that reaches the colon vary and have been based on indirect measurements of breath hydrogen concentrations. Probably less than 20% of ingested lactose reaches the colon, but a much smaller proportion is lost in the stool because of bacterial hydrolysis and absorption of the products.

The glucose/galactose transporter in the apical membrane of villous enterocytes is well developed in full-term infants but may be suboptimal in premature ones. This is unlikely, however, to pose a significant barrier to nutrition.

Protein Digestion and Absorption in Infants

Although acid and pepsinogens are secreted in neonates, little intragastric proteolysis occurs during the first 2 to 6 weeks of life. A renin-like protease is secreted during the first 10 days of life, which causes protein precipitation.[266]

Pancreatic proteolytic enzymes are secreted at birth, although at slower rates than in adults. Trypsinogen secretion is low and, particularly in preterm infants, does not respond to feeding. Furthermore, stimulation with pancreozymin has little effect on pancreatic enzyme secretion for the first 1 to 2 months of life.[177] Enterokinase (enteropeptidase) is present at birth and is capable of activating trypsinogen. Despite the apparent immaturity of the proteolytic machinery, it has been estimated that duodenal proteolysis can cope with as much as 3 or 4 g of protein per kg of body weight of casein, and infants seem not to be prone to defective nitrogen nutrition.

A number of proteases have been found in breast milk, including plasmin, which is most active against casein.[272] The importance of these milk-derived proteases, or the protease inhibitors also found in milk,[273] in overall nutrition is not known. Transport systems for amino acids and small peptides appear to be well developed in neonates.

The infant intestine has greater capacity than the adult intestine to absorb intact macromolecules, including proteins. Transport by pinocytosis or receptor-mediated endocytosis probably accounts for the ability of infants to take in biologically important whole proteins, such as the immunoglobulins, during this phase of life. This mechanism disappears after the first 3 months of life, when "closure" is said to have occurred[274]; however, uptake of intact proteins continues throughout life, albeit in trace amounts, and the role of M cells on Peyer's patches is of major importance in this process. It is likely to be an important mechanism by which dietary antigens are presented for immune surveillance later in life but is of little nutritional significance.

REFERENCES

1. Alpers D: Digestion and a absorption of carbohydrates and proteins. In Johnson L (ed): Physiology of the Gastrointestinal Tract. New York, Raven Press, 1987, p 1469.
2. McNeil M: Nutritional implications of human and mammalian large intestinal function. World Rev Nutr Diet 56:1, 1988.
3. Fallstrom SP, Nygren CO, Olegard R: Plasma triglyceride increase after oral fat load in malabsorption during early childhood. Acta Paediatr Scand 66:111, 1977.
4. Fomon SJ, Ziegler EE, Thomas LN, et al: Excretion of fat by normal full-term infants fed various milks and formulas. Am J Clin Nutr 23: 1299, 1970.
5. Buddington RK, Diamond JM: Ontogenetic development of intestinal nutrient transporters. Annu Rev Physiol 51:601, 1989.
6. Karasov W, Diamond J: Adaptation of intestinal nutrient transport. In Johnson L (ed): Physiology of the Gastrointestinal Tract. New York, Raven Press, 1987, p 1489.
7. Sarles H, et al: Cephalic phase of pancreatic secretion in man. Gut 9: 214, 1968.
8. Brown JC, Harper AA, Scratcherd T: Potentiation of secretin stimulation of the pancreas. J Physiol 190:519, 1967.
9. DiPalma J, et al: Lipase and pepsin activity in the gastric mucosa of infants, children, and adults. Gastroenterology 101:116, 1991.
10. Carriere F, et al: Secretion and contribution to lipolysis of gastric and pancreatic lipases during a test meal in humans. Gastroenterology 105: 876, 1993.
11. Lieverse RJ, et al: Satiety effects of a physiological dose of cholecystokinin in humans. Gut 36:176, 1995.
12. Gibbs J, Smith GP, Kirkham TO: Gastrin-releasing peptide and satiety. Gastroenterology 106:1374, 1994.
13. Apo A-I: A new satiety signal. Nutr Rev 51:273, 1993.
14. Malagelada J-R, Azpiroz F: Determinants of gastric emptying and transit in the small intestine. In Schultz S (ed): Handbook of Physiology—The Gastrointestinal System. Bethesda, Md, American Physiological Society, 1989, p 909.
15. Meyer JH, et al: Sieving of solid food by the canine stomach and sieving after gastric surgery. Gastroenterology 76:804, 1979.
16. Cooke A: Localisation of receptors inhibiting gastric emptying in the gut. Gastroenterology 72:875, 1977.
17. Meeroff JC, Go VL, Phillips SF: Control of gastric emptying by osmolality of duodenal contents in man. Gastroenterology 68:1144, 1975.
18. Hunt JN, Smith JL, Jiang CL: Effect of meal volume and energy density on the gastric emptying of carbohydrates. Gastroenterology 89: 1326, 1985.
19. Mayer E: The physiology of gastric storage and emptying. In Johnson L (ed): Physiology of the Gastrointestinal Tract. New York, Raven Press, 1994, p 929.
20. Read NW, McFarlane A, Kinsman RI, et al: Effect of infusion of nutrient solutions into the ileum on gastrointestinal transit and plasma levels of neurotensin and enteroglucagon. Gastroenterology 86:274, 1984.
21. Nightingale JM, Kamm MA, van der Sijp JR, et al: Disturbed gastric emptying in the short bowel syndrome. Evidence for a 'colonic brake.' Gut 34:1171, 1993.
22. Pironi L, Stanghellini V, Miglioli M, et al: Fat-induced ileal brake in humans: A dose-dependent phenomenon correlated to the plasma levels of peptide YY. Gastroenterology 105:733, 1993.
23. Tso P: Intestinal lipid absorption. In Johnson L (ed): Physiology of the Gastrointestinal Tract. New York, Raven Press, 1994, p 1873.
24. Wright JP, Barbezat GO, Clain JE: Jejunal secretion in response to a duodenal mixed nutrient perfusion. Gastroenterology 76:94, 1979.
25. Greenwood B, Davison JS: The relationship between gastrointestinal motility and secretion. Am J Physiol 252:G1, 1987.
26. Winne D: Influence of blood flow on intestinal absorption of drugs and nutrients. Pharmacol Ther 6:333, 1979.
27. Northfield TC, Hofmann AF: Biliary lipid output during three meals and an overnight fast. I. Relationship to bile acid pool size and cholesterol saturation of bile in gallstone and control subjects. Gut 16: 1, 1975.
28. Household Food Consumption and Expenditure: Annual Report of the National Food Survey Committee. London, Fisheries and Food, Ministry of Agriculture, 1989.
29. Rizek R, Friend B, Page L: Fat in today's food supply; Level of use and source. J Am Oil Chem Soc 51:244, 1974.
30. Davidson S, et al (eds): Human Nutrition and Dietetics. Edinburgh, Churchill Livingstone, 1979.
31. Kern F Jr: Normal plasma cholesterol in an 88-year-old man who eats 25 eggs a day. Mechanisms of adaptation. N Engl J Med 324:896, 1991.

32. Report of the Task Force on Trans Fatty Acids. London, British Nutrition Foundation, 1987.
33. Enig MG, Munn RJ, Keeney M: Dietary fat and cancer trends—a critique. Fed Proc 37:2215, 1978.
34. Borel P, Lairon D, Senft M, et al: Wheat bran and wheat germ: Effect on digestion and intestinal absorption of dietary lipids in the rat. Am J Clin Nutr 49:1192, 1989.
35. Thomson AB, Keelan M, Gary M, et al: Dietary effects of omega 3-fatty acids on intestinal transport function. Can J Physiol Pharmacol 66:985, 1988.
36. Abrams CK, Hamosh M, Lee TC, et al: Gastric lipase: Localization in the human stomach. Gastroenterology 95:1460, 1988.
37. Thomson AB, et al: Lipid absorption: Passing through the unstirred layers, brush-border membrane, and beyond. Can J Physiol Pharmacol 71:531, 1993.
38. Hernell O, Blackberg L, Bernback S: Digestion of human milk fat in early infancy. Acta Paediatr Scand 351:57, 1989.
39. Blow D: Enzymology. Lipases reach the surface. Nature 351:444, 1991.
40. Sims HF, Lowe ME: The human colipase gene: Isolation, chromosomal location, and tissue- specific expression. Biochemistry 31:7120, 1992.
41. Renaud W, Dagorn JC: cDNA sequence and deduced amino acid sequence of human preprocolipase. Pancreas 6:157, 1991.
42. Erlanson-Albertsson CLA: A possible physiological function of pancreatic pro-colipase activation peptide in appetite regulation. Biochemie 70:1245, 1988.
43. Bosner MS, Gulick T, Riley DJ: Heparin-modulated binding of pancreatic lipase and uptake of hydrolyzed triglycerides in the intestine. J Biol Chem 264:2021, 1989.
44. Carey MC, Small DM: The characteristics of mixed micellar solutions with particular reference to bile. Am J Med 49:590, 1970.
45. Holt PR, Fairchild BM, Weiss J: A liquid crystalline phase in human intestinal contents during fat digestion. Lipids 21:444, 1986.
46. Hernell O, Staggers JE, Carey MC: Physical-chemical behavior of dietary and biliary lipids during intestinal digestion and absorption. 2. Phase analysis and aggregation states of luminal lipids during duodenal fat digestion in healthy adult human beings. Biochemistry 29:2041, 1990.
47. Rigler MW, Honkanen RE, Patton JS: Visualization by freeze fracture, in vitro and in vivo, of the products of fat digestion. J Lipid Res 27: 836, 1986.
48. Strocchi A, Levitt MD: A reappraisal of the magnitude and implications of the intestinal unstirred layer. Gastroenterology 101:843, 1991.
49. Shiau YF: Mechanism of intestinal fatty acid uptake in the rat: The role of an acidic microclimate. J Physiol 421:463, 1990.
50. DeSchryver-Kecskemeti K, Eliakim R, Carroll S, et al: Intestinal surfactant-like material. A novel secretory product of the rat enterocyte. J Clin Invest 84:1355, 1989.
51. Hofmann AB, Borgstrom B: The intraluminal phase of fat digestion in man: The lipid content of the micellar and oil phases of intestinal content obtained during fat digestion and absorption. J Clin Invest 43: 247, 1964.
52. Carey MC, Small DM, Bliss CM: Lipid digestion and absorption. Annu Rev Physiol 45:651, 1983.
53. Phan CT, Tso P: Intestinal lipid absorption and transport. Front Biosci 6:299, 2001.
54. Ling KY, Lee HY, Hollander D: Mechanisms of linoleic acid uptake by rabbit small intestinal brush border membrane vesicles. Lipids 24: 51, 1989.
55. Stremmel W: Uptake of fatty acids by jejunal mucosal cells is mediated by a fatty acid binding membrane protein. J Clin Invest 82:2001, 1988.
56. Sylven C: Influence of blood supply on lipid uptake from micellar solutions by the rat small intestine. Biochim Biophys Acta 203:365, 1970.
57. Thurnhofer H, Hauser H: Uptake of cholesterol by small intestinal brush border membrane is protein-mediated. Biochemistry 29:2142, 1990.
58. Wouters FS, Markman M, de Graaf P, et al: The immunohistochemical localization of the non-specific lipid transfer protein (sterol carrier protein-2) in rat small intestine enterocytes. Biochim Biophys Acta 1259:192, 1995.
59. Patel SB, Salen G, Hidaka H, et al: Mapping a gene involved in regulating dietary cholesterol absorption. The sitosterolemia locus is found at chromosome 2p21. J Clin Invest 102:1041, 1998.
60. Berge KE, Tian H, Graf AA, et al: Accumulation of dietary cholesterol in sitosterolemia caused by mutations in adjacent ABC transporters. Science 290:1771, 2000.
61. Moestrup SK, Cui S, Vorum H, et al: Evidence that epithelial glycoprotein 330/megalin mediates uptake of polybasic drugs. J Clin Invest 96:1404, 1995.
62. Schulthess G, Compassi S, Werder M, et al: Intestinal sterol absorption mediated by scavenger receptors is competitively inhibited by amphipathic peptides and proteins. Biochemistry 39:12623, 2000.
63. Farquhar M: The unfolding story of megalin (gp 330): Now recognized as a drug receptor. J Clin Invest 96:1184, 1995.
64. Abumrad NA, Sfeir Z, Connelly MA, Coburn C: Lipid transporters: Membrane transport systems for cholesterol and fatty acids. Curr Opin Clin Nutr Metab Care 3:255, 2000.
65. Murata M, Peranen J, Schreiner A, et al: VIP21/caveolin is a cholesterol-binding protein. Proc Natl Acad Sci U S A 92:10339, 1995.
66. Subbaiah PV, Ganguly J: Studies on the phospholipases of rat intestinal mucosa. Biochem J 118:233, 1970.
67. Kumar BV, Aleman-Gomez JA, Colwell N, et al: Structure of the human pancreatic cholesterol esterase gene. Biochemistry 31:6077, 1992.
68. DiPersio LP, Fontaine RN, Hui DY: Identification of the active site serine in pancreatic cholesterol esterase by chemical modification and site-specific mutagenesis. J Biol Chem 265:16801, 1990.
69. DiPersio LP, Fontaine RN, Hui DY: Site-specific mutagenesis of an essential histidine residue in pancreatic cholesterol esterase. J Biol Chem 266:4033, 1991.
70. DiPersio LP, Hui DY: Aspartic acid 320 is required for optimal activity of rat pancreatic cholesterol esterase. J Biol Chem 268:300, 1993.
71. Storch J, Thumser AE: The fatty acid transport function of fatty acid-binding proteins. Biochim Biophys Acta 1486:28, 2000.
72. Noland BJ, Arebalo RE, Hansbury E, et al: Purification and properties of sterol carrier protein2. J Biol Chem 255:4282, 1980.
73. Scallen TJ, et al: Sterol carrier protein 2 and fatty acid-binding protein. Separate and distinct physiological functions. J Biol Chem 260: 4733, 1985.
74. Shiau YF: Mechanisms of intestinal fat absorption. Am J Physiol 240: G1, 1981.
75. Lehner R, Kuksis A: Triacylglycerol synthesis by purified triacylglycerol synthetase of rat intestinal mucosa. Role of acyl-CoA acyltransferase. J Biol Chem 270:13630, 1995.
76. Smith SJ, et al: Obesity resistance and multiple mechanisms of triglyceride synthesis in mice lacking Dgat. Nat Genet 25:87, 2000.
77. Oelkers P, Tinkelenberg A, Erdeniz N, et al: A lecithin cholesterol acyltransferase-like gene mediates diacylglycerol esterification in yeast. J Biol Chem 275:15609, 2000.
78. Field FJ, Cooper AD, Erickson SK: Regulation of rabbit intestinal acyl coenzyme A-cholesterol acyltransferase in vivo and in vitro. Gastroenterology 83:873, 1982.
79. Chang CC: Immunological quantitation and localization of ACAT-1 and ACAT-2 in human liver and small intestine. J Biol Chem 275: 28083, 2000.
80. Miyazaki AS, Lee N: Expression of ACAT-1 protein in human arteriosclerotic lesions in cultured human monocyte-macrophages. Arterioscler Thromb Vasc Biol 18:1568, 1998.
81. Buhman KK, Accad M, Novak S, et al: Resistance to diet-induced hypercholesterolemia and gallstone formation in ACAT2-deficient mice. Nat Med 6:1341, 2000.
82. Go MF, Schonfeld G, Pfleger B, et al: Regulation of intestinal and hepatic apoprotein synthesis after chronic fat and cholesterol feeding. J Clin Invest 81:1615, 1988.
83. Davidson NO, Magun AM, Brasitus TA, et al: Intestinal apolipoprotein A-I and B-48 metabolism: Effects of sustained alterations in dietary triglyceride and mucosal cholesterol flux. J Lipid Res 28:388, 1987.
84. Hayashi H, Fujimoto K, Cardelli JA, et al: Fat feeding increases size, but not number, of chylomicrons produced by small intestine. Am J Physiol 259:G709, 1990.
85. Ohashi K, Ishibashi S, Osuga S, et al: Novel mutations in the microsomal triglyceride transfer protein gene causing abetalipoproteinemia. J Lipid Res 41:1199, 2000.
86. Glickman RM, et al: Apolipoprotein synthesis in normal and abetalipoproteinemic intestinal mucosa. Gastroenterology 101:749, 1991.
87. Bouma ME, Beucler A, Aggerbeck LP, et al: Hypobetalipoproteinemia

with accumulation of an apoprotein B-like protein in intestinal cells. Immunoenzymatic and biochemical characterization of seven cases of Anderson's disease. J Clin Invest 78:398, 1986.

88. Dannoura AB-V, Amati N, V: Anderson's disease: Exclusion of apolipoprotein and intracellular lipid transport genes. Arterioscler Thromb Vasc Biol 19:2494, 2000.
89. Sabesin SM, Frase S: Electron microscopic studies of the assembly, intracellular transport, and secretion of chylomicrons by rat intestine. J Lipid Res 18:496, 1977.
90. Dietary Reference Values for Food Energy and Nutrients for the United Kingdom. Report of the Panel on Dietary Reference Values of the Committee on Medical Aspects of Food Policy. London, Department of Health, 1991, HMSO, p 72.
91. McNeil NI: The contribution of the large intestine to energy supplies in man. Am J Clin Nutr 39:388, 1984.
92. Gumucio DL, Wiebauer K, Dranginis A, et al: Evolution of the amylase multigene family. YBR/Ki mice express a pancreatic amylase gene which is silent in other strains. J Biol Chem 260:13483, 1985.
93. Horii A, Kobayashi T, Tomita N, et al: Primary structure of human pancreatic alpha-amylase gene: Its comparison with human salivary alpha-amylase gene. Gene 60:57, 1987.
94. Nishide T, et al: Corrected sequences of cDNAs for human salivary and pancreatic alpha-amylases [corrected]. Gene 28:263, 1984.
95. Layer P, Zinsmeister AR, DiMagno EP: Effects of decreasing intraluminal amylase activity on starch digestion and postprandial gastrointestinal function in humans. Gastroenterology 91:41, 1986.
96. Heitlinger LA, Lee PC, Dillen WP, et al: Mammary amylase: A possible alternate pathway of carbohydrate digestion in infancy. Pediatr Res 17:15, 1983.
97. Van Beers E, Buller H, Grand R: Intestinal brush border blycohydrolases: Structure, function, and development [review]. Crit Rev Biochem Molec Biol 30:197, 1995.
98. Dahlquist A, Semenza G: Disaccharidases of small-intestinal mucosa. J Pediatr Gastroenterol Nutr 4:857, 1985.
99. Sterchi EE, Lentze MJ, Naim HY: Molecular aspects of disaccharidase deficiencies. Baillieres Clin Gastroenterol 4:79, 1990.
100. Naim HY, Sterchi EE, Lentze MJ: Biosynthesis and maturation of lactase-phlorizin hydrolase in the human small intestinal epithelial cells. Biochem J 241:427, 1987.
101. Naim HY, Sterchi EE, Lentze MJ: Structure, biosynthesis, and glycosylation of human small intestinal maltase-glucoamylase. J Biol Chem 263:19709, 1988.
102. Leeper LL, Henning SJ: Development and tissue distribution of sucrase-isomaltase mRNA in rats. Am J Physiol 258:G52, 1990.
103. Wu GD, Wang W, Traber PG: Isolation and characterization of the human sucrase-isomaltase gene and demonstration of intestine-specific transcriptional elements. J Biol Chem 267:7863, 1992.
104. West LF, Davis MB, Green FR, et al: Regional assignment of the gene coding for human sucrase-isomaltase (SI) to chromosome 3q25-26. Ann Hum Genet 52:57, 1988.
105. Traber PG, Silberg DG: Intestine-specific gene transcription. Annu Rev Physiol 58:275, 1996.
106. Traber PG: Epithelial cell growth and differentiation. V. Transcriptional regulation, development, and neoplasia of the intestinal epithelium. Am J Physiol 273:G979, 1997.
107. Markowitz AJ, Wu GD, Bader A, et al: Regulation of lineage-specific transcription of the sucrase-isomaltase gene in transgenic mice and cell lines. Am J Physiol 269:G925, 1995.
108. Tung JM, Silberg AJ: Developmental expression of SI in transgenic mice is regulated by an evolutionary conserved promoter. Am J Physiol G83:273, 1997.
109. Wu GD, Chen L, Forslund K, et al: Hepatocyte nuclear factor-1 alpha (HNF-1 alpha) and HNF-1 beta regulate transcription via two elements in an intestine-specific promoter. J Biol Chem 269:17080, 1994.
110. Suh E, et al: A homeodomain protein related to caudal regulates intestine-specific gene transcription. Mol Cell Biol 14:7340, 1994.
111. Cezard JP, Broyart JP, Cuisinier-Gleizes P, et al: Sucrase-isomaltase regulation by dietary sucrose in the rat. Gastroenterology 84:18, 1983.
112. Rodolosse A, Chantret I, Locasa M, et al: A limited upstream region of the human sucrase-isomaltase gene confers glucose-regulated expression on a heterologous gene. Biochem J 315:301, 1996.
113. Boll W, Wagner P, Mantei N: Structure of the chromosomal gene and cDNAs coding for lactase-phlorizin hydrolase in humans with adult-type hypolactasia or persistence of lactase. Am J Hum Genet 48:889, 1991.
114. Kruse TA, Bolund L, Byskov A: Mapping of the human lactase-phlorizin hydrolase gene to chromosome 2. Cytogenet Cell Genet 51: 1026, 1989.
115. Troelsen JT, Mitchelmore C, Spodsberg N: Regulation of lactase-phlorizin hydrolase gene expression by the caudal-related homeodomain protein Cdx-2. Biochem J 322:833, 1997.
116. Gordon JI: Intestinal epithelial differentiation: New insights from chimeric and transgenic mice. J Cell Biol 108:1187, 1989.
117. Dahlqvist A, Nordstrom C: The distribution of dissacharidases in the villi and crypts of the small intestinal mucosa. Biochim Biophys Acta 113:624, 1966.
118. Traber PG, et al: Sucrase-isomaltase gene expression along crypt-villus axis of human small intestine is regulated at level of mRNA abundance. Am J Physiol 262:G123, 1992.
119. Hoffman LC, EB: Regional expression and regulation of intestinal sucrase-isomaltase. J Nutr Biochem 4:130, 1992.
120. Hoffman LR, Chang EB: Determinants of regional sucrase-isomaltase expression in adult rat small intestine. J Biol Chem 266:21815, 1991.
121. Das B, Gray C: Intestinal sucrase: In vivo synthesis and degradation. Clin Res 18:378, 1970.
122. Stevens BR, Kaunitz JD, Wright EM: Intestinal transport of amino acids and sugars: Advances using membrane vesicles. Annu Rev Physiol 46:417, 1984.
123. Desjeux J (ed): Metabolic Basis of Inherited Diseases. New York, McGraw-Hill, 1989.
124. Ferraris RP, Yasharpour S, Lloyd KC, et al: Luminal glucose concentrations in the gut under normal conditions. Am J Physiol 259:G822, 1990.
125. Birnir B, Lee HS, Hediger MA, et al: Expression and characterization of the intestinal Na+/glucose contransporter n COS-7 cells. Biochim Biophy Acta 1048:100, 1990.
126. Umbach JA, Coady MJ, Wright EM: Intestinal Na+/glucose cotransporter expressed in *Xenopus oocytes* is electrogenic. Biophys J 57: 1217, 1990.
127. Stevens BR, et al: Intestinal brush border membrane Na+/glucose cotransporter functions in situ as a homotetramer. Proc Natl Acad Sci U S A 87:1456, 1990.
128. Hediger MA, Coady MJ, Ikeda TS, Wright EM: Expression cloning and cDNA sequencing of the Na+/glucose co-transporter. Nature 330: 379, 1987.
129. Turk E, Zabel B, Mundlos S, et al: Glucose/galactose malabsorption caused by a defect in the Na+/glucose cotransporter. Nature 350:354, 1991.
130. Wright EM, et al: Regulation of Na+/glucose cotransporters. J Exp Biol 200:287, 1997.
131. Dyer J, Hosie KB, Shirazi-Beechey SP: Nutrient regulation of human intestinal sugar transporter (SGLT1) expression. Gut 41:56, 1997.
132. Burant CF, Takeda J, Brot-Lároche E, et al: Fructose transporter in human spermatozoa and small intestine is GLUT5. J Biol Chem 267: 14523, 1992.
133. Kellet G: The facilitated component of intestinal glucose absorption. J Physiol 531:585, 2001.
134. Pappenheimer JR, Reiss KZ: Contribution of solvent drag through intercellular junctions to absorption of nutrients by the small intestine of the rat. J Membr Biol 100:123, 1987.
135. Ferraris RP, Diamond JM: Specific regulation of intestinal nutrient transporters by their dietary substrates. Annu Rev Physiol 51:125, 1989.
136. Kellett GL: The facilitated component of intestinal glucose absorption. J Physiol 531:585, 2001.
137. Thorens B: Facilitated glucose transporters in epithelial cells. Annu Rev Physiol 55:591, 1993.
138. Samloff IM: Pepsins, peptic activity, and peptic inhibitors. J Clin Gastroenterol 3:91, 1981.
139. Nordstrom C: Release of enteropeptidase and other brush border enzymes from the small intestinal wall in the rat. Biochim Biophys Acta 289:376, 1972.
140. Nixon SE, Mawer GE: The digestion and absorption of protein in man. 2. The form in which digested protein is absorbed. Br J Nutr 24: 241, 1970.
141. Adibi S: Glycyl-dipeptides: New substrates for protein nutrition. J Lab Clin Med 113:665, 1989.
142. Adibi S: Peptide absorption and hydrolysis. In Johnson L (ed): Physiology of the Gastrointestinal Tract. New York, Raven Press, 1981, p 1073.

143. Tobey N, Heizer W, Yeh R, et al: Human intestinal brush border peptidases. Gastroenterology 88:913, 1985.
144. Erickson R, Bella A, Brophy E: Purification and molecular characterization of rat intestinal brush border membrane dipeptidyl aminopeptidase IV. Biochim Biophys Acta 756:258, 1983.
145. Ferraci H, Maroux S: Rabbit intestinal amino peptidase N. Purification and molecular properties. Biochim Biophys Acta 448:599, 1980.
146. Erickson RH, Song IS, Yoshioka M, et al: Identification of proline-specific carboxypeptidase localized to brush border membrane of rat small intestine and its possible role in protein digestion. Dig Dis Sci 34:400, 1989.
147. Duggan KA, Mendelsohn FA, Levens NR: Angiotensin receptors and angiotensin I-converting enzyme in rat intestine. Am J Physiol 257: G504, 1989.
148. Ahnen D, Mircheff A, Santiago N: Intestinal surface amino-oligopeptidase. Distint molecular forms during assembly in intra-cellular membranes in vivo. J Biol Chem 258:5960, 1983.
149. Danielson E, Cowell GH, Noren O, Sjostrom H: Biosynthesis of microvillar proteins. Biochem J 221:1, 1984.
150. Kenny AJ, Maroux S: Topology of microvillar membrane hydrolases of kidney and intestine. Physiol Rev 62:91, 1982.
151. Doumeng C, Maroux S: Aminotripeptidase, a cytosol enzyme from rabbit intestinal mucosa. Biochem J 177:801, 1979.
152. Crampton RF, Gangolli SD, Simpson P, Matthews DM: Rates of absorption by rat intestine of pancreatic hydrolysates of proteins and their corresponding amino acid mixtures. Clin Sci 41:409, 1971.
153. Silk D, Marrs T, Addison J: Absorption of amino acids from an amino acid mixture simulating casein and a tryptic hydrolysate of casein in man. Clin Sci Molec Med 45:715, 1973.
154. Asatoor A, Chadra A, Milne MB, Prosser DI: Intestinal absorption of sterioisomers of dipeptides in the rat. Clin Sci Molec Med 45:199, 1973.
155. Miyamoto Y, Thompson YG, Howard EF, et al: Functional expression of the intestinal peptide-proton co-transporter in *Xenopus laevis* oocytes. J Biol Chem 266:4742, 1991.
156. Liang R, Fei YJ, Prasad PD, et al: Human intestinal H+/peptide cotransporter. Cloning, functional expression, and chromosomal localization. J Biol Chem 270:6456, 1995.
157. Fei YJ, Kanai Y, Nussberger S, et al: Expression cloning of a mammalian proton-coupled oligopeptide transporter. Nature 368:563, 1994.
158. Amasheh S, Wenzel U, Boll M, et al: Transport of charged dipeptides by the intestinal H+/peptide symporter PepT1 expressed in *Xenopus laevis* oocytes. J Membr Biol 155:247, 1997.
159. Steel A, Nussberger S, Romero MF, et al: Stoichiometry and pH dependence of the rabbit proton-dependent oligopeptide transporter PepT1. J Physiol 498:563, 1997.
160. Leibach FH, Ganapathy V: Peptide transporters in the intestine and the kidney. Annu Rev Nutr 16:99, 1996.
161. Mackenzie B, Loo DD, Fei Y, et al: Mechanisms of the human intestinal H+-coupled oligopeptide transporter hPEPT1.J Biol Chem 271:5430, 1996.
162. Nussberger S, Steel A, Trotti D, et al: Symmetry of H+ binding to the intra- and extracellular side of the H+-coupled oligopeptide cotransporter PepT1. J Biol Chem 272:7777, 1997.
163. Kekuda R, Torres-Zamorano V, Fei YJ, et al: Molecular and functional characterization of intestinal Na(+)-dependent neutral amino acid transporter BO. Am J Physiol 272:G1463, 1997.
164. Calonge MJ, Gasparini P, Chillaron J, et al: Cystinuria caused by mutations in rBAT, a gene involved in the transport of cystine. Nat Genet 6:420, 1994.
165. Hoshide R, Ikeda Y, Karashima S, et al: Molecular cloning, tissue distribution, and chromosomal localization of human cationic amino acid transporter 2 (HCAT2). Genomics 38:174, 1996.
166. Brandsch M, Miyamoto Y, Ganapathy V, Leibach FH: Expression and protein kinase C-dependent regulation of peptide/H+ co- transport system in the Caco-2 human colon carcinoma cell line. Biochem J 299:253, 1994.
167. Muller U, Brandsch M, Prasad PD, et al: Inhibition of the H+/peptide cotransporter in the human intestinal cell line Caco-2 by cyclic AMP. Biochem Biophys Res Commun 218:461, 1996.
168. Erickson RH, Gum JR Jr, Lindstrom MM, et al: Regional expression and dietary regulation of rat small intestinal peptide and amino acid transporter mRNAs. Biochem Biophys Res Commun 216:249, 1995.
169. Ganapathy V, Brandsch M, Lelbach F: Intestinal transport of amino acids and peptides. In Johnson L (ed): Physiology of the Gastrointestinal Tract. New York, Raven Press, 1994, p 1782.
170. Chung YC, Kim YS, Shadchehr A, et al: Protein digestion and absorption in human small intestine. Gastroenterology 76:1415, 1979.
171. Siliprandi L, Vanni P, Kessler M, Semenza G: Na+-dependent, electroneural L-ascorbate transport across brush border membrane vesicles from guinea pig small intestine. Biochim Biophys Acta 552:129, 1979.
172. Halsted C: The intestinal absorption of dietary folates in health and disease. J Am Col Nutr 8:651, 1989.
173. Rosenberg IH: 1989 Herman Award lecture. Folate absorption: Clinical questions and metabolic answers. Am J Clin Nutr 51:531, 1990.
174. Seetharam B: Gastrointestinal absorption and transport of coobalamin. In Johnson L (ed): Physiology of the Gastrointestinal Tract. New York, Raven Press, 1994, p 1997.
175. Marcoullis G, Parmentier Y, Nicolas JP, et al: Cobalamin malabsorption due to nondegradation of R proteins in the human intestine. Inhibited cobalamin absorption in exocrine pancreatic dysfunction. J Clin Invest 66:430, 1980.
176. Allen RH, Seetheram B, Podell E, Alpers DH: Effect of proteolytic enzymes on the binding of cobalamin to R protein and intrinsic factor. In vitro evidence that a failure to partially degrade R protein is responsible for cobalamin malabsorption in pancreatic insufficiency. J Clin Invest 61:47, 1978.
177. Kolhouse JF, Allen RH: Absorption, plasma transport, and cellular retention of cobalamin analogues in the rabbit. Evidence for the existence of multiple mechanisms that prevent the absorption and tissue dissemination of naturally occurring cobalamin analogues. J Clin Invest 60:1381, 1977.
178. Hagedorn C, Alpers D: Distribution of intrinsic factor vitamin B_{12} receptors in human intestine. Gastroenterology 73:1010, 1977.
179. Donaldson R, Small DM, Robbins S, Mathan VI: Receptors for vitamin B_{12} related to ileal surface area and absorptive capacity. Biochim Biophys Acta 311:477, 1973.
180. Robertson JA, Gallagher ND: Effect of placental lactogen on the number of intrinsic factor receptors in the pregnant mouse. Gastroenterology 77:511, 1979.
181. Rose R: Intestinal absorption of water soluble vitamins. In Johnson L (ed): Physiology of the Gastrointestinal Tract. New York, Raven Press, 1987, p 1581.
182. Said HM, Arianas P: Transport of riboflavin in human intestinal brush border membrane vesicles. Gastroenterology 100:82, 1991.
183. Goodman DS, Blomstrand R, Werner B, et al: The intestinal absorption and metabolism of vitamin A and beta-carotene in man. J Clin Invest 45:1615, 1966.
184. Hollander D: Intestinal absorption of vitamins A, E, D, and K. J Lab Clin Med 97:449, 1981.
185. Hollander D, Rim E, Morgan D: Intestinal absorption of 25-hydroxyvitamin D_3 in unanesthetized rat. Am J Physiol 236:E441, 1979.
186. Hollander D, Muralidhara KS, Zimmerman A: Vitamin D-3 intestinal absorption in vivo: Influence of fatty acids, bile salts, and perfusate pH on absorption. Gut 19:267, 1978.
187. Hollander D, Rim E, Muralidhara KS: Mechanism and site of small intestinal absorption of alpha-tocopherol in the rat. Gastroenterology 68:1492, 1975.
188. Nakamura T, Aoyama Y, Fujita T, Katsni G: Studies on tocopherol derivatives: V. Intestinal absorption of several d,1-3,4-3H2-alpha-tocopheryl esters in the rat. Lipids 10:627, 1975.
189. Hollander D: Vitamin K1 absorption by everted intestinal sacs of the rat. Am J Physiol 225:360, 1973.
190. Hollander D, Rim E, Ruble PE Jr: Vitamin K2 colonic and ileal in vivo absorption: Bile, fatty acids, and pH effects on transport. Am J Physiol 233:E124, 1977.
191. Armbrecht H: Effect of age and the milk sugar lactose on calcium absorption by the small intestine. Adv Exp Med Biol 249:185, 1989.
192. Wasserman RH, Fullmer CS: Vitamin D and intestinal calcium transport: Facts, speculations and hypotheses. J Nutr 125:1971S, 1995.
193. Bronner F: Intestinal calcium transport: The cellular pathway. Miner Electrolyte Metab, 16:94, 1990.
194. Calcium phosphate and magnesium absorption. In Johnson L (ed): Physiology of the Gastrointestinal Tract. New York, Raven Press, 1994, p 2175.
195. Krejs GJ, Nicar MJ, Zerwekh JE, et al: Effect of 1,25-dihydroxyvitamin D3 on calcium and magnesium absorption in the healthy human jejunum and ileum. Am J Med 75:973, 1983.
196. Karbach U: Segmental heterogeneity of cellular and paracellular calcium transport across the rat duodenum and jejunum. Gastroenterology 100:47, 1991.

197. Madara JL: Loosening tight junctions. Lessons from the intestine. J Clin Invest 83:1089, 1989.
198. Feher JJ: Facilitated calcium diffusion by intestinal calcium-binding protein. Am J Physiol 244:C303, 1983.
199. Carafoli E, James P, Strehler E: Structure-function relationship in the calcium pump of plasma membrane. In Peterlik M, Bronner R (eds): Molecular and Cellular Regulation of Calcium and Phosphate Metabolism. 1990, p 181.
200. Bronner F, Pansu D: Nutritional Aspects of Calicium Absorption. J Nutr 129:9, 1999.
201. Walters JR, Weiser, MM: Calcium transport by rat duodenal villus and crypt basolateral membranes. Am J Physiol 252:G170, 1987.
202. Favus MJ, Kathpalia SC, Coe FL: Kinetic characteristics of calcium absorption and secretion by rat colon. Am J Physiol 240:G350, 1981.
203. Hylander E, Ladefoged K, Jarnum S: Calcium absorption after intestinal resection. The importance of a preserved colon. Scand J Gastroenterol 25:705, 1990.
204. Freund T, Bronner F: Regulation of intestinal calcium-binding protein calcium intake in the rat. Am J Physiol 228:861, 1975.
205. Karbach U, Rummel W: Cellular and paracellular magnesium transport across the terminal ileum of the rat and its interaction with the calcium transport. Gastroenterology 98:985, 1990.
206. Cox T, Mazurier G, Spik G: Iron binding proteins and influx across the duodenal brush border. Evidence for specific lactotransferrin receptors in human intestine. Biochim Biophys Acta 588:120, 1969.
207. Davidson LA, Lonnerdal B: Fe-saturation and proteolysis of human lactoferrin: Effect on brush- border receptor-mediated uptake of Fe and Mn. Am J Physiol 257:G930, 1989.
208. Conrad M: Iron absorption. In Johnson L (ed): Physiology of the Gastrointestinal Tract. New York, Raven Press, 1987, p 1437.
209. Parmley R, Barton J, Conrad M: Ultrastructural cytochemistry and radio-autography of hemoglobin iron absorption. Exp Mole Pathol 34: 131, 1981.
210. Raffin SB, Woo CH, Roost KT, et al: Intestinal absorption of hemoglobin iron-heme cleavage by mucosal heme oxygenase. J Clin Invest 54:1344, 1974.
211. Simpson R, Raja K, Peters T: Mechanisms of intestinal brush border iron transport. Adv Exp Med Biol 149:1989, 1989.
212. Riedel HD, Remus AJ, Fitscher BA: Characterization and partial purification of a ferrireductase from human duodenal microvillus membrane. Biochem J 309:745, 1995.
213. Wessling-Resnick M: Iron transport. Annu Rev Nutr 20:129, 2000.
214. Nunez MT, Alvarez X, Smith M, Tapia V: Role of redox systems on Fe3+ uptake by transformed human intestinal epithelial (Caco-2) cells. Am J Physiol 267:C1582, 1997.
215. Umbreit JN, Conrad ME, Moore EG: Iron aborption and cellular transport: The mobilferrin/paraferritin paradigm. Semin Hematol 35: 13, 1998.
216. Andrews N: Disorders of iron metabolism. N Engl J Med 341:1986, 1999.
217. Gunshin H, Mackensie B, Berger UV: Cloning and characterization of a mammalian proton-coupled metal-ion transporter. Nature 388:482, 1997.
218. Bacon B: Hemochromatosis: Diagnosis and management. Gastroenterology 120:718, 2001.
219. Vulpe CD, Kuo YM, Murphy TL: Hephaestin, a ceruloplasmin homologue implicated in intestinal iron transport, is defective in the sla mouse. Nat Genet 21:195, 1999.
220. Barrett JF, Whittaker PG, Williams JG, Lind T: Absorption of non-haem iron from food during normal pregnancy. Br Med J 309:79, 1994.
221. Miyoshi H, Ashida K, Hirata I, et al: Transferrin is not involved in initial uptake process of iron in rat duodenal mucosa. Ultrastructural study by x-ray energy spectrometry. Dig Dis Sci 40:1484, 1995.
222. Wheby M, Jones L, Crosby W: Studies on iron absorption. Intestinal regulatory mechanisms. J Clin Invest 43:1433, 1964.
223. Cox TM, Peters TJ: Cellular mechanisms in the regulation of iron absorption by the human intestine: Studies in patients with iron deficiency before and after treatment. Br J Haematol 44:75, 1980.
224. Sandstrom B: Factors influencing the uptake of trace elements from the digestive tract. Proc Nutr Soc 47:161, 1988.
225. Taylor CM, et al: Homeostatic regulation of zinc absorption and endogenous losses in zinc- deprived men. Am J Clin Nutr 53:755, 1991.
226. Tacnet F, Watkins D, Ripoche P: Studies of zinc transport into brush border membrane vesicles isolated from pig small intestine. Biochim Biophys Acta 1024:1990, 1990.
227. Krebs N: Overview of zinc absorption and excretion in the human gastrointestinal tract. J Nutr 130:1374S, 2000.
228. McMahon RJ, Cousins RJ: Mammalian zinc transporters. J Nutr 128: 667, 1998.
229. McMahon RJ, Cousins RJ: Regulation of the zinc transporter ZnT-1 by dietary zinc. Proc Natl Acad Sci 95:4841, 1998.
230. Menard MP, McCormick CC, Cousins RJ: Regulation of intestinal metallothionein biosynthesis in rats by dietary zinc. J Nutr 111:1353, 1981.
231. Steel L, Cousins RJ: Kinetics of zinc absorption by luminally and vascularly perfused rat intestine. Am J Physiol 248:G46, 1985.
232. Davies NT, Williams RB: The effect of pregnancy and lactation on the absorption of zinc and lysine by the rat duodenum in situ. Br J Nutr 38:417, 1977.
233. Davis SM, McMahon RJ, Cousins RJ: Metallothionein knockout and transgenic mice exhibit altered intestinal processing of zinc with uniform zinc-dependent zinc transporter-1 expression. J Nutr 128:825, 1998.
234. Stuart MA, Johnson PE: Copper absorption and copper balance during consecutive periods for rats fed varying levels of dietary copper. J Nutr 116:1028, 1986.
235. Davies T, Williams R: The effects of pregnancy on uptake and distribution of copper in the rat. Proc Nutr Soc 35:4A, 1976.
236. Zhou B, Gitschier J: hCTR1: A human gene for copper uptake identified by complementation in yeast. Proc Natl Acad Sci 94:7481, 1997.
237. Pena MM, Lee J, Thiele DJ: A delicate balance: Homeostatic control of copper uptake and distribution. J Nutr 129:1251, 1999.
238. Chelly J, Turner Z, Tonnesen T: Isolation of a candidate gene for Menkes disease that encodes a potential heavy metal binding protein. Nat Genet 3:14, 1993.
239. Rucker R, Lonnerdal B, Keen C: Intestinal absorption of nutritionally important trace elements. In Johnson L (ed): Physiology of the Gastrointestinal Tract. New York, Raven Press, 1994, p 2195.
240. Yan G, Ge K, Chen J, Chen X: Selenium-related endemic diseases and the daily requirements of humans. World Rev Nutr Dietet 55:98, 1988.
241. Thomson CD, Rea HM, Doesburg VM, Robinson MF, et al: Selenium concentrations and glutathione peroxidase activities in whole blood of New Zealand residents. Br J Nutr 37:457, 1977.
242. Reasbeck PG, Barbezat GO, Weber FL Jr, et al: Selenium absorption by canine jejunum. Dig Dis Sci 30:489, 1985.
243. Heubi JE, Fellows JL: Postnatal development of intestinal bile salt transport. Relationship to membrane physico-chemical changes. J Lipid Res 26:797, 1985.
244. Cripps AW, Williams VJ: The effect of pregnancy and lactation on food intake, gastrointestinal anatomy and the absorptive capacity of the small intestine in the albino rat. Br J Nutr 33:17, 1975.
245. Olsen WA, Rosenberg IH: Intestinal transport of sugars and amino acids in diabetic rats. J Clin Invest 49:96, 1970.
246. Jacobs L, Bloom S, Harsoulis P, Dowling RH: Intestinal adaptation to hypothermic hyperphagia. Clin Sci Molec Med 48:14, 1975.
247. Weser E, Heller R, Tawil T: Stimulation of mucosal growth in the rat ileum by bile and pancreatic secretions after jejunal resection. Gastroenterology 73:524, 1977.
248. Bloom S, Polak J: The hormonal pattern of intestinal adaptation: A major role for enteroglucagon. Scand J Gastroenterol 115:2176, 1984.
249. Johnson LR: The trophic action of gastrointestinal hormones. Gastroenterology 70:278, 1976.
250. Goodlad RA, Wilson TJ, Lenton W, Gregory H, et al: Intravenous but not intragastric urogastrone-EGF is trophic to the intestine of parenterally fed rats. Gut 28:573, 1987.
251. Lund PK, Ulshen MH, Rountree DB, et al: Molecular biology of gastrointestinal peptides and growth factors: Relevance to intestinal adaptation. Digestion 46:66,(Suppl 2) 1990.
252. Dowling RH: Polyamines in intestinal adaptation and disease. Digestion 46(Suppl 2):331, 1990.
253. Bamba T, Bamba T, Vaja S, et al: Effect of fasting and feeding on polyamines and related enzymes along the villus:crypt axis. Digestion 46(Suppl 2):424, 1990.
254. Johnson L: Regulation of gastrointestinal growth. In Johnson L (ed): Physiology of the Gastrointestinal Tract. New York, Raven Press, 1987, p 301.
255. Scheele G: Regulation of gene expression in the exocrine pancreas. In Do V, et al (eds): The Exocrine Pancreas; Biology, Pathobiology, and Diseases. New York, Raven Press, 1986, p 55.

256. Rausch U, Rudiger K, Vasiloudes P, et al: Lipase synthesis in the rat pancreas is regulated by secretin. Pancreas 1:522, 1986.
257. Borel P, Armand M, Senft M, et al: Gastric lipase: Evidence of an adaptive response to dietary fat in the rabbit. Gastroenterology 100: 1582, 1991.
258. Renaud W, Giorgi D, Iovanna J, Dagorn JC: Regulation of concentrations of mRNA for amylase, trypsinogen I and chymotrypsinogen B in rat pancreas by secretagogues. Biochem J 235:305, 1986.
259. Goda T, Koldivsky O: Dietary regulation of small intestinal disaccharidases. World Rev Nutr Dietet 57:275, 1988.
260. Flatz G: Genetics of lactose digestion in humans. Adv Human Gen 177:487, 1987.
261. Diamond J: Evolutionary design of intestinal nutrient absorption: Enough but not too much. Perspectives, News Physiol Sci 6:92, 1991.
262. Solberg DH, Diamond JM: Comparison of different dietary sugars as inducers of intestinal sugar transporters. Am J Physiol 252:G574, 1987.
263. Stein ED, Chang SD, Diamond JM: Comparison of different dietary amino acids as inducers of intestinal amino acid transport. Am J Physiol 252:G626, 1987.
264. Maenz D, Cheeseman C: Effect of hyperglycemia on D-glucose transport across the brush border and basolateral membranes of rat small intestine. Biochim Biophys Acta 860:277, 1986.
265. Hernell O: Specificity of human milk bile salt stimulated lipase. J Pediatr Gastroenterol Nutr 4:1985, 1985.
266. Britton J, Koldovsky O: Development of luminal protein digestion: Implications for biologically active dietary polypeptides. J Paediatr Gastroenterol Nutr 9:144, 1989.
267. Scheele G, Kern H: Selective regulation of gene expression in the exocrine pancreas. In Schultz S (ed): Handbook of Physiology—The Gastrointestinal System, Section 6. Bethesda, MD, American Physiological Society, 1989, p 499.
268. Kien C, Heitlinger LA, Li BU, Murray RD: Digestion, absorption, and fermentation of carbohydrates. Semin Perinatol 13:78, 1989.
269. Zoppi G, Andreotti G, Pajno-Ferrara F, et al: Exocrine pancreas function in premature and full term neonates. Pediatr Res 6:880, 1972.
270. Moreau H, Laugier R, Gargouri Y, et al: Human preduodenal lipase is entirely of gastric fundic origin. Gastroenterology 95:1221, 1988.
271. Antonowicz I, Lebenthal E: Developmental pattern of small intestinal enterokinase and disaccharidase activities in the human fetus. Gastroenterology 72:1299, 1977.
272. Korychka-Dahl M, Ribadeau DB, Chene N, Martal J: Plasmin activity in milk. J Dairy Sci 66:704, 1983.
273. McGilligan KM, Thomas DW, Eckhert CD: Alpha-1-antitrypsin concentration in human milk. Pediatr Res 22:268, 1987.
274. Udall JN, Walker WA: The physiologic and pathologic basis for the transport of macromolecules across the intestinal tract. J Pediatr Gastroenterol Nutr 1:295, 1982.

Chapter 89

MALDIGESTION AND MALABSORPTION

Christoph Högenauer, MD, and Heinz F. Hammer, MD

Whereas in the past it was believed that most malabsorptive diseases present clinically with diarrhea and steatorrhea, it has been recently recognized that many malabsorptive disorders, like celiac disease, may have subtle clinical presentations. Extraintestinal manifestations of malabsorption, like anemia, bone loss, or menstrual disturbances, may even be the presenting symptom. In other cases gastrointestinal symptoms, like bloating or changes in bowel habits, may be subtle, so that other much more common disorders, like irritable bowel syndrome, may be erroneously diagnosed. At the same time, there is an increasing awareness that subtle malabsorption of single nutrients, like calcium or cobalamin (vitamin B_{12}), may, if unrecognized, lead to complications that may be difficult to reverse or may not be reversible at all.

The classic distinction between maldigestion and malabsorption defines maldigestion as a defective hydrolysis of nutrients and malabsorption as a defective mucosal absorption. Although this distinction may be useful on pathophysiologic grounds, the clinical presentation and the complications of maldigestion and malabsorption are similar. In addition, physiologic processes other than digestion and absorption, like solubilization, intestinal motility, or hormone secretion, are involved in normal absorption of various nutrients, vitamins, and minerals. Therefore, the classic definitions of maldigestion and malabsorption do not cover the pathophysiologic spectrum of malabsorption syndrome.

In this chapter the terms digestion and absorption, or maldigestion and malabsorption, are only used separately in the discussion of pathophysiology. When the distinction between these terms does not seem to be of clinical importance, only the terms absorption and malabsorption are used.

Malabsorption can be caused by many diseases of the small bowel and by diseases of the pancreas, the liver, the biliary tract, and the stomach (Table 89–1). Whereas in some of these diseases malabsorption may be the presenting feature, in other diseases malabsorption may only be a minor clinical problem or may only be detected as a laboratory abnormality.

The scope of this chapter is as follows: to provide an understanding of basic pathophysiologic mechanisms leading to symptoms or complications of maldigestion or malabsorption, including the discussion of compensating mechanisms; to describe the clinical manifestations and complications of maldigestion and malabsorption; to describe tests that can be used clinically to evaluate digestive and absorptive function and to provide a rational diagnostic approach to the individual patient; to describe malabsorptive diseases that are not covered in other chapters of this book; and to describe general measures of the treatment of malabsorption syndrome.

ETIOLOGY AND PATHOPHYSIOLOGY OF MALABSORPTION SYNDROMES

From the pathophysiologic point of view, mechanisms causing malabsorption could be divided into premucosal (lu-

Table 89–1 | **Diseases Causing Nutrient, Vitamin, and Mineral Malabsorption**

- Gastric diseases
  - Autoimmune gastritis (pernicious anemia)
  - Atrophic gastritis
  - Gastric resections
- Pancreatic diseases
  - Pancreatic insufficiency
    - Chronic pancreatitis
    - Cystic fibrosis
    - Johanson-Blizzard syndrome
    - Pearson's marrow-pancreas syndrome
    - Shwachman's syndrome
  - Congenital pancreatic enzyme deficiencies
    - Colipase deficiency
    - Lipase deficiency
    - Trypsinogen deficiency
  - Pancreatic tumors
- Liver diseases
  - Inborn errors in bile acid biosynthesis and transport
  - Liver cirrhosis
  - Parenchymal liver diseases
- Obstructive biliary diseases
  - Biliary tumors
  - Primary and secondary sclerosing cholangitis
  - Primary biliary cirrhosis
- Intestinal diseases
  - Amyloidosis
  - Autoimmune enteropathy
  - Celiac sprue
  - Collagenous sprue
  - Congenital enterocyte defects (Table 89–14)
  - Crohn's disease
  - Enterokinase deficiency
  - Eosinophilic gastroenteritis
  - Fistulas
  - Food allergy
  - Graft-versus-host disease
  - Hypogammaglobulinemia
  - Ileal bile acid malabsorption
  - Immunoproliferative small intestinal disease
  - Intestinal infections
    - Whipple's disease
    - Giardiasis
    - Cryptosporidiosis
    - Bacterial overgrowth syndrome
    - Helminthic infections
    - Tuberculosis
    - Acquired immunodeficiency syndrome (human immunodeficiency virus infection)
    - *Mycobacterium avium* complex infections
    - Virus infections
  - Intestinal ischemia
  - Intestinal lymphoma
  - Intestinal resections or bypass
  - Lactose intolerance
  - Mastocytosis
  - Microvillus inclusion disease
  - Nongranulomatous ulcerative jejunitis
  - Postinfectious malabsorption
  - Radiation enteritis
  - Refractory sprue
  - Sarcoidosis
  - Tropical sprue
- Neuroendocrine tumors
  - Carcinoid
  - Gastrinoma
  - Glucagonoma
  - Somatostatinoma
- Lymphatic disease
  - Intestinal lymphangiectasia
    - Primary
    - Secondary
      - Infiltrations
      - Lymphoma
      - Solid tumors
      - Trauma, damage, or obstruction to thoracic duct
- Cardiac and vascular diseases
  - Congestive heart failure
  - Constrictive pericarditis
  - Portal hypertension
- Endocrine causes
  - Addison's disease
  - Autoimmune polyglandular syndrome type 1
  - Diabetes mellitus
  - Hyperthyroidism
- Systemic diseases
  - Cronkhite-Canada syndrome
  - Mixed connective tissue disease
  - Neurofibromatosis type 1
  - Protein calorie malnutrition
  - Scleroderma
  - Systemic lupus erythematosus

minal) factors, mucosal factors, and postmucosal factors (vascular and lymphatic). For clinical purposes, this approach is of limited value because the variety of clinical pictures caused by malabsorption syndromes is mainly characterized by the nature of the substrates malabsorbed. We therefore discuss the mechanisms causing malabsorption on the basis of the malabsorbed substrate. A separate section discusses the role of mechanisms compensating for the consequences of malabsorption.

Normal uptake of nutrients, vitamins, and minerals by the gastrointestinal tract requires several steps, which can be compromised in diseases, which are as follows.

Solubilization is a prerequisite for the absorption of nutrients like fat or calcium. Fat and fat-soluble vitamins are solubilized through the formation of micelles, and calcium is solubilized through the acidification of the gastrointestinal lumen. On the other hand, increased solubilization of components of intestinal chyme may be a contributing factor to the manifestation of gastrointestinal diseases (e.g., the increased absorption of oxalate, which may result in the development of kidney stones in patients with short bowel syndrome).

Liberation of substrate, like cobalamin, from binding sites in food, or, conversely, *binding* to factors such as intrinsic factor, allows absorption to take place.

Chemical changes to nutrients may be required for absorption, as is the case for changing the charge of iron.

Digestion of macromolecular compounds, like polysaccharides, triglycerides, and proteins, to their molecular components, like monosaccharides, fatty acids, and amino acids, is achieved by soluble or membrane bound digestive enzymes. Absorption of undigested or partially digested macromolecular compounds occurs to a very minor degree in health and may be increased slightly in various intestinal diseases. Although this does not play a nutritive role, it may be important for the normal function of the immune system and for the pathogenesis of diseases like food allergies (see Chapter 101).

Intestinal sensory and motor function detects the presence of nutrients and facilitates adequate mixing of nutrients with intestinal secretions, delivery to absorptive sites, and providing adequate time for nutrient absorption.

Neural and hormonal functions are required to stimulate and coordinate digestive secretions, mucosal absorption, and intestinal motility.

Mucosal absorption may be by active or passive carrier-mediated transport or by diffusion.

Postmucosal transport of absorbed substrates occurs. An overview of pathophysiologic mechanisms of maldigestion and malabsorption is provided in Table 89–2. This table also shows the ingested substrates primarily affected by the individual pathophysiologic mechanisms and the principal disease etiologies of these mechanisms.

Fat Malabsorption

Defective Mixing

For sufficient digestion and absorption of lipids, dietary fat must be adequately mixed with digestive secretions. Gastric resections or gastrointestinal motility disorders that result in rapid gastric emptying and/or rapid intestinal transit, like autonomic neuropathy due to diabetes mellitus or amyloidosis, may cause fat malabsorption due to impaired gastrointestinal mixing of dietary fat.[1]

Reduced Solubilization of Fat

Fat malabsorption due to decreased micelle formation occurs if the luminal concentrations of conjugated bile acids are lower than the critical concentration required for micelle formation.[2, 3] Table 89–3 shows causes of luminal bile acid deficiency.

Decreased Lipolysis (Lipid Hydrolysis)

If exocrine pancreatic function is severely reduced, impaired pancreatic lipase and colipase secretion result in decreased luminal hydrolysis of dietary fat.[4] Chronic pancreatitis or cystic fibrosis, pancreatic duct obstructions by pancreatic and ampullary tumors, and pancreatic resections are the most common causes of pancreatic insufficiency.[1] Even when pancreatic enzyme concentrations are normal, reduced pancreatic lipase *activity* due to a low luminal pH,[5] excessive calcium ingestion,[6, 7] or the specific lipase inhibitor orlistat[8] also

Table 89–2 | **Pathophysiologic Mechanisms of Malabsorption, the Substrates Affected (Substrates in Bold Are Mainly Affected), and Etiologies**

PATHOPHYSIOLOGIC MECHANISM	MALABSORBED SUBSTRATE(S)	ETIOLOGIES
Maldigestion		
Conjugated bile acid deficiency	**Fat**	Hepatic parenchymal disease
	Fat-soluble vitamins	Obstructive biliary disease
	Calcium	Bacterial overgrowth in small bowel with deconjugation
	Magnesium	Ileal bile acid malabsorption
		Cholecystokinin deficiency
Pancreatic insufficiency	**Fat**	Congenital defects
	Protein	Chronic pancreatitis
	Carbohydrate	Pancreatic tumors
	Fat-soluble vitamins	Inactivation of pancreatic enzymes (Zollinger-Ellison syndrome)
	Vitamin B_{12} (cobalamin)	
Reduced mucosal digestion	**Carbohydrate**	Congenital defects (Table 89–14)
	Protein	Acquired lactase deficiency
		Generalized mucosal disease (e.g., celiac sprue, Crohn's disease)
Intraluminal consumption of nutrients	**Vitamin B_{12} (cobalamin)**	Bacterial overgrowth
		Helminthic infections
Malabsorption		
Reduced mucosal absorption	**Fat**	Congenital transport defects (Table 89–14)
	Protein	Generalized mucosal diseases (e.g., celiac sprue, Crohn's disease)
	Carbohydrate	Intestinal resections or bypass
	Vitamins	Infections
	Minerals	Intestinal lymphoma
Decreased transport from the intestine	**Fat**	Intestinal lymphangiectasia
	Protein	Primary
		Obstruction by, e.g., solid tumors, Whipple's disease, or lymphomas
		Venous stasis (e.g., congestive heart failure)
Other mechanisms		
Decreased gastric acid and/or intrinsic factor secretion	**Vitamin B_{12}**	Pernicious anemia
	Iron	Atrophic gastritis
		Gastric resections
Decreased gastric mixing and/or rapid gastric emptying (other mechanisms?)	Fat	
	Calcium	Gastric resections
	Protein	Autonomic neuropathy
Rapid intestinal transit	Fat	Autonomic neuropathy
		Hyperthyroidism

Table 89–3 | **Pathophysiologic Mechanisms Resulting in Deficiency of Luminal Conjugated Bile Acids**

PATHOPHYSIOLOGIC MECHANISM	DISEASES
Decreased synthesis and/or secretion of conjugated bile acids	Parenchymal liver diseases (e.g., liver cirrhosis) Biliary obstruction (e.g., primary biliary cirrhosis, tumors) Biliary fistulas Inborn errors of bile acid synthesis Cholecystokinin deficiency
Intestinal loss of conjugated bile acids	Ileal resection Severe ileal mucosal disease Congenital defects of the ileal sodium/bile acid cotransporter
Luminal deconjugation of bile acids	Bacterial overgrowth syndrome
Binding of bile salts or insolubilization of bile salts by a low luminal pH	Cholestyramine (binding) Zollinger-Ellison syndrome (low pH) Exocrine pancreatic insufficiency (low pH)

Data from references 1 and 249.

causes pancreatic steatorrhea. Finally, selective congenital lipase or colipase deficiency are rare causes of pancreatic fat malabsorption.[9]

Decreased Mucosal Absorption and Chylomicron Formation

Generalized mucosal diseases, like celiac disease or tropical sprue, are often associated with fat malabsorption. Defective uptake of free fatty acids and monoglycerides are due to a reduction of the mucosal surface by villous shortening, reduced enterocyte function, and mucosal inflammation.[1] Intestinal fat absorption is also impaired in diseases that result in disturbance of intracellular formation of chylomicrons and accumulation of lipids within the enterocytes, as in abetalipoproteinemia, hypobetalipoproteinemia, and chylomicron retention disease.[10]

Defective Lymphatic Transport of Chylomicrons

Impairment of lymphatic transport of chylomicrons can be a cause for postmucosal malabsorption of dietary fat. Decreased lymphatic transport can be caused by congenital diseases like primary intestinal lymphangiectasia or by obstruction of lymphatic vessels due to metastatic solid tumors, lymphomas, Whipple's disease, retroperitoneal fibrosis, or trauma[5] (see Chapter 25). Usually, lymphatic vessels in the mucosa become dilated (lymphangiectasia) and chylomicrons are lost into the intestinal lumen postprandially and also in the fasting state.[11] Steatorrhea is usually only mild to moderate.[1]

Protein and Amino Acid Malabsorption

Defective absorption and/or digestion of dietary proteins has to be differentiated from excessive loss of serum proteins into the gastrointestinal tract, which is termed protein-losing enteropathy (see Chapter 25).

Defective Intraluminal Proteolysis (Protein Hydrolysis)

Protein digestion may be impaired in patients with partial or total gastric resections,[12] presumably due to poor mixing with digestive secretions, although gastric pepsin deficiency could contribute. Defective proteolysis also occurs in various causes of exocrine pancreatic insufficiency.[1, 4, 13] In congenital diseases pancreatic proteolysis can be impaired by either inborn errors in synthesis of proteolytic enzymes (trypsinogen deficiency)[14] or by defective activation of pancreatic proenzymes due to congenital deficiency of intestinal enterokinase (see subsequent text).[15]

Defective Mucosal Hydrolysis of Peptides and Decreased Absorption of Oligopeptides and Amino Acids

Generalized mucosal diseases, such as celiac disease and tropical sprue, result in global malabsorption, which includes malabsorption of oligopeptides and amino acids due to lack of mucosal hydrolysis of oligopeptides and defective mucosal absorption.[14] Furthermore, reduction of intestinal absorptive surface, as in short bowel syndrome or jejunoileal bypass, also results in protein and amino acid malabsorption.[14, 16] Congenital defects of amino acid transporters on the enterocytes (e.g., Hartnup's disease, lysinuric protein intolerance) can lead to selective malabsorption of a subgroup of amino acids (see below).

Carbohydrate Malabsorption

Defective Intraluminal Hydrolysis of Carbohydrates

Pancreatic α-amylase is normally secreted in excess into the intestinal lumen. In mild forms of pancreatic insufficiency, carbohydrate digestion is usually at least partially preserved,[17] whereas severe pancreatic insufficiency results in clinically apparent carbohydrate malabsorption and diarrhea due to decreased luminal hydrolysis of ingested starch.[18, 19]

Mucosal Defects of Carbohydrate Digestion and Absorption

The most common cause for carbohydrate malabsorption is late-onset lactose malabsorption due to decreased levels of the intestinal brush border enzyme lactase (acquired primary lactase deficiency). Depending on the ethnic background, lactase is present in less than 5% to more than 90% of the adult population, and its deficiency results in a selective malabsorption of lactose. Acquired malabsorption of carbohydrates occurs commonly after extensive intestinal resections, in diffuse mucosal diseases such as celiac disease or Crohn's disease, or temporarily after gastrointestinal infections (postinfectious carbohydrate malabsorption).[17, 18, 20] The pathophysiologic mechanisms are reduction of the intestinal mucosal surface area and a reduced activity or expression of intestinal oligo- and disaccharidases or transport proteins for monosaccharides.[17] Finally, congenital disaccharidase deficiencies (lactase, sucrase-isomaltase, and trehalase)[21] and congenital deficiency or malfunction of transport molecules as in congenital glucose-galactose malabsorption[22] can cause early onset of malabsorption of mono- or disaccharides (see subsequent text). Fructose intolerance is discussed later in this chapter.

Vitamin Malabsorption

Fat-Soluble Vitamins (Vitamins A, D, E, and K)

Diseases causing malabsorption of dietary fat commonly cause malabsorption of fat-soluble vitamins, because they require similar absorptive mechanisms. This is especially important in diseases that result in impaired micelle formation due to bile salt deficiency.[23] Fat-soluble vitamins are also malabsorbed in diffuse diseases of the mucosal surface area and in diseases affecting chylomicron formation and transport.[12, 24] Malabsorption of fat-soluble vitamins also may occur in exocrine pancreatic insufficiency, resulting in steatorrhea.[25] However, some authors have suggested that absorption of fat-soluble vitamins is less affected by exocrine pancreatic insufficiency than by small intestinal diseases resulting in steatorrhea.[26]

Vitamin B_{12} (Cobalamin)

Decreased release of dietary vitamin B_{12} due to impaired pepsin and acid secretion in atrophic gastritis[27] or due to acid inhibitory drugs[28] usually results in only mild cobalamin malabsorption. Deficiency of gastric intrinsic factor secretion, as occurs in autoimmune gastritis of pernicious anemia or after gastric resections or due to secretion of an abnormal intrinsic factor in congenital diseases, results in severe and clinically apparent vitamin B_{12} malabsorption.[27] Autoimmune gastritis is the most common cause of vitamin B_{12} malabsorption.[29] Cobalamin malabsorption in this disease is caused both by decreased intrinsic factor secretion due to parietal cell destruction in the stomach and by blocking autoantibodies, which inhibit intrinsic factor binding to vitamin B_{12}.[29] Mild cobalamin malabsorption is also found in patients with pancreatic insufficiency, including patients with Zollinger-Ellison syndrome, due to decreased proteolytic release of vitamin B_{12} from its complex with R-binding protein[27, 30] (see Chapter 38). In bacterial overgrowth syndrome (see Chapter 90) or helminthic infections like *Diphyllobothrium latum* (see Chapter 99), dietary cobalamin is consumed by the microorganisms or parasites in the intestinal lumen and is therefore not available for intestinal absorption.[27] Diseases affecting the ileal mucosa, such as Crohn's disease or ileal resection, lead to a reduction of specific absorptive sites for the intrinsic factor–vitamin B_{12} complex.[27] Ileal resections of more than 60 cm usually result in clinically significant vitamin B_{12} malabsorption. Imerslund-Gräsbeck syndrome, an autosomal recessive disease, is characterized by selective ileal malabsorption of the intrinsic factor–vitamin B_{12} complex despite normal ileal morphology.[27] Finally, congenital diseases affecting transcobalamin II also result in malabsorption of cobalamin.[27, 31] In previously healthy persons it usually takes several years of vitamin B_{12} malabsorption before cobalamin deficiency develops, because the body stores contain large amounts of cobalamin.

Folate

Folate malabsorption occurs in mucosal diseases affecting the proximal small intestine, such as celiac disease, Whipple's disease, and tropical sprue.[32, 33] Folate deficiency, a common feature in chronic alcoholism, is postulated to be mainly caused by decreased dietary intake in these patients. However, decreased intestinal absorption of folate in chronic alcoholics has also been demonstrated.[34] As discussed later in this chapter, several drugs result in impaired intestinal uptake of folate, and an inherited form of selective folate malabsorption has been described. As compared with cobalamin, the body folate stores are small relative to the daily requirements; therefore, folate deficiency states develop faster in the presence of malabsorption.

Other Water-Soluble Vitamins

Other water-soluble vitamins, like ascorbic acid and the B vitamins complex, are absorbed in the small intestine by either carrier-mediated transport or by passive diffusion. Generalized malabsorption syndromes of intestinal etiology impair the absorption of these vitamins and can therefore lead to deficiency states.[35] Deficiency of these vitamins also occurs in chronic alcoholism, probably due to decreased oral intake and also reduced intestinal absorption.[34]

Mineral Malabsorption

Calcium

Severe calcium malabsorption may occur in diseases affecting the small intestinal mucosa, such as celiac disease. In these disease states, calcium absorption is impaired directly due to the reduction of the intestinal surface area and indirectly due to formation of insoluble calcium soaps with malabsorbed long-chain fatty acids.[36] Therefore, diseases causing malabsorption of long-chain fatty acids by other mechanisms, such as bile acid deficiency, may also result in calcium malabsorption.[24] Calcium malabsorption occurs commonly after gastric resections (see subsequent section, Malabsorption after Gastric Resection). In many of these diseases, malabsorption and deficiency of vitamin D contribute to intestinal calcium malabsorption.[24] Selective intestinal malabsorption of calcium (i.e., without fat malabsorption) may occur in renal disease, hypoparathyroidism, and inborn defects in either $1\alpha,25(OH)_2$ vitamin D formation or the intestinal vitamin D receptor.[24, 37]

Magnesium

In many generalized malabsorptive disorders, magnesium malabsorption may result in magnesium deficiency.[38] Malabsorption is due to the reduction of mucosal absorptive surface area and luminal binding of magnesium by malabsorbed fatty acids. A congenital form of selective intestinal magnesium malabsorption has been reported.[39]

Iron

Iron deficiency is common in patients with gastric resections. Reduction of the mucosal surface area of the small intestine due to diffuse mucosal diseases, intestinal resections, or intestinal bypass may also result in impaired iron absorption and lead to iron deficiency.[40] Chronic intestinal loss of iron due to gastrointestinal bleeding is, however, the most common gastrointestinal cause of iron deficiency.[41]

Zinc

Zinc, like other minerals, is malabsorbed in generalized mucosal diseases of the small intestine.[42] A congenital selective defect of zinc absorption has been postulated to be the cause of acrodermatitis enteropathica.[43]

Other Minerals

Generalized malabsorption can cause deficiency of copper.[44] In Menkes' disease (kinky hair disease), an inherited disorder of cellular copper transport, selective intestinal copper malabsorption is observed (see subsequent text). It remains uncertain whether or not malabsorptive diseases result in deficiencies of chromium, selenium, and manganese.[42]

Mechanisms Compensating for Malabsorption

Role of the Colon

Although the primary function of the colon is absorption of water and electrolytes, the colon also has the capacity to absorb a limited variety of nutrients and minerals. Although nutrient absorption does not play a major role in health, the nutritive role of the colon in patients with severe malabsorption is increasingly appreciated.[45] On the other hand, colonic preservation of malabsorbed nutrients may also result in symptoms and complications of malabsorption,[46] and colonic hyperabsorption of oxalate contributes to renal stone formation (see subsequent text).

Colonic Salvage of Incompletely Absorbed Carbohydrates

In healthy people, between 2% and 20% of ingested starch escapes absorption in the small intestine.[47] Pancreatic insufficiency or severe intestinal disorders further increase this amount.[18] Carbohydrates that reach the colon cannot be absorbed by the colonic mucosa but can be metabolized by the bacterial flora. Anaerobic bacterial metabolism results in the breakdown of oligosaccharides and polysaccharides to mono- and disaccharides. These small carbohydrates are further metabolized to lactic acid and short-chain (C2-C4) fatty acids, such as acetate, propionate, and butyrate, as well as to odorless gases, like hydrogen, methane, and carbon dioxide.[48]

Studies in normal subjects have suggested that the bacterial metabolism of starch to small carbohydrate moieties is a rapid process in the normal colon. The rate-limiting step in the overall conversion of polysaccharides to short-chain fatty acids appears to be the conversion of monosaccharides to short-chain fatty acids.[18] Colonic absorption of short-chain fatty acids[49] results in a reduction of the osmotic load and, as a result, in mitigation of osmotic diarrhea. For example, in normal subjects more than 45 g of carbohydrates have to reach the colon to cause diarrhea, and up to 80 g of carbohydrates can be metabolized by bacteria to short-chain fatty acids per day.[50] Chronic carbohydrate malabsorption causes adaptive changes in bacterial metabolic activity, which result in an even higher efficiency of the bacterial flora to digest carbohydrates,[51] although at the expense of increased flatus production (see below).

Because short-chain fatty acids have caloric values between 3.4 and 5.95 kcal/g,[52] colonic absorption of these acids may contribute to overall calorie balance. In patients with short bowel syndrome, colonic salvage of malabsorbed carbohydrates can contribute up to 700 to 950 kcal/day, provided that a substantial part of the colon remains in continuity to the small bowel.[53] Not all short-chain fatty acids are absorbed by the colon, and those that are not absorbed contribute to osmotic diarrhea.

The beneficial effects of colonic bacterial carbohydrate metabolism may be accompanied by side effects due to gas production (see Chapter 10). Large interindividual differences in the volume of gas produced in the colon have been observed. The colon can also absorb gas. If intracolonic gas volumes are low, up to 90% of the volume of intracolonic gas can be absorbed. However, if gas volumes are high, this proportion decreases to 20%.[54] Therefore, those individuals who have the disadvantage of producing more gas in their colon have the second disadvantage of absorbing a smaller fraction of gas. Gas produced from bacterial carbohydrate metabolism is odorless. The odor of flatus is due to volatile sulfur-containing substrates, which result from bacterial metabolism of protein.[55]

Impaired colonic salvage of carbohydrates has been suggested to contribute to diarrhea in Crohn's disease[56] or ulcerative colitis.[57] Bacterial carbohydrate metabolism may be inhibited by antibiotic treatment,[58, 59] and in some patients antibiotic-associated diarrhea may be the result of impaired colonic salvage of carbohydrates that are normally not absorbed or dietary fibers.[60]

Colon in Fat Malabsorption

Long-chain triglycerides or fatty acids, which constitute most dietary fat, cannot be absorbed by the human colon. Long-chain fatty acids bind calcium in the colon, thereby increasing the amount of free oxalate that can be absorbed.[61] Fatty acids with chain lengths larger than C-12 may cause diarrhea, because they increase mucosal permeability and inhibit colonic absorption of fluid and electrolytes.[62] An increase in colonic permeability due to long-chain fatty acids may also be a contributing factor for increased colonic oxalate absorption seen in patients with steatorrhea and hyperoxaluria.[63]

Patients with short bowel syndrome can gain more caloric energy from medium-chain triglyceride supplementation if they have at least part of the colon in continuity with the remaining small bowel as compared with patients without remaining colon.[64] This suggests that medium-chain triglycerides can be digested and absorbed in the colon, although the metabolic and absorptive pathways have not been elucidated.

Colonic Salvage of Calcium

Although most unabsorbed calcium is insoluble when it reaches the terminal ileum,[65] preservation of at least half of the colon in patients with extensive small bowel resection improves calcium absorption by about 40% as compared with patients with ileostomy.[66] Absorption of calcium requires solubilization of calcium salts. Bacterial metabolism of dietary fibers, incompletely absorbed carbohydrates, or malabsorbed carbohydrates may play a role in solubilizing calcium by causing a decrease in the pH of luminal contents in the colon. Once calcium is solubilized, it may contact the cecal mucosa, which in the rat has been demonstrated to be the site with the highest calcium absorption rate per surface area in the whole intestine.[67] Colonic calcium solubilization due to bacterial fermentation of malabsorbed lactose may also occur in patients with lactose malabsorption, because in this condition the bioavailability of calcium from milk is greater than that from mineral water.[68] In addition to their effect on luminal pH, the short-chain fatty acids acetate and propionate, which are products of bacterial metabolism of lactose, have been shown to directly enhance calcium absorption in the human colon.[69]

Role of Intestinal Transit in the Salvage of Malabsorbed Nutrients

The lower parts of the gastrointestinal tract do not normally contact nutrients, and when they do, intestinal transit time is prolonged.[70–74] This delay in transit could contribute to the compensation mechanisms in malabsorptive disease. However, the nutritional salvage by this mechanism has not been quantitated.

CLINICAL PRESENTATION AND EVALUATION OF MALABSORPTION AND MALDIGESTION

Diagnosis of malabsorption requires, first, suspecting its presence; second, confirming its existence; and third, demonstrating its cause. Malabsorption is usually suspected on the basis of the patient's history, signs and symptoms, or routine laboratory evaluations. Malabsorption of an ingested nutrient or substrate can be confirmed by measuring its increased stool concentration or its decreased serum concentration or urinary output. Finding the cause of malabsorption often requires structural tests like endoscopy, small intestinal biopsies, or radiographic tests, although under certain clinical circumstances noninvasive tests may be helpful in providing a specific diagnosis.

Table 89–4 | **Symptoms and Signs of Malabsorption and Their Pathophysiologic Background**

SYMPTOM OR SIGN	PATHOPHYSIOLOGIC BACKGROUND
Gastrointestinal symptoms	
Diarrhea	Osmotic activity of carbohydrates or short-chain fatty acids Secretory activity of bile acids, fatty acids Decreased absorptive surface
Abdominal distension, flatulence	Bacterial gas production from carbohydrates in the colon or small bowel bacterial overgrowth
Foul smelling flatulence or stool	Malabsorption of proteins or intestinal protein loss
Pain	Flatulence
Ascites	Protein loss or malabsorption
Musculoskeletal symptoms	
Tetany, muscle weakness, paresthesias	Malabsorption of vitamin D, calcium, magnesium, and phosphate
Bone pain, osteomalacia, fractures	Protein, calcium, or vitamin D deficiency; secondary hyperparathyroidism
Skin and mucous membranes	
Easy bruisability, ecchymoses, petechiae	Vitamin K and C deficiency
Glossitis, cheilosis, stomatitis	Deficiency of vitamin B complex, B_{12}, C, folate, and iron
Edema	Protein loss or malabsorption
Acrodermatitis, scaly dermatitis	Zinc and essential fatty acid deficiency
Follicular hyperkeratosis	Vitamin A deficiency
Hyperpigmented dermatitis	Niacin deficiency (pellagra)
Thin nails with spoon-shaped deformity	Iron deficiency
Finger clubbing	Severe nutrient malabsorption
Other symptoms	
Weight loss, hyperphagia	Nutrient malabsorption
Growth and weight retardation and/or infantilism	Nutrient malabsorption in children and adolescents
Anemia	Iron, folate, or vitamin B_{12} deficiency
Kidney stones	Increased colonic oxalate absorption
Amenorrhea, impotence, infertility	Multifactorial (including protein malabsorption, secondary hypopituitarism, anemia)
Night blindness, xerophthalmia	Vitamin A deficiency
Peripheral neuropathy	Vitamin B_{12} or thiamin deficiency
Tiredness, fatigue, weakness	Calorie depletion, iron and folate deficiency, anemia

Raising the Suspicion and Confirming the Presence of Malabsorption

History and Physical Examination

Table 89–4 lists symptoms and signs suggestive of malabsorption. Virtually all the symptoms and signs may have causes other than malabsorption. For example, greasy stools may be indicative of malabsorption, but a greasy appearance can also be due to mucus in stool. Floating of stool in the toilet water can be due to high fat content but can also be caused by high gas content. Nevertheless, these symptoms and signs may be helpful in raising the suspicion and guiding the physician in ordering specific laboratory tests, structural evaluations, or function tests.

Laboratory Findings

Certain blood tests may be abnormal in malabsorption, but with rare exceptions they are not specific for malabsorptive diseases. Blood tests can also be used as a screening tool to help the physician decide on how vigorously he or she should evaluate malabsorption. Table 89–5 lists blood tests in which abnormal results should raise the suspicion of malabsorption. Table 89–5 also lists stool tests that should be used to confirm the suspicion of malabsorption.

Quantitative fecal fat measurement followed by measurement of fecal chymotrypsin or elastase concentration may be helpful, both in establishing malabsorption and in differentiating between pancreatic and intestinal causes. Low levels of serum β-carotene, cholesterol, triglycerides, and calcium and a prolonged prothrombin time suggest malabsorption of fat and fat-soluble vitamins. Low levels of vitamin B_{12}, folate, iron, and albumin suggest malabsorption of water-soluble substances and therefore indicate intestinal disease rather than pancreatic or biliary disease. Severe deficiency of fat-soluble vitamins may indicate intestinal or biliary disorders.

Table 89–5 | **Laboratory Tests Useful for Raising the Suspicion of Malabsorption and for Establishing Possible Nutrient Deficiencies and Consequences of Malabsorption**

TEST	COMMENT
Blood cell count	
Hematocrit, hemoglobin	Decreased in iron, vitamin B_{12}, folate malabsorption, or blood loss
Mean corpuscular hemoglobin or mean corpuscular volume	Decreased in iron malabsorption, increased in folate and vitamin B_{12} malabsorption
White blood cells, differential	Low lymphocyte count in lymphangiectasia
Biochemical tests (*serum*)	
Triglycerides	Decreased in severe fat malabsorption
Cholesterol	Decreased in bile acid malabsorption or severe fat malabsorption
Albumin	Decreased in severe malnutrition, lymphangiectasia, protein-losing enteropathy
Alkaline phosphatase	Increased in calcium and vitamin D malabsorption (severe steatorrhea)
Calcium, phosphorus, magnesium	Decreased in extensive mucosal disease, intestinal resection, or vitamin D deficiency
Zinc	Decreased in extensive mucosal disease, intestinal resection
Iron, ferritin	Decreased in celiac sprue, other extensive mucosal diseases, blood loss
Other blood tests	
Prothrombin time	Prolonged in vitamin K malabsorption
β-Carotene	Decreased in fat malabsorption due to hepatobiliary or intestinal diseases
Immunoglobulins	Decreased in lymphangiectasia, diffuse lymphoma
Folic acid	Decreased in extensive small bowel mucosal diseases, anticonvulsants, pregnancy
Vitamin B_{12}	Decreased in postgastrectomy, pernicious anemia, terminal ileal disease
Methylmalonic acid	Markedly elevated in vitamin B_{12} deficiency
Homocysteine	Markedly elevated in vitamin B_{12} or folate deficiency
Stool tests	
Fecal fat	Qualitative or quantitative parameter for fat malabsorption
Elastase, chymotrypsin	Decreased concentration and output in exocrine pancreatic insufficiency
pH	Below 5.5 in carbohydrate malabsorption

Diagnostic Approach to Establish the Cause of Malabsorption

Clinical Clues for the Presence of Specific Diseases Causing Malabsorption

Clinical clues (Table 89–6) or results of laboratory tests (Table 89–7) may indicate the presence of a specific underlying disease or may help in the differential diagnosis of malabsorption.

History and Physical Examination

The following questions should be asked:

- Has the patient undergone previous surgery, such as gastric or small bowel resection or gastrointestinal bypass operations?
- Is there a family or childhood history of celiac disease?
- Is there a history of travel to endemic areas of tropical sprue, giardiasis, or other gastrointestinal infections?
- Is there excessive alcohol consumption?
- Does the patient have a history of chronic pancreatitis or symptoms suggestive of a pancreatic tumor?
- Does the patient have clinical features of thyrotoxicosis, Addison's disease, Whipple's disease, biliary or liver disease, or diabetic neuropathy?
- Does the patient eat a diet high in poorly absorbable carbohydrates (sweeteners like sorbitol or fructose) or fat substitutes or an unbalanced diet that could result in malnutrition?
- Is there an increased likelihood of human immunodeficiency virus infection?
- Is the patient on current therapy with a drug that may cause malabsorption?
- Does the patient have a history of organ transplantation or abdominal radiation exposure?

A rational approach to establishing the cause of malab-

Table 89–6 | **Cardinal Clinical Features of Specific Malabsorptive Diseases**

DISEASE	CARDINAL FEATURES
Adrenal insufficiency	Skin darkening, hyponatremia, hyperkalemia
Amyloidosis	Renal disease, cardiomyopathy, neuropathy, carpal tunnel syndrome, macroglossia, hepatosplenomegaly
Bacterial overgrowth	Previous surgery, scleroderma, pseudo-obstruction, diverticula, strictures
Bile acid deficiency	Ileal resection or disease, liver disease
Carcinoid	Flush, cardiac murmur
Celiac sprue	Variable symptoms, from mono- or oligosymptomatic (e.g., mild iron deficiency) to life-threatening malnutrition, dermatitis herpetiformis, alopecia, aphthous mouth ulcers, arthropathy, neurologic symptoms
Crohn's disease	Arthritis, aphthous mouth ulcers, episcleritis, erythema nodosum, laboratory signs of inflammation, abdominal mass, fistulas, pyoderma gangrenosum, primary sclerosing cholangitis
Cystic fibrosis	Chronic sinopulmonary disease, meconium ileus, distal intestinal obstruction syndrome, elevated sweat chloride
Cystinuria, Hartnup's disease	Kidney stones, dermatosis
Diabetic malabsorption	Long history of diabetes and diabetic complications
Disaccharidase deficiency	Dominant bloating and cramping, intermittent diarrhea
Fistulas	Previous surgery or trauma, Crohn's disease
Glucagonoma	Migratory necrolytic erythema
Hyperthyroidism	Specific symptoms of thyroid disease
Hypogammaglobulinemia	Recurrent infections
Intestinal ischemia	Other ischemic organ manifestations, abdominal pain
Lymphoma	Mesenteric or retroperitoneal lymph nodes, abdominal mass, abdominal pain, fever
Mastocytosis	Skin changes, peptic ulcers
Mycobacterium avium complex	Acquired immunodeficiency syndrome
Pancreatic insufficiency	History of pancreatitis, abdominal pain, or alcoholism; large fatty stools
Parasitic infection	Travel history to endemic areas
Primary biliary cirrhosis	Jaundice, itching
Scleroderma	Raynaud's phenomenon, skin tightening
Tropical sprue	Travel history to endemic areas
Tuberculosis	Specific history of exposure, endemic areas, immunosuppression, abdominal mass
Whipple's disease	Lymphadenopathy, fever, arthritis, cerebral symptoms
Zollinger-Ellison syndrome	Peptic ulcers

sorption may require several diagnostic steps. Depending on the care provider's background, the availability of different tests, and the patient's preferences, different diagnostic approaches may be used. If there are no time constraints, a stepwise approach may be used starting with noninvasive evaluations that may guide further invasive procedures or may even provide a diagnosis. In other instances the physician may choose a more invasive test, in hopes of reaching a diagnosis with the fewest possible tests in the shortest possible time. Diagnostic approaches differ, depending on the epidemiologic or ethnic background of an individual patient. For example, if parasitic infections are a likely possibility, stool examination may provide a rapid diagnosis by noninvasive testing. In populations with a high prevalence of celiac disease, serologic testing may make small intestinal biopsies or evaluation of intestinal function unnecessary. In populations with a very low prevalence of lactose intolerance, a secondary cause of lactose malabsorption is more likely, which requires further tests, than in populations with a high prevalence of acquired primary lactase deficiency.

The sequence of tests therefore depends on symptoms and patient history, as well as results of previous testing (Table 89–8). Tests that may detect the most common causes of malabsorption or are noninvasive or inexpensive usually should be performed initially (first-line tests). In some patients, testing for rarer etiologies of malabsorption and use of more invasive or more expensive tests may be necessary to establish the diagnosis (second-line tests). For unusually difficult cases, additional tests may be required that may only be available in specialized centers (third-line tests).

In some clinical circumstances, like bile acid malabsorption, lactose malabsorption, and bacterial overgrowth, it may be difficult to establish a causal link between symptoms and the malabsorbed substrate. In these conditions, observation of the response to therapy may be an important tool to prove or disprove a causal relationship.

ANATOMIC INVESTIGATIONS

Endoscopic examination of the stomach, duodenum, or ileum and histologic examination of mucosal biopsies can establish a diagnosis of the conditions causing malabsorption listed in Table 89–9. The role for radiographic examinations is mostly limited to answering questions about abdominal regions not accessible to endoscopy, like parts of the small intestine, parenchymatous organs, the peritoneal cavity, the mesentery, or the retroperitoneum. However, gastrointestinal x-rays can show evidence of stasis, blind loops, diverticula, fistulas, rapid transit, and other abnormalities that may assist in diagnosis (see subsequent text).

Endoscopic Examination, Mucosal Biopsy, and Aspiration of Intestinal Secretions

Endoscopic inspection of the duodenal mucosa may provide clues to some causes of malabsorption. Aphthae may be suggestive of Crohn's disease, and white punctate lesions can be seen in primary or secondary lymphangiectasia. Mosaic or nodular mucosa, scalloping of duodenal folds, and reduction in number of duodenal folds are highly suggestive of villous atrophy in celiac disease, although these abnormalities may be seen in other diseases.[75] However, a normal

Table 89–7 | **Laboratory Tests that Can Aid in the Differential Diagnosis of Malabsorption**

TEST	COMMENT
Blood cell count	
Acanthocytes	Abetalipoproteinemia
Nuclear remnants in erythrocytes (Howell-Jolly bodies)	Splenic atrophy in celiac sprue, inflammatory bowel disease, radiation, amyloidosis
White blood cells, differential	Eosinophilia in eosinophilic gastroenteritis and parasitic disease Low lymphocyte count in lymphangiectasia, tuberculosis Low $CD4^+$ count in AIDS complex
Platelets	Increased in inflammatory diseases
Other tests	
Erythrocyte sedimentation rate, C-reactive protein	Increased in Crohn's disease, Whipple's disease, lymphoma
Ferritin	Increased in inflammatory diseases
Liver enzymes, bilirubin	Increased in primary biliary cirrhosis and liver diseases, celiac sprue
Serum sodium, potassium	Abnormal in adrenal insufficiency
Immunologic markers	
EMA/anti-tissue TG, gliadin antibodies	Celiac sprue
Immunoglobulins	IgA deficiency, immunodeficiency syndromes
Allergen-specific IgE	IgE mediated hypersensitivity
Autoantibodies (e.g., antinuclear antibodies and subtypes)	Connective tissue diseases
HLA DQ2 or DQ8	Celiac sprue, refractory sprue
Anti-mitochondrial autoantibodies	Primary biliary cirrhosis
HIV antibodies	AIDS
Neuroendocrine markers	
ACTH, cortisol	Abnormal values in Addison's disease
Basal TSH	Decreased in hyperthyroidism
Chromogranin	Elevated in neuroendocrine tumors
5-OH-indole acetic acid in urine	Elevated in carcinoid syndrome
Gastrin*	Elevated in Zollinger-Ellison syndrome (gastrinoma)
Glucagon*	Elevated in glucagonoma
Somatostatin*	Elevated in somatostatinoma
Stool tests	
Occult blood test	Erosive or ulcerative intestinal disease, tumor, or celiac sprue
Ova and parasites	Repeated samples may be needed to detect *Giardia lamblia*
Leukocytes	Elevated in some inflammatory diseases
Chymotrypsin, elastase	Decreased exocrine pancreatic insufficiency

*Only to be performed if there is a high suspicion of an underlying neuroendocrine tumor.[250]

ACTH, adrenocorticotropic hormone; AIDS, acquired immunodeficiency syndrome; EMA, endomysial antibody; HIV, human immunodeficiency virus; TG, transglutaminase; TSH, thyroid-stimulating hormone.

duodenal fold pattern should not deter the endoscopist from taking mucosal biopsies. Endocrine tumors causing malabsorption such as duodenal gastrinomas or somatostatinomas or ampullary tumors obstructing the pancreatic duct sometimes can also be detected during endoscopy. If malabsorption is suspected to be caused by ileal disease, visual examination and biopsies from the ileal mucosa may be required to establish a diagnosis.

Examination of endoscopic biopsies obtained at the level of the duodenal ampulla may be diagnostic or highly suggestive of a variety of small bowel disorders resulting in malabsorption. Repeat small intestinal biopsy can be used to assess treatment effects. Endoscopic biopsies are an adequate substitute for jejunal suction biopsies,[76] and their advantage over capsule biopsy[77, 78] is that focal or patchy lesions can be seen and biopsied.[79] Adequacy of mucosal biopsies is a function of size and numbers of biopsies obtained.[80] If large biopsies can be obtained using "jumbo" biopsy forceps, they can be oriented on a piece of paper before they are put into a fixing solution.[81] This allows histologic sectioning parallel to the villi and crypts. Nevertheless, biopsies also may be obtained with smaller forceps, although in this case the number of biopsies taken has to be increased to four to six. Biopsies can be inspected with a low-power dissecting microscope to get an initial impression of the villous architecture.

The diagnostic yield of biopsies is influenced by the distribution of histologic abnormalities, which in some diseases is diffuse but in other diseases is patchy. Tropical diarrhea malabsorption syndrome (tropical sprue; see Chapter 94), Whipple's disease (see Chapter 95), abetalipoproteinemia, and immunodeficiency usually result in a diffuse alteration of small intestinal mucosa, and thus a completely normal proximal mucosal biopsy rules out these disorders. Primary lymphangiectasia has a patchy distribution, so that a single mucosal biopsy may not rule out the disorder (see Chapter 25). Patchy distribution has also been described for the histologic changes in some patients with celiac disease, although this disorder usually affects the small intestine diffusely.[82] Other possible sources of error and misdiagnosis include poorly orientated specimens and biopsies obtained too proximally, where peptic injury can be the cause of mucosal alterations. Distortion of villous architecture over Brunner's glands or lymphoid aggregates, common in the duodenum, should be interpreted with caution.

Specific histologic features may be diagnostic for some rare causes of malabsorption (see Table 89–9), like Whipple's disease, abetalipoproteinemia-hypobetalipoproteinemia, intestinal lymphangiectasia, giardiasis, lymphoma, or collagenous sprue. However, in most patients with small bowel disorders, histologic features are not diagnostic (Table 89–10). Histology may reveal a spectrum of mucosal responses

Table 89–8 | **Tests to Establish the Cause of Malabsorption Based on Main Symptoms**

A. TESTS IN PATIENTS WITH WEIGHT LOSS, OSTEOMALACIA/OSTEOPENIA, DIARRHEA, SUSPECTED STEATORRHEA, OR DEFICIENCY OF FAT-SOLUBLE VITAMINS

First-line tests
- Laboratory tests (whole blood cell count, white blood cell differential, cholesterol, triglycerides, electrolytes, calcium, magnesium, ALT, AST, AP, bilirubin, prothrombin time, albumin, erythrocyte sedimentation rate/C-reactive protein, TSH)
- Endomysial antibodies/tissue transglutaminase antibodies and antigliadin antibodies
- Gastroduodenoscopy and small intestinal biopsies
- Ova, parasites, and leukocytes in stool
- Chymotrypsin and/or elastase concentration in stool
- Abdominal ultrasonogram
- Plain abdominal x-ray

Second-line tests
- Small bowel x-ray
- Abdominal computed tomography
- Special staining of small intestinal biopsies (e.g., Congo red, staining for lymphomas, chromogranin A)
- Endoscopic examination of the terminal ileum, including ileal biopsies
- Quantitative small intestinal culture or breath tests for bacterial overgrowth
- More extensive laboratory investigation (immunoglobulins, human immunodeficiency virus antibodies, antinuclear antibodies and subtypes, ferritin, food allergen-specific IgE, adrenocorticotropic hormone, cortisol, chromogranin, gastrin, urinary 5-HIAA)
- Quantitative fecal fat
- Endoscopic retrograde cholangiopancreatography/MRCP
- Therapeutic trial of pancreatic enzymes, antibiotics (tetracycline, metronidazole,) or a gluten-free diet

Tests in unusually difficult cases (third-line tests)
- Glucagon, somatostatin in serum/plasma
- Tube test for exocrine pancreatic secretion (secretin, cholecystokinin, or Lundh test)
- Tests for bile acid malabsorption
- Thin section computed tomography of the pancreas for tumor
- Enteroscopy, including biopsies
- Endoscopic ultrasound
- Somatostatin scan
- Positron emission tomography
- Abdominal angiogram
- Magnetic resonance angiography

B. TESTS IN PATIENTS WITH BLOATING, WITH OR WITHOUT DIARRHEA

First-line tests
- Lactose H_2 breath test
- Lactose tolerance test
- Fructose H_2 breath test
- Stool pH (in patients with diarrhea)

Second-line tests
- Gastroduodenoscopy plus duodenal biopsies
- Endomysial antibodies/tissue transglutaminase antibodies and antigliadin antibodies
- Quantitative small intestinal culture or breath tests for bacterial overgrowth
- Chymotrypsin and/or elastase concentration in stool

C. TESTS IN PATIENTS WITH ANEMIA AND SUSPECTED MALABSORPTION

Microcytic or hypochromic anemia (low MCV, MCH)
- Iron, ferritin, and transferrin in serum
- Exclude gastrointestinal and extragastrointestinal blood loss
- Endomysial antibodies/tissue transglutaminase antibodies and antigliadin antibodies
- Gastroduodenoscopy plus duodenal biopsies
- Ova and parasites in stool

Macrocytic anemia (high MCV, MCH)
- First-line tests
  - Folic acid in serum or red blood cells
  - Vitamin B_{12} in serum
- Second-line tests in cases of vitamin B_{12} deficiency
  - Schilling test (with and without intrinsic factor)
  - Ova and parasites in stool
  - Evaluation of ileum
    - Endoscopy
    - Computed tomography, small bowel series, enteroclysis
  - Gastroduodenoscopy plus gastric and duodenal biopsies
  - Endomysial antibodies/tissue transglutaminase antibodies and antigliadin antibodies
  - Quantitative small intestinal culture or breath tests for bacterial overgrowth
- Second-line tests in cases of folate deficiency
  - Endomysial antibodies/tissue transglutaminase antibodies and antigliadin antibodies
  - Gastroduodenoscopy plus duodenal biopsies

ALT, alanine aminotransferase; AP, alkaline phosphatase; AST; aspartate aminotransferase; HIAA, hydroxyindole acetic acid; MCH, mean corpuscular hemoglobin; MCV, mean corpuscular volume; MRCP, magnetic resonance cholangiopancreatography; TSH, thyroid-stimulating hormone.

Table 89–9 | **Causes of Malabsorption in which the Diagnosis Can Be Established by Small Bowel Biopsy**

	MAIN HISTOLOGIC FEATURE
Generalized histologic abnormalities	
Abetalipoproteinemia-hypobetalipoproteinemia	Lipid accumulation and vacuolization of enterocytes
Collagenous sprue	Collagenous band below atrophic mucosa
Mycobacterium avium complex	Acid-fast bacilli, foamy cells
Whipple's disease (see Chapter 95)	Foamy macrophages with periodic acid–Schiff–positive inclusion bodies
Patchy histologic abnormalities	
Amyloidosis	Deposits, Congo red stain: apple green birefringence in polarized light
Crohn's disease (see Chapter 103)	Epithelioid granulomas
Eosinophilic gastroenteritis (see Chapter 100)	Eosinophilic infiltration
Lymphangiectasia	Ectatic lymph vessels
Lymphoma (see Chapter 26)	Clonal expansion of lymphocytes
Mastocytosis	Diffuse infiltration with mast cells
Parasites (*Giardia lamblia*, strongyloides, coccidia) (see Chapters 98 and 99)	Parasites may be seen on histology

From Riddell RH. Small intestinal biopsy: Who? How? What are the findings? *In* Barkin JS, Rogers AI (eds.): Difficult Decisions in Digestive Diseases. Chicago, Year Book Medical Publishers, 1989, p 326. Riley SA, Marsh MN. Maldigestion and malabsorption. *In* Feldman M, Scharschmidt BF, Sleisenger MH (eds.): Sleisenger & Fordtran's Gastrointestinal and Liver Disease, 6th ed. Philadelphia, WB Saunders, 1998, p 1501.

ranging from infiltration by lymphocytic cells to a flat mucosa with villous atrophy and crypt hyperplasia. In many parts of the world celiac disease is by far the most common cause of this type of histologic alteration. Nevertheless, a definite diagnosis of celiac disease cannot be established by mucosal biopsy alone (see Chapter 93).

Some disease states can only be identified by special histologic stains, such as a Congo red stain for intestinal amyloidosis, use of anti-heavy chain antisera, and special immunohistochemical staining for small intestinal lymphomas, or immunohistochemical staining for chromogranin A to detect enteroendocrine insufficiency (see subsequent text). Polymerase chain reaction analysis of intestinal biopsies for *Tropheryma whippelii* performed in special laboratories may be helpful in patients suspected of having Whipple's disease.[83] In cases in which these diseases are a possibility, the clinician has to request these specific tests. Measurement of mucosal enzyme activities in a jejunal biopsy can be used to confirm the diagnosis of disaccharidase deficiency, although this is neither recommended nor available for routine clinical use.

Fluid aspirated from the descending part of the duodenum may be examined microscopically for *Giardia lamblia* (see Chapter 98) or cultured to detect bacterial overgrowth in diffuse small bowel motility disorders (see Chapter 90).

Radiographic Imaging of the Abdomen

Small Bowel Series

The principal roles of small bowel radiographic series in the evaluation of malabsorption are to identify alterations that predispose to bacterial overgrowth, like diverticula, stagnant loops of the intestine, or generalized intestinal hypomotility or dilatation; intestinal fistulas; and tumors. Alterations associated with diffuse, localized, or distal mucosal disease, which might have been missed by proximal mucosal biopsy, may also be identified. Normal results of a small bowel series do not rule out intestinal causes of malabsorption and should not dissuade the clinician from obtaining small bowel biopsies.

Ulcerations and strictures may be seen in different causes of malabsorption, such as Crohn's disease, radiation enteritis, celiac disease, intestinal lymphoma, and tuberculosis. Aphthous ulcers or cobblestoning of mucosa either alone or with thickened and distorted folds are features of Crohn's disease or radiation enteritis, but they can be also present in other conditions. Reduced numbers of jejunal folds may be present in celiac disease. Mass lesions can be found in intestinal lymphoma or, rarely, in hormone-producing tumors. Double contrast techniques, in which intubation of the upper jejunum is used to apply contrast material directly into the upper jejunum, have a higher sensitivity for detecting mucosal changes, although they are less acceptable to the patient

Table 89–10 | **Malabsorptive Diseases with Abnormal but not Diagnostic Small Intestinal Histology**

- Lymphocyte infiltration with or without crypt hypertrophy
  - Acquired immunodeficiency syndrome enteropathy (see Chapter 28)
  - Celiac sprue (see Chapter 93)
  - Graft-versus-host disease (see Chapter 27)
  - Infection (*Giardia lamblia*, cryptosporidia, viral enteritis)
  - Prolonged folate or cobalamin deficiency
  - Tropical sprue (see Chapter 94)
- Flat destructive lesion
  - Celiac sprue (see Chapter 93)
  - Drug induced (nonsteroidal anti-inflammatory drugs, colchicine, neomycin)
  - Food protein hypersensitivity (rye, barley, egg, fish, rice, poultry) (see Chapter 101)
  - Immunodeficiency (hypogammaglobulinemia) (see Chapter 2)
  - Immunoproliferative small intestinal disease (see Chapter 26)
  - Infection (*Giardia lamblia*, cryptosporidia) (see Chapter 98)
  - Lymphoma (see Chapter 26)
  - Protein calorie malnutrition
  - Transplantation
  - Traumatic
  - Tropical sprue (see Chapter 94)
  - Zollinger-Ellison syndrome (see Chapter 41)
- Atrophic lesion
  - Chronic radiation damage (see Chapter 102)
  - Cicatrizing Crohn's disease (see Chapter 103)
  - Diffuse lymphoma (see Chapter 26)
  - Idiopathic diarrhea of infancy (microvillus inclusion disease)
  - Unresponsive gluten sensitivity (lymphoma or ulcerative jejunitis)

From Riddell RH. Small intestinal biopsy: Who? How? What are the findings? *In* Barkin JS, Rogers AI (eds.): Difficult Decisions in Digestive Diseases. Chicago, Year Book Medical Publishers, 1989, p 326. Riley SA, Marsh MN. Maldigestion and malabsorption. *In* Feldman M, Scharschmidt BF, Sleisenger MH (eds.): Sleisenger & Fordtran's Gastrointestinal and Liver Disease, 6th ed. Philadelphia, WB Saunders, 1998, p 1501.

and may miss focal changes in the duodenum, like diverticula.

Abdominal Computed Tomography

Abdominal computed tomography is useful for detecting focal intestinal lesions like thickening of the small bowel wall in Crohn's disease or small intestinal lymphoma, intestinal fistula, and dilated bowel loops. Computed tomography is a sensitive test to detect enlarged abdominal lymph nodes, which are commonly present in disorders like Whipple's disease, small bowel lymphoma, or small intestinal inflammatory diseases such as Crohn's disease. Evidences for pancreatic disease that may be detected on computed tomography are calcifications of the pancreas, dilatation of the pancreatic duct, and an atrophic pancreas. Furthermore, tumors obstructing the pancreatic duct or hormone-secreting neuroendocrine tumors can be located by computed tomography.

Other Radiographic Studies

A *plain film of the abdomen* may be helpful to detect pancreatic calcifications if exocrine pancreatic insufficiency is suspected. It should be noted, however, that morphologic signs of chronic pancreatitis alone do not prove a pancreatic cause of malabsorption, because the function of the exocrine pancreas must be severely impaired before malabsorption becomes evident. A plain film of the abdomen may also document stagnant loops of intestine, predisposing to small bowel bacterial overgrowth or suggesting the presence of an obstruction.

Endoscopic retrograde pancreatography may be helpful in establishing the cause of pancreatic insufficiency (see Chapter 49). It can help to distinguish between chronic pancreatitis and pancreatic tumor or document pancreatic duct stones. *Endoscopic retrograde cholangiography* is the method of choice for documenting various causes of biliary obstruction. Noninvasive *magnetic resonance cholangiography* is increasingly used to replace diagnostic endoscopic retrograde cholangiography (see Chapter 61). Magnetic resonance imaging of the abdomen is also useful to demonstrate complications of Crohn's disease, like fistulas.

If malabsorption is suspected to be caused by a neuroendocrine tumor (e.g., gastrinoma, somatostatinoma), *an indium-111 octreotide scintigraphic scan* or an *endoscopic ultrasound examination* of the pancreas may be helpful in establishing the diagnosis or demonstrating the extent of the disease (see Chapter 51).

Transabdominal ultrasound examinations are very popular in some countries, although they are very operator dependent. They have the advantage of having no radiation exposure and therefore can also be used in pregnant patients. Ultrasonography is frequently used to investigate the pancreas, although the sensitivity for the detection of tumors is lower compared with endoscopic retrograde cholangiopancreatography or computed tomography. Nevertheless, obstruction of the biliary tract, pancreatic calcifications, dilatation of the pancreatic duct, or stones within the pancreatic duct may be demonstrated. Ultrasound may also be used to document thickening of the bowel wall, abscesses, and fistula in Crohn's disease.

NONINVASIVE EVALUATION OF GASTROINTESTINAL ABSORPTIVE AND DIGESTIVE FUNCTION

Some conditions causing malabsorption can be diagnosed by the use of noninvasive tests, although, as pointed out in Table 89–11, diagnostic accuracy may be limited, and further tests may be necessary to identify underlying diseases or to differentiate between primary and secondary causes. Apart from providing a diagnosis, tests evaluating gastrointestinal absorptive and digestive function may be helpful in the evaluation of complex disease presentations. For most or all of the following tests, the potential benefits with regard to the costs of workup or to patient acceptability have not been established. Because test procedures and analytical

Table 89–11 | **Malabsorptive Diseases or Conditions in which Noninvasive Tests Can Establish Malabsorption or Provide a Diagnosis**

DISEASE, CONDITION	DIAGNOSTIC TESTS*	COMMENTS
Lactose malabsorption	Lactose hydrogen breath test	Tests do not differentiate among primary and secondary lactose malabsorption.
	Lactose tolerance test	Questionable clinical relevance
Fructose malabsorption	Fructose hydrogen breath test	
Small bowel bacterial overgrowth (see Chapter 90)	^{14}C D-xylose breath test	Search for predisposing factor if either one of the tests is positive
	Glucose hydrogen breath test	
	Schilling test plus antibiotics	
Bile acid malabsorption	SeHCAT test, ^{14}C TCA test	No differentiation between primary and secondary causes
Exocrine pancreatic insufficiency	Quantitative fecal fat	To establish malabsorption in chronic pancreatitis
	Fecal elastase or chymotrypsin	Variable sensitivity and specificity, depending on type of test and stage of the disease
	Tubeless tests†	
Vitamin B_{12} malabsorption	Schilling test	Appropriate interventions needed to differentiate among gastric, intestinal, or pancreatic causes; diagnostic for pernicious anemia; further tests are needed if small bowel bacterial overgrowth, terminal ileal disease, and pancreatic disease are suspected

*See text for diagnostic accuracy of the different tests mentioned.
†See chapter 46.
^{14}C TCA test; ^{14}C-labeled taurocholic acid test; SeHCAT, selenium-75 labeled homotaurocholic acid test.

methods may vary,[84] laboratories that offer the following tests should establish their own reference values.

Tests for Fat Malabsorption

Quantitative Fecal Fat Analysis

The *van de Kamer method*, which is the titrimetric measurement of fatty acid equivalents and the expression of results as fecal fat output in grams per 24 hours, is considered to be the gold standard.[85] Modifications in which the extracted fats are weighed rather than titrated[86, 87] have an excellent correlation with the results of the titrimetric method.[86] *Near-infrared reflectance analysis* may be a less cumbersome method to quantify fecal fat output in quantitative stool collections,[88] because it requires less handling of stool by the laboratory personnel, but it still requires a 48- to 72-hour stool collection to exclude the influence of day to day variability and mixing of the stool before a sample is obtained for analysis. In our own unpublished experience, the accuracy of the near-infrared reflectance analysis technology is influenced by stool consistency—in watery stools the accuracy of the method decreases.

Fecal fat excretion of less than 7 g/day on a 100-g/day fat diet is usually considered to be normal. It is, however, important to note that the volume effect of diarrhea by itself increases fecal fat output to levels of up to 14 g/day (secondary fat malabsorption)[89]; this latter normal value could be used in patients with diarrhea.

Quantitative fecal fat analysis is routinely available only in a few centers. Reasons for the limited clinical use of quantitative fecal fat measurements are as follows. First, if the main symptom of malabsorption is chronic diarrhea, measurement of fecal fat may not influence the subsequent workup because the diagnostic tests performed to establish the etiology of diarrhea are similar to the tests for the workup of steatorrhea. Second, an elevated fecal fat level cannot be used to differentiate between biliary, pancreatic, and enteric causes of malabsorption. Third, on clinical grounds, in many patients with severe steatorrhea, the porridge-like appearance of the stools is characteristic, and quantitative studies are not necessary to establish fat malabsorption. Fourth, fat absorption may be normal despite malabsorption of other nutrients. Therefore, a normal fat balance does not imply normal absorptive function of the gastrointestinal tract. Finally, accuracy depends on quantitative stool collections for 48 to 72 hours, adherence to an 80- to 100-g fat diet, and a diet diary to determine fat intake.

Keeping the limitations of quantitative fecal fat analysis in mind, it is nevertheless still useful in several clinical circumstances: to establish malabsorption when there are no overt features of intestinal or pancreatic disorders, like in cases of osteoporosis, osteomalacia, anemia, or weight loss; to monitor treatment in patients with established malabsorptive disorders, like exocrine pancreatic insufficiency or short bowel syndrome; to estimate fecal calorie loss in patients with severe malabsorption syndromes; and to quantitate fecal fat excretion in patients with diarrhea and ileal resections to help distinguish patients with steatorrhea due to bile acid deficiency from patients with secretory diarrhea caused by bile acid loss, because treatments for these conditions differ.[90] Falsely elevated fecal fat values (pseudo-steatorrhea) can be observed in patients consuming a diet rich in the fat substitute olestra.[86]

Semiquantitative Fat Analysis

For the *acid steatocrit test*,[91] a sample of stool is diluted to a 1:3 concentration with distilled water in a test tube. The diluted stool is homogenized, and a 500-μL aliquot is pipetted into a tube. Then 100 μL of 5 M $HClO_4$ is added. An aliquot of the diluted stool–$HClO_4$ mixture is put into a nonheparinized microcapillary tube and sealed on one end. After centrifugation at 13,000 rpm for 15 minutes, the fatty layer (FL) and the solid layer (SL) are measured and the acid steatocrit (AS) is determined according to the following equation: $AS\ (\%) = [FL/(FL + SL)] \times 100$. An acid steatocrit of less than 31% is considered to be normal. In a small study, the acid steatocrit performed on random spot stool samples had a high sensitivity and specificity to detect steatorrhea, as compared with the van de Kamer method, which was performed on a 72-hour stool collection. There was also a linear correlation between results obtained with the acid steatocrit and results of the van de Kamer method, although there were quite divergent results in some patients.[91] Considering the fact that quantitative fecal fat measurements are usually based on 48- to 72-hour stool collections to minimize the effect of day to day variability in fecal fat excretion, it cannot be expected that the acid steatocrit can replace quantitative measurement of fat output in borderline cases or in cases in which exact measurements of fecal fat loss are required.

Qualitative Fecal Fat Analysis

Fat analysis by *microscopic examination* of random stool samples may provide a clue to the presence of steatorrhea, although it cannot be used to exclude steatorrhea. Its advantage is that it is easy to perform. A sample of stool is placed on a glass slide to which several drops of glacial acetic acid and Sudan III stain are added. Acidification of stool samples improves fat extraction and separation of the lipid layer.[91] The acidified mixture is heated to boiling and examined while still warm for presence of orange fat globules. Up to 100 globules with a diameter less than 4 μm per high-power field are considered to be normal.[5] Results of the Sudan stain and of quantitative fat analysis do not correlate very well.[92] In a small study, Sudan staining of spot stool samples had a sensitivity of 78% and a specificity of 70% for the detection of steatorrhea.[91] Recently, a new quantitative microscopic method of counting and measuring fat globules has been shown to correlate with chemically measured fecal fat output.[93]

Breath Tests for Fat Malabsorption

The test principle of the *^{14}C-triolein breath test* is to measure $^{14}CO_2$ in breath after ingestion of a triglyceride that has been radiolabeled with ^{14}C. Fat malabsorption results in decreased pulmonary excretion of $^{14}CO_2$.[94] Because of erroneous results in a variety of metabolic and pulmonary diseases, lack of sensitivity in mild malabsorption, the radiation exposure of the patient, cost of the substrate, or the need for expensive equipment, this test has not found widespread acceptance for clinical use. Recently, the nonradioactive isotope ^{13}C has been used to label triglycerides (see below).

Serum Tests for Fat Malabsorption

Experience with the measurement of the serum concentration of β-carotene for the qualitative assessment of fat malabsorption is limited. It has been suggested to be a useful screening test for steatorrhea, with values below 100 μg/100 mL suggestive of the presence of steatorrhea and values of less than 47 μg/100 mL strongly indicative of steatorrhea. β-Carotene can be measured photometrically at 456 nm.[95] Concentrations in excess of 100 μg/100 mL do not exclude mild steatorrhea, although they make steatorrhea in excess of 16 g fat loss per day very unlikely. Normal values have also been established in the pediatric population.[96] β-Carotene can be falsely low in liver diseases or in alcoholics who eat a β-carotene deficient diet. Disorders in lipoproteins or intake of carotene-containing food additives can also influence the results.

Tests for Carbohydrate Malabsorption

The *hydrogen breath test* is a noninvasive test that takes advantage of the fact that in most people bacterial carbohydrate metabolism results in accumulation of hydrogen, which then is absorbed by the intestinal mucosa and excreted in breath. Using different carbohydrates, like lactose or fructose, the hydrogen breath test can be used to detect whether malabsorption of these carbohydrates is present. Measurement of hydrogen excretion in breath after ingestion of lactulose has been used to assess orocecal transit time, and glucose has been used as a substrate to detect small bowel bacterial overgrowth, although sensitivity and specificity are poor. Unfortunately, up to 18% of persons are hydrogen nonexcretors.[97] In these persons hydrogen breath tests may be falsely negative because hydrogen is metabolized by bacteria to methane.

The diagnosis of lactose malabsorption is established if there is an increase in breath hydrogen concentration of more than 20 parts per million over baseline after ingestion of 50 g of lactose. An increase within the first 30 minutes after ingestion of lactose has to be disregarded, because it may be due to bacterial degradation of lactose in the oral cavity. It may take up to 4 hours until the increase in breath hydrogen concentration occurs. Breath hydrogen measurements obtained before and at 30, 60, 90, 180, and 240 minutes after ingestion of 50 g of lactose provide the best diagnostic yield at the least possible number of measurements.[97]

Lactose hydrogen breath test is still considered to be the gold standard for the diagnosis of lactose malabsorption by many researchers, but this test may miss the disorder in hydrogen nonexcretors. In these patients a *lactose tolerance test*, that is, measurements of blood glucose before and 30 minutes after ingestion of 50 g of lactose, can be used. An increase in glucose concentration of less than 20 mg/dL over baseline within 30 minutes of ingestion of 50 g of lactose is indicative of lactose malabsorption. The lactose tolerance test has a lower sensitivity as compared with lactose hydrogen breath test.[97]

In patients with diarrhea, a *stool test* to detect a fecal pH lower than 5.5 can serve as a qualitative indicator of carbohydrate malabsorption.[98] In the research setting, fecal carbohydrates can be measured by the anthrone method, which measures carbohydrates on a weight basis.[99] In contrast, the reducing sugar method gives results on a molar basis. Therefore, in contrast to the anthrone method, the reducing sugar method provides information about the osmotic activity of malabsorbed carbohydrates.[18] Total short-chain fatty acids and lactic acid, which are the products of bacterial carbohydrate metabolism, can be measured in stool by titration.[100] Individual short-chain fatty acids can be determined by gas chromatography.[101]

Tests for Protein Malabsorption

The classic test to quantify protein malabsorption, measurement of fecal nitrogen content in a quantitatively collected stool specimen,[13] is rarely used today. For research purposes, a combined ^{14}C octanoic acid/^{13}C egg white breath test accompanied by measurement of the urinary output of phenol and *p*-cresol, which are specific metabolites of tyrosine, has been used to assess the effect of gastric acid on protein digestion.[102]

Tests for Cobalamin (Vitamin B_{12}) Malabsorption

Schilling Test

The Schilling test is used clinically to distinguish between gastric and ileal causes of vitamin B_{12} deficiency and to evaluate the function of the ileum in patients with diarrhea or malabsorption. The results of the test are not influenced by vitamin B_{12} replacement therapy. The Schilling test does not have an important clinical role for the assessment of pancreatic insufficiency or bacterial overgrowth, because more direct approaches to diagnose these disorders are available. Because in humans both intrinsic factor and hydrochloric acid are produced by parietal cells, alternative approaches to diagnosing pernicious anemia are to document atrophic gastritis by endoscopy and biopsy, to confirm achlorhydria by acid secretion analysis to detect increased gastrin levels, or to look for antibodies directed against parietal cells or intrinsic factor in the serum.[29, 33, 103]

The Schilling test is performed by administering a small oral dose of radiolabeled vitamin B_{12} and, simultaneously or within 1 to 2 hours, a large intramuscular "flushing dose" of nonradiolabeled vitamin B_{12}. The latter saturates vitamin B_{12} carriers; thus, radioactive vitamin B_{12} absorbed by the intestine is excreted in the urine. If less than 7% to 10% of the administered dose is recovered in urine within 24 hours, vitamin B_{12} malabsorption is confirmed. To specify the site of vitamin B_{12} malabsorption, a second phase of the Schilling test has to be performed subsequently with oral administration of intrinsic factor. In patients with pernicious anemia, the results of the Schilling test normalize after oral administration of intrinsic factor.[27, 103]

Patients with pancreatic exocrine insufficiency may have abnormal results of the Schilling test, with or without added intrinsic factor, but they normalize with the addition of pancreatic enzymes (see Chapters 38 and 46). In ileal disease or resection, abnormal results of the Schilling test persist despite use of intrinsic factor. The Schilling test is normal in patients with dietary vitamin B_{12} deficiency, protein-bound (food-bound) vitamin B_{12} malabsorption,[27, 33] and sometimes in congenital transcobalamin II deficiency.[104] In patients with food-bound cobalamin malabsorption, a modified Schilling test using cobalamin bound to eggs, chicken serum, or various meats can be used to detect cobalamin malabsorption.[33]

False-positive results of the Schilling test may be due to renal dysfunction or inadequate urine collections.[103] The value of this test is diminished by the need for accurately timed urine collections. Results in the 5% to 10% excretion range are often difficult to interpret. A variation of the standard Schilling test is the dual-isotope or "single-stage" Schilling test, using two different cobalamin isotopes simultaneously, one of them bound to intrinsic factor. This makes it possible to perform the first two phases of the Schilling test in one day. However, the results of this test are not as accurate as the standard protocol.[27, 103]

Serum Test for Vitamin B_{12} and Folate Deficiency

Measurements of serum cobalamin and folate concentrations are commonly used to detect deficiency states of these vitamins. The sensitivity and specificity of these tests are unknown, because there is no established gold standard and because serum levels do not always correlate with body stores.[27, 105] Some authors suggest that the disappearance of symptoms after cobalamin or folate replacement is probably the most sensitive marker for deficiency of these vitamins.[103] Several causes of misleading serum cobalamin levels have been established. Serum vitamin B_{12} levels can be normal although body stores are depleted in small intestinal bacterial overgrowth (due to production of inactive cobalamin analogs by the bacteria), in liver disease, in myeloproliferative disorders, and in congenital transcobalamin II deficiency. In contrast, use of oral contraceptives, pregnancy, and folate deficiency can cause low serum cobalamin levels despite normal body stores.[103] Serum folate concentrations decrease within a few days of dietary folate restriction even if tissue stores are normal. Feeding also influences serum folate levels, and therefore determination of folate in the fasting state is recommended. Measurement of red blood cell folate has been considered a better estimate of folate tissue stores by some authors.[33, 103]

In cobalamin deficiency, serum concentrations of methymalonic acid and total homocysteine are elevated.[33, 103, 105] Folate deficiency results only in an increase in serum homocysteine concentration.[33, 103, 105] In cases of patients with slightly low or borderline serum cobalamin levels, determination of methymalonic acid and homocysteine may therefore be helpful in establishing the diagnosis of a deficiency state. These metabolites tend to normalize within 1 to 2 weeks after replacement therapy, and some authors have suggested that the measurement of these metabolites can be used to distinguish between cobalamin and folate deficiency states.[105] The distinction is important because in cobalamin-deficient patients supplemental replacement of folate may correct hematologic changes, despite progression of neurologic disease.

Tests for Bacterial Overgrowth

Tests for the diagnosis of bacterial overgrowth are covered in more detail in Chapter 90. Briefly, tests used to diagnose bacterial overgrowth are the quantitative culture of a small intestinal aspirate (which is considered to be the gold standard) and several breath tests, including the ^{14}C-glycocholate breath test, the ^{14}C-D-xylose breath test, the lactulose-H_2 breath test, and the glucose-H_2 breath test. The rationale for the breath tests is the production of volatile metabolites, that is, $^{14}CO_2$ or H_2, from the administered substances by intraluminal bacteria, which can be measured in the exhaled air. Details about the sensitivity and specificity of the various tests are provided in Chapter 89.

Tests for Exocrine Pancreatic Function

Pancreatic function tests are discussed in detail in Chapter 46. Invasive pancreatic function tests require duodenal intubation and measurement of pancreatic enzyme, volume, or bicarbonate output after pancreatic stimulation by a liquid test meal (Lundh test) or by injection of cholecystokinin and/or secretin. Noninvasive tests include measurement of fecal chymotrypsin or elastase concentration, the fluorescein dilaurate test, and the *N*-benzoyl-L-tyrosyl para-aminobenzoic acid (NBT-PABA) test. In many clinical settings the measurement of fecal concentration of chymotrypsin or elastase may be sufficient for the diagnosis or exclusion of exocrine pancreatic insufficiency. Elastase may have a higher sensitivity for the detection of exocrine pancreatic insufficiency as compared with chymotrypsin.[106]

Tests for Bile Salt Malabsorption

In patients with steatorrhea due to ileal disease or resection, bile salt malabsorption is usually present, but measurement of bile acid malabsorption is of limited clinical value in these patients. In some patients with diarrhea without steatorrhea, bile salt malabsorption may be present in the absence of overt ileal disease, and in these cases measurement of bile salt absorption may be helpful.

Measurement of Fecal Bile Acid Output

Elevated fecal bile acid concentrations and/or output can indicate intestinal bile acid malabsorption.[107] Under steady-state conditions, the increased fecal bile acid output reflects increased hepatic synthesis of bile acids.[108] However, in severe bile acid malabsorption, fecal bile acid output theoretically can be reduced if hepatic synthesis of bile acids is impaired. The measurement can be performed by either enzymatic methods or by gas chromatography. This test requires a quantitative stool collection, and the analytic techniques are time consuming and require considerable expertise.

^{14}C-Taurocholate Bile Acid Absorption Test

This test requires a 72-hour stool collection after ingestion of a radioactively labeled bile acid. The rate of intestinal bile acid absorption is calculated from the fecal recovery of ^{14}C-labeled taurocholic acid (^{14}C-TCA). Normal values for this test have been established in normal subjects with laxative-induced diarrhea, because diarrhea by itself can increase fecal losses of bile acids.[108] Clinical limitations of this test are that it requires substantial analytical work, access to a gamma camera, and a time-consuming stool collection.

Therapeutic Trial of Bile Acid Binding Resins (Cholestyramine)

A therapeutic trial of cholestyramine or other bile acid binding resins can be used to diagnose bile acid malabsorption as a cause of diarrhea. It is, however, controversial to what extent a clinical response to cholestyramine correlates with the presence of bile acid malabsorption, because cholestyramine may have a nonspecific effect in patients with diarrhea from other causes. Failure to improve diarrhea significantly within 3 days of starting cholestyramine makes bile acid malabsorption as a cause of diarrhea unlikely; however, it has been reported that some patients respond only to large doses of cholestyramine.

In patients with established bile acid malabsorption in whom there is no improvement on bile acid binding resins, it is very unlikely that bile acid malabsorption is the cause of diarrhea. In these patients, bile acid malabsorption is considered to be a secondary phenomenon due to the "washout effect."[108] It should be noted that in patients with severe bile acid malabsorption resulting in steatorrhea, cholestyramine may even aggravate fat malabsorption and diarrhea.[3] Therefore, without further testing for bile acid malabsorption, neither a positive nor a negative result of a therapeutic trial are a proof for the presence or absence of bile acid malabsorption.

Selenium-75 Labeled Homotaurocholic Acid Test

The radioactive taurocholic acid analog used for this test is resistant to bacterial deconjugation. After oral administration, the patient undergoes serial gamma scintigraphy to measure whole-body bile acid retention or, as suggested by some authors, bile acid retention in the gallbladder.[109] The limitations of this test are that normal values for bile acid retention, which are used to compare between normal and abnormal bile acid absorption, were obtained only in healthy subjects without diarrhea.[110] However, as mentioned above, "secondary" bile acid malabsorption can be induced by diarrhea itself and is proportional to the stool weight, as demonstrated with the ^{14}C-TCA test.[108] To be of clinical usefulness, adequate normal values need to be established for patients with diarrhea for this test. This test is very time consuming because bile acid retention needs to be measured, depending on the protocol, 4 or 7 days after the bile acid administration.

D-Xylose Test

The D-xylose test was introduced in the 1950s to distinguish small intestinal from pancreatic causes of malabsorption.[111] Most verification studies have involved patients with celiac disease or inflammatory bowel disease. The test is of limited clinical value today and has mostly been replaced by a small bowel biopsy.[112]

Absorption of D-xylose, a pentose, is facilitated by passive diffusion. About 50% of the absorbed D-xylose is metabolized, and the remainder is excreted in urine. After an overnight fast, a 25-g dose of D-xylose is swallowed and the patient is encouraged to drink to maintain good urine output. Urine is collected for the next 5 hours. As an alternative, 1 hour after ingestion of D-xylose a venous sample may be taken.[113] Less than 4 g (16% excretion) of D-xylose in the urine collection or a serum xylose concentration below 20 mg/dL is indicative of abnormal intestinal absorption. In direct comparisons, the traditional urine test appears to be more reliable than the 1-hour blood test.

False-positive results occur if the duration of urine collection is too short or if the patient is dehydrated or has renal dysfunction, significant ascites, delayed gastric emptying, and portal hypertension. D-Xylose absorption may be normal in patients with only mild impairment of mucosal function or with predominantly distal small bowel disease. Because D-xylose is susceptible to bacterial metabolism, absorption is diminished in patients with bacterial overgrowth, although the test has a poor sensitivity for detection of this condition.[114]

Intestinal Permeability Tests

Intestinal permeability tests are mostly used in studies of the pathophysiology of intestinal disorders. They do not provide a specific diagnosis.[115]

Most current permeability tests are based on the differential absorption of mono- and disaccharides. Mucosal damage results in an increased permeability for disaccharides and oligosaccharides due to epithelial damage and a decreased permeability of monosaccharides due to reduction of mucosal surface area.[116] Absorption is measured by urinary excretion. The expression of results as the absorption ratio of the mono- and disaccharide minimizes the influence of gastric emptying, intestinal transit, renal and hepatic function, and variations in time of urine collections.[117]

Increased intestinal permeability has been shown to predict the development of Crohn's disease or relapse in patients with this disease.[118, 119] In celiac disease, permeability tests are a sensitive marker for advanced disease and have also been used to assess response to a gluten-free diet.[120] Hypertransaminasemia in patients with celiac disease correlates with increased intestinal permeability.[121] Disturbances of intestinal permeability have been documented in users of nonsteroidal anti-inflammatory drugs,[122] in inflammatory joint disease,[123] and in diabetic diarrhea.[124]

^{13}C Breath Tests

The increasing availability of methods for analyzing stable isotopes has raised interest in replacing the radioactive ^{14}C by nonradioactive ^{13}C.[125–127] With regard to malabsorption, ^{13}C-labeled substrates have been evaluated for the diagnosis of steatorrhea,[128] evaluation of the digestibility of egg protein,[102] and the diagnosis of small bowel bacterial overgrowth and exocrine pancreatic insufficiency.[129] In general, because of concerns about diagnostic accuracy, costs of the substrates, and the equipment and limited availability, these tests have not gained widespread acceptance.

Table 89–12 | **Prevalence of Acquired Primary Lactase Deficiency**

Examples of groups among whom lactase deficiency predominates
(60–100% lactase deficient)
Near East and Mediterranean: Arabs, Jews, Greek Cypriots, southern Italians
Asia: Thais, Indonesians, Chinese, Koreans
Africa: South Nigerians, Hausa, Bantu
North and South America: Eskimos, Canadian and U.S. Indians, Chami Indians
Examples of groups among whom lactase persistence predominates
(2–30% lactase deficient)
Northern Europeans
Africa: Hima, Tussi, Nomadic Fulani
India: Punjab and New Delhi areas

From Johnson JD. The regional and ethnic distribution of lactose malabsorption. *In* Paige DM, Bayless TM (eds.): Lactose Digestion. Clinical and Nutritional Implications, 1st ed. Baltimore, The Johns Hopkins University Press, 1981, p 11.

MALABSORPTION IN SPECIFIC DISEASE STATES

Lactose Malabsorption and Intolerance

Deficiency of the intestinal brush border enzyme lactase may lead to lactose malabsorption, which may result in lactose intolerance. Lactase deficiency in infants may have several causes. Unlike other intestinal disaccharidases, which develop early in fetal life, lactase levels remain low until the 34th week of gestation.[130] *Transient lactase deficiency in premature infants* may lead to symptoms of lactose malabsorption, like diarrhea, until normal intestinal lactase activity develops. In rare cases, in which enzyme deficiency is manifest at the time of birth and is permanent, *congenital lactase deficiency* has to be considered. *Reversible lactase deficiency* may occur at every age as a result of transient small bowel injury associated with acute diarrhea illnesses.

Acquired primary lactase deficiency is the most common form of lactase deficiency worldwide. Most populations lose considerable lactase activity in adulthood.[131] The decline in lactase activity is a multifactorial process that is regulated at the gene transcription level[132] and leads to decreased biosynthesis or retardation of intracellular transport or maturation of the enzyme lactase-phlorizin hydrolase.[133] This "normal" form of lactase deficiency usually manifests symptoms only in adulthood, although lactase levels in these persons start to decline during childhood.[134]

Lactase activity persists in most adults of western European heritage (Table 89–12). Even in adults with preserved lactase activity, the activity of lactase is only about half the activity of sucrase and less than 20% the activity of maltase.[134] This makes lactose digestion much more susceptible to a reduction of mucosal digestive function in acute or chronic gastrointestinal illnesses.

In lactose malabsorbers it may remain unclear whether lactose malabsorption is due to acquired primary lactase deficiency or is the consequence of another small bowel disorder. Therefore, in the individual lactose malabsorber, especially if he or she has an ethnic background with a low prevalence of acquired primary lactase deficiency, it may be necessary to exclude other malabsorptive small bowel disorders, like celiac disease.

The main symptoms of lactose intolerance are bloating, abdominal cramps, increased flatus, and diarrhea. The development of bloating and abdominal cramps is presumably associated with increased perception of luminal distension by gas.[135] There is no clear relation between the amount of lactose ingestion and the severity of these symptoms.[136] Ingestion of as little as 3 g of lactose to as high as 96 g of lactose may be required to induce symptoms in individuals with lactose malabsorption.[137] Severity of gastrointestinal symptoms, including diarrhea, has been shown to be greater in adults with shorter small bowel transit time,[138] but there is no such relation between intestinal transit and symptoms in children.[139] Also, in pregnant women and in thyrotoxic patients with Graves' disease, changes in intestinal motility play a role in the clinical manifestation of lactose malabsorption.[140, 141]

Considering the poor correlation between lactose malabsorption and lactose intolerance, it is very important to monitor symptoms during a lactose hydrogen breath test and to confirm with the patient that symptoms during the test are representative of the patient's symptoms.

Patients in whom a clear association between symptoms and lactose malabsorption can be established should be educated about a lactose-reduced or lactose-free diet. Yogurts may be better tolerated by these patients,[142] and they provide a good source of calcium. Consumption of whole milk or chocolate milk, rather than skim milk, and consuming milk with meals may reduce symptoms of lactose intolerance, presumably due to prolongation of gastric emptying. Alternatively, supplementation of dairy products with lactase of microbiologic origin may be suggested.[143] Furthermore, because many carbohydrates other than lactose are incompletely absorbed by the normal small intestine[47] and because dietary fibers also may be metabolized by colonic bacteria, persistence of some symptoms of "lactose intolerance" while the patient is on a lactose-free diet is not uncommon. It also has to be kept in mind that symptoms after ingestion of dairy products may also be due to milk protein allergy or to intolerance of fat.

Fructose Malabsorption and Intolerance

Fructose is found in modern diets either as a constituent of the disaccharide sucrose or as the monosaccharide, which is used as a sweetener in a variety of food items. Fructose as the constituent of sucrose is absorbed by a well-characterized absorptive system integrating enzymatic hydrolysis of the disaccharide by sucrase and transfer of the resulting two monosaccharides through the apical membrane of the epithelial cell. In contrast, the absorptive capacity for fructose, which is not accompanied by glucose, is relatively small.[144]

Ingestion of food that contains fructose may result in symptoms like abdominal bloating or diarrhea[145] and may also provoke symptoms in irritable bowel syndrome.[146] It has been suggested that as little as 3 g of fructose may provoke symptoms in functional bowel disorders.[147] Fructose malabsorption is usually identified by a positive breath hydrogen test after ingestion of 25 or 50 g of fructose. Because fructose content in fruit and in soft drinks is usually below 8 g/100 g of fruit or drink, the amounts of fructose used in the breath hydrogen test are unphysiologic, and there are no data on how many asymptomatic people would have a positive test result. Nevertheless, fructose contents of 30 to 40 g/100 g can be present in chocolate or hard nougat.[148]

Most studies on fructose malabsorption are limited to patients who presented with symptoms of fructose intolerance, which in this context means development of gastrointestinal symptoms after ingestion of fructose-containing food. In a group of patients with isolated fructose malabsorption, no defect of the gene encoding for the luminal fructose transporter (*GLUT5*) could be detected.[149] It is therefore currently unclear whether patients who present with symptoms of fructose malabsorption really have a defect of intestinal fructose absorption or belong to a subset of people in whom ingestion of foods rich in fructose provokes symptoms related to other disorders, like irritable bowel syndrome. Patients who develop symptoms after ingestion of fructose-rich food may also represent a subset of persons with special, and not necessarily abnormal, colonic bacterial activity.[150]

In conclusion, testing for fructose malabsorption by the hydrogen breath test may be useful in identifying a subset of patients in whom dietary restriction of foods with excessive fructose content may be useful for the treatment of bloating and diarrhea. Symptoms most likely are the result of ingestion of unphysiologic amounts of fructose rather than the consequence of a defect in fructose absorption.

Steatorrhea due to Ileal Bile Acid Malabsorption

Bile acid malabsorption is usually present in patients with resections, bypass operations, or severe diseases of the ileum, where specific bile acid transport proteins are normally located. The clinical consequences of bile acid malabsorption depend on whether bile acid loss can or cannot be compensated by increased synthesis by the liver.[151] Ileal resection of more than 100 cm usually results in severe bile acid malabsorption that cannot be compensated by increased hepatic synthesis and therefore causes steatorrhea by impaired micelle formation due to decreased luminal concentrations of conjugated bile acids.[3, 151] In ileal resections of less than 100 cm, bile acid malabsorption can usually be compensated by increased hepatic synthesis, and malabsorbed bile acids cause secretory diarrhea rather than steatorrhea.[3, 151] Secretory diarrhea caused by or associated with bile acid malabsorption is discussed in detail in Chapter 9.

The different pathophysiology of steatorrhea and secretory diarrhea due to bile acid malabsorption not only determines the clinical picture but also is important for choosing the appropriate therapy. In patients with compensated bile acid malabsorption, binding of bile salts in the lumen of the intestine by cholestyramine reduces diarrhea. In contrast, in decompensated bile acid malabsorption, cholestyramine further increases depletion of the bile acid pool and therefore results in worsening of steatorrhea. In several cases of decompensated bile acid malabsorption after extensive ileal resections, intestinal fat absorption was markedly improved by the oral administration of conjugated bile acids.[90, 152, 153]

A syndrome of primary bile acid malabsorption with normal ileal morphology has been reported in children. In these patients, bile acid malabsorption results in severe diarrhea and steatorrhea (which starts at the time of birth), failure to thrive, and reduced plasma cholesterol levels.[154, 155] A recent study in an index case has shown that bile acid malabsorption is caused by mutations in the ileal sodium–bile acid cotransporter gene.[156]

Amyloidosis

Malabsorption has been reported in AL-amyloidosis, AA-amyloidosis, and familial amyloidosis.[157–159] Fat malabsorption occurs in less than 5% of patients with AL-amyloidosis,[157] whereas fat malabsorption was present in 58% of Swedish patients with familial amyloidosis.[158] Fecal fat excretion can reach levels up to 60 g/day.[158] Gastrointestinal absorption of D-xylose and vitamin B_{12} can be reduced,[158, 160] and protein losing enteropathy may occur.[161] Amyloid deposits are found in the muscle layers, the stroma of the lamina propria and the submucosa, the wall of mucosal and submucosal vessels of the gastrointestinal tract, and in enteric and extraenteric nerves.[162, 163]

In many amyloidosis patients with diarrhea and/or malabsorption, symptoms suggestive of autonomic neuropathy are present.[158] Diarrhea and malabsorption in an individual patient with amyloidosis are most likely of multifactorial origin. Diarrhea and malabsorption may be mediated by rapid intestinal transit due to autonomic neuropathy and intestinal myopathy,[158] decreased absorption due to a physical barrier effect of amyloid deposits,[164] or small intestinal bacterial overgrowth.[160] Bile acid malabsorption, which is found in many amyloidosis patients with autonomic neuropathy, may be a contributing factor.[165] Barium studies in amyloidosis patients are usually normal, but they may show thickened folds, nodular lesions, filling defects, dilatation of bowel segments, or altered transit of the gastrointestinal tract.[159, 166] The endoscopic appearance of the gastrointestinal mucosa can show a fine granular appearance, polypoid protrusions, erosions, ulcerations, atrophic changes, and mucosal friability, but in many affected patients there are no macroscopic changes.[159, 163] Histologic examination demonstrates amyloid deposits in 72% of esophageal, 75% to 95% of gastric, 83% to 100% of small intestinal, and 75% to 95% of colorectal biopsies.[157, 163, 167] Subcutaneous fat pad aspirate/biopsies may more safely make the diagnosis without having to resort to endoscopic biopsy and its risks (e.g., bleeding). Amyloid deposits may not be seen on routine histologic stains and may only be revealed by a Congo red stain. Therapy of diarrhea in amyloidosis includes attempts to prolong intestinal transit time by opioids or octreotide and to avoid further amyloid deposition in the tissue.[168]

Malabsorption Caused by Drugs and Food Supplements

Table 89–13 lists drugs and food supplements reported to induce malabsorption of vitamins, minerals, or nutrients, as well as the suggested pathophysiologic mechanisms.

Malabsorption after Gastric Resection

Severe steatorrhea after total and partial gastric resections has been a long-observed complication of these operations (see also Chapter 42).[12] Fecal fat excretion rates are usually between 15 and 20 g/day,[1] but values of up to 60 g/day have been reported.[169, 170] Suggested mechanisms include defective mixing of nutrients with digestive secretions, lack of gastric acid and gastric lipase secretion, decreased small bowel transit time, small intestinal bacterial overgrowth, and pancreatic insufficiency.[1, 171] Recent studies showed that pancreatic enzyme supplements[172] and antibiotic treatment[171] did not improve fat malabsorption or symptoms after gastric

Table 89–13 | **Drugs and Dietary Products Causing Malabsorption**

SUBSTANCE	SUBSTRATE MALABSORBED	SUGGESTED MECHANISM	REFERENCE(S)
Acarbose	Carbohydrates	Inhibition of α-glucosidase	254
Antacids	Phosphate, iron, vitamin A	Luminal binding of substrates	255
Biguanides (metformin, phenformin)	Cobalamin, folate, glucose	Inhibition of intestinal glucose or folate absorption, reduced ileal absorption of cobalamin–IF complex	255–257
Carbamazepine	Folate	Inhibition of intestinal folate absorption	258
Cholestyramine	Fat, fat-soluble vitamins	Binding of conjugated bile salts	255
Colchicine	Fat, xylose, nitrogen, cobalamin, carotene	Mucosal damage and villous atrophy at high doses (impaired processing of IF-cobalamin receptor, cubilin)	27, 255, 259
Contraceptives, oral*	Folate	Inhibition of pteroylpolyglutamate hydrolase (folate conjugase)	255
Ethanol	D-Xylose, fat, glucose, nitrogen, thiamine, cobalamin, folate	Mucosal damage, decreased disaccharidase activity, decreased pancreatic exocrine function and bile secretion	34, 255
Fiber, phytates	Iron, calcium, magnesium, zinc	Chelating agents	260
Glucocorticoids	Calcium	Inhibition of calcium absorption	24
Histamine 2 receptor antagonists*	Cobalamin	Impaired release of food-bound vitamin B_{12} due to reduced gastric acid and pepsin secretion (and reduced IF secretion)	261
Irritant laxatives (phenolphthalein, bisacodyl, anthraquinones)	Fat, glucose, xylose	Washout effect, toxic effect on the mucosa	89, 255
Methotrexate	Folate, fat, cobalamin, xylose	Mucosal damage, inhibition of intestinal folate transport	255, 260
Methyldopa†	Generalized malabsorption	Mucosal damage	262
Neomycin	Fat, nitrogen, fat-soluble vitamins, cobalamin, mono- and disaccharides, iron	Mucosal damage, disruption of micelle formation	255, 259, 260
Olestra*	Fat-soluble vitamins	Binding of fat-soluble vitamins	263, 264
Orlistat	Fat, fat-soluble vitamins	Inhibition of pancreatic lipase	254
Para-aminosalicylate	Fat, cobalamin, folate	Unknown	27, 255
Phenytoin	Folate, calcium	Inhibition of folate and calcium absorption due to luminal alkalinization, impaired vitamin D metabolism	24, 260, 265
Proton pump inhibitors*	Cobalamin	Impaired release of food-bound cobalamin due to reduced gastric acid secretion, small bowel bacterial overgrowth	28
Pyrimethamine	Folate	Competitive inhibition of intestinal folate absorption	266
Somatostatin analogs (Octreotide)	Fat	Inhibition of hepatobiliary bile acid secretion, inhibition of pancreatic enzyme secretion, inhibition of cholecystokinin release	267, 268
Sulfonamides, including sulfasalazine	Folate	Inhibition of pteroylpolyglutamate hydrolase and folate transport	103, 260
Tetracycline	Calcium	Precipitation of luminal calcium	269
Thiazides	Calcium	Decreased $1,25(OH)_2$ vitamin D synthesis	270
Trimamterene*	Folate	Competitive inhibition of intestinal folate absorption	266, 271

*Malabsorption usually does not result in deficiency states.
†Findings in case reports.
IF, intrinsic factor.

resections. Although less appreciated in the more recent literature, total and partial gastric resections can also result in significant protein malabsorption.[12] The absorption of carbohydrates seems not to be significantly impaired. Nutrient malabsorption in these patients can result in gastrointestinal symptoms such as diarrhea and severe weight loss.[173, 174]

Loss of parietal cells after total gastric resection results in diminished intrinsic factor secretion, which in turn leads to malabsorption of vitamin B_{12} and, in about 30% of patients, vitamin B_{12} deficiency. Lack of release of food-bound cobalamin by diminished gastric acid and pepsin secretion and bacterial overgrowth have been implicated as additional pathogenetic factors. Iron malabsorption resulting in iron deficiency anemia is also commonly present in patients with gastric resections. The mechanisms for iron malabsorption are not fully established. Lack of acid secretion resulting in decreased solubilization of iron salts has been suggested as one of the responsible factors. Calcium absorption can be severely impaired in patients with gastric resections, which may result in reduced bone density.[175] The mechanisms for calcium malabsorption are probably various, including decreased solubilization of calcium salts by the loss of gastric acid secretion, rapid intestinal transit, low calcium intake resulting from milk intolerance, and malabsorption of vitamin D. Recent studies in gastrectomized rats have suggested that diminished calcium absorption after gastric resections is mainly, if not entirely, due to decreased calcium solubilization.[176] In contrast, studies in humans have shown that calcium absorption is normal in subjects with atrophic gastritis and in subjects in whom acid secretion was inhibited by acid-inhibiting drugs.[177] Treatment of patients with gastric resections should include the adequate supplementation of malabsorbed vitamins and minerals to prevent serious long-term complications.[178]

Malabsorption in the Elderly

Malabsorption in elderly persons should not be ascribed to the aging process; it should be evaluated like malabsorption occurring in younger patients. In healthy elderly persons, small bowel histology is normal despite a decline in cell turnover and continual cell renewal.[179, 180] Malabsorption of fat has been described in chronic congestive heart failure[181] and in chronic intestinal ischemia (see Chapter 119), but this is not due to aging per se. Elderly persons may be more susceptible to insult and subsequent decompensation of gastrointestinal function.[182]

Nutrient deficiencies, presumably caused by malabsorption, may be present in elderly persons with no overt gastrointestinal disease. An increased risk of deficiency of folate and vitamin B_{12}, despite adequate intake of these vitamins, has been reported in the elderly.[183] Malnutrition in the elderly can considerably contribute to morbidity and mortality, although it may be difficult to ascertain whether weight loss is due to altered appetite, increased catabolism, or malabsorption.

Small bowel bacterial overgrowth in elderly persons with gastric hypochlorhydria secondary to atrophic gastritis or treatment with a proton pump inhibitor is usually not associated with clinically significant malabsorption,[184] but an improvement in nutritional status after antibiotic treatment has been described in some elderly patients.[185]

Connective Tissue Diseases

Scleroderma

Various degrees of gastrointestinal involvement occur in most patients with systemic sclerosis. Early pathology is characterized by vasculopathy, which results in ischemia and progressive organ dysfunction.[186] The typical histologic findings include atrophy of the muscle layers with increased deposition of elastin and collagen in the submucosa and serosa and between smooth muscle bundles of the muscularis externa.[35] Small bowel biopsy may reveal an increased number of plasma cells within the lamina propria and collagen deposits around and between lobules of Brunner's glands in the submucosa of the duodenum.[187]

Malabsorption in scleroderma is usually due to bacterial overgrowth secondary to ineffective motility in the small bowel,[188] but other factors, like decreased mucosal blood flow,[189] may also contribute. Malabsorption and bacterial overgrowth are not limited to patients with diffuse disease but may also occur in patients with long-standing limited cutaneous systemic sclerosis.[190] Elevations of serum concentrations of motilin and cholecystokinin have been described in patients with fat malabsorption[191] but are thought to be secondary to myogenic or neurogenic disturbances of intestinal or gallbladder contractions.[192] In addition to antibiotic treatment of bacterial overgrowth, low doses of octreotide (50 μg subcutaneously every evening over 3 weeks) have been shown to induce intestinal migrating motor complexes, reduce bacterial overgrowth, and improve abdominal symptoms.[188]

Lupus Erythematosus and Other Connective Tissue Diseases

Excessive fecal fat excretion associated with abnormal results of a D-xylose test may be found in some patients with lupus erythematosus. These findings may be accompanied by flattened and deformed villi with an inflammatory infiltrate on duodenal biopsy.[193] Malabsorption that resolved after treatment with prednisolone has also been described in association with hypereosinophilic syndrome in lupus erythematosus.[194] Malabsorption is an uncommon feature of mixed connective tissue disease and polymyositis.[195, 196]

Congenital Defects Causing Malabsorption

Table 89–14 lists congenital intestinal diseases that result in malabsorption of specific substrates or in generalized malabsorption syndrome. Most of these diseases are very rare, but some occur with an increased frequency in certain ethnic groups.

Amino Acid Transport Defects

Amino acids are absorbed by the enterocyte as oligopeptides, dipeptides, and free amino acids. In several inborn diseases, transport defects for different groups of amino acids have been identified in the intestine and kidney (see

Table 89–14 | **Congenital Disorders of the Gastric and Intestinal Mucosa Resulting in Malabsorption**

	SUGGESTED MODE OF INHERITANCE	MALABSORBED SUBSTRATES	SUGGESTED MECHANISM OF MALABSORPTION	CLINICAL PRESENTATION	REFERENCE(S)
Amino acids					
Hartnup disorder	AR	Neutral amino acids (leucine, methionine, phenylalanine, tyrosine, valine, histidine?, lysine?)	Decreased intestinal absorption of free neutral amino acids	Most patients are asymptomatic; in some patients photosensitive skin rash, intermittent ataxia, psychotic behavior, mental retardation, diarrhea may occur	198
Cystinuria (types 1–3)	AR and incomplete AR	Cystine and dibasic amino acids (lysine, ornithine, arginine)	Decreased intestinal absorption of specific free amino acids; the defect is probably located at the brush border membrane. *Type 1*: no transport of cystine, lysine, or arginine. *Type 2*: no transport of lysine and arginine and reduced cystine transport. *Type 3*: reduced or normal cystine transport and reduced lysine and arginine transport	Aminoaciduria, cystine stones in the urinary tract	197
Lysinuric protein intolerance	AR	Dibasic amino acids (lysine, ornithine, arginine)	Defect of the transporter on the basolateral membrane for cationic amino acids (also malabsorption of di- and oligopeptides)	Hyperammonemia, nausea, vomiting, diarrhea, protein malnutrition, failure to thrive, aversion to protein-rich food, sparse hair	200
Isolated lysinuria*	?	Lysine	Decreased intestinal absorption of lysine	Mental retardation, malnutrition, failure to thrive	200
Iminoglycinuria	AR	L-Proline	Impaired intestinal absorption of L-proline in a subgroup of subjects	Aminoaciduria, benign disorder	199
Blue diaper syndrome*	AR	Tryptophan	Intestinal tryptophan absorption defect	Blue discoloration of diapers, failure to thrive, hypercalcemia, nephrocalcinosis	272
Oasthouse syndrome*	AR	Methionine	Intestinal methionine absorption defect	Mental retardation, convulsions, diarrhea, white hair, hyperpnea, characteristic sweet smell	273
Lowe's syndrome	XR	Lysine, arginine	Impaired intestinal lysine and arginine absorption	Aminoaciduria, mental retardation, cataracts, rickets, choreoathetosis, renal disease	274
Carbohydrates					
Congenital lactase deficiency	AR	Lactose	Permanent very low lactase activity	Diarrhea, bloating, dehydration starting in the first days of life	201, 275
Sucrase-isomaltase	AR	Sucrose, starch	Sucrase activity absent, isomaltase activity absent or reduced, reduced maltase activity	Osmotic diarrhea, failure to thrive starting after starch or sucrose ingestion	21, 275
Trehalase deficiency	AR	Trehalose	Lack of intestinal trehalase activity	Diarrhea and/or vomiting after mushroom ingestion	21, 201
Glucose galactose malabsorption	AR	Glucose, galactose	Defect of the brush border sodium-glucose cotransporter (SGLT1)	Neonatal onset of osmotic diarrhea, dehydration, intermittent or constant glycosuria	22, 202, 276
Fat					
Abetalipoproteinemia	AR	Fat, fat-soluble vitamins	Triglyceride accumulation in the enterocytes, no chylomicron formation	Steatorrhea, diarrhea, neurologic symptoms, retinitis pigmentosa, failure to thrive, absence of chylomicrons and VLDL in the blood, acanthocytosis	10
Familial hypobetalipoproteinemia	Incomplete AD	Fat, fat-soluble vitamins	Triglyceride accumulation in the enterocytes in homozygotes	*Homozygotes*: similar clinical manifestations as in abetalipoproteinemia. *Heterozygotes*: fat absorption probably normal, hypolipidemia, neurologic manifestations	10
Chylomicron retention disease (Anderson's disease)	AR	Fat	Accumulation of chylomicrons in the enterocytes	Steatorrhea, failure to thrive, absence of chylomicrons and reduced LDL levels in the blood, neurologic symptoms may occur	10

Table 89–14 | **Congenital Disorders of the Gastric and Intestinal Mucosa Resulting in Malabsorption** *Continued*

	SUGGESTED MODE OF INHERITANCE	MALABSORBED SUBSTRATES	SUGGESTED MECHANISM OF MALABSORPTION	CLINICAL PRESENTATION	REFERENCE(S)
Wolman's disease	AR	Fat	Deficient activity of the lysosomal acid lipase, causing accumulation of cholesteryl esters and triglycerides in various body tissues, infiltration of intestinal mucosa with foamy cells, intestinal damage	Steatorrhea, hepatosplenomegaly, abdominal distension, failure to thrive, adrenal calcification	277
Vitamins					
Congenital intrinsic factor deficiency (congenital pernicious anemia)	AR	Cobalamin (Vit B_{12})	Defective synthesis of IF or synthesis of an abnormal IF	Megaloblastic anemia, neurologic symptoms, delayed development	31, 104
Imerslund-Gräsbeck syndrome (ileal Vit B_{12} malabsorption)	AR	Cobalamin (Vit B_{12})	Defective ileal absorption of IF-Cbl complex (probably several different molecular mechanisms: decreased affinity of IF-Cbl receptor [cubilin] or expression of an unstable IF-Cbl receptor)	Megaloblastic anemia, neurologic symptoms, proteinuria	27, 31, 104
Transcobalamin II deficiency	AR	Cobalamin (Vit B_{12})	Defective transport of Cbl out of the enterocytes into portal blood due to total absence or malfunction of transcobalamin II	Vomiting, diarrhea, failure to thrive, anemia, immunodeficiency, neurologic symptoms	31, 104, 278
Congenital folate malabsorption	AR	Folate	Defective folate transport across the intestinal mucosa	Megaloblastic anemia, diarrhea, failure to thrive, neurologic symptoms	276, 279, 280
Minerals					
Acrodermatitis enteropathica	AR	Zinc	Defective zinc absorption in the small intestine	Diarrhea, scaling erythematous dermatitis, alopecia, neuropsychatric symptoms (onset of symptoms after weaning)	43
Isolated magnesium malabsorption	AR	Magnesium	Selective defect in intestinal magnesium absorption	Tetany, convulsion, diarrhea	39, 281
Menkes disease	XR	Copper	General copper transport disorder, intestinal copper malabsorption with copper accumulation in the intestinal mucosa	Cerebral degeneration, diarrhea, abnormal hair, hypopigmentation, arterial rupture, thrombosis, hypothermia, bone changes	276, 282, 283
Occipital horn syndrome (X-linked cutis laxa)	XR	Copper	Probably mild form of same defect as in Menkes disease	Inguinal hernias, bladder and ureteric diverticula, skin and joint laxiety, chronic diarrhea, bone changes	283
Hereditary selective deficiency of $1\alpha,25(OH)_2D$	AR	Calcium	Defective 25(OH)D 1α hydroxylase resulting in $1\alpha,25(OH)_2D$ deficiency and reduced intestinal calcium absorption	Bone pain, deformities and fractures, muscle weakness	37
Hereditary generalized resistance to $1\alpha,25(OH)_2D$	AR	Calcium	Defects in the vitamin D receptor resulting in malabsorption of calcium	Bone pain, deformities and fractures, muscle weakness, alopecia	37
Other defects					
Enterokinase deficiency	AR	Protein, fat	Defective activation of pancreatic proenzymes due to lack of enterokinase	Diarrhea, failure to thrive, hypoproteinemia, edema, anemia	15, 206
Congenital bile acid malabsorption	AR	Bile acids, fat	Defect of the ileal sodium bile acid cotransporter	Steatorrhea, diarrhea, failure to thrive	154–156
Microvillus inclusion disease	AR	Carbohydrates, fat, cobalamin, electrolytes, water	Villous atrophy with microvillus inclusions in enterocytes, absent or shortened brush border microvilli	Severe watery diarrhea, steatorrhea, requiring total parenteral nutrition	284

*Only reported in a few case reports.

AD, autosomal dominant; AR, autosomal recessive; Cbl, cobalamin (vitamin B_{12}); IF, intrinsic factor; LDL, low-density lipoprotein; Vit B_{12}, vitamin B_{12}; VLDL, very-low-density lipoprotein; XR, X-linked recessive.

Table 89–14). In *iminoglycinuria, Hartnup disorder,* and *cystinuria* the intestinal transport defect seems to be of no or only minor clinical significance, because the amino acids affected by the transporter defects can still be absorbed as oligo- and dipeptides, avoiding protein malnutrition.[197–199] The manifestations in these diseases are therefore mainly due to amino acid transport defects in the kidneys. However, in *lysinuric protein intolerance* the transport defect is located on the basolateral membrane of the enterocytes, leading to malabsorption of cationic amino acids in both their mono- and dipeptide forms.[200] Patients with lysinuric protein intolerance are therefore intolerant to high protein foods and develop protein malnutrition. Malabsorption of lysine resulting in deficiency of this essential amino acid is thought to be an important factor in the development of several disease manifestations in these patients (see Table 89–14).[200]

Disaccharidase Deficiency and Transport Defects for Monosaccharides

In *sucrase-isomaltase deficiency*, symptoms usually start after weaning with the introduction of starch and sucrose to the diet. Symptoms include osmotic diarrhea, failure to thrive, excess flatus, and occasional vomiting. The diagnosis can be established by an oral sucrose absorption test. Treatment includes dietary avoidance of starch and sucrose.[201] Patients with this disease tend to show spontaneous improvement of their symptoms with age. Patients with *glucose-galactose malabsorption* suffer from severe diarrhea, leading to dehydration in the first days of life. The diarrhea stops only if glucose and galactose are eliminated from the diet. Older children and adults tolerate the offending carbohydrates better, but the transport defect is life long. The diagnosis can be established with an oral glucose tolerance test or by *in vitro* glucose absorption tests of intestinal biopsies. Therapy consists of a fructose-based diet free of glucose and galactose. After the age of 3 months it is considered to be safe to add foods containing low quantities of glucose or galactose (e.g., vegetables, fruits, cheese).[202]

Congenital Disorders of Lipid Absorption

Abetalipoproteinemia is an autosomal recessive disorder characterized by triglyceride accumulation in the enterocytes. Although the pathophysiology of this disease is not fully understood, suggested mechanisms include defective processing of B apoproteins or a defect in the assembly of triglyceride-rich lipoproteins.[10] In the homozygous state, the autosomal dominant disorder *familial hypobetalipoproteinemia* has similar clinical manifestations as abetalipoproteinemia (see Table 89–14). This disease seems to be caused by mutations of the apolipoprotein B gene in most cases.[10] *Chylomicron retention disease* is caused by defective secretion of chylomicrons by enterocytes due to an unknown mechanism. General measures of treatment in all three diseases include the replacement of triglycerides containing long-chain fatty acids by medium-chain triglycerides and supplementation with tocopherol.[10]

Congenital Disorders of Cobalamin Absorption

Several different congenital diseases can result in vitamin B_{12} malabsorption. Absence of intrinsic factor synthesis is the most common cause of congenital cobalamin deficiency; abnormal Schilling tests normalize by the coadministration of intrinsic factor.[27, 104] In some patients an abnormal (nonfunctional) intrinsic factor is secreted. In these cases, the abnormal intrinsic factor has a decreased affinity for cobalamin, a decreased affinity for the ileal intrinsic factor cobalamin receptor (cubulin), or an increased susceptibility to proteolysis.[27, 104] *Imerslund-Gräsbeck syndrome* is a congenital disease characterized by malabsorption of the cobalamin–intrinsic factor complex despite normal ileal morphology. Recent data suggest that this syndrome can be caused by several different pathophysiologic mechanisms. Reported mechanisms include decreased activity of the intrinsic factor-cobalamin receptor, cubilin;[203] expression of an unstable receptor;[204] and decreased affinity of cubilin for binding of the cobalamin–intrinsic factor complex.[205] In some patients the receptor appears to be normal as measured in homogenates of ileal biopsies.[206] In *transcobalamin II deficiency*, serum levels of cobalamin are commonly normal, although in most patients intestinal cobalamin absorption is abnormal.[104] A diagnosis can be established by demonstrating the absence of transcobalamin II in the plasma.[104] All congenital disorders in cobalamin malabsorption are treated by the parenteral administration of cobalamin, although high dose oral cobalamin may also suffice (see Chapter 38).

Intestinal Enterokinase Deficiency

Enterokinase is an enzyme secreted by the intestinal mucosa initiating the activation of pancreatic proenzymes. Several patients have been reported to have an inborn deficiency of this enzyme, leading to diarrhea, failure to thrive, and hypoproteinemia mainly due to protein malabsorption. These patients respond well to pancreatic enzyme replacement, and some patients show a tendency to improve with age.[207] Secondary enterokinase deficiency has also been reported in patients with villous atrophy, although patients with celiac disease seem not to be affected.[15]

Malabsorption Associated with Primary Immunodeficiency Diseases

Malabsorption commonly occurs in different entities that are characterized by deficiencies in humoral and/or cellular immunity (see Chapter 2).[208] The immunodeficiency syndromes most commonly associated with malabsorption are *selective IgA deficiency, common variable immunodeficiency (CVID),* and *severe combined immunodeficiency*. The etiologies for malabsorption are different in the separate syndromes.

Selective IgA Deficiency

This is the most common primary immunodeficiency disorder and is characterized by a selective near-absence of secretory and serum IgA, leading to susceptibility to respiratory, urogenital, and gastrointestinal infections. Affected patients also commonly develop autoimmune and allergic diseases. An increased incidence of gluten-sensitive enteropathy has also been reported.[209, 210] However, at least a subgroup of patients have sprue-like small intestinal lesions, leading to severe diarrhea and malabsorption, that are unresponsive to a gluten-free diet.[209] Improvement on immunosuppressive therapy has been described in one case report.[211] Pernicious anemia, giardiasis, and secondary disaccharidase deficiencies are also seen with increased incidence in these patients.[209, 210]

Common Variable Immunodeficiency (Acquired Hypogammaglobulinemia)

This syndrome is composed of a group of immunodeficiency disorders characterized by decreased serum IgG levels. Decreased serum levels of other immunoglobulin subclasses and T-cell defects are commonly present. The onset of the disease is usually in adults, with recurrent respiratory and gastrointestinal infections. Affected patients also have tendencies for autoimmune and neoplastic diseases. Malabsorption and diarrhea occur in 9% to 40% of patients with CVID.[209, 211] Malabsorption involves dietary fat, carbohydrates, vitamin B_{12}, and folate.[208, 212] Small intestinal biopsies show either sprue-like histologic features, including villous shortening with increased numbers of lymphocytes in the epithelium and in the lamina propria, or a pattern similar to graft-versus-host disease.[209, 213] There are some specific histologic features, namely a near absence of plasma cells. There is no response to a gluten-free diet. Therefore, it appears that the sprue-like syndrome in CVID is a distinct entity,[213] and it is sometimes referred to as hypogammaglobulinemic sprue.[214] In some patients with CVID, foamy macrophages are present, as found in Whipple's disease, but in contrast to Whipple's disease the macrophages do not contain periodic–acid–Schiff-positive material.[213] In addition, nodular lymphoid hyperplasia can be detected in the gastrointestinal tract in a high proportion of CVID patients. However, the presence of nodular lymphoid hyperplasia does not correlate with the presence of malabsorption. The increased incidence of small bowel lymphoma in CVID also has to be considered as a cause of malabsorption in these patients. *Giardia* organisms are often isolated in CVID, and small bowel bacterial overgrowth is also frequently present. Unfortunately, only some of these patients respond to antimicrobial treatment.[213] Some patients with sprue-like intestinal changes have responded to glucocorticoids[210] or immunoglobulins. Patients with CVID have a higher prevalence of atrophic gastritis causing cobalamin malabsorption, although antibodies against parietal cells and intrinsic factor are absent.[209, 212]

X-Linked Infantile Agammaglobulinemia (Bruton's Agammaglobulinemia)

This disease usually manifests after the first 6 months of life and is characterized by recurrent severe bacterial infections. The incidence of severe gastrointestinal problems seems to be less common than in CVID.[213] The prevalence of chronic gastroenteritis was 10% in one large series.[215] In these patients, giardiasis and bacterial overgrowth need to be considered.[213, 215]

Other Congenital Immunodeficiency Syndromes

In *severe combined immunodeficiency*, diarrhea and malabsorption are common. Symptoms are associated with stunting of intestinal villi or their complete absence. The pathophysiology of malabsorption is unknown, and patients usually fail to respond to antimicrobial treatment.[209, 210] Malabsorption has also been reported in *DiGeorge's syndrome* (thymic hypoplasia) and *chronic granulomatous disease of childhood*, but little is known about its etiology.[209]

Neurofibromatosis Type 1 (Von Recklinghausen's Disease)

Malabsorption can be an intestinal complication of neurofibromatosis type 1. Mechanisms include periampullary duodenal tumors, which are mainly somatostatin-containing neuroendocrine tumors, or pancreatic carcinomas causing pancreatic duct obstruction. Tumors may result in exocrine pancreatic insufficiency and biliary obstruction.[216, 217] Duodenal somatostatinomas in von Recklinghausen's disease have not been demonstrated to increase plasma somatostatin levels or cause a somatostatinoma syndrome. Infiltrating mesenteric plexiform neurofibromas and vascular damage caused by proliferation of nerves can cause lymphatic and/or vascular obstruction resulting in abdominal pain, protein-losing enteropathy, diarrhea, steatorrhea, and bowel ischemia.[218, 219] In patients with von Recklinghausen's disease there is an increased incidence of neuroendocrine tumors also in other locations. Gastrinomas have been reported in two patients.[220, 221]

Malabsorption in Endocrine and Metabolic Disorders

Adrenal Insufficiency (Addison's Disease)

Fat malabsorption is observed in some patients with adrenal insufficiency, independent of its etiology. Fecal fat values of up to 30 g/day have been observed.[222] Fat malabsorption is also observed in rats after adrenalectomy.[223] The pathophysiologic mechanism of malabsorption in this disease is unknown. Fat absorption normalizes after steroid replacement.

An association between isolated autoimmune Addison's disease with pernicious anemia[224, 225] or celiac disease[226] has been reported. An increased incidence of celiac disease and pernicious anemia is also found in autoimmune polyglandular syndrome type 2 (Schmidt's syndrome), which is characterized by the association of autoimmune Addison's disease with other autoimmune endocrine disorders, except hypoparathyroidism.[227, 228]

Malabsorption Associated with Hypoparathyroidism (Autoimmune Polyglandular Syndrome Type 1)

This disease is characterized by failure of multiple endocrine organs due to autoimmune destruction (especially hypoparathyroidism and adrenal insufficiency), ectodermal dystrophy, and susceptibility to chronic candida infections.[227] About 20% of autoimmune polyglandular syndrome type 1 patients develop severe malabsorption, which tends to occur periodically. It was recently demonstrated that malabsorption in a patient with autoimmune polyglandular syndrome type 1 was caused by a transient and selective destruction of small intestinal enteroendocrine cells, leading to a transient deficiency of enteroendocrine hormones (especially cholecystokinin).[229] The long-known association between hypoparathyroidism and steatorrhea may also be caused by the same mechanism, because most reported patients with this association fulfill the diagnostic criteria for autoimmune polyglandular syndrome type 1.[230, 231] Selective absence of small intestinal enteroendocrine cells can be diagnosed by special immunohistochemical stains for these cells (e.g., immunohistochemical stains for chromogranin A or cholecystokinin) or by measurements of postprandial serum levels of the affected hormones. Patients with autoimmune polyglandular syndrome type 1 also have an increased incidence of vitamin B_{12} malabsorption due to autoimmune gastritis.[227]

Hyperthyroidism and Autoimmune Thyroid Disease

Some reports suggest that up to 25% of hyperthyroid patients have at least some degree of fat malabsorption, but data from large series of patients are lacking. Fecal fat values in hyperthyroid patients can reach 35 g/day.[232] The mechanism of steatorrhea in this entity has not been established. Motility studies in hyperthyroid patients (including patients with and without diarrhea) demonstrated accelerated small bowel transit time and whole gut transit time.[233] However, fecal fat values were not reported in these patients. It can be hypothesized that more pronounced disturbances of intestinal transit may lead to decreased mixing of food and digestive secretions and reduced intestinal absorption of nutrients. Some of the steatorrhea in hyperthyroid patients might be due to hyperphagia with increased dietary intake of fat.[234] An increased number of lymphocytes and plasma cells and some degree of edema in small intestinal biopsies have been found in patients with steatorrhea and hyperthyroidism; villous architecture is normal, however.[232] Absorption of glucose and D-xylose is normal in hyperthyroid patients with and without malabsorption.[234] Fat malabsorption tends to normalize when patients reach a euthyroid state.[232, 234, 235]

In patients with autoimmune thyroid diseases there is an increased prevalence of celiac disease[228] and primary biliary cirrhosis,[225] both of which can result in fat malabsorption. Cobalamin malabsorption due to autoimmune gastritis is found in a considerable number of patients with thyrotoxicosis and hypothyroidism.[29, 225]

Diabetes Mellitus

Chronic diarrhea is a common feature in patients with diabetes mellitus, especially in patients with long-standing diabetes mellitus type I. Mild steatorrhea is often present in patients with diabetic diarrhea and in patients who do not complain of diarrhea.[236, 237] However, in a subgroup of patients steatorrhea can be substantial, with fecal fat levels of up to 70 g/day,[237] suggesting a different etiology in these patients. The exact pathophysiologic mechanism of malabsorption and diarrhea in patients with diabetes mellitus is unknown. Most patients have signs of autonomic neuropathy such as orthostatic hypotension, impotence, bladder dysfunction, incontinence, decreased heart rate variability, and abnormal sweating.[236] Therefore, the etiology of diarrhea and malabsorption has been attributed to rapid gastric emptying and rapid intestinal transit causing impaired mixing of nutrients with digestive secretions and decreased contact time between nutrients and the intestinal mucosa. The clinician has to be aware that certain treatable diseases, like celiac disease,[238] small intestinal bacterial overgrowth,[239] and pancreatic insufficiency,[240] can be associated with diabetes mellitus. These diseases therefore should be excluded in every patient with diabetes mellitus and malabsorption. Furthermore, cobalamin malabsorption caused by autoimmune atrophic gastritis is more prevalent in patients with diabetes mellitus type I.[241, 242]

In patients receiving acarbose as an antidiabetic treatment, ingested carbohydrates are malabsorbed, which in turn can lead to symptoms of diarrhea and malabsorption. Dietary foods rich in fructose or sorbitol may also result in bloating and diarrhea.

Metabolic Bone Disease

Special consideration has to be given to osteoporosis and osteomalacia in malabsorptive diseases. Patients with these metabolic bone diseases do not usually present with symptoms or abnormal findings on physical examination or routine laboratory examinations. Reduced bone mineral density is a common feature in patients with gastric resection[243] or in celiac disease.[244] Osteoporosis has been suggested to result from calcium malabsorption, which leads to secondary hyperparathyroidism, which in turn increases bone turnover and cortical bone loss. Vitamin D malabsorption is probably of less importance. Although up to one half of patients on a gluten-free diet may have osteoporosis,[245] other studies have shown significant improvement of bone mineral density 1 year after starting a gluten-free diet.[246] In inflammatory bowel diseases such as Crohn's disease, which may be accompanied by malabsorption, other features such as corticosteroid use or testosterone deficiency[247] may contribute to the decrease in bone mass. In addition to treating the underlying cause of malabsorption, calcium supplements should be used to ensure a daily intake of 1500 mg of calcium, and vitamin D deficiency has to be corrected. If there is osteoporosis, as detected by bone densitometry, bisphosphonate treatment is suggested.[244] Nutritional management is discussed in more detail in Chapter 15.

GENERAL APPROACH TO THE MANAGEMENT OF MALABSORPTION

Treatment of malabsorptive diseases has to be directed against the underlying condition, if possible. In addition, nutritional deficits have to be corrected. As far as the treatment of specific diseases and the nutrition management are concerned, the reader is referred to the respective chapters of this book.

In severe pancreatic diseases, in disorders of intestinal fat absorption, and in short bowel syndrome, medium-chain triglycerides can be used as a source of dietary calories.[60] In patients with short bowel syndrome and remaining colon, colonic salvage capacity can be used to regain calories from carbohydrates.[248] Therefore, these patients should eat a diet rich in carbohydrates and medium-chain triglycerides.

In patients with malabsorption and an intact colon, fluid depletion has to be avoided in order to prevent kidney stones associated with hyperoxaluria.[249] In patients with malabsorption syndrome, special care should be given to the replacement of vitamins, iron, calcium, and trace elements in order to avoid deficiency syndromes (see Chapter 15).

Acknowledgment

We thank Dr. John S. Fordtran for his valuable advice.

REFERENCES

1. Wilson RA, Dietschy JM. Differential diagnostic approach to clinical problems of malabsorption. Gastroenterology 61:911, 1971.
2. Van Deest BW, Fordtran JS, Morawski SG, et al. Bile salt and micellar fat concentration in proximal small bowel contents of iliectomy patients. J Clin Invest 47:1314, 1968.
3. Hofmann AF, Poley JR. Role of bile acid malabsorption in pathogenesis of diarrhea and steatorrhea in patients with ileal resection. Gastroenterology 62:918, 1972.
4. Di Magno EP, Go VLW, Summerskill WHJ. Relations between pancreatic enzyme outputs and malabsorption in severe pancreatic insufficiency. N Engl J Med 288:813, 1973.
5. Ryan ME, Olsen WA. A diagnostic approach to malabsorption syndromes: a pathophysiological approach. Clin Gastroenterol 12:533, 1983.
6. Graham DY. Pancreatic enzyme replacement. The effect of antacids or cimetidine. Dig Dis Sci 27:485, 1982.
7. Graham DY, Sackman JW. Mechanism of increase in steatorrhea with calcium and magnesium in exocrine pancreatic insufficiency: an animal model. Gastroenterology 83:638, 1982.
8. Heck AM, Yanovski JA, Calis KA. Orlistat, a new lipase inhibitor for the management of obesity. Pharmacotherapy 20:270, 2000.
9. Gaskin KJ, Durie PR, Hill RE, et al. Colipase and maximally activated pancreatic lipase in normal subjects and patients with steatorrhea. J Clin Invest 69:427, 1982.
10. Kane JP, Havel RJ. Disorders of the biogenesis and secretion of lipoproteins containing the B apolipoproteins. In Scriver CR, Beaudet AL, Sly WS, et al. (eds.): The Metabolic and Molecular Bases of Inherited Disease, 7th ed. New York, McGraw-Hill, 1995, p 1853.
11. Mistilis SP, Skyring AP, Stephen DD. Intestinal lymphangiectasia: mechanism of enteric loss of plasma-protein and fat. Lancet 1:77, 1965.
12. Volwiler W. Gastrointestinal malabsorptive syndromes. Am J Med 23: 250, 1957.
13. Comfort MW, Wollaeger EE, Power MH. Total fecal solids, fat and nitrogen. A study of patients with chronic relapsing pancreatitis. Gastroenterology 11:691, 1948.
14. Freeman HJ, Sleisenger MH, Kim YS. Human protein digestion and absorption: normal mechanisms and protein-energy malnutrition. Clin Gastroenterol 12:357, 1983.
15. Lebenthal E, Antonowicz I, Shwachman H. Enterokinase and trypsin activities in pancreatic insufficiency and diseases of the small intestine. Gastroenterology 70:508, 1976.
16. Ladefoged K, Nicolaidou P, Jarnum S. Calcium, phosphorus, magnesium, zinc, and nitrogen balance in patients with severe short bowel syndrome. Am J Clin Nutr 33:2137, 1980.
17. Ravich WJ, Bayless TM. Carbohydrate absorption and malabsorption. Clin Gastroenterol 12:335, 1983.
18. Hammer HF, Fine KD, Santa Ana CA, et al. Carbohydrate malabsorption. Its measurement and its contribution to diarrhea. J Clin Invest 86:1936, 1990.
19. Finkelstein JD. Malabsorption. Med Clin North Am 52:1339, 1968.
20. Ushijima K, Riby JE, Kretchmer N. Carbohydrate malabsorption. Pediatr Clin North Am 42:899, 1995.
21. Gudmand-Hoyer E, Skovbjerg H. Disaccharide digestion and maldigestion. Scand J Gastroenterol 31(Suppl 216):111, 1996.
22. Wright EMI. Glucose galactose malabsorption. Am J Physiol 275: G879, 1998.
23. Sokol RJ. Fat-soluble vitamins and their importance in patients with cholestatic liver diseases. Gastroenterol Clin North Am 23:673, 1994.
24. Bilke DD. Calcium absorption and vitamin D metabolism. Clin Gastroenterol 12:379, 1983.
25. Marotta RB, Floch MH. Dietary therapy of steatorrhea. Gastroenterol Clin North Am 18:485, 1989.
26. Evans WB, Wollaeger EE. Incidence and severity of nutritional deficiency states in chronic exocrine pancreatic insufficiency: comparison with nontropical sprue. Am J Dig Dis 11:594, 1966.
27. Seetharam B. Gastrointestinal absorption and transport of cobalamin (vitamin B_{12}). In Johnson LR (ed.): Physiology of the Gastrointestinal Tract, 3rd ed. New York, Raven, 1994, p 1997.
28. Howden CW. Vitamin B12 levels during prolonged treatment with proton pump inhibitors. J Clin Gastroenterol 30:29, 2000.
29. Toh BH, van Driel I, Gleeson PA. Pernicious anemia. N Engl J Med 337:1441, 1997.
30. Glasbrenner B, Malfertheiner P, Büchler M, et al. Vitamin B12 and folic acid deficiency in chronic pancreatitis: a relevant disorder? Klin Wochenschr 69:168, 1991.
31. Rosenblatt DS, Whitehead VM. Cobalamin and folate deficiency: acquired and hereditary disorders in children. Semin Hematol 36:19, 1999.
32. Gallagher ND. Importance of vitamin B12 and folate metabolism in malabsorption. Clin Gastroenterol 12:437, 1983.
33. Zittoun J, Zittoun R. Modern clinical testing strategies in cobalamin and folate deficiency. Semin Hematol 36:35, 1999.
34. Green PHR. Alcohol, nutrition and malabsorption. Clin Gastroenterol 12:563, 1983.
35. Hoskins LC, Norris HT, Gottlieb LS, et al. Functional and morphologic alterations of the gastrointestinal tract in progressive systemic sclerosis (scleroderma). Am J Med 33:459, 1962.
36. Pak CYC, Fordtran JS. Disorders of mineral metabolism. In Sleisenger MH, Fordtran JS (eds.): Gastrointestinal Disease, 2nd ed. Philadelphia, WB Saunders, 1978, p 251.
37. Marx SJ. Vitamin D and other calciferols. In Scriver CR, Beaudet AL, Sly WS, et al. (eds.): The Metabolic and Molecular Bases of Inherited Disease, 7th ed. New York, McGraw-Hill, 1995, p 3091.
38. Booth CC, Barbouris S, Hanna S, et al. Incidence of hypomagnesaemia in intestinal malabsorption. Br Med J 2:141, 1963.
39. Milla PJ, Aggett PJ, Wolff OH, et al. Studies in primary hypomagnesaemia: evidence of defective carrier-mediated small intestinal transport of magnesium. Gut 20:1028, 1979.
40. de-Vizia B, Poggi V, Conenna R, et al. Iron absorption and iron deficiency in infants and children with gastrointestinal diseases. J Pediatr Gastroenterol Nutr 14:21, 1992.
41. Goddard AF, McIntyre AS, Scott BB. Guidelines for the management of iron deficiency anaemia. Gut 46(Suppl IV):iv1, 2000.
42. Goldschmid S, Graham M. Trace element deficiencies in inflammatory bowel disease. Gastroenterol Clin North Am 18:579, 1989.
43. van Wouwe JP. Clinical and laboratory diagnosis of acrodermatitis enteropathica. Eur J Pediatr 149:2, 1989.
44. Goyens P, Brasseur D, Cadranel S. Copper deficiency in infants with active celiac disease. J Pediatr Gastroenterol Nutr 4:677, 1985.
45. Basilisco G, Phillips SF. Colonic salvage in health and disease. Eur J Gastroenterol Hepatol 5:777, 1993.

46. Nightingale JMD, Lennard-Jones JE, Gertner DJ, et al. Colonic preservation reduces need for parenteral therapy, increases incidence of renal stones, but does not change high prevalence of gall stones in patients with short bowel. Gut 33:1493, 1992.
47. Stephen AM, Phillips SF. Passage of carbohydrate into the colon. Direct measurements in humans. Gastroenterology 85:589, 1983.
48. Cummings JH, Macfarlane GT. Role of intestinal bacteria in nutrient metabolism. JPEN J Parenter Enteral Nutr 21:357, 1997.
49. Ruppin H, Bar Meir S, Soergel KH, et al. Absorption of short-chain fatty acids by the colon. Gastroenterology 78:1500, 1980.
50. Hammer HF, Santa Ana CA, Schiller LR, et al. Studies of osmotic diarrhea induced in normal subjects by ingestion of polyethylene glycol and lactulose. J Clin Invest 84:1056, 1989.
51. Florent C, Flourie B, Leblond A, et al. Influence of chronic lactulose ingestion on the colonic metabolism of lactulose in man (an in vivo study). J Clin Invest 75:608, 1985.
52. Yang MG, Manoharan K, Mickelsen O. Nutritional contribution of volatile fatty acids from the cecum of rats. J Nutrition 100:545, 1970.
53. Jeppesen PB, Mortensen PB. Significance of a preserved colon for parenteral energy requirements in patients receiving home parenteral nutrition. Scand J Gastroenterol 33:1175, 1998.
54. Hammer HF. Colonic hydrogen absorption: quantification of its effect on hydrogen accumulation caused by bacterial fermentation of carbohydrates. Gut 34:818, 1993.
55. Moore JG, Jessop LD, Osborne DN. A gas chromatographic and mass spectrometric analysis of the odor of human feces. Gastroenterology 93:1321, 1987.
56. el-Yamani J, Mizon C, Capon C, et al. Decreased faecal exoglycosidase activities identify a subset of patients with active Crohn's disease. Clin Sci Colch 83:409, 1992.
57. Rao SS, Read NW, Holdsworth CD. Is the diarrhoea in ulcerative colitis related to impaired colonic salvage of carbohydrate? Gut 28: 1090, 1987.
58. Högenauer C, Hammer HF, Krejs GJ, et al. Mechanisms and management of antibiotic-associated diarrhea. Clin Infect Dis 27:702, 1998.
59. Hove H, Tvede M, Brobech-Mortensen P. Antibiotic-associated diarrhoea, *Clostridium difficile*, and short chain fatty acids. Scand J Gastroenterol 31:688, 1996.
60. Kurpad AV, Shetty PS. Effects of antimicrobial therapy on faecal bulking. Gut 27:55, 1986.
61. Hatch M, Freel RW. Alterations in intestinal transport of oxalate in disease states. Scanning Microsc 9:1121, 1995.
62. Ammon HV, Phillips SF. Inhibition of colonic water and electrolyte absorption by fatty acids in man. Gastroenterology 65:744, 1973.
63. Dobbins JW, Binder HJ. Effect of bile salts and fatty acids on the colonic absorption of oxalate. Gastroenterology 1096, 1976.
64. Jeppesen PB, Mortensen PB. The influence of a preserved colon on the absorption of medium chain fat in patients with small bowel resection. Gut 43:478, 1998.
65. Sheikh MS, Schiller LR, Fordtran JS. In vivo intestinal absorption of calcium in humans. Miner Electrolyte Metab 16:130, 1990.
66. Hylander E, Ladefoged K, Jarnum S. Calcium absorption after intestinal resection. The importance of a preserved colon. Scand J Gastroenterol 25:705, 1990.
67. Karbach U, Feldmeier H. The cecum is the site with the highest calcium absorption in rat intestine. Dig Dis Sci 38:1815, 1993.
68. Halpern GM, Van-de-Water J, Delabroise AM, et al. Comparative uptake of calcium from milk and a calcium-rich mineral water in lactose intolerant adults: implications for treatment of osteoporosis. Am J Prev Med 7:379, 1991.
69. Trinidad TP, Wolever TM, Thompson LU. Effects of calcium concentration, acetate, and propionate on calcium absorption in the human distal colon. Nutrition 15:529, 1999.
70. Hammer J, Hammer K, Kletter K. Lipids infused into the jejunum accelerate small intestinal transit but delay ileocolonic transit of solids and liquids. Gut 43:111, 1998.
71. Spiller RC, Trotman IF, Higgins BE. The ileal brake-inhibition of jejunal motility after ileal fat perfusion in man. Gut 25:365, 1984.
72. Jain NK, Boivin M, Zinsmeister AR, et al. Effect of perfusing carbohydrates and amylase inhibitor into the ileum on gastrointestinal hormones and gastric emptying of homogenized meal. Gastroenterology 96:377, 1989.
73. Hammer J, Pruckmayer M, Bergmann H, et al. The distal colon provides reserve storage capacity during colonic fluid overload. Gut 41:658, 1997.
74. Read NW. The relationships between colonic motility and transport. Scand J Gastroenterol 19 (Suppl 93):35, 1984.
75. Shah VH, Rotterdam H, Kotler DP, et al. All that scallops is not celiac disease. Gastrointest Endosc 51:717, 2000.
76. Mee A, Burke M, Vallon AG, et al. Small bowel biopsy for malabsorption: comparison of the diagnostic accuracy of endoscopic forceps and capsule biopsy specimens. Br Med J 291:769, 1985.
77. Crosby WH, Kugler HW. Intraluminal biopsy of the small intestine. Am J Dig Dis 2:236, 1957.
78. Flick AL, Quinton WE, Rubin CE. A peroral hydraulic biopsy tube for multiple sampling at any level of the gastrointestinal tract. Gastroenterology 40:120, 1961.
79. Dickey W, Hughes D. Prevalence of celiac disease and its endoscopic markers among patients having routine upper gastrointestinal endoscopy. Am J Gastroenterol 94:2182, 1999.
80. Dandalides SM, Cavey W, Petras R, et al. Endoscopic small bowel mucosal biopsy: a controlled trial evaluating forceps size and biopsy location in the diagnosis of normal and abnormal mucosal architecture. Gastrointest Endosc 35:197, 1989.
81. Ladas SD, Tsamouri M, Kouvidou C, et al. Effect of forceps size and mode of orientation on endoscopic small bowel biopsy evaluation. Gastrointest Endosc 40:51, 1994.
82. Siegel LM, Stevens PD, Lightdale CJ, et al. Combined magnification endoscopy with chromoendoscopy in the evaluation of patients with suspected malabsorption. Gastrointest Endosc 46:226, 1997.
83. Ramzan NN, Loftus E, Burgart LJ, et al. Diagnosis and monitoring of Whipple disease by polymerase chain reaction. Ann Intern Med 126: 520, 1997.
84. Fine KD, Schiller LR. AGA technical review on the evaluation and management of chronic diarrhea. Gastroenterology 116:1464, 1999.
85. Van de Kamer JH, Ten Bokkel Huinink H, Weyers HA. Rapid method for the determination of fat in feces. J Biol Chem 177:347, 1949.
86. Balasekaran R, Porter JL, Santa AC, et al. Positive results on tests for steatorrhea in persons consuming olestra potato chips. Ann Intern Med 132:279, 2000.
87. Jeejeebhoy KN, Ahmad S, Kozak G. Determination of fecal fats containing both medium and long chain triglycerides and fatty acids. Clin Biochem 3:157, 1970.
88. Picarelli A, Greco M, DiGiovambattista F. Quantitative determination of faecal fat, nitrogen and water by the means of a spectrophotometric technique: near infrared reflectance analysis (NIRA). assessment of accuracy and reproducibility compared with chemical methods. Clin Chim Acta 234:147, 1995.
89. Fine KD, Fordtran JS. The effect of diarrhea on fecal fat excretion. Gastroenterology 102:1936, 1992.
90. Gruy-Kapral C, Little KH, Fordtran JS, et al. Conjugated bile acid replacement therapy for short-bowel syndrome. Gastroenterology 116: 15, 1999.
91. Amann ST, Josephson SA, Toskes PP. Acid steatocrit: a simple, rapid gravimetric method to determine steatorrhea. Am J Gastroenterol 92: 2280, 1997.
92. Romano TJ, Dobbins JW. Evaluation of the patient with suspected malabsorption. Gastroenterol Clin North Am 18:467, 1989.
93. Fine KD, Ogunji F. A new method of quantitative fecal fat microscopy and its correlation with chemically measured fecal fat output. Am J Clin Pathol 113:528, 2000.
94. Pedersen NT, Halgreen H. Simultaneous assessment of fat maldigestion and fat malabsorption by a double-isotope method using fecal radioactivity. Gastroenterology 88:47, 1985.
95. Lembcke B, Geibel K, Kirchhoff S, et al. Serum beta-carotene: a simple static laboratory parameter for the diagnosis of steatorrhea. Dtsch Med Wochenschr 114:243, 1989.
96. Leung AK, Siu TO, Chiu AS, et al. Serum carotene concentrations in normal infants and children. Clin Pediatr Phila 29:575, 1990.
97. Hammer HF, Petritsch W, Pristautz H, et al. Assessment of the influence of hydrogen nonexcretion on the usefulness of the hydrogen breath test and lactose tolerance test. Wien Klin Wochenschr 108:137, 1996.
98. Eherer AJ, Fordtran JS. Fecal osmotic gap and pH in experimental diarrhea of various causes. Gastroenterology 103:545, 1992.
99. Ameen VZ, Powell GK. A simple spectrophotometric method for quantitative fecal carbohydrate measurement. Clin Chim Acta 152:3, 1985.
100. Collin DP, McCormick PG. Determiantion of short chain fatty acids in stool ultrafiltrate and urine. Clin Chem 20:1173, 1974.
101. Hoverstad T, Fausa O, Bjorneklett A, et al. Short-chain fatty acids in the normal human feces. Scand J Gastroenterol 19:375, 1984.
102. Evenepoel P, Claus D, Geypens B, et al. Evidence for impaired

assimilation and increased colonic fermentation of protein, related to gastric acid suppression therapy. Aliment Pharmacol Ther 12:1011, 1998.
103. Snow CF. Laboratory diagnosis of vitamin B_{12} and folate deficiency. Arch Intern Med 159:1289, 1999.
104. Fenton WA, Rosenberg LE. Inherited disorders of cobalamin transport and metabolism. In Scriver CR, Beaudet AL, Sly WS, et al. (eds.): The Metabolic and Molecular Bases of Inherited Disease, 7th ed. New York, McGraw-Hill, 1995, p 3129.
105. Allen RH, Stabler SP, Savage DG, et al. Diagnosis of cobalamin deficiency I: usefulness of serum methylmalonic acid and total homocysteine concentrations. Am J Hematol 34:90, 1990.
106. Loeser C, Moellgaard A, Foelsch UR. Faecal elastase 1: a novel, highly sensitive, and specific tubeless pancreatic function test. Gut 39: 580, 1996.
107. Schiller LR, Bilhartz LE, Santa Ana CA, et al. Comparison of endogenous and radiolabeled bile acid excretion in patients with idiopathic chronic diarrhea. Gastroenterology 98:1036, 1990.
108. Schiller LR, Hogan RB, Morawski SG, et al. Studies of the prevalence and significance of radiolabeled bile acid malabsorption in a group of patients with idiopathic chronic diarrhea. Gastroenterology 92:151, 1987.
109. Hofmann AF, Bolder U. Detection of bile acid malabsorption by the SeHCAT test. Principles, problems, and clinical utility. Gastroenterol Clin Biol 18:847, 1994.
110. Sciarretta G, Vicini G, Fagioli G, et al. Use of 23-selena-25-homocholyltaurine to detect bile acid malabsorption in patients with ileal dysfunction or diarrhea. Gastroenterology 91:1, 1986.
111. Benson JA, Culver PJ, Ragland S, et al. The D-xylose absorption test in malabsorption syndromes. N Engl J Med 256:335, 1957.
112. Uil JJ, van-Elburg RM, van-Overbeek FM, et al. Clinical implications of the sugar absorption test: intestinal permeability test to assess mucosal barrier function. Scand J Gastroenterol 23(Suppl 223), 70, 1997.
113. Peled Y, Doron O, Laufer H, et al. D-Xylose absorption test. Urine or blood? Dig Dis Sci 36:188, 1991.
114. Riordan SM, McIver CJ, Duncombe VM, et al. Factors influencing the 1-g ^{14}C-D-xylose breath test for bacterial overgrowth. Am J Gastroenterol 90:1455, 1995.
115. Bjarnason I, Macpherson A, Hollander D. Intestinal permeability: an overview. Gastroenterology 108:1566, 1995.
116. Bai JC. Malabsorption syndromes. Digestion 59:530, 1998.
117. Cobden I, Hamilton I, Rothwell J, et al. Cellobiose/mannitol test: physiological properties of probe molecules and influence of extraneous factors. Clin Chim Acta 148:53, 1985.
118. Wyatt J, Vogelsang H, Hubl W, et al. Intestinal permeability and the prediction of relapse in Crohn's disease. Lancet 341:1437, 1993.
119. Meddings JB. Review article: intestinal permeability in Crohn's disease. Aliment Pharmacol Ther 11:47, 1997.
120. Smecuol E, Bai JC, Vazquez H, et al. Gastrointestinal permeability in celiac disease. Gastroenterology 112:1129, 1997.
121. Novacek G, Miehsler W, Wrba F, et al. Prevalence and clinical importance of hypertransaminasemia in coeliac disease. Eur J Gastroenterol Hepatol 11:283, 1999.
122. Sigthorsson G, Tibble J, Hayllar J, et al. Intestinal permeability and inflammation in patients on NSAIDs. Gut 43:506, 1998.
123. Rooney PJ, Jenkins RT, Buchanan WW. A short review of the relationship between intestinal permeability and inflammatory joint disease. Clin Exp Rheumatol 8:75, 1990.
124. Cooper BT, Ukabam SO, O'Brien IA, et al. Intestinal permeability in diabetic diarrhoea. Diabet Med 4:49, 1987.
125. Kato M, Asaka M, Ohara S, et al. Clinical studies of ^{13}C urea breath test in Japan. J Gastroenterol 33:36, 1998.
126. Braden B, Caspary WF, Lembcke B. Nondispersive infrared spectrometry for $^{13}CO_2/^{12}CO_2$ measurements: a clinically feasible analyzer for stable isotope breath tests in gastroenterology. Z Gastroenterol 37:477, 1999.
127. de Meer K, Roef MJ, Kulik W, et al. In vivo research with stable isotopes in biochemistry, nutrition and clinical medicine: an overview. Isotopes Environ Health Stud 35:19, 1999.
128. Loser C, Brauer C, Aygen S, et al. Comparative clinical evaluation of the ^{13}C mixed triglyceride breath test as an indirect pancreatic function test. Scand J Gastroenterol 33:327, 1998.
129. Braden B, Picard H, Caspary WF, et al. Monitoring pancreatin supplementation in cystic fibrosis patients with the ^{13}C-Triolein breath test: evidence for normalized fat assimilation with high dose pancreatin therapy. Z Gastroenterol 35:123, 1997.
130. Antonowicz I, Lebenthal E. Developmental patterns of small intestinal enterokinase and disaccharidase activities in the human fetus. Gastroenterology 72:1299, 1977.
131. Welsh JD, Poley JR, Bhatia M, et al. Intestinal disaccharidase activities in relation to age, race, and mucosal damage. Gastroenterology 75:847, 1978.
132. Sahi T. Genetics and epidemiology of adult-type hypolactasia. Scand J Gastroenterol 29(Suppl 202):7, 1994.
133. Escher JC, de Koning ND, van Engen CG, et al. Molecular basis of lactase levels in adult humans. J Clin Invest 89:480, 1992.
134. Sterchi EE, Mills PR, Fransen JA, et al. Biogenesis of intestinal lactase-phlorizin hydrolase in adults with lactose intolerance. J Clin Invest 86:1329, 1990.
135. Hammer HF, Petritsch W, Pristautz H, et al. Evaluation of the pathogenesis of flatulence and abdominal cramps in patients with lactose malabsorption. Wien Klin Wochenschr 108:175, 1996.
136. Gudmand-Hoyer E, Simony K. Individual sensitivity to lactose in lactose malabsorption. Am J Dig Dis 22:177, 1977.
137. Bedine MS, Bayless TM. Intolerance of small amounts of lactose by individuals with low lactase levels. Gastroenterology 65:735, 1973.
138. Ladas SD, Papanikos J, Arapakis G. Lactose malabsorption in Greek adults: correlation of small bowel transit time with the severity of lactose intolerance. Gut 23:968, 1982.
139. Roggero P, Offredi ML, Mosca F, et al. Lactose absorption and malabsorption in healthy Italian children: do the quantity of malabsorbed sugar and the small bowel transit time play a role in symptom production? J Pediatr Gastroenterol Nutr 4:82, 1985.
140. Szilagyi A, Salomon R, Martin M, et al. Lactose handling by women with lactose malabsorption is improved during pregnancy. Clin Invest Med 19:416, 1996.
141. Szilagyi A, Lerman S, Barr RG, et al. Reversible lactose malabsorption and intolerance in Graves' disease. Clin Invest Med 14:188, 1991.
142. Kolars JC, Levitt MD, Aouji M, et al. Yogurt: an autodigesting source of lactose. N Engl J Med 310:1, 1984.
143. Moskovitz M, Curtis C, Gavaler J. Does oral enzyme replacement therapy reverse intestinal lactose malabsorption? Am J Gastroenterol 82:632, 1987.
144. Riby JE, Fujisawa T, Kretchmer N. Fructose absorption. Am J Clin Nutr 58:748S, 1993.
145. Hoekstra JH, van-Kempen AA, Kneepkens CM. Apple juice malabsorption: fructose or sorbitol? J Pediatr Gastroenterol Nutr 16:39, 1993.
146. Evans PR, Piesse C, Bak YT, et al. Fructose-sorbitol malabsorption and symptom provocation in irritable bowel syndrome: relationship to enteric hypersensitivity and dysmotility. Scand J Gastroenterol 33: 1158, 1998.
147. Rumessen JJ, Gudmand-Hoyer, E. Functional bowel diseases: malabsorption and abdominal distress after ingestion of fructose, sorbitol, and fructose-sorbitol mixtures. Gastroenterology 95:694, 1988.
148. Mishkin D, Sablauskas L, Yalovsky M, et al. Fructose and sorbitol malabsorption in ambulatory patients with functional dyspepsia. Dig Dis Sci 42:2591, 1997.
149. Wasserman D, Hoekstra JH, Tolia V, et al. Molecular analysis of the fructose transporter gene (*GLUT5*) in isolated fructose malabsorption. J Clin Invest 98:2398, 1996.
150. Born P, Zech J, Lehn H, et al. Colonic bacterial activity determines the symptoms in people with fructose-malabsorption. Hepatogastroenterology. 42:778, 1995.
151. Fromm H, Malavolti M. Bile acid–induced diarrhoea. Clin Gastroenterol 15:567, 1986.
152. Fordtran JS, Bunch F, Davis GR. Ox bile treatment of severe steatorrhea in an ileectomy-ileostomy patient. Gastroenterology 82:564, 1982.
153. Little KH, Schiller LR, Bilhartz LE, et al. Treatment of severe steatorrhea with ox bile in an ileectomy patient with residual colon. Dig Dis Sci 37:929, 1992.
154. Balistreri WF, Partin JC, Schubert WK. Bile acid malabsorption — a consequence of terminal ileal dysfunction in protracted diarrhea of infancy. J Pediatr 89:21, 1977.
155. Heubi JE, Balistreri WF, Partin JC, et al. Refractory infantile diarrhea due to primary bile acid malabsorption. J Pediatr 94:546, 1979.
156. Oelkers P, Kirby LC, Heubi JE, et al. Primary bile acid malabsorption caused by mutations in the ileal sodium-dependent bile acid transporter gene (*SLC10A2*). J Clin Invest 99:1880, 1997.
157. Kyle RA, Gertz MA. Primary systemic amyloidosis: clinical and laboratory features in 474 cases. Semin Hematol 32:45, 1995.
158. Steen LE, Ek BO. Familial amyloidosis with polyneuropathy. Aspects of the relationship between gastrointestinal symptoms, EMG findings, and malabsorption studies. Scand J Gastroenterol 19:480, 1984.

159. Lovat LB, Pepys MB, Hawkins PN. Amyloid and the gut. Dig Dis 15: 155, 1997.
160. Feurle GE. Pathophysiology of diarrhea in patients with familial amyloid neuropathy. Digestion 36:13, 1987.
161. Hunter AM, Campbell IW, Borsey DQ, et al. Protein-losing enteropathy due to gastro-intestinal amyloidosis. Postgrad Med J 55:822, 1979.
162. Carrizosa J, Lin KY, Myerson RM. Gastrointestinal neuropathy in familial amyloidosis. Report of a case with severe diarrhea without steatorrhea or malabsorption. Am J Gastroenterol 59:541, 1973.
163. Tada S, Iida M, Iwashita A, et al. Endoscopic and biopsy findings of the upper digestive tract in patients with amyloidosis. Gastrointest Endosc 36:10, 1990.
164. Herskovic T, Bartholomew LG, Green PA. Amyloid and malabsorption syndrome. Arch Intern Med 114:629, 1964.
165. Suhr O, Danielsson A, Steen L. Bile acid malabsorption caused by gastrointestinal motility dysfunction? An investigation of gastrointestinal disturbances in familial amyloidosis with polyneuropathy. Scand J Gastroenterol 27:201, 1992.
166. Steen LE, Öberg L. Familial amyloidosis with polyneuropathy: roentgenological and gastroscopic appearance of gastrointestinal involvment. Am J Gastroenterol 78:417, 1983.
167. Steen L, Börje E. Familial amyloidosis with polyneuropathy. A long-term follow-up of 21 patients with special reference to gastrointestinal symptoms. Acta Med Scand 214:387, 1983.
168. Stone MJ. Amyloidosis: a final common pathway for protein deposition in tissues. Blood 75:531, 1990.
169. Bragelmann R, Armbrecht U, Rosemeyer D, et al. Nutrient malassimilation following total gastrectomy. Scand J Gastroenterol 31(Suppl 218):26, 1996.
170. Wollaeger EE, Comfort MW, Weir JF, et al. The total solids, fat and nitrogen in the feces. II. A study of persons who had undergone partial gastrectomy with anastomosis of the entire cut end of the stomach and the jejunum (polya anastomosis). Gastroenterology 6:93, 1946.
171. Griffiths A, Taylor RH. Postgastrectomy pancreatic malabsorption: is there a case for intervention? Eur J Gastroenterol Hepatol. 11:219, 1999.
172. Bragelmann R, Armbrecht U, Rosemeyer D, et al. The effect of pancreatic enzyme supplementation in patients with steatorrhoea after total gastrectomy. Eur J Gastroenterol Hepatol 11:231, 1999.
173. Bae JM, Park JW, Yang HK, et al. Nutritional status of gastric cancer patients after total gastrectomy. World J Surg 22:254, 1998.
174. Steffes C, Fromm D. Postgastrectomy syndromes. In Zuidema GD (ed.): Shackelford's Surgery of the Alimentary Tract, 4th ed. Philadelphia, WB Saunders, 1996, p 166.
175. Nilas L, Christiansen C, Christiansen J. Regulation of vitamin D and calcium metabolism after gastrectomy. Gut 26:252, 1985.
176. Hara H, Suzuki T, Kasai T, et al. Ingestion of guar gum hydrolysate, a soluble fiber, increases calcium absorption in totally gastrectomized rats. J Nutr 129:39, 1999.
177. Bo-Linn GW, Davis GR, Buddrus DJ, et al. An evaluation of the importance of gastric acid secretion in the absorption of dietary calcium. J Clin Invest 73:640, 1984.
178. Eagon JC, Miedema BW, Kelly KA. Postgastrectomy syndromes. Surg Clin North Am 72:445, 1992.
179. Lipski PS, Bennett MK, Kelly PJ, et al. Ageing and duodenal morphometry. J Clin Pathol 45:450, 1992.
180. Madjumdar AP, Jaszewski R, Dubick MA. Effect of aging on the gastrointestinal tract and the pancreas. Proc Soc Exp Biol Med 215: 134, 1997.
181. King D, Smith ML, Chapman TJ, et al. Fat malabsorption in elderly patients with cardiac cachexia. Age Ageing 25:144, 1996.
182. Lovat LB. Age related changes in gut physiology and nutritional status. Gut 38:306, 1996.
183. Quinn K, Basu TK. Folate and vitamin B_{12} status of the elderly. Eur J Clin Nutr 50:340, 1996.
184. Saltzman JR, Kowdley KV, Pedrosa MC, et al. Bacterial overgrowth without clinical malabsorption in elderly hypochlorhydric subjects. Gastroenterology 106:615, 1994.
185. Haboubi NY, Montgomery RD. Small-bowel bacterial overgrowth in elderly people: clinical significance and response to treatment. Age Ageing 21:13, 1992.
186. Sjogren RW. Gastrointestinal features of scleroderma. Curr Opin Rheumatol 8:569, 1996.
187. Rosson RS, Yesner R. Peroral duodenal biopsy in progressive systemic sclerosis. N Engl J Med 272:391, 1965.
188. Soudah HC, Hasler WL, Owyang C. Effect of octreotide on intestinal motility and bacterial overgrowth in scleroderma. N Engl J Med 325: 1461, 1991.
189. Kaye SA, Seifalian AM, Lim SG, et al. Ischaemia of the small intestine in patients with systemic sclerosis: Raynaud's phenomenon or chronic vasculopathy? QJM 87:495, 1994.
190. Kaye SA, Lim SG, Taylor M, et al. Small bowel bacterial overgrowth in systemic sclerosis: detection using direct and indirect methods and treatment outcome. Br J Rheumatol 34:265, 1995.
191. Akesson A, Ekman R. Gastrointestinal regulatory peptides in systemic sclerosis. Arthritis Rheum 36:698, 1993.
192. Folwaczny C, Rothfuss U, Riepl RL, et al. Gastrointestinal involvement in progressive systemic scleroderma. Z Gastroenterol 33:654, 1995.
193. Mader R, Adawi M, Schonfeld S. Malabsorption in systemic lupus erythematosus. Clin Exp Rheumatol 15:659, 1997.
194. Markusse HM, Schravenhoff R, Beerman H. Hypereosinophilic syndrome presenting with diarrhoea and anaemia in a patient with systemic lupus erythematosus. Neth J Med 52:79, 1998.
195. Marshall JB, Kretschmar JM, Gerhardt DC, et al. Gastrointestinal manifestations of mixed connective tissue disease. Gastroenterology 98:1232, 1990.
196. Narayanaswamy AS, Akhtar M, Kumar N, et al. Polymyositis—a review and follow up study of 24 cases. J Assoc Physicians India 41: 354, 1993.
197. Segal S, Thier SO. Cystinuria. In Scriver CR, Beaudet AL, Sly WS, et al. (eds.): The Metabolic and Molecular Bases of Inherited Disease, 7th ed. New York, McGraw-Hill, 1995, p 3581.
198. Levy HL. Hartnup disorder. In Scriver CR, Beaudet AL, Sly WS, et al. (eds.): The Metabolic and Molecular Bases of Inherited Disease, 7th ed. New York, McGraw-Hill, 1995, p 3629.
199. Chesney RW. Iminoglycinuria. In Scriver CR, Beaudet AL, Sly WS, et al. (eds.): The Metabolic and Molecular Bases of Inherited Disease, 7th ed. New York, McGraw-Hill, 1995, p 3643.
200. Simell O. Lysinuric protein intolerance and other cationic aminoacidurias. In Scriver CR, Beaudet AL, Sly WS, et al. (eds.): The Metabolic and Molecular Bases of Inherited Disease, 7th ed. New York, McGraw-Hill, 1995, p 3603.
201. Auricchio S. Genetically determined disaccharidase deficiencies. In Walker WA (ed.): Pediatric Gastrointestinal Disease, 2nd ed. St. Louis, Mosby, 1996, p 761.
202. Desjeux JF, Turk E, Wright E. Congenital selective Na+ D-glucose cotransport defects leading to renal glycosuria and congenital selective intestinal malabsorption of glucose and galactose. In Scriver CR, Beaudet AL, Sly WS, et al. (eds.): The Metabolic and Molecular Bases of Inherited Disease, 7th ed. New York, McGraw-Hill, 1995, p 3563.
203. Gueant JL, Saunier M, Gastin I, et al. Decreased activity of intestinal and urinary intrinsic factor receptor in Grasbeck-Imerslund disease. Gastroenterology 108:1622, 1995.
204. Eaton DM, Livingston JH, Seetharam B, et al. Overexpression of an unstable intrinsic factor-cobalamin receptor in Imerslund-Grasbeck syndrome. Gastroenterology 115:173, 1998.
205. Kristiansen M, Aminoff M, Jacobsen C, et al. Cubilin P1297L mutation associated with hereditary megaloblastic anemia 1 causes impaired recognition of intrinsic factor-vitamin B(12) by cubilin. Blood 96:405, 2000.
206. Mac Kenzie IL, Donaldson RMJ, Trier JS, et al. Ileal mucosa in familial selective vitamin B_{12} malabsorption. N Engl J Med 286:1021, 1972.
207. Ghishan FK, Lee PC, Lebenthal E, et al. Isolated congenital enterokinase deficiency. Recent findings and review of the literature. Gastroenterology 85:727, 1983.
208. Spickett GP, Misbah SA, Chapel HM. Primary antibody deficiency in adults. Lancet 337:281, 1991.
209. Ament ME. Immunodeficiency syndromes and gastrointestinal disease. Pediatr Clin North Am 22:807, 1975.
210. Doe WF, Hapel AJ. Intestinal immunity and malabsorption. Clin Gastroenterol 12:415, 1983.
211. McCarthy DM, Katz SI, Gazze L, et al. Selective IgA deficiency associated with total villous atrophy of the small intestine and an organ-specific anti-epithelial cell antibody. J Immunol 120:932, 1978.
212. Cunningham-Rundles C. Clinical and immunologic analyses of 103 patients with common variable immunodeficiency. J Clin Immunol 9: 22, 1989.

213. Washington K, Stenzel TT, Buckley RH, et al. Gastrointestinal pathology in patients with common variable immunodeficiency and X-linked agammaglobulinemia. Am J Surg Pathol 20:1240, 1996.
214. Lewin KJ, Riddell RH, Weinstein WM. Gastrointestinal Pathology and Its Clinical Implications, 1st ed. New York, Igaku-Shoin, 1992.
215. Lederman HM, Winkelstein JA. X-linked agammaglobulinemia: an analysis of 96 patients. Medicine (Baltimore) 64:145, 1985.
216. Wormsley KG, Logan WF, Sorrell VF, et al. Neurofibromatosis with pancreatic duct obstruction and steatorrhoea. Postgrad Med J 43:432, 1967.
217. Dayal Y, Tallberg KA, Nunnemacher G, et al. Duodenal carcinoids in patients with and without neurofibromatosis. A comparative study. Am J Surg Pathol 10:348, 1986.
218. Partin JS, Lane BP, Partin JC, et al. Plexiform neurofibromatosis of the liver and mesentery in a child. Hepatology 12:559, 1990.
219. Tatemichi M, Nagata H, Morinaga S, et al. Protein-losing enteropathy caused by mesenteric vascular involvement of neurofibromatosis. Dig Dis Sci 38:1549, 1993.
220. Chagnon JP, Barge J, Henin D, et al. Recklinghausen's disease with digestive localizations associated with gastric acid hypersecretion suggesting Zollinger-Ellison syndrome. Gastroenterol Clin Biol 9:65, 1985.
221. Garcia JC, Carney JA, Stickler GB, et al. Zollinger-Ellison syndrome and neurofibromatosis in a 13-year-old boy. J Pediatr 93:982, 1978.
222. McBrien DJ, Vaughan Jones R, Creamer B. Steatorrhea in Addison's disease. Lancet 1:26, 1963.
223. Rodgers JB, Riley EM, Drummey GD, et al. Lipid absorption in adrenalectomized rats: the role of altered enzyme activity in the intestinal mucosa. Gastroenterology 53:547, 1967.
224. Orth DN, Kovacs WS, DeBold CR. The adrenal cortex. In Wilson JD, Foster DW (eds.): Williams Textbook of Endocrinology, 8th ed. Philadelphia, WB Saunders, 1992, p 489.
225. Su AY, Bilhartz LE. Endocrine-related gut dysfunction. Semin Gastrointest Dis 6:217, 1995.
226. Heneghan MA, McHugh P, Stevens FM, et al. Addison's disease and selective IgA deficiency in two coeliac patients. Scand J Gastroenterol 32:509, 1997.
227. Brosnan P, Riley WJ. Autoimmune polyglandular syndrome. In Sperling MA (ed.): Pediatric Endocrinology. Philadelphia, WB Saunders, 1996, p 509.
228. Kaukinen K, Collin P, Mykkanen AH, et al. Celiac disease and autoimmune endocrinologic disorders. Dig Dis Sci 44:1428, 1999.
229. Högenauer C, Meyer RL, Netto GJ, et al. Malabsorption due to cholecystokinin deficiency in a patient with autoimmune polyglandular syndrome type 1. N Engl J Med 344:270, 2001.
230. Jackson WPU. Steatorrhea and hypoparathyroidism. Lancet 272: 1086, 1957.
231. Sjoberg KH. Moniliasis—an internal disease? Three cases of idiopathic hypoparathyroidism with moniliasis, steatorrhea, primary amenorrhea and pernicious anemia. Acta Med Scand 179:157, 1966.
232. Hellesen C, Friis T, Larsen E, et al. Small intestinal histology, radiology and absorption in hyperthyroidism. Scand J Gastroenterol 4:169, 1969.
233. Wegener M, Wedmann B, Langhoff T, et al. Effect of hyperthyroidism on the transit of a caloric solid-liquid meal through the stomach, the small intestine, and the colon in man. J Clin Endocrinol Metab 75: 745, 1992.
234. Thomas FB, Caldwell JH, Greenberger NJ. Steatorrhea in thyrotoxicosis. Relation to hypermotility and excessive dietary fat. Ann Intern Med 78:669, 1973.
235. Goswami R, Tandon RK, Dudha A, et al. Prevalence and significance of steatorrhea in patients with active Graves' disease. Am J Gastroenterol 93:1122, 1998.
236. Schiller LR, Santa Ana CA, Schmulen AC, et al. Pathogenesis of fecal incontinence in diabetes mellitus: evidence for internal-anal-sphincter dysfunction. N Engl J Med 307:1666, 1982.
237. Whalen GE, Soergel KH, Greenen JE. Diabetic diarrhea. Gastroenterology 56:1021, 1969.
238. Rensch MJ, Merenich JA, Lieberman M, et al. Gluten-sensitive enteropathy in patients with insulin-dependent diabetes mellitus. Ann Intern Med 124:564, 1996.
239. Goldstein F, Wirts CW, Kowlessar D. Diabetic diarrhea and steatorrhea. Microbiologic and clinical observations. Ann Intern Med 72:215, 1970.
240. Blumenthal HT. Interrelationships of diabetes mellitus and pancreatitis. Arch Surg 87:844, 1963.
241. De-Block CE, De-Leeuw I, Van-Gaal LF. High prevalence of manifestations of gastric autoimmunity in parietal cell antibody-positive type 1 (insulin-dependent) diabetic patients. The Belgian Diabetes Registry. J Clin Endocrinol Metab 84:4062, 1999.
242. Irvine WJ, Clarke BF, Scarth L, et al. Thyroid and gastric autoimmunity in patients with diabetes. Lancet 2:163, 1970.
243. Klein KB, Orwoll ES, Lieberman DA, et al. Metabolic bone disease in asymptomatic men after partial gastrectomy with Billroth II anastomosis. Gastroenterology 92:608, 1987.
244. Scott EM, Gaywood I, Scott BB. Guidelines for osteoporosis in coeliac disease and inflammatory bowel disease. British Society of Gastroenterology. Gut(Suppl 1)46: il, 2000.
245. McFarlane XA, Bhalla AK, Reeves DE, et al. Osteoporosis in treated adult coeliac disease. Gut 36:710, 1995.
246. Valdimarsson T, Lofman O, Toss G, et al. Reversal of osteopenia with diet in adult coeliac disease. Gut 38:322, 1996.
247. Farthing MGJ, Dawson AM. Impaired semen quality in Crohn's disease—drugs, ill health or undernutrition? Scand J Gastroenterol 18:57, 1983.
248. Jeppesen PB, Mortensen PB. Colonic digestion and absorption of energy from carbohydrates and medium-chain fat in small bowel failure. JPEN J Parenter Enteral Nutr 23:S101, 1999.
249. Wharton R, D'Agati V, Magun AM, et al. Acute deterioration of renal function associated with enteric hyperoxaluria. Clin Nephrol 34:116, 1990.
250. Westergaard H. Duodenal bile acid concentrations in fat malabsorption syndromes. Scand J Gastroenterol 12:115, 1977.
251. Schiller LR, Rivera L, Santangelo WC, et al. Diagnostic value of fasting plasma peptide concentrations in patients with chronic diarrhea. Dig Dis Sci 39:2216, 1994.
252. Riddell RH. Small intestinal biopsy: Who? How? What are the findings? In Barkin JS, Rogers AI (eds.): Difficult Decisions in Digestive Diseases. Chicago, Year Book Medical Publishers, 1989, p 326.
253. Riley SA, Marsh MN. Maldigestion and malabsorption. In Feldman M, Scharschmidt BF, Sleisenger MH (eds.): Sleisenger & Fordtran's Gastrointestinal and Liver Disease, 6th ed. Philadelphia, WB Saunders, 1998, p 1501.
254. Johnson JD. The regional and ethnic distribution of lactose malabsorption. In Paige DM, Bayless TM (eds.): Lactose Digestion. Clinical and Nutritional Implications, 1st ed. Baltimore, The Johns Hopkins University Press, 1981, p 11.
255. Chassany O, Michaux A, Bergmann JF. Drug-induced diarrhoea. Drug Saf 22:53, 2000.
256. Longstreth GF, Newcomer AD. Drug-induced malabsorption. Mayo Clin Proc 50:284, 1975.
257. Adams JF, Clark JS, Ireland JT, et al. Malabsorption of vitamin B_{12} and intrinsic factor secretion during biguanide therapy. Diabetologia 24:16, 1983.
258. Bauman WA, Shaw S, Jayatilleke E, et al. Increased intake of calcium reverses vitamin B_{12} malabsorption induced by metformin. Diabetes Care 23:1227, 2000.
259. Hendel J, Dam M, Gram L, et al. The effects of carbamazepine and valproate on folate metabolism in man. Acta Neurol Scand 69:226, 1984.
260. Race TF, Paes IC. Intestinal malabsorption induced by oral colchicine. Am J Med Sci 259:32, 1970.
261. Lembcke B, Caspary WF. Malabsorption syndromes. Baillieres Clin Gastroenterol 2:329, 1988.
262. Force RW, Nahata MC. Effect of histamine H_2-receptor antagonists on vitamin B_{12} absorption. Ann Pharmacother 26:1283, 1992.
263. Shneerson JM, Gazzard BG. Reversible malabsorption caused by methyldopa. Br Med J 2:1456, 1977.
264. Peters JC, Lawson KD, Middleton SJ, et al. Assessment of the nutritional effects of olestra, nonabsorbed fat replacement: summary. J Nutr 127:1719, 1997.
265. Thornquist MD, Kristal AR, Patterson RE, et al. Olestra consumption does not predict serum concentrations of carotenoids and fat-soluble vitamins in free-living humans: early results from the sentinel site of the olestra post-marketing surveillance study. J Nutr 130:1711, 2000.
266. Shafer RB, Nuttall FQ. Calcium and folic acid absorption in patients taking anticonvulsant drugs. J Clin Endocrinol Metab 41:1125, 1975.
267. Zimmerman J, Selhub J, Rosenberg IH. Competitive inhibition of folate absorption by dihydrofolate reductase inhibitors, trimethoprim and pyrimethamine. Am J Clin Nutr 46:518, 1987.
268. Nakamura T, Kudoh K, Takebe K, et al. Octreotide decreases biliary

and pancreatic exocrine function, and induces steatorrhea in healthy subjects. Intern Med 33:593, 1994.
269. Witt K, Pedersen NT. The long-acting somatostatin analogue SMS 201-995 causes malabsorption. Scand J Gastroenterol 24:1248, 1989.
270. Oliver MR, Scott RB. Drug-induced bowel injury. In Walker WA (ed.): Pediatric Gastrointestinal Disease, 2nd ed. St. Louis, Mosby, 1996, p 882.
271. Zerwekh JE, Pak CY. Selective effects of thiazide therapy on serum 1 alpha,25-dihydroxyvitamin D and intestinal calcium absorption in renal and absorptive hypercalciurias. Metabolism 29:13, 1980.
272. Mason JB, Zimmerman J, Otradovec CL, et al. Chronic diuretic therapy with moderate doses of triamterene is not associated with folate deficiency. J Lab Clin Med 117:365, 1991.
273. Thier SO, Alpers DH. Disorders of intestinal transport of amino acids. Am J Dis Child 117:13, 1969.
274. Hooft C, Timmermans J, Snoeck J, et al. Methionine malabsorption in a mentally defective child. Lancet 2:20, 1964.
275. Desjeux JF. Congenital transport defects. In Walker WA (ed.): Pediatric Gastrointestinal Disease, 2nd ed. St. Louis, Mosby, 1996, p 792.
276. Semenza G, Auricchio S. Small-intestinal disaccharidases. In Scriver CR, Beaudet AL, Sly WS, et al. (eds.): The Metabolic and Molecular Bases of Inherited Disease, 7th ed. New York, McGraw-Hill, 1995, p 4451.
277. Desjeux JF. The molecular and genetic base of congenital transport defects. Gut 46:585, 2000.
278. Assmann G, Seedorf U. Acid lipase deficiency: Wolman disease and cholesteryl ester storage disease. In Scriver CR, Beaudet AL, Sly WS, et al. (eds.): The Metabolic and Molecular Bases of Inherited Disease, 7th ed. New York, McGraw-Hill, 1995, p 2563.
279. Hitzig WH, Dohmann U, Pluss HJ, et al. Hereditary transcobalamin II deficiency: clinical findings in a new family. J Pediatr 85:622, 1974.
280. Chanarin I. Disorders of vitamin absorption. Clin Gastroenterol 11:73, 1982.
281. Muller DPR, Millo PJ. Selective inborn errors of absorption. In Muller DRR, Millo PJ: Harries's Pediatric Gastroenterology, 2nd ed. New York, Churchill Livingstone, 1988, p 211.
282. Romero R, Meacham LR, Winn KT. Isolated magnesium malabsorption in a 10-year-old boy. Am J Gastroenterol 91:611, 1996.
283. Danks DM. Copper transport and utilization in Menkes' syndrome and in mottled mice. Inor Perspect Biol Med 1:73, 1977.
284. Danks DM. Disorders of copper transport. In Scriver CR, Beaudet AL, Sly WS, et al. (eds.): The Metabolic and Molecular Bases of Inherited Disease, 7th ed. New York, McGraw-Hill, 1995, p 2211.
285. Davidson GP. Enteropathies of unknown origin. In Walker WA (ed.): Pediatric Gastrointestinal Disease, 2nd ed. St. Louis, Mosby, 1996, p 862.

Chapter 90

Enteric Bacterial Flora and Small Bowel Bacterial Overgrowth Syndrome

Clark R. Gregg and Phillip P. Toskes

When overgrowth of bacteria occurs in the small bowel upstream to the distal ileum, symptoms of vitamin malabsorption, malnutrition, and weight loss may occur. This clinical condition is known as the stagnant or blind loop syndrome, or more generally, small bowel bacterial overgrowth syndrome (SBBOS). SBBOS may be an underappreciated cause of malnutrition, especially in the elderly.

A comprehensive understanding of SBBOS is based on knowledge of the indigenous microbial flora of the gastrointestinal tract. Classic investigations have thoroughly described the acquisition, evolution, and functions of the normal gastrointestinal flora beginning in the neonatal period.[1] This flora has been shown to have key roles not only in the intraluminal processing or modification of nutrients, drugs, and host-derived products of metabolism, but also in the normal development of the gastrointestinal immune system.[2] Control of the dense and diverse population of enteric microbial flora depends not only on the normal anatomic, physiologic, and immunologic traits of the gastrointestinal tract, but also on competitive behavior among different microbial species.

Bacterial overgrowth in segments of the intestinal tract not normally inhabited by high concentrations of microbes is implicated in the pathogenesis of diverse clinical problems such as biliary tract infection, spontaneous bacterial peritonitis complicating cirrhosis, exacerbations of inflammatory bowel disease, and infections that complicate major trauma or surgery. These disorders are considered in other chapters.

This chapter focuses on the development of the normal indigenous flora of the gastrointestinal tract, the mechanisms by which this flora is normally controlled, and the pathogenesis and clinical aspects of the small bowel bacterial overgrowth syndrome. Emphasis is placed on pitfalls in the diagnosis of SBBOS and on recent trends in the management of this clinical entity.

INDIGENOUS MICROBIAL FLORA OF THE ALIMENTARY TRACT

The acquisition of a normal resident enteric microbial population has been extensively investigated for decades and has been the subject of comprehensive reviews.[1–3] The quality of these studies rests on the contemporary technologies for collecting, culturing, identifying, and counting the complex array of species of microorganisms found in the gastrointestinal tract. Only recently have molecular diagnostic techniques been used to identify and recategorize the intestinal microflora.[4]

At birth the mammalian alimentary canal is sterile, and animals raised in a germ-free environment do not acquire an enteric flora. Within hours after birth, however, animals, including humans, in an ordinary environment become colonized perorally by coliforms and streptococci from their nursery surroundings and their mother's fecal flora.[5, 6] As these facultative bacteria multiply in the intestinal lumen, they consume oxygen and lower the redox potential in the gut lumen, thereby creating a receptive environment for growth of strictly anaerobic bacteria during the first weeks of life. At this time bifidobacteria, clostridia, and *Bacteroides* proliferate. Rates and patterns of acquisition of enteric flora differ with the mode of delivery (vaginal vs. cesarean section), the level of hygiene in the neonatal environment, the exposure to antibiotics and neonatal intensive care, and whether the neonate is breast-fed or bottle-fed.[6]

Anaerobic bacteria destined for static autochthonous residence in the gut of adults, including peptostreptococci, peptococci, eubacteria, and lactobacilli, are acquired later in infancy.[6] In parallel with the establishment of a predominantly anaerobic microflora of the lower intestinal tract, the number of facultative bacteria declines, and they are ultimately outnumbered as much as 10,000 : 1 by strict anaerobes in adult feces.

Table 90–1 | **Microbiologic and Physicochemical Ecology of the Normal Human Intestinal Tract**

PARAMETER	STOMACH	JEJUNUM	ILEUM	COLON
Total bacterial count*	0–3	0–4	5–9	10–12
Aerobes, facultative anaerobes*	0–3	0–4	2–5	2–9
Anaerobes*	0	0	3–7	9–12
Redox potential (mV)	+150	−50	−150	−200
pH	2.0–4.0	6.0–7.0	7.5	6.8–7.3

*Log_{10} CFU/g or mL contents (CFU, colony-forming units).

Because of peristalsis and the antimicrobial effects of gastric acidity, the stomach and proximal small bowel normally contain relatively small numbers of bacteria in most adults.[1, 7] Some healthy people will harbor microbes at concentrations exceeding 10^5 colony-forming units (CFU)/mL in the jejunum. When organisms are present, they are usually lactobacilli, oral streptococci, and other gram-positive aerobes or facultative anaerobes. Low concentrations of Enterobacteriaceae, yeasts, or swallowed oral or nasopharyngeal gram-negative microorganisms may be detected in the jejunum of 10% or more of healthy adults. The concentrations of microorganisms that normally populate the various portions of alimentary canal, the intraluminal pH, and the corresponding redox potential (i.e., the potential difference generated by the relative state of oxidation or reduction) are illustrated in Table 90–1 An increasingly negative redox potential corresponds to an increasingly anaerobic environment.

Proceeding aborally through the small intestine, acid is neutralized and the redox potential becomes strongly negative. The ileum is a zone of microbiologic transition from the sparse jejunal populations of predominantly aerobic flora to the dense anaerobic bacterial colonization of the colon. Bacterial colony counts are commonly 10^5 to 10^9 CFU/mL in the ileum and include coliforms and other typical fecal flora as well as strict anaerobes. An intact ileocecal valve seems to be an important barrier to backflow of colonic bacteria into the ileum.

The number and variety of enteric flora increase dramatically in the colon (Table 90–2). Bacteria reach concentrations of 10^{12} CFU/mL in feces and consist of as many as several hundred different species. The most common are *Bacteroides*, *Porphyromonas*, bifidobacteria, lactobacilli, *Escherichia coli* and other coliforms, enterococci, and clostridia.[1–3, 8]

Effects on Morphology and Function of the Intestine

Our knowledge of the consequences of having a normal enteric flora derives from studies comparing germ-free and conventionally reared animals. Recent studies have attempted to categorize these differences as microflora-associated characteristics (MAC) or germ-free animal characteristics (GAC) to determine the influence of the intestinal microflora.[9] In the small bowel mucosa of germ-free animals, villi are slender and uniform, and crypts are shallow compared with those in conventional animals. There are also dramatic reductions in leukocytic infiltration of the lamina propria, the size and number of Peyer's patches, the number of mitoses in crypt epithelium, and the rate of mucosal regeneration in germ-free animals.[9, 10]

Colonization of the intestinal tract of germ-free animals with even a single strain of bacteria is followed by the rapid development of physiologic inflammation of the mucosa resembling that of conventional animals. Other MAC consequences of acquisition of an enteric flora include stimulation of the spatial and temporal spread of migrating motor complexes (MMCs) in the small intestine; expression of enteroendocrine cells; reduction in the cecum size; and establishment of a physicochemical milieu that permits the survival of a strictly anaerobic microflora in the colon.[9]

Biochemical Functional Activities

A variety of intestinal functions are influenced by the presence of an autochthonous symbiotic microflora in the intestinal tract. These biochemical functions are summarized in Table 90–3.

The principal mechanisms by which bacteria influence bile acid metabolism are deconjugation, oxidation, dehydroxylation, and hydroxylation. In humans, the primary bile acids cholic acid and chenodeoxycholic acid are excreted in bile as conjugates with taurine, glycine, sulfate, or glucuronide and participate in dietary lipid absorption (see Chapter 88). In the colon, bacterial enzymes convert cholic acid and chenodeoxycholic acid to the secondary bile acids deoxycholic acid and lithocholic acid, respectively, which are poorly reabsorbed and are then eliminated in the stool. In SBBOS, bile acids are deconjugated and metabolized more proximally in the small bowel and removed from further participation in the normal enterohepatic circulation (see Chapter 54), resulting in bile acid malabsorption and steatorrhea.[3, 9]

Intestinal bacteria also metabolize biologically active sterols such as androgens and estrogens. Conjugates of these hormones are excreted in bile into the gut, where bacterial

Table 90–2 | **Human Colonic Bacterial Flora**

BACTERIAL GENUS	PREVALENCE (%)
Anaerobes	
Bacteroides	100
Porphyromonas	100
Bifidobacterium	30–70
Lactobacillus	20–60
Clostridium	25–35
Peptostreptococcus	*
Peptococcus	*
Various methanogens	*
Facultative aerobes	
Enterococcus	100
E. coli	100
Enterobacteriaceae other than *E. coli*	40–80
Staphylococcus	30–50

*Although exact prevalence is unknown, these are very common in fecal flora.

Modified from Levy J: The effects of antibiotic use on gastrointestinal function. Am J Gastroenterol 95(suppl. 1):S8, 2000.

Table 90–3 | **Intraluminal Biochemical Functions Influenced by Enteric Flora**

FUNCTION	MECHANISM OR PRODUCT	IMPORTANCE TO HOST
Bile acid metabolism	Deconjugation Dehydrogenation Dehydroxylation	Enterohepatic circulation Steatorrhea in SBBOS
Bilirubin metabolism	Deconjugation Urobilin formation	Bilirubin excretion
Cholesterol metabolism	Coprostanol	Excretion of cholesterol
Mucin metabolism	Degradation	Sustenance of flora
Lipid metabolism	Fatty acids and hydroxylated fatty acids	Diarrhea
Protein metabolism	Ammonia, amines	Metabolic encephalopathy
Carbohydrate metabolism	Organic acids	Calorie conservation by colon Water and electrolyte conservation by colon ?Role in hepatic coma, colon cancer, IBD
	CO_2, H_2	Breath tests for malabsorption
	Methane	Explosions at colonoscopy
	D-Lactate	Encephalopathy

IBD, inflammatory bowel disease; SBBOS, small bowel bacterial overgrowth syndrome.

Adapted from Toskes PP, Kumar A: Enteric bacterial flora and bacterial overgrowth syndrome. Midtvedt T: Microbial functional activities. In Hanson LA, Yolken RH (eds): Probiotics, Other Nutritional Factors, and Intestinal Microflora. Philadelphia, Lippincott-Raven, 1999, p 79.

β-glucuronidase and sulfatase hydrolyze the conjugate. This deconjugation is necessary for reabsorption and conservation of the sterol hormones. Exogenous and endogenous cholesterol are metabolized by anaerobic intestinal bacteria to form coprostanol, a sterol that is excreted in feces without being absorbed.[9] This pathway could be a component in the normal regulation of circulating cholesterol levels.

As unabsorbed dietary lipids, proteins, carbohydrates and fiber reach the colon, they are rapidly metabolized by enteric bacteria.[1, 3, 11] Short-chain fatty acids (SCFAs) are produced by microbial degradation of exogenous or endogenous lipids via complex mechanisms that are influenced by diet and antibiotic exposure.[12] Microbial production of SCFA is of interest because of the role SCFA may play not only in regulation of the normal enteric flora but also in normal mucosal physiology and the pathogenesis of cancer.[1, 9] Hydroxy fatty acids produced by bacteria cause diarrhea in some patients with steatorrhea.[3]

Degradation of protein and urea to form ammonia is a function of intestinal bacteria. Absorption of ammonia is important in hepatic encephalopathy and in metabolic defects in the urea cycle.[3] Enteric flora also inactivate trypsin, but the clinical or physiologic consequences of this effect are poorly understood.[9]

Short-chain fatty acids such as acetic, propionic, and butyric acids are also products of enteric microbial fermentation of unabsorbed dietary carbohydrates. Absorption of these SCFAs supports the normal integrity of the colonic mucosa and conserves energy even in patients with substantial malabsorption. Antibiotic-associated diarrhea, especially that encountered with enteral alimentation, may in many cases result from interruption of this fermentation process, leading to increased intraluminal osmolality and osmotic diarrhea.[13] Bacterial fermentation of carbohydrates to form D-lactate can lead to D-lactic acidosis in patients with malabsorption or intestinal bypass surgery[14] and may be influenced by the dietary intake of nutrient substrates.[11]

The bacterial flora of the intestinal tract are also important in the metabolism of some drugs and other xenobiotics. Drugs for which this interface is a key to their pharmacologic effect include sulfasalazine and the prodrugs balsalazide and olsalazine. Digoxin, chloramphenicol, rifampin, morphine, colchicine, conjugated estrogens, and levodopa are also metabolized in part by enteric bacteria.[1, 3] Dietary cyclamates are converted by enteric bacteria to the carcinogen cyclohexylamine, and mutagenic nitrosamines are produced by bacterial metabolism of nitrate food preservatives.[1, 3]

Homeostasis

In the healthy human host, control of the growth of enteric bacterial populations is multifactorial. The most important control mechanisms are the ability of gastric acid to inhibit or kill swallowed microorganisms (even in immunocompromised hosts) and the cleansing effects of normal intestinal motility.[1, 3] Immunoglobulins in intestinal secretions and an intact ileocecal valve are also important.

Achlorhydria resulting from gastric mucosal atrophy, gastric resection or vagotomy, or highly effective antacid or acid antisecretory therapies permits viable swallowed bacteria to pass into the small intestine.[3, 15, 16] In the small bowel, the cleansing action of antegrade peristalsis, especially the interdigestive migrating motor complex (MMC),[17, 18] is responsible for sweeping bacteria into the colon at a rapid rate.[3] Conditions that result in dysmotility of the small bowel are frequently complicated by bacterial overgrowth, which may not necessarily be symptomatic.[15, 16] Interception of bacteria by the mucous layer may further retard their ability to gain a foothold in the proximal small bowel.

Stagnation of intraluminal flow and incomplete competence of the ileocecal sphincter account for the ordinarily higher bacterial counts in the distal ileum.[3] In the colon, bacterial interaction, competition for nutrients, and the anaerobic environment attributable to bacterial metabolism are significant factors that control microbial populations.[1, 3] Other modulating factors that are less well understood include the bacterial production of bacteriocins and toxic metabolites, microbial sharing of metabolic factors, transfer of antibiotic resistance, and the role of the mucosa in elaboration of growth factors and secretory immunoglobulins.[2, 19]

Antibiotic therapy is widely recognized to alter the microflora of the intestinal tract by suppressing or eradicating selected populations of bacteria while permitting resistant microbes to flourish. These effects depend on the composition of the enteric flora and the spectrum of activity, route of administration, dose, duration, and pharmacokinetics of the antibiotic.[8] Selective antibiotic suppression of intestinal bacteria may be important in the use of these drugs for preventing infections in patients compromised by surgery, trauma, or granulocytopenia.[3] Treatment of SBBOS generally includes oral antibiotics, but the broader effects of these drugs on the balance of intestinal flora are complex.[8]

Some studies support a contributing role of the immune system in regulation of the intestinal flora. There may be altered levels of intraluminal secretory IgA[20, 21] or increased mucosal IgA immunocytes[22] in patients with small bowel bacterial overgrowth. Patients with chronic lymphocytic leukemia and bacterial overgrowth have had undetectable secretory component of IgA in jejunal aspirate specimens.[23] Deficiencies of immunoglobulins or specific secretory IgA as well as T cell defects have been associated with SBBOS.[24] However, bacterial overgrowth in the elderly seems not to be related to immunosenescence.[25, 26]

There is little evidence indicating a significant role of dietary composition or manipulation on regulation of the microbial population of the normal bowel.[3] Moreover, pancreatic and biliary secretions do not likely influence the intestinal flora significantly.

MECHANISMS OF MALABSORPTION AND DIARRHEA IN SMALL BOWEL BACTERIAL OVERGROWTH SYNDROME

In the small bowel of patients or experimental animals with SBBOS, the microbial population is variable but complex and usually resembles the bacterial composition of the colon. Bacterial colony counts may reach 10^{10} CFU/mL and consist of *Bacteroides*, anaerobic lactobacilli, facultative Enterobacteriaceae, enterococci, clostridia, and diphtheroids. Small bowel bacterial overgrowth syndrome is associated with various nonspecific abdominal symptoms and malassimilation of nutrients including cobalamin (vitamin B_{12}), fats, carbohydrates, and protein.

In general, malabsorption in SBBOS can be attributed to the intraluminal effects of proliferating bacteria combined with damage to mucosal enterocytes. A patchy microscopic small bowel mucosal lesion can be readily identified and consists of villus blunting, loss of structural integrity of epithelial cells, and inflammatory infiltration of the lamina propria.[27] Functional consequences of this damage that have been detected include diminished disaccharidase activity; decreased transport of monosaccharides, amino acids, and fatty acids; and protein-losing enteropathy.[3, 28, 29]

Cobalamin deficiency that cannot be corrected by intrinsic factor, but improves after antibiotic administration, is a classic manifestation of SBBOS. At the resident pH of the proximal small bowel, gastric intrinsic factor normally binds tightly to cobalamin, and the vitamin is then absorbed from the distal ileum (see Fig. 38–10). Bacteria prevalent in SBBOS, especially various anaerobes and facultative gram-negative aerobes, competitively utilize dietary cobalamin. Intrinsic factor inhibits cobalamin utilization by aerobic bacteria but has no effect on the ability of gram-negative anaerobic flora to take up dietary cobalamin.[30] Although enteric bacteria also synthesize some cobalamin, they retain the vitamin, so it does not become sufficiently available to the host for absorption. Thus, paradoxically, cobalamin deficiency develops in patients with SBBOS even though they harbor large quantities of the vitamin in bacteria in their small bowel. In patients whose predisposition to SBBOS is achlorhydria, the defects in cobalamin absorption are even more complex (see Chapter 38); nonetheless, the principal factor responsible for its malabsorption seems to be intraluminal bacterial utilization of cobalamin.[31, 32]

These same bacteria synthesize folic acid and liberate it into the small bowel lumen from which it is absorbed. Thus, patients with SBBOS rarely become folate deficient and, in fact, may have high rather than low folate levels.[3]

Fat malabsorption (steatorrhea) in SBBOS is a consequence of small intestinal bacterial deconjugation of bile salts. Water-soluble conjugated bile salts normally are secreted to form mixed micelles with partially digested dietary lipids. These conjugated bile salts are not readily reabsorbed until they reach the ileum. When bacteria overgrow the proximal small bowel, they deconjugate bile salts to form free bile acids, which are readily reabsorbed by the jejunum. If this effect is rapid, there is impaired formation of bile salt–lipid mixed micelles, and dietary fat is malabsorbed. Additionally, the free bile acids formed in SBBOS may be toxic for the mucosa and contribute directly to the patchy mucosal lesion of SBBOS.[33] Malaborption of fat-soluble vitamins (vitamins A, D, E, and K) may occur in SBBOS as a consequence of general fat malabsorption. In rare cases, these deficiencies may be clinically significant.[31]

Carbohydrate malassimilation may also be a consequence of SBBOS. This may result from a combination of intraluminal carbohydrate degradation by bacteria and damage to the brush border disaccharidase functions of the small bowel mucosa. D-Xylose absorption is often reduced in SBBOS, and excessive intraluminal carbohydrate metabolism by bacteria is the basis for the ^{14}C-xylose breath test sometimes used to diagnose SBBOS.[3] Furthermore, malabsorbed carbohydrates can be catabolized by small bowel and colonic bacteria to form short-chain organic acids that increase the osmolarity of intestinal fluid and contribute to diarrhea.

Protein depletion in SBBOS is also multifactorial. Protein malnutrition results from a combination of impaired absorption of amino acids,[28] intraluminal utilization of dietary proteins by bacteria,[34] and an antibiotic-reversible protein-losing enteropathy resulting from mucosal damage and leakage of protein into the lumen.[3, 29, 31] The cobalamin deficiency of SBBOS may aggravate small bowel mucosal damage and protein malabsorption.[31]

Two additional factors may contribute to the diarrhea and other features of SBBOS. First, bacterial metabolites, such as free bile acids,[35] hydroxylated fatty acids, and other organic acids, stimulate secretion of water and electrolytes into the bowel lumen. This effect may result in a component of secretory diarrhea in SBBOS. Second, experimental bacterial overgrowth in rats results in further dysmotility of the bowel, which may encourage additional bacterial overgrowth.[36]

Clinical Aspects

Predisposition

Various clinical disorders predispose patients to SBBOS. Unifying features of many of these conditions include most prominently (1) small intestinal stagnation and dysmotility, or (2) compromise of the gastric acid barrier to survival of swallowed bacteria.

Prior to the recognition and management of *Helicobacter pylori* infection as a common cause of duodenal ulcer disease, aggressive surgical management of this disease was common. The most frequent operation was the Billroth II gastrojejunostomy, which created a stagnant afferent loop that often resulted in bacterial overgrowth. Similarly, stagnant loops of intestine and bacterial overgrowth result from enteroenteric fistulas that complicate Crohn's disease or the surgical enterostomies often used to manage this disease. The ileo-anal pouch procedure, used to treat ulcerative colitis and familial adenomatous polyposis, inevitably results in some degree of SBBOS, which may be severe.[37] Other gastroduodenal surgeries have also been associated with postoperative SBBOS.[38–42] Similarly, in patients with gastrocolic or gastrojejunocolic fistulas, massive overgrowth and severe malabsorption may develop.[3]

Obstruction or dysmotility of the small bowel caused by diverse problems such as Crohn's disease, radiation enteropathy, adhesions, lymphoma, or tuberculosis may result in SBBOS.[3, 43] Other intestinal motility disorders, often coupled with hypochlorhydria, also predispose to SBBOS. Reported examples include scleroderma (Fig. 90–1),[44, 45] chronic intestinal pseudo-obstruction,[46] diabetes mellitus,[47] cystic fibrosis,[48] and disordered migrating motor complex.[17] Duodenal and jejunal diverticula (Fig. 90–2) may also be overgrown, especially in patients with hypochlorhydria or achlorhydria.[3]

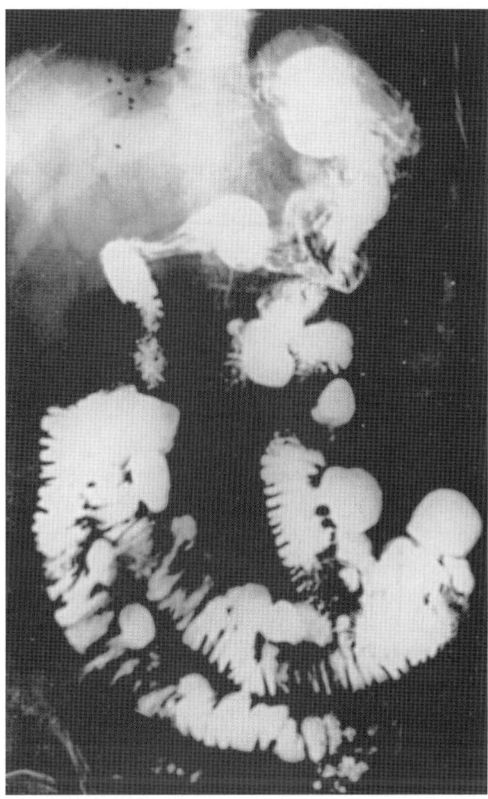

Figure 90–2. An upper gastrointestinal and small bowel series in an elderly man with small bowel bacterial overgrowth syndrome due to numerous small bowel diverticula.

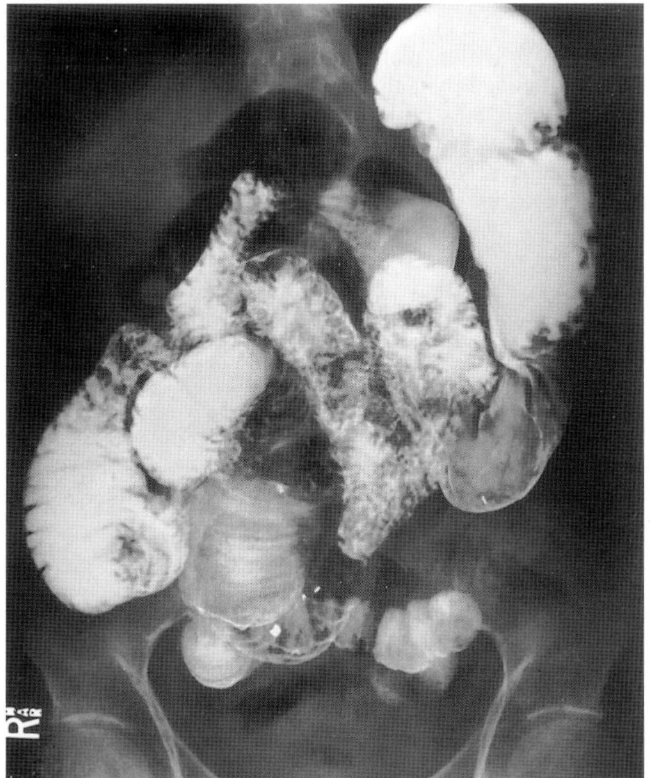

Figure 90–1. An upper gastrointestinal and small bowel series in a woman with scleroderma who presented with severe weight loss, cobalamin (vitamin B_{12}) deficiency, and marked steatorrhea. These abnormalities were corrected by broad spectrum antibiotics. Note the marked dilation of intestinal segments throughout the entire small bowel.

Several other clinical entities with which there has been a possible association of SBBOS include chronic pancreatitis,[49] end-stage renal disease,[50] myotonic muscular dystrophy,[51] fibromyalgia,[52] and chronic fatigue syndrome.[53] The underlying pathophysiologic mechanisms of bacterial overgrowth described with these diseases has not been fully elucidated. Small intestinal bacterial overgrowth has been described in cirrhosis,[54–56] likely related to intestinal dysmotility, but this finding has seemed more relevant to the occurrence of spontaneous bacterial peritonitis rather than malabsorption.

Healthy elderly subjects have been found to have small bowel bacterial overgrowth without recognized problems with nutrient absorption, a condition known as simple colonization.[15, 57, 58] However, symptomatic SBBOS may develop in the aged as a consequence of achlorhydria or other predisposing diseases. Some authorities think that SBBOS is perhaps the most common discernible cause of malabsorption in geriatric populations.[3, 59–62]

The importance of both normal gastric acidity and normal intestinal motility is highlighted by experience with patients with scleroderma and reflux esophagitis in whom symptomatic malabsorption developed only after proton pump inhibitor treatment was substituted for less effective antacid therapy.[3] Indeed the impact of highly effective antacid therapies, including histamine H_2 blockers[63] and especially proton pump inhibitors,[64–66] on the subsequent occurrence of SBBOS is beginning to be appreciated.

Bacterial overgrowth has been described in patients with various immunodeficiency syndromes including chronic lymphocytic leukemia,[23] immunoglobulin deficiencies,[67] and selective T cell deficiency.[24] Although epidemiologic studies have not been reported, symptomatic SBBOS appears to be less common than simple colonization of the small bowel in these immunodeficiency diseases.

Clinical Features

The clinical consequences of SBBOS are similar regardless of the underlying predisposition to overgrowth (Table 90–4). However, individual symptoms may vary depending on the nature of the primary small bowel abnormality.

Small bowel diverticula, which may be multiple in elderly patients, are generally asymptomatic for many years before sufficient bacterial overgrowth occurs, often as a consequence of acquired achlorhydria, to cause malabsorption (see Chapter 19). Patients with strictures, obstruction, motility disorders, or surgically formed blind loops of bowel typically complain of variable abdominal discomfort, bloating, or periumbilical cramps, which may herald by months or years the development of diarrhea and malabsorption. In patients with Crohn's disease, scleroderma, chronic intestinal pseudo-obstruction, radiation enteritis, short bowel syndromes, or intestinal lymphoma, it may be difficult to determine the extent to which symptoms and malabsorption are attributable to the primary disease or to SBBOS.

In one third of patients with SBBOS severe enough to cause cobalamin deficiency, weight loss occurs that is associated with clinically demonstrable steatorrhea.[68] Malabsorption of fat-soluble vitamins can cause night blindness (vitamin A), osteomalacia (vitamin D), hypocalcemic tetany (vitamin D), coagulopathy (vitamin K), or vitamin E deficiency syndromes (neuropathy, retinopathy, T cell abnormalities).[31]

Cobalamin malabsorption caused by SBBOS results in macrocytic and megaloblastic anemia. If the cobalamin deficiency is severe and prolonged, characteristic neurologic damage including posterolateral spinal cord demyelinization, peripheral neuropathy, and cerebral cognitive defects can occur. Additionally, iron deficiency may result from intestinal blood loss, perhaps secondary to ulcerations within stagnant bowel loops. Thus patients with SBBOS may have detectable fecal occult blood and hypochromic microcytic anemia coincident with megaloblastic anemia.[3, 69]

Table 90–4 | **Clinical Features of Small Bowel Bacterial Overgrowth Syndrome**

SYMPTOMS	Abdominal discomfort Bloating sensation Diarrhea Weight loss Weakness Neuropathy

CLINICAL FINDINGS	Vitamin deficiencies
	  Cobalamin (vitamin B_{12})
	  Fat-soluble vitamins (A, D, E, K)
	Fat and carbohydrate malabsorption
	Hypoproteinemia or hypoalbuminemia
	Iron deficiency

Hypoproteinemia and hypoalbuminemia are common consequences of SBBOS and can be severe enough to cause edema. These mucosal and intraluminal abnormalities of protein digestion and assimilation, as well as protein-losing enteropathy, are reversible with successful management of bacterial overgrowth.

Similarly, SBBOS results in intraluminal catabolism of carbohydrates and dysfunction of mucosal disaccharidases and malabsorption of sugars.[28, 70] Short-chain organic acids, which are products of this disorder of carbohydrate digestion, may contribute to osmolar and pH changes in the colon. These factors combine with other intraluminal disturbances (deconjugated bile acids, hydroxylated fatty acids) and intestinal dysmotility to aggravate watery diarrhea in SBBOS.

Approaches to Diagnosis of SBBOS

With the recent decline in surgery for management of peptic ulcer disease, the diagnosis of SBBOS is now considered most commonly in patients with problems other than those associated with gastrointestinal surgery. Dysmotility syndromes (especially gastroparesis and irritable bowel syndrome) and chronic pancreatitis with symptoms suggestive of malabsorption have been frequent reasons for referral to centers that specialize in testing for small bowel bacterial overgrowth.[71] Differentiation of the symptoms of these disorders from similar symptoms that might be caused by superimposed SBBOS is critical to these patients' treatment and requires sophisticated testing.

Symptoms of diarrhea, weight loss, bloating, and flatulence in patients with coexisting predispositions to SBBOS, regardless of whether malabsorption has been demonstrated, are reasons to consider testing for bacterial overgrowth, especially if patients have failed to respond to empirical measures.[3] Certainly any patient with a known predisposition to bacterial overgrowth who has diarrhea, steatorrhea, weight loss, or cobalamin deficiency should be evaluated for SBBOS (Fig. 90–3).

A history of gastrointestinal surgery in patients with symptoms of SBBOS should prompt a review of whether that surgery resulted in construction of an afferent loop (Billroth II procedure), or end-to-side or side-to-side small bowel anastomosis. Recurrent symptoms of small bowel obstruction might result from strictures, adhesions, dysmotility, or intestinal pseudo-obstruction, which can cause stasis and bacterial overgrowth. Dysphagia and other symptoms of systemic sclerosis should suggest that scleroderma might explain symptoms of malabsorption resulting from bacterial overgrowth. The barium small bowel series radiograph is an appropriate noninvasive study for these conditions as well as for small bowel diverticula or enteric fistulas.

Basic laboratory evaluations should optimally include quantitative stool fat measurement to document steatorrhea, and a differential Schilling test to detect cobalamin malabsorption. In clinically significant SBBOS, cobalamin absorp-

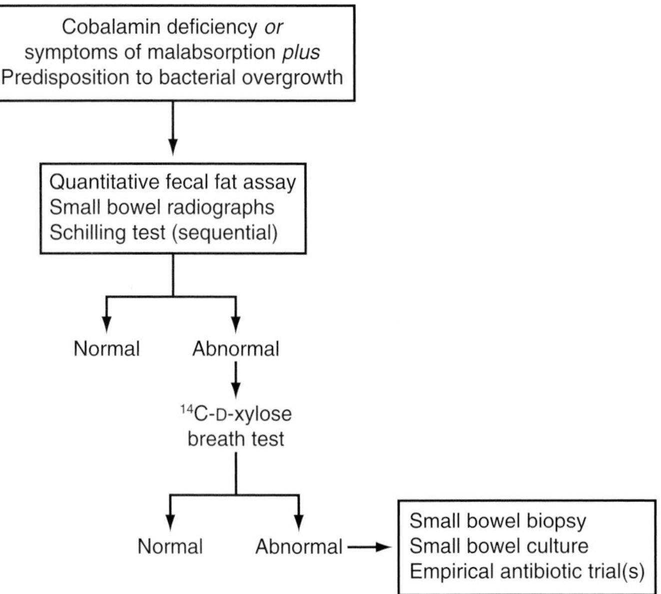

Figure 90–3. Diagnostic algorithm for small bowel bacterial overgrowth syndrome (SBBOS).

tion in the Schilling test, part 1 is often significantly impaired even though anemia, neurologic disease, and abnormal serum levels of vitamin B_{12} and methylmalonate may not yet be apparent. Administration of intrinsic factor (Schilling test, part 2) does not correct this absorptive defect, but a course of broad-spectrum oral antibiotic therapy is followed by normalization of cobalamin absorption in SBBOS.[72] In some patients with SBBOS, the D-xylose absorption test result is also abnormal, and the serum folate level may be elevated.

Following documentation of abnormal functional tests that suggest SBBOS, a small intestine biopsy may be useful to exclude primary mucosal diseases such as celiac sprue as causes of malabsorption. Unlike the diffuse mucosal abnormality in celiac sprue, a similar but patchy inflammatory lesion is often found in SBBOS. This lesion characteristically consists of infiltration of the lamina propria with lymphocytes, plasma cells, and neutrophils. Mean villus height is significantly reduced,[27] and villi are thickened and blunt. The mucosal histologic morphology often returns to normal in SBBOS following successful antibiotic treatment.[27] More thorough differentiation of SBBOS from celiac sprue ideally will include quantitative and qualitative small bowel culture specimens obtained by endoscopy or intestinal intubation.

For several decades, the gold standard for confirming a diagnosis of bacterial overgrowth has been a properly collected culture specimen of fluid aspirated from the proximal small intestine. These techniques are cumbersome, time-consuming, and expensive, and they require the services of a dedicated microbiology laboratory highly skilled with quantitative culture techniques and anaerobic bacteriology. Specimens are collected anaerobically, serially diluted, and cultured quantitatively on a variety of routine and selective bacteriologic media. In patients with clinically significant bacterial overgrowth, a mixed variety of anaerobic and facultative bacteria are detected, and bacterial colony counts are expected to exceed 10^5 CFU/mL of aspirate. In SBBOS, satisfactory cultures are generally obtained nonselectively from the proximal jejunum, but occasionally an isolated or more distal nidus of bacterial colonization can be missed by sampling a single site.

Positive small bowel culture results may be found in asymptomatic patients with simple colonization, which seems to be common in elderly patients.[15, 73] However, one study has shown that the finding of Enterobacteriaceae of nonsalivary origin in culture specimens of small bowel fluid is sufficient evidence for intestinal hypomotility.[74] Culture results must be interpreted in the context of the patients' other clinical and laboratory findings.

Because small intestinal intubation for quantitative culture is inconvenient, expensive, and not widely available, a variety of surrogate tests for bacterial overgrowth have been devised based on the metabolic actions of enteric bacteria (Table 90–5). Measurement of urinary excretion of indican, phenols, drug metabolites, and deconjugated para-aminobenzoic acid[75] are not sufficiently sensitive or specific to distinguish SBBOS from other causes of malabsorption. Quantitation of deconjugated bile acids[35] and short-chain fatty acids[76] in jejunal fluid requires intestinal intubation and thus is hampered by methodologic drawbacks that are similar to those of intestinal cultures.

Breath Tests

The ongoing search for less cumbersome alternatives to jejunal aspiration and culture for the diagnosis of SBBOS has led to the development of a variety of tests that measure the excretion in expired breath of volatile metabolites produced by intraluminal bacteria. The most successful and popular methods analyze either expired isotope-labeled CO_2 after timed oral administration of ^{14}C- or ^{13}C-enriched substrates or breath hydrogen following feeding of a nonlabeled fermentable carbohydrate substrate.

The first promising breath test technique for bacterial overgrowth was the bile acid or ^{14}C-cholylglycine test, based on the premise that small bowel bacteria in high concentrations would deconjugate this bile salt. This test was only moderately sensitive for detecting bacterial overgrowth, with a false-negative rate of 30% to 40%.[77, 78] Furthermore, the specificity of this breath test was poor because of colonic bacterial deconjugation of unabsorbed bile salt when there was ileal damage or resection.

A more sensitive and specific breath test has been the ^{14}C-D-xylose breath test.[79] Xylose is catabolized by aerobic gram-negative overgrowth flora, and both $^{14}CO_2$ produced by

Table 90–5 | **Tests for Small Bowel Bacterial Overgrowth**

TEST	SENSITIVITY	SPECIFICITY	SIMPLICITY
Jejunal culture	Excellent	Excellent	Poor
Urinary indican	Poor	Poor	Fair
Jejunal bile acids	Fair	Excellent	Poor
^{14}C-bile acid BT	Fair	Poor	Excellent
^{14}C-xylose BT	Good	Excellent	Excellent
Fasting H_2 BT	Poor	Good	Excellent
Lactulose-H_2 BT	Poor	Fair	Excellent
Glucose-H_2 BT	Fair	Fair	Excellent

BT, breath test; H_2, hydrogen.

bacterial fermentation of xylose and unmetabolized xylose are absorbed by the proximal small bowel, which thus avoids confusion of results caused by metabolism of substrate downstream by colonic bacteria. Following a 1-g oral dose of ^{14}C-xylose, elevated $^{14}CO_2$ levels are detected in the breath within 60 minutes in 85% of patients with SBBOS. The sensitivity and specificity of the ^{14}C-xylose breath test are superior to those of the ^{14}C-bile acid test.[77] Consequently, the ^{14}C-xylose test became a popular and reliable surrogate test for bacterial overgrowth.[80–82] Although more recent studies have raised doubts as to the accuracy of this test,[15] especially in severe disorders of intestinal motility,[83, 84] refinement of the ^{14}C-xylose breath test to include a transit marker for intestinal motility may enhance its specificity.[85]

A drawback of breath tests utilizing a ^{14}C-labeled substrate is that the use of the radioactive isotope is not recommended for study of children or fertile women. Xylose and cholyl-1-glycine labeled with ^{13}C, a nonradioactive isotope that is measured in breath as $^{13}CO_2$ by mass spectrometry, have been studied recently in adults and children.[86, 87] These tests show some promise in evaluating malabsorption but are not yet sufficiently validated to recommend widespread acceptance.[88]

Since mammalian tissue does not generate hydrogen, the detection of hydrogen in expired breath is considered a measure of the metabolic activity of enteric bacteria. This observation has suggested that measurement of breath hydrogen could circumvent the administration of a radioactive isotope in testing for bacterial overgrowth. In patients with bacterial overgrowth, excessive breath hydrogen production has been detected in some fasting patients[89] and also following oral administration of 50 to 80 g of glucose or 10 to 12 g of lactulose.[90]

Despite the simplicity of breath hydrogen testing, there are numerous factors that influence the results of this test, and these factors are not always controlled for in published studies or clinical application. Antibiotics and laxatives must be avoided perhaps for weeks prior to breath hydrogen testing. Bread, pasta, and fiber must not be consumed the night before the test because these foods cause prolonged hydrogen excretion. Cigarette smoking and exercise must be avoided before and during the test. Chlorhexidine mouthwash must be used before the test to try to eliminate oral bacteria, which might otherwise contribute to an early hydrogen peak after the substrate is given. Also, strict interpretive criteria, such as requiring two consecutive breath hydrogen values more than 10 ppm above the baseline reading, and recording a clear distinction of the small bowel peak from the subsequent colonic peak (double peak criterion), are recommended.[3] Poor sensitivity of breath hydrogen testing may result from inadequate fermentation by enteric flora (approximately 25%–40% of subjects harbor bacteria that do not ferment lactulose)[3, 48]; rapid absorption of the glucose substrate in the proximal small bowel; a washout effect of concomitant diarrhea; loss of bacterial flora because of recent antibiotic therapy; or an acidic bowel lumen, which inhibits hydrogen generation.[91] The specificity of breath hydrogen testing is compromised when hydrogen is produced by colonic bacteria, especially when transit times are accelerated by the osmotic load of the substrate dose.

A recent study examined the diagnostic value of the 10-g lactulose breath hydrogen test and of a scintigraphic orocecal transit study compared with the value of small bowel cultures.[92] The sensitivity of the breath test alone to detect small bowel bacterial overgrowth was only 16.7% and the specificity 70%. Combination of breath testing with scintigraphy increased specificity to 100% but sensitivity was only 38.9%. Application of the double peak criterion alone for interpretation of the lactulose breath hydrogen test was thus inadequately sensitive, even with scintigraphy, to diagnose bacterial overgrowth.

Other investigators have encountered similar problems with the sensitivity and specificity of either the lactulose or glucose hydrogen breath test compared to intestinal culture.[93, 94] One controlled trial compared the glucose and lactulose hydrogen breath tests with the 1-g ^{14}C-D-xylose breath test in 10 control subjects and 20 patients with culture-proven bacterial overgrowth. The ^{14}C-D-xylose test was 95% sensitive and 100% specific. In contrast, the breath hydrogen test results were often uninterpretable or nondiagnostic.[90]

Despite the attractions of ease of performance and the avoidance of a radioactive tracer, breath hydrogen tests are not sufficiently sensitive or specific to justify their substitution for the ^{14}C-D-xylose breath test for the noninvasive detection of intestinal bacterial overgrowth.[3, 91] Furthermore, many authorities still regard small bowel aspiration for quantitative and qualitative culture specimens the reference standard for diagnosis of SBBOS.[3, 85, 91, 92]

Treatment

A primary goal of managing SBBOS should be to try *to correct the underlying small intestinal abnormality*, when possible. Unfortunately, surgical intervention is often impractical (e.g., in patients with scleroderma or multiple jejunal diverticula) or unacceptable.

When surgical correction of the primary condition leading to stasis is not feasible, management efforts must concentrate on *long-term antibiotic therapy* and adjunctive treatment of dysmotility. Although bacterial overgrowth may be asymptomatic in many patients, the occurrence of compatible symptoms supported by positive results of testing for overgrowth (see Fig. 90–3) should lead to a decision to treat.[3] Theoretically, the choice of antimicrobial agent should be based on in vitro susceptibility testing of the bacteria in the small bowel of the individual patient.[35] This information is, however, impractical to obtain in most cases, and therefore choices of antibiotics are largely empirical and based on the results of published series in which small intestinal cultures have been done[95] or successful outcomes of therapies obtained. Whereas most patients with SBBOS have anaerobic overgrowth, in others malabsorption has been associated with overgrowth of purely aerobic flora.[35] Therefore, the most effective antibiotic regimens generally include one or more drugs with activity against both aerobic and anaerobic bacteria.

Historically, the treatment of first choice was tetracycline 250 mg orally four times a day, with which improvement in symptoms and signs of malabsorption was expected within a week.[3] Although recent experience suggests that up to 60% of patients with SBBOS do not respond to tetracycline, studies are still published in which doxycycline[58] or minocycline[96] was effective as first-line therapy.

Amoxicillin-clavulanic acid (Augmentin), by virtue of its broad spectrum of antimicrobial activity[95] and a convenient twice-daily dosing regimen, has become a popular choice for empirical treatment of SBBOS. Small uncontrolled trials have demonstrated the effectiveness of this antibiotic in improving symptoms and objective abnormalities in SBBOS.[27, 47] Alternative combination regimens that have also been successful include (1) cephalexin, 250 mg four times a day plus metronidazole, 250 mg three times a day[3]; (2) colistin, 250,000 IU/kg per day, plus metronidazole[35, 97]; and (3) trimethoprim-sulfamethoxazole.[35] Chloramphenicol, 250 mg four times a day has also been a successful alternative therapy,[44] which might be acceptable in refractory cases. Antibiotics whose activity is largely limited to anaerobes such as metronidazole[35] or clindamycin have limited value as monotherapy. Conversely, antibiotics whose activity against enteric anaerobes such as *Bacteroides* is poor, such as penicillin and oral aminoglycosides, should also be avoided.

Recent successful experience with the quinolone ciprofloxacin treatment of SBBOS[45] has been followed by a placebo-controlled randomized crossover trial that compared treatment of ten symptomatic patients with the quinolone norfloxacin (800 mg per day), amoxicillin-clavulanic acid (1500 mg per day), or *Saccharomyces boulardii* (1500 mg per day).[98] Both norfloxacin and amoxicillin-clavulanic acid treatment resulted in modest but significant short-term decreases in stool frequency and substantial improvement in the results of glucose-hydrogen breath testing. Probiotic treatment with *S. boulardii* did not result in any improvement in these outcome measures.[98]

For most patients, a single 7- to 10-day course of antibiotics may relieve symptoms for months. In others, symptoms recur promptly following cessation of antibiotics. Satisfactory management of recurrent SBBOS can often be achieved with cyclic (e.g., 1 week of 4) or continuous longer term antibiotic therapy. No controlled trials offer guidance as to duration of therapy or management of refractory or stubbornly recurrent cases. Decisions on management must be individualized and weigh the risks of long-term antibiotic therapy such as diarrhea, *Clostridium difficile* colitis, patient intolerance, bacterial resistance, and expense.

Prokinetic agents that might help propel bacteria through the stagnant small bowel would be attractive adjuncts to antibiotic treatment of SBBOS. Animal studies suggest that enteric bacterial overgrowth might be favorably affected by prokinetic drugs.[99, 100] In a small study of humans with cirrhosis, orocecal transit time was decreased, and, in four of five patients, bacterial overgrowth was abolished by cisapride treatment.[100] Cisapride has, however, been withdrawn from the U.S. market due to cardiotoxicity.

In one study of five patients with SBBOS, low doses of octreotide (50 μg), given at bedtime so as not to impair the motor response to daytime feeding, stimulated motor activity evoking phase 3 motor complexes that propagated the same velocity as that of spontaneous complexes in healthy subjects.[101] In addition, that dose of octreotide decreased nausea, vomiting, bloating, and abdominal pain in these patients and cleared bacterial overgrowth as demonstrated by complete normalization of abnormal breath hydrogen tests. Thus, low doses of octreotide given at bedtime may be useful adjunctive treatment for SBBOS in patients who do not respond to antibiotics, cannot tolerate them, or develop complications with antibiotics. Encouraging results have also been obtained with octreotide and erythromycin therapy in scleroderma-associated dysmotility syndromes and SBBOS.[102] However, relatively few patients have been studied with octreotide, and questions remain about the long-term side effects, the maintenance of remission, the length of treatment needed, the likelihood of recurrence, and whether combining octreotide therapy with antibiotics is reproducibly beneficial.

There has been recent interest in the concept that some enteric diseases might be ameliorated as a result of manipulating the intestinal flora by feeding live "probiotic" microbial supplements that change the enteric microbial balance. Probiotics have been actively studied in the management of inflammatory bowel disease, *C. difficile* colitis, and now SBBOS. Unfortunately, studies of probiotic therapy for SBBOS have so far shown disappointing or inconclusive results.[50, 98, 102, 103]

In parallel with antibiotic treatments for SBBOS, nutritional support is a crucial early and ongoing component of management. Mucosal enterocyte damage may be incompletely reversible, and bacterial overgrowth may be refractory to antibiotic treatments. Dietary modifications might include a lactose-free diet or substitution of medium-chain triglycerides for a large part of dietary fat. Cobalamin deficiency is managed using monthly intramuscular injections of 100 μg of vitamin B_{12}. Correction of deficiencies of other nutrients such as calcium, magnesium, iron, and fat-soluble vitamins may also be necessary.[104]

REFERENCES

1. Simon GL, Gorbach SL: The human intestinal microflora. Dig Dis 30(suppl 9):147S, 1986.
2. Hanson LA, Dahlman-Höglund A, Karlsson M, et al: Normal microbial flora of the gut and the immune system. In Hanson LA, Yolken RH (eds): Probiotics, other Nutritional Factors, and Intestinal Microflora. Philadelphia, Lippincott-Raven, 1999, p 217.
3. Toskes PP, Kumar A: Enteric bacterial flora and bacterial overgrowth syndrome. In Feldman M, Scharschmidt BF, Sleisenger MH (eds): Sleisenger & Fordtran's Gastrointestinal and Liver Disease, 6th ed. Philadelphia, WB Saunders, 1998, p 1523.
4. Wilson KH, Ikeda JS, Blitchington RB: Phylogenetic placement of community members of human colonic biota. Clin Infect Dis 25(suppl 2):S114, 1997.
5. Rolfe RD: Interactions among microorganisms of the indigenous intestinal flora and their influence on the host. Rev Infect Dis 6 (suppl 1): S73, 1984.
6. Adlerberth I: Establishment of a normal intestinal microflora in the newborn infant. In Hanson LA, Yolken RH (eds): Probiotics, Other Nutritional Factors, and Intestinal Microflora. Philadelphia, Lippincott-Raven, 1999, p 63.
7. Justesen T, Nielsen OH, Jacobsen IE, et al: The normal cultivable microflora in upper jejunal fluid in healthy adults. Scand J Gastroenterol 19:279, 1984.
8. Levy J: The effects of antibiotic use on gastrointestinal function. Am J Gastroenterol 95(suppl 1):S8, 2000.
9. Midtvedt T: Microbial functional activities. In Hanson LA, Yolken RH (eds): Probiotics, Other Nutritional Factors, and Intestinal Microflora. Philadelphia, Lippincott-Raven, 1999, p 79.
10. Savage DC: Gastrointestinal microflora in mammalian nutrition. Ann Rev Nutr 6:155, 1986.
11. Heile M, Ghoss Y, Rutgeerts P, et al: Influence of nutritional substrates on the formation of volatiles by fecal flora. Gastroenterology 100:1597, 1991.

12. Hoeverstad T, Carlstedt-Duke B, Lingaas E, et al: Influence of oral intake of 7 different antibiotics upon faecal short chain fatty acid excretion in healthy subjects. Scand J Gastroenterol 21:997, 1986.
13. Clausen MR, Bonnen H, Tuede M, et al: Colonic fermentation to short-chain fatty acids is decreased in antibiotic-associated diarrhea. Gastroenterology 101:1497, 1991.
14. Halverson J, Gale A, Lazarus C, et al: D-Lactic acidosis and other complications of intestinal bypass surgery. Arch Intern Med 144:357, 1984.
15. Saltzman JR, Kowdley KV, Pedrosa MC, et al: Bacterial overgrowth without clinical malabsorption in elderly hypochlorhydric patients. Gastroenterology 106:615, 1994.
16. Husebye E, Skar V, Hoeverstad T, et al: Fasting hypochlorhydria with gram positive gastric flora is highly prevalent in healthy old people. Gut 33:1331, 1992.
17. Vantrappen G, Janssens J, Hellemans J, et al: The interdigestive motor complex of normal subjects and patients with bacterial overgrowth of the small intestine. J Clin Invest 59:1158, 1977.
18. Nieuwenhuijs VB, Verheem A, van Duijvenbode-Beumer H, et al: The role of interdigestive small bowel motility in the regulation of gut microflora, bacterial overgrowth, and bacterial overgrowth in rats. Ann Surg 228:188, 1998.
19. van der Waaij D: Microbial ecology of the intestinal microflora: Influence of interactions with the host organism. In Hanson LA, Yolken RH (eds): Probiotics, Other Nutritional Factors, and Intestinal Microflora. Philadelphia, Lippincott-Raven, 1999, p 1.
20. Riordan SM, McIver CJ, Wakefield D, et al: Luminal antigliadin antibodies in small intestinal bacterial overgrowth. Am J Gastroenterol 92:1335, 1997.
21. Riordan SM, McIver CJ, Wakefield D, et al: Serum immunoglobulin and soluble IL-2 receptor levels in small intestinal overgrowth with indigenous gut flora. Dig Dis Sci 44:939, 1999.
22. Kett K, Baklien K, Bakken A, et al: Intestinal B-cell isotype response in relation to local bacterial load: evidence for immunoglobulin A subclass adaptation. Gastroenterology 109:819, 1995.
23. Smith GM, Chesner IM, Asquith P, et al: Small intestinal bacterial overgrowth in patients with chronic lymphocytic leukaemia. J Clin Pathol 43:57, 1990.
24. Pignata C, Budillon G, Monaco G, et al: Jejunal bacterial overgrowth and intestinal permeability in children with immunodeficiency syndromes. Gut 31:879, 1990.
25. Arranz E, O'Mahoney S, Barton JR, et al: Immunosenescence and mucosal immunity: Significant effects of old age on secretory IgA concentrations and intraepithelial lymphocyte counts. Gut 33:882, 1992.
26. Riordan SM, McIver CJ, Wakefield D, et al: Luminal immunity in small-intestinal bacterial overgrowth and old age. Scand J Gastroenterol 31:1103, 1996.
27. Haboubi NY, Lee GS, Montgomery RD: Duodenal mucosal morphometry of elderly patients with small intestinal bacterial overgrowth: Response to antibiotic treatment. Age Ageing 20:29, 1991.
28. Giannella RA, Rout WR, Toskes PP: Jejunal brush border injury and impaired sugar and amino acid uptake in the blind loop syndrome. Gastroenterology 67:965, 1974.
29. King CE, Toskes PP: Protein-losing enteropathy in the human and experimental rat blind loop syndrome. Gastroenterology 80:504, 1981.
30. Welkos SA, Toskes PP, Baer H, et al: Importance of anaerobic bacteria in the cobalamin malabsorption of experimental rat blind loop syndrome. Gastroenterology 80:313, 1981.
31. Saltzman JR, Russell RM: Nutritional consequences of intestinal bacterial overgrowth. Comp Ther 20:523, 1994.
32. Suter PM, Golner BB, Goldin BR, et al: Reversal of protein-bound vitamin B_{12} malabsorption with antibiotics in atrophic gastritis. Gastroenterology 101:1039, 1991.
33. Wanitschke R, Ammon HV: Effects of dihydroxy bile acids and hydroxy fatty acids on the absorption of oleic acid in the human jejunum. J Clin Invest 61:178, 1978.
34. Varcoe R, Holliday D, Tavill A: Utilization of urea nitrogen for albumin synthesis in the stagnant loop syndrome. Gut 15:898, 1974.
35. Kocoshis SA, Schletewitz K, Lovelace G, et al: Duodenal bile acids among children: Keto derivatives and aerobic small bowel bacterial overgrowth. J Pediatr Gastroenterol Nutr 6:686, 1987.
36. Justus PG, Fernandez A, Martin JL, et al: Altered myoelectric activity in the experimental blind loop syndrome. J Clin Invest 72:1064, 1983.
37. Levitt MD, Kuan M: The physiology of ileo-anal pouch function. Am J Surg 176:384, 1998.
38. Bragelmann R, Armbrecht U, Rosemeyer U, et al: Small bowel bacterial overgrowth in patients after total gastrectomy. Eur J Clin Invest 27:409, 1997.
39. Casellas F, Guarner L, Vaquero E, et al: Hydrogen breath test with glucose in exocrine pancreatic insufficiency. Pancreas 16:481, 1998.
40. Corrodi P: Jejunoileal bypass: Change in the flora of the small intestine and its clinical impact. Rev Infect Dis 6(suppl 1):S80, 1984.
41. Trespi E, Ferrieri A: Intestinal bacterial overgrowth during chronic pancreatitis. Curr Med Res Opin 15:47, 1999.
42. Iivonen MK, Ahola TO, Matikainen MJ: Bacterial overgrowth, intestinal transit, and nutrition after total gastrectomy. Comparison of a jejunal pouch with Roux-en-Y reconstruction in a prospective random study. Scand J Gastroenterol 33:63, 1998.
43. Husebye E, Skar V, Hoeverstad T, et al: Abnormal intestinal motor patterns explain enteric colonization with gram-negative bacilli in late radiation enteropathy. Gastroenterology 109:1078, 1995.
44. Shindo K, Machida M, Koide K, et al: Deconjugation ability of bacteria isolated from the jejunal fluid of patients with progressive systemic sclerosis and its gastric pH. Hepatogastroenterology 45:1643, 1998.
45. Kaye SA, Lim SG, Taylor M, et al: Small bowel bacterial overgrowth in systemic sclerosis: Detection using direct and indirect methods and treatment outcome. Br J Rheumatol 34:265, 1995
46. Pearson AJ, Brzechwa-Adjukiewicz A, McCarthy CF: Intestinal pseudo-obstruction with bacterial overgrowth in the small intestine. Am J Dig Dis 14:200, 1969.
47. Virally-Monod M, Tielmans D, Kevorkian JP, et al: Chronic diarrhoea and diabetes mellitus: Prevalence of small intestinal bacterial overgrowth. Diab Metab 23:530, 1998.
48. Lewindon PJ, Robb TA, Moore DJ, et al: Bowel dysfunction in cystic fibrosis: Importance of breath testing. J Paediatr Child Health 34:79, 1998.
49. Lembeke B, Kraus B, Lankisch PG: Small intestinal function in chronic relapsing pancreatitis. Hepatogastroenterology 32:149, 1985.
50. Dunn SR, Simenhoff ML, Ahmed KE, et al: Effect of oral administration of freeze-dried *Lactobacillus acidophilus* on small bowel bacterial overgrowth in patients with end stage kidney disease: Reducing uremic toxins and improving nutrition. Int Dairy J 8:545, 1998.
51. Ronnblom A, Andersson S, Danielsson A: Mechanisms of diarrhoea in myotonic dystrophy. Eur J Gastroenterol Hepatol 10:607, 1998.
52. Pimentel M, Chow EJ, Bonorris G, et al: Eradication of small intestinal bacterial overgrowth decreases the gastrointestinal symptoms in fibromyalgia. Abstract 2143. Annual Meeting of the American Gastroenterological Society. Gastroenterology 118:A413, 2000.
53. Pimentel M, Hallegua D, Chow EJ, et al: Eradication of small intestinal bacterial overgrowth decreases symptoms in chronic fatigue syndrome: A double blind, randomized study. Abstract 2144. Annual Meeting of the American Gastroenterological Society. Gastroenterology 118:A414, 2000.
54. Morencos F, de las Heras Castano G, Martin Ramos L, et al: Small bowel bacterial overgrowth in patients with alcoholic cirrhosis. Dig Dis Sci 41:552, 1996.
55. Yang C-Y, Chang C-S, Chen G-H: Small-intestinal bacterial overgrowth in patients with liver cirrhosis diagnosed with glucose H_2 or CH_4 breath tests. Scand J Gastroenterol 33:867, 1998.
56. Chang C-S, Chen G-H, Lien H-C, et al: Small intestine dysmotility and bacterial overgrowth in cirrhotic patients with spontaneous bacterial peritonitis. Hepatology 28:1187, 1998.
57. Lipski P, Kelly P, James F: Bacterial contamination of the small bowel in elderly people: Is it necessarily pathological? Ageing 21:5, 1992.
58. Lewis SJ, Potts LF, Malhotra R, et al: Small bowel bacterial overgrowth in subjects living in residential care homes. Age Ageing 28: 181, 1999.
59. McEvoy A, Dutton J, James OF: Bacterial contamination of the small intestine is an important cause of occult malabsorption in the elderly. Br Med J 287:789, 1983.
60. Haboubi NY, Montgomery RD: Small bowel bacterial overgrowth in elderly people: Clinical significance and response to treatment. Age Ageing 21:13, 1992.
61. Riordan SM, McIver CJ, Wakefield D, et al: Small intestinal bacterial overgrowth in the symptomatic elderly. Am J Gastroenterol 92:47, 1997.
62. Baik HW, Russell RM: Vitamin B_{12} deficiency in the elderly. Annu Rev Nutr 19:357, 1999.

63. Shindo K, Yamazaki R, Koide K, et al: Alteration of bile acid metabolism by cimetidine in healthy humans. J Invest Med 44:462, 1996.
64. Fried M, Slegrish H, Frei R, et al: Duodenal bacterial overgrowth during treatment with omeprazole in outpatients. Gut 35:23, 1996.
65. Hutchinson S, Logan R: The effect of long-term omeprazole on the glucose-hydrogen breath test in elderly patients. Age Ageing 26:87, 1997.
66. Shindo K, Machida M, Fukumura M, et al: Omeprazole induces altered bile acid metabolism. Gut 42:266, 1998.
67. Parkin DM, McClelland DBL, O'Moore RR, et al: Intestinal bacterial flora and bile salt studies in hypogammaglobulinemia. Gut 13:182, 1972.
68. Tabaquchali S: The pathophysiological role of the small intestinal bacterial flora. Scand J Gastroenterol 5(suppl 6):139, 1970.
69. Giannella RA, Toskes PP: Gastrointestinal bleeding and iron absorption in the experimental blind loop syndrome. Am J Clin Nutr 29:754, 1976.
70. Toskes PP, King CE, Spivey JC, et al: Xylose catabolism in experimental rat blind loop syndrome: Studies including newly developed D-[^{14}C] xylose breath test. Gastroenterology 74:691, 1978.
71. Kumar A, Forsmark C, Toskes P: Small bowel bacterial overgrowth, the changing face of an old disease. Gastroenterology 110:A340, 1996.
72. Toskes P: Malabsorption. In Bennett JC, Plum F (eds): Cecil Textbook of Medicine, 20th ed. Philadelphia, WB Saunders, 1996, p 695.
73. Donald IP, Kitchingmam G, Donald F, et al: The diagnosis of small bowel bacterial overgrowth in elderly patients. J Am Geriatr Soc 40: 692, 1992.
74. Riordan SM, McIver CJ, Walker BM, et al: Bacteriological method for detecting small intestinal hypomotility. Am J Gastroenterol 91: 2399, 1996.
75. Kiss ZF, Wolfling J, Csati S, et al: The ursodeoxycholic acid-p-aminobenzoic acid deconjugation test, a new tool for the diagnosis of bacterial overgrowth syndrome. Eur J Gastroenterol Hepatol 9:679, 1997.
76. Hoeverstad T, Bjorneklett A, Fausa O, et al: Short-chain fatty acids in the small bowel bacterial overgrowth syndrome. Scand J Gastroenterol 20:492, 1985.
77. King CE, Toskes PP, Guilarte TR, et al: Comparison of the one gram ^{14}C-xylose breath test to the ^{14}C-bile acid breath test in patients with small intestine bacterial overgrowth. Dig Dis Sci 25:53, 1980.
78. Ferguson J, Walker K, Thomson AB: Limitations in the use of ^{14}C-glycocholate breath and stool bile acid determinations in patients with chronic diarrhea. J Clin Gastroenterol 8:258, 1986.
79. King CE, Toskes PP, Spivey JC, et al: Detection of small intestine overgrowth by means of a ^{14}C-D-xylose breath test. Gastroenterology 77:75, 1979.
80. Schneider A, Novis B, Chen V, et al: Value of the ^{14}C-D-xylose breath test in patients with intestinal bacterial overgrowth. Digestion 32:86, 1985.
81. Rumessen JJ, Gudmand-Hoyer E, Bachmann E, et al: Diagnosis of bacterial overgrowth of the small intestine. Scand J Gastroenterol 20: 1267, 1985.
82. Pruthi HS, Mehta SK, Pathak CM: Evaluation of ^{14}C-D-xylose breath test in the diagnosis of small intestinal bacterial overgrowth. Indian J Med Res 80:598, 1984.
83. Valdovinos M, Camilleri M, Thomforde G, et al: Reduced accuracy of ^{14}C-D-xylose breath test for detecting bacterial overgrowth in gastrointestinal motility disorders. Scand J Gastroenterol 28:963, 1993.
84. Riordan S, McIver C, Duncombe V, et al: Factors influencing the 1-gram ^{14}C-D-xylose breath test for bacterial overgrowth. Am J Gastroenterol 90:1455, 1995.
85. Lewis SJ, Young G, Mann M, et al: Improvement in specificity of [^{14}C]D-xylose breath test for bacterial overgrowth. Dig Dis Sci 42: 1587, 1997.
86. Lim H, Wagner DA, Toskes PP: A ^{13}C-xylose breath test for bacterial overgrowth. Gastroenterology 104:A259, 1993.
87. Dellert SF, Nowicki MJ, Farell MK, et al: The ^{13}C-xylose breath test for the diagnosis of small bowel bacterial overgrowth in children. J Pediatr Gastroenterol Nutr 25:153, 1997.
88. Swart GR, van den Berg JWO: ^{13}C breath tests in gastroenterological practice. Scand J Gastroenterol 225(suppl.):13, 1998.
89. Perman SA, Modler S, Barr RG, et al: Fasting breath hydrogen concentration: Normal values and clinical application. Gastroenterology 87:1358, 1984.
90. King CE, Toskes PP: Comparison of the 1-gram [^{14}C]xylose, 10-gram lactulose-H_2, and 80-gram glucose-H_2 breath tests in patients with small intestine bacterial overgrowth. Gastroenterology 91:1447, 1986.
91. Bishop WP: Breath hydrogen testing for small bowel bacterial overgrowth—a lot of hot air? J Pediatr Gastroenterol Nutr 25:245, 1997.
92. Riordan SM, McIver CJ, Walker BM, et al: The lactulose breath hydrogen test and small intestinal bacterial overgrowth. Am J Gastroenterol 91:1795, 1996.
93. Corazza GR, Menozzi MG, Strocchi A, et al: The diagnosis of small bowel bacterial overgrowth. Gastroenterology 98:302, 1990.
94. MacMahon M, Gibbons N, Mullins E, et al: Are hydrogen breath tests valid in the elderly? Gerontology 42:40, 1996.
95. Bouhnik Y, Alain S, Attar A, et al: Bacterial populations contaminating the upper gut in patients with small intestinal bacterial overgrowth syndrome. Am J Gastroenterol 94:1327, 1999.
96. Funayama Y, Sasaki I, Naito H, et al: Monitoring and antibacterial treatment for postoperative bacterial overgrowth in Crohn's disease. Dis Colon Rectum 42:1072, 1999.
97. de Boissieu D, Chaussain M, Badoual J, et al: Small-bowel bacterial overgrowth in children with chronic diarrhea, abdominal pain, or both. J Pediatr 128:203, 1996.
98. Attar A, Flourie B, Rambaud JC, et al: Antibiotic efficacy in small intestinal bacterial overgrowth-related chronic diarrhea: A crossover, randomized trial. Gastroenterology 117:794, 1999.
99. Wang X, Soltesz V, Axelson J, et al: Cholecystokinin increases small intestinal motility and reduces enteric bacterial overgrowth and translocation in rats with surgically induced acute liver failure. Digestion 57:67, 1996.
100. Pardo A, Bartoli R, Lorenzo-Zuniga V, et al: Effect of cisapride on intestinal bacterial overgrowth and bacterial translocation in cirrhosis. Hepatology 31:858, 2000.
101. Soudah HC, Hasler WL, Owyang C: Effect of octreotide on intestinal motility and bacterial overgrowth in scleroderma. N Engl J Med 325: 1461, 1991.
102. Verne GN, Eaker EY, Hardy E, et al: Effect of octreotide and erythromycin on idiopathic and scleroderma-associated intestinal pseudoobstruction. Dig Dis Sci 40:1892, 1995.
103. Stotzer P-O, Blomberg L, Conway PL, et al: Probiotic treatment of small intestinal bacterial overgrowth by Lactobacillus fermentum KLD. Scand J Infect Dis 28:615, 1996.
104. Meyers JS, Ehrenpreis ED, Craig RM: Small intestinal bacterial overgrowth syndrome. Curr Treatment Options Gastroenterol 4:7, 2001.

Chapter 91

IRRITABLE BOWEL SYNDROME

Nicholas W. Read

DEFINITION AND CLINICAL FEATURES

Irritable bowel syndrome (IBS) is a chronic continuous or remittent gastrointestinal illness characterized by frequent unexplained symptoms that include abdominal pain, bloating, and bowel disturbance, which may be either diarrhea or constipation or an erratic bowel habit that has features of both. These symptoms are common. Everybody experiences them from time to time, but more than 40% of IBS patients have symptoms that are so frequent and severe that they have to take time off from work, curtail their social life, avoid sexual intercourse, cancel appointments, stop traveling, take medication, and even stay confined to their house for fear of embarrassment.[1] It is this reduction in quality of life, rather than the specific symptoms, that most determines how patients rate the severity of IBS.[2] IBS should not be dismissed as a trivial condition. Patients often state that their symptoms completely dominate their lives. Difficulty in confirming the diagnosis may lead to further worry and doubt, resulting in numerous visits to doctors and repeated, unpleasant tests. Unnecessary operations such as cholecystectomy and hysterectomy may complicate the condition with scar pain, adhesions, and further alteration in bowel habit. The estimated health care cost of IBS in the United States is $8 billion per year.[3]

IBS is heterogeneous in nature. Patients with IBS experience not only abdominal discomfort and bowel symptoms, but also, in many cases, tiredness, breathlessness, indigestion, heartburn, back pain, headache, dizziness, urinary frequency, muscle pains, arthritis, palpitations, anorexia, sleeplessness, menorrhagia, dyspareunia, panic attacks, anxiety, and depression.[4] The symptoms that IBS patients exhibit are so variable that they can appear to be a unique expression of the individual.

IBS is an illness—a state of mental and visceral disharmony—rather than a specific medical disease. Unlike many of the conditions described in this book, IBS has no recognized abnormality and no specific cause; diagnosis is at best arbitrary and at worst spurious; and medical treatment is often ineffective. The Rome Committee for the Classification of Functional Gastrointestinal Disorders has defined IBS on the basis of abdominal and bowel symptoms that occur with sufficient frequency in affected patients (Table 91–1).[5]

Other groups of "functional" symptoms have been similarly defined, but there is a growing opinion that illnesses that have no pathologic basis, such as IBS, chronic fatigue syndrome, fibromyalgia syndrome, eating disorders, and premenstrual syndrome, should be grouped together as a distinct type of illness,[6] not only because they have considerable overlap in presentation, but also because they all share distinctive features, such as a female preponderance, high prevalence in youth and middle age, and strong association with psychopathologic disorders. Yunus has called this illness phenomenon the "third disease paradigm"—a condition that is neither purely mental nor physical, but a reaction of the whole organism to life situations.[7] Nevertheless, the age and sex distribution and the waxing and waning nature of the symptoms are similar to the pattern seen in psychiatric disorders, such as generalized anxiety disorder, panic disorder, dysthymic disorder, and major depression.[8]

EPIDEMIOLOGY

Epidemiologic studies are designed to identify possible causes of disease by demonstrating associations between a particular disease and demographic and life-style characteristics. Such studies are difficult to interpret in illnesses with no clear pathologic features, like IBS, because the data are fundamentally influenced by an arbitrary definition of disease. The population under investigation may vary not only according to the nature and interpretation of the diagnostic criteria, but also according to the beliefs of both patients and their health care providers as to what constitutes a disease. Cultural differences in health care seeking behavior may explain why IBS appears to be more common in Western industrialized countries than in some developing countries,[9] in rural Africa than in African cities,[10] and among Asians living in American cities than among whites or Hispanics.[11] In India, gastrointestinal symptoms often are seen as manifestations of depression.[12] In the past gastrointestinal symptoms resembling IBS were a common feature of what was known as "hysterical" or "hypochondriacal" illness[13] and were understood in terms appropriate to contemporary beliefs, such as barrenness in antiquity, demonic possession in the Middle Ages, and overcrowded cities and foreign imports in 18th-century England.

Table 91–1 | **Diagnostic Criteria for Irritable Bowel Syndrome***

At least 12 weeks or more, which need not be consecutive, in the preceding 12 months of abdominal discomfort or pain that has two of the following three features:
- Relief by defecation
- Onset associated with a change in the frequency of stool
- Onset associated with a change in the form (appearance) of stool

Symptoms that cumulatively support the diagnosis of irritable bowel syndrome:
- Abnormal stool frequency (>3 bowel movements per day or <3 bowel movements per week)
- Abnormal stool form (lumpy/hard or loose/watery)
- Abnormal stool passage (straining, urgency, or feeling of incomplete evaluation)
- Passage of mucus
- Bloating or feeling of abdominal distention

*In the absence of structural or metabolic abnormalities to explain the symptoms.

From Drossman DA: Rome II: The Functional Gastrointestinal Disorders. McLean, Va, Degnan Associates, 2000.

Early epidemiologic studies of IBS were carried out on chronic clinic attenders with abdominal discomfort and bowel upset that could not be explained by any obvious organic disease. These were really studies of the epidemiologic characteristics of illness behavior rather than of the illness itself. With the advent of strict diagnostic criteria the emphasis has shifted to the community. Although community studies focus on the illness, epidemiologic studies are still confined by what the Rome Committee has decided by consensus should constitute the disease.

Gender Differences

In Western countries approximately four times as many women as men report IBS to a physician. Female patients also seem to have more frequent and severe symptoms and more interference with daily activities and are less likely to attribute their symptoms to stress than male patients. The situation appears to be very different in Asia; studies from both India and Sri Lanka have shown that more men than women seek help from doctors for IBS.[14] Sociologists suggest that women are more prepared to report abdominal symptoms to their doctors in Western cultures because of patterns of socialization learned during childhood,[15] but the female preponderance of both IBS[16] and erratic bowel habits[17] still exists in community samples from Western countries, a factor that indicates that these characteristics cannot be explained solely by health care–seeking behavior. Thus, either women experience more or frequent gastrointestinal symptoms than men, or they are more likely to remember and report them. Talley has suggested that cognitive processing of visceral sensations is amplified to a greater extent in women than men,[18] but physiologic evidence shows that healthy women have greater rectal sensitivity,[19] slower bowel transit, and smaller stool output[20] than men. To some extent the female preponderance may depend on the bias given to certain symptoms, because straining and passage of hard stool are more frequent in women, whereas frequent and loose stools are more common in men.[16, 17]

Age

IBS can affect people at any age, although epidemiologic surveys conducted in the community as well as in clinic samples suggest a greater prevalence of IBS in younger than older adults, and a notable decline in prevalence in people age 50 and older, when chronic organic diseases of the gut increase in prevalence.[18, 21] IBS tends to occur for the first time in the young and is even common in schoolchildren.[22]

Psychopathology

Early studies showed that the prevalence of psychiatric disorders and psychiatric symptoms was three times as high among clinic patients with IBS as among those with organic gastrointestinal conditions.[23] Anxiety and depression were the most common psychiatric symptoms, but phobias, obsessional behavior, sleep disturbance, multiple somatic symptoms, hostile feelings, panic attacks, and alcohol abuse were also more common than in healthy control subjects.[24] At least one study has challenged the association between psychopathologic disorders and IBS,[25] but IBS was diagnosed according to specific diagnostic criteria that excluded patients who experienced multiple unexplained symptoms referable to the gut and other organ systems on a daily basis for most of their lives. Those are the patients who have very high rates of psychiatric disorders. Moreover, the prevalence of IBS in psychiatric clinics varies from 13% to 71% according to whether restrictive or clinical diagnostic criteria are used to make the diagnosis.[26] Retrospective studies have indicated that psychopathologic disorders may precede the onset of IBS, but such reports are influenced by biases resulting from selective recall and the need to find meaning for symptoms. The only prospective studies have been conducted on patients with IBS triggered by an attack of gastroenteritis, in whom psychological disturbance occurring at the time of the gastroenteritis episode appeared to predict the development of chronic bowel symptoms that resembled IBS.[27]

Illness Behavior

Patients with IBS who seek medical attention are more disturbed psychologically than nonconsulters.[28, 29] They also are more likely to have abnormal personality profiles, are more concerned about their health and fearful of illness, and appear to experience a greater number of negative life events. These observations suggest that anxiety about their health led them to seek medical help. In support of this conclusion, studies have shown that people who consult their doctor about IBS also are more likely to consult their doctor about colds, headaches, and other relatively minor complaints.[30] They also are more likely than healthy control subjects to report poor health in childhood, greater parental attention to illness, the receipt of gifts and rewards for being ill,[31] and school absences,[32] all of which may have programmed them to a pattern of illness behavior. If a child only gains real attention when he or she is ill, then he or she quickly learns the advantage of being ill. The relationship between psychosocial disorders and frequent medical visits is true, however, for many disorders, not just IBS.[33]

The first studies on illness behavior and IBS were carried out in the United States, where most health care was based on a private insurance–based, fee-paying, consultation-on-demand system. Studies conducted in the United Kingdom[34] have indicated that consultation for functional abdominal symptoms is related not only to anxiety, depression, difficult life situations, and concern about health, but also to the severity and chronicity of the symptoms.

Although some studies have suggested that nonconsulters do not exhibit more psychopathologic conditions than healthy subjects, the findings also appear to be influenced heavily by the application of diagnostic criteria. People with unexplained bowel and abdominal symptoms that do not necessarily fulfill strict diagnostic criteria for IBS are more likely than healthy control subjects to experience depression, alcohol abuse, panic disorder, agoraphobia, and a range of unexplained physical symptoms,[35] and they tend to be members of households with lower incomes.

Diary records indicate that everybody experiences some symptoms of IBS over the course of a month.[36] Most people forget about them, however. Remembering of symptoms is related to the emotional significance of the symptoms,[37] which relates both to context and to severity. It is tempting to speculate that the variability in IBS symptoms throughout the menstrual cycle that is observed by some women is explainable by corresponding fluctuations in emotional arousal.[38]

PATHOPHYSIOLOGY

Motility

For many years, IBS was regarded as a disturbance of gastrointestinal motility. Studies claimed to have identified abnormal patterns of contractile activity and electrical activity in the distal colon of patients with IBS. With further investigation, however, it has become clear that these patterns are not necessarily abnormal but exaggerated. They are perhaps better regarded as "gut reactions": disturbances of gastrointestinal function that occur in everybody from time to time in response to dietary indiscretions or psychosocial upheaval, but present to a greater extent and with greater frequency and severity in patients with IBS.

Recordings of the electrical and pressure activity of the distal colon, in studies conducted in 1978, showed that patients with IBS exhibited a regular three-cycle-a-minute oscillation.[39] This pattern, it was suggested, might be a marker of IBS, but the same pattern could be observed in normal subjects, especially when the rectum was distended with a balloon or was not cleansed of feces, and in psychoneurotic patients without bowel symptoms. These observations suggested that three-cycle-a-minute activity might be related to a state of emotional, autonomic, and visceral arousal.[40] This interpretation was consistent with observations that patients with IBS, particularly those with abdominal pain and constipation, demonstrate exaggerated rectosigmoid contractile activity in response to a meal, injections of cholecystokinin (CCK), local infusion of bile acids, and distention of the rectum.[41]

It is not only the colon that shows abnormal patterns of motor activity. Several studies have shown an abnormally high frequency of discrete clusters of contractions (DCCs) in the jejunum and prolonged propagated contractions in the ileum.[42] Like three-cycle-a-minute activity in the distal colon, these characteristics initially were considered to be specific abnormalities in IBS. However, DCCs are a feature of patients with mechanical intestinal obstruction and pseudo-obstruction of the small intestine and also can be generated by noxious stimuli such as ionizing radiation.[41] The increased frequency of this adaptive pattern of motor activity in patients with IBS, in whom there is no obvious source of irritation or obstruction, and the involvement of parts of the small intestine where these patterns are not normally seen also suggest a state of increased arousal and responsiveness of the gut to stimuli.[43] This interpretation is supported by the occurrence of exaggerated small intestinal contractile activity during sleep, during stress tests, and after injection of CCK in patients with IBS.[41, 43]

IBS is associated with a wide range of visceral hyperreactivity. There is evidence of exaggerated intestinal secretory responses to stimuli, increased frequency of strong nonpropulsive esophageal contractions, increased frequency of disturbances in gastric emptying, altered reactivity of the gallbladder, urodynamic abnormalities, increased responsiveness of bronchiolar smooth muscle, and enhanced vasomotor reactivity[44] in patients with IBS as compared with normal subjects.

Visceral Sensitivity

The exaggerated visceral reactivity in IBS patients is related to and may be a consequence of increased visceral sensitivity. Patients with IBS exhibit more symptoms during transit of a standard meal[45] and during transit of gases[46] than do normal subjects. They also show greater sensitivity to rectal distention, even at levels that cause no change in motility.[44] The rectum is not the only segment of the gut that is hypersensitive to distention in patients with IBS. Distention of other regions of the gut also gives rise to pain at volumes that are lower than those that cause pain in normal volunteers,[47] and the pain is distributed over a much wider area—to the upper gut, back, and even thigh. These changes are specific to visceral stimulation, because somatic pain thresholds have been normal and even higher in patients with IBS in some studies.[48]

Gastrointestinal sensitization may be regarded as an alarm signal that stops the normal unconscious processes of digestion and puts the gut on alert, ready to evacuate its contents at a moment's notice, either downward by diarrhea or upward by vomiting. However, this explanation does not account for IBS patients who experience constipation.

The Relationship between Gastrointestinal Symptoms and Physiologic Disturbance

The disturbances in colonic physiologic processes observed in patients with IBS are not diagnostic markers for IBS but are related to particular disturbances in bowel habit. Measurements of colonic transit and multichannel manometric or myoelectric recordings have shown that IBS patients whose primary sympton is diarrhea have more rapid colonic transit and a greater prevalence of propagated pressure or myoelectrical sequences than do more constipated patients, who have slow transit and more nonpropagated and retrograde motor events.[41, 44, 45] Corresponding changes in small bowel transit time also have been reported.[45] One study described delayed ileal emptying and impaired ileocecal clearance in patients with IBS whose predominant symptom was bloating,[49] a symptom that is often associated with constipation.

Visceral sensitization is much more frequently observed in patients with diarrhea than in those with constipation, whereas some patients with constipation show a reduction in rectal sensitivity.[50] Constipated patients with a sensitive rectum may be distinguished from those with an insensitive rectum by their frequent frustrated desire to defecate and their positive scores for anxiety.[51] It is possible that the frustrated need to defecate may be caused by the retention in a sensitive rectum of fecal pellets that are too small to evacuate.[52]

The relationship between colonic physiologic characteristics and abdominal or pelvic pain is less clear. Some prolonged recordings have shown a clear temporal association between pain and strong contractile events in the sigmoid colon[53] or ileum.[54] However, similarly powerful motor events can occur in normal subjects, but they rarely give rise to pain. The implication is that compression and tension forces associated with gastrointestinal contractile activity and the transient ischemia that they produce are associated with pain in IBS because the bowel is more sensitive than the normal bowel. The relationship between visceral sensitivity and symptoms, however, is less straightforward than the gastrointestinal physiologic findings would suggest. The reporting of pain by patients appears to be more closely associated with a psychopathologic condition than with rectal sensitivity.[27] The sensation of pain is generated in the brain. Although pain may be given form and expression by physiologic changes that take place in a specific part of the gut, the pain is greatly enhanced by emotional connotations of panic and dread. Once generated, pain can persist as a memory that can be evoked by associations with the conditions under which the pain was first experienced.[55] Thus, it is quite possible for pain to be generated in the absence of any change in visceral physiologic condition and even when the organ to which the pain is referred has been removed, as in phantom limb or phantom gallbladder pain.

What Is Responsible for Sensitization?

Local Inflammation

Inflammatory disease of the colon such as ulcerative colitis is associated with visceral sensitivity and reactivity,[56] similar to that seen in IBS. Although IBS is not associated with obvious inflammatory change, several studies have drawn attention to the increase in inflammatory cells, notably mast cells, in the colons of patients with IBS,[44] and a 1999 study showed increases in proinflammatory cytokines in patients with diarrhea-predominant IBS.[57]

Inflammation is associated with the release of cytokines from damaged tissue, white blood cells, and other cells in the vicinity. Cytokines orchestrate the inflammatory and immune processes and enhance sensitivity and reactivity by stimulating sensory nerve endings and by encouraging the proliferation and degranulation of local mast cells. Once stimulated, a cycle of sensitization may be maintained by several possible mechanisms.[57, 58]

1. One popular theory involves local proliferation of mast cells, which produce potent inflammatory mediators that enhance tissue sensitivity and reactivity. The classic stimulus for mast cell discharge is an allergic, or type I, hypersensitivity reaction, but nonspecific release of mast cell products can occur in response to cell injury, ischemia, infection, some foods, drugs, alcohol, and stress. When mast cells degranulate, they also encourage the proliferation of more mast cells and establish linkages with nerves. Mast cell degranulation can be conditioned by psychic stimuli to respond to audiovisual and stressful stimuli,[59] a finding that suggests a mechanism whereby an acute reaction to gut irritants or damage might be conditioned by anxiety and fear. A few studies have reported mast cell hyperplasia in patients with IBS,[60] and disodium cromoglycate, a mast cell stabilizer, can improve symptoms in some patients with diarrhea-predominant IBS.[61]
2. The excitation of sympathetic afferent nerves as a result of visceral inflammation or trauma results in the production of neuropeptides in the cell bodies of these nerves. These neuropeptides amplify the sensory experience centrally by enhancing sensory transmission in the dorsal horn of the spinal cord[58] and locally by exciting axon reflexes that cause changes in blood flow, smooth muscle contraction, immune reactivity, and degranulation of mast cells, which in turn may recruit other sensory nerves.
3. Inflammation causes not only white cells but also smooth muscle cells and fibroblasts to elaborate cytokines, other transmitters, and growth factors, which amplify the inflammatory process and tend to consolidate the potential for a longer-lasting state of hyperreactivity through the proliferation of neuromuscular elements.[57]

In the ways outlined, sensitization of the gut can persist in the form of a tissue memory[58] that can be activated by behavioral and stressful stimuli, such as eating and emotion.

Postinfective Sensitization

There is a well-documented relationship between an attack of gastroenteritis and chronic symptoms compatible with the diagnosis of IBS.[62] A 1999 prospective study of more than 500,000 patients showed that a bout of culture-positive gastroenteritis was the strongest predictor of IBS, with a relative risk of 11.9.[63] IBS does not develop in all gastroenteritis patients but is more likely to do so in hospitalized patients than in those treated at home. There is no evidence for persistent infection; prospective studies have shown that compared with those whose bowel habits return to normal, patients in whom IBS develops are predominantly women, experience more severe acute illness, and, most notably, exhibit more psychological disturbance and higher scores for neuroticism on psychometric tests conducted at the time of the initial illness.[27] They also have experienced more traumatic life events during the 6 months preceding the attack of gastroenteritis. Nevertheless, both groups of patients have increased colonic transit, enhanced rectal sensitivity, and evidence of a mild ongoing inflammatory process, which is greater in the group with IBS.[27] These findings suggest that an attack of gastroenteritis may sensitize the bowel, but that development of symptoms of IBS depends on the coexistence of psychosocial factors, which may act via psychoneuroendocrine mechanisms to induce an increase in intestinal inflammatory cellularity. In support of this interpretation is the observation that psychological stress can reactivate inflammation in the gut of animals predisposed by a previous episode of acute inflammation.[57]

Bile Acid Malabsorption

Bile acids are intensely irritating to the colonic mucosa; they induce a mild inflammatory reaction, stimulate secretion and propulsive motility,[64] and may exacerbate diarrhea and rectal urgency. Several studies have shown that diarrhea-predominant IBS is associated with rapid small bowel transit and impaired intestinal absorption of bile acids[65] and that symptoms may resolve with administration of the bile acid binding agent cholestyramine.

Hysterectomy

IBS develops for the first time in some patients after a hysterectomy.[66] Physiologic studies have shown that hysterectomy is associated with an increase in rectal and bladder sensitivity. Surgical trauma to the pelvis could sensitize adjacent organs by stimulating the production of neuropeptides in primary sympathetic afferents, thus enhancing spinal transmission of afferent impulses (as discussed earlier[58]).

Food Allergy and Food Intolerance

Acute hypersensitivity reactions are mediated by mast cells and result in dramatic gut reactions (see Chapter 101). Affected patients often have other "atopic" conditions, such as eczema, asthma, angioedema, urticaria, and rhinorrhea,[67] and they respond well to elimination diets and disodium cromoglycate.[60] Nevertheless, acute hypersensitivity reactions are rare causes of IBS.

Although studies of dietary restriction followed by the sequential reintroduction of single foods have suggested that food intolerance exists in up to two thirds of patients with IBS,[68] few studies have confirmed the findings immunologically or biochemically. It seems likely, therefore, that the link between food and symptoms of IBS may be explained by autonomic arousal in relation to aversions to or fears of certain foods or of eating in general.[69] Lactose intolerance as well as intolerance to sorbitol or fructose[70] have been implicated in IBS, but it is likely that the specific enzyme deficiency is not the cause of IBS but that the hypersensitive and hyperreactive guts of patients with IBS show exaggerated responses to the gaseous and fluid distention caused by incomplete absorption of the carbohydrate. A similar mechanism may explain the exacerbation of abdominal pain, bloating, borborygmi, flatulence, and diarrhea by dietary fiber.[71]

A 1998 study demonstrated altered colonic fermentation in patients with diarrhea-predominant IBS,[72] but this finding may be the result of the diarrhea, which may flush out the colonic microbial ecosystem, thereby altering the fermentative mix of bacterial colonies. More convincing is the contention that foods rich in sulfur compounds, such as meat and preserved foods, encourage the growth of sulfate-reducing bacteria at the expense of methanogenic bacteria.[73] Hydrogen sulfide is quite toxic and may cause colonic inflammation and irritation by impairing the utilization of butyrate, the preferred energy source of colonocytes. These discoveries have stimulated a renewed interest in using either probiotics to seed the colon with healthy bacteria (e.g., lactobacilli and *Bifidobacterium* species) or oligosaccharide prebiotics to encourage a more healthy ecosystem. However, there is little convincing evidence to date of the long-term efficacy of this approach in patients with IBS.[74]

Central Mechanisms of Sensitization

The association between emotion and gut motility has been recognized for years. Physiologic studies have shown that anger is associated with exaggerated contractile activity in the rectosigmoid colon, whereas sadness or fear is associated with lack of motility.[41] Anxiety is associated with rapid small bowel transit and increased bowel frequency, whereas delays in small bowel and whole gut transit occur in people who are depressed and those who exercise great control over their anger.[75, 76]

The effects of emotion on gastrointestinal function are mediated by the autonomic nervous system (see also Chapters 85 and 86). Eating and the presence of food in the gut activate the vagus nerve, which, in concert with gastrointestinal peptides, promotes digestive secretions and induces a pattern of gastrointestinal motor activity that is exquisitely tuned to the process of digestion. With the body at rest and under the gentle control of the parasympathetic nervous system, digestion proceeds in a peaceful and painless manner. Any threat to the person induces a state of arousal, which interrupts gut function by stimulating the sympathetic nervous system. Measurements of autonomic nerve activity have shown that constipation is associated with low vagal tone[77, 78] and diarrhea is associated with increased sympathetic activity.[79] Moreover, patients with acute autonomic neuropathy can report typical symptoms of IBS.[80]

The use of experimental stressors to induce a state of tension and arousal has been associated with enhanced visceral sensitivity, irregular contractility in the small intestine, and accelerated small bowel and colonic transit.[81, 82] These changes are similar to those seen in patients with diarrhea-predominant IBS, suggesting that this condition may be characterized by an abnormal degree of autonomic arousal. In support of this concept is the observation that sleep disturbance is common in patients with IBS, who also show a remarkable increase in rapid eye movements during sleep as compared with normal subjects.[83] Similar observations have been made in depressed patients. Poor quality of sleep is also associated with an increased reporting of IBS symptoms.[84] Recordings of small intestinal contractile activity during sleep in IBS patients have shown a greater preponderance of irregular or phase II activity, indicative of arousal, and less regular phase III activity.[85] Therefore, it seems that during sleep both the brain and the gut in IBS patients are in enhanced states of arousal. The notion of hyperarousal in IBS is supported by experimental studies that show exaggerated responses to stressors[41] and by clinical observations that indicate exaggerated responses to minor life events.

The normal physiologic response to acute stress involves the linked activation of the hypothalamopituitary axis and the sympathetic nervous system. In humans an infusion of corticotropin releasing hormone (CRH) increases contractile activity in the descending colon and induces abdominal pain.[86] These responses are greater in patients with IBS, who, like depressed patients, exhibit elevated cerebrospinal fluid levels of CRH and high serum levels of cortisol.

The brain can influence the transmission of nociceptive information from the gut and the activation of visceral reflexes by means of descending inhibitory and excitatory pathways that terminate via synapses within the dorsal horn at the secondary sensory neuron.[58] During relaxed and peaceful digestion, the inhibitory signals damp down sensory transmission and ensure that normal gut events do not reach consciousness. Anxiety, anger, and other causes of emotional arousal alter the balance of these descending cerebrospinal influences in the direction of excitation. Thus, not only do more gastrointestinal events reach consciousness, but also events that normally cause slight discomfort may cause severe pain, and the pain is distributed over a wider area as impulses entering through one nerve root spread to involve adjacent segments. Patients with IBS often experience pain over a wide somatic distribution, including the thigh, shoulder blade, and back.[47] "Up-regulation" of afferent nerve traffic also reduces the threshold stimulation required to induce gastrointestinal reflexes, thereby increasing contractile responses to stimuli and, as a result, diarrhea, vomiting, and disturbances in eating behavior. Furthermore, the extensive convergence of afferent spinal input from different viscera explains why gastrointestinal sensitization induced by emotional arousal is associated with increases in bronchiolar tone and reactivity, urinary frequency, and vasomotor instability.[44, 58] Finally, sensitization of sympathetic afferents increases sympathetic tone[87] and accounts for the sweaty palms, cardiac palpitations, increased tendon jerks, and nervousness so common in patients with IBS. Thus, anxiety could be the consequence of gastrointestinal sensitization rather than its cause. States of diminished emotional arousal may enhance descending inhibition from the brain and reduce intestinal sensitivity and reactivity, thereby causing constipation and a state of helplessness and inertia.

Psychoneural modulation of gastrointestinal sensorimotor function may explain why the symptoms of IBS are not constant but can vary from day to day and at different times of the day, why diarrhea alternates with constipation, and why IBS sufferers experience dramatic changes in mood. Even in normal subjects, rectal sensitivity and motility can be increased by sleep deprivation, stress, focused attention, and anger and can be reduced by relaxation, sadness, and distraction[43, 88–91]

THE IMPACT OF LIFE EVENTS

(See also Chapter 122)

Experimental stressors may provide important insights into brain-gut physiologic characteristics but can never reproduce the long-term effects of the "gut-wrenching" incidents that patients experience, such as bereavement, loss of a job, or physical or sexual abuse. A sense of loss or injustice that cannot be properly grieved tends to reverberate for years as a state of grievance, creating a chronic relentless drain on the personality, converting mild upsets into major catastrophes, and causing physical disease. IBS sufferers, irrespective of whether they seek medical help, report more loss, separation, and familial disruption both during childhood and in adult life than normal control subjects.[31]

Changes always disrupt the harmony of existence and require some degree of mental tension to adjust to them, but the events people find stressful always involve the loss or the threat of the loss of "objects" that are essential to the sense of identity.[92] Examples include the death of a parent, marital separation and divorce, unemployment, relocation, retirement, failure to receive an expected promotion, the shame of being "found out," or the drastic loss of personal integrity and self-esteem consequent to abuse; in fact, anything, either external or internal, that leads to a sense of loss of who one is as a person can cause a descent into illness. Not only negative events, but also positive changes, such as marriage or the birth of a child, involve losses and can trigger IBS in susceptible people.

It is important to understand the meaning of an event in the context of the patient's personal history. For example, in 10% to 15% of women IBS develops for the first time after hysterectomy.[66] Although there may be physiologic reasons for the onset of IBS in this setting, hysterectomy represents a loss of femininity, motherhood, and family to which it is difficult for some women to adjust. Persons with IBS are more likely than peptic ulcer disease patients to report life events as negative.[93] Many find it difficult to cope with change. Instead of seeing an opportunity, they sense that something might go wrong and feel threatened by it. For many people the threat of what might happen is worse than the actual event. Patients with IBS experience an abnormally high prevalence of chronic threats.[94] Such people are constantly "on the edge," dreading the consequences of a loss that has not yet occurred but probably will.

Although external losses can result in disease in susceptible people, the effect of these losses on the internal integration of the self is the crucial determinant of health and illness. The most serious events are those that result in negative feelings, such as isolation, guilt, shame, loss of security, and the kind of embarrassment that leaves a scar on the psyche. Nothing can be more threatening and damaging to the self than the experience of physical or sexual abuse. The feeling of being invaded, overpowered, penetrated, and controlled leaves the victim feeling dirty, humiliated, used, vulnerable, depersonalized, and shamed and is frequently associated with the development of psychiatric and psychosomatic conditions. If abuse occurs in childhood before the achievement of a full sense of autonomy, then the effects are likely to be more serious. Chronic disturbances in gastrointestinal function, many of which would satisfy the diagnostic criteria for IBS, have been documented in survivors of the Nazi Holocaust, former hostages, and victims of sexual abuse.[95, 96] Furthermore, the prevalence of previous physical or sexual abuse has been reported in 32% to 44% of patients with IBS, much higher than the rate in people with organic gastrointestinal disorders.[97] Gastrointestinal symptoms do not develop immediately after the abusive event but occur after a period of phobias and denial as sufferers use different strategies to block out the experience.[98] They often do not realize that there is an association between the physical symptoms and the traumatic experience, and physical symptoms tend to emerge when recollection of the abusive experience diminishes. It would be a mistake, however, to presume that severe symptoms of IBS indicate a hidden history of sexual abuse, and physicians should avoid zealous inquisition, which may be considered by the patient to be a damaging and disturbing intrusion, as may a rectal examination.

Coping with Loss

People who have been brought up with a sense of self-confidence and integrity respond to loss with an appropriate sense of grief or sorrow and are able to work through the loss in a way that leaves the personality intact and able to cope. Vulnerable people, who have experienced deficiency in their emotional development and rely on family, friends, home, job, political convictions, grievances, and religious beliefs to maintain a coherent and stable sense of self, experience loss or the threat of loss as catastrophic. For such people, loss seems to remove an essential regulator that may have been acting to hold body and mind together,[99] and the ensuing emotional tension may be expressed as intolerable psychological or physical illness. Under these circumstances, the presence of social support can be essential for recovery.

Some people seem to express a hopeless and helpless response to loss. They depend on and idealize the impression of catastrophe, deny psychological disturbance, and project blame onto others.[100] If feelings are so intense that they cannot be expressed without intolerable emotional tension and the risk of disintegration, then the terror, grievance, or desolation is expressed through the body as the catastrophic symptom that controls their lives, whereas the remainder of the personality appears in ostensibly good order and denies any emotional distress. The patient's sense of fragility and need for validation create a highly suggestible personality that is said to require a mission, sense of purpose, and focus of identification to hold it together. Many IBS patients identify strongly with environmental pollution and food contamination. They also readily identify with the sick role. Illness, especially an illness that "baffles doctors and is unique to medical science," provides a sense of identity that is difficult to dislodge.[100] Often such patients do not seem to want to get better; they need instead to feel validated, supported, and cared for, and perhaps the only way they can achieve these goals is by being ill. Failure of the doctor to recognize the true needs of the patient can lead to mutual frustration and a breakdown in communication.

Other patients exhibit a high degree of emotional control. For them, emotional expression seems so dangerous that it cannot be risked. Some of these patients seem to have the personality defect known as *alexithymia* (literally, "absence of word emotion"[101]). They do not seem to be in touch with their feelings, show little imagination, think in a very rigid concrete way, and have an impoverished dream life. Communication with them can seem sterile and lifeless. They cannot see that their symptoms have any meaning other than that of a complex biologic disease. Tension, therefore, remains locked in a mind-body circuit and cannot be expressed except through physical illness.

Neuroendocrine Mediators of Psychovisceral Tension

Events or thoughts that give rise to psychovisceral tension are relayed to the body via the hypothalamic-pituitary-adrenal axis and the locus ceruleus noradrenergic system. As discussed earlier, the tension is thought to cause changes in visceral function, which feed back to the brain via afferent nerves and, when combined with contextual information, generate "emotions."[102] Emotions demand resolution through thought, communication, and action. When the source of the tension cannot be recognized, acknowledged, or communicated, it tends to persist and may lead to functional illnesses, such as IBS or psychiatric illnesses such as panic and depression.

Exaggerated and prolonged activation of the hypothalamic-pituitary-adrenal axis may arise through chronic unremitting stress, a failure to adapt to the same stressful situation, and an inability to suppress the stress response.[103] These responses are determined both by genetic predisposition and by the previous experience of the person. An exaggerated stress response is associated with increased vigilance; feelings of fatigue, irritability, demoralization, and exhaustion; and increases in colonic motility that lead to an increased frequency of defecation. Exaggerated hypothalamic-pituitary-adrenal responses were reported in 1998 in a small group of patients with IBS characterized by diarrhea and constipation.[86]

In contrast, abnormal suppression of the hypothalamic-pituitary-adrenal axis implies a resistance and control of emotional reactions to stressful situations and is more likely to be associated with constipation and enhancement of inflammation caused by the unrestrained release of cytokines.[103] This type of neurohumoral dysregulation may correlate with the inflammatory changes observed in some patients with IBS.[44, 57]

Collectively these observations suggest that bowel function may act as a sensitive visceral marker of emotional expression. This idea is supported by neuroanatomic evidence that different regions of the prefrontal cortex and brainstem periaqueductal gray matter may mediate active and passive coping strategies.[100] These observations appear to correspond with concepts of control or chaos, sympathetic or parasympathetic dominance, and visceral expression of either constipation or diarrhea. For example, control and resistance are expressed by constipation, whereas diarrhea and rectal urgency are associated with a more uncontained hopeless and helpless style of emotional expression.[100] Seen from this perspective, it is not surprising that there often is a connection between constipation and anorexia ("nothing in, nothing out")[104] and between diarrhea and binge eating, whereas patients with alternating diarrhea and constipation or those with bulimia nervosa can seem to be on an emotional roller coaster—up one moment and down the next. The suggested link between emotional expression and bowel symptoms also is supported by the published association between larger and more frequent bowel movements and high scores for extroversion.[105]

Developmental Determinants of Responses to Stress

Growing up is a graded process of increasing separation and autonomy and is achieved through the constancy of the primal relationship of the child and parent and the allocation of tolerable separations.[99, 106] Failure of the parent-child relationship can leave a child without sufficient internal resources to cope with separation and overdependence on "external regulators" such as family, friends, home, institutions, ideas, and symptoms to hold the personality together.[99] The subsequent loss of these external regulators then leaves the personality open to psychobiologic dysregulation, expressed though feelings of tension and depression, and alterations in the functioning of the autonomic nervous system and hypothalamic-pituitary-adrenal axis. This theory may explain why psychosomatic disorders such as IBS are often triggered by loss and cluster at ages associated with separation, such as adolescence, the early 20s, and the mid-40s.

THE MEANING OF IBS SYMPTOMS

Psychobiologic dysregulation does not explain why one patient may express emotional tension as IBS, another as headaches, and a third as asthma. The predominant symptom may carry a meaning for the patient.[100] The association between emotional distress and postgastroenteritis IBS suggests that a visceral memory is recruited to express the unresolved emotional tension.[27] This visceral memory may not necessarily be the experience of the acute infection but may emanate from a generalized stress response to an emotional upset, such as the diarrhea caused by severe apprehension or the memory of a particular disease in a close relative. Finally, the visceral memory could arise through "identification" with a disease that is "in fashion," such as food allergy, environmental pollution, or yeast infection.[106] In some cases the symptom may represent emotional tension in symbolic form, for example, fecal incontinence as shame, borborygmi as guilty secrets, constipation as fear of exposure, and diarrhea as destructive anger.[100]

Studies using positron emission tomography (PET) have suggested that the anterior cingulate and prefrontal cortices may provide the neuroanatomic source of specific visceral symptoms from an unpleasant idea or memory.[100] The prefrontal cortex receives signals from all sensory brain regions in which the images that constitute our thoughts are formed and serves as a vast personal memory bank that combines meaning and emotional significance with personal experience. The anterior cingulate cortex (ACC) is thought to respond to emotionally laden ideas, memories, and stimuli and to generate visceral responses. For example, pain induced by colonic distention is associated with emotional changes and activation of these regions of the brain. Moreover, both the activity of the ACC and the unpleasantness of pain[107] can be reduced by hypnosis without any change in the activation of the somatosensory cortex, a finding that implies that we can create the unpleasantness of symptoms by the way we think about them.[108] Thus, if a person has had the experience of being hospitalized for severe abdominal pain caused by appendicitis, the abdominal symptom and the frightening experience of separation create a psychovisceral connection that can be reactivated by any experience that recalls the memory. Phenomena such as phantom limb or phantom gallbladder syndrome suggest that the sensation of pain in any part of the body can be determined internally from its representation in the central nervous system. It would appear, then, that the ACC can actually generate symptoms that bear a symbolic relationship with life events and feelings and that thought can give rise to the symptom.[109]

DIAGNOSIS

Although symptoms that are said to support a positive diagnosis of IBS[5] (see Table 91–1) also can be found in patients with inflammatory bowel disease, diverticular disease, solitary rectal ulcer syndrome, and many other conditions and patients with IBS have symptoms referable to other organ systems, IBS is not necessarily a diagnosis of exclusion. The diagnosis of IBS and similar illnesses that have no clear pathologic conditions and no clear cause relies on the clinician's art and understanding, rather than the results of diagnostic tests. Features that lead the clinician to make a diagnosis of IBS, apart from the absence of signs of organic disease such as rectal bleeding and precipitous weight loss, include the chronicity of the history, relationship between exacerbations of symptoms and life events, variability of symptoms, association with symptoms in other organ systems, presence of anxiety and depression, and distress that may seem out of proportion to the nature of the symptoms (Table 91–2).

Patients who have IBS, like those who have chronic fatigue syndrome, fibromyalgia, and eating disorders, are recognized as much by the way they behave when reporting their illness as by the combination of physical symptoms they experience. The patient's complaints may be dramatic, and the patient may have an extreme degree of distress and air of catastrophe. Although the physical symptoms may appear to an outsider to be relatively mild, the patient may assert that they are interfering with his or her life. The patient may believe that the condition is caused by food allergy, candidiasis, environmental pollution, food additives,

Table 91–2 | **Clinical Features Supporting the Diagnosis of Irritable Bowel Syndrome**

- Rome II criteria (see Table 91–1)
- Long history with relapsing and remitting course
- Exacerbations triggered by life events and difficult life situations
- Variability of symptoms
- Association with symptoms in other organ systems
- Coexistence of anxiety and depression
- Distress that seems out of proportion to the nature of the symptom
- Symptoms that are exacerbated by eating
- Conviction of the patient that the disease is caused by "popular" concerns (e.g., allergy, pollution, candidiasis, food toxicity)

allergies, dental amalgam, or any of a number of factors. The patient may be desperate to find someone who will take control of his or her life in a way that the patient cannot. These features resemble classic descriptions of hysterical illness.[100]

The diagnosis of an illness such as IBS is made most confidently by a physician who has established a relationship with the patient over the course of many years and is in a position to observe the illness in the context of the vicissitudes of the patient's life. The onus on the doctor is not necessarily to make a positive diagnosis of IBS but to be sensitive to changes in the patient's symptoms that may indicate a coexistent organic disease that requires investigation and treatment[110] (Table 91–3). If the patient is young (below age 45 years); the symptoms are typical and commensurate with life situations and the patient's life events; there are no sinister features such as weight loss, rectal bleeding, or fever; and findings of physical examination including sigmoidoscopy are normal, then no further investigations are necessary to make a working diagnosis of IBS. Nongastroenterologic features such as lethargy, poor sleep, fibromyalgia, backache, urinary frequency and urgency, nocturia, incomplete bladder emptying, an unpleasant taste in the mouth, early satiety, and dyspareunia are more common in IBS patients than in healthy subjects and support the diagnosis.

A change in the patient's dietary habits or therapeutic regimens may trigger the development of symptoms of IBS or cause symptoms suggestive of IBS. Particular attention should be given to an abnormally low or excessive intake of dietary fiber or excess ingestion of poorly absorbed sugars, such as fructose or sorbitol, or stimulants, such as coffee. Angiotensin converting enzyme inhibitors, β blockers, antibiotics, chemotherapeutic agents, proton pump inhibitors, and nonsteroidal anti-inflammatory drugs can cause diarrhea, whereas constipation may result from opiate analgesics, calcium channel blockers, or antidepressants with anticholinergic effects, for example.

Because there is considerable overlap between the symptoms of IBS and those of organic disease, diagnoses based on clinical features alone misdiagnose some patients, particularly middle-aged or elderly persons who have a higher risk of organic disease. However, studies in which extensive investigations have been carried out in persons with suspected IBS have produced a low yield of organic diagnoses, which are frequently chance findings and not responsible for the symptoms.[111] The danger of missing a diagnosis needs to be balanced against the cost of performing unnecessary investigations and the potent risk of reinforcing illness behavior.

Table 91–3 | **Clinical and Laboratory Features That Suggest Diseases Other Than Irritable Bowel Syndrome**

- Onset in old age
- Course characterized by progressive deterioration
- Fever
- Progressive weight loss
- Rectal bleeding from causes other than anal fissures and hemorrhoids
- Steatorrhea
- Dehydration

Table 91–4 | **Recommended Laboratory Investigations in Patients Suspected of Having Irritable Bowel Syndrome**

All patients
- Hemoglobin or hematocrit, white blood cell count, erythrocyte sedimentation rate
- Protoscopy/sigmoidoscopy

If diarrhea is persistent or severe
- Malabsorption screen (fecal fat, serum B_{12}, red cell folate, plasma ferritin, serologic tests for celiac sprue)
- Stool cultures, *Clostridium difficile* toxin, ova and parasites
- Colonoscopy
- Small bowel follow-through
- Lactose tolerance test

Constipated patients and those with severe rectal urgency or fecal incontinence
- Colonic transit study
- Anorectal function tests (e.g., manometry and electrophysiology)
- Endoanal ultrasonography

The most important diagnosis not to be overlooked is cancer, and the decision to investigate depends on the age of the patient and a family history. In patients with chronic persistent diarrhea, screening investigations, such as measurement of serum vitamin B_{12}, red blood cell folate, ferritin, thyroid function, antiendomysial or tissue transglutaminase antibodies, and plasma albumin; stool microscopy; and sigmoidoscopy with rectal biopsy, should be performed. Colonoscopy to exclude microscopic and collagenous colitis also should be considered. Patients who have rectal urgency and fecal incontinence may require anorectal function tests (Table 91–4).

TREATMENT

There is no cure for IBS, but effective management may lessen the symptoms and lead to remission for many years. The management of patients with IBS should be individualized and based on an integrated philosophy that combines measures to relieve the predominant symptoms with insight into the way symptoms express emotional tension related to life situations and changes. The therapeutic attitude of the physician during the first interview is of paramount importance. The physician should acknowledge the distress caused by the illness. Careful attention to the way in which the assessment interview is conducted makes the patient feel heard and builds an atmosphere of trust and confidence that encourages healing. The physician should allow the patient sufficient time to tell his or her story and comment on particular associations between symptoms and life events. Time spent building the therapeutic relationship at this stage can pay enormous dividends in the long run for both the patient and doctor. It is important to ask the patient to describe his or her fears and beliefs. Many patients with IBS believe that they have some serious disease, especially cancer. Direct explanations of the symptoms should be provided. Abdominal cramps and spasms are easily accepted as causes of pain, and mechanisms whereby a "sensitive gut," for example, reacts excessively to food and mood can allay the patient's anxiety and promote an understanding of links with life events.[111]

Most drugs used in IBS aim to relieve the dominant symptoms (Table 91–5). Antispasmodics are prescribed for abdominal cramps, opiate-like antidiarrheal agents and cholestyramine are prescribed for diarrhea, and bulk laxatives are prescribed for consipation. However, what may be useful for one symptom may make another worse. For example, loperamide may relieve diarrhea at the expense of worsening abdominal pain and bloating. Similarly, constipation may be relieved by dietary fiber or bulk laxatives, but patients frequently experience an increase in bloating and abdominal pain that makes the treatment unacceptable. Abdominal pain may be dulled temporarily by antispasmodics, but these drugs may cause constipation, and the pain may return with increased intensity. Many patients with IBS appear to be intolerant of drugs of any sort. Recent efforts at drug development have been directed toward modifying visceral sensitivity and reactivity by using ligands for specific intestinal serotonin receptors. The long-term benefit of such agents remains to be determined. Antidepressants may be effective by relieving underlying emotional tension expressed in mental and visceral symptoms.[112]

In a much-quoted review, Klein concluded that "there is no therapeutic trial that has ever convincingly demonstrated the efficacy of any drug in IBS."[113] One of the problems in demonstrating the efficacy of drug treatment for IBS is that the placebo response is high, more than 60% for pain, for example. The same applies to dietary restrictions, which probably work on the basis of avoidance of food that the patient feels anxious about rather than circumvention of any biochemical or immunologic sensitivity. Dietary exclusion should be confined to specific foods that the patient believes contribute to his or her symptoms and should not extend to other dietary constituents, because the nervous patient may readily accept a nutritionally deficient diet. Similar considerations apply to psychotherapies, hypnosis, relaxation, and complementary therapies. However, such therapies should not be dismissed as useless simply because they have not been verified in randomized controlled trials. If diseases such as IBS are caused by unresolved tension related to life situations that cannot be resolved or talked about, then anything that allays those fears, relaxes the patient, and provides time to work things out may relieve the symptoms.

Table 91–5 | **Drugs That Are Useful in the Treatment of Irritable Bowel Syndrome**

Drug	Dose
Antispasmodics (for abdominal pain)	
Dicyclomine hydrochloride	10–20 mg tid, before meals
Hyoscyamine butylbromide	10–20 mg qid
Mebeverine hydrochloride	135 mg bid 20 min before meals
Alverine citrate	60–120 mg tid, before meals
Peppermint oil	1–2 capsules, 30–60 min before meals
Antidiarrheal agents	
Loperamide hydrochloride	2–8 mg/day in divided doses
Diphenoxylate hydrochloride	2–6 pills per day
Cholestyramine	1–3 packets per day, 30 min before meals
Anticonstipating agents	
Methylcellulose	1–3 packets or tbsp/day in divided doses
Isphagula husk	1–9 sachets in divided doses
Antidepressants	
Imipramine hydrochloride	10–100 mg/day
Amitryptyline hydrochloride	10–75 mg/day
Fluoxetine hydrochloride	20–60 mg/day
Paroxetine hydrochloride	20–50 mg/day

The "placebo effect" underlies the importance of faith and confidence in healing.[114] Placebos work by suggestion. Treatments must be commensurate with the patient's beliefs and attitudes. If the patient has faith in the therapy, the ensuing feelings of self-confidence and control may normalize the activities of the autonomic nervous system and the hypothalamic-pituitary-adrenal axis, thereby reducing emotional tension and restoring visceral function.

Similarly, complementary and alternative remedies may restore a sense of harmony and balance that is essential for health by providing time, relaxation, understanding, and confidence that allow the patient to recover.[115] Such therapies have been shown to reduce the secretion of stress hormones and exert positive modifications in other physiologic functions. Different therapies emphasize different aspects of the healing process. Physical therapies such as massage, acupuncture, reflexology, and shiatsu work on the release of emotional tension. Meditation and hypnotherapy induce a trancelike state of focused relaxation in which the person can accept and act on healthy ideas. In IBS, psychotherapies enable the patient to gain insight into the relationship between the symptoms and life events, understand the meaning of the symptoms, discover the source of emotional tension, correct dysfunctional thoughts, and gain a sense of control of life.[116] Hypnotherapy and cognitive behavioral therapy work well with people who are receptive to change. Biofeedback and homeopathy may work better for more resistant patients who need to be convinced of the need to gain control over their symptoms.[117] Self-help groups are available for patients with IBS in many countries. The dedication of such organizations is unquestionable, and the quality of the information they provide is high. Many patients are helped by joining such groups. The web address of the IBS Network is www.ibsnetwork.org.uk; the address of the International Federation for Functional Gastrointestinal Disorders (IFFGD) is www.iffgd.org; and the address of the Irritable Bowel Information and Support Association of Australia (IBIS) is www.powerup.com.au/~ibis.

PROGNOSIS

Once the diagnosis of IBS is established it rarely needs to be revised, and the incidence of new significant diagnoses is extremely low. In fact, the chance of remaining free of serious disease in IBS is excellent.[112] However, the prognosis for abdominal symptoms is not so good. Although a proportion of patients experience loss of symptoms of IBS over 12 months, other functional symptoms such as dyspepsia or fatigue may develop. Factors that have been shown to worsen prognosis include more prominent psychological symptoms, a longer history of illness, and previous abdominal surgery.[118]

REFERENCES

1. Corney RH, Stanton R: Physical symptom severity, psychological and social dysfunction in a series of outpatients with irritable bowel syndrome. J Psychosom Res 34:483–491, 1990.

2. Hahn BA, Kirchdoerfer LJ, Fullerton S, Mayer E: Patient-perceived severity of irritable bowel syndrome in relation to symptoms, health resource utilization and quality of life. Aliment Pharmacol Ther 11: 553–559, 1997.
3. Talley NJ, Gabriel SE, Mannsen WS, et al: Medical costs in community subjects with irritable bowel syndrome. Gastroenterology 109: 1736, 1995.
4. Talley NJ, Phillips SF, Bruce B, et al: J. Multi-system complaints in patients with the irritable bowel syndrome and functional dyspepsia. Eur J Gastroenterol Hepatol 3:71–77, 1991.
5. Drossman DA: Rome II: The Functional Gastrointestinal Disorders. McLean, Va, Degnon Associates, 2000.
6. Wessley S, Nimnuan C, Sharpe M: Functional somatic syndromes: One or many. Lancet 354:936–939, 1999.
7. Yunus MB: Central sensitivity syndromes: A unified concept of fibromyalgia and other similar maladies. J Indian Med Assoc (in press).
8. Walker EA, Roy-Byrne PP, Katon WJ: Irritable bowel syndrome and psychiatric illness. Am J Psychiatry 147:565–572, 1990.
9. Danivat D, Tankeyoon M, Sriratanaban A: Prevalence of irritable bowel syndrome in a non-Western population. BMJ 296:1710, 1988.
10. Olubuyide IO, Olawuyi F, Fasanmade AA: A study of irritable bowel syndrome diagnosed by Manning criteria in an African population. Dig Dis Sci 40:983–985, 1995.
11. Zuckerman MJ, Guerra LG, Drossman DA, et al: Comparison of bowel patterns in Hispanics and non-Hispanic whites. Dig Dis Sci 40: 1761–1769, 1995.
12. Wolpert L: Malignant Sadness: The Anatomy of Depression. London, Faber and Faber, 1999, pp 31–38.
13. Veith I: Hysteria: The History of a Disease. Chicago, University of Chicago Press, 1965.
14. Kapoor KK, Nigam P, Rastogi CK, et al: Clinical profile of the irritable bowel syndrome. Indian J Gastroenterol 4:15–16, 1985.
15. Mechanic D: Sex, illness, illness behavior and the use of health services. Soc Sci Med 12:207–214, 1978.
16. Drossman DA, Li Z, Andruzzi E, et al: US householder survey of functional gastrointestinal disorders: Prevalence, sociodemography and health impact. Dig Dis Sci 38:1569–1580, 1993.
17. Heaton KW, Radvan J, Cripps H, et al: Defaecation frequency and timing and stool pattern in the general population—a prospective study. Gut 33:818–824, 1992.
18. Talley NJ: Diagnosing irritable bowel syndrome: Does sex matter? Gastroenterology 100:834–837, 1991.
19. Sun WM, Donnelly TC, Read NW: Anorectal function in normal volunteers: The effect of gender. Int J Colorectal Dis 4:188–196, 1989.
20. Davies GJ, Crowder M, Reid B, Dickerson JTW: Bowel function measurements of individuals with different eating patterns. Gut 27: 164–169, 1989.
21. Talley NJ, O'Keefe EA, Zinsmeister AR, Melton L II: Prevalence of gastrointestinal symptoms in the elderly: A population-based study. Gastroenterology 102:895–901, 1992.
22. Thompson S, Dancey CP: Symptoms of irritable bowel syndrome in schoolchildren: Prevalence and psychological effects. J Paediatr Health Care 10:280–285, 1996.
23. Langeluddecke PM: Psychological aspects of irritable bowel syndrome. Aust N Z J Psychiatry 19:218–226, 1985.
24. Whitehead WE, Crowell MD: Psychologic considerations in the irritable bowel syndrome. Gastroenterol Clin North Am 20:249–267, 1991.
25. Bleijenberg G, Furness JFN: Anamnestic and psychological features in diagnosis and prognosis of functional abdominal complaints: A prospective study. Gut 30:1076–1081, 1989.
26. North CS, Alpers DN: Prevalence of irritable bowel syndrome in a psychiatric patient population. In Goebell H, Hoffman G, Talley NJ (eds): Functional Dyspepsia and Irritable Bowel Syndrome Concepts and Controversies: Falk Symposium 99. Dordrecht, Netherlands, Kluwer, 1998.
27. Gwee KA, Leong YL, Graham C, et al: The role of psychological and biological factors in postinfective gut dysfunction. Gut 44:400–406, 1999.
28. Drossman DA, McKee DC, Sandler RS, et al: Psychosocial factors in the irritable bowel syndrome: A multivariate study of patients and non-patients with irritable bowel syndrome. Gastroenterology 95:701–708, 1988.
29. Whitehead WE, Basmajian L, Zonderman AB, et al: Symptoms of psychologic distress associated with irritable bowel syndrome: Comparison of community and medical clinic samples. Gastroenterology 95:709–714, 1988.
30. Sandler RS, Drossman DA, Nathan HP, McKee DC: Symptom complaints and health care seeking behavior in subjects with bowel dysfunction. Gastroenterology 87:314–318, 1984.
31. Lowman BC, Drossman DA, Kramer EM, et al: Recollection of childhood events in adults with irritable bowel syndrome. J Clin Gastroenterol 9:324–330, 1987.
32. Whitehead WE, Winget C, Fedoravicius AS, Blackwell B: Learned illness behavior in patients with irritable bowel syndrome and peptic ulcer. Dig Dis Sci 27:202–208, 1982.
33. Smith RC, Greenbaum DS, Vancouver JB, et al: Psychosocial factors are associated with health care seeking rather than diagnosis in irritable bowel syndrome. Gastroenterology 98:293–301, 1990.
34. Heaton KW, O'Donnell LJD, Braddon FEM, et al: Symptoms of irritable bowel syndrome in a British urban community, consulters and nonconsulters. Gastroenterology 102:1962–1967, 1992.
35. Jones R, Lydeard S: Irritable bowel syndrome and the general population. BMJ 304:87–90, 1992.
36. Heaton KW, Chosh S, Braddon FEM: How bad are the symptoms and bowel dysfunction of patients with irritable bowel syndrome? A prospective, controlled study with emphasis on stool form. Gut 32(1):73–79, 1991.
37. Bower GH: Mood and memory. Am Psychol 6:129–148, 1981.
38. Heitkemper MM, Jowett M: Pattern of gastrointestinal and somatic symptoms across the menstrual cycle. Gastroenterology 102:505–513, 1992.
39. Snape WJ, Carlson GM, Maturazzo SA, et al: Evidence that abnormal myoelectrical activity produces colonic motor dysfunction in the irritable bowel syndrome. Gut 19:391–395, 1978.
40. Latimer P, Sarna S, Campbell D, et al: Colonic motor and myoelectrical activity: A comparative study of normal subjects, psychoneurotic patients and patients with the irritable bowel syndrome. Gastroenterology 80:893–901, 1981.
41. McKee DP, Quigley EMM: Intestinal motility in irritable bowel syndrome: Is IBS a motility disorder? Dig Dis Sci 38:1761–1782, 1993.
42. Kellow JE, Gill RC, Wingate DL: Prolonged ambulant recordings of small bowel motility demonstrate abnormalities in the irritable bowel syndrome. Gastroenterology 98:1208–1218, 1990.
43. Kellow J, Miller LJ, Phillips SF, Zinsmeister AR: Dysmotility of the small intestine is provoked by stimuli in the irritable bowel syndrome. Gut 29:1236–1243, 1988.
44. Read NW: Visceral afferent information and functional bowel disease: Evidence for dyssensation and altered reflex function. In Mayer EA, Raybould NE (eds): Basic and Clinical Aspects of Chronic Abdominal Pain. Amsterdam, Elsevier, 1993, pp 87–96.
45. Cann PA, Read NW, Brown C, et al: The irritable bowel syndrome (IBS) relationship of disorders in the transit of a single solid meal to symptom patterns. Gut 24:405–411, 1983.
46. Lasser RB, Bond JH, Levitt ND: The role of intestinal gas and functional abdominal pain. New Engl J Med 293:524–526, 1975.
47. Swarbrick ET, Haggerty JE, Bat L: Site of pain from the irritable bowel syndrome. Lancet 2:443–446, 1980.
48. Cook IJ, Van Eeden A, Collins SM: Patients with irritable bowel syndrome have a greater pain tolerance than normal subjects. Gastroenterology 93:727–733, 1987.
49. Trotman IF, Price CC: Bloated irritable bowel syndrome defined by dynamic ^{99}Tc brain scan. Lancet 2:364–366, 1986.
50. Bannister JJ, Timms JM, Barfield L, Read NW: Physiological studies in young women with chronic constipation. Int J Colorectal Dis 1: 175–182, 1986.
51. Prior A, Sorial E, Sun WM, Read NW: Irritable bowel syndrome: Differences between patients who show rectal sensitivity and those who do not. Eur J Gastroenterol Hepatol 5:343–349, 1993.
52. Bannister JJ, Dawson P, Timms JM, et al: Effect of stool size and consistency on defaecation. Gut 28:1246–1250, 1987.
53. Ritchie J: Mechanisms of pain in the irritable bowel syndrome. In Read NW (ed:) Irritable Bowel Syndrome. Philadelphia, Grune & Stratton, 1985, pp 163–172.
54. Kellow JE, Phillips SF: Altered small bowel motility in irritable bowel syndrome is correlated with symptoms. Gastroenterology 92:1885–1893, 1987.
55. Wall P: Pain: The Science of Suffering. London, Weidenfeld and Nicolson, 1999.
56. Rao SCC, Holdsworth CD, Read NW: Anorectal sensitivity and reac-

tivity in patients with ulcerative colitis. Gastroenterology 93:1270–1275, 1987.

57. Collins SM: Putative inflammatory and immunological mechanisms in functional bowel disorders. Clin Gastroenterol 13:429–436, 1999.
58. Mayer EA, Gebhart GF: Basic and clinical aspects of visceral hyperalgesia. Gastroenterology 107:271–293, 1994.
59. MacQueen G, Marshall J, Perdue M, Siegel S: Pavlovian conditioning of the rat muscosal mast cells to secrete rat mast cell protease II. Science 243:83–85, 1989.
60. Weston AP, Biddle WL, Bhatia PS, Miner PB: Terminal ileal mucosal mast cells in irritable bowel syndrome. Dig Dis Sci 38:1590–1595, 1993.
61. Stephanini GP, Saggioro A, Alvisi V, et al: Oral chromolyn sodium in comparison with elimination diet in the irritable bowel syndrome diarrhea type: Multicentre study of 428 patients. Scand J Gastroenterol 30: 535–541, 1995.
62. McKendrick MW, Read NW: Irritable bowel syndrome—post salmonella infection. J Infect 29:1–3, 1994.
63. Rodriguez LA, Ruigomez A: Increased risk of irritable bowel syndrome after bacterial gastroenteritis. BMJ 318:565–566, 1999.
64. Edwards CA, Baxter J, Brown S, et al: Effect of bile acids on anorectal function in humans. Gut 30:383–386, 1989.
65. Merrick MV, Eastwood MA, Ford MJ: Is bile acid malabsorption under-diagnosed? An evaluation of diagnosis by measurement of SeHcat retention. Br J Med 290:665–668, 1985.
66. Prior A, Stanley K, Smith ARB, Read NW: The relationship between hysterectomy and the irritable bowel: A prospective study. Gut 33: 814–817, 1992.
67. Smith MA, Youngs GR, Finn R: Food intolerance, atopy, and irritable bowel syndrome. Lancet 2:1064, 1985.
68. Nanda R, James R, Smith H, et al: Food intolerance and the irritable bowel syndrome. Gut 30:1099–1104, 1989.
69. Pearson DJ: Pseudo-food allergy. BMJ 292:221–222, 1986.
70. Rumessen JJ, Gudmund Hoyer E: Functional bowel disease: The role of fructose and sorbitol. Gastroenterology 101:1452–1453, 1991.
71. Francis CY, Whorwell PJ: Bran and the irritable bowel syndrome: Time for reappraisal. Lancet 344:39–40, 1994.
72. King TS, Elia M, Hunter JO: Abnormal colonic fermentation in irritable bowel syndrome. Lancet 352:1187–1189, 1998.
73. Gibson G, MacFarlane S, MacFarlane G: Metabolic interactions involving sulphate reducing and methanogenic bacteria in the human large intestine. FEMS Microbiology Ecology 12:117, 1993.
74. Hamilton-Miller JMT: Prebiotics, panacea or nostrum. Nutrit Bull 21: 199–201, 1996.
75. Gorard DA, Gomborone JE, Libby GW, Farthing MJG: Intestinal transit in anxiety and depression. Gut 39:551–555, 1996.
76. Bennett EJ, Evans P, Scott AM, et al: Psychological and gender features of impaired gut transit in functional gastrointestinal disorder. Gut 46:83–87, 2000.
77. Lee CT, Chuang TY, Lu CL, Chen CY: Abnormal vagal cholinergic function and psychological behaviors in irritable bowel syndrome patients: A hospital-based Oriental study. Dig Dis Sci 43:1794–1799, 1998.
78. Heitkemper M, Burr RL, Jarrett M, Hertig V: Evidence for autonomic nervous system imbalance in women with irritable bowel syndrome. Dig Dis Sci 43:2093–2098, 1999.
79. Aggarwal A, Cutts TF, Abell TL, et al: Predominant symptoms in irritable bowel syndrome correlate with specific autonomic nervous system abnormalities. Gastroenterology 106:945–950, 1994.
80. Camilleri M, Fealey RD: Idiopathic autonomic denervation in eight patients presenting with functional gastrointestinal disease: A causal association? Dig Dis Sci 35:609–616, 1990.
81. Narducci F, Snape WJJ, Battle WM: Increased colonic motility during exposure to a stressful situation. Dig Dis Sci 30:40–44, 1985.
82. Bharucha AE, Camilleri M, Ford JJ, et al: Hyperventilation alters colonic motor and sensory function: Effects and mechanisms in humans. Gastroenterology 111:368–377, 1996.
83. Orr WC, Crowell MD, Lin B, et al: Sleep and gastric function in irritable bowel syndrome: Derailing the brain gut axis. Gut 41:390–393, 1997.
84. Goldsmith G, Levin JS: Effect of sleep quality on symptoms of irritable bowel syndrome. Dig Dis Sci 38:1809–1814, 1993.
85. Kellow JE, Gill RC, Wingate DL: Prolonged ambulant recordings of small bowel motility demonstrate abnormalities in the irritable bowel syndrome. Gastroenterology 98:1208–1218, 1990.
86. Fukudo S, Nomura T, Hongo M: Impact of corticotropin-releasing hormone on gastrointestinal motility and adrenocorticotropic hormone in normal controls and patients with irritable bowel syndrome. Gut 42: 845–849, 1998.
87. Svensson TH: Peripheral, autonomic regulation of locus coeruleus noradrenergic neurones in the brain. Psychopharmacology 92:1–7, 1987.
88. Connell ALN, Jones FA, Rowlands EN: Motility of the pelvic colon, pain associated with colonic hypermotility after meals. Gut 6:105–112, 1965.
89. Welgan P, Meshkinpour H, Beeler J: The effect of anger on colon motor and myoelectrical activity in irritable bowel syndrome. Gastroenterology 94:1150–1156, 1988.
90. Accarino AM, Azpiroz F, Malagelada JR: Attention and distraction: Effects on gut perception. Gastroenterology 113:415–422, 1997.
91. Whorwell PJ, Houghton LA, Taylor EE, et al: Physiological effects of emotion: Assessment via hypnosis. Lancet 340:69–72, 1992.
92. Rahe RH, Meyer M, Smith M, et al: Social stress and illness onset. J Psychosom Res 8:25, 1964.
93. Dinan TG, O'Keane V, O'Boyle C, et al: A comparison of the mental status, personality profiles and life events of patients with irritable bowel syndrome and peptic ulcer disease. Acta Psychiatr Scand 84: 26–28, 1991.
94. Bennett EJ, Tennant CC, Piesse C, et al: Level of chronic life stress predicts clinical outcome in irritable bowel syndrome. Gut 43:256–261, 1998.
95. Stermer E, Bar H, Levy N: Chronic functional gastrointestinal symptoms in Holocaust survivors. Am J Gastroenterol 86:417–422, 1991.
96. Rimsza ME, Berg RA, Locke C: Sexual abuse: Somatic and emotional reactions. Child Abuse Negl 12:201–208, 1988.
97. Walker EA, Katon WJ, Ray-Byrne PP: Histories of sexual victimization in patients with irritable bowel syndrome or inflammatory bowel disease. Am J Psychiatry 150:1502, 1993.
98. Felice M, Grant J, Reynolds B, et al: Follow-up observations of adolescent rape victims: Rape may be one of the more serious afflictions of adolescence with respect to long term psychological effects. Clin Pediatr 17:311–315, 1978.
99. Taylor GJ: Psychobiological disregulation: A new model of disease. In Taylor GJ (ed): Psychosomatic Medicine in Contemporary Psychoanalysis. IUP Stress and Health Series Monograph 3. Madison, Conn, International Universities Press, 1987, pp 279–319.
100. Read NW: Bridging the gap between mind and body: Do cultural and psychoanalytical concepts of visceral disease have an explanation in contemporary neuroscience? In Mayer EA, Soper CB (eds): Progress in Brain Research, vol 122. Amsterdam, Elsevier, 2000, pp 425–443.
101. Sifneos PE: The prevalence of alexithymic characteristics in psychosomatic patients. Psychother Psychosom 22:255–262, 1973.
102. Dimasio A: The Feeling of What Happens: Body, Emotion and the Making of Consciousness. London, Heinemann, 1999.
103. McEwen BS: Protective and damaging effects of stress mediators. New Engl J Med 338:171–179, 1998.
104. Guthrie EA, Creed FA, Whorwell PJ: Eating disorders in patients with irritable bowel syndrome. Eur J Gastroenterol Hepatol 2:471–473, 1994.
105. Tucker DM, Sandstead NM, Logan GM: Dietary fiber and personality factors in determinants of stool output. Gastroenterology 81:879–883, 1981.
106. Showater E: Hysteries: Hysterical Epidemics and Modern Culture. London, Picador, 1997.
107. Rainville P, Duncan GH, Price DD, et al: Pain affect encoded in human anterior cingulate but not somatosensory cortex. Science 277: 968–971, 1997.
108. Read NW: Rectal distension: From sensation to feeling. Gastroenterology 118:972–974, 2000.
109. Read NW: Psychodynamic aspects of bowel dysfunction. In Ewe K, Ekhardt VF, Enck P (eds): Constipation and Anorectal Insufficiency. Dordrecht, Netherlands, Kluwer Press, 1997, pp 19–32.
110. Jones J, Boorman J, Cann P, et al: British Society of Gastroenterology Guidelines for the Management of Functional Bowel Disorders with Special Reference to the Irritable Bowel Syndrome. Gut 47 (suppl II): 1–19, 2000.
111. Harvey RF, Mauad EC, Brown AM: Prognosis in the irritable bowel syndrome: A 5-year prospective study. Lancet 1:963–965, 1987.
112. Myren J, Lovland B, Larssen S-E, Larsen S: A double-blind study of the effect of trimipramine in patients with the irritable bowel syndrome. Scand J Gastroenterol 19:835–843, 1984.

113. Klein KB: Controlled treatment trails in irritable bowel syndrome: A critique. Gastroenterology 95:232–241, 1988.
114. Read NW: Placebo and panacea: The healing effect of nutritional supplements. In Ransley JK, Donnelly JK, Read NW (eds): Food and Nutritional Supplements in Health and Disease. London, Springer Verlag, 2001, pp 45–64.
115. Graham H: Complementary Therapies in Context: The Psychology of Healing. London, Jessica Kingsley, 1999.
116. Read NW: Harnessing the patient's powers of recovery: The role of psychotherapies in the irritable bowel syndrome. Clin Gastroenterol 13:473–487, 1999.
117. Wickramakesere I: How does biofeedback reduce clinical symptoms and do memories and beliefs have biological consequences? Towards a model of mind body healing. Appl Psychophysiol Biofeedback 24: 91–103, 1999.
118. Lembo T, Fullerton S, Diehl D, et al: Symptom duration in patients with irritable bowel syndrome. Am J Gastroenterol 91:898–905, 1996.

Chapter 92

Short Bowel Syndrome

Arshad Malik and Henrik Westergaard

Short bowel syndrome can be defined as a malabsorption syndrome that results from extensive intestinal resection (see Chapter 89). The spectrum of short bowel syndrome ranges from limited ileocolonic resections with moderate nutritional compromise to extensive small intestinal and colonic resections, leading to either high jejunostomy or jejunocolonic anastomosis with severe nutritional consequences. In practice, a small bowel length of less than 200 cm is commonly used as an anatomic definition of short bowel syndrome.[1] Intestinal failure is a functional definition of the syndrome that denotes the inability of the remnant intestine to maintain nutritional balance.

ETIOLOGY

The major causes of short bowel syndrome in adults are inflammatory bowel disease, particularly Crohn's disease, mesenteric infarction, and radiation injury (Table 92–1). The series in Table 92–1 includes a total of 356 patients followed at three European centers that specialize in the treatment of short bowel syndrome.[2–4] The causes of short bowel syndrome in the pediatric population are congenital abnormalities (see Chapter 84) including gastroschisis, intestinal atresia, malrotation, and aganglionosis, and necrotizing enterocolitis, an acquired condition.[5] More than 90% of infants now survive the extensive intestinal resections required for these conditions and need to be observed as adults for their short bowel syndrome. Finally, the jejunoileal bypass operation (previously used in the treatment of morbid obesity) should be mentioned. This operation has been abandoned because of severe side effects, but there are still an unknown number of patients with this operation who may present with complications from induced short bowel syndrome.

INCIDENCE AND PREVALENCE

The incidence of short bowel syndrome is difficult to assess because of a lack of prospective studies in defined populations of patients who have undergone extensive intestinal resections. The incidence of severe short bowel syndrome requiring long-term parenteral nutrition was estimated to be 2 per 1 million per year in the United Kingdom.[6] The prevalence of patients with short bowel syndrome is also unknown. It is estimated that between 10,000 and 20,000 patients in the United States are on home parenteral nutrition for this syndrome.[7] The prevalence is undoubtedly increasing due to advances in surgical techniques, postoperative care, and increasing experience with nutritional management, including long-term parenteral nutrition (see Chapter 16).

PATHOPHYSIOLOGY

The major consequence of extensive intestinal resections is loss of absorptive surface area, which results in malabsorption of macronutrients, micronutrients, electrolytes, and water.[8, 9] The degree of malabsorption is determined by the length of the remnant intestine, the specific parts of small and large intestine resected causing loss of site-specific transport processes and endocrine cells, and adaptive processes over time in the remaining intestine. Three types of intestinal resections are typically encountered: limited ileal resection for Crohn's disease, often accompanied by cecectomy or right hemicolectomy; extensive ileal resections with or without partial colectomy with jejunocolonic anastomosis; and extensive small intestinal resection and total colectomy resulting in a high jejunostomy (Fig. 92–1). Patients in the two latter groups commonly suffer from Crohn's disease or had mesenteric infarction.

Loss of Absorptive Surface Area

Nutrient Malabsorption

The specific areas of absorption in the small intestine of nutrients, minerals, vitamins, and trace elements were summarized in Chapters 87 and 88 and are illustrated in Figure 92–2. The estimated length of the small intestine varies between 3 and 8 m.[2, 4] Removal of up to one half of the small intestine is generally well tolerated in terms of nutrient absorption, which underscores its large reserve capacity. The

Table 92–1 | **Causes of Short Bowel Syndrome in Adult Patients**

	NIGHTINGALE ET AL.[2] (*N* = 84)	NORDGAARD ET AL.[3] (*N* = 148)	MESSING ET AL.[4] (*N* = 124)
Crohn's disease	49	91	11
Ulcerative colitis	5	16	—
Mesenteric infarction	8	17	50
Radiation enteritis	8	2	28
Other*	14	22	35

*Other causes include volvulus, postsurgical complications, jejunoileal bypass, and benign tumors.

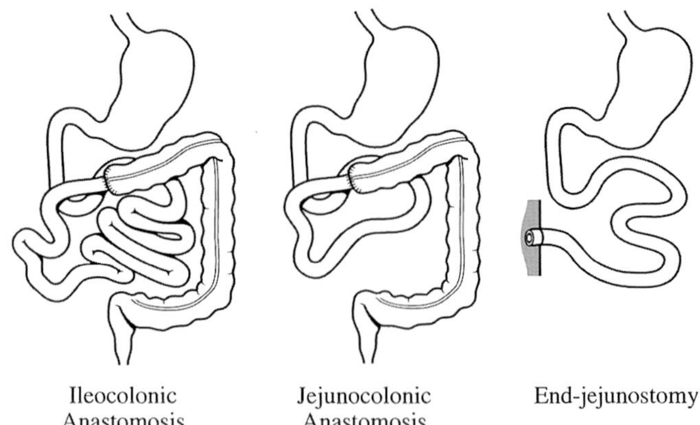

Figure 92–1. The three common types of intestinal resection—ileocolonic anastomosis, jejunocolonic anastomosis, and end-jejunostomy—observed in patients with short bowel.

enterocytes lining the small intestine appear uniform from the duodenum to the ileocecal valve, but there is a distinct proximal to distal gradient in both morphology and function.[10] The villi are taller and the crypts are deeper in the jejunum than in the ileum, and the activity of microvillus enzymes and nutrient absorptive capacity per unit length of intestine is several-fold higher in the proximal than in the distal small intestine. Thus, loss of part of jejunum will initially compromise nutrient absorption more than loss of an ileal segment of similar length because of these morphologic and functional differences. Normal digestion and absorption depend on gradual gastric emptying of partially digested nutrients, mixing with bile and pancreatic enzymes in the duodenum, and rapid digestion and absorption of the digestive products in the proximal small intestine. Patients with high jejunostomy have rapid gastric emptying of liquids and rapid intestinal transit, which may compromise the gastric digestive phase and result in inadequate mixing with biliary and pancreatic secretions with insufficient time for enzymatic digestion and cause nutrient maldigestion. In normal humans, the digestion and absorption of nutrients is more than 90% complete within the first 100 cm of jejunum.[11, 12] These observations are corroborated by the fact that patients with short bowel syndrome in general can maintain nutritional balance on oral feeding when more than 100 cm (≈3 feet) of jejunum is preserved.[13] Conversely, most patients with a jejunal length of less than 100 cm and no colon will require long-term parenteral nutrition. Preservation of partial or full colonic function at surgery is highly beneficial for nutrient absorption. Malabsorbed carbohydrates and proteins are degraded by bacterial enzymes in the colon to short-chain fatty acids and lactate, which are readily absorbed by colonic epithelium. It has been estimated that this colonic digestive process can generate up to 1000 kcal/day in energy supply.[3, 14, 15]

Water and Electrolyte Malabsorption

The gastrointestinal tract serves an important role in electrolyte and water conservation. Loss of absorptive surface area may result in significant stomal or fecal losses of electrolytes and water. The proximal small bowel receives about 9 L/day of water and electrolytes from food and secretions, of which nearly 8 L is reabsorbed in the small intestine (see Chapter 87). Patients with high jejunostomies cannot reabsorb such a large volume of water and electrolytes and develop large volume diarrhea and may experience hypovolemia, hyponatremia, and hypokalemia on unrestricted diets. For example, the diarrheal volume in six jejunostomy patients with a mean jejunal length of 50 cm ranged from 3.2 to 8.3 L/day when they were allowed free access to food and water.[16] All six patients were in a negative sodium and water balance, and four of the six were also in a negative potassium balance. These six patients required parenteral nutrition with electrolyte replacement to maintain a stable condition and restriction of their oral intake of food and water to avoid unacceptable stomal losses. Seven of nine other jejunostomy patients, included in the same study,[16] with a mean jejunal length of 120 cm were able to maintain a positive water and sodium balance under the same conditions. The absorption of water, sodium, and potassium in these 15 jejunostomy patients was significantly correlated to jejunal length. At least 100 cm of intact jejunum was required to maintain a positive water and

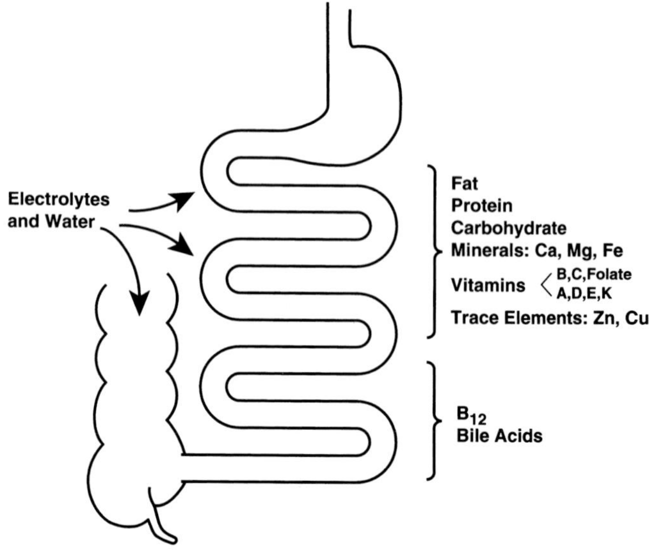

Figure 92–2. Specific areas of absorption of constituents of diet and secretions in the gastrointestinal tract. Macronutrients and micronutrients are predominantly absorbed in the proximal jejunum. Bile acids and cobalamin (vitamin B_{12}) are only absorbed in the ileum. Electrolytes and water are absorbed in both the small and the large intestine.

electrolyte balance, which is similar to the length required for nutrient absorption.

In general, high jejunostomy patients lose 90 to 100 mEq sodium and 10 to 20 mEq potassium/L of stomal effluent.[17] Some of these patients will require long-term parenteral electrolyte and water supplements, often administered overnight, whereas others can maintain a positive balance by sipping a glucose–saline solution throughout the day. The tight junctions in the jejunum are relatively leaky compared with tight junctions in the ileum and colon, and thus a high sodium chloride concentration (>100 mmol) is required in the glucose–saline solution to achieve net sodium and water absorption.[18, 19] A mixture of 120 mmol sodium chloride and 50 mmol glucose is recommended, and such a solution is not that tasteful to drink. Another approach is to give sodium chloride capsules (1 g [~17 mmol]) with meals. Both approaches take advantage of the coupled active transport of sodium with glucose and amino acids in the jejunum (see Chapter 87). Electrolyte and water absorption continues in the colon, and in normal humans only 100 to 150 mL of water is lost in the stool each day. The colon has a large reserve absorptive capacity for electrolytes and water, estimated to be 3 to 4 L of isotonic salt solution per day. Preservation of colon or part of the colon can significantly reduce fecal electrolyte and water losses in patients with short bowel syndrome. A comparison of patients with similar jejunal length ending either in a jejunostomy or anastomosed to colon showed that patients in the latter group were less likely to require oral or intravenous supplements.[2]

Loss of Site-Specific Transport Processes

Although nutrient absorption may potentially take place at any level of the small intestine, albeit at different rates due to the proximal to distal gradient in functional activity of microvillus enzymes and transporters, the absorption of some compounds is restricted to certain areas of the small intestine (see Fig. 92–2). The minerals calcium, magnesium, phosphorus, and iron and the water- and fat-soluble vitamins are predominantly absorbed in the duodenum and proximal jejunum (see Chapter 88). Most patients with short bowel syndrome have an intact duodenum and a variable length of jejunum, and the risk of developing iron, phosphorus, or vitamin deficiency even in patients with a high jejunostomy is not well documented. Calcium absorption was found to be highly variable in a large study of patients with small intestinal resections.[20] The net absorption of calcium (intake minus fecal loss) ranged from +573 to −268 mg/day with a median of +65 mg/day. However, 64% of the patients were in a negative calcium balance (balance = intake minus fecal and urinary loss). The risk of developing symptomatic hypocalcemia or hypomagnesemia is illustrated by a study of 25 patients with a mean jejunal length of 128 cm and large volume diarrhea (2 to 6 L/day) and steatorrhea.[21] Thirteen patients developed hypocalcemia and 18 developed hypomagnesemia during a therapeutic trial of enteral hyperalimentation despite supplementation with calcium, magnesium, and vitamin D. The malabsorption of calcium and magnesium is a consequence of fat malabsorption because these minerals are precipitated intraluminally by unabsorbed long-chain fatty acids. Both calcium and magnesium absorption improve on a low-fat diet in patients with small intestinal resections.[22]

The active absorption of cobalamin (vitamin B_{12}) and bile acids is restricted to the ileum. Cobalamin–intrinsic factor complexes and bile acids are taken up by specific transport proteins in ileal enterocytes (see Chapters 54 and 88). Most patients with short bowel syndrome have lost part or all of the ileum and develop cobalamin and bile acid malabsorption. The degree of malabsorption depends on the length of resected ileum. Resection of less than 100 cm of ileum causes moderate bile acid malabsorption and increased bile acid loss to the colon or in stomal effluents.[23] The increased loss of bile acids to the colon induces electrolyte and water secretion and may exacerbate diarrhea. More extensive ileal resections (>100 cm) cause severe bile acid malabsorption. This in turn may result in a reduced bile acid pool size, if bile acid loss exceeds hepatic synthesis, and insufficient micellar solubilization of lipolytic products. Thus, these patients develop fat malabsorption. The loss of unabsorbed long-chain fatty acids to the colon may further exacerbate diarrhea if the fatty acids are hydroxylated by colonic bacteria. Hydroxylated fatty acids stimulate colonic electrolyte and water secretion.[24] Cobalamin malabsorption is usually demonstrable when more than 60 cm of ileum has been resected.[9]

Loss of Site-Specific Endocrine Cells and Gastrointestinal Hormones

The synthesis of gastrointestinal hormones in the intestinal mucosa is distributed in a site-specific manner along the gastrointestinal tract (see Chapter 1). Gastrin, cholecystokinin, secretin, gastric inhibitory polypeptide, and motilin are produced by endocrine cells in the proximal gastrointestinal tract and regulate secretory processes and motility. The area of synthesis of these hormones is usually intact in patients with short bowel syndrome, and the hormonal profiles are normal. However, about 50% of patients with extensive intestinal resections temporarily develop hypergastrinemia and increased gastric acid secretion in the early postoperative phase.[25, 26] The cause of hypergastrinemia is not known but could be due to loss of inhibitory signals because hypergastrinemia resolves spontaneously. Glucagon-like peptide 1 and 2 (GLP1 and GLP2), neurotensin, and peptide YY (PYY) are produced in the ileum and proximal colon, and these intestinal segments are frequently lost in short bowel patients. GLP1 and GLP2 and PYY are released by intraluminal fat and carbohydrates and cause a delay in gastric emptying and slowing of intestinal transit (ileal brake).[27, 28] Jejunostomy patients have impaired release of these hormones in response to a meal and have rapid gastric emptying and rapid intestinal transit of liquids.[29, 30] Short bowel patients with preserved colon have increased GLP1 and GLP2 concentrations and normal gastric emptying.[31] Of note, these three hormones have also been shown to inhibit gastric acid secretion and to promote intestinal growth.

Loss of Ileocecal Valve

The primary functions of the ileocecal valve are to separate ileal and colonic contents and thus minimize bacterial colonization of the small intestine and to regulate emptying of ileal contents into the colon. The ileocecal valve is removed in most ileal resections, and these patients have decreased intestinal transit time and are at risk of bacterial overgrowth of the small intestine if the ileum is anastomosed to the colon. Bacterial overgrowth may worsen nutrient and cobalamin malabsorption (see Chapters 89 and 90). However, rapid intestinal transit in these patients may counteract the risk of bacterial colonization. Studies to document the role of bacterial overgrowth in malabsorption in short bowel syndrome patients are lacking.

Intestinal Adaptation to Resection

The adaptive changes in the remaining intestine after intestinal resection have been extensively studied in animal models and to a limited extent in humans.[32, 33] The adaptive changes are more pronounced in the ileum than in the jejunum. After jejunectomy and duodenoileal anastomosis, the ileum attains the morphologic characteristics of the jejunum with taller villi and deeper crypts.[34] With time, there is also an increase in ileal diameter and length. The result of these changes is an increase in absorptive surface area with an increase in microvillous enzyme activity and absorptive capacity per unit length.[35] In humans, the adaptive changes may take 1 to 2 years to fully develop. The adaptive changes depend on the presence of food and biliary and pancreatic secretions in the intestinal lumen.[36] Jejunectomized animals fed only by parenteral alimentation fail to develop adaptive hyperplasia of the ileum.[37] Short bowel syndrome patients are therefore encouraged to start oral feeding as early as possible in the postoperative phase to induce adaptive processes.

Adaptive hyperplasia is the result of an increase in crypt cell production rate presumably mediated by growth factors released by the presence of food and secretions in the intestinal lumen. So far, GLP2 and L-glutamine have been shown to stimulate intestinal growth in experimental animals.[38, 39] The extracellular growth factors stimulate polyamine synthesis in crypt cells, which in turn induces increased DNA synthesis and mitotic activity.[40] Inhibition of polyamine synthesis in jejunectomized animals prevents adaptive changes in the ileum.[41] Elucidation of the mediators regulating enterocyte proliferation may eventually lead to development of pharmacologic interventions that can accelerate intestinal adaptation in patients with short bowel syndrome.

Morphologic and functional adaptation has also been documented in patients with short bowel syndrome. A prospective study of seven patients with jejunoileal bypass operation (20 cm of jejunum anastomosed to 25 cm of ileum) showed an increase in jejunal (80%) and ileal length (128%) and diameter (40% and 50%, respectively) after 18 months of observation.[42] The same study also demonstrated a gradual increase in intestinal transit time, which was most pronounced for ileal transit. The impressive increase in intestinal length, diameter, and transit may be the result of maintained ileocolonic function and hence release of intestinotrophic hormones. An increase in absorptive capacity was demonstrated in a French study of 41 patients with short bowel syndrome (mean jejunal length, 119 cm) in whom the mean stool volume decreased from 2.5 to 0.9 L/day over a period of 3 months on constant oral intake.[43] The patients gained weight, and nitrogen balance increased from +3.2 g in the first month to +7.8 g in the second month.

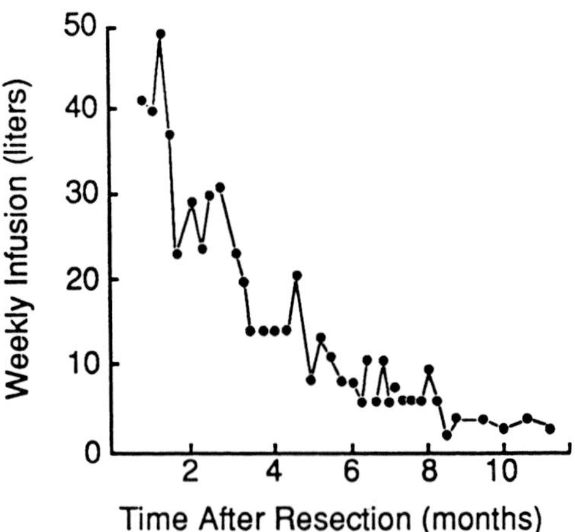

Figure 92–3. The decrease in weekly infusion requirements due to intestinal adaptation as a function of time after surgery in a 51-year-old man with a severe short bowel syndrome after anastomosis of 25 cm of jejunum to sigmoid colon after resection for bowel infarction. (From Griffin GE, Fagan EF, Hodgson HJ, et al. Enteral therapy in the management of massive gut resection complicated by chronic fluid and electrolyte depletion. Dig Dis Sci 27:902, 1982.)

An example of the capacity to increase intestinal electrolyte and water absorption with time is illustrated in a patient who was left with 25 cm of jejunum anastomosed to the descending colon (Fig. 92–3).[44] Over a period of 10 months, his weekly infusion requirements decreased from nearly 50 to only 4 L, presumably due to adaptive changes in the remaining intestine. An improvement in mineral absorption with time has also been observed in a series of 30 patients with short bowel syndrome (mean jejunal length, 81 cm) in whom fractional calcium absorption was positively correlated with time after surgery.[45] Thus, there is convincing evidence that the human small intestine undergoes morphologic and functional adaptive changes after resection and that adaptive changes are most pronounced in the ileum. Finally, patients with short bowel syndrome with colon in continuity have qualitative and quantitative changes in colonic flora that result in an increased capacity to metabolize carbohydrate and in an increased fecal bacterial mass.[46]

CLINICAL MANIFESTATIONS AND DIAGNOSIS

The clinical manifestations in patients with short bowel syndrome are primarily determined by the extent of the intestinal resection. The degree of malabsorption in the three common types of resection, illustrated in Figure 92–1, varies from mild in the first type to severe panmalabsorption in patients with high jejunostomy. The predominant clinical symptoms in all three types of short bowel syndrome are diarrhea or steatorrhea or both. These patients may develop significant weight loss, mineral and trace element deficiencies, and hypovolemia with hyponatremia and hypokalemia due to malabsorption of macronutrients, micronutrients, and water and electrolytes. The common symptoms of patients with malabsorption and the assessment of the degree and type of malabsorption are discussed in Chapter 89.

The diagnosis of short bowel syndrome is straight forward because these patients have undergone resection of a

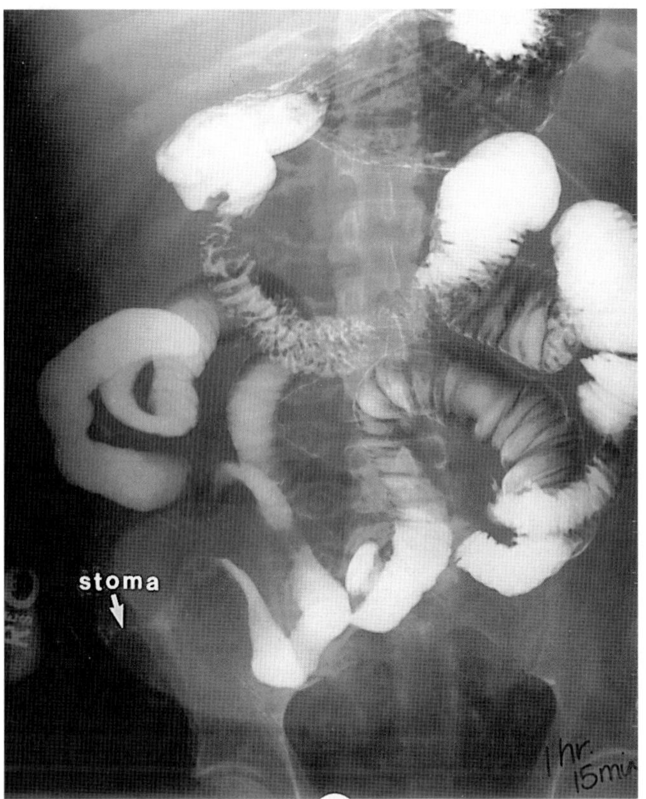

Figure 92–4. Small bowel follow-through in a 51-year-old man after small bowel resection and right hemicolectomy due to an acute superior mesenteric artery thrombosis. Note the ischemic changes of the distal loops ending in a stoma with narrowing and effacement of the circular folds. The patient subsequently underwent a second small bowel resection of these loops that left him with 3 feet of functional jejunum. (Courtesy of J.D. Eisner, M.D., Hampton, VA.)

variable length of intestine. During laparotomy, the surgeon should attempt to preserve as much viable intestine as possible and measure the length of the remaining small and large intestine, as well as the amount resected. The estimated length of short bowel from a small bowel radiograph is in good agreement with measured length at surgery.[47] A small bowel follow-through from a patient with short bowel syndrome is shown in Figure 92–4.

MANAGEMENT

In the immediate postoperative phase, most patients with extensive intestinal resections are kept fasting and are supported with total parenteral nutrition with careful monitoring of weight and volume status and measurement of stomal, fecal, and urinary losses of water, sodium, and potassium to ensure optimal electrolyte and water balance. H_2 receptor blockers are given intravenously to suppress gastric acid hypersecretion secondary to possible hypergastrinemia and also to limit volume losses. Patients with jejunostomies have large stomal effluents of up to several liters per day in this early phase, with obligatory losses of sodium, potassium, and possibly magnesium.

Oral feeding is begun in the late postoperative phase. Patients with extensive resections are kept fasting up to 10 days to allow healing of enteric anastomoses and to assess basal losses of water and electrolytes. Patients with a high jejunostomy are often started on an oral isotonic glucose–saline solution sipped throughout the day or administered 24 hours a day through a nasogastric tube to stimulate jejunal electrolyte and water absorption.[1] These patients are warned against consuming water and any drink with a low sodium content because they cause jejunal sodium and water secretion and an increase in stomal losses. Patients with less extensive resections (jejunal length >150 cm) and those with colon in continuity are fed a liquid polymeric diet (such as Ensure), either sipped or as a continuous nasogastric drip, to maximally utilize the available absorptive surface area.[43] The response to intake of this solution in terms of weight balance and magnitude of stomal or fecal volume losses allows an assessment of how a more complex diet will be tolerated. Oral nutrient intake is also a prerequisite for induction of adaptive changes. At this early stage, it is difficult to predict how an individual patient ultimately will fare because adaptation evolves at a slow rate and the change in needs of calories, minerals, vitamins, electrolytes, and water must be monitored on a regular basis. The needs and medical management beyond the postoperative phase are mainly determined by the type of intestinal resection.[48–50]

Limited Ileal Resection

Patients with limited ileal resection (<100 cm) with or without right hemicolectomy can resume intake of solid food in the late postoperative phase. The response to solid food is mainly determined by the length of removed ileum and whether the right colon was resected. These patients may develop diarrhea or steatorrhea on a regular diet. The diagnostic approach to these patients is quantitative stool collection with measurement of fecal fat, electrolytes, and osmolality. Secretory diarrhea without steatorrhea is the typical finding in limited ileal resections. Treatment with a bile acid-binding resin, such as 2 to 4 g of cholestyramine taken with meals, will often ameliorate diarrhea if bile acid malabsorption is the main cause. The diarrhea of some patients with limited ileal resection and right hemicolectomy does not respond to cholestyramine despite documented bile acid malabsorption. The diarrhea in these patients is presumably due to loss of intestinal absorptive capacity for sodium chloride.[51] The medical management of patients with documented fat malabsorption on a regular diet is best accomplished by a change to a low-fat (40 g) high-carbohydrate diet. Patients maintained on such a diet have a decrease in diarrhea and steatorrhea and improve their net absorption of calcium, magnesium, and zinc.[9] If necessary, medium-chain triglycerides, which do not require micellar solubilization, can be added as a fat calorie source. The possibility of cobalamin malabsorption should be assessed with a Schilling test with intrinsic factor. Patients with documented cobalamin malabsorption will require parenteral cobalamin, usually as 1 mg intramuscularly every 1 to 3 months for life.

Malabsorption of fat-soluble vitamins and of calcium and magnesium is a definite risk in patients with fat malabsorption. Fourteen of 27 patients with ileal resections of 50 to 150 cm with colon in place were in negative calcium balance when studied on a fixed calcium intake of 800 mg/day and supplemented with 400 to 800 IU of vitamin D per

Table 92–2 | **Mean Caloric Intake, Fecal Loss, Caloric Absorption, and Coefficient of Absorption in 10 Patients with Short Bowel Syndrome**

	INTAKE (KCAL/DAY)	FECAL LOSS (KCAL/DAY)	ABSORPTION (KCAL/DAY)	COEFFICIENT OF ABSORPTION (%)
Carbohydrate	1427	272	1155	79
Fat	962	448	514	52
Protein	714	253	461	61
Total	3103	973	2130	67
Total per kg body weight	57.9	18.2	39.7	

Modified from Messing B, Pigot F, Rongier M, et al. Intestinal absorption of free oral hyperalimentation in the very short bowel syndrome. Gastroenterology 100:1502, 1991, with permission.

day.[20] Supplementation with vitamins, calcium, and possibly magnesium should be initiated before overt signs of vitamin deficiency or hypocalcemia and hypomagnesemia develop. The tests to assess vitamin and mineral balance and recommended dosages in malabsorption are discussed in Chapter 15. The absorption of water-soluble vitamins and of carbohydrates and proteins is, in general, not compromised in patients with limited ileal resections.

Extensive Small Intestinal Resection and Partial Colectomy

Patients in this group typically have Crohn's disease and are left with a variable length of proximal small bowel anastomosed to the remaining colon. The loss of ileum results in obligatory bile acid and cobalamin malabsorption, but these patients are also at risk for more pronounced nutrient, mineral, vitamin, and electrolyte and water malabsorption than patients with limited ileal resection, due to greater loss of absorptive surface area and rapid intestinal transit. The loss of the ileocecal valve increases the risk of bacterial overgrowth of the small intestine, which may worsen nutrient absorption. Thus, these patients pose a more difficult management problem. The ultimate goal is to ensure a stable condition in which all their needs are met, preferably by oral intake alone. In a series of 38 patients with a jejunal length less than 200 cm in continuity with colon, all patients with a jejunal length of more than 100 cm could be managed on oral intake alone.[2]

Table 92–3 | **Therapeutic Agents Used to Decrease Intestinal Transit and Diarrheal Volume**

AGENT	DOSAGES
Loperamide (Imodium)*	4–6 mg
Diphenoxylate/atropine (Lomotil)*	2.5–5 mg
Codeine phosphate*	30 mg
Ranitidine (Zantac)†	300 mg bid
Omeprazole (Prilosec)‡	40 mg qd
Octreotide (Sandostatin)§	50–100 μg sc bid

*The antidiarrheals loperamide, diphenoxylate, and codeine phosphate are given 1 hour before meals and at bedtime. The dosages may be increased over the recommended dosage due to incomplete absorption in patients with short bowel syndrome.

†Cimetidine, famotidine, or nizatidine in appropriate doses are alternatives.

‡Lansoprazole, rabeprazole, and pantoprazole are alternatives.

§A long-acting once-a-month preparation (Sandostatin LAR) may also be used.

In the late postoperative phase, the liquid diet is replaced by solid food, and the absorptive capacity of the remaining intestine is assessed by measurement of fecal fat, volume, and electrolytes while on a known nutrient and liquid intake. Fat absorption is, in general, more compromised than protein and carbohydrate absorption in these patients. The optimal diet composition for patients with short bowel syndrome has been debated, but a low-fat high-carbohydrate diet is of documented advantage in patients with colon in continuity. In eight such patients, the energy absorption increased from 49% on a high-fat low-carbohydrate diet to 69% on a low-fat high-carbohydrate diet.[15] The major problem with a low-fat diet is its palatability, which makes it difficult for patients to adhere to the diet. Because these patients have significant energy malabsorption, to maintain a stable weight they must increase total nutrient intake by eating many meals per day to compensate for fecal losses. The measured intake, fecal loss, and absorption of calories from carbohydrates, fat, and protein in 10 patients with short bowel syndrome (mean small intestinal length, 75 cm; mean colonic percent, 67%) during a 3-day study are shown in Table 92–2.[52] Five patients maintained a stable weight on only oral intake but had increased caloric intake to two and one-half times their basal energy expenditures. The other five patients required parenteral nutrition. The coefficient of carbohydrate absorption (79%) was significantly higher than the coefficient of protein (61%) and fat absorption (52%), presumably because part or all of the colon was preserved in 9 of 10 patients. The range in stool output was 317 to 3,812 g/day and was not correlated with length of remaining intestine or any coefficient of absorption.

Lactose malabsorption due to substantial loss of jejunal length may worsen diarrhea, but a study of 14 short bowel patients on either a lactose-free diet or a diet with 20 g lactose/day showed no significant differences in stool volumes.[53] Rapid intestinal transit contributes to malabsorption and diarrhea, and antidiarrheal drugs are commonly used (Table 92–3). These medications should be taken 1 hour before meals, and their effect on diarrheal volume should be evaluated before they are administered on a long-term basis. The possibility of bacterial overgrowth can be evaluated with one of the breath tests discussed in Chapter 90. Patients with a positive breath test should receive a therapeutic trial with tetracycline, 250 mg three times a day, or metronidazole, 500 mg three times a day, for 2 weeks. Fat-soluble vitamin and mineral deficiencies may develop because of fat malabsorption, and these patients need supplementation with multivitamins, calcium, magnesium, and possibly zinc.[54] The development of zinc deficiency is mainly observed in patients with large diarrheal volumes. Longitudinal studies of bone density may be of value to detect early manifestations of metabolic bone disease.[20, 55] The long-term nutritional management of malabsorption in the short bowel syndrome patient is also discussed in Chapter 15.

Extensive Small Bowel Resection and Colectomy

Patients in this group are left with only the duodenum and a short segment of jejunum ending in a jejunostomy and have the most severe short bowel syndrome. The length of the remaining jejunum is of critical importance. In general, patients with jejunal length of less than 100 cm cannot maintain adequate nutrient absorption on oral feeding and will require long-term parenteral nutrition. Moreover, they often have excessive secretory responses to food and drink and therefore restrict oral intake to avoid the risk of volume depletion. Patients with a longer jejunal segment (>100 cm) can usually maintain nutritional balance but may have large stomal losses of water and electrolytes. Patients with losses up to 2 L/day can usually maintain a positive salt and water balance by sipping 1 to 2 L of glucose–saline solution during the day.[1] Patients with larger losses (3 to 4 L/day) require intravenous saline infusion, usually administered overnight. These guidelines are naturally not absolute, and the need for continued parenteral nutrition or electrolyte infusions must be assessed in the individual patient in the late postoperative phase and during regular follow-up visits. Patients who lose weight rapidly or have large stomal losses when switched to oral feeding need continued parenteral alimentation. In a study of energy absorption in patients with short bowel syndrome, it was found that patients who needed parenteral nutrition absorbed less than 35% of ingested calories, whereas jejunostomy patients without a need for parenteral nutrition absorbed on average 67% of caloric intake.[13]

The experience with long-term parenteral nutrition has mainly been gained in patients with severe short bowel syndrome (see Chapter 16). Despite the limited adaptive capacity of the jejunum, about 50% of patients on home parenteral nutrition are able to switch to oral intake after 1 to 2 years.[6] The diet composition in jejunostomy patients on oral intake can be more liberal because the percent of energy absorption is similar on a low-fat high-carbohydrate and a high-fat low-carbohydrate diet.[56, 57] However, one study in five jejunostomy patients documented net calcium, magnesium, zinc, and copper losses on a high-fat diet that were reversed to net absorption on a low-fat diet.[58] The average daily stomal losses of electrolytes, minerals, and trace elements in severe short bowel syndrome are listed in Table 92–4.[22, 56, 58–61] Patients whose stomal losses exceed liquid intake secondary to excessive secretion (gastric, biliary, pancreatic) benefit from reduction of gastric secretion by the use of either H_2 receptor blockers, proton pump inhibitors, or the somatostatin analog octreotide (see Table 92–3). Most studies have shown a reduction in stoma output by up to 50% by the use of these inhibitors, but a positive water and electrolyte balance is rarely achieved.[62–64] Octreotide and omeprazole were found to have equivalent effects when compared in the same patient. A new dietary approach to improve fat absorption in jejunostomy patients is oral administration of bile acids with meals. Both ox bile and the synthetic bile acid, cholylsarcosine, in a dose of 2 g per meal increased fat absorption by 20 to 40 g/day without an increase in stomal volume.[65, 66] The mineral, vitamin, and trace element requirements are administered intravenously in patients on parenteral nutrition and orally in malabsorption dosages in patients on oral intake (see Chapters 15 and 16). Patients with high jejunostomies should be observed at regular intervals to monitor nutritional balance and adjust the treatment according to identified needs.

Table 92–4 | **Average Daily Stomal or Fecal Losses of Electrolytes, Minerals, and Trace Elements in Severe Short Bowel Syndrome**

Sodium*	90–100 mEq/L
Potassium*	10–20 mEq/L
Calcium	772 (591–950) mg/day
Magnesium	328 (263–419) mg/day
Iron	11 (7–15) mg/day
Zinc	12 (10–14) mg/day
Copper	1.5 (0.5–2.3) mg/day

*Average concentration of sodium and potassium per liter of stomal effluent. The values for minerals and trace elements are mean 24-hour losses in milligrams (n = 37), with range in parentheses. See text for details.

COMPLICATIONS

Cholesterol Gallstones

Interruption of the enterohepatic circulation of bile acids by ileal resection results in a decrease of hepatic bile acid secretion and an altered composition of hepatic bile in terms of the organic components: bile acid, cholesterol, and phospholipids (see Chapter 54). Hepatic bile becomes supersaturated with respect to cholesterol with subsequent formation of cholesterol crystals and gallstones in gallbladder bile (see Chapter 55). A very high prevalence of 44% of asymptomatic gallstones was documented in a study of 84 patients with severe short bowel syndrome.[2] Formation of biliary sludge and gallbladder hypomotility probably contributed to the high prevalence because many of these patients were on long-term parenteral nutrition.[67]

Oxalate Kidney Stones

Fat malabsorption secondary to bile acid deficiency in patients with extensive ileal resections is associated with an increased risk of formation of oxalate kidney stones when the colon is preserved. Oxalate in food is usually precipitated out as calcium oxalate in the intestinal lumen and lost in the stool. Lipolysis in short bowel syndrome patients with fat malabsorption is normal, and unabsorbed long-chain fatty acids compete with oxalate for available calcium. Consequently, a larger amount of free oxalate is lost to the colon, where it is absorbed and ultimately excreted in the kidney. These patients may develop hyperoxaluria and calcium oxalate kidney stones. Patients without colon in continuity are not at increased risk. Nine of 38 patients (24%) with short bowel syndrome and preserved colon developed symptomatic kidney stones within 2 years.[2] These patients should be monitored with regular assessment of urinary oxalate excretion. Treatment of hyperoxaluria consists of restriction of oxalate-containing food products (tea, chocolate, cola beverages, certain fruits, and vegetables). If hyperoxaluria persists, then oral administration of calcium citrate should be tried. Citracal Liquitabs, which contain 500 mg elemental calcium per tablet, may be given as one tablet twice a day. The extra calcium precipitates dietary oxalate, and citrate prevents stone growth in the urine.

D-Lactic Acidosis

D-Lactic acidosis is a rare complication of short bowel syndrome and is only observed in patients with preserved colon. The episodes of acidosis are usually precipitated by increased oral intake of refined carbohydrates and can be induced in the short bowel syndrome patient by carbohydrate overfeeding.[68] Malabsorbed carbohydrate is metabolized by colonic bacteria to short-chain fatty acids and lactate, which lower the colonic pH. A lower pH inhibits the growth of the predominant *Bacteroides* species and promotes the growth of acid-resistant gram-positive anaerobes (*Bifidobacterium, Lactobacillus*, and *Eubacterium*), which have the capacity to produce D-lactate. D-Lactate is absorbed from the colon and is only metabolized to a limited extent by humans due to lack of D-lactate dehydrogenase. The main excretory route is by the kidney.[69] Absorbed D-lactate results in the development of a metabolic acidosis and characteristic neurologic symptoms with nystagmus, ophthalmoplegia, ataxia, confusion, and inappropriate behavior. These patients are often suspected of being inebriated, but their blood alcohol levels are normal. Blood tests will confirm a metabolic acidosis and a normal D-lactate. The constellation of specific neurologic symptoms and metabolic acidosis in a patient with short bowel syndrome should raise the suspicion of possible D-lactic acidosis. The diagnosis is confirmed by measurement of D-lactate in the blood, which will be significantly elevated (>3 mmol/L; normal, <0.5 mmol/L).

Treatment consists primarily of correcting the acidosis with sodium bicarbonate and stopping oral intake, which usually results in rapid improvement of the neurologic symptoms. The potential benefit of antibiotic treatment to change the colonic flora is still debated. Replacement of refined carbohydrates with starch in the diet has prevented recurrent D-lactic acidosis in a few patients.[70] The mediator of the neurologic symptoms is still unknown. Infusion of D-lactic acid in normal subjects to blood levels commonly observed in D-lactic acidosis does not cause any neurologic symptoms.[67] Some patients with short bowel syndrome may have a latent deficiency of a cofactor required for D-lactate production. The neurologic symptoms have a striking resemblance to Wernicke's encephalopathy, and it is of some interest that recurrent D-lactic acidosis was prevented by thiamine supplementation in one short bowel syndrome patient.[71]

Reoperations

About 50% of short bowel syndrome patients will require reoperation because of complications from the initial operation (strictures or adhesions) or for recurrent Crohn's disease.[72] A number of surgical procedures, such as tapering enteroplasty, reversal of a short intestinal segment, or colonic interposition, have been attempted to increase intestinal transit time. Generation of recirculating loops to increase contact time and tapering and lengthening of an intestinal segment to increase surface area are newer surgical interventions. These procedures have only been used in a small number of patients, mainly in the pediatric population, and with limited success and thus should still be considered experimental.

INTESTINAL TRANSPLANTATION

Intestinal transplantation is performed by an increasing number of centers worldwide. The main indication for transplantation in children and adults is total parenteral nutrition–dependent short bowel syndrome complicated by progressive liver disease. The most recent report from the Intestinal Transplant Registry has data on 474 transplants in 446 patients from 46 centers.[73] The surgical procedures used were isolated small bowel transplant (46%), combined intestinal and liver transplant (40%), and multivisceral transplant (14%). The 1-year graft survival was 50% to 60% for all three procedures. The major causes of death and graft failure in intestinal transplantation are rejection, sepsis, multiorgan failure, and lymphoproliferative disease. Thus, intestinal transplantation has reached a stage where it is a feasible, but still not a practical, alternative to conservative treatment of the patient with severe short bowel syndrome.

NEW TREATMENTS (GROWTH FACTORS)

The growing knowledge of growth factors has stimulated several clinical studies in short bowel patients. The promising results of the use of growth hormone and dietary L-glutamine in a large uncontrolled study of total parenteral nutrition–dependent short bowel patients raised hopes that intestinal mucosal growth can be enhanced beyond the adaptive period.[7] However, two placebo-controlled studies of identical growth hormone and L-glutamine supplementation failed to show any absorptive benefit of this regimen.[74, 75]

GLP2 is intestinotrophic and has been used in a small uncontrolled study of eight short bowel patients who received GLP2 400 μg subcutaneously twice a day for 35 days.[76] The treatment resulted in an increase of several absorptive parameters, body weight, and mucosal growth. The rapid advance in knowledge of epithelial growth factors will undoubtedly lead to discovery of still other growth factors that can stimulate intestinal epithelial growth and thus benefit these patients.

PROGNOSIS

The prognosis of patients with short bowel syndrome is primarily determined by the type and extent of intestinal resection and by the underlying disease. Patients with limited small intestinal resections in general have an excellent prognosis with careful management of their specific malabsorptive defects. Patients with high jejunostomies and severe malabsorption present difficult management problems and are a challenge for surgeons, gastroenterologists, and dietitians in their long-term care. The rate of survival, prognosis, and quality of life are, however, steadily improving even in this group of patients because of increasing experience with long-term parenteral nutrition and better methods to assess nutritional needs.

The probability of survival and total parenteral nutrition dependence has been assessed in a prospective study of 124 short bowel patients.[4] A majority of these patients had intestinal resection for either mesenteric infarction or radiation enteritis. The probability of survival and total parenteral nutrition dependence was 86% and 49% at 2 years and 75% and 45% at 5 years, respectively. In a multivariate analysis, survival was negatively related to high jejunostomy, to small bowel length of less than 50 cm, and to mesenteric infarction as a cause for intestinal resection. Total parenteral nutrition dependence was primarily related to small bowel length. A remnant bowel length of less than 100 cm was highly predictive of permanent intestinal failure and life-long total parenteral nutrition dependence. Fortunately, most patients with short bowel syndrome have a good quality of life and can work full time.[2]

REFERENCES

1. Lennard-Jones JE. Review article: Practical management of the short bowel. Aliment Pharmacol Ther 8:563, 1994.
2. Nightingale JMD, Lennard-Jones JE, Gertner DJ, et al. Colonic preservation reduces need for parenteral therapy, increases incidence of renal stones, but does not change high prevalence of gall stones in patients with a short bowel. Gut 33:1493, 1992.
3. Nordgaard I, Hansen BS, Mortensen PB. Importance of colonic support for energy absorption as small-bowel failure proceeds. Am J Clin Nutr 64:222, 1996.
4. Messing B, Crenn P, Beau P, et al. Long-term survival and parenteral nutrition dependence in adult patients with the short bowel syndrome. Gastroenterology 117:1043, 1999.
5. Grosfeld JL, Rescorla FJ, West KW. Short bowel syndrome in infancy and childhood. Am J Surg 151:41, 1986.
6. Lennard-Jones JE. Indications and need for long-term parenteral nutrition: implications for intestinal transplantation. Transplant Proc 22: 2427, 1990.
7. Byrne TA, Persinger RL, Young LS, et al. A new treatment for patients with short-bowel syndrome-growth hormone, glutamine, and a modified diet. Ann Surg 222:243, 1995.
8. Jeejeebhoy KN. Nutrition: the changing scene. Lancet 1:1427, 1983.
9. Andersson H, Bosaeus I, Brummer R-J, et al. Nutritional and metabolic consequences of extensive bowel resection. Dig Dis 4:193, 1986.
10. Clarke RM. Mucosal architecture and epithelial cell production rate in the small intestine of the albino rat. J Anat 107:519, 1970.
11. Johansson C. Studies of gastrointestinal interactions. Scand J Gastroenterol 10:33, 1975.
12. Ruppin H, Bar-Meir S, Soergel KH, et al. Effects of liquid formula diets on proximal gastrointestinal function. Dig Dis Sci 26:202, 1981.
13. Rodrigues CA, Lennard-Jones JE, Thompson DG, et al. Energy absorption as a measure of intestinal failure in the short bowel syndrome. Gut 30:176, 1989.
14. Royall D, Wolever TMS, Jeejeebhoy KN. Evidence for colonic conservation of malabsorbed carbohydrate in short bowel syndrome. Am J Gastroenterol 87:751, 1992.
15. Nordgaard I, Hansen BS, Mortensen PB. Colon as a digestive organ in patients with short bowel. Lancet 343:373, 1994.
16. Nightingale JMD, Lennard-Jones JE, Walker ER, et al. Jejunal efflux in short bowel syndrome. Lancet 336:765, 1990.
17. Ladefoged K, Olgaard K. Fluid and electrolyte absorption and renin-angiotensin-aldosterone axis in patients with severe short-bowel syndrome. Scand J Gastroenterol 14:729, 1979.
18. Spiller RC, Jones BJM, Silk DBA. Jejunal water and electrolyte absorption from two proprietary enteral feeds in man: importance of sodium content. Gut 28:681, 1987.
19. Lennard-Jones JE. Oral rehydration solutions in short bowel syndrome. Clin Ther 12:129, 1990.
20. Hylander E, Ladefoged K, Madsen S. Calcium balance and bone mineral content following small-intestinal resection. Scand J Gastroenterol 16:167, 1981.
21. Cosnes J, Gendre J-P, Evard D, et al. Compensatory enteral hyperalimentation for management of patients with severe short bowel syndrome. Am J Clin Nutr 41:1002, 1985.
22. Hessov I, Andersson H, Isaksson B. Effects of a low-fat diet on mineral absorption in small-bowel disease. Scand J Gastroenterol 18:551, 1983.
23. Andersson H. Effects of a fat-reduced diet on the faecal excretion of radioactivity following administration of ^{14}C-cholic acid and on the duodenal concentration of bile salts in patients with ileal disease. Nutr Metab 20:254, 1976.
24. Bright-Asare P, Binder H. Stimulation of colonic secretion of water and electrolytes by hydroxy fatty acids. Gastroenterology 64:81, 1973.
25. Williams NS, Evans P, King RFGJ. Gastric acid secretion and gastrin production in the short bowel syndrome. Gut 26:914, 1985.
26. Hyman PE, Everett SL, Harada T. Gastric acid hypersecretion in short bowel syndrome in infants: association with extent of resection and enteral feeding. J Pediatr Gastroenterol Nutr 5:191, 1986.
27. Spiller RC, Trotman IF, Higgins BE. The ileal brake-inhibition of jejunal motility after ileal perfusion in man. Gastroenterology 25:365, 1984.
28. Holgate AM, Read NW. Effect of ileal infusion of intralipid on gastrointestinal transit, ileal flow rate and carbohydrate absorption in humans after ingestion of a liquid meal. Gastroenterology 88:1005, 1985.
29. Nightingale JMD, Kamm MA, van der Sijp JRM, et al. Disturbed gastric emptying in the short bowel syndrome: evidence for a "colonic brake." Gut 34:1171, 1993.
30. Jeppesen PB, Hartmann B, Hansen BS, et al. Impaired meal stimulated glucagon-like peptide 2 response in ileal resected short bowel patients with intestinal failure. Gut 45:559, 1999.
31. Jeppesen PB, Hartmann B, Thulesen J, et al. Elevated plasma glucagon-like peptide 1 and 2 concentrations in ileum resected short bowel patients with a preserved colon. Gut 47:370, 2000.
32. Williamson RCN, Chir M. Intestinal adaptation. I. Structural, functional and cytokinetic changes. N Engl J Med 298:1393, 1978.
33. Williamson RCN, Chir M. Intestinal adaptation. II. Mechanisms of control. N Engl J Med 298:1444, 1978.
34. Appleton GVN, Bristol JB, Williamson RCN. Proximal enterectomy provides a stronger systemic stimulus to intestinal adaptation than distal enterectomy. Gut 28:165, 1987.
35. Chaves M, Smith MW, Williamson RCN. Increased activity of digestive enzymes in ileal enterocytes adapting to proximal small bowel resection. Gut 28:981, 1987.
36. Dowling RH. Small bowel adaptation and its regulation. Scand J Gastroenterol 17:53, 1982.
37. Johnson LR, Copeland EM, Diedrich SJ. Structural and hormonal alterations in the gastrointestinal tract of parenterally fed rats. Gastroenterology 68:1177, 1975.
38. Drucker DJ, Ehrlich P, Asa SL, et al. Induction of intestinal epithelial proliferation by glucagon-like peptide 2. Proc Natl Acad Sci USA 93: 7911, 1996.
39. Rhoads JM, Argenzio RA, Chen W, et al. L-Glutamine stimulates intestinal cell proliferation and activates mitogen-activated protein kinases. Am J Physiol 272:G943, 1997.
40. Luk G, Baylin SB. Polyamines and intestinal growth-increased polyamine biosynthesis after jejunectomy. Am J Physiol 245:G656, 1983.
41. Luk G, Baylin SB. Inhibition of intestinal epithelial DNA synthesis and adaptive hyperplasia after jejunectomy in the rat by suppression of polyamine biosynthesis. J Clin Invest 74:698, 1984.
42. Solhaug JH, Tvete S. Adaptive changes in the small intestine following bypass operation for obesity. Scand J Gastroenterol 13:401, 1978.
43. Levy E, Frileux P, Sandrucci S, et al. Continuous enteral nutrition during the early adaptive stage of the short bowel syndrome. Br J Surg 75:549, 1988.
44. Griffin GE, Fagan EF, Hodgson HJ, et al. Enteral therapy in the management of massive gut resection complicated by chronic fluid and electrolyte depletion. Dig Dis Sci 27:902, 1982.
45. Gouttebel MC, Saint Aubert B, Colette C, et al. Intestinal adaptation in patients with short bowel syndrome. Dig Dis Sci 34:709, 1989.
46. Briet F, Flourie B, Achour L, et al. Bacterial adaptation in patients with short bowel and colon in continuity. Gastroenterology 109:1446, 1995.

47. Nightingale J, Bartram C, Lennard-Jones J. Length of residual small bowel after partial resection: correlation between radiographic and surgical measurements. Gastrointest Radiol 16:305, 1991.
48. Ladefoged K, Hessov I, Jarnum S. Nutrition in short-bowel syndrome. Scand J Gastroenterol 31(Suppl 216):122, 1996.
49. Buchman AL. The clinical management of short bowel syndrome: steps to avoid parenteral nutrition. Nutrition 13:907, 1997.
50. Nightingale JMD. Management of patients with a short bowel. Nutrition 15:633, 1999.
51. Arrambide KA, Santa Ana CA, Schiller LR, et al. Loss of absorptive capacity for sodium chloride as a cause of diarrhea following partial ileal and right colon resection. Dig Dis Sci 34:193, 1989.
52. Messing B, Pigot F, Rongier M, et al. Intestinal absorption of free oral hyperalimentation in the very short bowel syndrome. Gastroenterology 100:1502, 1991.
53. Marteau P, Messing B, Arrigoni E, et al. Do patients with short-bowel syndrome need a lactose-free diet? Nutrition 13:13, 1997.
54. Selby PL, Peacock M, Bambach CP. Hypomagnesaemia after small bowel resection: treatment with 1 alpha-hydroxylated vitamin D metabolites. Br J Surg 71:334, 1984.
55. Hessov I, Mosekilde L, Melsen F, et al. Osteopenia with normal vitamin D metabolites after small-bowel resection for Crohn's disease. Scand J Gastroenterol 19:691, 1984.
56. McIntyre PB, Fitchew M, Lennard-Jones JE. Patients with a high jejunostomy do not need a special diet. Gastroenterology 91:25, 1986.
57. Woolf GM, Miller C, Kurian R, et al. Nutritional absorption in short bowel syndrome. Dig Dis Sci 32:8, 1987.
58. Ovesen L, Chu R, Howard L. The influence of dietary fat on jejunostomy output in patients with severe short bowel syndrome. Am J Clin Nutr 38:270, 1983.
59. Ladefoged K, Nicolaidou P, Jarnum S. Calcium, phosphorus, magnesium, zinc, and nitrogen balance in patients with severe short bowel syndrome. Am J Clin Nutr 33:2137, 1980.
60. Ladefoged K. Intestinal and renal loss of infused minerals in patients with severe short bowel syndrome. Am J Clin Nutr 36:59, 1982.
61. Engels LGJ, van den Hamer CJA, van Tongeren JHM. Iron, zinc, and copper balance in short bowel patients on oral nutrition. Am J Clin Nutr 40:1038, 1984.
62. Nightingale JMD, Waler ER, Farthing MJG, et al. Effect of omeprazole on intestinal output in the short bowel syndrome. Aliment Pharmacol Ther 5:405, 1991.
63. Farthing MJG. Octreotide in dumping and short bowel syndromes. Digestion 54:47, 1993.
64. O'Keefe SJD, Peterson ME, Fleming CR. Octreotide as an adjunct to home parenteral nutrition in the management of permanent end-jejunostomy syndrome. J Parenter Enter Nutr 18:26, 1994.
65. Gruy-Kapral C, Little KH, Fordtran JS, et al. Conjugated bile acid replacement therapy for short-bowel syndrome. Gastroenterology 116: 15, 1999.
66. Heydorn S, Jeppesen PB, Mortensen PB. Bile acid replacement therapy with cholylsarcosine for short-bowel syndrome. Scand J Gastroenterol 34:818, 1999.
67. Roslyn JJ, Pitt HA, Mann LL, et al. Gallbladder disease in patients on long-term parenteral nutrition. Gastroenterology 84:148, 1983.
68. Dahlquist NR, Perrault J, Callaway CW, et al. D-Lactic acidosis and encephalopathy after jejunoileostomy: response to overfeeding and to fasting in humans. Mayo Clin Proc 59:141, 1984.
69. Oh MS, Uribarri J, Alveranga D, et al. Metabolic utilization and renal handling of D-lactate in men. Metabolism 34:621, 1985.
70. Mayne AJ, Handy DJ, Preece MA, et al. Dietary management of D-lactic acidosis in short bowel syndrome. Arch Dis Child 65:229, 1990.
71. Hudson M, Pocknee R, Mowat AG. D-Lactic acidosis in short bowel syndrome—an examination of possible mechanisms. Q J Med 74:157, 1990.
72. Thompson JS, Langnas AN. Surgical approaches to improving intestinal function in the short-bowel syndrome. Arch Surg 134:706, 1999.
73. Kumar N, Grant D. Gastrointestinal transplantation: an update. Liver Transplant 6:515, 2000.
74. Scolapio JS, Camilleri M, Fleming CR, et al. Effect of growth hormone, glutamine, and diet on adaptation in short bowel syndrome: a randomized, controlled study. Gastroenterology 113:1074, 1997.
75. Szkudlarek J, Jeppesen PB, Mortensen PB. Effect of high dose growth hormone with glutamine and no change in diet on intestinal absorption in short bowel patients: a randomised, double blind, crossover, placebo controlled study. Gut 47:199, 2000.
76. Jeppesen PB, Hartmann B, Thulesen J, et al. Treatment of short bowel patients with glucagon-like peptide 2 (GLP-2), a newly discovered intestinotrophic, anti-secretory, and transit modulating peptide. Gastroenterology 118:A178, 2000.

Chapter 93

Celiac Sprue and Refractory Sprue

Richard J. Farrell, MD, and Ciarán P. Kelly, MD

DEFINITIONS

Celiac sprue is characterized by small intestinal malabsorption of nutrients after the ingestion of wheat gluten or related proteins from rye and barley; a characteristic, though not specific, villous atrophy of the small intestinal mucosa; prompt clinical and histologic improvement after adherence to a strict gluten-free diet; and clinical relapse when gluten is reintroduced.[1] The many other names used to identify patients with this condition (nontropical sprue, celiac syndrome, adult celiac disease, idiopathic steatorrhea, primary malabsorption, and others) is testimony to the confusion of the past. The term celiac sprue is widely recognized and is used in this chapter; the terms *celiac disease* or *gluten-sensitive enteropathy* are acceptable alternatives. Although the spectrum of celiac sprue includes *classic* or *typical* celiac sprue (fully expressed gluten-sensitive enteropathy found in association with the classic features of malabsorption), most patients have either *atypical* celiac sprue (fully expressed gluten-sensitive enteropathy found in association with atypical manifestations, including short stature, anemia, and infertility) or *silent* celiac sprue (fully expressed gluten-sensitive enteropathy found after serologic screening in asymptomatic patients) (Fig. 93–1).

A combination of serologic, genetic, and histologic data has also led to the identification of two other classes of celiac sprue. The term *latent celiac sprue* refers to patients who have normal villous architecture on a gluten-containing diet but in whom small bowel villous atrophy compatible with celiac sprue later develops. Two variants of latent celiac sprue have been identified. In the first, celiac sprue was present previously, often in childhood; the patient recovered completely with a gluten-free diet, but the disease remains "latent" even when a normal diet is adopted. In the second, a normal mucosa was diagnosed at an earlier occasion while the patient was ingesting a normal diet, but celiac sprue developed later. *Potential celiac sprue* refers to patients who have never had a small bowel biopsy consistent with celiac sprue but show immunologic abnormalities characteristic for the disease, for example, a positive immunoglobulin (Ig)A antibody to endomysium or increased intraepithelial lymphocytes (IELs) in the small intestine. These patients often have a genetic predisposition to celiac sprue, especially human leukocyte antibody (HLA)-DQ2, or an affected first-degree relative, or both, and their probability of developing celiac sprue may be as high as 50%.[2] *Refractory sprue*, also known as unclassified or intractable celiac sprue, is defined as symptomatic severe small-intestinal villous atrophy mimicking celiac sprue but not responding primarily or secondarily to at least 6 months of a strict gluten-free diet. Refractory sprue is a diagnosis of exclusion that cannot be explained by inadvertent gluten ingestion, other causes of villous atrophy, or overt intestinal lymphoma.[1, 3] The precise link between celiac sprue, refractory sprue, and enteropathy-associated T-cell lymphoma continues to evolve (see also Chapters 26 and 106).

HISTORY

Celiac sprue was first recognized as a clinical entity by Aretaeus the Cappadocian in the first century A.D.[4] The name "sprue" was coined in the 18th century and is derived from the Dutch word "spruw," which means aphthous disease, so named because of the high prevalence of aphthous mouth ulcers in these patients. In 1888, Samuel Gee described many of the clinical features of celiac sprue in patients of all age groups and stated, "If the patient can be cured at all it must be by means of the diet."[5] However, it was not until the middle of this century that the link between certain cereals and celiac sprue was made by Dicke, a Dutch pediatrician. He became convinced that the consump-

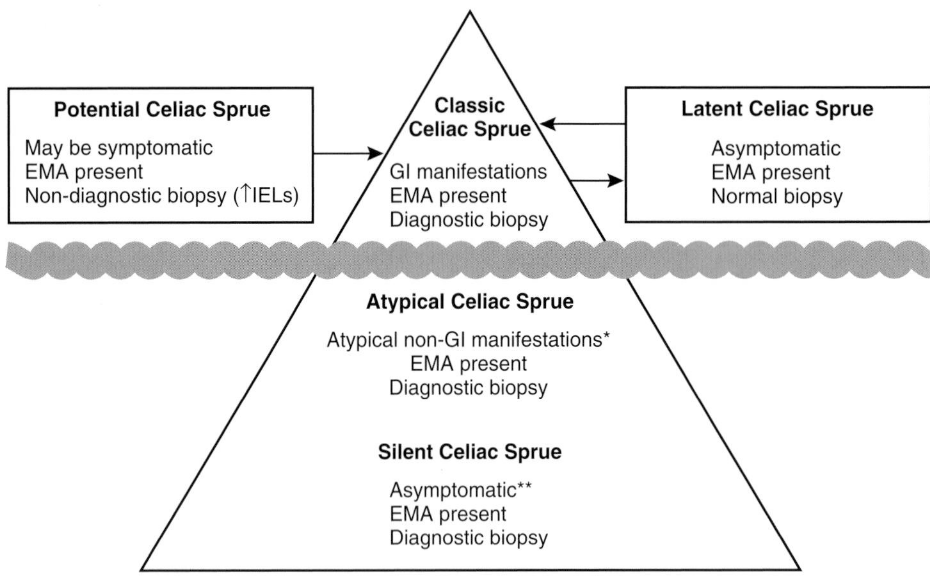

Figure 93–1. The celiac iceberg and the spectrum of celiac sprue. *Insulin-dependent diabetes mellitus, infertility, seizures, ataxia, bone pain. **May be identified through a positive family history, hematologic, or biochemical abnormalities. GI, gastrointestinal; EMA, endomysial antibodies; IELs, intraepithelial lymphocytes. (From Farrell RJ, Kelly CP: Diagnosis of celiac sprue. Am J Gastroenterol 96:3237–3246, 2001.)

tion of bread and wheat flour was directly responsible for the deterioration in patients with this condition.[6] During World War II in the Netherlands, cereals used to make bread were particularly scarce. During this time, children with celiac sprue improved, only to relapse after the replenishment of the cereal supply at the end of the war. It was this serendipitous observation that led to the finding that wheat exacerbates celiac sprue. Subsequent work by Dicke and coworkers[7] showed that it was the water-insoluble portion, or gluten moiety, of wheat that produced malabsorption in patients with celiac sprue. In 1954, Paulley[8] provided the first accurate description of the characteristic intestinal lesion in patients with celiac sprue. With the development of effective peroral suction biopsy instruments in the late 1950s, Rubin et al.[9] demonstrated that celiac sprue in children and idiopathic or nontropical sprue in adults were identical diseases with the same clinical and pathologic features.

The past 15 years has seen substantial advances in our understanding of the genetic, immune, and molecular mechanisms fundamental to the pathogenesis of celiac sprue. In 1986, Howell et al.[10] observed that celiac sprue was associated with specific HLA class II DQ haplotypes. In 1993, Lundin and colleagues[11] demonstrated that the DQ gene products preferentially present gluten-derived gliadin peptides to intestinal mucosal T cells in celiac patients. More recently, the search for the "celiac autoantigen" has focused on the enzyme tissue transglutaminase (tTG) and has led to more accurate serologic diagnostic tests.[12] In 1998, Molberg et al.[13] reported that host tTG modification of gliadin enhances gliadin-specific celiac sprue T-cell responses. The recent identification of a single tTG-modified peptide as the dominant alpha-gliadin T-cell epitope[14] has highlighted the pivotal role played by tTG in the pathogenesis of celiac sprue and may pave the way for antigen-specific immunotherapy in the future.

EPIDEMIOLOGY

Many patients with celiac sprue have minimal or no symptoms and consequently remain undiagnosed. Therefore, the true prevalence of the disease is not known. Most studies probably underestimate the prevalence of the disease, a phenomenon known as the "celiac iceberg." Celiac sprue shows a marked geographic variation with the highest incidence in Western Europe. The prevalence in most of Europe is estimated to be about 1 : 1000[15] but higher in Western Europe. The condition is significantly more common in Celtic populations, including those in the west of Ireland and Northern Ireland, where the prevalence has been reported to be 1 : 300[16] and 1 : 122[17], respectively. The prevalence is similarly high in Italy,[18] Sweden,[19] and the southeastern region of Austria.[20] The prevalence in Denmark is 40-fold lower than that in Sweden,[21] suggesting considerable variation in prevalence among geographically proximate populations. Factors such as the predominant HLA haplotype, timing of introduction of gluten into the diet, differences in the gliadin concentration of infant formulas, and interobserver variation in interpreting small intestinal biopsy findings may explain the differences in prevalence.[21]

Celiac sprue also is found in countries to which Europeans have emigrated, notably North America and Australia. However, celiac sprue remains a rare diagnosis in North America, with an estimated prevalence of 1 : 3000.[22] Whether celiac sprue is truly rare among North Americans compared with genetically similar populations in Western Europe or simply underdiagnosed remains to be established. Possible differences in the antigenicity or tTG substrate specificity of Irish and American wheat gliadins has recently been discounted.[23] In a recent study of 2000 healthy blood donors in Baltimore, MD who were screened for anti-gliadin (AGA) and IgA endomysial antibodies (EMA), the estimated prevalence of celiac sprue was approximately 1 : 300,[24] suggesting that a large number of Americans with celiac sprue are undiagnosed.

Although celiac sprue is rare in the predominantly rice-eating area of southern India, it is prevalent in the Bengal and Punjab provinces of northwest India, where wheat rather than rice has formed part of the staple diet for many generations. The condition has been reported in blacks, Arabs, Hispanics, Israeli Jews, Sudanese of mixed Arab-black descent, and Cantonese.[25] However, the condition rarely if ever affects people of purely Afro-Caribbean, Chinese, or Japanese descent. Celiac sprue affects women more commonly than men. Some authors have suggested a female-to-male ratio of 2 : 1, whereas others have reported ratios as low as 1.3 : 1.

PATHOLOGY

Celiac sprue affects the mucosa of the small intestine; the submucosa, muscularis, and serosa are usually not involved. The mucosal lesion may vary considerably in both severity and extent.[9] This spectrum of pathologic involvement helps explain the striking variability of the clinical manifestations of the disease. Examination of the mucosal surface of biopsy specimens from untreated patients with severe celiac sprue with a hand lens or a dissecting microscope reveals a flat mucosal surface with complete absence of normal intestinal villi. Histologic examination of tissue sections confirms the loss of normal villous structure (Fig. 93–2*A*). The intestinal crypts are markedly elongated and open onto a flat absorptive surface. The total thickness of the mucosa is only slightly reduced in most cases, because crypt hyperplasia compensates for the absence or shortening of the villi. These architectural changes decrease the amount of epithelial surface available for digestion and absorption.[9] The remaining absorptive cells, which appear columnar in normal biopsy specimens, are cuboidal or at times squamoid in celiac sprue biopsy specimens. Their cytoplasm is more basophilic (RNA-rich), the basal polarity of the nuclei is lost, and the brush border is markedly attenuated. When viewed with the electron microscope, the microvilli of the absorptive cells appear shortened and often fused. The number of free ribosomes is increased, reflecting impaired differentiation and resulting in increased cytoplasmic basophilia on histologic examination. Degenerative changes include cytoplasmic and mitochondrial vacuolization and the presence of many large lysosomes. Structural abnormalities of tight junctions between damaged absorptive cells[26] provide a morphologic explanation for the observed increase in permeability of the mucosal barrier.[26] The endoplasmic reticulum is sparse, reflecting the low level of synthesis of digestive enzymes, including disaccharidases and peptidases. Thus, mature absorptive cells are reduced in number and functionally compromised.

Unlike the absorptive cells, the undifferentiated crypt cells are increased markedly in number in patients with severe untreated celiac sprue, and the crypts are therefore lengthened. Moreover, the number of mitoses in the crypts is strikingly increased. The cytologic features and histochemistry of the crypt cells are normal by both light and electron microscopy. Studies of epithelial cell kinetics in untreated celiac sprue suggest that "villous atrophy" is a misnomer, because there is evidence of an increase in "enteropoiesis" in the crypts. Wright and colleagues[27] estimated that intestinal mucosa from patients with celiac sprue produces six times as many cells per hour per crypt as the normal small intestine, and the cell cycle time is halved, reflecting premature shedding. The experimental evidence suggests, therefore, that the central mechanism of villous shortening in celiac sprue is a gliadin-associated toxic effect on maturing enterocytes that results in their premature loss into the intestinal lumen and a compensatory increase in enterocyte replication in the crypts.

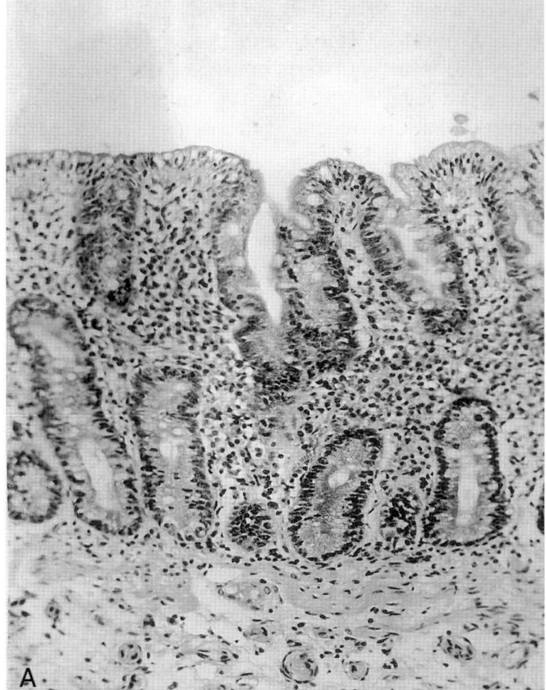

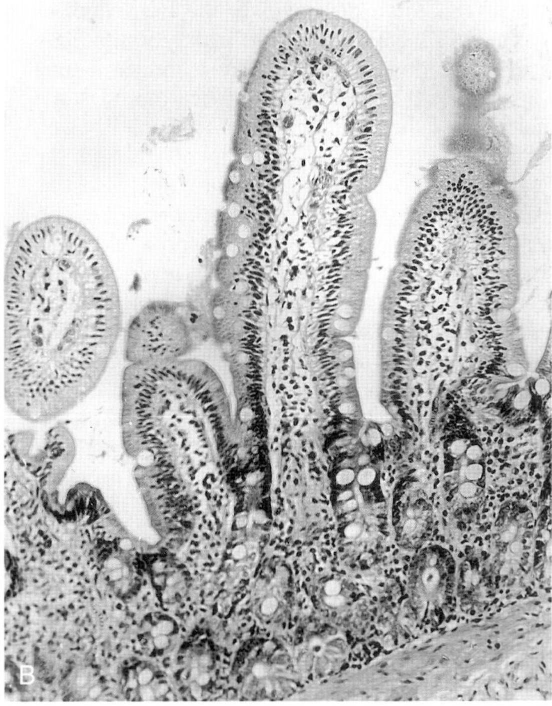

Figure 93–2. Mucosal pathology in celiac sprue. *A*, Duodenal biopsy specimen of a patient with untreated celiac sprue. The histologic features of severe villous atrophy, crypt hyperplasia, enterocyte disarray, and intense inflammatory infiltrate of the lamina propria and epithelial cell layer are evident. *B*, Repeat duodenal biopsy after 6 months on strict gluten-free diet. There is marked improvement with well-formed villi and a return of mucosal architecture toward normal.

Such a mechanism would explain many of the histologic abnormalities described above.

The cellularity of the lamina propria is increased in the involved small intestine. The cellular infiltrate consists largely of plasma cells and lymphocytes. The number of IgA-, IgM-, and IgG-producing cells is increased two- to sixfold, but as in normal mucosa, IgA-producing cells predominate.[28] Polymorphonuclear leukocytes, eosinophils, and mast cells also may contribute substantially to the increased cellularity of the lamina propria. Although the number of IELs per unit length of absorptive epithelium is increased in untreated celiac sprue, the total number of IELs may not be increased, because the absorptive surface is markedly reduced.[9] In the normal small intestinal mucosa, lamina propria T cells are predominantly CD4+ positive (helper/inducer cells), whereas the IELs are mainly CD8+ positive (cytotoxic/suppressor) cells. In untreated celiac sprue, this distribution of T cells is maintained, but the density of cells in both compartments is increased.

Marsh[29] pioneered the theory that there is a sequence of progression of the celiac lesion in the small intestinal mucosa. Starting with a preinfiltrative (stage 0) mucosa, the initial event is an increase in IELs, followed by infiltration of the lamina propria with lymphocytes (stage 1). Crypt hyperplasia (stage 2) precedes villous atrophy (stage 3) and is observed only in the presence of lamina propria lymphocytosis. This finding suggests that IELs are not sufficient to induce intestinal architectural changes in celiac sprue. Finally, total mucosal atrophy (stage 4) is seen and is characterized by complete loss of villi, enhanced apoptosis, and crypt hyperplasia.

The length of small intestinal involvement by the celiac sprue lesion in untreated patients varies from patient to patient and correlates with the severity of clinical symptoms. Patients with a severe lesion that involves the full length of the small intestine will have more severe malabsorption than patients with a severe duodenal lesion but a milder jejunal lesion and a histologically normal ileum. When the intestinal lesion does not involve the entire length of the small bowel, the proximal intestine is most severely involved, and the severity decreases distally. Sparing of the proximal intestine with involvement of the distal small intestine does not occur. In some untreated patients with mild celiac sprue, even the proximal intestine may not show the typical severe flat lesion. Rather, some villous structure remains, and the absorptive surface, although less than normal, is largely preserved.[9] However, some shortening of the villi, crypt hyperplasia, cytologically abnormal surface cells, and increased lamina propria cellularity must be present to establish the diagnosis.

Treatment with a gluten-free diet results in significant improvement in intestinal structure (Fig. 93–2*B*). The cytologic appearance of the surface absorptive cells improves first, often within a few days. Tall columnar absorptive cells with basal nuclei and well-developed brush borders replace the abnormal and immature cuboidal surface cells, and the ratio of IELs to absorptive cells decreases. Subsequently, villous architecture reverts toward normal, the villi lengthen, the crypts shorten, and the lamina propria decreases in cellularity. The mucosa of the distal small intestine improves more rapidly than that of the severely involved proximal bowel.[30] In some patients months or even years of gluten withdrawal may be required before the mucosa reverts to normal; indeed, some residual abnormality, which may be striking or subtle, often persists, possibly because of inadvertent gluten ingestion.[31] In the debilitated patient with severe untreated celiac sprue and associated nutritional deficiencies, pathologic changes may be present in other organ systems besides the digestive tract. Moreover, the mucosal lesion of celiac sprue can be identical histologically to the mucosal response to injury seen in a wide range of other enteropathies.

PATHOGENESIS

The interaction of the water-insoluble protein moiety (gluten) of certain cereal grains with the mucosa of the small intestine in susceptible persons is central to the pathogenesis of celiac sprue. Although the exact molecular mechanism by which gluten damages the mucosa has not been established, our knowledge of the pathogenesis of celiac sprue has accelerated recently. Celiac sprue is now considered to be an immune disorder that is triggered by an environmental agent (gliadin) in genetically predisposed persons. The wide spectrum of clinical manifestations is the result of a complex interplay of variable environmental, genetic, and immune factors.

Environmental Factors

The wheat fraction responsible for celiac sprue is known to be protein, because gliadin that has been chemically processed to remove fat will still induce the disease. Wheat protein exists in a number of storage forms, which can be categorized into four general groups based on their solubility characteristics: prolamins (soluble in ethanol), glutenins (partially soluble in dilute acid or alkali solutions), globulins (soluble in 10% NaCl), and minor albumins (soluble in water). The term *gluten* encompasses the prolamins and glutenins. Although most toxicity studies have been performed with prolamins, recent data suggest that glutenins also can damage the celiac intestinal mucosa.[32] The prolamins of wheat are referred to as gliadins. Prolamins from other cereals are also considered to be gluten and are named according to their source (secalins from rye, hordeins from barley, avenins from oats, and zeins from celiac nontoxic corn). The taxonomic relationships among the major cereal grains provides a framework on which their toxicity in celiac sprue can be predicted (Fig. 93–3). Wheat, rye, and barley belong to the tribe known as Triticeae, whereas oats belong to a neighboring tribe known as Aveneae. Avenin is genetically less similar to gliadin than gliadin is to secalin and hordein. However, despite the genetic differences, the prolamins from oats, barley, wheat, and rye have immunologic cross-reactivity, because of their common ancestry.[33] Grains that do not activate disease (rice, corn, sorghum, and millet) are separated still further from wheat, rye, and barley in terms of their derivation from the primitive grasses.

Gliadin can be separated electrophoretically into four major fractions that range in molecular weight from 20 to 75 kDa and exist as single polypeptide chains. These fractions have been designated alpha, beta, gamma, and omega gliadins,[34] and all four appear to be toxic to patients with celiac sprue.[35] The complete amino acid sequence of several of the

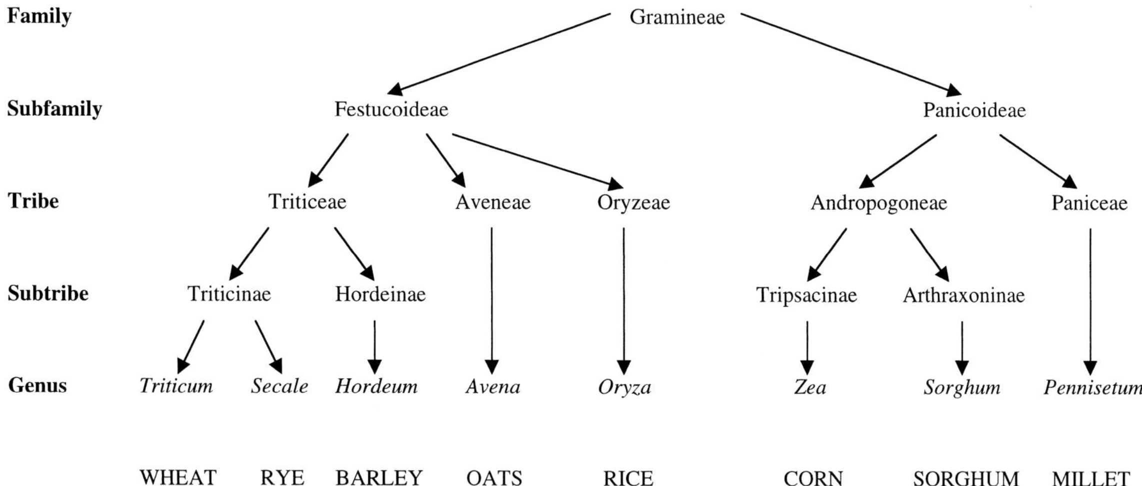

Figure 93–3. Taxonomic relationships of the major cereal grains. (From Kasarda DD, Okita TW, Bernardin JE, et al: Nucleic acid [cDNA] and amino acid sequences of α-type gliadin from wheat *[Triticum aestivum]*. Proc Natl Acad Sci U S A 181:4712–4716, 1984.)

gliadins and related prolamins in other grains is known.[36] A variety of gliadin peptides has been identified as potential epitopes for gliadin-specific T-cell clones and has been implicated in the pathogenesis of celiac sprue through their bioactivity in feeding studies or in *ex vivo* celiac sprue intestinal biopsy challenges. Anderson and colleagues[14] recently identified a partially deamidated peptide consisting of amino acids 56–75 of alpha gliadin as the dominant epitope responsible for the T-cell response in celiac sprue (see later).

It is possible that immunologic similarities between gliadin protein motifs and enteric pathogens may be involved in the pathogenesis of an immunologic response to gluten antigens. This hypothesis was supported by a study in which analysis of alpha gliadin demonstrated an amino acid region that was homologous to the 54-kDa E1b protein coat of adenovirus 12, thereby suggesting that exposure to the virus in a susceptible person could be involved in the pathogenesis of celiac sprue.[37] Furthermore, patients with celiac sprue have been reported to have a significantly higher prevalence of past adenovirus 12 infection than control subjects,[38] a finding that suggests molecular mimicry may be involved in the pathogenesis of celiac sprue.

The reason why oats may be tolerated by patients with celiac sprue is not obvious, because the prolamin fraction of oats contains the same amino acid sequences (QQQPF) that have been shown to be toxic in wheat gliadin.[39] A possible explanation is that oats contain a relatively smaller proportion of this toxic prolamin moiety than do other gluten-containing cereals. Although a common feature of prolamins of wheat, rye, and barley is a high content of glutamine (>30%) and proline (>15%), the prolamins of oats have an intermediate content of these amino acids, and the nontoxic prolamins of rice, corn, and millet have a lower content of them.[40] Studies on oat challenges in patients with celiac sprue suggest that tolerance to oats depends at least in part on the total amount consumed.[41] Oat consumption of less than 40 to 60 g/day by patients with celiac sprue in remission appears to be well tolerated, whereas a larger daily intake may be associated with relapse.[41] The data on oats also highlight the important relationship between the amount of gluten consumed and the severity of disease. A 5- to 10-fold higher incidence of overt celiac sprue in children from Sweden compared with Denmark (two populations with similar genetic backgrounds) has long been cited as evidence of the importance of environmental factors in the pathogenesis of celiac sprue. Subsequent studies found as much as a 40-fold difference in the gliadin concentration of Swedish compared with Danish infant formulas.[21] This finding suggests that early exposure of the immature immune system to substantial amounts of gliadin is a prominent cofactor for the development of overt celiac sprue, possibly by skewing the intestinal immune response to gliadin toward a T helper 1 T-cell response.

Genetic Factors

Family studies reflect the importance of genetic factors in the pathogenesis of celiac sprue.[40] Concordance for celiac sprue in first-degree relatives of affected persons ranges from 8% to 18% and reaches 70% in monozygotic twins.[42] Our understanding of the nature of this genetic predisposition began with the observation by Howell and colleagues[10] that celiac sprue is associated with specific HLA class II DQ haplotypes. HLA class II molecules are glycosylated transmembrane heterodimers (α and β chains), which are organized into three related subregions—DQ, DR, and DP—and are encoded within the HLA class II region of the major histocompatibility complex on chromosome 6p. The HLA-DQ(α1*501,β1*02) heterodimer, known as HLA-DQ2, is found in 95% of patients with celiac sprue, and the related DQ(α1*0301,β1*0302) heterodimer, known as HLA-DQ8, is found in most of the remaining patients. An important link to genetic predisposition was provided by the isolation of gliadin-specific HLA-DQ2–restricted T-cell clones from celiac sprue mucosa.[11] A further advance was the finding that the HLA-DQ2 heterodimer is encoded in either the *cis* or *trans* position with respect to HLA-DR3 or HLA-DR5/7, respectively.[43] It is now known that after gluten is absorbed, lamina propria antigen presenting cells, probably dendritic cells that express HLA-DQ2 or DQ8, present gliadin peptides on their α/β heterodimer antigen presenting grooves to sensitized T lymphocytes that express the α/β T-cell receptor. These lymphocytes then activate B lymphocytes to generate immunoglobulins and other T lymphocytes to secrete cytokines, predominantly interferon-γ and to a lesser degree interleukin (IL)-4, IL-5, IL-6, IL-10, tumor necrosis factor (TNF)-α, and transforming growth factor-β.[44] These cytokines not only damage enterocytes but also induce expression of aberrant HLA class II cell-surface antigens on the luminal surface of enterocytes, possibly facilitating additional direct antigen presentation by these cells to the sensitized lymphocytes (Fig. 93–4).

Celiac sprue develops in only a minority of persons who express DQ2. In fact, HLA-DQ2 is common in Europeans and is expressed in 25% to 30% of the normal population. Consequently, the estimated HLA contribution to the development of celiac sprue among siblings is only 36%.[45] Thus, another gene (or genes) at an HLA-unlinked locus must also participate and is likely to be a stronger determinant of disease susceptibility than the HLA locus.[46] In Irish patients with celiac sprue, an additional predisposing role of TNF genes, an association independent of DQ2, has been demonstrated using a microsatellite polymorphism situated near the TNF genes.[47] Moreover, a polymorphism of the TNF-α gene promoter has been demonstrated to be a component of the DR3-DQ2 haplotype.[48] Although a Finnish study failed to reproduce the finding of a DQ2-independent association of the TNF microsatellites,[49] these discrepant results may relate to population differences. Other associations have been reported with chromosome 15q26, which contains a type I diabetes susceptibility locus,[46] chromosome 5q, and possibly chromosome 11q.[50] The non-HLA locus appears to be inherited as an autosomal recessive trait.[46] One major site has

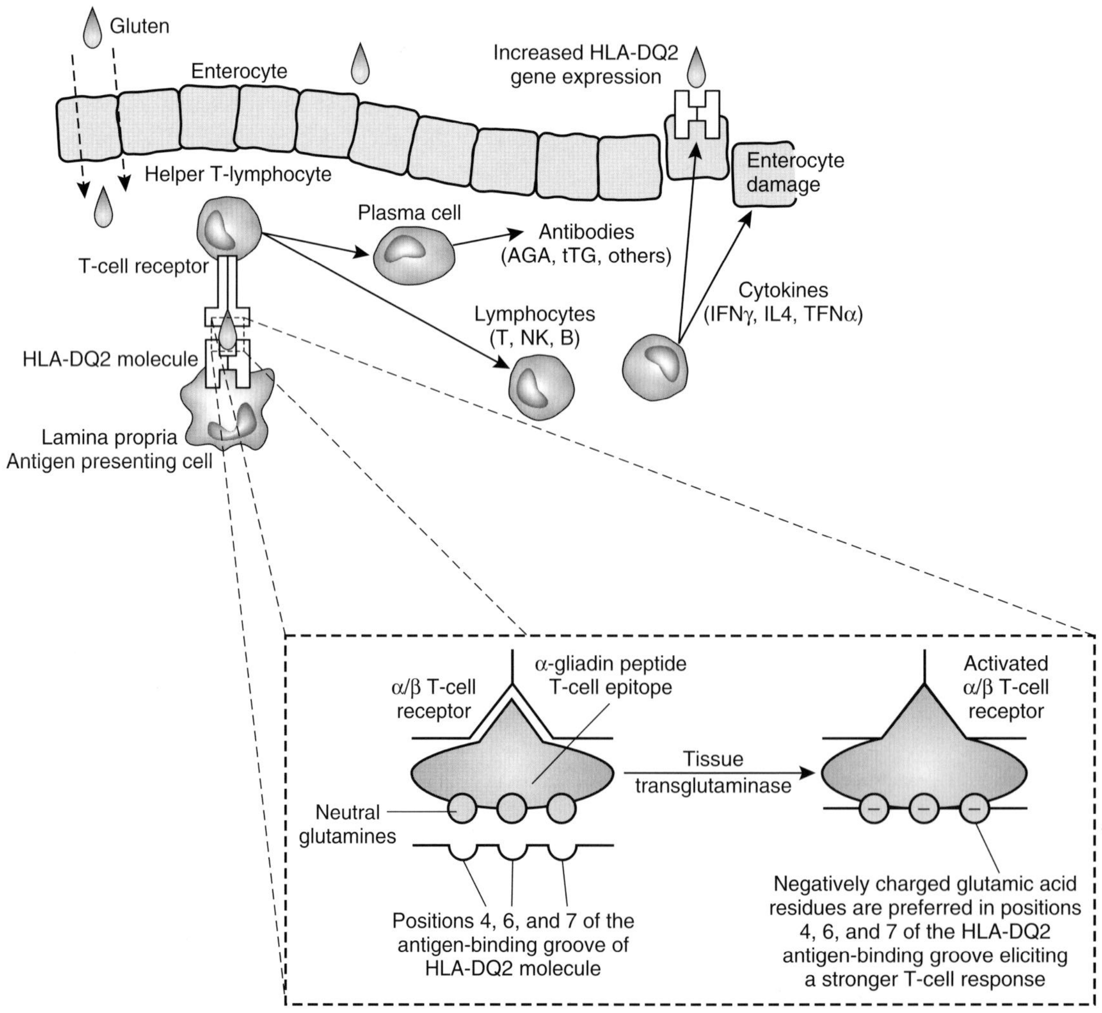

Figure 93–4. Proposed pathogenesis of celiac sprue. Gluten is absorbed into the lamina propria and presented in conjunction with human leukocyte antigen (HLA)-DQ2 or DQ8 cell-surface antigens by antigen presenting cells, probably dendritic cells, to sensitized T lymphocytes expressing the α/β T-cell receptor (afferent limb). Tissue transglutaminase deamidates gliadin peptides generating acidic negatively charged glutamic acid residues from neutral glutamines *(inset)*. Because negatively charged residues are preferred in positions 4, 6, and 7 of the antigen-binding groove of HLA-DQ2, deamidated gliadin elicits stronger T-lymphocyte responses. These lymphocytes then activate other lymphocytes to generate immune products that damage the enterocytes, resulting in villous atrophy (efferent limb). Induction of aberrant HLA-class II cell-surface antigens on the enterocytes may permit additional antigen presentation by these cells to the sensitized lymphocytes. AGA, antigliadin antibody; HLA, human leucocyte antigen; IFNγ, interferon gamma; NK, natural killer; tTG, tissue transglutaminase. (Adapted with permission from Farrell RJ, Kelly CP: Celiac sprue. N Engl J Med 346:180–188, 2002.)

also been found on chromosome 6p, although the gene has not been identified.[46]

Immune Factors

Evidence implicating both humoral and cell-mediated immune responses to gliadin and related prolamins in the pathogenesis of celiac sprue is substantial. There is a two- to sixfold increase in the number of immunoglobulin-producing B cells in the lamina propria of the small intestine in untreated patients with celiac sprue.[28] In addition, IgA and IgG to purified gliadin and to all major fractions of gliadin can be detected in the sera of most patients with untreated celiac sprue, some patients with treated celiac sprue, and some patients with subclinical disease.[51, 52] However, AGAs do not appear to be essential for the pathogenesis of celiac sprue and may simply reflect a nonspecific response to the passage of incompletely digested antigenic gluten proteins across an abnormally permeable intestinal epithelium.[53] Furthermore, many normal persons have increased serum IgA or IgG antigliadin levels or both.[54] Many persons with celiac sprue have increased levels of serum antibodies against other food proteins such as β-lactoglobulin, casein, and ovalbumin.[55] It is unclear whether the presence of such antibodies reflects a general aberrant immune responsiveness to food antigens in celiac patients or enhanced systemic exposure to these proteins because of increased small intestinal permeability.

The recent identification of more specific autoantibody responses has altered our understanding of the pathogenesis of celiac sprue. IgA antibodies to endomysium, a connective tissue structure surrounding smooth muscle, are virtually pathognomonic of celiac sprue and are rarely found in the absence of the disease.[56] It is now known that the target autoantigen contained within the endomysium is the enzyme tissue transglutaminase (tTG).[12] Gliadin is a preferred substrate for this ubiquitous calcium-dependent intracellular enzyme, and it has been shown that tTG deamidates key neutral glutamine residues in gliadin and converts them into negatively charged glutamic acid residues, which are preferred in positions 4, 6, and 7 of the nonapeptide antigen-binding groove of the HLA-DQ2 heterodimer (see Fig. 93–4).[13, 57] Thus, tTG-mediated modification of gliadin plays a pivotal role in eliciting a stronger proliferative response by gliadin-specific T cell clones, or, stated differently, tTG makes “gliadin tastier for the T cells.” With gliadin serving as a glutamine-donor, tTG also can generate additional novel antigenic epitopes by cross-linking molecules of the extracellular matrix with gliadin or with tTG–gliadin complexes.[58] As evidence of the fundamental role of tTG in the pathogenesis of celiac sprue, the dominant epitope responsible for the T-cell response has recently been reported to contain a deamidated glutamine residue (Q65E) of alpha gliadin.[14] It also has been observed that tTG is necessary for the bioactivation of transforming growth factor-β, which is required for epithelial differentiation, and in a T-84 crypt epithelial cell culture system autoantibodies to tTG block transforming growth factor-β-mediated enterocyte differentiation.[59] This finding suggests not only that release of tTG from cells during inflammation may potentiate gliadin presentation by HLA-DQ2 and HLA-DQ8, as noted above, but also that local production of autoantibodies to tTG may contribute to the lack of epithelial differentiation observed in the active celiac lesion.

Cell-mediated immune responses also appear to be important in the pathogenesis of celiac sprue. In untreated celiac sprue, many of the T cells in the mucosa of the small intestine are activated and release potent proinflammatory mediators such as interferon-γ and TNF-α.[44] Activated T lymphocytes are abundant in the lamina propria of the small intestine; most of these are CD4+ cells.[60] In contrast, IELs, which are present in large numbers in untreated celiac sprue, are CD8+ T cells.[61] The increased expression of CD45RO on T cells in the mucosa of untreated patients has led to the suggestion that there is an influx of primed memory cells.[62] Whereas in healthy persons over 90% of IELs express the α/β T-cell receptor, expression of the γ/δ T-cell receptor by IELs in patients with untreated celiac sprue is increased as much as sixfold (to 35%) and is considered a hallmark of the disease.[63] These primitive lymphocytes recognize bacterial nonpeptide antigens and unprocessed stress-related proteins. They appear to act as mucosal guardians and may protect the intestinal mucosa from chronic exposure to dietary gluten in gluten-tolerant persons by secreting IL-4, which dampens T helper 1 in favor of T helper 2 reactivity.[64] Their continuous presence in patients on a gluten-free diet may indicate inadvertent gluten ingestion. Although patients with refractory sprue also have aberrant IELs with restricted γ/δ T-cell receptor gene rearrangements (see discussion of Refractory Sprue later), the pathogenetic role of these lymphocytes, as compared with the lamina propria lymphocytes, remains controversial.[65]

CLINICAL FEATURES

Samuel Gee’s classic and evocative description of celiac sprue was concerned largely with the gross manifestations of the disorder.[5] However, this florid presentation is now unusual in the Western world and constitutes only the extreme tip of the “celiac iceberg.” Although some patients still present with severe illness, most patients have few, subtle, or no symptoms at diagnosis. Such cases may be identified by screening relatives of patients during research studies or screening patients with associated disorders, such as diabetes mellitus, hypothyroidism, or Down’s syndrome. Incidental hematologic or biochemical abnormalities also may lead to a diagnosis of celiac sprue.

Childhood Presentation

The classic presentation of celiac sprue in infancy is not easily missed. The typical history is that of steatorrhea with or without vomiting and occasional crampy abdominal pain occurring anytime after weaning, when cereals are first introduced into the diet, especially in the first and second years of life. Classically, the child fails to thrive and is apathetic and irritable, with muscle wasting, hypotonia, and abdominal distention. Watery diarrhea or occasionally constipation may be reported. Diagnosis is more difficult when gastrointestinal features are less prominent. The possibility of gluten sensitivity should be considered in all children of relevant ethnic background who present with short stature or failure to thrive, even when there are no other symptoms to suggest an enteropathy. Once a gluten-free diet is commenced, catch-up growth is well documented.[66] Nutritional deficiencies, particularly anemia, are another common mode of presentation, especially in older children. With earlier diagnosis, clinical rickets is now an uncommon complication but is seen occasionally, especially among Asian children with untreated celiac sprue. Many childhood patients experience a temporary spontaneous remission of symptoms during adolescence, and it is unusual for celiac sprue to present during the teen years.

Considerable debate continues as to why celiac sprue tends to be diagnosed later and with milder symptoms and signs than in the past. Early work suggested that breast-feeding could delay the onset of symptoms.[67] However, a more recent study found that neither breast-feeding, age at introduction of cow's milk products, nor gluten consumption had any bearing on the onset of symptoms.[68] Although the impact of changes in infant feeding practices remains unclear, the variable effect of gluten on the immature gastrointestinal system also may be an important factor.

Adult Presentation

In the past celiac sprue was perceived to be a pediatric disorder. However, the diagnosis is now often made in adult life. The unmasking of asymptomatic disease by surgery that induces rapid gastric emptying (gastric resection, pyloroplasty) or the finding of the typical lesion in an asymptomatic relative of a patient with celiac sprue suggests that adults may have clinically inapparent celiac sprue for some time. A proportion of these adult patients are short in stature or give a history consistent with unrecognized gluten-sensitive enteropathy in childhood. In many cases, however, there is nothing to suggest previous disease, and it is possible that celiac sprue may develop for the first time in adult life. Occasionally, celiac sprue may present de novo in elderly patients.[69]

Gastrointestinal Features

The clinical manifestations of celiac sprue vary greatly from patient to patient. Because most symptoms result from intestinal malabsorption, they are not specific for celiac sprue but resemble those seen in other disorders that cause malabsorption. Many adult patients present with gastrointestinal symptoms, including diarrhea, steatorrhea, flatulence, and weight loss, which are similar to those seen in childhood celiac sprue. Diarrhea is often episodic rather than continuous. Nocturnal or early morning diarrhea is common. Patients with extensive intestinal involvement may have in excess of 10 stools per day. Because of their high fat content, the stools of patients with celiac sprue may be light tan or grayish and greasy in appearance, with a tendency to float, and difficult to flush from the toilet bowl. Steatorrhea is often absent in patients with disease limited to the proximal small intestine.

Several factors contribute to the diarrhea associated with celiac sprue. The stool volume and osmotic load delivered to the colon are increased by the malabsorption of fat,[70] carbohydrate, protein, electrolytes, and other nutrients. In addition, the delivery of excessive dietary fat into the large bowel probably results in the production by bacteria of hydroxy fatty acids, which are potent cathartics. In symptomatic patients electrolytes are actually secreted into, rather than absorbed from, the lumen of the severely damaged upper small intestine. This secretion further increases luminal fluid in an intestine with already compromised absorptive capacity. There also is evidence that the release of secretin and cholecystokinin in response to a meal is impaired in celiac sprue, thereby diminishing delivery of bile and pancreatic secretions into the gut lumen and possibly compromising intraluminal digestion.[71, 72] Alterations in the secretion of other gut peptides also may contribute to the observed diarrhea. Finally, if the disease extends to and involves the ileum, patients may experience the direct cathartic action of malabsorbed bile salts on the colon.[70]

The amount of weight loss in a patient with celiac sprue depends on the severity and extent of the intestinal lesion and on the ability of the patient to compensate for the malabsorption by increasing dietary intake. Some patients with substantial malabsorption have enormous appetites and lose little or no weight. Rarely, in severe disease, anorexia may develop with associated rapid and severe weight loss. In such debilitated patients, some of the weight loss may be masked by fluid retention caused by hypoproteinemia. Malaise, lassitude, and fatigue are also common even when anemia is absent. Occasionally, severe hypokalemia resulting from the loss of potassium in the stool may cause severe muscle weakness.

Vague abdominal discomfort and abdominal bloating are common and may lead to a mistaken diagnosis of irritable bowel syndrome. Severe abdominal pain may occur but is uncharacteristic in uncomplicated celiac sprue. However, abdominal distention with excessive amounts of malodorous flatus is a common complaint. Nausea and vomiting are uncommon in uncomplicated celiac sprue. Recurrent severe aphthous stomatitis affects a significant proportion of patients and may be the sole presenting complaint. It is important to exclude celiac sprue in patients with recurrent aphthous stomatitis, because many of these patients respond well to dietary treatment for sprue.[73]

Extraintestinal Features

Many patients with celiac sprue present with complaints not directly referable to the gastrointestinal tract. These extraintestinal symptoms and clinical findings often result from nutrient malabsorption and may involve virtually all organ systems (Table 93–1). Extraintestinal features, including anemia, osteopenic bone disease, neurologic symptoms, and menstrual abnormalities, often prove more distressing to the patient than do the gastrointestinal symptoms.

Anemia is common in both children and adults with celiac sprue and usually is caused by impaired iron or folate absorption from the proximal intestine; in severe disease with ileal involvement, vitamin B_{12} absorption also is impaired. Patients with extensive disease may bleed into the skin or mucous membranes or have hematuria, epistaxis, and vaginal or gastrointestinal bleeding. Bleeding may further aggravate preexisting anemia and is most often caused by a coagulopathy resulting from impaired intestinal absorption of vitamin K. Evidence of hyposplenism of unknown cause

Table 93–1 | **Extraintestinal Manifestations of Celiac Sprue**

ORGAN SYSTEM	MANIFESTATION	PROBABLE CAUSE(S)
Hematopoietic	Anemia	Iron, folate, vitamin B_{12}, or pyridoxine deficiency
	Hemorrhage	Vitamin K deficiency; rarely, thrombocytopenia because of folate deficiency
	Thrombocytosis, abnormal red blood cells	Hyposplenism
Skeletal	Osteopenia	Malabsorption of calcium and vitamin D
	Pathologic fractures	Osteopenia
	Osteoarthropathy	Unknown
Muscular	Atrophy	Malnutrition due to malabsorption
	Tetany	Calcium, vitamin D, or magnesium malabsorption
	Weakness	Generalized muscle atrophy, hypokalemia
Nervous	Peripheral neuropathy	Vitamin deficiencies such as vitamin B_{12} and thiamine
	Ataxia	Cerebellar and posterior column damage
	Demyelinating central nervous system lesions	Unknown
	Seizures	Unknown
Endocrine	Secondary hyperparathyroidism	Calcium/vitamin D malabsorption causing hypocalcemia
	Amenorrhea, infertility, impotence	Malnutrition, hypothalamic–pituitary dysfunction
Integument	Follicular hyperkeratosis and dermatitis	Vitamin A malabsorption, vitamin B complex malabsorption
	Petechiae and ecchymoses	Vitamin K deficiency; rarely, thrombocytopenia
	Edema	Hypoproteinemia
	Dermatitis herpetiformis	Unknown

From Trier JS. Celiac sprue and refractory sprue. In Feldman M, Scharschmidt BF, Sleisenger MH (eds): Gastrointestinal and Liver Disease. Philadelphia; W.B. Saunders, 1998:1557, with permission.

with thrombocytosis, deformed erythrocytes, and splenic atrophy occurs in up to 50% of adults with celiac sprue but only rarely in children.[74] In most cases, evidence of hyposplenism disappears with elimination of gluten from the diet.[74]

Bone mineral density is almost invariably low in patients with untreated celiac sprue, and osteoporosis occurs in more than one fourth of patients.[75] Osteopenic bone disease develops as a result of impaired calcium absorption secondary to defective calcium transport by the diseased small intestine, vitamin D deficiency caused by impaired absorption of this fat-soluble vitamin, and binding of intraluminal calcium and magnesium to unabsorbed dietary fatty acids to form insoluble soaps, which are then excreted in the feces. Whereas bone disease is generally more severe among patients with symptomatic celiac sprue, severe osteopenia has been reported in up to one third of symptom-free adults with celiac sprue diagnosed during childhood and resumption of a normal diet during adolescence.[76] Patients may present with bone pain, especially in the lower back, rib cage, and pelvis. Calcium and magnesium depletion may cause paresthesias, muscle cramps, and even tetany. Although pathologic fractures are thought to be unusual, a recent study reported peripheral bone fractures in 25% of patients with celiac sprue; most of these fractures occurred before the diagnosis of sprue was made or in patients who were noncompliant with a gluten-free diet.[77] With prolonged calcium malabsorption, patients may develop secondary hyperparathyroidism, resulting in mobilization of calcium from bones and further exacerbation of osteopenia.

Neurologic symptoms caused by lesions of the central or peripheral nervous system occur occasionally in patients with severe celiac sprue, but the pathogenesis is poorly understood. Ataxia is the commonest neurologic manifestation, and progressive gait and limb ataxia may be the sole manifestation in some patients. These abnormalities are thought to result from immunologic damage to the cerebellum, posterior columns of the spinal cord, and peripheral nerves, and the term "gluten ataxia" has been proposed to describe this disorder.[78] Muscle weakness and paresthesias with sensory loss also are occasionally encountered, and pathologic evidence of peripheral neuropathy and rarely patchy demyelinization of the spinal cord, cerebellar atrophy, and capillary proliferation suggestive of Wernicke's encephalopathy have been described. Although potential causative roles for specific deficiencies of vitamin B_{12}, thiamine, riboflavin, and pyridoxine have not been established, neurologic symptoms have been reported to improve in some patients receiving multivitamins, including vitamins A, B, and E, or calcium. Night blindness is a clear indication for vitamin A therapy. Peripheral neuropathy and ataxia, however, often appear to be unrelated to specific vitamin deficiencies and usually do not respond to gluten withdrawal.[79] The association between celiac sprue and both epilepsy (complex partial seizures) and bilateral parieto-occipital cerebral calcification is well recognized.[80] In one series, epilepsy was reported in approximately 5% of children and young adults with celiac sprue.[81] The cause of the epilepsy remains unclear, but the prognosis appears to depend on how early in the course of the disease a gluten-free diet is started. Although most celiac patients do not appear to be psychologically abnormal, many report a striking improvement in mood, irritability, and depression shortly after commencing a gluten-free diet.[79]

Gynecologic and obstetric problems are common in women with untreated celiac sprue.[82] Amenorrhea occurs in one third of female patients of childbearing age, and there frequently is a delay in menarche (typically by 1 year) in untreated persons. Women with untreated celiac sprue may present with infertility, and it is common for infertile women with celiac sprue to become pregnant shortly after beginning a gluten-free diet.[83] Because spontaneous and recurrent abortions, low-birth-weight babies, and an unfavorable outcome of pregnancy are more frequent in untreated patients and may be prevented by a gluten-free diet, it has been suggested that in areas where celiac sprue is prevalent, pregnant women should be screened routinely with EMA.[84] Infertility secondary to impotence or an abnormally low sperm count is common in adult men with untreated celiac sprue.[85] Although malnutrition related to malabsorption may contribute to male infertility, abnormalities in hypothalamic-pituitary regulation of gonadal function and gonadal androgen resistance that disappears on gluten withdrawal also have been incriminated.[85]

Physical Findings

Physical findings, like symptoms, vary considerably among patients with celiac sprue. Patients with mild disease frequently have a normal physical examination. In more severe disease the physical abnormalities are usually the result of malabsorption and are not specific for celiac sprue. Growth retardation occurs commonly in children, but when a gluten-free diet is begun before puberty, a compensatory growth spurt occurs, and the effect on adult height is minimized. Persons with celiac sprue are on average 3 inches shorter than their peers. Tall patients are seen, however, and a height of more than 6 feet does not preclude the diagnosis. In patients with severe celiac sprue, emaciation with evidence of recent weight loss, including loose skinfolds and muscle wasting, may be prominent. Adults with celiac sprue commonly experience a weight gain of more than 6 kg after institution of a gluten-free diet. Clubbing of the fingers occurs occasionally, and koilonychia may be associated with long-standing iron deficiency anemia. Pitting edema of the lower extremities may result from hypoproteinemia. Hypotension may be related to fluid and electrolyte depletion, and the skin may be dry with poor turgor if there is dehydration. Occasionally, a low-grade fever associated with anemia is found in patients with untreated celiac sprue, but this finding may indicate a concurrent complication, such as infection or malignancy, particularly lymphoma. Increased skin pigmentation may be obvious in severely ill patients. In addition to dermatitis herpetiformis (see later), other dermatologic findings may include spontaneous ecchymoses related to hypoprothrombinemia, hyperkeratosis follicularis caused by vitamin A deficiency, and pallor caused by anemia.

Examination of the mouth may show aphthous stomatitis, angular cheilosis, and glossitis with decreased papillation of the tongue. Defects in dental enamel are common.[86] The abdomen may be protuberant and tympanitic with a characteristic doughy consistency on palpation due to distention of intestinal loops with fluid and gas. Hepatomegaly and abdominal tenderness are uncommon, but ascites may be detected in patients with hypoproteinemia. Peripheral lymphadenopathy is unusual in the absence of complicating lymphoma. Rarely, lymphadenitis or cavitating abdominal mesenteric lymph nodes that resolve with a gluten-free diet have been reported. On computed tomography, low-grade lymphadenopathy sometimes can be found and frequently is associated with hyposplenism.

The extremities may reveal loss of various sensory modalities, including light touch, vibration, and position, usually resulting from peripheral neuropathy and rarely demyelinating spinal cord lesions. If neuropathy is severe, deep tendon reflexes are diminished or even absent. Hyperpathia may be present. A positive Chvostek or Trousseau sign may be elicited in patients with severe calcium and magnesium depletion. In such persons, bone tenderness related to osteopenia may be present, especially if collapsed vertebrae or other fractures are present.

DIAGNOSTIC STUDIES

The laboratory findings in celiac sprue, like symptoms and signs, vary with the extent and severity of the intestinal lesion. Serum IgA EMA or tTG antibody and small bowel biopsy are the most accurate diagnostic tests for celiac sprue. Stool studies, hematologic and biochemical tests, and radiologic studies may be abnormal but seldom provide a specific diagnosis, because similar abnormalities may be seen in patients with other diseases that produce intestinal malabsorption (see Chapter 89).

Stool Examination

If malabsorption is sufficient to produce significant steatorrhea, watery or bulky, semiformed, light tan or grayish, malodorous, greasy-appearing stools are characteristic. Microscopic evaluation of the fat content of a stool suspension stained with Sudan III or IV after hydrolysis with acetic acid and heat is a helpful screening test. To document steatorrhea unequivocally, the amount of fat in a 3-day collection of stool may be determined quantitatively, using the reliable van de Kamer chemical method.

Hematologic and Biochemical Tests

A variety of hematologic and biochemical abnormalities may be found in persons with untreated celiac sprue, including iron deficiency, folic acid deficiency, and vitamin D deficiency. These abnormalities reflect nutritional deficiencies secondary to enteropathy-induced malabsorption. Iron deficiency anemia is common in both children and adults with celiac sprue. A combination of iron and folate defiency is characteristic in children. Except during pregnancy, severe anemia is uncommon, usually occurs with extensive disease, and should raise the suspicion of a complication such as lymphoma. The peripheral blood film may reveal target cells, siderocytes, Heinz bodies, and crenated red cells. Howell-Jolly bodies, which suggest splenic atrophy, are frequently seen.[74] Although relevant to patient management, none of these hematologic or biochemical tests is sufficiently sensitive or specific to serve as a useful screening or diagnostic tool.[87] Similarly, although an oral D-xylose tolerance test and fecal fat evaluation may be abnormal in patients with untreated celiac sprue, they will not provide a specific diagnosis and no longer have a place as routine investigations in suspected celiac sprue. Furthermore, the absorption and urinary excretion of D-xylose can be normal in up to 20% of patients with untreated celiac sprue, and a 3-day fecal fat estimation is a relatively crude test that is subject to errors because of varying dietary fat intake and incomplete stool collection. Chronically elevated serum aminotransferase levels have been reported in 9% to 40% of patients with untreated celiac sprue, presumably because of increased intestinal permeability. In most patients, the elevations resolve on a gluten-free diet.

Serologic Tests

In current clinical practice, four serologic studies are used to aid in the diagnosis of celiac sprue. IgA EMA and IgA tTG antibody are based on the target antigen tTG, whereas IgA AGA and IgG AGA are based on the target antigen gliadin.[53] The approximate sensitivities and specificities of these serum antibody tests are shown in Table 93–2. In addition to laboratory variation, the reported sensitivity and specificity rates for these tests depend on the prevalence of the disease in the tested population and the severity of the disease. In one study of 101 patients with biopsy-proven celiac sprue,[88] the sensitivity of IgA EMA among patients with total villous atrophy was 100% compared with only 31% in those with partial villous atrophy.

IgA Endomysial Antibodies

EMAs bind to connective tissue surrounding smooth muscle cells.[53, 56] Frozen sections of monkey esophagus were used initially for the assay. Currently, most laboratories use sections of human umbilical cord, which are more readily available.[89] Serum IgA EMA binds to the endomysium to produce a characteristic staining pattern, which is visualized by indirect immunofluorescence. The test result is reported simply as positive or negative, because even low titers of serum IgA EMA are highly specific for celiac sprue. As mentioned earlier, the target antigen has been identified as tTG. IgA EMA has a sensitivity of 90% or greater and a specificity approaching 100% in untreated celiac sprue.[53, 56, 90] Antibody levels fall on a gluten-free diet, and the test often becomes negative in treated patients.[91] The clinical application of EMA and other serologic tests is discussed below.

Anti-Tissue Transglutaminase Antibodies

The epitope against which EMA is directed has been identified as tTG.[12] IgA anti-tTG assays are proving to be highly sensitive and specific for the diagnosis of celiac sprue.[92, 93] In one study, anti-tTG were present in 98% of patients with biopsy-proven celiac sprue compared with 5% of control subjects.[92] In another study that included 136 patients with celiac sprue and 207 control subjects, the sensitivity and specificity of anti-tTG were 95% and 94%, respectively.[93] Enzyme-linked immunosorbent assay tests for IgA anti-tTG are now widely available, less costly, and easier to perform than the immunofluorescence assay used to detect IgA EMA.

Table 93–2 | **Sensitivity and Specificity of Serologic Tests in Celiac Sprue**

SERUM TESTS	SENSITIVITY*	SPECIFICITY*
IgA endomysial antibodies	85–98%	97–100%
IgA tissue transglutaminase antibodies†	90–98%	94–97%
IgA anti-gliadin antibodies	75–90%	82–95%
IgG anti-gliadin antibodies	69–85%	73–90%

*Wide variations in test sensitivity and specificity are reported among different laboratories.[53]

†Data on tissue transglutaminase antibodies based on two recent large studies.[92, 93]

From Farrell RJ, Kelly CP: Diagnosis of celiac sprue. Am J Gastroenterol 96: 3237–3246, 2001.

Anti-Gliadin Antibodies

Purified gliadin, a component of the wheat storage protein gluten, is readily available and is used as the antigen for enzyme-linked immunosorbent assays to detect serum AGA. Although serum IgA and IgG AGA levels are frequently elevated in untreated celiac sprue and AGA assays have been used for some years as a diagnostic aid, unfortunately, these tests have only moderate sensitivity and specificity.[52, 53, 87, 96] The sensitivity and specificity of IgA AGA is marginally superior to that of IgG AGA. However, many clinicians test simultaneously for both IgA and IgG AGA, an approach that gives a small incremental increase in sensitivity but reduces specificity further. IgG AGA testing is particularly useful in the 1% to 2% of patients with celiac sprue who have IgA deficiency. Unfortunately, the positive predictive value of AGA in a general population is relatively poor. In one series, the positive predictive value of IgG AGA corrected for its expected prevalence in the general population was less than 2%.[94] AGA test results are reported as a titer; a high titer of AGA is somewhat more specific for celiac sprue than a low titer, but as mentioned earlier, some normal persons have high AGA levels.[54]

Clinical Application of Serologic Tests

Clinical applications of serologic tests include evaluating patients with suspected celiac sprue depending on their pretest probability of having the disease, monitoring adherence and response to a gluten-free diet, and possibly screening asymptomatic persons for the disease.

An approach to diagnosing celiac sprue is outlined in Figure 93–5. When the index of suspicion for celiac sprue is low (i.e., the pretest probability is $<5\%$), a negative result for either IgA EMA or IgA anti-tTG has a high negative predictive value and may obviate the need for small bowel biopsy. In this setting, IgA EMA has the highest diagnostic accuracy but is more expensive and less widely available than the test for IgA anti-tTG. The AGA tests have a lower diagnostic accuracy.[53, 90] Because the specificities of IgA EMA and IgA anti-tTG tests are very high, their positive predictive values are high even in low-risk populations.[90, 95] In contrast, the specificities of IgA and IgG AGA are lower, and positive results have a low positive predictive value in low-risk populations.[54, 95]

When the index of suspicion for celiac sprue is moderate to high (i.e., the pretest probability is $>5\%$), the high specificities of IgA EMA and IgA anti-tTG have led to a debate as to whether a positive result in the appropriate clinical setting can be considered diagnostic of celiac sprue and eliminate the need for a small bowel biopsy. However, we recommend that both IgA EMA (or anti-tTG) and a small bowel biopsy are performed before dietary treatment is recommended. This approach provides the best means of making a definitive diagnosis of celiac sprue at the outset. In contrast, AGA tests are not helpful when there is a moderate or high probability of celiac sprue. A positive or negative result will not alter the need for a small bowel biopsy.

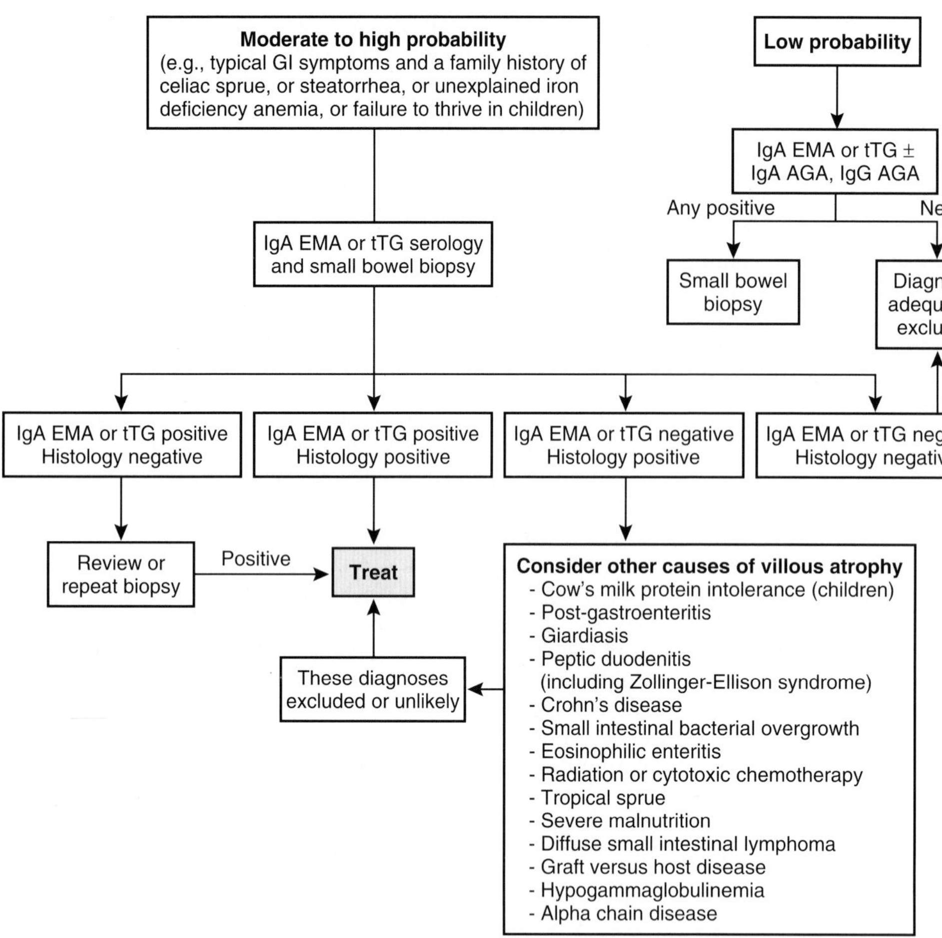

Figure 93–5. Diagnosis of celiac sprue. GI, gastrointestinal; EMA, endomysial antibody; tTG, tissue transglutaminase; AGA, anti–gliadin antibody. False-positive EMA and anti-tTG are rare; false-negative EMA and anti-tTG can occur in mild enteropathy, children younger than 2 years of age, and patients with IgA deficiency. (From Farrell RJ, Kelly CP: Diagnosis of celiac sprue. Am J Gastroenterol 96:3237–3246, 2001.)

Because AGA tests have a high false-positive rate, there is no role for a trial of a gluten-free diet for presumed celiac sprue based on the finding of an elevated IgA or IgG AGA antibody level.

AGA levels decrease during treatment with a gluten-free diet and are useful in assessing dietary compliance and excluding inadvertent gluten ingestion.[52] IgA AGA is currently the most widely used test for monitoring adherence and response to a gluten-free diet among patients whose antibody levels are elevated before therapy.[96] Hence, a pretreatment antibody level should be determined at the time of diagnosis. Serial samples should be sent to a single laboratory for testing to keep interassay variation to a minimum. A normal baseline value is typically reached within 3 to 6 months of treatment (Fig. 93–6). If the levels do not fall as anticipated, the patient may be continuing to ingest gluten either intentionally or inadvertently. However, minor fluctuations in IgA AGA levels are typical, and their importance should not be overinterpreted. Serum IgG AGA, IgA EMA, and anti-tTG antibody levels also fall to normal when patients adhere to a strict gluten-free diet. The decline in IgG AGA is more gradual than that for IgA AGA,[52, 96] whereas the IgA EMA test is more expensive and results more difficult to quantify. There is less experience with IgA anti-tTG assays, but these also may prove to be useful for monitoring adherence to gluten-free diet.

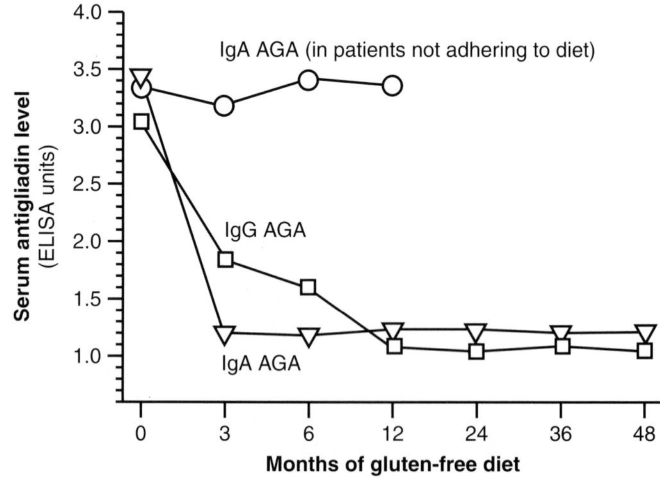

Figure 93–6. Anti–gliadin antibody (AGA) levels decrease during treatment with a gluten-free diet and are useful in assessing dietary compliance and excluding inadvertent gluten ingestion. IgA AGA is the most widely used test for monitoring adherence and response to gluten-free diet among patients whose antibody levels are elevated before therapy. Hence, a pretreatment antibody level should be determined at the time of diagnosis. A normal baseline value is typically reached within 3 to 6 months. If the levels do not fall as anticipated, the patient may be continuing to ingest gluten either intentionally or inadvertently. The decline in IgG AGA is more gradual than that for IgA AGA.[52]

The advent of highly sensitive and specific serologic tests

has led to debate on the merits of screening asymptomatic persons for celiac sprue. To date, the benefit of screening for asymptomatic celiac sprue, usually using IgA EMA, has not been demonstrated.[54, 95, 97] The potential advantages of screening for asymptomatic celiac sprue include a reduction in risk for enteropathy-associated T-cell lymphoma, reversal of unrecognized nutritional deficiencies, resolution of mild or ignored intestinal symptoms, avoidance of other autoimmune disorders, and improvement in general well-being. However, all these hypothetical benefits depend on compliance with a difficult dietary regimen. Asymptomatic persons may not be sufficiently motivated to adhere to a strict gluten-free diet. There also may be adverse psychologic effects when asymptomatic persons receive a diagnosis of celiac sprue. For these reasons, widespread screening of asymptomatic persons is generally not advocated at this time, even in populations in which the prevalence of celiac sprue is high. In contrast, case-finding among at-risk groups, such as first- and second-degree relatives of affected patients or persons with anemia, insulin-dependent diabetes mellitus, autoimmune thyroid disease, connective tissue disease, liver disease, Down's syndrome, or IgA deficiency, is widely accepted.

Radiology

Small bowel barium studies are helpful in evaluating patients suspected of having untreated celiac sprue. Abnormal findings include dilatation of the small intestine, replacement of the normal delicate feathery mucosal pattern with either marked thickening or complete obliteration of the mucosal folds, and straightening of the valvulae conniventes. Even with modern less viscous barium preparations, flocculation, segmentation, and clumping of contrast occasionally may be seen in severe cases. In patients with mild or moderate disease, the distorted mucosal pattern is usually confined to the proximal small intestine, whereas patients with severe disease have an abnormal mucosal pattern throughout the entire small intestine. Excessive secretion of fluid into the proximal small intestine, coupled with defective absorption of intraluminal contents, causes dilution of the barium, resulting in decreased contrast in the distal small intestine. Small bowel studies are most useful in suggesting diagnoses other than celiac sprue, such as Crohn's disease (terminal ileitis), scleroderma (hypotonicity), bacterial overgrowth (small bowel diverticulosis), or collagenous sprue (bowel wall rigidity). Patients with mild celiac sprue may have a normal small bowel barium study, and the study is not as sensitive as small intestinal biopsy or serology in providing diagnostic information. Routine small bowel barium studies are unnecessary in most patients with celiac sprue and may be considered primarily to exclude complications such as lymphoma, carcinoma, ulcerative jejunoileitis, or stricture. Abdominal computed tomography or magnetic resonance imaging may provide diagnostic clues to the presence of celiac sprue or refractory sprue by revealing hyposplenism, ascites, lymphadenopathy, and cavitating mesenteric lymph nodes. Radiographic films of the bones may reveal diffuse demineralization with a generalized decrease in bone density. Occasionally, the secondary effects of osteopenic bone disease, including vertebral compression fractures and pseudofractures (Milkman's lines), are seen.

Small Intestinal Biopsy

Although the diagnosis of celiac sprue may be suspected on clinical grounds or as a result of serologic tests, confirmation of the diagnosis requires a small intestinal biopsy. Since its introduction in the mid-1950s, small intestinal biopsy has remained the standard test to establish a diagnosis of celiac sprue. Originally, biopsy specimens were obtained with a suction biopsy tube using a Crosby-Krugler, Watson, or similar suction biopsy capsule.[9] Although capsule biopsy has the advantage of obtaining relatively large distal duodenal or proximal jejunal biopsies, correct positioning of the capsule is difficult and often time consuming, requires x-ray verification, and is not always successful. Consequently, the technique has generally been abandoned in favor of endoscopic biopsy, particularly for older children and adults. Endoscopic biopsy is now widely available and is indicated anyway for investigation of iron deficiency anemia.[98] Biopsies should be obtained from the distal duodenum (second or third parts) to avoid the mucosal architectural distortion produced by Brunner's glands and changes caused by peptic duodenitis, both of which can confound histopathologic diagnosis of celiac sprue.[9] That endoscopic biopsies are smaller than capsule biopsies can be offset by taking multiple samples. Scalloping or absence of duodenal folds has been noted in some patients with celiac sprue[99] and, if present, should alert the endoscopist to the possible diagnosis. However, scalloping is not specific for celiac sprue. Other conditions that can cause duodenal scalloping include eosinophilic enteritis, giardiasis, tropical sprue, and human immunodeficiency virus enteropathy.[100]

Once obtained, biopsy tissue should be handled carefully so as to avoid artefactual damage. By gently floating the tissue in a small amount of saline, an experienced observer can examine even small endoscopic biopsies using a dissecting microscope or magnifying lens. The villous structure of normal small intestinal mucosa is readily apparent, whereas in severe untreated celiac sprue, a flat featureless mucosa is easily recognized. The mosaic pattern of less complete forms of villous atrophy also may be recognized, although differentiation from normal tissue is difficult and requires experience.

Gluten Challenge

In the past, gluten challenge (discontinuation of treatment with a gluten-free diet) followed by biopsy of the small intestine was considered an important confirmatory step in the diagnosis of celiac sprue. However, current practice is to reserve a gluten challenge for some patients in whom the diagnosis remains doubtful after a period of treatment with a gluten-free diet. Gluten challenge is seldom necessary for patients who present with typical signs or symptoms of celiac sprue and have documented abnormalities consistent with a celiac lesion on small bowel biopsy. A positive IgA EMA or IgA anti-tTG test before treatment lends further support to the diagnosis of celiac sprue and makes a gluten challenge superfluous.

A gluten challenge should be considered in patients who commenced a gluten-free diet empirically without documentation of a characteristic intestinal lesion or the presence of IgA EMA or anti-tTG antibody. In such persons a symptomatic response to a gluten-free diet may indicate the presence of gluten-sensitive enteropathy or may simply reflect a change in gastrointestinal function in response to a major dietary change. Persons with irritable bowel syndrome, for example, may experience improvement in abdominal bloating, cramping, or diarrhea after commencing a gluten-free diet. Such changes in mild nonspecific gastrointestinal symptoms are not a reliable method to diagnose celiac sprue. Gluten challenge also should be considered if a diagnosis of celiac sprue was made during childhood based on small intestinal biopsy abnormalities in the absence of a positive IgA EMA, because a number of transient childhood enteropathies can mimic the celiac lesion (see later).

Before embarking on a gluten challenge, the patient should be evaluated to determine the current response to treatment with a gluten-free diet. The evaluation should include a careful nutritional history, including the symptomatic response to previous episodes of inadvertent or purposeful ingestion of gluten-containing foods. Patients who experience substantial symptoms after ingestion of gluten are unlikely to tolerate a formal gluten challenge and usually prefer to remain on a gluten-free diet despite diagnostic uncertainty. Serologic studies should be performed and a small bowel biopsy obtained as a baseline. A gluten challenge must be initiated with caution because occasional patients are exquisitely sensitive to small amounts of gluten.[101] Other patients may require a prolonged challenge before symptoms or significant histologic abnormalities recur. If a small amount of gluten, such as a cracker or a quarter of a slice of bread, is well tolerated, the amount can be doubled every 3 days until the equivalent of at least four slices of bread is ingested daily. The challenge should then be continued for at least 6 weeks or until symptoms redevelop, at which time both serum IgA EMA and small bowel biopsy should be performed. Ten grams of gluten daily for a period of 6 to 8 weeks is usually sufficient to result in definite histologic deterioration. If the IgA EMA and small bowel biopsy are both negative, the patient should be monitored for symptoms and signs of celiac sprue on a normal diet for at least 6 months, after which IgA EMA should be determined again and repeat biopsy considered.

DIFFERENTIAL DIAGNOSIS

The differential diagnosis of celiac sprue includes other causes of malabsorption and other gastrointestinal disorders that are associated with changes in proximal small bowel morphology. Malabsorption and steatorrhea may result from pancreatic insufficiency, cholestatic liver disease, terminal ileal disease or resection, or small intestinal bacterial overgrowth. In some patients, pancreatic insufficiency may be present concurrently with celiac sprue. Patients who do not respond to a gluten-free diet should be evaluated for this possibility.[102] In adults, celiac sprue is easily distinguished from *Whipple's disease,* which is a multisystem disease, and malabsorption secondary to infiltration of the mucosa with *Mycobacterium avium* complex, because the histologic findings on small intestine biopsy are distinctly different in these diseases.

Although changes in mucosal morphology also can be seen in parasitic infections besides giardia, such as strongyloidiasis, coccidiosis, and hookworm, these changes rarely include villous atrophy. Although villous atrophy is characteristic of untreated celiac sprue, it is by no means pathognomonic and may be seen to varying degrees in a wide variety of other enteric disorders (see Fig. 93–5). Therefore, the finding of villous atrophy on small intestinal biopsy is not sufficient for a diagnosis of celiac sprue. Crypt cell activity, enterocyte characteristics, and the nature of the inflammatory infiltrate also must be examined and in some instances will point toward another diagnosis. For example, patients with *hypogammaglobulinemia* may have an architectural lesion that resembles celiac sprue, but plasma cells are absent or markedly diminished in the lamina propria, not increased as in celiac sprue. After an *acute viral gastroenteritis* the morphologic abnormalities may be indistinguishable from those seen in celiac sprue. In infants and young children, *cow's milk* or *soy protein intolerance* also may result in biopsy findings identical to those of celiac sprue.[103, 104] For this reason morphologic improvement on gluten withdrawal, with subsequent deterioration on gluten rechallenge, forms the basis for a definitive diagnosis of celiac sprue in children. Although soy protein is frequently used as a substitute for milk protein in cow's milk protein intolerance, mucosal abnormalities resembling those of celiac sprue may develop in some children after ingestion of soy protein.[104] In adults, the differential diagnosis is less challenging, and consequently gluten challenge is performed less commonly.

A rare condition that may cause diagnostic confusion with celiac sprue is *collagenous sprue* (see later discussion of refractory sprue). Patients with collagenous sprue may present initially with symptoms and biopsy findings consistent with celiac sprue. However, they fail to respond to gluten withdrawal, and with time extensive deposition of collagen develops in the lamina propria just beneath the absorptive epithelium.[105] The relationship between celiac sprue and both collagenous sprue and the microscopic colitides *(lymphocytic* and *collagenous colitis)* is discussed later.

Finally, in some patients with *potential celiac sprue* diarrhea develops on gluten ingestion, but the small intestinal mucosa is normal or only mildly edematous, with a minimal infiltrate of inflammatory cells. Such gluten-sensitive diarrhea responds to a gluten-free diet, and in many of these patients classic celiac sprue develops subsequently.[106] Other patients have characteristic findings of celiac sprue but fail to respond to a gluten-free diet. In most cases, the problem is the inadvertent presence of gluten in the diet or failure to adhere to a strict gluten-free diet. However, a small number of these patients have refractory sprue or a complication such as lymphoma, ulcerative jejunitis, or collagenous sprue (see later).

DISEASES ASSOCIATED WITH CELIAC SPRUE

A large number of diseases occur with increased frequency among patients with celiac sprue and are outlined in Table 93–3. In addition to an association with autoimmune disorders, many diseases associated with celiac sprue have similar HLA haplotype associations.

Table 93–3 | **Celiac Sprue and Associated Disorders**

DEFINITE ASSOCIATION	POSSIBLE ASSOCIATION
Dermatitis herpetiformis	Congenital heart disease
Insulin-dependent diabetes mellitus	Lung cavities
Thyroid disease	Sjögren's syndrome
IgA deficiency	Systemic and cutaneous vasculitis
Epilepsy with cerebral calcification	Systemic lupus erythematosus
Inflammatory bowel disease	Polymyositis
Microscopic colitides	Myasthenia gravis
IgA mesangial nephropathy	Iridocyclitis or choroiditis
Rheumatoid arthritis	Cystic fibrosis
Sarcoidosis	Macroamylasemia
Down syndrome	Addison's disease
Bird-fancier's lung	Autoimmune thrombocytopenic purpura
Fibrosing alveolitis	Autoimmune hemolytic anemia
Recurrent pericarditis	Schizophrenia
Idiopathic pulmonary hemosiderosis	

From Mulder CJ, Tytgat GN. Coeliac disease and related disorders. Neth J Med 1987;31:286, with permission.

Dermatitis Herpetiformis

Dermatitis herpetiformis (DH) is a skin disease characterized by papulovesicular lesions that occur symmetrically on the extensor surfaces of the extremities and the buttocks, trunk, neck, and scalp. Unlike celiac sprue, DH is rarely diagnosed in childhood but usually presents in early or middle adult life and affects both sexes equally. The rash is intensely pruritic, and intact vesicles may not be present except for the earliest lesions. The diagnosis of DH requires the demonstration by immunoflouoresence studies of granular or speckled IgA deposits in an area of normal skin not affected by blistering.[107] Two thirds of patients have a patchy enteropathy indistinguishable from celiac sprue that may require multiple small intestinal biopsies to demonstrate; the remaining one third have associated features of gluten sensitivity (increased IELs and γ/δ T cells[107] or the induction of villous atrophy with a gluten challenge).[107] DH-associated enteropathy tends to be less severe than that seen in patients with celiac sprue, and less than 10% of patients have intestinal symptoms.[107, 108] However, a 10- to 40-fold increased risk of lymphoma has been reported, similar to the risk in celiac sprue,[109] and most lymphomas occur in patients in whom DH is not controlled by a strict gluten-free diet or in those who have been treated with a gluten-free diet for less than 5 years.[110]

From 5% to 15% of patients with DH-like skin lesions have linear IgA deposits along the dermal–epidermal junction. This condition has been termed linear IgA disease and is distinguished from DH on the basis of its unique immunofluorescent finding, the presence of circulating IgA anti-basement membrane antibody, which binds to a 97-kDa protein found in normal human skin,[111] the absence of circulating IgA EMA[56] or antibodies to tTG,[112] different HLA susceptibility genes, and, most importantly, the lack of an associated gluten-sensitive enteropathy.

The pathogenesis of DH remains unknown. It has been suggested that antibodies form in the small intestinal mucosa as a result of stimulation by gluten and that these antibodies are carried through the circulation and bind at the dermoepidermal junction, resulting in the characteristic skin lesions. Elevated circulating levels of IgA, lowered levels of IgM, and variable changes in IgG occur in DH, as in celiac sprue. Similarly, the frequency of HLA-DQ2, HLA-B8, and HLA-DR3 and of circulating AGA, anti-reticulin antibody, and EMA parallels those observed in patients with celiac sprue without DH.[107] Although patients with DH have IgA antibodies to tTG confirming the pathogenic relationship between DH and celiac sprue, the frequency of antibodies to tTG in DH (75%) is lower than that found in celiac sprue (95% to 98%) and, as for EMA, reflects the milder enteropathy in DH.[113]

Thus, DH and celiac sprue appear to be distinct diseases with the curious relationship that more than 80% of patients with DH also have at least latent celiac sprue, whereas less than 10% of patients with celiac sprue have DH. Treatment with dapsone in a dose of 1 to 2 mg/kg/day is effective in DH and often diagnostic in its ability to heal the associated rash and relieve the pruritus rapidly, but the enteropathy associated with DH does not improve with dapsone. However, 6 to 12 months of gluten withdrawal usually reverses both the intestinal and skin lesions in most patients with DH, and a strict gluten-free diet allows most patients to reduce or discontinue dapsone.[114] As for celiac sprue, patients with DH can include moderate amounts of oats in their gluten-free diet without deleterious effects to the skin or intestine.[115]

Other Disease Associations

There is an established association between celiac sprue and insulin-dependent diabetes mellitus (IDDM), reflecting in part the increased frequency of the DQ alleles in patients with IDDM. The frequency of celiac sprue in patients with IDDM ranges from 3% to 6%.[116–118] One Irish study reported a frequency of 8%,[119] suggesting that in areas where celiac sprue is particularly prevalent, consideration should be given to screening patients with IDDM for EMA. Although most patients with celiac sprue and IDDM are asymptomatic with regard to the sprue, unexpected episodes of hypoglycemia or diarrhea should alert clinicians to the possibility of coexisting celiac sprue. Unfortunately, control of diabetes in these persons can be difficult because of variable nutrient absorption. There also is a high frequency of autoimmune thyroid disease among patients with celiac sprue; hypothyroidism is seen more commonly than hyperthyroidism.[120] Celiac sprue also may be associated with a variety of other connective tissue diseases,[121] including systemic lupus erythematosus,[122] Sjögren's syndrome,[123] and polymyositis.[124] Although the relationship between celiac sprue and many autoimmune disorders has been explained by shared genetic factors, a recent multicenter study demonstrated that the frequency of autoimmune disorders increases with increasing age at diagnosis of celiac sprue, a finding that suggests that the duration of exposure to gluten is an important factor in the development of associated autoimmune diseases.[125]

Although many patients with celiac sprue exhibit lactose and sucrose intolerance at the time of diagnosis, only a small percentage have persistent disaccharidase deficiency after gluten withdrawal. These patients experience abdominal

Table 93–4 | **Principles of Initial Dietary Therapy for Patients with Celiac Sprue**

Avoid all foods containing wheat, rye, and barley gluten.
Avoid all oats initially.
Use only rice, corn, maize, buckwheat, potato, soybean, or tapioca flours, meals, or starches.
Wheat starch from which gluten has been removed can be tried after the diagnosis is established.
Read all labels and study ingredients of processed foods.
Beware of gluten in medications, food additives, emulsifiers, or stabilizers.
Limit milk and milk products initially.
Avoid all beers, lagers, ales, and stouts.
Wine, liqueurs, ciders, and spirits, including whiskey and brandy, are allowed.

From Trier JS. Celiac sprue and refractory sprue. In Feldman M, Scharschmidt BF, Sleisenger MH (eds): Gastrointestinal and Liver Disease. Philadelphia; W.B. Saunders, 1998:1557; with permission.

pain and diarrhea with lactose or sucrose intake and usually can be diagnosed by a sugar tolerance test or hydrogen breath test. If concomitant disaccharidase deficiency is present, the relevant disaccharide should be excluded from the diet. Selective IgA deficiency occurs 10 times as often in patients with celiac sprue as in the general population, and as many as 2% of patients are IgA deficient.[126] Hyposplenism and splenic atrophy have been noted in approximately 50% of patients with celiac sprue; the frequency increases with advancing age, duration of exposure to dietary gluten, and disease activity.[74] The underlying mechanism is unknown, but affected patients are at increased risk of developing bacterial infections[127] and should take antibiotics prophylactically for invasive manipulations, including dental procedures, and may benefit from pneumococcal vaccination.

Evidence also supports associations between celiac sprue and inflammatory bowel disease, particularly ulcerative proctitis,[128] chronic hepatitis,[129] sclerosing cholangitis,[129] primary biliary cirrhosis,[129] IgA nephropathy,[130] interstitial lung disease including chronic fibrosing alveolitis[131] and idiopathic pulmonary hemosiderosis,[132] and Down's syndrome.[133]

Finally, there is the curious but well-established relationship between celiac sprue and the microscopic colitides (see also Chapter 118).[134] Mild to moderate small intestinal lymphocytosis, and occasionally partial or subtotal villous atrophy, is common in patients with either lymphocytic or collagenous colitis,[135] whereas mild colonic lymphocytosis occurs in patients with untreated celiac sprue.[136] Rectal gluten challenge in patients with celiac sprue has been shown to induce a mild proctitis characterized by lymphocytosis of the rectal lamina propria and epithelium.[137] Furthermore, a gluten-free diet has been reported to be an effective therapy in some patients with refractory collagenous colitis.[138] The recent demonstration that patients with celiac sprue and microscopic colitis share a set of predisposing HLA-DQ genes[139] underscores the overlap between both diseases. However, in most patients with celiac sprue, colonic lymphocytosis can be distinguished from lymphocytic colitis by the lack of surface epithelial abnormalities, lack of increased cellularity of the lamina propria, and lack of ongoing watery diarrhea after treatment with a gluten-free diet. Confusion also can arise because patients with refractory sprue have a higher frequency of colonic lymphocytosis than do patients with celiac sprue. Although these changes are virtually indistinguishable histologically from lymphocytic colitis, important immunohistochemical differences exist: Most colonic IELs in lymphocytic colitis are CD8+, whereas those in the colonic lymphocytosis of refractory sprue rarely are CD8+.[102]

TREATMENT

Gluten-Free Diet

Removal of gluten from the diet is essential for patients with celiac sprue (Table 93–4). The importance of gluten withdrawal was established in the early 1950s when the toxicity of wheat protein in children with celiac sprue was demonstrated.[6, 7] In 1962, Rubin and colleagues[30] showed that instillation of wheat, barley, and rye flour into histologically normal-appearing small intestine of persons with treated celiac sprue rapidly induced sprue-like symptoms, which were accompanied by the development of the typical lesions of celiac sprue in the exposed mucosa.

In reality, complete dietary elimination of all gluten-containing cereal grains is difficult for most patients to achieve and maintain. Gluten is present in a wide variety of processed foods, because wheat flour is widely used in the food industry as a thickener and inexpensive filler in many commercial products, precooked meals, and convenience foods, including ice cream, pasta, sausages, fish sticks, cheese spreads, salad dressings, soups, sauces, mixed seasonings, mincemeat for mince pies, and some medications[140] and vitamin preparations. Wheat flour also is contained in some brands of instant coffee, ketchup, mustard, and most candy bars, to give only a few examples (Table 93–5). Listings of gluten-free products have been drawn up, and a gluten-free symbol (a crossed ear of wheat) has been devised and is widely used by food manufacturers in Europe but, unfortunately, less often in the United States. Although gluten-free wheat is available for baking, grains that are naturally free of gluten can become contaminated with wheat, particularly when mills use the same production lines and equipment to process both gluten-containing and gluten-free products. All beers, lagers, ales, and stouts should be avoided, but wines, liqueurs, ciders, and spirits, including brandy as well as malt and scotch whiskey, can be consumed. Helpful recipes and

Table 93–5 | **Representative Foods that May or May Not Contain Gluten, Depending on Manufacturer**

Ice cream	Chip and dip mixes
Nondairy creamer	Luncheon meats
Yogurts and fruit	Wieners and sausage products
Hot chocolates	Processed canned meats and poultry
Instant coffee and tea	Meat sauces (soy, Worcestershire, etc.)
Bouillon cubes	Mustard
Soup mixes	Ketchup
Canned soups	Tomato sauce
Salad dressings	Peanut butter
Cheese spreads	Mixed seasonings

From Trier JS. Celiac sprue and refractory sprue. In Feldman M, Scharschmidt BF, Sleisenger MH (eds): Gastrointestinal and Liver Disease. Philadelphia; W.B. Saunders, 1998:1557; with permission.

detailed instructions regarding gluten-free diets have been published in excellent inexpensive books that are of great value to patients with celiac sprue.[141] National celiac societies in many countries publish regularly updated handbooks that list the available gluten-free products, but it is important for patients to remember that food lists are applicable for use only in the country in which they were compiled. Similar foods with well-known brand names may be made under franchise using slightly different recipes in different countries and may be gluten-free in one country but not in others. Consequently, patient education is crucial, and the institution of an effective gluten-free diet requires extensive and repeated instruction of the patient by the physician and dietitian, as well as motivated and discerning label-reading by the patient (see www.celiac.com).

There is considerable variation in the ability of patients with celiac sprue to tolerate gluten. Some patients can ingest small amounts of gluten without developing symptoms. Others are exquisitely sensitive to the ingestion of even minute amounts of gluten and may develop massive watery diarrhea reminiscent of acute cholera within hours of eating a small piece of bakery bread. Occasionally, the diarrhea may be so severe that it can induce acute dehydration, termed *gliadin shock*.[101]

Patients with untreated celiac sprue may have accompanying lactase deficiency secondary to damage to the surface epithelial cells. Therefore, milk and milk products should be avoided at the initiation of a gluten-free diet. However, after a response to the diet, these products can be reintroduced, if they are tolerated. It is now apparent that moderate amounts of oats, at least in the short term, are not toxic in patients with celiac sprue. In a carefully conducted randomized, controlled, clinical trial, adults with celiac sprue who consumed 50 to 70 g oats/day for 6 to 12 months did not differ with regard to symptoms, nutritional status, or duodenal mucosal histology from patients maintained on an oat-restricted gluten-free diet.[142] Patients with DH also can include moderate amounts of oats in their gluten-free diet without deleterious effects to the skin or intestine.[115] A recent open-label study showed that a 6-month trial of commercial oat breakfast cereal was safe for children beginning a gluten-free diet for newly diagnosed celiac sprue.[143] However, oat products obtained from the grocery store shelf may be contaminated with small amounts of other grains, especially wheat. Therefore, oats should be avoided initially in all newly diagnosed patients until remission is achieved on a strict gluten-free diet. Subsequently, up to 2 ounces of oats per day from a reliable source can be introduced and continued if tolerated. The long-term safety of oats in patients with celiac sprue is unknown.

Because a gluten-free diet represents a life-long commitment for patients with celiac sprue, is more expensive than a normal diet, and carries a social liability, especially in children and teenagers, such a diet should not be undertaken casually as a therapeutic trial. Rather, the diagnosis of celiac sprue should be established first by serologic studies and small intestinal biopsy. Thereafter, institution of a gluten-free diet serves two functions: treatment, followed by clinical improvement, and confirmation of the histologic diagnosis of celiac sprue.

After starting a gluten-free diet, most patients improve symptomatically within a few weeks. In many, symptomatic improvement is noticed within 48 hours, although weeks or months may be needed for full clinical remission. Pink and Creamer[144] reported that 70% of patients with celiac sprue begun on a gluten-free diet returned quickly to normal health and reported improvement in their symptoms within 2 weeks. The speed and ultimate degree of histologic improvement are unpredictable but invariably lag behind the clinical response. Although an increase in enterocyte height may be evident within one week of gluten withdrawal, the return of villous architecture toward normal takes considerably longer and may not be evident on repeat biopsy for 2 or 3 months. In some patients, histologic improvement may take up to 2 years.[31] Although a return to normal is common in children, in approximately 50% of adults on a gluten-free diet, biopsies show a partial improvement, and the less severely damaged distal intestine recovers more rapidly than the maximally damaged proximal intestine.[145]

If a patient fails to improve on a gluten-free diet, either the diet is inadequate or the mucosal lesion is a result of another disease that causes villous atrophy. A less likely explanation is that the patient has refractory sprue. Dietary failure is not always the cause of persistent symptoms. Other disorders such as irritable bowel syndrome, lactose intolerance, or pancreatic insufficiency may coexist with celiac sprue.[102] In the study by Pink and Creamer,[144] 30% of patients who failed to respond to a gluten-free diet fell into three groups. Patients in the first group experienced progressive clinical deterioration, which was halted in some cases by treatment with glucocorticoids, but which progressed to death in others. Patients in the second group had an associated pancreatic disorder. Those in the third group were poorly compliant with a strict gluten-free diet, but even when this problem was addressed, their minor abdominal symptoms, including diarrhea, persisted in some cases.

Immunosuppressive Therapy

In vitro studies have shown that the addition of glucocorticoids prevents the harmful effects of gluten on biopsies from patients with celiac sprue.[146] In addition to anti-inflammatory effects, glucocorticoids may also exert a local beneficial effect on the mucosal transport of water and sodium.[147] Although patients with celiac sprue can be treated with glucocorticoids with rapid improvement in symptoms, the effect rarely persists once the drug is stopped.[148] Therefore, glucocorticoids are not indicated in the routine management of celiac sprue but are reserved for severely ill patients who present with acute celiac crisis manifested by severe diarrhea, dehydration, weight loss, acidosis, hypocalcemia, and hypoproteinemia.[149] These few patients may benefit from a short course of glucocorticoids until the gluten-free diet takes effect. Glucocorticoids also can be used in rare instances of gliadin shock that occur in occasional treated patients who are subjected to a gluten challenge.[101]

Glucocorticoids may also be necessary in patients with refractory sprue (see later). Azathioprine or 6-mercaptopurine can be used as glucocorticoid-sparing agents if a dose of 10 mg prednisone or more per day is required to keep the condition under control.[150] Although cyclosporine therapy has been reported to be life-saving in occasional patients with refractory sprue-like disease and may result in reversal of glucocorticoid resistance, its efficacy remains unproven.[151, 152]

Supplemental Therapy

In addition to a gluten-free diet, patients with severe celiac sprue should receive appropriate supplemental therapy to help correct nutritional deficiencies caused by malabsorption. Anemic patients should receive supplemental iron and folate. Rarely, treatment with vitamin B_{12} may be required. Patients with purpura, bruising, or bleeding may have a prolonged prothrombin time and may require supplemental vitamin K. Patients with severe diarrhea and dehydration require vigorous intravenous replacement of fluids and electrolytes. Intravenous calcium gluconate, 1 to 2 g, should be administered promptly to patients with tetany. If there is no response, the tetany may be caused by hypomagnesemia and require magnesium replacement.

All patients with hypocalcemia or with clinical or radiologic evidence of osteopenic bone disease should receive oral calcium supplementation equivalent to 2 to 3 g of elemental calcium per day and oral vitamin D or 25-hyroxyvitamin D. All patients with significant steatorrhea should receive supplemental calcium and vitamin D to help prevent mobilization of skeletal calcium until the malabsorption has responded to gluten withdrawal. There is evidence that strict adherence to a gluten-free diet protects against further bone loss and is associated initially with an increase in bone mineral denisty.[153] However, although gluten withdrawal for 1 year has been shown to reverse osteopenia in most patients, including postmenopausal women and patients with incomplete mucosal recovery,[154] patients who have secondary hyperparathyroidism at the time celiac sprue is diagnosed tend to have more refractory osteopenic bone disease, and their bone mineral density may not normalize even after several years of gluten withdrawal.[155] The serum calcium level must be monitored in patients on supplemental calcium, and supplementation must be discontinued promptly if hypercalcemia develops. There are no specific data on the role of bisphosphonates in osteopenic bone disease complicating celiac sprue.

Vitamin A, thiamine, riboflavin, niacin, pyridoxine, vitamin C, and vitamin E, in the form of a multivitamin preparation, should probably be administered to patients with newly diagnosed celiac sprue and clinically evident malabsorption. However, there is no need for long-term supplementation of these vitamins once intestinal absorption has normalized. Some patients have experienced symptomatic improvement with correction of magnesium, copper, and zinc deficiency.[156] Finally, drugs, like nutrients, may be absorbed inconsistently by the intestine in patients with severe celiac sprue. Medications considered essential for the patient's well-being may need to be administered parenterally until intestinal absorption improves in response to treatment with a gluten-free diet.

COMPLICATIONS

Malignancy, ulcerative jejunoileitis, and collagenous sprue are major complications of celiac sprue. The incidence of *malignant disease* is approximately twofold greater in adults with celiac sprue than in the general population. Although two early studies reported that malignancy develops in approximately 10% to 15% of patients with celiac sprue,[157, 158] a more recent study of 335 adults with celiac sprue reported that the incidence of malignancy was closer to 3% during a mean follow-up of 5 years.[118] Small intestinal lymphoma, often multifocal and diffuse, accounts for more than one half of these malignancies and typically occurs after 20 to 40 years of celiac sprue (see Chapter 26).[159] Whereas most small intestinal lymphomas in the general population are of B-cell origin, intestinal lymphoma complicating celiac sprue is usually of T-cell origin,[160] and the term enteropathy-associated T-cell lymphoma (EATL) was coined to describe both intestinal and extraintestinal lymphomas that complicate celiac sprue. The clinical onset of EATL may be insidious, and the initial presentation and small bowel biopsy appearance mimic those of untreated celiac sprue. EATL is commonly accompanied by nonspecific mucosal ulceration, similar to that seen in *ulcerative jejunoileitis,* and these ulcers may be the only endoscopic manifestation of lymphoma (see Chapter 106). Although some patients with EATL may have a partial or temporary response to a strict gluten-free diet, most are unresponsive to gluten withdrawal. In patients previously controlled on a gluten-free diet, the recurrence of gastrointestinal symptoms such as abdominal pain, weight loss, diarrhea, and intestinal bleeding should raise the clinical suspicion of lymphoma. In some patients with frank lymphoma, mucosal histology adjacent to and distant from the lymphoma is indistinguishable from that of untreated celiac sprue yet unresponsive to gluten withdrawal.[161] There is a long-standing controversy as to whether such patients have latent celiac sprue that becomes evident after lymphoma has developed, refractory sprue complicated by lymphoma, or refractory enteropathy induced by primary intestinal T-cell lymphoma and indistinguishable by histologic criteria from celiac sprue.[162] Recent molecular and immunohistochemical studies that have advanced our understanding of the relationship between celiac sprue, refractory sprue, and EATL are discussed in the section on refractory sprue.

Other features that suggest lymphoma include intestinal obstruction or bleeding, fever, hypoalbuminemia, lymphadenopathy, and erythrophagocytosis. Small bowel radiology, small bowel enteroscopy with biopsy of the mucosa at multiple levels, and computed tomography may help confirm the diagnosis. Mesenteric lymphadenopathy with central cavitation has been described in patients with celiac sprue, both with[163] and without[164] concurrent lymphoma. If the index of suspicion for lymphoma is high and the studies listed above are not diagnostic, full-thickness biopsy specimens of the small intestine should be obtained at laparoscopy or laparotomy with careful examination of the entire length of the small bowel and examination of mesenteric lymph nodes. Even with such an aggressive approach, EATL can be extremely difficult to diagnose. EATL is commonly fatal, with overall 1-year and 5-year survival rates of 31% and 11%, respectively, reported in one small series; long-term survival was confined almost exclusively to patients treated with chemotherapy.[165]

Carcinoma, particularly of the oropharynx, esophagus, and small intestine, accounts for more than one half of the remaining malignancies that may complicate celiac sprue. The average age of affected patients is greater than 50

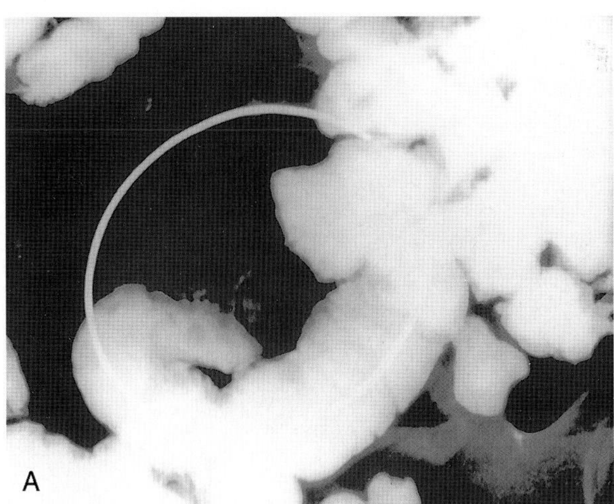

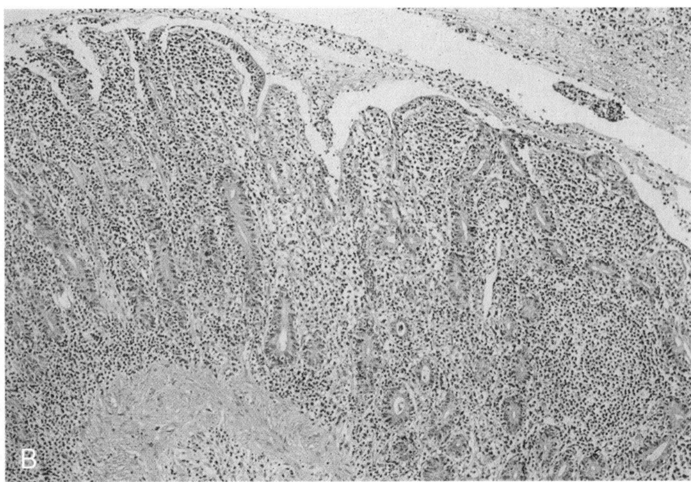

Figure 93–7. Ulcerative jejunoileitis complicating celiac sprue. *A,* Small bowel barium contrast study from a patient with celiac sprue showing a segmental area of fixed narrowing with associated mucosal distortion and ulceration in the distal jejunum/proximal ileum. *B,* Resection specimen histology showing ulcerated mucosa with adjacent diffuse villous atrophy with lymphocytic infiltrate consistent with celiac sprue. Lymphocyte infiltrate within the epithelium and lamina propria were positive for T cell antigen (CD3). Histology from the ulcerated area did not identify overt lymphoma. Southern blot analysis revealed clonal TCR gene rearrangements in both the involved and uninvolved small intestine and an adjacent mesenteric lymph node consistent with cryptic enteropathy-associated T cell lymphoma. (TCR, T cell receptor.)

years. The mechanisms responsible for the increased frequency of malignancy are unknown. Increased intestinal crypt mitotic activity, increased turnover of lymphoid cells in the mucosa, penetration of the damaged jejunal mucosa by carcinogens, infection with oncogenic viruses, and underlying abnormalities in the mucosal immune system and surface epithelium are all potential factors. Evidence that strict adherence to a gluten-free diet reduces the risk of all malignancies, not just EATL, is provided by a single study.[109] Although further studies are awaited, it seems prudent to recommend life-long strict adherence to gluten-free diet in all patients with celiac sprue, hopefully to reduce the risk of malignancy.

Ulcerative jejunoileitis, also known as chronic nongranulomatous ulcerative enterocolitis or nongranulomatous jejunitis, is a rare but serious complication of celiac sprue and is characterized by ulceration and strictures of the small intestine (see Chapter 106). Whether ulcerative jejunoileitis is truly a discrete entity has been questioned, because lymphoma is ultimately diagnosed in many patients with ulcerative jejunoileitis.[167] Indeed, ulcerative jejunoileitis in association with EATL was previously designated malignant histiocytosis. Ulcerative jejunoileitis should be suspected in patients with celiac sprue who present with abdominal pain, weight loss, and diarrhea that does not respond to a gluten-free diet. Typically, patients experience recurrent episodes of intestinal ulceration and obstruction with gradual weight loss despite surgery and strict adherence to a gluten-free diet. Areas of intestinal ulceration and stricture formation typically cause obstruction and hemorrhage (Fig. 93–7). Intestinal perforation with peritonitis may also occur. The diagnosis is made by small bowel radiography, abdominal CT, or, most frequently, laparotomy. Although some patients may respond to a gluten-free diet, surgical excision of the most severely affected segments of small bowel has proved to be the most effective treatment. There is a high risk of transition to diffuse or multifocal EATL, and there are few well-documented cases of celiac sprue and localized jejunoileitis in which no evidence of malignant disease develops and which respond to either surgical resection or therapy with glucocorticoids and azathioprine.[168] However, even in the absence of malignant transformation, the 5-year survival rate for patients with ulcerative jejunoileitis is less than 50%.

Collagenous sprue is characterized by the development of a subepithelial collagen band thicker than 10 μm in the small intestine (Fig. 93–8). Although collagenous sprue has been regarded as an entity distinct from celiac sprue,[105] deposition of collagen under the intestinal epithelial cells has been noted in up to 36% of patients with classic celiac sprue.[169] Furthermore, there are several reports of patients with collagenous sprue who have EMA[170] and complications of refractory sprue, specifically ulcerative jejunoileitis[171] and lymphoma.[162] Although persons with collagenous sprue are frequently refractory to therapy for celiac sprue, the presence of subepithelial collagen does not a priori preclude a successful response to gluten withdrawal.[169, 172] Collagenous sprue should be distinguished from collagenous colitis, which rarely may accompany celiac sprue and should be considered in the differential diagnosis of refractory sprue.[173] In contrast to both celiac sprue and collagenous colitis, the prognosis in collagenous sprue is grim; most reported patients die of the disease.

REFRACTORY SPRUE

Refractory sprue, also known as unclassified or intractable celiac sprue, is defined as symptomatic severe small intestinal villous atrophy that mimics celiac sprue but does not respond primarily or secondarily to a strict gluten-free diet for at least 6 months and is not explained by other causes of villous atrophy or overt intestinal lymphoma.[3] Refractory sprue is uncommon and is largely a diagnosis of exclusion (Fig. 93–9). Symptoms may persist in patients with treated

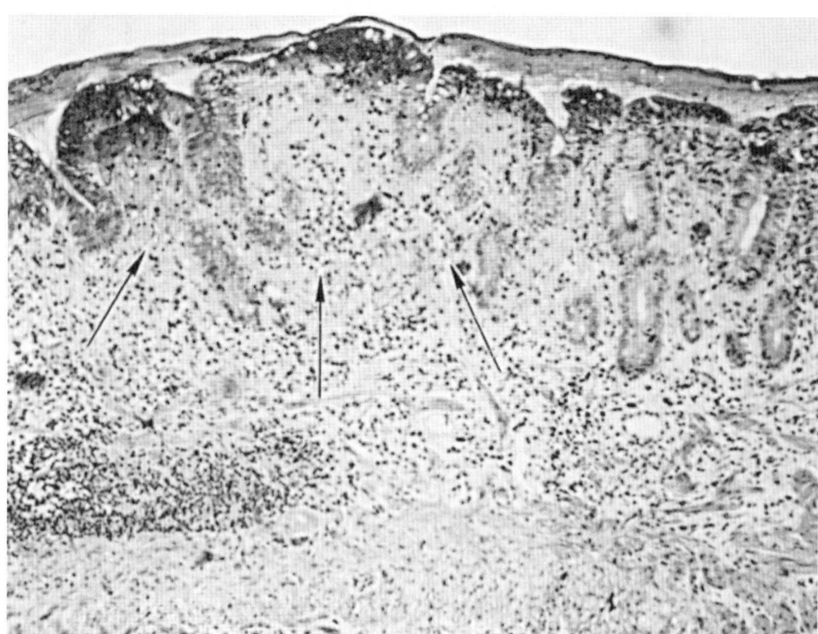

Figure 93–8. The histologic appearance of jejunal mucosa from a patient with collagenous sprue. Note the deposition of collagen in the lamina propria, particularly beneath the absorptive epithelium *(arrows)*. Crypts are decreased in number. Masson trichrome stain. (Magnification, ×80.) (Reprinted with permission. Courtesy of the late L.L. Brandborg, M.D., San Francisco.)

celiac sprue for a variety of reasons, the commonest of which is lack of strict adherence to a gluten-free diet, often because of inadvertent ingestion of dietary gluten.[174] Other causes of villous atrophy should be excluded, as should coexisting conditions such as disaccharidase deficiency, bacterial overgrowth, pancreatic insufficiency, inflammatory bowel disease, and the microscopic colitides. Trials of exclusion diets should be considered to uncover protein enteropathies to milk, egg, or soy.[175]

In patients with celiac sprue and no demonstrable cause for nonresponsiveness to a gluten-free diet, a variety of treatments (based mostly on small uncontrolled studies) have been described, including elimination diets, dietary supplementation with zinc and copper,[156] and immunosuppressive therapy. Evidence supporting the use of immunosuppressive therapy in the treatment of refractory sprue is based mainly on anecdotal reports, and to date no controlled trials have been performed.[176] Some patients with refractory sprue have responded to treatment with glucocorticoids, whereas others have responded to immunosuppressive drugs such as azathioprine[150] and cyclosporine.[152, 177] In a recent open pilot study in 13 adult patients with refractory celiac sprue treated for 2 months with oral cyclosporine in doses titrated to achieve serum levels of 100 to 200 ng/mL, small intestinal histology improved in 8 patients (61%), with normalization of villi in 5 (38%). Although a trial of immunosuppressive therapy is worth considering in all patients with refractory sprue, caution must be used, because these patients are often malnourished, have hyposplenism, and may be prone to opportunistic infections.[150] Unfortunately, in some patients, there is only a partial or no response to immunosuppressive therapy, and the clinical course is characterized by progressive malabsorption necessitating total parenteral nutrition.

It has long been appreciated that patients with refractory sprue are at high risk for uncommon but frequently fatal complications, such as lymphoma, ulcerative jejunoileitis, and collagenous sprue. Until recently, the precise link between refractory sprue and these complications and between refractory sprue and celiac sprue was controversial. The spectrum of autoimmune enteropathy was implicated in a handful of adult patients with refractory sprue by the presence of anti-enterocyte antibodies.[152, 178] However, it is now becoming clear that refractory sprue, EATL, ulcerative jejunoileitis, and possibly collagenous sprue represent a heterogeneous but related group of clinical conditions at the extreme end of the celiac sprue spectrum. There is a growing realization that many patients with refractory sprue have a cryptic intestinal T-cell lymphoma characterized by phenotypically abnormal IELs that have monoclonal rearrangements of the T-cell receptor γ gene (see also Chapters 26 and 106).[162]

Early immunophenotypic studies demonstrated that the normal cellular counterpart of EATL was the IEL.[161] However, not until 1995 did Murray and colleagues[179] make the remarkable observation that nonlymphomatous mucosa in patients with overt EATL contains histologically undetected cells with a monoclonal T cell receptor gene rearrangement identical to that seen in overt lymphoma, and the term *cryptic intestinal T-cell lymphoma* was coined. Ashton-Key and colleagues[180] later confirmed this finding and showed that both the inflammatory ulcers and the intact (nonlymphomatous) mucosa in cases of ulcerative jejunoileitis harbor a monoclonal T-cell population and that lymphomas that later develop in these patients consist of the identical T-cell clone. Cellier and colleagues[65] showed that the IELs in patients with refractory sprue make up a monoclonal population that lack the expression of CD8+ found consistently on most normal or celiac sprue IELs. Subsequent work showed that the monoclonal IELs in ulcerative jejunoileitis and nonlymphomatous mucosa in EATL share not only the genotype but also the immunophenotype of the lymphoma.[181] Recently, Cellier and colleagues[162] detected aberrant clonal IELs (similar to those in most cases of EATL) in 16 of 19 (84%) patients with refractory sprue, 7 (37%) of whom had collagenous sprue, 6 (32%) of whom had ulcerative jejunoileitis, 6 (32%) of whom had mesenteric lymph node cavitation, and 3 (16%) of whom developed overt EATL that was clonally identical to the IELs of the preexisting refractory

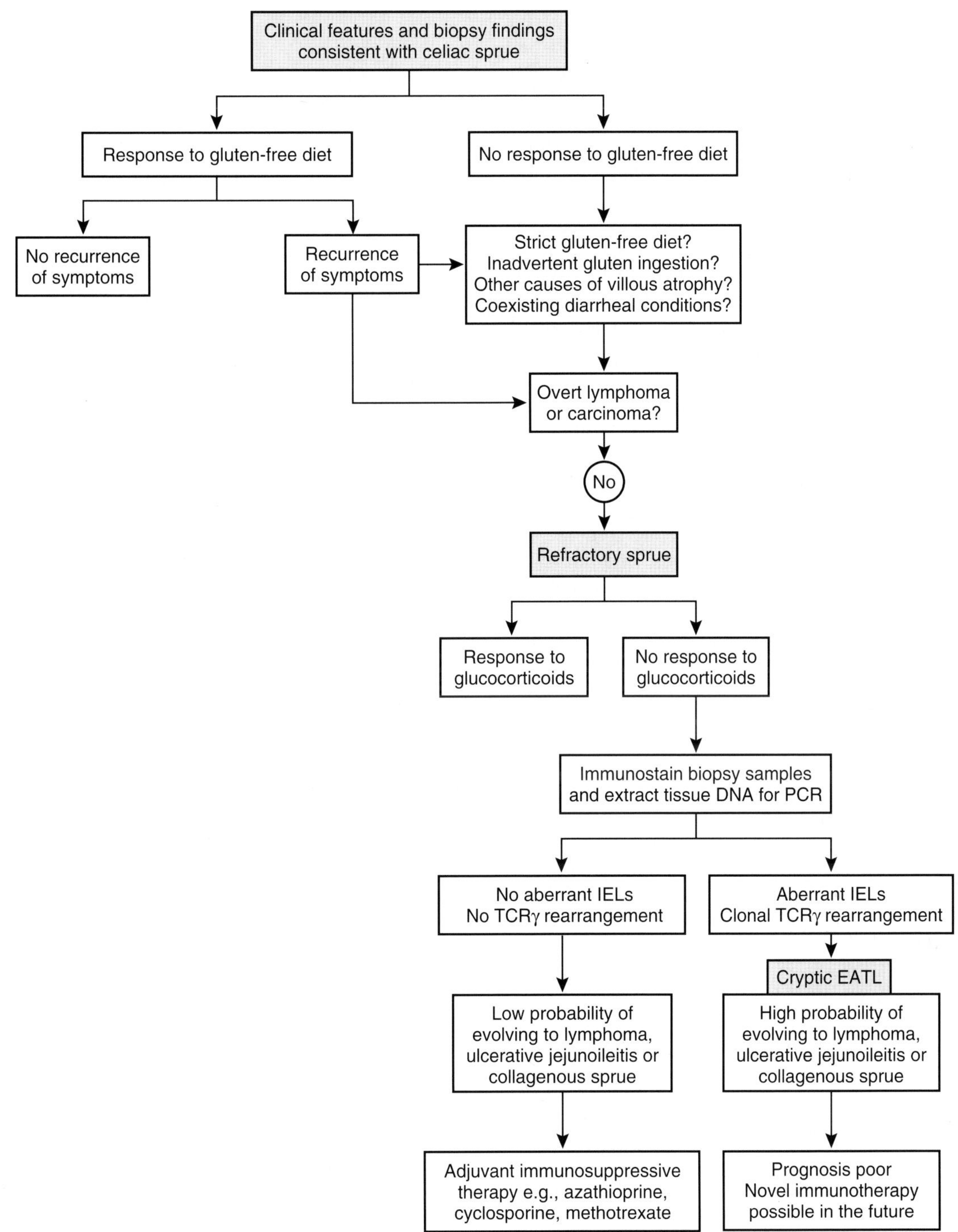

Figure 93–9. Approach to diagnosis and management of refractory sprue. TCR, T-cell receptor; PCR, polymerase chain reaction; IEL, intraepithelial lymphocyte; EATL, enteropathy-associated T-cell lymphoma.

sprue. All three (16%) patients without aberrant clonal IELs made a complete clinical and histologic recovery with glucocorticoid therapy and a gluten-free diet. Thus, the cumulative evidence suggests that refractory sprue is a manifestation of an aberrant clonal IEL-mediated neoplastic process. These clonal IEL cells have destructive properties, possibly related to their cytotoxic phenotype, which leads to mucosal ulceration and lymph-node cavitation. Sometimes, but not always, the cells undergo molecular and clinical progression to lymphoma. On the basis of this evidence, T-cell receptor and monoclonal antibody studies should be performed on small bowel biopsy samples from patients with refractory sprue (see Fig. 93–9). In the future, early recognition of the malignant potential of the intestinal infiltrate may permit curative surgery or the development of effective chemotherapeutic regimens.

PROGNOSIS

Celiac sprue has an excellent prognosis if patients are diagnosed early and adhere to a life-long gluten-free diet. Conversely, if the disease is not recognized and treated properly, marked malnutrition and debilitation may develop, and patients may die of complications such as intercurrent infection or hemorrhage. Earlier studies reported 1.9-fold[182] and 3.4-fold[183] increases in mortality in patients with celiac sprue, but these studies lacked patients with latent celiac sprue and included patients who were not adhering to a gluten-free diet or who had refractory sprue and intestinal lymphoma. A study of 335 adults from Finland with celiac sprue, at least 83% of whom adhered strictly to a gluten-free diet, showed that 5-year survival was comparable with that of the general population.[118] Growth and development in infants and children proceed normally with continued gluten withdrawal. In adults, intestinal absorptive function usually returns to normal, and many manifestations of disease disappear after a gluten-free diet is initiated. However, complications of the disease, such as peripheral neuropathy, ataxia, or pathologic fractures secondary to severe osteopenic bone disease, particularly in the setting of secondary hyperparathyroidism, may not be completely reversible.

Several lines of evidence suggest that celiac sprue is not always a life-long condition. First, among children with proven celiac sprue who are followed long term, latent celiac sprue develops in 10% to 20% who become "tolerant" (defined on clinical, biologic, and histologic grounds) to gluten during adolescence. Second, the mucosal lesions typical of celiac sprue may appear de novo during adulthood.[184] However, the factors leading to the appearance or disappearance of gluten-sensitive enteropathy are still unknown. Although adolescent patients may stray from a gluten-free diet, often without apparent ill effects, they remain unable to tolerate gluten, and many asymptomatic adolescent patients have persistent hematologic, biochemical, and morphologic abnormalities.[76] If ingestion of gluten continues into adult life, clinical evidence of celiac sprue recurs in most of these patients. Therefore, patients with unequivocal evidence of celiac sprue in childhood should be encouraged to remain on a gluten-free diet indefinitely, if recurrent clinical disease is to be avoided during adult life.

REFERENCES

1. Trier JS. Diagnosis of celiac sprue. Gastroenterology 115:211, 1998.
2. Arranz E, Ferguson A. Intestinal antibody pattern of celiac disease: occurrence in patients with normal jejunal biopsy histology [see comments]. Gastroenterology 104:1263, 1993.
3. Trier JS, Falchuk ZM, Carey MC, et al. Celiac sprue and refractory sprue. Gastroenterology 75:307, 1978.
4. Adams F. The Extant Works of Aretaeus of Cappodocian. London, Sydenham Society, 1856.
5. Gee S. On the coeliac affection. St Barth Hosp Rep 24:17, 1888.
6. Dicke W. Coeliac Disease: Investigation of Harmful Effects of Certain Types of Cereal on Patients with Coeliac Disease. The Netherlands, University of Utrecht, 1950.
7. van de Kamer JH, Weijers HA, Dicke WK. Coeliac disease. IV. An investigation into the injurious constituents of wheat in connection with their action in patients with coeliac disease. Acta Paediatr 42: 223, 1953.
8. Paulley L. Observations on the aetiology of idiopathic steatorrhea. BMJ 2:1318, 1954.
9. Rubin CE, Brandborg LL, Phelps PC, et al. Studies of celiac disease. I. The apparent identical and specific nature of the duodenal and proximal jejunal lesion in celiac disease and idiopathic sprue. Gastroenterology 38:28, 1960.
10. Howell MD, Austin RK, Kelleher D, et al. An HLA-D region restriction fragment length polymorphism associated with celiac disease. J Exp Med 164:333, 1986.
11. Lundin KE, Scott H, Hansen T, et al. Gliadin-specific, HLA-DQ (alpha 1*0501, beta 1*0201) restricted T cells isolated from the small intestinal mucosa of celiac disease patients. J Exp Med 178:187, 1993.
12. Dieterich W, Ehnis T, Bauer M, et al. Identification of tissue transglutaminase as the autoantigen of celiac disease. Nat Med 3:797, 1997.
13. Molberg O, McAdam SN, Korner R, et al. Tissue transglutaminase selectively modifies gliadin peptides that are recognized by gut-derived T cells in celiac disease. Nat Med 4:713, 1998.
14. Anderson RP, Degano P, Godkin AJ, et al. In vivo antigen challenge in celiac disease identifies a single transglutaminase-modified peptide as the dominant A-gliadin T-cell epitope. Nat Med 6:337, 2000.
15. Logan RF, Tucker G, Rifkind EA, et al. Changes in clinical features of coeliac disease in adults in Edinburgh and the Lothians 1960–79. Br Med J (Clin Res Ed) 286:95, 1983.
16. Mylotte M, Egan-Mitchell B, McCarthy CF, et al. Coeliac disease in the West of Ireland. Br Med J 3:498, 1973.
17. Johnston SD, Watson RG, McMillan SA, et al. Coeliac disease detected by screening is not silent—simply unrecognized. Q J Med 91: 853, 1998.
18. Catassi C, Ratsch IM, Fabiani E, et al. Coeliac disease in the year 2000: Exploring the iceberg. Lancet 343:200, 1994.
19. Cavell B, Stenhammar L, Ascher H, et al. Increasing incidence of childhood coeliac disease in Sweden. Results of a national study. Acta Paediatr 81:589, 1992.
20. Rossipal E. Incidence of coeliac disease in children in Austria. Z Kinderheilkd 119:143, 1975.
21. Weile B, Cavell B, Nivenius K, et al. Striking differences in the incidence of childhood celiac disease between Denmark and Sweden: A plausible explanation. J Pediatr Gastroenterol Nutr 21:64, 1995.
22. Fasano A. Where have all the American celiacs gone? Acta Paediatr Suppl 412:20, 1996.
23. Keaveny AP, Offner GD, Bootle E, et al. No significant difference in antigenicity or tissue transglutaminase substrate specificity of Irish and US wheat gliadins. Dig Dis Sci 45:755, 2000.
24. Not T, Horvath K, Hill ID, et al. Celiac disease risk in the USA: High prevalence of antiendomysium antibodies in healthy blood donors. Scand J Gastroenterol 33:494, 1998.
25. Misra RC, Kasthuri D, Chuttani HK. Adult coeliac disease in tropics. Br Med J 2:1230, 1966.
26. Madara JL, Trier JS. Structural abnormalities of jejunal epithelial cell membranes in celiac sprue. Lab Invest 43:254, 1980.
27. Wright NA, Watson AJ, Morley AR, et al. Cell production rate in mucosa of untreated coeliac disease. Gut 13:846, 1972.
28. Baklien K, Brandtzaeg P, Fausa O. Immunoglobulins in jejunal mucosa and serum from patients with adult coeliac disease. Scand J Gastroenterol 12:149, 1977.
29. Marsh MN. Gluten, major histocompatibility complex, and the small intestine. A molecular and immunobiologic approach to the spectrum of gluten sensitivity ("celiac sprue"). Gastroenterology 102:330, 1992.
30. Rubin CE, Brandborg LL, Flick AL, et al. Biopsy studies on the pathogenesis of celiac sprue. In Wolstenholme GEW, Cameron MC (eds): Intestinal Biopsy. Boston, Little, Brown & Co., 67, 1962.
31. Grefte JM, Bouman JG, Grond J, et al. Slow and incomplete histological and functional recovery in adult gluten sensitive enteropathy. J Clin Pathol 41:886, 1988.
32. De Vincenzi M, Luchetti R, Peruffo AD, et al. In vitro assessment of acetic-acid-soluble proteins (glutenin) toxicity in celiac disease. J Biochem Toxicol 11:205, 1996.
33. Troncone R, Auricchio S, De Vincenzi M, et al. An analysis of cereals that react with serum antibodies in patients with coeliac disease. J Pediatr Gastroenterol Nutr 6:346, 1987.
34. Autran JC, Ellen J, Law L, et al. N-terminal amino acid sequencing of prolamins of wheat and related species. Nature 282:527, 1979.
35. Ciclitira PJ, Ellis HJ. Investigation of cereal toxicity in coeliac disease. Postgrad Med J 63:767, 1987.
36. Kasarda DD, Okita TW, Bernardin JE, et al. Nucleic acid (cDNA) and amino acid sequences of alpha-type gliadins from wheat *(Triticum aestivum).* Proc Natl Acad Sci USA 81:4712, 1984.
37. Kagnoff MF, Paterson YJ, Kumar PJ, et al. Evidence for the role of a human intestinal adenovirus in the pathogenesis of coeliac disease. Gut 28:995, 1987.
38. Arato A, Kosnai I, Szonyi L, et al. Frequent past exposure to adenovirus 12 in coeliac disease. Acta Paediatr Scand 80:1101, 1991.

39. Shidrawi RG, Day P, Przemioslo R, et al. In vitro toxicity of gluten peptides in coeliac disease assessed by organ culture. Scand J Gastroenterol 30:758, 1995.
40. Schuppan D. Current concepts of celiac disease pathogenesis. Gastroenterology 119:234, 2000.
41. Schmitz J. Lack of oats toxicity in coeliac disease. BMJ 314:159, 1997.
42. Ellis A. Coeliac disease: Previous family studies. In: McConnell RB (ed): The Genetics of Coeliac Disease. Lancaster, MTP Press, 1981 p 197.
43. Sollid LM, Markussen G, EK J, et al. Evidence for a primary association of celiac disease to a particular HLA-DQ alpha/beta heterodimer. J Exp Med 169:345, 1989.
44. Nilsen EM, Lundin KE, Krajci P, et al. Gluten specific, HLA-DQ restricted T cells from coeliac mucosa produce cytokines with Th1 or Th0 profile dominated by interferon gamma. Gut 37:766, 1995.
45. Petronzelli F, Bonamico M, Ferrante P, et al. Genetic contribution of the HLA region to the familial clustering of coeliac disease. Ann Hum Genet 61:307, 1997.
46. Houlston RS, Tomlinson IP, Ford D, et al. Linkage analysis of candidate regions for coeliac disease genes. Hum Mol Genet 6:1335, 1997.
47. McManus R, Wilson AG, Mansfield J, et al. TNF2, a polymorphism of the tumour necrosis-alpha gene promoter, is a component of the celiac disease major histocompatibility complex haplotype. Eur J Immunol 26:2113, 1996.
48. McManus R, Moloney M, Borton M, et al. Association of celiac disease with microsatellite polymorphisms close to the tumor necrosis factor genes. Hum Immunol 45:24, 1996.
49. Polvi A, Maki M, Collin P, et al. TNF microsatellite alleles a2 and b3 are not primarily associated with celiac disease in the Finnish population. Tissue Antigens 51:553, 1998.
50. Greco L, Corazza G, Babron MC, et al. Genome search in celiac disease. Am J Hum Genet 62:669, 1998.
51. Friis SU, Gudmand-Hoyer E. Screening for coeliac disease in adults by simultaneous determination of IgA and IgG gliadin antibodies. Scand J Gastroenterol 21:1058, 1986.
52. Kelly CP, Feighery CF, Gallagher RB, et al. Mucosal and systemic IgA anti-gliadin antibody in celiac disease. Contrasting patterns of response in serum, saliva, and intestinal secretions. Dig Dis Sci 36: 743, 1991.
53. Maki M. The humoral immune system in coeliac disease. Baillieres Clin Gastroenterol 9:231, 1995.
54. Uibo O, Uibo R, Kleimola V, et al. Serum IgA anti-gliadin antibodies in an adult population sample. High prevalence without celiac disease. Dig Dis Sci 38:2034, 1993.
55. Hvatum M, Scott H, Brandtzaeg P. Serum IgG subclass antibodies to a variety of food antigens in patients with coeliac disease. Gut 33:632, 1992.
56. Chorzelski TP, Beutner EH, Sulej J, et al. IgA anti-endomysium antibody. A new immunological marker of dermatitis herpetiformis and coeliac disease. Br J Dermatol 111:395, 1984.
57. van de Wal Y, Kooy Y, van Veelen P, et al. Selective deamidation by tissue transglutaminase strongly enhances gliadin-specific T cell reactivity. J Immunol 161:1585, 1998.
58. Szabolcs M, Sipka S, Csorba S. In vitro cross-linking of gluten into high-molecular-weight polymers with transglutaminase. Acta Paediatr Hung 28:215, 1987.
59. Halttunen T, Maki M. Serum immunoglobulin A from patients with celiac disease inhibits human T84 intestinal crypt epithelial cell differentiation. Gastroenterology 116:566, 1999.
60. Halstensen TS, Scott H, Fausa O, et al. Gluten stimulation of coeliac mucosa in vitro induces activation (CD25) of lamina propria CD4+ T cells and macrophages but no crypt-cell hyperplasia. Scand J Immunol 38:581, 1993.
61. Brandtzaeg P, Halstensen TS, Kett K, et al. Immunobiology and immunopathology of human gut mucosa: humoral immunity and intraepithelial lymphocytes. Gastroenterology 97:1562, 1989.
62. Halstensen TS, Scott H, Brandtzaeg P. Human CD8+ intraepithelial T lymphocytes are mainly CD45RA-RB+ and show increased co-expression of CD45R0 in celiac disease. Eur J Immunol 20:1825, 1990.
63. Halstensen TS, Scott H, Brandtzaeg P. Intraepithelial T cells of the TcR gamma/delta+CD8- and V delta 1/J delta 1+ phenotypes are increased in coeliac disease. Scand J Immunol 30:665, 1989.
64. Mak TW, Ferrick DA. The gammadelta T-cell bridge: Linking innate and acquired immunity. Nat Med 4:764, 1998.
65. Cellier C, Patey N, Mauvieux L, et al. Abnormal intestinal intraepithelial lymphocytes in refractory sprue. Gastroenterology 114:471, 1998.
66. Damen GM, Boersma B, Wit JM, et al. Catch-up growth in 60 children with celiac disease. J Pediatr Gastroenterol Nutr 19:394, 1994.
67. Ansaldi N, Tavassoli K, Dell'Olio D, et al. Clinical data on celiac disease with an early or late onset. Minerva Pediatr 43:377, 1991.
68. Ascher H, Krantz I, Rydberg L, et al. Influence of infant feeding and gluten intake on coeliac disease. Arch Dis Child 76:113, 1997.
69. Beaumont DM, Mian MS. Coeliac disease in old age: "a catch in the rye." Age Ageing 27:535, 1998.
70. Vuoristo M, Miettinen TA. The role of fat and bile acid malabsorption in diarrhoea of coeliac disease. Scand J Gastroenterol 22:289, 1987.
71. Rhodes RA, Tai HH, Chey WY. Impairment of secretin release in celiac sprue. Am J Dig Dis 23:833, 1978.
72. Maton PN, Selden AC, Fitzpatrick ML, et al. Defective gallbladder emptying and cholecystokinin release in celiac disease. Reversal by gluten-free diet. Gastroenterology 88:391, 1985.
73. O'Farrelly C, O'Mahony C, Graeme-Cook F, et al. Gliadin antibodies identify gluten-sensitive oral ulceration in the absence of villous atrophy. J Oral Pathol Med 20:476, 1991.
74. O'Grady JG, Stevens FM, Harding B, et al. Hyposplenism and gluten-sensitive enteropathy. Natural history, incidence, and relationship to diet and small bowel morphology. Gastroenterology 87:1326, 1984.
75. Kemppainen T, Kroger H, Janatuinen E, et al. Osteoporosis in adult patients with celiac disease. Bone 24:249, 1999.
76. Cellier C, Flobert C, Cormier C, et al. Severe osteopenia in symptom-free adults with a childhood diagnosis of coeliac disease. Lancet 355: 806, 2000.
77. Vasquez H, Mazure R, Gonzalez D, et al. Risk of fractures in celiac disease patients: A cross-sectional, case-control study. Am J Gastroenterol 95:183, 2000.
78. Hadjivassiliou M, Grunewald RA, Chattopadhyay AK, et al. Clinical, radiological, neurophysiological, and neuropathological characteristics of gluten ataxia. Lancet 352:1582, 1998.
79. Pallis CA, Lewis LP. Neurological Complications of Coeliac Disease and Tropical Sprue. The Neurology of Gastrointestinal Disease. Vol. 138. London, W.B. Saunders, 1974.
80. Gobbi G, Bouquet F, Greco L, et al. Coeliac disease, epilepsy, and cerebral calcifications. The Italian Working Group on Coeliac Disease and Epilepsy. Lancet 340:439, 1992.
81. Ferroir JP, Fenelon G, Billy C, et al. Epilepsy, cerebral calcifications and celiac disease. Rev Neurol (Paris) 153:354, 1997.
82. Molteni N, Bardella MT, Bianchi PA. Obstetric and gynecological problems in women with untreated celiac sprue. J Clin Gastroenterol 12:37, 1990.
83. Collin P, Vilska S, Heinonen PK, et al. Infertility and coeliac disease. Gut 39:382, 1996.
84. Martinelli P, Troncone R, Paparo F, et al. Coeliac disease and unfavourable outcome of pregnancy. Gut 46:332, 2000.
85. Farthing MJ, Rees LH, Dawson AM. Male gonadal function in coeliac disease. III. Pituitary regulation. Clin Endocrinol (Oxf) 19:661, 1983.
86. Aine L, Maki M, Collin P, et al. Dental enamel defects in celiac disease. J Oral Pathol Med 19:241, 1990.
87. Kelly CP, Feighery CF, Gallagher RB, et al. Diagnosis and treatment of gluten-sensitive enteropathy. Adv Intern Med 35:341, 1990.
88. Rostami K, Kerckhaert J, Tiemessen R, et al. Sensitivity of antiendomysium and antigliadin antibodies in untreated celiac disease: Disappointing in clinical practice. Am J Gastroenterol 94:888, 1999.
89. Volta U, Molinaro N, de Franceschi L, et al. IgA anti-endomysial antibodies on human umbilical cord tissue for celiac disease screening. Save both money and monkeys. Dig Dis Sci 40:1902, 1995.
90. Ferreira M, Davies SL, Butler M, et al. Endomysial antibody: Is it the best screening test for coeliac disease? Gut 33:1633, 1992.
91. Kapuscinska A, Zalewski T, Chorzelski TP, et al. Disease specificity and dynamics of changes in IgA class anti-endomysial antibodies in celiac disease. J Pediatr Gastroenterol Nutr 6:529, 1987.
92. Dieterich W, Laag E, Schopper H, et al. Autoantibodies to tissue transglutaminase as predictors of celiac disease. Gastroenterology 115: 1317, 1998.
93. Sulkanen S, Halttunen T, Laurila K, et al. Tissue transglutaminase autoantibody enzyme-linked immunosorbent assay in detecting celiac disease. Gastroenterology 115:1322, 1998.
94. Corrao G, Corazza GR, Andreani ML, et al. Serological screening of coeliac disease: Choosing the optimal procedure according to various prevalence values. Gut 35:771, 1994.

95. Grodzinsky E, Hed J, Skogh T. IgA antiendomysium antibodies have a high positive predictive value for celiac disease in asymptomatic patients. Allergy 49:593, 1994.
96. Kilander AF, Nilsson LA, Gillberg R. Serum antibodies to gliadin in coeliac disease after gluten withdrawal. Scand J Gastroenterol 22:29, 1987.
97. Unsworth DJ, Brown DL. Serological screening suggests that adult coeliac disease is underdiagnosed in the UK and increases the incidence by up to 12%. Gut 35:61, 1994.
98. Achkar E, Carey WD, Petras R, et al. Comparison of suction capsule and endoscopic biopsy of small bowel mucosa. Gastrointest Endosc 32:278, 1986.
99. Jabbari M, Wild G, Goresky CA, et al. Scalloped valvulae conniventes: An endoscopic marker of celiac sprue. Gastroenterology 95:1518, 1988.
100. Shah VH, Rotterdam H, Kotler DP, et al. All that scallops is not celiac disease. Gastrointest Endosc 51:717, 2000.
101. von Krainick HG, Debatin F, Gautier F, et al. Additional research on the injurious effect of wheat flour in coeliac disease. Acute gliadin reactions (gliadin shock). Helv Paediatr Acta 13:432, 1958.
102. Fine KD, Lee EL, Meyer RL. Colonic histopathology in untreated celiac sprue or refractory sprue: Is it lymphocytic colitis or colonic lymphocytosis? Hum Pathol 29:1433, 1998.
103. Walker-Smith J, Harrison M, Kilby A, et al. Cows' milk-sensitive enteropathy. Arch Dis Child 53:375, 1978.
104. Ament ME, Rubin CE. Soy protein—another cause of the flat intestinal lesion. Gastroenterology 62:227, 1972.
105. Weinstein WM, Saunders DR, Tytgat GN, et al. Collagenous sprue—an unrecognized type of malabsorption. N Engl J Med 283:1297, 1970.
106. Cooper BT, Holmes GK, Ferguson R, et al. Gluten-sensitive diarrhea without evidence of celiac disease. Gastroenterology 79:801, 1980.
107. Otley C, Hall RP III. Dermatitis herpetiformis. Dermatol Clin 8:759, 1990.
108. Brow JR, Parker F, Weinstein WM, et al. The small intestinal mucosa in dermatitis herpetiformis. I. Severity and distribution of the small intestinal lesion and associated malabsorption. Gastroenterology 60: 355, 1971.
109. Holmes GK, Prior P, Lane MR, et al. Malignancy in coeliac disease—effect of a gluten free diet. Gut 30:333, 1989.
110. Lewis HM, Renaula TL, Garioch JJ, et al. Protective effect of gluten-free diet against development of lymphoma in dermatitis herpetiformis. Br J Dermatol 135:363, 1996.
111. Smith EP, Zone JJ. Dermatitis herpetiformis and linear IgA bullous dermatosis. Dermatol Clin 11:511, 1993.
112. Rose C, Dieterich W, Brocker EB, et al. Circulating autoantibodies to tissue transglutaminase differentiate patients with dermatitis herpetiformis from those with linear IgA disease. J Am Acad Dermatol 41: 957, 1999.
113. Porter WM, Unsworth DJ, Lock RJ, et al. Tissue transglutaminase antibodies in dermatitis herpetiformis. Gastroenterology 117:749, 1999.
114. Garioch JJ, Lewis HM, Sargent SA, et al. 25 years' experience of a gluten-free diet in the treatment of dermatitis herpetiformis. Br J Dermatol 131:541, 1994.
115. Hardman CM, Garioch JJ, Leonard JN, et al. Absence of toxicity of oats in patients with dermatitis herpetiformis. N Engl J Med 337:1884, 1997.
116. Sjoberg K, Eriksson KF, Bredberg A, et al. Screening for coeliac disease in adult insulin-dependent diabetes mellitus. J Intern Med 243: 133, 1998.
117. Talal AH, Murray JA, Goeken JA, et al. Celiac disease in an adult population with insulin-dependent diabetes mellitus: Use of endomysial antibody testing. Am J Gastroenterol 92:1280, 1997.
118. Collin P, Reunala T, Pukkala E, et al. Coeliac disease—associated disorders and survival. Gut 35:1215, 1994.
119. Cronin CC, Feighery A, Ferriss JB, et al. High prevalence of celiac disease among patients with insulin-dependent (type I) diabetes mellitus. Am J Gastroenterol 92:2210, 1997.
120. Counsell CE, Taha A, Ruddell WS. Coeliac disease and autoimmune thyroid disease. Gut 35:844, 1994.
121. Collin P, Maki M. Associated disorders in coeliac disease: Clinical aspects. Scand J Gastroenterol 29:769, 1994.
122. Rustgi AK, Peppercorn MA. Gluten-sensitive enteropathy and systemic lupus erythematosus. Arch Intern Med 148:1583, 1988.
123. Iltanen S, Collin P, Korpela M, et al. Celiac disease and markers of celiac disease latency in patients with primary Sjögren's syndrome. Am J Gastroenterol 94:1042, 1999.
124. Henriksson KG, Hallert C, Norrby K, et al. Polymyositis and adult coeliac disease. Acta Neurol Scand 65:301, 1982.
125. Ventura A, Magazzu G, Greco L. Duration of exposure to gluten and risk for autoimmune disorders in patients with celiac disease. Gastroenterology 117:297, 1999.
126. Collin P, Maki M, Keyrilainen O, et al. Selective IgA deficiency and coeliac disease. Scand J Gastroenterol 27:367, 1992.
127. O'Donoghue DJ. Fatal pneumococcal septicaemia in coeliac disease. Postgrad Med J 62:229, 1986.
128. Shah A, Mayberry JF, Williams G, et al. Epidemiological survey of coeliac disease and inflammatory bowel disease in first-degree relatives of coeliac patients. Q J Med 74:283, 1990.
129. Freeman HJ. Hepatobiliary tract and pancreatic disorders in celiac disease. Can J Gastroenterol 11:77, 1997.
130. Fornasieri A, Sinico RA, Maldifassi P, et al. IgA-antigliadin antibodies in IgA mesangial nephropathy (Berger's disease). Br Med J (Clin Res Ed) 295:78, 1987.
131. Smith MJ, Benson MK, Strickland ID. Coeliac disease and diffuse interstitial lung disease. Lancet 1:473, 1971.
132. Reading R, Watson JG, Platt JW, et al. Pulmonary haemosiderosis and gluten. Arch Dis Child 62:513, 1987.
133. Simila S, Kokkonen J. Coexistence of celiac disease and Down syndrome. Am J Ment Retard 95:120, 1990.
134. DuBois RN, Lazenby AJ, Yardley JH, et al. Lymphocytic enterocolitis in patients with "refractory sprue." JAMA 262:935, 1989.
135. Moayyedi P, O'Mahony S, Jackson P, et al. Small intestine in lymphocytic and collagenous colitis: Mucosal morphology, permeability, and secretory immunity to gliadin. J Clin Pathol 50:527, 1997.
136. Wolber R, Owen D, Freeman H. Colonic lymphocytosis in patients with celiac sprue. Hum Pathol 21:1092, 1990.
137. Loft DE, Marsh MN, Crowe PT. Rectal gluten challenge and diagnosis of coeliac disease. Lancet 335:1293, 1990.
138. McCashland TM, Donovan JP, Strobach RS, et al. Collagenous enterocolitis: A manifestation of gluten-sensitive enteropathy. J Clin Gastroenterol 15:45, 1992.
139. Fine KD, Do K, Schulte K, et al. High prevalence of celiac sprue-like HLA-DQ genes and enteropathy in patients with the microscopic colitis syndrome. Am J Gastroenterol 95:1974, 2000.
140. Miletic ID, Miletic VD, Sattely-Miller EA, et al. Identification of gliadin presence in pharmaceutical products. J Pediatr Gastroenterol Nutr 19:27, 1994.
141. Hagman B. The Gluten-Free Gourmet. New York, Henry Holt, 1990.
142. Janatuinen EK, Pikkarainen PH, Kemppainen TA, et al. A comparison of diets with and without oats in adults with celiac disease. N Engl J Med 333:1033, 1995.
143. Hoffenberg EJ, Haas J, Drescher A, et al. A trial of oats in children with newly diagnosed celiac disease. J Pediatr 137:361, 2000.
144. Pink IJ, Creamer B. Response to a gluten-free diet of patients with the coeliac syndrome. Lancet 1:300, 1967.
145. MacDonald WC, Brandborg LJ, Flick AL, et al. Studies of celiac sprue. IV. The response of the whole length of the small bowel to a gluten-free diet. Gastroenterology 47:573, 1964.
146. Katz AJ, Falchuk ZM, Strober W, et al. Gluten-sensitive enteropathy. Inhibition by cortisol of the effect of gluten protein in vitro. N Engl J Med 295:131, 1976.
147. Sandle GI, Keir MJ, Record CO. The effect of hydrocortisone on the transport of water, sodium, and glucose in the jejunum. Perfusion studies in normal subjects and patients with coeliac disease. Scand J Gastroenterol 16:667, 1981.
148. Mitchison HC, al Mardini H, Gillespie S, et al. A pilot study of fluticasone propionate in untreated coeliac disease. Gut 32:260, 1991.
149. Lloyd-Still JD, Grand RJ, Khaw KT, et al. The use of corticosteroids in celiac crisis. J Pediatr 81:1074, 1972.
150. Vaidya A, Bolanos J, Berkelhammer C. Azathioprine in refractory sprue. Am J Gastroenterol 94:1967, 1999.
151. Longstreth GF. Successful treatment of refractory sprue with cyclosporine. Ann Intern Med 119:1014, 1993.
152. Rolny P, Sigurjonsdottir HA, Remotti H, et al. Role of immunosuppressive therapy in refractory sprue-like disease. Am J Gastroenterol 94:219, 1999.
153. Valdimarsson T, Lofman O, Toss G, et al. Reversal of osteopenia with diet in adult coeliac disease. Gut 38:322, 1996.

154. Sategna-Guidetti C, Grosso SB, Grosso S, et al. The effects of 1-year gluten withdrawal on bone mass, bone metabolism and nutritional status in newly-diagnosed adult coeliac disease patients. Aliment Pharmacol Ther 14:35, 2000.
155. Valdimarsson T, Toss G, Lofman O, et al. Three years' follow-up of bone density in adult coeliac disease: Significance of secondary hyperparathyroidism. Scand J Gastroenterol 35:274, 2000.
156. Jones PE, Peters TJ. Oral zinc supplements in non-responsive coeliac syndrome: Effect on jejunal morphology, enterocyte production, and brush border disaccharidase activities. Gut 22:194, 1981.
157. Holmes GK, Stokes PL, Sorahan TM, et al. Coeliac disease, gluten-free diet, and malignancy. Gut 17:612, 1976.
158. Selby WS, Gallagher ND. Malignancy in a 19-year experience of adult celiac disease. Dig Dis Sci 24:684, 1979.
159. Cooper BT, Holmes GK, Cooke WT. Lymphoma risk in coeliac disease of later life. Digestion 23:89, 1982.
160. Isaacson PG, O'Connor NT, Spencer J, et al. Malignant histiocytosis of the intestine: A T-cell lymphoma. Lancet 2:688, 1985.
161. Spencer J, Cerf-Bensussan N, Jarry A, et al. Enteropathy-associated T cell lymphoma (malignant histiocytosis of the intestine) is recognized by a monoclonal antibody (HML-1) that defines a membrane molecule on human mucosal lymphocytes. Am J Pathol 132:1, 1988.
162. Cellier C, Delabesse E, Helmer C, et al. Refractory sprue, coeliac disease, and enteropathy-associated T-cell lymphoma. French Coeliac Disease Study Group. Lancet 356:203, 2000.
163. Freeman HJ, Chiu BK. Small bowel malignant lymphoma complicating celiac sprue and the mesenteric lymph node cavitation syndrome. Gastroenterology 90:2008, 1986.
164. Matuchansky C, Colin R, Hemet J, et al. Cavitation of mesenteric lymph nodes, splenic atrophy, and a flat small intestinal mucosa. Report of six cases. Gastroenterology 87:606, 1984.
165. Egan LJ, Walsh SV, Stevens FM, et al. Celiac-associated lymphoma. A single institution experience of 30 cases in the combination chemotherapy era. J Clin Gastroenterol 21:123, 1995.
166. Mills PR, Brown IL, Watkinson G. Idiopathic chronic ulcerative enteritis. Report of five cases and review of the literature. Q J Med 49:133, 1980.
167. Baer AN, Bayless TM, Yardley JH. Intestinal ulceration and malabsorption syndromes. Gastroenterology 79:754, 1980.
168. Enns R, Lay T, Bridges R. Use of azathioprine for nongranulomatous ulcerative jejunoileitis. Can J Gastroenterol 11:503, 1997.
169. Bossart R, Henry K, Booth CC, et al. Subepithelial collagen in intestinal malabsorption. Gut 16:18, 1975.
170. Freeman HJ. Hyposplenism, antiendomysial antibodies and lymphocytic colitis in collagenous sprue. Can J Gastroenterol 13:347, 1999.
171. Guller R, Anabitarte M, Mayer M. Collagenous sprue and ulcerative jejuno-ileitis in a patient with gluten-induced enteropathy. Schweiz Med Wochenschr 116:1343, 1986.
172. Holtmann M, von Herbay A, Galle PR, et al. Long-term collagenous sprue—remission with a gluten-free diet. Z Gastroenterol 37:1163, 1999.
173. O'Mahony S, Nawroz IM, Ferguson A. Coeliac disease and collagenous colitis. Postgrad Med J 66:238, 1990.
174. Ciacci C, Mazzacca G. Unintentional gluten ingestion in celiac patients. Gastroenterology 115:243, 1998.
175. Baker AL, Rosenberg IH. Refractory sprue: Recovery after removal of nongluten dietary proteins. Ann Intern Med 89:505, 1978.
176. Ryan BM, Kelleher D. Refractory celiac disease. Gastroenterology 119:243, 2000.
177. Wahab PJ, Crusius JB, Meijer JW, et al. Cyclosporin in the treatment of adults with refractory coeliac disease—an open pilot study. Aliment Pharmacol Ther 14:767, 2000.
178. Corazza GR, Biagi F, Volta U, et al. Autoimmune enteropathy and villous atrophy in adults. Lancet 350:106, 1997.
179. Murray A, Cuevas EC, Jones DB, et al. Study of the immunohistochemistry and T cell clonality of enteropathy-associated T cell lymphoma. Am J Pathol 146:509, 1995.
180. Ashton-Key M, Diss TC, Pan L, et al. Molecular analysis of T-cell clonality in ulcerative jejunitis and enteropathy-associated T-cell lymphoma. Am J Pathol 151:493, 1997.
181. Bagdi E, Diss TC, Munson P, et al. Mucosal intra-epithelial lymphocytes in enteropathy-associated T-cell lymphoma, ulcerative jejunitis, and refractory celiac disease constitute a neoplastic population. Blood 94:260, 1999.
182. Logan RF, Rifkind EA, Turner ID, et al. Mortality in celiac disease. Gastroenterology 97:265, 1989.
183. Nielsen OH, Jacobsen O, Pedersen ER, et al. Non-tropical sprue. Malignant diseases and mortality rate. Scand J Gastroenterol 20:13, 1985.
184. Schmitz J. Is celiac disease a lifelong disorder? Clin Invest Med 19: 352, 1996.
185. Trier JS. Celiac sprue and refractory sprue. In Feldman M, Scharschmidt BF, Sleisenger MH (eds): Gastrointestinal and Liver Disease. Philadelphia; W.B. Saunders, 1998:1557.
186. Mulder CJ, Tytgat GN. Coeliac disease and related disorders. Neth J Med 31:286, 1987.

Chapter 94

TROPICAL MALABSORPTION AND TROPICAL DIARRHEA

Michael J.G. Farthing

Malabsorption of dietary nutrients by the small intestine has special relevance for people living in the tropics and subtropics. The causes of intestinal malabsorption differ from those commonly seen in the industrialized world, and the clinical impact is often substantially greater because many persons in the developing world, particularly infants and young children, often exist in a state of borderline undernutrition. Tropical malabsorption and diarrhea are not limited to the indigenous population but commonly affect travelers, particularly those from the industrialized world.[1] Acute infective diarrhea, most commonly caused by enterotoxigenic *Escherichia coli,* is the most common affliction of travelers, although chronic diarrhea and malabsorption also occur as a result of specific infections and tropical sprue.

Tropical malabsorption can be considered to be caused either by *specific* causes, such as infections of known etiology and inflammatory and neoplastic disorders, or *nonspecific* conditions, such as tropical enteropathy and tropical sprue, for which the etiology has not been determined (Table 94–1). Acute diarrhea in the tropics without overt intestinal malabsorption is usually caused by acute infection with one or more of a variety of enteropathogens that include bacteria, viruses, protozoa, and helminths (Table 94–2). These organisms are not discussed in detail and are dealt with in Chapters 28, 96, 98, and 99.

SPECIFIC CAUSES OF TROPICAL MALABSORPTION

Intestinal Infection

The majority of infections that cause intestinal malabsorption in the tropics produce an enteropathy in the small intestine with varying degrees of villus atrophy, crypt hyperplasia, and inflammatory infiltrates in the lamina propria and in some cases in the epithelium.[2] *Giardia lamblia* is the most common human protozoan enteropathogen and is well recognized to cause chronic diarrhea and intestinal malabsorption. *G. lamblia* is considered to be a contributory factor in the retardation of growth and development in infants and young children. *Isospora belli* also produces chronic diarrhea and enteropathy but is geographically restricted to the tropics and subtropics, unlike *Giardia,* which is found worldwide. *Cyclospora cayetanensis* is a recently recognized intracellular protozoan that has been identified in a number of tropical and subtropical locations as a cause of chronic diarrhea and enteropathy in both immunocompetent and immunocompromised persons.[3] It was first recognized in travelers in Nepal who presented with diarrhea that persisted for many weeks, often in association with profound weight loss. The more commonly recognized intracellular protozoan, *Cryptosporidium parvum,* is a well-established cause of chronic diarrhea worldwide in immunocompetent persons, in whom the diarrhea is usually self-limiting. *C. parvum* is, however, a major cause of chronic, intractable diarrhea in patients with human immunodeficiency virus (HIV) infection or acquired immunodeficiency syndrome (AIDS), although in the developed world, where highly active antiretroviral therapy (HAART) is available, the clinical impact of infection with *C. parvum* has declined dramatically; cryptosporidiosis continues to be a major cause of morbidity and mortality in patients with AIDS in the tropics. The *Microsporidium* species have emerged as important causes of persistent diarrhea in HIV-infected patients in the tropics. *Enterocytozoon bieneusi* was the first microsporidium to be identified as an important cause of human diarrheal disease, followed by *Encephalitozoon intestinalis,* which occurs in the tropics and is notable for its susceptibility to albendazole.[4]

Helminths are not a major cause of intestinal malabsorption, although heavy infection with *Strongyloides stercoralis,* including the hyperinfection syndrome, should be included in the differential diagnosis. *Capillaria philippinensis* is an important cause of intestinal malabsorption in a highly restricted geographic area in Southeast Asia.

Rotavirus, enteric adenoviruses, and the small, round,

Table 94–1 | **Tropical Malabsorption**

SPECIFIC CAUSES	
Infection:	
Protozoa	*Giardia lamblia*
	Isospora belli
	Cryptosporidium parvum
	Enterocytozoon bieneusi
	Encephalitozoon intestinalis
	Cyclospora cayetanensis
Helminths	*Capillaria philippinensis*
	Strongyloides stercoralis
Bacteria	Enteropathogenic *E. coli*
	Mycobacterium tuberculosis
Viruses	Rotavirus
	Enteric adenoviruses (types 40, 41)
	Small, round, structured viruses (e.g., Norwalk virus)
	Measles virus
	Human immunodeficiency virus
Celiac sprue	
Lymphoma	
Severe undernutrition (kwashiorkor and marasmus)	
Primary hypolactasia	
NONSPECIFIC CAUSES	
Tropical enteropathy	
Tropical sprue	

structured viruses such as Norwalk virus all produce small bowel enteropathy, but the illness is usually self-limiting, and a chronic malabsorptive state virtually never occurs. The relationship of HIV to small intestinal enteropathy is controversial, although there is some evidence to suggest that the virus itself may be responsible for small intestinal damage, even in the absence of other defined enteropathogens. The precise mechanisms responsible have not been fully elucidated, although T-cell activation does not appear to play a major role, as it does in other forms of enteropathy such as celiac sprue.[5] HIV-related enteropathy appears to be more severe in Africa than in Western Europe, suggesting that background tropical enteropathy may be a risk factor for enteropathy in AIDS (see Chapter 28).

Table 94–2 | **Tropical Diarrhea: Major Enteropathogens**

BACTERIA		Enterotoxigenic *E. coli* (ETEC)
		Enteropathogenic *E. coli* (EPEC)
		Enteroaggregative *E. coli* (EAggEC)
		Enteroinvasive *E. coli* (EIEC)
		Salmonella spp.
		Shigella spp.
		Campylobacter jejuni
		Mycobacterium tuberculosis (and M. bovis)
		Aeromonas spp. and *Plesiomonas* spp.
VIRUSES		Rotavirus
		Enteric adenoviruses (types 40, 41)
		Measles virus
		Human immunodeficiency virus
PROTOZOA	Ciliophora	*Balantidium coli*
	Mastigophora	*Giardia lamblia*
	Coccidia	*Cryptosporidium parvum*
		Isospora belli
	Microspora	*Enterocytozoon bieneusi*
		Encephalitozoon intestinalis
	Cyclospora	*Cyclospora cayetanensis*
HELMINTHS		*Strongyloides stercoralis*
		Schistosoma spp.

Most bacterial infections of the small intestine produce acute diarrhea and a self-limiting illness. However, some enteropathogenic *E. coli* strains produce chronic diarrhea and malabsorption in infants and young children, as can diffuse small intestinal involvement with *Mycobacterium tuberculosis*.

Celiac Sprue

Celiac sprue (gluten-sensitive enteropathy) is uncommon in the tropics but is described in India, particularly northern India, where wheat-containing foods form an important part of the diet, and Africa. Celiac sprue may present for the first time in the tropics in European and North American expatriates and thus should be included in the differential diagnosis of such persons who develop persistent diarrhea. Distinguishing celiac sprue from tropical sprue can be difficult in the tropical setting. The morphologic changes in the jejunum are usually more profound in celiac sprue than in tropical sprue and will almost inevitably respond to gluten withdrawal but not to broad-spectrum antibiotics. Testing for antiendomysial or antitissue transglutaminase antibodies is now recognized to be a sensitive and specific screen for celiac sprue and should be performed in travelers returning with chronic diarrhea with or without overt malabsorption. If the antibody test is positive, the diagnosis of celiac sprue should be confirmed by jejunal biopsy. In most instances it is advisable to take the diagnostic process a step further by confirming histologic resolution on a second biopsy after gluten withdrawal, followed in some cases by a gluten challenge and a third biopsy to show morphologic relapse following reintroduction of gluten. Clearly, a patient with tropical malabsorption should not be committed to a life-long gluten-free diet unless the diagnosis of celiac sprue is absolutely secure (see Chapter 93).

Lymphoma

Immunoproliferative small intestinal disease (IPSID) and primary upper small intestinal lymphoma (PUSIL) are found predominantly in areas of socioeconomic deprivation (see also Chapter 26). Although commonly known as Mediterranean lymphoma, the condition has been described in other parts of the world, including the Middle East, South Africa, and South America. Current evidence suggests that these conditions are related, with IPSID progressing to PUSIL, and that IPSID is therefore a premalignant condition. These disorders usually occur in a younger age group, in contrast to primary intestinal lymphoma, which occurs worldwide, mostly in elderly people.

Severe Undernutrition

Although it is clearly established that luminal nutrients are vital for maintaining mucosal integrity in the gut, the role of undernutrition in the pathogenesis of intestinal malabsorption and small intestinal enteropathy remains controversial. Steatorrhea and villus atrophy have been described in children with severe kwashiorkor and marasmus, with reversion toward normal following nutritional rehabilitation. Current

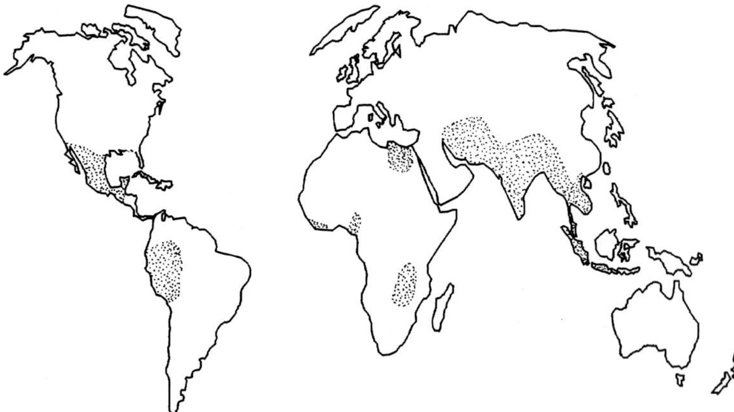

Figure 94–1. Geographic distribution of tropical enteropathy *(shaded areas)*.

evidence suggests, however, that less severe degrees of undernutrition do not have a major impact on small intestinal structure and function and are unlikely to explain the abnormalities of villus architecture commonly seen in the tropics.

Primary Hypolactasia

Lactose activity in the small intestine is high in neonates in all ethnic groups, but in many, particularly those indigenous to the tropics, lactase activity declines rapidly within 3 to 4 months after weaning. Adult hypolactasia is found throughout most countries in Southeast Asia, but it is less common in the Middle East and uncommon in Northern Europe. The practical importance of hypolactasia is small, because African and Asian adults avoid milk unless they wish to use it as a purgative. However, milk-based products cannot be used reliably in these regions as a nutritional supplement. Secondary hypolactasia occurs after small intestinal infections that produce enteropathy but is usually short-lived and self-limiting (see also Chapters 88 and 89).

Sucrase activity is also reduced in black South Africans living in Johannesburg but not to the same degree to which lactase levels are reduced.[6] These healthy persons have normal villus and crypt morphology, and this abnormality cannot be attributed to tropical enteropathy. Whether it is acquired or genetically determined remains to be established.

NONSPECIFIC TROPICAL MALABSORPTION

In addition to the specific causes of intestinal absorption in the tropics, malabsorption occurs in association with two conditions of unknown etiology, tropical enteropathy and tropical sprue. Although it has been suggested that tropical enteropathy and tropical sprue may represent the two ends of a clinical and pathologic spectrum, the evidence to support this view is far from compelling. Tropical enteropathy, for example, occurs in Africa, where tropical sprue is extremely uncommon. Thus, the widespread nature of tropical enteropathy and the geographic restriction of tropical sprue continue to challenge epidemiologists and clinical investigators. Despite intensive investigation during the latter half of the 20th century, the cause of both conditions remains obscure.

TROPICAL ENTEROPATHY

Definition

Enteropathy is characterized by a variable reduction in villus height, usually in association with a hyperplastic response in the crypt.[2] There is, therefore, a decrease in the villus-crypt ratio that is inevitably accompanied by a decrease in the surface area of the small intestine. There may also be evidence of damage to the surface epithelial cells with a reduction in the height of the cell, thereby changing its shape from columnar to cuboidal. The changes in villus morphology and enterocyte height are almost invariably associated with inflammatory cell infiltrates in the lamina propria and within the epithelium.

Epidemiology

Tropical enteropathy has been detected in most tropical regions of Asia, Africa, the Middle East, the Caribbean, and Central and South America (Fig. 94–1). The defect is acquired; newborn infants in the developing world have villi of a height similar to that of infants in the industrialized world, but by 4 to 6 months the villus architectural abnormalities and inflammatory infiltrates begin to appear. The onset at 4 to 6 months is consistent with the view that the postweaning environment in many countries in the developing world is relatively hostile to the small intestinal epithelium and leads to abnormalities of the villus and crypt architecture. It has been argued, however, that these features are the "normal state" for persons living in these locations. Tropical enteropathy is not limited to the indigenous population but may be acquired by travelers from the industrialized world and seen in expatriates living and working in the tropics.

Evidence from migrant studies of people traveling from the developed to the industrialized world have suggested that tropical enteropathy is a reversible process. However, a survey of small bowel morphology in British Indian and British African-Caribbean subjects who have lived in the United Kingdom for more than 30 years, in some instances, has raised the question of genetic predisposition to the development of enteropathy.[7] In both immigrant groups, villus height was reduced compared with indigenous British whites, although there was no obvious correlation between the reduction in villus height and the duration of residence in the United Kingdom. However, in the British Indian subjects, there was a relationship between villus height and the time since the last visit to the Indian subcontinent, suggesting that re-exposure to the tropical environment was involved in maintaining the enteropathy. Such a relationship was not apparent in the African-Caribbean subjects, suggesting that the persisting mild abnormality of villus architecture is more likely to be related to genetic factors rather than to re-exposure to the tropical environment.

Pathophysiology

Formal investigation of small intestinal absorption in apparently healthy persons in India, Africa, and Central and South America has revealed reduced absorption of D-xylose, glucose, vitamin B_{12}, and fat compared with healthy Western controls. In addition, intestinal perfusion studies of the transport of glucose, amino acids, and small peptides have confirmed reduced absorption rates, compared with healthy Europeans.[8, 9] For example, 50% of healthy Southern Indian adults had reduced D-xylose absorption, 10% had mild impairment of fat absorption, and 3% had reduced vitamin B_{12} absorption. It should be stressed, however, that these functional abnormalities were mild, were indicative only of a subclinical malabsorptive state, and did not correlate with overt manifestations of clinical disease. These minor abnormalities appear to be more common in persons living in rural or poor periurban locations than in more affluent city dwellers. We have recently demonstrated a clear difference between healthy black residents in a Johannesburg township, in whom mean villus height was indistinguishable from that of healthy Johannesburg whites or British whites, and relatively deprived blacks living in a poor periurban development in Lusaka, Zambia, in whom the mean villus height was substantially lower (Fig. 94–2).

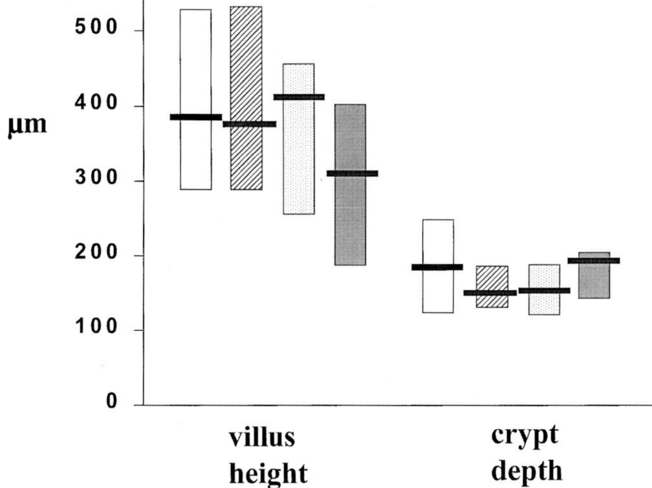

Figure 94–2. Villus height and crypt depth in black Zambians with tropical enteropathy *(gray bars)* and black South Africans *(dotted bars)* from Johannesburg with normal villus-crypt architecture. *Open bars,* white British subjects; *hatched bars,* white South Africans.

Theories of Etiopathogenesis

Current epidemiologic evidence indicates that tropical enteropathy occurs as a result of environmental factors. Climate alone cannot explain these abnormalities, because tropical enteropathy has not been found in locations like Singapore where water quality, sanitation, and nutritional status are similar to those of industrialized countries. The major contributors to the production of enteropathy appear to be (1) intestinal infection or continuing bacterial contamination of the upper small intestine, and (2) nutritional insufficiency. In the developing world, it is difficult to separate these factors and to explore in a controlled way their independent and combined effects on intestinal structure and function. Evidence from human and animal studies indicates, however, that the small intestine is relatively resistant to nutritional insufficiency, except when it is severe, although insufficiency of riboflavin in utero can program villus and crypt architecture in the fetus and result in an irreversible, riboflavin-resistant defect in the neonatal small intestinal epithelium. These relatively subtle influences of micronutrient deficiency on small intestinal structure require further evaluation.

The major emphasis in the study of the pathogenesis of tropical enteropathy has been on the microbiologic milieu of the small intestine. Studies in southern Indians have identified a number of "infective factors" that may be important. Apparently healthy, asymptomatic persons have heavy colonization of the small intestine by aerobic and anerobic organisms and, in addition, excrete a range of established, classic enteropathogens in their feces.[10] This finding suggests that the persistence of either established enteropathogens or the colonization of the small intestine by excessive numbers of commensal bacteria can result in subclinical small intestinal damage (see Chapter 90). Studies in germ-free animals have clearly shown the importance of the luminal and mucosal bacterial flora in modulating villus architecture and the inflammatory infiltrate, and there is compelling circumstantial evidence to support the view that the increased bacterial load of commensal and pathogenic microorganisms leads to the mucosal abnormalities in many parts of the developing world.

We have tested the hypothesis that the inflammatory response in the epithelium and submucosa is important in the pathogenesis of villus atrophy, specifically the presence of activated T cells. The T-cell activation marker CD69 was increased in black Zambians with tropical enteropathy and was associated with human leukocyte antigen (HLA)-DR expression.[11, 12] These findings suggest that T-cell activation in the lamina propria may be involved in the genesis of the villus architectural abnormalities in tropical enteropathy.

The mucosal abnormalities in tropical enteropathy are not limited to the small intestine. There also are subclinical abnormalities of colonocyte structure and function, which can be called *tropical colonopathy.*[13]

The broad geographic distribution of tropical enteropathy indicates that environmental factors are most important in its etiology, and there is little support for a genetic basis for this condition. Still, the recent description of mild, persisting enteropathy in British African-Caribbean subjects who have not returned to their country of origin for many years suggests that there also may be a genetic component.[7]

TROPICAL SPRUE

Although few would dispute the existence of the clinical entity of idiopathic chronic malabsorption in the tropics, commonly referred to as *tropical sprue,* the condition continues to be surrounded by epidemiologic, clinical, and etiopathogenetic controversies.[14] The epidemiology is perplexing because of the restrictive geographic distribution of tropical sprue within the tropics and, unlike most other diarrheal diseases, its prevalence is relatively low in children. Its etiology is unknown, but there is no lack of hypotheses. However, the varied clinical presentation makes it difficult to establish a unifying hypothesis on etiology. One of the problems has been the failure to agree on a universally accepted definition of the syndrome.

Definition

The Wellcome Trust collaborative study "Tropical Sprue and Megaloblastic Anaemia," published in 1971, concluded that "tropical sprue is a syndrome of intestinal malabsorption which occurs among residents in or visitors to certain regions of the tropics."[15] The definition was further modified by Baker and Mathan, working in Vellore, southern India, by including "malabsorption of two or more substances in people in the tropics when other known causes have been excluded."[15] Cook noted that tropical sprue often followed an acute diarrheal illness, and on the basis of this observation and the evidence that the small intestine in sprue was colonized by aerobic and anerobic bacteria, he recommended that the term *postinfective tropical malabsorption* be used in preference to tropical sprue.[16] Booth opposed this change on the basis that not all episodes of tropical sprue follow an acute diarrheal illness and that the syndrome may remain latent for many years, even after an expatriate has returned to his or her homeland.[17] He proposed the definition "malabsorption in defined areas of the tropics in which no bacterial, viral, or parasitic infection can be detected," which carefully excludes any assumptions about etiopathogenesis. Although the etiology of tropical sprue remains unknown, it would seem wise to resist including speculation on its etiology in the definition.

Historical Aspects

A malabsorptive illness in the tropics was described in an ancient treatise on medicine, "The Charakasamhida," which was written before 600 BC. William Hillary published the first clear clinical description of the disease in the European literature in 1759, when he described his observations on chronic diarrhea and malabsorption in Barbados in the Caribbean.[18] Reports of a similar illness soon followed, largely associated with the colonization of India and Southeast Asia by the European maritime powers. British military physicians referred to the illness as *the white flux, diarrhea alba,* or *chronic diarrhea of the tropics.* The disorder was subsequently described among the Dutch in Java, the French in Indochina, and Europeans in China. In 1880, Manson introduced the word "sprue," which was derived from the Dutch term *Indische sprouw,* which describes the oral aphthous ulceration often associated with this form of chronic diarrhea in children.[19] It became apparent that tropical sprue was not confined to Asia when, following the Spanish-American War, it was seen among American expatriates in the Philippines and Puerto Rico. By the beginning of the 20th century, it became evident that tropical sprue was associated with morphologic abnormalities in the small intestine, although all the early observations were made at autopsy, and the significance of the abnormalities remained controversial. Sir Philip Manson-Bahr, in 1924, was convinced that the primary lesion in sprue was in the small intestinal mucosa,[20] and this speculation was confirmed when per oral jejunal biopsy was introduced in the 1950s.

Epidemiology

Unlike the majority of infective diarrheas in the tropics, tropical sprue is markedly geographically restricted. It is predominantly a disease of southern and Southeast Asia, the Caribbean islands, and, to a much lesser extent, Central and South America (Fig. 94–3).[21–23] It almost never occurs in expatriates in Africa, although there have been sporadic reports from South Africa, Zimbabwe, and Nigeria.[24–26] Thus, *endemic* tropical sprue is not found universally in tropical and subtropical regions, a finding that strongly suggests that the etiologic factor or factors are geographically restricted.

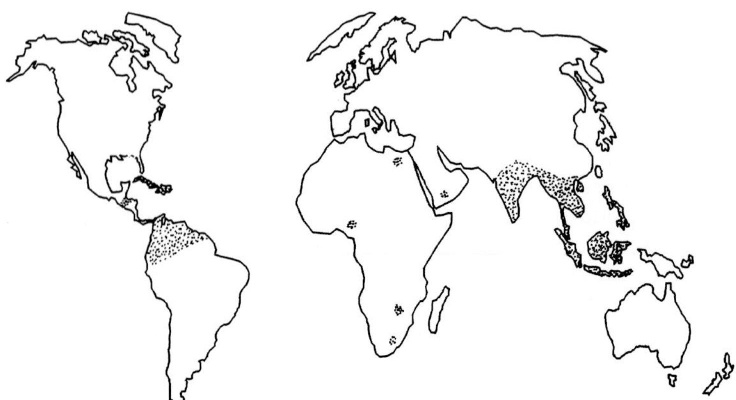

Figure 94–3. Geographic distribution of tropical sprue *(shaded areas).*

The prevalence of endemic tropical sprue has not been clearly defined, although in Europeans living in Ceylon, the prevalence was estimated to be 0.5%, and in North Americans living in Puerto Rico, the prevalence is 8%.[27] During World War II, tropical sprue was a major cause of morbidity among British troops serving in India and Burma[28] but rare among American forces operating in the islands of the Pacific. Subsequently, it was noted to be common among British troops serving in Malaya and Hong Kong.[29] Tropical sprue was common among Europeans traveling overland in Asia,[30] although an unexpectedly low prevalence was found in American forces serving in Vietnam[31] and Peace Corps volunteers working in tropical areas. These data and the apparent decline in the incidence of tropical sprue in European overland travelers have been attributed to the widespread, early use of antibiotics for acute traveler's diarrhea.

Epidemic tropical sprue has been documented most clearly in villages around Vellore in southern India.[32–34] Epidemics differ from other causes of acute diarrhea, because the epidemic evolves over many months, with new cases continuing to appear after a year or more. Attack rates are high in adults but relatively low in children; exposure during the first wave of an epidemic appears to offer protection during subsequent waves. Epidemics also have been described in northern India and Burma. During the major epidemics in southern India between 1960 and 1962, an estimated 100,000 people were affected, and tropical sprue was directly related to the deaths of at least 30,000 people.[34] In southern India, epidemics do not exhibit seasonality, although in Puerto Rico, cases commonly present during the first 3 months of the year, which is not a time of high rainfall. Clinical impressions worldwide suggest that the incidence of tropical sprue is declining in both the indigenous population and visitors to endemic areas.

Clinical Features

Tropical sprue is a syndrome consisting of chronic diarrhea often with clinical features of steatorrhea, anorexia, abdominal cramps, bloating, and prominent bowel sounds.[15, 17, 35–38] In expatriates and during epidemics in the indigenous population, the illness often begins with an acute attack of watery diarrhea associated with fever and malaise. After 1 week, the acute symptoms resolve and are followed by milder chronic diarrhea or overt steatorrhea, usually accompanied by progressive weight loss.[39] This particular form of the illness is found most commonly in persons who travel overland from Europe to India. Lactose intolerance is commonly described as part of this illness and may be associated with deficiencies of vitamin B_{12} and folic acid and occasionally hypocalcemia and hypomagnesemia. Physical findings during the early phase of the illness are usually limited to signs of weight loss and hyperactive bowel sounds.

In some persons, the acute phase of tropical sprue evolves into a chronic phase with persistent diarrhea and steatorrhea. After months or even years, the clinical picture becomes dominated by nutritional deficiencies that result in anemia, stomatitis, glossitis, pigmentation of the skin, and edema caused by hypoproteinemia. In southern India, 1% of patients with endemic tropical sprue present with nutritional deficiencies in the absence of diarrhea. Occasionally, vitamin B_{12} deficiency produces subacute combined degeneration of the spinal cord. Vitamin A deficiency may manifest as night blindness. In general, the long-term nutritional impact of chronic tropical sprue is more evident in the indigenous population than in visitors, because the natives are more likely already to be borderline undernourished.

A number of case reports have described patients in whom the initial presentation of tropical sprue involved only a mild or subclinical illness and in whom chronic diarrhea and nutritional deficiencies develop months or even years after leaving the tropics.[17, 27] This form of the illness has been called *latent sprue.* It has been described in Puerto Ricans living in New York and in Anglo-Indians in London, who typically present with steatorrhea and megaloblastic anemia.

Pathology

The morphologic changes in the gastrointestinal tract in tropical sprue are highly variable but generally correlate with the duration and severity of the clinical presentation.

CHRONIC ATROPHIC GASTRITIS. Chronic atrophic gastritis is a common finding in tropical sprue, particularly in subjects studied in southern India. Affected persons have reduced secretion of gastric acid and intrinsic factor, resulting in vitamin B_{12} malabsorption, which can be corrected by administration of intrinsic factor. The gastritis may persist even after the enteropathy has resolved and clinical symptoms have improved markedly. However, these observations were made before the discovery of *Helicobacter pylori,* and in view of the extremely high prevalence of *H. pylori* in the developing world, it is possible that the abnormalities observed in the stomach of patients with tropical sprue are not specific to sprue but related to co-infection with *H. pylori.*

ENTEROPATHY. Tropical sprue is noted for the broad spectrum of histopathologic abnormalities that can be observed in the jejunal mucosa.[15, 40, 41] In the early stages, the jejunal mucosa may be normal, but in persons with persistent diarrhea, there usually is a reduction in villus height, increase in crypt depth, and an associated inflammatory cell infiltrate in both the lamina propria and epithelium (Fig. 94–4). The changes are similar to those in tropical enteropathy but generally more severe. There is a moderately close relationship between abnormalities of intestinal structure and function, in that the extent of nutrient malabsorption increases with the severity of the villus architectural abnormalities. Ultrastructural studies have suggested that an abnormality in stem cells in the small intestinal crypts may be the primary lesion in tropical sprue.[42, 43] Thus, although the rates of crypt cell production and enterocyte migration up the villus are increased in tropical sprue,[44] the cells that are produced are damaged and thus extruded more rapidly than normal from the villus.

Electron microscopy shows distortion and grouping of the microvilli, fragmentation of the terminal web, an increased number of lysosomes, and mitochrondrial changes in the enterocytes. In the crypts, cell nuclei show megalocytic changes and argentaffin cells are increased, but Paneth's

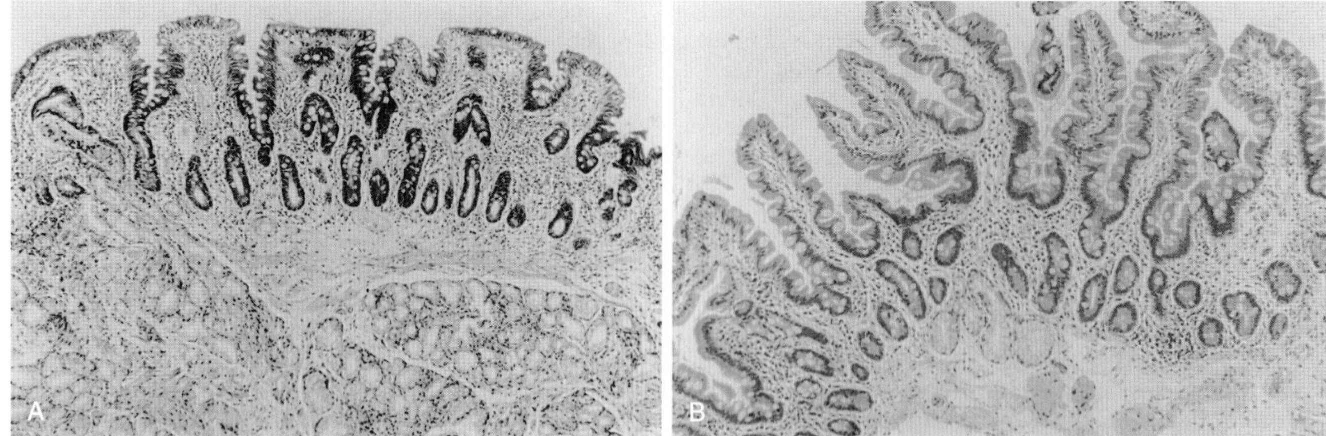

Figure 94–4. Jejunal morphology in a traveler from the United Kingdom with tropical sprue. *A*, Before, and *B*, after treatment with tetracycline and folic acid.

cells are normal in number. The basement membrane usually appears thickened and stains as collagen on light microscopy. Light and electron microscopy demonstrate an accumulation of lipid droplets immediately adjacent to the surface epithelium. The pattern of lipid accumulation in tropical sprue is different from that in normal subjects and patients with celiac sprue but reverts to normal following clinical recovery. The precise significance of this abnormality in tropical sprue is uncertain.

COLONOPATHY. Colonic epithelial cells show structural abnormalities similar to those described in the small intestine. Sodium and water absorption by the colon are impaired, in part because of increased concentrations of unsaturated free fatty acids in the stool.[45] The free fatty acids have a variety of effects on colonic structure and function, including inhibition of sodium-potassium adenosine triphosphatase, which promotes sodium and water absorption by the colonic epithelium.

Pathophysiology

Although tropical sprue is generally considered to be a disease primarily of the proximal small intestine, pathophysiologic disturbances also occur in the stomach and colon. The mechanisms by which gastric acid secretion and intrinsic factor production are reduced is not clear, and it is uncertain as to whether these changes are primary manifestations of the disease or merely secondary phenomena resulting from severe undernutrition. *H. pylori* is likely to be extremely common in the indigenous populations with endemic tropical sprue and is well recognized to cause acute gastritis, which generally progresses to gastric atrophy and impaired gastric acid secretion. The relationship between *H. pylori* infection and tropical sprue has not been investigated. Similarly, the mechanisms of colonic dysfunction in tropical sprue are not entirely clear and may also be related to the secondary effects of undernutrition and impaired absorption of long-chain fatty acids by the small intestine. The major pathophysiologic disturbances in tropical sprue occur predominantly in the small intestine.

IMPAIRMENT OF SMALL INTESTINAL TRANSPORT. Perfusion studies of the small intestine indicate that some patients with tropical sprue in Puerto Rico have a net secretory state for water in the jejunum that is reversed by treatment with antibiotics.[46] However, patients with tropical sprue in southern India were not found to have a secretory state, and they absorb water and electrolytes to the same extent as local healthy control subjects.[47] Impaired absorption of amino acids and dipeptides has been shown in proximal small intestine.[48, 49] D-Xylose absorption is commonly reduced in patients with tropical sprue from all geographic locations, as are disaccharidase activity and lactose absorption. One of the most consistent findings in tropical sprue from both Asia and the Caribbean is impaired fat absorption; more than 90% of subjects in southern India have increased fecal fat excretion. Absorption of micronutrients, particularly folic acid, is also impaired, and as the enteropathy progresses to involve the ileum, vitamin B_{12} malabsorption often follows.

DISTURBANCE OF INTESTINAL MOTILITY. Small bowel transit time is increased in some patients with tropical sprue,[50] but in others it has been found to be normal. However, in a small group of patients, transit time returned toward normal after treatment with tetracycline and folic acid. It is unclear whether the increase in small intestinal transit is part of the primary pathophysiology of tropical sprue or whether it is secondary to bacterial colonization of the small intestine. Fat malabsorption, which leads to increased concentrations of fat in the distal ileum and colon, is known to increase small intestinal transit time and may be an important factor in modulating small intestinal transit in tropical sprue.

GASTROINTESTINAL PEPTIDE HORMONE ABNORMALITIES. Fasting serum concentrations of motilin and enteroglucagon are increased in patients with acute tropical sprue.[51] Following a standard test meal, there is a marked increase in the concentrations of both gut hormones. There also is a relationship between the plasma enteroglucagon concentration and mouth-to-cecum transit time, indicating that enteroglucagon is a candidate hormonal mediator of the increase in small intestinal transit time. Infusion of triglyceride or oleic acid into the distal small intestine increases plasma concentrations of enteroglucagon, neurotensin, and peptide YY (PYY). PYY concentrations correlate closely with changes in small intestinal transit, and PYY is now considered to have a major role in mediating the effects of fat on small intestinal transit, via the so-called "ileal brake." However, serum PYY concentrations have not been measured in patients with tropical sprue.

Theories of Etiopathogenesis

The cause of tropical sprue has not been clearly defined, although epidemiologic evidence indicates that, like tropical enteropathy, it relates to factors in the tropical environment.[16, 52, 53] Nutritional insufficiency and intestinal infection, possibly with the liberation of secretory or cytopathic toxins, have been implicated as causes. Nutritional deficiencies of folate, vitamin B_{12}, or protein, which can cause small bowel abnormalities under certain circumstances, do not appear to play a primary role in the pathogenesis of the disease, which commonly develops in well-nourished persons as well as those with varying degrees of undernutrition. Thus, although the disease can have a major effect on macro- and micronutrient status, there is little evidence to suggest that undernutrition has a major role in initiating the disease process. Considerable evidence, however, favors the concept that tropical sprue is an infectious disease caused by persistent, chronic intestinal contamination with one or more enteropathogens.

In most instances, either in isolated individual cases or in epidemic outbreaks, tropical sprue follows an episode of acute diarrhea for which no enteric pathogen can be identified. In epidemic outbreaks in southern Indian villages, the acute diarrhea often involves multiple persons within the same household, with evidence of propagation within families.[34] Chronic diarrhea develops in approximately 50% of such persons but remits spontaneously within 3 months of onset in most persons. However, diarrhea persists in approximately 10% and develops into overtly recognizable tropical sprue. In similar annual seasonal epidemics of acute diarrhea among American military personnel in the Philippines, many affected persons develop chronic diarrhea with abnormalities of intestinal structure and function.[54] The illness resolves spontaneously in some but persists in others to become tropical sprue. The studies of epidemics in the Vellore in southern India are entirely consistent with an infective etiology, and in one outbreak, there was epidemiologic evidence that protection against the condition appeared to emerge during the later phases of the epidemic, consistent with the development of protective immunity.[34]

A variety of bacteria have been isolated from the jejunums of patients with tropical sprue.[55–58] In northern India, Puerto Rico, and Haiti and in Europeans traveling to India, coliforms are present in increased numbers in the jejunum. In the Europeans, *Alcaligenes fecalis, Enterobacter aerogenes,* and *Hafnia* species have been found. In patients from India and the Caribbean, *Klebsiella pneumoniae, E. coli,* and *Enterobacter cloacae* are common. In southern India, however, the prevalence of coliforms in patients with tropical sprue is the same as in healthy controls. Thus, in some geographic areas, there is bacterial colonization of the proximal small intestine with coliforms, but no single species has emerged to explain tropical sprue in all geographic locations. Colonization of the small intestine with coliforms can change villus architecture in animal models, and similar histopathologic lesions have been described in patients with bacterial overgrowth of other causes. *Klebsiella* and other coliform bacteria isolated from patients with tropical sprue in Puerto Rico have been found to produce secretory enterotoxins and to induce structural abnormalities in the small intestine in experimental models.[57, 59, 60] Although these organisms might be incriminated in the structural and functional disturbances seen in patients in the Caribbean, it seems unlikely that they account for the disease in southern India, where coliform contamination is uncommon.

Viruses have been sought as a cause of tropical sprue, and viral particles resembling orthomyxo- and coronaviruses have been found in the feces of patients with tropical sprue[62]; however, these viruses were also found in similar numbers of asymptomatic control subjects.

It seems possible that the syndrome of tropical sprue may have more than one cause. In the Caribbean, tropical sprue is always associated with vitamin B_{12} malabsorption, is strongly linked to the presence of enterotoxin-producing coliforms, and responds well to broad-spectrum antibiotics. Disease patterns and the bacterial profile in the small intestine differ in patients from southern India and in overland travelers, and the response of these patients to treatment is less predictable than that of patients with Caribbean sprue.

A POSSIBLE MODEL FOR ETIOPATHOGENESIS. Although the etiology of tropical sprue is unknown, it is difficult to develop a clear model of pathogenesis. Cook has suggested that the primary event in the pathogenesis of tropical sprue is acute intestinal infection involving the small and possibly large intestine.[16] He has proposed that this infection produces nonspecific mucosal injury, which leads to the elevated plasma levels of enteroglucagon,[51] which is responsible for slowing small intestinal transit, thereby resulting in bacterial overgrowth. The transit abnormality amplifies the mucosal injury, which slows the transit cycle. Although attractive, this hypothesis does not explain all cases of tropical sprue. It is not always possible, for example, to identify an acute diarrheal illness in cases of tropical sprue. It would, however, be possible to postulate that subclinical infection had occurred. In addition, the relationship between the raised plasma enteroglucagon levels and retardation of small intestinal transit is not a universally accepted concept. Finally, the effect of bacterial overgrowth on the small intestine is not clear-cut, and some studies have demonstrated that motility actually may be increased by bacterial overgrowth.

Whatever the initial injury or predisposing factor is, an increased number of coliforms in the small intestine does seem to be a consistent observation in many patients studied.[55–58] The response to broad-spectrum antibiotics, at least in some patients, would support the clinical importance of this finding. The importance of fat malabsorption, with respect to the "ileal brake," slowing of intestinal transit, and the effect of fatty acids on colonocyte function, would appear to be possible mechanisms in the pathogenetic cascade. Possible routes by which these factors may interact to perpetuate the chronic diarrhea-malabsorption cycle are outlined in Figure 94–5.

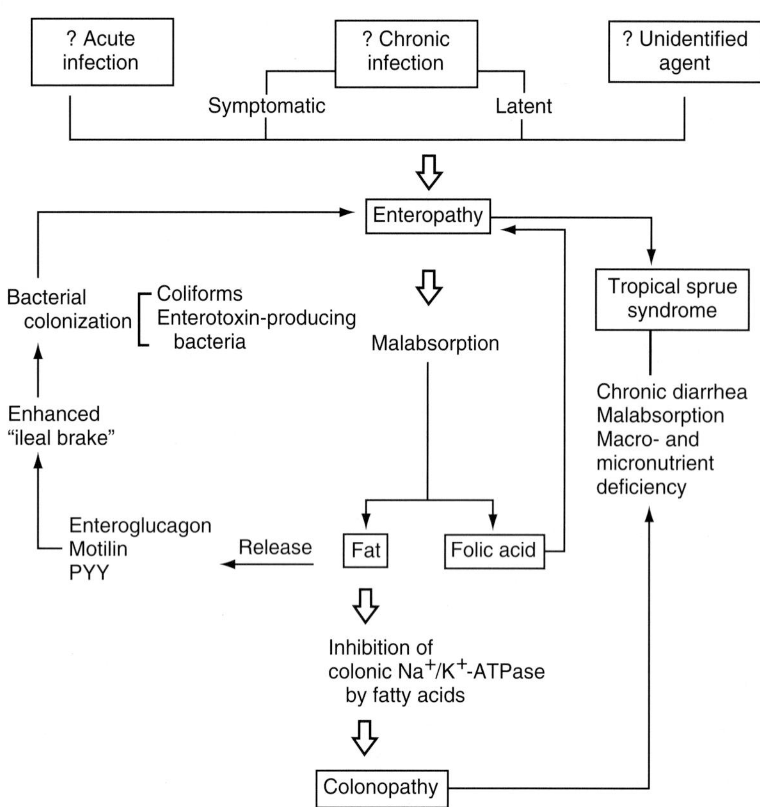

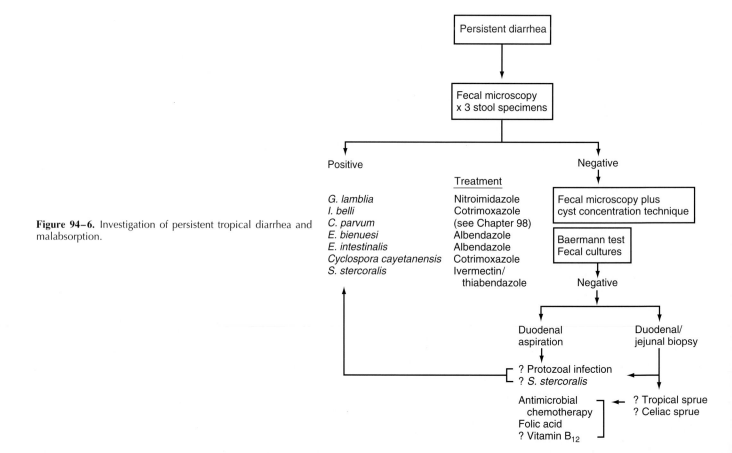

Figure 94–5. A possible model that relates the many factors that have been proposed to explain the pathogenesis of tropical sprue. PYY, peptide YY.

Persistent diarrhea

Fecal microscopy x 3 stool specimens

Positive

Negative

	Treatment
G. lamblia	Nitroimidazole
I. belli	Cotrimoxazole
C. parvum	(see Chapter 98)
E. bienuesi	Albendazole
E. intestinalis	Albendazole
Cyclospora cayetanensis	Cotrimoxazole
S. stercoralis	Ivermectin/ thiabendazole

Fecal microscopy plus cyst concentration technique

Baermann test
Fecal cultures

Negative

Duodenal aspiration

Duodenal/ jejunal biopsy

? Protozoal infection
? *S. stercoralis*

? Tropical sprue
? Celiac sprue

Antimicrobial chemotherapy
Folic acid
? Vitamin B_{12}

Figure 94–6. Investigation of persistent tropical diarrhea and malabsorption.

Diagnosis

Investigation of chronic diarrhea with or without overt clinical malabsorption in persons who have recently returned from the tropics must be targeted at excluding specific causes of malabsorption, namely intestinal infections (Fig. 94–6). At least three stool specimens obtained on separate days should be examined by light microscopy, using appropriate stains to search for the parasites *G. lamblia, C. parvum,* and *Cyclospora cayetanensis;* in an immunocompromised person, special attention should be paid to the identification of *C. parvum,* the microsporidia (*Enterocytozoon bieneusi* and *Encephalitozoon intestinalis*), and *Isospora belli.* Stool microscopy should include cyst and oocyst concentration techniques if fecal saline wet mounts are negative. Fecal examination is a relatively insensitive method to detect *Strongyloides stercoralis,* but detection of larvae can be improved by using the Baermann test or fecal culture.

If fecal microscopy is negative and any of these infections are strongly suspected, then it is often worthwhile to perform jejunal aspiration and jejunal mucosal biopsy to search for parasites in intestinal fluid or associated with the small intestinal mucosa. *Giardia* often can be identified in fluid or in mucosal smears produced from jejunal biopsies, whereas the intracellular protozoa (*C. parvum, I. belli,* and the microsporidia) can be seen in Giemsa-stained specimens of small intestinal mucosa examined by light microscopy. Occasionally celiac sprue presents for the first time in persons returning from the tropics, and this disease can now be screened for serologically by testing for the presence of antiendomysial or antitissue transglutaminase antibodies. Confirmation of the diagnosis by jejunal biopsy is usually required, and if diagnostic uncertainty between celiac sprue and tropical sprue persists, then it may be wise to perform a gluten challenge after recovery of the jejunal mucosa with gluten withdrawal (see Chapter 93).

A barium follow-through examination of the small intestine and multiple small bowel biopsies by endoscopy or enteroscopy will be necessary to exclude small intestinal lymphoma or immunoproliferative small intestinal disease (IPSID).

Once the specific causes of diarrhea and malabsorption have been excluded, fat, vitamin B_{12}, and possibly D-xylose malabsorption are established, and a jejunal biopsy shows partial villus atrophy, the diagnosis can be assumed to be tropical sprue. The barium small bowel follow-through examination in tropical sprue usually shows an increase in the caliber of the small intestine and thickening of the folds (Fig. 94–7).[62] These changes are present throughout the small intestine, and the examination is usually notable for the slow transit of the barium column through the gut.

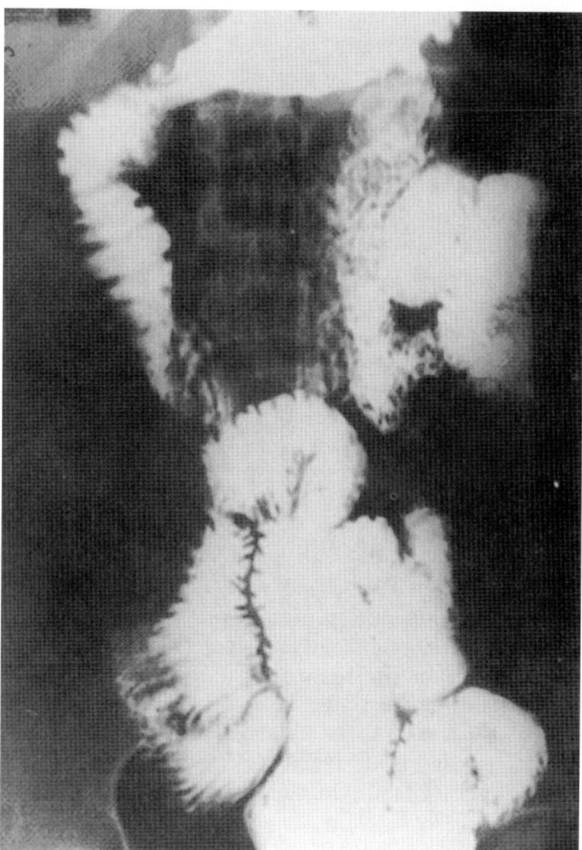

Figure 94–7. Barium follow-through examination of the small intestine in a patient from southern India with chronic tropical sprue shows jejunal dilatation and fold thickening.

Treatment

General Measures

Restoration of water and electrolyte balance and replacement of nutritional deficiencies are the priorities in the initial management of persons with tropical sprue. These interventions alone are thought to have been responsible for the marked decrease in mortality in epidemic sprue in southern India. Vitamin B_{12} should be given parenterally, but iron and folic acid are effective when provided orally. These interventions usually result in a prompt hematologic remission of the megaloblastic anemia, disappearance of glossitis, and return of appetite, which results in the onset of weight gain even before improvements in intestinal absorption are apparent.[63–67] Improvement in jejunal structural abnormalities, particularly in the crypts, is evident within 3 to 6 days in those who have marked abnormalities but may be delayed for as long as several weeks in those who have mild abnormalities. The results of treatment with folic acid appear to depend on the chronicity of the intestinal lesions.[29, 68] Treatment can be curative in those who have had the disease for only a few months, whereas in those with chronic disease, notably indigenous residents, folic acid alone usually does not correct the intestinal abnormalities.[63]

Antimicrobial Chemotherapy

The role of broad-spectrum antibiotics in the treatment of tropical sprue remains controversial. Overland travelers, such as those from the United Kingdom, and patients in Puerto Rico are reported to improve on tetracycline, 250 mg four times daily, usually given over a period of several months.[28, 69, 70] In a controlled trial in southern India, the addition of antibiotics to vitamin B_{12} and folic acid supplementation did not appear to improve the rate of recovery. Spontaneous recovery does occur, possibly related to a change in environment and the oral bacterial load. Symptomatic treatment with an antidiarrheal preparation such as loperamide is often advised. However, if intestinal stasis and bacterial colonization are important in the pathogenesis of this syndrome, one might argue that slowing small intestinal transit with an antidiarrheal preparation may delay recovery.

The prognosis in expatriates is good, with the vast majority experiencing complete and permanent recovery.[27] Recovery may be more rapid in expatriates who leave the tropics and return to a temperate climate. There is some evidence, however, that recurrence of tropical sprue can occur in treated patients of the indigenous population in the tropics. Significant malabsorption was detected in 50% of a group of Puerto Ricans examined 5 years after their intestinal abnormalities apparently had been cured by antimicrobial chemotherapy.[71]

Prevention

Other than the usual advice to travelers regarding the avoidance of contaminated food and water, there are no specific preventive measures for tropical sprue. The incidence appears to be declining in overland travelers and expatriates, perhaps because of the more liberal use of antibiotics for traveler's diarrhea. The epidemics of tropical sprue in southern India also appear to be on the decline, presumably because of improving water quality and sanitary conditions and the widespread availability of antibiotics.

REFERENCES

1. Thielman NM, Guerrant RL: Persistent diarrhea in the returned traveler. Infect Dis Clin North Am 12:489, 1998.
2. Farthing MJG, Kelly MP, Veitch AM: Recently recognised microbial enteropathies in HIV infection. J Antimicro Chemother 37(suppl B):61, 1996.
3. Hoge CW, Shlim DR, Ghimire M, et al: Placebo-controlled trial of co-trimoxazole for cyclospora infections among travellers and foreign residents in Nepal. Lancet 345:691, 1995.
4. Kelly MP, McPhail J, Ngwenya B, et al: *Septata intestinalis*: A new microsporidian in Africa. Lancet 344:271, 1994.
5. Veitch A, Kelly P, Luo N, et al: Small intestine mucosal T-cell expression in Africans with HIV infection. Gastroenterology 108:A936, 1995.
6. Veitch AM, Kelly P, Segal I, et al: Does sucrase deficiency in black South Africans protect against colonic disease [research letter]? Lancet 351:183, 1998.
7. Wood GM, Gearty JC, Cooper BT: Small bowel morphology in British Indian and Afro-Caribbean subjects: Evidence of tropical enteropathy. Gut 32:256, 1991.
8. Cook GC: Impairment of D-xylose absorption in Zambian patients with systemic intestinal infection. Am J Clin Nutr 25:490, 1972.
9. Cook GC: Tropical Gastroenterology. Oxford, Oxford University Press, 1980, pp 271–324.
10. Bhat P, Shantakumari S, Rajan D, et al: Bacterial flora of the gastrointestinal tract in Southern Indian control subjects and patients with tropical sprue. Gastroenterology 62:11, 1972.
11. Veitch AM, Kelly P, Pobee JOM, et al: Small intestinal mucosal T cell activation in African tropical enteropathy. Gastroenterology 110:A038, 1996.
12. Veitch AM, Kelly P, Luo N, et al: Small intestinal crypt hyperplasia and T cell activation in African tropical enteropathy. Gastroenterology 114(suppl Part 2):G4536, 1998.
13. Ramakrishna BS, Mathan VI: Absorption of water and sodium and activity of adenosine triphosphatases in the rectal mucosa in tropical sprue. Gut 29:665, 1988.
14. Haghighi P, Wolf PL: Tropical sprue and subclinical enteropathy: A vision for the nineties. Crit Rev Clin Lab Sci 34:313, 1997.
15. Baker SJ, Mathan VI: Tropical sprue in Southern India. In Wellcome Trust Collaboration Study 1961–1969. London, Churchill Livingstone, 1970, pp 453–467.
16. Cook GC: Aetiology and pathogenesis of post-infective tropical malabsorption (tropical sprue). Lancet 1:721, 1984.
17. Tomkins A, Booth CC: (1985). Tropical sprue. In Disorders of the Small Intestine. Oxford, Blackwell Scientific Publications, 1985, pp 311–332.
18. Booth CC: The first description of tropical sprue. Gut 5:45, 1964.
19. Manson P: Notes on sprue. Med Rep China Imp Marit Customs 19:33, 1880.
20. Manson-Bahr PH: The morbid anatomy and pathology of sprue and their bearing upon aetiology. Lancet 1:1148, 1924.
21. Mathan VI, Baker SJ: The epidemiology of tropical sprue. In Wellcome Trust Collaborative Study 1961–1969. London, Churchill Livingstone 1971, pp 159–188.
22. Klipstein FA, Beauchamp I, Corcino JJ, et al: Nutritional status and intestinal function among rural populations of the West Indies. II. Barrio Nuevo, Puerto Rico. Gastroenterology 63:758, 1971.
23. Klipstein FA, Samloff IM, Smarth G, Schenk EA: Malabsorption in rural Haiti. Am J Clin Nutr 21:1042, 1968.
24. Moshal MG, Hirst W, Kallicburum S, Pillay K: Enteric tropical sprue in Africa. J Trop Med Hyg 78:2, 1975.
25. Thomas G, Clain DJ: Endemic tropical sprue in Rhodesia. Gut 12:877, 1976.
26. Falaiye JM: Tropical sprue in Nigeria. J Trop Med Hyg 73:119, 1970.
27. Klipstein FA, Falaiye JM: Tropical sprue in expatriates from the tropics living in the continental United States. Medicine 48:475, 1969.
28. Keele KD, Bound JP: Sprue in India: Clinical survey of 600 cases. Br Med J 1:77, 1946.
29. O'Brien W, England NWJ: Tropical sprue amongst British servicemen and their families in South-East Asia. In Tropical Sprue and Megaloblastic Anaemia. London, Churchill Livingstone, 1971, pp 25–60.
30. Walters AM, James WPT, Cole ACE, Walters JH: Malabsorption in overland travellers to India. Br Med J 3:380, 1974.
31. Sheehy TW: Digestive disease as a national problem. VI. Enteric disease among United States troops in Vietnam. Gastroenterology 55:105, 1968.
32. Mathan VI, Baker SJ: An epidemic of tropical sprue in Southern India. I. Clinical features. Ann Trop Med Parasitol 64:439, 1970.
33. Baker SJ, Mathan VI: Epidemic tropical sprue. Pt. II. Epidemiology. Ann Trop Med Parasitol 64:453, 1970.
34. Mathan VI, Baker SJ: Epidemic tropical sprue and other epidemics of diarrhea in South Indian villages. Am J Clin Nutr 21:1077, 1968.
35. Baker SJ: Idiopathic small-intestinal disease in the tropics. In Critical Reviews in Tropical Medicine. New York, Plenum Publishing, 1982, pp 197–245.
36. Klipstein FA, Falaiye JM: Tropical sprue in expatriates from the tropics living in the continental United States. Medicine 48:475, 1969.
37. Klipstein FA: Tropical sprue in travellers and expatriates living abroad. Gastroenterology 80:590, 1981.
38. Mathan VI: Tropical sprue in Southern India. Trans R Soc Trop Med 82:10, 1988.
39. Klipstein FA, Corcino JJ: Factors responsible for weight loss in tropical sprue. Am J Clin Nutr 30:1703, 1977.
40. Swanson VL, Thomassen RW: Pathology of the jejunal mucosa in tropical sprue. Am J Pathol 46:511, 1963.
41. Wheby MS, Swanson VL, Bayless TM: Comparison of ileal and jejunal biopsies in tropical sprue. Am J Clin Nutr 24:117, 1971.
42. Mathan M, Mathan VI, Baker SJ: An electron microscope study of jejunal mucosal morphology in control subjects and in patients with tropical sprue in Southern India. Gastroenterology 68:17, 1975.
43. Brunser O, Eidelman S, Klipstein FA: Intestinal morphology of rural Haitians. A comparison between overt tropical sprue and asymptomatic subjects. Gastroenterology 58:655, 1970.
44. Mathan MM, Ponniah J, Mathan VI: Epithelial cell renewal and turnover and relationship to morphologic abnormalities in jejunal mucosa in tropical sprue. Dig Dis Sci 31:586, 1986.
45. Ramakrishna BS, Mathan VI: Water and electrolyte absorption by the colon in tropical sprue. Gut 23:843, 1982.
46. Corcino JJ, Maldonado M, Klipstein FA: Intestinal perfusion studies in tropical sprue. I. Transport of water, electrolytes, and D-xylose. Gastroenterology 65:192, 1983.
47. Hellier MD, Bhat P, Albert J, Baker SJ: Intestinal perfusion studies in tropical sprue. 2. Movement of water and electrolytes. Gut 18:480, 1977.

48. Hellier MD, Radhakrishnan AN, Ganapathy V, et al: Intestinal perfusion studies in tropical sprue. 1. Aminoacid and dipeptide absorption. Gut 17:511, 1976.
49. Hellier MD, Ganapathy C, Gammon A, et al: Impaired intestinal absorption of dipeptide in tropical sprue patients in India. Clin Sci 58: 431, 1980.
50. Cook GC: Delayed small intestinal transit in tropical malabsorption. Br Med J 2:238, 1978.
51. Besterman HS, Cook GC, Sarson DL: Gut hormones in tropical malabsorption. Br Med J 2:1252, 1979.
52. Glynn J: Tropical sprue—its aetiology and pathogenesis. J Roy Soc Med 79:599, 1986.
53. Tomkins A: Tropical malabsorption: Recent concepts in pathogenesis and nutritional significance. Clin Sci 60:131, 1981.
54. Jones TC, Dean AG, Parker GW: Seasonal gastroenteritis and malabsorption at an American military base in the Philippines. II. Malabsorption following the acute illness. Am J Epidemiol 95:128, 1972.
55. Gorbach SL, Mitra R, Jacobs B, et al: Bacterial contamination of the upper small bowel in tropical sprue. Lancet 1:74, 1969.
56. Gorbach SL, Banwell JG, Jacobs B, et al: Tropical sprue and malnutrition in West Bengal. I. Intestinal microflora and absorptions. Am J Clin Nutr 23:1545, 1970.
57. Klipstein FA, Haldeman LV, Corcino JJ, Moore WEC: Enterotoxigenic intestinal bacteria in tropical sprue. Ann Intern Med 79:632, 1973.
58. Tomkins AM, Drasar BS, James WPT: Bacterial colonisation of jejunal mucosa in acute tropical sprue. Lancet 1:59, 1975.
59. Klipstein FA, Engert RF, Short HB: Enterotoxigenicity of colonising coliform bacteria in tropical sprue and blind-loop syndrome. Lancet 2: 342, 1978.
60. Klipstein FA, Horowitz IR, Engert RF, Schenk EA: Effect of *Klebsiella pneumoniae* enterotoxin on intestinal transport in the rat. J Clin Invest 56:799, 1975.
61. Baker SJ, Mathan M, Mathan VI, Swaminathan SP: Chronic enterocyte infection with coronavirus. One possible cause of the syndrome of tropical sprue? Dig Dis Sci 11:1039, 1982.
62. McLean AM, Farthing MJG, Kurian G, Mathan VI: The relationship between hypoalbuminaemia and the radiological appearances of the jejunum in tropical sprue. Br J Radiol 55:725, 1982.
63. Sheehy TW, Baggs B, Perez-Santiago E, Floch MH: Prognosis of tropical sprue. A study of the effect of folic acid on the intestinal aspects of acute and chronic sprue. Ann Intern Med 57:892, 1962.
64. Klipstein FA, Schenk EA, Samloff IM: Folate repletion associated with oral tetracycline therapy in tropical sprue. Gastroenterology 51:317, 1966.
65. Tomkins AM, Smith T, Wright SG: Assessment of early and delayed responses in vitamin B_{12} absorption during antibiotic therapy in tropical malabsorption. Clin Sci Mol Med 55:533, 1978.
66. Spies TD, Milanes F, Menandez A, et al: Observations on treatment of tropical sprue with folic acid. J Lab Clin Med 31:223, 1946.
67. Spies TD, Suarez RM: Responses of tropical sprue to vitamin B_{12}. Blood 3:1213, 1948.
68. Sheehy TW, Cohen WH, Wallace DK, Legtens LJ: Tropical sprue in North Americans. JAMA 194:1069, 1965.
69. Guerra R, Whelby MS, Bayless TM: Long-term antibiotic therapy in tropical sprue. Ann Intern Med 63:619, 1965.
70. Sheehy TW, Perez-Santiago E: Antibiotic therapy in tropical sprue. Gastroenterology 41:208, 1961.
71. Rickles FR, Klipstein FA, Tomasini J, et al: Long-term follow-up of antibiotic-treated tropical sprue. Ann Intern Med 76:203, 1972.

Chapter 95

WHIPPLE'S DISEASE

Matthias Maiwald, Axel von Herbay, and David A. Relman

Whipple's disease is a chronic systemic infection by a gram-positive bacterium, *Tropheryma whippelii*. The small intestine is most often affected, but a variety of other organs may also be involved, including the joints, the cardiovascular system, and the central nervous system (CNS). The clinical symptoms and findings are protean, including weight loss, diarrhea, malabsorption, fever, arthralgias, skin hyperpigmentation, and dementia. The disease was considered to be uniformly fatal in the preantibiotic era, but today treatment with antibiotics usually leads to clinical remission. Many open questions still surround the pathogenesis of this disease; it is presumed that host genetic factors increase susceptibility to disease.

HISTORY

In 1907, the pathologist George H. Whipple reported in detail the case of a 36-year-old male physician-missionary who had died after a 5-year illness involving arthritis, chronic cough, weight loss, and chronic diarrhea.[1] At autopsy, Whipple found lipid deposits in the intestinal mucosa and in mesenteric and retroperitoneal lymph nodes. Microscopic examination further revealed a large number of macrophages with foamy cytoplasm in the lamina propria of the small intestine. Whipple suspected a disorder of fat metabolism and proposed the term "intestinal lipodystrophy" for this disease. In a silver-stained mesenteric lymph node, he also described rod-shaped bacteria, with the approximate thickness of a syphilis spirochete and a length of approximately 2 μm, but did not interpret this finding as related to the causation of the disease.

In the following decades, only a few cases were reported and the diagnosis was uniformly made at autopsy. The first antemortem diagnosis was made in 1947, based on findings in a mesenteric lymph node removed at laparotomy[2] and the first diagnosis by peroral intestinal biopsy was made in 1958.[3] In 1949, Black-Schaffer[4] introduced the periodic acid–Schiff (PAS) stain to the histopathologic diagnosis of Whipple's disease. Inclusions in macrophages stained red using this stain, thus documenting that intracellular material was glycoprotein rather than lipid.

Further advances came in 1952 with the first observation of successful antibiotic treatment of a case (using chloramphenicol)[5] and in 1961 when two groups independently visualized bacteria by electron microscopy in affected tissues.[6, 7] Subsequent reports confirmed these observations. Bacteria associated with Whipple's disease were rod shaped and of uniform size. Consistent positive therapeutic effects were achieved with antibiotic treatment.[8] These findings and those of Black-Schaffer[4] suggested that the disease was unlikely to be a primary disorder of fat metabolism, as previously suspected, and that instead it was a bacterial disease. Efforts to cultivate this bacterium before 2000 failed to yield reproducible or consistent results.

The nature of the bacterium remained obscure until the early 1990s, when its 16S ribosomal DNA (rDNA) sequence was determined and phylogenetic analysis established a relationship of the Whipple's disease bacterium to the actinomycetes.[9, 10] The name *Tropheryma whippelii* was proposed.[10] More recent efforts to cultivate this bacterium in coculture with human cells have been successful, albeit with long generation times.[11] Colocalization of the unique *T. whippelii* 16S rDNA sequence with areas of pathology in cases of Whipple's disease establishes the relevance of this sequence and the inferred phylogeny.[12] This novel 16S rDNA sequence also provides the basis for sensitive diagnostic testing using the polymerase chain reaction (PCR).

EPIDEMIOLOGY

Whipple's disease is a rare disorder. The first comprehensive epidemiologic survey was performed by Dobbins,[8] in which he compiled information on 696 patients, comprising 617 published and 79 unpublished cases recorded through 1986. According to this meta-analysis, Whipple's disease is a sporadic disease with a predilection for middle-aged white men. Data on age and sex were available for 664 patients; 86% were male, and the mean age at diagnosis was 49 years. Only very few cases (4%) were reported in patients in the age group of 30 years or younger. Most patients were white, only 10 were African, one was a native American, 3 patients were from India, and 1 was Japanese. Most of the patients originated from Europe (373 patients) or from the United States (246 patients). Within Europe, Germany (114 patients) and France (91 patients) were strongly represented. Relatively few cases originated from South America (11 patients) and Australia (13 patients).

A small epidemiologic study from western Switzerland calculated the incidence of Whipple's disease to be approximately 0.4 per million of inhabitants per year.[13] An epidemiologic analysis of 110 patients in Germany noted a relatively stable incidence of cases of Whipple's disease over three decades and a relatively even geographic distribution of the patients' residences.[14] There are only few observations of geographically confined case clusters (up to seven cases).[15–17]

Several studies[14, 18, 19] indicate an increase in the age of patients in recent decades; this is statistically significant.[14] Presently, patients are diagnosed at a mean age of 56 years, with approximately 80% male.[20] It has been speculated that the increasing use of antibiotics for unrelated complaints in medical practice may be a contributing factor in delaying the age at onset of Whipple's disease.

One remarkable epidemiologic feature in Dobbins' analysis[8] was the strong representation of patients with occupations in the farming and building trades; of 191 patients for whom data were available, 43 (22%) were farmers and 10 (5%) were carpenters. Patients in all farming-related trades accounted for 34% of the total. By comparison, the proportion of farm workers among the total workforce in the analyzed countries was approximately 10%. These occupations may be described as involving work outdoors or frequent contact with animals or soil.

MICROBIOLOGY, IMMUNOLOGY, AND PATHOGENESIS

Many attempts have been undertaken to cultivate the bacterium associated with Whipple's disease, a significant number of which have probably not been reported in the literature.[8] Most reports of "successful" cultivation have been nonreproducible or due to the isolation of contaminants.[8] In one study,[21] heart valve tissue of two infected patients was inoculated onto primary human monocytes that were treated with interleukin-4 in culture. Accumulation of PAS-positive intracellular particles and the persistence of PCR signals after several culture passages were interpreted to indicate growth of *T. whippelii*. However, subsequent attempts by others using this method failed to confirm growth of the organism.[22]

In 2000, the cultivation of *T. whippelii* from infected heart valve tissue using human fibroblast-like cells was reported.[11] Seven culture passages were performed, over a period of 285 days, and the 16S rDNA sequence of *T. whippelii* was detected after each passage. The doubling time of the bacteria was estimated to be 18 days, which is slower than that of any other known pathogenic bacterium. The associated data provided good evidence that *T. whippelii* does replicate under these conditions *in vitro*, although the reported doubling time renders the method impractical for routine diagnostic use. The organism has also been cultivated from an intestinal mucosal biopsy specimen.[22a]

Phylogenetic analysis of the *T. whippelii* 16S rDNA sequence, based on a cultivation-independent approach, established that this bacterium is an actinomycete and a previously unrecognized member of the Actinobacteria bacterial division.[9, 10] A subsequent more detailed analysis placed the organism in an intermediate position between the genus *Cellulomonas* and a rare group of actinomycetes with group B peptidoglycan.[23] Both of these groups of organisms are predominantly environmental bacteria and are found in soil, water, and on plants, although the relationships of *T. whippelii* to any of the other known actinomycetes are relatively distant (<92% 16S rRNA sequence similarity).

To establish a molecular typing system for different *T. whippelii* strains, the 16S–23S rRNA intergenic spacer of this bacterium has been determined[23]; six different sequence types have been described so far.[24, 25] The two most common spacer types, "1" and "2," are found in a similar ratio (approximately 1:2) in the United States, Germany, and Switzerland. The same spacer type is found in different anatomic compartments (e.g., intestine, blood, cerebrospinal fluid [CSF]) of any given patient.[25] The latter finding argues for systemic dissemination of a single bacterial strain in an individual with Whipple's disease. The numbers of patients studied in this manner are insufficient to address the possible association of different clinical features with different strain types.

Transient (during active disease) and persistent (after therapy) abnormalities of immune function have been observed in patients with Whipple's disease.[8, 26, 27] The persistent defects are presumed to serve as predisposing factors for development of disease. However, precisely defined immune defects, such as the absence of specific cell types, mediators, or receptors, have not been identified. Small case series[28, 29] have described an over-representation of the HLA-B27 haplotype in patients with Whipple's disease, whereas others[30] have not supported this association. Humoral immunity grossly appears to be normal, although patient antisera have failed to react with areas of pathology in tissue sections of the intestinal mucosa.[8, 31]

During active disease, reduced CD4/CD8 T-cell ratios (both in the lamina propria and in peripheral blood), reduced proliferation of peripheral T cells to stimulating agents (e.g., phytohemagglutinin, concanavalin A), and reduced delayed-type hypersensitivity reactions to common antigens in skin tests have been observed.[26, 28, 32] The extent to which these immune disturbances are a consequence of malnutrition in active Whipple's disease, rather than preexisting factors, remains unclear. The monocytes of one patient exhibited an impaired ability to degrade bacterial antigens after ingestion,[33] which would be consistent with the prolonged persistence of bacterial remnants in intestinal macrophages after therapy, as observed in histologic studies of Whipple's disease.[8, 34] Other abnormalities have been found that persist after therapy: reduced numbers of peripheral blood monocytes that express the α chain of complement receptor 3 (CD11b)[26] and a reduced capability of peripheral blood monocytes to produce interleukin-12 upon stimulation with bacterial antigens.[27] These features and activities play roles in microbial phagocytosis, antigen processing, and the regulation of a cellular immune response.[26, 27]

Several reports describe opportunistic infections in patients with Whipple's disease, but this is not a generally observed phenomenon. Secondary or opportunistic agents have included *Giardia lamblia, Pneumocystis carinii, Cryptosporidium parvum, Nocardia* spp., *Mycobacterium tuberculosis, Serratia marcescens, Candida* spp., dermatophytes, and *Strongyloides stercoralis*.[34–36] In addition, *T. whippelii* infection has been detected in a patient with acquired immunodeficiency syndrome on one occasion.[37] A role of the immune system for clearing a *T. whippelii* infection was further suggested by the report of one patient without adequate response to treatment with various antibiotics who eventually benefitted from adjuvant interferon-γ treatment.[38] Taken together, these observations and laboratory findings suggest that host immunologic factors play a role in determining the occurrence of Whipple's disease.

Because of the prominence of intestinal manifestations, an oral route of acquisition is generally assumed,[8] but this has not been proven. Current concepts hold that once *T. whippelii* has been acquired, it passes through the stomach and enters the proximal small intestine where the bacteria invade the mucosa. Evidence for this is provided by electron microscopy.[39–41] Fluorescent *in situ* hybridization techniques indicate that most viable bacteria are extracellular and located just below the epithelial basement membrane (see later).[12] From the intestinal mucosa, bacteria are thought to spread via the lymphatic drainage into the mesenteric lymph nodes[40] and from there into the mediastinal lymph nodes, the thoracic duct, and the blood.

The natural habitats of *T. whippelii* are unknown. Only humans seem to be affected, with outdoor workers more strongly represented than other professional groups.[8] A PCR-based search in German sewage treatment plant effluent, which constitutes a rich polymicrobial environment, revealed positive results for *T. whippelii* in 25 of 38 samples from five different plants; this is the only published evidence of bacterial localization outside of a human host and suggests a possible environmental source of infection.[42] From within the human host, some investigators have detected *T. whippelii* DNA in saliva,[43] gastric juice, and intestinal biopsies[44] of asymptomatic persons. However, other PCR-based studies of intestinal biopsy samples provide little or no evidence of infection in persons without typical histologic features of Whipple's disease (see later).[45–49] The preponderance of available data argues against the human intestine serving as a significant reservoir for *T. whippelii* in nature. There is also no evidence for person-to-person transmission of Whipple's disease,[8] and there are only a few reports of the disease in close relatives.[50–52]

CLINICAL MANIFESTATIONS

Whipple's disease is a systemic disorder, and almost any organ or organ system can be affected.[8] Manifestations in the intestinal tract are most commonly reported; they are largely responsible for the "classic" clinical features of Whipple's disease.[16, 53] In many cases, arthralgias precede intestinal symptoms by several years (1 to 10 years; up to 30 years reported), and in some cases, low-grade intermittent fever also occurs for years before the diagnosis is made.[19, 54] More recent reports provide a wider spectrum of manifestations, especially those that are extraintestinal. This probably reflects advances in diagnostic procedures. As a result, patients tend to be diagnosed with less advanced disease.[8, 19]

Intestines and Lymphatic System

Bacterial and macrophage-predominant inflammatory cell infiltration of the small intestinal mucosa and obstruction of mesenteric lymph nodes lead to a malabsorption syndrome with weight loss, diarrhea, and abdominal pain as the dominant signs and symptoms.[16, 19, 53–55] Weight loss occurs gradually, usually over a period of at least 1 year and in amounts of 5 to 15 kg, sometimes leading to severe cachexia in the terminal stage of untreated disease.[8, 16, 54] Diarrhea may consist of voluminous steatorrheic stools or may be watery.[16] Occult gastrointestinal bleeding is common, and in some cases gross gastrointestinal bleeding occurs.[8, 16]

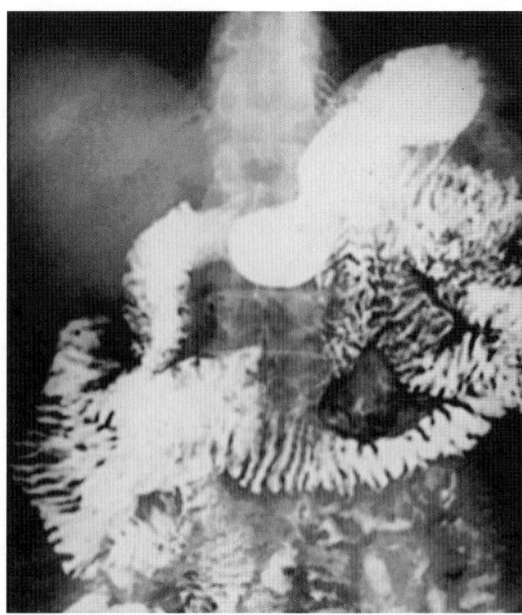

Figure 95–1. Barium contrast study of the small intestine from a patient with Whipple's disease. There is marked thickening of the plicae circulares and a loss of the normal delicate mucosal relief pattern. There is some dilatation of the small intestine. (Courtesy of Elihu Schimmel, MD, Boston, MA.)

Abdominal (mesenteric and retroperitoneal) and peripheral lymphadenopathy are common,[16, 19, 54, 55] and in some instances enlarged abdominal lymph nodes raised the suspicion of malignancy.[55] In rare instances, malignant lymphomas have occurred in patients with Whipple's disease.[56–58]

Radiographic examination of the intestinal tract with barium contrast may reveal nonspecific abnormalities that are also found in other malabsorption syndromes,[8, 54] such as prominent and edematous duodenal and jejunal folds and dilatation (Fig. 95–1). Computed tomography (Fig. 95–2) or magnetic resonance imaging may detect retroperitoneal or paraaortic lymphadenopathy.[54, 59] Enlarged abdominal lymph nodes have a hypodense appearance on CTs and are hyperechoic on ultrasonograms.[36, 60]

Laboratory examinations in patients with intestinal Whipple's disease often reveal increased erythrocyte sedimentation rates, decreased serum carotene levels, decreased serum iron concentration, anemia, decreased serum protein levels, proteinuria, and elevated stool fat content.[8, 54]

Central Nervous System

Symptomatic CNS manifestations have been reported in 10% to 43% of patients with intestinal Whipple's disease.[16, 19, 54, 55] Neurologic disease can occur concurrently with intestinal

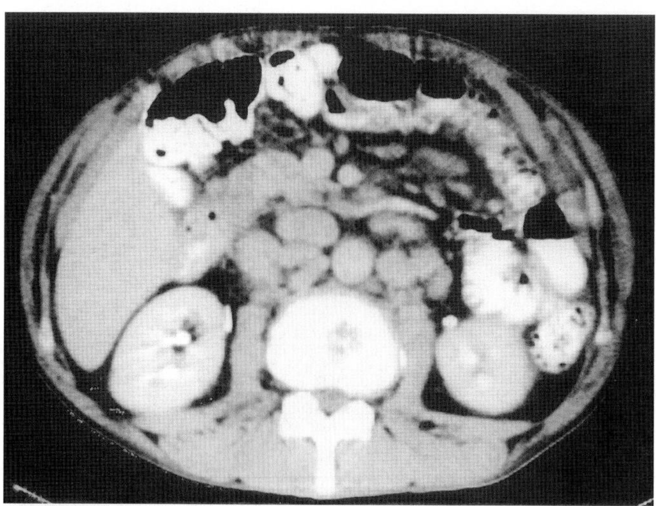

Figure 95–2. CT scan showing extensive retroperitoneal and mesenteric adenopathy in Whipple's disease, simulating lymphoma. (Courtesy of Mark Feldman, MD, Dallas, TX.)

manifestations at the time of diagnosis, but it is more frequent at the time of clinical relapse during or after treatment.[8, 61] Relapses affecting the CNS are ominous, because they can be refractory to renewed antibiotic treatment.[8, 62] Although rare, several cases of neurologic Whipple's disease have been reported in patients without intestinal manifestations.[63, 64]

According to a meta-analysis of 84 published cases,[65] common neurologic findings are progessive dementia and cognitive changes (71%), supranuclear opthalmoplegia (51%), and altered level of consciousness (50%). Other less frequent signs are psychiatric symptoms, hypothalamic manifestations (e.g., polydipsia, hyperphagia, insomnia[66]), cranial nerve abnomalities, nystagmus, seizures, and ataxia. Two signs are considered to be characteristic of CNS Whipple's disease: oculomasticatory myorhythmia and oculofacial skeletal myorhythmia. These have not yet been documented in other CNS diseases.[65] Both consist of slow rhythmic and synchronized contractions (~1/sec) of ocular, facial, or other muscles. However, both occur in less than 20% of patients with CNS Whipple's disease.[65]

Results of neuroimaging (computed tomography or magnetic resonance imaging) may be normal or may reveal mild to moderate brain atrophy or focal lesions without a predilection for specific sites.[65, 67] These abnormalities are not specific for Whipple's disease, but focal lesions may be used to guide stereotactic biopsies, which in most cases reveal characteristic histology.[65] Results of standard CSF examinations are most often normal, although sometimes there is mild pleocytosis.[8, 65] CSF cytology reveals PAS-positive sickleform particle-containing cells, and PCR often yields positive results for *T. whippelii* DNA, even in a considerable proportion of neurologically asymptomatic patients.[68]

Cardiovascular System

Cardiac manifestations of Whipple's disease comprise endocarditis, myocarditis, and pericarditis.[19] In one autopsy series from the preantibiotic era,[53] valvular endocarditis with vegetations was noted in 58% of cases. In contrast, in a more recent series,[19] clinically apparent endocarditis was less frequent (3 of 52 patients). All valves may be affected, with the mitral valve most frequently altered pathologically and the aortic valve leading to the most significant symptoms.[8] Some patients require valve replacement.[69] PAS-positive macrophages and bacteria have been documented on valve tissue by histology and electron microscopy, respectively,[70] including on a porcine prosthetic valve[71] and in the myocardium.[72] Recent reports of patients with *T. whippelii* endocarditis have described a syndrome of "blood culture-negative endocarditis" with only minor or no apparent intestinal Whipple's disease.[73–75]

Musculoskeletal System

Oligo- or polyarthralgias, usually involving the ankles, knees, elbows, or fingers, are a common complaint of patients with Whipple's disease.[8] Rheumatoid factor is usually absent. Destructive joint changes or synovial fluid accumulation are rare, but, if present, PAS-positive macrophages (by histology), bacteria (by electron microscopy), or DNA of *T. whippelii* (by PCR) can be found in synovial tissue or joint fluid.[8, 76, 77] Sacroiliitis and spondylitis may occur, but ankylosing forms are rare and there does not seem to be a strong association of these manifestations with HLA-B27.[8] Rare manifestations are infectious spondylodiscitis[78] and prosthetic joint infection.[79]

Other Manifestations

One common feature of Whipple's disease is skin hyperpigmentation, which has been found in 17% to 66% of patients in different series.[16, 19, 53–55] This finding tends to occur in light-exposed areas of the skin and is unrelated to adrenal dysfunction or hyperbilirubinemia. Histopathologic changes in the skin are, however, extremely rare.[80]

Diverse ocular manifestations of Whipple's disease have been described but are rare. These include uveitis, vitritis, retinitis, retrobulbar neuritis, and papilledema.[8] They are usually associated with CNS disease, and almost all reported patients had clinical or histologic evidence of intestinal involvement. PAS-positive macrophages or DNA of *T. whippelii* may be detected in vitrectomy specimens.[81] A case of uveitis has been reported in which the vitreous fluid and one intestinal biopsy specimen yielded positive PCR results, although intestinal histology was normal.[82]

Chronic cough was a symptom in Whipple's original patient and was reported relatively frequently in earlier series[53] but has been reported less frequently since then.[19] Some patients have pleuritis with effusion or granulomatous pulmonary disease resembling sarcoidosis.[8]

PATHOLOGY

Small Intestine

The histopathologic features of intestinal Whipple's disease are quite distinctive. At gross inspection, most patients have abnormal mucosa in the distal duodenum and jejunum.

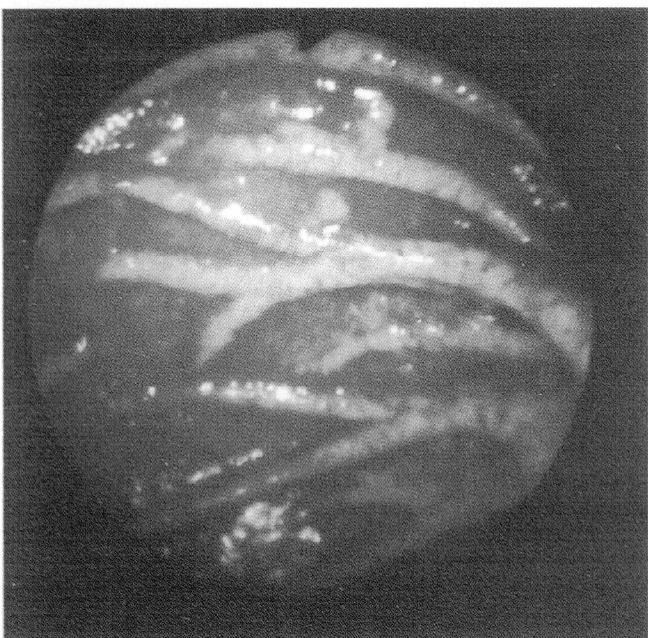

Figure 95–3. Endoscopic view of the distal duodenum in a patient with untreated Whipple's disease. The plicae appear swollen, and the mucosal surface is intact. Numerous whitish patches are present within the mucosa, reflecting lipid deposits. (Courtesy of Hans Jörg Meier-Willersen, MD, Heidelberg, Germany.)

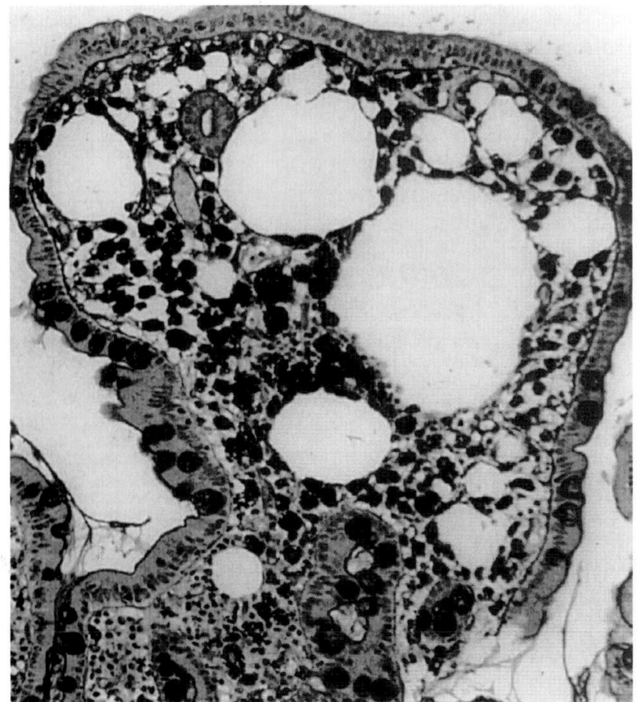

Figure 95–4. Histology of the small intestinal mucosa (biopsy from the same patient as in Fig. 95–3). A villus is distended by an infiltrate of macrophages that contain PAS-positive granular particles (type 1 cells), and by lipid droplets. The epithelial layer is intact. PAS stain; original magnification ×84.

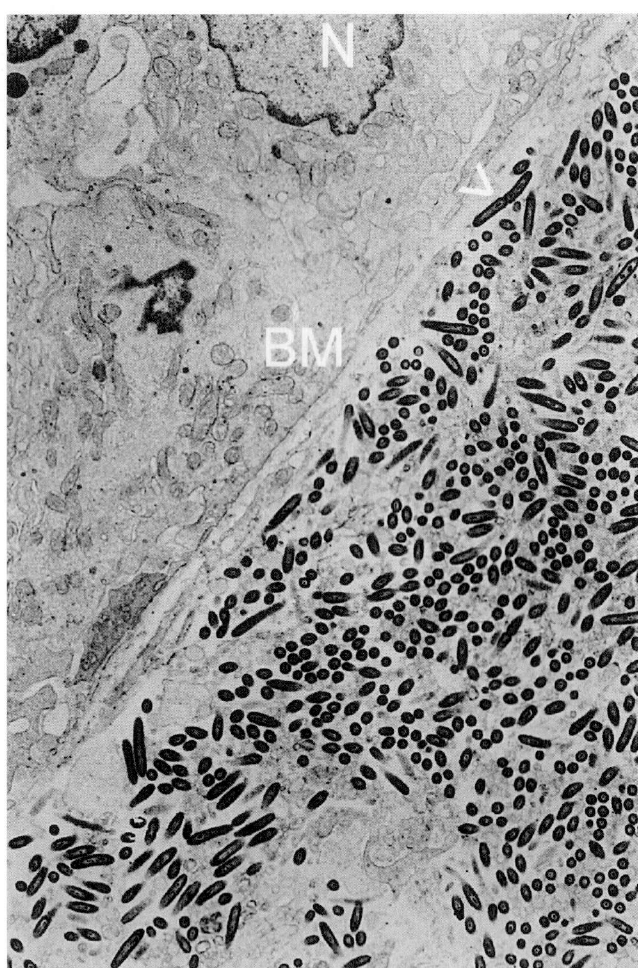

Figure 95–5. Electron microscopy of a small intestinal biopsy in a patient with untreated Whipple's disease. Just beneath the epithelial basement membrane, the lamina propria is densely infiltrated by extracellular rod-shaped bacteria. Bacteria have uniform size and structure. Some of them are dividing. BM, basement membrane; N, nucleus of enterocyte; arrowhead, dividing bacterium.

Whitish to yellow plaque-like patches are observed in approximately three fourths of patients (Fig. 95–3); alternatively, the mucosa may appear pale yellow.[34, 83] Abnormal villous structure and mild mucosal flattening become evident using magnifying optics. Viewed with light microscopy, the visible patches reflect lipid deposits or lymphangiectasia, whereas villous distension results from infiltration by macrophages in the lamina propria (Fig. 95–4). The swollen cytoplasm of macrophages appears foamy when stained with hematoxylin-eosin, but numerous granular particles become visible when the PAS stain is used (Fig. 95–4). These particles correspond to lysosomes filled with numerous *T. whippelii*, and the positive reaction with PAS reflects the glycoprotein content of the bacterial cell walls. Single extracellular bacteria are barely visible with conventional light microscopy due to their size, but they become evident in the mucosal stroma with high-resolution light microscopy and electron microscopy (Fig. 95–5). Their number varies greatly among patients.

Electron microscopic studies have revealed uniformity in the size of the rod-shaped bacteria, with an external diameter

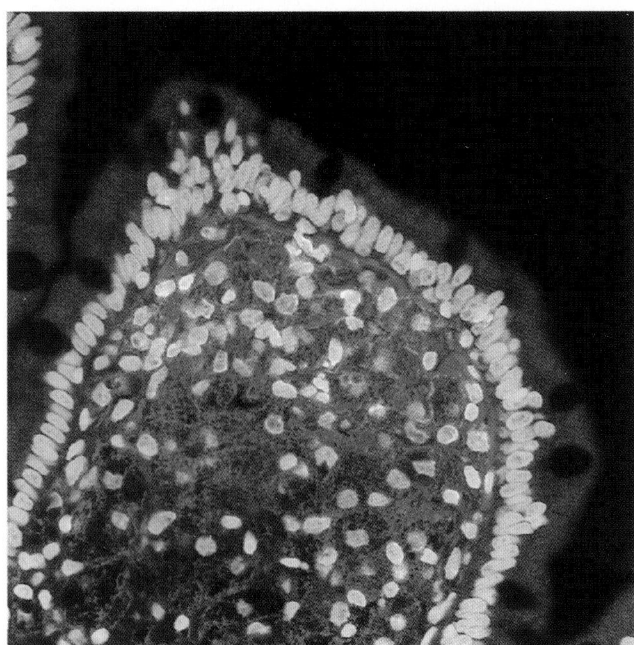

Figure 95–6. Fluorescent in situ hybridization of a small intestinal biopsy in a case of Whipple's disease. In this confocal micrograph, nuclei of human cells are green, the intracellular cytoskeletal protein vimentin is red, and *T. whippelii* rRNA is blue. The *T. whippelii* rRNA signal is most intense in the extracellular spaces of the lamina propria, immediately subjacent to the basement membrane. Magnification approximately ×200. (Courtesy David N. Fredricks, MD, Stanford University, Palo Alto, CA.)

of 0.2 to 0.25 μm and a length of up to 2.5 μm.[41, 84] There is an electron-dense outer layer that is not found in other bacteria; some have speculated this unusual membrane may be of host origin.[84] Most of the structurally intact bacteria, including dividing forms, are found outside of host cells in the lamina propria (see Fig. 95–5).[8, 84] In contrast, the intracellular bacteria in macrophages are often found in various stages of degradation. Findings based on fluorescent *in situ* hybridization using specific *T. whippelii* 16S rDNA probes support and extend the findings derived from electron microscopy[12]; the 16S rRNA signal from metabolically active bacteria is found in the intestinal lamina propria, just beneath the basement membrane, but is absent from the PAS-positive macrophages. (Fig. 95–6). Thus, *T. whippelii* appears to prefer extracellular environments within the host, despite its association with eukaryotic cells.

Mucosal infiltration is usually diffuse, but in some patients patchy lesions may be present.[85] The inflammatory reaction is generally dominated by macrophages, whereas neutrophils and eosinophils are more scarce, as are lymphocytes and plasma cells.[34, 86] This cellular composition is unusual for an invasive bacterial infection, a feature that suggests a disturbance of mobilization and chemotaxis of leukocytes.[34]

Variants of the usual histologic findings occur in some patients. These include rare cases with PAS-positive macrophages that are located exclusively in the submucosa and rare cases with epithelioid granulomas in the affected mucosa.[34] Taken together, the intestinal histopathology of Whipple's disease demonstrates some heterogeneity.

During treatment, the histologic findings in the intestinal mucosa change substantially but slowly over several months or more.[34, 40, 87] In addition to a continuous decrease in the number of PAS-positive macrophages, the pattern of cellular infiltration of the mucosa changes with time from diffuse to patchy. This feature demands multiple biopsies during follow-up examinations. Mucosal infiltration shifts from the upper portion (i.e., involving villi) to the lower part of the mucosa (i.e., pericryptal lamina propria) and submucosa. More significantly, the cytologic aspects of the PAS-positive macrophages undergo changes.[34] Before treatment, most macrophages have numerous granular particles in the cytoplasm that stain intensely red with PAS (type 1 macrophages; see Fig. 95–2). Within 1 to 6 months of treatment, the percentage of type 1 macrophages gradually decreases, and in parallel, cells prevail with only some coarse granular inclusions and a background of diffuse or fine granular more faintly PAS-positive cytoplasm (type 2 macrophages). After 6 to 15 months, most macrophages that are still present have diffuse and faintly PAS-positive material in their cytoplasm but lack granular inclusions (type 3 macrophages). Type 3 macrophages contain only filamentous remnants of bacteria.[34] Thus, their positive PAS reaction reflects the presence of glycoprotein residue of degraded bacterial cell wall. In patients with adequate therapy, some type 3 macrophages usually persist, even for more than 10 years; in fact, the finding of type 3 macrophages alone is consistent with intestinal remission. On the other hand, despite documented clinical remission of intestinal disease, some patients may still harbor *T. whippelii* and may later develop extraintestinal Whipple's disease. Thus, the prognostic value of intestinal histology during the follow-up of patients is limited.[34]

Extraintestinal Pathology

Autopsy reports in untreated patients have illustrated involvement of virtually any organ and tissue in Whipple's disease.[53, 88] As with intestinal disease, the histologic hallmark of extraintestinal involvement is the presence of intracellular PAS-positive granular particles. However, the diagnostic significance of these lesions in extraintestinal tissues is limited, and additional evidence is required for the diagnosis of Whipple's disease. Rod-shaped bacteria have been documented by electron microscopy in many extraintestinal organs, including colon, liver, heart, lung, brain, eye, lymph node, bone marrow, and spleen.[8]

Two different types of lymph node lesions are common in Whipple's disease. Abdominal nodes generally contain lipid deposits that induce a granulomatous foreign body type of reaction.[1] Peripheral lymph nodes (inguinal, axillary, cervical) generally do not contain lipids but feature a toxoplasmosis-like lymphadenitis with small clusters of epithelioid macrophages, some of which have PAS-positive particles that correspond to inclusions with *T. whippelii*. Rarely, a third type of lymph node reaction may be observed that resembles sarcoidosis; it occurs most commonly in the mediastinum.

Whipple's disease affects diverse regions of the brain. Most commonly, perivascular infiltrates of PAS-positive macrophages are present, as well as tumor-like granulomas of variable size, consisting of glial cells with intensely PAS-positive granular particles.[8] Occasionally, granulomas in the ventricular system cause occlusive hydrocephalus. Floating PAS-positive macrophages can frequently be detected in the CSF, even in patients without neurologic or psychiatric symptoms (see later).

DIAGNOSIS

Almost all patients with Whipple's disease have involvement of the intestinal tract by this infection, regardless of whether gastrointestinal symptoms are present.[19, 54, 55] Thus, the primary diagnostic approach to a patient with clinical suspicion of possible Whipple's disease is upper endoscopy (see Fig. 95–1) with mucosal biopsy. To avoid sampling errors in patients with patchy lesions of Whipple's disease, one should obtain approximately five biopsy specimens from regions as far distal as possible within the small intestines.[89] Histologic examination with use of routine and PAS stains is usually sufficient to reach a diagnosis (see earlier). In some cases, the findings may be corroborated with silver stains[1]; in contrast, the Gram stain is less useful in this infection. Immunocytochemistry with cross-reactive antisera directed against other bacteria may show positive reactions that colocalize with PAS-positive inclusions,[90, 91] but this has not found practical use in histopathology. It remains to be seen whether specific antisera raised against *T. whippelii*[11] will prove useful in histopathologic practice. Traditionally, electron microscopy has been used as the "gold standard" for confirming the diagnosis of Whipple's disease.[8] Currently, PCR analysis serves in this capacity.[45, 46]

After the molecular characterization of *T. whippelii*, several PCR-based assays have been developed for diagnostic purposes.[10, 45–47, 78, 82, 92–94] However, many of these assays have not been thoroughly validated with measurement of performance characteristics and adequate identification of amplified products. In almost all patients with a histologic diagnosis of Whipple's disease, well-standardized PCR assays detect *T. whippelii* DNA in the intestinal mucosa.[45, 46] In contrast, intestinal biopsies with normal histology are almost always negative for DNA of *T. whippelii*.[49] In practical terms, a normal intestinal histology in the absence of extraintestinal disease suggestive of Whipple's disease *bona fide* rules out the diagnosis, provided that multiple biopsy specimens are evaluated.

Extraintestinal manifestations warrant the examination of specimens from affected sites. Histology and cytology with PAS staining, electron microscopy, and PCR are all useful for this purpose. Since the introduction of PCR for *T. whippelii*,[10] some patients have been reported with a PCR-based diagnosis of *T. whippelii* infection in extraintestinal samples, whereas intestinal histology (when tested) was negative for PAS-positive macrophages. Examples of such patients are a case of febrile illness with erythrocyte-associated bacteria,[95] a case of uveitis,[82] and cases of valvular heart disease.[75] The small number of reported cases suggests that these are rare events, although there have been few prospective studies of extraintestinal syndromes suggestive of Whipple's disease. PCR testing of peripheral blood samples has been proposed as a potential noninvasive screening method,[96] but its diagnostic usefulness has been questioned.[97]

Considering the systemic nature of this disorder, it is important to evaluate commonly involved organ systems when a new diagnosis of Whipple's disease has been reached. Ultrasound examination may reveal enlarged mesenteric lymph nodes that have unusually high echogenicity due to lipid deposits.[36] Neurologic examination is indicated, including routine sampling of CSF.[68] Based on cytologic or PCR analysis, 70% of patients with intestinal Whipple's disease in one study were found to have CNS infection with *T. whippelii*, even though they had no neurologic or psychiatric symptoms.[68] Imaging studies of the brain are generally not helpful in patients without neurologic symptoms.

During treatment, one should repeat diagnostic assessments at regular intervals. Endoscopic lesions usually resolve within some months but may last for up to a year.[83] Intestinal histology improves within several months,[34] and PCR assays on intestinal biopsy tissues convert to negative within a wide time range (1 to 12 months) after institution of appropriate therapy.[45] Some PAS-positive macrophages may persist for years,[34] even while the patient remains in clinical remission (see earlier). Regression of enlarged abdominal lymph nodes may require more than a year and may result in fibrosis. Follow-up examination of the CSF is most effectively performed with inclusion of PCR analysis.[68]

DIFFERENTIAL DIAGNOSIS

Almost all symptoms and findings of Whipple's disease are nonspecific. The broad spectrum of possible clinical presentations generates a wide differential diagnosis, involving several subspecialities of medicine: gastroenterology, rheumatology, hematology, neurology, psychiatry, and ophthalmology.

Disorders that mimic the histology of Whipple's disease are uncommon.[20] PAS-positive cells in intestinal biopsies may include mucosal smooth muscle cells that are rich in glycogen or plasma cells that contain immunoglobulin (Russell bodies) in the setting of chronic duodenitis. Rarely, these cells reflect intestinal infection with *Mycobacterium avium* complex, histoplasmosis, macroglobulinemia, intestinal xanthelasmas, or pseudomelanosis duodeni. Differentiation from Whipple's disease is usually possible by means of histochemical stains (e.g., stains for acid-fast bacteria and use of diastase) and by immunocytochemistry.[20]

Sarcoid-like granulomas are rare in Whipple's disease but may occur in the stomach,[98] small intestine,[34, 99] liver,[100] and lymph nodes. A possible relationship between Whipple's disease and sarcoidosis remains unresolved.[101] By means of PCR analysis, thoracic sarcoidosis[102] and intestinal sarcoidosis[103] tissues were both found to be negative for *T. whippelii* DNA.

Most patients with Whipple's disease have enlarged abdominal lymph nodes. This became more apparent with the advent of abdominal ultrasonography and computed tomography.[56] Only rare cases of Whipple's disease associated with metachronous or synchronous malignant lymphomas have been observed.[56–58] The relationship between *T. whippelii* infection and lymphoma, if any, remains unclear.

TREATMENT AND PROGNOSIS

The initial response of Whipple's disease to antibiotic treatment is usually prompt.[104] Diarrhea often resolves within several days, arthralgias within a few weeks, and significant

Table 95–1 | **Overview of Antibiotics Used for the Treatment of Whipple's Disease**

DRUG(S)	DOSAGE	COMMENTS	REFERENCES
Penicillin G + streptomycin	6–24 million U IV qd + 1 g IM qd	Induction therapy (first 10–14 days)	8, 16, 61
Ceftriaxone	2 g IV qd	Induction therapy (first 10–14 days) or salvage therapy; less widely used than PcnG + Str	68, 111, 112
Trimethoprim-sulfamethoxazole	160 mg/800 mg PO bid	Long-term therapy; first-line drug; good CNS penetration, but CNS relapses may occur	61, 104, 106, 107
Penicillin VK	500 mg PO qid	Alternative for long-term therapy; limited experience	8, 61
Doxycycline (or tetracycline)	100 mg PO bid (500 mg PO qid)	Used for many years; but well-described clinical relapses, including CNS	16, 61, 104
Cefixime	400 mg PO bid	Alternative for long-term therapy; limited experience	108
Rifampin	600 mg PO qd	Second-line drug; good CNS penetration	64, 109, 113
Chloramphenicol	500 mg PO qid	Second-line drug; worrisome side effects	5, 8, 64
Erythromycin	500 mg PO qid	Second-line drug; limited experience	8, 105, 111, 113
Pefloxacin	400 mg PO qd	Second-line drug; very limited experience	113

PcnG, penicillin G; Str, streptomycin.

weight gain occurs within a few months.[16] In the 1970s and early 1980s, long-term tetracycline therapy was usually provided[19, 55]; however, it later became increasingly clear that patients treated in this manner frequently suffered from relapses, many of which affected the CNS.[105, 106] CNS relapses have a poor prognosis, because they are often refractory to renewed treatment.[61] It was therefore suggested that the initial treatment of Whipple's disease includes antibiotics that cross the blood–brain barrier. Since the mid-1980s, trimethoprim-sulfamethoxazole has been commonly used.[61, 107]

Current recommendations for treatment of Whipple's disease are based on observations from case reports,[8] several clinical series,[19, 54, 55] and retrospective analyses of antibiotic regimens.[61, 104] Evidence from a randomized prospective study is not available to date. In an analysis of 88 patients,[61] relapses were most common after monotherapy with tetracyclines. Of 49 patients treated with tetracycline alone, 21 relapsed, including 9 with CNS relapses. Only a small number of relapses (2 of 15 patients treated), and none in the CNS, were observed after initial parenteral treatment with penicillin plus streptomycin, followed by long-term oral tetracycline (the "Duke regimen"). Tetracyclines and trimethoprim-sulfamethoxazole were compared in another series of 30 patients.[104] Trimethoprim-sulfamethoxazole was significantly superior to tetracyclines in inducing remission (12 of 13 vs. 13 of 22 treatment courses, respectively). Relapses in the CNS occurred in 2 of 22 patients receiving tetracycline and in 1 of 13 receiving trimethoprim-sulfamethoxazole. Despite its clinical efficacy and ability to cross the blood–brain barrier, several other reports indicate that relapses can occur after use of trimethoprim-sulfamethoxazole, including CNS relapses.[108–110] Some patients appear to have benefited from repeated intravenous courses of third-generation cephalosporins[68] and one patient from adjuvant interferon-γ treatment.[38]

Based on these observations, the current recommendation for treatment of Whipple's disease is to begin with an induction phase using either penicillin G plus streptomycin or a third-generation cephalosporin, such as ceftriaxone, followed by treatment with at least one drug that efficiently crosses the blood–brain barrier (e.g., trimethoprim-sulfamethoxazole), for at least 1 year. An overview of antibiotic treatment, including suggested doses, is given in Table 95–1.

FUTURE PROSPECTS

Whipple's disease remains an enigmatic disorder, producing a wide spectrum of clinical manifestations and associated with a poorly understood bacterium. The true prevalence of the disease is unknown, but its apparent rarity, its epidemiology, and circumstantial evidence that the causative agent occupies a niche in a soil-based environment suggest that as yet unknown host genetic defects predispose toward development of Whipple's disease. Rapidly unfolding developments in human and microbial genomics suggest that these puzzles may be solved in the next decade. Regardless of the magnitude of the burden imposed by this organism on human health, the study of *T. whippelii* and Whipple's disease will reveal important principles in intestinal pathophysiology, actinomycete biology, bacterial cultivation, and the human immune system.

REFERENCES

1. Whipple GH. A hitherto undescribed disease characterized anatomically by deposits of fat and fatty acids in the intestinal and mesenteric lymphatic tissues. Bull Johns Hopkins Hosp 18:382, 1907.
2. Oliver-Pascual E, Galan J, Oliver-Pascual A, et al. Un caso de lipodistrofia intestinal con lesions gangliones mesentericas de granulomatosis lipofagica (Enfermedad de Whipple). Rev Esp Enferm Apar Digest 6: 213, 1947.
3. Bolt RJ, Pollard HM, Standaert L. Transoral small-bowel biopsy as an aid in the diagnosis of malabsorption states. N Engl J Med 259:32, 1958.
4. Black-Schaffer B. The tinctoral demonstration of a glycoprotein in Whipple's disease. Proc Soc Exp Biol Med 72:225, 1949.
5. Paulley JW. A case of Whipple's disease (intestinal lipodystrophy). Gastroenterology 22:128, 1952.
6. Chears WC, Ashworth CT. Electron microscopic study of the intestinal mucosa in Whipple's disease. Demonstration of encapsulated bacilliform bodies in the lesion. Gastroenterology 41:129, 1961.
7. Yardley JH, Hendrix TR. Combined electron and light microscopy in Whipple's disease. Bull Johns Hopkins Hosp 109:80, 1961.
8. Dobbins WO, III. Whipple's Disease. Springfield, Charles C Thomas, 1987.
9. Wilson KH, Blitchington R, Frothingham R, et al. Phylogeny of the Whipple's disease-associated bacterium. Lancet 338:474, 1991.
10. Relman DA, Schmidt TM, Macdermott RP, et al. Identification of the

uncultured bacillus of Whipple's disease. N Engl J Med 327:293, 1992.
11. Raoult D, Birg ML, LaScola B, et al. Cultivation of the bacillus of Whipple's disease. N Engl J Med 342:620, 2000.
12. Fredricks DN, Relman DA. Localization of *Tropheryma whippelii* rRNA in Whipple's disease tissues. J Infect Dis 183:1229, 2001.
13. Salomoni I. La maladie de Whipple en Suisse occidentale entre 1960 et 1983. Rev Med Suisse Romande 104:655, 1984.
14. von Herbay A, Otto HF, Stolte M, et al. Epidemiology of Whipple's disease in Germany: analysis of 110 patients diagnosed in 1965–95. Scand J Gastroenterol 32:52, 1997.
15. Capron JP, Thevenin A, Delamarre J, et al. Whipple's disease: study of 3 cases and epidemiological and radiological remarks. Lille Med 20:842, 1975.
16. Maizel H, Ruffin JM, Dobbins WO, III. Whipple's disease: a review of 19 patients from one hospital and a review of the literature since 1950. Medicine (Baltimore) 49:175, 1970.
17. Lopatin RN, Grossman ET, Horine J, et al. Whipple's disease in neighbors. J Clin Gastroenterol 4:223, 1982.
18. Ectors NL, Geboes KJ, Devos RM, et al. Whipple's disease: a histological, immunocytochemical, and electron-microscopic study of the small-intestinal epithelium. J Pathol 172:73, 1994.
19. Vital Durand D, Lecomte C, Cathébras P, et al. Whipple disease: clinical review of 52 cases. Medicine (Baltimore) 76:170, 1997.
20. von Herbay A. Morbus Whipple. Histologische Diagnostik nach der Entdeckung von *Tropheryma whippelii*. Pathologe 22:82, 2001.
21. Schoedon G, Goldenberger D, Forrer R, et al. Deactivation of macrophages with interleukin-4 is the key to the isolation of *Tropheryma whippelii*. J Infect Dis 176:672, 1997.
22. Zaaijer H, Savelkoul P, Vandenbroucke-Grauls C. *Tropheryma whippelii* is easily ingested by interleukin-4-deactivated macrophages, but does not multiply [abstract 141]. Clin Infect Dis 27:947, 1998.
22a. Raoult D, LaScola B, Lecocq P, et al. Culture and immunological detection of *Tropheryma whippelii* from the duodenum of a patient with Whipple disease. JAMA 285:1039, 2001.
23. Maiwald M, Ditton HJ, von Herbay A, et al. Reassessment of the phylogenetic position of the bacterium associated with Whipple's disease and determination of the 16S-23S ribosomal intergenic spacer sequence. Int J Syst Bacterial 46:1078, 1996.
24. Hinrikson HP, Dutly F, Nair S, et al. Detection of three different types of "*Tropheryma whippelii*" directly from clinical specimens by sequencing, single-strand conformation polymorphism (SSCP) analysis and type-specific PCR of their 16S-23S ribosomal intergenic spacer region. Int J Syst Bacteriol 49:1701, 1999.
25. Maiwald M, von Herbay A, Lepp PW, et al. Organization, structure, and variability of the rRNA operon of the Whipple's disease bacterium (*Tropheryma whippelii*). J Bacteriol 182:3292, 2000.
26. Marth T, Roux M, von Herbay A, et al. Persistent reduction of complement receptor 3 alpha-chain expressing mononuclear blood cells and transient inhibitory serum factors in Whipple's disease. Clin Immunol Immunopathol 72:217, 1994.
27. Marth T, Neurath M, Cuccherini BA, et al. Defects of monocyte interleukin 12 production and humoral immunity in Whipple's disease. Gastroenterology 113:442, 1997.
28. Feurle GE, Dörken B, Schopf E, et al. HLA B27 and defects in the T-cell system in Whipple's disease. Eur J Clin Invest 9:385, 1979.
29. Dobbins WO, III. HLA antigens in Whipple's disease. Arthritis Rheum 30:102, 1987.
30. Bai JC, Mota AH, Maurino E, et al. Class I and class II HLA antigens in a homogeneous Argentinean population with Whipple's disease: lack of association with HLA-B27. Am J Gastroenterol 86: 992, 1991.
31. Kirkpatrick PM, Kent SP, Mihas A, et al. Whipple's disease: case report with immunological studies. Gastroenterology 75:297, 1978.
32. Martin FF, Vilseck J, Dobbins WO, III, et al. Immunological alterations in patients with treated Whipple's disease. Gastroenterology 63: 6, 1972.
33. Bjerknes R, Odegaard S, Bjerkvig R, et al. Whipple's disease. Demonstration of a persisting monocyte and macrophage dysfunction. Scand J Gastroenterol 23:611, 1988.
34. von Herbay A, Maiwald M, Ditton HJ, et al. Histology of intestinal Whipple's disease revisited: a study of 48 patients. Virchows Arch 429:335, 1996.
35. Bassotti G, Pelli MA, Ribacchi R, et al. *Giardia lamblia* infestation reveals underlying Whipple's disease in a patient with longstanding constipation. Am J Gastroenterol 86:371, 1991.
36. Meier-Willersen HJ, Maiwald M, von Herbay A. Morbus Whipple in Assoziation mit opportunistischen Infektionen. Dtsch Med Wochenschr 118:854, 1993.
37. Maiwald M, Meier-Willersen HJ, Hartmann M, et al. Detection of *Tropheryma whippelii* DNA in a patient with AIDS. J Clin Microbiol 33:1354, 1995.
38. Schneider T, Stallmach A, von Herbay A, et al. Treatment of refractory Whipple disease with interferon-gamma. Ann Intern Med 129: 875, 1998.
39. Kent TH, Layton JM, Clifton JA, et al. Whipple's disease: light and electron microscopic studies combined with clinical studies suggesting an infective nature. Lab Invest 12:1163, 1963.
40. Dobbins WO, III, Ruffin JM. A light- and electron-microscopic study of bacterial invasion in Whipple's disease. Am J Pathol 51:225, 1967.
41. Dobbins WO, III, Kawanishi H. Bacillary characteristics in Whipple's disease: an electron microscopic study. Gastroenterology 80:1468, 1981.
42. Maiwald M, Schuhmacher F, Ditton HJ, et al. Environmental occurrence of the Whipple's disease bacterium (*Tropheryma whippelii*). Appl Environ Microbiol 64:760, 1998.
43. Street S, Donoghue HD, Neild GH. *Tropheryma whippelii* DNA in saliva of healthy people. Lancet 354:1178, 1999.
44. Ehrbar HU, Bauerfeind P, Dutly F, et al. PCR-positive tests for *Tropheryma whippelii* in patients without Whipple's disease. Lancet 353: 2214, 1999.
45. von Herbay A, Ditton HJ, Maiwald M. Diagnostic application of a polymerase chain reaction assay for the Whipple's disease bacterium to intestinal biopsies. Gastroenterology 110:1735, 1996.
46. Ramzan NN, Loftus E, Burgart LJ, et al. Diagnosis and monitoring of Whipple disease by polymerase chain reaction. Ann Intern Med 126: 520, 1997.
47. Müller C, Petermann D, Stain C, et al. Whipple's disease: comparison of histology with diagnosis based on polymerase chain reaction in four consecutive cases. Gut 40:425, 1997.
48. Pron B, Poyart C, Abachin E, et al. Diagnosis and follow-up of Whipple's disease by amplification of the 16S rRNA gene of *Tropheryma whippelii*. Eur J Clin Microbiol Infect Dis 18:62, 1999.
49. Maiwald M, von Herbay A, Persing DH, et al. *Tropheryma whippelii* DNA is rare in the intestinal mucosa of patients without other evidence of Whipple disease. Ann Intern Med 134:115, 2001.
50. Puite RH, Tesluk H. Whipple's disease. Am J Med 19:383, 1955.
51. Gross JB, Wollaeger EE, Sauer WG, et al. Whipple's disease: a report of four cases, including two in brothers, with observations on pathologic physiology, diagnosis, and treatment. Gastroenterology 36:65, 1959.
52. Dykman DD, Cuccherini BA, Fuss IJ, et al. Whipple's disease in a father-daughter pair. Dig Dis Sci 44:2542, 1999.
53. Enzinger FM, Helwig EB. Whipple's disease. A review of the literature and report of fifteen patients. Virchows Arch 336:238, 1963.
54. Fleming JL, Wiesner RH, Shorter RG. Whipple's disease: clinical, biochemical, and histopathologic features and assessment of treatment in 29 patients. Mayo Clin Proc 63:539, 1988.
55. von Herbay A, Otto HF. Whipple's disease: a report of 22 patients. Klin Wochenschr 66:533, 1988.
56. von Herbay A, Otto HF. Abdominale Lymphome beim Morbus Whipple. Dtsch Med Wochenschr 114:2028, 1989.
57. Gillen CD, Coddington R, Monteith PG, et al. Extraintestinal lymphoma in association with Whipple's disease. Gut 34:1627, 1993.
58. Gruner U, Goesch P, Donner A, et al. Morbus Whipple disease and non-Hodgkin lymphoma. Z Gastroenterol 39:305, 2001.
59. MacDermott RP, Shephard JAO. Whipple's disease. Case record 37-1997. N Engl J Med 337:1612, 1997.
60. Albrecht T. Computertomographie abdominaler Lymphome bei Morbus Whipple. Rofo Fortschr Geb Röntgenstr Neuen Bildgeb Verfahr 160:487, 1994.
61. Keinath RD, Merrell DE, Vlietstra R, et al. Antibiotic treatment and relapse in Whipple's disease. Long-term follow-up of 88 patients. Gastroenterology 88:1867, 1985.
62. Schnider PJ, Reisinger EC, Gerschlager W, et al. Long-term follow-up in cerebral Whipple's disease. Eur J Gastroenterol Hepatol 8:899, 1996.
63. Johnson L, Diamond I. Cerebral Whipple's disease. Diagnosis by brain biopsy. Am J Clin Pathol 74:486, 1980.
64. Adams M, Rhyner PA, Day J, et al. Whipple's disease confined to the central nervous system. Ann Neurol 21:104, 1987.

65. Louis ED, Lynch T, Kaufmann P, et al. Diagnostic guidelines in central nervous system Whipple's disease. Ann Neurol 40:561, 1996.
66. Lieb K, Maiwald M, Berger M, et al. Insomnia for 5 years. Lancet 354:1966, 1999.
67. Verhagen WIM, Huygen PLM, Dalman JE, et al. Whipple's disease and the central nervous system: a case report and a review of the literature. Clin Neurol Neurosurg 98:299, 1996.
68. von Herbay A, Ditton HJ, Schuhmacher F, et al. Whipple's disease: staging and monitoring by cytology and polymerase chain reaction analysis of cerebrospinal fluid. Gastroenterology 113:434, 1997.
69. Schneider T, Salamon-Looijen M, von Herbay A, et al. Whipple's disease with aortic regurgitation requiring aortic valve replacement. Infection 26:178, 1998.
70. Jeserich M, Ihling C, Holubarsch C. Aortic valve endocarditis with Whipple disease. Ann Intern Med 126:920, 1997.
71. Ratliff NB, McMahon JT, Naab TJ, et al. Whipple's disease in the porcine leaflets of a Carpentier-Edwards prosthetic mitral valve. N Engl J Med 311:902, 1984.
72. Silvestry FE, Kim B, Pollack BJ, et al. Cardiac Whipple disease: Identification of Whipple bacillus by electron microscopy in the myocardium of a patient before death. Ann Intern Med 126:214, 1997.
73. Célard M, de Gevigney G, Mosnier S, et al. Polymerase chain reaction analysis for diagnosis of *Tropheryma whippelii* infective endocarditis in two patients with no previous evidence of Whipple's disease. Clin Infect Dis 29:1348, 1999.
74. Elkins C, Shuman TA, Pirolo JS. Cardiac Whipple's disease without digestive symptoms. Ann Thorac Surg 67:250, 1999.
75. Gubler JGH, Kuster M, Dutly F, et al. Whipple endocarditis without overt gastrointestinal disease: report of four cases. Ann Intern Med 131:112, 1999.
76. Rubinow A, Canoso JJ, Goldenberg DL, et al. Arthritis in Whipple's disease. Isr J Med Sci 17:445, 1981.
77. O'Duffy JD, Griffing WL, Li CY, et al. Whipple's arthritis: direct detection of *Tropheryma whippelii* in synovial fluid and tissue. Arthritis Rheum 42:812, 1999.
78. Altwegg M, Fleisch-Marx A, Goldenberger D, et al. Spondylodiscitis caused by *Tropheryma whippelii*. Schweiz Med Wochenschr 126: 1495, 1996.
79. Frésard A, Guglielminotti C, Berthelot P, et al. Prosthetic joint infection caused by *Tropheryma whippelii* (Whipple's bacillus). Clin Infect Dis 22:575, 1996.
80. Balestrieri GP, Villanacci V, Battocchio S, et al. Cutaneous involvement in Whipple's disease. Br J Dermatol 135:666, 1996.
81. Williams JG, Edward DP, Tessler HH, et al. Ocular manifestations of Whipple disease: an atypical presentation. Arch Ophthalmol 116:1232, 1998.
82. Rickman LS, Freeman WR, Green WR, et al. Uveitis caused by *Tropheryma whippelii* (Whipple bacillus). N Engl J Med 332:363, 1995.
83. Geboes K, Ectors N, Heidbuchel H, et al. Whipple's disease: endoscopic aspects before and after therapy. Gastrointest Endosc 36:247, 1990.
84. Silva MT, Macedo PM, Moura Nunes JF. Ultrastructure of bacilli and the bacillary origin of the macrophagic inclusions in Whipple's disease. J Gen Microbiol 131:1001, 1985.
85. Moorthy S, Nolley G, Hermos JA. Whipple's disease with minimal intestinal involvement. Gut 18:152, 1977.
86. Ectors N, Geboes K, Devos R, et al. Whipple's disease: a histological, immunocytochemical and electron-microscopic study of the immune-response in the small intestinal mucosa. Histopathology 21:1, 1992.
87. Dvorak AM. Ultrastructural monitoring of progress of Whipple's disease therapy. Dig Dis Pathol 2:81, 1989.
88. Sieracki JC, Fine G. Whipple's disease—observations on systemic involvement. II. Gross and histologic observations. Arch Pathol 67:81, 1959.
89. von Herbay A. Whipple's disease online. URL: http://www.WhipplesDisease.net.
90. Keren DF, Weisburger WR, Yardley JH, et al. Whipple's disease: demonstration by immunofluorescence of similar bacterial antigens in macrophages from three cases. Johns Hopkins Med J 139:51, 1976.
91. Evans DJ, Ali MH. Immunocytochemistry in the diagnosis of Whipple's disease. J Clin Pathol 38:372, 1985.
92. Dauga C, Miras I, Grimont PAD. Strategy for detection and identification of bacteria based on 16S rRNA genes in suspected cases of Whipple's disease. J Med Microbiol 46:340, 1997.
93. Gross M, Jung C, Zoller WG. Detection of *Tropheryma whippelii* DNA (Whipple's disease) in faeces. Ital J Gastroenterol Hepatol 31: 70, 1999.
94. Hinrikson HP, Dutly F, Altwegg M. Evaluation of a specific nested PCR targeting domain III of the 23S rRNA gene of "*Tropheryma whippelii*" and proposal of a classification system for its molecular variants. J Clin Microbiol 38:595, 2000.
95. Lowsky R, Archer GL, Fyles G, et al. Diagnosis of Whipple's disease by molecular analysis of peripheral blood. N Engl J Med 331:1343, 1994.
96. Müller C, Stain C, Burghuber O. *Tropheryma whippelii* in peripheral blood mononuclear cells and cells of pleural effusion. Lancet 341:701, 1993.
97. Marth T, Fredricks D, Strober W, et al. Limited role for PCR-based diagnosis of Whipple's disease from peripheral blood mononuclear cells. Lancet 348:66, 1996.
98. Ectors N, Geboes K, Wynants P, et al. Granulomatous gastritis and Whipples disease. Am J Gastroenterol 87:509, 1992.
99. Babaryka I, Thorn L, Langer E. Epithelioid cell granulomata in the mucosa of the small intestine in Whipple's disease. Virchows Arch 382:227, 1979.
100. Saint-Marc Girardin MF, Zafrani ES, Chaumette MT, et al. Hepatic granulomas in Whipple's disease. Gastroenterology 86:753, 1984.
101. Donaldson RM. Whipple's disease: rare malady with uncommon potential. N Engl J Med 327:346, 1992.
102. von Herbay A, Ditton HJ, Schuhmacher F, et al. Molecular screening of DNA of *Tropheryma whippelii* in sarcoidosis [abstract]. Pathol Res Pract 193:87, 1997.
103. Abdelmalek MF, Procop GW, Mitchell PS, et al. Lack of association of sarcoidosis and intestinal lymphoma with *T. whippelii* infection [abstract]. Gastroenterology 114:G1410, 1998.
104. Feurle GE, Marth T. An evaluation of antimicrobial treatment for Whipple's disease. Tetracycline versus trimethoprim-sulfamethoxazole. Dig Dis Sci 39:1642, 1994.
105. Knox DL, Bayless TM, Pittman FE. Neurologic disease in patients with treated Whipple's disease. Medicine (Baltimore) 55:467, 1976.
106. Feurle GE, Volk B, Waldherr R. Cerebral Whipple's disease with negative jejunal histology. N Engl J Med 300:907, 1979.
107. Ryser RJ, Locksley RM, Eng SC, et al. Reversal of dementia associated with Whipple's disease by trimethoprim-sulfamethoxazole, drugs that penetrate the blood-brain barrier. Gastroenterology 86:745, 1984.
108. Cooper GS, Blades EW, Remler BF, et al. Central nervous system Whipple's disease: relapse during therapy with trimethoprim-sulfamethoxazole and remission with cefixime. Gastroenterology 106:782, 1994.
109. Singer R, von Herbay A, Willig F. Successful treatment of cerebral Whipple's disease with rifampicin. Med Klinik 90:117, 1995.
110. Garas G, Cheng WS, Abrugiato R, et al. Clinical relapse in Whipple's disease despite maintenance therapy. J Gastroenterol Hepatol 15:1223, 2000.
111. Adler CH, Galetta SL. Oculo-facial-skeletal myorhythmia in Whipple disease: treatment with ceftriaxone. Ann Intern Med 112:467, 1990.
112. Simpson DA, Wishnow R, Gargulinski RB, et al. Oculofacial-skeletal myorhythmia in central nervous system Whipple's disease: additional case and review of the literature. Mov Disord 10:195, 1995.
113. Amarenco P, Roullet E, Hannoun L, et al. Progressive supranuclear palsy as the sole manifestation of systemic Whipple's disease treated with pefloxacine. J Neurol Neurosurg Psychiatry 54:1121, 1991.

Chapter

96

Infectious Diarrhea and Bacterial Food Poisoning

Davidson H. Hamer and Sherwood L. Gorbach

Our knowledge of infectious diarrheal diseases has expanded exponentially in the past two decades. Advances have come from a number of disciplines, with an integration of epidemiologic, clinical, and laboratory studies to produce new understandings of this ancient group of diseases.

Diarrhea is the first or second cause of death in most developing countries; its greatest impact is seen in infants and children. In the United States, there is an average of two episodes of diarrhea per year in children under 5 years of age. In developing countries, diarrhea rates are two to three times higher. Overall, physicians in the United States are consulted annually for 8.2 million diarrheal episodes.[1] Also in the United States, an average rate of 300 deaths per year is recorded for children younger than 5 years of age, mostly related to dehydration.[2] A miscellany of complications, some mild and others life-threatening, can accompany infectious diarrhea (Table 96–1). Medical costs and loss of productivity resulting from infectious diarrhea amount to $23 billion a year in the United States.

CHANGES IN NORMAL FLORA CAUSED BY DIARRHEA

The proximal small bowel, including the stomach, duodenum, jejunum, and upper ileum, has a sparse microflora. The concentrations of bacteria are generally less than 10^4/mL.[3] Most organisms are derived from the oropharynx, come down with each meal, and pass through the upper bowel in a wave-like manner. Colonization of the upper intestine by Gram-negative bacilli is an abnormal event and is characteristic of disease caused by pathogens such as *Vibrio cholerae* and *Escherichia coli*. The colon contains a luxuriant microflora, with total concentrations of 10^{11} bacteria per gram. Anaerobes, such as *Bacteroides*, anaerobic *Streptococcus*, and *Clostridium*, outnumber aerobic bacteria, such as coliforms, by 1000-fold. During an episode of acute diarrhea, regardless of the etiology, the colonic flora change and become less anaerobic because of the rapid transit. As a result, strict anaerobic bacteria decrease in number, with an increase in coliforms, which often are aberrant types such as *Klebsiella*, *Enterobacter*, and *Proteus*. The pathogen itself rises to ascendancy in the flora, so that the major isolate from the feces may be *V. cholerae* or *Shigella*, for example.

There is not only a longitudinal distribution of bacteria in the gastrointestinal tract, but also a cross-sectional arrangement with regard to the mucosal surface. The microflora is found within the lumen, overlying the epithelial cells, and adherent to the mucous layer. Penetration of bacteria through the mucosal surface is an abnormal event that can be caused by invasive agents such as *Shigella*, *Salmonella*, *Campylobacter*, and *Yersinia*.

Control Mechanisms

The same mechanisms that control the normal flora also serve to protect the bowel from invasion by pathogens. At the portal of entry, gastric acid suppresses most organisms

Table 96–1 | **Complications of Infectious Diarrhea**

COMPLICATION	SEEN IN
Dehydration	Cholera; enterotoxigenic *Escherichia coli* (ETEC); rotavirus; *Salmonella* (rare)
Severe vomiting	Food poisoning (staphylococcal); rotavirus; Norwalk virus
Hemorrhagic colitis	Enterohemorrhagic *E. coli* O157:H7 (EHEC); *Shigella; Vibrio parahaemolyticus; Campylobacter, Salmonella*
Toxic megacolon, intestinal perforation	*Shigella,* EHEC, *Clostridium difficile* (rare); *Campylobacter* (rare); *Yersinia* (rare); *Salmonella* (rare)
Hemolytic-uremic syndrome, thrombotic thrombocytopenia	EHEC; *Shigella; Campylobacter* (rare)
Reactive arthritis	*Shigella; Salmonella; Yersinia; Campylobacter*
Distant metastatic infection	*Salmonella; Yersinia* (rare); *Campylobacter* (rare)
Malnutrition (wasting)	Various infectious diarrheas
Guillain-Barré syndrome	*Campylobacter jejuni* (rare)

that are swallowed. Persons with reduced or absent gastric acid have a high frequency of bacterial colonization in the upper small bowel and are more susceptible to diarrheal diseases. Bile has antibacterial properties, which may help control flora. A key element in maintaining the sparse flora of the upper bowel is forward propulsive motility. Finally, the microflora, by producing its own antibacterial substances, maintains the stability of the normal bacterial populations and prevents implantation of pathogens.

CLASSIFICATIONS OF BACTERIAL DIARRHEA

Acute bacterial diarrhea can be classified into *toxigenic* types, in which an enterotoxin is the major if not exclusive pathogenic mechanism, and *invasive* types, in which the organism penetrates the mucosal surface as the primary event, but enterotoxin may be produced as well. Many organisms elaborate enterotoxins that cause fluid and electrolyte secretion in the gut. That an organism produces an enterotoxin is established in the laboratory by in vivo tests, such as the rabbit ileal loop model and the suckling mouse model, or by in vitro tests involving a tissue culture line, such as Y-1 adrenal cells or Chinese hamster ovary cells.[4]

The recognized diarrheal toxins can be grouped broadly into two categories: *cytotonic*, producing fluid secretion by activation of intracellular enzymes such as adenylate cyclase without any damage to the epithelial surface, and *cytotoxic*, causing injury to the mucosal cell and inducing fluid secretion, but not primarily by activation of cyclic nucleotides.

TOXIGENIC DIARRHEAS

The prototypical organisms in this group are *V. cholerae* and enterotoxigenic *Escherichia coli* (ETEC). These pathogens elaborate enterotoxins of the cytotonic type that cause dehydrating diarrhea.

Diarrheal disease caused by *V. cholerae* and ETEC has the following characteristics:

1. The entire disease consists of intestinal fluid loss, which is related to the action of the enterotoxin on the small bowel epithelial cells.
2. The organism itself does not invade the mucosal surface; rather, it colonizes the upper small bowel, "sticks" to the epithelial cells, and elaborates an enterotoxin. The mucosal architecture remains intact, with no evidence of cellular destruction. Bacteremia is not a complication.
3. The fecal effluent is watery and often voluminous, producing clinical features of dehydration. The origin of the fluid is the upper small bowel, where the enterotoxin has its greatest activity.

Cholera

Cholera is a severe diarrheal disorder that can cause dehydration and death within 3 to 4 hours of onset. Stool output can exceed 1 L/hr, with daily fecal outputs of 15 to 20 L, if parenteral fluid replacement is kept up. The acutely ill patient has marked signs of dehydration, poor skin turgor, "washerwoman's hands," absent pulses, reduced renal function, and hypovolemic shock. It has been said that cholera is a disease that begins where other diseases end—with death.

Cholera is the prototypical toxigenic diarrhea. Its importance derives not necessarily from its incidence, because cholera is confined to certain areas of the world and tends to occur in epidemics, but from its role as a model of secretory diarrhea. More has been learned about pathophysiology—and normal intestinal function—from cholera than from any other intestinal disease. Treatment programs have been devised, including an oral rehydration regimen; the enterotoxin has been purified; the immunology and epidemiology have been clarified; and vaccines have been developed.

Our interest in cholera was renewed as a result of a massive epidemic that arose in Peru in January 1991 and caused more than 300,000 cases within the year. The epidemic rapidly involved many countries in South and Central America, with cases reported as far north as Mexico. Cholera has become endemic in much of Latin America. The North American continent had not experienced epidemic cholera since 1895, as recounted by Gabriel García Márquez in his novel *Love in the Time of Cholera.*

Microbiology

V. cholerae is a Gram-negative, short, curved rod that looks like a comma. It is actively motile by means of a single polar flagellum. The organisms are strongly aerobic and prefer alkaline and high salt environments. Toxigenic *V. cholerae* that agglutinate in 01 antiserum are the main cause of epidemic cholera. There are two major biotypes of *V. cholerae* 01, *classic* and *El Tor*. The latter strain, first isolated at the El Tor Quarantine Station on the Sinai Peninsula, is responsible for the current pandemic that began in 1961. It is differentiated from classic strains by its ability to hemolyze sheep and goat red blood cells, reactivity to certain phages, and resistance to polymyxin. El Tor vibrios are somewhat hardier than others in nature. The clinical disease is similar with both biotypes, although on average, El Tor infections are milder. Antigenic serotypes are identified by the somatic antigen. The major serotypes associated with clinical disease are Inaba and Ogawa; a rare third type is Hikojima. The El Tor Inaba type is responsible for the current outbreak in South America. There are also unique 01 cholera strains that cause endemic disease along the Gulf Coast of the United States.[5]

A newly described toxigenic non-01 strain, now designated *V. cholerae* 0139 Bengal, was responsible for an epidemic that started in southern India and Bangladesh in late 1992 and spread rapidly to many other countries in Southeast Asia.[6, 7] This strain was classified as a new serogroup because it did not react with antisera to the previously known 138 serogroups.[7] Although closely related to *V. cholerae* 01 El Tor, the Bengal strain differs by the expression of a polysaccharide capsule, presence of a distinct O antigen, and in vitro resistance to killing with normal human serum.[8]

Cholera Toxin

All wild strains of *V. cholerae*, including 0139, elaborate the same enterotoxin, a protein molecule with a molecular weight of 84,000 Da.[8] The structural genes for the cholera toxin are encoded by a filamentous bacteriophage.[9] Like the diphtheria toxin, the cholera toxin is composed of two types of subunits. Each toxin molecule contains five "B" subunits that encircle a single "A" subunit. The B subunit is responsible for binding to the receptor on the mucosa. The A subunit is responsible for binding and activation of adenylate cyclase located on the inner cellular membrane. A second 10- to 30-kDa heat-labile toxin has been described. This toxin alters intestinal permeability by acting on intestinal epithelial cell tight junctions; it has been called zonula occludens toxin.[10]

Epidemiology

For many centuries, the Bay of Bengal has been considered the "cradle of cholera." The disease has raged in the Indian subcontinent and Asia since recorded history. Western countries were relatively free of cholera epidemics until the 19th century. Since then, when cholera spread worldwide, six pandemics have been reported, and we are currently in the seventh. This outbreak started in 1961, initially in the Celebes Island in Indonesia, then made its way to the Philippines, Hong Kong, Japan, Korea, Thailand, India, Pakistan, and the Middle East, and finally passed across the African continent to engulf the entire region. In 1991, it spread to South America. Although the overall number of cases of cholera in Latin America has subsided since 1991, outbreaks of *V. cholerae* have continued to occur sporadically throughout sub-Saharan Africa. In fact, during 1999, more than 200,000 cases of cholera were reported from Africa, and these cases accounted for 81% of the global total.[11]

The organism associated with the current pandemic is an El Tor biotype. The disease is, in general, milder than that seen with "classic" strains, and there is a higher frequency of inapparent infection.

Cholera occurs sporadically along the Gulf Coast of the United States, primarily in Texas and Louisiana.[12] Among the millions of American travelers to endemic areas in foreign countries, only 41 imported cases of cholera were reported in the United States from 1961 to 1990, and none was associated with secondary spread. The current epidemic in South America resulted in 26 cases in 1991, 103 in 1992, and 22 in 1993 in the United States; one death was reported.[13]

The South American epidemic that began in Peru in January 1991 caused over one million cases in the first 3 years. The disease occurred in all age groups because the population had no protective antibody. From 15,000 to 20,000 cases of cholera were reported each week during the peak of the epidemic, for a national incidence of 1 in 1000 persons. Unboiled drinking water, unwashed fruits or vegetables, and food or water from street vendors were implicated risk factors in this explosive outbreak.[14, 15]

The epidemic of *V. cholerae* 0139 Bengal that began in southern India and Bangladesh in late 1992 affected adults predominantly.[7] The clinical features of infection with the 0139 Bengal strain were virtually indistinguishable from infection caused by *V. cholerae* 01.[16, 17]

Contaminated water and food are the major vehicles for the spread of cholera. Infection by person-to-person contact is uncommon, and rarely do physicians, nurses, ward attendants, and laboratory workers who come in contact with the microorganism acquire clinical disease. The inoculum required to cause acute cholera is large, approximately 10^9 organisms. Even this number cannot cause disease in a healthy person without bicarbonate or some other substance to buffer the acidity of the stomach. In nature, people with low gastric acidity, often associated with malnutrition, are more easily infected than those with normal acidity.

Humans are the only host for cholera vibrios. The carrier rate is approximately 5% after acute exposure, although long-term carriers are much less common. Cholera vibrios are harbored in the gallbladder.

Pathogenesis

The clinical syndrome of cholera is caused by the action of the toxin on intestinal epithelial cells. Fluid loss in cholera originates in the small intestine. The most sensitive areas are the upper bowel, particularly the duodenum and upper jejunum; the ileum is less affected; and the colon is usually in a state of absorption and is relatively insensitive to the toxin. The diarrhea is an "overflow" type, with a large volume of fluid produced in the upper intestine that overwhelms the capacity of the lower bowel to absorb it. Cholera toxin increases adenylate cyclase activity to result in elevated levels of cyclic AMP in the intestinal mucosa. There appears to be differential action on mucosal cells, with a direct secretory effect on crypt cells and an antiabsorptive effect on villous cells.

Attachment of *V. cholerae* to the intestinal mucosa is mediated by various surface components, including a fimbrial colonization factor, known as *toxin-coregulated pilus*. The toxin-coregulated pilus attachment protein may play an important role in producing protective antibodies.[18]

The visual appearance of cholera stools resembles "rice water," that is, the stool has lost all pigment and becomes a clear fluid with small flecks of mucus. The electrolyte composition is isotonic with plasma, and the effluent has a low protein concentration (Table 96–2). On microscopic examination there are no inflammatory cells, only small numbers of shed mucosal cells.

Table 96–2 | **Fluid Compositions in Infectious Diarrhea**

	ELECTROLYTE CONCENTRATIONS (MMOL/L)			
	Sodium	**Potassium**	**Chloride**	**Bicarbonate**
Stool				
Cholera, adult	124	16	90	48
Cholera, child	101	27	92	32
Nonspecific, child	56	25	55	14
Intravenous therapy				
Lactated Ringer's solution	130	4	109	28*
5:4:1 solution	129	11	97	44
2:1 solution	141	—	94	47

*Equivalent from lactate conversion.
†Add glucose, 110 mmol (20 g/L).

Cholera vibrios do not invade the mucosal surface, and bacteremia is virtually unknown in this disease. A biopsy specimen of the mucosa during acute cholera shows evidence of dehydration, with maintenance of normal architecture, in sharp contrast to the invasive and ulcerating lesions associated with *Salmonella* and *Shigella.*

Clinical Features

Like many other infectious diseases, there is a spectrum of clinical manifestations—from an asymptomatic carrier state to a desperately ill patient with severe dehydration. The initial stage is characterized by vomiting and abdominal distention. This stage is followed rapidly by diarrhea, which accelerates over the next few hours to frequent purging of large volumes of rice water stools. All the clinical symptoms and signs can be ascribed to the fluid and electrolyte losses. Patients present with profound dehydration and hypovolemic shock, usually leading to renal failure. The stool is isotonic with plasma, although there is an inordinate loss of potassium and bicarbonate, thereby producing hypokalemic acidosis (see Table 96–2). Mild fever may be present, but there are no signs of sepsis.

Immunologic Responses

After acute cholera, two serum antibodies can be demonstrated: a vibriocidal antibody directed against somatic antigen and an antitoxin antibody against the enterotoxin. Vibriocidal titers rise and fall rapidly during infection, and by 6 months only 1% of patients have high levels. In areas of high endemnicity, such as the Indian subcontinent, the level of vibriocidal titer rises with age; by the 10th year of life, 50% of people have measurable titers. Protection is related to the presence and actual level of vibriocidal antibody. From these observations, it follows that acute cholera in endemic areas is a disease largely of young children, primarily those who lack vibriocidal antibody. Antitoxin titers rise somewhat slowly after acute infection and remain elevated for many months. The susceptibility of adults in areas endemic for the 0139 Bengal strain of cholera indicates that the afflicted populations are immunologically naive and that prior exposure to *V. cholerae* 01 does not provide cross-protective immunity. Nevertheless, volunteer challenge studies indicate that an initial infection with 0139 Bengal provides protection against recurrent disease.[16]

Exposure to vibrios, by either actual infection or asymptomatic carriage, causes an elevation in titers of vibriocidal antibody. In field situations, the clinical case rate is approximately 0.26%; that is, for every clinical case of cholera there are approximately 400 asymptomatic people who have contact with the organism, as demonstrated by a rise in vibriocidal antibody titer.

Treatment

Fluid and electrolyte replacement is the mainstay of therapy for cholera. Fluid repletion was first advocated in 1830, by two workers at the Institute for Artificial Mineral Waters in Moscow. Dr. William O'Shaughnessy, working in Scotland in 1831, measured stool electrolyte losses in cholera and echoed the suggestion that fluids and electrolytes should be effective treatment for cholera. In the next 120 years, however, irrational therapy prevailed. Misdirected suggestions for "abstraction of blood" or exchange transfusions set back the application of rational effective management.

Treatment of acute cholera is based on physiologic principles of restoring fluid and electrolyte balance and maintaining intravascular volume. These objectives can be accomplished with intravenous solutions or oral fluids that contain electrolytes in isotonic concentrations. Particular attention is paid to administration of bicarbonate and potassium, which are lost excessively in cholera stool. An oral rehydration solution (ORS) has been developed for treating mild-to-moderate cases and is especially useful in developing countries[19] (Table 96–2 and Table 96–3).

Antimicrobial agents are useful as ancillary measures to treat cholera because their use leads to reductions in stool output, duration of diarrhea, fluid requirements, and *Vibrio* excretion.[20] The dose of tetracycline is 40 mg/kg/day orally, up to a maximum of 4 g/day, in four divided doses for 2 days (Table 96–4). Intravenous therapy is indicated for patients unable to take medication by mouth. There is no proven value in lengthening the duration of treatment to 4 days. In fact, single-dose therapy with ciprofloxacin results in a successful clinical response in 94% of patients infected with *V. cholerae*.[21, 22] As a result of rising rates of resistance, tetracycline and doxycyline are often less effective than the fluoroquinolones.[22, 23] Alternative drugs include trimethoprim-sulfamethoxazole (TMP-SMX) and furazolidone.

The simple therapeutic principles of fluid replacement and antibiotics can save many lives. This knowledge has been available only in the past 30 years; before then the mortality for cholera was 50% to 75%. Application of these physiologic principles reduces the mortality rate in adults to less than 1%. Indeed, the mortality rate in the current epidemic in Peru is less than 1%. Children with cholera still have a mortality rate of 3% to 5% because of a lack of fluid reserve in the young child.

Vaccines

A commercial cholera vaccine is available and consists of the somatic antigen of the two major serotypes of *V. cholerae*. Most countries no longer require cholera vaccine for

Table 96–3 | **Oral Rehydration Solutions**

COMPONENTS	WHO FORMULA*	RICELYTE†	PEDIALYTE‡	REHYDRALYTE§	CERALYTE‖
Sodium (mEq/L)	90	50	45	75	70
Potassium (mEq/L)	20	25	20	20	20
Chloride (mEq/L)	80	45	35	65	60
Citrate (mEq/L)	30	34	30	30	30
Glucose (g/L)	20	—	25	25	—
Rice syrup solid (g/L)		30			40
Average cost¶	NA	$4.09	$4.06	NA	$1.00**

*WHO, World Health Organization; Not available at most pharmacies but may be ordered in bulk from IDE Interstate Drug Exchange, Amityville, NY 11701 (800-666-8100).
†Mead Johnson Nutritionals, Evansville, IN.
‡Ross Laboratories, Columbus, OH.
§Not available at most pharmacies; may be special ordered in cases of 8-oz. bottles from Ross Laboratories, Columbus, OH.
‖Available as packets of powder that must be reconstituted in 1 L drinking water; manufactured by Cera products, Columbia, MD (301-490-4941).
¶Cost is average of retail prices at two or three Baltimore pharmacies for a 1-L bottle.
**Average cost per packet.
Modified from Santosham M, Greenough WB. Oral rehydration therapy: a global perspective. J Pediatr 118:544, 1991, with permission.

Table 96–4 | **Antimicrobial Drug Therapy for Infectious Diarrhea**

	ANTIBIOTIC OF CHOICE	ALTERNATIVE DRUGS
Recommended in symptomatic cases		
Shigella	Ampicillin, 500 mg PO q.i.d. or 1 g IV q6h; 50–100 mg/kg/day for children Ampicillin-resistant strains: TMP-SMX, 10 mg/kg/day TMP and 50 mg/kg/day SMX × 5 days	Fluoroquinolones, nalidixic acid
Clostridium difficile	Metronidazole, 500 mg PO t.i.d. or vancomycin, 125–500 mg PO q.i.d. × 10 days	
Traveler's diarrhea	Ciprofloxacin, 500 mg PO b.i.d. × 3 days	TMP-SMX, other fluoroquinolones
EPEC, EAggEC, and DAEC in infants; EIEC	TMP-SMX, as for *Shigella*	
Typhoid fever	Chloramphenicol, 500 mg PO or IV q.i.d. × 14 days	Amoxicillin, 1 g PO q.i.d. × 14 days; ciprofloxacin, 500 mg PO b.i.d. × 10 days; TMP-SMX; third-generation cephalosporins
Cholera	Tetracycline, 40 mg/kg/day in four doses (max. 4 g/day) × 2 days	TMP-SMX, norfloxacin, furazolidone
Salmonella (unusual cases)	Ampicillin, 50–100 mg/kg/day in four doses × 10–14 days Ampicillin-resistant strains: TMP-SMX, 8 mg/kg/day TMP and 40 mg/kg/day SMX (max. of 320 mg/1600 mg/day) × 14 days	Ciprofloxacin, 500 mg PO b.i.d. × 14 days
Amebiasis†	Metronidazole, 750 mg PO t.i.d. × 10 days then iodoquinol, 650 mg PO t.i.d. × 20 days, or paromomycin, 500 mg PO t.i.d. × 7 days	Tetracycline, 500 mg PO q.i.d. × 14 days and dehydroemetine, 0.5–0.75 mg/kg (max. of 90 mg/day) IM q12h × 5 days
Giardiasis†	Metronidazole, 250 mg PO t.i.d. × 5 days	Quinacrine HCl,* 100 mg PO t.i.d. × 5 days; furazolidone, paromomycin
Not generally recommended due to inconclusive findings or no studies except for immunocompromised, bacteremic, or seriously ill patients and when microbiologic diagnosis is established in 72 h		
Campylobacter	Erythromycin, 250–500 mg PO q.i.d. × 7 days	Ciprofloxacin, 500 mg PO b.i.d. × 7 days
Yersinia‡	Fluoroquinolones, TMP-SMX, chloramphenicol	Aminoglycosides, tetracycline
Aeromonas‡	TMP-SMX, third-generation cephalosporins, fluoroquinolones	Tetracyline, chloramphenicol
Vibrio, noncholera species‡	Tetracycline	
EPEC, EAggEC, or DAEC in adults, EHEC	TMP-SMX	
Not recommended		
ETEC		
Viral diarrhea		

*No longer available in the United States.
†See Chapter 98 for details.
‡Dosages same as under Recommended in symptomatic cases.
TMP-SMX, trimethoprim-sulfamethoxazole; EPEC, enteropathogenic *Escherichia coli*; EAggEC, enteroaggregative *E. coli*; DAEC, diffusely adhering *E. coli*; EIEC, enteroinvasive *E. coli*; EHEC, enterohemorrhagic *E. coli*; ETEC, enterotoxigenic *E. coli*.

entering tourists because of its limited efficacy. Studies in Bangladesh have shown that the effectiveness of the vaccine is only 70% for 3 to 5 months.[24] After vaccination, an elevation in antibody titer can be seen within 8 days in persons who previously had a demonstrable antibody titer; this rise indicates an anamnestic response. Young children, presumably having had no prior contact with the vibrio, show a more delayed antibody response and often do not develop significant titers until a second injection is administered, approximately 3 to 4 weeks later. Thus, the vaccine has limited effectiveness in epidemics because by the time the initial cases are seen, the infection is already widely spread in the community. Vaccination at this stage requires days to weeks before immunity is produced in children.

The B subunit of cholera toxin has been used in a newer cholera vaccine; two to three doses of this oral vaccine have provided protective efficacy rates of 61% to 86% against symptomatic cholera, especially for illness requiring hospitalization.[25, 26] Several novel oral vaccines, which use genetic engineering to delete the toxin gene, have been developed.[27] The most extensively studied of these live attenuated vaccines, CVD 103 HgR, is immunogenic and well tolerated and provides good protective efficacy against challenge with *V. cholerae*.[28] However, a recently completed field trial in Indonesia failed to show meaningful protective efficacy of the vaccine even though vibriocidal seroresponses developed in most vaccinees after one dose.[29]

Other Vibrios

In addition to the cholera vibrios, at least nine other vibrios have important pathogenic significance.[12, 30, 31] These organisms are halophilic (prefer high salt concentration) and are associated primarily with mollusks such as oysters, crabs, and mussels. Strains within the same species may produce different toxins, including enterotoxins, cytotoxins, and hemolysins. The diversity of toxin production is matched by the diversity of clinical symptoms, which range from watery dehydrating diarrhea to frank dysentery. Some strains penetrate the intestinal mucosa and produce bacteremia, whereas others have been incriminated in wound infections after exposure to ocean water or handling raw seafood.[32]

The incidence of vibrio intestinal infections was studied among participants at an antimicrobial conference in New Orleans, many of whom consumed raw oysters. Of 479 persons surveyed, 11% had a positive stool culture for vibrios, mainly *V. parahaemolyticus*, and approximately one third of those with a positive culture had diarrhea. Samples of local seafood, especially oysters, were found to harbor five different species of vibrios.[33] In the Chesapeake Bay the annual incidence of vibrio infections related to consuming seafood is estimated to be 1.6 per 100,000 persons.[34]

Vibrio parahaemolyticus

V. parahaemolyticus causes an acute diarrheal disease after consumption of raw fish or shellfish. Recognized as an important pathogen in the Far East, *V. parahaemolyticus* also has been isolated in the United States, although the exact incidence is unknown. Strains of *V. parahaemolyticus* produce a number of distinct hemolysins, the most significant of which appears to be responsible for the "Kanagawa phenomenon," which causes hemolysis of human red blood cells in Wagatsuma bacteriologic medium. Kanagawa-positive isolates are pathogenic for humans, whereas Kanagawa-negative strains are nonpathogenic and isolated from marine sources as part of their flora.

Pathogenic strains produce a number of other toxins, including a lethal toxin, which is also hemolytic. In some studies, these organisms produce an enterotoxin that causes fluid accumulation in the rabbit ileal loop model and a cytotoxic toxin that causes damage to HeLa cells. Some strains have the ability to invade the intestinal mucosa and cause bacteremia in experimental animals.[35]

Epidemiology

Many outbreaks of *V. parahaemolyticus* gastroenteritis have been reported in Japan; during the warm months, when the incidence is higher, this organism is responsible for most episodes of bacterial food poisoning in that country. Infections also have been documented in other countries in Asia, as well as Australia and Great Britain. In the United States, there is a striking geographic association, with most cases occurring in coastal states such as Maryland, Massachusetts, Louisiana, New Jersey, and Washington. The organism is ubiquitous in marine waters and can be found along the coastline of most countries in which cases have been reported.

The attack rate in epidemics varies from 24% and 86% of exposed persons. The mean incubation period for most outbreaks has been 13 to 23 hours, with a range of 4 to 48 hours.

Most infections have been associated with seafish or seawater. Occasionally, boiled sardines, salted vegetables (contaminated from saltwater), or crabs, shrimp, and oysters (both cooked and uncooked) have been incriminated. The common factor in most outbreaks appears to be a hiatus of several hours without proper refrigeration.

Clinical Features

The diversity in toxins and virulence mechanisms is reflected in the variation in symptoms and signs observed in laboratory-confirmed outbreaks in the United States.[36, 37] Explosive watery diarrhea is the cardinal manifestation in over 90% of the cases. Abdominal cramps, nausea, vomiting, and headaches are common. Fever and chills occur in 25% to 50% of cases. Clinically, this illness resembles that produced by nontyphoidal *Salmonella*. However, in some cases a bloody dysenteric syndrome is observed, with fecal leukocytes and superficial mucosal ulcerations on sigmoidoscopic examination.

The duration of illness generally is short, with a median of 6 days (range, less than 1 to 30 days). Fatalities are rare and usually occur in persons with preexisting medical conditions. The diarrhea usually is not as profuse as in *V. cholerae*, but hypotension and shock have been noted in some patients.

Subclinical cases have been demonstrated in less than 1% of healthy persons. The infection is rare in the winter, suggesting that the carrier state is probably transient. The organism is no longer detectable in the stool once symptoms have resolved.

Therapy

Although explosive in onset, this disease is generally rather short-lived. Patients generally are treated symptomatically. The organism is sensitive to several antibiotics, including tetracycline, but there is no evidence that antimicrobial therapy has a role in the management of this infection.

Vibrio cholerae *Non-01*

These strains represent a diverse group of organisms that are identical morphologically and biochemically to *V. cholerae*, but they do not agglutinate with the 0-group antiserum of the three cholera serotypes.[31, 38] The non-01 cholera vibrios produce several toxins in vitro and cause a wider range of infection than do cholera vibrios, including watery diarrhea, dysentery, wound infections, ear infections, and septicemia.[12, 31]

The non-01 cholera vibrios can be isolated from salty coastal waters of the United States, most commonly in the summer and fall when the temperature rises. Mollusks, particularly oysters, have a reported contamination rate of 10% to 15% and are the major source; clams, mussels, and crabs also have been implicated.

In the Far East, non-01 cholera vibrios have been associated mainly with severe dehydrating diarrhea. In Peru, serogroups 010 and 012 were isolated from patients with liquid diarrhea associated with mild to moderate dehydration.[39] Although these isolates did not have genes encoding cholera toxin, they were capable of inducing diarrhea in an animal model. In the United States, reported cases of disease caused by non-01 cholera vibrios include wound and ear infections, septicemia, and infections of the lung and biliary tract.[31] The most common antecedent history is consumption of raw oysters within the previous 72 hours. In outbreaks, there is a high attack rate, with incubation periods that range from as short as 6 to 12 hours to as long as 3 days. A 1-week course of diarrheal illness is common. Because the gastrointestinal disease is self-limited and relatively benign in the United States, antibiotics are not recommended. However, septicemia, wound infections, and deep organ infections should be treated with appropriate antibiotics.

V. vulnificus is perhaps the most important noncholera vibrio in the United States because of its severity of illness, especially in patients with underlying liver disease. The infection can be acquired as a wound infection in people swimming in salt waters or by direct consumption of seafood, usually raw oysters; the mortality rate of resulting septicemia is 50%. Because this infection can be lethal in patients with underlying liver disease, such persons should be warned to avoid eating raw seafood, especially oysters.[40]

V. mimicus acquires its name from its similarity to cholera vibrios, even in producing an enterotoxin that resembles cholera toxin.[41] The organism has been isolated from patients in the United States with diarrhea, septicemia, or wound infections.[30] *V. hollisae*, also known as enteric EF-13, is a rare isolate from stool and, occasionally, blood cultures. *V. furnissii* is found in the Orient. Its most celebrated outbreak was an air flight from Tokyo to Seattle, in which 23 passengers developed severe diarrhea, resulting in one death and two hospitalizations.

V. fluvialis, previously designated as enteric group EF-6, has been isolated from patients with severe watery diarrhea in the Orient and the coastal United States.[30, 31, 34] The isolates produced a range of toxins, including an enterotoxin similar to classic cholera toxin. The organism is found only rarely in other parts of the world, including the United States. Bacteremia caused by *V. metschnikovii* has been described in a limited number of cases and may be more common in patients with an underlying disease.[42] *V. alginolyticus* is a rare cause of wound or ear infections and gastroenteritis.[30] *V. damsela* is encountered rarely in wound infections.

Aeromonas

Aeromonas species are ubiquitous environmental organisms found principally in fresh and brackish water, especially in the summer months. These organisms are often mistaken for coliforms in the laboratory, and as a result reported incidence rates are falsely low. *Aeromonas* spp. are divided into two groups: psychrophilic aeromonads, which grow optimally at temperatures ranging from 22°C to 28°C, and mesophilic aeromonads, which grow best between 35°C and 37°C.[43] Psychrophilic strains are usually isolated from environmental water sources and fish; *A. salmonicida* is the most common strain in this group. Based on their phenotypic features, the mesophilic aeromonads are grouped into three complexes: *A. hydrophila*, *A. caviae*, and *A. veronii*. All three of these *Aeromonas* spp. have been associated with human infections.[43, 44] *Aeromonas* strains produce an array of toxins, including heat-labile enterotoxin, hemolysin, and cytotoxin.[45]

Epidemiology

Aeromonas infections are often associated with drinking untreated water, such as well water or spring water, just before the onset of symptoms.[46] Several studies have reported a high incidence of isolation of the organism from the stools of children with diarrhea; for example, the incidence of *Aeromonas* isolations in Western Australia was 10.2% in more than 1000 cases of childhood diarrhea, compared with 0.06% in control subjects.[47] Other studies have found a high carrier rate in healthy people, with a range of 0.7% to 3.2% and up to 27% in Thailand. The high carrier rate has raised some question about the pathogenicity of these organisms.[48]

Clinical Features

Aeromonas has long been recognized as a cause of wound infections after swimming in fresh or brackish water and of bacteremic or deep organ infections in immunocompromised hosts. However, in recent years most isolates have come from intestinal infections. There is a range of illness, from mild diarrhea seen mostly in children to more severe cases that can require hospitalization. In a study from Western Australia, 22% of patients had blood and mucus in their stools, and one third required hospitalization for severe illness.[47] Most cases resolved within 1 week, but 37% of these children had symptoms for 2 or more weeks. In adults, chronic diarrhea is even more common, lasting an average of 42 days in the United States.[46]

Treatment

These organisms are consistently resistant to β-lactam antibiotics, such as penicillin, ampicillin, and first- or second-generation cephalosporins.[49] In fact, some cases of *Aeromonas* diarrhea have been activated apparently by prior treatment with ampicillin. The organisms tend to be sensitive to TMP-SMX, third-generation cephalosporins, fluoroquinolones, tetracycline, and chloramphenicol. There is no convincing evidence that mild cases are improved by antibiotic treatment, but the duration of a chronic infection may be shortened by appropriate use of these drugs.

Plesiomonas shigelloides

P. shigelloides is also a member of the family *Vibrionaceae* but is isolated less frequently than *Aeromonas* in the United States.[43, 48, 50] Most cases have been associated with consumption of raw oysters or recent travel to Mexico or to the Orient.[51] Diarrhea ranges from mild and watery to severe colitis with visible blood. Abdominal pain is often prominent. The antibiotic sensitivity pattern is similar to that of *Aeromonas*, but little information is available on the efficacy of treatment.

Escherichia coli

These organisms are major components of the normal intestinal microflora in humans and animals. Although most strains are relatively harmless in the bowel, others possess virulence factors that are related to diarrheal disease. At least six types of *E. coli* intestinal pathogens have been recognized (Table 96–5). Their virulence factors include toxin production, adherence to epithelial cells, and invasiveness, each encoded by specific genetic elements (plasmids or chromosomal genes) that determine pathogenicity.

Enteropathogenic E. coli *(EPEC)*

Severe epidemics of diarrhea raged in neonatal nurseries for decades, starting in the 1920s. Although uncommon in recent years, such outbreaks had a high mortality in infants. Approximately 14 serotypes were associated epidemiologically with neonatal diarrhea, including the well-known types 055, 0111, and 0119.[52] An analysis of published case-controlled studies and longitudinal surveys found that EPEC designated by serotype was recovered more frequently from sick children than from healthy control subjects.[52]

Virulence is related to the mechanism of colonization in the bowel. EPEC attaches to the intestinal mucosa in a characteristic manner, producing ultrastructural changes known as attachment-effacement lesions; these lesions lead to elongation and destruction of microvilli. The laboratory counterpart of mucosal colonization is adherence in tissue culture to cells such as Hep-2 and HeLa lines. A characteristic form of *localized adherence* is observed only with classic EPEC serotypes. These events occur in three phases as follows[4]: (1) nonintimate attachment of EPEC to intestinal epithelial cells—attachment is mediated by a bundle-forming pilus associated with a large plasmid common to EPEC isolates; (2) a signal transduction event that leads to cytoskeletal changes in the enterocyte via the activation of protein kinase and the release of intracellular calcium; and (3) intimate attachment of the bacterium to the host cell membrane—attachment is mediated by an outer membrane protein called intimin, which is encoded by the *eaeA* gene cluster on the EPEC chromosome.[53] EPEC strains with localized adherence produce acute diarrhea when these strains are administered to normal volunteers.[54] The role of the *eaeA* gene as a virulence factor in human EPEC infection has been confirmed in volunteer challenge studies.[55]

The presence of a plasmid in EPEC serves to increase intimin production; this process is needed for localized adherence to occur.[56] A probe constructed from this plasmid, known as enteropathogenic *E. coli* adherence factor, has been used to identify EPEC strains rapidly in stools of patients with diarrhea.[57] In a study from São Paulo, Brazil, EAF-positive classic EPEC was found in 26% of children with acute diarrhea; these organisms were the most common pathogens isolated from these children and exceeded rotavirus isolations in frequency.[58] EPEC strains are less frequent causes of diarrhea in industrialized countries but seem to be

Table 96–5 | **Types of *E. coli* Intestinal Pathogens**

STRAINS	MECHANISMS	TYPES OF PATIENTS	CLINICAL FEATURES
Enteropathogenic (EPEC)	Localized adherence O serogroups	Children Newborn nursery outbreaks	Watery diarrhea
Enterotoxigenic (ETEC)	Heat-labile toxin (LT) and/or heat-stable toxin (ST) Adherence	Children (developing countries); travelers	Watery diarrhea
Enteroinvasive (EIEC)	Shiga-like toxin Epithelial cell adherence O serogroups (related to *Shigella*)	Children and adults Food and water outbreaks	Dysentery (white and red blood cells in feces)
Enterohemorrhagic (EHEC)	Shiga-like toxin (large quantities) O serogroups (usually O157:H7)	Children and adults Food (hamburger) outbreaks	Bloody diarrhea Hemolytic-uremic syndrome
Enteroaggregative (EAggEC)	Aggregative adherence to Hep-2 and HeLa cells	Children (developing countries)	Watery diarrhea (acute) and persistent diarrhea
Diffusely adhering (DAEC)	Diffuse adherence to Hep-2 cells	Children (developing countries)	Acute and persistent diarrhea

important pathogens in many developing countries, especially in children in the first 2 years of life.[59, 60]

Resistance to antimicrobial drugs is common in *E. coli* adherence factor-positive classic EPEC strains.[58] Because most of these infections appear to be self-limited, there is no indication for antibiotic treatment, although nonabsorbable antibiotics such as neomycin have been used in the past for neonates with severe EPEC diarrhea.

Enterotoxigenic E. coli

Inspired by the discoveries in cholera, investigators directed their attention to *E. coli* as a cause of acute toxigenic diarrheal disease. Originally in India, and thereafter in many parts of the world, strains of *E. coli* were found to elaborate an enterotoxin similar to the toxin of *V. cholerae*.[61] ETEC is a group of *E. coli* not belonging to serotypes previously recognized as EPEC. ETEC infections are mostly sporadic but may cause large outbreaks.

Pathologic Mechanism of Infection

ETEC is acquired by consuming contaminated food and liquids. The organisms must pass the acid barrier of the stomach. They then colonize the surface of the small bowel epithelium without penetrating the epithelial layer. As in cholera, there is neither mucosal damage nor bacteremia. The process of colonization is related to specific protein antigens on the surface of the bacterial cell known as pili or fimbriae. These pili are capable of hemagglutination in the presence of mannose. They are variously known as adherence antigens or colonization factor antigens.[62]

The antigenic structure of the adherence pili determines the host specificity of the ETEC strains. For example, those bearing a K88 antigen are pathogenic for piglets, whereas others bearing K99 antigen cause disease in calves and lambs. The ETEC that are pathogenic for humans has another group of antigens.[62] The enterotoxins, on the other hand, are similar in the human and animal strains.

Enterotoxins

Two types of enterotoxins are produced by ETEC.[4] The *heat-labile* toxin (LT) is a protein that is destroyed by heat and acid and has a molecular weight of approximately 80. It acts pathophysiologically like cholera toxin by activating adenylate cyclase, thereby causing secretion of fluid and electrolytes into the intestinal lumen. LT also shares antigenic components with cholera toxin. The second toxin is *heat stable* (ST) and is able to withstand heating to 100°C. This toxin has a low molecular weight of approximately 4500, activates guanylate cyclase, and has no biochemical similarity to cholera toxin. ST is really a family of toxins; the forms that cause disease most commonly in humans are ST1a and ST1b. A trivalent probe for these two STs and LT has been described.[63] ETEC strains may elaborate LT only, ST only, or both forms of toxins. Not only do these toxins cause diarrhea in humans, but similar types of toxigenic *E. coli* also cause dehydrating diarrhea in domestic animals such as pigs, cows, and sheep.

Epidemiology

ETEC infections are acquired from other humans; animal strains of ETEC are rather host specific. The major vehicles of infection appear to be contaminated food and beverages. Infection occurs primarily in children, with the highest incidence in the tropics. There have been varying reports of ETEC infection in the United States, with high incidences in Chicago and Dallas but low figures in other American cities and Canada. Even in developing countries, the frequency of ETEC infection in children has varied from 15% to 50% of all diarrheal episodes. ETEC is the most common cause of diarrhea in travelers from North America and Northern Europe to areas of the developing world where diarrheal disease is prevalent. This pathogen has also become the leading bacterial etiology of outbreaks of gastroenteritis on cruise ships; water stored at overseas ports is the probable source of these ETEC infections.[64]

Clinical Features

ETEC infections are among the most common causes of diarrhea in children living in developing countries and travelers to these regions.[59] There is nothing distinctive about the clinical presentation of ETEC diarrhea. The incubation period is 24 to 48 hours, and the disease often begins with upper intestinal distress, followed shortly by watery diarrhea. The infection can be mild, with only a few loose bowel movements, or quite severe, mimicking cholera, with severe dehydration and even rice water stools. Indeed, the initial demonstration of toxigenic diarrhea came from studies in Calcutta of a serious form of diarrheal disease called "acute undifferentiated diarrhea." Affected patients were admitted to the cholera ward until it was determined that vibrios were not present in their stools. ST-only strains cause a milder attack of diarrhea than LT-producing strains, but affected patients have more vomiting and constitutional complaints.[65]

Immunologic Responses

Antibodies to the enterotoxins and colonization factors have been demonstrated in persons infected with ETEC. It appears that people residing in areas at high risk for ETEC infection acquire some mucosal immunity over time.[4] Thus, the risk that ETEC diarrhea will develop in students at a college in Mexico depends on their country of origin; those from South America have a relatively low risk of ETEC diarrhea, whereas those from North America have a high risk.[66]

Treatment

Most patients with ETEC diarrhea have only mild dehydration, but in children and older people even small amounts of intestinal purging can have serious consequences. The stool electrolyte losses in ETEC diarrhea are similar to those in cholera, and fluid replacement should follow the same principles. Although these organisms are often sensitive to many antimicrobial drugs, including ampicillin, tetracycline, and TMP-SMX, resistant isolates are being encountered increasingly.[64] Studies of patients with acute traveler's diarrhea have demonstrated shortening of the duration of diarrhea when effective antimicrobial therapy is initiated early in the course of illness.[67] Nevertheless, because most episodes of ETEC diarrhea are self-limited, treatment with antibiotics is generally not necessary.

Enteroinvasive E. coli *(EIEC)*

Originally described in Asia, EIEC is recognized as a rare cause of the dysentery syndrome. During 1971, there was an EIEC outbreak in the United States that was related to contaminated imported cheese.[68] Most episodes of EIEC infections are characterized by watery diarrhea; some patients experience a dysenteric syndrome, which is manifested as bloody mucoid diarrhea, tenesmus, fever, intestinal cramps, and multiple polymorphonuclear leukocytes in the fecal effluent. EIECs have been recognized in at least eight *E. coli* serogroups, most of which are related biochemically and antigenically to *Shigella*. Other similarities to *Shigella* include the ability to invade epithelial cells and production of a Shiga-like toxin. An enterotoxin also has been identified in EIEC strains. Diagnosis of EIEC in a routine bacteriologic laboratory is difficult and generally impractical. Surveys of EIEC in the United States have shown low isolation rates, except in a few celebrated outbreaks. Low rates of infection have been observed in some less developed countries,[59] although in Thailand the organism is common in children with diarrhea.[69]

Enterohemorrhagic E. coli *(EHEC)*

Acute hemorrhagic colitis, which was first recognized in two separate outbreaks in Michigan and Oregon in 1982,[70] has been associated mainly with a specific serotype of *E. coli*, O157 : H7. This organism is estimated to be responsible for 0.6% to 2.4% of all cases of diarrhea and 15% to 36% of cases of hemorrhagic colitis in Canada, the United Kingdom, and the United States.[71] The spectrum of disease associated with *E. coli* O157 : H7 includes bloody diarrhea, which is seen in as many as 95% of patients, nonbloody diarrhea, hemolytic-uremic syndrome (HUS), and thrombotic thrombocytopenic purpura.

Epidemiology

EHEC has become the most commonly isolated pathogen from the stools of patients with bloody diarrhea in the United States.[72] The disease is most common in northern climates such as Massachusetts, Minnesota, the Pacific Northwest, Canada, and Great Britain. Infections occur sporadically or as large outbreaks. The leading vehicle of infection is hamburger meat, although outbreaks have been associated with precooked meat patties, roast beef, salami, fresh-pressed apple cider, lettuce, alfalfa sprouts, and unpasteurized milk.[4, 73–76] Water-borne outbreaks have also been associated with contaminated swimming pools, other recreational water bodies, well water, and municipal water systems.[4] Person-to-person transmission has probably played a role in outbreaks in day-care centers and nursing homes.[71, 77, 78] Infection rates vary seasonally with a peak incidence from June to September.

Shiga-like cytotoxin-producing *E. coli* are found in the fecal flora of a wide variety of animals, including cattle, sheep, pigs, goats, chickens, dogs, and cats. Many of these strains are of serotypes other than *E. coli* O157 : H7. The most important reservoir of infection is cattle, especially younger animals.

A striking association has been noted between intestinal infection with EHEC and HUS. In Minnesota, the incidence of HUS increased progressively during the 1980s to a current rate of 2.0 cases per 100,000 child-years. *E. coli* O157 : H7 was isolated in 46% of children presenting with HUS. Risk factors for HUS include age under 5 years, attendance at a large day-care center, presence of bloody diarrhea, and high white blood cell count.[73] Another study from the British Isles showed that 95% of the cases of HUS had a prodromal diarrheal illness. The disease was seen most commonly in the summer. Most EHEC strains were O157 : H7 or H-, although approximately 30% of the isolates belonged to nine other serogroups of *E. coli*.[79, 80]

Virulence Factors

EHEC strains possess at least two virulence factors: an adherence mechanism causing attachment-effacement lesions similar to those seen with EPEC (see earlier) and two Shiga-like cytotoxins (Stx I and II).[71, 81] The toxins, which are identified either in stool samples or from the organism itself, cause characteristic lesions in tissue culture lines such as Vero cells and HeLa cells. Some EHEC strains produce only Stx I or II, whereas others produce both toxins. Most strains of *E. coli* O157 : H7 possess the *eaeA* gene, which is associated with intimate attachment to the intestinal mucosa, as in EPEC (see earlier). They also produce enterohemolysin and are capable of using both heme and hemoglobin, a property that may enhance their virulence as well.[82]

Clinical Features

After an incubation period of 1 to 14 days (mean, 3 to 4 days), there is the onset of watery nonbloody diarrhea associated with severe abdominal cramping and progression often to visibly bloody stools. Other related symptoms include nausea, vomiting, low grade fever, and chills. The development of frankly bloody diarrhea frequently results in admission to the hospital. Examination of the colon by endoscopy demonstrates a friable inflamed mucosa with patchy erythema, edema, and superficial ulcerations. Plain radiographs of the abdomen show mucosal involvement with submucosal edema and "thumbprinting" in the ascending and transverse colon. Leukocytosis with a shift to the left is usually present, but anemia is uncommon unless infection is complicated by the development of HUS or thrombotic thrombocytopenic purpura.[71] Microscopic examination of the stool reveals red blood cells, whereas white blood cells are present in low to moderate amounts. The median duration of diarrhea is 3 to 8 days, with longer durations in children and persons with bloody diarrhea.[71]

Diagnosis

Several laboratory methods are used to diagnose EHEC infections. Stx testing has been widely used but requires special facilities. Newer tests, including DNA probes, polymerase chain reaction, and enzyme immunoassays, can detect Stx I and II directly in stool specimens. Because most isolates of *E. coli* O157:H7 do not ferment D-sorbitol, screening for this pathogen can be done with sorbitol-MacConkey agar. Sorbitol-negative colonies should be sent to a reference laboratory for serotyping and toxin testing. The chances of obtaining a positive culture in stool depend on the time between the onset of symptoms and collection of the stool. Within 2 days of onset, virtually all stool specimens are positive for EHEC, whereas after 7 days only one third are positive.[83] In contrast, other studies have found that the median duration of excretion of EHEC is 17 to 29 days, with some patients shedding the bacterium for as long as 124 days.[4, 84, 85]

Treatment

The desire to treat EHEC infections is understandable because of the presence of bloody diarrhea and concern that HUS will develop. However, several reports have raised concern that the risk of HUS is increased by antimicrobial therapy. In a murine model, certain antibiotics, notably ciprofloxacin, caused enhanced Stx production by *E. coli* O157:H7 in vitro via the induction of bacteriophage encoded gene; this occurrence was associated with an increased death rate in treated mice.[86]

Antimicrobial therapy in humans does not appear to provide much benefit and may even be harmful. A randomized controlled trial of TMP-SMX in children with *E. coli* O157:H7 enteritis found no effect of therapy on the duration of symptoms, pathogen excretion, or incidence of HUS.[87]

A recent prospective cohort study identified 71 children with acute *E. coli* O157:H7 gastroenteritis of whom only 9 had been treated with antibiotics; however, 5 of the 10 children in whom HUS developed had received either TMP-SMX or a cephalosporin.[88] In this study, antibiotic therapy was associated with a significantly increased risk of HUS.

Because the use of antibiotics has not been shown to decrease morbidity resulting from EHEC and appears to increase the risk of HUS, *we strongly recommend against antibiotic treatment of gastroenteritis if* E. coli *O157:H7 is the known or suspected cause*. In cases of confirmed *E. coli* O157:H7, patients should be followed closely for manifestations of HUS. Thorough cooking of ground beef is an important preventive measure.

Enteroaggregative E. coli *(EAggEC)*

Unlike the localized adherence to Hep-2 cells seen with EPEC, some *E. coli* strains have been observed to adhere in an aggregative pattern with the bacteria clumping in a "stacked brick" pattern to the cell surface.[4] Although some investigations have implicated EAggEC as a cause of acute and persistent diarrhea in children in developing countries,[4, 89] other investigations have failed to find a significant association with diarrhea.[58, 59, 90] Up to one third of infected children have grossly bloody diarrhea. EAggEC also has been associated with diarrhea in patients infected with human immunodeficiency virus.[91]

Volunteer challenge studies with different strains of EAggEC have yielded mixed results, suggesting that certain strains may be more virulent than others.[92] As yet, there have been no studies documenting the need for or efficacy of treatment of EAggEC infections. EAggEC include numerous serogroups that are largely distinct from those of EPEC. Certain serotypes such as O44:H18 appear to be more pathogenic than others. Rabbit ileal loop models of EAggEC infection have demonstrated histopathologic evidence of villous shortening, hemorrhagic necrosis of villous tips, and mild inflammation associated with aggregates of bacteria on the mucosal surface.[93] A 65-Mda plasmid associated with EAggEC appears to be necessary for expression of a heat-stable enterotoxin and aggregative adherence to Hep-2 cells in vitro, which may occur via an outer membrane protein.[4, 94]

Although there have been no controlled trials of therapy for EAggEC infections in children, a recent study of human immunodeficiency virus–positive patients with diarrhea caused by EAggEC found a 50% reduction in stool output, fewer intestinal symptoms, and microbiologic eradication of the organism during treatment with ciprofloxacin.[95] Similarly, ciprofloxacin therapy of EAggEC resulted in a reduction of the duration of diarrhea in patients with traveler's diarrhea.[96]

Diffusely Adhering E. coli *(DAEC)*

Another type of *E. coli* infection is characterized by *diffuse adherence* of bacteria to Hep-2 cells in a uniform manner and has been associated with diarrhea in children in some developing countries.[59, 90] DAEC strains appear to be more pathogenic for older than younger children.[59, 90] DAEC strains were also associated with diarrhea in a study of hospitalized patients of all ages in France, thus suggesting that this pathogen may be common in developed countries as well.[97] On the other hand, studies in Brazil and Thailand failed to find an association between DAEC and childhood diarrhea.[58, 98] Volunteers infected with diffuse adherent strains failed to develop diarrhea.[99] However, a retrospective case-control study found that most patients infected with DAEC had watery nonbloody diarrhea with fecal leukocytes.[100] Specific virulence factors have not been elucidated for this class of *E. coli*; the variability in recognizing DAEC strains with DNA probes suggests that this group also may be heterogeneous.

INVASIVE PATHOGENS

Invasive organisms make their main impact on the host by invading the intestinal epithelium. Whereas the toxigenic organisms characteristically involve the upper intestine, the invasive pathogens target the lower bowel, particularly the distal ileum and colon. The main histologic finding is mucosal ulceration with an acute inflammatory reaction in the lamina propria. The principal pathogens in this group are *Salmonella*, *Shigella*, invasive *E. coli* (EIEC), *Campylobacter*, and *Yersinia*. There are important differences among these organisms, but they all share the property of mucosal invasion as the initiating event.

The precise mechanism of fluid production in invasive diarrhea is not known, but three theories have been invoked:

1. An enterotoxin may be responsible for fluid production, at least in the initial phase of the illness. Most *Shigella* strains elaborate an enterotoxin that differs significantly from cholera toxin but does cause fluid and electrolyte secretion by the intestine.[101] A similar toxin has been proposed for *Salmonella*, and there is suggestive evidence that *Campylobacter* and *Yersinia* elaborate enterotoxins.
2. Invasive organisms increase local synthesis of prostaglandins at the site of the intense inflammatory reaction. In experimental animals, fluid secretion can be blocked by prostaglandin inhibitors such as indomethacin.[102] This theory suggests that prostaglandins are responsible for fluid secretion and subsequent diarrhea.
3. Damage to the epithelial surface may prevent reabsorption of fluids from the lumen. Transudation of fluid from the colon does not appear to be a significant factor; however, colonic malabsorption of fluid, with a constant level of secretion, would produce net accumulation of luminal fluid, thereby resulting in diarrhea.

Shigella

Shigella organisms cause bacillary dysentery, a disease that has been described since early recorded history. The inhabitants of Athens in the second year of the Peloponnesian War were ravaged by dysentery: "The disease descended to the bowels, producing violent ulceration and uncontrollable diarrhea." In the American Civil War, over 1,700,000 soldiers suffered from dysentery, with 44,500 deaths. World War I also produced a high incidence of dysentery: 3.7 per 1000 total casualties in France and up to 486 per 1000 casualties in East Africa. Although dysentery is a disease that becomes more prevalent in wartime, there is a constant endemic incidence in tropical countries as well as in temperate zones.

Microbiology

Shigellae comprise a group of Gram-negative enteric organisms that are included in the *Enterobacteriaceae* and most closely resemble *E. coli*. They are differentiated from *E. coli* by being nonmotile, not producing gas from glucose, and generally being lactose negative. There are four major subgroups:

Group A: *S. dysenteriae*, 10 serotypes
Group B: *S. flexneri*, 14 serotypes
Group C: *S. boydii*, 18 serotypes
Group D: *S. sonnei*, 1 serotype

Group A (*S. dysenteriae* 1), also known as the *Shiga bacillus*, produces the severest form of dysentery. An outbreak in Central America in the late 1960s and early 1970s caused over 10,000 deaths, mostly in young children. This organism has caused outbreaks in many developing countries in recent years. *S. sonnei* produces the mildest disease.

There have been recent shifts in the incidence of dysentery and in the prevalence of specific serotypes. In the tropics, dysentery occurs mostly in late summer. In developed countries, such as the United States and those in Europe, the occurrence of dysentery has increased steadily, and the seasonal prevalence has shifted to winter. *S. flexneri* is the most common organism in tropical countries; however, in the United States and Europe, *S. flexneri* has decreased in prevalence, and *S. sonnei* is now the most common serotype. In the United States, for example, 60% to 80% of cases of bacillary dysentery are caused by *S. sonnei*.

Pathogenicity

All strains of *Shigella* cause dysentery, a term that refers to a diarrheal stool that contains an inflammatory exudate composed of polymorphonuclear leukocytes and blood. The exudative character of the stool is a point to be emphasized: This is not mere watery diarrhea but rather a loose bowel movement that contains pus. The inflammatory exudate is related to the main pathologic event—invasion of the colonic epithelium.

Humans are the only natural host for the dysentery organism, although monkeys and chimpanzees can become infected in captivity. Experimental infections can be produced in monkeys and guinea pigs. Mucosal invasion is demonstrated in the conjunctival sac of guinea pigs (Sereny test), and direct invasion of HeLa cells is observed in tissue culture. In experimental animal infections, the disease is made worse by starving the animals, feeding them antibiotics, or administering opium to reduce forward propulsive motility of the bowel.

The major site of attack of *Shigella* is the colon; scattered ulcerations can be seen in the terminal ileum as well. Although involvement of the stomach and small bowel has been noted in animal experiments and occasionally in fatal human infections, these organs are usually spared in clinical cases.

Invasion by *Shigella* is associated with a constellation of virulence factors that are related to various stages of invasion and lead eventually to death of the intestinal epithelial cell, focal ulcers, and inflammation of the lamina propria. These virulence factors are encoded by both chromosomal and plasmid genes, all of which are needed for the full expression of virulence. All virulent *Shigella*, as well as EIEC, contain large 120- to 140-Mda plasmids, which are related to outer membrane proteins. Various loci encode for an invasion plasmid antigen (ipa), which seems to determine recognition of the epithelial cell; invasion factors (inv); and a series of vir proteins that are involved in regulation within the cell.[103]

Having penetrated the mucosal surface, the organisms multiply within the epithelial cells and extend the infected area by "cell-to-cell transfer" of bacilli. Time-lapse phase-contrast cine-microscopy of HeLa cells infected with *Shigella* has shown bacilli moving vigorously throughout the cytoplasm and migrating to adjacent cells by filopodium-like protrusions. Shigellae rarely penetrate beyond the intestinal mucosa and generally do not invade the bloodstream. However, bacteremia can occur in malnourished children and immunocompromised patients.

Although the initial lesions are confined to the epithelial layer, the local inflammatory response is severe, consisting of polymorphonuclear leukocytes and macrophages. There is edema, microabscess formation, loss of goblet cells, degeneration of normal cellular architecture, and mucosal ulceration. These events give rise to the characteristic clinical picture of bloody mucopurulent diarrhea. As the disease progresses, the lamina propria is involved extensively with the inflammatory response. Crypt abscess is a prominent feature (Fig. 96–1).

Cytotoxins

Until recently, only *S. dysenteriae* 1 was known to elaborate an enterotoxin. This toxin, first identified by Shiga, has since been shown to display a variety of biologic effects, depending on the experimental model used. In brief, these include cytotoxicity (but not adenylate cyclase activation, as with cholera toxin), neurotoxicity in mice, and enterotoxicity (secretion of fluid and electrolytes). The toxin, which is a 75,000-Mda protein composed of two subunits, inhibits protein synthesis by irreversible inactivation of the 60S ribosomal subunit.[104] A toxin with similar antigenic and physiologic effects has been found in strains of *S. flexneri* and *S. sonnei*.[105]

Epidemiology

Shigellosis is a major diarrheal disease throughout the world. The frequency of 10% to 20% of all cases of diarrhea is remarkably similar from country to country. Dysentery occurs mostly in children between the ages of 6 months and 5 years, among whom the disease tends to be less severe than in adults; it is rare in infants less than 6 months of age.

During infection, Shigellae are present in large numbers in feces. The route of infection is oral. The organisms survive best in alkaline conditions and are highly sensitive to heat and drying. Fecal specimens are the best source of a positive culture; blood and urine are only rarely positive in acute cases. Most transmission is person-to-person and is related to close human contact. There also have been dramatic epidemics related to ingestion of milk, ice cream, other foods, and occasionally water. A high incidence of infection occurs among laboratory workers who come in contact with this organism.

Measurements of inoculum size in volunteers reveal that 10^5 organisms produce an attack rate of 75%.[106] Increasing the inoculum size above this number does not increase the attack rate. There is not a good dose–response curve with *Shigella* (in contrast to *Salmonella*); indeed, dysentery can be produced with as few as 200 bacteria. The ability of *Shigella* species to survive in acidic conditions, a property that depends on the growth phase of the organism, may account for the low inoculum that can produce disease.[107] Person-to-person transmission, facilitated by the low infective dose, accounts for rapid spread of *Shigella* in day-care centers and among people living in conditions of poor hygiene. These factors also explain the high frequency of dysentery among male homosexuals.

Clinical Features

The classic presentation of bacillary dysentery is with crampy abdominal pain, rectal burning, and fever, associated with multiple small-volume bloody mucoid bowel movements.[104] However, this full array is seen in only some patients. The most constant findings are lower abdominal pain and diarrhea. Fever is present in approximately 40% of patients, and the typical dysentery stool, consisting of blood and mucus, is present in only one third. Many patients demonstrate a biphasic illness. The initial symptoms are fever, abdominal pain, and watery diarrhea without gross blood; this stage may be related to the action of the enterotoxin. The second phase, which starts 3 to 5 days after onset, is characterized by tenesmus and small-volume bloody stools. This period corresponds to invasion of the colonic epithelium and acute colitis. A few patients have a toxic highly febrile illness associated with more severe colitis; even in this setting, bacteremia is distinctly uncommon. Malnutrition, especially in young children, and infection with *S.*

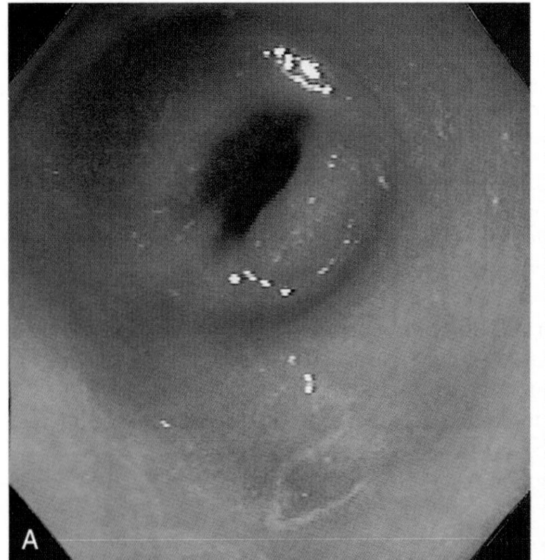

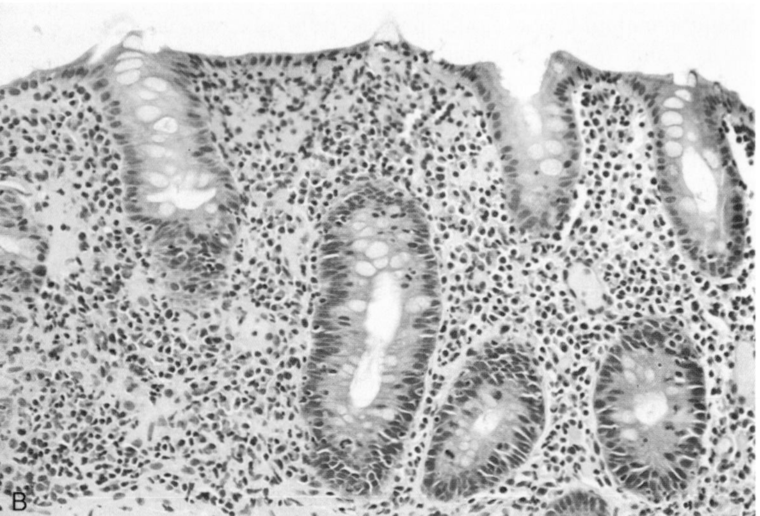

Figure 96–1. Shigellosis. *A,* The view of the rectum on sigmoidoscopy shows narrowing and mucosal inflammation similar to that seen in ulcerative colitis. *B,* Histologic features include a severe inflammatory infiltrate of polymorphonuclear leukocytes and macrophages of the mucosa and submucosa. (From Wilcox CM: Atlas of Clinical Gastrointestinal Endoscopy. Philadelphia, WB Saunders, 1995, pp 214–215.)

dysenteriae type 1 are associated with a more severe course. Among the intestinal complications are intestinal perforation and severe protein loss.

An extensive list of extraintestinal complications is associated with bacillary dysentery.[108] Many patients complain of respiratory symptoms, such as cough and coryza, although pneumonia is rare. In young children, hypoglycemia may occur, and several neurologic findings can dominate the clinical picture, even before the diarrheal symptoms. Meningismus (the cerebrospinal fluid is normal) and seizures have been noted with shigellosis, although there is no direct involvement of the central nervous system.[109, 110] These findings have been related to the high fever, but there seems to be something unusual about their occurrence in dysentery, because they can occur when the fever is not extraordinarily high. During the acute phase, HUS may occur.[111] Thrombocytopenia and a severe leukemoid reaction also have been reported.[112] Several types of rash have been noted during the acute phase of shigellosis.

After an acute attack of dysentery, usually 2 to 3 weeks after the onset, arthritis may appear. The presentation of joint pain or effusion is usually asymmetric, involving large joints. The joint complaints are present by themselves, not necessarily with other signs of Reiter's syndrome. Joint complaints are usually associated with human leukocyte antigen B27; autoantibodies to this antigen cross-react with *Shigella* proteins, thereby resulting in circulating antibody-antigen complexes.[113]

The course of shigellosis is variable. Children tend to have mild infections, lasting no more than 1 to 3 days. The average length of symptoms in adults is approximately 7 days. In more severe cases symptoms persist for 3 to 4 weeks and often are associated with relapses. Untreated bacillary dysentery, particularly with a more prolonged course, can be confused with ulcerative colitis.

Chronic carriers of *Shigella* have been identified; they may pass this organism in their feces for 1 year or more. Such carriers are distinctly uncommon, and they usually lose the organism spontaneously. Carriers of *Shigella* are prone to intermittent attacks of the disease, in contrast to *Salmonella* carriers, who rarely become reinfected with the strain they carry.

Diagnosis

The diagnosis of shigellosis should be suspected by the triad of lower abdominal pain, rectal burning, and diarrhea. Microscopic examination of the fecal effluent is extremely useful and reveals multiple polymorphonuclear leukocytes and red blood cells. This information is often sufficient to make a diagnosis of bacillary dysentery, although the identification of the specific bacterial pathogen must await culture, because other microorganisms can cause the dysentery syndrome (e.g., *Campylobacter*, *V. parahaemolyticus*, *Salmonella*). Because *Shigella* species are fastidious, stool specimens or rectal swabs should be inoculated rapidly into appropriate media. Sigmoidoscopy can confirm the diagnosis of colitis but is not necessary in most cases of shigellosis and is extremely uncomfortable in the setting of dysentery. If there is an urgent need to distinguish dysentery from the acute presentation of idiopathic ulcerative colitis, a colonic biopsy may be useful when taken within 4 days of the onset of symptoms.[114] Serologic and molecular tests are not useful for diagnosing acute cases of dysentery, although they are available for epidemiologic investigations.

A subacute presentation of dysentery can masquerade as ulcerative colitis. The patient may have endured bloody diarrhea, cramps, and rectal pain for 2 to 4 weeks. At this stage, sigmoidoscopy, barium enema, and even mucosal biopsy specimens are indistinguishable from those of patients with idiopathic ulcerative colitis (see Fig. 96–1*B*). The two major differences are a positive stool culture for *Shigella* and dramatic improvement in symptoms after treatment with appropriate antimicrobial agents.

Deaths are rare in healthy persons, particularly adults, with bacillary dysentery; mortality is usually seen in young often malnourished children or in debilitated patients, either the elderly or those with an immunodeficiency disease. A decreased level of consciousness and documented seizures are associated with a poor outcome in children.[109]

Treatment

The following general principles apply to the therapeutic approach to bacillary dysentery:

1. Rehydration must be managed appropriately in any diarrheal disease, regardless of etiology; this maxim holds for dysentery.
2. General supportive measures require attention; in the case of dysentery, children may have seizures related to high fever and electrolyte imbalance or meningismus.
3. Narcotic-related drugs should be avoided, including tincture of opium, paregoric, diphenoxylate with atropine (Lomotil), and loperamide (Imodium).
4. Antibiotic treatment is indicated for most patients with shigellosis.

Fluid and Electrolyte Therapy

Most patients with dysentery can be managed with oral rehydration. The indications for parenteral fluid replacement are marked diarrhea that leads to dehydration and severe vomiting that prevents oral replacement. High-volume diarrhea is seen occasionally with shigellosis, even to the point of severe dehydration and hypovolemia. Intravenous fluid replacement is indicated in this situation. Fluid losses can be repaired within a few hours by intravenous solutions (see Table 96–2), and oral replacement should be encouraged as soon as possible (see Table 96–3).

High fever in children should be treated with tepid water sponges or baths. Phenobarbital is recommended (short-term) for children with seizures or meningismus. Antidiarrheal remedies are generally worthless and may even aggravate a case of bacillary dysentery. Kaolin and pectate and other "water-binding" agents do not diminish stool volume or frequency. Narcotic-containing drugs are interdicted because they can prolong the diarrhea and even provoke toxic megacolon, a dire complication of dysentery.

Antimicrobial Agents

The major determinant in the decision to use antibiotics is the severity of the illness. In practice, patients with moderate and severe cases of dysentery should receive antibiotic therapy. Mild cases often pass as self-limited events, without coming to a physician's attention. If such cases are seen in the clinic or in the doctor's office, antibiotic therapy may not be required in view of the relatively benign course. A reappraisal should be made when the culture report returns as positive for *Shigella*. In many cases, diarrhea has already ceased. Patients with persistent diarrhea should receive antibiotics.

Ampicillin is preferred for drug-sensitive strains when a decision has been made to begin therapy (see Table 96–4). When isolates in a community are known to be resistant to ampicillin, an alternative antibiotic in the United States is TMP-SMX, which also should be used for patients with a penicillin allergy. Plasmid-mediated resistance of *Shigella* strains, particularly *S. dysenteriae* type 1, *S. sonnei*, and *S. flexneri*, to ampicillin is widespread in some geographic areas. Although the rates of resistance to ampicillin or TMP-SMX of *Shigella* strains identified in the United States were relatively low in the past, recent data from Oregon reveal a changing picture. Of more than 400 isolates identified using active surveillance for shigellosis, susceptibility testing revealed that 59% were resistant to TMP-SMX and 63% were resistant to ampicillin.[115] *Shigella* strains acquired during travel outside the United States had a higher frequency of antibiotic resistance. Quinolone resistance was found in less than 1% of strains.[116] The rate of antibiotic resistance among *Shigella* strains is high in certain countries; for example, 100% of strains in Catania, Sicily are resistant to TMP-SMX, and in Pakistan more than 90% are resistant to both TMP-SMX and ampicillin.[117]

The fluoroquinolone (quinolone) antibiotics, such as ciprofloxacin, ofloxacin, and norfloxacin, are highly active in vitro against *Shigella* and should be used in patients with highly resistant organisms, particularly those acquired in developing countries. In a clinical trial of ciprofloxacin versus ampicillin conducted in adult men with shigellosis in Bangladesh, resistance to ampicillin was seen in 60% of isolates, and not surprisingly ampicillin treatment failed in two thirds of these persons. All strains were sensitive to ciprofloxacin, which produced better clinical results than ampicillin, even in patients infected with ampicillin-sensitive strains. A more recent study found that single-dose therapy with 1.0 g of ciprofloxacin was as effective as two doses or a 5-day standard regimen in patients with *Shigella* infection; however, single-dose therapy proved less effective than multiple-dose regimens for patients with *S. dysenteriae* type 1.[118] Problems with using quinolones in the treatment of *Shigella* include the high cost of the drugs and concern about cartilage damage in young children. Nalidixic acid is an alternative therapeutic agent that has produced good results, although resistance develops rapidly with widespread use of this drug.[117]

Because there is now increasing evidence of the skeletal safety of quinolones in children,[119] these drugs are being studied increasingly in pediatric populations. With single-dose pefloxacin therapy of infected children during an outbreak of multidrug resistant *S. dysenteriae* type 1 in Burundi, 91% of treated children became symptom free by day 5, and the remainder were substantially improved.[120] None of the children experienced any joint problems during the 4-week period of follow-up. Similarly, a double-blind trial of pivmecillinam versus ciprofloxacin suspension for childhood shigellosis found that ciprofloxacin resulted in clinical responses in 80% of children, with no associated arthropathy.[121]

Although early animal and human volunteer studies indicated that the use of antimotility agents in the treatment of invasive diarrhea might lead to prolonged fever and pathogen carriage, a recent study has challenged this dictum. Treatment of dysenteric patients with a combination of the synthetic antidiarrheal agent loperamide and ciprofloxacin resulted in a significantly shortened duration of diarrhea and decreased number of stools when compared with ciprofloxacin alone.[122] The use of loperamide did not lead to prolonged fever or excretion of the pathogenic bacilli.

Antibiotics for shigellosis must be absorbed from the bowel to reach organisms within the intestinal wall and lamina propria, and the only effective delivery system is the bloodstream.[123] Nonabsorbable drugs, such as neomycin, kanamycin, paromomycin, colistin, and polymyxin, are clinically ineffective, despite in vitro sensitivity. Intravenous cefamandole also has proved disappointing. Curiously, amoxicillin, which is well-absorbed and achieves higher serum levels than ampicillin, is not effective therapy for shigellosis.[124]

Chronic carriers of *Shigella* are rare. Postinfection carriage generally lasts less than 3 to 4 weeks and rarely exceeds 3 to 4 months. In circumstances in which eradication of the carrier state is deemed necessary, TMP-SMX is effective and eliminates the carrier state in approximately 90% of patients. The dose of trimethoprim is 5 mg/kg body weight/day and that of sulfamethoxazole is 25 mg/kg body weight/day, for 28 days.

Mild grinding diarrhea and cramps may continue for days to weeks after treatment of bacillary dysentery, even when the organism is no longer present and the acute episode seems to have passed. These symptoms are not necessarily a cause for alarm, because the bowel may have sustained severe mucosal injury that requires time for repair.

Instances of *chronic ulcerative colitis* have been traced to a proven attack of dysentery, but such cases are rare. Certain antibiotics, especially ampicillin, have a high incidence of intestinal side effects, including *Clostridium difficile*-associated diarrhea, and persistent diarrhea must be evaluated in terms of a possible untoward drug reaction.

Finally, shigellosis is highly contagious. Spread within a family is common. Secondary cases can occur in hospitals among other patients, nurses, and physicians. Careful hand washing and stool precautions should prevent dissemination of this disease.

Nontyphoidal Salmonellosis

Nontyphoidal salmonellosis refers to disease caused by any serotype of the genus *Salmonella*, with the exception of *S. typhi* and *S. paratyphi*. Approximately 2000 serotypes and variants are potentially pathogenic for animals and humans.

Microbiology

Salmonella is a large group of Gram-negative bacilli that comprise one of the divisions in the family *Enterobacteriaceae*. Most strains are motile and produce acid and gas from glucose, mannitol, and sorbitol (except *S. typhi* and rare strains that produce only acid); they are active producers of hydrogen sulfide; and they are closely related to each other by somatic and flagellar antigens. These organisms are primarily intestinal parasites, although some can be found in the bloodstream and internal organs of invertebrates; they are frequently isolated in sewage, river and seawater, and certain foods. Most salmonellae have a wide range of hosts.

These bacteria grow on several types of artificial media. They can be separated on differential media by the inclusion of certain chemicals that favor their growth and suppress that of other coliforms (i.e., brilliant green, selenite, tetrathionate, lithium, and bile salts). Most strains die at 55°C in 1 hour or at 60°C in 15 to 20 minutes.

The initial separation of *Salmonella* from other bacteria is based on biochemical characteristics. The biochemically positive organisms have antigenic similarity to other *Salmonella* strains, and the antigenic structure confers the species designation. The possession of *Salmonella* antigens does not automatically qualify an organism for inclusion in this group; to qualify as a *Salmonella*, the organism must have the proper antigens and biochemical characteristics.

The typing scheme is based on the antigenic structure, but in recent years the name of the strain has been derived from the city in which it was first isolated (e.g., Montevideo, Heidelberg, Dublin, Newport). Most salmonellae are flagellated; utilizing the proper growth conditions, the H (flagellar) and O (somatic) antigens can be tested separately.

In addition to H and O antigens, some strains, notably typhoid bacilli, have an additional somatic antigen associated with virulence (Vi). The Vi antigen prevents agglutination with O antigen. A positive correlation exists between virulence in mice and the amount of Vi antigen in a specific strain. However, this correlation does not carry over completely to humans, because even typhoid bacilli without measurable Vi antigen can be pathogenic for humans. A bacteriophage typing system against the Vi antigen is used for epidemiologic investigation of typhoid outbreaks. More than 70 anti-Vi phage types have been identified.

For convenience in the laboratory, a series of Kauffmann-White serogroups that contain several serotypes was developed; these serotypes were based on shared antigens among the most common *Salmonella* types. Ninety percent of *Salmonella* pathogenic for humans falls into groups A to E, which contain 40 serotypes. The application of newer molecular methods to the taxonomy of salmonellae has revealed that all serotypes of *Salmonella* belong to one species that includes seven subspecies, which can be differentiated with biochemical tests. To avoid confusion with previous nomenclature, the new species *S. enterica* was proposed.[125] Using this approach, the typhoid bacillus would be named *S. enterica* ssp. *enterica* serotype typhi. However, because this lengthy name is cumbersome, simpler acceptable versions are *S. typhi* or *S. enterica* serotype typhi.

Epidemiology

Salmonella is one of the great food-borne infections.[126] The major route of passage is by "5 Fs": flies, food, fingers, feces, and fomites. The disease can cause large outbreaks, which often are associated with common-source routes of spread. A frequent setting is an institutional supper or barbecue. Community outbreaks may persist for several months. For example, Riverside, California experienced an epidemic involving 16,000 persons that raged for months and was related to a contaminated municipal water supply. The two most common serotypes in the United States are *S. enteritidis* and *S. typhimurium*. Salmonellae are so ubiquitous in our environment that it is extraordinary that so few human infections are encountered.

Attack rates of *Salmonella* show a strong relationship to age. Children younger than 1 year of age have the highest attack rate, especially in the subset of infants 3 to 5 months old. The susceptibility of infants may be related to immunologic immaturity. There is also a high attack rate and increased mortality in elderly persons.

The marked similarity in the frequency of serotypes isolated from human and animal sources suggests that nonhuman reservoirs play a crucial role in the transmission of the disease. By examining common-source outbreaks, the importance of animal reservoirs is easily discerned. In 500 outbreaks investigated over a 10-year period, almost 50% were related to animals or animal products. Poultry, meats, eggs, and dairy products were involved most frequently (Fig. 96–2).

Salmonellae have a tendency to colonize domestic animals. Poultry has the highest incidence of *Salmonella* carriage, particularly hens, chickens, and ducks. Vertical transmission via the transovarian route can occur in chickens, so even normal-appearing eggs can be contaminated with *Salmonella*. Pigs and cattle also are heavily contaminated. Many of these animals can cohabit peacefully with salmonellae and are usually asymptomatic. Other creatures known

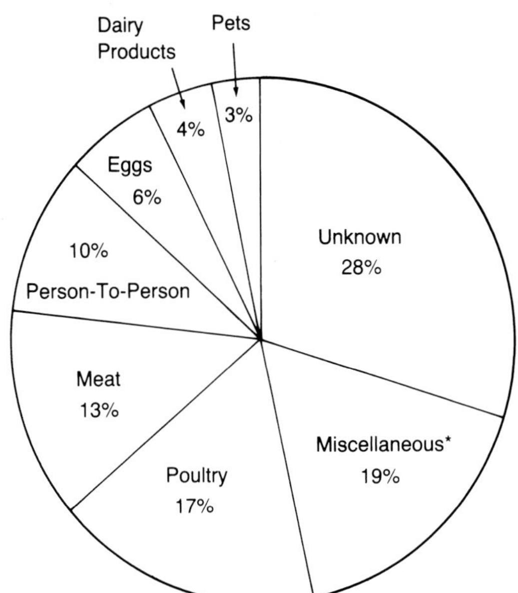

Figure 96–2. Mode of transmission in 500 human salmonellosis outbreaks between 1966 and 1975. (Redrawn from the Centers for Disease Control, Salmonella Surveillance, Annual Summary, 1976. Washington, D.C., U.S. Department of Health, Education and Welfare, Public Health Service, 1977.)

to harbor *Salmonella* include buffalo, sheep, dogs, cats, rats, mice, guinea pigs, hamsters, seals, donkeys, turkeys, doves, pigeons, parrots, sparrows, lizards, whales, tortoises, house flies, ticks, lice, fleas, and cockroaches, to name a few.

Commercially prepared food may be contaminated with salmonellae: 40% of turkeys examined in California, 50% of chickens in Massachusetts, and 20% of commercial egg whites have been shown in surveys to harbor these organisms. Large national and international outbreaks have been traced to commercially prepared chocolate balls, precooked roast beef, smoked whitefish, frozen eggs, ice cream, raw-milk cheese, alfalfa sprouts, cantaloupe, and powdered milk. Other commercial products not directly related to foods, such as carmine dye or brewer's yeast, can be contaminated. Infected pets, especially turtles and lizards, have been implicated in the transmission of salmonellosis.

Salmonella infections have been increasing in incidence in recent years in the United States. During the 1970s, approximately 25,000 cases were reported annually, with an increase to 45,000 cases annually by the mid-1980s. Even these numbers reflect vast under-reporting, and it is estimated that 1.4 million cases of *Salmonella* food poisoning occur each year.[126] A recent pandemic of *S. enteritidis* infections has been noted, particularly in Great Britain and the United States. Eggs and poultry are the major sources of this upsurge.

Pathogenic Mechanisms

Although many serotypes of *Salmonella* are restricted to animals and have narrow host preferences, some strains are less fastidious and can cause serious human infection. *S. typhimurium* causes a spectrum of disease ranging from gastroenteritis to bacteremia. On the other hand, *S. newport* causes septicemia, and *S. typhi*, *S. paratyphi*, *S. schottmülleri*, and *S. hirschfeldii* (the last three known formerly as *S. paratyphi* A, B, and C, respectively) cause enteric (typhoid) fever.

Salmonellae are unique in attacking the ileum and, to a lesser extent, the colon. They cause mild mucosal ulcerations and rapidly make their way through the epithelial surface to the lamina propria and then to the lymphatics and bloodstream. Histologic sections show edematous shortened crypts, invasion of the lamina propria by polymorphonuclear leukocytes, and rapid spread of infection to other organs by hematogenous dissemination.

A series of pathogenic factors, each controlled by plasmids or chromosomal loci, are required for a fully pathogenic *Salmonella* strain. Specific plasmids encode for bacterial spread from Peyer's patches to other sites in the body.[127] Another virulence factor determines the ability of the strain to survive within macrophages after phagocytosis.[128] The outer membrane lipopolysaccharide and the Vi antigen are additional virulence factors. Another recently described virulence factor imparts the ability of salmonellae to elicit transepithelial signaling to neutrophils.[129] Finally, there have been suggestions, as yet not fully substantiated, that *Salmonella* strains produce enterotoxins which play a role in diarrhea.[130]

The infectivity of a specific strain is related to its serotype and the inoculum size. For example, 10^5 *S. newport* produces illness in some volunteers, whereas 10^9 *S. pullorum* is unable to do so. The latter strain is poorly adapted to humans, as suggested by its rarity in clinical infections, but is well adapted to chickens, from which it is frequently isolated. A dose–response curve has been determined for certain strains of *Salmonella*. An approximately 50% infection rate is seen with 10^7 organisms, whereas the infectivity rate rises to 90% at 10^9 organisms.

In experimental animals, the number of bacteria required to produce infections can be reduced by pretreating the animals with antibiotics. Antibiotic exposure in humans also increases susceptibility to *Salmonella* infection.[131] In addition, reduced or absent gastric acid is known to increase the susceptibility to infection, because acid in the stomach kills many of the challenge organisms.[107]

Immunology

Antibody is formed to both somatic and flagella antigens. In experimental animals such antibody production correlates strongly with survival. Titers of the anti-O antibody are the first to rise, reaching a peak in the third week of infection and falling off during subsequent weeks. H antibody titers rise more slowly after several weeks of infection but maintain a high level for many months after infection. The laboratory examination for H and O antibody is called the *Widal test*. These humoral antibodies, although impressively high in titer in some people, do not correlate well with protection against *Salmonella* infection.

Clinical Features

Five clinical syndromes are seen with *Salmonella*[132] (Table 96–6): (1) *gastroenteritis*, noted in 75% of *Salmonella* infections; (2) *bacteremia*, with or without gastrointestinal involvement, seen in approximately 10% of cases; (3) *typhoidal* or *enteric fever*, seen with all typhoid and paratyphi strains and in approximately 8% of other *Salmonella* infections; (4) *localized infections* (e.g., bones, joints, and meninges), seen in approximately 5%; and (5) a carrier state in

Table 96–6 | **Clinical Syndromes of *Salmonella* Infection**

SYNDROME	FREQUENCY (%)
Gastroenteritis	75
Mild	
Dehydrating	
Colitis ("dysenteric")	
Bacteremia	5–10
With or without gastroenteritis	
Endocarditis	
Arteritis	
Acquired immunodeficiency syndrome	
Typhoidal ("enteric fever")	5–10
With or without gastroenteritis	
Localized	5
Meninges	
Bones, joints	
Wounds	
Abscesses	
Gallbladder	
Carrier state (>1 year)	<1

asymptomatic people (the organism is usually harbored in the gallbladder).

The most common syndrome is *gastroenteritis*. The incubation period is usually 6 to 48 hours but can last as long as 7 to 12 days. The initial symptoms are nausea and vomiting, followed by abdominal cramps and diarrhea. The diarrhea usually lasts 3 or 4 days and is accompanied by fever in approximately 50% of persons. In general, the pain of *Salmonella* gastroenteritis is located in the periumbilical area or the right lower quadrant. The diarrhea can vary from a few loose stools to dysentery with grossly bloody and purulent feces to a cholera-like syndrome, which has been described in patients who are achlorhydric.[133] Persistent fever or specific findings on physical examination suggest bacteremia or focal infection. *Salmonella* bacteremia is similar to sepsis caused by other Gram-negative bacteria, although there is an impression that it is less severe. A recurrent form of *Salmonella* bacteremia is seen in patients with the acquired immunodeficiency syndrome (AIDS) (see Chapter 28).[134]

Once the organism invades the bloodstream, almost any organ can become involved. *Meningitis*, *arteritis*, *endocarditis*, *osteomyelitis*, *wound infections*, *septic arthritis*, and *focal abscesses* all have been reported.[132]

Patients become *chronic carriers* (defined as persistence for more than 1 year) of nontyphoidal *Salmonella* as a consequence of either symptomatic or asymptomatic infections. The overall carrier rate is between 2 and 6 per 1000 infected persons. Children, especially neonates, and patients older than 60 years tend to become carriers more frequently than others. Also, structural abnormalities in the biliary tract, such as cholelithiasis, or the urinary tract, such as nephrolithiasis, predispose to and perpetuate the carrier state.[135]

Predisposing Conditions

A number of associated conditions seem to increase the risk of salmonellosis (Table 96–7). The relationship between sickle cell anemia and *Salmonella* osteomyelitis is well known. Indeed, several forms of hemolytic anemia predispose to this infection, including *malaria*, *bartonellosis*, and *louse-borne relapsing fever*. The presumed mechanism of increased susceptibility is blockage of the reticuloendothelial system by macrophages that have ingested breakdown products of red blood cells, thereby reducing their ability to phagocytize salmonellae.[136] Patients with sickle cell anemia also have a decreased capacity to opsonize salmonellae because of defective activation of the alternative complement pathway.[137]

Table 96–7 | **Predisposing Conditions in *Salmonella* Infection**

Hemolytic anemia
Sickle cell anemia
Malaria
Bartonellosis
Malignancy
Lymphoma
Leukemia
Disseminated carcinoma
Immunosuppression
Acquired immunodeficiency syndrome
Glucocorticoid therapy
Chemotherapy
Radiation
Achlorhydria
Gastroduodenal surgery
Idiopathic
Ulcerative colitis
Schistosomiasis

Neoplastic disease has been associated with an increased risk of salmonellosis. *Leukemia*, *lymphomas*, and *disseminated malignancy* appear to predispose patients to bloodstream invasion by this organism.[138] Use of *glucocorticoids*, *chemotherapy*, or *radiotherapy* also is associated with *Salmonella* sepsis (see Chapter 27). In AIDS patients, persistent *Salmonella* bacteremia, only temporarily yielding to antibiotic therapy, is related to the profound suppression of cell-mediated immunity (see Chapter 28).[134] *Gastric surgery* appears to be an important predisposing condition in the development of *Salmonella* infection. The obvious implication is that destruction of the gastric acid barrier enhances the host's susceptibility to infection.

All three forms of *schistosomiasis* have been associated with invasive salmonellosis.[139] Salmonellae, as well as other Gram-negative bacteria, are capable of penetrating and multiplying within the parasites, which then serve as a source for recurrent bacteremia or bacilluria.

Ulcerative colitis may predispose to *Salmonella* infection and the carrier state, although this implication is based on only a few retrospective studies. One such analysis found that 5% of patients with idiopathic ulcerative colitis harbored *Salmonella* in their stools.[140]

Salmonella *Colitis*

Involvement of the colon in the course of *Salmonella* gastroenteritis probably is common, at least on the basis of animal studies and sigmoidoscopic examinations in selected patients.[141] Although most patients with *Salmonella* present with mild diarrhea and watery bowel movements, in a small but important group, colonic involvement dominates the clinical picture. Indeed, toxic megacolon and perforation due to *Salmonella* can develop in an occasional patient.[142] Patients with *Salmonella* colitis typically have diarrhea for 10 to 15 days before the diagnosis is established. In contrast, patients with the usual form of gastroenteritis are symptomatic for 5 days or less. In the colonic form, diarrhea is more persistent, even though the organism may have disappeared from the feces. Bowel movements are grossly bloody in approximately one half of the patients. Sigmoidoscopic findings include hyperemia, granularity, friability, and ulcerations. Rectal biopsy specimens reveal mucosal ulcerations, hemorrhage, and crypt abscesses. Barium enema films confirm these findings and usually show a patchy global colitis. In the acute period, there is no reliable method to distinguish idiopathic ulcerative colitis from *Salmonella* colitis, except by a positive stool culture. Any patient with an acute onset of colitis and no past history of colitis and with a duration of symptoms of 3 weeks or less should be considered to have infectious colitis, and *Salmonella*, as well as EHEC, *Shigella*, *Campylobacter*, and *C. difficile*, are important diagnostic considerations.

The course of *Salmonella* colitis is variable and can be as short as 1 week or as long as 2 to 3 months. The average duration of illness is 3 weeks. Complications include toxic megacolon, bleeding, and overwhelming sepsis.

It is important to recognize *Salmonella* colitis, so that inappropriate therapy is not administered. Glucocorticoids can exacerbate *Salmonella* colitis and result in silent perforation and septicemia. Finally, patients can be reassured of the self-limited course of *Salmonella* colitis as opposed to the chronic relapsing course of idiopathic ulcerative colitis.

Treatment

Although many antibiotics have been used to treat nontyphoidal *Salmonella* gastroenteritis, all have failed to alter the rate of clinical recovery. In fact, antibiotic therapy increases the frequency and duration of intestinal carriage of these organisms. In one report,[143] 185 patients with *S. typhimurium* gastroenteritis were treated with either chloramphenicol or ampicillin; stools from 65.4% were still positive for the organism 12 days after exposure, and 27% were positive at 31 days. In contrast, among 87 patients who were not treated, only 42.5% and 11.5% of stool cultures were positive at 12 and 31 days, respectively. *Salmonella* strains resistant to one or more antibiotics were isolated from 9.7% of patients treated with antibiotics, whereas no resistant strains were obtained from untreated patients. A review of 12 randomized trials found no differences in the duration of illness, diarrhea, or fever between patients treated with antibiotics and those treated with placebo.[144] Relapses were more common in those treated with antimicrobial agents, as were adverse drug reactions. It is thus apparent that antimicrobial therapy should not be used in most cases of *Salmonella* gastroenteritis.

Despite this general rule, antibiotics should be used when *Salmonella* gastroenteritis complicates certain conditions (Table 96–8): *lymphoproliferative disorders*; *malignant disease*; *immunosuppressed states* (AIDS and congenital or acquired forms); *transplantation*; known or suspected *abnormalities of the cardiovascular system* such as prosthetic heart valves, vascular grafts, aneurysms, and rheumatic or congenital valvular heart disease; *foreign bodies implanted* in the skeletal system; *hemolytic anemias*; and the *extreme ages* of life. In addition, patients with *Salmonella* gastroenteritis should be treated with antibiotics when they exhibit findings of *severe sepsis*—that is, high fever, rigors, hypotension, decreased renal function, and systemic toxicity.

If a decision is made to initiate therapy in these selected patients, the choice of drug may be problematic because of high levels of antibiotic resistance to ampicillin or TMP-SMX. For patients with sensitive strains, ampicillin or TMP-SMX can be used (see Table 96–4).

The quinolones, particularly ciprofloxacin, which has been studied most intensely, are highly active in vitro and have shown good results in patients with enteric fever[145] and in chronic carriers.[146] However, ciprofloxacin therapy in patients with uncomplicated *Salmonella* gastroenteritis has led to an unacceptably high relapse rate that is associated with more prolonged fecal excretion of salmonellae than seen in placebo-treated control subjects.[147] As might be expected, resistance to ciprofloxacin has been observed during therapy.[148]

During the past decade there has been an increase in the isolation of quinolone-resistant *Salmonella* isolates in Europe, especially from cattle.[149] The use of quinolones for veterinary use has been blamed for this rise in resistance. The strain of *S. typhimurium* known as definitive phage type 104 (DT104) is often multidrug resistant, but until recently, this strain has remained susceptible to the quinolones. In 1998, a community outbreak of salmonellosis in Denmark that appeared to arise from a Danish swine herd was caused by a strain of DT104 that was resistant to nalidixic-acid and showed decreased susceptibility to fluoroquinolones in vitro.[150] The epidemiologic investigation of this outbreak suggested that the clinical effectiveness of the quinolones was decreased in the treatment of these *Salmonella* infections. Resistance to ceftriaxone of a *Salmonella* strain from livestock also has been observed recently in the United States.[151] As a consequence of the increasing levels of drug resistance, both domestically and internationally, antimicrobial therapy of *Salmonella* infections must be limited to high-risk patients and should be based on sensitivity testing.

Table 96–8 | **Indications for Therapy in *Salmonella* Gastroenteritis**

Lymphoproliferative disorders
Leukemia
Lymphoma
Malignant disease
Immunosuppression
Acquired immunodeficiency syndrome
Congenital and other acquired forms
Glucocorticoids
Transplant patients
Abnormal cardiovascular system
Prosthetic heart valves
Vascular grafts
Aneurysms
Valvular heart disease
Prosthetic orthopedic devices
Hemolytic anemia
Extreme ages of life
Severe sepsis, toxicity

Typhoid Fever

Typhoid ("cloudy") fever is a febrile illness of prolonged duration, marked by hectic fever, delirium, persistent bloodstream infection, enlargement of the spleen, abdominal pain, and a variety of systemic manifestations. The illness caused by this pathogen differs from the nontyphoidal *Salmonella* infections in several respects. Typhoidal disease is not truly an intestinal disease and has more systemic than intestinal symptoms; it clearly differs from the usual form of gastroenteritis produced by nontyphoidal strains of *Salmonella. S. typhi* is remarkably adapted to humans, who represent the only natural reservoir; the other salmonellae are associated by and large with animals.

Although *S. typhi* is the main cause of typhoid fever, other *Salmonella* serotypes occasionally produce a similar clinical picture, known variously as typhoidal disease, enteric fever, or paratyphoid fever. These serotypes are *S.*

paratyphi, *S. schottmülleri* (formerly *S. paratyphi B*), and *S. hirschfeldii* (formerly *S. paratyphi C*), as well as others such as *S. typhimurium*.

Microbiology

S. typhi is biochemically similar to other salmonellae and is distinguished primarily by its specific antigens. As a rule, this organism produces little or no gas from carbohydrates, elaborates only small amounts of hydrogen sulfide, and bears the Vi antigen on its surface. These markers should alert the laboratory to the possibility of this pathogen; confirmation of *S. typhi* is accomplished by serotyping.

Pathogenic Mechanisms

The pathologic events of typhoid fever are initiated in the intestinal tract after oral ingestion of typhoid bacilli.[152] The organism spares the stomach, penetrates the small bowel mucosa, and makes its way rapidly to the lymphatics, the mesenteric nodes, and, within minutes, the bloodstream. There is a paucity of local inflammatory findings, which explains the lack of intestinal symptoms at this stage. This sequence of events is in marked contrast to that of other forms of salmonellosis and shigellosis, in which intestinal findings are prominent at the onset.

After the initial bacteremia, the organism is sequestered in macrophages and monocytic cells of the reticuloendothelial system. It undergoes multiplication and re-emerges several days later in recurrent waves of bacteremia, an event that initiates the symptomatic phase of infection. Now in great numbers, the organism is spread throughout the host and infects many organ sites. The intestinal tract may be seeded by direct bacteremic spread to Peyer's patches in the terminal ileum or via drainage of contaminated bile from the gallbladder, which often harbors large numbers of organisms.

Hyperplasia of the reticuloendothelial system, including lymph nodes, liver, and spleen, is characteristic of typhoid fever. The liver contains discrete micronodular areas of necrosis surrounded by macrophages and lymphocytes. Inflammation of the gallbladder is common and may lead to acute cholecystitis. Patients with preexisting gallbladder disease have a penchant for becoming carriers, because the bacillus becomes intimately associated with the chronic infection and may be incorporated within gallstones. Lymphoid follicles in the gut, such as Peyer's patches, become hyperplastic, with infiltration of macrophages, lymphocytes, and red blood cells. Subsequently, a follicle may ulcerate, penetrate through the submucosa to the intestinal lumen, and discharge large numbers of typhoid bacilli in its wake. As the bowel wall is progressively involved, it becomes paper thin, most commonly in the terminal ileum, and is susceptible to transmural perforation into the peritoneal cavity. Erosion into blood vessels produces severe intestinal hemorrhage.

An analogy has been drawn between the biologic effects of endotoxin and typhoid fever.[152] Both cause chills, fever, headache, nausea, and vomiting, as well as leukopenia and thrombocytopenia. With endotoxin, however, increasing doses produce a state of tolerance in which further administration has no effect. By contrast, typhoid fever is a relentless and sustained state of febrile illness. Administration of viable typhoid organisms to volunteers rendered tolerant to endotoxin still produce symptoms. Thus, typhoid fever cannot be explained merely as a reaction to endotoxin, although endotoxin may play some role in the disease state.

Epidemiology

Improvements in environmental sanitation have reduced the incidence of typhoid fever in industrialized nations. Approximately 400 to 500 cases occur each year in the United States, chiefly in young people. Large-scale epidemics of typhoid occur on a regular basis in developing countries; they are usually traced to contaminated food that is imported from an endemic area or to contaminated water supplies.[153]

Because *S. typhi* cohabits exclusively with humans, the appearance of a case could indicate the presence of a carrier. An investigation by public health authorities should be instituted to determine the source and the presence of other cases. As they are discovered, chronic carriers are registered with the health authorities, and the microorganism is phage typed so that it can be traced in the event of an outbreak. However, the registered carriers represent only some of the potential reservoir and do not take into account imported cases of typhoid, which represent more than 70% of the acute infections in the United States.[154]

Clinical Features

In its classic form without treatment, typhoid fever lasts about 4 weeks and evolves in a manner consistent with the pathologic events. The illness is described traditionally as a series of 1-week stages, although this pattern may be altered in mild cases and by antibiotic treatment.[155] The *incubation period* is generally 7 to 14 days, with wide variations at either extreme. During the *first week,* high fever, headache, and abdominal pain are common. The pulse is often slower than would be expected for the degree of fever. Abdominal pain is localized to the right lower quadrant in most cases but can be diffuse. In approximately 50% of patients, there is no change in bowel habits; in fact, constipation is more common than diarrhea in children with typhoid fever. Near the end of the first week, enlargement of the spleen is noticeable, and an evanescent classic rash, "rose spots," becomes manifest, most commonly on the chest.

During the *second week,* the fever becomes more continuous, and the patient looks sick and withdrawn. During the *third week,* the patient's illness evolves into the "typhoidal state," with disordered mentation and, in some cases, extreme toxemia. In this period there is often intestinal involvement, manifested clinically by greenish "pea-soup" diarrhea and the dire complications of intestinal perforation and hemorrhage. The *fourth week* brings slackening of the fever and improvement in the clinical status.

Typhoid fever is a less severe illness in previously healthy adults who seek medical attention for the earliest symptoms of fever, lassitude, and headache than in those who wait. Prompt diagnosis and appropriate therapy interrupt the classic 4-week scenario and produce an aborted illness consisting of little more than a few days of fever and malaise.

Because the typhoid bacillus is widely disseminated through recurrent waves of bacteremia, many organ sites are involved. Patients with typhoid fever can have *pneumonia*, *pyelonephritis*, and *metastases* to *bone*, *large joints*, and the *brain*. The gallbladder and liver are involved with inflammatory changes. Acute cholecystitis can occur during the initial 2 to 3 weeks, and jaundice, resulting from diffuse hepatic inflammation, has been observed in some patients.

The preeminent complications are *intestinal hemorrhage* and *perforation*.[156] These events are most likely to occur in the third week and during convalescence and are not related to the severity of the disease. However, they tend to occur in the same patient, with bleeding serving as a harbinger of possible perforation. Bleeding may be sudden and severe or a slow ooze. Before the availability of antibiotics, the frequency of hemorrhage was 20% in various series; it is less frequent since specific treatment has been available. Approximately 3% of patients with typhoid fever experience intestinal perforation, which commonly occurs in the ileum.[157] The onset may be sudden, with signs of an acute abdomen, or there may be a leak of intraluminal contents to form an abscess in the lower quadrant or pelvis, producing a more chronic insidious course.

After defervescence has occurred and the patient has apparently "ridden through the storm," a potential for recurrence remains. The relapse generally occurs 8 to 10 days after cessation of drug therapy and consists of a reenactment of the major manifestations. The organism is the same as the one that caused the original infection, with the identical antimicrobial susceptibility pattern.

Carriers

After 6 weeks, approximately 50% of typhoid victims are still shedding the organism in their feces. This figure declines progressively, and after 3 months only 5% to 10% are excreters; by 1 year the frequency is 1% to 3%.[158] The chronic carrier is identified by positive stool cultures for *S. typhi* at least 1 year after the acute episode or, in some cases, positive stool cultures without a documented history of disease. The probability of spontaneously aborting the carrier state is highly unlikely after this time. Chronic carriers are more common in older age groups, women (a 3:1 ratio of women to men), and persons with biliary disease. The organism is usually harbored in the gallbladder, although occasionally it is carried in the large intestine without involvement of the biliary tract.

Diagnosis

The diagnosis of typhoid fever is established by isolating the organism. Blood culture is the primary diagnostic test and is positive in 90% of patients during the first week and remains positive for several weeks thereafter if the patient is untreated. Bone marrow culture also has a high yield, even in treated patients.[159] Stool cultures become positive in the second and third weeks. Sampling duodenal contents by a "string test" yields a positive culture in 70% of patients. By the third week, urine cultures reveal the organism in approximately 25% of patients. The titer of agglutinins against somatic (O) antigen (Widal test) rises during the second and third week of illness. An O titer of 1:80 or more in a nonimmunized person is suggestive of typhoid fever, and a titer of 1:320 is usually diagnostic in the appropriate clinical setting. A fourfold rise in titer provides stronger evidence. Although the H antigen is less specific than an O titer and is likely to be elevated from prior immunization or by infection with other enteric bacteria, an initial H antigen titer of 1:640 is strongly suggestive of typhoid fever. There are many false-positive and occasional false-negative Widal reactions, so that a diagnosis based on a rise in titer alone is tenuous. Serologic tests have become available and permit rapid diagnosis of typhoid fever with a higher sensitivity and specificity relative to blood culture than the Widal test.[140] Polymerase chain reaction assays for the diagnosis of *S. typhi* have been developed, but these are still research tools.

Treatment

Drug resistance, mediated by plasmids, occurs among typhoid bacilli. Most strains are susceptible to chloramphenicol and ampicillin, although notable epidemics with strains resistant to either or both of these drugs have been reported in recent years. Hence, a great effort should be made in each case to isolate the organism and perform drug susceptibility tests. Chloramphenicol has high activity against most clinical isolates of typhoid bacilli. The response to therapy is remarkably constant, and defervescence regularly occurs 3 to 5 days after treatment is begun.[156] The clinical condition improves within 1 to 2 days, with decreased toxemia and slowly declining fever. In adults, chloramphenicol should be given in a total daily dose of 2 g, administered in four equally divided doses by mouth. Occasionally, in very sick patients it may be necessary to give the drug by the intravenous route in the same total daily dose. Oral medication can be given after improvement in the clinical status. Chloramphenicol is well absorbed from the intestinal tract but is rather poorly absorbed from intramuscular sites. Thus, the intramuscular route is to be avoided. The duration of treatment is 2 weeks; prolongation of this treatment does not reduce the frequency of complications or carriers. Intestinal perforation and hemorrhage can occur during apparently successful treatment. Relapse may follow an otherwise uneventful course and should be treated with the same drug.

Ampicillin has been recommended as alternative therapy but has been disappointing in comparison with chloramphenicol.[155, 161] The dose is 6 g/day intravenously in four to six divided doses. Amoxicillin, a closely related drug, provides better absorption and increased efficacy. Several studies have shown that amoxicillin, in doses of 4 g/day in four divided doses, has good activity. TMP-SMX also has been used in the therapy of typhoid fever with good results.

The advent of plasmid-mediated multidrug resistance and newer potentially more effective antimicrobial agents, such as the quinolones and third-generation cephalosporins, has led to a reevaluation of the treatment of typhoid fever. The fluoroquinolones, ciprofloxacin and ofloxacin, have been found to be highly effective therapy for infections caused by multidrug-resistant *S. typhi* and *paratyphi*. Long-term fecal carriage of *S. typhi* is a rare event in patients treated with quinolones. A 10- to 14-day course of a quinolone has proved highly effective for the treatment of enteric fever, with cure rates consistently close to 100%.[23] The only exception has been norfloxacin, which has provided slightly lower cure rates of 83% to 90%.[23] Defervescence generally occurs within 3 to 5 days of initiating therapy. When treatment of enteric fever with a quinolone was compared with chloramphenicol, TMP-SMX, or azithromycin, no significant difference in clinical or microbiologic efficacy was found.

The optimal length of fluoroquinolone therapy for typhoid fever has not been fully elucidated. A number of studies have shown that courses of therapy ranging from 7 to 14 days provide a high degree of success. However, courses of therapy shorter than 5 to 6 days have been associated with unacceptable levels of failure.[23] The duration of fever before treatment, severity of infection at the time of presentation, and time to defervescence are factors that must be considered when determining the duration of fluoroquinolone therapy in a patient with enteric fever.

Certain caveats should be made regarding the fluoroquinolones. The frequency of resistance of *S. typhi* to ciprofloxacin has been increasing gradually, especially in the Indian subcontinent, central Asia, and Vietnam.[153, 162, 163] Although in a study conducted in India no isolates of *S. typhi* or *S. paratyphi* had a mean inhibitory concentration for ciprofloxacin of 0.25 μg/mL or greater in 1991, from 1998 to 1999 60% of the isolates tested had a mean inhibitory concentration of 2 μg/mL or greater.[162] In association with the rise in nalidixic acid resistance and decreased in vitro susceptibility to ciprofloxacin, clinicians in India and Vietnam have observed a longer time to defervescence and an increase in the number of patients who require treatment in recent years.[162, 163]

Third-generation cephalosporins such as cefotaxime, ceftriaxone, and cefoperazone also have been used successfully to treat typhoid fever; courses as short as 3 days have been shown to be as effective as the usual 10- to 14-day regimens.[164, 165] On the other hand, a recent trial that compared a 5-day course of ofloxacin to a 7-day course of cefixime found that the median fever clearance time was significantly longer and the rate of treatment failure was higher in children treated with cefixime.[166]

Glucocorticoids are administered for severe toxemia and fever and may produce a dramatic response in patients with profound sepsis.[167] The treatment should be given in high doses, 60 mg/day of prednisone divided into four doses, and tapered rapidly over the next 3 days. The wide experience with glucocorticoid treatment has failed to show any adverse effects, although the potential for masking intestinal perforation is always present. Glucocorticoids should be reserved for patients with severe toxicity.

Recent studies have emphasized the importance of aggressive surgical intervention in typhoid fever.[157, 168, 169] Indications for surgery are progressive peritoneal signs or localization of an abscess. Double-layer closure of the perforation coupled with broad-spectrum antibiotics have resulted in reduced mortality from this dreaded complication.[169] However, the ileum may be riddled with multiple perforations, and resection or exteriorization of an intestinal loop may be required.

Good nursing care plays a major role in the recovery from typhoid fever. The pyrexia can be managed with tepid baths and sponging. Salicylates and antipyretics should be avoided, because they cause severe sweating and lower the blood pressure.

A chronic carrier who has been discharging *S. typhi* for longer than 1 year can be treated with antimicrobials in an attempt to eliminate the infection. The quinolone antibiotics, such as ciprofloxacin and norfloxacin, have become the treatment of choice in eradicating the carrier state.[170] Reappearance of the carrier state after such treatment is generally associated with gallbladder disease. Cholecystectomy eliminates the carrier state in 85% of carriers with gallstones or chronic cholecystitis but is recommended only for persons whose profession is incompatible with the typhoid carrier state, such as food handlers and health care providers.

Vaccines

Three types of typhoid vaccine are currently available in the United States. An acetone-inactivated vaccine affords 55% to 85% protection for 2 to 5 years. This relative immunity can be overcome by a large inoculum of bacilli. Local pain at the injection site and mild systemic reactions are common with this vaccine. A slightly less effective phenol-inactivated vaccine is available in the United States, whereas the acetone-inactivated vaccine is not. A live attenuated *S. typhi* strain, Ty21a, which is given by mouth, produced 96% protection in an initial field trial in Alexandria,[171] but subsequent studies showed less impressive results.[172, 173] Although the evidence is inconclusive, it appears that the live attenuated oral vaccine is protective. Because of its low toxicity and ease of administration, this vaccine should be used for travelers to high-risk areas particularly in the developing world, although the protective efficacy of the oral vaccine has not yet been established in travelers. The third typhoid vaccine consists of purified Vi capsular polysaccharide and has demonstrated 75% efficacy in a large trial in Nepal.[174] This vaccine has fewer adverse effects than the killed whole cell parenteral vaccines, but its efficacy has not been established in travelers.

Campylobacter

The most important *Campylobacter* species found in human infections are *C. jejuni*, a major cause of diarrhea; *C. fetus*, which is generally found in immunocompromised patients; *C. coli*, a rare cause of gastroenteritis; and two new species, *C. cinaedi* and *C. fennelliae*, which are found in male homosexuals. Other species cause diarrhea on rare occasions: *C. hyointestinalis*, *C. upsaliensis*, and *C. laridis*.

The incidence and importance of human *Campylobacter* gastroenteritis have been recognized increasingly. It is estimated that 4% to 11% of all cases of diarrhea in the United States are caused by *C. jejuni*, and the isolation of *Campylobacter* often exceeds that of *Salmonella* and *Shigella*.[175]

The organism is isolated only rarely from fecal samples of asymptomatic persons, except in the tropics, where the

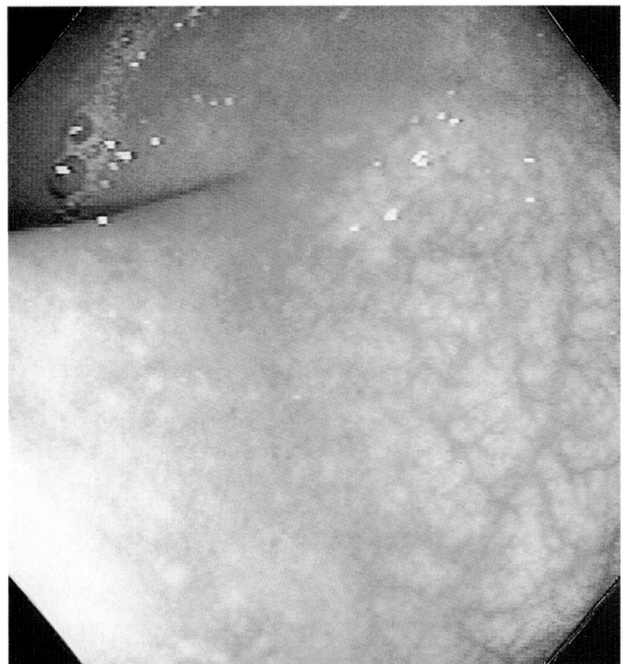

Figure 96–3. *Campylobacter* colitis. The colitis is patchy, with areas of erythema and erosion (*left*). The rectal mucosa on the right is hyperemic, without loss of the mucosal vascular pattern. *Campylobacter jejuni* was identified on stool culture. (From Wilcox CM: Atlas of Clinical Gastrointestinal Endoscopy. Philadelphia, WB Saunders, 1995, p 215.)

incidence of *Campylobacter* infections is higher and there are many asymptomatic carriers.

Epidemiology

Transmission appears to occur most commonly from infected animals and their food products to humans. The reservoir for *Campylobacter* is enormous, because many animals can be infected: cattle, sheep, swine, birds, including poultry, and dogs. Furthermore, the organism has been isolated from fresh and salt water. Most human infections are related to consumption of improperly cooked or contaminated foodstuffs. As for *Salmonella*, chickens seem to be the major source, accounting for 50% to 70% of infections in some surveys.[176]

Clinical Features

The incubation period is 24 to 72 hours after organisms are ingested but can extend as long as 10 days. There is a wide spectrum of clinical illness, from frank dysentery to watery diarrhea to asymptomatic excretion.[177] Diarrhea and fever are almost invariable (90%). Abdominal pain is usually present (70%), and the patient may note bloody stools (50%). Constitutional symptoms such as headache, myalgia, backache, malaise, anorexia, and vomiting are frequent. The duration of illness usually is less than 1 week, although symptoms can persist for 2 weeks or more, and relapses occur in as many as 25% of patients. Prolonged carriage of *Campylobacter* for 2 to 10 weeks after the onset of illness occurs in 16% of patients.[178]

Infections rarely may be complicated by gastrointestinal hemorrhage, toxic megacolon, pancreatitis, cholecystitis, HUS, bacteremia, meningitis, and purulent arthritis.[177] Postinfectious complications include reactive arthritis, usually in patients with the human leukocyte antigen B27 phenotype, and Guillain-Barré syndrome.[177, 179]

Diagnosis

Stool examination confirms colitis on the basis of fecal leukocytes on methylene blue staining and occult blood.[177] Endoscopy may reveal an inflammatory colitis (Fig. 96–3). Although certain clinical features suggest the diagnosis of *Campylobacter* rather than other pathogens, the diagnosis can only be established by culture. Features suggestive of *Campylobacter* infection are (1) a prodrome consisting of constitutional symptoms with coryza, headache, and generalized malaise; (2) a prolonged, often biphasic diarrheal illness presenting initially with diarrhea, followed by slight improvement and then by increasing severity; and (3) many white and red blood cells on microscopic examination of the stool (Fig. 96–4).

The most reliable way to diagnose *Campylobacter* gastroenteritis is by stool culture. A selective isolation medium containing antibiotics must be used because campylobacters grow more slowly than other enteric bacteria; the plates are grown at 42°C under CO_2 and reduced oxygen conditions. Dark-field or phase-contrast microscopy of fresh diarrheal stool shows the organism as a curved highly motile rod, with darting corkscrew movements.

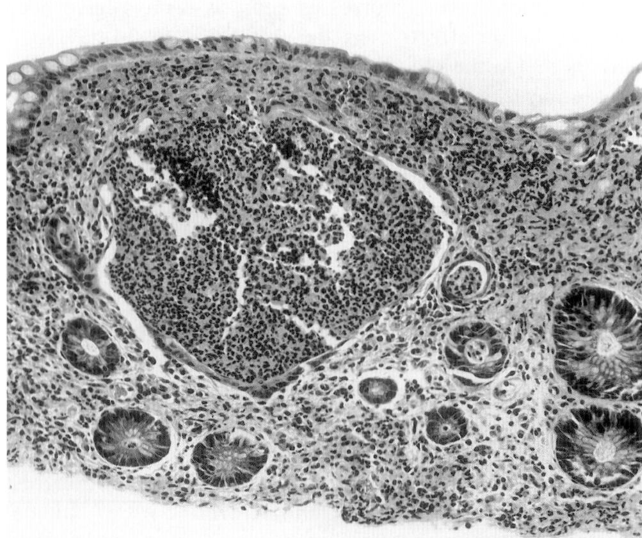

Figure 96–4. Colonic biopsy specimen showing histologic features of acute infectious colitis caused by *Campylobacter jejuni* with acute and chronic inflammation of the lamina propria and a large crypt abscess, but no distortion of the crypt architecture. (Hematoxylin-eosin, low power. Courtesy of Edward Lee, MD, Dallas VA Medical Center, Dallas, TX.)

Treatment

Although *C. jejuni* is sensitive to erythromycin in vitro, three controlled therapeutic trials with this drug have shown no effect on the clinical course when compared with placebo.[180] One study showed some clinical benefit when the antibiotic was started within 3 days of the onset of symptoms. A delay in therapy beyond 4 days produces no clinical improvement. However, fecal excretion of the organism is reduced by erythromycin (see Table 96–4). The fluoroquinolone antibiotics, such as ciprofloxacin, are also active against these organisms, and clinical trials have shown encouraging results.[181] Resistance to fluoroquinolones has been observed during the course of treatment for *Campylobacter* diarrhea.[182, 183] The penicillins, cephalosporins, and sulfonamides have little effect on *Campylobacter*.

Resistance to the fluoroquinolones is a major problem in some parts of the developing world. In Thailand, a study of United States military personnel found that 50% of isolates were resistant to ciprofloxacin, whereas none were resistant to azithromycin.[184] A large study of human *Campylobacter* isolates in Minnesota found a rise in quinolone resistance from 1.3% to 10.2% between 1992 and 1998.[185] Factors associated with resistance of *Campylobacter* species to the quinolones include foreign travel and local patterns of fluoroquinolone use, especially if these agents are used in animal husbandry.[185, 186] In locales where quinolone resistance is common, azithromycin has been shown to be superior to ciprofloxacin in decreasing the excretion of *Campylobacter* species and equivalent in terms of reducing the duration of symptoms.[184]

Mild cases of *Campylobacter* do not benefit from antibiotic therapy, but treatment should be given, early if possible, to patients with dysentery and those with high fever suggestive of bacteremia. Because of the difficulty in making an etiologic diagnosis on clinical grounds, a quinolone antibiotic should be used empirically because it would be active against *Campylobacter*, *Shigella*, and other enteric pathogens.

Yersinia

Yersinia enterocolitica is an important intestinal pathogen that causes a spectrum of clinical illnesses from simple gastroenteritis to invasive ileitis and colitis.[187] It is a nonlactose-fermenting, urease-positive, Gram-negative rod. More than 50 serogroups and 5 biotypes have been identified.[187] The pathogenic mechanisms include the ability to invade epithelial cells and the production of a heat-stable enterotoxin, which is elaborated at 25°C but not at 37°C. Not all strains have these pathogenic properties.

The organism targets for invasion the epithelium overlying Peyer's patches, after which it proliferates within the follicles and spreads to the lamina propria. The ability to attach to and penetrate epithelial cells is determined by the *inv* gene, which encodes a 103-kDa protein known as *invasin*.[188]

Epidemiology

Yersinia gastroenteritis has been reported more frequently in Scandinavian and other European countries than in the United States. Several epidemics have been related to the consumption of contaminated milk and ice cream. The organism can be found in stream and lake water and has been isolated from many animals, including puppies, cats, cows, pigs, chickens, and horses. Animals, either as pets or food sources, are believed to be involved in the transmission of this disease.[189]

The serotypes most frequently involved in Scandinavia and Europe are 03 and 09, and Canada has many serotype 03 isolates.[190] Most of the isolates in the United States are serotype 08. Serogroups O:8 and O:5,27 have been responsible for most episodes of invasive disease in the United States.

Clinical Features

Several clinical syndromes have been described with *Yersinia* and tend to vary with the age of the patient and the underlying disease state.[187, 191] Enterocolitis is the most common clinical condition, accounting for two thirds of all reported cases. This illness occurs most frequently in children younger than 5 years.[188, 191] The presentation is nonspecific, with fever, abdominal cramps, and diarrhea, usually lasting 1 to 3 weeks. Microscopic examination of the fecal effluent reveals leukocytes and red blood cells in most instances. Profuse watery diarrhea, possibly related to the enterotoxin, also can occur. The diarrheal condition can persist for several weeks and may raise the possibility of inflammatory bowel disease. Radiographic findings, particularly in prolonged cases, are most intense in the terminal ileum and may resemble Crohn's disease.[192] However, most patients have normal findings on endoscopy, intestinal biopsy, and barium x-ray studies.[190]

In children over age 5 years, mesenteric adenitis and associated ileitis have been described. Accompanying symptoms include nausea, vomiting, and aphthous ulcers in the mouth. Affected children often undergo a laparotomy, at which time enlarged mesenteric nodes and an ulcerated ileitis are observed. The condition may be confused clinically with acute appendicitis, although ultrasonography can be useful in separating these processes.[193] *Yersinia* is less likely to cause severe disease in adults, in whom acute diarrhea may be followed 2 to 3 weeks later by joint symptoms and rash (erythema nodosum or erythema multiforme), reminiscent of Reiter's syndrome. Reactive polyarthritis occurs in 2% of patients with yersiniosis, usually in persons positive for human leukocyte antigen B27. *Yersinia* antigens can be detected in synovial fluid cells[194] and in intestinal mucosal biopsies, and specific IgA antibodies are found in the blood.[195]

Yersinia bacteremia is a relatively uncommon condition that is seen in patients with underlying diseases such as malignancy, diabetes mellitus, anemia, and liver disease. Metastatic foci can occur in bones, joints, and lungs.

The diagnosis of yersiniosis is established by culture of stool or body fluids. Because the organism is easily missed on the culture plate, the laboratory should be advised of the suspicion of this infection. Serologic tests have proved useful in Europe and Canada[196] but have not provided much help for the cases reported in the United States.[197]

Treatment

Y. enterocolitica strains are susceptible to several antimicrobial agents, including chloramphenicol, gentamicin, tetracycline, TMP-SMX, and fluoroquinolones, but they are resistant to penicillins and cephalosporins. There is no substantial evidence that antibiotics alter the course of the gastrointestinal infection[187, 197]; indeed, the diagnosis often is established late in the course when the patient is improving spontaneously. However, antibiotics should be used in more severe intestinal infections, particularly those masquerading as appendicitis. For the chronic relapsing form of diarrhea, antibiotic therapy has not proved useful. Septicemia in the immunocompromised patient is associated with a high mortality, with no apparent benefit from antibiotics, although treatment is mandatory in this setting.

VIRAL DIARRHEA

The major causes of gastroenteritis in the United States and in the rest of the world are viruses, which account for 30% to 40% of acute episodes of diarrhea. The leading human pathogens can be grouped into five categories: rotavirus, enteric adenovirus, calicivirus including Norwalk virus, astrovirus, and torovirus (Table 96–9).[198]

Rotavirus

This group of viruses was discovered in 1973, in studies of Australian children with diarrhea in which the viral particles were visualized in duodenal biopsy specimens by electron microscopy. Rotavirus infection is now recognized to be cosmopolitan in distribution, occurring in virtually every part of the world where it has been studied.

Microbiology

The virus measures 70 to 75 nm in diameter and contains a double-walled outer capsid and segmented double-stranded RNA with specific gene functions. The virus has an icosahedral structure resembling the spokes of a wheel, hence the name "rota." Highly stable to heat, ether, and mild acids, the virus can be maintained in prolonged storage; indeed, an

Table 96–9 | **Medical Importance, Clinical and Epidemiologic Characteristics, and Diagnosis of Human Gastroenteritis Viruses**

VIRUS	MEDICAL IMPORTANCE DEMONSTRATED	EPIDEMIOLOGIC CHARACTERISTICS	CLINICAL CHARACTERISTICS	LABORATORY DIAGNOSTIC TESTS*
Rotavirus				
Group A	Yes	Major cause of endemic severe diarrhea in infants and young children worldwide (in winter in temperate zone)	Dehydrating diarrhea for 5–7 days; vomiting and fever very common	Immunoassay, electron microscopy, PAGE
Group B	Partially	Large outbreaks in adults and children in China	Severe watery diarrhea for 3–5 days	Electron microscopy, PAGE
Group C	Partially	Sporadic cases in young children worldwide	Similar to characteristics of group A rotavirus	Electron microscopy, PAGE
Calicivirus	Yes	Usually pediatric diarrhea; associated with shellfish and other food in adults	Rotavirus-like illness in children; Norwalk-like in adults	Immunoassay, electron microscopy
Norwalk virus	Yes	Epidemics of vomiting and diarrhea in older children and adults; occurs in families, communities, and nursing homes; often associated with shellfish, other food, or water	Acute vomiting, diarrhea, fever, myalgia, and headache lasting 1–2 days	Immunoassay, immune electron microscopy
Norwalk-like viruses (small, round structured viruses)	Partially	Similar to characteristics of Norwalk virus	Acute vomiting, diarrhea, fever, myalgia, and headache lasting 1–2 days	Immunoassay, immune electron microscopy
Enteric adenovirus	Yes	Endemic diarrhea of infants and young children	Prolonged diarrhea lasting 5–12 days; vomiting and fever	Immunoassay, electron microscopy with PAGE
Astrovirus	Yes	Pediatric diarrhea; reported in nursing homes	Watery diarrhea, often lasting 2–3 days, occasionally longer	Immunoassay, electron microscopy
Torovirus	Yes	Pediatric diarrhea; acute and persistent; increased in immunocompromised children; occurs in community and hospital settings	Dehydrating, watery, occasionally bloody diarrhea with vomiting and abdominal pain; usually lasts 5–7 days	Immunoassay, electron microscopy

*Laboratory diagnostic tests, other than those for rotavirus group A, are usually available only in specialized research or diagnostic referral laboratories. Immunoassays are usually enzyme-linked immunosorbent assays or radioimmunoassays.

PAGE, polyacrylamide-gel electrophoresis and silver staining of viral nucleic acid in stool.

Modified from Blacklow NR, Greenberg HB. Viral gastroenteritis. N Engl J Med 325:252, 1991, with permission.

unknown viral agent isolated by Hodes in 1943 from an infection in infants was maintained in a freezer until 1977, when it was shown by electron microscopy to contain rotavirus particles.

Three groups of rotavirus, A, B, and C, cause disease in humans. Group A rotavirus contains four common serotypes, which are the leading pathogens and cause severe gastroenteritis in young children worldwide.[198, 199] Group B rotavirus is responsible for large outbreaks of diarrhea in children and adults in China but is otherwise a rare isolate. Group C rotavirus causes disease in various parts of the world infrequently.

Pathology and Pathogenesis

Duodenal biopsy specimens of young children with rotavirus infection have demonstrated a patchy abnormality that is confined mostly to the epithelial cells of the upper intestine.[200] In its severe form, the infection can produce denuded villi and flattening of the epithelial surface. These changes persist for 3 to 8 weeks. The morphologic changes are accompanied by physiologic abnormalities such as decreased xylose absorption and reduced brush border levels of disaccharidases. Although the precise mechanism by which rotavirus causes diarrhea has not been defined, there is evidence that the virus activates the enteric nervous system, which then stimulates the intestinal epithelial cells to increase fluid secretion.[201]

Epidemiology

Rotavirus is responsible for childhood diarrhea in 35% of hospitalized and 10% to 30% of community-based cases.[199, 202] The virus appears to be spread by the fecal–oral route. In temperate zones, the disease is more common in winter, but in the tropics it is endemic year-round. Within a family, the young child is often afflicted with the clinical illness, whereas older siblings and adults can excrete the virus asymptomatically.

Clinical Features

Rotavirus causes a range of clinical illness from asymptomatic carriage to severe dehydration and even fatality.[203] The disease occurs principally in children aged 3 to 15 months; infections continue into the second year of life but are less common thereafter. Mild infections with group A rotaviruses can develop in adults and usually are acquired from a sick child in the household. Vomiting often heralds the illness and is followed shortly by watery diarrhea. The incubation period is 1 to 3 days, and the average duration of illness is 5 to 7 days, although some instances of chronic diarrhea have been noted. Loss of fluids and electrolytes appears to be the main pathophysiologic event. Excretion of virus for as long as 3 to 8 weeks occurs in approximately one third of infected children.[204]

Diagnosis

Rapid diagnosis is achieved by detection of rotavirus antigen in the feces with several commercial immunoassays. Polymerase chain reaction and nucleic acid probes also are available to detect the virus and identify its serogroups.[205, 206]

Immunity

After infection with rotavirus, antibody develops in serum and intestinal secretions.[207] The antibody is active against the specific serotype and crosses over to other serotypes.[208, 209] Natural rotavirus infection has a protective efficacy of 93% against recurrent rotavirus disease.[209] Levels of antibody in either serum or intestinal fluids do not correlate precisely with protection, a finding that has raised the possibility that cellular immunity plays a role as well.

Infants are protected for at least the first 3 months of life by maternal antibodies, although there is no convincing evidence that breast-feeding provides complete protection against this infection.[210] In addition to the possible protective role of maternal antibodies in breast milk, human milk mucin appears to have a potent antirotaviral activity in vitro and in a mouse model of infection.[211] The glycoprotein lactadherin binds specifically to all human rotavirus strains and inhibits their infectivity. Higher breast milk concentrations of lactadherin have been associated with protection against symptomatic rotavirus infection.[212]

Rotavirus vaccines are derived from related animal rotaviruses or genetic reassortments of various human and animal strains.[213] A tetravalent rhesus–human reassortant rotavirus, which provided moderate protection against all severities of rotavirus gastroenteritis and excellent protection against severe dehydrating disease, was licensed for use among infants in the United States in 1998.[213] However, the postlicensing recognition of intussusception as an uncommon serious complication of the live attenuated rotavirus vaccine led to the withdrawal of recommendations for its use.[214]

Treatment

Rehydration is the mainstay of therapy for this infection. Field studies have established that the oral rehydration solutions consisting of glucose and electrolytes (see Table 96–3) are effective in restoring fluid balance.[215] Antirotavirus immunoglobulin of bovine colostral origin has been found to be effective in reducing the duration of rotavirus infection and the amount of oral rehydration therapy required.[216]

Calicivirus

Caliciviruses are single-stranded RNA viruses that are responsible for human and animal infections. The characteristic "Star of David" appearance when visualized by electron microscopy served in the past to differentiate caliciviruses from small round enteric viruses such as the Norwalk virus and the Snow Mountain agent. However, recent molecular studies have demonstrated that the similar genetic composition of these enteric viruses places them in the taxonomic family of caliciviruses.[217]

The typical caliciviruses cause disease mainly in infants and young children.[218, 219] The disease is particularly common in day-care centers, where it accounts for more diarrhea than is attributed to bacterial infections.[219] The illness is generally mild and indistinguishable from rotavirus or even epidemic Norwalk disease.

Norwalk and Norwalk-like Virus

Named for a 1968 outbreak of "winter vomiting disease" in Norwalk, Ohio, this group of viruses is recognized as the pathogen in approximately 40% of nonbacterial epidemics of diarrhea in the United States. The virus also has been encountered in Hawaii, England, Australia, and Japan.[198]

Microbiology

Because these viruses have defied growth in cell cultures, our current knowledge is based on electron microscopic studies of viral particles and purification of viral material in feces.[220] These small viral agents measure 27 to 35 nm. The group includes many small viruses named after the site of an outbreak of gastroenteritis: Norwalk, Hawaii, Snow Mountain, Montgomery, Taunton, Otofuke, and Sapporo. These viruses all contain a single structural protein with single-stranded RNA.

Pathology and Pathogenesis

Intestinal biopsies have been performed in volunteers who have received a challenge of the infective agent. The upper small intestine is the focus of attack, and the stomach and colon are spared. Patchy mucosal lesions are noted in the proximal small bowel in all symptomatic volunteers and some asymptomatic subjects. Because the virus is so small, viral particles cannot be observed in electron microscopic sections, in contrast to the rotavirus. Among the physiologic abnormalities observed during illness caused by these agents are malabsorption of fat and xylose, diminished activity of intestinal disaccharidases, and delayed gastric emptying. Both the morphologic and physiologic abnormalities reverse within 1 to 2 weeks.

Epidemiology

The Norwalk virus causes explosive epidemics of diarrhea that sweep through a community and have a high attack rate. The virus shows no respect for age and preys on virtually all age groups, except infants. Transmission occurs by person-to-person contact, primarily by the fecal–oral route. Raw shellfish is a major source of infection; during an 8-month period in 1982, 103 outbreaks of Norwalk virus infection in New York State were related to ingestion of raw clams or oysters.[221] This virus is a major cause of outbreaks of gastroenteritis in camps, cruise ships, nursing homes, and hospitals.[222] It can also contaminate drinking water supplies.[223]

Clinical Features

The disease has a spectrum of symptoms and signs, all mild. In one outbreak of the Norwalk agent, diarrhea was noted in 92% of proven cases, nausea in 88%, abdominal cramps in 67%, vomiting in 66%, and muscle aches in 56%.[224] Generally, the clinical illness lasts no longer than 24 to 48 hours.

Because the virus cannot be grown in the laboratory, the diagnosis can be established only by identifying viral antigen in the stool, and these tests currently are available only in research laboratories. The virus can also be seen in fecal effluent by using the immune electron microscopy technique with the aid of serum from a convalescent subject (Fig. 96–5). A monoclonal antibody-based enzyme-linked, immunoabsorbent assay (ELISA) and a polymerase chain reaction assay have been developed and can detect Norwalk virus in stool specimens, but these assays are not yet commercially available.[225, 226] Another option is an ELISA that can mea-

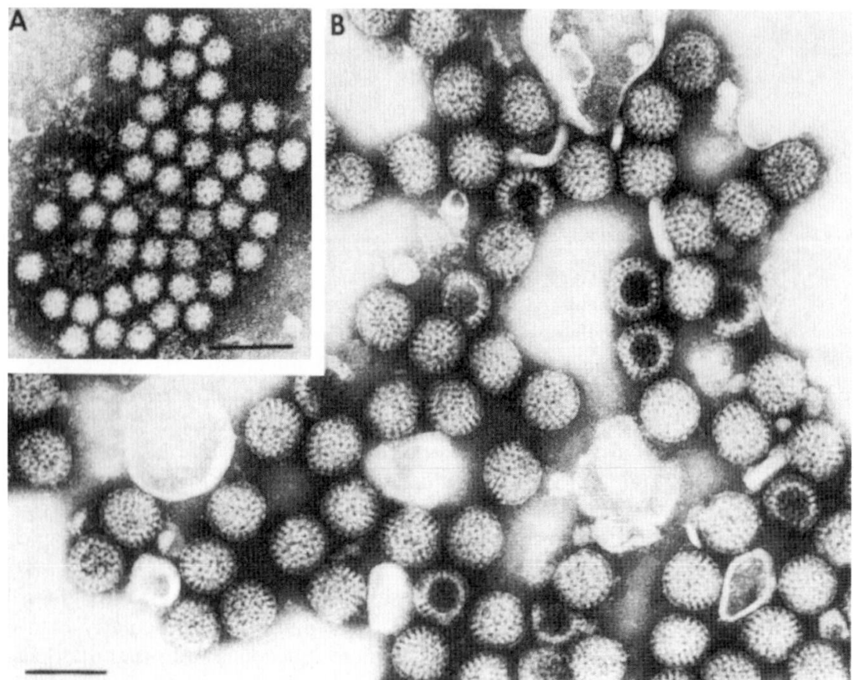

Figure 96–5. *A,* The Norwalk virus particle and aggregate from the stool of a volunteer administered the Norwalk agent. Bar equals 100 nm. *B,* Human rotavirus particles from the stool of an infant with gastroenteritis. The particles appear to have a double-shelled capsid. Occasional "empty" particles are seen. Bar equals 100 nm. (Courtesy of A. Kapikian, MD. Previously published in Lennete EH, Schmidt NJ. Diagnostic Procedures for Viral, Rickettsial, and Chlamydial Infections, 5th ed. New York, American Public Health Association, 1979, p 933.)

sure an IgM antibody response in serum, thereby suggesting a recent infection.

Immunity

Serum antibody titers are low in children, increase in adolescents, and are present in 60% of adults. Volunteer studies have revealed an unusual form of immunity that apparently is not related to antibody formation.[227] Volunteers who became sick during initial challenge were the same ones who became ill when rechallenged 24 to 42 months later. In contrast, those who resisted the initial challenge also resisted the subsequent challenge. Measurement of antibody in serum and intestinal juice showed higher levels of antibody in the volunteers who became ill on both the initial and subsequent challenge. This antibody had some protective value, albeit short-lived, because early rechallenge at 6 to 14 weeks after the initial dose produced protection in the subjects with antibody. Yet this protection did not persist, because the same group with antibody became ill when rechallenged several months later. Thus, it is postulated that nonimmune mechanisms in the intestine resist infection by this virus; repeated infections produce some protection, which is not permanent.

Treatment

No specific treatment is available. The disease is usually mild, but it can produce dehydration in elderly patients, who may require hospitalization. Bismuth subsalicylate was unimpressive in a controlled trial of infected volunteers; there was some decrease in abdominal cramps, but vomiting episodes, the rate of purging, and other symptoms were unaffected.[228]

Enteric Adenovirus

Most adenoviruses cause upper respiratory infections, but a new group of fastidious strains, known as serotypes 40 and 41, which constitute subgenus F, are responsible for gastroenteritis in children less than 2 years of age.[229] From 5% to 10% of childhood diarrhea is associated with enteric adenovirus. There is no seasonal occurrence.[199] Unlike rotavirus or Norwalk virus, infection with enteric adenovirus has a long incubation period of 8 to 10 days, and the illness can be prolonged for up to 2 weeks. Nosocomial and day-care center outbreaks are common and associated with high rates of asymptomatic infections.[230, 231] Adults are generally protected from this infection. The virus cannot be cultured in available cell lines but can be visualized in stool by electron microscopy or with dot-blot hybridization or immunoassays. An enzyme immunoassay licensed by the Food and Drug Administration (Adenoclone, Meridian Diagnostics, Cincinnati) is available for detection of enteric adenoviruses in stool specimens.

Astrovirus

Astrovirus is a small, nonenveloped, single-stranded RNA virus similar in structure to calicivirus.[232] In adults the disease has relatively low infectivity, but in children it is a major cause of diarrheal illness. In a study from Thailand, astrovirus was second only to rotavirus as a cause of diarrhea in children.[233] There are at least seven viral serotypes. Antibody develops to many of these serotypes by 4 years of age, indicating that they probably cause infections frequently in childhood.

Astroviruses are responsible for outbreaks of diarrhea in day-care centers and communities with children less than 12 months old.[231, 234, 235] The disease is characterized by watery or mucoid stools, nausea, vomiting, and occasionally fever but tends to be milder than rotavirus diarrhea, with less than 6% of children developing dehydration.[233, 235] Coinfections with other pathogens are common, and repeated infections may occur as a result of a lack of cross-protective immunity to the multiple serotypes of astrovirus. The virus can be recognized in stool specimens by means of electron microscopy, specific immunoassays, RNA probe hybridization, and polymerase chain reaction methodology, although all these tests remain research tools.[234, 236] Treatment is supportive with an emphasis on oral rehydration.

Torovirus

Toroviruses are enveloped single-stranded RNA viruses that cause enteric infections in animals.[237] Recent case-control studies have demonstrated the role of toroviruses as causes of diarrhea in children.[238, 239] In a large prospective study of pediatric viral diarrhea, toroviruses accounted for 3% of episodes, a greater percentage than that for either the caliciviruses or astrovirus.[199] Although most diarrhea due to toroviruses occurs in children under the age of 2 years, older children, especially those who are immunocompromised, are at risk for symptomatic infections.[239]

Toroviruses have been associated with both acute and persistent (lasting longer than 14 days) diarrhea in children.[238, 239] When torovirus has been encountered in children with persistent diarrhea, it often is found in association with other potential pathogens such as EAggEC. When compared with infection with rotavirus, children infected with torovirus have less vomiting and more bloody diarrhea, although the latter symptom occurs in only 11% of patients. Toroviruses can be detected in stool specimens by electron microscopy or ELISA. As in other viral diarrheas, treatment is supportive. Fluid replacement is often required for as long as one week.[239]

TRAVELER'S DIARRHEA

Diarrheal illness has plagued travelers for centuries. It has given rise to numerous theories of causation and has achieved worldwide fame by its various euphemisms. Within the glossary of descriptive epithets that have been applied to the intestinal agonies of travelers are GI trots, gyppy (Egyptian) tummy, Casablanca crud, Aden gut, Barsa belly, Turkey trot, Hong-Kong dog, Delhi belly, Aztec two-step, Montezuma's revenge, and turista. Most recently, a disease associated with *Giardia* infection acquired by travelers to Russia has been called "the Trotskys."

Annually, more than 500 million people travel from one country to another, with an ever growing number traveling from industrialized countries to developing countries. Travelers from the United States to Mexico alone number over 15 million annually. With an attack rate of 25% to 50%, diarrheal illness may affect upward of 1 million United States visitors to Mexico yearly, nearly 30% of whom are ill enough to require confinement to bed and another 40% of whom must alter their scheduled activities.[240]

Microbiology

As improved laboratory methods became available, particularly testing for ETEC, it became apparent that traveler's diarrhea is caused mainly by infectious microorganisms that are acquired from food and drink.[241–244] Several studies have isolated specific microbial pathogens from the feces of sick tourists. The causal link between infection and clinical disease has been solidified by field trials that have demonstrated that antibacterial drugs are effective in preventing and treating traveler's diarrhea.[244] Indeed, prevention rates of 80% or more, which have been achieved with a variety of antimicrobial drugs, strongly implicate bacterial pathogens, especially Gram-negative enteric organisms, as the cause in most cases. Although an array of pathogens have been found, the leading culprits are various forms of *E. coli*, particularly ETEC (Table 96–10). *Shigella* species have been encountered in approximately 10% of cases of traveler's diarrhea, although the rate of isolation varies from 0 to more than 20%. The disease caused by *Shigella* tends to be more severe than the usual form. Strains of *Campylobacter* are encountered in as many as 41% of cases, with the higher rates during cooler seasons.[244–246] Salmonella organisms are found in fewer than 5% of cases, although the frequency is higher among travelers to Asia than elsewhere. Rotavirus has been encountered in approximately 10% of episodes of traveler's diarrhea when this pathogen is sought.[243, 247] Among the parasites, *Giardia lamblia* and *Cryptosporidium* are hazards to travelers in Leningrad but not necessarily in Latin America and Asia (see Chapter 98). Amebiasis, which has been characterized by Elsdon Dew as the "refuge of the diagnostically destitute," is a relatively uncommon cause of diarrhea in travelers to Mexico and Asia. The newly described protozoan parasite *Cyclospora cayetanensis* is responsible for traveler's diarrhea in visitors to a number of less developed countries, especially Nepal[248] (see Chapter 98). *G. lamblia*, *C. cayetanensis*, and, rarely, *Shigella*, *Salmonella*, *Isospora belli*, or *C. jejuni* may be responsible for rare cases of persistent diarrhea in travelers.[249] A causative agent will not be identified in many travelers with prolonged diarrhea.

More than one pathogen may be found in travelers with acute diarrhea (up to 15% in Mexico and 33% in Thailand). To confuse the issue further, no pathogens have been identified, despite careful laboratory study, in more than 40% of cases from all parts of the world.

Table 96–10 | **Microbial Pathogens in Traveler's Diarrhea**

	FREQUENCY	
	Average (%)	Range (%)
Enterotoxigenic *E. coli*	40–60	0–72
Enteroadherent *E. coli*	15	—
Campylobacter	10	0–41
Shigella	10	0–30
Invasive *E. coli*	<5	0–5
Salmonella	<5	0–15
Vibrio	<5	0–30
Aeromonas	<5	0–30
Rotavirus	5	0–36
Giardia lamblia	<5	0–6
Entamoeba histolytica	<5	0–6
Cryptosporidium	<5	—
Cyclospora cayetanensis	<5	—
Hafnia alvei	<5	0–16
No pathogen identified	40	22–83

Epidemiology

The major determinant of risk is the destination of the traveler. According to studies of nearly 20,000 European tourists to various locations, three zones of risk have been defined. High-risk destinations, where the frequency of traveler's diarrhea ranges from 20% to 50%, include Latin America, Africa, the Middle East, and Asia. Intermediate-risk destinations, with a 10% to 20% frequency, include southern European countries, Israel, and a few Caribbean islands. Low-risk areas, where the frequency is below 8%, include Canada, the United States, northern Europe, Australia, New Zealand, and a number of the Caribbean islands.[247] However, these estimates are based on questionnaires filled out by returning travelers. In summarizing the experience from 34 prospective studies, a somewhat greater risk emerges: median traveler's diarrhea rates of 53% (21% to 100%) in Latin America, 54% (21% to 100%) in Asia, and 54% (36% to 62%) in Africa.[250]

The national origin of the traveler is another important factor. At an international conference in Mexico held in 1968, participants from the United States and northern Europe had a 36% attack rate, compared with only 8% for colleagues from developing countries and 2% for local Mexicans.[251] Longer residence in a tropical country also leads to increased resistance to traveler's diarrhea, although a high risk of diarrhea persists during the first 2 years of residence.[248] Previous short-term travel to areas of high risk does not necessarily lead to protection.

The purpose of travel and the style of eating are both important factors that influence the risk of developing this illness. The greatest frequency of diarrhea occurs in people traveling as students or itinerant tourists, the lowest risk in those visiting relatives, and an intermediate risk in business travelers.[247] Young travelers—particularly those aged 20 to 29 years—have the highest risk, whereas the rates are lowest in persons over 55 years of age.

Traveler's diarrhea is acquired through ingestion of fecally contaminated food or beverages. Especially risky foods include uncooked vegetables, meat, and seafood. Tap water, ice, unpasteurized milk and dairy products, and unpeeled fruits are also associated with an increased risk. Bottled carbonated beverages (especially flavored beverages), beer, wine, hot coffee, hot tea, and water boiled or appropriately treated with chlorine are relatively safe. However, some studies show that drinking bottled uncarbonated mineral water increases the risk of water-borne infection.[252]

Dietary indiscretion is penalized by an increased risk of

diarrhea. Yet even the most conscientious travelers were unable to resist such temptations; 98% of Swiss travelers consumed unsafe food and beverages during the first 3 days of an overseas journey, 71% consumed salads or uncooked vegetables, and 53% accepted ice cubes in drinks.[253] Hence, dietary advice, although universally recognized as important and of proven efficacy, is rarely heeded by even the most informed responsible travelers.

Clinical Features

The disease does not begin immediately after the traveler's arrival but generally 2 to 3 days later.[241, 247] Although most people have three to five loose stools per day, about 20% can have 6 to 15 watery bowel movements.[241, 249] The average duration of illness in untreated subjects is 3 to 5 days, but a few unfortunate ones have persistent diarrhea throughout their stay.

Watery loose stools are the most common complaint, with an array of associated symptoms (Table 96–11). From 2% to 10% of patients have fever, bloody stools, or both, and they are more likely to have shigellosis.[242] In general, persons with a milder clinical presentation, regardless of the pathogen, experience more rapid resolution of disease than those with more severe symptoms, but even mild disease can produce an illness that lasts 4 to 5 days. Despite the impressive list of symptoms, fewer than 1% of travelers are admitted to a local hospital, and no reports of death due to diarrhea have been recorded among several hundred thousand travelers from Switzerland.[247] Diarrhea persists in 1% to 3% of travelers for as long as 30 days or more.[249]

Treatment

As for all forms of diarrhea, treatment entails fluid replacement and appropriate drugs. In cases of traveler's diarrhea, severe dehydration seldom is encountered, and fluid losses generally can be replaced with soft drinks, fruit juices, and clear fluids. Drug treatment is directed at either suppressing the pathogen with antibiotics or reducing fluid and electrolyte losses with antisecretory agents.

Several antibiotics have been used successfully to treat traveler's diarrhea. TMP-SMX or TMP alone reduced the duration of diarrhea from 93 hours to approximately 30 hours.[254] Ciprofloxacin was as effective as TMP-SMX[255]; results with a single dose of fluoroquinolones are encouraging.[256] However, the development of ciprofloxacin resistance in patients with *Campylobacter* enteritis has been associated with clinical relapse after treatment.[246] In areas where fluoroquinolone resistant *C. jejuni* has become more common, azithromycin, rather than ciprofloxacin, should be used to treat traveler's diarrhea.[184]

Antimotility drugs have enjoyed considerable support among tourists for providing relief from the intestinal indignities of travel, and their approbation is supported by good scientific studies.[257] Loperamide induces rapid improvement that is demonstrable even on the first day of therapy, when the results are significantly better than those of either placebo or bismuth subsalicylate.[257] Bismuth subsalicylate is an effective alternative treatment for mild-to-moderate traveler's diarrhea.[258] The most effective relief has been provided by a combination of an antimicrobial drug and an antimotility drug. In a study of travelers to Mexico, the combined use of loperamide and TMP-SMX curtailed diarrhea in 1 hour, compared with 30 hours when either drug was used alone or 59 hours with placebo.[259] However, another study from Egypt failed to show much benefit for the combination over the antibiotic alone.[260]

Current recommendations for treatment differ somewhat from those made by a 1986 National Institutes of Health Consensus Conference.[240] For mild-to-moderate diarrhea, generally less than four bowel movements per day without blood or fever, either loperamide or bismuth subsalicylate can be used effectively. For more severe diarrhea, the optimal therapy seems to be a combination of an antimotility drug and an effective antimicrobial drug.[261]

Travelers with persistent diarrhea in whom a specific pathogen cannot be identified should be treated with an antibiotic directed at common bacterial pathogens if the drug has not been tried previously. If this approach does not alleviate the symptoms, an empiric course of antiprotozoal therapy should be used. Finally, if this agent fails, an endoscopic evaluation may be needed.

Prevention

It is certainly beneficial to prevent an attack of diarrhea, especially one that can interfere with an overseas journey, but prevention is not easy to accomplish unless one travels with sterile hermetically sealed containers of food and drink. Four approaches to preventing traveler's diarrhea can be conceived: avoidance of unsafe foods and beverages, use of anti-infective drugs, use of other medications, and immunization.

Certain precautions about eating habits should be observed, to prevent not only diarrhea but other food- and water-borne diseases as well. Bottled beverages are generally safe, although some epidemics have been associated with contaminated bottled drinks.[252] Carbonated beverages are safer than noncarbonated ones, due to the low pH (generally 4.0 to 5.0), which has antibacterial properties. Tea or coffee prepared with boiling water generally is safe when consumed while still hot. Because the venue of food consumption determines the risk of traveler's diarrhea, travelers are advised not to eat food from street vendors. Despite these recommendations, most travelers are unable to maintain perfect vigilance during a pleasure trip; thus this approach, although universally recommended, does not in reality provide complete protection.[262]

Table 96–11 | **Associated Symptoms in Traveler's Diarrhea**

SYMPTOM	%	SYMPTOM	%
Gas	79	Headache	39
Fatigue	74	Chills	38
Cramps	68	Backache	35
Nausea	61	Dizziness	34
Fever	56	Vomiting	29
Abdominal pain	55	Malaise	24
Anorexia	53	Arthralgia	23

Antimicrobial drugs have been used extensively to prevent traveler's diarrhea. Protection rates have varied from 28% to 100%; the lower rates have been seen with what are now recognized to be poorly effective antimicrobial drugs, such as sulfonamides and streptomycin, or with a high level of resistance to the drug in ETEC isolated in an area. In more recent studies using TMP-SMX, protection rates have ranged from 71% to 95%; with norfloxacin or ciprofloxacin, the protection rates are 68% to 94%.

Bismuth subsalicylate has been used for prevention, based on its antimicrobial and antisecretory activities[258]; however, it provides modest protection only when the traveler is conscientious about taking higher doses.

Among drugs other than antimicrobials, halogenated hydroxyquinolines have enjoyed popular use. Some studies have shown benefit, whereas others have failed to find any salutary effect.[262] Notwithstanding its questionable efficacy for prophylaxis of traveler's diarrhea, this class of drug should not be used in travelers, nor in other situations, because of the reported association with subacute myelotic neuropathy.[263]

DIARRHEA IN THE ELDERLY

Diarrheal disease is a major cause of morbidity and mortality in adults over age 65 years.[264, 265] The elderly are at increased risk for diarrhea and associated complications as a consequence of hypochlorhydria, intestinal motility disorders, underlying chronic medical diseases, immune senescence, and exposure to multiple medications, including antibiotics. A review of national mortality data found that most diarrheal deaths in the United States between 1979 and 1987 occurred in people over age 74 years (51%) and in adults aged 55 to 74 years (27%).[264] Although these data did not allow the evaluation of specific causes, diarrhea-associated mortality in the elderly tended to peak in winter months, a finding suggestive of an underlying infectious etiology. Elderly people living in chronic care facilities are at greater risk of death from diarrhea than are independent elderly.[264, 266] Infectious diarrhea was the fourth most common infectious disease in residents of long-term care facilities.[267]

Microbiology

A number of infectious bacterial, viral, and parasitic agents can cause diarrhea in the elderly. In addition, noninfectious causes of diarrhea need to be considered in the elderly, including medications such as laxatives or antacids, intestinal tumors that cause obstruction or secrete hormones, inflammatory bowel disease, malabsorption, and systemic illnesses including diabetes mellitus and thyrotoxicosis.[266]

A consistent association has been noted between advanced age and *C. difficile* infection.[268, 269] Given the frequent need for hospitalization and the use of antimicrobial agents in the elderly, it is not surprising that *C. difficile* is the most commonly identified cause of diarrhea in the elderly. Older adults are more likely than younger people to have a severe event when exposed to enterohemorrhagic *E. coli*[270] and *C. perfringens*.[271] In an outbreak of *E. coli* O157 : H7 in a chronic care facility in Toronto in 1985, one third of the nursing home residents were infected, whereas only 13% of the employees developed diarrhea.[78] The elderly residents were also at substantially increased risk for mortality from EHEC in this study; 35% of the infected residents died, primarily from complications of HUS, whereas none of the infected staff members died. Elderly persons represented the only fatalities in a large outbreak of *E. coli* O157 : H7 in Missouri.[270] As was recently demonstrated in Washington,[88] the use of antibiotics for treatment of EHEC infections in the nursing home residents was associated with a threefold increased risk of death.[78]

Norwalk-like viruses are a common source of nursing home outbreaks and are responsible for substantial morbidity in the institutionalized elderly.[272] The elderly are also more likely than younger persons to have severe infections and to die from nontyphoidal salmonellosis and campylobacteriosis. Among the parasitic causes of diarrhea, *Cryptosporidium parvum* is a cause of morbidity in the elderly. In a Rhode Island hospital, a retrospective chart review of stool studies for *C. parvum* over a 5-year period showed that 36% of positive smears were in elderly patients, whereas 50% were in patients with human immunodeficiency virus.[273] Most of the elderly with positive stool specimens acquired the infection in an institutional setting, and nearly one half were coinfected with *C. difficile*.

Clinical Features

Although the clinical manifestations of gastrointestinal infections in the elderly vary by pathogen, there are few major differences between the young and the old. However, the elderly are more likely to experience complications resulting from volume depletion. Dehydration may exacerbate other age-related complications such as delirium, electrolyte disturbances, renal insufficiency, malnutrition, and micronutrient deficiencies. If hemorrhagic colitis develops, the new blood loss superimposed on preexisting anemia can precipitate congestive heart failure, angina, or a myocardial infarction.

Whereas the elderly clearly have increased rates of *C. difficile* colitis, this population does not appear to have more severe disease or higher mortality rates than in younger populations.[274] In addition, the response to therapy appears to be equivalent in older adults when compared with younger adults.

Diagnosis

Because many episodes of infectious diarrhea in the elderly are self-limited, supportive therapy is often all that is necessary. Signs of dehydration that are useful for evaluating young adults and children are often less reliable indicators of an elderly patient's hydration status. Older adults often have decreased skin elasticity, dry oral mucosa because of mouth breathing, and sunken eyes. Although it is important to take orthostatic vital signs, orthostatic changes generally do not occur until there has been substantial volume loss ($\geq$10%). Laboratory tests also are not especially helpful for diagnosing dehydration in the elderly. Although the ratio of blood urea nitrogen to creatinine, if elevated, suggests dehydration, this ratio is only a crude indicator of a patient's underlying volume status.

Noninfectious causes of diarrhea, such as use of magnesium-containing antacids, laxatives, and stool softeners, should be eliminated before embarking on a diagnostic workup. If diarrhea persists, disorders of intestinal motility such as fecal impaction should be excluded. Although stool cultures are often not helpful, except in outbreaks, stool studies for *C. difficile* toxin should be obtained, especially if the patient has recently received chemotherapy or antimicrobial treatment. Endoscopic procedures should be done if fecal occult blood tests are positive and invasive pathogens have been excluded. Persistent or recurrent symptoms also should prompt consideration of colonoscopy or upper endoscopy, or both.

Treatment

If an elderly patient with diarrhea and deyhdration is not severely dehydrated and is able to tolerate fluids by mouth, oral rehydration therapy is preferred (see later). Patients who are severely dehydrated or unable to tolerate oral therapy should be rehydrated by the parenteral route. Antimicrobial therapy generally should be reserved for the treatment of specific infections such as shigellosis, invasive salmonellosis, or *C. difficile*.

DIAGNOSIS OF INFECTIOUS DIARRHEAL DISEASE (see also Chapter 9)

A pathophysiologic approach can be used to make a presumptive etiologic diagnosis in patients with infectious diarrhea (Table 96–12). Perhaps the most convenient method is to separate pathogens that target the upper small intestine from those that attack the large bowel. Toxigenic bacteria (*E. coli*, *V. cholerae*), viruses, and the parasite *Giardia* are examples of small bowel pathogens. These organisms produce watery diarrhea, which may lead to dehydration. Abdominal pain, although often diffuse and poorly defined, is generally periumbilical. Microscopic examination of the stool fails to reveal formed cellular elements such as erythrocytes and leukocytes.

A large bowel pathogen, the major one being *Shigella*, is an invasive organism that causes the clinical syndrome of dysentery. Characteristic rectal pain, or tenesmus, strongly implicates colonic involvement. Although the fecal effluent initially may be watery, by the second or third day of illness the stool becomes relatively small in volume and often bloody and mucoid. Microscopic examination usually reveals abundant erythrocytes and leukocytes. Proctoscopy shows a diffusely ulcerated, hemorrhagic, and friable colonic mucosa. Other organisms that fit into this category are *Campylobacter* and *E. coli* (EIEC and EHEC).

Certain pathogens involve principally the lower small bowel but may invade the colon as well; *Salmonella* and *Yersinia* make up this group. Although watery diarrhea is the usual presentation, depending on the focus of infection, the spectrum extends from dehydrating diarrhea to frank colitis. Vibrios produce varying clinical presentations, apparently related to the virulence factors in each infecting strain. *Entamoeba histolytica* attacks the large bowel and produces an invasive disease (see Chapter 98). Curiously, there is a paucity of polymorphonuclear leukocytes in the stool, although occasional macrophages are present.

Table 96–12 | **Clinical Features of Diarrheal Diseases**

FEATURE	LOCATION OF INFECTION	
	Small Bowel	**Large Bowel**
Pathogens	*Vibrio cholerae* *Escherichia coli* (ETEC, EPEC) Rotavirus Norwalk virus *Giardia*	*Shigella* *E. coli* (EIEC, EHEC) *Entamoeba histolytica*
Location of pain	Midabdomen	Lower abdomen, rectum
Volume of stool	Large	Small
Type of stool	Watery	Mucoid
Blood in stool	Rare	Common
Leukocytes in stool	Rare	Common (except in amebiasis)
Proctoscopy	Normal	Mucosal ulcers; hemorrhage; friable mucosa

EHEC, enterohemorrhagic *E. coli;* EIEC, enteroinvasive *E. coli;* EPEC, enteropathogenic *E. coli;* ETEC, enterotoxigenic *E. coli.*

Laboratory Diagnosis

Infectious diarrhea is a major cause of illness throughout the world. It leads to high morbidity with loss of time from school and work in Western countries and high mortality in developing countries. As a consequence of the substantial morbidity and mortality caused by episodes of diarrhea, a specific laboratory diagnosis is useful epidemiologically, diagnostically, and therapeutically.

An etiologic diagnosis of infectious diarrhea is obtained mainly through study of fecal specimens, by using bacteriologic culture, viral culture or direct electron microscopy for viral particles, and identification of microbial antigens (viruses, bacteria, parasites, or toxins). DNA probes and polymerase chain reaction methodology can now be used to identify several pathogens in stool specimens.[275] Immunodiagnostic tests have been developed that allow for the rapid detection of both *V. cholerae* 01 and *V. cholerae* 0139 and group A rotavirus in stool samples.[276, 277] Although some diseases can be diagnosed on the basis of rising serum antibody titers, this method is usually retrospective and inaccurate.

Standard stool cultures for pathogens cost $50 to $70, depending on the laboratory and the need for antibiotic sensitivities or special tests. Fecal examinations for ova and parasites cost an additional $60 to $100. Ordering the full range of diagnostic tests for a stool specimen could easily cost $150 to $200. Yet the yield of positive results is disappointingly paltry. At the Massachusetts General Hospital, the isolation rate of bacterial pathogens from 2000 fecal cultures in 1980 was 2.4%, producing a cost per positive test of $952.[278] In patients with severe diarrhea requiring hospitalization, the isolation rate in feces is somewhat higher, ranging from 27% to 43%,[279, 280] and up to 58% in a study using more advanced techniques.[281] Even in hospitalized dysentery cases, the rate of positivity for microbiologic diagnosis is only 40% to 60%. In community patients with severe acute gastroenteritis (more than four fluid stools per day lasting at least 3 days with at least one associated symptom), the yield of a stool culture and ova and parasite examination increases

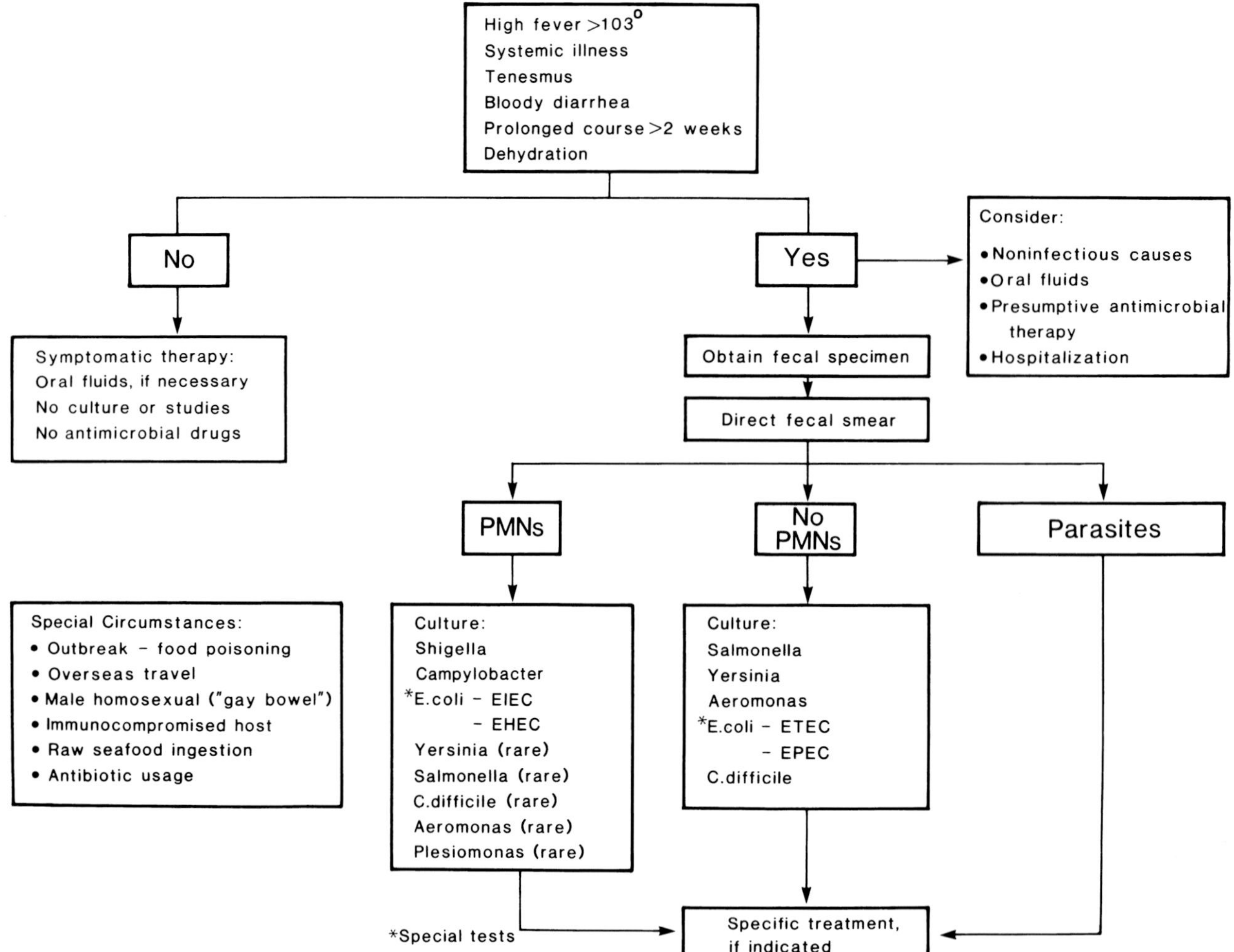

Figure 96–6. Algorithm for the diagnosis and treatment of infectious diarrhea. EHEC, enterohemorrhagic *E. coli;* EIEC, enteroinvasive *E. coli;* EPEC, enteropathogenic *E. coli;* ETEC, enterotoxigenic *E. coli;* PMNs, polymorphonuclear leukocytes.

to 88%.[282] In outbreaks of gastroenteritis in the United States, only one half of the cases have a confirmed etiology, of which two thirds are bacterial in origin. These unimpressive figures suggest that many cases of acute diarrhea are caused by as yet unidentified pathogens.

The yield of a stool culture and ova and parasite examination in patients in whom diarrhea develops 3 or more days after hospitalization is close to nil. On the other hand, the yield of *C. difficile* toxin assays is high in this group of patients (see Chapter 97).

An algorithm for the diagnosis of acute diarrhea is presented to help decide which patients should be treated symptomatically and which require further diagnostic studies and treatment (Fig. 96–6). Approximately 90% of cases of acute diarrhea fall into the "no studies–no treatment" category.

Fecal Leukocytes

A particularly useful technique to establish a presumptive diagnosis in infectious diarrhea is microscopic examination of the stool (Table 96–13). Using two drops of Loeffler's methylene blue mixed with a small amount of stool on a slide, a search for leukocytes and erythrocytes is undertaken. (An experienced observer can do the examination without the stain, thereby looking for protozoa and other parasites on the same slide.) Invasive pathogens, such as *Shigella* and *Campylobacter*, produce a "sea of polys," easily visible in every field, as well as red blood cells. The toxigenic organisms, viruses, and food-poisoning bacteria cause a watery stool that harbors few formed elements. A latex agglutination test for lactoferrin in fecal specimens is available (Techlab Inc., Blacksburg, VA) and provides a rapid and sensitive alternative to microscopy for the identification of inflammatory diarrhea.[283]

Several organisms produce variable findings on microscopic stool examination, depending on the invasive properties of the strain and the degree of colonic involvement. This category, which includes *Salmonella*, *Yersinia*, *V. parahaemolyticus*, and pseudomembranous colitis and antibiotic-associated diarrhea caused by *C. difficile*, has unpredictable findings with regard to cellular elements in the stool. Most cases show a profusion of sloughed epithelial and red blood cells but only occasional polymorphonuclear leukocytes. An acute exacerbation of ulcerative colitis can produce a great discharge of leukocytes and erythrocytes into the stool, thereby resulting in an exudative microscopic appearance that resembles bacillary dysentery.

Although the fecal microscopic examination is neither infallible nor even helpful in all cases, it is inexpensive and

Table 96–13 | **Fecal Leukocytes in Intestinal Infections**

Present
- *Shigella*
- *Campylobacter*
- EIEC
- EHEC

Variable
- EAggEC
- *Salmonella*
- *Yersinia*
- *V. parahaemolyticus*
- *C. difficile* (antibiotic-associated colitis)
- *Aeromonas*

Absent
- *V. cholerae*
- ETEC
- EPEC
- DAEC
- Rotavirus
- Calicivirus, including Norwalk virus
- *Giardia lamblia*
- *Entamoeba histolytica*
- Food poisoning
  - *Staphylococcus aureus*
  - *Clostridium perfringens*
  - *Bacillus cereus*
  - Viruses

DAEC, diffusing adhering *E. coli;* EAggEC, enteroaggregative *E. coli;* EHEC, enterohemorrhagic *E. coli;* EIEC, enteroinvasive *E. coli;* EPEC, enteropathogenic *E. coli;* ETEC, enterotoxigenic *E. coli.*

yields immediate information that can guide antibiotic therapy, especially in cases of bacillary dysentery. Although the latex agglutination test for fecal lactoferrin is slightly more expensive than microscopy for fecal leukocytes, the lactoferrin assay has several advantages, including ease, rapidity, and the absence of a requirement for a fresh stool specimen.

Dysentery versus Ulcerative Colitis

Two features distinguish dysentery from an acute attack of idiopathic ulcerative colitis (see also Chapter 104): a positive culture for a pathogen and a self-limited course without relapse. However, a positive bacteriologic culture has a relatively poor record in dysentery, a condition also known as acute self-limited colitis, because positive cultures are encountered in only 40% to 60% of reported cases.[114, 281] The diagnostic criterion of "self-limited course without relapse" is useful when a patient has had a history of repeated attacks, but it is a retrospective consideration in a patient with a first attack.

Histopathologic examination of colonic mucosa obtained by endoscopic biopsy can be helpful if obtained within 4 days of the onset of symptoms. Both the microbial form (dysentery) and the idiopathic form of acute colitis show edema, neutrophils in the lamina propria, and superficial cryptitis with preservation of the normal crypt pattern. However, idiopathic ulcerative colitis shows signs of chronicity such as crypt distortion and plasmacytosis in the lamina propria, which may extend to the base of the mucosa. Focal cryptitis and a mild increase in the cellularity of the lamina propria are found in both the microbial and idiopathic forms and can lead to confusion.[114]

In clinical practice, the main diagnostic problem is illustrated by a patient with severe acute colitis, generally present for several days, who has not responded to antibiotic therapy. Presumptive treatment should include a fluoroquinolone for bacterial pathogens and metronidazole for protozoa. The decision to use other treatment, such as glucocorticoids, rests on the distinction between these diseases, and it may not be possible to make this distinction based on culture or histopathologic findings.

TREATMENT OF INFECTIOUS DIARRHEA

Fluid Therapy

The most devastating consequences of acute infectious diarrhea result from fluid losses. Toxigenic organisms, such as *V. cholerae* and certain strains of *E. coli* (ETEC), are associated with extreme dehydration resulting from the production of large amounts of isotonic fluid in the small bowel; this fluid overwhelms the ability of the lower intestine to reabsorb it (see Table 96–2). Children with toxigenic diarrhea lose somewhat less sodium and bicarbonate in their feces than do adults, but they excrete significantly more potassium. "Nonspecific" diarrhea, usually caused by viruses, causes less fluid loss and a lower electrolyte concentration in the fecal effluent than toxigenic diarrhea.

The major aim of treatment is to replace fluid and electrolytes. The traditional route of administration has been intravenous, but in recent years ORS have proved to be as effective physiologically and more practical logistically in developing countries.[19, 20, 284] Even in the United States, ORS is the treatment of choice for mild-to-moderate diarrhea in both children and adults and can be used in severe diarrhea after initial parenteral fluid replacement.[285] ORS is based on the sound physiologic principle that glucose enhances sodium absorption in the small intestine, even in the presence of secretory losses caused by bacterial toxins (see Chapter 87).

Although there is agreement on the value of ORS in treating dehydrating diarrhea, the formulation of electrolytes remains in dispute, particularly in treating well-nourished children with mild-to-moderate diarrhea in industrialized countries. Specifically, some authorities have voiced concern that the concentration of sodium (90 mmol) in the standard ORS formulation may be high and could cause hypernatremia and seizures.[215, 284, 286] This issue was examined in a study from Scotland in which children with acute diarrhea with mild dehydration were treated in a randomized fashion with solutions containing sodium concentrations of 35, 50, or 90 mmol and dextrose concentrations of 200, 111, and 110 mmol, respectively; all three formulations proved to be equally safe and effective.[287] On the basis of these and other studies, several authorities have recommended lower concentrations of sodium and a reduced osmolarity in ORS for children with diarrhea in a developed country.[215, 284, 286] A recently completed multicenter study of male children with acute noncholera diarrhea found that treatment of dehydration with a reduced-osmolarity reduced-sodium ORS (see Table 96–3) was associated with a lower total stool output, less total ORS intake, and a shortened duration of diarrhea than treatment with the standard ORS.[288] Patients treated with the reduced-osmolarity ORS had a lower mean serum sodium concentration after treatment, but this was not associated with any adverse clinical events.

Additional criticisms of the traditional glucose-based ORS

are that it fails to decrease the quantity and duration of diarrhea and provides only minimal nutrition with the rehydration. An inexpensive alternative to glucose-based ORS is the substitution of starch derived from rice or cereals for glucose. Treatment with rice-based salt solutions produces lower stool losses, a shorter duration of diarrhea, and greater fluid and electrolyte absorption and retention than does glucose-based ORS in children and adults with diarrhea.[289] Improved growth and weight gain are also observed with rice-based ORS. More recently, the addition of an amylase-resistant starch to ORS has been demonstrated to be even more effective in reducing the duration of diarrhea and fecal weight than a rice flour–based ORS in patients with cholera.[290]

Diet

The traditional approach to any diarrheal illness is dietary abstinence, which restricts the intake of necessary calories, fluids, and electrolytes. Certainly, during an acute attack, the patient often finds it more comfortable to avoid high-fiber foods, fats, and spices, all of which can increase stool volume and intestinal motility; any oral consumption can provide a stimulus to defecation. Although giving the bowel a rest provides symptomatic relief, the patient must maintain intake with oral fluids containing calories and some electrolytes. On balance, it is better to eat judiciously during an attack of diarrhea than to restrict oral intake severely. In children, it is particularly important to restart feeding immediately after the child is able to accept oral intake.

It is wise to avoid milk and dairy products during the acute episode of diarrhea because ingestion of such items in this setting could potentiate fluid secretion and increase stool volume. Beverages that contain caffeine or methylxanthine products should be avoided because these agents increase intestinal motility. Thus, coffee, strong tea, cocoa, and soft drinks such as the colas all contain chemicals that can potentiate abdominal cramps and diarrhea. Alcohol has similar actions on the gut, and abstinence is recommended. In addition to the oral rehydration therapy outlined above, acceptable beverages for mildly dehydrated adults include fruit juices and various bottled soft drinks. It is advisable to "defizz" a carbonated drink by letting it stand in a glass before it is consumed. Soft easily digestible foods are most acceptable to a patient with acute diarrhea.

Antimicrobial Drugs

Less than 10% of cases of acute diarrhea are benefitted by treatment with antimicrobial drugs.[291] Among the causes that should be treated with such drugs are shigellosis, cholera, typhoid fever, symptomatic traveler's diarrhea, *E. coli* diarrhea in infants, and *C. difficile* diarrhea (see Table 96–4). There are conflicting reports concerning the efficacy of antimicrobial drugs in several important infections, such as those caused by *Campylobacter*, and insufficient data for infections caused by *Yersinia*, *Aeromonas*, vibrios, and several forms of *E. coli*.

The issue of when antimicrobial therapy is appropriate for the management of acute diarrhea has been a vexing problem. This issue was addressed in a placebo-controlled study of empiric treatment of severe, acute, community-acquired gastroenteritis with ciprofloxacin that included patients with more than four stools per day for more than 3 days and at least one associated symptom.[282] Treatment with ciprofloxacin, 500 mg twice a day for 5 days, was associated with a reduction in the duration of diarrhea and other symptoms by more than 2 days, fewer failures, and significant clearing of pathogens when compared with placebo. Six weeks later there was no difference in stool carriage of the pathogen (12%) nor any demonstrable antibiotic resistance. A study from Chicago of outpatient treatment of adults with acute diarrhea compared ciprofloxacin, TMP-SMX, and placebo and found that ciprofloxacin, but not TMP-SMX, shortened the duration of diarrhea.[292] Similar findings have been noted in other studies of the empiric therapy of diarrhea.[293]

Based on these studies, a patient with severe community-acquired diarrhea, defined as a previously healthy person with diarrhea (more than four watery stools per day) lasting at least 3 days and at least one of the following symptoms: abdominal pain, fever, vomiting, myalgia, or headache, should receive an antimicrobial drug, preferably a fluoroquinolone. In this subset of patients with acute diarrhea, there is a high likelihood that a bacterial pathogen will be isolated and treatment with an antibiotic will provide prompt relief of symptoms with a low risk of adverse effects. In patients with bloody diarrhea, it is not possible to distinguish among *Shigella*, *Campylobacter*, and EHEC on clinical grounds. If symptoms of dysentery predominate, quinolone therapy is indicated. If dysentery is not present and if there is a reasonable possibility, based on epidemiologic evidence, that EHEC is the responsible pathogen, then antimicrobial therapy should be withheld until a microbiologic diagnosis can be established.[88]

The choice of antimicrobial drugs, when indicated, is based on in vitro sensitivity patterns, which are related to geographic prevalence. The fluoroquinolones, including norfloxacin, ciprofloxacin, and ofloxacin, possess broad-spectrum activity against virtually all important diarrheal pathogens (except *C. difficile*) and thus represent one of the best choices for treatment. (There are few data on the efficacy of levofloxacin.)

The optimal duration of antimicrobial therapy has not been defined with precision. Some authors recommend 3 days of treatment for diarrhea, others 5 days, and others 10 days. Yet there are several studies of patients with severe diarrhea which suggest that a *single* dose is as effective as more prolonged therapy. For example, single-dose tetracycline produced the same results in treating cholera as the standard 2-day treatment.[294] Similarly, a single dose of trimethoprim has the same efficacy in shigellosis as a standard 5-day course.[295] Single-dose fluoroquinolone therapy is highly effective for infections caused by *V. cholerae*, *V. parahaemolyticus*, and most *Shigella* species.[118, 296] On the other hand, short-course treatment of gastroenteritis caused by *Salmonella* with fleroxacin has not been found to be clinically beneficial.[296]

Nonspecific Therapy

The first line of therapeutic defense against acute diarrhea is nonspecific therapy (Table 96–14). Antimotility drugs are

Table 96–14 | **Nonspecific Therapy for Infectious Diarrhea**

Effective
Fluid
Intravenous
Oral rehydration therapy
Food
Continue nutrition intake
Avoid lactose, caffeine, and methylxanthines
Antimotility drugs
Codeine, paregoric, tincture of opium
Loperamide
Diphenoxylate
Bismuth subsalicylate
Lactobacillus GG (may be effective in children with rotaviral diarrhea)
Antisecretory drugs (zaldaride maleate)
Not effective
Lactobacilli
Kaolin, pectin, charcoal
Anticholinergics
Cholestyramine
Hydroxyquinolones (enterovioform, diiodohydroxyquin)

particularly useful in controlling moderate to severe diarrhea. These agents decrease jejunal motor activity, thereby disrupting forward propulsive motility. Opiates may decrease fluid secretion, enhance mucosal absorption, and increase rectal sphincter tone. The overall effect is to normalize fluid transport, slow transit time, reduce fluid losses, and ameliorate abdominal cramping.

Loperamide is arguably the best agent for acute diarrhea because it does not cross the blood–brain barrier, thereby reducing the risk for habituation and for depressing the respiratory center. Treatment with loperamide produces rapid improvement, often within the first day of therapy.[259] Racecadotril, an enkephalinase inhibitor that has both antisecretory and antidiarrheal properties, has been shown to be effective and safe for the treatment of acute watery diarrhea.[297] The concern that an antimotility drug may exacerbate a case of dysentery[298] has largely been dispelled by clinical experience; patients with shigellosis, even a case of *S. dysenteriae* type 1, have been treated inadvertently with loperamide as the only drug and have had a normal resolution without evidence that the illness was prolonged or excretion of the pathogen was delayed.[257] However, these drugs generally should not be used in a patient with acute severe colitis, either infectious or noninfectious in origin, as suggested by bloody mucoid diarrhea or by endoscopy.

Bismuth subsalicylate is effective in treating mild-to-moderate diarrhea.[258] Bismuth subsalicylate is an insoluble complex of trivalent bismuth and salicylate. The drug possesses antimicrobial properties on the basis of the bismuth and antisecretory properties related to the salicylate moiety. In various trials of diarrhea among travelers in Mexico or West Africa, bismuth subsalicylate reduced the frequency of diarrhea significantly over placebo, but results were generally better when a high dose (4.2 g/day) was used.[299]

The combination of an antimicrobial drug and an antimotility drug provides the most rapid relief of diarrhea. In a study of travelers to Mexico, the combined use of loperamide and TMP-SMX curtailed diarrhea in 1 hour, compared with 30 hours with either drug alone or 59 hours with placebo.[259] Even with the severest diarrhea with fecal leukocytes or blood-tinged stool, the median duration of illness was 4.5 hours, a remarkable result in this setting. In a similar study involving U.S. military personnel in Egypt, loperamide added little to the efficacy of ciprofloxacin except in the initial 24 hours, when the combination was slightly better than the antibiotic alone.[260] Yet, the addition of loperamide to ciprofloxacin for the treatment of invasive diarrhea led to a significantly shorter duration of diarrhea and a reduction in the median number of diarrheal stools.[122]

Literally hundreds of antidiarrheal nostrums can be found in pharmacies, apothecary shops, herbal stands, homeopathy stores, soothsayers' booths, witchcraft dispensaries, and assorted medical establishments throughout the world. Each country has its own brand names and labeling requirements. Many products contain a combination of drugs, most of them therapeutically worthless and others potentially dangerous. Various starches, talcs, and chalks have been prescribed for diarrheal illnesses for as long as recorded history. Kaolin and pectin, alone or in combination, are popular remedies. Theoretically, they absorb water and convert a loose stool into a mushy one with lumps. Although this effect may have some aesthetic appeal and perhaps produces a more formed stool, there is no evidence that these preparations diminish intestinal fluid losses.

Because most patients with infectious diarrhea, even with a recognized pathogen, have a mild self-limited course, it follows that neither a stool culture nor specific treatment is required for such cases. For more severe cases, as defined above, empiric antimicrobial therapy with a fluoroquinolone should be instituted, pending results of stool and blood cultures.

TUBERCULOSIS OF THE GASTROINTESTINAL TRACT

Any region of the gastrointestinal tract can be involved with tuberculosis. This complication is still prevalent in the developing countries where tuberculosis is a common health problem. In recent years there has been an upsurge of gastrointestinal tuberculosis in the United States as a result of the influx of immigrants and the AIDS epidemic.[292–295] Unfortunately, the older literature does not separate Crohn's disease from tuberculosis, so there is some confusion about the incidence and clinical course in earlier studies.

Pathogenesis

Mycobacterium tuberculosis is the pathogen responsible for most cases of intestinal tuberculosis, although in some parts of the world cases caused by *M. bovis*, an organism found in dairy products, are still reported. However, *M. bovis* is an uncommon human pathogen in Western countries. The usual route of infection is direct penetration of the intestinal mucosa by swallowed organisms. In the past, intestinal tuberculosis was associated with active pulmonary infection and especially with active laryngeal involvement. Autopsies of patients with pulmonary tuberculosis, before the era of effective treatment, demonstrated intestinal involvement in 55% to 90% of fatal cases. The frequency of intestinal disease was related to the severity of pulmonary involvement: 1% in patients with minimal pulmonary tuberculosis, 4.5% in those with moderately advanced pulmonary disease, and 25% in those with advanced disease. There was also a higher risk of intestinal involvement with pulmonary cavitation and positive sputum smears, again reflecting the risk of a high inoculum of swallowed organisms. In modern series, however, pulmonary involvement is seen in less than 50% of patients with intestinal tuberculosis.[300–302] Indeed, the chest x-ray is unremarkable in most patients now seen with intestinal tuberculosis.

Classification and Distribution of Disease

The most frequent sites of intestinal involvement (75% of cases) are the ileocecum and jejunum. Both sides of the ileocecal valve are usually involved, leading to incompetence of the valve, a finding that distinguishes tuberculosis from Crohn's disease. The other locations of involvement, in order of frequency, are the ascending colon, jejunum, appendix, duodenum, stomach, esophagus, sigmoid colon, and rectum. Multiple areas of the bowel can be affected.

Pathology

The gross appearance of intestinal tuberculosis has been divided into three categories.[300, 301] (1) *Ulcerative* lesions are seen in 60% of patients. There are multiple superficial lesions confined largely to the epithelial surface. The process is highly virulent and in the past was associated with a high mortality rate. (2) *Hypertrophic* lesions occur in 10% of patients. The condition consists of scarring, fibrosis, and heaped-up mass lesions that mimic carcinoma. (3) *Ulcerohypertrophic* lesions are seen in 30% of patients. In this type, mucosal ulcerations are combined with healing and scar formation.

At operation, tuberculous lesions can be recognized by an experienced surgeon. The bowel wall appears thickened, and there is an inflammatory mass surrounding the ileocecal region. Active inflammation is apparent, as are strictures and even fistula formation. The serosal surface is covered with multiple tubercles. The mesenteric lymph nodes frequently are enlarged and thickened; on sectioning, caseous necrosis is seen. The mucosa itself is hyperemic, cobblestoned, edematous, and, in some cases, ulcerated. In contrast to Crohn's disease, the superficial ulcers tend to be circumferential, with the long axis perpendicular to the lumen. When these ulcers heal, the associated fibrosis causes stricture and stenosis of the lumen.

Histologically, the distinguishing lesion is a granuloma (Fig. 96–7). Caseation is not always seen, especially in the mucosa, although caseating granulomas are found with regularity in regional lymph nodes. The muscularis usually is spared. Sections of the involved region show acid-fast bacilli using the Ziehl-Neelsen stain in approximately one third of patients. The organism also can be recovered in a culture of the involved tissues.

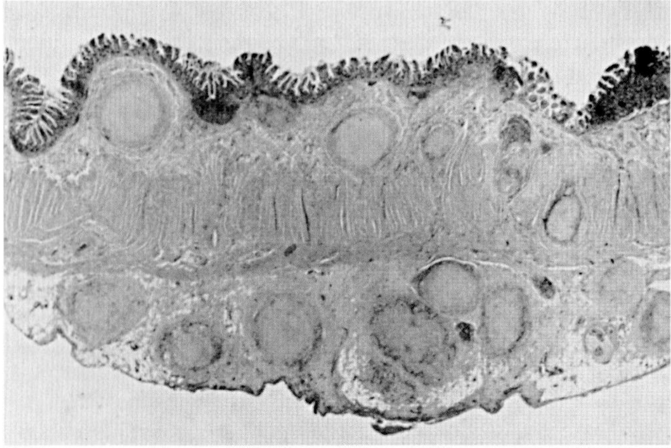

Figure 96–7. Low-power histologic view of tuberculosis of the terminal ileum, showing transmural distribution of multiple caseating granulomas. (Hematoxylin and eosin stain, ×10.)

Clinical Features

Only some patients with intestinal tuberculosis have specific symptoms. The most common complaint is chronic abdominal pain, which is nonspecific in character and is reported in 80% to 90% of patients. Weight loss, fever, diarrhea or constipation, and blood in the stool may be present.[300, 301, 303] An abdominal mass, usually deep and posterior in the right lower quadrant of the abdomen, can be appreciated in approximately two thirds of patients.

Laboratory findings include mild anemia with a normal white blood cell count. The tubercle bacillus can be isolated from the stool in one third of patients, but this finding is not helpful in patients with coexisting pulmonary tuberculosis, in whom it may represent only swallowed organisms.

Complications include intestinal hemorrhage, perforation, obstruction, fistula formation, and malabsorption.[301, 304] Perforation is uncommon but can occur even during treatment. Intestinal obstruction is a more common finding and is typically segmental and stenotic. Surgical intervention may be required to relieve obstruction despite appropriate drug therapy. Malabsorption can occur when obstruction leads to proximal bacterial overgrowth. In the past, involvement of the mesenteric lymphatic system, known as "tabes mesenterica," also was associated with malabsorption.

Diagnosis

The definitive diagnosis of intestinal tuberculosis is made by identification of the organism in tissue, either by direct visualization with an acid-fast stain, by culture of the excised tissue, or by a polymerase chain reaction assay.[302] A presumptive diagnosis can be established in a patient with active pulmonary tuberculosis and radiographic and clinical findings that suggest intestinal involvement. Colonoscopic findings, although nonspecific, consist of superficial areas of ulceration and a nodular friable mucosa.[302, 303] At laparotomy, an experienced surgeon may have a strong suspicion of tuberculosis, although the disease can simulate several other disorders. The tuberculin skin test is less helpful, because a positive test does not necessarily mean active disease. In addition, many patients, especially older persons with weight loss and inanition and those with AIDS, have a negative skin test in the face of active intestinal tuberculosis.

Radiographic examination of the bowel reveals a thickened mucosa with distortion of the mucosal folds, ulcerations, varying degrees of thickening and stenosis of the bowel, and pseudopolyp formation[305, 306] (Fig. 96–8). Computed tomography may show preferential thickening of the ileocecal valve and medial wall of the cecum, extension to the terminal ileum, and massive lymphadenopathy with central necrosis.[305] The cecum is contracted with disease on both sides of the valve, and the valve itself is often distorted and incompetent. Tuberculosis tends to involve short segments of the intestine with stenosis and fistula formation. In the hypertrophic form a mass can be seen that resembles a cecal carcinoma. Calcified mesenteric lymph nodes and an abnormal chest x-ray are other signs that aid in the diagnosis of intestinal tuberculosis.

Several diseases can resemble intestinal tuberculosis. Crohn's disease gives virtually all of the changes of intestinal tuberculosis, except for the presence of the organism, which makes the definitive diagnosis of mycobacterial infection. *Yersinia enterocolitica* can produce mesenteric adenopathy, ulcerations, and thickening of the bowel mucosa. Usually, this infection has a shorter history and resolves spontaneously. Involvement of the cecum with carcinoma or amebiasis can be confused with the tuberculosis. Syphilis and lymphogranuloma venereum should be considered, but intestinal involvement with these infections is now uncommon.

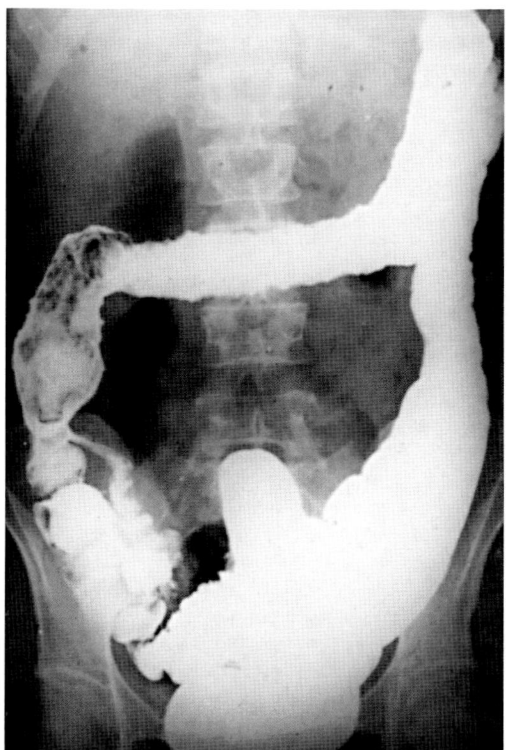

Figure 96–8. A barium enema of a tuberculous colon showing extensive involvement of the cecum and ascending and transverse colon. The ulcerated, narrowed, ahaustral appearance is typical of granulomatous infiltration of the bowel. (Courtesy of H. I. Goldberg, MD, University of California, San Francisco.)

Treatment

Standard antituberculosis treatment gives a high cure rate for intestinal tuberculosis. There are no controlled studies to determine the optimal therapy or duration, but extrapolation from other forms of extrapulmonary tuberculosis suggests that a three-drug regimen for a period of 12 months would be adequate treatment. The drugs are isoniazid (300 mg/day), pyrazinamide (15 to 30 mg/kg/day), and rifampin (600 mg/day). This regimen has not been studied in intestinal tuberculosis. In AIDS patients the course of intestinal tuberculosis is more prolonged and may need treatment with "second-line" drugs because of the high frequency of resistant organisms.

In the past, surgical intervention often was required for intestinal tuberculosis, especially in cases involving the ileocecal region.[307, 308] Obstruction and fistula formation were the leading indications for surgery. In the current era, most fistulas respond to medical management, as do the ulcerative complications. However, mass lesions associated with the hypertrophic form still may necessitate an operative approach, because they can lead to compromise of the lumen, strictures, and eventually complete obstruction.[300, 304] Surgery also may be necessary when free perforation, confined perforation with abscess formation, or massive hemorrhage occur. Because of its similarity to carcinoma of the cecum, undiagnosed ileocolonic tuberculous disease may prompt exploratory laparotomy and right hemicolectomy, although minimal resection is required for tuberculous disease because the condition often improves dramatically with appropriate drug therapy. Complications of surgery for intestinal tuberculosis include obstruction, enterocutaneous fistula, perforation, wound infection, and bleeding.[300, 308] Postoperative pulmonary complications are more common in patients with than without concomitant active pulmonary tuberculosis.[308]

BACTERIAL FOOD POISONING

Bacterial food poisoning is defined as an illness caused by the consumption of food contaminated with bacteria or bacterial toxins. Food poisoning also can be related to parasites (e.g., trichinosis), viruses (e.g., hepatitis), and chemicals (e.g., mushrooms). Food poisoning caused by bacteria constitutes 75% of the outbreaks and 86% of cases in the United States for which an etiology can be determined.[309] However, only 42% of such outbreaks fulfill the microbiologic standards for a confirmed etiology (Table 96–15).

A food-borne disease outbreak is defined by two criteria: similar illness, usually gastrointestinal, in two or more persons and epidemiologic or laboratory investigation that implicates food as the source. The major recognized causes of bacterial food poisoning are limited to 12 bacteria: *Clostridium perfringens*, *Staphylococcus aureus*, *Vibrio* (including *V. cholerae* and *V. parahaemolyticus*), *Bacillus cereus*, *Salmonella*, *Clostridium botulinum*, *Shigella*, toxigenic *E. coli*, and certain species of *Campylobacter*, *Yersinia*, *Listeria*, and *Aeromonas*. Other bacteria, such as group A *Streptococcus* and *Listeria monocytogenes*, have been implicated in some outbreaks (Table 96–16).

In the 1993–1997 reporting period in the United States, 2751 food-borne outbreaks affected more than 86,000 people.[309] Surveillance suggests that the true scope of infection related to food is probably 10 to 100 times more frequent. *Salmonella* outbreaks predominate and constitute over one half of confirmed cases of food-borne illness, in part because of the ease of recognition and awareness of general physicians and the public. *E. coli* is the next most frequent cause of food-borne outbreaks, followed closely by *S. aureus*, *C. perfringens*, and *Shigella*. Several pathogens are rarely reported, namely *Bacillus cereus* and *V. parahaemolyticus*, but have been well studied in other parts of the world. Their contribution to food-borne diarrheal illness in the United States has been recognized only recently, and their recovery from stool or food requires special laboratory procedures.

This section deals with *C. perfringens*, *S. aureus*, *Listeria*, *B. cereus*, and botulism; the other bacterial agents are discussed in previous sections. The causative agents are summarized in Table 96–16.

Clostridium perfringens

C. perfringens is a major food-borne pathogen that produces vomiting and diarrhea in a high percentage of exposed persons. The disease is caused by an enterotoxin elaborated by strains of *C. perfringens* type A. A more severe and often lethal food-borne illness, known variously as enteritis necroticans (Darmbrand) and pigbel, is caused by *C. perfringens* type C. (This group of diseases is discussed later.)

Microbiology

Clostridia are Gram-positive, spore-forming, obligate anaerobes that can be found in the intestinal flora of humans and animals and in the soil. Although all species of clostridia grow better under anaerobic conditions, *C. perfringens* is remarkably aerotolerant and survives exposure to oxygen for as long as 72 hours. It was originally thought that food poisoning strains were heat resistant and hemolytic, but it is now clear that heat-sensitive and nonhemolytic strains can cause this illness as well.

C. perfringens produces 12 toxins, which are mostly ac-

Table 96–15 | **Estimates of Rates of Food-borne Illnesses and Mortality in the United States**

PATHOGEN	ESTIMATED TOTAL CASES	FOOD-BORNE TRANSMISSION (%)	NO. OF DEATHS	CASE FATALITY RATE
Bacterial				
Brucella spp.	1554	50	11	0.05
Campylobacter spp.	2,453,926	80	124	0.001
E. coli O157:H7 (EHEC)	73,480	85	61	0.0083
E. coli, non-O157:H7 (EHEC)	36,740	85	30	0.0083
Listeria monocytogenes	2,518	99	504	0.2
Salmonella typhi	824	80	3	0.004
Salmonella, nontyphoidal	1,412,498	95	582	0.0078
Shigella spp.	448,240	20	70	0.0016
Noncholera *Vibrio* spp.	7,880	65	20	0.025
Vibrio vulnificus	94	50	37	0.39
Yersinia enterocolitica	96,368	90	3	0.0005
Toxin mediated				
Bacillus cereus	27,360	100	0	0
Clostridium botulinum (food botulism)	58	100	4	0.0769
Clostridium perfringens	248,520	100	7	0.0005
Staphylococcal food poisoning	185,060	100	2	0.0002
Streptococcal food poisoning	50,920	100	0	0.0000
Parasitic				
Cryptosporidium parvum	300,000	10	66	0.005
Cyclospora cayetanensis	16,264	90	0	0.0005
Giardia lamblia	2,000,000	10	10	<0.0001
Toxoplasma gondii	225,000	50	750	<0.0001
Trichinella spiralis	52	100	0	0.003
Viral				
Norwalk-like viruses	23,000,000	40	310	<0.0001
Rotavirus	3,900,000	1	30	<0.0001
Astrovirus	3,900,000	1	10	<0.0001
Hepatitis A virus	83,391	5	83	0.003
Grand Total	38,629,641		1809	

EHEC, enterohemorrhagic *E. coli.*
From Mead PS, Slutsker L, Dietz V, et al. Food-related illness and death in the United States. Emerg Infect Dis 5:607, 1999, with permission.

Table 96–16 | **Characteristics of Bacterial Food Poisoning**

ORGANISM	COMMON VEHICLES	MEDIAN INCUBATION IN HOURS (RANGE)	TOXIN, PRIMARY IN PATHOGENESIS	CLINICAL FEATURES	MEDIAN DURATION, DAYS (RANGE)	SECONDARY ATTACK RATE (%)	SOURCES OF DIAGNOSTIC MATERIAL	LABORATORY DIAGNOSIS
Bacillus cereus	Fried rice, vanilla sauce, cream, meatballs, boiled beef, barbecued chicken	2 (1–16) 9 (6–14)	Heat-stable Heat-labile	V, C, D (33%) D, C, V	0.4 (0.2–0.5) 1 (1–2)	— —	Vomitus, stool, food	>10^5 Colonies on peptone-beef extract egg yolk agar; need controls for stool analysis (may be normal flora), serotyping
Clostridium perfringens	Beef, turkey, chicken	12 (8–22)	Heat-labile	D, C (N, V, F rare)	1 (0.3–3)	—	Stool, rectal swab; food, food-contact surfaces	Egg yolk–free tryptose-sulfite-cycloserine agar; Hobbs or bacteriocin typing
Vibrio parahaemolyticus	Seafood, rarely salt water or salted vegetables	12 (2–48)	?	D, C, N, V, H, F (25%), B (rare)	3 (2–10)	—	Stool, rectal swab; food, food-contact surfaces; seawater	TCBS agar; test for Kanagawa phenomenon (see text), serotyping
Staphylococcus aureus	Ham, pork, canned beef, cream-filled pastry	3 (1–6)	Heat-stable	V, N, C, D, F (rare)	1 (0.3–1.5)	—	Stool, vomitus; food or food-contact surfaces; nose, hands, purulent lesion on food preparer	Egg yolk–tellurite–glycine–pyruvate agar or mannitol salt; phage type isolates; enterotoxin testing
Yersinia enterocolitica	Chocolate milk or raw milk, pork	72 (2–144)	Heat-stable	F, C, D, V, pharyngitis, arthritis, mesenteric adenitis, rashes	7 (2–30)	20	Stool from food preparer	Cold enrichment; serotyping, serology
Listeria monocytogenes	Milk, raw vegetables, cole slaw, dairy products, poultry, beef	?	?	D, F, C, N, V, B	?	10	Stool, rectal swab	Cold enrichment, nutrient broth potassium thiocyanate and nalidixic acid
Campylobacter jejuni	Milk, chicken, pet animals, beef	48 (24–240)	?	D, F, C, B, H, M, N, V	7 (2–30)	25	Stool, rectal swab	*Brucella* agar base with vancomycin, polymixin, and trimethoprim grown in reduced oxygen
Escherichia coli	Salads, beef	24 (8–44) 96 (24–120)	Heat-labile Heat-stable Verotoxin	D, C, N, H, F, M F, M, D, C B, C, F, hemolytic-uremic syndrome	3 (1–4)	0	Stool, rectal swab	MacConkey media: *E. coli* must be tested for toxin production: serotyping
Salmonella	Eggs, meat, poultry	24 (5–72)	—	D, C, N, V, F, H, B (rare), enteric fever	3 (0.5–14)	30–50	Stool, rectal swab from patients and food-preparation workers; raw food	*Salmonella-Shigella* (SS), deoxycholate-citrate, Hektoen enteric, or xylose-lysine-deoxycholate; phage typing for *S. typhimurium*
Shigella	Milk, salads (potato, tuna, turkey)	24 (7–168)	—	C, F, D, B, H, N, V	3 (0.5–14)	40–60	Stool, rectal swab from patients, food workers; food	Same media as for *Salmonella;* colicin typing

B, bloody diarrhea; C, crampy abdominal pain; D, diarrhea; F, fever; H, headache; M, myalgia; N, nausea; V, vomiting; TCBS, thiosulfate citrate bile salts sucrose.
From Snydman DR. Food poisoning. In Gorbach SL, Bartlett JG, Blacklow NR (eds): Infectious Diseases. Philadelphia, WB Saunders, 1992, p. 771 with permission.

tive in tissues, as well as several enterotoxins. Food poisoning is caused by a heat-labile protein enterotoxin with a molecular weight of 35,000. The enterotoxin is a structural component of the spore coat and is formed during sporulation; it causes fluid accumulation in the rabbit ileal loop model.[310] Although both cholera vibrios and *C. perfringens* produce enterotoxins, the enterotoxins differ in several respects. Clostridial enterotoxin has its maximum activity in the ileum and minimal activity in the duodenum, opposite to that of cholera toxin. Clostridial enterotoxin inhibits glucose transport, damages the intestinal epithelium, and causes protein loss into the intestinal lumen, none of which is observed with cholera toxin.[311]

Epidemiology

Epidemics are characterized by high attack rates, with a large number of affected persons, usually 40 to 50 per outbreak. The incubation period in most outbreaks varies from 8 to 14 hours but can be as long as 22 hours. Such outbreaks are most frequently reported from institutions or after large gatherings. The pathogenesis of infection requires a meat or poultry dish to be precooked and then reheated to be served. Beef, turkey, and chicken are the most frequent vehicles of infection.

Pathogenic Mechanisms

In almost every outbreak of clostridial food poisoning, roasted, boiled, stewed, or steamed meats or poultry is the vehicle of infection. Usually, the meat is cooked in bulk so that heat gain and internal pressure are insufficient to kill the spores. The implicated food invariably undergoes a period of inadequate cooling, at which time the food is in a reduced rather than oxidized state that allows the spores to germinate, usually below 50°C. Unless the food is reheated to a very high temperature, it will contain many viable organisms.

Once the organisms endure the initial heating, they must be ingested in large quantities to cause disease. It also appears that older cultures are more readily able to withstand the acid pH of the stomach than younger cultures. Therefore, food that has been allowed to cool for some period of time may be a better medium for producing disease.

Clinical Features

C. perfringens food poisoning is characterized by watery diarrhea and severe crampy abdominal pain, usually without vomiting, beginning 8 to 24 hours after the incriminating meal. Fever, chills, headache, or other signs of infection usually are absent. The illness is of short duration—usually less than 24 hours. Rare fatalities have been recorded in debilitated or hospitalized patients.[312]

Treatment

No specific treatment is required for this illness. The symptoms last no longer than 24 to 36 hours.

Enteritis Necroticans

This disease was described originally in post–World War II Germany, in an outbreak affecting over 400 people who consumed rancid meat. Similar outbreaks, associated with the consumption of poorly cooked pork, have been described in New Guinea and are labeled pigbel.[313] The disease is caused by strains of *C. perfringens* type C, which elaborate an enterotoxin similar, and possibly identical, to that of type A strains.

Outbreaks of pigbel have been related to orgiastic consumption of pig in large native feasts. The pig is improperly cooked, and large quantities are consumed over 3 or 4 days. Other cases, most often in children under 10 years of age, occur in villages. Enteritis necroticans associated with the consumption of chitterlings is encountered rarely in the United States.[314]

Compared with the usual form of clostridial food poisoning seen in the United States and Europe, pigbel is a more severe necrotizing disease of the small intestine with a high mortality rate. After a 24-hour incubation period, the illness ensues, with intense abdominal pain, distention, bloody diarrhea, vomiting, and shock. The mortality rate in this disease is approximately 40%, usually resulting from intestinal perforation.

Staphylococcus aureus

Coagulase-positive strains of *S. aureus* is the third most common cause of food poisoning in the United States, and before 1973, it was the leading cause.

Microbiology

Five immunologically distinct enterotoxins have been associated with food-poisoning strains of *S. aureus*. These enterotoxins, termed A, B, C, D, and E, are heat-resistant single polypeptide chains that range in molecular weight from 28,000 to 34,000. When tested in a rat intestinal loop model, net secretion of water and electrolytes is observed.[315] Vomiting is induced in monkeys and in human volunteers with the enterotoxins or culture filtrates of the organism.

Epidemiology

Staphylococcal food poisoning has a short incubation period, approximately 3 hours with a range of 1 to 6 hours. The disease usually is clustered within a family or group, with a high attack rate. Many foods have been implicated in this form of food poisoning. However, foods with a high salt concentration, such as ham or canned meat, or a high sugar content, such as custard and cream, selectively favor the growth of staphylococci. A multistate outbreak of staphylococcal food poisoning was found to originate from imported canned mushrooms.[316] The major mode of transmission is from a food handler to the food product. Involved foods usually have been cut, sliced, grated, mixed, or ground by workers who are carriers of toxin-producing strains of *S. aureus*.

Pathogenic Mechanisms

Three requisites for staphylococcal food poisoning are (1) contamination of a food with enterotoxin-producing staphylococci, (2) suitable growth requirements of the food for the organism, and (3) a suitable time and temperature for the organism to multiply.

The emetic dose of enterotoxin A or B for human beings has been estimated to be between 1 and 25 μg (assuming 100 g of food is consumed). Clearly, people have different sensitivities to the enterotoxins, because studies in volunteers show a varying dose response among individuals. However, in outbreaks in which the concentration of toxin is high in the implicated food, the attack rate approaches 100%.

Clinical Features

The symptoms of staphylococcal food poisoning are primarily profuse vomiting, nausea, and abdominal cramps, often followed by diarrhea. Vomiting is the dominant initial symptom and can lead to a severe metabolic alkalosis. Rarely, hypotension and marked prostration occur. Fever is not common, but a low-grade fever may be present in severe cases. Fatalities are unusual, and recovery is complete within 24 to 48 hours.

Treatment

Most people with staphylococcal food poisoning suffer in silence, without reporting their symptoms to a physician. More severe cases may require supportive care, particularly rehydration and correction of alkalosis. No specific therapy is available.

Listeria

Listeria are Gram-positive highly motile bacilli that are relatively heat resistant. They have been isolated from the intestinal tract of humans and animals and from sewage and well water. Cases can occur as part of an outbreak or on a sporadic basis. In reported epidemics, the vehicles of infection have been raw and pasteurized milk, soft cheeses, cole slaw, shrimp, rice salad, pork dishes, and raw vegetables.[317, 318] *Listeria* can be cultured from raw poultry, beef, or pork; prepackaged meat products; cheeses; and raw vegetables.[319]

Listeriosis is usually a systemic disease associated with bacteremia that can seed the meninges, heart valves, or various organs. Intestinal symptoms such as diarrhea and cramping often precede fever and bacteremia. Immunocompetent hosts occasionally develop gastroenteritis characterized by fever, headache, abdominal pain, nausea, and diarrhea; this form of listeriosis usually is not complicated by bacteremia.[320]

Among the food-borne pathogens, *Listeria* have been associated with the highest mortality rates; 70 deaths were reported from 1983 to 1987, for a case-fatality rate of 27%. Neurologic sequelae may occur in a sizeable proportion of survivors of central nervous system listeriosis. The propensity of the organism to attack immunosuppressed persons and pregnant women may account for the severity of the infection.

Bacillus cereus

B. cereus is an aerobic, spore-forming, Gram-positive rod that has been associated with two clinical types of food poisoning—a *diarrhea* syndrome and a *vomiting* syndrome.[321] The organisms responsible for the two syndromes produce distinct toxins and have different epidemiologies.

Diarrhea Syndrome

The original report of *B. cereus* as a cause of diarrheal disease was associated with consumption of contaminated meatballs in a sanatorium. Subsequent studies have demonstrated that an enterotoxin produced by this organism causes fluid accumulation in the rabbit ileal loop. The mechanism appears to be activation of adenylate cyclase in intestinal epithelial cells, similar to the action of cholera toxin. Cultures of the strains elaborating this enterotoxin cause diarrhea when fed to rhesus monkeys.

The median incubation period appears to be 9 hours, with a range of 6 to 14 hours. The clinical illness is characterized by diarrhea (96%), generalized cramps (75%), and vomiting (23%).[321] Fever is uncommon. The duration of illness ranges from 20 to 36 hours, with a median of 24 hours. The strains of *B. cereus* associated with diarrhea are found in approximately 25% of many foodstuffs sampled, including cream, pudding meat, spices, dried potatoes, dried milk, vanilla sauces, and spaghetti sauces, all of which are contaminated before cooking.[322] If the food is prepared so that the temperature is maintained at 30°C to 50°C, vegetative growth is permitted. Spores can survive extreme temperatures, and when allowed to cool relatively slowly, they germinate, multiply, and elaborate toxin. There is no evidence that human carriage of the organism or other means of contamination plays a role in transmission.

Whether the diarrheogenic heat-labile enterotoxin is actually ingested or produced in vivo is not known; however, several pieces of evidence favor the latter mechanism. The incubation of diarrheal illness is too long for preformed toxin, and a large inoculum (10^6) is required to cause illness, an observation which suggests that intestinal colonization is required.

Vomiting Syndrome

Although the organism associated with the vomiting disease appears to be the same, a different type of toxin has been implicated.[323] Cell-free culture filtrates from these strains do not produce fluid accumulation in the rabbit ileal loop nor do they stimulate adenylate cyclase; however, they produce vomiting when fed to rhesus monkeys. This vomiting toxin is stable to heat.

The vomiting syndrome has a short incubation period of approximately 2 hours. Virtually all affected persons have vomiting and abdominal cramps. Diarrhea is present in only one third. The duration of illness ranges from 8 to 10 hours with a median of 9 hours; the illness usually is mild and self-limited. Nearly all reported cases involving the vomiting toxin have implicated fried rice as the vehicle.[321]

In England, almost 90% of uncooked rice was found to be colonized by *B. cereus*, although the number of organisms was relatively low.[324] The disease has been ascribed to the common practice in Chinese restaurants of allowing large portions of boiled rice to drain unrefrigerated to avoid clumping. Flash-frying during the final preparation of the fried rice does not produce enough heat to destroy apparently preformed heat-stable toxin. It appears that the emetic illness is caused by preformed toxin, because the incubation period is short, and there is an extremely high attack rate approaching 100% in outbreaks.

Botulism

Botulism is a rare food-borne disease resulting from exposure to neurotoxins secreted by strains of *Clostridium botulinum*. Between 1993 and 1997, there were 13 outbreaks of botulism in the United States, accounting for 56 cases and 1 death.[309] Although food-borne botulism is relatively uncommon, it is the most lethal of all the bacterial toxin-mediated food-borne diseases and the only one for which specific effective therapy is available.

Epidemiology

During the past few decades, food-borne botulism has become the least common form of botulism, behind wound and infant botulism. Food-borne botulism develops after the ingestion of preformed toxin in inadequately preserved canned vegetables, salsas, meats, and fish. A disproportionate number of recent cases have occurred in the Pacific Northwest and Alaska, and cases have been associated with native American foods such as whale or seal that have been fermented or preserved with traditional methods. Recent outbreaks in the United States have been associated with baked potatoes, cheese sauce, beef stew, and garlic cooking oil.[325]

Infant botulism develops in infants whose gastrointestinal tract becomes colonized with live *C. botulinum* bacteria, which secrete small amounts of botulinum toxin. Absorption of low concentrations of the toxin leads to lethargy, poor feeding, constipation, diminished muscle tone, and a weak cry. The source of the botulinum toxin is not clear; household dust, soil, and honey in feedings have been suggested as possible sources.

Pathogenic Mechanisms

C. botulinum and closely related species of clostridia produce heat-resistant spores that are capable of surviving food preservation techniques that destroy nonsporulating organisms. The seven serologically distinct botulinum toxins are designated with the letters A to G. Neutralization by type-specific serologic reagents is used to differentiate the different serotypes. Types A, B, and E are responsible for most human cases of botulism.[326] Neurotoxin-producing strains of *C. butyricum* and *C. baratii* are less commonly responsible for human botulism. Toxin production occurs in the presence of anaerobic, low solute, and low acid conditions.

C. botulinum is usually unable to replicate in the mature human gut, although the toxin is acid-stable and easily traverses the gastric barrier intact. After absorption, the botulinum toxin binds irreversibly to presynaptic cholinergic nerve endings of the cranial and peripheral nerves, thereby resulting in inhibition of the release of acetylcholine and the characteristic clinical syndrome that results from the blockade of voluntary motor and autonomic cholinergic junctions.

Clinical Features

The ingestion of botulinum toxin results initially in gastrointestinal symptoms, including nausea, vomiting, abdominal pain, and diarrhea, usually within 18 to 36 hours after toxin ingestion.[325] Once neurologic symptoms develop, constipation is common. Dry mouth, diplopia, and blurred vision are followed by dysarthria, dysphonia, dysphagia, and peripheral muscle weakness. The typical symmetric descending paralysis starts with the cranial nerves and then affects the upper extremities, respiratory muscles, and finally lower extremities. Respiratory muscle paralysis may result in respiratory failure and death if mechanical ventilation is not instituted; higher cortical functions are unaffected.

Diagnosis

Botulism should be suspected in any patient with the acute onset of gastrointestinal, autonomic nervous system, and cranial nerve dysfunction, especially if the patient has recently consumed foods that were home-canned. Results of magnetic resonance imaging or computed tomography of the brain and lumbar puncture are normal in patients with botulism, whereas electromyography may show characteristic abnormalities. If food-borne botulism is suspected, stool, serum, and implicated foods should be tested for botulinum neurotoxin by the mouse inoculation test.

Treatment

Supportive therapy with mechanical ventilation has helped to reduce mortality rates from botulism greatly during the past several decades. The diagnosis of botulism must be considered early in any case of unexplained paralysis, and antitoxin should be administered if the diagnosis is credible. The trivalent equine botulinum antitoxin is available only through the Centers for Disease Control and Prevention, which maintains supplies of antitoxin at sites around the country for immediate release in case of an emergency. To obtain the antitoxin, physicians need to contact their state health department's emergency hotline or the CDC directly (telephone no. 404-639-2206).

Speed is of the essence, because the antitoxin cannot displace the toxin once it has bound to the presynaptic nerve terminal but serves only to bind free toxin in circulation. Once symptoms have developed, the utility of the antitoxin is greatly reduced. In a large retrospective analysis of 134 cases of botulinum toxin A–mediated disease, patients who received antitoxin therapy early in the course had a mortality rate of 10%, as opposed to 15% in those who received the antitoxin more than 24 hours after the onset of symptoms and 46% in those who did not receive antitoxin at all.[327] Moreover, patients who received antitoxin stayed in the hospital an average of 10 days, compared with 56 days for the untreated group.

The current recommendation is to administer a single 10-mL dose of intravenous antitoxin to each exposed person. This recommendation is based on the calculation that each vial has enough neutralizing antibody (for types A, B, and E) to bind a titer of toxin that is 100 times greater than the highest titer documented to date by the CDC. Multidose protocols are no longer recommended, because they have been associated with hypersensitivity reactions in 9% of patients; it is hoped (although as yet unproven) that the single-dose protocol will decrease the rate of this complication.

Bacillus anthracis

Although most anthrax infections are the result of cutaneous exposure to or inhalation of infected spores, the ingestion of infected animal tissue can lead to gastrointestinal disease.

Microbiology

B. anthracis is an aerobic, gram-positive spore-forming, nonmotile bacillus that is found in soil. Endospores can remain dormant in soil for many years. Anthrax spores germinate in nutrient rich environments. Vegetative anthrax bacilli elaborate an antiphagocytic polyglutamyl capsule and a toxin complex that is composed of protective antigen, lethal factor, and edema factor.[328] Protective antigen acts as the binding site for the lethal and edema factors. The lethal toxin stimulates macrophages to release TNF-α and interleukin-1. The release of these cytokines contributes to death from toxemia in anthrax infections characterized by high-grade bacteremia. The edema factor is a calmodulin-dependent adenylate cyclase, which is responsible for the development of edema at the site of infection and for inhibition of neutrophil function.

Epidemiology

The consumption of endospore-contaminated meat from infected animals is the primary mode of transmission of gastrointestinal anthrax. Point source outbreaks within households are common. This form of anthrax has never been conclusively documented in the United States, presumably because livestock are vaccinated for anthrax in regions endemic for the disease and because animals are routinely inspected by federal and state meat inspectors. Interestingly, a recent outbreak of gastrointestinal illness characterized by diarrhea, abdominal pain, and fever was identified in two family members who had consumed meat from a carcass that was found to be contaminated with *B. anthracis*.[329] Fortunately, the infections were mild and self-limited.

Pathogenic Mechanisms

Entry of endospores through the gastrointestinal mucosa initiates infection. Macrophages phagocytose ingested endospores, which then germinate to form vegetative bacteria in mesenteric lymph nodes. The bacteria are then released from the macrophages, multiply in the local lymphatic systems, and enter the bloodstream. The release of the exotoxin complexes results in local tissue damage with massive edema, mucosal ulcerations, and the development of systemic toxemia.

Clinical Features

Approximately 1 to 7 days after the ingestion of raw or undercooked meat from infected animals, gastrointestinal anthrax develops. Initial symptoms include nausea, vomiting, abdominal pain, and fever. Patients often rapidly develop worsening manifestations characterized by bloody diarrhea, diffuse abdominal pain with rebound tenderness, and, occasionally, hematemesis. Ascites, which may be purulent, develops 2 to 4 days later. More than 50% of episodes are fatal, with death occurring as a consequence of toxemia, intestinal perforation, or shock from hemorrhage and fluid losses.

Oropharygeal anthrax is a less common form of infection that develops when spores are deposited in the oropharynx. Symptoms include fever, a severely sore throat, and dysphagia, which may progress to respiratory distress. Examination often reveals swelling of the neck, lymphadenitis, and pharyngeal ulcers covered by a pseudomembrane. Despite the relatively severe symptoms, this form of infection tends to be milder than gastrointestinal disease and is rarely fatal.

Treatment and Prevention

Because some strains of *B. anthracis* contain an inducible beta-lactamase, initial therapy should consist of ciprofloxacin. Because the risk of mortality is elevated in severe cases, the addition of rifampin or clindamycin, or both, is recommended. Penicillin and doxycycline are both highly active against *B. anthracis* in the absence of resistance. An anthrax vaccine, consisting of a sterile filtrate of an attenuated strain of the organism, is available to the U.S. military but not to civilians. The vaccine's protective component is the protective antigen. Although the vaccine has been shown to be effective in protecting monkeys in challenge experiments, the six-dose regimen with yearly boosters is cumbersome.

REFERENCES

1. Garthright WE, Archer DL, Kvenberg JE. Estimates of incidence and costs of intestinal infectious diseases in the United States. Public Health Rep 103:107, 1988.
2. Glass RI, Lew JF, Gangarosa RE, et al. Estimates of morbidity and mortality rates for diarrheal diseases in American children. J Pediatr 118:S27, 1991.
3. Simon GL, Gorbach SL. Normal alimentary tract microflora. In Blaser MJ, Smith PD, Ravdin JI, et al. (eds): Infections of the Gastrointestinal Tract. New York, Raven Press, 1995, p 53.
4. Nataro JP, Kaper JB. Diarrheagenic *Escherichia coli*. Clin Microbiol Rev 11:142, 1998.
5. Blake PA, Allegra DT, Snyder JD, et al. Cholera—a possible endemic focus in the United States. N Engl J Med 310:305, 1980.
6. Ramamurthy T, Garg S, Sharma R, et al. Emergence of novel strain of *Vibrio cholerae* with epidemic potential in southern and eastern India. Lancet 341:703, 1993.
7. Cholera Working Group. Large epidemic of cholera-like disease in Bangladesh caused by *Vibrio cholerae* 0139 synonym Bengal. Lancet 342:387, 1993.
8. Johnson JA, Salles CA, Panigrahi P, et al. *Vibrio cholerae* 0139 synonym Bengal is closely related to *Vibrio cholerae* El Tor but has important differences. Infect Immun 62:2108, 1994.
9. Waldor MK, Mekalanos J. Lysogenic conversion by a filamentous phage encoding cholera toxin. Science 272:1910, 1996.
10. Fasano A, Baudry B, Pumplin DW, et al. *Vibrio cholerae* produces a second enterotoxin which affects intestinal tight junctions. Proc Natl Acad Sci U S A 88:5242, 1991.
11. World Health Organization. Cholera, 1999. Wkly Epidemiol Rec 75: 249, 2000.
12. Morris JG, Black RE. Cholera and other vibrios in the United States. N Engl J Med 312:343, 1985.
13. Update: *Vibrio cholerae* 01-Western hemisphere, 1991–1994, and *V. cholerae* 0139-Asia, 1994. MMWR Morb Mortal Wkly Rep 44:215, 1995.
14. Ries AA, Vugia DJ, Beingolea L, et al. Cholera in Piura, Peru: a modern urban epidemic. J Infect Dis 166:1429, 1992.
15. Mujica OJ, Quick RE, Palacios AM, et al. Epidemic cholera in the Amazon: the role of produce in disease risk and prevention. J Infect Dis 169:1381, 1994.
16. Morris JG, Losonsky GE, Johnson JA, et al. Clinical and immunologic characteristics of *Vibrio cholerae* 0139 Bengal infection in North American volunteers. J Infect Dis 171:903, 1995.
17. Basu A, Garg P, Datta S, et al. *Vibrio cholerae* 0139 in Calcutta,

1992–1998: incidence, antibiograms, and genotypes. Emerg Infect Dis 6:139, 2000.
18. Herrington DA, Hall RH, Losonsky G, et al. Toxin, toxin-coregulated pili and the toxR regulon are essential for *Vibrio cholerae* pathogenesis in humans. J Exp Med 168:1487, 1989.
19. World Health Organization. Guidelines for cholera control. Geneva, Switzerland, World Health Organization, Programme for control of diarrhoeal disease. WHO/CCD/SER/80.4 Rev. 2, 1991.
20. Centers for Disease Control and Prevention. Update: cholera—Western Hemisphere, and recommendations for treatment of cholera. MMWR Morb Mortal Wkly Rep 40:562, 1991.
21. Gotuzzo E, Seas C, Echevarria J, et al. Ciprofloxacin for the treatment of cholera: a randomized, double-blind, controlled clinical trial of a single daily dose in Peruvian adults. Clin Infect Dis 20:1485, 1995.
22. Khan WA, Bennish ML, Seas C, et al. Randomised controlled comparison of single-dose ciprofloxacin and doxycycline for cholera caused by *Vibrio cholerae* 01 or 0139. Lancet 348:296, 1996.
23. Hamer DH, Gorbach SL. Use of the quinolones for the treatment and prophylaxis of bacterial infections. In Andriole VT (ed): The Quinolones, 3rd ed. San Diego, Academic Press, 2000.
24. Joo I. Cholera vaccines. In Barua D, Burrows W (eds): Cholera. Philadelphia, WB Saunders, 1975, p 335.
25. Sanchez JL, Vasquez B, Begue RE, et al. Protective efficacy of oral whole-cell/recombinant-B-subunit cholera vaccine in Peruvian military recruits. Lancet 344:1273, 1994.
26. Taylor DN, Cárdenas V, Sanchez JL, et al. Two-year study of the protective efficacy of the oral whole cell plus recombinant B subunit cholera vaccine in Peru. J Infect Dis 181:1667, 2000.
27. Tacket CO, Losonsky G, Nataro JP, et al. Initial clinical studies of CVD 112 *Vibrio cholerae* 0139 live oral vaccine: safety and efficacy against experimental challenge. J Infect Dis 172:883, 1995.
28. Tacket CO, Cohen MB, Wasserman SS, et al. Randomized, double-blind, placebo-controlled, multicentered trial of a single dose of live oral cholera vaccine CVD 103-HgR in preventing cholera following challenge with *Vibrio cholerae* O1 El Tor Inaba three months after vaccination. Infect Immun 67:6341, 1999.
29. Richie E, Punjabi NH, Sidharta Y, et al. Efficacy trial of single-dose live oral cholera vaccine CVD 103-HgR in North Jakarta, Indonesia, a cholera-endemic area. Vaccine 18:2399, 2000.
30. Hlady WG, Klontz KC. The epidemiology of *Vibrio* infections in Florida, 1981–1993. J Infect Dis 173:1176, 1996.
31. Blake PA, Weaver RE, Hollis DG. Diseases of humans (other than cholera) caused by vibrios. Annu Rev Microbiol 34:341, 1980.
32. Shapiro RL, Altekruse S, Hutwagner L, et al. and the Vibrio Working Group. The role of Gulf Coast oysters harvested in warmer months in *Vibrio vulnificus* infections in the United States, 1988–1996. J Infect Dis 178:752, 1998.
33. Lowry PW, McFarland LM, Peltier BH, et al. Vibrio gastroenteritis in Louisiana: a prospective study among attendees of a scientific congress in New Orleans. J Infect Dis 160:978, 1989.
34. Hoge CW, Watsky D, Peeler RN, et al. Epidemiology and spectrum of vibrio infections in a Chesapeake Bay community. J Infect Dis 160: 985, 1989.
35. Calia FM, Johnson DE. Bacteremia in suckling rabbits after oral challenge with *Vibrio parahaemolyticus*. Infect Immun 11:1222, 1975.
36. Daniels NA, MacKinnon L, Bishop R, et al. *Vibrio parahaemolyticus* infections in the United States, 1973–1998. J Infect Dis 181:1661, 2000.
37. Daniels NA, Ray B, Easton A, et al. Emergence of a new *Vibrio parahaemolyticus* serotype in raw oysters. A prevention quandary. J Am Med Assoc 284:1541, 2000.
38. Hughes JM, Hollis DG, Gangarosa EJ, et al. Non-cholera vibrio infections in the United States. Ann Intern Med 88:602, 1978.
39. Dalsgaard A, Albert MJ, Taylor DN, et al. Characterization of *Vibrio cholerae* non-01 serogroups obtained from an outbreak of diarrhea in Lima, Peru. J Clin Microbiol 33:2715, 1995.
40. Klontz KC, Lieb S, Schreiber M, et al. Syndromes of *Vibrio vulnificus* infections: clinical and epidemiologic features in Florida cases, 1981–1987. Ann Intern Med 109:318, 1988.
41. Shandera WX, Johnston JM, Davis BR, et al. Disease from infection with *Vibrio mimicus*, a newly recognized vibrio species. Ann Intern Med 99:169, 1983.
42. Hansen W, Freney J, Benyagoub H, et al. Severe human infections caused by *Vibrio metschnikovii*. J Clin Microbiol 31:2529, 1993.
43. Janda JM, Abbott SL. Unusual food-borne pathogens. *Listeria monocytogenes*, *Aeromonas*, *Plesiomonas*, and *Edwardsiella* species. Clin Lab Med 19:553, 1999.
44. Namdari H, Bonnone EJ. Microbiologic and clinical evidence supporting the role of *Aeromonas caviae* as a pediatric enteric pathogen. J Clin Microbiol 28:837, 1990.
45. Namdari H, Bottone EJ. Cytotoxin and enterotoxin production as factors delineating enteropathogenicity of *Aeromonas caviae*. J Clin Microbiol 28:1796, 1990.
46. Holmberg SD, Schell WL, Fanning GR, et al. *Aeromonas* infections in the United States. Ann Intern Med 105:683, 1986.
47. Gracey M, Burke V, Robinson J. *Aeromonas*-associated gastroenteritis. Lancet 2:1304, 1982.
48. Holmberg SD, Farmer JJ III. *Aeromonas hydrophila* and *Plesiomonas shigelloides* as causes of intestinal infections. Rev Infect Dis 6:633, 1984.
49. Jones BL, Wilcox MH. Aeromonas infections and their treatment. J Antimicrob Chemother 35:453, 1995.
50. Brenden RA, Miller A, Janda JM. Clinical disease spectrum and pathogenic factors associated with *Plesiomonas shigelloides* infections in humans. Rev Infect Dis 10:303, 1988.
51. Holmberg SD, Wachsmuth K, Hickman-Brenner FW, et al. *Blake PA and Farmer JJ III*. Plesiomonas enteric infections in the United States. Ann Intern Med 105:690, 1986.
52. Levine MM, Edelman R. Enteropathogenic *Escherichia coli* of classic serotypes associated with infant diarrhea: epidemiology and pathogenesis. Epidemiol Rev 6:31, 1984.
53. Donnenberg MS, Kaper JB. Enteropathogenic *Escherichia coli*. Infect Immun 60:3953, 1992.
54. Levine MM, Nataro JP, Karch H, et al. The diarrheal response of humans to some classic serotypes of enteropathogenic *Escherichia coli* is dependent on a plasmid encoding an enteroadhesiveness factor. J Infect Dis 152:550, 1985.
55. Donnenberg MS, Tacket CO, James SP, et al. Role of the *eaeA* gene in experimental enteropathogenic *Escherichia coli* infection. J Clin Invest 92:1412, 1993.
56. Jerse AE, Kaper JB. The *eae* gene of enteropathogenic *Escherichia coli* encodes a 94-kilodalton membrane protein, the expression of which is influenced by the EAF plasmid. Infect Immun 59:4302, 1991.
57. Jerse AE, Martin WC, Galen JE, et al. Oligonucleotide probe for detection of the enteropathogenic *Escherichia coli* (EPEC) adherence factor of localized adherent EPEC. J Clin Microbiol 28:2842, 1990.
58. Tardelli TA, Rassi V, MacDonald KL, et al. Enteropathogens associated with acute diarrheal disease in urban infants in Sao Paulo, Brazil. J Infect Dis 164:331, 1991.
59. Levine MM, Ferreccio C, Prado V, et al. Epidemiologic studies of *Escherichia coli* diarrheal infections in a low socioeconomic level peri-urban community in Santiago, Chile. Am J Epidemiol 138:849, 1993.
60. Germani Y, Bégaud E, Duval P, et al. Prevalence of enteropathogenic, enteroaggregative, and diffusely adherent *Escherichia coli* among isolates from children with diarrhea in New Caledonia. J Infect Dis 174: 1124, 1996.
61. Clements JD, Finkelstein RA. Immunological cross-reactivity between a heat-labile enterotoxin of *Escherichia coli* and subunits of *Vibrio cholerae* enterotoxin. Infect Immun 21:1036, 1978.
62. Evans DG, Silver RP, Evans DJ Jr, et al. Plasmid-controlled colonization factor associated with virulence in *Escherichia coli* enterotoxigenic for humans. Infect Immun 12:656, 1975.
63. Abe A, Komase K, Bangtrakulnonth A, et al. Trivalent heat-labile and heat-stable enterotoxin probe conjugated with horseradish peroxidase for detection of enterotoxigenic *Escherichia coli* by hybridization. J Clin Microbiol 28:2616, 1990.
64. Daniels NA, Neimann J, Karpati A, et al. Traveler's diarrhea at sea: three outbreaks of waterborne enterotoxigenic *Escherichia coli* on cruise ships. J Infect Dis 181:1491, 2000.
65. Merson MH, Sack RB, Islam S, et al. Disease due to enterotoxigenic *Escherichia coli* in Bangladeshi adults: clinical aspects and a controlled trial of tetracycline. J Infect Dis 141:702, 1980.
66. Evans DJ Jr, Ruiz-Palacios G, Evans DG, et al. Humoral immune response to the heat-labile enterotoxin of *Escherichia coli* in naturally acquired diarrhea and antitoxin determination by passive immune hemolysis. Infect Immun 16:781, 1977.
67. Mattila L, Peltola H, Siitonen A, et al. Short-term treatment of traveler's diarrhea with norfloxacin: a double-blind, placebo-controlled study during two seasons. Clin Infect Dis 17:779, 1993.

68. Tulloch EF, Ryan KJ, Formal SB. Invasive enteropathic *Escherichia coli* dysentery: an outbreak in 28 adults. Ann Intern Med 79:13, 1973.
69. Taylor DN, Echeverria P, Sethabutr O, et al. Clinical and microbiologic features of *Shigella* and enteroinvasive *Escherichia coli* infections detected by DNA hybridization. J Clin Microbiol 26:1362, 1988.
70. Riley LW, Remis RS, Helgerson SD, et al. Hemorrhagic colitis associated with a rare *Escherichia coli* serotype. N Engl J Med 308:681, 1983.
71. Su C, Brandt LJ. *Escherichia coli* O157:H7 infection in humans. Ann Intern Med 123:698, 1995.
72. Slutzker LA, Ries AA, Green JG, et al. *Escherichia coli* O157:H7 diarrhea in the United States: clinical and epidemiological features. Ann Intern Med 126:505, 1997.
73. Martin DL, MacDonald KL, White KE, et al. The epidemiology and clinical aspects of the hemolytic uremic syndrome in Minnesota. N Engl J Med 323:1161, 1990.
74. Bell BP, Goldoft M, Griffin PM, et al. A multistate outbreak of *Escherichia coli* O157:H7-associated bloody diarrhea and hemolytic uremic syndrome from hamburgers. The Washington experience. J Am Med Assoc 272:1349, 1994.
75. Keene WE, Hedberg K, Herriot DE, et al. A prolonged outbreak of *Escherichia coli* O157:H7 infections caused by commercially distributed raw milk. J Infect Dis 176:815, 1997.
76. Besser RE, Lett SM, Weber JT, et al. An outbreak of diarrhea and hemolytic uremic syndrome from *Escherichia coli* O157:H7 in fresh-pressed apple cider. J Am Med Assoc 269:2217, 1993.
77. Belongia EA, Osterholm MT, Soler JT, et al. Transmission of *Escherichia coli* O157:H7 infection in Minnesota child day-care facilities. J Am Med Assoc 269:883, 1993.
78. Carter AO, Borczyk AA, Carlson JAK, et al. A severe outbreak of *Escherichia coli* O157:H7-associated hemorrhagic colitis in a nursing home. N Engl J Med 317:1496, 1987.
79. Milford DV, Taylor CM, Guttridge B, et al. Haemolytic uraemic syndromes in the British Isles 1985–1988: association with verocytotoxin-producing *Escherichia coli*. Part 1. Clinical and epidemiological aspects. Arch Dis Child 65:716, 1990.
80. Kleanthous H, Smith HR, Scotland SM, et al. Haemolytic uraemic syndromes in the British Isles, 1985–1988: association with verocytotoxin-producing *Escherichia coli*. Part 2. Microbiological aspects. Arch Dis Child 65:722, 1990.
81. Karmali MA. Infection by verocytotoxin-producing *Escherichia coli*. Clin Microbiol Rev 2:15, 1989.
82. Law D, Kelly J. Use of heme and hemoglobin by *Escherichia coli* O157 and other Shiga-like toxin-producing *E. coli* serogroups. Infect Immun 63:700, 1995.
83. Tarr PI, Neill MA, Clausen CR, et al. *Escherichia coli* O157:H7 and the hemolytic uremic syndrome: importance of early cultures in establishing the etiology. J Infect Dis 162:553, 1990.
84. Shah S, Hoffman R, Shillam P, et al. Prolonged fecal shedding of *Escherichia coli* O157:H7 during an outbreak at a day care center. Clin Infect Dis 23:835, 1996.
85. Karch H, Russman H, Schmidt H, et al. Long-term shedding and clonal turnover of enterohemorrhagic *Escherichia coli* O157 in diarrheal disease. J Clin Microbiol 33:1602, 1995.
86. Zhang X, McDaniel AD, Wolf LE, et al. Quinolone antibiotics induce Shiga toxin-encoding bacteriophages, toxin production, and death in mice. J Infect Dis 181:664, 2000.
87. Proulx F, Turgeon JP, Delage G, et al. Randomized, controlled trial of antibiotic therapy for *Escherichia coli* O157:H7 enteritis. J Pediatr 121:299, 1992.
88. Wong CS, Srdjan J, Habeeb RL, et al. The risk of hemolytic uremic infections. N Engl J Med 342:1930, 2000.
89. Cravioto A, Tello A, Navarro A, et al. Association of *Escherichia coli* Hep-2 adherence patterns with type and duration of diarrhoea. Lancet 337:262, 1991.
90. Gunzberg ST, Chang BJ, Elliott SJ, et al. Diffuse and enteroaggregative patterns of enteric *Escherichia coli* isolated from aboriginal children from the Kimberley region of Western Australia. J Infect Dis 167:755, 1993.
91. Wanke CA, Mayer H, Weber R, et al. Enteroaggregative *Escherichia coli* as a potential cause of diarrheal disease in adults infected with human immunodeficiency virus. J Infect Dis 178:185, 1998.
92. Nataro JP, Yikang D, Cookson S, et al. Heterogeneity of enteroaggregative *Escherichia coli* virulence demonstrated in volunteers. J Infect Dis 171:465, 1995.
93. Vial PA, Robins-Browne R, Lior H, et al. Characterization of entero-adherent-aggregative *Escherichia coli*, a putative agent of diarrheal disease. J Infect Dis 158:70, 1988.
94. Debroy C, Yealy J, Wilson RA, et al. Antibodies raised against the outer membrane protein interrupt adherence of enteroaggregative *Escherichia coli*. Infect Immun 63:2873, 1995.
95. Wanke CA, Gerrior J, Blais V, et al. Successful treatment of diarrheal disease with enteroaggregative *Escherichia coli* in adults infected with human immunodeficiency virus. J Infect Dis 178:1369, 1998.
96. Glandt M, Adachi JA, Mathewson JJ, et al. Enteroaggregative *Escherichia coli* as a cause of traveler's diarrhea: clinical response to ciprofloxacin. Clin Infect Dis 29:335, 1999.
97. Jallat C, Livrelli V, Darfeuille-Michaud A, et al. *Escherichia coli* strains involved in diarrhea in France: high prevalence and heterogeneity of diffusely adhering strains. J Clin Microbiol 31:2031, 1993.
98. Echeverria P, Serichantalerg O, Changchawalis S, et al. Tissue culture-adherent *Escherichia coli* in infantile diarrhea. J Infect Dis 165: 141, 1992.
99. Tacket CO, Moseley SL, Kay B, et al. Challenge studies in volunteers using *Escherichia coli* strains with diffuse adherence to HEp-2 cells. J Infect Dis 162:550, 1990.
100. Poitrineau P, Forestier C, Meyer M, et al. Retrospective case-control study of diffusely adhering *Escherichia coli* and clinical features in children with diarrhea. J Clin Microbiol 33:1961, 1995.
101. Keusch GT, Grady GF, Mata LJ, et al. Pathogenesis of shigella diarrhea. I. Enterotoxin production by *Shigella dysenteriae* I. J Clin Invest 51:1212, 1972.
102. Gots RE, Formal SB, Giannela RA. Indomethacin inhibition of *Salmonella typhimurium*, *Shigella flexneri*, and cholera-mediated rabbit ileal secretion. J Infect Dis 130:280, 1974.
103. Keusch GT, Bennish ML. Shigellosis: recent progress, persisting problems and research issues. Pediatr Infect Dis J 8:713, 1989.
104. Acheson DWK, Keusch GT. *Shigella* and enteroinvasive *Escherichia coli*. In Blaser MJ, Smith PD, Ravdin JI, et al. (eds): Infections of the Gastrointestinal Tract. New York, Raven Press, 1995, p 763.
105. Keusch GT, Jacewicz M. The pathogenesis of shigella diarrhea. VI. Toxin and antitoxin in *Shigella flexneri* and *Shigella sonnei* infections in humans. J Infect Dis 135:552, 1977.
106. DuPont HL, Levine MM, Hornick RB, et al. Inoculum size in shigellosis and implications for expected mode of transmission. J Infect Dis 159:1126, 1989.
107. Gorden J, Small PLC. Acid resistance in enteric bacteria. Infect Immun 61:364, 1993.
108. Barrett-Connor E, Conner JD. Extra-intestinal manifestations of shigellosis. Am J Gastroenterol 52:234, 1970.
109. Khan WA, Dhar U, Salam MA, et al. Central nervous system manifestations of childhood shigellosis: prevalence, risk factors, and outcome. Pediatrics 103:E18, 1999.
110. Daoud AS, Zaki M, al-Mutari G, et al. Childhood shigellosis: clinical and bacteriological study. J Trop Med Hyg 93:275, 1990.
111. Koster FT, Boonpuncknavig V, Sujaho S, et al. Renal histopathology in the hemolytic-uremic syndrome following shigellosis. Clin Nephrol 21:126, 1984.
112. Butler T, Islam M, Bardhan PK. The leukemoid reaction in shigellosis. Am J Dis Child 138:162, 1984.
113. Tsuchiya N, Husby G, Williams RC, et al. Autoantibodies to the HLA-B27 sequence cross-react with the hypothetical peptide from the arthritis-associated *Shigella* plasmid. J Clin Invest 86:1193, 1990.
114. Nostrant TT, Kumar NB, Appleman HD. Histopathology differentiates acute self-limited colitis from ulcerative colitis. Gastroenterology 92: 318, 1987.
115. Replogle ML, Fleming DW, Cieslak PR. Emergence of antimicrobial-resistant shigellosis in Oregon. Clin Infect Dis 30:515, 2000.
116. Tauxe RV, Puhr ND, Wells JG, et al. Antimicrobial resistance of *Shigella* isolates in the USA: the importance of international travelers. J Infect Dis 162:1107, 1990.
117. Khalil K, Khan SR, Mazhar K, et al. Occurrence and susceptibility to antibiotics of *Shigella* species in stools of hospitalized children with bloody diarrhea in Pakistan. Am J Trop Med Hyg 58:800, 1998.
118. Bennish ML, Salam MA, Khan WA, et al. Treatment of shigellosis. III. Comparison of one- or two-dose ciprofloxacin with standard 5-day therapy. A randomized, blinded trial. Ann Intern Med 117:727, 1992.
119. Burkhardt JE, Walterspiel JN, Schaad UB. Quinolone arthropathy in animals versus children. Clin Infect Dis 25:1196, 1997.
120. Gendrel D, Moreno JL, Nduwimana M, et al. One-dose treatment of

pefloxacin for infection due to multidrug-resistant *Shigella dysenteriae* type 1 in Burundi. Clin Infect Dis 24:83, 1997.
121. Salam MA, Dhar U, Khan AK, et al. Randomised comparison of ciprofloxacin suspension and pivmecillinam for childhood shigellosis. Lancet 352:522, 1998.
122. Murphy GS, Bodhidatta L, Echeverria P, et al. Ciprofloxacin and loperamide in the treatment of bacillary dysentery. Ann Intern Med 118:582, 1993.
123. Haltalin KC, Nelson JD, Hinton LV, et al. Comparison of orally absorbable and nonabsorbable antibiotics in shigellosis. J Pediatr 2: 708, 1968.
124. Nelson JD, Haltalin KC. Amoxicillin less effective than ampicillin against *Shigella in vitro* and *in vivo*: relationship of efficacy to activity in serum. J Infect Dis 129:S222, 1974.
125. Le Minor L, Popoff MY. Designation of *Salmonella* enterica sp. nov., non. Rev., as the type and only species of the genus *Salmonella*. Int J Sys Bacteriol 37:465, 1987.
126. Mead PS, Slutsker L, Dietz V, et al. Food-related illness and death in the United States. Emerg Infect Dis 5:607, 1999.
127. Finley BB, Heffron F, Falkow S. Epithelial cell surfaces induce *Salmonella* proteins required for bacterial adherence and invasion. Science 243:940, 1989.
128. Fields PI, Groisman EA, Heffron F. A *Salmonella* locus that controls resistance to microbial proteins from phagocytic cells. Science 243: 1059, 1989.
129. McCormick BA, Miller SI, Carnes D, et al. Transepithelial signaling to neutrophils by salmonellae: a novel virulence mechanism for gastroenteritis. Infect Immun 63:2302, 1995.
130. Wallis TS, Starkey WG, Stephen J, et al. Enterotoxin production by *Salmonella typhimurium* strains of different virulence. J Med Microbiol 21:19, 1986.
131. Pavia AT, Shipman LD, Wells JG, et al. Epidemiologic evidence that prior antimicrobial exposure decreases resistance to infection by antimicrobial-sensitive *Salmonella*. J Infect Dis 161:255, 1990.
132. Rubin HR, Weinstein L. Salmonellosis: Microbiologic, Pathologic, and Clinical Features. New York, Stratton Intercontinental Medical Book Corporation, 1977.
133. Gray JI, Trueman AM. Severe salmonella gastroenteritis associated with hypochlorhydria. Scot Med J 16:255, 1971.
134. Glaser JB, Morton-Kute L, Berger SR. Recurrent *Salmonella typhimurium* bacteremia associated with the acquired immune deficiency syndrome. Ann Intern Med 102:189, 1985.
135. Musher DN, Rubenstein AD. Permanent carriers of nontyphosa salmonellae. Arch Intern Med 132:869, 1973.
136. Kaye D, Gill FA, Hook EW. Factors influencing host resistance to salmonella infections: the effects of hemolysis and erythrophagocytosis. Am J Med Sci 254:205, 1967.
137. Hand WL, King NL. Serum opsonization of salmonella in sickle cell anemia. Am J Med 64:388, 1977.
138. Han T, Sokal JE, Neter E. Salmonellosis in disseminated malignant diseases. N Engl J Med 276:1045, 1967.
139. Rocha H, Brazil S, Kirk JW, et al. Prolonged salmonella bacteremia in patients with *Schistosoma mansoni* infection. Arch Intern Med 128: 254, 1971.
140. Lindeman RJ, Weinstein L, Levitan R, et al. Ulcerative colitis and intestinal salmonellosis. Am J Med Sci 254:855, 1967.
141. Mandal BK, Mani V. Colonic involvement in salmonellosis. Lancet 1: 887, 1976.
142. Deppisch LM, Grans CA. Salmonellosis: a cause of toxic megacolon. J Clin Gastroenterol 12:605, 1990.
143. Askerkoff B, Bennett JV. Effect of antibiotic therapy in acute salmonellosis on the fecal excretion of salmonellae. N Engl J Med 281:636, 1969.
144. Sirinavin S, Garner P. Antibiotics for treating *Salmonella* gut infections. The Cochrane Library 2000.
145. Stanley PJ, Flegg PJ, Mandal BK, et al. Open study of ciprofloxacin in enteric fever. J Antimicrob Chemother 23:789, 1989.
146. Cherubin CE, Kowalski J. Nontyphoidal *Salmonella* carrier state treated with norfloxacin. Ann Intern Med 85:100, 1990.
147. Neill MA, Opal SM, Heelan J, et al. Failure of ciprofloxacin in convalescent fecal excretion after acute salmonellosis: experience during an outbreak in health care workers. Ann Intern Med 114:195, 1991.
148. Piddock LJV, Whale K, Wise R. Quinolone resistance in salmonella: clinical experience. Lancet 1:1459, 1990.
149. Malorny B, Schroeter A, Helmuth R. Incidence of quinolone resistance over the period 1986 to 1998 in veterinary *Salmonella* isolates from Germany. Antimicrob Agents Chemother 43:2278, 1999.
150. Molbak K, Baggesen DL, Aarestrup FM, et al. An outbreak of multidrug-resistant, quinolone-resistant *Salmonella enterica* serotype typhimurium DT104. N Engl J Med 341:1420, 1999.
151. Fey PD, Safranek TJ, Rupp ME, et al. Ceftriaxone-resistant *Salmonella* infection acquired by a child from cattle. N Engl J Med 342: 1242, 2000.
152. Hornick RB, Greisman SE, Woodward TE, et al. Typhoid fever: pathogenesis and immunologic control. N Engl J Med 283:686, 1970.
153. Tarr PE, Kuppens L, Jones TC, et al. Considerations regarding mass vaccination against typhoid fever as an adjunct to sanitation and public health measures: potential use in an epidemic in Tajikistan. Am J Trop Med Hyg 61:163, 1999.
154. Mermin JH, Townes JM, Gerber M, et al. Typhoid fever in the United States, 1985–1994. Changing risks of international travel and antimicrobial resistance. Arch Intern Med 158:633, 1998.
155. Stuart BM, Pullen RL. Typhoid: clinical analysis of 360 cases. Arch Intern Med 78:629, 1946.
156. Woodward TE, Smadel JE. Management of typhoid fever and its complications. Ann Intern Med 60:144, 1964.
157. Butler T, Knight J, Nath SK, et al. Typhoid fever complicated by intestinal perforation: a persisting fatal disease requiring surgical management. Rev Infect Dis 7:244, 1985.
158. Kaye D, Merselis JG, Connolly CS, et al. Treatment of chronic carriers of *Salmonella typhosa* with ampicillin. Ann N Y Acad Sci 145: 429, 1967.
159. Gilman RH, Terminel M, Levine MM, et al. Relative efficacy of blood, urine, rectal swab, bone-marrow, and rose-spot cultures for recovery of *Salmonella typhi* in typhoid fever. Lancet 1:1211, 1975.
160. Bhutta ZA, Mansurali N. Rapid serologic diagnosis of pediatric typhoid fever in an endemic area: a prospective comparative evaluation of two dot-enzyme immunoassays and the Widal test. Am J Trop Med Hyg 61:654, 1999.
161. Robertson RP, Wahab MFA, Raasch FO. Evaluation of chloramphenicol and ampicillin in *Salmonella* enteric fever. N Engl J Med 278:171, 1968.
162. Chitnis V, Chitnis D, Verma S, et al. Multidrug-resistant *Salmonella typhi* in India. Lancet 354:514, 1999.
163. Wain J, Hoa NTT, Chinh NT, et al. Quinolone-resistant *Salmonella typhi* in Vietnam: molecular basis of resistance and clinical response to treatment. Clin Infect Dis 25:1404, 1997.
164. Soe GB, Overturf GD. Treatment of typhoid fever and other systemic salmonelloses with cefotaxime, ceftriaxone, cefoperazone, and other new cephalosporins. Rev Infect Dis 9:719, 1987.
165. Acharya G, Butler T, Ho M, et al. Treatment of typhoid fever: randomized trial of a three-day course of ceftriaxone versus a fourteen-day course of chloramphenicol. Am J Trop Med Hyg 52:162, 1995.
166. Phuong CXT, Kneen R, Anh NT, et al. A comparative study of ofloxacin and cefixime for treatment of typhoid fever in children. Pediatr Infect Dis J 18:245, 1999.
167. Hoffman SL, Punjabi NH, Kumala S, et al. Reduction of mortality in chloramphenicol-treated severe typhoid fever by high-dose dexamethasone. N Engl J Med 310:83, 1984.
168. Bitar R, Tarpley J. Intestinal perforation in typhoid fever: an historical and state-of-the-art review. Rev Infect Dis 7:257, 1985.
169. Mock CN, Amaral J, Visser LE. Improvement in survival from typhoid ileal perforation. Results of 221 operative cases. Ann Surg 215: 244, 1992.
170. Rodriguez-Noriega E, Andrade-Villanueva J, Amaya-Tapia G. Quinolones in the treatment of *Salmonella* carriers. Rev Infect Dis 11: S1179, 1989.
171. Wahdan MH, Serie C, Cerisier Y, et al. A controlled field trial of live *Salmonella typhi* Ty 21a oral vaccine against typhoid: three-year results. J Infect Dis 145:292, 1982.
172. Levine MM, Ferreccio C, Black RE, et al. Chilean Typhoid Committee: Large-scale field trial of Ty21a live oral typhoid vaccine in enteric-coated capsule formulation. Lancet 1:1049, 1987.
173. Hirschel B, Wurthrich R, Somaini B, et al. Inefficacy of the commercial live oral Ty 21a vaccine in the prevention of typhoid: three-year results. J Infect Dis 145:292, 1982.
174. Acharya IL, Lowe CU, Thapa R, et al. Prevention of typhoid fever in Nepal with the Vi capsular polysaccharide of *Salmonella typhi*. N Engl J Med 317:1101, 1987.

175. Altekruse SF, Stern NJ, Fields PI, et al. *Campylobacter jejuni*—an emerging foodborne pathogen. Emerg Infect Dis 5:28, 1999.
176. Deming MS, Tauxe RV, Blake PA, et al. *Campylobacter* enteritis at a university: transmission from eating chicken and from cats. Am J Epidemiol 126:526, 1987.
177. Mishu Allos B, Blaser MJ. *Campylobacter jejuni* and the expanding spectrum of related infections. Clin Infect Dis 20:1092, 1995.
178. Kapperud G, Lassen J, Ostroff SM, et al. Clinical features of sporadic *Campylobacter* infections in Norway. Scand J Infect Dis 24:741, 1992.
179. Rees JH, Soudain SE, Gregson NA, et al. *Campylobacter jejuni* infection and Guillain-Barré syndrome. N Engl J Med 333:1374, 1995.
180. Levine MM. Antimicrobial therapy for infectious diarrhea. Rev Infect Dis 8:S207, 1986.
181. Pichler HET, Diridl G, Stickler K, et al. Clinical efficacy of ciprofloxacin compared with placebo in bacterial diarrhea. Am J Med 82(S4A): 329, 1987.
182. Segreti J, Gootz TD, Goodman LJ, et al. High-level quinolone resistance in clinical isolates of *Campylobacter jejuni*. J Infect Dis 165: 667, 1992.
183. Wretlind B, Stromberg A, Ostlund L, et al. Rapid emergence of quinolone resistance in *Campylobacter jejuni* in patients treated with norfloxacin. Scand J Infect Dis 24:685, 1992.
184. Kuschner RA, Trofa AF, Thomas RJ, et al. Use of azithromycin for the treatment of *Campylobacter* enteritis in travelers to Thailand, an area where ciprofloxacin resistance is prevalent. Clin Infect Dis 21: 536, 1995.
185. Smith KE, Besser JM, Hedberg CW, et al. Quinolone-resistant *Campylobacter jejuni* infections in Minnesota, 1992–1998. N Engl J Med 340:1525, 1999.
186. Talsma E, Goettsch WG, Nieste HLJ, et al. Resistance in *Campylobacter* species: increased resistance to fluoroquinolones and seasonal variation. Clin Infect Dis 29:845, 1999.
187. Naktin J, Beavis KG. *Yersinia enterocolitica* and *Yersinia pseudotuberculosis*. Clin Lab Med 19:523, 1999.
188. Isberg RR, Leong JM. Cultured mammalian cells attach to the invasion protein of *Yersinia* pseudotuberculosis. Proc Natl Acad Sci U S A 85:6682, 1988.
189. Ackers M-L, Schoenfeld S, Markman J, et al. An outbreak of *Yersinia enterocolitica* O:8 infections associated with pasteurized milk. J Infect Dis 181:1834, 2000.
190. Simmonds SD, Noble MA, Freeman HJ. Gastrointestinal features of culture-positive *Yersinia enterocolitica* infection. Gastroenterology 92: 112, 1987.
191. Ostroff SM, Kapperud G, Lassen J, et al. Clinical features of sporadic *Yersinia enterocolitica* infections in Norway. J Infect Dis 166:812, 1992.
192. Vantrappen G, Pouette E, Geboes K. *Yersinia enteritis* and enterocolitis: gastroenterological aspects. Gastroenterology 72:220, 1977.
193. Puylaert JBCM, Cermeijden RJ, Van Der Werf SDJ, et al. Incidence and sonographic diagnosis of bacterial ileocaecitis masquerading as appendicitis. Lancet 2:84, 1989.
194. Granforb K, Jalkanan S, Von Essen R, et al. *Yersinia* antigens in synovial fluid cells from patients with reactive arthritis. N Engl J Med 320:216, 1989.
195. DeKoning J, Heesemann J, Hoogkamp-Korstanje JAA, et al. *Yersinia* in intestinal biopsy specimens from patients with seronegative spondyloarthropathy: correlation with specific serum IgA antibodies. J Infect Dis 159:109, 1989.
196. Bottone EJ, Sheehan DJ. *Yersinia enterocolitica*: guidelines for serologic diagnosis of human infections. Rev Infect Dis 5:898, 1982.
197. Paim CH, Gillis F, Tuomanen E, et al. Placebo-controlled double-blind evaluation of trimethoprim-sulfamethoxazole treatment of *Yersinia enterocolitica* gastroenteritis. J Pediatr 104:308, 1984.
198. Blacklow NR, Greenberg HB. Viral gastroenteritis. N Engl J Med 325:252, 1991.
199. Waters V, Ford-Jones EL, Petric M, et al. Etiology of community-acquired pediatric viral diarrhea: a prospective longitudinal study in hospitals, emergency departments, pediatric practices, and child care centers during the winter rotavirus outbreak, 1997 to 1998. Pediatr Infect Dis J 19:843, 2000.
200. Davidson GP, Barnes GL. Structural and functional abnormalities of the small intestine in infants and young children with *Rotavirus* enteritis. Acta Paediatr Scand 68:181, 1979.
201. Lundgren O, Peregrin AT, Persson K, et al. Role of the enteric nervous system in the fluid and electrolyte secretion of rotavirus diarrhea. Science 287:491, 2000.
202. Rodriguez WJ, Kim HW, Brandt CD, et al. Longitudinal study of rotavirus infection and gastroenteritis in families served by a pediatric medical practice: clinical and epidemiologic observations. Pediatr Infect Dis J 6:170, 1987.
203. Zheng BJ, Lo SKF, Tam JSL, et al. Prospective study of community-acquired rotavirus infection. J Clin Microbiol 27:2083, 1989.
204. Richardson S, Grimwood K, Gorrell R, et al. Extended excretion of rotavirus after severe diarrhoea in young children. Lancet 351:1844, 1998.
205. Wilde J, Yolken R, Willoughby R, et al. Improved detection of rotavirus shedding by polymerase chain reaction. Lancet 337:323, 1991.
206. Gouvea V, Allen JR, Glass RI, et al. Detection of group B and C rotaviruses by polymerase chain reaction. J Clin Microbiol 29:519, 1991.
207. Matson DO, O'Ryan ML, Herrera I, et al. Fecal antibody responses to symptomatic and asymptomatic rotavirus infections. J Infect Dis 167: 577, 1993.
208. Brussow H, Wechau H, Lerner L, et al. Seroconversion patterns to four human rotavirus serotypes in hospitalized infants with acute rotavirus gastroenteritis. J Infect Dis 161:1105, 1990.
209. Ward RL, Bernstein DI, for the US Rotavirus Vaccine Efficacy Group. Protection against rotavirus disease after natural rotavirus infection. J Infect Dis 169:900, 1994.
210. Glass RI, Stoll BJ, Wyatt RG, et al. Observations questioning a protective role for breast-feeding in severe rotavirus diarrhea. Acta Paediatr Scand 75:713, 1986.
211. Yolken RH, Peterson JA, Vonderfecht SL, et al. Human milk mucin inhibits rotavirus replication and prevents experimental gastroenteritis. J Clin Invest 90:1984, 1992.
212. Newburg DS, Peterson JA, Ruiz-Palacios GM, et al. Role of human-milk lactadherin in protection against symptomatic rotavirus infection. Lancet 351:1160, 1998.
213. Centers for Disease Control and Prevention. Rotavirus vaccine for the prevention of rotavirus gastroenteritis among children. MMWR Morb Mortal Wkly Rep 48(Suppl. RR2):1, 1999.
214. Centers for Disease Control. Intussusception among recipients of rotavirus vaccine United States, 1998–1999. MMWR Morb Mortal Wkly Rep 48:577, 1999.
215. Santosham M, Burns B, Nadkarni V, et al. Oral rehydration therapy for acute diarrhea in ambulatory children in the United States: a double-blind comparison of four different solutions. Pediatrics 76:159, 1985.
216. Sarker SA, Casswall TH, Mahalanabis D, et al. Successful treatment of rotavirus diarrhea in children with immunoglobulin from immunized bovine colostrum. Pediatr Infect Dis J 17:1149, 1998.
217. Green KY, Ando T, Balayan MS, et al. Taxonomy of the caliciviruses. J Infect Dis 181(Suppl. 2):S322, 2000.
218. Matson DO, Estes MK, Glass RI, et al. The occurrence of calicivirus-associated diarrhea in children attending day care centers. J Infect Dis 159:71, 1989.
219. O'Ryan ML, Mamani N, Gaggero A, et al. Human caliciviruses are a significant pathogen of acute sporadic diarrhea in children of Santiago, Chile. J Infect Dis 182:1519, 2000.
220. Jiang X, Graham DY, Wang K, et al. Norwalk virus genome cloning and characterization. Science 250:1580, 1990.
221. Morse DL, Guzewich JJ, Hanrahan JP, et al. Widespread outbreaks of clam- and oyster-associated gastroenteritis: role of Norwalk virus. N Engl J Med 314:678, 1986.
222. Fankhauser RL, Noel JS, Monroe SS, et al. Molecular epidemiology of Norwalk-like viruses in outbreaks of gastroenteritis in the United States. J Infect Dis 178:1571, 1998.
223. Kukkula M, Maunula L, Silvennoinen E, et al. Outbreak of viral gastroenteritis due to drinking water contaminated by Norwalk-like viruses. J Infect Dis 180:1771, 1999.
224. Kuritsky JN, Osterhold MT, Greenberg HB, et al. Norwalk gastroenteritis: a community outbreak associated with bakery product consumption. Ann Intern Med 100:519, 1984.
225. Moe CL, Gentsch J, Grohmann G, et al. Application of PCR to detect Norwalk virus in fecal specimens from outbreaks of gastroenteritis. J Clin Microbiol 32:642, 1994.
226. Herrmann JE, Blacklow NR, Matsui SM, et al. Monoclonal antibodies for detection of Norwalk virus antigen in stools. J Clin Microbiol 33: 2511, 1995.

227. Johnson PC, Mathewson JJ, DuPont HL, et al. Multiple-challenge study of host susceptibility to Norwalk gastroenteritis in U.S. adults. J Infect Dis 161:18, 1990.
228. Steinhoff MC, Douglas RG, Greenberg HB, et al. Bismuth subsalicylate therapy of viral gastroenteritis. Gastroenterology 78:1495, 1980.
229. Kotloff KL, Losonsky GA, Morris JG Jr, et al. Enteric adenovirus infection and childhood diarrhea: an epidemiologic study in three clinical settings. Pediatrics 84:219, 1989.
230. Van R, Wun CC, O'Ryan ML, et al. Outbreaks of human enteric adenovirus types 40 and 41 in Houston day care centers. J Pediatr 120:516, 1992.
231. Lew JF, Moe CL, Monroe SS, et al. Astrovirus and adenovirus associated with diarrhea in children in day care settings. J Infect Dis 164: 673, 1991.
232. Kurtz JB, Lee TW. Astroviruses: human and animal. In Novel Diarrhoea Viruses. CIBA Foundation Symposium 128. Chichester, England, John Wiley, 1987, p 92.
233. Herrmann JE, Taylor DN, Echeverria P, et al. Astroviruses as a cause of gastroenteritis in children. N Engl J Med 324:1757, 1991.
234. Mitchell DK, Monroe SS, Jiang X, et al. Virologic features of an astrovirus diarrhea outbreak in a day care center revealed by reverse transcriptase-polymerase chain reaction. J Infect Dis 172:1437, 1995.
235. Naficy AB, Rao MR, Holmes JL, et al. Astrovirus diarrhea in Egyptian children. J Infect Dis 182:685, 2000.
236. Moe CL, Allen JR, Monroe SS, et al. Detection of astrovirus in pediatric stool samples by immunoassay and RNA probe. J Clin Microbiol 29:2390, 1991.
237. Koopmans M, Horzinek MC. Toroviruses of animals and humans: a review. Adv Virus Res 43:233, 1994.
238. Koopmans MPG, Goosen ESM, Lima AM, et al. Association of torovirus with acute and persistent diarrhea in children. Pediatr Infect Dis J 16:504, 1997.
239. Jamieson FB, Wang EEL, Bain C, et al. Human torovirus: a new nosocomial gastrointestinal pathogen. J Infect Dis 178:1263, 1998.
240. Gorbach SL, Edelman R (eds). Travelers' diarrhea: National Institutes of Health Consensus Development Conference. Rev Infect Dis 8(Suppl. 2):S109, 1986.
241. Gorbach SL, Kean BH, Evans DG, et al. Travelers' diarrhea and toxigenic *Escherichia coli*. N Engl J Med 292:933, 1975.
242. Black RE. Pathogens that cause travelers' diarrhea in Latin America and Africa. Rev Infect Dis 12(S1):S131, 1990.
243. Steffen R, Collard F, Tornieporth N, et al. Epidemiology, etiology, and impact of traveler's diarrhea in Jamaica. JAMA 281:811, 1999.
244. Dupont HL, Ericsson CD. Prevention and treatment of traveler's diarrhea. N Engl J Med 328:1821, 1993.
245. Mattila L, Siitonen A, Kyronseppa H, et al. Seasonal variation in etiology of travelers' diarrhea. J Infect Dis 165:385, 1992.
246. Petruccelli BP, Murphy GS, Sanchez JL, et al. Treatment of traveler's diarrhea with ciprofloxacin and loperamide. J Infect Dis 165:557, 1992.
247. Steffen R. Epidemiologic studies of travelers' diarrhea, severe gastrointestinal infections, and cholera. Rev Infect Dis 8(Suppl. 2):S122, 1986.
248. Shlim DR, Hoge CW, Rajah R, et al. Persistent high risk of diarrhea among foreigners in Nepal during the first 2 years of residence. Clin Infect Dis 29:613, 1999.
249. DuPont HL, Capsuto EG. Persistent diarrhea in travelers. Clin Infect Dis 22:124, 1996.
250. Black RE. Epidemiology of travelers' diarrhea and relative importance of various pathogens. Rev Infect Dis 12(S1):S73, 1990.
251. Lowenstein MS, Balows A, Gangarosa EJ. Turista at an international congress in Mexico. Lancet 1:529, 1973.
252. Harris JR. Are bottled beverages safe for travelers [editorial]? Am J Public Health 72:787, 1982.
253. Kozicki M, Steffen R, Schar M. "Boil it, cook it, peel it, or forget it." Does this rule prevent travelers' diarrhoea? Int J Epidemiol 14:169, 1985.
254. DuPont HL, Evans DG, Rios N, et al. Prevention of travelers' diarrhea with trimethoprim-sulfamethoxazole. Rev Infect Dis 4:533, 1982.
255. Ericsson CD, Johnson PC, DuPont HL, et al. Ciprofloxacin or trimethoprim-sulfamethoxazole as initial therapy for travelers' diarrhea. Ann Intern Med 106:216, 1987.
256. Salam I, Katelaris P, Leigh-Smith S, et al. Randomised trial of single-dose ciprofloxacin for travellers' diarrhoea. Lancet 344:1537, 1994.
257. Johnson PC, Ericsson CD, DuPont HL, et al. Comparison of loperamide with bismuth subsalicylate for the treatment of acute travelers' diarrhea. JAMA 255:757, 1986.
258. Gorbach SL. Bismuth therapy in gastrointestinal diseases. Gastroenterology 99:863, 1990.
259. Ericsson CD, DuPont HL, Mathewson JJ, et al. Treatment of travelers' diarrhea with sulfamethoxazole and trimethoprim and loperamide. JAMA 263:257, 1990.
260. Taylor DN, Sanchez JL, Candler W, et al. Treatment of travelers' diarrhea: ciprofloxacin plus loperamide compared with ciprofloxacin alone. Ann Intern Med 114:731, 1991.
261. Adachi JA, Ostrosky-Zeichner L, DuPont HL, et al. Empirical antimicrobial therapy for traveler's diarrhea. Clin Infect Dis 31:1079, 2000.
262. Steffen E, Heusser R, DuPont HL. Prevention of travelers' diarrhea with nonantibiotic drugs. Rev Infect Dis 8(S2):S151, 1986.
263. Tsubaki T, Honma Y, Hoshi M. Neurologic syndrome associated with clioquinol. Lancet 1:696, 1971.
264. Lew JF, Glass RI, Gangarosa RE, et al. Diarrheal deaths in the United States, 1979 through 1987. A special problem for the elderly. JAMA 265:3280, 1991.
265. Gangarosa RE, Glass RI, Lew JF, et al. Hospitalizations involving gastroenteritis in the U.S., 1985: the special burden of the disease among the elderly. Am J Epidemiol 135:281, 1992.
266. Bennett RG, Greenough WB. Approach to acute diarrhea in the elderly. Gastroenterol Clin North Am 22:517, 1993.
267. Garibaldi RA, Brodine S, Matsumiya S, et al. Infections among patients in nursing homes. N Engl J Med 305:731, 1981.
268. Aronsson B, Mollby R, Nord CE. Antimicrobial agents and *Clostridium difficile* in acute enteric disease: epidemiological data from Sweden, 1980–1982. J Infect Dis 151:476, 1985.
269. Brown E, Talbot G, Axelrod P, et al. Risk factors for *Clostridium difficile* toxin-associated diarrhea. Infect Control Hosp Epidemiol 11: 283, 1990.
270. Swerdlow DL, Woodruff BA, Brady RC, et al. A waterborne outbreak in Missouri of *Escherichia coli* O157:H7 associated with bloody diarrhea and death. Ann Intern Med 117:812, 1992.
271. Borriello SP, Barclay FE, Welch AR, et al. Epidemiology of diarrhoea caused by enterotoxigenic *Clostridium perfringens*. J Med Microbiol 20:363, 1985.
272. Gordon SM, Oshiro LS, Jarvis WR, et al. Foodborne Snow Mountain agent gastroenteritis with secondary person-to-person spread in a retirement community. Am J Epidemiol 131:702, 1990.
273. Neill MA, Rice SK, Ahmad NV, et al. Cryptosporidiosis: an unrecognized cause of diarrhea in elderly hospitalized patients. Clin Infect Dis 22:168, 1996.
274. Brandt LJ, Kosche KA, Greenwald DA, et al. *Clostridium difficile*-associated diarrhea in the elderly. Am J Gastroenterol 94:3263, 1999.
275. Gaudio P, Sethabutr O, Echeverria P, et al. Utility of a polymerase chain reaction diagnostic system in a study of the epidemiology of shigellosis among dysentery patients, family contacts, and well controls living in a shigellosis-endemic area. J Infect Dis 176:1013, 1997.
276. Qadri F, Hasan JAK, Hossain J, et al. Evaluation of the monoclonal antibody-based kit Bengal SMART for rapid detection of *Vibrio cholerae* 0139 synonym Bengal in stool samples. J Clin Microbiol 33:732, 1995.
277. Dennehy PH, Hartin M, Nelson SM, et al. Evaluation of the immunoCardSTAT rotavirus assay for detection of group A rotavirus in fecal specimens. J Clin Microbiol 37:1977, 1999.
278. Koplan JP, Fineberg HV, Ferraro MJB, et al. Value of stool cultures. Lancet 2:413, 1980.
279. Rowland MG, Davies H, Patterson S, et al. Viruses and diarrhea in West Africa and London: a collaborative study. Trans R Soc Trop Med Hyg 72:95, 1978.
280. Watson B, Ellis M, Mandal B, et al. A comparison of the clinic-pathological features with stool pathogens in patients hospitalized with the symptom of diarrhoea. Scand J Infect Dis 18:553, 1986.
281. Jewkes J, Larson HE, Price AB, et al. Aetiology of acute diarrhea in adults. Gut 22:388, 1981.
282. Dryden MS, Gabb RJ, Wright SK. Empirical treatment of severe acute community-acquired gastroenteritis with ciprofloxacin. Clin Infect Dis 22:1019, 1996.
283. Guerrant RL, Araujo V, Soares E, et al. Measurement of fecal lactoferrin as a marker of fecal leukocytes. J Clin Microbiol 30:1238, 1992.
284. Avery ME, Snyder JD. Oral therapy for acute diarrhea: the underused simple solution. N Engl J Med 13:891, 1990.
285. Santosham M, Daum AS, Dillman L, et al. Oral rehydration therapy of infantile diarrhea. A controlled study of well-nourished children hospitalized in the United States and Panama. N Engl J Med 306: 1071, 1982.

286. Santosham M, Greenough WB. Oral rehydration therapy: a global perspective. J Pediatr 118:544, 1991.
287. Cutting WA, Belton NR, Gray JA, et al. Safety and efficacy of three oral rehydration solutions for children with diarrhoea (Edinburgh 1984–1985). Acta Paediatr Scand 78:253, 1989.
288. International Study Group on Reduced-Osmolarity ORS solutions. Multicentre evaluation of reduced-osmolarity oral rehydration salts solution. Lancet 345:282, 1995.
289. Gore SM, Fontaine O, Pierce NF. Impact of rice based oral rehydration solution on stool output and duration of diarrhoea: meta-analysis of 13 clinical trials. Br Med J 304:287, 1992.
290. Ramakrishna BS, Venkataraman S, Srinivasan P, et al. Amylase-resistant starch plus oral rehydration solutions for cholera. N Engl J Med 342:308, 2000.
291. Savarino SJ, Levine MM. Specific and nonspecific treatment of diarrhea. In Gorbach SL, Bartlett JG, Blacklow NR (eds): Infectious Diarrhea. Philadelphia, WB Saunders 1992, p 638.
292. Goodman LJ, Trenholme GM, Kaplan RL, et al. Empiric antimicrobial therapy of domestically acquired acute diarrhea in urban adults. Arch Intern Med 150:541, 1990.
293. Wistrom J, Norrby SR. Fluoroquinolones and bacterial enteritis, when and for whom? J Antimicrob Chemother 36:23, 1995.
294. Islam MR. Single dose tetracycline in cholera. Gut 28:1029, 1987.
295. Oldfield EC III, Bourgeois AL, Omar AK, et al. Empirical treatment of *Shigella* dysentery with trimethoprim: five-day course vs. single dose. Am J Trop Med Hyg 37:616, 1986.
296. Butler T, Lolekha S, Rasidi C, et al. Treatment of acute bacterial diarrhea: a multicenter international trial comparing placebo with fleroxacin given as a single dose or once daily for 3 days. Am J Med 94(Suppl. 3A): 187S, 1993.
297. Salazar-Lindo E, Santisteban-Ponce J, Chea-Woo E, et al. Racecadotril in the treatment of acute watery diarrhea in children. N Engl J Med 343:463, 2000.
298. DuPont HL, Hornick RB. Adverse effect of lomotil therapy in shigellosis. JAMA 226:1525, 1990.
299. DuPont HL, Sullivan P, Pickering LK, et al. Symptomatic treatment of diarrhea with bismuth subsalicylate among students attending a Mexican university. Gastroenterology 73:715, 1977.
300. Horvath KD, Whelan RL. Intestinal tuberculosis: return of an old disease. Am J Gastroenterol 93:692, 1998.
301. Marshall JB. Tuberculosis of the gastrointestinal tract and peritoneum. Am J Gastroenterol 88:989, 1993.
302. Kim KM, Lee A, Choi YK, et al. Intestinal tuberculosis: clinicopathologic analysis and diagnosis by endoscopic biopsy. J Gastroenterol 93: 606, 1998.
303. Shah S, Thomas V, Mathan M, et al. Colonoscopic study of 50 patients with colonic tuberculosis. Gut 33:347, 1992.
304. McGee GS, Williams LF, Potts J, et al. Gastrointestinal tuberculosis: resurgence of an old pathogen. Am Surg 55:16, 1989.
305. Balthazar EJ, Gordon R, Hulnick D. Ileocecal tuberculosis: CT and radiologic evaluation. AJR Am J Roentgenol 154:499, 1990.
306. Park SJ, Han JK, Kim JS, et al. Tuberculous colitis: radiologic-colonoscopic correlation. AJR Am J Roentgenol 175:121, 2000.
307. Bentley G, Webster JHH. Gastrointestinal tuberculosis: a 10-year review. Br J Surg 54:90, 1967.
308. Chen W-S, Su W-J, Wang H-S, et al. Large bowel tuberculosis and possible influencing factors for surgical prognosis: 30 years' experience. World J Surg 21:500, 1997.
309. Olson SJ, MacKinnon LC, Goulding JS, et al. Surveillance for foodborne-disease outbreaks—United States, 1993–1997. MMWR Morb Mortal Wkly Rep 49 (Suppl. SS-1):1, 2000.
310. Duncan CL, Strong DH. *Clostridium perfringens* type A food poisoning. I. Response of the rabbit ileum as an indication of enteropathogenicity of strains of *Clostridium perfringens* in monkeys. Infect Immun 3:167, 1971.
311. McDonel JL, Duncan CL. Regional localization of activity of *Clostridium perfringens* type A enterotoxin in the rabbit ileum, jejunum, and duodenum. J Infect Dis 136:661, 1977.
312. Thomas M, Noah ND, Male GE, et al. Hospital outbreak of *Clostridium perfringens* food poisoning. Lancet 1:1046, 1977.
313. Murrell TGC, Egerton JR, Rampling A, et al. The ecology and epidemiology of the pigbel syndrome in man in New Guinea. J Hyg Camb 64:375, 1966.
314. Petrillo TM, Beck-Sagué CM, Songer JG, et al. Enteritis necroticans (pigbel) in a diabetic child. N Engl J Med 342:1250, 2000.
315. Sullivan R, Asano T. Effects of staphylococcal enterotoxin B on intestinal transport in the rat. Am J Physiol 222:1793, 1971.
316. Levine WC, Bennett RW, Choi Y, et al. Staphylococcal food poisoning caused by imported canned mushrooms. J Infect Dis 173:1263, 1996.
317. Schlech WF III. Foodborne listeriosis. Clin Infect Dis 31:770, 2000.
318. Schuhat A, Deaver KA, Wenger JD, et al. Role of foods in sporadic listeriosis. I. Case-control study of dietary risk factors. J Am Med Assoc 267:2041, 1992.
319. Pinner RW, Schuchat A, Swaminathan B, et al. Role of foods in sporadic listeriosis. II. Microbiologic and epidemiologic investigation. J Am Med Assoc 267:2046, 1992.
320. Aureli P, Fiorucci GC, Caroli D, et al. An outbreak of febrile gastroenteritis associated with corn contaminated by *Listeria monocytogenes*. N Engl J Med 342:1236, 2000.
321. Terranoca W, Blake PA. *Bacillus cereus* food poisoning. N Engl J Med 298:143, 1978.
322. Gilbert RJ, Parry JM. Serotypes of *Bacillus cereus* from outbreaks of food poisoning and from routine foods. J Hyg Camb 78:69, 1977.
323. Melling J, Capel BJ, Turnbull PCB, et al. Identification of a novel enterotoxigenic activity associated with *Bacillus cereus*. J Clin Pathol 29:938, 1976.
324. Mortimer PR, McCann G. Food poisoning episodes associated with *Bacillus cereus* in fried rice. Lancet 1:1043, 1974.
325. Crane JK. Preformed bacterial toxins. Clin Lab Med 19:583, 1999.
326. Shapiro RL, Hatheway C, Swerdlow DL. Botulism in the United States: a clinical and epidemiologic review. Ann Intern Med 129:221, 1998.
327. Tacket CO, Shandera WX, Mann JM, et al. Equine antitoxin use and other factors that predict outcome in type A foodborne botulism. Am J Med 76:794, 1984.
328. Dixon TC, Meselson M, Guillemin J, Hanna PC. Anthrax. N Engl J Med 341:815, 1999.
329. Human ingestion of *Bacillus anthracis*-contaminated meat—Minnesota, August 2000. MMWR 49:813, 2000.

Chapter 97

Pseudomembranous Enterocolitis and Antibiotic-Associated Diarrhea

John G. Bartlett

Pseudomembranous enterocolitis was first described in the nineteenth century and has subsequently been recognized with increasing frequency as a serious, sometimes lethal, gastrointestinal disease. The common thread, regardless of clinical setting, is gross or histologic evidence of pseudomembranous exudative plaques attached to the mucosal surface of the small intestine, colon, or both. A variety of seemingly unrelated risk factors have been identified, suggesting that this condition represents a nonspecific response to heterogeneous insults; however, the vast majority of cases reported during the past three decades have occurred in association with antibiotic exposure. Antibiotic-associated pseudomembranous enterocolitis was commonly ascribed to *Staphylococcus aureus* in the 1950s, but by 1978, the toxin or toxins produced by *Clostridium difficile* were implicated in the great majority of cases.

HISTORICAL PERSPECTIVE

Current knowledge of pseudomembranous enterocolitis, which has evolved over a century, involves three different areas of investigation: the anatomy of the lesion, studies of antibiotic-associated colitis in rodent models, and studies of *C. difficile* (Table 97–1).[1]

Anatomic Studies

Anatomic studies began with the original report of pseudomembranous lesions of the intestinal tract in a case report published by Finney in 1893.[2] The patient was a 22-year-old woman described preoperatively by her physician, Dr. William Osler, as a "miserable, emaciated creature in wretched physical condition." Surgery performed by Finney in 1892 involved resection of a tumor in the gastric pylorus. After the operation, diarrhea developed and became progressively more severe, leading to her death on the 15th postoperative day. The autopsy showed a "diphtheritic membrane" in the small bowel.

Pseudomembranous enterocolitis was a relatively rare condition in the preantibiotic era; only about four cases were recognized annually at the Mayo Clinic.[3] In the early 1950s, however, it became a common complication of antibiotic use, especially after surgery in patients given prophylactic antibiotics. In some surgical reports the rate was as high as 14%,[4] or even 27%.[5] *S. aureus*, the principal nosocomial pathogen at that time, was implicated as the agent of this condition on the basis of results of gram stain and culture of stool specimens.[4–7] During this period, the terms *pseudomembranous colitis* (PMC), *postoperative enterocolitis*, *antibiotic-associated colitis*, and *staphylococcal enterocolitis* were often used interchangeably. On the assumption that *S. aureus* was the putative agent, orally administered vancomycin became the standard treatment and seemed to work.[8]

The etiologic role of *S. aureus* was not seriously challenged until interest in the disease was renewed during the 1970s. The most important report described the investigation of what came to be known as *clindamycin colitis* by Tedesco and colleagues at Barnes Hospital in St. Louis in 1974.[9] This study was the first in which endoscopy was used routinely in patients with antibiotic-associated diarrhea. The results showed that, among the 200 patients treated with clindamycin, diarrhea developed in 42 (21%) and 20 (10%)

Table 97–1 | **History of *Clostridium difficile*–Associated Colitis**

ANATOMY	ANIMAL STUDIES	STUDIES OF *C. DIFFICILE*
Early Studies		
Initial report of pseudomembranous enterocolitis (Finney, 1893)[2]	Penicillin-induced death in guinea pigs (Hambre et al, 1943)[10]	Initial detection and recognition of toxigenic potential (Hall and O'Toole, 1935)[13]
1950s–1960s		
"Antibiotic-associated colitis," "pseudomembranous enterocolitis," or "Staphylococcus enterocolitis"	Theories of causation: hypersensitivity, gram-positive bacteria (*S. aureus*)	Review of clinical studies suggests it is not a human pathogen (Smith and King, 1962)[83]
1974		
Endoscopy for detection of antibiotic-associated PMC or "clindamycin colitis" (Tedesco et al., 1974)[9]	"Latent virus" postulated, based on cytotoxicity noted with tissue cultures (Green, 1974)[11]	Extensive review of lethal toxin production in vitro and demonstration that it is widespread in environment (Hafiz, Ph.D. thesis, 1974)[15]
1978		
Demonstration that the gut pathology (pseudomembranous colitis) described by Tedesco's group[9] is caused by the toxin or toxins described by Green[11] that are produced by *C. difficile*, as reviewed by Hafiz.[15]		

exhibited PMC at endoscopy. The report by the Barnes group shocked the medical community because it implied an extraordinarily high rate of a life-threatening complication associated with the use of the drug that, in the United States, had become the gold standard for treatment of anaerobic infections. It was also noted that *S. aureus* could not be recovered from the stools of affected persons. Subsequent studies of eight stool specimens collected by Tedesco's group and tested 5 years later in the author's laboratory showed that all contained both *C. difficile* and its cytopathic toxin. This series is now viewed as the first microbiologically confirmed hospital epidemic of *C. difficile* colitis.

Studies of a Rodent Model

The second series of relevant experiments in the history of PMC concerns the early observation that antibiotics caused a similar disease in guinea pigs and hamsters. The toxicity of penicillin for guinea pigs was initially reported by Hamre and associates in 1943, during attempts to determine its potential use for the treatment of gas gangrene in an animal model, a vitally important issue in World War II.[10] The authors found that penicillin per se was even more lethal than the *Clostridium* challenge. At necropsy, the only finding in the penicillin-treated guinea pigs was large cecums filled with hemorrhagic fluid. Subsequent work showed that most antibiotics were similarly lethal to guinea pigs and that hamsters were also susceptible. Multiple mechanisms of death were postulated, but an important report by Green in 1974 was clearly overlooked.[11] This investigator examined the role of viruses in the guinea pig model by using tissue-cultured cells and noted cytopathic changes. The postulated agent could not be propagated, and consequently, he concluded that it was a latent virus. Presumably, this report is the first demonstration of *C. difficile* toxin. A similar observation was made in 1977 by Larson and coworkers,[12] who used stool specimens from patients with PMC.

Studies of *Clostridium difficile*

C. difficile initially was reported to be a component of the normal intestinal flora of newborn infants by Hall and O'Toole in 1935.[13] These investigators noted that the bacterium produced a "neurotoxin," so defined because the cell-free supernatant of broth cultures was lethal when injected into guinea pigs or rabbits. Subsequent work in the pre-antibiotic era showed that the toxin produced by *C. difficile* was extraordinarily potent on parenteral challenge to multiple animal species.[14] Nevertheless, the clinical significance of this organism escaped detection until 1977, when its role in antibiotic-associated colitis was elucidated. The most comprehensive report on *C. difficile* before that time was the 1974 doctoral thesis of Hafiz at the University of Leeds, who noted that the organism was widespread in nature and that most strains of *C. difficile* produced the lethal toxin.[15]

This historical review concerns three quite different lines of investigation, including studies of the anatomy of PMC that culminated in the report by Tedesco's group,[9] studies of the animal model that culminated in the first recognition of a cytopathic toxin by Green,[11] and studies of *C. difficile* that culminated in its comprehensive review by Hafiz.[15] All three of these landmark studies were published in 1974. Nevertheless, at that time it was not possible to know that the lesions described by Tedesco and colleagues involved the toxin reported by Green as a product of the organism described in elaborate detail by Hafiz.

The work that eventually elucidated the relevance of these three seemingly diverse lines of investigation initially was conducted in the hamster model, and the lessons were then applied to the clinical setting. It was first noted that clindamycin and many other antibiotics were lethal to hamsters. The animals had a characteristic inflammatory lesion of the cecum, and the cecal contents contained a filterable toxin that was cytopathic in a cell culture assay and reproduced the typical lesion when injected intracecally into healthy recipients.[16] The source of the toxin proved to be *C. difficile*; both the organism and its cytopathic toxin could be detected in nearly all patients with antibiotic-associated PMC, and the toxin was not found in healthy controls.[17, 18] Koch's postulates were satisfied.

PATHOLOGY

Pseudomembranous enterocolitis is a pathologic diagnosis that can take a variety of forms, depending on the nature of the associated condition and the time frame in which the patient is examined. The common denominator is the pres-

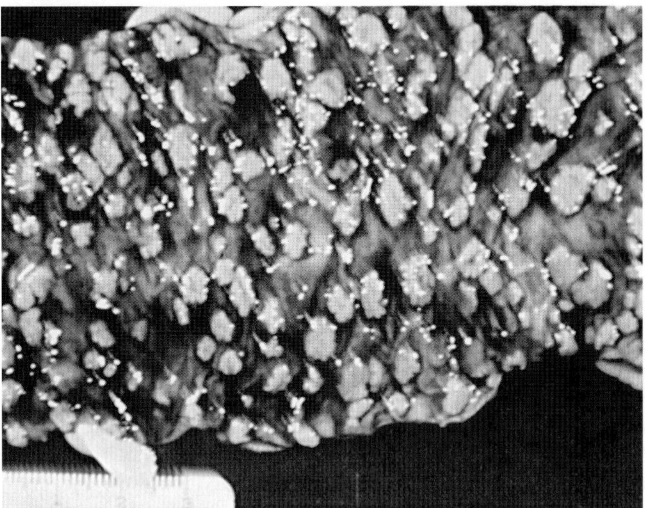

Figure 97–1. Pseudomembrane formation in colon. Note the flat, raised lesions that vary in size from a few millimeters to 8 mm. The intervening mucosa is hyperemic.

ence of pseudomembranes on the intestinal mucosa, which may be located in the small bowel (pseudomembranous enteritis), colon (PMC), or both (pseudomembranous enterocolitis). Early studies showed high rates of small bowel involvement.[19–21] Nearly all cases reported in the past two decades have followed antibiotic use and have shown changes restricted to the colon (eg, antibiotic-associated PMC). Rare cases with small bowel involvement have been reported, both with and without antecedent antibiotic exposure.[22, 23] On gross inspection there are multiple elevated yellowish white plaques, which vary in size from a few millimeters to 10 to 20 mm (Figs. 97–1 and 97–2).[9, 24, 25] The intervening mucosa appears normal or shows hyperemia and edema. Early lesions are punctate, and with advanced disease the pseudomembranes may coalesce and eventually slough, leaving large denuded areas. Antibiotic-associated PMC is rarely a segmental disease, and pseudomembranes are often distributed throughout the colon.

Histologic studies show that the pseudomembrane typically arises from a point of superficial ulceration and is accompanied by an acute or chronic inflammatory infiltrate in the lamina propria (Figs. 97–3 and 97–4).[24, 25] The pseudomembrane is composed of fibrin, mucin, sloughed mucosal epithelial cells, and acute inflammatory cells. The spectrum of changes has been classified by Price and Davies into three categories, which appear to be uniform in any individual patient.[25] The earliest and mildest form consists of focal necrosis with polymorphonuclear cells that forms a characteristic "summit lesion." The second category, which appears to represent more advanced disease, shows glandular disruption and a focal polymorphonuclear cell infiltrate surmounted by typical pseudomembranes, which may appear as a volcanic eruption (see Figs. 97–3*A* and 97–4). With both lesions there are areas of intervening mucosa that appear normal, and the inflammatory infiltrate is generally limited to the superficial portion of the lamina propria, predominantly the subepithelium. The third and most advanced form of the disease shows complete structural necrosis with extensive involvement of the lamina propria, which is overlaid by a thick, confluent pseudomembrane (Fig. 97–3*B*).

Bacterial invasion of the bowel mucosa by *C. difficile* is not seen because the disease is toxin-mediated. Studies in

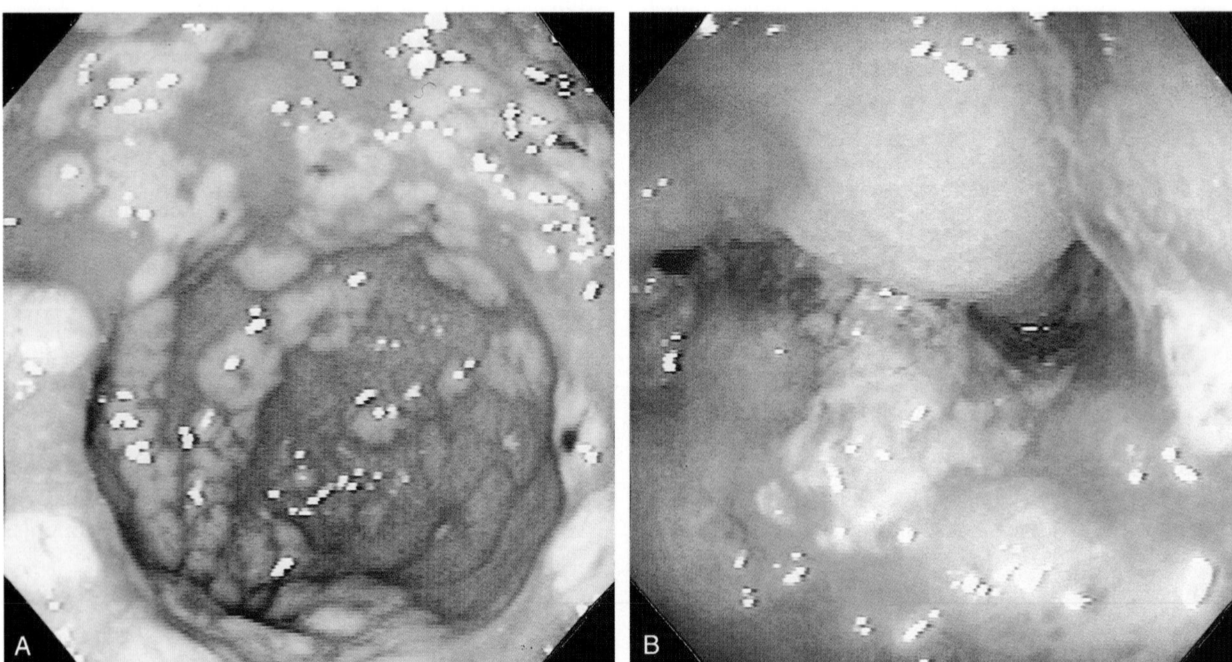

Figure 97–2. Colonoscopic findings in *Clostridium difficile* colitis. *A,* Multiple yellow coalescent plaques throughout the rectum. In some areas around the yellow plaques, edema is present, manifested by loss of the normal vascular pattern. In other areas, the vascular pattern is preserved. *B,* Severe colitis with diffuse edema (loss of vascularity) and yellow plaques with ulcer. The severe edema compromised the colonic lumen. (From Wilcox CM: Atlas of Clinical Gastrointestinal Endoscopy. Philadelphia, W.B. Saunders, 1995, p 216.)

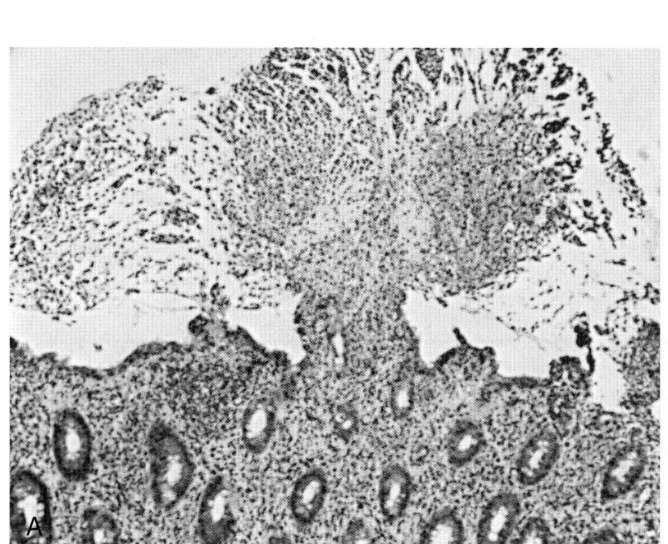

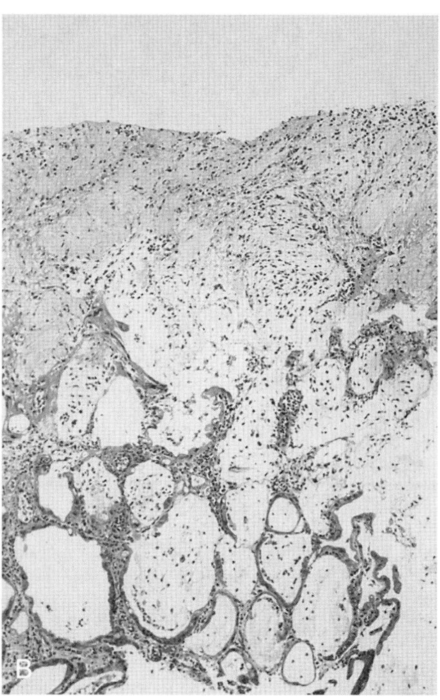

Figure 97–3. Microscopic pathologic appearance of pseudomembranous colitis. *A,* A homosexual man had received ampicillin and developed toxic megacolon. A mushroom-shaped pseudomembrane is seen. (Courtesy of M.H. Sleisenger, MD.) *B,* In this case, the pseudomembrane is at the top and underneath it are dilated crypts filled with mucin and acute inflammatory cells. (Courtesy of Edward Lee, MD, Dallas, TX.)

animals show complete structural necrosis of the intestine following intraluminal challenge with cell-free supernatant or purified toxin A from *C. difficile*. Similarly, no typical bacterial morphotype is seen within the pseudomembrane. The presumed reason is that *C. difficile* represents a relatively minor component of the colonic flora, even in patients with advanced disease.

UNDERLYING AND ASSOCIATED CONDITIONS

The initial reports of pseudomembranous enteritis antedated the antibiotic era, and a number of risk factors have been identified. The most common clinical setting in cases that are not associated with antimicrobial agents is surgery, usually colonic, gastric, or pelvic.[2–5, 19–21] Other risk factors include spinal fracture, intestinal obstruction, colon carcinoma, leukemia, severe burns, shock, uremia, heavy metal poisoning, hemolytic-uremic syndrome, ischemic cardiovascular disease, Crohn's disease, shigellosis, severe infection, neonatal necrotizing enterocolitis, ischemic colitis, and Hirschsprung's disease.[26–32] Occasional cases have been encountered in previously healthy persons who reported no recent antimicrobial exposure and no other identifiable risk factor.[33–35]

Despite the diversity of clinical settings noted above, the vast majority of PMC cases observed during the past four decades have occurred in association with antimicrobial use.[1, 3–9, 24, 25, 31, 36–41] Nearly all antimicrobial agents with an antibacterial spectrum of activity have been implicated in PMC-causing *C. difficile*–associated colitis in both patients and hamsters. The following antibiotics cause lethal hemorrhagic cecitis in hamsters: ampicillin, carbenicillin, essentially all cephalosporins, clindamycin, oral gentamicin, imipenem, metronidazole, nafcillin, penicillin, ticarcillin, and vancomycin.[42–46] Antimicrobial agents that failed to cause this complication or showed inconsistent results include chloramphenicol, tetracyclines, and sulfonamides, including trimethoprim-sulfamethoxazole.[46]

Clinical reports in the 1970s emphasized the role of clindamycin and its parent compound lincomycin.[9, 37–41] The prevalence of PMC with clindamycin or lincomycin varies from 0.01% to 10%, depending to a large extent on the frequency with which endoscopy is performed and the epidemiologic patterns of *C. difficile*.[9, 37, 41] It is important to recognize, however, that many other antimicrobial agents may be associated with this disease (see later section).

CLINICAL FEATURES

In the preantibiotic era, pseudomembranous enterocolitis was regarded as a catastrophic complication, but the high mortality rate may reflect the fact that the diagnosis was usually established only at autopsy examination.[3–5, 19–21, 31] During the early antibiotic era, when *S. aureus* was commonly implicated, this condition was regarded as a relatively serious complication in which patients often presented with diarrhea and fever, but the course and outcome were variable. The anatomic diagnosis was not established in most cases, so clinical descriptions and mortality data must be considered unreliable. The extensive use of endoscopy in the 1970s permitted much more accurate assessment of the clinical spectrum observed in patients with an established diagnosis

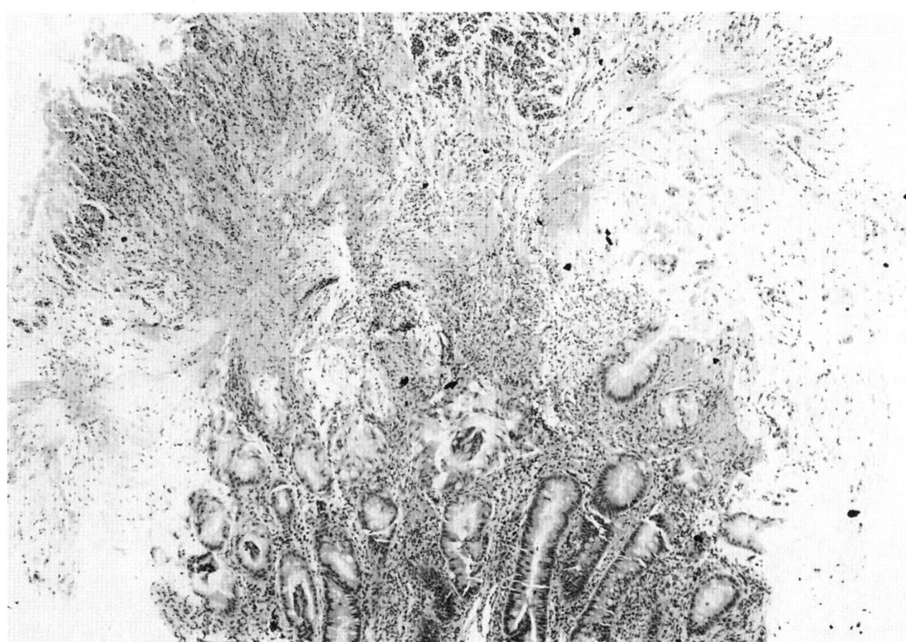

Figure 97–4. Microscopic pathologic appearance of severe pseudomembranous colitis with acute and chronic inflammatory cells, edema, and a mushroom-shaped pseudomembrane. The colonic architecture is preserved. (From Wilcox CM: Atlas of Clinical Gastrointestinal Endoscopy. Philadelphia, W.B. Saunders, 1995, p 216.)

of PMC. The single symptom found in nearly all patients is diarrhea, with the rare exception of patients with ileus.

Early work in the 1970s focused attention on the prominent role of clindamycin as an inducing agent in PMC. Most studies done after 1980 showed that cephalosporins have become the most common agents implicated in both community and nosocomially acquired cases of *C. difficile* colitis.[47–55] Ampicillin, amoxicillin, or amoxicillin-clavulanate (Augmentin) are also common causes, especially in outpatients. These three classes of drugs (cephalosporins, ampicillin/amoxicillin, and clindamycin) are considered the "big three" of *C. difficile*–associated enteric disease. Less commonly implicated are macrolides (erythromycin, clarithromycin, and azithromycin), penicillins other than ampicillin, fluoroquinolones, trimethoprim-sulfamethoxazole, metronidazole, rifampin, tetracyclines, and chloramphenicol. It has not been clearly established that the following drugs are associated with this complication: sulfonamides, parenteral aminoglycosides, parenteral vancomycin, urinary antiseptics (mendalamine, fosfomycin, or nitrofurantoin), or antimicrobial agents with activity restricted to fungi, mycobacteria (except rifampin), parasites, or viruses. Antineoplastic agents occasionally have been implicated, principally methotrexate.[32, 56]

The incidence of diarrhea ascribed to antimicrobial agents is obviously variable, depending on the agent and the host, as well as the definition of diarrhea. The usual criteria vary from two loose stools for at least 2 days to three loose stools for 3 days. By applying the former definition to clindamycin, the rate of diarrhea with clindamycin is 20% to 30%; by applying the latter, it is 5% to 10%.[57–59] With regard to other agents, the frequency of antibiotic-associated diarrhea is variously reported as follows: ampicillin 5% to 10%, amoxicillin-clavulanate 10% to 25%, cefixime 15% to 20%, other cephalosporins 2% to 5%, fluoroquinolones 1% to 2%, trimethoprim-sulfamethoxazole less than 1%, azithromycin 3% to 5%, clarithromycin 3% to 5%, erythromycin 2% to 5%, and tetracycline 2% to 5%.[60–62]

During the past decade there has been a reduction in the use of endoscopy in patients with suspected *C. difficile*–associated enteric disease, owing to increasing dependence on *C. difficile* toxin assays, which are now readily available and often are used relatively early in the course of the disease. The result is a substantial increase in the recognition of *C. difficile*–associated disease and relatively rare recognition of PMC; this decrease in the detection of PMC is ascribed to both a true decrease in frequency secondary to early therapy and a possibly artifactual decrease because of reduced use of endoscopy to characterize anatomic changes. Nevertheless, the number of recognized cases of *C. difficile* diarrhea has escalated greatly during the past 25 years to the point that this organism is now the leading recognized cause of bacterial diarrhea[63, 64] and possibly an important unrecognized cause of serious enteric disease as well.[65]

In nearly all cases of PMC, *C. difficile* is the pathogen, although most patients with antibiotic-associated diarrhea do not have *C. difficile* toxin. The issue confronting the clinician is to identify the clinical features or clues that suggest that a patient has *C. difficile*–associated disease in the setting of antibiotic-associated diarrhea, because this determination dictates the efficient use of the *C. difficile* toxin assay and the possible need for empiric treatment. These clinical clues are summarized in Table 97–2.

Compared to other forms of diarrhea, *C. difficile*–associated diarrhea usually occurs in association with use of clindamycin, ampicillin, or a cephalosporin, although nearly any antimicrobial agent with antibacterial activity may be responsible. The frequency of this complication is not clearly dose related. Diarrhea often persists or begins after the antibiotic has been discontinued; it is more likely to be severe than antibiotic-associated diarrhea in the absence of *C. difficile* toxin; it is most common in the nosocomial setting, where it may be endemic or epidemic; and there is more likely to be evidence of colitis with cramps, fever, leukocytosis, and fecal leukocytes. The pathogenesis of antibiotic-associated diarrhea without *C. difficile* toxin assays is usually enigmatic because no agent or clear mechanism can be de-

Table 97–2 | **Comparison of Antibiotic-Associated Diarrhea/Colitis Caused by *C. difficile* and Enigmatic Cases**

	CAUSES OF ANTIBIOTIC-ASSOCIATED DIARRHEA/COLITIS	
VARIABLE	***C. difficile***	**Cause Unknown**
Drugs most often implicated	Clindamycin, ampicillin, cephalosporins	Clindamycin, cefixime, cefoperazone, amoxicillin-clavulanate
Relationship of illness to dose	Usually not dose related	Dose related
Response to drug withdrawal	Symptoms often persist	Symptoms usually resolve
Clinical features		
Intestinal	Watery diarrhea and cramps	Loose stools
Constitutional	Fever and leukocytosis	Systemic symptoms are unusual
History	Usually noncontributory	History of diarrhea with same antibiotics or others
Complications	Toxic megacolon, ileus, high fever, leukemoid reaction, dehydration, hypoalbuminemia with anasarca, arthritis (rare)	Rarely serious ("nuisance diarrhea")
Evidence of colitis	Cramps, fecal leukocytes; colitis or PMC evident with endoscopy or CT	Colitis uncommon
Epidemiology	Epidemic or endemic in hospitals and nursing homes	Sporadic
Treatment	Discontinue implicated drug; oral vancomycin or metronidazole for severe cases	Discontinue implicated drug or reduce dose

PMC, pseudomembranous colitis; CT, computed tomography.

tected in most cases. This form is usually dose related. The patient often gives a history of diarrhea associated with use of the same antibiotic or others on previous occasions. The diarrhea is usually mild and usually resolves when the dose is reduced or the implicated drug is discontinued. Systemic signs of infection are usually absent, and there is usually no evidence of an epidemic or colitis. Although toxin-negative cases are enigmatic in pathogenesis, some of these cases are caused by false-negative toxin results, and 2% to 3% are ascribed to enterotoxin-producing strains of *Clostridium perfringens*[66] or to *Salmonella* organisms.[67] The roles of *Candida albicans* and *Staphylococcus aureus* in antibiotic-associated diarrhea are controversial.[68]

C. difficile–induced enteric disease includes a spectrum of clinical and pathologic findings. At one end is the asymptomatic carrier state, which, in the absence of antibiotic exposure in persons older than age 1 year, is not associated with detectable toxin. With antibiotic exposure, the range of findings includes asymptomatic carriage, trivial diarrhea, colitis that may resemble idiopathic ulcerative colitis, and, in its most severe and most characteristic form, PMC (see Table 97–2). Most cases of *C. difficile*–induced enteric disease are manifested by modest diarrhea that resolves when the inducing antibiotic is simply stopped; PMC represents a relatively unusual complication. On the other hand, 75% to 90% of patients with antibiotic-associated diarrhea have a negative *C. difficile* toxin assay, whereas PMC is nearly always caused by *C. difficile*.

Typical features of *C. difficile*–associated colitis in advanced stages include watery diarrhea with as many as 15 to 30 stools per day.[1, 9, 69–76] Most patients complain of abdominal pain or cramps, and they often have lower quadrant tenderness in association with fever and leukocytosis. These findings may suggest intraabdominal sepsis and occasionally lead to unwarranted laparotomy.[70] Fever, when present, is usually low grade but may be as high as 106° F, and the peripheral leukocyte count is usually in the range of 10,000 to 20,000/mm^3 but may be 40,000/mm^3 or greater. Unexplained leukocytosis may be a useful clue to this diagnosis.[77] There is protein-losing enteropathy, so hypoalbuminemia is a characteristic feature, even early in the disease course. Stool examination may show occult blood, but grossly bloody stools are unusual. Microscopic examination of the stool for white blood cells is positive in approximately one half of the cases; lactoferrin assays are preferred.[78–80] Serious complications include severe dehydration, electrolyte imbalance, hypotension, hypoalbuminemia with anasarca, and toxic megacolon. Colonic perforation is rare. Extraintestinal symptoms are also rare with antibiotic-associated colitis, except for the complications noted previously that are ascribed to fluid, albumin, or electrolyte losses. Polyarthritis involving large joints has been reported[81, 82]; the diagnostic criteria proposed by Putterman and Rubinow are arthritis following *C. difficile*–associated diarrhea with no alternative explanation for either the diarrhea or the arthritis.[81]

PATHOPHYSIOLOGY

C. difficile organisms have been known to produce a toxin that is highly lethal on systemic challenge to all animals tested since 1935.[13] This organism is occasionally found in diverse types of infections but does not appear to produce toxin at extraintestinal sites.[83–85] Thus, the role of *C. difficile* as a cause of a histotoxic *Clostridia* syndrome in humans remained enigmatic until the studies that implicated *C. difficile* as the cause of PMC. A striking feature of *C. difficile* in this setting is its intimate association with antibiotics. *C. difficile* toxin has been sought in stool in numerous other puzzling medical conditions, including sudden infant death syndrome,[86, 87] neonatal necrotizing enterocolitis,[88, 89] and relapses of idiopathic inflammatory bowel disease.[90–92] None of these associations has withstood the test of time. The conclusion of these studies is that *C. difficile* toxin is important only as an enteric toxin and *C. difficile* causes disease almost exclusively in association with exposure to antimicrobial agents.

Contributing factors in the pathogenesis of *C. difficile*–associated enteric disease are the requirements for 1) a source of the organism, presumably from the host's normal flora or from an environmental source; 2) altered normal

Table 97–3 | **Rates of *C. difficile* Isolation and *C. difficile* Cytotoxin in Stools**

PATIENT CATEGORY	CULTURE-POSITIVE RATES (%)	TOXIN-POSITIVE RATES (TISSUE CULTURE ASSAYS) (%)
Antibiotic-associated diarrhea or colitis with positive toxin assay	95–100	—
Antibiotic-associated PMC	95–100	90–100
Antibiotic-associated diarrhea	15–25	10–20
Antibiotic exposure without diarrhea	10–20	2–8
Hospitalized patients	10–25	?
Nursing home patients	5–15	?
Gastrointestinal disease unrelated to antibiotic exposure	2–3	0.5
Healthy adults	2–3	0
Healthy neonates	5–70	5–63

PMC, pseudomembranous colitis.

flora, which is the apparent role of antibiotics; 3) toxin production that appears to reflect rapid growth of toxigenic strains at a time that the competing flora are suppressed; 4) age-related susceptibility; and 5) immunologic susceptibility.

Colonization Rates

Culture of *C. difficile* using selective media[93, 94] to determine carrier rates shows considerable variation depending on the population studied (Table 97–3). When data from multiple investigations are combined, the recovery rate from healthy adults is 2% to 3%; from patients with antibiotic-associated diarrhea or colitis with positive toxin assays, 90% to 100%; from hospitalized patients without diarrhea, 15% to 30%; and from adults who have recently received antimicrobials but do not have diarrhea, 5% to 15%.[1, 93–102] The isolation rate in infants ranges from 5% to 70%; controlled studies show that the rate of carriage is similar in children with and without enteric disease.[92–96] Relatively high carriage rates persist during the first 8 months of life, until the "normal flora" become established.[13, 102–107]

In Vitro Susceptibility

It is commonly assumed that *C. difficile*–induced diarrhea or colitis in association with antibiotic exposure represents a superinfection with a resistant microbe; however, experiments in hamsters have shown little correlation between activity in vitro against *C. difficile* and the propensity to cause lethal colitis.[42–46] A similar observation appears to apply to patients. In vitro sensitivity tests show most strains of *C. difficile* to be susceptible to vancomycin, metronidazole, bacitracin, rifampin, penicillins, and tetracyclines. Cephalosporins are less active; results with clindamycin and quinolones are variable.[108–115] All of these drugs induce lethal *C. difficile* cecitis in hamsters, and most are known to induce *C. difficile*–associated enteric disease in humans, although the rates vary substantially. The paradox of in vitro sensitivity correlations is illustrated well by the observation that the minimum inhibitory concentrations (MIC) of ampicillin and vancomycin are approximately the same, although the former is one of the most frequent inducing agents and the latter is standard treatment. Some of these inconsistencies presumably are explained by the fact that activity in vitro is judged by serum levels, but relevant risk factors, such as the potential to alter the colonic flora and the activity against *C. difficile*, depend on antibiotic levels in the colonic lumen. Thus, vancomycin is poorly absorbed and reaches levels that are 100 to 10,000 times higher than the MIC in the colon; by contrast, ampicillin is better absorbed and largely destroyed by beta-lactamases of the fecal flora, so that activity against colonic *C. difficile* is poor.

Disruption of the fecal flora is assumed to be the critical factor in *C. difficile*-associated enteric disease; activity against anaerobic bacteria is particularly important because these organisms account for more than 99% of the fecal flora and appear to be responsible for population control in the colonic lumen.[116, 117] The major inducing agents—clindamycin, ampicillin, and cephalosporins—obey this rule; sulfonamides, trimethoprim-sulfamethoxazole, parenteral aminoglycosides, and quinolones have less impact on the fecal flora and are less frequently implicated. Thus, a simplistic explanation is that antibiotics alter the flora, thereby providing a suitable environment for conversion of *C. difficile* spores to vegetative forms, with rapid replication and toxin production.

Epidemiology

C. difficile is a sporulating organism that survives well in nature and, like other clostridia, is distributed widely in the environment.[15, 118–122] Unlike other anaerobes, including other clostridia, there is compelling evidence that *C. difficile* is a transferrable pathogen that poses a threat to hospitalized patients who are exposed to a nosocomial source of the organism and are rendered susceptible by antibiotic administration. The result is that *C. difficile* is by far the most common identifiable microbial pathogen in nosocomial diarrhea, and it is also responsible for multiple outbreaks of diarrheal disease in hospitals and nursing homes.[9, 78, 99, 123–129] Early reports dealt with epidemics marked by extensive morbidity and mortality.[38–41, 69–72] More recent reports deal primarily with higher attack rates and modest disease. This change reflects the combined effects of increased cephalosporin use, more aggressive testing, and early intervention.[121–129]

Evaluation of epidemics includes case surveillance, stool cultures to identify carriers, typing of strains, and cultures of environmental sources. Surveillance cultures have shown environmental sources of *C. difficile*, especially in case-associated areas.[118–131] Mulligan and colleagues isolated the organism in environmental samplings from 37 of 114 (32%) case-associated sites, as compared with 6 of 445 (1.3%) control sites.[119] Similar findings were reported by Fekety and coworkers.[120] In both investigations, the principal sources for positive culture results were toilets, bedpans, and floors. *C. difficile* was also found in hand and stool culture specimens from asymptomatic hospital personnel who worked in case-associated areas.[122] Culture specimen results of air, food, and walls were uniformly negative.

Epidemiologic studies have also involved a variety of methods for typing strains in an effort to monitor epidemics and to correlate the strain with virulence according to clinical severity and with production of toxin in vitro. The methods of strain typing used are diverse and include "plasmid fingerprinting," antibiotic sensitivity tests, protein profile analysis, immunoblotting, polyacrylamide gel electrophoresis (PAGE) typing, PAGE after incorporation of ^{35}S methionine, serotyping, restriction endonuclease analysis, slide agglutination for flagellar antigens, polymerase chain reaction (PCR) ribotyping, bacteriocin typing, and restriction fragment length polymorphism.[132–139] These are considered research methods and are not available for routine use. There is no consensus on which method is best. Furthermore, specific strains have not been shown consistently to correlate with clinical features because host factors appear to be more important than strain type in clinical expression[137, 139]; an exception is one report of a correlation between strain type, toxin production in vitro, and clinical disease.[140]

Clostridium difficile Toxins

C. difficile–associated colitis is a toxin-mediated disease that requires production of toxin for clinical expression. At least two toxins are recognized: toxin A, or enterotoxin, and toxin B, or cytotoxin.[140–143] These toxins are large molecular weight, heat-labile proteins that are neutralized by *C. difficile* and *C. sordellii* antitoxin. The genes for toxin A and B have been cloned.[144, 145] They are separated by only 1.2 kb on the *C. difficile* chromosome.[146, 147] Strains that produce one toxin in vitro produce both, with rare exceptions,[148–151] and both are expressed under identical culture conditions.[141, 142] As expected, nontoxigenic strains lack both toxin A and toxin B genes.[152]

Both toxins are lethal in systemic challenge to mice in concentrations about 1/100th of the lethal dose of botulinum toxin.[141] The mechanism of death is not known, although both toxins induce proinflammatory monokines, including interleukin-1 (IL-1) and tumor necrosis factor (TNF).[153] Both toxins inconsistently elicit a systemic humoral response with immunoglobulins A and G (IgA and IgG).[154] Toxins A and B differ on the basis of their separation by anion exchange chromatography, antigenic differences, and variations in biologic properties.[141, 143]

Toxin B, a 270- to 279-kd protein, is a highly potent cytopathic toxin to virtually all cell lines examined. With fibroblasts there are characteristic actinomorphic changes, reflecting nonlethal disruption of actin microfilaments of the cytoskeleton.[155–157] As little as 0.2 pg of toxin B causes typical changes, an observation that may account for the acute sensitivity of tissue culture assay for disease detection.

Toxin A is a 308-kd protein that also causes identical nonlethal cytoskeletal changes in tissue-cultured cells but is substantially less potent than toxin B. The major difference is that toxin A induces a fluid flux and causes intense mucosal inflammation in animal loop assays using small bowel or colon of guinea pigs, hamsters, rats, mice, and rabbits.[141–143, 158] In rabbit distal colon loops, toxin A induces increased myoelectric activity, significant neutrophil infiltration, and increased production of prostaglandin E_2 and leukotrienes.[159] Toxin B has no activity in these assays.[141, 143, 160] These observations have led some investigators to conclude that toxin B is most useful for disease detection but that toxin A may be principally responsible for clinical expression of the disease. More recent studies of human intestinal cells (T84) in Ussing chambers have shown that toxin B is approximately 10 times more potent than toxin A in inducing permeability and morphologic changes.[161] These observations suggest that, in contrast to animal models, both toxin A and B play roles in the pathogenesis of *C. difficile*–associated enteric disease in humans. Support for this conclusion comes from cases involving toxin A−, toxin B+ strains.[148–151]

Age-Related Risk

Studies cited above show that infants and children younger than 1 year of age commonly harbor *C. difficile* and its toxin without experiencing deleterious consequences. The reason is not known. Older children may develop antibiotic-associated PMC,[89, 161, 162] but it is clear that the incidence is less than that in adults. Population-based studies in Sweden have shown that the incidence of *C. difficile* toxin-positive stools increases 20- to 100-fold when persons aged 10 to 20 years are compared with those over 60 years.[63, 100] Multivariate analysis of hospitalized patients who are colonized with *C. difficile* also show that increased age correlates significantly with clinical expression.[100]

Immunologic Susceptibility

Prior studies have shown that about one half of adults have circulating IgG that neutralizes toxin A, toxin B, or both[154] and that *C. difficile* infection may be associated with serum and fecal IgA antibody.[154, 162] The relevence of these observations was shown in studies by Kyne and associates,[162] who examined the correlation between IgG, IgA, and IgM antibodies to toxin A or B and clinical expression among hospitalized carriers of *C. difficile*. They showed that an anamnestic response with serum IgG antibody against toxin A correlated with protection from clinical disease, that is, asymptomatic carriage. A subsequent report by the same group showed that the development of serum IgG antibody against toxin A also provides protection against relapse.[163]

DIAGNOSIS

Laboratory Tests

Laboratory tests that are nonspecific but suggest *C. difficile* as a cause of diarrhea or colitis include leukocytosis, with a mean peripheral leukocyte count of about 15,000/mm^3 [1, 31, 73, 77]; hypoalbuminemia, which is nearly always present, even early in the course[1, 31, 73]; and positive assay results for fecal leukocytes, which are found in approximately one half of all patients with *C. difficile*–associated diarrhea and nearly all with *C. difficile*–associated colitis.[49, 78–80]

Anatomic Diagnosis

Radiologic findings are usually nonspecific but may be helpful in suggesting PMC in as many as one half of patients

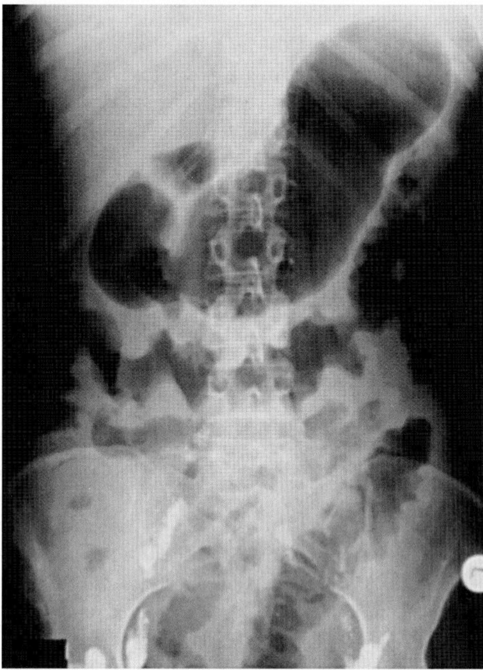

Figure 97–5. Plain abdominal film of antibiotic-associated pseudomembranous colitis. Note the involvement of the entire colon, the markedly edematous folds, and the lack of dilatation. The small bowel is normal. Severe edema and thickness of the colon wall are indicated by the distance between the gastric air shadow above and the colon below.

with advanced disease.[164–166] Plain radiographs of the abdomen may show a markedly edematous colon, distorted haustral markings, and distention of the entire colon (Fig. 97–5). Occasionally, small irregularities represent pseudomembranous plaques in profile. Barium contrast studies may show rounded filling defects that outline the plaques, but the findings are often nondiagnostic due to underpenetration of barium, excessive mucus secretion, confluence of the pseudomembranes, or minimal involvement (Fig. 97–6). The diagnostic accuracy is improved with air-contrast studies, which must be performed with caution because of the potential complication of colonic perforation. Computed tomography (CT) often shows a thickening of the colonic wall, averaging 10 to 15 mm, that may be focal or pancolonic (Fig. 97–7).[167, 168] Almost invariably, changes are restricted to the colon. There is often evidence of ascites, and contrast trapped in the thickened folds shows a characteristic "accordion sign." Nevertheless, nearly one half of patients with *C. difficile* disease have normal CT findings.[168]

The preferred method of establishing the diagnosis of PMC is endoscopy to detect typical mucosal plaquelike lesions (see Fig. 97–2). The distal colon is involved in most patients, so sigmoidoscopy is usually adequate, but as many as one third of patients have lesions restricted to the right colon, necessitating colonoscopy for detection.[169, 170] Endoscopy often requires an experienced endoscopist. Copious amounts of mucus must be removed cautiously to reveal the plaques without separating the loosely adherent stalks. Similar precautions are necessary for preprocedure colon preparation, for the same reasons. Care must also be taken to include the entire lesion in any biopsy, because the stalk attachment may be narrow, fragile, and easily dislodged. Mucosal changes other than PMC that may be observed on endoscopy in patients with antibiotic-associated diarrhea include erythema, edema, friable mucosa, colonic ulceration, or hemorrhage. In some instances, the changes noted on both gross inspection and biopsy specimens may be highly suggestive of idiopathic ulcerative colitis.[171–173]

Identifying the Pathogen

C. difficile has been implicated in enteric disease almost exclusively as a complication of antibiotic exposure (see Table 97–3). An exception is the occasional case of PMC that occurs in the absence of antibiotic exposure.[33–35] With antibiotic-associated diarrhea, the frequency with which *C. difficile* is implicated correlates directly with the severity of the disease. Thus, for patients with uncomplicated diarrhea the frequency is 15% to 25%; for antibiotic-associated colitis it is 50% to 70%; and for antibiotic-associated PMC it is 90% to 100%.

The "gold standard" for *C. difficile* detection is the cytotoxicity assay using tissue-cultured cells, as originally described in 1978 (Fig. 97–8).[17, 18] The recommended method is to test undiluted watery stool or a 1:4 dilution of solid stool after passage through a 0.45-μm filter. The criterion for a positive test is demonstration of a cytopathic toxin that is neutralized by *C. sordellii* or *C. difficile* antitoxin.[174, 175] This assay has problems: 1) Most laboratories do not offer tissue culture assays; 2) results are not available for 24 to 28 hours; and 3) some investigators report relatively poor clinical correlations.[176, 177] Sequential analysis of hamster stools following antimicrobial challenge shows virtually 100% sensitivity and specificity; additionally, there is a gradual increase in toxin titer to consistent levels of 10^{-5} to 10^{-7} dilutions at death.[16, 42, 43] In contrast, toxin titers in patients show no clear correlation with disease severity. Despite the variations noted in clinical reports, many authorities consider this to be the most accurate diagnostic test, provided that stool is not diluted more than 1 : 4 and that clinical correlations are made.[1, 76, 178, 179] This test can detect 10 pg of toxin, thereby making it the most sensitive test currently available for toxin detection.[179]

Multiple alternative tests are now available to detect *C. difficile*, and these are advocated because of possible advantages in technical ease, speed of results, or cost. The relative merits of these assays are summarized in Table 97–4.

The first commercially available test was the latex particle agglutination assay, which was initially designed to detect toxin A, but later work showed that the assay recognized another protein product produced by other microbial species and by both toxigenic and nontoxigenic strains of *C. difficile*.[180–182] Other methods that are used or are under development are enzyme immunoassays (EIAs), dot immunoblotting, culture, and PCR. A preferred method for most laboratories is EIA.[183–188] This test shows good specificity, but requires 100 to 1000 pg of either toxin, so that the sensitivity is reduced compared with the cytotoxin assay.[179] The reported frequency of false-negative results compared to the tissue culture assay is 10% to 30%, so that repeated testing is sometimes required.[49, 183–187] Commercially available reagents for the EIA will detect toxin A or toxins A and B;

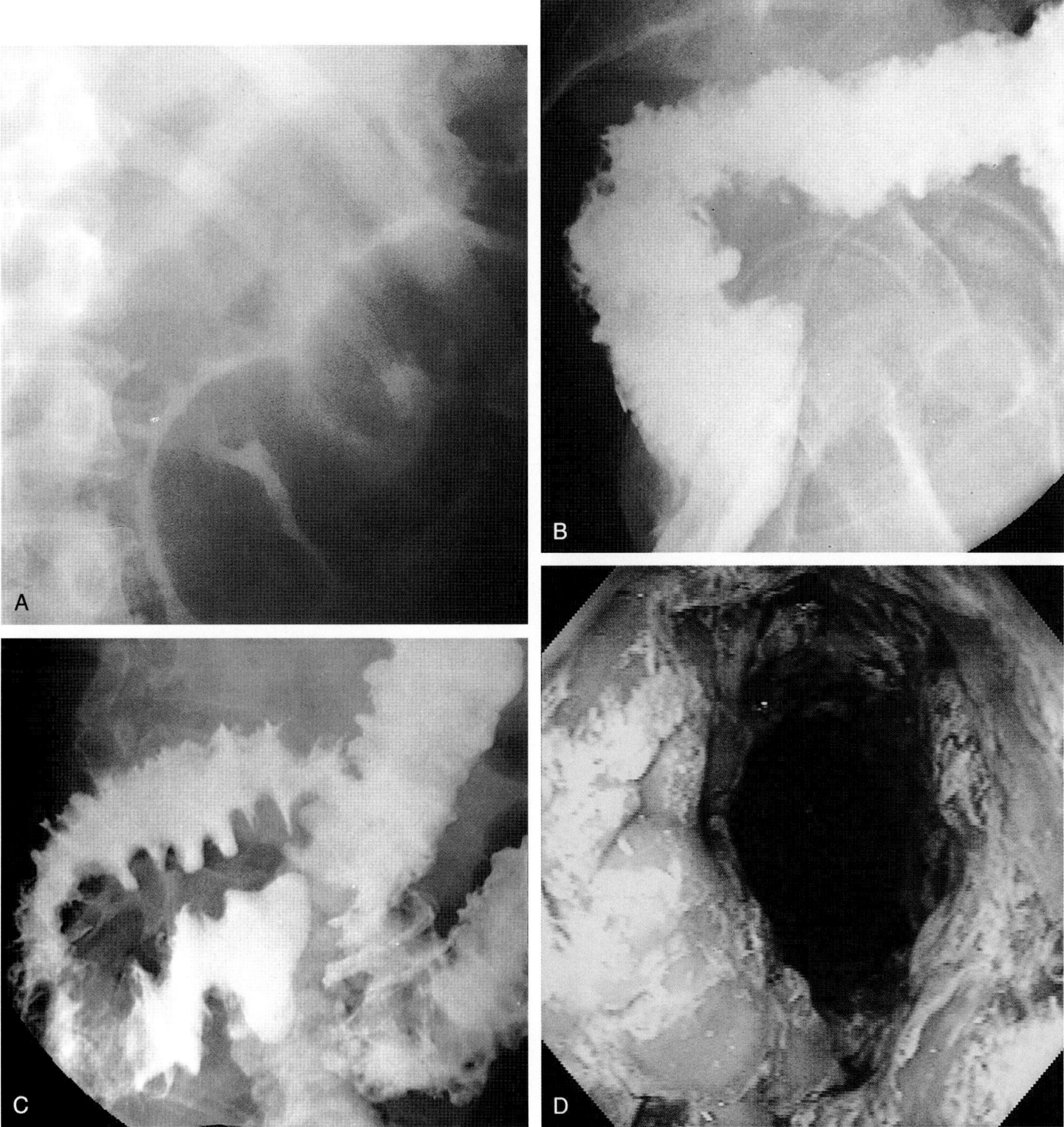

Figure 97–6. Severe *Clostridium difficile* colitis. *A,* Abdominal radiograph shows subtle nodularity of the colon. *B,* Barium enema film shows marked irregularity of the rectal wall. *C,* The more proximal colon demonstrates marked nodularity (thumb-printing) of the wall. The mucosa in some areas is poorly coated by the barium. *D,* Colonoscopy shows that the colonic wall is covered by a thick, tenacious membrane. The rectum had multiple well-circumscribed yellow plaques characteristic of *C. difficile* colitis. (From Wilcox CM: Atlas of Clinical Gastrointestinal Endoscopy. Philadelphia, W.B. Saunders, 1995, p 217.)

many authorities now prefer tests that detect both toxins, because of reports of a few cases involving *C. difficile* strains that produce only toxin B.[148–151] An alternative rapid test is a dot immunobinding assay (*C. difficile*-CUBE) for detection of toxin A in stool.[189] PCR technology has been developed to amplify gene fragments that encode for either toxin A or B, and results of preliminary tests appear promising.[190, 191]

Some authorites advocate stool cultures for *C. difficile* by using selective media, with or without toxin assays of broth cultures of isolated strains, to identify toxigenic strains.[192–195] Advantages are the high degree of sensitivity and the opportunity for strain typing in epidemics. Potential problems are the lack of specificity, delays in the availability of results, and difficulties encountered in recovering *C. difficile*, which is easy for research laboratories with extensive experience but difficult for clinical laboratories where such experience—or commitment—is not available.

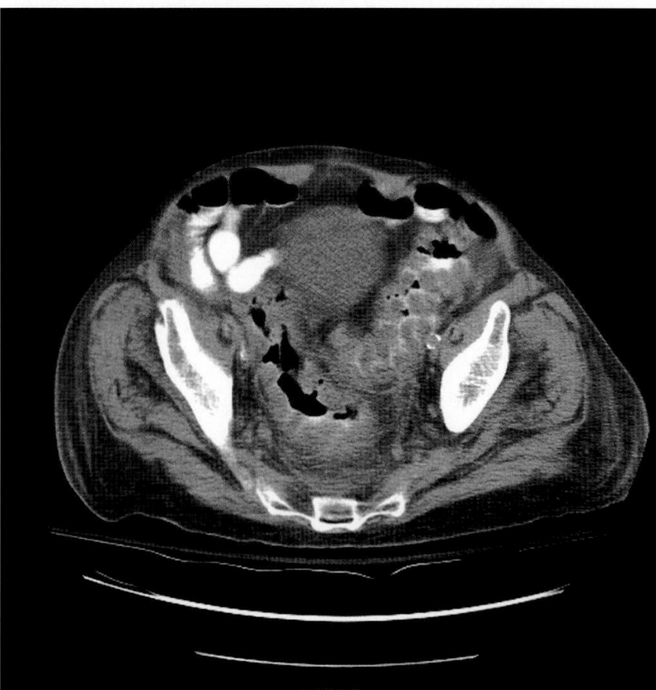

Figure 97–7. CT image showing pseudomembranous colitis with marked thickening of the colonic wall.

Recommendations of the Society for Hospital Epidemiology and Infection Control (SHEA) for *C. difficile* detection are[196]: (1) test only diarrheal stools, unless there is ileus; 2) do not perform a "test of cure" except for epidemiologic investigation; 3) test stools only from persons over 1 year of age (because of a lack of clinical correlations in infants); 4) the preferred test for sensitivity is culture (although most laboratories do not offer it); and 5) EIA is an acceptable alternative to the cytotoxin assay but is less sensitive. Patients who have nosocomial diarrhea, defined as diarrhea with an onset after day 3 of hospitalization, usually have *C. difficile*–associated enteric disease or no detectable pathogen.[197] For this reason, the Infectious Diseases Society of America recommends "the 3-day rule," which means initial testing for microbial pathogens in patients with nosocomial diarrhea is done only for *C. difficile*.[78] Possible exceptions are patients older than 65 years of age or with comorbid disease, neutropenia, and human immunodeficiency virus infections.[198]

TREATMENT

Therapy for PMC includes discontinuation of implicated antimicrobial agents, nonspecific supportive measures, and, in some cases, antimicrobial agents directed against *C. difficile* (Table 97–5). Supportive measures include intravenous fluids to correct fluid losses, electrolyte imbalance, and hypoalbuminemia. Parenteral nutrition is sometimes required. Antiperistalsis agents such as diphenoxylate with atropine (Lomotil) should be avoided because they have been observed to increase the frequency of antibiotic-associated diarrhea and to exacerbate symptoms among patients with established disease.[199–201] Systemic administration of glucocorticoids is sometimes advocated for critically ill patients, although treatment with methylprednisolone in an animal model of antibiotic-induced colitis failed to delay death, and the clinical experience is limited.[202, 203] When antimicrobial treatment must be continued despite *C. difficile*–associated complications, the recommendation is to treat the enteric complication with oral metronidazole or vancomycin and to use systemic antibiotics that were not implicated in the individual case and are unlikely to produce this complication: aminoglycosides, metronidazole, sulfonamides, trimethoprim-sulfamethoxazole, macrolides, parenteral vancomycin, and quinolones.

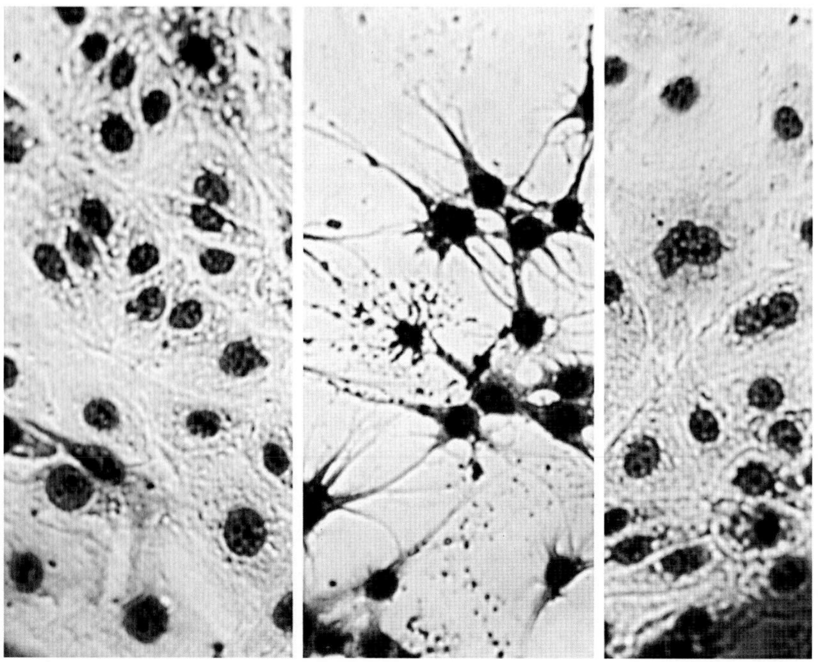

Figure 97–8. Results of tissue culture assay for *C. difficile* toxin, with use of primary human amnion cells. The left panel shows normal cells; the center panel shows typical actinomorphic changes after application of stool containing *C. difficile* toxin; and the right panel shows the tissue cultured cells with the same specimen after neutralization with *C. sordellii* antitoxin. Identical changes are noted with inocula of stools from experimental animals that have antibiotic-induced cecitis, stools from patients with pseudomembranous colitis, cell-free supernatant fluid of *C. difficile* in broth culture, and *C. difficile* purified toxin A or toxin B. Toxin B is approximately 1000 times more active than toxin A in the tissue culture assay.

Table 97–4 | **Diagnostic Tests for *Clostridium difficile* Toxins**

VARIABLE	TISSUE CULTURE ASSAY[1, 72, 73, 75, 178, 183, 184, 186–188]	LATEX PARTICLE AGGLUTINATION[180–182]	ENZYME IMMUNOASSAY[49, 183–188]	DOT IMMUNOBLOT[189]	PCR[190, 191]	CULTURE[83, 84, 192, 195–198]
Source	Microliter wells often preferred	Commercially available	Four suppliers	Commercially available	Experimental	CCFA media, etc.
Product detected	Toxin B	Glutamate dehydrogenase	Toxin A or Toxin A plus Toxin B	Toxin A	Toxin B gene, Toxin A gene, or both	Organism
Time required	28–48 hr	30 min	2–4 hr	30 min	2–4 hr	24–72 hr
Clinical correlations	Best sensitivity with proper dilutions; good specificity	Least sensitive and least specific	Good specificity; fair sensitivity	Results of initial studies promising	Good sensitivity; fair specificity	Good sensitivity; poor specificity

CCFA, cycloserine, cefoxitin, fructose, and egg yolk agar.[93, 197]

Antibiotics

Antimicrobial treatment options include vancomycin, metronidazole, teicoplanin, fusidic acid, and bacitracin[204–211] (see Table 97–5). The most extensive clinical experience is with oral metronidazole and oral vancomycin, which appear to be comparable in terms of response rates, time to response, and relapse rates.[210–215] Particularly important was the report by Wenisch and associates[212] because it included 36 patients with established PMC; results with metronidazole and vancomycin showed that each group had a 94% response rate, a mean duration of diarrhea of three days after treatment, and a 16% relapse rate. Despite comparability of metronidazole and vancomycin in therapeutic trials, theoretical advantages of oral vancomycin are the facts that colonic levels are extremely high, all strains of *C. difficile* are highly sensitive in vitro, and vancomycin is more effective in the hamster model.[42] Specifically, levels in the colon after oral doses of 125 mg are 350 to 500 μg/g stool,[108, 206, 214] and testing of over 200 strains has shown that most strains have an MIC of 1 μg/mL or less and none have an MIC greater than 16 μg/mL.[108–112] (The reason colonic levels are relevant is that *C. difficile* does not invade the mucosa, and the disease is restricted to the colon.) By contrast, metronidazole is well absorbed when taken orally so that colonic levels and in vitro activity are less predictable.[110, 212, 216, 217] Nevertheless, most authorities favor metronidazole because it has performed well in clinical trials, the price is 20-fold less than that of oral vancomycin, and there is concern that oral vancomycin in hospitalized patients will promote vancomycin-resistant strains.[218] Exceptions are pregnancy and metronidazole intolerance. Some authorities prefer vancomycin for initial therapy in seriously ill patients on the basis of the theoretical issues summarized previously.

In response to therapy, fever usually resolves in 24 to 48 hours and diarrhea in 1 to 13 days, with a mean of 3 to 4 days.[204, 209–213, 219] Failure to respond is usually the result of ileus or an alternative or concurrent cause of enteric disease such as inflammatory bowel disease. The only antibiotic treatments with established merit are those administered orally; patients with ileus may be treated with installations of vancomycin or metronidazole into the small intestine by long tubes, although the reported experience with this approach is limited. The experience with intravenous therapy is variable,[220] but if required, intravenous metronidazole is rec-

Table 97–5 | **Treatment of *C. difficile*–Induced Diarrhea and Colitis**

NONSPECIFIC MEASURES

Discontinue implicated antimicrobial agent (alternatives are to change to another agent that is infrequently associated with this complication or continue implicated agent while giving oral vancomycin)
Supportive measures: Correct fluid losses and electrolyte imbalance
Avoid antiperistaltic agents
Enteric isolation precautions for hospitalized patients

SPECIFIC TREATMENT

Antimicrobial Agents (Only If Symptoms Are Severe or Persistent)

Oral agent (preferred)
- Vancomycin: 125 mg PO q.i.d. × 7–14 days*
- Metronidazole: 250 mg PO t.i.d. × 7–14 days*
- Bacitracin: 25,000 U PO q.i.d. × 7–14 days*

Parenteral agents (to be used only until oral agents are tolerated): metronidazole, 500 mg IV q6h

Alternative Treatments

Anion-exchange resins
- Cholestyramine, 4-g packet PO t.i.d. × 5–10 days*
- Colestipol, 5-g packet PO t.i.d. × 5–10 days*

Alter fecal flora
Lactinex (or alternative *Lactobacillus* preparation): 1-g packet PO q.i.d. × 7–14 days

MULTIPLE RELAPSES

Vancomycin or metronidazole PO × 10–14 days, followed by
- Cholestyramine (above dose), plus *Lactobacillus* (above doses), × 4–6 weeks
- Vancomycin, 125 mg PO q.o.d. × 4–6 weeks

Vancomycin plus rifampin × 7–14 days
Experimental
- *Saccharomyces boulardii:* Vancomycin or metronidazole (per above doses) ≥4 days with addition of *S. boulardii* as two 250-mg capsules b.i.d. × 4 weeks[225–227]
- *Lactobacillus GG* 10^{10}/day × 7–10 after course of vancomycin or metronidazole[228–230]
- Intravenous immunoglobulin: 400 mg/kg q3wk (reported primarily in pediatric patients and an adult with IgA deficiency)[231, 232]
- Rectal instillation of feces: 50 g fresh stool from healthy donor in 500 mg saline delivered by enema[236]
- Rectal instillations of broth cultures of bacterial isolates from healthy donors: Strains selected for in vitro inhibition of *C. difficile*, cultured to 10^9/mL, 2 mL of each mixed in anaerobic glovebox with 180 mL saline and given by enema[237]

*Efficacy is established.
Do not give vancomycin and *Lactobacillus* preparations together because vancomycin kills lactobacilli.

ommended because therapeutic levels of the drug are achieved in the colon.[217]

Most patients have self-limited disease with spontaneous resolution if the implicated antibiotic is simply discontinued. A major complication of antibiotic therapy for *C. difficile*–associated disease is relapse, which is noted in 15% to 25% of patients treated with antimicrobial agents. Therefore, the main indications for antibiotic therapy are severe disease (severe diarrhea or evidence of colitis) and persistent diarrhea despite discontinuation of the implicated drug.

Relapses

Relapses occur only with antibiotic treatment, and they appear to occur with nearly equal frequency regardless of drug, dose, or duration of treatment with metronidazole, vancomycin, fucidic acid, bacitracin or teicoplanin.[204–211, 221] Thus, one principle in management is that prevention of relapses is unlikely to be promoted by changes in the dose, duration, or selection of antimicrobial agent for treatment.

The frequency of relapses is reported to be 5% to 50%.[204, 208, 212, 221] The largest reported series concerned 189 patients, including 100 with PMC. Following treatment with oral vancomycin 46 (24%) had relapses; all responded to retreatment with oral vancomycin, but 22 (23%) experienced a second relapse, and 4 (2%) had six or more relapses.[209] Relapses are thought to occur because *C. difficile* is not eliminated by antimicrobial therapy[222] owing to sporulation; spores revert to vegetative forms that produce toxin when antibiotics directed against *C. difficile* are discontinued; and the normal fecal flora is ineffective in controlling *C. difficile* replication because of the impact of the antibiotic used to treat *C. difficile*. This concept is supported by experiments with *C. difficile* treated with vancomycin in a chemostat; the drug controls growth of vegetative forms, but spores persist, and when the drug is removed, growth of vegetative forms and production of toxin resume.[223] The immune response with serum IgG levels is another factor that renders the host vulnerable.[163]

The clinical features of relapses are essentially identical to those of the prior episode except for the severity, which may be milder or more severe. The characteristic pattern is clinical recovery followed by recurrence of the same symptoms, usually diarrhea and cramps, 3 to 10 days after vancomycin or metronidazole is discontinued. *C. difficile* toxin assay results at the time of relapse are positive, but are usually not necessary because the patient's history provides the diagnosis.

Most relapses are managed simply by repeating a course of treatment with metronidazole or vancomycin, with success in 60% to 70% of cases.[209] The major challenge has been the management of patients with multiple relapses. Several options have been tried with variable success:

- Antimicrobial agents: A repeat course of vancomycin or metronidazole, which is often successful. An alternative approach is a standard course for 10 to 14 days to control the acute episode followed by "pulse-dose" vancomycin (125 mg every day) for 6 weeks to keep *C. difficile* in the spore state while the normal flora becomes reestablished.
- Biotherapy (use of microorganisms with therapeutic properties): The major interest has been with *Lactobacillus* and *Saccharomyces boulardii*.[224] *S. boulardii* is a nonpathogenic fungus that produces a protease that blocks attachment of *C. difficile* toxins to colonic mucosa.[225, 226] *S. boulardii* has been found to reduce the frequency of relapses when given for 1 month after completion of a 7 to 10 day course of oral vancomycin.[225, 227] Another use of biotherapy is *Lactobacillus casei ss rhamosum*, which has inhibitory activity against *C. difficile*,[228] persists in the colon after ingestion,[229] and appears to reduce the frequency of relapses.[230] *Lactobacillus acidophilus* (Lactinex) is another option but is not a component of the normal colonic flora, so persistence is potentially problematic; also, it has not been extensively studied. Neither *S. boulardii* nor *Lactobacillus GG* are approved by the Food and Drug Administration in the United States, but both may be available in health food stores and in other countries.
- Antibody: Studies showing the critical role of the humoral immune response in controlling the clinical expression of *C. difficile* infection support the role of immunoglobulin therapy in a dose of 200 to 300 mg/kg.[162, 163] A limited experience with intravenous immune globulin (IVIG) is encouraging.[231, 232]
- Anion exchange resins: Cholestyramine and colestipol have been used to treat *C. difficile*–associated diarrhea and relapsing diarrhea with variable success.[233, 234] These drugs bind the toxins of *C. difficile*.[235] Potency is limited, and the major interest is for prolonged use of these agents to prevent relapses after an initial response or as prototypes for new products with greater toxin-binding properties. If used, these anion exchange resins should not be given with vancomycin because they bind this antibiotic.
- Fecal therapy: Human feces may be administered via a Fleet enema bottle to replenish the normal flora.[236, 237] This approach has demonstrated efficacy but lacks esthetic appeal and risks transmission of potentially hazardous viruses (hepatitis, retroviruses) unless reconstituted fecal strains are used.[238]

Surgery

Seriously ill patients who have fulminant or intractable symptoms may require intestinal surgery. In our experience, surgical intervention is needed in approximately 0.4% of cases.[239] The major indications are failure to respond to medical management with progressive organ failure, toxic megacolon, worsening of findings on CT scan, or signs of peritonitis. The preferred procedure is usually total colectomy. Some authorities recommend intraluminal instillation of vancomycin at the time of surgery.

Infection Control

C. difficile has been implicated in epidemics, or it may be endemic in hospitals, long-term care facilities, and, to a lesser extent, day-care centers.[9, 53, 69, 99, 101, 102, 118–120, 124–126, 240–247] The organism is the only major anaerobe for which person-to-person transmission is important. Contributing factors are the proximity of patients, widespread environmental contamination, and extensive use of antimicrobial agents, especially those likely to cause this complication. *C. difficile* is widespread in the environment, with positive culture results reported in 2.2% of residencies, 2.4% of raw vegetables, 0.1%

of farm animals, and 2% of cats.[248] The frequency of positive cultures is much higher in the hospital environment, especially in case-associated areas,[118–131] where the yield is as high as 32%.[119] The frequency of stool colonization in adults is 2% to 3% in the community and 15% to 30% in hospitalized patients and residents of long-term care facilities.[93, 95, 99, 101, 102, 128] It is estimated that approximately one third of all patients receive antibiotics during hospitalization. These observations provide the basis for long-term care facilities and hospitals as the major foci of endemic and epidemic *C. difficile* cases.

Recommendations of SHEA[196] to control *C. difficile* in hospitals and long-term care facilities especially in epidemics are 1) restrict antibiotic use/abuse with particular attention to clindamycin[249–251] and possibly cephalosporins[50]; 2) handwashing with soap; 3) use of vinyl gloves[252]; 4) cleaning of environmental surfaces with sporicidal agents, especially in case-associated areas[253, 254]; 5) isolation of symptomatic patients, especially those incontinent of stool, in private rooms; and 6) avoidance of rectal thermometers.[255]

PREVENTION

The major methods for prevention that are currently available are restraint in the use of antibiotics and infection control in acute and chronic care facilities. There has been interest in the prophylactic use of *S. boulardii* and *Lactobacillus GG* concurrently with antibiotics.[256, 257] Problems with this approach are a lack of impressive results in clinical trials and limited availability of these products from commercial sources. There is increasing interest in a vaccine, on the basis of studies showing the important role of the humoral antibody response in the clinical expression of disease,[165, 166] preliminary studies showing response to IVIG therapy,[230, 231] promising results in the hamster model,[258] and preliminary success in preparing an immunogen.[259]

REFERENCES

1. Bartlett JG: Clostridium difficile: Clinical considerations. Rev Infect Dis 12:S244, 1990.
2. Finney JMT: Gastro-enterostomy for cicatrizing ulcer of the plyorus. Bull Johns Hopkins Hosp 4:53, 1893.
3. Penner A, Bernheim A: Acute postoperative enterocolitis. Arch Pathol 27:966, 1939.
4. Hummel RP, Altemeier WA, Hill EQ: Iatrogenic staphylococcal enterocolitis. Ann Surg 160:551, 1964.
5. Wakefield RD, Sommers Sd: Fatal membranous staphylococcal enteritis in surgical patients. Ann Surg 138:249, 1953.
6. Altemeier WA, Hummel RP, Hill EO: Staphylococcal enterocolitis following antibiotic therapy. Ann Surg 157:847, 1963.
7. Azar H, Drapanas T: Relationship of antibiotics to wound infection and enterocolitis in colon surgery. Am J Surg 115:209, 1968.
8. Khan MY, Hall WH: Staphylococcal enterocolitis: Treatment with oral vancomycin. Ann Intern Med 65:1, 1966.
9. Tedesco FJ, Barton RW, Alpers DH: Clindamycin-associated colitis: A prospective study. Ann Intern Med 81:429, 1974.
10. Hambre DM, Rake G, McKee CM, MacPhillamy HB: The toxicity of penicillin as prepared for clinical use. Am J Med Sci 206:642, 1943.
11. Green RH: The association of viral activation with penicillin toxicity in guinea pigs and hamsters. Yale J Biol Med 47:166, 1974.
12. Larson HE, Parry JV, Price AB, et al: Undescribed toxin in pseudomembranous colitis. Br Med J 1:1246, 1977.
13. Hall IC, O'Toole E: Intestinal flora in newborn infants: With a description of a new pathogenic anaerobe, Bacillus difficilis. Am J Dis Child 49:390, 1935.
14. Snyder MD: Further studies on Bacillus difficilis. J Infect Dis 60:223, 1937.
15. Hafiz S: Clostridium difficile and Its Toxins. PhD dissertation, Leeds, UK, University of Leeds, 1974.
16. Bartlett JG, Onderdonk AB, Cisneros AB, Kapser DL: Clindamycin-associated colitis due to toxin-producing species of Clostridium in hamsters. J Infect Dis 136:701, 1977.
17. Bartlett JG, Chang TW, Gurwith M, et al: Antibiotic-associated pseudomembranous colitis due to toxin-producing clostridia. N Engl J Med 298:531, 1978.
18. George RH, Symonds JM, Dimock F, et al: Identification of Clostridium difficile as a cause of pseudomembranous colitis. Br Med J 1:695, 1978.
19. Dixon CF, Weismann RE: Acute pseudomembranous enteritis or enterocolitis: A complication following intestinal surgery. Surg Clin North Am 28:999, 1948.
20. Kay AW, Richards RL, Watson AM: Acute necrotizing (pseudomembranous) enterocolitis. Br J Surg 46:45, 1958.
21. Kleckner MS Jr, Bargen JA, Baggenstoss AH: Pseudomembranous enterocolitis: Clinicopathologic study of fourteen cases in which the disease was not preceded by an operation. Gastroenterology 21:212, 1952.
22. Tsutaoka B, Hansen J, Johnson D, Holodniy M: Antibiotic-associated pseudomembranous enteritis due to Clostridium difficile. Clin Infect Dis 18:982, 1994.
23. Wiesen S, Gregg PA, Kershenobich D, et al: Pseudomembranous enteritis: Rediscovery of a previously well-described entity? Am J Gastroenterol 87:1631, 1992.
24. Summer HW, Tedesco FJ: Rectal biopsy in clindamycin-associated colitis. Arch Pathol 99:237, 1975.
25. Price AB, Davies DR: Pseudomembranous colitis. J Clin Pathol 30:1, 1977.
26. Kelber M, Ament ME: Shigella disenteriae. I. A forgotten cause of pseudomembranous colitis. J Pediatr 89:595, 1976.
27. Hardaway RM, McKay DG: Pseudomembranous enterocolitis. Arch Surg 78:446, 1959.
28. Prolla JC, Kirsner JB: The gastrointestinal lesions and complications of the leukemias. Ann Intern Med 67:1084, 1964.
29. Dosik GM, Luna M, Valdivieso M, McCredie KB: Necrotizing colitis in patients with cancer. Am J Med 67:646, 1979.
30. Margaretten W, McKay DG: Thrombotic ulceration of the gastrointestinal tract. Arch Intern Med 127:250, 1971.
31. Bartlett JG, Gorbach SL: Pseudomembranous enterocolitis (antibiotic-related colitis). In Stollerman GH (ed): Advances in Internal Medicine. Chicago, Year Book Medical Publishers, 1977, p 455.
32. Cudmore MA, Silva J, Fekety R, et al: Clostridium difficile colitis associated with cancer chemotherapy. Arch Intern Med 142:333, 1982.
33. Moskovitz M, Bartlett JG: Recurrent pseudomembranous colitis unassociated with prior antibiotic therapy. Arch Intern Med 141:663, 1981.
34. Peikin SR, Galdibini J, Bartlett JG: Role of Clostridium difficile in a case of nonantibiotic-associated pseudomembranous colitis. Gastroenterology 79:949, 1980.
35. Wald A, Mendelow H, Bartlett JG: Nonantibiotic-associated pseudomembranous colitis due to toxin-producing clostridia. Ann Intern Med 92:798, 1980.
36. Cummins AJ: Pseudomembranous enterocolitis and the pathology of nosology. Am J Dig Dis 6:429, 1961.
37. Keusch GT, Present DH: Summary of workshop on clindamycin colitis. J Infect Dis 133:578, 1976.
38. Totten MA, Gregg JA, Fremont-Smith P, Legg M: Clinical and pathologic spectrum of antibiotic-associated colitis. Am J Gastroenterol 69: 311, 1978.
39. LeFrock JL, Klainer AS, Chen S, et al: The spectrum of colitis associated with lincomycin and clindamycin therapy. J Infect Dis 131: S108, 1975.
40. Slagle GW, Boggs HW: Drug-induced pseudomembranous enterocolitis. Dis Colon Rectum 19:253, 1976.
41. Ramirez-Ronda CH: Incidence of clindamycin-associated colitis. Ann Intern Med 81:860, 1974.
42. Bartlett JG, Chang TW, Moon N, Onderdonk AB: Antibiotic-induced lethal enterocolitis in hamsters. Am J Vet Res 39:1525, 1978.
43. Ebright JR, Fekety R, Silva J, Wilson K: Evaluation of eight cephalosporins in hamster colitis model. Antimicrob Agents Chemother 19: 980, 1981.
44. Kemp G: Therapy of experimental leptospirosis. In Sylvester JC (ed): Antimicrobial Agents and Chemotherapy—1964. Washington, DC, American Society of Microbiologists, 1965, pp 746–750.

45. Fekety R, Silva J, Toshniwal R, et al: Antibiotic-associated colitis: Effects of antibiotics on Clostridium difficile and the disease in hamsters. Rev Infect Dis 1:386, 1979.
46. Small JD: Drugs used in hamsters with a review of antibiotic-associated colitis. In Van Hoosier GL Jr, McPherson CW (eds): The Laboratory Hamster. Orlando, Academic Press, 1987, pp 179–199.
47. Bartlett JG: Antimicrobial agents implicated in Clostridium difficile toxin-associated diarrhea or colitis. Johns Hopkins Med J 149:6, 1981.
48. Golledge CL, McKenzie T, Riley TV: Extended spectrum cephalosporins and Clostridium difficile. J Antimicrob Chemother 23:929, 1989.
49. Manabe YC, Vinetz JM, Moore RD, et al: Clostridium difficile colitis: An efficient clinical approach to diagnosis. Ann Intern Med 123:835, 1995.
50. Anand A, Bashey B, Mir T, Glatt AE: Epidemiology, clinical manifestations, and outcome of Clostridium difficile-associated diarrhea. Am J Gastroenterol 89:519, 1994.
51. Mulligan ME, Citron D, Gabay E, et al: Alterations in human fecal flora, including ingrowth of Clostridium difficile, related to cefoxitin therapy. Antimicrob Agents Chemother 26:343, 1984.
52. Chachaty E, Despitre C, Mario N, et al: Presence of Clostridium difficile and antibiotic and B-lactamase activities in feces of volunteers treated with oral cefixime and cefpodoxime proxetil or placebo. Antimicrob Agents Chemother 36:2009, 1992.
53. Mody LR, Smith SM, Dever LL: Clostridium difficile-associated diarrhea in a VA medical center: Clustering of cases, association with antibiotic usage, and impact on HIV-infected patients. Infect Control Hosp Epid 22:42, 2001.
54. Hirschborn LR, Trnka Y, Onderdonk A, Lee MLT, Platt R: Epidemiology of community-acquired Clostridium difficile-associated diarrhea. J Infect Dis 169:127, 1994.
55. Levy DG, Stergachis A, McFarland LV, et al: Antibiotics and Clostridium difficile diarrhea in the ambulatory care setting. Clin Ther 22: 91, 2000.
56. Anand A, Glatt AE: Clostridium difficile infection associated with antineoplastic chemotherapy: A review. Clin Infect Dis 17:109, 1993.
57. Swartzberg JE, Maresca RM, Remington JW: Gastrointestinal side effects associated with clindamycin. Arch Intern Med 136:876, 1976.
58. Neu HC, Prince A, Neu CO, Garvey GJ: Incidence of diarrhea and colitis associated with clindamycin therapy. J Infect Dis 135:S120, 1977.
59. Gurwith M, Rabin HR, Love K: Diarrhea associated with clindamycin and ampicillin therapy. J Infect Dis 135:S104, 1977.
60. Gilbert DN: Aspects of the safety profile of oral antimicrobial agents. Infect Dis Clin Pract 4(suppl 2):S103, 1995.
61. Tedesco FJ: Ampicillin-associated diarrhea: A prospective study. Dig Dis 20:295, 1975.
62. Gilligan PH, McCarthy LR, Genta VM: Relative frequency of Clostridium difficile in patients with diarrheal disease. J Clin Microbiol 14: 26, 1981.
63. Karlstrom O, Fryklund B, Tullus K, et al: A prospective nationwide study of Clostridium difficile-associated diarrhea in Sweden. Clin Infect Dis 26:141, 1998.
64. Svenungsson B, Lagergren A, Ekwall E, et al: Enteropathogens in adult patients with diarrhea and healthy control subjects: A one year prospective study in a Swedish clinic for infectious diseases. Clin Infect Dis 30:770, 2000.
65. Frost F, Craun GG, Calderon RL: Increasing hospitalization and death possibly due to Clostridium difficile diarrheal disease. Emerg Infect Dis 4:619, 1998.
66. Borriello SP, Larson HE, Welch AR: Enterotoxigenic Clostridium perfringens: A possible cause of antibiotic-associated diarrhoea. Lancet 1: 305, 1984.
67. Sun M: In search of Salmonella's smoking gun. Science 226:30, 1984.
68. Danna PL, Urban D, Bellin E, Rahall JJ: Role of Candida in pathogenesis of antibiotic-associated diarrhea in elderly inpatients. Lancet 337:511, 1991.
69. Mogg GM, Keighley M, Burdon D, et al: Antibiotic-associated with colitis—A review of 66 cases. Br J Surg 66:738, 1979.
70. Tedesco FJ, Anderson CB, Ballinger WF: Drug-induced colitis mimicking an acute surgical condition of the abdomen. Arch Surg 100: 481, 1975.
71. Stroehlein JB, Sedlack RE, Hoffman HN, Newcomer AD: Clindamycin-associated colitis. Mayo Clin Proc 49:240, 1974.
72. Keighley MRB: Antibiotic-associated pseudomembranous colitis: Pathogenesis and management. Drugs 20:49, 1990.
73. Bartlett JG: Antibiotic-associated diarrhea. Clin Infect Dis 15:573, 1992.
74. Seppal K, Hjelt L, Sipponen P: Colonoscopy in the diagnosis of antibiotic-associated colitis: A prospective study. Scand J Gastroenterol 16:465, 1981.
75. Kelly CP, Pothoulakis C, LaMont JT: Clostridium difficile colitis. N Engl J Med 330:257, 1994.
76. Mylonakis E, Ryan ET, Calderwood SB: Clostridium difficile-associated diarrhea. Arch Intern Med 161:525, 2001.
77. Bulusu M, Narayan S, Shetler K, Triadafilopoulos G: Leukocytosis as a harbinger and surrogate marker of Clostridium difficile infection in hospitalized patients with diarrhea. Am J Gastroenterol 95:3137, 2000.
78. Guerrant RL: Practice guidelines for the management of infectious diarrhea. Clin Infect Dis 32:331, 2001.
79. Yong WH, Mattia AR, Ferraro MJ: Comparison of fecal lactoferrin latex agglutination assay and methylene blue microscopy for detection of fecal leukocytes in Clostridium difficile-associated disease. J Clin Microbiol 32:1360, 1994.
80. Schleupner MA, Garner DC, Sosnowski KM, et al: Concurrence of Clostridium difficile toxin A enzyme-linked immunosorbent assay, fecal lactoferrin assay, and clinical criteria with C. difficile cytotoxin titer in two patient cohorts. J Clin Microbiol 33:1755, 1995.
81. Putterman C, Rubinow A: Reactive arthritis associated with Clostridium difficile pseudomembranous colitis. Semin Arthritis Rheum 22: 420, 1993.
82. Mermel LA, Osborn TG: Clostridium difficile-associated reactive arthritis in an HLA-B27 positive female: Report and literature review. J Rheumatol 16:133, 1989.
83. Smith LDS, King EO: Occurrence of Clostridium difficile in infections of man. J Bacteriol 84:65, 1962.
84. Feldman RJ, Kallich M, Weinstein MP: Bacteremia due to Clostridium difficile: Case report and review of extraintestinal C. difficile infections. Clin Infect Dis 20:1560, 1995.
85. Jacobs A, Barnard K, Fischel R, Gradon J: Extra-colonic manifestations of Clostridium difficile infection: Presentation of 2 cases and review of the literature. Medicine 80:88, 2001.
86. Scopes JW, Smith MF, Beach RC: Pseudomembranous colitis and sudden infant death syndrome. Lancet 1:1144, 1980.
87. Laughon B, Kozakewich H, Vawter GF, et al: The role of Clostridium difficile in sudden infant death syndrome. In Tildon JT, Roeder LM, Steinschneider A (eds): Sudden Infant Death Syndrome. New York, Academic Press, 1983, p 557.
88. Han VKM, Sayed H, Chance GW, et al: An outbreak of Clostridium difficile necrotizing enterocolitis: A case of oral vancomycin therapy? Pediatrics 71(6):935, 1983.
89. Cashore WJ, Peter G, Lauermann M, et al: Clostridia colonization and clostridial toxin in neonatal necrotizing enterocolitis. J Pediatr 98:30, 1981.
90. LaMont JT, Trnka YM: Therapeutic implications of Clostridium difficile toxin during relapse of chronic inflammatory bowel disease. Lancet 1:381, 1980.
91. Bolton RP, Sherriff RJ, Read AE: Clostridium difficile-associated diarrhoea. A role in inflammatory bowel disease? Lancet 1:383, 1990.
92. Bartlett JG, Laughon BE, Bayless TM: Role of microbial agents in relapses of idiopathic inflammatory bowel disease. In Bayless TM (ed): Current Management of Inflammatory Bowel Disease. Toronto, BC Decker, 1989, pp 86–93.
93. George WL, Sutter VL, Citron D, Finegold SM: Selective and differential medium for isolation of Clostridium difficile. J Clin Microbiol 9:214, 1979.
94. Willey SH, Bartlett JG: Cultures for Clostridium difficile in stools containing a cytotoxin neutralized by Clostridium sordellii antitoxin. J Clin Microbiol 10:880, 1979.
95. Viscidi R, Willey S, Bartlett JG: Isolation rates and toxigenic potential for Clostridium difficile isolates from various patient populations. Gastroenterology 81:5, 1981.
96. Barbut F, Leluan P, Antoniotti G, et al: Value of routine stool cultures in hospitalized patients with diarrhea. Eur J Clin Microbiol Infect Dis 14:346, 1995.
97. Varki NM, Aquino TJ: Isolation of C. difficile from hospitalized patients without antibiotic-associated diarrhea or colitis. J Clin Microbiol 16:659, 1982.
98. Gilligan PH, McCarthy LR, Genta VM: Relative frequency of Clostridium difficile in patients with diarrhea disease. J Clin Microbiol 14: 26, 1981.

99. McFarland LV, Surawicz CM, Stamm WE: Risk factors for Clostridium difficile carriage and C. difficile-associated diarrhea in a cohort of hospitalized patients. J Infect Dis 162:678, 1990.
100. Aronsson B, Mollby R, Nord CE: Antimicrobial agents and Clostridium difficile in acute disease: Epidemiological data from Sweden, 1980–1982. J Infect Dis 151:476, 1985.
101. Samore MH, DeGirolami PC, Tlucko A, et al: Clostridium difficile colonization and diarrhea at a tertiary care hospital. Clin Infect Dis 18:181, 1994.
102. Simor AE, Yake SL, Tsimidis K: Infection due to Clostridium difficile among elderly residents of a long-term care facility. Clin Infect Dis 17:672, 1993.
103. Holst E, Helin I, Mardh PA: Recovery of Clostridium difficile from children. Scand J Infect Dis 13:41, 1981.
104. Larson HE, Barclay FE, Honour P, Hill ID: Epidemiology of Clostridium difficile in infants. J Infect Dis 146:727, 1982.
105. Welch DF, Marks MI: Is Clostridium difficile pathogenic in infants? J Pediatr 100:393, 1982.
106. Snyder ML: The normal fecal flora of infants between two weeks and one year of age. I. Serial studies. J Infect Dis 65:1, 1940.
107. Hardy SP, Bayston R, Spitz L: Prolonged carriage of Clostridium difficile in Hirschsprung's disease. Arch Dis Child 69:221, 1993.
108. Burdon DW, Brown JD, Youngs D, et al: Antibiotic susceptibility of Clostridium difficile. J Antimicrob Chemother 5:307, 1979.
109. George WL, Sutter VL, Finegold SM: Toxicity and antimicrobial susceptibility of Clostridium difficile, a cause of antimicrobial agent-associated colitis. Curr Microbiol 1:55, 1978.
110. Dzink JA, Bartlett JG: In vitro susceptibility of Clostridium difficile isolates from patients with antibiotic-associated diarrhea or colitis. Antimicrob Agents Chemother 17:695, 1980.
111. Shuttleworth R, Taylor M, Jones DM: Antimicrobial susceptibilities of Clostridium difficile. J Clin Pathol 33:1002, 1980.
112. Brazier JS, Levett PN, Stannard KD, et al: Antibiotic susceptibility of clinical isolates of clostridia. J Antimicrob Chemother 15:181, 1985.
113. Lettau LA: Oral fluoroquinolone therapy in Clostridium difficile enterocolitis. JAMA 260:2216, 1988.
114. Chow AW, Cheng N, Bartlett KH: In vitro susceptibility of Clostridium difficile to new betalactam and quinolone antibiotics. Antimicrob Agents Chemother 28:842, 1985.
115. Wexler HM, Mditoris E, Molitoris D, Finegold SM: In vitro activity of moxifloxacin against 179 strains of anaerobic bacteria found in pulmonary infections. Anaerobe 6:227, 2000.
116. Van der Waaji D, Berghuis-de Vries JM: Selective elimination of Enterobacteriaceae species from the digestive tract in mice and monkeys. J Hyg 72:205, 1974.
117. Donskey CJ, et al: Effect of antibiotic therapy on the density of vancomycin-resistant Enterococci in the stool of colonized patients. N Engl J Med 343:1925, 2000.
118. Kim KH, Fekety R, Botts DH, Brown D: Isolation of Clostridium difficile from the environment and contacts of patients with antibiotic-associated colitis. J Infect Dis 143:42, 1981.
119. Mulligan ME, George WL, Rolfe RD, Finegold SM: Epidemiological aspects of Clostridium difficile-induced diarrhea and colitis. Am J Clin Nutr 33:2533, 1981.
120. Fekety R, Kim KH, Brown D, et al: Epidemiology of antibiotic-associated colitis. Am J Med 70:906, 1981.
121. Thibault A, Miller MA, Gaese C: Risk factors for the development of Clostridium difficile-associated diarrhea during a hospital outbreak. Infect Control Hosp Epidemiol 12:345, 1991.
122. Samore MH, Venkataraman L, De Girolami PC, et al: Clinical and molecular epidemiology of sporadic and clustered cases of nosocomial Clostridium difficile diarrhea. Am J Med 100:32, 1996.
123. Asnis DS, Bresciani A, Ryan M, et al: Cost-effective approach to evaluation of diarrheal illness in hospitals [letter to the editor]. J Clin Microbiol 31:1675, 1993.
124. Cirisano FD, Greenspoon JS, Stenson R, et al: The etiology and management of diarrhea in the gynecologic oncology patient. Gynecol Oncol 50:45, 1993.
125. Pear SM, Williamson TH, Bettin KM, et al: Decrease in nosocomial Clostridium difficile-associated diarrhea by restricting clindamycin use. Ann Intern Med 120:272, 1994.
126. Gerding DN, Olson M, Peterson R, et al: Clostridium difficile-associated diarrhea and colitis in adults. A prospective case controlled epidemiologic study. Arch Intern Med 146:95, 1986.
127. Johnson S, Gerding DN: Clostridium difficile-associated diarrhea. Clin Infect Dis 26:1027, 1998.
128. McFarlan LV, Mulligan ME, Kwok RYY, Stamm WE: Nosocomial acquisition of Clostridium difficile infection. N Engl J Med 320:204, 1989.
129. Lai KK, Melvin ZS, Menard MJ, et al: Clostridium difficile-associated diarrhea: Epidemiology, risk factors, and infection control. Infect Control Epidemiol 18:628, 1997.
130. Cohen SH, Tang YJ, Rahmani D, et al: Persistence of an endemic (toxigenic) isolate of Clostridium difficile in the environment of a general medical ward. Clin Infect Dis 30:952, 2000.
131. Chang VT, Nelson K: The role of physical proximity in nosocomial diarrhea. Clin Infect Dis 31:717, 2000.
132. Clabots CR, Peterson LR, Gerding DN: Characterization of a nosocomial Clostridium difficile outbreak by using plasmid profile typing and clindamycin susceptibility testing. J Infect Dis 158:4:731, 1988.
133. Pantosti A, Cerquetti M, Gianfrilli PM: Electrophoretic characterization of Clostridium difficile strains isolated from antibiotic-associated colitis and other conditions. J Clin Microbiol 26:540, 1988.
134. Mulligan ME, Halebian S, Kwok RYY, et al: Bacterial agglutination and polyacrylamide gel electrophoresis for typing Clostridium difficile. J Infect Dis 153:267, 1986.
135. Kuijper EJ, Oudbier JH, Stuifbergen WNHM, et al: Application of whole-cell DNA restriction endonuclease profiles to the epidemiology of Clostridium difficile-induced diarrhea. J Clin Microbiol 25:751, 1987.
136. Delmee M, Avesani V, Delferriere N, Burtonboy G: Characterization of flagella of Clostridium difficile and their role in serogrouping reactions. J Clin Microbiol 28(10):2210, 1990.
137. McFarland LV, Elmer GW, Stamm WE, Mulligan ME: Correlation of immunoblot type, enterotoxin production, and cytotoxin production with clinical manifestations of Clostridium difficile infection in a cohort of hospitalized patients. Infect Immun 59:2456, 1991.
138. Clabots CR, Johnson S, Bettin KM, et al: Development of a rapid and efficient restriction endonuclease analysis typing system for Clostridium difficile and correlation with other typing systems. J Clin Microbiol 31:1870, 1993.
139. Brazier JS: An international study on the unification of nomenclature for typing Clostridium difficile. Clin Infect Dis 20(Suppl 2):S325, 1995.
140. Wren BW, Heard S, Tabaqchali S: Association between production of toxins A and B and types of Clostridium difficile. J Clin Pathol 40: 1297, 1987.
141. Taylor NS, Thorne G, Bartlett JG: Comparison of two toxins produced by Clostridium difficile. Infect Immun 34:1036, 1981.
142. Sullivan NM, Pettett S, Wilkins TD: Purification and characterization of toxins A and B of Clostridium difficile. Infect Immun 35:1032, 1982.
143. Lima AAM, Lyerly DM, Wilkins TD, et al: Effects of Clostridium difficile toxins A and B in rabbit small and large intestine in vivo and on cultured cells in vitro. Infect Immun 56:582, 1988.
144. Barroso LA, Wang SZ, Phelps CJ, et al: Nucleoside sequence of Clostridium difficile toxin B gene. Nucleic Acids Res 18:4004, 1990.
145. Dove CH, Wang AZ, Price SB, et al: Molecular characteristic of the Clostridium difficile toxin A gene. Infect Immun 58:480, 1990.
146. Phelps CJ, Lyerly D, Johnson J, Wilkins TD: Construction and expression of the complete Clostridium difficile toxin A gene in Escherichia coli. Infect Immun 59:150, 1991.
147. Johnson JL, et al: Cloning and expression of the toxin B gene of Clostridium difficile. Curr Microbiol 20:397, 1990.
148. Limaye AP, Turgeon DK, Cookson BT, Fritsche TR: Pseudomembranous colitis caused by a toxin A− B+ strain of Clostridium difficile. J Clin Microbiol 38:1696, 2000.
149. Kato H, Kato N, Watanabe K, et al: Identification of a toxin-negative toxin B-positive Clostridium difficile by PCR. J Clin Microbiol 36: 2178, 1998.
150. Lyerly DM, Barroso LA, Wilkins TD, et al: Characterization of a toxin A-negative, toxin B-positive strain of Clostridium difficile. Infect Immun 60:4633, 1992.
151. Borriello SP, Wren BW, Hyde S, et al: Molecular, immunological, and biological characterization of a toxin A-negative, toxin B-positive strain of Clostridium difficile. Infect Immun 60:4192, 1992.
152. Fluit AC, Wolfhagen MJHM, Verdonk GPHT, et al: Nontoxigenic strains of Clostridium difficile lack the genes for both toxin A and toxin Br J Clin Microbiol 29:2666, 1991.
153. Flegel WA, Miller F, Daubener W, et al: Cytokine response by human monocytes to Clostridium difficile toxin A and toxin B. Infect Immun 59:3659, 1991.

154. Viscidi R, Laughon BE, Yolken R, et al: Serum antibody response to toxins A and B of Clostridium difficile. J Infect Dis 148:93, 1983.
155. Fiorentini C, Malorni W, Paradisi S, et al: Interaction of Clostridium difficile toxin A with cultures' cells: Cytoskeletal changes and nuclear polarization. Infect Immun 58:2329, 1990.
156. Ottlinger MD, Lin S: Clostridium difficile toxin B induces reorganization of actin, vinculin, and talin in cultured cells. Exp Cell Res 174: 215, 1988.
157. Just I, Selzer J, Wilm M, et al: Glucosylation of Rho proteins by Clostridium difficile toxin B. Nature 375:500, 1995.
158. Burakoff R, Zhao L, Celifarco AJ, et al: Effects of purified Clostridium difficile toxin A on rabbit distal colon. Gastroenterology 190(2): 348, 1995.
159. Rocha MF, Soares AM, Ribeiro RA, Lima AA: Absence of intestinal secretion on supernatants from macrophages stimulated with Clostridium difficile toxin B on rabbit ileum. Toxicon 39:335, 2001.
160. Riegler M, Sedivy R, Pothoulakis C, et al: Clostridium difficile toxin B is more potent that toxin A in damaging human colonic epithelium in vitro. J Clin Invest 95:2004, 1995.
161. Viscidi RP, Bartlett JG: Antibiotic-associated pseudomembranous colitis in children. Pediatrics 67:381, 1981.
162. Kayne L, Warny M, Qamar A, Kelly CP: A symptomatic carriage of *Clostridium difficile* and serum levels of IgG antibody against toxin A. N Engl J Med 342:390, 2000.
163. Kayne L, Warny M, Qamar A, Kelly CP: Association between antibody response to toxin A and protection against recurrent *Clostridium difficile* diarrhea. Lancet 357:189, 2001.
164. Stanley RJ, Melson GL, Tedesco FJ: The spectrum of radiographic findings in antibiotic-related pseudomembranous colitis. Radiology 111:519, 1974.
165. Stanley RJ, Melson GL, Tedesco FJ, Saylor JL: Plain-film findings in severe pseudomembranous colitis. Radiology 118:7, 1976.
166. Rubesin SE, Levine MS, Glick SN, et al: Pseudomembranous colitis with rectosigmoid sparing on barium studies. Radiology 170:811, 1989.
167. Fishman E, Kavuru M, Kulzlman JE, et al: CT of pseudomembranous colitis: Radiologic, clinical and pathologic correlation. Radiology 180: 57, 1991.
168. Boland GW, Lee MJ, Cats AM, et al: Antibiotic-induced diarrhea: Specificity of abdominal CT for the diagnosis of Clostridium difficile disease. Radiology 191:103, 1994.
169. Tedesco FJ, Corless JK, Brownstein RE: Rectal sparing in antibiotic-associated pseudomembranous colitis: A prospective study. Gastroenterology 83:1259, 1982.
170. Burbige EJ, Radigan JJ: Antibiotic-associated colitis with normal-appearing rectum. Dis Colon Rectum 23:198, 1981.
171. Pittman FE, Pitman JC, Humphrey CD: Colitis following oral lincomycin therapy. Arch Intern Med 134:368, 1974.
172. Manashil GB, Kern JA: Nonspecific colitis following oral lincomycin therapy. Am J Gastroenterol 60:394, 1973.
173. Koltz AP, Palmer WL, Kirsner JB: Aureomycin proctitis and colitis: A report of five cases. Gastroenterology 25:44, 1953.
174. Chang TW, Lauermann M, Bartlett JG: Cytotoxicity assay in antibiotic-associated colitis. J Infect Dis 140:765, 1979.
175. Bartlett JG: Laboratory diagnosis of antibiotic-associated colitis. Lab Med 12:347, 1981.
176. Lashner BA, Todsrczuk J, Staim DF, Hanauer SB: Clostridium difficile culture-positive toxin negative diarrhea. Am J Gastroenterol 81: 940, 1986.
177. Gerding DN: Disease associated with Clostridium difficile infection. Ann Intern Med 110:255, 1989.
178. Fekety R, Shah AB: Diagnosis and treatment of Clostridium difficile colitis. JAMA 269:71, 1993.
179. Kelly C, Pothoulakis C, LaMont JT: Clostridium difficile colitis. N Engl J Med 330:257, 1994.
180. Shahrabadi MS, Bryan LE, Gaffney D, et al: Latex agglutination test for detection of Clostridium difficile toxin in stool samples. J Clin Microbiol 20:339, 1984.
181. Lyerly DM, Ball DW, Toth J, Wilkins TD: Characterization of cross-reactive proteins detected by Culturette-brand rapid latex test for Clostridium difficile. J Clin Microbiol 26:397, 1988.
182. Lyerly DM, Barroso LA, Wilkins TD: Identification of the latex test-reactive protein of Clostridium difficile as glutamate dehydrogenase. J Clin Microbiol 29:2639, 1991.
183. Laughon BE, Viscidi RP, Gdovin SL, et al: Enzyme immunoassays for detection of Clostridium difficile toxins A and B in fecal specimens. J Infect Dis 149:781, 1984.
184. Walker RC, Ruane PJ, Rosenblatt JE, et al: Comparison of culture, cytotoxicity assays, and linked immunosorbent assay for toxin A and toxin B in the diagnosis of Clostridium difficile-related enteric disease. Diagn Microbiol Infect Dis 5:61, 1986.
185. DiPersio JP, Varga FJ, Conwell DL, et al: Development of a rapid enzyme immunoassay for Clostridium difficile toxin A and its use in the diagnosis of C. difficile-associated disease. J Clin Microbiol 29: 2724, 1991.
186. Woods GL, Iwen Pd: Comparison of a dot immunobinding assay, latex agglutination, and cytotoxin assay for laboratory diagnosis of Clostridium difficile-associated diarrhea. J Clin Microbiol 28:855, 1990.
187. Barbut F, Kajzer C, Planas N, Petit J-C: Comparison of three enzyme immunoassays, a cytotoxicity assay, and toxigenic culture for diagnosis of Clostridium difficile-associated diarrhea. J Clin Microbiol 31: 963, 1993.
188. Merz CS, Kramer C, Forman M, et al: Comparison of four commercially available rapid enzyme immunoassays with cytotoxin assay for detection of Clostridium difficile toxin(s) from stool specimens. J Clin Microbiol 32:1142, 1994.
189. Kurzynski TA: Evaluation of C. difficile CUBE test for detection of Clostridium difficile-associated diarrhea. Diagn Microbiol Infect Dis 15:493, 1992.
190. Kato N, Ou C-Y, Kato H, et al: Detection of toxigenic Clostridium difficile in stool specimens by the polymerase chain reaction. J Infect Dis 167:455, 1993.
191. Kuhl SJ, Tang YJ, Navarro L, et al: Diagnosis and monitoring of Clostridium difficile infections with the polymerase chain reaction. Clin Infect Dis 16(Suppl 4):S234, 1993.
192. Mundy LS, Shanholtzer CJ, Willard KE, et al: Laboratory detection of Clostridium difficile. A comparison of media and incubation systems. Am J Clin Pathol 103:52, 1995.
193. Bond F, Payne G, Borriello SP, Humphreys H: Usefulness of culture in the diagnosis of Clostridium difficile infection. Eur J Clin Microbiol Infect Dis 14:223, 1995.
194. Gerding DN, Johnson S, Peterson LR, et al: Clostridium difficile-associated diarrhea and colitis. Infect Control Hosp Epidemiol 16:459, 1995.
195. Riley TV, Cooper M, Bell B, Golledge CL: Community-acquired Clostridium difficile-associated diarrhea. Clin Infect Dis 20(Suppl 2): S263, 1995.
196. Gerding DN, Johnson S, Peterson LR, et al: Clostridium difficile-associated diarrhea and colitis. Infect Control Hosp Epidemiol 16:459, 1995.
197. Hines J, Nachamkin I: Effective use of the microbiology laboratory for diagnosing diarrheal diseases. Clin Infect Dis 23:1292, 1996.
198. Bauer TM, Lalvani A, Fahrenbach J, et al: Derivation and validation of guidelines for stool cultures for Enteropathogenic bacteria other than Clostridium difficile in hospitalized adults. JAMA 285:313, 2001.
199. Novak E, Lee JE, Seckman CE, et al: Unfavorable effect of atropine-diphenoxylate (Lomotil) therapy in lincomycin-caused diarrhea. JAMA 235:1451, 1976.
200. Pittman EF: Lomotil and antibiotic colitis. Ann Intern Med 83:124, 1975.
201. Fekety R: Guidelines for the diagnosis and management of Clostridium difficile-associated diarrhea and colitis. Am J Gastroenterol 92: 739, 1997.
202. Bartlett JG, Chang TW, Onderdonk AB: Comparison of five regimens of treatment of experimental clindamycin-associated colitis. J Infect Dis 138:81, 1978.
203. Viteri AL, Howard PH, Dyck WP: The spectrum of colitis associated with lincomycin and clindamycin therapy. J Infect Dis 131:S1135, 1974.
204. Bartlett JG: Treatment of Clostridium difficile colitis. Gastroenterology 89:1192, 1985.
205. Fekety R, Silva J, Armstrong J, et al: Treatment of antibiotic-associated enterocolitis with vancomycin. Rev Infect Dis. 3:S273, 1981.
206. Young GP, Ward PB, Bayley N: Antibiotic-associated colitis due to Clostridium difficile: Double-blind comparison of vancomycin with bacitracin. Gastroenterology 89:1038, 1985.
207. Dudley MN, McLaughlin JC, Carrington G, et al: Oral bacitracin vs. vancomycin therapy for Clostridium difficile-induced diarrhea. Arch Intern Med 146:1101, 1986.

208. Bartlett JG, Tedesco FJ, Shull S, et al: Symptomatic relapse after oral vancomycin therapy of antibiotic-associated pseudomembranous colitis. Gastroenterology 78:431, 1980.
209. Bartlett JG: Treatment of antibiotic-associated pseudomembranous colitis. Rev Infect Dis 6:S235, 1984.
210. Mogg GAG, Arabi Y, Youngs D, et al: Therapeutic trials of antibiotic-associated colitis. Scand J Infect Dis 23(Suppl):41, 1980.
211. Teasley DG, Olson MM, Gebhard RL, et al: Prospective randomized trial of metronidazole versus vancomycin for Clostridium difficile-associated diarrhoea and colitis. Lancet 2:1444, 1983.
212. Wenisch C, Parschalk B, Hasenhundl M, et al: Comparison of vancomycin, metronidazole, and fusidic acid for the treatment of Clostridium difficile-associated diarrhea. Clin Infect Dis 22:813, 1996.
213. Wilcox MH, Howe R: Diarrhoea caused by Clostridium difficile: Response time for treatment with metronidazole and vancomycin. J Antimicrob Chemother 36:673, 1995.
214. Johnson S, Homann SR, Bettin KM, et al: Treatment of asymptomatic Clostridium difficile carriers (fecal excretors) with vancomycin or metronidazole: A randomized, placebo-controlled study. Ann Intern Med 117:297, 1992.
215. Fekety R, Shah AB: Diagnosis and treatment of Clostridium difficile colitis. JAMA 269:71, 1993.
216. Johnson S, Sanchez JL, Gerding DN: Metronidazole resistance in Clostridium difficile. Clin Infect Dis 31:625, 2000.
217. Bolton RP, Culshaw MA: Fecal metronidazole concentrations during oral and intravenous therapy for antibiotic associated colitis due to Clostridium difficile. Gut 27:1169, 1986.
218. Centers for Disease Control: Recommendations for preventing the spread of vancomycin resistance. MMWR 44 RR-12:1, 1995.
219. Fekety R, Silva J, Kauffman C, et al: Treatment of antibiotic-associated Clostridium difficile colitis with oral vancomycin: Comparison of two dosage regimens. Am J Med 86:15, 1989.
220. Oliva SL, Guglielmo BJ, Jacobs R, Pons VG: Failure of intravenous vancomycin and intravenous metronidazole to prevent or treat antibiotic-associated pseudomembranous colitis. J Infect Dis 159:1154, 1989.
221. Fekety R, McFarland LV, Surawicz CM, et al: Recurrent Clostridium difficile diarrhea: Characteristics of and risk factors for patients in a prospective randomized study, double-blind trial. Clin Infect Dis 24: 324, 1997.
222. Walters BAJ, Roberts R, Stafford R, Senevirantne E: Relapse of antibiotic-associated colitis: Endogenous persistence of Clostridium difficile during vancomycin therapy. Gut 24:206, 1983.
223. Onderdonk AB, Lowe BR, Bartlett JG: Effect of environmental stress on Clostridium difficile toxin levels during continuous cultivation. Appl Environ Microbiol 38:637, 1979.
224. Elmer GW, Surawicz CM, McFarland LV: Biotherapeutic agents. A neglected modality for the treatment and prevention of selected intestinal and vaginal infections. JAMA 276:870, 1996.
225. Elmer GW, McFarland LV: Suppression by Saccharomyces boulardii of toxigenic Clostridium difficile overgrowth after vancomycin treatment in hamsters. Antimicrob Agents Chemother 31:129, 1987.
226. Castigliuolo I, Riegler MF, Valenick L: Saccharomyces boulardii protease inhibits the effects of Clostridium difficile toxins A and B in human colonic mucosa. Infection Immun 67:3021, 1999.
227. McFarland LV, Surawicz CM, Greenberg RN, et al: A randomized, placebo-controlled trial of Saccharomyces boulardii in combination with standard antibiotics for Clostridium difficile disease. JAMA 271: 1913, 1994.
228. Silva M, Jacobus N, Deneke C, Gorbach S: Antimicrobial substance from a human Lactobacillus strain. Antimicrob Ag Chemother 31: 1231, 1987.
229. Goldin BR, Gorbach SL, Saxelin M, et al: Lactobacillus species (strain GG) in human gastrointestinal tract. Dig Dis Sci 37:121, 1992.
230. Gorbach S, Chang T-W, Goldin B: Successful treatment of relapsing C. difficile colitis with Lactobacillus GG. Lancet 2:1519, 1987.
231. Leung DY, Kelly CP, Boguniewicz M, et al: Treatment with intravenously administered gammaglobulin of chronic relapsing colitis induced by C. difficile toxin. J Pediatr 118:633, 1991.
232. Salcedo J, Keates S, Pothoulakis C, et al: Intravenous immunoglobulin therapy for severe Clostridium colitis. Gut 41:366, 1997.
233. Kreutzer EW, Milligan FD: Treatment of antibiotic-associated pseudomembranous colitis with cholestyramine resin. Johns Hopkins Med J 143:67, 1978.
234. Tedesco FJ, Napier J, Gamble W, et al: Therapy of antibiotic-associated pseudomembranous colitis. J Clin Gastroenterol 1:51, 1979.
235. Taylor NS, Bartlett JG: Binding of Clostridium difficile cytotoxin and vancomycin by anion exchange resins. J Infect Dis 141:92, 1980.
236. Bowden TA, Mansberger AR, Lykins LE: Pseudomembranous enterocolitis: Mechanism of restoring floral homeostasis. Am Surg 47:178, 1981.
237. Schwan A, Sjolin S, Trottestam U, et al: Relapsing Clostridium difficile enterocolitis cured by rectal infusion of normal feces. Scand J Infect Dis 16:211, 1984.
238. Tvede M, Rask-Madsen J: Bacteriotherapy for chronic relapsing Clostridium difficile diarrhoea in six patients. Lancet 6:1156, 1989.
239. Lipsett PA, Samantaray DK, Tam ML, et al: Pseudomembranous colitis: A surgical disease? Surgery 116:491, 1994.
240. Walker KJ, Gilliland SS, Vance-Bryan K, et al: Clostridium difficile colonization in residents of long-term care facilities: Prevalence and risk factors. J Am Geriatr Soc 41:940, 1993.
241. Kaatz GW, Gitlin SD, Schaberg DR, et al: Acquisition of Clostridium difficile from the hospital environment. Am J Epidemiol 127:1289, 1988.
242. Bender BS, Laughon BE, Gaydos G, et al: Is Clostridium difficile endemic in chronic-care facilities. Lancet 2:11, 1986.
243. Johnson S, Clabots CR, Linn FV, et al: Nosocomial Clostridium difficile colonization and disease. Lancet 336:97, 1990.
244. Silva J, Lezzi C: Clostridium difficile as a nosocomial pathogen. J Hosp Infect 2(Suppl A):378, 1988.
245. Samore MH: Epidemiology of nosocomial Clostridium difficile diarrhoea. J Hosp Infect 43(Suppl S):183, 1999.
246. Chang VT, Nelson K: The role of physical proximity in nosocomial pneumonia diarrhea. Clin Infect Dis 31:717, 2000.
247. Johnson S, Samore MH, Farrow KA, et al: Epidemics of diarrhea caused by a clindamycin-resistant strain of Clostridium difficile in four hospitals. N Engl J Med 341:1645, 1999.
248. Saif N, Brazier JS: The distribution of Clostridium difficile in the environment of South Wales. J Med Microbiol 45:133, 1996.
249. Pear SM, Williamson TH, Bettin KM, et al: Decrease in nosocomial Clostridium difficile-associated diarrhea by restricting clindamycin use. Ann Intern Med 120:272, 1994.
250. McNulty C, Logan M, Donald IP, et al: Successful control of Clostridium difficile infection in an elderly care unit through use of a restrictive antibiotic policy. J Antimicrob Chemother 40:707, 1997.
251. Climo MN, Israel DS, Wong ES, et al: Hospital-wide restriction of clindamycin: Effect on the incidence of Clostridium difficile-associated diarrhea and cost. Ann Intern Med 128:989, 1998.
252. Johnson S, Gerding DS, Olson MM, et al: Prospective controlled study of vinyl glove use to interrupt Clostridium difficile nosocomial transmission. Am J Med 88:187, 1990.
253. Mayfield JL, Leet T, Miller J, Mundy L: Environmental control to reduce transmission of Clostridium difficile. Clin Infect Dis 31:995, 2000.
254. Rutula W, Gergen M, Weber D: Inactivation of Clostridium difficile spores by disinfectants. Infect Control Hosp Epidemiol 14:36, 1993.
255. Brooks SE, Veal RO, Kramer M, et al: Reduction in the incidence of Clostridium difficile-associated diarrhea in an acute care hospital and a skilled nursing facility following replacement of electronic thermometers with single-use disposables. Infect Control Hosp Epidemiol 13:98, 1992.
256. Vanderhoof JA, Whitney DB, Antonson DL, et al: Lactobaccillus GG in the prevention of antibiotic-associated diarrhea in children. J Pediatr 135:564, 1999.
257. McFarland LV, Surawicz CM, Greenberg RN, et al: Prevention of betalactam-associated diarrhea by Saccharomyces boulardii compared to placebo. Am J Gastroenterol 90:439, 1995.
258. Giannasea PJ, Zhang ZX, Lei WD, et al: Serum antitoxin antibodies mediate systemic and mucosal protection from Clostridium difficile disease in hamsters. Infect Immun 67:527, 1999.
259. Genth H, Selzer J, Busch C, et al: New method to generate enzynamically deficient Clostridium difficile toxin B as an antigen for immunization. Infect Immun 68:1094, 2000.

Chapter 98

INTESTINAL PROTOZOA

Christopher D. Huston and Richard L. Guerrant

ENTAMOEBA HISTOLYTICA

Epidemiology

Entamoeba histolytica was first linked causally to amebic colitis and liver abscess by Lösch in 1875, and was named by Schaudinn in 1903 for its ability to destroy host tissues. In 1925, to explain why only a minority of individuals infected with what was then termed *E. histolytica* develop invasive disease, Emil Brumpt proposed the existence of a second, nonpathogenic *Entamoeba* species, *Entamoeba dispar*, that is morphologically indistinguishable from *E. histolytica.* Although Brumpt's hypothesis was not accepted during his lifetime, it is now clear that he was correct. In 1993, based on cumulative clinical, biochemical, immunologic, and genetic data, *E. histolytica* (Schaudinn, 1903) was redefined to include two morphologically indistinguishable, but genetically distinct species: *E. histolytica*, the cause of invasive amebiasis, and *E. dispar*, a nonpathogenic intestinal commensal parasite (see later section).[1]

Entamoeba histolytica is a parasite of global distribution, but the preponderance of the morbidity and mortality due to amebiasis occurs in Central and South America, Africa, and the Indian subcontinent.[2] Fortunately, the majority of the 500 million individuals worldwide previously believed to be asymptomatic *E. histolytica* cyst passers are actually infected with *E. dispar*, which has not been shown to cause human disease. The best current estimate is that *E. histolytica* causes 34 to 50 million symptomatic infections annually worldwide, resulting in between 40 and 100 thousand deaths each year.[3, 4] In Dhaka, Bangladesh, where diarrheal diseases are the leading cause of childhood death, approximately 50% of children have serologic evidence of exposure to *E. histolytica* by 5 years of age.[5]

E. histolytica has a simple, two-stage life cycle consisting of an infectious cyst and a motile trophozoite (Fig. 98–1). The cyst form measures 5 to 20 μm in diameter and contains four or fewer nuclei. The amoeboid trophozoite, which is responsible for tissue invasion, measures 10 to 60 μm (Fig. 98–2) and contains a single nucleus with a central karyosome (Fig. 98–3). The cysts are relatively resistant to chlorination and desiccation, and survive in a moist environment for several weeks. Infection occurs following ingestion of cysts in fecally contaminated food or water. Within the lumen of the small intestine, the quadrinucleate cyst undergoes nuclear followed by cytoplasmic division, giving rise to eight trophozoites.[6] Approximately 90% of infected individuals become asymptomatic cyst passers, completing the organism's life cycle. In the remaining 10%, trophozoites invade the colonic epithelium and cause colitis.[1] Trophozoites that gain access to the bloodstream may spread hematogenously to establish infection at distant sites (most commonly liver abscess, as discussed in Chapter 69).

Pathogenesis, Pathology, and Immunology

Following infection with *E. histolytica*, microscopy studies suggest a well-defined sequence of adherence, tissue inva-

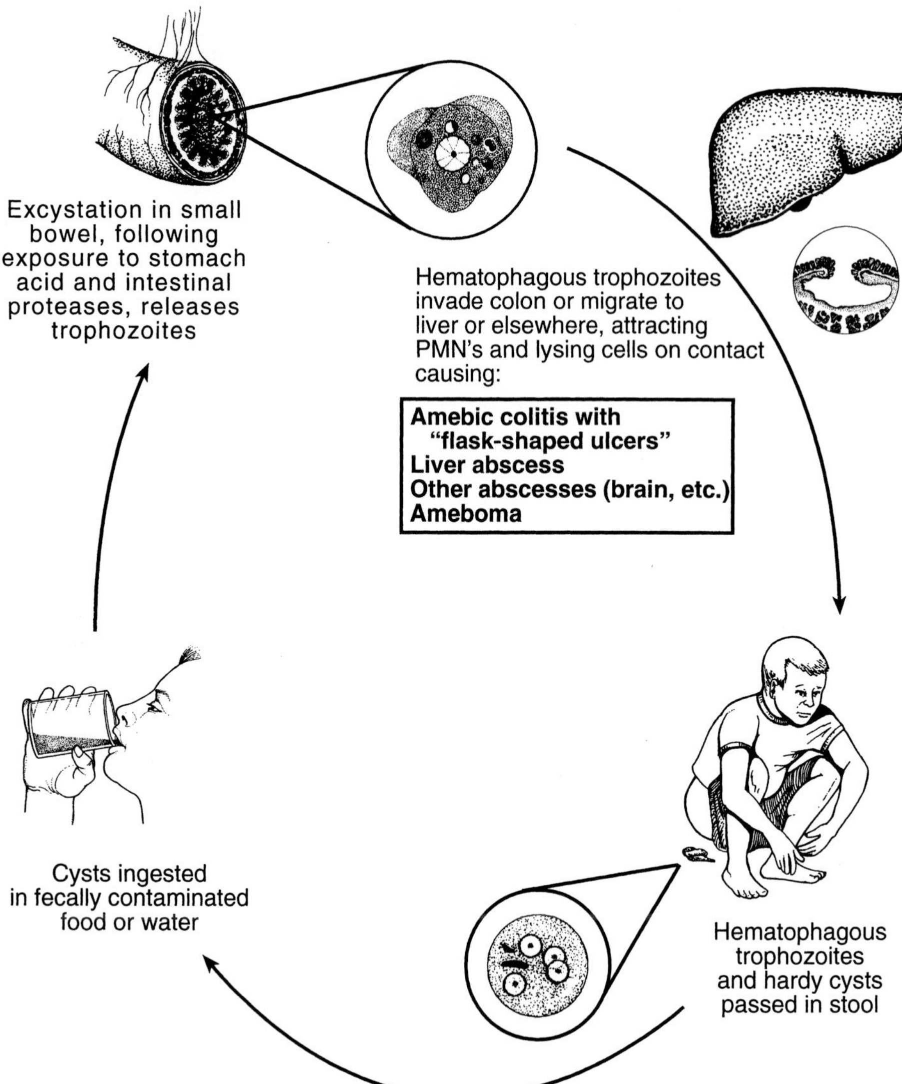
Entamoeba histolytica
Excystation in small bowel, following exposure to stomach acid and intestinal proteases, releases trophozoites
Hematophagous trophozoites invade colon or migrate to liver or elsewhere, attracting PMN's and lysing cells on contact causing:
Amebic colitis with "flask-shaped ulcers"
Liver abscess
Other abscesses (brain, etc.)
Ameboma
Hematophagous trophozoites and hardy cysts passed in stool
Cysts ingested in fecally contaminated food or water

Figure 98–1. Life cycle of *Entameba histolytica.* (From Petri WA, Sing U, Ravdin JI: Enteric amebiasis. In Guerrant RL, Walker DH, Weller PF: Tropical Infectious Diseases, Principles, Pathogens, & Practice. Philadelphia, WB Saunders, 1999, p 687.)

sion, cytolysis, and inflammation leading to disease.[7–10] After excystation within the lumen of the small intestine, trophozoites first adhere to colonic mucins and epithelial cells via an amebic galactose/N-acetyl-D-galactosamine inhibitable surface lectin.[11–14] Secreted cysteine proteinases then facilitate tissue invasion by degrading extracellular matrix proteins, thereby disrupting the colonic mucous and epithelial barrier.[15–18] During tissue invasion, trophozoites kill epithelial and immune cells by a contact-dependent mechanism that requires amebic adherence to host cells via the galactose inhibitable lectin.[11] Finally, killed epithelial cells release pro-interleukin-1-β which is processed by the amebic cysteine proteinases to its active form, resulting in the tissue inflammation and edema seen during early disease.[19]

The cecum and ascending colon are affected most commonly, although in severe disease the entire colon may be involved. On gross examination, pathology can range from mucosal thickening to multiple punctate ulcers with normal intervening tissue (Fig. 98–4), to frank necrosis. The downward invasion of amebic trophozoites is often halted at the level of the muscularis mucosa. Subsequent lateral spread of amebae undermines the overlying epithelium resulting in the clean-based, flask-shaped ulcers (see Fig. 98–1) that characterize amebic colitis.[20, 21] Early in infection, an influx of neutrophils is typical, but, in well-established ulcers, few inflammatory cells are seen.[10, 20–22] Organisms may be seen ingesting red blood cells (erythrophagocytosis). At distant sites of infection (eg, liver abscess), similar pathologic characteristics include central liquefaction of tissue surrounded by a minimal mononuclear cell infiltrate.[21–23]

The evidence for acquired immunity to *E. histolytica* infection is limited. In a retrospective study of 1021 Mexican patients cured of amebic liver abscess between 1963 and 1968, only three patients were readmitted to the study hospital with recurrent liver abscess.[24] Although this number is substantially fewer than expected, no control population was included in the study. Better evidence of immunity comes from the natural history of asymptomatic infection. Greater

	Human pathogen	Estimated frequency	Trophozoite [usual size μm (range)]	Cyst (usual size in μm)	Characteristic features
Entamoeba histolytica	+	1–10%	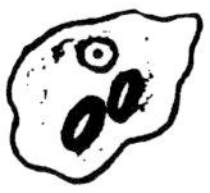 10–20 (10–60)	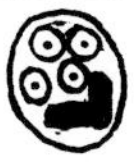 5–20	Central punctate karyosome, erythrophagocytosis Indistinguishable from *E. dispar*
E. coli	–	3–20%	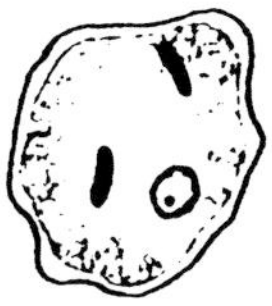 15–25 (10–50)	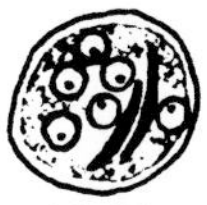 10–30	Larger, 5 to 8 nuclei; splinter-like chromatoid bodies Eccentric karyosome distinguishes trophozoite from *E. histolytica* and *dispar*
E. hartmanni	–	?	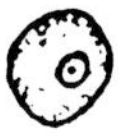 < 10	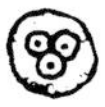 4–10	Small size ("Small race")
E. gingivalis	–	10–90% (mouth)	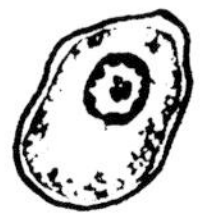 15 (3–35)	none	Oral trophozoite only
E. polecki	±	rare	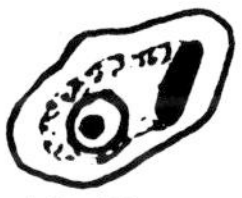 16–18	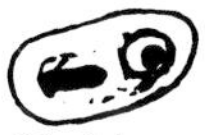 12–14	Uninucleate cyst with large karyosome
Endolimax nana	–	10–33%	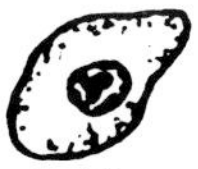 8–12	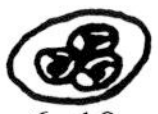 6–10	Vesiculate nucleus
Iodamoeba butschlii	–	5–8%	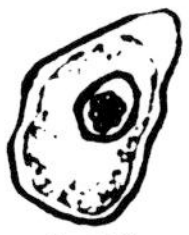 9–20	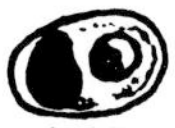 6–15	"I" cyst (see text)
Dientamoeba fragilis	+	4–10%	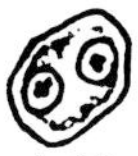 4–12	none	Binucleate trophs with connecting thread

Figure 98–2. Amebae that infect the human gastrointestinal tract. (From Ravdin JI, Guerrant RL: Current problems in the diagnosis and treatment of amebic infections. Curr Clin Trop Inf Dis 7:82–111, 1986.)

than 90% of individuals colonized with *E. histolytica* spontaneously clear the infection within 1 year.[25] Furthermore, although intestinal colonization following invasive disease occurs, individuals with serum anti-amebic antibodies indicating prior infection are less likely to become colonized than seronegative controls.[26]

The contributions of humoral and cellular immunity to protection from amebiasis remain unclear. Nearly everyone with invasive amebiasis develops a systemic and a mucosal humoral immune response.[26–31] Antibodies alone are unable to clear established infection, since asymptomatic cyst passers remain infected for months after anti-amebic antibodies develop.[25, 26] Passive immunization experiments in a severe combined immunodeficient (SCID) mouse model of liver abscess, however, demonstrate an important role for preexisting humoral immunity in protection from infection.[32] Reports that individuals receiving corticosteroids may be at increased risk of severe amebic colitis suggest that cellular immunity also plays an important role in control of *E. histolytica* infection.[33] To date, however, no increase in the severity of disease in patients with the acquired immunodeficiency syndrome (AIDS) has been observed.

Clinical Presentation

Infection with *E. histolytica* results in one of three outcomes. Approximately 90% of infected individuals remain asymptomatic. The other 10% of infections result in invasive amebiasis characterized by dysentery (amebic colitis) or, in a mi-

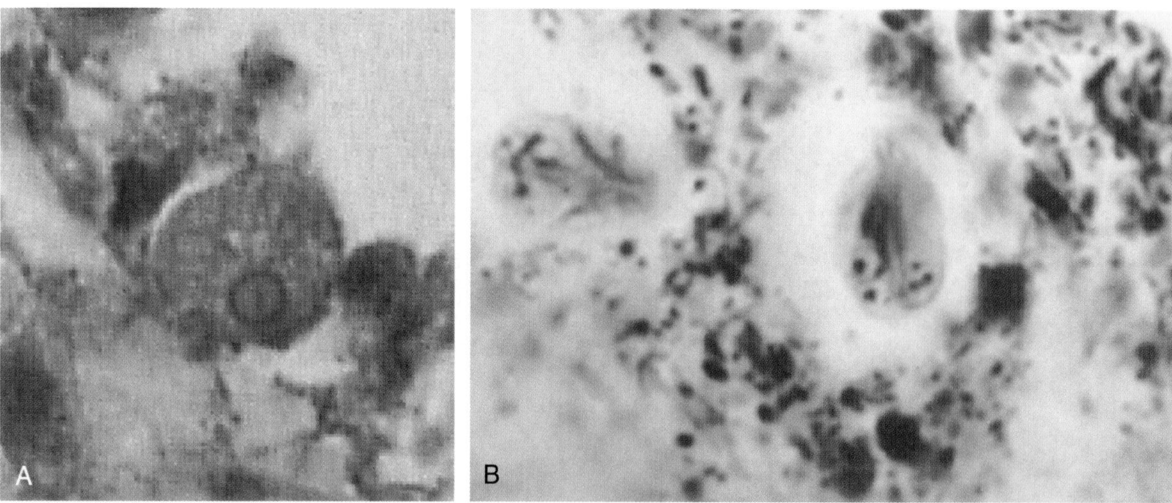

Figure 98–3. *A,* An *E. histolytica* trophozoite in stool. Note the nucleus with prominent central karyosome. *B, Giardia lamblia* cyst in stool (original magnification ×400).

nority of cases, extraintestinal disease (most commonly amebic liver abscess; see Chapter 69).[1, 25]

When epidemiologic risk factors are present, amebic dysentery should be considered in the differential diagnosis of occult or grossly bloody diarrhea. In the United States, immigrants from or travelers to endemic regions, male homosexuals, and institutionalized individuals are at greatest risk for amebiasis. In addition, malnourished patients, infants, the elderly, pregnant women, and patients receiving corticosteroids may be at increased risk for fulminant disease.[2, 33, 34]

The major diagnostic challenge for the clinician seeing a patient with amebic colitis is to distinguish the illness from other causes of bloody diarrhea. The *differential diagnosis* includes causes of bacterial dysentery (eg, *Shigella*, *Salmonella*, and *Campylobacter* species and enteroinvasive or enterohemorrhagic *Escherichia coli*), and noninfectious diseases, including inflammatory bowel disease, and ischemic colitis.[2, 35] In contrast to bacterial dysentery, which typically begins abruptly, amebic colitis begins gradually over 1 to several weeks (Table 98–1). Although greater than 90% of patients with amebic colitis present with diarrhea, abdominal pain without diarrhea may occur. The presence or absence of abdominal pain, tenesmus, and fever is highly variable. Weight loss is common because of the chronicity of the illness, and only microscopic blood is present in the stool of a majority of patients.[2, 35, 36]

The most lethal manifestation of amebic dysentery is acute necrotizing colitis with toxic megacolon, which occurs in 0.5% of cases. This complication manifests as an acute dilatation of the colon, and 40% of patients die from sepsis unless it is promptly recognized and treated surgically.[37, 38] Other unusual complications of amebic colitis include the formation of enterocutaneous, rectovaginal, and enterovesicular fistulas (see Chapter 24) and ameboma. Ameboma, due to intraluminal granulation tissue, can cause bowel obstruction and mimic carcinoma of the colon.[2, 35]

Amebic liver abscess is discussed in detail in Chapter 69. Although a history of dysentery is often obtained, the majority of patients do not have coexistent dysentery.[39–41] Other extraintestinal sites of infection rarely occur, and typically result either from direct extension of liver abscesses (eg, amebic pericarditis or lung abscess) or hematogenous spread (eg, brain abscess).[2, 35, 42]

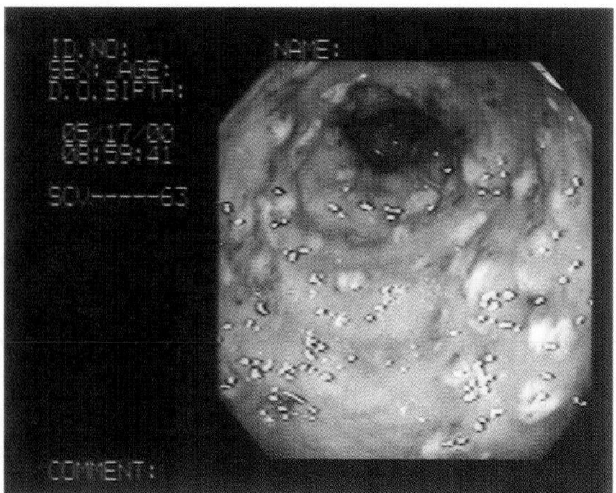

Figure 98–4. Colonoscopy findings in a patient with amebic colitis. Multiple punctate ulcers are visible.

Diagnosis

Since amebiasis patients erroneously treated with corticosteroids for inflammatory bowel disease may develop fulminant colitis, accurate initial diagnosis is critical.[33, 34] The gold standard for diagnosis of amebic colitis remains colonoscopy with biopsy, and colonoscopy should be performed when noninfectious causes of bloody diarrhea are strong considerations in the differential diagnosis (eg, ulcerative colitis). Since the cecum and ascending colon are most frequently affected, colonoscopy is preferred to sigmoidoscopy. Classically, multiple punctate ulcers measuring 2 to 10 mm are seen with essentially normal intervening tissue (see Fig. 98–4); however, the colonic epithelium may simply appear indurated with no visible ulcerations, and, in severe cases where the ulcers have coalesced, the epithelium may appear necrotic. Histologic examination of a biopsy specimen of the

Table 98–1 | **Comparison of Amebic Colitis and Bacterial Dysentery**

CHARACTERISTIC	AMEBIC COLITIS	BACTERIAL DYSENTERY
Immigration from or travel to an endemic area	Yes	No
Usual duration of symptoms	>7 d	2–7 d
Diarrhea	94–100%	100%
Positive fecal occult blood test	100%	40%
Abdominal pain	12–80%	~50%
Weight loss	Common	Unusual
Fever >38°C	Minority	Majority

Adapted from Huston CD, Petri WA: Amebiasis. In Rakel R (ed): Conn's Current Therapy 2001. Philadelphia, WB Saunders, 2001.

edge of an ulcer reveals amebic trophozoites and a variable inflammatory infiltrate (Figs. 98–5, 98–6).[21] The identification of amebae can be aided by periodic acid-schiff staining of biopsy tissue, which stains trophozoites magenta.

Microscopic examination of stool samples to diagnose amebiasis, which for decades has been used as the initial diagnostic test of choice for amebic colitis, has low sensitivity (30%–60%).[43, 44] More importantly, light microscopy cannot distinguish *E. histolytica* infection from infection with the intestinal commensal parasite *E. dispar*, which appears to be approximately ten times more common.[1, 4] The presence of erythrophagocytic trophozoites in stool samples suggests *E. histolytica* infection, but these are rarely seen.[45] Confusion between *E. histolytica*, other nonpathogenic amebae (eg, *Entamoeba coli*), and white blood cells also contributes to overdiagnosis of amebiasis.[43] Thus, stool examination for ova and parasites should no longer be relied on to diagnose amebiasis.[4] In evaluating a patient with diarrhea, the primary utility of stool microscopy for ova and parasites is to evaluate for other parasitic causes of diarrhea.

Entamoeba histolytica can be differentiated accurately from *E. dispar* infection using culture with isoenzyme analysis, and with molecular diagnostic tests including serum antibody titers, polymerase chain reaction (PCR), and an enzyme-linked immunosorbant assay (ELISA) against the amebic lectin antigen. In the absence of invasive amebic trophozoites in biopsy tissue, stool culture followed by isoenzyme analysis is considered to be the "gold standard" for diagnosis of amebiasis. However, culture takes 1 to several weeks and requires special laboratory facilities, making it unsuitable for use in all but research settings. Moreover, culture specimens must be inoculated rapidly since delays in stool sample processing dramatically reduce sensitivity.[46] Numerous investigators have developed PCR-based tests with sensitivities and specificities greater than 90%.[47–51] Cur-

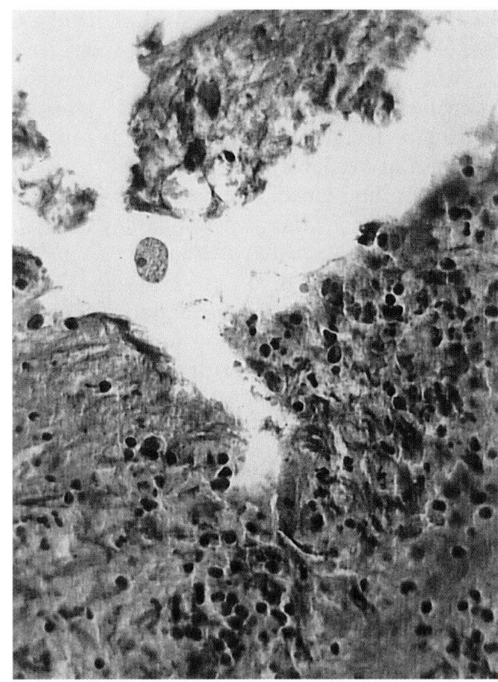

Figure 98–6. Colonic biopsy from a patient with amebic colitis. Note amebic trophozoite and ulcer with surrounding inflammatory infiltrate (H&E stain, original magnification ×100).

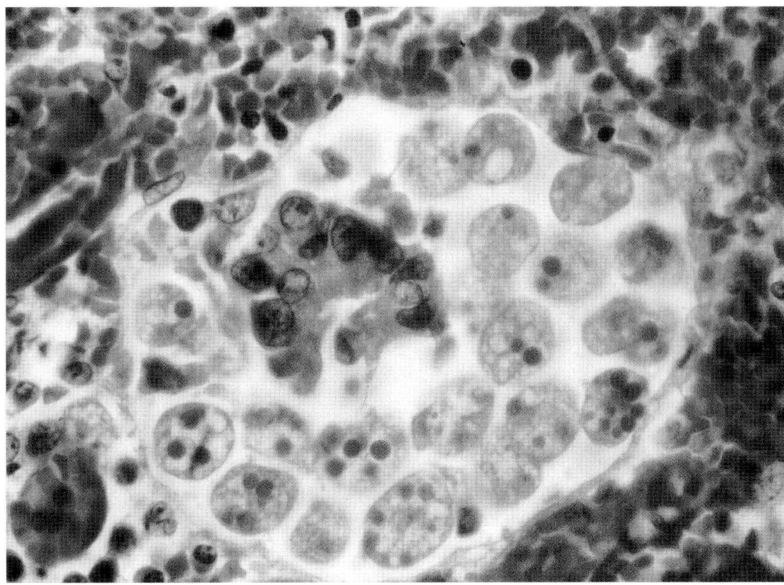

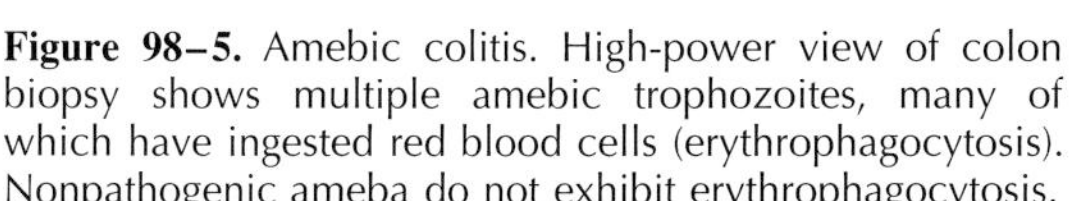

Figure 98–5. Amebic colitis. High-power view of colon biopsy shows multiple amebic trophozoites, many of which have ingested red blood cells (erythrophagocytosis). Nonpathogenic ameba do not exhibit erythrophagocytosis.

rently, these tests are most suitable for use in research settings where their ability to differentiate between strains of *E. histolytica* will make them very useful. In the clinical setting, anti-amebic antibody titers and an ELISA test to detect amebic adherence lectin antigen in stool and serum samples are the most useful available tests.

Because serum anti-amebic antibodies do not develop in patients infected with *E. dispar*, serologic tests for amebiasis accurately distinguish *E. histolytica* and *E. dispar* infection. Seventy-five percent to 85% of patients with acute amebic colitis have detectable anti-amebic antibodies on presentation, and convalescent titers develop in greater than 90% of patients.[27, 28, 52] For amebic liver abscess, 70% to 80% of patients have detectable antibody titers on presentation, and convalescent titers develop in greater than 90% of patients. Because anti-amebic antibodies can persist for years, however, a positive result must be interpreted with care.[27] For individuals with known epidemiologic risks (eg, emigration from or prior travel to an endemic region), a positive result may simply represent infection in the distant past. In the setting of recent travel to an endemic region and a positive antibody titer, diagnosis is confirmed by an appropriate response to anti-amebic treatment.

The most specific clinically available test for diagnosis of amebiasis is an ELISA to detect *E. histolytica* adherence lectin antigen (*E. histolytica* II test, TechLab, Blacksburg, VA). Of the many ELISA tests developed thus far, this is the only commercially available test capable of accurately distinguishing *E. histolytica* from *E. dispar*.[44, 53–59] The sensitivity of this method for detection of amebic antigen in the stool of patients with colitis is greater than 85%, and its specificity when compared to the "gold standard" of stool culture followed by isoenzyme analysis is greater than 90%.[56] Prior to initiation of treatment, amebic lectin antigen can also be detected in the serum of greater than 90% of patients with amebic liver abscess.[60]

Treatment

The agents for treatment of amebiasis can be categorized as luminal or tissue amebicides on the basis of the location of their anti-amebic activity (Table 98–2). The luminal amebicides include iodoquinol, diloxanide furoate, and paromomycin.[61, 62] Of these, paromomycin, a nonabsorbable aminoglycoside, is preferred because of its safety and the short duration of required treatment. Its major side effect is diarrhea.[35] Because paromomycin is nonabsorbable and has moderate activity against trophozoites that have invaded the colonic mucosa, it may also be useful for single-drug treatment of mild invasive disease during pregnancy.[63] The tissue amebicides include metronidazole, tinidazole, erythromycin, and chloroquine.[4, 64] Of these, metronidazole is the drug of choice, with cure rates greater than 90%.[64] Erythromycin has no activity against amebic liver disease, and chloroquine has no activity against intestinal disease.[65]

Because an estimated 10% of asymptomatic cyst passers will develop invasive disease, *E. histolytica* carriers should be treated.[1, 4] For noninvasive disease, treatment with a luminal agent alone is adequate (eg, paromomycin 25–35 mg/kg/day in three divided doses for 7 days).[62] Patients with amebic colitis should be treated with oral metronidazole (500–750 mg three times daily for 10 days) followed by a luminal agent such as paromomycin to prevent recurrent disease.[62, 64, 65] At the doses of metronidazole required, gastrointestinal side effects develop in approximately 30% of patients.[64] Because of severe gastrointestinal side effects, simultaneous treatment with metronidazole and a luminal agent is generally not recommended. Most patients with colitis respond promptly to metronidazole with resolution of diarrhea in 2 to 5 days.[2] Despite conflicting reports on the safety of metronidazole for the developing fetus during pregnancy, women with severe disease during pregnancy should probably be treated without delay. As discussed in Chapter 69, metronidazole (750 mg three times a day for 10 days) followed by a luminal agent is also the treatment of choice for amebic liver abscess.[62, 65]

Control and Prevention

Prevention and control of *E. histolytica* infection depends on interruption of fecal-oral transmission. Water can be made safe for drinking and food preparation by boiling (for 1 minute), halogenation (with chlorine or iodine), or filtration.[6] In the United States and Europe, modern water treatment facilities effectively remove *E. histolytica*. The importance of safe drinking water is highlighted by a recent outbreak of amebiasis in Tblissi, Republic of Georgia, where there is an ongoing waterborne epidemic due to decay of water treatment facilities following the demise of the Soviet Union.[66] More importantly, in the vast majority of the developing world, no modern water treatment facilities exist and none are likely to be constructed in the foreseeable future. This has led many investigators to focus on developing a vaccine for amebiasis. Because humans and some higher non-human primates are the only known hosts for *E. histolytica*, a vaccine that successfully prevents colonization might enable eradication of the disease.[74]

OTHER INTESTINAL AMEBAE

Seven species of commensal amebae infect the human gastrointestinal tract (see Fig. 98–2). These include *Entamoeba dispar*, *Entamoeba coli*, *Entamoeba hartmanni*, *Entamoeba gingivalis*, *Entamoeba polecki*, *Endolimax nana*, and *Iodamoeba butschlii*. *Dientamoeba fragilis* (discussed in following section), previously thought to be an ameba, is more closely related to the flagellated protozoan *Trichomonas vaginalis* than to the true amebae.[6] With the exception of *E. gingivalis*, which has no known cyst stage, all of these true amebae have simple two-stage life cycles, consisting of an infectious cyst form and a motile trophozoite form.[6] All but *E. dispar* can be differentiated from *E. histolytica* using light microscopy based on characteristic features of the cyst and trophozoite forms (see Fig. 98–2). *E. dispar* must be differentiated from *E. histolytica* based on antigenic or genetic differences.[1]

Entamoeba dispar is a nonpathogenic protozoan parasite that is morphologically indistinguishable from *Entamoeba histolytica* by light microscopy (see Fig. 98–2).[1] An estimated 450 million people worldwide are infected with *E. dispar*, and infection with *E. dispar* is approximately 10 times more prevalent than *E. histolytica* infection.[1, 3, 4] Al-

Table 98–2 | **Current Amebicidal Agents Available in the United States**

AMEBICIDAL AGENT	ADVANTAGES	DISADVANTAGES
Luminal Amebicides		
Paromomycin (Humatin)	7-day treatment course; may be useful during pregnancy	Frequent GI disturbances; rare ototoxicity and nephrotoxicity
Iodoquinol (Yodoxin)	Inexpensive and effective	20-day treatment course; contains iodine; rare optic neuritis and atrophy with prolonged use
Diloxanide furoate (Furamide)		Available in United States only from CDC; frequent GI disturbances; rare diplopia
For Invasive Intestinal Disease Only		
Tetracyclines, erythromycin		Not active for liver abscesses; frequent GI disturbance; tetracyclines should not be administered to children or pregnant women
For Invasive Intestinal and Extraintestinal Amebiasis		
Metronidazole (Flagyl)	Drug of choice for amebic colitis and liver abscess	Anorexia, nausea, vomiting, and metallic taste in nearly one third of patients at dosages used; disulfiram-like reaction with alcohol; rare seizures
Chloroquine (Aralen)	Useful only for amebic liver abscess	Occasional headache, pruritus, nausea, alopecia, and myalgias; rare heart block and irreversible retinal injury

CDC, Centers for Disease Control and Prevention; GI, gastrointestinal. Adapted from Huston CD, Petri WA: Amebiasis. In Rakel R (ed): Conn's Current Therapy 2001. Philadelphia, WB Saunders, 2001.

though *E. dispar* has been demonstrated to cause mucosal ulcerations in animal models, it has not been demonstrated to cause human disease and does not require treatment.[1] The primary clinical significance of *E. dispar* infection is that it must be distinguished from *E. histolytica* to enable accurate diagnosis of invasive amebiasis. Polymerase chain reaction to amplify small ribosomal RNA (not clinically available), and enzyme-linked immunosorbant assays (ELISAs) using monoclonal anti-amebic antibodies to detect specific *E. histolytica* antigens make accurate diagnosis possible (see *E. histolytica* diagnosis).[44, 47–51, 53–59]

Besides *E. dispar*, *Entamoeba coli* is the intestinal commensal most frequently mistaken for *E. histolytica*. *Entamoeba coli* trophozoites contain a single nucleus with a prominent karyosome that is usually eccentric in location, distinguishing them from *E. histolytica/E. dispar* trophozoites, which have a centrally located karyosome. In addition, the cyst form of *E. coli* typically contains from five to eight nuclei (see Fig. 98–2). *Entamoeba coli* is nonpathogenic, and requires no specific treatment. However, it is a valuable marker of fecal-oral exposure, and can be found concurrently with *E. histolytica* in 10% to 30% of patients in endemic regions.[6]

Entamoeba hartmanni was classified as "small race" *E. histolytica* for many years. It is now recognized as a nonpathogen, and requires no treatment. The trophozoites resemble those of *E. histolytica* except for their small size (<10 μm).[6]

Entamoeba gingivalis is the only ameba found in the oral cavity, where it lives in the anaerobic environment of the gingival crease. The trophozoite is identical in size to E. histolytica's and contains a single nucleus with a prominent central karyosome (see Fig. 98–2). No cyst form of *E. gingivalis* has been identified, and oral-oral contact is believed to be the mode of transmission.[6, 68] *Entamoeba gingivalis* is associated with poor dental hygiene and periodontal disease, but no causal relationship to periodontitis has been proven.[68] The increased frequency of colonization in this setting may simply reflect a more hospitable host environment. *Entamoeba gingivalis* is also frequently associated with periodontal disease in AIDS patients, in whom treatment with metronidazole has been reported to be effective.[69]

Entamoeba polecki is a parasite of pigs and monkeys that on rare occasions infects humans.[6] In Papua, New Guinea, one study found that 19% of children were colonized. At present, specific treatment for *E. polecki* is not routinely recommended, but persons with heavy burdens of this parasite may develop nonspecific gastrointestinal symptoms and might benefit from treatment. Good clinical responses to metronidazole and diloxanide furoate have been reported.[77]

Endolimax nana is an additional nonpathogenic intestinal ameba that frequently infects humans.[6] The distribution of *E. nana* is worldwide, but it is most common in the tropics where 5% to 33% of individuals are infected.[68, 71, 72] Infection requires no specific treatment, but serves as a useful marker for fecal-oral exposure. *Endolimax nana* trophozoites can be distinguished from *E. histolytica* by their vesiculate nucleus, large irregular karyosome, and relatively small size (8–12 μm).[6, 68] *Iodamoeba butschlii* is a final nonpathogenic intestinal ameba passed by the fecal-oral route. The trophozoites contain a single nucleus with a large karyosome (which is distinct from the punctate karyosome of *E. histolytica*). *Iodamoeba butschlii* cysts contain a single nucleus, and a large, eccentric glycogen mass that stains with iodine (hence the name *Iodamoeba*). *Iodamoeba butschlii* infection also requires no treatment.[6]

GIARDIA LAMBLIA

Epidemiology

Giardia lamblia is a ubiquitous flagellated intestinal protozoan. Van Leeuwenhoek accurately described its motile trophozoite form in 1681, but it was not until 1915 that Stiles named the species.[6] The life cycle of *Giardia* consists of an infectious cyst form and a motile trophozoite (Fig. 98–7). The cyst is oval (8–12 μm long by 7–10 μm wide), contains four nuclei, and has a rigid outer wall that protects it from dehydration, extremes of temperature, and

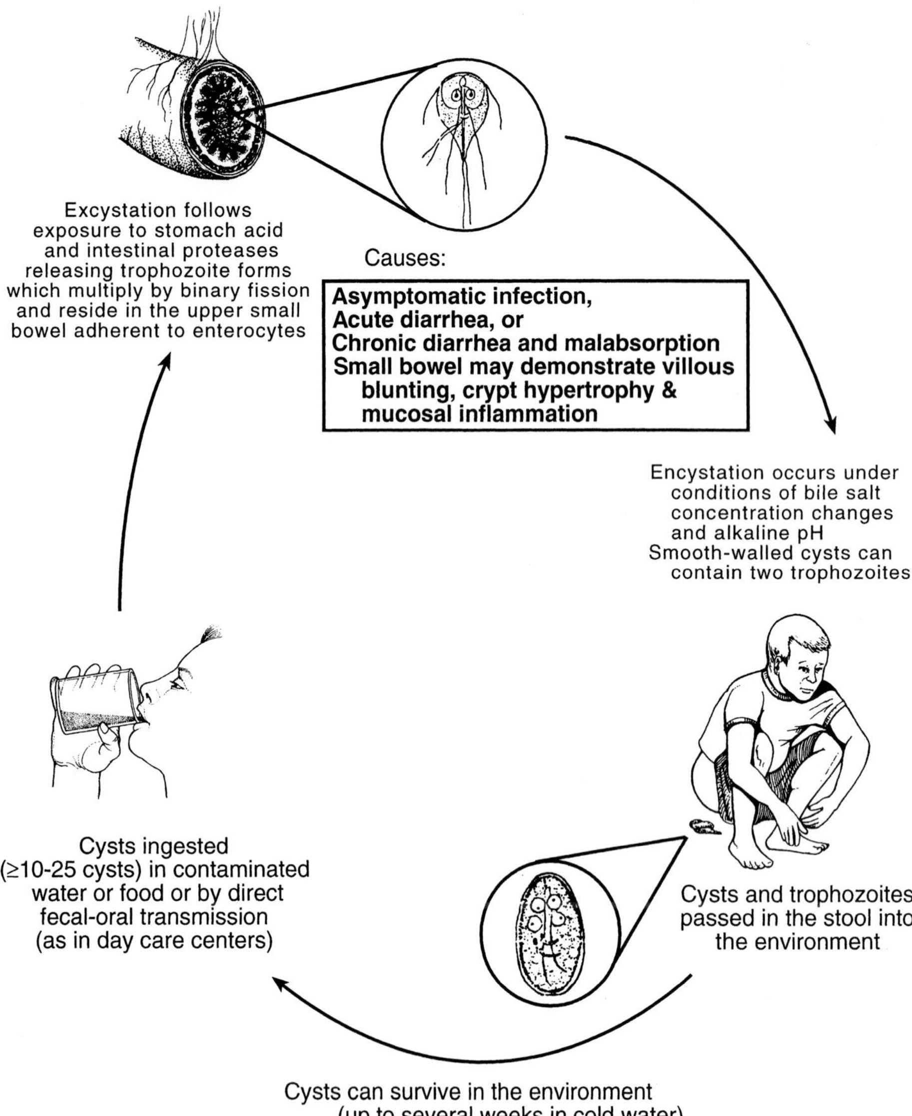

Giardia lamblia
Excystation follows exposure to stomach acid and intestinal proteases releasing trophozoite forms which multiply by binary fission and reside in the upper small bowel adherent to enterocytes
Causes:
Asymptomatic infection,
Acute diarrhea, or
Chronic diarrhea and malabsorption
Small bowel may demonstrate villous blunting, crypt hypertrophy & mucosal inflammation
Encystation occurs under conditions of bile salt concentration changes and alkaline pH
Smooth-walled cysts can contain two trophozoites
Cysts ingested (≥10-25 cysts) in contaminated water or food or by direct fecal-oral transmission (as in day care centers)
Cysts and trophozoites passed in the stool into the environment
Cysts can survive in the environment (up to several weeks in cold water)
May also infect non-human mammalian species

Figure 98–7. Life cycle of *Giardia lamblia.* (From Hill DR, Nash TE: Intestinal flagellate and ciliate infections. In Guerrant RL, Walker DH, Weller PF: Tropical Infectious Diseases, Principles, Pathogens, & Practice. Philadelphia, WB Saunders, 1999, p 706.)

chlorination (Fig. 98–8). *Giardia* cysts can survive in cold water for several weeks.[6, 73] Ingestion of as few as 10 to 25 cysts can result in infection.[73] Excystation occurs after ingestion following exposure to stomach acid and intestinal proteases, with each cyst giving rise to two trophozoites. Giardia trophozoites (see Fig. 98–3*B*)are pear-shaped (10–20 μm long by 7–10 μm wide), contain two nuclei, have eight flagellae for locomotion, and replicate by binary fission. The trophozoites live in the duodenum where they adhere to enterocytes. Trophozoites eventually encyst following exposure to alkaline conditions or bile salts, and are excreted in the stool to complete the life cycle.[73]

Analysis of DNA restriction fragment length polymorphisms has demonstrated tremendous variability of *Giardia* isolates from humans and other mammals, and different *Giardia lamblia* isolates have been shown to have very different pathogenicity in experimental human infections.[74, 75] Common patterns are observed among *Giardia* isolates from humans, beavers, and other mammals, however, suggesting that these animals do not have their own species of *Giardia* and can serve as a reservoir for human disease.[74]

Giardia lamblia is the most frequently identified intestinal parasite in the United States, and was identified in 7.2% of stool samples examined by state health departments in 1987.[83] Giardiasis occurs in both endemic and epidemic forms via waterborne, foodborne, and person-to-person transmission.[76–82] Worldwide, *Giardia* infects infants more commonly than adults and in highly endemic regions, essentially all children are infected by 2 to 3 years of age.[84, 85] In the developing world, it is likely that recurrent infantile diarrhea due to giardiasis contributes significantly to malnutrition.[84] In the United States, children in day care and sexually active homosexual men have the greatest risk of infection.[83, 86] During a yearlong longitudinal study at a US day care cen-

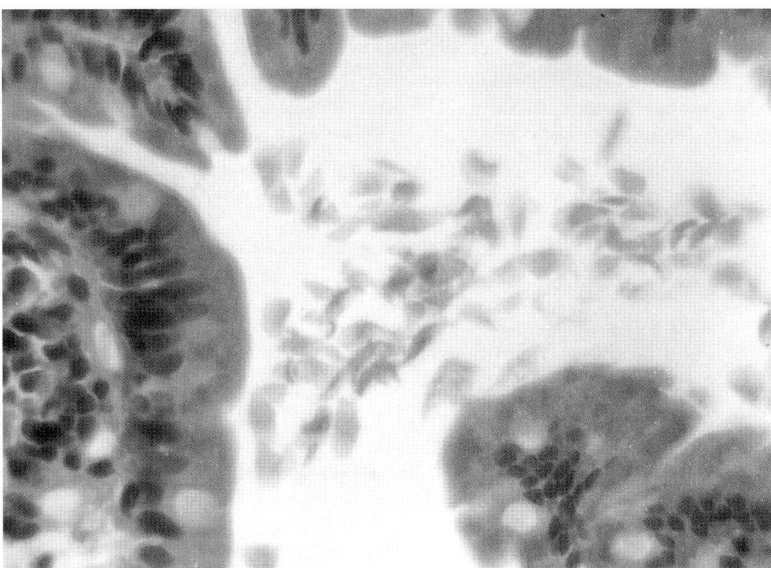

Figure 98–8. Giardiasis. High-power view of duodenal biopsy showing many trophozoites near the surface of the epithelium between the villi.

ter, *Giardia* cysts were identified at some time in the stool of more than 30% of children.[82] Additional risk factors for infection include drinking untreated surface water, a shallow dug well as a residential water source, swimming in any natural body of fresh water, and contact with a person with giardiasis or a child in day care.[77]

Pathogenesis, Pathology, and Immunology

Giardia causes malabsorptive diarrhea by an unknown mechanism. Trophozoites adhere (perhaps by suction) to the epithelium of the upper small intestine using a disk structure located on their anterior ventral surface.[6, 73] There is no evidence that trophozoites invade the mucosa.[87] Studies using electron microscopy have shown damage to the mucosal brush border.[73, 88] On biopsy, pathologic changes range from an entirely normal appearing duodenal mucosa (except for adherent trophozoites), as was found in more than 96% of biopsy specimens in one large study, to severe villous atrophy with a mononuclear cell infiltrate that resembles celiac sprue.[87, 89, 90] The severity of diarrhea appears to correlate with the severity of the pathologic change.[73]

The host immune response plays a critical role in limiting the severity of giardiasis. When infected with *Giardia*, individuals with common variable immunodeficiency develop severe, protracted diarrhea and malabsorption with sprue-like pathologic changes that resolve with treatment.[90] Both a systemic and mucosal humoral immune response can consistently be measured following *Giardia* infection. High serum IgM, IgG, and IgA titers can be detected, and secretory IgA (s-IgA) can be detected in saliva and in breast milk of infected mothers.[91–93] In a B cell-deficient transgenic mouse model, mice do not resolve the parasite infection, confirming the importance of the humoral immune response.[94] Interestingly, *Giardia* vary expression of a group of cysteine-rich surface proteins (termed variant surface proteins) in culture, and, in experimental human infections, *G. lamblia* isolates have been shown to undergo antigenic variation after approximately 2 weeks (roughly the time required to mount an initial antibody response).[95] Although the role of the variant surface proteins remains unproven, antigenic variation may enable Giardia to evade the host immune response.[96]

The importance of a cellular immune response is also clear from animal studies. Athymic nude mice are unable to control Giardia muris infection, but reconstitution with immune spleen cells results in partial control. Upon immune reconstitution, however, severe inflammatory changes and villous atrophy develop in the intestine, suggesting that the immune response to infection may contribute to pathology.[97] Despite the importance of cellular immunity for controlling infection in animal models, no increase in the severity of illness has been observed in patients with the acquired immunodeficiency syndrome (AIDS).[98]

Table 98–3 | **Frequency of Symptoms in Patients with Giardiasis** [87, 94, 98]

Symptom	Frequency
Diarrhea	32–100%
Fatigue	22–97%
Abdominal pain/cramps	75–83%
Weight loss	60%
Flatulence/bloating	58–79%
Anorexia	45%
Vomiting	17–26%
Fever	12–21%

Clinical Presentation

The clinical manifestations of *Giardia* are highly variable, ranging from asymptomatic infection to severe, chronic diarrhea with malabsorption. In one large study of biopsy-proven giardiasis, only 32% of patients had diarrhea. The majority of patients had nonspecific gastrointestinal complaints.[87] Reported symptoms in order of decreasing frequency include diarrhea, fatigue, abdominal cramps, bloating, malodorous stool, flatulence, weight loss, fever, and vomiting (Table 98–3).[80, 91] During a foodborne outbreak, the mean duration of diarrhea was 16 days, but symptoms resolved spontaneously in nearly one half of infected individuals after 7 to 8 days.[80]

As mentioned above, the severity of illness depends upon both host and parasite factors. Different *Giardia* isolates have dramatically different abilities to cause disease during experimental human infections.[75] Furthermore, certain populations, including children less than 2 years of age and patients with hypogammaglobulinemia, are more likely to develop serious disease.[84, 90]

Diagnosis

Examination of concentrated, iodine-stained wet stool preparations and modified-trichrome stained permanent smears has been the conventional approach to identifying *Giardia* infections (see Fig. 98–3*B*). Because cysts and trophozoites are only present intermittently in the stool, however, even with examination of multiple specimens, the sensitivity is only around 50%.[80, 89] With direct sampling of duodenal contents (eg, duodenal aspiration or the "string test"), sensitivity can be improved to approximately 80% (see Fig. 98–8).[89] Even on small intestinal biopsy specimens identification of trophozoites requires careful examination of multiple microscope fields to ensure accuracy.[87]

Numerous molecular tests based on enzyme-linked immunosorbant assays (ELISAs) or direct immunofluorescent antibody (DFA) microscopy are now widely commercially available to diagnose giardiasis in stool samples.[99–101] These assay kits all work well, with sensitivities greater than 90% and specificities approaching 100%.[101] Given the inability to rule out giardiasis even with repeated conventional stool examinations for ova and parasites and the difficulties of duodenal sampling, the first diagnostic test performed to evaluate for *Giardia* infection should be a stool ELISA or DFA. The primary role of endoscopy is evaluation for other pathologic conditions.

Treatment

Metronidazole (250 mg orally three times a day for 5 days) is the preferred treatment for giardiasis.[62] At this relatively low dosage, metronidazole is generally well tolerated, and is 80% to 95% effective at eradicating *Giardia*.[102] The most common side effects are nausea, a metallic taste, and a disulfiram-like reaction with alcohol. Alternative regimens include 1) tinidazole (2 g orally for one dose), 2) furazolidone (100 mg orally four times a day for 7–10 days), or 3) paromomycin (25–35 mg/kg/day in three divided doses for 7 days). Because paromomycin is not absorbed and there have been conflicting reports regarding the safety of metronidazole for the developing fetus, paromomycin may be useful for treatment of giardiasis during pregnancy. Single-dose treatment with tinidazole, though simple and effective, is not available in the United States.[62]

Many patients have prolonged lactose intolerance following *Giardia* infection, which can mimic ongoing infection. Therefore, the diagnosis should be reconfirmed prior to repeating therapy. For people who fail therapy, repeat therapy with the same drug (eg, with higher doses of metronidazole) or combination therapy with metronidazole and quinacrine may work.[102] Patients who repeatedly fail treatment should be evaluated for common variable immunodeficiency.[90, 102]

Control and Prevention

Control of giardiasis relies on interruption of fecal-oral transmission. Water can be made safe for drinking and food preparation by boiling (for 1 minute), halogenation (with chlorine or iodine preparations), or filtration.[6, 102] Because of the low infectious dose of *Giardia* cysts and the poor hygiene of infants and children, person-to-person spread in day care centers is much more difficult to control. Temporarily removing infected children who are ill from day care is ineffective, perhaps because many infected children remain asymptomatic and go unrecognized.[102] In the developing world, endemic giardiasis is unlikely to be controlled until facilities for adequate filtration of water and disposal of sewage become available. There are currently no *Giardia* vaccine candidates in development.

DIENTAMOEBA FRAGILIS

Dientamoeba fragilis is a binucleate organism with an ameboid trophozoite that measures 4 to 12 μm in diameter (see Fig. 98–2). There is no cyst form. The organism was initially classified as an ameba, but is more closely related to the flagellates (trichomonads) based on structural and antigenic studies. Transmission is presumed to be via the fecal-oral route, although the trophozoite is killed by stomach acid.[6] Because of an association with *Enterobius vermicularis* (pinworm), some have hypothesized that it is carried in pinworm eggs.[102] Infection with *D. fragilis* is common throughout the world. *D. fragilis* was identified in 0.5% of all stool samples examined in a large US study, and the prevalence has been as high as 20% to 50% in selected populations.[83, 104–107]

The role of *D. fragilis* as a pathogen has been controversial. *D. fragilis* trophozoites do not invade tissue, and many individuals infected with *D. fragilis* remain asymptomatic.[6] Furthermore, the organism is often identified in the presence of other intestinal parasites, making its role in disease unclear.[104, 106, 107] Several studies of patients infected only with *D. fragilis* have found an association with diarrhea, abdominal pain, nausea, weight loss, anorexia, flatus, and malaise.[105, 108, 109] Treatment with iodoquinol, metronidazole, and tetracycline has been effective.[105, 109, 110]

BLASTOCYSTIS HOMINIS

Blastocystis hominis is an intestinal protozoan parasite that commonly infects the human colon. It is of uncertain taxonomic classification and its significance as a pathogen remains controversial. Diameter ranges from 3 to 30 μm and, in culture, *B. hominis* has ameboid, vacuolated, and granular forms.[6, 111] Recently, a cyst form has also been identified.[111]

The distribution of *B. hominis* is worldwide, but infection is most common in the tropics.[72, 83, 112–114] In a large study of intestinal parasitism in the United States, *B. hominis* was identified in 2.6% of stool specimens submitted to state health departments. Greater than 70% of positive samples were from California.[83] Among American travelers and expatriates, the prevalence often exceeds 30%.[79, 114]

B. hominis infection is not more common among patients with gastrointestinal complaints (eg, abdominal pain, constipation, diarrhea, alternating diarrhea and constipation, and vomiting) than among asymptomatic control subjects.[72, 114, 115] In addition, the parasite burden does not correlate with symptoms.[72, 112] Nevertheless, multiple studies have used iodoquinol (650 mg orally three times a day for 20 days) or metronidazole (750 mg orally three times a day for 10 days) for treatment of symptomatic patients, with an overall improvement rate of about 50%.[71, 116] This clinical improvement may actually be due to treatment of unrecognized infections due to other organisms, since many people infected with *B. hominis* simultaneously harbor known pathogens.[104, 117, 118]

CRYPTOSPORIDIUM PARVUM

Epidemiology

First recognized by Tyzzer as a gastric infection in mice in 1907, Cryptosporidium is a tiny, intracellular sporozoan protozoan parasite (2–5 μm) that was brought to prominent medical attention only in the early 1980s because of the devastating disease it causes in patients with advanced HIV infection. However, it is increasingly recognized as a cause of self-limited diarrhea, usually lasting 1 to 4 weeks in immunocompetent patients as well. Because cryptosporidial oocysts are small and highly chlorine-resistant, they are spread in chlorinated water such as in the largest waterborne outbreak ever recorded that occurred in Milwaukee in 1993[119] and in numerous chlorinated swimming pool outbreaks. It also has a low infectious dose and is readily spread person-to-person in hospitals or in day care centers.

Besides the gastric species of *C. muris* and *C. serpentis* that infect mice and snakes, the smaller intestinal species of *C. parvum* and *C. baileyi* infect a wide range of mammals (including humans) and chickens, respectively. Most infections are type 1 (human) or type 2 (bovine) *C. parvum* infections, although related *C. felis* (from cats) and *C. meleagridis* (from turkeys) may infect patients with AIDS.[120, 121]

Pathogenesis, Pathology, and Immunology

Upon ingestion of an infectious dose that may be as low as 1 to 10 hardy oocysts, excystation and release of sporozoa occurs in the presence of bile salts in the small bowel. The sporozoites then invade the intestinal epithelium, where they develop into asexual merozoites, then into sexual gametes and zygotes before meiosis and returning to naked sporozoites in oocysts to complete the life cycle. However, sporozoites only invade to a uniquely extracytoplasmic edge of the enterocyte where a special feeder organelle enables the parasite to develop. Rarely multiplication has been seen in the biliary, respiratory or even conjunctival sites in immunocompromised patients, probably from luminal and not hematogenous spread.

Both animal and human studies suggest that both humoral and cellular immune responses aid in the control of *Cryptosporidium* infections. Cryptosporidial diarrhea is clearly much more severe, if not intractable, in patients with immunoglobulin deficiency, lymphocytic malignancies or low CD4 counts associated with HIV infection.

Clinical Presentation

Following a 1-week incubation period (range, 2–14 days), a watery, relatively noninflammatory diarrheal illness typically lasts for 10 to 14 days in immunocompetent hosts. Nausea, vomiting, abdominal pain, and mild fever may also be seen. Rarely, respiratory symptoms, pancreatitis, and biliary tract involvement have been reported, the latter in HIV-infected individuals (see Chapter 28). Brief recurrence of diarrhea may be seen after improvement.

In immunocompromised patients, particularly those with very low CD4 lymphocyte counts, the diarrheal illness with cryptosporidial infection can be cholera-like, protracted (often for the duration of severe immune compromise) and may be fatal.

Diagnosis

Since cryptosporidial infection will not usually be identified in the laboratory unless specifically requested, the most important element in diagnosis is to consider it in patients with diarrhea lasting longer than 5 to 7 days and to request special fecal studies for *Cryptosporidium*. Because *Cryptosporidium* is also spread in water, it is reasonable to consider cryptosporidiosis in the same clinical settings when one considers the diagnosis of giardiasis. In addition, it should certainly be considered in persistent diarrhea in immunocompromised patients.

Traditionally, cryptosporidial oocysts have been detected with a modified acid-fast stain of the stool (which can also detect *Cyclospora* as well as *Isospora*). As with giardiasis, ELISA or direct fluorescence antibody tests of the stool are increasingly useful in the diagnosis of cryptosporidiosis. However, one should remember that these immunodiagnostic tests may be of limited value in testing of environmental samples since there is some cross-reactivity with nonhuman cryptosporidial oocysts as well.[101] Occasionally, cryptosporidiosis is diagnosed with intestinal biopsy.

Serologic tests are primarily helpful in epidemiologic studies, especially since they may be negative at the time of initial clinical presentation and often persist after infection is resolved. Finally, abdominal ultrasound, CT scans, and ERCP may be helpful in diagnosis of acalculous cholecystitis and cholangiopathies.

Treatment

Although over 100 antimicrobial and antiparasitic drugs have been tested, none have been consistently curative of cryptosporidial infection, especially in immunocompromised individuals. However, some clinical improvement and reduction in oocycts shedding has been seen with the nonabsorbable aminoglycoside paromomycin, paromomycin in combination with azithromycin, or with nitazoxanide.[101, 122]

Most important in treating HIV-infected patients with cryptosporidiosis is highly active antiretroviral therapy (HAART), since ultimate improvement of cryptosporidial illnesses is dependent upon improvement in CD4 lymphocyte counts and immune compromise. Finally, papillotomy may be required for biliary obstruction with papillary stenosis with cryptosporidiosis in immunocompromised patients (see Chapter 28).

Control and Prevention

Most important in control and prevention of this difficult protozoan parasitic infection is education regarding boiling or careful filtration of water (ie, filter pores must be less than 1 μm in diameter). In addition, scrupulous enteric precautions are required in institutions such as hospitals, day care centers, or extended care facilities for the elderly. These precautions are especially important since chlorine is ineffective in reducing oocyst viability. Other means for disinfection that are being studied include ultraviolet light and irradiation. Challenges are also presented for sterilization of endoscopes.[123, 124]

Finally, because of the potential substantial long-term impact of cryptosporidial infection on growth and development,[125, 126] control of cryptosporidiosis is critical to child development in developing areas and must receive appropriate high priority in programs directed at improved water and sanitation worldwide.

CYCLOSPORA CAYETANENSIS

Epidemiology

Although recognized by Schaudinn as a cause of enteritis in moles in 1901,[127] *Cyclospora* was first described (although not named) by Ashford in 1979 in three patients in Papua, New Guinea (where he also described its sporulation).[128] *Cyclospora* was then seen increasingly in AIDS patients with protracted diarrhea and in nonimmunocompromised patients with persistent diarrhea in New York City, the Caribbean, among expatriots in Nepal, and in an outbreak among house staff in a Chicago hospital.[129–131] Finally, its definitive sporulation and naming as *Cyclospora cayetanensis* was reported by Ortega and associates in 1993.[132] Ribosomal DNA analysis of phylogenetic relationships suggest that *Cyclospora* is closely related to *Eimeria*.[132]

Like *Cryptosporidium*, *Cyclospora* is increasingly recognized in immunocompetent as well as immunocompromised individuals. The infection is probably spread via contaminated water, and is usually highly seasonal (in summer or wet months). *Cyclospora* was brought to prominent attention throughout the United States and Canada with repeated outbreaks of diarrheal illnesses occurring in over 2000 patients every year from 1996 through 2000 in association with consumption of the late spring shipment (but not the fall shipment) of Guatemalan raspberries.[134, 135]

Pathogenesis, Pathology, and Immunology

The apparent pathogenesis, pathology and immunology, although not as thoroughly studied, appears to be similar to that described for *Cryptosporidium*. One important distinction is that, unlike *Cryptosporidium*, which is promptly infectious when it is excreted in the stool, *Cyclospora* requires development outside the host before it becomes infectious. Consequently, the risk of secondary person-to-person spread, which is very common with cryptosporidial infections, is not described with *Cyclospora* infections. An additional difference is that, unlike the numerous mammalian hosts for cryptosporidial infections that may also infect humans, the animal reservoir(s) for *Cyclospora* are very poorly understood at present.

The histopathologic changes seen in *Cyclospora* infections are, again, similar to those seen with cryptosporidiosis, with villous blunting and mild inflammatory infiltrate in the lamina propria predominately in the small bowel.[136]

Clinical Presentation

The clinical presentation of *Cyclospora* infection is also indistinguishable with that described earlier with *Cryptosporidium* infections. Perhaps more prominent is the description of severe generalized fatigue and malaise with *Cyclospora* infections (even in immunocompetent individuals). *Cyclospora* diarrhea typically lasts for 1 to 3 weeks and may be associated with significant weight loss as well.

Finally, also as seen with cryptosporidiosis, protracted diarrhea and acalculous cholecystitis may also be seen with *Cyclospora* infection in HIV-infected individuals.

Diagnosis

As with *Cryptosporidium*, one must consider the diagnosis of *Cyclospora*. Because it is readily treatable, even in immunocompromised patients, the diagnosis of *Cyclospora* infection is even more important. This is best done at present with the acid-fast stain. *Cyclospora* oocysts are nearly twice the size of *Cryptosporidium* (4–10 μm). In addition, *Cyclospora* exhibits striking blue-green autofluorescence when examined under fluorescence microscopy, a characteristic that may have contributed to its initial confusion with cyanobacteria. Improved diagnostic methods using immunologic and PCR techniques are under current active development.

Treatment

In contrast to *Cryptosporidium* infections, *Cyclospora* infections are readily treatable even in immunocompromised patients. The drug of choice is trimethoprim/sulfamethoxazole at a dosage of 160/800 mg twice daily for 1 week. This treatment promptly eradicates the organism and relieves symptoms.[138, 139] This treatment is similarly effective in patients with AIDS, although maintenance therapy with a single dose of trimethoprim-sulfamethoxazole three times per week may be needed to prevent relapse.[140] Recent data also show that ciprofloxacin provides a reasonable alternative in patients unable to tolerate trimethoprim/sulfamethoxazole.[141]

Control and Prevention

Although they are readily treatable as previously noted, *Cyclospora* infections are proving to be extremely difficult to control or prevent. This is especially because of our limited ability to detect low infectious doses (for humans) of oocysts, which may contaminate products such as raspberries from which it is extremely difficult to eradicate. From limited studies, the organism also appears to be relatively chlorine-resistant as well and thus poses challenges to effective water treatment much like those seen with *Cryptosporidium*. Finally, elucidation of the reservoir of *Cyclospora* will also undoubtedly enhance our ability to prevent and control the spread of this highly infectious parasite. For example, it remains unclear why it is only the spring rather than the fall shipment of raspberries from Guatemala that has consistently posed problems with spread of *Cyclospora* infections. Whether this is related to migration of an avian reservoir has been postulated but not proven.[142]

ISOSPORA BELLI

Epidemiology

A relative of *Cyclospora* and *Eimeria*, *Isospora belli* is much larger, with elliptical oocysts measuring 20 to 30 μm long containing two visible sporocysts that are acid-fast. Like *Cyclospora*, *Isospora* oocysts appear to require sporulation outside of the human host before they are infectious. Although there are no known nonhuman hosts for *Isospora belli*, its distribution appears to be throughout tropical areas around the world. However, it appears to be less common as a cause of diarrhea in children in developing areas than *Cryptosporidium* and is seen more often in older children, immunocompromised patients, and in institutionalized children in North America.[143, 144]

Pathogenesis, Pathology, and Immunology

The pathogenesis, pathology, and immunology of *Isospora* infections, while less thoroughly studied, appears to be similar to that seen with *Cryptosporidium* and *Cyclospora* infections already discussed.

Clinical Presentation

Similar to *Cryptosporidium* and *Cyclospora* infections, *Isospora* characteristically produces a self-limiting diarrheal illness in immunocompetent individuals and in travelers to tropical areas, with watery diarrhea and abdominal pain lasting 2 to 4 weeks. In immunocompromised patients, *Isospora* may produce protracted sprue-like illnesses with malabsorption, weight loss, and prolonged diarrhea. As with *Cryptosporidium* and *Cyclospora*, acalculous cholecystitis has also been reported in patients with AIDS and *Isospora* infections.

Diagnosis

The diagnosis of *Isospora* should be suspected in immunocompetent patients with persistent diarrhea, especially following travel to tropical or developing areas, and in immunocompromised patients with persistent diarrhea. Unlike other protozoan infections, *Isospora* infections may be associated with peripheral eosinophilia and with Charcot-Leyden crystals in the stool. The diagnosis of *Isospora* is documented with acid-fast staining of characteristic oocysts seen in stool or rarely on small bowel biopsy. In contrast to *Cryptosporidium* and *Cyclospora* infections, *Isospora* organisms have been observed invading beyond the epithelium into the lamina propria.[145]

Treatment

As with *Cyclospora*, *Isospora* infections are readily treated with trimethoprim/sulfamethoxazole at a dosage of 160/800 mg orally four times a day for 10 days, and then two times a day for 3 weeks, with both symptomatic and parasitologic responses, even in patients with AIDS. As previously described with *Cyclospora*, maintenance suppressive therapy may be required in patients with AIDS. Alternatives to trimethoprim/sulfamethoxazole may include ciprofloxacin.[141]

Control and Prevention

Prevention and control of *Isospora* infections will likely require improved sanitation in tropical areas.

MICROSPORIDIA

Epidemiology

Microsporidia, the nontaxonomic term for *Enterocytozoan bieneusi*, *Encephalitozoan* (old *Septata*) *intestinalis*, and several nonintestinal members of the Microspora family are important causes of diarrhea, primarily in immunocompromised patients with AIDS or post-transplant around the globe.[146] Their role in immunocompetent persons is less clear, but appears distinctly less common. Likewise, the reservoir and modes of transmission of microsporidial infections are uncertain. Even in tropical developing areas where cryptosporidial infections are highly seasonal, microsporidial infections in HIV-infected individuals occur throughout the year.[147]

Pathogenesis, Pathology, and Immunology

While *E. bieneusi* enters only the cytoplasm of enterocytes, *E. intestinalis* enters parasitophorous vacuoles in enterocytes, endothelial cells, fiboblasts and macrophages, and may disseminate to the kidney, prostate gland, and upper respiratory tract. Typically intestinal pathosis involves villous atrophy, crypt hyperplasia and mild inflammation in the lamina propria. The importance of cellular immunity in determining both infection and illness with intestinal microsporidia is indicated by its striking predominance in immunocompromised individuals after organ transplant or in those with AIDS.

Clinical Presentation

Although primarily limited to immunocompromised patients, microsporidia (much like *Cryptosporidium* and *Cyclospora*) cause watery, relatively noninflammatory diarrhea and weight loss, occasionally with abdominal pain, nausea, vomiting, fever, and acalculous cholecystitis or even sclerosing cholangitis.[146, 148] *E. intestinalis* may also cause colitis and dissemination especially to the kidneys or less often to sinuses, bronchi, conjunctiva or prostate. Rarely cases of self-limited diarrhea in travelers or health professionals have also been reported.[149, 150]

Diagnosis

After considering the diagnosis in any immunocompromised patient with persistent unexplained diarrhea, microsporidial spores can be identified in the stool or, with *E. intestinalis*, in the urine using special chromotrope stains. With Weber's modified chromotrope stain, for example, microsporidial spores stain as bright pink, tiny ovoid, refractile organisms measuring only 1 to 1.5 μm (*E. intestinalis* are slightly larger), often with a pink beltlike band. In intestinal biopsy specimens, gram stain or electron microscopy is needed to identify the organisms inside the enterocyte or (with *E. intestinalis*) macrophage cytoplasm, the latter in a parasitophorous vacuole.

Treatment

Although responses of *E. bieneusi* are less clear, *E. intestinalis* infections appear to respond well to albendazole, 400 mg twice or three times daily for 2 weeks to 3 months. As with all opportunistic infections in patients with AIDS, effective antiretroviral therapy (HAART) is key to controlling microsporidial infections and illnesses.

Control and Prevention

As the reservoir and transmission of microsporidia remain unclear, control measures are primarily directed toward appropriate sanitary precautions and handwashing.

TRYPANOSOMA CRUZI (AMERICAN TRYPANOSOMIASIS OR CHAGAS' DISEASE)

Epidemiology

Although symptomatic Chagas' disease has been confined to South and Central America, at least four autochthonous (indigenous) cases, as well as occasional laboratory-acquired and imported cases of acute Chagas' disease have occurred in the United States. However, increasing numbers of immigrants are presenting with chronic Chagas' disease and pose distinct risks for transmission of Chagas' disease.[151] In patients surviving acute infection with *Trypanosoma cruzi* in whom the chronic form of illness develops, myocardial disease is the most common manifestation. Megaesophagus and megacolon are the most common intestinal manifestations of American trypanosomiasis. Small intestinal dilatation and aperistalsis also are seen. At post-mortem examination, even in patients with asymptomatic *T. cruzi* involvement of the intestine, the small intestine has a significant reduction in submucosal and myenteric autonomic plexuses.

American trypanosomiasis could prove to be a significant health problem in the United States. There is a large reservoir of *T. cruzi* infection in animals in the southern United States. Infection has been detected in animals in Arizona, California, New Mexico, Texas, Louisiana, Georgia, Florida, and Maryland. The epidemiologically important insects, the reduviid bugs of the Triatominae group, also have the same wide geographic distribution. Infection is transmitted when the reduviid bug infected with *T. cruzi* bites the victim. On biting, the arthropod discharges feces. The parasite is then introduced through the skin by the patient's scratching the bite. The apparent difference between the South American reduviid bugs and those found in the United States is that the species in the United States do not defecate on biting.

Pathogenesis, Pathology, and Immunology

Metacyclic trypanosomes are deposited from the feces of the bug during the time it is taking a blood meal. Characteristically, deposition occurs on or near mucous membranes, particularly on the outer canthus of the eye or around the nose or lips. The invading organisms are phagocytosed by histiocytes in the corium and invade the adipose and subcutaneous muscle cells. They multiply in this location in the amastigote forms, previously called *Leishmania* forms because of their similarity in appearance to intracellular amastigote forms of *Leishmania*, a related hemoflagellate (see Chapter 69). When the histiocytes and other parasitized cells rupture on the fourth or fifth day, the amastigote forms are taken up by regional lymph nodes, from where, at variable intervals, they are discharged through the blood and lymphatic circulation and spread to diverse areas of the body.

The signs and symptoms of Chagas' disease are caused by the intracellular amastigote forms. When the host cell ruptures, large numbers escape and temporarily enter the circulation as trypanosome forms. In the intestine, tissue injury may occur acutely or may trigger autoimmune damage to nerve or cardiac epitopes that cross react with *T. cruzi* antigens to destroy the submucosal and the myenteric plexuses. The end result is enteromegaly, which at times may be massive. Immunosuppression as a consequence of chemotherapy or AIDS can reactivate chronic *T. cruzi* infection, causing acute disease or brain abscesses.

Clinical Presentation

Acute Chagas' disease occurs most often in children. It is characterized by high fever and marked edema, particularly with a periorbital distribution and often involving the entire body. In patients with acute Chagas' disease, the periorbital edema of one or both eyes is striking. The victim may appear to be suffering from myxedema. There usually is enlargement of the thyroid gland, lymph nodes, and salivary glands and hepatosplenomegaly is present. The acute stage lasts about 20 to 30 days.

Chronic Chagas' disease depends on the major organ involvement within the body. Most commonly the symptoms are cardiac, manifested primarily as arrhythmias and congestive heart failure. With megaesophagus, the history is indistinguishable from that of achalasia. With megacolon, infrequent bowel movements and chronic constipation are the cardinal symptoms. With dilatation of the small intestine, diarrhea or constipation may be part of the picture. There may be evidence of weight loss and abdominal distention caused by the markedly dilated bowel.

Diagnosis

Routine laboratory data provide no clue to the diagnosis of Chagas' disease. Diagnosis of acute disease depends on demonstration of the trypanosome forms on blood smears during periods when the amastigotes rupture cells. During febrile periods, if the blood smear results are negative, inoculation of a patient's blood into a guinea pig leads to proliferation of trypanosomes that frequently can be recovered and identified. Amastigote forms may be detected in bone marrow, the spleen, or enlarged lymph nodes.

The most usual immunologic method for diagnosis of American trypanosomiasis is complement fixation. Other immunologic tests are under investigation but not widely applied. Xenodiagnosis has been used but is relatively insensitive, identifying fewer than 50% of patients infected with chronic Chagas' disease. In this technique, trypanosome-free laboratory reduviid bugs are allowed to bite suspected victims. The trypanosomes multiply rapidly in the intestinal tract of the insect, and examination of the intestine reveals flagellated trypanosomes in 10 to 30 days. Immunologic and PCR-based assays have also been developed.[151]

Treatment

Nifurtimox, available from the Centers for Disease Control and Prevention Parasitic Disease Drug Service, Atlanta, Georgia, may be given in a dose of 8 to 10 mg/kg orally in four divided doses.[152] Patients with achalasia caused by Chagas' disease may be treated with either brusque pneumatic dilation of the esophagus or esophagomyotomy (see Chapter 32). Occasionally, aperistaltic segments of intestine that are responsible for symptoms may be resected.

Control and Prevention

Control and prevention require improved housing, use of insecticides and netting, and screening blood for antibody in endemic areas.

Acknowledgment
We acknowledge Dr. Owen's chapter in the previous edition from which the *T. cruzi* section was adapted.

REFERENCES

1. Diamond LS, Clark CG: A redescription of Entamoeba histolytica Schaudinn, 1903 (amended Walker, 1911) separating it from Entamoeba dispar Brumpt, 1925. J Eukaryot Microbiol 40(3):340–344, 1993.
2. Petri WA, Jr: Recent advances in amebiasis. Crit Rev Clin Lab Sci 33(1):1–37, 1996.
3. Walsh JA: Problems in recognition and diagnosis of amebiasis: Estimation of the global magnitude of morbidity and mortality. Rev Infect Dis 8(2):228–238, 1986.
4. WHO/PAHO/UNESCO report:. A consultation with experts on amoebiasis. Mexico City, Mexico 28–29 January, 1997. Epidemiol Bull 18(1):13–14, 1997.
5. Haque R, Ali IM, Petri WA, Jr: Prevalence and immune response to Entamoeba histolytica infection in preschool children in Bangladesh. Am J Trop Med Hyg 60(6):1031–1034, 1999.
6. Katz M, Despommier DD, Gwadz R: Parasitic Diseases, 2nd ed. New York, Springer-Verlag, 1989.
7. Ravdin JI: Amebiasis now. Am J Trop Med Hyg 41(3 Suppl):40–48, 1989.
8. Takeuchi A, Phillips BP: Electron microscope studies of experimental Entamoeba histolytica infection in the guinea pig. I. Penetration of the intestinal epithelium by trophozoites. Am J Trop Med Hyg 24(1):34–48, 1975.
9. Beaver PC, Blanchard JL, Seibold HR: Invasive amebiasis in naturally infected New World and Old World monkeys with and without clinical disease. Am J Trop Med Hyg 39(4):343–352, 1988.
10. Chadee K, Meerovitch E: Entamoeba histolytica: Early progressive pathology in the cecum of the gerbil (Meriones unguiculatus). Am J Trop Med Hyg 34(2):283–291, 1985.
11. Ravdin JI, Guerrant RL: Role of adherence in cytopathogenic mechanisms of Entamoeba histolytica. J Clin Invest 68:1305–1313, 1981.
12. Ravdin JI, Murphy CF, Salata RA, Guerrant RL, Hewlett EL: N-acetyl-D-galactosamine-inhibitable adherence lectin of Entamoeba histolytica. I. Partial purification and relation to amoebic virulence in vitro. J Infect Dis 151(5):804–815, 1985.
13. Chadee K, Petri WA, Jr., Innes DJ, Ravdin JI: Rat and human colonic mucins bind to and inhibit adherence lectin of Entamoeba histolytica. J Clin Invest 80(5):1245–1254, 1987.
14. Petri Jr. WA, Smith RD, Schlesinger PH, et al: Isolation of the galactose binding adherence lecting of Entamoeba histolytica. J Clin Invest 80:1238–1244, 1987.
15. McKerrow JH, Sun E, Rosenthal PJ, Bouvier J: The proteases and pathogenicity of parasitic protozoa. Annu Rev Microbiol 47:821–853, 1993.
16. Keene WE, Petitt MG, Allen S, McKerrow JH: The major neutral proteinase of Entamoeba histolytica. J Exp Med 163(3):536–549, 1986.
17. Luaces AL, Barrett AJ: Affinity purification and biochemical characterization of histolysin, the major cysteine proteinase of Entamoeba histolytica. Biochem J 250(3):903–909, 1988.
18. Lushbaugh WB, Hofbauer AF, Pittman FE: Entamoeba histolytica: Purification of cathepsin B. Exp Parasitol 59(3):328–336, 1985.
19. Zhang Z, Wang L, Seydel KB, et al: Entamoeba histolytica cysteine proteinases with interleukin-1 beta converting enzyme (ICE) activity cause intestinal inflammation and tissue damage in amoebiasis. Mol Microbiol 37(3):542–548, 2000.
20. Brandt H, Tamayo RP: Pathology of human amebiasis. Hum Pathol 1(3):351–385, 1970.
21. Cotran RS, Cotran RS, Kumar V, Robbins SL: Robbins' Pathologic Basis of Disease, 4th ed. Philadelphia, WB Saunders, 1989.
22. Chadee K, Meerovitch E: The pathology of experimentally induced cecal amebiasis in gerbils (Meriones unguiculatus). Liver changes and amebic liver abscess formation. Am J Pathol 119(3):485–494, 1985.
23. Chadee K, Meerovitch E: The mongolian gerbil (Meriones unguiculatus) as an experimental host for Entamoeba histolytica. Am J Trop Med Hyg 33(1):47–54, 1984.
24. DeLeon A: Archives of Investigative Medicine (Mex). Suppl 1:S205, 1970.
25. Gathiram V, Jackson TF: A longitudinal study of asymptomatic carriers of pathogenic zymodemes of Entamoeba histolytica. S Afr Med J 72(10):669–672, 1987.
26. Choudhuri G, Prakash V, Kumar A, Shahi SK, Sharma M: Protective immunity to entamoeba histolytica infection in subjects with antiamoebic antibodies residing in a hyperendemic zone. Scand J Infect Dis 23(6):771–776, 1991.
27. Krupp IM: Antibody response in intestinal and extraintestinal amebiasis. Am J Trop Med Hyg 19(1):57–62, 1970.
28. Ortiz-Ortiz L, Zamacona G, Sepulveda B, Capin NR: Cell-mediated immunity in patients with amebic abscess of the liver. Clin Immunol Immunopathol 4(1):127–134, 1975.
29. del Muro R, Acosta E, Merino E, Glender W, Ortiz-Ortiz L: Diagnosis of intestinal amebiasis using salivary IgA antibody detection. J Infect Dis 162:1360–1364, 1990.
30. Aceti A, Pennica A, Celestino D, et al: Salivary IgA antibody detection in invasive amebiasis and in asymptomatic infection [letter; comment]. J Infect Dis 164(3):613–615, 1991.
31. Abou-el-Magd I, Soong CJ, el Hawey AM, Ravdin JI: Humoral and

mucosal IgA antibody response to a recombinant 52-kDa cysteine-rich portion of the Entamoeba histolytica galactose-inhibitable lectin correlates with detection of native 170-kDa lectin antigen in serum of patients with amebic colitis. J Infect Dis 174(1):157–162, 1996.
32. Cieslak PR, Virgin HW, Stanley SL Jr: A severe combined immunodeficient (SCID) mouse model for infection with Entamoeba histolytica. J Exp Med 176(6):1605–1609, 1992.
33. Kanani SR, Knight R: Relapsing amoebic colitis of 12 year's standing exacerbated by corticosteroids. BMJ 2(657):613–614, 1969.
34. Kanani SR, Knight R: Amoebic dysentery precipitated by corticosteroids. BMJ 3(662):114, 1969.
35. Huston CD, Petri WA: Amebiasis. In Conn HF, Rakel RE (eds): Conn's Current Therapy, 2000. Philadelphia, WB Saunders, 2000, pp 56–59.
36. Speelman P, McGlaughlin R, Kabir I, Butler T: Differential clinical features and stool findings in shigellosis and amoebic dysentery. Trans R Soc Trop Med Hyg 81(4):549–551, 1987.
37. Ellyson JH, Bezmalinovic Z, Parks SN, Lewis FR Jr: Necrotizing amebic colitis: A frequently fatal complication. Am J Surg 152(1):21–26, 1986.
38. Aristizabal H, Acevedo J, Botero M: Fulminant amebic colitis. World J Surg 15(2):216–221, 1991.
39. Kapoor OP, Joshi VR: Multiple amoebic liver abscesses. A study of 56 cases. J Trop Med Hyg 75(1):4–6, 1972.
40. Katzenstein D, Rickerson V, Braude A: New concepts of amebic liver abscess derived from hepatic imaging, serodiagnosis, and hepatic enzymes in 67 consecutive cases in San Diego. Medicine (Baltimore) 61(4):237–246, 1982.
41. Nordestgaard AG, Stapleford L, Worthen N, Bongard FS, Klein SR: Contemporary management of amebic liver abscess. Am Surg 58(5): 315–320, 1992.
42. Kapoor OP, Shah NA: Pericardial amoebiasis following amoebic liver abscess of the left lobe. J Trop Med Hyg 75(1):7–10, 1972.
43. Krogstad DJ, Spencer HC Jr, Healy GR, Gleason NN, Sexton DJ, Herron CA: Amebiasis: Epidemiologic studies in the United States, 1971–1974. Ann Intern Med 88(1):89–97, 1978.
44. Haque R, Neville LM, Hahn P, Petri WA Jr: Rapid diagnosis of Entamoeba infection by using Entamoeba and Entamoeba histolytica stool antigen detection kits. J Clin Microbiol 33(10):2558–2561, 1995.
45. Gonzalez-Ruiz A, Haque R, Aguirre A, et al: Value of microscopy in the diagnosis of dysentery associated with invasive Entamoeba histolytica. J Clin Pathol 47(3):236–239, 1994.
46. Strachan WD, Chiodini PL, Spice WM, Moody AH, Ackers JP: Immunological differentiation of pathogenic and non-pathogenic isolates of Entamoeba histolytica. Lancet 1(8585):561–563, 1988.
47. Tannich E, Burchard GD: Differentiation of pathogenic from nonpathogenic Entamoeba histolytica by restriction fragment analysis of a single gene amplified in vitro. J Clin Microbiol 29(2):250–255, 1991.
48. Acuna-Soto R, Samuelson J, De Girolami P, et al: Application of the polymerase chain reaction to the epidemiology of pathogenic and nonpathogenic Entamoeba histolytica. Am J Trop Med Hyg 48(1):58–70, 1993.
49. Katzwinkel-Wladarsch S, Loscher T, Rinder H: Direct amplification and differentiation of pathogenic and nonpathogenic Entamoeba histolytica DNA from stool specimens. Am J Trop Med Hyg 51(1):115–118, 1994.
50. Britten D, Wilson SM, McNerney R, Moody AH, Chiodini PL, Ackers JP: An improved colorimetric PCR-based method for detection and differentiation of Entamoeba histolytica and Entamoeba dispar in feces. J Clin Microbiol 35(5):1108–1111, 1997.
51. Troll H, Marti H, Weiss N: Simple differential detection of Entamoeba histolytica and Entamoeba dispar in fresh stool specimens by sodium acetate-acetic acid-formalin concentration and PCR. J Clin Microbiol 35(7):1701–1705, 1997.
52. Ravdin JI, Jackson TF, Petri WA Jr, et al: Association of serum antibodies to adherence lectin with invasive amebiasis and asymptomatic infection with pathogenic Entamoeba histolytica. J Infect Dis 162(3):768–772, 1990.
53. Petri WA Jr, Jackson TF, Gathiram V, et al: Pathogenic and nonpathogenic strains of Entamoeba histolytica can be differentiated by monoclonal antibodies to the galactose-specific adherence lectin. Infect Immun 58(6):1802–1806, 1990.
54. Haque R, Kress K, Wood S, et al: Diagnosis of pathogenic Entamoeba histolytica infection using a stool ELISA based on monoclonal antibodies to the galactose-specific adhesin [see comments]. J Infect Dis 167(1):247–249, 1993.
55. Haque R, Faruque AS, Hahn P, Lyerly DM, Petri WA Jr: Entamoeba histolytica and Entamoeba dispar infection in children in Bangladesh. J Infect Dis 175(3):734–736, 1997.
56. Haque R, Ali IK, Akther S, Petri WA Jr: Comparison of PCR, isoenzyme analysis, and antigen detection for diagnosis of Entamoeba histolytica infection. J Clin Microbiol 36(2):449–452, 1998.
57. Ong SJ, Cheng MY, Liu KH, Horng CB: Use of the ProSpecT microplate enzyme immunoassay for the detection of pathogenic and non-pathogenic Entamoeba histolytica in faecal specimens. Trans R Soc Trop Med Hyg 90(3):248–249, 1996.
58. Jelinek T, Peyerl G, Loscher T, Nothdurft HD: Evaluation of an antigen-capture enzyme immunoassay for detection of Entamoeba histolytica in stool samples. Eur J Clin Microbiol Infect Dis 15(9):752–755, 1996.
59. Mirelman D, Nuchamowitz Y, Stolarsky T: Comparison of use of enzyme-linked immunosorbent assay-based kits and PCR amplification of rRNA genes for simultaneous detection of Entamoeba histolytica and E. dispar. J Clin Microbiol 35(9):2405–2407, 1997.
60. Haque R, Mollah NU, Ali IK, et al: Diagnosis of amebic liver abscess and intestinal infection with the TechLab entamoeba histolytica II antigen detection and antibody tests [in process citation]. J Clin Microbiol 38(9):3235–3239, 2000.
61. McAuley JB, Herwaldt BL, Stokes SL, et al: Diloxanide furoate for treating asymptomatic Entamoeba histolytica cyst passers: 14 years' experience in the United States [see comments]. Clin Infect Dis 15(3): 464-468, 1992.
62. Drugs for parasitic infections [published erratum appears in Med Lett Drugs Ther Feb 27,40(1021):28, 1998]. Med Lett Drugs Ther 40(1017):1–12, 1998.
63. McAuley JB, Juranek DD: Paromomycin in the treatment of mild-to-moderate intestinal amebiasis [letter]. Clin Infect Dis 15(3):551–552, 1992.
64. Bassily S, Farid Z, el Masry NA, Mikhail EM: Treatment of intestinal E. histolytica and G. lamblia with metronidazole, tinidazole and ornidazole: A comparative study. J Trop Med Hyg 90(1):9–12, 1987.
65. Powell SJ, Wilmot AJ, Elsdon-Dew R: Further trials of metronidazole in amoebic dysentery and amoebic liver abscess. Ann Trop Med Parasitol 61(4):511–514, 1967.
66. Barwick RS, Uzicanin A, Lareau S, et al: Program and Abstracts of the American Society of Tropical Medicine and Hygiene Annual Meeting, Washington DC, January 1999.
67. Huston CD, Petri WA Jr: Host-pathogen interaction in amebiasis and progress in vaccine development. Eur J Clin Microbiol Infect Dis 17(9):601–614, 1998.
68. Petri WA, Jr., Singh U, Ravdin JI: Enteric amebiasis. In Guerrant RL, Walker DH, Weller PF (eds): Tropical Infectious Diseases: Principles, Pathogens, and Practice. Philadelphia, Churchill Livingstone, 2000, pp 685–702.
69. Lucht E, Evengard B, Skott J, Pehrson P, Nord CE: Entamoeba gingivalis in human immunodeficiency virus type 1-infected patients with periodontal disease. Clin Infect Dis 27(3):471–473, 1998.
70. Salaki JS, Shirey JL, Strickland GT: Successful treatment of symptomatic Entamoeba polecki infection. Am J Trop Med Hyg 28(2):190–193, 1979.
71. Qadri SM, al Okaili GA, al Dayel F: Clinical significance of Blastocystis hominis [see comments]. J Clin Microbiol 27(11):2407–2409, 1989.
72. Herwaldt BL, de Arroyave KR, Wahlquist SP, du Pee LJ, Eng TR, Juranek DD: Infections with intestinal parasites in Peace Corps volunteers in Guatemala. J Clin Microbiol 32(5):1376–1378, 1994.
73. Hill DR: *Giardia lambtia*. In Mandell GL, Douglas RG, Bennett JE, Dolin R (eds): Mandell, Douglas, and Bennett's Principles and Practice of Infectious Diseases. Philadelphia, Churchill Livingstone, 2000, pp 2888–2894.
74. Nash TE, McCutchan T, Keister D, Dame JB, Conrad JD, Gillin FD: Restriction-endonuclease analysis of DNA from 15 Giardia isolates obtained from humans and animals. J Infect Dis 152(1):64–73, 1985.
75. Nash TE, Herrington DA, Losonsky GA, Levine MM: Experimental human infections with Giardia lamblia. J Infect Dis 156(6):974–984, 1987.
76. Moore GT, Cross WM, McGuire D, et al: Epidemic giardiasis at a ski resort. N Engl J Med 281(8):402–407, 1969.
77. Dennis DT, Smith RP, Welch JJ, et al: Endemic giardiasis in New Hampshire: A case-control study of environmental risks. J Infect Dis 167(6):1391–1395, 1993.

78. Isaac-Renton JL, Cordeiro C, Sarafis K, Shahriari H: Characterization of Giardia duodenalis isolates from a waterborne outbreak. J Infect Dis 167(2):431–440, 1993.
79. Isaac-Renton JL, Lewis LF, Ong CS, Nulsen MF: A second community outbreak of waterborne giardiasis in Canada and serological investigation of patients. Trans R Soc Trop Med Hyg 88(4):395–399, 1994.
80. Osterholm MT, Forfang JC, Ristinen TL, et al: An outbreak of foodborne giardiasis. N Engl J Med 304(1):24–28, 1981.
81. White KE, Hedberg CW, Edmonson LM, Jones DB, Osterholm MT, MacDonald KL: An outbreak of giardiasis in a nursing home with evidence for multiple modes of transmission. J Infect Dis 160(2):298–304, 1989.
82. Pickering LK, Woodward WE, DuPont HL, Sullivan P: Occurrence of Giardia lamblia in children in day care centers. J Pediatr 104(4):522–526, 1984.
83. Kappus KD, Lundgren RG Jr, Juranek DD, Roberts JM, Spencer HC: Intestinal parasitism in the United States: Update on a continuing problem. Am J Trop Med Hyg 50(6):705–713, 1994.
84. Farthing MJ, Mata L, Urrutia JJ, Kronmal RA: Natural history of Giardia infection of infants and children in rural Guatemala and its impact on physical growth. Am J Clin Nutr 43(3):395–405, 1986.
85. Fraser D, Dagan R, Naggan L, et al: Natural history of Giardia lamblia and Cryptosporidium infections in a cohort of Israeli Bedouin infants: A study of a population in transition. Am J Trop Med Hyg 57(5):544–549, 1997.
86. Peters CS, Sable R, Janda WM, Chittom AL, Kocka FE: Prevalence of enteric parasites in homosexual patients attending an outpatient clinic. J Clin Microbiol 24(4):684–685, 1986.
87. Oberhuber G, Kastner N, Stolte M: Giardiasis: A histologic analysis of 567 cases. Scand J Gastroenterol 32(1):48–51, 1997.
88. Chavez B, Gonzalez-Mariscal L, Cedillo-Rivera R, Martinez-Palomo A: Giardia lamblia: In vitro cytopathic effect of human isolates. Exp Parasitol 80(1):133–138, 1995.
89. Kamath KR, Murugasu R: A comparative study of four methods for detecting Giardia lamblia in children with diarrheal disease and malabsorption. Gastroenterology 66(1):16–21, 1974.
90. Ament ME, Rubin CE: Relation of giardiasis to abnormal intestinal structure and function in gastrointestinal immunodeficiency syndromes. Gastroenterology 62(2):216–226, 1972.
91. Soliman MM, Taghi-Kilani R, Abou-Shady AF, et al: Comparison of serum antibody responses to Giardia lamblia of symptomatic and asymptomatic patients. Am J Trop Med Hyg 58(2):232–239, 1998.
92. Nayak N, Ganguly NK, Walia BN, Wahi V, Kanwar SS, Mahajan RC: Specific secretory IgA in the milk of Giardia lamblia-infected and uninfected women. J Infect Dis 155(4):724–727, 1987.
93. Rosales-Borjas DM, Diaz-Rivadeneyra J, Dona-Leyva A, et al: Secretory immune response to membrane antigens during Giardia lamblia infection in humans. Infect Immun 66(2):756–759, 1998.
94. Stager S, Muller N: Giardia lamblia infections in B-cell-deficient transgenic mice. Infect Immun 65(9):3944–3946, 1997.
95. Nash TE, Herrington DA, Levine MM, Conrad JT, Merritt JW Jr: Antigenic variation of Giardia lamblia in experimental human infections. J Immunol 144(11):4362–4369, 1990.
96. Nash TE: Antigenic variation in Giardia lamblia and the host's immune response. Philos Trans R Soc Lond B Biol Sci 352(1359):1369–1375, 1997.
97. Hill DR: Giardiasis. Issues in diagnosis and management. Infect Dis Clin North Am 7(3):503–525, 1993.
98. Smith PD, Lane HC, Gill VJ, et al: Intestinal infections in patients with the acquired immunodeficiency syndrome (AIDS). Etiology and response to therapy. Ann Intern Med 108(3):328–333, 1988.
99. Alles AJ, Waldron MA, Sierra LS, Mattia AR: Prospective comparison of direct immunofluorescence and conventional staining methods for detection of Giardia and Cryptosporidium spp. in human fecal specimens. J Clin Microbiol 33(6):1632–1634, 1995.
100. Zimmerman SK, Needham CA: Comparison of conventional stool concentration and preserved-smear methods with Merifluor Cryptosporidium/Giardia Direct Immunofluorescence Assay and ProSpecT Giardia EZ Microplate Assay for detection of Giardia lamblia. J Clin Microbiol 33(7):1942–1943, 1995.
101. Garcia LS, Shimizu RY: Evaluation of nine immunoassay kits (enzyme immunoassay and direct fluorescence) for detection of Giardia lamblia and Cryptosporidium parvum in human fecal specimens. J Clin Microbiol 35(6):1526–1529, 1997.
102. Hill DR, Nash TE: Intestinal flagellate and ciliate infections. In Guerrant RL, Walker DH, Weller PF (eds): Tropical Infectious Diseases: Principles, Pathogens, and Practice. Philadelphia, Churchill Livingstone, 2000, pp 703–720.
103. Bartlett AV, Englender SJ, Jarvis BA, Ludwig L, Carlson JF, Topping JP: Controlled trial of Giardia lamblia: control strategies in day care centers [published erratum appears in Am J Public Health 81(10): 1251, 1991]. Am J Public Health 81(8):1001–1006, 1991.
104. Markell EK, Udkow MP: Blastocystis hominis: Pathogen or fellow traveler? Am J Trop Med Hyg 35(5):1023–1026, 1986.
105. Millet V, Spencer MJ, Chapin M, et al: Dientamoeba fragilis, a protozoan parasite in adult members of a semicommunal group. Dig Dis Sci 28(4):335–339, 1983.
106. Millet VE, Spencer MJ, Chapin MR, Garcia LS, Yatabe JH, Stewart ME: Intestinal protozoan infection in a semicommunal group. Am J Trop Med Hyg 32(1):54–60, 1983.
107. Spencer MJ, Millet VE, Garcia LS, Rhee L, Masterson L: Parasitic infections in a pediatric population. Pediatr Infect Dis 2(2):110–113, 1983.
108. Shein R, Gelb A: Colitis due to Dientamoeba fragilis. Am J Gastroenterol 78(10):634–636, 1983.
109. Spencer MJ, Garcia LS, Chapin MR: Dientamoeba fragilis. An intestinal pathogen in children? Am J Dis Child 133(4):390–393, 1979.
110. Dardick KR: Tetracycline treatment of Dientamoeba fragilis. Conn Med 47(2):69–70, 1983.
111. Keystone JS, Kozarsky P: *Isospora belli, Sarcocystis* species, *Blastocystis hominis,* and *Cyclospora*. In Mandell GL, Douglas RG, Bennett JE, Dolin R (eds): Mandell, Douglas, and Bennett's Principles and Practice of Infectious Diseases. Philadelphia, Churchill Livingstone, 2000, pp 2915–2920.
112. Doyle PW, Helgason MM, Mathias RG, Proctor EM: Epidemiology and pathogenicity of Blastocystis hominis. J Clin Microbiol 28(1): 116–121, 1990.
113. Nimri LF: Evidence of an epidemic of Blastocystis hominis infections in preschool children in northern Jordan. J Clin Microbiol 31(10): 2706–2708, 1993.
114. Shlim DR, Hoge CW, Rajah R, Rabold JG, Echeverria P: Is Blastocystis hominis a cause of diarrhea in travelers? A prospective controlled study in Nepal [see comments]. Clin Infect Dis 21(1):97–101, 1995.
115. Udkow MP, Markell EK: Blastocystis hominis: Prevalence in asymptomatic versus symptomatic hosts. J Infect Dis 168(1):242–244, 1993.
116. Grossman I, Weiss LM, Simon D, Tanowitz HB, Wittner M: Blastocystis hominis in hospital employees. Am J Gastroenterol 87(6):729–732, 1992.
117. Markell EK, Udkow MP: Association of Blastocystis hominis with human disease? [letter; comment]. J Clin Microbiol 28(5):1085–1086, 1990.
118. Markell EK: Is there any reason to continue treating Blastocystis infections? [editorial; comment]. Clin Infect Dis 21(1):104–105, 1995.
119. MacKenzie WR, Hoxie NJ, Proctor ME, et al: A massive outbreak in Milwaukee of Cryptosporidium infection transmitted through the public water supply. N Engl J Med 331(3):161–167, 1994.
120. Xiao L, Morgan UM, Fayer R, Thompson RC, Lal AA: Cryptosporidium systematics and implications for public health. Parasitol Today 16(7):287–292, 2000.
121. Sterling CR, Guerrant RL: Cryptosporidium. In Blaser MJ, Smith PD, Ravdin JI, Greenberg HB, Guerrant RL (eds): Infections of the Gastrointestinal Tract. New York, Raven Press, 2001.
122. Rossignol JF, Hidalgo H, Feregrino M, et al: A double-'blind' placebo-controlled study of nitazoxanide in the treatment of cryptosporidial diarrhoea in AIDS patients in Mexico. Trans R Soc Trop Med Hyg 92(6):663–666, 1998.
123. Casemore DP, Blewett DA, Wright SE: Cleaning and disinfection of equipment for gastrointestinal flexible endoscopy: Interim recommendations of a Working Party of the British Society of Gastroenterology [letter; comment]. Gut 30(8):1156–1157, 1989.
124. Cleaning and disinfection of equipment for gastrointestinal flexible endoscopy: Interim recommendations of a Working Party of the British Society of Gastroenterology [see comments]. Gut 29(8):1134–1151, 1988.
125. Guerrant DI, Moore SR, Lima AAM, Patrick P, Schorling JB, Guerrant RL: Association of early childhood diarrhea and cryptosporidiosis with impaired physical fitness and cognitive function four–seven years later in a poor urban community in Northeast Brazil. Am J Trop Med Hyg 61(5):707–713, 1999.

126. Checkley W, Epstein LD, Gilman RH, Black RE, Cabrera L, Sterling CR: Effects of Cryptosporidium parvum infection in Peruvian children: Growth faltering and subsequent catch-up growth. Am J Epidemiol 148(5):497–506, 1998.
127. Schaudinn F: Studien über krankheitserregende Protozoen I. Cyclospora carolytica Schaud., de Erreger der perniciösen Enteritis des Maulwurfs. Arbeit Kaiserl Gesundh 18[378]:416, 1901.
128. Ashford RW: Occurrence of an undescribed coccidian in man in Papua New Guinea. Ann Trop Med Parasitol 73(5):497–500, 1979.
129. Huang P, Weber JT, Sosin DM, et al: The first reported outbreak of diarrheal illness associated with Cyclospora in the United States. Ann Intern Med 123(6):409–414, 1995.
130. Long EG, Ebrahimzadeh A, White EH, Swisher B, Callaway C: Alga associated with diarrhea in patients with acquired immunodeficiency syndrome and in travelers. J Clin Microbiol 28(6):1101–1104, 1990.
131. Centers for Disease Control: Update: Outbreaks of Cyclospora cayetenensis Infection—United States. MMWR 45(26):611–612, 1996.
132. Ortega YR, Sterling CR, Gilman RH, Cama VA, Diaz F: Cyclospora sp—a new protozoan pathogen of humans. N Engl J Med 328:1308–1312, 1993.
133. Relman DA, Schmidt TM, Gajadhar A, et al: Molecular phylogenetic analysis of Cyclospora, the human intestinal pathogen, suggests that it is closely related to Eimeria species. J Infect Dis 173(2):440–445, 1996.
134. Herwaldt BL, Ackers ML: An outbreak in 1996 of cyclosporiasis associated with imported raspberries. The Cyclospora Working Group [see comments]. N Engl J Med 336:1548–56, 1997.
135. Herwaldt BL, Beach MJ: The return of Cyclospora in 1997: Another outbreak of cyclosporiasis in North America associated with imported raspberries. Cyclospora Working Group [see comments]. Ann Intern Med 130(3):210–220, 1999.
136. Connor BA, Shlim DR, Scholes JV, Rayburn JL, Reidy J, Rajah R: Pathologic changes in the small bowel in nine patients with diarrhea associated with a coccidia-like body. Ann Intern Med 119(5):377–382, 1993.
137. Berlin OG, Novak SM, Porschen RK, Long EG, Stelma GN, Schaeffer FW III: Recovery of Cyclospora organisms from patients with prolonged diarrhea. Clin Infect Dis 18(4):606–609, 1994.
138. Hoge CW, Shlim DR, Ghimire M, et al: Placebo-controlled trial of co-trimoxazole for Cyclospora infections among travellers and foreign residents in Nepal [see comments] [published erratum appears in Lancet 345(8956):1060, 1995]. Lancet 345(8951):691–693, 1995.
139. Pape JW, Verdier RI, Johnson WD Jr: Treatment and prophylaxis of Isospora belli infection in patients with the acquired immunodeficiency syndrome [see comments]. N Engl J Med 320(16):1044–1047, 1989.
140. Pape JW, Verdier RI, Boncy M, Boncy J, Johnson WD Jr: Cyclospora infection in adults infected with HIV. Clinical manifestations, treatment, and prophylaxis. Ann Intern Med 121(9):654–657, 1994.
141. Verdier RI, Fitzgerald DW, Johnson WD Jr, Pape JW: Trimethoprim-sulfamethoxazole compared with ciprofloxacin for treatment and prophylaxis of Isospora belli and Cyclospora cayetanensis infection in HIV-infected patients. A randomized, controlled trial. Ann Intern Med 132(11):885–888, 2000.
142. Osterholm MT: Cyclosporiasis and raspberries—Lessons for the future. N Engl J Med 336:1597–1598, 1997.
143. Godiwala T, Yaeger R: Isospora and traveler's diarrhea [letter]. Ann Intern Med 106(6):908–909, 1987.
144. DeHovitz JA, Pape JW, Boncy M, Johnson WD Jr: Clinical manifestations and therapy of Isospora belli infection in patients with the acquired immunodeficiency syndrome. N Engl J Med 315:87–90, 1986.
145. Brandborg LL, Goldberg SB, Briedenbach WC: Human coccidiosis—a possible cause of malabsorption. The life cycle in small-bowel mucosal biopsies as a diagnostic feature. N Engl J Med 283:1306–1313, 1970.
146. Bryan RT, Weber R, Schwartz DA: Microsporidiosis. In Guerrant RL, Walker DH, Weller PF (eds): Tropical Infectious Diseases: Principles, Pathogens, & Practice. Philadelphia, Churchill Livingstone, 2000, pp 840–851.
147. Wuhib T, Silva TM, Newman RD, et al: Cryptosporidial and microsporidial infections in human immunodeficiency virus-infected patients in northeastern Brazil. J Infect Dis 70(2):494–497, 1994.
148. Guerrant RL, Thielman NM. Emerging enteric protozoa: Cryptosporidium, Cyclospora, and Microsporidia. In Scheld MW, Armstrong D, Hughes JM (eds): Emerging Infections. Washington DC, ASM Press, 1998, pp 233–245.
149. Sandfort J, Hannemann A, Gelderblom H, Stark K, Owen RL, Ruf B: Enterocytozoon bieneusi infection in an immunocompetent patient who had acute diarrhea and who was not infected with the human immunodeficiency virus. Clin Infect Dis 19(3):514–516, 1994.
150. Sobottka I, Albrecht H, Schafer H, et al: Disseminated Encephalitozoon (Septata) intestinalis infection in a patient with AIDS: novel diagnostic approaches and autopsy-confirmed parasitological cure following treatment with albendazole. J Clin Microbiol 33(11):2948–2952, 1995.
151. Kirchhoff LV: American trypanosomiasis. In Guerrant RL, Walker DH, Weller PF (eds): Tropical Infectious Diseases: Principles, Pathogens and Practice. New York, Churchill Livingstone, 1999.
152. Upcroft JA, Upcroft P, Boreham PF: Drug resistance in Giardia intestinalis. Int J Parasitol 20(4):489–496, 1990.

Chapter 99

Intestinal Infections by Parasitic Worms

David E. Elliott

Parasitic worms colonize people worldwide. Travel, emigration, and exotic cuisine allow intestinal helminths to appear in any locale. Travel history is a critical but often overlooked aspect of the patient interview. Many helminths survive for decades within a host so even remote visits to endemic countries is important. The same is true for emigration. Fresh food is flown around the world and frequently consumed raw. Patients can now acquire tropical helminths without leaving their industrialized temperate city. Physicians need to remain alert for these organisms as some cause severe disease that can take years to develop. Patients may have occult *Strongyloides stercoralis* until treatment with glucocorticoids causes fulminant disease. Patients may have occult *Clonorchis sinensis* until cholangiocarcinoma develops. Patients may have occult *Schistosoma mansoni* until portal hypertension and esophageal varices develop.

In developed countries, we usually stumble across the diagnosis of an intestinal helminth rather than pursue it. Helminths are complex organisms well adapted to their hosts. Like quiet house guests, most cause no symptoms. Athough worms almost never cause diarrhea, many medical laboratories do not perform a routine assay on formed stool for parasite eggs. Physicians need to communicate their concerns to laboratory personnel. A telephone call to the local laboratory before the sample is sent can dramatically improve diagnostic results. Occasionally, alarmed patients may bring proglottids or whole worms that they passed with their stools. These specimens should be fixed in 5% aqueous formalin and sent for identification.[1] All specimens should be handled carefully with full precautions.

Some helminths are difficult to diagnose. *S. stercoralis* eggs do not appear in the stool; diagnosis is best made serologically. *Ancylostoma caninum* causes eosinophilic enteritis but does not lay eggs when infecting people. Also, light infections with helminths are difficult to detect. Diagnosis may require serologic evaluation, analysis of multiple stool samples, or use of concentration techniques.

While some helminths can cause severe disease, this is unusual. The vast majority of individuals colonized with these organisms have no symptoms or illness attributable to the parasites. Only with heavy infections does disease result. Well-adapted worms appear to act more as commensals than as pathogens. Helminths often induce a strong Th2 (IL-4 predominant) response that serves to limit their numbers.[2] Strong Th2 responses also can impede development of excessive Th1 (IFN-γ predominant) reactions. Many immune illnesses such as Crohn's disease and multiple sclerosis appear to result from excessive Th1 reactions. These Th1-mediated immune diseases appear to be rare in regions where parasitic helminths are common. It is possible that exposure to helminths affords some protection against disease due to excessive immune reactions.[3] If this hypothesis proves to be true, some individuals actually may benefit from certain types of helminthic parasite exposure.

This chapter is divided into three sections: the nematodes or roundworms, the cestodes or tapeworms, and the trematodes or flukes (flatworms). For the most part, each worm is addressed separately, noting its epidemiology, life cycle, clinical manifestations, diagnosis, and treatment. Hepatic manifestations of some of these infestations are also discussed in Chapter 69.

NEMATODES

Ascaris lumbricoides

A. lumbricoides is the largest of the nematode parasites that colonize people. Females can grow to 49 cm (19 inches).[4] The name "lumbricoides" alludes to its resemblance to earthworms (*Lumbricus* sp.). The parasite is acquired by ingesting eggs. *Ascaris* can cause intestinal obstruction and biliary symptoms. Treatment is with albendazole.

Epidemiology

A. lumbricoides is distributed worldwide. The parasites are most numerous in less-developed countries and in areas with

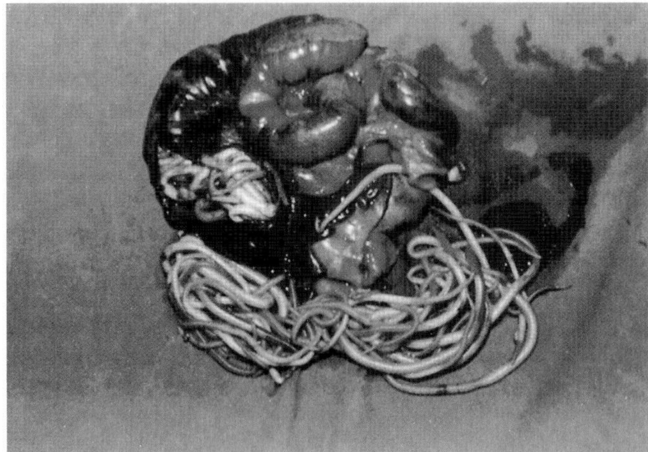

Figure 99–1. Bowel obstruction caused by *Ascaris lumbricoides.* (From Wasadikar, PP, Kulkarni, AB: Intestinal obstruction due to ascariasis. Br J Surg 84(3):410–412, 1997.)

poor sanitation. Recent estimates predict that 25% of the world's population (1.5 billion people) harbor *A. lumbricoides.*[5] Children acquire the parasite playing in dirt contaminated with eggs. Adults most often acquire the infection by farming or eating raw vegetables from plants fertilized with untreated sewage.

Life Cycle

People obtain the parasite by ingesting embryonated eggs that contain third stage larva. Freshly deposited fertilized eggs incubate in the soil for 10 to 15 days while the embryo develops and molts twice. The eggs become infective after this incubation period. The eggs are remarkably stable, survive freezing, and can remain viable for 7 to 10 years. The eggs are resistant to most chemical treatments including pickling but rapidly die in boiling water.

Once ingested, eggs hatch in the duodenum, releasing larva. The larva penetrate the intestinal wall and enter the mesenteric venules and lymphatics. Larvae migrating with portal blood pass to the liver, through sinusoids to the hepatic veins, then through the right heart and enter the lungs. Larva migrating via the lymphatics pass through mesenteric lymph nodes, to the thoracic duct and enter the superior vena cava to arrive in the lungs. The larva lodge in the pulmonary capillaries and break into the alveoli. They molt twice while growing to 1.5 mm in length then ascend the tracheobronchial tree. Upon arriving in the hypopharynx, they are again swallowed, and pass with the gastric chyme to the small intestine where they molt again and finally mature.

Mature *A. lumbricoides* are sexually dimorphic. Males are smaller (10–30 cm) than females (20–49 cm). The worms mate in the small intestine and females deposit about 200,000 eggs a day. Adult worms live for about 1 year (6–18 months). Because their eggs require incubation in the soil to become infective, *Ascaris* do not multiply in the host. Continued infection requires repeat ingestion of embryonated eggs.

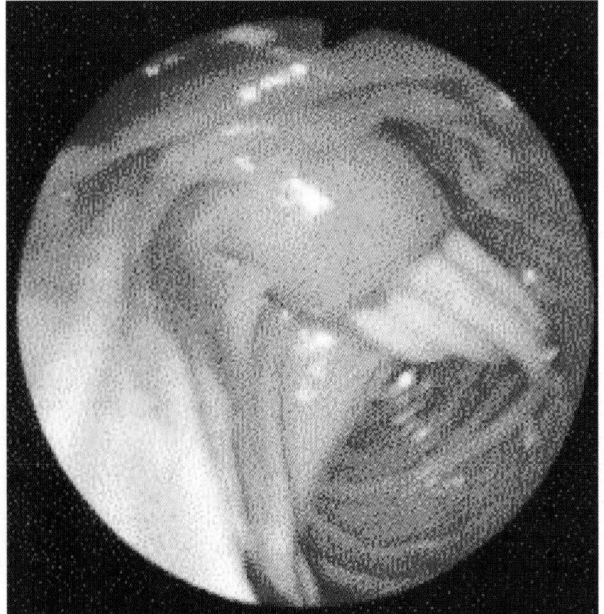

Figure 99–2. Four *Ascaris lumbricoides* in the ampulla. (From van den Bogaerde JB, Jordaan M: Intraductal administration of albendazole for biliary ascariasis. Am J Gastroenterol 92:1531–1533, 1997.)

Clinical Features/Pathophysiology

A. lumbricoides produces no symptoms in most patients. Often worms are found unexpectedly on endoscopy or eggs are identified in stool specimens of patients with symptoms not directly attributable to *A. lumbricoides.* Disease usually develops only in those with heavy worm burdens. Three diseases, pulmonary, intestinal, and hepatobiliary ascariasis are well described.

Pulmonary ascariasis (*Ascaris* pneumonia) develops 4 to 16 days after ingesting infective eggs as the larva migrate into the alveoli. This elicits an inflammatory response that can cause consolidation. The pneumonia is self-limited but can be life-threatening.

Large numbers of mature worms can cause severe intestinal symptoms. The most common complication is intestinal obstruction. Patients present with partial or complete small bowel obstruction and often have a history of passing mature worms in stool or vomitus. Patients with intestinal obstruction generally have more than 60 worms.[6] Rare fatal cases often have more than 600 worms. Fatality results from obstruction, intussusception, or volvulus, producing intestinal necrosis[7] (Fig. 99–1).

A. lumbricoides are highly motile. Mature worms may enter the ampulla of Vater and migrate into the bile or pancreatic ducts[8] (Fig. 99–2). The worms can cause biliary colic, obstructive jaundice, ascending cholangitis, acalculous cholecystitis, or acute pancreatitis.[4] The worms may move in and out of the papilla, producing intermittent symptoms. Recurrent ascending cholangitis or acute pancreatitis due to ascariasis is rare in highly developed western countries but can be fatal if the diagnosis is not entertained.[9]

Diagnosis

Often it is an alarmed patient who initially discovers *Ascaris* after passing a motile adult worm with a bowel movement.

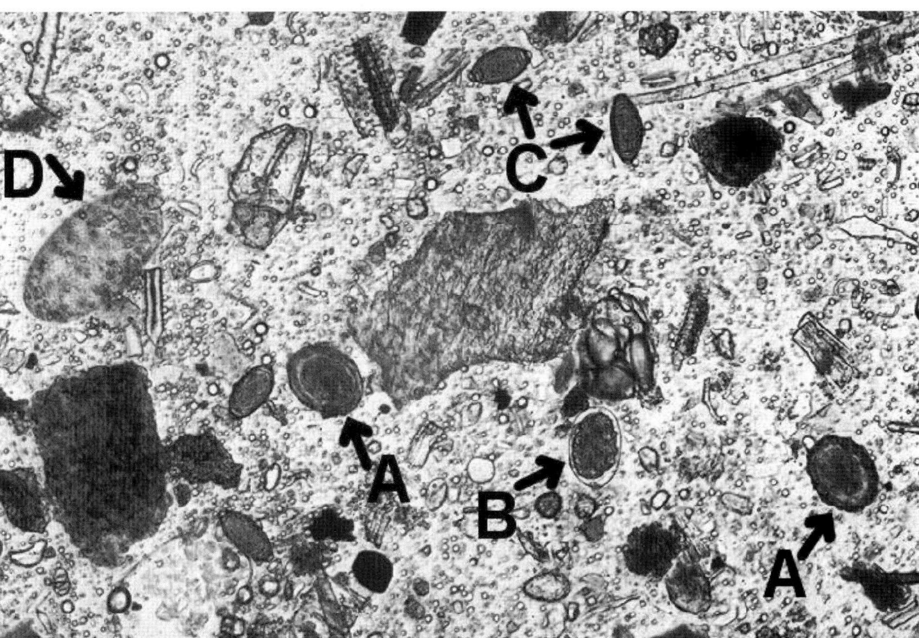

Figure 99–3. Stool specimen containing helminth eggs. *A, Ascaris lumbricoides. B,* Hookworm. *C, Trichuris trichiura. D, Fasciolopsis buski.*

The worms usually do not cause diarrhea. Most patients do not have specific symptoms or eosinophilia.

Ascaris eggs are visible in direct smears of stool (Fig. 99–3). The eggs begin to appear in the stool about 2 months after initial exposure. Fertilized eggs are 35 by 55 μm and have a thick shell and outer layer. Females also lay unfertilized eggs that are larger (90 × 44 μm) and have a thin shell and outer layer. *Ascaris* eggs that lose the outer layer resemble the eggs of hookworms.

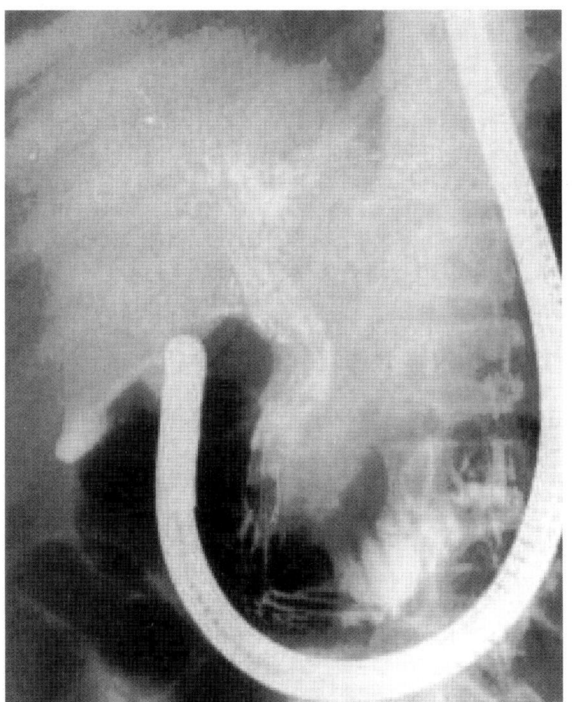

Figure 99–4. ERCP showing multiple *Ascaris lumbricoides* in the common bile duct. (From van den Bogaerde JB, Jordaan M: Intraductal administration of albendazole for biliary ascariasis. Am J Gastroenterol 92:1531–1533, 1997.)

Adults worms may be visualized endoscopically, or on an upper gastrointestinal (GI) series as linear filling defects within the small bowel. The worms will retain barium after it has cleared from the patient's GI tract, producing linear opacities. Similar findings are seen on endoscopic retrograde cholangiopancreatography (ERCP) if a worm is in the bile duct (Fig. 99–4). The worms have a characteristic appearance on ultrasound of the biliary tree or pancreas. They appear as long linear echogenic strips that do not cast acoustic shadows. In cross section, they have a "bull's eye" appearance.[10, 11]

Treatment

Asymptomatic colonization with *A. lumbricoides* is easily treated with a single 400 mg oral dose of albendazole. Albendazole inhibits glucose uptake and microtubule formation, effectively paralyzing the worms. Albendazole is poorly absorbed but is teratogenic and cannot be used in pregnant women. Patients with pulmonary ascariasis should be treated with steroids to reduce the pneumonitis and given two 400 mg doses of albendazole 1 month apart to kill worms that were migrating through tissues.

Intestinal ascariasis often can be treated conservatively with fluid resuscitation, nasogastric decompression, antibiotics, and one dose of albendazole. If signs of volvulus, intussusception, or peritonitis develop, then surgery is warranted. If the bowel is viable, then an enterotomy allows intraoperative removal of worms.

Hepatobiliary ascariasis also can be treated conservatively with fluid resuscitation, bowel rest, and antibiotics. Worms in the bile duct are not effectively treated with albendazole that is poorly absorbed and not concentrated in the bile. However, this is beneficial. Paralyzed worms, unable to pass through the sphincter of Oddi, can become trapped in the bile duct. Patients should be treated with albendazole 400 mg each day for several days because the worms become susceptible when they migrate out of the duct. Ascending cholangitis, acute obstructive jaundice, or acute pancreatitis requires emergent ERCP. Worms can be extracted from the ducts by balloon or forceps.

Strongyloides stercoralis

S. stercoralis is a free-living tropical and semi-tropical soil helminth that has a larval form that penetrates intact skin. As a parasite, *Strongyloides* lives in the intestine and lays eggs that hatch while still in the gut. Filariform larvae develop within the intestine, migrate, and mature to increase the number of adult parasites. Immunosuppression or corticosteroid treatment cause a fulminant reproduction of parasites that can prove fatal. Treatment is with ivermectin.

Epidemiology

S. stercoralis is endemic in tropical and semi-tropical regions. The parasite also can be acquired in rural southeastern United States and northern Italy. *Strongyloides* exists as a free-living organism that does not require a host to replicate. Improved sanitation does not remove the risk of acquiring the parasite from soil. Patients from endemic areas, military veterans who served in Asia, and prisoners of war are at high risk of having subclinical strongyloidiasis.

Life Cycle

Adult male and female *S. stercoralis* can live in the soil and lay eggs that hatch rhabditiform larvae. Rhabditiform larvae develop in the soil into mature adult worms. Rhabditiform larvae also may develop into longer (500 μm) infective filariform larvae. Filariform larvae can penetrate any intact skin that contacts the soil. They migrate through the dermis to enter the vasculature. The larvae circulate with the venous blood flow until they reach the lungs where they break into the alveoli and ascend the bronchial tree. The worms are swallowed with bronchial secretions and pass with gastric chyme into the small bowel. The worms embed in the jejunal mucosa where they mature. Female *S. strongyloides* can lay fertile eggs by parthenogenesis so do not require males to reproduce. The eggs hatch within the small bowel and rhabditiform larvae migrate into the lumen. Rhabditiform larvae, not eggs, are passed in the stool.

A critical feature of *S. stercoralis* infection is that rhabditiform larvae can develop into infective filariform within the intestine. These filariform larvae are able to reinfect (autoinfect) the patient, increasing the parasite burden and permitting prolonged colonization. Subclinical strongyloidiasis may exist for many decades after the host has left an endemic area.

Clinical Features/Pathophysiology

Most patients with *S. stercoralis* have no abdominal symptoms. Patients may have a serpiginous uticarial rash (larva currens) caused by rapid (5–10 cm/hour) dermal migration of filariform larvae. The rash often occurs on the buttocks from larvae entering the perianal skin. A study of prisoners of war found this creeping eruption to be a far more common symptom of chronic strongyloidiasis than gastrointestinal complaints.[12] Occasionally, patients do have nausea, abdominal pain, or unexplained occult GI blood loss due to *S. stercoralis*. The parasite may also cause colonic inflammation that resembles ulcerative colitis but is more right-sided and strongly eosinophilic.[13, 14]

While the parasite burden remains balanced, symptoms are minimal or absent. Immunosuppression or corticosteroid administration upsets this balance. Fulminant, potentially fatal strongyloidiasis develops in previously asymptomatic but chronically infected patients due to massive autoinfection. The mechanisms that permit massive autoinfection are unknown but chemotherapy or immunosuppression decreases local eosinophils, which may help constrain the parasites. In addition, corticosteroids may act directly on the parasites to increase development of infective filariform larvae.[15] Cyclosporin A may be partially toxic for *S. stercoralis* and appears to suppress autoinfection until it is discontinued.[16]

Massive autoinfection produces disseminated fulminant strongyloidiasis. Migrating filariform larvae injure the intestinal mucosa and carry luminal bacteria into the bloodstream. Polymicrobial sepsis with enteric organisms often develops. *Streptococcal bovis* endocarditis or meningitis[17] may result. Numerous larvae migrating through the lungs cause pneumonitis. Worms may arrive in unique locations such as the brain. Fulminant strongyloidiasis is frequently fatal.

Diagnosis

Patients with chronic strongyloidiasis are often asymptomatic. The peripheral blood eosinophil level may be elevated but a normal eosinophil count does not argue against infection with the parasite. The best current method for detecting exposure is enzyme-linked immunoassay for IgG antibodies against *S. stercoralis*. This assay as performed by the Centers for Disease Control in the United States is 84% to 92% sensitive in detecting infection. False-positive results occur in patients exposed to other helminthic parasites but this may improve with newer recombinant protein-based assays. Serologic positivity demonstrates prior exposure to *S. stercoralis* but not necessarily active infection. However, because chronic strongyloidiasis can remain subclinical and difficult to detect for decades, treatment of seropositive patients is warranted. Indeed, some argue that patients even suspected of having strongyloidiasis should be treated empirically prior to corticosteroid therapy.[18]

Active infection can be diagnosed by finding rhabditiform larvae in direct smears of the stool, though this is insensitive. A tenfold more sensitive technique is to spread stool on an agar plate and look for serpentine tracks left by migrating larvae.[19] Intestinal biopsy is very insensitive.

Treatment

Chronic strongyloidiasis is best treated with ivermectin 200 μg/kg orally one dose only. This dose applies to both adult and pediatric patients. Ivermectin is better tolerated than thiabendazole. Ivermectin is active against the intestinal worms, not the migrating larvae. Recurrent infection from migrating larvae can develop. A repeat dose after 2 weeks reduces this concern. Patients with fulminant disseminated strongyloidiasis complicating acquired immune deficiency syndrome (AIDS) require repeat doses on days 2, 15, and 16.

Aonchotheca (Capillaria) philippinensis

Capillariasis is acquired by eating raw fish that have the parasite.[20] Recently, the parasite causing capillariasis has been renamed from *Capillaria philippinensis* to *Aonchotheca philippinensis*. By any name, it is deadly. The parasite replicates in the host, creating an ever-increasing number of intestinal worms. Protein-losing spruelike diarrhea develops with progressive emaciation and anasarca ultimately leading to death. Treatment is with albendazole.

Epidemiology

The first known human case of capillariasis was reported in 1964. It remains a rare but deadly parasitic infection. In 1965 through 1968, an epidemic in the rural Philippines involved 229 cases with an overall 30% mortality rate.[21] As the name implies, *Aonchotheca philippinensis* is endemic to the Philippines. It also is endemic in Thailand and cases have occurred in Japan, Taiwan, Egypt, and Iran.

Life Cycle

Birds, not humans, are the natural hosts for *A. philippinensis*. People acquire *A. philippinensis* by eating raw or undercooked fresh and brackish water fish that contain parasite larvae. In the small intestine, the larvae mature into adults. The adults are very small, measuring up to 3.9 mm for males and 5.3 mm for females. Adult worms mate and produce eggs. Eggs deposited with feces (normally bird droppings) into ponds and rivers are swallowed by fish to complete the life cycle.

Some female adult *A. philippinensis* are larviparous, producing infective larvae instead of eggs. These larvae then mature in the small intestine and increase the parasite burden. This pathway of autoinfection permits a massive increase in parasite numbers. A rhesus monkey originally fed 27 larvae had more than 30,000 worms by 162 days of infection.[22]

Clinical Features/Pathophysiology

Capillariasis produces a progressive spruelike illness. Symptoms begin with vague abdominal pain and borborygmi. After 2 or 3 weeks, patients begin to have diarrhea. Initially intermittent, diarrhea becomes persistent and then voluminous. Rapid wasting due to escalating steatorrhea and protein-losing enteropathy develops. Eventually emaciation, anasarca, and hypotension occur. Diarrhea produces severe hypokalemia. If untreated, patients die of cardiac failure or secondary bacterial sepsis about 2 months after initial onset of symptoms.

The progressive disease is believed to result from an increasing number of poorly adapted intestinal parasites. In autopsy studies, the jejunal intestinal mucosa showed flattened denuded villi with numerous plasma cells, lymphocytes, macrophages, and neutrophils infiltrating the lamina propria.[20]

Diagnosis

Diagnosis is made by finding eggs and larvae in stool specimens. No serologic tests are available. Symptomatic patients will have detectable eggs in their stool. The eggs are easily confused with those of *Trichurius trichiura*. *T. trichiura* eggs (see Fig. 99–3*C*) have prominent bipolar plugs that appear cut off in *C. philippinensis*.[20]

Treatment

Capillariasis requires extended treatment with antihelminthic agents. Albendazole 200 mg orally twice daily for 10 days or mebendazole 200 mg orally twice daily for 20 days is needed to prevent recurrence. Albendazole is better tolerated. The extended treatment is necessary because larvae are resistant to these agents. Both albendazole and mebendazole are teratogenic in rats. No increase in birth defects was noted in pregnant women inadvertently treated with mebendazole; however, neither agent should be used in pregnant women.

HOOKWORMS

An estimated 1 billion people are infected with hookworm worldwide. Most hookworm infections are by *Necator americanus*, *Ancylostoma duodenale*, or a mixture of these two. Hookworm is acquired by skin contact with contaminated soil. The most common result of moderate infection is iron deficiency. Hookworm should be suspected in patients with eosinophilia and iron deficiency anemia. The dog and cat parasite, *Ancylostoma caninum*, is a cause of eosinophilic enteritis. Treatment is with albendazole.

Necator americanus and *Ancylostoma duodenale*

Epidemiology

N. americanus and *A. duodenale* infect about one fifth (20%) of the world population. The geographic distribution of the two species extensively overlaps: *N. americanus* predominates in the Americas, South Pacific, Indonesia, southern India, and central Africa; *A. duodenale* is more common in northern Africa, the Middle East, Europe, Pakistan, and northern India. *Ancylostoma ceylonicum* usually infects cats but also causes some human hookworm infections. Infections are acquired by contacting soil contaminated with human waste. Hookworm is endemic in tropical to warm temperate areas that lack sufficient sewage facilities. Indigenous hookworm infection has been largely eradicated in the United States although small areas with transmission may still exist.[23]

Life Cycle

Infective third-stage hookworm larvae penetrate intact skin, for example, between the toes of bare feet walking on contaminated ground. Larvae migrate through the dermis to reach blood vessels. This migration can cause a pruritic serpiginous rash (Fig. 99–5). *A. braziliense* normally infects

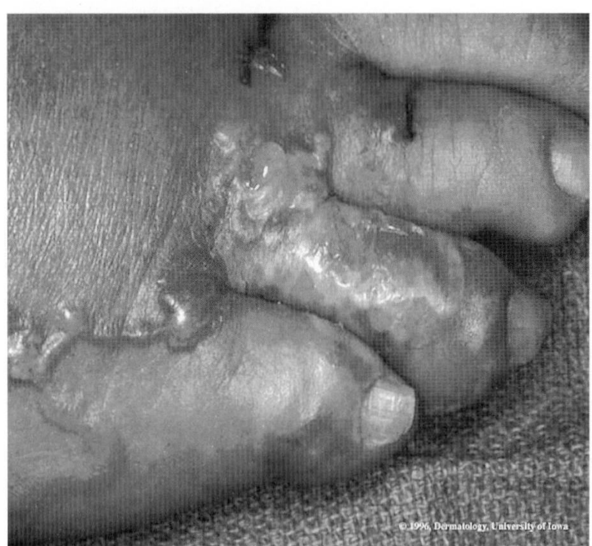

Figure 99–5. Serpiginous rash caused by hookworm larva migrating through dermis. (From the University of Iowa Dermatology website *http://tray.dermatology.uiowa.edu/LarvMi02.htm.*)

dogs and cats but produces a similar rash, cutaneous larva migrans, during its ineffective dermal wandering in people. Larvae of *N. americanus* and *A. duodenale* enter blood vessels and migrate with venous flow through the right heart to the lungs. *A. duodenale* larvae may arrest migration and become dormant for many months before proceeding to the lungs.[24] In the lungs, larvae penetrate the alveoli and enter the air space. They migrate up the pulmonary tree and are swallowed with saliva. The larvae pass with the gastric chyme into the small intestine, where they mature. Adult worms develop large buccal cavities and graze on the intestinal mucosa, ingesting epithelial cells and blood (Figs. 99–6, 99–7). Adults are about 1 cm long and can live for up to 14 years. Mature worms mate and lay eggs. Each female *N. americanus* lays about 10,000 and *A. duodenale* 20,000 eggs a day. Eggs are deposited with feces in moist shady soil where they hatch to release larvae. The larvae molt twice, then move to the soil surface seeking a suitable host. Patients also can acquire *A. duodenale* by directly ingesting larvae crawling on contaminated fresh vegetables.

Clinical Features/Pathophysiology

Light infections with *N. americanus* and *A. duodenale* cause no symptoms. The major consequence of moderate and heavy hookworm infection is iron deficiency. Adult worms feed on intestinal epithelial cells and blood. The closely related *A. caninum* (see later section) secretes anticoagulant peptides that inhibit clotting factors[25] and platelet aggregation.[26] This prevents hemostasis, permitting the hematophagous parasites to feed on host blood. Intestinal blood loss is estimated to be 0.01 to 0.04 mL/day per adult *N. americanus* and 0.05 to 0.3 mL/day per adult *A. duodenale*.[27] With a moderate number of worms, this blood loss becomes appreciable (Table 99–1). Iron deficiency results if iron loss outstrips absorption.[28] Males with a diet high in iron (>20 mg/day) can tolerate up to 800 adult hookworms without anemia. The average North American diet is high in iron, so anemia may not develop.

Diagnosis

Hookworms produce numerous eggs that can be identified on direct smears of formalin-fixed stool (see Fig. 99–3*B*). Evaluation of three stool specimens obtained on separate days should permit diagnosis of hookworm. However, light infections may require concentration techniques. Eggs mature rapidly at room temperature and may hatch to release larvae. It is difficult to distinguish *N. americanus* eggs from *A. duodenale* eggs based on morphologic studies. The eggs of *Trichostrongylus orientalis* can be mistaken as hookworm eggs.

Treatment

Albendazole 400 mg orally as a single dose treats hookworm; however, albendazole is teratogenic. Mebendazole 100 mg orally twice a day for 3 days is also effective but not as well tolerated. *A. duodenale* larvae can remain in a dormant state for months then proceed to mature causing apparent relapse. This is treated with a repeat course of albendazole or mebendazole.

Ancylostoma caninum

Epidemiology/Life Cycle

A. caninum is a common hookworm of dogs and cats. It is distributed worldwide and is prevalent in the northern hemisphere. The parasite exists in areas with adequate sanitation because cats and dogs indiscriminately defecate in yards, parks, and sandboxes. The life cycle of *A. caninum* is simi-

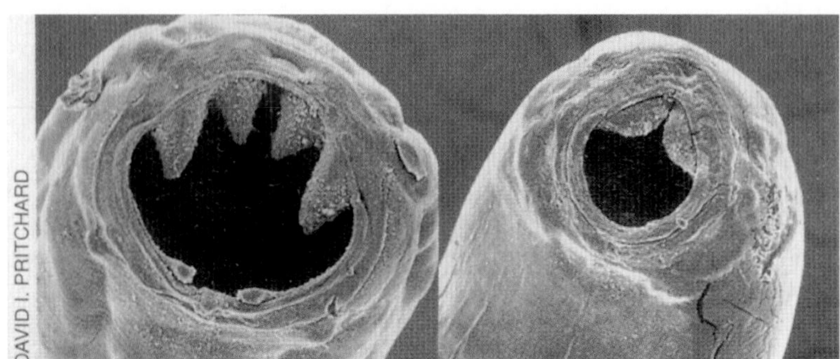

Figure 99–6. Buccal cavities of *A. duodenale* and *N. americanus.* (From Hotez PJ, Pritchard DI: Hookworm infection. Sci Am 272:70–74, 1995.)

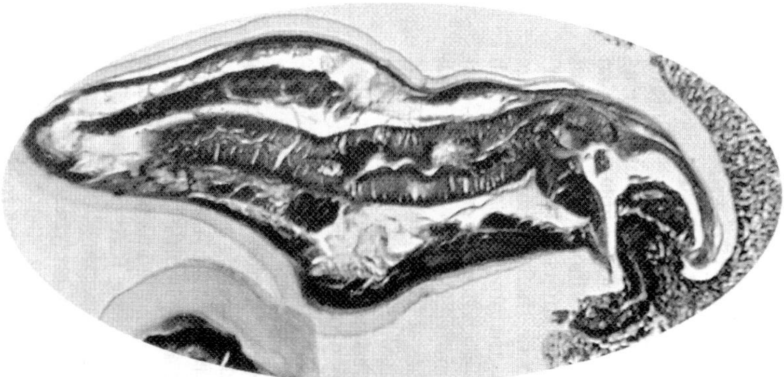

Figure 99–7. Hookworm grazing on intestinal mucosa. (Photo Courtesy of Wayne Meyers, A.F.I.P.)

lar to that of *A. duodenale* and can be acquired orally. However, *A. caninum* does not fully mature in a human host so no eggs are produced.

Clinical Features/Pathophysiology

The dog and cat hookworm, *A. caninum*, is a well-recognized cause of cutaneous larva migrans. This is a distinctive serpiginous rash caused by an abortive migration of the parasite in an unsupportive host. Recently, *A. caninum* has been identified as a cause of eosinophilic enteritis.[29] Patients with *A. caninum* eosinophilic enteritis are often dog owners, and present with colicky midabdominal pain and peripheral eosinophilia.[30] Most patients did not recall cutaneous larva migrans. Intestinal biopsy specimens show high numbers (>45/high-power field) of mucosal eosinophils.[31] Eosinophilic inflammation is most prevalent in distal small bowel and, unlike eosinophilic gastroenteritis, is absent in the stomach. On endoscopy of the terminal ileum, patients may have scattered small superficial apthous ulcers and mucosal hemorrhages.[32] Serologic evidence suggests that *A. caninum* is also a cause of abdominal pain without eosinophilia or eosinophilic enteritis.[30]

Diagnosis

Diagnosis of *A. caninum* infection is difficult. The parasite never fully matures, does not lay eggs, and is hard to detect. Serologic tests for *A. caninum* are research tools not routinely available at the time of this writing.

Table 99–1 | **Comparison of Hookworm with Typical Sources of Iron Loss in Women**

SOURCE	IRON LOSS (mg/day)
Basal	0.72
Menstruation	0.44
Pregnancy	2.14
Lactation	0.23
Moderate hookworm infection	
N. americanus (60–200 worms)	1.10
A. duodenale (20–100 worms)	2.30

Adapted from Stoltzfus RJ, Dreyfuss ML, Chwaya HM, Albonico M: Hookworm control as a strategy to prevent iron deficiency. Nutr Rev 55(6): 223–32, 1997.

Treatment

Albendazole 400 mg as a single oral dose or mebendazole 100 mg orally twice daily for 3 days treats *A. caninum*. These drugs given for brief periods are quite safe. Patients with distal small bowel eosinophilic enteritis not attributable to another cause may benefit from empiric treatment for *A. caninum*.

Whipworm (*Trichuris trichiura*)

T. trichiura, commonly called whipworm, is distributed worldwide. People acquire *Trichuris* by ingesting embryonated parasite eggs. Most individuals have no symptoms, although heavy infections are associated with a dysentery-like syndrome. Treatment is with mebendazole.

Epidemiology

An estimated 800 million people have *T. trichuria*. Colonization with *T. trichiura* was very common prior to the industrial revolution. It occurs in temperate as well as tropical countries and remains prevalent in areas with suboptimal sanitation. In one equatorial Cameroon province, 97% of school-age children had *T. trichiura*.[33] Whipworm eggs are sensitive to desiccation so prevalence is low in desert climates.

Life Cycle

T. trichiura has a simple life cycle. Colonization occurs by ingesting parasite eggs. Each infective egg contains a developed larva. The eggs hatch in the intestine. Larvae migrate to the cecum, mature, mate, and lay eggs. This process takes approximately 8 to 12 weeks. Adults worms are approximately 3 cm long and have a thin tapered anterior region so that the worm resembles a whip (Fig. 99–8). A mature female worm lays approximately 20,000 eggs/day and can live for 3 years. Eggs are deposited with feces into the soil. Over the next 2 to 6 weeks, larva develop within the eggs.

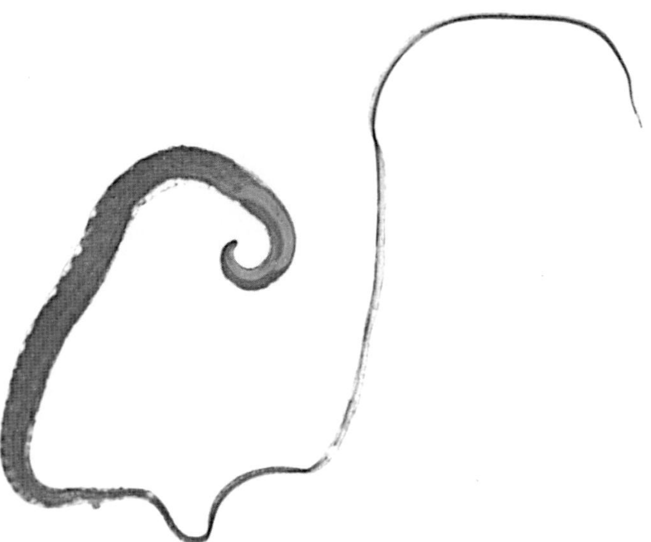

Figure 99–8. *Trichuris trichiura,* adult male whipworm. (Photomicrograph by Zane Price. From Markell EK, Voge M: Medical Parasitology, 3rd ed. Philadelphia, WB Saunders, 1971.)

The egg is not infective until it has fully embryonated. Therefore, *T. trichiura* does not multiply in the host and is not directly transmitted to other persons.

Clinical Features/Pathophysiology

Most individuals with *T. trichiura* infection have no symptoms attributable to the parasite. The majority of people in an endemic area are colonized by small numbers (less than 15) of worms. For these people, the parasite is a commensal rather than a pathogen. But several will harbor hundreds or even thousands of worms.[34] The bimodal distribution persists after patients are treated but then naturally become re-infected. This suggests that unique host factors (genetic or behavioral) help determine the number of worms in an individual.

Rectal prolapse can occur in children with extremely high numbers of *T. trichiura* worms.[35] Some individuals with numerous worms have mucoid diarrhea and occasional bleeding. This combination is called the trichuris dysentery syndrome. Children with this condition appear to have growth retardation.[36] However, studies attributing these symptoms to *T. trichiura* are complicated because individuals with trichuris dysentery syndrome are often socioeconomically deprived and may be coinfected with other pathogens.

Colonic biopsy specimens from patients with trichuris dysentery syndrome show little or no pathosis compared to those of local children[37] other than an increase in mast cells.[38] There also is an increase in the number of cells that express tumor necrosis factor α and calprotectin in children with trichuris dysentery syndrome.[39]

A different but closely related species, *Trichuris muris*, infects mice. Mouse strains that react to the parasite with a strong Th2 response, characterized by production of interleukins 4, 5, and 13, are able to expel the worms. Strains that respond with a Th1 response (interferon gamma [IFNγ]) have difficulty expelling the worms.[40] Blocking IL4 makes resistant strains susceptible and blocking IFNγ makes susceptible strains resistant to chronic infection with *T. muris*.[41] The type of immune response developed by inbred mice to *T. muris* is an important factor in determining length and intensity of infection. This may explain why some people repeatedly acquire heavy infections while others carry only a few worms.

Diagnosis

Diagnosis is made by identifying *T. trichiura* eggs in stool specimens. Trichuris eggs are 23 μm by 50 μm in size and have characteristic "plugs" at each end (Fig. 99–3*C*).

Treatment

T. trichiura is treated with mebendazole 100 mg twice a day for 3 days. Alternatively, patients can take albendazole 400 mg each day for 3 days. Single dose treatment with a combination of albendazole (400 mg) and ivermectin (200 μg/kg) appears quite effective with cure rates of 80% and egg reduction rates of 94%.[42]

Pinworm (*Enterobius vermicularis*)

E. vermicularis, commonly called pinworm, is the most common helminthic parasite encountered by primary care providers in developed nations. It is acquired by ingesting parasite eggs. Most people have no symptoms from the parasite. Diagnosis is made by the cellophane tape test. Treatment is with mebendazole, and all family members require treatment.

Epidemiology

E. vermicularis is the quintessential intestinal parasite and has no geographic constraints. It is transmissible by close contact with colonized individuals. Prior to the industrial revolution and modern sanitation, colonization by pinworm was probably universal. People have had pinworm for thousands of years. *E. vermicularis* eggs were identified in a 10,000-year-old human stool (coprolite) found in Utah.[43]

Recently, another pinworm species, *E. gregorii*, has been distinguished in France[44] and England.[45] The two species can coexist. There is no apparent clinical difference between species; this section will focus on *E. vermicularis*.

People of every socioeconomic group may acquire pinworm and it remains quite prevalent. School-age children are most commonly colonized, permitting other household members to acquire the parasite. Crowding and institutionalization promote acquisition. Eggs can survive in the environment for approximately 15 to 20 days and are resistant to chlorinated water (e.g., swimming pools).

Pinworm remains common in many areas but appears to be decreasing in prevalence. A survey of positive cellophane tape tests (see later section) in New York City documented a sharp decline from 57 positive of 248 tests in 1971, to 17 positive of 165 in 1978, to 0 positive of 38 in 1986.[46] Similar trends are reported in California.

Life Cycle

E. vermicularis has a simple life cycle with a "hand to mouth" existence. The worm is acquired by ingesting parasite eggs. Most often these eggs are on the hands of the host. However, the small eggs also may become airborne, inhaled, and then swallowed.

Eggs hatch in the duodenum, releasing larvae that molt twice as they mature and migrate to the cecum and ascending colon (Fig. 99–9). Adult parasites are small; males measure 0.2 mm by 2 to 5 mm, females measure 0.5 mm by 8 to 13 mm. The worms mate and gravid females migrate to the rectum. During the night, egg-laden females migrate out of the anal canal and onto the perianal skin. Each female deposits up to 17,000 eggs. The eggs rapidly mature and become infective within 6 hours. Pinworm frequently causes perianal itching. Scratching gathers eggs onto the hands, promoting reinfection and easy transmission to others.

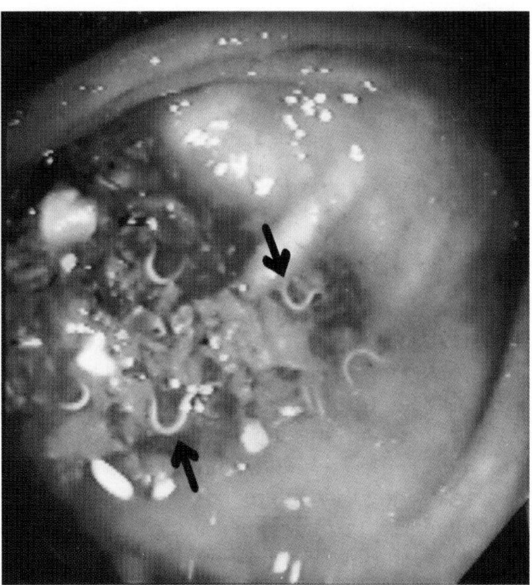

Figure 99–9. Pinworm infection (*Enterobius vermicularis, arrows*) found on screening colonoscopy of an institutionalized male.

Clinical Features/Pathophysiology

E. vermicularis is an extremely well adapted parasite that produces no specific symptoms in the vast majority of persons. Most symptoms are minor such as pruritis ani and restless sleeping. Pinworm does not cause eosinophilia or appendicitis. A case report implicates a heavy synchronous *E. vermicularis* exposure with development of eosinophilic colitis in a homosexual man.[47]

Vulvovaginitis is more frequent in girls with pinworm than without. This may be caused by migration of the worms into the introitus and genital tract. Dead worms and eggs encased in granulomas have been found in the cervix, endometrium, fallopian tubes, and peritoneum, attesting to the migratory effort of female worms.[48] Ectopic enterobiasis remains rare, causing no or very little overt pathosis.

Diagnosis

E. vermicularis eggs are not plentiful in stool. This may account for the low prevalence rates determined by studies that use only stool specimens. The National Institutes of Health cellophane tape test is the classic diagnostic test for pinworm. A 2- to 3-inch piece of clear tape is serially applied to several perianal areas in the morning before washing. The tape is then applied to a glass slide. Microscopic evaluation demonstrates parasite eggs that measure 30 by 60 μm, have a thin shell, and appear flattened on one side. Three to seven daily samples are needed to exclude pinworm infection.

Treatment

Pinworm actually requires no treatment unless the patient has symptoms. However, it is highly transmittable and for that reason should be expunged. *E. vermicularis* is readily treated with a single 100 mg dose of mebendazole or a 400 mg dose of albendazole. Re-infection is common and patients should receive a second treatment after 15 days. All members of the family should be treated and clothes and bed linens washed. Albendazole and mebendazole are teratogens and should not be given to pregnant women.

Trichinella sp.

Trichinosis is a systemic illness caused by any of the five closely related *Trichinella* species. People acquire the parasite by ingesting larvae present in raw or undercooked meat such as pork. Trichinosis has both intestinal and systemic phases characterized by nausea, diarrhea, fever, myalgia, and periorbital edema. Intense exposure can cause death due to severe myositis, neuritis, and thrombosis. Treatment is with albendazole and glucocorticoids.

Epidemiology

Trichinosis is acquired by eating raw or undercooked meat that contains parasite larva. Domestic pigs are the most common carriers. Human disease is caused by the closely related *T. spiralis*, *T. pseudospiralis*, *T. britovi*, *T. nelsoni*, or *T. nativa*, which can be distinguished using molecular approaches.[49] Trichinella has worldwide distribution with *T. spiralis* and *T. pseudospiralis* in the Americas, Europe, and Russia; *T. britovi* in Europe, northern Africa, the Middle East, and Asia; *T. nelsoni* in equatorial Africa; and *T. nativa* in the Arctic and subarctic regions. *T. nativa* is resistant to freezing. Each of the Trichinella can infect any mammal. *T. pseudospiralis* also can infect birds.

Previously, trichinosis was common in the United States. In the late 1940s, about 400 cases/year of symptomatic trichinosis were reported to health agencies in the United States. This dropped to 13 cases/year in 1996.[50] Germany shows a similar pattern.[51] This decrease is due to two major factors. First is the strong admonition to thoroughly cook all pork products. Second is a change in farming practice to now feed pigs only grain.

Currently, most reported cases involve a discrete exposure. For example, a 1991 outbreak in Wisconsin involved 40 people who ate pork sausage from one shop. A 1995 outbreak in Idaho involved 10 people who ate cougar jerky.[50] In France, several outbreaks have resulted from eating raw horse meat.[52] This emphasizes that all mammals, including herbivores, can transmit *Trichinella*.

Life Cycle

The same host harbors both the adult and larval form of *Trichinella*.[53] People acquire the parasite by eating raw or undercooked meat that contains encapsulated parasite larvae. Each cyst dissolves in the digestive tract releasing one larva that invades the small intestinal mucosa. The larva enters enterocytes on a villus living within the cytoplasm of about 45 cells. Larvae rapidly mature and mate within 30 hours. Adults are minute with males measuring 60 μm by 1.2 mm and females measuring 90 μm by 2.2 mm. Females are viviparous, and begin releasing larvae approximately 1 week after initial ingestion. Adults are short-lived, producing larvae for only 4 weeks by which time they are expelled by the host.

The larvae live longer. Larvae measure 6 by 100 μm and enter the blood and lymphatic vessels. They are distributed through the body but develop only within striated muscle. The larva enters a striated muscle fiber but does not kill the myocyte. Instead, it induces the cell to transform into a novel "nurse cell" that houses and feeds the parasite. The larva grows and develops into the infective stage in about 5 weeks. A capsule forms around the coiled larvae as it awaits ingestion by another carnivore. The encapsulated larva remain viable for many years.

Clinical Features/Pathophysiology

While most infections with *Trichinella* are asymptomatic, significant exposure produces illness and even death.[54] Clinical trichinosis has two phases caused by the enteral (adult) and parenteral (larval) stages of the parasite. Intestinal symptoms result from enteritis due to adult worms embedded in the intestinal epithelium. Enteritis produces abdominal pain, nausea, vomiting, diarrhea, and low-grade fever. Intestinal symptoms begin about 2 days to 1 week and peak at 2 weeks after ingestion of contaminated meat. The timing and severity of symptoms vary with intensity of exposure. The intestinal phase of trichinosis is often misdiagnosed as viral gastroenteritis or food poisoning.

T. spiralis also infects mice and rats, permitting detailed study of the intestinal phase.[2] Mice begin to expel adult worms about 2 weeks after initial infection. Type 2 (Th2) cytokines (IL-4 and IL-5) promote worm expulsion. Expulsion of adult worms results from focal immune attack, increased secretions, and enhanced intestinal motility. T lymphocytes, eosinophils, and mast cells assist this primary response. Rats previously exposed to *T. spiralis* rapidly expel the parasite on rechallenge. This protection may result from an immediate-type hypersensitivity response to the parasite triggered by IgE-armed mast cells.

The parenteral phase of trichinosis begins with the birth of migratory larvae about 1 week after ingestion of contaminated meat. Larvae migrate into muscle and other organs such as the brain, spinal cord, and heart, evoking inflammatory responses. High fever, myalgia, periorbital edema, dysphagia, headache, and paresthesia result. Symptoms peak about 4 to 5 weeks after initial exposure and can take months to resolve. The severity and timing of symptoms vary with the intensity of exposure. Systemic complaints develop in many patients without prior intestinal symptoms.

The inflammatory response to migrating larvae produces myositis. Patients have eosinophilia and an elevated creatinine phosphokinase level. An intense exposure can cause fatal myocarditis, neuritis, and vasculitis or thrombosis. Patients are at highest risk of death between the 3rd and 6th week after exposure. Because trichinosis is rare, index cases often are initially misdiagnosed. Multiple individuals presenting with similar symptoms prompts consideration of trichinosis.

Diagnosis

Trichinella cannot be diagnosed with stool examination or intestinal biopsy. *Trichinella* do not lay eggs. No larvae are present in stool specimens. Even in heavy infections, adult worms are too infrequent to be found with random biopsy. Diagnosis is made by muscle biopsy demonstrating larvae within nurse cells. Diagnosis also can be made with serologic studies. Acute and convalescent serum samples confirm a rise in anti-*Trichinella* antibody.

Treatment

Although adults are short-lived, treatment with albendazole 400 mg/day for 3 days is warranted. Mebendazole 200 mg/day for 5 days also is effective. Treatment abbreviates the production of larvae by adult worms. Glucocorticoids reduce inflammation and systemic symptoms. However, glucocorticoids given in the absence of a benzimidazole can prolong the intestinal phase, increasing the number of larvae released.

Anisakis simplex

A. simplex can transiently infect people, causing abdominal pain, hematemesis, or intestinal inflammation. It is also a cause of food allergy. It is acquired by eating raw or undercooked fish. No treatment is necessary.

Epidemiology/Life Cycle

A. simplex infects fish and marine mammals. People become accidental hosts by eating raw or pickled fish. Instances of anisakiasis have become more common with the increased popularity of eating raw fish (e.g., sushi). Many species of salt-water fish harbor *A. simplex*, including herring, mackerel, salmon, plaice, and even squid (a cephalopod). The parasite initially infects crustaceans that are consumed by fish. The fish are then eaten by marine mammals that serve as definitive hosts for the intestinal worm. Adult intestinal worms lay eggs that are passed with feces. The eggs hatch to release larvae that infect crustaceans.

Clinical Features/Pathophysiology

A. simplex causes a transient infection in people. It does not reach full maturity so produces no eggs. The most common gastrointestinal symptom is stomach pain, nausea, and hematemesis occurring shortly after eating raw fish. Endoscopy may demonstrate a small larva partially penetrating the gastric or intestinal wall.[55, 56] Rarely, *A. simplex* can enter into the intestinal wall and cause a strong inflammatory reaction that may mimic acute appendicitis.[57]

A. simplex is a potent allergen. Many cases of seafood (fish) allergy may be reactions to *A. simplex*.[58] This includes anaphylaxis from well-cooked marine fish.

Diagnosis/Treatment

Diagnosis is made by finding larvae on endoscopy or in surgically excised specimens. Infections are transient; the parasite does not survive in people. No drug therapy is needed.

Trichostrongylus sp.

Epidemiology/Life Cycle

Trichostrongylus sp. are intestinal worms that infect ruminants such as sheep, goats, and cattle. People also may acquire these parasites by eating raw vegetables fertilized with animal excrement. *T. orientalis* appears to be a natural parasite for humans.

Parasite eggs deposited in the soil release free-living larvae that molt twice before becoming the ensheathed infective larvae that coat local plants. Ingested larvae enter the small intestinal wall and develop into adolescent worms. They exit into the lumen and mature into 4- to 7-mm long adults that attach to the duodenal and jejunal mucosa. They mate and lay eggs that closely resemble those of hookworms.

Clinical Features/Diagnosis

Most people have low level colonization and no symptoms. Mild eosinophilia may develop.[59] The eggs of *Trichostrongylus* sp. are often mistaken for those of *N. americanus* or *A. duodenale*.

Treatment

Trichostrongyliasis is treated with a single 400 mg dose of albendazole. A single dose of pyrantel pamoate (11 mg/kg) also is effective.

CESTODES

Diphyllobothrium latum

Fish tapeworm is the largest parasite of humans, reaching lengths of up to 40 feet (12 m). People acquire the parasite by eating raw or undercooked fresh water fish. *D. latum* absorbs dietary cobalamin and can cause vitamin B_{12} deficiency over time. Treatment is with albendazole.

Epidemiology

D. latum is most common but other *Diphyllobothrium* species also can colonize people. *D. latum* is endemic in northern Europe, Russia, and Alaska. Fish tapeworm (*Diphyllobothrium* sp.) has been reported in Africa, Japan, Taiwan, Australia, South America, North America, and Canada.[60]

Life Cycle

Fish tapeworm has a complex life cycle with two intermediate hosts. Parasite eggs that reach fresh water embryonate, then release free-swimming larvae called coracidia. Coracidia are ingested by water fleas (Cyclops and Diaptomus) and develop into procercoid larvae. Freshwater fish eat these small crustaceans and the parasite changes into the infective pleroceroid form. If an infected fish is consumed by another fish, the plerocercoid larva simply migrates into the flesh of the second fish. Trout, salmon, pike, perch, and whitefish can harbor *D. latum*. The plerocercoid larva embed in fish muscle and organs growing to 2 cm in length. People acquire the parasite by eating raw or undercooked fish. *D. latum* also can colonize many other mammals such as dogs, cats, bears, and seals. In mammals, the ingested plerocercoid larva attaches to the wall of the small intestine and matures into an adult worm. A long chain of proglottids, called the stroblia, develops off of the scolex. The proglottids release eggs into the lumen that pass with the feces.

Clinical Features/Pathophysiology

Fish tapeworm is not invasive and causes no direct symptoms. The worm obtains nutrients by absorbing luminal contents through its surface. *D. latum* avidly absorbs vitamin B_{12} effectively competing with its host for limited cobalamin. The worm is very long-lived and can cause significant B_{12} deficiency over time. Rarely, severe B_{12} deficiency results in megaloblastic anemia and neurologic symptoms.

Diagnosis/Treatment

Fish tapeworm is diagnosed by identifying *D. latum* eggs in stool specimens. Occasionally, proglottids are passed that also are diagnostic. Praziquantel is effective as a single oral dose of 10 mg/kg. Patients should be warned that they may pass a rather long worm 2 to 5 hours after taking the medication. Albendazole 400 mg each day for 3 days also kills the tapeworms.

Taenia saginata and *T. solium*

An estimated 50 million people are colonized with beef (*T. saginata*) or pork (*T. solium*) tapeworm. Colonization occurs by eating raw or undercooked meat infested with cysticerci. Tapeworms usually cause no symptoms and may surprise an endoscopist who finds the unsuspected jejunal inhabitant.

Ingestion of *T. solium* eggs causes cysticercosis, a potentially fatal disease. Treatment is with praziquantel or albendazole.

Epidemiology

Beef and pork tapeworm occur where livestock are exposed to untreated human waste and people eat raw or undercooked meat. Both parasites have a worldwide distribution, although infections originating in the United States and Europe are rare. Beef tapeworm is endemic in Africa, the Middle East, Eastern Europe, Asia, and Latin America. Pork tapeworm is endemic in Africa, India, China, Asia, and Latin America. *T. solium* is rare in Muslim countries where pork consumption is prohibited. *T. solium* is considered an eradicable parasite.[61]

Life Cycle

Adult tapeworms release gravid proglottids each containing up to 100,000 eggs. Proglottids and eggs are passed with the stool. Proglottids of *T. saginata* remain motile and may crawl out of the feces prompting patient alarm. Untreated human waste used to fertilize fields allows cattle to eat infective eggs on vegetation. Free ranging pigs are coprophagous and directly consume poorly disposed human waste. Ingested eggs release an embryo (oncosphere) that penetrates the intestinal wall and enters the blood vessels or lymphatics. The parasites are carried to subcutaneous tissue, muscle, and organs where they develop into cysticerci. The cysticerci can live for several years awaiting human consumption of infected meat. Once in a person's intestine, the cysticercus evaginates to form a scolex that serves as the anterior attachment point of the tapeworm. The scolex attaches to the intestinal mucosa in the proximal jejunum. The worm develops over several months as proglottids form and mature in a chain behind the scolex. This long tapelike chain is called the strobila. Beef tapeworms can reach 4 to 10 m and pork 2 to 4 m in length. Mature gravid proglottids break away from the distal end of the worm and pass with the stool to complete the life cycle. Adult worms can live in the small intestine for 25 years.

Clinical Features/Pathophysiology

Most people colonized with adult *T. saginata* or *T. solium* are asymptomatic. Colonization is usually limited to one worm that obtains nutrients by absorbing luminal contents through its surface. Motile proglottids may crawl out of the anus or swim in the toilet, eliciting immediate concern. Rarely, acute biliary or pancreatic duct obstruction can occur if proglottids migrate into these sites.

The most feared complication of *T. solium* infection is cysticercosis.[62] This occurs when people inadvertently consume *T. solium* eggs. Just as in pigs, the eggs release oncospheres that penetrate the intestinal wall, disseminate through the body, and form cysticerci. Cysticerci produce localized inflammation in the brain, spinal cord, eye, and heart with dire consequences. Neurocysticercosis is a common cause of epilepsy in countries where *T. solium* is endemic. An estimated 50,000 people die of neurocysticercosis each year. Because the disease occurs after ingestion of parasite eggs, neurocysticercosis in a patient who has not visited or emigrated from an endemic country should prompt an effort to identify local carriers.

Diagnosis

Beef and pork tapeworm is diagnosed by identifying eggs or proglottids in stool specimens. The eggs of the two species are microscopically indistinguishable. The proglottids of *T. saginata* are 2 cm long and have more than 12 uterine branches while those of *T. solium* measure 1.2 cm and have less than 10 uterine branches.[60] Egg and proglottid production can be sporadic necessitating repeated stool tests. Cystericercosis is usually diagnosed with computed tomography or magnetic resonance imaging and confirmed with serologic studies.

Treatment

Praziquantel is effective as a single oral dose of 10 mg/kg. Albendazole 400 mg each day for 3 days also kills the tapeworms. The worms usually break apart and are passed as sections of disintegrating strobila. Patients with cysticercosis should be treated with albendazole 5 mg/kg every 8 hours for 1 to 4 weeks to kill the cysticerci. Local inflammation transiently increases as cysticerci die. The addition of corticosteroids prevents exacerbation of neurocysticercosis during therapy.

Hymenolepis nana and *H. diminuta*

Hymenolepis nana (dwarf tapeworm) is the smallest but most common tapeworm that colonizes people. It can be transmitted directly from person to person. Self-inoculation or internal autoinfection permits accumulation of a large number of worms, which can cause anorexia, abdominal pain, and diarrhea. *H. diminuta* (rodent tapeworm) is larger but rarely colonizes people. It is acquired by ingesting infected insects and usually causes no symptoms. Treatment is with praziquantel.

Epidemiology

H. nana is the most common tapeworm of humans. Unlike other tapeworms, it can be transmitted from person to person without need of an intermediate host. Dwarf tapeworm has a worldwide distribution. Prevalence is highest in warm and arid regions. A survey of Egyptian children found that 16% carried *H. nana*.[63] Recently, *H. nana* was found in 54% of individuals within a coastal Australian Aboriginal community.[64] In the United States, a 1987 survey of state diagnostic laboratories found that 900 of 216,000 submitted stool specimens demonstrated *H. nana* with 34 states reporting positive specimens.[23] *H. nana* also colonizes mice and rats. However, the strains that colonize people appear to differ from those of rodents.

Human colonization with *H. diminuta* is rare but also enjoys a worldwide distribution. Rats and mice are the parasite's usual hosts. People acquire rodent tapeworm by ingesting fleas, grain beetles, mealworms, or cockroaches infested with larval forms of the parasite. Most cases involve young children. The incorporation of beetles in traditional oriental medications also permits transmission.[65]

Life Cycle

H. nana do not require an intermediate insect host. Ingested eggs release oncospheres that invade the mucosa of the small bowel. They lodge within the lymphatics of the villi and develop into cysticercoid larvae. Each cysticercoid larva then ruptures into the lumen and evaginates to form a scolex that attaches to the mucosa of the ileum. The worms mature growing a strobila or chain of developing proglottids. Adult worms average 2 cm in length and have about 200 proglottids. Each proglottid contains about 150 eggs. The most distal proglottids disintegrate to release eggs into the lumen. About 20 to 30 days after initial ingestion the worm begins to shed eggs in the stool. *H. nana* adults live for only 4 to 6 weeks. However, eggs shed in the stool are immediately infective. Self-inoculation or internal autoinfection allows colonization to persist for years. Limited sanitation or poor handwashing permits transmission to others.

Like other *Hymenolepis* sp., *H. nana* can infect insects, forming cysticercoid larvae. Ingestion of infected fleas, beetles, mealworms, or cockroaches allows transmission of *H. nana*. However, acquisition by this pathway is rare. Most transmission is by direct ingestion of eggs.

H. diminuta requires intermediate insect hosts. Insects ingest eggs as they consume rodent droppings. The eggs release oncospheres that penetrate into the insect's viscera and form cysticercoid larvae. Rats and mice that eat infected insects acquire the tapeworm. People acquire rodent tapeworm the same way. Once in the intestine, the cysticercoid larva evaginates to form a scolex that attaches to the ileal mucosa. The worm matures growing a strobila of proglottids and reaches a length of up to 90 cm. The most distal proglottids disintegrate, releasing eggs into the intestinal lumen.

Clinical Features/Pathophysiology

Most people colonized with *H. nana* or *H. diminuta* have no symptoms. However, self-inoculation or internal autoinfection can cause heavy infections with *H. nana*. Enteritis results as numerous cysticercoid larvae damage intestinal villi. In heavy infections, anorexia, abdominal pain, and diarrhea may develop.

Mice can harbor *H. nana*, permitting investigation of the mechanisms that limit worm density. It appears that a Th1 cell IFNγ response provides protective immunity against cysticerciod larvae,[66, 67] and a Th2 response involving IgE and mast cells assist expulsion of adult worms.[68, 69]

Diagnosis/Treatment

Dwarf or rodent tapeworm is diagnosed by finding parasite eggs in the stool. *H. nana* eggs measure 30 to 47 μm in diameter. The eggs of the less prevalent *H. diminuta* are larger, measuring 56 to 86 μm in diameter. Examination of several stool specimens obtained on different days are needed to identify low level colonization. Adults of both parasites can be killed with a single oral dose of praziquantel at 25 mg/kg. However, eggs escape this treatment. Therefore, patients with *H. nana* should be retreated in 1 week. Family members should also be examined and considered for treatment.

Dipylidium caninum

Dipylidium caninum (dog tapeworm) is a common parasite of household pets that rarely colonizes children. It is acquired by eating fleas that contain parasite cysticercoid larvae. Dog tapeworm causes no symptoms but parents who find crawling proglottids in a diaper prompt a medical evaluation. Treatment is with praziquantel.

Echinococcus sp. also are tapeworms of dogs. Ingestion of *E. granulosus, E. multilocularis*, or *E. vogeli* eggs causes severe disease due to formation of hydatid cysts. For information on *Echinococcus*, see Chapter 69.

Epidemiology

D. caninum is the most common tapeworm of domesticated dogs and cats. People acquire dog tapeworm by inadvertently ingesting fleas infected with the parasite. It is distributed worldwide. Most cases involve infants and young children who have close contact with their pets.

Life Cycle

Parasite eggs are ingested by the larval form of fleas that inhabit dogs or cats. Each egg releases an oncosphere that penetrates the gut wall and develops into a cysticercoid larva within the insect's viscera. The insect larva then develops into an adult flea that can distribute the cysticercoid larva to other animals. Dogs, cats, and occasionally children ingest infected adult fleas. Once in the intestine, the cysticercoid larva evaginates to form a scolex, which attaches to the mucosa of the small intestine. The worm matures, forming a strobila or chain of developing proglottids that trails behind the scolex. The adult worm measures 10 to 70 cm long. Gravid proglottids detach from the distal end of the worm and pass with the stool. The proglottids look like cucumber seeds (12 $\times$ 3 mm), are motile, and occasionally crawl out of the anus. They can be mistaken for maggots. As they dry, they release small packets that contain 5 to 15 eggs.

Clinical Features/Pathophysiolgy

Because people usually do not eat fleas, colonization is limited. Low numbers of dog tapeworms cause no symptoms. *D. caninum* is discovered when patients or their parents find motile proglottids crawling in a diaper, underwear, or stool.

Diagnosis/Treatment

D. caninum is identified by a characteristic proglottid that looks like a moving cucumber seed. The proglottids are often mistaken for adult pinworms (*E. vermicularis*) because that parasite is much more common. Stool examination for egg packets is usually unrewarding.

D. caninum causes a self-limited colonization that should spontaneously clear. Therefore, dog tapeworm requires no treatment. However, most patients and their families prefer that the parasite be expunged. Treatment is with a single oral dose of praziquantel 10 mg/kg or *niclosamide 500 mg* (chewable tablet).

TREMATODES

Intestinal Flukes

Fasciolopsis buski, Heterophyes sp., and Echinostoma sp.

Most intestinal trematodes have a broad host range and more than 50 different species are capable of colonizing people.[70] Many of these are geographically restricted and are acquired due to specific indigenous dietary behaviors. The more common intestinal trematodes are *Fasciolopsis buski*, *Heterophyes* sp., and *Echinostoma* sp.

Fasciolopsis buski

F. buski is the largest intestinal trematode that colonizes people. Adult worms are 7.5 cm long and 2 cm wide. It is endemic in southeast Asia and Indonesia. People acquire the parasite by ingesting metacercariae encysted on freshwater plants. The metacercariae excyst in the duodenum and attach to the small intestinal mucosa. Within 3 months, they mature to adult flat worms and begin to lay eggs. The eggs pass with feces into freshwater and embryonate. Each egg releases a ciliated miracidium that hunts for a suitable snail to infect. The miracidium enters the snail and develops into a sporocyst that asexually multiplies, releasing numerous cercariae. The cercariae swim to a freshwater plant and encyst on the wall, awaiting ingestion by a mammal.

Adult *F. buski* live for about 1 year and cause no symptoms in most people.[71] Histologic findings of jejunal biopsy specimens along with carbohydrate, fat, and protein absorption were normal in one study of patients harboring *F. buski*.[72] However, in 1952, a 15-year-old Thai girl, hospitalized for diarrhea and abdominal pain, died of anasarca with more than 470 adult worms in her small intestine.[73] Diagnosis is by finding parasite eggs in the stool (see Fig. 99–3*D*). Treatment is with praziquantel 25 mg/kg orally every 8 hours for 1 day.

Heterophyes sp.

Heterophyes sp. and the closely related *Metagonimus yokogawai* are small flat worms approximately 1.0 to 1.7 mm long and 0.3 to 0.6 mm wide. *H. heterophyes* is endemic in west Africa, Egypt, Israel, Turkey, China, Japan, Taiwan, and the Philippines. *H. nocens* is endemic to Japan and Korea. *M. yokogawai* is endemic in Siberia, the Balkans, China, Korea, and Japan. People acquire these parasites by eating raw or undercooked fish that contain metacercariae. In the United States, a case of *H. heterophyes* involved a Pennsylvanian woman who ate sushi flown in from the Orient.[74] The metacercariae ingested with raw fish excyst in the intestine, attach to the small intestinal mucosa, and develop into adults. The adults lay eggs that are deposited with the feces into freshwater or brackish water. The eggs release miracidia that swim in search of a suitable snail. Each miracidium enters a snail and develops into a sporocyst that asexually multiplies, releasing numerous cercariae. The cercariae swim away from the snail in search of a fish to infect. Either freshwater fish or saltwater fish feeding in brackish outlets can become infected.

These parasites produce no specific symptoms in most people. Occasional heavy infections will cause mild abdominal pain and mucoid diarrhea. The worms attach at the crypts and produce a localized eosinophilic inflammation. Rarely, parasite eggs may enter blood vessels and lymphatics, producing distant granulomatous reactions. Diagnosis is by finding eggs in the stool. This may require concentration techniques. The eggs of *Heterophyes* sp. appear similar to those of *M. yokogawai*. Treatment of the trematodes is with 25 mg/kg of praziquantel every 8 hours for 1 day.

Echinostoma sp.

There are at least 16 species of *Echinostoma* that can colonize people.[75] Adults are 2 to 6 mm long and 1 to 1.5 mm wide, depending on species. *Echinostoma* sp. are endemic in Taiwan, Korea, Thailand, Japan, Indonesia, and the Philippines. One outbreak of probable echinostomiasis involved 18 of 20 American travelers returning from Kenya.[76] People acquire *Echinostoma* by eating raw or undercooked freshwater mollusks or fish infected with metacercariae. The ingested metacercariae excyst in the intestine, attach to the small intestinal mucosa, and develop into adults. The adults lay eggs that are deposited into freshwater with the feces. The eggs embryonate and then hatch, each releasing a miracidium that swims in search of a suitable snail. Each miracidium enters a snail and develops into a sporocyst that asexually multiplies, releasing numerous cercariae. Depending on the species, the *Echinostoma* cercariae swim away from the snail in search of another mollusk or fish to infect.

While *Echinostoma* sp. produce no symptoms in most people, the parasites may cause epigastric pain, abdominal cramps, and diarrhea.[76] Diagnosis is by finding eggs in the stool. *Echinostoma* eggs resemble those of *F. buski* but are smaller. Treatment is with one oral dose of praziquantel at 25 mg/kg.

Liver Flukes

Clonorchis sinensis, Opisthorchis viverrini, and *O. felineus*

C. sinensis and *Opisthorchis* sp. are closely related parasites that have similar life cycles and cause similar disease. *C. sinensis* is endemic to China, Hong Kong, Taiwan, and North Vietnam (see Chapter 69, Fig. 69–6). *O. viverrini* is endemic to Thailand and Laos. *O. felineus* is endemic in Russia and the Ukraine. People acquire these parasites by eating metacercariae present in raw or undercooked fish. The metacercariae excyst in the stomach and duodenum as the meat is digested. The worms migrate along the mucosa to the ampulla of Vater and into the biliary tree. They grow into adults. Leaf-shaped adult *C. sinensis* measure 5 mm wide by 2.5 cm long by 1 mm thick. *Opisthorchis* are smaller. The adult parasites lay eggs that pass with the bile into the intestinal lumen and are excreted. The eggs are ingested by freshwater snails where they hatch, releasing miracidia that develop into sporocysts. Each sporocyst asexually reproduces within the snail eventually producing numerous cercariae. The cercariae exit the snail and swim in search of a suitable fish that they invade. The parasites encyst as metacercariae in the muscles of the fish, awaiting ingestion by a mammalian host.

Most infections with *C. sinensis* or *Opisthorchis* are asymptomatic. With heavy exposures, the parasites acutely cause fever, malaise, hepatic tenderness, and eosinophilia.[77] These symptoms and signs abate as the worms mature and begin laying eggs in the bile ducts. In a minority of patients, the parasites may cause relapsing cholangitis (see Chapter 59). The worms elicit a fibrotic and adenomatous reaction in the smaller branches of the biliary ducts. This can produce a localized obstruction and hepatic absess. The flukes may also migrate into the pancreatic duct and cause pancreatitis.

The most important complication of chronic infection with *C. sinesis* or *O. viverrini* is cholangiocarcinoma (see Chapter 60). Infection with these parasites dramatically increases the risk of developing this otherwise rare cancer (Table 99–2).[78–83] The parasites damage the bile duct causing desquamation followed by hyperplasia, adenomatous hyperplasia, periductal fibrosis, dysplasia, and finally cholangiocarcinoma.[84] Cancer may result from increased sensitivity to carcinogens. Cholangiocarcinoma develops in hamsters infected with *O. viverrini* when treated with subcarcinogenic doses of dimethylnitrosamine. *C. sinensis* and *O. viverrini* may sensitize patients to dietary or endogenously produced N-nitroso-compounds and increase the risk for developing cholangiocarcinoma.[85] This is an important consideration in Western countries as well. A 1977 study found that 26% of Chinese immigrants relocating to New York had *C. sinensis*.[86] Because of the increased cancer risk, it is advisable to look for these parasites in patients from endemic areas.[87]

Diagnosis is by finding parasite eggs in the stool or duodenal aspirate specimen. Symptomatic patients may have curvilinear lucencies in the bile and pancreatic ducts on ERCP.[88] The recommended treatment is praziquantel 25 mg/kg every 8 hours for a total of three doses. Heavy infections may require 2 days of therapy.[89] An alternative treatment is albendazole 10 mg/kg twice a day for 7 days. Albendazole is teratogenic and should not be given to pregnant women.

Table 99–2 | **Relative Risk of Cholangiocarcinoma in Patients Colonized with *Clonorchis* or *Opisthorchis***

PARASITE	RELATIVE CANCER RISK (REF)	95% CI
C. sinensis		
	3.1[79]	0.13–8.4
	6.5[80]	3.7–12
	6.0[81]	2.8–13
O. viverrini		
	5.0[82]	2.3–11.0
	Light* 1.7[83]	0.2–16.3
	Medium* 3.2[83]	0.4–30
	Heavy* 14.0[83]	1.7–119

*Light, <1500; medium, 1501–6000; heavy, 6000+ eggs/g stool.

Fasciola hepatica and *F. gigantica*

F. hepatica has a worldwide distribution while *F. gigantica* is endemic in Hawaii, Asia, India, the Middle East, and Africa. Both species infect sheep, goats, and cattle as their normal hosts. People acquire the parasites by ingesting metacercariae encysted on freshwater plants such as watercress. The metacercariae excyst in the small intestine, penetrate through the bowel wall, and enter the peritoneal cavity. They migrate to the liver, penetrate the capsule, and travel through the hepatic parenchyma in search of a bile duct. They reside within the bile ducts, reach maturity within 3 or 4 months, and lay eggs. Adult *F. hepatica* are 1.3 cm by 4.0 cm in size; *F. gigantica* are up to 7.0 cm long. Adults of both species are only 1 mm thick and therefore resemble leaves. Fasciola are long-lived—one documented infection persisted for 16 years.[90] Adults lay eggs that pass with the bile into the intestinal lumen and are excreted. On reaching freshwater, *Fasciola* eggs embryonate, hatch, and release miracidia that swim in search of a suitable snail. The miracidium enters the snail and develops into a sporocyst that asexually multiplies eventually releasing numerous cercariae. The cercariae swim to a freshwater plant and encyst on the wall awaiting ingestion by a mammal.

Fasciola infections are usually asymptomatic. In the acute phase, patients can have abdominal pain and hepatomegaly as the parasites penetrate the intestinal wall and hepatic capsule. Abdominal computed tomography may show low-density areas in the periphery of the liver. Symptoms may develop from migration of the parasites to other sites such as subcutaneous fat.[91] Acute symptoms wane as the parasites enter the bile ducts. During the chronic phase of fascioliasis, patients may have symptoms of intermittent biliary obstruction and cholangitis. Rarely, pancreatitis develops. ERCP may show curvilinear lucencies in the bile duct (Fig. 99–10).[92]

Diagnosis is by finding eggs in the stool. However, *Fasciola* release low numbers of eggs, making this test insensitive. Duodenal or bile aspirates also can demonstrate eggs. The most sensitive method to detect *Fasciola* infection is testing for the presence of antibodies against the worms by ELISA.[93] Antibody titer drops after successful drug treatment.

Unlike other trematodes, *Fasciola* are resistant to praziquantel. Triclabendazole is the drug of choice for fascioliasis. In one study, a single oral dose of triclabendazole (10 mg/kg) cured 79% of patients as measured by fecal egg counts and ELISA.[94]

Blood Flukes

The majority of visceral (hepatosplenic and intestinal) schistosomiasis is due to *S. mansoni* or *S. japonicum*. *S. mekongi* and *S. intercalatum* also cause visceral schistosomiasis. Schistosomes infect about 200 million people worldwide. People acquire the parasite through contact with contaminated water. Visceral schistosomiasis can cause fibrosis of the portal vein, producing portal hypertension. Treatment is with praziquantel.

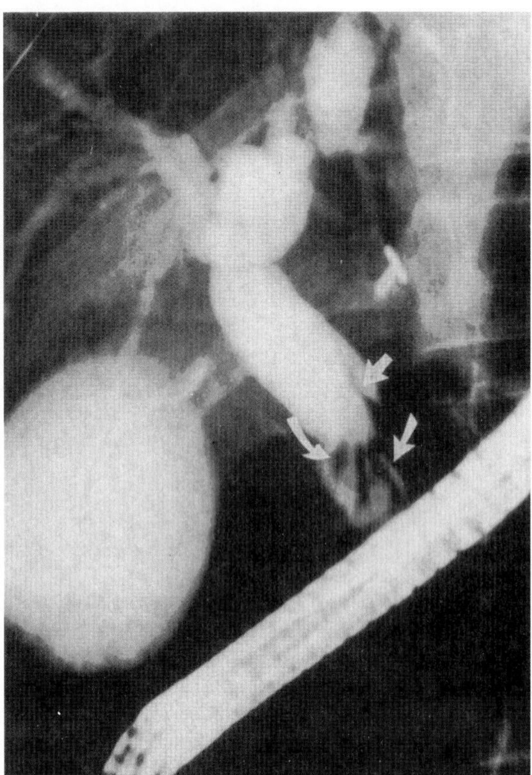

Figure 99–10. *Fasciola hepatica* showing curvilinear lucencies *(arrows)* in the distal bile duct on endoscopic retrograde cholangiogram. Leaf-shaped fluke was extracted from bile duct. (From Veerappan A, Siegel JH, Podany J, et al. *Fasciola hepatica* pancreatitis: Endoscopic extraction of live parasites. Gastrointest Endosc 37:473–475, 1991.)

Epidemiology

Schistosomes are tropical parasites with a worldwide distribution. *S. mansoni* is endemic in regions of Africa, the Middle East, Puerto Rico, the Dominican Republic, Central America, and South America. *S. japonicum* is endemic in China, Indonesia, the Philippines and Thailand. *S. mekongi* is endemic in Loa and Cambodia. *S. intercalatum* is endemic in Africa. In most countries, some regions have a high prevalence of infection while in other areas the parasite is absent. Schistosomes live in tropical snails for part of their life cycle. It is the distribution of these snails that helps define the geographic limits of schistosomes.

Construction of water reservoirs and irrigation canals has expanded the snail habitat in many countries. This has increased the risk of acquiring schistosomiasis. Mice and other mammals can harbor schistosomes and may allow spread of the parasite even with improved sanitation.[95] This makes it difficult to eradicate. However, Japan successfully eradicated *S. japonicum* and recent evidence suggests that *S. mansoni* is vanishing from some areas of Puerto Rico.[96]

Life Cycle

Schistosome worms are acquired by contacting fresh water infested with parasite cercariae (also see Chapter 69, Fig. 69–4). Cercariae are fork-tailed, microscopic larva that swim through the water in search of a suitable host. They penetrate through intact skin, shed their tails, and transform into schistosomules that are covered with a double lipid-bilayer tegument. This tegument thwarts most immunologic attacks. The schistosomules migrate into blood vessels where they are swept with the venous flow through the right heart into the lungs. They migrate through the pulmonary capillaries, flow through the left heart into the systemic circulation, and eventually reach the liver. The worms mature in the liver, mate, and migrate up the portal venous system. The 2-cm long female is partly ensheathed by the shorter male. The couple reside together within the mesenteric veins. *S. mansoni* and *S. intercalatum* prefer to dwell in the vessels drained by the inferior mesenteric vein. *S. japonicum* and *S. mekongi* prefer the vessels drained by the superior mesenteric vein.

The worms remain in the mesenteric vessels, consuming blood and nutrients, and depositing eggs. *S. mansoni* lay 250 eggs and *S. japonicum* lay 3500 eggs per worm pair each day. Many of the eggs pass through the intestinal wall and enter the lumen of the bowel. The eggs pass with the stool, and if deposited in freshwater, hatch to release ciliated miracidia. Miracidia swim in search of a suitable tropical snail to infect. After penetrating into the snail's foot process, a miracidium transforms into a primary (mother) sporocyst. Secondary sporocysts bud off of the primary sporocyst, migrate to the snail's liver, and mature. Cercariae bud off the secondary sporocysts, exit the snail, and swim in search of a permissive mammalian host.

Clinical Features/Pathophysiology

Dermal invasion and migration by infecting cercariae usually produce no symptoms. A mild papular rash may develop in patients with repeated contact. This contrasts with the intensely pruritic papular rash that develops after exposure to avian schistosomes such as *Trichobilharzia ocellata*. These trematodes infect water fowl but are unable to live in mammals. The cercariae/schisosomules die in a person's skin, eliciting an immunologic response that produces swimmer's itch. Swimmer's itch is common in the Great Lakes region and has been found as far north as Iceland.[97] Swimmer's itch is not dangerous but scratching can cause a secondary cellulitis.

Schistosomules migrate through the body without producing symptoms. Juvenile and adult worms elegantly evade immune attack. Their tegument is coated with histocompatibility and blood group antigens confiscated from the host. The tegument contains immunoglobulin receptors and proteases that may help cleave any bound antibody. Furthermore, schistosomes produce several proteins that prevent complement, neutrophils, macrophages, or lymphocytes from injuring the worms.[98] This immune evasion allows the adult worms to survive in the blood vessels without causing much direct damage. The average life span of worms is thought to be about 5 years, but there are documented cases of adult worms surviving for more than 35 years after individuals left an endemic area.[99]

Schistosome worms release eggs each day throughout their long life. It is the parasite's eggs that cause pathosis. While the adult worms evade an immune response, the eggs invite one. The eggs exude antigens that trigger a strong cell-mediated Th2 immune response.

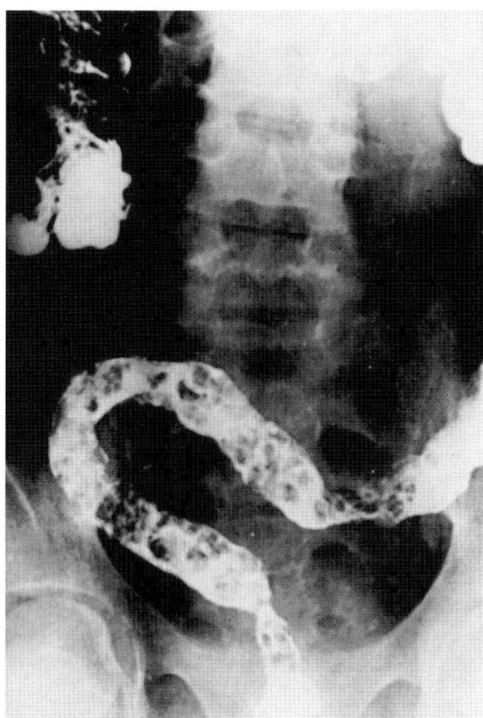

Figure 99–11. Barium enema from a 20-year-old Egyptian man with bloody diarrhea and tenesmus. Multiple polypoid lesions due to *Schistosoma mansoni* are seen throughout the rectosigmoid colon, which is displaced out of the pelvis by a large pericolic abscess. (From Reeder MM, Hamilton LC: Radiologic diagnosis of tropical diseases of the gastrointestinal tract. Radiol Clin North Am 7:57, 1969.)

Katayama fever is the classic presentation of acute schistosomiasis. It results from a brisk early immune response to schistosome eggs that occurs within the first 2 weeks of egg deposition or from about 35 to 50 days after contacting water heavily infested with cercariae. Symptoms are caused by circulating immune complexes and resemble those due to serum sickness. Patients have fever, malaise, arthralgia, myalgia, cough and diarrhea with the additional finding of a marked eosinophilia. Transaminase levels are normal and eggs are usually absent from the stool. *S. japonicum* releases the largest number of eggs and causes the most intense acute schistosomiasis with fatality rates approaching 25%. Yet, acute schistosomiasis does not develop in most people. In those in whom schistosomiasis develops and who survive, the symptoms resolve as the infection enters the chronic phase.

Each schistosome egg secretes antigens that provoke a focal granulomatous reaction. This inflammation helps move the egg from the inside of a capillary, through the intestinal wall, and out into the lumen.[100] Thus, inflammation actually benefits the parasite. Passage of eggs through the bowel wall causes intestinal schistosomiasis with hemoccult-positive stools or even bloody diarrhea. Patients also may have tenesmus and tenderness over the sigmoid colon. Patients with *S. mansoni* can develop inflammatory polyps (Fig. 99–11) that have numerous eosinophils and occasional eggs.[101] *S. japonicum* prefers to dwell in veins drained by the superior mesenteric vein and lays thousands of eggs at a time. *S. japonicum* can produce upper abdominal pain unrelated to meals, gastric bleeding, and pyloric obstruction due to inflammation and fibrosis.

About half of the eggs pass out of the body, the other half lodge in the host's tissues and cause the pathosis of chronic schistosomiasis. Eggs are carried by the portal flow and lodge in the liver. Other eggs lodge in the mesenteric and portal veins or remain in the intestinal wall. In these locations, the eggs elicit granulomas composed of eosinophils, macrophages, lymphocytes, fibroblasts, and mast cells (Fig. 99–12). Eosinophils account for 50% of the schistosome egg granuloma cell population. Eosinophils degranulate depositing major basic protein that produces an eosinophilic halo around the eggs termed the Slendore-Hoeppli phenomenon. Eosinophils likely assist in killing the miracidia that is protected by the tough egg shell. After 1 or 2 weeks the miracidium dies, antigen release wanes, and the granuloma involutes to leave a fibrotic scar.

Over the years, the daily production of eggs, granulomas, and scars accumulates enough damage to produce disease. Eggs that lodge in the hepatic and portal vessels produce a unique pattern of scarring called *Symmers' pipe stem fibrosis* (see Fig. 69–5). The vessels become fibrotic, resembling pipe stems on cross section. This causes the presinusoidal venous obstruction and portal hypertension characteristic of hepatosplenic schistosomiasis. Patients have an enlarged left hepatic lobe, splenomegaly, and thrombocytopenia due to platelet sequestration. Hepatocellular function remains normal as the blood supply to the liver is maintained by increased hepatic artery flow. Patients have normal serum transaminase levels and mildly elevated alkaline phospatase and gamma-glutamyl transferase levels. Cirrhosis does not develop in patients with hepatosplenic schistosomiasis unless coinfected with hepatisis B or C, and so lack stigmata of hepatic insufficiency such as palmar erythema, spider angiomata, testicular atrophy, gynecomastia, or encephalopathy. The classic presentation of decompensated hepatosplenic schistosomiasis is variceal hemorrhage.

Hepatosplenic schistosomiasis results from accumulated injury and requires prolonged, moderately intense infection. Patients are usually adolescent to late 20s and have had

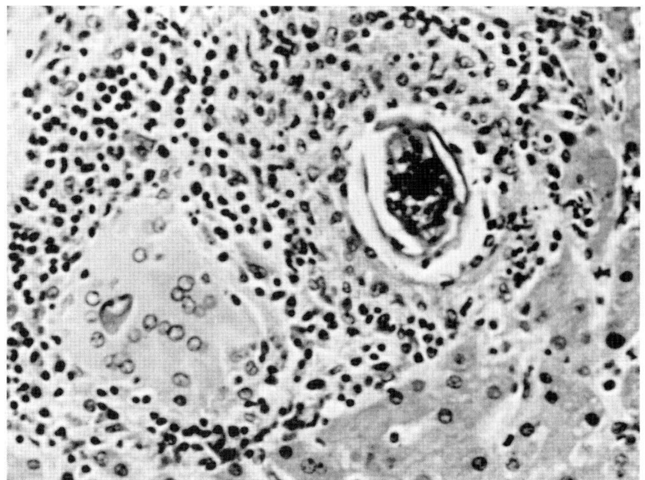

Figure 99–12. Schistosome egg granuloma in the liver of a patient. Note the ovum on the right and foreign body giant cell on the left. Magnification, ×150. (Courtesy of SH Choy, MD, San Francisco.)

schistosomiasis for 5 to 15 years. However, compensated disease improves after schistosomes are killed by drug therapy, permitting the portal tributaries to heal and remodel.[102]

Schistosome eggs also can lodge in other sites. Eggs may percolate through portocaval collateral vessels and lodge in the pulmonary capillaries. Over time, this can cause pulmonary hypertension and cor pulmonale. Eggs may enter the vertebral venous plexus and travel as emboli to the spinal cord or brain. Granulomatous inflammation in the central nervous system can result in conus equinus syndrome, transverse myelitis, or schistosomal cerebritis.

Patients with schistosomiasis may present with recurrent bacteremia. Adult schistosome worms accidentally ingest enteric bacteria transiently present in the portal circulation. They can harbor these bacteria and serve as reservoirs for infection. Recurrent salmonella infections are particularly common.[103]

Schistosomiasis may cause proteinuria, nephrotic syndrome, and end-stage renal disease. This schistosomal nephropathy is caused by deposition of immune complexes of parasite antigens and antibodies. Renal biopsy specimens show membranoproliferative glomerulonephritis or focal glomerulosclerosis. The renal disease can be progressive even if the parasites are killed with drug therapy.[104]

Diagnosis

Schistosome eggs are present in stool but not in high numbers. The classic test for detecting eggs is the Kato-Katz thick smear (for method, see reference 105). This is not performed as part of the standard ova and parasite test.

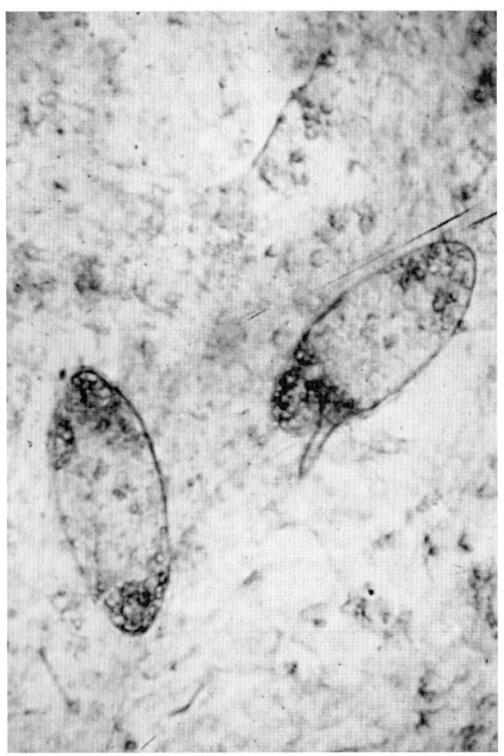

Figure 99–13. Schistosoma mansoni egg as it appears microscopically in the bowel wall. Magnification, ×200. (Courtesy of CM Knauer, MD, San Jose, CA.)

Table 99–3 | **Ultrasonographic Parameter Values Summed Together to Score Hepatosplenic Schistosomiasis (see text for details)**

PARAMETER	PARAMETER VALUE 0	1	2	3
Peripheral periportal tract thickening	<3 mm	3–5 mm	>5–7 mm	>7 mm
Portal vein diameter*	<14 mm	14–19 mm	>20 mm	
Spleen length above normal†	Normal	>0–5 cm	>5 cm	
Dilated collateral veins	None	Noncoronary‡	Coronary	

*Measured midway between entrance at porta hepatis and the bifurcation.
†Length below left costal margin on deep inspiration.
‡Dilated splenic hilum or umbilical veins.
Adapted from Abdel-Wahab MF, Esmat G, Farrag A, et al: Ultrasonographic prediction of esophageal varices in Schistosomiasis mansoni. Am J Gastroenterol 88(4): 560–3, 1993.

Standard evaluation is not sensitive enough to find the relatively rare schistosome eggs. Even Kato-Katz thick smears are not highly sensitive and are unlikely to detect low level infection.[105]

The vast majority of intestinal schistosome infections are asymptomatic. These patients come to medical attention during evaluation of mild anemia, hemoccult-positive stools, or unexpected variceal hemorrhage. On endoscopy, a patient may have inflammatory polyps that contain eggs.[101] But usually, the intestinal mucosa appears normal. Subtle changes in the vascular pattern may result from egg emboli producing a terminal curling of small blood vessels.[106] A biopsy specimen of the rectum can demonstrate eggs. Crushing the biopsy specimen between two glass slides and microscopically surveying the whole biopsy specimen increases the chance of finding eggs (Fig. 99–13). Evaluation of six crush biopsies is more sensitive than two Kato-Katz smears for *S. mansoni*.[107]

Although eggs lodge in the liver and cause portal hypertension, liver biopsy is an insensitive method for detecting schistosomiasis. Liver biopsy should not be used solely to test for schistosomiasis but rather to stage comorbid disease such as hepatitis B or C.

Exposure to schistosomes is detectable with serologic studies. Antischistosome antibodies are detected with ELISA using adult microsomal antigens. Sensitivity varies depending on if the infecting schistosome is the same species as that used to prepare the antigens. The ELISA uses *S. mansoni* microsomal antigens so immunoblot tests employing antigens from *S. japonicum* and *S. hematobium* (urinary schistosomiasis) also are performed.[108] The antibody assay also is useful to diagnose acute schistosomiasis (Katayama fever) as there are few or no eggs in the stool during the peak of the reaction. The ELISA does not distinguish active from prior infections. Therefore, it is most useful for recent travelers rather than expatriates. However, schistosomes can be long-lived so one-time treatment of antibody-positive patients is reasonable.

If needed, active infection can be demonstrated by detecting circulating parasite antigens in the patient's serum.[109] These antigens are schistosome gut-associated proteins, named CCA and CAA, that are copiously released into the bloodstream by adult worms. Serologic detection of CCA and CAA has an equivalent or higher sensitivity than the Kato-Katz thick smear but each test individually misses some low level infections.[110] Measurement of circulating antigens also may prove useful to document response to treatment.[111] However, these tests are not yet commercially available in the United States.

Abdominal ultrasound is an important additional test in hepatosplenic schistosomiasis. Ultrasound evaluation documents periportal fibrosis, splenomegaly, portal blood flow and collateral vessels. Periportal fibrosis has the characteristic appearance of multiple echogenic areas each with central echolucency.[112] A scoring system exists that uses the sum of four parameters determined by ultrasound (Table 99–3). An ultrasound score of 5 or greater correlates with the presence of esophageal varices grade 2 or greater.[113]

Treatment

Praziquantel is the drug of choice for treating schistosomiasis. It is the safest schistosomicide in current use. Best cure rates are obtained with praziquantel given orally in three doses of 20 mg/kg, each 4 hours apart (total dose, 60 mg/kg). This gives cure rates of 60% to 98%, depending on the series. Note that eggs will continue to be shed in the stool for up to 2 weeks after drug treatment. This is because eggs that were deposited before treatment can take this long to work through the intestinal wall. Patients who are not cured with a single course have dramatic decrease in egg counts and will respond to a second course of praziquantel. Periportal fibrosis improves after the worms are killed, halting the daily deluge of eggs and permitting the portal tributaries to heal and remodel.[102]

REFERENCES

1. Little MD: Laboratory diagnosis of worms and miscellaneous specimens. Clin Lab Med 11(4):1041–50, 1991.
2. Finkelman FD, Shea-Donohue T, Goldhill J, et al: Cytokine regulation of host defense against parasitic gastrointestinal nematodes: lessons from studies with rodent models. Annu Rev Immunol 15:505–33, 1997.
3. Elliott DE, Urban JF, Argo CK, Weinstock JV: Does the failure to acquire helminthic parasites predispose to Crohn's disease? FASEB J 14(12):1848–55, 2000.
4. Khuroo MS: Ascariasis. Gastroenterol Clin North Am 25(3):553–77, 1996.
5. Chan MS, Medley GF, Jamison D, Bundy DA: The evaluation of potential global morbidity attributable to intestinal nematode infections. Parasitology 109(Pt 3):373–87, 1994.
6. de Silva NR, Guyatt HL, Bundy DA: Worm burden in intestinal obstruction caused by Ascaris lumbricoides. Trop Med Int Health 2(2):189–90, 1997.
7. Wasadikar PP, Kulkarni AB: Intestinal obstruction due to ascariasis. Br J Surg 84(3):410–2, 1997.
8. van den Bogaerde JB, Jordaan M: Intraductal administration of albendazole for biliary ascariasis. Am J Gastroenterol 92(9):1531–3, 1997.
9. Maddern GJ, Dennison AR, Blumgart LH: Fatal ascaris pancreatitis: An uncommon problem in the west. Gut 33(3):402–3, 1992.
10. Khuroo MS, Zargar SA, Mahajan R, et al: Sonographic appearances in biliary ascariasis. Gastroenterology 93(2):267–72, 1987.
11. Schulman A: Ultrasound appearances of intra- and extrahepatic biliary ascariasis. Abdom Imaging 23(1):60–6, 1998.
12. Gill GV, Bell DR: Strongyloides stercoralis infection in former Far East prisoners of war. Br Med J 2(6190):572–4, 1979.
13. Weight SC, Barrie WW: Colonic Strongyloides stercoralis infection masquerading as ulcerative colitis. J R Coll Surg Edinb 42(3):202–3, 1997.
14. Al Samman M, Haque S, Long JD: Strongyloidiasis colitis: A case report and review of the literature. J Clin Gastroenterol 28(1):77–80, 1999.
15. Genta RM: Dysregulation of strongyloidiasis: A new hypothesis. Clin Microbiol Rev 5(4):345–55, 1992.
16. Palau LA, Pankey GA: Strongyloides hyperinfection in a renal transplant recipient receiving cyclosporine: Possible Strongyloides stercoralis transmission by kidney transplant. Am J Trop Med Hyg 57(4):413–5, 1997.
17. Link K, Orenstein R: Bacterial complications of strongyloidiasis: Streptococcus bovis meningitis. South Med J 92(7):728–31, 1999.
18. Klein RA, Cleri DJ, Doshi V, Brasitus TA: Disseminated Strongyloides stercoralis: A fatal case eluding diagnosis. South Med J 76(11):1438–40, 1983.
19. Jongwutiwes S, Charoenkorn M, Sitthichareonchai P, et al: Increased sensitivity of routine laboratory detection of Strongyloides stercoralis and hookworm by agar-plate culture. Trans R Soc Trop Med Hyg 93(4):398–400, 1999.
20. Cross JH: Intestinal capillariasis. Clin Microbiol Rev 5(2):120–9, 1992.
21. Detels R, Gutman L, Jaramillo J, et al: An epidemic of intestinal capillariasis in man. A study in a Barrio in Northern Luzon. Am J Trop Med Hyg 18(5):676–82, 1969.
22. Cross JH, Banzon T, Clarke MD, et al: Studies on the experimental transmission of Capillaria philippinensis in monkeys. Trans R Soc Trop Med Hyg 66(6):819–27, 1972.
23. Kappus KD, Lundgren RGJ, Juranek DD, et al: Intestinal parasitism in the United States: Update on a continuing problem. Am J Trop Med Hyg 50(6):705–13, 1994.
24. Nawalinski TA, Schad GA: Arrested development in Ancylostoma duodenale: Course of a self-induced infection in man. Am J Trop Med Hyg 23(5):895–8, 1974.
25. Stassens P, Bergum PW, Gansemans Y, et al: Anticoagulant repertoire of the hookworm Ancylostoma caninum. Proc Natl Acad Sci USA 93(5):2149–54, 1996.
26. Chadderdon RC, Cappello M: The hookworm platelet inhibitor: functional blockade of integrins GPIIb/IIIa (alphaIIbbeta3) and GPIa/IIa (alpha2beta1) inhibits platelet aggregation and adhesion in vitro. J Infect Dis 179(5):1235–41, 1999.
27. Roche M, Layrisse M: The nature and causes of "hookworm anemia." Am J Trop Med Hyg 15(6):1029–102, 1966.
28. Stoltzfus RJ, Dreyfuss ML, Chwaya HM, Albonico M: Hookworm control as a strategy to prevent iron deficiency. Nutr Rev 55(6):223–32, 1997.
29. Khoshoo V, Schantz P, Craver R, et al: Dog hookworm: A cause of eosinophilic enterocolitis in humans. J Pediatr Gastroenterol Nutr 19(4):448–52, 1994.
30. Croese J, Loukas A, Opdebeeck J, Prociv P: Occult enteric infection by Ancylostoma caninum: A previously unrecognized zoonosis. Gastroenterology 106(1):3–12, 1994.
31. Walker NI, Croese J, Clouston AD, et al: Eosinophilic enteritis in northeastern Australia. Pathology, association with Ancylostoma caninum, and implications. Am J Surg Pathol 19(3):328–37, 1995.
32. Croese J, Fairley S, Loukas A, et al: A distinctive aphthous ileitis linked to Ancylostoma caninum. J Gastroenterol Hepatol 11(6):524–31, 1996.
33. Ratard RC, Kouemeni LE, Ekani BM, et al: Ascariasis and trichuriasis in Cameroon. Trans R Soc Trop Med Hyg 85(1):84–8, 1991.
34. Bundy DA, Cooper ES, Thompson DE, et al: Predisposition to Trichuris trichiura infection in humans. Epidemiol Infect 98(1):65–71, 1987.
35. Jung RC, Beaver PC: Clinical Observations on Trichocephalus trichiurus (whipworm) infestation in children. Pediatrics 85:48–57, 1951.
36. Cooper ES, Bundy DA, MacDonald TT, Golden MH: Growth suppression in the Trichuris dysentery syndrome. Eur J Clin Nutr 44(4):285–91, 1990.
37. MacDonald TT, Choy MY, Spencer J, et al: Histopathology and immunohistochemistry of the caecum in children with the Trichuris dysentery syndrome. J Clin Pathol 44(3):194–9, 1991.
38. Cooper ES, Spencer J, Whyte-Alleng CA, et al: Immediate hypersensitivity in colon of children with chronic Trichuris trichiura dysentery. Lancet 338(8775):1104–7, 1991.

39. MacDonald TT, Spencer J, Murch SH, et al: Immunoepidemiology of intestinal helminthic infections. 3. Mucosal macrophages and cytokine production in the colon of children with Trichuris trichiura dysentery. Trans R Soc Trop Med Hyg 88(3):265–8, 1994.
40. Else KJ, Hultner L, Grencis RK: Cellular immune responses to the murine nematode parasite Trichuris muris. II. Differential induction of TH-cell subsets in resistant versus susceptible mice. Immunology 75(2):232–7, 1992.
41. Else KJ, Finkelman FD, Maliszewski CR, Grencis RK: Cytokine-mediated regulation of chronic intestinal helminth infection. J Exp Med 179(1):347–51, 1994.
42. Ismail MM, Jayakody RL: Efficacy of albendazole and its combinations with ivermectin or diethylcarbamazine (DEC) in the treatment of Trichuris trichiura infections in Sri Lanka. Ann Trop Med Parasitol 93(5):501–4, 1999.
43. Fry GF, Moore JG: Enterobius vermicularis: 10,000 year old human infection. Science 166:1620, 1969.
44. Hugot JP: Enterobius gregorii (Oxyuridae, Nematoda), a new human parasite. Ann Parasitol Hum Comparee 358(4):403–4, 1983.
45. Chittenden AM, Ashford RW: Enterobius gregorii Hugot 1983; first report in the U.K. Ann Trop Med Parasitol 81(2):195–8, 1987.
46. Vermund SH, MacLeod S: Is pinworm a vanishing infection? Laboratory surveillance in a New York City medical center from 1971 to 1986. Am J Dis Child 142(5):566–8, 1988.
47. Liu LX, Chi J, Upton MP, Ash LR: Eosinophilic colitis associated with larvae of the pinworm Enterobius vermicularis. Lancet 346(8972):410–2, 1995.
48. Sinniah B, Leopairut J, Neafie RC, et al: Enterobiasis: A histopathological study of 259 patients. Ann Trop Med Parasitol 85(6):625–35, 1991.
49. Appleyard GD, Zarlenga D, Pozio E, Gajadhar AA: Differentiation of Trichinella genotypes by polymerase chain reaction using sequence-specific primers. J Parasitol 85(3):556–9, 1999.
50. Moorhead A, Grunenwald PE, Dietz VJ, Schantz PM: Trichinellosis in the United States, 1991–1996: Declining but not gone. Am J Trop Med Hyg 60(1):66–9, 1999.
51. Hinz E: Trichinellosis and trichinellosis control in Germany. Southeast Asian J Trop Med Public Health 22 Suppl:329–33, 1991.
52. Ancelle T, Dupouy-Camet J, Desenclos JC, et al: A multifocal outbreak of trichinellosis linked to horse meat imported from North America to France in 1993. Am J Trop Med Hyg 59(4):615–9, 1998.
53. Despommier DD: Trichinella spiralis and the concept of niche. J Parasitol 79(4):472–82, 1993.
54. Capo V, Despommier DD: Clinical aspects of infection with Trichinella spp. Clin Microbiol Rev 9(1):47–54, 1996.
55. Ikeda K, Kumashiro R, Kifune T: Nine cases of acute gastric anisakiasis. Gastrointest Endosc 35(4):304–8, 1998.
56. Deardorff TL, Kayes SG, Fukumura T: Human anisakiasis transmitted by marine food products. Hawaii Med J 50(1):9–16, 1991.
57. Kark AE, McAlpine JC: Anisakiasis ('herring worm disease') as a cause of acute abdominal crisis. Br J Clin Pract 48(4):216–7, 1994.
58. del Pozo MD, Moneo I, de Corres LF, et al: Laboratory determinations in Anisakis simplex allergy. J Allergy Clin Immunol 97(4):977–84, 1996.
59. Boreham RE, McCowan MJ, Ryan AE, et al: Human trichostrongyliasis in Queensland. Pathology 27(2):182–5, 1995.
60. Schantz PM: Tapeworms (cestodiasis). Gastroenterol Clin North Am 25(3):637–53, 1996.
61. Centers for Disease Control and Prevention: Recommendations of the International Task Force for Disease Eradication. MMWR 421–46, 1993.
62. Garcia HH, Del Brutto OH: Taenia solium cysticercosis. Infect Dis Clin North Am 14(1):97–119, 2000.
63. Khalil HM, el Shimi S, Sarwat MA, et al: Recent study of Hymenolepis nana infection in Egyptian children. J Egypt Soc Parasitol 21(1): 293–300, 1991.
64. Reynoldson JA, Behnke JM, Pallant LJ, et al: Failure of pyrantel in treatment of human hookworm infections (Ancylostoma duodenale) in the Kimberley region of north west Australia. Acta Trop 68(3):301–12, 1997.
65. Chu GS, Palmieri JR, Sullivan JT: Beetle-eating: A Malaysia folk medical practice and its public health implications. Tropical Geographical Medicine 29(4):422–7, 1977.
66. Asano K, Okamoto K: Murine T cell clones specific for Hymenolepis nana: Generation and functional analysis in vivo and in vitro. Int J Parasitol 21(8):891–6, 1991.
67. Asano K, Muramatsu K: Importance of interferon-gamma in protective immunity against Hymenolepis nana cysticercoids derived from challenge infection with eggs in BALB/c mice. Int J Parasitol 27(11): 1437–43, 1997.
68. Watanabe N, Nawa Y, Okamoto K, Kobayashi A: Expulsion of Hymenolepis nana from mice with congenital deficiencies of IgE production or of mast cell development. Parasite Immunol 16(3):137–44, 1994.
69. Conchedda M, Bortoletti G, Gabriele F, et al: Immune response to the cestode Hymenolepis nana: Cytokine production during infection with eggs or cysts. Int J Parasitol 27(3):321–7, 1997.
70. Liu LX, Harinasuta KT: Liver and intestinal flukes. Gastroenterol Clin North Am 25(3):627–36, 1996.
71. Plaut AG, Kampanart-Sanyakorn C, Manning GS: A clinical study of Fasciolopsis buski infection in Thailand. Trans R Soc Trop Med Hyg 63(4):470–8, 1969.
72. Jaroonvesama N, Charoenlarp K, Areekul S: Intestinal absorption studies in Fasciolopsis buski infection. Southeast Asian J Trop Med Public Health 17(4):582–6, 1986.
73. Sadun EH, Maiphoom C: Studies on the epidemiology of the human intestinal fluke, Fasciolopsis buski (Lankester) in central Thailand. Am J Trop Med Hyg 2:1070–84, 1953.
74. Adams KO, Jungkind DL, Bergquist EJ, Wirts CW: Intestinal fluke infection as a result of eating sushi. Am J Clin Pathol 86(5):688–9, 1986.
75. Huffman JE, Fried B: Echinostoma and echinostomiasis. Adv Parasitol 29:215–69, 1990.
76. Poland GA, Navin TR, Sarosi GA: Outbreak of parasitic gastroenteritis among travelers returning from Africa. Arch Intern Med 145(12):2220–1, 1985.
77. Koenigstein RP: Observations on the epidemiology of infections with Clonorchis sinensis. Trans R Soc Trop Med Hyg 42:503–6, 1949.
78. Anonymous: Infection with liver flukes (Opisthorchis viverrini, Opisthorchis felineus and Clonorchis sinensis). IARC Monographs on the Evaluation of Carcinogenic Risks to Humans 61:121–75, 1994.
79. Gibson JB: Parasites, liver disease and liver cancer. IARC Scientific Publications 1971, pp 142–50.
80. Kim YI, Yang DH, Chang KR: Relationship between Clonorchis sinensis infestation and cholangiocarcinoma of the liver in Korea. Seoul J Med 15:247–53, 1974.
81. Chung CS, Lee SK: An epidemiological study of primary liver carcinomas in Busan area with special reference to clonorchiasis. Korean J Pathol 10:33–46, 1976.
82. Parkin DM, Srivatanakul P, Khlat M, et al: Liver cancer in Thailand. I. A case-control study of cholangiocarcinoma. Int J Cancer 48(3):323–8, 1991.
83. Haswell-Elkins MR, Mairiang E, Mairiang P, et al: Cross-sectional study of Opisthorchis viverrini infection and cholangiocarcinoma in communities within a high-risk area in northeast Thailand. Int J Cancer 59(4):505–9, 1994.
84. Kim YI: Liver carcinoma and liver fluke infection. Arzneimittel-Forschung 34(9B):1121–6, 1984.
85. Haswell-Elkins MR, Satarug S, Elkins DB: Opisthorchis viverrini infection in northeast Thailand and its relationship to cholangiocarcinoma. J Gastroenterol Hepatol 7(5):538–48, 1992.
86. Kammerer WS, Van Der Decker JD, Keith TB, Mott KE: Clonorchiasis in New York City Chinese. Trop Doc 7(3):105–6, 1977.
87. Schwartz DA: Cholangiocarcinoma associated with liver fluke infection: a preventable source of morbidity in Asian immigrants. Am J Gastroenterol 81(1):76–9, 1986.
88. Leung JW, Sung JY, Chung SC, Metreweli C: Hepatic clonorchiasis—a study by endoscopic retrograde cholangiopancreatography. Gastrointest Endosc 35(3):226–31, 1989.
89. Harinasuta T, Pungpak S, Keystone JS: Trematode infections. Opisthorchiasis, clonorchiasis, fascioliasis, and paragonimiasis. Infect Dis Clin North Am 7(3):699–716, 1993.
90. Reinhard GH, Graf V, Augustin HJ: Chronic fascioliasis with destructive cholangitis. Fortschr Med 109(36):737–8, 1991.
91. Arjona R, Riancho JA, Aguado JM, et al: Fascioliasis in developed countries: A review of classic and aberrant forms of the disease. Medicine 74(1):13–23, 1995.
92. Veerappan A, Siegel JH, Podany J, et al: Fasciola hepatica pancreatitis: endoscopic extraction of live parasites. Gastrointest Endosc 37(4): 473–5, 1991.
93. Hillyer GV, Soler de Galanes M, Rodriguez-Perez J, et al: Use of the

Falcon assay screening test—enzyme-linked immunosorbent assay (FAST-ELISA) and the enzyme-linked immunoelectrotransfer blot (EITB) to determine the prevalence of human fascioliasis in the Bolivian Altiplano. Am J Trop Med Hyg 46(5):603–9, 1992.
94. Apt W, Aguilera X, Vega F, et al: Treatment of human chronic fascioliasis with triclabendazole: Drug efficacy and serologic response. Am J Trop Med Hyg 52(6):532–5, 1995.
95. Sene M, Bremond P, Herve JP, et al: Comparison of human and murine isolates of Schistosoma mansoni from Richard-Toll, Senegal, by isoelectric focusing. J Helminthol 71(2):175–81, 1997.
96. Hillyer GV, Soler DG: Seroepidemiology of schistosomiasis in Puerto Rico: Evidence for vanishing endemicity. Am J Trop Med Hyg 60(5): 827–30, 1999.
97. Kolarova L, Skirnisson K, Horak P: Schistosome cercariae as the causative agent of swimmer's itch in Iceland. J Helminthol 73(3):215–20, 1999.
98. Fishelson Z: Novel mechanisms of immune evasion by Schistosoma mansoni. Mem Inst Oswaldo Cruz 90(2):289–92, 1995.
99. Hornstein L, Lederer G, Schechter J, et al: Persistent Schistosoma mansoni infection in Yemeni immigrants to Israel. Israel J Med Sci 26(7):386–9, 1990.
100. Doenhoff MJ, Hassounah O, Murare H, et al: The schistosome egg granuloma: Immunopathology in the cause of host protection or parasite survival? Trans R Soc Trop Med Hyg 80(4):503–14, 1986.
101. el-Masry NA, Farid Z, Bassily S, et al: Schistosomal colonic polyposis: clinical, radiological and parasitological study. J Trop Med Hyg 89(1):13–7, 1986.
102. Doehring-Schwerdtfeger E, Abdel-Rahim IM, Kardorff R, et al: Ultrasonographical investigation of periportal fibrosis in children with Schistosoma mansoni infection: Reversibility of morbidity twenty-three months after treatment with praziquantel. Am J Trop Med Hyg 46(4):409–15, 1992.
103. Rocha H, Kirk JW, Hearey CD Jr: Prolonged Salmonella bacteremia in patients with Schistosoma mansoni infection. Arch Intern Med 128(2):254–7, 1971.
104. Martinelli R, Pereira LJ, Brito E, Rocha H: Clinical course of focal segmental glomerulosclerosis associated with hepatosplenic schistosomiasis mansoni. Nephron 69(2):131–4, 1995.
105. Elliott DE: Schistosomiasis. Pathophysiology, diagnosis, and treatment. Gastroenterol Clin North Am 25(3):599-625, 1996.
106. Sanguino J, Peixe R, Guerra J, et al: Schistosomiasis and vascular alterations of the colonic mucosa. Hepato-Gastroenterology 40(2):184–7, 1993.
107. Abdel-Hafez MA, Bolbol AH: Fibre-optic sigmoidoscopy compared with the Kato technique in diagnosis and evaluation of the intensity of Schistosoma mansoni infection. Trans R Soc Trop Med Hyg 86(6): 641–3, 1992.
108. Tsang VC, Wilkins PP: Immunodiagnosis of schistosomiasis. Immunol Invest 26(1–2):175–88, 1997.
109. de Jonge N, Kremsner PG, Krijger FW, et al: Detection of the schistosome circulating cathodic antigen by enzyme immunoassay using biotinylated monoclonal antibodies. Trans R Soc Trop Med Hyg 84(6):815–8, 1990.
110. van Lieshout L, Panday UG, de Jonge N, et al: Immunodiagnosis of schistosomiasis mansoni in a low endemic area in Surinam by determination of the circulating antigens CAA and CCA. Acta Trop 59(1):19–29, 1995.
111. De Clercq D, Sacko M, Vercruysse J, et al: Assessment of cure by detection of circulating antigens in serum and urine, following schistosomiasis mass treatment in two villages of the Office du Niger, Mali. Acta Trop 68(3):339–46, 1997.
112. Abdel-Wahab MF, Esmat G, Milad M, et al: Characteristic sonographic pattern of schistosomal hepatic fibrosis. Am J Trop Med Hyg 40(1):72–6, 1990.
113. Abdel-Wahab MF, Esmat G, Farrag A, et al: Ultrasonographic prediction of esophageal varices in Schistosomiasis mansoni. Am J Gastroenterol 88(4):560–3, 1993.

Chapter 100

Eosinophilic Gastroenteritis

Nicholas J. Talley

Eosinophilic gastroenteritis is a disease characterized by tissue eosinophilia that can involve any layer or layers of the gut wall. The term, however, is a misnomer; eosinophilic gastroenteritis, like Crohn's disease, may involve any segment of the gastrointestinal (GI) tract, from the esophagus to the rectum. Because therapy is available, it is an important disease to recognize.[1–4]

DEFINITION AND INCIDENCE

Kaijser[5] is credited with the first description of eosinophilic gastroenteritis in 1937; localized jejunal swelling attributed to an allergy to neoarsphenamine developed in two patients with syphilis. In one of the two patients, eosinophilic infiltration was demonstrated, whereas a third patient with a history of allergy to onions presented with pyloric channel disease. Since the first description by Kaijser, the definition of eosinophilic gastroenteritis has been refined. A definite diagnosis must fulfill the following criteria: (1) the presence of GI symptoms, (2) demonstration of eosinophilic infiltration of one or more areas of the GI tract on biopsy, (3) absence of eosinophilic involvement of multiple organs outside the GI tract, and (4) absence of parasitic infestation.[4] Peripheral blood eosinophilia is absent in at least 20% of patients and should not be considered a diagnostic criterion.[4] Furthermore, food intolerance or allergy is not required for the diagnosis, because many patients have no objective evidence of these problems.[4]

The disease is rare; although increasing numbers of cases have been reported in the medical literature,[1–4, 6–8] the incidence is difficult to estimate, because some patients are probably undiagnosed and surely unreported.[4] Patients typically present in the third through fifth decades of life, but the disease can affect any age group. An equal gender distribution or a slight male preponderance has been reported.[4]

PATHOGENESIS

The cause of eosinophilic gastroenteritis is unknown, and the pathogenesis is poorly understood. It is conceivable that this is not one but rather several disorders that manifest similar histopathologic features. Recent data suggest that in eosinophilic gastroenteritis, eosinophils may directly damage the GI tract wall. Tissue eosinophilia is the hallmark of eosinophilic gastroenteritis. Normally, after eosinophils leave the circulation, they preferentially distribute to the stomach and small bowel. In health, eosinophils are part of the normal inflammatory cells that populate the entire gut. It is likely that eosinophils play a role in the upper gut in immediate hypersensitivity reactions.[9, 10] Eosinophil granules contain a number of cationic proteins, including the major basic protein (MBP), eosinophil-derived neurotoxin, eosinophil cationic protein, and eosinophil peroxidase.[9–11] MBP, a low-molecular-weight polypeptide that has been localized to the cores of both the guinea pig and the human eosinophil granules, accounts for more than 50% of the eosinophil granule protein.[12]

Substantial data indicate that once released, the cationic granular proteins of eosinophils can produce tissue destruction directly and perhaps through the synthesis of leukotrienes.[13] In parasitic disease, release of eosinophil granules disrupts the external membrane of the parasite, probably by activating powerful membrane effector systems.[14] In the presence of specific antibody, eosinophils also can lyse mammalian cells.[9, 10] In guinea pigs, these proteins are toxic to intestinal epithelial cells.[15]

In one study, use of a monoclonal antibody to the secreted form of eosinophil cationic protein demonstrated that the presence of activated degranulating eosinophils in the small bowel of two teenage siblings with eosinophilic gastroenteritis correlated with the degree of histologic damage.[16] In another patient, the electron core density of eosinophil granules had inverted or disappeared (suggesting release of the toxic cationic proteins) in damaged areas of the duodenum.[17] Striking but variable release of MBP into the damaged gut in patients with eosinophilic gastroenteritis has been confirmed in controlled studies,[18, 19] although eosinophils can degranulate modestly in normal intestinal mucosa.[18, 20] In humans, degranulated eosinophils also have been demonstrated in tissue granulomas in patients with the Churg-Strauss syndrome[21] and in organs affected by the hypereosinophilic syndrome.[22]

What triggers eosinophilic infiltration and degranulation with subsequent tissue damage is largely unknown. An allergic cause has been postulated.[3, 4, 23–26] The tissue and blood eosinophilia, increased incidence of allergic disorders, elevated IgE levels, and response to glucocorticoids in affected patients support the hypothesis of a type I hypersensitivity reaction to certain foods. In sensitized people, IgE is bound to mast cells at the Fc receptor sites; specific food antigens could react with these mast cells, thereby resulting in degranulation, and the released mast cell products such as eosinophil chemotactic factor of anaphylaxis and platelet-activating factor could in turn attract eosinophils to these sites (see Chapter 101).[3] There is also evidence that eosinophil degranulation can directly initiate mast cell degranulation; thus, by noncytotoxic mechanisms, MBP stimulates histamine release from mast cells and basophils.[27, 28] Eosinophil peroxidase also can induce the release of histamine from mast cells.[29] Eosinophils contain interleukin-3 and -5 and granulocyte-macrophage colony stimulating factor; release of these cytokines in eosinophilic gastroenteritis appears to lead to further recruitment and activation of eosinophils.[30, 31] Finally, the cytokine tumor necrosis factor-α has been identified in the secretory granules of eosinophils and may promote tissue inflammation.[32] Therefore, a vicious cycle may be induced whereby specific food antigens induce mast cell degranulation, activated eosinophils are attracted to the area, and eosinophil degranulation products are released and not only damage the gut wall, but also cause further mast cell degranulation (Fig. 100–1).

Many patients with eosinophilic gastroenteritis report food intolerance or allergy or a past or family history of allergy. To firmly establish food allergy as a cause of eosinophilic gastroenteritis, certain criteria must be fulfilled, first defined by Ingelfinger and associates.[33] Symptoms must invariably follow contact with a specific food substance that is harmless to most people, immune mechanisms should be evident, other possible pathogenetic mechanisms should be absent, and lesions or functional abnormalities should be demonstrable after contact. In adults with eosinophilic gastroenteritis, only occasional patients with an unequivocal allergy to dietary allergens have been reported,[2, 34–38] although young children may have a different disease process in which allergy to food plays a key role (see Chapter 101).[39] Indeed, Leinbach and Rubin[40] described a 23-year-old man with eosinophilic gastroenteritis in whom symptoms could be reproduced by food but tissue eosinophilia was not identifiable. In support of the notion that mast cell degranulation contributes to the pathogenesis, immunohistochemical studies in the stomach of a 50-year-old Japanese man with eosinophilic gastroenteritis and food allergy revealed many IgE-staining mast cells scattered among the eosinophilic infiltrate.[37] However, other investigators have not shown an increased number of mast cells in the eosinophilic infiltrates of patients with idiopathic eosinophilic gastroenteritis.[41–43] Furthermore, the removal of implicated dietary factors seldom leads to total resolution of the disease.[4, 40] Therefore, it is possible

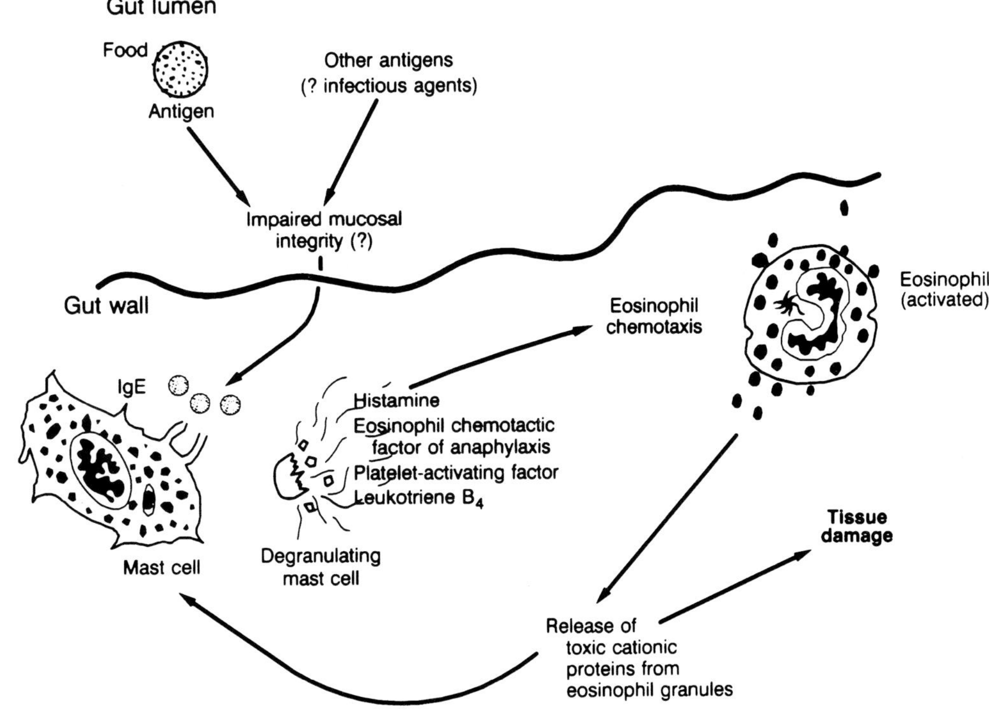

Figure 100–1. Hypothetical scheme of the pathophysiology of eosinophilic gastroenteritis. In the predisposed patient with a loss of integrity of the mucosal lining, food (or other) antigen passes through the mucosa and binds to two molecules of mast cell–bound IgE. Mast cell degranulation occurs, and the cell products attract activated eosinophilis to the site. Degranulation of eosinophils releases toxic cationic granular proteins that directly damage the host tissue and lead to further mast cell degranulation. (Adapted from Cello JP: Eosinophilic gastroenteritis—a complex disease entity. Am J Med 67:1097, 1979; and Talley NJ, Kephart GM, McGovern TW, et al. Deposition of eosinophil granule major basic protein in eosinophilic gastroenteritis and celiac disease. Gastroenterology 103:137, 1992.)

that the primary defect in eosinophilic gastroenteritis is a disturbance of epithelial integrity that permits the entry of many types of food and nonfood antigens, which induce eosinophilia in the gut wall and peripheral blood (see Fig. 100–1).

Unrecognized parasitic infestation may explain some cases of eosinophilic gastroenteritis.[44–46] In Queensland, Australia, the canine hookworm *Ancylostoma caninum* has been implicated in a major outbreak of eosinophilic enteritis; unlike classic eosinophilic gastroenteritis, almost all patients had ileal or colonic disease, few had proximal small bowel involvement, and none had gastric disease. Occult infestation, as determined by enzyme-linked immunosorbent assay, was detected in 71% of patients with documented disease compared with 8% of control subjects, despite the absence of parasitic disease on routine testing.[44] Of note, 80% of affected patients in this study were dog owners. *A. caninum* is present worldwide, and cases in the United States have now been reported.[47] *Enterobius vermicularis* was implicated as the cause of eosinophilic colitis in a homosexual male patient, based on cloning of nematode RNA.[48] Enterobiasis is widely prevalent but has not been implicated previously as a cause of eosinophilic gastroenteritis. Other undiscovered zoonoses also may conceivably play a role (see Chapters 98 and 99). Human immunodeficiency virus associated eosinophilic gastroenteritis, possibly resulting from disordered IgE regulation, has been reported.[49]

Exposure to a drug or toxin is the cause in a few cases of eosinophilic gastroenteritis.[50–54] Two cases in children on cyclosporine after liver transplantation have been reported, despite concurrent use of prednisone.[55] The *toxic-oil syndrome*, linked to an unlabeled illegally marketed cooking oil in Spain, was associated with striking tissue eosinophilia.[56] Similarly, some patients with the *eosinophilic-myalgia syndrome* associated with ingestion of L-tryptophan had GI tract eosinophilia.[57]

CLASSIFICATION AND CLINICAL FEATURES

Any segment of the GI tract may be involved, including the esophagus[58–60] or colon,[61, 62] but most commonly the stomach or small bowel is affected.[1–4, 6, 7, 41, 58] The clinical features typically are intermittent but often long-standing; cases have been reported in which disease was present for over 30 years.[63, 64] Up to one third of patients have self-limited disease (4 weeks or less) and do not require treatment.[7]

A pathologic and clinical classification of eosinophilic gastroenteritis has been proposed based on the predominant layer of the gut wall involved.[2] Although the clinical and pathologic features often overlap, because multiple layers of the gut wall can be affected,[4] it seems conceptually useful to separate the disease into that affecting the mucosal, muscle, or subserosal layer (Table 100–1).

The most prevalent form is characterized by predominantly *mucosal (and submucosal) disease* (Fig. 100–2).[2, 4, 65] Symptoms typically include colicky abdominal pain, nausea, vomiting, diarrhea, and weight loss. About 50% of patients have a past or family history of allergy (including atopy, asthma, nasal polyps, or hay fever), and 50% report a history of food intolerance or allergy. There may be evidence of iron-deficiency anemia, protein-losing enteropathy, or malabsorption. Acute pancreatitis secondary to swelling of the region of the duodenum around the ampulla of Vater has been described.[66]

In children, an allergic history is even more common, and the condition has been termed *allergic gastroenteropathy*.[39] Children or adolescents can present with growth failure, delayed puberty, or amenorrhea, and physical examination may

Table 100–1 | **Classification of Eosinophilic Infiltrations Confined to the Gastrointestinal Tract**

Eosinophilic gastroenteritis
Predominant mucosal layer disease
Pain, nausea, vomiting, diarrhea, weight loss
Iron-deficiency anemia
Malabsorption
Protein-losing enteropathy
Predominant muscle layer disease
Obstruction
Predominant subserosal layer disease
Eosinophilic ascites
Parasitic infestations
Drugs
Connective tissue disease or vasculitis
Systemic mastocytosis
Crohn's disease
Celiac sprue
Cancer
Cow's milk protein sensitivity

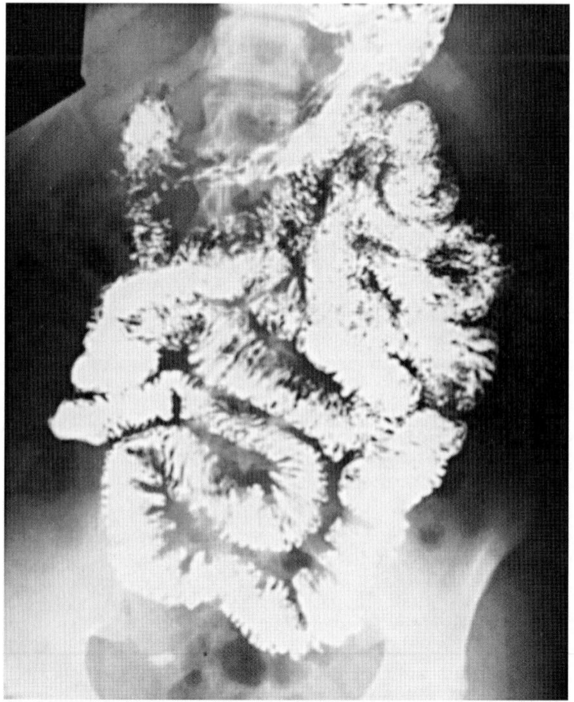

Figure 100–2. Upper gastrointestinal series with small bowel follow-through showing diffusely thickened small bowel folds with nodularity in eosinophilic gastroenteritis. Note concomitant gastric involvement. (From MacCarty RL, Talley NJ: Barium studies in diffuse eosinophilic gastroenteritis. Gastrointest Radiol 15:183, 1990.)

reveal evidence of nutritional deficiencies. Atopic dermatitis or urticaria are uncommon. Disease characterized by increased numbers of eosinophils, mast cells, and IgE-containing plasma cells has been described in the colon and rectum of young children; this disorder is termed *allergic proctitis* and is probably a different disease process that responds to a change in diet (see Chapter 101).[67, 68]

Patients with disease predominantly affecting the *muscle layer* typically present with pyloric or upper intestinal obstruction; associated mucosal or serosal involvement is not uncommon. Cecal obstruction also has been reported.[69] Involvement of the muscle layer most often is localized but sometimes diffuse, involving the stomach and small bowel. Crampy abdominal pain associated with nausea and vomiting is frequent and is related to the thickened and rigid bowel, which may obstruct the lumen. Food intolerance or allergy is unusual, and a past or family history of allergy is less common than with mucosal disease.[2, 4, 35]

The rarest form is *serosal disease*; all layers of the bowel wall usually are involved, and patients typically present with eosinophilic ascites.[2, 4, 70] Serosal and visceral peritoneal inflammation (perhaps secondary to the destructive effects of released eosinophil granule proteins) leads to weeping of fluid, as occurs in peritoneal carcinomatosis. Only rarely is mucosal involvement absent when serosal disease is present.[70] An allergic history appears to be common in this group.[70]

DIAGNOSIS

Laboratory Studies

Peripheral blood eosinophilia is found in about 80% of patients; the absolute eosinophil count (normal range, 0 to 500 cells/μL) averages 2000 cells/μL in patients with mucosal disease and 1000 cells/μL in patients with disease of the muscle layer, although the count may fluctuate markedly over time.[4] Patients with serosal disease almost always have marked blood eosinophilia, averaging 8000 cells/μL, although rarely the peripheral eosinophil count is normal.[4, 71] The differential diagnosis of a peripheral blood eosinophilia in association with GI symptoms includes *drugs* (e.g., aspirin, sulfonamides, penicillin, cephalosporins), *parasites, vasculitis, lymphoma*, and *Addison's disease*. Asthma and allergic rhinitis are common in the general population, frequently cause peripheral eosinophilia, and may confound the clinical picture of a patient with suspected eosinophilic gastroenteritis.

Iron-deficiency anemia can develop, probably from blood loss with mucosal disease. The serum albumin level also may be low in 20% to 30% of cases, usually in patients with predominantly mucosal disease.[4, 38] Protein loss from the gut can be measured by ^{51}Cr-labeled albumin or α_1-antitypsin clearance[72]; severe protein loss in eosinophilic gastroenteritis can result in low immunoglobulin levels (see Chapter 25). The serum IgE level may be elevated, particularly in children.[55] The erythrocyte sedimentation rate is not always normal, as some have suggested,[3] but may be moderately elevated.[4]

Stool Studies

In all cases, stool studies must be done to exclude parasitic infestation. A wet mount or stained smear should be obtained first; the diagnostic yield is maximized if three separate specimens are collected at intervals of 2 to 3 days. Charcot-Leyden crystals (caused by the release from eosinophils of a plasma membrane lysophospholipase enzyme that crystallizes) may be seen in the stools, but their sensitivity and specificity in detecting eosinophilic gastroenteritis are unknown; they often are present with severe mucosal disease. The stools may be positive for occult blood, but this finding is not of discriminating value. Mild-to-moderate steatorrhea is present in up to 30% of cases.[4]

Radiographic Studies

The radiographic changes found in eosinophilic gastroenteritis are variable, nonspecific, and absent in at least 40% of patients.[73, 74] Abnormalities predominate in the stomach and small intestine. The gastric folds can be enlarged, with or without nodular filling defects (see Fig. 100–2). The differential diagnosis includes *granulomatous gastritis, Ménétrier's disease, gastric hypersecretory states, lymphoma*, and *carcinoma* (see Chapters 26, 39, 41, 43, and 44). In disease of the muscle layer, there may be localized involvement of the antrum and pylorus, with narrowing of the distal antrum and occasionally gastric retention.

Thickening of the folds with or without nodules may be seen with small intestinal disease (see Fig. 100–2). The differential diagnosis includes *lymphoma, Whipple's disease, amyloidosis, giardiasis, paraproteinemia*, and *intestinal lymphangiectasia* (see Chapters 25, 26, 29, 95, 99, and 113). The small intestine also may be dilated. Occasionally, the ileum resembles the jejunum because of an increase in the thickness of the ileal folds, as is seen also in some patients with celiac sprue. Prominent mucosal folds may also be seen in the colon. Rarely, diffuse esophageal narrowing, at times with motor incoordination or an achalasia-like picture, has been observed.[75]

Computed tomography may demonstrate a thickened intestinal wall and localized mesenteric lymphadenopathy; with serosal involvement, ascitic fluid usually is detected.[76]

Endoscopy and Biopsy

At endoscopy, the mucosa may be normal or there may be prominent mucosal folds, hyperemia, ulceration, or nodularity.[65] Histologic evaluation of samples from involved areas represents the best way to make a firm diagnosis. Because the disease may affect different layers of the gut wall and tends to be patchy,[4, 40] it is recommended that, in suspected cases, multiple endoscopic biopsies be obtained from the stomach and small bowel, the areas most likely to have pathologic abnormalities (see also Fig. 43–7*B*). The biopsies should be taken from normal and, if present, abnormal areas; at least six specimens should be obtained.[3, 4] If small bowel parasitic infection, such as giardiasis or strongyloidiasis, is suspected, a duodenal aspirate also should be obtained, be-

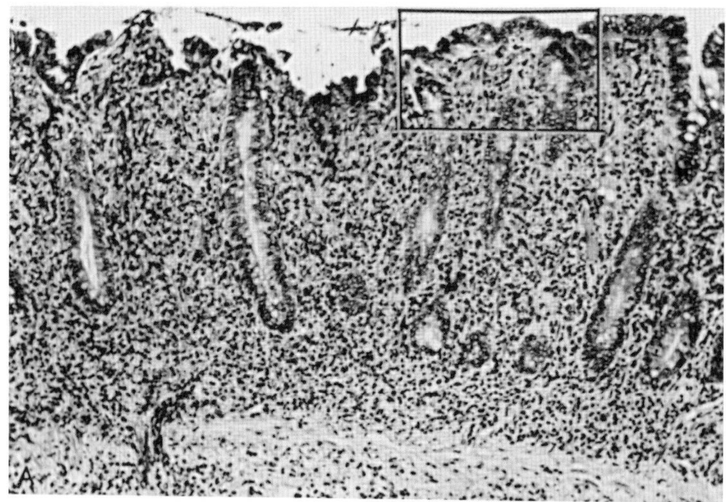

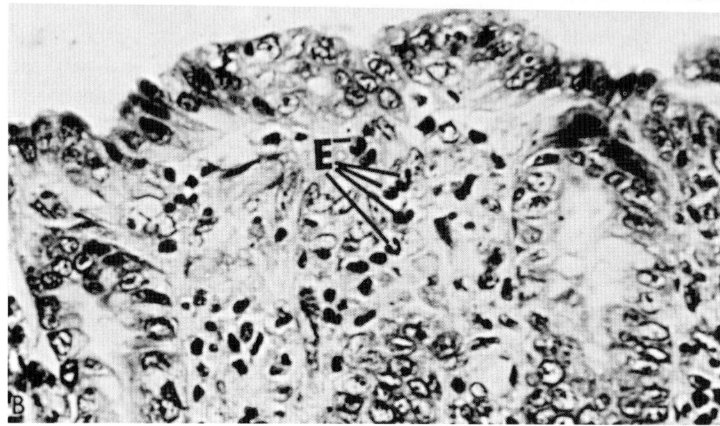

Figure 100–3. *A,* Small bowel suction biopsy specimen revealing absence of villi and massive infiltration of the lamina propria with eosinophils (eosinophilic enteritis). Hematoxylin and eosin stain; magnification ×100. *B,* Enlargement of boxed area in *A.* Note the surface epithelial abnormalities and the eosinophils (*E*). (From Lienbach GE, Rubin CE: Eosinophilic gastroenteritis: A simple reaction to food allergens? Gastroenterology 59:874, 1970. Copyright by the American Gastroenterological Association.)

cause at times it is the only way to establish the diagnosis of a parasitic disease.

In patients with esophageal or colonic symptoms, diagnosis may require additional biopsies from the relevant sites.[77] Gastroesophageal reflux is the most common cause of tissue eosinophilia in the distal esophagus, especially in children. Eosinophilic infiltration in distal esophageal biopsies occurs in both gastroesophageal reflux and true eosinophilic esophagitis, but superficial clumping of eosinophils histologically and involvement of the mid- or upper esophagus strongly support the latter diagnosis.[60] If the colon or terminal ileum is the site of the disease, aphthous ulcers may be seen; these lesions are found most often in the cecum and ascending colon and may sometimes be caused by worm bites.[45, 46] Rarely, intact hookworms may be observed at colonoscopy.[46]

With sufficient tissue sampling, most cases of eosinophilic gastroenteritis can be identified, and other diseases that may be confused with eosinophilic gastroenteritis can be excluded. In patients with chronic unexplained GI symptoms and peripheral eosinophilia in whom initial biopsies and other tests have not provided a diagnosis, biopsies should be repeated.

Mucosal biopsies are sometimes not helpful, particularly in patients with eosinophilic gastroenteritis confined to the muscle layer. Full-thickness biopsies at laparoscopy may then be required to establish the diagnosis. However, if the clinical, laboratory, and radiologic findings make eosinophilic gastroenteritis highly likely, surgical intervention should be avoided, unless cancer is suspected or persistent pyloric outlet or small bowel obstruction require treatment.

Histology

Histologically, eosinophilic gastroenteritis is characterized by edema and an *inflammatory cell infiltrate that is almost entirely composed of eosinophils*; the eosinophils may occur in clumps.[41, 58] Maximum infiltration of eosinophils is commonly in the submucosa. (Fewer than 25 eosinophils per high-power field are present normally.[4]) There also may be necrosis and regeneration of the surface and glandular epithelium (Fig. 100–3). Immunofluorescent staining for MBP may demonstrate eosinophil degranulation when intact eosinophils are not visible, but this technique is not routinely available.[18] It must be remembered that eosinophils may be a predominant component of almost any inflammatory process; therefore, a substantial increase in the numbers of other inflammatory cells makes the diagnosis of eosinophilic gastroenteritis unlikely.

Abdominal Paracentesis and Laparoscopy

Patients with ascites should have a diagnostic abdominal paracentesis performed. In serosal disease with ascites, the fluid usually is a sterile exudate that contains a high eosinophil count (a smear is needed to differentiate eosinophils from neutrophils); sometimes the fluid is bloody.[4, 70] Serosal eosinophilic gastroenteritis rarely presents as ascites with few eosinophils.[71] An associated pleural effusion may be present. The differential diagnosis of eosinophilic ascites includes *vasculitis, lymphoma, chronic peritoneal dialysis, Toxocara canis* or *Strongyloides stercoralis* infection, a *ruptured hydatid cyst, spontaneous bacterial peritonitis* in cirrhosis, and the *hypereosinophilic syndrome*.[71, 78] Findings at laparoscopy vary from hyperemia to a picture resembling peritoneal carcinomatosis. When the diagnosis is uncertain, laparoscopy is useful, because biopsy material can be obtained.[79]

Other Studies

Hepatic granulomas infiltrated with eosinophils,[63, 64] gallbladder involvement,[80] and cholangitis[62] have been reported in association with eosinophilic gastroenteritis. In rare instances, eosinophilic cystitis may coexist with eosinophilic gastroenteritis.[81] A serologic test for *A. caninum* has been developed, but the diagnostic utility of this enzyme-linked immunosorbent assay has not been established in view of an apparently low sensitivity; furthermore, it has not been evaluated outside Australia.[44]

DIFFERENTIAL DIAGNOSIS

Parasitic Infestations

Helminthic infections characteristically are associated with peripheral eosinophilia, which reflects an immunologic response to tissue migration; however, when migration ceases, the eosinophilia often resolves. Hookworms may present with tissue eosinophilia; eosinophilic ileocolitis is caused by the dog hookworm *A. caninum*.[44–47] The pinworm *Enterobius vermicularis* also may cause eosinophilic colitis.[48] *Eustoma rotundtum*, a herring parasite, has been implicated in GI tract eosinophilic infiltration in a few patients who ate raw herrings.[82] Eosinophilic ascites has occurred with *T. canis*[83] and *S. stercoralis*.[84] *Giardia lamblia* can be associated with a dense eosinophilic infiltration of the jejunum but without peripheral eosinophilia. Stool studies will isolate only some infestations, but sometimes *Giardia* can be recognized by careful examination of histologic sections. The diagnostic yield is highest (90%) with a duodenal aspirate. People who eat raw fish can be infected with *Anisakis*. The larvae may be identified at endoscopy in the stomach in an area of mucosal edema and, in some cases, ulceration.[85] This parasitic infestation may be underdiagnosed; a Spanish study suggested that up to 8 of 10 patients thought to have idiopathic eosinophilic gastroenteritis had evidence of exposure to *Anisakis*, compared with 10% of control subjects.[86] In persons who eat contaminated raw meat, *Trichinella spiralis* can cause eosinophilia and intestinal inflammation; the serum level of creatine kinase, a muscle enzyme, may be elevated, and the disease can be diagnosed serologically. *Schistosomiasis* should be considered in patients with eosinophilia and colonic disease, particularly in those with a history of overseas travel to Africa, the Far East, or South America. *Ascaris* and *Trichuris* can cause eosinophilia and abdominal pain, whereas *Fasciola hepatica* can cause eosinophilia, right upper quadrant pain, fever, and hepatomegaly (see Chapter 99).

Drugs

A drug allergy may result in eosinophilic involvement of the gut. For example, an association between gold salts and the onset of eosinophilic gastroenteritis has been reported.[50] Azathioprine or gemfibrozil may cause intestinal eosinophilia,[51] co-trimoxazole has been linked to eosinophilic ascites,[52] and carbamazepine or clofazimine may induce eosinophilic colitis.[53, 54]

Connective Tissue Disease

Patients with *scleroderma, dermatomyositis*, or *polymyositis* may have a band-like infiltrate of eosinophils and mast cells between the small intestinal crypts and the muscularis mucosae.[42, 43] Cytotoxic changes in the smooth muscle cells, with hyperplasia and scarring of the muscularis mucosae, have been observed in infiltrated areas, but epithelial changes were absent. Episodic peripheral eosinophilia can also occur in scleroderma and dermatomyositis.[42] The other clinical features of these diseases usually allow their differentiation from eosinophilic gastroenteritis (see Chapter 29).

Vasculitis

In *allergic angiitis and granulomatosis* (the *Churg-Strauss syndrome*), an eosinophilic infiltrate involves the small arteries and veins; granulomas can be found in the lungs, heart, kidneys, and subcutaneous tissues and also may occur in the stomach, small bowel, and colon. Patients typically have a long history of asthma and peripheral eosinophilia; the chest radiograph may show diffuse interstitial disease or nodular masses. *Polyarteritis nodosa* also may be associated with eosinophilic infiltration of the bowel.[6, 86] Often there is mucosal thickening from edema. Peripheral eosinophilia is common, the erythrocyte sedimentation rate usually is elevated, and there may be extraintestinal manifestations of the disease, with involvement of the kidney (e.g., hematuria, hypertension), lung (e.g., pneumonitis, effusion), nervous system (e.g., mononeuritis multiplex), or skin. The diagnosis of vasculitis often can be made by biopsy of involved organs (e.g., skin, muscle) (see Chapter 29).

Systemic Mastocytosis

In systemic mastocytosis, a rare disease of mast cell proliferation, mast cells typically infiltrate most intensely into the submucosa and serosa of the GI tract; in some cases, the mucosa alone may be infiltrated with eosinophils. Intestinal edema with a sprue-like picture may supervene, but usually there is *urticaria pigmentosa* (widely scattered brown-red macules, like small freckles, which often are slightly raised and pruritic) (see Chapter 29).

Inflammatory Bowel Disease

Numerous eosinophils are seen in the mucosa involved in *Crohn's disease* and *ulcerative colitis*; indeed, in Crohn's disease, eosinophil degranulation has been reported,[87] and secretions from eosinophils have been implicated in the pathogenesis of *pouchitis*.[88] Crohn's disease of the terminal ileum in particular can be confused with eosinophilic gastroenteritis, because the radiographic appearances may be similar and patients with either disease respond to glucocorticoids; the histologic features should clearly differentiate the two diseases (see Chapters 2, 103, and 104).

Celiac Sprue

In celiac sprue, there is increased cellularity in the lamina propria of involved small intestine, with eosinophils commonly constituting one of the cellular components.[18] Although subtotal villous atrophy is found in some patients with established eosinophilic gastroenteritis,[4, 40, 58] the clinical and histologic features of celiac sprue and the response to a gluten-free diet usually allow clear discrimination between it and eosinophilic gastroenteritis (see Chapter 93).

Cancer

Gastric infiltration of eosinophils may be striking in *gastric adenocarcinoma*; peripheral eosinophilia and a history of allergy are unusual.[6] *Lymphoma* also may cause diagnostic confusion. Eosinophilic gastroenteritis as a possible paraneoplastic manifestation of large cell lung cancer has been reported.[89]

Cow's Milk Protein Sensitivity

This disorder typically presents in the first year of life after the introduction of cow's milk into the diet and may affect the upper or lower GI tract. Most children with small bowel disease have enteropathy with a degree of villous atrophy, but not all have mucosal eosinophilia. Removal of cow's milk from the diet leads to resolution of the symptoms, particularly in patients with large bowel disease (see Chapter 101).

Inflammatory Fibroid Polyps

These benign localized lesions should not be confused with eosinophilic gastroenteritis. They originate in the submucosa and typically appear as polyps or nodules; peripheral eosinophilia is absent, and a history of allergy is unusual.[6, 90] Many other terms have been used to refer to these lesions, including fibroma, inflammatory pseudotumor, submucosal granuloma, and, incorrectly, "localized" eosinophilic gastroenteritis. Histologically, the stroma in these lesions is characterized by a concentric arrangement of proliferating spindle cells (which may be fibroblasts or endothelial cells, although their exact nature remains controversial) surrounding arborizing capillaries, with a variable eosinophilic infiltration. These lesions are relatively rare, with a slight male preponderance; although they may appear at any age, they are most common in the sixth and seventh decades. They typically are found in the gastric antrum (~70% of cases) and the small bowel (20%), but they rarely may be in the esophagus or colon. Most patients present with obstructive symptoms that depend on the site of the lesion; pyloric-outlet obstruction and small bowel intussusception are common manifestations. Surgical excision is curative in symptomatic patients, and recurrence has not been reported. Glucocorticoids are not indicated.

Hypereosinophilic Syndrome

Occasionally, multisystem disorders can involve the gut and can be confused with eosinophilic gastroenteritis. By definition, eosinophilic infiltration of multiple organs outside the abdomen excludes the diagnosis of eosinophilic gastroenteritis. In the *hypereosinophilic syndrome*, a persistent and prolonged unexplained blood eosinophilia (defined as an absolute eosinophil count > 1500 cells/μL, present for longer than 6 months[91]) is associated with bone marrow and tissue infiltration by relatively mature eosinophils. The eosinophil count can be as high as 50,000 to 100,000 cells/μL, and the heart, lungs, liver, spleen, kidneys, skin, and central nervous system typically are affected. There often is anemia and thrombocytopenia. Congestive heart failure with endocardial fibrosis (and valvular incompetence), venous and arterial thromboembolism, neuropsychiatric disturbances, mononeuritis multiplex, and fever are common clinical features. The prognosis is poor in patients with prominent organ involvement, with a 75% 3-year survival rate without treatment. The prognosis tends to be better in patients who have angioedema. Treatment may include glucocorticoids (about one third respond), hydroxyurea, and, in resistant cases, interferon-α.[91]

TREATMENT

A management algorithm is presented in Figure 100–4. All relevant drugs should be discontinued, if possible, to exclude a drug reaction.

Diet

In patients with mucosal disease and no clinical evidence of muscle layer or serosal involvement, it is reasonable to attempt dietary manipulation, particularly in those who report a history consistent with food intolerance or food allergy.[36, 38] Any benefit obtained, however, is usually temporary.[4, 40] Measurement of specific IgE antibodies directly in the skin has a high false-positive rate; also, a negative skin test does not exclude food allergy on the basis of a delayed hypersensitivity reaction. Therefore, skin testing results must be interpreted cautiously.[40, 92] The radioallergosorbent test measures serum IgE antibodies to specific antigens, but it is even less specific than skin testing. If a specific food sensitivity is not suspected, the sequential elimination of milk (especially in children), beef, pork, eggs, and gluten can be

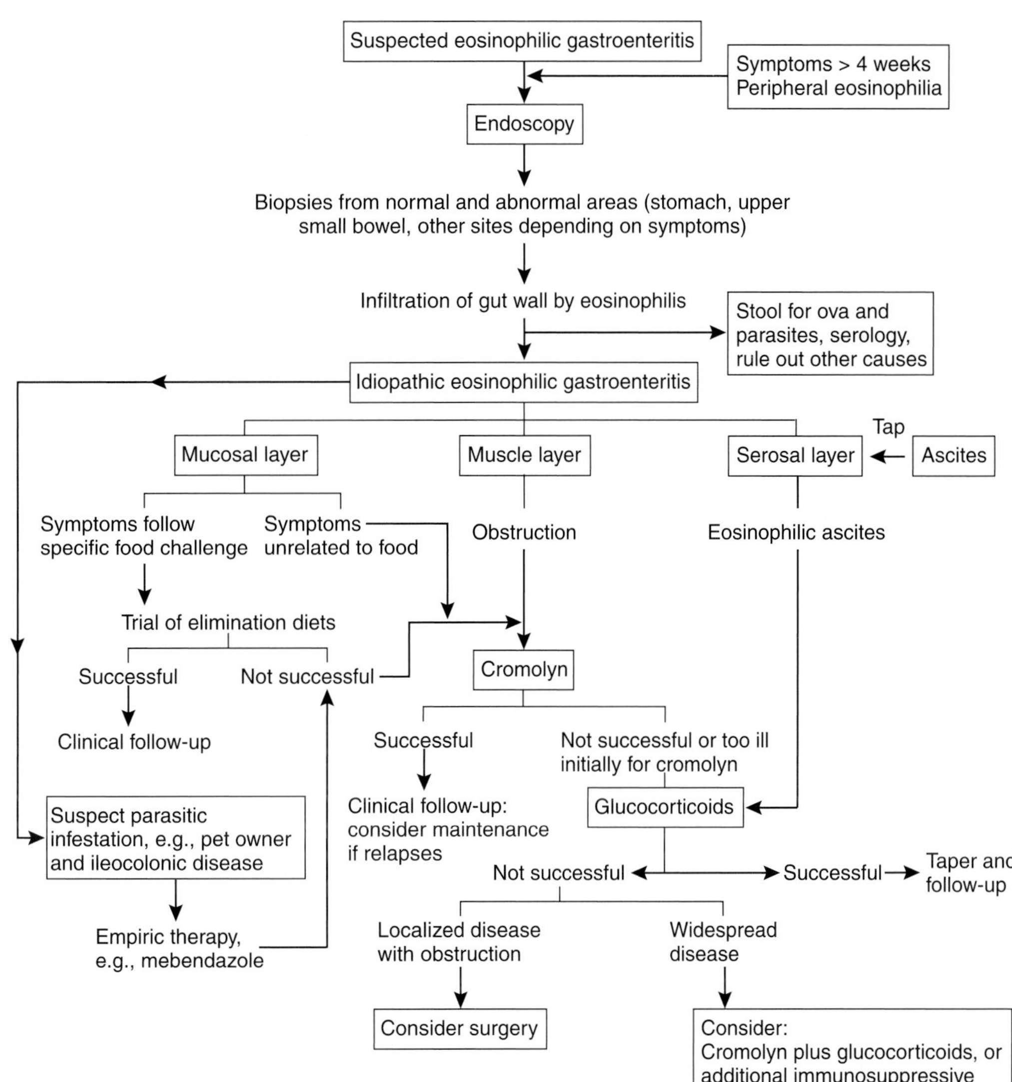

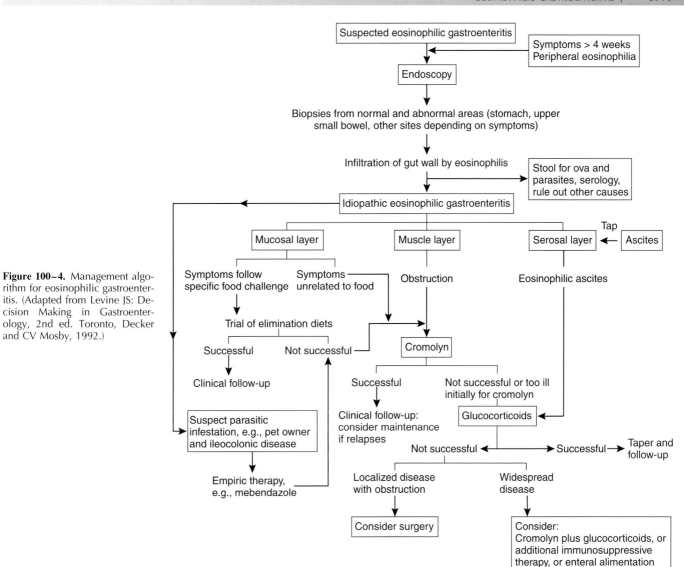

Figure 100–4. Management algorithm for eosinophilic gastroenteritis. (Adapted from Levine JS: Decision Making in Gastroenterology, 2nd ed. Toronto, Decker and CV Mosby, 1992.)

tried. Children with "allergic proctitis" typically have a good response to dietary manipulation; the allergen in such cases usually is milk protein (see Chapter 101). It is important to ensure that adequate nutrition is given regardless of the diet that is recommended. Enteral alimentation with an elemental diet, or even total parenteral nutrition, may be considered for the few patients in whom any food induces severe symptoms that cannot be controlled with the use of glucocorticoids or in whom glucocorticoids produce unacceptable adverse effects.[93, 94]

Antihelminthics

Patients who have traveled to or live in areas that put them at high risk for parasitic infestation should be offered an empirical trial of antiparasitic therapy (e.g., mebendazole 100 mg twice a day for 3 consecutive days in patients with ileocolitis, in whom canine hookworm or pinworm is a possibility). Such a trial is justified because frequently the parasite cannot be detected despite careful stool collections and other studies.[44]

Sodium Cromoglycate

There are scattered reports of patients with eosinophilic gastroenteritis who respond to sodium cromoglycate (cromolyn).[4, 16, 95, 96] The drug prevents the release of toxic mast cell mediators, such as histamine, platelet-activating factor, and leukotrienes; it also can reduce absorption of antigens by the small intestine.[97] Less than 1% of orally administered drug is absorbed from the gut.[95] Sodium cromoglycate has been used to treat milk allergy and other GI allergic reactions in children and adults, as well as malabsorption caused by systemic mastocytosis. Although only some may benefit,[4, 95] a therapeutic trial should be considered initially because the drug is safe; later glucocorticoids can be added, if necessary. The dose of sodium cromoglycate that should be prescribed is not well established, and up to 300 mg four times a day has been given; 200 mg three or four times a day is usually required to obtain sustained benefit and is well tolerated. If the patient relapses after successful treatment, consider maintenance therapy.

Glucocorticoids and Immunosuppressive Agents

Although no controlled trials are available, glucocorticoids are the mainstay of therapy in patients who fail to respond to dietary manipulation, antihelminthics, and sodium cromoglycate, and in those with obstructive symptoms or eosinophilic ascites. Most patients with serosal disease respond dramatically to glucocorticoids.[4] Prednisone should be initiated at a dose of 20 to 40 mg in adults and may be given as a single dose in the morning. Approximately 90% of patients will respond quickly, and after 7 to 14 days, the dose frequently can be tapered slowly over several weeks. About 15% of responders will relapse when the dose is tapered, and one half to one third will relapse on stopping glucocorticoids.[65] Low-dose maintenance prednisone (5 to 10 mg/day) is needed to keep symptoms under acceptable control in up to 50% of patients; alternate-day therapy (10 to 20 mg every other day) is probably less effective.

If high-dose glucocorticoids are required to maintain remission, azathioprine can be added for its steroid-sparing effects, but its efficacy is unknown. Although hydroxyurea has been used in the hypereosinophilic syndrome,[91] its role in eosinophilic gastroenteritis has not been defined. In severe disease, additional immunosuppressive therapy using cyclophosphamide or cyclosporine may be considered, but there is no published experience with these agents. The use of interferon-α or antibodies to tumor necrosis factor has not been examined in this disease.

Surgery

Surgery should be avoided if possible; significant gastrointestinal bleeding or perforation is rare,[98, 99] and patients in whom bowel obstruction develops usually respond to conservative measures and glucocorticoids. Even patients with localized muscle layer disease often have recurrences after surgical excision.

Other Treatments

In patients with malabsorption, it is important to exclude secondary bacterial overgrowth from stasis, because it is potentially reversible with antibiotic therapy. Ketotifen, an H_1-antihistamine, has been reported to reduce symptoms and the tissue eosinophil count, but its role is not established, and it is not available in the United States.[100]

PROGNOSIS

Eosinophilic gastroenteritis has a good prognosis; excluding patients who have multisystem disease (hypereosinophilic syndrome), vasculitis, or cancer, fatal outcomes have been reported only rarely.[98, 99] Intestinal obstruction is the most common acute complication, and chronic malnutrition can occur. There is no increased risk of GI cancer.[2–4]

REFERENCES

1. Ureles AL, Alschibaja T, Lodico D, et al. Idiopathic eosinophilic infiltration of the gastrointestinal tract, diffuse and circumscribed: A proposed classification and review of the literature, with two additional cases. Am J Med 30:899, 1961.
2. Klein NC, Hargrove R, Sleisenger MH, et al. Eosinophilic gastroenteritis. Medicine (Baltimore) 49:299, 1970.
3. Cello JP. Eosinophilic gastroenteritis—a complex disease entity. Am J Med 67:1097, 1979.
4. Talley NJ, Shorter RG, Phillips SF, et al. Eosinophilic gastroenteritis: a clinicopathological study of patients with disease of the mucosae, muscle layer, and subserosal tissues. Gut 31:54, 1990.
5. Kaijser R. Zur Kenntnis der allergischen Affektionen des Verdauungskanals vom Standpunkt des Chirurgen aus. Arch Klin Chir 188:36, 1937.
6. Blackshaw AJ, Levison DA, Eosinophilic infiltrates of the gastrointestinal tract. J Clin Pathol 39:1, 1986.
7. Naylor AR. Eosinophilic gastroenteritis. Scott Med J 35:163, 1990.
8. Lee C-M, Changshien CS, Chen P-C, et al. Eosinophilic gastroenteritis: 10 years experience. Am J Gastroenterol 88:70, 1993.
9. Altman LC, Gleich GJ. Eosinophils. Immunol Aller Clin North Am 10:263, 1990.
10. Weller PF. The immunobiology of eosinophils. N Engl J Med 324: 110, 1991.
11. Gleich GJ, Adolphson CR. The eosinophilic leukocyte: structure and function. Adv Immunol 39:177, 1986.
12. Peters MS, Rodriguez M, Gleich GJ. Localization of human eosinophil granule major basic protein, eosinophil cationic protein, and eosinophil-derived neurotoxin by immunoelectron microscopy. Lab Invest 54:656, 1986.
13. Shaw RJ, Walsh GM, Cromwell O, et al. Activated human eosinophils generate SRS-A leukotrienes following IgG-dependent stimulation. Nature 316:150, 1985.
14. Ackerman SJ, Gleich GJ, Loegering DA, et al. Comparative toxicity of purified human eosinophil granule cationic proteins for schistosomula of *Schistosoma mansoni*. Am J Trop Med Hyg 34:735, 1985.
15. Gleich GJ, Frigas E, Loegering DA, et al. Cytotoxic properties of the eosinophil major basic protein. J Immunol 123:2925, 1979.
16. Keshavarizian A, Saverymuttu SH, Tai P-C, et al. Activated eosinophils in familial eosinophilic gastroenteritis. Gastroenterology 88:1041, 1985.
17. Torpier G, Colombel JF, Mathieu-Chandelier C, et al. Eosinophilic gastroenteritis: ultrastructural evidence for a selective release of eosinophil major basic protein. Clin Exp Immunol 74:404, 1988.
18. Talley NJ, Kephart GM, McGovern TW, et al. Deposition of eosinophil granule major basic protein in eosinophilic gastroenteritis and celiac disease. Gastroenterology 103:137, 1992.
19. Bischoff SC, Mayer J, Nguyen QT, et al. Immunohistological assessment of intestinal eosinophil activation in patients with eosinophilic gastroenteritis and inflammatory bowel disease. Am J Gastroenterol 94:3521, 1999.
20. Kato M, Kephart GM, Talley NJ, et al. Eosinophil infiltration and degranulation in normal human tissue. Anat Rec 252:418, 1998.
21. Tai P-C, Holt ME, Denny P, et al. Deposition of eosinophil cationic protein in granulomas in allergic granulomatosis and vasculitis: the Churg-Strauss syndrome. BMJ 289:400, 1984.
22. Spry C, Tai P-C. Eosinophils in disease. J Soc Med 77:152, 1984.
23. Jaffe JS, James SP, Mullins GE, et al. Evidence for an abnormal profile of interleukin-4 (IL-4), IL-5 and gamma-interferon (gamma-IFN) in peripheral blood T cells from patients with eosinophilic gastroenteritis. J Clin Immunol 14:299, 1994.
24. Verdaguer J, Corominas M, Bas J, et al. IgE antibodies against bovine serum albumin in a case of eosinophilic gastroenteritis. Allergy 48: 542, 1993.
25. Fang J, Viksman MY, Ebisawa M, et al. Increased circulating levels of interleukin-5 in a case of steroid-resistant hypereosinophilic syndrome with ileal involvement. J Allergy Clin Immunol 94:129, 1994.
26. Jaffe JS, Metcalfe DD. Cytokines and their role in the pathogenesis of severe food hypersensitivity reactions. Ann Allergy 71:362, 1993.

27. O'Donnell MC, Ackerman SJ, Gleich GJ, et al. Activation of basophil and mast cell histamine release by eosinophil granule major basic protein. J Exp Med 157:1981, 1983.
28. Zheutlin LM, Ackerman SJ, Gleich GJ, et al. Stimulation of basophil and rat mast cell histamine release by eosinophil granule-derived cationic proteins. J Immunol 133:2180, 1984.
29. Henderson WR, Chi EY, Klebanoff SJ. Eosinophil peroxidase-induced mast cell secretion. J Exp Med 152:265, 1980.
30. Desreumaux P, Bloget F, Seguy D, et al. Interleukin 3, granulocyte-macrophage colony-stimulating factor, and interleukin 5 in eosinophilic gastroenteritis. Gastroenterology 110:768, 1996.
31. Levy AM, Kita K. The eosinophil in gut inflammation: effector or director? Gastroenterology 110:952, 1996.
32. Beil WJ, Weller PF, Tzizik DM, et al. Ultrastructural immunogold localization of tumour necrosis factor-alpha to the matrix compartment of eosinophil secondary granules in patients with idiopathic hypereosinophilic syndrome. J Histochem Cytochem 41:1611, 1993.
33. Inglefinger FJ, Lowell FC, Franklin W. Gastrointestinal allergy. N Engl J Med 241:303, 1949.
34. Caldwell JH, Sharma HM, Hurtubise PE, et al. Eosinophilic gastroenteritis in extreme allergy: immuonpathological comparison with nonallergic gastrointestinal disease. Gastroenterology 77:560, 1979.
35. Caldwell JH, Mekhjian HS, Hurtubise PE, et al. Eosinophilic gastroenteritis with obstruction: immunologic studies of seven patients. Gastroenterology 74:825, 1978.
36. Scudamore HH, Philips SF, Swedlund HA, et al. Food allergy manifested by eosinophilia, elevated immunoglobulin E level, and protein-losing enteropathy: the syndrome of allergic gastroenteropathy. J Allergy Clin Immunol 70:129, 1982.
37. Oyaizu N, Uemura Y, Isumi H, et al. Eosinophilic gastroenteritis: immunohistochemical evidence for IgE mast cell-mediated allergy. Acta Pathol Jpn 35:759, 1985.
38. Greenberger NJ, Tennebaum JI, Ruppert RD. Protein-losing enteropathy associated with gastrointestinal allergy. Am J Med 43:777, 1967.
39. Moon A, Kleinman RE. Allergic gastroenteropathy in children. Ann Allergy 74:5, 1995.
40. Leinbach GE, Rubin CE. Eosinophilic gastrenteritis: a simple reaction to food allergens? Gastroenterology 59:874, 1970.
41. Johnstone JM, Morson BC. Eosinophilic gastroenteritis. Histopathology 2:335, 1978.
42. DeSchryver-Kecskemeti K, Clouse RE. A previously unrecognized subgroup of "eosinophilic gastroenteritis": association with connective tissue diseases. Am J Surg Pathol 8:171, 1984.
43. Clouse RE, Alpers DH, Hockenbery DM, et al. Pericrypt eosinophilic enterocolitis and chronic diarrhea. Gastroenterology 103:168, 1992.
44. Croese J, Loukas A, Opdebeeck J, et al. Occult enteric infection by *Ancylostoma caninum*: a previously unrecognized zoonosis. Gastroenterology 106:3, 1994.
45. Croese J, Loukas A, Opdebeeck J, et al. Human enteric infection with canine hookworms. Ann Intern Med 120:369, 1994.
46. Prociv P, Croese J. Human eosinophilic enteritis caused by dog hookworm *Ancylostoma caninum*. Lancet 335:1299, 1990.
47. Khoshoo V, Schantz P, Craver R, et al. Dog hookworm: a cause of eosinophilic enterocolitis in humans. J Pediatr Gastroenterol 19:448, 1994.
48. Liu LX, Chi J, Upton MP, et al. Eosinophilic colitis associated with pinworm *Enterobius vermicularis*. Lancet 2:410, 1995.
49. Mazza DS, O'Sullivan M, Grieco MH. HIV-1 infection complicated by food allergy and allergic gastroenteritis: a case report. Ann Allergy 66:436, 1991.
50. Michet CJ Jr, Rakela J, Luthra HS. Auranofin associated with colitis and eosinophilia. Mayo Clin Proc 62:142, 1987.
51. Lee JY, Medellin MV, Tumpkin C. Allergic reaction to gemfibrozil manifesting as eosinophilic gastroenteritis. South Med J 93:807, 2000.
52. Wienand B, Sanner B, Liersch M. Eosiniphile gastroenteritis als allergische realoction auf ein sulfonamid-praparat. Dtsch Med Wochenschr 116:371, 1991.
53. Anttila VJ, Valtonen M. Carbamazepine-induced eosinophilic colitis. Epilepsia 33:119, 1992.
54. Ravi S, Holubka J, Veneri R, et al. Clofazimine-induced eosinophilic gastroenteritis in AIDS [Letter]. Am J Gastroenterol 88:612, 1993.
55. Dhawan A, Seemayer TA, Pinsinski C, et al. Post transplant eosinophilic gastroenteritis in children. Liver Transpl Surg 3:591, 1997.
56. Killbourne EM, Rigau-Perez JG, Heath CW Jr, et al. Clinical epidemiology of toxic-oil syndrome: manifestations of a new illness N Engl J Med 309:1408, 1983.
57. Hertzman PA, Blevias WL, Mayer J, et al. Association of the eosinophilia-myalgia syndrome with the ingestion of tryptophan. N Engl J Med 322:869, 1990.
58. Katz AJ, Goldman H, Grand RJ. Gastric mucosal biopsy in eosinophilic (allergic) gastroenteritis. Gastroenterology 72:1312, 1977.
59. Dobbins JW, Sheahan DG, Behar J. Eosinophilic gastroenteritis with esophageal involvement. Gastroenterology 72:1312, 1977.
60. Walsh SV, Antonioli DA, Goldman H, et al. Allergic esophagitis in children: a clinicopathological entity. Am J Surg Pathol 23:390, 1999.
61. Naylor AR, Pollet JE. Eosinophilic colitis. Dis Colon Rectum 28:615, 1985.
62. Schoonbroodt D, Horsmans Y, Laka A, et al. Eosinophilic gastroenteritis presenting with colitis and cholangitis. Dig Dis Sci 40:308, 1995.
63. Weisberg SC, Crosson JT. Eosinophilic gastroenteritis: report of case of 32 years' duration. Am J Dig Dis 18:1005, 1973.
64. Everett GD, Mitros FA. Eosinophilic gastroenteritis with hepatic eosinophilic granulomas: report of a case with 30-year follow-up. Am J Gastroenterol 74:519, 1980.
65. Kalantar SJ, Marks R, Lambert JR, et al. Dyspepsia due to eosinophilic gastroenteritis. Dig Dis Sci 42:2327, 1997.
66. Maeshima A, Murakami H, Sadakata H, et al. Eosinophilic gastroenteritis presenting with acute pancreatitis. J Med 28:265, 1997.
67. Thomas DW, Talley NJ, Mahnovski V, et al. Rectal mucosal major basic protein in infants with dietary protein-induced colitis. Ann Allergy 71:66, 1993.
68. Goldman H, Proujansky R. Allergic proctitis and gastroenteritis in children. Clinical and mucosal biopsy features in 53 cases. Am J Surg Pathol 10:75, 1986.
69. Shweiki E, West JC, Klena JW, et al. Eosinophilic gastroenteritis presenting as an obstructing cecal mass—a case report and review of the literature Am J Gastroenterol 94:3644, 1999.
70. McNabb PC, Fleming CR, Higgins JA, et al. Transmural eosinophilic gastroenteritis with ascites. Mayo Clin Proc 54:119, 1979.
71. Fortman LM, Johanson JF, Baskin WN, et al. Eosinophilic ascites without eosinophilia: a unique presentation of serosal eosinophilic gastroenteritis. Am J Gastroenterol 88:1280, 1993.
72. Perrault J, Markowitz H. Protein-losing gastroenteropathy and the intestinal clearance of serum alpha-l-antitrypsin. Mayo Clin Proc 59:278, 1984.
73. MacCarty RL, Talley NJ. Barium studies in diffuse eosinophilic gastroenteritis. Gastrointest Radiol 15:183, 1990.
74. Stallmeyer MJ, Chew FS. Eosinophilic gastroenteritis. AJR Am J Roentgenol 161:296, 1993.
75. Landres RT, Kuster GGR, Strum WB. Eosinophilic esophagitis in a patient with vigorous achalasia. Gastroenterology 74:1298, 1978.
76. Van Hoe L, Vanghillewe K, Baert AL, et al. CT findings in nonmucosal eosinophilic gastroenteritis. J Comput Assist Tomogr 18:818, 1994.
77. Carpenter HA, Talley NJ. The importance of clinicopathological correlation in the diagnosis of inflammatory conditions of the colon: histological patterns with clinical implications. Am J Gastroenterol 95:878, 2000.
78. Lambroza A, Dannenberg AJ. Eosinophilic ascites due to infection with *Strongyloides stercoralis*. Am J Gastroenterol 86:89, 1991.
79. Solis-Herruzo J, de Cuenca B, Munoz-Yagüe MT. Laparoscopic findings in serosal eosinophilic gastroenteritis: report of two cases. Endoscopy 20:152, 1988.
80. Kerstein MD, Sheahan DG, Gudjonsson B, et al. Eosinophilic cholecystitis. Am J Gastroenterol 66:349, 1976.
81. Gregg JA, Utz DC. Eosinophilic cystitis associated with eosinophilic gastroenteritis. Mayo Clin Proc 49:185, 1974.
82. Ashby BS, Appleton PJ, Dawson I. Eosinophilic granuloma of gastro-intestinal tract caused by herring parasite *Eustoma rotundatum*. BMJ 1:1141, 1964.
83. Van Laethem JL, Jacobs F, Braude P, et al. *Toxacara canis* infection presenting as eosinophilic ascites and gastroenteritis. Dig Dis Sci 39: 1370, 1994.
84. Lambroza A, Dannenberg AJ. Eosinophilic ascites due to hyperinfection with *Strongyloides stercoralis*. Am J Gastroenterol 82:89, 1991.
85. Kakizoe S, Kakizoe H, Kakizoe K, et al. Endoscopic findings and clinical manifestations of gastric anisakiasis. Am J Gastroenterol 90: 761, 1995.
86. Gomez B, Tabar Al, Tunon T, et al. Eosinophilic gastroenteritis and *Anisakis*. Allergy 53:1148, 1998.

87. McGovern TW, Talley NJ, Kephart GM, et al. Eosinophil infiltration and degranulation in *Helicobacter pylori*-associated chronic gastritis. Dig Dis Sci 36;435, 1991.
88. Dvorak AM, Onderdonk AB, McLeod RS, et al. Ultrastructural identification of exocytosis of granules from human gut eosinophils *in vivo*. Int Arch Allergy Immunol 102:33, 1993.
89. Stefanni GF, Addolorato G, Marsigli L, et al. Eosinophilic gastroenteritis in a patient with large-cell anaplastic lung carcinoma: a paraneoplastic syndrome? Ital J Gastroenterol 26:354, 1994.
90. Johnstone JM, Morson BC. Inflammatory fibroid polyp of the gastrointestinal tract. Histopathology 2:349, 1978.
91. Butterfield JH, Gleich GJ. Interferon-alpha treatment of six patients with the idiopathic hypereosinophilic syndrome. Ann Intern Med 121: 648, 1994.
92. Sampson HA, Albergo R. Comparison of results of skin tests. RAST, and double-blind placebo-controlled food challenges in children with atopic dermatitis. J Allergy Clin Immunol 72:26, 1984.
93. Justinich C, Katz A, Gurbindo C, et al. Elemental diet improves steroid-dependent eosinophilic gastroenteritis and reverses growth failure. J Pediatr Gastroenterol Nutr 23:81, 1996.
94. Pfaffenbach G, Adamek RJ, Bethke B, et al. Eosinophilic gastroenteritis in food allergy. Z Gastroenterol 34:490, 1996.
95. Van Dellen RG, Lewis JC. Oral administration of cromolyn in a patient with protein-losing enteropathy, food allergy, and eosinophilic gastroenteritis. Mayo Clin Proc 69:441, 1994.
96. Perez-Millan A, Martin-Lorente JL, Lopez-Morante A, et al. Subserosal eosinophilic gastroenteritis treated efficaciously with sodium cromoglycate. Dig Dis Sci 42:342, 1997.
97. Paganelli R, Levinsky RJ, Brostoff J, et al. Immune complexes containing food proteins in normal and atopic subjects after oral challenge and effect of sodium cromoglycate on antigen absorption. Lancet 1: 1270, 1979.
98. Fraile G, Rodriguez-Carcia JL, Beni-Perez R, et al. Localized eosinophilic gastroenteritis with necrotizing granulomas presenting as acute abdomen. Postgrad Med J 70:510, 1994.
99. Felt-Bersma RJF, Meuwissen SGM, van Velzen D. Perforation of the small intestine due to eosinophilic gastroenteritis. Am J Gastroenterol 79:442, 1984.
100. Melamed I, Feanny SF, Sherman PM, et al. Benefit of ketotifen in patients with eosinophilic gastroenteritis. Am J Med 90:310, 1991.

FOOD ALLERGIES

Chapter 101

Hugh A. Sampson, MD

BACKGROUND

Food allergy has been recognized since the time of Hippocrates, but not until 1921, with the classic experiment of Prausnitz and Kustner, was food allergy addressed on a scientific level. In 1950, Loveless[1] demonstrated the inaccuracy of diagnosing food allergy by history in a report of the first blinded placebo-controlled food trials in patients with milk allergy. In a study of milk allergy, Goldman and colleagues[2] stated that three successive challenges that duplicated the presenting symptoms were necessary to make a diagnosis of food allergy. However, in 1976, Charles May[3] introduced the use of the double-blind placebo-controlled oral food challenge (DBPCFC), which is now accepted as the gold standard for the diagnosis of food allergy.

DEFINITIONS

An *adverse food reaction* is a generic term that indicates any untoward reaction that occurs after the ingestion of a food and may be the result of *toxic* or *nontoxic* reactions. *Toxic reactions* will occur in any exposed person provided the dose is sufficiently high. *Nontoxic reactions* depend on individual susceptibilities and may be either immune mediated (*food allergy* or *food hypersensitivity*) or nonimmune mediated (*food intolerance*). Food intolerances are believed to comprise most adverse food reactions and are categorized as *enzymatic*, *pharmacologic*, and *idiopathic food intolerances*. Secondary lactase deficiency, an enzymatic intolerance, affects most adults, whereas most other enzyme deficiencies are rare inborn errors of metabolism. Pharmacologic food intolerances are present in persons who are abnormally reactive to substances, such as vasoactive amines, that are normally present in some foods (e.g., tyramine in aged cheeses). Confirmed adverse food reactions for which the mechanism is not known are generally classified as intolerances.

PREVALENCE OF FOOD ALLERGY

The prevalence of food allergy is greatest in the first few years of life. Up to 8% of infants under the age of 3 years are affected and the rate then falls to approximately 2.5% of the population after the first decade. In the first 3 years of life, gastrointestinal hypersensitivities comprise approximately one half of all allergic reactions. Bock[4] followed 480 newborns from a general pediatric practice prospectively through their third birthday and found that 8% had food allergic reactions, as confirmed by oral food challenge or a convincing history. Gastrointestinal symptoms included diarrhea in 63%, vomiting in 38%, and colic in infancy in 19% of sensitized children. In four prospective studies from four different countries, appropriately performed milk challenges revealed that ~2.5% of infants have cow's milk allergy in the first 1 to 2 years of life.[5] However, follow-up studies revealed that approximately 80% of these milk-sensitive infants lost their reactivity to milk by their third birthday.[6] Comparable controlled studies have not been performed in adults, and the prevalence of food-induced gastrointestinal hypersensitivity in adults is unknown.

PATHOGENESIS OF FOOD ALLERGY

The gut-associated lymphoid tissue (GALT), a component of the mucosal immune system, lies juxtaposed to the external environment and is required to differentiate organisms and foreign proteins that are potentially harmful from those that are not. All foods are comprised of foreign proteins and carbohydrates, which would serve as excellent antigens if injected subcutaneously or intramuscularly. However, unlike the systemic immune system, the general immunologic tone of the mucosal immune system is characterized by suppressed or down-regulated immune responses. A single-cell layer of columnar intestinal epithelial cells (IECs) separates the external environment from the loosely organized lymphoid tissue of the lamina propria. Overlying the epithelium is the glycocalyx, comprised of complex glycoproteins and mucins. This mucous coat provides an important physical barrier to potential pathogens by trapping organisms, which are then passed out in the stool. The epithelial cells provide a second level of physical protection. The cell membrane prevents noninvasive bacteria and viruses from entering the underlying lymphoid tissue. Invasive organisms and certain viruses, however, have the ability to bind to the epithelial cell membrane and enter the cell, thereby often provoking the development of disease. A third level of physical protection consists of the "tight junctions" joining adjacent IECs, which prevent even small peptides from passing through to the lamina propria. As outlined in Table 101–1, there are a number of immunologic and nonimmunologic mechanisms present in the gastrointestinal (GI) tract to prevent immunologically intact proteins from entering the systemic immune system.

Despite this elegant barrier, approximately 2% of ingested food antigens are absorbed, even in the mature gut, and transported throughout the body in an "immunologically" intact form.[6, 7] Increased stomach acidity and the presence of other food in the gut decrease the absorption of antigens, whereas decreased stomach acidity (e.g., use of histamine H_2-receptor antagonists or proton pump inhibitors) and ingestion of alcohol increase absorption.[8] The immunologically intact proteins that elude the gut barrier normally do not cause adverse reactions because most persons have developed *tolerance*, but in the sensitized host, these proteins can provoke a variety of hypersensitivity responses. Although more common in the developing GALT of young children, both cellular and immunoglobulin (Ig) E-mediated hypersensitivity responses to foods can develop at any age.

The dominant response in the GALT is suppression, or tolerance. The means by which the immune system is "educated" to avoid sensitization to ingested food antigens is not well understood. Early studies suggested that M cells, specialized epithelial cells overlying the Peyer's patches, were the major sites of immune antigen sampling in the intestine.[9] More recent studies, however, indicate that IECs may be the central antigen-presenting cells (APCs) for generating immunosuppression in the gut.[10] These "nonprofessional" APCs have been shown to express major histocompatibility complex (MHC) class II molecules, take up soluble protein from the apical end and transport it basolaterally, and selectively activate CD8+ suppressor cells. Activation of CD8+ suppressor cells appears to be regulated by nonclassical class I molecules (CD1d) and other novel membrane molecules that interact with CD8+ T cells. Studies suggest that soluble antigens in the gut lumen are sampled and presented primarily by IECs, leading to suppression of the immune response, whereas particulate antigens and intact bacteria, viruses, and parasites are sampled by M cells, leading to active immunity and generation of IgA (Fig. 101–1). In persons in whom food allergies develop, the normal immunosuppressive response of the GALT breaks down and hypersensitivity responses, both IgE mediated and cell mediated, develop.

Table 101–1 | **Physiologic and Immunologic Barriers of the Gastrointestinal Tract**

Physiologic barriers
Block penetration of ingested antigens
Epithelial cells—one cell layer of columnar epithelium
Glycocalyx—coating of complex glycoprotein and mucins that traps particles
Intestinal microvillus membrane structure—prevents penetration
Tight junctions joining adjacent enterocytes—prevent penetration even of small peptides
Intestinal peristalsis—flushes "trapped" particles out in the stool
Break down ingested antigens
Salivary amylases and mastication
Gastric acid and pepsins
Pancreatic enzymes
Intestinal enzymes
Intestinal epithelial cell lysozyme activity
Immunologic barriers
Block penetration of ingested antigens
Antigen-specific s-IgA in gut lumen
Clear antigens penetrating GI barrier
Serum antigen-specific IgA and IgG
Reticuloendothelial system

GI, gastrointestinal; s-IgA, secretory immunoglobulin A.

Recent studies indicate that IECs also play a central regulatory role in determining the rate and pattern of uptake of ingested antigens. Studies in sensitized rats indicate that intestinal antigen transport proceeds in two phases.[11] In the first phase, transepithelial transport occurs via endosomes, is antigen specific and mast cell independent, and occurs 10 times faster in sensitized rats than in nonsensitized controls.[12] Antigen-specific IgE antibodies bound to the mucosal surface of IECs via Fc_ε II receptors are responsible for this accelerated allergen entry.[13] In the second phase, paracellular transport predominates. "Loosening" of the tight junctions occurs secondary to factors released by mast cells that are activated in the first phase. Whereas the first antigen-specific pathway involves antibody, the second nonspecific pathway most likely involves cytokines. Consistent with this concept, IECs express receptors for a number of different cytokines (interleukin [IL]-1, IL-2, IL-6, IL-10, IL-12, IL-15, granulocyte–macrophage colony stimulating factor) and interferon-γ), and IECs have been shown to be functionally altered by exposure to these cytokines.

Although the development and mechanistic features of cell-mediated hypersensitivity responses are poorly understood, the development of IgE-mediated responses has been well characterized. Sensitivity to allergens (generally a glycoprotein) is the result of a series of molecular and cellular interactions involving APCs, T cells, and B cells.[14] APCs present small peptide fragments (T-cell epitopes) in conjunction with MHC class II molecules to T cells. T cells that bear the appropriate complementary T-cell receptor will bind to the peptide–MHC complex. This interactive "first signal" leads to T-cell proliferation and cytokine generation and the generation of a "second" signal, which promotes an IgE response (Th2-like cell activation). These cells and their products, in turn, interact with B cells that bear appropriate antigen-specific receptors, leading to isotype switching and the generation of antigen-specific IgE. At all stages, a number of specific cytokines are secreted and modulate the cell interactions. The antigen-specific IgE then binds to surface receptors of mast cells, basophils, macrophages, and other APCs, thereby arming the immune system for an allergic reaction with the next encounter of the specific antigen. A breakdown in mucosal integrity, caused by infection or other inflammatory processes, leads to increased intestinal permeability; as a result, antigens bypass the normal tolerogenic presentation by IECs, leading to systemic presentation and consequent sensitization.

Oral tolerance of both humoral and cellular immunity has been demonstrated in rodents, and recently Husby[15] demonstrated that the feeding of keyhole limpet hemocyanin to human volunteers resulted in T-cell tolerance but priming of B cells at both mucosal and systemic sites. The failure of human infants to develop oral tolerance or the "breakdown" of oral tolerance in older persons results in the development

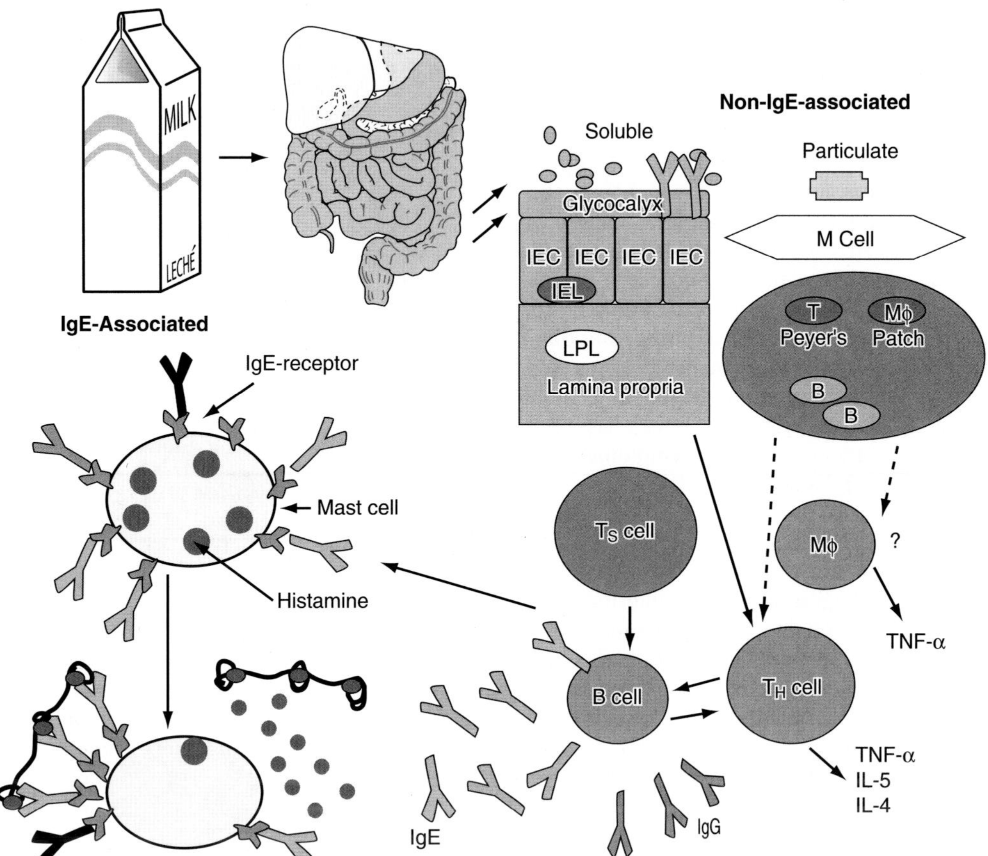

Figure 101–1. Immunopathogenesis of food hypersensitivities. Massive quantities of food proteins are processed in the intestinal tract to nonimmunogenic peptides and amino acids. However, as described in the text, a small amount of immunogenic protein passes through the gut barrier. Intestinal epithelial cells (IECs) normally process soluble proteins for presentation to appropriate helper (T_H) and suppressor T (T_s) cells. Protective IgA and IgG antibody responses are generated, and systemic T-cell responses are down-regulated. In IgE-associated disorders, food-specific IgE-producing B cells are activated. IgE antibodies adhere to the surface of mast cells, which will release histamine and other mediators if surface-bound IgE encounters the food antigen. IgE also binds to $Fc_{\varepsilon}R$ on gut IECs, expediting antigen transfer through IECs. In non–IgE-associated disorders, antigen-presenting (M) cells and/or T cells are activated to secrete TNF-$_{\alpha}$ (dietary protein-induced enterocolitis syndrome) or IL-4 and/or IL-5 (allergic eosinophilic gastroenteritis). M cells overlying Peyer's patches are believed to play a major role in processing particulate protein and pathogens. (TNF, tumor necrosis factor; IL, interleukin; $Fc_{\varepsilon}R$, Fc epsilon receptor.)

of food hypersensitivity.[16] Young infants are more prone to food allergic reactions because of the immaturity of their immunologic functions and, to some extent, of their GI tracts (see Table 101–1). Among a number of immature immunologic functions, newborns lack IgA and IgM in salivary and exocrine secretions at birth, and secretion of these antibodies remains low during the early months of life. Exclusive breast-feeding promotes the development of oral tolerance and may prevent some food allergy and atopic dermatitis.[17] The protective effect of breast milk appears to be the result of several factors, including a decreased content of foreign proteins, the presence of secretory (s)-IgA, which provides passive protection against foreign proteins and pathogens, and the presence of soluble factors that may induce earlier maturation of the gut barrier and the infant's immune response.[18] The antibacterial activity of breast milk is well established, but the ability of breast milk s-IgA to prevent food antigen penetration is less clear. Low concentrations of food-specific IgG, IgM, and IgA antibodies commonly are found in the serum of normal persons. Serum levels of food protein-specific IgG antibodies tend to rise in the first months after the introduction of a food and then generally decline, even though the food protein continues to be ingested.[15] Persons with various inflammatory bowel disorders (e.g., celiac sprue, food allergy) frequently have high levels of food-specific IgG and IgM antibodies, but there is no evidence that these antibodies are pathogenic. Increased lymphocyte proliferation or IL-2 production after food antigen stimulation in vitro is frequently seen in patients with inflammatory bowel disorders but also occurs in normal persons.[5] Antigen-specific T-cell proliferation in vitro alone does not represent a marker of immunopathogenicity but simply reflects response to antigen exposure.

In genetically predisposed persons, as noted above, antigen presentation leads to excessive Th2 responsiveness (lymphocytes secreting IL-4, IL-5, IL-10, and IL-13), resulting in increased IgE production and expression of Fc_{ε} receptors on a variety of cells.[14, 19] These IgE antibodies bind high-affinity $Fc_{\varepsilon}I$ receptors on mast cells and basophils as well as low-affinity $Fc_{\varepsilon}II$ receptors on macrophages, monocytes, lymphocytes, eosinophils, and platelets. When food allergens penetrate mucosal barriers and reach IgE antibodies bound to mast cells or basophils, the cells are activated and mediators are released (e.g., histamine, prostaglandins, and leukotrienes), which induce vasodilatation, smooth muscle contraction, and mucus secretion and lead to symptoms of immediate hypersensitivity. These activated mast cells also may release a variety of cytokines (e.g., IL-4, IL-5, IL-6, tumor necrosis factor-α, platelet-activating factor), which may induce the IgE-mediated late-phase inflammation. A variety of symptoms has been associated with IgE-mediated allergic reactions—*generalized*: shock; *cutaneous*: urticaria, angioedema, and a pruritic morbilliform rash; *oral and GI*: lip, tongue, and palatal pruritus and swelling, vomiting, and diarrhea; and *upper and lower respiratory*: ocular pruritus and tearing associated with nasal congestion, laryngeal edema, and wheezing. A rise in plasma histamine levels has been associated with the development of these symptoms after blinded food challenges.[20] In IgE-mediated GI reactions, endoscopic observation has revealed local vasodilatation, edema, mucous secretion, and petechial hemorrhaging.[21] Cell-mediated hypersensitivity reactions are believed to be responsible for allergic eosinophilic esophagitis and gastroenteritis. It is believed that activated T cells secrete IL-5, and other cytokines attract eosinophils and induce the inflammatory response responsible for the delayed onset of symptoms. Expansion of T cells from biopsy specimens of patients with milk-induced allergic eosinophilic gastroenteritis reveals large numbers of CD4+ Th2 T cells (unpublished data).

The GI tract processes ingested food into a form that can be absorbed and used for energy and cell growth. During this process, nonimmunologic and immunologic mechanisms are used to help destroy or block foreign antigens (e.g., bacteria, virus, parasites, food proteins) from entering the body proper. Despite this GI barrier, antigenically intact food proteins enter the circulation and are distributed throughout the body. In a classic series of experiments, Walzer[8] used sera from food-allergic patients to passively sensitize cutaneous mast cells in nonallergic volunteers. As seen in the classic experiment of Prausnitz and Kustner, a wheel-and-flare response was noted at the sensitized site within 5 to 90 minutes in more than 90% subjects who ingested the relevant food antigen. Through the introduction of food into specific locations along the GI tract, it was shown that food antigens are absorbed most readily from the small intestine, colon, and rectum and somewhat more slowly from the esophagus and stomach.[22] Through the passive sensitization of rectal, colonic, and ileal mucosa in volunteers with ileostomies and colostomies, ingestion of food allergen was shown initially to provoke pallor at the sensitized site, followed by edema, hyperemia, petechiae, and marked mucus secretion. An allergen introduced to the sensitized tissues by a vascular route provoked a greater mucosal reaction than larger quantities of antigen applied topically to the sensitized site. Collectively, these studies demonstrated that food antigens are absorbed rapidly from the GI tract and transported by the circulation to intestinal and extraintestinal mast cells.

CLINICAL MANIFESTATIONS OF GASTROINTESTINAL FOOD ALLERGY

As depicted in Table 101–2, a number of GI food hypersensitivity disorders have been described. Clinically, these disorders generally are divided into two main categories: IgE/Th2-mediated and non–IgE-mediated hypersensitivities. However, a number of other disorders may result in symptoms similar to food allergic reactions, and these disorders must be excluded during the evaluation, as noted in Table 101–3.

Table 101–2 | **Gastrointestinal Food Hypersensitivities**

IgE-mediated food hypersensitivities
- Oral allergy syndrome
- Gastrointestinal anaphylaxis
- Allergic eosinophilic esophagitis/gastritis/gastroenteritis (some cases)
- Infantile colic (some cases)

Non–IgE-mediated food hypersensitivity
- Dietary protein-induced enterocolitis syndrome
- Dietary protein-induced eosinophilic proctocolitis
- Dietary protein-induced enteropathy
  - Celiac sprue
  - Dermatitis herpetiformis
- Allergic eosinophilic esophagitis
  - Gastroesophageal reflux
- Allergic eosinophilic gastritis
- Allergic eosinophilic gastroenteritis

Mechanism unknown
- Cow's milk–induced occult gastrointestinal blood loss and iron-deficiency anemia of infancy
- Infantile colic (some cases)
- ? Inflammatory bowel disease

IgE-Mediated Food-Induced GI Hypersensitivity

Even before IgE antibodies had been identified, studies of food hypersensitivity focused on radiographic changes associated with "immediate" hypersensitivity reactions. In one of the first reports, hypertonicity of the transverse and rectosigmoid colon and hypotonicity of the cecum and ascending colon were noted after wheat was fed to an allergic patient.[23] In a later report, gastric retention, hypermotility of the small intestine, and colonic spasm were observed in four patients studied after the administration of barium that contained specific food allergens.[24] In a third study, fluoroscopy was used to compare the effect of barium contrast with and without food allergens in 12 food-allergic children.[25] Gastric hypotonia and retention of the allergen test meal, prominent pylorospasm, and increased or decreased peristaltic activity of the intestines were noted.

In the late 1930s, the rigid gastroscope was used to observe reactions in the stomachs of allergic patients. In one study, patients with gastrointestinal food allergy, patients with wheezing exacerbated by food ingestion, and control subjects were evaluated.[26] Thirty minutes after a food allergen was placed on the gastric mucosa, patients with gastrointestinal food allergy had markedly hyperemic and edematous patches of thick gray mucus and scattered petechiae at these sites, similar to those reported earlier by Walzer.[8] Only mild hyperemia of the gastric mucosa was noted in patients with wheezing provoked by food ingestion. More recent studies have confirmed these earlier observations and established an IgE-mediated mechanism.[21] They demonstrated food-specific IgE antibodies and increased numbers of intestinal mast cells before challenge in food-allergic patients

Table 101–3 | **Disorders That Must Be Differentiated from Food Hypersensitivities**

Food intolerances
- **Postinfectious malabsorption** (secondary disaccharidase deficiency, villous atrophy, bile salt deconjugation)
  - Viral: *Rotavirus*
  - Parasitic: *Giardia, Cryptosporidium*
  - Bacterial: *Shigella, Clostridium difficile*
- **Metabolic disorders**
  - Transient fructose or sorbitol malabsorption
  - Primary carbohydrate malabsorption (lactase deficiency, sucrase deficiency)
  - Hypo- or abetalipoproteinemia
  - Acrodermatitis enteropathica
- **Bacterial enterotoxins**
  - *Vibrio cholerae,* toxigenic *Escherichia coli, C. difficile*

Other disorders
- Cystic fibrosis
- Chronic inflammatory bowel disease
- "Chronic nonspecific diarrhea of infancy"
- Tumors: neuroblastoma (produces catecholamines or vasoactive inhibitory peptide)
- Zollinger-Ellison syndrome (produces gastrin)

Anatomic abnormalities
- Intestinal lymphangiectasia
- Short bowel syndrome
- Hirschsprung's disease (especially with enterocolitis)
- Ileal stenosis

compared with normal control subjects and significant decreases in stainable mast cells and tissue histamine content after a positive food challenge.

Several symptom complexes comprise the IgE-mediated food-induced gastrointestinal hypersensitivities: oral allergy syndrome, gastrointestinal anaphylaxis, and subgroups of allergic eosinophilic gastroenteritis and infantile colic. These disorders are characterized by a rapid onset, usually within minutes to an hour. In addition, simple laboratory tests that detect food-specific IgE antibodies, such as prick skin tests and radioallergosorbent tests, are useful in determining which foods are responsible for the patient's symptoms.

Oral Allergy Syndrome

This syndrome is a form of immediate contact hypersensitivity confined predominantly to the oropharynx and rarely involving other target organs. Symptoms include the rapid onset of pruritus and angioedema of the lips, tongue, palate, and throat, generally followed by rapid resolution of symptoms and most commonly associated with the ingestion of various fresh (uncooked) fruits and vegetables. Symptoms are caused by local IgE-mediated reactions to "conserved homologous proteins," which are heat labile (i.e., readily destroyed by cooking) and shared by certain fruits, vegetables, and some plant pollens.[5] Patients with allergic rhinitis secondary to ragweed or birch pollen sensitivity are most frequently afflicted with this syndrome. For example, in up to 50% of patients with ragweed-induced allergic rhinitis, oral symptoms are provoked by ingestion of melons (watermelon, cantaloupe, honeydew, etc.) and bananas,[27, 28] whereas in birch pollen-allergic patients, symptoms may develop after the ingestion of raw potatoes, carrots, celery, apples, hazelnuts, and kiwi.[29–31] Diagnosis is based on a classic history and positive prick skin tests ("prick and prick," i.e., pricking the implicated fresh fruit or vegetable with a needle and then pricking the skin of the patient).[32]

Gastrointestinal Anaphylaxis

This presentation is a relatively common form of IgE-mediated hypersensitivity that generally accompanies allergic manifestations in other target organs (i.e., skin, airway) and results in a variety of symptoms.[33] Symptoms typically develop within minutes to 2 hours of consuming a food and consist of nausea, abdominal pain, cramps, vomiting, or diarrhea. In some infants, the frequent ingestion of a food allergen appears to induce partial desensitization of gastrointestinal mast cells, thereby resulting in a subclinical reaction, and the only symptoms reported are poor appetite and periodic abdominal pain. The diagnosis is established by clinical history, evidence of food-specific IgE antibodies (positive prick skin tests or radioallergosorbent tests), resolution of symptoms after complete elimination of the suspected food, and recurrence of symptoms after oral food challenges. GI anaphylaxis is common in IgE-mediated food allergies; more than 50% of affected children experience GI symptoms during DBPCFC.[34]

Allergic Eosinophilic Esophagitis, Gastritis, and Gastroenteritis

These disorders are characterized by infiltration of the esophageal, gastric, or intestinal walls with eosinophils, an absence of vasculitis, and peripheral eosinophilia in up to 50% of patients (see Chapter 100). The eosinophilic infiltrate may involve the mucosal, muscular, or serosal layers (or more than one layer) of the stomach or small intestine.[35–37] Eosinophilic invasion of the muscular layer leads to thickening and rigidity of the stomach and small intestine, whereas infiltration of the serosa commonly results in ascites that contains eosinophils. Patients with this syndrome commonly present with postprandial nausea and vomiting, abdominal pain, diarrhea, occasional steatorrhea, and weight loss in adults or failure to thrive in infants. In a subset of patients with allergic eosinophilic esophagitis and gastroenteritis, food-induced IgE-mediated reactions have been implicated in the pathogenesis of this disorder. Patients with food-induced symptoms generally have atopic disease (atopic dermatitis, allergic rhinitis, or asthma), elevated serum IgE concentrations, positive prick skin tests to a variety of foods and inhalants, peripheral blood eosinophilia, iron-deficiency anemia, and hypoalbuminemia. In some infants, generalized edema secondary to hypoalbuminemia may result from marked protein-losing enteropathy, often in the presence of minimal gastrointestinal symptoms such as occasional vomiting and diarrhea.[38] Rarely, allergic eosinophilic gastroenteritis may present as pyloric stenosis in infants with gastric outlet obstruction and postprandial projectile emesis.[39] The diagnosis depends on the demonstration of a characteristic eosinophilic infiltration on gastrointestinal biopsy. Elimination of the responsible food allergen from the diet for up to 10 weeks may be necessary to bring about resolution of symptoms and normalization of intestinal histology.[40]

Infantile Colic

This disorder is an ill-defined syndrome of paroxysmal fussiness characterized by inconsolable "agonized" crying, drawing up of the legs, abdominal distention, and excessive gas. It generally develops in the first 2 to 4 weeks of life and persists through the third to fourth month of life.[41] A variety of psychosocial and dietary factors has been implicated in the etiology of infantile colic, but trials in bottle-fed and breast-fed infants suggest that IgE-mediated hypersensitivity occasionally may be a pathogenic factor, possibly in 10% to 15% of colicky infants.[42] Diagnosis of food-induced colic is established by the implementation of several brief trials of a hypoallergenic formula. In infants with food allergen-induced colic, symptoms are generally short-lived, so periodic rechallenges every 3 to 4 months should be carried out.

Non–IgE-Mediated Food-Induced Gastrointestinal Hypersensitivities

Most food hypersensitivity disorders are not IgE mediated but are believed to be the result of various cell-mediated mechanisms. Consequently, tests for evidence of food-specific IgE antibodies are of no value in identifying the responsible food. Although a number of laboratory tests have been suggested, none has proved useful in identifying foods that provoke these disorders. These non–IgE-mediated hypersensitivities are believed to be the result of abnormal antigen processing or cell-mediated mechanisms and may be divided into the following syndromes: dietary protein-induced enterocolitis, dietary protein-induced eosinophilic proctocolitis, dietary protein-induced enteropathy, and most cases of allergic eosinophilic esophagitis, gastritis, and gastroenteritis.[43]

Dietary Protein-Induced Enterocolitis Syndrome

This disorder is seen most commonly in infants presenting between 1 week and 3 months of age who present with protracted vomiting and diarrhea, which frequently result in dehydration.[44, 45] About one third of affected infants with severe diarrhea develop acidosis and transient methemoglobinemia. Cow's milk and soy protein are most often responsible, but enterocolitis secondary to egg, wheat, rice, oat, nut (including peanut), chicken, turkey, and fish sensitivities also have been reported in older persons.[46] Similar reactions to seafood (e.g., shrimp, crab, lobster), with symptoms that develop 2 to 4 hours after ingestion, often are reported in adults. The stools of affected persons frequently contain occult blood, polymorphonuclear neutrophils, and eosinophils. Jejunal biopsies classically reveal flattened villi, edema, and increased numbers of lymphocytes, eosinophils, and mast cells. Food challenges generally result in vomiting and diarrhea within 1 to 3 hours and result in hypotension in approximately 15% of cases. The immunopathogenesis of this syndrome remains unknown. Recent evidence suggests that food antigen-induced secretion of tumor necrosis factor-α from local mononuclear cells (e.g., macrophages, dendritic cells) may account for the reaction.[47, 48]

The diagnosis can be established when elimination of the responsible allergen leads to resolution of symptoms within 72 hours and oral challenge provokes symptoms.[44, 46] However, secondary disaccharidase deficiency may persist longer and may result in ongoing diarrhea for up to 2 weeks. Oral food challenges consist of administering 0.3 to 0.6 g/kg body weight of the suspected protein allergen while the peripheral blood white count is monitored. Vomiting generally develops within 1 to 4 hours of administering the challenge food. Diarrhea or loose stools often develop after 4 to 8 hours. In conjunction with a positive food challenge, the absolute neutrophil count in the peripheral blood will increase at least 3500 cells/mm^3 within 4 to 6 hours of the onset of symptoms, and neutrophils and eosinophils may be found in the stools. Approximately 15% of food antigen challenges lead to profuse vomiting, dehydration, and hypotension, so they must be performed under medical supervision.

Dietary Protein-Induced Eosinophilic Proctocolitis

This disorder also generally presents in the first few months of life and is most often secondary to cow's milk or soy protein hypersensitivity. More than one half of reported cases are in breast-fed infants and result from food antigens passed in maternal breast milk.[49–51] These infants usually appear healthy, often have normally formed stools, and generally are evaluated because of the presence of gross or occult blood in their stools. Blood loss is typically minor but occasionally can produce anemia. Lesions generally are confined to the distal colon and consist of mucosal edema with infiltration of eosinophils in the epithelium and lamina propria. In severe lesions with crypt destruction, neutrophils also are prominent. The diagnosis can be established when elimination of the responsible allergen leads to resolution of hematochezia, generally with dramatic improvement within 72 hours; complete resolution of mucosal lesions may take up to 1 month.[51] Reintroduction of the allergen leads to recurrence of symptoms within several hours to days. Findings on sigmoidoscopy are variable and range from areas of patchy mucosal injection to severe friability with small aphthoid ulcerations and bleeding. Colonic biopsy reveals a prominent eosinophilic infiltrate in the surface and crypt epithelia and the lamina propria. Allergies to cow's milk or soy protein that lead to proctocolitis are usually outgrown within 6 months to 2 years of avoidance of the allergen, but occasional refractory cases are seen.

Dietary Protein-Induced Enteropathy (Excluding Celiac Sprue)

This disorder frequently presents in the first several months of life as diarrhea (with mild to moderate steatorrhea in about 80% of cases) and poor weight gain.[52, 53] Symptoms include protracted diarrhea, vomiting in up to two thirds of patients, failure to thrive, and malabsorption, demonstrated by the presence of reducing substances in the stools, increased fecal fat, and abnormal D-xylose absorption. Cow's milk sensitivity is the most frequent cause, but the syndrome also has been associated with sensitivities to soy, egg, wheat, rice, chicken, and fish. The diagnosis is established by identifying and excluding the responsible allergen from the diet; symptoms should resolve within several days to weeks. On endoscopy, a patchy villous atrophy is evident, and biopsy reveals a prominent mononuclear round cell infiltrate and a small number of eosinophils, not unlike the findings seen in celiac sprue but generally much less extensive.[54] Colitic features usually are absent, but anemia occurs in approximately 40% of affected infants and protein loss occurs in most. Complete resolution of the intestinal lesions may require 6 to 18 months of allergen avoidance. In contrast to celiac sprue, loss of clinical reactivity occurs frequently, but the natural history of this disorder has not been well studied.

Celiac Sprue

Celiac sprue is a more extensive enteropathy leading to malabsorption and is reviewed in detail in Chapter 93. Total villous atrophy and an extensive cellular infiltrate are associated with sensitivity to gliadin, the alcohol-soluble portion of gluten found in wheat, oat, rye, and barley. Celiac sprue is strongly associated with HLA-DQ2 (α1*0501, β1*0201), which is present in more than 90% of patients.[55] The prevalence of celiac sprue is reported to be 1 in 250 in the United States (Celiac Disease Foundation). The recent striking increase in the incidence of celiac sprue in Sweden compared with genetically similar Denmark[56] and the variation in prevalence associated with changes in patterns of gluten feeding in Sweden[57] strongly implicate environmental factors (i.e., feeding practices) in the etiology of this disorder. The intestinal inflammation in celiac sprue is precipitated by exposure to gliadin and is associated with increased mucosal activity of tissue transglutaminase, which deamidates gliadin in an ordered and specific fashion to create epitopes that bind efficiently to DQ2 and are recognized by T cells.[58] Initial symptoms often include diarrhea or frank steatorrhea, abdominal distention and flatulence, weight loss, and occasionally nausea and vomiting. Oral ulcers and other extraintestinal symptoms secondary to malabsorption are common. Villous atrophy of the small bowel is a characteristic feature of patients with celiac sprue who ingest gluten. IgA antibodies to gluten are present in more than 80% of adults and children with untreated celiac sprue.[59] In addition, patients generally have increased levels of IgG antibodies to a variety of foods, presumably because of increased absorption of food antigens. The diagnosis depends on demonstrating biopsy evidence of villous atrophy and the characteristic inflammatory infiltrate, resolution of biopsy findings 6 to 12 weeks after gluten is eliminated, and recurrence of biopsy changes after another gluten challenge.[60] Revised diagnostic criteria have been proposed that include a greater dependency on serologic studies. Quantitation of IgA antigliadin antibodies may be used for screening, along with IgA antiendomysium and anti-tissue transglutaminase antibodies in patients over 2 years of age.[61] Once the diagnosis of celiac sprue is established, life-long elimination of gluten-containing foods is necessary to control symptoms and avoid an increased risk of malignancy.

Dermatitis Herpetiformis

Dermatitis herpetiformis (DH) is a chronic blistering skin disorder associated with a gluten-sensitive enteropathy (see Chapter 93). It is characterized by a chronic, intensely pruritic papulovesicular rash symmetrically distributed over the extensor surfaces and buttocks.[62] The histology of the intestinal lesion is virtually identical to that seen in celiac sprue, although the villous atrophy and inflammatory infiltrate are generally milder and T-cell lines isolated from intestinal biopsy specimens of patients with DH produce significantly more IL-4 than T-cell lines isolated from patients with celiac sprue.[63] The diagnosis of DH depends on the presence of the characteristic skin lesions and demonstration of IgA deposition at the dermal–epidermal junction of the skin. Although many patients have minimal or no gastrointestinal complaints, biopsy of the small bowel generally reveals intestinal involvement. Elimination of gluten from the diet generally leads to resolution of skin symptoms and normalization of intestinal findings over several months. Administration of sulfones, the mainstay of therapy, leads to rapid resolution of skin symptoms but has virtually no effect on intestinal symptoms.

Allergic Eosinophilic Esophagitis, Gastritis, and Gastroenteritis

These disorders are characterized by prominent infiltration of the stomach or small intestinal mucosa, muscular layer, or serosa with eosinophils. Clinical symptoms correlate with the extent of eosinophilic infiltration of the esophagus [EEG], gastric [AEG], or intestinal [AEGE] wall (see Chapter 100).[35, 36, 40, 43] Infiltration of the mucosal layer corresponds to a syndrome of malabsorption, whereas infiltration of the muscular layer leads to thickening and rigidity of the stomach and small intestine and may present as a clinical picture of obstruction. The immunopathogenic mechanism(s) responsible for AEG are not known but are believed to involve primarily cell-mediated mechanisms. As discussed earlier, a subset of patients have exacerbations of symptoms after the ingestion of food to which they have specific IgE antibodies. Peripheral blood T cells from all patients with AEG have been shown to secrete excessive amounts of IL-4 and IL-5 as compared with normal control subjects.[64] Most children and adolescents with food-induced AEG, especially those who have AEG and gastroesophageal reflux, have non–IgE-mediated food hypersensitivity.

Food-induced AEE was described in a group of 10 children with postprandial abdominal pain, early satiety or food refusal, vomiting or retching, failure to thrive, and refractoriness to standard medical therapy (6 of 10 had undergone Nissen fundoplication).[40] After 6 to 8 weeks of an amino acid-based formula (Neocate) plus rice, symptoms resolved in eight patients and were markedly improved in two. Biopsies revealed a marked reduction or clearing of the eosino-

Table 101–4 | **Foods Responsible for Most Food Hypersensitivity Disorders**

IgE-MEDIATED FOOD HYPERSENSITIVITIES	NON–IgE-MEDIATED FOOD HYPERSENSITIVITIES
Milk	Milk
Egg	Egg
Peanut	Soy
Wheat	Wheat
Soy	Barley
Fish	White potato
Shellfish	Banana
Nuts	Fish
	Shellfish

philic infiltrate in the esophagus and significant improvement in the basal zone hyperplasia and length of the vascular papillae.[40] Symptoms could be reproduced with the introduction of certain foods.

The diagnosis of EEG, AEG, and AEGE is based on a suggestive history and the demonstration of an eosinophilic infiltrate in the gastrointestinal wall. Because the eosinophilic infiltrate may be patchy, multiple sites should be biopsied. Elimination of suspect foods for 6 to 12 weeks should lead to normalization of gut histology, although clinical symptoms should improve substantially in 3 to 6 weeks. Challenge consists of reintroducing the suspect food allergen and demonstrating recurrence of symptoms and an eosinophilic infiltrate on biopsy. If food allergens are not identified as provoking agents, oral glucocorticoids (e.g., prednisone 1 to 2 mg/kg/day) are generally required to alleviate symp-

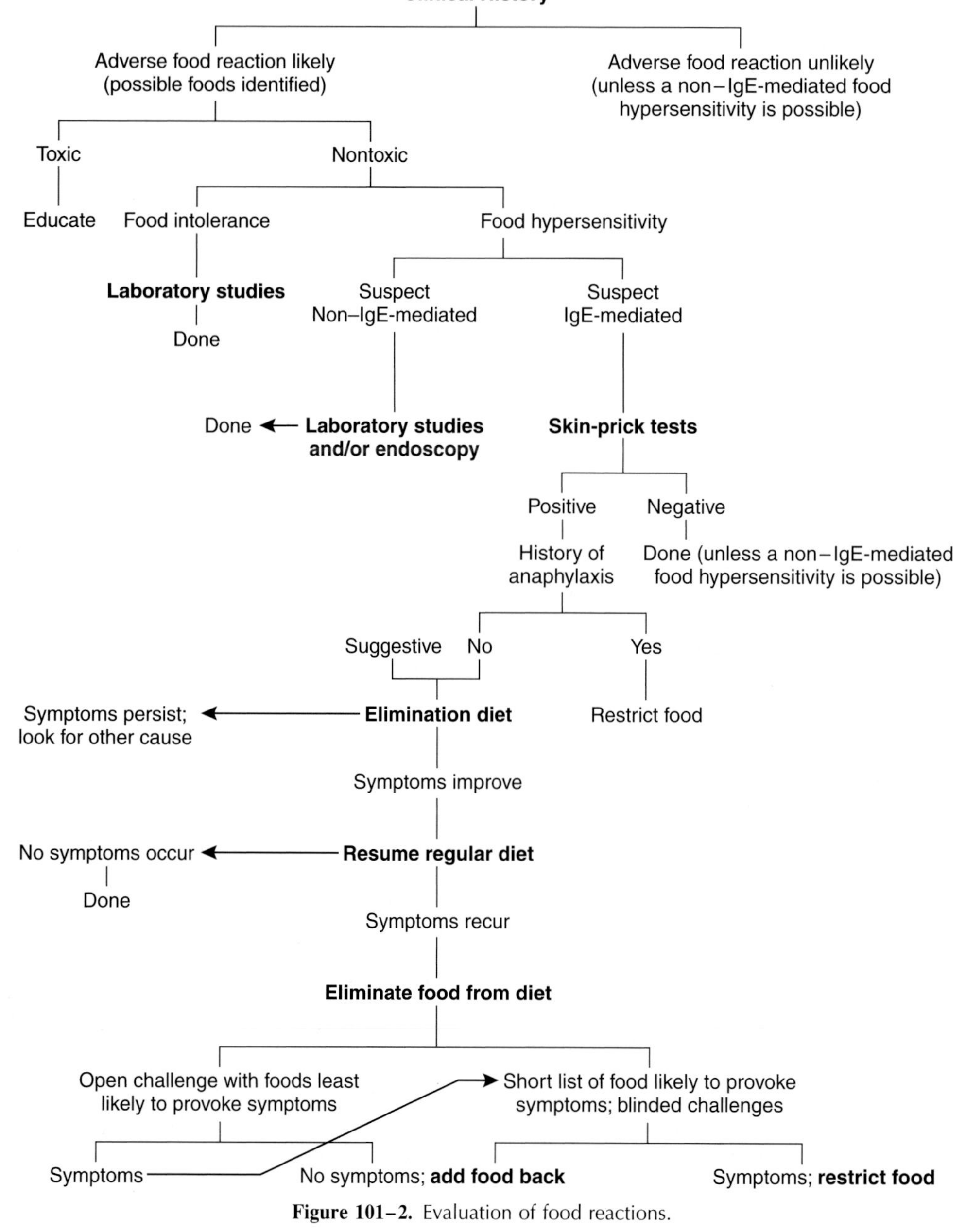

Figure 101–2. Evaluation of food reactions.

Table 101–5 | **Differences among the Non–IgE-Mediated Food Hypersensitivities**

	DIETARY PROTEIN-INDUCED ENTEROCOLITIS	DIETARY PROTEIN-INDUCED PROCTOCOLITIS	DIETARY PROTEIN INDUCED ENTEROPATHY	AEE AEG AEGE
Age at onset	2 wk–9 mo	1 wk–3 mo	1–18 mo	≥1 mo
Duration	9–36 mo	6–18 mo	18–36 mo	≥1 yr
Food proteins implicated	Cow's milk Soy	Cow's milk Soy Breast milk*	Cow's milk Soy Wheat Barley	Cow's milk Egg, Soy Wheat Barley
Clinical features				
FTT or weight loss	Moderate	No	Moderate	Moderate to severe
Vomiting	Prominent	No	Variable	Prominent†
Diarrhea	Severe	Rare	Moderate	Minimal
Hematochezia	Moderate	Moderate to severe	Moderate	Minimum to moderate

*Food proteins in breast milk (most often cow's milk or egg protein).
†Retching or gastroesophageal reflux.
AEE, allergic eosinophilic esophagitis; AEG, allergic eosinophilic gastritis; AEGE, allergic eosinophilic gastroenteritis; FTT, failure to thrive.

toms. Although symptoms usually respond to glucocorticoid therapy, exacerbations are not infrequent when therapy is discontinued. If exacerbations recur, prednisone given in a low dose or every other day may suppress symptoms.[35]

Gastroesophageal Reflux Disease

In young infants, gastroesophageal reflux disease may be the result of food-induced AEE. In a study of 204 infants < 1 year of age with gastroesophageal reflux disease (diagnosed by 24-pH probe and esophageal biopsy), 85 (42%) were found to have cow's milk-induced reflux by blinded milk challenges. These infants experienced resolution of gastroesophageal reflux disease once cow's milk was eliminated from the diet.[65]

Other GI Disorders

Several other disorders have been suggested to be secondary to food protein hypersensitivity. Ingestion of pasteurized whole cow's milk by infants less than 6 months of age may lead to occult GI blood loss and occasionally to iron-deficiency anemia.[66] Substitution of heat-processed infant formula (including cow's milk-derived formulas) for whole cow's milk generally leads to resolution of symptoms within 3 days. Circumstantial evidence suggests a possible role for food allergy in inflammatory bowel disease (Crohn's disease and ulcerative colitis), but convincing evidence of an immunopathogenic role remains to be established.

DIAGNOSING ADVERSE FOOD REACTIONS

The diagnosis of food allergy is a clinical exercise involving careful history-taking, physical examination, and selective laboratory studies. A variety of tests is used in the evaluation of food hypersensitivity, as discussed fully elsewhere.[67] In some cases, the medical history may be useful in diagnosing food allergy (e.g., acute anaphylaxis after the isolated ingestion of peanuts). However, fewer than 50% of reported food allergic reactions can be verified by DBPCFC. Information useful in establishing that a food allergic reaction occurred and in constructing an appropriate food challenge includes the following: (1) the food presumed to have provoked the reaction, (2) the quantity of the suspect food ingested, (3) the length of time between the ingestion and development of symptoms, (4) the type of symptoms provoked, and (5) a history of similar symptoms (if any) on other occasions when the food was eaten. Although any food may induce an allergic reaction, a few foods are responsible for most reactions (Table 101–4).

Figure 101–2 depicts a standard approach for evaluating adverse food reactions. If an IgE-mediated disorder is suspected, selected skin-prick tests or radioallergosorbent tests followed by an appropriate exclusion diet and blinded food challenge are warranted. If a non–IgE-mediated GI hypersensitivity disorder is suspected, laboratory and endoscopic studies (with or without oral food challenges) are required to arrive at the correct diagnosis. Table 101–5 compares the main features of four non–IgE-mediated food allergic disorders. An exclusion diet that excludes all foods suspected by history or skin testing should be prescribed for 1 to 2 weeks in suspected IgE-mediated disorders, food-induced enterocolitis, and eosinophilic proctocolitis. Exclusion diets may need to be extended for as long as 12 weeks in other suspected GI hypersensitivity disorders and may require the use of elemental diets to exclude all allergens (e.g., Vivonex, Neocate 1+, or Elocare). If no improvement is noted and dietary compliance is assured, it is unlikely that food allergy is involved. Before undertaking blinded food challenges (single or double blind), suspect foods should be eliminated from the diet for 7 to 14 days before challenge and even longer in some disorders when secondary disaccharidase deficiency may have developed. Elimination diets, like medications, may have adverse effects (e.g., malnutrition or eating disorders) and should not be done in the absence of solid diagnostic criteria.

THERAPY AND NATURAL HISTORY OF FOOD-ALLERGIC DISORDERS

Once the diagnosis of food hypersensitivity is established, strict elimination of the offending allergen is the only proven therapy. Patients must be taught to scrutinize food labels to detect potential sources of hidden food allergens.[68] Drugs such as H_1-antihistamines and H_2-receptor antagonists and glucocorticoids modify symptoms to food allergens but have minimal overall efficacy or unacceptable side effects.

The prevalence of food hypersensitivity is greatest in the first few years of life, but most young children outgrow their food hypersensitivity within 3 to 5 years, except possibly for sensitivities to peanuts, nuts, and seafood.[5] Although younger children are more likely to outgrow their food hypersensitivity, older children and adults may lose their food hypersensitivity if the responsible food allergen can be identified and completely eliminated from the diet.[69, 70]

REFERENCES

1. Loveless MH. Milk allergy: a survey of its incidence; experiments with a masked ingestion test. J Allergy 21:489–499, 1950.
2. Goldman AS, Anderson DW, Sellers WA, et al. Milk allergy. I. Oral challenge with milk and isolated milk proteins in allergic children. Pediatrics 32:425–443, 1963.
3. May CD. Objective clinical and laboratory studies of immediate hypersensitivity reactions to food in asthmatic children. J Allergy Clin Immunol 58:500–515, 1976.
4. Bock SA. Prospective appraisal of complaints of adverse reactions to foods in children during the first 3 years of life. Pediatrics 79:683–688, 1987.
5. Sampson HA. Food allergy. Part 1. Immunopathogenesis and clinical disorders. J Allergy Clin Immunol 103:717–728, 1999.
6. Host A. Cow's milk protein allergy and intolerance in infancy. Pediatr Allergy Immunol 5:5–36, 1994.
7. Wilson SJ, Walzer M, Absorption of undigested proteins in human beings. IV. Absorption of unaltered egg protein in infants. Am J Dis Child 50:49–54, 1935.
8. Walzer M. Allergy of the abdominal organs. J Lab Clin Med 26:1867–1877, 1941.
9. Wolf JL, Bye WA. The membranous epithelial (M) cell and the mucosal immune system. Annu Rev Med 35:95–112, 1984.
10. Mayer L. Mucosal immunity and gastrointestinal antigen processing. J Pediatr Gastroenterol Nutr 30:S4–S12, 2000.
11. Berin MC, Kiliaan AJ, Yang PC, et al. Rapid transepithelial antigen transport in rat jejunum: impact of sensitization and the hypersensitivity reaction. Gastroenterology 113:856–864, 1997.
12. Berin MC, Kiliaan AJ, Yang PC, et al. The influence of mast cells on pathways of transepithelial antigen transport in rat intestine. J Immunol 161:2561–2566, 1998.
13. Yang PC, Berin MC, Yu LC, et al. Enhanced intestinal transepithelial antigen transport in allergic rats is mediated by IgE and CD23 (FcepsilonRII) J Clin Invest 106:879–886, 2000.
14. Vercelli D, Geha R. Regulation of IgE synthesis in humans: a tale of two signals. J Allergy Clin Immunol 88:285–295, 1991.
15. Husby S. Normal immune responses to ingested foods. J Pediatr Gastroenterol Nutr 30:S13–S19, 2000.
16. Crowe SE, Perdue MH. Gastrointestinal food hypersensitivity: basic mechanisms of pathophysiology. Gastroenterology 103:1075–1095, 1992.
17. Zeiger R, Heller S. The development and prediction of atopy in high-risk children: follow-up at seven years in a prospective randomized study of combined maternal and infant food allergen avoidance. J Allergy Clin Immunol 95:1179–1190, 1995.
18. Zeiger R. Breast-feeding and dietary avoidance. In de Weck A, Sampson HA (eds): Intestinal Immunology and Food Allergy. New York, Raven Press, 1995, pp 203–222.
19. Bacharier LB, Geha RS. Molecular mechanisms of IgE regulation. J Allergy Clin Immunol 105:S547–S558, 2000.
20. Sampson HA, Jolie PL. Increased plasma histamine concentrations after food challenges in children with atopic dermatitis. N Engl J Med 311: 372–376, 1984.
21. Reimann HJ, Lewin J. Gastric mucosal reactions in patients with food allergy. Am J Gastroenterol 83:1212–1219, 1988.
22. Gray I, Walzer M, Studies in absorption of undigested protein in human beings. VIII. Absorption from the rectum and a comparative study of absorption following oral, duodenal, and rectal administrations. J Allergy 11:245–250, 1940.
23. Eyermann C. X-ray demonstration of colonic reaction in food allergy. J Miss State Med Assoc 24:129–132, 1927.
24. Rowe AH. Roentgen studies of patients with gastrointestinal food allergy. JAMA 100:394–400, 1933.
25. Fries JH, Zizmor J. Roentgen studies of children with alimentary disturbances due to food allergy. Am J Dis Child 54:1239–1251, 1937.
26. Pollard H, Stuart G. Experimental reproduction of gastric allergy in human beings with controlled observations on the mucosa. J Allergy 13:467–473, 1942.
27. Amlot PL, Kemeny DM, Zachary C, et al. Oral allergy syndrome (OAS): symptoms of IgE-mediated hypersensitivity to foods. Clin Allergy 17:33–42, 1987.
28. Ortolani C, Ispano M, Pastorello EA, et al. Comparison of results of skin prick tests (with fresh foods and commercial food extracts) and RAST in 100 patients with oral allergy syndrome. J Allergy Clin Immunol 83:683–690, 1989.
29. Andersen K, Lowenstein H. An investigation of the possible immunological relationship between allergen extracts from birch pollen, hazelnut, potato, and apple. Contact Dermatitis 4:73–78, 1970.
30. Ortolani C, Ispano M, Pastorello EA, et al. The oral allergy syndrome. Ann Allergy 61:47–52, 1988.
31. Pastorello EA, Incorvaia C, Pravetonni V, et al. New allergens in fruits and vegetables. Allergy 53:48–51, 1998.
32. Dreborg S, Foucard T. Allergy to apple, carrot, and potato in children with birch-pollen allergy. Allergy 38:167–172, 1983.
33. Sampson HA. Food allergy. JAMA 278:1888–1894, 1997.
34. Sampson HA. Food allergy. In Kay AB (ed): Allergy and Allergic Diseases. London, Blackwell Science, 1997, pp 1517–1549.
35. Lee C, Changchien C, Chen P, et al. Eosinophilic gastroenteritis: 10 years experience. Am J Gastroenterol 88:70–74, 1993.
36. Min K-U, Metcalfe D. Eosinophilic gastroenteritis. Immunol Allergy Clin North Am 11:799–813, 1991.
37. Moon A, Kleinman R. Allergic gastroenteropathy in children. Ann Allergy Asthma Immunol 74:5–12, 1995.
38. Waldman T, Wochner R, Laster R, et al. Allergic gastroenteropathy. A cause of excessive gastrointestinal protein loss. N Engl J Med 276: 761–769, 1967.
39. Snyder JD, Rosenblum N, Wershil B, et al. Pyloric stenosis and eosinophilic gastroenteritis in infants. J Pediatr Gastroenterol Nutr 6:543–547, 1987.
40. Kelly KJ, Lazenby AJ, Rowe PC, et al. Eosinophilic esophagitis attributed to gastroesophageal reflux: improvement with an amino-acid based formula. Gastroenterology 109:1503–1512, 1995.
41. Hill DJ, Hosking CS. Infantile colic and food hypersensitivity. J Pediatr Gastroenterol Nutr 30(Suppl):S67–S76, 2000.
42. Sampson HA. Infantile colic and food allergy: fact or fiction? J Pediatr 115:583–584, 1989.
43. Sampson HA, Anderson JA. Summary and recommendations: classification of gastrointestinal manifestations due to immunologic reactions to foods in infants and young children. J Pediatr Gastroenterol Nutr 30: S87–S94, 2000.
44. Powell GK. Enterocolitis in low-birth-weight infants associated with milk and soy protein intolerance. J Pediatr 88:840–844, 1976.
45. Sicherer SH. Food protein-induced enterocolitis syndrome: clinical perspectives. J Pediatr Gastroenterol Nutr 30:S45–S49, 2000.
46. Sicherer SH, Eigenmann PA, Sampson HA. Clinical features of food protein-induced enterocolitis syndrome. J Pediatr 133:214–219, 1998.
47. Heyman M, Darmon N, Dupont C, et al. Mononuclear cells from infants allergic to cow's milk secrete tumor necrosis factor alpha, altering intestinal function. Gastroenterology 106:1514–1523, 1994.
48. Benlounes N, Candahl C, Matarazzo P, et al. The time course of milk-antigen induced TNF-alpha secretion differs according to the clinical symptoms in children with cow's milk allergy. J Allergy Clin Immunol 104:863–869, 1999.
49. Machida H, Smith A, Gall D, et al. Allergic colitis in infancy: clinical and pathologic aspects. J Pediatr Gastroenterol Nutr 19:22–26, 1994.
50. Odze R, Wershil B, Leichtner A. Allergic colitis in infants. J Pediatr 126:163–170, 1995.
51. Lake AM. Food-induced eosinophilic proctocolitis. J Pediatr Gastroenterol Nutr 30:S58–S60, 2000.
52. Kosnai I, Kuitunen P, Savilahti E, et al. Mast cells and eosinophils in

the jejunal mucosa of patients with intestinal cow's milk allergy and celiac disease of childhood. J Pediatr Gastroenterol Nutr 3:368–374, 1984.
53. Savilahti E. Food-induced malabsorption syndromes. J Pediatr Gastroenterol Nutr 30:S61–S66, 2000.
54. Nagata S, Yamashiro Y, Ohtsuka Y, et al. Quantitative analysis and immunohistochemical studies on small intestinal mucosa of food-sensitive enteropathy. J Pediatr Gastroenterol Nutr 20:44–48, 1995.
55. Sollid LM, Thorsby E. HLA susceptibility genes in celiac disease: genetic mapping and role in pathogenesis. Gastroenterology 105:910–922, 1993.
56. Weile B, Cavell B, Nivenius K, et al. Striking differences in the incidence of childhood celiac disease between Denmark and Sweden: a plausible explanation. J Pediatr Gastroenterol Nutr 21:64–68, 1995.
57. Ivarsson A, Persson LA, Nystrom L, et al. Epidemic of coeliac disease in Swedish children. Acta Paediatr 89:165–171, 2000.
58. Anderson RP, Degano P, Godkin AJ, et al. In vivo antigen challenge in celiac disease identifies a single transglutaminase-modified peptide as the dominant A-gliadin T-cell epitope. Nat Med 6:337–342, 2000.
59. Scott H, Fausa V, EK J, et al. Immune response patterns in coeliac disease: serum antibodies to dietary antigens measured by an enzyme-linked immunosorbent assay. Clin Exp Immunol 57:25–32, 1984.
60. McNeish AS, Harms HK, Rey T, et al. Re-evaluation of diagnostic criteria for coeliac disease. Arch Dis Child 54:783–786, 1979.
61. Grodzinsky E, Jansson G, Skogh T, et al. Anti-endomysium and anti-gliadin antibodies as serological markers for coeliac disease in childhood: a clinical study to develop a practical routine. Acta Paediatr 84: 294–298, 1995.
62. Hall RP. Dermatitis herpetiformis. J Invest Dermatol 99:873–881, 1992.
63. Hall RP, Smith AD, Streilein RD. Increased production of IL-4 by gut T-cell lines from patients with dermatitis herpetiformis compared to patients with isolated gluten-sensitive enteropathy. Dig Dis Sci 45: 2036–2043, 2000.
64. Jaffe J, James S, Mullins G, et al. Evidence for an abnormal profile of interleukin-4 (IL-4), IL-5, and gamma interferon in peripheral blood T cells from patients with allergic eosinophilic gastroenteritis. J Clin Immunol 14:299–309, 1994.
65. Iacono G, Carroccio A, Cavataio F, et al. Gastroesophageal reflux and cow's milk allergy in infants: a prospective study. J Allergy Clin Immunol 97:822–827, 1996.
66. Ziegler EE, Fomon SJ, Nelson SE, et al. Cow milk feeding in infancy: further observations on blood loss from the gastrointestinal tract. J Pediatr 116:11–18, 1990.
67. Sampson HA. Food allergy. Part 2. Diagnosis and management. J Allergy Clin Immunol 103:981–999, 1999.
68. Barnes Koerner C, Sampson HA. Diets and nutrition. In Metcalfe DD, Sampson HA, Simon RA (eds): Food Allergy: Adverse Reactions to Foods and Food Additives. Boston, Blackwell Scientific, 1996, pp 461–484.
69. Sampson HA, Scanlon SM. Natural history of food hypersensitivity in children with atopic dermatitis. J Pediatr 115:23–27, 1989.
70. Pastorello EA, Stocchi L, Pravetonni V, et al. Role of the food elimination diet in adults with food allergy. J Allergy Clin Immunol 84:475–483, 1989.

Chapter 102

RADIATION ENTERITIS

Nam P. Nguyen and John E. Antoine

Fractionated external beam radiation therapy is an effective modality for the cure of many pelvic malignancies. It can be used alone as in the treatment of cervical carcinoma and prostate carcinoma or in combination with chemotherapy and surgery as adjuvant therapy for rectal carcinoma.[1–3] The current trend toward combined radiation with chemotherapy has resulted in an increased incidence of acute toxicity and late effects on normal tissues.[4] Bowel injury resulting in fistula, stricture, and malabsorption are potential life-threatening complications and also impact the patient's quality of life. A thorough understanding of the mechanism of radiation-induced enteritis is necessary for the clinician to manage the patient's side effects during radiation treatment or its late sequelae.

PHYSICS OF MEGAVOLTAGE IRRADIATION

Pelvic and abdominal irradiation is usually delivered by the use of a high energy linear accelerator (>10 MeV photon). The high photon energy allows skin and small bowel sparing because the depth of penetration of the photons increases with the photon energy. In a radiation field, there are anatomic areas that receive a greater amount of radiation compared with the dose prescribed for the tumor. For obese individuals with a large pelvic thickness, dose distribution improves with high energy photons, and consequently a large volume of small intestines receives less radiation.

Photons interact with normal tissues through three mechanisms: photoelectric effect, Compton effect, and pair production.[5] In the photoelectric effect, the total energy of the photon is transferred to an orbital electron. The photon disappears, and the electron is ejected from the atom with an energy equal to the photon energy minus the binding energy of the electron. The Compton effect results from the partial transfer of the photon energy to the electron, which is also ejected from its orbit. The photon is deviated from its trajectory with a lesser amount of energy because of the transfer. Pair production is observed only for photons with high energy (>1.02 MeV photon). When the photon approaches the atomic nucleus, it disappears and transforms to a pair of positron (positively charged electron) and electron. The sum of the positron and electron energy created equals the energy of the incident photon.

Photons are electromagnetic waves that by themselves do not produce chemical or biologic effects. When the photons get absorbed in the medium, they release their energy to produce fast-moving electrons that in turn induce damage to the normal tissues. In the photon high-energy range used in therapeutic radiation, Compton effects predominate. The amount of energy absorbed after interaction of photon and biologic material is quantified as the gray (Gy) by the Systeme International. One Gy is defined as an energy absorption of 1 joule per kilogram. One Gy is the equivalent of 100 cGy (cGy).

The radiation dose given in 1 day is defined as a fraction. The fraction dose in therapeutic radiology is usually 180 to 200 cGy. The total dose to the pelvis ranges from 4500 to 5000 cGy because of the limit of tolerance of the small bowels to radiation. One fraction may be delivered by the use of multiple fields.

BIOLOGIC EFFECTS OF RADIATION

The electron produced by the Compton effect of photons induces the formation of free radicals. A free radical is a charged particle carrying an unpaired electron in the outer shell of the atom. Because of the abundance of water in the cell, the most important radical produced is the hydroxyl radical (OH·). The free radicals in turn cause single or double DNA strand breaks. The cell has the enzymatic ability to repair single-strand DNA damage using the opposite strand as a template.[6] However, if both strands break occur, the cell usually dies.[7] This is thought to be the principal mechanism of radiation-induced cell death. Recent evidence also shows interaction of radiation with the cell membrane, which may contribute to cell death.[8] The importance of this mechanism of cell killing is still controversial.

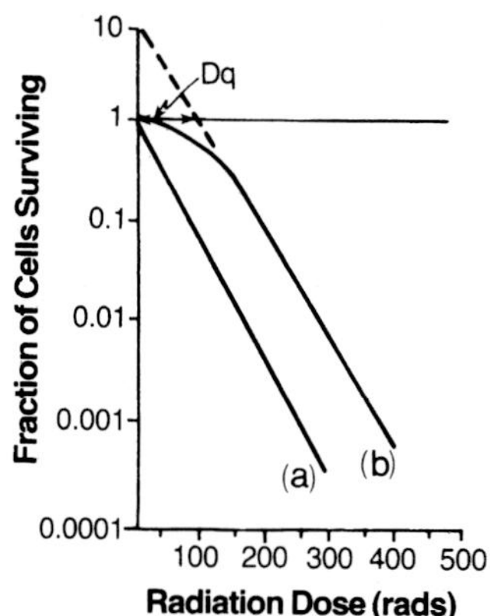

Figure 102–1. Typical cell survival curve in response to radiation exposure. Densely ionizing radiation, line (a), can produce cell death from each radiation hit. Less dense radiation, line (b), produces sublethal damage at low radiation doses. This results in a shoulder on the cell survival curve reflecting cell repair. Radiation doses below the quasi-threshold (Dq) for cell death kill few cells, whereas radiation doses above the Dq kill more cells per unit dose.

CELL SURVIVAL CURVES

The ability of the cell to survive after irradiation is described as the conservation of their reproductive integrity. Radiation experiments are conducted with single cells plating after graded dose of radiation (usually from 0 to 11 Gy). The number of macroscopic colonies formed after radiation are plotted on a logarithmic scale against the dose of radiation on a linear scale. In the ranges of dose in radiation therapy, the survival fraction appears to be an exponential function of dose. As the dose increases, the curve bends and becomes progressively steeper (Fig. 102–1). This linear quadratic form is described through a mathematic model: $S = e^{-\alpha D-\beta D^2}$, where S is the fraction of cells surviving a dose (D) and α and β are constants.

RADIOSENSITIVITY OF THE CELL THROUGH CELL CYCLE

Using autoradiography with the incorporation of tritiated thymidine into the cell, the cell cycle is divided into four stages (see Fig. 102–2). The interval between mitosis (M) and DNA synthesis where no label incorporation occurs is defined as gap phase, or G_1. The phase during which the cell incorporates thymidine is the DNA synthetic phase, or S phase. After DNA synthesis is complete, there is a second gap phase, or G_2. All proliferating mammalian cells go through these four consecutive phases (M, G_1, S, and G_2). However, the relative lengths of the four constituents of the cell cycle depend on the specific tissue. The G_1 period varies considerably between different tissues and accounts mainly for the difference in cell cycle time.

The radiosensitivity of the cell changes with the phase of the cell cycle. The cells are most vulnerable to the killing effect of radiation during G_2 and M phases.[9] Therefore, actively dividing tissues such as the small intestinal epithelium crypts are particularly sensitive to radiation. Rapid depletion of stem cells is responsible for the acute clinical manifestation of toxicity during radiation treatment. This effect can be exacerbated by the concurrent administration of chemotherapy.

MECHANISM OF REGENERATION OF THE INTESTINAL EPITHELIUM

The epithelial lining of the small intestine is replaced every 5–6 days in humans (see Chapter 84). The stem cells are located at the base of the crypts of Lieberkühn and have multipotential capacities to differentiate into various epithelial lineages (enterocytes, goblet cells, endocrine cells, Paneth cells, and M cells). They actively divide to produce a daughter stem cell and another cell that migrates upward to the surface of the villus and undergoes differentiation to fulfill the function of nutrient digestion and absorption and mucus secretion. Afterward the differentiated cell undergoes apoptosis (programmed cell death) and is shed.[10]

Apoptosis is a Greek term used to describe the falling of the leaves from the tree. It is an active mode of cell death characterized by distinctive morphologic and biochemical features. The chromatin of cells undergoing apoptosis aggregates into compact granular masses and the cytoplasm also condenses. The affected cells shrink in volume and detach from adjacent cells. Rupture of the cells follows and results in the formation of fragments called apoptotic bodies. The bodies undergo phagocytosis by macrophages or are shed into adjacent lumina. These morphologic changes are initiated by a rise in the cytosolic Ca^{+2} that activates DNA endonucleases and transglutaminases, enzymes that result in DNA fragmentation and crosslinking of cytosolic proteins, respectively. Apoptosis is activated by regulatory genes like *ced-3*, *ced-4*, and *p53* and suppressed by *ced-9* and *bcl-2*. Apoptosis is distinguished from necrosis, which is another mode of cell death resulting from physical injury.[11]

The epithelial cells of the intestines undergo apoptosis after stimulation by a polypeptide, transforming growth factor $\beta 1$ (TGF-$\beta 1$).[12] Immunohistochemical studies show the

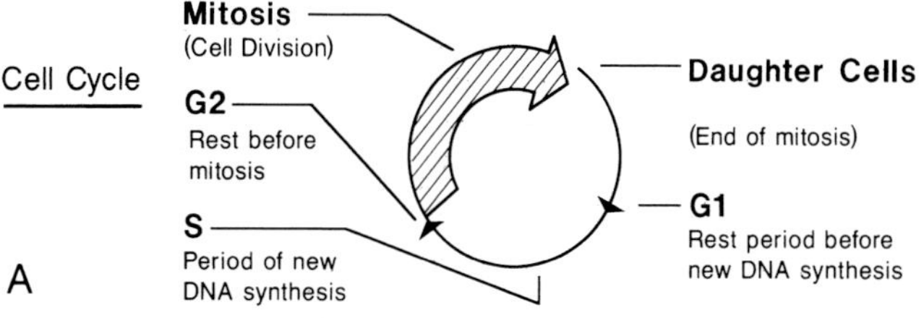

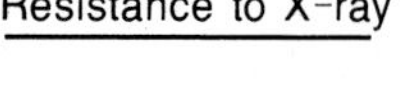

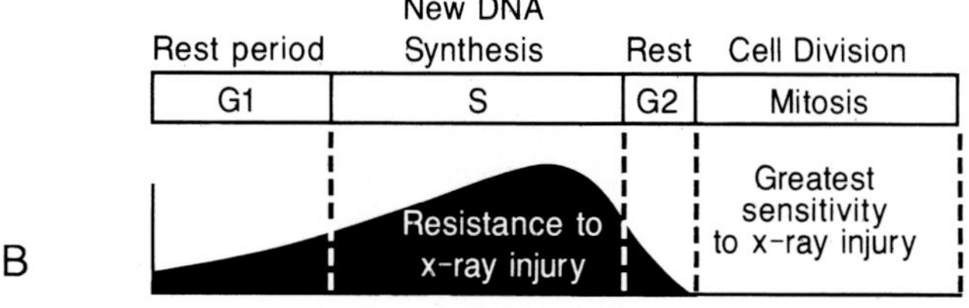

Figure 102–2. *A*, The cell division cycle showing the stages at which synthesis of new DNA and mitosis (cell division) occur. *B*, Relative sensitivity to radiation injury according to the stage of the cell cycle. Greatest sensitivity to injury is during mitosis.

location of TGF-β1 primarily in the intestinal villus. Under normal conditions, there is an equilibrium between the production of the differentiated cells from stem cells and the rate of apoptosis to maintain epithelial integrity.

In the colonic mucosa, TGF-β1 is present predominantly at the top of the colonic crypts. In addition, stem cells in the colon express the anti-apoptotic protein Bcl-2, a protein which is absent in small intestine epithelial cells.

Under normal physiologic conditions, both small intestine and colonic epithelium undergo a low rate of spontaneous apoptosis. In the colon the apoptotic rate is very low because of the presence of Bcl-2.[13]

MOLECULAR BIOLOGY OF RADIATION DAMAGE TO THE INTESTINAL OR COLONIC MUCOSA

In animal experiments, a rapid increase in the rate of apoptosis of the intestinal crypts occurs dramatically when the animals are exposed to low dose radiation (1–5 cGy). The apoptosis is observed mainly in the stem cells of the crypts. The rate of apoptosis is dose dependent and reaches a plateau at 1 Gy.

Parallel to the increase rate of apoptosis is a radiation-induced increase in the expression of the tumor suppressor gene *p53* in the stem cell region. The apoptosis induced by radiation is dependent on the presence of *p53*. In animals devoid of *p53* (*p53* null mice), there is no increase in the rate of apoptosis after irradiation in both small intestinal and colonic mucosa.

In addition to the increased level of *p53*, an increased expression of *bcl-2* is also observed in radiated colon mucosa. The rate of spontaneous and radiation-induced apoptosis is significantly increased in animals lacking *bcl-2* (*bcl-2* knockout mice), suggesting a protective effect of *bcl-2* against radiation damage.[14] It is postulated that *p53* produces apoptosis after intestinal irradiation and *bcl-2* protects the colonic mucosa from the radiation-induced apoptosis. The expression of *bcl-2* explains a higher tolerance of the colonic and rectal mucosa to radiation as compared with the small intestine. The 5% risk of complications at 5 years is estimated to be 4500 to 5000 cGy for the small intestines and 6000 to 6500 cGy for the colonic and rectal mucosa.[15] This is only an approximation because the long-term complications also depend on the volume of tissue irradiated.

Ionizing radiation also activates the translation of the gene coding for TGF-β in the small intestine and colon. TGF-β is a potent fibrogenic and pro-inflammatory cytokine, leading to hyperplasia of connective tissue mast cells and leukocyte migration into the intestinal wall. TGF-β promotes fibrosis by stimulating the expression of collagen and fibronectin genes and the chemotaxis of fibroblasts. The extracellular matrix is also increased as TGF-β inhibits its degradation. The increased expression of TGF-β is particularly enhanced in areas with histopathologic changes consistent with radiation damage: mucosal ulceration, mucosal and serosal thickening, inflammatory cell infiltrates, and vascular sclerosis (see later).[16, 17]

Experimental studies also revealed the existence of TGF-β in three isoforms (TGF-β1, TGF-β2, and TGF-β3). All three isoforms are overexpressed in the early postradiation phase, but by 26 weeks after radiation, only isoform β1 remains elevated. In the first 2 weeks after radiation, TGF-β1 messenger RNA is increased in epithelial cells, fibroblasts of the submucosa and subserosa, vascular endothelial cells and smooth muscle cells of the intestinal wall. However, at 26 weeks, the expression of TGF-β1 of epithelial cells has returned to baseline but remains elevated in vascular endothelial cells, fibroblasts, and smooth muscles cells.[18] Compared with sham-irradiated mouse intestine, the TGF-β1 immunoreactivity increased strongly in areas of radiation-induced injury. The expression of TGF-β1 also increased with fraction size.[19] These observations may have clinical significance. For example, pathological examination of bowel specimens from patients undergoing surgery for radiation enteropathy shows an increased immunoreactivity of TGF-β in areas with vascular sclerosis and fibrotic areas of the serosa and muscularis propria as compared with patients who have surgery for other causes.[20]

Other cytokines besides TGF-β, like epidermal growth factors, interleukins, and tumor necrosis factors, are currently being investigated for their effects in chronic radiation injury.[21]

INCIDENCE

Acute Radiation Enteritis

Acute radiation enteritis usually appears during the third week of a fractionated course of irradiation but may also occur a few hours after the first fraction because of abnormal motility. The incidence of acute radiation enteritis varies between 20% and 70% and depends on many factors: radiation therapy technique, volume irradiated, total dose and fractionation, and concurrent chemotherapy. The severity of radiation enteritis may require a break during the treatment or even hospitalization for the treatment of dehydration and electrolyte imbalances.[22] It is rarely life-threatening except when chemotherapy is administered concurrently and the patient's demise is usually related to sepsis and pancytopenia secondary to chemotherapy.[23] The symptoms of radiation enteritis usually improve and resolve within 2 to 6 weeks after completion of radiation.

Chronic Radiation Enteritis

The incidence of chronic radiation enteritis is unknown.[24] Retrospective series suggest a prevalence of 5% to 15%. However, in these reports a large number of patients were lost to follow-up or died between the end of radiation therapy and the completion of the study. A recent literature search for randomized trials of adjuvant therapy for rectal cancer shows severe long-term complications as low as 1.2% and as high as 15%.[25] Factors predisposing to complications are older age, postoperative irradiation, collagen vascular disease, combined chemotherapy, and poor radiation technique.[24, 25] Adhesions of small bowel loops prolapsing in the pelvis after surgery expose a large volume of intestine to radiation as compared with preoperative irradiation where the bowels are freely mobile and move out of the radiation field. The use of anterior and posterior radiation portals leads to "hot spots" (areas of higher doses of radiation) and a larger volume of bowel being irradiated. A three- or four-field technique gives a better dose distribution and significant sparing of the intestines from radiation.[25]

HISTOPATHOLOGY

Acute Radiation Enteritis

There is a dense cellular infiltrate of leukocytes and plasma cells within the intestinal crypts, resulting in edema and hyperemia. Depletion of intestinal crypts cells occur. The villi become shortened and the total epithelial surface area is reduced subsequently. In severe cases denudation and ulceration of the mucosa ensue.[26] These epithelial changes are generally reversible (Fig. 102–3). In the colonic mucosa, crypt abscesses may occur (Fig. 102–4).

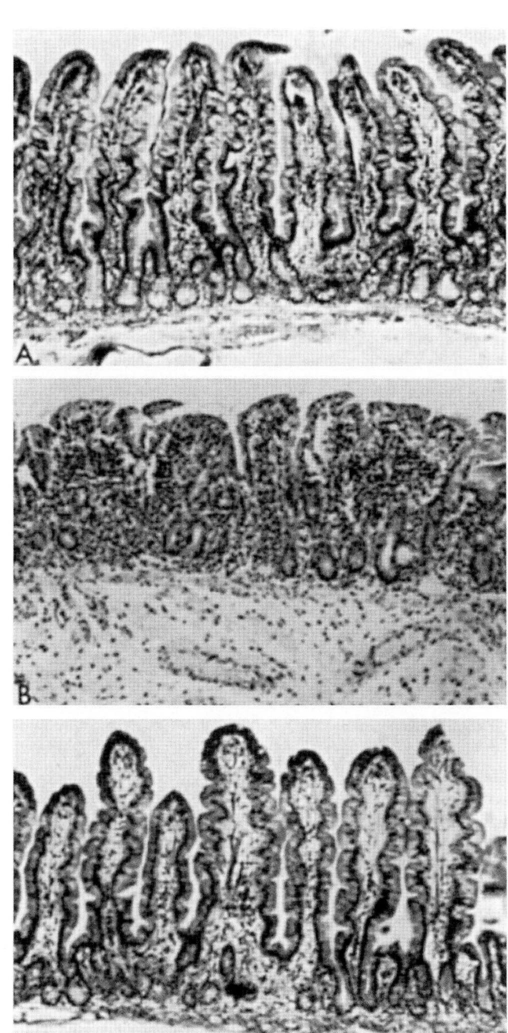

Figure 102–3. Three biopsies from the duodenojejunal junction of a patient undergoing abdominal X-ray therapy. *A*, Before treatment, the villous architecture is normal. *B*, After 3300 cGy (33 Gy) of X-ray therapy, the villi are shortened, there is increased infiltration of the lamina propria with inflammatory cells, and submucosal edema is present. *C*, Twelve days after cessation of therapy, villous architecture has returned to normal. Hematoxylin-eosin stain. Magnification, ×75. (From Trier JS, Browning, TH: Morphologic response of the human small intestine to X-ray exposure. J Clin Invest 45:194, 1966. By permission of the American Society for Clinical Investigation.)

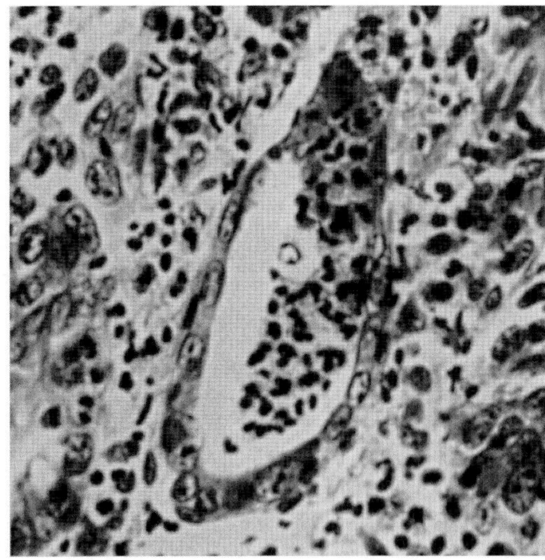

Figure 102–4. A crypt abscess in a biopsy of small bowel in a patient given 3300 cGy (33 Gy) of X-ray therapy. The surrounding epithelial cells are flattened and contain megaloblastic nuclei. The crypt abscess consists primarily of polymorphonuclear leukocytes, which are also seen in the lamina propria. Eosinophils may be prominent. Hematoxylin-eosin stain. Magnification, ×500. (From Trier JS, Browning, TH: Morphologic response of human small intestine to X-ray exposure. J Clin Invest 45:194, 1966. By permission of the American Society for Clinical Investigation.)

Chronic Radiation Enteritis

Progressive occlusive vasculitis and diffuse collagen deposition with fibrosis are the prominent features (Fig. 102–5). Large foam cells appear beneath the intima along with hyaline ring-like thickening of the arteriolar walls. The vasculitis progresses over time, resulting in mucosal ulceration, necrosis, and occasionally perforation of the intestinal wall (Fig. 102–6). Fistulas and abdominal abscesses may occur. The fibrosis leads to lumen narrowing with dilation of the bowel proximal to the stricture (Fig. 102–7). The affected segments of intestine and serosa appear thickened with areas of telangiectasis.[27] It is important to understand that once these complications occur, the vasculitis and fibrosis progress over time and all therapeutic measures should take into consideration this relentless evolution.

CLINICAL SYMPTOMS AND SIGNS

Acute Radiation Enteritis

Abdominal cramps, diarrhea, and nausea are common and result from increased intestinal motility. The loss of intestinal crypt cells and the decreased surface area for absorption may lead to malabsorption. The terminal ileum lies within the radiation field for most commonly treated pelvic malignancies. As a consequence, decreased absorption of vitamin B_{12}, bile acids, and steatorrhea may occur. Most symptoms are transient and usually subside after the discontinuation of radiation.[28, 29]

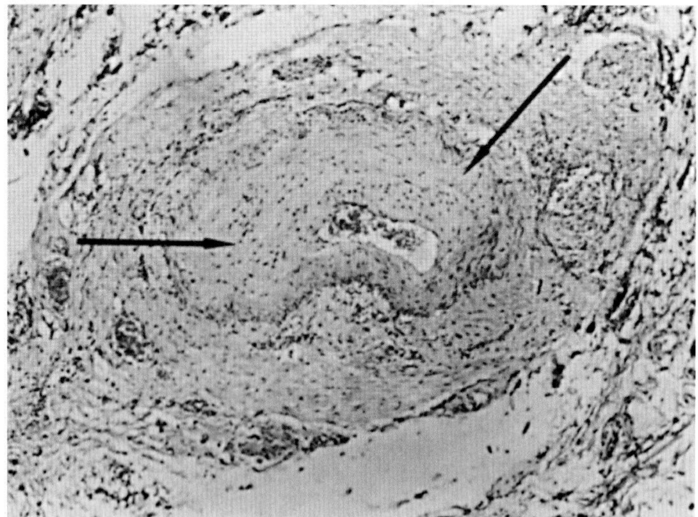

Figure 102–5. Characteristic radiation-induced change in a small submucosal arteriole. There is marked thickening of the vessel wall (*arrows*) and hydropic change of the subintimal cells. Luminal occlusion, thrombosis, and recanalization may occur. This progressive vascular lesion leads to tissue ischemia. Hematoxylin-eosin stain. Magnification, ×100.

Chronic Radiation Enteritis

The fibrosis and vasculitis of the bowel may lead to stricture and malabsorption. Bacterial overgrowth may be an indirect complication in a dilated loop of bowel proximal to the stricture (see Chapter 90). Fistula and abdominal abscess formation are serious complications requiring surgical interventions (see Chapter 24). The combination of intra-abdominal infection and malnutrition carries a poor prognosis and may result in patient demise. The severity of complications varies, and one clinical syndrome may predominate. The manifestations are usually insidious in onset, and the latency period ranges from 6 months to 25 years.[28]

There are numerous manifestations of chronic phase radiation enteritis[30] (Table 102–1).

Severe rectal damage may occur when the rectal mucosa receives a high dose of radiation from the use of intracavitary radioactive implants (e.g., in gynecologic malignancies). A high index of suspicion is required for the diagnosis of intra-abdominal abscess, because the fibrotic loops of bowel may wall off the abscess, masking symptoms of peritonitis, and delaying diagnosis.[28]

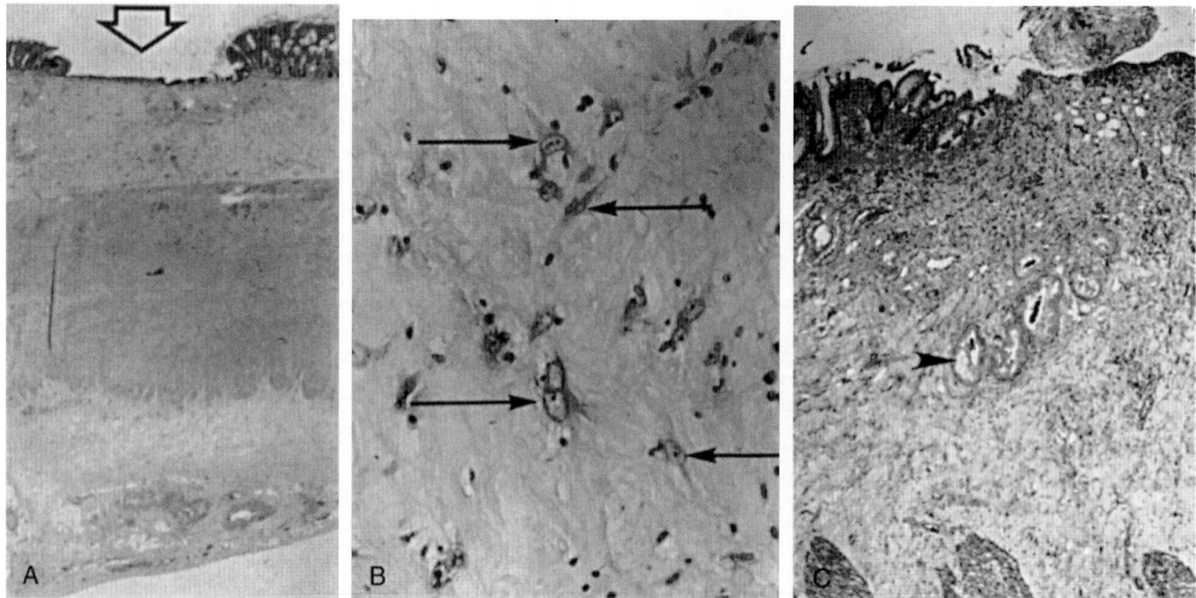

Figure 102–6. *A*, Full-thickness section (magnification, ×13) of the sigmoid colon from a patient six years after radiation therapy for carcinoma of the cervix. There is mucosal ulceration (*arrow*), thickening and scarring in both submucosa and serosa, and narrowing of the lumen of arterioles, especially in the subserosa. *B*, A high-power (magnification, ×250) view of the subserosa showing the characteristic large, bizarre radiation fibroblasts (*arrows*). *C*, Section from a similar patient with a radiation-induced colon ulceration. The ulcer surface (upper right) is covered by granulation tissue. There are residual and regenerating glands in the upper left quadrant. The submucosa is greatly thickened and contains clusters of thick-walled, small arteries (*arrowhead*) with mural aggregates of lipid-filled histiocytes. The resultant arteriolar narrowing causes progressive ischemia. (*C*, Courtesy of David C. White, M.D.)

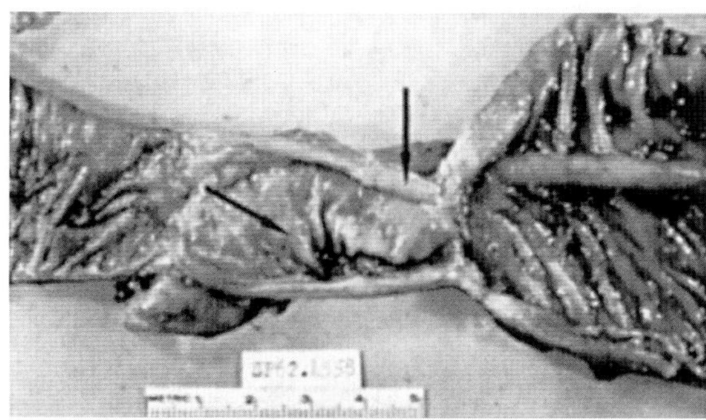

Figure 102–7. Narrow stricture (*arrows*) of the ileum 1 year after radiation therapy for carcinoma of the urinary bladder. The patient presented with symptomatic small bowel obstruction.

DIAGNOSIS

Consultation with the radiation oncology department should be requested if the clinical presentation is consistent with radiation enteritis. Review of the patient's previous radiation treatment record should reveal the total dose, fractionation, volume of treatment, and radiation technique. Analysis of the treatment plan and dose distribution may show areas of high dose, especially if the patient had an intracavitary implant. Lesions subsequently found on endoscopy or x-ray studies are usually localized in the area of high dose, exceeding the limit of tolerance of the normal organs to radiation.

Acute Radiation Enteritis

The diagnosis is straightforward based on the history. No diagnostic test is necessary unless the patient presents with the manifestation of an acute abdomen that would require the investigation of the underlying etiology, as the patient may have another condition coexisting with the cancer. Colonoscopic exam should be avoided unless necessary because of the risk of perforation secondary to insufflation and the friability of the rectal mucosa during radiation.[28]

Chronic Radiation Enteritis

Recurrence of the cancer should be excluded because the clinical manifestations of chronic radiation enteritis are nonspecific. A barium contrast study such as an enteroclysis (small bowel enema produced through the introduction of a nasoduodenal tube) may reveal a stricture with dilation of the small bowels proximal to the stricture. The enteroclysis is superior to the conventional small bowel follow-through because it provides better intestinal distension, therefore allowing a greater visualization of any intestinal abnormality.[31, 32] In one review of 1465 patients, the sensitivity and specificity of the small bowel enema was over 90%.[33]

Ulceration of the mucosa, thickening of jejunal folds, and thickening of the intestinal loops are radiologic signs that suggest radiation damage to the small bowel (Fig. 102–8). When combined with endoscopy as a one-step procedure, enteroclysis provides a safe and better localization of the occult bleeding source.[34]

Computed tomography (CT) of the abdomen is not helpful in the precise diagnosis of radiation enteritis because the CT findings are nonspecific. However, it is a valuable procedure to diagnose high-grade bowel obstruction resulting from abdominal metastases. Despite some controversy, CT enteroclysis may be the best single test when the clinical presentation is an acute or intermittent obstruction.[35] The contrast product (methylcellulose, diatrizoate solution, or 1% barium solution) is infused through a nasoenteric tube that is positioned under fluoroscopic guidance in the duodenojejunal region. Opacification and distension of the small bowels are produced with a pump producing continuous pressure. It is very sensitive for detection of low grade or intermittent obstruction (sensitivity, 88%; specificity, 82%).[36] Cross-sectional imaging with CT is obtained after the entire small bowels are opacified and provides a high accuracy in the diagnosis of high-grade obstruction from tumor recurrence (Fig. 102–9). CT enteroclysis has been reported to have a greater sensitivity (89%) and specificity (100%) than CT in patients suspected to have a partial small bowel obstruction.[37] The nasoenteric tube may also be used for suction and decompression of the obstruction. CT enteroclysis is particularly helpful in locating the obstruction when surgical intervention is contemplated or in avoiding surgery altogether if tumor recurrence is found (such as diffuse peritoneal metastases). CT enteroclysis may also be helpful for detection of the source of occult bleeding, as a vascular malformation may be shown on helical CT with contrast bolus or a small bowel neoplasm may be detected with the enteroclysis.

Barium enema may reveal stricture of the rectum or sigmoid colon in addition to a haustral segment.[38] In addition, the barium studies may show tumor recurrence or a second primary tumor. A colonoscopy may be helpful for the investigation of rectal bleeding to locate the lesion and may complement the barium enema for the detection of recurrence.[39]

Barium studies and endoscopy are not helpful for the diagnosis of abdominal abscess. A CT of the abdomen should be performed in this setting,[40] and if it is still inconclusive and the index of suspicion is high, a gallium scan may aid in the diagnosis.[41] Laparotomy and surgical exploration rather than radiologic procedures are indicated in the presence of an acute abdomen.

Table 102–1 | **Manifestations of Chronic Radiation Enteritis**

MANIFESTATION	LESION(S)	SYMPTOMS
Obstruction	Stricture	Constipation, nausea, vomiting, postprandial abdominal pain
Infection	Abscess	Abdominal pain, fever, chills, sepsis, peritonitis
Fistulization	Fistula	Fecal, vaginal, or bladder discharge; pneumaturia
Bleeding	Ulceration	Rectal pain, tenesmus, rectal bleeding, anemia
Malabsorption	Small bowel damage	Diarrhea, steatorrhea, weight loss, malnutrition, cachexia

From Girvent M, Carlson GL, Anderson I, et al. Intestinal failure after surgery for complicated radiation enteritis. Ann R Coll Surg Engl 82:198, 2000, with permission.

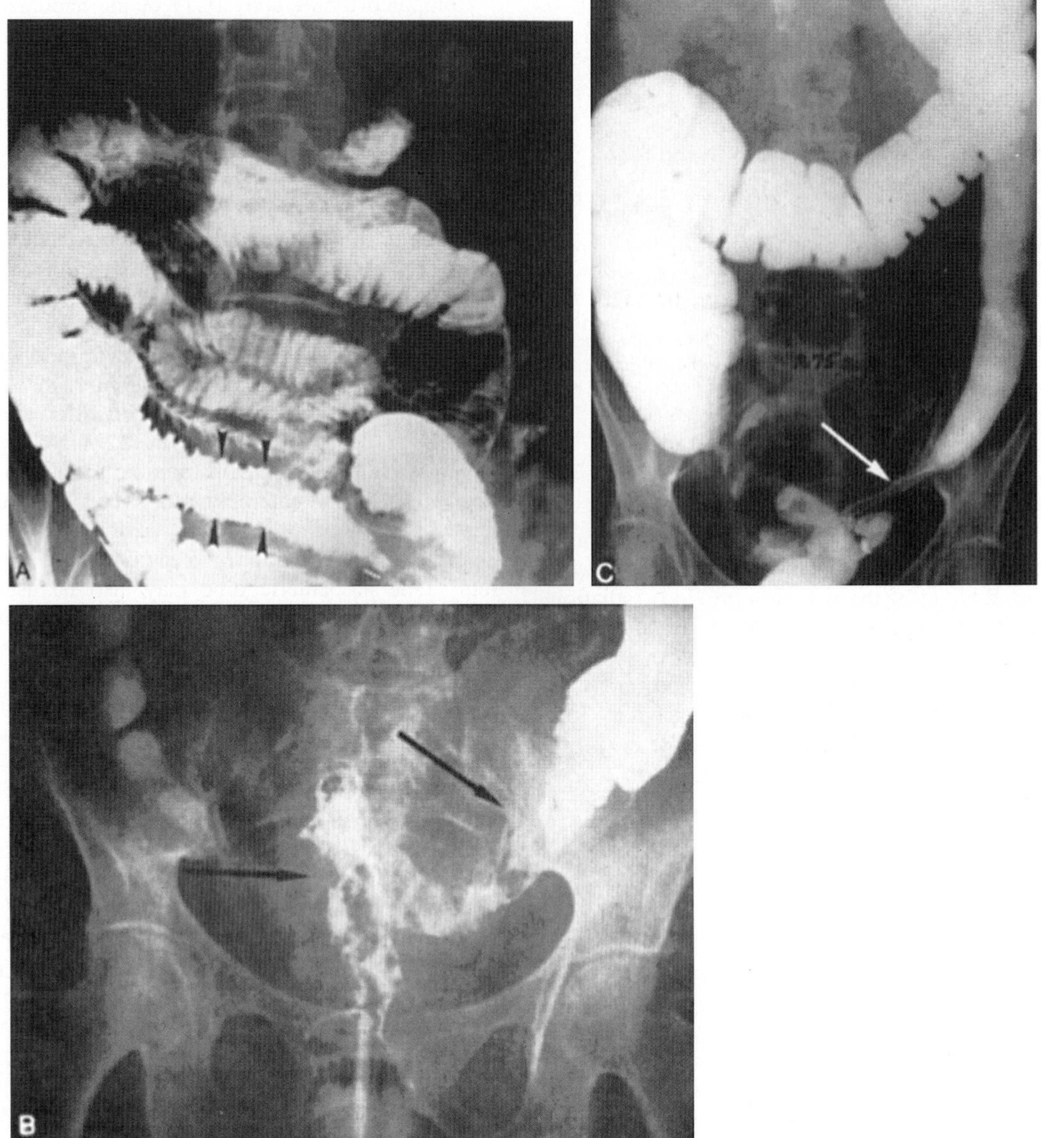

Figure 102–8. *A*, In early radiation injury of the small intestine, edema may cause separation of intestinal loops, lead to thickening and straightening of mucosal folds, and impart a spiked appearance (*arrowheads*) to the mucosa. *B*, Severe radiologic abnormalities of the rectosigmoid colon are present on this barium enema performed 2 months after the patient underwent radiation therapy for cervical carcinoma. Subacute radiation injury of the colon may present radiologically as edematous, occasionally ulcerated mucosa, with asymmetrical areas of narrowing suggestive of Crohn's colitis or recurrent tumor (*arrow*). *C*, Late radiation change in the colon after approximately 55 Gy (5500 cGy). A postirradiation stricture such as this in the proximal sigmoid colon (*arrows*) may be difficult to differentiate radiologically from malignancy.

MANAGEMENT

Acute Radiation Enteritis

Most cases of acute radiation enteritis are self-limiting, and the treatment is only supportive. Diarrhea usually resolves with antidiarrheal medications and a reduction of fat and lactose in the diet. The severity of the diarrhea rarely requires a break in the treatment unless chemotherapy is given concurrently with radiation.[42] Intractable diarrhea during the combined treatment may result in the need for hospital admission and the use of parenteral fluid administration. Severe neutropenia from chemotherapy may require cytokines such as filgrastim to shorten the period of neutropenia and avoiding excessive delay in the treatment from the bone marrow depression.[43]

Chronic Radiation Enteritis

The management of chronic radiation enteritis remains a challenge because of the progressive evolution of the lesion, mainly obstructive endarteritis and fibrosis. The treatment should be as conservative as possible because of the diffuse nature of the lesion and the high morbidity associated with surgery.

A faster intestinal transit and reduced bile acid and lactose absorption are observed in patients with chronic radia-

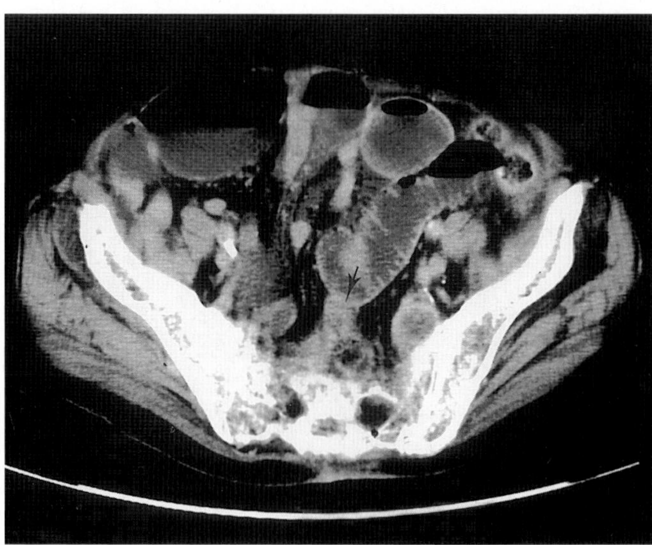

Figure 102–9. CT scan of small bowel obstruction secondary to radiation therapy of pelvis. The arrow points to the area of obstruction that corresponds to the region that received the highest dose.

tion enteritis.[44] These effects are improved after the administration of loperamide, a peripheral opiate agonist. Antibodies are indicated if there is small bowel bacterial overgrowth syndrome (see Chapter 90).[45, 46] In severe cases of malnutrition, total parenteral nutrition should be considered. The 5-year survival for patients undergoing total parenteral nutrition ranges from 36% to 54%.[47, 48]

An innovative approach to treatment of chronic radiation enteritis is the application of hyperbaric oxygen, which is currently under investigation in Europe.[49, 50] The rationale for hyperbaric oxygen is the creation of an oxygen gradient in hypoxic tissue that stimulates the formation of new vessels. Neoangiogenesis improves the blood supply and decreases the ischemia and necrosis responsible for severe complications such as fistula and bowel perforations. In a retrospective study of 36 patients with severe radiation enteritis refractory to medical management, improvement of clinical symptoms was observed in two thirds of the patients.[51] However, the optimal number of hyperbaric treatments remains unclear. Despite the limitations of such a retrospective study, this is an interesting concept that should be tested in a prospective study given the poor outcome of surgical treatment.

It is difficult to perform surgery for chronic radiation enteritis because of the diffuse fibrosis and adhesions between the bowel loops. The risk of anastomotic leak is high (up to 50%) if the anastomosis is performed using irradiated tissue because of its poor healing qualities.[30] It is difficult to distinguish between the area of normal tissue and the irradiated part of the intestines by gross examination even when the tissue is sent for fresh frozen section. The accuracy of the determination of the injured bowel may be improved by intraoperative endoscopic exam, which can detect radiation-induced mucosal injury.[52]

Another method the surgeon may use to circumvent this technical difficulty is to perform the anastomosis with colonic tissue that is located outside the pelvis and usually has not been radiated (unless the patient had whole abdominal irradiation). When one end of the anastomosis is normal tissue, the risk of an anastomotic leak is considerably reduced.[53] It is still controversial which operative procedure is optimal for the management of radiation enteritis.[54–56] Surgical resection of the diseased intestines may lead to short bowel syndrome and the need for total parenteral nutrition if the lesion is extensive (see Chapter 92). Furthermore, because of the progressive evolution of the fibrosis, the patient may require additional surgery. Surgical bypass of the injured bowel is associated with a blind loop syndrome (see Chapter 90) and does not address the risk of perforation, bleeding, abscess, and fistulas that may develop after surgery because the affected bowels are still present.

There are no randomized studies comparing surgical resection with bypass procedures. In the absence of data, surgery should be performed by an experienced team familiar with the management of radiation enteritis. Limited resection of the diseased intestine is the goal, but if the lesion is too diffuse a bypass procedure may be attempted.

Management of a pelvic fistula (e.g., vaginal or bladder fistula) is also complex and requires fecal diversion before the corrective surgery (see Chapter 24). A thorough radiographic investigation such as barium enema, small bowel follow-through, or enteroclysis to delineate the extent of the fistula should be performed before surgery. Patients with fistulas usually have electrolyte imbalance, malnutrition, and infections that make their management a challenge. Many surgical techniques have been described to repair the fistula, but they are best done when the patient is medically stable and enough time has elapsed after the surgical diversion to allow the healing and decreased inflammation of the affected tissues.[57, 58]

Hemorrhage due to radiation enteritis rarely requires surgery. Bleeding is usually minor and controlled with conservative measures like cauterization of the telangiectasis or application of formalin.[59] If the bleeding is uncontrolled, resection or ligation of the affected area(s) is preferred over a bypass procedure, because the latter will allow the hemorrhage to continue and may result in a higher mortality rate.[60]

An innovative surgical approach is small bowel transplantation, which may be considered for a pediatric population with radiation enteritis. A 5-year survival of 68% was observed with restoration of the nutrition needed for growth in patients between 2 and 18 years undergoing bowel transplant for various indications.[61] The feasibility of this approach for radiation enteritis should be investigated in this subset of patients because they usually have stunted growth and this surgical procedure is potentially a curative modality.

PREVENTION

Because the treatment of radiation enteritis is complex and rarely curative, measures should be taken to decrease its incidence. The main risk factor is surgery, which leads to the prolapse of the small intestines into the pelvis, exposing them to a full dose of radiation. The adhesions observed after surgery also increase the volume of bowel irradiated because normal intestines are usually mobile and move out of the radiation field. With adhesions, the intestines are trapped, exposing them to a high dose of radiation. If radiation therapy is anticipated after surgery, every attempt

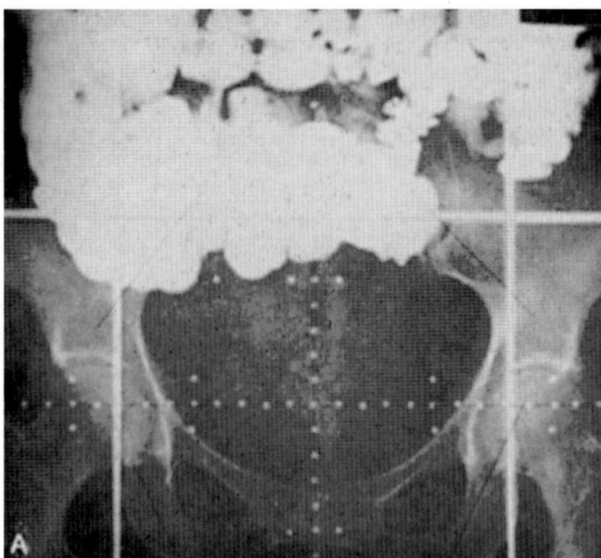

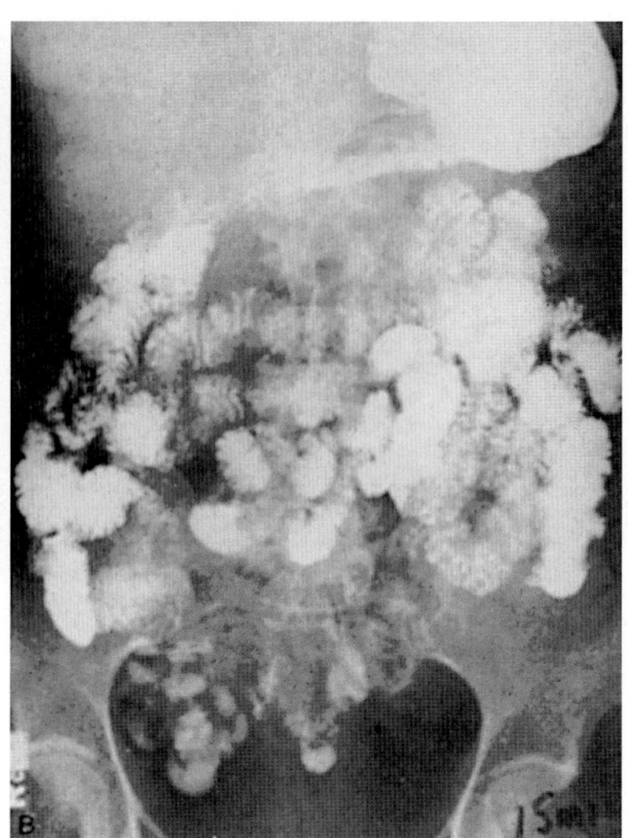

Figure 102–10. *A,* Small bowel radiograph from a patient with a biodegradable mesh sling surgically placed to keep the small intestine out of the radiation field during X-ray therapy for a pelvic malignancy. The small bowel roentgenogram shows protection of the small bowel from the pelvic area. *B,* Repeat small bowel barium radiograph 16 weeks after completion of the radiation therapy shows descent of the intestine into the pelvis after absorption of the mesh. (From Dasmahapatra KS and Swaminathan AP. The use of a biodegradable mesh to prevent radiation-associated small bowel injury. Arch Surg 126:366, 1991. By permission of the American Medical Association.)

should be made to displace the bowel outside the radiation field.[62]

One simple technique is the surgical placement of a polyglycolic biodegradable mesh that supports the intestines out of the pelvis (Fig. 102–10).[63, 64] The procedure has little morbidity, does not increase significantly the operating time, and does not require a second operation to remove the mesh because it is absorbed 3 to 4 months after surgery. Magnetic resonance imaging is used after surgery to verify the position of the mesh, the small bowel, and its disappearance. A reduction of 50% of the volume of the small bowel exposed to the radiation was demonstrated, allowing a high dose of radiation to be given when there was gross residual tumor after surgery.[65, 66] Other techniques, such as pelvic reconstruction, omentoplasty, and transposition of the colon, also decrease the volume of bowel irradiated up to 60%.[67–70] The surgical technique used is more likely linked to the experience and training of the surgeon.

Radiation therapy technique also plays an important role in the reduction of complications. The use of only anterior and posterior fields for pelvic radiation (as opposed to using three or four fields) should be avoided if possible because of the high dose and large volume of bowel irradiated. A higher rate of operative mortality was reported in trials using this technique preoperatively for rectal cancers.[71, 72] The toxicity of radiation is directly related to the volume of small bowels irradiated.[73] In obese patients, treatment in the prone position and with a belly board allows the protrusion of the small intestines out of the radiation field.[74, 75] Patients should be instructed to maintain a full bladder, which mechanically displaces the intestines out of the pelvis.[76] Modern radiation treatment techniques, like three-dimensional treatment planning, also optimize the treatment plan by developing accurate dose distributions. A three-dimensional treatment algorithm allows the sparing of excessive radiation dose to normal tissues while maximizing target dose with judicious use of multiple fields to the pelvis.[77] Appropriate packing to push the rectum and bladder away from the radioactive sources will decrease the risk of complications in brachytherapy gynecologic implants.

Among all the pharmacologic agents investigated for radiation protection and the prevention of chronic radiation enteritis, amifostine (WR-2721) is the most promising. It is a sulfhydryl compound that is converted intracellularly to an active metabolite, WR-1065, which in turn binds to free radicals and protects the cell from radiation injury.[78] The drug is well tolerated and decreases the acute side effects of radiation in clinical trials without affecting the treatment efficacy.[79] In one randomized study, the late effects of radiation were significantly reduced in the group receiving amifostine. However, the median follow-up was quite short (24 months) and longer follow-up is needed to confirm the benefits of the medication, because the incidence of late complications increases with time.[80] Other agents such as glutamine and sucralfate have been tried, but their efficacy has not been confirmed in clinical trials.[81]

It is clear that the best treatment for radiation enteritis is its prevention. Anticipation for the need of radiation and chemotherapy after surgery requires close collaboration of the surgical, radiation, and medical oncology departments. If residual disease is expected after surgery, preoperative chemotherapy and radiation may be considered to allow a curative resection. However, if gross residual tumor is found unexpectedly at surgery, outlining the tumor bed with surgical clips and surgical technique to keep the small intestine outside the pelvis (such as polyglycolic mesh) will significantly decrease the rate of complications and allow the patient a chance for a cure through the use of postoperative radiation with multiple fields, high energy beam, and three-dimensional treatment planning.

The current treatment of radiation enteritis is often only partially successful, and management should be as conservative as possible because of the relentless progression of the disease. Molecular biology studies, further understanding of the mechanism of fibrosis, and the interaction of the genes controlling apoptosis and fibrosis may assist in the identification of the patient at risk for radiation complications and in the development of new therapeutic approaches.

REFERENCES

1. Coucke PA, Maingon P, Ciernik IF, et al. A survey on staging and treatment in uterine cervical carcinoma in the Radiotherapy Cooperative Group of the European Organization for Research and Treatment of Cancer. Radiother Oncol 54:221, 2000.
2. Vicini FA, Kestin LL, Martinez AA. The correlation of serial prostate specific antigen measurement with clinical outcome after external beam radiation therapy of patients for prostate carcinoma. Cancer 88:2305, 2000.
3. Coia LR, Gunderson LL, Haller D, et al. Outcomes of patients receiving radiation for carcinoma of the rectum. Results of the 1988–1989 patterns of care study. Cancer 86:1952, 1999.
4. Ooi BS, Tjandra JJ, Green MD. Morbidities of adjuvant chemotherapy and radiotherapy for resectable rectal cancer. An overview. Dis Colon Rectum 42:403, 1999.
5. Khan FM. The physics of radiation therapy. In: Interaction of Ionizing Radiation. Baltimore, Williams & Wilkins, 1994, p 79.
6. Leadon SA. Repair of DNA damage produced by ionizing radiation: a minireview. Semin Radiat Oncol 6:295, 1996
7. Hall EJ. Radiobiology for the radiologist. In: DNA Strand Breaks and Chromosal Aberrations. Philadelphia, JB Lippincott, 1994, p 15.
8. Haimovitz-Friedman A. Radiation-induced signal transduction and stress response. Radiat Res 150:S102, 1998.
9. Bernhard EJ, McKenna WG, Muschel RJ. Radiosensitivity and the cell cycle. Cancer J Sci Am 5:194, 1999.
10. Potten CS, Booth C, Pritchard DM. The intestinal epithelial stem cell: the mucosal governor. Int J Exp Pathol 78:219, 1997.
11. Milas L, Stephens LC, Meyn RE. Relation of apoptosis to cancer therapy. In Vivo 8:665, 1994.
12. Jones BA, Gores GJ. Physiology and pathophysiology of apoptosis in epithelial cells of the liver, pancreas, and intestine. Am J Physiol 273: G1174, 1997.
13. Metcalfe A, Streuli C. Epithelial apoptosis. Bioessays 19:711, 1997.
14. Potten CS, Booth C. The role of radiation induced and spontaneous apoptosis in the homeostasis of the gastrointestinal epithelium. Comp Biochem Physiol 3:473, 1997.
15. Cohen L, Creditor M. Iso-effect tables for tolerance of irradiated normal human tissue. Int J Radiat Oncol Biol Phys 2:233, 1983.
16. Landberg CW, Hauer-Jensen M, Sung CC, et al. Expression of fibrogenic cytokines in rat small intestine after fractionated irradiation. Radiother Oncol 32:29, 1994.
17. Richter KK, Langberg CW, Sung CC, et al. Increased transforming growth factor β (TGF-β) immunoreactivity is independently associated with chronic injury in both consequential and primary radiation enteropathy. Int J Radiat Oncol Biol Phys 19:187, 1997.
18. Wang J, Zheng H, Sung CC, et al. Cellular sources of transforming grow factor-β isoforms in early and chronic radiation enteropathy. Am J Pathol 5:1531, 1998.
19. Wang J, Richter KK, Sung CC, et al. Upregulation and spatial shift in the localization of the mannose 6-phosphate/insulin-like growth factor II receptor during radiation enteropathy development in the rat. Radiother Oncol 50:205, 1999.
20. Richter KK, Fink LM, Hughes BM, et al. Is the loss of endothelial thrombomodulin involved in the mechanism of chronicity in late radiation enteropathy? Radiother Oncol 44:65, 1997.
21. Herskind C, Bamberg M, Roderman HP. The role of cytokines in the development of normal tissue reactions after radiotherapy. Strahlenther Onkol 174:12, 1998.
22. Claben J, Belka C, Paulsen F, et al. Radiation induced gastrointestinal toxicity. Strahlenther Onkol 174:82, 1998.
23. Nguyen NP, Sallah S, Karlsson U, et al. Combined preoperative chemotherapy and radiation for locally advanced rectal carcinoma. Am J Clin Oncol 23:442, 2000.
24. Rodier JF. Radiation enteropathy—incidence, aetiology, risk factors, pathology and symptoms. Tumori 81:122, 1995.
25. Ooi BS, Tjandra JJ, Green MD. Morbidities of adjuvant chemotherapy and radiotherapy for resectable rectal cancer. An overview. Dis Col Rect 42:403, 1999.
26. Carr KE, Hume SP, Ettarh R, et al. Radiation-induced changes to epithelial and non-epithelial tissue. In Dubois A, King GL, Livengood D (eds): Radiation and the Gastrointestinal Tract. Boca Raton, CRC Press, 1994, p 113.
27. Hasleton PS, Carr N, Schofield PF. Vascular changes in radiation bowel disease. Histopathology 9:517, 1985.
28. Nussbaum ML, Campana TJ, Wees JL. Radiation induced intestinal injury. Clin Plast Surg 20:573, 1993.
29. McNaughton WK. Review article: new insights into the pathogenesis of radiation induced intestinal dysfunction. Aliment Pharmacol Ther 14: 523, 2000.
30. Girvent M, Carlson GL, Anderson I, et al. Intestinal failure after surgery for complicated radiation enteritis. Ann R Coll Surg Engl 82:198, 2000.
31. Maglinte DDT, Kelvin FM, O'Connor K, et al. Current status of small bowel radiography. Abdom Imaging 21:247, 1996.
32. Nolan DJ. The true yield of the small intestinal barium study. Endoscopy 29:447, 1997.
33. Dixon PM, Roulston ME, Nolan DJ. The small bowel enema: a ten year review. Clin Radiol 47:46, 1993.
34. Willis JR, Chokshi HR, Zuckeman GR, et al. Enteroscopy-enteroclysis: experience with a combined endoscopic–radiographic technique. Gastrointest Endosc 45:163, 1997.
35. Bender GN, Maglinte DDT, Kloppel VR, et al. CT enteroclysis: a superfluous diagnostic procedure or valuable when investigating small-bowel disease? AJR Am J Roentgenol 172:373, 1999.
36. Bender GN, Timmons JH, Williard WC, et al. Computed tomographic enteroclysis: one methodology. Invest Radiol 31:43, 1996.
37. Walsh DW, Bender GN, Timmons JH. Comparison of computed tomography–enteroclysis and traditional computed tomography in the setting of suspected partial small bowel obstruction. Emerg Radiol 5:29, 1998.
38. Den Hartos-Jager FC, Cohen P, van Hasstert M. Late radiation injury of the rectum and sigmoid colon: barium enema findings in 92 patients. Br J Radiol 62:807, 1989.
39. Strom E, Larsen JL. Colon cancer at barium enema examination and colonoscopy: a study from the county of Hordaland, Norway. Radiology 211:211, 1999.
40. Freed KS, Lo JY, Baker JA, et al. Predictive model for the diagnosis of intra-abdominal abscess. Acad Radiol 5:473, 1998.
41. Lantto E. Investigation of suspected intra-abdominal sepsis: the contribution of nuclear medicine. Scand J Gastroenterol 203(Suppl):11, 1994.
42. Classen J, Belka C, Paulsen F, et al. Radiation induced gastrointestinal toxicity. Pathophysiology, approaches to treatment and prophylaxis. Strahlenther Onkol 174:82, 1998.
43. Lyman GH. A novel approach to maintain planned dose chemotherapy on time: a decision-making tool to improve patient care. Eur J Cancer 36:S15, 2000.
44. Yeoh EK, Horowitz M, Russo A, et al. Gastrointestinal function in chronic radiation enteritis-effects loperamide-N-oxide. Gut 34:476, 1993.
45. Meyers JS, Ehrenpreis ED, Craig RM. Small intestinal bacterial overgrowth syndrome. Curr Treat Options Gastroenterol 4:7–14, 2001.
46. Attar A, Flourie B, Rambaud JC, et al. Antibiotic efficacy in small intestinal bacterial overgrowth-related chronic diarrhea: a crossover, randomized trial. Gastroenterology 117:794, 1999.
47. Silvain C, Besson I, Ingrand P, et al. Long term outcome of severe

radiation enteritis treated by total parenteral nutrition. Dig Dis Sci 37: 1065, 1992.
48. Van Gossum A, Bakker H, Bozetti F, et al. Home parenteral nutrition in adults: a European multicentre survey in 1997. Clin Nutr 18:135, 1999.
49. Neurath MF, Branbrink A, Meyer K, et al. A new treatment for severe malabsorption due to radiation enteritis. Lancet 347:1302, 1996.
50. Hamour AA, Denning DW. Hyperbaric oxygen therapy in a woman who declined colostomy. Lancet 348:197, 1996.
51. Gouello JP, Bouachour G, Person B, et al. Interet de l'oxygenotherapie hyperbare dans la pathologie digestive post radique. La Presse Med 28: 1053, 1993.
52. Kuroki F, Iida M, Matsui T, et al. Intraoperative endoscopy for small intestinal damage in radiation enteritis. Gastroenterol Endosc 38:196, 1992.
53. Galland RB, Spencer J. Surgical management of radiation enteritis. Surgery 99:133, 1986.
54. Hendrix P, Cahow E. Chronic radiation enteritis. Gastroenterologist 2: 70, 1994.
55. Nakashima H, Ueo H, Shibuta K, et al. Surgical management of patients with radiation enteritis. Int Surg 81:415, 1996.
56. Joyeux H, Matias J, Gouttebel MC, et al. Strategie therapeutique dans 46 cas d'intestin radique. Chirurgie 120:129, 1994.
57. Frileux P, Berger A, Zinzindohoue F, et al. Fistules recto-vaginales de l'adulte. Ann Chir 48:412, 1994.
58. Mann WJ. Surgical management of radiation enteropathy. Surg Clin North Am 71:977, 1991.
59. Seow-Choen F, Goh HS, Eu KW, et al. A simple and effective treatment for hemorrhagic radiation proctitis using formalin. Dis Colon Rectum 36:135, 1993.
60. Libotte F, Autier P, Delmelle M, et al. Survival of patients with radiation enteritis of the small and large intestine. Acta Chir Belg 95:190, 1995.
61. Abu-Elmagd K, Reyes J, Todo S, et al. Clinical intestinal transplantation: new perspectives and immunologic consideration. J Am Coll Surg 5:512, 1998.
62. Waddell BE, Rodriguez MA, Lee RJ, et al. Prevention of chronic radiation enteritis. J Am Coll Surg 189:611, 1999.
63. Meric F, Hirschl RB, Womer RB, et al. Prevention of radiation enteritis in children, using a pelvic mesh sling. J Pediator Surg 29:917, 1994.
64. Rodier JF, Janser JC, Rodier J, et al. Prevention of radiation enteritis by an absorbable polyglycolic acid mesh sling. Cancer 68: 2545, 1991.
65. Dasmahapatra KS, Swaminathan AP. The use of a biodegradable mesh to prevent radiation associated small bowel injury. Arch Surg 126:366, 1991.
66. Rodier J, Janser J, Rodier D, et al. Prevention of radiation enteritis by an adsorbable polyglycolic acid mesh sling: A 60-case multicentric study. Cancer 68:2545, 1991.
67. Logmans A, van Lent M, van Geel AN, et al. The pedicled omentoplasty, a simple and effective surgical technique to acquire a safe pelvic radiation field: theoretical and practical aspects. Radiat Oncol 33:269, 1994.
68. Logmans A, Trimbos JB, van Lent M. The omentoplasty: a neglected ally in gynecologic surgery. Eur J Obstet Gynecol 58:167, 1995.
69. Smedh K, Moran BJ, Heald RJ. Fixed rectal cancer at laparotomy: a simple operation to protect the small bowel from radiation enteritis. Eur J Surg 163:547, 1997.
70. Chen JS, Changchien CR, Wang JY, et al. Pelvic peritoneal reconstruction to prevent radiation enteritis in rectal carcinoma. Dis Colon Rectum 35:897, 1992.
71. Stockholm Rectal Cancer Study Group. Preoperative short term radiation therapy in operable rectal cancer: a prospective randomized trial. Cancer 66:49, 1990.
72. Goldberg PA, Nicholls RJ, Porter NH, et al. Long term results of a randomized trial of short course low dose adjuvant preoperative radiotherapy for rectal cancer: reduction in local treatment failure. Eur J Cancer 30A:1602, 1994.
73. Letschert JG, Lebesque JV, de Boer RW, et al. Dose-volume correlation in radiation induced late small bowel complications: a clinical study. Radiother Oncol 18:307, 1990.
74. Caspars RJL, Hop WCJ. Irradiation of true pelvis for bladder and prostatic carcinoma in supine, prone or Trendelenburg position. Int J Radiat Oncol Biol Phys 9:589, 1983.
75. Shanahan TJ, Mehta MP, Berterud KL, et al. Minimization of small bowel volume within treatment fields utilizing customized belly boards. Int J Radiat Oncol Biol Phys 19:469, 1990.
76. Green N. The avoidance of small intestine injury in gynecologic cancer. Int J Radiat Oncol Biol Phys 9:1385, 1983.
77. Kolbl O, Richter S, Flentje M. Influence of treatment technique on dose-volume histogram and normal tissue complication probability for small bowel and bladder. A prospective study using a 3-D planning system and a radiobiological model in patients receiving postoperative pelvic irradiation. Strahlenther Onkol 176:105, 2000.
78. Door RT. Radioprotectants: pharmacology and clinical applications of Amifostine. Semin Radiat Oncol 8:10, 1998.
79. Brizel D, Sauer R, Wannenmacher M, et al. Randomized phase III trial of radiation and amifostine in patients with head and neck cancer. Proc Am Soc Clin Oncol 17:386, 1998.
80. Liu T, Liu Y, He S, et al. Use of radiation with or without WR-2721 in advanced rectal cancer. Cancer 69:2820, 1992.
81. Henriksson R, Franzen L, Littbrand B. Effects of sucralfate on acute and late bowel discomfort following radiotherapy of pelvic cancer. J Clin Oncol 10:969, 1992.

Chapter 103

CROHN'S DISEASE

Bruce E. Sands

Idiopathic inflammatory bowel disease (IBD) comprises those conditions characterized by a tendency for chronic or relapsing immune activation and inflammation within the gastrointestinal tract. Crohn's disease and ulcerative colitis are the two major forms of idiopathic IBD. Less common but increasingly recognized are the atypical, microscopic colitides, primarily collagenous colitis and lymphocytic colitis. Other chronic inflammatory conditions of the intestine share some features of presentation and pathogenesis but have identifiable etiologies. These disorders include diversion colitis, bypass enteropathy, radiation colitis, and drug-induced colitides. The two major forms of IBD share many clinical and epidemiologic characteristics, suggesting that underlying causation may be similar. Indeed, more than occasionally Crohn's disease cannot be distinguished from ulcerative colitis on clinical grounds. Yet Crohn's disease and ulcerative colitis are distinct syndromes with divergent treatment and prognosis.

Crohn's disease is a condition of chronic inflammation potentially involving any location of the alimentary tract from mouth to anus but with a propensity for the distal small bowel and proximal large bowel. Inflammation in Crohn's disease is often discontinuous along the longitudinal axis of the gut but may involve all layers from mucosa to serosa. Affected persons usually experience the cardinal symptoms of diarrhea, abdominal pain, and, often, weight loss. Frequent complications include stricture and fistula, which often necessitate surgery. Numerous extraintestinal manifestations also may be present. The etiology of Crohn's disease is incompletely understood, and therapy, although generally effective in alleviating the symptoms, is not curative.

HISTORY

Although the eponymous "Crohn's disease" has gained general acceptance in recent years, clear clinicopathologic reports of the same process date back at least two centuries. Morgagni provided a description of intestinal inflammation characteristic of Crohn's disease in 1761.[1] Only after the identification of the tubercle bacillus by Koch in 1882 was it possible to describe persons with ileocecal disease similar to intestinal tuberculosis but lacking the organism. Such reports were provided by Fenwick (1889),[1] Dalziel (1913),[2] Weiner (1914), Moschcowitz and Wilensky (1923 and 1927), and Goldfarb and Suissman (1931).[3] The landmark publication of Crohn, Ginzburg, and Oppenheimer in 1932 called attention to "terminal ileitis" as a distinct and chronic entity.[4] This term was soon deemed unsuitable when it became apparent that the disease process might also involve the colon. Patients, too, misunderstood the "terminal" nature of their illness. The term "regional enteritis" embraced the focal nature of the process but failed to incorporate knowledge of the possibility of disparate sites of involvement within the gastrointestinal tract, including the small and large bowel in combination[5] and large bowel in isolation.[6] The term "granulomatous enterocolitis" lost acceptance when it became clear that granulomas were not a *sine qua non* of the diagnosis. In the end, the name "Crohn's disease" has been adopted to encompass the many clinical presentations of this pathologic entity. But for the alphabetical priority these authors chose, Crohn's disease might well have been "Ginzburg's" or "Oppenheimer's" disease.

EPIDEMIOLOGY

Accurate comparisons of epidemiologic data on the incidence and prevalence of Crohn's disease are hampered by a lack of gold standard criteria for diagnosis and inconsistent case ascertainment. The invasiveness and expense of diagnostic modalities ensures that diagnosed cases represent only a fraction of the diseased population. Studies relying on the observations of large referral centers may be biased toward reporting more aggressive forms of the disease while underestimating the incidence.

Misclassification of disease is also problematic. Historically, unidentified infections, later recognized with improving culture and diagnostic techniques, may have accounted for some portion of cases, particularly among persons with a single episode of disease. At times, differentiating Crohn's disease from ulcerative colitis may be difficult, particularly at the time of diagnosis, before the passage of time has allowed distinctive disease characteristics to become manifest. Reassignment of a diagnosis of Crohn's disease or ulcerative colitis may be as high as 10% in the first 2 years after diagnosis.[7]

Despite these methodologic limitations, distinct and reproducible geographic and temporal trends in incidence have been observed. In both Europe and North America, higher incidence rates have been noted in more northern latitudes. For example, age-adjusted annual incidence rates of 6.0 and 10.0 cases per 100,000 persons have been reported in Northern Alberta[8] and Southeastern Norway,[7] respectively, whereas estimates of incidence rates reached only 0.9 in Spain[9] and 3.4 in Italy.[10] In the United States, recent estimates of incidence rates ascertained by various methodologies have ranged from 3.6 to 8.8 per 100,000.[11, 12] A north–south gradient similar to that observed in Europe has been noted within the United States[13] and even within the state of California itself, with estimated incidence rates of 7.0 in northern California and 3.6 in southern California.[11, 14] Recent estimates of incidence across Europe have confirmed prior observations of a north–south gradient, but the differential is now less than previously observed, perhaps because of increasing rates in the south and stabilization of rates in the north.[15]

In Japan, the incidence rate has remained low, with estimates between 0.08 and 0.5 per 100,000,[16, 17] whereas in Australia and New Zealand, incidence rates have ranged from 1.75 to 2.1 per 100,000.[18, 19] Crohn's disease is thought to be extremely rare in much of South America and Africa,[20] with the exception of South Africa, where the most recent estimate of the incidence rate for the white population is 2.6 per 100,000 and is considerably lower among nonwhite populations.[21] Estimates from less affluent nations, however, are likely to be influenced by decreased access to health care. Genetic and environmental factors in these regions are therefore difficult to disentangle.

In regions where incidence estimates have been ascertained over long periods of time, a sharp rise in incidence has been observed from the mid-1950s to the early 1970s, followed by stabilization of the rate since the 1980s. This trend has been shown most clearly in population-based studies in the United States and Denmark. In Olmsted County, Minnesota, the incidence rate rose from approximately 3 per 100,000 in 1954–1963 to nearly 8 per 100,000 in 1964–1973.[22] In Copenhagen County, Denmark, the rise has been even more precipitous, with a sixfold increase in incidence between 1962 and 1987, from less than 1 to 4.1 per 100,000 per year.[23] The factors contributing to this trend have not been completely elucidated but probably do not merely reflect improved diagnostic capabilities and the discovery of greater numbers of mild cases. This possibility is negated by the observation that death rates from Crohn's disease in six geographically diverse countries also increased through the 1950s to the 1970s.[24] These trends are best explained by one or more environmental factors, although which of these has been the driving force remains elusive (see later).

Studies throughout the world and at different times have shown a small excess risk of Crohn's disease among women. Most reports show a female-to-male ratio between unity and 1.2:1. Some studies have noted a trend from unity to increasing female risk over the past five decades.[22] This slight difference in risk may be explained by hormonal or life-style factors and stands in contrast to the nearly equal or even slight male predominance seen in ulcerative colitis.

Crohn's disease is diagnosed most frequently among persons aged 15 to 30, although the age of diagnosis may range from early childhood through the entire lifespan. Population-based studies from recent years have shown the median age of diagnosis to be approximately 30 years.[22, 25] Conflicting information may be found regarding trends in the age of diagnosis. In Olmsted County, Minnesota, younger age groups, particularly between ages 20 and 29, account for the rise in incidence over the 1960s and 1970s.[22] In contrast, population-based studies in Uppsala, Sweden[26] and Copenhagen, Denmark[25] have observed a trend toward increasing median age at diagnosis. In Stockholm, the median age of diagnosis has increased from 25 in 1960–1964 to 32 in 1985–1989. These findings reflect a larger proportion of patients diagnosed when older than age 60 years. Indeed, many, though not all, studies have shown a smaller second peak in incidence later in life, generally in the seventh decade.[27] This second peak may be the result of ascertainment bias because of more frequent contact with medical care and more frequent evaluation of older patients. Differences in clinical presentation among younger and older patients suggest that distinct risk factors are operative at different ages at onset.[28] The pathologic findings in young and old patients are not discernibly different, yet some studies have identified a greater proportion of colonic disease among older patients,[27] whereas younger patients tend to have ileal disease with greater frequency.[29] The tendency for small intestinal localization in younger patients may correlate with familial Crohn's disease, suggesting that additional nongenetic factors play a greater role in disease of later onset.

ETIOLOGY AND PATHOGENESIS

Initiating Events

In light of the nature of the pathologic findings in Crohn's disease (see later) and ulcerative colitis, it has long been clear that IBD represents a state of sustained immune response. The question arises as to whether this is an appropriate response to an unrecognized pathogen or an inappropriate response to an innocuous stimulus. Over the decades, many infectious agents have been proposed as the causative organism of Crohn's disease. Candidate agents have included chlamydia, *Listeria monocytogenes*, cell-wall deficient *Pseudomonas* species, reovirus, and many others. Paramyxovirus (measles virus) has been implicated etiologically in Crohn's disease as a cause of granulomatous vasculitis and microinfarcts of the intestine.[30] However, a proposed association between early measles vaccination and Crohn's disease has been largely disproved.[31] Another suggestion has been that the commensal flora, although normal in speciation, possess more subtle virulence factors, such as enteroadherence, that cause or contribute to IBD.[32]

Among the most enduring hypotheses is that *Mycobacterium paratuberculosis* is the causative agent of Crohn's disease. This notion dates to Dalziel's observation in 1913 that idiopathic granulomatous enterocolitis in humans is similar to Johne's disease, a granulomatous bowel disease of ruminants caused by *M. paratuberculosis*.[33] *M. paratuberculosis* is extremely fastidious in its culture requirements, and some proponents of this hypothesis have speculated that the presence of *M. paratuberculosis* as a spheroplast may confound efforts to confirm the theory. Efforts to confirm this hypothesis have included attempts to culture the organism directly, indirect demonstration of the organism by immunohistochemistry, in situ hybridization, and polymerase chain reaction methodology, and empiric treatment with anti-mycobacterial antibiotics. Most investigation in this area has been inconclusive, providing insufficient evidence to either prove or reject the hypothesis.

Experiments in genetic animal models of IBD have strongly suggested that in a genetically susceptible host, one need not invoke a classic pathogen as the cause of IBD, but rather the nonpathogenic commensal enteric flora is sufficient to induce a chronic inflammatory response. In diverse models, animals grown under germ-free conditions show diminished or delayed expression of the IBD phenotype.[34] On introduction of defined bacterial flora, however, the expected phenotype of bowel inflammation becomes manifest (Fig. 103–1).[34]

In light of the diversity of substances and bacteria within the intestinal lumen, it is remarkable that the gut is not perpetually inflamed. The presence of low-level physiologic inflammation within the healthy intestinal mucosa represents a state of preparedness to deal with potentially harmful agents, but a more vigorous response would not be appropriate if directed toward the innocuous commensal flora of the gut. Inflammation is kept in check through an active process of *immune tolerance*. Tolerance is mediated in part by subsets of CD4+ helper T cells that are generated in the intestinal mucosa and characterized by the secretion of the down-regulatory cytokines transforming growth factor-β_1 and interleukin (IL)-10. Two specific populations, T regulatory 1 and T helper 3 (Th3) cells, appear to have similar roles in maintaining mucosal tolerance in the intestine.[35] As with the animal models, evidence in humans points to an over-responsiveness of mucosal T cells to the enteric flora in IBD.[36]

When an antigenic challenge occurs, or when tolerance is broken, the immune response may be skewed toward cell-mediated immunity or toward humoral immunity and production of characteristic cytokine profiles by CD4+ T-cell populations. T helper 1 (Th1) cells are characterized by production of a typical cytokine profile of IL-2 and interferon-γ. Th1 responses support cell-mediated immunity and a delayed hypersensitivity-type response. T helper 2 (Th2) cells, in contrast, evoke humoral immunity and antibody production and elaborate IL-4, IL-5, IL-10, and other cytokines.[37] In normal hosts, the nature of the response, Th1 or Th2, depends on the characteristics of the pathogen and of the antigen-presenting cell, as well as intrinsic characteristics of the host. In the dysregulated immune response of IBD, however, the response is sustained. Most animal models of IBD are Th1 models. These models include the IL-2 −/− mouse, the IL-10 −/− mouse, and the CD45RB^{hi} SCID (severe combined immune deficiency) mouse transfer model.

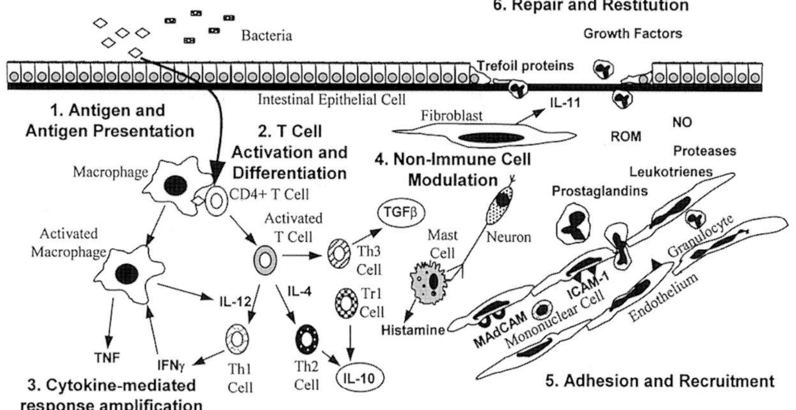

Figure 103–1. Pathogenesis of Crohn's disease. Mucosal inflammation in IBD is triggered by antigen (1) believed to be bacterial in origin. Antigen-presenting cells, which include macrophages, process antigen and present it in the context of a major histocompatibility complex class II molecule to CD4+ T cells, leading to activation and differentiation (2). T cells may differentiate as T helper 1 (Th1), T helper 2 (Th2), T helper 3 (Th3), or T regulatory 1 (Tr1) cells. Interleukin-10 (IL-10) produced by Th2 and Tr1 cells and transforming growth factor-β (TGF-β) released locally by Th3 cells down regulate inflammation. The T cell–derived cytokine IL-4 leads to Th2 differentiation, whereas the macrophage-derived cytokine IL-12 promotes Th1 differentiation of T cells. Macrophages are stimulated by interferon gamma (IFN$_\gamma$), produced by Th1 cells, leading to further release of IL-12, as well as tumor necrosis factor (TNF) and other proinflammatory cytokines (3). Nonimmune cells also modulate the immune response (4). Fibroblasts produce IL-11 and other regulatory cytokines, whereas neurons help regulate the immune reponse by stimulating release of histamine from mast cells and by secreting substance P, both of which may increase vascular permeability locally. Granulocytes and mononuclear cells are recruited into the mucosa in a highly coordinated fashion through the expression of integrins on the leukocyte and adhesion molecules, such as mucosal addressin cellular adhesion molecule (MAdCAM) and intercellular adhesion molecule-1 (ICAM-1) (5). Once present in the mucosa, these cells release directly injurious and proinflammatory substances, including prostaglandins, leukotrienes, proteases, reactive oxygen metabolites (ROM), and nitric oxide (NO). Finally, mucosal healing may occur through a process of restitution and repair (6). (From Sands BE: Novel therapies for inflammatory bowel disease. Gastroenterol Clin North Am 28:323–351, 1999. Adapted with permission.)

In Crohn's disease, CD4+ T cells have a clear-cut Th1 cytokine profile, whereas in ulcerative colitis the cytokine profile is similar to what is expected in a Th2 response, although lacking in IL-4 expression.[38, 39]

Animal models have demonstrated that a broad array of genetic alterations may result in the stereotypic responses of Th1-like or Th2-like IBD. In these models, the sustained nature of the inflammation is the result of either abnormal barrier function (dominant negative N-cadherin mouse,[40] intestinal trefoil factor −/− mouse,[41] mdr1a −/− mouse[42]) or immune dysregulation (IL-2 −/− mouse,[43] IL-10 −/− mouse,[44] HLA-B27 rat,[45] and others). It seems likely that the same phenomenon will apply in human IBD, namely, that diverse genetic perturbations may result in two main disease phenotypes characterized as Crohn's disease or ulcerative colitis. In addition, the animal models point to the likelihood that interactions among many genes will be important in disease expression because the expression of the IBD phenotype is specific to the strain of animal onto which the genetic variant is bred. An intriguing observation in humans is that bone marrow transplantation may cure Crohn's disease,[46] whereas small bowel transplantation may not.[47] This observation suggests that immunologic defects, rather than defects intrinsic to the bowel, may be paramount.

The sustained nature of the immune response in IBD may have diverse causes. Poor barrier function may permit continued exposure of lamina propria lymphocytes to antigenic stimuli from the lumen. Poor barrier function may be a factor in the onset of Crohn's disease, because patients have discernibly increased intestinal permeability preceding clinical relapse of disease.[48] Abnormally increased intestinal permeability is also found in a subset of apparently healthy family members, suggesting a possible genetic susceptibility.[49] Alternatively, a sustained exaggerated inflammatory reaction may result from an ineffective immune response—resulting from a variety of defects—to an ever-present stimulus, as occurs in a number of conditions in humans in which there is a known immunologic defect. For example, patients with chronic granulomatous disease have a defect in oxidative metabolism of granulocytes that results in a Crohn's-like inflammatory response in the bowel. Finally, the sustained nature of the inflammation may result from a programmed over-responsiveness to a persistent stimulus. Consistent with this theory is the finding that the mucosal T cells in patients with Crohn's disease have defective apoptosis. This finding could account for the sustained nature of inflammation in IBD, because programmed cell death of lymphocytes is a normal mechanism for dampening the immune response. Preliminary work suggests that IL-6 may be central to this defect in apoptosis. Increased *trans*-signaling by soluble IL-6 receptor bound to IL-6 may contribute to this failure in apoptosis, because antibodies against soluble IL-6 receptor restore apoptosis and effectively treat the disease in Th1 animal models of IBD.[50]

The interaction between T cells and macrophages is also critical to the pathogenesis of Crohn's disease. Both cell types are found together in the earliest lesions of Crohn's disease. Whatever the nature of the antigen driving the immune response, antigen is taken up by macrophages. Degradation of antigen within proteosomes in macrophages results in presentation of an epitope in the context of the class II major histocompatibility complex (MHC). Interaction between MHC class II and the T-cell receptor (CD3) results in antigen-specific interaction between the macrophage and the CD4+ T cell. This event is necessary but not sufficient to activate the T cell. A second costimulatory signal is needed as well, because binding of CD3 to MHC class II without a costimulatory signal may result in anergy or apoptosis. Important costimulatory signals include the binding of tumor necrosis factor (TNF) to TNF receptor, CD40 to CD40 ligand, and B7 to CD28. Activation of T cells leads to production of IL-2, an important growth factor for T cells. The nature of the costimulatory signal also influences the differentiation of T cells into Th1, Th2, or Th3 cells.

Amplification and Tissue Reaction

On activation, macrophages further shape and amplify the immune response by producing IL-2 and the proinflammatory cytokines IL-1 and TNF. IL-12 is likely to be a master cytokine in shaping Th1 responses and may be a highly effective target for future therapies.[51] Within mononuclear cells, the key nuclear transcription factor is NF-κB, which regulates the transcription of IL-1, IL-6, IL-8, TNF, and other peptides central to the inflammatory response.[52] NF-κB is tightly regulated within the cell. In the inactive state, NF-κB is held in the cytoplasm, bound to inhibitory κBα. During cell activation after receptor binding, various kinases phosphorylate inhibitory κBα, thereby leading to its degradation. NF-κB is then released, permitting translocation to the nucleus, where it binds to the promoter regions of numerous genes that support the inflammatory response. Such genes include those that encode proinflammatory cytokines such as TNF, adhesion molecules, and chemokines.[53] In addition to being essential to the formation of granulomas, TNF causes neutrophil activation and, along with interferon-γ, induces the expression of MHC class II on intestinal epithelial cells. Finally, TNF and other proinflammatory cytokines contribute to the expression of adhesion molecules on the endothelial cells of the intestinal vasculature.

The last step is critical for the amplification of the immune response, because the resident population of granulocytes and mononuclear cells alone do not account for the vigorous inflammatory reaction seen in IBD. Adhesion molecules on the leukocyte surface and their ligands on the high endothelial venules interact in a coordinated multistep process that permits trafficking of inflammatory cells into the mucosa. First, a weak interaction between selectins on the leukocyte surface and the endothelium leads to rolling of the leukocytes along the endothelium. Second, in the presence of chemokines such as IL-8, activation occurs, and integrins are expressed on the leukocyte surface. Third, interactions between leukocyte integrins and immunoglobulin-like cellular adhesion molecules on the endothelial surface lead to spreading of the cell and diapedesis.[54] Specificity is conferred by the presence of tissue-specific cellular adhesion molecules. The integrins $\alpha4\beta7$ and $\alpha E\beta7$ are of special importance in IBD, because the corresponding ligands—mucosal addressin cellular adhesion molecule and E-cadherin—are gut specific. Mucosal addressin cellular adhesion molecule is constitutively expressed on the high endothelial venules of the lamina propria,[55] whereas binding of $\alpha E\beta7$ on intestinal lymphocytes to E-cadherin on intestinal epithelium permits localization of intraepithelial lymphocytes. Antibodies to the $\alpha 4$ subunit of integrin,[56] to $\alpha 4\beta 7$[57], or to $\alpha E\beta 7$[58] all have proven to be therapeutic in animal models of IBD.

Once recruited to the lamina propria, mononuclear cells and granulocytes elaborate a variety of injurious and proinflammatory substances that are the ultimate cause of tissue destruction. These substances include prostaglandins, reactive oxygen metabolites, nitric oxide, leukotrienes, and proteases. Collagenase and matrix metalloproteinases play a pivotal role in the tissue destruction seen in IBD.[59] Counterbalancing these destructive substances are others that promote epithelial restitution and repair. These substances include IL-11, trefoil peptides, and growth factors, such as epidermal growth factor and keratinocyte growth factor.

Genetics

The argument for a genetic predisposition in IBD begins with the observation that family members of affected persons are at greatly increased risk of developing IBD. The relative risk among first-degree relatives is 14 to 15 times higher than that of the general population.[60] Roughly one of five patients with Crohn's disease will report having at least one affected relative. Many families have more than one affected member, and although there is a tendency within families for either ulcerative colitis or Crohn's disease to be present exclusively, mixed kindreds also occur, suggesting the presence of some shared genetic traits as a basis for both diseases. Ethnicity plays a role as well. Eastern European (Ashkenazi) Jews are at a two- to fourfold higher risk of developing IBD than non-Jews in the same geographic location and are at greater risk of having multiple affected family members. Studies of monozygotic and dizygotic twins suggest that genetic composition is a more powerful determinant of disease for Crohn's disease than for ulcerative colitis: The concordance rate among monozygotic twins is as high as 67% for Crohn's disease but only 13% to 20% for ulcerative colitis. Most studies have suggested that concordance of disease location[49, 61, 62] and disease behavior[63] are higher than one would expect by chance. Some have also noted a tendency for earlier age of diagnosis of Crohn's disease with each succeeding generation.[64] This phenomenon is called genetic anticipation and is thought to result from expansion of trinucleotide repeats in the genome over successive generations. This observation has been disputed, however, and attributed by some investigators to ascertainment bias.[65] Others have found this phenomenon to be limited to Jewish populations, particularly when the father is the transmitting parent.[66] Finally, some subclinical markers of Crohn's disease, including anti-*Saccharomyces cerevisiae* antibodies[67] and pancreatic antibodies,[68] are more frequent among apparently healthy family members of Crohn's disease probands than among the general population.

Although it is clear that the influence of genetics is more important in Crohn's disease than in ulcerative colitis, neither disease is inherited as a simple mendelian trait; rather, both are complex genetic disorders. Two complementary methods are used to unravel the genetic basis of IBD. The first method is the *genome-wide scan for linkage.* This method involves a search for shared chromosomal segments among affected family members. Genome-wide scans for linkage do not require a prior hypothesis regarding the location or nature of the responsible genes, and relatively large chromosomal segments can be searched efficiently through the use of evenly dispersed markers. The second approach is exploration of the *association of candidate genes* with the disease. This method specifically tests a hypothesis regarding the magnitude of the effect of a given gene on the phenotype. Therefore, the overall approach is to conduct broad genome-wide screens by linkage, refine the chromosomal localization successively to smaller regions, and then identify specific alleles of a candidate gene by testing for an association with the disease.

With the sequencing of the entire human genome, as well as remarkable progress in genome-wide scans for regions of IBD linkage, specific IBD genes have been identified. The presence of a locus on chromosome 16 (the so-called IBD1 locus) had been confirmed repeatedly to be linked to Crohn's disease, indicating the presence of a Crohn's disease gene in this region.[69] Two independent groups have identified the IBD1 locus as the *NOD2* gene.[69a, 69b] NOD2 mediates the innate immune response to microbial pathogens, leading to activation of NF-κB. Persons with allelic variants on both chromosomes have a 40-fold relative risk of Crohn's disease compared to those without variant *NOD2* genes.[69b] In contrast to the IBD1 locus, a locus on chromosome 12 (IBD2)[70] has been observed less consistently, in both Crohn's disease and ulcerative colitis families. Other loci suggested to have linkage to IBD include regions on chromosomes 1p,[71] 1q, 3p, 3q, 6p, and 7. The 6p region, though not as strongly associated as IBD1 or IBD2, is of interest because it is the site of the human leukocyte antigen (HLA) genes and the TNF gene. Crohn's disease has been associated with a variety of HLA class II genes, albeit inconsistently.

Environment

Although the greatest relative risk of Crohn's disease is found among first-degree relatives of affected persons, particularly siblings of the proband, environmental factors also clearly play a role. As noted earlier, the rising incidence of Crohn's disease over many decades is highly suggestive of an environmental contribution to the expression of disease. Epidemiologic studies have examined numerous risk factors for Crohn's disease. Most studies have found breast-feeding to be protective for IBD, presumably by playing a role in early programming of immune responses in the developing gastrointestinal tract. Occupations associated with outdoor physical labor are relatively under-represented among patients with Crohn's disease, and Crohn's has been associated with higher socioeconomic status,[72] presumably because of relative underexposure to diverse environmental antigens in the course of childhood. Many, but not all, studies have discerned an increased risk of Crohn's disease among women who use oral contraceptives. Nonsteroidal anti-inflammatory drugs (NSAIDs) have been implicated not only in exacerbations of IBD, but also as a potential precipitant of new cases, perhaps by increasing intestinal permeability. Increased intake of refined sugars and a paucity of fresh fruits and vegetables in the diet have been associated with the development of Crohn's disease. It is conceivable that this observation may be confounded by exacerbation of symptoms in patients with mild disease by increased dietary fiber intake, leading to avoidance of these food items before diagnosis. Another intriguing potential association is with titanium oxide in the diet, primarily as an ingredient of toothpaste. It has been shown that ultrafine particles of titanium oxide may act as an adsorbent for lipopolysaccharide and may lead to markedly heightened lymphocyte responses.[73]

One of the more notable environmental factors in IBD is smoking. Ulcerative colitis is largely a disease of ex-smokers and nonsmokers, whereas Crohn's disease is associated with smoking. Crohn's disease is more prevalent among smokers, and smokers have more surgery for their disease and a greater risk of relapse after resection. The reasons for the divergent effect of smoking on Crohn's disease and ulcerative colitis are poorly understood but may include effects on intestinal permeability, cytokine production, and clotting of the microvasculature.

Many patients report a correlation between disease exacerbations and stress. Although depression and anxiety are common in reaction to the illness, Crohn's disease is clearly not caused by stress or by an anxious personality.[74] The mind–body connection between emotional states or stress and intestinal inflammation in IBD is only slowly being revealed.[75] For example, in animal models of IBD, animals under stress are more prone to exacerbation of gut inflammation.[76]

A virtually unexplored area is the connection between environmental and genetic factors in the expression of disease. One initial foray into this area includes the finding of a differential increase in intestinal permeability among first-degree relatives of Crohn's disease probands when given NSAIDs, as compared with control subjects given NSAIDs.[77]

PATHOLOGY

Focal intestinal inflammation is the hallmark pathologic finding in Crohn's disease. This tendency for focal inflammation is evident in focal crypt inflammation, focal areas of marked chronic inflammation, the presence of aphthae and ulcers on a background of little or no chronic inflammation, and the interspersing of segments of involved bowel with segments of uninvolved bowel. Even within a single biopsy specimen one may see a pronounced variability in the degree of inflammation. The presence of focally enhanced gastritis, characterized by a focal perifoveolar or periglandular lymphomonocytic infiltrate, is a common finding in Crohn's disease that occurs in 43% of unselected patients.[78] This finding underscores the focal nature of the inflammation, despite the strong potential for inflammation to occur anywhere along the entire longitudinal axis of the gut. To a certain extent, the nature of the findings and the depth of inflammatory changes depend on the chronicity of the inflammation.

Early Findings

Because of the variable and often long delay between the onset of the disease process and diagnosis, it is rarely possible to observe the evolution of pathology from the earliest events. Studies of recurrent Crohn's disease after ileal resection have offered a window into the sequence of pathologic changes in Crohn's disease.[79] The earliest lesion characteristic of Crohn's disease is the *aphthous ulcer*. These superficial ulcers are minute, ranging in size from barely visible to 3 mm, and are surrounded by a halo of erythema.[80] In the small intestine, aphthous ulcers arise most often over lymphoid aggregates with destruction of the overlying M cells. In the colon, aphthae may occur without a central erosion and may be associated with lymphoepithelial complexes.[81] Aphthae in Crohn's disease most typically arise in the midst of normal mucosa, although villus blunting may be seen in the surrounding mucosa.[80] Aphthous ulcers represent focal areas of immune activation. The M cells and underlying lymphoid aggregates are primary locations for antigen sampling and antigen presentation, so it is not surprising that human leukocyte antigen (HLA)-DR is strongly expressed on the follicle-associated epithelium of the aphthous ulcer.[82] Furthermore, contact with luminal contents is a key factor in the development of aphthous ulcers in Crohn's disease. Aphthous ulcers heal in bowel excluded from the fecal stream by ileostomy, whereas re-establishing intestinal continuity leads to their recurrence.[83] This provides strong evidence for the role of luminal factors in the early pathogenesis of Crohn's disease.

The presence of *granulomas* (Fig. 103–2), while highly characteristic of Crohn's disease, is neither unique to Crohn's disease nor universally found. Noncaseating granulomas, like aphthous lesions, are believed to be an early finding.[84] Estimates of the prevalence of granulomas in Crohn's disease have varied greatly, ranging from 15% in endoscopic series[81] to as high as 70% in surgical series.[85] Whether granulomas are found appears to be in part a matter of how hard one looks and how much tissue is available to examine: The more tissue sampled, the larger the specimen, and the more levels taken for histopathology, the more likely granulomas are to be found. Granulomas may be discovered

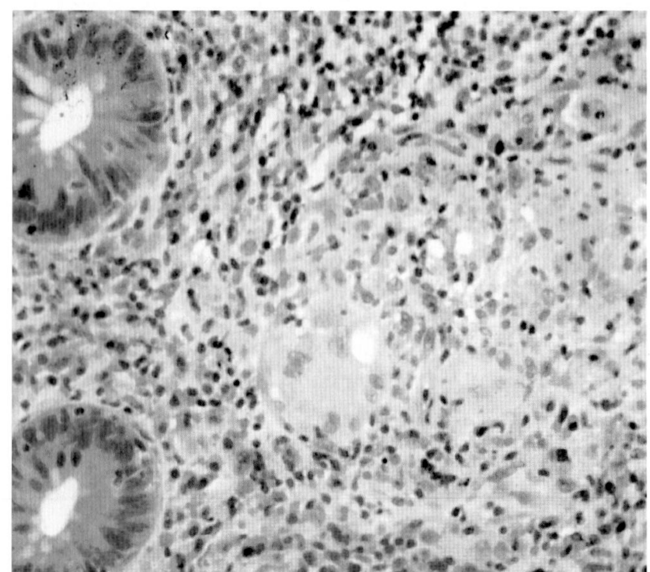

Figure 103–2. Photomicrograph of a Crohn's disease granuloma. A typical granuloma found in an endoscopic biopsy. Note the loosely formed collection of cells, consisting of multinucleated giant cells (not always observed) and mononuclear cells, including T cells and epithelioid macrophages. No central caseation is noted. (Courtesy of Dr. Gregory Lauwers.)

in involved and uninvolved bowel, in any layer of the gut, and in mesenteric lymph nodes. Occasionally, they may be recognized as serosal nodularity at laparotomy. The granulomas of Crohn's disease are sarcoid-like, consisting of collections of epithelioid histiocytes and a mixture of other inflammatory cells such as lymphocytes and eosinophils. Giant cells are occasionally seen. The granulomas are usually sparse, scattered, and not well formed. In contrast to the granulomas of tuberculosis, little or no central necrosis is present, and acid-fast stains and mycobacterial cultures are negative. It is also important to discriminate between the granulomas of Crohn's disease and those that may occasionally occur in association with an injured crypt. The latter represent a response to mucin released from injured goblet cells and may be found in ulcerative colitis and other conditions.

Regardless of whether granulomas are found, the granulomatous inflammation of Crohn's disease represents a particular process involving characteristic cell types and regulation by specific cytokines and adhesion molecules. TNF is the key cytokine in the formation of granulomas. Appreciation of this fact led to the concept of anti-TNF therapies as a treatment for Crohn's disease (see later).

Later Findings

At times, localized foci of architectural distortion unaccompanied by chronic inflammation may be observed in resected intestinal specimens. This observation suggests that early superficial lesions such as aphthae may be transient and reversible.[86] However, when the disease becomes chronic, aphthae may coalesce into larger ulcers with a stellate appearance. Linear or serpiginous ulcers may form when multiple ulcers fuse in a longitudinal direction. With transverse coalescence of ulcers, the classic cobblestoned appearance may arise, representing a network of ulcers surrounding relatively normal mucosa and prominent submucosal edema.[86] Ulcers may extend to the muscularis propria.

A prevailing generalization is that intestinal inflammation in Crohn's disease is a transmural process, as opposed to the mucosal and submucosal process characteristic of ulcerative colitis. The transmural nature of the inflammation is poorly appreciated on superficial endoscopic biopsy, but even in resected specimens the transmural aspect of the disease tends to be focal. Transmural involvement is observed less commonly than disease of the mucosa and submucosa, but to the extent that transmural disease is noted, it is highly consistent with a diagnosis of Crohn's disease. Dense lymphoid aggregates may enlarge the submucosa. At times lymphoid aggregates may also be seen just outside the muscularis propria. The presence of lymphoid aggregates in both the submucosa and external to the muscularis propria are an accurate sign of Crohn's disease even when granulomas are not seen.[86] Lymphoid aggregates occasionally may be seen within the muscularis propria, most often along the myenteric plexus.

Large ulcers, sinus tracts, and strictures are late features of Crohn's disease. Sinuses and fistulous tracts represent extensions of fissures; sinus tracts end blindly, and fistulas communicate with other organs. Intramural sinus tracts are easily recognized on barium studies. With penetration of inflammation to the serosa, serositis may occur, resulting in adhesion of bowel to other loops of large or small bowel or other adjacent organs. As a result of the chronicity of the inflammatory process, free perforation is much less common than walled-off or contained intra-abdominal abscesses or fistulas to bowel, skin, bladder, or vagina. Fissures and fistulas are lined by neutrophils and surrounded by histiocytes and a mononuclear cell infiltrate. Partial epithelialization is also frequently observed, perhaps reflecting partial healing.

Fibrosis is another transmural aspect of the disease. Fibrosis may be evident grossly as irregular thickening of the bowel wall and, along with hypertrophy of the muscularis mucosa, may contribute to the development of stricture. Transforming growth factor-β (TGF-β) is released locally in the presence of inflammation and is a cytokine critical for restitution and healing. However, TGF-β may be a double-edged sword in Crohn's disease. Fibroblasts isolated from the lamina propria produce primarily type III collagen in response to TGF-β_1, and in inflamed tissues of Crohn's disease, significantly greater amounts of type III collagen are produced in response to this cytokine.[87] Thus, a cytokine essential to the healing process is also implicated in fibrogenesis in Crohn's disease.

Other Findings

At the anatomic level, one of the most characteristic findings of Crohn's disease is the presence of *fat wrapping*. This finding, virtually pathognomonic of Crohn's disease, is the encroachment of mesenteric fat onto the serosal surface of the bowel. Surgeons have long taken fat wrapping as a reliable indicator of the presence of diseased tissue, an observation born out by careful study. Findings of adipose tissue hypertrophy of the mesentery and fat wrapping may be recognized at diagnosis. Locally, the presence of fat wrapping correlates with the presence of underlying acute and chronic inflammation, as well as transmural inflammation in the form of lymphoid aggregates.[88] A recent study demonstrated that expression of peroxisome proliferator activated receptor γ, a pivotal mediator in the regulation of adipose tissue homeostasis, is increased greatly in Crohn's tissues.[89] In turn, adipocytes may participate in the inflammatory process of Crohn's disease by producing TNF and other inflammatory mediators.

At the microscopic level, the finding of *pyloric metaplasia*, normally a response to peptic ulcer disease when found in the duodenum, strongly suggests a diagnosis of Crohn's disease when found in the terminal ileum. Careful descriptive immunopathology of areas of pyloric metaplasia reveals the presence of an ulcer-associated cell lineage. Bud-like glandular structures arise adjacent to areas of ulceration and are distinguished by production of epidermal growth factor in acinar cells of the nascent gland and by trefoil proteins in the more superficial cells lining the tract. Epidermal growth factor and trefoil proteins, in turn, may promote restitution of the epithelium in adjacent mucosal ulceration.[90]

CLINICAL MANIFESTATIONS

Disease Location

Crohn's disease has a predilection for the distal small bowel and proximal large bowel. Nearly one half of all patients have disease affecting both ileum and colon. Another one third have disease confined to the small bowel, primarily the terminal ileum and in some cases including the jejunum as well.[25] Gross involvement of the esophagus, stomach, or duodenum is rare and almost always seen in association with disease of the more distal small bowel or large bowel. Focally enhanced acute and chronic inflammation may be seen in gastric biopsies in patients with Crohn's disease either with or without gross involvement of the stomach.[91] From 20% to 25% of patients have disease confined to the colon. The discontinuous nature of the disease makes possible many variations in disease location, leading to considerable differences in the clinical presentation. Anatomic localization may also vary over time, generally by involvement of additional segments of the alimentary tract, reflecting gross involvement with a disease that has the potential to affect any segment of the gastrointestinal tract.

Clinical Presentation

The presentation of Crohn's disease may be subtle and varies considerably. Factors contributing to this variability include the location of disease within the gastrointestinal tract, intensity of inflammation, and presence of specific intestinal and extraintestinal complications. Compared with ulcerative colitis, abdominal pain is a more frequent and persistent complaint. Pain may be intermittent and colicky in nature or sustained and severe. Some patients may experience symptoms that are mild but long-standing or that are atypical. Such patients are more likely to experience a delay in diagnosis in excess of 1 year. In the past, a mean delay in diagnosis of 3.3 years from the onset of symptoms was reported,[92] but with improved diagnostic methods, and perhaps heightened awareness of the disease, more recent series have described delays of under 1 year. Occasionally, radiographic and endoscopic findings are subtle, precluding definitive diagnosis even among patients with typical symptoms. Fecal occult blood may be found in roughly one half of patients, but in contrast to ulcerative colitis, gross rectal bleeding is uncommon, and acute hemorrhage is rare.[93] Constitutional symptoms, particularly weight loss and fever, or growth retardation in children may also be prominent and are occasionally the sole presenting features of Crohn's disease.

Typical Presentations

Disease of the ileum, often accompanied by involvement of the *cecum*, may present insidiously. Some patients may present initially with a small bowel obstruction, perhaps precipitated by impaction of indigestible foods such as raw vegetables or fruit. Many years of subclinical inflammation may progress to fibrotic stenosis, with the subsequent onset of intermittent colicky pain, sometimes accompanied by nausea and vomiting. Physical examination may reveal fullness or a tender mass in the right hypogastrium during obstructive episodes. Patients with an active inflammatory component to their disease more often present with anorexia, loose or frequent stools, and weight loss. Examination may reveal fever or evidence of malnutrition. Occasionally, a patient may present with a more acute onset of right lower quadrant pain, mimicking appendicitis.

In addition to involvement of the ileum and right colon, *colonic disease* may involve primarily the right colon or may extend distally to involve most or all of the colon (*extensive or total colitis*). In patients with Crohn's colitis, tenesmus is a less frequent complaint than in patients with ulcerative colitis, because the rectum is often not involved or may be less severely inflamed than other colonic segments. The typical presenting symptom is diarrhea, occasionally with passage of obvious blood. The severity of the diarrhea tends to correlate with both the extent of colitis and the severity of inflammation, and the presentation may range from minimally altered bowel habits to fulminant colitis. Abdominal pain may be present to a greater extent than is seen in ulcerative colitis. Systemic manifestations such as weight loss and malaise may also be prominent.

Although most patients with Crohn's colitis have relative or complete sparing of the rectum, *proctitis* may be the initial presentation in some cases of Crohn's disease. Among a series of 96 patients with idiopathic proctitis, 13.6% progressed to develop Crohn's disease, usually within 3 years of initial presentation.[94]

Perianal disease is another common presentation. In as many as 24% of patients with Crohn's disease, perianal disease may precede the intestinal manifestations of Crohn's disease with a mean lead time of 4 years.[95] More often, the onset of perianal disease occurs concomitantly with or after the onset of the symptoms of luminal disease. The findings may be categorized as skin lesions, anal canal lesions, and perianal fistulas.[96] Skin lesions include maceration, superficial ulcers, and abscesses. Anal canal lesions include fissures, ulcers, and stenosis. The anal fissures of Crohn's disease tend to be placed more eccentrically than idiopathic fissures, which tend to occur along the midline. In most cases, anal stricture is asymptomatic, but occasionally obstruction may occur, particularly if the anal canal is stenotic and stool consistency improves in the course of treatment. Deeper abscesses may arise secondary to fistulas, especially when the internal os is located high in the rectum.

Unusual Presentations

Upper gastrointestinal tract Crohn's disease is uncommon in the absence of disease beyond the ligament of Treitz. Approximately one third of patients with proximal Crohn's disease do not have evidence of distal Crohn's disease at the time of diagnosis, but virtually all develop distal disease in time.[97] Patients with proximal Crohn's disease tend to be younger at the time of diagnosis and more often present with abdominal pain and malaise.[97] Patients with upper tract disease do not undergo surgery more often than patients with lower tract disease alone, but the length of bowel resected tends to be greater.[97] *Gastroduodenal Crohn's disease* presents as *Helicobactor pylori*-negative peptic ulcer disease, with dyspepsia or epigastric pain as the primary symptoms. When outflow obstruction occurs because of stricture formation or edema, early satiety, nausea, vomiting, and weight loss may predominate.

Esophageal Crohn's disease is rare, occurring in less than 2% of patients. The presenting symptoms may include dysphagia, odynophagia, substernal chest pain, and heartburn. These symptoms may be progressive and lead to profound weight loss.[98] Aphthous ulcers may sometimes be found in the mouth and posterior pharynx. Esophageal stricture and even esophagobronchial fistula may complicate the course. An intriguing observation is that HLA-DR expression is frequently seen in the esophageal epithelium in patients with Crohn's disease even when the disease is located more distally in the gastrointestinal tract, perhaps indicating widespread immunologic activation of the gastrointestinal mucosa.[99]

Crohn's disease confined solely to the jejunum and ileum is unusual and may be impossible to differentiate from *ulcerative jejunoileitis*, a distinct condition that may occasionally respond to a gluten-free diet (see Chapter 106). Frank malabsorption and steatorrhea often occur. When the disease is confined to a short segment of intestine or has other features consistent with Crohn's disease, then the management should be predicated on the diagnosis of Crohn's disease.

Controversy continues to surround the diagnosis of *Crohn's disease of the appendix*. When idiopathic granulomatous inflammation is confined to the appendix, the presentation most often resembles acute appendicitis and occasionally periappendiceal abscess. The condition is rare, but the lack of disease in other locations of bowel portends a favorable prognosis, with a postoperative recurrence rate as low as 6%.[100] Therefore, some authors suggest that granulomatous appendicitis should be considered an entity separate from Crohn's disease.[100]

Disease Behavior

Clinical observation suggests that disease behavior in Crohn's disease may be divided roughly into two categories: aggressive fistulizing disease and indolent cicatrizing disease denoted by fibrostenotic stricture.[101] A third subset of patients appear to develop neither behavior over long periods of observation. Moreover, these distinctions are not always neat. Both fistula and stricture may occur simultaneously in the same patient, as in the patient with a fistula arising behind a terminal ileal stricture, or at different times. Nevertheless, a distinctive cytokine profile of increased IL-1β and IL-1 receptor antagonist levels in intestinal tissues from patients with nonpenetrating noncicatrizing disease suggests that distinct pathogenetic mechanisms operate among these groups.[102]

Fistula and Abscess

Fistulas are frequent manifestations of the transmural nature of Crohn's disease. Immune activation triggers the release of a variety of proteases and matrix metalloproteinases[103] that may contribute directly to tissue destruction, sinus tract formation, and, finally, penetration to adjacent tissue planes. *Perianal fistulas* are common, estimated to occur among 15% to 35% of patients. When the fistula arises from an anal gland, a low-lying perianal fistula develops. Such fistulas are often minimally symptomatic and may resolve with local care alone. Surprisingly, not all perianal fistulas occur in the setting of active rectal inflammation. In some cases, perianal fistulization may be extensive, forming a network of passages and extending to multiple openings that may include not only the perianal region but also the labia or scrotum, buttocks, or thighs.

Fistulas from one segment of the gastrointestinal tract to another also occur frequently. Enteroenteric, enterocolonic, and colocolonic fistulas are often asymptomatic. Much more rarely, diseased colon penetrates normal duodenum or stomach to form a coloduodenal or cologastric fistula. Affected patients may have feculent vomiting. When the fistula tracks posteriorly from the terminal ileum to the retroperitoneum, the phlegmon may ensnare the ureter, causing noncalculous right-sided hydronephrosis. Deeper penetration yields the classic, but fortunately rare, circumstance of a psoas abscess. Affected patients typically present with right flank discomfort, fever, and a limping gait.

Fistula to the vagina may occur with penetration from a severely inflamed rectal vault anteriorly as a *rectovaginal fistula* or from the small bowel. *Enterovaginal fistulas* tend to occur among women who have had a hysterectomy, permitting direct extension to the adjacent vaginal cuff. Patients present with foul, persistent vaginal discharge and occasionally with passage of flatus or frank stool per vagina. Patients may also complain of dyspareunia or perineal pain. The vaginal os of the fistula may be difficult to visualize, but palpation may elicit tenderness of the posterior vaginal wall. Fistulas arising from terminal ileal disease often occur in the setting of an ileal stricture, where back pressure and stasis may contribute to the process. *Enterovesicular* or *colovesicular fistulas* may present as recurrent polymicrobial urinary tract infection or as frank pneumaturia and fecaluria. These fistulas are notoriously difficult to heal by nonsurgical means. *Enterocutaneous fistulas* to the anterior abdomen, often occurring after surgery, may be especially troublesome. A classic presentation of Crohn's disease is the onset of an enterocutaneous fistula after appendectomy for what had been presumed to be appendicitis. Often the tract of the fistula will follow the planes of dissection to the abdominal surface.

It has been estimated that as many as one fourth of all patients with Crohn's disease will present with an intra-abdominal abscess at some time in their lives.[104] This figure is much less than one would imagine in light of the high frequency of fistulas. For the most part, the inflamed serosal surface adheres to the innocent serosa, thereby containing an otherwise free perforation. The classic presentation of an intra-abdominal abscess is that of a patient with spiking fevers and focal abdominal tenderness or localized peritoneal signs. Unfortunately, many patients at highest risk for perforation or abscess are also on glucocorticoids, which are notorious for suppressing peritoneal signs and fever and masking the presentation. Therefore, a high level of suspicion must be maintained. When free perforation and peritonitis do occur, the situation is life-threatening.

Stricture

Stricture is another characteristic complication of Crohn's disease. Strictures represent long-standing inflammation and may occur in any segment of the gastrointestinal tract in which inflammation has been active. Nevertheless, strictures do not develop in all patients with inflammatory disease, whereas strictures are likely to recur, most often at the anastomosis, in patients who undergo bowel resection for a stricture. These observations suggest that additional unidentified factors play a role in stricture formation. Strictures are usually silent until the luminal caliber is small enough to cause relative obstruction. Symptoms may include colicky postprandial abdominal pain and bloating, punctuated by more severe episodes, and often culminating in complete obstruction. It is important to note, however, that not all obstructive presentations represent a fibrotic stricture. The classic radiographic "string sign" of a markedly narrowed bowel segment in a widely spaced bowel loop is a result of spasm and edema associated with active inflammation rather than fibrostenosis. Short of demonstrating a clearcut response to anti-inflammatory therapy or reviewing a surgical specimen, the clinician may find it extremely difficult to differentiate a fibrostenotic from an inflammatory stricture. All strictures must be considered with suspicion, and biopsies of a stricture need to be pursued vigorously because some strictures will harbor cancer.

Classification of Disease

A major need in the clinical investigation of Crohn's disease is the ability to define subgroups of patients with distinct characteristics. The ability to define such subgroups of patients with distinct prognoses could add tremendous power to the investigation of new therapies and to genetic studies. However, in light of the wide heterogeneity of demographic, anatomic, and disease behavior characteristics, distilling the numerous possible phenotypes into simple categories is a formidable task. One classification scheme that is gaining acceptance is the Vienna Classification of Crohn's Disease, which incorporates the patient's age at onset, disease location, and disease behavior into a schema with 24 potential subgroups (Table 103–1).[105] It is not surprising that in this scheme, significant associations between age at diagnosis and location and between disease behavior and location are observed, along with a trend toward an association between age at diagnosis and disease behavior.[105] The result is a clustering of patients in some subgroups (e.g., 20.4% in A1B1L2) and virtually none in others.

Pathophysiology of Common Symptoms and Signs

Diarrhea is the most common complaint among patients with Crohn's disease. Increased stool frequency and decreased stool consistency arise through alterations in mucosal function and intestinal motility.[106] In any given patient, multiple factors are likely to contribute to diarrhea. Altered fluid and electrolyte absorption and secretion may decrease stool consistency. Increased mucosal permeability from mucosal inflammation may result in exudation of protein and fluids. Increased production of prostaglandins, biogenic amines, cytokines, neuropeptides, and reactive oxygen metabolites all contribute to these alterations. An imbalance in the luminal concentration of bile acids relative to dietary fat may result in either bile salt-induced diarrhea or steatorrhea in the setting of ileal dysfunction or resection. Bacterial overgrowth may occur behind strictured bowel and contribute to malabsorption. Disordered colonic motility is seen in the setting of chronic inflammation and also contributes to diarrhea. Occasionally, medications used to treat Crohn's disease may exacerbate diarrhea. Diarrhea can occur with olsalazine, which may induce a secretory diarrhea, and any of the 5-aminosalicylates, which rarely may induce a paradoxical flare of Crohn's disease.

Table 103–1 | **Vienna Classification of Crohn's Disease**

Age at diagnosis	A1, <40 yr
	A2, ≥40 yr
Location	L1, terminal ileum
	L2, colon
	L3, ileocolon
	L4, upper gastrointestinal
Behavior	B1, nonstricturing, nonpenetrating
	B2, stricturing
	B3, penetrating

From Gasche C, Scholmerich J, Brynskov J, et al. A simple classification of Crohn's disease: report of the Working Party for the World Congresses of Gastroenterology, Vienna 1998. Inflam Bowel Dis 6:11, 2000, with permission.

The pathophysiology of *abdominal pain* in Crohn's disease is less well understood. Multiple lines of investigation have provided tantalizing clues about the connection between the nervous system and Crohn's disease. Stretch receptors in the bowel wall may be stimulated as a food bolus passes through stenotic bowel, leading to abdominal pain and possibly vomiting. Visceral pain may result from inflammation of the serosa. However, the relationship among the enteric nervous system, inflammation, and immune activation in Crohn's disease appears to be much more complex. The ganglia of the myenteric plexuses in the intestine in Crohn's disease have been noted to be increased in both size and number, possibly indicating neural dysfunction.[107] Substance P binding may participate in the expression of pain. Substance P receptors have been found in increased numbers around the lymphoid follicles in the microvasculature and on enteric neurons in Crohn's disease, even in locations distant from active inflammation.[108] Enteroglia, support cells of the enteric nervous system, express MHC class II antigens in Crohn's disease, raising the possibility that they participate in the inflammatory process directly as antigen presenting cells.[109]

Weight loss and *malnutrition* are also often seen in patients with Crohn's disease and contribute to the complaints of weakness, irritability, malaise, and easy fatiguability that are so common. In children, malnutrition may manifest as growth retardation. A host of specific nutritional deficiencies may be found even among patients in long-standing remission.[110, 111] There may be deficiencies in iron, folic acid, vitamin B_{12}, calcium, magnesium, zinc, and, particularly in the setting of malabsorption from small bowel disease, fat-soluble vitamins. Potential contributing factors are numerous and include inadequate intestinal absorption among patients with extensive small bowel disease or resection; increased protein losses through exudation from inflamed bowel; specific medications (e.g., decreased calcium absorption with glucocorticoids; malabsorption of fat, fat-soluble vitamins, and calcium with cholestyramine; folate malabsorption with sulfasalazine); and increased energy and protein requirements resulting from the catabolic state induced by intense inflammation. Moreover, unrecognized infection can be a major contributing factor beyond the catabolism induced by the disease itself. Bypassing of small bowel by enteroenteric or enterocolonic fistulas may rarely contribute to undernutrition. The most important factor in weight loss, however, is poor oral intake. Most often, poor intake results from fear of eating induced by postprandial abdominal pain or diarrhea and restriction of activities associated with meals. Decreased intake occasionally may be a consequence of unnecessarily restrictive diets imposed by the physician or the patient in an effort to control symptoms. Weight loss disproportionate to the burden of disease should raise the suspicion of occult malignancy.

Anorexia, nausea, and vomiting may also contribute to weight loss and poor nutrition. As with other symptoms of Crohn's disease, diverse mechanisms may contribute. TNF was originally discovered as a cytokine capable of inducing cachexia in malignancy and sepsis. Serum levels of TNF in severely ill patients with Crohn's disease may be high enough to contribute to anorexia. Delayed gastric emptying may be a factor in as many as one third of children with Crohn's disease.[112] Delayed gastric emptying appears to reflect an unexpectedly high rate of gastroduodenal Crohn's disease. Anorexia, nausea, or vomiting also may be caused by drugs used to treat the disease, including metronidazole, sulfasalazine, 6-mercaptopurine, azathioprine, and methotrexate.

Fever associated with active disease is usually low grade and may occasionally be the presenting complaint in Crohn's disease. Increased production of pro-inflammatory cytokines, including IL-1, IL-6, and TNF, likely contribute to this manifestation. When spiking or persistent fevers occur, the clinician needs to consider an infectious etiology and undertake an evaluation appropriate to the clinical picture.

Anemia is found in one third of patients, primarily as a consequence of iron deficiency from losses. Macrocytic anemia may also result from vitamin B_{12} deficiency because of ileal disease or resection or, less commonly, from folate deficiency because of proximal small bowel disease or sulfasalazine therapy. Overproduction of interferon-γ, TNF, or IL-1 may inhibit erythropoietin production, contributing to anemia resistant to iron supplementation.[113]

Extraintestinal Manifestations

In addition to penetrating and cicatrizing complications that may arise in patients with Crohn's disease, numerous complications may occur distant from the bowel. It is estimated that one fourth of all patients with Crohn's disease will have an extraintestinal manifestation of IBD.[114] Many of these complications are common to both Crohn's disease and ulcerative colitis and indeed to other nonidiopathic inflammatory conditions of the bowel. For example, patients with ileal Crohn's disease are at increased risk of cholelithiasis, but patients with extensive ulcerative colitis are at nearly the same risk.[115] In Crohn's disease, however, the major risk factor appears to be the number of prior ileal resections.[116] In large series, extraintestinal manifestations are found to occur more frequently in Crohn's disease than in ulcerative colitis. One fourth of those affected will have more than one manifestation.[117, 118] Conceptually, these extraintestinal manifestations may be categorized as those associated with small bowel disease or large bowel disease and those that occur in association with active bowel disease or independent of the state of inflammation. Some complications occur as a direct result of the bowel disease, such as nephrolithiasis resulting from oxalate malabsorption. In the case of inflammatory mucocutaneous, joint, and ocular manifestations, the pathogenesis is an influx of mononuclear cells activated in the gut but homing aberrantly to the involved extraintestinal organs.[119]

Musculoskeletal Manifestations

Among the most common extraintestinal manifestations are disorders of the bone and joints. Clubbing of the fingernails is a common, although innocuous, finding. More consequential are arthritic manifestations, which are observed more frequently in patients with Crohn's disease than in those with ulcerative colitis. In a study of 976 patients with ulcerative colitis and 483 with Crohn's disease, pauciarticular arthropathy (type I, affecting four or fewer joints) occurred in 3.6% of patients with ulcerative colitis and in 6.0% of those with Crohn's disease.[120] In most, joint symptoms occurred in the setting of a relapse of bowel symptoms. Polyarticular arthropathy (type II, with five or more joints affected) occurred in 2.5% of patients with ulcerative colitis and 4.0% of those with Crohn's disease.[120] Among patients with Crohn's disease, nearly one half had joint symptoms in association with a relapse in bowel disease. Intriguingly, distinct HLA genotypes are associated with these two types of peripheral arthropathy.[121]

Other investigators have reported that peripheral arthralgias occur among 16% to 20% of patients with Crohn's disease,[122] most strongly in association with colonic disease.[118] Patients tend to have waxing and waning joint pain and stiffness in association with flares of bowel disease. Joints may be involved in an asymmetric or migratory fashion. With rare exception, the disease is nondeforming and is often accompanied by skin complications (erythema nodosum) and eye complications (uveitis). Patients are seronegative for rheumatoid factor. Knee and ankle joints are often affected first, but elbows, wrists, proximal interphalangeal, metacarpophalangeal, and metatarsophalangeal joints may also be involved.[122] Ileocecal resection tends to reduce the number of episodes of joint symptoms.[123]

Axial arthropathies are less common, occurring by most estimates in 3% to 6% of patients with IBD. Spondylitis associated with IBD, like idiopathic ankylosing spondylitis, presents as insidious low back pain and morning stiffness improved by exercise. As many as 75% of patients with Crohn's disease and spondylitis may be positive for HLA-B27. Iritis may occur in association with this manifestation. A symmetric sacroiliitis without progression to spondylitis is more common and is reported to occur in 4% to 18% of patients.[122] In one study, radiographic findings of sacroiliitis were detected in 29% of patients with Crohn's disease, although only 3% had symptoms of sacroiliitis.[124]

More rare rheumatologic complications include granulomatous vasculitis,[125] periostitis, and amyloidosis. (It has been suggested that the basis of the intestinal disease is in fact the direct result of a granulomatous vasculitis affecting the intestinal microvasculature.[125]) A septic joint, although a rare complication of Crohn's disease, should be kept in mind. A septic hip joint is a striking, devastating, and fortunately rare complication of a psoas abscess that extends directly to the acetabular capsule.

Glucocorticoids used to treat Crohn's disease may be a cause of joint pain. Withdrawal of glucocorticoids may lead to pseudoarthritis, with diffuse joint aches that resolve gradually over time. Adrenal insufficiency should be considered in such patients. Aseptic necrosis of the hip and other joints may occur with or without the use of glucocorticoids and may be disabling.[126] Osteomyelitis may occur as a result of direct extension by a fistula, usually to the pelvis, or may be a recurrent problem distant to the site of inflammation, presumably through hematogenous spread of bacteria.[127]

Metabolic bone disease is common in Crohn's disease; osteopenia (T score on dual energy x-ray absorptiometry between −2.49 and −1.0) or osteoporosis (T score no more than −2.5) occurs in 30% to 60% of patients. Morbidity occurs as a consequence of increased susceptibility to bone fractures, including debilitating and painful vertebral crush fractures, which may occur even among children with Crohn's disease. Although glucocorticoid use is the main risk factor for this complication in ulcerative colitis, low bone mineral density is a feature of Crohn's disease even at diagnosis.[128] Contributing factors include malabsorption of calcium and vitamin D, smoking,[129] and perhaps the effects of pro-inflammatory cytokines such as TNF, IL-1, and IL-6 on osteoclasts, some of which may be genetically determined.[130]

Mucocutaneous Manifestations

The most common skin lesions associated with IBD are *pyoderma gangrenosum* and *erythema nodosum*. Neither condition is found solely in IBD, and the finding of one or the other lesion is not specific for either major form of IBD.[131] Pyoderma gangrenosum appears first as a papule, pustule, or nodule, most often on the leg or occasionally around a stoma, that progresses to an ulcer with undermined borders. The ulcer typically has a violaceous rim and crater-like holes pitting the base. The phenomenon of pathergy, or the development of large ulcers in response to minor trauma, is highly characteristic and common to pyoderma gangrenosum and the skin lesions of Behçet's syndrome.[132] Healing is associated with a classically cribiform, or pocked, scar. In Crohn's disease the presentation of pyoderma gangrenosum often occurs without an associated flare of bowel symptoms.

In contrast to pyoderma gangrenosum, erythema nodosum is much more frequently seen in women than in men. Like pyoderma gangrenosum, many other diseases are associated with erythema nodosum, including streptococcal or *Yersinia* infection, tuberculosis, leprosy, fungal infections, Behçet's syndrome, and sarcoidosis. The classic appearance is of tender subcutaneous nodules with an erythematous or dusky appearance, most often seen on the pretibial region. There is a strong association with arthropathy. Erythema nodosum often presents during exacerbations of bowel disease and tends to improve with treatment of the underlying bowel disease.

Aphthous ulcers of the mouth are common among patients with Crohn's disease and ulcerative colitis but are also frequently seen among otherwise healthy persons.[133] As the most cephalad point of the gastrointestinal tract, the mouth may rarely be involved directly by the granulomatous inflammation of Crohn's disease. Angular cheilitis may be seen in nearly 8% of patients with Crohn's disease.[133]

A rare manifestation is *metastatic Crohn's disease*, granulomatous inflammation of the skin remote from the gastrointestinal tract and identical to the primary bowel lesion.[134] Described cases have included lesions on the legs, penis, or vulva. Other rare skin manifestations of Crohn's disease include leukocytoclastic vasculitis,[135] Sweet's syndrome (neutrophilic dermatosis),[136] cutaneous polyarteritis nodosa, and epidermolysis bullosa acquisita. Some reports have suggested an increased occurrence of psoriasis among patients with Crohn's disease.[137]

Ocular Manifestations

Ocular manifestations are estimated to occur in 6% of patients with Crohn's disease.[138] *Episcleritis*, more common in Crohn's disease than in ulcerative colitis, consists of injection of the sclera and conjunctiva and does not affect visual acuity. Episodes tend to occur in association with active bowel disease. *Scleritis* involves deeper layers of the eye and also occurs most often in parallel with active bowel disease but may cause lasting damage if untreated. *Uveitis* usually presents with headache, blurred vision, photophobia, and iridospasm. Visual acuity is preserved unless the posterior segment becomes involved. However, in contrast to uveitis associated with ankylosing spondylitis, the presentation in patients with IBD is often insidious, with bilateral involvement and extension to the posterior segment.[139] Slit-lamp examination demonstrates an inflammatory "flare" in the anterior chamber. At least one report suggests that children with Crohn's colitis frequently have asymptomatic anterior chamber inflammation.[140] Other ocular complications of Crohn's disease include keratopathy and night blindness resulting from malabsorption of vitamin A.

Hepatobiliary Manifestations

Gallstones are found in over 25% of both men and women with Crohn's disease, representing a relative risk of 1.8 compared with the general population.[116] Aysmptomatic and mild elevations of liver biochemical tests are often seen in Crohn's disease but rarely progress to cirrhosis. Primary sclerosing cholangitis is most often associated with ulcerative colitis but may occur in 4% of patients with Crohn's disease, usually in those with colonic disease.[141] In patients with Crohn's disease, the inflammatory changes are most often confined to the small biliary radicals. Therefore, the presentation is usually one of abnormal liver biochemical tests, *pericholangitis* on liver biopsy, but an essentially normal cholangiogram.[141] Other hepatobiliary complications of Crohn's disease include fatty liver and autoimmune hepatitis.

Renal and Genitourinary Manifestations

In addition to the direct complications of perforating Crohn's disease with encroachment on the bladder and other genitourinary structures, *uric acid* and *oxalate stones* are common in patients with Crohn's disease. In the setting of fat malabsorption resulting from intestinal resection or extensive small bowel disease, luminal calcium binds free fatty acids, thereby decreasing calcium available to bind and clear oxalate. Increased oxalate is absorbed, resulting in hyperoxaluria and calcium oxalate stone formation. Uric acid stones are believed to result from volume depletion and a hypermetabolic state. More rare complications include membranous nephropathy, glomerulonephritis, and renal amyloidosis. Penile and vulvar edema have been reported.

Coagulation and Vascular Complications

A *prothrombotic tendency* has been noted in both major forms of IBD. Patients may present with venous thromboembolism or, much less commonly, arterial thrombosis. The hypercoagulable state may arise from many possible causes. Contributing factors may include thrombocytosis, increased levels of fibrinogen, fibrinopeptide A, factor V, and factor VIII, antithrombin III deficiency, and free protein S deficiency, all related to active bowel inflammation. Circulating immune complexes, increased levels of plasminogen activator inhibitors, decreased levels of tissue plasminogen activator, and spontaneous platelet aggregation may be present independent of bowel inflammation. Increased prevalence of the factor V Leiden mutation has been observed by some[142] but not other investigators.[143] Defective methylenetetrahydrofolate reductase is more prevalent among patients with IBD than the general population.[144] This finding, along with folate and vitamin B_{12} deficiency, is linked to hyperhomocysteinemia, which in turn predisposes to thrombosis. In more than one half of patients who experience thrombosis, however, no predisposing factor can be identified.[145]

Other Manifestations

Clinically significant disease of the lungs,[146, 147] heart, pancreas, and nervous system[148, 149] in association with Crohn's disease is unusual but reported. Subclinical lung involvement may be much more common than is apparent, perhaps reflecting the commonality of bronchus-associated lymphoid tissue and gut-associated lymphoid tissue.[146] Cardiomyopathy may result from a variety of nutrient deficiencies in patients with marked malabsorption. Pleuropericarditis, myocarditis, and endocarditis may rarely occur.[150] Acute pancreatitis,[151] granulomatous pancreatitis,[152] and pancreatic insufficiency[153] have also been reported.

DIFFERENTIAL DIAGNOSIS

Establishing a diagnosis of Crohn's disease is usually straightforward once it is considered. Nevertheless, a large number of alternative diagnoses may be considered during various stages of the evaluation. Reports of other diseases mistakenly diagnosed as Crohn's disease and of Crohn's disease mistaken for other diseases are legion (Table 103–2). Misdiagnoses may be attributed to the protean presentations of Crohn's disease, which include considerable variability among patients with distinct anatomic distributions of disease, different degrees of inflammation, and the variable presence of intestinal complications and extraintestinal manifestations. There are a number of clinical situations in which Crohn's disease should enter the differential diagnosis. These clinical presentations include abdominal pain, especially when localized to the right lower quadrant pain, or diarrhea; evidence of intestinal inflammation on radiography or endoscopy; the discovery of a bowel stricture or fistula arising from the bowel; and evidence of inflammation or granulomas on intestinal histology. Categories of causation that overlap with Crohn's disease in clinical presentation include functional bowel disorders, primarily irritable bowel syndrome; immune-mediated diseases, particularly other colitides and most importantly ulcerative colitis (see Chapter 104); drug-related causes, especially NSAIDs; vascular causes, notably ischemic bowel disease and collagen vascular diseases; neoplasia, including carcinoma and lymphoma; infectious causes of diarrhea, gut inflammation, or granulomas; and miscellaneous other diseases and syndromes, including diverticular disease (see Table 103–2).

ESTABLISHING THE DIAGNOSIS AND EVALUATION OF DISEASE

No single symptom, sign, or diagnostic test establishes the diagnosis of Crohn's disease. Rather the diagnosis is established through a total assessment of the clinical presentation with confirmatory evidence from radiographic, endoscopic, and, in most cases, pathologic findings. The initial evaluation includes a thorough history-taking and physical examination and simple laboratory tests. History-taking focuses on the key symptoms and their severity and duration. Specific points to be covered should include recent travel history, antibiotic use, diet, and sexual activity. Family history of IBD may raise the level of suspicion but, when found, does not guarantee the diagnosis. The review of systems should focus on eliciting extraintestinal manifestations and weight loss. Fever may be associated with the underlying disease or a suppurative complication. A careful examination of the abdomen for signs of obstruction, tenderness, or a mass should be undertaken. Thorough inspection of the perianal region and rectal examination may disclose perianal disease highly suggestive of the underlying diagnosis or gross or occult blood loss.

Laboratory data may be normal, but evidence of anemia and hypoalbuminemia should be sought. Anemic patients should undergo further evaluation to define the contributions of iron, folate, or vitamin B_{12} deficiencies. The white blood cell count may be normal or elevated; an increased number of band forms should suggest the possibility of a pyogenic complication. In the patient with vague symptoms suggestive of irritable bowel syndrome, an elevated C-reactive protein or erythrocyte sedimentation rate, although not specific for IBD, may prompt further investigation. Stool studies should include culture, examination for ova and parasites, and testing for *Clostridium difficile* toxin and should be performed before endoscopy or barium studies. Serology for *Entamoeba histolytica* should be considered in selected patients.

Ultimately, a diagnosis of Crohn's disease is confirmed by findings on barium radiography, endoscopy, and usually histopathology. Barium studies accurately define the anatomic location of disease and can discern evidence of active

Table 103–2 | **Differential Diagnosis of Crohn's Disease**

- Infection
  - **Bacterial**
    - Intestinal tuberculosis
    - Atypical mycobacteria
    - *Clostridium difficile*
    - *Yersinia enterocolitica*
    - *Yersinia pseudotuberculosis*
    - Enterohemorrhagic *Escherichia coli* (EHEC), including *E. coli* O157:H7
    - *Salmonella*
    - *Shigella*
    - *Campylobacter jejuni*
    - Spirochetosis
    - *Chlamydia trachomatis* (lymphogranuloma venereum and nonlymphogranuloma venereum)
    - *Aeromonas hydrophilia*
    - *Plesiomonas hydrophilia*
    - Acute self-limited colitis
  - **Viral**
    - Cytomegalovirus
    - Herpes simplex virus
  - **Helminthic**
    - Anisakiasis
    - Whipworm (trichiuriasis)
    - *Strongyloides stercoralis*
    - *Angiostrongylus costaricensis* enterocolitis
  - **Fungal**
    - Histoplasmosis
    - Actinomycosis
    - Cryptococcosis
    - Basidiobolomycosis
  - **Protozoa**
    - Amebiasis
    - *Giardia lamblia*
    - *Endolimax nana*
    - *Cryptosporidia*
    - *Entameba coli*
    - *Isospora beli*
    - Schistosomiasis
- Neoplasia
  - Carcinoma
    - Primary
    - Metastatic
  - Lymphoma
  - Carcinoid
  - Mycosis fungoides
  - Malignant histiocytosis (histiocytosis X)
- Functional/psychiatric disorders
  - Irritable bowel syndrome
  - Anorexia nervosa (children, adolescents)
  - Sexual abuse (children)
- Vascular
  - Ischemic bowel of various causes
  - Superior mesenteric venous thrombosis
  - Collagen vascular disease (see immune mediated below)
  - Solitary rectal ulcer syndrome (localized colitis cystica profunda)
  - Radiation enteritis/colitis
- Drug related
  - Nonsteroidal anti-inflammatory drugs
  - Oral contraceptives
  - Gold
  - Cathartic colon
  - Phosphosoda bowel preparation
  - Enteric-coated potassium chloride
  - Pancreatic enzyme supplements in cystic fibrosis (fibrosing colonopathy)
- Immune mediated
  - Congenital immunodeficiency
    - X-linked agammaglobulinemia
    - Common variable immunodeficiency
    - Glycogen storage disease type Ib
    - Chronic granulomatous disease
    - Turner's syndrome
    - Hermansky-Pudlak syndrome
    - Chediak-Higashi syndrome
    - C1 inhibitor deficiency and angioedema
  - HIV-related (see infections)
  - Collagen vascular disease
    - Polyarteritis nodosa
    - Systemic lupus erythematosus
    - Rheumatoid arthritis
    - Progressive systemic sclerosis
    - Necrotizing angiitis
    - Essential mixed cryoglobulinemia
    - Dermatomyositis
    - Henoch-Schönlein purpura
    - Seronegative spondyloarthropathy-related enteritis
    - Sarcoidosis
    - Graft-versus-host disease
    - Castleman's disease and neutropenic enterocolitis
    - Small bowel angioedema
    - Linear IgA disease
    - Extranodal angioimmunoblastic lymphadenopathy
    - Paroxysmal nocturnal hemoglobinuria
  - Other enterocolitidies
    - Ulcerative colitis
    - Eosinophilic gastroenteritis
    - Collagenous colitis
    - Allergic colitis
    - Nongranulomatous ulcerative jejunoileitis
    - Segmental colitis
    - Diversion colitis
    - Bypass enteritis
  - Celiac sprue
- Miscellaneous
  - Nodular lymphoid hyperplasia
  - Diverticular disease
  - Pneumatosis cystoides intestinalis
  - Peptic ulcer disease
  - Adhesions
  - Ileocolonic anastomotic ulcers
  - Endometriosis
  - Conditions of the ovary or fallopian tube
    - Abscess
    - Cysts
    - Tumors
    - Ectopic pregnancy
    - Pelvic inflammatory disease
  - Conditions of the ileum, appendix, and cecum
    - Acute appendicitis
    - Periappendiceal abscess
    - Infarction of the appendiceal epiploica
    - Mucocele
    - Cecal diverticulitis
    - Meckel's diverticulum
    - Lipomatosis of ileocecal valve
  - Blunt trauma injury
  - Amyloidosis
  - Malakoplakia
  - Hidradenitis suppurativa
  - Melkersson-Rosenthal syndrome
  - Infected urachal cyst
  - Foreign body perforation and abscess (e.g., toothpick)
  - Thermal injury from colostomy irrigation
  - Phytobezoar
  - Zollinger-Ellison syndrome
  - Mesenteric panniculitis

inflammation. A small bowel follow-through study is the primary modality when small bowel disease is suspected (Fig. 103–3). For most situations, small bowel enema, or enteroclysis, adds little additional information and may in fact miss gastroduodenal findings but increases the cost and morbidity considerably.[154] Barium studies are especially useful in delineating the late transmural complications of Crohn's disease, but typical findings may be seen early in the disease as well. Early findings include aphthous ulcers, a coarse villous pattern of the mucosa, and thickened folds.[155] Submucosal edema may be evident as thickening or flattening of the valvulae conniventes, whereas transmural edema manifests as widening of the separation between loops of bowel. Ulcers most often occur on the mesenteric border with consequent pseudosacculation of the antimesenteric border because of shortening of the mesenteric portion.[155] Later findings include a cobblestone appearance resulting from edema in relatively spared islands of mucosa that are separated by longitudinal and transverse knife-like clefts of ulceration.[155] Still later, one may discern fistulas, sinus tracts, and fixed strictures.

Other radiographic studies may provide adjunctive information. Computed tomography (CT) studies do not demonstrate mucosal detail and often appear normal early in the course of the disease (Fig. 103–4). Nevertheless, CT is of great value in discerning extraluminal features.[156] As the disease progresses, mesenteric lymphadenopathy and transmural thickening of the bowel are usually seen. CT is highly sensitive for detecting differences in tissue densities. Therefore, the detection on CT of even small amounts of air in the bowel wall or adjacent structures is highly suggestive of perforating disease. Fibrofatty proliferation of the mesentery, the radiographic correlate of creeping fat seen at laparotomy, may be noted.[157] CT is the essential study for identifying suppurative complications of Crohn's disease, such as intra-abdominal and retroperitoneal abscess.

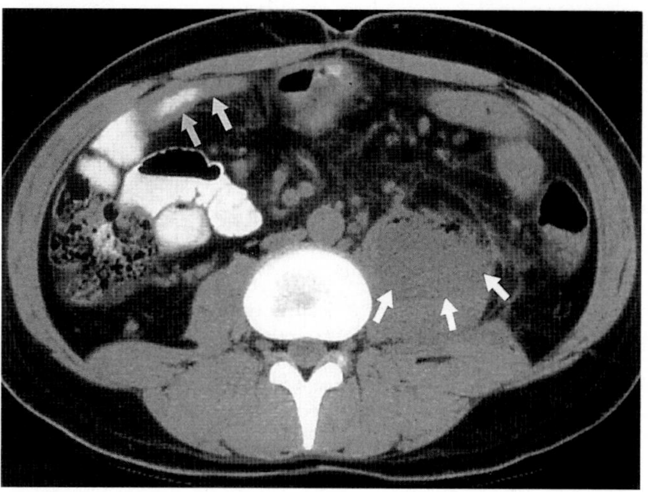

Figure 103–4. Abdominal CT in Crohn's disease. Cross-sectional imaging by computed tomography plays a complementary role in the evaluation of Crohn's disease. This image was obtained from the same patient whose small bowel follow through is seen in Figure 103–3. The left psoas muscle abscess (*white arrows*), arising from penetrating disease from overlying bowel, is completely missed on small bowel follow through. Thickened small bowel (*gray arrows*) is also seen, along with minor retroperitoneal lymphadenopathy and fatty proliferation of the mesentery. (Courtesy of Dr. Jack Wittenberg, Massachusetts General Hospital, Boston, MA.)

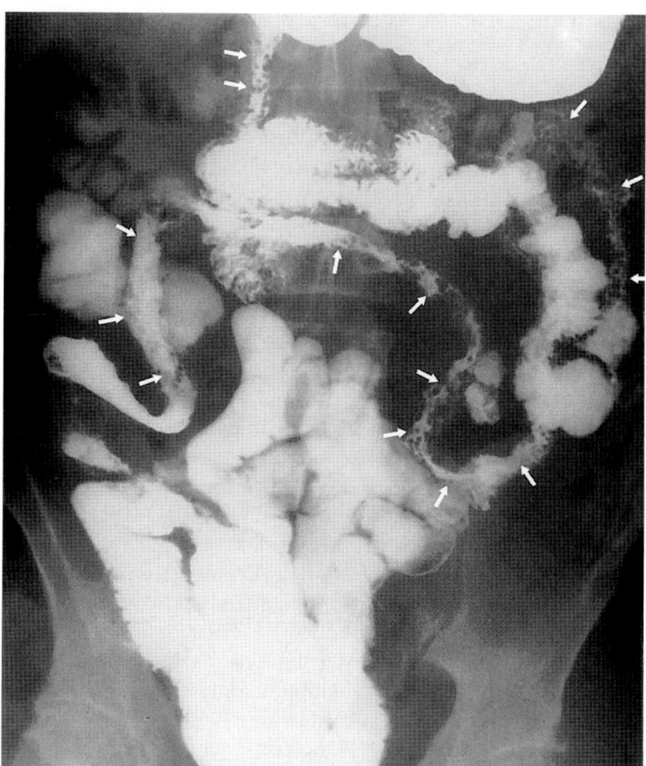

Figure 103–3. Small bowel follow through in Crohn's disease. Barium studies continue to play an important role in the evaluation of Crohn's disease. Multiple areas of narrowed small bowel are noted (*white arrows*) with classic cobblestone appearance of the mucosa. Note also separation of the loops of bowel. (Courtesy of Dr. Jack Wittenberg, Massachusetts General Hospital, Boston, MA.)

Other potentially useful modalities include ultrasound, magnetic resonance imaging, and scintigraphy. Ultrasound is useful primarily in excluding other causes of abdominal pain, including biliary and gynecologic causes. Continuing advances in transabdominal ultrasound,[158] endosonography,[159] and vascular flow studies[160] may in time provide improved diagnostic accuracy and grading of activity in Crohn's disease. Magnetic resonance imaging may provide visualization of complex perianal fistulas superior to that of pelvic CT.[161] As technology improves, magnetic resonance imaging may provide imaging of the abdomen equal or superior to CT without exposure to ionizing radiation[162] and may also prove useful in demonstrating response to treatment.[163] Ultrasound- and CT-guided percutaneous drainage of intra-abdominal abscesses is a safe and effective alternative to surgical drainage in well-selected patients.[164] A growing body of evidence suggests that leukocyte scintigraphy may be a useful diagnostic study in Crohn's disease. Among children with suspected IBD, ^{99m}Tc leukocyte scintigraphy is highly sensitive in identifying patients with mild inflammation on biopsy and a normal small bowel follow-through.[165] Lower radiation exposure is an advantage of this technique over barium studies.

Because of its ability to visualize the mucosa directly and permit biopsy for histopathology, endoscopy complements radiographic techniques. Many of the same mucosal features

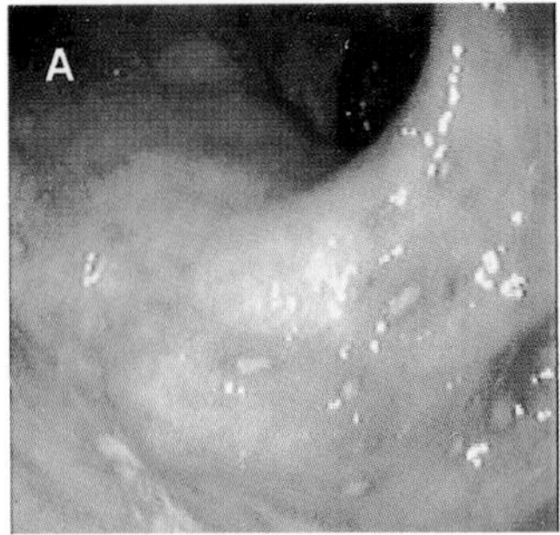

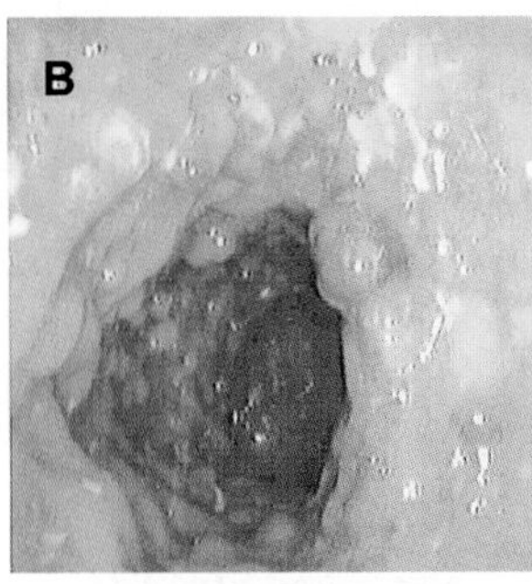

Figure 103–5. Endoscopic appearance of Crohn's disease. A wide variety of findings may be visualized on endoscopy, in part depending on the duration and severity of the inflammation. *A,* Typical aphthous ulcers, consisting of a central white depression surrounded by a slightly elevated, erythematous rim only a few millimeters in diameter. *B,* Findings more typical of advanced disease, with erythema, edema, and a cobblestone appearance.

seen on barium studies are also recognized on endoscopy, including aphthous ulcers, mucosal edema, cobblestoning, and luminal narrowing (Fig. 103–5.) The visual impression of demarcated lesions on a background of normal mucosa is most easily recognized in early or mild disease. Rectal sparing is also more specific before treatment has been initiated. The discontinuous segmental nature of the disease is an important clue to the diagnosis and has a high positive predictive value.[166] Intubation and biopsy of the terminal ileum should be attempted in all patients and greatly increase the sensitivity and specificity of the examination.[167] In general, the diagnostic accuracy of colonoscopy and histologic interpretation is increased substantially by obtaining multiple biopsies from both involved and uninvolved sites. The use of jumbo forceps should be considered to improve sampling of the submucosa. Balloon dilation of strictures is another application of endoscopy in Crohn's disease that may delay or spare the need for surgery.

Differentiating Crohn's Disease from Ulcerative Colitis

When IBD is confined to the colon, the main diagnostic distinction is between Crohn's colitis and ulcerative colitis. As noted earlier, ulcerative colitis and Crohn's disease share many similarities in epidemiology and manifestation. The distinction between these diseases is increasingly important in the choice of surgical and medical therapies. Patients with features of both diseases are said to have indeterminate colitis, a vague term applied in various ways among different centers. As many as 10% of patients presenting with IBD are considered to have indeterminate colitis. A diagnosis of indeterminate colitis has particular implications for surgical therapy, because patients undergoing ileoanal pouch construction for indeterminate colitis have a relatively high likelihood of developing Crohn's-like complications of the pouch.[168] Histology, when applied without attention to clinical features, has a high likelihood of yielding a diagnosis of indeterminate colitis.[169, 170] Therefore, the entire clinical picture must be considered (Table 103–3). Discriminating features include small bowel disease, predominantly right colonic disease, rectal sparing, fistulization (with the exception of rare rectovaginal fistulas in ulcerative colitis), major perianal complications, and granulomas, all of which are strongly indicative of Crohn's disease. In the few cases initially labeled as indeterminate, the true diagnosis usually becomes clear with the passage of time.

In the absence of knowledge of the precise environmental and genetic determinants that produce a clinical phenotype of Crohn's disease or ulcerative colitis, immunologic markers are being explored as a means of differentiating the two diseases. The presence in serum of perinuclear anti-neutrophil cytoplasmic antibody (pANCA) and antiglycan antibodies to mannan, a constituent of the cell wall of baker's yeast (anti-*Saccharomyces cerevisiae* antibody [ASCA]), correlate with diagnoses of ulcerative colitis and Crohn's disease, respectively.[171–173] The specificity of each of these serologic markers is approximately 85%, but sensitivity is considerably lower at 50% to 65%, with considerable variation among assays performed in different laboratories. In addition, pANCA may be found in approximately 15% of patients with Crohn's disease, particularly among patients with an ulcerative colitis-like phenotype.[174] Combining the two assays improves specificity but at the further expense of sensitivity.[171] Thus, serologic testing for pANCA and ASCA may be considered at this time to be an adjunct to diagnosis in selected cases—one additional piece of evidence to be considered but not definitive in establishing the diagnosis.

Measuring Disease Activity

For the purposes of daily practice, it is usually sufficient to follow the patient's symptoms and signs in response to treatment. Rarely is it necessary to subject the patient to repeated radiographic studies or colonoscopies to ascertain disease activity, and disease location tends to be stable over time. Repeat studies are best undertaken when symptoms have changed substantially or are suspected to arise not from persistent intestinal inflammation but from other causes such an infection, complication, or functional disorder. In clinical research, however, more quantitative evaluations are needed. Composite scoring systems, most commonly the Crohn's Disease Activity Index (CDAI, Table 103–4), are used in an attempt to integrate the many possible features of the disease. Other disease activity indices include the van Hees index,[175] the Cape Town index,[176] the Harvey-Bradshaw index,[177] the International Organization of IBD (or Oxford) index,[178] the St. Marks Crohn's index,[179] De Dombal's index,[180] the Talstad index,[181] and a Crohn's disease activity index for survey research.[182] Specialized indices have been developed for use in children.[183, 184] These indices vary in the features included in the scoring system, but most include a combination of subjective symptoms and objective findings on examination and laboratory testing. A great deal of interobserver variation has been noted,[185] and in fibrostenotic disease those indices relying more heavily on subjective measurements may poorly reflect bowel inflammation as a cause of symptoms.[186] Other approaches have included use of disease activity indices that focus on a specific outcome, such as perianal disease,[187, 188] endoscopic findings,[189] or

Table 103–3 | **Differentiating Crohn's Disease from Ulcerative Colitis**

FEATURE	CROHN'S DISEASE	ULCERATIVE COLITIS
Abdominal pain	Frequent and prominent complaint but may not be present	Primarily cramping associated with bowel movement
Diarrhea	Watery or voluminous stools common but may not be present	Usually; occasionally constipation with proctitis
Gross blood in stool	Occasionally; primarily with colonic disease	Frequently
Mucus in stool	Occasionally	Frequently
Abdominal mass	Frequently, particularly with ileocecal disease	Rarely
Abdominal tenderness	Frequently	Rarely
Intestinal obstruction	Frequently	Rarely
Perianal disease	Frequently	Rarely
Perianal fistulas	Frequently	No
Rectovaginal fistulas	Occasionally	Rarely
Abscess	Occasionally	No
Recurrence after surgery	Yes	No recurrence after total proctocolectomy, though pouchitis may occur in ileal pouch
Toxic megacolon	Rare	Infrequent
Current smoker	Frequently	Rarely
Former smoker	Rarely	Frequently
Previous appendectomy	Occasionally (for misdiagnosed right lower quadrant pain)	Rarely
Macrocytic anemia	Occasionally (from malabsorption of cobalamin)	Rarely (from folate deficiency secondary to sulfasalazine use)
Perinuclear antineutrophil cytoplasmic antibodies (pANCA)	20%	70%
Anti-*Saccharomyces cerevisiae* antibodies (ASCA)	65%	15%
Distribution of disease	May involve any segment of gastrointestinal tract	Contiguous involvement of colon from rectum proximally
Abnormalities proximal to terminal ileum	Sometimes	No
Abnormal terminal ileum	Frequently	Occasionally, from backwash ileitis
Ileocecal valve	Often narrowed	Normal or gaping
Rectal involvement	25–50%	95–100% (before treatment)
Continuous colitis	Rarely	Yes
Symmetry of inflammation	Eccentric inflammation	Circumferential inflammation
Bowel wall thickening	Marked	None to moderate
Cobblestone appearance	Frequent	Rare
Background mucosa	Normal	Abnormal
Fistula	Often	Rarely (rectovaginal)
Mesenteric inflammation	Frequent	Rare, except with toxic megacolon
Segmental inflammation	Yes, skip areas frequently seen	No, except for cecal inflammation adjacent to appendiceal orifice
Stricture	Often	Rarely
Ulceration	Depth: aphthous to deep Shape: linear, serpiginous, stellate	Superficial
Mesenteric proliferation of fat	Frequent	No

Adapted from Marion JF, Rubin PH, Present DH. Differential diagnosis of chronic ulcerative colitis and Crohn's disease. In Kirsner JB (ed): Inflammatory Bowel Disease, 5th ed. Philadelphia: WB Saunders, 2000, with permission.

achieving an individual goal of therapy.[190] Whereas each of these approaches has advantages and disadvantages, all have their application in research rather than clinical practice.

Another approach with some merit is the measurement of biologic markers of disease inflammation. The erythrocyte sedimentation rate and acute phase response proteins such as C-reactive protein and orosomucoid, measured in serum, may be somewhat useful in tracking disease activity but lack sensitivity and specificity. Another approach is to measure the serum levels of cytokines, cytokine receptors, and adhesion molecules that are proximate to the expression of acute phase reactants. Examples include IL-6, IL-1, soluble IL-2 receptor, and soluble intercellular adhesion molecule-1.[191] As with the acute phase reactants, these tests lack sensitivity and specificity. Direct measurements of intestinal immune activation in a mucosal sample could enhance sensitivity and specificity but are inconvenient, invasive, and, if dependent on biopsy, subject to variability and poor standardization. Quantification of radiolabeled leukocytes in stool appears to be a sensitive and fairly specific indicator of mucosal inflammation but is cumbersome to perform and exposes the patient to radiation. More recently, fecal excretion of calprotectin, a protein found in neutrophils, has been shown to be a sensitive marker of bowel inflammation and may also correlate with relapse of quiescent disease.[192]

Ultimately, it is desirable to measure the patient's overall state of well-being, or subjective health status. Health-related quality of life may be measured with generic instruments, which focus on various domains of health common to many disease states, or with disease-specific instruments, which focus on specific domains relevant to the disease of interest. The Inflammatory Bowel Disease Questionnaire is the most

Table 103–4 | **Crohn's Disease Activity Index**

VARIABLE	SCALE	WEIGHT
Liquid or very soft stools	Stool count summed daily for 7 days	2
Abdominal pain	Sum of 7 days of daily ratings as: 0 = none, 1 = mild, 2 = moderate, 3 = severe	6
General well-being	Sum of 7 days of daily ratings as 0 = generally well, 1 = slightly below par, 2 = poor, 3 = very poor, 4 = terrible	6
Features of extraintestinal disease	Any of the following present during the previous 7 days: a. Arthritis or arthralgias b. Skin or mouth lesions, including pyoderma gangrenosum, erythema nodosum, aphthous stomatitis c. Iritis or uveitis d. Anal fissure, fistula, or perirectal abscess e. Other external fistula f. Fever > 100°F	20 each
Opiates for diarrhea	0 = no, 1 = yes	30
Abdominal mass	0 = none, 2 = questionable, 5 = definite	10
Hematocrit	47−hematocrit (males) 42−hematocrit (females)	6
% Body weight below standard	100 × [1 − (body weight/ standard weight)]	1

From Best WR, Becktel JM, Singleton JW, et al. Development of a Crohn's disease activity index. National Cooperative Crohn's Disease Study. Gastroenterology 70:439, 1976, with permission.

widely accepted disease-specific instrument and measures separate domains for bowel, social, systemic, and emotional function.[193]

TREATMENT

Goals of Therapy

Because neither medical nor surgical therapy provides a cure, the primary goals of therapy are to induce and maintain remission. In achieving these goals, the intention is to ameliorate symptoms and improve the patient's quality of life. Therefore, it is essential to consider the adverse consequences of therapy, particularly with regard to any durable consequences of short-term treatment and adverse effects of maintenance therapy. Other goals may be specific to the problems or characteristics of the patient, such as healing a fistula or achieving normal growth in a child. Maintaining adequate nutrition may at times be a challenge and is an important goal in all patients.

Medical Therapy

Aminosalicylates

In the United States, aminosalicylates are often used in the treatment of ulcerative colitis and in mild to moderate Crohn's disease. Sulfasalazine, the parent compound of all aminosalicylates used in IBD, was developed as a treatment for rheumatoid arthritis but was serendipitously found to improve the bowel symptoms of patients with colitis who where treated for associated arthropathy. Later, a classic experiment by Azad Khan and colleagues implicated 5-aminosalicylate (mesalamine) rather than sulfapyridine as the therapeutic moiety of sulfasalazine.[194] Many adverse effects of sulfasalazine are due to the sulfapyridine moiety. However, the beneficial effects of 5-aminosalicylates depend on topical delivery to the affected mucosa, and almost the entire dose of the compound is absorbed in the upper gastrointestinal tract when given orally. Functionally, the sulfapyridine moiety serves as a carrier for 5-aminosalicylate, with release of 5-aminosalicylate depending on the azoreductase activity of the colonic flora, thereby ensuring delivery to the colon. Diverse means of overcoming proximal intestinal absorption of 5-aminosalicylate have been developed. These delivery systems include enemas or suppositories, which provide the drug to the left colon or rectum; encoating with protective materials that release the drug in a pH-dependent manner to achieve controlled (Pentasa) or delayed (Asacol) delivery; and diazo-bonding the drug to a second 5-aminosalicylate molecule (olsalazine) or to an inert carrier (balsalazide). The site of delivery of coated preparations depends largely on the properties of the coating material used and its pH sensitivity. Some preparations (Pentasa) release half of the dose in the small bowel and the remainder in the colon, whereas other preparations release mesalamine in the distal terminal ileum and beyond. Diazo-bonded preparations have release profiles closely resembling that of sulfasalazine.

Numerous therapeutic mechanisms have been attributed to aminosalicylates, including inhibition of T-cell proliferation, presentation of antigen to T cells, and antibody production by B cells; inhibition of the adhesion of macrophages and neutrophils; and decreased production of IL-1 and TNF. The aminosalicylates are excellent free radical scavengers and inhibit cyclooxygenase and production of prostaglandin E_2.[195] Many of these effects appear to be mediated through down-regulation of NF-κB activity.[196]

Most studies have shown sulfasalazine to be superior to placebo in inducing remission in active Crohn's disease when the colon is the primary site affected.[197] Efficacious doses, as used in the National Cooperative Crohn's Disease Study (NCCDS), are in the range of 4 to 6 g/day (1 g/15 kg body weight),[197] whereas the European Cooperative Crohn's Disease Study (ECCDS) found sulfasalazine 3 g/day to provide no significant benefit in achieving remission.[198] Early studies with controlled-release mesalamine (Pentasa) at doses less than 2 g/day failed to show efficacy in the treatment of mild to moderately active Crohn's disease.[199, 200] A much larger study of 466 patients with mild to moderate Crohn's disease compared daily doses of 1, 2, and 4 g to placebo for 16 weeks. The 43% remission rate on 4 g mesalamine was statistically and clinically superior to the placebo response rate of 18%.[201] Notably, ileal disease responded best to the 4 g/day dose, thereby suggesting that mesalamine provides a potential benefit over sulfasalazine in treating this subgroup of patients. Subsequent trials of similar design, however, failed to show benefit over placebo; although the treatment effect was of similar magnitude, the placebo response was larger than the originally observed 18%. A more recent study compared two different preparations of mesalamine in a dose of 4 g/day with methylprednisolone 40 mg/day in a 12-week course of therapy for patients with mild to moderate ileal disease.[202] The mesalamine preparations were not significantly different from methylprednisolone in the magnitude of response or the proportion of patients achieving remission.[202] A study of delayed release mesalamine (Asacol) 3.2 g/day for 16 weeks showed a 28% margin of benefit over placebo in achieving partial or complete response in mild to moderately active Crohn's disease.[203] In summary, sulfasalazine 4 to 6 g/day may be useful in the treatment of mild to moderate colonic Crohn's disease, whereas mesalamine in doses greater than 3 g/day may be efficacious in mild to moderate Crohn's disease, particularly in ileal disease. The small margin of benefit and relatively slow onset of effect (4–8 weeks) must be weighed against the excellent safety profile of these agents (Table 103–5).

The benefits of aminosalicylates are less clear with regard to maintenance of remission. Numerous studies with a variety of preparations have failed to demonstrate prevention of relapse with doses of mesalamine below 3 g/day.[204] The most recent meta-analysis examining prevention of relapse with mesalamine demonstrated a significant benefit but primarily for patients receiving prophylactic treatment after surgical resection.[205] Other factors predictive of benefit were ileal disease and prolonged disease duration.[205] However, when put to the test in a recent prospective, randomized, controlled trial of postsurgical prophylaxis, controlled-release mesalamine 4 g/day for 18 months was not superior to placebo.[206] Therefore, although maintenance therapy with mesalamine is often prescribed, little data justify the expense and inconvenience of this practice.

Antibiotics

Antibiotics have a clear role in treating pyogenic complications of Crohn's disease. On the basis of relatively little evidence, antibiotics are also used to treat perianal disease, fistulas, and active Crohn's disease. Most reported experience has related to the use of metronidazole. The anaerobic flora affected by metronidazole may have particular importance in the pathogenesis of Crohn's disease.[36] Perhaps the clearest demonstration of this principle is a study of postsurgical prophylaxis after ileal resection. In this disease model, which in some ways may replicate the earliest events in the initiation of Crohn's disease, high-dose metronidazole (20 mg/kg/day for 3 months) demonstrated a prophylactic effect on endoscopic and clinical recurrence at 1 year, with numerical but not statistical advantages at 2 and 3 years of follow-up.[207] In this study, as in clinical usage, side effects—including gastrointestinal upset, nausea, dysgeusia, and peripheral neuropathy—were common.

Open-label experience suggests that metronidazole 1 to 2 g/day is beneficial in healing simple perianal fistulas.[208] Fistulas tend to recur with cessation of therapy, but long-term use is limited by side effects. Studies of metronidazole in active Crohn's disease have generally not demonstrated benefit but have suggested better outcomes in subgroups of patients with a colonic component to their disease.[209, 210]

Ciprofloxacin is also used increasingly to treat Crohn's disease. One study compared the combined use of ciprofloxacin and metronidazole, 1 g each, against methylprednisolone for active Crohn's disease. The antibiotic combination was comparable with glucocorticoids in achieving remission over 12 weeks.[211] Another study found ciprofloxacin 1 g/day to be equivalent to mesalamine 4 g/day in achieving remission of mild to moderately active Crohn's disease at week 6, with more than one half of the patients in each group achieving remission.[212]

Preliminary evidence suggests that clarithromycin monotherapy may also be useful in treating active disease.[213] Additional interest in clarithromycin attaches to its role as part of a highly effective treatment for atypical mycobacterial infection. Studies of antimycobacterial therapy, however, have not shown consistent benefit. A study of quadruple therapy (rifampicin, ethambutol, dapsone, and clofazimine) showed significantly fewer relapses when compared with placebo among patients with inactive disease treated for 9 months.[214] Radiographic or endoscopic healing was not observed, however, suggesting that this therapy was not curative. Other antimycobacterial regimens have failed to produce either short-term or durable benefit, thus far failing to fulfill Koch's postulates for disease causation.

In summary, antibiotics may play an adjunctive role in the treatment of Crohn's disease and in selected patients may be useful in treating perianal disease, enterocutaneous fistulas, or active colonic disease. As the antigenic determinants of the intestinal flora are further elucidated, more directed antibiotic approaches may be feasible.

Glucocorticoids

Glucocorticoids play a central yet vexing role in the treatment of Crohn's disease. Early favorable series of glucocorticoid treatment led to the validation of their short-term efficacy in the NCCDS (prednisone 0.5–0.75 mg/kg/day for initial treatment of active disease with the dose adjusted according to CDAI)[197] and the ECCDS (6-methylprednisolone 48 mg/day in the first week, tapered to 12 mg by week 6, and held at 8 mg for remission up to 2 years).[198] In usual practice, patients with mild to moderate disease that does not respond to primary therapy and those with moderately severe symptoms are treated initially with 40 to 60 mg of prednisone and then tapered off the drug over a period of 6 to 12 weeks. Response rates are high, approximately 80% by 1 month.[215] When doses are pushed as high as 1 mg/kg/day for up to 7 weeks, 92% of patients may achieve clinical remission.[216] The onset of response is rapid, usually within the first 3 weeks of treatment. Patients with severely active disease usually respond to intravenous administration of glucocorticoids.[217]

Numerous anti-inflammatory and immunosuppressive effects have been attributed to glucocorticoids to account for their efficacy. These effects include inhibition of the expression of proinflammatory cytokines, adhesion molecules, MHC class II molecules, leukotrienes, elastase, collagenase, and nitric oxide synthase. Glucocorticoids bind to a cytoplasmic receptor found in all cells and then enter the nucleus to bind glucocorticoid-response elements on the chromosomal DNA, thereby producing a variety of downstream physiologic effects.[218] The anti-inflammatory effects of glucocorticoids may follow from down-regulation of NF-κB and induction of inhibitory κB.[219] Direct cellular effects may

Table 103–5 | **Safety Profiles of Drugs Used to Treat Crohn's Disease**

AGENT	ADVERSE EFFECTS	PREGNANCY*	NURSING*
5-Aminosalicylates (5-ASA)			
Sulfasalazine	Anorexia, dyspepsia, nausea/vomiting; hemolysis; neutropenia, agranulocytosis; folate deficiency; reversible male infertility; neuropathy; see also sulfa-free 5-ASAs	No evidence of teratogenicity; normal fetal growth; give with folic acid	Negligible amounts; safe for term neonates
Sulfa-free (mesalamine, olsalazine, balsalazide)	Headache; drug fever, rash; paradoxical exacerbation; pancreatitis; hepatitis; pericarditis; pneumonitis; nephritis; secretory diarrhea (olsalazine)	No evidence of teratogenicity, normal fetal growth	Found in breast milk in low concentrations; rare watery diarrhea in fed infants
Antibiotics			
Metronidazole	Anorexia, nausea/vomiting, dysgeusia; disulfiram-like effect; peripheral neuropathy; reversible neutropenia	Questionable teratogenicity, normal fetal growth	Found in breast milk; with rare exception, should not be used
Ciprofloxacin	Nausea/vomiting; headache; restlessness; rash; pseudomembranous colitis; elevated aminotransferases; spontaneous tendon rupture	Theoretical teratogenic potential; insufficient data in humans	Found in breast milk, should not be used
Glucocorticoids			
Classic	Sleep and mood disturbance; acne, striae, hirsutism, adrenal suppression, proximal myopathy, glucose intolerance, hypertension, narrow angle glaucoma, cataracts, pseudotumor cerebri, infection, edema, impaired wound healing, growth retardation, bone loss, aseptic necrosis	No evidence of teratogenicity in humans. More frequent stillbirths and reduced fetal birthweight when used for other diseases; may be used as indicated by severity of disease	Safe for breast-feeding
Novel	Controlled ileal release budesonide; adrenal suppression at doses of 9mg/day in two divided doses and higher, but occurrence of classic glucocorticoid adverse effects similar to placebo	No data available	No data available
Immune modulators			
6-Mercaptopurine, azathioprine	Nausea; drug fever, rash, arthralgias; leukopenia; thrombocytopenia; bone marrow suppression; pancreatitis; hepatitis; infection; lymphoma?	Teratogenic in animals, but large series in renal transplantation and other diseases do not demonstrate significant increase in birth defects; evidence for fetal growth retardation and prematurity; isolated cases of neonatal immune and bone marrow suppression; limited series in IBD appear favorable; may be used where indicated by severity of disease.	Small amounts excreted in breast milk; not recommended
Methotrexate	Anorexia, nausea/vomiting; leukopenia; megaloblastic anemia; alopecia; hepatic fibrosis; interstitial pneumonitis; neuropathy	Highly teratogenic, particularly in first trimester; abortifacient	Small amounts excreted in breast milk; not recommended
Cyclosporine	Reversible or irreversible decrease in renal function; hypertension; tremor, headache, paresthesias, seizure; hypertrichosis; hepatotoxicity; infection; lymphoma; gingival hyperplasia	Significant levels in fetal circulation; does not appear to be teratogenic; intrauterine growth retardation and premature delivery increased, especially at higher doses; little reported experience in IBD	Excreted in breast milk; not recommended
Biologic response modifiers			
Infliximab	Upper respiratory tract and other infections; disseminated tuberculosis; acute or delayed hypersensitivity reactions; anti-nuclear antibody, anti-double-stranded DNA antibody, lupus-like reaction; ?lymphoma	May enter fetal circulation; no data available; effects unknown	No data available; not recommended

*From Connell WR. Safety of drug therapy for inflammatory bowel disease in pregnant and nursing women. Inflam Bowel Dis 2, 33, 1996, with permission.
Adapted from Sands BE. Therapy of inflammatory bowel disease. Gastroenterology 118(2 Suppl 1):S72, 2000, with permission.

also occur, with reduced phagocytic activity of neutrophils and, in some situations, apoptosis of lymphocytes.[218]

Unfortunately, the beneficial effects of glucocorticoids come at the expense of frequent and often severe adverse effects (see Table 103–5). The most common side effects are troubling neuropsychiatric symptoms (mood disturbance and insomnia) and cosmetic effects (acne, cushingoid appearance, hair loss, and hirsutism). Still more serious are metabolic consequences, such as adrenocortical suppression, glucose intolerance, myopathy, and bone loss. The risk of infectious complications is increased, particularly at doses of prednisone higher than 40 mg, whereas doses lower than 10 mg confer no appreciable increased risk of infection.[220] This unfavorable risk profile makes prolonged use of glucocorticoids hazardous.

Furthermore, glucocorticoids are not effective as long-term therapy. A meta-analysis of maintenance glucocorticoid therapy in Crohn's disease failed to detect benefit at 6, 12, or 24 months in the prevention of relapse.[221] On the other hand, many patients, once introduced to glucocorticoids, are unable to taper them off without recurrent symptoms, a problem that has been called *glucocorticoid dependence*. Among patients with Crohn's disease who receive glucocorticoids for the first time, no response (*glucocorticoid resistance*) was seen in 20% in the first 30 days.[215] Among the 80% who were complete or partial responders, 55% had a prolonged response, whereas 45% relapsed or were unable to taper off treatment within 1 year.[215] Clinical factors associated with glucocorticoid dependence include smoking, younger age at onset, colonic location, and nonfibrostenotic disease.[222] Mechanisms that may contribute to glucocorticoid resistance may include up-regulation of the multidrug resistance (*mdr*) gene[223] and increased serum levels of glucocorticoid binding globulin.[224] Also relevant to the phenomenon of glucocorticoid dependence is the finding that only 29% of patients who achieve clinical remission on glucocorticoids also achieve endoscopic remission.[216] This finding suggests that the effect of glucocorticoids in most patients is to suppress symptoms when given in doses above a threshold that may vary among patients and even in the same patient over time.

Principles of glucocorticoid use in Crohn's disease include the following. First, *use an effective dose*. Underdosing at the start of therapy typically leads to dose escalation and prolonged dosing to achieve a response. Second, *do not overdose*. Patients who do not benefit from 40 to 60 mg are unlikely to benefit from increased or prolonged oral dosing. Such patients require intravenous dosing or treatment with another rapidly acting agent, such as infliximab (see later). Third, *do not treat for excessively short periods*. Very brief courses of glucocorticoids (3 weeks or less) are likely to result in a rebound flare. Fourth, *do not treat for excessively long periods*. Patients who fail a second glucocorticoid taper shortly after a first should be considered candidates for glucocorticoid-sparing immune modulators. Glucocorticoids should not be begun without a strategy in mind for terminating treatment. Finally, *anticipate side effects*. Bone loss in particular may be anticipated with even short-term use. Strategies to preserve bone density should be undertaken early (Fig. 103–6).

In an attempt to limit the unintended systemic effects of glucocorticoid therapy, novel glucocorticoids have been developed. These include fluticasone propionate, tixocortol pivalate, beclomethasone dipropionate, and budesonide. These agents possess glucocorticoid receptor affinity equal or superior to that of traditional glucocorticoids and may also take advantage of enhanced first-pass metabolism by the liver to limit systemic exposure. *Budesonide* has been investigated primarily as a controlled ileal-release formulation that targets the terminal ileum and right colon. Studies have demonstrated 9 mg/day of this preparation to be superior to placebo and mesalamine[225, 226] and nearly as effective as prednisolone in achieving remission but with fewer side effects. Pushing the dose higher results in better efficacy but at the expense of increasing adrenocortical suppression and side effects.[226] Budesonide treatment in asymptomatic patients delays the time to relapse slightly, but the rate of relapse at 1 year is not superior to that for placebo.[227, 228] Similarly, budesonide 3 or 6 mg/day after ileal or ileocecal resection does not improve the recurrence rate at 1 year.[229, 230] Therefore, lack of a maintenance effect is consistent among novel and traditional glucocorticoids. In light of the superior response to mesalamine and its relative safety, budesonide may be considered an alternative to mesalamine as first-line therapy for patients with active ileal, ileocecal, or right colonic disease.

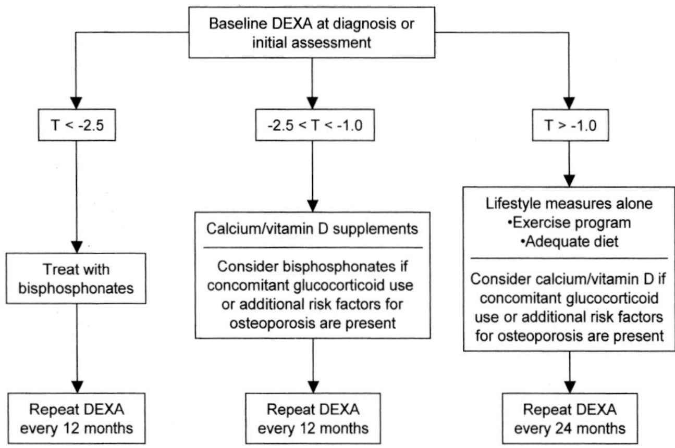

Figure 103–6. Management of metabolic bone disease in Crohn's disease. T, T score. DEXA, dual energy X-ray absorptiometry. (From Silverberg MS, Steinhart AH. Bone density in inflammatory bowel disease. Clin Perspect Gastroenterol 3:117–125, 2000, with permission.

Thiopurine Agents

The thiopurine antimetabolites *azathioprine* and *6-mercaptopurine* have been considered treatments for Crohn's disease since the initial report of Brooke and colleagues describing healing of fistulas with azathioprine.[231] Another decade would pass before the efficacy of this class of drugs was demonstrated in a randomized controlled trial by Present and colleagues.[190] Earlier studies were marred by either insufficient power or incomplete understanding of adequate dosing and the slow onset of action of these agents.

A meta-analysis of studies of azathioprine and 6-mercaptopurine in Crohn's disease has provided the best summary of the effects of these drugs. For active disease, treatment produced an odds ratio of response of 3.09 (95% CI, 2.45–3.91) compared with placebo, with improved response when treatment was continued for at least 17 weeks.[232] Convincing evidence of benefit was also seen in maintenance of remission (odds ratio over placebo 2.27, 95% CI 1.76–2.93),[232] glucocorticoid sparing[233, 234] (odds ratios for active disease 3.69, 95% CI 2.12–6.42; for quiescent disease, 4.64, 95% CI 1.00–21.54),[232] and improvement in fistulas (odds ratio 4.64, 95% CI 1.50–13.20).[232] Overall, approximately one half to two thirds of patients may respond to therapy. In contrast to glucocorticoids, mucosal healing is frequently seen with adequate dosing of thiopurine agents.[235]

In clinical practice, azathioprine and 6-mercaptopurine are used virtually interchangeably with the exception of dosing. Azathioprine is generally used in doses of 2.0 to 2.5 mg/kg/day, whereas 6-mercaptopurine is given in doses of 1.0 to 1.5 mg/kg/day. Much is known about the metabolism of 6-mercaptopurine and azathioprine (Fig. 103–7). Azathioprine is a prodrug that is converted in part to 6-mercaptopurine through nonenzymatic means and into a variety of other immunologically active and inert metabolites. Xanthine oxidase converts 6-mercaptopurine to 6-thiouric acid, in competition with hypoxanthine phosphoribosyltransferase. The former pathway accounts for an important drug reaction with allopurinol, a xanthine oxidase inhibitor. Concurrent treatment with allopurinol and a thiopurine agent necessitates a dose reduction of at least one third if leukopenia is to be avoided.

Thiopurine methyltransferase (TPMT) plays a key role in the metabolic pathway. Variations in TPMT activity, which are largely determined genetically, account for preferential shunting of 6-mercaptopurine to the production of 6-methylmercaptopurine when enzyme activity is normal or high. Persons who are homozygous for a recessive mutation that results in inactivation of TPMT (approximately 1 in 300 persons) produce exceedingly high levels of 6-thioguanine nucleotides. These persons are unlikely to tolerate thiopurine agents at all and tend to have profound leukopenia and other limiting adverse effects. In contrast, persons who are TPMT heterozygous (approximately 10% of the population) are likely to have moderately high levels of 6-thioguanine nucleotides. They usually require lower doses of drug but are much more likely to respond. A steady state in the production of erythrocyte 6-thioguanine nucleotides is reached 2 weeks after dosing.[236] The reported positive correlation between erythrocyte 6-thioguanine nucleotides and therapeutic response offers the possibility of both monitoring adherence to the drug regimen and optimizing dosing of these agents.[237] Correlations between higher levels of 6-thioguanine nucleotides and leukopenia on the one hand and between metabolite levels and response to therapy on the other may explain the clinical observation that patients who achieve mild leukopenia are more likely to respond to therapy.[238] Conversely, leukopenia is not necessary to achieve a therapeutic response.

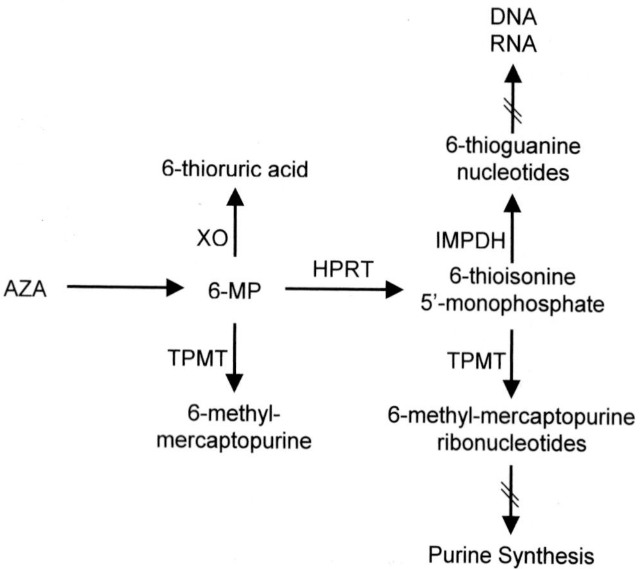

Figure 103–7. Metabolism of azathioprine and 6-mercaptopurine. Azathioprine is converted to 6-mercaptopurine non-enzymatically. (AZA, azathioprine; 6-MP, 6-mercaptopurine; XO, xanthine oxidase; HPRT, hypoxanthine phosphoribosyltransferase; TPMT, thiopurine methyltransferase; IMPDH, inosine monophosphate dehydrogenase.) (From Dubinsky M, et al: Pharmacogenomics and metabolite measurement for 6-mercaptopurine therapy in inflammatory bowel disease. Gastroenterology 118:705–713, 2000, with permission.)

Not all the immunologic effects of azathioprine and 6-mercaptopurine may be ascribed to 6-thioguanine nucleotides alone. A preliminary study of the drug 6-thioguanine in IBD has shown evidence of efficacy, but the erythrocyte 6-thioguanine nucleotide concentrations seen with effective doses are many-fold higher than those observed with 6-mercaptopurine and azathioprine.[239] The relevant mechanisms of action of azathioprine and 6-mercaptopurine are also not clearly understood. Metabolites of both agents inhibit de novo synthesis of purine ribonucleotides and thereby inhibit cell proliferation. Azathioprine and its metabolites may have immunosuppressive properties beyond those of the metabolites produced in common with 6-mercaptopurine. Both drugs inhibit cell-mediated immunity. The thiopurine agents cause a reduction in the number of circulating natural killer cells over many months, perhaps accounting for the slow onset of action.[240]

A recent study found no acceleration of the time to response with intravenous loading of azathioprine. Unexpectedly, the oral dosing arm of the study with azathioprine 2 mg/kg/day achieved a maximum rate of remission of 24% (discontinuation of prednisone and CDAI < 150) by week 8. The remission rate did not increase over an additional 8 weeks of follow-up, thereby contradicting the long-held notion of a prolonged time to response. The study did not, however, address improvement beyond the 16th week of treatment.

In clinical trials, adverse events severe enough to result in withdrawal have been seen in 8.9% of patients.[232] Nausea is often reported in the first weeks of treatment but gradually subsides. Allergic reactions consisting of fever, rash, or arthralgias, usually within a few weeks of introducing the drug, are seen in 2% of patients. Pancreatitis, observed in 3% to 7%, is another idiosyncratic reaction and usually occurs in the first month of therapy. The presentation may be subtle, with nausea and vague dyspepsia, or may be one of classic epigastric pain with radiation to the back. If serum amylase and lipase levels are followed closely, symptoms may sometimes be noted to precede the discovery of laboratory abnormalities. When recognized promptly, discontinuation of the drug leads to resolution of pancreatitis. Rechallenge with either drug should not be attempted because recurrent pancreatitis is certain to occur. Elevated serum aminotransferase levels develop in as many as 9% of patients and have been correlated with the presence of very high levels of 6-methylmercaptopurine.[237] More serious cholestatic hepatitis is rare, occurring in less than 1% of patients.[241]

Bone marrow suppression is another concern with thiopurine agents. A 27-year, retrospective, single-center study of 739 IBD patients treated with azathioprine found 28 patients (3.8%) to have developed leukopenia (white blood cell count $< 3 \times 10^9/mm^3$), 9 of whom (1.2%) had severe leukopenia (white blood cell count $< 2 \times 10^9/mm^3$).[242] Three of these patients became pancytopenic, and two died of sepsis. In another retrospective report of 396 patients treated with 6-mercaptopurine, 2% experienced leukocyte counts below $3.5 \times 10^9/mm^3$.[241] Although leukopenia occurs early among patients with low TPMT activity, it may not be related solely to TPMT genotype and may occur at any time during therapy.[243] For this reason, it is advisable to continue monthly monitoring of the complete blood count for the duration of therapy and more frequently in the weeks after introducing the drug or increasing the dose. Temporary cessation of therapy for a week or two and an adjustment in the dose are usually sufficient to bring the leukocyte count within the normal range. Careful monitoring of the leukocyte count should also be performed during a tapering regimen of glucocorticoids. Concurrent treatment with glucocorticoids may raise the leukocyte count, but as the glucocorticoid is discontinued, leukopenia may arise.

Infections may also occur in the setting of thiopurine therapy. With long-term therapy as many as 1.8% of patients may experience a severe infection, not necessarily in the setting of leukopenia.[241] Patients treated concurrently with glucocorticoids may be at greater risk of serious infection, including cytomegalovirus. Treatment should be interrupted when serious infections occur, although the effect of the drug will endure for weeks.

The question of whether patients with IBD who are treated with 6-mercaptopurine or azathioprine are at increased risk of malignancy is unresolved. Immunosuppressive regimens given to patients after organ transplantation and for other immune-mediated conditions are associated with an excess risk of malignancy, particularly non-Hodgkin's lymphoma. Such regimens have included azathioprine, often administered in high doses and in conjunction with other immunosuppressive agents. The combined long-term experience at two centers involving treatment of 1151 patients with IBD failed to reveal an excess risk of cancer but did include a single case of diffuse histiocytic lymphoma of the brain.[241, 244] Most cancers in treated patients were colorectal cancers assumed to be a consequence of the underlying IBD itself. Such studies cannot formally confirm or exclude a possible association with non-Hodgkin's lymphoma, however, because of the rarity of lymphoma and the unsettled question of whether Crohn's disease itself confers an increased risk of lymphoma. Nevertheless, if there is an increased risk of lymphoma with immunosuppressive therapy, studies suggest that the absolute risk is small.[245] For the properly selected patient, the small risk of lymphoma does not outweigh the benefits of improved quality of life and possibly of increased life expectancy.[246]

Azathioprine and 6-mercaptopurine should be considered for patients with active Crohn's disease who fail to respond to first-line therapies or who fail to taper off glucocorticoids successfully. Patients who are treated with antibiotics for a fistula and who fail to tolerate or respond to these agents also may be considered for treatment with a thiopurine agent. The introduction of thiopurine medications should be timed with their slow onset of action in mind. Many patients require an initial tapering regimen of glucocorticoids as a fast-acting agent to complement azathioprine or 6-mercaptopurine. Thiopurine therapy may also be considered for the postsurgical prophylaxis of Crohn's disease. Compared with placebo, 6-mercaptopurine significantly decreases the risk of endoscopic and clinical relapse after bowel resection[247] and may be considered in patients who are deemed at high risk of future resections. Given the favorable efficacy of thiopurine agents and their relative safety, there is increasing interest in introducing these agents earlier in the course of the disease. Recent evidence suggests that the addition of 6-mercaptopurine is advantageous for children who require even a first course of glucocorticoids shortly after diagnosis.[248] It is unclear whether thiopurine therapy prevents or delays the occurrence of fibrostenotic complications of Crohn's disease, and it is possible to see the slow progression of a stricture in patients who otherwise have been asymptomatic on such therapy for many years.

Once treatment has begun and proved to be effective, the question of how long to continue therapy inevitably arises. Some data suggest that after 4 years of remission on thiopurine therapy, the risk of relapse is similar regardless of whether or not treatment is continued.[249] Nevertheless, it is common to see patients relapse on cessation of therapy after remission has been maintained for long periods, only to remit again on resuming treatment. For this reason, most large referral centers follow numerous patients treated with azathioprine or 6-mercaptopurine for many years.

Methotrexate

Methotrexate has long been used to treat psoriasis and rheumatoid arthritis. A promising open-label study of methotrexate in IBD[250] led to a randomized controlled trial in Crohn's disease. Patients with chronic active Crohn's disease despite at least 3 months of prednisone 12.5 mg/day or more and with at least one failed attempt to taper off treatment were enrolled.[251] All patients were brought to a common dose of prednisone 20 mg/day to standardize therapy, with separate stratification for patients in whom the dose of prednisone was increased and for those in whom the dose had dropped to 20 mg before entry. Subjects then received either weekly injections of methotrexate 25 mg intramuscularly or placebo while executing a tapering prednisone regimen over 16 weeks. Overall, 39.4% of patients assigned to methotrexate achieved remission off prednisone compared with 19.1% of placebo-treated patients.[251] Most patients responded by the 8th week of treatment. Although the remission rates in the methotrexate-treated high- and low-prednisone group were nearly equal (39.0% and 40.0%, respectively), the remission rate for placebo-treated patients in the high-dose group was 10.0%, compared with 35.3% in the low-dose group.[251] This result is often misconstrued as showing that methotrexate works well for patients on high doses of prednisone but not for those on low doses of prednisone, but it merely shows an unexpectedly high placebo response rate among patients dependent on low doses of glucocorticoids.

Methotrexate is also beneficial in maintaining remission. A follow-up study randomized patients who achieved remission on methotrexate 25 mg intramuscularly once weekly to receive either placebo injections or weekly injections of methotrexate 15 mg. At week 40, 65% of patients treated with methotrexate were still in remission, compared with 39% of placebo-treated patients ($P = .04$).[252] Treatment was well tolerated. Among patients who relapsed on the lower maintenance dose, more than one half were able to achieve remission again with resumption of a 25-mg dose. If the 16 weeks of induction therapy are included, the combined duration of therapy was nearly 1 year, with some patients in selected practices treated successfully for more than 4 years. Although oral dosing would be more convenient for long-term administration, this route is unreliable because of variable intestinal absorption, particularly in the presence of small bowel disease.

Although methotrexate is a folate antagonist, the drug is often given with folic acid 1 to 2 mg/day to prevent nausea and stomatitis. Therefore, other modes of action are likely responsible for its efficacy. The drug possesses a variety of other immune-modulating and anti-inflammatory effects, including inhibition of IL-1, IL-2, IL-6, and IL-8 and induction of adenosine, which has direct immunosuppressive properties.[253]

In addition to stomatitis and nausea, diarrhea, hair loss, and mild leukopenia may occur with methotrexate. Serum aminotransferase elevations sometimes may be seen but correlate poorly with the more serious complication of hepatic fibrosis. Liver biopsy is performed routinely in patients with psoriasis after cumulative doses of 1.5, 3, and 5 g have been administered, but these guidelines have not been widely adopted in patients with rheumatoid arthritis, in whom the risk of hepatic fibrosis appears to be lower. Obesity and alcohol intake correlate with fibrosis. Methotrexate interacts with sulfa medications and with azathioprine and 6-mercaptopurine to cause severe leukopenia. Rare but potentially life-threatening interstitial pneumonitis may present as cough and dyspnea of insidious onset. Early detection, cessation of methotrexate, and treatment with glucocorticoids is essential. Finally, methotrexate is a potent abortifacient and is strongly teratogenic. Women of childbearing capacity must use methotrexate only with highly effective contraception.

Methotrexate may be considered as an alternative to the thiopurine analogs, particularly among patients who do not tolerate these drugs. Some patients who fail to respond to 6-mercaptopurine may respond to methotrexate.[254] In addition to its proven role as a glucocorticoid-sparing agent, methotrexate may be considered as a treatment for active disease, although its value for this indication is less clear.[255]

Other Immune Modulators

In contrast to ulcerative colitis, for which *cyclosporine* may be considered for the treatment of severe glucocorticoid-refractory disease, there appears to be little role for cyclosporine in Crohn's disease. A series of uncontrolled and randomized controlled trials has shown high doses of cyclosporine to be efficacious in treating inflammatory disease and fistulas but at an unacceptably high cost in adverse effects. Moreover, lower doses, although somewhat safer, are not effective in maintaining remission.[256] For virtually all indications, equally effective and less hazardous medications are available. *Tacrolimus* is more reliably absorbed from the intestine than is cyclosporine and has a similar mode of action via inhibition of calcineurin, thereby diminishing T-cell activation.[257] Preliminary data suggest that tacrolimus may be useful in treating glucocorticoid-resistant and fistulizing disease.[258, 259] The drug may also be effective as a topical agent for oral or perineal disease.[260] *Mycophenolate mofetil*, like azathioprine and 6-mercaptopurine, inhibits purine synthesis. Because of the similarity of these agents in mode of action, mycophenolate mofetil has been considered primarily as an alternative treatment for patients intolerant of or resistant to treatment with azathioprine. The efficacy of mycophenolate mofetil in Crohn's disease remains unclear, and further trials are needed.[261, 262]

Infliximab

Infliximab is the first biologic response modifier shown to be effective in Crohn's disease. This chimeric monoclonal anti-TNF antibody had an unsuccessful history as an investigational antisepsis agent before its use in Crohn's disease was explored. Despite conflicting reports regarding the importance of TNF in IBD, the Dutch investigator van Deventer posited that in light of the critical role of TNF in granuloma formation, an anti-TNF agent might prove efficacious for granulomatous bowel disease. Open-label trials demonstrated rapid and prolonged improvement in disease activity, accompanied in many cases by mucosal healing.[263–265]

A randomized controlled trial provided strong confirmation of the initial impression of efficacy. Patients with moderate to severe Crohn's disease were randomized to an initial infusion of placebo or 5, 10, or 20 mg/kg infliximab (then called cA2).[266] Qualifying patients had moderate to severe Crohn's disease (CDAI, 220 to 400) despite treatment with aminosalicylates (59%), oral glucocorticoids (59%), or 6-mercaptopurine or azathioprine (37%). Approximately one half of the studied patients had prior segmental intestinal resections, and the group had a mean duration of disease in excess of 10 years. The major end point was clinical response, defined as a decrease in the CDAI of 70 or more points at week 4.

All treatment groups had results significantly better than placebo (placebo response rate of 17%), with the highest rate of response seen in the 5-mg/kg group (81%).[266] A smaller but still significant proportion of patients had a clinical response by week 12 (48% for 5 mg/kg vs. 12% for placebo). The proportion of patients in clinical remission (CDAI $<$ 150 and a decrease in CDAI of 70 or more points) at week 4 was also significantly higher among the 5-mg/kg group (33%) compared with placebo (4%). Time to response for nearly all patients was 2 weeks. Clinical improvement was accompanied by improvement in health-related quality of life and decreases in serum C-reactive protein levels.

Coincidental healing of enterocutaneous fistulas in some patients led to a separate randomized controlled trial of infliximab for this indication. Patients with draining enterocutaneous fistula were enrolled and followed for closure of

50% or more of the fistulas at two successive visits 1 month apart. More than one half of the patients had more than one fistula, and 90% of the fistulas were perianal. Infliximab in a dose of 5 or 10 mg/kg or placebo was infused at weeks 0, 2, and 6. Among patients assigned to infliximab 5 mg/kg, 68% achieved the primary end point, compared with 26% of those given placebo ($P = 0.0002$).[267] Complete closure of all fistulas was observed in 55% of patients given infliximab 5 mg/kg but only 13% of placebo-treated patients. Among patients who achieved the primary end point, the median duration of response was 3 months.[267]

Limited information regarding the efficacy of repeated dosing was available before the commercial release of infliximab in the United States. A second phase of the initial randomized controlled trial accepted patients who had a clinical response by week 8 and rerandomized them to infliximab 10 mg/kg or placebo at week 12.[268] Patients received four infusions 8 weeks apart and were followed for continued response. In contrast to the placebo group, patients assigned to repeated dosing with infliximab maintained their response through roughly 8 weeks after the last infusion given. These data, which await confirmation in long-term trials, suggest that infliximab may be useful for maintaining remission.

The mode of action of infliximab is likely to be more involved than its nominal binding of TNF. The antibody may bind and clear soluble TNF but also binds to cell-bound TNF. Through the latter mechanism, infliximab may induce antibody-dependent cell-mediated cytotoxicity or, by virtue of its IgG1 isotype, complement fixation and lysis of cells bearing TNF on their surface.[269] These mechanisms may account for a response that may occasionally extend well beyond the 10-day half-life of the drug. Downstream effects from the inhibition of TNF include decreased expression of IL-2, interferon-γ, and other proinflammatory cytokines; down-regulation of adhesion molecules, inducible nitric oxide synthetase, and acute phase proteins; and inhibition of proteolysis and bone resorption.[270]

Although highly effective, not all patients respond to infliximab. In the first controlled trial, patients who failed to respond to the initial blinded infusion were permitted to receive an open-label infusion of infliximab 10 mg/kg 4 weeks later. Among patients originally assigned to placebo, the response rate to open-label treatment was similar to that seen among patients who received drug during the initial blinded infusion.[266] However, patients who had failed to respond to an initial infusion of drug were about one half as likely to respond to a second open-label treatment. This result suggests that specific characteristics of the patient or features of the patient's disease may be predictive of a response. Although it is tempting to speculate that genetic determinants might predict response, studies to date have failed to identify specific TNF genotypes that account for infliximab responsiveness. Clinical features such as age at onset, location of disease, or prior therapies also fail to identify persons likely to respond to or fail infliximab therapy.

Treatment with infliximab is usually well tolerated. In clinical trials, human anti-chimeric antibodies (HACA) developed in 13% of patients with Crohn's disease. Patients in whom HACA develop are more likely—although not uniformly so—to experience acute infusion reactions, which may include chest tightness, dyspnea, rash, and hypotension. HACA are less likely to develop in patients treated concomitantly with glucocorticoids or immune modulators, providing a justification for continuing methotrexate, azathioprine, or 6-mercaptopurine even when the patient has failed these treatments. Delayed hypersensitivity reactions, consisting of severe polyarthralgia, myalgia, facial edema, urticaria, or rash, are an unusual complication occurring from 3 to 12 days after an infusion.[271] High HACA titers appear in such patients after the occurrence of delayed hypersensitivity but are not necessarily found before reinfusion. The major risk factor for delayed hypersensitivity appears to be a long delay (probably 6 months or more) between infusions, thereby priming an anamnestic antibody response.[271] Delayed hypersensitivity appears to be less common when the induction regimen is a series of three infusions, as is used to treat a fistula, and when an immune modulator is given concurrently.[271] Anti-double-stranded DNA antibodies develop in 9% of treated patients, but lupus-like reactions are rare. As with HACA, anti-double-stranded DNA antibodies are less likely to occur if an immune modulator is continued with infliximab. Upper respiratory infections occur with greater frequency during treatment with infliximab. In the course of treatment of enterocutaneous fistulas, perianal abscesses may arise from superficial healing, with closing of an infected pocket. Any patient suspected of having a pyogenic complication of Crohn's disease or any serious infection should undergo adequate drainage and treatment with antibiotics before starting or continuing infliximab. Reactivation of tuberculosis has been observed with anti-TNF therapies, including infliximab, and has resulted in disseminated disease and death. Therefore, all patients should be screened for pulmonary tuberculosis before starting therapy. In clinical trials totaling roughly 500 patients, lymphoma developed in 4 patients with rheumatoid arthritis and 1 with Crohn's disease. It remains difficult to disentangle the potential confounding effects of other drugs and baseline risk in assessing causality and magnitude of risk for non-Hodgkin's lymphoma with infliximab. It is not yet known whether infliximab is teratogenic, and its use in pregnant women should be avoided.

Selection of patients is the key to using infliximab safely, effectively, and appropriately (Fig. 103–8) Patients without objective findings of inflammation or with fibrostenotic disease are unlikely to benefit, whereas treating patients with an undrained abscess is likely to be unsafe. Appropriate patients will generally have failed other therapies, including immune modulators, if the urgency of the patient's symptoms permits an adequate trial of these agents. Patients selected in this way are likely to require repeated dosing with infliximab to control disease over long periods of time. For the occasional patient who has a prolonged response to induction therapy with infliximab, repeated dosing at roughly 6 months may be considered to maintain tolerance to the drug. Maintenance dosing trials, soon to be completed, should illuminate the best course of action. Although not yet demonstrated in prospective trials, clinical experience shows infliximab to be useful as a glucocorticoid-sparing agent as well.

Adjunctive Therapies

Many other therapies are used to control the symptoms and adverse consequences of Crohn's disease. Antidiarrheal and

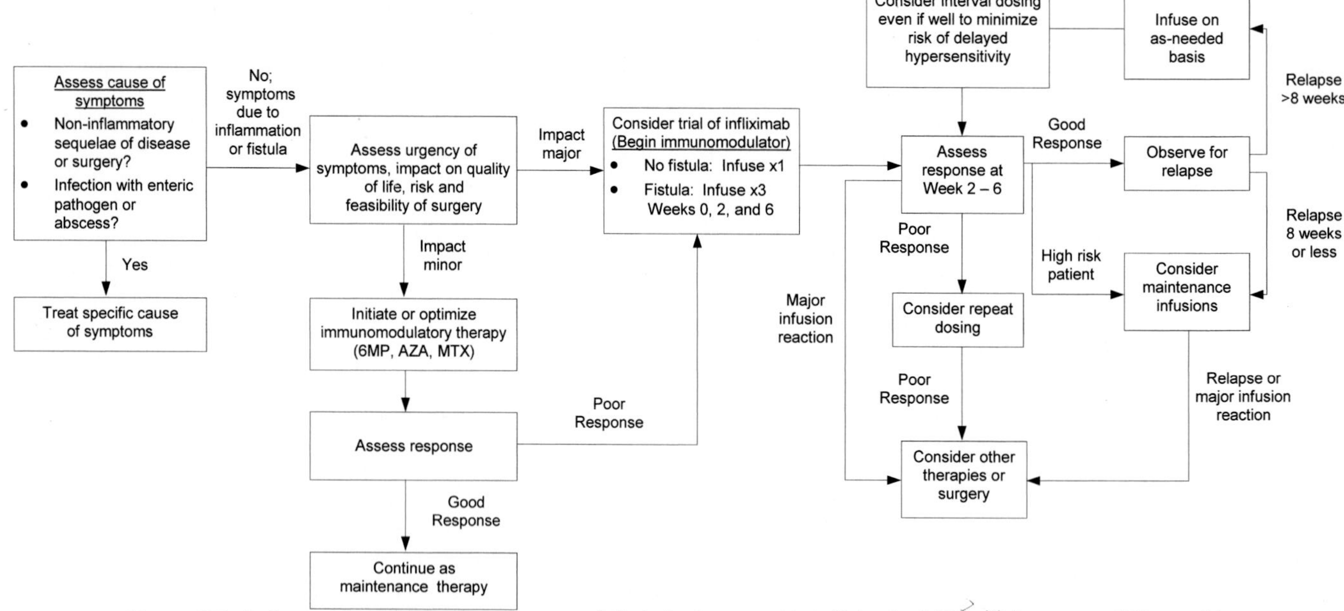

Figure 103–8. Proposed guidelines for treatment of Crohn's disease with infliximab. (MTX, methotrexate; AZA, azathioprine; 6MP, 6-mercaptopurine.) (Adapted from Sands BE. Therapy of inflammatory bowel disease. Gastroenterology 118: S68–S82, 2000, with permission.)

anticholinergic agents may help to alleviate symptoms. Patients with ileal disease or resection may require parenteral vitamin B_{12} supplementation or cholestyramine 1 to 4 g/day to control bile salt diarrhea. Iron supplementation may also be needed. Smoking cessation should be vigorously pursued as a means of improving long-term outcomes.[272] Bone loss should be anticipated as a potentially serious complication in all patients. Bone density should be checked at diagnosis and at regular intervals thereafter with appropriate medical management of bone loss (see Fig. 103–6).

Novel Therapies

Promising agents under investigation include anti-IL-12 antibodies, inhibitors of NF-κB, anti-adhesion molecule antibodies and compounds, and growth factors.[273] Human growth hormone given with a high protein diet has shown preliminary efficacy but cannot be recommended without further evaluation of safety and efficacy.[274] Alternative approaches to TNF inhibition are being explored, including CDP-571, a humanized anti-TNF antibody.[275] Open-label studies with thalidomide, which has anti-angiogenic properties in addition to destabilizing TNF mRNA, are promising, but the potent teratogenicity of this agent precludes widespread use.[276, 277] Probiotic therapies are being examined as a safe means of modulating the intestinal immune response in IBD.[278]

Nutritional Therapy

Nutritional therapy in Crohn's disease may target two purposes: repletion of nutrients and treatment of the primary disease (see Chapter 16). Specific deficits should be identified and repleted. Protein-calorie malnutrition should be addressed, preferably with enteral supplementation. Many, but not all, patients with Crohn's disease are lactose intolerant and may require increased calcium supplementation. Total parenteral nutrition may be considered for patients with severe malnutrition before surgery or for selected patients with severe Crohn's disease as a primary therapy in combination with bowel rest.[111] Patients with short bowel syndrome from multiple small bowel resections may require enteral nutrition with defined diets. Rare patients with severe short bowel syndrome may require life-long total parenteral nutrition.

A meta-analysis has found defined enteral diets to be inferior to glucocorticoids in achieving clinical response,[279] but defined enteral diets may still be useful for children in whom glucocorticoids are undesirable.[111] Elemental diets do not appear to be superior to polymeric diets.[279] Children may learn to receive nocturnal feedings after self-intubation with a nasogastric tube. Long-term tolerance may be poor, however, and disease tends to recur when the patient's usual diet is reintroduced. Self-reported food intolerances are common among patients with Crohn's disease,[280] but exclusion diets have not been shown to be beneficial.[281] Elimination of multiple food items may lead to serious malnutrition. Patients with a stricture may tolerate roughage poorly or may experience complete intestinal obstruction. Increasingly, specific nutrients are being considered for their therapeutic properties. Examples include a delayed release formulation of fish oil,[282] in which the active component is eicosapentaenoic acid, and so-called prebiotic nutrients, which facilitate the growth of beneficial flora.

Surgical Therapy

Surgery plays an integral role in the treatment of Crohn's disease, both to control symptoms and treat complications. By the 20th year from the onset of symptoms, roughly three fourths of patients will have had surgery.[283] Depending on the prevalent medical culture in the country of study, the rate of surgery within 3 years of diagnosis varies from 25% to 45%. From 25% to 38% of patients require a second surgery by 5 years after the first, and about one third of patients who need a second surgery eventually require a third.[284] Because of the high likelihood of recurrence after segmental resection, the guiding principle of surgery in Crohn's disease is the preservation of length and function. Taking wide margins does not reduce the likelihood of recurrent disease but with repeated resection may contribute to intestinal failure. Procedures may be categorized as resections with or without anastomosis, external (i.e., stoma) or internal bypass surgery, and a variety of surgical approaches for repair or resection of a fistula.[285] Stricturoplasty rather than resection may be appropriate for patients with multiple fibrotic nonphlegmonous strictures of the small bowel and for patients with short bowel syndrome or at risk for this complication from prior resections.[285] Although 80% of patients who undergo ileocecal resection have evidence of endoscopic recurrence in the neoterminal ileum within 1 year of surgery,[79] the time to symptomatic recurrence is usually several years. Recurrent disease almost always occurs proximal to the anastomosis. Recurrence after proctocolectomy and permanent ileostomy is relatively uncommon.

Indications for surgery include complications such as intra-abdominal abscess, medically intractable fistula, fibrotic stricture with obstructive symptoms, toxic megacolon, hemorrhage, and cancer.[286] Patients with symptoms refractory to medical therapy should also be considered for surgery, particularly when the patient remains glucocorticoid-dependent or refractory despite optimal medical therapy. Among children, a well-timed bowel resection may be indicated for growth failure. In patients with indeterminate colitis for whom colectomy and ileal pouch/anal anastomosis is being considered, there is a high rate of pouch failure. Therefore, thorough preoperative assessment should be completed to ascertain the correct diagnosis.[287] In selected cases with rectal sparing and lack of fistulizing behavior, ileal pouch/anal anastomosis or ileorectal anastomosis may be considered (see Chapter 105).[288, 289] Increasing facility with laparoscopic approaches to Crohn's disease may reduce the morbidity and improve the safety of surgery.[290, 291]

Costs of Care

Substantial medical and societal costs are incurred in the course of Crohn's disease. A recent study from Sweden showed that although ulcerative colitis is twice as prevalent as Crohn's disease, the total combined medical and societal costs of Crohn's disease are twice that of ulcerative colitis.[292] A recent analysis of data from a population-based cohort in the United States found projected lifetime costs of medical care to exceed $40,000 when median charges were applied.[293] Surgery generated the largest proportion of costs (44%), but nearly two thirds of patient time was spent off medical therapies, largely reflecting surgically induced remission.[293] Short of a cure, safe, well-tolerated, effective, and inexpensive means of maintaining remission should provide the greatest economic impact in the care of patients with the disease.

CROHN'S DISEASE IN THE LIFE CYCLE

Children and Adolescents

Approximately 25% of new Crohn's disease diagnoses are made in persons younger than 20 years of age. In most respects, Crohn's disease has the same pathophysiology and clinical features in children as it does in adults. The special consequences of Crohn's disease in children and adolescents relate to the vulnerability of this population to disturbances in physical growth, sexual maturation, and psychosocial development. Deceleration of growth velocity may precede gastrointestinal symptoms in as many as 20% of children.[294] Correction of nutritional deficits and vigorous treatment of inflammation will lead to normal growth and development in most patients. The potential for glucocorticoids to cause mood disturbances and cosmetic side effects may have dire implications for the child's psychosocial development, but their role in decreased height velocity has been questioned.[295] Increasingly, immune modulators are being incorporated into pediatric treatment regimens as a means of minimizing glucocorticoid use.[248, 296]

In evaluating disease, medical personnel must be particularly sensitive to the trauma of intrusive and sometimes painful examinations and procedures that are done routinely in adults. Sadly, children with Crohn's disease are also subject to the vicissitudes of their social circumstances; underinsured children are more likely to present with more severe disease, undoubtedly because of poor access to medical care and prolonged delays in diagnosis.[297] As much as possible, children with Crohn's disease should be permitted to function normally in school and extracurricular activities, although special accommodations may sometimes need to be arranged.

Sexuality, Fertility, and Pregnancy

Crohn's disease affects many persons in the peak of their reproductive years. Studies have varied in the assessment of female fertility in Crohn's disease, showing either no difference from the general population or a slight decrease. Studies that have detected diminished fertility have generally correlated this finding with increased disease activity. Contributing factors may include true infertility or a conscious decision to avoid childbearing. In men and women, decreased libido from symptoms such as diarrhea, abdominal pain, fatigue, or dyspareunia from rectovaginal fistula may play a role. Except for reversible sperm abnormalities caused by sulfasalazine, men with Crohn's disease are anticipated to have normal fertility.

The effect of pregnancy on the course of the disease depends on the status of the disease at conception. Women with quiescent disease at conception have the same rate of relapse as nonpregnant women. Among women with active disease at conception, the "one-third rule" applies: one third improve, one third worsen, and one third have unchanged symptoms during their pregnancy.[298] Postpartum relapses are uncommon and tend to be mild.

Most pregnancies carried by women with Crohn's disease are normal. Among the small number of women who experience stillbirth, spontaneous abortion, or premature labor, two thirds had active disease during the pregnancy. The rate of cesarean section is not increased compared with that of the general population, and perianal complications occur infrequently among women who deliver vaginally with an episiotomy.[299] For a review of the safety of medical therapies in pregnancy and nursing, see Table 103–5.

The Aging Patient

Compared with younger patients diagnosed with Crohn's disease, older patients are more likely to have colonic disease. As with children, the presentation may be subtle; extraintestinal symptoms may predominate, and diagnosis may be delayed. Medical management is essentially no different for the older patient, but the clinician more often must consider the variety of other conditions prevalent among older patients when choosing therapies. Older patients treated with glucocorticoids are at increased risk for hypertension, hypokalemia, and confusion.[300] Glucocorticoids may also complicate the management of diabetes. Antibiotics may diminish vitamin K production by intestinal flora and cause an excessively prolonged prothrombin time with warfarin therapy. Anticholinergic drugs may induce urinary retention, altered mental status, or glaucoma.

PROGNOSIS

Morbidity

The natural history of Crohn's disease is a moving target, continuously changing as therapeutic strategies improve. The course is highly variable and difficult to predict for a given patient. Population-based studies from Scandinavia provide the best information regarding the course of disease. In the first year after diagnosis, the cumulative relapse rate is high, approaching 50%, with 10% of patients having a chronic relapsing course.[301] Thereafter, patients are generally true to their own history: The rate of relapse in the first 1 or 2 years of the disease correlates with the risk of relapse in the ensuing 5 years.[302] Symptomatically active disease in the preceding year yields a high likelihood of active disease in the next year. Conversely, a year in which symptoms are quiescent has an 80% probability of being followed by another year without exacerbation.[302] Over a 4-year period, the same analysis has shown that 22% of patients remain in remission, 25% experience chronically active symptoms, and 53% have a course that fluctuates between active and inactive disease.[302] Although most persons continue to lead productive lives, the course of the disease may be punctuated by periods of poor productivity. Over time, approximately 10% of patients may be disabled by their disease.

Cancer

The estimated risk of colorectal cancer in Crohn's disease has varied widely, ranging from no risk above that of the general population to an estimated standardized incidence ratio as high as 26.6.[303] When Crohn's disease involves the large bowel, the excess risk of colorectal cancer appears to be similar to that in ulcerative colitis of similar extent.[303] The characteristics and prognosis of colorectal cancer in Crohn's disease are also similar to those for colorectal cancer in ulcerative colitis.[304] For these reasons, surveillance colonoscopies have been recommended as a means of early detection.[305] A thinner caliber colonoscope may be required to traverse narrowed bowel. Segments of bowel excluded by diversion procedures are at greatly increased risk of developing cancer and also present a great challenge to early detection.

Little controversy surrounds the increased risk of small bowel adenocarcinoma associated with long-standing disease or bypassed loops of the small intestine. Despite a roughly 12-fold relative risk, small bowel cancers remain rare, because of the extremely low incidence of this disease in the general population.[303]

The association between Hodgkin's and non-Hodgkin's lymphoma and Crohn's disease remains unclear. Studies relying on cases at referral centers have found an increased risk of lymphoma, whereas population-based studies have not. The most likely explanations are either a referral bias or an increased risk confined to patients with more severe disease.[303]

Squamous cell carcinomas may arise in association with a chronic fistula to the skin. Some studies also have found an association between Crohn's disease and respiratory cancers,[306] perhaps attributable to increased smoking behavior.

Mortality

Population-based studies have generally shown a modestly increased mortality rate in Crohn's disease.[307–311] Mortality appears to be highest in the first 4 or 5 years after diagnosis, with a 15-year survival rate that is 93.7% of that of the general population.[309, 310] Patients with proximal small bowel disease may have a higher risk of mortality, whereas those with ileal or ileocecal disease have a lower risk.[309, 311] The excess mortality may be ascribed to complications of Crohn's disease, including colorectal cancer.

Coping with Crohn's Disease

Although the old myths surrounding psychopathology as an underlying cause of IBD have long been debunked, coping with diarrhea, pain, malaise, and decreased energy takes a toll on all who suffer from Crohn's disease and their families. Depression and anxiety often diminish daily functioning that is already impaired by the physical manifestations of the disease, and psychosocial functioning has a large impact on the patient's quality of life.[312] Patients cite concerns about lack of energy, loss of control, body image, fear and isolation, feeling unclean, and not reaching their full potential.[313] The medical provider can help greatly in alleviating these concerns by providing accurate and plentiful information. Lay organizations such as the Crohn's and Colitis Foundation of America provide valuable resources in support of affected persons and their families (http://www.ccfa.org). An attitude of hopefulness is warranted, as an astounding number of therapeutic innovations—and someday perhaps a cure—unfold.

REFERENCES

1. Kirsner JB. Historical aspects of inflammatory bowel disease. J Clin Gastroenterol 10:286, 1988.
2. Dalziel TK. Thomas Kennedy Dalziel 1861–1924. Chronic interstitial enteritis [classical article]. Dis Colon Rectum 32:1076, 1989.
3. Baron JH. Inflammatory bowel disease up to 1932. M Sinai J Med 67: 174, 2000.
4. Crohn BB, Ginzburg L, Oppenheimer GD. Regional ileitis, a pathological and clinical entity. JAMA 99:1923, 1932.
5. Brooke BN. Granulomatous disease of the intestine. Lancet 2:745, 1959.
6. Lockhart-Mummery HE, Morson BC. Crohn's disease of the large intestine and its distinction from ulcerative colitis. Gut 1:87, 1960.
7. Moum B, Ekbom A, Vatn MH, et al. Inflammatory bowel disease: re-evaluation of the diagnosis in a prospective population based study in south eastern Norway. Gut 40:328, 1997.
8. Pinchbeck BR, Kirdeikis J, Thomson AB. Inflammatory bowel disease in northern Alberta. An epidemiologic study. J Clin Gastroenterol 10: 505, 1988.
9. Martinez-Salmeron JF, Rodrigo M, de Teresa J, et al. Epidemiology of inflammatory bowel disease in the Province of Granada, Spain: a retrospective study from 1979 to 1988. Gut 34:1207, 1993.
10. Ranzi T, Bodini P, Zambelli A, et al. Epidemiological aspects of inflammatory bowel disease in a north Italian population: a 4-year prospective study. Eur J Gastroenterol Hepatol 8:657, 1996.
11. Kurata JH, Kantor-Fish S, Frankl H, et al. Crohn's disease among ethnic groups in a large health maintenance organization. Gastroenterology 102:1940, 1992.
12. Nunes GC, Ahlquist RE, Jr. Increasing incidence of Crohn's disease. Am J Surg 145:578, 1983.
13. Sonnenberg A, McCarty DJ, Jacobsen SJ. Geographic variation of inflammatory bowel disease within the United States. Gastroenterology 100:143, 1991.
14. Hiatt RA, Kaufman L. Epidemiology of inflammatory bowel disease in a defined northern California population. West J Med 149:541, 1988.
15. Shivananda S, Lennard-Jones J, Logan R, et al. Incidence of inflammatory bowel disease across Europe: is there a difference between north and south? Results of the European Collaborative Study on Inflammatory Bowel Disease (EC-IBD). Gut 39:690, 1996.
16. Morita N, Toki S, Hirohashi T, et al. Incidence and prevalence of inflammatory bowel disease in Japan: nationwide epidemiological survey during the year 1991. J Gastroenterol 30(Suppl 8):1, 1995.
17. Yoshida Y, Murata Y. Inflammatory bowel disease in Japan: studies of epidemiology and etiopathogenesis. Med Clin North Am 74:67, 1990.
18. Eason RJ, Lee SP, Tasman-Jones C. Inflammatory bowel disease in Auckland, New Zealand. Austr N Z J Med 12:125, 1982.
19. Anseline PF. Crohn's disease in the Hunter Valley region of Australia. Austr N Z J Surg 65:564, 1995.
20. Mayberry J, Mann R. Inflammatory bowel disease in rural sub-Saharan Africa: rarity of diagnosis in patients attending mission hospitals. Digestion 44:172, 1989.
21. Wright JP, Froggatt J, O'Keefe EA, et al. The epidemiology of inflammatory bowel disease in Cape Town 1980–1984. S Afr Med J 70:10, 1986.
22. Loftus EV, Jr, Silverstein MD, Sandborn WJ, et al. Crohn's disease in Olmsted County, Minnesota, 1940–1993: incidence, prevalence, and survival. Gastroenterology 114:1161, 1998.
23. Munkholm P, Langholz E, Nielsen OH, et al. Incidence and prevalence of Crohn's disease in the county of Copenhagen, 1962–87: a sixfold increase in incidence. Scand J Gastroenterol 27:609, 1992.
24. Delco F, Sonnenberg A. Commonalities in the time trends of Crohn's disease and ulcerative colitis. Am J Gastroenterol 94:2171, 1999.
25. Munkholm P. Crohn's disease—occurrence, course and prognosis. An epidemiologic cohort-study. Dan Med Bull 44:287, 1997.
26. Ekbom A, Helmick C, Zack M, et al. The epidemiology of inflammatory bowel disease: a large, population-based study in Sweden. Gastroenterology 100:350, 1991.
27. Andres PG, Friedman LS. Epidemiology and the natural course of inflammatory bowel disease. Gastroenterol Clin North Am 28:255, 1999.
28. Sandler RS, Eisen GM. Epidemiology of inflammatory bowel disease. In Kirsner JB (ed): Inflammatory Bowel Disease. Philadelphia, WB Saunders, 2000, p 89.
29. Polito JM, 2nd, Childs B, Mellits ED, et al. Crohn's disease: influence of age at diagnosis on site and clinical type of disease. Gastroenterology 111:580, 1996.
30. Wakefield AJ, Pittilo RM, Sim R, et al. Evidence of persistent measles virus infection in Crohn's disease. J Med Virol 39:345, 1993.
31. Organization WH. Association between measles infection and the occurrence of chronic inflammatory bowel disease. Wkly Epidemiol Rec 73:33, 1998.
32. Schultsz C, Moussa M, van Ketel R, et al. Frequency of pathogenic and enteroadherent Escherichia coli in patients with inflammatory bowel disease and controls. J Clin Pathol 50:573, 1997.
33. Van Kruiningen HJ. Lack of support for a common etiology in Johne's disease of animals and Crohn's disease in humans. Inflam Bowel Dis 5:183, 1999.
34. Fiocchi C. Inflammatory bowel disease: etiology and pathogenesis. Gastroenterology 115:182, 1998.
35. MacDonald TT. Effector and regulatory lymphoid cells and cytokines in mucosal sites. Curr Top Microbiol Immunol 236:113, 1999.
36. Duchmann R, May E, Heike M, et al. T cell specificity and cross reactivity towards enterobacteria, bacteroides, bifidobacterium, and antigens from resident intestinal flora in humans. Gut 44:812, 1999.
37. Romagnani S. T-cell subsets (Th1 versus Th2). Ann Allerg Asthma Immunol 85:9, 2000.
38. Strober W, Ludviksson BR, Fuss IJ. The pathogenesis of mucosal inflammation in murine models of inflammatory bowel disease and Crohn disease. Ann Intern Med 128:848, 1998.
39. Fuss IJ, Neurath M, Boirivant M, et al. Disparate CD4+ lamina propria (LP) lymphokine secretion profiles in inflammatory bowel disease. Crohn's disease LP cells manifest increased secretion of IFN-gamma, whereas ulcerative colitis LP cells manifest increased secretion of IL-5. J Immunol 157:1261, 1996.
40. Hermiston ML, Gordon JI. Inflammatory bowel disease and adenomas in mice expressing a dominant negative N-cadherin. Science 270:1203, 1995.
41. Mashimo H, Wu DC, Podolsky DK, et al. Impaired defense of intestinal mucosa in mice lacking intestinal trefoil factor. Science 274:262, 1996.
42. Panwala CM, Jones JC, Viney JL. A novel model of inflammatory bowel disease: mice deficient for the multiple drug resistance gene, mdrla, spontaneously develop colitis. J Immunol 161:5733, 1998.
43. Sadlack B, Merz H, Schorle H, et al. Ulcerative colitis-like disease in mice with a disrupted interleukin-2 gene. Cell 75:253, 1993.
44. Kuhn R, Lohler J, Rennick D, et al. Interleukin-10-deficient mice develop chronic enterocolitis. Cell 75:263, 1993.
45. Hammer RE, Maika SD, Richardson JA, et al. Spontaneous inflammatory disease in transgenic rats expressing HLA-B27 and human beta 2m: an animal model of HLA-B27-associated human disorders. Cell 63:1099, 1990.
46. Lopez-Cubero SO, Sullivan KM, McDonald GB. Course of Crohn's disease after allogeneic marrow transplantation. Gastroenterology 114: 433, 1998.
47. Sustento-Reodica N, Ruiz P, Rogers A, et al. Recurrent Crohn's disease in transplanted bowel. Lancet 349:688, 1997.
48. D'Inca R, Di Leo V, Corrao G, et al. Intestinal permeability test as a predictor of clinical course in Crohn's disease. Am J Gastroenterol 94: 2956, 1999.
49. Peeters M, Nevens H, Baert F, et al. Familial aggregation in Crohn's disease: increased age-adjusted risk and concordance in clinical characteristics. Gastroenterology 111:597, 1996.
50. Atreya R, Mudter J, Finotto S, et al. Blockade of interleukin 6 trans signaling suppresses T-cell resistance against apoptosis in chronic intestinal inflammation: evidence in Crohn disease and experimental colitis in vivo. Nat Med 6:583, 2000.
51. Neurath MF, Fuss I, Kelsall BL, et al. Antibodies to interleukin 12 abrogate established experimental colitis in mice. J Exp Med 182: 1281, 1995.
52. Neurath MF, Pettersson S. Predominant role of NF-kappa B p65 in the pathogenesis of chronic intestinal inflammation. Immunobiology 198:91, 1997.
53. Barnes PJ, Karin M. Nuclear factor-kappaB: a pivotal transcription factor in chronic inflammatory diseases. N Engl J Med 336:1066, 1997.

54. Walzog B, Gaehtgens P. Adhesion molecules: the path to a new understanding of acute inflammation. News Physiol Sci 15:107, 2000.
55. Briskin M, Winsor-Hines D, Shyjan A, et al. Human mucosal addressin cell adhesion molecule-1 is preferentially expressed in intestinal tract and associated lymphoid tissue. Am J Pathol 151:97, 1997.
56. Podolsky DK, Lobb R, King N, et al. Attenuation of colitis in the cotton-top tamarin by anti-alpha 4 integrin monoclonal antibody. J Clin Invest 92:372, 1993.
57. Hesterberg PE, Winsor-Hines D, Briskin MJ, et al. Rapid resolution of chronic colitis in the cotton-top tamarin with an antibody to a gut-homing integrin alpha 4 beta 7. Gastroenterology 111:1373, 1996.
58. Ludviksson BR, Strober W, Nishikomori R, et al. Administration of mAb against alpha E beta 7 prevents and ameliorates immunization-induced colitis in IL-2−/− mice. J Immunol 162:4975, 1999.
59. von Lampe B, Barthel B, Coupland SE, et al. Differential expression of matrix metalloproteinases and their tissue inhibitors in colon mucosa of patients with inflammatory bowel disease. Gut 47:63, 2000.
60. Binder V. Genetic epidemiology in inflammatory bowel disease. Dig Dis 16:351, 1998.
61. Satsangi J, Grootscholten C, Holt H, et al. Clinical patterns of familial inflammatory bowel disease. Gut 38:738, 1996.
62. Bayless TM, Tokayer AZ, Polito JM, 2nd, et al. Crohn's disease: concordance for site and clinical type in affected family members–potential hereditary influences. Gastroenterology 111:573, 1996.
63. Colombel JF, Grandbastien B, Gower-Rousseau C, et al. Clinical characteristics of Crohn's disease in 72 families. Gastroenterology 111: 604, 1996.
64. Polito JMD, Rees RC, Childs B, et al. Preliminary evidence for genetic anticipation in Crohn's disease. Lancet 347:798, 1996.
65. Lee JC, Bridger S, McGregor C, et al. Why children with inflammatory bowel disease are diagnosed at a younger age than their affected parent. Gut 44:808, 1999.
66. Heresbach D, Gulwani-Akolkar B, Lesser M, et al. Anticipation in Crohn's disease may be influenced by gender and ethnicity of the transmitting parent. Am J Gastroenterol 93:2368, 1998.
67. Sendid B, Quinton JF, Charrier G, et al. Anti-Saccharomyces cerevisiae mannan antibodies in familial Crohn's disease. Am J Gastroenterol 93:1306, 1998.
68. Seibold F, Mork H, Tanza S, et al. Pancreatic autoantibodies in Crohn's disease: a family study. Gut 40:481, 1997.
69. Hugot JP, Laurent-Puig P, Gower-Rousseau C, et al. Mapping of a susceptibility locus for Crohn's disease on chromosome 16. Nature 379:821, 1996.
69a. Ogura Y, Bonen DK, Inohara N, et al. A frameshift mutation in *NOD2* associated with susceptibility to Crohn's disease. Nature 411: 603, 2001.
69b. Hugot JP, Chamaillard M, Zouali H, et al. Association of NOD2 leucine-rich repeat variants with susceptibility to Crohn's disease. Nature 411:599, 2001.
70. Duerr RH, Barmada MM, Zhang L, et al. Linkage and association between inflammatory bowel disease and a locus on chromosome 12. Am J Hum Genet 63:95, 1998.
71. Cho JH, Nicolae DL, Ramos R, et al. Linkage and linkage disequilibrium in chromosome band 1p36 in American Chaldeans with inflammatory bowel disease. Hum Mol Genet 9:1425, 2000.
72. Sonnenberg A. Occupational distribution of inflammatory bowel disease among German employees. Gut 31:1037, 1990.
73. Powell JJ, Harvey RS, Ashwood P, et al. Immune potentiation of ultrafine dietary particles in normal subjects and patients with inflammatory bowel disease. J Autoimmun 14:99, 2000.
74. Addolorato G, Capristo E, Stefanini GF, et al. Inflammatory bowel disease: a study of the association between anxiety and depression, physical morbidity, and nutritional status. Scand J Gastroenterol 32: 1013, 1997.
75. Anton PA. Stress and mind-body impact on the course of inflammatory bowel diseases. Semin Gastrointest Dis 10:14, 1999.
76. Qiu BS, Vallance BA, Blennerhassett PA, et al. The role of CD4+ lymphocytes in the susceptibility of mice to stress-induced reactivation of experimental colitis. Nat Med 5:1178, 1999.
77. Zamora SA, Hilsden RJ, Meddings JB, et al. Intestinal permeability before and after ibuprofen in families of children with Crohn's disease. Can J Gastroenterol 13:31, 1999.
78. Parente F, Cucino C, Bollani S, et al. Focal gastric inflammatory infiltrates in inflammatory bowel diseases: prevalence, immunohistochemical characteristics, and diagnostic role. Am J Gastroenterol 95: 705, 2000.
79. Rutgeerts P, Geboes K, Vantrappen G, et al. Natural history of recurrent Crohn's disease at the ileocolonic anastomosis after curative surgery. Gut 25:665, 1984.
80. Rickert RR, Carter HW. The "early" ulcerative lesion of Crohn's disease: correlative light- and scanning electron-microscopic studies. J Clin Gastroenterol 2:11, 1980.
81. Okada M, Maeda K, Yao T, et al. Minute lesions of the rectum and sigmoid colon in patients with Crohn's disease. Gastrointest Endosc 37:319, 1991.
82. Fujimura Y, Kamoi R, Iida M. Pathogenesis of aphthoid ulcers in Crohn's disease: correlative findings by magnifying colonoscopy, electron microscopy, and immunohistochemistry. Gut 38:724, 1996.
83. Rutgeerts P, Goboes K, Peeters M, et al. Effect of faecal stream diversion on recurrence of Crohn's disease in the neoterminal ileum. Lancet 338:771, 1991.
84. Kelly JK, Sutherland LR. The chronological sequence in the pathology of Crohn's disease. J Clin Gastroenterol 10:28, 1988.
85. Chambers TJ, Morson BC. The granuloma in Crohn's disease. Gut 20: 269, 1979.
86. Riddell RH. Pathology of idiopathic inflammatory bowel disease. In Kirsner JB (ed): Inflammatory Bowel Disease. Philadelphia, WB Saunders, 2000, p 427.
87. Stallmach A, Schuppan D, Riese HH, et al. Increased collagen type III synthesis by fibroblasts isolated from strictures of patients with Crohn's disease. Gastroenterology 102:1920, 1992.
88. Borley NR, Mortensen NJ, Jewell DP, et al. The relationship between inflammatory and serosal connective tissue changes in ileal Crohn's disease: evidence for a possible causative link. J Pathol 190:196, 2000.
89. Desreumaux P, Ernst O, Geboes K, et al. Inflammatory alterations in mesenteric adipose tissue in Crohn's disease. Gastroenterology 117:73, 1999.
90. Wright NA, Poulsom R, Stamp G, et al. Trefoil peptide gene expression in gastrointestinal epithelial cells in inflammatory bowel disease. Gastroenterology 104:12, 1993.
91. Oberhuber G, Puspok A, Oesterreicher C, et al. Focally enhanced gastritis: a frequent type of gastritis in patients with Crohn's disease [comment]. Gastroenterology 112:698, 1997.
92. Higgens CS, Allan RN. Crohn's disease of the distal ileum. Gut 21: 933, 1980.
93. Belaiche J, Louis E, D'Haens G, et al. Acute lower gastrointestinal bleeding in Crohn's disease: characteristics of a unique series of 34 patients. Belgian IBD Research Group. Am J Gastroenterol 94:2177, 1999.
94. Langevin S, Menard DB, Haddad H, et al. Idiopathic ulcerative proctitis may be the initial manifestation of Crohn's disease. J Clin Gastroenterol 15:199, 1992.
95. Baker WN, Milton-Thompson GJ. The anal lesion as the sole presenting symptom of intestinal Crohn's disease. Gut 12:865, 1971.
96. Buchmann P, Alexander-Williams J. Classification of perianal Crohn's disease. Clin Gastroenterol 9:323, 1980.
97. Wagtmans MJ, Verspaget HW, Lamers CB, et al. Clinical aspects of Crohn's disease of the upper gastrointestinal tract: a comparison with distal Crohn's disease. Am J Gastroenterol 92:1467, 1997.
98. D'Haens G, Rutgeerts P, Geboes K, et al. The natural history of esophageal Crohn's disease: three patterns of evolution. Gastrointest Endosc 40:296, 1994.
99. Oberhuber G, Puspok A, Peck-Radosavlevic M, et al. Aberrant esophageal HLA-DR expression in a high percentage of patients with Crohn's disease. Am J Surg Pathol 23:970, 1999.
100. Richards ML, Aberger FJ, Landercasper J. Granulomatous appendicitis: Crohn's disease, atypical Crohn's or not Crohn's at all? J Am Coll Surg 185:13, 1997.
101. Greenstein AJ, Lachman P, Sachar DB, et al. Perforating and nonperforating indications for repeated operations in Crohn's disease: evidence for two clinical forms. Gut 29:588, 1988.
102. Gilberts EC, Greenstein AJ, Katsel P, et al. Molecular evidence for two forms of Crohn disease. Proc Nat Acad Sci USA 91:12721, 1994.
103. Heuschkel RB, MacDonald TT, Monteleone G, et al. Imbalance of stromelysin-1 and TIMP-1 in the mucosal lesions of children with inflammatory bowel disease. Gut 47:57, 2000.
104. Ribeiro MB, Greenstein AJ, Yamazaki Y, et al. Intra-abdominal abscess in regional enteritis. Ann Surg 213:32, 1991.
105. Gasche C, Scholmerich J, Brynskov J, et al. A simple classification of Crohn's disease: report of the Working Party for the World Con-

gresses of Gastroenterology, Vienna 1998. Inflam Bowel Dis 6:8, 2000.
106. Urayama S, Chang EB. Mechanisms and treatment of diarrhea in inflammatory bowel diseases. Inflam Bowel Dis 3:114, 1997.
107. Dvorak AM, Silen W. Differentiation between Crohn's disease and other inflammatory conditions by electron microscopy. Ann Surg 201: 53, 1985.
108. Mantyh CR, Vigna SR, Bollinger RR, et al. Differential expression of substance P receptors in patients with Crohn's disease and ulcerative colitis. Gastroenterology 109:850, 1995.
109. Geboes K, Collins S. Structural abnormalities of the nervous system in Crohn's disease and ulcerative colitis. Neurogastroenterol Motil 10: 189, 1998.
110. Geerling BJ, Badart-Smook A, Stockbrugger RW, et al. Comprehensive nutritional status in patients with long-standing Crohn disease currently in remission. Am J Clin Nutr 67:919, 1998.
111. Han PD, Burke A, Baldassano RN, et al. Nutrition and inflammatory bowel disease. Gastroenterol Clin North Am 28:423, 1999.
112. Gryboski JD, Burger J, McCallum R, et al. Gastric emptying in childhood inflammatory bowel disease: nutritional and pathologic correlates. Am J Gastroenterol 87:1148, 1992.
113. Schreiber S, Howaldt S, Schnoor M, et al. Recombinant erythropoietin for the treatment of anemia in inflammatory bowel disease. N Engl J Med 334:619, 1996.
114. Veloso FT, Carvalho J, Magro F. Immune-related systemic manifestations of inflammatory bowel disease. A prospective study of 792 patients. J Clin Gastroenterol 23:29, 1996.
115. Lorusso D, Leo S, Mossa A, et al. Cholelithiasis in inflammatory bowel disease. A case-control study. Dis Colon Rectum 33:791, 1990.
116. Lapidus A, Bangstad M, Astrom M, et al. The prevalence of gallstone disease in a defined cohort of patients with Crohn's disease [see comments]. Am J Gastroenterol 94:1261, 1999.
117. Danzi JT. Extraintestinal manifestations of idiopathic inflammatory bowel disease. Arch Intern Med 148:297, 1988.
118. Farmer RG, Hawk WA, Turnbull RB, Jr. Clinical patterns in Crohn's disease: a statistical study of 615 cases. Gastroenterology 68:627, 1975.
119. Salmi M, Jalkanen S. Endothelial ligands and homing of mucosal leukocytes in extraintestinal manifestations of IBD. Inflam Bowel Dis 4:149, 1998.
120. Orchard TR, Wordsworth BP, Jewell DP. Peripheral arthropathies in inflammatory bowel disease: their articular distribution and natural history. Gut 42:387, 1998.
121. Orchard TR, Thiyagaraja S, Welsh KI, et al. Clinical phenotype is related to HLA genotype in the peripheral arthropathies of inflammatory bowel disease. Gastroenterology 118:274, 2000.
122. Gravallese EM, Kantrowitz FG. Arthritic manifestations of inflammatory bowel disease. Am J Gastroenterol 83:703, 1988.
123. Orchard TR, Jewell DP. The importance of ileocaecal integrity in the arthritic complications of Crohn's disease. Inflam Bowel Dis 5:92, 1999.
124. Scott WW, Jr, Fishman EK, Kuhlman JE, et al. Computed tomography evaluation of the sacroiliac joints in Crohn disease. Radiologic/ clinical correlation. Skel Radiol 19:207, 1990.
125. Wakefield AJ, Sankey EA, Dhillon AP, et al. Granulomatous vasculitis in Crohn's disease. Gastroenterology 100:1279, 1991.
126. Freeman HJ, Freeman KJ. Prevalence rates and an evaluation of reported risk factors for osteonecrosis (avascular necrosis) in Crohn's disease. Can J Gastroenterol 14:138, 2000.
127. Bousvaros A, Marcon M, Treem W, et al. Chronic recurrent multifocal osteomyelitis associated with chronic inflammatory bowel disease in children. Dig Dis Sci 44:2500, 1999.
128. Ghosh S, Cowen S, Hannan WJ, et al. Low bone mineral density in Crohn's disease, but not in ulcerative colitis, at diagnosis. Gastroenterology 107:1031, 1994.
129. Dresner-Pollak R, Karmeli F, Eliakim R, et al. Increased urinary N-telopeptide cross-linked type 1 collagen predicts bone loss in patients with inflammatory bowel disease. Am J Gastroenterol 95:699, 2000.
130. Schulte CM, Dignass AU, Goebell H, et al. Genetic factors determine extent of bone loss in inflammatory bowel disease. Gastroenterology 119:909, 2000.
131. Lebwohl M, Lebwohl O. Cutaneous manifestations of inflammatory bowel disease. Inflam Bowel Dis 4:142, 1998.
132. Finkel SI, Janowitz HD. Trauma and the pyoderma gangrenosum of inflammatory bowel disease. Gut 22:410, 1981.
133. Lisciandrano D, Ranzi T, Carrassi A, et al. Prevalence of oral lesions in inflammatory bowel disease. Am J Gastroenterol 91:7, 1996.
134. Hackzell-Bradley M, Hedblad MA, Stephansson EA. Metastatic Crohn's disease. Report of 3 cases with special reference to histopathologic findings. Arch Dermatol 132:928, 1996.
135. Zlatanic J, Fleisher M, Sasson M, et al. Crohn's disease and acute leukocytoclastic vasculitis of skin. Am J Gastroenterol 91:2410, 1996.
136. Travis S, Innes N, Davies MG, et al. Sweet's syndrome: an unusual cutaneous feature of Crohn's disease or ulcerative colitis. The South West Gastroenterology Group. Eur J Gastroenterol Hepatol 9:715, 1997.
137. Lee FI. Bellary SV, Francis C. Increased occurrence of psoriasis in patients with Crohn's disease and their relatives. Am J Gastroenterol 85:962, 1990.
138. Hopkins DJ, Horan E, Burton IL, et al. Ocular disorders in a series of 332 patients with Crohn's disease. Br J Ophthalmol 58:732, 1974.
139. Lyons JL, Rosenbaum JT. Uveitis associated with inflammatory bowel disease compared with uveitis associated with spondyloarthropathy. Arch Ophthalmol 115:61, 1997.
140. Hofley P, Roarty J, McGinnity G, et al. Asymptomatic uveitis in children with chronic inflammatory bowel diseases. J Pediatr Gastroenterol Nutr 17:397, 1993.
141. Rasmussen HH, Fallingborg JF, Mortensen PB, et al. Hepatobiliary dysfunction and primary sclerosing cholangitis in patients with Crohn's disease. Scand J Gastroenterol 32:604, 1997.
142. Over HH, Ulgen S, Tuglular T, et al. Thrombophilia and inflammatory bowel disease: does factor V mutation have a role? Eur J Gastroenterol Hepatol 10:827, 1998.
143. Zauber NP, Sabbath-Solitare M, Rajoria G, et al. Factor V Leiden mutation is not increased in patients with inflammatory bowel disease. J Clin Gastroenterol 27:215, 1998.
144. Mahmud N, Molloy A, McPartlin J, et al. Increased prevalence of methylenetetrahydrofolate reductase C677T variant in patients with inflammatory bowel disease, and its clinical implications. Gut 45:389, 1999.
145. Jackson LM, O'Gorman PJ, O'Connell J, et al. Thrombosis in inflammatory bowel disease: clinical setting, procoagulant profile and factor V Leiden. QJM 90:183, 1997.
146. Fireman Z, Osipov A, Kivity S, et al. The use of induced sputum in the assessment of pulmonary involvement in Crohn's disease. Am J Gastroenterol 95:730, 2000.
147. Mansi A, Cucchiara S, Greco L, et al. Bronchial hyperresponsiveness in children and adolescents with Crohn's disease. Am J Respir Crit Care Med 161:1051, 2000.
148. Elsehety A, Bertorini TE. Neurologic and neuropsychiatric complications of Crohn's disease. South Med J 90:606, 1997.
149. Lossos A, River Y, Eliakim A, et al. Neurologic aspects of inflammatory bowel disease. Neurology 45:416, 1995.
150. Levine JB. Extraintestinal manifestations of inflammatory bowel disease. In Kirsner JB (ed): Inflammatory Bowel Disease. Philadelphia, WB. Saunders, 2000, p 397.
151. Weber P, Seibold F, Jenss H. Acute pancreatitis in Crohn's disease. J Clin Gastroenterol 17:286, 1993.
152. Barthet M, Hastier P, Bernard JP, et al. Chronic pancreatitis and inflammatory bowel disease: true or coincidental association? Am J Gastroenterol 94:2141, 1999.
153. Hegnhoj J, Hansen CP, Rannem T, et al. Pancreatic function in Crohn's disease. Gut 31:1076, 1990.
154. Bernstein CN, Boult IF, Greenberg HM, et al. A prospective randomized comparison between small bowel enteroclysis and small bowel follow-through in Crohn's disease. Gastroenterology 113:390, 1997.
155. Scotiniotis I, Rubesin SE, Ginsberg GG. Imaging modalities in inflammatory bowel disease. Gastroenterol Clin North Am 28:391, 1999.
156. Gore RM, Balthazar EJ, Ghahremani GG, et al. CT features of ulcerative colitis and Crohn's disease. AJR Am J Roentgenol 167:3, 1996.
157. Herlinger H, Furth EE, Rubesin SE. Fibrofatty proliferation of the mesentery in Crohn disease. Abdom Imag 23:446, 1998.
158. Gasche C, Moser G, Turetschek K, et al. Transabdominal bowel sonography for the detection of intestinal complications in Crohn's disease. Gut 44:112, 1999.
159. Cho E, Mochizuki N, Ashihara T, et al. Endoscopic ultrasonography in the evaluation of inflammatory bowel disease. Endoscopy 30 (Suppl 1):A94, 1998.
160. Ludwig D, Wiener S, Bruning A, et al. Mesenteric blood flow is related to disease activity and risk of relapse in Crohn's disease: a prospective follow-up study. Am J Gastroenterol 94:2942, 1999.
161. Hussain SM, Outwater EK, Joekes EC, et al. Clinical and MR imag-

ing features of cryptoglandular and Crohn's fistulas and abscesses. Abdom Imag 25:67, 2000.
162. Low RN, Francis IR, Politoske D, et al. Crohn's disease evaluation: comparison of contrast-enhanced MR imaging and single-phase helical CT scanning. J Magn Reson Imag 11:127, 2000.
163. Madsen SM, Thomsen HS, Schlichting P, et al. Evaluation of treatment response in active Crohn's disease by low-field magnetic resonance imaging. Abdom Imag 24:232, 1999.
164. Sahai A, Belair M, Gianfelice D, et al. Percutaneous drainage of intra-abdominal abscesses in Crohn's disease: short and long-term outcome. Am J Gastroenterol 92:275, 1997.
165. Charron M, Di Lorenzo C, Kocoshis S. Are 99mTc leukocyte scintigraphy and SBFT studies useful in children suspected of having inflammatory bowel disease? Am J Gastroenterol 95:1208, 2000.
166. Pera A, Bellando P, Caldera D, et al. Colonoscopy in inflammatory bowel disease. Diagnostic accuracy and proposal of an endoscopic score. Gastroenterology 92:181, 1987.
167. Marshall JK, Hewak J, Farrow R, et al. Terminal ileal imaging with ileoscopy versus small-bowel meal with pneumocolon. J Clin Gastroenterol 27:217, 1998.
168. Koltun WA, Schoetz DJ, Jr, Roberts PL, et al. Indeterminate colitis predisposes to perineal complications after ileal pouch-anal anastomosis. Dis Colon Rectum 34:857, 1991.
169. Shivananda S, Hordijk ML, Ten Kate FJ, et al. Differential diagnosis of inflammatory bowel disease. A comparison of various diagnostic classifications. Scand J Gastroenterol 26:167, 1991.
170. Riegler G, Arimoli A, Esposito P, et al. Clinical evolution in an outpatient series with indeterminate colitis. Dis Colon Rectum 40:437, 1997.
171. Quinton JF, Sendid B, Reumaux D, et al. Anti-*Saccharomyces cerevisiae* mannan antibodies combined with antineutrophil cytoplasmic autoantibodies in inflammatory bowel disease: prevalence and diagnostic role. Gut 42:788, 1998.
172. Ruemmele FM, Targan SR, Levy G, et al. Diagnostic accuracy of serological assays in pediatric inflammatory bowel disease. Gastroenterology 115:822, 1998.
173. Sutton CL, Yang H, Li Z, et al. Familial expression of anti-*Saccharomyces cerevisiae* mannan antibodies in affected and unaffected relatives of patients with Crohn's disease. Gut 46:58, 2000.
174. Vasiliauskas EA, Plevy SE, Landers CJ, et al. Perinuclear antineutrophil cytoplasmic antibodies in patients with Crohn's disease define a clinical subgroup. Gastroenterology 110:1810, 1996.
175. van Hees PA, van Elteren PH, van Lier HJ, et al. An index of inflammatory activity in patients with Crohn's disease. Gut 21:279, 1980.
176. Wright JP, Marks IN, Parfitt A. A simple clinical index of Crohn's disease activity–the Cape Town index. S Afr Med J 68:502, 1985.
177. Harvey RF, Bradshaw M. A simple index of Crohn's-disease activity. Lancet 1:514, 1980.
178. Myren J, Bouchier IA, Watkinson G, et al. The O.M.G.E. Multinational inflammatory bowel disease survey 1976–1982. A further report on 2,657 cases. Scand J Gastroenterol 95(Suppl):1, 1984.
179. Willoughby JM, Kumar P, Beckett J, et al. A double-blind trial of azathioprine in Crohn's disease. Gut 12:864, 1971.
180. De Dombal FT, Burton IL, Clamp SE, et al. Short-term course and prognosis of Crohn's disease. Gut 15:435, 1974.
181. Talstad I, Gjone E. The disease activity of ulcerative colitis and Crohn's disease. Scand J Gastroenterol 11:403, 1976.
182. Sandler RS, Jordan MC, Kupper LL. Development of a Crohn's index for survey research. J Clin Epidemiol 41:451, 1988.
183. Hyams JS, Ferry GD, Mandel FS, et al. Development and validation of a pediatric Crohn's disease activity index. J Pediatr Gastroenterol Nutr 12:439, 1991.
184. Lloyd-Still JD, Green OC. A clinical scoring system for chronic inflammatory bowel disease in children. Dig Dis Sci 24:620, 1979.
185. de Dombal FT, Softley A. IOIBD report no 1: observer variation in calculating indices of severity and activity in Crohn's disease. International Organisation for the Study of Inflammatory Bowel Disease. Gut 28:474, 1987.
186. Papi C, Ciaco A, Bianchi M, et al. Correlation of various Crohn's disease activity indexes in subgroups of patients with primarily inflammatory or fibrostenosing clinical characteristics. J Clin Gastroenterol 23:40, 1996.
187. Allan A, Linares L, Spooner HA, et al. Clinical index to quantitate symptoms of perianal Crohn's disease. Dis Colon Rectum 35:656, 1992.
188. Irvine EJ. Usual therapy improves perianal Crohn's disease as measured by a new disease activity index. McMaster IBD Study Group. J Clin Gastroenterol 20:27, 1995.
189. Mary JY, Modigliani R. Development and validation of an endoscopic index of the severity for Crohn's disease: a prospective multicentre study. Groupe d'Etudes Therapeutiques des Affections Inflammatoires du Tube Digestif (GETAID). Gut 30:983, 1989.
190. Present DH, Korelitz BI, Wisch N, et al. Treatment of Crohn's disease with 6-mercaptopurine. A long-term, randomized, double-blind study. N Engl J Med 302:981, 1980.
191. Nielsen OH, Vainer B, Madsen SM, et al. Established and emerging biological activity markers of inflammatory bowel disease. Am J Gastroenterol 95:359, 2000.
192. Tibble JA, Sigthorsson G, Bridger S, et al. Surrogate markers of intestinal inflammation are predictive of relapse in patients with inflammatory bowel disease. Gastroenterology 119:15, 2000.
193. Guyatt G, Mitchell A, Irvine EJ, et al. A new measure of health status for clinical trials in inflammatory bowel disease. Gastroenterology 96:804, 1989.
194. Azad Khan AK, Piris J, Truelove SC. An experiment to determine the active therapeutic moiety of sulphasalazine. Lancet 2:892, 1977.
195. MacDermott RP. Progress in understanding the mechanism of action of 5-aminosalicylic acid. Am J Gastroenterol 95:3343, 2000.
196. Bantel H, Berg C, Vieth M, et al. Mesalazine inhibits activation of transcription factor NF-B in inflamed mucosa of patients with ulcerative colitis. Am J Gastroenterol 95:3452, 2000.
197. Summers RW, Switz DM, Sessions JT, Jr, et al. National Cooperative Crohn's Disease Study: results of drug treatment. Gastroenterology 77:847, 1979.
198. Malchow H, Ewe K, Brandes JW, et al. European Cooperative Crohn's Disease Study (ECCDS): results of drug treatment. Gastroenterology 86:249, 1984.
199. Mahida YR, Jewell DP. Slow-release 5-amino-salicylic acid (Pentasa) for the treatment of active Crohn's disease. Digestion 45:88, 1990.
200. Rasmussen SN, Lauritsen K, Tage-Jensen U, et al. 5-Aminosalicylic acid in the treatment of Crohn's disease. A 16-week double-blind, placebo-controlled, multicentre study with Pentasa. Scand J Gastroenterol 22:877, 1987.
201. Singleton JW, Hanauer SB, Gitnick GL, et al. Mesalamine capsules for the treatment of active Crohn's disease: results of a 16-week trial. Pentasa Crohn's Disease Study Group. Gastroenterology 104:1293, 1993.
202. Prantera C, Cottone M, Pallone F, et al. Mesalamine in the treatment of mild to moderate active Crohn's ileitis: results of a randomized, multicenter trial. Gastroenterology 116:521, 1999.
203. Tremaine WJ, Schroeder KW, Harrison JM, et al. A randomized, double-blind, placebo-controlled trial of the oral mesalamine (5-ASA) preparation, Asacol, in the treatment of symptomatic Crohn's colitis and ileocolitis. J Clin Gastroenterol 19:278, 1994.
204. Lang KA, Peppercorn MA. Medical therapy for Crohn's disease. In Kirsner JB (ed): Inflammatory Bowel Disease. Philadelphia, WB Saunders, 2000, p 557.
205. Camma C, Giunta M, Rosselli M, et al. Mesalamine in the maintenance treatment of Crohn's disease: a meta-analysis adjusted for confounding variables. Gastroenterology 113:1465, 1997.
206. Lochs H, Mayer M, Fleig WE, et al. Prophylaxis of postoperative relapse in Crohn's disease with mesalamine: European Cooperative Crohn's Disease Study VI. Gastroenterology 118:264, 2000.
207. Rutgeerts P, Hiele M, Geboes K, et al. Controlled trial of metronidazole treatment for prevention of Crohn's recurrence after ileal resection. Gastroenterology 108:1617, 1995.
208. Brandt LJ, Bernstein LH, Boley SJ, et al. Metronidazole therapy for perineal Crohn's disease: a follow-up study. Gastroenterology 83:383, 1982.
209. Sutherland L, Singleton J, Sessions J, et al. Double blind, placebo controlled trial of metronidazole in Crohn's disease. Gut 32:1071, 1991.
210. Ursing B, Alm T, Barany F, et al. A comparative study of metronidazole and sulfasalazine for active Crohn's disease: the cooperative Crohn's disease study in Sweden. II. Result. Gastroenterology 83:550, 1982.
211. Prantera C, Zannoni F, Scribano ML, et al. An antibiotic regimen for the treatment of active Crohn's disease: a randomized, controlled clinical trial of metronidazole plus ciprofloxacin. Am J Gastroenterol 91:328, 1996.

212. Colombel JF, Lemann M, Cassagnou M, et al. A controlled trial comparing ciprofloxacin with mesalazine for the treatment of active Crohn's disease. Groupe d'Etudes Therapeutiques des Affections Inflammatoires Digestives (GETAID). Am J Gastroenterol 94:674, 1999.
213. Leiper K, Morris AI, Rhodes JM. Open label trial of oral clarithromycin in active Crohn's disease. Aliment Pharmacol Therap 14:801, 2000.
214. Prantera C, Kohn A, Mangiarotti R, et al. Antimycobacterial therapy in Crohn's disease: results of a controlled, double-blind trial with a multiple antibiotic regimen. Am J Gastroenterol 89:513, 1994.
215. Munkholm P, Langholz E, Davidsen M, et al. Frequency of glucocorticoid resistance and dependency in Crohn's disease. Gut 35:360, 1994.
216. Modigliani R, Mary JY, Simon JF, et al. Clinical, biological, and endoscopic picture of attacks of Crohn's disease. Evolution on prednisolone. Groupe d'Etude Therapeutique des Affections Inflammatoires Digestives. Gastroenterology 98:811, 1990.
217. Shepherd HA, Barr GD, Jewell DP. Use of an intravenous steroid regimen in the treatment of acute Crohn's disease. J Clin Gastroenterol 8:154, 1986.
218. Rubin RH, Ikonen T, Gummert JF, et al. The therapeutic prescription for the organ transplant recipient: the linkage of immunosuppression and antimicrobial strategies. Transplant Infect Dis 1:29, 1999.
219. Thiele K, Bierhaus A, Autschbach F, et al. Cell specific effects of glucocorticoid treatment on the NF-kappaBp65/IkappaBalpha system in patients with Crohn's disease. Gut 45:693, 1999.
220. Stuck AE, Minder CE, Frey FJ. Risk of infectious complications in patients taking glucocorticosteroids. Rev Infect Dis 11:954, 1989.
221. Steinhart AH, Ewe K, Griffiths AM, et al. Corticosteroids for maintaining remission of Crohn's disease. Cochrane Database of Systematic Reviews [computer file]:CD000301, 2000.
222. Franchimont DP, Louis E, Croes F, et al. Clinical pattern of corticosteroid dependent Crohn's disease. Eur J Gastroenterol Hepatol 10: 821, 1998.
223. Farrell RJ, Murphy A, Long A, et al. High multidrug resistance (P-glycoprotein 170) expression in inflammatory bowel disease patients who fail medical therapy. Gastroenterology 118:279, 2000.
224. Mingrone G, DeGaetano A, Pugeat M, et al. The steroid resistance of Crohn's disease. J Invest Med 47:319, 1999.
225. Thomsen OO, Cortot A, Jewell D, et al. A comparison of budesonide and mesalamine for active Crohn's disease. International Budesonide-Mesalamine Study Group. N Engl J Med 339:370, 1998.
226. Greenberg GR, Feagan BG, Martin F, et al. Oral budesonide for active Crohn's disease. Canadian Inflammatory Bowel Disease Study Group. N Engl J Med 331:836, 1994.
227. Greenberg GR, Feagan BG, Martin F, et al. Oral budesonide as maintenance treatment for Crohn's disease: a placebo-controlled, dose-ranging study. Canadian Inflammatory Bowel Disease Study Group. Gastroenterology 110:45, 1996.
228. Lofberg R, Rutgeerts P, Malchow H, et al. Budesonide prolongs time to relapse in ileal and ileocaecal Crohn's disease. A placebo controlled one year study. Gut 39:82, 1996.
229. Hellers G, Cortot A, Jewell D, et al. Oral budesonide for prevention of postsurgical recurrence in Crohn's disease. The IOIBD Budesonide Study Group. Gastroenterology 116:294, 1999.
230. Ewe K, Bottger T, Buhr HJ, et al. Low-dose budesonide treatment for prevention of postoperative recurrence of Crohn's disease: a multicentre randomized placebo-controlled trial. German Budesonide Study Group. Eur J Gastroenterol Hepatol 11:277, 1999.
231. Brooke BN Hoffmann DC, Swarbrick ET. Azathioprine for Crohn's disease. Lancet 2:612, 1969.
232. Pearson DC, May GR, Fick GH, et al. Azathioprine and 6-mercaptopurine in Crohn disease. A meta-analysis. Ann Intern Med 123:132, 1995.
233. Candy S, Wright J, Gerber M, et al. A controlled double blind study of azathioprine in the management of Crohn's disease. Gut 37:674, 1995.
234. Ewe K, Press AG, Singe CC, et al. Azathioprine combined with prednisolone or monotherapy with prednisolone in active Crohn's disease. Gastroenterology 105:367, 1993.
235. D'Haens G, Geboes K, Ponette E, et al. Healing of severe recurrent ileitis with azathioprine therapy in patients with Crohn's disease. Gastroenterology 112:1475, 1997.
236. Sandborn WJ, Tremaine WJ, Wolf DC, et al. Lack of effect of intravenous administration on time to respond to azathioprine for steroid-treated Crohn's disease. North American Azathioprine Study Group. Gastroenterology 117:527, 1999.
237. Dubinsky MC, Lamothe S, Yang HY, et al. Pharmacogenomics and metabolite measurement for 6-mercaptopurine therapy in inflammatory bowel disease. Gastroenterology 118:705, 2000.
238. Colonna T, Korelitz BI. The role of leukopenia in the 6-mercaptopurine-induced remission of refractory Crohn's disease. Am J Gastroenterol 89:362, 1994.
239. Dubinsky MC, Hassard PV, Abreu MT, et al. Thioguanine (6-TG): a therapeutic alternative in a subgroup of IBD patients failing 6-mercaptopurine (6-MP). Gastroenterology 118:A891, 2000.
240. Pedersen BK, Beyer JM. A longitudinal study of the influence of azathioprine on natural killer cell activity. Allergy 41:286, 1986.
241. Present DH, Meltzer SJ, Krumholz MP, et al. 6-Mercaptopurine in the management of inflammatory bowel disease: short- and long-term toxicity. Ann Intern Med 111:641, 1989.
242. Connell WR, Kamm MA, Ritchie JK, et al. Bone marrow toxicity caused by azathioprine in inflammatory bowel disease: 27 years of experience. Gut 34:1081, 1993.
243. Colombel JF, Ferrari N, Debuysere H, et al. Genotypic analysis of thiopurine S-methyltransferase in patients with Crohn's disease and severe myelosuppression during azathioprine therapy. Gastroenterology 118:1025, 2000.
244. Connell WR, Kamm MA, Dickson M, et al. Long-term neoplasia risk after azathioprine treatment in inflammatory bowel disease. Lancet 343:1249, 1994.
245. Farrell RJ, Ang Y, Kileen P, et al. Increased incidence of non-Hodgkins lymphoma in inflammatory bowel disease patients on immunosuppressive therapy but overall risk is low. Gut 47:514, 2000.
246. Lewis JD, Schwartz JS, Lichtenstein GR. Azathioprine for maintenance of remission in Crohn's disease: benefits outweigh the risk of lymphoma. Gastroenterology 118:1018, 2000.
247. Korelitz B, Hanauer S, Rutgeerts P, et al. Post-operative prophylaxis with 6-MP, 5-ASA or placebo in Crohn's disease: a 2 year multicenter trial. Gastroenterology 114:A1011, 1998.
248. Markowitz J, Grancher K, Kohn N, et al. A multicenter trial of 6-mercaptopurine and prednisone in children with newly diagnosed Crohn's disease. Gastroenterology 119:895, 2000.
249. Bouhnik Y, Lemann M, Mary JY, et al. Long-term follow-up of patients with Crohn's disease treated with azathioprine or 6-mercaptopurine. Lancet 347:215, 1996.
250. Kozarek RA, Patterson DJ, Gelfand MD, et al. Methotrexate induces clinical and histologic remission in patients with refractory inflammatory bowel disease. Ann Intern Med 110:353, 1989.
251. Feagan BG, Rochon J, Fedorak RN, et al. Methotrexate for the treatment of Crohn's disease. The North American Crohn's Study Group Investigators. N Engl J Med 332:292, 1995.
252. Feagan BG, Fedorak RN, Irvine EJ, et al. A comparison of methotrexate with placebo for the maintenance of remission in Crohn's disease. North American Crohn's Study Group Investigators. N Engl J Med 342:1627, 2000.
253. Cronstein BN, Naime D, Ostad E. The antiinflammatory mechanism of methotrexate. Increased adenosine release at inflamed sites diminishes leukocyte accumulation in an in vivo model of inflammation. J Clin Invest 92:2675, 1993.
254. Mack DR, Young R, Kaufman SS, et al. Methotrexate in patients with Crohn's disease after 6-mercaptopurine. J Pediatr 132:830, 1998.
255. Lemann M, Chamiot-Prieur C, Mesnard B, et al. Methotrexate for the treatment of refractory Crohn's disease. Aliment Pharmacol Therap 10:309, 1996.
256. Feagan BG, McDonald JW, Rochon J, et al. Low-dose cyclosporine for the treatment of Crohn's disease. The Canadian Crohn's Relapse Prevention Trial Investigators. N Engl J Med 330:1846, 1994.
257. Gerber DA, Bonham CA, Thomson AW. Immunosuppressive agents: recent developments in molecular action and clinical application. Transplant Proc 30:1573, 1998.
258. Fellermann K, Ludwig D, Stahl M, et al. Steroid-unresponsive acute attacks of inflammatory bowel disease: immunomodulation by tacrolimus (FK506). Am J Gastroenterol 93:1860, 1998.
259. Sandborn WJ. Preliminary report on the use of oral tacrolimus (FK506) in the treatment of complicated proximal small bowel and fistulizing Crohn's disease. Am J Gastroenterol 92:876, 1997.
260. Casson DH, Eltumi M, Tomlin S, et al. Topical tacrolimus may be effective in the treatment of oral and perineal Crohn's disease. Gut 47: 436, 2000.

261. Fellermann K, Steffen M, Stein J, et al. Mycophenolate mofetil: lack of efficacy in chronic active inflammatory bowel disease. Aliment Pharmacol Therap 14:171, 2000.
262. Neurath MF, Wanitschke R, Peters M, et al. Randomised trial of mycophenolate mofetil versus azathioprine for treatment of chronic active Crohn's disease. Gut 44:625, 1999.
263. Derkx B, Taminiau J, Radema S, et al. Tumour-necrosis-factor antibody treatment in Crohn's disease [letter]. Lancet 342:173, 1993.
264. van Dullemen HM, van Deventer SJ, Hommes DW, et al. Treatment of Crohn's disease with anti-tumor necrosis factor chimeric monoclonal antibody (cA2). Gastroenterology 109:129, 1995.
265. Baert FJ, D'Haens GR, Peeters M, et al. Tumor necrosis factor alpha antibody (infliximab) therapy profoundly down-regulates the inflammation in Crohn's ileocolitis. Gastroenterology 116:22, 1999.
266. Targan SR, Hanauer SB, van Deventer SJ, et al. A short-term study of chimeric monoclonal antibody cA2 to tumor necrosis factor alpha for Crohn's disease. Crohn's Disease cA2 Study Group. N Engl J Med 337:1029, 1997.
267. Present DH, Rutgeerts P, Targan S, et al. Infliximab for the treatment of fistulas in patients with Crohn's disease. N Engl J Med 340:1398, 1999.
268. Rutgeerts P, D'Haens G, Targan S, et al. Efficacy and safety of retreatment with anti-tumor necrosis factor antibody (infliximab) to maintain remission in Crohn's disease. Gastroenterology 117:761, 1999.
269. Scallon BJ, Moore MA, Trinh H, et al. Chimeric anti-TNF-alpha monoclonal antibody cA2 binds recombinant transmembrane TNF-alpha and activates immune effector functions. Cytokine 7:251, 1995.
270. Eigler A, Sinha B, Hartmann G, et al. Taming TNF: strategies to restrain this proinflammatory cytokine. Immunol Today 18:487, 1997.
271. Hanauer SB, Rutgeerts PJ, D'Haens G, et al. Delayed hypersensitivity to infliximab (Remicade) re-infusion after 2–4 year interval without treatment. Gastroenterology 116:A731, 1999.
272. Cosnes J, Carbonnel F, Carrat F, et al. Effects of current and former cigarette smoking on the clinical course of Crohn's disease. Aliment Pharmacol Therap 13:1403, 1999.
273. Sands BE. Novel therapies for inflammatory bowel disease. Gastro Clin North Am 28:323, 1999.
274. Slonim AE, Bulone L, Damore MB, et al. A preliminary study of growth hormone therapy for Crohn's disease. N Engl J Med 342:1633, 2000.
275. Stack WA Mann SD, Roy AJ, et al. Randomised controlled trial of CDP571 antibody to tumour necrosis factor-alpha in Crohn's disease. Lancet 349:521, 1997.
276. Ehrenpreis ED, Kane SV, Cohen LB, et al. Thalidomide therapy for patients with refractory Crohn's disease: an open-label trial. Gastroenterology 117:1271, 1999.
277. Vasiliauskas EA, Kam LY, Abreu-Martin MT, et al. An open-label pilot study of low-dose thalidomide in chronically active, steroid-dependent Crohn's disease. Gastroenterology 117:1278, 1999.
278. Malchow HA. Crohn's disease and *Escherichia coli*. A new approach in therapy to maintain remission of colonic Crohn's disease? J Clin Gastroenterol 25:653, 1997.
279. Griffiths AM, Ohlsson A, Sherman PM, et al. Meta-analysis of enteral nutrition as a primary treatment of active Crohn's disease. Gastroenterology 108:1056, 1995.
280. Ballegaard M, Bjergstrom A, Brondum S, et al. Self-reported food intolerance in chronic inflammatory bowel disease. Scand J Gastroenterol 32:569, 1997.
281. Pearson M, Teahon K, Levi AJ, et al. Food intolerance and Crohn's disease. Gut 34:783, 1993.
282. Belluzzi A, Brignola C, Campieri M, et al. Effect of an enteric-coated fish-oil preparation on relapses in Crohn's disease. N Engl J Med 334: 1557, 1996.
283. Mekhjian HS, Switz DM, Watts HD, et al. National Cooperative Crohn's Disease Study: factors determining recurrence of Crohn's disease after surgery. Gastroenterology 77:907, 1979.
284. Whelan G, Farmer RG, Fazio VW, et al. Recurrence after surgery in Crohn's disease. Relationship to location of disease (clinical pattern) and surgical indication. Gastroenterology 88:1826, 1985.
285. Strong S, Fazio VW. The surgical management of Crohn's disease. In Kirsner JB, (ed): Inflammatory Bowel Disease. Philadelphia, WB Saunders, 2000, p 658.
286. Hurst RD, Molinari M, Chung TP, et al. Prospective study of the features, indications, and surgical treatment in 513 consecutive patients affected by Crohn's disease. Surgery 122:661, 1997.
287. Sagar PM, Dozois RR, Wolff BG. Long-term results of ileal pouch-anal anastomosis in patients with Crohn's disease. Dis Colon Rectum 39:893, 1996.
288. Panis Y, Poupard B, Nemeth J, et al. Ileal pouch/anal anastomosis for Crohn's disease. Lancet 347:854, 1996.
289. Pastore RL, Wolff BG, Hodge D. Total abdominal colectomy and ileorectal anastomosis for inflammatory bowel disease. Dis Colon Rectum 40:1455, 1997.
290. Alabaz O, Iroatulam AJ, Nessim A, et al. Comparison of laparoscopically assisted and conventional ileocolic resection for Crohn's disease. Eur J Surg 166:213, 2000.
291. Wu JS, Birnbaum EH, Kodner IJ, et al. Laparoscopic-assisted ileocolic resections in patients with Crohn's disease: are abscesses, phlegmons, or recurrent disease contraindications? Surgery 122:682, 1997.
292. Blomqvist P, Ekbom A. Inflammatory bowel disease: health care and costs in Sweden in 1994. Scand J Gastroenterol 32:1134, 1997.
293. Silverstein MD, Loftus EV, Sandborn WJ, et al. Clinical course and costs of care for Crohn's disease: Markov model analysis of a population-based cohort. Gastroenterology 117:49, 1999.
294. Kanof ME, Lake AM, Bayless TM. Decreased height velocity in children and adolescents before the diagnosis of Crohn's disease. Gastroenterology 95:1523, 1988.
295. Motil KJ, Grand RJ, Davis-Kraft L, et al. Growth failure in children with inflammatory bowel disease: a prospective study. Gastroenterology 105:681, 1993.
296. Markowitz J, Grancher K, Mandel F, et al. Immunosuppressive therapy in pediatric inflammatory bowel disease: results of a survey of the North American Society for Pediatric Gastroenterology and Nutrition. Subcommittee on Immunosuppressive Use of the Pediatric IBD Collaborative Research Forum. Am J Gastroenterol 88:44, 1993.
297. Spivak W, Sockolow R, Rigas A. The relationship between insurance class and severity of presentation of inflammatory bowel disease in children. Am J Gastroenterol 90:982, 1995.
298. Korelitz BI. Inflammatory bowel disease and pregnancy. Gastroenterol Clin North Am 27:213, 1998.
299. Brandt LJ, Estabrook SG, Reinus JF. Results of a survey to evaluate whether vaginal delivery and episiotomy lead to perineal involvement in women with Crohn's disease. Am J Gastroenterol 90:1918, 1995.
300. Akerkar GA, Peppercorn MA, Hamel MB, et al. Corticosteroid-associated complications in elderly Crohn's disease patients. Am J Gastroenterol 92:461, 1997.
301. Moum B, Ekbom A, Vatn MH, et al. Clinical course during the 1st year after diagnosis in ulcerative colitis and Crohn's disease. Results of a large, prospective population-based study in southeastern Norway, 1990–93. Scand J Gastroenterol 32:1005, 1997.
302. Munkholm P, Langholz E, Davidsen M, et al. Disease activity courses in a regional cohort of Crohn's disease patients. Scand J Gastroenterol 30:699, 1995.
303. Lewis JD, Deren JJ, Lichtenstein GR. Cancer risk in patients with inflammatory bowel disease. Gastroenterol Clin North Am 28:459, 1999.
304. Ribeiro MB, Greenstein AJ, Sachar DB, et al. Colorectal adenocarcinoma in Crohn's disease. Ann Surg 223:186, 1996.
305. Friedman S, Rubin PH, Bodian C, et al. Screening and surveillance colonoscopy in chronic Crohn's colitis. Gastroenterology 120:820, 2001.
306. Persson PG, Karlen P, Bernell O, et al. Crohn's disease and cancer: a population-based cohort study. Gastroenterology 107:1675, 1994.
307. Ekbom A, Helmick CG, Zack M, et al. Survival and causes of death in patients with inflammatory bowel disease: a population-based study. Gastroenterology 103:954, 1992.
308. Gollop JH, Phillips SF, Melton LJD, et al. Epidemiologic aspects of Crohn's disease: a population based study in Olmsted County, Minnesota, 1943–1982. Gut 29:49, 1988.
309. Munkholm P, Langholz E, Davidsen M, et al. Intestinal cancer risk and mortality in patients with Crohn's disease. Gastroenterology 105: 1716, 1993.
310. Persson PG, Bernell O, Leijonmarck CE, et al. Survival and cause-specific mortality in inflammatory bowel disease: a population-based cohort study. Gastroenterology 110:1339, 1996.
311. Probert CS, Jayanthi V, Wicks AC, et al. Mortality from Crohn's disease in Leicestershire, 1972–1989: an epidemiological community based study. Gut 33:1226, 1992.
312. Turnbull GK, Vallis TM. Quality of life in inflammatory bowel disease: the interaction of disease activity with psychosocial function. Am J Gastroenterol 90:1450, 1995.
313. Casati J, Toner BB, de Rooy EC, et al. Concerns of patients with inflammatory bowel disease: a review of emerging themes. Dig Dis Sci 45:26, 2000.

ULCERATIVE COLITIS

Chapter 104

Derek P. Jewell

Ulcerative colitis is an inflammatory disorder that affects the rectum and extends proximally to affect a variable extent of the colon. The cause of the disease and the factors determining its chronic course are unknown.

HISTORY

The disease was first recognized as an entity distinct from bacillary dysentery by Samuel Wilks, a physician at Guy's Hospital. In 1859, he lectured on "simple idiopathic colitis" and distinguished it from ulceration caused by congestion, mercurial poisoning, diphtheritic inflammation, and bacillary dysentery.[1] In the same year, he described "the morbid appearances in the intestines of Miss Bankes."[2] The colon was dilated and thin and showed severe universal inflammation, which he regarded as typical of idiopathic colitis. Additional cases were reported, and it was noted that, although the disease was rare, mild cases that did not come to post mortem might be overlooked or misdiagnosed. By 1909, Hawkins[3] was able to give an excellent account of the disease and its natural history. He recognized that the course of the disease may be either intermittent or chronic, and that first attacks carried the highest mortality. He also described the "stealthy hemorrhage" onset of distal disease in which bleeding often occurred in the presence of constipation. Also in 1909, the London Teaching Hospitals were able to collate their experience of about 300 cases, most of which had been diagnosed since 1888. In an account of this symposium,[4] held at the Royal Society of Medicine in London, the debate on the etiology of the disease makes for interesting reading. It was obviously a spirited evening with intense disagreement among those who considered the disease to have resulted from the introduction of tinned foods and the use of preservatives, those who still thought the disease was an atypical dysentery, and those who believed it to be psychosomatic. Perhaps the first complete description of ulcerative colitis was given by Sir Arthur Hurst, who also described associated sigmoidoscopic appearances and gave a clear differentiation from bacillary dysentery.[5]

Nevertheless, Hurst considered the disease to be primarily an infective dysentery in which other factors had occurred secondarily, thus establishing a chronic disease process.[6] He based this view on the identical sigmoidoscopic features of ulcerative colitis and dysentery, the isolation of dysenteric organisms from the feces of some patients with ulcerative colitis, and the apparent effectiveness of polyvalent antidysenteric sera in the treatment of ulcerative colitis. This view found support in the epidemiologic association between ulcerative colitis and dysentery,[7, 8] and the finding of raised agglutination titers to *Shigella* in the sera of patients with ulcerative colitis.[7] Claims were made that specific organisms could be isolated from the stools of patients with ulcerative colitis, but these claims were not substantiated.

EPIDEMIOLOGY

Ulcerative colitis is a worldwide disorder, although its precise incidence varies. Diagnosis may be difficult in areas where infective colitis is common, but with better diagnostic facilities and increasing medical awareness, the disease is now recognized in most countries.[9]

High-incidence areas (Table 104–1) include the United Kingdom, the United States, Northern Europe, and Australia. Among whites, the incidence ranges from 3 to 15 cases per 100,000 persons per year, with a prevalence of 80 to 120 per 100,000. In countries in which time trends have been studied, the incidence has remained remarkably steady between the 1950s and the 1980s. This stability is in sharp contrast to Crohn's disease, which has shown up to a six-fold increase in incidence over a similar period. Low-incidence areas include Asia, Japan, and South America. It is difficult to obtain accurate figures but the incidence rates are probably about 10-fold less in low-incidence areas than in high-incidence areas. The incidence in Southern Europe, previously thought to be low, is probably not too different from that in Northern Europe, now that vigorous epidemiologic studies have been performed.

Age and Sex

Ulcerative colitis primarily affects young adults (20 to 40 years of age) but may present at all ages, from younger than 1 year of life to the 80s. Many series show a secondary peak in incidence among the elderly. Women tend to be affected more commonly than men, although many more recent series have failed to find a sex difference for occurrence of this disorder.

Ethnic Variation

In the United States, Jews are more prone to ulcerative colitis than are non-Jews. In Baltimore, the incidence among Jews was 13 per 100,000 persons compared with 3.8 per 100,000 among non-Jewish whites.[9] Similar findings have been reported in Cape Town. Within Israel, Ashkenazi Jews have a higher incidence than Sephardic Jews but a lower incidence than in the United States and Northern Europe, suggesting that environmental factors play a role. Low incidence rates are found among blacks in the United States (1.4 per 100,000) and Cape Town (0.6 per 100,000).

Table 104–1 | **Incidence of Ulcerative Colitis**

	PERIOD OF STUDY	INCIDENCE (PER 100,000)
USA		
Minnesota	1935–64	7.2
Baltimore	1960–63	4.6
UK		
Oxford	1951–60	6.5
Wales	1968–77	7.2
Aberdeen	1967–76	11.3
Denmark		
Copenhagen	1962–78	8.1
	1981–88	9.5
Holland		
Leiden	1979–83	6.8
Sweden		
Stockholm County	1975–79	4.3
Israel		
Tel-Aviv	1961–70	3.6

Urban-Rural Differences

Minor variations in incidence have been found among urban as opposed to rural populations, but these differences have not been consistent, and there is probably no true difference.

Socioeconomic Factors

There may be a slightly higher incidence of ulcerative colitis among the higher salaried or better educated members of a population, at least in Denmark and the United States, but these differences are slight.

GENETICS

The familial incidence of ulcerative colitis has been recognized for many years but has proved difficult to quantify. Figures vary widely among series, probably in part because of referral bias, but about 10% to 20% of patients have at least one other affected family member.[10] Data from New York and Cleveland suggest a preponderance of parent-sibling combinations, but in the United Kingdom the disease is more commonly shared by siblings. There is general agreement that most of the familial association is noted in first-degree relatives. Furthermore, the other affected family members may have either ulcerative colitis or Crohn's disease, although the majority have ulcerative colitis.

This familial association contrasts with the low incidence among spouses of patients with inflammatory bowel disease in the majority of series, although in New York 19 couples have been reported in which both husband and wife were affected by either ulcerative colitis or Crohn's disease.[11]

Studies on the clinical characteristics of familial disease have shown that the onset of disease in a child is noted at a much earlier age than in the affected parent, but there is a high degree of concordance between affected siblings for age of onset. The reasons for the younger age of onset in the offspring of an affected patient are not known but probably include bias from case ascertainment as well as genetic reasons, such as inheritance from parents of a greater number of putative susceptibility genes. For all affected first-degree relatives within a family, there is a high concordance for type of disease (ulcerative colitis or Crohn's disease), extent of disease, and occurrence of extraintestinal manifestations.[12]

Twin studies are helpful in assessing the interaction between genetic susceptibility and environmental factors because twins normally are raised together and therefore share the same environment. For Crohn's disease, concordance rates among monozygotic twin pairs are 30% to 67% compared with about 4% for dizygotic pairs. For ulcerative colitis, the concordance rates are lower—13% and 2% for monozygotic and dyzygotic twins, respectively. Thus genetic susceptibility seems to play a minor role in overall pathogenesis and is more marked in Crohn's disease than in ulcerative colitis.

The inheritance of ulcerative colitis cannot be described by a simple mendelian model, and it seems likely that several genes are involved in determining disease susceptibility.[13] Linkage studies using dinucleotide repeats (highly polymorphic markers that are distributed throughout the genome) have suggested that there are susceptibility genes for ulcerative colitis on chromosomes 2, 3, 6, 7, and 12. The finding of a locus on chromosome 12 has been replicated by more than one center.[14] Some of these loci may be shared with Crohn's disease, and it seems possible on the basis of present evidence that there may be a pool of genes conferring overall susceptibility to inflammatory bowel disease but that other genes determine which type of disease develops. The current challenge is to narrow these regions of linkage, which are large (10 to 20 cM), in order to allow gene identification studies to begin.

There are also genes that appear to influence disease behavior independently of susceptibility genes. The best studied of these are the human leukocyte antigen (HLA) alleles. One allele of HLA-DR2 (*DRB1*1502*) appears to be involved in disease susceptibility in Japanese and Jewish populations. Several centers have reported an association between severe disease and a rare allele of HLA-DR1 (*DRB1*0103*). Furthermore, this allele is found in approximately 35% of patients in whom an acute reactive arthropathy develops during a severe attack of colitis, compared with a frequency of 3% for a healthy control population and 8% in patients with colitis as a group. In some studies, the HLA-DR3, DQ2 haplotype is associated with extensive colitis, especially among women.

Among the Jewish population, the perinuclear antineutrophil antibody (p-ANCA) is a marker for the *DRB*1502* allele of HLA-DR2, but in non-Jewish Caucasians, the antibody is associated with the HLA-DR3 DQ2-tumor necrosis factor (TNF)-α2 haplotype.

ETIOLOGY

The etiology of ulcerative colitis remains unknown. The major hypotheses have included infection, allergy to dietary components, immune responses to bacterial or self-antigens, and the psychosomatic theory. There also is the possibility that the epithelial cell may be abnormal and the basis for susceptibility to the disease.

Infection

Despite many attempts, no specific infective organism has been isolated consistently from patients with ulcerative colitis. Therefore, ulcerative colitis is unlikely to be a simple infective disorder unless caused by an as yet unrecognized class of microorganism. The failure to identify an infective agent and the recognition that the strains of *Escherichia coli* in the normal colon are changing continually[15] led to the suggestion that patients might harbor specific strains that may release enzymes or other products that would damage the mucosa. Thus Cooke and her colleagues found that the *E. coli* strains isolated from patients with ulcerative colitis were more likely to produce hemolysins and necrotoxins than were strains isolated from a normal colon.[16] Unfortunately, it was then shown that this difference tended to occur following rather than before a relapse. More recently, it has been reported that *E. coli* from patients in complete remission express adhesins more frequently than do *E. coli* from healthy controls.[17] This finding implies that *E. coli* from colitic patients have a greater potential for adhering to the epithelial cell of the colon and therefore may initiate damage. This interesting hypothesis led to a clinical trial of tobramycin, an antibiotic that is highly effective against *E. coli*. The results showed that tobramycin was significantly better than placebo in treating active ulcerative colitis.[18] Recent trials suggesting that certain nonpathogenic strains of *E. coli* may be beneficial in treating ulcerative colitis further suggest that luminal microflora are highly relevant to the pathogenesis of the disease.[19, 20]

Food Allergy

Andresen[21] first suggested that ulcerative colitis may be caused by an allergy to milk, and in 1942, claimed that two thirds of his patients had a food allergy; the majority (84%) of them were sensitive to milk. There followed many anecdotal case reports of food allergy, with milk again being the most common allergen. Truelove[22] reintroduced milk into the diets of a small group of patients with ulcerative colitis who had responded previously to a milk-free diet and found that they relapsed soon after the challenge. This observation led to a controlled therapeutic trial of a milk-free diet, which suggested that approximately 20% of patients might benefit from this diet.[23] Many studies have shown increased serum levels of antibodies to milk proteins in these patients, although no immunoglobulin E (IgE) antibodies have been demonstrated. However, no correlation has been shown between the height of an antibody titer and any clinical feature such as extent or severity of disease; it seems as if antibodies to dietary proteins are an epiphenomenon. Skin tests to dietary proteins have not been helpful, although an interesting unconfirmed report on allergens injected into the rectal mucosa apparently found a good correlation between the local response and the effect on disease activity of removing those allergens from the diet.

Two clinical observations suggest that a dietary allergy is unlikely, although they by no means disprove that such an allergy is possible. First, the outcome of a severe attack of ulcerative colitis is not influenced by whether the patient is fed orally or intravenously.[24] Second, anecdotal experience has shown that ulcerative colitis does not remit if the colon is defunctioned by a split ileostomy.

Therefore, there is little evidence that milk, or any other food, plays a primary role in the etiology of the disease. Even the results of the controlled trial[23] could possibly be confounded, not only by relatively small numbers of patients studied, but by other factors such as lactase deficiency.

Environmental Factors

In addition to infective agents and diet, two other environmental factors have been proposed as contributing factors to the etiology of ulcerative colitis. These are smoking and the use of oral contraceptives.

Many studies have found consistently that ulcerative colitis is more common among nonsmokers than smokers; the relative risk of ulcerative colitis in nonsmokers ranges from 2 to 6. The risk is particularly high for ex-smokers, especially within the first 2 years of giving up smoking; it is higher for ex–heavy smokers than for ex–light smokers.[25]

This apparent protective effect of smoking is intriguing, especially because smoking increases the risk for Crohn's disease (see Chapter 103). The mechanisms underlying these effects are not clear. Smoking may have an effect on mucus production by the colonic mucosa because less mucous glycoprotein is synthesized by nonsmoking patients with ulcerative colitis than by controls, but patients who smoke produce amounts of mucous glycoprotein similar to amounts produced by controls.[26] Further, smoking can alter colonic mucosal blood flow[27] and decrease mucosal permeability as measured by chromium-51 ethylenediaminetetraacetic acid (^{51}Cr-EDTA).[28] Thus, smoking has the potential to alter the function of the colonic epithelium. However, further work is required before it can be concluded that this is the mechanism by which smoking influences susceptibility to intestinal inflammation.

Oral contraceptive use was reported initially to be more common in young women with Crohn's disease of the colon than in controls. In a prospective study, there was also a slight increase in ulcerative colitis among contraceptive users, but the association is weak and becomes insignificant when the data are corrected for social class and smoking habits.[29]

Another consistent finding is the low appendectomy rate among patients with ulcerative colitis compared with controls, but the explanation for this finding is obscure.[30, 31]

IMMUNOPATHOGENESIS

Immunologic mechanisms within the colonic lamina propria are involved in the pathogenesis of the inflammation in ulcerative colitis and involve both humoral and cellular responses. The difficulty is to know whether these responses are appropriate to an increased antigenic challenge secondary to an inflammatory response, whether they represent a response to a specific etiologic agent, or whether they indicate an underlying defect in mucosal immunoregulation. These proposed mechanisms provide little explanation for the predominantly left-sided nature of the colonic disease in ulcerative colitis. However, the left colon differs from the right in many aspects (e.g., permeability, ion transport, mucus composition, and immunologic epitopes), some of which may be relevant to disease distribution.

Humoral Responses

Histologic examination of the inflamed colon indicates a marked increase in plasma cells, and quantitative immunohistochemical studies have shown that the largest proportional increase occurs in cells that produce immunoglobulin G (IgG). Much of the increased IgG synthesis results from an increase in the IgG_1 and IgG_3 subclasses, in contrast to Crohn's disease, in which there is a more marked increase in IgG_2 synthesis.[32, 33] An IgG_1/IgG_3 response suggests that protein antigens may be the predominant triggers in ulcerative colitis. These subclasses of IgG are particularly effective in fixing complement, and there is considerable evidence for complement activation in active ulcerative colitis, as a result of the formation of antigen-antibody complexes.[34]

Much of the increased IgG synthesis may represent polyclonal stimulation. However, patients with ulcerative colitis frequently have circulating antibodies to dietary, bacterial, and self-antigens that are mostly of the IgG isotype, usually of the IgG_1 subclass. Many of these antibodies are thought to be epiphenomena because the height of the antibody titer shows no correlation with any clinical parameter (e.g., length of history, extent or activity of disease). Nevertheless, the known cross-reaction between enterobacterial antigens and colonic epithelial epitopes may be an important triggering event, even though, later in the course of the disease, the serum antibody titer to either the bacterial or the colonic antigen may be unimportant.

Ulcerative colitis has been considered to be an autoimmune disease. There is an increased association with other autoimmune disorders (e.g., thyroid disease, diabetes, pernicious anemia),[35] and in addition to autoantibodies to colonic epithelium, patients may have autoantibodies to lymphocytes and ribonucleic acid, as well as low titers of smooth muscle, gastric parietal cell, and thyroid antibodies. Antibodies to epithelial cell–associated components (ECACs) have been described, as have antibodies to a 40-kd epithelial antigen.[36] This latter antigen is found in normal colonic epithelial cells and is distinct from the lipopolysaccharide antigen of the goblet cells, which cross-reacts with enterobacterial antigens and reacts with the classic anticolon antibody. Das and colleagues[37] have reported that antibody to this 40-kd molecule can be eluted from the inflamed colonic mucosa of patients with ulcerative colitis and that a radioimmunoassay detects the circulating antibody. The antibody response to the 40-kd protein appears to be unique to ulcerative colitis and is not found in Crohn's disease or other inflammatory conditions. The specificity of this response is interesting, as is the finding that the antigen is found only in the colon, skin, and bile duct,[37] because the latter two sites are frequently affected by the extraintestinal manifestations of ulcerative colitis. Why immune tolerance to this self-antigen should break down specifically is unknown, but knowledge of the mechanisms involved may provide a clue to the pathogenesis of the inflammation.

Another autoantibody that occurs in 60% to 85% of patients is p-ANCA,[38] which appears to be synthesized within the lamina propria and is of the IgG_1 subclass. The p-ANCA titer is not affected by disease activity but may decline in patients with long-standing remission or in those who have had a colectomy at least 10 years previously. However, there is considerable controversy about these findings.

The antigen to which the p-ANCA is directed has not yet been determined with certainty. A variety of antigens have been proposed, including nuclear histone and nonhistone proteins. The most recent evidence suggests that the antigen is a 50-kd nuclear envelope protein that is specific to myeloid cells.[39]

Cellular Responses

T Cells

Studies on T cells have resulted in many discrepant results and have produced considerable confusion, especially in terms of T cell function. Most investigators have found that the distribution of T cell subsets (CD4+, CD8+) in both ulcerative colitis and Crohn's disease is similar when compared with that in controls. This finding is particularly true for peripheral blood, although studies on isolated lamina propria cells suggest a possible increase in CD8+ (suppressor cytotoxic) T cells in patients with Crohn's disease.[40] T cell function has been assessed in terms of cytotoxicity, help, and suppression. Major histocompatibility complex–restricted T cell cytotoxicity has not yet been demonstrated in either peripheral blood or the lamina propria. Lymphocytes from both compartments have been reported to be cytotoxic to autologous colonic epithelial cells, but the exact mechanisms are obscure and the results have not been confirmed.[41] It is unlikely that this phenomenon is T cell mediated, even if it does occur in vivo. Helper function has mainly involved the effect of T cells on immunoglobulin production by B cells. The results have been varied and do not provide firm evidence for an underlying immune abnormality in ulcerative colitis. The suppressor function of T cells has received more attention, mainly because it is postulated that many of the immune responses directed toward specific antigens in ulcerative colitis may arise because of failure to control or suppress the immune system. Many reports, but not all, have found diminished suppressor activity during active disease only, suggesting that the effect is secondary to inflammation. These studies have involved nonspecific suppression in which stimulation with nonspecific mitogens has been used to generate the suppression. An antigen-driven suppressor assay has shown that patients with either ulcerative colitis or Crohn's disease show suppressor defects to a range of mycobacterial and enterobacterial antigens.[42] These defects were present when patients were in remission and correlated with a poor response to skin testing with purified protein derivative. Furthermore, the phenomenon is mediated predominantly by CD8+ cells. This finding could explain much of the immunologic activity seen in these patients, but it appears to be confined to the systemic immune system. Lymphocytes from the lamina propria have not shown a similar defect in antigen-driven suppression.

Regardless of their functional status, both peripheral blood and mucosal T cells show phenotypic evidence of activation. Expression of the early activation markers (4F2, OKT9)[43, 44] is increased, although there is little increase in the late markers (interleukin [IL]-2R, HLA-DR).[40] Studies of T cell receptors have shown restricted Vβ usage, but there is no distinct pattern when compared with T cells from healthy lamina propria.

Intraepithelial Lymphocytes

Most (>90%) intraepithelial lymphocytes (IELs) in the human intestine are T cells (CD3+) and, of these, the majority (>80%) are CD8+ cells. In the inflamed intestines of patients with ulcerative colitis, the absolute number of IELs is normal or reduced and the CD4+/CD8+ ratio is unchanged. However, the proportion of cells using the $\gamma\delta$ T cell receptor may increase. This population is 5% or less in healthy controls but may rise to 30% to 40% in patients with ulcerative colitis.[45] However, the function and significance of $\gamma\delta$ T cells are unknown. The function of IELs is also unknown, although they can be activated by colon epithelial cells bearing HLA-DR molecules[46] and can behave as suppressor cells.[47]

Monocytes and Macrophages

In patients with active disease, there is a circulating monocytosis and the cells are stimulated, as is shown by increased chemotaxis, phagocytosis, and respiratory burst activity. The same is true for mucosal macrophages, which, in addition, appear to provide help for immunoglobulin synthesis by B cells.[48] Mucosal macrophages in particular show a specific pattern of phenotype. In active ulcerative colitis, as well as Crohn's disease, there is a population of cells that exhibit a low-affinity FcγR (3G8+, CD14) and a population that expresses RFD9, a marker for epithelioid cells. Although 3G8+ macrophages are seen in intestinal infections, the presence of 3G8+ and RFD9+ populations appears to be unique for ulcerative colitis and Crohn's disease. CD14+ macrophages (3G8+) are exquisitely sensitive to lipopolysaccharide,[49] and this finding may be highly relevant to the pathogenesis of these diseases. The RFD9+ cells occur in clusters deep in the lamina propria, but the function and origin of these cells are unknown. RFD9 is not simply an activation marker, and these cells seem to appear in response to a specific local stimulus.

Consequences of T Cell and Macrophage Activation

Activation of immune cells leads to the release of an extensive number of cytokines and inflammatory mediators, which mediate tissue damage and serve to amplify the immune response and hence promote further inflammation. Macrophages in the inflamed colon of patients with active ulcerative colitis are known to synthesize IL-1β, TNF, and IL-6, which are cytokines that cause fever and stimulate an acute phase response. There is some dispute about the ability of lamina propria T cells to produce IL-2 and interferon-γ, but there is strong class II expression on colonic epithelial cells in an inflamed colon,[50] a finding that suggests that interferon-γ must be present locally.

In vitro data suggest that epithelial cells bearing class II antigens may present antigen to lymphocytes. Epithelial cells isolated from healthy mucosa present antigen to CD8+ cells and hence initiate a down-regulatory signal. However, epithelial cells from an inflamed colon appear to present antigen to CD4+ cells and may therefore lead to up-regulation of the mucosal immune response.[51] Whether this occurs in vivo is uncertain, and it is possible that non-HLA molecules, such as CD1d, also may be involved in antigen presentation by epithelial cells.[52]

Other features of ulcerative colitis may also be explained on the basis of cytokine release. Epithelial cell permeability is altered by interferon-γ; collagen synthesis is stimulated by transforming growth factor (TGF)-β, IL-1, and IL-6; and endothelium is altered by many cytokines, including IL-1, TNF, IL-6, and interferon-γ. This last phenomenon may lead to local ischemia within the bowel and may explain the vascular abnormalities that have been demonstrated.[53] Elevated cytokine concentrations within the mucosa also lead to the release of metalloproteinase from fibroblasts, which causes matrix degradation.

In addition to cytokine release, leukotrienes (LTs), thromboxane, platelet-activating factor, nitric oxide, and reactive oxygen metabolites are released from activated mucosal cells, predominantly from neutrophils and macrophages. Increased mucosal concentrations of these mediators have been shown to be associated with active disease.[54] These mediators not only contribute to tissue damage and inflammation (e.g., LTB4 is a potent chemoattractant for neutrophils), but they also profoundly affect epithelial cell permeability and ion transport. These effects contribute, in turn, to diarrhea. The release of kinins and other inflammatory mediators from the degranulation of mast cells and eosinophils, as well as the activation of complement by antigen-antibody complexes, also contributes to diarrhea. (For a more complete discussion of the immunologic responses and inflammation of the gut, see Chapter 2.)

The Epithelial Cell

The turnover rate of epithelial cells of the colon is increased when ulcerative colitis is active, but even when there is histologic remission, proliferation is still increased.[55] Whether the increased proliferation is a consequence of the disease process or a basic abnormality of the epithelium is unclear. Other lines of evidence also demonstrate that the biology of the epithelium may be abnormal in patients with ulcerative colitis, even when there is no increase in the inflammatory infiltrate. Thus epithelial cells from patients with colitis show a reduced metabolism of short-chain fatty acids, especially butyrate, and their membranes are abnormally permeable to labeled chromium.[56] Furthermore, mucus production by the epithelium differs in patients and controls,[57] a phenomenon that may be genetically determined.[58]

The hypothesis that the basic abnormality rendering persons susceptible to ulcerative colitis lies within the epithelial cell is attractive. However, the current evidence is tenuous but sufficiently interesting to warrant further investigation.

PSYCHOSOMATIC ASPECTS

Despite early claims that ulcerative colitis was caused by psychosomatic factors, there is no good evidence for this concept. Indeed, there is little hard evidence that psychological factors influence the disease, although this notion is widely believed by both patients and physicians.[59] Undoubtedly, the presence of chronic symptoms such as diarrhea, the fear of incontinence, abdominal discomfort, and a general lack of well-being have a major impact on patients. Thus, many of the psychological features associated with ulcerative colitis are largely secondary to the disease process. It is essential for physicians to be aware of this effect when managing these patients. Patients are able to adjust to their disease much more readily when they become informed about the nature of the disease and its effects, and when they know that they are free to discuss their problems with their physician.[60] The complex interaction between personality and disease has been well reviewed by Drossman.[59] (See also Chapter 122, in which Dr. Drossman puts this complex and important interaction into perspective.)

PATHOLOGY

Macroscopic Features

Approximately 20% of patients have total colitis, 30% to 40% have disease extending beyond the sigmoid but not involving the whole colon, and 40% to 50% have disease limited to the rectum and rectosigmoid. The changes are usually most severe in the rectum and extend for a variable extent around the colon, although there are several exceptions to this general rule. Apparent rectal sparing may be seen as a result of topical treatment (glucocorticoids or mesalamine) and rarely in acute severe disease when the proximal colon tends to be much more severely involved than the rectum.[61] Although skip lesions are characteristic of Crohn's disease, there are two situations in which skip lesions may be seen in ulcerative colitis: evidence of appendiceal inflammation and areas of cecal inflammation have both been described in patients with left-sided ulcerative colitis.

With mild inflammation, the mucosa is hyperemic, edematous, and granular (Fig. 104–1). As the disease becomes more severe, the mucosa becomes intensely hemorrhagic, and small punctate ulcers become visible, which may enlarge and extend deeply into the lamina propria. These ulcers are often irregular with overhanging edges and give rise to the "collar-stud" or "collar-button" effect seen on a barium study. The ulceration may be linear along the line of the teniae coli (Fig. 104–2). In long-standing disease, inflammatory polyps (pseudopolyps) may be present as a result of exuberant regeneration of the epithelium (Fig. 104–3). Why pseudopolyps are found in the colon, as opposed to the rectum, is not clear.

In remission, the mucosa appears normal, but in patients who have had recurrent attacks over several years, the mucosa becomes atrophic and featureless. This development is

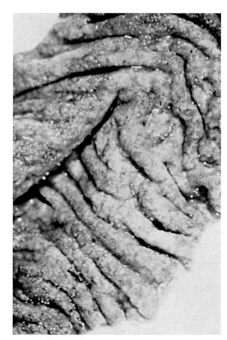

Figure 104–1. Gross resection specimen of active ulcerative colitis showing mucosal edema and granularity.

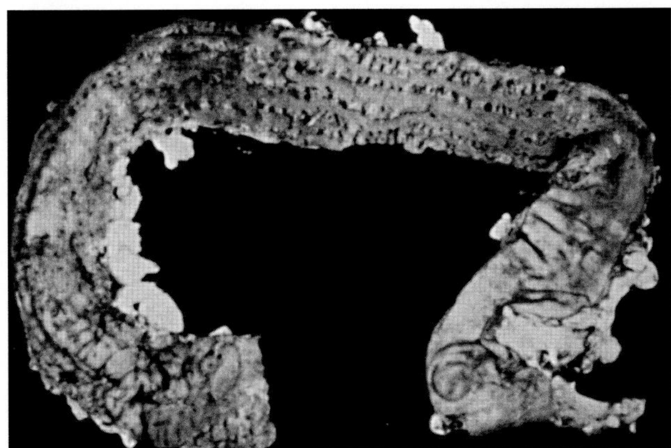

Figure 104–2. Colectomy specimen of severe ulcerative colitis affecting the whole colon with linear ulceration.

usually accompanied by shortening and narrowing of the colon as a result of abnormalities in the muscle layers. In contrast to Crohn's disease, fibrosis is uncommon, and smooth strictures only rarely occur in long-standing chronic disease.

An acute dilatation of the colon may develop in patients with severe disease. In these cases, the bowel wall becomes thin, and the mucosa is grossly ulcerated with only small fragments or islands of mucosa remaining. Acute dilatation may be complicated by perforation, in which case a fibrinopurulent exudate may be seen on the serosal surface.

Microscopic Features

The inflammation is predominantly confined to the mucosa. The lamina propria becomes edematous and the capillaries are dilated and congested, often with extravasation of red cells. There is an inflammatory infiltrate of neutrophils, lymphocytes, plasma cells, and macrophages. Eosinophils and mast cells are also present in increased numbers. The neutrophils invade the epithelium, usually in the crypts, giving rise to cryptitis and ultimately to crypt abscesses (Fig. 104–4). The stimulus for this very striking migration of neutrophils

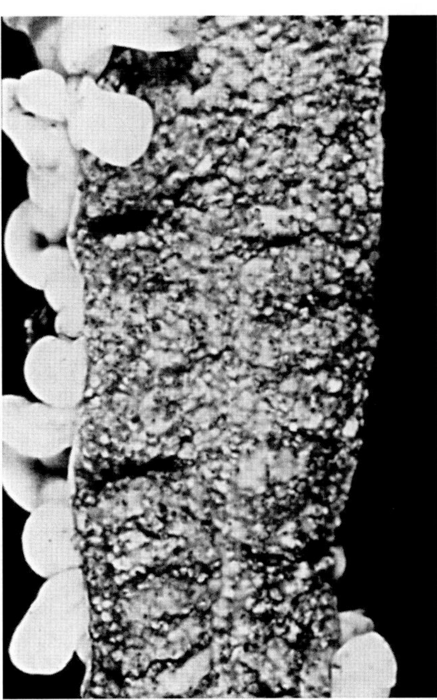

Figure 104–3. Gross resection specimen of active ulcerative colitis with multiple small inflammatory polyps.

is unknown but may be the potent chemotactic peptides of colonic bacteria (e.g., formyl-methionyl-leucyl-phenylalanine [FMLP]). The role of IL-8, another powerful chemoattractant for neutrophils, is currently being investigated. Activated complement, platelet-activating factor, and LTB4 are other chemoattractants that are present within the inflamed mucosa and may be responsible for promoting migration of neutrophils from the circulation into the lamina propria. The cryptitis is associated with discharge of mucus from goblet cells and increased epithelial cell turnover. Histologically, the goblet cells are depleted of mucin and epithelial cells become more basophilic, which is an indicator of young, immature cells.

The marked increase in lamina propria plasma cells is accompanied by changes in isotype distribution. Although

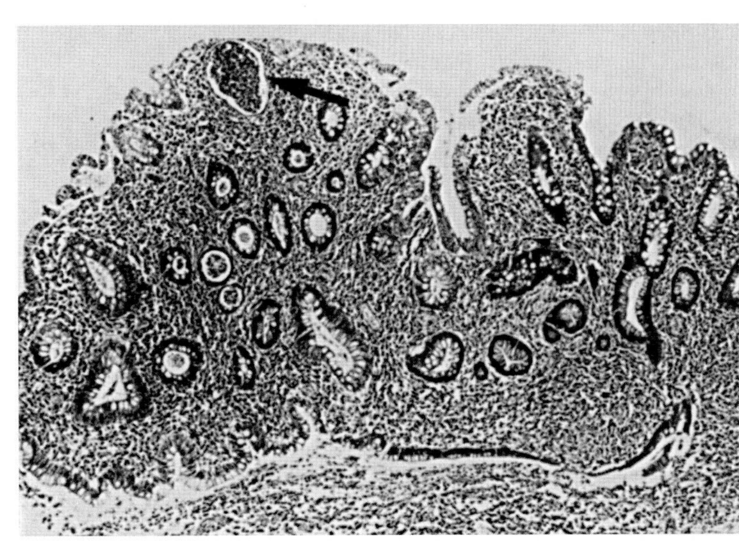

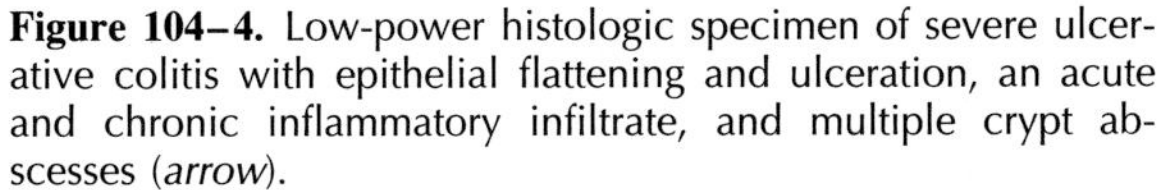

Figure 104–4. Low-power histologic specimen of severe ulcerative colitis with epithelial flattening and ulceration, an acute and chronic inflammatory infiltrate, and multiple crypt abscesses (*arrow*).

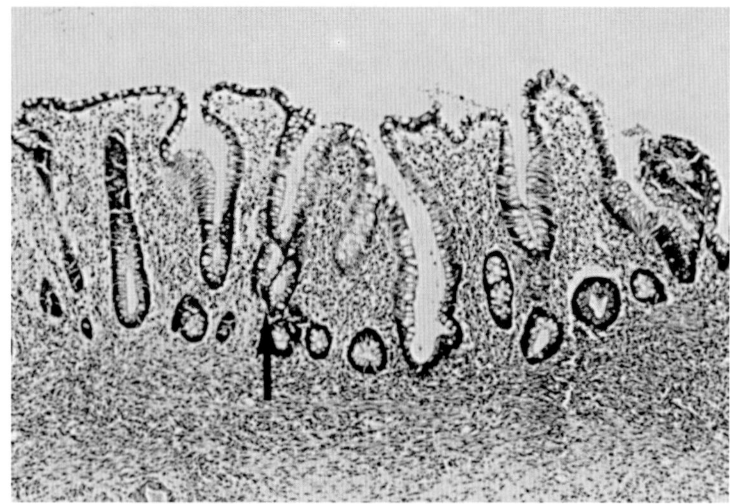

Figure 104–5. Low-power histologic specimen of chronic ulcerative colitis showing a bifid gland (*arrow*) and a mild increase in chronic inflammatory cells.

IgA-containing cells predominate, the greatest percentage increase occurs in IgG-containing cells and, to a lesser extent, in IgM-containing cells. Furthermore, the rise in IgG is largely the result of an increase in IgG_1 and IgG_3, which contrasts with Crohn's disease in which the predominant rise occurs in IgG_2.

Many of these changes are nonspecific and may be confused with an infective or acute self-limiting colitis. Features that suggest chronicity may help to make the diagnosis of ulcerative colitis with a probability of more than 80%; these features include distorted crypt architecture, crypt atrophy, increased intercrypt spacing to fewer than 6 crypts per millimeter, an irregular mucosal surface, basal lymphoid aggregates, and a chronic inflammatory infiltrate.[62, 63]

With increasing inflammation, the surface epithelial cells become flattened and eventually ulcerate. The ulcers can be deep and undermine the surrounding epithelium. At this stage of the disease, some inflammation and vascular congestion may be seen in the submucosa. In acute dilatation, ulceration may extend to the muscle, which may undergo ischemic necrosis. When the inflammatory infiltrate extends into the muscularis propria in ulcerative colitis, it does so in a diffuse pattern with myocytolysis. This pattern is in contrast to the transmural inflammation of Crohn's disease, which is in the form of discrete lymphoid aggregates.

Once the disease has gone into remission, the histologic appearances may revert to normal, especially after mild attacks early in the course of the disease. However, there is usually evidence of altered crypt architecture or actual dropout of glands (Fig. 104–5). Architectural changes include bifid glands and shortened glands that do not extend down to the muscularis mucosae. If there is persistent evidence of acute inflammation, despite clinical remission, there is said to be a high risk of relapse. Other chronic changes that are sometimes seen are neuronal hypertrophy and fibromuscular hyperplasia of the muscularis mucosae. In some patients, a double muscularis mucosae develops and may provide diagnostic confusion because, in biopsy specimens, the inflammation may appear to spread below the muscularis mucosae. Paneth cell metaplasia is frequently seen, although the significance of this finding is uncertain.

CLINICAL FEATURES

The major symptoms of ulcerative colitis include diarrhea, rectal bleeding, the passage of mucus, and abdominal pain. The symptom complex tends to differ according to the extent of disease,[64] but generally the severity of the symptoms correlates with the severity of the disease. Active disease may be found at sigmoidoscopy in patients who are otherwise asymptomatic. Symptoms have usually been present for weeks, or even months, by the time a patient presents to a physician; the slow, insidious onset is characteristic of the disease. Ulcerative colitis may present much more acutely and may then mimic an infective etiology. Indeed, it is not uncommon to find a patient whose illness began with a documented infection (e.g., *Salmonella* spp or *Campylobacter* spp), which raises the question as to whether the infection merely revealed preexisting but silent disease or was actually the initiating factor. Yet another presentation is a history of intermittent episodes of diarrhea and bleeding that have been sufficiently mild that the patient has not sought medical attention.

Rectal Bleeding

Patients with a hemorrhagic proctitis (i.e., inflammation confined to the rectum) usually complain of passing fresh blood, either separately from the stool or streaked on the surface of a normal or hard stool.[65] This symptom is often mistaken for hemorrhoidal bleeding, but the patient with proctitis often passes, and may even be incontinent of, a blood-stained mucus. When the disease extends beyond the rectum, blood is usually mixed with stool or there may be grossly bloody diarrhea. The passage of clots is unusual (unless the patient has a massive hemorrhage) and suggests other diagnoses such as a tumor or angiodysplasia. When the disease is severe, patients pass liquid stool containing blood, pus, and fecal matter. This stool is often likened to anchovy sauce, and some patients with this symptom do not actually recognize that they are passing blood.

Active ulcerative colitis that is sufficient to cause diarrhea is almost always associated with macroscopic blood. If blood is absent, the diagnosis must be questioned (e.g., Could the patient have Crohn's disease?). The patient may have either not looked at the stool or not recognized the blood if it is altered in color.

Diarrhea

Diarrhea is not always present in patients with ulcerative colitis. For example, patients with proctitis or proctosigmoiditis may complain of constipation and hard stools.[65] However, most patients with active disease complain of diarrhea—the frequent passage of loose or liquid stool—and may have nocturnal diarrhea. Postprandial diarrhea is common. Urgency, with a feeling of incomplete evacuation, is also common, especially when the rectum is severely inflamed. Patients may be distressed by incontinence. The diarrhea is often associated with passing large quantities of mucus, often with blood and pus.

The pathophysiology of the diarrhea involves several mechanisms, but the failure to absorb salt and water is perhaps the predominant factor.[66] This failure results from reduced Na^+/K^+-ATPase pump activity, increased mucosal permeability, and altered membrane phospholipids. By contrast, high mucosal concentrations of lipid inflammatory mediators, which are detected in ulcerative colitis, have been shown to stimulate chloride secretion in normal colon; it is possible that these mediators contribute to diarrhea by increasing mucosal permeability. Urgency and tenesmus, which are common symptoms when the rectum is inflamed, are caused by poor compliance and loss of the reservoir capacity of the inflamed rectum.[67] With severe inflammation, the urgency can be sufficiently acute as to cause incontinence.

Colonic motility is altered by inflammation, and there is rapid transit through the inflamed colon. With left-sided disease, distal transit is rapid, but there is actual slowing of proximal transit,[68] which may explain the proximal constipation that is commonly seen in patients with distal colitis. Prolonged transit times in the small intestine also occur in the presence of active colonic inflammation.[68]

Abdominal Pain

For most patients with ulcerative colitis, pain is not a prominent symptom. Some patients with active disease may experience vague lower abdominal discomfort, an ache in the left iliac fossa, or mild central abdominal cramping. Severe cramping and abdominal pain can occur in association with severe attacks of the disease.

The cause of the pain is unclear but may relate to increased tension within the inflamed colonic wall during muscular contraction. It is not uncommon for patients with mild distal colitis to have the symptoms of irritable bowel syndrome, which presumably reflects altered motility between the proximal and distal segments of the colon (see Chapter 91).

Other Symptoms

Disease of moderate or severe activity may often be associated with systemic symptoms. Patients may become anorectic and nauseated and, in severe attacks, may vomit. These symptoms, as well as protein loss through inflamed mucosa, hypercatabolism, and down-regulation of albumin synthesis caused by the inflammation, account for weight loss and hypoalbuminemia, which may be profound. Fever, an additional catabolic factor, usually accompanies severe attacks. Patients also may complain of the symptoms of anemia, such as breathlessness, ankle swelling, and fatigue. The anemia is secondary to blood loss, but bone marrow suppression resulting from chronic inflammation may contribute, and drug-induced causes (6-mercaptopurine, azathioprine, sulfasalazine) should be considered for patients on treatment.

Signs

Patients with mild or even moderately severe disease exhibit few abnormal physical signs. They are usually well nourished and not anemic and show no signs of chronic disease. Indeed, these patients can appear deceptively well. Weight should always be recorded and, for children and adolescents, both height and weight should be plotted on development charts. The affected portion of the colon may be tender on abdominal palpation, but tenderness is frequently absent. Bowel sounds are normal. Digital examination of the rectum is also frequently normal, but the mucosa may feel "velvety" and edematous, the anal canal may be sore, and there may be blood on the finger.

Patients with severe attacks also may look well, and tachycardia or a tender colon may be the only abnormal sign. However, many of them look ill, with evidence of weight loss and depletion of salt and water. They may be clinically anemic, with signs of iron deficiency, and may be febrile. Dependent edema secondary to anemia or hypoproteinemia may occur. There may be oral candidiasis or aphthoid ulceration of the oral mucosa. Clubbing of the fingernails is a frequent manifestation of chronic disease. The abdomen may be distended and tympanitic, the colon tender, and the bowel sounds reduced. Minor perianal disease may be present but is never as severe as is often seen in patients with Crohn's disease. Signs of extraintestinal manifestations may be present.

ASSESSMENT OF DISEASE SEVERITY

The severity of disease can be ascertained by various criteria, as follows.

Clinical

The original criteria of Truelove and Witts[69] are simple, easy to use, and of proven value as a guide to disease severity:

Mild—fewer than four stools daily, with or without blood, with no systemic disturbance and a normal erythrocyte sedimentation rate (ESR).

Moderate—more than four stools daily but with minimal systemic disturbance.

Severe—more than six stools daily with blood and with evidence of systemic disturbance, as shown by fever, tachycardia, anemia, or an ESR greater than 30.

Although this classification is still used, it lacks precision, especially in the definition of "severe," because it is not clear how many systemic features are required. Furthermore, an attack can be regarded mistakenly as less than severe because the patient looks well despite fever, tachycardia, or anemia. Sometimes the term *fulminant* is used to describe a particularly severe attack, but this term is best avoided because its meaning is ambiguous. Despite these problems, the classification is still useful, and attempts to create a numerical index[70] have not been widely accepted. Some clinicians use the modified Crohn's Disease Activity Index. However, because it has not been validated for ulcerative colitis, this index cannot be recommended.

Sigmoidoscopic

Sigmoidoscopic assessment is useful for describing the macroscopic appearance of the colonic mucosa, not only for clinical trials, but also for clinical practice when the patient is being followed at regular intervals. Nevertheless, there is considerable interobserver variation.[71] A convenient grading system is as follows:

0—Normal mucosa
1—Loss of vascular pattern
2—Granular, nonfriable mucosa
3—Friability on rubbing
4—Spontaneous bleeding, ulceration

Histologic

Because the histologic features change more slowly than do clinical symptoms or sigmoidoscopic appearances, microscopic assessment is less useful in decision-making about therapy. However, a histologic assessment is still valuable over the long term and can be graded as follows[72]:

1. No significant inflammation—possibly architectural changes of chronic disease and small foci of lymphocytes but no acute inflammation, crypt abscesses, or epithelial destruction.
2. Mild to moderate inflammation—edema, vascularity, increased acute and chronic inflammatory cells but intact epithelium.
3. Severe inflammation—heavy infiltrate of acute and chronic inflammatory cells, crypt abscesses, ulceration of surface epithelium, purulent exudate.

Laboratory Data

Active disease may be associated with a rise in levels of acute phase reactants in serum (C-reactive protein [CRP], orosomucoid), platelet count, and ESR, and a fall in hemoglobin and serum albumin levels.[73] There may be a neutrophilic leukocytosis, but because the white blood cell count rises during glucocorticoid therapy, it can be an unreliable indicator of disease activity. The presence of band cells (young neutrophils) is often seen in peripheral blood in patients with severe attacks and may predict a poor response to medical treatment. Disease limited to the rectum, or even the rectosigmoid, rarely causes a rise in CRP,[74] unless the disease is particularly severe.

DIAGNOSIS

The diagnosis of ulcerative colitis relies on the clinical picture (mainly the history), a stool examination, the sigmoidoscopic or colonoscopic appearance, and the histologic assessment of rectal or colonic biopsy specimens.

Stool Samples

Stool samples from patients with ulcerative colitis contain many pus cells, red blood cells, and frequently eosinophils. Routine cultures should be obtained to exclude *Salmonella* spp and *Shigella* spp infections; special culture conditions are needed to exclude *Campylobacter* spp, *Clostridium difficile*, and *Yersinia* spp. The presence of *C. difficile* toxin also must be excluded. When appropriate, fresh warm stool may be examined for the presence of amebae (see Chapter 98). In patients who are suspected of being immunosuppressed (from chemotherapy, following transplantation, or from human immunodeficiency virus infection or acquired immunodeficiency syndrome), the possibility of opportunistic infections of the colon must be excluded (e.g., cytomegalovirus, herpes, *Mycobacterium avium* complex). Special cultures for gonococcus or *Chlamydia* also may be necessary. The possibility of an infection with *E. coli* O157:H7 also must be considered in patients with an acute onset of symptoms, especially if blood loss and abdominal pain are prominent (see Chapters 96 and 116).

Sigmoidoscopic Appearance

Sigmoidoscopy is best performed in the unprepared bowel so the earliest signs of ulcerative colitis can be detected without the hyperemia that so frequently follows preparative enemas. If the patient is examined in the knee-chest position, little, if any, air insufflation is required, which is comfortable for the patient. However, some air is required if sigmoidoscopy is performed in the left lateral position; care must be taken to avoid excessive distention if severe inflammation is present.

The earliest sign of ulcerative colitis is blurring or loss of the vascular pattern with hyperemia and edema of the mucosa (Fig. 104–6). Edema often is manifested by thickened and blunted valves of Houston, which normally are sharp, crescentic folds. With more severe inflammation, the mucosa becomes granular; friability is detected by the occurrence of small bleeding points when the mucosa is rubbed. Finally, severe ulcerative colitis is associated with a mucosa that bleeds spontaneously and with the presence of ulceration (see Fig. 104–6). These changes are diffuse and extend proximally from the rectum.

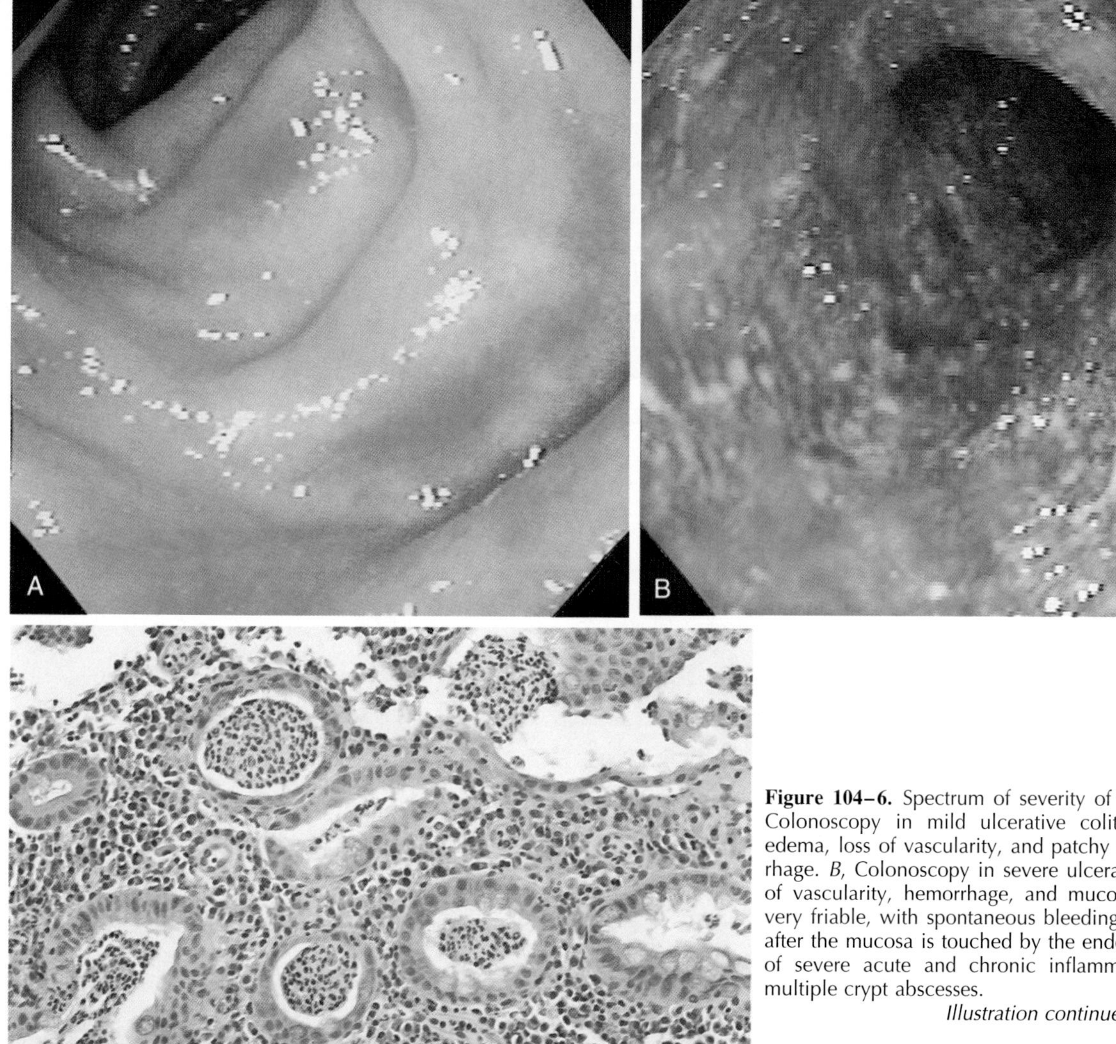

Figure 104–6. Spectrum of severity of ulcerative colitis. *A*, Colonoscopy in mild ulcerative colitis demonstrated by edema, loss of vascularity, and patchy subepithelial hemorrhage. *B*, Colonoscopy in severe ulcerative colitis with loss of vascularity, hemorrhage, and mucopus. The mucosa is very friable, with spontaneous bleeding as well as bleeding after the mucosa is touched by the endoscope. *C*, Histology of severe acute and chronic inflammatory process, with multiple crypt abscesses.

Illustration continued on following page

In patients with long-standing ulcerative colitis, pseudopolyps may be present. Following remission, the mucosa can return to normal, but in patients who have had repeated attacks, it may become thin, pale, and atrophic.

Interpretation of sigmoidoscopic appearances is subject to considerable interobserver variation, especially with regard to milder changes of hyperemia, edema, and granularity.[71] Thus, any assessment of disease severity is always strengthened by a rectal biopsy specimen. More extensive inspection of the distal colon is afforded by flexible as compared with rigid sigmoidoscopy.

Colonoscopy

Colonoscopy is not necessary for diagnosis in most patients but is useful for determining the extent of disease. Multiple biopsy specimens throughout the colon should be taken to map the histologic extent of disease and to confirm the diagnosis if there is concern about Crohn's disease.[75] Colonoscopy has been used increasingly in severe attacks of ulcerative colitis on the grounds that colonoscopy provides a better assessment of severity than does clinical assessment.[76] In referral centers, colonoscopy has been a safe procedure, but it cannot be recommended for general use. For most patients, colonoscopy for confirming the diagnosis and determining the extent of disease should be performed when active disease has been controlled. Preparation must be mild (osmotic purgatives such as GoLYTELY or Picolax are usually safe), and the examination must be gentle.

Colonoscopy is especially useful for assessing patients whose symptoms seem out of proportion to the known radiologic extent of disease. In one study, 14% of patients with total colitis on colonoscopy had had a normal barium enema.[77] Colonoscopy is essential for cancer surveillance (see later) and for the assessment of strictures and polyps.

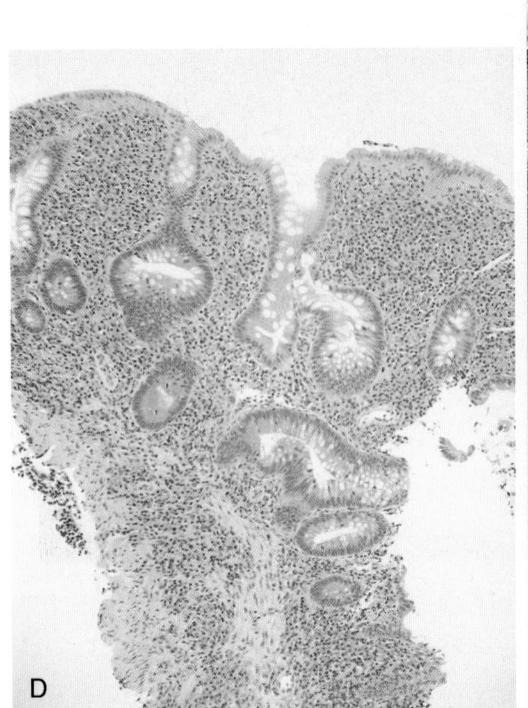

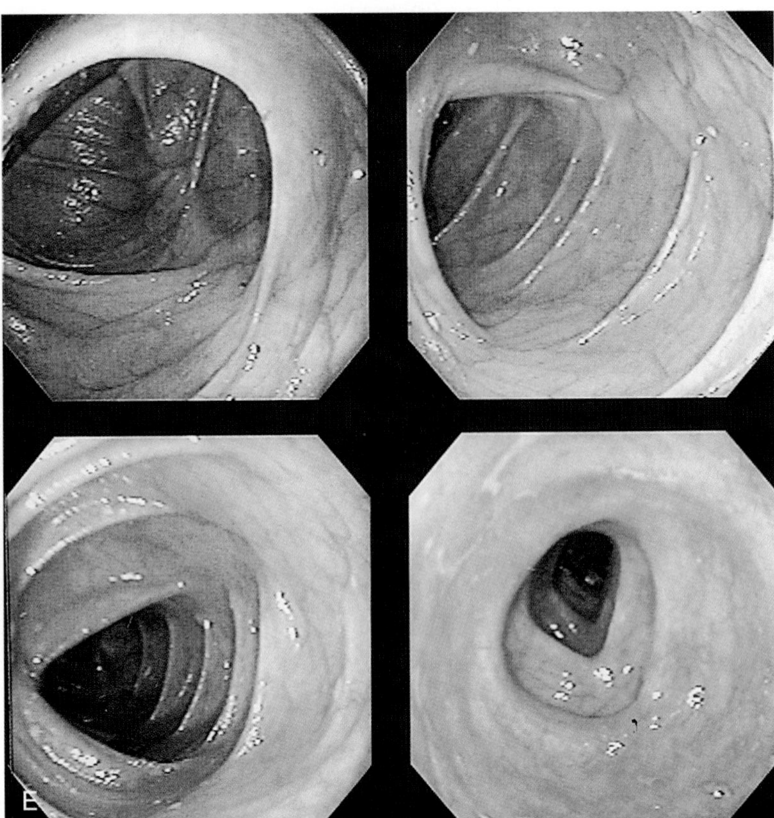

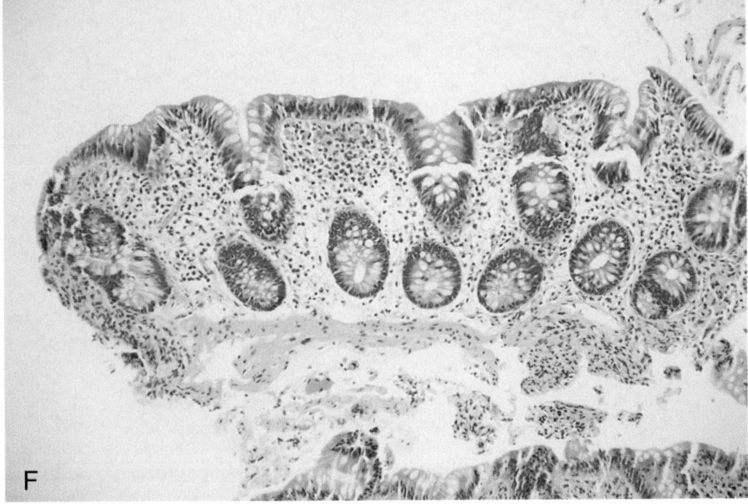

Figure 104–6 *Continued. D,* The colonic architecture is distorted, with a loss of crypts and abnormal branching of the crypts. The disordered architecture is useful in differentiating acute from chronic colitis. *E,* Surveillance colonoscopy in a patient with chronic ulcerative colitis. The ascending colon (*top left*), transverse colon (*top right*), and descending colon (*bottom left*) are normal, with active disease of the sigmoid colon (*bottom right*). *F,* Biopsy samples of the normal-appearing colon demonstrate abnormal architecture consisting of shortened crypts, but no active colitis.

Radiology

Patients with a severe attack of ulcerative colitis must have a plain supine film of the abdomen.[78] In the presence of severe disease, the margin of the colon (i.e., the interface between the colonic mucosa and the luminal gas) becomes edematous and irregular. Thickening of the wall of the colon is often apparent on a plain radiograph, and prognostic signs (see later) such as mucosal islands, small bowel distention, and colonic dilatation can be detected (Fig. 104–7). Plain films are also useful for detecting the presence of fecal material. Inflamed colon seldom contains feces; therefore, no fecal material is present when the whole colon is involved. However, it is common for a patient with left-sided disease to have proximal constipation (Fig. 104–8). Thus, a plain film can give considerable information with respect to the extent of disease.

If the diagnosis is in doubt, an "instant" enema can be performed. Barium is run into the unprepared colon at low pressure, without the use of a balloon catheter, and only a single-contrast study is performed. This technique may give useful information (especially if Crohn's disease of the colon is suspected) but is best avoided. The information gained can be misleading, there are risks of perforating the colon or exacerbating the colitis, and much of the information can be obtained from a plain film. The procedure is contraindicated

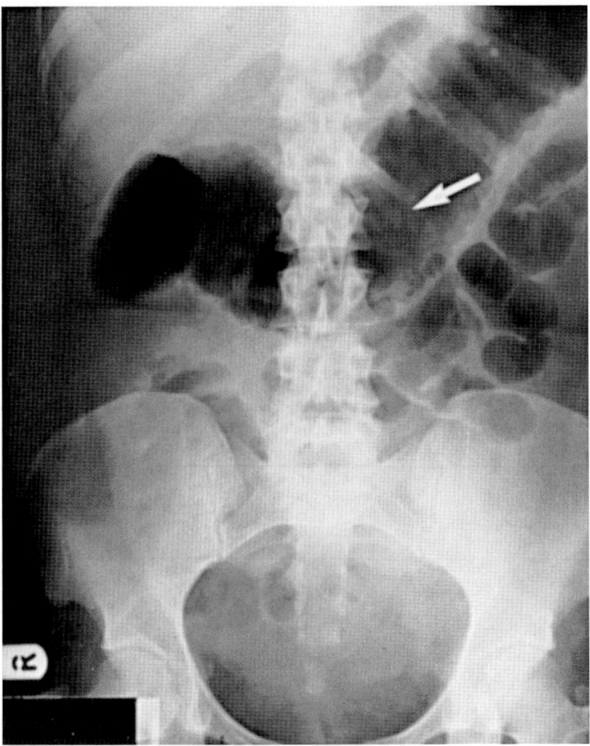

Figure 104–7. Plain abdominal radiograph of a patient with severe ulcerative colitis. The transverse colon is dilated (*arrow*), there is thickening of the abdominal wall, and mucosal islands are visible. In addition, there are distended loops of small bowel.

if the colon is dilated. In patients with mild to moderate disease, a diagnostic double-contrast barium enema is safe, provided the radiologist is aware of the diagnosis. Overinflation of the colon must be avoided, and the procedure must be stopped if the patient experiences pain.

The earliest radiologic change of ulcerative colitis seen on a double-contrast barium enema is fine mucosal granularity (Fig. 104–9). The mucosal line becomes irregular and is not as sharp as that seen in a normal colon. With increasing severity, the mucosal line becomes thickened and irregular, and superficial ulcers are well shown "en face." Deep ulceration can appear as "collar-stud" or "collar-button" ulcers in tangent, which indicates that the ulceration has gone through the mucosa (Fig. 104–10).

The haustral folds show a range of appearances in patients with ulcerative colitis. They may be normal in mild disease, but as activity progresses, they become edematous and thickened. These findings are often visible on a plain abdominal radiograph. Loss of haustrations also can occur, especially in patients with long-standing disease (see Fig. 104–9), but it must be remembered that lack of haustrations can be a normal appearance for the left colon. Thus, this sign is relevant for only the ascending and transverse colon. Another feature of long-standing disease is shortening and narrowing of the colon, and there may be widening of the presacral space, the space between the posterior wall of the rectum and the sacrum, as seen on a lateral film of the rectum; this space is normally less than 1 cm.

Polyps in the colon may be postinflammatory or pseudopolyps, adenomatous polyps, or carcinoma. The postinflammatory polyps are common and may take a variety of forms. Many of them are filiform, but in the presence of active inflammation (especially when partial healing has occurred), the polypoid change can resemble a cobblestone pattern (Fig. 104–11).

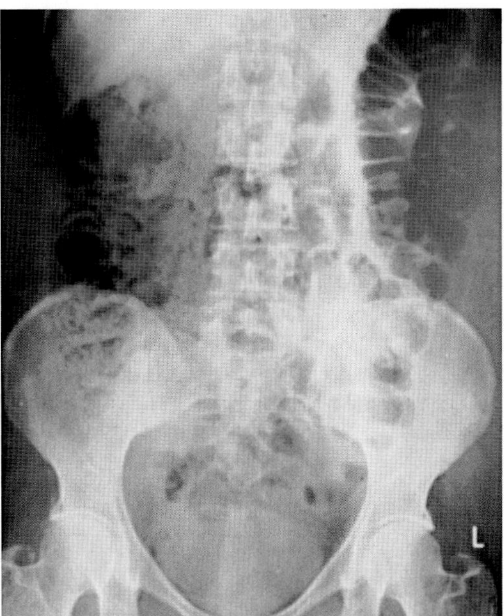

Figure 104–8. Plain abdominal radiograph of a patient with a mild left-sided ulcerative colitis showing marked proximal constipation (stool-filled colon).

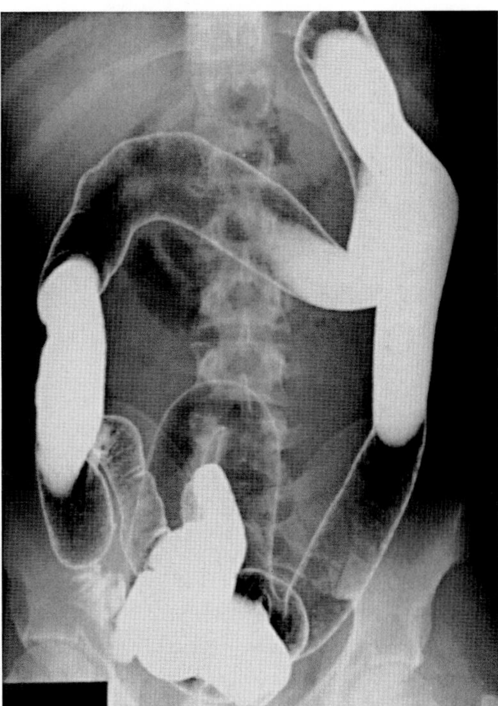

Figure 104–9. A double-contrast barium enema in a patient with long-standing ulcerative colitis indicated by a marked loss of haustration. The mucosa is finely granular throughout the colon, consistent with mildly active disease. The terminal ileum is normal.

Biopsy Specimens

Biopsy specimens always should be taken at the first sigmoidoscopy or colonoscopy. Indeed, it is good practice to obtain a biopsy specimen whenever an endoscopic procedure is performed because there is often disparity between the macroscopic and histologic appearances. If a rigid sigmoidoscopy is performed, biopsy specimens should be taken on the posterior wall within 10 cm of the anal canal (i.e., below the peritoneal reflection) to minimize the risk of perforation. The other major complication of rigid sigmoidoscopy is hemorrhage from a biopsy site. If small-cup forceps are used and hemostasis is ensured before the instrument is removed, the risk of hemorrhage is small. Perforation or hemorrhage rarely occurs as a complication of biopsy if flexible instruments are used (see Chapters 30 and 117).

Laboratory Data

Laboratory data are required for two reasons: first, to document hematologic or biochemical abnormalities and, second, to assist in assessing disease activity.

Many patients become iron deficient because of chronic blood loss, and iron deficiency can be exacerbated if an attack is severe because 0.5 g of elemental iron can be lost during the attack.[79] A hypochromic, microcytic anemia is therefore commonly found. Serum iron and total iron binding capacity should be measured intermittently, especially if there are no signs of iron deficiency on the blood smear. Other hematologic changes—thrombocytosis, leukocytosis, eosinophilia, monocytosis—may simply reflect active disease.

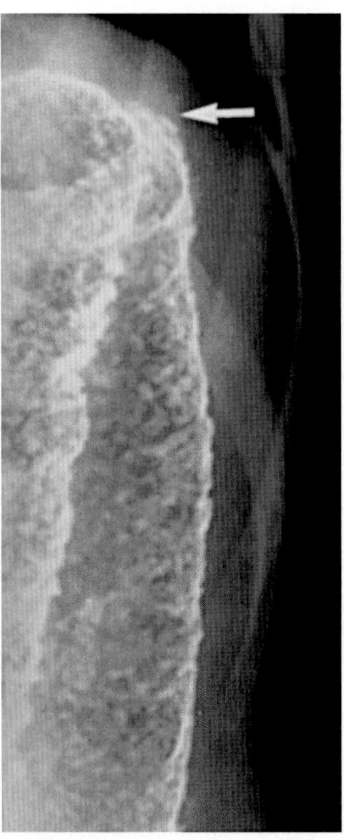

Figure 104–10. A double-contrast barium enema in a patient with active ulcerative colitis. This localized view of the splenic flexure shows multiple ulcers. At the flexure itself there is deep ulceration appearing as "collar-stud" ulcers (*arrow*).

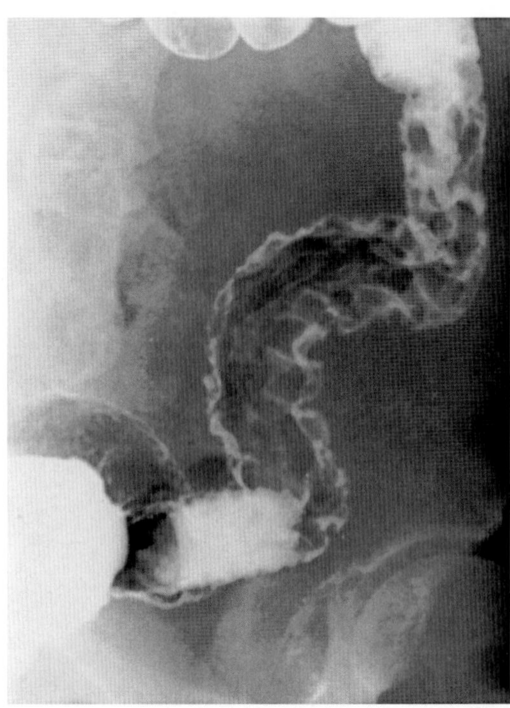

Figure 104–11. Postinflammatory polyps seen in a shortened sigmoid and descending colon in a patient with active ulcerative colitis.

Mild or moderate attacks are rarely associated with any biochemical disturbance, but hypokalemia, hypoalbuminemia, and a rise in serum gamma 2-globulin levels are common in patients with a severe attack. Minor elevations in serum levels of aspartate aminotransferase or alkaline phosphatase are also frequently associated with severe disease, but these changes are transient and return to normal when the disease goes into remission. They probably reflect a fatty liver and the effects on the liver of toxemia, sepsis, or poor nutrition. Persistently abnormal liver biochemical tests, especially serum alkaline phosphatase, are seen in about 3% of patients with ulcerative colitis and should lead to further investigation. The majority of these patients will have sclerosing cholangitis (see Chapter 59).

Serum immunoglobulins usually rise during active disease and fall in remission. They are rarely elevated out of the normal range.[80]

DIFFERENTIAL DIAGNOSIS

The differential diagnosis differs according to the rapidity of onset of significant symptoms. If a patient gives a history of several months of altered bowel habits with blood and mucus and has diffuse inflammation on sigmoidoscopy, the diagnosis of ulcerative colitis is highly probable. The major differential diagnosis is Crohn's disease, and colonoscopy with multiple biopsy specimens is necessary to reach the correct diagnosis (see Chapter 103). It is not uncommon for patients with ileal Crohn's disease to have a proctitis, and they may present with symptoms of proctitis rather than symptoms of small intestinal involvement. Thus it is advis-

Table 104–2 | **Differential Diagnosis of Ulcerative Colitis**

	CLINICAL	RADIOLOGIC	HISTOLOGIC
Ulcerative colitis	Bloody diarrhea	Extends proximally from rectum; fine mucosal ulceration	Distortion of crypts; acute and chronic diffuse inflammatory infiltrate; goblet cell depletion; crypt abscesses; lymphoid aggregates
Crohn's colitis	Perianal lesions common; frank bleeding less frequent than in ulcerative colitis	Segmental disease; rectal sparing; strictures, fissures, ulcers, fistulas; small bowel involvement	Focal inflammation; submucosal involvement; granulomas; goblet cell preservation; transmural inflammation; fissuring
Ischemic colitis	Older age groups; vascular disease; sudden onset, often painful	Splenic flexure; "thumb printing"; rectal involvement rare	Mucosal necrosis; ballooning of capillaries; red blood cell congestion; hemosiderin and fibrosis (chronic disease)
Collagenous colitis	Watery diarrhea; rectal bleeding rare	Usually normal	$>$10-μm-thick subepithelial collagen band; chronic inflammatory infiltrate
Microscopic (lymphocytic) colitis	Watery diarrhea; often in older women; macroscopically normal colonic mucosa	Normal	Chronic inflammatory infiltrate; increased intraepithelial lymphocytes; crypt distortion unusual
Infective colitis	Sudden onset usual; identifiable source with other cases (e.g., *Salmonella*); pain may predominate (e.g., *Campylobacter*); pathogens present in stool	Usually normal	Crypt architecture usually normal Edema, superficial neutrophil infiltrate, crypt abscesses
Pseudomembranous colitis	May be a history of antibiotics; "membrane" may be seen on sigmoidoscopy; *C. difficile* toxin detectable in stools	Edematous; shaggy outline	Similar to acute ischemic colitis but may show "summit" lesions of fibrinopurulent exudate
Amebic colitis	Travel in endemic area; amebae in fresh stool	Discrete ulcers; ameboma or strictures	Similar to ulcerative colitis; amebae in lamina propria or in flask-shaped ulcers, identified by periodic acid-Schiff stain
Gonococcal proctitis	Rectal pain; pus	Granular changes in rectum	Intense neutrophil infiltration; purulent exudate; Gram-negative cocci

able to obtain radiologic assessment of the small intestine in all patients with colonic disease. This is particularly true for patients in whom inflammation is limited to the rectum, but laboratory data show a raised CRP or ESR, or a low serum albumin level. If Crohn's disease is confined to the colon, an accurate diagnosis can be made in the majority of patients (95%) if clinical, radiologic, endoscopic, and histologic data are considered together. Other forms of segmental colitis (e.g., ischemia) must be excluded. If there is diffuse inflammation of the colon, distinguishing Crohn's disease of the colon from ulcerative colitis may be exceptionally difficult. These cases are called *indeterminate colitis.* Affected patients should be followed at regular intervals and treated as for ulcerative colitis, unless more characteristic features of Crohn's disease appear. Tables 104–2 and 104–3 summarize the key points in the differential diagnosis between ulcerative colitis and Crohn's disease.

Table 104–3 | **Endoscopic Differentiation Between Ulcerative Colitis and Crohn's Disease**

	ULCERATIVE COLITIS	CROHN'S DISEASE
Distribution	Diffuse inflammation extending from rectum	Rectal sparing, frequent skip lesions
Inflammation	Diffuse, with mucosal granularity or friability	Focal and asymmetrical, cobblestoning; granularity and friability less common
Ulceration	Small ulcers in a diffusely inflamed mucosa; deep, ragged ulcers in severe disease	Aphthoid ulcers, linear/ serpiginous ulceration; intervening mucosa often normal
Colonic lumen	Often narrowed in long-standing chronic disease; strictures very rare	Strictures common

Other diagnoses that must also be considered in patients with a history extending for several months include ischemia, radiation, collagenous colitis, lymphocytic colitis, and drug-induced colitis. Ischemic colitis classically is segmental and centered around the splenic flexure (the watershed between the superior and inferior mesenteric arteries). However, ischemic proctitis has been described, usually in elderly people. If ischemic proctitis occurs acutely, the mucosa becomes intensely hemorrhagic and edematous. More commonly, ischemic proctitis is chronic, and the diagnosis is made on histologic criteria (see Chapter 119). Radiation colitis usually occurs in women receiving radiotherapy for uterine or cervical carcinoma, especially if cesium rods are used. The sigmoid colon is the usual site of damage, which is segmental. The rectum can be involved, as is also the case for men receiving radiotherapy to the prostate. The diagnosis of radiation colitis is usually straightforward if symptoms begin just after the irradiation, but for some patients the symptoms of radiation colitis may not appear for months or even several years (see Chapter 102).

A drug history must always be taken in a patient with colitis. Nonsteroidal anti-inflammatory drugs, gold, and penicillamine all have been implicated in causing a mild diffuse colitis. Salicylates may also rarely cause a colitis[81]; affected patients may be diagnosed incorrectly as having ulcerative colitis and treated with drugs containing 5-aminosalicylic acid, which invariably makes their condition worse. A history of antibiotic ingestion suggests pseudomembranous colitis associated with *C. difficile*. However, *C. difficile* colitis can occur in the absence of antibiotics, especially in elderly people. Occasionally, ulcerative colitis appears to be initiated by an infective colitis, including *C. difficile* colitis, but whether the infection actually triggers the chronic colitis or merely reveals preexisting but asymptomatic inflammation is uncertain. In some patients with established ulcerative colitis, infective colitis may develop and can be misinterpreted as a relapse of ulcerative colitis unless appropriate stool cultures are obtained.

Microscopic (lymphocytic and collagenous) colitis is becoming more widely recognized (see Chapter 118). Lymphocytic colitis is associated with a normal endoscopic appearance of the colon and is readily distinguished from ulcerative colitis. Collagenous colitis also may show a normal endoscopic appearance but often causes a granular or even a friable mucosa on sigmoidoscopy and is distinguished from ulcerative colitis by the histologic appearance of a subepithelial collagen band ($>$10 μ thick).

For patients with a more acute history, the major differential diagnosis is an infective cause of colitis. The commonest organisms are *Salmonella* spp, *Shigella* spp, and *Campylobacter* spp. Clinical clues to an infective cause are the suddenness of onset, evidence of diarrheal disease in contacts, and prominence of abdominal pain (see Chapter 96). The sigmoidoscopic appearance is indistinguishable from that of ulcerative colitis, but the histologic appearance may be very helpful in differentiating infective from a more chronic colitis. The presence of a chronic inflammatory infiltrate, architectural disturbances, and basal lymphoid aggregates favor a diagnosis of ulcerative colitis. These features distinguish infective colitis from ulcerative colitis with a probability of 80%, but there is considerable interobserver variation.[62, 63] *E. coli* O157:H7 has been recognized as a cause of bloody diarrhea in adults, especially in institutions. Associated disease is normally acute in onset, blood loss is usually considerable, and patients, particularly children, may develop hemolytic-uremic syndrome. Diagnosis is difficult because many clinical microbiology laboratories are not equipped to identify the organism or to measure specific antibody (see Chapter 96). *Yersinia* infections may cause enterocolitis or colitis and may last for several months before resolving spontaneously. The diagnosis is made on the basis of stool culture or a rising titer of serum antibody. Amebic colitis must be excluded in any patient whose symptoms began in an endemic area. The course of the infection is more prolonged than that of most bacterial colitides, but amebiasis is not a cause of chronic colitis. In severe cases of acute bloody diarrhea in which glucocorticoids may be prescribed, amebiasis must be excluded because such therapy may disseminate this protozoal infection and may even cause death (see Chapter 98). Schistosomal colitis (*Schistosoma mansoni*, *S. japonicum*) may be diffuse and involve the rectum. The presence of ova in a biopsy specimen confirms the diagnosis (see Chapter 99).

Other infective causes of a bloody diarrhea include opportunistic infections of the colon in immunosuppressed patients (see Chapters 27 and 28). *Cytomegalovirus* infections are often associated with characteristic endoscopic appearances but can cause diffuse inflammation. *Herpes simplex virus* usually gives rise to a vesicular appearance in the colon. *Mycobacterium avium* complex usually causes patchy rather than diffuse inflammation. Sexually transmitted causes of proctitis, including *gonorrhea*, *chlamydia*, and *lymphogranuloma venereum*, usually do not cause diarrhea and, especially with gonorrhea, are associated with large volumes of watery pus. The diagnosis is made clinically and is confirmed by appropriate cultures as well as histologic appearance on a rectal biopsy specimen (see Chapter 116).

Symptomatically, ulcerative colitis has to be differentiated from the irritable bowel syndrome, colonic carcinoma or polyps, solitary rectal ulcer syndrome, diverticular disease, and factitious diarrhea. These diagnoses do not give rise to diffuse inflammation in the colon and therefore should be readily distinguished from ulcerative colitis, but there are some exceptions. Many patients with acute diverticulitis of the sigmoid colon have rectal inflammation, although the inflammation tends to be patchy and to involve the upper rectum, an appearance that is more likely to be confused with Crohn's disease than ulcerative colitis. The second exception is factitious illness because proctitis can result when patients insert foreign objects into the rectum. Finally, solitary rectal ulcer syndrome can be mistaken for ulcerative colitis if the ulceration extends circumferentially around the rectum. On examination, there is usually a rectal prolapse, and the histologic appearance should clarify the diagnosis. Prolapse may also be associated with "cap polyposis." This condition is associated with diarrhea, blood, and mucus. Endoscopically, small areas of intense hemorrhage, often with ulceration, are found on edematous valves of Houston.[82] The areas of involvement may have a polypoid appearance. Biopsy specimens show an intense inflammatory infiltrate on the crest of the mucosal folds with ulceration, ballooning of glands, and a cap of purulent exudate (see Chapters 91, 108, 114, 117, and 118).

EXTRAINTESTINAL MANIFESTATIONS

Extraintestinal manifestations are commonly present in patients with ulcerative colitis[83] and can be classified as shown in Table 104–4. This classification is useful because the manifestations that are related to the activity of the colitis usually settle when the colonic inflammation is brought into remission.

Skin

The most common rashes are related to therapy and include hypersensitivity or photosensitivity rashes to sulfasalazine

Table 104–4 | **Extraintestinal Manifestations of Ulcerative Colitis**

Related to activity of colitis
Peripheral arthropathy
Erythema nodosum
Episcleritis
Aphthous ulceration of the mouth
Fatty liver
Usually related to activity of colitis
Pyoderma gangrenosum
Anterior uveitis
Unrelated to colitis
Sacroiliitis
Ankylosing spondylitis
Primary sclerosing cholangitis
Rare
Pericarditis
Acute febrile neutrophilic dermatosis (Sweet's syndrome)
Amyloidosis

and urticarial reactions to 5-aminosalicylic acid (mesalamine).

Erythema nodosum also may occur as a reaction to sulfasalazine (specifically, the sulfapyridine component) but can also occur in 2% to 4% of patients with active ulcerative colitis. Erythema nodosum presents as multiple tender and inflamed nodules, mostly on the anterior aspect of the lower legs.

Pyoderma gangrenosum is rare and occurs in only 1% to 2% of patients. It is usually related to active colonic inflammation, although rarely the pyoderma may persist despite inactive colitis. The lesions are usually multiple and may occur on the trunk or the limbs. They begin as pustules (but the pus, if aspirated, is sterile), which then break down, ulcerate, and may coalesce with surrounding lesions. Ulceration leads to considerable necrosis. Histopathologically, pyoderma has the features of a sterile abscess with a marked neutrophilic infiltration. The etiology is unknown. Even less common is the association of ulcerative colitis with *pyodermite végétante Hallopeau*, which has some similarity with pyoderma but also involves the mouth. *Sweet's syndrome* (acute febrile neutrophilic dermatosis) also can occur with active ulcerative colitis.

Mouth

Crops of oral *aphthous ulcers* occur in at least 10% of patients with ulcerative colitis and rapidly resolve once the disease goes into remission. A *sore tongue* and *angular stomatitis* are frequent in patients with associated iron deficiency.

Eyes

Episcleritis or *anterior uveitis* occurs in 5% to 8% of patients with active colitis. Mild conjunctivitis is also common, although direct questioning may be needed to elicit the symptoms of sore, gritty, and watering eyes. Topical glucocorticoids are useful for controlling symptoms.

Joints

An *acute arthropathy* occurs in 5% to 10% of patients with an acute attack of ulcerative colitis.[84] The arthropathy has an asymmetrical distribution and affects the larger joints (knees, hips, ankles, wrists, and elbows). The joints usually become hot and swollen. The condition is nonerosive and resolves as the colitis goes into remission.

A small joint arthropathy also may occur in approximately 5% of patients. This arthropathy is symmetrical and is unrelated to the activity of the intestinal inflammation. It is nondeforming and seronegative.[84]

Sacroiliitis, determined radiologically, occurs in 12% to 15% of patients but in an even higher percentage if isotopic scans are performed. Sacroiliitis may be asymptomatic but can cause low back pain. The majority of patients with sacroiliitis are negative for HLA-B27 and do not progress to ankylosing spondylitis.

Ankylosing spondylitis affects 1% to 2% of patients, and approximately 60% of these have the HLA-B27 phenotype. Men predominate, but the gender ratio seems less marked than that for ankylosing spondylitis in the absence of intestinal disease. The natural history of the spondylitis is independent of the ulcerative colitis, and symptoms of the spinal disease may appear long before the colitis becomes manifest or may develop after the onset of the intestinal symptoms. Spondylitis should be treated with nonsteroidal anti-inflammatory drugs and physiotherapy. Proctocolectomy does not affect the course of the ankylosing spondylitis. The spondylitis is often associated with uveitis and, less commonly, with aortitis or aortic valve disease. The cause of spondylitis is unknown, but the possibility that there may be molecular mimicry between HLA-B27 and a peptide sequence of a nitrogenase enzyme carried by *Klebsiella pneumoniae* is intriguing. Because patients with ulcerative colitis tend to have heightened immune responses to the gut flora, it is possible that persons who are also positive for HLA-B27 are particularly susceptible to developing spinal disease.

Liver Disease

Minor elevations in serum aminotransferase and alkaline phosphatase levels are common in patients with severe attacks of ulcerative colitis, but the levels return to normal once remission is achieved. The reasons for these changes may include malnutrition, sepsis, and fatty liver. An excess of fat in the hepatocytes is found in 60% of patients who undergo urgent colectomy for severe colitis.

The major liver complication of ulcerative colitis is *primary sclerosing cholangitis,* which occurs in approximately 3% of all patients (see Chapter 59). Primary sclerosing cholangitis is a chronic inflammatory disease of the biliary tree and is diagnosed by endoscopic or magnetic resonance cholangiography. Both intrahepatic and extrahepatic ducts may be involved, leading to the characteristic radiologic features of beading, irregularity, and stricturing of the ducts. Some patients show only intrahepatic involvement and, rarely, only extrahepatic duct changes are seen. Histologically, the appearances on liver biopsy specimens can be variable. Classically, there is concentric fibrosis around the bile ductules and ultimately obliteration of the ducts. There is a variable chronic inflammatory infiltrate in the portal tracts and, in some patients, a marked lymphocytic infiltration of the liver cell plates, leading to an interface hepatitis and an appearance resembling that of autoimmune hepatitis. In others, there is frank cirrhosis, and it may be difficult to see the classic biliary changes. Therefore, it seems likely that the majority of chronic liver disease associated with ulcerative colitis is caused by sclerosing cholangitis. All patients with persistently abnormal liver tests or clinical evidence of chronic liver disease must undergo cholangiography for accurate diagnosis. Early studies of liver disease associated with ulcerative colitis claimed associations with portal triaditis, chronic hepatitis, and cirrhosis. However, the biliary tree was not visualized in these studies; therefore, these appearances may well have reflected the histologic diversity seen in sclerosing cholangitis. Although autoimmune hepatitis may occasionally occur in patients with ulcerative colitis, it is uncommon.

The cause of the liver disease in ulcerative colitis is unknown. The majority (70%) of patients have the HLA-DR3, B8 haplotype, and low titers of autoantibodies to smooth muscle, parietal cells, and nuclear antigens are common. High serum titers of antibodies to neutrophils (p-ANCAs) have been described.[85] These antibodies show a perinuclear pattern of staining and are therefore different from ANCA associated with vasculitic disorders. Most patients with sclerosing cholangitis have total colitis, which is often mild. The colitis may go undetected in patients presenting primarily with liver disease unless sigmoidoscopy and rectal biopsy are performed. The possibility that there are cross-reacting epitopes between the colonic and biliary epithelium remains an attractive hypothesis that has received some recent support. Das and colleagues[37] have demonstrated that a monoclonal antibody to the colonic epithelial 40-kd protein also reacts with bile duct epithelium as well as skin. It is possible that patients who are HLA-DR3, B8 mount an immune response to epithelial antigens because they are susceptible to autoimmune disease in general. The trigger for the response remains unknown but may be a bacterial peptide.

Most patients with ulcerative colitis and sclerosing cholangitis remain well with regard to their liver disease for many years. However, the liver disease is progressive and independent of the outcome of the colitis. Ultimately, all the complications of portal hypertension and chronic liver failure develop. Furthermore, the well-recognized association between bile duct carcinoma and ulcerative colitis appears to result from underlying sclerosing cholangitis, which is a premalignant condition.

There is no satisfactory treatment for sclerosing cholangitis, although ursodeoxycholic acid may delay disease progression. Most patients do not require specific treatment, although a few may benefit from glucocorticoids if there is active liver cell damage as shown by fever, malaise, and a rise in serum aspartate aminotransferase levels. Patients with steatorrhea should receive fat-soluble vitamins intramuscularly at regular intervals (see Chapter 89). Some patients may have cholestasis that is caused largely by a single extrahepatic biliary stricture. In these patients, endoscopic dilatation or insertion of a stent may be useful. For patients with end-stage liver disease, liver transplantation should be considered and can be highly successful.[86] Mathematical models have been developed that help predict prognosis and promise to be useful in decision-making about when to consider transplantation.[87, 88]

Thromboembolism

Deep vein thromboses and pulmonary emboli are well-recognized complications of ulcerative colitis and may be causes of mortality. The cause of the thromboembolism is multifactorial. Undoubtedly, hospitalization, immobility, and malnutrition contribute, but in severe disease, usually there are an elevated platelet count and an increased concentration of many clotting factors that behave as acute phase proteins. In populations of patients with ulcerative colitis, there is no increase in the frequency of the factor V Leiden mutation, although in the small groups of patients that have been studied in whom thromboembolic complications developed in association with ulcerative colitis, there is an increased frequency of this mutation. Patients with these complications should be treated with anticoagulants, initially heparin or low molecular weight heparin, followed by warfarin. Anticoagulation is safe and is rarely complicated by colonic bleeding.

Other Rare Associations

Pericarditis with or without an effusion has been described in a few patients with ulcerative colitis, but whether this is a true association is uncertain. In most cases, colitis has been active at the time of the pericarditis.

Amyloidosis is occasionally associated with Crohn's disease and rarely with ulcerative colitis.

MEDICAL MANAGEMENT

The introduction of glucocorticoids in the early 1950s has had a dramatic effect on the management of active ulcerative colitis. For a severe attack, the mortality rate has fallen from 37% to less than 1%, including mortality associated with emergency colectomy (Fig. 104–12). This impressive fall in the death rate, although due partly to glucocorticoids, is also the result of better management of fluids and electrolytes

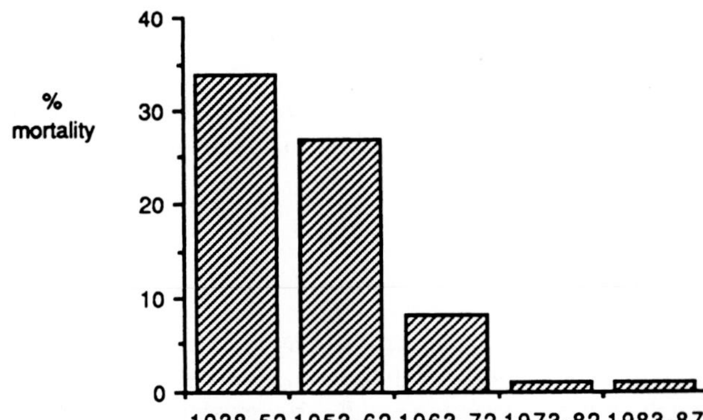

Figure 104–12. The change in mortality from a severe attack of ulcerative colitis in Oxford, United Kingdom. Glucocorticoids were introduced in 1952.

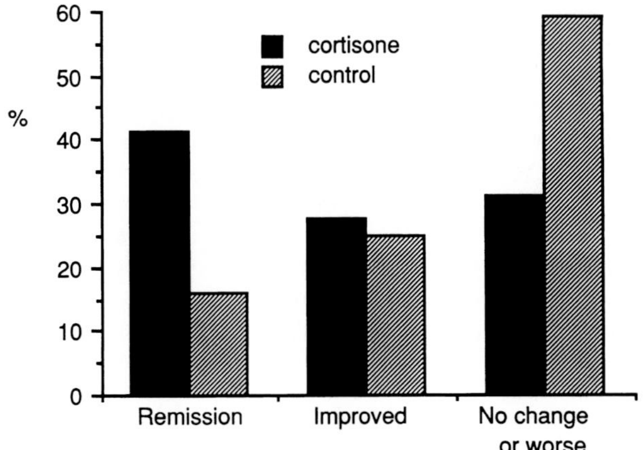

Figure 104–13. The results of a double-blind trial of oral cortisone acetate compared with a placebo (control) for active ulcerative colitis. (Drawn from the data of Truelove and Witts.[69])

and improved surgical technique. The collaborative approach, in which gastroenterologists and surgeons assess patients and make decisions jointly, is also a factor in the improved prognosis. Realization of the basic principles of managing severe attacks has ensured that these low mortality figures also can be achieved in community hospitals.[89]

The other major milestone in the management of ulcerative colitis was the introduction of sulfasalazine by Dr. Nana Svartz in 1942. The use of this drug as maintenance therapy has reduced the relapse rate fourfold and has improved the quality of life for many patients. The introduction of new 5-aminosalicylic acid formulations and attempts to find new glucocorticoid compounds with low systemic bioavailability promise to continue this trend.

Glucocorticoids

The classic trial of cortisone acetate by Truelove and Witts[69] was the first controlled evidence that glucocorticoids were of benefit in treating active disease. Figure 104–13 summarizes the outcome after 6 weeks of treatment with either cortisone 37.5 mg daily by mouth or placebo. Forty-one percent of patients who received the steroid achieved remission, compared with only 15% of those who received a placebo. Correspondingly, only 32% on active therapy deteriorated, compared with 60% on placebo. The beneficial effect of glucocorticoids for active colitis was confirmed in a trial of oral prednisolone (prednisone). This study also demonstrated a dose-response effect using 20, 40, and 60 mg.[90] There was greater benefit to 40 mg over 20 mg daily, but the use of 60 mg daily, although showing some additional benefit, was associated with a marked increase in the frequency of adverse effects. Glucocorticoids are also effective for active distal disease when used as topical treatment in the form of retention enemas, foams, or suppositories. Both oral cortisone and prednisone have been shown to be ineffective in maintaining remission. Thus, glucocorticoids should be used to treat active disease, and prolonged therapy is contraindicated not only because of long-term adverse effects, but also because it is ineffective as maintenance therapy in the vast majority of patients.[91]

Whether or not the use of corticotropin (ACTH) is of value is not entirely clear. Earlier studies suffered from small numbers of patients, and comparisons between studies are difficult because of differing trial designs and routes of administration (intramuscular or intravenous). However, the most recent trial suggested that intravenous ACTH is more effective than intravenous hydrocortisone in patients who have not previously received oral glucocorticoids.[92]

There is considerable interest in the possibility of a corticosteroid with low systemic bioavailability. When given as a retention enema, betamethasone 17-valerate, beclomethasone, and prednisolone metasulfobenzoate have been shown to be therapeutically effective for active distal colitis but with minimal effects on the hypothalamic-pituitary-adrenal axis.[91] These steroid compounds are all in use as topical treatment. Budesonide also has been shown to be effective when given as a retention enema[93]; a colonic-release preparation for oral use has become available.

Aminosalicylates

Sulfasalazine was introduced initially for the treatment of rheumatoid arthritis but was quickly found to be effective for ulcerative colitis. The drug consists of 5-aminosalicylic acid (5-ASA) linked to sulfapyridine by an azo bond, which is poorly absorbed in the upper gastrointestinal tract. Once sulfasalazine reaches the colon after oral ingestion, bacterial azoreductases split the azo bond to release the two components. Sulfapyridine is absorbed rapidly, metabolized in the liver, and excreted in the urine. The aminosalicylate moiety, however, is largely excreted in the feces (approximately 70%). Approximately 25% is absorbed from the colon, and the majority appears in the blood as *N*-acetyl-5-ASA. Some acetylation takes place in the lumen by bacterial acetyltransferases, but most 5-ASA is acetylated in the cytosol of colonic epithelial cells.[94] Both acetylated and nonacetylated 5-ASA are excreted in the urine.

For active disease, sulfasalazine is less effective than glucocorticoids; its principal use is to maintain remission once active inflammation has subsided. This effect was shown initially by Misiewicz and associates[95] and has subsequently been confirmed in other studies. The suppressive effect of sulfasalazine on the disease is maintained over many years.[95] Nevertheless, the incidence of adverse effects is high.[96] These adverse reactions may be divided into those that are dose dependent and those that are not (Table 104–5). After

Table 104–5 | **Adverse Effects of Sulfasalazine**

Dose-Related
Nausea
Vomiting
Anorexia
Folate malabsorption
Headache
Alopecia
Non–Dose-Related
Hypersensitivity skin rashes (occasionally with photosensitivity)
Hemolytic anemia (Heinz bodies)
Agranulocytosis
Hepatitis
Fibrosing alveolitis, pulmonary eosinophilia
Male infertility
Colitis

a dose-dependent adverse effect (headache, nausea, vomiting, diarrhea), intolerance often can be overcome by starting the dose at 0.5 g daily and gradually increasing it over 6 to 8 days. Patients with hypersensitivity rashes can be desensitized by starting with a few milligrams and gradually increasing the dose over several weeks. Infertility in men is usually reversible once the sulfasalazine is stopped. Patients with the nonacetylator phenotype are especially prone to the dose-dependent adverse effects.[97, 98]

The dose-dependent adverse effects and male infertility are now known to be caused by the sulfapyridine component of the sulfasalazine molecule. Most hypersensitivity rashes, especially those that are photosensitive, as well as Heinz body hemolytic anemia, are induced by the sulfapyridine. Thus, the demonstration by Azad Khan and colleagues[99] that the beneficial effect of the drug was mediated by the aminosalicylate moiety allowed the development of new drugs that deliver 5-ASA to the colon without using sulfapyridine as a carrier molecule.

When given by mouth, 5-ASA is absorbed rapidly from the jejunum and does not reach the colon. Therefore, two types of delivery systems have been used to obtain high concentrations of drug in the colonic lumen.[96] The first is to coat 5-ASA with a resin or a semipermeable membrane that is pH sensitive. The second is to link 5-ASA with another molecule by an azo bond. Table 104–6 lists the 5-ASA drugs that have been developed. The generic name for enteric-coated or delayed-release preparations is mesalamine (mesalazine in Europe). Asacol is coated with Eudragit S, which dissolves at pH 7.0 or above, whereas Salofalk and Claversal are coated with Eudragit L and release the active ingredient at pH 6.0 and above. Pentasa is mesalamine within a semipermeable membrane that releases the drug at luminal pH values greater than 6.0 in a timed-release manner. The two prodrugs are olsalazine (two molecules of 5-ASA linked by an azo bond) and balsalazide (5-ASA linked to a peptide). The pharmacodynamics of these two prodrugs is similar to that of sulfasalazine.

Many clinical trials have shown that these newer salicylate drugs are as effective as sulfasalazine, both for treating active ulcerative colitis and for maintaining remission.[96, 100] Adverse effects have been minimal and occur in less than 5% of patients. Furthermore, the majority of patients who are intolerant to sulfasalazine are able to tolerate these newer preparations. Increasing the dose of these drugs increases their therapeutic efficacy without causing adverse effects. Which of these new compounds should be given? There is no clear answer to this question at the present time. One trial has shown that the relapse rate with olsalazine is lower than that with mesalamine, but this study was small and not totally blind.[101] Loose stools and occasionally frank diarrhea occur with all the 5-ASA drugs but especially with olsalazine. However, diarrhea is rarely a problem if the dose is built up gradually and the drug is taken with food. There is concern that 5-ASA may affect renal function adversely. Because the resin-coated mesalamine drugs may be released rapidly in the small intestine, blood concentrations of 5-ASA tend to be higher than those associated with olsalazine. It is therefore wise to check renal function at occasional intervals in patients receiving the mesalamine preparations.

Table 104–6 | **5-Aminosalicylic Acid (5-ASA) Drugs**

MESALAMINE PREPARATIONS	
Enteric-coated	Asacol
	Claversal
	Salofalk
	Rowasa
Controlled-release	Pentasa
PRODRUGS	Sulfasalazine
	Olsalazine
	Balsalazide

Topical treatment with sulfasalazine or mesalamine (as an enema, foam, or suppository) also can be used and is effective both for active disease and for maintenance therapy.[102, 103] It has been shown that topical mesalamine is at least as effective as, and possibly better than, topical glucocorticoids for treating active distal disease.[104] The combination of a topical glucocorticoid and mesalamine appears to be better than either alone.[105]

Immunosuppressive Agents

Azathioprine and 6-mercaptopurine (6-MP) have been the most widely used immunosuppressive agents. Azathioprine is converted to 6-MP in the liver and then to thioguanine. This latter compound impairs purine biosynthesis and thus inhibits cellular proliferation. The major use of these drugs in ulcerative colitis is for the management of chronic active disease (in these cases, their use can lead to a glucocorticoid-sparing effect)[105] and for the maintenance of remission.[106] This latter indication is usually for patients who have experienced repeated relapses of their disease once glucocorticoids have been stopped. When used in moderate doses (2.0 to 2.5 mg/kg for azathioprine), adverse effects are minimal but include nausea, fever, myalgia, diarrhea, pancreatitis, and hepatic dysfunction. Patients who experience nausea and headaches on azathioprine can sometimes tolerate 6-MP. Bone marrow suppression occurs rarely and usually in patients who are deficient in the enzyme thiopurine methyltransferase, which occurs in about 1 in 300 of a white population.

Cyclosporine is being used increasingly in severe ulcerative colitis. Favorable results have been reported for intravenous use (4 mg/kg) and have been confirmed in a small placebo-controlled trial.[107] From 50% to 80% of patients with severe attacks who fail to respond to intravenous glucocorticoids may avoid colectomy during the attack if given a slow, continuous infusion of cyclosporine. Adverse effects have been minimal, but patients with a low serum cholesterol concentration may be at risk for seizures, which can be induced by the cremophor carrier.[108] The other indication for cyclosporine is as a retention enema for resistant distal colitis or proctitis.[109] Anecdotally, patients appear to respond well but tend to relapse soon after treatment is stopped. Blood concentrations of cyclosporine following rectal administration are low, suggesting that absorption from the colon is poor.

Other Drugs

Antibiotics have no place in the management of ulcerative colitis unless there is a specific indication, such as an abscess or positive blood cultures. Antibiotics are indicated, of course, if perforation occurs.

Anecdotal evidence suggests that weekly administration of methotrexate is effective for patients with refractory disease. A randomized controlled trial was negative, but a low dose of methotrexate was used. Most clinicians have used 20 to 25 mg IM weekly. No formal trial of infliximab, the chimeric anti-tumor necrosis factor antibody, has been reported, and anecdotal experience in severe colitis has been variable.

TREATMENT REGIMENS

There is a range of opinion concerning the precise regimens for the treatment of ulcerative colitis, but, in general, physicians use glucocorticoids to control active disease because they are more effective than sulfasalazine.[110] Once disease is controlled, remission is maintained by using a 5-ASA drug. The following discussion reviews the regimens that are effective and that allow rapid control of disease in the majority of patients.

Active Colitis

Proctitis

Most patients respond to topical treatment with glucocorticoids or 5-ASA, which should be given in the form of a suppository. A combination of both treatments can be particularly useful.[105] One of the commonest reasons that patients fail to respond is that they receive foams or enemas; these preparations travel up into the sigmoid or even the descending colon and leave little active drug in the rectum. Changing to twice-daily suppositories often leads to an improved response. If symptoms continue, oral treatment should be instituted with glucocorticoids and 5-ASA. There is anecdotal evidence that cyclosporine enemas (containing 250 mg of cyclosporine) are beneficial, although the disease usually relapses once treatment is stopped. Unfortunately, a negative randomized trial[111] has largely been interpreted as concluding that topical cyclosporine should not be used. However, the trial included patients with a relapse of left-sided colitis, conceivably a different disease from refractory proctitis.

In many patients with proctitis, severe constipation develops above the level of the inflammation and can cause bloating, abdominal discomfort, and nausea. Relief of constipation, initially with osmotic purgation, provides considerable relief and may be associated with a marked improvement in the inflammation.

Mildly Active Disease

Patients who have inflammation extending beyond the limits of the rigid sigmoidoscope, who are systemically well, and who have no more than an average of four bowel movements daily should be treated with prednisone 20 mg orally daily and topical glucocorticoids. This regimen can be continued for 4 weeks and then tapered if remission has occurred. Many physicians use 5-ASA compounds before starting glucocorticoids, but for those not responding to 5-ASA, it may be weeks before symptoms are controlled.

Moderately Active Disease

Patients with more than four bowel movements daily but no evidence of systemic illness are best given higher doses of oral glucocorticoids, such as 40 or 60 mg daily, which is reduced to 20 mg over 2 to 3 weeks. The regimen then follows that described for mild disease.

Severe Disease

Severe attacks, as have been described earlier, are those in which severe bloody diarrhea is associated with evidence of systemic disturbance (e.g., fever, tachycardia, anemia). These patients should be admitted to the hospital, and fluid and electrolyte replacement should be given intravenously. Patients are given intravenous glucocorticoids (e.g., hydrocortisone 100 mg every 6 hours or methylprednisolone 16 mg every 6 hours) together with twice-daily rectal glucocorticoids; a rectal drip of hydrocortisone 100 mg in 100 mL water given over 20 to 30 minutes is usually well tolerated.[112, 113] Patients who are poorly nourished should receive parenteral nutrition. Continuing oral nutrition appears not to affect the outcome of a severe attack, but many patients feel better receiving only clear fluids. Furthermore, if oral feeding is withheld, a food challenge can be a useful means of assessing whether the disease has resolved (see later).

Treatment is continued for 5 to 7 days if the patient continues to improve. A good response is one in which, at the end of this time, the patient feels well, there is no fever or tachycardia, the colon is not tender on abdominal palpation, and the diarrhea has largely resolved, usually to fewer than four bowel movements daily. The stools are rarely formed at this stage, but macroscopic bleeding has stopped. These patients can then be started on oral prednisone (e.g., 40 mg daily) plus a 5-ASA drug and a light diet.

Patients whose condition deteriorates during the first few days of intravenous therapy require surgery, as do those who fail to improve.[114] Management decisions become difficult for patients who show some improvement after a few days of treatment but are still anorectic, with tachycardia, continuing bloody diarrhea, and a tender colon. Medical therapy can be continued for a longer period, but many patients require urgent surgery. It is in this group of patients that the introduction of a light diet toward the end of the first week of intravenous treatment provides a useful guide to future management. If the patient's pulse rate rises or a fever develops in response to feeding, urgent colectomy is required. As indicated earlier, the addition of intravenous cyclosporine induces remission in many of these patients who do not improve rapidly with intravenous glucocorticoids.

There are many unresolved questions about the use of cyclosporine. There are differences in opinion about when cyclosporine should be introduced. It should probably be considered toward the end of the first week of glucocorticoid treatment (5 to 7 days) for patients who responded rapidly. Although 4 mg/kg has become the accepted intravenous dose of cyclosporine, dose-response trials have not been performed. Anecdotal evidence suggests that a dose of 2 mg/kg

Table 104–7 | **Prognostic Indicators for the Outcome of Medical Therapy for Severe Ulcerative Colitis**

		% FAILURE
Clinical and Laboratory Parameters		
Number of bowel movements > 9	in the first 24 hr	33
Pulse > 100/min	in the first 24 hr	36
Maximum temperature > 38°C	in the first 24 hr	56
Serum albumin < 3.0 mg/dL (30 g/L)		42
Radiologic Signs		
Mucosal islands		75
Colonic dilatation		75
Small intestinal distention		73

may be as effective, and it is possible that oral cyclosporine (as Neoral) may be as effective as intravenous administration. One of the most controversial issues is how to continue management in patients who respond well to cyclosporine. Many clinicians will continue with oral cyclosporine (5 mg/kg), taper glucocorticoids over 6 to 8 weeks, and then stop the cyclosporine at 3 to 6 months. Others will not use oral cyclosporine but will add azathioprine, whereas others will use a combination of cyclosporine and azathioprine for 6 to 8 weeks and then stop the cyclosporine.

One of the major concerns regarding cyclosporine is toxicity. In many centers that have reported their experiences, major toxicity has not been seen, but renal impairment, hypertension, opportunistic infection, and even deaths have occurred. Early introduction and short periods of treatment are probably the best ways of avoiding toxicity. Most patients who respond to cyclosporine do so within 3 to 4 days, and it is questionable whether longer periods of treatment can be justified.

From 20% to 30% of patients with a severe attack of ulcerative colitis will require urgent colectomy, and it is helpful to identify patients at risk early in the course (Table 104–7). Indicators of a poor prognosis include the passage of more than nine stools per day, a pulse rate higher than 100/min, and a temperature greater than 38°C in the first 24 hours of treatment.[115] A serum albumin level of less than 3.0 mg/dL (30 g/L) over the first 4 days and failure of the CRP and other acute phase proteins to fall are also poor prognostic signs.[73] Seventy-five percent of patients who have mucosal islands in the colon or more than three loops of distended small bowel on a plain abdominal radiograph will require urgent surgery.[115, 116]

A prospective study of patients with severe colitis showed that the need for colectomy could be predicted in 85% if stool frequency was greater than eight per day on day 3 of glucocorticoid therapy, or if the CRP was greater than 45 mg/L (normal < 8 mg/L) in patients who were still passing three to eight stools daily.[117] These parameters may allow an early decision about introducing cyclosporine and identifying those patients who need to be educated about surgical treatment.

Chronic Active Disease

Some patients relapse repeatedly once oral glucocorticoids are tapered or the dose of prednisone drops to less than 10 to 15 mg daily. It may be worth admitting these patients to the hospital for intravenous glucocorticoids. Otherwise, immunosuppressive therapy can be used and may allow prednisone to be discontinued. Azathioprine and 6-MP act slowly, over 3 to 6 weeks or more and, if clinical benefit occurs, are usually continued for several months. Most physicians do not prolong treatment with these drugs for longer than 18 to 24 months. Persistent chronic active disease in patients who are receiving glucocorticoids and immunosuppressive therapy, especially if adverse effects occur or the patient's lifestyle is impaired, is an indication for surgery.

Maintenance Therapy

Once the disease is in remission, patients are maintained on a 5-ASA drug. The mesalamine preparations, olsalazine and balsalazide, are as effective as sulfasalazine and have fewer adverse effects but are more expensive. Whichever drug is used, it should be used indefinitely because 5-ASA exerts its suppressive effect on the disease over many years.[95] This point is illustrated in Figure 104–14, which shows that the risk of relapse in patients randomized to sulfasalazine or placebo is just as great for patients who had previously been on sulfasalazine for longer than 3 years as it is for those who had been on sulfasalazine for much shorter periods. If patients are maintained on olsalazine, the dose should be increased gradually to 1 g twice daily for patients with distal

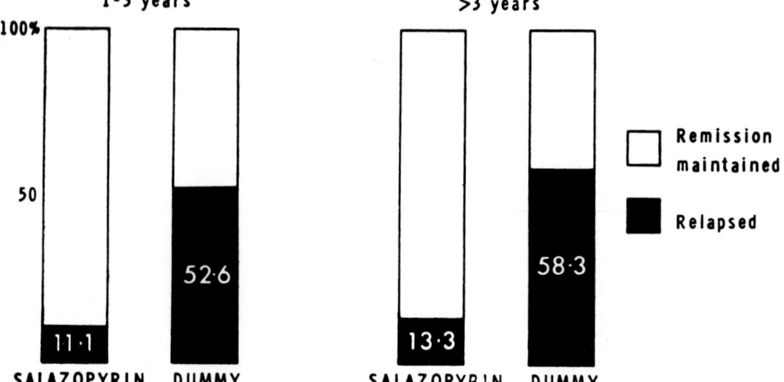

Figure 104–14. The results of a double-blind maintenance trial comparing sulfasalazine (Salazopyrin) with placebo (dummy). The figures give relapse rates over a 6-month period. Patients who had been receiving sulfasalazine for more than 3 years before the trial still had a high chance of relapsing if they were randomized to a placebo compared with continuing sulfasalazine. The relapse rates were similar to those who had received only sulfasalazine for less than 3 years before randomization. (From Dissanayake AS, Truelove SC: A controlled therapeutic trial of long-term maintenance treatment of ulcerative colitis with sulphasalazine. Gut 14: 923, 1973. Reproduced by the kind permission of Dr. S.C. Truelove and the Editor of Gut.)

colitis because this dose is more effective than lower doses. Similarly, Pentasa 1 g twice daily provides a better therapeutic response than is provided by 500 mg twice daily.

LOCAL COMPLICATIONS

Perianal Lesions

Patients with ulcerative colitis occasionally develop anal fissures, perianal abscesses, or hemorrhoids, but the occurrence of extensive perianal lesions should suggest Crohn's disease. For fissures, treatment of the active rectal inflammation is essential, and operative intervention should be avoided if possible.

Massive Hemorrhage

Massive hemorrhage occurs in association with severe attacks of the disease. Transfusion combined with treatment of the attack usually allows the bleeding to stop. However, if patients require 6 to 8 units of blood within 24 to 48 hours and are still bleeding, urgent colectomy must be considered.

Perforation

Perforation is the most dangerous local complication, and the physical signs of peritonitis may not be obvious, especially if the patient is already receiving glucocorticoids. Malaise, tachycardia, and reduced bowel sounds may be the only clinical features. Plain abdominal radiographs, including erect or decubitus films, usually show free peritoneal air. Perforation may complicate an acute dilatation but can occur in its absence. Fortunately, it is a rare complication. Management consists of medical therapy to correct metabolic disturbances, intravenous antibiotics, and glucocorticoids. As soon as the patient's general condition improves, urgent colectomy is performed within a few hours.

The mortality rate for perforation complicating toxic megacolon is high; 16% was reported from the Mount Sinai Hospital.[118] Thus, there should be a low threshold for surgery, but it is imperative to spend time improving the general state of the patient with fluids, potassium, and antibiotics before operating.

Acute Dilatation

An acute dilatation of the colon ("toxic megacolon") is defined as a transverse colon diameter of greater than 6 cm with loss of haustrations in a patient with a severe attack of ulcerative colitis.[119] This complication occurs in approximately 5% of severe attacks and may be triggered by hypokalemia or the administration of opiates. Many affected patients have a rise in arterial pH, indicating a metabolic alkalosis.[120] As with perforation, physical signs can be minimal, but the abdomen may be distended (the dilated transverse colon may be visible in thin patients), bowel sounds are reduced, there is tachycardia, and the patient may or may not be obtunded. If the dilatation occurs during treatment of the acute attack, emergency colectomy is required. However, if dilatation is present when the patient is first seen for that attack, medical therapy with fluid and potassium replacement and intravenous glucocorticoids should be started. Approximately 50% of acute dilatations resolve with medical therapy.[121, 122] Urgent colectomy is required for patients who do not improve or who continue to deteriorate. The trial period for improvement before surgery is performed is 24 hours in our clinic; others are willing to wait 48 to 72 hours. For patients who achieve remission on medical therapy, subsequent management is more controversial. Data from the Mayo Clinic suggest that 42% of such patients achieve satisfactory long-term results, although 58% either will have continuing symptoms of active disease or will require surgery.[121] Thus, some clinicians advise an elective colectomy for patients who have recovered from acute dilatation of the colon, whereas others adopt a more expectant policy.

Strictures

Fibrous strictures are rare in patients with long-standing ulcerative colitis with a shortened, narrowed colon. The diagnosis requires a high index of suspicion for carcinoma, and multiple biopsy specimens must be obtained at colonoscopy. The strictures rarely cause frank obstruction; therefore, colectomy is not necessarily indicated. When surgery is not done, close colonoscopic surveillance with multiple biopsies is advised.

Pseudopolyps

Pseudopolyps also are known as inflammatory polyps because they occur as a result of exuberant granulation tissue that subsequently becomes epithelialized. They are highly variable in shape and size but are usually less than 1.5 cm long. They may be filiform or sessile or may form bridges. They can occur in all parts of the colon, although the rectum is often spared.[123] They are not premalignant and occasionally may regress (see Fig. 104–11).

Colorectal Cancer

The risk of colonic cancer as a complication of ulcerative colitis has been recognized since the 1930s, but there has been considerable variation in the estimated risk.[124] Most studies have agreed that the risk is highest in patients with extensive or total colitis, and it only becomes appreciable once the patient has had the disease for 10 years. The cancers tend to be distributed more evenly around the colon in patients with, than in those without, ulcerative colitis; multiple tumors can be present. Patients whose disease began at an early age or who have pursued a chronic continuous course also may have a higher risk, but these have not been identified as independent risk factors in all studies.

The risk of cancer in patients with proctitis is not increased, and the risk for those with left-sided disease is minimally increased, although there is some discrepancy among study results. For extensive disease, the variable risk

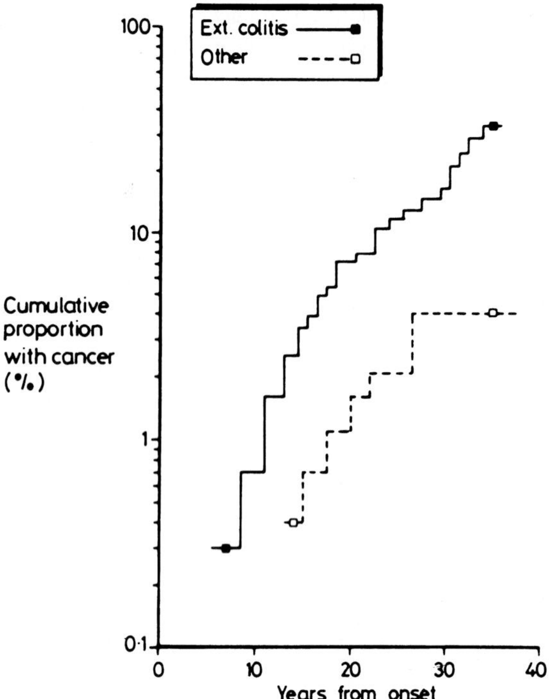

Figure 104–15. The cumulative risk of colorectal cancer with length of history in a primary cohort of patients with ulcerative colitis. A higher risk is seen for patients with extensive colitis (Ext. colitis) than for those with left-sided or distal disease (Other). Note that the vertical axis is logarithmic. (From Gyde SN, Prior P, Allan RN, et al: Colorectal cancer in ulcerative colitis: A cohort study of primary referrals from three centers. Gut 29:206, 1988. Reproduced by the kind permission of the Editor of Gut.)

among studies is due largely to methodologic problems.[124] Most reports have been based on hospital series, which can be a source of considerable bias because they select more severely ill patients, there may be referral bias, and the reason for referral may be the complicating carcinoma. Population studies are difficult to do because ulcerative colitis is relatively uncommon, and the incidence of carcinoma is low; this incidence only becomes appreciable when a population is studied prospectively over at least 20 years.

Two series from Europe, based on hospital patients, have attempted to overcome the problems of selection bias by studying primary cohorts, that is, patients living near the hospital where the diagnosis was made and those in whom the diagnosis was made soon after the onset of symptoms. In a collaborative study among Birmingham, Oxford, and Stockholm, the cumulative risk of cancer in patients with extensive disease was 7.2% at 20 years and 16.5% at 30 years after the onset of colitis (Fig. 104–15).[125] In the other study, also from Sweden, the cumulative risk was 16% at 20 years from onset in patients who were over age 40 years at onset, but only 13% at 25 years in patients who were younger than 40 years of age at onset.[126] There appeared to be a much greater cancer risk when the colitis began in childhood than in adulthood. Nearly all studies of cumulative incidence tend to show an annual increment of 0.8% to 1.0% in the risk of colon cancer after 15 to 20 years of colitis. There is increasing evidence that long-term maintenance therapy with 5-ASA drugs may diminish the cancer risk.[127]

In the past, some clinicians have favored prophylactic colectomy for patients at high risk of developing cancer (i.e., extensive disease for many years, especially in those with frequent relapses or chronic continuous disease). However, the recognition that dysplasia could be identified histologically by colonoscopic surveillance has altered the management of this group of patients.[128, 129] Nevertheless, the histologic recognition of dysplasia is not always easy, especially in small biopsy specimens with active inflammation, because regenerating glands can look like low-grade dysplasia. Therefore, it is always wise to obtain further biopsies after the inflammation is treated if low-grade dysplasia is reported when the disease is active. Differentiating regenerative changes from dysplasia requires well-orientated biopsy specimens. The most reliable histologic feature of low-grade dysplasia is the failure of maturation of nuclear changes from the crypts toward the surface. In regenerating mucosa, maturation occurs with an increase in the cytoplasmic/nuclear ratio.

The classification of dysplasia recommended by an international working party[129] is as follows: negative; indefinite; definite; low grade (Fig. 104–16); and high grade (Fig. 104–17).

Because colonoscopic surveillance for dysplasia may select patients in whom the risk of cancer is sufficiently high to justify a prophylactic proctocolectomy, a number of questions arise to which there is no consensus. The natural history of dysplasia, especially when it is of low grade, is not known, and dysplasia can disappear. Nevertheless, a number of reports have suggested that low-grade dysplasia may be associated with cancer and cannot be regarded as a "benign" lesion, as was originally thought. Dysplasia is patchy, and there is considerable sampling error at colonoscopy. The time intervals between colonoscopic examinations also are not well defined. Finally, large numbers of colonoscopies are involved in a surveillance program, and issues of cost versus benefit arise. Even with colonoscopic surveillance, a high proportion of cancers detected will be Dukes' stage B or C, and the value of prophylactic colectomy for high-grade dysplasia can never be really assessed without a controlled trial. However, two studies have suggested that the outcome with respect to cancer is worse in patients who are not under regular surveillance than in those who are under regular surveillance.[130, 131]

Despite these uncertainties, patients with extensive colitis for longer than 8 to 10 years should be offered colonoscopic surveillance. Multiple biopsy specimens should be taken at 10-cm intervals around the colon with additional biopsy specimens from suspicious areas (so-called dysplasia-associated lesion or mass, DALM). If dysplasia is not found, colonoscopy should be repeated every 1 to 3 years with the precise frequency determined largely by local facilities and resources, although annual surveillance is probably the ideal. High-grade dysplasia, if found, should be confirmed by a second pathologist and possibly a repeat examination, and then prophylactic surgery should be advised. If low-grade dysplasia is reported, a colonoscopy with multiple biopsies should also be repeated within 3 months. If low-grade dysplasia is confirmed, the patient should probably be examined

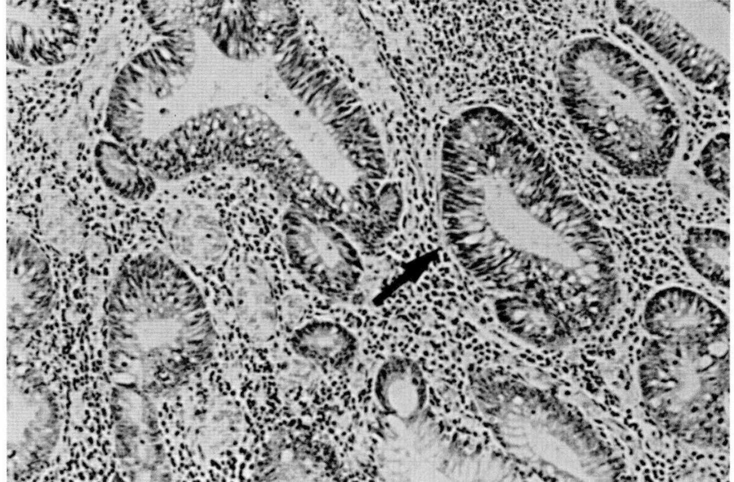

Figure 104–16. Rectal biopsy specimen from a patient with extensive ulcerative colitis for 18 years showing low-grade dysplasia. There is marked nuclear stratification and hyperchromasia (*arrow*).

at 6-monthly intervals until either the dysplasia disappears (but this could merely be a sampling problem) or high-grade dysplasia is seen. However, some physicians now recommend colectomy even for low-grade dysplasia.

One study examined the role of flow cytometry as a means of detecting DNA aneuploidy in a rectal biopsy.[132] The correlation between aneuploidy and dysplasia is good, but the number of patients who show aneuploidy in the absence of histologic dysplasia seems to be small. However, once aneuploidy occurs, it appears to persist and may therefore be more readily detectable than dysplasia on repeat colonoscopy.

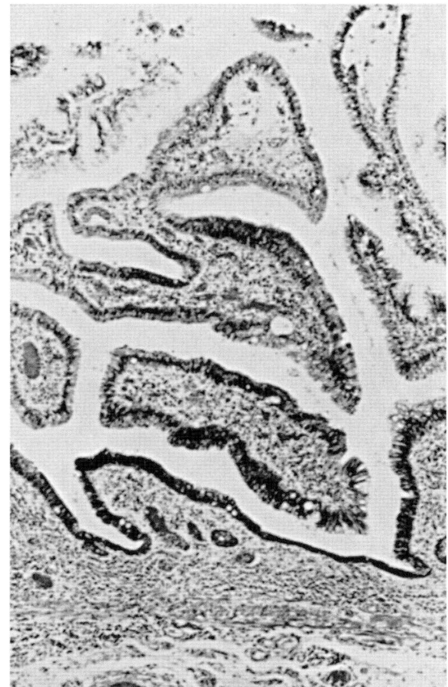

Figure 104–17. High-grade dysplasia in a patient with a 22-year history of ulcerative colitis. There is loss of glands. hyperchromasia, and nuclear stratification. The mucosa shows a marked villous pattern.

INDICATIONS FOR SURGERY AND CHOICE OF OPERATION

The indications for colectomy are as follows:

1. Severe attacks that fail to respond to medical therapy.
2. Complications of a severe attack (e.g., perforation, acute dilatation).
3. Chronic continuous disease with an impaired quality of life.
4. Dysplasia or carcinoma.

The choice of operation includes proctocolectomy with a permanent Brooke ileostomy, proctocolectomy with an ileoanal pouch, or colectomy with an ileorectal anastomosis. This last operation is rarely performed now, largely because many patients continue to have attacks of colitis with urgency and fear of incontinence; in addition, they usually have frequency of stooling and are at risk of carcinoma in the rectal stump. Proctocolectomy with a permanent ileostomy is the operation of choice for elderly persons, those with impaired anal sphincter pressures, and those who do not wish to have a restorative proctocolectomy. Restorative proctocolectomy with an ileoanal pouch is now the operation of choice for most patients with colitis who require colectomy, but it is best performed in centers with considerable experience in the operation and the management of pouch dysfunction (see Chapter 105).

COURSE AND PROGNOSIS

Most patients (80%) with ulcerative colitis have intermittent attacks of their disease, but the length of remission varies considerably from a few weeks to many years. From 10% to 15% of patients pursue a chronic continuous course, and the remainder have a severe first attack requiring urgent colectomy.[133] Few, if any, patients have only one attack. In a large study from Copenhagen, a relapse-free course was found in only 1% of patients after 18 years from the time of presentation.[134]

The extent of disease determines in part the severity and

therefore the course of disease. Patients with extensive or total colitis are more likely to have severe attacks than are those with more limited disease, and the colectomy rate is correspondingly higher. In the Copenhagen series,[134] one third of patients presenting with total colitis had a colectomy within the first year compared with less than 8% of patients with more limited disease. However, once the first year has passed, the subsequent course of the disease seems similar for all patients regardless of the extent of involvement. The colectomy rate then appears to be about 1% per year.

Patients with proctitis (i.e., disease limited to the rectum) are a special group. In general, they have a benign course, but in many of them, more extensive disease develops with time. Powell-Tuck and coworkers[135] showed that 11% of patients with proctitis had extended disease after 5 years, 19% after 10 years, and 29% after 19 years of follow-up. However, 70% continued to have only rectal involvement. Similar data have been published from Copenhagen. The Danish study also recognized that extensive disease can regress to more distal involvement.

Despite having a chronic intermittent disease, the majority of patients (90%) are able to work and miss only a few days each year. Nevertheless, quality of life is impaired, at least to a degree, in many patients.[136] During episodes of active disease, urgency of defecation, lassitude, and pain (abdominal and rectal) are the major symptoms that limit everyday living activities. Sexual problems and marriage difficulties are also common, although a carefully controlled study from Denmark showed little difference in marital problems or physical or social activity between patients with colitis and those with other acute illnesses.[137] When colitis is in remission, most of these problems disappear. However, many patients remain anxious because of the fear of relapse and the need for continuing treatment and medical supervision. Many alter their life-styles with respect to daily activity, travel, and diet. Nevertheless, with supportive medical care and prompt treatment of active disease, the majority of patients are able to live a normal life most of the time. Patient self-help groups have proved of tremendous value, not only for education and fundraising, but also for providing an environment where patients can regain their confidence and overcome the problem of isolation engendered by an uncommon disease with unpleasant and unsociable symptoms. The development of indices to measure quality of life[138] may provide additional useful information in the assessment of new therapies.

Mortality from ulcerative colitis has diminished dramatically since the introduction of glucocorticoids and the use of maintenance therapy with sulfasalazine. Figure 104–12 shows that the mortality rate for a severe attack of ulcerative colitis has fallen from about 37% in the preglucocorticoid era to less than 2% at the present time, a figure that includes mortality from urgent colectomy. In the longer term, survival differs little from expected in the United States and Europe.[139–141] One large study from Sweeden[142] showed a trend toward excess mortality, especially from unrelated disease, but this finding has not been noted in other series and may be explained by an unusually low mortality rate in the Swedish control population. Unfortunately, these low mortality rates and a consequent normal life expectancy for the great majority of patients with ulcerative colitis have not been accepted by life insurance companies, which continue to charge excessively high premiums to these patients. Patients frequently need strong support from their physicians to obtain more realistic premiums.

ULCERATIVE COLITIS IN PREGNANCY

There is considerable concern about pregnancy in young women with ulcerative colitis. However, when large populations of women with ulcerative colitis have been studied, a reassuring picture emerges.[143–146] The women appear to have no difficulty conceiving and are not at increased risk of having a spontaneous abortion. Moreover, there is no good evidence that pregnancy is a risk factor for relapse nor that relapse is frequent in the puerperium. Women with ulcerative colitis usually produce healthy babies, and the disease has no adverse effect on the developing fetus. Furthermore, glucocorticoids, sulfasalazine, and even azathioprine appear to be safe during pregnancy. Therefore, there is no medical indication to stop maintenance therapy if a female patient becomes pregnant. Methotrexate, however, is teratogenic and contraindicated. Relapses of the disease during pregnancy must be treated aggressively if a quick remission is to be attained.

ULCERATIVE COLITIS IN CHILDHOOD

The incidence of ulcerative colitis in children is considerably lower than that in adults and, for the United Kingdom, is about 10 per 100,000.[147] The mean age of presentation is around 10 years, but the disease can present within the first few months of life. Usual symptoms include diarrhea, rectal bleeding, abdominal pain, and failure to thrive.[148, 149] Poor growth as the predominant presenting symptom seems less common than in Crohn's disease. Unfortunately, diagnosis is often delayed especially in babies and toddlers because symptoms are often attributed to milk allergy or toddler's diarrhea without proper investigation of the child. The diagnostic process should be identical to that described earlier for adults.

The clinical picture and course of ulcerative colitis in children are the same as those in adults, although the proportion of children having total colitis is higher, approximately 50% compared with only 25% to 30% of adults. The spectrum of extraintestinal manifestations is also similar to that in adults, although these manifestations are said to be less common in children.

Treatment should be guided by the same principles as described above for adults, although drug doses require adjustments according to weight.[148, 150] Active disease must be treated aggressively using systemic and topical glucocorticoids, and remission then should be maintained with a 5-ASA drug. Immunosuppressive therapy should be reserved for patients with chronic active disease who require repeated courses of glucocorticoids. One of the major problems of management is to establish satisfactory growth. Control of the disease achieves this, but in children with chronic "grumbling" disease, growth can be suppressed not only by the disease, but also by the prolonged use of glucocorticoids. An alternate-day regimen of glucocorticoids can be helpful. Because it is important to identify children with growth retardation, both height and weight must be plotted on appropriate growth charts at every outpatient visit.

One of the most important emphases in management is nutrition.[151] Many children have been shown to be deficient in the intake of calories, as well as of vitamins and minerals. Therefore, it is essential for a dietitian to interview the child's primary caregiver to have a precise analysis of dietary intake. Supplements should be given as required, and for adolescents, a total caloric intake of at least 3000 kcal should be achieved.

The course of the disease in children is similar to that in adults and is therefore partly dependent on extent, severity, and duration of disease. Because a greater proportion of children have total colitis, the colectomy rate tends to be higher than in adults. In the St. Bartholomew series, 24% of children with ulcerative colitis had colectomy by 17 years of age.[151] Indications for surgery are similar to those described in adults, with the addition of growth failure, although this is an uncommon indication. Children do well with a restorative proctocolectomy, which should be the operation of choice.[152]

REFERENCES

1. Wilks S: Lectures on Pathological Anatomy. London, Longmans, 1859.
2. Wilks S: Morbid appearances in the intestines of Miss Bankes. Med Times Gazette 264:1859.
3. Hawkins HP: An address on the natural history of ulcerative colitis and its bearing on treatment. BMJ 765:1909.
4. Allchin WH: Ulcerative colitis—symposium and discussion based on 314 cases reported by the London Hospitals. R Soc Med II2:59–82, 1909.
5. Hurst AF: Ulcerative colitis. Guy's Hosp Rep 71:26, 1909.
6. Hurst AF: Ulcerative colitis. Guy's Hosp Rep 85:317, 1935.
7. Felsen J: The relation of bacilliary dysentery to distal iliitis, chronic ulcerative colitis and non-specific intestinal granuloma. Ann Intern Med 10:645, 1936.
8. Felsen J, Wolarsky W: Acute and chronic bacilliary dysentery and chronic ulcerative colitis. JAMA 153:1069, 1953.
9. Mendeloff AI, Calkins BM: The epidemiology of idiopathic inflammatory bowel disease. In Kirsner JB, Shorter RG (eds): Inflammatory Bowel Disease, 4th ed. Philadelphia, Lea and Febiger, 1995, p 31.
10. Satsangi J, Jewell DP, Rosenberg WMC, Bell JI: Genetics of inflammatory bowel disease. Gut 35:696, 1994.
11. Bennett RA, Rubin PH, Present DH: Frequency of inflammatory bowel disease in offspring of couples both presenting with inflammatory bowel disease. Gastroenterology 100(6):1638, 1991.
12. Satsangi J, Grootscholten C, Holt H, Jewell DP: Clinical patterns of familial inflammatory bowel disease. Gut 38:738, 1996.
13. van Heel DA, Satsangi J, Carey AH, Jewell DP: Inflammatory bowel disease: Progress toward a gene. Can J Gastroenterol 14(3):207, 2000.
14. Parkes M, Barmada MM, Satsangi J, et al: The IBD2 locus shows linkage heterogeneity between ulcerative colitis and Crohn's disease. Am J Hum Genet 67:1605, 2000.
15. Cooke EM, Ewins S, Shooter RA: Changing faecal population of *Escherichia coli* in hospital medical patients. BMJ 4(683):593, 1969.
16. Cooke EM, Ewins SP, Hywel Jones J, Lennard-Jones JE: Properties of strains of *Escherichia coli* carried in different phases of ulcerative colitis. Gut 15:143, 1974.
17. Burke DA, Axon AT: Ulcerative colitis and *Escherichia coli* with adhesive properties. J Clin Pathol 40(7):782, 1987.
18. Burke DA, Axon ATR, Clayden SA, et al: The efficacy of tobramycin in the treatment of UC. Aliment Pharmacol Ther 4:123, 1990.
19. Rembacken BJ, Snelling AM, Hawkey PM, et al: Non-pathogenic *Escherichia coli* versus mesalazine for the treatment of ulcerative colitis: A randomised trial. Lancet 354(9179):635, 1999.
20. Shanahan F: Probiotics and inflammatory bowel disease: Is there a scientific rationale? Inflamm Bowel Dis 6(2):107, 2000.
21. Andresen AFR: Ulcerative colitis—an allergic phenomenon. Am J Dig Dis 9:91, 1942.
22. Truelove SC: Ulcerative colitis provoked by milk. BMJ 1:154, 1961.
23. Wright R, Truelove SC: A controlled therapeutic trial of various diets in ulcerative colitis. BMJ ii:138, 1965.
24. McIntyre PB, Powell-Tuck J, Wood SR, et al: Controlled trial of bowel rest in the treatment of severe ulcerative colitis. Gut 27:481, 1986.
25. Lindberg E, Tysk C, Andersson K, Jarnerot G: Smoking and inflammatory bowel disease. A case control study. Gut 29(3):352, 1988.
26. Cope GF, Heatley RV, Kelleher J, Axon ATR: In vitro mucus glycoprotein production by colonic tissue from patients with ulcerative colitis. Gut 29:229, 1986.
27. Srivastava ED, Russell MA, Feyerabend C, Rhodes J: Effect of ulcerative colitis and smoking on rectal blood flow. Gut 31(9):1021, 1990.
28. Prytz H, Benoni C, Tagesson d: Does smoking tighten the gut? Scand J Gastroenterol 24(9):1084, 1989.
29. Vessey M, Jewell DP, Smith A, et al: Chronic inflammatory bowel disease, cigarette smoking and use of oral contraceptives: Findings in a large cohort study of women of childbearing age. BMJ 292:1101, 1986.
30. Rutgeerts P, D'Haens G, Hiele M, et al: Appendectomy protects against ulcerative colitis. Gastroenterology 106(5):1251, 1994.
31. Smithson JE, Radford-Smith G, Jewell DP: Appendectomy and tonsillectomy in patients with inflammatory bowel disease. J Clin Gastroenterol 21(4):283, 1995.
32. Scott MG, Nahm MH, Macke K, et al: Spontaneous secretion of IgG subclasses by intestinal mononuclear cells: Differences between ulcerative colitis, Crohn's disease, and controls. Clin Exp Immunol 66(1): 209, 1986.
33. Kett K, Rognum TO, Brandtzaeg P: Mucosal subclass distribution of immunoglobulin G–producing cells is different in ulcerative colitis and Crohn's disease of the colon. Gastroenterology 93(5):919, 1987.
34. Halstensen TS, Mollnes TE, Garred P, et al: Epithelial deposition of immunoglobulin G1 and activated complement (C3b and terminal complement complex) in ulcerative colitis. Gastroenterology 98(5 Pt 1):1264, 1990.
35. Snook JA, Silva HJD, Jewell DP: The association of autoimmune disorders with inflammatory bowel disease. Q J Med New Series 72(269):835, 1989.
36. Takahasi F, Das d: Isolation and characterisation of a colon autoantigen specifically recognised by colon tissue bound immunoglobulin from idiopathic ulcerative colitis. J Clin Invest 76:311, 1985.
37. Das KM, Vecchi M, Sakamaki S: A shared and unique epitope(s) on human colon, skin, and biliary epithelium detected by a monoclonal antibody. Gastroenterology 98(2):464, 1990.
38. Shanahan F: Neutrophil autoantibodies in inflammatory bowel disease: Are they important? Gastroenterology 107(2):586, 1994.
39. Terjung B, Spengler U, Sauerbruch T, Worman HJ: "Atypical p-ANCA" in IBD and hepatobiliary disorders react with a 50-kilodalton nuclear envelope protein of neutrophils and myeloid cell lines. Gastroenterology 119(2):310, 2000.
40. Senju M, Wu KC, Mahida YR, Jewell DP: Two-colour immunofluorescence and flow cytometry analysis of lamina propria lymphocyte subsets in ulcerative colitis and Crohn's disease. Dig Dis Sci 36:1453, 1991.
41. Gibson PR, van de Pol E, Pullman W, Doe WF: Lysis of colonic epithelial cells by allogeneic mononuclear and lymphokine activated killer cells derived from peripheral blood and intestinal mucosa: Evidence against a pathogenic role in inflammatory bowel disease. Gut 29(8):1076, 1988.
42. Dalton HR, Hoang P, Jewell DP: Antigen-induced suppression in peripheral blood and lamina propria mononuclear cells in inflammatory bowel disease. Gut 33:324, 1992.
43. Fais S, Pallone F, Squarcia O, et al: T cell early activation antigens expressed by peripheral lymphocytes in Crohn's disease. J Clin Lab Immunol 16(2):75, 1985.
44. Raedler A, Fraenkel S, Klose G, Thiele HG: Elevated numbers of peripheral T cells in inflammatory bowel diseases displaying T9 antigen and Fc alpha receptors. Clin Exp Immunol 60(3):518, 1985.
45. Trejdosiewicz LK, Smart CJ, Oakes DJ, et al: Expression of T-cell receptors TcR1 (gamma/delta) and TcR2 (alpha/beta) in the human intestinal mucosa. Immunology 68(1):7, 1989.
46. Hoang P, Crotty B, Dalton HR, Jewell DP: Epithelial cells bearing Class II molecules stimulate allogeneic human colonic intraepithelial lymphocytes. Gut 33:1089, 1992.

47. Hoang P, Dalton HR, Jewell DP: Human colonic intra-epithelial lymphocytes are suppressor cells. Clin Exp Immunol 85:498, 1991.
48. Mahida YR: Macrophage function in inflammatory bowel disease. Eur J Gastroenterol Hepatol 2:251, 1990.
49. Grimm MC, Pavli P, Van de Pol E, Doe WF: Evidence for a CD14+ population of monocytes in inflammatory bowel disease mucosa—implications for pathogenesis. Clin Exp Immunol 100(2):291, 1995.
50. Selby WS, Janossy G, Mason DY, Jewell DP: Expression of HLA-DR antigens by colonic epithelium in inflammatory bowel disease. Clin Exp Immunol 53:614, 1983.
51. Mayer L, Schlien R: Evidence for function of Ia molecule on gut epithelial cells in man. J Exp Med 166:1471, 1987.
52. Panja A, Blumberg R, Balk S, Mayer L: CDId is involved in T-cell–epithelial cell interactions. J Exp Med 178:1115, 1993.
53. Wakefield AJ, Sankey EA, Dhillon AP, et al: Granulomatous vasculitis in Crohn's disease. Gastroenterology 100(5 Pt 1):1279, 1991.
54. Boughton-Smith N, Pettipher R: Lipid mediators and cytokines in inflammatory bowel disease. Eur J Gastroenterol Hepatol 2:241, 1990.
55. Allan A, Bristol JB, Williamson Rd: Crypt cell production rate in ulcerative proctocolitis: Differential increments in remission and relapse. Gut 26(10):999, 1985.
56. Gibson PR, van de Pol E, Barratt PJ, Doe WF: Ulcerative colitis—a disease characterised by the abnormal colonic epithelial cell? Gut 29(4):516, 1988.
57. Podolsky DK, Isselbacher KJ: Glycoprotein composition of colonic mucosa. Specific alterations in ulcerative colitis. Gastroenterology 87: 991, 1984.
58. Tysk C, Riedesel H, Lindberg E, et al: Colonic glycoproteins in monozygotic twins with inflammatory bowel disease. Gastroenterology 100:419, 1991.
59. Drossman DA: Psychological aspects of ulcerative colitis and Crohn's disease. In Kirsner JB, Shorter RG (eds): Inflammatory Bowel Disease. Philadelphia, Lea & Febiger, 1988, p 209.
60. Olbrisch ME, Ziegler SW: Psychological adjustment to inflammatory bowel disease: Informational control and private self-consciousness. J Chronic Dis 35(7):573, 1982.
61. Whitehead R: Ulcerative colitis. In Whitehead R (ed): Gastrointestinal and Oesophageal Pathology. Edinburgh, Churchill Livingstone, 1989, p 522.
62. Surawicz CM, Belic L: Rectal biopsy helps to distinguish acute self-limited colitis from idiopathic inflammatory bowel disease. Gastroenterology 86(1):104, 1984.
63. Allison MC, Hamilton-Dutoit SJ, Dhillon AP, Pounder RE: The value of rectal biopsy in distinguishing self-limited colitis from early inflammatory bowel disease. Q J Med 65(248):985, 1987.
64. Both H, Torp-Pedersen K, Kreiner S, et al: Clinical appearance at diagnosis of ulcerative colitis and Crohn's disease in a regional patient group. Scand J Gastroenterol 18(7):987, 1983.
65. Rao SS, Holdsworth CD, Read NW: Symptoms and stool patterns in patients with ulcerative colitis. Gut 29(3):342, 1988.
66. Sandle GI, Higgs N, Crowe P, et al: Cellular basis for defective electrolyte transport in inflamed human colon. Gastroenterology 99(1): 97, 1990.
67. Rao SS, Read NW, Davison PA, et al: Anorectal sensitivity and responses to rectal distention in patients with ulcerative colitis. Gastroenterology 93(6):1270, 1987.
68. Rao SS, Read NW, Brown C, et al: Studies on the mechanism of bowel disturbance in ulcerative colitis. Gastroenterology 93(5):934, 1987.
69. Truelove SC, Witts LJ: Cortisone in ulcerative colitis—final report on a therapeutic trial. BMJ 2:1041, 1955.
70. Rachmilewitz D: Coated mesalazine (5-aminosalicylic acid) versus sulphasalazine in the treatment of active ulcerative colitis: A randomised trial. BMJ 298:82, 1989.
71. Baron JH, Connell AM, Lennard-Jones JE: Variation between observers in describing mucosal appearances in proctocolitis. BMJ 1:89, 1964.
72. Truelove SC, Richards WRD: Biopsy studies in ulcerative colitis. BMJ 1:1315, 1956.
73. Buckell NA, Lennard-Jones JE, Hernandez MA, et al: Measurement of serum proteins during attacks of UC as a guide to patient management. Gut 20:22, 1979.
74. Prantera C, Davoli M, Lorenzetti R, et al: Clinical and laboratory indicators of extent of ulcerative colitis. Serum C-reactive protein helps the most. J Clin Gastroenterol 10(1):41, 1988.
75. Pera A, Bellando P, Caldera D, et al: Colonoscopy in inflammatory bowel disease. Diagnostic accuracy and proposal of an endoscopic score. Gastroenterology 92(1):181, 1987.
76. Carbonnel F, Lavergne A, Lemann M, et al: Colonoscopy of acute colitis: A safe and reliable tool for assessment of severity. Dig Dis Sci 39(7):1550, 1994.
77. Loose HW, Williams CB: Barium enema versus colonoscopy. Proc R Soc Med 67(10):1033, 1974.
78. Buckell NA, Williams GT, Bartram CI, Lennard-Jones JE: Depth of ulceration in acute colitis. Correlation with outcome and clinical and radiological features. Gastroenterology 79:19, 1980.
79. Stack BH, Smith T, Jones JH, Fletcher J: Measurement of blood and iron loss in colitis with a whole-body counter. Gut 10(10):769, 1969.
80. Hodgson HJF, Jewell DP: The humoral immune system in inflammatory bowel disease. II. Immunoglobulin levels. Am J Dig Dis 23:123, 1978.
81. Austin CA, Cann PA, Jones TH, Holdsworth CD: Exacerbation of diarrhoea and pain in patients treated with 5-aminosalicylic acid for ulcerative colitis [letter]. Lancet 1(8382):917, 1984.
82. Campbell AP, Cobb CA, Chapman RW, et al: Cap polyposis—an unusual cause of diarrhoea. Gut 34(4):562, 1993.
83. Snook J, Jewell DP: Management of the extra-intestinal manifestations of ulcerative colitis and Crohn's disease. Semin Gastrointest Dis 2: 115, 1991.
84. Orchard TR, Wordsworth BP, Jewell DP: Peripheral arthropathies in inflammatory bowel disease: Their articular distribution and natural history. Gut 42(3):387, 1998.
85. Duerr RH, Targan SR, Landers CJ, et al: Neutrophil cytoplasmic antibodies: A link between primary sclerosing cholangitis and ulcerative colitis. Gastroenterology 100:1385, 1991.
86. Narumi S, Roberts JP, Emond JC, et al: Liver transplantation for sclerosing cholangitis. Hepatology 22(2):451, 1995.
87. Wiesner RH, Grambsch PM, Dickson ER, et al: Primary sclerosing cholangitis: Natural history, prognostic factors and survival analysis. Hepatology 10(4):430, 1989.
88. Farrant JM, Hayllar KM, Wilkinson ML, et al: Natural history and prognostic variables in primary sclerosing cholangitis. Gastroenterology 100(6):1710, 1991.
89. Jones HW, Grogono J, Hoare AM: Acute colitis in a district general hospital. BMJ (Clin Res Ed) 294(6573):683, 1987.
90. Baron JH, Connell AM, Kanaghinis TG, et al: Outpatient treatment of ulcerative colitis: Comparison between three doses of oral prednisolone. BMJ 2:441, 1962.
91. Jewell DP: Corticosteroids for the management of ulcerative colitis and Crohn's disease. Gastroenterol Clin North Am 18(1):21, 1989.
92. Meyers S, Sachar DB, Goldberg JD, Janowitz Hd: Corticotropin versus hydrocortisone in the intravenous treatment of ulcerative colitis. A prospective, randomized, double-blind clinical trial. Gastroenterology 85(2):351, 1983.
93. Danielsson A, Hellers G, Lyrenas E, et al: A controlled randomized trial of budesonide versus prednisolone retention enemas in active distal ulcerative colitis. Scand J Gastroenterol 22(8):987, 1987.
94. Ireland A, Priddle JD, Jewell DP: Acetylation of 5-aminosalicylic acid by human colonic epithelial cells. Gastroenterology 90:1471, 1986.
95. Misiewicz JJ, Lennard-Jones JE, Connell AM, et al: Controlled trial of sulphasalazine in maintenance therapy of ulcerative colitis. Lancet 1: 185, 1965.
96. Dissanayake AS, Truelove SC: A controlled therapeutic trial of long-term maintenance treatment of ulcerative colitis with sulphasalazine (Salazopyrin). Gut 14:923, 1973.
97. Ireland A, Jewell DP: Sulphasalazine and the new salicylates. Eur J Gastroenterol Hepatol 1:43, 1989.
98. Das KM, Eastwood MA, McManus JP, Sircus W: Adverse reactions during salicylazosulfapyridine therapy and the relation with drug metabolism and acetylator phenotype. N Engl J Med 289(10):491, 1973.
99. Azad Khan AK, Howes DT, Piris J, Truelove SC: Optimum dose of sulphasalazine for maintenance treatment in ulcerative colitis. Gut 21(3):232, 1980.
100. Azad Khan AK, Piris J, Truelove SC: An experiment to determine the active therapeutic moiety of sulphasalazine. Lancet 2(8044):892, 1977.
101. Sutherland LR, May GR, Shaffer EA: Sulphasalazine revisited: A meta-analysis of 5-aminosalicylic acid in the treatment of ulcerative colitis. Ann Intern Med 118:540, 1993.
102. Courtney MG, Nunes DP, Bergin CF, et al: Randomised comparison of olsalazine and mesalazine in prevention of relapses in ulcerative colitis [see comments]. Lancet 339(8804):1279, 1992.

103. Campieri M, Gionchetti P, Belluzzi A, et al: Optimum dosage of 5-aminosalicylic acid as rectal enemas in patients with active ulcerative colitis. Gut 32:929, 1991.
104. Marshall JK, Irvine EJ: Rectal aminosalicylate therapy for distal ulcerative colitis: A meta-analysis. Aliment Pharmacol Ther 9(3):293, 1995.
105. Mulder CJ, Fockens P, Meijer JW, et al: Beclomethasone dipropionate (3 mg) versus 5-aminosalicylic acid (2 g) versus the combination of both (3 mg/2 g) as retention enemas in active ulcerative proctitis. Eur J Gastroenterol Hepatol 8(6):549, 1996.
106. Biddle WL, Greenberger NJ, Swan JT, et al: 5-Aminosalicylic acid enemas: Effective agent in maintaining remission in left-sided ulcerative colitis [published erratum appears in Gastroenterology 96(6):1630, 1989]. Gastroenterology 94(4):1075, 1988.
107. Campieri M, Lanfranchi GA, Bazzocchi G, et al: Treatment of ulcerative colitis with high-dose 5-aminosalicylic acid enemas. Lancet 2(8241):270, 1981.
108. Kirk AP, Lennard-Jones JE: Controlled trial of azathioprine in chronic ulcerative colitis. BMJ (Clin Res Ed) 284(6325):1291, 1982.
109. Jewell DP, Truelove SC: Azathioprine in ulcerative colitis: Final report on a controlled therapeutic trial. BMJ IV:627, 1974.
110. Lichtiger S: Cyclosporin therapy in inflammatory bowel disease: Open label experience. Mt Sinai J Med 57:315, 1990.
111. Sandborn WJ, Tremaine WJ, Schroeder KW, et al: A placebo-controlled trial of cyclosporine enemas for mildly to moderately active left-sided ulcerative colitis. Gastroenterology 106(6):1429, 1994.
112. Lichtiger S, Present DH: Preliminary report: Cyclosporin in treatment of severe active ulcerative colitis. Lancet 336:16, 1990.
113. Winter TA, Dalton HR, Merrett NM, et al: Cyclosporin A retention enemas in refractory distal ulcerative colitis and "pouchitis." Scand J Gastroenterol 28:701, 1993.
114. Truelove SC, Watkinson G, Draper G: Comparison of corticosteroid and sulphasalazine in ulcerative colitis. BMJ 2:1708, 1962.
115. Truelove SC, Jewell DP: Intensive intravenous regimen for severe attacks of ulcerative colitis. Lancet i:1067, 1974.
116. Jarnerot G, Rolny P, Sandberg Gertzen N: Intensive intravenous treatment of ulcerative colitis. Gastroenterology 89:1005, 1985.
117. Travis SPL, Farrant JM, Ricketts C, et al: Predicting outcome in severe ulcerative colitis. Gut 38:905, 1996.
118. Jewell DP, Caprilli R, Mortensen N, et al: Indications and timing for surgery for severe ulcerative colitis. Gastroenterol Int 4(4):161, 1991.
119. Lennard-Jones JE, Ritchie JR, Hilder W, Spicer CC: Assessment of severity in colitis: A preliminary study. Gut 16:579, 1975.
120. Chew CN, Nolan DN, Jewell DP: Small bowel gas in severe ulcerative colitis. Gut 32:1535, 1991.
121. Greenstein AJ, Aufses AH Jr: Differences in pathogenesis, incidence and outcome of perforation in inflammatory bowel disease. Surg Gynecol Obstet 160(1):63, 1985.
122. Bartram CI: Ulcerative colitis. In Radiology in Inflammatory Bowel Disease. New York, Marcel Decker, 1983, p 31.
123. Caprilli R, Vernia P, Latella G, Torsoli A: Early recognition of toxic megacolon. J Clin Gastroenterol 9(2):160, 1987.
124. Grant CS, Dozois RR: Toxic megacolon: Ultimate fate of patients after successful medical management. Am J Surg 147(1):106, 1984.
125. Present DH, Wolfson D, Gelernt IM, et al: Medical decompression of toxic megacolon by "rolling." A new technique of decompression with favorable long-term follow-up. J Clin Gastroenterol 10(5):485, 1988.
126. De Dombal FT, Watts JM, Watkinson G, Goligher JC: Local complications of ulcerative colitis: Stricture, pseudopolyposis, and carcinoma of colon and rectum. BMJ 5501:1442, 1966.
127. Eaden J, Abrams K, Ekbom A, et al: Colorectal cancer prevention in ulcerative colitis: A case-control study. Aliment Pharmacol Ther 14(2):145, 2000.
128. Gyde SN: Cancer in ulcerative colitis: What is the risk and is screening effective in saving lives? In O'Morain C (ed): Ulcerative Colitis. Boca Raton, Fla, CRC Press, 1991, p 169.
129. Gyde SN, Prior P, Allan RN, et al: Colorectal cancer in ulcerative colitis: A cohort study of primary referrals from three centres. Gut 29(2):206, 1988.
130. Ekbom A, Helmick C, Zack M, Adami HO: Ulcerative colitis and colorectal cancer. A population-based study. N Engl J Med 323(18): 1228, 1990.
131. Morson BC, Pang LS: Rectal biopsy as an aid to cancer control in ulcerative colitis. Gut 8(5):423, 1967.
132. Collins RH Jr, Feldman M, Fordtran JS: Colon cancer, dysplasia, and surveillance in patients with ulcerative colitis. A critical review. N Engl J Med 316(26):1654, 1987.
133. Riddell RH, Goldman H, Rasnsohoff DF, et al: Standardised nomenclature, terminology and criteria for dysplasia in inflammatory bowel disease with recommendations for patient management. Hum Pathol 14:931, 1983.
134. Hendrikson C, Kreiner S, Binder V: Long-term prognosis in ulcerative colitis based on results from a regional patient group from the Country of Copenhagen. Gut 26:158, 1985.
135. Powell-Tuck J, Ritchie JK, Lennard-Jones JE: The prognosis of idiopathic proctitis. Scand J Gastroenterol 12(6):727, 1977.
136. Mallett SJ, Lennard-Jones JE, Bingley J, Gilon E: Colitis. Lancet 2(8090):619, 1978.
137. Hendriksen C, Binder V: Social prognosis in patients with ulcerative colitis. BMJ 281(6240):581, 1980.
138. Irvine EJ, Feagan B, Rochon J, et al: Quality of life: A valid and reliable measure of therapeutic efficacy in the treatment of inflammatory bowel disease. Canadian Crohn's Relapse Prevention Trial Study Group. Gastroenterology 106(2):287, 1994.
139. Stonnington CM, Phillips SF, Zinsmeister AR, Melton LJD: Prognosis of chronic ulcerative colitis in a community. Gut 28(10):1261, 1987.
140. Sinclair TS, Brunt PW, Mowat NA: Nonspecific proctocolitis in northeastern Scotland: A community study. Gastroenterology 85(1):1, 1983.
141. Ritchie JK, Powell-Tuck J, Lennard-Jones JE: Clinical outcome of the first ten years of ulcerative colitis and proctitis. Lancet 1(8074):1140, 1978.
142. Brostrom O, Monsen U, Nordenwall B, et al: Prognosis and mortality of ulcerative colitis in Stockholm County, 1955–1979. Scand J Gastroenterol 22(8):907, 1987.
143. Willoughby CP, Truelove SC: Ulcerative colitis and pregnancy. Gut 21(6):469, 1980.
144. Baiocco PJ, Korelitz BI: The influence of inflammatory bowel disease and its treatment on pregnancy and fetal outcome. J Clin Gastroenterol 6(3):211, 1984.
145. Nielsen OH, Andreasson B, Bondesen S, Jarnum S: Pregnancy in ulcerative colitis. Scand J Gastroenterol 18(6):735, 1983.
146. Willoughby CP: Inflammatory bowel disease and pregnancy. In Allan RN, Keighley MRB, Alexander-Williams J, Hawkins CF (eds): Inflammatory Bowel Diseases. Edinburgh, Churchill Livingstone, 1990, p 547.
147. Evans CM, Beattie RM, Walker-Smith JA: Inflammatory bowel disease in children. In Allan RN, Rhodes JM, Hanauer SB, et al (eds): Inflammatory Bowel Diseases, 3rd ed. Edinburgh, Churchill Livingstone, 1997, pp 647–670.
148. Grand RJ, Ramakrishna J, Calenda KA: Inflammatory bowel disease in the pediatric patient. Gastroenterol Clin North Am 24(3):613, 1995.
149. Chong SK, Walker-Smith JA: Ulcerative colitis in childhood. J R Soc Med 77(suppl 3):21, 1984.
150. Evans CM, Walker-Smith JA: Inflammatory bowel disease in childhood. In Allan RN, Keighley MRB, Alexander-Williams J, Hawkins CF (eds): Inflammatory Bowel Diseases. Edinburgh, Churchill Livingstone, 1990, p 523.
151. Motil KJ, Grand RJ: Nutritional management of inflammatory bowel disease. Pediatr Clin North Am 32(2):447, 1985.
152. Telander RL, Spencer M, Perrault J, et al: Long-term follow-up of the ileoanal anastomosis in children and young adults [discussion 23-5]. Surgery 108(4):717, 1990.

Chapter 105

Ileostomy and Its Alternatives

John H. Pemberton and Sidney F. Phillips

Proctocolectomy and permanent ileostomy return most patients with chronic ulcerative colitis to excellent health and remove premalignant mucosa in patients with either chronic ulcerative colitis or familial adenomatous polyposis (FAP). Many of the former inconveniences and dangers associated with an ileal stoma have been eliminated by improved surgical techniques, a wider range of better stomal appliances, and more effective education of patients.[1]

Between 1930 and 1950, the metabolic consequences of ileostomy became more apparent, as did the frequent mechanical complications caused by "ileostomy dysfunction." Better understanding of fluid, electrolyte, and blood replacement provided answers to the first problem; new construction of ileostomies resolved the second problem.[2, 3] Before these advances, ileostomies were made by withdrawal of the intestine through the abdominal wall, with suturing of the serosal surface to the skin. Ileostomy dysfunction resulted from the (not unexpected) serositis that follows exposure of ileal serosa to stomal effluent. However, the *mucosa* of the ileum should not be susceptible to such inflammation, and a solution was therefore conceptually simple: Evert the mucosal surface of the bud and suture the mucosa to the skin. Described simultaneously in the United Kingdom and the United States, this modification is commonly referred to as a *Brooke ileostomy* (Fig. 105–1). Development of new ileostomy appliances quickly led to better acceptance by patients and, ultimately, to the excellent long-term results provided by an ileostomy that are now expected.[4] Enterostomal therapy was introduced in the 1960s as an additional allied health support, and ileostomy societies have blossomed in most countries and provide a lay component of support to treatment.

Of course, Brooke ileostomies were incontinent by definition. During the 1960s, the first effective alternative to the incontinent ileostomy was developed.[5] This "Kock pouch" procedure featured an ileal pouch, a nipple valve, and an ileal conduit, which led to a cutaneous stoma that, because an appliance was not needed, could be made flush with the skin. Sufficient clinical experience accumulated, and the technique was used in selected patients with ulcerative colitis and FAP.[6]

Stimulated by patients' acceptance, surgeons explored other alternatives to the incontinent ileal stoma, with its ever-present bag. The ileoanal pull-through operation was resurrected,[7] with an important technical modification—the addition of an ileal reservoir.[8] This procedure offered the advantages of a normal flow of stool and preservation of the anal sphincters. Several forms of the ileoanal pouch anastomosis (IPAA) are now advocated by different surgical groups. Indeed, the nearly universal use of this procedure in thousands of patients has actually elevated IPAA past the Brooke ileostomy as the procedure of choice in most patients who require proctocolectomy for ulcerative colitis or FAP.

Although the Brooke ileostomy had become the usual operation after a colectomy in the United Kingdom and the United States, in continental Europe and South America, ileorectostomy was standard. Indeed, these different attitudes continue to influence approaches to the newer operations. This chapter details the pathophysiologic and clinical implications of colectomy per se and describes the options for control of enteric content. Thus, three different operations constitute the realistic surgical options for total colectomy in patients with ulcerative colitis and FAP: (1) proctocolectomy with the terminal Brooke ileostomy, (2) one of the varieties of IPAA, and (3) ileorectostomy. These recommendations are modified when the diagnosis is Crohn's colitis, for which the Kock pouch and IPAA are contraindicated but the option of segmental colectomy is available.

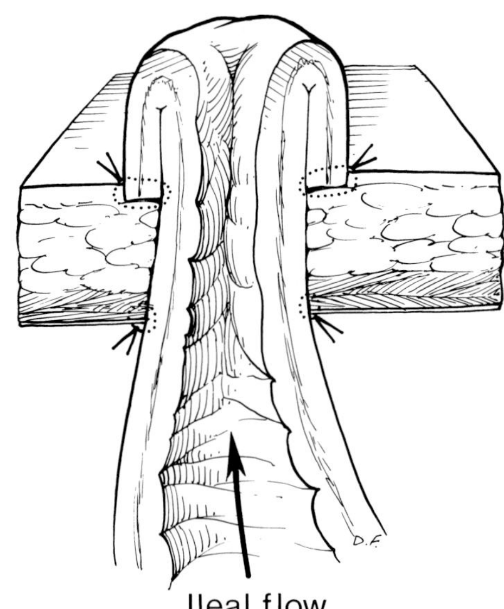

Figure 105–1. Anatomy of the Brooke ileostomy. The mucosa is everted and sewn to the skin. No serosal surface is therefore exposed to intestinal content.

PATHOPHYSIOLOGIC CONSEQUENCES OF PROCTOCOLECTOMY

Fecal Output After Proctocolectomy

After a colectomy and any form of ileostomy, the capacity of the colon to reabsorb electrolytes and water is lost. Usually, this creates no major pathophysiologic disturbance, but some important principles should be remembered. A normal colon absorbs at least 1000 mL (1 L) of water and 100 mEq of sodium chloride each day.[9] More important, these amounts can be augmented; when overloaded progressively, the healthy colon absorbs more than 5 L/day[10] (see Chapter 9). Also, the colon responds to salt depletion by conserving NaCl avidly, but the small intestine has a lesser capacity to adapt in this manner. For example, under conditions of extremely low salt intake, fecal losses of sodium in normal stools can be reduced to 1 or 2 mEq/day,[11] whereas patients with ileostomies have obligatory losses of sodium of 30 to 40 mEq/day.[12, 13]

Well-functioning conventional (Brooke) ileostomies discharge 300 to 800 g of material daily; 90% of this output is water.[12, 13] Continent ileostomies and IPAAs have similar volumes of effluent.[14] Foods that contain much unabsorbable residue increase the total output by increasing the quantity of solids that are discharged. Although many anecdotal effects of certain foods on the volume and consistency of effluents have been reported, the response to specific foods varies from one patient to another, and changes are usually minimal.[15]

Functional Sequelae

When oral intake of sodium, chloride, and fluid is adequate, patients with ileostomies do not become depleted; however, negative sodium balance may follow periods of diminished oral intake, vomiting, or excessive perspiration.[16] In addition, chronic oliguria is to be anticipated because normal stools contain approximately 100 mL of water,[16, 17] whereas ileostomies lose 500 to 600 mL/day. Patients with ileostomies also have lower Na^+/K^+ ratios in urine owing to compensatory renal conservation of sodium and water. These changes in the composition of urine presumably contribute to the increased frequency of urolithiasis (probably around 5%) in these patients.[18] The stones are composed predominantly of urate or calcium salts.

When an ileostomy is accompanied by resection of the terminal ileum, abnormalities of bile acid reabsorption (see Chapter 9) and malabsorption of vitamin B_{12} may result. Steatorrhea and greater daily losses of fluid (1 L/day or more) also may be seen. However, these abnormalities usually do not follow a colectomy that is performed for ulcerative colitis or FAP because the ileum, being free of disease, is preserved. Resection for Crohn's colitis may require removal of additional diseased ileum with the possible consequences of malabsorption, depending on the length of small bowel removed (see Chapter 92).

Lack of a colon also reduces the exposure of bile acids to the metabolic effects of the fecal flora. After ileostomy, secondary bile acids largely disappear from bile,[19, 20] but no important metabolic consequences have been recognized. The flora of ileostomy effluents has quantitative (10^4 to 10^7 organisms/mL) and qualitative characteristics that are intermediate between those of feces and those of normal ileal contents.[21–23] Moreover, the presence of a reservoir, Kock pouch, or IPAA predisposes to a more fecal-like flora.

The principal pathophysiologic sequelae of colectomy with ileostomy are therefore mainly the potential consequences of a salt-losing state; patients should be advised to use salt liberally and to increase their fluid intake, especially at times of stress, particularly in extremely hot weather and after vigorous exercise. A balanced salt solution (e.g., Gatorade® or Powerade®) is a great source of balanced electrolytes. Clearly, however, the limited ability of the small intestine to absorb sodium and water means that stomal volumes also will increase when oral intake is increased.[13]

OVERALL CLINICAL CONSEQUENCES OF PROCTOCOLECTOMY

After successful surgery, life expectancy is slightly below normal for the first few years owing to complications of the stoma and to intestinal obstruction. After ileorectostomy for FAP or chronic ulcerative colitis, particularly the former, cancer may develop in the retained rectum (see Chapters 104 and 114). In general, however, the long-term mortality rate of patients after proctocolectomy and conventional ileostomy is virtually the same as that of a matched normal population.[24] Ninety percent of patients with conventional ileostomies who responded to a survey rated the results of their operation as excellent and claimed little inconvenience.[4] Almost all were able to lead normal lives and enjoy normal sexual relationships. Certain strenuous physical activities were avoided by a few patients.

The metabolic consequences of a proctocolectomy per se should be no different regardless of whether a conventional ileostomy or an alternative procedure is performed. Patients in whom an ileostomy alternative achieves an excellent result will have a better quality of life than will patients with a stoma because the former will not need to wear a bag constantly. Indeed, when the Brooke ileostomy and IPAA were compared,[25] patients with an IPAA experienced significant advantages in performing daily activities and appeared to experience a better quality of life. However, there are certain special complications of the newer operations, which are discussed later.[14, 26]

COMPLICATIONS AND MANAGEMENT OF CONVENTIONAL ILEOSTOMIES

Major long-term complications of ileostomies relate to malfunctioning, prestomal ileitis, and irritation of the peristomal skin. If the ileostomy was improperly constructed (a less frequent problem with newer techniques), the stoma may become obstructed. *Obstruction* leads to cramping, abdominal pain, increased ileal discharge (up to 4 L/day), and fluid and electrolyte depletion. Excessive ileal output arises, at least in part, from increased intestinal secretion as a result of dilatation of the intestine proximal to the obstructed stoma. Stomal obstruction can usually be demonstrated by examining the stoma with the little finger or by endoscopy with a small sigmoidoscope. X-rays reveal a dilated ileum proximal to the point of obstruction. Many affected ileostomies require reconstruction. At operation, ulcerations are often found in the resected terminal ileum; their pathogenesis is unclear but probably relates in some way to the mechanical consequences of obstruction.

Prestomal ileitis is a much less common problem.[27] Patients with this syndrome exhibit the features of mechanical obstruction but, in addition, have signs of systemic toxicity (e.g., fever, tachycardia, and anemia). The ileal mucosa has numerous punched-out ulcers, sometimes extending to the serosa. It is not clear whether prestomal ileitis has a different pathogenesis from the changes that follow simple mechanical obstruction of the stoma. Both complications may develop in a segment of ileum that was normal histologically at the time of colectomy. "Backwash ileitis" does not seem to predispose the patient to the development of either problem. On the other hand, in patients who have had a colectomy and ileostomy for Crohn's disease, subsequent problems with the ileal stoma are more common and may arise from the spread of transmural inflammation to the new terminal ileum. In some instances, it may be difficult to determine with certainty whether stomal dysfunction is caused by mechanical obstruction or recurrent Crohn's disease.

Most people with an ileostomy lead a normal life and eat a normal diet[4]; poorly digested foods (e.g., nuts, corn, some fruits, lightly cooked vegetables) may obstruct the stoma and should be eaten in moderation, after careful chewing. However, a few patients experience continuing problems with management of the ileostomy. These problems vary in severity; some are minor inconveniences, and others are significant drawbacks to the success of the operation. Mechanical difficulties with a poorly fitting appliance on the stoma may cause excoriation of the skin around the ileostomy or may even erode the stoma to produce a fistula. Occasionally, a peristomal abscess or peristomal hernia may develop, and in a small number of pregnant women, prolapse of the stoma occurs. Some patients have unpleasant odors in the ileostomy bag, especially after eating certain foods such as onions and beans. However, because most odor arises from bacterial action on the contents of the bag, the problem can be controlled by emptying the bag frequently and by adding sodium benzoate or chlorine tablets to the bag. Orally administered bismuth subgallate also controls odor,[28] but doubts exist as to whether its long-term use is justified because questions of toxicity have been raised.[29]

In the handling of these numerous aspects of postoperative care, trained stomal therapists and lay societies of ileostomy patients can be most helpful. Education of the patient is best started before surgery, when meetings with others who have undergone ileostomy and referral to specialized texts can allay many fears and uncertainties.[30, 31]

The United Ostomy Association (19772 MacArthur Blvd., Suite 200, Irvine, CA 92612-2405; telephone 800-826-0826; http://www.uoa.org) publishes an excellent series of booklets dealing with all aspects of life for the ileostomy patient. These materials are also of great help to nursing staffs when registered enterostomal therapists are not available. The locations of therapists can be obtained from the Wound Ostomy and Continence Nurses Society (1550 South Coast Highway, Suite 201, Laguna Beach, CA 92651; telephone 888-224-WOCN; http://www.wocn.org).

CONTINENT ILEOSTOMY (KOCK POUCH)

Clearly, one of the major social drawbacks to an ileostomy could be eliminated if a continent stoma were possible. Nils Kock reasoned that a pouch and nipple valve constructed of terminal ileum could store ileal content internally until emptied voluntarily by passage of a large, soft catheter several times daily,[5] obviating the need for an external appliance (Fig. 105–2). The first such operations were reported in 1969, and the results were promising.[5] However, the nipple valve sometimes failed, usually by slipping out of the pouch,

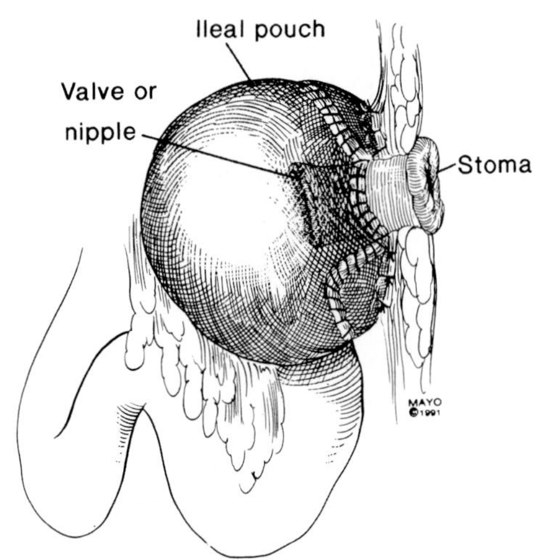

Figure 105–2. The continent ileostomy. The pouch is formed from a loop of ileum, folded on itself as a U, and sutured along the antimesenteric borders. The limbs are then incised, exposing the mucosa, and the nipple valve is fashioned. The pouch is closed and positioned as shown underneath the abdominal wall. Note that the stoma is flush with the skin. (Copyright 1991 by the Mayo Clinic, Rochester, MN.)

thereby leading to incontinence.[32] Techniques gradually improved, and the most recent approaches have been more successful,[33] providing continence in the majority of patients. Two surgical groups with much experience have reported their results.[6, 32] In both series, well over 90% of patients were continent of gas and feces (i.e., they never required a bag). However, this success rate is achieved at the price of additional operations in most patients for nipple or pouch dysfunction, fistula, or stricture.

Long-term follow-up has shown excellent acceptance by the majority of patients with functioning pouches.[6, 32, 33] In as many as one half of all pouches, however, incontinence develops, usually during the first year. Risk factors for incontinence have been examined by the Mayo Clinic group; older, overweight men who have had a conventional ileostomy converted to a pouch are most at risk. Young, nonobese women who have a pouch fashioned as a primary procedure have a risk of nipple valve failure estimated at less than 10%.[6] Nonspecific inflammation, or "pouchitis," developed in as many as 30% of patients with the Kock pouch.[22, 34] The symptoms and signs of Kock pouch pouchitis include abdominal cramps, difficult intubation, increased output, and bleeding from the pouch; these features are comparable with those of pouchitis after IPAA (see the following discussion). Moreover, antibiotics usually relieve symptoms promptly.[22] In the 27 years since the Kock procedure was first performed, there has been only one report of cancer occurring in the pouch.[35] Today, the continent ileostomy operation is primarily of historical interest and is performed rarely. Its use is restricted to patients who have had a proctocolectomy and ileostomy and who desire enteric continence. However, the contributions of Nils Kock to the current surgical approaches to proctocolectomy are legion; they provide the foundation for the current major alternative to ileostomy, the IPAA.

ILEAL POUCH–ANAL ANASTOMOSIS

IPAA is now the procedure of choice for most patients requiring proctocolectomy for either chronic ulcerative colitis or FAP. The procedure is not suitable for patients with Crohn's disease, although this recommendation is now being questioned.[35a] The operation has several major advantages: (1) nearly all mucosal disease is removed (in contrast to ileorectostomy); (2) the normal route of elimination is maintained (a stoma is not required); (3) the anal sphincters are undisturbed; and (4) the pelvic dissection, which is less extensive than that for cancer operations, should not endanger innervation of the sexual organs. The general principle was first described in 1947, and its revival was influenced by the success of local resections performed by pediatric surgeons for Hirschsprung's disease.[7] Early approaches used only a straight pull-through whereby the ileum was sutured directly to the anal verge.[36] Although results in children were encouraging,[37] excessive stool frequency and anal seepage were unacceptable to many adult patients. Subsequently, the operation was modified to include one of several forms of ileal pouch (Fig. 105–3). The principles are as follows: An abdominal colectomy is performed; the distal rectal mucosa is excised from the underlying upper internal anal sphincter and lower rectal muscular cuff, which is left in place; an ileal pouch is fashioned; and the reservoir is sutured to the midanal canal, with the ileal mucosa anastomosed to the anoderm. A diverting ileostomy is usually required for 2 to 3 months until the anastomosis heals completely. At a second operation 8 to 12 weeks later, the diverting ileostomy is closed.

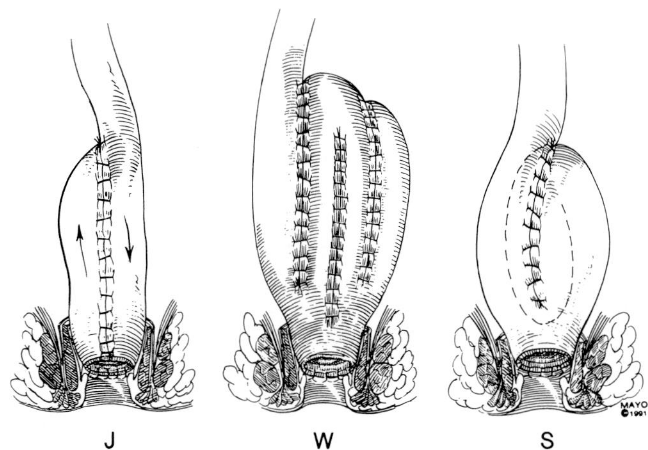

Figure 105–3. Anatomy of the major forms of ileal pouch used for anastomosis to the anal canal (ileal pouch-anal anastomosis). (Copyright 1991 by the Mayo Clinic, Rochester, MN.)

The Mayo Clinic has acquired considerable experience with IPAA. The experience is now at more than 2200 patients.[38, 39, 40] Although pouches of different configurations have been advocated by various surgical groups, techniques are still evolving, and differences among the procedures are likely to be minimal. The most used types—J, W, and S—are shown in Figure 105–3.

Long-Term Results

IPAA is a complex, sophisticated operation, and complications occur frequently. The overall rate of morbidity for all patients still hovers between 25% and 30%. Failure, however, is rare, even in patients who experience a postoperative complication. At the Mayo Clinic, 94% of patients have a successful outcome. It is just as important to understand the complications of restorative proctocolectomy, how to avoid them, and what to do if they occur as it is to know how to select appropriate patients and how to perform the procedure rapidly and accurately. The key to a successful outcome is a surgeon who performs the operation effortlessly; the operation struggled through is the one fraught with complications and sometimes failure.

Complications

Pelvic infection is a serious complication that occurs in the early postoperative period in approximately 5% of patients with ulcerative colitis. Computed tomography (CT) is useful for demonstrating a pelvic fluid collection or phlegmon. Patients with pelvic phlegmon usually respond to conservative treatment with broad-spectrum antibiotics and bowel rest. Patients with a pelvic abscess should undergo CT-guided drainage, if technically feasible, or laparotomy and drainage. The frequency of pelvic abscess is declining owing to increased experience with the procedure and the construction of a shorter rectal muscular cuff.

The frequency of *abdominal sepsis*, which is an ominous development, is 6%. Ultimately, 41% of patients who undergo laparotomy for control of abdominal sepsis require pouch excision. Moreover, normal function is achieved in only 29% of patients who require a reoperation. However, among septic patients who do not require reoperation, but rather undergo aggressive nonsurgical management, 92% have satisfactory pouch function over the long term.

Small bowel obstruction occurs in 17% of patients, 8% of whom require surgical intervention.

Closure of temporary ileostomies is also associated with complications. *Peritonitis* occurs in 4% of patients, and postoperative obstruction occurs in 12%. Proximal and distal *serosal tears* during mobilization of the stoma, in addition to *anastomotic leaks*, are important causes of peritonitis. If all extraperitoneal bowel (afferent and efferent limbs and the stoma itself) is resected, however, the chance of leaving an unrecognized perforation is nearly eliminated.

Nearly all patients have a weblike *stricture* of the ileoanal anastomosis on returning for ileostomy closure. This stricture generally is dilated digitally without difficulty. If the pouch retracts under anastomotic tension, heavy scarring and a long, fibrotic stricture result. This type of stricture is manifested by straining at stool, a sensation of incomplete pouch evacuation, or a high stool frequency (>10 to 12 stools/day). Repeated anal dilatation may prevent progression of the stricture.

Impotence and *retrograde ejaculation* develop in 1.5% and 4% of men, respectively. *Dyspareunia* develops in 7% of women postoperatively. Although 49% of women note sexual dysfunction preoperatively, sexual activity increases dramatically after IPAA because of an improvement in general health.

Clinical Results

Following an IPAA, the average stool frequency during the day is 6 stools, with 1 stool at night. Importantly, daytime and nocturnal stool frequency and the ability to discriminate flatus from stool remain stable over time, whereas the need for stool bulking and hypomotility agents declines. The lower stool frequencies 6 months after surgery compared with the frequency in the early postoperative period are likely attributable to increased pouch capacity over time.

Major fecal incontinence (more than twice per week) occurs in 5% of patients during the day and 12% during sleep. In contrast, minor episodes of nocturnal incontinence occur in up to 30% of patients at least 1 year after the operation. A pad must be worn by 28% of patients for protection against seepage. Minor perianal skin irritation is reported by 63% of patients.

Patients over 50 years of age have a higher daytime stool frequency (8/day) than do patients younger than age 50 (6/day). Men and women have similar stool frequencies postoperatively, but women have more episodes of fecal soilage during the day and night.

Seventy-eight percent of patients with excellent continence at 1 year after surgery remain unchanged at 10 years, 20% experience minor incontinence, and 2% have poor control. Of patients with minor incontinence at 1 year, 40% remain unchanged, 40% improve, and 20% worsen by 10 years. Nocturnal fecal spotting increases during the 10-year period but not significantly.

Pouchitis

A wide range of quoted incidences suggests that the level of clinical suspicion and diagnostic criteria for pouchitis vary greatly.[23, 41, 42] Indeed, most patients with apparent pouchitis have intermittent symptoms or respond well to therapy. However, in a minority, symptoms are severe and persistent enough to lead to surgical removal of the pouch. Patients present with increased volumes of output, bleeding, discomfort from the pouch, and general symptoms similar to those of the initial disease. Fecal incontinence is also common. Classic extraintestinal manifestations in the skin and joints are seen occasionally.[42]

Endoscopy shows the pouch mucosa to be reddened, swollen, and often ulcerated. The mucosa is friable and bleeds readily from minor trauma during endoscopy; inflammatory changes are usually confined to the pouch but also can be seen in the adjacent ileum. Histologically, biopsies show a range of acute and chronic inflammatory changes depending on severity; fever, anemia, and dehydration as a result of diarrhea may be present. A disease activity index combining clinical, endoscopic, and histologic features has been developed (Table 105–1).[43]

Exclusion of other possible etiologies is essential. Patients with ileal pouches are not immune to superimposed specific

Table 105–1 | **Pouchitis Disease Activity Index***

CRITERIA	SCORE
Clinical	
Postoperative stool frequency	
Usual	0
1–2 stools/day more than usual	1
3 or more stools/day more than usual	2
Rectal bleeding	
None or rare	0
Present daily	1
Fecal urgency/abdominal cramps	
None	0
Occasional	1
Usual	2
Fever (temperature >100°F)	
Absent	0
Present	1
Endoscopic	
Edema	1
Granularity	1
Friability	1
Loss of vascular pattern	1
Mucus exudate	1
Ulceration	1
Acute histologic	
Polymorphonuclear leukocyte infiltration	
Mild	1
Moderate + crypt abscess	2
Severe + crypt abscess	3
Ulceration per low-power field (average)	
<25%	1
≥25%, ≤50%	2
>50%	3

***Pouchitis is defined as a total score of ≥7.**

Adapted and reprinted with permission from Sandborn WJ, Tremaine WJ, Batts KP, et al. Mayo Clin Proc 69:409, 1994.[43]

enteric infections, and stool culture and examination for parasites are appropriate. Recurrent Crohn's disease is always a major concern. The clinical features of the underlying inflammatory bowel disease need to be reviewed carefully, including further pathologic examination of the resected bowel. Because a small but definite proportion of colitis falls into an "unclassifiable" group, some patients with previously unrecognized Crohn's disease will present with pouchitis as a manifestation of recurrent Crohn's disease. Surgical complications, such as a strictured anastomosis with partial obstruction to outflow from the pouch, need to be looked for carefully and treated by dilatation if present.

Treatment

If diarrhea alone is the major complaint, treatment with simple antidiarrheal measures may be all that is required. For more severely symptomatic patients, a variety of empirical treatments have emerged. When the condition was first encountered in patients with continent ileostomies,[22] anecdotal evidence suggested that constant drainage would help, on the basis of the assumption that stasis is an important predisposing factor. Stasis should be a lesser factor after IPAA, although incomplete emptying (e.g., with the S pouch) or a persistent anastomotic stricture may need to be excluded. Metronidazole has been used often as a first line of treatment. The response to metronidazole and other broad-spectrum antibiotics is usually dramatic. Some patients relapse after initial therapy with antibiotics and require subsequent courses of treatment. In general, antibacterial agents that have activity against anaerobes have been most successful.

When antibiotics are ineffective, treatment should consist of regimens that are effective in inflammatory bowel disease: glucocorticoid enemas, aminosalicylates, mesalamine enemas, and even systemic glucocorticoids. There is evidence that bismuth subsalicylate (Pepto-Bismol®) is effective in patients with antibiotic-resistant pouchitis. Most patients who are unresponsive to antibiotics will improve on one of these regimens. Severe recurrent disease or major extraintestinal symptoms rarely require removal of the pouch. Patients with preoperative extraintestinal manifestations of chronic ulcerative colitis have significantly higher rates of pouchitis than do patients without such manifestations (39% vs. 26%).[42]

Possible Etiologies

Acute, nonspecific inflammation of ileal pouches apparently reflects the propensity of the patient for inflammatory bowel disease. Thus, pouchitis is much more common in patients for whom the pouch was constructed as treatment for inflammatory bowel disease than it is in patients with FAP. Still, patients operated on for FAP are not completely immune to pouchitis. The nonspecific pathologic features of pouchitis suggest that pouchitis may be an expression of multiple conditions of different etiologies.[44]

The histopathology of healthy and diseased pouches has only recently been examined systematically.[45, 46] Chronic inflammation is usual, even in asymptomatic pouches. The villous architecture is distorted, and colonic metaplasia is present in biopsies from most pouches. Thus, these changes must be considered natural sequelae of the altered anatomy. By analogy with experimental and clinical blind-loop syndromes, these histologic changes have been attributed to bacterial overgrowth (see Chapter 90). These changes develop in experimental pouches of the ileum in the absence of severe, acute inflammation.

Other possible etiologies have little support. Some investigators hypothesize that pouchitis is the result of ischemic changes. Damage by bile acids or their bacterial metabolites is a possibility, because dihydroxy bile acids are intestinal secretagogues and cellular toxins.[47] Short-chain fatty acids (SCFAs) have also been implicated in pouchitis, although the mechanism is unclear. There is an increasing body of evidence that normal colonic mucosa uses SCFAs as a source of energy, and some authors have proposed that inflammatory bowel disease can result when the colon is deprived of SCFAs.[48] The clearest clinical experiment that tests this hypothesis is "diversion colitis." Harig and coworkers proposed that diversion colitis is caused by deprivation of SCFAs.[49] Support for this proposal is provided by the observation that diversion colitis improves in response to enemas of SCFA (see Chapter 118). On the other hand, ileal pouches contain high concentrations of SCFAs (up to 100 mM), and a state of deprivation seems unlikely. Indeed, pouchitis has worsened or shown no predictable response to SCFA enemas.[50] Pouchitis has no relationship to the presence or absence of backwash ileitis at the time of proctocolectomy.[51] In a detailed evaluation of luminal factors, fecal concentrations of bacteria, bile acids, and SCFAs were similar in patients with and without pouchitis.[47]

The overall experience with pouchitis is that 40% of patients with a pouch will never have pouchitis, 40% will have a single episode, 15% will have intermittently recurring episodes, and 5% or fewer will develop chronic pouchitis.[44]

Possible Sequelae

Although the prevalence of chronic pouchitis is low, the possible consequences of chronic inflammation of the neorectum, especially dysplasia and malignant change, arouse concern. Cancer has been reported in the pouch and in the pelvis after IPAA; the likely sequence in patients with pelvic cancer is malignant degeneration of a dysplastic rectal cuff.[52] Morphologic and biochemical changes in the ileal mucosa of pouches include villous blunting, chronic inflammatory infiltrates, variable transition to production of a colonic type of mucus (sulfomucins), and increased cellular proliferation.[53] Observation based on the longest follow-up (mean of 6.3 years) to date suggests that there are three patterns of mucosal adaptation.[46] Approximately one half of the patients show mild villous atrophy and minimal inflammation, slightly fewer have transient moderate or severe atrophy and inflammation with intervals of recovery, and approximately 10% have permanent subtotal or total villous atrophy with chronic inflammation. In this study,[46] low-grade dysplasia developed in three of eight patients in the last group, as early as 2 years postoperatively in one patient. The patients at risk of dysplasia are those with chronic pouchitis.

Pouch Failure

Six percent of patients ultimately require pouch excision or construction of a permanent ileostomy. Other large series have reported failure rates of 2% to 12%. The most frequent causes of failure, either alone or in combination, include pelvic sepsis, high stool volumes, Crohn's disease, and uncontrollable fecal incontinence. Pouchitis is the sole cause in 2% of all patients. Importantly, of the patients in whom the pouch fails, 75% fail within 1 year, 12% by 2 years, and 12% by 3 years. Thus, failure after IPAA is manifested within several years of the operation and is the result of a combination of early or late complications of the procedure.

Quality of Life

Often, the quality of life is the deciding factor for patients choosing a particular operation for ulcerative colitis. Several studies that analyzed the outcome of surgery for ulcerative colitis have demonstrated that most patients are satisfied with the operation and lead a normal life-style regardless of the choice of procedure.

In a study of the quality of life after a Brooke ileostomy or IPAA for ulcerative colitis and FAP, patients were highly satisfied with either operation (Brooke ileostomy, 93%; IPAA, 95%). However, daily activities (e.g., sexual life, participation in sports, social interaction, work, recreation, family relationships, and travel) were more likely to be affected adversely by a Brooke ileostomy than by an IPAA.

Controversies

Which Pouch Design is Best?

Of all the pouch designs championed in the literature S, H, W, K, and J, the J-shaped pouch is easiest to construct and has functional outcomes identical to those of the more complex designs. It is the pouch design of choice at the Mayo Clinic.

Two Stages or One? Role of Defunctioning Ileostomy

The most feared complication of IPAA is pelvic sepsis, and therefore, a defunctioning ileostomy after pouch construction usually is performed to minimize the risk of pelvic sepsis.[54] Whereas pelvic sepsis complicates 6% of IPAA procedures at the Mayo Clinic, the rates reported in the literature vary between 0% and 25%. Moreover, disturbingly high rates of pelvic sepsis have been reported in patients who undergo a one-stage procedure (no ileostomy). Although the incidence of pelvic sepsis is low at the Mayo Clinic, when it occurs, it is responsible for a substantial proportion of the failed pouches.[55]

Protagonists of defunctioning ileostomies argue that diverting stomas allow the anal sphincter and ileal mucosa to recover before restoration of intestinal continuity. Moreover, because patients have the experience, albeit short-lived, of a stoma, they will fully appreciate the ultimate benefit of IPAA. Use of a loop ileostomy does not appear to protect the patient fully from pelvic sepsis; however, it is easier to manage a patient with sepsis if an ileostomy is in place. Among the patients at the Mayo Clinic who required laparotomy to control sepsis, 41% ultimately lost the pouch, and only 29% ever recovered ileoanal function. However, if no reoperation was required, 92% of patients with sepsis eventually had a functioning pouch.[55]

A reasonable approach is to use a defunctioning ileostomy in those patients who are receiving glucocorticoid treatment at the time of surgery, are nutritionally compromised, or undergo an urgent operation. Additionally, if there are concerns about the blood supply of the pouch or anastomotic tension, a diverting ileostomy is almost mandatory. Using these criteria, 56 of 1800 patients who underwent IPAA at the Mayo Clinic between 1980 and 1996 had a one-stage procedure performed.

Double-Stapled Versus Hand-Sewn Anastomosis

Much of the debate as to whether to staple the anastomosis or not has evolved because functional outcomes should be improved if the anal transition zone (or more recently "columnar cuff" [CC]) is preserved. Does preserving the CC enhance continence after IPAA? In nonrandomized trials, stapled anastomosis has been equated with a better outcome, which in turn has been attributed to less injury to the anal sphincters, with preservation of the CC and hence anal sensory discrimination and with preservation of the rectoanal inhibitory reflex. In order to determine if a stapled IPAA confers any advantage over a hand-sewn IPAA, we randomized 41 patients at the Mayo Clinic to double-stapled (n = 17 patients) or hand-sewn (n = 15 patients) techniques.[56] In the stapled group, 1.5 to 2.0 cm of CC was preserved, whereas in the hand-sewn group, complete mucosectomy was performed. Overall, the rate of complications was the same in the two groups. Stool frequency and rates of fecal incontinence during the day and night were similar between the groups. However, fewer patients treated with the double-stapled technique had incontinence at night. Moreover, resting and squeeze anal pressures were better preserved after double stapling. Both hand-sewn and double-stapled IPAA improved the quality of life dramatically. Double-stapled IPAA has further benefits because it may preserve the anal canal better than the hand-sewn anastomosis and thus enable older and perhaps overweight patients to be candidates for IPAA.

Additional Issues

Risk of Cancer

Patients with chronic ulcerative colitis are at risk of developing adenocarcinoma of the colon. This risk increases with the duration of disease and the extent of colonic involvement. Any surgery that leaves behind diseased colonic mucosa puts the patient at risk of developing dysplasia or neoplasia in the residual colonic mucosa. The risk of developing a carcinoma in the residual colonic mucosa may be related directly to the amount of residual mucosa remaining in situ.

Complete excision of the rectum during IPAA decreases the risk of dysplasia significantly. With the widespread acceptance of stapled IPAA, the residual cuff epithelium (CE) is reduced to less than 1 cm or eliminated nearly completely.

Studies, such as that by Tsunoda and associates,[57] which demonstrated the presence of dysplasia in mucosectomy specimens, have been used as evidence to support the use of routine complete mucosal resection. Opposite conclusions were drawn by Ziv and colleagues after stapled IPAA.[58]

To make this issue even more complex, several studies have reported that viable mucosa is present in the rectal muscular cuff *after* mucosal resection. In one study, islands (rests) of mucosa were present despite "complete" mucosal resection.[59] The frequency of dysplasia in the retained rectal mucosa, or distal rectal doughnut, after double-stapled ileoanal anastomosis is approximately 1%. Histologic analysis of mucosectomy specimens includes one report of a carcinoma, which had been undetected clinically, in a patient who had dysplasia in the rectal mucosa. Despite this, no patient has developed a rectal cancer in the retained rectal muscular cuff after IPAA and endorectal mucosal resection. Patients have developed adenocarcinoma in the retained CE. The residual CE has the potential for dysplasia, neoplasia, and continuing inflammation after IPAA. However, the four patients with carcinoma reported in a pouch all have been patients who underwent total mucosectomy as part of their original surgery.

The question of follow-up of the residual CE has been addressed by several investigators. The Cleveland Clinic reported its experience with 254 patients who underwent double-stapled IPAA and annual postsurgical CE biopsy.[58] During a mean follow-up of 2 years, low-grade dysplasia was found in eight patients (3%). Repeat biopsies confirmed dysplasia in only two of these eight patients. A significant correlation was seen between CE dysplasia and dysplasia or cancer of the large bowel *before* surgery. There was no association with age, sex, duration of the disease, anastomotic technique, or length of rectal cuff. The risk of dysplasia in the residual CE was 25% in patients who had cancer in the original proctocolectomy specimen, but only 10% in patients who had dysplasia in the original specimen.

Reports of dysplasia and carcinoma in the pouch mucosa have prompted some investigators to perform endoscopic surveillance and pouch biopsy regularly in all patients with a pouch. A subgroup of patients has been identified in whom the mucosa of the pouch develops severe villous atrophy and who have a significantly higher incidence of dysplasia compared with patients without villous atrophy (71% vs. 0%).[59] The former group may be at greater risk of developing carcinoma and may require more intensive follow-up with regular pouch endoscopy and biopsy.

Dysplasia

The presence of dysplasia in the pouch, rectal cuff, or CE should not be ignored. Routine endoscopic surveillance with biopsy after IPAA shows dysplastic changes in as many as 3% of patients. Low-grade dysplasia should prompt the close follow-up of the patient and repeated multiple endoscopic biopsies of the cuff. Repeat biopsies are likely to be normal in the majority of patients, and continued surveillance of these patients is likely to be sufficient. Persistence of dysplastic mucosa or the presence of high-grade dysplasia is an indication for more aggressive intervention. Completion mucosectomy or laser ablation may be sufficient if the dysplastic mucosa involves only the CE. In more refractory cases, pouch excision may be considered, but this is uncommon.

Pregnancy

We and several other centers have observed that women who become pregnant and deliver a child after IPAA have few long-term problems with pouch function. However, the fertility rate of women after IPAA is unknown.[39, 61, 62]

IPAA and "Indeterminate Colitis"

Among 1519 consecutive patients with chronic ulcerative colitis who underwent IPAA between January, 1981 and December, 1995, 82 (5%) had features of indeterminate colitis, characterized by an unusual distribution of inflammation, deep linear ulcers, neural proliferation, transmural inflammation, fissures, and creeping fat.[63] We found that Crohn's disease developed in 12 of 82 (15%) patients with indeterminate colitis during follow-up compared with only 26 of 1437 patients with ulcerative colitis. The probability of remaining free of Crohn's disease at 10 years was 98% among patients with ulcerative colitis but only 81% among those with indeterminate colitis. Interestingly, after IPAA, patients with indeterminate colitis in whom Crohn's disease did not develop experienced long-term outcomes nearly identical to those of patients with a diagnosis of ulcerative colitis; that is, nearly 85% had functioning pouches 10 years after IPAA. However, Crohn's disease, whether it eventually develops and is diagnosed after surgery for apparent ulcerative colitis or indeterminate colitis, is associated with a poor long-term outcome. Whether patients with indeterminate colitis need to be managed expectantly for the development of Crohn's disease needs further study.

Psychological Factors

Some progress has been made toward identifying subgroups of patients who are at increased risk for developing pouch dysfunction or complications. Several studies have confirmed that during long-term follow-up, functional results are poor in patients who had adverse personality factors before surgery. Personality traits were measured before surgery in 53 patients who underwent surgery for ulcerative colitis, and the traits were correlated with psychological adjustment at a mean of 17 months after surgery. The patient's long-term sexual functioning and satisfaction before surgery, the importance attached to his or her appearance, the level of alexithymia, and the general capacity to tolerate frustration and setbacks in life were factors that affected the patient's adjustment after surgery.

ABDOMINAL COLECTOMY AND ILEORECTAL ANASTOMOSIS

The aim of a colectomy with an ileorectal anastomosis (ileorectostomy) is to extirpate *most* of the diseased colonic mucosa, thus reducing the risks of hemorrhage, dilatation, perforation, and malignant degeneration, while allowing the rectum to retain continence for stool and gas. The rationale for an ileorectostomy is that the operation avoids a permanent stoma, minimizes or eliminates injury to the pelvic nerves, and is easy to perform; other operations, if they become necessary, are not precluded.[64–66] However, the arguments against the operation are nearly as convincing. Subsequent proctectomy is required in 6% to 37% of patients; poor results have been reported in up to 50% of cases[67]; and the risk of developing carcinoma in the retained rectum approaches 17% after 27 years.[67] In patients with Crohn's disease and minimal or no rectal involvement, ileorectostomy with excision of the diseased colon is a favorable situation, and, accordingly, this procedure unquestionably has a central role in the management of Crohn's disease with rectal sparing.

Patient Selection

Patients are candidates for ileorectostomy if the rectum is distensible, the disease (ulcerative colitis or Crohn's disease) involves the rectum only minimally, and patients are willing to undergo follow-up screening for rectal cancer. Patients up to age 70 years and of any body type may undergo ileorectostomy.

Complications

Operative mortality for elective ileorectostomy has been reported to vary from 2% to 8%.[68] Almost all deaths have been caused by *anastomotic leakage*, which affects 3% of patients; *small bowel obstruction* complicates the recovery of about 15%. Although sexual function in men is usually preserved postoperatively, up to 50% of women experience *dyspareunia*.

Physiology

The primary attraction of ileorectostomy is that the major anatomic mechanisms responsible for maintaining continence are retained: The rectal reservoir, pelvic floor, and internal and external anal sphincters are preserved. However, the absorptive capacity of the proximal colon has been lost, and ileal content is presented continuously to the rectal remnant.

To accommodate passively, the rectum should be compliant and large. Compliance depends on rectal wall elasticity, and in active inflammatory disease, compliant accommodation is impaired.[70] Moreover, the smaller the rectum, the greater the elasticity coefficient; patients with active ulcerative colitis have a smaller rectum than do controls.[71] Therefore, the less the mucosal inflammation and elasticity coefficient, the better the compliance, with fewer stools per day. Sphincteric function in patients with ileorectal anastomosis differs little from that in normal people.

After ileorectostomy, patients with *quiescent* rectal disease should be able to absorb water and sodium in the rectal segment. Moreover, the rectum is capacious and distensible, resulting in low stool frequency and little or no incontinence. On the other hand, if the mucosa of the rectum is inflamed, absorption is impaired and fecal volume is greater. Moreover, the more inflamed the mucosa, the less capacious and distensible the rectum; increased stool frequency, urgency, and incontinence will follow.

The best measure of a successful clinical outcome after an ileorectostomy is the rate of subsequent proctocolectomy for persistent or recurrent disease or rectal cancer. The reported late proctectomy rate for persistent or recurrent disease varies greatly, from 5% to 58%. The probability that a patient with ulcerative colitis will have a good result after ileorectostomy—will not require glucocorticoids but will be in good general health and have an acceptable stool frequency with no incontinence—is approximately 50%. The risk that cancer will develop in the retained rectum is approximately 5% at 15 years after the operation; this rate increases to 15% by 30 years.[65, 68, 69] Unfortunately, these cancers are usually advanced in grade and stage compared with usual colorectal cancer. Those operated on for FAP must, of course, undergo close surveillance for cancer (see Chapter 114).

The quality of life after ileorectal anastomosis has been reported to be good[72]; patient satisfaction is high, and an active, productive life-style can be preserved. Overall satisfaction is tempered, however, by the patient's belief that the underlying disease has not been cured because of the need for frequent follow-up examinations.

COLOSTOMY IN THE MANAGEMENT OF INFLAMMATORY BOWEL DISEASE

For patients with ulcerative colitis, colostomy has no role in elective or emergency surgery. Resection of the rectosigmoid,[73] coloanal anastomosis,[74] and cecoanal anastomosis[75] are operations mentioned here only to be condemned in patients with ulcerative colitis. Urgent or emergency intervention for decompensating or fulminant ulcerative colitis is best managed by abdominal colectomy, Brooke ileostomy, and either oversewing of the rectum or establishing a rectal mucous fistula.

Colostomy is only a slightly better choice for patients with Crohn's colitis than for those with ulcerative colitis. Segmental resection, although fraught with higher recurrence rates, is an acceptable alternative to abdominal colectomy and ileorectostomy, if there is a significant length of normal colon proximal to the diseased segment. Conventional wisdom is to remove the involved segment together with the colon proximal to this segment and to perform an ileocolostomy. In a patient with Crohn's disease of the distal sigmoid colon alone, it makes better sense to resect the sigmoid colon only and anastomose the descending colon to the rectum, rather than to perform an abdominal colectomy and ileorectostomy.

SUMMARY OF RISK-BENEFIT ANALYSIS

Conventional Ileostomy

The Brooke ileostomy is safe and reliable and has broad applicability to patients with inflammatory bowel disease who require proctocolectomy; however, it is not entirely free

Table 105–2 | **Comparison of Surgical Options After Colectomy**

	STOMA	CONTI-NENT	MOR-TALITY (%)	OVERALL MORBID-ITY (%)	SMALL BOWEL OBSTRUC-TION (%)	PERINEAL WOUND COMPLI-CATION (%)	STOOLS/ 24 HOUR	FAILURE (%)	ALL DISEASE REMOVED?	CANCER RISK (%)	DISEASE INDICA-TION
Brooke ileos-tomy	Yes	No	<1.0	19–70	15	33	NA	—	Yes	0	CD (?UC, FAP)
Ileorectostomy	No	Yes	2.5–8.0	16–20	15	NA	1–3	24–60	No	15 (30 yr)	CD, UC
Continent ileostomy	Yes	Yes	<1.0	15–60	7	35	3–5	50	Yes	*	UC, FAP
Ileal pouch–anal anasto-mosis	No	Yes	<1.0	30–50	22	NA	5–7	8	Yes*	†	UC, FAP

Maximum follow-up time is 13 years.
Disease indication: CD, Crohn's disease; FAP, familial adenomatous polyposis; UC, ulcerative colitis.
*10 reports of neoplasia in the cuff or pouch after ileal pouch–anal anastomosis have been reported in > 12,000 cases.
†2 cancers in Kock pouches (continent ileostomies) have been reported.

of complications (Table 105–2). Up to 30% of patients have a septic complication, 20% to 25% require stomal revision, 15% have recurrent small bowel obstruction, and stomal dysfunction can occur in up to 30% of cases. These data should be kept in mind when alternative procedures are evaluated.

Ileorectal Anastomosis

The primary benefit of an ileorectostomy is that the rectum is undisturbed by the operative dissection; the normal pathway of defecation is left intact; and the frequency of bladder or sexual problems is low. Moreover, there is no perineal wound (see Table 105–2). In many patients, the overall functional results are reasonably good. The major problem with an ileorectostomy is that actual or potentially diseased mucosa is left intact. In a few patients, inflammatory changes resolve, but in most, the disease process continues unabated. The sequelae of leaving disease behind include: (1) poor anastomotic healing, which is responsible for the relatively higher mortality rate after ileorectal anastomosis than after continent ileostomy and IPAA; (2) continued need for anti-inflammatory therapy; (3) continued bleeding and mucous discharge; (4) incontinence and high stool frequency when inflammation flares; and (5) the possibility of malignant degeneration.

Continent Ileostomy

The major benefit of the Kock pouch is that, although a stoma is constructed, discharge is controlled without the need for an external appliance (see Table 105–2). Moreover, in patients with ulcerative colitis, all disease is removed. The principal problem with a continent ileostomy is the impressively high rate of complications. Most complications involve the nipple valve and lead invariably to incontinence or complete outflow obstruction. These complications, in turn, almost always require another operation. As with the Brooke ileostomy, a perineal wound accompanies this operation; the wound fails to heal promptly in approximately one third of patients. In general, this operation is not performed electively anymore.

Ileal Pouch–Anal Anastomosis

The major benefit of IPAA is that fecal continence is restored in most patients, but the major problem is that the complication rate is approximately 30%. Occasional incontinence appears early in almost all patients after the operation, particularly at night. Major episodes of daytime incontinence affect approximately 10% of patients, but the frequency declines to almost zero after 4 years. Other complications are pelvic infection, stricture, fistula, sinus tracts, pouch leakage, and small bowel obstruction. As surgeons' experience with the operation has broadened, however, these surgical complications have decreased in frequency. Although nonspecific inflammation of the pouch, or pouchitis, is the most important current drawback, this entity is treated effectively and simply with antibiotics. When severe and recurrent, pouchitis can lead to failure of the operation; fortunately, this occurrence is uncommon. Despite these problems, the benefits of IPAA are clear: All disease is removed, the patient does not have a stoma, and anal defecation is voluntary and controlled.

REFERENCES

1. Hill GL: Historical introduction. In Hill GL (ed): Ileostomy: Surgery, Physiology and Management. New York, Grune & Stratton, 1976, p 1.
2. Brooke BN: Management of ileostomy including its complications. Lancet 2:102, 1952.
3. Turnbull RB: Symposium on ulcerative colitis; management of ileostomy. Am J Surg 86:617, 1953.
4. Roy PH, Sauer WG, Beahrs OH, Farrow GN: Experience with ileostomies: Evaluation of long-term rehabilitation in 497 patients. Am J Surg 119:77, 1970.
5. Kock NG: Intra-abdominal reservoir in patients with permanent ileostomy: Preliminary observations on a procedure resulting in fecal continence in five ileostomy patients. Arch Surg 99:223, 1969.
6. Dozois RR, Kelly KA, Beart RW Jr, Beahrs OH: Continent ileostomy: The Mayo Clinic experience. In Dozois RR (ed): Alternatives to Continent Ileostomy. Chicago, Year Book Medical Publishers, 1985.

7. Ravitch MM, Sabiston Dd: Anal ileostomy with preservation of the sphincter. Surg Gynecol Obstet 84:1095, 1947.
8. Beart RW Jr, Metcalf AM, Dozois RR, Kelly KA: The J ileal pouch–anal anastomosis: The Mayo Clinic experience. In Dozois RR (ed): Alternatives to Conventional Ileostomy. Chicago, Year Book Medical Publishers, 1985.
9. Phillips SF, Giller J: Contribution of the colon to electrolyte and water conservation in man. J Lab Clin Med 81:733, 1973.
10. Debongnie JC, Phillips SF: Capacity of the human colon to absorb fluid. Gastroenterology 74:698, 1978.
11. Dole VP, Dahle LK, Cotzias G, et al: Dietary treatment of hypertension: Clinical and metabolic studies of patients on the rice-fruit diet. J Clin Invest 29:1189, 1950.
12. Kramer P: The effect of varying sodium loads on the ileal excreta of human ileostomized subjects. J Clin Invest 45:1710, 1966.
13. Kanaghinis T, Lubran M, Coghill NF: The composition of ileostomy fluid. Gut 4:322, 1963.
14. Metcalf AM, Phillips SF: Ileostomy diarrhea. Clin Gastroenterol 15: 705, 1986.
15. Kramer P, Kearney MS, Ingelfinger FJ: The effect of specific foods and water loading on the ileal excreta of ileostomized human subjects. Gastroenterology 42:535, 1962.
16. Gallagher ND, Harrison DD, Skyring AP: Fluid and electrolyte disturbances in patients with long established ileostomies. Gut 3:219, 1962.
17. Clarke AM, Chirnside A, Hill GL, et al: Chronic dehydration and sodium depletion in patients with established ileostomies. Lancet 2:740, 1967.
18. Clarke AM, McKenzie RG: Ileostomy and the risk of urinary uric acid stones. Lancet 2:395, 1969.
19. Morris JS, Low-Beer TS, Heaton KW: Bile salt metabolism and the colon. Scand J Gastroenterol 8:425, 1973.
20. Gadacz TR, Kelly KA, Phillips SF: The Kock ileal pouch: Absorptive and motor characteristics. Gastroenterology 72:1287, 1977.
21. Gorbach SL, Nahas L, Weinstein L: Studies of intestinal microflora: IV. The microflora of ileostomy effluent: A unique microbial etiology. Gastroenterology 53:874, 1967.
22. Kelly DG, Phillips SF, Kelly KA, et al: Dysfunction of the continent ileostomy: Clinical features and bacteriology. Gut 24:193, 1983.
23. O'Connell PR, Rankin DR, Weiland LH, Kelly KA: Enteric bacteriology, absorption, morphology and emptying after ileal pouch–anal anastomosis. Br J Surg 73:909, 1986.
24. Watts JM, de Dombal FT, Goligher Jd: Long-term complications and prognosis following major surgery for ulcerative colitis. Br J Surg 53: 1014, 1966.
25. Pemberton JH, Phillips SF, Ready RR, et al: Quality of life after Brooke ileostomy and ileal pouch–anal anastomosis. Ann Surg 209: 620, 1989.
26. Phillips SF: Metabolic consequences of a stagnant loop at the end of the small bowel. World J Surg 11:763, 1987.
27. Knill-Jones RP, Morson B, Williams R: Prestomal ileitis: Clinical and pathological findings in five cases. Q J Med 39:287, 1970.
28. Sparberg M: Bismuth subgallate as an effective means for control of ileostomy odor: A double-blind study. Gastroenterology 66:476, 1974.
29. Report from the Australian Drug Evaluation Committee: Adverse effects of bismuth subgallate. Med J Aust 2:664, 1974.
30. Lennenberg E, Rowbotham JL: The ileostomy patients: A descriptive study of 1425 persons. Springfield, IL, Charles C Thomas, 1970.
31. Sparberg M: The Ileostomy Case. Springfield, IL, Charles C Thomas, 1971.
32. Koch NG, Mynvold HE, Nilsson LO, Phillipson BN: Continent ileostomy: The Swedish experience. In Dozois RR (ed): Alternatives to Conventional Ileostomy. Chicago, Year Book Medical Publishers, 1985, p 163.
33. Mullen P, Behrens D, Chalmers T, et al: Barnett continent intestinal reservoir. Multicenter experiences with an alternative to the Brooke ileostomy. Dis Colon Rectum 38:573, 1995.
34. Kelly DG, Branon ME, Phillips SF, Kelly KA: Diarrhea after continent ileostomy. Gut 21:711, 1980.
35. Cox CL, Butts DR, Roberts MP, et al: Development of invasive adenocarcinoma in a long-standing Kock continent ileostomy: Report of a case. Dis Colon Rectum 40:500, 1997.
35a. Regimbeau JM, Panic Y, Pocard M, et al: Long-term results of ileal pouch–anal anastomosis for colorectal Crohn's disease. Dis Colon Rectum 44:769, 2001.
36. Stryker SJ, Dozois RR: The ileoanal anastomosis: Historical perspectives. In Dozois RR (ed): Alternatives to the Conventional Ileostomy. Chicago, Year Book Medical Publishers, 1985, p 225.
37. Coran AG: Straight endorectal pull-through of the ileum for the management of benign disease of the colon and rectum in children and adults. In Dozois RR (ed): Alternatives to the Conventional Ileostomy. Chicago, Year Book Medical Publishers, 1985, p 335.
38. Pemberton JH, Kelly KA, Beart RW Jr, et al: Ileal pouch–anal anastomosis for chronic ulcerative colitis: Long-term results. Ann Surg 206: 504, 1987.
39. Farouk R, Pemberton JH, Wolff BG, et al: Functional outcomes after ileal pouch–anal anastomosis for chronic ulcerative colitis. Ann Surg 231:919, 2000.
40. Dozois RR, Kelly KA: J ileal pouch–anal anastomosis for chronic ulcerative colitis—complications and long-term outcome in 1310 patients. Br J Surg 85:800, 1998.
41. Fleshman JW, Cohen A, McLeod RS, et al: The ileal reservoir and ileo-anal anastomosis procedure: Factors affecting technical and functional outcome. Dis Colon Rectum 31:10, 1988.
42. Lohmuller JL, Pemberton JH, Dozois RR, et al: Pouchitis and extraintestinal manifestations of inflammatory bowel disease after ileal pouch–anal anastomosis. Ann Surg 211:622, 1990.
43. Sandborn WJ, Tremaine WJ, Batts KP, et al: Pouchitis after ileal pouch–anal anastomosis: A pouchitis disease activity index. Mayo Clin Proc 69:409, 1994.
44. Sandborn WJ: Pouchitis following ileal pouch–anal anastomosis: Definition, pathogenesis, and treatment. Gastroenterology 107:1856, 1994.
45. Apel R, Cohen Z, Andrews CW, et al: Prospective evaluation of early morphological changes in pelvic ileal pouches. Gastroenterology 107: 435, 1994.
46. Veress B, Reinholt FP, Lindquist K, et al: Long-term histomorphological surveillance of the pelvic ileal pouch: Dysplasia develops in a subgroup of patients. Gastroenterology 109:1090, 1995.
47. Sandborn WJ, Tremaine WJ, Batts KP, et al: Fecal bile acids, short-chain fatty acids, and bacteria after ileal pouch–anal anastomosis do not differ in patients with pouchitis. Dig Dis Sci 40:1474, 1995.
48. Roediger WEW: The colonic epithelium in ulcerative colitis—An energy deficiency disease? Lancet 2:712, 1980.
49. Harig JM, Soergel KH, Komorowski RA, Wood CM: Treatment of diversion colitis with short chain fatty acid irrigation. N Engl J Med 320:23, 1989.
50. DeSilva HJ, Ireland A, Kettlewell M, et al: Short-chain fatty acids irrigation in severe pouchitis [letter]. N Engl J Med 321:1416, 1989.
51. Gustavsson S, Weiland LH, Kelly KA: Relationship of backwash ileitis to ileal pouchitis after ileal pouch–anal anastomosis. Dis Colon Rectum 30:25, 1987.
52. Stern H, Walfisch S, Mullen B, et al: Cancer in an ileoanal reservoir: A new late complication. Gut 31:473, 1990.
53. DeSilva HJ, Millaro PR, Kettlewell M, et al: Mucosal characteristics of pelvic ileal pouches. Gut 32:61, 1991.
54. Galandiuk S, Wolff BG, Dozois RR, Beart RW Jr: Ileal pouch–anal anastomosis without ileostomy. Dis Colon Rectum 34:870, 1991.
55. Galandiuk S, Scott NA, Dozois RR, et al: Ileal pouch–anal anastomosis. Reoperation for pouch-related complications. Ann Surg 212:446-452, 1990.
56. Reilly WT, Pemberton JH, Wolff BG, et al: Randomized prospective trial comparing ileal pouch–anal anastomosis (IPAA) performed by excising the anal mucosa to IPAA performed by preserving the anal mucosa. Ann Surg 225:666, 1997.
57. Tsunoda A, Talbot IC, Nicholls RJ: Incidence of dysplasia in the anorectal mucosa in patients having restorative proctocolectomy. Br J Surg 77:506, 1990.
58. Ziv Y, Fazio VW, Sirimarco MT, et al: Incidence, risk factors, and treatment of dysplasia in the anal transition zone after ileal pouch–anal anastomosis. Dis Colon Rectum 37:1281, 1994.
59. Haray PN, Amamath B, Weiss EG, et al: Low malignant potential of the double-stapled ileal pouch–anal anastomosis. Br J Surg 83:1406, 1996.
60. Veress B, Reinholt FP, Lindquist K, et al: Long-term histomorphological surveillance of the pelvic ileal pouch: Dysplasia develops in a subgroup of patients. Gastroenterology 109:1090, 1995.
61. Nelson H, Dozois RR, Kelly KA, et al: The effect of pregnancy and delivery on ileal pouch–anal anastomosis functions. Dis Colon Rectum 32:384, 1989.
62. Juhasz ES, Fozard B, Dozois RR, et al: Ileal pouch–anal anastomosis function following childbirth. An extended evaluation. Dis Colon Rectum 38:59, 1995.

63. Yu CS, Pemberton JH, Larson D: Ileal pouch–anal anastomosis in patients with indeterminate colitis: Long-term results. Dis Colon Rectum 43:1487, 2000.
64. Aylett SO: Three hundred cases of diffuse ulcerative colitis treated by total colectomy and ileo-rectal anastomosis. Br Med J 1:1001, 1966.
65. Grundfest SF, Fazio V, Weiss RA, et al: The risk of cancer following colectomy and ileorectal anastomosis for extensive mucosal ulcerative colitis. Ann Surg 193:9, 1981.
66. Watts J McK, Hughes SR: Ulcerative colitis and Crohn's disease: Results after colectomy and ileorectal anastomosis. Br J Surg 64:77, 1977.
67. Adson MA, Cooperman AM, Farrow GM: Ileorectostomy for ulcerative disease of the colon. Arch Surg 104:424, 1972.
68. Johnson WR, McDermott FT, Hughes ESR, et al: The risk of rectal carcinoma following colectomy in ulcerative colitis. Dis Colon Rectum 26:44, 1983.
69. Baker WNW, Glass RE, Ritchie JK, Aylett SO: Cancer of the rectum following colectomy and ileorectal anastomosis for ulcerative colitis. Br J Surg 65:862, 1978.
70. Denis PH, Colin R, Galmiche JP, et al: Elastic properties of the rectal wall in normal adults and in patients with ulcerative colitis. Gastroenterology 77:45, 1979.
71. Farthing MJG, Lennard-Jones JE: Sensibility of the rectum to distension and the anorectal distension reflex in ulcerative colitis. Gut 19:64, 1978.
72. Mignon M, Bonfils S: Altered physiology in ulcerative colitis patients with ileorectal anastomosis. In Dozois RR (ed): Alternative to Conventional Ileostomy. Chicago, Year Book Medical Publishers, 1985, p 61.
73. Clark CG, Ward MWM: The place of isolated rectal excision in the treatment of ulcerative colitis. Br J Surg 67:653, 1980.
74. Roediger WEW, Pihl E, Hughes E: Preserving the ascending colon as an alternative support option in ulcerative colitis. Surg Gynecol Obstet 54:348, 1982.
75. Varma JS, Browning GGP, Smith AW, et al: Mucosal proctectomy and colo-anal anastomosis for distal ulcerative proctocolitis. Br J Surg 74: 381, 1987.

Chapter 106

Isolated and Diffuse Ulcers of the Small Intestine

Deborah D. Proctor and Lisa Ann Panzini

Although rare, ulcers of the jejunum and ileum are responsible for a broad spectrum of disease. Clinical presentations range from anemia and hypoproteinemia to abdominal pain, hemorrhage, obstruction, and perforation. Ulcers may be solitary or multiple with intervening mucosa that is normal or diseased. This chapter first discusses isolated ulcers of the small intestine, including nonspecific solitary ulcers and drug-induced ulceration, with an emphasis on the pathogenesis of nonsteroidal anti-inflammatory drug (NSAID)-induced ulcers. The second part of this chapter discusses syndromes of diffuse intestinal ulceration. These include ulcerative enteritis, refractory celiac sprue, and enteropathy-associated T cell lymphoma. The syndromes of diffuse intestinal ulceration have a poor prognosis, and, recently, abnormal monoclonal intestinal intraepithelial T lymphocytes have been demonstrated in these patients. Because of the great length and relative inaccessibility of the small intestine, the diagnosis of these syndromes remains challenging.

ISOLATED ULCERS

Nonspecific or Idiopathic Small Intestinal Ulceration

Solitary ulcers of the small intestine can result from a wide variety of causes (Table 106–1). Solitary ulcers beyond the duodenum that cannot be explained on the basis of a known etiology are referred to as nonspecific or idiopathic intestinal ulcers. Solitary nonspecific ulcers are rare, with an incidence of 4 in 100,000.[1]

Clinical Presentation

Patients with nonspecific ulcers of the small intestine present most commonly with symptoms of intermittent small bowel obstruction, but they may also present with abdominal pain, perforation, or acute or chronic gastrointestinal blood loss. Symptoms may be present from a few days to many years before a diagnosis is made. In a review of the Mayo Clinic experience of 59 cases of small intestinal ulcers over the 22 years ending in 1979, Boydstun and associates[1] identified only six patients who had used potassium supplements, which were probably the etiology of their ulcers. The remaining 53 patients had no identifiable cause of ulceration. They ranged in age from 17 to 77 years, and the majority were in their fifth and sixth decades of life. Solitary ulcers were equally likely in men and women. The most common presenting symptom was intermittent small bowel obstruction (63%). Physical findings ranged from abdominal tenderness and distention to an acute abdomen in those with perforation. Laboratory evaluation was notable only for anemia in one half the patients. Radiographic evaluation was not specific for small bowel ulcerations. Of 108 gastrointestinal contrast studies obtained, only five identified an ulcer. However, 66% of patients had some radiographic abnormality that led to surgical management.[1]

Pathology

In the Mayo Clinic series,[1] the ileum was the most common location of nonspecific ulceration (78%), whereas perforation (13 cases) occurred more commonly in the jejunum (78%). At the time of laparotomy, 41 patients were found to have solitary ulcers, five patients had two ulcers, and six patients had more than three. Ulcer size varied between 0.3 and 5.0 cm. At pathologic examination, the ulcers were predominantly anti-mesenteric and in some cases were associated with a fibrous scar that narrowed the lumen. Microscopic examination revealed nonspecific chronic inflammation, which ended abruptly at the ulcer edge. The intervening bowel and vasculature were normal.[1]

Management

The patients reported in the Mayo series[1] were treated with segmental resection; only two had recurrent ulceration 2 and 10 years after initial diagnosis and resection. Vascular disease, central nervous system disease, infection, trauma, and hormonal influences have all been postulated as possible causes of primary nonspecific ulceration. However, the etiol-

Table 106–1 | **Causes of Small Intestinal Ulceration**

Infectious	Bacteria, virus, fungus, parasites, protozoa, worms
Inflammatory	Crohn's disease, Behçet's syndrome, granulomatous enteritis, sarcoidosis
Collagen vascular and other immune-mediated diseases	Vasculitis, polyarteritis nodosa, systemic lupus erythematosus, giant cell arteritis, polymyositis-dermatomyositis, thrombotic thrombocytopenic purpura, mixed connective tissue disease, Churg-Strauss syndrome, Henoch-Schönlein purpura, reactive arthritis
Drugs	Aspirin, nonsteroidal anti-inflammatory drugs, potassium, antimetabolites, chemotherapeutic agents, antibiotics
Celiac sprue	Refractory celiac sprue, ulcerative enteritis
Hypersensitivity	Food allergies
Ischemia	Mesenteric ischemia, vascular abnormalities
Radiation	Therapeutic, accidental
Traumatic	Incarcerated hernia, stomal ulceration, intussusception, foreign body ingestion
Toxic	Heavy metal poisoning, Pasini's regional jejunitis
Neoplastic	Primary, metastatic Angiocentric T cell lymphoma
Congenital	Duplications, stenoses
Metabolic	Uremia
Malnutrition	
Gastric hyperacidity	Zollinger-Ellison syndome, heterotopic gastric mucosa
Tropical sprue	
Mucosal lesions	Lymphocytic enterocolitis, eosinophilic gastroenteritis
Miscellaneous	Hypogammaglobulinemia, nongranulomatous chronic idiopathic enterocolitis, cryptogenic multifocal ulcerous stenosing enteritis

ogy (or etiologies) remains unknown. In the absence of more recent reviews of solitary nonspecific ulcers, it is impossible to determine the current incidence rate of these ulcers.

Drug-Induced Small Intestinal Ulceration

Several drugs, most notably potassium chloride and nonsteroidal anti-inflammatory drugs (NSAIDs), have been noted to cause small intestinal ulceration that cannot be distinguished from the idiopathic ulcers described earlier. The causative mechanism for NSAID-induced ulcerations is an area of active study.

Potassium Chloride Ulceration

In the early 1960s, enteric-coated potassium chloride was used either alone or in combination with thiazide diuretics. During this period, it was noted that the incidence of ulcerative obstructive lesions of the small intestine appeared to be rising. Lawrason and coworkers[2] published a retrospective review of 440 cases of small intestinal ulceration gleaned from chart reviews in selected hospitals in the United States, Canada, South America, and Europe and incorporated previously published cases, for a total of 484. They noted that of this group, 275 patients had been receiving potassium chloride, an oral diuretic, or both. Potassium chloride was established as the causative agent when experimental studies showed that small intestinal ulcerations developed in monkeys *(Macaca mulatta)* given potassium preparations, but not those given diuretics. Further, the site of injury appeared to be determined by the site of release of the potassium chloride in the gastrointestinal tract, rather than the type of preparation used.[3] These enteric-coated potassium preparations were withdrawn from the market in the mid-1960s, and the incidence of small intestinal ulceration at the Mayo Clinic declined from 3.6 cases per year between 1960 and 1969 to 1.2 cases per year between 1970 and 1979.[1] Potassium chloride was the first drug implicated as a cause of small bowel ulceration on the basis of strong clinical and experimental evidence.

Nonsteroidal Anti-inflammatory Drug Ulceration

NSAIDs are among the most frequently prescribed drugs, with a world market in excess of $6 billion per year. Their side effects largely involve the gastrointestinal tract. Their effect on the stomach is well documented, with gastric erosions and ulcerations occurring in 10% to 30% of NSAID users. Suppression of prostaglandin synthesis appears to be a major mechanism underlying gastric damage (see Chapter 23). NSAIDs have been noted increasingly to cause damage to the small bowel distal to the duodenum via both cyclooxygenase (COX)-dependent and independent mechanisms and are a source of considerable morbidity. The spectrum of NSAID-associated disease in the small intestine varies from a subtle enteropathy to small bowel ulcerations and diaphragm-like strictures.

Clinical Presentation

The spectrum of small intestinal disease caused by NSAIDs varies from occult blood and protein loss in the absence of symptoms to hypoalbuminemia, anemia, diarrhea, and weight loss. Symptoms of partial small bowel obstruction, such as vomiting and colicky abdominal pain, may be seen. Laboratory evaluation is often notable for hypoalbuminemia and anemia. Recently, it has been recognized that a variety of NSAIDs can cause jejunal and ileal inflammation and ulceration.[4] Osmosin, a long-acting preparation of indomethacin, was withdrawn from the market in 1983 because of its propensity to cause small bowel ulceration and perforation.[5]

In addition to the clinically apparent syndromes described previously, NSAIDs may cause more subtle changes in the small intestine known as "NSAID enteropathy." Increased intestinal permeability, inflammation, and subtle bleeding can be demonstrated by nuclear medicine techniques in many patients on NSAIDs, in whom anemia and hypoalbuminemia can develop. To date, there is no gross pathologic correlate to this syndrome, and the responsible changes may be apparent only at the cellular and subcellular levels.

Pathology

In an autopsy study, Allison and associates[6] established that small intestinal ulcerations distal to the duodenum are prevalent in NSAID users. Of 713 patients studied, NSAIDs had been prescribed to 249 in the 6 months before death; 8.4% of the NSAID users had ulcerations of the small intestine, compared with only 0.6% of the NSAID nonusers. Although no information is available regarding morbidity caused by NSAIDs in these patients, three of the NSAID users had died of small intestinal perforation.[6]

The pathologic appearance of NSAID-induced ulceration is nonspecific. Ulcerations can be single or multiple and range from tiny punched-out ulcers to confluent areas of deep ulceration with stricture formation. The intervening mucosa is normal. These ulcers cannot be distinguished from nonspecific or idiopathic intestinal ulcerations on the basis of gross or microscopic pathologic appearance. In patients with long-standing NSAID use, ulcerations are sometimes associated with diaphragm-like strictures, referred to as "diaphragm disease." The "diaphragms" found in these patients are thin, concentric strictures that comprise mucosa and submucosa with or without submucosal fibrosis.

Mechanism of Injury

The mechanisms of NSAID-induced injury to the small bowel are not completely understood and may involve both a systemic and a local effect (Fig. 106–1). In a rat model of jejunal ulceration caused by indomethacin, Anthony and colleagues[7] observed that the ulcers are localized to the mesenteric margin of the bowel, an area that is relatively poorly perfused in rats. Indomethacin may selectively cause ischemia-reperfusion injury at these sites. Trevethick and coworkers[8] suggested that indomethacin-induced damage to the rat intestine is histologically similar to that found in man and, in the rat, can be limited by treatment with misoprostol and sulfasalazine.

Bjarnason and associates[9] demonstrated that NSAIDs cause increased intestinal permeability in humans, as measured by loss of chromium-51–labeled proteins into the intestine. In another study, 111 patients were given oral NSAIDs, and within 4 hours of ingestion, 70% were found to have intestinal inflammation, as measured by indium-111–labeled white blood cell accumulation in the small bowel by scintigraphy, as well as by fecal excretion of indium-111.[10] Nineteen of the 32 patients who also underwent scanning with ^{99m}Tc-labeled red blood cells showed blood loss at the sites where intestinal inflammation was demonstrated. Quantitation of blood loss in eight patients was comparable to that seen in colorectal cancer.

Bjarnason and coworkers[10] have suggested that topical injury to the small intestine is a COX-independent mechanism and is due to the ability of NSAIDs to uncouple mitochondrial oxidative phosphorylation at the time of drug absorption. This leads to a reduction of adenosine triphosphate (ATP) production and leakage of calcium (Ca^{2+}) from mitochondria. Sequelae of this process include increased cytosolic Ca^{2+}, damage to mitochondria with increased production of reactive oxygen species, and disturbed sodium/potassium (Na^+/K^+) ratios with cellular osmotic imbalance. The result is a loss of control of intercellular junctions, leading to increased permeability. Inappropriate contact of luminal contents, such as bile acids, pancreatic secretions, bacteria, and food antigens, with enterocytes results in neutrophil chemotaxis, causing nonspecific inflammation and ulceration as a systemic response to the initial injury. In addition, the concomitant cyclooxygenase inhibition that occurs with all COX-nonselective NSAIDs regardless of the route of administration may result in decreased prostaglandin synthesis and an alteration in mucosal blood flow, which may potentiate ulceration[11] (see Fig. 106–1). The enterohepatic circulation of NSAIDs also appears to contribute to mucosal injury in both animal models and humans.[12]

Diagnosis

Despite the use of esophagogastroduodenoscopy (EGD), colonoscopy, and barium contrast x-ray studies, no source of blood loss is found in one half the patients with iron-deficiency anemia who are taking NSAIDs. In one reported case, intraoperative use of Sonde enteroscopy revealed an ulcerated and strictured area of the ileum in a transfusion-dependent patient in whom prior conventional investigations had been uninformative.[13] Recently, Tibble and associates[14] demonstrated that fecal excretion of calprotectin, a nonde-

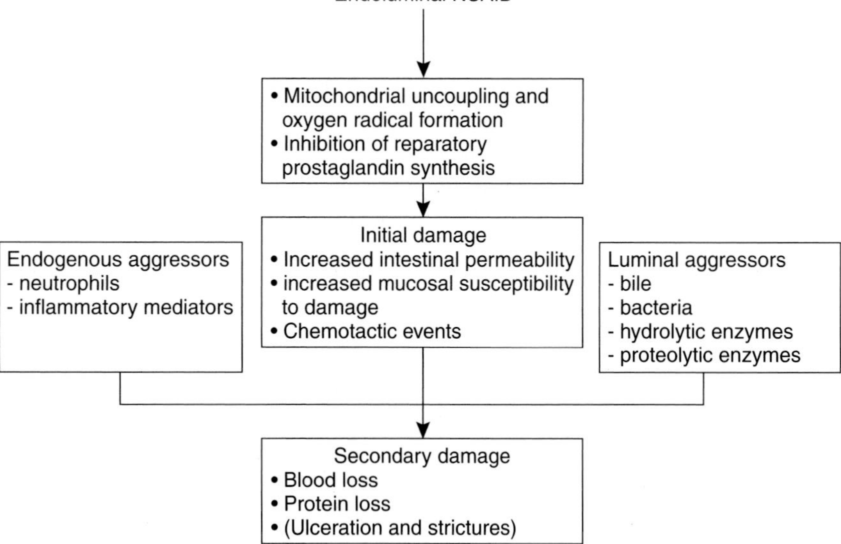

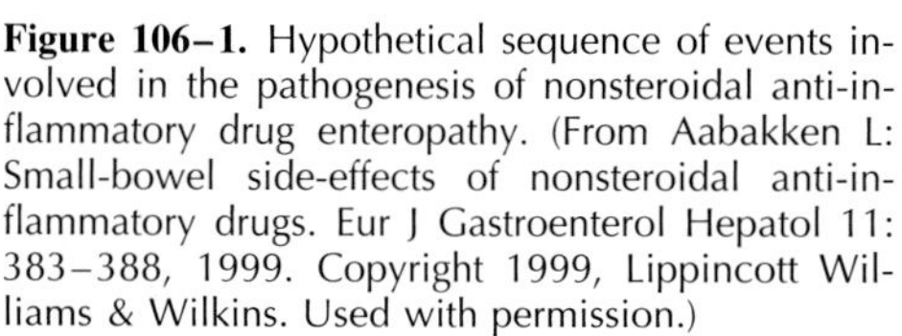
Figure 106–1. Hypothetical sequence of events involved in the pathogenesis of nonsteroidal anti-inflammatory drug enteropathy. (From Aabakken L: Small-bowel side-effects of nonsteroidal anti-inflammatory drugs. Eur J Gastroenterol Hepatol 11: 383–388, 1999. Copyright 1999, Lippincott Williams & Wilkins. Used with permission.)

graded neutrophil cytosolic protein, can be used to assess intestinal inflammation and may prove to be a practical method for diagnosing NSAID enteropathy.

Management

Although avoidance of NSAIDs is the most effective therapy for NSAID enteropathy, experimental studies show that administration of metronidazole reduces inflammation and occult blood loss without changing intestinal permeability.[15] Sulfasalazine has also been shown to reduce intestinal inflammation, as measured by fecal indium-labeled neutrophil excretion,[16] thereby suggesting that active mediators of inflammation as well as anaerobes found normally in the small intestine may play a role in the pathogenesis of NSAID injury to the small bowel.

DIFFUSE ULCERATIONS

Ulcerative Enteritis, Refractory Celiac Sprue, and Enteropathy-Associated T Cell Lymphoma

Diffuse small intestinal ulcerations can complicate celiac sprue and can occur in patients without previously known celiac sprue who present with spruelike symptoms and have either flat or normal intervening intestinal mucosa but are refractory to gluten withdrawal. These syndromes have been called *ulcerative jejunitis, chronic ulcerative (nongranulomatous) jejunoileitis,* or *idiopathic chronic ulcerative enteritis.*[17–19] The term *ulcerative enteritis* will be used in this discussion. *Refractory celiac sprue* itself encompasses a heterogeneous group of patients and is discussed more fully in Chapter 93. The most common cause of "refractoriness" is inadvertent or deliberate gluten ingestion. However, for the purposes of this discussion, refractory celiac sprue will refer to those patients with small intestinal histology consistent with celiac sprue and severe, persistent malabsorption, often with diffuse small intestinal ulcerations, despite strict adherence to a gluten-free diet, but as yet without histologically evident lymphoma.[20–23]

In addition, T cell lymphoma can complicate the course of previously established celiac sprue or can present de novo with multiple intestinal ulcerations and malabsorption in patients without known underlying celiac sprue but with small intestinal biopsies that demonstrate villous atrophy. The term *enteropathy-associated T cell lymphoma (EATL)* has been given to this syndrome (see also Chapter 26).[24]

The subject is confusing because, even though the various groups of patients share clinical and histologic similarities and ulcerative enteritis and refractory celiac sprue have an increased risk of progressing to T cell lymphoma, the clinical syndromes are rare, there is no well-defined etiology or pathogenesis, and the diagnoses have been based on varying criteria. Until recently, it was not possible to link them together, and in many patients, the relationship to celiac sprue was unclear. Over the past 15 years, evidence has emerged to suggest that some patients with the clinical syndromes mentioned previously can be linked by the presence of intestinal intraepithelial T cell lymphocyte abnormalities.[20, 21, 23, 25, 26] The relationship to celiac sprue is still unclear, but it appears that many of these patients have previously undiagnosed celiac sprue.[21, 24, 27]

Background

The association of celiac sprue and lymphoma was first reported in 1937.[28] In 1949, two patients with small intestinal ulcerations and spruelike symptoms were described, and the term *ulcerous jejunoileitis* was coined.[29] Over the next four decades, several case reports appeared and a registry was established noting clinical and histologic similarities among patients with ulcerative enteritis, refractory celiac sprue, and intestinal lymphoma.[17–19]

Beginning in the 1980s, evidence in favor of underlying celiac sprue as the predisposing factor for ulcerative enteritis, refractory celiac sprue, and EATL in many patients began emerging from both registries[19, 27] and genotyping studies.[24] It is impossible to determine the exact relationship of ulcerative enteritis and refractory celiac sprue to celiac sprue itself, because before the availability of serologic testing for antiendomysial and antigliadin antibodies, some studies included patients who had intestinal biopsies consistent with celiac sprue but who were refractory to gluten withdrawal.[19] Further confusing the issue, refractory celiac sprue had largely been a diagnosis of exclusion (that is, exclusion of gluten ingestion, lymphoma, and collagenous sprue). More recently, patients with ulcerative enteritis and refractory celiac sprue have been identified as having evidence of underlying celiac sprue based on genotyping studies or serum antibodies, even though they may be nonresponsive to gluten withdrawal, either from the outset or after a period of gluten sensitivity.[20, 21, 23, 25] The relationship of EATL to celiac sprue is now somewhat clearer, as an exhaustive genotyping study has shown that EATL arises against the same genetic background as that predisposing to celiac sprue.[24] In this context, even though gluten sensitivity is almost certainly present at birth, its clinical expression is highly variable, and symptoms may be masked until the onset of a secondary event such as ulcerative enteritis or overt lymphoma. Therefore, it is now thought that most patients with ulcerative enteritis, refractory celiac sprue, and EATL have underlying celiac sprue, even if it is not possible to prove this conclusively by demonstration of histologic resolution of sprue on repeat intestinal biopsy after a gluten-free diet.

In 1985, DNA analysis was used to show that, in four patients with celiac sprue, multiple small intestinal ulcers, and lymphoma, the intestinal intraepithelial T cells were monoclonal.[30] Subsequently, using the polymerase chain reaction (PCR), several groups demonstrated that in EATL, ulcerative enteritis, and refractory celiac sprue, the intestinal intraepithelial T cells consist of a monoclonal population of cells.[20, 21, 23, 25, 26] In 1995, Murray and colleagues[26] used PCR amplification in patients with EATL to show that the neoplastic T cells share the same monoclonal T cell receptor gene rearrangements as the T cell population in the nonlymphomatous adjacent intestinal mucosa. In 1997, Ashton-Key and coworkers[25] used PCR amplification of the T cell receptor γ-chain gene in six patients with EATL and 7 patients with ulcerative enteritis to confirm the findings of Murray and associates, and demonstrated further that the intraepithelial T cell population is monoclonal both in the ulcers and in the nonulcerated intervening intestinal mucosa in patients with ulcerative enteritis. In the two patients with ulcerative enteritis in whom lymphoma subsequently developed, the same clone was detected in the ulcers and in the malignant lymphoma. Forty control subjects, including eight patients with uncomplicated celiac sprue and 12 patients with Crohn's disease, had polyclonal T cell receptor gene rearrangements.[25] In 1998, Carbonnel and associates[20] demonstrated the monoclonality of intraepithelial T cells in four patients with refractory celiac sprue, two with ulcerative enteritis, and three in whom T cell lymphoma subsequently developed. Seven patients with responsive celiac disease and four control patients had either a polyclonal or an oligoclonal population of intraepithelial T cells.[20] Cellier and colleagues[23] further demonstrated that, in six patients with refractory celiac sprue (two of whom had diffuse ulcerations and none with histologic evidence of lymphoma), the intestinal intraepithelial T cells were not only monoclonal but also phenotypically abnormal.[23] In 1999, Bagdi and colleagues[21] confirmed these observations and also showed the monoclonality of intraepithelial T cells in six patients with refractory celiac sprue, five with ulcerative enteritis, and nine with EATL. Seventeen patients with uncomplicated celiac sprue had polyclonal T cell receptor gene rearrangements. These investigators concluded that patients with ulcerative enteritis, refractory celiac sprue, and EATL have a fundamental neoplastic T cell disorder and that the accumulation of phenotypically aberrant, monoclonal T cells is potentially the first step in the genesis of EATL.[21]

The origin of the abnormal intestinal intraepithelial T cells remains controversial. Because normal human small intestinal intraepithelial T lymphocytes have been shown to be oligoclonal,[31] one possibility is that the abnormal, monoclonal T cells represent an expansion of mature clones that were prevalent in the intestinal epithelium before the onset of disease. Alternatively, T cells could be recruited into the epithelium and could undergo monoclonal expansion after antigenic stimulation. A third hypothesis is that the monoclonal population of T cells is derived from the expansion of T cell precursors that are present normally in a small percentage of the gut epithelium in mice and humans. Finally, abnormal lymphocytes with a restricted repertoire may undergo proliferation and eventually develop into overt lymphoma.[23, 31]

In summary, many patients with ulcerative enteritis, refractory celiac sprue, and EATL have underlying celiac sprue that precedes their presentation with diffuse small intestinal ulcerations and malabsorption. The underlying gluten sensitivity provides an antigenic stimulus for the activation of intestinal T cells, whose origin is unclear at this time.[32] It appears likely that refractory celiac sprue, ulcerative enteritis, or lymphoma can supervene when a dominant clone of T lymphocytes from this stimulated pool undergoes neoplastic transformation. The precise relationship between the monoclonal intraepithelial T cells seen in ulcerative enteritis and refractory celiac sprue and the lymphocytes seen in fully developed T cell lymphoma is unknown. However, at this time, it seems appropriate to consider these diseases as part of an overlapping spectrum of abnormal T cell proliferation syndromes that occur in patients with a predisposition toward gluten sensitivity (or possibly other antigenic stimuli).[20, 21, 23, 25, 26]

Clinical Presentation

The age of patients with ulcerative enteritis, refractory celiac sprue, and EATL ranges from 18 to 80 years, with the majority presenting in the fifth and sixth decades of life. Women are affected slightly more commonly than men. Patients with either the new onset of or long-standing celiac sprue can present with worsening malabsorption and abdominal pain that are increasingly unresponsive to a gluten-free diet. Another group of patients present with unexplained malabsorption and abdominal pain and either a flat or an otherwise normal appearing small intestinal biopsy, but with no response to a gluten-free diet. Malabsorption, diarrhea, and weight loss are conspicuous and often severe. Symptoms can be present for days to years. In addition, patients can present with complications, including gastrointestinal hemorrhage, perforation, or intestinal obstruction secondary to strictures. Patients with ulcerative enteritis and refractory celiac sprue have an increased risk of progression to overt lymphoma.[18–21, 23, 25, 26]

Physical examination reveals signs of severe malabsorption with steatorrhea and a protein-losing enteropathy. There is often significant weight loss and cachexia. Fever and signs of dehydration can be present. Abdominal tenderness can be present and can be mild, diffuse, and crampy or severe. Hepatomegaly and splenic atrophy can occur. Lymphadenopathy is unusual, even in patients in whom lymphoma has developed. Symptoms and signs of anemia can be present as a result of chronic nutritional deficiency or acute gastrointestinal hemorrhage. Intestinal perforation typically leads to signs of peritonitis. When intestinal obstruction has occurred, there can be acute vomiting and abdominal distention.[17–21, 23, 25, 26]

Laboratory Diagnosis

The laboratory abnormalities reflect the diarrhea, severe malabsorption, and complications of the disease. Findings include iron deficiency or macrocytic anemia, prolongation of the prothrombin time, electrolyte abnormalities consistent with the degree of dehydration, hypoalbuminemia, hypocalcemia, hypomagnesemia, hypocholesterolemia, and low serum carotene levels. The white blood cell count is usually normal unless a complication, such as intestinal perforation or obstruction, has occurred. Acute gastrointestinal bleeding is reflected in the hematocrit value.[18–21, 23, 25, 26] Serum antigliadin and antiendomysial antibodies, which are typically present in celiac sprue, can be either present or absent in ulcerative enteritis, refractory sprue, or EATL. Stool abnormalities include increased volume, mild to severe steatorrhea, increased fecal α_1-antitrypsin excretion, and a positive fecal occult blood test. The D-xylose absorption test is usually abnormal.[17, 20, 21, 23]

Pathology

In ulcerative enteritis and refractory celiac sprue, the histologically benign appearing ulcers are diffuse and may be present in the duodenum but are more commonly located in the jejunum and ileum. Rarely, gastric and colonic ulcers also develop. The ulcers range in size from 1 mm to 3.5 cm, are rarely solitary, and are well circumscribed. Some ulcers are superficial, extending to the muscularis mucosa, but usually they extend to the muscularis propria and occasionally through it, thus causing a perforation. The inflammatory infiltrate at the base of the ulcer is usually mixed and consists of both acute and chronic inflammatory cells. The T cells are monoclonal. Muscular hypertrophy and fibrosis may be present.[19–21, 23]

Overt T cell lymphoma can present either as multiple intestinal ulcers or as an ulcerated mass. Tumor cells can be demonstrated in intestinal ulcerations, as well as in nonulcerated areas of the intestine. The tumor cells can vary in appearance from well-differentiated lymphocytes to sheets of blast cells with large, vesicular nuclei and prominent nucleoli in high-grade tumors. A dense infiltrate of inflammatory cells may accompany the tumor cells.[19–21, 25, 30] Tumor cells can disseminate to lymph nodes, bone marrow, liver, spleen, and lung.[17, 18, 26]

The grossly normal appearing intervening intestinal mucosa adjacent to or distant from either a benign or a malignant-appearing ulcer can show either normal villous architecture or partial or total villous atrophy with crypt hyperplasia (Fig. 106–2). The lamina propria may contain inflammatory infiltrates consisting of a mixture of plasma cells, lymphocytes, polymorphonuclear cells, and macrophages. Epithelioid granulomas and other features of inflammatory bowel disease are absent. There is no evidence of an infectious process. There usually is an increased number of intraepithelial lymphocytes. As has been discussed earlier, the intraepithelial T lymphocytes are monoclonal.[17–21, 23, 25, 30]

Endoscopic Features

Because the ulcers are located most commonly distal to the duodenum, small bowel enteroscopy is the diagnostic procedure of choice in patients with ulcerative enteritis, refractory celiac sprue, and EATL. Direct small intestinal visualization can be accomplished via operative enteroscopy, Sonde enteroscopy, or push enteroscopy. Push enteroscopy has advantages over the other two methods in that procedure time is usually less than 1 hour, and mucosal biopsies can be obtained through a standard 2.8-mm biopsy channel. The chief limitation of push enteroscopy is that the depth of insertion is generally only to the mid- or distal jejunum. However, the availability of longer scopes (250 cm) will likely increase this distance.

Enteroscopic features include multiple erosions, ulcerations, and loss of vascular markings (Fig. 106–3). Biopsies should be taken of both the ulcerated areas and the grossly normal-appearing intervening intestinal mucosa.[20, 22, 23] Occasional patients will also have gastric or colonic ulcers, which can be identified on routine esophagogastroduodenoscopy or colonoscopy.

In one study, eight patients with refractory celiac sprue were evaluated prospectively by push videoenteroscopy, and examination of the duodenum and jejunum showed discordant results in four patients.[22] These four patients had no duodenal ulcers, but did have multiple jejunal ulcers, none of which had been detected by barium contrast radiography of the small intestine during the preceding year. The authors concluded that, in these patients with celiac sprue that was not responding to a strict gluten-free diet, push enteroscopy was a good diagnostic tool that identified multiple ulcerations in the jejunum that had not been detected by other diagnostic studies.[22]

Radiographic Features

Radiologic abnormalities are common in these clinical syndromes. Plain abdominal films may show a normal intestinal gas pattern or a pattern suggestive of small bowel obstruction. If perforation has occurred, free air may be present on the upright film. A barium contrast study of the small bowel or an enteroclysis study may show separation and thickening of small intestinal loops, ulcerations, or a mass (Fig.

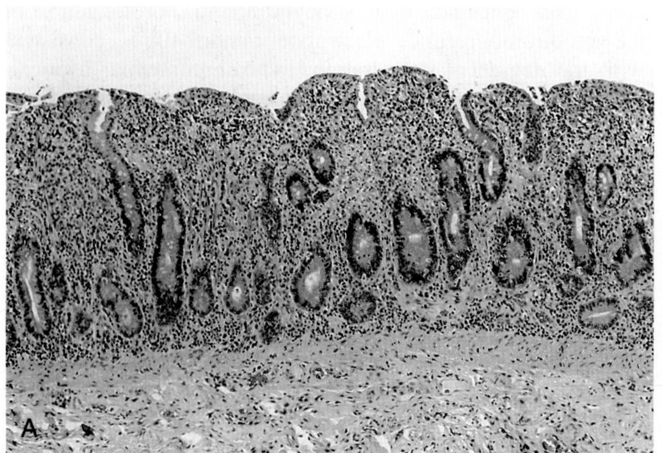

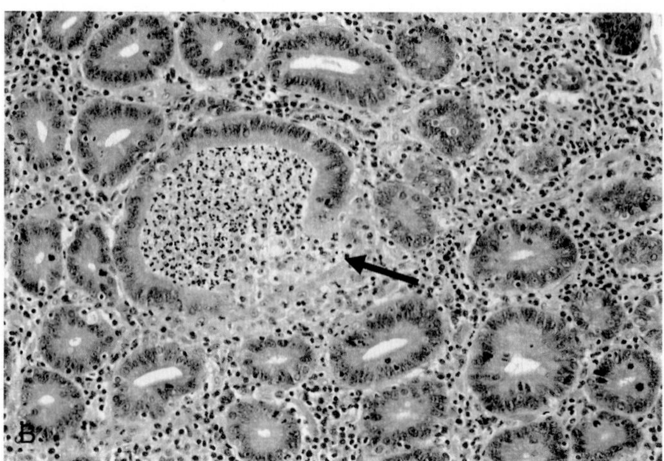

Figure 106–2. Full-thickness biopsy of the jejunum in a patient with long-standing, severe refractory celiac sprue. *A*, Low-power view. The mucosal architecture shows complete villous flattening with crypt hyperplasia (severe mucosal lesion). There is an increase in the number of intraepithelial lymphocytes. The lamina propria is expanded by inflammatory cells that extend beneath the base of the crypts. *B*, High-power view. Neutrophils are destroying an epithelial crypt *(arrow)*. In other areas small ulcers were present. (Courtesy of Marie E. Robert, M.D., Yale University School of Medicine, Department of Pathology, New Haven, Connecticut.)

106–4). Strictures may be single or multiple and appear as areas of luminal narrowing alternating with more dilated portions of small bowel.[17, 19, 33] Computed tomography may show nonspecific thickening and separation of small bowel loops, enlarged mesenteric lymph nodes, or metastatic disease.[23]

Management and Prognosis

There have been no reported controlled therapeutic trials for these rare diseases. Prognosis has been uniformly poor, with patients dying from severe malnutrition, hemorrhage, perforation, or T cell lymphoma. Although the magnitude is difficult to assess, patients with ulcerative enteritis and refractory celiac sprue have a significantly increased risk of progressing to frank lymphoma. Currently, there are no recommendations for screening patients with celiac disease for these disorders.

All patients initially should be treated with fluid and electrolyte replacement and supportive therapy. Total parenteral nutrition can improve nutritional status in severely malnourished patients. If small intestinal biopsies show villous atrophy and there is no evidence of overt lymphoma, patients should be placed on a gluten-free diet. However, it is impossible to predict which patients will respond to gluten withdrawal. After gluten withdrawal has failed, oral glucocorticoids are often tried, with varying success. Patients who do respond to glucocorticoids often remain steroid dependent.[17–20, 23, 25] Treatment with immunosuppressants, such as azathioprine or cyclosporine, has been successful in a few patients.*[23] Exploratory laparotomy may be considered in selected cases, for either diagnosis or therapy, because surgical resection of the involved bowel, especially if the disease is localized to one part of the intestine, offers the greatest chance for survival.[19, 25]

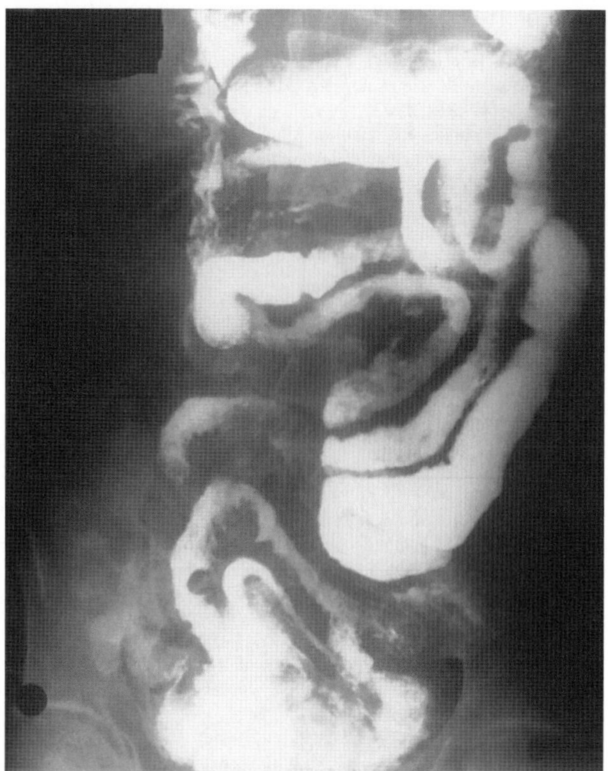

Figure 106–4. Barium radiograph of the small bowel showing diffuse small intestinal ulceration in a patient with refractory celiac sprue (ulcerative enteritis). There is diffuse involvement of the small intestine with multiple ulcerations and separation and thickening of the loops of jejunum and ileum. (Courtesy of Christophe Cellier, MD, PhD, Laennec and European Hospital Georges Pompidou, Paris, France.)

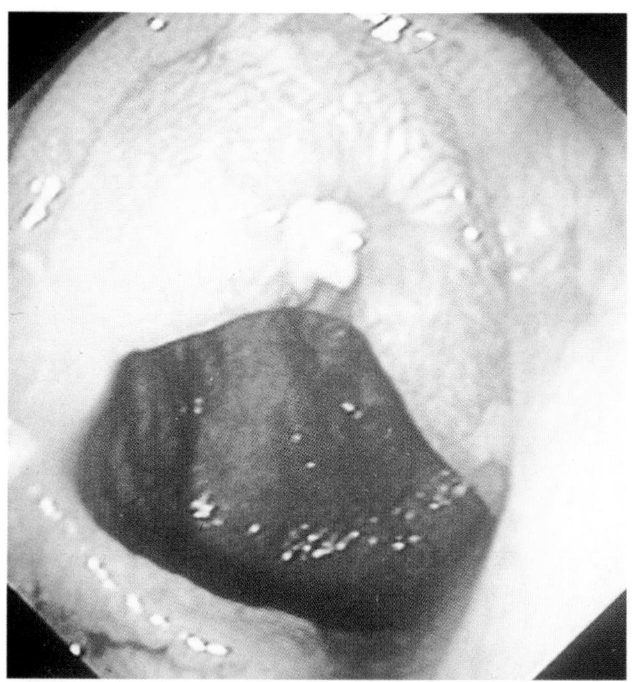

Figure 106–3. Push enteroscopy findings in ulcerative enteritis. The endoscopic photograph shows multiple small ulcers located in the midjejunum. (Courtesy of Christophe Cellier, MD, PhD, Laennec and European Hospital Georges Pompidou, Paris, France.)

In patients with overt lymphoma, surgical resection and chemotherapy have been attempted. Prognosis appears to be better in the recent literature compared with the prognosis reported 20 or 30 years ago. However, because of the rarity of this disease, there are no published controlled trials, only case reports.[18, 25, 26, 30]

With the recent recognition that refractory celiac sprue, ulcerative enteritis, and EATL are all characterized by the proliferation of an aberrant monoclonal population of T cells, therapy targeted to the abnormal T cell population will no doubt be possible in the future.[21]

REFERENCES

1. Boydstun JS, Gaffey TA, Bartholomew LG: Clinicopathologic study of nonspecific ulcers of the small intestine. Dig Dis Sci 26:911–916, 1981.
2. Lawrason FD, Alpert E, Mohr FL, et al: Ulcerative-obstructive lesions of the small intestine. JAMA 191:105–108, 1965.
3. Diener RM, Shoffstall DH, Earl AE: Production of potassium-induced gastrointestinal lesions in monkeys. Toxicol Appl Pharmacol 7:746–755, 1965.
4. Bjarnason I, Hayllar J, Macherson AJ, et al: Side effects of nonsteroidal anti-inflammatory drugs on the small and large intestine in humans. Gastroenterology 104:1832–1847, 1993.

*Personal communication, Christopher Cellier MD, PhD, 2000

5. Cree IA, Walker MA, Wright M, Forrester JC: Osmosin and ileal ulceration: A case report. Scot Med J 30:40–41, 1985.
6. Allison MC, Howatson AG, Torrance CJ, et al: Gastrointestinal damage associated with the use of nonsteroidal anti-inflammatory drugs. N Engl J Med 327:749–754, 1992.
7. Anthony A, Pounder RE, Dhillon AP, Wakefield AJ: Vascular anatomy defines sites of indomethacin induced jejunal ulceration along the mesenteric margin. Gut 41:763–770, 1997.
8. Trevethick MA, Clayton N, Strong P, et al: Indomethacin induced small intestinal damage in rats resembles NSAID induced enteropathy of the human small intestine. Gut 32:A1224, 1991.
9. Bjarnason I, Zanelli G, Prouse P, et al: Blood and protein loss via small intestinal inflammation induced by non-steroidal anti-inflammatory drugs. Lancet 2(8561):711–714, 1987.
10. Bjarnason I, Williams P, So A, Zanelli GD: Intestinal permeability and inflammation in rheumatoid arthritis: Effects of non-steroidal anti-inflammatory drugs. Lancet 2(8413):1171–1174, 1984.
11. Somasundaram S, Hayllar H, Rafi S, et al: The biochemical basis of non-steroidal anti-inflammatory drug-induced damage to the gastrointestinal tract: A review and a hypothesis. Scand J Gastroenterol 30:289–299, 1995.
12. Wallace JL: Nonsteroidal anti-inflammatory drugs and gastroenteropathy: The second hundred years. Gastroenterology 112:1000–1016, 1997.
13. Achanta KK, Petros JG, Cave DR, et al: Use of intraoperative enteroscopy to diagnose nonsteroidal anti-inflammatory drug injury to the small intestine. Gastrointest Endosc 49:544–546, 1999.
14. Tibble JA, Sigthorsson G, Foster R, et al: High prevalence of NSAID enteropathy as shown by a simple faecal test. Gut 45:362–366, 1999.
15. Bjarnason I, Hayllar J, Smethurst P, et al: Metronidazole reduces intestinal inflammation and blood loss in non-steroidal anti-inflammatory drug induced enteropathy. Gut 33:1204–1208, 1992.
16. Bjarnason I, Hopkinson N, Zanelli G, et al: Treatment of non-steroidal anti-inflammatory drug induced enteropathy. Gut 31:777–780, 1990.
17. Jeffries GH, Steinberg H, Sleisenger MH: Chronic ulcerative (nongranulomatous) jejunitis. Am J Med 44:47–59, 1968.
18. Isaacson P, Wright DH: Malignant histiocytosis of the intestine. Its relationship to malabsorption and ulcerative jejunitis. Hum Pathol 9: 661–677, 1978.
19. Baer AN, Bayless TM, Yardley JH: Intestinal ulceration and malabsorption syndromes. Gastroenterology 79:754–765, 1980.
20. Carbonnel F, Grollet-Bioul L, Brouet JC, et al: Are complicated forms of celiac disease cryptic T-cell lymphomas? Blood 92:3879–3886, 1998.
21. Bagdi E, Diss TC, Munson P, et al: Mucosal intra-epithelial lymphocytes in enteropathy-associated T-cell lymphoma, ulcerative jejunitis, and refractory celiac disease constitute a neoplastic population. Blood 94:260–264, 1999.
22. Cellier C, Cuillerier E, Patey-Mariaud de Serre N, et al: Push enteroscopy in celiac sprue and refractory sprue. Gastrointest Endosc 50:613–617, 1999.
23. Cellier C, Patey N, Mauvieux L, et al: Abnormal intestinal intraepithelial lymphocytes in refractory sprue. Gastroenterology 114:471–481, 1998.
24. Howell WM, Leung ST, Jones DB, et al: HLA-DRB, -DQA, and -DQB polymorphism in celiac disease and enteropathy-associated T-cell lymphoma. Common features and additional risk factors for malignancy. Hum Immunol 43:29–37, 1995.
25. Ashton-Key M, Diss TC, Pan L, et al: Molecular analysis of T-cell clonality in ulcerative jejunitis and enteropathy-associated T-cell lymphoma. Am J Pathol 151:493–498, 1997.
26. Murray A, Cuevas EC, Jones DB, et al: Study of the immunohistochemistry and T cell clonality of enteropathy-associated T cell lymphoma. Am J Pathol 146:509–519, 1995.
27. Swinson CM, Slavin G, Coles EC, et al: Coeliac disease and malignancy. Lancet I:111–115, 1983.
28. Fairley NH, Mackie FP: The clinical and biochemical syndrome in lymphadenoma and allied diseases involving the mesenteric lymph glands. BMJ i:375–380, 1937.
29. Nyman E: Ulcerous jejuno-ileitis with symptomatic sprue. Acta Med Scand 84:275–283, 1949.
30. Isaacson PG, O'Connor NTJ, Spencer J, et al: Malignant histiocytosis of the intestine: A T-cell lymphoma. Lancet 2(8457):688–691, 1985.
31. Gross GG, Schwartz VL, Stevens C, et al: Distribution of dominant T cell receptor β chains in human intestinal mucosa. J Exp Med 180: 1337–1344, 1994.
32. Godkin A, Jewell D: The pathogenesis of celiac disease. Gastroenterology 115:206–210, 1998.
33. Brunton FJ, Guyer PB: Malignant histiocytosis and ulcerative jejunitis of the small intestine. Clin Radiol 34:291–295, 1983.

Chapter 107

APPENDICITIS

George A. Sarosi, Jr. and Richard H. Turnage

HISTORICAL PERSPECTIVE

Although the appendix has been a likely source of intra-abdominal pathology for most of human history, the recognition of its role in acute abdominal syndromes is a recent event in the history of medicine. The first anatomic mention of the appendix was made by Leonardo da Vinci in the early 15th century. The first clearly recognizable case report of appendicitis was recorded in 1711 by the German surgeon Lorenz Heister.[1] Throughout the 18th and 19th centuries the prevailing medical opinion was that acute right lower quadrant pain and inflammation was a consequence of inflammation of the cecum or its surrounding tissues. The modern description of the pathophysiology of appendicitis and the role of the appendix in acute abdominal syndromes dates to 1886. In that year Reginald Fitz presented a paper in which he coined the term *appendicitis* and espoused early surgical intervention as the appropriate course of treatment.[2] The first appendectomy for acute appendicitis had been performed by Lawson Tait in 1880, but he did not report the case until 1890.[3]

EPIDEMIOLOGY

Appendicitis is the most common acute abdominal emergency seen in developed countries. The crude incidence of appendicitis in the United States for all age groups is 11 per 10,000 population per year.[4] Similar rates are noted in other developed countries. It is interesting that the rates of appendicitis are up to ten times lower in many less-developed African countries, although the reasons for the difference in incidence rates between developed and less-developed countries are not clear.[5] The incidence of the disease peaks between age 15 and 19 years, with a rate of 48.1 per 10,000 population per year. The rate falls to approximately 5 per 10,000 population per year by age 45 years and remains constant thereafter.[4] Men are at a significantly greater risk than women, with a case ratio in most series of 1.4:1. The lifetime risk of appendicitis has been estimated to be 8.6% in men and 6.7% in women.[4] Approximately 250,000 appendectomies are performed for acute appendicitis each year in the United States. Including incidental appendectomies, the lifetime risk of appendectomy is estimated to be approximately 15%. However, the rates of appendicitis have been declining over the past half-century. From 1975 to 1995, a 36% decrease in the overall incidence of appendicitis has been noted in the United States[4] and England.[6] The explanation for this decrease has not yet been elucidated.

ANATOMY AND EMBRYOLOGY

The vermiform appendix and cecum, the first portion of the colon, can be thought of as a single anatomic unit. Developmentally, the appendix and cecum are part of the midgut and form between the 8th and 12th weeks of gestation as a bud arising from the midgut loop. Congenital malformations of the appendix, such as agenesis and duplication, have been reported but are rare. The appendix is a tubular segment of bowel extending from the posteromedial border of the cecum. With an average length of 9 cm,[7] the appendix is found at the pole of the cecum where the 3 taenia coli intersect. Unlike the rest of the colon, the appendix has a complete longitudinal muscle layer. The blood supply of the appendix is found in its own mesentery, the mesoappendix, and consists of an appendicular branch of the ileocolic trunk of the superior mesenteric artery. The lymphatic drainage of the appendix occurs via the ileocolic lymph nodes, which are shared with the terminal ileum and right colon.

Although the right colon is fixed in the retroperitoneum, the appendix and cecum have a more variable position within the abdomen. A variety of classifications exist to describe the position of the appendix, but in general, the appendix is retrocecal, pelvic, subcecal, or paraileal (Fig. 107–1). The position of the appendix has important clinical implications, because the classic progression of symptoms requires irritation of the parietal peritoneum by a mobile appendix. In some series as many as 60% of cases of appendicitis may be associated with a retrocecal position, which may result in an atypical clinical presentation.

The classic surface anatomy of the appendix was described by McBurney in the late 19th century.[8] McBurney's point is located at the junction of the lateral and middle thirds of a line drawn from the right anterior superior iliac spine to the umbilicus. This surface marking is important in both the diagnosis and treatment of acute appendicitis. However, two recent studies have shown that the appendix is

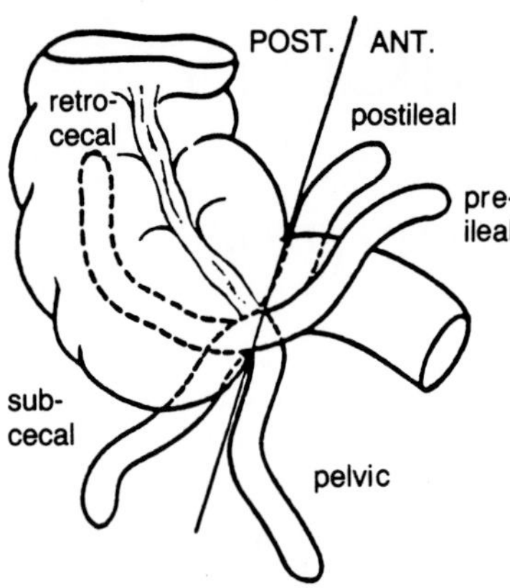

Figure 107–1. Positions of the appendix. (From Buschard K, Kjaeldgaard A: Investigation and analysis of the position, fixation, length and embryology of the vermiform appendix. Acta Chir Scand 139:293, 1973.)

located within 5 cm of McBurney's point less than 50% of the time.[9, 10] This anatomic finding helps explain why pain and tenderness located at McBurney's point are not found in all cases of acute appendicitis.

PATHOLOGY

Acute appendicitis is classified as acute, gangrenous, or perforated. Grossly, the earliest findings of acute appendicitis are injection of the serosal blood vessels and edema of the appendiceal wall. In more advanced cases, the serosal surface is dull in appearance, a fibrinopurulent exudate appears, and focal areas of gangene marked by greenish and black discoloration of the wall develop. In the presence of perforation, focal necrosis of the appendiceal wall is present, with purulence and adjacent abscesses.[11]

Microscopically, each of the forms of acute appendicitis has distinctive characteristics. In acute or suppurative appendicitis, a neutrophilic infiltrate involves the muscularis propria in a circumferential fashion. In addition, there often is inflammation and ulceration of the mucosa, edema and microabscesses in the appendicular wall, and vascular thrombosis. The hallmarks of gangrenous appendicitis are transmural inflammation of the wall of the appendix in association with focal areas of necrosis. Vascular thrombosis is more prominent in gangrenous than in suppurative appendicitis. Pathologically, perforating appendicitis and gangrenous appendicitis are similar in appearance. Intraluminal or mucosal inflammation (catarrhal inflammation) alone is more characteristic of infectious enteritis or colitis and is not considered evidence of acute appendicitis.[12]

PATHOGENESIS

Despite more than 100 years of study, there is still no single hypothesis that explains the etiology of appendicitis in all cases. The classic hypothesis holds that obstruction of the appendiceal lumen by either a fecolith or lymphoid hyperplasia results in increased intraluminal pressure, which results eventually in venous hypertension, ischemia of the appendiceal wall, and subsequent bacterial invasion of the appendix with necrosis and perforation. Experimental evidence in animal models supports this hypothesis.[13]

Despite this experimental evidence, there is reason to doubt that luminal obstruction is the precipitating event in all cases of appendicitis. Review of pathologic series shows that luminal obstruction is found in a minority of cases. Rates of fecoliths in acute appendicitis range from 8% to 44%, with the majority at the lower end of the range.[11, 12, 14] Lymphoid hyperplasia, the other putative source of luminal obstruction in appendicitis, is more common in noninflamed appendices than in acute appendicitis.[15] Other causes of luminal obstruction such as foreign bodies, tumors, and fibrous bands are uncommon pathologic findings. Finally, direct measurement of intraluminal pressure at appendectomy for appendicitis reveals an elevated pressure in only a minority of cases.[16]

An alternative hypothesis for the etiology of appendicitis is based on the concept that either bacterial or viral enteric infection leads to mucosal ulceration of the appendix, with subsequent bacterial invasion from the normal colonic flora. This theory is supported by the finding that up to 75% of cases of appendicitis demonstrate well-defined superficial mucosal ulceration. Furthermore, mucosal ulceration is a more consistent finding than dilation of the appendix or fecoliths and is found earlier in the course of appendicitis.[17] Additional support for the role of infection in the etiology of appendicitis is found in two lines of epidemiologic evidence. The first line of evidence is based on the hygiene theory of appendicitis advocated by Barker[18] in the mid-1980s. According to this theory, changes in sanitation tied to the Industrial Revolution resulted in a decrease in enteric infections in infants, with a subsequent decrease in immunity to the same infections in children and young adults. Acquisition of these infections later in life is thought to predispose people to appendicitis. As a result, the rates of appendicitis rose in the first half of the 20th century. The decrease in the overall rate of enteric infections over the past half-century has resulted in an overall decline in the incidence of appendicitis.[18] The second line of epidemiologic evidence to support the role of infection in the etiology of appendicitis is the seasonal variance in rates of appendicitis and the temporal and spatial clustering of appendicitis, both hallmarks of infectious diseases.[19] However, no specific infectious agent has been clearly linked with appendicitis, and infection is not the complete story.

A decrease in the intake of dietary fiber (the fiber hypothesis) also has been proposed as the cause of appendicitis. According to this hypothesis, decreased dietary fiber causes firmer stool with an increased enteric transit time that results in more fecoliths and more appendicitis. This hypothesis was felt to explain both the rise in appendicitis rates in the early 20th century and the marked differences in appendicitis rates between developed Western countries and undeveloped African countries. However, doubt has been cast on this hypothesis. First, despite falling dietary fiber intake in urban Africans, appendicitis rates have not risen markedly.[20] Second, the rates in the Western world have fallen without changes in dietary fiber intake. Third and most important, a recent prospective series from Africa demonstrates continued high-fiber intake even in patients with appendicitis.[21]

It is likely that one of several different inciting events, such as luminal obstruction, infection, or trauma, causes breakdown of the appendiceal mucosa and secondary bacterial invasion. The end result is appendicitis.

DIAGNOSIS

The diagnosis of appendicitis remains a clinical challenge because of the broad differential diagnosis of acute abdominal pain and the relatively nonspecific presentation of patients with appendicitis. Because the natural history of appendicitis is a progression to perforation, there is some urgency in making a prompt and accurate diagnosis. However, not all causes of the acute abdomen require surgical intervention, and a negative appendectomy carries some risk for the patient. Table 107–1 illustrates the common diagnoses that may mimic acute appendicitis. Compounding the diagnostic challenge is that there is no single symptom, sign, or laboratory test that is completely sensitive or specific for the diagnosis of appendicitis.[22] This diagnostic challenge makes appendicitis a fascinating clinical problem.

Table 107–1 | **Differential Diagnosis of Right Lower Quadrant Abdominal Pain and Clinical Factors Opposing Acute Appendicitis**

DIAGNOSIS	DIFFERENTIATION FROM APPENDICITIS
Bacterial or viral enteritis	Nausea, vomiting, and diarrhea severe, pain develops after vomiting
Mesenteric adenitis	Fever uncommon, WBC usually normal, duration of symptoms longer, RLQ physical findings less pronounced
Pyelonephritis	High fever and rigors common, marked pyuria or bacteriuria, urinary symptoms, abdominal rigidity less marked
Renal colic	Pain radiates to right groin, significant hematuria, character of pain clearly colic
Acute pancreatitis	Pain and vomiting more severe, tenderness less well localized, amylase elevated
Inflammatory bowel disease	History of similar attacks, diarrhea more common, palpable mass more common
Cholecystitis	Pain and tenderness higher, radiation of pain to right shoulder, nausea more extensive, liver biochemical tests abnormal, history of prior attacks common
Meckel's diverticulitis	Difficult to distinguish preoperatively from appendicitis
Cecal diverticulitis	Difficult to distinguish preoperatively, symptoms milder and of longer duration, CT scan helpful
Sigmoid diverticulitis	Older patient, radiation of pain to suprapubic area (not RLQ), fever and WBC higher, change in bowel habits more common
Small bowel obstruction	Prior abdominal surgery, colicky pain, vomiting and distention more marked, RLQ localization uncommon
Ectopic pregnancy	Positive pregnancy test, menstrual irregularity, characteristic progression of symptoms absent; syncope
Ruptured ovarian cyst	Occurs midmenstrual cycle, WBC normal, nausea and vomiting less common, sudden onset of pain
Ovarian torsion	Vomiting more marked, occurs at same time as pain, progression of symptoms absent, mass often palpable
Acute salpingitis or tubo-ovarian abscess	Longer duration of symptoms, pain begins in lower abdomen, history of STD, vaginal discharge, and marked cervical tenderness

CT, computed tomography; RLQ, right lower quadrant; STD, sexually transmitted disease; WBC, white blood cell.

Clinical Presentation

Detailed history-taking and a careful physical examination remain the cornerstones of the diagnosis of acute appendicitis. Although no single item of the history in isolation will make the diagnosis reliably, the combination of classic symptoms and typical progression of symptoms, coupled with right lower quadrant tenderness, allows diagnostic accuracy. The classic presentation of acute appendicitis is well known to all physicians and medical students. Generally patients first note vague, poorly localized epigastric or periumbilical discomfort. This pain typically is not severe and often is attributed to "gastric upset." Patients commonly report feeling that a bowel movement should relieve the pain, a sensation known as the "downward urge."[23] Diarrhea is sometimes seen with appendicitis but is not a common symptom.

Within 4 to 12 hours most patients also note nausea, anorexia, vomiting, or some combination of these 3 symptoms. The nausea is usually mild to moderate, and most patients have only a few episodes of emesis. If vomiting is the major symptom, the diagnosis of appendicitis should be questioned. Similarly, emesis before the onset of abdominal pain suggests another diagnosis.[22] Many patients report a mild fever or chills; high fevers or rigors are uncommon. The patient's abdominal pain typically increases in intensity, and a characteristic shift in the pain to the right lower quadrant occurs over 12 to 24 hours. The character of the pain becomes achy and more localized. The localization of the pain to the right lower quadrant is a valuable finding when present and occurs in more than 80% of patients with appendicitis.[22]

On physical examination, most patients will appear slightly ill. Tachycardia is uncommon with simple appendicitis but may be seen with complicated appendicitis. The majority of patients with simple appendicitis have a temperature of less than 100.5°F. The presence of a temperature greater than 100.5° is often associated with a perforated or gangrenous appendicitis.[14] Patients with appendicitis, like other patients with peritonitis, tend to lie still rather than move about. Right lower quadrant tenderness and rigidity, both voluntary and involuntary, are common findings on abdominal palpation. Localized right lower quadrant tenderness is an important finding when present, but its absence does not exclude appendicitis. There are a variety of methods to elicit localized right lower quadrant peritonitis. Commonly used methods include the cough sign (the presence of point tenderness with a cough), percussion tenderness, and formal elicitation of rebound tenderness. Although all these techniques are reasonably sensitive, in a recent small study rebound tenderness was found to be the most accurate predictor of localized peritonitis associated with appendicitis.[24]

Additional findings that may be helpful in diagnosing appendicitis accurately include the psoas sign, the obturator sign, Rosvig's sign, and rectal tenderness. The psoas sign is sought by having a supine patient flex the right hip against resistance or by having the patient passively flex and extend the right hip while in the left lateral decubitus position. Pain with either of these maneuvers is thought to be a result of irritation of the underlying psoas muscle by an inflamed retroperitoneal appendix. The obturator sign is elicited by rotating the flexed right hip internally and externally. Pain is thought to arise from irritation of the obturator internus muscle by an inflamed pelvic appendix. Rosvig's sign is the finding of right lower quadrant pain with the elicitation of left-sided rebound tenderness. Although these findings all are valuable when present, their absence does not exclude appendicitis.[22]

The typical presentation of appendicitis can be easy to detect but is encountered in only 50% to 60% of cases. An atypical presentation of appendicitis can occur for various reasons. The classic migration of periumbilical pain to the right lower quadrant is thought to result from irritation of the parietal peritoneum in the right lower quadrant by the inflamed appendix. In cases of retrocecal or pelvic appendicitis, this irritation may not occur. Atypical presentations of appendicitis are particularly common in patients who are at the extremes of age, pregnant, or immunosuppressed, including those infected with human immunodeficiency virus (HIV).

Appendicitis in the young remains a diagnostic challenge because of difficulties in obtaining an accurate history from the patient. In infants and young children, the characteristic history of pain is difficult to elicit; nonspecific findings such as vomiting, lethargy, and irritability predominate. Physical examination is difficult to perform because of poor patient cooperation. Localized right lower quadrant tenderness is found in less than 50% of cases.[25] In addition, the characteristic laboratory findings often are not present; leukopenia is as common as leukocytosis in young infants.[26] As a result, errors in diagnosis are common, and the frequency of complicated appendicitis has been reported to be as high as 40%.

The diagnosis of appendicitis in older patients also is a challenge. The classic pattern of pain migration is less common in older than in younger patients. Furthermore, localized right lower quadrant tenderness is less common in patients over age 65 years. Fever and leukocytosis also are observed less frequently.[26] Finally, older patients tend to present to medical attention late in the course relative to younger patients. For all these reasons, the complication and perforation rates can be as high as 63% in patients over age 50 years.[27]

The presentation of appendicitis during pregnancy also is associated with an atypical clinical presentation, particularly as the pregnancy progresses. In one recent series, only 57% of pregnant women with appendicitis had the classic progression of pain.[28] Nausea and vomiting tend to be more common in pregnant patients with appendicitis than in nonpregnant patients but also are common during normal pregnancy. Fever and leukocytosis are less common in pregnant women than in other patients, and the value of leukocytosis is clouded by the physiologic leukocytosis seen with pregnancy. Although right-sided abdominal pain and tenderness are found in over 90% of pregnant women, the pain is located in the right lower quadrant only 75% of the time.[28]

Immunocompromised patients in general, and HIV-infected patients in particular, also represent a challenging group in which to diagnose appendicitis. Abdominal pain is common in patients with the acquired immunodeficiency syndrome (AIDS), with reported incidence rates of 12% to 50%. The number of potential diagnoses responsible for the pain is significantly greater than that in non-HIV-infected patients. Although HIV-infected patients usually present with classic symptoms of appendicitis, there often is a history of chronic abdominal pain. Diarrhea is a more common presenting symptom of appendicitis in HIV-positive patients than in non-HIV patients, and leukocytosis is relatively uncommon. Declining $CD4^+$ counts are associated with delays in presentation for medical attention and increased appendiceal perforation rates.[29] Nevertheless, the reported surgical outcomes with appropriate treatment are quite good, with low mortality and morbidity rates.[29]

Laboratory Studies

The laboratory findings in patients with acute appendicitis include a variety of markers of acute inflammation. An elevated total white blood cell count in the range of 11,000 to 17,000/mm^3 is seen in approximately 80% of patients, but the specificity of leukocytosis for acute appendicitis is poor.[14, 30] An elevated proportion of or total number of polymorphonuclear leukocytes also is seen in the majority of patients with appendicitis. However, these findings are not specific for appendicitis.[30] C-reactive protein (CRP), an acute-phase reactant synthesized by the liver, is thought to rise within 12 hours of the development of an acute inflammatory process. Although elevated in 50% to 90% of cases of appendicitis, CRP is nonspecific when cut-off values of 5 to 25 mg/L are used.[31] A urinalysis frequently is checked in patients with acute appendicitis, primarily to exclude a urinary tract infection, but mild abnormalities, either pyuria or hematuria, are seen in about 50% of cases of appendicitis.[32]

The value of laboratory investigations in making the diagnosis of acute appendicitis is a matter of some debate. In patients with a classic presentation by history and physical examination, little additional information is obtained from laboratory studies. However, when all cases of appendicitis are considered, the addition of laboratory studies such as the white blood cell count, "left shift," and CRP has been shown to improve diagnostic accuracy.[30, 33] Direct comparison of the white blood cell count and CRP suggests that the total white blood cell count is more sensitive and accurate than CRP for detecting acute appendicitis.[31] In particular, the inflammatory markers are useful in identifying patients with either gangrenous or perforated appendicitis.

A complete blood count should be checked in all patients suspected of having acute appendicitis, and a pregnancy test should be obtained in women of childbearing age. The value of other laboratory tests such as amylase, liver biochemical tests, or urinalysis lies in helping exclude other diagnoses that may mimic acute appendicitis.

Imaging Studies

Traditionally there has been little role for routine imaging studies in patients suspected of having acute appendicitis. As stated in the classic work *Cope's Early Diagnosis of the Acute Abdomen*, "Overreliance on laboratory tests and radiological evaluations will very often mislead the clinician, especially if the history and physical examination are less than diligent and complete."[23] In 50% to 60% of cases, the diagnosis of appendicitis will require no imaging studies and can be made on clinical grounds alone.[34, 35] When the diagnosis is less certain, a variety of imaging tests can help confirm the diagnosis of acute appendicitis: plain abdominal radiographs, abdominal ultrasound, radionuclide scans, and abdominal and pelvic computed tomography (CT).

Plain abdominal radiography often is the initial imaging study for patients with acute abdominal pain. Findings on plain x-rays of the abdomen consistent with appendicitis include a radiopaque right lower quadrant fecolith, focal right lower quadrant ileus, and loss of the right psoas shadow. All these findings are suggestive but not definitive for appendicitis. In a recent prospective study in which plain abdominal x-rays were ordered on all patients suspected of having appendicitis, the radiographs changed clinical management in only 6% of cases.[36] A role for plain abdominal x-rays in acute appendicitis exists only when intestinal obstruction or perforation is thought to be a likely diagnosis. Routine use of plain x-rays in the evaluation of appendicitis should be discouraged.

Abdominal ultrasound has been used in the imaging of the acute abdomen for about 20 years. Although ultrasound is considered the imaging test of choice for biliary and gynecologic diseases, its importance in the diagnosis of acute appendicitis remains controversial. The ultrasound characteristics of appendicitis are well defined. With a 5- or 7.5-MHz transducer, a technique of graded compression is used to displace the mobile loops of bowel in the right lower quadrant. The diagnosis of appendicitis can be confidently made if a 7-mm or thicker noncompressible blind-ended loop of bowel is identified (Fig. 107–2). A shadowing fecolith, pericecal inflammation, or localized pericecal fluid collection is suggestive of appendicitis.[37] A normal appendix is visualized in only 4% of cases. The reported sensitivity and specificity rates of ultrasound for the diagnosis of appendicitis in adults are 85% and 92%, respectively, in a recent collected review.[38] Ultrasound appears to be more sensitive and specific in children than in adults.

There are some important limitations to ultrasound in the diagnosis of appendicitis. All ultrasound-based techniques are operator-dependent. The excellent results just described were achieved in dedicated trials performed by interested and experienced ultrasonographers. In a recent multicenter trial focused on the diagnosis of the acute abdomen, the "real-world" sensitivity of ultrasound fell to 55%.[39] Ultrasound also is less useful in obese patients and those with perforated appendicitis.[37]

Radionuclide scanning also has been advocated for the diagnosis of uncertain cases of appendicitis. Two major techniques are used: 99mTc-hexamethylpropyleneamine oxime (HMPAO)-labeling of the patient's own leukocytes or technetium-99m-labeled antigranulocyte antibodies. With both techniques, an accumulation of the radionuclide in the right lower quadrant is considered to be a positive scan for appendicitis. The reported sensitivity and specificity rates of radionuclide scanning are 91% to 94% and 82% to 94%, respectively.[40, 41] Limitations of these techniques are their lack of universal availability in all hospitals, the relatively long time required to perform them, and operator dependence in the interpretation of the scans.

Abdominal CT scans also have been advocated as the imaging study of choice in atypical cases of appendicitis. With the development and proliferation of rapid helical CT scanners, CT imaging is being applied increasingly to the evaluation of acute abdominal pain. CT has long been considered valuable in confirming a diagnosis of appendiceal abscess, and CT-guided therapy of such abscesses has become common. Over the past few years, a number of investigators have advocated broadening the use of CT scans to include assistance in the diagnosis of atypical appendicitis. Various techniques that are used for appendiceal protocol CT scans differ in terms of the amount of the abdomen scanned, thickness of the individual cuts, and types of contrast used. Several conclusions have emerged from these studies: thin (5-mm) cuts are better than thick (10-mm) cuts,[42] and luminal contrast improves accuracy.

CT findings consistent with appendicitis include a distended (>6 mm) appendix that fails to fill with contrast or air (Fig. 107–3). In addition, an appendicolith or appendiceal wall thickening is often seen. Periappendiceal inflammation, cecal apical thickening, and pericecal fluid collections are associated findings.[43] Visualization of a normal appendix or alternative intra-abdominal pathology constitutes a negative study.

The reported performance of appendiceal CT has been impressive (Table 107–2), with sensitivity rates ranging

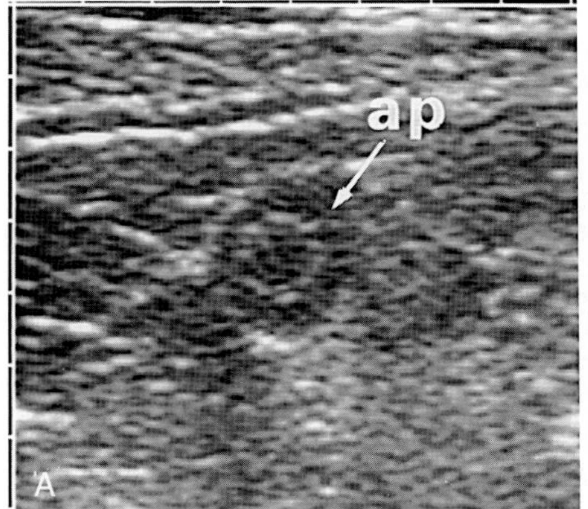

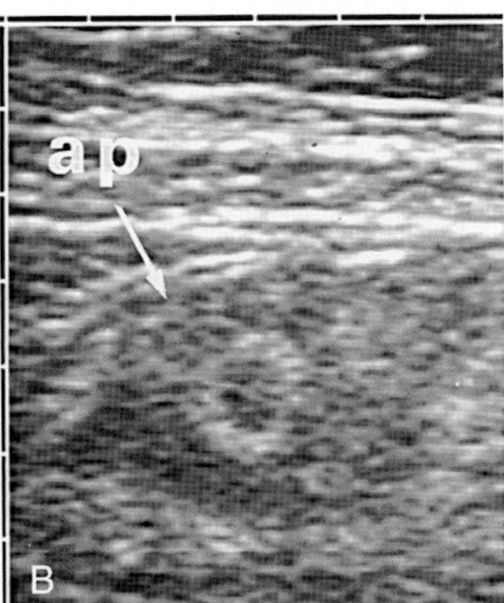

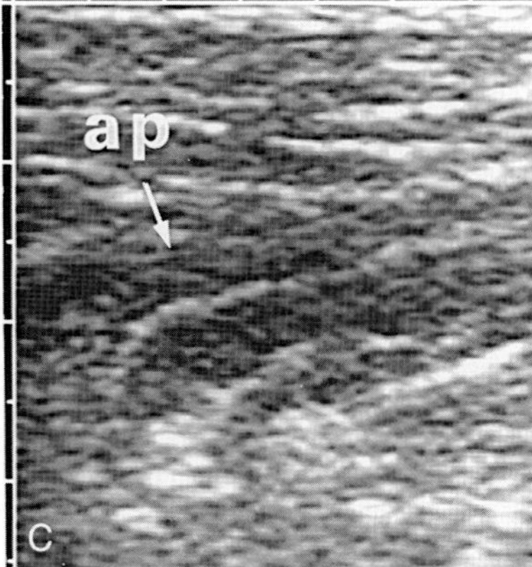

Figure 107–2. Transverse (*A* and *B*) and longitudinal (*C*) ultrasonograms of the right lower quadrant demonstrating a swollen, noncompressible appendix (ap) proved at operation to be acute appendicitis. (Courtesy of Roy A. Filly, M.D.)

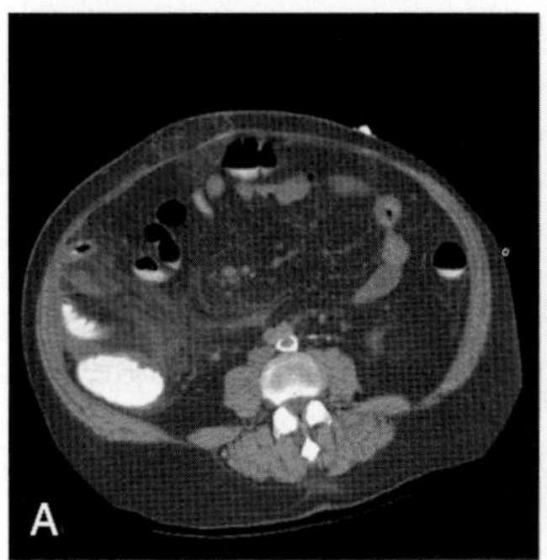

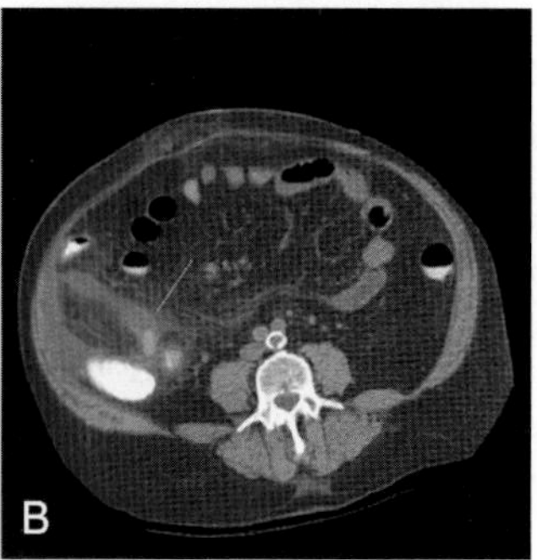

Figure 107–3. *A*, Diffuse inflammatory changes in the mesentery surrounding the distal ileum and cecum. *B*, The coned down view demonstrates a fecolith in the appendix lumen (thin arrow). (Courtesy of Dr. William Brugge, Boston, MA.)

from 87% to 100% and specificity rates ranging from 83% to 99%. The best results occur when contrast is administered both by mouth and per rectum and contrast opacification of the cecum is good. Limitations of CT scanning for appendicitis include the preparation time required for luminal contrast administration, decreased sensitivity in patients with a low body fat content, cost, risk of an allergic reaction to intravenous contrast, and exposure of the patient to ionizing radiation.

In patients in whom a diagnosis of appendicitis cannot be confirmed based on clinical history, physical examination, and laboratory findings, the appropriate imaging study has not been clearly determined. However, based on the current evidence, it appears that CT scanning is more sensitive, more specific, and less operator-dependent in adult patients than other techniques. In pregnant patients and very thin patients, especially in institutions with experienced ultrasonographers, abdominal ultrasonography is an alternative initial imaging study in atypical cases of appendicitis.

Clinical Scoring Systems and Computer-Aided Diagnosis

Based on data that suggest that the experience of the examiner correlates with diagnostic accuracy in acute appendicitis, a variety of scoring systems have been devised since the mid-1980s to aid in the diagnosis of appendicitis. Most of these scoring systems assign numerical weights to findings from the history, physical examination, and laboratory studies in an attempt to predict the probability of appendicitis. More than 10 different scoring systems have been published, and all have purported to reduce errors in diagnosis and negative appendectomy rates. However, in a recent examination of all the published scores to a master data set, the performance of the scores was disappointing when applied to a patient population different from the group for which they were developed.[44] Other studies have reported similar results looking at individual scores.[45, 46] Therefore, at this time no universally applicable scoring system for the diagnosis of acute appendicitis exists.

Diagnostic Laparoscopy

An additional investigation proposed to assist in making the diagnosis of acute appendicitis in equivocal cases is diagnostic laparoscopy. Laparoscopy allows direct visualization of the appendix without appendectomy if the appendix is normal. The appeal of this approach is greatest in women of childbearing age in whom the presence of gynecologic causes of acute abdominal pain may cloud the diagnosis and may be amenable to laparoscopic treatment. In addition, there is weak evidence to suggest that appendectomy may predispose women to tubal infertility,[47] making avoidance of unnecessary appendectomies desirable. Diagnostic laparoscopy has been found in prospective series to eliminate almost completely negative appendectomies in women of childbearing age.[48] Despite these promising results, some cautionary notes must be sounded. Most studies of diagnostic laparoscopy have reported examinations performed under general anesthesia; therefore, the test is resource-intensive when compared with imaging studies. Although diagnostic laparoscopy can be performed under local anesthesia, technical constraints reduce the success rate. When gynecologic pelvic laparoscopy is performed under local anesthesia, visualization of the pelvis is incomplete in up to 15% of cases.[49] This incomplete examination rate compares poorly with CT scanning. At this time, diagnostic laparoscopy cannot be recommended over appendiceal protocol CT scanning.

DIAGNOSTIC ACCURACY

Not all patients with a preoperative diagnosis of acute appendicitis are found to have appendicitis at operation. Because of the time-dependent risk of appendiceal perforation and resulting complications, there is some urgency in making the diagnosis of appendicitis. As a result, treatment decisions are made in the face of incomplete information. An appendectomy is termed negative when a normal appendix is found at exploration for acute appendicitis. Traditionally, an inverse relationship has been found between the rate of neg-

Table 107–2 | **Comparison and Outcomes of Contrast Techniques in Appendiceal Protocol Computed Tomography Scans**

CONTRAST TECHNIQUE	ACCURACY (%)	SENSITIVITY (%)	SPECIFICITY (%)	ALTERNATIVE DIAGNOSIS (%)
No contrast[77]	93–97	87–96	89–99	35
PO & IV[78]	93–94	96–98	83–89	48–55
PO & rectal[79]	98	100	95	80
Rectal[80]	98	98	98	62

IV, intravenous; PO, oral.

ative appendectomies and the rate of perforation at operation. Studies have shown that an increase in the diagnostic accuracy rate results in an increase in the perforation rate.[50] This tradeoff has been thought to be a consequence of the increased time required to confirm the etiology of acute abdominal pain in the absence of a specific test for appendicitis. In the interest of avoiding complications, the standard teaching has been to accept a certain negative appendectomy rate in order to improve patient outcomes.[51] In most series in which diagnostic imaging was not used, a negative appendectomy rate of 10% to 30% and a perforation rate of 10% to 25% were felt to represent a good balance.[4, 14, 35] In these series, the negative appendectomy rate was higher in women than men.

In recent years there appears to be a trend toward improved diagnostic accuracy without a concomitant increase in the risk of perforation because of the use of imaging studies to aid in the diagnosis of appendicitis. In several recent series in which CT scanning was used selectively or universally in cases of presumed appendicitis, negative appendectomy rates have been reduced to 4% to 7% without an increase in the perforation rate.[35, 52, 53] The improvement in diagnostic accuracy has been observed in all patient groups, especially women and children. These results suggest that with the judicious use of new diagnostic techniques it may be possible to increase diagnostic certainty without exposing patients to an increased risk of perforation. Whether a policy of increased utilization of imaging studies in the diagnosis of appendicitis will prove to be cost-effective is not yet clear, but early arguments suggest that enough negative explorations can be avoided to justify the added cost.[53, 54] As a result of the new diagnostic modalities, a new approach to the patient with acute abdominal pain and suspected appendicitis is emerging. A suggested management approach that takes into consideration these new technologies is outlined in Figure 107–4. The goal of this approach using imaging techniques and laparoscopy is to eliminate in-hospital observation as a tool for improving diagnostic accuracy, because the time required to increase diagnostic certainty also may increase the likelihood of complications.

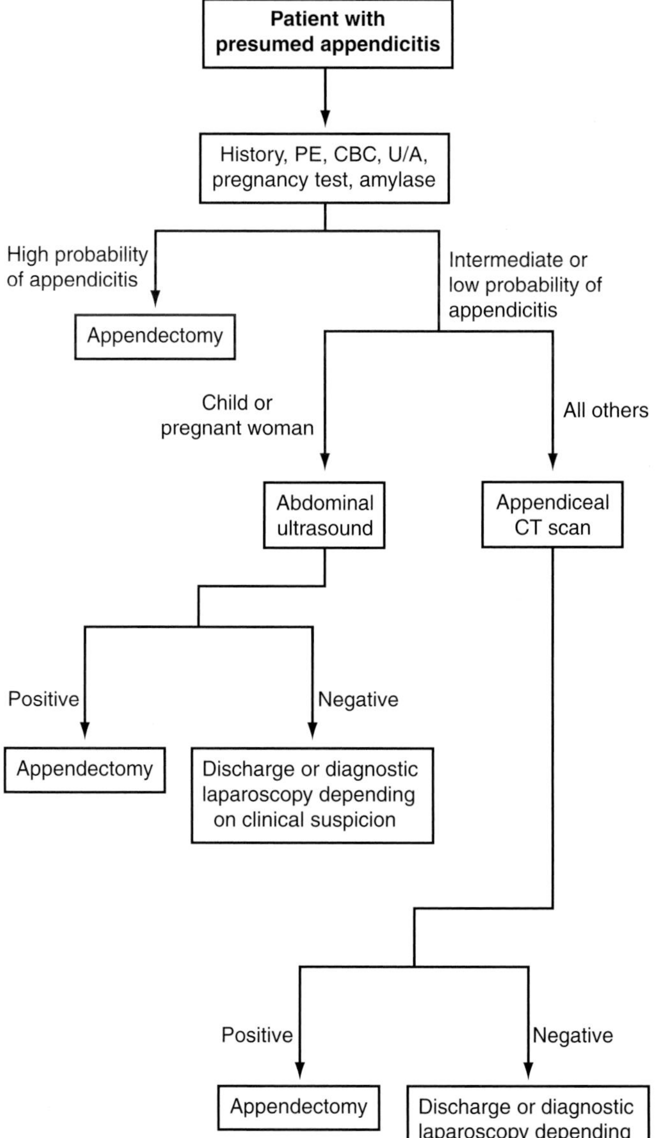

Figure 107–4. A proposed diagnostic and therapeutic algorithm for the patient with presumed appendicitis that uses diagnostic imaging to avoid hospital admissions for observation. CBC, complete blood count; CT, computed tomography; PE, physical examination; U/A, urinalysis.

A strong incentive beyond diagnostic pride exists for avoiding negative appendectomies. Important complications can occur as a consequence of removing a normal appendix. Complication rates of 5% to 15% have been reported for normal appendectomies. The majority of complications are infectious—either wound, pulmonary, or urinary tract infections. However, a 1% risk of small bowel obstruction is reported in the series with the longest follow-up.[55] Of patients found to have a normal appendix at operation, approximately 12% are found to have another surgical disease. An additional 18% to 20% have intra-abdominal findings that can explain the symptoms but are nonsurgical, the most common being ileocolitis or ileitis, mesenteric adenitis, or right ovarian cystic disease. An additional advantage of utilizing CT scanning in atypical appendicitis is that many of these diagnoses can be made by CT scan.[35] In as many as 60% of patients with a negative appendectomy, no diagnosis is made even on subsequent evaluation.

COMPLICATIONS

The major complication of untreated appendicitis is perforation, which can result in peritonitis, abscess, and portal pylephlebitis. The overall perforation rate is between 10% and 30% in most series. The rate of perforation varies widely with age and is most common at the extremes of age. Perforation rates as high as 90% have been reported in children under 2 years of age.[25] At the other end of the age spectrum, patients over age 70 years have perforation rates of 50% to 70%.[27, 50] Patients between the ages of 10 and 30 years have the lowest perforation rates, generally from 10% to 20%. The risk of perforation appears to increase as the duration of illness increases, particularly after 24 hours. Perforation of the appendix is a consequence of a delay in diagnosis. Several studies have shown that patients with a perforation have symptoms for 30 hours longer on average than patients with simple appendicitis.[56] Much of this delay appears to be a consequence of a delay in presentation for medical attention rather than a delay in medical decision-making. Patients with a perforation tend to have atypical presentations of appendicitis.

Patients with perforation are more likely to have significant fever, elevated white blood cell count, and physical signs of peritonitis than are patients with uncomplicated appendicitis. Although perforation often can be predicted preoperatively based on the presence of these findings, not all patients with these findings will have a perforation.[57] Free perforation into the peritoneal cavity will result in findings of diffuse peritonitis and can be associated with free intraperitoneal air on abdominal radiographs. Patients with generalized peritonitis from appendicitis are difficult to distinguish preoperatively from patients with other causes of diffuse peritonitis.

An abscess will develop after perforation if the perforated appendix is walled off from the remainder of the peritoneal cavity by a retroperitoneal location, loops of small bowel, or omentum. Initially a localized collection of inflammatory tissue, or phlegmon, will form. Subsequently a true abscess will form. On physical examination, patients with an abscess often present with a palpable right lower quadrant mass.

The most severe complication of perforation of the appendix is septic thrombophlebitis of the portal vein, or portal pylephlebitis. Although more common early in the 20th century, cases of this disease still occur today. This rare complication should be considered in a patient with appendicitis who presents with high fevers and mild jaundice. Diverticular disease is now the most common cause of portal pylephlebitis.[58] The treatment of pylephlebitis is control of the inciting infection and long-term (4 to 6 weeks) antibiotic therapy. The major organisms are gram-negatives and anaerobes. Even with aggressive therapy, the frequency of hepatic abscesses following pylephlebitis is 50%, and mortality rates of 30% to 50% have been reported.[59]

TREATMENT

The treatment of acute appendicitis remains appendectomy. Little has changed since Fitz and McBurney advocated for early operative treatment of appendicitis in the late 19th century. Appendectomy is recommended even though some cases of appendicitis may resolve spontaneously. At this time, however, we have no prospective ability to identify self-limited cases, and to wait for resolution places patients at risk for perforation and the resulting complications. Although small studies have demonstrated that the majority of patients will improve with intravenous antibiotics alone, more than 35% of patients treated in this manner will relapse in 1 year.[60] Appendectomy is a surgical urgency, not a true emergency. Patients with appendicitis should be given intravenous fluids to correct dehydration and electrolyte imbalances and intravenous antibiotics to decrease wound infection rates and should be taken to the operating room when they are stable. A short amount of time may be used to optimize a patient's concomitant medical conditions for surgery, but long delays will increase the rate of perforation and compromise the patient's outcome.

There are two standard surgical approaches for performing an appendectomy, either open appendectomy or laparoscopic appendectomy. The gold standard is the open appendectomy, an operation that has changed little since McBurney's original description. The operation is performed though a muscle-splitting, right lower quadrant incision. Either an oblique or a transverse skin incision may be used. The appendix is identified and removed even if it is found to be normal, to prevent future diagnostic confusion. In advanced cases with severe inflammation, a cecectomy may be required.[61] If a normal appendix is found, an exploration is carried out to identify other intra-abdominal causes of the patient's symptoms. If other surgical pathology is found at exploration, the incision may be extended or a separate incision made to address the process at hand. Any abscesses must be drained, and the abdomen should be irrigated and closed.

The other approach to appendectomy is laparoscopic appendectomy. First described by Semm in 1983,[62] laparoscopic appendectomy has been the subject of considerable study since that time. The technique has become standardized and is typically performed via a three-trocar technique. After access to the abdomen is gained, the appendix and then the entire abdomen are inspected. If the appendix is inflamed, an appendectomy is performed. If other intra-abdominal surgical pathology is found, laparoscopic treatment can be carried out, or an appropriate open surgical procedure can be performed.

Whether laparoscopic appendectomy is superior to open appendectomy remains controversial. There have now been more than 20 randomized controlled trials and 4 meta-analyses comparing the two procedures.[63-67] All these studies have had remarkably similar conclusions. Both procedures are safe and effective in the treatment of nonperforated appendicitis. After laparoscopic appendectomy, patients require less pain medication and return to normal activity approximately 1 week sooner than after open appendectomy. The wound infection rate is 50% lower after laparoscopic than after open appendectomy, but there may be an increased rate of intra-abdominal abscesses. The hospital stay is 0.6 days shorter after the laparoscopic procedure, and patients resume a normal diet at about the same time as they do after open appendectomy. Laparoscopic appendectomy takes 40% more time to perform and is associated with higher equipment costs. At this time it is not possible to conclude that one procedure is superior to the other for all patients. However, for some patients, particularly those who need to return to work rapidly and those with an uncertain diagnosis, laparoscopic appendectomy is clearly preferable.

An exception to the statement that all patients with appendicitis require urgent appendectomy is the patient with perforation and a palpable right lower quadrant mass. These patients usually have extensive periappendiceal inflammation or an abscess. In patients with a palpable mass but without diffuse peritonitis or toxicity, initial management can be operative or nonoperative. Although data are limited, there is a suggestion that early operative intervention may be associated with a higher complication rate.[68] With nonoperative management, patients are placed on bowel rest and given intravenous fluids and antibiotics, and a CT scan of the abdomen is obtained. If a single abscess that is 3 cm in size or larger is discovered, percutaneous drainage of the abscess under CT guidance is performed. If multiple abscesses are found or the patient does not improve with 24 to 48 hours of conservative therapy, operative drainage of the abscess is performed. Success rates of 88% to 95% have been reported with initial nonoperative management.[69, 70]

Following resolution of the acute illness in older patients in whom a perforated cecal cancer is a possibility, a colonoscopy or barium enema should be performed to exclude a cancer. Most investigators recommend interval appendectomy once the acute inflammation has resolved (6 to 12 weeks later). However, the role of interval appendectomy remains controversial because the rate of recurrent appendicitis is less than 20% at 1 year.

TREATMENT OUTCOMES

Simple acute appendicitis is associated with excellent outcomes. The mortality rate from acute appendicitis in a recent large series was 0.08%, with a complication rate of 5%.[14] Other older series have reported mortality rates of 0.2%, with a complication rate of 6%.[4] Patients are typically hospitalized for 24 to 48 hours after open appendectomy and 24 to 36 hours after laparoscopic appendectomy. Patients will usually return to full activity 2 weeks after laparoscopic appendectomy and 3 weeks after open appendectomy.[64]

Morbidity and mortality attributable to appendicitis increase markedly with complicated and in particular perforated appendicitis. Mortality rates of 1% to 2% and complication rates of 12% to 20% have been reported for perforated appendicitis. In patients over age 70 years in whom both perforation and significant medical comorbidity are common, the mortality rate has been reported to be as high as 32%.[27] Patients with perforated appendicitis often have a stormy postoperative course, with frequent intra-abdominal abscesses and the need for reoperation.

MISCELLANEOUS TOPICS

APPENDIX AND ULCERATIVE COLITIS (see also Chapter 104). There are now at least 9 epidemiologic studies that suggest that appendectomy may be inversely related to the development of ulcerative colitis. The majority of these case-control studies show a risk of ulcerative colitis in patients with an appendectomy of 0.2 to 0.5 relative to patients without an appendectomy.[71] Although these data come from case-control studies and questions can be raised about the appropriateness of the controls, the finding is remarkably consistent. A similar relationship is not seen in patients with Crohn's disease. Some researchers have suggested that appendectomy may attenuate the course of active ulcerative colitis.[72] In a mouse model of autoimmune colitis similar to human ulcerative colitis, removal of the appendix early in life causes significant attenuation of the colonic inflammation.[73] Although these findings are far from conclusive, they provide important insights into both ulcerative colitis and the potential function of the appendix.

RECURRENT AND CHRONIC APPENDICITIS. Recurrent appendicitis is the clinical scenario in which a patient with pathologically confirmed acute appendicitis relates one or more prior episodes of identical symptoms that resolved without surgical intervention. This diagnosis remains somewhat controversial but has been documented in clinical series.[74] The diagnosis of recurrent appendicitis presupposes that some cases of appendicitis can resolve without medical intervention. Series of such cases exist in the radiologic literature, in which patients with imaging findings consistent with appendicitis have had rapid resolution of their symptoms without treatment. The percentage of cases of appendicitis that resolve spontaneously is unknown, but estimates of 6% to 8% have been made. In small series of patients with spontaneous resolution of appendicitis, the recurrence rate is approximately 40%.[75] There are no prospective means to identify spontaneously resolving appendicitis, and as a consequence, all cases of appendicitis should be treated surgically. The existence of recurrent appendicitis serves as a reminder not to discount the diagnosis of appendicitis in patients with a previous episode of similar abdominal pain.

Chronic appendicitis is the pathologic finding of fibrosis and chronic inflammation of the appendix in the presence of a clinical syndrome consistent with appendicitis. Many affected patients report previous episodes of pain and the relief of their symptoms after appendectomy.[76] This problem is not common, and caution should be used in applying the diagnosis of chronic appendicitis to patients with poorly characterized chronic abdominal pain, because many of these patients are unlikely to improve with appendectomy.

INCIDENTAL OR PROPHYLACTIC APPENDECTOMY. The lifetime risk of appendicitis at birth is about 1 in 12; the risk declines to 1 in 35 by age 35 years. The greatest risk of appendicitis in a given year occurs during the second decade of life, when the risk is approximately 0.25% per year.[4] Although appendicitis is the most common cause of emergency abdominal surgery, in light of the low lifetime risk of appendicitis, elective prophylactic appendectomy cannot be recommended. Incidental appendectomy, the removal of a normal appendix at the time of other abdominal surgery, was once the leading cause of appendectomy in women. In light of the falling incidence of appendicitis, the enthusiasm for incidental appendectomy has declined. However, during operations in which appendectomy will not add morbidity, a case may be made for incidental appendectomy in patients under age 30 years. In older patients, the low residual lifetime risk of appendicitis makes incidental appendectomy difficult to defend.

REFERENCES

1. Williams GR: Presidential Address: A history of appendicitis. With anecdotes illustrating its importance. Ann Surg 197:495, 1983.
2. Golden RL: Reginald H. Fitz, appendicitis, and the Osler connection—a discursive review. Surgery 118:504, 1995.
3. Seal A: Appendicitis: A historical review. Can J Surg 24:427, 1981.
4. Addiss DG, Shaffer N, Fowler BS, Tauxe RV: The epidemiology of appendicitis and appendectomy in the United States. Am J Epidemiol 132:910, 1990.
5. Walker AR, Segal I: Appendicitis: An African perspective. J R Soc Med 88:616, 1995.
6. Williams NM, Jackson D, Everson NW, Johnstone JM: Is the incidence of acute appendicitis really falling? Ann R Coll Surg Engl 80:122, 1998.
7. Schumpelick V, Dreuw B, Ophoff K, Prescher A: Appendix and cecum. Embryology, anatomy, and surgical applications. Surg Clin North Am 80:295, 2000.
8. McBurney C: Experience with early operative interference in cases of diseases of the vermiform appendix. NY Med J 21:676, 1889.

9. Ramsden WH, Mannion RA, Simpkins KC, deDombal FT: Is the appendix where you think it is—and if not does it matter? Clin Radiol 47:100, 1993.
10. Karim OM, Boothroyd AE, Wyllie JH: McBurney's point—fact or fiction? Ann R Coll Surg Engl 72:304, 1990.
11. Gray GF, Jr, Wackym PA: Surgical pathology of the vermiform appendix. Pathol Annu 21 Pt 2:111, 1986.
12. Carr NJ: The pathology of acute appendicitis. Ann Diagn Pathol 4:46, 2000.
13. Pieper R, Kager L, Tidefeldt U: Obstruction of appendix vermiformis causing acute appendicitis. An experimental study in the rabbit. Acta Chir Scand 148:63, 1982.
14. Hale DA, Molloy M, Pearl RH, et al: Appendectomy: A contemporary appraisal. Ann Surg 225:252, 1997.
15. Chang AR: An analysis of the pathology of 3003 appendices. Aust NZ J Surg 51:169, 1981.
16. Arnbjornsson E, Bengmark S: Obstruction of the appendix lumen in relation to pathogenesis of acute appendicitis. Acta Chir Scand 149:789, 1983.
17. Sisson RG, Ahlvin RC, Harlow MC: Superficial mucosal ulceration and the pathogenesis of acute appendicitis. Am J Surg 122:378, 1971.
18. Barker DJ: Rise and fall of Western diseases. Nature 338:371, 1989.
19. Andersson R, Hugander A, Thulin A, et al: Clusters of acute appendicitis: Further evidence for an infectious aetiology. Int J Epidemiol 24: 829, 1995.
20. Walker AR, Segal I: Effects of transition on bowel diseases in sub-Saharan Africans. Eur J Gastroenterol Hepatol 9:207, 1997.
21. Naaeder SB, Archampong EQ: Acute appendicitis and dietary fibre intake. West Afr J Med 17:264, 1998.
22. Wagner JM, McKinney WP, Carpenter JL: Does this patient have appendicitis? JAMA 276:1589, 1996.
23. Silen W: Cope's Early Diagnosis of the Acute Abdomen. New York, Oxford University Press, 1991.
24. Golledge J, Toms AP, Franklin IJ, et al: Assessment of peritonism in appendicitis. Ann R Coll Surg Engl 78:11, 1996.
25. Rothrock SG, Pagane J: Acute appendicitis in children: Emergency department diagnosis and management. Ann Emerg Med 36:39, 2000.
26. Paajanen H, Mansikka A, Laato M, et al: Are serum inflammatory markers age-dependent in acute appendicitis? J Am Coll Surg 184:303, 1997.
27. Franz MG, Norman J, Fabri PJ: Increased morbidity of appendicitis with advancing age. Am Surg 61:40, 1995.
28. Anderson B, Nielsen TF: Appendicitis in pregnancy: Diagnosis, management and complications. Acta Obstet Gynaecol Scand 78:758, 1999.
29. Flum DR, Steinberg SD, Sarkis AY, Wallack MK: Appendicitis in patients with acquired immunodeficiency syndrome. J Am Coll Surg 184:481, 1997.
30. Andersson RE, Hugander AP, Ghazi SH, et al: Diagnostic value of disease history, clinical presentation, and inflammatory parameters of appendicitis. World J Surg 23:133, 1999.
31. Hallan S, Asberg A: The accuracy of C-reactive protein in diagnosing acute appendicitis—a meta-analysis. Scand J Clin Lab Invest 57:373, 1997.
32. Puskar D, Bedalov G, Fridrih S, et al: Urinalysis, ultrasound analysis, and renal dynamic scintigraphy in acute appendicitis. Urology 45:108, 1995.
33. Hallan S, Asberg A, Edna TH: Additional value of biochemical tests in suspected acute appendicitis. Eur J Surg 163:533, 1997.
34. Horton MD, Counter SF, Florence MG, Hart MJ: A prospective trial of computed tomography and ultrasonography for diagnosing appendicitis in the atypical patient. Am J Surg 179:379, 2000.
35. Rao PM, Rhea JT, Rattner DW, et al: Introduction of appendiceal CT: Impact on negative appendectomy and appendiceal perforation rates. Ann Surg 229:344, 1999.
36. Boleslawski E, Panis Y, Benoist S, et al: Plain abdominal radiography as a routine procedure for acute abdominal pain of the right lower quadrant: Prospective evaluation. World J Surg 23:262, 1999.
37. Birnbaum BA, Jeffrey RB Jr: CT and sonographic evaluation of acute right lower quadrant abdominal pain. AJR Am J Roentgenol 170:361, 1998.
38. Orr RK, Porter D, Hartman D: Ultrasonography to evaluate adults for appendicitis: Decision-making based on meta-analysis and probabilistic reasoning. Acad Emerg Med 2:644, 1995.
39. Franke C, Bohner H, Yang Q, et al: Ultrasonography for diagnosis of acute appendicitis: Results of a prospective multicenter trial. Acute Abdominal Pain Study Group. World J Surg 23:141, 1999.
40. Barron B, Hanna C, Passalaqua AM, et al: Rapid diagnostic imaging of acute, nonclassic appendicitis by leukoscintigraphy with sulesomab, a technetium 99m-labeled antigranulocyte antibody Fab′ fragment. LeukoScan Appendicitis Clinical Trial Group. Surgery 125:288, 1999.
41. Rypins EB, Kipper SL: 99mTc-hexamethylpropyleneamine oxime (Tc-WBC) scan for diagnosing acute appendicitis in children. Am Surg 63: 878, 1997.
42. Weltman DI, Yu J, Krumenacker J Jr et al: Diagnosis of acute appendicitis: Comparison of 5- and 10-mm CT sections in the same patient. Radiology 216:172, 2000.
43. Rao PM, Rhea JT, Novelline RA: Helical CT of appendicitis and diverticulitis. Radiol Clin North Am 37:895, 1999.
44. Ohmann C, Yang Q, Franke C: Diagnostic scores for acute appendicitis. Abdominal Pain Study Group. Eur J Surg 161:273, 1995.
45. Macklin CP, Radcliffe GS, Merei JM, Stringer MD: A prospective evaluation of the modified Alvarado score for acute appendicitis in children. Ann R Coll Surg Engl 79:203, 1997.
46. Jahn H, Mathiesen FK, Neckelmann K, et al: Comparison of clinical judgment and diagnostic ultrasonography in the diagnosis of acute appendicitis: Experience with a score-aided diagnosis. Eur J Surg 163: 433, 1997.
47. Coste J, Job-Spira N, Fernandez H, et al: Risk factors for ectopic pregnancy: A case-control study in France, with special focus on infectious factors. Am J Epidemiol 133:839, 1991.
48. Lamparelli MJ, Hoque HM, Pogson CJ, Ball AB: A prospective evaluation of the combined use of the modified Alvarado score with selective laparoscopy in adult females in the management of suspected appendicitis. Ann R Coll Surg Engl 82:192, 2000.
49. Zupi E, Marconi D, Sbracia M, et al: Is local anesthesia an affordable alternative to general anesthesia for minilaparoscopy? J Am Assoc Gynecol Laparosc 7:111, 2000.
50. Wen SW, Naylor CD: Diagnostic accuracy and short-term surgical outcomes in cases of suspected acute appendicitis. Can Med Assoc J 152:1617, 1995.
51. Velanovich V, Satava R: Balancing the normal appendectomy rate with the perforated appendicitis rate: Implications for quality assurance. Am Surg 58:264, 1992.
52. Balthazar EJ, Rofsky NM, Zucker R: Appendicitis: The impact of computed tomography imaging on negative appendectomy and perforation rates. Am J Gastroenterol 93:768, 1998.
53. Schuler JG, Shortsleeve MJ, Goldenson RS, et al: Is there a role for abdominal computed tomographic scans in appendicitis? Arch Surg 133:373, 1998.
54. Rao PM, Rhea JT, Novelline RA, et al: Effect of computed tomography of the appendix on treatment of patients and use of hospital resources. N Engl J Med 338:141, 1998.
55. Lau WY, Fan ST, Yiu TF, et al: Negative findings at appendectomy. Am J Surg 148:375, 1984.
56. Temple CL, Huchcroft SA, Temple WJ: The natural history of appendicitis in adults. A prospective study. Ann Surg 221:278, 1995.
57. Oliak D, Yamini D, Udani VM, et al: Can perforated appendicitis be diagnosed preoperatively based on admission factors? J Gastrointes Surg 4:470, 2000.
58. Drabick JJ, Landry FJ: Suppurative pylephlebitis. South Med J 84: 1396, 1991.
59. Plemmons RM, Dooley DP, Longfield RN: Septic thrombophlebitis of the portal vein (pylephlebitis): Diagnosis and management in the modern era. Clin Infect Dis 21:1114, 1995.
60. Eriksson S, Granstrom L: Randomized controlled trial of appendicectomy versus antibiotic therapy for acute appendicitis. Br J Surg 82:166, 1995.
61. Sarkar R, Bennion RS, Schmit PJ, Thompson JE: Emergent ileocecectomy for infection and inflammation. Am Surg 63:874, 1997.
62. Semm K: Endoscopic appendectomy. Endoscopy 15:59, 1983.
63. Garbutt JM, Soper NJ, Shannon WD, et al: Meta-analysis of randomized controlled trials comparing laparoscopic and open appendectomy. Surg Laparosc Endosc Percutan Tech 9:17, 1999.
64. Hellberg A, Rudberg C, Kullman E, et al: Prospective randomized multicentre study of laparoscopic versus open appendicectomy. Br J Surg 86:48, 1999.
65. Temple LK, Litwin DE, McLeod RS: A meta-analysis of laparoscopic versus open appendectomy in patients suspected of having acute appendicitis. Can J Surg 42:377, 1999.
66. Sauerland S, Lefering R, Holthausen U, Neugebauer EA: Laparoscopic vs. conventional appendectomy—a meta-analysis of randomised controlled trials. Langenbecks Arch Surg 383:289, 1998.
67. Golub R, Siddiqui F, Pohl D: Laparoscopic versus open appendectomy: A meta-analysis. J Am Coll Surg 186:545, 1998.

68. Hurme T, Nylamo E: Conservative versus operative treatment of appendicular abscess. Experience of 147 consecutive patients. Ann Chir Gynaecol 84:33, 1995.
69. Yamini D, Vargas H, Bongard F, et al: Perforated appendicitis: Is it truly a surgical urgency? Am Surg 64:970, 1998.
70. Nitecki S, Assalia A, Schein M: Contemporary management of the appendiceal mass. Br J Surg 80:18, 1993.
71. Sandler RS: Appendicectomy and ulcerative colitis. Lancet 352:1797, 1998.
72. Russel MG, Stockbrugger RW: Is appendectomy a causative factor in ulcerative colitis? Eur J Gastroenterol Hepatol 10:455, 1998.
73. Mizoguchi A, Mizoguchi E, Chiba C, Bhan AK: Role of appendix in the development of inflammatory bowel disease in TCR-alpha mutant mice. J Exp Med 184:707, 1996.
74. Barber MD, McLaren J, Rainey JB: Recurrent appendicitis. Br J Surg 84:110, 1997.
75. Cobben LP, de Van Otterloo AM, Puylaert JB: Spontaneously resolving appendicitis: Frequency and natural history in 60 patients. Radiology 215:349, 2000.
76. Mattei P, Sola JE, Yeo CJ: Chronic and recurrent appendicitis are uncommon entities often misdiagnosed. J Am Coll Surg 178:385, 1994.
77. Lane MJ, Liu DM, Huynh MD, et al: Suspected acute appendicitis: Nonenhanced helical CT in 300 consecutive patients. Radiology 213:341, 1999.
78. Balthazar EJ, Birnbaum BA, Yee J, et al: Acute appendicitis: CT and US correlation in 100 patients. Radiology 190:31, 1994.
79. Rao PM, Rhea JT, Novelline RA, et al: Helical CT technique for the diagnosis of appendicitis: Prospective evaluation of a focused appendix CT examination. Radiology 202:139, 1997.
80. Rao PM, Rhea JT, Novelline RA, et al: Helical CT combined with contrast material administered only through the colon for imaging of suspected appendicitis. AJR Am J Roentgenol 169:1275, 1997.

Chapter

108 DIVERTICULAR DISEASE OF THE COLON

Clifford L. Simmang and G. Thomas Shires III

DIVERTICULAR DISEASE OF THE COLON

Diverticular disease of the colon includes a constellation of symptoms that range from mild irregularities in defecatory function to severe bleeding and the consequences of severe intra-abdominal inflammation. The earliest pathologic description of chronic diverticula is traditionally attributed to Cruveilhier in 1849.[1] However, an earlier description by Sir Erasmus Wilson was noted in an editorial comment in *Lancet* in 1840.[2] Other 19th-century surgeons and pathologists made occasional reports of the condition.[3] Mayo and coworkers defined the role of surgery in the treatment of acute inflammation due to diverticulitis by 1907.[4] The presence of uncomplicated pseudodiverticula, herniations of the mucosa and submucosa through the muscular coat of the colon, was defined as *diverticulosis* from radiographic studies by Case in 1914.[5]

Epidemiology

Clinical reports of diverticular disease were uncommon until the 20th century. It is now clear that the incidence of diverticula rises within a society as it reduces its intake of dietary fiber. Historically, geographic location has been an important predictor of the prevalence of this illness. As economic development and the adoption of a Western diet increase, the prevalence of diverticular disease rises as well.[6, 7] Diverticula are common in Western countries, less common in South America, and exceedingly rare in Africa and the Orient. The true prevalence of diverticular disease is not known. In the United States and other developed countries, the prevalence approaches 10%.

Common to many acquired abnormalities, age is an important variable. Diverticulosis is uncommon before age 40 and increases in frequency with age.[8] Autopsy reports suggest that it is found in up to one half of adults above the age of 60.[9]

The anatomic distribution of diverticula also varies with geographic location. In general, industrialized regions with a Western diet, including North America, Europe, and Australia have predominantly left-sided diverticula. Right-sided diverticulosis is much more common in the Orient[10] and appears to have fewer clinical complications than left-sided disease in Japan.[11] As the clinical importance of diverticular disease increases in societies of previously low prevalence, right-sided colonic diverticulosis appears to persist.[12] These variations in anatomic distribution among ethnic groups support the concept of a multifactorial basis for this disease (Table 108–1).

In the United States, the most frequent anatomic site of diverticular disease is the sigmoid colon. This pattern has been noted since 1930, when Renkin reported that the Mayo Clinic experience found that diverticulosis spared the sigmoid colon in only 3% of cases. This pattern has persisted, with most reports noting sigmoid colon involvement, either alone or in combination with more proximal regions, in about 95% of cases.[8, 13]

Pathogenesis

The pathogenesis of diverticular disease is multifactorial, as the population and pathologic studies suggest. The anatomic features intrinsic to the colon, alterations in colonic wall with aging, motor dysfunction, abnormal increases in intraluminal pressure, and dietary fiber may all contribute to the development of diverticulosis in ill-defined interrelationships.

Pathology

Most diverticula in the colon are actually pseudodiverticula, consisting of herniations of the mucosa and submucosa through the muscular coat of the colon. Although true diverticula, containing all layers of the bowel wall, do occur as congenital anomalies, the more common pulsion pseudodiverticula are acquired (Fig. 108–1). The outer longitudinal

Table 108–1 | **Incidence of Diverticulitis in Various Populations**

COUNTRY	POPULATION SERVED		DIVERTICULITIS Mean Age	DIVERTICULITIS Cases/10^6/Yr
Scotland	European	400,000	68	12.88
Nigeria	African	400,000	53	0.17
Singapore	European	15,000	59	5.41
	Chinese	1,014,000	58	0.14
	Malay	190,500	53	0.10
	Indian	111,000	49	0.18
Fiji	European	7,500	60	7.62
	Indian	165,000	51	0.34

muscle fibers form discrete teniae, leaving the colonic wall predominantly a single layer of circular muscle fibers. Diverticula develop in rows between the mesenteric and the two (antimesenteric) lateral teniae. The points of greatest muscular weakness are where the intramural vasa recta penetrate the circular muscle to the submucosa. Vessels arising from the main circumferential arterial supply to the muscularis course along the neck of the diverticulum.[14] This relationship between the herniated sac and the arterial supply may be important in pathophysiologic processes of diverticular hemorrhage.[15] In most sigmoid diverticulosis patients, both longitudinal (teniae) and circular muscle layers are greatly increased in thickness. This thickening is associated with shorting of the teniae that produces a deformity called myochosis, which narrows the colonic lumen, allowing muscle contractions to obliterate the lumen and divide the bowel into isolated segments. Neither hypertrophy nor hyperplasia of the colonic muscular wall has been documented.[16] The histologic abnormality has been attributed to the presence of excess elastin within the teniae, which is not seen in the circular muscle.[17] Increased elastin deposition in the teniae occurs via an unknown mechanism.[18] Luminal narrowing may be secondary to the shortening of the sigmoid musculature as well as pericolic fibrosis.[10]

Structural Abnormalities

To allow mucosal herniation, the integrity of the muscular layer of the bowel wall must be breached by differential pressure between the lumen and the serosa of the bowel. The myochosis described previously is seen in patients who have spastic colon diverticulosis,[19] most commonly in the descending and sigmoid colon. However, pseudodiverticula may occur throughout the colon, in the absence of a thickened muscular layer. In this condition, segmentation of the bowel into closed regions of extremely high pressure leading to the development of pulsion diverticula seems less likely.

The histologic abnormality of elastosis may contribute to sacculation and contraction of the sigmoid colon, as elastin fibers in the remaining circular muscle deteriorate with age. Tensile strength in the bowel wall may also decrease with senescence.[20] Alterations in collagen structure appear to be due to increases in the crosslinking of colonic collagen with age, rather than a decrease in the total collagen content.[21] Any structural changes that lead to decreased compliance would facilitate transmission of higher pressures to mucosa in the interteniae regions transversed by the intramural vasa recta.

Functional Abnormalities

Extensive studies by Painter have implicated the interplay of hypersegmentation resulting in intraluminal hypertension and the low-bulk Western diet as the primary cause of diverticular disease.[22] Intraluminal manometry has shown that intracolonic pressures may exceed 90 mm Hg when segmentation allows the motor work of the colonic musculature to be transmitted to the bowel wall rather than producing transit of feces. Painter postulated that the formation of these "little bladders," in myochosis patients, generated very high pressures and resulted in mucosal herniation (Fig. 108–2).

Measurements of myoelectrical activity and intracolonic pressure patterns in patients have yielded confusing data. Painter found that diverticulosis patients may have normal resting pressure patterns in the sigmoid colon yet have an exaggerated pressure responses to morphine in the diverticula-bearing segments. Connell likewise found an exaggerated response to pharmacologic stimulation in patients who have diverticular disease, compared with that in normal control subjects.[23] Further supporting the concept that diverticular disease represents a spectrum of underlining causes, alterations in colonic motor activity and the presence of intraluminal hypertension are not found in all diverticular disease patients.[24]

Painter and Burkett are responsible for the current fiber hypothesis regarding the development of diverticula. Fiber increases stool weight, lowers colonic pressures, and improves transit time.[25] These processes may prevent muscular hypertrophy and decrease the likelihood of segmentation and resulting intraluminal hypertension. This hypothesis is supported in epidemiologic studies by the inverse relationship between dietary fiber and the presence of colonic diverticula.[26] Vegetarians living in Oxford, England, have a 12% incidence of diverticular disease, compared with non-vegetarians with one half the mean daily intake of dietary fiber, who have a 33% incidence. This importance of dietary fiber

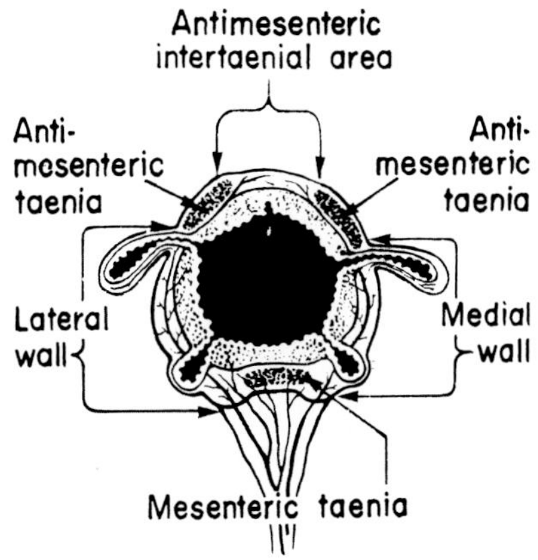

Figure 108–1. Cross-sectional drawing of the colon showing principal points of diverticular formation between mesenteric and antimesenteric teniae. (From Goligher JC: Surgery of the Anus, Rectum, and Colon, 4th ed. London, Baillière Tyndall, 1980, p 883.)

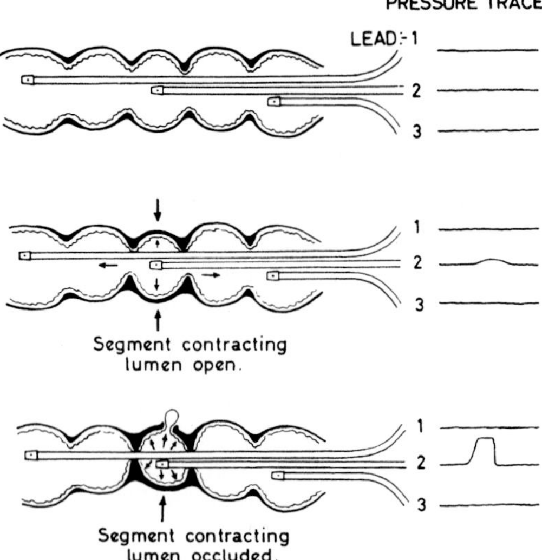

Figure 108–2. Painter's conception of the formation of "little bladders" in the sigmoid colon with myochosis. Manometric traces from three sites show that intraluminal pressure rises higher when contractions occlude the lumen and form isolated segments. (From Painter NS: The etiology of diverticulosis of the colon with special reference to the action of certain drugs on behavior of the colon. Ann R Coll Surg 34: 98, 1964.)

in the pathogenesis of diverticulosis has been noted in other societies as well.[27]

DIVERTICULOSIS

Clinical Manifestations

Most diverticulosis patients have no symptoms or such minor symptoms that they never seek medical attention.[28] Some patients have symptoms such as intermittent abdominal pain, bloating, excessive flatulence, and irregular defecation. Nausea, anorexia, passage of pellet-like stools, or attacks of diarrhea may also be present. Rectal bleeding is uncommon in uncomplicated diverticular disease.[29] Patients who have a history of rectal bleeding for whom a barium study has shown only diverticular disease should be investigated for other diseases as though the diverticula were not present. Some patients report a history of narrow-caliber stools that may suggest a neoplasm.[30] The cause of these symptoms is unknown and could well be secondary to coexistent irritable bowel.[31]

Differential Diagnosis

Many conditions, especially those associated with altered intestinal motility, may be confused with diverticular disease. The most common of these is irritable bowel syndrome, although the most important entity to consider is carcinoma.

Both diverticular disease and colorectal carcinoma have many similarities. Both conditions are common and are most frequently seen in the elderly. Any segment of the colon can be involved, but most commonly the left side of the colon, especially the sigmoid, is. Late manifestations of both diseases can result in luminal narrowing, and complications of these conditions may progress to obstruction, perforation, or development of a fistula. Also, both may be clinically silent for a long period.

Irritable bowel syndrome patients exhibit intestinal symptoms; however, evaluation reveals no anatomic abnormality. It has been suggested that irritable bowel syndrome may proceed to development of diverticular disease, but no evidence of a causal relationship between these two conditions has been found.[30] Whether the pain is intrinsic to diverticulosis or is caused by coexisting irritable bowel syndrome is unknown. Either way, the management of diverticular disease is similar to management of irritable bowel syndrome.

Diagnostic Studies

The diagnosis is most often established with a barium enema examination, which is also the best way to determine the extent and severity of diverticulosis. Diverticula may be distributed through the entire colon (Fig. 108–3). The left colon, particularly the sigmoid, is most often affected. Predominantly right-sided diverticula may be seen, particularly in Asians (Fig. 108–4). Common radiographic findings include colonic spasm, sacculation, and retained contrast material within diverticula.

Colonic evaluation is performed as much to rule out neoplasm as to confirm the diagnosis. In diverticulosis patients, barium enema is probably more reliable and accurate than colonoscopy in documenting the presence or absence of diverticula as well as the distribution. However, the accuracy of barium enema in diagnosing concomitant lesions has been reported to be as low as 50% in some series.[32, 33] Reasons

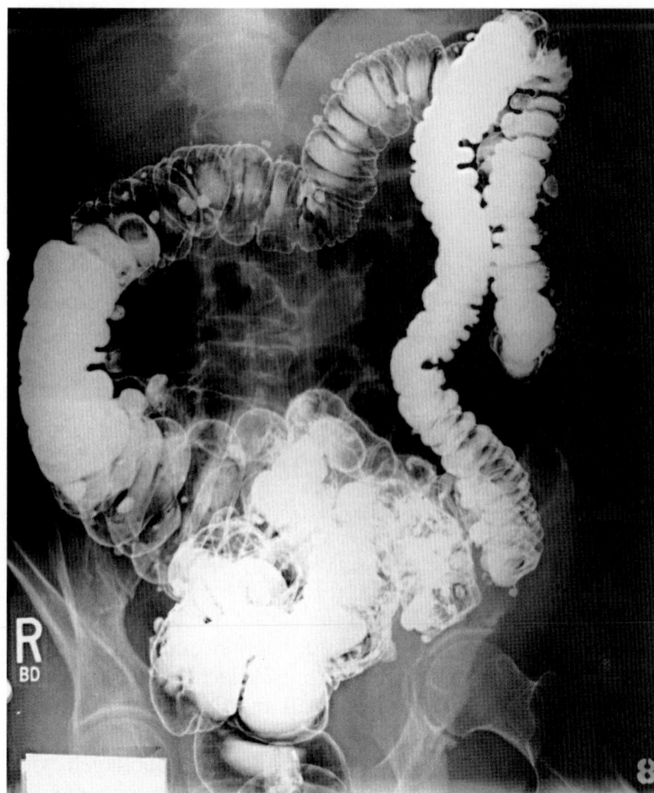

Figure 108–3. Pancolonic diverticula with marked redundancy and overlapping of the sigmoid colon obscuring intraluminal definition.

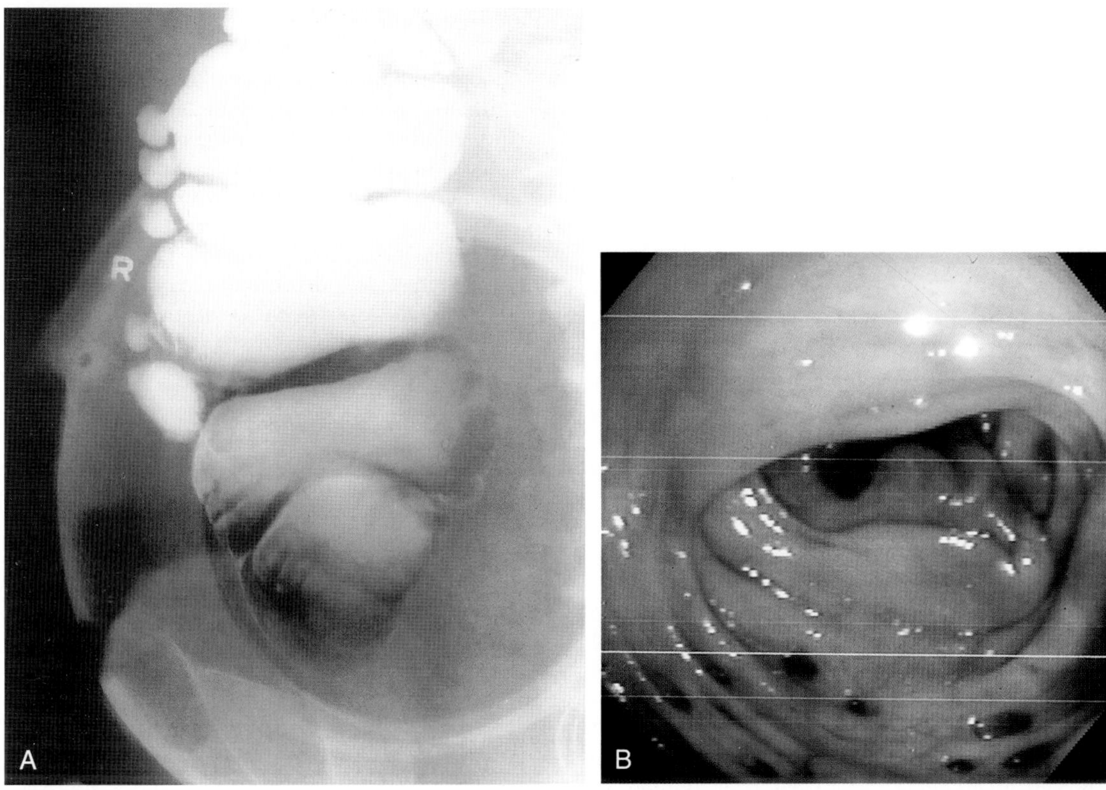

Figure 108–4. *A,* A barium enema showing right-sided diverticulosis. (Courtesy of Mark Feldman, MD.) *B,* Endoscopic appearance of a diverticulum in the right colon.

for this include a redundant and overlapping sigmoid obscuring visualization (see Fig. 108–3) or a narrowed, spastic zigzag segment in which the intraluminal outline is difficult to visualize (Fig. 108–5). Diverticula may also masquerade as polyps either by inversion or as a result of an adherent ball of stool.[34, 35] Multiple views along with compression spot films and postevacuation film help to improve the diagnostic accuracy. As digital radiography, which allows gray scale enhancement by using computerized techniques, becomes more widespread, it may further improve diagnostic accuracy.

Lower gastrointestinal endoscopy is probably more useful for evaluating the large bowel for concomitant abnormality than for actually diagnosing diverticular disease. The rigid sigmoidoscope usually cannot be advanced beyond the rectosigmoid junction and only rarely visualizes diverticular orifices. The flexible sigmoidoscope may allow identification of diverticular orifices. The examination may be limited by patient discomfort and difficulty of advancement of the endoscope. Sigmoid tortuosity and thickened rugae suggest previous episodes of diverticulitis.[36]

Colonoscopy has proved to be useful in differentiating diverticular disease from carcinoma. The endoscopist must be certain that the area of narrowing has been traversed to rule out malignancy. Attempts to visualize colonoscopically the diseased segments demonstrated on barium enema have been successful in only 50% to 73% of patients.[37, 38] An evaluation of 125 patients who had complicated diverticular disease identified an associated carcinoma in 17% and an additional diagnosis in 32%.[39] The presence of bleeding is a significant risk factor for the presence of a concomitant lesion. In a group of 135 patients with persistent bleeding for whom barium enema examination showed only diverticular disease, 11% had carcinoma and an additional diagnosis was made in 37%.[30] These findings strongly suggest that colonic

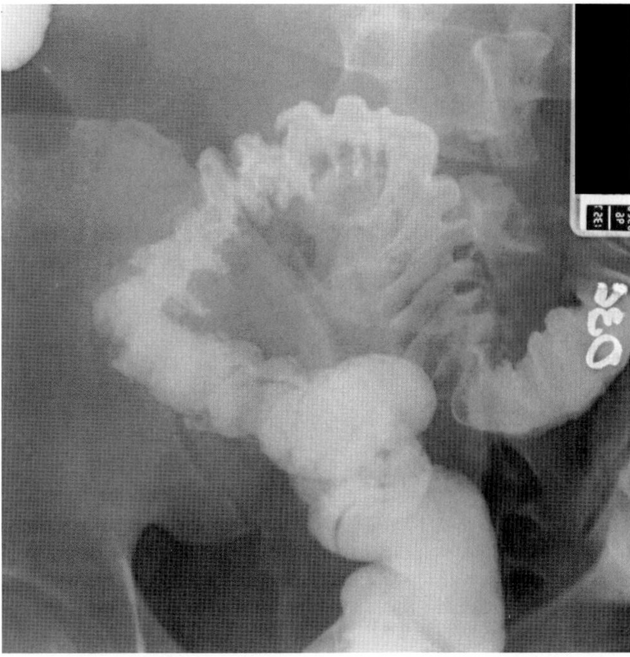

Figure 108–5. Barium enema, diverticular disease. Classic zigzag pattern of a sigmoid colonic spasm in a patient recovering from a recent episode of diverticulitis.

evaluation of patients who have diverticular disease, especially complicated diverticular disease, should be performed. In those patients who have associated bleeding endoscopic evaluation is recommended; if the examination cannot be completed because of stricture and tortuosity, surgical resection of the diseased segment should be considered.

Treatment

The principal treatment of diverticular disease patients has been a high-fiber diet. A diet with a high bulk content reduces colonic pressure and should correct the underlying disorder that precipitates the development of diverticulosis. In fact, the use of bulk-forming agents has been associated with prevention of the development of diverticula.[26, 40] The ingestion of 20 to 30 g of bran is necessary to achieve a therapeutic effect.[41] Coarse bran has been shown to be more effective than fine bran in increasing stool weight, speeding transit time, and reducing intraluminal pressure in the colon.[42]

Many patients find it difficult to ingest the needed 20 to 30 g of fiber per day from dietary foods. The addition of bulk-forming agents provides a suitable substitute. Many of the commercial preparations contain psyllium, which provides an effective supplement to dietary fiber.

The performance of surgical procedures for the patient with uncomplicated diverticular disease has been limited. In 1964, Reilly recommended sigmoid myotomy in the treatment of diverticular disease.[43] This procedure involves division of the antimesenteric tenia (see Fig. 108–1) and underlying circular muscle from the rectosigmoid junction to "whatever distance is necessary." In 1973, transverse tenia-myotomy was proposed by Hodgson.[44] In this procedure the two antimesenteric teniae were transversely incised at 2-cm intervals from the rectosigmoid junction to normal colon proximally. Neither procedure has gained acceptance. At the present time surgical treatment for diverticulosis, whether symptomatic or asymptomatic, is not indicated and should be reserved for complicated diverticular disease.[36]

DIVERTICULAR BLEEDING

Painless rectal bleeding is associated with diverticulosis in 15% to 40% of patients. Although this bleeding is usually of minor clinical significance, massive bleeding from colonic diverticula may occur in 5% of patients who have diverticulosis.[45] Because most rectal bleeding in these patients does not require therapy, the importance of the evaluation of bleeding in patients with known diverticular disease lies in its ability to facilitate diagnosis of concurrent and treatable causes, including colitis and carcinoma. Diverticulosis is so common in the adult population that the attribution of bleeding to diverticular disease must be a diagnosis of exclusion.

Until the 1980s, massive lower gastrointestinal bleeding was usually attributed to diverticular disease. Angiodysplasia of the right colon has now been recognized as having near-equal importance in causing severe lower gastrointestinal hemorrhage.[46] Particularly in the elderly population,[47] the most frequent location of massive bleeding is the right colon, a common site for angiodysplasia, although a less common site for diverticula. Fortuitously, most bleeding diverticula are also found in the right colon.

Pathogenesis

Although inflammation was the presumed mechanism for diverticular bleeding, little or no inflammation has been found in most resected specimens. The cause appears to be chronic injury to the vasa recta adjacent to the lumen of the diverticulum.[48] The mechanism leading to intimal thickening with fragmentation of the internal elastic lamina and thinning of the media is not known. The predilection for bleeding of right-sided diverticula may be related to a larger lumen, which exposes more of the vasa recta to potential disruption.[48]

Differential Diagnosis

Patients who experience profuse rectal bleeding often have no antecedent history of diverticular complications. In an elderly patient, the sudden onset of painless, brisk hematochezia may quickly lead to hypotension, which demands a prompt and organized evaluation concurrent with resuscitation. Although physical examination may be unrewarding, proctosigmoidoscopy may reveal the rare rectal cancer or identify the patient who has colitis due to ischemia, infection, or inflammatory bowel disease resulting in massive bleeding. Vascular lesions such as angiodysplasia may be accompanied by acute rectal bleeding (see Chapters 13 and 120). Of more importance is the evaluation of comorbid factors, which may influence the treatment plan, because frail, elderly patients who have cardiopulmonary or renal disease have little tolerance for uncontrolled hemorrhage.

The usual resuscitative measures, establishing large-bore intravenous access and placement of a Foley catheter, should also include passage of a nasogastric tube to rule out massive bleeding from an upper gastrointestinal source.[49] Blood should be obtained for typing and crossmatching, determination of serum electrolyte concentrations, and coagulation studies. Further invasive diagnostic techniques depend on the rate of blood loss, the medical condition of the patient, and the prompt availability of these procedures. A barium enema is no longer considered a useful initial study, because its sensitivity and specificity are both inadequate for this purpose. In addition, residual barium obscures subsequent urgent angiographic imaging and endoscopic assessment (discussed later).

Diagnostic Studies

Emergency angiography has become the initial procedure of choice for patients who experience brisk bleeding. Angiography is both specific and highly sensitive if the rate of bleeding is sufficient (0.5–1.0 mL/minute).[45] The superior mesenteric artery is studied first, as the incidence of acute bleeding is highest from the right side. Next, the inferior mesenteric artery is studied, to be followed by the celiac axis injection, which may show an unsuspected upper intestinal bleeding site. The positive predictive value of angiography is quite high if the study result is positive and may reveal tumors, diffuse mucosal bleeding, or the characteristic angiographic signs of angiodysplasia, including delayed venous emptying, vascular tufts, or an early filling vein (see Chapter 120).[50]

Nuclear scanning techniques using technetium 99m sulfur

colloid (^{99m}TcSC) and technetium-tagged red blood cells may be useful for patients who experience a slower rate of bleeding (Fig. 108–6). The cost, limited availability, and associated morbidity of emergency arteriography initially prompted enthusiasm for radionuclide imaging, at least as a screening test prior to angiography.[51] In animal studies, bleeding scans can detect very low bleeding rates (0.1 mL/minute) and are more likely to detect intermittent bleeding.[52] A patient who has a negative arteriogram result but a positive radionuclide scan result should be a good candidate for prompt colonoscopy, as scanning techniques may be sensitive but are relatively nonspecific.

Controversy exists as to whether a bleeding scan can be used to guide surgical colon intervention accurately to perform a segmental resection. Suzman and associates retrospectively reviewed 224 patients who had lower gastrointestinal (GI) bleeding who were evaluated through radionuclide red blood cell scanning. Bleeding was demonstrated in 115 scans (51%). Abnormal scan findings were then classified as positive/localizing when activity was visible at a specific locus (n = 90) or positive/nonlocalizing (n = 19) when the precise focus of initial hemorrhage could not be identified. About 80% of the patients had spontaneous cessation of bleeding. Fifty patients had surgery; of these, 37 (74%) had had the bleeding site localized preoperatively. Thirty-three of the 50 patients had segmental resection prompted by bleeding scan findings. None of these patients continued to bleed postoperatively. These data suggest that when performed correctly and interpreted conservatively, scintigraphy is a useful and safe diagnostic tool to guide segmental resection.[53]

The early use of colonoscopy is warranted for the acutely bleeding but hemodynamically stable patient. In such patients, total colonoscopy is the procedure of choice after the usual colonic lavage via the oral route. Bleeding sites have been identified in up to 85% of patients.[54] The technical difficulty of performing emergency colonoscopy can be overcome when the bowel preparation and procedure are performed in the intensive care unit by expert endoscopists.[55]

Treatment

In most patients who have diverticular hemorrhage, the bleeding stops spontaneously. Supportive medical care, in-

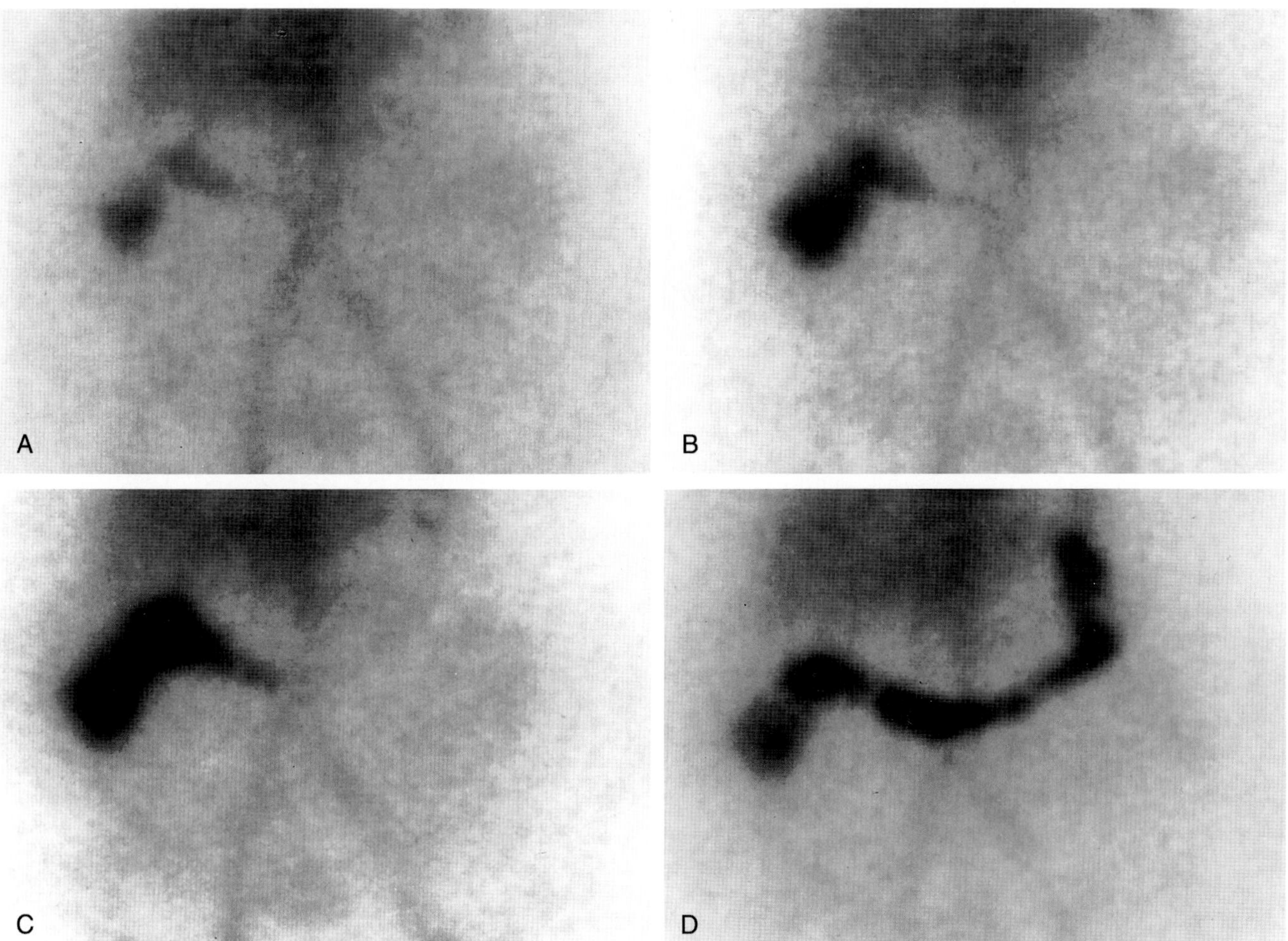

Figure 108–6. Tagged red blood cell scans demonstrating the site of bleeding in the area of the hepatic flexure (anterior view). *A,* Scanning at 1 minute demonstrating extravasation of radionuclide at the site of bleeding. *B,* Scanning at 11 minutes demonstrating continued enhancement in the area of the hepatic flexure. *C,* Scanning at 21 minutes with continued enhancement at the hepatic flexure and beginning transit of radionuclide into the transverse colon. *D,* Scanning at 36 minutes clearly demonstrating continued extravasation with the origin of the bleeding site at the hepatic flexure in transit outlining the transverse colon and splenic flexure.

cluding volume resuscitation and component therapy of coagulation abnormalities, stabilizes the condition of those patients who have a low transfusion requirement. The subset of patients who have hypotension or an ongoing transfusion requirement need prompt intervention, as these frequently elderly patients have significant morbidity and mortality rates, even when arteriography or surgical intervention controls bleeding.

One advantage of diagnostic angiography is the option to attempt therapy by either infusion of vasospastic substances or selective embolization. Intra-arterial vasopressin can be temporarily effective in controlling diverticular hemorrhage.[47] Unfortunately, rebleeding occurs in up to half of these patients after withdrawal of vasopressin.[45] In addition, the use of vasopressin by these patients has several disadvantages, including reduced coronary perfusion, hypertension, and cardiac arrhythmias. Embolization of the affected vessel with autologous blood or absorbable gelatin powder (Gelfoam) is also effective. However, postembolic colonic infarction is a significant risk.[56] In patients for whom angiographic treatment fails, the mortality rate is increased, probably because of delay in eventual surgical treatment.[57] Consequently, transcatheter embolization should likely be reserved for those patients at prohibitive surgical risk.

Colonoscopic intervention is useful when the bleeding site can be visualized with this technique. Success has been reported with electrocoagulation of associated arterial venous malformations.[58] Similarly to angiography, colonoscopic localization is extremely valuable in planning definitive surgical treatment, even if endoscopic therapy ultimately proves unsuccessful.

Emergency surgery is clearly indicated in the treatment of persistent or recurrent diverticular bleeding. The most important factor in both safety and efficacy of emergency surgery is a clear definition of the bleeding site during preoperative investigations. Appropriate segmental colectomy yields a very low rebleeding rate.[45, 47, 57, 59] Considerable controversy is related to the selection of operation for the declining number of patients who have massive presurgical bleeding without preoperative localization. Historically, total abdominal colectomy with ileorectal anastomosis was the procedure of choice, as a rebleeding rate of 30% was noted to follow blind segmental resection.[60] The high operative morbidity and potential long-term morbidity rates of emergency subtotal colectomy have limited its current use to patients who experience continued severe bleeding and a negative arteriography result. The high mortality rate associated with total colectomy may reflect other surgical risk factors such as multiple transfusions, age, and coagulopathy in this difficult-to-manage subset of patients, rather than the technical aspects of the procedure. Both blind left colectomy and blind right colectomy have been advocated after retrospective analysis of failure of therapy. Most surgeons have concluded that subtotal colectomy remains the procedure of choice in this subset of patients.[60]

The indications for elective colonic resection, to prevent recurrent bleeding in patients who avoid initial operation, are poorly defined. The incidence of rebleeding is not known. Recurrence of bleeding after one episode has been estimated at 20% to 30%,[59] with a readmission rate for further bleeding of 5% per year.[61] Patients with a second diverticular bleed have a risk of further recurrences greater than 50%.[62] A conservative approach is likely warranted for most patients who have a single bleed with a low transfusion requirement. However, resection after two or more episodes of bleeding requiring transfusion may be considered if the source of bleeding has been clearly identified and the operative risk is acceptable, as the probability of recurrent hemorrhage is high in this group. The morbidity and mortality rates of elective colon resection are much lower than the risks of emergency surgery, which continues to have a mortality rate above 20% in bleeding patients.[57, 63, 64]

DIVERTICULITIS

Diverticulitis results from inflammation of a colonic diverticulum with subsequent perforation. Diverticulitis is the most common complication of diverticulosis, occurring in 10% to 25% of patients. The initial event is a microperforation of the bowel through a diverticulum, which results in a peridiverticulitis and/or phlegmon and is referred to as *uncomplicated diverticulitis.* Complicated diverticulitis ensues if continuation of the inflammatory and septic process is associated with obstruction, free perforation, fistula, or abscess.[65]

Pathogenesis

Diverticulitis is thought to be a result of fecal matter that has become inspissated within a diverticulum, producing a fecolith. This fecolith then abrades the mucosal lining to produce a low-grade chronic inflammation or becomes impacted.[10] Commonly only one diverticulum is involved, and the location is most often in the sigmoid colon. This inflammatory process then proceeds to either a microperforation or a macroperforation.[30] After a microperforation, peridiverticulitis ensues and remains locally contained by pericolonic fat, mesentery, or adjacent organs. This is an extramural pericolonic process, which results in the localized phlegmon. With repeated episodes the phlegmonous reaction becomes more extensive, and with healing, the fibrotic reaction may ensheathe the colon and produce segmental narrowing, stricture, or even obstruction.[66]

A more complicated form of diverticulitis results from a macroperforation. Either free perforation with generalized peritonitis or a walled off pericolonic abscess may occur. The septic process may erode into adjacent structures and produce a fistula. The most common is the colovesical fistula.[67] Other common fistulas are colocutaneous, colovaginal, and coloenteric fistulas.[67–69] Uncommon fistulas that have been reported include fistulas between the colon and the ureter, uterus, fallopian tube, perineum,[70] and even the venous system.[71]

Clinical Features

The most common symptoms include left lower quadrant abdominal pain (93% to 100%), fever (57% to 100%), and leukocytosis (69% to 83%). Associated symptoms may include nausea, vomiting, constipation, diarrhea, dysuria, and urinary frequency. If there has been progression of the disease process the patient may report symptoms of complicated diverticulitis such as recurrent urinary tract infections, pneumaturia that results from a colovesical fistula, or a feculent vaginal discharge from a colovaginal fistula. The patient with free perforation and peritonitis exhibits acute peritoneal signs and abdominal wall rigidity consistent with a perforated viscus.

The most common physical examination finding is tenderness in the left lower quadrant. Signs of localized peritoneal inflammation may be present with involuntary guarding and percussion tenderness localized in this area. A tender mass representing the phlegmon can occasionally be palpated. Rectal examination reveals some tenderness in the pelvis. Occasionally a mass may be palpated.

Differential Diagnosis

Conditions that can mimic diverticulitis include gastroenteritis, appendicitis, perforated colon cancer, inflammatory bowel disease, and urinary tract infections.

Diagnostic Studies

Initial laboratory studies include complete blood count, urinalysis, and abdominal flat and upright radiography. The white blood cell count is usually elevated with a predominance of polymorphonuclear leukocytes; band forms may be present. Urinalysis may reveal pyuria if the inflammatory process is adjacent to either the ureter or the bladder. Finding bacteria in the urine sample consistent with urinary infection is suggestive of a colovesical fistula, especially if urine culture findings reveal multiple enteric organisms. If the clinical picture is clear, the diagnosis can be made on the basis of clinical criteria and results of the initial laboratory studies. If the diagnosis is in doubt, however, additional diagnostic testing should be considered. Computed tomography (CT) scanning of the abdomen and pelvis, ultrasonography, and contrast enema have been used to help confirm the diagnosis of diverticulitis.

CT with intravenous (IV) and oral contrast medium is usually the test of choice to confirm the suspected diagnosis of diverticulitis.[72] CT reliably detects the location of the inflammation and provides valuable accessory information such as the presence of an abscess (Fig. 108–7), thickened colonic wall, urethral obstruction, or a fistula between the colon and the urinary bladder.[73, 74] Air in the bladder of a patient who has not had urinary tract manipulations is diagnostic of a fistula from the intestinal tract.[74] If an abscess is present, percutaneous drainage under CT guidance is a valuable therapeutic procedure.[73, 75]

Ultrasonography can reveal thickened, hypoechoic inflamed colonic wall, as well as abscesses and diverticula. Percutaneous drainage of an abscess can also be accomplished with ultrasonic guidance.[76]

The performance of a contrast enema for the evaluation of acute diverticulitis has diminished since the introduction of CT. Although water-soluble contrast material is used, the injection of contrast material under pressure into the colon carries the risk of spreading infection by extension through the perforated diverticulum. If the infection has not been well contained, a localized infection may be converted to generalized peritonitis. Although colonic wall thickening, diverticula, fistula formation, or displacement of the colon by abscess may be detected by contrast study, these findings can generally be demonstrated more safely by abdominal CT.

Treatment

UNCOMPLICATED DIVERTICULITIS. Severity of the inflammatory and infectious process determines the treatment for diverticulitis. Patients can be treated on an outpatient basis if they have minimal symptoms or signs of inflammation. A clear liquid diet is recommended, and broad-spectrum antibiotics such as metronidazole plus ciprofloxacin are continued for 7 to 10 days. Opiate analgesics, especially morphine, which has been shown to increase intracolonic pressure, should be avoided.

Signs of significant inflammation indicate that the patient should be hospitalized for bowel rest, intravenous fluids, and broad-spectrum intravenous antibiotics, such as ampicillin sodium/sulbactam sodium (Unasyn); metronidazole plus a

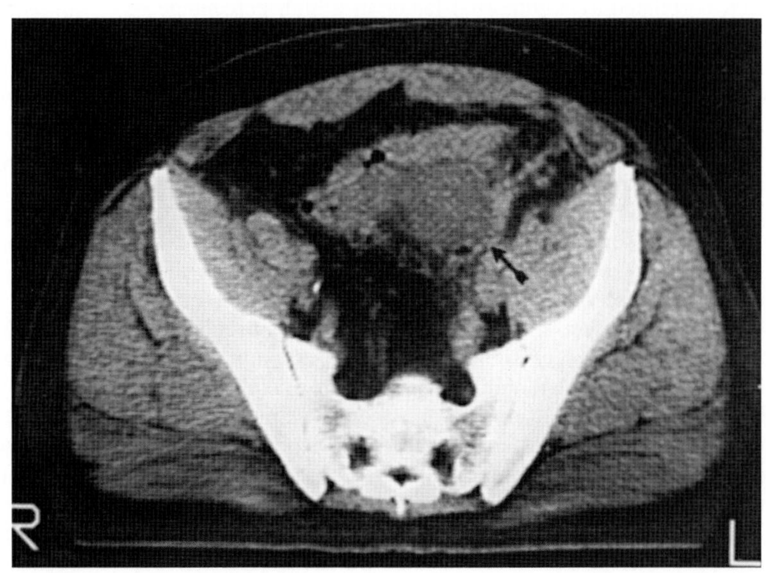

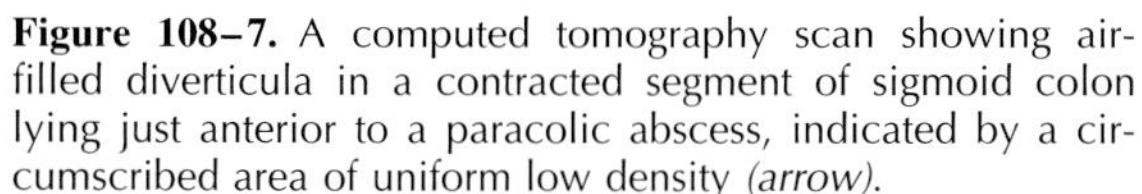
Figure 108–7. A computed tomography scan showing air-filled diverticula in a contracted segment of sigmoid colon lying just anterior to a paracolic abscess, indicated by a circumscribed area of uniform low density *(arrow)*.

cephalosporin (such as cefotetan) or less commonly an aminoglycoside such as gentamicin; ticarcillin disodium/clavulanate potassium (Timentin); or pipericillin sodium/tazobactam sodium (Zosyn). If pain medication is required, parenteral meperidine hydrochloride is an appropriate analgesic as it has been shown to decrease intraluminal pressure.[77] Unless there is a significant ileus or obstructive component, nasogastric suction is usually not required.

Improvement in most patients occurs in the first 48 to 72 hours. As the inflammatory process continues to resolve, diet is resumed and the person may be discharged to complete a 7- to 10-day course of oral antibiotics as an outpatient. Investigative studies are usually performed 4 to 6 weeks after resolution of symptoms. The patient's colon should be evaluated by either colonoscopy or barium enema. A barium enema more clearly demonstrates the extent and anatomic distribution of diverticulosis but is less accurate in identifying other disease in a segment of numerous diverticula.[78, 79] Colonoscopy may be preferable if the inflammatory process was associated with a mass effect of the colon and exclusion of cancer is mandated.

After recovery from the first episode of simple uncomplicated diverticulitis, surgery is seldom indicated because only 20% to 30% of patients have a recurrent episode of diverticulitis. A high-fiber diet often supplemented with psyllium is recommended. If the patient suffers a second attack of diverticulitis requiring treatment with antibiotic therapy as described, surgical treatment should be considered. After a second episode of diverticulitis, the probability of a third episode is greater than 50%. For this reason, elective resection should be performed approximately 4 to 6 weeks after resolution of the inflammation.[66]

Patients below 40 to 50 years of age who have acute diverticulitis are an exception to the preceding recommendation. In such patients a more aggressive course of diverticulitis has been reported. The initial diagnosis is correct in only 50% to 60% of cases.[80, 81] Because the sigmoid colon may loop to the right, in young patients who have right-sided abdominal pain appendicitis is the most common mistaken diagnosis. Young patients exhibit a complicated diverticulitis requiring urgent surgery in 50% to 75%, compared with only 15% to 30% of older patients.[80, 81] Obesity has been correlated as a comorbid factor in a high percentage of young patients with acute diverticulitis. For young patients who have completed a successful treatment for a first episode of acute diverticulitis, elective surgery is strongly recommended, to prevent a later urgent operation that may require a temporary colostomy and to decrease the overall morbidity and mortality rates, allowing a single-stage resection.[80, 81]

Although several surgical options are available, the extent of resection should be the same in all. It is believed that a major cause of recurrent diverticulitis after sigmoidectomy is failure to resect the abnormal thickened muscular wall completely at the rectosigmoid junction. Although it is seldom necessary to mobilize the rectum distally beyond 2 cm below the sacral promontory, the distal line of transection must be below the confluence of the tenia of the colon onto the rectum.[82] The proximal margin of resection is determined by the abnormally thickened colon wall. Although diverticula may be present throughout the colon, it is not necessary to remove all colon that contains diverticula. The proximal line of transection should be through the bowel wall with a normal thickness and proximal to the hypertrophied thickened muscular wall of the abnormal colon.

Resection and Primary Anastomosis. Resection and primary anastomosis is the most common operation employed for patients who can have bowel preparation prior to surgery. This is a one-stage procedure in which the diseased segment of bowel is removed and intestinal continuity is restored. For patients who have recurrent uncomplicated diverticulitis, this procedure is the standard operation performed. It is also commonly used when patients have fistula or preoperative percutaneous drainage of an abscess when intraoperative contamination is minimized. Relative contraindications include significant intra-abdominal contamination and inability to perform bowel preparation of the proximal colon.

Resection with Sigmoid Colostomy and Closure of the Rectal Stump (Hartmann's Procedure). Hartmann's procedure was named for Henri Hartmann, the French surgeon who described it as the treatment for proximal rectal cancer in 1923.[83] This procedure has become the most common operation for the emergency treatment of diverticulitis. The advantage of this two-stage procedure is that the septic focus is removed by the primary operation and the source of continued contamination is eliminated. The wisdom of resection of the perforated segment is underlined by a review of 57 publications describing 1282 patients who had emergency surgery for perforated diverticulitis. Of these, 61% had some form of conservative operation (drainage, perforation closure, proximal colostomy), with a 25% mortality rate. In contrast, those patients who had resection of the perforated segment had a mortality rate of 11%.[84] After a sufficient period to allow the intra-abdominal inflammatory process to subside, the colostomy can be taken down and anastomosed to the rectal stump to restore intestinal continuity, most commonly 3 to 6 months later.

Transverse Colostomy and Drainage. Although transverse colostomy and drainage, as the first step of a three-stage procedure, was the traditional recommendation for patients with perforated sigmoid diverticulitis and abscess formation, with rare exceptions it has been supplanted by one of the procedures described previously. There are several disadvantages to this operative approach. Most importantly, the mortality rate is higher, primarily because the continued presence of the perforated sigmoid colon with a column of stool remaining in the left colon provides a continuing focus of sepsis. Progressive disease may persist and lead to the formation of a fistula even with an adequate diverting colostomy. This procedure should only be performed when peritonitis and the inflammatory process are so severe that resection of the perforated segment cannot be safely accomplished.

Laparoscopic Colectomy. Laparoscopic colorectal surgery has been performed since 1991, but acceptance and application by surgeons have been slow. One reason is that laparoscopic colorectal surgery is significantly more difficult than most other advanced laparoscopic procedures. Recently, there has been increasing interest among surgeons to learn and implement laparoscopic colectomy in their practice. Laparoscopically assisted anterior resection for diverticular disease has been demonstrated to have acceptable morbidity and mortality rates with a shorter hospital stay and improved cosmetic and functional results.[85] Most surgeons who perform laparoscopic colectomy for both benign and malignant conditions have commented that colectomy for diverticulitis is often much more difficult than colectomy for cancer. This is because the inflammatory process promotes adherence of colon to adjacent structures and obliterates the normal tissue plane between associated organs, making it more difficult to identify and prevent injury. Several series have documented that laparoscopic surgical techniques for diverticular disease are safe, although challenging, with a conversion rate to a standard open laparotomy from laparoscopic technique of less than 10%.[85–88] Even in cases of complicated diverticular disease with fistula, laparoscopically assisted colectomy has been shown to be an effective means of treatment.[89] Another major concern has been the increased cost because of longer operating times and the significant cost associated with operating room charges. Although operating room charges were higher in laparoscopic patients, the total hospital charges and costs were markedly lower in one series.[90]

Laparoscopic colectomy is gaining acceptance, which will increase in the future. It is important that the surgeon who performs this operation is performing the same operation that he or she would perform if this were an open procedure, with no compromise of the procedure. Also, the more complicated conditions should be reserved for those surgeons who have gained significant experience. Laparoscopic colectomy for diverticulitis is safe and has benefits for patients, especially an improved postoperative course and more rapid return to normal activity.

GENERALIZED PERITONITIS. Free perforation from diverticulitis into the peritoneal cavity results in generalized peritonitis. Intra-abdominal findings are classified as purulent peritonitis or the more devastating form of feculent peritonitis. Purulent peritonitis may arise from the sudden rupture of a previously walled-off pericolic or pelvic abscess or from a persistently leaking diverticular perforation. The site of perforation may not be identified. Patients report severe abdominal pain, often acute in onset. Voluntary and involuntary guarding is present throughout the abdomen. Abdominal radiography may reveal intraperitoneal free air, but the absence of free air does not exclude the diagnosis. Leukocytosis with a left shift is generally observed, although in some cases leukopenia may accompany instances of severe sepsis, especially among elderly or immunocompromised patients. Prompt resuscitation and preoperative preparation are begun. Urgent celiotomy is then performed.

Guidelines for emergency operations for patients who have generalized peritonitis secondary to perforated diverticulitis include limiting the extent of resection to the perforated segment, to prevent opening of further avenues of sepsis from extensive peritoneal dissection or colonic mobilization. The distal colon can be stapled and a mucous fistula prevented. Before closure of the abdomen the specimen should be opened so that if a malignancy is found a wider resection can be considered if the patient's overall condition is satisfactory. After resection the peritoneal cavity should be copiously irrigated with warm saline solution. If an abscess cavity is present, drains should be used. An end-descending colostomy is usually performed. Primary resection and anastomosis have been used on selected patients in recent years but are not widely accepted.[91] The principles concerning the extent of the resection as previously described should be applied during the second stage at a later date when the colostomy is taken down and intestinal continuity restored.

The most catastrophic but least common manifestation of perforated diverticulitis is feculent peritonitis. In this situation a generalized peritonitis rapidly develops from the spillage of fecal material. The mortality rate for feculent peritonitis patients has been reported at 35% compared with 6% for those with diffuse purulent peritonitis.[84, 92] Factors identified with an increased mortality risk include persistent sepsis, fecal peritonitis, preoperative hypotension, and prolonged duration of symptoms. Aggressive resuscitation followed by emergency resection without anastomosis remains the preferred treatment.[86]

ABSCESS. As a result of perforation an abscess may develop as either a localized abscess or a pelvic abscess. The localized abscess is a walled-off perforation contained within the pericolic region or within the intramesenteric portion of the colon (see Fig. 108–7). This is the most common complication of sigmoid diverticulitis. A pelvic abscess results from a perforation that is contained and walled off within the pelvis by adjacent organ structures.

The localized pericolic or intramesenteric abscess is associated with clinical manifestations confined to the left lower quadrant. Left lower quadrant pain and localized peritoneal signs are present. Tachycardia and leukocytosis also occur and correlate with degree of inflammation. Abdominal examination may reveal a tender fullness or mass in the left lower quadrant. Initial management consists of intravenous broad-spectrum antibiotic therapy (see the earlier discussion of the treatment of uncomplicated diverticulitis) and bowel rest. If clinical improvement does not occur in the first 48 to 72 hours or the patient's symptoms worsen, then an undrained abscess should be suspected. An abscess may be diagnosed and differentiated from a phlegmon by ultrasonography or CT scanning. CT scanning is especially useful as both a diagnostic and a therapeutic intervention. Previously when an abscess was suspected or diagnosed, operative intervention was performed; the most common procedure was a Hartmann procedure, leading to the two-stage operative approach. More recently the application of CT scanning to localize and drain these abscesses percutaneously has been successful in converting an emergency situation to a semi-elective one.[75, 93, 94] Detection followed by successful drainage of diverticular abscesses has also been performed with ultrasonography.[76] Once the abscess is drained, water-soluble contrast medium can be injected to evaluate for resolution of the abscess cavity as well as to detect a fistula to the colon. Early resection is performed 10 to 14 days after drainage of the abscess cavity. During this period no oral intake is permitted, the patient receives total parenteral nutrition (TPN) for nutritional support, and administration of antibiotics continues. This time frame is needed to allow the inflammatory process to resolve and permit a safer operative procedure more likely to be completed in one stage with restoration of intestinal continuity. If no fistula is demonstrated and a delayed operative procedure is selected, the patient is then allowed to resume oral intake. The catheter is left within the collapsed abscess cavity in the event that resumption of oral intake might result in recurrence of colonic leakage with development of a fistula. If no new drainage is noted, the catheter may be removed. The operation is then performed about 3 months later to allow the inflammatory process to subside and yield a safer operative procedure.

Pelvic abscess results when the perforation is contained by the adjacent structures surrounding the pelvic cavity. The clinical presentation is similar to that already described. However, the symptoms and signs may be diminished if protection from the contiguous structures masks the presence of an abscess. Rectal or vaginal examination may reveal a tender, bulging mass. If the abscess is located in the mid- to upper pelvis, no mass may be palpable. The management of a pelvic abscess is the same as that described previously. In the event that transabdominal drainage of the pelvic abscess is technically difficult, transrectal or transvaginal drainage may be performed. This procedure may be guided by either transvaginal or transrectal ultrasound to localize the abscess cavity clearly and permit safe drainage. Subsequent patient management and operative intervention are the same as described previously. Early operative intervention while the patient remains on TPN and bowel rest is preferred.

FISTULA. Diverticular fistula results from diverticulitis with an associated abscess that erodes into an adjacent organ. A tract is established between the source of the abscess (perforated sigmoid diverticulum) and the secondarily involved adjacent organ. This is a relatively frequent complication of diverticulitis and has been reported in 5% to 33% of diverticular disease patients requiring an operation. Diverticulitis is the most common cause of a colovesical fistula.[67, 70] The second most common cause is sigmoid carcinoma, which should also be considered during the evaluation and management process. Colonoscopy should be used to visualize the sigmoid mucosa directly and exclude carcinoma because the potentially curative surgical treatment of a colovesical fistula from cancer involves wider surgical resection, especially of the bladder, than would be recommended for a patient with diverticulitis. Crohn's disease is another cause of fistula that would be discovered by colonoscopy (see Chapter 103).

A large variety of fistulas have been described in diverticular disease patients. Colovesical fistula is the most common variety, followed by colocutaneous, colovaginal, and coloenteric fistulas.[70] Other fistulas include the coloureteral, colouterine, colosalpingeal, coloperianeal, coloappendiceal, and colovenous. Colovesical fistulas are far more common in men than in women, with ratios ranging from 2:1 to 6:1.[67, 95] In women the uterus is interposed between the bladder and the colon and presumably acts as a protective shield. This protective effect is highlighted by the high percentage (83%) of patients who have had a previous hysterectomy in whom colovaginal fistula develops.[67]

Diverticulitis with a fistula may show signs and symptoms of diverticulitis preceding the development of a fistula or may exhibit signs and symptoms related to the fistula itself; when this happens, the symptoms are related to the organ involved with the fistula. Patients who have a colovesical fistula often have symptoms of urinary tract infection (75%) and pneumaturia (60%). Rarely does the patient pass urine from the rectum.[30] Ninety-five percent of colocutaneous fistulas associated with diverticulitis develop after an operation, whereas only 5% develop spontaneously.[68] The presence of a diverting stoma was not shown to prevent the formation of a fistula, but morbidity was decreased.[68] The diagnosis of a colonic fistula associated with diverticulitis may be either simple or difficult, depending upon the size of the fistula and the organ to which the fistula communicates. CT scanning most accurately confirms a colovesical fistula by demonstrating air within the bladder. This test is also useful in assessing the extent and degree of pericolonic inflammation, aiding both diagnosis and preoperative surgical planning. Barium enemas have been reported to demonstrate the communication in only 50% of cases but confirm the presence of diverticular disease. Cystograms have been shown to demonstrate the fistula in approximately 30% of cases.[30] Cystoscopy demonstrates the internal opening in less than 50% of patients, although some abnormality has been demonstrated in 90% of patients with the finding of bullous edema or localized cystitis in the area of the fistula.[67] Coloenteric fistulas can usually be demonstrated by a barium enema. A vaginogram may demonstrate a colovaginal fistula and hysterogram may demonstrate a colouterine fistula.

Emergency surgical intervention is seldom required when a fistula is caused by diverticulitis. Often the formation of a fistula results in improvement in the patient's condition because it allows natural drainage of an abdominal abscess. The initial treatment should be directed to identification and control of associated sepsis, which may be present in the patient who has a persistent and only partially drained abscess cavity. Sepsis in a patient with a sigmoid-vesical fistula and distal urinary tract obstruction should be treated by relief of the obstruction with Foley catheter drainage or a suprapubic cystostomy along with appropriate intravenous antibiotics.

The general principle of treating fistulas is to remove the offending organ of origin. Most of these patients can undergo preoperative bowel preparation after control of sepsis and are suitable candidates for a one-stage resection.[67] The sigmoid colon is usually adherent to the viscus to which it has communicated. Adherence to both the bladder and the left ureter may be present with a colovesical fistula. The colon usually can be pinched off the bladder, and seldom is it necessary to resect a portion of the bladder. Although the wall of the bladder surrounding the fistula connection is often indurated, the fistula is pinhead-sized and the actual opening not clearly seen. It is unnecessary to resect the indurated portion of the bladder because this resolves once the colon has been excised. If an opening is present, it can be closed in two layers. Careful and meticulous dissection must be performed when mobilizing the left colon to prevent injury to the left ureter. The preoperative placement of a ureteral stent may help prevent ureteral damage. Postoperative urinary drainage usually using a Foley catheter should be continued for at least 7 days. A cystogram may be performed prior to removing the Foley catheter to ensure that there is no leakage from the bladder. After the diseased bowel is resected, a primary anastomosis is constructed, attempting to leave the site of the anastomosis separated from the region of the prior fistula and inflammation. Omental interposition can be performed to further segregate the new anastomosis from the area of inflammation if suitable omentum is available.

Similarly, in the case of a colouterine fistula no treatment of the uterus is required. However, for appropriate indications an elective hysterectomy may be performed as a concomitant procedure. After resection of a colovaginal fistula the apex of the vaginal vault may be closed or left open as closure is often unnecessary. Again, omental interposition should be considered. In resecting a coloenteric fistula the small bowel may be primarily closed if the bowel surrounding the fistula is soft and supple.[67] If the surrounding bowel is indurated, a segmental small bowel resection with primary anastomosis should be performed.

REFERENCES

1. Cruveilhier J: Traite d'anatomie pathologique generale, 1:593, 1849.
2. Nathan BN: Who first described colonic diverticula? Can J Surg 34: 203, 1991.
3. Painter NS, Burkitt DP: Diverticular disease of the colon: A deficiency disease of Western civilization. BMJ 1:450, 1971.
4. Mayo WJ, Wilson LB: Acquired diverticulitis of the large intestine. Surg Gynecol Obstet 5:8, 1907.
5. Case JT: The roentgen demonstration of multiple diverticula of the colon. AJR Am J Roentgenol 2:654, 1914.
6. Madiba TE, Mokoena T: Pattern of diverticular disease among Africans. East Afr Med J 71:644, 1994.
7. Sugihara K, Muto T, Morioka Y, et al: Diverticular disease of the colon in Japan: A review of 615 cases. Dis Colon Rectum 27:531, 1984.
8. Parks TG: Natural history of diverticular disease of the colon. J Clin Gastroenterol 4:53, 1975.
9. Painter NS, Burkitt DP: Diverticular disease of the colon, a 20th century problem. Clin Gastroenterol 4:3, 1975.
10. Morson BC: Pathology of diverticular disease of the colon. Clin Gastroenterol 4:37, 1975.
11. Nakada I, Ubukata H, Goto Y, et al: Diverticular disease of the colon at a regional general hospital in Japan. Dis Colon Rectum 38:755, 1995.
12. Goenka MK, Nagi, B, Kochar R, et al: Colonic diverticulosis in India: The changing scene. Indian J Gastroenterol 13:86, 1994.
13. Rodkey GV, Welch CE: Changing patterns in the surgical treatment of diverticular disease. Ann Surg 200:466, 1984.
14. Slack WW: The anatomy, pathology, and some clinical features of diverticulitis of the colon. Br J Surg 50:185, 1962.
15. Meyers MA, Volberg F, Katzen B, et al: The angio-architecture of colonic diverticula: Significance in bleeding diverticulosis. Radiology 108:249, 1973.
16. Whiteway J, Morson BC: Pathology of the aging—diverticular disease. Clin Gastroenterol 14:829, 1985.
17. Whiteway J, Morson BC: Elastosis in diverticular disease of the sigmoid colon. Gut 26:158, 1985.
18. Watters DAK, Smith AN: Strength of the colon wall in diverticular disease. Br J Surg 77:257, 1990.
19. Fleischner FG: Diverticular disease of the colon: New observations and revised concepts. Gastroenterology 60:316, 1971.
20. Bornstein, P: Disorders of connective tissue function and the aging process: A synthesis and review of current concepts and findings. Mech Ageing Dev 5:305, 1976.
21. Wess L, Eastwood MA, Wess TJ, et al: Cross linking of collagen is decreased in colonic diverticulosis. Gut 37:91, 1995.
22. Painter NS: The cause of diverticular disease of the colon: Its symptoms and its complications. J R Coll Surg Edinb 30:118, 1985.
23. Connell AM: Applied physiology of the colon: Factors relevant to diverticular disease. Clin Gastroenterol 4:23, 1975.
24. Weinreich J, Anderson D: Intraluminal pressure in the sigmoid colon. II. Patients with sigmoid diverticula and related conditions. Scand J Gastroenterol 11:581, 1976.
25. Burkitt DP, Walker ARP, Painter NS: Dietary fiber and disease. JAMA 229:1068, 1974.
26. Gear JSS, Ware A, Fursdon, et al: Symptomless diverticular disease and intake of dietary fibre. Lancet 1:511, 1979.
27. Manousos O, Day NE, Tzanou A, et al: Diet and other factors in the etiology of diverticulosis: An epidemiological study in Greece. Gut 26: 544, 1985.
28. Thompson WG: Do colonic diverticula cause symptoms? Am J Gastroenterol 81:613, 1968.
29. Kewenter J, Hellezen-Ingemarsson A, Kewenter G, et al: Diverticular disease and minor rectal bleeding. Scand J Gastroenterol 20:922–924, 1985.
30. Gordon PH: Diverticular disease of the colon. In Gordon PH, Nivatrongs S (eds): Principles and Practice of Surgery for the Colon, Rectum, and Anus. St. Louis, Quality Medical, 1992, pp 739–797.
31. Otte JJ, Lanses L, Andersen R: Irritable bowel syndrome and symptomatic diverticular disease—different diseases? Am J Gastroenterol 81: 529–531, 1986.
32. Schnyden P, Moss AA, Thoeni RF, et al: A double-blind study of radiologic accuracy in diverticulitis, diverticulosis, and carcinoma of the sigmoid colon. J Clin Gastroenterol 1:55, 1979.
33. Boulos PB, Cowen AP, Karamoils PG, et al: Early detection of carcinoma in sigmoid diverticular disease. Ann Surg 202:607, 1985.
34. Freeny PC, Walker JH: Inverted diverticula of the gastrointestinal tract. Gastrointest Radiol 4:57, 1979.
35. Lappas JC, Maglinte DD, Kopecky KK, et al: Diverticular disease: Imaging with post contrast sigmoid flush. Radiology 168:35, 1988.
36. Pemberton JH, Armstrong DN, Dietzer CD: Diverticulitis. In: Textbook of Gastroenterology, 2nd ed. Philadelphia, JB Lippincott, 1992, pp 1876–1890.
37. Dean ACB, Newell JP: Colonoscopy in the differential diagnosis of carcinoma from diverticulitis of the sigmoid colon. Br J Surg 60:633–635, 1973.
38. Max MH, Knudson CO: Colonoscopy in patients with inflammatory colonic strictures. Surgery 84:551–556, 1978.
39. Hunt HR: The role of colonoscopy in complicated diverticular disease: A review. Acta Chir Belg 78:349–353, 1979.
40. Hodgson WJB: An interim report on the production of colonic diverticula in the rabbit. Gut 13:802, 1972.
41. Thompson WG, Patel DG: Clinical picture of diverticular disease of the colon. Clin Gastroenterol 15:903–916, 1986.
42. Smith AN, Drummond E, Eastwood MA: The effect of coarse and fine Canadian red spring wheat and French soft white bran on colonic motility in patients with diverticular disease. Am J Clin Nutr 34:2460–2463, 1981.
43. Reilly MCT: Sigmoid myotomy: A new operation. Proc R Soc Med 57: 56, 1964.
44. Hodgson WJB: Transverse teniamyotomy for diverticular disease. Dis Colon Rectum 16:283, 1973.
45. Browder W, Cerise EJ, Litwin MS: Impact of emergency angiography in massive lower gastrointestinal bleeding. Ann Surg 204:530, 1986.
46. Welch CE, Athanasoulis CSA, Galdabini JJ: Hemorrhage from the large bowel with special reference to angiodysplasia and diverticular disease. World J Surg 2:73, 1978.
47. Boley SJ, DiBiase A, Brandt LJ: Lower intestinal bleeding in the elderly. Am J Surg 137:57, 1979.
48. Meyers MA, Alonso DR, Gray GF, et al: Pathogenesis of bleeding diverticulosis. Gastroenterology 71:577, 1976.
49. Jensen DM, Machicado GA: Emergent colonoscopy in patients with severe lower gastrointestinal bleeding. Gastroenterology 80:1184, 1981.
50. Boley SJ, Brandt LJ, Frank MS: Severe lower intestinal bleeding: Diagnosis and treatment. Clin Gastroenterol 10:65, 1981.
51. Winzelberg GG, Froelich JW, McKusick KA, et al: Radionuclide localization of lower gastrointestinal hemorrhage. Radiology 139:465, 1981.
52. Gupta S, Luna E, Kingsley S, et al: Detection of gastrointestinal bleeding by radionuclide scintigraphy. Am J Gastroenterol 79:26, 1984.
53. Suzman MS, Talmor M, Jennis R, et al: Accurate localization and surgical management of active lower gastrointestinal hemorrhage with technetium-labeled erythrocyte scintigraphy. Ann Surg 224:29, 1996.
54. Forde KA: Colonoscopy in acute rectal bleeding. Gastrointest Endosc 27:219, 1981.
55. Jensen DM, Machicado AM: Diagnosis and treatment of severe hematochezia: The role of urgent colonoscopy after purge. Gastroenterology 95:1569, 1988.
56. Rosenkrantz H, Bookstein JJ, Rosen RJ, et al: Postembolic colonic infarction. Radiology 142:47, 1982.
57. Leitman M, Paull DE, Shires GT III: Evaluation and management of massive lower gastrointestinal hemorrhage. Ann Surg 209:175, 1989.
58. Brandt LJ, Boley SJ: The role of colonoscopy in the diagnosis and management of lower intestinal bleeding. Scand J Gastroenterol 19:61, 1984.
59. McGuire HH: Bleeding colonic diverticula: A reappraisal of natural history and management. Ann Surg 220:653, 1994.
60. Drapanas T, Pennington DG, Kappelman M, et al: Emergency subtotal

colectomy: Preferred approach to management of massive bleeding diverticular disease. Ann Surg 177:519, 1973.
61. Sarin S, Boulos PB: Long-term outcome of patients presenting with acute complications of diverticular disease. Ann R Coll Surg Eng 76: 117, 1994.
62. McGuire HH Jr, Haynes BW Jr: Massive hemorrhage from diverticulosis of the colon: Guidelines for therapy based on bleeding patterns observed in fifty cases. Ann Surg 175:847, 1972.
63. Britt LG, Warren L, Moore OF: Selective management of lower gastrointestinal bleeding. Am Surg 49:121, 1983.
64. Irvin GL, Hersley JS, Caruanci JA: The morbidity and mortality of emergent operations for colorectal disease. Ann Surg 199:598, 1984.
65. Roberts P, Abel M, Rosen L: Practice parameters for sigmoid diverticulitis. Dis Colon Rectum 38:125, 1995.
66. Rege RV, Nahrwald DL: Diverticular disease. Curr Probl Surg 26:138–189, 1989.
67. Woods RJ, Lave IC, Fazio VW, et al: Internal fistulas in diverticular disease. Dis Colon Rectum 31:591–596, 1988.
68. Fazio VW, Church JM, Jagelman DG, et al: Colocutaneous fistula complicating diverticulitis. Dis Colon Rectum 30:89–94, 1987.
69. Grissom R, Snyder TE: Colovaginal fistula secondary to diverticular disease. Dis Colon Rectum 34:1043–1049, 1991.
70. Colcock BP, Stahlman FD: Fistulas complicating diverticular disease of the sigmoid colon. Ann Surg 175:838–846, 1972.
71. Sonnernshein MA, Cone LA, Alexander RM: Diverticulitis with colovenous fistula and portal venous gas. J Clin Gastroenterol 8:195–198, 1986.
72. Cho KC, Morehouse HT, Alterman DD, et al: Sigmoid diverticulitis: Diagnostic role of CT—comparison with barium enema studies. Radiology 176:111, 1990.
73. Birnbaum BA, Balthazar EJ: CT of appendicitis and diverticulitis. Radiol Clin North Am 32:885, 1994.
74. Labs JD, Sarr MG, Fishman EK, et al: Complications of acute diverticulitis of the colon: Improved early diagnosis with computerized tomography. Am J Surg 155:331, 1988.
75. Stabile BE, Puccio E, van Sonnenberg E, et al: Preoperative percutaneous drainage of diverticular abscesses. Am J Surg 159:99, 1990.
76. Schwerk WB, Schwarz S, Rothmud M: Sonography in acute colonic diverticulitis. Dis Colon Rectum 35:1077, 1992.
77. Almy TP, Howell DA: Diverticula of the colon. N Engl J Med 302: 324, 1980.
78. Fork FT: Double contrast enema and colonoscopy in polyp resection. Gut 22:971, 1981.
79. Stefansson T, Bergman A, Ekbom R, et al: Accuracy of double contrast barium enema and sigmoidoscopy in the detection of polyps in patients with diverticulosis. Acta Radiol 35:442, 1994.
80. Konvolinka CW: Acute diverticulitis under age forty. Am J Surg 167: 562, 1994.
81. Schauer PR, Ramos R, Ghiatas AA, et al: Virulent diverticular disease in young obese men. Am J Surg 164:443, 1992.
82. Benn PL, Woltt BG, Ilstrop DM: Level of anastomosis and recurrent colonic diverticulitis. Am J Surg 151:269, 1986.
83. Hartmann H: Nouveau procédé d'ablation des cancers de la partie terminale du colo pelvien. Congres Fr Chir 29:662, 1923.
84. Krukowski ZH, Matheson NA: Emergency surgery for diverticular disease complicated by generalized and faecal peritonitis. Br J Surg 7:921, 1984.
85. Stevenson AR, Stitz RW, Lumley JW, et al: Laparoscopically assisted anterior resection for diverticular disease. Ann Surg 227:335, 1998.
86. Smadja C, Sbai I, Tahrat M, et al: Elective sigmoid colectomy for diverticulitis: Results of a prospective study. Surg Endosc 13:645, 1999.
87. Berthou JC, Charbonneau P: Elective laparoscopic management of sigmoid diverticulitis: Results in a series of 110 patients. Surg Endosc 13: 457, 1999.
88. Bouillot JH, Aouad K, Badawy A, et al: Elective laparoscopic-assisted colectomy for diverticular disease: A prospective study in 50 patients. Surg Endosc 12:1393, 1998.
89. Hewett PJ, Stitz R: The treatment of internal fistulae that complicate diverticular disease of the sigmoid colon by laparoscopically assisted colectomy. Surg Endosc 9:411, 1995.
90. Liberman MA, Phillips EH, Carroll BJ, et al: Laparoscopic colectomy vs. traditional colectomy for diverticulitis: Outcome and costs. Surg Endosc 10:15, 1996.
91. Alanis A, Papanicolaou GK, Tadros R, et al: Primary resection and anastomosis for treatment of acute diverticulitis. Dis Colon Rectum 32: 933, 1989.
92. Tudor RG, Keighley MRB: The options in surgical treatment of diverticular disease. Surg Annu 19:135, 1987.
93. Mueller PR, Saini S, Wittenburg J, et al: Sigmoid diverticular abscesses: Percutaneous drainage as an adjunct to surgical resection in 24 cases. Radiology 164:321, 1987.
94. Neff CC, van Sonneberg E, Casola G, et al: Diverticular abscesses: Percutaneous drainage. Radiology 163:15, 1987.
95. Krompier A, Howard R, Macewen A, et al: Vesicocolonic fistulas in diverticulitis. J Urol 115:664, 1976.

Chapter 109

INTESTINAL OBSTRUCTION AND ILEUS

Richard H. Turnage and Patricia C. Bergen

DEFINITIONS

Impairment to the aboral passage of intestinal contents may result from either a mechanical obstruction or the failure of normal intestinal motility in the absence of an obstructing lesion (ileus). Intestinal obstruction may be categorized according to the degree of obstruction to the flow of intestinal contents (partial or complete), the absence or presence of intestinal ischemia (simple or strangulated), and the site of obstruction (small intestinal or colonic). These distinctions have prognostic and therapeutic relevance. For example, complete or strangulated obstruction requires urgent operative management, whereas partial small intestinal obstruction may, in selected cases, be successfully managed without laparotomy. A closed loop obstruction refers to a mechanical obstruction in which both the proximal and distal parts of the involved intestinal segment are occluded. This condition has a particularly high risk of strangulation, necrosis, and perforation.

SMALL INTESTINAL OBSTRUCTION

Etiology

The most common causes of small intestinal and colonic obstruction are illustrated in Figure 109–1, and the overall causes are shown in Table 109–1. The three most common causes of small bowel obstruction (SBO) are postoperative intra-abdominal adhesions, hernias, and neoplasms.

Intra-abdominal Adhesions

By far, the most common etiology of SBO is intra-abdominal adhesions following laparotomy, accounting for about 66% to 75% of cases.[1–3] Peritoneal adhesions are common following laparotomy and may be exacerbated by intra-abdominal infection, ischemia, and the presence of foreign bodies, including suture material.

Adhesive SBO is a relatively frequent complication following various commonly performed operative procedures such as colectomy, appendectomy, and gynecologic procedures. The frequency of adhesive obstruction after colectomy may be as high as 18%.[4, 5] Following hysterectomy, the incidence is between 1% and 2%, and it is much less following cesarean deliveries (1 per 2000).[6] Lower abdominal or pelvic procedures have a higher risk of postoperative adhesive obstruction than do upper abdominal procedures, such as cholecystectomy or gastric or pancreatic operations.[4–7]

Patients are at risk for intestinal obstruction anytime following laparotomy. Nieuwemhuijzen and associates reported that the 1-year risk of adhesive SBO during the first year following colectomy was 11%. By 10 years postoperatively, the risk had increased to 30%.[5] An earlier study found the interval between laparotomy and the development of adhesive obstruction ranged from 7 months to 65 years and averaged 6 years.[8]

Hernias

Hernias are the second most common cause of SBO, accounting for about 25% of all cases.[3, 8–10] The relative frequency of various types of hernias causing small intestinal obstruction is shown in Table 109–2. With the more frequent performance of laparoscopic procedures in recent years, various authors have reported the herniation of a portion of the intestinal wall (Richter's hernia[11]), or of a whole segment of the intestine through a laparoscopic trocar site with resultant obstruction.[12, 13]

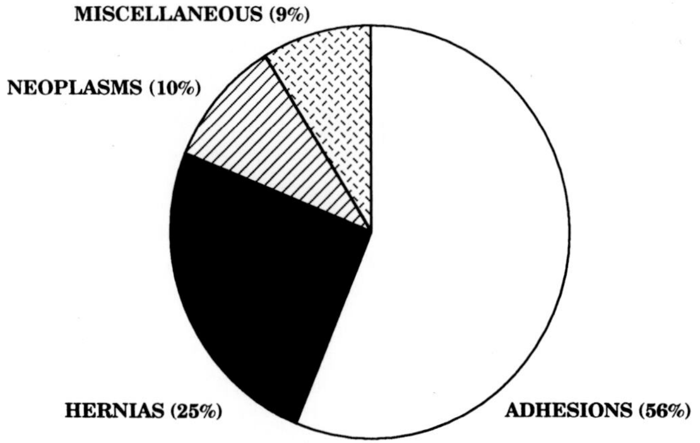

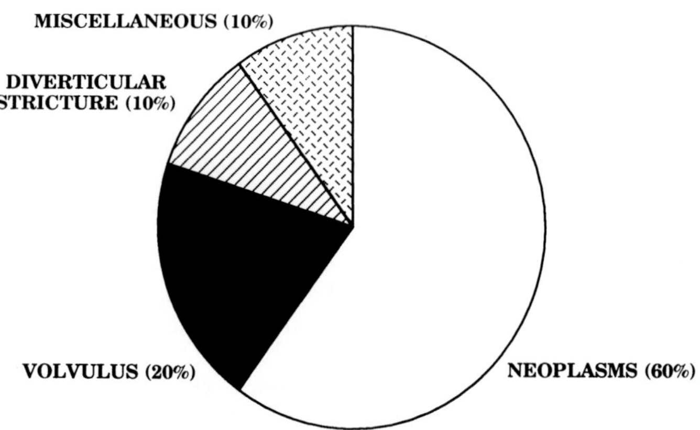

Figure 109–1. Relative frequency of the most common causes of small intestinal obstruction (*a*) and colonic obstruction (*b*). (See Table 109–1 for some of the miscellaneous causes of obstruction.)

Mucha reported that strangulated obstruction occurred in one third of cases due to hernias whereas only 8% of patients with adhesive obstruction had strangulated bowel.[8] Brolin and colleagues[10] found that each of the 22 cases of intestinal obstruction due to hernias was complete, whereas only 38% of patients with obstruction due to intra-abdominal adhesions were complete. The high risk of complete obstruction and strangulation in instances of SBO due to hernias is related to the rigid fascial defect through which the herniated intestine passes. The femoral hernia is a quintessential example. The herniated intestine passes through the femoral canal bound anteriorly and medially by the ileopubic tract as it inserts into the pectineus fascia, posteriorly by the pectineus fascia and the superior ramus of the pubis, and laterally by the femoral vessels. In one study, three fourths of patients with intestinal obstruction due to femoral hernias had gangrenous bowel within the hernia sac.[3]

The occurrence of SBO in a patient without a prior laparotomy should suggest a hernia as the cause. If no hernia is discovered on physical examination, internal hernias such as paraduodenal and obturator hernias must also be considered. Retro-anastomotic and paracolostomy hernias are also important causes of intestinal obstruction in patients who have had operative procedures in which mesenteric defects may be present. Hernias are discussed in greater detail in Chapter 20.

Table 109–1 | **Causes of Intestinal Obstruction**

I. Intrinsic Bowel Lesions
- A. Congenital atresia / stenosis
- B. Inflammatory
  - Diverticulitis
  - Inflammatory bowel disease, e.g., Crohn's disease
  - Ischemia
  - Radiation injury
  - Chemical (e.g., potassium chloride)
  - Endometriosis
  - Postanastomotic
- C. Intussusception
- D. Obturation
  - Polypoid neoplasms
  - Gallstones
  - Foreign bodies
  - Bezoars
  - Feces
- E. Neoplastic strictures

II. Extrinsic Bowel Lesions
- A. Congenital bands
- B. Adhesions
- C. Hernias
- D. Volvulus
- E. Carcinomatosis
- F. Abscess

Neoplasms

In contrast to colonic obstruction, neoplasms are a relatively unusual cause of SBO, accounting for about 10% of cases.[8] Most commonly, the small intestine is obstructed by extrinsic compression or local invasion by advanced gastrointestinal (pancreatic, colonic, gastric) or gynecologic (ovarian) malignancies. This mechanism accounted for 92% of neoplastic SBO in a Mayo Clinic series.[8] Hematogenous metastases from breast adenocarcinoma and melanoma may also involve the intestine with subsequent obstruction.

Primary neoplasms of the small intestine are the cause of obstruction in less than 3% of cases. Carcinoid tumors (see Chapter 112) and adenocarcinoma (see Chapter 113) have been variably reported as the most common malignancy of the small intestine. Within the small intestine, carcinoid tumors are found in the ileum about ten times more frequently than in the jejunum. Adenocarcinoma of small intestine

Table 109–2 | **Relative Frequency of Specific Types of Hernias Associated with Small Intestinal Obstruction in 4 Series**

	STEWARDSON[3] (N = 57)	MUCHA[8] (N = 47)	MCENTEE[9] (N = 59)	GREENE[1] (N = 106)
Inguinal	54%	26%	46%	54%
Femoral	14%	9%	37%	24%
Incisional	14%	21%	10%	7%
Umbilical	16%	8%	3%	9%
Internal	—	34%	—	4%

arises more frequently in the duodenum and jejunum than in the ileum.

Pathophysiology

The duration and degree of obstruction and the presence and severity of ischemia determine the local and systemic pathophysiologic consequences of intestinal obstruction. Intestinal obstruction causes the profound accumulation of fluid and swallowed air within the intestinal lumen proximal to the obstruction. Impaired water and electrolyte absorption and enhanced secretion result in the net movement of isotonic fluid from the intravascular space into the intestinal lumen.[14] The accumulation of swallowed air, and to a much lesser extent H_2, CO_2, and CH_4 generated by bacterial overgrowth within the obstructed lumen, also contribute to intestinal distention.[15]

The failure of normal intestinal motility results in the overgrowth of bacteria within the small intestine and the loss of the normally increasing concentration gradient of bacteria from the jejunum to the ileum. In one study using a porcine model of ileal obstruction, there was a 10,000-fold increase in the concentration of *Escherichia coli* in the ileum and a 40 million–fold increase in the jejunum when compared with normal controls.[16] Data in humans and in animals suggest that the overgrowth of enteric flora occurs within a few hours of obstruction and is maximal by 24 hours.[17] Temporally, this has been related to the presence of endotoxin within the portal and systemic circulation.[16]

Experimental and clinical evidence suggests that bacterial overgrowth is an important part of the pathophysiology of intestinal obstruction. Disruption of the ecologic balance of the normal enteric microflora is associated with the translocation of bacteria to mesenteric lymph nodes and systemic organs in laboratory and clinical situations.[18–20] In one study by Deitch, enteric organisms, particularly *E. coli*, were cultured from mesenteric lymph nodes in nearly 60% of patients with simple intestinal obstruction compared with only 4% of controls.[20] These data[18–20] are consistent with a hypothesis that translocating enteric bacteria contribute to the systemic infections and septic consequences associated with intestinal obstruction and other serious illnesses. Bacterial overgrowth within the obstructed intestine may also contribute to the hypersecretion of fluid by the intestinal mucosa. Heneghan and coworkers[21] found that ileal obstruction in germ-free animals caused intestinal distention without hypersecretion, suggesting that a bacterially derived enterotoxin may be the mediator of intestinal hypersecretion.

The systemic manifestations of intestinal obstruction are related, at least in part, to hypovolemia and the inflammatory response incited by ischemic or gangrenous intestine. Hypovolemia is due primarily to the loss of fluid into the intestinal lumen, the bowel wall, and the peritoneal cavity. When such fluid loss is combined with anorexia and vomiting, a marked reduction in the intravascular volume results. Intestinal ischemia or infarction markedly exacerbates the loss of intravascular fluid both locally into the bowel and systemically through a generalized microvascular "leak." The generation and activation of numerous proinflammatory mediators (such as neutrophils, complement, cytokines, eicosanoids, and oxygen-derived free radicals) have been related to remote organ failure and mortality associated with intestinal ischemia and reperfusion injury.

CLINICAL PRESENTATION

History

Patients with small intestinal obstruction classically present with an acute onset of cramping midabdominal pain, vomiting, obstipation, and abdominal distention. The magnitude of symptoms depends on the degree of obstruction (i.e., complete or partial) and the site and duration of the obstruction. Typically, patients describe paroxysms of periumbilical pain occurring at 4- to 5-minute intervals for proximal obstruction and less frequently for more distal sites of obstruction. With prolonged obstruction, the cramping pain subsides as the motility in the distended intestine is inhibited. The development of continuous severe pain, particularly when localized, strongly suggests the presence of strangulated obstruction. Closed loop obstructions may be associated with the sudden onset of severe unremitting abdominal pain. Proximal obstructions are associated with profuse vomiting, pain, and minimal abdominal distention, whereas more distally located obstruction typically produces less frequent vomiting and greater abdominal distention. The emesis of patients with SBO is often feculent due to the increased bacterial count in the obstructed gut.

Although obstipation is considered the sine qua non of SBO, patients with partial obstruction may continue to pass flatus and stool. Even patients with complete SBO will evacuate the intestine distal to the obstruction. Timing of the duration of obstruction is best judged by determining the time lapsed since the last passage of flatus, if known, because the transit time of swallowed air is much less than that of solid intestinal contents.

Physical Examination

Auscultation of the abdomen may reveal periods of increasing bowel sounds separated by intervals of relative quiet. The quality of the bowel sounds is usually described as high-pitched or musical. *Borborygmi* may be audible in these patients and may correspond with paroxysms of abdominal cramping pain (see Bowel Sounds, which follows Chapter 4 [Volume 1]). In the setting of prolonged obstruction, bowel sounds disappear as intestinal motility decreases.

Abdominal tenderness with guarding or other evidence of peritonitis suggests the presence of strangulated obstruction and necessitates urgent laparotomy. Closed loop obstruction may present with pain out of proportion to the physical findings much like that of acute mesenteric ischemia. Occult rectal bleeding suggests the presence of mucosal ulceration, which may be the result of intestinal ischemia or a mucosal lesion such as adenocarcinoma. The presence of a tender mass at the site of an inguinal, femoral, or umbilical hernia strongly suggests that this is the etiology of the obstruction. Erythema of the overlying skin suggests the presence of strangulation.

The patient's heart rate, blood pressure, and temperature

may provide insight into the systemic response to the obstruction and may give evidence of strangulation. The most common systemic manifestations of intestinal obstruction are related to hypovolemia (e.g., tachycardia, tachypnea, altered mental status, oliguria, and hypotension). The presence of these findings, particularly when unresponsive to volume repletion, suggests strangulated obstruction. With the exception of clinical evidence of a complete obstruction, none of these physical findings is sufficiently reliable to predict the presence of early intestinal strangulation.

RADIOLOGIC FINDINGS

Abdominal Radiographs

After history and physical examination, plain abdominal radiographs should be obtained on patients suspected of having intestinal obstruction. Abdominal radiographs, taken with the patient in the supine position and in the upright (or lateral decubitus) position, will: (1) confirm the diagnosis of intestinal obstruction; (2) localize the obstruction to the small intestine or colon; and (3) provide evidence of the degree of obstruction, that is, partial or complete. Radiographs taken with the patient in a supine position may demonstrate distended small intestine with an abnormal gas pattern (see Fig. 109–2*A*). Abdominal radiographs in the upright position often show multiple air-fluid levels with loops of distended bowel resembling an inverted "U" (Fig. 109–2*B*). The presence of gas within the colon above the peritoneal reflection in an otherwise obstructed-appearing small intestine suggests a partial obstruction, whereas its absence is consistent with a complete SBO. Abdominal radiographs may also demonstrate an abnormal, thickened intestinal wall or even *pneumatosis intestinalis* (a finding diagnostic of gangrenous bowel).

The limitations of plain abdominal radiographs in determining the presence of intestinal obstruction are well recognized. Twenty to thirty percent of patients with SBO will have equivocal or normal abdominal radiographs (i.e., sensitivity = 70% to 80%).[8, 22] False-negative radiographs are particularly likely to occur with proximal or closed loop obstructions.

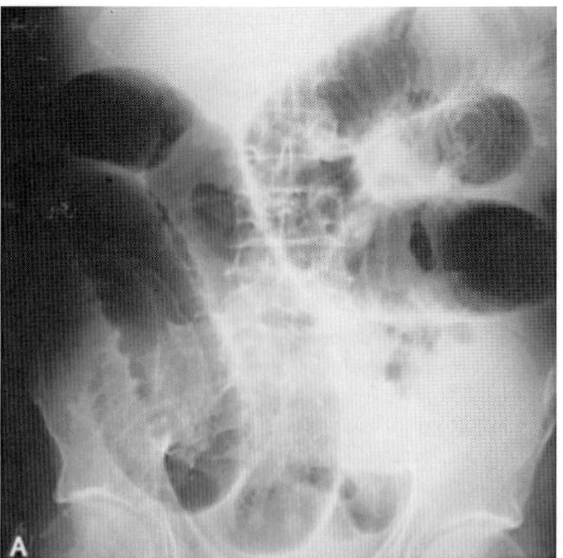

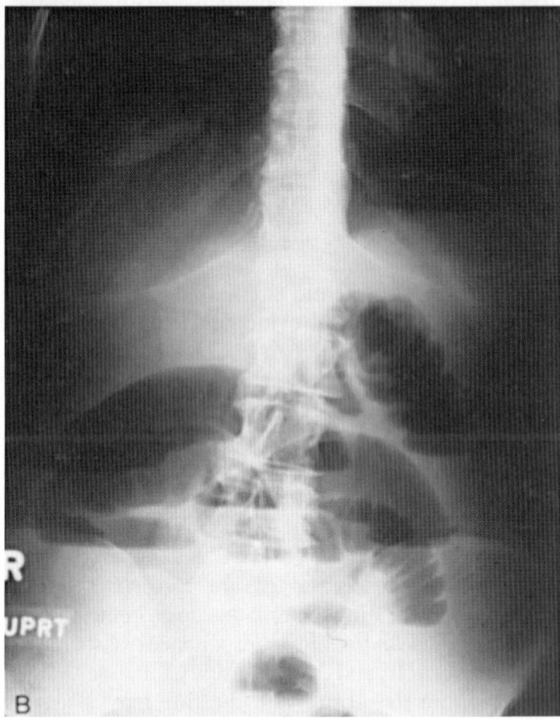

Figure 109–2. Abdominal radiograph of a patient with a distal small bowel obstruction in the supine (*A*), and upright (*B*) position. The supine abdominal radiograph demonstrates centrally located dilated loops of small intestine with prominent valvulae conniventes. No colonic gas is present. The upright abdominal radiograph demonstrates multiple air-fluid levels, intestinal wall thickening, and effacement of mucosal detail in several areas, suggesting progression to ischemia.

Contrast Studies

Radiographic studies using barium sulfate as a contrast agent may be helpful in evaluating patients with atypical clinical presentations and nondiagnostic plain abdominal films. Contrast radiography has been shown to provide "useful" information (i.e., definite diagnosis, no obstruction, high-grade or complete obstruction) in 50% to 80% of patients studied.[22–24] In our practice, barium sulfate is the preferred contrast agent for oral or gastric administration to patients suspected of having SBO because the large amount of fluid present within the obstructed bowel dilutes aqueous contrast agents and hence prevents adequate definition of the site of obstruction. Others have suggested that water-soluble contrast agents may be of value in determining the presence or absence of small intestinal obstruction.[25] Water-soluble contrast agents are preferred for contrast enema studies in patients suspected of having colonic obstruction. In these instances, there is minimal fluid distal to the colonic obstruction. Furthermore, the reflux of barium above an obstructing colon lesion may promote the development of a complete obstruction.

Computed Tomography

Many recent studies have supported the use of abdominal computed tomography (CT) in the evaluation of patients with possible intestinal obstruction but with atypical clinical presentations and equivocal abdominal radiographs. Abdominal CT with enteral and intravenous contrast may be particularly helpful in differentiating mechanical obstruction from paralytic ileus. The findings suggestive of mechanical SBO are shown in Table 109–3. The demonstration of a transition zone with dilated fluid or gas-filled loops of bowel proximal to an obstruction and collapsed loops of bowel distal to an obstruction strongly supports the diagnosis of intestinal obstruction (Fig. 109–3). CT is 80% to 90% sensitive, 70% to 90% specific, and 80% to 90% accurate in determining the presence of SBO.[26–30]

Computed tomography may also provide evidence of a closed loop obstruction or strangulation (see Table 109–3). A U-shaped or C-shaped dilated bowel loop with a radial distribution of stretched mesenteric vessels converging toward a torsion point is characteristic of a closed loop obstruction. Strangulation is suggested by bowel wall thickening, *pneumatosis intestinalis*, or inflammatory changes and hemorrhage in the mesentery.[27] The sensitivity, specificity, and accuracy of these criteria to predict strangulated obstruction range from 83% to 94%.[31–33] It should be noted that, although radiographic contrast studies and abdominal CT may demonstrate SBO, it is the rare patient who requires these tests. In general, the diagnosis, including that of strangulated SBO, is based on the clinical presentation of the patient and plain abdominal radiographs.

Table 109–3 | **Computed Tomography Findings in Patients with Simple Complete, Closed Loop and Strangulated Small Intestinal Obstruction**

Simple Complete Intestinal Obstruction[26, 27, 29]
Proximal bowel dilatation, discrete transition zone, with collapsed distal small bowel and no passage of oral contrast beyond the transition zone
Colon with little gas or fluid
Closed Loop Obstruction[27, 32, 33]
Bowel Wall Changes
U-shaped, distended, fluid-filled bowel loop
Whirl sign—tightly twisted mesentery around a collapsed bowel segment
Beak sign—fusiform tapering in the longitudinal section at the site of obstruction
Two adjacent collapsed round, oval, or triangular loops of bowel at the site of obstruction
Mesenteric Changes
Fixed radial distribution of several dilated bowel loops with stretched and thickened mesenteric vessels converging toward the point of obstruction
Strangulated Intestinal Obstruction[27, 32, 33]
Bowel Wall Changes
Bowel wall thickening (>5 mm) with increased attenuation on unenhanced images
Target or halo sign—concentric rings of slightly different densities
Pneumatosis intestinalis
Poor or lack of enhancement of the bowel wall with IV contrast
Serrated beak configuration of the obstructed bowel loop
Mesenteric Changes
Mesentery changes ranging from haziness and blurring of the mesenteric vessels to obliteration of the fatty mesentery and its vessels caused by mesenteric congestion and hemorrhage
Diffuse engorgement of mesenteric vasculature
Unusual course of the mesenteric vasculature
Other Changes
Large amount of ascites

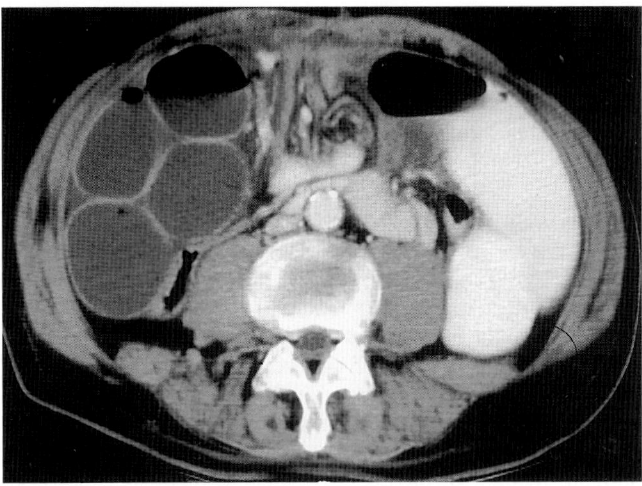

Figure 109–3. Computed tomographic image of the abdomen of a patient with a closed loop obstruction. Note the massively dilated loops of contrast-filled proximal intestine on the right and the fluid filled loops of bowel containing no contrast on the left. In the center of the abdomen is tightly twisted segment of bowel (whirl sign) consisting of the site of torsion with obstruction of the afferent and efferent limbs of the intestine.

LABORATORY FINDINGS

The complete blood count in patients with intestinal obstruction often reveals a slight leukocytosis. Although significant neutrophilia and immature white cellular forms (e.g., bands) are more common among patients with strangulated obstruction than among patients with simple obstruction, the predictive value of this parameter is too low for it to be useful as a sole determinant of strangulation.[34] Vomiting and the profound loss of fluid from the intravascular space that accompanies intestinal obstruction may alter serum electrolyte composition and impair renal function. Serum levels of amylase, lipase, lactate dehydrogenase, phosphate, and potassium may be elevated in patients with strangulated bowel; however, these parameters lack sufficient predictive value to allow differentiation between simple intestinal obstruction and strangulated obstruction, particularly at a stage prior to frank intestinal necrosis and peritonitis.[34]

TREATMENT AND OUTCOME

Resuscitation and Initial Management

Restoration of intravascular volume should be initiated by the infusion of isotonic fluids. A Foley catheter is placed to allow rapid and ongoing assessment of the adequacy of fluid resuscitation. Central venous catheterization or even Swan-Ganz catheterization may ultimately be required to accurately guide fluid management, especially in patients with cardiac or renal disease. Serum electrolytes should be measured and abnormalities corrected. Metabolic acidosis suggests profound intravascular volume depletion with or without gangrenous bowel. Metabolic acidosis refractory to fluid resuscitation strongly suggests strangulated obstruction. A nasogastric tube should be placed to decompress the stomach and minimize further intestinal distention. Decompression of the stomach may also reduce the discomfort associated with gastric distention and the risk of aspiration. Following these initial measures, subsequent therapeutic decisions depend primarily on the presence of complete or partial obstruction or evidence of strangulation.

Complete Small Intestinal Obstruction

Complete SBO necessitates early laparotomy. Broad-spectrum antibiotics directed toward gram-negative aerobes and anaerobes should be administered intravenously. Second-generation cephalosporins such as cefoxitin or cefotetan are commonly used agents. The rationale for early laparotomy in patients with complete obstruction is based on three observations: (1) the low likelihood of spontaneous resolution of complete SBO with nonoperative management; (2) the high risk of strangulation for complete SBO; and (3) the difficulty of detecting strangulated obstruction through the use of clinical parameters, until very late in the course of the disease.

In a series of 149 patients with complete small intestinal obstruction, 84% required laparotomy owing to either failure to resolve the obstruction or clinical evidence of strangulation.[10] In a series in which 24 patients with complete SBO and no initial signs of strangulation were managed nonoperatively, 18 came to operation within 48 hours—13 for persistence of symptoms and 5 for suspected strangulation. Of note, half of the patients with suspected strangulation had gangrenous bowel, and two patients without clinical evidence of strangulation were found at laparotomy to have necrotic bowel.[35]

The overall incidence of intestinal strangulation in patients with SBO (complete or partial) ranges from 8% to 22%.[2, 3, 10] However nearly half of patients with complete SBO have strangulated bowel.[34] Patients with SBO due to hernias are at particularly high risk of strangulation.[8] This high risk, combined with the very low likelihood of spontaneous resolution, mandates an operative approach to patients with SBO related to hernias.[8]

Differentiating patients with early strangulated SBO from those with simple complete bowel obstruction is not possible with currently available clinical parameters. The classic features of strangulated obstruction include leukocytosis, tachycardia, localized abdominal tenderness, and fever. The greater the number of these findings that are present, the greater the probability of gangrenous bowel.[3] However, 5% to 15% of patients with gangrenous bowel have none of these classical features.[35] In Sarr's study of 51 patients with complete SBO,[34] no preoperative clinical parameter (including continuous abdominal pain, fever, peritoneal signs, leukocytosis, and acidosis) or any combination of these findings was predictive of strangulation. Even the clinical judgment of experienced senior surgeons predicted the presence of strangulation in only 10 of 21 patients. Furthermore, only one of these 10 patients who were correctly predicted to have strangulation had an early, reversible ischemic lesion. In this study, the preoperative assessment of simple complete bowel obstruction was correct in only 69% of cases, and nonoperative treatment of complete intestinal obstruction was associated with a 31% risk of delayed definitive treatment of strangulated bowel.[34]

The operative management of complete SBO entails relief of the obstruction and resection of gangrenous bowel. The point of obstruction can often be identified by a transition zone of dilated intestine proximal, and decompressed bowel distal, to the point of obstruction. In the absence of frankly necrotic intestine, viability should be assessed several minutes following the release of the obstruction. Return of normal color and peristalsis, as well as arterial pulsation in the vasa recta and arterial bleeding at a resection margin, suggests that the involved segment is viable. The detection of blood flow at the antimesenteric surface with a Doppler flowmeter and inspection of the bowel using Wood's lamp following intravenous injection of fluorescein are also useful techniques for assessing the viability of a segment of intestine.

Partial Small Intestinal Obstruction

Selected patients with partial SBO due to intra-abdominal adhesions may be treated nonoperatively provided that there is no clinical evidence of gangrenous bowel and there is significant clinical improvement within 48 hours of presentation. Patients managed nonoperatively should receive intravenous fluid and electrolyte restoration and gastric decompression, as was described earlier. It is imperative that these patients be examined frequently and that evidence of clinical deterioration, or even the failure to promptly improve, should mandate urgent operative management.

Although the likelihood of gangrenous bowel in patients with partial SBO is very low (0/91 patients in one series[36]) when compared with instances of complete SBO (21/51 in one series[34]), patients with partial obstruction who present with severe abdominal pain or with physical findings suggestive of peritonitis should be resuscitated and then should undergo urgent laparotomy. A similar approach should be taken for those patients who develop these symptoms during a period of nonoperative management.

The success of nonoperative management of patients with partial SBO has been well documented. In two series, 65% and 81% were managed successfully without an operation.[10, 35] Patients managed in this manner should demonstrate substantial clinical improvement within 24 hours of treatment. If, after 48 hours of nonoperative treatment, resolution has not occurred, operative management is indicated.[10, 35] Only 5% to 15% of patients whose partial obstructions ultimately resolved without operation did not significantly improve within the first 48 hours of treatment.[10, 35]

Laparoscopic Management of Small Bowel Obstruction

Several recent reports have documented the use of laparoscopy to treat adhesive small bowel obstruction. Observations emerging from this early experience include the following: (1) At the present time, about 45% to 60% of cases of adhesive obstruction may be managed exclusively by laparoscopy[37–40]; (2) Patients managed laparoscopically are discharged from the hospital about 3 to 6 days earlier than those treated by laparotomy[37, 38, 41]; and (3) Patients managed laparoscopically required urgent reoperation more often than did those treated with laparotomy. For example, five of 35 patients (14%) treated laparoscopically by Bailey and associates required early unplanned reoperation, compared with only 4 of 88 patients (5%) treated with laparotomy.[37] A similar frequency was reported by Suter and associates.[39] Moreover, bowel injuries are not uncommon in patients with adhesive SBO managed laparoscopically. In a series by Navez and colleagues,[40] injuries occurred in 9 of 68 patients (13%), although all these injuries were recognized at the time of operation.

SPECIAL CONSIDERATIONS

Early Postoperative Obstruction

Intestinal obstruction during the early postoperative period may be very difficult to distinguish from normal postoperative ileus. The incidence of early postoperative obstruction was shown by Stewart and associates to be 0.7% in 8098 patients undergoing laparotomy.[42] The operations associated with the highest incidence of postoperative obstruction were those performed on the small intestine, including enterolysis for SBO (3.0%), left colectomy or proctectomy (2.9%), and appendectomy for perforated appendicitis (1.7%). Upper abdominal operations, such as hepatobiliary procedures, had the lowest risk of early postoperative obstruction (0.06%).[42]

The most important clinical feature differentiating early postoperative SBO from postlaparotomy ileus is the occurrence of obstructive symptoms after the initial return of bowel function and the resumption of oral intake.[42] Patients with early postoperative obstruction present with nausea and vomiting, abdominal distention, and abdominal pain. It is relatively unusual for these patients to have a complete obstruction.[42–44] Symptoms of obstruction may occur as early as the fourth to seventh postoperative day.[42, 44] Plain abdominal radiographs often demonstrate dilated loops of small intestine with air-fluid levels. However, the study will be interpreted as normal or nonspecific in as many as 10% to 27% of cases.[43, 44] Barium contrast studies[43, 44] and abdominal CT will successfully define the obstruction in 65% to 70% of cases.[43, 44] Abdominal CT will define the site of obstruction, and hence will confirm the diagnosis, as well as demonstrate the presence of an intra-abdominal abscess that may be either the cause of a mechanical obstruction or a contributor to the development of paralytic ileus.

Management of patients with early postoperative obstruction begins with intravascular volume resuscitation and nasogastric aspiration. In one series, nearly 80% of 101 patients had spontaneous resolution of their symptoms after an average of 6 days. Only 4% of patients required more than 2 weeks of treatment.[44] Strangulated obstruction is very uncommon.[43, 44] Patients who develop SBO following laparoscopy are less likely to be successfully managed nonoperatively. These patients must be suspected of having had a portion of their intestine herniate through a trocar site; they require urgent operative relief of their obstruction.[13]

Small Bowel Obstruction in Patients with Malignancies

About 25% to 33% of patients with a history of carcinoma who present with intestinal obstruction have adhesions as the etiology of their obstruction.[45] Even in those instances in which the obstruction is related to recurrent malignancy, many patients may be successfully palliated by bypassing the obstructing lesion with an enteroenterostomy. This palliative approach is associated with greater-than-1-year survival in as many as 40% to 60% of instances.[45, 46]

Intussusception

Intussusception is defined as the invagination of a proximal segment of bowel (intussusceptum) into an adjacent distal segment (intussuscipiens). This is illustrated in Figure 109–4. Although it is more likely to be recognized as a cause of intestinal obstruction in the pediatric population, about 5% of cases of intussusception occur in adults.[47] In contrast to children, in whom there is rarely an anatomic abnormality of the intestine, intussusception in adults is associated with an underlying pathologic process in more than 90% of cases.[47, 48] The most common lesions associated with intussusception are neoplasms, inflammatory lesions, and Meckel's diverticula. In one review of 48 adults with intus-

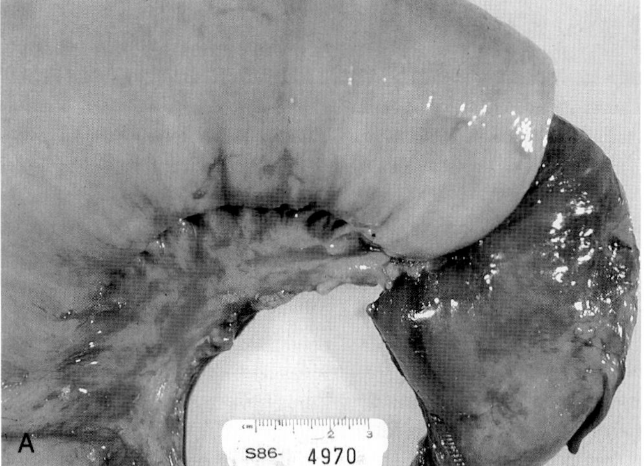

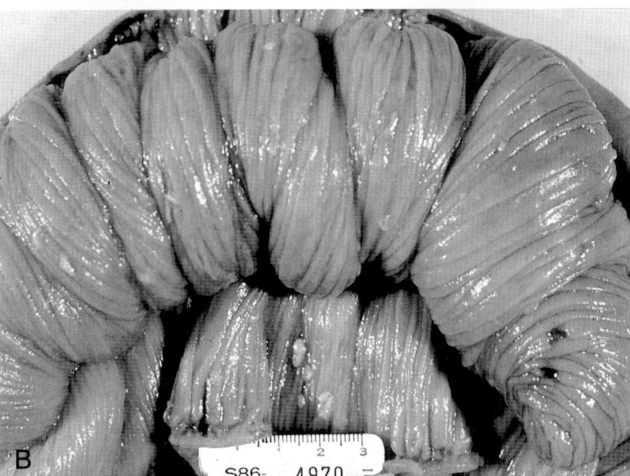

Figure 109–4. Small bowel intussusception presenting as small bowel obstruction. *A,* On the right, the proximal loop of bowel (intussusceptum) is discolored and hemorrhagic and has telescoped into the normal distal segment of bowel (intussuscipiens). *B,* Opened specimen shows a corkscrew gross pattern of the intussusceptum as well as the normal small bowel mucosa of the intussuscipiens.

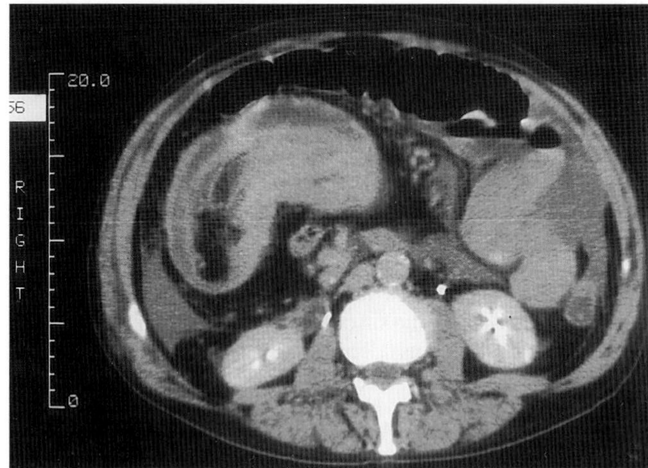

Figure 109–5. Computed tomographic image of the abdomen of a patient with an ileocolic intussusception due to adenocarcinoma of the cecum. As described by Merine and colleagues,[49] this image demonstrates a large, reniform shaped mass with alternating areas of low and high attenuation representing closely spaced bowel wall, mesenteric fat, or intestinal fluid and gas.

susception, 36 were related to neoplasms.[48] Malignant neoplasms were found in 54% to 65% of patients with colocolic intussusceptions and in 29% to 48% of enteroenteric intussusceptions.[47, 48]

The clinical presentation of adults with intussusception is generally that of partial intestinal obstruction. Most patients experience intermittent cramping abdominal pain, vomiting, and to a lesser extent, diarrhea. Patients may have occult or overt rectal bleeding. Often symptoms are present for several weeks prior to presentation. In one series, an abdominal mass was palpable in 42% of patients.[48]

The diagnosis can be confirmed with barium enema, ultrasonography, or CT. CT patterns include (1) *target lesion,* characterized by an intraluminal soft-tissue density mass with an eccentrically placed fatty area of CT attenuation that represents the intussusception and the intussuscepted mesentery, respectively; (2) *reniform mass,* with a high attenuation peripherally and lower attenuation centrally (Fig. 109–5) (this appearance is due to the invaginated intussusception surrounded by thickened small bowel); and (3) *sausage-shaped mass,* with alternating areas of low and high attenuation representing closely spaced bowel wall, mesenteric fat, or intestinal fluid and gas.[49]

The association of neoplasms and other intestinal pathology with intussusception in adults mandates resection of the involved bowel and makes hydrostatic or pneumatic reduction untenable. Primary resection without attempt at reduction represents the treatment of choice for colonic intussusception, including ileocecal intussusception in which the ileocecal valve is the lead point for the intussusception.[47, 48] For lesions involving the right colon, a right hemicolectomy is the procedure of choice. When the intussusception involves only the small intestine, resection remains the preferred operative approach, although manual reduction of the intussusception with careful palpation of the intestinal wall may allow the surgeon to limit the amount of intestine resected.

Sixty to eighty percent of children with ileocolic intussusception may be successfully managed by hydrostatic reduction with contrast enema at the time of diagnosis. The success of this approach diminishes substantially after the duration of symptoms exceeds 24 hours. In those settings in which hydrostatic reduction is unsuccessful or unavailable, manual reduction of the intussusception with careful inspection of the involved intestine is necessary. Intestinal resection is reserved for those instances in which the bowel is nonviable.

Gallstone Ileus

Gallstone ileus is an unusual cause of intestinal obstruction, accounting for about 1% to 4% of all cases.[50, 51] This complication of cholelithiasis is more common among the elderly (see Chapter 55). The term "gallstone ileus" is a misnomer as this condition represents a true mechanical obstruction of the intestine by a gallstone or gallstones within the lumen of the bowel (Fig. 109–6). Most commonly, gallstones large enough to cause obstruction enter the gastrointestinal tract via a cholecystoduodenal fistula.[50] Rarely do stones large enough to obstruct the bowel pass

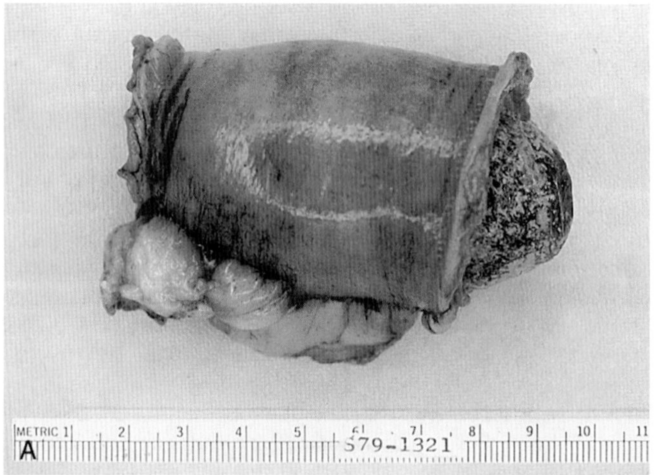

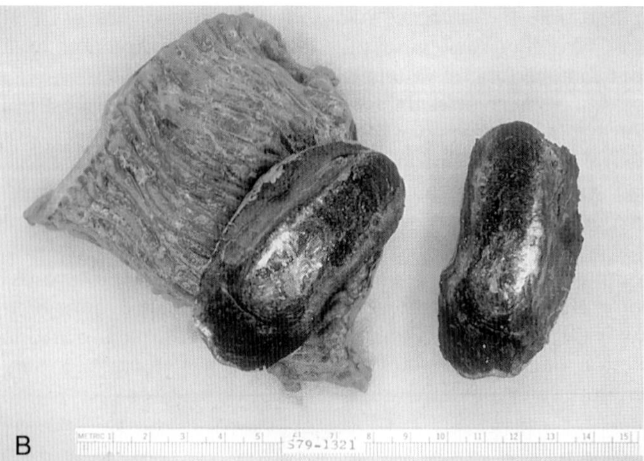

Figure 109–6. Gallstone ileus. *A,* A large gallstone has impacted in this loop of small bowel, causing small bowel obstruction. *B,* Opened specimen showing a discolored mucosal surface and a large (4.2 cm) barrel-shaped gallstone. Note that the diameter of the bowel at the site of the gallstone impaction (*A*) was also 4.2 cm.

spontaneously through the ampulla of Vater. As the stone migrates through the GI tract, it produces intermittent obstruction with resultant waxing and waning of symptoms, making early diagnosis difficult. The most common site of obstruction is the ileum, representing about 60% of instances. Jejunal or gastric obstruction occurs in about 15% of cases and the gallstone obstructs the colon or duodenum in less than 5% of cases. In the absence of an intestinal stricture, a gallstone of at least 2 centimeters is usually required to cause intestinal obstruction (see Fig. 109–6), and stones as large as $7 \times 4 \times 3$ centimeters have been reported.

The diagnosis is delayed in as many as half of patients because of nonspecific and inconsistent symptoms. Only 50% to 70% of patients have clinical features of SBO. Some may present with diarrhea.[52] The classical radiographic features of gallstone ileus include pneumobilia, intestinal obstruction, aberrant gallstone location, and changing the location of a previously observed stone.[53, 54] Only about 10% of gallstones are sufficiently calcified to be visualized radiographically.

The treatment of gallstone ileus is focused on removing the obstructing stone. This is usually accomplished by operative enterolithotomy.[53] Endoscopic removal of stones with or without lithotripsy has also been reported.[54, 55] In general, enterolithotomy alone is the appropriate initial treatment given the emergent nature of this procedure, the advanced age of many of these patients, and the frequent occurrence of a complex right upper quadrant mass containing the cholecystoenteric fistula. Together these factors oppose identification and repair of the fistula at the time of emergent laparotomy for intestinal obstruction. Up to 17% of patients will develop recurrent gallstone ileus or other biliary complications after enterolithotomy alone. Therefore, "open" cholecystectomy with repair of the fistula should be undertaken at an elective setting when the patient has recovered from his/her initial operative procedure.[52]

Midgut Volvulus

As was discussed in greater detail in Chapter 84, midgut volvulus due to intestinal rotational anomalies is an important cause of intestinal obstruction, particularly among neonates. Fifty to 75% of intestinal malrotations are discovered during the first month of life, and about 90% occur in children younger than 1 year of age.[56, 57] The discovery of malrotation at this time usually results from clinical evidence of duodenal obstruction from Ladd's bands, or midgut volvulus. Infants with duodenal obstruction from Ladd's bands present with the clinical signs and symptoms of gastric and proximal duodenal obstruction, including bilious vomiting with minimal abdominal distention. Midgut volvulus may also present with obstructive symptoms, as well as those of intestinal ischemia. Occult gastrointestinal bleeding is a common early finding and, if transmural necrosis develops, acidosis, thrombocytopenia, and frank sepsis may ensue.

The high risk of intestinal ischemia and necrosis from midgut volvulus and the associated high mortality rate mandate aggressive diagnosis and management of neonatal intestinal obstruction. A plain abdominal radiograph will demonstrate a distended stomach and a proximal duodenal bulb with a paucity of small bowel gas. An upper gastrointestinal contrast study will be diagnostic by demonstrating malpositioning of the duodenojejunal junction to the right of the midline with the small intestine on the right and the cecum and ascending colon to the left. The contrast study may also demonstrate a characteristic corkscrew or coiled appearance in the third or fourth portion of the duodenum.

The treatment of intestinal malrotation, whether manifested by duodenal obstruction from Ladd's bands or by midgut volvulus, is surgical. In the latter case, the diagnosis should be followed immediately by laparotomy because a delay of even hours may mean the difference between viable or infarcted intestine. Operative repair of malrotation is achieved by performance of the Ladd procedure, which consists of two parts: (1) relief of the midgut volvulus and division of the peritoneal bands that tether the cecum, small bowel mesentery, mesocolon, and duodenum around the base of the SMA (this allows the mesenteric leaves to open widely and is associated with a very low incidence of recurrent volvulus); (2) division of the Ladd peritoneal bands to relieve the extrinsic compression and obstruction of the distal duodenum. This is accomplished by meticulous and complete mobilization of the entire duodenum with division of all anterior, lateral, and posterior attachments.

COLONIC OBSTRUCTION

Etiology

As is shown in Figure 109–1*B*, the three most common causes of colonic obstruction are malignancy, volvulus, and strictures secondary to diverticulitis.

Adenocarcinoma

Malignant disease accounts for more than 50% of all cases of colonic obstruction, with nearly all of these due to adenocarcinoma (see Chapter 115). About 20% of patients with colorectal cancer present with obstructive symptoms; half of these patients will require emergency operative decompression. Patients requiring emergent management of obstructing colorectal cancer have a worse prognosis than do those undergoing elective operations.[58, 59] This poorer prognosis appears to be related to a more advanced stage of disease with completely obstructing lesions.

Seventy-five percent of obstructing adenocarcinomas occur distal to the splenic flexure, many of which are within reach of a flexible sigmoidoscope. Carcinomas of the left colon most commonly present as a scirrhous tumor that produces progressive stenosis of the lumen, whereas those located within the right colon grow as a polypoid or fungating mass that obstructs the colon either by reaching a size that occludes the lumen or by acting as a lead point of a colocolic intussusception.

Volvulus

Volvulus is an abnormal twisting of a segment of bowel on itself along its longitudinal axis, resulting in occlusion of the intestinal lumen. A closed loop obstruction is often produced, accounting for a high incidence of strangulation.[60–62]

In the United States and other western countries, colonic volvulus causes 1% to 4% of all cases of intestinal obstruction and 10% to 15% of colonic obstructions. In Eastern Europe and parts of Africa and Asia, volvulus accounts for 20% to 50% of all intestinal obstructions.[61]

The sigmoid colon and cecum are the most frequent sites of colonic volvulus, accounting for about 75% and 22% of all cases, respectively. Rare sites for colonic volvulus include the transverse colon (2%) and the splenic flexure (<1%).[61–63] The anatomic factors necessary for the development of volvulus include a redundant segment of bowel that is freely moveable within the peritoneal cavity and close approximation of the points of fixation of the bowel.

Diverticulitis and Other Causes of Benign Colonic Strictures

Benign colonic strictures occur as a consequence of diverticulitis, ischemia, and postoperative anastomotic strictures. Obstruction accounts for about 10% of the complications related to diverticular disease. This complication is discussed in more detail in Chapter 108.

Pathophysiology

The competency of the ileocecal valve is of great importance to the pathophysiology of colonic obstruction. When the ileocecal valve is competent, the cecum cannot decompress fluid and gas into the small bowel, resulting in a closed loop obstruction. As fluid and gas accumulate, intraluminal pressure rises, and when it exceeds capillary pressure, the colonic wall becomes ischemic. Because the cecal diameter is greater than that of other segments of the colon, at any given intraluminal pressure, the greatest wall tension occurs within the cecum (LaPlace's law). As a generic guide, acute dilatation of the cecum to 10 cm suggests colonic wall ischemia, and a diameter greater than 13 cm suggests imminent perforation. Of note, the necessity for emergency operation is dictated by the presence of complete colonic obstruction and not by the measurement of cecal diameter.

Clinical Presentation

Many of the clinical manifestations of colonic obstruction are similar, regardless of the etiology. Periumbilical or hypogastric pain and abdominal distention are the two most common presenting features. The pain may vary from a vague discomfort to the excruciating pain of peritonitis. Severe unremitting pain suggests gangrenous bowel and requires urgent laparotomy. Patients may experience either diarrhea (reflecting the passage of liquid stool around an obstructing lesion) or obstipation, depending on the degree and location of the obstruction.

Benign and Malignant Colonic Strictures

Patients with left-sided colonic tumors or benign fibrotic strictures often have noted a change in stool caliber over the past several months. The presence of blood in the stool (or an iron-deficiency anemia) is highly suggestive of a neoplastic etiology as is the occurrence of weakness, weight loss, and anorexia. Vomiting, when present, is usually a late finding. The symptoms of malignant and diverticular-associated colonic obstruction are often insidious in onset, with a median duration of 3 months. One fourth of patients have symptoms for 6 to 24 months.[64, 65]

Colonic Volvulus

Patients with sigmoid volvulus are often in the seventh or eighth decade of life and frequently have a variety of comorbid illnesses.[60–63, 66] In one of the largest series of patients, 30% had a history of psychiatric disease and 13% were institutionalized at the time of diagnosis.[66] The duration of symptoms is significantly less than that of patients with a malignant or diverticular stricture. In one report, patients with sigmoid volvulus had had symptoms for an average of 5 days prior to presentation.[66] Abdominal tenderness occurs in less than one third of patients who present with colonic volvulus. Significant tenderness with signs of peritonitis suggests impending or actual colonic necrosis and perforation.

Patients with cecal volvulus tend to be younger than patients with sigmoid volvulus and often have a history of prior abdominal operations or distal obstruction. Of interest, nearly one third of patients with cecal volvulus will have a concomitant partially obstructing lesion located more distally in the colon. A history of chronic constipation and laxative use is a frequent finding in patients with either cecal or sigmoid volvulus.

Diagnostic Evaluation

The initial diagnostic approach to patients suspected of having colonic obstruction is similar to that for patients with SBO, which was discussed earlier. Plain abdominal radiographs in the supine and upright or decubitus positions should be obtained to localize the site of the obstruction, determine whether the obstruction is partial or complete, and allow differentiation between Olgilvie's syndrome, ileus, and mechanical small or large bowel obstruction. Small bowel distention may or may not be present depending on the competency of the ileocecal valve.

The abdominal radiograph of patients with sigmoid volvulus will demonstrate a markedly dilated sigmoid colon and proximal bowel with minimal gas in the rectum. As was described by Agrez and Cameron,[67] the standard radiographic feature of sigmoid volvulus is a distended ahaustral sigmoid loop, that is, "bent inner-tube" appearance, the apex of which is often directed toward the right shoulder (Fig. 109–7). The classical radiographic features of cecal volvulus include: (1) a massively dilated cecum located in the epigastrium or left upper quadrant; (2) the distended cecum, which assumes a kidney bean shape; (3) distended loops of small bowel, suggesting SBO; and (4) a single, long air-fluid level present on upright or decubitus films (Fig. 109–8).[68] In these instances, the massively distended cecum extends across the abdominal midline and is "directed" toward the left upper quadrant or left midabdomen. These "classical" radiographic findings are seen in 40% to 60% of cases.[60–62, 66, 68]

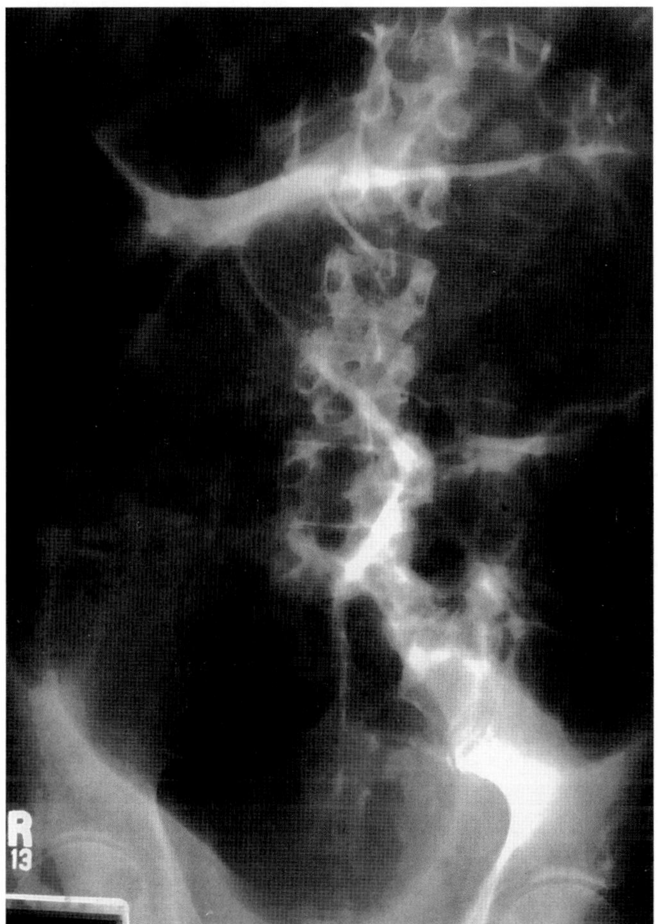

Figure 109–7. Abdominal radiograph of sigmoid volvulus. Note the massively dilated colon with a classic bent inner tube appearance emanating from the pelvis toward the right upper quadrant of the abdomen.

The diagnostic approach to patients with colonic obstruction is predicated on the presence or absence of peritonitis and the degree of obstruction (i.e., partial or complete). Patients with peritonitis should undergo resuscitation and urgent laparotomy without diagnostic procedures, whereas patients without evidence of strangulated bowel and an abdominal radiograph suggestive of a distal complete obstruction should first undergo rigid proctosigmoidoscopy. This procedure will demonstrate the site and nature of distal strictures and in the case of sigmoid volvulus may allow decompression.

If the obstruction is proximal to the area visualized by proctosigmoidoscopy, a water-soluble contrast enema will confirm the diagnosis of colonic obstruction and delineate the site of obstruction (Fig. 109–9). In patients with sigmoid or cecal volvulus and an equivocal plain abdominal radiograph, a water-soluble contrast enema may be helpful by demonstrating a point of torsion (e.g., a mucosal spiral pattern, or "bird's beak" sign; Fig. 109–10). The use of water-soluble contrast media obviates the risk of barium impaction at the site of obstruction and barium peritonitis in the case of unrecognized perforation. The sole purpose of this study is to determine the presence or absence of obstruction. The fine mucosal detail provided by air contrast barium studies is not required in these patients.

Although colonoscopy may be useful in patients with partial colonic obstructions, it has little role in the initial evaluation of patients suspected of having complete obstruction. The insufflation of air or CO_2 through the endoscope into the obstructed bowel may exacerbate colonic distention and precipitate perforation. Brothers and associates highlight the risk of perforation and the danger of missing a segment of ischemic bowel, thus delaying definitive treatment.[69]

Treatment and Outcome

Benign and Malignant Colonic Strictures

The resuscitative phases of treatment of colonic obstruction are the same as those described earlier for small intestinal obstruction (i.e., restoration of intravascular volume, correction of electrolyte abnormalities, and nasogastric aspiration). The urgency with which the obstruction must be decompressed is dependent on the degree of obstruction (partial or complete) and the clinical presentation of the patient (evidence of strangulation or not).

Patients with partially obstructing benign or malignant strictures without evidence of peritonitis who demonstrate prompt improvement with intravenous hydration and nasogastric aspiration may undergo semielective resection of the

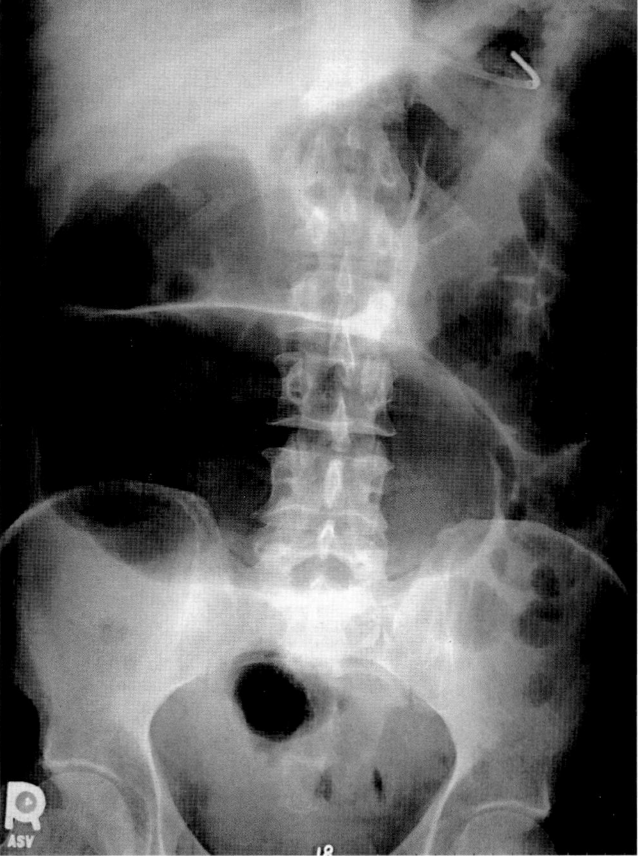

Figure 109–8. Abdominal radiograph of a patient with a cecal volvulus in the supine position. Note the massively dilated cecum extending from the right lower abdomen across the midline toward the left side. This particular patient had a cecal bascule in which the cecum folds on itself in an anterior-cephalad direction.

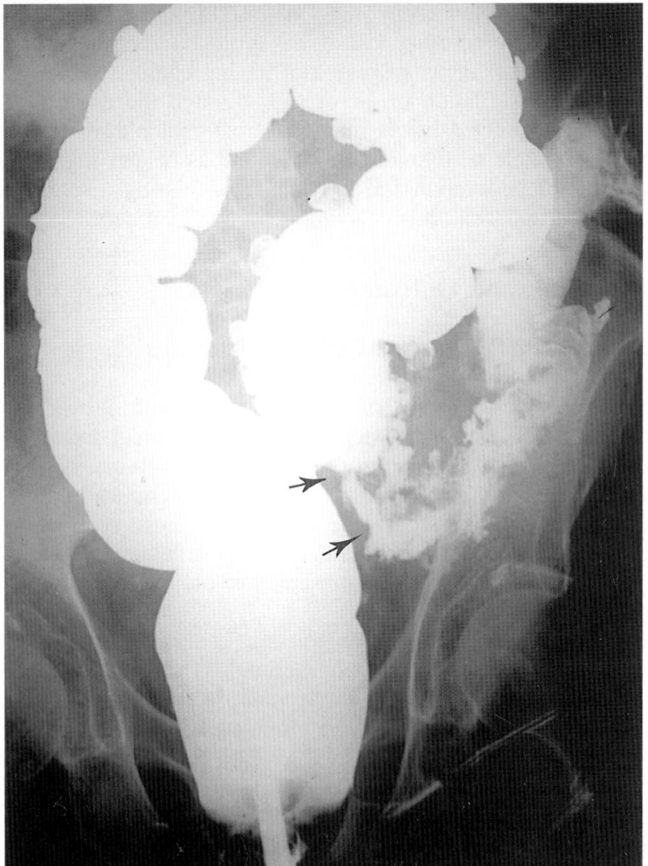

Figure 109–9. Contrast enema of patient with a high-grade sigmoid obstruction. Although this patient has multiple diverticula within the sigmoid colon, differentiation of this benign diverticular stricture from a malignant stricture is not possible based on this study alone.

stricture. The conversion of an emergency operation to a semielective procedure allows preparation of the colon for primary anastomosis and substantially lowers operative risk. If improvement is not seen within 24 hours, the nonoperative approach should be abandoned and the patient should undergo operative decompression of the obstructed colon.

Complete colonic obstruction necessitates emergency operative decompression. The goals of operative management are three-fold: (1) to quickly decompress the obstructed colon; (2) to definitively treat the obstructing lesion; and (3) to reestablish intestinal continuity. All three of these goals may or may not be obtainable at the initial operation.

Obstructions located proximal to the splenic flexure are most frequently adenocarcinomas and can be treated with right hemicolectomy and primary ileocolic anastamosis in all but the most unfit patients.[70] This operation accomplishes all three goals of treatment and can be performed in unprepared bowel with minimal increase in postoperative septic complications. Operative options in obstructed patients who are medically unable to withstand resection include tube cecostomy and loop ileostomy. The authors prefer loop ileostomy because it (1) permits complete diversion of the fecal stream; (2) allows access to all parts of the colon for bowel preparation preceding subsequent definitive resection; and (3) allows for the easy fitting of appliances, thus minimizing local wound complications. The presence of nonviable colon necessitates resection, even in the most severely compromised patient. In this instance, resection with end ileostomy and distal mucous fistula obviates the risk of performing an anastomosis in a grossly contaminated field or in a critically ill patient in whom the risk of anastomotic dehiscence may be particularly high.

Obstruction located at or distal to the splenic flexure may be either adenocarcinomas or diverticular strictures. Differentiation of these two entities may be very difficult at the time of emergent laparotomy. The approach to patients with complete obstruction of the left colon or rectum depends on the precise location of the lesion and the clinical status of the patient. Medically compromised patients and those with large bulky masses are best managed by emergent proximal diversion followed by definitive resection, and then by reanastomosis at a later date (3-stage approach). A transverse loop colostomy can be performed quickly and will effectively decompress the obstructed left colon. The advantages of this procedure are as indicated previously for diverting loop ileostomy.

Patients that are medically fit and who have relatively small tumors or inflammatory masses may undergo resection of the lesion with end colostomy and with closure of the distal bowel or the creation of a distal mucous fistula. In

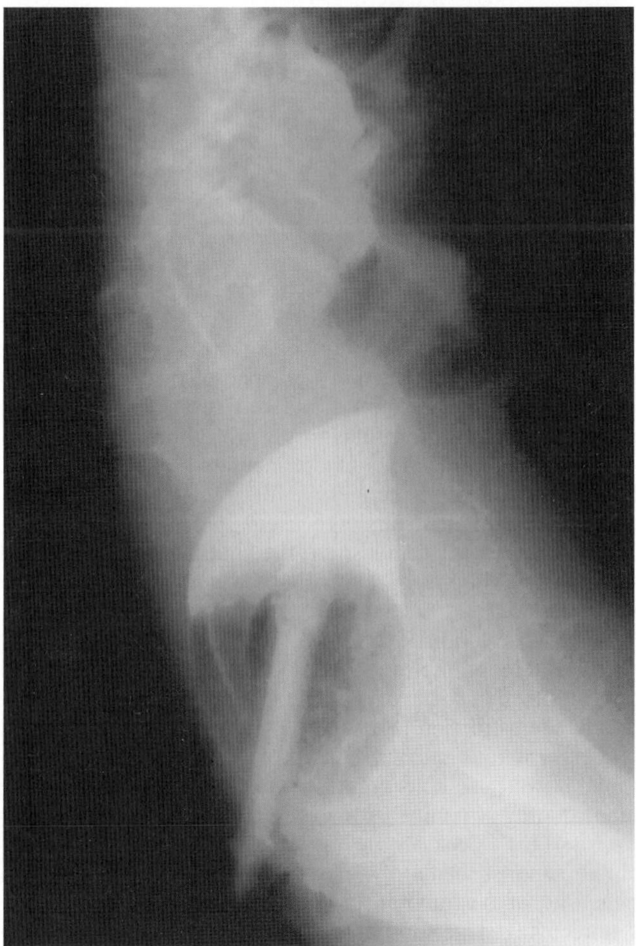

Figure 109–10. Water-soluble contrast enema in a 66-year-old patient with a sigmoid volvulus demonstrating characteristic "bird's beak" obstruction at the junction between the sigmoid colon and the rectum.

those instances in which the lesion is located in the sigmoid colon, Hartmann's procedure is often performed in which the involved bowel is resected with the performance of an end-sigmoid colostomy and closure of the rectal stump. The advantages of this approach are two-fold: (1) Immediate resection of the tumor or the inflammatory mass may promote a more rapid convalescence than if the lesion had been left in situ, and (2) avoidance of an anastomosis in an unprepared left colon reduces postoperative complications such as wound infection, anastomotic dehiscence, and sepsis.[70] The disadvantage of this approach is that it requires a subsequent laparotomy to restore intestinal continuity (i.e., second or third stage). In a review of seven series containing more than 300 patients, Deans and colleagues found that the mortality rate for this approach was 8.7%. This was similar to the mortality rates of patients undergoing initial diverting colostomy with subsequent colonic resection (9.2%).[70] Two less commonly employed operative approaches to patients with inflammatory or neoplastic obstruction of the left colon are (1) primary resection, on-table colonic lavage, and immediate anastomosis; and (2) subtotal colectomy with ileoproctostomy.[70–72] These approaches allow resection of the tumor with immediate restoration of intestinal continuity. The mortality rates and rates of anastomotic leak have been similar to those of primary resection with colostomy, or the three-stage approach.

Recent studies have reported the successful use of endoscopically placed self-expanding metallic endoprostheses to relieve malignant obstruction prior to definitive resection and to palliate patients with advanced disease.[73–75] In one study of 25 patients, the procedure was effective in relieving the obstruction in 14 of 15 patients with advanced disease who were undergoing palliation, and in 9 of 10 patients who ultimately were resected for cure. In the palliative group, the average stent duration was 17.3 weeks and ranged from 2 to 64 weeks. Major complications occurred in 7 of the 25 stented patients (28%).[75]

Colonic Volvulus

The initial management of patients with sigmoid volvulus without evidence of peritonitis is proctoscopic decompression of the obstruction, often assisted by placing a rectal tube into the obstructed bowel. Ballantyne[60–62] compiled the results of 19 American series containing 595 sigmoid volvulus patients treated nonoperatively. Proctoscopy, either alone or combined with a rectal tube, successfully reduced the volvulus in 70% to 80% of attempts, representing 60% of patients.[60, 63, 66] The placement of a rectal tube for 48 hours may minimize the possibility of early recurrence. Successful reduction of sigmoid volvulus has also been reported with colonoscopy[69, 76]; however the procedure must be performed with limited manipulation and minimal insufflation of air or CO_2 in order to minimize the risk of perforation of the distended, inflamed bowel. Brothers and coworkers warn of the difficulty in adequately examining the colonic mucosa in the emergent setting, thus possibly delaying appropriate management.[69]

The risk of recurrence following nonoperative reduction of a sigmoid volvulus is 40% to 50%.[60, 63, 66, 69] Thus, following proctoscopic decompression, the patient should undergo mechanical cleansing of the bowel, followed by elective sigmoid resection. This approach allows time for optimization of the patient's condition prior to laparotomy, resection, and the performance of a primary anastomosis. Recurrence rates following this approach are below 3%.[69] Patients requiring emergent laparotomy for strangulated sigmoid volvulus require sigmoid resection with an end colostomy and Hartmann pouch.

The role of initial nonoperative management of patients with cecal volvulus is less well defined than that of sigmoid volvulus. Although colonoscopy has been successfully employed to reduce the volvulus, the risk of perforation of the thinned, often ischemic cecum is substantial, as is the danger of missing a segment of necrotic bowel with delay of definitive resection.[69] Current options for the operative management of cecal volvulus include cecopexy, cecostomy, and resection. The optimal approach in patients with nongangrenous cecal volvulus has yet to be determined. Detorsion alone or when combined with appendectomy is associated with a very high recurrence rate.[77] Others have favored the performance of a cecopexy in which the right colon is anchored to the peritoneum of the right paracolic gutter, with or without a cecostomy.[78, 79] Right colectomy with primary ileotransverse colostomy effectively prevents recurrent volvulus and is the procedure of choice of a number of surgeons. Ballantyne reported 27 patients with cecal volvulus who were treated with resection and primary anastomosis with no operative mortality and no recurrences in 5 years of follow-up.[61]

Overall, the mortality rate for patients with colonic volvulus is about 8%, with the major predictive factor for mortality being the presence of gangrenous bowel.[69] The incidence of gangrenous bowel in patients with either cecal or sigmoid volvulus is 15% to 20%.[60, 61, 69] In a review of 18 American studies totaling 299 patients with sigmoid volvulus, the mortality rate for patients with gangrenous colons was 80%, whereas only 10% of patients without colonic necrosis died.[60] In a more recent study, the mortality rate for patients with gangrenous colonic volvulus was 25%.[63, 69]

ILEUS

Etiology

As was indicated earlier, *ileus* refers to the failure of aboral passage of intestinal contents in the absence of mechanical obstruction. Ileus may be categorized into postoperative, inflammatory, metabolic, neurogenic, and drug-related causes (Table 109–4). Each of these general categories is a relatively common cause of ileus in hospitalized patients.

Following most abdominal surgeries or injuries, the motility of the gastrointestinal tract is transiently impaired. The return of normal motility following uncomplicated abdominal operations follows a consistent temporal sequence with small intestinal motility and function generally returning to normal within the first 24 hours after laparotomy and gastric and colonic motility has been restored to normal by 48 hours and 3 to 5 days, respectively. The clinical and physiologic consequences of ileus include postoperative discomfort, increased metabolic demands, delay in nutrition, and prolongation of immobilization. Return of normal gastrointestinal

Table 109–4 | **Causes of Ileus**

Laparotomy
Electrolyte derangements
e.g., Hypokalemia, hyponatremia, hypomagnesemia, hypermagnesemia
Drugs
e.g., Narcotics, phenothiazines, diltiazem, anticholinergic agents, clozapine
Intra-abdominal inflammation
e.g., Appendicitis, diverticulitis, perforated duodenal ulcer
Retroperitoneal inflammation or hemorrhage
e.g., Lumbar compression fracture, acute pancreatitis, pyelonephritis
Intestinal ischemia
e.g., Mesenteric arterial embolus or thrombosis, mesenteric venous thrombosis, chronic mesenteric ischemia
Thoracic diseases
e.g., Lower rib fractures, lower lobe pneumonia, myocardial infarction
Systemic sepsis

function may be delayed by the presence of intra-abdominal infection, systemic conditions (e.g., sepsis), or drugs (e.g., narcotics). The duration of the operation, degree of intestinal manipulation, performance of an enterotomy or even vagotomy, does not appear to influence the duration of postoperative ileus.[80–82] The effective duration of ileus is mainly dependent on the return of colonic motility, particularly that of the left colon.[83, 84]

Pathophysiology

Postoperative ileus is thought to result from the loss of normal coordination of intestinal contraction by the intrinsic electrical activity of the bowel. Laparotomy decreases the amplitude of the duodenal pacesetter without altering the frequency of gastric or small intestinal pacesetter potentials. In the stomach and small bowel, there is transient suppression in the migrating action potentials and contractions that normally sweep through the gut during fasting. By 24 to 48 hours after operation, these action potentials and contractions have returned to normal. This return of normal intrinsic electrical activity and contractions occurs last in the left colon.

Numerous neurohormonal factors also likely contribute to the development and persistence of ileus. The interactions are, as yet, poorly understood. The pathogenic mechanisms include sympathetic inhibitory reflexes, inhibitory mediators of the inflammatory response, humoral agents, and anesthetic/analgesic effects. Recent reports have demonstrated that continuous thoracic epidural local anesthetic blockade with limitation or elimination of opioid analgesia reduces postoperative ileus. The use of NSAIDs such as ketorolac (Toradol) in the postoperative period is an important component of epidural/nonopioid regimens. The reduction in ileus after laparoscopic surgery may be related to reduced inflammatory response and decreased bowel dysmotility.[85, 86]

Clinical Presentation and Diagnostic Evaluation

The principal clinical findings include poorly localized abdominal pain, abdominal distention, nausea, vomiting, and obstipation. These clinical manifestations, including the abdominal pain, may be very difficult to distinguish from those associated with mechanical bowel obstruction. The absence of bowel sounds is not a consistent feature of nonobstructive ileus, although "rushes and tinkles" and borborygmi are not usually heard (see Bowel Sounds, which follows Chapter 4 [Volume 1]).

Differentiation of ileus from mechanical obstruction is usually possible based on the entire clinical scenario and the presence of gas in the stomach, small intestine, and colon on plain abdominal radiography. In the past, a contrast study in which barium is administered orally was sometimes useful in ruling out mechanical obstruction in cases in which plain abdominal radiographs are equivocal. Prompt passage of barium through the small intestine and colon confirmed the absence of mechanical obstruction and was consistent with the diagnosis of ileus.[23, 24, 26] More recently, CT scanning has proved useful in this situation. CT offers the additional benefit of delineating other intra-abdominal inflammatory processes, such as abscess, pancreatitis, or retroperitoneal hemorrhage, that may contribute to nonmechanical bowel dysfunction. The passage of CT contrast into the colon within 4 hours excludes small bowel obstruction and favors ileus as the etiology of a patient's intestinal dysmotility.[29]

Management and Outcome

The treatment of ileus following uncomplicated laparotomy involves limiting oral intake, maintaining intravascular volume, and correcting electrolyte abnormalities, particularly hypokalemia. If accompanied by abdominal distention, nausea, or vomiting, a nasogastric tube should be placed. If ileus is prolonged (more than 3 to 5 days), a thorough search for an underlying cause must be undertaken (see Table 109–4). Review of the patient's medications may reveal drugs known to be associated with impaired intestinal motility, especially opiates. Measurement of serum electrolytes may demonstrate hypokalemia, hypocalcemia, hypomagnesemia, or hypermagnesemia, or other electrolyte disturbances commonly associated with ileus. CT may demonstrate the presence of an intra-abdominal abscess or other evidence of peritoneal sepsis, as well as the presence of postoperative obstruction.

Supportive treatment of patients with ileus includes meticulous management of volume and electrolytes, as well as parenteral nutritional support until the ileus resolves (see Chapter 16). Prokinetic agents including erythromycin and somatostatin analogs have not been helpful.[87] Recently, a poorly absorbed opioid antagonist has been shown to shorten the time of ileus following hysterectomy or colectomy and to shorten hospital stay.[88] Additional studies of this potentially promising therapy are awaited.

REFERENCES

1. Greene WW: Bowel obstruction in the aged patient. Am J Surg 118: 541, 1969.
2. Bizer LS, Liebling RW, Delany HM, et al: Small bowel obstruction: The role of non-operative treatment in simple intestinal obstruction and predictive criteria for strangulation obstruction. Surgery 89:407, 1981.
3. Stewardson RH, Bombech CT, Nyhus LM: Critical operative management of small bowel obstruction. Ann Surg 187:189, 1978.
4. Edna TH, Bjerkeset T: Small bowel obstruction in patients previously operated on for colorectal cancer. Eur J Surg 164:587, 1998.

5. Nieuwemhuijzen M, Reijnen MM, Kuijpers JH, et al: Small bowel obstruction after total or subtotal colectomy: A 10-year retrospective review. Br J Surg 85:1242, 1998.
6. Al-Took S, Platt R, Tulandi T: Adhesion-related small-bowel obstruction after gynecologic operations. Am J Obstet Gynecol 180:313, 1999.
7. Matter I, Khalemsky L, Abrahamson J, et al: Does the index operation influence the course and outcome of adhesive intestinal obstruction? Eur J Surg 163:767, 1997.
8. Mucha P Jr: Small intestinal obstruction. Surg Clin North Am 67:597, 1987.
9. McEntee G, Pender D, Mulvin D, et al: Current spectrum of intestinal obstruction. Br J Surg 74:976, 1987.
10. Brolin RE, Krasna MJ, Mast BA: Use of tubes and radiographs in the management of small bowel obstruction. Ann Surg 206:126, 1987.
11. Hass BE, Schrager RE: Small bowel obstruction due to Richter's hernia after laparoscopic procedures. J Laparosc Surg 3:421, 1993.
12. Tsang S, Normand R, Karlin R: Small bowel obstruction: A morbid complication after laparoscopic herniorrhaphy. Am Surg 60:332, 1994.
13. Velasco JM, Vallina VL, Bonomo SR, et al: Post-laparoscopic small bowel obstruction: Rethinking its management. Surg Endosc 12:1043, 1998.
14. Shields R: The absorption and secretion of fluid and electrolytes by the obstructed bowel. Br J Surg 52:774, 1965.
15. Levitt MD: Volume and composition of intestinal gas determined by means of an intestinal wash out technique. N Engl J Med 284:1394, 1971.
16. Roscher R, Oettinger W, Beger HG: Bacterial microflora, endogenous endotoxin, and prostaglandins in SBO. Am J Surg 155:348, 1988.
17. Bishop RF, Allcock EA: Bacterial flora of the small intestine in acute intestinal obstruction. Br Med J 1:766, 1960.
18. Berg RD, Garlington AW: Translocation of certain indigenous bacteria from the gastrointestinal tract to the mesenteric lymph nodes and other organs in a gnotobiotic mouse model. Infect Immun 23:403, 1979.
19. Deitch EA, Maejima K, Berg RD: Effect of oral antibiotics and bacterial overgrowth on the translocation of the gastrointestinal tract microflora in burned rats. J Trauma 25:385, 1985.
20. Deitch EA: Simple intestinal obstruction causes bacterial translocation in man. Arch Surg 124:699, 1989.
21. Heneghan JB, Robinson JWL, Menge H, et al: Intestinal obstruction in germ-free dogs. Eur J Clin Invest 11:285, 1981.
22. Dunn JT, Halls JM, Berne TV: Roentgenographic contrast studies in acute small bowel obstruction. Arch Surg 119:1305, 1984.
23. Riveron FA, Obeid FN, Horst HM, et al: The role of contrast radiography in presumed bowel obstruction. Surgery 106:496, 1989.
24. Zer M, Kaznelson D, Fergenberg Z, et al: The value of gastrografin in the differential diagnosis of paralytic ileus versus mechanical intestinal obstruction. Dis Colon Rectum 20:573, 1979.
25. Blackmon S, Lucius C, Wilson JP, et al: The use of water-soluble contrast in evaluating clinically equivocal small bowel obstruction. Am Surg 66:238, 2000.
26. Megibow AJ, Balthazar EJ, Cho KC, et al: Bowel obstruction: Evaluation with computed tomography. Radiology 180:313, 1991.
27. Balthazar EJ: Computed tomography of small bowel obstruction. Am J Radiol 162:255, 1994.
28. Suri S, Gupta S, Sudhakar PJ, et al: Comparative evaluation of plain films, ultrasound and CT in the diagnosis of intestinal obstruction. Acta Radiol 40:422, 1999.
29. Peck JJ, Milleson T, Phelan J: The role of computed tomography with contrast and small bowel follow-through in management of small bowel obstruction. Am J Surg 177:375, 1999.
30. Daneshmand S, Hedley CG, Stain SC: The utility and reliability of computed tomography scan in the diagnosis of small bowel obstruction. Am Surg 65:922, 1999.
31. Makita O, Ikushima I, Matsumoto N, et al: CT differentiation between necrotic and non-necrotic small bowel in closed loop and strangulating obstruction. Abdom Imaging 24:120, 1999.
32. Ha HK, Kim JS, Lee MS, et al: Differentiation of simple and strangulated small bowel obstruction: Usefulness of known CT criteria. Radiology 204:507, 1997.
33. Balthazar EJ, Liebeskind ME, Macari M: Intestinal ischemia in patients in whom small bowel obstruction is suspected: Evaluation of accuracy, limitations and clinical implications of CT in diagnosis. Radiology 205:519, 1997.
34. Sarr MG, Bulkley GB, Zuidema GD: Preoperative recognition of intestinal strangulation obstruction: Prospective evaluation of diagnostic capability. Am J Surg 145:176, 1983.
35. Peetz DJ, Gamelli RL, Pilcher DB: Intestinal intubation in acute, mechanical small-bowel obstruction. Arch Surg 117:334, 1982.
36. Brolin RE: Partial small bowel obstruction. Surgery 95:145, 1984.
37. Bailey IS, Rhodes M, O'Rourke N, et al: Laparoscopic management of acute small bowel obstruction. Br J Surg 85:84, 1998.
38. Strickland P, Lourie DJ, Suddleson EA, et al: Is laparoscopy safe and effective for treatment of acute small-bowel obstruction? Surg Endosc 13:695, 1999.
39. Suter M, Zermatten P, Halkic N, et al: Laparoscopic management of mechanical small bowel obstruction: Are there predictors of success or failure? Surg Endosc 14:478, 2000.
40. Navez B, Arimont JM, Guiot P: Laparoscopic approach in acute small bowel obstruction. A review of 68 patients. Hepatogastroenterology 45:2146, 1998.
41. Leon EL, Metzger A, Tsiotos GG, et al: Laparoscopic management of small bowel obstruction: Indications and outcome. J Gastrointest Surg 2:132, 1998.
42. Stewart RM, Page CP, Brender J, et al: The incidence and risk of early postoperative small bowel obstruction: A cohort study. Am J Surg 154:643, 1987.
43. Quatromoni JC, Rosoff L, Halls JM, et al: Early postoperative small bowel obstruction. Ann Surg 191:72, 1980.
44. Pickleman J, Lee RM: The management of patients with suspected early postoperative small bowel obstruction. Ann Surg 210:216, 1989.
45. Walsh HPJ, Schofield PF: Is laparotomy for small bowel obstruction justified in patients with previously treated malignancy? Br J Surg 71:933, 1984.
46. Ketcham AS, Hoye RC, Pilch YH, et al: Delayed intestinal obstruction following treatment for cancer. Cancer 25:406, 1970.
47. Weilbaecher D, Bolin JA, Hearn D, et al: Intussusception in adults: Review of 160 cases. Am J Surg 121:531, 1971.
48. Nagorney DM, Sarr MG, McIlrath DC: Surgical management of intussusception in the adult. Ann Surg 193:230, 1981.
49. Merine D, Fishman EK, Jones B: Enteroenteric intussusception: CT findings in nine patients. Am J Roentgenol 148:1129, 1987.
50. Lobo DL, Jobling JC, Balfour TW: Gallstone ileus: Diagnostic pitfalls and therapeutic successes. J Clin Gastroenterol 30:72, 2000.
51. Clavien PA, Richon J, Burgan S, et al: Gallstone ileus. Br J Surg 77:737, 1990.
52. Reisner RM, Cohen JR: Gallstone ileus: A review of 1001 reported cases. Am Surg 60:441, 1994.
53. van Hillo M, van der Vliet JA, Wiggers T, et al: Gallstone obstruction of the intestine. An analysis of ten patients and a review of the literature. Surgery 101:273, 1987.
54. Franklin ME Jr, Dorman JP, Schuessler WW: Laparoscopic treatment of gallstone ileus: A case report and review of the literature. J Laparoendosc Surg 4:265, 1994.
55. Lubbers H, Mahlke R, Lankisch PG: Gallstone ileus: Endoscopic removal of a gallstone obstructing the upper jejunum. J Int Med 246:593, 1999.
56. Andrassy RJ, Mahour GH: Malrotation of the midgut in infants and children. Arch Surg 215:179, 1981.
57. Oldham KT, Coran AG, Wesley JR: Pediatric abdomen. In Greenfield L, Mulholland M, Oldham K, et al (eds): Surgery: Scientific Principles and Practice, 2nd ed. Philadelphia, Lippincott-Raven, 1997, p 2028.
58. Brown SC, Walsh S, Abraham JS, et al: Risk factors and operative mortality in surgery for colorectal cancer. Ann Roy Coll Surg Engl 73:269, 1991.
59. Phillips RK, Hittinger R, Fry JS, et al: Malignant large bowel obstruction. Br J Surg 72:296, 1985.
60. Ballantyne GH: Review of sigmoid volvulus: History and results of treatment. Dis Colon Rectum 25:494, 1982.
61. Ballantyne GH, Brandner MD, Beart RW Jr, et al: Volvulus of the colon: Incidence and mortality. Ann Surg 202:83, 1985.
62. Ballantyne GH: Review of sigmoid volvulus: Clinical patterns and pathogenesis. Dis Colon Rectum 25:823, 1982.
63. Grossman EM, Longo WE, Stratton MD, et al: Sigmoid volvulus in Department of Veterans Affairs Medical Centers. Dis Colon Rectum 43:414, 2000.
64. Glenn F, McSherry CK: Obstruction and perforation in colorectal cancer. Ann Surg 173:983, 1971.
65. Carson SN, Poticha SM, Shields TW: Carcinoma obstructing the left side of the colon. Arch Surg 112:523, 1977.
66. Arnold GJ, Nance FC: Volvulus of the sigmoid colon. Ann Surg 177:527, 1973.
67. Agrez M, Cameron D: Radiology of sigmoid volvulus. Dis Colon Rectum 24:510, 1981.

68. Haskin PH, Teplick SK, Teplick JG, et al: Volvulus of the cecum and right colon. JAMA 245:2433, 1981.
69. Brothers TE, Strodel WE, Eckhauser FE: Endoscopy in colonic volvulus. Ann Surg 206:1, 1987.
70. Deans GT, Krukowski ZH, Irwin ST: Malignant obstruction of the left colon. Br J Surg 81:1270, 1994.
71. Murray JJ, Schoetz DJ Jr, Coller JA, et al: Intraoperative colonic lavage and primary anastomosis in nonelective colon resection. Dis Colon Rectum 34:527, 1991.
72. Brief DK, Brener BJ, Goldenkranz R, et al: Defining the role of subtotal colectomy in the treatment of carcinoma of the colon. Ann Surg 213:248, 1991.
73. Boorman P, Soonawalla Z, Sathananthan N, et al: Endoluminal stenting of obstructed colorectal tumors. Ann Roy Coll Surg Engl 81:251, 1999.
74. Lo SK: Metallic stenting for colorectal obstruction. Gastrointest Endosc Clin North Am 9:459, 1999.
75. Baron TH, Dean PA, Yates MR III, et al: Expandable metal stents for the treatment of colonic obstructions: Techniques and outcomes. Gastrointest Endosc 47:277, 1998.
76. Procaccino J, Labow SB: Transcolonoscopic decompression of sigmoid volvulus. Dis Colon Rectum 32:349, 1989.
77. Burke JB, Ballantyne GH: Cecal volvulus: Low mortality at a city hospital. Dis Colon Rectum 27:737, 1984.
78. Todd GJ, Forde KA: Volvulus of the cecum: Choice of operation. Am J Surg 138:632, 1979.
79. Anderson JR, Welch GH: Acute volvulus of the right colon: An analysis of 69 patients. World J Surg 10:336, 1986.
80. Graber JN, Schulte WJ, Condon RE, et al: Relationship of duration of postoperative ileus to extent and site of operative dissection. Surgery 92:87, 1982.
81. Condon RE, Cowles VE, Schulte WJ, et al: Resolution of postoperative ileus in humans. Ann Surg 203:574, 1986.
82. Ross B, Watson BW, Kay AW: Studies on the effect of vagotomy on small intestinal motility using the radio-telemetering capsule. Gut 4:77, 1963.
83. Waldhausen JH, Shaffrey ME, Skenderis BS, II, et al: Gastrointestinal myoelectric and clinical patterns of recovery after laparotomy. Ann Surg 211:777, 1990.
84. Condon RE, Cowels VE, Ferraz AA, et al: Human colonic smooth muscle electrical activity during and after recovery from postoperative ileus. Am J Physiol 269:G408, 1995.
85. Kehlet H: Postoperative ileus. Gut 47:iv85, 2000.
86. Holte K, Kehlet H: Postoperative ileus: A preventable event. Br J Surg 87:1480, 2000.
87. Bungard TJ, Kale-Pradhan PP: Prokinetic agents for the treatment of postoperative ileus in adults: A review of the literature. Pharmacotherapy 19:416, 1999.
88. Taguchi A, Sharma N, Saleem RM, et al: Selective postoperative inhibition of gastrointestinal opioid receptors. N Engl J Med 345:935, 2001.

Chapter 110

MEGACOLON: CONGENITAL AND ACQUIRED

Elizabeth J. McConnell and John H. Pemberton

CLASSIFICATION OF MEGACOLON

Megacolon and *megarectum* are descriptive terms that carry no etiologic or pathophysiologic implication. The terms *megacolon* and *megarectum*, as defined by Preston and associates,[1] are used when the radiographic diameter of the rectosigmoid region or descending colon is greater than 6.5 cm, the ascending colon is wider than 8 cm, or the cecal diameter is greater than 12 cm. Megacolon can be a sign of clinical disorders as diverse as congenital megacolon (Hirschsprung's disease), idiopathic megacolon (occurring with chronic constipation of any cause), or intestinal pseudo-obstruction (a manifestation of diffuse gastrointestinal dysmotility). Toxic megacolon, a feared complication of idiopathic inflammatory bowel disease and severe infectious colitis, is not considered in this chapter (see Chapter 104). A classification of the causes of megacolon is shown in Table 110–1.

Congenital megacolon is the term often applied to Hirschsprung's disease, in which colonic dilatation (Fig. 110–1) results from a functional obstruction (usually of the rectum) caused by congenital absence of the intramural neural plexus ("aganglionosis"). The aganglionosis results in a "narrower segment" of distal colon (i.e., one that fails to relax). Hirschsprung's disease can be present in a number of disorders such as multiple endocrine neoplasia (MEN) type IIb. Variants of Hirschsprung's disease include other congenital neuromuscular disorders and a spectrum of diseases, including piebaldism–Waardenburg's syndrome,[2] associated with autonomic denervation such as hypoganglionosis and neuronal intestinal dysplasia.[3] Even Chagas' disease acquired in utero can result in a Hirschsprung's-like disease.[4, 5] In fact, animal studies suggest that the aganglionosis that occurs in Hirschsprung's disease may be the result of not one, but several genetic malfunctions that result in the expression of Hirschsprung's disease.[6, 7] Intriguing is the recent demonstration by Basilova and associates[8] that almost 70% of the histologic changes in the intramural nervous system in idiopathic megacolon in adults may be considered congenital in origin. These more recent studies suggest that most, if not all, megacolon has a congenital basis.

Acquired megacolon can be associated with any of the many causes of constipation (see Chapter 12), and megacolon may be assumed to be acquired when it can be ascertained that colonic dilatation was not present on an earlier examination. The distinction between congenital and acquired megacolon is confusing in light of the histopathologic demonstration of hypoganglionosis, hyperganglionosis, and hypoplasia in the ganglia of the muscular-enteric plexus of patients with acquired megacolon.[8] The most common background for acquired megacolon is colonic inertia, which is common at both extremes of life. In children, this form of megacolon can be confused with a congenital condition (Table 110–2).

Infection with *Trypanosoma cruzi* (Chagas' disease) is the most common and best documented cause of acquired megacolon. In this condition, the dilated segment of colon is abnormal, owing to autoimmune cell–mediated destruction[9] of the enteric nervous system by the organism's neurotoxin. Although the infection was originally confined to South America, there are now an estimated 350,000 seropositive persons in the United States; among these, one third are thought to have chronic Chagas' disease.[5] Although intestinal denervation is a late manifestation of the illness, Chagas' megacolon will certainly be seen more frequently in the United States.

A subset of patients acquire megacolon as part of a generalized chronic intestinal pseudo-obstruction (see Chapter 111). When colonic pseudo-obstruction is acute and associated with another medical condition (abdominal or orthopedic surgery, spinal cord injuries, and serious cardiovascular or other medical problems), the term *Ogilvie's syndrome* is often applied.

PATHOPHYSIOLOGY OF COLONIC DILATATION

The large intestine is susceptible to dilatation, and thus to megacolon, and the most dramatic example of this occurrence is Ogilvie's syndrome. As is discussed later, even in

Table 110–1 | **Classification of Megacolon**

Congenital Megacolon (Hirschsprung's Disease)
"Classic" type
Short-segment
Ultrashort-segment
Total colonic aganglionosis, zonal loss of ganglia, other variants (neuronal intestinal dysplasia)
Acquired Megacolon (Associated with Constipation)
Idiopathic
In children
In adults
Acute form (Ogilvie's syndrome)
Neurologic diseases
Chagas' disease
Parkinson's disease and central nervous system dysfunction
Myotonic dystrophy
Diabetic neuropathy
Others (gangliomatosis, familial autonomic dysfunction)
Intestinal pseudo-obstruction ("neurogenic" forms)
Diseases involving intestinal smooth muscle
Scleroderma and other "collagen diseases"
Amyloidosis
Intestinal pseudo-obstruction ("myogenic" forms)
Metabolic diseases
Hypothyroidism
Hypokalemia, porphyria
Pheochromocytoma (with ganglioneuromatosis)
Drugs
Mechanical obstruction

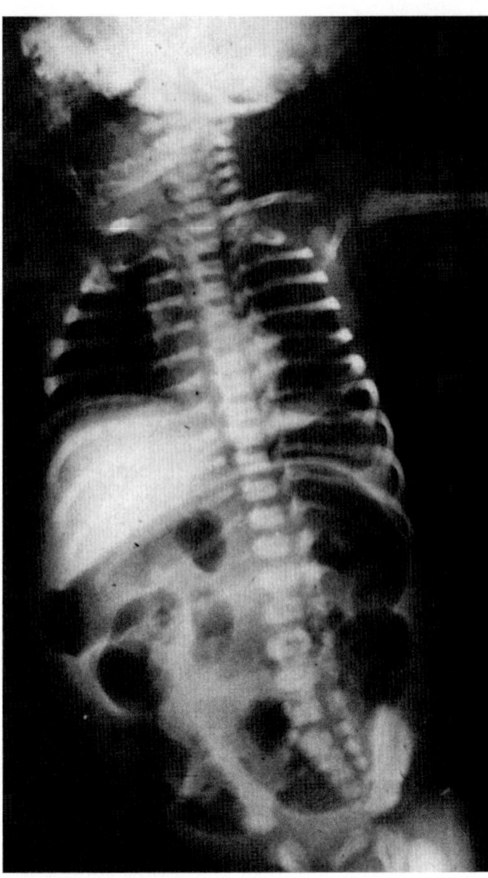

Figure 110–1. Plain abdominal radiograph of neonate with megacolon caused by aganglionosis. (Courtesy of H. J. Goldberg.)

the absence of mechanical obstruction, the large bowel may dilate, often to alarming dimensions. Evidence to suggest that dilatation is a characteristic pathophysiologic reaction of the colon also is provided by the clinical syndrome of toxic megacolon. Once thought to be restricted to chronic ulcerative colitis, it is now clear that Crohn's colitis, amebic colitis, pseudomembranous colitis, and specific infectious colitides can all lead to this life-threatening complication.

Does the large intestine thus have a special property of dilatation? Is dilatation one phenomenologic expression of the colon's physiology? This concept has been explored experimentally. The proximal large bowel is able to react to its luminal contents by dramatically expanding or constricting its capacity. When fatty acids are infused into the healthy human cecum, the volume accommodated by the right colon is markedly reduced.[10] Moreover, pharmacologic agents, notably morphine sulfate, reduce the propensity of the colon to constrict. The canine colon has been shown to be under inhibitory control by adrenergic, cholinergic-nicotinic, and nitrergic transmitters; however, reflex colonic dilatation, which was stimulated by ileal distention, is not mediated solely by any of these mechanisms.[7]

The animal model of Hirschsprung's disease, megacolon in the piebald rat, has also provided insights.[11] Pressure-volume relationships have been studied in the dilated segment of colon and the narrowed, aganglionic region. The dilated colon has been shown to be markedly compliant, but the aganglionic segment is much less so. Electrophysiologic studies have suggested that inhibitory innervation is lacking in the aganglionic bowel. The obstructed colon develops a hypertrophic circular muscle layer, and the muscle cells develop higher stress forces.[12]

Two models of pathogenesis have emerged. One model, associated with mutations in genes encoding endothelin-3 or its receptor endothelin B, proposes that the premature differentiation of migrating neural crest–derived progenitors

Table 110–2 | **Differentiating Types of Megacolon in Children**

	CONGENITAL	ACQUIRED
Early history		
Neonatal failure of bowel movement	+	±
Passage of small hard stools	±	+
Visible straining with bowel movement	−	+
Presence of early enterocolitis	+	−
Later history		
Evidence of voluntary withholding	−	+
Overflow soiling	−	+
Physical and laboratory findings		
Palpable stool at internal sphincter	−	+
Fecal impaction (on physical examination and x-ray)	+	+
Dilated colon on barium enema	+	+
Transition zone on x-ray view	+	−
Aganglionosis on biopsy	+	−
Abnormal motility responses	+	−
Absent internal sphincter reflex	+	−
Inconsistent response to parasympathomimetic agents	+	−

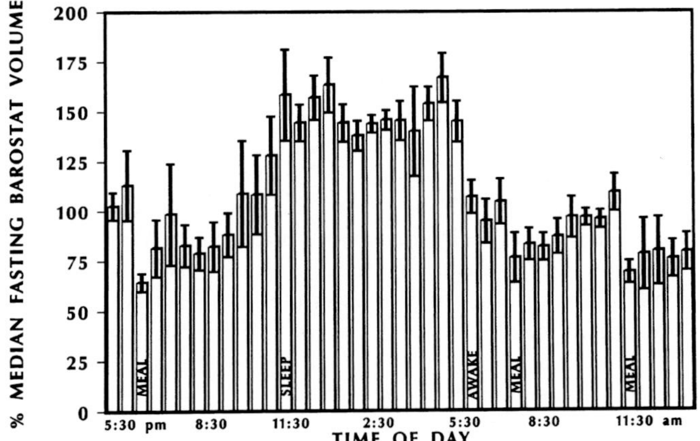

Figure 110–2. Histogram shows mean volume of a segment of colon, recorded overnight by an electromechanical barostat. When subjects slept, the volume of the colonic segment always increased, reflecting diminished tone in the wall of the colon.[7]

causes the precursor pool of progenitor cells to become depleted before the bowel has been fully colonized. The second model, associated with mutations in genes encoding glial cell line–derived neurotrophic factor (GDNF), its preferred receptor GFR alpha-1, or their signaling component RET, proposes that the GDNF-dependent common progenitor is deprived of adequate support or mitogenic stimulation. In both cases, the terminal bowel becomes aganglionic when the number of colonizing neuronal precursors is inadequate.[7]

The human colon's capacity to alter the tone in its wall has been studied more directly with the electromechanical "barostat."[13] When subjected to a low-pressure distending force (intraluminal pressures usually less than 8 mm Hg), the human colon demonstrates major fluctuations of tone (i.e., resistance of the wall to distention). The large bowel is shown to relax its wall tone often; relaxation is most obvious during sleep (Fig. 110–2) but also after atropine and in response to morphine.

HIRSCHSPRUNG'S DISEASE: CONGENITAL MEGACOLON

Pathophysiology

Aganglionosis is thought to result from arrest of the caudal migration of cells from the neural crest; these are the cells that are destined to develop as the gut's intramural plexuses.[14] The pathogenesis of Hirschsprung's disease favors the "abnormal microenvironment" hypothesis, wherein the developing and migrating normal neural crest cells confront a segmentally abnormal and hostile microenvironment in the colon, thereby accounting for both the congenital absence of ganglion cells in the wall of colon and the range of enteric neuronal abnormalities encountered, including neuronal dysplasia, hypoganglionosis, and zonal aganglionosis.[15] A separate, caudal origin for ganglion cells is also possible.[15] In Hirschsprung's disease, the aganglionic segment always extends proximally from the internal anal sphincter for some distance. In most instances, the aganglionic segment is in the rectum and sigmoid colon; involvement of very short segments, affecting only the region of the anal sphincters, has also been described. The aganglionic segment is permanently contracted and causes dilatation proximal to it. A longer aganglionic segment occurs in fewer than 20% of patients. Involvement of the entire colon is infrequent, and reports of aganglionosis extending proximally throughout the entire small intestine are rare. Thus, the hallmark of the diagnosis of Hirschsprung's disease is the absence of ganglion cells from the myenteric and submucosal plexuses, as seen on a full-thickness or suction (mucosal-submucosal) biopsy of the rectum. Proximal contents fail to enter the unrelaxed, aganglionic segment. Although longer aganglionic segments tend to produce more dramatic syndromes, some patients with even short-segment disease deteriorate rapidly.

Morphologically, ganglion cells are absent from the narrowed segment and for some distance (1 to 5 cm usually) into the dilated segment. The pattern of nerve fibers is also abnormal; the nerve fibers are hypertrophic with abundant, thickened bundles. Specific stains for acetylcholinesterase are used to highlight the abnormal morphology. Adrenergic denervation of the dilated segment is another prominent but inconsistent finding, as is decreased innervation by peptidergic nerves (containing vasoactive intestinal peptide [VIP], substance P, enkephalins, and other peptides). The functional role of these neuropeptides in the control of gut motility is unclear. Nevertheless, a synergistic effect on the control of intestinal motility between VIP and nitric oxide (NO) has been shown,[16] which suggests that a lack of NO and VIP in nerve fibers in the aganglionic segment in Hirschsprung's disease may contribute to or be responsible for the inability of the smooth muscle to relax, thereby preventing peristaltic waves.[14]

Experimentally, the inherited aganglionosis in piebald mice is thought to be mediated by loss of spontaneous active inhibitory neurons.[11, 17] Inhibitory innervation of the gut is provided by intrinsic nonadrenergic, noncholinergic (NANC) fibers and to a lesser extent extrinsic adrenergic fibers. The key neurotransmitter in the NANC inhibitory control system is nitric oxide (NO); aganglionic colon is deficient in NO synthase–containing nerves. This deficiency could prevent smooth muscle relaxation in the aganglionic colon of patients with Hirschsprung's disease.[14] NO has been identified as an important mediator of relaxation of the gut musculature (see Chapter 1).[18]

Studies in the 1990s have demonstrated that NO is absent in the aganglionic segment in Hirschsprung's disease.[19–21] Further evidence that lack of NANC nerves is the specific defect that induces bowel obstruction in patients with Hirschsprung's disease was provided in an elegant study by Bealer and colleagues.[14] A 70% reduction in resting tension was demonstrated after electrical field stimulation of isolated smooth muscle from aganglionic colon after exposure to an exogenous source (S-nitroso-N-acetylpenicillamine) of NO.[14] This and other work, in which topically applied NO (nitrate paste) has been used successfully in the treatment of achalasia,[22] also points to potential future therapeutic advances in the management of Hirschsprung's disease.

The most characteristic functional abnormality of aganglionosis is failure of the internal anal sphincter to relax following rectal distention.[23] In health, a "rectal (or rectoanal) inhibitory reflex" is almost always demonstrable (Fig. 110–3). Transient distention of a balloon in the rectum decreases the intraluminal pressure at the level of the internal anal

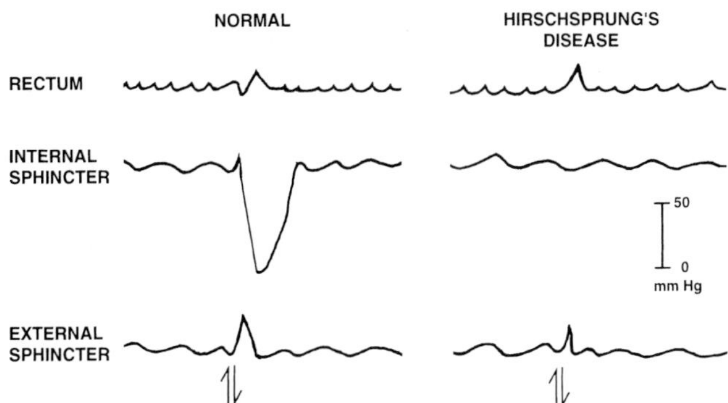

Figure 110–3. Schematic diagram of anorectal manometry in Hirschsprung's disease. On inflation-deflation of a rectal balloon, *bottom arrows,* the normal internal sphincter relaxes and the external sphincter contracts. In Hirschsprung's disease, the internal sphincter does not relax with rectal distention.

sphincter; this decrease is often accompanied by reflex contractions of the external anal sphincter. As many as 20% of normal children may have a falsely absent reflex, especially if they are premature or of low birth weight, but presence of the reflex is strong evidence against Hirschsprung's disease. Resting pressure in the internal anal sphincter is normal or slightly elevated in aganglionosis, and in some instances, the response of the internal anal sphincter to rectal distention is an inappropriate contraction. Another pathophysiologic aspect of colorectal motility in aganglionosis is failure of the contracted segment to relax after parasympathomimetic agents; by contrast, the innervated or dilated segment was able to relax in four of six patients and most healthy control subjects.[24]

A final abnormality described in Hirschsprung's disease is a stiff rectal wall. This increased resistance to stretch has been noted even in the dilated, uncontracted bowel; moreover, the greater the degree of stiffness, the more severe the clinical picture.[25] These changes relate to properties of connective tissue and the inability of the smooth muscle to relax. The abnormal constitution of the mesenchymal and basement membrane extracellular matrix in the affected segment of colon is presumably determined genetically.

Incidence and Genetics

Hirschsprung's disease, defined as congenital absence of enteric innervation with resulting intestinal obstruction,[26] occurs in approximately one in 5000 live births and can be sporadic or familial.[27] When it is familial, the trait can be autosomal dominant or recessive, and its penetrance is relatively low, around 30%. In one series, 17 of 326 index male cases and 13 of 88 female cases had affected siblings; overall, the prevalence was 3.6% among siblings of all index cases.[27] The risk of short-segment disease was 5% in brothers and 1% in sisters of index cases; for long-segment disease, the risk was 10% regardless of sex. Because the disease was highly lethal until the introduction of curative surgery in the 1950s, accurate assessment of the incidence in offspring of successfully treated patients is incomplete. Consanguinity of parents is exceptional, and only three such instances have been reported in a study of more than 300 patients. The disease is reported to be discordant in dizygotic twins and concordant in monozygotic twins.

Association of congenital aganglionosis of the colon with Down's syndrome is ten times more frequent than would be expected by chance.[27] Approximately 2% of patients with congenital megacolon have Down's syndrome. Other anomalies reported to be associated with congenital megacolon include hydrocephalus, ventricular septal defect, cystic deformities and agenesis of the kidney, cryptorchidism, diverticulum of the urinary bladder, imperforate anus, Meckel's diverticulum, hypoplastic uterus, polyposis of the colon, ependymoma of the fourth ventricle, the Laurence-Moon-Biedl-Bardet syndrome, and congenital central hypoventilation syndrome (Ondine's curse). Hirschsprung's disease should be considered as one feature of more generalized developmental abnormalities of the neural crest, the neurocristopathies. Mutations of four different genes have been implicated in the pathogenesis of Hirschsprung's disease: the RET tyrosine kinase receptor gene; one of its ligands, the glial cell line–derived neurotrophic factor (GDNF) gene; the endothelin receptor B (EDNRB) gene; and its ligand, endothelin-3 (EDN3). Recently, combinations of mutations in two of these genes (RET and GDNF) have been reported in patients with Hirschsprung's disease. This finding illustrates the complexity of the molecular background of Hirschsprung's disease.[28, 29] In addition, the RET oncogene (on chromosome 10q11x2) has been associated with Hirschsprung's disease, MEN type IIb, and sporadic medullary thyroid cancer.[30, 31] From a clinical point of view, it would be wise to screen a child with Hirschsprung's disease for MEN-II–associated tumors.[30]

The types of mutations found in the RET gene that have been implicated in Hirschsprung's disease can be placed loosely into two groups: either frameshift or missense mutations that disrupt the structure of the intracellular tyrosine kinase domain,[29] or missense mutations in exon 2, 3, 5, or 6 of the extracellular domain.[32] Patients in whom mutations of the intracellular domain of RET were studied[29] had either short-segment or long-segment Hirschsprung's disease, and patients in whom mutations of the extracellular domain of RET were studied[32] had long-segment Hirschsprung's disease. It is not yet known whether mutations in RET are also implicated in total colonic aganglionosis.[33]

Close clinicopathologic relationships between Hirschsprung's disease and neuronal intestinal dysplasia (NID) are also apparent. NID is recognized most widely in Europe, where at least two types have been described. Type A mimics Hirschsprung's disease, and type B has a somewhat later onset and better prognosis,[30, 31] even without surgical treatment. Subtle histopathologic differences between Hirschsprung's disease and NID have been recorded,[16] although overlap is prominent, and controversy still exists over the appropriate nosology for this spectrum of neuropathies.

Clinical Features

Hirschsprung's disease becomes apparent shortly after birth, when the infant (usually male, in a ratio of 5:1) passes little meconium and the abdomen is distended. Digital examination of the rectum, insertion of a rectal tube, or administration of a small enema may result in a gush of retained fecal material with apparent relief of symptoms, but this respite is short lived. Signs of partial intestinal obstruction return, with persistent vomiting and distention as the major features. In approximately 20% of patients, diarrhea persists and is caused by pseudomembranous enterocolitis, which develops as a complication of the obstruction.

Later in life, the presentation is often less dramatic and may not mimic acute intestinal obstruction. Severe constipation and recurrent fecal impactions are common. Children occasionally show evidence of anemia, malnutrition, and even hypoproteinemia resulting from protein-losing enteropathy; their resistance to infection can be impaired. Although most children have major difficulties before the second month of life, very short segment aganglionosis may not cause severe symptoms until after infancy.

Diagnosis and Differential Diagnosis

Hirschsprung's disease in the neonate must be distinguished from other causes of intestinal obstruction such as intestinal atresias and imperforate anus (see Chapter 84). Later in life, acquired (secondary) megacolon is the other major consideration (see Table 110–1). The diagnosis of congenital megacolon is usually not difficult after the immediate neonatal period, and the better diagnostic methods now available should lead to a positive diagnosis in 75% of cases. Obstipation, with infrequent spontaneous passage of stool, dates from infancy, and the rectal examination reveals an empty ampulla. Overflow incontinence is not a feature of Hirschsprung's disease. In extreme instances, the abdominal wall is stretched and the venous pattern is prominent; large fecal masses may be palpable over the left colon.

A barium enema study confirms the diagnosis if the characteristic transition from the narrowed distal rectal or rectosigmoid segment to the dilated proximal colon is seen (Fig. 110–4). This finding is usually best demonstrated in a lateral view; however, when the aganglionic segment is very short, a narrowed segment is not seen radiologically. In patients with acquired megacolon, encopresis is common, dilatation extends to the anus, and a narrowed zone is not seen.

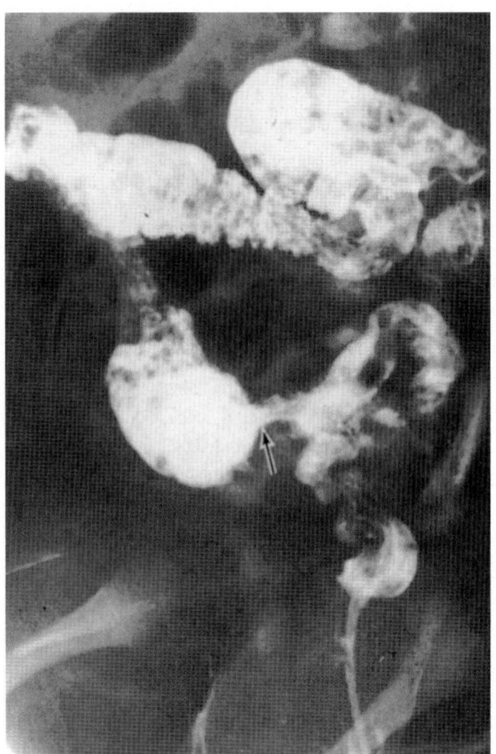

Figure 110–4. Barium enema in an 11-month-old with Hirschsprung's disease shows transition zone *(arrow)* between dilated proximal and narrowed distal segments.

Proctosigmoidoscopy reveals a normal but empty rectum. The dilated proximal bowel, if within the range of the endoscope, is easily traversed, except for feces in the dilated lumen; occasionally, stercoral ulcers may be noted. The key findings are the empty lower segment and absence of organic obstruction.

In doubtful cases, the diagnosis requires full-thickness biopsy of the rectum. The presence of a normal number of ganglion cells excludes the diagnosis (Fig. 110–5). Mucosal suction biopsy, which is satisfactory in many instances, is the initial procedure of choice because it can be performed easily and requires no anesthesia. If the depth of the examination is sufficient to show the presence of ganglia in Meissner's (submucosal) plexus, the classic form of Hirschsprung's disease is ruled out. Absence of ganglion cells in such a specimen does not establish the diagnosis and should be followed by a full-thickness biopsy obtained at least 3 cm proximal to the pectinate line.[1] Diminution or absence of ganglion cells distal to this point is difficult to interpret. Careful measurements proximal to the internal anal sphincter have suggested that myenteric ganglia may be absent in normal infants over a distance of 4 to 5 mm in this segment; ganglia may be absent in the deep submucosal layer for 7 to 10 mm and in the superficial submucosal layer for 10 to 20 mm. Immunohistochemical techniques can be helpful in highlighting the morphologic abnormalities, which feature an abundance of hyperplastic axons but an absence of ganglion cells. Several approaches have been described, mostly using acetylcholinesterase but also neuron-specific enolase, neural filament antibodies, and neuropeptides.[13, 16, 21, 33, 34, 35]

Physiologic tests complement the diagnosis in doubtful cases, and may be crucial when the aganglionic segment is short. Such cases are less easily detectable by x-ray and are also likely to be missed by biopsy. The most important pathophysiologic test is the response of the anal sphincter to distention of the rectum. In contrast to normal persons and to patients with acquired megacolon, the internal anal sphincter in patients with congenital aganglionosis fails to relax (or even contracts) after distention of the rectum (see Fig. 110–3).

One group of investigators[36] compared anorectal manometry and histochemistry of a superficial rectal biopsy stained for acetylcholinesterase and found that all nine patients with proven aganglionosis had increased staining for acetylcholinesterase, whereas all 15 unaffected controls had normal staining. In a larger study, 1 of 18 patients with Hirschsprung's disease had a falsely present rectal inhibitory reflex, and 11 of 104 controls had an absent reflex. When the results of the two studies were combined, the authors found that the need for deep rectal biopsy to make a positive diagnosis was virtually eliminated. However, other authors

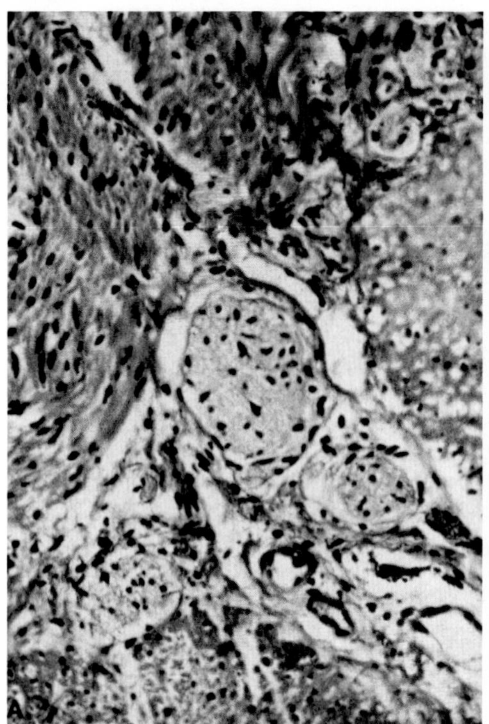

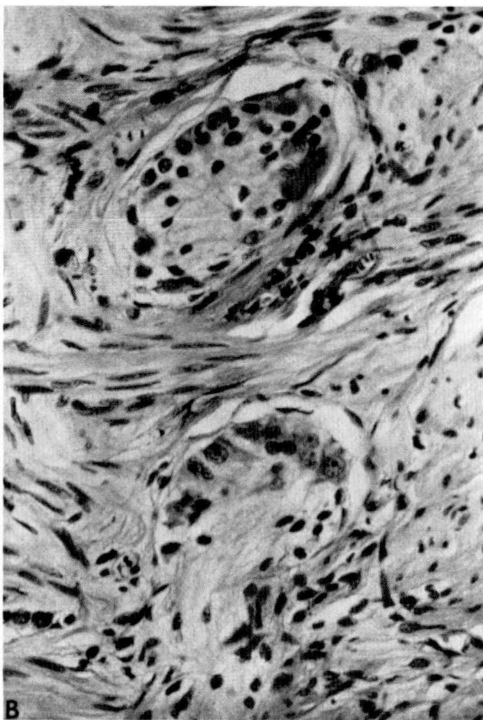

Figure 110–5. *A,* Biopsy of rectum in a patient with Hirschsprung's disease shows Auerbach's plexus at center with neural elements but absence of ganglion cells. Hematoxylin-eosin stain; original magnification, ×200. *B,* Normal specimen at same magnification and staining techniques shows ganglion cells within plexus.

maintain that deep rectal biopsy is required to exclude the diagnosis of Hirschsprung's disease.

The diagnosis of Hirschsprung's disease is often made in stages. Superficial suction biopsies done on an outpatient basis may need to be followed by deeper mucosal and muscular biopsies under anesthesia. Infants and children suspected of having Hirschsprung's disease on the basis of a negative rectal inhibitory reflex are subjected first to suction biopsy. If the biopsy shows ganglion cells, the patient does not have Hirschsprung's disease. If the biopsy yields no ganglion cells but shows hypertrophic nerve trunks, the diagnosis of Hirschsprung's disease is confirmed. If there are no ganglion cells and no hypertrophic nerve trunks, the next step is deep mucosal biopsy of the rectum under general anesthesia; the submucosal plexus is examined for lack of ganglion cells. The prenatal diagnosis of colonic obstruction presumed to be caused by Hirschsprung's disease has been reported with use of ultrasonography.[37]

Treatment

Once the diagnosis of Hirschsprung's disease is established, definitive surgical cure is the treatment of choice. Preliminary decompression by colostomy is still sometimes necessary to relieve obstruction or when definitive surgery is postponed. In general, the goal should be early diagnosis and a one-stage operative approach.

The main goals of surgery are to establish regular and spontaneous defecation, maintain normal continence, and not interfere with sexual potency. The surgical procedure should have essentially no mortality and minimal morbidity. A number of different approaches have been used successfully to remove or counterbalance the obstructing effect of the aganglionic segment (Fig. 110–6). Long-term results are good in the great majority of patients, but approximately 12% experience residual problems with fecal soiling over time.[38]

Further understanding of the pathogenesis of Hirschsprung's disease will emerge as molecular geneticists characterize the specific genes and gene products associated with the disease, thereby permitting gene probes to be developed

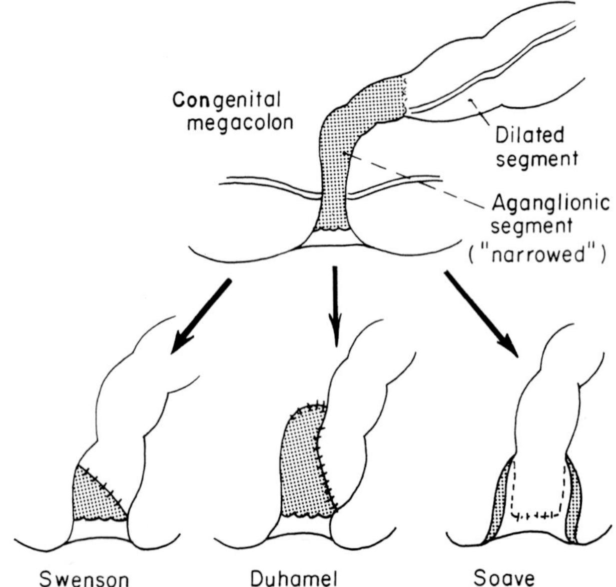

Figure 110–6. The Swenson procedure removes the aganglionic segment up to the dentate line posteriorly, leaving a short segment of abnormal bowel anteriorly. The Duhamel operation excises the aganglionic segment above the peritoneal reflection only. The Soave procedure is an endorectal mucosal proctectomy with the rectal muscle layer left in place.

to facilitate prenatal and postnatal diagnosis and possibly treatment.[8]

VARIANTS OF CONGENITAL MEGACOLON

The spectrum of Hirschsprung's disease has widened considerably beyond its original description. Patients with a compatible clinical picture may have an ultrashort segment of aganglionosis, involving only the internal anal sphincter.[39] Morphologic confirmation of the diagnosis may be quite difficult, and these patients therefore require physiologic testing. Patchy or zonal loss of ganglia ("ladder pattern") and abnormal or dysplastic neurons also have been described.[40, 41] Other investigators have emphasized the continuing uncertainty with which these variants can be diagnosed; they note that the presence of morphologically normal, or even hypertrophic,[16, 30, 31] ganglia does not necessarily imply normal function. These reports merely highlight the vagaries attendant with superficial, mucosal-submucosal suction biopsies and the difficulties encountered in their histologic interpretation. Indeed, cases classified as "acquired aganglionosis" have been reported in which ganglia have been seen in tissues removed at initial operation, but, when clinical failure led to further surgery, an aganglionic segment was clearly demonstrable. Rather than being an acquired disease, it seems just as likely that a short aganglionic segment was missed on the initial evaluation. Further, with greater awareness of the more subtle morphologic and physiologic abnormalities, it is not surprising that previously undiagnosed Hirschsprung's disease is being detected increasingly in adults.[42] The clinical, physiologic, and morphologic features in adults are usually similar to those of the milder form of the disease recognized earlier in life. Thus, congenital megacolon (Hirschsprung's disease) should be subdivided into the classic form, short-segment types, ultrashort-segment types, and other variants (see Table 110–1).

These findings, which greatly expand the spectrum of congenital megacolon, also raise questions about the etiopathogenesis of some examples of acquired megacolon and even of the less well-defined syndrome of functional constipation in children.[30] Possibly, some subgroups of patients with these conditions represent additional variants or forme frustes of Hirschsprung's disease.

ACQUIRED MEGACOLON AND MEGARECTUM

The best proof that megacolon in a given patient has an acquired basis is radiographic evidence that at some earlier point in time, the colon was not dilated. Unfortunately, this information is not usually available, and megacolon must be assumed to be acquired if there is no detectable congenital abnormality (aganglionosis, atresia, or stricture) or when symptoms of constipation did not appear early in infancy. Once megacolon can be designated as the acquired type, it is necessary to establish whether or not an underlying, and possibly treatable, cause exists (see Table 110–1).

The basis of chronic dilatation of the colon and rectum that is not caused by Hirschsprung's disease is not well understood. By contrast, the presentation, symptoms, and treatment are rather straightforward; however, because the cause of both conditions is unknown, separating patients with acquired megacolon from those with congenital megacolon can sometimes be difficult. Moreover, it is never entirely clear when to assign megacolon to the general category of chronic idiopathic intestinal pseudo-obstruction.[43] The heterogeneity of the patient population designated as having pseudo-obstruction is impressive, and the spectrum is expanding (see Chapter 111).

It is of some interest to define terms. *Megacolon* denotes a dilatation of the abdominal colon that is not caused by mechanical obstruction.[1] In this condition, the rectum is normal in size. *Megarectum* implies that the rectal vault is enlarged, often massively. *Megabowel* implies that the patient has an enlarged colon and rectum. It is clear that not all patients with megarectum have megacolon,[42] and vice versa.[44] It is, therefore, important that the anatomy of the colon be visualized adequately and that the patient be categorized accurately, because medical and surgical options differ depending on the extent of colon or rectum that is involved. Acquired megarectum and megacolon, as strictly defined, are not common conditions.[45] It is important to note that the terms do not refer to elongation of the colon (dolichocolon) often encountered in a patient with (but also in those without) chronic constipation.

Etiology

Although the precise cause of acquired megabowel is often unknown, no segment of colon can be shown to be aganglionic; this finding is the principal feature that differentiates congenital from acquired disease. A generalized hollow visceral myopathy or neuropathy[43, 46] may be the cause of megabowel, but patients with megabowel do not usually exhibit abnormalities of gastric or small bowel motility. On the other hand, patients with chronic intestinal pseudo-obstruction involving the stomach and small intestine may have slow colonic transit but often do not have a dilated colon or rectum (see Chapter 111).

Clinical Features

Whereas Hirschsprung's disease occurs predominantly in boys, acquired megacolon is more equally distributed between the sexes.[4] Moreover, the general health of patients with megabowel is often good, as compared with the more serious clinical features of Hirschsprung's disease.

Two groups of adult patients with megabowel are identifiable.[1, 42] One experiences the onset of constipation in childhood, usually before age 1 year, whereas the other group develops symptoms after age 10 or even in adulthood.[1, 42, 45] In the former group, constipation, rectal impaction, and fecal soiling occur during early childhood; in the latter group, constipation and abdominal pain predominate, but fecal soiling does not occur. Encopresis also does not occur in patients with Hirschsprung's disease. In patients whose symptoms begin early in life, the condition of acquired megacolon is considered to be "organic" (rather than "functional") because (1) the history often begins in infancy, (2) the family history is often positive, and (3) related psychopathology is absent. On the other hand, chronic acquired megabowel beginning later in childhood can sometimes result merely from refusal to stool during toilet training.[30, 47, 48]

The predominant symptom of both early- and late-onset megabowel is constipation; weeks may pass between bowel movements. In some patients, a fecal mass impacted in the rectal vault is actually palpable low in the abdomen. A hard mass of stool resides, sometimes rather permanently, just above the anorectal ring. This mass, in turn, causes the anus to gape open because the internal anal sphincter is inhibited by chronic rectal distention.[49] In some patients with megarectum, fecal incontinence (of an "overflow" type), and not constipation, may be the predominant presenting symptom.[50]

Diagnosis

The primary diagnostic dilemma is to differentiate congenital megabowel from the acquired type; history taking and physical examination may be inadequate to distinguish between the two types. The approach to a patient who is suspected on physical examination to have a dilated colon and who has long-standing constipation is first to demonstrate the anatomy. Water-soluble contrast media are of great value in evaluating patients with severe constipation. Although Hypaque has been criticized as a contrast medium because mucosal detail is lacking with its use, in the present context, this limitation is unimportant because only the gross dimensions of bowel need to be determined. Preston and coworkers[1] have differentiated reliably between control subjects and patients with megacolon by measuring the width of the bowel at the level of the pelvic brim. Among normal controls, the range of widths of the colon at this level is 2.4 to 6 cm. The range in patients with megacolon is 6.9 to 14.7 cm. Thus, the authors recommend a diagnosis of megacolon if the diameter of the bowel at the pelvic brim is 6.5 cm or greater.

Additionally, contrast enemas display gross fecal loading of the rectum and of the colon for a variable distance. A lateral view of the pelvis best visualizes the narrowed segment characteristic of Hirschprung's disease (see Fig. 110–4).

Anorectal Manometry

Anorectal manometry demonstrates the presence of a rectoanal inhibitory response as the most useful method of distinguishing acquired from congenital megacolon. An intact reflex is dependent on intact ganglia, and, if present, the patient does not have Hirschsprung's disease. If the reflex is absent, however, the patient still may not have Hirschsprung's disease. Sometimes a response cannot be elicited because the internal anal sphincter has been chronically inhibited by a fecal bolus. If the response is absent and there is no fecal impaction, biopsy of the rectal muscular wall above the anorectal ring should be performed.

Transit

Patients with diffuse megacolon usually have delayed colonic transit, but those with megarectum alone may have normal colonic transit to the rectum. On the other hand, it has been claimed that patients with an enlarged colon or rectum who do not have delayed colonic transit have simple constipation and rarely need surgery.[44]

Total and regional colonic transit are measured most conveniently by the radiopaque marker technique.[51] Twenty-four radiopaque markers are ingested at the same time of day on three successive days. A plain abdominal radiograph is obtained, again at the same time of day, on days four and seven. Normal values have been well established,[51] and the results can be analyzed for total or segmental colonic inertia. This approach has been used to evaluate large numbers of patients with severe constipation, even in the absence of dilatation of the colon or rectum.[52] Transit measurements are refined by employing radioscintigraphy using the gamma camera,[53] and these techniques are now being applied in larger clinical series.[54]

Management

Medical

The goal of medical treatment of megacolon or megarectum is to empty the bowel of stool and keep it empty. Disimpaction (even manually under anesthesia) is indicated to render the large intestine clean. The patient is placed on a strict program of bowel habit retraining, not unlike that prescribed for patients with spinal cord injury. Bulking agents and large volumes of water assist in daily defecation. The simplest laxatives are used first, and saline cathartics are nearly always required. In addition, sodium docusate or a similar wetting agent often helps. Preparations that contain senna, cascara, bisacodyl, and other "stimulant" laxatives should be avoided. Patients are encouraged to try to pass stool at the same time every day, usually after meals. Sometimes irritation of the rectum by glycerine suppositories or a small tap water enema prompts defecation. Central to the goal of retraining the bowel is providing enough residue to produce stools of sufficient bulk and appropriate consistency to stimulate the desire to evacuate, which should be centered around mealtimes, to take advantage of the gastrocolic reflex (see Chapter 86).

The final goal of treatment is to reduce the strictness of the program. Although this is rarely achieved, most patients with megabowel can be treated effectively according to the general guidelines described earlier. Of central importance to the success of medical treatment is the patient's desire to be relieved of symptoms and to gain understanding of and adhere to the guidelines.

Surgical

For patients in whom medical management fails, surgery is a viable option. The most important question is, which operation is best. It is crucial that patients be categorized accurately because surgical options are driven by the diagnostic categories. For example, for patients with megabowel and slow colonic transit, ileostomy or ileoanal anastomosis can be considered, depending on the patient's age, life-style, and body habitus.[55, 56] In general, ileorectal anastomosis needs to be considered carefully in this setting because some patients continue to be constipated, especially if disorders of pelvic floor function ("obstructed defecation" or dyschezia) have not been excluded (see Chapter 12).[52] After ileoanal anastomosis patients have an excellent functional response, and their pattern of stooling is frequently controlled.[56] Ileostomy is also a good operation for older patients, who often are restored rapidly to excellent health.[57]

For patients with megacolon, a normal-sized rectum, and a normal mechanism of defecation, as determined by the tests of pelvic floor function,[52] ileorectostomy is the operation of choice even in older people.[45] These patients usually establish a relatively normal bowel habit. Patients with megarectum, a normal-sized colon, and a defecation abnormality are candidates for the Duhamel operation (see Fig. 110–6) or perhaps a coloanal anastomosis. The enlarged rectum is resected in its entirety; fecaliths in the rectal remnant, which are so common in patients after a Duhamel operation, are avoided.

Various operative procedures have been proposed for the chagasic colon (Chagas' disease), from sigmoidectomy to subtotal colectomy; however, longer follow-up has led most experts to conclude that leaving a diseased rectum in place often leads to unsatisfactory results. Abdominoperineal endoanal pull-through with variants on the Duhamel procedure are now preferred.[58]

ACUTE MEGACOLON

Acute megacolon occurs in patients with severe, fulminant inflammatory bowel disease or infectious colitis (see Chapters 96, 103, and 104) and in response to acute distal obstruction (e.g., volvulus; see Chapter 109). Acute megacolon also occurs in patients without obvious colonic disease or mechanical obstruction. In these instances, the pseudo-obstruction is localized to the colon (Ogilvie's syndrome).[59] The characteristic time course is an acute or subacute process that may be caused by trauma, orthopedic surgery, obstetric procedures, pelvic and abdominal surgery, metabolic imbalance (e.g., hypokalemia), or a neurologic condition.[60, 61]

Pathophysiology

The precise cause of acute colonic pseudo-obstruction is unknown; however, most patients have a coexisting problem such as recent trauma or surgery, and Ogilvie's syndrome is the clearest example of dilatation of the human colon in response to nonmechanical factors. This propensity of the colon to dilate has been explored experimentally,[7, 10, 17] and with similar techniques, the tone of the rectal wall also has been studied.[62] In these experiments, rectal tone decreased (the rectal wall relaxed) in response to glucagon and increased in response to neostigmine. This concept—that the wall of the colon and rectum is able to relax in response to physiologic and pharmacologic stimulus—is one that Ogilvie recognized in proposing autonomic imbalance of intrinsic control as a basis for the syndrome.[59] More recently, symptomatic relief has been obtained from adrenergic blockade followed by cholinergic stimulation[63, 64] or by neostigmine alone.[65]

Clinical Presentation

The typical patient is an older person who is often recovering quite uneventfully from orthopedic surgery performed a few days previously and who is already eating a regular diet. The abdomen becomes grossly distended, breathing becomes labored, but, early in the course, no peritoneal signs are present, and the white blood cell count is normal. An abdominal x-ray shows massive gaseous distention of the colon (Fig. 110–7). Usually, the small bowel is not seen. The cecal diameter at this point in the course is often 9 to 10 cm.

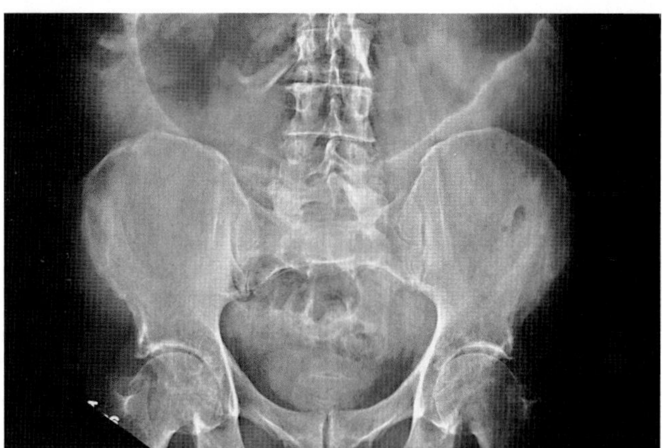

Figure 110–7. Plain abdominal radiograph of a patient with idiopathic megacolon shows enormous dilatation of the transverse colon.

Initial Management

Oral feedings should be withheld, parenteral fluids started, and a nasogastric tube passed. A Hypaque (water-soluble contrast) enema is administered to exclude mechanical obstruction and confirm pseudo-obstruction. As an added benefit, the hyperosmolar Hypaque usually evacuates the colon. Once confirmed, acute colonic pseudo-obstruction is treated aggressively with a rectal decompression tube and enemas. Any associated metabolic or electrolyte abnormalities (e.g., hypokalemia) should be corrected, but such abnormalities are not usually prominent. If the patient responds incompletely, treatment with cisapride (which is no longer available in the United States),[66] erythromycin,[67] or neostigmine[64, 65] has been reported to help. Indeed, Pronec and associates[64] reported on the results of a prospective randomized study of neostigmine compared with placebo and found an immediate response rate of 91% in the patients treated with neostigmine and a 0% response rate in those treated with placebo. There is little question that many patients will respond to simple medical treatment alone,[68] but neostigmine appears to be a powerful new tool in the management of acute pseudo-obstruction. Our recommended protocol for the use of neostigmine, which is successful in the majority of patients, is 2.5 mg intravenously given over 1 to 3 minutes. The patient should be on electrocardiographic monitor, and atropine should be available. Treatment is successful in 2 to 20 minutes. The regimen may be repeated up to three consecutive times until success is achieved.

Subsequent Management

There are few patients who do not respond to enemas, nasogastric decompression, and drug therapy. For those patients who do not respond but continue to have a normal white blood cell count and no fever or peritoneal signs, the next step is colonoscopic decompression if the cecum measures greater than 11 cm.[69–71] The Hypaque enema given previously often empties the colon, facilitating endoscopy.[72] Gas and liquid stool are aspirated continuously while little additional air (or carbon dioxide) is insufflated. Mucosal detail is often obscured, but an obstructing lesion can be seen easily. It is not necessary to reach the cecum to accomplish adequate decompression; positioning the endoscope at the hepatic flexure with aspiration of proximal contents usually collapses the right colon. A decompression tube can be left behind,[73] but its efficacy is controversial. An abdominal film is then obtained; if a collapsed cecum can be documented, the patient can be kept on enemas until stool and flatus pass spontaneously. Although colonoscopic decompression is commonly repeated, more than 80% of patients respond to the treatment[69–71] and require no further management. As many as 20%, however, require operation because of cecal dilatation refractory to colonoscopic decompression.

An operation is advisable for patients with a cecal diameter greater than 11 or 12 cm and intractability to medical and endoscopic management. The most useful and efficacious approach is tube cecostomy, either by conventional open, percutaneous, or, more recently, laparoscopic techniques.[74] Moreover, if at any time a patient manifests fever, leukocytosis, or peritoneal signs, abdominal exploration is mandatory. In these situations, the right colon is frequently nonviable or has perforated. For perforation, combined right hemicolectomy, ileostomy, and mucous fistula is the operation of choice. In patients with nonviable bowel but without perforation, right hemicolectomy and primary anastomosis can be performed with little risk of serious complications.

Acknowledgement

The authors and editors are grateful to Sidney F. Phillips, MD, our mentor, for his valuable contributions to this and previous versions of this chapter.

REFERENCES

1. Preston DM, Lennard-Jones JE, Thomas BM: Towards a radiologic definition of idiopathic megacolon. Gastrointest Radiol 10:167, 1985.
2. Kaplan P, de Chaderevian JP: Piebaldism-Waardenburg syndrome: Histopathologic evidence for a neural crest syndrome. Am J Med Genet 31:679, 1988.
3. Doig CM: Hirschsprung's disease and mimicking conditions. Dig Dis Sci 12:106, 1994.
4. de Almeida MAC, Barbosa HS: Congenital Chagas megacolon. Report of a case. Rev Soc Bras Med Trop 19:167, 1986.
5. Holbert RD, Magiris E, Hirsch CP, Nunenmacher SJ: Chagas' disease: A case in south Mississippi. J Miss State Med Assoc 36:1, 1995.
6. Gershon MD: Lessons from genetically engineered animal models. II. Disorders of enteric neuronal development: Insights from transgenic mice. Am J Physiol 277:G262, 1999.
7. Basilisco G, Phillips SF: Ileal distention relaxes the canine colon: A model of megacolon? Gastroenterology 106:606, 1994.
8. Basilova TI, Vorob'ev GI, Nasyrina TA: Changes in the intramural nervous system in idiopathic megacolon in adults. Arkh Patol 57:28, 1995.
9. Fernandez A, Hontebeyrie M, Said G: Autonomic neuropathy and immunological abnormalities in Chagas' disease. Clin Auton Res 2:409, 1992.
10. Kamath PS, Phillips SF, O'Connor MK, et al: Colonic capacitance and transit in man: Modulation by luminal contents and drugs. Gut 31:443, 1990.
11. Wood JD, Brann LR, Vermillion DL: Electrical and contractile behavior of large intestinal musculature of piebald mouse model for Hirschsprung's disease. Dig Dis Sci 31:638, 1986.
12. Hillemeier C, Biancani P: Mechanical properties of obstructed muscle in Hirschsprung's model. Gastroenterology 99:995, 1990.
13. Steadman CJ, Phillips SF, Camilleri M, et al: Variation of muscle tone in the human colon. Gastroenterology 101:373, 1991.
14. Bealer JF, Natuzzi ES, Buscher C, et al: Nitric oxide synthase is deficient in the aganglionic colon of patients with Hirschsprung's disease. Pediatrics 93:647, 1994.
15. Tam PKH: An immunochemical study with neuro-specific-enolase and substance P of human enteric innervation. The normal developmental pattern and abnormal deviations in Hirschsprung's disease and pyloric stenosis. J Pediatr Surg 21:227, 1986.
16. Holschneider AM, Meier-Ruge W, Ure BM: Hirschsprung's disease and allied disorders: A review. Eur J Pediatr Surg 4:260, 1994.
17. Hosoda K, Hammer RE, Richardson RE, et al: Targeted and natural (piebald-lethal) mutations of entotherlin-B receptor gene produce megacolon associated with spotted coat color in mice. Cell 79:1267, 1994.
18. Huizenga JD, Tomlinson J, Pintin-Quezada J: Involvement of nitric oxide in nerve-mediated inhibition and action of vasoactive intestinal peptide in colonic smooth muscle. J Pharmacol Exp Ther 260:803, 1992.
19. Vanderwinden JM, De Laet MH, Schiffmann SN, et al: Nitric oxide synthase distribution in the enteric nervous system of Hirschsprung's disease. Gastroenterology 105:969, 1993.
20. O'Kelly TJ, Davies JR, Tam PK, et al: Abnormalities of nitric-oxide–producing neurons in Hirschsprung's disease: Morphology and implications. J Pediatr Surg 29:294, 1994.
21. Larsson LT, Sundler F: Neuronal markers in Hirschsprung's disease with special reference to neuropeptides. Acta Histochem Suppl 38:115, 1990.
22. Gelfond M, Rozen P, Gilat T: Isosorbide dinitrate and nifedipine treatment of achalasia: A clinical, manometric and radionuclide evaluation. Gastroenterology 83:963, 1992.
23. Tobon F, Rein NCRW, Talbert JL, Schuster MM: Nonsurgical test for the diagnosis of Hirschsprung's disease. N Engl J Med 278:188, 1968.
24. Davidson M, Sleisenger MH, Steinberg H, Almy TP: Studies of distal colonic motility in children. III. The pathologic physiology of congenital megacolon (Hirschsprung's disease). Gastroenterology 29:803, 1955.
25. Arhan P, Devroede GJ, Danis K, et al: Viscoelastic properties of the rectal wall in Hirschsprung's disease. J Clin Invest 62:82, 1978.
26. Okamotao E, Ueda T: Embryogenesis of intramural ganglia of the gut and its relation to Hirschsprung's disease. J Pediatr Surg 2:437, 1967.
27. Passarge E: The genetics of Hirschsprung's disease. Evidence for heterogeneous etiology and a study of sixty-three families. N Engl J Med 276:138, 1967.
28. Hofstra RMW, Lanesvater RM, Ceccherini I, et al: A mutation in the RET proto-oncogene associated with multiple endocrine neoplasia type 2B and sporadic medullary thyroid carcinoma. Nature 367:375, 1994.
29. Edery P, Lyonnet S, Mulligan LM, et al: Mutations on the RET procto-oncogene in Hirschsprung's disease. Nature 367:378, 1994.
30. Loening-Bauke V: Functional constipation. Semin Pediatr Surg 4:26, 1995.
31. Ryan DP: Neuronal intestinal dysplasia. Semin Pediatr Surg 4:22, 1995.
32. Romeo G, Ronchetto P, Luo Y, et al: Point mutations affecting the tyrosine kinase domain of the RET proto-oncogene in Hirschsprung's disease. Nature 367:377, 1994.
33. Wartiovaara K, Salo M, Sariola H: Hirschsprung's disease genes and the development of the enteric nervous system. Ann Med 30:66, 1998.
34. Ikawa H, Kim SH, Hendren WH, Donahoe PK: Acetyl cholinesterase and manometry in the diagnosis of the constipated child. Arch Surg 121:435, 1986.
35. Vinores SA, May E: Neuron-specific enolase as an immunohistochemical tool for the diagnosis of Hirschsprung's disease. Am J Surg Pathol 9:281, 1985.
36. Morikawa Y, Donahoe PK, Hendren WH: Manometry and histochemistry in the diagnosis of Hirschsprung's disease. Pediatrics 63:865, 1979.
37. Vermesh J, Mayden KL, Confino E, et al: Prenatal sonographic diagnosis of Hirschsprung's disease. J Ultrasound Med 5:37, 1986.
38. Marty TL, Leo T, Matlak ME, et al: Gastrointestinal function after surgical correction of Hirschsprung's disease: Long-term follow-up in 135 patients. J Pediatr Surg 30:655, 1995.

39. Neilson IR, Yazbeck S: Ultrashort Hirschsprung's disease: Myth or reality. J Pediatr Surg 25:1135, 1990.
40. McMahon RA, Moore CCM, Cussen LJ: Hirschsprung's-like syndromes in patients with normal ganglion cells on suction rectal biopsy. J Pediatr Surg 16:835, 1981.
41. Nixon HH, Lake B: "Not Hirschsprung's disease"—rare conditions with some similarities. S Afr J Surg 29:97, 1982.
42. Barnes PRH, Lennard-Jones JE, Hawley PR, Todd IP: Hirschsprung's disease and idiopathic megacolon in adults and adolescents. Gut 27: 534, 1986.
43. Krishnamurthy S, Heng Y, Schuffler MD: Chronic intestinal pseudo-obstruction in infants and children caused by diverse abnormalities of the myenteric plexus. Gastroenterology 104:1398, 1993.
44. Verduron A, Devroede G, Bouchoucha M, et al: Megarectum. Dig Dis Sci 33:1164, 1988.
45. Stabile G, Kamm MA, Hawley PR, Lennard-Jones JE: Colectomy for idiopathic megarectum and megacolon. Gut 32:1538, 1991.
46. Camilleri M, Phillips SF: Acute and chronic intestinal pseudo-obstruction. In Strollerman GH, LaMonth JT, Lenard JJ, Siperstein MD (eds): Advances in Internal Medicine, vol 36. Chicago, Year Book Medical Publishers, 1990, p 287.
47. Pinkerton P: Psychogenic megacolon in childhood: The implication of bowel negativism. Arch Dis Child 33:371, 1958.
48. Nixon HH: Megarectum in the older child. Proc R Soc Med 60:3, 1967.
49. Porter HH: Megacolon: A physiological study. Proc R Soc Med 54: 1043, 1961.
50. Lane RHS, Todd IP: Idiopathic megacolon: A review of 42 cases. Br J Surg 64:305, 1977.
51. Metcalf AM, Phillips SF, Zinsmeister AR, et al: A simplified assessment of segmental colonic transit. Gastroenterology 92:40, 1987.
52. Pemberton JH, Rath DM, Ilstrup DM: Evaluation and surgical treatment of severe chronic constipation. Ann Surg 214:403, 1991.
53. Stivaland T, Camilleri M, Vassallo M, et al: Scintigraphic measurement of regional gut transit in severe idiopathic constipation. Gastroenterology 101:107, 1991.
54. Charles F, Camilleri M, Phillips SF, et al: Scintigraphy of the whole gut: Clinical evaluation of transit disorders. Mayo Clin Proc 70:113, 1995.
55. Nicholls RJ, Kamm MA: Proctocolectomy with restorative ileoanal reservoir for severe idiopathic constipation. Report of two cases. Dis Colon Rectum 31:968, 1988.
56. Hosie KB, Kmiott WA, Keighley MR: Constipation: Another indication for restorative proctocolectomy. Br J Surg 77:801, 1990.
57. Stryker SJ, Pemberton JH, Zinsmeister AR: Long-term results of ileostomy in older patients. Dis Colon Rectum 28:844, 1985.
58. Cutait DE, Cutait R: Surgery of chagasic megacolon. World J Surg 15: 188, 1991.
59. Ogilvie H: Large intestinal colic due to sympathetic deprivation: A new clinical syndrome. Br Med J 2:671, 1948.
60. Vanek VW, Al-Salti M: Acute pseudoobstruction of the colon (Ogilvie's syndrome): An analysis of 400 cases. Dis Colon Rectum 29:203, 1986.
61. Dorudi S, Berry AR, Rettlewell MG: Acute colonic pseudoobstruction. Br J Surg 79:99, 1992.
62. Bell AM, Pemberton JH, Hanson RB, Zinsmeister AR: Variations in muscle tone of the human rectum: Recordings with an electromechanical barostat. Am J Physiol 260:G17, 1991.
63. Hutchinson R, Griffiths C: Acute colonic pseudo-obstruction: A pharmacological approach. Ann R Coll Surg Engl 74:364, 1992.
64. Pronec RJ, Saunders MD, Kimmey MB: Neostigmine for the treatment of acute colonic pseudo-obstruction. N Engl J Med 341:137, 1999.
65. Stephenson BM, Morgan AR, Salaman JR, Wheeler MH: Ogilvie's syndrome: A new approach to an old problem. Dis Colon Rectum 38: 424, 1995.
66. MacColl C, MacConnell KL, Baylis B, Lee SS: Treatment of acute colonic pseudoobstruction (Ogilvie's syndrome) with cisapride. Gastroenterology 98:773, 1990.
67. Armstrong DN, Ballantyne GH, Modlin IM: Erythromycin for reflex ileus in Ogilvie's syndrome. Lancet 337:378, 1991.
68. Sloyer AF, Panella VS, Demas BE, et al: Ogilvie's syndrome. Successful management without colonoscopy. Dig Dis Sci 33:1391, 1988.
69. Bode WE, Beart RW Jr, Spencer RJ, et al: Colonoscopic decompression for acute pseudo-obstruction of the colon (Ogilvie's syndrome). Report of 22 cases and review of the literature. Am J Surg 147:243, 1984.
70. Strodel WE, Brothers T: Colonoscopic decompression of pseudo-obstruction and volvulus. Surg Clin North Am 69:1327, 1989.
71. Jetmore AB, Timmcke AE, Gathright JB Jr, et al: Ogilvie's syndrome: Colonoscopic decompression and analysis of predisposing factors. Dis Colon Rectum 35:1135, 1992.
72. Chapman AH, McNamara M, Porter G: The acute contrast enema in suspected large bowel obstruction: Volumes and techniques. Clin Radiol 46:273, 1992.
73. Stephenson KR, Rodriguez-Bigas MA: Decompression of the large intestine in Ogilvie's syndrome by a colonoscopically placed long intestinal tube. Surg Endosc 8:116, 1994.
74. Duh QY, Way LW: Diagnostic laparoscopy and laparoscopic cecostomy for colonic pseudo-obstruction. Dis Colon Rectum 36:65, 1993.

Chapter 111

CHRONIC INTESTINAL PSEUDO-OBSTRUCTION

Michael D. Schuffler

Chronic intestinal pseudo-obstruction is a clinical syndrome caused by ineffective intestinal propulsion and characterized by symptoms and signs of intestinal obstruction in the absence of an occluding lesion of the intestinal lumen.[1] It is caused by a large number of disorders of the smooth muscle, myenteric plexus, or extraintestinal nervous system.[2] The criteria for the diagnosis should include definite symptoms and signs of obstruction, with documentation of an ileus or air-fluid levels on plain radiographs of the abdomen, or a dilated duodenum, small intestine, or colon on barium radiographs. Even though severe dysmotility may otherwise be present, the term *pseudo-obstruction* should not be used when such radiographic findings are absent.

Chronic intestinal pseudo-obstruction may be secondary to systemic illnesses such as progressive systemic sclerosis, or it may be primary. *Chronic idiopathic intestinal pseudo-obstruction* (CIIP) is a term that has been often used to denote the primary syndrome. It is now recognized as a heterogeneous syndrome that has multiple causes.[2]

Chronic intestinal pseudo-obstruction is often associated with structural changes in the gut wall that result in marked enlargement anywhere along the gastrointestinal tract, as in *megaesophagus, megaduodenum, megajejunum,* and *megacolon.*[3, 4] Megacolon is discussed in Chapter 110. Patients with megaduodenum are sometimes misdiagnosed as having the "superior mesenteric artery syndrome."[3] In fact, patients with megaduodenum usually have a primary structural problem of the duodenal wall that causes the duodenum to enlarge. As the duodenum enlarges, the superior mesenteric artery holds down the third part of the duodenum, producing a picture of apparent, but not real, obstruction.

Another structural change is *jejunal diverticulosis* or *small intestinal diverticulosis.*[2] These multiple diverticula result from one of several types of disorders of the smooth muscle or myenteric plexus. Patients may present with symptoms of pseudo-obstruction, the stagnant loop syndrome, small intestinal diverticulitis, perforation, or hemorrhage.

Chronic intestinal pseudo-obstruction should not be confused with a related motility disorder—severe idiopathic constipation. In this syndrome, the radiographic findings of chronic intestinal pseudo-obstruction and megacolon are absent. Severe idiopathic constipation is discussed in Chapter 12.

CAUSES AND PATHOLOGY

A classification of chronic intestinal pseudo-obstruction is shown in Table 111–1. *Visceral myopathies* constitute a group of diseases characterized by degeneration and fibrosis of the muscularis propria.[5, 6] The smooth muscles of the bladder, uterus, and iris of the eyes may also be involved.[7, 8] Visceral myopathies occur at any age, including infancy, and either are transmitted genetically or occur sporadically. The *familial* visceral myopathies are transmitted as autosomal dominant or recessive traits.[7–9]

A variety of other forms of visceral myopathy exist, including the mitochondrial neurogastrointestinal encephalopathy (MNGIE) syndrome, characterized by pseudo-obstruction, peripheral neuropathy, myopathy, and ophthalmoplegia associated with mitochondrial abnormalities in smooth muscle and neurons.[10] Others are characterized by inclusions consisting of degenerating myofibrils within smooth muscle[11] and absence of smooth muscle actin.[12]

Systemic disorders involving the smooth muscle are also characterized by fibrosis and muscle atrophy. This is typical of *progressive systemic sclerosis*[6] and *progressive muscular dystrophy.*[2] *Amyloidosis* is most often characterized by deposition of amyloid within the smooth muscle.[13] Additional types of muscle disorders are characterized by *diffuse lymphoid infiltration* of the smooth muscles.[14]

Visceral neuropathies encompass a number of degenerative disorders of the myenteric plexus and, occasionally, the submucosal plexus.[2] The pathology of these disorders is best identified by using the silver technique of Barbara Smith.[15] Familial and sporadic forms of visceral neuropathies are characterized by a variety of degenerative changes of neurons, axons, and dendrites. These changes are occasionally accompanied by inflammatory cells in the myenteric plexus. One type of inflammatory visceral neuropathy, *paraneoplas-*

Table 111–1 | **Clinicopathologic Classification of Chronic Intestinal Pseudo-Obstruction**

I. Disorders of the smooth muscle
  A. Primary
    1. Familial visceral myopathies
      a. Type I (autosomal dominant)
      b. Type II (autosomal recessive, with ptosis and external ophthalmoplegia)
      c. Type III (autosomal recessive, with total gastrointestinal tract dilatation)
    2. Sporadic visceral myopathy
    3. Congenital, in infants
  B. Secondary
    1. Progressive systemic sclerosis/polymyositis
    2. Muscular dystrophy syndromes
    3. Systemic lupus erythematosus
    4. Amyloidosis
    5. Radiation injury
    6. Ehlers-Danlos syndrome
    7. Mitochondrial myopathy
  C. Diffuse lymphoid infiltration
  D. Others (muscle cell inclusions; absence of actin)
II. Disorders of the myenteric plexus
  A. Familial visceral neuropathies
    1. Recessive, with intranuclear inclusions (neuronal intranuclear inclusion disease)
    2. Recessive (familial steatorrhea with calcification of the basal ganglia and mental retardation)
    3. Dominant, with neither of the above
    4. POLIP syndrome (*P*olyneuropathy, *O*phthalmoplegia, *L*euko-encephalopathy, *I*ntestinal *P*seudo-obstruction)
    5. Infantile short bowel, malrotation, and pyloric hypertrophy
    6. With progressive neurologic disease at young age
  B. Sporadic visceral neuropathies
    1. Degenerative, noninflammatory (at least two types)
    2. Degenerative, inflammatory (with lymphocytes and/or plasma cells in the myenteric and, sometimes, submucosal plexus)
      a. Paraneoplastic
      b. Infectious (Chagas' disease, cytomegalovirus)
      c. Idiopathic
      d. Isolated axonopathy
  C. Developmental abnormalities
    1. Total colonic aganglionosis (sometimes with small intestinal aganglionosis)
    2. Maturational arrest
      a. Isolated to myenteric plexus
      b. With mental retardation
      c. With other neurologic abnormalities
    3. Neuronal intestinal dysplasia
      a. Isolated to intestine
      b. With neurofibromatosis
      c. With multiple endocrine neoplasia, Type IIb
  D. Myotonic dystrophy
III. Neurologic disorders
  A. Parkinson's disease
  B. Autonomic dysfunction, familial and sporadic
  C. Total autonomic or selective cholinergic dysfunction after Epstein-Barr viral infection
  D. Brainstem tumor
IV. Small intestinal diverticulosis
  A. With muscle resembling visceral myopathy
  B. With muscle resembling progressive systemic sclerosis
  C. With visceral neuropathy and neuronal intranuclear inclusions
  D. Secondary to Fabry's disease
V. Endocrine and metabolic disorders
  A. Myxedema
  B. Pheochromocytoma
  C. Hypoparathyroidism
  D. Acute intermittent porphyria
VI. Drugs
  A. Opiates (narcotic bowel syndrome)
  B. Anticholinergics
  C. Phenothiazines
  D. Clonidine
  E. Tricyclic antidepressants
  F. Vinca alkaloids, e.g., vincristine
  G. Calcium channel blockers
  H. Fetal alcohol syndrome
VII. Miscellaneous
  A. Jejunoileal bypass
  B. Sclerosing mesenteritis
  C. Celiac sprue
  D. Ceroidosis?

tic visceral neuropathy, is a complication of small cell carcinoma or carcinoid of the lung.[16] Another, Chagas' disease, is a late complication of infection with *Trypanosoma cruzi*.[2] Others are idiopathic. Amyloid can also infiltrate the myenteric plexus.

Developmental abnormalities of the myenteric plexus usually present in infancy or early childhood. The abnormalities range from aganglionosis of the entire colon and part of the small intestine to maturational arrest of the myenteric plexus, the latter varying from near absence of the plexus to a plexus that contains a deficient number of argyrophilic neurons.[2] Another developmental abnormality is *neuronal intestinal dysplasia*.[2]

Neurologic disorders can sometimes be complicated by chronic intestinal pseudo-obstruction,[17] as in Parkinson's disease, brain tumors, neuronal intranuclear inclusion disease (NIID),[18] and paraneoplastic visceral neuropathy.[16] All components of the enteric and extraintestinal nervous systems can be involved in the latter two syndromes, and the intranuclear inclusions of NIID are found within the central, peripheral, autonomic, and enteric nervous systems. Viral infections, such as those associated with cytomegalovirus and Epstein-Barr virus, can be followed by pseudo-obstruction,[19] and in rare patients, evidence of viral infection of the myenteric plexus has been found using polymerase chain reaction amplification and in situ staining.[20]

Small intestinal diverticulosis is often associated with abnormalities of the smooth muscle or myenteric plexus.[2] Atrophy and fibrosis of smooth muscle may produce weak areas that protrude as diverticula of the full intestinal wall. In other cases, an abnormal myenteric plexus leads to disordered muscle function and smooth muscle hypertrophy. Disordered muscle contractions produce protrusions of mucosa and submucosa through the weakest part of the intestinal wall, adjacent to penetrating blood vessels.

Other causes of intestinal pseudo-obstruction include the fetal alcohol syndrome,[21] endocrine disorders such as myxedema,[22] and drugs, particularly opiates. The latter can produce the "narcotic bowel syndrome," which is usually seen in patients who abuse opiates for chronic pain.[23] Although diabetes mellitus is a not infrequent cause of gastroparesis, severe constipation, esophageal dysmotility, diarrhea, and fecal incontinence, and is listed as a cause of pseudo-obstruction in many review articles, I have never personally diagnosed a case of pseudo-obstruction caused by diabetes.

Abnormal distribution of c-kit immunoreactive cells in an infant[24] and a deficiency of c-kit immunoreactive cells in adults with pseudo-obstruction have recently been reported.[25]

Because c-kit is a marker for the interstitial cells of Cajal and these cells are regarded as being the pacemaker cells of the intestine, it is possible, but unproved, that their absence may be important in the pathogenesis of pseudo-obstruction in some patients. At the very least, an abnormality of c-kit immunoreactivity could serve as a readily available histologic marker for confirming the diagnosis of a severe motility disorder.

CLINICAL MANIFESTATIONS

Intestinal pseudo-obstruction may present at any age.[3, 9, 26, 27] Developmental abnormalities almost always present in infancy or childhood, whereas degenerative disorders usually present later. Intestinal pseudo-obstruction secondary to progressive systemic sclerosis, amyloidosis, or small cell carcinoma of the lung presents at ages characteristic of these disorders. Visceral myopathy may occur at any age and may also involve the genitourinary tract; some patients present with genitourinary symptoms, megacystis, or megaloureters.[26, 27]

Patients have variable amounts of abdominal pain, distention, and vomiting. One type of pain is directly related to intestinal distention and improves or temporarily disappears if intestinal distention decreases. A second type is probably secondary to smooth muscle spasm or visceral hyperalgesia and is independent of intestinal distention. Abdominal distention varies from almost none to the equivalent of a 9-month pregnancy, depending on the nature and extent of the underlying pathology. Visceral myopathies and neuropathies both may produce enormous distention when the entire small intestine and colon are involved, whereas patients with visceral myopathy limited to the duodenum may have little distention. An audible succussion splash and loud borborygmi may be present. Pain and distention may be almost continuous or separated by periods of clinical improvement. The vomitus frequently consists of food ingested 12 or more hours previously and may be feculent.

In patients with predominant small intestinal involvement, bacterial overgrowth and the stagnant loop syndrome often develop and may lead to steatorrhea and diarrhea. Predominant colonic involvement usually results in constipation or megacolon, or both. Patients with both types of involvement may cycle from diarrhea to constipation, depending on the severity of steatorrhea and the relative involvement of each organ.

Many patients have involvement of the esophagus, which may be asymptomatic or may produce dysphagia, chest pain, regurgitation, reflux, and heartburn.[3] Visceral neuropathies may present with symptoms resembling achalasia or diffuse esophageal spasm.

Gastric involvement produces gastroparesis. The abdominal distention and pain produced by any combination of gastric, small intestine, and colonic involvement result in decreased food intake, weight loss, and malnutrition, especially when combined with malabsorption. Patients with involvement limited to the colon and distal small bowel may have relatively normal weights because their unaffected proximal bowel allows for normal absorption.

Physical examination findings may disclose cachexia and abdominal distention. Patients with small intestinal involvement usually have a succussion splash located in the midabdomen, whereas patients with gastric involvement may have a splash in the left upper quadrant. Hypertympany to percussion is usually present, and, occasionally, contracting bowel loops are observed pushing up against the abdominal wall. Bowel sounds are of no value in making a diagnosis of pseudo-obstruction. Evidence for central and peripheral nervous system disease should be sought, and autonomic nervous system testing should be done, when indicated. The coexistence of digital arches (ascertained by fingerprinting), mitral valve prolapse, and joint laxity may serve as a marker for the presence of chronic intestinal pseudo-obstruction in some patients, especially if constipation was present before age 10.[28]

LABORATORY FINDINGS

Laboratory abnormalities reflect the degree of malabsorption and malnutrition,[3] as well as the presence of underlying disorders. Thyroid function tests diagnose myxedema; antinuclear antibodies (SCL-70, anticentromere, and antitopoisomerase) and proliferating cell nuclear antigen suggest the presence of connective tissue disorders[29]; enteric neuronal autoantibodies may be present in the paraneoplastic visceral neuropathy of small cell carcinoma of the lung.[30]

Patients with diarrhea usually have steatorrhea due to small bowel bacterial overgrowth, and many of these patients also have vitamin B_{12} malabsorption. Evaluation of diarrhea or steatorrhea may lead to small intestinal biopsy, which can show mucosal damage.[2] The damage is often patchy, with some biopsies appearing normal or only mildly abnormal. On the other hand, mucosal damage may be se-

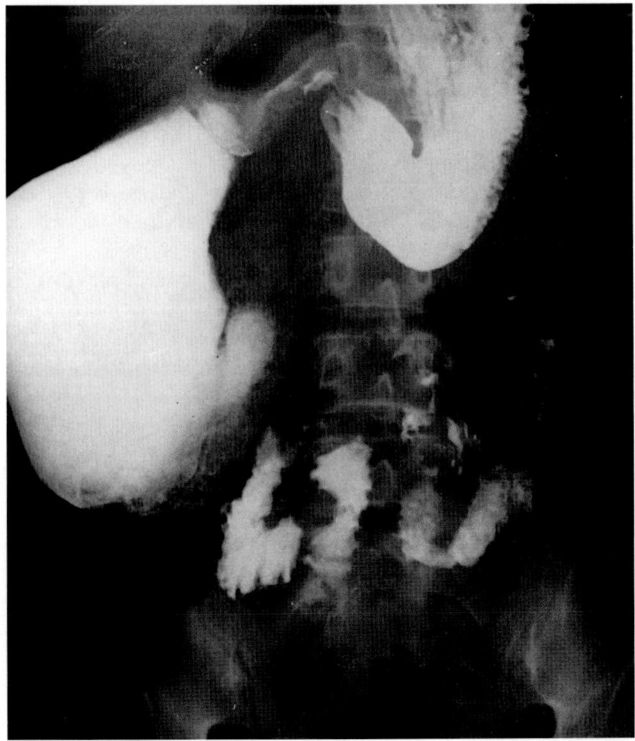

Figure 111–1. Megaduodenum in a patient with type I familial visceral myopathy. (From Schuffler M, Rohrmann CA Jr, Templeton FE: The radiologic manifestations of idiopathic intestinal pseudo-obstruction. Am J Roentgenol 127:734, 1976.)

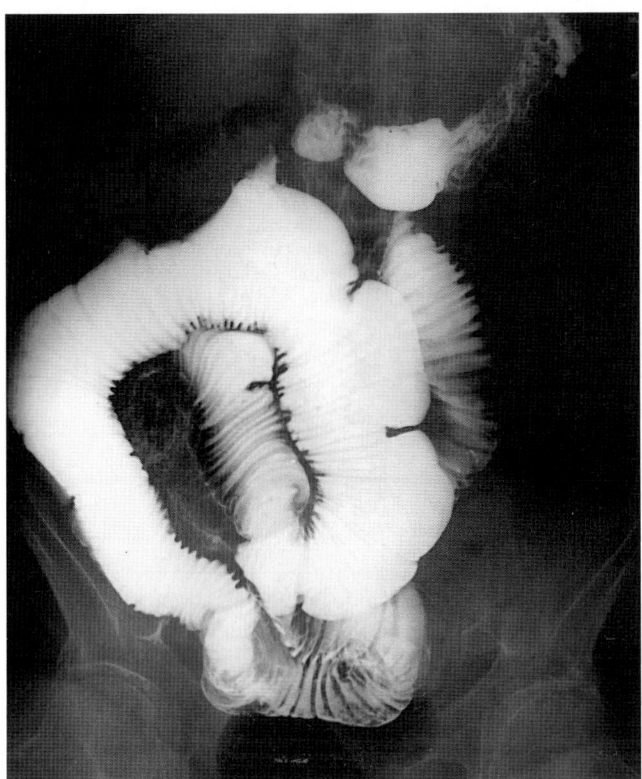

Figure 111–2. The jejunum in one patient with progressive systemic sclerosis showing packing and sacculation of the valvulae conniventes. (From Rohrmann CA Jr, Ricci MJ, Krishnamurthy S, Schuffler MD: Radiologic and histologic differentiation of neuromuscular disorders of the gastrointestinal tract. AJR Am J Roentgenol 143:939, 1984.)

vere enough to mimic celiac sprue. This finding may complicate the differential diagnosis because, rarely, celiac sprue may actually be complicated by pseudo-obstruction. Small bowel mucosal biopsy is of no value in diagnosing the pathologic basis of pseudo-obstruction because neither the muscularis propria nor the myenteric plexus is sampled.

RADIOGRAPHIC FINDINGS

Findings on plain abdominal films may resemble paralytic ileus or may mimic true mechanical obstruction.[4] In approximately 20% of patients, the films are normal, and abnormalities are apparent only on barium radiographs. Additional findings may include pneumatosis intestinalis and benign pneumoperitoneum.

Barium contrast studies of the entire gastrointestinal tract should be done whenever intestinal pseudo-obstruction is suspected. The identification of multiple sites of abnormality increases the likelihood of this diagnosis. Although pseudo-obstruction can be limited to the small intestine or colon, abnormalities isolated to the small intestine should raise the concern that there is a mechanical obstruction of the small intestine or ileocecal valve. The most important goal of the small bowel series is to exclude mechanical obstruction.

Many patients have an esophageal motor abnormality. Disorders of the esophageal smooth muscle produce hypocontractility, dilatation, and gastroesophageal reflux. Esophageal strictures are not uncommon in progressive systemic sclerosis. Visceral neuropathies may be characterized by uncoordinated hyperactive muscle contractions, and the detection of aperistalsis, esophageal dilatation, and delayed transit may mimic the radiographic findings in achalasia or diffuse esophageal spasm.

About one third of patients have a distended stomach and delayed gastric emptying. The duodenum is usually, but not invariably, abnormal. Megaduodenum is characteristic of the autosomal dominant form of visceral myopathy (Fig. 111–1).[5] Visceral myopathy may be limited to the duodenum or may involve up to all of the small intestine. Contractions are weak or absent, and there is markedly prolonged transit of barium. In progressive systemic sclerosis, the valvulae conniventes are often "packed," and there may be wide-mouthed sacculations (Fig. 111–2).

Visceral neuropathies are often characterized by only mild to moderate dilatation of the duodenum and small intestine, and there may be uncoordinated contractions and slow transit. On the other hand, some patients have enormous dilatation (Fig. 111–3). Diffuse small intestinal diverticulosis may be present in either visceral myopathies or neuropathies.

In visceral myopathy, the colon usually lacks haustrations and has an increased width and length. In visceral neuropathy, the colon is more likely to have fairly normal haustrations and length, but there can be extreme degrees of colonic dilatation and elongation. Both visceral myopathies and neuropathies can result in megacolon, and diffuse and extensive diverticular disease may occur in neuronal intranuclear inclusion disease.[18]

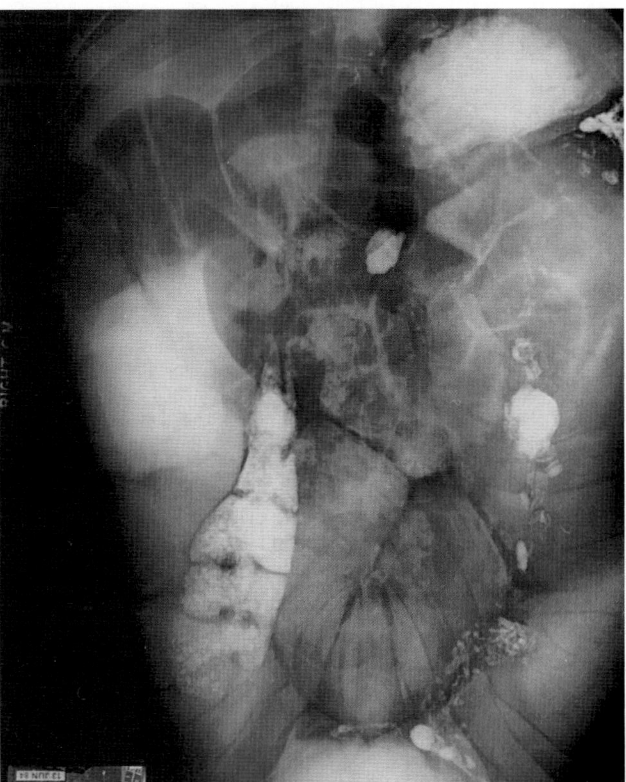

Figure 111–3. Small bowel radiograph in a patient with a degenerative visceral neuropathy showing diluted barium within massively dilated loops of jejunum. (From Schuffler MD, Leon SH, Krishnamurthy S: Intestinal pseudo-obstruction caused by a new form of visceral neuropathy: Palliation by radical small bowel resection. Gastroenterology 89:1153, 1985.)

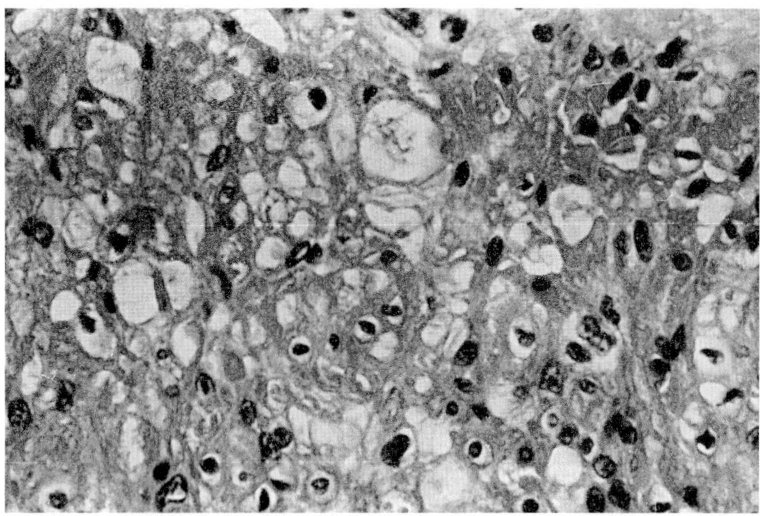

Figure 111–4. Circular muscle from a patient with familial visceral myopathy showing vacuolar degeneration and fibrosis. Masson's trichrome, ×1280.

MANOMETRIC ABNORMALITIES

Approximately 75% of patients with primary intestinal pseudo-obstruction have esophageal aperistalsis.[3] Patients with visceral myopathy tend to have simultaneous waves of low amplitude. Those with progressive systemic sclerosis have low-amplitude peristaltic waves or absent contractions, low to absent lower esophageal sphincter pressure, and gastroesophageal reflux. Visceral neuropathy may mimic achalasia or diffuse esophageal spasm.

Abnormalities of the migrating motor complex (MMC) occur in both visceral myopathies and neuropathies (see

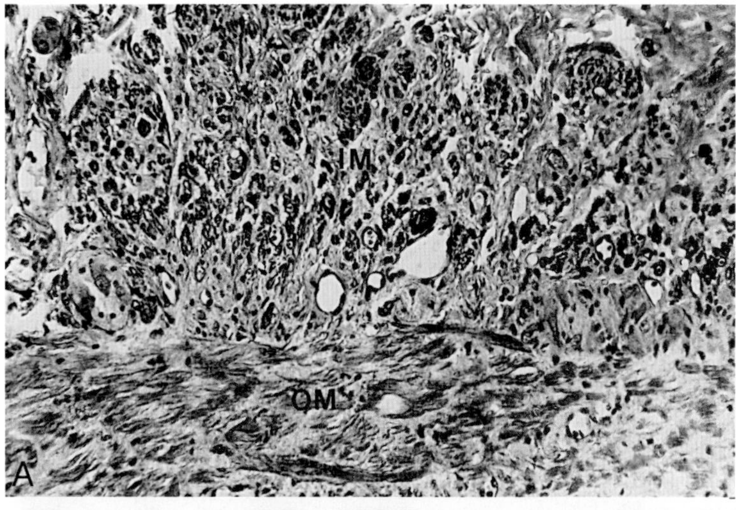

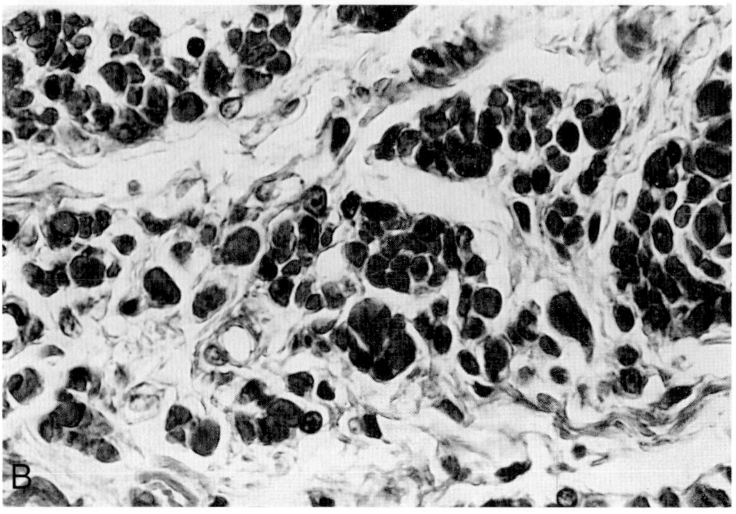

Figure 111–5. *A*, Small intestinal smooth muscle layers in a patient with progressive systemic sclerosis, showing extensive fibrosis. IM, inner circular muscle; OM, outer longitudinal muscle. Masson's trichrome, ×320. *B*, Smooth muscle at higher magnification, showing that residual muscle cells are normal in appearance. Masson's trichrome, ×1280. (From Schuffler MD, Beegle RG: Progressive systemic sclerosis of the gastrointestinal tract and hereditary hollow visceral myopathy. Gastroenterology 77:669, 1979.)

Chapter 85).[1] Gastroduodenal manometry is not invariably abnormal, however, because some patients lack involvement of the stomach and duodenum.[31] In *visceral myopathies*, the MMCs are either of low amplitude or, in severe disease, absent. In *visceral neuropathies*, the MMCs may be absent or associated with a variety of abnormalities, including (1) abnormal propagation or configuration of the MMCs; (2) uncoordinated bursts of phasic pressure activity; (3) sustained (>30 min) uncoordinated intestinal pressure activity; and (4) failure of a meal to induce a fed pattern or premature resumption of MMCs after a meal. Mechanical obstruction is associated with prolonged simultaneous contractions and repeated clustered contractions, especially after a test meal.[32] Although manometry does not always differentiate mechanical obstruction from pseudo-obstruction, the presence of such abnormal motility makes it mandatory to exclude mechanical obstruction. However, gastroduodenal manometry is still not widely available, and the diagnosis of pseudo-obstruction and the exclusion of mechanical obstruction must usually be made without it.

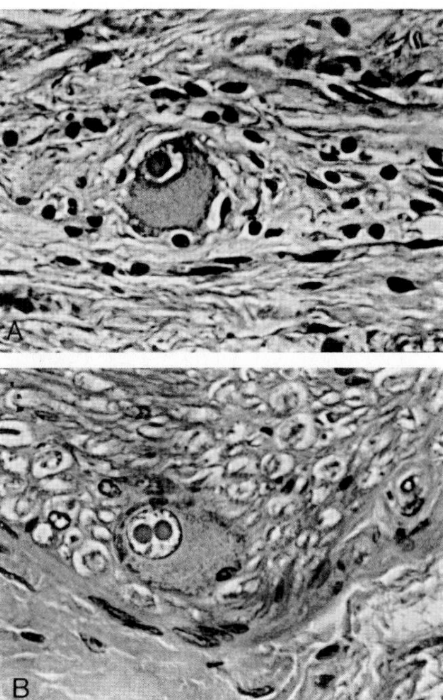

Figure 111–6. *A,* Single intranuclear inclusion within an enteric neuron of a patient with neuronal intranuclear inclusion disease. *B,* Two inclusions within an enteric neuron of the patient's sibling. H & E, ×460. (From Schuffler MD, Bird TD, Sumi SM, Cook A: A familial neuronal disease presenting as intestinal pseudo-obstruction. Gastroenterology 75:892, 1978.)

EXAMPLES OF SPECIFIC SYNDROMES

Familial Visceral Myopathies

At least three types of familial visceral myopathy have been distinguished genetically and by different patterns of involvement, both systemically and within the gastrointestinal and genitourinary tracts.[5, 7, 9] All three types are characterized by muscle cell degeneration, atrophy, and fibrosis of the muscularis propria without inflammatory cells (Fig. 111–4). The pathology usually, but not always, can be distinguished from that of progressive systemic sclerosis (Fig. 111–5).[6] Type I familial visceral myopathy is an autosomal dominant disorder characterized by esophageal dilatation, megaduodenum, a redundant or enlarged colon, and megacystis.[5] The stomach is not usually involved. Mydriasis may occur, and females can have uterine inertia. Type II familial visceral myopathy is an autosomal recessive disorder characterized by ptosis and external ophthalmoplegia, gastric dilatation, and mild dilatation and diverticulosis of the entire small intestine.[7] Type III familial visceral myopathy is probably an autosomal recessive disorder, with marked dilatation of the entire gastrointestinal tract.[9]

Visceral myopathy also exists as a sporadic disorder, and a congenital form, infantile visceral myopathy, may be fatal within the first 2 years of life.[27]

Familial Visceral Neuropathies

Familial visceral neuropathies encompass a number of syndromes with descriptive names (see Table 111–1). They differ with regard to inheritance, extraintestinal manifestations, and patterns of involvement within the gastrointestinal tract. The most frequently reported familial visceral neuropathy is neuronal intranuclear inclusion disease.[18] This disorder is transmitted as an autosomal recessive trait, and neurologic symptoms generally begin in childhood. Clinical findings may include mental deterioration, central and peripheral nerve abnormalities, autonomic dysfunction, and intestinal pseudo-obstruction. Neurons within both the myenteric and submucosal plexuses contain the intranuclear inclusions (Fig. 111–6), so that the diagnosis can be made by rectal biopsy into the submucosa.[33] Widespread neuronal degeneration and loss are noted throughout the myenteric plexus (Fig. 111–7).

In another form of familial visceral neuropathy, characterized by a short small bowel, malrotation, and pyloric hypertrophy, and associated with a deficiency of argyrophilic neurons in the myenteric plexus, genetic studies have shown an X-linked recessive inheritance pattern, and linkage analysis has localized the gene to chromosome Xq28.[34]

Sporadic Visceral Neuropathies

Sporadic visceral neuropathies include a number of disorders characterized by different types of neuron degeneration and loss, sometimes accompanied by glial cell proliferation and scars of the myenteric plexus (Fig. 111–8).[2] Smith's silver technique is necessary to make the diagnosis. In most cases of sporadic visceral neuropathy, the myenteric plexus does not contain inflammatory cells. However, one particular form, *paraneoplastic visceral neuropathy*, is characterized by an inflammatory destruction of the myenteric plexus (Fig. 111–9),[16] with striking degeneration and dropout of neurons. Symptoms of paraneoplastic visceral neuropathy often precede the diagnosis of cancer and may include intestinal pseudo-obstruction, constipation or obstipation, esophageal dysmotility, peripheral neuropathy, central nervous system dysfunction, autonomic insufficiency, and bladder dysfunction.

The diagnosis of small cell carcinoma can be extremely difficult, even when it is suspected. The presence of immunoglobulin G antibodies reactive to neurons of the submuco-

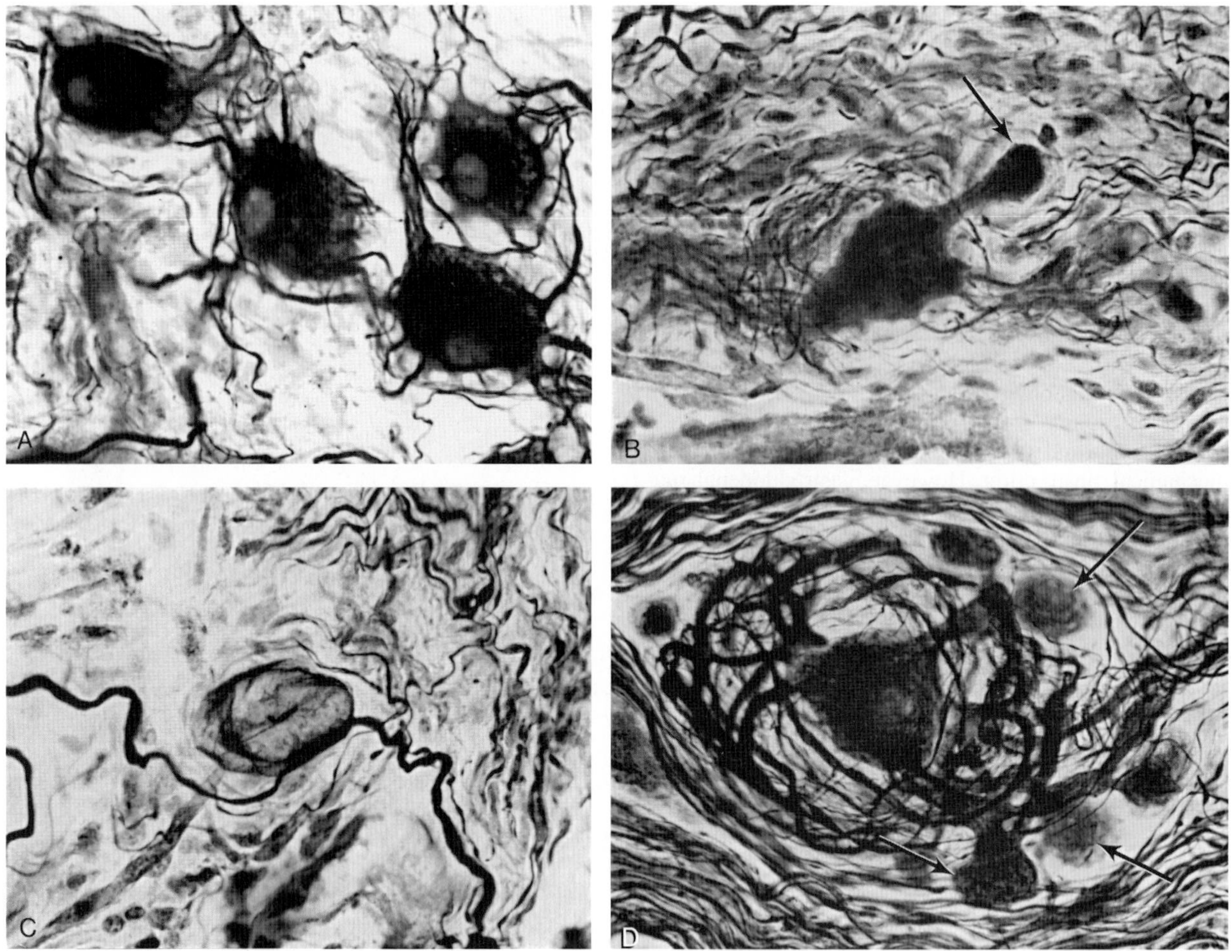

Figure 111–7. *A.* Four normal control esophageal neurons with multiple delicate processes. *B,* An abnormal esophageal neuron with clubbed dendrite *(arrow)* from a patient with neuronal intranuclear inclusion disease. *C,* Degenerated esophageal neuron. *D,* Abnormal esophageal neuron with multiple swollen dendrites *(arrows)* from same case. Silver, ×460. (From Schuffler MD, Bird TD, Sumi SM, Cook A: A familial neuronal disease presenting as intestinal pseudo-obstruction. Gastroenterology 75:894, 1978.)

sal and myenteric plexus (enteric neuronal autoantibodies) suggests that an autoimmune process is responsible for the neuropathy.[30]

Inflammatory visceral neuropathy can also be a consequence of infections. The most common is Chagas' disease.[2] *Cytomegalovirus,* a rare cause of pseudo-obstruction, produces an inflammatory neuropathy with typical viral inclusions within neurons.[2] Rarely, *infectious mononucleosis* is followed by dysautonomia and pseudo-obstruction.[19]

Developmental Disorders of the Myenteric Plexus

Intestinal pseudo-obstruction in infants and children usually results from abnormal development of the enteric nervous system. The most extreme form is absence of the plexuses, or "aganglionosis."[2] It is possible for the development of the myenteric plexus to halt at any stage. In the most common developmental arrest, normal numbers of neurons are present on hematoxylin and eosin (H & E) stains, but they are qualitatively abnormal based on the lack of argyrophilia on silver stains.[35] The lack of neuronal argyrophilia is related to a deficiency of neurofilaments.

Pseudo-Obstruction Associated with Neurologic Disorders

A wide variety of neurologic diseases may result in intestinal pseudo-obstruction because of involvement of the extrinsic nerve supply, the enteric nervous system, or both.[17] Pseudo-obstruction may be associated with Parkinson's disease, myotonic dystrophy, brainstem lesions, such as medullary astrocytoma, and acute encephalitis.

DIAGNOSIS

The diagnosis of intestinal pseudo-obstruction is made through a combination of history-taking, physical examination, laboratory tests, radiology, and esophageal and small intestinal manometry (Table 111–2). A positive family history will be elicited in about 30% of patients, and a number of patients will have had previous laparotomies, at which no

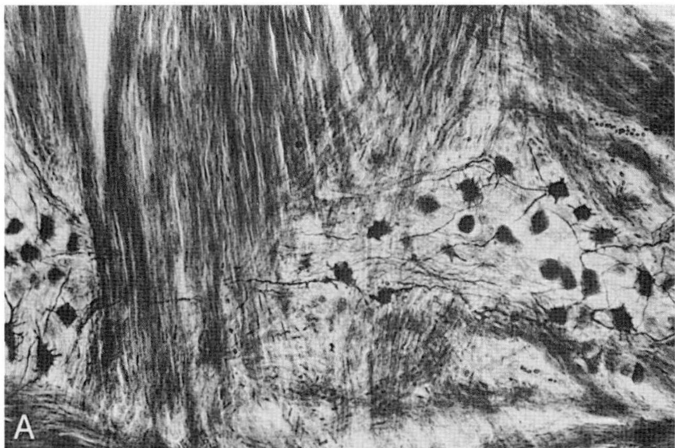

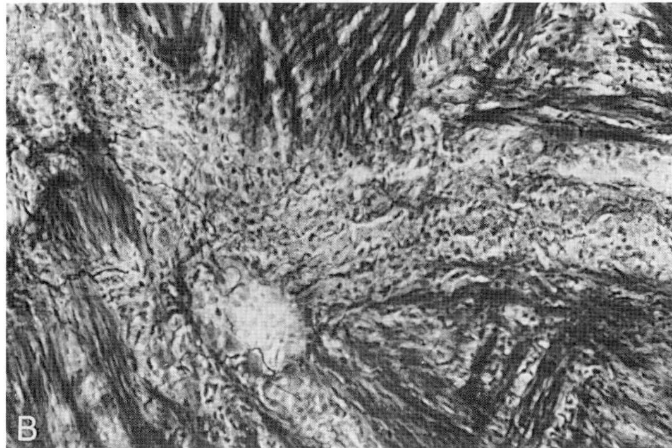

Figure 111–8. *A,* Control colonic myenteric plexus showing numerous neurons and nerve fibers. *B,* Colonic myenteric plexus from a patient with sporadic visceral neuropathy showing replacement by a glial cell scar, denoted by the multiple small nuclei. Silver, ×340. (From Schuffler MD, Jonak Z: Chronic idiopathic intestinal pseudo-obstruction caused by a degenerative disorder of the myenteric plexus. Gastroenterology 82:484, 1982.)

Table 111–2 | **Diagnostic Approach***

History

Months to years of symptoms consistent with partial intestinal obstruction; diarrhea, steatorrhea, constipation; weight loss; previous laparotomies with distended intestine but no obstructing lesions. Positive family history

Physical Examination

Signs of weight loss

Abdominal distention, hypertympany, succussion splash, visible bowel loops, loud borborygmi, palpable bladder; positive neurologic findings (central, peripheral, and autonomic); signs of systemic diseases (e.g., progressive sclerosis, amyloidosis, myxedema, etc.)

Imaging

(To exclude mechanical obstruction and to look for findings of pseudo-obstruction)

Plain x-rays of the abdomen

Barium contrast studies of esophagus, stomach, small intestine, and colon; enteroclysis; intravenous pyelography, voiding cystogram, or ultrasonography of urinary system; esophagogastroduodenoscopy

Functional Studies

(To document impaired transit and abnormal contractility)

Radionuclide gastric emptying and small bowel transit studies; esophageal manometry; gastroduodenal manometry; cystometrogram

Laboratory and Other Imaging Tests

(To evaluate for underlying causes)

Thyroid functions and thyroid-stimulating hormone

Antinuclear antibody and SCL-70 antibody; serum enteric antineuronal antibody; urinary porphobilinogen and porphyrins; serum porphobilinogen deaminase; serum creatine phosphokinase and aldolase; serologic tests for Chagas' disease; chest film and computed tomography of chest

Other Tests

(To evaluate for underlying causes)

Autonomic function tests

Electromyogram and nerve conduction velocity

Striated muscle biopsy

Magnetic resonance imaging of brain

Diagnostic laparoscopy or laparotomy, with full-thickness biopsy or resection, using hematoxylin and eosin, Masson's trichrome, Smith's silver technique, and immunohistochemistry for c-kit-positive cells

*Although many diagnostic tests are listed, note that relatively few are needed in any one patient. Tests should be selected on the basis of clinical judgment; for example, tests for porphyria should be done only when porphyria is suspected; autonomic function tests when patients have symptoms or signs of autonomic insufficiency; and nerve conduction velocities when peripheral nerve dysfunction is suspected. Diagnostic laparotomy is indicated whenever the diagnosis is in doubt after all other studies prove inconclusive.

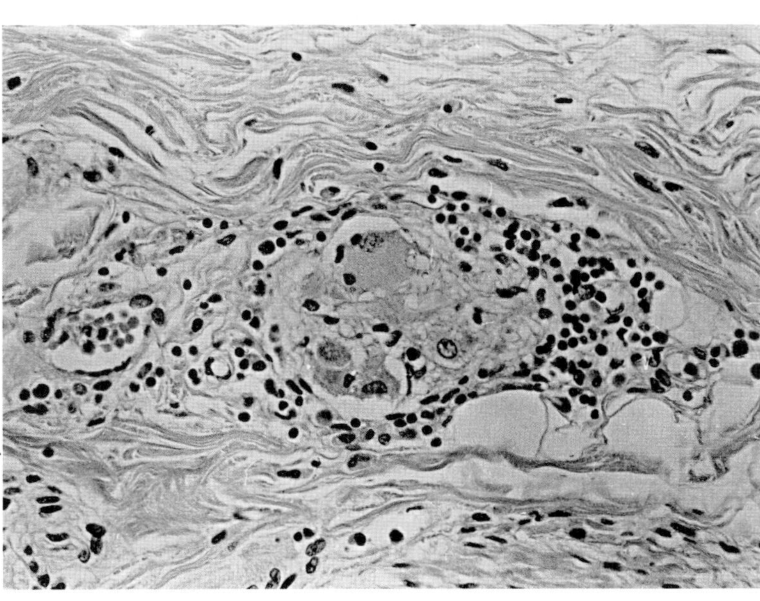

Figure 111–9. Myenteric plexus from a patient with paraneoplastic visceral neuropathy showing infiltration with lymphocytes and plasma cells. H & E, ×320. (From Krishnamurthy S, Schuffler MD: Pathology of neuromuscular disorders of the small intestine and colon. Gastroenterology 93:623, 1987.)

evidence of intestinal obstruction was found. Symptoms and signs of systemic illnesses and of neurologic and autonomic nervous system dysfunction should be sought.

In patients with neurologic findings, further tests could include magnetic resonance imaging to search for a brainstem tumor; electromyography and nerve conduction velocity to determine the presence of a systemic muscle disease or peripheral neuropathy, as in amyloidosis; and autonomic nervous system testing.[18] Because visceral neuropathies may be associated with autonomic dysfunction in the absence of clinical neurologic findings,[36] autonomic testing may be useful in many patients with chronic intestinal pseudo-obstruction.

The evaluation should include contrast studies of the entire gastrointestinal tract. The urinary tract should also be studied to look for evidence of megacystis or megaloureters. The finding of multiple sites of abnormality within the gastrointestinal tract and urinary system provides strong evidence for chronic intestinal pseudo-obstruction. Exploratory laparotomy should be considered if abnormalities are limited to the small intestine and do not exclude mechanical obstruction. Two exceptions are small intestinal diverticulosis and diffuse lymphoid infiltration, both of which may be limited to the small intestine. In situations that are unclear, an enteroclysis with barium should be done to exclude an obstruction. If obstruction is detected in the terminal ileum, a barium enema or colonoscopy should be done to visualize the area.

Gastroduodenal manometry is not available at most medical centers and is rarely necessary for diagnosis in adults who have adequate radiographic examinations. Small bowel manometry does not always differentiate mechanical obstruction from pseudo-obstruction, and its sensitivity and specificity are unknown. When the diagnosis of pseudo-obstruction remains uncertain, small bowel manometry can be used to increase the evidence that a visceral myopathy or neuropathy is present. Occasionally, rectal mucosal biopsy may be useful for diagnosing neuronal intranuclear inclusion disease,[34] neuronal intestinal dysplasia,[37] amyloidosis, and inflammatory neuropathies, which involve the submucosal plexus. The role of full-thickness rectal biopsy remains to be defined; it might reveal pathologic abnormalities of the muscularis propria and myenteric plexus.

If there is continuing uncertainty as to the correct diagnosis, laparoscopy or laparotomy should be undertaken to exclude mechanical obstruction and obtain tissue for pathologic diagnosis.

A full-thickness biopsy of the small intestine can be obtained via laparoscopy, with or without placement of a feeding jejunostomy tube. Full-thickness biopsies should be examined for muscle disease, inflammatory infiltrates of the myenteric plexus, neuronal intranuclear and intracytoplasmic inclusions, neuronal destruction, and absent or deficient c-kit immunoreactivity.[24, 25]

If laparotomy is done, two sites should be biopsied, with tissue obtained from both dilated and nondilated segments of intestine and processed for conventional light microscopy and by Smith's method, if available. Conventional full-thickness biopsy is large enough for conventional light microscopy and immunohistochemistry but not large enough for Smith's method, which requires a sample measuring close to 2 × 2 cm when opened and flattened out. Palliative resections, of course, will yield adequate tissue.

TREATMENT

No treatment is curative or halts the natural history of any of the disorders that cause intestinal pseudo-obstruction. The goal of treatment is to alleviate symptoms and restore and maintain nutrition and fluid and electrolyte balance (Table 111–3). Drug therapy with metoclopramide and domperidone (not available in the United States) appears to be ineffective. Cisapride has had limited success, although few controlled studies are available. However, because of cardiac toxicity and reported deaths, the manufacturer has restricted cisapride for compassionate use only, and it remains available only by special request. In single-administration studies in patients with pseudo-obstruction, cisapride increased contractility and hastened transit, but a controlled trial of outpatient use failed to show improvement in symptoms.[38] By contrast, an uncontrolled trial of cisapride in 106 patients resulted in improved symptoms in the majority.[39] A response is more likely in the subgroup of patients with intact vagal function.[40] The dose is 20 mg three times daily in adults. Tachyphylaxis may occur, but effectiveness may be restored by discontinuing the drug for 2 to 3 weeks.

Erythromycin has been used in just a few patients to date. There is no evidence that, when used alone, erythromycin is effective beyond a few weeks of use. Octreotide in small doses can induce migrating motor complexes in the small intestine. A bedtime octreotide dose of 50 mcg subcutaneously, with or without a daily dose of erythromycin suspension, 200 mg orally three times daily, can sometimes result in clinical improvement, especially in patients with progressive systemic sclerosis.[41, 42]

Broad-spectrum antibiotics are useful in treating patients with the stagnant loop syndrome.[43] A 7-day course of an

Table 111–3 | **Summary of Treatment Options**

Drugs (inconsistent efficacy, but worth trying)
Metoclopramide 10–20 mg tid–qid PO, SC, IM, or IV
Cisapride 10–20 mg bid–qid PO (Compassionate use only; beware of contraindications)
Domperidone 10–20 mg tid–qid PO (Not available in U.S.)
Octreotide 50–100 mcg SC qhs
Erythromycin 250 mg tid PO
Intermittent broad-spectrum antibiotics, e.g., ciprofloxacin 500 mg bid ×7 days.

Diet
Low in fat, lactose, residue, and gas-producing foods
Frequent, small feedings
Blenderized, pureed foods
Liquid formula supplementation
Vitamin and mineral supplements to maintain blood levels

Palliative Surgery
To decompress, remove, or bypass bowel:
- Duodenojejunostomy
- Duodenoplasty
- Limited or extensive small bowel resections
- Abdominal colectomy and ileorectal anastomosis
- Decompressive gastrostomy, jejunostomy, and/or ileostomy
- Feeding jejunostomy
- Small intestinal transplantation

Home Parenteral Nutrition

antibiotic such as tetracycline, doxycycline, ampicillin, norfloxacin, ciprofloxacin, or metronidazole may induce a gain in weight and remission of diarrhea that lasts weeks to months. It is not usually necessary to re-treat the patient until diarrhea recurs, and in fact, continuous use of antibiotics may result in the emergence of resistant organisms. Alternatively, a rotating cycle of antibiotics for 1 week every month may be tried. The optimal length of treatment, timing of antibiotic administration, and best way of preventing symptomatic recurrences are unknown.[43] Antibiotics do not usually alter the long-term course of pseudo-obstruction, and they do not seem to be of value in patients who primarily have obstructive symptoms and constipation.

Patients should be instructed to follow a diet low in fat, lactose, and residue with small frequent meals six to eight times per day; each meal should provide about 200 to 300 kcal.[44] Gas-producing foods should be avoided, and blenderized pureed foods may be better tolerated than solids. A variety of liquid dietary supplements have been used. Ideally, such supplements should be palatable and lactose-free, with only small quantities of long-chain fats. Consultation with a dietitian will provide the patient with a number of options. Liquid formulas do not work well for long-term management but may be beneficial during short periods of symptomatic exacerbation.

Specific deficiencies of vitamins and minerals should be corrected and prevented. Treatment may involve injections of vitamin B_{12} and oral supplementation of iron, calcium, folic acid, water-soluble vitamins, vitamins A, D, E and K, and trace elements. A multivitamin, such as Centrum Silver, should be taken daily.

Palliative surgery may be of value in selected patients who are incapacitated by their intestinal symptoms and who should be considered for an operation to decompress, remove, or bypass nonfunctioning intestine.[45, 46] Before deciding on a particular operation, it is extremely important to determine which symptoms are being palliated and from which area of the intestine these symptoms emanate. Side-to-side duodenojejunostomy may be done to palliate an isolated megaduodenum[47] but will probably be ineffective if the patient also has gastroparesis or involvement of the small intestine distal to the duodenum. If the duodenum is huge, a duodenoplasty can be done to reduce the size of the duodenum.[5] Extensive, sometimes radical, small bowel resection may be necessary in rare patients with unrelenting intestinal obstruction and massive intestinal fluid secretion that makes it impossible to keep up with fluid losses or to control severe obstructive symptoms.[46, 48] In such cases, the patient is invariably on home parenteral nutrition and deriving no benefit from the small bowel anyway.

A total abdominal colectomy with ileorectal anastomosis may be necessary in patients who have a megacolon and severe abdominal distention.[15, 45] However, even with this procedure, some patients continue to have severe symptoms from coexistent small intestinal disease. In addition, colectomy may exacerbate diarrhea. Thus, palliative surgery should be undertaken only after careful thought.

Laparoscopic placement of a feeding jejunostomy tube may be helpful, especially in patients who have predominantly gastric and duodenal involvement and a fairly normal distal bowel and who cannot maintain their nutrition by oral intake. The jejunostomy tube should be placed surgically because there are too many technical problems after placement of a jejunal tube via a percutaneous endoscopic gastrostomy tube. In order to prove that a jejunal feeding tube will work, the patient should first be fed successfully by a nasojejunal tube for several days at a rate sufficient to provide adequate calories. Some patients may be nourished from a combination of enteral and parenteral feedings while utilizing a gastrostomy to vent the proximal bowel. Jejunostomies and ileostomies can also be created to vent the more distal segments of the bowel.[45]

Unnecessary surgery should be avoided at all costs. Once any abdominal procedure is performed, it may be difficult to exclude mechanical obstruction caused by adhesions when the patient returns with symptoms of intestinal obstruction. On the other hand, surgery may be quite necessary for acute problems, such as intestinal volvulus, perforation, or herniation, all of which can occur in patients with pseudo-obstruction.

If the patient is unable to maintain nutrition or continues to have severe symptoms despite palliative treatment, long-term home parenteral nutrition may be necessary.[49] Although this approach usually provides nutritional repletion and correction of vitamin and mineral deficiencies, some patients continue to have abdominal pain or such copious intestinal secretion that vomiting and fluid and electrolyte losses remain substantial. These patients may require a decompressive gastrostomy or an extended small bowel resection to remove the abnormal intestine. Many patients on home parenteral nutrition seem to do well, although some fall victim to septic and thrombotic complications of the central intravenous catheter, depression, prolonged suffering, and analgesic dependence. Support groups, such as the American Association of Gastrointestinal Motility Disorders, Inc. (www.digestivemotility.org) and the American Pseudo-obstruction and Hirschsprung's Society, Inc., (www.tiac.net/users/aphs) provide advice, information, educational meetings, and psychological support to patients and their families.

The advent of small intestinal transplantation has increased the therapeutic options available to patients with pseudo-obstruction.[50] However, the more widespread use of this still experimental operation in patients with severe pseudo-obstruction awaits improved rates of survival of both grafts and patients. Steady progress has been made, and improved survival has occurred over the past 5 years.

PROGNOSIS

The natural history of chronic intestinal pseudo-obstruction depends on the underlying cause. Patients with progressive systemic sclerosis usually die within 5 to 10 years from renal, cardiac, or pulmonary complications of the disease. Patients with small cell carcinoma of the lung usually die within 1 year of the onset of extraintestinal manifestations.[16] Patients with other forms of visceral myopathy and visceral neuropathy may live for prolonged periods, as long as they continue to maintain their nutrition and do not have life-threatening complications from indwelling catheters.[3] Some patients with visceral neuropathy have had symptoms for over 40 years, and some patients with visceral myopathy have had symptoms for over 30 years. Infants and young children who are born with visceral myopathy or developmental abnormalities of the myenteric plexus may die at a young age, although many have survived for years on home parenteral nutrition.[27]

REFERENCES

1. Verne G, Sninsky C: Chronic intestinal pseudo-obstruction. Dig Dis Sci 13:163, 1995.
2. Krishnamurthy S, Schuffler M: Pathology of neuromuscular disorders of the small intestine and colon. Gastroenterology 93:610, 1987.
3. Schuffler M, Rohrmann C, Chaffee R, et al: Chronic intestinal pseudo-obstruction: A report of 27 cases and review of the literature. Medicine 60:173, 1981.
4. Rohrmann C, Ricci M, Krishnamurthy S, et al: Radiologic and histologic differentiation of neuromuscular disorders of the gastrointestinal tract: Visceral myopathies, visceral neuropathies and progressive systemic sclerosis. Am J Roentgenol 143:933, 1984.
5. Schuffler M, Lowe M, Bill A: Studies of idiopathic intestinal pseudo-obstruction. I. Hereditary hollow visceral myopathy: Clinical and pathological studies. Gastroenterology 73:327, 1977.
6. Schuffler M, Beegle R: Progressive systemic sclerosis of the gastrointestinal tract and hereditary hollow visceral myopathy: Two distinguishable disorders of intestinal smooth muscle. Gastoenterology 77:664, 1979.
7. Anuras S, Mitros F, Nowak T, et al: A familial visceral myopathy with external ophthalmoplegia and autosomal recessive transmission. Gastroenterology 84:346, 1983.
8. Schuffler M, Pope C: Studies of idiopathic intestinal pseudo-obstruction. II. Hereditary hollow visceral myopathy: Family studies. Gastroenterology 73:339, 1977.
9. Anuras S, Mitros F, Milano A, et al: A familial visceral myopathy with dilatation of the entire gastrointestinal tract. Gastroenterology 90:385, 1986.
10. Perez-Atayde P, Fox V, Teitelbaum J, et al: Mitochondrial neurogastrointestinal encephalopathy. Diagnosis by rectal biopsy. Am J Surg Pathol 22:1141, 1998.
11. Fogel S, DeTar M, Shimada H, et al: Sporadic visceral myopathy with inclusion bodies. Am J Surg Pathol 17:473, 1993.
12. Smith V, Lake B, Kamm M, et al: Intestinal pseudo-obstruction with deficient smooth muscle α-actin. Histopathology 21:535, 1992.
13. Tada S, Iida M, Yao T, et al: Intestinal pseudo-obstruction in patients with amyloidosis: Clinicopathologic differences between chemical types of amyloid protein. Gut 34:1412, 1993.
14. McDonald G, Schuffler M, Kadin M, et al: Intestinal pseudo-obstruction caused by diffuse lymphoid infiltration of the small intestine. Gastroenterology 89:882, 1985.
15. Schuffler M, Jonak Z: Chronic idiopathic intestinal pseudo-obstruction caused by a degenerative disorder of the myenteric plexus: The use of Smith's method to define the neuropathology. Gastroenterology 82:476, 1982.
16. Chinn J, Schuffler M: Paraneoplastic visceral myopathy as a cause of severe gastrointestinal motor dysfunction. Gastroenterology 95:1279, 1988.
17. Camilleri M: Disorders of gastrointestinal motility in neurologic diseases. Mayo Clin Proc 65:825, 1990.
18. Schuffler M, Bird T, Sumi S, et al: A familial neuronal disease presenting as intestinal pseudo-obstruction. Gastroenterology 75:889, 1978.
19. Besnard M, Faure C, Fromont-Hankard G, et al: Intestinal pseudo-obstruction and acute pandysautonomia associated with Epstein-Barr infection. Am J Gastroenterol 95:280, 2000.
20. Debinski H, Kamm M, Talbot I, et al: DNA viruses in the pathogenesis of sporadic chronic intestinal pseudo-obstruction. Gut 41:100, 1997.
21. Uc A, Vasiliauskas E, Piccoli D, et al: Chronic intestinal pseudo-obstruction associated with fetal alcohol syndrome. Dig Dis Sci 42: 1163, 1997.
22. Salerno N, Grey N: Myxedema pseudoobstruction. AJR Am J Roentgenol 130:175, 1978.
23. Rogers M, Cerda J: The narcotic bowel syndrome. J Clin Gastroenterol 11:132, 1989.
24. Yamataka A, Ohshiro K, Kobayashi H, et al: Abnormal distribution of intestinal pacemaker (C-Kit positive) cells in an infant with chronic intestinal pseudo-obstruction. J Pediatr Surg 33:859, 1998.
25. Moussa K, Proctor D, Jain D, et al: Absence of c-Kit$^+$ cells in resected segments of patients with chronic intestinal pseudo-obstruction (CIIP). Gastroenterology 118:A866, 2000.
26. Stangellini V, Camillieri M, Malagelada J: Chronic idiopathic intestinal pseudo-obstruction: Clinical and intestinal manometric findings. Gut 28: 5, 1987.
27. Schuffler M, Pagon R, Schwartz R, et al: Visceral myopathy of the gastrointestinal and genitourinary tracts in infants. Gastroenterology 94: 892, 1988.
28. Pulliam T, Schuster M: Congenital markers for chronic intestinal pseudo-obstruction. Am J Gastroenterol 90:922, 1995.
29. Nojima Y, Mimura T, Hamasaki K, et al: Chronic intestinal pseudo-obstruction associated with autoantibodies against proliferating cell nuclear antigen. Arthritis Rheum 39:877, 1996.
30. Lennon V, Sas D, Busk M, et al: Enteric neuronal autoantibodies in pseudo-obstruction with small-lung carcinoma. Gastroenterology 100: 137, 1991.
31. Mayer E, Schuffler M, Rotter J, et al: A familial visceral neuropathy with autosomal dominant transmission. Gastroenterology 91:1528, 1989.
32. Frank J, Sarr M, Camilleri M: Use of gastroduodenal manometry to differentiate mechanical and functional intestinal obstruction: An analysis of clinical outcome. Am J Gastroenterol 89:339, 1994.
33. Barnett J, McDonnell W, Appleman H, et al: Familial visceral neuropathy with neuronal intranuclear inclusions: Diagnosis by rectal biopsy. Gastroenterology 102:684, 1992.
34. Auricchio A, Brancolini V, Casari G, et al: The locus for a novel syndromic form of neuronal intestinal pseudo-obstruction maps to Xq28. Am J Hum Genet 58:743, 1996.
35. Krishnamurthy S, Heng Y, Schuffler M: Chronic intestinal pseudo-obstruction in infants and children caused by diverse abnormalities of the myenteric plexus. Gastroenterology 104:1398, 1993.
36. Khurana R, Schuster M: Autonomic dysfunction in chronic intestinal pseudo-obstruction. Clin Auton Res 8:335, 1998.
37. Achem S, Owyang C, Schuffler M, et al: Neuronal dysplasia and chronic idiopathic intestinal pseudo-obstruction: Rectal biopsy as an aid to diagnosis. Gastroenterology 92:805, 1987.
38. Camilleri M, Malagelada J, Abell T, et al: Effect of six weeks of treatment with cisapride in gastroparesis and intestinal pseudo-obstruction. Gastroenterology 96:704, 1989.
39. Reyntjens A, Verlinden M, Schuermans V: Cisapride in the treatment of chronic intestinal pseudo-obstruction. Gastroenterology 28(suppl 1): 79, 1990.
40. Camilleri M, Balm R, Zinsmeister A, et al: Determinants of response to a prokinetic agent in neuropathic chronic intestinal motility disorder. Gastroenterology 106:916, 1994.
41. Soudah H, Hasler W, Owyang C: Effect of octreotide on intestinal motility and bacterial overgrowth in scleroderma. N Engl J Med 325: 1461, 1991.
42. Verne G, Eaker E, Hardy E, et al: Effect of octreotide and erythromycin on idiopathic and scleroderma-associated intestinal pseudo-obstruction. Dig Dis Sci 40:1892, 1995.
43. Attar A, Flourie B, Rambaud J-C, et al: Antibiotic efficacy in small intestinal bacterial overgrowth-related diarrhea: A crossover, ramdomized trial. Gastroenterology 117:794, 1999.
44. Scolapio J, Ukleja A, Bouras E, et al: Nutritional management of chronic intestinal pseudo-obstruction. J Clin Gastroenterol 28:306, 1999.
45. Murr M, Sarr M, Camilleri M: The surgeon's role in the treatment of chronic intestinal pseudoobstruction. Am J Gastroenterol 90:2147, 1995.
46. Noel R, Schuffler M, Helton W: Small bowel resection for relief of chronic intestinal pseudo-obstruction. Am J Gastroenterol 90:1142, 1995.
47. Anuras S, Shirazi S, Faulk D, et al: Surgical treatment in familial visceral myopathy. Ann Surg 189:306, 1979.
48. Schuffler M, Leon S, Krishnamurthy S: Intestinal pseudo-obstruction caused by a new form of visceral neuropathy. Palliation by radical small bowel resection. Gastroenterology 89:1152, 1985.
49. Warner E, Jeejeebhoy K: Successful management of chronic intestinal pseudo-obstruction with home parenteral nutrition. J Parenter Enter Nutr 9:173, 1985.
50. Niv Y, Mor E, Tzakis A: Small bowel transplantation—a clinical review. Am J Gastroenterol 94:3126, 1999.

Chapter 112

Gastrointestinal Carcinoid Tumors and the Carcinoid Syndrome

Thomas Anthony and Lawrence Kim

Carcinoid tumors are among the most interesting and challenging tumors encountered in clinical practice. Historically, the term *carcinoid* was first applied in 1907 by Oberndorfer,[1] but the tumor was first described in 1888 by Lubarsch.[2] Because of their neuroendocrine origin, carcinoid tumors are equipped with neurosecretory capability, which produces one of their defining clinical characteristics: the ability to secrete a variety of peptides and bioactive amines. Chief among these is 5-hydroxytryptamine (5-HT) or serotonin. A wide variety of other secretory products have also been described, including corticotropin (ACTH), histamine, and dopamine (Table 112–1).

Because carcinoids arise from cells of the diffuse neuroendocrine system, they are therefore related to medullary carcinoma of the thyroid, pheochromocytoma, and pancreatic neuroendocrine tumors. Carcinoids occur in about 9% of patients who have multiple endocrine neoplasia (MEN), predominantly MEN type 1.[3] Carcinoids belong to the family of tumors known as *tumor of amine precursor uptake and decarboxylation cells* (APUD cells). The term *APUD* has fallen somewhat out of favor because many of the secretory products of these tumors are peptides rather than amines. Cells of the diffuse neuroendocrine system are found throughout the gastrointestinal (GI) tract. Although once thought to arise from the neural crest, they now appear to differentiate within the gut itself.[4, 5]

An extensive analysis of the anatomic location of carcinoid tumors used data from the Surveillance, Epidemiology, and End Results (SEER) program of the National Cancer Institute.[6] Carcinoid tumors occur most frequently in the GI tract (74%). They also occur in the bronchopulmonary system (25%).[6] The remaining 1% occur in a variety of locations, including the ovary,[7] gallbladder,[8] extrahepatic bile ducts,[9] thymus,[10] testis,[11] liver,[12] cervix,[13] spleen,[14] breast,[15] and larynx.[16] This chapter considers only carcinoid tumors of the GI tract and digestive organs (Table 112–2).

The overall incidence of carcinoid tumors is difficult to determine because many are asymptomatic. One autopsy study estimated the incidence to be 8.4/100,000 people annually; about 90% of these were incidental autopsy findings.[17] The incidence of clinical cases of carcinoid is in the range of 1 to 2/100,000 per year. There is a slightly increased incidence in African Americans as compared with white Americans, and there is a slight female predominance during the reproductive years.[6, 18]

CLINICAL PRESENTATION

Carcinoid tumors are often discovered incidentally during surgery, endoscopic procedures, or imaging studies. They cause symptoms either through their mass effect or through their secretory products. The mass effect may occasionally cause pain but more commonly causes luminal obstruction. Obstruction may be due to direct tumor growth or to scarring caused by the intense desmoplastic reaction associated with these lesions. Symptoms are often nonspecific, consisting of malaise, vague abdominal pain, or weight loss.

Carcinoid syndrome is an unusual presentation of GI carcinoids. Because most primary carcinoids of the GI tract are drained by the portal venous system, most bioamines such as serotonin and histamine are cleared by the liver prior to entry into the systemic circulation. Thus, even tumors that secrete high levels of these amines may be asymptomatic. On the other hand, if the primary tumor secretes ACTH or other peptide hormones, symptoms due to these products may develop when the tumor is still quite small. Symptoms caused by secretory products vary according to the substance produced. The classic product, serotonin, may produce flushing and diarrhea (see "Carcinoid Syndrome"). ACTH producing tumors cause Cushing's syndrome; gastrin producing tumors may cause Zollinger-Ellison syndrome (see Chapter 41).

Table 112–1 | **Secretory Products of Carcinoids**

Bioactive amines
Serotonin (5-hydroxytryptamine [5-HT])
Histamine
Dopamine
Norepinephrine
Peptides
Corticotropin (ACTH)
Calcitonin
Pancreatic polypeptide
Bradykinin
Neurotensin
Tachykinins
Chromogranin
Secretin
Cholecystokinin
Kallikrein
Gastrin
Insulin
Parathyroid hormone–related protein
Fatty acids
Prostaglandins

PATHOLOGY

Grossly carcinoid tumors appear as solid yellow-tan lesions. Except those in the stomach and ileum, which may be multicentric, they are usually solitary. In the GI tract they are often submucosal but may cause ulceration. A striking feature of carcinoids is the intense desmoplasia within and surrounding the tumor. This may in some cases lead to GI obstruction or vascular occlusion secondary to anatomic distortion caused by the surrounding tissue reaction.[19]

Carcinoid tumors appear histologically as uniform small, round cells with rare mitotic figures (Fig. 112–1). Two types of silver staining are commonly used to identify neuroendocrine cells. In argyrophil reactions, silver salts are bonded to cytoplasmic granules in an aqueous medium and then reduced to metallic silver. In argentaffin staining, the endogenous reducing power of the cells converts ammoniacal silver nitrate to silver.[20] Classically foregut and hindgut carcinoids are typically argyrophil, and midgut serotonin secreting carcinoids are argentaffin.[21] There are many exceptions to these generalities, however, because the type of silver staining does not always correlate with the site of origin, clinical outcome, or secretory product. These stains are less important in the pathologic evaluation of carcinoids.[22]

Immunohistochemical stains of carcinoid tumors usually yield positive results for markers of neuroendocrine differentiation. Among these stains are chromogranins A, B, and C; synaptophysin; and neuron specific enolase. Under electron microscopy, dense membrane-bound core secretory vesicles can be visualized, along with small, clear vesicles that correspond to neuronal synaptic vesicles (Fig. 112–2).[23]

Chromogranins have been found to be reliable serum markers for the detection of neuroendocrine tumors.[24] Although serum chromogranin A appears to be most useful for gastrinomas, about 80% of patients who have carcinoids have an elevation of the serum chromogranin A concentration.[25, 26] A number of non-neuroendocrine tumors may also secrete chromogranin A. One group has suggested that measurement of both chromogranins A and B resulted in superior discriminatory ability as compared with measurement of chromogranin A alone.[27] A very high serum level of chromogranin A is a poor prognostic indicator in individuals with metastatic disease.[28]

CLASSIFICATION

Williams and Sandler classified carcinoid tumors according to their embryologic region of origin—foregut, midgut, or hindgut.[29] Foregut carcinoids include those arising in the esophagus, stomach, pancreas, and duodenum. Midgut carcinoids comprise tumors arising in the superior mesenteric artery distribution, including the ileum and appendix, the two most common sites of carcinoids. Hindgut carcinoids arise in the distribution of the inferior mesenteric artery, including the rectum. Williams and Sandler suggested that midgut tumors were more likely to secrete 5-HT than foregut or hindgut tumors. Foregut and hindgut tumors were more likely to metastasize than midgut lesions. Several differences in protein expression have also been identified among the types; these include differences in neural cell adhesion molecule (NCAM), S-100, and chromogranin.[30]

Table 112–2 | **Site-Specific Characteristics of Gastrointestinal Carcinoid Tumors***

	FRACTION OF ALL CARCINOIDS	AVERAGE AGE AT DIAGNOSIS†	SYNCHRONOUS OR METACHRONOUS NONCARCINOID TUMORS	REGIONAL SPREAD†, ‡	DISTANT METASTASES†, ‡	5-YEAR SURVIVAL† RATE
All carcinoids	—	—	13.0	25.7	19.6	50.35
Stomach	3.19	63.8	7.8	10.3	20.6	48.6
Small bowel	26.48	65.1	16.6	39.3	31.4	55.4
Appendix	18.9	42.2	14.6	26.8	8.5	85.9
Colon	9.95	65.6	13.1	33.4	37.8	41.6
Rectum	11.38	58.2	9.2	7.1	7.1	72.2

*Values (other than age in column 2) are given as percentages.
†Surveillance, Epidemiology, and End Results (SEER) data 1973–1991.
‡At presentation.
Information adapted from Modlin IM, Sandor A: An analysis of 8305 cases of carcinoid tumors. Cancer 79: 813–829, 1997.

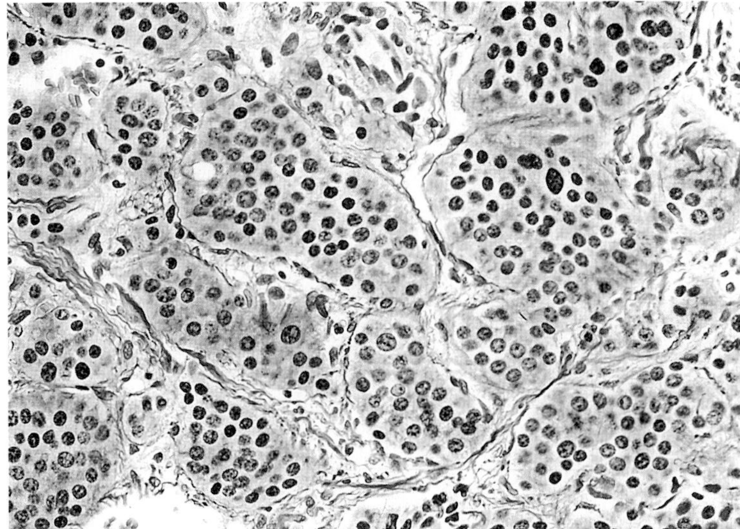

Figure 112–1. Typical histologic appearance of carcinoid on hematoxylin and eosin staining. Note the uniform, small, round cells with rare mitotic figures.

Modlin and Sandor, in their analysis of 8305 cases of carcinoid tumors, attempted to correlate embryologic site of origin with survival.[6] Foregut (GI only) lesions appeared to have a generally worse prognosis than midgut or hindgut lesions. However, these authors found that the differences between groups were not sufficient to validate Williams and Sandler's classification of carcinoids as a major predictor of outcome.[29] Although Modlin and Sandor's analysis of this classification system was compromised because SEER data did not allow survival analysis based on the anatomic location of colonic lesions,[6] other authors also have questioned the utility of the Williams and Sandler system because of the variability of behavior of tumors within these broad divisions.[23] Because of the diverse biologic behavior of carcinoids within each embryologic division, grouping carcinoids in such a manner tends to overlook distinct behavior unique to tumors of specific organs. Therefore, we have chosen to base the present discussion on the organ of origin.

Esophagus

Carcinoid tumors of the esophagus are extremely rare. Lindberg in a review[31] identified only 14 cases in the world literature. These were usually located in the distal portion of the esophagus. There is a distinct male predominance. Dysphagia is the most common symptom. Most have been treated by esophagogastrectomy.[31]

Stomach

The stomach is the most common foregut location for carcinoid tumors. Gastric carcinoids account for approximately 3% of all carcinoid tumors, but carcinoids are responsible for only about 0.5% of gastric malignancies.[6] Gastric carcinoids have increased in incidence since the 1980s, although it is unclear whether that incidence represents a true increase or simply increases in awareness and accuracy of detection.[32]

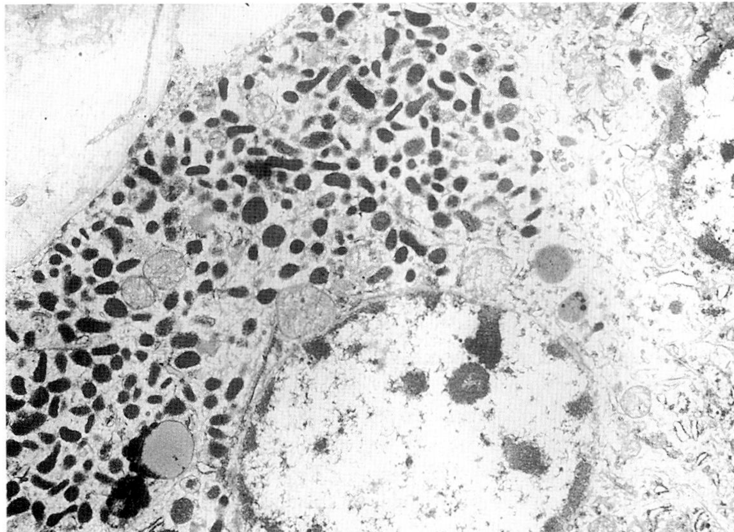

Figure 112–2. Electron micrograph of a carcinoid cell with a large number of densely packed neurosecretory granules.

Overall, the 5-year survival rate for gastric carcinoids is 49% if localized, 40% with regional nodal metastases, and 10% with distant metastases. A complete discussion of gastric carcinoids is found in the chapter on gastric malignancies (see Chapter 44).

Pancreas

The distinction between pancreatic carcinoids and other neuroendocrine tumors of the pancreas is primarily a matter of definition. Maurer and associates defined a pancreatic carcinoid as a tumor with the histologic features of a neuroendocrine tumor and obviously increased serotonin metabolism. Using this definition, these authors found only 29 cases in the world literature published between 1966 and 1996.[33] Likewise, in Modlin and Sandor's review of SEER data, only 46 cases of carcinoid tumor of the pancreas are reported.[6] Because these cases were gathered from those reported to the SEER database, the original pathologic findings were not reviewed. Therefore, it is possible that some, if not most, of these cases represent other neuroendocrine tumors such as pancreatic islet cell tumors.[6]

Pancreatic carcinoids, like other pancreatic tumors, tend to appear later than carcinoids in other locations. In Maurer's review, tumors ranged in size from 2 to 12 cm with a mean of 4 cm. Abdominal pain, diarrhea, and weight loss were the most common symptoms. Nineteen of 29 patients (66%) exhibited metastases, and in 2 others metastases developed during follow-up. The median survival of metastatic disease patients was only 7 months.[33] Similarly, SEER data showed that pancreatic carcinoids were nonlocalized in 76% of cases, and 5-year survival was only 34%. This is a better survival rate than those of other pancreatic malignancies but worse than those of carcinoids in other sites.[6] Another study confirmed the poor outcome of pancreatic carcinoids as compared with other foregut carcinoids.[34] Treatment is by surgical resection if possible. A pancreaticoduodenectomy (Whipple procedure) is often required, but lesser resections are occasionally possible.

Duodenum and Ampulla of Vater

Carcinoids of the duodenum represent approximately 2% of carcinoids.[6] Carcinoids of the ampulla of Vater are even more rare: in 1999 fewer than 100 cases had been reported.[35, 36] Subclinical ampullary carcinoids may be much more common.[37] Although they are usually discussed together, duodenal and ampullary carcinoids appear to be significantly different.

Duodenal carcinoids are discovered most commonly during endoscopy. They are usually argyrophil, as contrasted with typical small bowel carcinoids, which are argentaffin.[38, 39] Duodenal carcinoids rarely secrete serotonin; therefore carcinoid syndrome resulting from duodenal or ampullary carcinoids is virtually unknown. One of the most significant products of duodenal carcinoids is gastrin, which is found in about half of cases.[35, 40] Although duodenal carcinoids are associated with Zollinger-Ellison syndrome (see Chapter 41), it has been emphasized that histochemical evidence of tumor production of gastrin does not necessarily correlate with documented Zollinger-Ellison syndrome. In fact most patients who have gastrin-producing duodenal carcinoids do not have Zollinger-Ellison syndrome.[40]

As might be expected, ampullary carcinoids frequently exhibit with jaundice. Ampullary carcinoids, particularly those associated with von Recklinghausen's disease (neurofibromatosis type 1), often exhibit psammoma bodies and express somatostatin.[35, 39] Approximately 25% of patients with a periampullary carcinoid have von Recklinghausen's disease.[35, 41]

The average sizes of ampullary and duodenal carcinoids are 1.7 and 1.8 cm, respectively. In general, the risk of metastasis increases with increased size of the primary tumor.[35] The treatment of ampullary or duodenal carcinoids is by resection. Too few cases have been documented in the literature to allow a definitive description of the optimal treatment for a given lesion. Endoscopic resection, local surgical excision, and pancreaticoduodenectomy have all been employed successfully. Tumor characteristics suggestive of increased metastatic risk are invasion into the muscularis propria, size greater than 2 cm, and presence of mitotic figures.[40] However, there are no data to show that more extensive surgical resection of high-risk lesions improves outcome. At present, local excision either endoscopically or surgically appears to be adequate treatment for small, low-risk tumors. More radical excision is occasionally needed for large primary tumors and in those in which regional nodal metastases are already evident.

Small Bowel

The small bowel, particularly the ileum, is the most common site of carcinoid tumors, accounting for almost 30% of all carcinoids.[6] Even a Meckel's diverticulum may harbor a carcinoid tumor occasionally. Because malignant small bowel tumors are uncommon, carcinoids form a relatively large fraction of the tumors, accounting for 28% to 38% of small bowel malignant tumors.[6, 42]

The mean age at presentation of small bowel carcinoid tumors is 62 to 65 years, but these tumors may occur at almost any age after childhood. In Burke and coworkers' series from the Armed Forces Institute of Pathology,[43] 86% expressed serotonin, a fraction that is higher than in other carcinoid sites. Small bowel carcinoids are multifocal in approximately one fourth of cases.[43, 44] X-chromosome inactivation analysis has suggested that multiple lesions are actually monoclonal and that they may therefore represent metastases from a single primary lesion.[45]

The most frequent clinical symptom of small bowel carcinoids is intermittent intestinal obstruction (46%). Vague abdominal pain is also common (41%). Bleeding is uncommon, as is carcinoid syndrome as an initial presentation.[44] As mentioned, carcinoid tumors have a remarkable propensity to incite a fibrotic reaction in surrounding tissue. Such fibrosis may kink the bowel, causing obstruction (Fig. 112–3), or in some cases it may obstruct vascular supply, causing ischemia of the involved segment. In some instances, complete infarction of the small bowel due to superior mesenteric artery occlusion may be the initial and/or terminal event in a case of a small bowel carcinoid. Al-

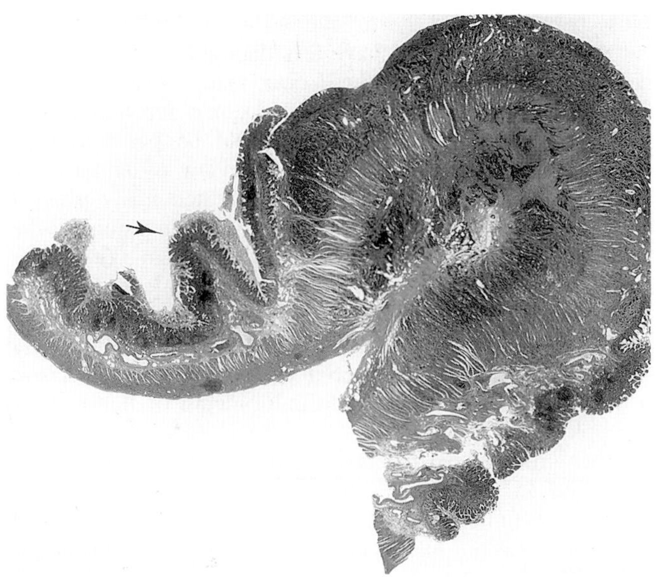

Figure 112–3. A whole mount through the small intestine, illustrating the angulation of the bowel secondary to an infiltrating carcinoid tumor that involves the mucosa, the muscularis propria, and the serosa with an associated dense desmoplastic reaction. Normal small intestine is noted on the left *(arrow)*.

though serotonin production is frequent in small bowel carcinoids, the overt carcinoid syndrome is uncommon as an initial presentation. Small bowel venous effluent enters the portal circulation, where 5-HT is metabolized on the first pass. Presence of the carcinoid syndrome usually indicates hepatic or retroperitoneal metastases and is an ominous indicator of an unfavorable outcome.[43]

The primary difficulty in treating small bowel carcinoids is their late presentation. Primary tumors often remain asymptomatic until bulky mesenteric nodal disease is present or until liver metastases occur with the resultant carcinoid syndrome. If they are found early (usually incidentally), the treatment is straightforward. The primary tumor and the associated mesenteric lymph nodes should be resected surgically. The fibrotic reaction caused by these lesions may complicate the resection by causing mesenteric shortening, even with small tumors. Bulky nodal metastases, with their associated fibrosis, may extend to the root of the superior mesenteric vessels, thereby precluding curative resection. Palliative debulking has been advocated by some and may provide significant symptomatic relief.[46, 47] The risk-to-benefit ratio needs to be weighed carefully for each patient.

Approximately one third of patients exhibit regional nodal metastases only, and another third show distant metastases.[6, 43] The prevalence of distant metastases increases with size of the primary tumor. In Moertel's series from 1961, the rate of metastases from tumors smaller than 1 cm was 2%; from tumors 1 to 2 cm, 50%; and from tumors larger than 2 cm, 80%.[44] In Burke's series,[43] tumors larger than 2 cm had only a 33% probability of distant metastasis. This series had a greater proportion of large tumors, which may reflect a different referral population. Other series have noted the high likelihood of distant metastases even with small primary tumors.[48] The 5-year survival rate for small bowel carcinoids is 55% to 60%.[6, 43]

Appendix

The appendix is the second most common site of GI carcinoids, accounting for almost 20% of the total.[6] As in the small bowel, primary tumors in the appendix are rare. Therefore, the proportion of tumors that are carcinoids is high, around one third to one half of all appendiceal tumors.[6, 49, 50]

Appendiceal carcinoids are diagnosed at an earlier age than other carcinoids. Most studies suggest a mean age of about 42 years, although considerable variation is possible.[6, 50] Several series report cases in children[50–53] the youngest child reported was age 3. Appendiceal carcinoids occur in women twice as often as in men.[54, 55] Most appendiceal carcinoids are less than 1 cm in diameter, and very few are more than 2 cm.[49, 50, 55, 56] The frequency of distant metastases increases with the size of the tumor. Moertel, in his seminal series from 1968,[50] found no metastatic spread from an appendiceal carcinoid less than 2 cm. A few reports have found lymph node metastases from primary tumors less than 2 cm in diameter. Distant metastases from an appendiceal carcinoid less than 1 cm have been reported in only one patient.[57] Conversely, metastatic disease in tumors more than 2 cm in diameter is common.[50–56]

On the basis of these findings, most authors advocate simple appendectomy for appendiceal carcinoids less than 1 cm and right hemicolectomy for appendiceal carcinoids greater than 2 cm. For tumors between 1 and 2 cm, most patients are adequately treated with simple appendectomy. Moertel and associates found no recurrences or metastases after appendectomy in 122 patients who had tumors less than 2 cm in a mean follow-up period of 26 years.[58] Some authors have used criteria such as lymphatic invasion and mesoappendiceal invasion as indicators for right hemicolectomy. The significance of these pathologic findings has not been validated, and most researchers consider them too common to warrant a second more extensive procedure.[59] Indeed, if a simple appendectomy is deemed adequate at initial exploration on the basis of size and absence of regional spread, tumor recurrence has not been documented.[58, 59] The published evidence to date would recommend simple appendectomy for all patients who have tumors less than 2 cm unless local or regional extension of the tumor is evident at initial exploration.

Appendiceal carcinoids have the most favorable prognosis of all carcinoids, probably a result of their tendency to cause symptoms early through appendiceal luminal obstruction and consequent appendicitis. There may also be biologic differences that contribute to the favorable prognosis, but this possibility has not been confirmed. In Modlin and Sandor's review, appendiceal carcinoids had an overall 5-year survival rate of 86%. In only 8.5% were distant metastases present at the time of diagnosis.[6]

Colon

Carcinoids of the colon account for just below 10% of carcinoid tumors. The average age at diagnosis, 65 years, is not significantly different from that of other colon cancers.[6] There appears to be an increasing female-to-male predominance of these lesions (1.5 : 1).[6, 60] Colon carcinoids occur more commonly in the right colon; about two thirds to three quarters occur in the ascending or proximal transverse colon.[60, 61] Colon carcinoids also tend to produce larger lesions, averaging about 5 cm, than most other carcinoids.[61, 62] One in five tumors has a positive silver staining result. These tumors tend to occur in the proximal colon and are probably closely related to typical argentaffin small bowel carcinoids, as both the small bowel and the right colon are derived from the midgut embryologically. The tumors that are argentaffin- and argyrophil-negative are distributed equally throughout the colon.[62]

Symptoms of colonic carcinoids are usually due to bulky, advanced lesions, which may cause malaise, anorexia, and weight loss before localizing symptoms are evident. Fecal occult blood is present in the minority of cases, probably as a result of the submucosal origin of these tumors. Advanced lesions may cause pain or colonic obstruction. Only about 5% initially have evidence of elevated serotonin metabolite levels or carcinoid syndrome.[60] Approximately one third of patients exhibit regional nodal metastases and another third already have distant metastatic disease.[6]

Therapy for colonic carcinoids is straightforward after the initial diagnosis is made. Surgical resection of the primary tumor and the regional lymph node drainage should be performed. No adjuvant treatment has been shown to be effective. The overall 5-year survival rate is 42%, which is slightly worse than the average for all carcinoids combined.[6]

Rectum

Rectal carcinoids constitute approximately 11% of carcinoid tumors. They appear at a slightly younger age than colonic carcinoids (58 years versus 65 years). Men and women are equally affected. Most (85%) are still localized at the time of diagnosis.[6]

Rectal carcinoids usually appear as single nodules, which can range in size from only a few millimeters to larger than 5 cm. Tumors may present with local symptoms of bleeding, pain, or decreased stool caliber, or may present with systemic signs. The systemic signs are usually nonspecific and may include weight loss, changes in bowel habits, or vague abdominal pain. Rectal carcinoids are also commonly detected incidentally.[63, 64] Carcinoid syndrome due to rectal lesions is distinctly uncommon despite the ability of low rectal tumors to secrete hormonal products directly into the systemic circulation.[20]

A study of rectal carcinoids from the Armed Forces Institute of Pathology found that approximately 45% of rectal carcinoids stain positively for serotonin. Pancreatic polypeptide is also commonly expressed (46%); glucagon, gastrin, somatostatin, and ACTH are less often expressed. Carcinoembryonic antigen (CEA) was found in 24%, and the prostatic acid phosphatase result was positive in 82%. Although hindgut carcinoids are often thought of as producing negative results on silver staining, this study found that 55% of tumors were argyrophil and 28% argentaffin.[65]

Rectal carcinoids have been treated by endoscopy by local excision, and by radical excision with either a low anterior or abdominoperineal resection. Rectal carcinoids greater than 2 cm have a 60% to 80% probability of metastasis. Those between 1 and 2 cm have a 10% to 15% probability, and those less than 1 cm have less than a 2% probability of metastatic spread.[20] From these data, many physicians have concluded that local treatment is adequate for lesions less than 2 cm but radical resection should be performed for lesions larger than 2 cm. However, a review of data on 595 patients found that this practice undertreated many patients with metastases. These authors found that invasion of the muscularis propria was a poor prognostic sign. Their data suggested that if all lesions larger than 2 cm, and any smaller lesions showing muscular invasion, were treated by radical excision, only 1.2% of patients would be initially treated inadequately.[66] Endorectal ultrasonography may prove to be a useful adjunct in determining depth of tumor invasion preoperatively.[67]

Other groups have reached a different conclusion regarding radical excision for rectal carcinoids. These authors suggest that if tumors are greater than 2 cm in diameter, if muscular invasion has occurred, or if atypical histologic findings are present, the prognosis is poor and aggressive surgery does not alter the outcome. In one series, all 20 patients who had tumors larger than 2 cm died of the disease. In another series, two out of four patients who had tumors greater than 2 cm survived, but both of these were treated with local excision alone. Both groups concluded that aggressive surgery did not improve outcome of these aggressive tumors.[68, 69] Schindl and associates also noted that small- to medium-sized T1 to T2 lesions (confined to submucosa or muscularis propria) are adequately treated with local excision, but more advanced lesions have a high mortality rate even if aggressive surgery is pursued.[63] These data suggest that underlying tumor biologic characteristics are the primary determinant of outcome in rectal carcinoids and question the utility of radical surgery unless local resection is technically unfeasible. The overall 5-year survival rate for rectal carcinoids is 72%, which is better than that of most GI carcinoids except those arising in the appendix.

METASTATIC CARCINOID AND CARCINOID SYNDROME

Carcinoid Syndrome

Since the description of carcinoid syndrome in the early 1950s, our understanding of this interesting and challenging disease entity has grown considerably.[70–72] The spectrum of disease encountered in carcinoid syndrome is a function of the secretory factors produced by the individual tumor. The factors that are produced vary according to the primary site of the tumor. For example, gastric carcinoids tend to produce more histamine, and midgut tumors mainly tend to produce serotonin.[73] Despite considerable potential variability, the classic or typical carcinoid syndrome is still by far the dominant type encountered clinically. Typically carcinoid syndrome is characterized by flushing, diarrhea, nonspecific abdominal pain, bronchospasm, pellagra-like skin reactions, and progressive right-sided congestive heart failure. In most cases, carcinoid syndrome is related to the presence of hepatic metastases from a midgut primary tumor. However, the disease may result from any carcinoid tumor, primary or metastatic, with a systemically draining blood supply.

TYPICAL CARCINOID SYNDROME. Typical carcinoid syndrome is the most common clinical pattern and is usually caused by metastatic midgut carcinoids. In typical carcinoid syndrome, the amino acid tryptophan is hydroxylated to 5-hydroxytryptophan (5-HTP) and then rapidly decarboxylated by dopa-decarboxylase to serotonin (5-HT). Serotonin is then stored in neurosecretory granules or released into the circulation. Once in the circulation, the enzymes monoamine oxidase and aldehyde dehydrogenase convert serotonin into 5-hydroxyindoleacetic acid (5-HIAA), which is excreted in urine. Patients who have typical carcinoids therefore have elevated plasma and platelet serotonin concentrations as well as increased 5-HIAA in urine.

The atypical carcinoid syndrome is most often associated with foregut carcinoids. In this type of carcinoid syndrome, patients are deficient in the enzyme dopa-decarboxylase, the enzyme responsible for the conversion of 5-HTP to serotonin. Thus, these individuals have high plasma levels of 5-HTP and normal levels of serotonin. Because the kidney is able to decarboxylate some of the excess 5-HTP, urine levels of serotonin may be elevated. 5-HIAA levels are typically normal to slightly elevated.

DIAGNOSIS. Although the diagnosis of carcinoid syndrome relies on an appropriate history of episodic flushing or diarrhea, nonspecific abdominal pain is often the first symptom. Thus, delays in diagnosis are common.[74] Early in the course of the disease, carcinoid syndrome is often misdiagnosed as irritable bowel syndrome, peptic ulcer disease, gastritis, or Crohn's disease.[74] Rarely, symptoms of right-sided heart failure or bronchospasm may be the first manifestation of the syndrome.[75]

To make the diagnosis, most physicians rely on the presence of diarrhea and flushing and a 24-hour urine collection for 5-HIAA. 5-HIAA is typically measured by using high-performance liquid chromatography. Reference values vary among laboratories; the upper limits of normal excretion vary between 6 and 15 mg/day.[76] Levels greater than 25 mg/day are diagnostic of carcinoid syndrome. False-positive results may occur with dietary intake of foods high in serotonin (e.g., walnuts, pecans, bananas, tomatoes); dietary supplements (melatonin or 5-HTP); medications (e.g., guaifenesin, methyldopa, isoniazid); and other disease processes (celiac sprue, tropical sprue, Whipple's disease, and other neuroendocrine tumors[76–78]). Elevations in urinary 5-HIAA excretion due to these noncarcinoid factors are usually mild. Despite these limitations, 5-HIAA urinary excretion remains the most useful test in this disease. Feldman and O'Dorisio reported a 73% sensitivity and a 100% specificity (upper limit of normal = 8 mg/day) in predicting the presence of a systemic draining carcinoid tumor.[79] The level of 5-HIAA generally correlates well with symptoms and provides a useful marker of tumor mass and thus becomes useful in follow-up and the assessment of objective response to treatment. Although serotonin is often the most prominent substance secreted, many others have been identified, including tachykinin, substance P, kallikrein, histamine, dopamine, corticotropin, neurotensin, and chromogranin (see Table 112–1).[22, 79–81] Much less experience in clinical measurement of these factors in carcinoid syndrome patients has been documented.

FLUSHING. The most distinctive feature of carcinoid syndrome is flushing, which is present in 30% to 94% of patients at some time in the course of the disease.[74, 82, 83] The particular pattern of flushing is dependent on tumor location. Flushing from a metastatic midgut carcinoid is characterized by the sudden appearance of a red to purple discoloration of the neck and face. The upper torso may also be involved. These episodes may last from several minutes to hours and are usually associated with an unpleasant sensation of warmth. More rarely, lacrimation, facial and conjunctival edema, palpitations, and hypo- or hypertension can occur in conjunction with flushing.[73] These episodes can be related to a variety of factors including emotional or physical stress, alcohol ingestion, use of medication (calcium, pentagastrin), large meals, or intake of certain foods (e.g., cheeses, chocolate). Bronchial carcinoids tend to produce a different type of flush, which is generally more widespread and intense. This type of flushing has been reported to result in a constant cyanotic hue after prolonged duration of disease. Gastric carcinoids (see Chapter 44) can also produce a unique type of flushing thought to be due to greater levels of histamine release.[84] In this type of flushing, the face and neck are typically involved in a patchy manner. The rash itself is typically erythematous with central clearing and is more frequently pruritic than the lesions associated with the typical foregut or midgut flush. Although flushing is a symptom commonly associated with carcinoid syndrome, the differential diagnosis also includes medullary thyroid carcinoma, pheochromocytoma, idiopathic flushing, anaphylaxis, and mastocytosis. When the cause of flushing is unclear, urinary 5-HIAA measurement can help distinguish carcinoid syndrome from other possible causes.[85, 86]

The biochemical basis of flushing is not completely understood. There are contradictory data concerning the role of serotonin in flushing. One study has observed an increased plasma level of serotonin and norepinephrine during flushing episodes associated with metastatic carcinoids. Furthermore, serotonin levels in the external jugular vein were higher than in the antecubital vein, possibly explaining the characteristic distribution of the flushing.[87] Elevations in serum serotonin concentrations have not, however, been universally observed, and several studies have suggested that serotonin antagonists such as methysergide, ondansetron, and cyproheptadine have little effect on flushing.[87, 88] Others have suggested a role of tachykinins such as substance P in flushing, but this possibility does not completely explain the phenomenon, because elevated levels of substance P have not been universally observed in pentagastrin stimulated flushing episodes.[85, 89]

DIARRHEA. Diarrhea is a common symptom of carcinoid syndrome, affecting 38% to 86% of patients at some time in the course of the disease.[73, 74] Diarrhea most often occurs in conjunction with flushing, but in 10% to 15% of cases it is present alone.[90] The cause of diarrhea in carcinoid syndrome is unclear. Both mechanical and neurohumoral factors (principally serotonin) have been implicated. Diarrhea has been associated with partial bowel obstruction, accelerated small bowel and colonic transit, reduced colonic capacitance, and exaggerated postprandial colonic tone.[91, 92] Unlike in the case of flushing, serotonin antagonists (methysergide maleate, cyproheptadine, ondansetron hydrochloride, ketanserin) are frequently helpful in alleviating diarrhea, suggesting a prominent role of serotonin in the pathogenesis of this portion of the carcinoid syndrome.[89] Ondansetron hydrochloride has

Table 112–3 | **Carcinoid Syndrome: Symptom Prevalence, Mediators of Symptoms, and Treatment**

SYMPTOM	FREQUENCY	PROPOSED MEDIATOR/CAUSE	TREATMENT
Flushing	30%–94%	Tachykinins* Norepinephrine Serotonin? Histamine Bradykinin	• Somatostatin analogs† • H_2 blockers • Parachlorophenylalanine‡ • Aprotinin
Diarrhea	38%–84%	Serotonin Prostaglandins	• Somatostatin analogs† • Serotonin antagonists§ • Loperamide
Abdominal pain	15%–72%	Partial obstruction? Serotonin?	• Surgical correction • Somatostatin analogs?†
Bronchoconstriction	2%–19%	Serotonin Tachykinins* Bradykinin	• Somatostatin analogs† • Glucocorticoids • Ipratropium bromide (inhaled)
Pellagra	2%–5%	Excessive tryptophan conversion	• Niacin supplementation

*Tachykinins include neurokinin A, neuropeptide K, substance P, and vasoactive intestinal polypeptide (VIP).
†Somatostatin analogs include octreotide, octreotide acetate long-acting formulation, and lanreotide acetate.
‡Inhibitor of tryptophan hydroxylase that converts tryptophan to 5-hydroxytryptamine (5-HT).
§Serotonin antagonists include cyproheptadine hydrochloride (Periactin), ketanserin, ondansetron hydrochloride (Zofran), and methysergide maleate.

been particularly effective in treating carcinoid-related diarrhea, apparently through restoration of normal colonic motility.[88, 93]

ADDITIONAL SYMPTOMS. Other symptoms experienced by carcinoid syndrome patients include nonspecific abdominal pain (15% to 72%), cardiac symptoms (45% to 77%), bronchospasm (2% to 19%), and pellagra-like skin reactions associated with niacin deficiency (2% to 5%).[73, 94] Rare manifestations of carcinoid syndrome include Cushing's syndrome caused by corticotropin secretion, depression, anorexia, arthritis, ophthalmologic changes, ureteral obstruction secondary to retroperitoneal fibrosis, and Peyronie's disease.[74, 90, 95, 96] The most common symptoms, their proposed mediators, and treatments are reviewed in Table 112–3.

Special Conditions Associated with Carcinoid Syndrome

CARCINOID HEART DISEASE. Through echocardiography, evidence of cardiac involvement can be identified in 45% to 77% of patients who have carcinoid syndrome.[97–101] Nearly all affected patients have tricuspid valvular lesions. Involvement of the pulmonary valve is also common but is more difficult to identify by two-dimensional echocardiography as a result of extreme shortening and retraction of the pulmonic valve leaflets. Doppler echocardiography, however, frequently identifies both regurgitant and stenotic physiologic characteristics of both right-sided valves. Left-sided cardiac involvement had been thought to occur rarely and primarily in the setting of a patent foramen ovale or pulmonary carcinoids.[97] A 1995 study, however, suggested that mitral and aortic valve involvement is more common than was originally thought.[102] The typical lesions seen in carcinoid heart disease are characterized by thickening and retraction of the involved valve. Histologically, fibrous plaques lacking elastic fibers cover normal endothelium on both chambers and valves, characteristically on the downstream side of the valve.[103] These fibrous plaques cause failure of leaflet coaptation that results in both stenosis and insufficiency.

The diagnosis of carcinoid heart disease may be suggested by signs of right-sided heart failure (jugular venous distention, hepatomegaly, ascites, and peripheral edema) in a patient with carcinoid syndrome. Occasionally, however, symptoms of left-sided heart failure may be the first manifestations of the disease. Rarely, angina pectoris associated with coronary vasospasm may occur.[104, 105] Clinically, carcinoid heart disease may be identified by the characteristic murmurs. One study identified heart murmurs in 92% of patients with echocardiographic evidence of cardiac involvement; 84% of these patients had the murmur of tricuspid regurgitation; 32% had a murmur consistent with pulmonary stenosis; and 31% had the murmur of pulmonary regurgitation.[97] Other studies such as chest radiography and electrocardiography often have abnormal results in these individuals, but the lack of specific findings does not aid in making the diagnosis. Clinical examination and echocardiography are the cornerstones in establishing a diagnosis.

Several authors have suggested a lower survival rate among carcinoid syndrome patients with heart disease than among those without heart disease. Ross and Roberts reported a cardiac mortality rate of 43% in patients with carcinoid heart disease and no cardiac mortality in those with carcinoid syndrome alone.[106] Pellikka and colleagues reported a 3-year survival rate of only 31% for those with carcinoid heart disease, versus 68% for those without heart involvement.[97] Most studies indicate no relationship between duration of symptoms of carcinoid syndrome and development of heart disease.[97, 107] This finding suggests that cardiac involvement in itself may be responsible for a reduced survival rate.

The dominance of right-sided abnormality suggests that carcinoid heart disease may be related to factors secreted by hepatic or nonportal sources of carcinoid tumor into the systemic circulation. Partial metabolism of these secreted factors in the pulmonary circulation would account for the lower incidence of left-sided lesions. Increased serotonin levels have been postulated to lead to valvular and endocardial damage and subsequent fibrosis.[108] In support of this theory, several studies have documented higher levels of either serotonin or urinary 5-HIAA in patients with carcinoid syndrome and carcinoid heart disease, compared with those without heart disease.[97, 100, 107, 109] Interestingly, a number of anorectic agents that increase serum serotonin levels have recently been implicated in valvular heart disease. However, studies of these agents indicate a predominance of left-sided heart valvular disease with prolonged ingestion.[110–112]

Therapy for carcinoid heart disease has been focused in two directions. First, studies have attempted to show that a reduction in circulating serotonin (as measured by decreased urinary 5-HIAA excretion) results in stabilization or regression of cardiac disease. Despite their effectiveness in reducing serotonin concentrations and 5-HIAA excretion, somatostatin analogs have not proved useful in patients followed by serial echocardiography.[97, 107] Second, therapy has been directed at the valves themselves, either replacement or valvuloplasty.[113] The principal indication for operative intervention is valvular dysfunction with signs of progressive right-sided heart failure. Numerous operative strategies have been described, including tricuspid valve replacement alone, combined replacement of both tricuspid and pulmonic valves, and tricuspid replacement combined with pulmonary valvectomy.[103, 109, 110] Several authors have suggested that the carcinoid fibrotic plaques also involve replaced bioprosthetic valves.[114, 115] Most authors recommend valve replacement with mechanical valves as a result of this concern. Although appealing for palliation of symptoms, attempts at surgical valve replacement have been characterized by high perioperative morbidity and mortality rates.[103, 109, 116, 117] Mortality is due primarily to postoperative bleeding or progressive right-sided heart failure. Selected patients have, however, had excellent palliation of symptoms and long-term survival. The right-sided heart failure associated with advanced carcinoid heart disease sometimes complicates surgical treatment of carcinoid disease at other sites. In 1999, two studies reported success with staged valve replacement followed by hepatic resection of carcinoid metastases.[118, 119]

CARCINOID CRISIS. Carcinoid crisis, or the acute exacerbation of carcinoid syndrome, may occur in a number of situations but most commonly in association with surgical or anesthetic stresses. These stresses may include scrubbing of the abdomen prior to surgery, induction of anesthesia, or intraoperative manipulation of the tumor. Hyperglycemia, flushing, hyper- or hypotension, tachyarrhythmias, and refractory bronchospasm, possibly resulting in patient death, may characterize these episodes.[82, 120] All patients with known carcinoid disease should receive somatostatin analogs before surgery. Although many of these patients are already being treated with somatostatin analogs, there is no consensus on the duration of pretreatment necessary for patients who have not been receiving a somatostatin analog preoperatively. Preoperative treatment to the point of symptom control would seem a reasonable end point. Occasionally, the diagnosis of carcinoid syndrome may not be clear before surgical intervention. For individuals in whom carcinoid crisis develops during the operation, early recognition and prompt treatment offer the best chance for successful resolution.

Although most of the symptoms of carcinoid crisis are effectively controlled by somatostatin analog therapy, some such as hyperglycemia may actually be exacerbated by this treatment. Hyperglycemia due either to increased levels of serotonin or treatment with somatostatin analogs is usually easily treated by insulin administration. Flushing by itself is not a problem but often presages other aspects of carcinoid crisis such as cardiovascular instability. Cardiovascular instability is very common in carcinoid syndrome patients undergoing operation. One study has found that 70% of patients whose anesthetic records were examined demonstrated perioperative cardiac instability.[121] Hypertension is usually successfully treated by β blockade, although successful treatment with octreotide and ketanserin has also been reported.[122, 123] Hypotension in individuals with carcinoid syndrome can be very difficult to treat. A study by Ahlman and colleagues has suggested that a provocative infusion of pentagastrin induces release of catecholamines by the adrenal. This in turn activates β adrenoreceptors on enterochromaffin cells, causing the release of large amounts of serotonin into the circulation.[124] This finding is also supported by a clinical observation: most pressors (which are sympathomimetic) are ineffective in treatment of hypotension during carcinoid crisis. These agents may actually aggravate hypotension by increasing peptide release from the tumor.[82] A combination of fluid replacement and intravenous octreotide (10 μg/mL, administered as a slow continuous infusion until symptoms resolve) is therefore the recommended therapy in this situation. Hypotension usually responds within 10 minutes.[82, 121] Patients already treated with octreotide who experience these symptoms seem to benefit from glucocorticoid administration.[124]

Bronchospasm also may be resistant to treatment in individuals with carcinoid crisis for similar reasons. β-Receptor agonists and theophylline may aggravate bronchospasm secondary to adrenergically mediated release of tumor peptides and should therefore be avoided. Nebulized ipratropium bromide, glucocorticoids, and intravenous octreotide are useful in treating such patients.[82]

METASTATIC CARCINOID TUMORS

Identification of Metastatic Disease

The patient who has appropriate signs and symptoms of carcinoid syndrome and an elevated 5-HIAA level should have abdominal imaging directed specifically at the likely primary site of the tumor as well as the liver, because most of these individuals harbor metastatic disease in this location. Conventional imaging, positron emission tomography, and radionuclide imaging are used for this purpose.

COMPUTED TOMOGRAPHY AND MAGNETIC RESONANCE IMAGING. Although computed tomograpy (CT) and magnetic resonance imaging (MRI) are occasionally useful in identifying large primary tumors and regionally involved lymph nodes, they are primarily used to identify metastatic disease. In one study of 80 patients who had histologically verified midgut carcinoids and elevated 5-HIAA levels, initial CT scan results were abnormal in 63 (78%). Hepatic metastases accounted for most of the abnormal scan findings. The CT appearance of these lesions was similar to that

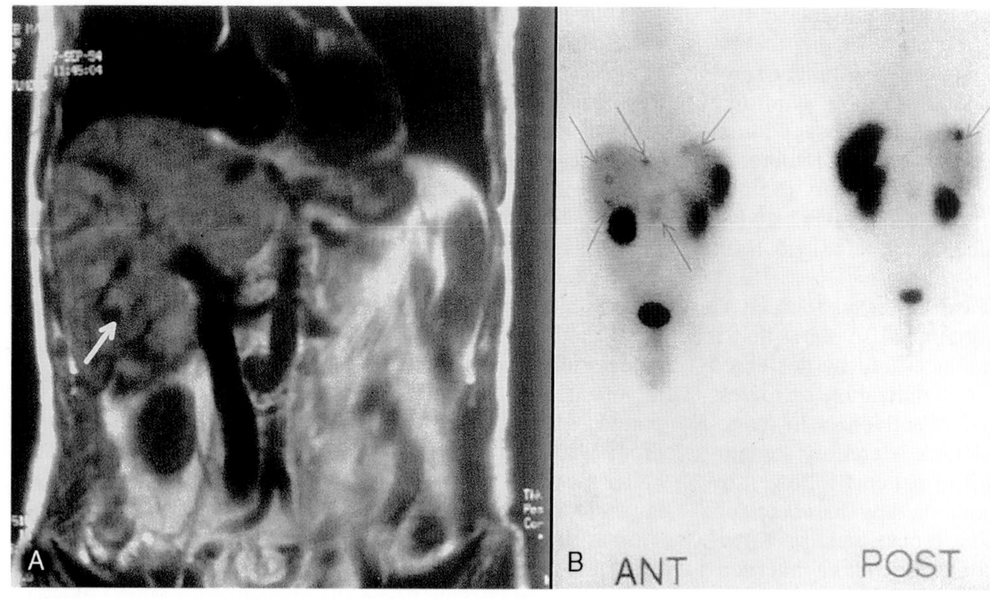

Figure 112–4. *A,* A magnetic resonance imaging scan showing a single focus of metastatic disease *(arrow)* in the right lobe of the liver in a patient with a carcinoid tumor and elevated 5-HIAA. *B,* ^{111}In-labeled pentreotide scan of the same patient, identifying multiple hepatic lesions and two involved para-aortic lymph nodes. These findings were confirmed at laparotomy. Radionuclide activity in the kidneys, spleen, and bladder is evident.

of other hepatic metastases: multiple low-density lesions that are rarely calcified and exhibit variable density after intravenous injection of contrast material.[125] Others have pointed out that carcinoid metastases in the liver are often hypodense compared with the surrounding parenchyma and are best seen on delayed imaging.[126] Some authors prefer to use MRI for abdominal imaging (Fig. 112–4*A*). Advocates of MRI cite improved definition of metastatic disease boundaries within the liver and the lack of need for oral contrast medium, which may aggravate diarrhea in some patients.[75]

POSITRON EMISSION TOMOGRAPHY. Few studies using positron emission tomography (PET) for imaging of patients with metastatic or regionally advanced carcinoid tumors have been reported. This modality is appealing because it allows the identification of disease throughout the body. Early reports are favorable, but more work is required to identify the optimal radiochemical.[127, 128] The expanding availability of PET imaging undoubtedly will lead to more studies in this area.

NUCLEAR MEDICINE. Eighty to 90 percent of carcinoid tumors express high levels of high-affinity receptors for somatostatin.[129] The presence of these high-affinity receptors allows excellent visualization of these tumors with radiolabeled somatostatin analogs. By using this technique it is possible to identify both primary and metastatic carcinoid tumors. Scintigraphy allows not only standard planar imaging, but also single photon emission computed tomography (SPECT). SPECT adds the ability to localize upper abdominal tumors that may be obscured on planar imaging secondary to physiologic uptake by the liver, kidneys, spleen, and bowel.[129, 130] First-generation somatostatin receptor scintigraphy using ^{123}I labeled tyrosine had sensitivity in the range of 50% for liver metastases and 60% for extrahepatic sites.[131] In the 1990s, indium 111 (^{111}In) labeled pentetreotide became available. This agent has several advantages: it is easier to prepare and causes less physiologic upper abdominal interference than ^{123}I labeled tyrosine.[132] Most studies report detection rates in the 80% to 90% range using ^{111}In labeled pentetreotide, which are considerably better than those for use of conventional imaging alone.[130, 133–137] Most studies also suggest that somatostatin receptor scintigraphy typically detects more lesions than conventional imaging and can often identify the correct number and location of lesions (see Fig. 112–4*B*) when conventional imaging fails. Nevertheless, most investigators believe that scintigraphy and conventional imaging with CT or MRI offer complementary information, and often both are used.[129, 130, 134, 135, 138]

False-negative somatostatin analog scintographic study results may occur occasionally, primarily in very small primary tumors (<1 cm), tumors with low numbers of somatostatin receptors, or tumors that have a reduced affinity for somatostatin. False-positive results are rare but may occur in areas of inflammation and occasionally in nonendocrine tumors.[139]

Metaiodobenzylguanidine (M^{131}IBG) is an amine precursor taken up by chromaffin cells and stored in neurosecretory granules. Imaging with M^{131}IBG may therefore theoretically complement somatostatin receptor imaging. A 1996 study of 20 patients examined the potential role of dual scintigraphy with both M^{131}IBG and ^{111}In pentetreotide in identifying carcinoid tumors.[132] Although either test was able to identify 84% of the sites of metastatic disease, the use of both tests increased the overall sensitivity to 95%.[132]

Somatostatin scintigraphy therefore improves the ability to localize sites of carcinoid tumors. Radiolabeled somatostatin analog scintigraphy is particularly helpful in (1) localization of primary occult tumors after failure of conventional imaging (provided that the tumors are larger than 1 cm in diameter); (2) staging of patients with known metastatic disease (because whole-body imaging is possible, it is especially useful for identifying occult disease outside the liver and therefore aids in staging of patients who are being evaluated for possible metastectomy); (3) circumstances in which findings of CT or MRI are equivocal; and (4) prediction of response (improvement in symptoms) to treatment with somatostatin analogs.[129, 133, 138]

RADIOLOGIC IDENTIFICATION OF THE PRIMARY TUMOR. Visualization of the primary tumor is in general more difficult than identification of metastatic disease. Plain abdominal film results are occasionally abnormal. Signs of partial obstruction, a thickened bowel wall, or a mass effect are sometimes noted but are nonspecific. GI contrast studies (enteroclysis or small bowel follow-through) are probably the best radiologic tests for identification of intraluminal disease. As tumors enlarge, CT becomes more useful; both the primary tumor and mesenteric lymph nodes have a characteristic "spokewheel" pattern secondary to desmoplasia.[140, 141] In general, primary tumors must be larger than 1 cm to be detected with any of the presently available scintigraphic studies. For tumors above this size, the ability to localize the primary site improves dramatically. Because of the hypervascular nature of these tumors, mesenteric angiography is sometimes useful when the diagnosis is uncertain after less invasive imaging studies. For patients suspected of having carcinoid syndrome undergoing angiography, pretreatment with somatostatin analogs is highly advisable to prevent incitement of carcinoid crisis.

Treatment of Metastatic Carcinoid Tumors

The diverse biologic behavior of carcinoid tumors is well known. This heterogeneity makes comparisons of survival rate of different treatments difficult outside the context of randomized controlled trials. Relatively few such trials have been performed, and given the infrequency of this tumor, there can be little expectation that such trials will be performed in the future. Interpretation of data on treatment and outcome is further complicated by the frequent grouping of all GI neuroendocrine tumors in reports of therapy. Nevertheless many case reports and series documenting different therapeutic options for metastatic disease patients appear in the literature.

Surgery is the only form of curative therapy for carcinoid syndrome. However, most patients are not candidates for curative treatment. For these individuals the focus of therapy is palliation of symptoms. Numerous therapies are available for this purpose, including surgery, pharmacologic therapy, interventional radiologic therapy, immunotherapy, chemotherapy, and in situ radionuclide therapy. The strategy pursued in treating a patient with carcinoid syndrome secondary to metastatic disease must take into account the location of the metastasis, the course of the patient's disease, and the severity and nature of the patient's symptoms. For the asymptomatic or minimally symptomatic patient, a course of close observation may be entirely appropriate. A treatment algorithm is presented in Table 112–4.

SURGERY FOR HEPATIC METASTASES. Most (50% to 95%) patients displaying symptoms of carcinoid syndrome have hepatic metastases.[74, 142] However, relatively few patients with metastatic carcinoid disease and/or carcinoid syndrome are candidates for curative resection (Fig. 112–5). Most studies indicate that only about 10% of these individuals have disease resectable for cure.[143–145] Suitable candidates for curative resection are those who are medically fit and who have disease confined to a portion or portions of the liver that can be completely resected. The operative mortality rate in most series is below 5%, with a morbidity rate in the 20% to 30% range.[146] These figures are similar to figures available for hepatic metastectomy for colorectal disease.[147] Successful resection, when possible, promises significant long-term palliation and survival.

A potentially attractive option, considering the large number of patients with unresectable, liver-only metastatic carcinoid disease, is orthotopic liver transplantation (OLT). Relatively little experience has been described for OLT for

Table 112–4 | **Algorithm for the Treatment of Metastatic Carcinoid Tumor**

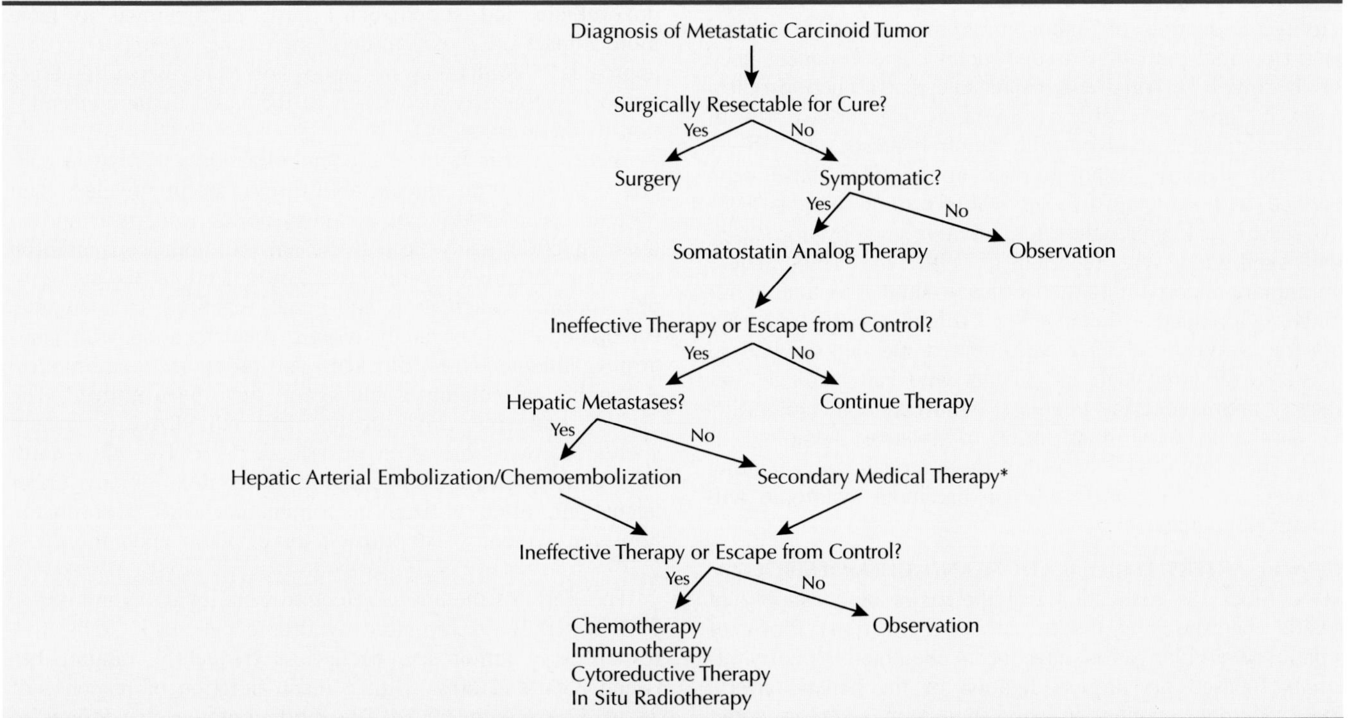

*Secondary medical therapy depends on predominant symptom(s) (see Table 112–3).

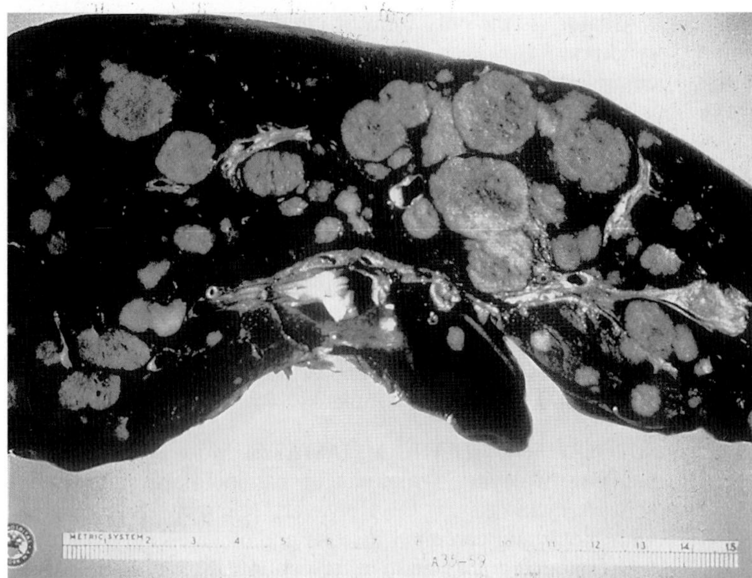

Figure 112–5. Autopsy specimen showing typical widespread hepatic involvement from metastatic midgut carcinoid.

neuroendocrine tumors generally and carcinoid tumors specifically.[143, 148, 149] Fewer than 50 cases of OLT for metastatic carcinoid disease have appeared in the literature.[149] Early series suggested relatively high surgical mortality and recurrence rates.[149–151] Reports in 1997 were more favorable.[148, 149] By 1997 the largest study reported, a multicenter report from France, showed a 69% 5-year survival rate among 15 patients with hepatic metastases from carcinoid tumors treated by OLT.[149]

CYTOREDUCTIVE THERAPY. A number of retrospective series have suggested that cytoreductive therapy, or debulking of carcinoid hepatic metastases, is useful in palliation in selected patients.[146, 152] This form of therapy is appealing because these tumors generally have a protracted course accompanied by disabling symptoms secondary to hormonal activity. Reduction of tumor mass may result in greater pharmacologic palliation or may delay the subsequent need for therapy.[75, 152] Most authors believe that reduction of tumor symptoms, to be effective, requires that at least 90% of the liver grossly involved with tumor be resected.[75, 152, 153] With this therapy, response rates up to 100% have been reported, with symptom-free survival of 6 to 36 months.[152, 153]

Cryosurgical approaches to palliative therapy for carcinoid syndrome were reported in 1997 and 1998. These preliminary reports suggested efficacy similar to that of resective cytoreductive therapy.[154–156] Bilchik reported a symptom-free survival of 10 months and a median survival in excess of 49 months in 19 patients who had medically refractory neuroendocrine tumors (8 with carcinoid tumors).[155] As familiarity with other forms of ablative therapies expands, more reports of the use of these modalities in treating unresectable hepatic metastases in carcinoid syndrome will undoubtedly appear.

HEPATIC ARTERY EMBOLIZATION AND CHEMOEMBOLIZATION. Since the realization that the major blood supply of hepatic metastases is the hepatic artery various forms of hepatic devascularization have been attempted.[157] Early attempts focused on surgical ligation of the hepatic artery. These attempts resulted in only short-term symptom relief and considerable morbidity rates. Interventional techniques now allow for more distal embolization, which limits the chance for rapid neovascularization, decreasing complications and increasing effectiveness.[158]

Given the slowly progressive nature of hepatic metastases from carcinoid tumors, most authors believe that embolization should be reserved for instances in which medical control of symptoms is failing. The primary goal of embolization is to control symptoms. Inhibited tumor growth and prolonged survival are secondary goals.[159] At least one study has suggested a greater response rate and longer duration of response for chemotherapy after hepatic artery occlusion than for occlusion alone. Thus, many of the current studies use a combination: chemotherapy immediately followed by occlusion.[158, 159] Several chemotherapeutic agents (such as doxorubicin and streptozocin) have been shown to have more impact on anoxic tumors, increasing the appeal of this approach.[160] Reduction in blood flow and increased target tissue hypoxia may also result in increased tissue concentration of these drugs.[161]

Inclusion criteria for chemoembolization vary, but in general a patient with unresectable disease occupying less than 50% of hepatic volume, a patent portal vein, near-normal liver function study results, serum bilirubin concentration less than 2.0 mg/dL, and no contraindications to angiography (normal coagulation and renal function) is a suitable candidate. Patients usually require premedication with analgesics, antiemetics, H_2 blockers, and prophylactic antibiotics. A number of techniques and agents have been utilized. The use of both polyvinyl alcohol and ethiodized oil-gelatin sponge particles has been described.[158, 162] The most commonly used chemotherapeutic agent is doxorubicin. Other agents are often utilized in conjunction with doxorubicin, however, including streptozocin or cisplatin and mitomycin C.[158, 159]

This form of therapy is effective in relieving symptoms in 73% to 100% of carcinoid syndrome patients.[162] Objective responses in tumor size occur less frequently, ranging between 33% and 60%, with a mean duration of response of 21 to 42.5 months.[163, 164] The most common side effects of the procedure include nausea, vomiting, pain, and increased serum transaminases.[158] Procedure-related complications are rare but may be life threatening; they include hepatic failure, hepatic abscess, cholecystitis, renal failure, and carcinoid crisis.[162, 165] In one large series of 251 hepatic artery chemoembolizations, there were five fatalities for a 2% mortality rate.[162]

PHARMACOLOGIC THERAPY. Many of the agents used in the control of carcinoid syndrome are directed at serotonin. Inhibitors of serotonin synthesis include methyldopa and parachlorophenylalanine. Parachlorophenylalanine blocks the conversion of tryptophan to 5-HTP; methyldopa partially blocks the conversion of 5-HTP to serotonin. Parachlorophenylalanine is partially effective in controlling symptoms of diarrhea and flushing, but hypersensitivity reactions and psychiatric side effects limit the feasibility of long-term use.[166] There is little clinical experience with use of methyldopa. It occasionally relieves flushing and has a minimal effect on diarrhea.[167] At least seven serotonin receptors have been characterized.[88] Although selective serotonin receptor blockade is possible, there is little consensus concerning which of the specific serotonin receptors it is most important to block to reduce carcinoid symptoms. Methysergide maleate (Sansert) (5-HT_1), cyproheptadine hydrochloride (Periactin) (5-HT_{1+2}), ketanserin (Sufrexal) ($5HT_2$), and ondansetron hydrochloride (Zofran) ($5HT_3$) have all been utilized with some success.[88, 168–170] These agents are generally more successful in controlling GI symptoms than flushing. For example, in a trial of 16 carcinoid syndrome patients, cyproheptadine hydrochloride (which also has antihistaminic and anticholinergic activity) was found to reduce diarrhea by 50% in 58% of patients, but only 17% of patients experienced a 50% improvement in flushing.[168] A 1998 report suggested improved short-term relief of diarrhea but no impact on flushing with ondansetron hydrochloride.[88] The clinical effectiveness of these agents occurs at the expense of considerable side effects. All are associated with dry mouth, sedation, and various psychiatric disturbances.[170]

The use of somatostatin to control flushing associated with carcinoid syndrome was first reported in 1978, and in 1980 a report suggested control of diarrhea as well.[171, 172] However, the short half-life of native somatostatin limited its clinical effectiveness. With the clinical availability of the longer-acting eight amino acid somatostatin analog octreotide, it became possible to treat patients with subcutaneous injections every 8 to 12 hours.

Somatostatin and its analogs are thought to affect carcinoid tumors by partially inhibiting synthesis and release of tumor-produced amines and peptides and by blocking their effect on target tissues.[170] These processes in turn decreases gut motility, blood flow, and both endocrine and exocrine function. Although five somatostatin receptor subtypes have been identified, the clinical efficacy of octreotide appears to be linked to binding of somatostatin receptor subtype 2.[173, 174]

Somatostatin analog therapy is the most effective palliative therapy for carcinoid syndrome patients. Octreotide is very effective in the control of flushing and diarrhea: it is effective in 50% to 87% of carcinoid syndrome patients who display these symptoms.[83, 175–177] Doses in these studies range from 100 to 1000 μg subcutaneously injected three times a day.[83, 175] In an extensive review of all available dose titration data, Harris and Redfern found that a biochemical response occurred with an octreotide dose range between 300 and 375 μg/day. For flushing, there was a direct relationship between control of symptoms and dose of octreotide over the entire range of doses reported (up to 2000 to 3000 μg/day). This same relationship was also observed for diarrhea at up to a 1000-μg/day dose. These findings led these authors to suggest a starting dose of 100 μg three times a day for cases of non–life-threatening carcinoid syndrome and titration of this dose according to relief of symptoms.[178]

Although beneficial in the treatment of diarrhea and flushing, somatostatin analogs have effects on the less frequent symptoms of carcinoid syndrome such as abdominal pain and bronchoconstriction that are unclear. There is also no information on the potential effect of somatostatin analogs on the development and progression of long-term complications of carcinoid syndrome such as carcinoid heart disease and retroperitoneal fibrosis. Studies have suggested that in a number of patients tachyphylaxis to this agent develops.[178, 179] Whether this effect is a function of receptor down-regulation, tumor growth, or changes in intracellular signaling is unclear.[178] Somatostatin analogs have also been associated with several side effects, including abdominal pain, nausea, headache, dizziness, diarrhea, steatorrhea, hyperglycemia, and cholelithiasis.[83, 170, 178]

Several trials have compared octreotide with even longer-acting agents (lanreotide acetate or octreotide acetate long-acting formulation [octreotide LAR, Sandostatin LAR Depot]). Lanreotide acetate, which is not yet available in the United States, may be administered intramuscularly (IM) every 10 to 14 days; octreotide LAR may be given as a monthly IM injection. These studies suggest similar efficacy for octreotide and longer-acting somatostatin analogs in the control of diarrhea and flushing.[83, 176] The longer-acting agents appear to be superior in terms of patient acceptance and cost-effectiveness.[176, 180]

The role of somatostatin analogs in the treatment of metastatic disease to reduce or forestall tumor growth is more controversial. Most studies suggest a modest effect in terms of reduction of tumor burden.[177, 180] However, stabilization of disease is commonly observed.[175, 177] Table 112–5 reviews the utility of somatostatin analog therapy in carcinoid syndrome in five studies.

IMMUNOTHERAPY. The use of interferon in carcinoid tumors was initially prompted by its role in stimulating natural killer cells and the observation that it controlled clinical symptoms in carcinoid syndrome patients.[181] However, the exact mechanism of action of interferon is unknown. Interferon alone has been shown to produce a measurable response in a small number of patients and to control symptoms of diarrhea and flushing in some patients. In a study of 111 patients who had metastatic carcinoids, a median dose of 6 million units of interferon-α was administered subcutaneously five times a week. Tumor size was reduced in 15% and stabilized in 39% of patients, and a biochemical response (reduction in urinary 5-HIAA levels) was observed in 42%. The median duration of response was 34 months.[182] Most other studies have also reported modest effects on tumor volume and control of symptoms.[75] Interferon therapy

Table 112–5 | **Somatostatin Analog in the Treatment of Carcinoid Syndrome**

AUTHOR/ YEAR (REF.)	NUMBER OF PATIENTS	DOSE	AGENT	SYMPTOM CONTROL		REDUCTION IN URINARY 5-HIAA	REGRESSION OF TUMOR/ STABILIZATION
				Flushing	Diarrhea		
Kvols et al., 1986 (177)	25	150 μg SC tid	Octreotide	79%	76%	72% (>50% Reduction)	0/13 Partial response; 61% stabilization
Ruszniewski et al., 1996 (180)	39	30 mg IM q 14 days	Lanreotide acetate	38%*	29%*	18% (>50% Reduction)	Not assessed
Eriksson et al., 1996 (194)	35 (32 Carcinoid syndrome)	1.5–3.0 mg/24 hr continuous SC	Octastatin (RC-160)	~20% Complete amelioration of carcinoid syndrome		20% (>50% Reduction)	2% Partial response; 76% stabilization at 3 months; 68% at 6 months
	19 (13 Carcinoid syndrome)	3.0 g SC qid	Lanreotide acetate	Not assessed		54% (>50% Reduction)	0/19 Partial responses; 90% stabilization
Rubin et al., 1999 (83)	26	100–300 μg SC tid	Octreotide	Complete or partial success† 58.3%		27%§	Not assessed
	22	10 mg IM q 4 wk	Octreotide LAR‡	Complete or partial success† 66.7%		5%§	Not assessed
	20	20 mg IM q 4 wk	Octreotide LAR‡	Complete or partial success† 71.4%		54%§	Not assessed
	25	30 mg IM q 4 wk	Octreotide LAR‡	Complete or partial success† 61.9%		7%§	Not assessed
O'Toole et al., 2000 (176)	33	200 μg SC bid or tid	Octreotide	68%	50%	50% (25% Reduction)	Not assessed
		30 mg IM q 10 days	Lanreotide acetate	54%	45%	58% (25% Reduction)	Not assessed

*Complete disappearance of symptom.
†Defined as control of symptoms with no rescue (additional SC octreotide) needed or less than two rescue doses per day for 5 days over a 3-week period.
‡Octreotide acetate long-acting formulation.
§Median percentage reduction from median 5-HIAA levels obtained during baseline washout.
5-HIAA, 5-hydroxyindoleacetic acid.

is associated with numerous side effects, including flulike symptoms, anorexia, fatigue, and autoimmune-like reactions resulting in a lupus-like syndrome and thyroiditis.[183, 184]

In 1999, a more favorable response rate using interferon combined with octreotide was reported. Twenty-one patients were enrolled in this trial; nine had carcinoid syndrome. Disease stabilization occurred in five of these latter nine patients, in whom tumor growth had been progressive prior to combined therapy. The median duration of this response was just under 20 months.[183] Oberg reported that combined therapy rarely resulted in reduction of tumor volume but had a significant effect on clinical symptoms and that interferon-α was better tolerated when given in combination with octreotide.[184] The exact role of interferon therapy for carcinoid syndrome remains to be determined.

CHEMOTHERAPY. Numerous studies in which chemotherapeutic agents were used in an attempt to control metastatic carcinoids have been reported. Interpretation of these studies is hampered by the inclusion of several types of neuroendocrine tumors in each study. Most reports, however, suggest response rates of less than 25%, with a short duration of response (<12 months)[166, 184–189] (Table 112–6). In an attempt to improve the modest gains observed with single-

Table 112–6 | **Selected Chemotherapy Trials for Treatment of Metastatic Carcinoid Tumors**

AUTHOR/YEAR (REF.)	NUMBER OF PATIENTS	AGENT(S)	OVERALL RESPONSE	MEDIAN DURATION OF RESPONSE
Moertel 1983 (166)	19	5-FU	26%	3 Months
Engstrom et al., 1984 (185)	81	Doxorubicin	21%	6.5 Months
	80	Streptozocin/5-FU	22%	7.75 Months
Bukowski et al., 1987 (186)	56	Streptozocin/cyclophosphamide/ Doxorubicin/5-FU	31%	5 Months
Moertel et al., 1991 (189)	13	Etoposide/cisplatin	0%	—
Oberg and Eriksson, 1991 (182)	111	Interferon-α	15% (Partial) 39% (Stable disease)	34 Months
Saltz et al., 1993 (187)	20	Carboplatin	0%	—
Bukowski et al., 1994 (188)	56	DTIC	16%	2.75 Months
Frank et al., 1999 (183)	9	Octreotide/interferon-α	56%	20 Months

DTIC, dimethyltriazenoimidfazole carboxamide (dacarbazine); 5-FU, 5-fluorouracil.

agent therapy, regimens of combination chemotherapy have also been employed. In many cases, when these regimens are compared with single agents, there is increased toxicity for very modest improvements in response rate, and the duration of response remains short. Because at present, chemotherapy has shown marginal benefit in patients who have metastatic carcinoids and there are excellent medications available for palliation of symptoms, chemotherapy should be reserved for symptomatic patients for whom more effective forms of palliative therapy are unsuccessful. Perhaps one exception is the case of anaplastic neuroendocrine carcinomas. These carcinomas are thought to be poorly differentiated variants of carcinoid tumors. Because of the observation that these tumors seem to be similar to small cell lung cancer and the favorable response rate to etoposide and cisplatin seen with this lung tumor, this regimen was used in a small series of patients with anaplastic neuroendocrine carcinoma. Therapy yielded a response rate of 67%, including three complete responses. For these patients, the median duration of response was 8 months.[189]

RADIOTHERAPY. External beam irradiation is rarely used as adjuvant therapy but has proved useful in palliation in cases of metastases to bone or central nervous system.[190] Given the high percentage of metastatic carcinoid tumors with somatostatin receptors and the generally high tumor-to-background ratios seen with diagnostic indium-labeled pentetreotide, it is not surprising that several centers are experimenting with in situ radiopharmaceutical treatment of these tumors.[191, 192] Although ^{111}In is a gamma emitter, its biologic effectiveness has been attributed to the emission of Auger electrons. The proposed mechanism of action is uptake of the radioligand into the tumor cell nucleus. In this location, ^{111}In Auger electron emissions cause critical deoxyribonucleic acid (DNA) damage, resulting in apoptosis.[191, 192] In addition to uptake by the tumor, ^{111}In is also concentrated in the kidney and spleen (Fig. 112-4*B*). The long-term effects of high doses of ^{111}In on these organs are unknown. Early studies have reported hematologic toxicities, especially thrombocytopenia, and recommend careful monitoring for bone marrow toxicity after therapy.[191, 192] Other radioligands are also being evaluated. Yttrium has been used with some success.[90, 193] The long-term outcomes for these patients are unknown, but this represents a new potential therapy for these difficult but fascinating tumors.

REFERENCES

1. Oberndorfer S: Karzinoide Tumoren des Dünndarms. Frankf Z Pathol 1:425–429, 1907.
2. Lubarsch O: Über den primären Krebs des Ileum, nebst Bemerkungen über das gleichzeitige Vorkommen von Krebs und Tuberkolose. Virchows Arch 111:280–317, 1888.
3. Janmohamed S, Bloom SR: Carcinoid tumours [review]. Postgrad Med J 73:207–214, 1997.
4. Delcore R, Friesen SR: Gastrointestinal neuroendocrine tumors [review]. J Am Coll Surg 178:187–211, 1994.
5. Caplin ME, Buscombe JR, Hilson AJ, et al: Carcinoid tumour [review]. Lancet 352:799–805, 1998.
6. Modlin IM, Sandor A: An analysis of 8305 cases of carcinoid tumors. Cancer 79:813–829, 1997.
7. Timmins PF, Kuo DY, Anderson PS, et al: Ovarian carcinoid: Management of primary and recurrent tumors. Gynecol Oncol 76:112–114, 2000.
8. Yokoyama Y, Fujioka S, Kato K, et al: Primary carcinoid tumor of the gallbladder: Resection of a case metastasizing to the liver and analysis of outcomes [review]. Hepatogastroenterology 47:135–139, 2000.
9. Chamberlain RS, Blumgart LH: Carcinoid tumors of the extrahepatic bile duct: A rare cause of malignant biliary obstruction. Cancer 86: 1959–1965, 1999.
10. Fukai I, Masaoka A, Fujii Y, et al: Thymic neuroendocrine tumor (thymic carcinoid): A clinicopathologic study in 15 patients. Ann Thorac Surg 67:208–211, 1999.
11. Glazier DB, Murphy DP, Barnard N, et al: Primary carcinoid tumour of the testis. BJU Int 83:153–154, 1999.
12. Kehagias D, Moulopoulos L, Smirniotis V, et al: Imaging findings in primary carcinoid tumour of the liver with gastrin production. Br J Radiol 72:207–209, 1999.
13. Koch CA, Azumi N, Furlong MA, et al: Carcinoid syndrome caused by an atypical carcinoid of the uterine cervix. J Clin Endocrinol Metab 84:4209–4213, 1999.
14. Ng JW, Liu KW, Mak KO: Carcinoid tumour of the spleen. Aust N Z J Surg 69:70–72, 1999.
15. Jablon LK, Somers RG, Kim PY: Carcinoid tumor of the breast: Treatment with breast conservation in three patients. Ann Surg Oncol 5:261–264, 1998.
16. Ferlito A, Barnes L, Rinaldo A, et al: A review of neuroendocrine neoplasms of the larynx: Update on diagnosis and treatment [review]. J Laryngol Otol 112:827–834, 1998.
17. Veenhof CH, de Wit R, Taal BG, et al: A dose-escalation study of recombinant interferon-alpha in patients with a metastatic carcinoid tumour. Eur J Cancer 28:75–78, 1992.
18. Newton JN, Swerdlow AJ, Dos SSI, et al: The epidemiology of carcinoid tumours in England and Scotland. Br J Cancer 70:939–942, 1994.
19. Cotran RS, Kumar V, Robbins SL: Robbins' Pathologic Basis of Disease, 5th ed. Philadelphia, WB Saunders, 1994, pp 818–820.
20. Mani S, Modlin IM, Ballantyne G, et al: Carcinoids of the rectum [review]. J Am Coll Surg 179:231–248, 1994.
21. Soga J, Tazawa K: Pathologic analysis of carcinoids: Histologic reevaluation of 62 cases. Cancer 28:990–998, 1971.
22. Yang K, Ulich T, Cheng L, et al: The neuroendocrine products of intestinal carcinoids: An immunoperoxidase study of 35 carcinoid tumors stained for serotonin and eight polypeptide hormones. Cancer 51:1918–1926, 1983.
23. Capella C, Heitz PU, Hofler H, et al: Revised classification of neuroendocrine tumors of the lung, pancreas and gut [review]. Digestion 55 (suppl 3):11–23, 1994.
24. O'Connor DT, Deftos LJ: Secretion of chromogranin A by peptide-producing endocrine neoplasms. N Engl J Med 314:1145–1151, 1986.
25. Goebel SU, Serrano J, Yu F, et al: Prospective study of the value of serum chromogranin A or serum gastrin levels in the assessment of the presence, extent, or growth of gastrinomas. Cancer 85:1470–1483, 1999.
26. Nobels FR, Kwekkeboom DJ, Coopmans W, et al: Chromogranin A as serum marker for neuroendocrine neoplasia: Comparison with neuron-specific enolase and the alpha-subunit of glycoprotein hormones. J Clin Endocrinol Metab 82:2622–2628, 1997.
27. Eriksson B, Arnberg H, Oberg K, et al: A polyclonal antiserum against chromogranin A and B—a new sensitive marker for neuroendocrine tumours. Acta Endocrinol (Copenh) 122:145–155, 1990.
28. Janson ET, Holmberg L, Stridsberg M, et al: Carcinoid tumors: Analysis of prognostic factors and survival in 301 patients from a referral center. Ann Oncol 8:685–690, 1997.
29. Williams ED, Sandler M: The classification of carcinoid tumours. Lancet 1:238–239, 1963.
30. Al-Khafaji B, Noffsinger AE, Miller MA, et al: Immunohistologic analysis of gastrointestinal and pulmonary carcinoid tumors. Hum Pathol 29:992–999, 1998.
31. Lindberg GM, Molberg KH, Vuitch MF, et al: Atypical carcinoid of the esophagus: A case report and review of the literature [review]. Cancer 79:1476–1481, 1997.
32. Modlin IM, Sandor A, Tang LH, et al: A 40-year analysis of 265 gastric carcinoids. Am J Gastroenterol 92:633–638, 1997.
33. Maurer CA, Baer HU, Dyong TH, et al: Carcinoid of the pancreas: Clinical characteristics and morphological features [review]. Eur J Cancer 32A:1109–1116, 1996.
34. Kirshbom PM, Kherani AR, Onaitis MW, et al: Foregut carcinoids: A clinical and biochemical analysis. Surgery 126:1105–1110, 1999.

35. Makhlouf HR, Burke AP, Sobin LH: Carcinoid tumors of the ampulla of Vater: A comparison with duodenal carcinoid tumors. Cancer 85: 1241–1249, 1999.
36. Hatzitheoklitos E, Buchler MW, Friess H, et al: Carcinoid of the ampulla of Vater: Clinical characteristics and morphologic features [review]. Cancer 73:1580–1588, 1994.
37. Noda Y, Watanabe H, Iwafuchi M, et al: Carcinoids and endocrine cell micronests of the minor and major duodenal papillae: Their incidence and characteristics. Cancer 70:1825–1833, 1992.
38. Attanoos R, Williams GT: Epithelial and neuroendocrine tumors of the duodenum [review]. Semin Diagn Pathol 8:149–162, 1991.
39. Burke AP, Federspiel BH, Sobin LH, et al: Carcinoids of the duodenum: A histologic and immunohistochemical study of 65 tumors. Am J Surg Pathol 13:828–837, 1989.
40. Burke AP, Sobin LH, Federspiel BH, et al: Carcinoid tumors of the duodenum: A clinicopathologic study of 99 cases. Arch Pathol Lab Med 114:700–704, 1990.
41. Klein A, Clemens J, Cameron J: Periampullary neoplasms in von Recklinghausen's disease [review]. Surgery 106:815–819, 1989.
42. North JH, Pack MS: Malignant tumors of the small intestine: A review of 144 cases. Am Surg 66:46–51, 2000.
43. Burke AP, Thomas RM, Elsayed AM, et al: Carcinoids of the jejunum and ileum: An immunohistochemical and clinicopathologic study of 167 cases. Cancer 79:1086–1093, 1997.
44. Moertel CG, Sauer WG, Dockerty MB, et al: Life history of the carcinoid tumor of the small intestine. Cancer 14:901–912, 1961.
45. Guo Z, Li Q, Wilander E, et al: Clonality analysis of multifocal carcinoid tumours of the small intestine by X-chromosome inactivation analysis. J Pathol 190:76–79, 2000.
46. Wangberg B, Westberg G, Tylen U, et al: Survival of patients with disseminated midgut carcinoid tumors after aggressive tumor reduction. World J Surg 20:892–899, 1996.
47. Makridis C, Rastad J, Oberg K, et al: Progression of metastases and symptom improvement from laparotomy in midgut carcinoid tumors. World J Surg 20:900–906, 1996.
48. Makridis C, Oberg K, Juhlin C, et al: Surgical treatment of mid-gut carcinoid tumors. World J Surg 14:377–383, 1990.
49. Connor SJ, Hanna GB, Frizelle FA: Appendiceal tumors: Retrospective clinicopathologic analysis of appendiceal tumors from 7,970 appendectomies. Dis Colon Rectum 41:75–80, 1998.
50. Moertel CG, Dockerty MB, Judd ES: Carcinoid tumors of the vermiform appendix. Cancer 21:270–278, 1968.
51. Jonsson T, Johannsson JH, Hallgrimsson JG: Carcinoid tumors of the appendix in children younger than 16 years: A retrospective clinical and pathologic study. Acta Chir Scand 155:113–116, 1989.
52. Parkes SE, Muir KR, al Sheyyab M, et al: Carcinoid tumours of the appendix in children 1957–1986: Incidence, treatment and outcome. Br J Surg 80:502–504, 1993.
53. Gorbon B, Taspinar AH: Bir appendiks karsinoidinin sebeb oldugu karaciger metastazi. Turk Tip Cem Mec 29:602–607, 1963.
54. Sandor A, Modlin IM: A retrospective analysis of 1570 appendiceal carcinoids. Am J Gastroenterol 93:422–428, 1998.
55. Roggo A, Wood WC, Ottinger LW: Carcinoid tumors of the appendix [review]. Ann Surg 217:385–390, 1993.
56. Bowman GA, Rosenthal D: Carcinoid tumors of the appendix. Am J Surg 146:700–703, 1983.
57. MacGillivray DC, Heaton RB, Rushin JM, et al: Distant metastasis from a carcinoid tumor of the appendix less than one centimeter in size. Surgery 111:466–471, 1992.
58. Moertel CG, Weiland LH, Nagorney DM, et al: Carcinoid tumor of the appendix: Treatment and prognosis. N Engl J Med 317:1699–1701, 1987.
59. Thirlby RC, Kasper CS, Jones RC: Metastatic carcinoid tumor of the appendix: Report of a case and review of the literature. Dis Colon Rectum 27:42–46, 1984.
60. Rosenberg JM, Welch JP: Carcinoid tumors of the colon: A study of 72 patients. Am J Surg 149:775–779, 1985.
61. Berardi RS: Carcinoid tumors of the colon (exclusive of the rectum): Review of the literature [review]. Dis Colon Rectum 15:383–391, 1972.
62. Spread C, Berkel H, Jewell L, et al: Colon carcinoid tumors: A population-based study. Dis Colon Rectum 37:482–491, 1994.
63. Schindl M, Niederle B, Hafner M, et al: Stage-dependent therapy of rectal carcinoid tumors. World J Surg 22:628–633, 1998.
64. Jetmore AB, Ray JE, Gathright JBJ, et al: Rectal carcinoids: The most frequent carcinoid tumor. Dis Colon Rectum 35:717–725, 1992.
65. Federspiel BH, Burke AP, Sobin LH, et al: Rectal and colonic carcinoids: A clinicopathologic study of 84 cases. Cancer 65:135–140, 1990.
66. Naunheim KS, Zeitels J, Kaplan EL, et al: Rectal carcinoid tumors—treatment and prognosis. Surgery 94:670–676, 1983.
67. Yoshida M, Tsukamoto Y, Niwa Y, et al: Endoscopic assessment of invasion of colorectal tumors with a new high-frequency ultrasound probe. Gastrointest Endosc 41:587–592, 1995.
68. Koura AN, Giacco GG, Curley SA, et al: Carcinoid tumors of the rectum: Effect of size, histopathology, and surgical treatment on metastasis free survival. Cancer 79:1294–1298, 1997.
69. Sauven P, Ridge JA, Quan SH, et al: Anorectal carcinoid tumors: Is aggressive surgery warranted? Ann Surg 211:67–71, 1990.
70. Thorson A, Bjork G, Bjorkman G, et al: Malignant carcinoid of the small intestine with metastasis to the liver, valvular disease of the right heart (pulmonary stenosis and tricuspid regurgitation without septal defect), peripheral vasomotor symptoms, bronchoconstriction and an unusual type of cyanosis. Am Heart J 47:794, 1954.
71. Isler P, Hedinger C: Metastasierendes Dunndarmcarcinom mit schweren vorwiegend das rechte Herz betreffenden Klappenfehlern und Pulmonalstenose ein eigenartiger Symptomkomplex. Schweiz Med Wochenschr 83:4, 1953.
72. Rosenbaum FF, Santer DG, Claudon DB: Essential telangiectasia, pulmonic and tricuspid stenosis, and neoplastic liver disease: A possible new clinical syndrome. J Lab Clin Med 42:941, 1953.
73. Creutzfeldt W: Carcinoid tumors: Development of our knowledge [review]. World J Surg 20:126–131, 1996.
74. Bax ND, Woods HF, Batchelor A, et al: Clinical manifestations of carcinoid disease [review]. World J Surg 20:142–146, 1996.
75. Kvols LK: Metastatic carcinoid tumors and the malignant carcinoid syndrome [review]. Ann N Y Acad Sci 733:464–470, 1994.
76. Nuttall KL, Pingree SS: The incidence of elevations in urine 5-hydroxyindoleacetic acid. Ann Clin Lab Sci 28:167–174, 1998.
77. Tormey WP, FitzGerald RJ: The clinical and laboratory correlates of an increased urinary 5-hydroxyindoleacetic acid [review]. Postgrad Med J 71:542–545, 1995.
78. Deacon AC: The measurement of 5-hydroxyindoleacetic acid in urine [review]. Ann Clin Biochem 31:215–232, 1994.
79. Feldman JM, O'Dorisio TM: Role of neuropeptides and serotonin in the diagnosis of carcinoid tumors. Am J Med 81:41–48, 1986.
80. Emson PC, Gilbert RF, Martensson H, et al: Elevated concentrations of substance P and 5-HT in plasma in patients with carcinoid tumors. Cancer 54:715–718, 1984.
81. Bergstrom M, Theodorsson E, Norheim I, et al: Immunoreactive tachykinins in 24-h collections of urine from patients with carcinoid tumours: Characterization and correlation with plasma concentrations. Scand J Clin Lab Invest 55:679–689, 1995.
82. Vaughan DJ, Brunner MD: Anesthesia for patients with carcinoid syndrome [review]. Int Anesthesiol Clin 35:129–142, 1997.
83. Rubin J, Ajani J, Schirmer W, et al: Octreotide acetate long-acting formulation versus open-label subcutaneous octreotide acetate in malignant carcinoid syndrome. J Clin Oncol 17:600–606, 1999.
84. Roberts LJ, Marney SRJ, Oates JA: Blockade of the flush associated with metastatic gastric carcinoid by combined histamine H1 and H2 receptor antagonists: Evidence for an important role of H2 receptors in human vasculature. N Engl J Med 300:236–238, 1979.
85. Vinik AI, Gonin J, England BG, et al: Plasma substance-P in neuroendocrine tumors and idiopathic flushing: The value of pentagastrin stimulation tests and the effects of somatostatin analog. J Clin Endocrinol Metab 70:1702–1709, 1990.
86. Metcalfe DD: Differential diagnosis of the patient with unexplained flushing/anaphylaxis [review]. Allergy Asthma Proc 21:21–24, 2000.
87. Matuchansky C, Launay JM: Serotonin, catecholamines, and spontaneous midgut carcinoid flush: Plasma studies from flushing and nonflushing sites. Gastroenterology 108:743–751, 1995.
88. Wymenga AN, De Vries EG, Leijsma MK, et al: Effects of ondansetron on gastrointestinal symptoms in carcinoid syndrome. Eur J Cancer 34:1293–1294, 1998.
89. Ahlman H, Dahlstrom A, Gronstad K, et al: The pentagastrin test in the diagnosis of the carcinoid syndrome: Blockade of gastrointestinal symptoms by ketanserin. Ann Surg 201:81–86, 1985.
90. Feldman JM: Carcinoid tumors and the carcinoid syndrome [review]. Curr Probl Surg 26:835–885, 1989.
91. Saslow SB, O'Brien MD, Camilleri M, et al: Octreotide inhibition of flushing and colonic motor dysfunction in carcinoid syndrome. Am J Gastroenterol 92:2250–2256, 1997.

92. von der Ohe MR, Camilleri M, Kvols LK, et al: Motor dysfunction of the small bowel and colon in patients with the carcinoid syndrome and diarrhea [published erratum appears in N Engl J Med 329(21): 1592, 1993]. N Engl J Med 329:1073–1078, 1993.
93. von der Ohe MR, Camilleri M, Kvols LK: A 5HT3 antagonist corrects the postprandial colonic hypertonic response in carcinoid diarrhea. Gastroenterology 106:1184–1189, 1994.
94. Arnold R: Medical treatment of metastasizing carcinoid tumors [review]. World J Surg 20:203–207, 1996.
95. Thorson A: Studies on carcinoid disease. Acta Med Scand 334:81, 1958.
96. Grahame-Smith DG: The carcinoid syndrome. London, William Heineman Medical Books, 1972.
97. Pellikka PA, Tajik AJ, Khandheria BK, et al: Carcinoid heart disease: Clinical and echocardiographic spectrum in 74 patients. Circulation 87:1188–1196, 1993.
98. Lundin L, Landelius J, Andren B, et al: Transoesophageal echocardiography improves the diagnostic value of cardiac ultrasound in patients with carcinoid heart disease. Br Heart J 64:190–194, 1990.
99. Howard RJ, Drobac M, Rider WD, et al: Carcinoid heart disease: Diagnosis by two-dimensional echocardiography. Circulation 66:1059–1065, 1982.
100. Lundin L, Norheim I, Landelius J, et al: Carcinoid heart disease: Relationship of circulating vasoactive substances to ultrasound-detectable cardiac abnormalities. Circulation 77:264–269, 1988.
101. Moyssakis IE, Rallidis LS, Guida GF, et al: Incidence and evolution of carcinoid syndrome in the heart. J Heart Valve Dis 6:625–630, 1997.
102. Jacobsen MB, Nitter-Hauge S, Bryde PE, et al: Cardiac manifestations in mid-gut carcinoid disease. Eur Heart J 16:263–268, 1995.
103. Roberts WC: A unique heart disease associated with a unique cancer: Carcinoid heart disease [review]. Am J Cardiol 80:251–256, 1997.
104. Mehta AC, Rafanan AL, Bulkley R, et al: Coronary spasm and cardiac arrest from carcinoid crisis during laser bronchoscopy. Chest 115: 598–600, 1999.
105. RuDusky BM: Carcinoid—a diagnostic and therapeutic dilemma [letter; comment]. Chest 116:1142–1143, 1999.
106. Ross EM, Roberts WC: The carcinoid syndrome: Comparison of 21 necropsy subjects with carcinoid heart disease to 15 necropsy subjects without carcinoid heart disease. Am J Med 79:339–354, 1985.
107. Denney WD, Kemp WEJ, Anthony LB, et al: Echocardiographic and biochemical evaluation of the development and progression of carcinoid heart disease. J Am Coll Cardiol 32:1017–1022, 1998.
108. Ferrans VJ, Roberts WC: The carcinoid endocardial plaque: An ultrastructural study. Hum Pathol 7:387–409, 1976.
109. Robiolio PA, Rigolin VH, Harrison JK, et al: Predictors of outcome of tricuspid valve replacement in carcinoid heart disease. Am J Cardiol 75:485–488, 1995.
110. Connolly HM, Crary JL, McGoon MD, et al: Valvular heart disease associated with fenfluramine-phentermine [published erratum appears in N Engl J Med 337(24):1783, 1997]. N Engl J Med 337:581–588, 1997.
111. Weissman NJ, Tighe JFJ, Gottdiener JS, et al: An assessment of heart-valve abnormalities in obese patients taking dexfenfluramine, sustained-release dexfenfluramine, or placebo: Sustained-Release Dexfenfluramine Study Group. N Engl J Med 339:725–732, 1998.
112. Jick H, Vasilakis C, Weinrauch LA, et al: A population-based study of appetite-suppressant drugs and the risk of cardiac-valve regurgitation. N Engl J Med 339:719–724, 1998.
113. Wright PW, Mulder DG: Carcinoid heart disease: Report of a case treated by open heart surgery. Am J Cardiol 12:864–868, 1963.
114. Ridker PM, Chertow GM, Karlson EW, et al: Bioprosthetic tricuspid valve stenosis associated with extensive plaque deposition in carcinoid heart disease. Am Heart J 121:1835–1838, 1991.
115. Ohri SK, Schofield JB, Hodgson H, et al: Carcinoid heart disease: Early failure of an allograft valve replacement [review]. Ann Thorac Surg 58:1161–1163, 1994.
116. Knott-Craig CJ, Schaff HV, Mullany CJ, et al: Carcinoid disease of the heart: Surgical management of ten patients. J Thorac Cardiovasc Surg 104:475–481, 1992.
117. Connolly HM, Nishimura RA, Smith HC, et al: Outcome of cardiac surgery for carcinoid heart disease. J Am Coll Cardiol 25:410–416, 1995.
118. McDonald ML, Nagorney DM, Connolly HM, et al: Carcinoid heart disease and carcinoid syndrome: Successful surgical treatment. Ann Thorac Surg 67:537–539, 1999.
119. Wu F, McCall J, Holdaway I: Surgical palliation of carcinoid syndrome [letter]. Aust N Z J Med 29:840, 1999.
120. Dougherty TB, Cronau LH Jr: Anesthetic implications for surgical patients with endocrine tumors. Int Anesthesiol Clin 36:31–44, 1998.
121. Veall GR, Peacock JE, Bax ND, et al: Review of the anaesthetic management of 21 patients undergoing laparotomy for carcinoid syndrome [review]. Br J Anaesth 72:335–341, 1994.
122. Warner RR, Mani S, Profeta J, et al: Octreotide treatment of carcinoid hypertensive crisis [review]. Mt Sinai J Med 61:349–355, 1994.
123. Hughes EW, Hodkinson BP: Carcinoid syndrome: The combined use of ketanserin and octreotide in the management of an acute crisis during anaesthesia. Anaesth Intensive Care 17:367–370, 1989.
124. Ahlman H, Nilsson O, Wangberg B, et al: Neuroendocrine insights from the laboratory to the clinic [review]. Am J Surg 172:61–67, 1996.
125. Sugimoto E, Lorelius LE, Eriksson B, et al: Midgut carcinoid tumours: CT appearance. Acta Radiol 36:367–371, 1995.
126. Woodard PK, Feldman JM, Paine SS, et al: Midgut carcinoid tumors: CT findings and biochemical profiles. J Comput Assist Tomogr 19: 400–405, 1995.
127. Hoegerle S, Nitzsche EU, Stumpf A, et al: Incidental appendix carcinoid: Value of somatostatin receptor imaging. Clin Nucl Med 22:467–469, 1997.
128. Sundin A, Eriksson B, Bergstrom M, et al: Demonstration of [11C]5-hydroxy-L-tryptophan uptake and decarboxylation in carcinoid tumors by specific positioning labeling in positron emission tomography. Nucl Med Biol 27:33–41, 2000.
129. Anthony LB, Martin W, Delbeke D, et al: Somatostatin receptor imaging: Predictive and prognostic considerations. Digestion 57(suppl 1): 50–53, 1996.
130. Krenning EP, Kooij PP, Pauwels S, et al: Somatostatin receptor: Scintigraphy and radionuclide therapy. Digestion 57(suppl 1):57–61, 1996.
131. Kwekkeboom DJ, Krenning EP, Bakker WH, et al: Somatostatin analogue scintigraphy in carcinoid tumours. Eur J Nucl Med 20:283–292, 1993.
132. Taal BG, Hoefnagel CA, Valdes OR, et al: Combined diagnostic imaging with ^{131}I-metaiodobenzylguanidine and ^{111}In-pentetreotide in carcinoid tumours. Eur J Cancer 32A:1924–1932, 1996.
133. Krausz Y, Bar-Ziv J, de Jong RB, et al: Somatostatin-receptor scintigraphy in the management of gastroenteropancreatic tumors. Am J Gastroenterol 93:66–70, 1998.
134. Kwekkeboom DJ, Krenning EP: Somatostatin receptor scintigraphy in patients with carcinoid tumors. World J Surg 20:157–161, 1996.
135. Ahlman H, Tisell LE, Wangberg B, et al: Somatostatin receptor imaging in patients with neuroendocrine tumors: Preoperative and postoperative scintigraphy and intraoperative use of a scintillation detector. Semin Oncol 21:21–28, 1994.
136. Olsen JO, Pozderac RV, Hinkle G, et al: Somatostatin receptor imaging of neuroendocrine tumors with indium-111 pentetreotide (Octreoscan) [review]. Semin Nucl Med 25:251–261, 1995.
137. Jamar F, Fiasse R, Leners N, et al: Somatostatin receptor imaging with indium-111-pentetreotide in gastroenteropancreatic neuroendocrine tumors: Safety, efficacy and impact on patient management. J Nucl Med 36:542–549, 1995.
138. Lobrano MB, McCarthy K, Adams L, et al: Metastatic carcinoid tumor imaged with CT and a radiolabeled somatostatin analog: A case report. Am J Gastroenterol 92:513–515, 1997.
139. Krenning EP, Bakker WH, Breeman WA, et al: Localisation of endocrine-related tumours with radioiodinated analogue of somatostatin. Lancet 1:242–244, 1989.
140. Wallace S, Ajani JA, Charnsangavej C, et al: Carcinoid tumors: Imaging procedures and interventional radiology [review]. World J Surg 20:147–156, 1996.
141. Buckley JA, Fishman EK: CT evaluation of small bowel neoplasms: Spectrum of disease. Radiographics 18:379–392, 1998.
142. Crasset V, Delcourt E: Facial flushes and diarrhoea. Postgrad Med J 73:337–338, 1997.
143. Frilling A, Rogiers X, Knofel WT, et al: Liver transplantation for metastatic carcinoid tumors. Digestion 55(suppl 3):104–106, 1994.
144. Ahlman H: The role of surgery in patients with advanced midgut carcinoid tumours. Digestion 57(suppl 1):86–87, 1996.
145. Ihse I, Persson B, Tibblin S: Neuroendocrine metastases of the liver [review]. World J Surg 19:76–82, 1995.
146. Que FG, Nagorney DM, Batts KP, et al: Hepatic resection for metastatic neuroendocrine carcinomas. Am J Surg 169:36–42, 1995.

147. Fong Y, Salo J: Surgical therapy of hepatic colorectal metastasis [review]. Semin Oncol 26:514–523, 1999.
148. Lang H, Oldhafer KJ, Weimann A, et al: Liver transplantation for metastatic neuroendocrine tumors [review]. Ann Surg 225:347–354, 1997.
149. Le Treut YP, Delpero JR, Dousset B, et al: Results of liver transplantation in the treatment of metastatic neuroendocrine tumors: A 31-case French multicentric report [review]. Ann Surg 225:355–364, 1997.
150. Anthuber M, Jauch KW, Briegel J, et al: Results of liver transplantation for gastroenteropancreatic tumor metastases. World J Surg 20:73–76, 1996.
151. Bechstein WO, Neuhaus P: Liver transplantation for hepatic metastases of neuroendocrine tumors. Ann N Y Acad Sci 733:507–514, 1994.
152. McEntee GP, Nagorney DM, Kvols LK, et al: Cytoreductive hepatic surgery for neuroendocrine tumors. Surgery 108:1091–1096, 1990.
153. Galland RB, Blumgart LH: Carcinoid syndrome: Surgical management. Br J Hosp Med 35:166–170, 1986.
154. Johnson LB, Krebs T, Wong YC, et al: Cryosurgical debulking of unresectable liver metastases for palliation of carcinoid syndrome. Surgery 121:468–470, 1997.
155. Bilchik AJ, Sarantou T, Foshag LJ, et al: Cryosurgical palliation of metastatic neuroendocrine tumors resistant to conventional therapy. Surgery 122:1040–1047, 1997.
156. Shapiro RS, Shafir M, Sung M, et al: Cryotherapy of metastatic carcinoid tumors. Abdom Imaging 23:314–317, 1998.
157. Markovitz J: The hepatic artery. Surg Gynecol Obstet 95:644, 1952.
158. Drougas JG, Anthony LB, Blair TK, et al: Hepatic artery chemoembolization for management of patients with advanced metastatic carcinoid tumors. Am J Surg 175:408–412, 1998.
159. Ruszniewski P, Malka D: Hepatic arterial chemoembolization in the management of advanced digestive endocrine tumors. Digestion 62(suppl 1):79–83, 2000.
160. Roche A: Hepatic chemo-embolization [in French] [review]. Bull Cancer 76:1029–1037, 1989.
161. Taourel P, Dauzat M, Lafortune M, et al: Hemodynamic changes after transcatheter arterial embolization of hepatocellular carcinomas. Radiology 191:189–192, 1994.
162. Gates J, Hartnell GG, Stuart KE, et al: Chemoembolization of hepatic neoplasms: Safety, complications, and when to worry [review]. Radiographics 19:399–414, 1999.
163. Ruszniewski P, Rougier P, Roche A, et al: Hepatic arterial chemoembolization in patients with liver metastases of endocrine tumors: A prospective phase II study in 24 patients. Cancer 71:2624–2630, 1993.
164. Diaco DS, Hajarizadeh H, Mueller CR, et al: Treatment of metastatic carcinoid tumors using multimodality therapy of octreotide acetate, intra-arterial chemotherapy, and hepatic arterial chemoembolization [review]. Am J Surg 169:523–528, 1995.
165. Sakamoto I, Aso N, Nagaoki K, et al: Complications associated with transcatheter arterial embolization for hepatic tumors. Radiographics 18:605–619, 1998.
166. Moertel CG: Treatment of the carcinoid tumor and the malignant carcinoid syndrome [review]. J Clin Oncol 1:727–740, 1983.
167. Jensen RT, Norton JA: Carcinoid tumors and the carcinoid syndrome. In DeVita VT Jr, Hellman S, Rosenberg SA (eds): Cancer: Principles and Practice of Oncology, 5th ed. Philadelphia, Lippincott-Raven, 1997, pp 1704–1723.
168. Moertel CG, Kvols LK, Rubin J: A study of cyproheptadine in the treatment of metastatic carcinoid tumor and the malignant carcinoid syndrome. Cancer 67:33–36, 1991.
169. Gustafsen J, Lendorf A, Raskov H, et al: Ketanserin versus placebo in carcinoid syndrome: A clinical controlled trial. Scand J Gastroenterol 21:816–818, 1986.
170. Gregor M: Therapeutic principles in the management of metastasising carcinoid tumors: Drugs for symptomatic treatment [review]. Digestion 55(suppl 3):60–63, 1994.
171. Frolich JC, Bloomgarden ZT, Oates JA, et al: The carcinoid flush: Provocation by pentagastrin and inhibition by somatostatin. N Engl J Med 299:1055–1057, 1978.
172. Dharmsathaphorn K, Sherwin RS, Cataland S, et al: Somatostatin inhibits diarrhea in the carcinoid syndrome. Ann Intern Med 92:68–69, 1980.
173. Patel YC, Srikant CB: Subtype selectivity of peptide analogs for all five cloned human somatostatin receptors (hsstr 1–5). Endocrinology 135:2814–2817, 1994.
174. Kubota A, Yamada Y, Kagimoto S, et al: Identification of somatostatin receptor subtypes and an implication for the efficacy of somatostatin analogue SMS 201-995 in treatment of human endocrine tumors. J Clin Invest 93:1321–1325, 1994.
175. di Bartolomeo M, Bajetta E, Buzzoni R, et al: Clinical efficacy of octreotide in the treatment of metastatic neuroendocrine tumors: A study by the Italian Trials in Medical Oncology Group. Cancer 77: 402–408, 1996.
176. O'Toole D, Ducreux M, Bommelaer G, et al: Treatment of carcinoid syndrome: A prospective crossover evaluation of lanreotide versus octreotide in terms of efficacy, patient acceptability, and tolerance. Cancer 88:770–776, 2000.
177. Kvols LK, Moertel CG, O'Connell MJ, et al: Treatment of the malignant carcinoid syndrome: Evaluation of a long-acting somatostatin analogue. N Engl J Med 315:663–666, 1986.
178. Harris AG, Redfern JS: Octreotide treatment of carcinoid syndrome: Analysis of published dose-titration data [review]. Aliment Pharmacol Ther 9:387–394, 1995.
179. Moertel CG: Karnofsky memorial lecture: An odyssey in the land of small tumors. J Clin Oncol 5:1502–1522, 1987.
180. Ruszniewski P, Ducreux M, Chayvialle JA, et al: Treatment of the carcinoid syndrome with the long-acting somatostatin analogue lanreotide: A prospective study in 39 patients. Gut 39:279–283, 1996.
181. Oberg K, Funa K, Alm G: Effects of leukocyte interferon on clinical symptoms and hormone levels in patients with mid-gut carcinoid tumors and carcinoid syndrome. N Engl J Med 309:129–133, 1983.
182. Oberg K, Eriksson B: The role of interferons in the management of carcinoid tumors. Acta Oncol 30:519–522, 1991.
183. Frank M, Klose KJ, Wied M, et al: Combination therapy with octreotide and alpha-interferon: Effect on tumor growth in metastatic endocrine gastroenteropancreatic tumors. Am J Gastroenterol 94:1381–1387, 1999.
184. Oberg K: Interferon-alpha versus somatostatin or the combination of both in gastro-enteropancreatic tumours. Digestion 57(suppl 1):81–83, 1996.
185. Engstrom PF, Lavin PT, Moertel CG, et al: Streptozocin plus fluorouracil versus doxorubicin therapy for metastatic carcinoid tumor. J Clin Oncol 2:1255–1259, 1984.
186. Bukowski RM, Johnson KG, Peterson RF, et al: A phase II trial of combination chemotherapy in patients with metastatic carcinoid tumors: A Southwest Oncology Group Study. Cancer 60:2891–2895, 1987.
187. Saltz L, Lauwers G, Wiseberg J, et al: A phase II trial of carboplatin in patients with advanced APUD tumors. Cancer 72:619–622, 1993.
188. Bukowski RM, Tangen CM, Peterson RF, et al: Phase II trial of dimethyltriazenoimidazole carboxamide in patients with metastatic carcinoid: A Southwest Oncology Group Study. Cancer 73:1505–1508, 1994.
189. Moertel CG, Kvols LK, O'Connell MJ, et al: Treatment of neuroendocrine carcinomas with combined etoposide and cisplatin: Evidence of major therapeutic activity in the anaplastic variants of these neoplasms. Cancer 68:227–232, 1991.
190. Schupak KD, Wallner KE: The role of radiation therapy in the treatment of locally unresectable or metastatic carcinoid tumors. Int J Radiat Oncol Biol Phys 20:489–495, 1991.
191. McCarthy KE, Woltering EA, Espenan GD, et al: In situ radiotherapy with ^{111}In-pentetreotide: Initial observations and future directions. Cancer J Sci Am 4:94–102, 1998.
192. Tiensuu JE, Eriksson B, Oberg K, et al: Treatment with high dose [(111)In-DTPA-D-PHE1]-octreotide in patients with neuroendocrine tumors—evaluation of therapeutic and toxic effects. Acta Oncol 38: 373–377, 1999.
193. Otte A, Mueller-Brand J, Dellas S, et al: Yttrium-90-labelled somatostatin-analogue for cancer treatment [letter]. Lancet 351:417–418, 1998.
194. Eriksson B, Janson ET, Bax ND, et al: The use of new somatostatin analogues, lanreotide and octastatin, in neuroendocrine gastro-intestinal tumours. Digestion 57(suppl 1):77–80, 1996.

Chapter 113

Small Intestinal Neoplasms

Anil K. Rustgi

EPIDEMIOLOGY

Small bowel neoplasms are uncommon. Benign and malignant neoplasms of the small bowel account for only a small fraction of all gastrointestinal neoplasms. Approximately two thirds of small bowel neoplasms are malignant and thus comprise 1.1% to 2.4% of gastrointestinal malignancies.[1–5] Fewer than 2500 cases of small bowel cancer are diagnosed annually in the United States, and fewer than 1000 patients succumb to their disease annually.[1–5] The most common malignant small bowel neoplasms are adenocarcinomas, carcinoids, lymphomas, and sarcomas.[6, 7] Adenocarcinoma, the most common small bowel malignancy, has an annual incidence in the United States of 3.9 cases per million persons.[7] The majority of patients are in their 50s or 60s at the time of diagnosis. Carcinoids (see Chapter 112) are the second most frequently diagnosed small intestinal malignancy, with an annual incidence of 2.9 cases per million persons in the United States and an average age at diagnosis of 55 to 60 years. The most common sites of extranodal lymphomas are the stomach and small intestine (see Chapter 26). Benign small bowel neoplasms include adenomas, lipomas, and leiomyomas, among others. Table 113–1 provides a classification of benign and malignant small bowel neoplasms.

PATHOLOGY

Neoplasms of the small intestine can arise from any of the cells that make up this organ. Adenomas and adenocarcinomas are derived from mucosal glands, leiomyomas and leiomyosarcomas arise from the smooth muscle, and carcinoids arise from argentaffin cells. Nerve sheath cells give rise to neurilemmomas and malignant schwannomas, and neurons are the site of origin of neurofibromas and neurofibrosarcomas. The vasculature gives rise to hemangiomas and angiosarcomas. Fibromas and fibrosarcomas are derived from fibroblasts. Finally, lymphomas originate from lymphocytes in the mucosa and Peyer's patches.

Adenocarcinomas comprise 35% to 50% of all primary malignant small intestinal neoplasms, followed by carcinoid tumors (20% to 40% of malignancies), lymphomas (14%), and sarcomas (11% to 13%).[8, 9] Small intestinal lymphomas (discussed in Chapter 26) are usually more common in the terminal ileum; adenocarcinomas more often arise proximally; carcinoid tumors (see Chapter 112) are almost always diagnosed in the ileum; and sarcomas are distributed evenly throughout the small intestine, with a slight predilection for the jejunum. Approximately 75% of primary small bowel carcinoids are less than 1.5 cm in diameter at the time of diagnosis. Approximately 30% of patients with carcinoid tumors have multifocal disease.

Benign neoplasms may be found throughout the small intestine, but some patterns are apparent. For example, adenomas are distributed evenly throughout the small intestine, although there is a slightly higher frequency of these lesions in the duodenum and ileum. Fibromas and lipomas are more common in the ileum, and 80% to 90% of hemangiomas and neurofibromas are distributed evenly between the jejunum and ileum. Adenomas arise from mucosal glands, and although they initiate as sessile growths, they become polypoid in most instances. Adenomas account for approximately one third of all benign small intestinal neoplasms. These lesions may be divided into tubular, villous, and tubulovillous adenomas on the basis of histologic examination. Villous adenomas are not as common as tubular neoplasms but are usually larger; they are more often sessile, located in the second portion of the duodenum, and have undergone malignant degeneration at the time of diagnosis in 40% to 45% of cases.

Leiomyomas are benign smooth muscle neoplasms that originate from the smooth muscle wall of the muscularis mucosa or muscularis propria. They account for up to 40% of benign small intestinal neoplasms. These lesions may grow intraluminally, extraluminally, or both. As they grow, leiomyomas may undergo necrosis and hemorrhage, which can be severe at times. Histologically, there are bundles of spindle-shaped smooth muscle cells with rare or absent mitoses; more than two mitoses per high-powered field or any nuclear pleomorphism is indicative of a leiomyosarcoma. Lipomas arise from the submucosa and tend to grow intraluminally, most often in the ileum. These lesions rarely bleed, but if large enough, they may cause intestinal obstruction and intussusception (Fig. 113–1).

Table 113–1 | **Small Intestinal Neoplasms**

BENIGN
Adenoma
Leiomyoma
Lipoma
Lymphangioma
Fibroma
Hemangioma
Neurofibroma
Neurilemmoma
MALIGNANT
Adenocarcinoma
Carcinoid
Sarcoma
Leiomyosarcoma
Liposarcoma
Fibrosarcoma
Neurofibrosarcoma
Angiosarcoma
Lymphoma
Low-grade B cell lymphoma
Immunoproliferative small intestinal neoplasms
Enteropathy-associated T-cell lymphoma
Metastatic

ETIOLOGY AND RISK FACTORS

Although the small intestine comprises nearly 75% of the entire gastrointestinal tract and approximately 90% of the mucosal surface, paradoxically only 1% of gastrointestinal adenocarcinomas arise from the small bowel. There is no single hypothesis or set of experimental data to explain the paucity of small bowel adenocarcinomas compared with colonic, gastric, and esophageal adenocarcinomas. Speculation has revolved around the following conditions in the small intestine that could reduce the rate of malignancy[10]: (1) less bacteria, especially anaerobic species, which convert bile acids to carcinogens; (2) increased luminal pH; (3) mucosal hydrolases, such as benzpyrene hydroxylase, which convert carcinogens into less active moieties; (4) rapid transit through the small bowel, which may limit contact between potential carcinogens and the mucosa; (5) dilution of carcinogens in the liquid chyme of the small intestine; (6) differential rates of mucosal cell turnover between the small and large intestines; and (7) higher concentrations of secretory IgA and mucosal T lymphocytes.

Experimental evidence supports the notion that the small intestine affords a protective milieu against malignant transformation. For example, in the BDF1 mouse, exposure to various carcinogens incites apoptosis (programmed cell death) in the stem cell compartment of small intestinal crypts, whereas damaged stem cells of colonic crypts survive and proliferate, with only limited apoptosis.[11] Moreover, comparison of specific DNA adducts (a reflection of DNA damage) from the mucosa of human small intestine and colon obtained at surgery has led to the observation that total DNA adducts are nearly 30 times greater in the large versus small intestine.[12] DNA adducts are crucial in malignant neoplastic development and progression. It has been noted that in the inbred mouse strain B10.O20, small intestinal adenocarcinomas develop after exposure in utero to *N*-ethyl-*N*-nitrosourea, whereas such neoplasms do not develop in other mouse strains. A putative gene that may account for this phenomenon, called *ssic1* (for susceptibility to small intestinal cancer), maps to the distal arm of mouse chromosome 4,[13] a locus that is in close proximity to the *Mom-1* (*mo*difer *o*f *m*in) gene.[14] *Mom-1* plays a role in the development of small and large intestinal tumors in mice with murine intestinal neoplasia,[15] a disorder somewhat analogous to human familial adenomatous polyposis (FAP). In contrast, in humans with FAP, colonic polyposis predominates and small intestinal neoplasms are less common.

Insights into the pathogenesis of malignant small intestinal neoplasms have been gained through molecular genetic approaches. Detailed analysis of small bowel adenocarcinomas reveals a profile reminiscent of colonic adenocarcinomas; specifically, Ki-ras and p53 mutations can be found in adenocarcinomas at both sites.[16–18] Small intestinal sarcomas, part of the spectrum of gastrointestinal stromal tumors (GISTs), harbor mutations in the c-kit oncogene, the functional consequence of which is aberrant cell growth.[19]

Small Bowel Adenocarcinoma

Despite the low incidence of malignant small intestinal neoplasms, several factors have been identified that contribute to

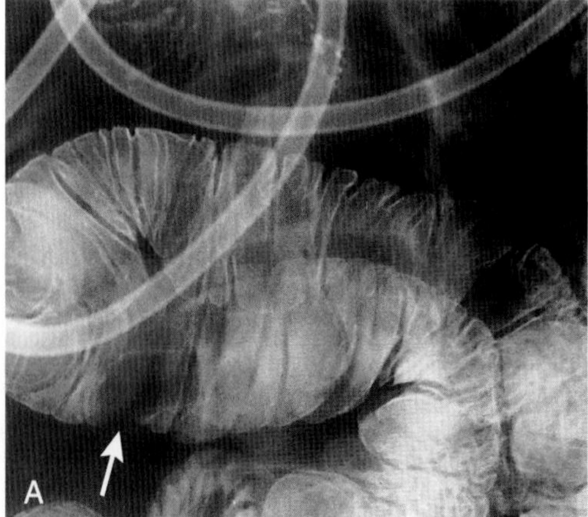

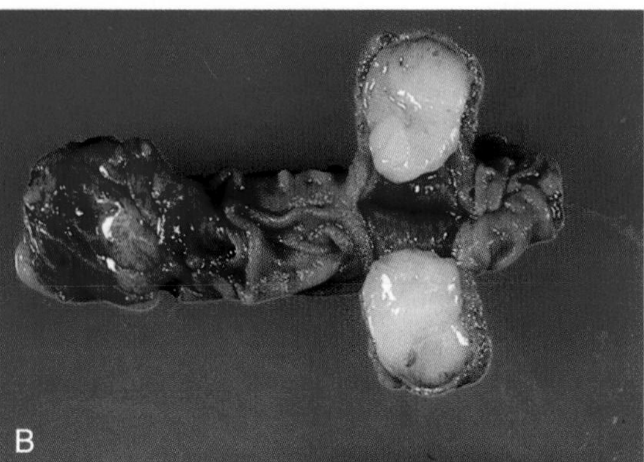

Figure 113–1. *A*, Enteroclysis demonstrating a smooth, submucosal lesion that was found to be lipoma *(arrow)*. *B*, Surgical resection specimen of a lipoma from another patient who presented with intussusception and bleeding. (Courtesy of Igor Laufer, MD, Hospital of the University of Pennsylvania, Philadelphia, PA.)

the development of these tumors. Small intestinal adenocarcinomas are more common in populations that consume diets high in animal fat and protein.[20, 21] There is a twofold increase in the relative risk of small bowel adenocarcinomas in patients who eat red meat at least once a week, although the risk does not increase with further increases in meat intake. There is a correlation between the occurrence of small bowel adenocarcinomas and ingestion of smoked or cured foods, with an odds ratio of 1.7:1 if such foods have been eaten one to three times per month and an odds ratio of 2.1:1 if they have been consumed daily. No association between fruit and vegetable consumption or use of tobacco or alcohol has been observed. Several carcinogens, including bracken fern, *N*-methyl-*N*-nitro-*N*-nitrosoguanidine, and 3-di-(hydroxymethyl)amino-6(5-nitro-2-furylethylanyl)-1,2,4-triazine, have been associated with the development of small bowel adenomas and adenocarcinomas in rodent models.[22] Bile acids may play a role in the development of small bowel adenocarcinoma, especially in the duodenum.[23] In patients with FAP, adenomatous polyps develop within the duodenum and around the ampulla of Vater. Adenocarcinomas of the proximal small bowel are the leading cause of cancer death in patients who have undergone colectomy for FAP.[24, 25]

Small bowel adenocarcinomas appear to progress through an adenoma-adenocarcinoma sequence, and all small bowel adenomas should be regarded as precancerous lesions.[26] Approximately one third of all spontaneous small bowel adenomas contain a malignant component, although the percentage varies greatly among published studies.[27] Those neoplasms located at the ampulla of Vater are larger, more likely to be villous rather than tubular, and more likely to undergo malignant transformation.[28–30] Other etiologic factors for the development of small bowel adenocarcinomas are Crohn's disease (Chapter 103),[31–33] celiac sprue (Chapter 93),[34] and hereditary nonpolyposis colorectal cancer (Chapter 114).[35]

Patients with Peutz-Jeghers syndrome develop hamartomatous polyps in the small and large intestines in addition to the hallmark orocutaneous melanin spots (Chapter 114).[36] These polyps are especially common in the jejunum, and adenocarcinoma can arise in adenomatous foci in such polyps.

CLINICAL PRESENTATION

Most small intestinal neoplasms are not associated with symptoms and are diagnosed either late in their course or incidentally at laparotomy or autopsy. The general absence of symptoms can be ascribed to the distensibility of the small bowel wall and the liquid nature of luminal contents. If a lesion (or lesions) leads to symptoms, the presentation depends on the pathology of the neoplasm and its location. At least 50% of benign lesions remain asymptomatic, whereas 70% to 90% of malignant lesions are associated with symptoms. However, no symptoms or signs are specific for either benign or malignant tumors, and even though the duration of symptoms tends to be shorter for patients with a malignancy, months may elapse before a diagnosis is made.

If a lesion becomes large enough, a patient may present with crampy periumbilical pain, bloating, and nausea with emesis resulting from mechanical small bowel obstruction. Small bowel obstruction is the most common presentation for benign lesions and occurs in as many as 70% of patients. Obstruction may result from either luminal constriction or intussusception. In fact, a benign small bowel neoplasm is the most common cause of intussusception in adults. Whereas adenomas, adenocarcinomas, and lymphomas tend to encroach on the lumen, other lesions may grow centripetally, often becoming large before a diagnosis is made; these lesions may also cause volvulus. As many as 80% of malignant tumors are associated with abdominal pain, although the pain is not caused by obstruction. Back pain in a patient with a primary malignant small bowel lesion suggests spread to the retroperitoneum.

Gastrointestinal bleeding, usually chronic, is the second most common symptom and occurs in 20% to 50% of patients with benign lesions but less commonly in patients with malignant lesions. Massive hemorrhage is more common with sarcomas than with carcinomas, carcinoid tumors, or lymphomas. Weight loss is rare in patients with benign lesions but is noted in 50% of patients with malignancies. Intestinal perforation is also rare in patients with benign lesions but occurs in 10% of patients with sarcomas and lymphomas. Periampullary lesions may result in jaundice or pancreatitis. In patients with carcinoid tumors, symptoms of the carcinoid syndrome typically do not develop in the absence of hepatic metastases, and even with hepatic lesions, 28% to 50% of patients with such tumors are free of the carcinoid syndrome (Chapter 112).

The physical examination may be unrevealing, although up to 25% of patients with small intestinal malignancies may have a palpable abdominal mass. Twenty-five percent of patients with malignancy may also present with the findings of obstruction—distention, loud borborygmi, a palpable mass, and diffuse mild to moderate abdominal tenderness. Some patients may have a positive fecal occult blood test result, and some may present with jaundice secondary to either biliary obstruction or hepatic replacement by metastases. Cachexia, hepatomegaly, and ascites may be present in patients with advanced metastatic disease.

DIAGNOSIS

Laboratory studies are of limited utility in the diagnosis of small intestinal neoplasms, especially in patients with localized disease. In patients with gastrointestinal blood loss, microcytic anemia eventually develops. Patients with biliary tract compromise have elevated serum alkaline phosphatase and bilirubin levels, and those with extensive hepatic disease have elevated lactate dehydrogenase and aminotransferase levels and decreased serum albumin levels. The only tumor marker that has been evaluated routinely in patients with small inestinal neoplasms, especially those with adenocarcinoma, is the serum carcinoembryonic antigen, which usually is not elevated in the absence of hepatic metastases. Similarly, for patients with carcinoid tumors, 5-hydroxyindole acetic acid (5-HIAA) is a useful marker but is cleared by the liver after the first pass from the primary tumor, and levels in urine are not elevated until hepatic metastases are extensive. There are specific immunoperoxidase (staining) and cell surface (flow cytometry) markers for lymphomas (see Chapter 26).

Abdominal plain films are usually nondiagnostic, although in patients with an acute presentation they may reveal obstruction or free subdiaphragmatic air. Barium contrast studies remain the primary radiographic means of diagnosing a small bowel neoplasm, and an upper gastrointestinal (UGI) series with a small bowel follow-through (SBFT) study is an optimal way to locate and possibly define small intestinal lesions.[37] The UGI with SBFT series is abnormal in approximately 50% to 80% of patients and can define neoplasms in 30% to 44% of cases; this figure increases to 90% if an enteroclysis study (small bowel enema) is performed.[38, 39] Barium enema may demonstrate abnormalities of the terminal ileum if there is sufficient reflux through the ileocecal valve.

Small bowel adenocarcinomas are associated with intraluminal lesions, often with an "apple-core" appearance similar to that seen with colorectal carcinomas, and with ulceration (Fig. 113–2). Sarcomas tend to produce an intraluminal "bulge," although the overlying mucosa is intact, and there is usually a large extraluminal component that displaces loops of bowel. A carcinoid tumor can have the appearance of focal mural nodularity, typically in the distal ileum. However, progressive disease is associated with fixation of bowel loops and loss of normal mucosal patterns, which may mimic Crohn's disease or fibrosis. Lymphomas may demonstrate a variety of appearances, including multiple nodules or polyps, a spruelike pattern, or intraluminal or extraluminal masses with possible fistula formation (see Chapter 26). Benign lesions typically appear as submucosal filling defects.

Abdominal computed tomography facilitates localization of small bowel abnormalities and is especially useful for detecting extraluminal disease. However, it is suboptimal for detecting small intraluminal or mucosal lesions. Ultrasound and magnetic resonance imaging do not have major roles in the diagnosis of small bowel lesions.

Angiography is of limited value except for delineating vascular lesions, such as carcinoids, hemangiomas, and smooth muscle tumors. A technetium-labeled red blood cell scan is also helpful in locating the source of gastrointestinal bleeding but alone cannot diagnose the presence of a neoplasm.

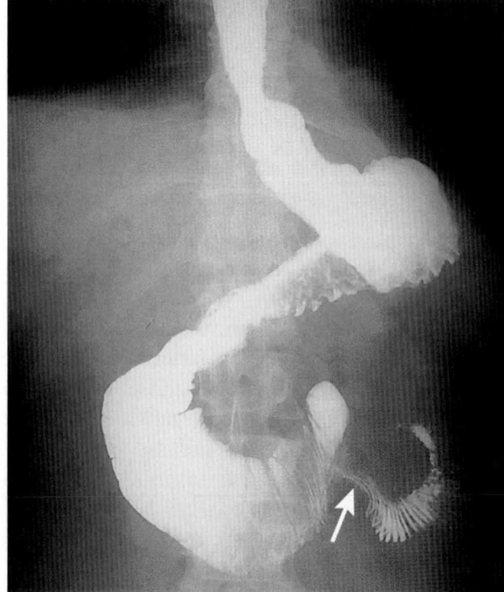

Figure 113–2. Small bowel follow-through series demonstrating an apple-core lesion *(arrow)* that was found to be adenocarcinoma. (Courtesy of Igor Laufer, MD, Hospital of the University of Pennsylvania, Philadelphia, PA.)

Endoscopic evaluation is usually limited to the duodenum, which may be visualized through either a forward or sideviewing endoscope.[40] Likewise, the terminal ileum may be visualized via colonoscopy. Small bowel enteroscopy is helpful as a supplement to barium studies. In addition, enteroscopy is useful in the evaluation of patients with gastrointestinal bleeding caused by a benign or malignant small bowel tumor. Intraoperative enteroscopy may be useful in selected cases. Future directions may involve use of swallowed radio-telemetry capsules that transmit images of the bowel wall.[41]

MANAGEMENT

Benign Neoplasms

Therapy of benign small intestinal neoplasms usually consists of resection, either via an endoscope or at laparotomy, as determined by the size, growth pattern, and location of the lesion. Most adenomas may be resected segmentally, although if there is any evidence of malignant degeneration, the margins of resection should be extended and draining lymph nodes should be excised. Pedunculated duodenal adenomas may be snared through the endoscope and removed. If an adenoma involves the ampulla, it may be necessary to perform a sphincterotomy or sphincteroplasty after local resection to reduce the risk of postoperative stricture formation of the biliary ductal tree. Larger periampullary or ampullary lesions, which are more likely to harbor malignancy, and any questionable lesions may require pancreaticoduodenectomy (Whipple's procedure). Patients must undergo periodic surveillance following removal of an adenoma, especially one of villous histology, because there is a significant chance of recurrence; however, survival is excellent for these patients. Endoscopic ultrasound is a useful supplement to the initial diagnosis of ampullary adenomas and for surveillance as well. The polyps of Peutz-Jeghers syndrome may be managed by either endoscopic or surgical resection. Hemangiomas and leiomyomas are best approached by segmental resection, if possible.

Malignant Neoplasms

Adenocarcinomas

In many patients, a preoperative diagnosis is made endoscopically, and most undergo surgical exploration and resection. Patients whose primary lesions arise in the first or second portion of the duodenum are usually treated by pancreaticoduodenectomy, although there is no evidence that the outcome with this procedure is superior to that with segmental resection, when technically feasible. Segmental resection is usually sufficient for patients with tumors arising from the third and fourth portions of the duodenum.

The prognosis is determined by resectability, pathologic status of the resection margins, histologic grade, and presence or absence of lymph node involvement.[26, 42] The overall

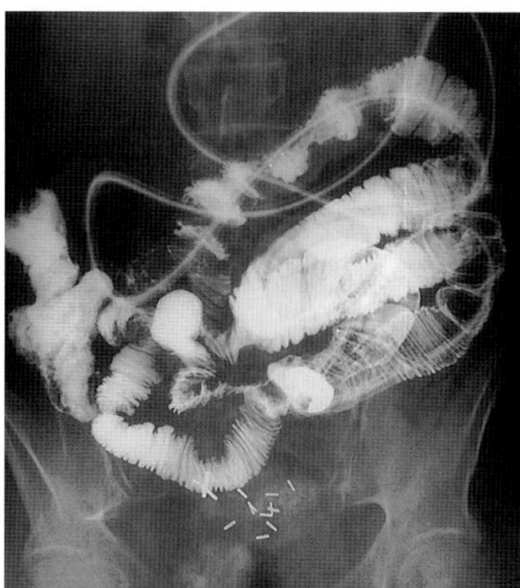

Figure 113–3. Contrast delivered through a Miller-Abbot tube in a patient with partial small bowel obstruction and extensive extramucosal disease caused by metastatic lung cancer. (Courtesy of Igor Laufer, MD, Hospital of the University of Pennsylvania, Philadelphia, PA.)

5-year survival rate ranges from 20% to 35%.[43–45] In one series of 67 patients, the 5-year survival rate for patients who underwent resection was 54%. Further analysis demonstrated that patients with tumor limited to the mucosa and submucosa had a 5-year survival rate of 100%, whereas 5-year survival rates for patients with disease extending to the serosa, regional lymph nodes, or distant sites were 52%, 45%, and 0%, respectively. In a separate study, patients with favorable prognostic features of negative lymph nodes and negative surgical margins, well-differentiated or moderately differentiated histologic grade, and a primary lesion limited to the duodenum or ampulla had an actuarial 5-year survival rate of 80%, whereas patients who lacked these features had a 5-year survival rate of 38%. Furthermore, although postoperative radiotherapy to the tumor bed increased local control of tumor, such therapy did not enhance survival, because patients still succumbed to distant metastatic disease.

The jejunum and ileum are the sites of small bowel adenocarcinomas in more than 50% of cases. The majority of tumors are technically resectable, although lymph node metastases are common. As for more proximal lesions, the overall 5-year survival rate is 20% to 30%. Prognostic factors are similar to those for duodenal lesions; 5-year survival rates are 45% to 70% in patients with negative lymph nodes but only 12% to 14% in those with lymph node involvement.

Although some patients may benefit from adjuvant therapy, the benefit of routine adjuvant chemotherapy or radiotherapy (or both) has yet to be confirmed. When chemotherapy is considered, 5-fluorouracil, doxorubicin (adriamycin), and mitomycin C are employed in the adjuvant setting and also for unresectable tumors.[46] Radiotherapy is fraught with the side effects caused by radiation-induced enteritis (see Chapter 102). Future directions may involve the correlation of genetic and biochemical abnormalities in tumors, with stratification of patients to different therapeutic modalities.[47, 48]

Sarcomas

The most common type of small intestinal sarcoma is a leiomyosarcoma. Gross inspection cannot distinguish a benign from a malignant smooth muscle neoplasm, so any such neoplasm requires wide excision. However, lymph node resection is usually unnecessary for leiomyosarcomas because they rarely metastasize to lymph nodes. The great majority of tumors can be resected. The 5-year survival rate is approximately 50%, and the major prognostic variables include tumor grade and surgical resectability. Even in the face of extensive disease, resection or bypass may offer considerable palliation. Rarely, isolated hepatic metastases are found and may be resected or embolized. Resection of isolated pulmonary disease may result in a 5-year survival rate of 20%. At 5 years, 25% of patients who underwent palliative resection are alive, and at 10 years 6% are alive. In comparison, 50% and 35% of patients who were resected with curative intent are still alive at 5 and 10 years, respectively. No benefit has yet been demonstrated for either adjuvant chemotherapy or radiotherapy. For patients with unresectable disease, doxorubicin-based regimens offer the best tumor response, although the median duration of the benefit is short, and the prognosis remains poor.

Lymphomas and Carcinoids

See Chapters 26 and 112.

Metastatic Cancer

Despite the rarity of primary small intestinal malignancies, the small bowel is frequently involved by metastatic disease. Metastatic lesions may produce symptoms of intestinal obstruction as well as bleeding and abdominal pain. The primary tumor that most often metastasizes to the small intestine is melanoma; 60% of patients with melanoma have metastases in the gastrointestinal tract. Virtually any other extra- or intra-abdominal malignancy (e.g., lung, breast, colon, stomach) may metastasize or extend directly to the small bowel (Figs. 113–3 and 113–4), and palliative resec-

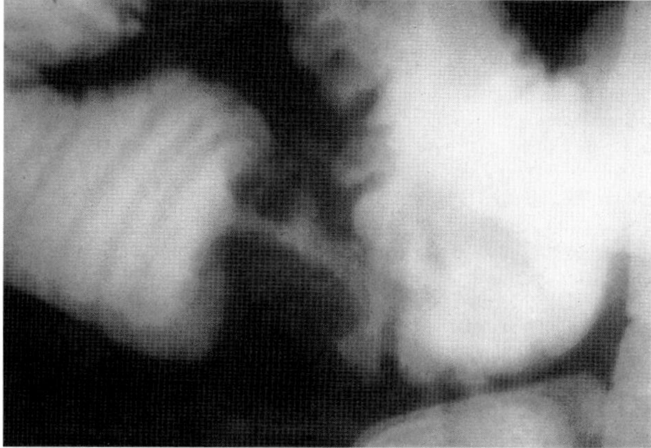

Figure 113–4. Small bowel follow-through series demonstrating metastic lesions to the small bowel from a scirrhous gastric cancer. (Courtesy of Igor Laufer, MD, Hospital of the University of Pennsylvania, Philadelphia, PA.)

tion may be considered in any but the most advanced cases. Systemic therapy may be offered if effective chemotherapy exists for the primary lesion; however, survival rates for these patients are poor because of the extensive tumor burden.

REFERENCES

1. Neugut AI, Marvin MR, Rella VA, et al: An overview of adenocarcinoma of the small intestine. Oncology 11:529–536, 1997.
2. Neugut AI, Jacobson JS, Suh S, et al: The epidemiology of cancer of the small intestine. Cancer Epidemiol Biomarkers Prev 7:243–251, 1998.
3. Chow JS, Chen CC, Ahsan H, et al: A population-based study of the incidence of malignant small bowel tumors: SEER, 1973–1990. Int J Epidemiol 25:722–728, 1996.
4. DiSario JA, Burt RW, Vargas H, et al: Small bowel cancer: Epidemiological and clinical characteristics from a population-based registry. Am J Gastroenterol 89:699–701, 1994.
5. Bhutani MS, Gopalswamy N: A multicenter experience in the United States with primary malignant tumors of the small intestine. Am J Gastroenterol 89:460, 1994.
6. Severson RK, Schenk M, Gurney JG: Increasing incidence of adenocarcinomas and carcinoid tumors of the small intestine in adults. Cancer Epidemiol Biomarkers Prev 5:81–84, 1996.
7. Howe JR, Karnell LH, Scott-Conner C: Adenocarcinoma of the small bowel. Cancer 86:2693–2706, 1999.
8. North JH, Pack MS: Malignant tumors of the small intestine: A review of 144 cases. Am Surg 66:46–51, 2000.
9. Lowenfels AB, Sonni A: Distribution of small bowel tumors. Cancer Lett 3:83–86, 1997.
10. Chow WH, Linet MS, McLaughlin JK, et al: Risk factors for small intestine cancer. Cancer Causes Control 4:163, 1993.
11. Potten CS, Li YQ, O'Connor PJ, Winton DJ: A possible explanation for the differential cancer incidence in the intestine, based on distribution of the cytotoxic effects of carcinogens in the murine large bowel. Carcinogenesis 12:2305, 1992.
12. Hamada K, Umemoto A, Kajikawa A, et al: Mucosa specific DNA adducts in human small intestine: A comparison with the colon. Carcinogenesis 15:2677, 1994.
13. Fineman RJA, Demant P: A gene for susceptibility to small intestinal cancer, *ssicl*, maps to the distal part of mouse chromosome 4. Cancer Res 55:3179, 1995.
14. Dietrich W, Lander ES, Smith J, et al: Genetic identification of Mom-1, a major modifier locus affecting MIN-induced intestinal neoplasia in the mouse. Cell 75:631, 1993.
15. Moser AR, Pitot HC, Dove WF: A dominant mutation that predisposes to mutiple intestinal neoplasia in the mouse. Science 247:322, 1990.
16. Arber N, Neugut AI, Weinstein IB, et al: Molecular genetics of small bowel cancer. Cancer Epidemiol Biomarkers Prev 6:745–748, 1997.
17. Rashid A, Hamilton SR: Genetic alterations in sporadic and Crohn's-associated adenocarcinomas of the small intestine. Gastroenterology 113:127–135, 1997.
18. Arber N, Shapira I, Ratan J, et al: Activation of c-K-*ras* mutations in human gastrointestinal tumors. Gastroenterology 118:1045–1050, 2000.
19. Hirota S, Isozaki K, Moriyama Y, et al: Gain-of-function mutations of *c-kit* in human gastrointestinal stromal tumors. Science, 279:577–580, 1998.
20. Negri E, Bosetti C, La Vecchia C, et al: Risk factors for adenocarcinoma of the small intestine. Int J Cancer 82:171–174, 1999.
21. Chow WH, Linet MS, McLaughlin JK, et al: Risk factors for small intestine cancer. Cancer Causes Control 4:164–169, 1993.
22. Martin MS, Martin F, Justabo E, et al: Susceptibility of inbred rats to gastric and duodenal carcinomas induced by *N*-methyl-*N*-nitro-*N'*-nitrosoguanidine. J Natl Cancer Inst 53:837, 1974.
23. Ross RK, Hartnett NM, Bernstein L, et al: Epidemiology of adenocarcinomas of the small intestine: Is bile a small bowel carcinogen? Br J Cancer 63:143–145, 1991.
24. Spigelman AD, Talbot IC, Penna C, et al: Evidence for adenoma-carcinoma sequence in the duodenum of patients with familial adenomatous polyposis. J Clin Pathol 47:709–710, 1994.
25. Offerhaus GJA, Giardiello FM, Krush AJ, et al: The risk of upper gastrointestinal cancer in familial adenomatous polyposis. Gastroenterology 102:1980–1982, 1993.
26. Rose DM, Hochwald SN, Klimstra DS, et al: Primary duodenal adenocarcinoma: A ten-year experience with 79 patients. J Am Coll Surg 182:89–96, 1996.
27. Weiss NS, Yang CP: Incidence of histologic types of cancer of the small intestine. J Natl Cancer Inst 78:653, 1987.
28. Wilson JM, Melvin DB, Gray GF: Primary malignancies of the small bowel: A report of 96 cases and a review of the literature. Ann Surg 180:175, 1974.
29. Shulten MF, Dyesu R, Beal JM: Villous adenoma of the duodenum: A case report and review of the literature. Am J Surg 130:90, 1976.
30. Bremer EH, Battaile WG, Bulle PH: Villous adenoma of the upper gastrointestinal tract: Clinical review and report of a case. Am J Gastroenterol 50:135, 1968.
31. Sigel JE, Petras RE, Lashner BA, et al: Intestinal adenocarcinoma in Crohn's disease. Am J Surg Pathol 23:651–655, 1999.
32. Munkholm P, Langholz E, Davidsen M, et al: Intestinal cancer risk and mortality in patients with Crohn's disease. Gastroenterology 105:1716–1723, 1993.
33. Lewis JD, Deren JJ, Lichtenstein GR: Cancer risks in patients with inflammatory bowel disease. Gastroenterol Clin North Am 28:459–477, 1999.
34. Pricolo VE, Mangi AA, Aswad B, et al: Gastrointestinal malignancies in patients with celiac sprue. Am J Surg 176:344–347, 1998.
35. Rodriguez-Bigas MA, Vasen HFA, Lynch HT, et al: Characteristics of small bowel carcinoma in hereditary nonpolyposis colorectal cancer. Cancer 83:240–244, 1998.
36. Hizawa K, Iida M, Matsumoto T, et al: Neoplastic transformation arising in Peutz-Jeghers polyposis. Dis Colon Rectum 36:953, 1993.
37. Ekberg O, Ekholm S: Radiography in primary tumors of the small bowel. Acta Radiol 21:79, 1980.
38. Maglinte DDT, Hall R, Miller RE, et al: Detection of surgical lesions of the small bowel by enteroclysis. Am J Surg 147:225, 1984.
39. Bessette JR, Maglinte DDT, Kelvin FM, Chernish SM: Primary malignant tumors in the small bowel: A comparison of the small bowel enema and conventional follow-through examination. AJR Am J Roentgenol 153:741, 1989.
40. Bowden TA: Endoscopy of the small intestine. Surg Clin North Am 69: 1237, 1989.
41. Iddan G, Meron G, Glukhovsky A, Swain P: Wireless capsule endoscopy. Nature 405:417, 2000.
42. Veyrieres M, Baillet P, Hay JM: Factors influencing long-term survival in 100 cases of small intestine primary adenocarcinoma. Am J Surg 173:237–239, 1997.
43. Lai ECS, Doty JE, Irving C, Tompkins RK: Primary adenocarcinoma of the duodenum: Analysis of survival. World J Surg 12:695, 1988.
44. Joesting DR, Beart RW, van Heerden JA, Weiland LH: Improving survival in adenocarcinoma of the duodenum. Am J Surg 141:228, 1981.
45. Barnes G Jr, Romero L, Hess KR, Curley SA: Primary adenocarcinoma of the duodenum: Management and survival in 67 patients. Ann Surg Oncol 1:73, 1994.
46. Crawey C, Ross P, Norman A, et al: The royal Marsden experience of small bowel adenocarcinoma treated with protracted venous infusion 5-fluorouracil. Br J Cancer 78, 508–510, 1998.
47. Boyle WJ, Brenner DA: Molecular and cellular biology of the small intestine. Curr Opin Gastroentrol 11:121–127, 1995.
48. Arber N, Hibshoosh H, Yasui W, et al: Abnormalities in the expression of cell cycle–related proteins in tumors of the small bowel. Cancer Epidemiol Biomarkers Prev 12:1101–1105, 1999.

Chapter 114

Colonic Polyps and Polyposis Syndromes

Steven H. Itzkowitz

A gastrointestinal (GI) polyp is a discrete mass of tissue that protrudes into the lumen of the bowel (Fig. 114–1). A polyp may be characterized by its gross appearance according to the presence or absence of a stalk, its overall size, and whether it is one of multiple similar masses elsewhere in the gut. Regardless of these features, specific definition rests on the histologic characteristics.

Because of their protrusion into the bowel lumen and the stresses of the fecal stream to which they are subject, polyps may cause symptoms. They may ulcerate and bleed; abdominal pain may result when a peristaltic wave propels a polyp downstream; large polyps rarely may even obstruct the intestine. Symptomatic polyps are uncommon; the greatest concern with polyps is their potential to become malignant (also see Chapter 115). The bulk of evidence supports the hypothesis that most colonic cancers arise within previously benign adenomatous polyps. However, only a small percentage of all colonic adenomas will progress to carcinoma, and because colonic polyps are so common in the industrialized world, universal detection and removal pose practical and economic problems. To manage colonic polyps, therefore, the physician must understand the differences in pathogenesis and natural history of the distinct pathologic categories of these lesions.

COLONIC POLYPS

Colonic polyps may be divided into two major groups: neoplastic (the adenomas and carcinomas) and non-neoplastic (Table 114–1). The adenomas and carcinomas share a common characteristic—cellular *dysplasia*—but they may be subdivided according to the relative contribution of certain microscopic features. The non-neoplastic polyps may be grouped into several distinct categories, including hyperplastic polyps, "mucosal polyps," juvenile polyps, inflammatory polyps, and others. Submucosal lesions also may impart a polypoid appearance to the overlying mucosa.

Neoplastic Polyps (Adenomatous and Malignant Polyps)

Pathology

HISTOLOGIC CHARACTERISTICS. Adenomatous polyps are tumors of benign neoplastic epithelium that may be either pedunculated (attached by a narrow stalk) or sessile (attached by a broad base with little or no stalk).[1, 2] The neoplastic nature of adenomas is apparent by histologic examination of their glandular architecture. *Tubular adenomas* are the most common subgroup, characterized by a complex network of branching adenomatous glands (Fig. 114–2*A*). In *villous adenomas,* the adenomatous glands extend straight down from the surface to the center of the polyp, thereby creating long, finger-like projections (Fig. 114–2*B*). *Tubulovillous* (villoglandular) *adenomas* manifest a combination of these two histologic types. A polyp is assigned a histologic type on the basis of its predominant glandular pattern, and in practice, pure villous adenomas are quite rare. According to the World Health Organization, adenomas are classified as tubular if at least 80% of the glands are the branching, tubule type and as villous if at least 80% of the glands are villiform.[3] Tubular adenomas account for 80% to 86% of adenomatous polyps, tubulovillous for 8% to 16%, and villous adenomas for 3% to 16%.[4, 5] Tubular adenomas usually are small and exhibit mild dysplasia, whereas villous architecture is more often encountered in large adenomas and tends to be associated with more severe degrees of dysplasia (Table 114–2).

By definition, all colorectal adenomas are dysplastic. Adenomatous epithelium is characterized by abnormal cellular differentiation and renewal, resulting in hypercellularity of colonic crypts with cells possessing variable amounts of mucin and hyperchromatic, elongated nuclei arranged in a picket-fence pattern. These cytologic alterations confer a more basophilic appearance to the adenomatous epithelium

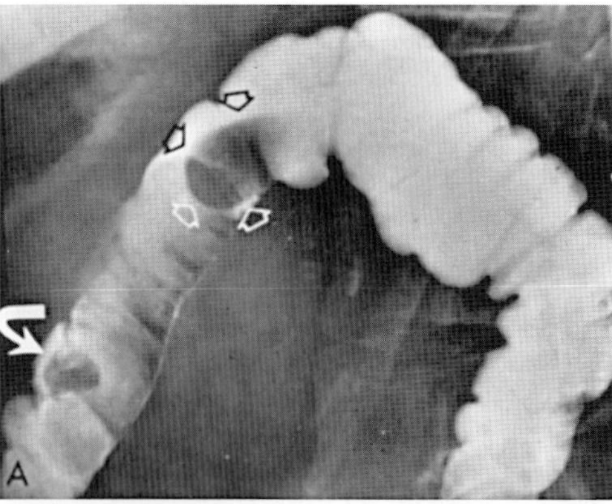

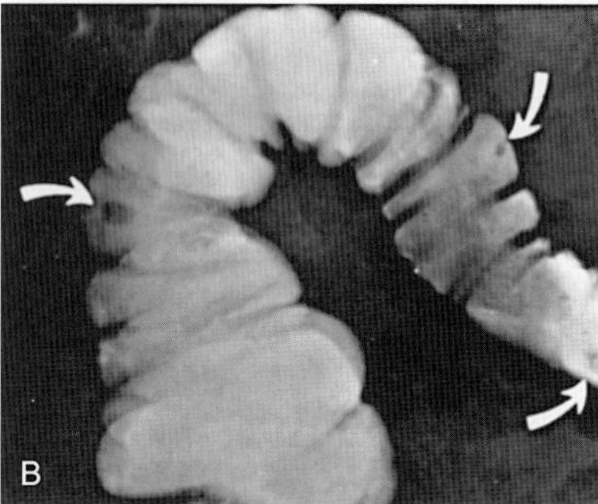

Figure 114–1. This barium enema demonstrates several polypoid lesions of the colon (*A*, splenic flexure; *B*, hepatic flexure). The largest polyp *(open arrows)* was a pedunculated lipoma. The other polyps *(white arrows)* were adenomas; the largest one contained tubular and villous elements and a focus of dysplasia. A total of eight polyps were removed from this patient.

Table 114–1 | **Classification of Colorectal Polyps**

NEOPLASTIC MUCOSAL POLYPS
Benign (adenoma)
- Tubular adenoma
- Tubulovillous adenoma
- Villous adenoma

Malignant (carcinoma)
- Noninvasive carcinoma
  - Carcinoma in situ
  - Intramucosal carcinoma
- Invasive carcinoma (through muscularis mucosae)

NON-NEOPLASTIC MUCOSAL POLYPS
Hyperplastic polyp (metaplastic polyp)
Normal epithelium (in a polypoid configuration)
Juvenile polyp (retention polyp)
Peutz-Jeghers polyp
Inflammatory polyps
- Inflammatory bowel disease
- In bacterial infections or amebiasis
- Schistosomiasis
- Cap polyposis

SUBMUCOSAL LESIONS
Colitis cystica profunda
Pneumatosis cystoides intestinalis
Lymphoid polyps (benign and malignant)
Lipomas
Carcinoids
Metastatic neoplasms
Other rare lesions

on conventional hematoxylin-eosin staining. Although the predominant cell type is an immature goblet cell or columnar cell, adenomas may contain other cell types, such as neuroendocrine cells, Paneth cells, squamous morules, and, rarely, melanocytes. On cross section, the inner contour of an adenomatous gland lumen is usually seen as smooth, in contrast to the serrated appearance of a hyperplastic gland lumen (see later).

The dysplasia exhibited by all adenomas can be graded subjectively on the basis of certain cytologic and architectural features into three categories: mild, moderate, and severe. Some polyps may contain the entire spectrum from mild to severe dysplasia, but in all cases, the adenoma is classified according to the most dysplastic focus within it. In cells that exhibit *mild dysplasia*, the nuclei maintain their basal polarity in the cell but are hyperchromatic and slightly enlarged and elongated yet uniform in size, without prominent nucleoli (Fig. 114–3*A*). There often is loss of goblet cell mucin. Architecturally, the glands manifest branching

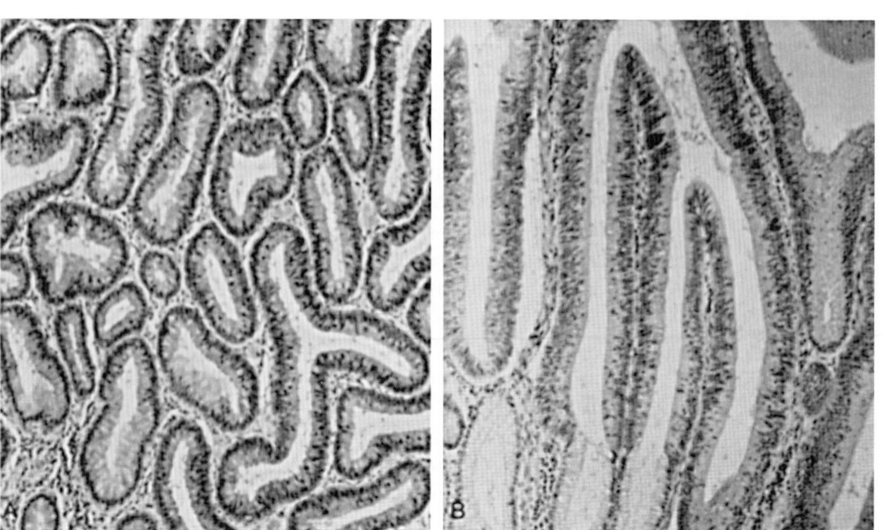

Figure 114–2. Comparison of tubular and villous histology. *A*, Tubular adenomas consist of branched, crowded glands arranged in a complex cerebriform pattern. *B*, Villous histology is marked by glands that are long, fingerlike fronds that typically project from the polyp stroma to the surface without much branching. In the center two crypts, the adenomatous epithelium at the top has not yet fully replaced the normal epithelium at the bottom.

Table 114–2 | **Frequency of Adenomas: Relation of Histologic Type to Adenoma Size and Degree of Dysplasia**

TYPE OF ADENOMA	ADENOMA SIZE*			DEGREE OF DYSPLASIA†		
	<1 cm (%)	1–2 cm (%)	>2 cm (%)	Mild (%)	Moderate (%)	Severe (%)
Tubular	77	20	4	88	8	4
Tubulovillous	25	47	29	58	26	16
Villous	14	26	60	41	38	21

*Adapted from Muto T, Bussey HJR, Morson BC: The evolution of cancer of the colon and rectum. Cancer 36:2251, 1975.
†Adapted from Konishi F, Morson BC: Pathology of colorectal adenomas: A colonoscopic survey. J Clin Pathol 35:830, 1989.

and budding and become more crowded. With *moderate dysplasia,* nuclei become stratified and pleomorphic with prominent nucleoli, along with further loss of goblet cell mucin and increased glandular crowding. *Severe dysplasia* (Fig. 114–3*B*) is characterized by further stratification and pleomorphism of nuclei, more numerous and prominent nucleoli, increased nuclear-cytoplasmic ratio, and extreme glandular crowding. With further cell proliferation within the crypt, cells pile up, lose polarity, and create glands-within-glands, giving a disorderly cribriform appearance termed *carcinoma in situ* (Fig. 114–4*A*). Many pathologists group severe dysplasia and carcinoma in situ together, considering them both as high-grade dysplasia,[4] in order to avoid using the term *carcinoma* for these lesions, which often can be managed endoscopically rather than surgically (see later). Indeed, it is now common practice to categorize dysplasia in colorectal adenomas into only two grades: *low-grade* dysplasia, which includes mild and moderate dysplasia, and *high-grade* dysplasia, which comprises severe dysplasia and carcinoma in situ.

Carcinoma in situ is characterized by intracryptal cell proliferation, leaving intact the basement membrane that surrounds the gland. If a focus of neoplastic cells grows beyond the basement membrane and into the lamina propria of the mucosa, the lesion has been termed *intramucosal carcinoma* (Fig. 114–4*B*). Both carcinoma in situ and intramucosal carcinoma are noninvasive lesions without metastatic potential because lymphatics are not present in the colonic mucosa above the level of the muscularis mucosae.[6] Because clinical confusion often arises on encountering these two entities, it has been suggested that both carcinoma in situ and intramucosal carcinoma be reported as "noninvasive carcinoma" to avoid unnecessarily aggressive management. Only when a focus of neoplastic cells has spread through the muscularis mucosae is the lesion considered *invasive carcinoma* (Fig. 114–4*C*). An adenoma that contains a focus of invasive carcinoma commonly is referred to as a *malignant polyp* (see later).

Mild dysplasia may be found in 70% to 86% of adenomatous polyps, moderate dysplasia in 18% to 20%, severe dysplasia (carcinoma in situ) in 5% to 10%, and invasive carcinoma in 5% to 7%.[5, 7, 8] Higher grades of dysplasia are more common in adenomas of larger size and greater villous content[4] (see Table 114–2), and adenomas with severe dysplasia are more likely to contain foci of invasive cancer.

ADENOMA SIZE. Adenomas have classically been categorized into three size groups: less than 1 cm, 1 to 2 cm, and greater than 2 cm.[7] Most adenomas are smaller than 1 cm, but the size distribution of adenomas may vary greatly between studies, depending on study design, age of the study population, and location of the adenomas within the colon. Thus, in autopsy series, which describe a predominantly asymptomatic population dying of other causes, only 13% to 16% of adenomas are larger than 1 cm,[9–11] whereas surgical and colonoscopic series that include symptomatic or higher-risk patients report a higher prevalence (26% to 40%) of adenomas larger than 1 cm.[4, 5, 7] In countries where the

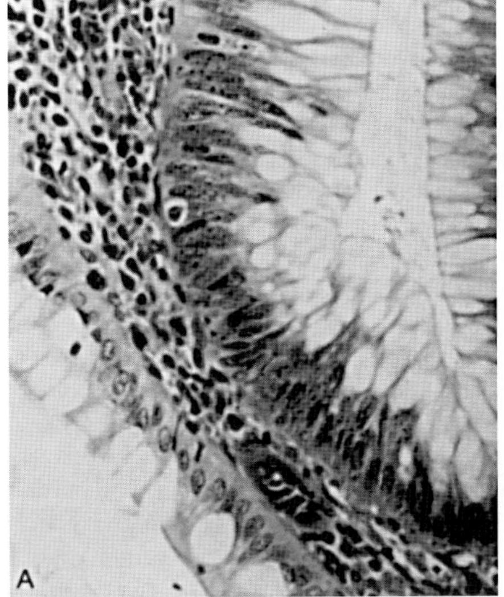

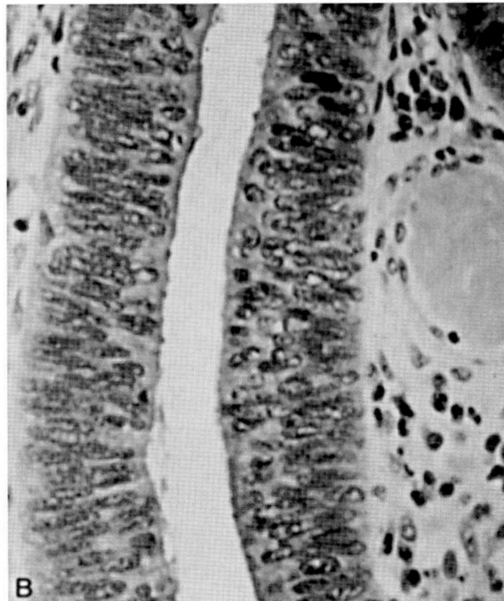

Figure 114–3. Examples of different degrees of dysplasia in adenomatous polyps. *A,* A relatively normal crypt *(lower left)* is characterized by well-formed goblet cells and nuclei that are small, round-ovoid, homogeneous, not stratified, and basally located in the cell. In contrast, the adenomatous crypt *(upper right)* with low-grade dysplasia is marked by nuclear abnormalities, consisting of elongated, crowded, cigar-shaped nuclei that are pleomorphic and exhibit occasional nucleoli. Mucin vacuoles also are distorted. *B,* High-grade dysplasia is characterized by loss of goblet cell vacuoles, extreme crowding and pleomorphism of nuclei, nuclear stratification with nuclei found at the apical surface of cells, and prominent nucleoli. The nuclear-cytoplasmic ratio is increased.

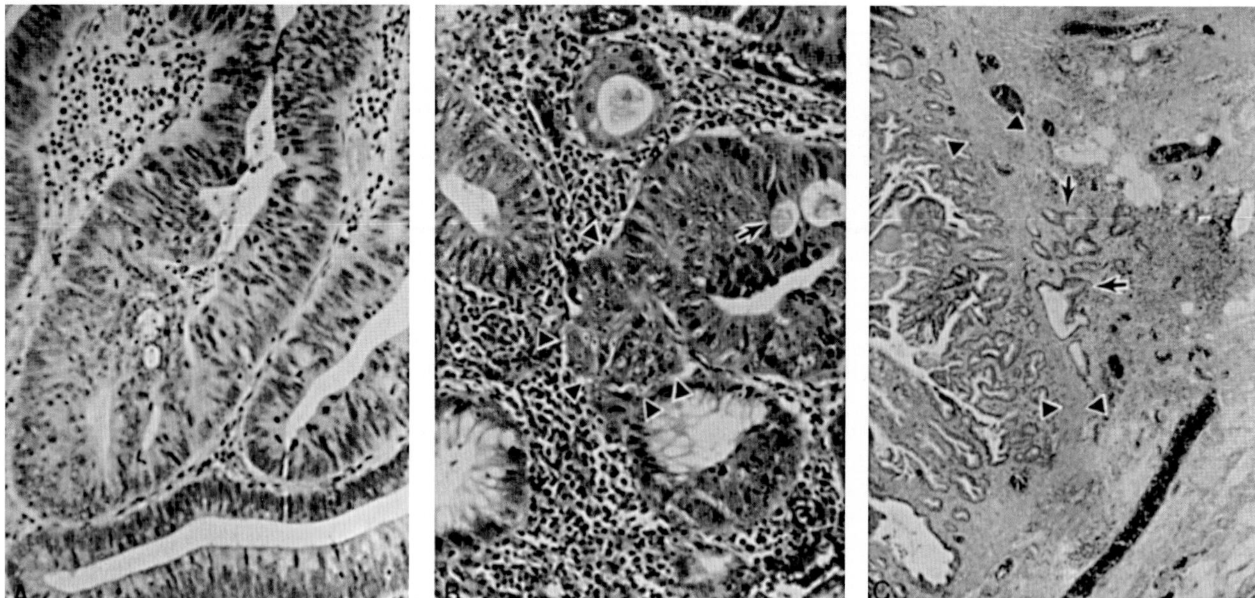

Figure 114–4. Examples of malignant transformation in adenomatous polyps. *A,* Carcinoma in situ. This lesion exhibits the same features as in severe dysplasia along with proliferation of cells into the crypt lumen. The basement membrane surrounding the crypt is intact. *B,* Intramucosal carcinoma *(enclosed in arrowheads)* shares the same features as in carcinoma in situ *(arrow),* but the malignant cells have grown beyond the basement membrane into the adjacent lamina propria. *C,* Invasive carcinoma in an adenomatous polyp. Cancer cells *(arrows)* have grown from the adenomatous tissue on the left, beyond the muscularis mucosae *(between arrowheads),* and reside in the submucosa.

prevalence of colon cancer is high, adenomas tend to be larger than in low-prevalence countries.[12, 13] Adenoma size increases as a function of age,[10, 14, 15] even in low-prevalence countries.[12] Larger adenomas are more common in distal colonic segments.[4, 7, 10]

DIMINUTIVE POLYPS. A *diminutive polyp* is one that measures 5 mm or less in diameter. Diminutive polyps have aroused much interest because they are so commonly encountered during endoscopy, but they are of little biologic or clinical significance. An earlier concept that these lesions were almost always non-neoplastic has been revised by several flexible sigmoidoscopy and colonoscopy studies in which 30% to 50% of diminutive polyps were found to be adenomatous.[16–20] Despite the frequency of adenomatous change, they represent little if any threat of cancer. In fact, fewer than 1% of diminutive polyps are villous or contain a focus of severe dysplasia, and they almost never harbor invasive carcinoma.[16–18, 20] Moreover, in a retrospective study of predominantly asymptomatic people with diminutive adenomas found on flexible sigmoidoscopy, full colonoscopy identified a synchronous proximal adenoma in only 33% of subjects, and most of the proximal lesions were also 5 mm or less.[21] Likewise, prospective colonoscopic studies confirm only a 24% to 34% prevalence of proximal adenomas in asymptomatic patients with distal diminutive polyps (of all histologic types)[22, 23]; the likelihood of finding proximal adenomas is greater when the distal polyp is larger than 5 mm.[22] Diminutive adenomas manifest little, if any, appreciable growth over time.[24, 25] A population-based study that involved fulgurating small polyps (even those up to 1 cm in size) without obtaining initial histologic identification reported that the subsequent risk for colorectal cancer and overall survival was no worse than in the general population.[26] Thus, taken together, these observations indicate that diminutive polyps, even when they prove to be adenomas, have little biologic or clinical significance. An exception to this rule is hereditary nonpolyposis colorectal cancer (HNPCC), in which even small adenomas may display villous features or high-grade dysplasia (see later).

MALIGNANT POTENTIAL OF ADENOMATOUS POLYPS. The three principal features that correlate with malignant potential for an adenomatous polyp are its size, histologic type, and degree of dysplasia (Table 114–3). Although higher rates of malignant transformation are found when the source of the pathologic material is mainly from surgical polypectomies[7] rather than colonoscopic polypectomies,[8] the malignant potential is directly correlated with larger adenoma size, more villous histology, and higher degrees of dysplasia. To be sure, these three histopathologic criteria are usually interdependent, so it is difficult to assign a primary premalignant role to any one of them. For example, although only 1.3% of all adenomas under 1 cm may harbor a cancer (see Table 114–3), if these small lesions have a predominant villous component or contain a focus of severe dysplasia the cancer rate rises to 10% or 27%, respectively (Table 114–4). Note, however, that a small (<1 cm), tubular, mildly dysplastic adenoma is very unlikely to harbor a focus of invasive cancer. This type of lesion not only is innocuous in itself, but, once removed, also is often considered a marker of an individual who is at low risk for developing a recurrent adenoma (discussed later). Since adenomas that are larger than 1 cm, have villous architecture, or manifest high-grade dysplasia or carcinoma represent a more biologically hazardous group, the term *adenoma with advanced pathology* (AAP) is often applied to them.

Table 114–3 | **Malignant Potential of Adenomatous Polyps**

	SURGICAL POLYPECTOMIES*		COLONOSCOPIC POLYPECTOMIES†	
	Total No.	**No. with Carcinoma (%)**	**Total No.**	**No. with Carcinoma (%)**
Adenoma Size				
<1 cm	1479	19 (1.3)	1661	8 (0.5)
1–2 cm	580	55 (9.5)	2738	125 (4.6)
>2 cm	430	198 (46.0)	1387	150 (10.8)
Histologic Type				
Tubular	1880	90 (4.8)	3725	104 (2.8)
Tubulovillous	383	86 (22.5)	1542	130 (8.4)
Villous	243	99 (40.7)	519	49 (9.5)
Degree of Dysplasia‡				
Mild	1734	99 (5.7)	N/A	N/A
Moderate	549	99 (18.0)	N/A	N/A
Severe	223	77 (34.5)	N/A	N/A

*Adapted from Muto T, Bussey HJR, Morson BC: The evolution of cancer of the colon and rectum. Cancer 36:2251, 1975.

†Adapted from Shinya H, Wolff WI: Morphology, anatomic distribution and cancer potential of colonic polyps. Ann Surg 190:679, 1979.

‡This category refers to the most extensive degree of dysplasia *outside* the area of carcinoma within the polyp. However, by convention, because an adenoma is classified according to the most severe grade of dysplasia, if carcinoma is present it is considered a malignant polyp regardless of the degree of surrounding dysplasia.

N/A, not available.

OTHER ADENOMA VARIANTS

Flat Adenomas. A subset of adenomas, termed *flat adenomas* by Muto and coworkers,[27] are receiving increasing attention as potentially important lesions. Macroscopically, a flat adenoma is completely flat or slightly raised, or may contain a central depression (so-called "depressed adenoma"). Typically smaller than 1 cm in diameter, these lesions can be easily missed by endoscopy. This has prompted investigators, particularly in Japan, to adapt novel methods of detection that involve the use of dye-spraying (chromoscopy), which generates a contrast relief-map image of the mucosa, or magnification colonoscopy to visualize these lesions better.[28] Flat adenomas may account for 8.5% to 12% of all adenomas[29–31] and can be multiple.[30] In a prospective study from the United States, 18 of 148 (12%) patients referred for colonoscopy within a 1-year period were found to have a flat adenoma without the use of special endoscopic techniques.[29] In a larger prospective study from the United Kingdom, however, specialized endoscopic techniques were used to demonstrate that 36% of detected adenomas were considered flat; four lesions were depressed, with three of the four depressed lesions already containing cancer or high-grade dysplasia.[32] Future studies may help define whether broader acceptance of chromoscopy or magnifying colonoscopy by endoscopists in Western countries will result in higher detection rates of flat adenomas and/or a lower colorectal cancer incidence following colonoscopy. A hereditary flat adenoma syndrome (HFAS) has been described by Lynch and colleagues in four families.[33] HFAS is now known by molecular genetic confirmation to be a variant of familial adenomatous polyposis (FAP) (see below).

The natural history of flat adenomas is not known. It is possible that they give rise to typical polypoid adenomas. On the other hand, the fact that residual flat adenoma tissue can be found adjacent to flat carcinomas, that some studies have observed a rather substantial incidence of high-grade dysplasia in these small lesions, and the finding that flat adenomas have a lower incidence of *k-ras* mutations compared with polypoid adenomas, suggest that malignant progression from flat adenomas may not necessarily involve a polypoid phase.[34] It is possible that flat adenomas are the precursors of the long-recognized but uncommon small de novo colon carcinomas.

Serrated Adenomas. Serrated adenomas are polyps that share features of both adenomatous and hyperplastic polyps. Originally called "mixed hyperplastic-adenomatous polyps," these lesions are characterized by having colonic crypts with a

Table 114–4 | **Relation of Adenoma Size, Histologic Type, and Degree of Dysplasia to Invasive Carcinoma**

	PERCENT WITH CARCINOMA					
	Histologic Type			**Degree of Dysplasia**		
ADENOMA SIZE	*Tubular*	*Tubulovillous*	*Villous*	*Mild*	*Moderate*	*Severe*
<1 cm	1	4	10	0.3	2	27
1–2 cm	10	7	10	3	14	24
>2 cm	35	46	53	42	50	48

Adapted from Muto T, Bussey HJR, Morson BC: The evolution of cancer of the colon and rectum. Cancer 36:2251, 1975.

sawtooth, serrated configuration resembling hyperplastic polyps, but because of nuclear atypia, they are considered to be adenomas. This is discussed later under hyperplastic polyps.

Aberrant Crypts. Investigations of human and carcinogen-treated rat colonic mucosa have disclosed a putative preneoplastic lesion called the *aberrant crypt*.[35] Found within macroscopically normal mucosa, aberrant crypts may occur individually or as small, slightly raised foci. They can be identified in methylene blue–stained whole mounts of colonic mucosa using a low-power lens (Fig. 114–5), or more recently with a magnifying endoscope.[36] When viewed from above, the lumens of aberrant crypts are elliptical and irregular rather than circular. Aberrant crypt foci have become useful biomarkers in animal studies of colon carcinogenesis and chemoprevention. It is not clear, however, whether these lesions are valid surrogate intermediate end-point markers for adenomas or whether the results of these experimental manipulations can be extrapolated to humans. Human aberrant crypts are often hyperplastic. However, dysplastic aberrant crypts may represent the earliest detectable preneoplastic lesions. This notion is supported by molecular studies indicating that dysplastic, but not hyperplastic, aberrant crypts manifest mutations in the adenomatous polyposis coli (*APC*) gene (see later).[37]

Pathogenesis

HISTOGENESIS. Adenomatous polyps are thought to arise from a failure in a step (or steps) of the normal process of cell proliferation and cell death (apoptosis). The initial aberration appears to arise in a single colonic crypt in which the proliferative compartment, instead of being confined to the crypt base, is expanded throughout the entire crypt. This disturbance results in a so-called *unicryptal adenoma*. The deoxyribonucleic acid (DNA)–synthesizing cells at the surface are not sloughed into the lumen normally and accumulate by downward infolding, interposing themselves between normal preexisting crypts. New adenomatous glands are then created either by further infolding or by branching. It is hypothesized that the histologic type of adenoma is then determined by the reaction of the underlying mesenchyme (connective tissue and capillaries). Thus, in tubular adenomas, mesenchymal proliferation is minimal, so that epithelial infolding develops against a tissue resistance, tending to limit the overall polyp size. In villous adenomas, mesenchymal proliferation accompanies epithelial proliferation, resulting in longer projections and, eventually, larger polyps.

The prevailing model of adenoma development holds that adenomas arise from a monoclonal expansion of an abnormal cell. However, recent studies applying Y chromosome probes to intestinal tissues from a very rare XO/XY mosaic individual (male Turner's syndrome) with FAP disclosed that whereas normal crypts of the small and large intestine and even unicryptal adenomas were monoclonal (either XO or XY), at least 76% of even very small microadenomas were polyclonal.[38] Whether the early onset of polyclonality also applies to sporadic adenoma development is not known at present.

ADENOMA-CARCINOMA HYPOTHESIS. It is universally accepted that most, if not all, colon cancers originate within previously benign adenomas (also see Chapter 115). Rarely, colon cancers may develop de novo in apparently flat, nonadenomatous epithelium,[39] although as noted, even these lesions may arise from preexisting flat adenomas. Evidence in support of the adenoma-carcinoma sequence comes from epidemiologic, clinical, pathologic, and molecular studies.

Epidemiologic Evidence. The prevalence of adenomas within a population, and the prevalence of people with multiple adenomas, geographically parallels the prevalence of colon cancer.[12] Indeed, adenoma prevalence increases in migrants from low-risk to high-risk colon cancer regions. The prevalence rates for both adenomatous polyps and cancer increase with age, and age distribution curves indicate that the development of adenomas precedes that of carcinomas by 5 to 10 years. Also, in the FAP syndromes, the appearance of benign adenomas antedates the development of carcinoma by

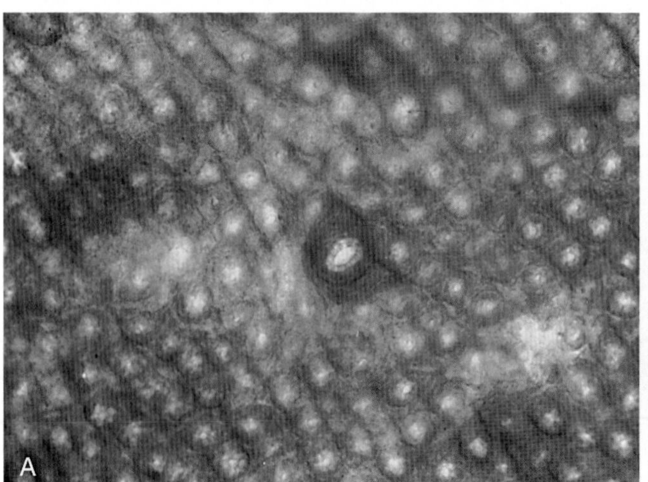

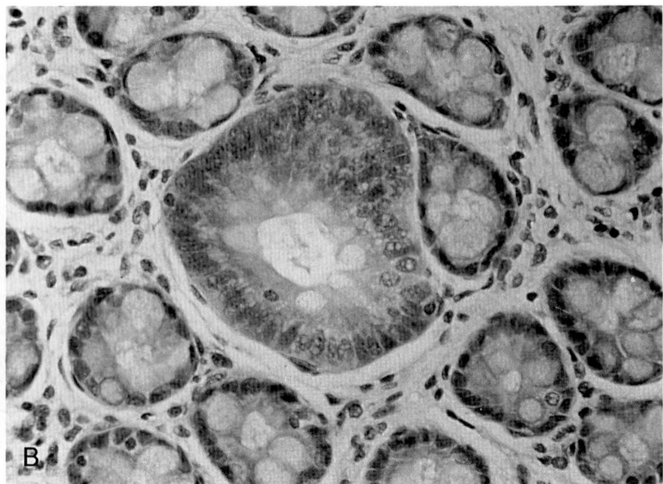

Figure 114–5. Aberrant crypt. *A*, Bird's-eye view of a whole mount of colonic mucosa stained with methylene blue and transilluminated from below. The aberrant crypt is readily seen in the center as a somewhat thickened crypt with an elliptical mouth. Foci of aberrant crypts (not shown) would comprise two or more of these aberrant crypts in a cluster. *B*, Histologic view of aberrant crypt showing loss of goblet cell mucin, increased nuclear to cytoplasmic ratio, and abnormal nuclei. (Courtesy Dr. Michael Wargovich, UT, M.D. Anderson Cancer Center.)

an average of 10 to 12 years.[7] Even with sporadic adenomas, the polyp-to-cancer interval is at least 4 years[7] and perhaps longer, depending on the degree of dysplasia.[40]

Clinicopathologic Evidence. The strongest proof of the concept that adenomas give rise to carcinomas comes from endoscopic interventional studies. The National Polyp Study (discussed later) demonstrated that colonoscopic removal of adenomas results in a much lower than expected incidence of subsequent colorectal cancer.[41] In addition, screening proctosigmoidoscopy can lower the expected incidence of[42, 43] and mortality from[44, 45] rectal cancer. Pathology-based studies describe the frequent presence of remnant adenoma tissue within colon cancers. Conversely, small foci of cancer are extremely rare in normal mucosa but commonly are found in adenomas, particularly in those that are larger, more dysplastic, and more highly composed of villous elements (see Tables 114–3 and 114–4). Furthermore, the site distribution within the colon is similar for large adenomas and colon cancers. In addition, adenomatous polyps are found in one third of surgical specimens that contain a single colon cancer and in more than two thirds of specimens that contain more than one synchronous cancer.

Molecular Genetic Evidence. Molecular genetic studies provide some of the strongest experimental support for the adenoma-carcinoma hypothesis. The progression from adenoma to carcinoma results from an accumulation of molecular genetic alterations involving, among other changes, activation of oncogenes and inactivation of tumor suppressor genes (see Chapter 3). The K-*ras* oncogene commonly undergoes point mutations at particular sites within the gene, thereby endowing it with the ability to transform cells. Only 9% of small adenomas exhibit *ras* gene mutations, compared with 58% of adenomas larger than 1 cm and 47% of colon cancers[46]; therefore, K-*ras* activation may act at an intermediate stage in tumorigenesis, perhaps contributing to a polypoid growth pattern. The fact that a large number of adenomas and cancers do not have *ras* gene mutations indicates that other genetic events also must play a role.

Tumor suppressor genes are frequently inactivated in colorectal neoplasms by mutation or allelic deletion, thereby promoting tumorigenesis. The loss of function of tumor suppressor genes located on chromosomes 5q, 18q, and 17p is critical for colorectal tumorigenesis. The *APC* gene, which resides on the long "q" arm of chromosome 5, is considered to be the "gatekeeper" for the process of colon carcinogenesis.[47] Mutation or loss of this gene confers susceptibility to colonic neoplasms in patients with FAP as well as in people with sporadic adenomas, and thus it qualifies as a tumor suppressor gene. The *APC* gene plays an important role in colonic epithelial cell homeostasis (see later). Other tumor suppressor genes are located on chromosome 18q in a region where the *DCC* (deleted in colon cancer) gene resides.[48] Loss of function of *DCC* or other nearby tumor suppressor genes seems to play a role in later stages of the adenoma-carcinoma sequence, since allelic deletion at this locus occurs in only 11% to 13% of small tubular or tubulovillous adenomas, but increases to 47% of adenomas with foci of cancer and to 73% of frank colon cancers.[46] Allelic deletion of chromosome 17p, at the locus that contains the *p53* gene, is the most common region of allelic loss in colorectal cancers. Because adenomas seldom manifest a 17p deletion,[46] this alteration probably occurs as a late step in the adenoma-carcinoma progression. Perhaps the most compelling evidence that colon carcinomas arise from previous adenomas is the observation that cancer cells in a malignant polyp share the identical pattern of molecular alterations as in the neighboring adenoma cells, but they acquire additional mutations that are presumably critical for malignant behavior.[49]

PATHWAYS OF COLON CARCINOGENESIS. The process of colon carcinogenesis can be considered in two general stages: the formation of the adenoma, termed *tumor initiation,* and the progression of the adenoma to carcinoma, termed *tumor promotion* (Fig. 114–6). It is believed that all adenomas arise from an initial loss of *APC* gene function. In the general population, sporadic adenomas arise as a consequence of acquired *somatic mutations* of both alleles of the *APC* gene. Because this so-called "two-hit" phenomenon is statistically uncommon and takes many years to occur, sporadic adenomas tend to occur later in life and are few in number.

In FAP, one *APC* allele is inherited in a mutated form from the affected parent *(germline mutation).* Adenomas arise after the second, normal copy of the *APC* gene (from the unaffected parent) is either lost or mutated (somatic mutation). Because individuals affected with FAP are already born with the first hit, they develop polyps at a much younger age and in much greater number than in the general population. As such, FAP can be considered a condition of accelerated tumor initiation. Despite this, once adenomas form in FAP patients, it is believed that each adenoma tends to display a typical rate of progression to carcinoma. Thus, the inevitable progression to cancer in FAP (see later) is more a consequence of the numerous polyps that exist rather than any increased premalignant potential of the individual adenoma.

Another major molecular pathway for colon carcinogenesis involves mutations in any one of several enzymes that control the DNA base mismatch repair process (see Chapters 3 and 115). This is the predominant pathway in patients

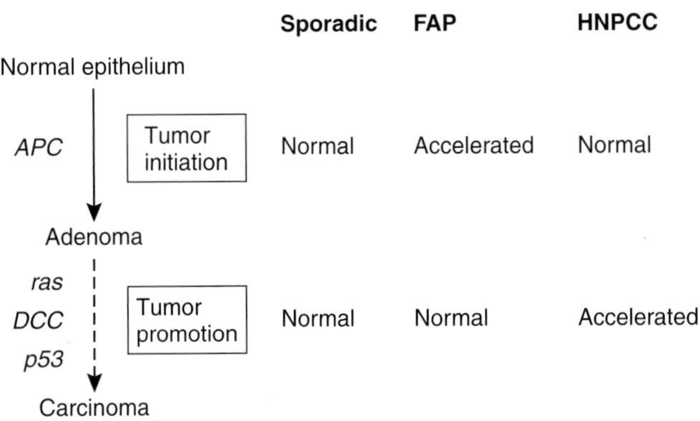

Figure 114–6. Pathways of colon carcinogenesis. Adenomatous polyps develop as a consequence of factors involved in tumor initiation. Adenomas progress to carcinomas by factors that act as tumor promoters. A simplified theory comparing the two hereditary colon cancer syndromes suggests that the tumor initiation phase is accelerated in FAP patients, accounting for numerous polyps, whereas the tumor promotion phase is accelerated in HNPCC patients, accounting for the often rapid progression of adenomas to carcinoma. FAP, familial adenomatous polyposis; HNPCC, hereditary nonpolyposis colorectal cancer.

with HNPCC. Mutations in these enzymes result in a characteristic molecular phenotype, termed *microsatellite instability,* a phenomenon that is observable in colon cancer cells from approximately 85% of HNPCC colon cancers, compared with 15% of sporadic colon cancers. Although its name implies a lack of polyps, HNPCC colon cancers do arise from preexisting adenomas. However, since HNPCC is not a condition of accelerated tumor initiation, the number of adenomas that occur is similar to that in the general population. Rather, HNPCC is marked by an accelerated tumor promotion stage, such that the few adenomas that do arise often manifest advanced pathology (villous features, high-grade dysplasia), even at small sizes.[50] Indeed, adenomas in patients with HNPCC often manifest microsatellite instability[51] even in their earliest stages of formation. Because these adenomas tend to progress more rapidly to carcinoma,[52, 53] surveillance intervals for colonoscopy following removal of adenomas in HNPCC patients should be shortened (see later and Chapter 115).

Epidemiology

PREVALENCE OF ADENOMAS. The prevalence of adenomatous polyps is affected by four major factors: the inherent risk for colon cancer in the population, age, gender, and family history of colorectal cancer. The frequency of colonic adenomas varies widely among populations, but it tends to be higher in populations at greater risk for colon cancer (Table 114–5).[12] One illustrative example is to compare the very high adenoma prevalence in Japanese living in Hawaii (a very high-risk area for colon cancer) with the much lower adenoma prevalence in Japanese who still reside in Japan—an area of much lower risk. Even within Japan itself, adenoma prevalence correlates quite well with colon cancer prevalence in different prefectures of the country. Adenoma prevalence also correlates with socioeconomic class, even in regions of low colon cancer risk, although this observation may be biased in favor of increased adenoma detection among those who can afford medical care.

Data from autopsy series provide an approximation of adenoma prevalence. In populations at low risk for colon cancer, adenoma prevalence rates are under 12% (see Table 114–5). In most intermediate- and high-risk populations, adenomas are found in 30% to 40% of the population, but rates as high as 50% to 60% have been observed.[9, 54, 55] One half to two thirds of people over age 65 years in high-risk areas may harbor colonic adenomas.[9, 54, 56]

The true prevalence rate of adenomatous polyps within an asymptomatic, living population is only now being elucidated because colonoscopy, until recently, was not performed on healthy, asymptomatic people. Recent studies indicate that asymptomatic average-risk individuals aged 50 years or more have colonoscopic adenoma prevalence rates ranging from 24% to 47%, with rates on the higher end coming from studies of predominantly male veterans.[23, 57–61] Indeed, colonoscopic series indicate that men have a 1.5 relative risk of adenomas compared with age-matched women,[60] confirming earlier observations in autopsy series.[10, 13]

The prevalence of adenomas is higher in older people, particularly those over age 60 years. In fact, age is perhaps the single most important independent determinant of adenoma prevalence.[9, 13, 14, 54–63] This is true of both high-risk and low-risk regions of the world (see Table 114–5). Not only is advancing age associated with a higher prevalence rate of adenomas, but it also correlates with a greater likelihood for multiple polyps, adenomas with more severe degrees of dysplasia, and, in some studies, larger adenoma size.

Adenoma prevalence is also higher in individuals with a positive family history of colorectal cancer and adenomas.[64–66] This is particularly true if more than one generation is affected with colorectal neoplasia, and if an affected relative is young.

Race, per se, does not appear to be an independent determinant of adenoma prevalence; adenomas seldom develop in blacks who reside in South Africa, whereas for African-Americans living in New Orleans, the adenoma prevalence rate is comparable to the prevalence rate for that city's high-risk white population.[12]

INCIDENCE OF ADENOMAS. Estimating the incidence rate of new adenomas requires examining the colon of individuals at more than one point in time. Two types of endoscopic studies lend themselves to this analysis: postpolypectomy (or postcancer resection) surveillance studies, and interval examinations in persons who had an initially negative examina-

Table 114–5 | **Prevalence of Adenomatous Polyps**

POPULATION	COLON CANCER FREQUENCY	PREVALENCE RATE (%)					
		Men			Women		
		Age *20–39*	Age *40–59*	Age *60+*	Age *20–39*	Age *40–59*	Age *60+*
Hawaiian-Japanese	Very high	50	69	64	0	71	58
New Orleans, white	High	0	39	47	0	10	35
New Orleans, black	High	19	26	52	0	27	41
Brazil (São Paulo)	Intermediate	5	14	30	8	14	23
Japan (Akita)	Intermediate	21	31	46	0	8	37
Japan (Miyagi)	Low	1	9	23	4	9	17
Costa Rica (San José)	Low	0	6	13	2	4	9
Colombia (Cali)	Low	2	7	18	2	10	15

From Correa P: Epidemiology of polyps and cancer. In Morson BC (ed): The Pathogenesis of Colorectal Cancer. Philadelphia, WB Saunders, 1978, p 126.

tion. Of course for both types of studies, the small but measurable (15% to 24%) miss rate of adenomas may contribute to the rate of apparent incident adenomas (see "Detection of Adenomas" later). For the purposes of this discussion, adenomas found in individuals after polypectomy are considered recurrences (see "Postpolypectomy Management: Polyp Recurrence Rates" later), whereas those that are found in individuals after an initial negative colonoscopy are considered incident adenomas. In this latter group of subjects, the incidence of new adenomas varies from 24% to 41%.[60] In one study, older male veterans who were at increased risk for colon adenomas underwent colonoscopy twice on the same day to clear the colon of potentially missed adenomas, and 38% were found to have new adenomas when re-colonoscoped 2 years later.[67] Only one study performed follow-up colonoscopy in average-risk, asymptomatic individuals who were originally negative for adenomas by colonoscopy.[68] At a mean interval of 5.5 years, the incidence rate of adenomas was 27%, although the rate for adenomas with advanced pathology was less than 1%.

ANATOMIC DISTRIBUTION. The distribution of adenomatous polyps within the colon differs, depending on the method of investigation (Table 114–6). In autopsy series that approximate the normal distribution in presumably asymptomatic subjects, adenomas are uniformly distributed throughout the colorectum. This even distribution has been confirmed in colonoscopic investigations of asymptomatic subjects.[23, 58] Large adenomas in autopsy series assume a distal predominance, in the region where most colon cancers arise, thereby supporting the adenoma-carcinoma hypothesis. Likewise, adenomas detected in surgical and colonoscopic studies of symptomatic people also display a left-sided predominance, indicating that distal adenomas are more likely to come to clinical attention. In older individuals, particularly those over age 60 years, adenoma distribution demonstrates a shift toward more proximal colonic locations. This phenomenon, which is based on both autopsy[13, 14, 55, 63] and colonoscopic studies of symptomatic[69] as well as asymptomatic subjects,[23, 57, 59, 61, 70, 71] has importance for choosing appropriate colon cancer screening approaches (see Chapter 115).

Risk Factors for Adenoma Susceptibility

Evidence is mounting to suggest that both heredity and environment contribute to colonic adenoma susceptibility. Indeed, the interplay between genetic predisposition and environmental factors finds support in a hypothesis proposed by Hill years ago concerning adenoma causation, which was based mainly on epidemiologic and histopathologic observations.[72] He postulated that an adenoma-prone genotype is extremely common throughout the world. For adenomas to form and then progress to cancer, several environmental factors, presumably dietary, must act in concert: one factor may be responsible for the initial development of adenomas, another may enhance the growth of adenomas that develop, and one or more carcinogens or tumor promoters may finally give rise to cancer.

INHERITED SUSCEPTIBILITY TO ADENOMATOUS POLYPS. There is certainly a strong genetic component to the well-defined hereditary polyposis and nonpolyposis colon cancer syndromes that exhibit a mendelian pattern of inheritance (see later). However, 95% of common (sporadic) adenomas or carcinomas arise in people who do not have these syndromes. In the past, this fact had been interpreted to mean that genetic predisposition played only a minor role in most colonic neoplasms. Epidemiologic studies, however, have revealed a twofold to threefold greater risk for colon cancer in probands who have a first-degree relative affected by colonic cancer or adenoma.[64, 73] Several studies have found a similar increase in risk for adenomas in first-degree relatives of people with adenomas.[64, 73] Moreover, data from the National Polyp Study indicate that siblings and parents of patients with adenomatous polyps are at an increased risk for colon cancer, particularly when the adenoma proband is younger than age 60 years.[74]

It is now estimated that as many as 10% to 30% of colon cancers are familial, implying the possibility of susceptibility genes that give rise to common colon cancers.[64] Indeed, several genes have been identified that may play a role in what has been referred to as *common familial risk.* These include a mutation in the *APC* gene on 5q at codon 1307 (I1307K), which appears to predispose Ashkenazi Jewish populations to colon cancer, mutations of the *MSH6* gene (a DNA mismatch repair gene; see Chapter 115), a type I transforming growth factor receptor allele-TβR-I(6A), and polymorphisms of certain genes involved in metabolism of nutrients and environmental agents, such as methylenetetrahydrofolate reductase and *N*-acetyltransferases 1 and 2.[64, 75]

DIETARY AND LIFE-STYLE RISK FACTORS. Although genetic predisposition clearly plays a role in colorectal carcinogenesis, diet and life-style factors also contribute. It is estimated that as much as a third to a half of colon cancer risk and a fourth to a third of distal colon adenoma risk might be avoidable by modification of dietary and life-style habits.[76] For the most part, dietary factors that correlate with a predisposition to colon cancer are also associated with a risk for colonic adenomas[76–78] (see Chapter 115). Dietary fiber, plant

Table 114–6 | **Anatomic Distribution of Adenomatous Polyps (Percentage of Patients with Adenomas)**

	CECUM AND ASCENDING	TRANSVERSE	DESCENDING	SIGMOID	RECTUM
Autopsy Series					
All adenomas[9, 11, 55]	34	26	10	19	10
Adenomas >1 cm[9]	34	11	14	16	21
Colonoscopy Series					
Asymptomatic[58]	23	24	24	24	5
Symptomatic[5]	8	14	19	47	12

foods, and carbohydrate have shown the most consistent protective effect against adenomas. Increased physical activity and high folate intake also have a protective effect. In contrast, factors that have each been correlated with an increased adenoma risk include excess dietary fat, excess alcohol intake, obesity, and cigarette smoking. It is curious that low calcium intake, despite being associated with increased risk for colon cancer, does not appear to confer risk for adenomas. Aspirin and nonsteroidal anti-inflammatory drugs (NSAIDs) have been shown to reduce colon carcinogenesis in epidemiologic studies as well as in animal models.[79] In addition, several interventional studies in patients with FAP demonstrate a marked reduction in adenoma size and number in response to NSAIDs (see later). Little is known about the effect of these agents on the natural history of sporadic adenomas. Two small interventional studies revealed little or no effect of NSAIDs on sporadic adenomas,[80, 81] whereas in two larger studies, aspirin use was associated with a considerably lower frequency of adenomas.[82, 83] Clinical trials are under way to determine the effect of selective cyclooxygenase-2 inhibitors on the recurrence rate of sporadic adenomas.

Based on leads from epidemiologic and observational studies, several prospective randomized studies were conducted during the last decade to test directly whether dietary or chemopreventive interventions could reduce adenomatous polyp formation. These studies share a fundamental experimental design: patients who have had an adenomatous polyp removed are randomly assigned to a nutritional intervention or to a control group, and then followed with repeat colonoscopy, usually 1 and 3 or 4 years later, to determine the efficacy of the intervention. Therefore, these studies investigate the ability of the intervention to prevent recurrent adenomas over a relatively short time. Nonetheless, this study design is the most feasible given the logistical and cost issues involved in performing alternative approaches, such as studies to prevent the first adenoma in healthy individuals or following adenoma patients for many more years using colon cancer as the end-point. With this polyp prevention clinical model, disappointing results were obtained from two large-scale prospective studies in the United States that tested the effects of dietary fiber on adenoma recurrence. Neither a low-fat, high-fiber/fruit/vegetable diet[84] nor a dietary supplement of wheat bran fiber[85] protected against recurrent adenomas. Likewise, the Australian Polyp Prevention Trial found that after a 1- to 2-year adherence to a low-fat, high-fiber diet, the total number of recurrent adenomas was unchanged from that in a control group.[86] In that study, however, the frequency of large (>1 cm) adenomas was in fact reduced. Unfortunately, no such reduction in large adenomas was reported in the two American studies.[84, 85] One interpretation of these apparently negative interventional studies is not that the intervention failed, but rather that the study design may not be able to demonstrate a positive effect of the intervention.[87]

Supplemental antioxidants, such as beta-carotene and vitamins C and E, also appear to have no effect on adenoma risk.[88] On the other hand, calcium supplementation (1200 mg per day of elemental calcium) has been shown to produce a modest (15%) reduction in recurrent adenomas.[89] The mechanism for this protective effect is likely to be multifactorial since calcium has been shown to decrease proliferation of colonic epithelial cells and to inhibit mucosal injury induced by bile acids and carcinogens in the fecal stream. Bearing in mind the limitations of polyp prevention clinical trials, results of additional studies of calcium, folate, and aspirin for polyp prevention are anxiously awaited.

CONDITIONS ASSOCIATED WITH ADENOMATOUS POLYPS. A variety of clinical circumstances have been associated with adenomatous polyps. Of the conditions discussed here, the predisposition to have or to develop adenomas is strongest for patients with ureterosigmoidostomies, those with acromegaly, and those with *Streptococcus bovis* bacteremia. These patients should undergo a thorough colorectal examination and, in the former two conditions, periodic surveillance (although the frequency of such examinations is not well defined). As for the other conditions, either the data are conflicting or the risk is not strong enough to recommend a policy of surveillance.

Polyps at Ureterosigmoidostomy Sites. Patients who have undergone a previous urinary diversion procedure with implantation of the ureters into the sigmoid colon are at particularly high risk for development of neoplastic lesions at the ureterosigmoidostomy sites.[90] The most important lesions are adenomatous polyps and carcinomas, which have been found after latent periods of 2 to 38 years, with mean latent periods of 20 and 26 years for adenomas and carcinomas, respectively. Lesions that resemble juvenile polyps and inflammatory polyps also have been reported at ureterosigmoidostomy sites. It appears that at least 29% of such patients develop colonic neoplasms after this procedure, usually close to the stoma. It has been suggested that these lesions are produced by the generation of *N*-nitrosamines from urinary amines in the presence of the fecal flora. In view of the extremely high frequency of neoplasia in this setting, these patients must undergo lifelong colonoscopic surveillance in keeping with the long latent period between the implantation of the ureters and the subsequent development of colonic neoplasia.

Acromegaly. Patients with acromegaly have an increased tendency to develop colon cancers and adenomas.[91–93] Although these studies inherently involve few subjects, consistently high prevalence rates of 5% to 25% for colon cancer and 14% to 35% for adenomatous polyps have been observed in acromegaly patients. The risk for colonic neoplasia may be higher in younger acromegalics,[91] those with a family history of colon cancer,[92] those with multiple skin tags (acrochordons),[93] and those with previous colorectal adenomas.[94] The mechanism for enhanced colonic neoplasia in this disease is not clear but probably relates to increased growth hormone and/or insulin-like growth factor-1 (IGF-1) levels. In non-acromegalics, high serum levels of IGF-1 have been correlated with an increased risk of colorectal cancer.[95] In acromegalics, high serum IGF-1 levels have been correlated with increased epithelial cell proliferation[96] and increased recurrence rates of colorectal adenomas.[94] Other studies in acromegalics, however, did not find that blood levels of growth hormone or IGF-1 correlated with the presence of neoplasms,[93] and the risk of neoplasia was actually greater in cured acromegalics than in those with active disease.[92]

***Streptococcus bovis* Bacteremia.** Bacteremia and endocarditis caused by *S. bovis* have been associated with colorectal carcinoma, adenomatous polyps, and even FAP.[97–99] In some studies, the fecal carrier rate of this organism is higher in people with adenomas or carcinomas than in those with benign colonic diseases or in normal controls.[99] In animal models, *S. bovis* or even an extract of its cell wall antigens increased the expression of markers associated with early colon carcinogenesis.[100] It has therefore been suggested that patients with *S. bovis* bacteremia undergo thorough colonic examination to exclude a neoplasm. Endocarditis caused by *Streptococcus agalactiae* (an organism that seldom is pathogenic in adults) also has been reported in two patients who each had a rectal villous adenoma with foci of carcinoma.[101]

Skin Tags. The correlation between colonic neoplasia and the presence and multiplicity of skin tags (acrochordons) in acromegalic patients led to the question of whether skin tags (usually located on the upper trunk or axillae) could serve as a cutaneous marker of colonic polyps in the general population. Although a significant correlation was found between the presence of skin tags and adenomatous polyps in prospective studies of symptomatic patients presenting for colonoscopy, no such correlation was found in asymptomatic patients and in members of familial polyposis kindreds.[102] Thus acrochordons do not appear to be useful markers for polyps in average-risk asymptomatic people.

Atherosclerosis and Cholesterol. An association between adenomatous polyps and atherosclerosis has been documented by necropsy studies,[103, 104] one of which noted a correlation between the degree of atherosclerosis and the multiplicity, size, and degree of dysplasia of adenomas.[104] This observation suggests that these two common conditions of Westernized populations share certain risk factors, possibly elevated serum cholesterol levels. However, a cause-and-effect relation between serum cholesterol concentration and adenomatous polyps has not been established. It is curious that patients with colon cancer often have low serum cholesterol levels, which apparently precede the development of cancer[105] and are therefore not simply a metabolic consequence of the cancer. If the cholesterol level does indeed gradually decline before the development of colon cancer, the apparent discrepancies between studies that attempt to correlate cholesterol level with the presence of adenomas may reflect differences in adenoma stage.

Breast Cancer. Epidemiologic investigations have found an association between cancers of the breast and colon in terms of prevalence and mortality rates.[106] Case-control studies, however, have found little or no increased risk for adenomatous polyps in women who have had breast cancer. Moreover, asymptomatic women whose only "risk factor" for colonic neoplasia was a personal history of breast cancer had an identical prevalence of adenomas compared with a control group.[107] Loss of the *BRCA1* tumor suppressor gene, which is important for predisposition to some hereditary breast and ovarian cancers, does not appear to play a role in colon carcinogenesis.[108] Therefore, unless future studies determine otherwise, a personal history of breast cancer should not be considered a risk factor for colonic adenomas.

Cholecystectomy. In some studies, cholecystectomy has been associated with an increased risk for colon cancer, although this increase is only modest and applies mainly to women and to proximal colonic lesions.[109] It is postulated that in the absence of the gallbladder, there is enhanced delivery of bile acids and possibly a shift from primary to secondary bile acids, which enhance the proliferative activity of the colonic mucosa. Case-control studies have not found an increased risk for adenomatous polyps among cholecystectomized patients in general.[110, 111]

Diagnosis of Adenomatous Polyps

SYMPTOMS AND SIGNS. Most patients with colonic polyps either have no symptoms referable to the gastrointestinal tract or have nonspecific intestinal symptoms. In individuals with symptoms that can be attributed to colonic polyps, the most common presenting symptom is occult or overt rectal bleeding. Histopathologic observations suggest that, in contrast with colonic carcinomas, which exhibit considerable surface erosion, the generally less rigid adenomas maintain the integrity of the surface epithelium but may bleed into the polyp stroma.[112] These findings help explain the clinical impression that bleeding from polyps is only intermittent and does not usually cause fecal occult blood loss or anemia.

Other symptoms that have been attributed to colonic polyps are constipation, diarrhea, and flatulence. Constipation or decreased stool caliber is more likely to be caused by bulky lesions in the distal colon. Large colonic polyps may be associated with cramping lower abdominal pain due to intermittent intussusception. Unless these widely prevalent symptoms disappear with the removal of the polyp, they must be attributed to other causes.

An uncommon syndrome of secretory diarrhea with considerable and sometimes life-threatening water and electrolyte depletion has occasionally been observed in patients with villous adenomas.[113] Tumors that produce this syndrome are typically larger than 3 to 4 cm in diameter and are almost always located in the rectum or rectosigmoid, providing little surface area distal to the tumor for reabsorption of fluid and electrolytes. In contrast to the absorption of water and sodium and secretion of potassium by normal colonic mucosa, secretory villous adenomas exhibit a net secretion of water and sodium and an exaggerated secretion of potassium.[114] A tumor-derived secretagogue has been postulated to account for the secretory diarrhea in this syndrome that mimics cholera. In one report, prostaglandin E_2 levels in rectal effluent were high and decreased in response to therapy with indomethacin, which produced partial symptomatic improvement.[115]

DETECTION OF ADENOMAS. Colorectal polyps usually are clinically silent. They typically are detected either in asymptomatic people being screened for colorectal neoplasia or incidentally during investigation for symptoms ostensibly referable to the colon or for unexplained iron deficiency anemia. A more complete discussion of colorectal cancer screening can be found in Chapter 115. This section will address the issue of adenoma detection using the various screening modalities available.

Fecal Occult Blood Testing. The actual frequency of bleeding from adenomas is difficult to determine. Fewer than 10% of people who report frank rectal bleeding will be found to have a significant adenoma (i.e., $\geq$1 cm or carcinoma in situ) as the cause.[116–118] In general, polyps under 1 cm do not bleed. This dictum is supported by quantitative measurements of fecal blood loss in people with known adenomas, which indicate that only those with adenomas larger than 1.5 to 2.0 cm lose more than the usual amounts of blood (regardless of the location of the polyp within the colon).[119] Likewise, when occult blood loss is detected qualitatively with Hemoccult cards, only 20% to 40% of patients with known adenomas show positive test results,[119–122] the rates being high primarily in patients with larger and distal polyps. Initial optimism that the more sensitive HemoQuant fecal occult blood test would improve detection of polyps has been dampened by the fact that this test detected only 20% of patients with polyps larger than 1 cm.[123] Newer immunochemical tests for fecal occult blood, particularly when combined with a more sensitive guaiac-based test, can enhance the sensitivity for detecting adenomas over 1 cm in size,[124] but their place in screening has not yet been established.

When asymptomatic individuals undergo colon cancer screening with guaiac-based fecal occult blood tests (see Chapter 115), about 1% to 3% of asymptomatic adults over age 40 years have a positive result.[125] Fewer than half of these people have a colorectal neoplasm; among the lesions found, adenomas outnumber carcinomas by 3:1. Thus the proportions of all positive guaiac tests attributable to colonic neoplasms (i.e., positive predictive values) are 30% to 35% for adenomas and 8% to 12% for cancer.[126] As mentioned earlier, because adenomas are usually asymptomatic, their detection in the context of colon cancer screening is serendipitous.[127] Despite the predominance of adenomas among lesions detected, 75% of adenomas may still be missed by guaiac testing (i.e., false-negative values) unless they are large or located in the distal portion of the colon. Positive test results for occult blood 1 to 2 years after a negative search will detect some of these missed polyps.[128] Because small polyps seldom bleed and their rate of detection by occult blood testing is meager, sigmoidoscopy is recommended to complement fecal occult blood testing.

Sigmoidoscopy. The flexible sigmoidoscope has essentially replaced the rigid sigmoidoscope in common practice. In symptomatic patients, the yield for detecting polyps (and cancer) is three times greater with the 60-cm flexible instrument than with the rigid one,[129] and this diagnostic advantage also applies to asymptomatic patients undergoing screening or surveillance sigmoidoscopy. The increased yield with the flexible instrument is due primarily to the fact that most of the polyps detected are located beyond the average depth of insertion of the rigid endoscope.[130] In asymptomatic people, rigid sigmoidoscopy will detect polyps (of all histologic types) in about 7% of people over age 40 years.[131] When used strictly for screening asymptomatic people over age 40 years, the flexible sigmoidoscope reveals polyps in 10% to 15%.[129, 132, 133] This yield is lower in screens of younger people[134] and higher in people with occult bleeding.[135]

Barium Enema. Although large polyps are readily detected by either the single-contrast or double-contrast method of barium enema, use of the latter technique maximizes the detection of small polyps.[136] A properly performed double-contrast barium enema examination can have a sensitivity as high as 85% to 95% for detecting colorectal polyps, although some studies report much lower rates of only 35% for all polyps and 39% for adenomas.[137] The detection of adenomas by barium enema is dependent upon size. In the National Polyp Study, the detection rates for adenomas 5 mm or less, 6 to 10 mm, and over 10 mm were 32%, 53%, and 48%, respectively.[137] Common sources of error include inadequate cleansing of the colon, which contributes to the 5% to 10% false-positive rate, and diagnostic difficulty caused by the presence of diverticulosis, redundant bowel, or poor mucosal coating, which results in a 10% false-negative rate at the least (see earlier).

Colonoscopy. Colonoscopy usually is preferred to double-contrast barium enema examination for adenoma detection because it has enhanced diagnostic accuracy as well as therapeutic capability. This diagnostic superiority has been demonstrated in studies of patients with known polyps,[137–139] as well as in symptomatic patients who have had negative findings on proctosigmoidoscopic and barium enema examinations.[140] Despite its reputation as the "gold standard" for adenoma detection, colonoscopy has some limitations. Colonoscopy fails to reach the cecum in up to 10% of cases; it usually requires patient sedation; and it carries a higher cost than barium enema. Colonoscopy can also miss neoplasms, especially those located at flexures or behind folds. In general, adenomas that are missed tend to be small. One study of tandem colonoscopy performed by two experienced endoscopists estimated that the first examination could "miss" up to 15% of small polyps (<8 mm), but none of the larger polyps.[141] A similar study reported an overall miss rate for adenomas of 24%, with miss rates for adenomas 5 mm or less, 6 to 9 mm, and 10 or more mm of 27%, 13%, and 6%, respectively.[142] In the National Polyp Study, the miss rate for adenomas was 20%, all of which were 1 cm or less in size.[137] These limitations notwithstanding, the use of colonoscopy as a primary screening method has gained acceptance, has been incorporated into colorectal cancer screening guidelines,[65] and is currently endorsed by governmental agencies.

The likelihood of finding an adenoma by colonoscopy for various clinical indications has been reviewed.[143] The baseline frequency of adenomas in asymptomatic individuals over age 50 years is a substantial 29%.

Newer Methods for Adenoma Detection. Performing colography by either helical computed tomography or magnetic resonance imaging (so-called *virtual colonoscopy*) holds promise as a noninvasive means for detecting colonic neoplasms. Compared with conventional colonoscopy, this method of imaging a prepped, air-insufflated colon typically identifies 91% to 100% of polyps ≥1 cm, 71% to 82% of polyps between 0.6 and 0.9 cm, but only up to 55% of polyps smaller than 0.5 cm.[144, 145] Further studies will help determine whether this promising modality will be incorporated into routine clinical practice. Endoscope-compatible optical fiber systems have been developed that permit the use of low-power laser illumination as a novel diagnostic tool. Without creating injury, this laser beam stimulates tissue to emit endogenous fluorescence, which can then be measured and analyzed by spectroscopy. The spectrum emitted by adenomatous polyps is distinct from that of hyperplastic polyps and normal mucosa.[146] Although this technology is intellectually tantalizing, its role in clinical diagnosis and management is not yet clear.

Based on our knowledge of molecular genetic alterations in colon carcinogenesis, a noninvasive method for detecting altered human DNA in stool has been developed.[147] Pilot studies indicate sensitivities of 91% and 82% for detecting cancers and adenomas greater than 1 cm, respectively, and a specificity of at least 93%. Because fecal occult blood testing is notoriously poor for detecting adenomas, this novel stool test holds promise as a screening modality and is currently undergoing further testing in larger studies.

Management of Adenomatous Polyps

Proper management of the patient with adenomatous polyps requires an understanding of the natural history of untreated adenomas, the relationship between multiple adenomas and carcinomas, and the course of patients after treatment (polypectomy).

NATURAL HISTORY OF ADENOMAS. Little is known about adenoma growth rate, primarily because with the advent of endoscopy, polyps are readily removed, thereby interrupting the natural history of their growth. Thus our limited knowledge about polyp growth rate has been pieced together from two main types of studies: (1) longitudinal follow-up studies on patients with unresected polyps, and (2) studies that compare the age distribution of people with adenomas with that of people with carcinomas.

The Untreated Adenoma. Longitudinal studies of people with untreated adenomas afford the most direct picture of the natural history of adenomas, although these people may not be representative of all polyp patients. In general, studies of this kind have been retrospective and either involved very few patients or suffered from a lack of histologic confirmation of the index polyp. Despite these drawbacks, it appears that the adenoma-to-carcinoma progression is rather slow, requiring several years to unfold. In 14 individuals with unresected polyps, it took at least 5 years and often more than 10 years for histologically proven adenomas to progress to cancer.[7] The size of the index polyp affects the interval to carcinoma, since larger adenomas are more likely than smaller ones to develop or already contain a focus of cancer. But even starting with a 1-cm polypoid tumor (histology unknown), serial barium enema measurements have suggested that it may take 2 to 5 years for cancer to develop[148] and that the cumulative risk of cancer at the polyp site is only 2.5% at 5 years, 8% at 10 years, and 24% at 20 years after diagnosis.[149] Other radiographic studies indicate that in adenomas with growth rates that are as rapid as those of cancer, doubling times are still longer than 4 to 6 months.[150, 151]

Smaller polyps are likely to require even more time to progress to cancer, and even after several years, many adenomas do not enlarge. For example, in a study involving 213 asymptomatic people with rectal polyps of unknown histology ranging in size from 0.2 to 1.5 cm, serial rigid sigmoidoscopies over 3 to 5 years detected only two cancers (1%), and only 4% of these polyps grew larger; the other 96% of polyps remained unchanged, got smaller, or disappeared.[152] A subsequent study reported that over a 3-year period, adenomas smaller than 1 cm did not significantly change size, and those that were 5 to 9 mm in size actually showed slight regression.[153] In another endoscopic study, histologically proven diminutive adenomas were left in place for 2 years, after which time only half of them enlarged, but none grew to more than 0.5 cm or developed severe dysplasia or cancer.[24] Other investigators measured 30 rectosigmoid polyps originally 3 to 9 mm in size every 6 months for two years; none regressed in size, and only 3 (10%) showed a fast growth rate (2 to 4 mm/yr).[154] A mathematical model using assumptions based on doubling-time calculations from serial barium enemas predicts that a diminutive polyp (less than 0.5 cm) requires 2 to 3 years to reach 1-cm size.[155]

Age Distribution Studies. Additional, albeit indirect support of the rather slow growth of adenomas comes from studies that have compared the mean age of people with adenomas with that of people with carcinomas. For instance, studies from St. Mark's Hospital in London and from the National Polyp Study in the United States indicate that the mean age of people with a single adenoma is about four to five years younger than those with a colon cancer.[7, 156] A similar analysis in FAP patients has shown that patients with adenomas are about 12 years younger than those with colon cancer.[7] Likewise, Kozuka and colleagues estimated that the transition period for adenomas with mild dysplasia to cancer is 8 years, whereas the interval for adenomas with severe dysplasia to become malignant is 3 to 4 years.[40] Eide[157] calculated that over a 10-year period, there is only a 2.5% risk that an adenoma-bearing person will develop colon cancer, but this risk would be greater if the adenoma is large or villous.

MULTIPLE ADENOMAS AND CARCINOMAS. For proper patient management and design of cancer screening and surveillance programs, it is important to know the frequency with which adenomas coexist with other adenomas or carcinomas. The term *multiple adenoma* (or carcinoma) simply means two or more neoplasms and should not be confused with the "multiple adenomatous polyposis syndromes" characterized by hundreds of polyps (see later). An adenoma or carcinoma that is diagnosed at the same time as an index colorectal neoplasm is called a *synchronous* lesion, but one that is diagnosed at least 6 months later (a somewhat arbitrary limit) is considered *metachronous*.

The adenomatous polyp itself commonly is regarded as a marker of a neoplasm-prone colon. Indeed, 30% to 50% of colons with one adenoma will contain at least one other synchronous adenoma, especially in older age groups.[7, 14, 18] In addition, the risk of colon cancer and of high-grade dysplasia both rise with the number of adenomas present (Table 114–7) and approach 100% in people with FAP.

A synchronous adenoma can be found in 30% of colons that harbor a carcinoma[7, 158–160] and in 50% to 85% of those that harbor two or more synchronous cancers.[7, 158, 161, 162] If the synchronous adenoma is diagnosed preoperatively and is distant from the carcinoma, the surgical approach may have to be adapted to the particular circumstances.[158] For this reason, preoperative colonoscopy is strongly recommended before the resection of any colorectal carcinoma. Also, the

Table 114–7 | **Correlation Between Number of Adenomas and Associated Carcinoma or High-Grade Dysplasia**

NO. OF ADENOMAS PER PATIENT	ST. MARK'S HOSPITAL[7]		NATIONAL POLYP STUDY[4]	
	No. of Patients	No. of Patients with Carcinoma (%)	No. of Patients	No. of Patients with High-Grade Dysplasia (%)
1	1331	395 (30)	1093	80 (7)
2	296	153 (52)	430	42 (10)
3	83	47 (57)	166	32 (19)
4	40	20 (50)	83	14 (17)
5	13	10 (77)	40	8 (20)
≥6	25	20 (80)	55	11 (20)

presence of a synchronous adenoma in a patient with colon cancer increases the risk for developing subsequent colon cancer.[7, 159] Similarly, a synchronous adenoma in a patient with a colonic polyp places that person at greater risk for developing metachronous polyps[163] and cancer.[163, 164]

INITIAL MANAGEMENT OF ADENOMAS. If a polyp is detected by barium enema, a colonoscopy is recommended to establish the histologic diagnosis of the polyp while simultaneously affording the opportunity to remove the polyp and search for synchronous neoplasms. When a polyp is encountered during sigmoidoscopy, it should be biopsied to establish its histologic type. If the polyp is hyperplastic, most authorities do not recommend a full colonoscopy[165] (see "Hyperplastic Polyps" later).

There is some debate as to whether rectosigmoid adenomas found at sigmoidoscopy are markers for proximal colonic neoplasia, thereby prompting the need for a full colonoscopy. This controversy particularly applies to patients who have only a single, small, tubular adenoma with low-grade dysplasia. Some studies indicate that in this subset of patients, colonoscopy does not discover a substantial number of proximal adenomas with advanced pathology (AAPs) or cancers,[166–168] nor is there a subsequent increased risk of developing proximal cancer among those who do not undergo colonoscopy.[169] In contrast, two screening colonoscopy studies suggest that the odds of finding advanced proximal neoplasia, even with a small, single, tubular adenoma, is 2.6-fold to fourfold that of finding no distal pathology.[61, 71] (Table 114–8). Likewise, some have estimated that by not doing colonoscopy for a distal, nonadvanced adenoma, 36% of advanced proximal neoplasms would be missed.[170] Furthermore, 52% of patients with advanced proximal neoplasia have no distal adenoma,[61] and 70% of proximal colon cancers lack a distal marker lesion.[171] These observations have increased the momentum to consider colonoscopy as a primary screening modality. For the time being, recommended guidelines are to individualize the approach to these patients.[165] Since risk factors for finding advanced proximal neoplasia are increasing age,[69–71] a positive family history of colorectal cancer,[69, 71] and male gender,[70] performing colonoscopy in these individuals on the basis of finding a distal, small, tubular adenoma would seem prudent.

There is little debate that if sigmoidoscopy reveals more than one adenoma, or a distal AAP, a full colonoscopy is warranted because of the higher likelihood of finding synchronous proximal advanced neoplasms (see Table 114–8). Because negative biopsy results from a fractional sample of a polyp cannot possibly rule out cancer, total excision of a polyp is the only method of providing a thorough and accurate histologic diagnosis. For larger polyps, this may require piecemeal excision, and for sessile growths, injection of saline into the polyp base can assist with complete endoscopic resection. After apparent complete removal of a large adenoma, it is advisable to repeat the colonoscopy in 3 to 6 months to document the completeness of the excision.[165] If a polyp cannot be completely excised after two or three endoscopic sessions, surgical therapy is recommended.

Based on the preceding discussion, screening colonoscopy

Table 114–8 | **Frequency of Advanced Proximal Neoplasia Related to Findings in the Distal Colon**

FINDING(S) IN DISTAL COLON	LIEBERMAN[61]*		IMPERIALE[70]*		LEVIN[71]†	
	Percent	*Odds Ratio (95% CI)*	*Percent*	*Relative Risk (95% CI)*	*Percent*	*Odds Ratio (95% CI)*
	← *Frequency of Advanced Proximal Neoplasia* →					
No distal polyps	2.7	1.0	1.5	1.0	5.3	1.0
Distal hyperplastic polyp	2.8	1.1 (0.6–2.1)	4.0	2.6 (1.1–5.9)	—	—
Distal adenoma	6.8	2.6 (1.7–4.1)	7.1	4.0 (1.9–8.3)	5.0	1.26 (0.81–1.98)
Distal advanced neoplasm	—		11.5	6.7 (3.2–16.6)	—	
Tubular adenoma >1 cm	8.6	3.2 (1.5–6.8)	—		4.5	1.66 ((1.10–2.52)
Villous features	12.5	4.7 (2.1–10.4)	—		12.1	2.46 (1.60–3.77)
High-grade dysplasia	11.4	4.5 (1.5–13.4)	—		—	
Invasive cancer	25.0	9.8 (3.6–26.4)	—		—	

*Screening colonoscopy study.
†Screening sigmoidoscopy followed by colonoscopy.
CI, confidence interval.

is gaining acceptance in the United States as a primary screening tool (see Chapter 115). However, many other countries with more limited resources do not yet subscribe to this philosophy. This has led to a large-scale screening flexible sigmoidoscopy trial based in the United Kingdom that will test whether a one-time sigmoidoscopy at around age 60 years, with selective colonoscopy only for high-risk adenomas, will be beneficial.[172] Results of this study, as well as the United States Prostate, Lung, Colorectal and Ovarian (PLCO) cancer screening trial[173] will provide additional data from prospective trials on the utility of screening sigmoidoscopy.

MANAGEMENT OF THE MALIGNANT POLYP. The term *malignant polyp* refers to an adenoma in which a focus of carcinoma has invaded beyond the muscularis mucosae into the submucosa. This term is not applied to adenomas containing either carcinoma in situ or intramucosal carcinoma because these lesions are not invasive and carry no metastatic potential. Rarely, polyps may consist entirely of carcinoma. These so-called polypoid carcinomas usually are considered a subset of malignant polyps, and they most likely represent a previous adenoma that is completely replaced by carcinoma. Sometimes islands of benign adenomatous epithelium are found beneath the muscularis mucosae, and care must be taken not to mistake such "pseudocarcinomatous invasion" for true invasive carcinoma; this important distinction may be particularly difficult in the rare instance when the ectopic benign epithelium exhibits features of high-grade dysplasia. Ectopic benign epithelium is seen more often in larger pedunculated polyps, particularly in the sigmoid colon. Because the distinction between carcinoma in situ and invasive carcinoma will influence both management and prognosis, it is crucial that tissue be properly oriented for pathologic examination and that close communication takes place among endoscopist, surgeon, and pathologist.

The endoscopic removal of the great majority of colorectal polyps raises two central questions: Is endoscopic polypectomy alone adequate therapy for the malignant polyp? If not, what features of the polyp can predict the presence of residual disease or subsequent recurrence? The answers are vital because on them rests the decision for subsequent surgical resection of bowel.

Complete endoscopic removal of an adenoma with noninvasive carcinoma represents curative therapy. The therapeutic dilemma becomes much more difficult when polyps contain invasive carcinoma (malignant polyp). Although most of these lesions are treated adequately by endoscopic polypectomy, about 10% of patients will experience an adverse outcome,[174] defined as residual cancer in the bowel wall or in lymph nodes either at the time of polypectomy or on follow-up. This rate of failure is comparable to that of the precolonoscopic era when adenomas were larger and underwent more complete surgical resection.[174] Because malignant polyps account for only 5% of all adenomas, and because not all patients who have had colonoscopic removal of malignant polyps have had surgical resection or are available for follow-up, conclusions often are based on small numbers.

Notwithstanding these limitations, combined experience has identified certain favorable and unfavorable histopathologic features of a colonoscopically resected malignant polyp that can be used to classify a patient as being at low or high risk for an adverse outcome (Table 114–9). If none of the four unfavorable risk factors is found, the patient is considered to have been cured by the endoscopic polypectomy alone. This principle applies even to endoscopically removed polypoid carcinomas, which have been associated with a surprisingly good outcome when not complicated by any unfavorable histopathologic features. If one or more unfavorable features are found in a malignant polyp (Fig. 114–7), the chance of an adverse outcome rises to about 10% to 25%.[175] In such cases, surgical resection usually should be performed, taking into account the risk of operative mortality in elderly patients with comorbid illnesses.[165]

Table 114–9 | **Risk Factors for Adverse Outcomes in Patients with Malignant Polyps**

	FAVORABLE (LOW RISK)	UNFAVORABLE (HIGH RISK)
Degree of differentiation	Well or moderate	Poor
Invasion of veins or lymphatics	Absent	Present
Polypectomy margin	Clear or >2-mm margin	Involved
Invasion of submucosa of bowel wall	Absent	Present

Several aspects of defining the risk factors just noted demand close collaboration between endoscopists and pathologists. First, some malignant polyps contain only a small focus of poorly differentiated carcinoma, so meticulous pathologic analysis is essential. Second, identification of vessel invasion by cancer cells in malignant polyps may be

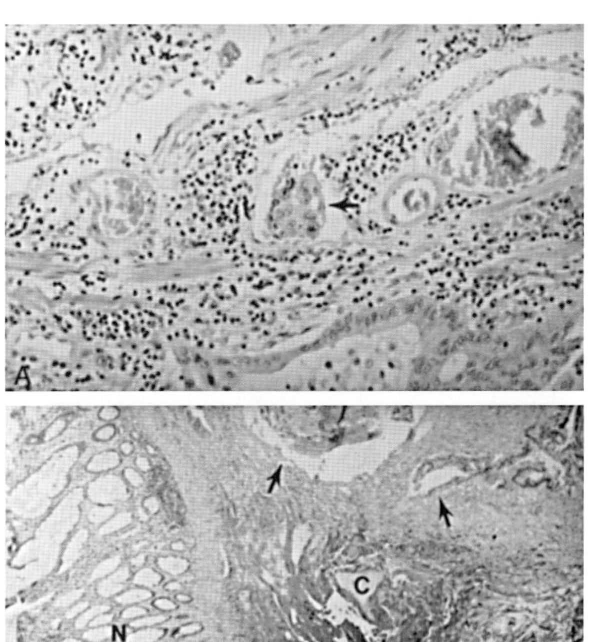

Figure 114–7. Unfavorable histopathologic features in a malignant polyp. *A,* Vascular invasion by a focus of cancer *(arrow). B,* Endoscopic polypectomy specimen illustrating the area of cautery (C) within adjacent normal (N) colonic mucosa. Cancer cells *(arrows)* are found within 1 mm of the line of cautery.

difficult, in which case special stains of vascular endothelium can be used for clarification. Third, although the polypectomy margin may be found microscopically to contain cancer cells, some studies suggest that if the endoscopist believes that a complete excision was achieved, surgical resection may not be necessary because the electrocautery may have effectively destroyed residual tumor in the bowel wall.[176] Finally, in judging the adequacy of endoscopic polypectomy, the issue of submucosal invasion is important. A pedunculated polyp differs anatomically from a sessile polyp in that the submucosa of the former projects up into the stalk, whereas the submucosa of the latter is in direct continuity with the bowel wall proper (Fig. 114–8). If cancer in a pedunculated polyp is confined to the submucosa of the stalk and all other histologic features are favorable, surgery is not indicated because the chance of an adverse outcome from endoscopic polypectomy is less than the operative mortality. Once the submucosa of the bowel wall (as opposed to the submucosa of the stalk) is involved with cancer (a situation that occurs more readily in sessile polyps), the chance of an adverse outcome often outweighs the operative mortality, thereby justifying surgical resection. Furthermore, because endoscopic technique purposely avoids cutting deep into the bowel wall submucosa, there are few published examples of sessile lesions that have been completely excised endoscopically with clear margins and no other unfavorable features.

Deciding on an optimal plan of management after polypectomy involves weighing the risks of morbidity and mortality from potential residual or recurrent cancer against the risks of morbidity and mortality from a surgical attempt to cure any such residual disease or lymph node metastasis. A few general recommendations may be offered. If adenoma excision is complete, endoscopic polypectomy alone is adequate therapy for adenomas that contain carcinoma in situ, pedunculated adenomas that harbor well-differentiated or moderately differentiated invasive carcinoma, and uncomplicated polypoid carcinomas. Resectional surgery is indicated for malignant polyps in which the invasive carcinoma (1) is poorly differentiated, (2) involves endothelium-lined channels (lymphatics, blood vessels), (3) extends to or within 2 mm of the polypectomy margin, or (4) involves the submucosa of the colonic wall (including all sessile adenomas). Clearly the ultimate plan of therapy must be individualized according to each patient's medical condition and the patient's wishes. For most patients with malignant polyps, polypectomy without surgical resection seems adequate, with the caveat that postpolypectomy endoscopic surveillance be incorporated into the patient's health care.

POSTPOLYPECTOMY MANAGEMENT

(see Chapter 30 for Complications of Colonoscopy and Polypectomy)

Polyp Recurrence Rates. Although patients in whom a colorectal adenoma has been completely excised are likely to develop subsequent (metachronous) neoplasms, the frequency and time course of this future transformation are not well understood. In long-term retrospective studies, the cumulative risk of adenoma recurrence is nearly linear, reaching 20% at 5 years after polypectomy and rising to 50% after 15 years (Fig. 114–9).[177] As noted earlier, recurrence rates tend to be somewhat inflated because lesions missed during the index colonoscopy may be considered metachronous lesions. It has been estimated that one third of people who have undergone polypectomy will develop recurrent adenomas.[178–181] The recurrence rate at 1 year is as low as 5%

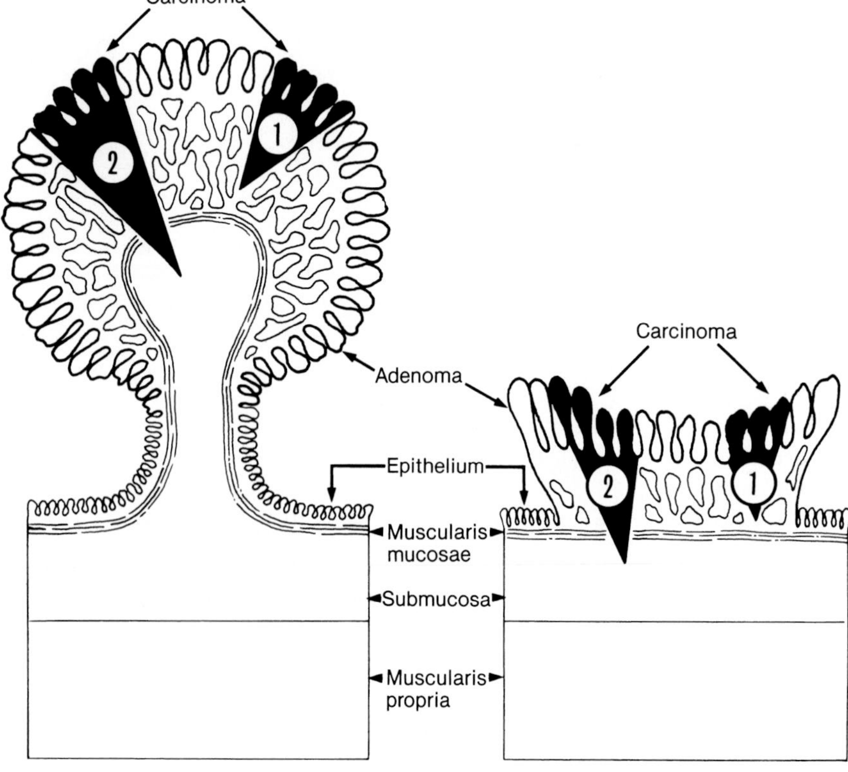

Figure 114–8. Carcinoma in situ versus invasive cancer. Carcinoma *(shaded dark)* is considered intramucosal or carcinoma in situ, as indicated by ① either in a pedunculated adenoma *(left)* or in a sessile adenoma *(right)*. This lesion, as a rule, does not metastasize. Carcinoma in an adenomatous polyp is considered invasive when it breaches the muscularis mucosae, as indicated by ②. Invasive cancer in a pedunculated polyp is unlikely to metastasize, but it is managed differently from invasive cancer in a sessile polyp, which often requires surgical resection. Some pathologists use the Haggitt classification for cancer within an adenomatous polyp. For the pedunculated polyp shown on the left, the cancer depicted as ① corresponds to Haggitt level 0, while the cancer depicted as ② would be Haggitt level 1. If the cancer extends to the junction of the polyp with the normal mucosa, the Haggitt level would be 2, whereas if the cancer involves the stalk, it would be level 3. If the cancer encroaches on the submucosa or extends to the cautery margin, it would be level 4. For the sessile polyp shown on the right, the cancer depicted as ① would be level two and as ② would be level 4.

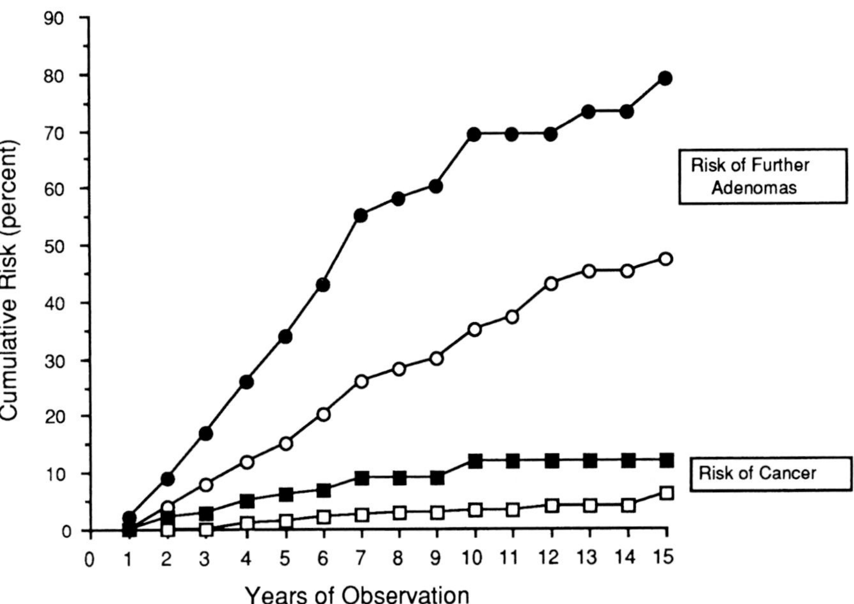

Figure 114–9. Recurrence rates of adenomas and colon cancers after adenoma removal. The risk of developing further adenomas *(circles)* or cancer *(squares)* is higher in patients who initially had removal of multiple lesions *(closed symbols)* rather than a single lesion *(open symbols)*. (Modified from Morson BC, Bussey HJR: Magnitude of risk for cancer in patients with colorectal adenomas. Br J Surg 1985;72(suppl): S23, by permission of the publishers Butterworth-Heineman Ltd.)

to 15%,[177, 180, 181] but more realistically ranges from 30% to 45% based on more recent prospective colonoscopy studies.[38, 84, 85, 178, 182, 183] There is general consensus that recurrent adenomas are typically smaller in size and less likely to harbor advanced pathology than are index adenomas. In the National Polyp Study, the overall adenoma recurrence rate was 42% for patients who underwent surveillance colonoscopy at 1 and 3 years after index polypectomy and 32% in the group that was examined only at 3 years.[41]

Can histopathologic features of adenomas at the time of the index polypectomy be used to help predict recurrence of adenomas? Virtually all studies agree that the presence of multiple index adenomas is an important predictor of subsequent adenoma (and carcinoma) recurrence[177, 178, 180, 181, 184, 185] (see Fig. 114–9). This dictum applies despite negative findings on colonoscopy 1 year after polypectomy.[182] Some studies suggest that polyp size greater than 1 cm,[179, 181, 185] severe dysplasia,[186] villous histology,[181, 184] and older age[178, 181] are also risk factors for adenoma recurrence, but the relative importance of each of these factors independently is uncertain.

It can be argued that the most clinically important recurrence is an adenoma with advanced pathology (AAP). Some studies have reported a 6% to 7% recurrence rate for AAP over a 4-year follow-up period.[84] In the National Polyp Study, the recurrence rate of advanced adenomas was 3.3%, regardless of whether patients underwent colonoscopy at 1 and 3 years or only 3 years after polypectomy. The cumulative incidence of AAP was 4% at 3 years and 8% at 6 years of follow-up. Independent predictors for AAP at follow-up were 3 or more adenomas at the index colonoscopy and age at adenoma diagnosis of 60 years or more with a parent with colorectal cancer.[187] In the presence of these two risk factors, cumulative AAP recurrence rates rose to 10% at 3 years and 20% at 6 years of follow-up. Those at lowest risk for developing AAP were patients with a single adenoma diagnosed and younger than 60 years of age. Another colonoscopic follow-up study reported that multiple adenomas at index colonoscopy increased the risk of AAP, but it also found that adenoma size greater than 1 cm and proximal location were additional risk factors.[185]

Effect of Polypectomy on Colorectal Cancer Incidence. If adenomas are the precursor to colon cancer, then removing them should decrease the subsequent incidence of colon cancer. Indeed, several uncontrolled and case-control series strongly suggest that distal colorectal cancers can be prevented and mortality reduced by screening proctosigmoidoscopy.[42–45] Other studies paradoxically found that adenomatous polypectomy was associated with an increased incidence of colon cancer.[188–90] However, since these retrospective studies did not establish a polyp-free colon (or always consider adenoma size and histology), the higher colon cancer rate may reflect malignant progression of other adenomas that had not been removed. Two studies from the Mayo Clinic also did not establish a polyp-free colon at the time of polypectomy.[26, 164] Despite this, if the removed polyps were small (<1 cm), there was no greater risk for subsequently developing colon cancer, whereas the removal of large adenomas was associated with a greater risk of subsequent colorectal cancer, supporting the concept that advanced neoplasms at index polypectomy are predictors of subsequent neoplasia. Important observations also come from the St. Mark's Hospital study in which rectal adenomas were removed without any subsequent examinations.[169] If the index polyp was a small, tubular adenoma, there was no greater risk of subsequent cancer anywhere in the colon, whereas the risk was significantly increased if the index adenoma was large or contained villous elements. Other studies have shown a marked reduction in colon cancer incidence related to polypectomy.[191]

The most valid study design to address this issue is a prospective colonoscopic study in which an adenoma-free colon is established, and patients are followed for subsequent development of colonic neoplasms. The National Polyp Study is a landmark in this regard. This was a prospective, multicenter trial in which a cohort of 1418 patients underwent a clearing colonoscopy to remove one or more adenomas and were then followed at specific intervals for a mean of 5.9 years. During the follow-up period, 5 early asymptomatic cancers were detected, which was only 10% to 24% of the expected incidence compared with three selected reference groups.[41] In other words, 20 to 50 cancers were anticipated had polypectomy not been performed. In a smaller study, the Funen Adenoma Follow-up Study found that although the incidence of subsequent colon cancers was not reduced by polypectomy, the mortality was reduced.[192] In summary, these studies indicate that the adenoma is a marker of a neoplasm-prone colon, and that colonoscopic clearing of all adenomas is of considerable benefit.

Frequency of Surveillance Colonoscopy. The National Polyp Study has taught us that performing follow-up colonoscopy at 1 year is a low-yield proposition, as others have observed using sigmoidoscopy.[191] It is also worth realizing that an endoscopic examination of the colorectum may afford protection against colon cancer for 6 to 10 years.[43, 44] Moreover, it has been proposed that a single lifetime sigmoidoscopy at about age 55 to 60 years could be standard policy for colon cancer sceening, with referral of patients for colonoscopy and subsequent surveillance only if the sigmoidoscopy discloses a distal adenoma with advanced features.[193]

A consensus statement for postpolypectomy surveillance guidelines has been generated by the major gastroenterology medical societies.[165] A complete colonoscopy should be performed at the time of polypectomy, clearing all existing adenomas. This may take more than one session for large or multiple polyps. The interval before the next surveillance colonoscopy is based upon the patient's category of recurrent adenoma risk (Table 114–10). If the patient is in the high-risk group for adenoma recurrence, repeat colonoscopy is performed in 3 years to check for metachronous adenomas. For low-risk patients, repeat colonoscopy should be performed in 5 years. After one negative follow-up surveillance colonoscopy, the subsequent surveillance interval can be increased to 5 years. Adherence to this plan is predicted to be cost-effective.[165]

Non-Neoplastic Polyps

Pathologically, all neoplastic polyps are part of an identifiable spectrum, but non-neoplastic polyps fall into several distinct and unrelated groups, including hyperplastic polyps, mucosal polyps, juvenile polyps, Peutz-Jeghers polyps, inflammatory polyps, and many other submucosal lesions (see Table 114–1).

Table 114–10 | **Risk for Developing Adenoma with Advanced Pathology (AAP) or Cancer After Colonoscopic Polypectomy**

Low risk for recurrence
- 1 or 2 small (<1 cm) tubular adenomas
- No family history of colorectal neoplasia

High risk for recurrence
- Multiple (≥3) adenomas
- Large adenoma (>1 cm)
- Adenoma with villous component
- Adenoma with high-grade dysplasia
- First-degree relative with colorectal cancer

Hyperplastic Polyps

The most common non-neoplastic polyp in the colon is the *hyperplastic polyp,* referred to by some pathologists as a metaplastic polyp. Hyperplastic polyps usually are small; their average size is less than 5 mm and they seldom are greater than 10 mm, although larger hyperplastic polyps have been reported.[194]

HISTOLOGIC CHARACTERISTICS. Hyperplastic polyps are small, usually sessile lesions that are grossly indistinguishable from small adenomatous polyps. Microscopically, the colonic crypts are elongated and the epithelial cells assume a characteristic papillary configuration (Fig. 114–10). The epithelium is made up of well-differentiated goblet and absorptive cells. The cytologic atypia that is characteristic of adenomatous polyps is not seen. Mitoses and DNA synthesis are limited to the base of the crypts, and orderly cell maturation is preserved. The epithelial cell and attendant pericryptal sheath fibroblast make up an epithelial-mesenchymal unit that migrates up the colonic crypt. In contrast to adenomatous polyps, in which the epithelium and fibroblast appear to be immature, this tissue is better differentiated, and abundant collagen is synthesized in the basement membrane.[195] It is thought that the migration of epithelial cells up the colonic crypt is slow and that hyperplastic polyps develop from the failure of mature cells to detach normally.[196] Hyperplastic polyps express several phenotypic markers in common with other types of metaplastic gastrointestinal lesions.[197]

Polyps that display features of both hyperplastic and adenomatous transformation have been described.[198] These mixed hyperplastic-adenomatous polyps are not rare, constituting about 13% of hyperplastic polyps.[196] When this type of polyp exhibits larger size, prominent architectural distortion, nuclear atypia, and upper crypt zone mitoses, they are usually considered more adenomatous than hyperplastic and are termed *serrated adenomas*. These lesions occasionally contain foci of dysplasia and even carcinoma,[199] and a syndrome marked by numerous serrated adenomas and even colon adenocarcinoma has been described (see later). It has been suggested that hyperplastic polyps give rise to serrated adenomas by a subtle form of genomic instability related to a specific type of DNA replication error, and that these lesions can then give rise to the approximate 10% of colon cancers that manifest low levels of microsatellite instability.[200]

For the most part, true sporadic hyperplastic polyps are considered to have little if any intrinsic malignant potential. The rare finding of cancer in a hyperplastic polyp probably results from malignant degeneration of the adenomatous component of a former mixed hyperplastic-adenomatous polyp.[199] Hyperplastic polyps and neoplastic lesions do appear in the same colons, suggesting that the two may be pathogenetically related. Indeed, a germline mutation of the *APC* gene (E1317Q) has been associated with an unusually large number of colorectal hyperplastic polyps occurring in association with adenomas.[201]

PREVALENCE OF HYPERPLASTIC POLYPS. The prevalence of hyperplastic polyps is not known with precision, but these growths are common. In colonoscopic examinations of asymptomatic patients over age 50 years, hyperplastic polyps

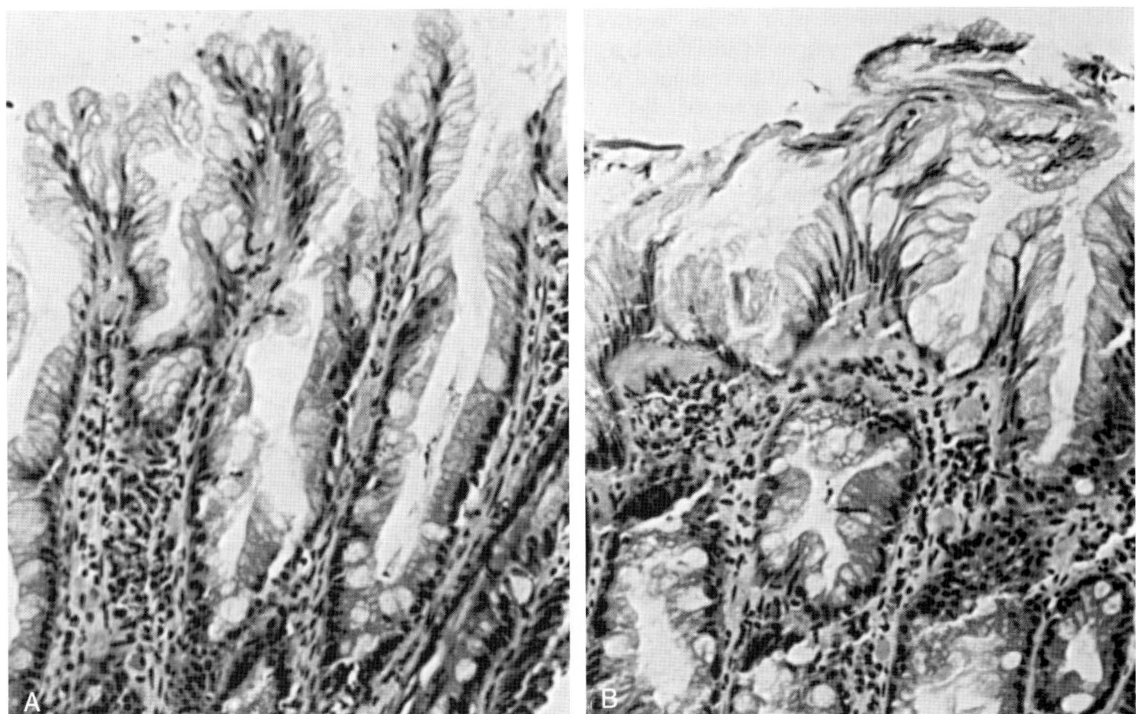

Figure 114–10. Hyperplastic polyp. *A,* This high-power photomicrograph demonstrates the papillary fronds of a hyperplastic polyp, consisting of elongated epithelial cells containing generous amounts of mucus. The nuclei retain their basal orientation and demonstrate no atypia. *B,* This photomicrograph demonstrates the characteristic "starfish" appearance of hyperplastic glands cut in cross section *(arrow).* Again, the orderly appearance of the nuclei, the generous cytoplasmic-nuclear ratio, and the abundance of secreted mucus at the surface of the polyp *(top)* can be readily appreciated.

were found in 9% to 10%,[57, 58] although this frequency may be higher (30% to 31%) among male veterans.[59, 202] Sigmoidoscopic screening of asymptomatic relatives of adenoma-prone kindreds revealed 26% with hyperplastic polyps—a prevalence that was essentially identical (28%) to that of asymptomatic spouse controls.[203] Autopsy data report a prevalence rate of 20% to 35%.[10, 14, 56]

The frequency of hyperplastic polyps depends largely on the site of the colon being examined and on the age of the patient. Autopsy studies repeatedly observe a distal predominance of hyperplastic polyps.[10, 13, 14, 61] Of course, sigmoidoscopic studies, which focus on the distal colon and rectum, often detect hyperplastic polyps, but even screening colonoscopy studies find more hyperplastic polyps in the distal colon.[70] Among all diminutive polyps (<5 mm) removed during colonoscopy, hyperplastic polyps outnumber adenomatous polyps in the rectum and sigmoid, whereas adenomas predominate in the remainder of the colon.[17, 204] The prevalence of hyperplastic polyps increases with age.[12, 50, 61] There also is an association between hyperplastic polyp prevalence and colon cancer prevalence (Table 114–11), although this correlation is not as firm as the association between adenomas and colon cancers, nor does it necessarily imply any premalignant potential for the hyperplastic polyp itself.

Table 114–11 | **Prevalence of Hyperplastic Polyps**

		PREVALENCE RATE (%)					
		Men			Women		
POPULATION	COLON CANCER FREQUENCY	Age *20–39*	*40–59*	*60+*	Age *20–39*	*40–59*	*60+*
Hawaiian-Japanese	Very high	50	69	84	0	57	73
New Orleans, white	High	11	19	13	—	25	30
New Orleans, black	High	10	18	14	6	7	9
Brazil (São Paulo)	Intermediate	14	26	40	12	23	31
Japan (Akita)	Intermediate	0	2	2	0	2	8
Japan (Miyagi)	Low	1	2	2	0	0	3
Costa Rica (San José)	Low	0	7	7	5	1	9
Colombia (Cali)	Low	6	14	11	2	9	16

From Correa P: Epidemiology of polyps and cancer. In Morson BC (ed): The Pathogenesis of Colorectal Cancer. Philadelphia, WB Saunders, 1978, p 126.

MANAGEMENT. Hyperplastic polyps remain small, usually are sessile, and seldom if ever cause symptoms. Inasmuch as they are not likely to give rise to cancer, little is gained by removing these polyps, but because they cannot be distinguished from neoplastic polyps simply by gross examination, they usually are removed anyhow. Given their usual predominance in the distal colorectum, finding hyperplastic polyps in this location (for example, by sigmoidoscopy) is not an alarming finding, particularly in elderly people. Therefore, the bulk of evidence does not support a policy of proximal polyp hunting by colonoscopy in patients with hyperplastic polyps in the rectosigmoid.[65, 67, 165, 205–207] However, some studies have suggested that finding a hyperplastic polyp in the distal colorectum is a harbinger of proximal adenomas,[202, 204, 208] and two recent screening colonoscopy studies found that distal hyperplastic polyps were associated with a 2.8% to 4.0% rate of advanced proximal neoplasia,[61, 70] which in one study represented a significantly greater risk for advanced proximal neoplasia than finding no distal polyps[70] (see Table 114–8). While we await additional data on this subject, current guidelines do not recommend performing colonoscopy for a distal hyperplastic polyp,[165] nor do such patients need to be entered into a regular surveillance program for detecting subsequent neoplasms.[165, 209]

Mucosal Polyps

The colon frequently harbors excrescences or mammillations of tissue that histologically are normal mucosa. In these instances, the submucosa has elevated the normal tissue overlying it. These lesions may be termed *mucosal polyps*, and their presence has no clinical significance. Mucosal polyps are almost always small and may constitute 8% to 20% of the material recovered in a collection of colonoscopic biopsies.

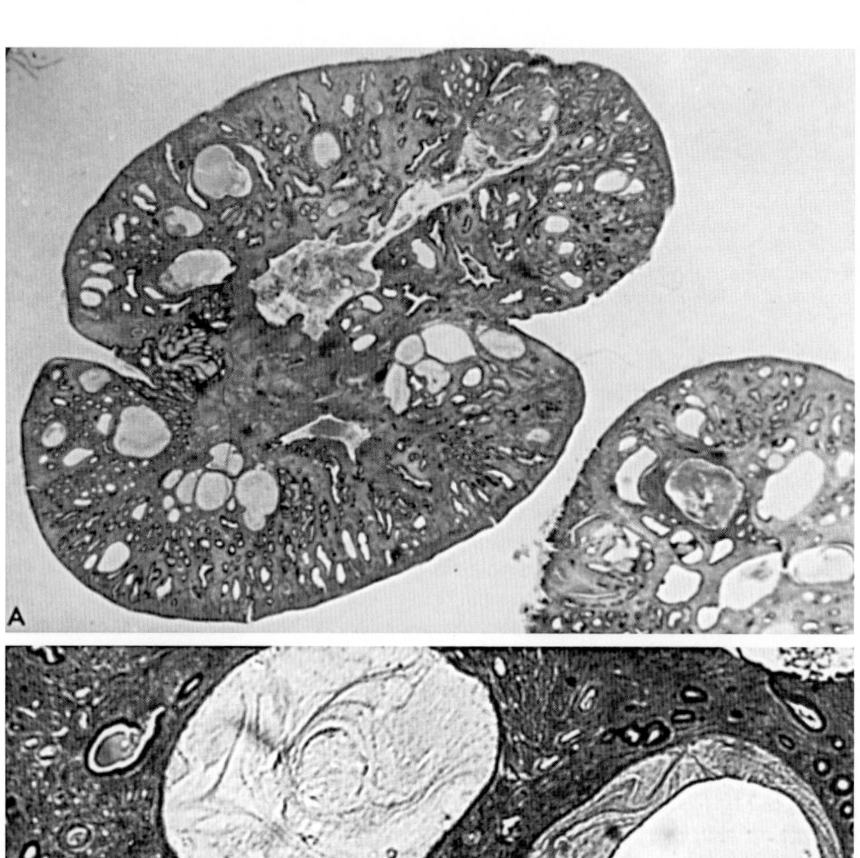

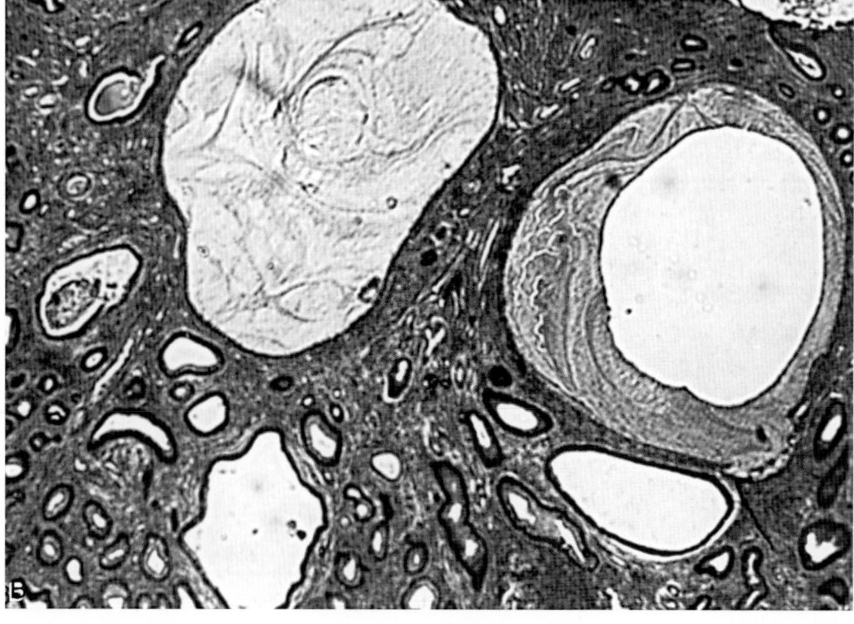

Figure 114–11. Juvenile polyp. *A*, This low-power photomicrograph demonstrates the dilated, mucus-filled glands and the extensive edema and inflammatory reaction in the lamina propria. *B*, This high-power view of a juvenile polyp demonstrates that in contrast to the adenomatous and hyperplastic polyps, the (darker) epithelial cells compose a relatively minor proportion of the total mass of the polyp, the majority of which consists of dilated glands and an expanded lamina propria.

Juvenile Polyps

Juvenile polyps (Fig. 114–11) are mucosal tumors that consist primarily of an excess of lamina propria and dilated cystic glands, rather than an overabundance of epithelial cells as seen in adenomatous and hyperplastic polyps, and they are therefore classified as *hamartomas*. The appearance of the distended, mucus-filled glands, inflammatory cells, and edematous lamina propria has prompted some observers to call these lesions *retention polyps*. Juvenile polyps appear to be acquired lesions because they seldom are seen in the first year of life and are most common from ages 1 to 7 years. They usually slough or regress spontaneously but occasionally are found in adults. Juvenile polyps more often are single than multiple, usually are pedunculated, and tend to range in size from 3 mm to 2 cm. Because these polyps tend to be rectal and develop a stalk, they may prolapse during defecation. In addition, the stroma contains a generous vascular supply, which explains the considerable blood loss suffered by some patients. Therefore, due to the high likelihood of bleeding and prolapse, removal of juvenile polyps is suggested.

Juvenile polyps have essentially no malignant potential when single,[210] and they tend not to recur. Although 18% to 20% of individual juvenile polyps in the rectum may be associated with proximal polyps, proximal adenomas are rare, and the subsequent risk of death from or the development of colorectal cancer is no greater than that of the general population even without specific surveillance.[210] However, when juvenile polyps are multiple (see "Juvenile Polyposis Syndrome" later), the risk of developing cancer is present, apparently because adenomatous epithelium may be present in some juvenile polyps.

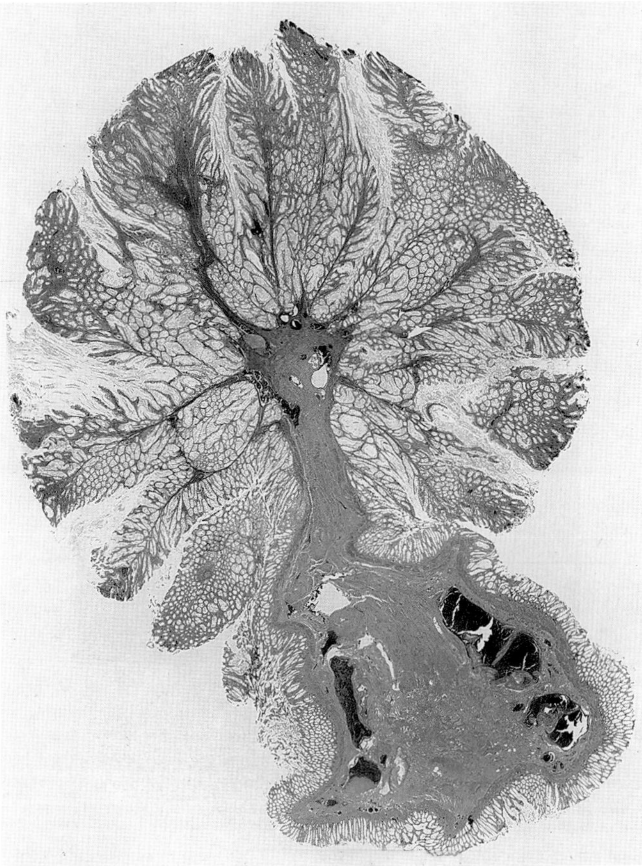

Figure 114–12. Peutz-Jeghers polyp. Low-power photomicrograph of a Peutz-Jeghers polyp of the small intestine. The central core, containing broad bands of smooth muscle not seen in other gastrointestinal polyps, arborizes and gives rise to the characteristic architecture of the lesion.

Peutz-Jeghers Polyps

The *Peutz-Jeghers polyp* is a unique hamartomatous lesion characterized by glandular epithelium that is supported by an arborizing framework of well-developed smooth muscle contiguous with the muscularis mucosae (Fig. 114–12). The smooth muscle bands fan out into the head of the polyp and become progressively thinner as they project toward the surface of the polyp. Unlike in the case of the juvenile polyp, the lamina propria is normal, and the characteristic architecture of the lesion appears to derive chiefly from the abnormal smooth muscle tissue. These polyps almost always are multiple, and their distinctive appearance, in association with the extraintestinal manifestations, makes Peutz-Jeghers syndrome easily identifiable. This type of polyp seldom is found in the colon in the absence of generalized polyposis (discussed further later).

Inflammatory Polyps (Pseudopolyps)

Inflammatory polyps are found in the regenerative and healing phases of inflammation. They are formed by full-thickness ulceration of epithelium followed by a regenerative process that leaves the mucosa in bizarre polypoid configurations. The lesions may be large and solitary, mimicking a neoplastic mass. Mucosal bridges may be formed across the lumen. Multiple lesions frequently are seen that may mimic a polyposis syndrome (Fig. 114–13). The term *pseudopolyp* is used to distinguish them from neoplastic lesions, but by definition, these are true polypoid protuberances. Histologically, inflammation and exuberant granulation tissue may be seen in the early postinflammatory period, but later the polyp may histologically resemble entirely normal mucosa.

Any form of severe colitis, including chronic inflammatory bowel disease (ulcerative colitis, Crohn's disease),[211] amebic colitis,[212] or bacterial dysentery, may give rise to inflammatory polyps. In chronic schistosomiasis, multiple inflammatory polyps that contain granulation tissue, eggs, or adult worms commonly are seen.[213] The significance of these polyps, which have no intrinsic neoplastic potential, is that they often appear in diseased colons that are at high risk for developing colon cancer (ulcerative colitis, schistosomiasis); therefore, they must be distinguished from neoplastic lesions that do carry premalignant potential.

Rare cases of multiple and recurrent inflammatory gastrointestinal polyps that produce pain and obstruction have been reported on a sporadic and even a familial basis.[214] These lesions are found primarily in the ileum, may be very large, and may even cause intussusception. Cap polyposis is another rare condition, characterized by inflammatory polyps with elongated crypts, a mixed inflammatory infiltrate in the lamina propria, and a surface cap of fibrinopurulent exu-

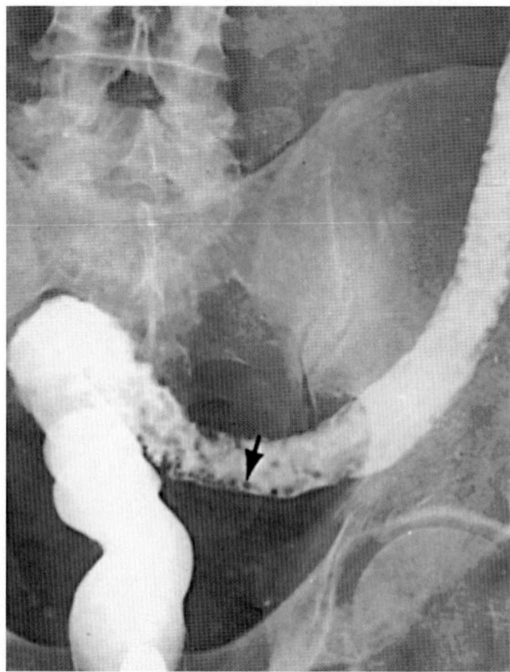

Figure 114–13. Pseudopolyps. *A,* This spot film from a barium enema from a patient with ulcerative colitis demonstrates numerous inflammatory polyps (pseudopolyps) in the sigmoid colon. From the barium enema, it can be concluded only that many polyps are present and a colonoscopic biopsy is required to identify the nature of the lesion. The associated mucosal abnormalities seen at colonoscopic examination assist in the proper identification of pseudopolyps; however, the physician must not overlook the possibility of a neoplastic lesion occurring in this setting.

date.[215] Although cap polyposis may be confused endoscopically with inflammatory bowel disease, mucosal prolapse has been suggested as a possible underlying etiology.

Submucosal Lesions

COLITIS CYSTICA PROFUNDA. Colitis cystica profunda is a rare lesion consisting of dilated, mucus-filled glands in the submucosa that may form solitary or multiple polyps (see Chapter 118).[216]

PNEUMATOSIS CYSTOIDES INTESTINALIS. Multiple air-filled cysts may be encountered within the submucosa of the colon (and small intestine) and may produce a polypoid appearance.[217–219] This entity is discussed in detail in Chapter 118.

OTHER SUBMUCOSAL LESIONS. Any lesion beneath the colonic mucosa may elevate the overlying epithelium to produce a polypoid appearance. Lymphoid tissue is present throughout the colon, and hypertrophied follicles may be mistaken for a pathologic mucosal process. *Benign lymphoid polyps* may even grow large enough to produce symptoms (pain, bleeding) or may become pedunculated. Multiple benign lymphoid polyps (nodular lymphoid hyperplasia) may be found as normal variants in children in particular (Fig. 114–14), but a malignant MALT lymphoma also may present with multiple polypoid lesions (see Chapter 26). Moreover, chronic lymphocytic leukemia may manifest as multiple colonic polyposis.[220] The principal importance of benign lymphoid polyps is, therefore, in their difficult distinction from the malignant lymphoid lesions.

The colon is the most common gastrointestinal site for *lipomas,* which tend to be solitary (but may be multiple) submucosal lesions. Lipomas usually are asymptomatic and detected incidentally. The low density of fat may give the lesions a characteristic radiographic appearance, and their soft, deformable nature is helpful to the colonoscopist in making the diagnosis grossly. Colonic lipomas are most frequent in the right colon and tend to occur on or near the ileocecal valve.[221] Removal of these lesions usually is unnecessary.

Important tumors such as *carcinoids* (Chapter 112), *metastatic neoplasms* (especially *melanoma*) (Chapter 29), and other rare cancers may produce submucosal lesions without distinctive identifying characteristics. Other submucosal lesions may be detected incidentally as curiosities, including leiomyomas,[222] granular cell tumors, fibromas, neurofibromas, hemangiomas, and endometriosis.

GASTROINTESTINAL POLYPOSIS SYNDROMES

Gastrointestinal polyposis refers to the presence of numerous polypoid lesions throughout the GI tract. The polyposis syndromes are distinctive entities clinically and pathologically that have been sorted into recognizable categories over the past century or so (Table 114–12). Most of these syndromes are inherited, and most are associated with an increased colon cancer risk, but all are classified on the basis of the histologic type of polyp and the clinical presentation. Recent advances in genetics not only have permitted a more accurate understanding of the relationship between these syndromes, but also the genes responsible for these conditions, particularly the adenomatous polyposis syndromes, have pro-

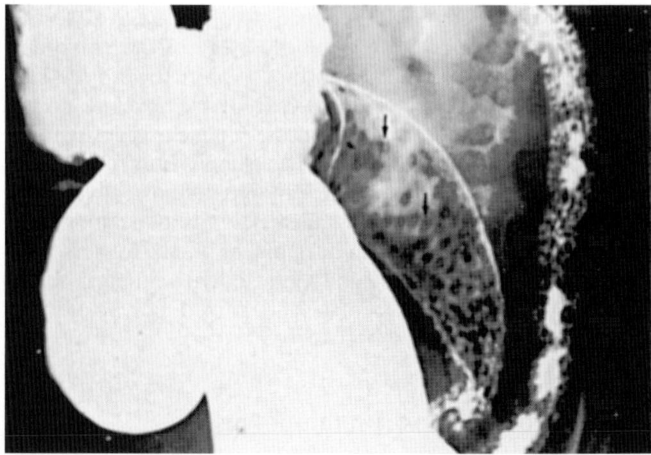

Figure 114–14. Lymphoid polyps. This spot film of the sigmoid colon demonstrates diffuse lymphoid hyperplasia throughout the colon of a child. Exuberant lymphoid hyperplasia may be a normal variant in some children; a malignant lymphoma also may rarely present a similar x-ray picture. On close examination of the radiograph, many of these polyps display characteristic umbilication.

Table 114–12 | **Classification of Gastrointestinal Polyposis Syndromes**

Inherited Polyposis Syndromes
- Adenomatous polyposis syndromes
  - Familial adenomatous polyposis
  - Variants of familial adenomatous polyposis
    - Gardner's syndrome
    - Turcot's syndrome
    - Attenuated adenomatous polyposis coli
- Hamartomatous polyposis syndromes
  - Peutz-Jeghers syndrome
  - Juvenile polyposis
  - Syndromes related to juvenile polyposis
    - Cowden's disease
    - Bannayan-Ruvalcaba-Riley syndrome
  - Rare hamartomatous polyposis syndromes
    - Hereditary mixed polyposis syndrome
    - Intestinal ganglioneuromatosis and neurofibromatosis
    - Devon family syndrome
    - Basal cell nevus syndrome

Noninherited Polyposis Syndromes
- Cronkhite-Canada syndrome
- Hyperplastic polyposis syndrome
- Lymphomatous polyposis
- Nodular lymphoid hyperplasia

vided insight into the genetic basis of sporadically occurring colon cancer.

Inherited Polyposis Syndromes

The inherited adenomatous polyposis syndromes include several entities that are characterized by the development of large numbers of adenomatous polyps in the colon. The identification of the *APC* gene permitted proper classification of Gardner's syndrome, attenuated adenomatous polyposis coli (AAPC), and many cases of Turcot's syndrome as variants of classic FAP (Table 114–13).

Familial Adenomatous Polyposis

GENETICS. FAP is the most common adenomatous polyposis syndrome. It is inherited as an autosomal dominant disease with 80% to 100% penetrance and an estimated prevalence of 1 in 5000 to 1 in 7500.[223] As described earlier, in this condition, one mutated *APC* allele is inherited as a germline mutation from the affected parent, and adenomas develop when the second allele (from the unaffected parent) becomes mutated or lost. The identification of the gene responsible for FAP began in 1986 with the investigation of a patient who had multiple congenital malformations and a deleted portion of the long arm of chromosome 5 that was identified cytogenetically.[224] Genetic mapping studies and restriction fragment length polymorphism (RFLP) analysis in 1987 led to the localization of the FAP gene in the 5q21-q22 region.[225, 226] At the same time, RFLP analysis suggested that one of the two normally occurring alleles for the FAP gene was frequently lost in sporadically occurring colorectal cancers. The fact that a lost gene might contribute to tumor progression suggested that the FAP locus may encode for a tumor suppressor gene.[227]

In 1991, the gene responsible for FAP was cloned by two collaborating groups and reported simultaneously.[228–230] The product of this gene, termed *APC* for adenomatous polyposis coli by geneticists, is quite large (2844 amino acids, with a molecular mass of 311,800 daltons), which may account for the relatively high frequency of new mutations at this locus. Germline mutations are found in patients with FAP and

Table 114–13 | **Familial Adenomatous Polyposis Syndromes: Clinical Variants**

SYNDROME	POLYPS	EXTRAINTESTINAL ABNORMALITIES	GENE MUTATION
Classic FAP	Colonic adenomas (thousands) Duodenal, periampullary adenomas Gastric fundic gland polyps Jejunal and ileal adenomas Ileal lymphoid polyps	Mandibular osteomas Dental abnormalities	*APC* gene (usually truncated protein)
Gardner's variant	Same as FAP	Osteomas of mandible, skull, long bones CHRPE Dental impactions, supernumerary teeth Desmoid tumors Epidermoid cysts Fibromas, lipomas Thyroid, adrenal tumors	*APC* gene
Turcot's variant	Colonic adenomas (sometimes fewer than in classic FAP)	Medulloblastoma Glioblastoma multiforme* CHRPE	*APC* gene DNA mismatch repair genes*
Attenuated APC (AAPC)	Colonic adenomas (<100; proximal colon) Duodenal, periampullary adenomas Gastric fundic gland polyps	Mandibular osteomas (rare)	*APC* gene 5′ and 3′ regions; E1317Q mutation

*May be more appropriately classified under hereditary nonpolyposis colon cancer (HNPCC) (see Chapter 115).
APC, adenomatous polyposis coli; CHRPE, congenital hypertrophy of the retinal pigment epithelium; FAP, familial adenomatous polyposis.

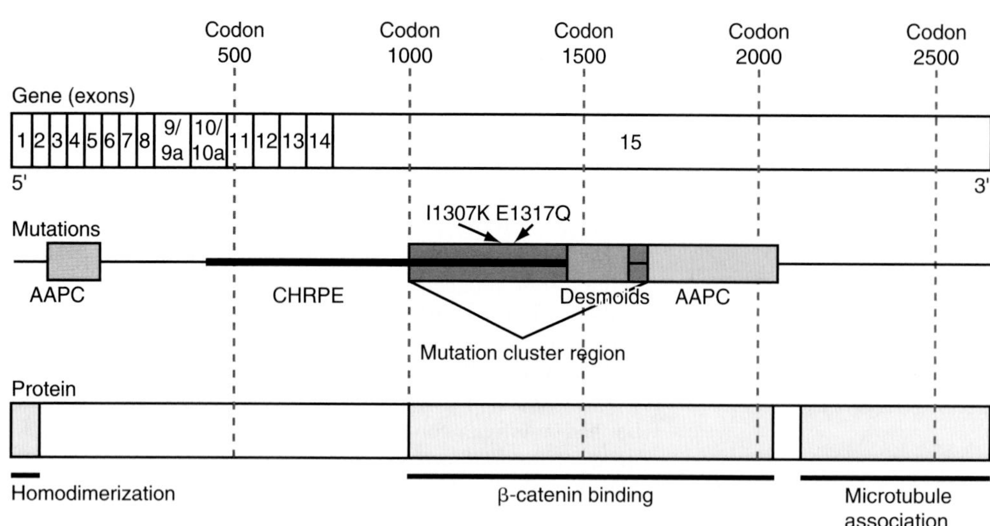

Figure 114–15. Schematic diagram of APC gene, its mutations, and functional domains of the protein. The gene consists of 15 exons. Mutations associated with attenuated adenomatous polyposis coli (AAPC) can occur in either the 5′ or 3′ region of the gene. Congenital hypertrophy of the retinal pigment epithelium (CHRPE) lesions are seen only with mutations downstream of exon 9. The mutation cluster region is in the center of the gene, where most mutations give rise to florid polyposis. Desmoid tumors are associated with the region shown. The I1307K and E1317Q mutations give rise to a milder phenotype. Domains of the APC protein responsible for homodimerization, β-catenin binding, and microtubule binding are shown along the bottom. (Modified from Goss KH, Groden J: Biology of the adenomatous polyposis coli tumor suppressor. J Clin Oncol 18:1967, 2000.)

Gardner's syndrome, and in most instances the mutations create a stop codon, resulting in a truncated protein. The germline mutations are dispersed throughout the 5′ half of the gene, whereas somatic mutations of *APC* tend to accumulate in the mutation cluster region near the center of the gene[231] (Fig. 114–15).

The APC protein is a multifaceted regulator of colonic epithelial cell homeostasis.[232] It functions as a tumor suppressor protein but also participates in processes of cell proliferation, migration, differentiation, and apoptosis. Because the vast majority of *APC* mutations result in the deletion of the carboxy-terminal portion of the protein, it is presumed that this region carries important tumor suppressor properties.[47] The carboxy-terminal portion of APC contains a domain that allows it to interact with microtubules, which may affect cell migration and/or adhesion. The proximal portion of the APC protein contains regions that enable homodimerization, suggesting that truncated APC can dimerize with wild-type APC to interfere with its function. In its central portion, the APC protein can bind to β-catenin, a protein that is important for maintaining normal cell-cell junctions through a cell surface adhesion molecule, E-cadherin. Normally, APC forms a complex with other proteins (axin and a serine-threonine kinase) to bind β-catenin. The β-catenin becomes phosphorylated and undergoes down-regulation in the cytoplasm. However, if the APC protein is mutated or lost, β-catenin is no longer down-regulated, allowing it to enter the nucleus where it acts in conjunction with other transcription factors to up-regulate target genes that then promote adenoma formation.

CLINICAL MANIFESTATIONS

Colonic Features. Classic FAP is characterized by the progressive development of hundreds to thousands of adenomatous polyps in the large intestine. If the colon is not removed, the development of colon cancer is virtually inevitable. A patient who inherits the gene for FAP is usually asymptomatic until puberty, at which time colonic polyps may begin to appear; rarely, however, polyps appear in the first decade of life. In one early series of FAP cases, the average age at onset of polyps was 25 years, but symptoms did not appear until the age of 33 years. The average age for the diagnosis of adenomas was 36 years, for cancer 39 years, and for death from cancer 42 years. Ninety percent of FAP cases have been identified by age 50 years.[233] However, a more recent study focused on early screening and reported that 50% of FAP gene carriers will have polyps at sigmoidoscopy by approximately age 15 years.[234]

The disease begins in younger patients with a small number of polyps, and the number increases progressively until the colon becomes studded with adenomas throughout its length (Figs. 114–16 and 114–17). All varieties of adenomatous polyps may be seen, including tubular, tubulovillous, and villous adenomas. The number of macroscopic polyps in a colectomy specimen averages a thousand but may be tens of thousands. Germline mutations of the mid-portion of the *APC* gene, between codons 1250 and 1464, have been associated with more profuse carpeting of the colon (see Fig. 114–15), whereas mutations elsewhere in the gene result in fewer colorectal polyps.[235] Histologic examination of the colon reveals numerous microscopic adenomas as well, the smallest of which may involve a single colonic crypt. The size and number of polyps correspond to the latent period between the onset of clinical disease and the time of colectomy; tumors tend to be more numerous in the symptomatic propositus cases than in asymptomatic younger relatives discovered by screening. The great majority of polyps are small (<1 cm), and individually, these polyps are identical to adenomatous polyps found in the general population.

Colorectal cancer should be considered an inevitable consequence in the natural history of FAP, appearing approximately 10 to 15 years after the onset of the polyposis. Colon cancer is unusual in adolescence, but it has been diagnosed as early as 9 years of age.[236] The cancers have the same pathologic grades of malignancy and the same distribution within the colon as are seen in the general population, except that multiple simultaneous (synchronous) cancers are

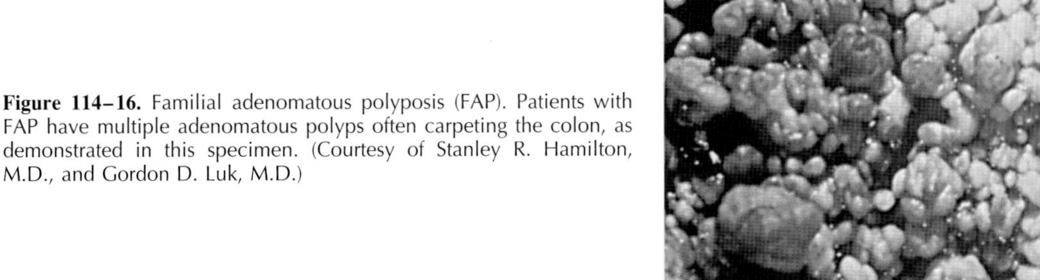

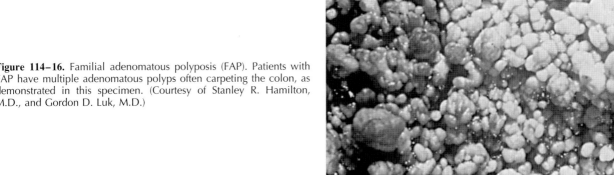

Figure 114–16. Familial adenomatous polyposis (FAP). Patients with FAP have multiple adenomatous polyps often carpeting the colon, as demonstrated in this specimen. (Courtesy of Stanley R. Hamilton, M.D., and Gordon D. Luk, M.D.)

much more frequent (48% of cases).[233] Despite attention to screening and surveillance, approximately 25% of patients with FAP will have colon cancer at the time of colectomy.[237]

Upper Gastrointestinal Polyps and Cancers. Because FAP patients are born with a germline *APC* mutation in all cells of the body, tumors frequently develop in other organs besides the colon. For example, polyps in the upper GI tract (stomach and small intestine) are present in almost all FAP patients.[238] Gastric polyps occur in 30% to 100% of patients, but curiously, most polyps in the stomach are non-neoplastic fundic gland polyps. These polyps are typically 1 to 5 mm sessile growths characterized microscopically by hyperplasia of fundic glands and microcysts. They may appear in the first decade of life, even before other GI adenomas develop. These lesions rarely show evidence of epithelial dysplasia and have little malignant potential. However, mutations of the *APC* gene are common in benign fundic gland polyps of FAP patients but quite rare in sporadic fundic gland polyps, implying that dysplasia can arise from these typically innocent lesions.[239] Microcarcinoids may also be found in the stomach.[240] Gastric adenomas are uncommon, occurring in approximately 5% of FAP patients, usually in the gastric antrum. The development of gastric adenocarcinoma in FAP patients is quite rare in the United States[241] but is higher in Japan, where the gastric cancer rate in the general population is higher.[242]

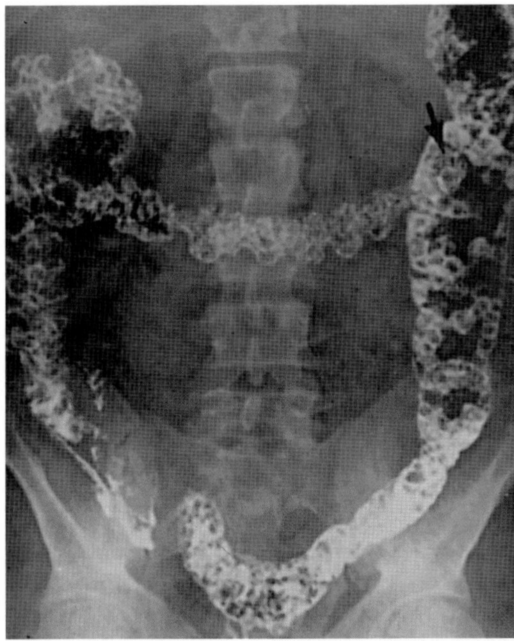

Figure 114–17. Familial adenomatous polyposis. This barium enema of a patient with FAP demonstrates the diffuse studding of the large bowel with the polyps. Note the variation in size and shape of the polyps.

Duodenal adenomas occur in 60% to 90% of FAP patients, and the incidence increases with age.[243] There is a propensity for adenomas to involve the periampullary region, and even obstruct the pancreatic or biliary drainage system and produce pancreatitis. As many as 50% to 85% of FAP patients manifest adenomatous change of the papilla of Vater.[238, 243] As a consequence, a 4% to 12% lifetime incidence of duodenal cancer (usually periampullary) has been reported,[238] with reported relative risks of 124 to 331.[241, 243] Collectively, these adenocarcinomas are a major cause of mortality after prophylactic colectomy in FAP patients. It is therefore advisable to perform screening and surveillance of the stomach and duodenum; although firm guidelines are not established, a suggested approach is outlined in Table 114–14. Jejunal adenomas have been detected in 40% and ileal adenomas in 20% of FAP patients. Fortunately, malignant transformation at these sites is rare,[238] but clinical vigilance is warranted. Likewise, attention should be given to surveillance of the distal ileum for neoplasia developing after subtotal colectomy or colectomy with ileoanal pull-through. Lymphoid hyperplasia may be present in the ileum in FAP patients and can be distinguished from adenomatous polyps only by biopsy.

Extraintestinal Features. Historically, intestinal polyposis with certain benign extraintestinal growths has been considered to constitute Gardner's syndrome. Gardner's syndrome is a familial disease consisting of gastrointestinal polyposis and *osteomas* associated with a variety of benign soft tissue tumors and other extraintestinal manifestations (see Table 114–13). We now know that FAP and Gardner's syndrome are variable manifestations of a disease traced to a single genetic locus, the *APC* gene. Bone abnormalities include

Table 114–14 | **Cancer Risks and Screening Recommendations in the Hereditary Polyposis Syndromes**

SYNDROME	ORGAN	LIFETIME RISK	SCREENING RECOMMENDATIONS
FAP, gene carriers	Colon cancer	Near 100%	Sigmoidoscopy annually; start at age 10–12 yr
	Duodenal/periampullary cancer	5–12%	Upper GI endoscopy q 1–3 yr; start at colectomy or age 20 yr
	Gastric cancer	~0.5%	Same as for duodenal
	Pancreatic cancer	~2%	Possibly periodic abdominal US after age 20 yr
	Thyroid cancer	~2%	Annual thyroid examination; start at age 10–12 yr
	CNS cancer	<1%	Annual physical examination; periodic head CT in affected families
	Hepatoblastoma	1.6% (<age 5)	Annual physical examination/hepatic US/α-fetoprotein for first decade of life
Peutz-Jeghers	Colon cancer	39%*	Colonoscopy at symptom onset, or late teens if asymptomatic; interval determined by number of polyps but at least q 3 yr
	Stomach cancer	29%	Upper GI endoscopy q 2 yr; start at age 10 yr
	Small bowel cancer	13%	Annual hemoglobin; small bowel series q 2 yr; start at age 10 yr
	Pancreatic cancer	36%	Endoscopic or abdominal US q 1–2 yr; start age 30 yr
	Breast cancer	54%	Annual breast examination; mammogram q 2–3 yr; start at age 25 yr
	Uterine; ovarian cancer	9–21%	Annual pelvic examination/PAP smear/ pelvic US; start at age 20 yr
	Sertoli cell tumor (testis)	9%	Annual testicular examination at age 10 yr; testis US if feminizing features
Juvenile polyposis	Colon cancer	<50%	Colonoscopy; start at symptoms or early teens if no symptoms; interval determined by number of polyps, but at least q 3 yr
	Gastric, duodenal cancer	Rare	Upper GI endoscopy q 3 yr; start in early teens
Cowden's	Colon cancer	Little–none	No recommendations given
	Thyroid cancer	3–10%	Annual thyroid examination; start in teens
	Breast cancer	25–50%	Annual breast examination at age 25 yr; annual mammogram at age 30 yr
	Uterine/ovarian cancer	?Increase	No recommendations given

*Figures for Peutz-Jeghers syndrome represent cumulative risks from age 15–64 yr; from Giardiello FM, Brensinger JD, Tersmette AC, et al: Very high risk of cancer in familial Peutz-Jeghers syndrome. Gastroenterology 119:1447, 2000.

Adapted from Burt RW: Colon cancer screening. Gastroenterology 2000;119:837, with permission.

CNS, central nervous system; CT, computed tomography; GI, gastrointestinal; PAP, Papanicolaou; US, ultrasound.

osteomas of the mandible, skull, and long bones; *exostoses;* and various *dental abnormalities* (including mandibular cysts, impacted teeth, and supernumerary teeth). When carefully sought, mandibular osteomas can be seen in up to 90% of patients with FAP even without other stigmata of Gardner's syndrome.[244, 245] Orthopantomography of the mandible is a simple and noninvasive means to screen for young carriers of the FAP gene; however, it is crucial to distinguish nonspecific sclerotic lesions in the mandible from true osteomas. Mandibular osteomas in FAP tend to be multiple, whereas nonspecific sclerotic bony lesions are usually single and located close to a diseased tooth. Osteomas can occur in children prior to the development of colonic polyposis. Because osteomas have no malignant potential, removal of them would be for symptomatic or cosmetic reasons.

Congenital hypertrophy of the retinal pigmented epithelium (CHRPE) has been reported in some families with FAP or Gardner's syndrome.[246–248] Over 90% of patients with Gardner's syndrome have pigmented ocular fundus lesions (versus 5% of controls), which are likely to be multiple (63% have four or more lesions) and are bilateral in 87% of those affected.[246] Pigmented ocular fundus lesions are found in approximately half of the unaffected but at-risk first-degree relatives and have been identified in infants as young as 3 months of age, suggesting that they are probably congenital. The presence of multiple, bilateral lesions appears to be a reliable marker for gene carriage in FAP, and their absence predicts lack of carriage if carrier relatives show CHRPE.[248] These marker lesions are asymptomatic curiosities that need not be sought in patients with an established diagnosis. CHRPE reflects the most accurate genotype-phenotype correlation in FAP patients; these lesions occur in patients with *APC* gene mutations distal to exon 9 up through the proximal portion of exon 15[249, 250] (see Fig. 114–15).

A particularly serious complication of the adenomatous polyposis syndromes is the development of diffuse mesenteric fibromatosis, also called *desmoid tumors*. Desmoid tumors are reported in 4% to 32% of patients and rank second, after metastatic carcinoma, among lethal complications of the disease.[251, 252] The absolute risk of desmoids in FAP patients has been estimated at 2.56 per 1000 person years, 825 times the risk in the general population.[252] Desmoid tumors often display familial aggregation; FAP patients who are first-degree relatives of an FAP patient with a desmoid have a 2.5-fold greater risk for developing desmoid tumors than that of FAP patients in general.[252] In this subset of patients, therefore, it would be prudent to incorporate abdominal imaging studies into their overall surveillance regimen, even though firm guidelines for desmoid tumor surveillance are not yet established.

Desmoids occur when the disease-causing mutation is distal to codon 1444 of the *APC* gene. It is curious that recurrent desmoid tumors may manifest a somatic mutation of *APC* gene different from that of the initial tumor.[231] Commonly, desmoid tumors are progressive growths of mesenteric fibroblasts after a laparotomy, but they occasionally appear spontaneously. They cause GI obstruction; constrict arteries, veins, or ureters; and are associated with a 10% to 50% mortality rate. Additional operative procedures are usually of no avail in this condition. They may respond to radiation when localized and accessible.[253] Unfortunately, most tumors are in the mesentery in these patients, making radiation therapy impractical. Systemic chemotherapy occasionally may be successful.[254] Attempts at medical therapy have resulted in some modestly encouraging results with this problem. The NSAID sulindac, which often can cause colonic adenoma regression in FAP (see later), has resulted in partial tumor shrinkage in some patients but no response in others.[255, 256] The antiestrogen drug tamoxifen has been effective in a few patients, as has progesterone.[257, 258] None of these approaches is reliably effective in most patients, and the mechanism for their actions awaits explanation. For desmoids that significantly compromise the small bowel mesentery, small intestinal transplantation should be considered.

In addition to desmoid tumors, other soft tissue tumors are well described in FAP and Gardner's syndrome, including *epidermoid cysts, fibromas,* and *lipomas*. The epidermoid cysts, also called inclusion cysts, have erroneously been referred to as sebaceous cysts in the past. Epidermoid cysts are lined with normal epithelium and contain no sebaceous glands. When multiple epidermoid cysts appear before puberty in these kindreds, this finding is a harbinger of polyposis. Neoplasms of the *thyroid, biliary tree, liver*, and *adrenals* also occur in these syndromes.[259–263] Hepatoblastoma may affect young children in FAP families.

GENOTYPE-PHENOTYPE CORRELATIONS. Drawing precise genotype-phenotype correlations in FAP is often difficult since the identical *APC* gene mutation may give rise either to isolated colonic polyposis or to the extracolonic manifestations.[229] Moreover, an identical *APC* gene mutation can manifest very different colonic and extracolonic phenotypic features among unrelated families.[264] Even within a single family, the disease may express itself variably in different individuals, including skipped generations and discordance in identical twins.[265] Some families even appear phenotypically to have FAP but do not have mutations of the *APC* gene.[266] Additional genetic or environmental disease-modifying factors appear to be responsible for generating phenotypic variation. For example, in an animal model of human FAP in which the mouse *APC* gene has a germline mutation, a second gene, phospholipase A_2, was found to modify the number of polyps.[266] So far, studies do not substantiate phospholipase A_2 as a genetic modifier of human FAP. In other animal experiments, crossing mice with FAP with those that lack the cyclooxygenase-2 (COX-2) gene resulted in a substantial decrease in intestinal polyposis.[267] Indeed, COX-2 inhibitors cause adenoma regression in FAP patients (see later). Thus, the FAP phenotype can be modified genetically and environmentally.

Despite the discrepancies in genotype-phenotype correlations, some general patterns have emerged (see Fig. 114–15).[266] Profuse polyposis is found in the midportion of the gene (between codons 1250 and 1464, but especially around codon 1300), whereas a mild colonic phenotype is observed for mutations that affect the extreme proximal (5′) and distal (3′) ends of the *APC* gene responsible for attenuated APC (AAPC) (see later) and for I1307K and E1317Q mutations. Desmoid tumors are seen with mutations just distal to the profuse polyposis region (between codons 1403 and 1578). CHRPE lesions are present only with mutations distal to exon 9 (codons 463 to 1387).

GENETIC TESTING AND COUNSELING. Genetic testing is an important component of the overall care of FAP patients and their families, not so much for the management of the affected individual but to detect mutant gene carriers. It is important to note that approximately 20% of FAP cases are associated with a negative family history and represent new mutations at the *APC* locus.[233] There are three types of genetic tests, all of which use DNA extracted from peripheral blood leukocytes. *Linkage testing* is based on using DNA markers near or in the *APC* locus to identify mutant gene carriers. With improved markers, a genetic diagnosis can now be made with a predicted accuracy of greater than 98%.[268] Despite this highly accurate method for diagnosing at-risk individuals, establishing linkage relationships requires that at least two individuals in a family already have a diagnosis of FAP, and this can present a problem. Since most mutations of the *APC* gene result in a truncated protein product, the in vitro *protein truncation test* offers a useful method for detecting gene carriers. This assay is successful in about 80% of families tested and has the advantage of only requiring one affected individual. If successful in one family member, this test carries a near 100% accuracy for identifying other gene carriers in that family. The third approach is to *sequence the APC gene* directly, which is theoretically the most accurate but logistically the most cumbersome and often reserved for research settings.

In most medical centers, the genetic test of choice is the commercially available protein truncation test. An affected individual is tested first. Absence of a mutation in the affected individual suggests that genetic testing of at-risk relatives is not likely to yield clinically useful information, so the family should be screened by clinical tests. A positive protein truncation test allows at-risk relatives to be tested in a more focused manner and at lesser cost. It is recommended that genetic testing of at-risk children be delayed until age 10 to 12 years, when clinical screening usually begins.[63] Genetic testing of other family members is best performed within the context of a comprehensive genetic counseling program because it raises many issues such as psychological denial, survivor guilt, premature worrying if tested too young, intrafamily strife, employment discrimination, and medical insurability.[269]

DIAGNOSIS AND SCREENING. Patients with FAP may present with nonspecific symptoms, such as hematochezia, diarrhea, and abdominal pain. However, the key to the diagnosis and management of this disease is to identify the presymptomatic individual, and this objective is achieved by the assiduous pursuit of the diagnosis in the relatives of affected patients. The diagnosis is easily made or excluded by colonoscopy or an air-contrast barium enema examination. In fact, the diffuse distribution of the polyps indicates that sigmoidoscopy is a suitable screening procedure. The presence of more than 100 polyps and the confirmation that these are adenomas establish the diagnosis of FAP, and further work-up of the colon usually is not required except to exclude the presence of carcinoma. The studies from St. Mark's Hospital in London on the natural history of FAP suggest that approximately 10 years elapses between the appearance of polyps and the development of cancer.[233] However, it is not advisable to delay surgery once the diagnosis is made, even in presymptomatic patients, except in individuals who have not completed puberty. Performing genetic testing at approximately age 10 to 12 years for at-risk individuals helps streamline the clinical evaluation. In a family with a known mutation, children who test positive can then undergo a screening sigmoidoscopy to determine the status of their disease. If the gene test is negative, the child can be spared sigmoidoscopy although it might still be prudent to perform sigmoidoscopy after adolescence for the rare possibility of laboratory error.

MANAGEMENT OF COLONIC DISEASE

Surgical Management. Surgery is the only reasonable management option in FAP, and the timing and extent of surgery are the major clinical considerations. Because any rectal mucosa that is left behind is at risk for developing subsequent carcinoma, the optimal treatment is to perform total proctocolectomy either with a conventional ileostomy or ileal pouch–anal anastomosis. For the most part, the latter operation in skilled hands is associated with very little morbidity and is preferred by patients. For some patients, a total proctocolectomy with conventional ileostomy is unacceptable, and they also do not want to chance the symptomatic complications of an ileoanal pouch. The decision to perform a subtotal colectomy with ileorectal anastomosis must be made on an individual basis, bearing in mind that the rectal segment will remain at risk and the patient will have to comply with periodic surveillance examinations. In contrast to older patients who undergo ileorectal anastomosis, about one fifth of younger patients (median age of 35 years) with many rectal polyps will develop cancer in 5 to 23 years. According to the Mayo Clinic experience, among those who are followed for more than 20 years, about three fifths will develop carcinoma in the rectal stump despite semiannual sigmoidoscopic surveillance and fulguration of all polyps.[270] The prognosis in patients who develop rectal cancers in this setting is dismal; the 5-year disease-free survival rate has been reported to be 25%. In patients with ileorectal anastomosis, the risk of subsequent rectal cancer was higher in patients who had an *APC* mutation between codons 1250 and 1464—a finding that awaits confirmation in other studies.[271] These data provide a strong case for total proctocolectomy for FAP patients.

In spite of this ominous warning, others have advocated rectum-sparing operations and have achieved a reasonable degree of success. The Memorial Sloan–Kettering group in New York has advocated that a subtotal colectomy is safe for those whose rectums are free of polyps. They also spare the rectum in patients with rectal polyps, carefully following them to perform additional surgery as soon as malignant change is found.[272] The St. Mark's group in London reports satisfaction with rectum-sparing procedures for all patients with FAP and, furthermore, fulgurates only adenomas 5 mm or more in diameter, at 3- to 6-month intervals. This group reported that 11 of 173 of their patients (6%) have developed carcinoma in the rectum, but that only 3 of the 11 (2% of the total) have died of rectal cancer.[273] The Cleveland Clinic group has advocated the use of colectomy with ileorectal anastomosis and reported an actuarial survivorship rate of 80% in 133 patients after 20 years, despite the presence of rectal polyps.[274] Other groups in the United States and Europe also prefer subtotal colectomy and ileoproctostomy, but approximately one quarter of patients treated this way have required a total proctectomy at a later date for cancer or intractable benign polyps.[275] It appears, therefore, that patients may elect the more limited procedure if they are willing to comply with rigorous follow-up (sigmoidoscopy every 3 to 6 months) and accept a risk of malignancy in the rectum of approximately 10%. The identification of effective medical therapy has provided new options for the surgical management of FAP, but as discussed in the next paragraph, rectal cancer can still occur despite adenoma regression.

Medical Management. Small adenomatous polyps in the rectum can be reversible lesions. Spontaneous regression of rectal polyps has been reported after subtotal colectomy and ileorectal anastomosis for FAP,[276] and this must be taken into account when one is evaluating the response of a rectal-sparing surgical procedure or medical treatment for this disease. Because of its antioxidant characteristics and its effects in experimental colon cancer, a trial of ascorbic acid (vitamin C, 3 g/day) was tried in patients with FAP who had undergone subtotal colectomy with ileorectal anastomosis at least 1 year earlier. A modest effect was observed, but it was neither consistent nor strong enough to advocate for general use.[277] Supplemental dietary calcium was similarly ineffective in polyposis patients.[278] A more ambitious trial has been reported in which 58 patients with FAP were treated with ascorbic acid (4 g/day), alpha-tocopherol (vitamin E, 400 mg/day), and supplemental fiber (22.5 g/day). Again, a modest effect was seen after 2 years of therapy.[279]

A higher degree of enthusiasm has been generated for the use of NSAIDs in the treatment of colorectal polyps in FAP (also see Chapter 23). Sulindac has been shown in both uncontrolled and controlled trials to decrease the number and size of colorectal adenomas in FAP patients.[79] This was applied to patients with intact colons as well as to those with subtotal colectomy and ileorectal anastomosis. Unfortunately, maintaining FAP patients on sulindac apparently does not protect them against the development of rectal cancer, and the effect on reducing adenomas is reversible upon discontinuing the drug. Furthermore, sulindac is less successful for controlling upper gastrointestinal neoplasia, and it has side effects (see Chapter 23).

The mechanism by which sulindac causes colorectal adenoma regression in FAP patients may relate in part to the ability of sulindac to inhibit cyclooxygenase (prostaglandin synthase) activity, thereby interfering with arachidonic acid metabolism. Since colorectal tumors (but not normal colonocytes) have high levels of COX-2 expression, it is possible that COX-2 inhibition by sulindac is responsible for adenoma regression.[280] Indeed, when mice carrying an *APC* mutation were bred with mice carrying a disrupted COX-2 gene, fewer polyps developed.[267] Sulindac is also capable of restoring the cell death program (apoptosis) that is deficient in colonocytes of FAP patients, even without affecting colonocyte proliferation.[281] Since COX-2 overexpression can prevent apoptosis, it is possible that the benefit from sulindac relates to its ability to inhibit COX-2.[280] Indeed, FAP patients with rectal adenomas treated with the selective COX-2 inhibitor celecoxib also demonstrated a significant reduction in the number and size of adenomas.[282] COX-2 may not be the entire story. The sulfone derivative of sulindac has no inhibitory effect on COX-2 (or COX-1), yet it has also been shown to cause rectal adenoma regression in

FAP patients.[283] Sulindac sulfone acts by enhancing apoptosis and is currently undergoing clinical trials in FAP patients to regress gastroduodenal polyps.

SCREENING OF EXTRACOLONIC ORGANS. Upper GI screening should be performed at the time multiple colonic adenomas are diagnosed, or at least by age 20 years (see Table 114–14).[63] A full evaluation of the entire small intestine should be performed at baseline, perhaps by performing intraoperative small bowel enteroscopy at the time of initial proctocolectomy. Upper GI polyps are rare prior to the onset of colonic disease. Side-viewing upper GI endoscopy should be performed because of its optimal visualization of the duodenal ampulla. The overall approach to upper GI polyps is one of conservatism. Gastric polyps should be sampled to see whether they are adenomas or fundic gland polyps with dysplasia. In the duodenum, villous adenomas, adenomas with high-grade dysplasia, large adenomas, and symptomatic adenomas regardless of histology should be removed. Endoscopic ablation of periampullary adenomas can be performed relatively safely by endoscopists skilled in this procedure, but regrowth of adenomatous tissue is common.[284] If duodenal polyps are small or few in number, surveillance can be performed every 1 to 3 years. The presence of worrisome duodenal adenomas or adenomatous change of the duodenal papilla warrants endoscopic inspection at more frequent intervals. Surgical resection of the duodenum, whether by local excision or pancreaticoduodenectomy, may be required in selected patients. Screening of other organs at risk for cancer is summarized in Table 114–14.

Variant Familial Adenomatous Polyposis Syndromes (see Table 114–13)

TURCOT'S SYNDROME (GLIOMA-POLYPOSIS). The term *Turcot's syndrome* applies to a syndrome of familial colonic polyposis with primary tumors of the central nervous system.[285, 286] The phenotypic spectrum may be broad, with colonic manifestations ranging from a single adenoma to profuse adenomatosis coli, and brain tumors representing different histopathologic types. Controversy exists as to whether this syndrome is inherited in an autosomal dominant or autosomal recessive manner. A comprehensive molecular diagnostic study of 14 Turcot's syndrome families has clarified that Turcot's syndrome kindreds fall into two groups, based on their types of brain tumor and particular genetic alteration.[287] The more common group has germline mutations of the *APC* gene, and these patients tend to have medulloblastomas. In several cases, the brain tumor preceded the diagnosis of polyposis. The *APC* mutations were heterogeneous, with no association between specific mutations and the development of brain tumors. The inactivation of both *APC* alleles in brain tumor tissue implicates the *APC* gene in the pathogenesis of these neoplasms. The risk of cerebellar medulloblastoma in FAP was calculated to be 92 times that of the general population. In contrast, the second group of patients, including the family originally described by Turcot, had glioblastoma multiforme tumors. These individuals were found to have germline mutations in DNA base mismatch repair genes typical of HNPCC (see Chapter 115). Thus, Turcot's syndrome can be considered a true variant of FAP, although as with Gardner's syndrome, maintaining a separate designation may be superfluous. To wit, CHRPE lesions have been described in a patient with Turcot's syndrome.[288] Because of familial clustering, once an individual with Turcot's syndrome has been identified, screening for affected family members should incorporate colonoscopy as well as imaging studies of the brain (see Table 114–14).

ATTENUATED ADENOMATOUS POLYPOSIS COLI (AAPC). Patients with classic FAP syndromes typically have tens to thousands of colonic adenomas. However, an attenuated form of FAP has been identified in which individuals manifest fewer adenomas, which often have a flat rather than polypoid growth pattern and tend to cluster in the proximal colon.[289, 290] As such, this condition may easily be confused with hereditary nonpolyposis colon cancer (see Chapter 115). Although previously termed *hereditary flat adenoma syndrome,* this syndrome is more aptly named *attenuated FAP* by virtue of the existence of germline mutations of the very proximal and distal portions of the *APC* gene.[291] Recent reports describe *APC* E1317Q mutation in individuals with multiple adenomas but without florid adenomatous polyposis.[266] Like classic FAP, patients with AAPC are prone to develop multiple fundic gland polyps, duodenal and gastric adenomas, and even periampullary carcinoma.[292] However, colorectal cancers arise at a later age (approximately 55 years) in AAPC patients compared with those with classic FAP.

OTHER SYNDROMES. Other familial syndromes, such as Torre-Muir syndrome, in which a high incidence of colonic cancer is associated with a small number of colonic adenomas, are probably part of the spectrum of HNPCC and should not be confused with FAP or Gardner's syndrome.[293] A single family with gastric hyperplastic polyposis and a high incidence of gastric cancer has been described.[294] This very rare condition is of interest because the gastric fundus may develop hyperplastic polyposis in FAP, but it is not known whether this syndrome is linked in any way to FAP. Other patients have been described with multiple hyperplastic polyposis of the colon, some of whom had coexisting adenomas or a vague family history of polyposis, but again any pathologic relationship to FAP is speculative.[295] In 1996, six patients with multiple serrated adenomas were described, four of whom had associated adenocarcinoma.[296] Further studies are needed to establish any genetic connection between serrated adenomatous polyposis and FAP.

Hamartomatous Polyposis Syndromes

Several discrete familial syndromes that are characterized by multiple hamartomatous polyps of the GI tract have been described. These include the Peutz-Jeghers syndrome, juvenile polyposis and related syndromes, and other rare syndromes (Table 114–15). Germline mutations of the *STK11/LKB1* gene account for Peutz-Jeghers syndrome, whereas the juvenile polyposis syndromes are associated with germline mutations of *PTEN* and *DPC4* (see later). Each of these syndromes is associated with an increased risk of colorectal cancer, presumably due to the fact that each of the genes responsible for the hamartomatous polyposis syndromes behave as tumor suppressor genes.

Table 114–15 | **Familial Hamartomatous Polyposis Syndromes**

SYNDROME	POLYPS	LOCATION OF GI POLYPS	OTHER MANIFESTATIONS	GENE MUTATION
Peutz-Jeghers	Hamartomas with bands of smooth muscle in lamina propria	Small intestine Stomach Colon	Pigmented lesions (mouth, hands, feet) Ovarian sex cord tumors Sertoli tumors of testis Airway polyps (nasal, bronchial) Pancreatic cancer Breast cancer Colon, esophageal cancer Urinary tract polyps	*STK11/LKB1*
Juvenile polyposis	Juvenile polyps; also adenomas and hyperplastic polyps	Colon Small Intestine Stomach	Colon cancer in some families Congenital abnormalities	*DPC4* (most) *PTEN* (some)
Cowden's disease	Hamartomas with disorganized muscularis mucosae	Stomach Colon	Trichilemmomas and papillomas Other hamartomas Benign and malignant breast disease Benign and malignant thyroid disease	*PTEN*
Bannayan-Ruvalcaba-Riley	Juvenile polyps	Colon Small intestine	Macrocephaly; developmental delay Penile pigmentation	*PTEN*
Neurofibromatosis	Neurofibromas	Small intestine Stomach Colon	von Recklinghausen's disease MEN type IIB	*NF1* *RET*

GI, gastrointestinal; MEN, multiple endocrine neoplasia.

PEUTZ-JEGHERS SYNDROME. Peutz in 1921 and Jeghers in 1949 described the familial syndrome consisting of mucocutaneous pigmentation and GI polyposis that now bears their names. Peutz-Jeghers syndrome (PJS) appears to be inherited as a single pleiotropic autosomal dominant gene with variable and incomplete penetrance.[297, 298] Germline mutations of *STK11/LKB1*, a serine-threonine kinase (STK) gene on chromosome 19p, cause this syndrome,[299, 300] but not all families with PJS are linked to this gene locus, suggesting genetic heterogeneity.

Early in infancy the characteristic mucocutaneous pigmentation of PJS may be noted. The melanin deposits are found most commonly around the mouth, nose, lips, buccal mucosa, hands, and feet, and they may also be present in the perianal and genital regions (Fig. 114–18). The macular lesions are brown to greenish-black, are glabrous, and, except for the buccal pigmentation, tend to fade at puberty. The clinician must distinguish these melanin deposits from ordinary freckles. Freckles are sparse near the nostrils and mouth, are absent at birth (but may occur in infancy), and never appear on the buccal mucosa. The presence of this pigmentation should alert the clinician to this syndrome, but the skin lesions and intestinal lesions occasionally are inherited separately.

Peutz-Jeghers polyps may increase in size progressively and cause small intestinal obstruction or intussusception,

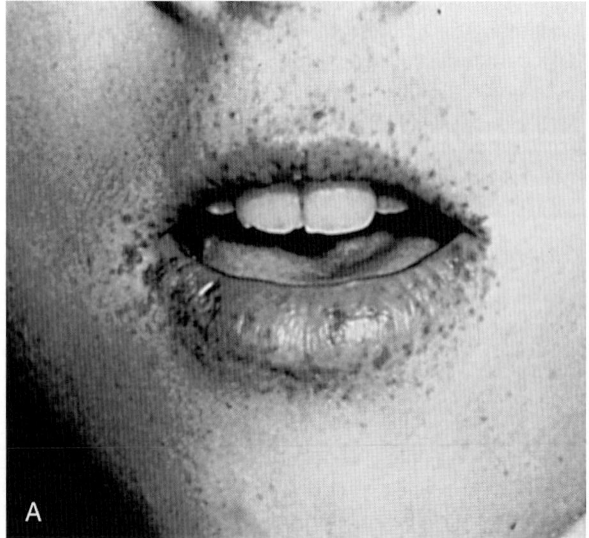

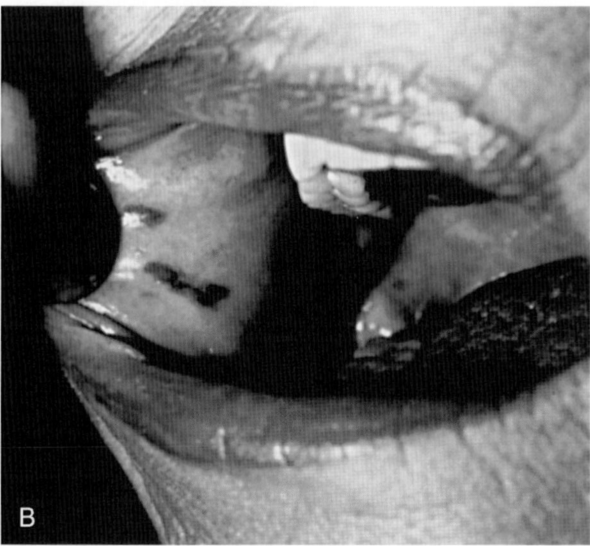

Figure 114–18. Peutz-Jeghers syndrome. *A*, Mucocutaneous pigmentation characteristic of Peutz-Jeghers syndrome. The "freckles" are seen around the lips and across the vermilion border. *B*, The pigmentation may also be seen on the buccal mucosa. Cutaneous pigmentation may also be found on the hands, fingers, palms, nostrils, and feet. The cutaneous pigmentation may fade with age, whereas the mucocutaneous pigmentation persists.

which may occur as early as infancy. The polyps may be found in the stomach, small intestine, or colon, but they tend to be most prominent in the small intestine. Acute upper GI bleeding and chronic fecal blood loss may complicate the disease. The average age at diagnosis in this syndrome is 23 to 26 years. Carcinomas of the colon, duodenum, jejunum, and ileum have been reported in these patients. Although it has been assumed that these cancers arise from rare foci of adenomatous epithelium that may develop within the Peutz-Jeghers polyps, recent evidence for loss of *STK11/LKB1* expression in Peutz-Jehgers polyps, even without dysplastic epithelium, raises the possibility that the *STK11/LKB1* gene itself might be the gatekeeper to carcinogenesis in this syndrome, much as the *APC* gene is the gatekeeper in FAP.[301, 302] The colonic polyps should be removed for histologic examination. The relative inaccessibility of small intestinal polyps and the unpredictability of neoplastic complications make a routine surveillance program for small intestinal cancer a difficult problem.

Cancers throughout the gastrointestinal tract and other organs are quite common in familial Peutz-Jeghers syndrome (see Table 114–15).[303] The mean age at diagnosis of cancer is approximately 40 to 50 years, with a 93% overall cumulative risk of developing cancer between ages 15 and 64 years. The cumulative risk of colon cancer is 39%, with similar rates for gastric and pancreatic cancer.[303] Ovarian cysts and distinctive ovarian sex cord tumors are seen in 5 to 12% of female patients with this syndrome.[304] The ovarian tumors are histologically unique and may occur in young patients. Hormonally active Sertoli cell testicular tumors with feminizing features may occur in young boys with Peutz-Jeghers syndrome.[305, 306] Breast cancers may be found in young women and may be bilateral[307]; indeed, the magnitude of breast cancer risk in this syndrome is similar to that in other hereditary forms of breast cancer caused by germline mutations of *BRCA1* and *BRCA2*.[303] Other tumors that may occur in this syndrome include pancreatic cancers in young patients, and polyps or cancers of the biliary tree and gallbladder.[308] Thus, Peutz-Jeghers syndrome confers an increased risk for cancer in a number of gastrointestinal and nonintestinal organs. Guidelines for screening are difficult to make, but it should be directed toward organs at risk, for which early detection and treatment are reasonable, such as the entire GI tract, gonads (in both sexes), and breasts (in women) (see Table 114–14).[308] Small bowel enteroscopy or intraoperative endoscopy of the entire GI tract should be considered.

Tuberous sclerosis is characterized by the presence of hamartomatous lesions, with the classic triad of mental retardation, epilepsy, and adenoma sebaceum.[309] Hamartomatous polyps resembling Peutz-Jeghers polyps, as well as adenomatous polyps, may occur and are often located in the distal colon.

JUVENILE POLYPOSIS SYNDROME. As discussed earlier, juvenile polyps are distinctive hamartomas that usually are solitary, located principally in the rectum of children and occasionally in adults. They have a smooth surface and are covered by normal colonic epithelium. Juvenile polyposis (i.e., the presence of multiple juvenile polyps) typically occurs in families; however, new mutations in patients with a negative family history also have been reported.[310] Juvenile polyposis syndrome (JPS) is defined by any one of the following criteria: 10 or more colonic juvenile polyps; juvenile polyps throughout the gastrointestinal tract; or any number of juvenile polyps with a family history of juvenile polyposis.[310–313] Often, JPS is considered when there is gastrointestinal polyposis in the absence of extraintestinal manifestations. However, juvenile polyposis can also occur as a component of Cowden's disease and of Bannayan-Riley-Ruvalcaba syndrome (BRRS; also known as Ruvalcaba-Myhre-Smith syndrome)[314–316]—two entities in which extraintestinal manifestations may predominate (see Tables 114–14 and 114–15). Cowden's disease and BRRS map primarily to chromosome 10q22-24, the locus for *PTEN,* a tumor suppressor gene with phosphatase activity, and germline mutations of *PTEN* have been described in some families with Cowden's disease (CD) and BRRS.[317, 318] In addition, some JPS families have *PTEN* mutations.[319, 320] Therefore, classifying a patient with a *PTEN* mutation can be problematic because, depending upon the syndrome (JPS, CD, BRRS), the risks for various cancers and hence appropriate management differ (see Table 114–14). Most JPS families in fact have germline mutations of the *DPC4* gene, a tumor suppressor gene that plays a role in signaling through the transforming growth factor-β cascade.[321, 322] The mechanism by which *PTEN* or *DPC4* contributes to juvenile polyp formation or transformation is not presently known.

Juvenile polyposis typically causes GI bleeding, intussusception, and obstruction. The clinical presentations of juvenile polyposis and the familial adenomatous polyposis syndromes differ. Juvenile polyps produce symptoms in childhood, whereas the adenomatosis syndromes rarely present in childhood and usually become evident in early adult life. In fact, the average age at onset of symptoms of juvenile polyposis is 4.5 years and 9.5 years in the nonfamilial and familial forms, respectively.[311] Congenital abnormalities of other organs are found in 20% of cases.

The risk of colon cancer is increased in familial juvenile polyposis,[323] with cancer occurring at an average age of 34 years. Although the juvenile polyps per se are not considered neoplastic, the synchronous adenomatous polyps and mixed juvenile-adenomatous polyps of these patients may give rise to concern.[324, 325] Thus, these polyps must be scrutinized by the pathologist for evidence of a mixed adenomatous appearance in the polyps or coexisting adenomas, and kindreds with colorectal cancer should be subjected to careful colonoscopic surveillance. Gastric cancer has developed in a patient with JPS whose gastric polyps had mixed juvenile, hyperplastic, and adenomatous features.[326]

The diagnosis is made by colonoscopy (see Table 114–14). Screening usually begins after 12 years of age if symptoms have not already occurred. Asymptomatic relatives should also be screened. If colonoscopy reveals polyps, upper GI endoscopy also should be performed. In general, juvenile polyps should be removed because of their tendency to bleed and obstruct. For a small number of polyps, periodic endoscopic polypectomy may be adequate. For individuals with numerous juvenile polyps, colectomy should be considered. If subtotal colectomy with ileorectal anastomosis is chosen, the rectal segment must remain under surveillance. Family history must be defined in patients with multiple juvenile polyps to determine the sites of involvement and the history of neoplastic lesions. Synchronous adenomatous polyps or mixed juvenile-adenomatous polyps are premalignant and must be excised. It has been suggested that surveillance endoscopy of the upper and lower GI tract be performed approximately every 1 to 3 years.[63]

SYNDROMES RELATED TO JUVENILE POLYPOSIS

Cowden's Disease (see Tables 114–14 and 114–15). Although reported in only a very small number of families, Cowden's disease, or the multiple hamartoma syndrome, consists of hamartomatous polyps of the stomach, small intestine, and colon, along with extraintestinal manifestations that include orocutaneous hamartomas, fibrocystic disease and cancer of the breast, nontoxic goiter, and thyroid cancer.[327] The hallmark of the disease is the presence of multiple facial *trichilemmomas*, which arise from follicular epithelium and typically occur around the eyes, nose, and mouth. Gastrointestinal symptoms and colorectal cancer appear to be uncommon in this syndrome. The colorectal polyps in Cowden's disease are distinctive lesions characterized by disorganization and proliferation of the muscularis mucosae, with nearly normal overlying colonic epithelium.[328] Ganglioneuromatosis of the colon and glycogenic acanthosis of the esophagus have been reported in association with Cowden's disease.[329] There does not appear to be an increased risk of gastrointestinal cancer; the major complication is breast cancer.

Bannayan-Ruvalcaba-Riley Syndrome (see Table 114–15). This rare syndrome consists of hamartomatous gastrointestinal polyposis with macrocephaly, developmental delay and other developmental abnormalities, and pigmented spots on the penis.[330, 331] Thyroiditis has also been described. Autosomal dominant inheritance has been suggested. As mentioned, BRRS, JPS, and Cowden's disease may represent different phenotypic manifestations of common genotypic abnormalities, much like the relationship between FAP and Gardner's syndrome.

RARE INHERITED HAMARTOMATOUS POLYPOSIS SYNDROMES

Hereditary Mixed Polyposis Syndrome. A large kindred with a tendency to develop colonic polyps of mixed histologic types has been identified.[332] The earliest age at onset of polyps was 23 years, the median age at onset of symptoms was 40 years, and the median age at colon cancer diagnosis was 47 years. The characteristic polyp was an atypical juvenile polyp, although some individuals had polyps of mixed histology and others had more than one histologic type of polyp. Linkage analysis maps the gene for this syndrome to a locus on chromosome 6, and not chromosome 10 (*PTEN* locus), distinguishing it from the juvenile polyposis syndromes.[333, 334]

Intestinal Ganglioneuromatosis and Neurofibromatosis (see also Chapter 29). Approximately 25% of patients with *von Recklinghausen's syndrome* (caused by *NF1* gene mutations) have neurofibromatosis involving the upper digestive tract, with multiple submucosal neurofibromas or, less commonly, ganglioneuromas, that may cause dyspepsia, abdominal pain, or hemorrhage.[335] The GI involvement is usually incidental and asymptomatic. Severe, uncontrolled symptoms have required surgical treatment in a few cases. Multiple intestinal ganglioneuromas have also been observed in families and individual cases unrelated to von Recklinghausen's disease.[336] Ganglioneuromas throughout the gastrointestinal tract can occur in patients with multiple endocrine neoplasia (MEN) type IIB, related to mutations of the *RET* gene.[337]

Devon Family Syndrome. Multiple and recurrent inflammatory "*fibroid polyps*" of the stomach and intestine have been reported in a family.[338] These lesions, histologically distinct from juvenile polyps, may cause gastrointestinal obstruction, with symptoms beginning in adult life.

Basal Cell Nevus Syndrome. The basal cell nevus syndrome has also been associated with multiple gastric hamartomatous polyps.[339] However, several kindreds have been reported without mention of gastrointestinal lesions.

Noninherited Gastrointestinal Polyposis Syndromes

Cronkhite-Canada Syndrome

In 1955, Cronkhite and Canada reported the first examples of an acquired, nonfamilial syndrome that now bears their names.[340] It is characterized by the presence of diffuse gastrointestinal polyposis, dystrophic changes in the fingernails, alopecia, cutaneous hyperpigmentation, diarrhea, weight loss, abdominal pain, and complications of malnutrition (Fig. 114–19).[341] Patients are typically middle-aged or older (average, 62 years) and present fairly acutely with a rapidly progressive illness consisting of chronic diarrhea and protein-losing enteropathy and the associated integumentary abnormalities. The diarrhea is attributable primarily to diffuse mucosal injury in the small intestine but may be complicated by bacterial overgrowth. Gastrointestinal polyps are found in 52% to 96% of patients, depending upon location, from the stomach to the rectum.[341] These polyps are hamartomas similar to the juvenile (retention) type, but unlike juvenile polyposis, the mucosa between polyps is histologically abnormal, with edema, congestion, and inflammation. As is the case with juvenile polyps, there may be foci of adenomatous epithelium, which may confer a risk of carcinoma. Although adenomatous epithelium has been reported in these polyps and carcinoma has been reported to complicate this syndrome, malignant degeneration is the exception rather than the rule in this disease.[342]

The *malabsorption syndrome* is progressive in most patients, and the prognosis is poor as there is no specific therapy. It has been suggested that complete symptomatic remission occasionally may be achieved with the appropriate supportive management. In some cases, a variety of medical and surgical measures have been employed, making it difficult to identify the essential therapeutic factor(s). Corticosteroids, anabolic steroids, antibiotics, and surgical resections have been tried in many of these patients in whom remissions have been reported. Despite this, aggressive nutritional support appears to be the most important factor influencing a favorable outcome. Enteral feeding (if possible) or parenteral feeding (if necessary) with sources of calories, nitrogen, and lipids, in addition to appropriate fluids, electrolytes, vitamins, and minerals, has resulted in complete symptomatic remissions with resolution of all of the ectodermal aberrations.[341] Antibiotics may be beneficial when bacterial over-

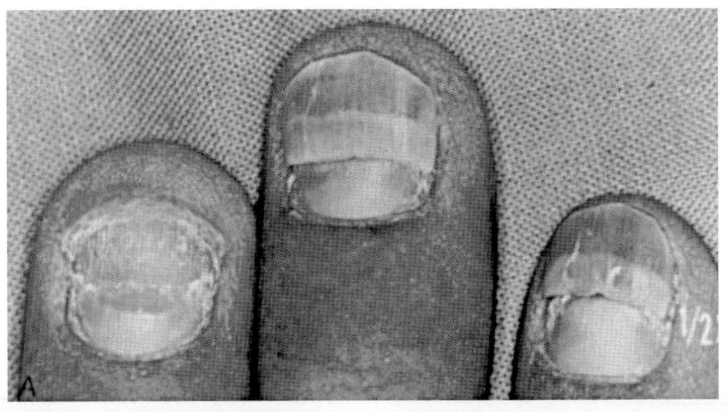

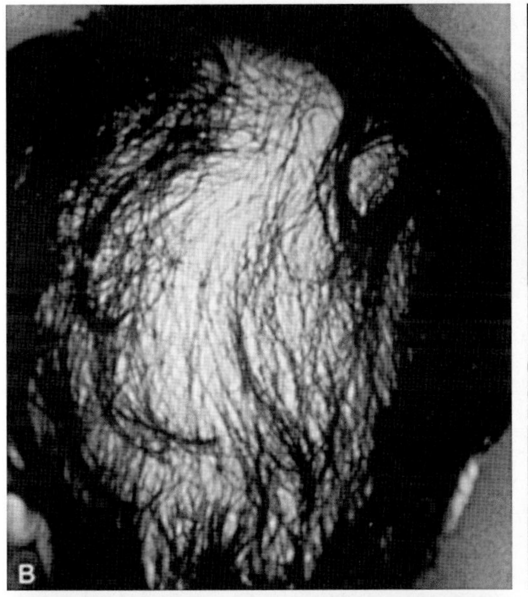

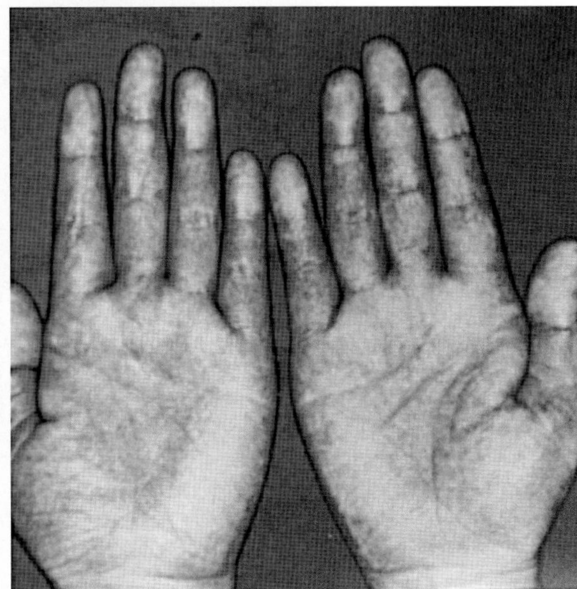

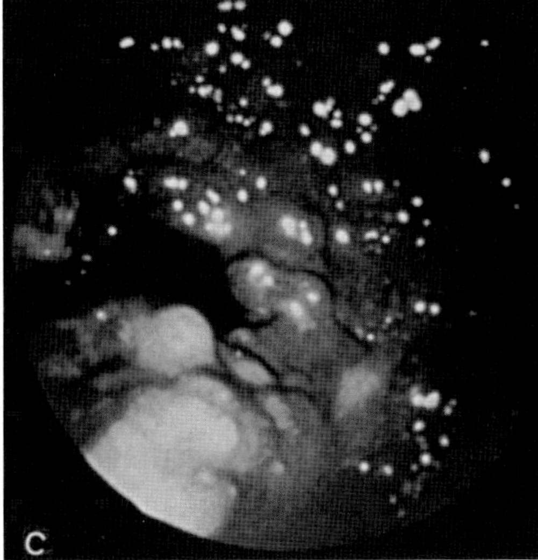

Figure 114–19. Manifestations of Cronkhite-Canada syndrome. *A*, Onycholysis, illustrating detachment of the fingernails from the nailbed. *B*, Alopecia *(left)* and hyperpigmentation of the palms *(right)*. Both of these abnormalities resolved in this patient after administration of corticosteroids and enteral alimentation. *C*, Colonoscopic appearance of colonic polyposis in the same patient as in *A* and *B*. Biopsy specimens of this lesion demonstrated cystic dilation of the glands and edema of the lamina propria, without neoplastic changes in the epithelium. (Courtesy of Chikao Shimamoto, M.D.)

growth contributes to the malabsorption. Although corticosteroids have been used in some of the cases of symptomatic remission, the evidence to support their use is weak. Surgical therapy offers less and is risky in such malnourished patients. One case of complete remission has been reported in a patient managed only with enteral administration of a nutritionally balanced complete liquid diet.[343] Attention should be paid to the possibility of secondary lactose or other disaccharide intolerance, or protein-losing enteropathy in patients with diffuse small intestinal disease. Specific management awaits a better understanding of this perplexing syndrome.

Hyperplastic Polyposis Syndrome

Initially described as a discrete entity in 1980,[261] the hyperplastic polyposis syndrome (HPS) is characterized by hyperplastic polyps that are often multiple (12 or more), large (often >1 cm, alternatively referred to as "giant hyperplastic polyps"), and more evenly distributed throughout the colon compared with sporadic hyperplastic polyps, which concentrate in the distal colon and rectum. In addition, the hyperplastic polyps in HPS seem to demonstrate more cytologic atypia while preserving their serrated appearance. This has led to the suggestion that the serrated adenomatous polyposis syndrome[296] may be a variant of HPS. Most cases of HPS are isolated, but a handful of families with HPS have been reported.[344, 345] About 35% of reported HPS cases have been associated with synchronous colorectal cancers,[344] suggesting an increased malignant potential of these otherwise innocent lesions. The mechanism by which colon cancers arise in this syndrome is controversial, with some investigators suggesting a novel pathway involving low-level microsatellite instability via a serrated adenoma precursor,[200] others suggesting the typical route involving chromosomal instability and p53 mutations,[344] and others implying frequent loss of chromosome 1p.[345] Patients with large hyperplastic polyps in the right colon have an increased risk of proximal colon cancer. In the absence of sufficient aggregate clinical experience with this entity, periodic colonoscopy with biopsies should be considered.

Lymphomatous Polyposis

As discussed and illustrated in Chapter 26, *lymphoma* may present as multiple lymphomatous polyps of the gastrointestinal tract.

Nodular Lymphoid Hyperplasia

Nodular lymphoid hyperplasia is a rare lymphoproliferative condition that is not related to a specific disease. It can be seen in healthy children (see Fig. 114–14) and has also been described in the terminal ileum of some patients with Gardner's syndrome and in some immunodeficiency syndromes. These polyps, which are more common in the small intestine and measure approximately 3 to 6 mm, do not typically cause symptoms.

REFERENCES

1. Itzkowitz SH: Gastrointestinal adenomatous polyps. Semin Gastrointest Dis 7:105, 1996.
2. Lev R: Adenomatous Polyps of the Colon: Pathological and Clinical Features. New York, Springer-Verlag, 1990.
3. Jass JR, Sobin LH (eds): World Health Organization: Histological Typing of Intestinal Tumours, 2nd ed. New York, Springer-Verlag, 1989.
4. O'Brien MJ, Winawer SJ, Zauber AG, et al: The National Polyp Study: Patient and polyp characteristics associated with high-grade dysplasia in colorectal adenomas. Gastroenterology 98:371, 1990.
5. Konishi F, Morson BCJ: Pathology of colorectal adenomas: A colonoscopic survey. J Clin Pathol 35:830, 1982.
6. Fenoglio CM, Kaye GI, Lane N: Distribution of human colonic lymphatics in normal, hyperplastic and adenomatous tissue. Gastroenterology 64:51, 1973.
7. Muto T, Bussey HJR, Morson BC: The evolution of cancer of the colon and rectum. Cancer 36:2251, 1975.
8. Shinya H, Wolff WI: Morphology, anatomic distribution, and cancer potential of colonic polyps. Ann Surg 190:679, 1979.
9. Rickert RR, Auerbach O, Garfinkel L, et al: Adenomatous lesions of the large bowel: An autopsy survey. Cancer 43:1847, 1979.
10. Williams AR, Balasooriya BAW, Day DW: Polyps and cancer of the large bowel: A necropsy study in Liverpool. Gut 23:835, 1982.
11. Arminski TC, McLean DW: Incidence and distribution of adenomatous polyps of the colon and rectum based on 1,000 autopsy examinations. Dis Colon Rectum 7:249, 1964.
12. Correa P: Epidemiology of polyps and cancer. In Morson BC (ed): The Pathogenesis of Colorectal Cancer. Philadelphia, WB Saunders, 1978, pp 126.
13. Clark JC, Collan Y, Eide TJ, et al: Prevalence of polyps in an autopsy series from areas with varying incidence of large-bowel cancer. Int J Cancer 36:179, 1985.
14. Eide TJ, Stalsberg H: Polyps of the large intestine in northern Norway. Cancer 42:2839, 1978.
15. Johannsen LGK, Momsen O, Jacobsen NO: Polyps of the large intestine in Aarhus, Denmark: An autopsy study. Scand J Gastroenterol 24: 799, 1989.
16. Granqvist S, Gabrielsson N, Sundelin P: Diminutive colonic polyps—clinical significance and management. Endoscopy 1:36, 1979.
17. Tedesco FJ, Hendrix JC, Pickens CA, et al: Diminutive polyps: Histopathology, spatial distribution, and clinical significance. Gastrointest Endosc 28:1, 1982.
18. Gottlieb LS, Winawer SJ, Sternberg S, et al: National Polyp Study (NPS): The diminutive colonic polyp. Gastrointest Endosc 30:143, 1984.
19. Ryan ME, Parent K, Wyman JB, et al: Significance of diminutive colorectal polyps in 3282 flexible sigmoidoscopic examinations. Gastrointest Endosc 31:149, 1985.
20. Weston AP, Campbell DR: Diminutive colonic polyps: Histopathology, spatial distribution, concomitant significant lesions, and treatment complications. Am J Gastroenterol 90:24, 1995.
21. Tripp MR, Morgan TR, Sampliner RE: Synchronous neoplasms in patients with diminutive colorectal adenomas. Cancer 60:1599, 1987.
22. Blue MG, Sivak MV Jr, Achkar E, et al: Hyperplastic polyps seen at sigmoidoscopy are markers for additional adenomas seen at colonoscopy. Gastroenterology 100:564, 1991.
23. Lieberman DA, Smith FW: Screening for colon malignancy with colonoscopy. Am J Gastroenterol 86:946, 1991.
24. Hoff G, Foerster A, Vatn MH, et al: Epidemiology of polyps in the rectum and colon. Recovery and evaluation of unresected polyps two years after detection. Scand J Gastroenterol 21:853, 1986.
25. Ueyama T, Kawamoto K, Iwashita I, et al: Natural history of minute sessile colonic adenomas based on radiographic findings. Dis Colon Rectum 38:268, 1995.
26. Spencer RJ, Melton LJ III, Ready RL, et al: Treatment of small colorectal polyps: A population-based study of the risk of subsequent carcinoma. Mayo Clin Proc 59:305, 1984.
27. Muto T, Kamiya J, Sawada T, et al: Small "flat adenoma" of the large bowel with special reference to its clinicopathologic features. Dis Colon Rectum 28:847, 1985.
28. Mitooka H: Flat neoplasms in the adenoma-carcinoma sequence in Japan. Semin Gastrointest Dis 11:238, 2000.

29. Lanspa SJ, Rouse J, Smyrk T, et al: Epidemiologic characteristics of the flat adenoma of Muto: A prospective study. Dis Colon Rectum 35: 543, 1992.
30. Wolber RA, Owen DA: Flat adenomas of the colon. Hum Pathol 22: 70, 1991.
31. Kubota O, Kino I, Kimura T, et al: Nonpolypoid adenomas and adenocarcinomas found in background mucosa of surgically resected colons. Cancer 77:621, 1996.
32. Rembacken BJ, Fujii T, Cairns A, et al: Flat and depressed colonic neoplasms: A prospective study of 1000 colonoscopies in the UK. Lancet 355:1211, 2000.
33. Lynch HT, Smyrk TC, Watson P, et al: Hereditary flat adenoma syndrome: A variant of familial adenomatous polyposis? Dis Colon Rectum 35:411, 1992.
34. Owen DA: Flat adenoma, flat carcinoma, and de novo carcinoma of the colon. Cancer 77:3, 1996.
35. Bird RP: Role of aberrant crypt foci in understanding the pathogenesis of colon cancer. Cancer Lett 93:55, 1995.
36. Takayama T, Katsuki S, Takahashi Y, et al: Aberrant crypt foci of the colon as precursors of adenoma and cancer. N Engl J Med 339:1277, 1998.
37. Jen J, Powell SM, Papadopoulos N, et al: Molecular determinants of dysplasia in colorectal lesions. Cancer Res 54:5523, 1994.
38. Novelli MR, Williamson JA, Tomlinson IPM, et al: Polyclonal origin of colonic adenomas in an XO/XY patient with FAP. Science 272: 1187, 1996.
39. Shamsuddin AM: Microscopic intraepithelial neoplasia in large bowel mucosa. Hum Pathol 13:510, 1982.
40. Kozuka S, Nogaki M, Ozeki T, et al: Premalignancy of the mucosal polyp in the large intestine. II. Estimation of the periods required for malignant transformation of mucosal polyps. Dis Colon Rectum 18: 494, 1975.
41. Winawer SJ, Zauber AG, Gerdes H, et al: Prevention of colorectal cancer by colonoscopic polypectomy. N Engl J Med 329:1977, 1993.
42. Gilbertsen VA, Nelms JM: The prevention of invasive cancer of the rectum. Cancer 41:1137, 1978.
43. Müller AD, Sonnenberg A: Prevention of colorectal cancer by flexible endoscopy and polypectomy: A case-control study of 32,702 veterans. Ann Intern Med 123:904, 1995.
44. Selby JV, Friedman GD, Quesenberry CP Jr, et al: A case-control study of screening sigmoidoscopy and mortality from colorectal cancer. N Engl J Med 326:653, 1992.
45. Newcomb PA, Norfleet RG, Storer BE, et al: Screening sigmoidoscopy and colorectal cancer mortality. J Natl Cancer Inst 84:1572, 1992.
46. Vogelstein B, Fearon ER, Hamilton S, et al: Genetic alterations during colorectal-tumor development. N Engl J Med 319:525, 1988.
47. Kinzler KW, Vogelstein B: Lessons from hereditary colorectal cancer. Cell 87:159, 1996.
48. Fearon ER, Cho KR, Nigro JM, et al: Identification of a chromosome 18q gene that is altered in colorectal cancers. Science 247:49, 1990.
49. Baker SJ, Preisinger AC, Jessup JM, et al: p53 gene mutations occur in combination with 17p allelic deletions as late events in colorectal tumorigenesis. Cancer Res 50:7717, 1990.
50. Ahlquist DA: Aggressive polyps in hereditary nonpolyposis colorectal cancer: Targets for screening. Gastroenterology 108:1590, 1995.
51. Jacoby RF, Marshall DJ, Kailas S, et al: Genetic instability associated with adenoma to carcinoma progression in hereditary nonpolyposis colon cancer. Gastroenterology 109:73, 1995.
52. Vasen HFA, Nagengast FM, Meera Khan P: Interval cancers in hereditary non-polyposis colorectal cancer (Lynch syndrome). Lancet 345: 1183, 1995.
53. Markowitz AJ, Winawer SJ, Zauber A, et al: Rapid appearance of colorectal cancer following negative colonoscopy in HNPCC. Gastroenterology 116:A458, 1999.
54. Stemmermann GN, Yatani R: Diverticulosis and polyps of the large intestine: A necropsy study of Hawaii Japanese. Cancer 31:1260, 1973.
55. Chapman I: Adenomatous polyps of large intestine: Incidence and distribution. Ann Surg 157:223, 1963.
56. Sato E, Ouchi A, Sasano N, et al: Polyps and diverticulosis of large bowel in autopsy population of Akita prefecture, compared with Miyagi. Cancer 37:1316, 1976.
57. Rex DK, Lehman GA, Hawes RH, et al: Screening colonoscopy in asymptomatic average-risk persons with negative fecal occult blood tests. Gastroenterology 100:64, 1991.
58. Johnson DA, Gurney MS, Volpe RJ, et al: A prospective study of the prevalence of colonic neoplasms in asymptomatic patients with an age-related risk. Am J Gastroenterol 85:969, 1990.
59. DiSario JA, Foutch PG, Mai HD: Prevalence and malignant potential of colorectal polyps in asymptomatic average-risk men. Am J Gastroenterol 86:941, 1991.
60. Villavicencio RT, Rex DK: Colonic adenomas: Prevalence and incidence rates, growth rates, and miss rates at colonoscopy. Semin Gastrointest Dis 11:185, 2000.
61. Lieberman DA, Weiss DG, Bond JH, et al: Use of colonoscopy to screen asymptomatic adults for colorectal cancer. N Engl J Med 343: 162, 2000.
62. Coode PE, Chan KW, Chan YT: Polyps and diverticula of the large intestine: A necropsy survey in Hong Kong. Gut 26:1045, 1985.
63. Vatn MH, Stalsberg H: The prevalence of polyps of the large intestine in Oslo: An autopsy study. Cancer 49:819, 1982.
64. Burt RW: Colon cancer screening. Gastroenterology 119:837, 2000.
65. Gaglia P, Atkin WS, Whitelaw S, et al: Variables associated with the risk of colorectal adenomas in asymptomatic patients with a family history of colorectal cancer. Gut 36:385, 1995.
66. Winawer SJ, Fletcher RH, Miller L, et al: Colorectal cancer screening: Clinical guidelines and rationale. Gastroenterology 112:594, 1997.
67. Hixson LJ, Fennerty MB, Sampliner RE, et al: Two-year incidence of colon adenomas developing after tandem colonoscopy. Am J Gastroenterol 89:687, 1994.
68. Rex DK, Cummings OW, Helper DJ, et al: 5-year incidence of adenomas after negative colonoscopy in asymptomatic average-risk persons. Gastroenterology 111:1178, 1996.
69. Granqvist S: Distribution of polyps in the large bowel in relation to age: A colonoscopic study. Scand J Gastroenterol 16:1025, 1981.
70. Imperiale TF, Wagner DR, Lin CY, et al: Risk of advanced proximal neoplasms in asymptomatic adults according to the distal colorectal findings. N Engl J Med 343:169, 2000.
71. Levin TR, Palitz A, Grossman S, et al: Predicting advanced proximal colonic neoplasia with screening sigmoidoscopy. JAMA 281:1611, 1999.
72. Hill M: Etiology of the adenoma-carcinoma sequence. In Morson BC (ed): The Pathogenesis of Colorectal Cancer. Philadelphia, WB Saunders, 1978, p 153.
73. Burt RW: Hereditary aspects of colorectal adenomas. Cancer 70:1296, 1992.
74. Winawer SJ, Zauber AG, Gerdes H, et al: Risk of colorectal cancer in the families of patients with adenomatous polyps. N Engl J Med 334: 82, 1996.
75. Potter JD: Colorectal cancer: Molecules and populations. J Natl Cancer Inst 91:916, 1999.
76. Tomeo CA, Colditz GA, Willett WC, et al: Harvard Report on Cancer Prevention. Vol 3: Prevention of colon cancer in the United States. Cancer Causes Control 10:167, 1999.
77. Potter JD: Epidemiologic, environmental and lifestyle issues in colorectal cancer. In Young GP, Rozen P, Levin B (eds): Prevention and Early Detection of Colorectal Cancer. London, WB Saunders, 1996, p 23.
78. Peipins LA, Sandler RS: Epidemiology of colorectal adenomas. Epidemiol Rev 16:273, 1994.
79. Giardiello FM, Offerhaus GJA, DuBois RN: The role of nonsteroidal anti-inflammatory drugs in colorectal cancer prevention. Eur J Cancer 31A:1071, 1995.
80. Hixson LJ, Earnest DL, Fennerty MB, et al: NSAID effect on sporadic colon polyps. Am J Gastroenterol 10:1647, 1993.
81. Ladenheim J, Garcia G, Titzer D, et al: Effect of sulindac on sporadic colonic polyps. Gastroenterology 108:1083, 1995.
82. Logan RFA, Little J, Hawtin PG, et al: Effect of aspirin and non-steroidal anti-inflammatory drugs on colorectal adenomas: Case-control study of subjects participating in the Nottingham faecal occult blood screening programme. Br Med J 307:285, 1993.
83. Giovannucci E, Rimm EB, Stampfer MJ, et al: Aspirin use and risk for colorectal cancer and adenoma in male health professionals. Ann Intern Med 121:241, 1994.
84. Schatzkin A, Lanza E, Corle D, et al: Lack of effect of a low-fat, high-fiber diet on the recurrence of colorectal adenomas. N Engl J Med 342:1149, 2000.

85. Alberts DS, Martinez E, Roe DJ, et al: Lack of effect of a high-fiber cereal supplement on the recurrence of colorectal adenomas. N Engl J Med 342:1156, 2000.
86. MacLennan R, Macrae F, Bain C, et al: Randomized trial of intake of fat, fiber, and beta carotene to prevent colorectal adenomas. J Natl Cancer Inst 87:1760, 1995.
87. Kim YI: AGA technical review: Impact of dietary fiber on colon cancer occurrence. Gastroenterology 118:1235, 2000.
88. Greenberg ER, Baron JA, Tosteson TD, et al: A clinical trial of antioxidant vitamins to prevent colorectal adenomas. N Engl J Med 331:141, 1994.
89. Baron JA, Beach M, Mandel JS, et al: Calcium supplements for the prevention of colorectal adenomas. N Engl J Med 340:101, 1999.
90. Stewart M, Macrae FA, Williams CB: Neoplasia and ureterosigmoidostomy: A colonoscopic survey. Br J Surg 69:414, 1982.
91. Delhougne B, Deneux C, Abs R, et al: The prevalence of colonic polyps in acromegaly: A colonoscopic and pathological study in 103 patients. J Clin Endocrinol Metab 80:3223, 1995.
92. Brunner JE, Johnson CC, Zafar S, et al: Colon cancer and polyps in acromegaly: Increased risk associated with family history of colon cancer. Clin Endocrinol 32:65, 1990.
93. Ezzat S, Strom C, Melmed S: Colon polyps in acromegaly. Ann Intern Med 114:754, 1991.
94. Jenkins PJ, Frajese V, Jones AM, et al: Insulin-like growth factor I and the development of colorectal neoplasia in acromegaly. J Clin Endocrinol Metab 85:3218, 2000.
95. Ma J, Pollak M, Giovannucci E, et al: Prospective study of colorectal cancer risk in men and plasma levels of insulin-like growth factor (IGF)-1 and IGF-binding protein-3. J Natl Cancer Inst 91:620, 1999.
96. Cats A, Dullaart RP, Kleibeuker JH, et al: Increased epithelial cell proliferation in the colon of patients with acromegaly. Cancer Res 56: 523, 1996.
97. Klein RS, Catalano MT, Edberg SC: *Streptococcus bovis* septicemia and carcinoma of the colon. Ann Intern Med 91:560, 1979.
98. Marshall JB, Gerhardt DC: Polyposis coli presenting with *Streptococcus bovis* endocarditis. Am J Gastroenterol 75:314, 1981.
99. Burns CA, McCaughey R, Lauter CB: The association of *Streptococcus bovis* fecal carriage and colon neoplasia: Possible relationship with polyps and their premalignant potential. Am J Gastroenterol 80:42, 1985.
100. Ellmerich S, Schöller M, Duranton B, et al: Promotion of intestinal carcinogenesis by *Streptococcus bovis*. Carcinogenesis 21:753, 2000.
101. Wiseman A, Rene P, Crelinsten GL: *Streptococcus agalactiae* endocarditis: An association with villous adenomas of the large intestine. Ann Intern Med 103:893, 1985.
102. Piette AM, Meduri B, Fritsch J, et al: Do skin tags constitute a marker for colonic polyps? A prospective study of 100 asymptomatic patients and metaanalysis of the literature. Gastroenterology 95:1127, 1988.
103. Correa P, Strong JP, Johnson WD, et al: Atherosclerosis and polyps of the colon. Quantification of precursors of coronary heart disease and colon cancer. J Chronic Dis 35:313, 1982.
104. Stemmermann GN, Heilbrun LK, Nomura A, et al: Adenomatous polyps and atherosclerosis: An autopsy study of Japanese men in Hawaii. Int J Cancer 38:789, 1986.
105. Winawer SJ, Flehinger BJ, Buchalter J, et al: Declining serum cholesterol levels prior to diagnosis of colon cancer. JAMA 263:2083, 1990.
106. Porter JB, Walker AM, Jick H: Cancer of the breast, colon, ovary, and testis in the United States: Rates 1970–1978 from a hospital reporting system. Am J Public Health 74:585, 1984.
107. Rex DK, Sledge GW, Harper PA, et al: Colonic adenomas in asymptomatic women with a history of breast cancer. Am J Gastroenterol 88:2009, 1993.
108. Peelen T, de Leeuw W, van Lent K, et al: Genetic analysis of a breast-ovarian cancer family, with 7 cases of colorectal cancer linked to BRCA1, fails to support a role for BRCA1 in colorectal tumorigenesis. Int J Cancer 88:778, 2000.
109. McFarlane MJ, Welch KE: Gallstones, cholecystectomy, and colorectal cancer. Am J Gastroenterol 88:1994, 1993.
110. Neugut AI, Murray TI, Garbowski GC, et al: Cholecystectomy as a risk factor for colorectal adenomatous polyps and carcinoma. Cancer 68:1644, 1991.
111. Sandler RS, Martin ZZ, Carlton NM, et al: Adenomas of the large bowel after cholecystectomy. A case-control study. Dig Dis Sci 33: 1178, 1988.
112. Sobin LH: The histopathology of bleeding from polyps and carcinomas of the large intestine. Cancer 55:577, 1985.
113. Shnitka TK, Friedman MHW, Kidd EG, et al: Villous tumors of the rectum and colon characterized by severe fluid and electrolyte loss. Surg Gynecol Obstet 112:609, 1961.
114. Duthie HL, Atwell JD: The absorption of water, sodium, and potassium in the large intestine with particular reference to the effects of villous papillomas. Gut 4:373, 1963.
115. Steven K, Lange P, Bukhave K, et al: Prostaglandin E_2-mediated secretory diarrhea in villous adenoma of rectum: Effect of treatment with indomethacin. Gastroenterology 80:1562, 1981.
116. Silman AJ, Mitchell P, Nicholls RJ, et al: Self-reported dark red bleeding as a marker comparable with occult blood testing in screening for large bowel neoplasms. Br J Surg 70:721, 1983.
117. Guillem JG, Forde KA, Treat MR, et al: The impact of colonoscopy on the early detection of colonic neoplasms in patients with rectal bleeding. Ann Surg 206:606, 1987.
118. Cheung PSY, Wong SKC, Boey J, et al: Frank rectal bleeding: A prospective study of causes in patients over the age of 40. Postgrad Med J 64:364, 1988.
119. Macrae F, St. John DJB: Relationship between patterns of bleeding and Hemoccult sensitivity in patients with colorectal cancers or adenomas. Gastroenterology 82:891, 1982.
120. Crowley ML, Freeman LD, Mottet MD, et al: Sensitivity of guaiac-impregnated cards for the detection of colorectal neoplasia. J Clin Gastroenterol 5:127, 1983.
121. Gabrielsson N, Granqvist S, Nilsson B: Guaiac test detection of occult faecal blood loss in patients with endoscopically verified colonic polyps. Scand J Gastroenterol 20:978, 1985.
122. Norfleet RG: Effect of diet on fecal occult blood testing in patients with colorectal polyps. Dig Dis Sci 31:498, 1986.
123. Ahlquist DA, Weiand HS, Moertel CG, et al: Accuracy of fecal occult blood screening for colorectal neoplasia: A prospective study using Hemoccult and HemoQuant tests. JAMA 269:1262, 1993.
124. Allison JE, Tekawa IS, Ransom LJ, et al: A comparison of fecal occult blood tests for colorectal-cancer screening. N Engl J Med 334: 155, 1996.
125. Simon JB: Occult blood screening for colorectal carcinoma: A critical review. Gastroenterology 88:820, 1985.
126. Winawer SJ, Schottenfeld D, Flehinger BJ: Colorectal cancer screening. J Natl Cancer Inst 83:243, 1991.
127. Ransohoff DF, Lang CA: Small adenomas detected during fecal occult blood test screening for colorectal cancer: The impact of serendipity. JAMA 264:76, 1990.
128. Hardcastle JD, Armitage NC, Chamberlain J, et al: Fecal occult blood screening for colorectal cancer in the general population: Results of a controlled trial. Cancer 58:397, 1986.
129. Marks G, Boggs HW, Castro AF, et al: Sigmoidoscopic examinations with rigid and flexible fiberoptic sigmoidoscopes in the surgeon's office: A comparative prospective study of effectiveness in 1,012 cases. Dis Colon Rectum 22:162, 1979.
130. Winnan G, Berci G, Panish J, et al: Superiority of the flexible to the rigid sigmoidoscope in routine proctosigmoidoscopy. N Engl J Med 302:1011, 1980.
131. Moertel CG, Hill JR, Dockerty MB: The routine proctoscopic examination: A second look. Mayo Clin Proc 41:368, 1966.
132. Rumans MC, Benner KG, Keeffe EB, et al: Screening flexible sigmoidoscopy by primary care physicians: Effectiveness and costs in patients negative for fecal blood. West J Med 144:756, 1986.
133. Bat L, Pines A, Ron E, et al: A community-based program of colorectal screening in an asymptomatic population: Evaluation of screening tests and compliance. Am J Gastroenterol 81:647, 1986.
134. Demers RY, Stawick LE, Demers P: Relative sensitivity in the fecal occult blood test and flexible sigmoidoscopy in detecting polyps. Prev Med 14:55, 1985.
135. Yarborough GW, Waisbren BA: The benefits of systematic fiberoptic flexible sigmoidoscopy. Arch Intern Med 145:95, 1985.
136. Ott DJ, Chen YM, Gelfand DW, et al: Single-contrast vs double-contrast barium enema in the detection of colonic polyps. AJR Am J Roentgenol 146:993, 1986.
137. Winawer SJ, Stewart ET, Zauber AG, et al: A comparison of colonoscopy and double-contrast barium enema for surveillance after polypectomy. N Engl J Med 342:1766, 2000.
138. Thoeni RF, Menuck L: Comparison of barium enema and colonoscopy in the detection of small colonic polyps. Radiology 124:631, 1977.

139. Williams CB, Macrae FA, Bartrum CI: A prospective study of diagnostic methods in adenoma follow-up. Endoscopy 14:74, 1982.
140. Aldridge MC, Sim AJW: Colonoscopy findings in symptomatic patients without X-ray evidence of colonic neoplasms. Lancet 2:833, 1986.
141. Hixson LJ, Fennerty MB, Sampliner RE, et al: Prospective blinded trial of the colonoscopic miss rate of large colorectal polyps. Gastrointest Endosc 37:125, 1991.
142. Rex DK, Cutler CS, Lemmel GT, et al: Colonoscopic miss rates of adenomas determined by back-to-back colonoscopies. Gastroenterology 112:24, 1997.
143. Rex DK: Colonoscopy: A review of its yield for cancers and adenomas by indication. Am J Gastroenterol 90:353, 1995.
144. Hara AK, Johnson CD, Reed JE, et al: Detection of colorectal polyps by computed tomographic colography: Feasibility of a novel technique. Gastroenterology 110:284, 1996.
145. Fenlon HM, Nunes DP, Schroy PC III, et al: A comparison of virtual and conventional colonoscopy for the detection of colorectal polyps. N Engl J Med 341:1496, 1999.
146. Kapadia CR, Cutruzola FW, O'Brien KM, et al: Laser-induced fluorescence spectroscopy of human colonic mucosa: Detection of adenomatous transformation. Gastroenterology 99:150, 1990.
147. Ahlquist DA, Skoletsky JE, Boynton KA, et al: Colorectal cancer screening by detection of altered human DNA in stool: Feasibility of a multitarget assay panel. Gastroenterology 119:1219, 2000.
148. Figiel LS, Figiel SJ, Wieterson FK: Roentgenologic observation of growth rates of colonic polyps and carcinoma. Acta Radiol Diagn 3: 417, 1965.
149. Stryker SJ, Wolff BG, Culp CE, et al: Natural history of untreated colonic polyps. Gastroenterology 93:1009, 1987.
150. Welin S, Youker J, Spratt JS Jr: The rates and patterns of growth of 375 tumors of the large intestine and rectum observed serially by double contrast enema study (Malmo technique). AJR Am J Roentgenol 90:673, 1963.
151. Tada M, Misaki F, Kawai K: Growth rates of colorectal carcinoma and adenoma by roentgenologic follow-up observations. Gastroenterol Jpn 19:550, 1984.
152. Knoernschild HE: Growth rate and malignant potential of colonic polyps: Early results. Surg Forum 14:137, 1963.
153. Hofstad B, Almendingen K, Vatn M, et al: Growth and recurrence of colorectal polyps: A double-blind 3-year intervention with calcium and antioxidants. Digestion 59:148, 1998.
154. Bersentes K, Fennerty B, Sampliner RE, et al: Lack of spontaneous regression of tubular adenomas in 2 years of follow-up. Am J Gastroenterol 92:1117, 1997.
155. Carroll RLA, Klein M: How often should patients be sigmoidoscoped? A mathematical perspective. Prev Med 9:741, 1980.
156. Winawer SJ, Zauber A, Diaz B: The National Polyp Study: Temporal sequence of evolving colorectal cancer from the normal colon. Gastrointest Endosc 33:167, 1987.
157. Eide TJ: Risk of colorectal cancer in adenoma-bearing individuals within a defined population. Int J Cancer 38:173, 1986.
158. Pagana TJ, Ledesman EJ, Mittelman A, et al: The use of colonoscopy in the study of synchronous colorectal neoplasms. Cancer 53:356, 1984.
159. Chu DZJ, Giacco G, Martin RG, et al: The significance of synchronous carcinoma and polyps in the colon and rectum. Cancer 57:445, 1986.
160. Langevin JM, Nivatvongs S: The true incidence of synchronous cancer of the bowel: A prospective study. Am J Surg 147:330, 1984.
161. Reilly JC, Rusin LC, Theuerkauf FJ Jr: Colonscopy: Its role in cancer of the colon and rectum. Dis Colon Rectum 25:532, 1982.
162. Greenstein AJ, Heimann T, Sachar DB, et al: A comparison of multiple synchronous colorectal cancer in ulcerative colitis, familial polyposis coli, and de novo cancer. Ann Surg 203:123, 1986.
163. Morson BC, Bussey HJR: Magnitude of risk for cancer in patients with colorectal adenomas. Br J Surg 72(Suppl):S23, 1985.
164. Lotfi AM, Spencer RJ, Ilstrup DM, et al: Colorectal polyps and the risk of subsequent carcinoma. Mayo Clin Proc 61:337, 1986.
165. Bond JH: Polyp guideline: Diagnosis, treatment, and surveillance for patients with colorectal polyps. Am J Gastroenterol 95:3053, 2000.
166. Grossman S, Milos ML, Tekawa IS, et al: Colonoscopic screening of persons with suspected risk factors for colon cancer. II. Past history of colorectal neoplasms. Gastroenterology 96:299, 1989.
167. Zarchy TM, Ershoff D: Do characteristics of adenomas on flexible sigmoidoscopy predict advanced lesions on baseline colonoscopy? Gastroenterology 106:1501, 1994.
168. Wallace MB, Kemp JA, Trnka YM, et al: Is colonoscopy indicated for small adenomas found by screening flexible sigmoidoscopy? Ann Intern Med 129:273, 1998.
169. Atkin WS, Morson BC, Cuzick J: Long-term risk of colorectal cancer after excision of rectosigmoid adenomas. N Engl J Med 326:658, 1992.
170. Schoen RE, Corle D, Cranston L, et al: Is colonoscopy needed for the nonadvanced adenoma found on sigmoidoscopy? Gastroenterology 115:533, 1998.
171. Dinning JP, Hixson LJ, Clark LC: Prevalence of distal colonic neoplasia associated with proximal colon cancers. Arch Intern Med 154:853, 1994.
172. Atkin WS, Edwards R, Wardle J, et al: UK flexible sigmoidoscopy screening trial: Compliance, yield, and adverse effects. Gastroenterology 118:A187, 2000.
173. Weissfeld JL, Ling BS, Schoen RE, et al: Repeat screening flexible sigmoidoscopy in the prostate, lung, colorectal, and ovarian (PLCO) cancer screening trial. Gastroenterology 118:A441, 2000.
174. Wilcox GM, Anderson PB, Colacchio TA: Early invasive carcinoma in colonic polyps: A review of the literature with emphasis on the assessment of the risk of metastasis. Cancer 57:160, 1986.
175. Coverlizza S, Risio M, Ferrari A, et al: Colorectal adenomas containing invasive carcinoma: Pathologic assessment of lymph node metastatic potential. Cancer 64:1937, 1989.
176. Morson BC, Whiteway JE, Jones EA, et al. Histopathology and prognosis of malignant colorectal polyps treated by endoscopic polypectomy. Gut 25:437, 1984.
177. Morson BC: The evolution of colorectal carcinoma. Clin Radiol 35: 425, 1984.
178. Neugut AI, Jacobson JS, Ahsan H, et al: Incidence and recurrence rates of colorectal adenomas: A prospective study. Gastroenterology 108:402, 1995.
179. Williams CB, Macrae FA: The St. Mark's neoplastic polyp follow-up study. Front Gastrointest Res 10:226, 1986.
180. Kirsner JB, Rider JA, Moeller HC, et al: Polyps of the colon and rectum: Statistical analysis of a long-term follow-up study. Gastroenterology 39:178, 1960.
181. Kronborg O, Hage E, Adamsen S, et al: Follow-up after colorectal polypectomy. II. Repeated examinations of the colon every 6 months after removal of sessile adenomas and adenomas with the highest degree of dysplasia. Scand J Gastroenterol 18:1095, 1983.
182. Waye JD, Braunfeld S: Surveillance intervals after colonoscopic polypectomy. Endoscopy 14:79, 1981.
183. Woolfson IK, Eckholdt GJ, Wetzel CR, et al: Usefulness of performing colonoscopy one year after endoscopic polypectomy. Dis Colon Rectum 33:389, 1990.
184. Van Stolk RU, Beck GJ, Baron JA, et al: Adenoma characteristics at first colonoscopy as predictors of adenoma recurrence and characteristics at follow-up. Gastroenterology 115:13, 1998.
185. Martinez ME, Sampliner R, Marshall JR, et al: Adenoma characteristics as risk factors for recurrence of advanced adenomas. Gastroenterology 120:1077, 2001.
186. O'Brien M, Winawer SJ, Gottlieb LS, et al: Analysis of multiple determinants of significant dysplasia in colorectal adenomas. Gastrointest Endosc 31:148, 1985.
187. Winawer SJ: Colon surveillance for neoplasia. Gastrointest Endosc 49: S63, 1999.
188. Kune GA, Kune S, Watson LF: History of colorectal polypectomy and risk of subsequent colorectal cancer. Br J Surg 74:1064, 1987.
189. Levi F, Randimbison L, La Vecchia C: Incidence of colorectal cancer following adenomatous polyps of the large intestine. Int J Cancer 55: 415, 1993.
190. Simons BD, Morrison AS, Lev R, et al: Relationship of polyps to cancer of the large intestine. J Natl Cancer Inst 84:962, 1992.
191. Murakami, R, Tsukuma H, Kanamori S, et al: Natural history of colorectal polyps and the effect of polypectomy on occurrence of subsequent cancer. Int J Cancer 46:159, 1990.
192. Jørgensen OD, Kronborg O, Fenger C: The Funen Adenoma Follow-up Study: Incidence and death from colorectal carcinoma in an adenoma surveillance program. Scand J Gastroenterol 28:869, 1993.
193. Atkin WS, Cuzick J, Northover JMA, et al: Prevention of colorectal cancer by once-only sigmoidoscopy. Lancet 341:736, 1993.
194. Warner AS, Glick ME, Fogt F: Multiple large hyperplastic polyps of

the colon coincident with adenocarcinoma. Am J Gastroenterol 89: 123, 1994.

195. Kaye GI, Pascal RP, Lane N: The colonic pericryptal fibroblast sheath: Replication, migration, and cytodifferentiation of a mesenchymal cell system in adult tissue. Gastroenterology 60:515, 1971.
196. Hayashi T, Yatani R, Apostol J, et al: Pathogenesis of hyperplastic polyps of the colon: A hypothesis based upon ultrastructural and in vitro cell kinetics. Gastroenterology 66:347, 1974.
197. Hanby AM, Poulsom R, Singh S, et al: Hyperplastic polyps: A cell lineage which both synthesizes and secretes trefoil-peptides and has phenotypic similarity with the ulcer-associated cell lineage. Am J Pathol 42:663, 1993.
198. Longacre TA, Fenoglio-Preiser CM: Mixed hyperplastic adenomatous polyps/serrated adenomas: A distinct form of colorectal neoplasia. Am J Surg Pathol 14:524, 1990.
199. Cooper HS, Patchefsky AS, Marks G: Adenomatous and carcinomatous changes within hyperplastic colonic epithelium. Dis Colon Rectum 27:152, 1979.
200. Iino H, Jass JR, Simms LA, et al: DNA microsatellite instability in hyperplastic polyps, serrated adenomas, and mixed polyps: A mild mutator pathway for colorectal cancer? J Clin Pathol 52:5, 1999.
201. Frayling IM, Beck NE, Ilyas M, et al: The APC variants I1307K and E1317Q are associated with colorectal tumors, but not always with a family history. Proc Natl Acad Sci USA 95:10722, 1998.
202. Foutch PG, DiSario JA. Pardy K, et al: The sentinel hyperplastic polyp: A marker for synchronous neoplasia in the proximal colon. Am J Gastroenterol 86:1482, 1991.
203. Cannon-Albright LA, Skolnick MH, Bishop DT, et al: Common inheritance of susceptibility to colonic adenomatous polyps and associated colorectal cancers. N Engl J Med 319:533, 1988.
204. Waye JD, Lewis BS, Frankel A, et al: Small colon polyps. Am J Gastroenterol 83:120, 1988.
205. Rex DK, Smith JJ, Ulbright TM, et al: Distal colonic hyperplastic polyps do not predict proximal adenomas in asymptomatic average-risk subjects. Gastroenterology 102:317, 1992.
206. Provenzale D, Garrett JW, Condon SE, et al: Risk for colon adenomas in patients with rectosigmoid hyperplastic polyps. Ann Intern Med 113:760, 1990.
207. Zauber AG, Winawer SJ, Diaz B, et al: The National Polyp Study: The association of colonic hyperplastic polyps and adenomas. Am J Gastroenterol 83:1060, 1988.
208. Pennazio M, Arrigoni A, Risio M, et al: Small rectosigmoid polyps as markers of proximal neoplasms. Dis Colon Rectum 36:1121, 1993.
209. Isbister WH: Hyperplastic polyps. Aust NZ J Surg 63:175, 1993.
210. Nugent KP, Talbot IC, Hodgson SV, et al: Solitary juvenile polyps: Not a marker for subsequent malignancy. Gastroenterology 105:698, 1993.
211. Teague RH, Read AE: Polyposis in ulcerative colitis. Gut 16:792, 1975.
212. Berkowitz D, Bernstein LH: Colonic pseudopolyps in association with amebic colitis. Gastroenterology 68:786, 1975.
213. Nebel OT, El Masry NA, Castell DO, et al: Schistosomal disease of the colon: A reversible form of polyposis. Gastroenterology 67:939, 1974.
214. Anthony PP, Morris DS, Vowles KDJ: Multiple and recurrent inflammatory fibroid polyps in three generations of a Devon family: A new syndrome. Gut 25:854, 1984.
215. Géhénot M, Colombel JF, Wolschies E, et al: Cap polyposis occurring in the postoperative course of pelvic surgery. Gut 35:1670, 1994.
216. Levine DS: "Solitary" rectal ulcer syndrome. Are "solitary" rectal ulcer syndrome and "localized" colitis cystica profunda analogous syndromes caused by rectal prolapse? Gastroenterology 92:243, 1987.
217. Shallal JA, van Heerden JA, Bartholomew LG, et al: Pneumatosis cystoides intestinalis. Mayo Clin Proc 49:180, 1974.
218. Mirables M, Hinojosa J, Alonso J, et al: Oxygen therapy of pneumatosis coli. What is minimum oxygen requirement? Dis Colon Rectum 26:458, 1983.
219. Born A, Inouye T, Diamant N: Pneumatosis coli. Case report documenting time from X-ray appearance to onset of symptoms. Dig Dis Sci 26:855, 1981.
220. Pescatore P, Benhamou Y, Raphael M, et al: Colonic polyposis as sole manifestation of chronic lymphocytic leukemia. J Clin Gastroenterol 18:248, 1994.
221. Pfeil SA, Weaver MG, Abdul-Karim FW, et al: Colonic lipomas: Outcome of endoscopic removal. Gastrointest Endosc 36:532, 1990.
222. Bjornsdottir H, Bjornsson J, Gudjonsson H: Leiomyomatous colonic polyp. Dig Dis Sci 38:1945, 1993.
223. Bussey HJR, Veale AMO, Morson BC: Genetics of gastrointestinal polyposis. Gastroenterology 74:1325, 1978.
224. Herrera L, Kakati S, Gibas L, et al: Brief clinical report: Gardner syndrome in a man with an interstitial deletion of 5q. Am J Med Genet 25:473, 1986.
225. Bodmer WF, Bailey CJ, Bodmer J, et al: Localization of the gene for familial adenomatous polyposis on chromosome 5. Nature 328:614, 1987.
226. Leppert M, Dobbs M, Scambler P, et al: The gene for familial polyposis coli maps to the long arm of chromosome 5. Science 238:1411, 1987.
227. Solomon E, Voss R, Hall V, et al: Chromosome 5 allele loss in human colorectal carcinomas. Nature 328:616, 1987.
228. Kinzler KW, Nilbert MC, Su LK, et al: Identification of FAP locus genes from chromosome 5q21. Science 253:661, 1991.
229. Nishisho I, Nakamura Y, Miyoshi Y, et al: Mutations of chromosome 5q21 genes in FAP and colorectal cancer patients. Science 253:665, 1991.
230. Groden J, Thliveris A, Samowitz W, et al: Identification and characterization of the familial adenomatous polyposis coli gene. Cell 66: 589, 1991.
231. Miyaki M, Tanaka K, Kikuchi-Yanoshita R, et al: Familial polyposis: Recent advances. Crit Rev Oncol/Hematol 19:1, 1995.
232. Goss KH, Groden J: Biology of the adenomatous polyposis coli tumor suppressor. J Clin Oncol 18:1967, 2000.
233. Bussey HJR: Familial Polyposis Coli. Baltimore, Johns Hopkins Press, 1975.
234. Petersen GM, Slack J, Nakamura Y: Screening guidelines and premorbid diagnosis of familial adenomatous polyposis using linkage. Gastroenterology 100:1658, 1991.
235. Nagase H, Miyoshi Y, Horii A, et al. Correlation between the location of germ-line mutations in the *APC* gene and the number of colorectal polyps in familial adenomatous polyposis patients. Cancer Res 52: 4055, 1992.
236. Naylor EW, Lebenthal E: Gardner's syndrome: Recent developments in research and management. Dig Dis Sci 25:945, 1980.
237. Jang YS, Steinhagen RM, Heimann TM: Colorectal cancer in familial adenomatous polyposis. Dis Colon Rectum 40:312, 1997.
238. Burt RW: Hereditary polyposis syndromes and inheritance of adenomatous polyps. Semin Gastrointest Dis 3:13, 1992.
239. Abraham SC, Nobukawa B, Giardiello FM, et al: Fundic gland polyps in familial adenomatous polyposis. Am J Pathol 157:747, 2000.
240. Watanabe H, Enjoji M, Yao T, et al: Gastric lesions in familial adenomatosis coli. Hum Pathol 9:269, 1978.
241. Offerhaus GJA, Giardiello FM, Krush AJ, et al: The risk of upper gastrointestinal cancer in familial adenomatous polyposis. Gastroenterology 102:1980, 1992.
242. Iwama T, Mishima Y, Utsunomiya J: The impact of familial adenomatous polyposis on the tumorigenesis and mortality at the several organs: Its rational treatment. Ann Surg 217:101, 1993.
243. Debinski HS, Spigelman AD, Hatfield A, et al: Upper intestinal surveillance in familial adenomatous polyposis. Eur J Cancer 31A:1149, 1995.
244. Bulow S, Sondergaard JO, Witt I, et al: Mandibular osteomas in familial polyposis coli. Dis Colon Rectum 27:105, 1984.
245. Utsunomiya J, Nakamura T: The occult osteomatous changes in patients with familial polyposis coli. Br J Surg 62:45, 1975.
246. Blair NP, Trempe CL: Hypertrophy of the retinal pigment epithelium associated with Gardner's syndrome. Am J Ophthalmol 90:661, 1980.
247. Traboulski EI, Krush AJ, Gardner EJ, et al: Prevalence and importance of pigmented ocular fundus lesions in Gardner's syndrome. N Engl J Med 316:661, 1987.
248. Burn J, Chapman P, Delhanty J, et al: The UK northern region genetic register for familial adenomatous polyposis coli: Use of age of onset, congenital hypertrophy of the retinal pigment epithelium, and DNA markers in risk calculations. J Med Genet 28:289, 1991
249. Olschwang S, Tiret A, Laurent-Puig P, et al: Restriction of ocular fundus lesions to a specific subgroup of *APC* mutations in adenomatous polyposis coli patients. Cell 75:959, 1993.
250. Wallis YL, Macdonald F, Hultén M, et al: Genotype-phenotype correlation between position of constitutional APC gene mutation and CHRPE expression in familial adenomatous polyposis. Hum Genet 94: 543, 1994.

251. Jones IT, Jagelman DG, Fazio VW, et al: Desmoid tumors in familial polyposis coli. Ann Surg 204:94, 1986.
252. Gurbuz AK, Giardiello FM, Petersen GM, et al: Desmoid tumors in familial adenomatous polyposis. Gut 35:377, 1994.
253. Kiel KD, Suit HD: Radiation therapy in the treatment of aggressive fibromatoses (desmoid tumors). Cancer 54:2051, 1984.
254. Tsukada K, Church JM, Jagelman DG, et al: Systemic cytotoxic chemotherapy and radiation therapy for desmoid in familial adenomatous polyposis. Dis Colon Rectum 34:1090, 1991.
255. Klein WA, Miller HH, Anderson M, et al: The use of indomethacin, sulindac, and tamoxifen for the treatment of desmoid tumors associated with familial polyposis. Cancer 12:2863, 1987.
256. Belliveau P, Graham AM: Mesenteric desmoid tumor in Gardner's syndrome treated by sulindac. Dis Colon Rectum 27:53, 1984.
257. Kingbrunner B, Ritter S, Domingo J, et al: Remission of rapidly growing desmoid tumors after tamoxifen therapy. Cancer 52:2201, 1983.
258. Lanari A: Effect of progesterone on desmoid tumors (aggressive fibromatosis). N Engl J Med 309:1523, 1983.
259. Plail RO, Bussey HJR, Glazer G, et al: Adenomatous polyposis: An association with carcinoma of the thyroid. Br J Surg 7:377, 1987.
260. Walsh N, Qizilbash A, Banerjee R, et al: Biliary neoplasia in Gardner's syndrome. Arch Pathol Lab Med 111:76, 1987.
261. LeSher AR, Castronuovo JJ Jr, Filippone AL Jr: Familial polyposis coli and hepatocellular neoplasms. Surgery 105:668, 1989.
262. Garber JE, Li FP, Kingston JE, et al: Hepatoblastoma and familial adenomatous polyposis. J Natl Cancer Inst 80:1616, 1988.
263. Painter TA, Jagelman DG: Adrenal adenomas and adrenal carcinomas in association with hereditary adenomatosis of the colon and rectum. Cancer 55:2001, 1985.
264. Giardiello FM, Krush AJ, Petersen GM, et al: Phenotypic variability of familial adenomatous polyposis in 11 unrelated families with identical *APC* gene mutation. Gastroenterology 106:1542, 1994.
265. Stevenson JK, Reid BJ: Unfamiliar aspects of familial polyposis coli. Am J Surg 152:81, 1986.
266. Houlston R, Crabtree M, Phillips R, et al: Explaining differences in the severity of familial adenomatous polyposis and the search for modifier genes. Gut 48:1, 2001.
267. Oshima M, Dinchuk JE, Kargman SL, et al: Suppression of intestinal polyposis in $APC^{\Delta 716}$ knockout mice by inhibition of cyclooxygenase 2 (COX-2). Cell 87:803, 1996.
268. Burt RW, Groden J: The genetic and molecular diagnosis of adenomatous polyposis coli. Gastroenterology 104:1211, 1993.
269. Lynch HT, Smyrk T, Lynch J, et al: Genetic counseling in an extended attenuated familial adenomatous polyposis kindred. Am J Gastroenterol 91:455, 1996.
270. Moertel CG, Hill JR, Adson MA: Management of multiple polyposis of the large intestine. Cancer 28:160, 1971.
271. Bertario L, Russo A, Radice P, et al: Genotype and phenotype factors as determinants for rectal stump cancer in patients with familial adenomatous polyposis. Ann Surg 231:538, 2000.
272. Harvey JC, Quan SHQ, Stearns WW: Management of familial polyposis with preservation of the rectum. Surgery 84:476, 1978.
273. Bussey HJR, Eyers AA, Ritchie SM, et al: The rectum in adenomatous polyposis: The St. Mark's policy. Br J Surg 72:529, 1985.
274. Jagelman DG: Clinical management of familial adenomatous polyposis. Cancer Surv 8:159, 1989.
275. Skinner MA, Tyler D, Branum GE, et al: Subtotal colectomy for familial polyposis. Arch Surg 125:621, 1990.
276. Feinberg SM, Jagelman DG, Sarre RG, et al: Spontaneous resolution of rectal polyps in patients with familial polyposis following abdominal colectomy and ileorectal anastomosis. Dis Colon Rectum 31:169, 1988.
277. Bussey HJR, DeCosse JJ, Deschner EE, et al: A randomized trial of ascorbic acid in polyposis coli. Cancer 50:1434, 1982.
278. Stern HS, Gregoire RC, Kashtan H, et al: Long-term effects of dietary calcium on risk markers for colon cancer in patients with familial polyposis. Surgery 108:528, 1990.
279. DeCosse JJ, Miller HH, Lesser ML: Effect of wheat fiber and vitamins C and E on rectal polyps in patients with familial adenomatous polyposis. J Natl Cancer Inst 81:1290, 1989.
280. Prescott SM, White RL: Self-promotion? Intimate connections between APC and prostaglandin H synthase-2. Cell 87:783, 1996.
281. Piazza GA, Kulchak Rahm AL, Krutzsch M, et al: Antineoplastic drugs sulindac sulfide and sulfone inhibit cell growth by inducing apoptosis. Cancer Res 55:3110, 1995.
282. Steinbach G, Lynch PM, Phillips RKS, et al: The effect of celecoxib, a cyclooxygenase-2 inhibitor, in familial adenomatous polyposis. N Engl J Med 342:1946, 2000.
283. Burke C, van Stolk R, Arber N, et al: Exisulind prevents adenoma formation in familial adenomatous polyposis. Gastroenterology 118: A657, 2000.
284. Norton ID, Geller A, Petersen BT, et al: Endoscopic surveillance and ablative therapy for periampullary adenomas. Am J Gastroenterol 96: 101, 2001.
285. Turcot J, Despres JP, St. Pierre T: Malignant tumors of the central nervous system associated with familial polyposis of the colon. Report of two cases. Dis Colon Rectum 2:465, 1959.
286. Baughman FA, List CF, Williams JR, et al: The glioma-polyposis syndrome. N Engl J Med 281:1345, 1969.
287. Hamilton SR, Liu B, Parsons RE, et al: The molecular basis of Turcot's syndrome. N Engl J Med 332:839, 1995.
288. Munden PM, Sobol WM, Weingeist TA: Ocular findings in Turcot syndrome (glioma-polyposis). Ophthalmology 98:111, 1991.
289. Lynch HT, Smyrk T, Lynch J, et al: Update on the differential diagnosis, surveillance and management of hereditary non-polyposis colorectal cancer. Eur J Cancer 31A:1039, 1995.
290. Leppert M, Burt R, Hughes JP, et al: Genetic analysis of an inherited predisposition to colon cancer in a family with a variable number of adenomatous polyps. N Engl J Med 322:904, 1990.
291. Spirio L, Olschwang S, Groden J, et al: Alleles of the APC gene: An attenuated form of familial polyposis. Cell 75:951, 1993.
292. Lynch HT, Smyrk TC, Lanspa SJ, et al: Upper gastrointestinal manifestations in families with hereditary flat adenoma syndrome. Cancer 71:2709, 1993.
293. Graham R, McKee P, McGibbon D, et al: Torre-Muir syndrome: An association with isolated sebaceous carcinoma. Cancer 55:2868, 1985.
294. Seruca R, Carneiro F, Castedo S, et al: Familial gastric polyposis revisited. Cancer Genet Cytogenet 53:97, 1991.
295. Williams GT, Arthur JF, Bussey HJR, et al: Metaplastic polyps and polyposis of the colorectum. Histopathology 4:155, 1980.
296. Torlakovic E, Snover DC: Serrated adenomatous polyposis in humans. Gastroenterology 110:748, 1996.
297. Burdick D, Prior JT: Peutz-Jeghers syndrome. A clinicopathologic study of a large family with a 27-year follow-up. Cancer 50:2139, 1982.
298. Foley TR, McGarrity TJ, Abt AB: Peutz-Jeghers syndrome: A clinicopathologic survey of the "Harrisburg Family" with a 49-year follow-up. Gastroenterology 95:1535, 1988.
299. Hemminki A, Markie D, Tomlinson I, et al: A serine/threonine kinase gene defect in Peutz-Jeghers syndrome. Nature 391:184, 1998.
300. Jenne DE, Reimann H, Nezu J, et al: Peutz-Jeghers Syndrome is caused by mutations in a novel serine threonine kinase. Nat Genet 18: 38, 1998.
301. Gruber SB, Entius MM, Petersen GM, et al: Pathogenesis of adenocarcinoma in Peutz-Jeghers syndrome. Cancer Res 58:5267, 1998.
302. Entius MM, Keller JJ, Westerman AM, et al: Molecular genetic alterations in hamartomatous polyps and carcinomas of patients with Peutz-Jeghers syndrome. J Clin Pathol 54:126, 2001.
303. Giardiello FM, Brensinger JD, Tersmette AC, et al: Very high risk of cancer in familial Peutz-Jeghers syndrome. Gastroenterology 119:1447, 2000.
304. Clement S, Efrusy ME, Dobbins WO III, et al: Pelvic neoplasia in Peutz-Jeghers syndrome. J Clin Gastroenterol 1:341, 1979.
305. Wilson DM, Pitts WC, Hintz RI, et al: Testicular tumors with Peutz-Jeghers syndrome. Cancer 57:2238, 1986.
306. Cantu JM, Rivera H, Ocampo-Campos R, et al: Peutz-Jeghers syndrome with feminizing Sertoli cell tumor. Cancer 46:223, 1980.
307. Trau H, Schewach-Millet M, Fisher BK, et al: Peutz-Jeghers syndrome and bilateral breast carcinoma. Cancer 50:788, 1982.
308. Pedersen IR, Hartvigsen A, Hansen B, et al: Management of Peutz-Jeghers syndrome: Experience with patients from the Danish Polyposis Registry. Int J Colorect Dis 9:177, 1994.
309. Devroede G, Lemieux B, Masse S, et al: Colonic hamartomas in tuberous sclerosis. Gastroenterology 94:182, 1988.
310. Beacham CH, Shields HM, Raffensperger EC, et al: Juvenile and adenomatous gastrointestinal polyposis. Am J Dig Dis 23:1137, 1978.
311. Grotsky HW, Rickert RR, Smith WD, et al: Familial juvenile polyposis coli. A clinical and pathologic study of a large kindred. Gastroenterology 82:494, 1982.
312. Watanabe A, Nagashima H, Motoi M, et al: Familial juvenile polyposis of the stomach. Gastroenterology 77:148, 1979.

313. Sachatello CR, Pickren JW, Grace JT: Generalized juvenile gastrointestinal polyposis. A hereditary syndrome. Gastroenterology 58:699, 1970.
314. Nelen MR, Padberg GW, Peeters EAJ, et al: Localization of the gene for Cowden's disease to chromosome 10q22–23. Nat Genet 13:114, 1996.
315. Zigman AF, Lavine JE, Jones MC, et al: Localization of the Bannayan-Riley-Ruvalcaba syndrome gene to chromosome 10q23. Gastroenterology 113:1433, 1997.
316. Arch EM, Goodman BK, Van Wesep RA, et al: Detection of PTEN in a patient with Bannayan-Riley-Ruvalcaba syndrome suggests allelism with Cowden disease. Am J Med Genet 71:489, 1997.
317. Liaw D, Marsh DJ, Li J, et al: Germline mutations of the PTEN gene in Cowden disease, an inherited breast and thyroid cancer syndrome. Nature Genet 16:64, 1997.
318. Marsh DJ, Dahia PLM, Zheng A, et al: Germline mutations in PTEN are present in Bannayan-Zonana syndrome. Nature Genet 16:333, 1997.
319. Jacoby RF, Schlack S, Sekhon G, et al: Del (10)(q22.3q24.1) associated with juvenile polyposis. Am J Med Genet 70:361, 1997.
320. Huang SC, Chen CR, Lavine JE, et al: Genetic heterogeneity in familial juvenile polyposis. Cancer Res 60:6882, 2000.
321. Howe JR, Roth S, Ringold JC, et al: Mutations in the SMAD4/DPC4 gene in juvenile polyposis. Science 280:1086, 1998.
322. Kim IJ, Ku JK, Yoon KA, et al: Germline mutations of the DPC4 gene in Korean juvenile polyposis patients. Int J Cancer 86:529, 2000.
323. Nugent KP, Talbot IC, Hodgson SV, et al: Solitary juvenile polyps: Not a marker for subsequent malignancy. Gastroenterology 105:698, 1993.
324. Goodman ZD, Yardley JH, Milligan FD: Pathogenesis of colonic polyps in multiple juvenile polyposis. Cancer 43: 1906, 1979.
325. O'Riordain DS, O'Dwyer PJ, Cullen AF, et al: Familial juvenile polyposis coli and colorectal cancer. Cancer 68:889, 1991.
326. Sassatelli R, Bertoni G, Serra L, et al: Generalized juvenile polyposis with mixed pattern and gastric cancer. Gastroenterology 104:910, 1993.
327. Salem OS, Steck WD: Cowden's disease (multiple hamartoma and neoplasia syndrome). J Am Acad Dermatol 8:686, 1983.
328. Carlson GJ, Nivatvongs S, Snover DC: Colorectal polyps in Cowden's disease (multiple hamartoma syndrome). Am J Surg Pathol 8:763, 1984.
329. Lashner BA, Riddell RH, Winans CS: Ganglioneuromatosis of the colon and extensive glycogenic acanthosis in Cowden's disease. Dig Dis Sci 31:213, 1986.
330. Ruvalcaba RHA, Myhre S, Smith DW: Sotos syndrome with intestinal polyposis and pigmentary changes of the genitalia. Clin Genet 18:413, 1980.
331. DiLiberti JH, Weleber RG, Budden S: Ruvalcaba-Myhre-Smith syndrome: A case with probably autosomal-dominant inheritance and additional manifestations. Am J Med Genet 15:491, 1983.
332. Whitelaw SC, Murday VA, Tomlinson IPM, et al: Clinical and molecular features of the hereditary mixed polyposis syndrome. Gastroenterology 112:327, 1997.
333. Thomas HUW, Whitelaw SC, Cottrell SE, et al: Genetic mapping of the hereditary mixed polyposis syndrome to chromosome 6q. Am J Hum Genet 58:770, 1996.
334. Tomlinson IPM, Cole CE, Jacoby RF, et al: Hereditary mixed polyposis syndrome: Exclusion of genetic linkage to the polyposis region of chromosome 10. Gastroenterology 114:A691, 1998.
335. Rutgeerts P, Hendricks H, Geboes K, et al: Involvement of the upper digestive tract by systemic neurofibromatosis. Gastrointest Endosc 27: 22, 1981.
336. Hirata K, Kitahara K, Momosaka Y, et al: Diffuse ganglioneuromatosis with plexiform neurofibromas limited to the gastrointestinal tract involving a large segment of small intestine. J Gastroenterol 32:263, 1996.
337. Marsh DJ, Mulligan LM, Eng C: RET proto-oncogene mutations in multiple endocrine neoplasia type 2 and medullary thyroid carcinoma. Horm Res 47:168, 1997.
338. Allibone RO, Nanson JK, Anthony PP: Multiple and recurrent inflammatory fibroid polyps in a Devon family ("Devon polyposis syndrome"): An update. Gut 33:1004, 1992.
339. Schwartz RA: Basal cell nevus syndrome and gastrointestinal polyposis. N Engl J Med 299:49, 1978.
340. Cronkhite LW, Canada WJ: Generalized gastrointestinal polyposis: An unusual syndrome of polyposis, pigmentation, alopecia and onychotrophia. N Engl J Med 252:1011, 1955.
341. Daniel ES, Ludwig SL, Lewin KJ, et al: The Cronkhite-Canada syndrome. An analysis of the pathologic features and therapy in 55 patients. Medicine 61:293, 1982.
342. Katayama Y, Kimura M, Konn M: Cronkhite-Canada syndrome associated with a rectal cancer and adenomatous changes in colonic polyps. Am J Surg Pathol 9:65, 1985.
343. Russell DM, Bhathal PS, St. John DJB: Complete remission in Cronkhite-Canada syndrome. Gastroenterology 85:180, 1983.
344. Hawkins NJ, Gorman P, Tomlinson IPM, et al: Colorectal carcinomas arising in the hyperplastic polyposis syndrome progress through the chromosomal instability pathway. Am J Pathol 157:385, 2000.
345. Rashid A, Houlihan PS, Booker S, et al: Phenotypic and molecular characteristics of hyperplastic polyposis. Gastroenterology 119:323, 2000.

Chapter 115

MALIGNANT NEOPLASMS OF THE LARGE INTESTINE

Robert S. Bresalier

Cancer of the colon and rectum (colorectal cancer) is a major cause of cancer-associated morbidity and mortality in North America, Europe, and other regions where life-styles and dietary habits are similar. The fourth most common newly diagnosed internal cancer overall in the United States (behind cancers of the breast, prostate, and lung), colorectal cancer currently constitutes 10% of new cancer cases in men and 11% in women. In 2001, there were an estimated 135,000 new cases in the United States and 57,000 related deaths (a rate second only to that of lung cancer).[1] Overall, incidence rates in men and women are similar in the United States, while there appears to be a slight male predominance worldwide. Approximately 6% of the American population will eventually develop invasive colon or rectal cancer, and over 6 million Americans who are alive today will die of the disease (an individual's lifetime risk of dying from colorectal cancer in the United States has been estimated to be 2.5%). Globally, it is the fourth most common cancer in men and the third most common in women, with mortality paralleling incidence.[2] Countries where colorectal cancer mortality was low before 1950 have reported substantial increases. Despite evidence that 5-year survival is 90% when colorectal cancer is diagnosed at an early stage, less than 40% of cases are diagnosed when the cancer is still localized.[3]

Rapid proliferation of knowledge about the molecular and biologic characteristics of colorectal cancer has provided useful insights into the pathogenesis of colonic neoplasms and cancer in general. New insights have also been gained in regard to primary prevention. Because these cancers arise over long periods as the result of interactions between genetic predisposition and environmental insults, it has become possible to identify preneoplastic and early neoplastic lesions better and to improve survival rates. Rapidly evolving knowledge of the pathogenesis of colorectal cancer, especially in high-risk groups, is leading to the development of new tools for identifying which persons will benefit most from cancer surveillance and from adjuvant therapy following potentially curative surgery.

Chapter 114 deals in detail with the principal premalignant colon lesion, the adenomatous polyp. In this chapter we examine what is known about factors that contribute to the further development of colorectal cancer, its predisposing conditions, biology, natural history, clinical presentation, diagnosis, and management. Current concepts and recent advances are stressed.

DESCRIPTIVE EPIDEMIOLOGY AND EPIDEMIOLOGIC PATTERNS

The frequency of colorectal cancer varies remarkably among different populations (Fig. 115–1).[4] Incidence rates are highest in the developed countries of North America, Australia, and New Zealand, intermediate in areas of Europe, and low in regions of Asia, South America, and especially sub-Saharan Africa. Internationally, the incidence of colon cancer

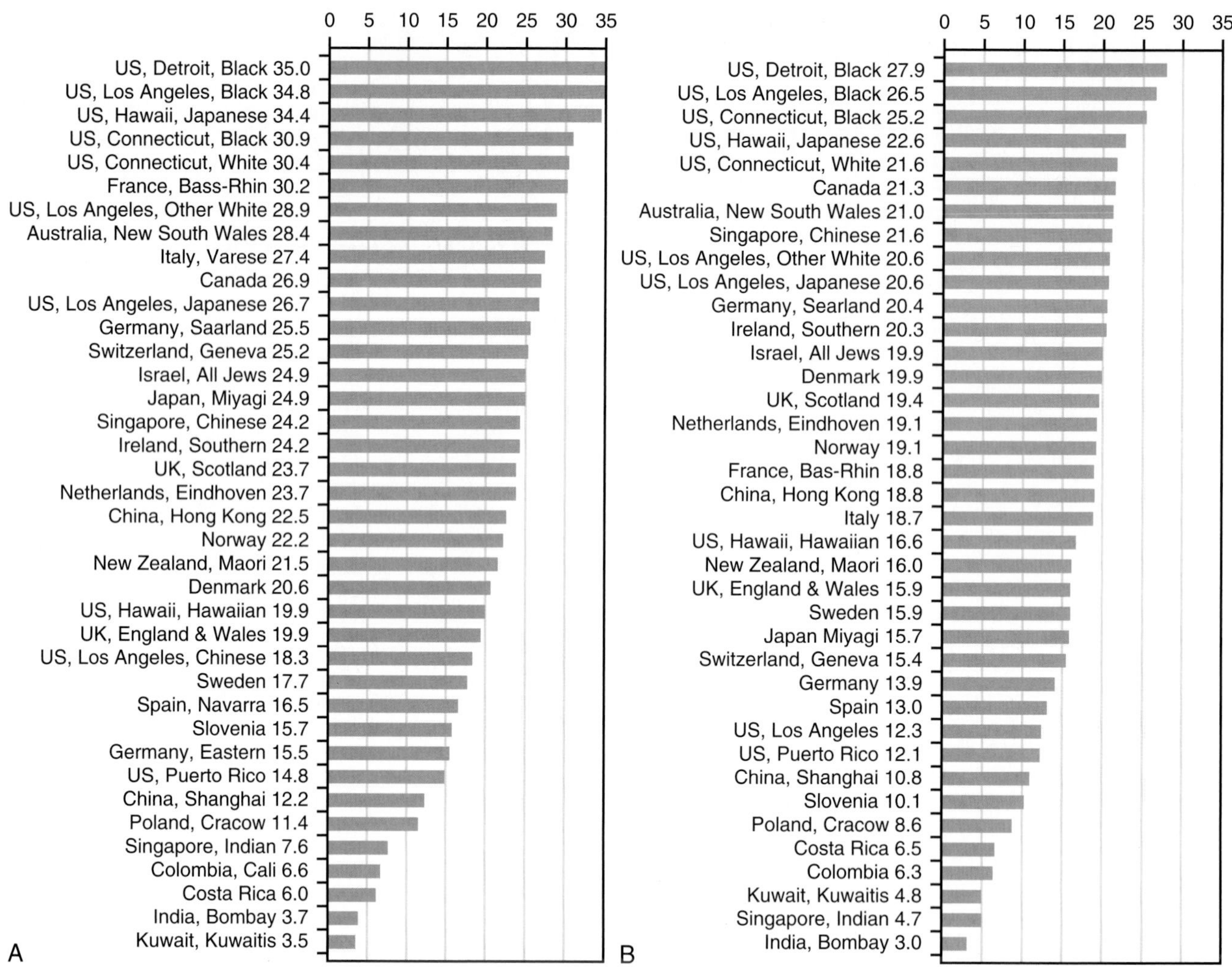

Figure 115–1. Age-standardized incidence of colon cancer per 100,000 population around the world. *A,* Men. *B,* Women. (Data from Parkin DM, Whelen SL, Ferlay J, et al: Cancer Incidence in Five Continents. [IARC Sci. Publ. No. 143]. Series. Lyon, International Agency for Research on Cancer, 1997.)

in men differs by a factor of almost 90 between areas with the extreme lowest and highest rates, and for rectal cancer (cancer within 11 cm of the anus), by a factor of 13. Colorectal cancer incidence also differs within countries, depending upon region and population (Fig. 115–2). These differences are most likely due to differences in environmental factors, including dietary patterns (discussed later).

Although the incidences of colon and rectal cancer overall are parallel, geographic variation is more pronounced for colon cancer than for rectal cancer. High ratios of colon to rectal cancer (2:1 or more) prevail in high-risk areas such as North America, whereas ratios below unity are often found in low-risk Asian and African populations. Women show a steeper rise in the incidence of colon cancer for each unit increase in the incidence of rectal cancer. Although part of the regional variation in the ratios of colon to rectal cancer may arise from local conventions for classifying rectosigmoid tumors, these differences nonetheless suggest that colon and rectal cancer have related, but not identical, causes.

In the United States, the incidence of colorectal cancer also varies regionally. In general, rates in Southern and Western United States (except the San Francisco Bay area and Hawaii) are lower than the United States' average, whereas rates are highest in the Northeast and the North Central states. Colorectal cancer incidence rates are also moderately higher for urban residents, although socioeconomic status is not a consistent risk factor for colorectal cancer in studies of the United States population. Although these regional differences in the United States have persisted over the long term, they are gradually fading, perhaps owing to the increasing homogeneity of dietary patterns across the country.

Between 1950 and the mid-1980s, the incidence of colon cancer in the United States rose in the white population, whereas that of rectal cancer remained fairly stable. Mortality rates from colorectal cancer were stable among white men but decreased in white women. Both incidence and mortality rates for colorectal cancer increased substantially among the nonwhite population during this period.[5] Colorectal cancer incidence and mortality have declined since 1985 in American adults at an average annual rate of 1.6% and 1.8%, respectively.[3] These trends are more evident in whites

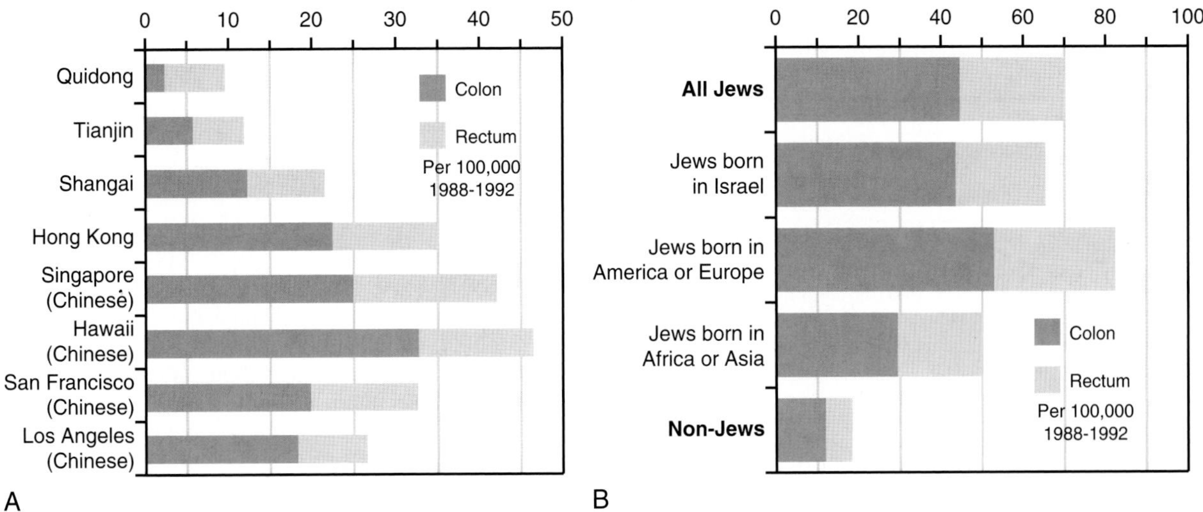

Figure 115–2. Age-standardized incidence of colon cancer in *A*, Ethnic Chinese; *B* populations in Israel. Colorectal cancer incidence differs considerably within countries, depending on region and population, and in ethnic groups who migrate to areas with different diets and lifestyles. (From Parkin DM, Whelen SL, Ferlay J, et al: Cancer Incidence in Five Continents [IARC Sci. Publ. No. 143.] Series. Lyon, International Agency for Research on Cancer, 1997.)

than blacks. Currently, both incidence and mortality rates for colorectal cancer are higher in the black population compared with the white population.[1, 6]

The risk of colorectal cancer rises rapidly in populations who migrate from areas of low risk to those of high risk. This was clearly demonstrated in Japanese immigrants to Hawaii and to the continental United States during the 1950s and 1960s. Cancer rates for Issei (the migrating generation) rose over a short period to exceed those of native Japanese living in Japan, and the incidence rates for Nissei (their United States–born offspring) rose progressively to approximate those of the native white population. A similar upward displacement of colorectal cancer risk was noted in Europeans who migrated to Australia after World War II and in Jews who migrated to Israel from low-risk areas in Yemen and North Africa. Longitudinal studies reveal that, in many countries where colorectal cancer mortality rates were low before 1950, rates have increased sharply, whereas in countries where rates were high or moderate, they have decreased, stabilized, or increased slightly. A good example is Japan. Once a low-risk region for colon cancer, incidence rates have risen to equal or exceed those in North America and Europe.[4]

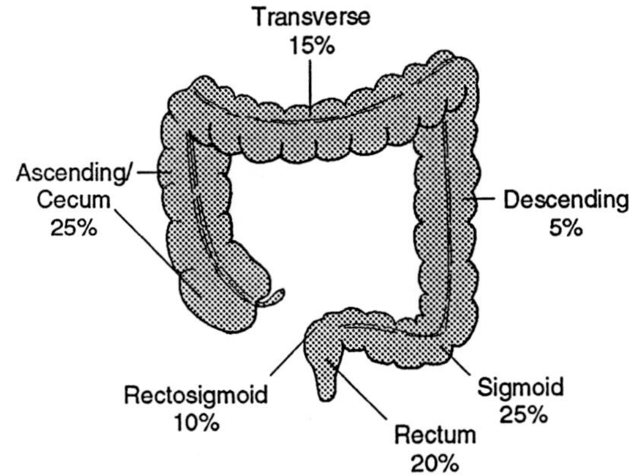

Figure 115–3. Distribution of colorectal cancers within the large intestine. Only half of cancers are within reach of the flexible sigmoidoscope.

Studies of temporal trends by subsite location of large bowel cancer demonstrate that, for both sexes, incidence rates have increased for cancers of the right colon (cecum, ascending colon) and sigmoid colon and have decreased for lesions in the rectum.[7] This may reflect differing susceptibilities to neoplastic transformation in the proximal and distal colon.[8] Currently in the United States, the prevalence of colorectal cancers in whites is higher in the cecum and ascending colon (22% in men, 27% in women) and in the sigmoid colon (25% in men, 23% in women). The percentages elsewhere in the large bowel are displayed in Figure 115–3.

Descriptive epidemiology, including the study of temporal trends in colorectal cancer incidence, has played an important role in formulating hypotheses about the causes and pathogenesis of these lesions. The alterations in the subsite location of these tumors also have implications for clinical cancer detection. The proportion of tumors beyond the reach of the sigmoidoscope increases with age, for example.[9] Subsite distribution also may differ according to race.[6, 10] These are discussed in subsequent sections.

THEORIES AND CLUES ABOUT CAUSATION

Interregional differences in the incidence of colorectal cancer, including differences among population groups who live in geographic proximity but with different life-styles, strongly suggest that environment plays a role in the development of this disease.[11] Migrant studies and rapid changes in incidence in countries assimilating Western practices support this concept. Strong circumstantial evidence exists for a link between diet and colorectal cancer. Population studies

Table 115–1 | **Environmental Factors Potentially Influencing Carcinogenesis in the Colon and Rectum**

PROBABLY RELATED
High fat and low fiber consumption*
POSSIBLY RELATED
Beer and ale consumption (especially rectal cancer)
Low dietary selenium
Environmental carcinogens and mutagens
Fecapentaenes (from colonic bacteria)
Heterocyclic amines (from charbroiled and fried meat and fish)
PROBABLY PROTECTIVE
High fiber consumption
Physical activity / low body mass
Aspirin and NSAIDs
Calcium
POSSIBLY PROTECTIVE†
Yellow-green cruciferous vegetables
Carotene (vitamin A)–rich foods
Vitamins C and E
Cyclooxygenase-2 (COX-2) inhibitors
Hormone replacement therapy (estrogen)

Based on epidemiologic observations.
*Dietary fats and fiber are heterogeneous in composition, and not all fats or fiber components may play a role in causation or protection.
†Based on limited data.
NSAIDs, Nonsteroidal anti-inflammatory drugs.

and animal studies have attempted to delineate the effects of various fats and proteins, carbohydrates, vegetable and fiber components, and micronutrients on the genesis of cancer of the large bowel (Table 115–1).

Fat, Bile Acids, and Bacteria

Several lines of evidence suggest that diets containing large proportions of fat predispose to colorectal cancer, especially in the descending and sigmoid colon. Colon cancer rates are high in populations whose total fat intake is high and are lower in those who consume less fat. On average, fat (saturated plus unsaturated) comprises 40% to 45% of total calorie intake in Western countries with high rates of colorectal cancer, whereas in low-risk populations fat accounts for only 10% to 15% of dietary calories.[12] Case-control and cohort studies have also suggested that the incidence and mortality rates from colon cancer, and in some cases rectal cancer, are positively correlated with dietary fat, but these findings are less convincing than data from descriptive epidemiologic studies. Differences may arise from methodologic limitations related to dietary history taking and a lack of sufficient variability in diet in communities from which subjects were drawn.

Early trials also often failed to take into account total energy intake. A prospective study assessed the relationship of meat, fat, and fiber intake among 88,751 women aged 34 to 59 years.[13] After adjustment for total energy intake, the intake of animal fat was significantly correlated with the risk of colon cancer. The intake ratio of red meat to chicken and fish was strongly associated with increased incidence of colon cancer, perhaps owing to differences in their fat composition. Similar findings have been reported that correlate the intake of saturated fat and the ratio of red meat to chicken and fish intake with both the incidence and recurrence of colorectal adenomas in women.[14] Recent cohort studies and a combined analysis of 13 case-control studies[15] that adjusted for total energy intake fail to provide clear-cut evidence for the association between dietary fat and colorectal cancer observed in earlier studies. Studies that specifically examine the association between intake of saturated/animal fat and colorectal cancer suggest a stronger association than with total fat.

An inverse relationship has been reported between physical activity and risk for colorectal cancer in men, whereas obesity is associated with elevated risk.[16] Serum cholesterol and beta-lipoprotein levels have been positively correlated with the development of colorectal adenomas and carcinomas, but this association has not been demonstrated consistently, and serum cholesterol levels may decline before the development of colon cancer.

Animal studies lend additional support for the role of dietary fat in the development of colon cancer. These studies usually involve the injection of carcinogens such as 1,2-dimethylhydrazine (DMH) or azoxymethane (AOM) into rodents fed various diets. Animals fed a variety of polyunsaturated and saturated fats develop greater numbers of carcinogen-induced colonic adenocarcinomas than do those on low-fat diets. The amount and source of dietary fat may affect tumor development in such studies[17]; fatty acids derived from polyunsaturated fish oils (omega-3 fatty acids) and monosaturated olive oil may not promote tumors to the extent that other polyunsaturated fats do.

It has been proposed that dietary fat enhances cholesterol and bile acid synthesis by the liver, increasing amounts of these sterols in the colon. Colon bacteria convert these compounds to secondary bile acids, cholesterol metabolites, and other potentially toxic metabolic compounds. Population studies demonstrate increased excretion of sterol metabolites and fecal bile acids in groups who consume a high-fat, low-fiber "Western" diet compared with other groups, and high fecal bile acid levels are found in some patients with colorectal cancer. Dietary fat also has been shown to increase the excretion of secondary bile acids in carcinogen-treated rats. Secondary bile acids do not act as primary carcinogens but as potent promoters of colon carcinogenesis in such animal models. Little is known about how lipid and sterol metabolites promote tumors, but both bile acids and free fatty acids have been shown to damage the colonic mucosa and increase the proliferative activity of the epithelium. Dietary consumption of high amounts of corn oil and beef fat increase colonic ornithine decarboxylase levels, which are associated with rapidly proliferating mucosa.

Activation of protein kinase C by bile acids in colonic mucosa may also represent an important intracellular event by which bile acids provoke a proliferative response. Bile acids may, in addition, induce release of arachidonate and conversion of arachidonic acid to prostaglandins in the mucosa, which may enhance cell proliferation.[18] Preclinical and clinical evidence indicate that nonsteroidal anti-inflammatory drugs (NSAIDs), which reduce prostaglandin synthesis, reduce the incidence of large bowel cancer (discussed later).[19–21] Inhibition of the inducible enzyme cyclooxygenase-2 (COX-2) may be particularly important in this regard.[21, 22] Certain fatty acids could promote carcinogenesis by altering membrane fluidity after being incorporated into cell membranes. Bacterial enzymes such as 7-alpha-dehydroxylase (which converts cholic to deoxycholic acid), beta-glucuronidase, nitroreductase, and azoreductase may be induced by a high-fat diet and could also convert compounds ingested in the diet to active carcinogens (see later).

Fiber

Epidemiologic, case-control, and animal studies suggest that dietary fiber protects against the development of colon cancer. Dietary fiber is plant material that resists digestion by the upper gastrointestinal tract and is composed of a heterogeneous mix of carbohydrates (cellulose, hemicellulose, pectin) and noncarbohydrates (e.g., lignin). Although the protective role of fiber is not completely clear (owing to the lack of definition of fiber components in some studies), epidemiologic studies correlate high-fiber intake with a lower incidence of colon cancer.[23–25] The majority of both observational-epidemiologic and case-control studies support the protective effect of fiber-rich diets; however, these data do not define the relationship between fiber-rich food and the importance of nonfiber vegetable components, nutrients, and micronutrients in fruits and vegetables. The effect of fiber components on different portions of the large bowel may also vary. This may explain, in part, the inability to demonstrate a protective effect of fiber in several recent randomized controlled trials that have examined the ability of fiber supplementation to prevent adenoma recurrence.[26, 27]

Investigators postulate that the protective mechanism of fibers such as cereal bran is increased stool bulk, which dilutes carcinogens and promoters of carcinogenesis, enhances their elimination, and minimizes duration of contact with mucosa by decreasing intestinal transit time. Increased fiber intake, in the form of whole wheat and rye bread, also reduces the concentration of fecal secondary bile acids and fecal mutagens in healthy subjects. Animal studies have also demonstrated a decreased incidence of colonic tumors in DMH-treated rats fed diets high in fibers and fiber components (wheat bran, cellulose, hemicellulose). Cellulose and hemicellulose decrease the levels of bacterial metabolic enzymes such as beta-glucuronidase in experimental animals and may diminish the activation of carcinogens or cocarcinogens. Further, some fiber components may bind to toxic or carcinogenic substances, perhaps decreasing their contact with the colonic mucosa. Fiber components are also fermented by fecal flora to short-chain fatty acids, decreasing colonic pH and potentially inhibiting carcinogenesis.

Carcinogens and Fecal Mutagens, Vitamins, and Micronutrients

The possibility that specific genotoxic carcinogens may play a role in the genesis of colorectal cancer was raised when it was noted that the stools of certain persons exhibited mutagenic activity for bacteria in vitro. Mutagenic activity is frequently present in the feces of populations at high risk for large bowel cancer and is low or absent in low-risk populations. A specific group of highly unsaturated reactive compounds synthesized by colonic bacteria, fecapentaenes, may play a role in large bowel carcinogenesis. It has also been recognized that "charbroiled" meat and fish—and to a lesser extent fried foods—contain powerful mutagenic compounds. The structures of these compounds resemble a heterocyclic amine known to cause colon cancer in rodents. Metabolites similar to those of fried meat and fish are actively being sought as mutagens in human stools. A possible association between rectal cancer and beer and ale drinking has also been noted.[28–30] A two- to threefold increase in colorectal cancer has also been observed in pattern and model makers in the automobile industry, but the specific carcinogenic agent has not yet been identified.

The exact nature of genotoxic carcinogens that may act in the human colon remains speculative, but the identification of such compounds could provide a basis for intervention and primary prevention of this disease. Limited data suggest that foods rich in carotene (vitamin A) and vitamin C could act as antioxidants in the chemoprevention of colon cancer. Other areas that merit further exploration include the role of yellow-green cruciferous vegetables and micronutrients, including selenium salts, vitamin E, and folic acid, in the prevention of colorectal cancer. Recently, a good deal of attention has been given to a possible role for dietary calcium in colon cancer prevention (discussed later).

Calcium and Vitamin D

Epidemiologic, clinical, and laboratory evidence suggest that calcium intake may protect against carcinogenesis in the colon. The potential chemopreventive activity of calcium was originally suggested by epidemiologic studies reporting an inverse relationship between intake of vitamin D and calcium and colorectal cancer.[31] A recent study demonstrated that dietary calcium supplementation in the form of low-fat dietary foods may affect a variety of "intermediate biomarkers" thought to be associated with tumor progression in the colon.[32] The relationship between calcium intake and a lower incidence of colonic adenomas and carcinomas has not, however, been uniformly demonstrated. These conflicting findings may have arisen because of the difficulties inherent in dietary assessment and differences in intake of potentially confounding factors, including dietary components and putative chemopreventive agents.

Further credence to the beneficial effect of calcium in preventing large bowel cancer comes from numerous animal studies. Abnormal proliferation occurs in both neoplastic and preneoplastic lesions in the colon. The increase in colonocyte proliferation stimulated by intrarectally instilled deoxycholate and free fatty acids or by dietary supplementation with cholic acid may be ameliorated by oral calcium supplementation in laboratory animals.[33] Studies in rodents fed high-fat diets also demonstrate a reduction in the number of carcinogen-induced tumors in animals receiving supplemental calcium in their diet. This may be especially true of tumors containing K-ras mutations, a finding also suggested by a recent study in humans.[34] Ornithine decarboxylase, an enzyme involved in polyamine biosynthesis and elevated in preneoplastic states, is reduced in rat colonic mucosa incubated with calcium in vitro, and supplemental calcium suppresses elevated levels of this enzyme in the mucosa of elderly patients with adenomatous polyps.

It has been suggested that dietary calcium binds to ionized fatty acids and bile acids in the intestine, converting them to insoluble calcium compounds incapable of stimulating epithelial proliferation. Calcium increases fecal excretion of both phosphate and bile acids and modifies relative amounts of bile acids in bile.[35] In addition, calcium in milk products is capable of precipitating luminal cytotoxic surfactants inhibiting their effects on the colonic mucosa. These potential beneficial effects of calcium have not been uniformly observed, however, and studies of the effects of calcium on the rectal mucosa have not always demonstrated a reduction in the rate of proliferation. In other studies, calcium supplementation normalized the distribution of proliferating cells in the colonic crypt without affecting the rate of proliferation in the colorectal mucosa.

Vitamin D_3 metabolites and analogs have recently been shown to play an important role in the regulation of a number of important cellular processes, including proliferation, differentiation, and apoptosis, in addition to their established role in mineral homeostasis. These steroid compounds have rapid effects that do not involve gene transcription or protein synthesis, as well as genomic effects involving the vitamin D receptor (VDR) and other transcription factors.[36] Effects of vitamin D and its metabolites have been demonstrated in normal and malignant colonocytes, and several potential mechanisms have been suggested by which these compounds might prevent carcinogenesis in the colon.

Arachidonic Acid, Eicosanoids, and Cyclooxygenase-2 (COX-2)

Clinical case-control and cohort studies have shown a 40% to 50% reduction in colorectal cancer-related mortality in individuals taking aspirin and other NSAIDs on a regular basis compared with those not taking these agents (see Chapter 23 and also later).[20] The mechanism for cancer protection is unknown but may relate to altered synthesis of arachidonic acid metabolites (eicosanoids) that include prostaglandins, thromboxanes, leukotrienes, and hydroxyeicosatetraenoic acids. These compounds modulate a number of signal transduction pathways that may affect cellular adhesion, growth, and differentiation.[37–39] Cyclooxygenase (COX or prostaglandin-endoperoxide synthase) oxidizes arachidonic acid to prostaglandin G_2, reduces prostaglandin G_2 to prostaglandin H_2, and is the key enzyme responsible for production of prostaglandins and other eicosanoids.

This enzyme exists in two isoforms: COX-1 and COX-2. COX-1, the constitutive form of the enzyme, is present in most tissues and is involved in the physiologic production of prostaglandins for maintaining normal homeostasis. COX-2 is induced by cytokines, mitogens, and growth factors, and its level has been shown to be elevated in both murine and human colorectal cancers.[22, 40–43] Expression of COX-2 is markedly increased in 85% to 95% of colorectal cancers,[40] and in experimental models. COX-2 inhibition prevents cancer development during both the initiation and promotion/progression stages of carcinogenesis.[44] Knockout of COX-2 results in suppression of intestinal polyposis in animal models of familial adenomatous polyposis (FAP).[22, 42] While it has been speculated that NSAIDs may reduce colon tumor formation through inhibition of prostaglandin-mediated proliferation, other evidence suggests that part of their effect may instead result from induction of programmed cell death or apoptosis. Overexpression of COX-2 has been demonstrated to decrease apoptosis, whereas COX-2 inhibition leads to an increase in apoptosis.[45]

One potential mechanism by which NSAIDs may induce apoptosis is through elevation of the prostaglandin precursor arachidonic acid. Increases in arachidonic acid after NSAID inhibition of cyclooxygenase stimulate conversion of sphingomyelin to ceramide, a mediator of apoptosis. NSAIDs may also inhibit the activation of genes by the nuclear hormone receptor peroxisome-proliferator-activated receptor δ (PPARδ) by disrupting the ability of this receptor to bind DNA.[38] PPARδ expression is elevated in colorectal cancers and repressed by the APC gene product in colorectal cancer cells. The inhibition of PPARδ function enhances the ability of NSAIDs to induce apoptosis in colon cancer cells. PPARδ activates a variety of genes, including those involved in cellular growth and differentiation after exposure to a variety of ligands, including eicosanoids. COX-2 inhibition could prevent production of those ligands and therefore activation of PPARδ.

Other potential mechanisms by which COX-2 inhibition may affect tumor formation include alterations of cell adhesion to extracellular matrix proteins,[45] inhibition of tumor neovascularization (angiogenesis),[43] and reduction in carcinogen activation. A recent study[43] using the $Apc^{\Delta 716}$ mouse, an animal model, of FAP, demonstrated that treatment with the COX-2 specific inhibitor rofecoxib (Vioxx) was associated with a significant dose-dependent reduction in polyp number and size (Fig. 115–4), as well as alterations in polyp morphology. COX-2 inhibition was associated with decreased levels of vascular endothelial growth factor (VEGF), and with lower rates of DNA replication.

In summary, environment and diet may affect the genesis of colorectal cancer, but their exact roles remain unclear. Their complex nature renders definition of the influence of individual environmental and dietary components difficult.

Chemoprevention of Colorectal Cancer

(See also Chapter 114)

Chemoprevention refers to the use of natural or synthetic agents to reverse, suppress, or prevent progression or recurrence of cancer.[11, 46, 47] This is a cornerstone of "primary prevention." Data on chemoprevention of colorectal cancer come from studies in laboratory animals (see earlier), observational epidemiologic studies, case-control studies, and randomized trials. Because the natural history of colorectal cancer is protracted, clinical randomized trials have often concentrated on prevention of colorectal adenomas, the precursors to carcinoma. The duration of the studies required, sample sizes necessary, cost, and ethical considerations make the use of cancer as an end-point impractical.

This has led to an increasing use of surrogate "biomarkers" to study chemoprevention of colorectal cancers. The hope is that use of such markers will lead to shorter, smaller, and less expensive trials.[48] To be valid, however, such biomarkers need to represent accurately the events involved in the process of carcinogenesis. When an intervention such as a chemopreventive agent is tested, there should be a clear relationship among the agent, modulation of the biomarker, and the development of cancer. Surrogate end-

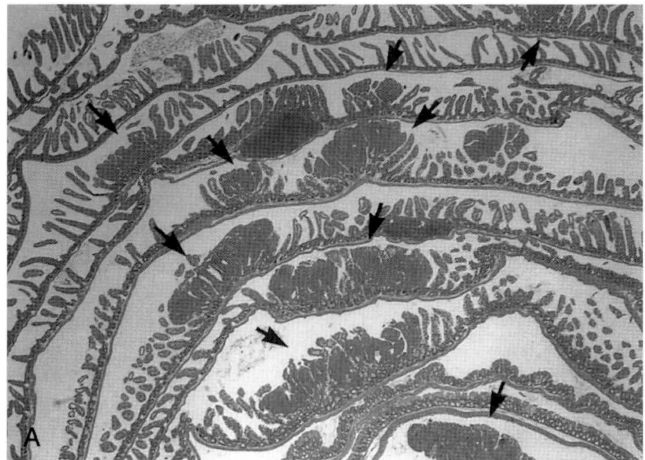

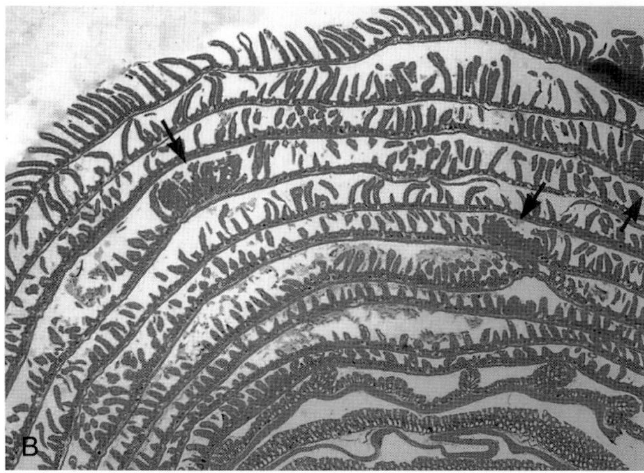

Figure 115–4. Effect of cyclooxygenase-2 (COX-2) inhibition on adenoma formation in the $Apc^{\Delta716}$ mouse, a model of familial adenomatous. *A*, Intestine from $Apc^{\Delta716}$ mouse fed a control diet exhibits hundreds of polyps (*arrows*). *B*, Mouse fed chow containing the specific COX-2 inhibitor rofecoxib shows a greatly reduced number of polyps with smaller size and flattened morphology. (From Oshima M, Murai(Hata) N, Kargman S, et al: Chemoprevention of intestinal polyposis in the $Apc^{\Delta716}$ mouse by rofecoxib, a specific cyclooxygenase-2 inhibitor. Cancer Res 61:1733, 2001.)

points for cancer ideally should be validated in the context of clinical studies that use cancer as the ultimate end-point. This is a difficult task because these are the very trials that such markers are designed to complement or replace.

There has been recent interest in the use of magnifying endoscopy to study aberrant crypt foci of the colon as possible markers in chemoprevention trials.[49] These consist of large, thick crypts in methylene blue-stained colonic mucosa. Aberrant crypt foci, particularly those that are large and have dysplastic features, are thought to be precursors of adenomas in the colon.[50] Standardization of techniques to identify and quantify these lesions will be crucial to the successful interpretation of data from these trials.

The potential benefit of low-fat, high-fiber diets based on descriptive epidemiology and case-control studies has already been discussed, but current data from prospective human trials are thus far equivocal[51] or negative.[52] Two large randomized trials were recently completed that examined the effects of fiber supplementation on adenoma recurrence. The Polyp Prevention Trial[27] randomized 2079 subjects with a history of colorectal adenomas to receive counseling together with a low-fat, high-fiber diet rich in fruits and vegetables, or to receive their usual diet alone. The incidence of recurrent adenomas at 1 and 4 years as determined by colonoscopy was similar in both groups. In a study conducted by the Phoenix Colon Cancer Prevention Physician's Network,[26] 1429 patients with a history of colorectal adenoma were randomized to receive 2.0 g or 13.5 g of supplemental wheat bran per day. Colonoscopy failed to show a difference in the incidence of recurrent adenomas at a median follow-up of 34 to 36 months.

A large body of observational and laboratory studies suggests a role for dietary calcium supplementation in chemoprevention (mentioned earlier). Recently, a prospective double-blind placebo-controlled trial showed that supplemental calcium (3000 mg of calcium carbonate per day, equivalent to 1200 mg of elemental calcium) reduced the incidence and number of recurrent adenomas in subjects chosen for a recent history of such lesions.[53] The effect of calcium was modest (19% reduction in adenoma recurrence and 24% reduction in the number of adenomas over 3 years). The effect was independent of age, sex, or dietary intake of calcium fat or fiber. Human trials using antioxidant vitamins A, C, and E have provided equivocal results, and current data do not support their routine use for colon cancer prevention in average-risk individuals.[54]

Epidemiologic studies have found a lower incidence of colorectal cancer among those with high compared with low dietary folate intakes.[30, 55, 56] This protective effect is also suggested by the Nurse's Health Study,[55] in which high doses of folate (as part of multivitamin supplementation) given over several years were protective against colorectal cancer. Prospective randomized trials designed to assess the effect of folate supplementation on adenoma recurrence are currently in progress. Folic acid and its metabolites play an important role in DNA synthesis and methylation. Folate supplementation prevented DNA strand breaks in certain areas of the p53 gene in the rat colon in one recent study,[56] suggesting one mechanism by which folate supplementation could suppress colorectal carcinogenesis.

Epidemiologic, case-control, and prospective cohort trials suggest a protective effect against the development of colorectal cancer in women taking hormone (estrogen) replacement therapy.[57] It has been postulated that estrogen may protect against colon cancer development by decreasing production of secondary bile acids, by decreasing levels of insulin-like growth factor I, or through as yet undetermined direct effects on colonic mucosal epithelial cells.

The most promising results come from trials utilizing aspirin and NSAIDs for colorectal cancer prevention. Case-control and cohort studies have suggested that the risk for development of adenoma and carcinoma may be substantially reduced (40% to 50%) among aspirin and NSAID users, compared with controls.[19, 20, 58] A prospective cohort study among male health professionals[19] demonstrated that persons who take aspirin more than two times per week were at lower risk for colorectal cancer (relative risk, 0.68) than controls, after accounting for a variety of potentially confounding factors. However, a randomized trial that assessed the effect of low-dose aspirin in an average-risk population demonstrated no significant reduction in the number of colorectal cancer cases during the first 6 years of follow-

Table 115–2 | **Chemopreventive Agents and Colorectal Neoplasia**

STRENGTH OF EVIDENCE	WEAK	◄ OBSERVATIONAL STUDIES		RANDOMIZED HUMAN TRIALS	►	STRONG
AGENT	**Animal Studies**	**Case Control**	**Cohort Studies**	**Mucosal Proliferation**	**Polyposis Patients**	**Sporadic Adenoma**
Aspirin/NSAID	↑	↑	↑		↑	⧗
COX-2 inhibitors*	↑				↑	⧗
Vitamins A, C, E	↑	↑	↑	↑ ↑	→	→
Calcium	↑	↑	↑	→		↑
Fiber	↑	↑	↑	↑	→	↓
Selenium	↑	↑	→			
Fish oil		↑			↑	
Organosulfur	↑					

*Cyclooxygenase-2.
↑, Most studies positive; ↓, most studies negative; →, studies equivocal; ⧗, studies ongoing.

up.[59] Longer follow-up may be necessary to demonstrate a significant aspirin effect, since a more recent study (The Nurses' Health Study) demonstrated that the benefits of aspirin may not be evident until after at least a decade of regular aspirin consumption.[20]

Given the long natural history of colorectal cancer, prevention of adenoma recurrence after endoscopic removal is often used as an intermediate or surrogate end-point in chemoprevention trials.[48] In FAP, where hundreds of adenomas occur in the colon and rectum, chemoprevention trials often use reductions of the number and size of adenomas as end-points in short-term studies. Such trials have suggested a potential role for NSAIDs as chemopreventive agents in this setting. There is a significant decrease in the mean number and size of polyps in patients treated with sulindac, a NSAID. In a small, randomized, double-blind, placebo-controlled trial of 22 patients with FAP, treatment with sulindac significantly reduced the number of colorectal polyps and their mean diameter during 9 months of treatment.[60] After 9 months of treatment, the number of polyps had decreased to 44% and the diameter of polyps to 35% of baseline values. Three months after treatment was stopped, however, both the number and size of polyps had increased.

Recently, a double-blind, placebo-controlled trial studied the effects of celecoxib (Celebrex), a selective COX-2 inhibitor, on colorectal polyps in patients with FAP.[61] Treatment with high doses of this agent for 6 months was associated with a significant reduction (28%) in the number of colorectal polyps compared with placebo (4.5%). This drug is now approved in the United States as an adjunct to standard therapy in patients with FAP.

It is unclear what the role of nonselective NSAIDs and COX-2 inhibitors will be in patients with sporadic adenomas and carcinomas. Trials are ongoing to determine their usefulness in preventing adenoma recurrence in this population. Table 115–2 summarizes the status of current studies that examine the effect of chemopreventive agents on colorectal neoplasia.

Observational studies from around the world that compare different populations continue to find the risk of colorectal cancer to be lower among populations with high intakes of fruits and vegetables, as well as some vitamins and micronutrients. Migration studies strongly suggest an influence of diet and environmental influences on the incidence of colorectal cancer. It has been difficult to demonstrate similar effects in randomized controlled chemoprevention trials. These trials ask narrowly defined questions and cannot easily assess complex interactions between dietary components or measure the effects of long-term alterations in dietary patterns on cancer per se. These trials have nonetheless provided exciting new data (e.g., calcium, COX-2 inhibitors) that may lead to primary prevention of colorectal cancer in the future.

BIOLOGY OF COLORECTAL CANCER

Current concepts concerning environmental causes for colorectal cancer have been discussed in the preceding sections. It has been suggested that carcinogens introduced into the bowel act in concert with other luminal factors (e.g., bile acid and other tumor promoters) to affect epithelial cells in the colonic mucosa; however, carcinogenesis is a multistage process. Cells must be genetically primed (through either hereditary disposition or genotoxic events), must be induced to proliferate, and must pass through a series of stages en route to immortalization and uncontrolled growth. Our knowledge of this sequence of events in the colon, though fragmentary, is growing rapidly (see also Chapter 3).

Abnormal Cellular Proliferation

Abnormal cellular proliferation is a hallmark of neoplasia (see Chapter 3). Actively proliferating cells are more susceptible to initiators of carcinogenesis (primary carcinogens) and genetic alterations. In the normal colon, DNA synthesis takes place and cells divide and proliferate only in the lower and middle regions of the crypts. As cells migrate "upward" from lower in the crypt, the number of cells that continue to proliferate decreases, and, upon reaching the upper crypt region, they become terminally differentiated and can no longer divide. A substantial body of literature indicates that this sequence of events is disordered during the evolution of neoplastic lesions in the colon. Increased proliferative activity and characteristic differences in the distribution of tritiated thymidine–labeled cells (i.e., those that actively synthesize DNA) within the colonic crypts have been demonstrated to distinguish both "at risk" and affected members of kindreds with familial polyposis, as well as "nonpolyposis"–inherited colon cancer from groups at lower risk. Correlations between rectal mucosal proliferation and the clinical and pathologic features of nonfamilial colorectal neoplasia have also been demonstrated.[62] On the other hand, populations at low risk of developing colon cancer, such as Seventh Day Adventist vegetarians, have relatively quiescent proliferative activity in their colonic mucosa.

Disordered proliferative activity can be found in the colonic mucosa of rodents treated with a variety of chemical carcinogens, and increased proliferative activity is seen in animals whose colonic or rectal mucosa is exposed to tumor promoters such as secondary bile acids. Colonic epithelial cells also fail to repress DNA synthesis during epithelial renewal in ulcerative colitis, a condition associated with an increased risk of colorectal cancer. Ornithine decarboxylase, an enzyme marker of rapid cellular proliferation, is present at high levels in the mucosa of family members of familial polyposis kindreds, and levels increase in the colonic mucosa during chemically induced colonic carcinogenesis in rats. This enzyme increases in the colonic mucosa with age and is elevated in elderly patients with colonic adenomas. Experimental evidence also suggests that protein kinase C may be involved in the stimulation of colonic epithelial cell proliferation by tumor promoters. These findings have led to speculation that inhibitors of cellular proliferation may prove useful as anticancer drugs. NSAIDs and COX-2 inhibitors, for example, decrease proliferation and increase apoptosis.[45]

A recent explosion of knowledge in the field of molecular genetics has demonstrated how alterations in proto-oncogenes and tumor suppressor genes may lead to disruption of mechanisms that regulate the normal cell cycle and cell proliferation. In some cases the cell is predisposed to abnormal proliferation by virtue of germline mutations (e.g., familial adenomatous polyposis). In other cases, somatic mutations occur as the result of complex interactions with environmental factors,[63] as detailed earlier.

Molecular Biology and Biochemical Changes (See Chapters 3 and 114)

Molecular Genetics

Tumor cells in the colon, as elsewhere, are characterized by heritable phenotypic changes that are the result of quantitative or qualitative alterations in gene expression. A large body of evidence demonstrates that colorectal cancers are associated with an accumulation of such genetic alterations (Table 115–3; Fig. 115–5). Genetic changes that may lead to the development of colorectal cancer can be generally categorized into three major classes: alterations in proto-oncogenes, loss of tumor suppressor gene activity, and abnormalities in genes involved in DNA mismatch repair.[64, 65] Adenomas and carcinomas arise in the context of genomic instability, by which epithelial cells acquire the number of mutations needed to attain a neoplastic state. Destabilization of the genome is a prerequisite to tumor formation. This most commonly involves chromosomal instability with subsequent allelic loss, chromosomal amplifications and translocations, or increased rates of intragenic mutation in tandemly repeated DNA sequences known as microsatellites (microsatellite instability).

Cellular proto-oncogenes are evolutionarily conserved human genes that contain DNA sequences homologous to those of acute transforming retroviruses. Many of these genes play a role in signal transduction and the normal regulation of cell growth. Inappropriate activation of these genes leads to abnormal transmission of regulatory messages from the cell surface to the nucleus, resulting in abnormal proliferation and, eventually, tumor formation. Three human *ras* genes—K-*ras*, N-*ras*, and H-*ras*—encode guanine nucleotide-binding proteins that regulate intracellular signaling pathways. Approximately 65% of sporadic colorectal carcinomas have activating point mutations in a *ras* gene, most in K-*ras*. Most *ras* mutations appear to occur during intermediate stages of adenoma growth (Chapter 114). *Ras* gene mutations were found to occur in 47% of carcinomas, 58% of adenomas larger than 1 cm,[66] but in only 10% of adenomas under 1 cm, suggesting that earlier events must contribute to neoplasia formation. Alterations in signal transduction may lead to abnormal cell growth and thus participate in neoplastic transformation, but activation of *ras* alone is not sufficient for progression to carcinoma. The exact functional relationship between *ras* mutations and carcinogenesis remains to be established, but understanding its role in stimulating proliferation may lead to the development of antitumor therapies aimed at interrupting signals that alter tumor cell growth.

Chromosomal abnormalities have been reported in colorectal carcinomas for more than a decade, and recent evidence has shown that allelic losses, particularly at chromosome locations 5q, 17p, and 18q, play major roles in the genesis of large bowel tumors.[64, 65, 67–74] A deletion within chromosome 5 in patients with familial adenomatous polyposis (FAP) led to the identification of the *APC* gene on the long arm of this chromosome (5q21). Positional cloning identified a single tumor suppressor gene, which is mutated in both the germline of FAP patients and in sporadic colorectal tumors. The protein encoded by *APC* consists of 2843 amino acids. It is located at the basolateral membrane in colorectal epithelial cells, with expression more pronounced as cells migrate up through the colonic crypt.

Somatic mutations of the *APC* gene occur in 60% to 80% of sporadic colorectal carcinomas and adenomas, including the smallest dysplastic lesions.[68] These mutations result in truncation of the *APC* protein in more than 98% of cases, a finding that has led to the development of clinically useful tests for genetic screening of FAP families.[75] Inactivation of both copies of the *APC* gene appears to be the "gate-keeping" event for the initiation of colorectal neoplasia. *APC* interacts with at least six other proteins, including glycogen synthetase 3β (GSK-3β) and axin in the cytoplasm. Inactivation of this gene is required for net cellular proliferation and initiation of neoplasia in the colon.

APC functions to modulate extracellular signals that are transmitted to the nucleus through the cytoskeletal protein β-catenin. One such pathway, the Wnt-1 signaling pathway,

Table 115–3 | **Genes Altered in Sporadic Colorectal Cancer**

GENE	CHROMOSOME	PERCENT OF TUMORS WITH ALTERATIONS	CLASS	FUNCTION
K-ras	12	50	Proto-oncogene	Encodes guanine nucleotide-binding protein that regulates intracellular signaling
APC	5	70	Tumor suppressor	Regulation of β-catenin involved in activation of Wnt/TcF signaling (activates c-myc, cyclin D1); * regulation of proliferation, apoptosis. Interaction with E-cadherin (? cell adhesion)
DCC	18	70	? Tumor suppressor	Netrin-1 receptor; caspase substrate in apoptosis; cell adhesion
SMAD4 (DPC4, MADH4)	18	?	Tumor suppressor	Nuclear transcription factor in *TGF-β1* signaling; regulation of angiogenesis; regulator of *WAF1* promoter; downstream mediator of *SMAD2*
p53	17	75	Tumor suppressor	Transcription factor; regulator of cell cycle progression after cellular stress, of apoptosis, of gene expression, and of DNA repair
hMSH2	2	†	DNA mismatch repair	Maintains fidelity of DNA replication
hMLH1	3	†	DNA mismatch repair	Maintains fidelity of DNA replication
hMSH6	2	†	DNA mismatch repair	Maintains fidelity of DNA replication
TGF-β1 RII	3	‡	Tumor suppressor	Receptor for signaling in the *TGF-β1* pathway; inhibitor of colonic epithelial proliferation, often mutated in tumors with MSI

*β-Catenin mutations (downstream of *APC*) are found in 16% to 25% of microsatellite instability (MSI) colon cancers, but not in microsatellite stable (MSS) cancers.

†Approximately 15% of sporadic colorectal cancers demonstrate microsatellite instability associated with alterations in mismatch repair genes (principally *hMSH2* and *hMLH1* but also *hMSH3, hMSH6, hPMS1* and *hPMS2*).

‡Mutated in 73% to 90% of MSI colon cancers. Up to 55% of MSS colon cancer cell lines may demonstrate a *TGF-β* signaling blockage distal to *TGF-β1 RII*.[89]

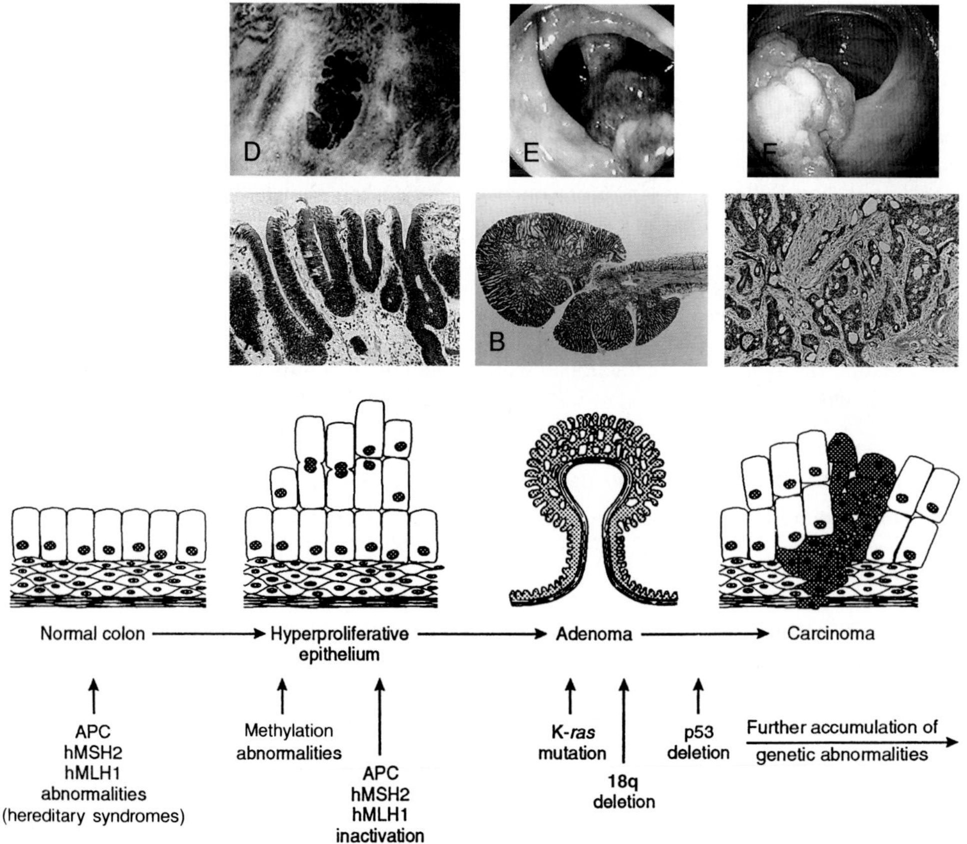

Figure 115–5. Proposed sequence of molecular genetic events in the evolution of colon cancer. Carcinomas arise from an accumulation of events whose sequence has been defined. Alterations in *APC* or DNA mismatch repair genes may be inherited in the germline (familial adenomatous polyposis, HNPCC) or may be acquired after birth (somatic mutations). Bottom row, (A-C) histology. Top row, (D-F) colonoscopic photographs. From left to right: Dysplastic aberrant crypt focus (A, D with methylene blue staining), adenomatous polyp (B, E), invasive carcinoma (C, F). (Aberrant crypt focus reproduced from Takayama T, Katsuki S, Takahashi Y, et al: Aberrant crypt foci of the colon as precursors of adenoma and cancer. N Engl J Med 339:1277, 1998.)

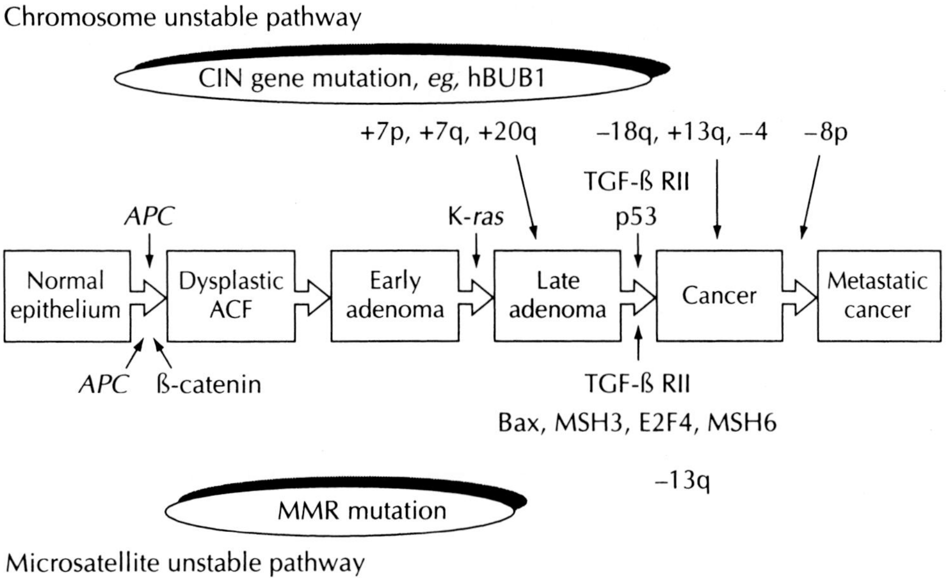

Figure 115–6. Model of colon cancer formation in tumors which progress through the adenoma-to-carcinoma sequence along pathways marked by chromosomal instability (CIN) or microsatellite instability. ACF, aberrant crypt focus; TGF, transforming growth factor. (From Grady WM, Markowitz S: Genomic instability and colorectal cancer. Curr Opin Gastroenterol 16:62, 2000.)

activates a protein (Tcf-4) in the nucleus, which in turn activates various target genes (e.g., c-myc, cyclin D1).[76, 77] *APC* is a tumor-suppressor gene that binds to β-catenin and causes its degradation through phosphorylation. Loss of *APC* function, therefore, leads to accumulation of β-catenin and unopposed stimulation through the Wnt-Tcf signaling pathway. This in turn leads to increased and unregulated proliferation and decreased programmed cell death (apoptosis). *APC* gene abnormalities may also lead to disruption of normal cell–cell adhesion through altered association with the cellular adhesion molecule *E-cadherin*. Disruption of *APC*-mediated regulation of transcriptional activation is critical for colorectal tumorigenesis. This is most commonly achieved through inactivating mutations of both *APC* alleles but can result through dominant mutations of the β-catenin gene that render β-catenin–Tcf-regulated transcription insensitive to the regulatory effects of normal wild-type *APC*.

Other genetic changes occur later in the adenoma-to-carcinoma sequence. Stepwise tumor progression is associated in more than 75% of cases with loss of the tumor-suppressor gene activity located on chromosome 18q. Several candidate genes are present on this chromosome, and loss of chromosome 18 is associated with a poor prognosis.[78, 79] One gene, designated *DCC* (deleted in colorectal cancer), was originally thought to be important because its loss from a stage II (Dukes B) cancer is associated in some studies with a significantly worse prognosis. Recent studies, however, have questioned its role as an important tumor-suppressor gene.[72] *DPC4* (*SMAD4*) is another candidate tumor suppressor gene whose inactivation may play a role in development of colorectal cancer. *DPC4* belongs to the *SMAD* gene family involved in signal transduction pathways activated through the transforming growth factor β (TGFβ) family receptors. Experimental inactivation of the mouse homologue *Dpc4* in a mouse model of adenomatous polyposis coli results in malignant progression of intestinal and colonic polyps initiated by loss of the *Apc* gene (the mouse homologue of *APC*).[80] Mutations in *SMAD4* and a related gene, *SMAD2*, have been reported in some sporadic colorectal cancers.[81] Deletions of chromosome 17p involve the *p53* tumor-suppressor gene, whose product normally prevents cells with damaged DNA from progressing from the G1 to the S phase in the cell cycle. Deletions within chromosome 17p are present in approximately 75% of colorectal cancers. Loss of *p53* may also be associated with reduced apoptosis (programmed cell death) of damaged cells. Inactivation of the *p53* gene mediates the conversion from adenoma to carcinoma. This is a late and important event in colon carcinogenesis. Distant metastases from colorectal cancers are significantly associated with high fractional allelic loss and deletions of 17p and 18q.[70, 71] A distinct set of "metastasis suppressor genes" has also been postulated.[82]

Genomic instability creates a permissive state in which a cell acquires enough mutations to be transformed to a cancer cell. This is a common mechanism central to the development of most, if not all, colon cancers.[65] Several forms of genomic instability are common in colon cancer, including chromosome instability (CIN) and chromosome translocations, and microsatellite instability (MSI) in which subtle sequence changes, including base substitutions, deletions, or

Table 115–4 | **Target Gene Mutations and Microsatellite Instability (MSI)**

TARGET GENE	INCIDENCE IN COLON CANCER WITH MSI (%)
TGF-β RII	73–90
Bax	41–52
Caspase 5	62
MSH 3	46–71
MSH 6	28–33
β-catenin	16–25
IGFIIR	6–8
APC	70
E2F4	65

Most mutations cause frame shifts that prematurely truncate the protein, leading to inactivation of the affected allele.

Modified from Grady WM, Markowitz S: Genomic instability and colorectal cancer. Current Opin Gastroenterol 16:62, 2000.

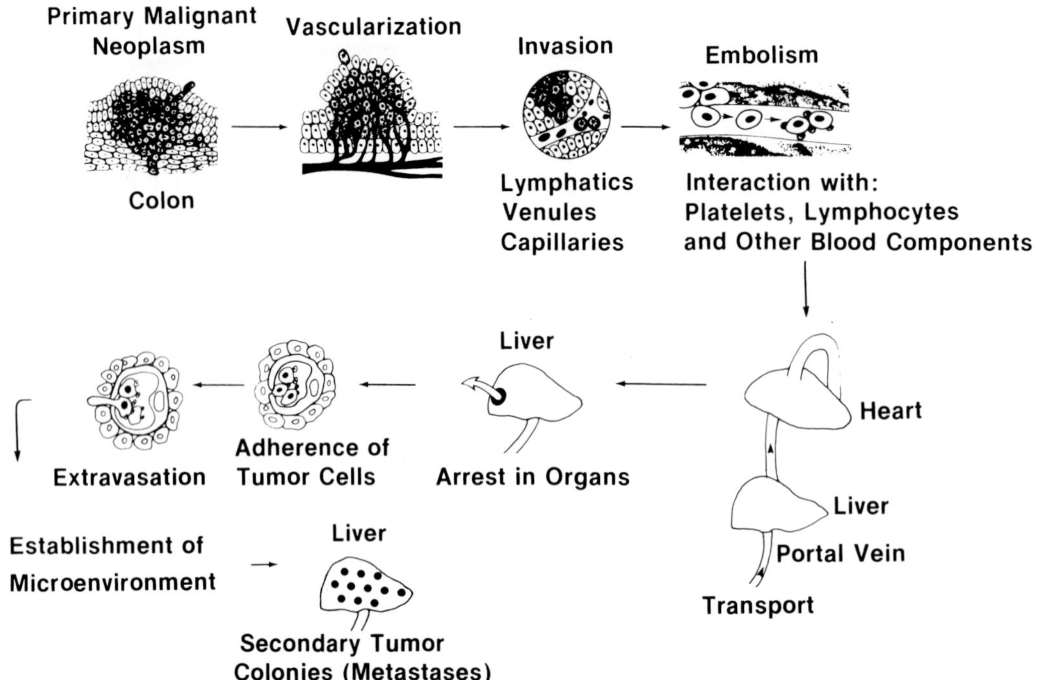

Figure 115–7. Colon cancer metastasis. Cancer cells metastasize through a complex, multistage process. In order for tumor cells to form metastatic foci at distant sites, they must complete all stages of this process.

insertions, lead to a hypermutable state (Fig. 115–6). Candidates responsible for CIN include genes responsible for the human mitotic checkpoint *hBUB1* and *hBUBR1*, genes involved in the DNA damage checkpoint *ATM, BRCA1* and *BRCA2, p53*, and *hRad17*, and genes that control centrosome number.

The significance of genomic instability in the pathogenesis of a subset of colon cancers became evident with the discovery of microsatellite instability (MSI) in colon cancers associated with hereditary nonpolyposis colorectal cancer (HNPCC). Alterations in genes that help maintain DNA fidelity during replication are characteristic of patients with HNPCC.83[65–88] Alterations in mismatch repair (MMR) genes

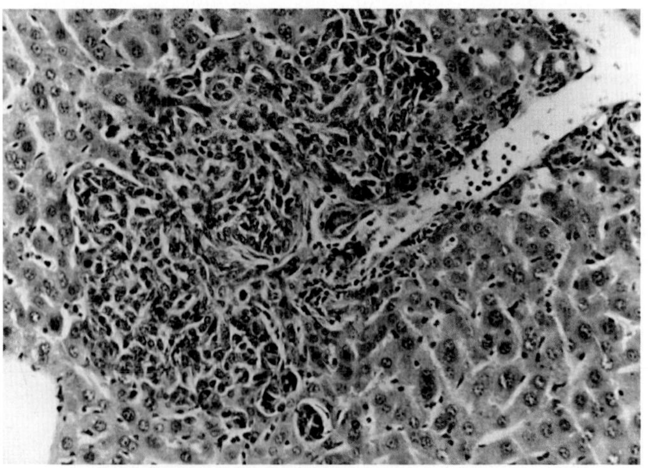

Figure 115–8. Colon cancer metastasis. On reaching the colon, cancer cells must adhere to the sinusoidal endothelium through specific interactions, and then invade the parenchyma. This photomicrograph shows tumor cells invading the liver after extravasation from a blood vessel.

designated *hMLH1, hPMS1* and *hPMS2*, and *hMSH2, hMSH3*, and *hMSH6* may lead to the inability to repair base pair mismatches and result in DNA replication errors or MSI. Inactivation of the MMR system causes genomic instability by increasing the rate of polymerase-generated replication errors, degrading the fidelity of DNA replication, particularly at microsatellite repeat sequences.[65, 89] MSI involves mutations or instability in short, tandemly repeated DNA sequences such as $(A)^n$, $(CA)^n$, and $(GATA)^n$. Such DNA sequences are found in several key genes that are important for maintaining normal cellular function (Table 115–4). The receptor for transforming growth factor-β (TGF-βRII), for example, is often mutated as the result of MSI.[89]

Multiple lines of evidence suggest that the TGF-β pathway is an important tumor-suppressing pathway in the colon, and that alterations in this pathway lead to tumor development. Less frequently targeted genes include the insulin growth factor 2 receptor (IGFIIR), Bax and caspase 5, proteins that regulate apoptosis; E2F4, a transcription factor, and MSH3 and MSH6, DNA mismatch repair proteins. β-Catenin mutations are present in up to 25% of MSI colon cancers. MSI therefore leads to accumulation of mutations in vulnerable genes, eventually resulting in the acquisition of the malignant phenotype. Although a high frequency of MSI (instability at 40% or more of microsatellite loci) is characteristic of HNPCC, similar alterations can be found in about 15% of sporadic colorectal cancers and also in premalignant lesions. MSI tumors remain diploid. Patients whose tumors demonstrate MSI may have a better prognosis than those whose tumors are characterized by chromosomal instability.[90, 91] MSI tumors may also respond differently to chemotherapy.[92, 93]

Most patients with MSI colon cancers do not possess mutations in the known mismatch repair genes. Recent evidence indicates that MSI in these tumors may arise through epigenetic mechanisms.[94] Hypermethylation of the *hMLH1* promoter has been reported in up to 70% of sporadic MSI tumors.[95, 96]

Biochemical and Other Changes

Chapter 3 deals in depth with the biologic and biochemical changes that occur during colorectal neoplasia. Alterations in cell surface and secreted proteins and glycoproteins, including a number of important cell adhesion molecules, are characteristic of colorectal cancers. Interactions between tumor cells themselves or between tumor cells and their environment may be homotypic (involving like molecules) or heterotypic (involving different adhesion molecules). Homotypic interactions often maintain the integrity of primary tumors by fostering adhesion between neighboring cells, whereas heterotypic interactions may occur between tumor cells and platelets, lymphocytes, vascular endothelial cells, and components of the basement membrane matrix. Most tumor-associated molecules represent quantitatively or qualitatively altered forms of molecules found on either normal tissues or during development (e.g., oncofetal antigens such as carcinoembryonic antigen). Many of these molecules appear to play a role in maintaining normal tissue homeostasis or targeting blood-borne cells to specific sites. Altered expression, therefore, may contribute to tumor invasion and metastasis.

Metastasis is a multistage process by which tumor cells escape the primary tumor and establish secondary foci at distant sites (Fig. 115–7). Cells in the primary tumor must become vascularized (angiogenesis via vascular endothelial growth factors), escape the primary tumor by overcoming adhesive interactions (e.g., loss of E-cadherin) and disrupting basement membranes (metalloproteinases such as type IV collagenase, matrilysin, loss of tissue inhibitors of collagenase), and enter lymphatics and the circulation. In the bloodstream they must survive interactions with blood components and the immune system and be transported to distant organ sites (principally the liver). At distant sites, tumor cells adhere to target endothelia via specific interactions (e.g., tumor-associated sialoglycoproteins and endothelial selectins) (Fig. 115–8), extravasate, interact with the microenvironment (e.g., growth factors) and establish secondary tumor foci.

Tumor cell subpopulations with different metastatic potential exist within the same primary tumor, and metastases result from the selective dissemination of those tumor cells possessing the ability to participate in all stages of this complex process. Several carbohydrate antigens have been studied in relation to their potential usefulness as diagnostic markers or in determining prognosis.[97–101]

FAMILIAL COLON CANCER

It has become increasingly clear that genetic predisposition plays a role in a substantial number of colorectal cancers. Although it is convenient to categorize colorectal cancers into hereditary (or familial) and nonhereditary (or sporadic) types, it is more appropriate to assume that all cancers have genetic components, which may be inherited or acquired, to varying degrees. Accordingly, persons with familial colon cancer are born with an altered genome, and the environment may contribute additional genotoxic events, leading to the malignant phenotype. In the case of "sporadic" cancers, multiple somatic mutations are contributed by the environment (see Chapter 3).

Table 115–5 | **Hereditary Nonpolyposis Colorectal Cancer***

At least three relatives with colorectal cancer (one must be first-degree relative of other two)
Colorectal cancer involving at least two generations
One or more colorectal cancer cases before age 50 years

*Criteria defined by the International Collaborative Group on Hereditary Nonpolyposis Colorectal Cancer ("Amsterdam Criteria").

The role of heredity in the genesis of colon cancer is most obviously manifested in those with the heritable polyposis syndromes (FAP, Gardner's syndrome) discussed in detail in Chapter 114. These syndromes are inherited in an autosomal dominant manner and are characterized by the presence of hundreds to thousands of colonic adenomas, with or without extracolonic tumors. Adenomas develop approximately a decade before the appearance of cancer, and virtually all affected persons eventually develop large bowel cancer if the colon is left in place. Nevertheless, these dramatic syndromes probably account for only a small fraction of cases of hereditary colorectal cancer (less than 1%).

HNPCC is an inherited disease in which colon cancers arise in discrete adenomas, but polyposis (i.e., hundreds of polyps) does not occur.[102–104] HNPCC accounts for approximately 6% of colonic adenocarcinoma. It is an autosomal dominant disorder with high penetration; approximately 80% are caused by germ-line mutations in genes responsible for repair of DNA errors called mismatches that occur during DNA replication (discussed earlier). During DNA synthesis, DNA polymerase may create single base-pair mismatches resulting in structural abnormalities (so-called "loop-outs") involving unpaired bases. These alterations tend to occur at repetitive DNA sequences termed microsatellites. These errors are repaired by enzymes coded for by "mismatch repair (MMR) genes." The majority of reported germ-line mutations in DNA mismatch repair genes have been associated with the *hMSH2* gene on chromosome 2 (40% to 50%) and *hMLH1* on chromosome 3 (20% to 30%).

Mutations in *hMSH6, hPMS1*, and *hPMS2* have also been reported in a small number of patients. No locus has been identified, however, for many HNPCC families. The definition of HNPCC was standardized and most strictly defined by the International Collaborative Group on Hereditary Nonpolyposis Colorectal Cancer. These "Amsterdam criteria"[103] (Table 115–5) include (1) at least three relatives with histologically verified colorectal cancer, one of them a first-degree relative of the other two (FAP excluded); (2) at least two successive generations affected; and (3) in one of the individuals, diagnosis of colorectal cancer before age 50 years. These criteria do not account, however, for the frequent occurrence of extracolonic cancers in such families, or for small kindreds. This has led to the development of broader clinical criteria, including guidelines published by a recent National Cancer Institute–sponsored workshop on HNPCC, the "Bethesda guidelines" (Table 115–6).[104]

Table 115–6 | **Bethesda Guidelines for Testing of Colorectal Tumors for Microsatellite Instability[104]**

1. Individuals with cancer in families that meet the Amsterdam Criteria (see Table 115–5)
2. Individuals with two HNPCC-related cancers, including synchronous and metachronous colorectal cancers or associated extracolonic cancers*
3. Individuals with colorectal cancers and a first-degree relative with colorectal cancer and/or HNPCC-related extracolonic cancer and/or a colorectal adenoma; one of the cancers diagnosed at age < 45 yr, and the adenoma diagnosed at age < 40 yr
4. Individuals with colorectal cancer or endometrial cancer diagnosed at age < 45 yr
5. Individuals with right-sided colorectal cancer with an undifferentiated pattern (solid/cribriform) on histopathology diagnosed at age < 45 yr†
6. Individuals with signet-ring-cell-type colorectal cancer diagnosed at age < 45 yr‡
7. Individuals with adenomas diagnosed at age < 40 yr

*Endometrial, ovarian, gastric, hepatobiliary, or small bowel cancer or transitional cell carcinoma of the renal pelvis or ureter.

†Solid/cribriform defined as poorly differentiated or undifferentiated carcinoma composed of irregular solid sheets of large eosinophilic cells and containing small glandlike spaces.

‡Composed of > 50% signet ring cells.

Table 115–7 | **Clinical Features of Hereditary Nonpolyposis Colorectal Cancer (HNPCC): Comparisons with Sporadic Cancer**

	HNPCC	SPORADIC CANCER
Mean age at diagnosis	45 yr	67 yr*
Multiple colon cancers	35%	4–11%
Synchronous	18%	3–6%
Metachronous	24%	1–5%
Proximal location†	72%	35%
Excess malignant tumors at other sites	Yes	No
Mucinous and poorly differentiated cancers	Common	Infrequent
Prognosis	Favorable‡	Variable

*Ninety percent of cancers in the general population are diagnosed in persons 50 years of age and older.

†Proximal to the splenic flexure. Location of the initial cancer.

‡Patients whose tumors demonstrate microsatellite instability have a more favorable prognosis than those with microsatellite-stable tumors.

Families include members whose heritable cancer is limited to the colon and rectum (site-specific HNPCC, HNPCC type a, Lynch syndrome I) and families whose members are also prone to cancer of the female genital tract and other sites (cancer family syndrome, HNPCC type b, Lynch syndrome II) (Fig. 115–9). In these syndromes, discrete polyps, but not polyposis, may antedate the cancers. Adenomas in the proximal colon may sometimes be flat or slightly raised lesions with foci of adenomatous change confined to the upper half of a crypt ("flat" adenomas). HNPCC is characterized by an autosomal dominant mode of genetic transmission, a tendency toward proximal sites of colon tumors, multiple primary malignancies (synchronous and metachronous), and a higher incidence of mucinous carcinomas (Table 115–7). These colorectal cancers usually appear at age 40 to 50 years, two decades earlier than colorectal cancer in the general population. In a study of a small, defined population

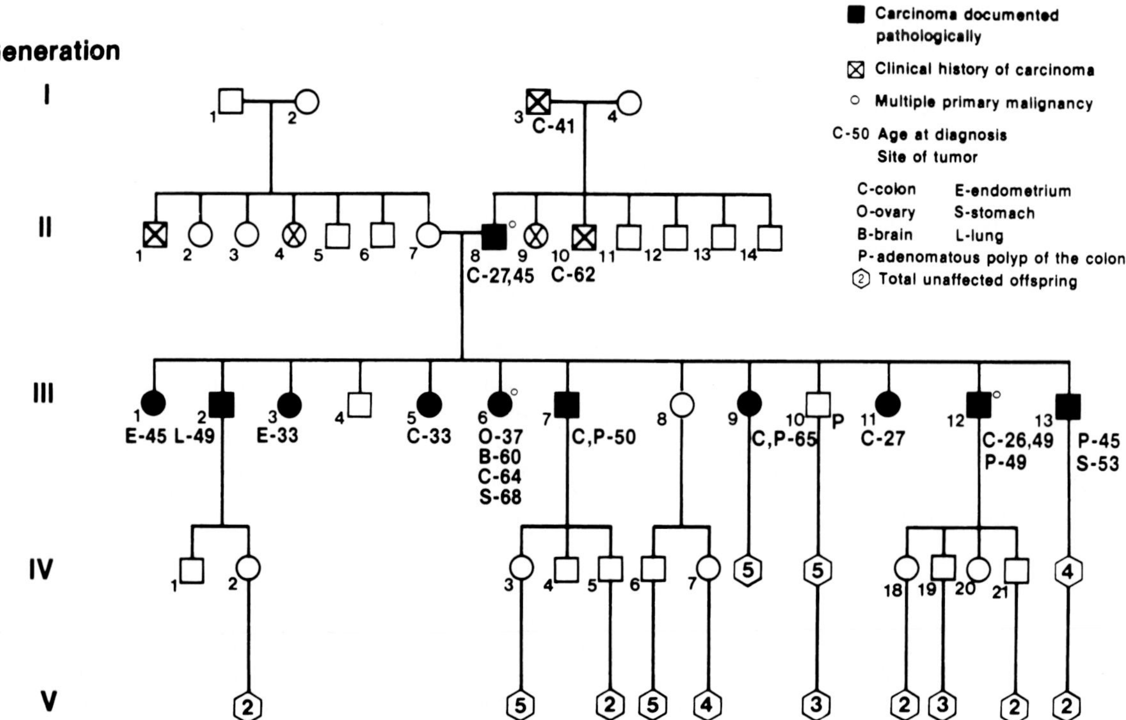

Figure 115–9. Pattern of inheritance of cancer in a familial aggregate with Lynch syndrome II (HNPCC type b). Affected members were found in generations I, II, and III; members of generations IV and V were still young and at risk for developing carcinomas when pedigree was obtained. (From Boland CR: Familial colonic cancer syndromes. West J Med 139:351, 1983.)

in central Finland, HNPCC accounted for 4% to 6% of colorectal cancers identified.[105] This figure is similar to estimates of Lynch and others.[103]

Both patients with HNPCC and some as yet unaffected family members have biologic markers that resemble those in patients with the familial adenomatous polyposis syndromes. These include abnormal proliferative activity of colonic crypt cells, increased tetraploidy (twice the normal DNA content) in vitro in cultured skin fibroblasts, decreased degradation of fecal cholesterol, and cell-mediated immune defects in vitro that might interfere in vivo with the recognition of killing of incipient tumor cells. The genetic defect in HNPCC, however, is due to loss of the *hMSH2* and *hMLH1* genes. Additional genes, such as *hPMS1, hPMS2*, and *hMSH6*, may also be involved. This leads to increased susceptiblity to mutation from failure to repair base pair mismatches.[83]

Although colorectal cancer syndromes with readily apparent patterns of inheritance currently account for only a small portion of total cancer cases in this organ, hereditary factors may be present in a larger proportion of cases.[106] Burt and colleagues studied the inheritance patterns of susceptibility to colorectal cancer in a large Utah pedigree with multiple cases of colorectal cancer but no recognizable inheritance pattern, and in 34 kindreds in which index cases were selected for a history of adenomatous polyps or clustering of colorectal cancer in close relatives.[107] These analyses, based on the systematic screening of pedigree members by flexible sigmoidoscopy, suggest that the excess of discrete adenomas and colorectal cancers in these families was the result of inherited defects transmitted in an autosomal dominant pattern. Another study by this same group further suggests that mutations at the genetic locus for FAP (*APC*) may be the cause of other, more subtle syndromes involving an inherited susceptibility to colonic adenomas and carcinomas.[108]

Genetic susceptibility to colorectal cancer in the general population is suggested by the two- to threefold increase in colorectal cancer in first-degree relatives of patients with "sporadic" adenomas and colorectal cancers.[106, 109–112] The relative risk is even stronger when cancer occurs in family members younger than age 50 years. The precise role of genetic factors in this group, and their interaction with the environment in the evolution of colorectal cancer, remain to be defined.

Table 115–8 | **Risk Factors for Colorectal Cancer**

High-fat, low-bulk diet*
Age above 40 yr
Personal history of:
Colorectal adenomas (synchronous or metachronous)
Colorectal carcinoma
Family history of:
Polyposis syndromes: familial polyposis coli; Gardner's syndrome; Turcot's syndrome (> 100 adenomas); Muir-Torre syndrome (scattered adenomas); Peutz-Jeghers' syndrome; familial juvenile polyposis (from adenomas, not hamartomas)
Nonpolyposis colon cancer; site-specific colon cancer; cancer family syndrome
First-degree relative with colorectal cancer
Inflammatory bowel disease
Ulcerative colitis } Especially with high-grade dysplasia
Crohn's disease } or dysplasia-associated mass lesions

*Based on descriptive epidemiology. Data from case-control, cohort, and randomized trials less convincing.

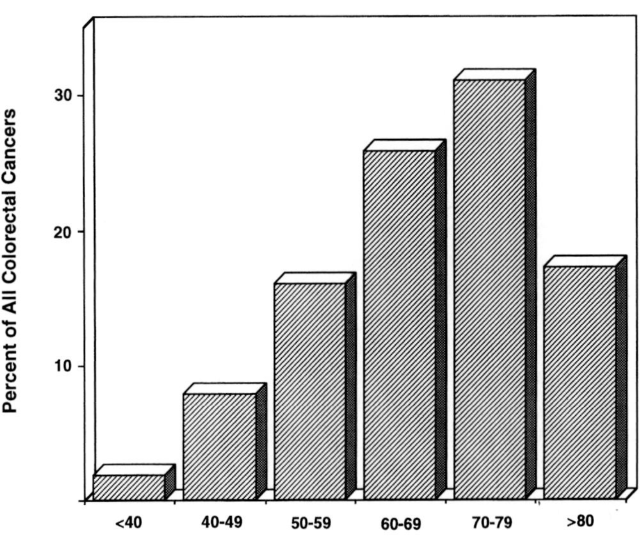

Figure 115–10. Colorectal cancer incidence by age at diagnosis in the United States. Ninety percent of cancers occur after age 50.

PREDISPOSITION TO COLORECTAL CANCER

The risk of developing colorectal cancer depends on a number of identified or suspected demographic factors (Table 115–8). The probable influence of diet and other environmental factors has been discussed (see Tables 115–1 and 2). Other factors include age, personal history of adenoma, of carcinoma, and of predisposing diseases (particularly inflammatory bowel disease), and family history (discussed earlier).

Age

The risk of developing colorectal cancer rises sharply after age 40 years in the general population, with 90% of cancers occurring in persons aged 50 years and older (Fig. 115–10). In fact, a 50-year-old person has approximately a 5% chance of developing colorectal cancer if he survives to age 80 and a 2.5% risk of dying from the disease. This has important implications for screening, as will be discussed later in the chapter. Sporadic colorectal cancers do arise in other age groups (third and fourth decades), however, and this diagnosis must be considered in younger persons with signs and symptoms characteristic of this disease, especially if they have a family history of colorectal neoplasia.

Prior Adenoma and Carcinoma

ADENOMA. (See also Chapter 114.) Present evidence strongly indicates that the majority of colorectal cancers arise from preexisting adenomas. The risk of colorectal cancer increases with the number of adenomas,[113] the most extreme example being the familial polyposis syndromes.

Clinical and morphologic evidence suggests that, as adenomas grow larger, they progressively dedifferentiate, become dysplastic, and then become malignant.[114] With increasing size or increasing villous architecture, the frequency of nuclear atypia, dysplasia, and in situ or invasive carcinoma increases. Despite the potential for adenomas to evolve to carcinomas, the actual risk is unknown.

Adenomatous polyps are common in populations who consume a "Western" diet, especially after age 50 years, but the prevalence of adenomas is high, compared with the incidence of cancer. In Norway it has been estimated that 29% of the living population older than 35 years have single or multiple colorectal adenomas.[115] The annual conversion rate in those with adenomas (based on cancer incidence from multiple tumor registries) is 0.25%, indicating a moderate risk for developing colorectal cancer. The malignancy rate is higher in large adenomas, adenomas with villous architecture, and adenomas with cytologic nuclear atypia or dysplasia.[114] In the Norwegian study cited, the estimated annual rate of conversion to invasive cancer for persons bearing adenomas greater than 1 cm, villous components, or severe dysplasia is 3%, 17%, and 37%, respectively.

CARCINOMA. People with colorectal carcinoma have an increased risk of harboring a second carcinoma (synchronous carcinomas) or of developing another one subsequently (metachronous carcinomas). The frequency of more than one carcinoma in the same person ranges between 2% and 6% (0.7% to 7.6% for synchronous cancers and 1.1% to 4.7% for metachronous ones).[116–118] In the minority of patients with synchronous cancers, the two lesions are located in the same colonic segment. Many patients with simultaneous cancers have one in the proximal and the other in the distal colon. The degree of invasiveness of synchronous cancers often differs, the prognosis depending on the "worst-stage" lesion. Five-year survival rates for patients with synchronous cancers who have had the cancers resected are similar to those with single lesions. The interval between an initial cancer and a metachronous one may be considerable (lesions separated by as much as 23 years have been reported), but several studies note that 50% of metachronous cancers arise within 5 to 7 years of the index lesion. Second cancers often occur at a site remote from the initial lesion.

Family History

The risk of colorectal cancer in first-degree relatives of those with sporadic colorectal cancer is increased two- to threefold (see earlier). The risk is higher when adenoma or carcinoma has occurred in a relative at an early age or when more than one relative has had carcinoma.[109–112] These factors have been taken into account in recent screening guidelines that stratify patients according to potential cancer risk.[106, 119–121] Familial adenomatous polyposis (FAP) and its variants are inherited in an autosomal dominant manner, and without colectomy virtually all affected members with polyps eventually develop carcinoma. Hereditary nonpolyposis colorectal cancer (HNPCC) also has an autosomal dominant pattern of inheritance.

Turcot's syndrome is defined by a rare combination of inherited adenomatous polyposis and malignant brain tumors. Patients with Turcot's syndrome have been described who have germline mutations in the *APC* gene or mutations of *hMLH1* and *hPMS2* characteristic of HNPCC.[122] Inheritance is autosomal dominant.

The *Muir-Torre syndrome* is a rare variant of HNPCC. Multiple skin lesions, including sebaceous adenomas and carcinomas, basal cell and squamous cell carcinomas, and keratoacanthomas occur in conjunction with the adenomas and adenocarcinomas of the colon.[123]

The Peutz-Jeghers syndrome and the familial form of juvenile polyposis have both been associated with an increased risk of small and large bowel cancer (see Chapter 114). Peutz-Jeghers syndrome is an autosomal dominant disease, which in most families has been mapped to chromosome 19 p13.3 and the *STK11* gene (serine threonine kinase 11). Adenomatous changes have been reported in 3% to 6% of hamartomas from these patients. Extracolonic cancers are common and have been reported to occur in 50% to 90% of patients with Peutz-Jeghers syndrome (relative risk for all cancers was 15.2).[124] A significant increase has been reported for a variety of cancers, including esophageal, stomach, small intestine, pancreas, lung, breast, uterus, and ovary.

Familial juvenile polyposis is a rare autosomal dominant disease that may be associated with polyps limited to the colon, limited to the stomach, or throughout the gastrointestinal tract. The genetic basis of this syndrome is not understood, but germline mutations in a gene (*SMAD4*) located on chromosome 18q21.1 that encodes an intracellular mediator in the TGF-β signaling pathway have been identified in some affected patients. The *PTEN* gene located on chromosome 10 also has been linked to some cases. The presence of mixed juvenile and adenomatous polyps indicates which lesions have malignant potential.

Inflammatory Bowel Disease

Patients with idiopathic inflammatory bowel disease (ulcerative colitis [UC], Crohn's disease) are at increased risk for developing adenocarcinoma of the colon (see also Chapters 103 and 104).[125–129] Actuarially derived (life table) cumulative cancer incidences from tertiary referral centers (Fig. 115–11) agree that the risk of cancer in patients with UC begins with a disease duration of 7 years and rises about 10% per decade, reaching approximately 30% at 25 years. Nonetheless, difficulties related to sources of referral, sampling, recognition and characterization of disease, differences in follow-up procedures, and methods used to detect neoplastic disease cloud many such studies. The assessed cancer risk for patients with UC followed in a private practice has been reported to be only 6.6% 26 years after onset of disease and 11.4% at 32 years.[129] The true risk of developing colorectal carcinoma in UC must lie between predictions from tertiary centers and the primary care setting.

The risk for patients with UC developing colorectal cancer correlates most closely with duration of disease. In a large group of patients with extensive disease who were followed prospectively, the risk of carcinoma per patient-year was zero before 10 years, and 1 in 86 after 20 years.[127] The risk is greatest in those with universal colitis.[128] Although it has been reported that the risk of cancer in left-sided disease (i.e., distal to the splenic flexure) begins approximately a decade later than with universal colitis, at least one surveillance study found no difference between

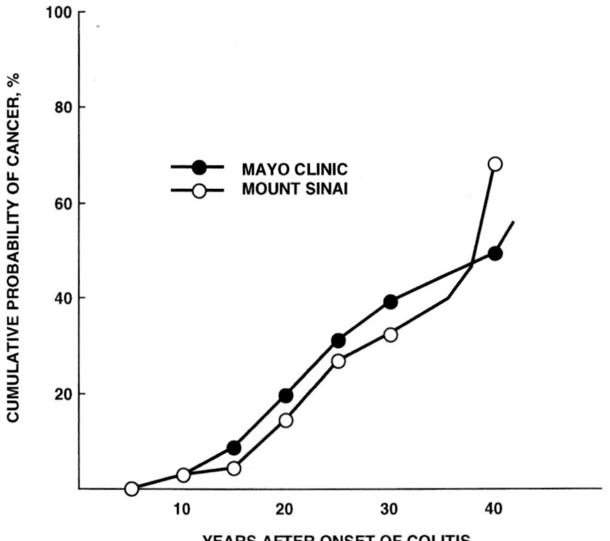

Figure 115–11. Cumulative probability of developing colorectal carcinoma in patients with ulcerative colitis seen at tertiary referral centers. Data from the primary care setting indicate a similar pattern but lower incidence rates (see text).

these groups in the temporal development of preneoplastic dysplasia.[126] The risk for patients with ulcerative proctitis is only slightly increased, compared with that in the general population.

The risk of cancer is not related to severity of the initial attack of colitis, disease activity, or age at onset of colitis (independent of duration of disease). Colorectal cancer in persons with UC appears to be a risk factor for colorectal cancer in their noncolitic relatives.[130] Similarly, cancer in relatives without UC is a risk factor for those with colitis. There is an association of backwash ileitis with colorectal cancer in patients with UC who undergo proctocolectomy.[131] Cancer arising in the setting of UC has traditionally been thought to be a highly malignant lesion with a poor prognosis, but studies using matched controls from colon cancer populations without colitis have failed to show a significant difference in survival between the two groups.

The increased risk for colorectal carcinoma in patients with Crohn's disease or ileocolitis has been reported to be as much as four to twenty times that in the general population,[132] but one cohort study failed to confirm an increased incidence of colon cancer in these patients.[133] Cancer may arise at an earlier age in these patients than in the general population. Many of these cancers are mucinous carcinomas and may be present in surgically bypassed or strictured segments of colon.

Carcinomas do not develop de novo from normal mucosa but from mucosa that has undergone a sequence of morphologic changes that culminate in invasive carcinoma. As in precancerous adenomas, dysplasia is a precursor to carcinoma in inflammatory bowel disease. Dysplasia includes abnormalities in crypt architecture and cytologic detail (Figs. 115–12 and 115–13). Epithelial crypts are reduced in number, irregularly branched, and crowded together ("back-to-back glands"). Cell nuclei may be enlarged and hyperchromatic, have increased numbers of mitoses, and be located at different levels in the cell, producing a "picket fence" appearance (pseudostratification). Dysplasia is classified by grade as mild (or low-grade) and severe (or high-grade) dysplasia.

Retrospective analyses report that 90% of resected colons from patients with UC and cancer somewhere contain dysplastic mucosa, and 30% of patients with severe rectal or colonic dysplasia on resection or biopsy have coexistent carcinoma. Colonoscopic studies suggest that 25% of colons that demonstrate severe (high-grade) dysplasia on biopsy harbor a carcinoma.[126, 127] The incidence of dysplasia is often patchy, and it may be present in the colon but absent from the rectum.

Since the lack of uniformity of the definition of dysplasia may make interpretation of such data difficult, a multidisciplinary Inflammatory Bowel Disease–Dysplasia–Morphology Study Group developed a standardized classification for dysplasia arising in the setting of inflammatory bowel disease.[134] Several large prospective studies have attempted to determine the true risk of cancer in patients with colonic dysplasia and UC and the impact of screening programs for dysplasia.[126–128]

Results thus far suggest that biopsy surveillance programs can be effective in helping control the risk of carcinoma in patients with long-standing UC. The risk of cancer appears highest in those with high-grade dysplasia that arises in

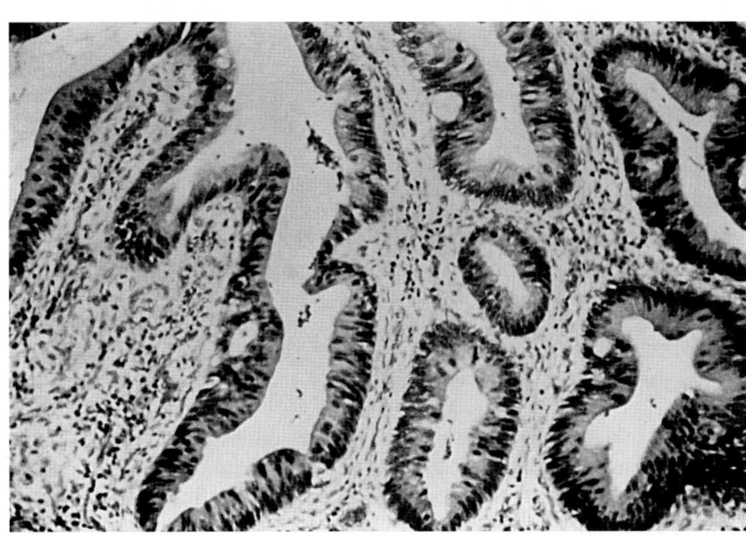

Figure 115–12. Dysplasia in the setting of ulcerative colitis. Goblet cells are decreased. Glands are branched, irregular, and crowded together. Cell nuclei are hyperchromatic and occur at different levels, producing a pseudopalisading or picket fence appearance.

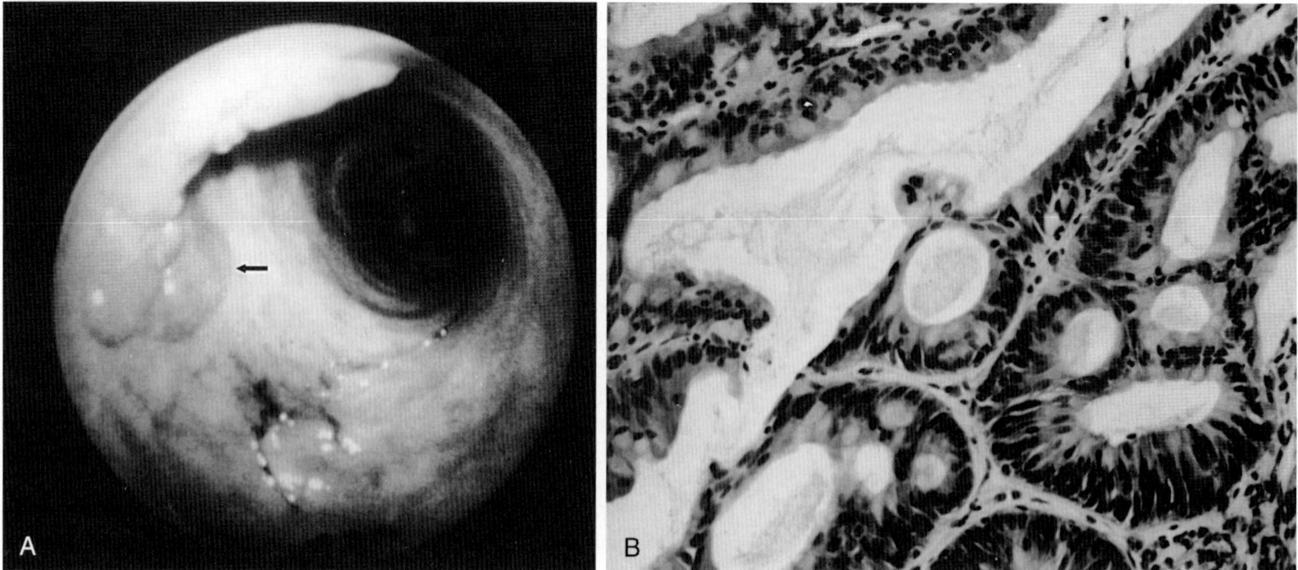

Figure 115–13. Plaquelike dysplasia-associated mass lesions (DAML) in a patient with long-standing ulcerative colitis. *A*, Lesions as seen through the colonoscope (*arrow*). *B*, Biopsy specimen reveals high-grade dysplasia.

visible plaques or masses (dysplasia-associated mass lesions, or DAML, as illustrated in Figure 115–13).[135] A computer cohort decision analysis suggested that surveillance should increase life expectancy for patients with UC.[125] Most investigators believe that patients who have UC longer than 7 to 8 years should undergo colonoscopy with multiple mucosal biopsies annually, to identify areas of dysplasia, and they advocate colectomy for severe dysplasia or DAML. Since the significance of low-grade or moderate dysplasia is less clear, immediate resection for patients with these levels of dysplasia is controversial. Others have advocated prophylactic colectomy as an option for those with disease of at least 10 years' duration.[125] Studies employing flow cytometry have detected aneuploid cell populations in colons resected for UC with dysplasia or early cancer. Flow cytometric analysis eventually may prove complementary to histology for identifying patients with UC who are at high risk of developing colorectal cancer.[134, 135] Chromosomal alterations may occur early in UC-related neoplastic progression[136] and appear to precede the histologic development of dysplasia. Relative loss of chromosome 18q may also be important in neoplastic progression.

Both dysplasia and increased risk of colon carcinoma have been reported in patients with Crohn's disease. As in UC, dysplasia appears in diseased colon segments, and its presence correlates with duration of disease. In a recent screening trial,[137] a finding of definite dysplasia was associated with age greater than 45 years and increased symptoms. By life table analysis, the probability of detecting dysplasia or cancer after a negative screening colonoscopy was 22% by the fourth surveillance examination.

Other Associated Disease States

Diverting bile to the lower small intestine, either surgically or by feeding cholestyramine, increases the yield of proximal colon tumors in carcinogen-treated animals. Since by analogy cholecystectomy in humans could lead to increased delivery of secondary bile acids to the proximal bowel, the possibility of an increase in colon cancer following cholecystectomy has been raised. However, the clinical evidence for such an association is contradictory. Increased proliferative activity in the distal colonic mucosa has been demonstrated in patients who have undergone cholecystectomy, and an increased frequency of tubular adenomas has been observed in patients older than 60 years of age with a postcholecystectomy interval of greater than 10 years, but an increased risk of colonic cancer for these patients has been both supported and refuted.

A Swedish population-based cohort study that followed a large group of patients for 14 to 17 years after cholecystectomy failed to show an association with colon cancer.[138] A more recent retrospective population-based cohort study that used the Swedish Inpatient Register studied almost 23,000 cholecystectomized persons for up to 31 years after surgery.[139] Patients with cholecystectomies had an increased risk of proximal intestinal adenocarcinoma, which declined with increasing distance from the common bile duct. The risk was significantly increased for adenocarcinoma of the small bowel and right colon, but not the remaining colon or rectum.

TUMOR PATHOLOGY, NATURAL HISTORY, AND STAGING

Gross Features

The gross morphologic features of adenocarcinoma in the large bowel depend on the tumor's site. Carcinomas of the proximal colon, particularly those of the cecum and ascending colon, tend to be large and bulky, often outgrowing their blood supply and undergoing necrosis (Fig. 115–14). This polypoid configuration may also be found elsewhere in the colon and rectum. In the more distal colon and rectum,

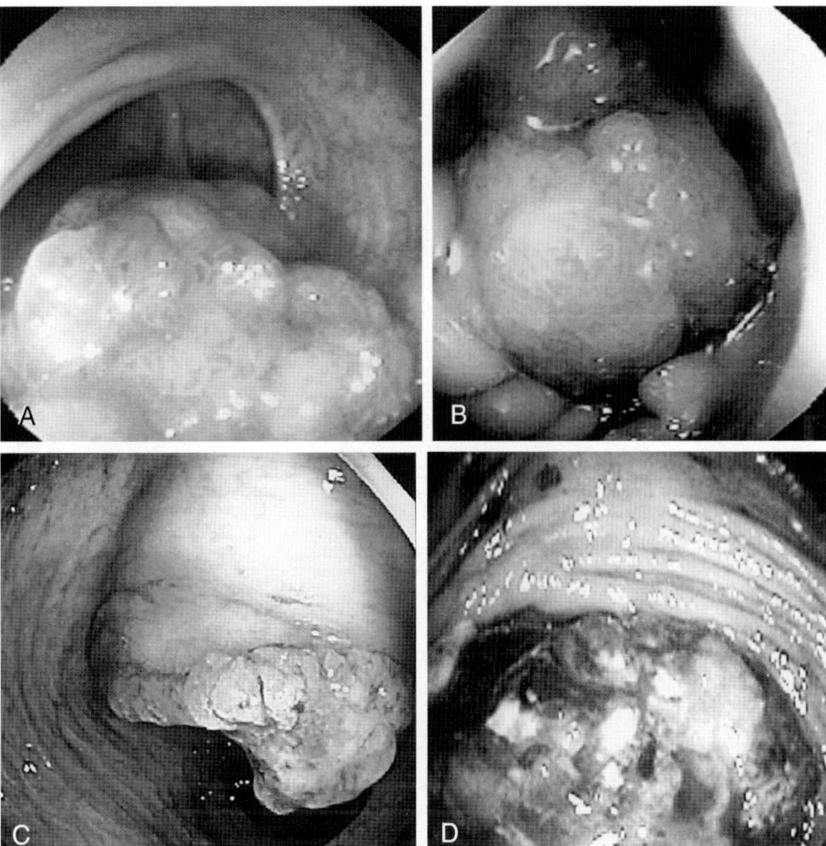

Figure 115–14. Carcinomas of the cecum seen at colonoscopy. Carcinomas of the proximal colon are often large and bulky polypoid lesions (*A, B*), involve the ileocecal valve (*C*), and may outgrow their blood supply and become necrotic (*D*).

tumors more frequently involve a greater circumference of the bowel, producing an annular constriction or "napkin-ring" appearance (Fig. 115–15). The fibrous stroma of these tumors accounts for constriction and narrowing of the bowel lumen, whereas the circular arrangement of colonic lymphatics (see Chapter 84) is responsible for their annular growth. These tumors may also become ulcerated. Occasionally, tumors have a flatter appearance with predominantly intramural spread (Fig. 115–16). The latter are seen most frequently in the setting of inflammatory bowel disease. The morphologic features of these carcinomas have clinical, diagnostic, and prognostic implications.

Histology

Carcinomas of the large bowel are characteristically adenocarcinomas, which form moderately to well-differentiated glands and secrete variable amounts of mucin (Fig. 115–17). Mucin, a high-molecular-weight glycoprotein, is the major product secreted by both normal and neoplastic glands of the colon and may be seen best with histochemical stains such as periodic acid–Schiff (PAS) (see Fig. 115–17*C*). In poorly differentiated tumors, gland formation and mucin production are present but are less prominent. "Signet-ring" cells, in which a large vacuole of mucin displaces the nucleus to one side, are a feature of some tumors (Fig. 115–18*A*). In approximately 15% of tumors, large lakes of mucin contain scattered collections of tumor cells (Fig. 115–18*B*). These mucinous or colloid carcinomas are most frequent in patients with HNPCC, in UC, and in patients whose carcinomas occur at an early age. Scirrhous carcinomas are uncommon and are characterized by sparse gland formation, with marked desmoplasia and fibrous tissue surrounding glandular structures. Sometimes tumors demonstrate a mixed histologic picture, with glands of varying degrees of differentiation (Fig. 115–19).

Cancers other than adenocarcinomas account for fewer than 5% of malignant tumors of the large bowel. Tumors arising at the anorectal junction include squamous cell carcinomas, cloacogenic or transitional cell carcinomas (see Chapter 117), and melanomas (see Chapters 29 and 117). Primary lymphomas and carcinoid tumors of the large bowel comprise fewer than 0.1% of all large bowel neoplasms (see Chapters 26 and 112).

Natural History and Staging

Colorectal cancers begin as intramucosal epithelial lesions, usually arising in adenomatous polyps or glands. As cancers grow, they become invasive, penetrating the muscularis mucosae of the bowel and invading lymphatic and vascular channels to involve regional lymph nodes, adjacent structures, and distant sites. Although adenocarcinomas of the colon and rectum grow at varying rates, they most often have long periods of silent growth before producing bowel symptoms. The mean doubling time of colon cancers determined radiographically in one study was 620 days. Patterns of spread depend on the anatomy of the individual bowel segment as well as its lymph and blood supplies.

Cancers of the rectum advance locally by progressive

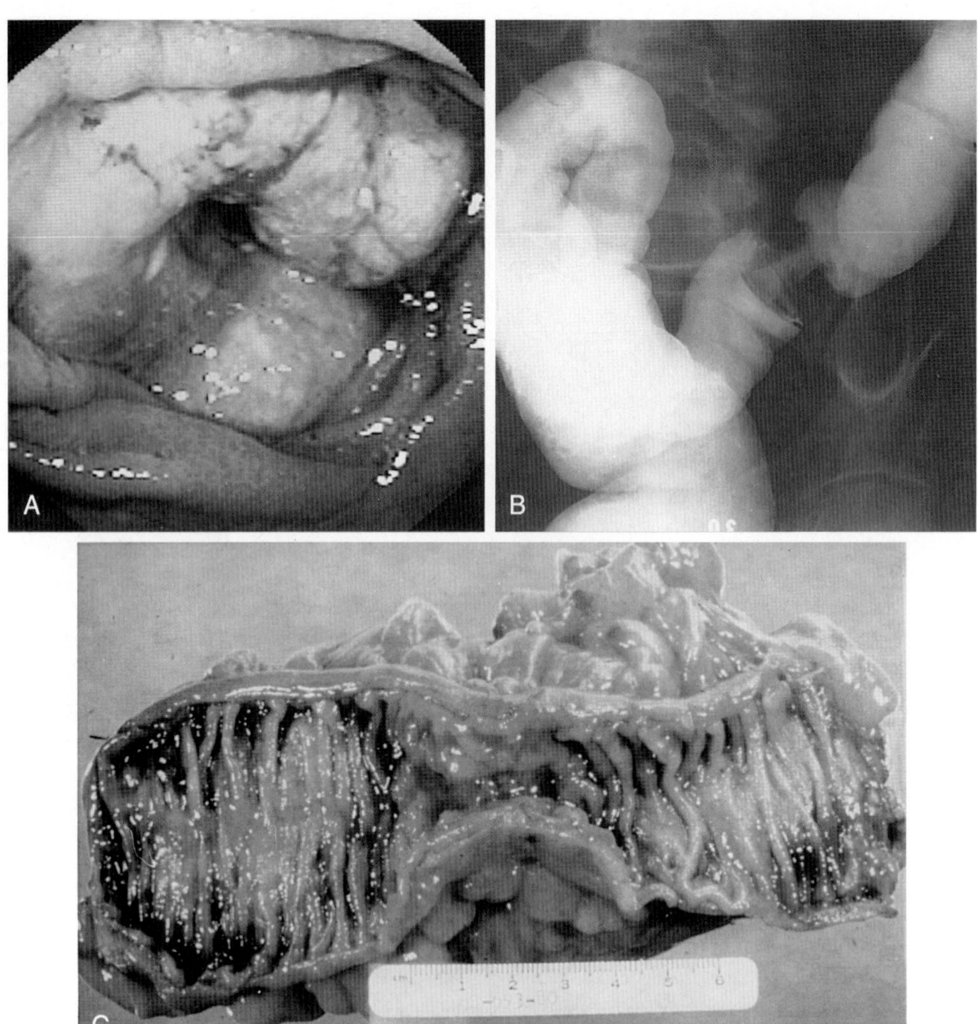

Figure 115–15. Obstructing carcinoma of the sigmoid colon. *A*, Colonoscopic view. *B*, Apple core lesion seen on full column barium enema. *C*, Surgical specimen demonstrates annular constriction or "napkin-ring" appearance.

penetration of the bowel wall. Extension of the primary tumor intramurally parallel to the long axis of the bowel is most often limited, and lymphatic and hematogenous spread are unusual before penetration of the muscularis mucosae. Exceptions appear to be poorly differentiated tumors, which may metastasize lymphatically or hematogenously before penetrating the bowel. Since the rectum is relatively immobile and lacks a serosal covering, rectal cancers tend to spread contiguously to progressively involve local structures. Transrectal ultrasonography can be useful in staging depth of rectal cancers. Because of the dual blood supply of the lower one third of the rectum, tumors arising here may metastasize hematogenously via the superior hemorrhoidal vein and portal system to the liver or by way of the middle hemorrhoidal vein and inferior vena cava to the lungs. The veins of the upper and middle thirds of the rectum drain into the portal system, and tumors in these segments first spread hematogenously to the liver. Occasionally, lumbar and thoracic vertebral metastases may result from hematogenous spread via portal-vertebral communications (Batson's vertebral venous plexuses).

Colon cancers also invade transmurally to penetrate the bowel wall and involve regional lymphatics and then distant nodes. As reviewed in Chapter 84, the lymphatic drainage generally parallels the arterial supply to a given bowel segment. The liver is the most common site of hematogenous spread from colon tumors via the portal venous system. Pulmonary metastases from colon cancer result, in general, from hepatic metastases.

On the basis of observations of what he believed to be an orderly progression of local-regional invasion by rectal cancers, Cuthbert Dukes proposed a classification in 1929, which has since been modified many times in attempts to increase its prognostic value for cancers of both the rectum and the colon (Table 115–9). The most commonly employed modification of Dukes' system is that of Astler and Coller in 1954 (see Table 115–9). This classification uses the following designations: A, tumors limited to the mucosa; B1, tumors extending into, but not through, the muscularis propria; B2, tumors penetrating the muscularis propria but without lymph node involvement; and C, tumors with regional lymph node involvement. Stage C tumors are further divided into primary tumors limited to the bowel wall (C1) and those that penetrate the bowel wall (C2). In contrast, in

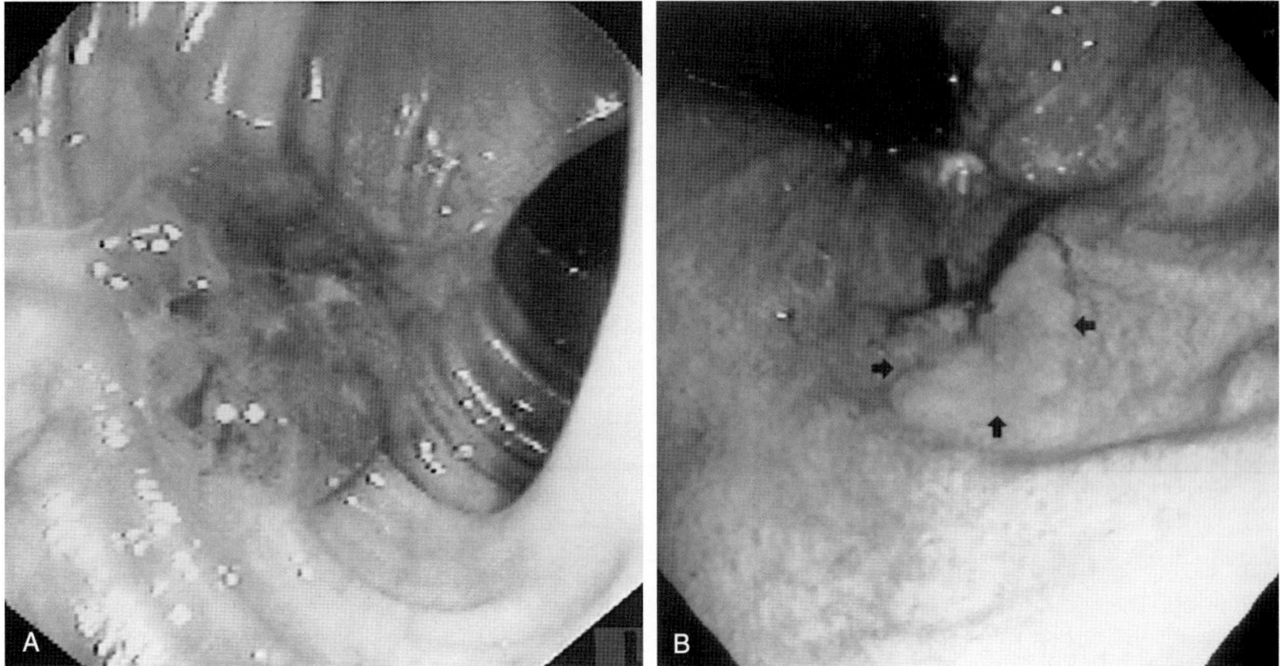

Figure 115–16. Flat, plaquelike carcinomas of the colon (*A*) and rectum (*B*) in patients with a history of inflammatory bowel disease.

the system proposed by the Gastrointestinal Tumor Study Group (GITSG) in 1975, C1 lesions are those in which 1 to 4 regional lymph nodes contain tumor, and C2 lesions are those in which more than 4 lymph nodes contain tumor (see Table 115–9). Another modification by Turnbull and associates in 1967 added a D category to account for distant metastases.

In an attempt to provide a uniform and orderly classification for colorectal cancers, the American Joint Committee (AJC) for Cancer Staging and End Results Reporting and the International Union Against Cancer (UICC) have introduced tumor–node–metastases (TNM) classifications for colorectal cancer.[140] These systems classify the extent of the primary tumor (T), the status of regional lymph nodes (N), and the presence or absence of distant metastases (M). Cases are assigned the highest value of TNM that describes the full extent of disease and are grouped into five stages (0 through IV). The five stages have become important in uniformly randomizing patients for therapeutic trials (Table 115–10) and have in many cases replaced the Dukes' classification for colorectal cancer.

PROGNOSTIC INDICATORS

Clinical and pathologic variables that may affect the prognosis of patients with colorectal cancer are outlined in Table 115–11. These variables are important in predicting clinical

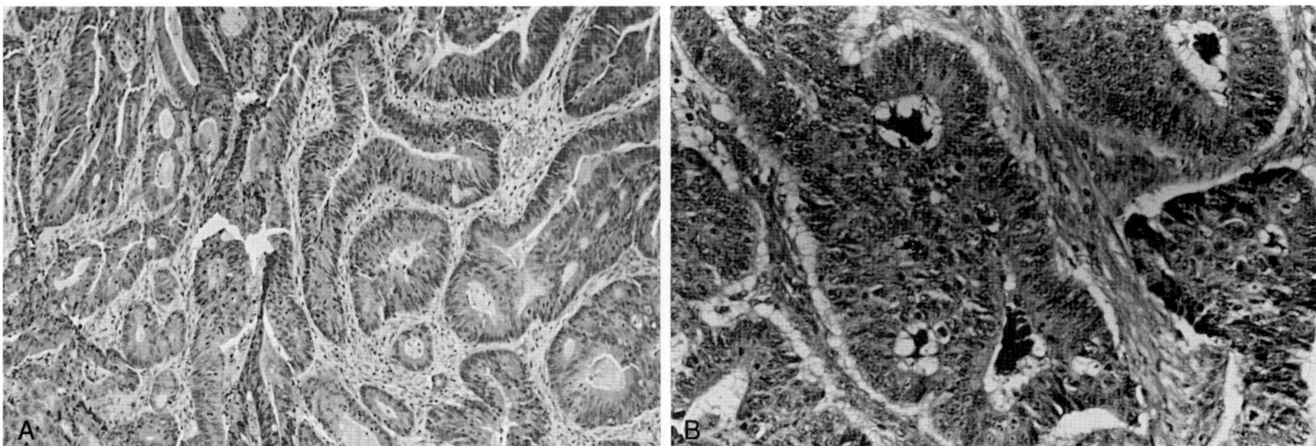

Figure 115–17. *A*, Well-differentiated adenocarcinoma of the colon. Histologic sections stained with hematoxylin and eosin demonstrate crowded neoplastic glands containing variable amounts of mucin. *B*, Section stained with periodic acid–Schiff (PAS) method better demonstrates mucin (dark material) in gland lumens.

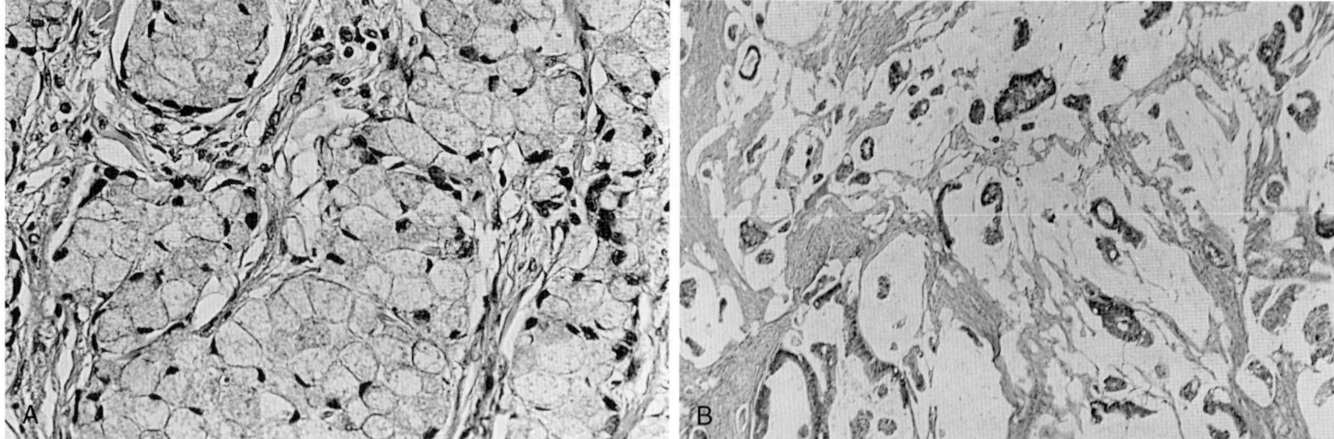

Figure 115–18. Mucinous carcinomas of the colon include signet-ring cell carcinomas in which a large vacuole of mucin displaces the nucleus (*A*) and colloid carcinomas with scattered nests of tumor cells floating in lakes of mucin (*B*).

outcome and in designing optimal strategies for treatment and follow-up. Their identification has led to a progressive modification of the staging classifications for colorectal cancer. The roles of histologic differentiation, tumor size, location, configuration, degree of invasion, and lymph node status must be evaluated on the basis of the prospective analysis of patients who undergo curative resections for colorectal cancer.

Surgical-Pathologic Stage of the Primary Tumor

The depth of transmural tumor penetration and the extent of regional lymph node spread are the most important determinants of prognosis (Fig. 115–20).[141–146] Further, the degree of bowel wall penetration affects prognosis, independently of lymph node status. The degree of tumor penetration correlates with the number of involved nodes[146] as well as with the incidence of local recurrence after surgical resection.[142, 144, 145] The number of involved regional lymph nodes also correlates independently with outcome (Fig. 115–20*B*).[142, 146, 147] The National Surgical Adjuvant Project for Breast and Bowel Cancer (NSABP) reported a significant difference in postresection survival for colorectal cancer in favor of patients with 1 to 4 involved nodes (GITSG stage C1; see Table 115–9) over those who have more than 4 nodes involved by tumor (GITSG stage C2; see Table 115–9), independent of degree of tumor penetration.[146] The GITSG similarly found that, at a median interval of 5.5 years after surgery, disease recurs in 35% patients with 1 to 4 positive nodes (C1) and in 61% of those with more than four such nodes (C2).[142]

Tumor Morphology and Histology

The TNM classification (see Table 115–10) for human carcinomas is based in part on the observation that, for most cancers, tumor size correlates with local and distant spread

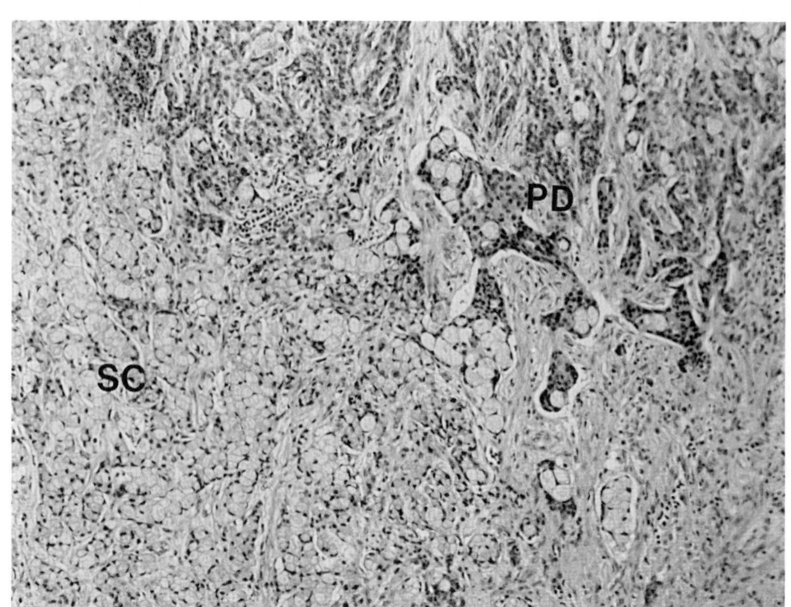

Figure 115–19. Carcinomas of the colon often demonstrate heterogeneity in histologic morphology. This specimen contains components of both signet ring cell (SC) and poorly differentiated (PD) carcinoma.

Table 115–9 | **Dukes' Classification for Carcinoma of the Rectum and Its Modifications for Colorectal Carcinoma**

STAGE	DUKES, 1932 (Rectum)	GABRIEL, DUKES, BUSSEY, 1935 (Rectum)	KIRKLIN ET AL, 1949 (Rectum & sigmoid)	ASTLER-COLLER, 1954 (Rectum & colon)	TURNBULL ET AL, 1967 (Colon)	MODIFIED ASTLER-COLLER (GUNDERSON & SOSIN, 1974) (Rectum & colon)	GITSG, 1975 (Rectum & colon)
A	Limited to bowel wall	Limited to bowel wall	Limited to mucosa	Limited to mucosa	Limited to mucosa	Limited to mucosa	Limited to mucosa
B	Through bowel wall	Through bowel wall	—	—	Tumor extension into pericolic fat	—	—
B1	—	—	Into muscularis propria	Into muscularis propria	—	Into muscularis propria	Into muscularis propria
B2	—	—	Through muscularis propria	Through muscularis propria (and serosa)	—	Through serosa m = microscopic; m + g = gross	Through serosa
B3	—	—	—	—	—	Adherent to or invading adjacent structures	—
C	Regional nodal metastases	—	Regional nodal metastases	—	Regional nodal metastases	—	—
C1	—	Regional nodal metastases near primary lesion	—	Same as B1 plus regional nodal metastases	—	Same as B1 plus regional nodal metastases	1–4 regional nodes positive
C2	—	Proximal node involved at point of ligation	—	Same as B2 plus regional nodal metastases	—	Same as B2 plus regional nodal metastases	> 4 regional nodes positive
C3	—	—	—	—	—	Same as B3 plus regional nodal metastases	—
D	—	—	—	—	Distant metastases (liver, lung, bone) or due to parietal or adjacent organ invasion	—	—

GITSG, Gastrointestinal Tumor Study Group.

and, thus, with prognosis. Numerous studies suggest that colorectal cancer is an exception and that the size of the primary tumor per se does not correlate with prognosis. Patients with exophytic or polypoid tumors appear to have a better prognosis than those with ulcerating or infiltrating tumors.

Tumor prognosis correlates with histologic grade: poor differentiation confers a worse prognosis than a high degree of differentiation.[144, 147–149] A comparison of poorly differentiated and well-differentiated tumors showed that the relative risk for survival was 1.68 in favor of well-differentiated cancers.[149] Since no uniform system for grading tumors exists, comparison between studies is difficult. Mucinous[150] and scirrhous carcinomas appear to be biologically more aggressive, and patients with these tumors do not survive as long as those who have other adenocarcinomas. Mucin-associated antigens may play a role in tumor progression and metastasis of colon cancer cells.[99, 100] Signet-ring carcinomas have been reported to present at an advanced stage and to be highly invasive tumors.[151]

Venous invasion by colorectal cancer (Fig. 115–21*A*) correlates in most studies with local recurrence after resection, visceral metastases, and decreased survival, but it may not be of independent prognostic value for tumors confined to the bowel wall. Although lymphatic invasion is associated with decreased survival, it is not clear whether this variable is independent of depth of tumor invasion and regional nodal metastasis. Perineural invasion (Fig. 115–21*B*) is also linked to increased local recurrence and decreased survival, but the data are limited. The degree of inflammatory response and lymphocytic infiltration in and around a cancer may be related to outcome, increased inflammation, and immune reaction conferring better prognosis, but, once again, the data are limited.

The prognosis of patients with colorectal cancer may be related to the DNA content of the primary tumor,[152, 153] since survival is shorter for patients with nondiploid or aneuploid tumors than for those whose tumor cells have a normal or diploid DNA content. Although the DNA content of the primary tumor may correlate with the potential for local or distant recurrence after primary resection, the value of routine flow cytometric measurements or image analysis of the DNA content of tumor cells for assessing clinical prognosis and planning treatment remains to be determined. Deletions in chromosomes 18q and 17p (p53) may be important indicators of prognosis, independent of stage.[70–73, 78, 79] As indi-

Table 115–10 | **Staging of Colorectal Cancer—American Joint Committee on Cancer (TNM Classification)**

STAGE 0
Carcinoma in situ intraepithelial or invasion of lamina propria* (Tis N0 M0)
STAGE I
Tumor invades submucosa (T1 N0 M0) Dukes' A
Tumor invades muscularis propria (T2 N0 M0)
STAGE II
Tumor invades through the muscularis propria into subserosa or into nonperitonealized pericolic or perirectal tissues (T3 N0 M0) Dukes' B
Tumor perforates the visceral peritoneum or directly invades other organs or structures and/or perforates visceral peritoneum** (T4 N0 M0)
STAGE III
Any degree of bowel wall perforation with regional lymph node metastasis
N1 Metastasis in 1 to 3 regional lymph nodes
N2 Metastasis in 4 or more regional lymph nodes
Any T N1 M0, Dukes' C
Any T N2 M0
STAGE IV
Any invasion of bowel wall with or without lymph node metastasis, but with evidence of distant metastasis.
Any T Any N, M1

Based on American Joint Committee on Cancer Manual for Staging of Cancer, 5th ed.[140] Dukes' B (corresponds to stage II) is a composite of better (T3, N0, M0) and worse (T4, N0, M0) prognostic groups, as is Dukes' C (corresponds to stage III) (Any T,N1, M0 and Any T, N2, M0).

Definitions: NX = regional lymph nodes cannot be assessed, N0 = no regional lymph node metastasis, MX = distant metastasis cannot be assessed, M0 = no distant metastasis, M1 = distant metastasis.

*Note: Tis includes cancer cells confined within the glandular basement membrane (intraepithelial) or lamina propria (intramucosal) with no extension through the muscularis mucosae into the submucosa.

**Note: Direct invasion in T4 includes invasion of other segments of the colorectum by way of the serosa; for example, invasion of the sigmoid colon by a carcinoma of the cecum.

Used with the permission of the American Joint Committee on Cancer (AJCC7), Chicago, Illinois. The original source for this material is the AJCC7 Cancer Staging Manual, 5th edition (1997) published by Lippincott-Raven Publishers, Philadelphia, Pennsylvania.

cated in Table 115–11, a growing number of other molecular markers also may predict prognosis or response to therapy.[79]

Clinical Features

Whereas screening programs for colorectal cancer suggest that tumors diagnosed in asymptomatic patients are less advanced, assessment of the impact of early diagnosis on survival of asymptomatic persons awaits the results of prospective, randomized, controlled studies such as the Prostate, Lung, Colorectal and Ovarian Cancer Screening Trial (PLCO).[154] Duration of symptoms may not correlate directly with prognosis, and some presenting symptoms (such as rectal bleeding) may be associated with better rates of survival.

Bowel obstruction or perforation has been linked with poor prognosis. Patients who present with obstructing lesions may not be candidates for curative surgery and have higher rates of operative morbidity and mortality. Recurrence following "curative" surgery is also higher in patients who present with obstruction or perforation.

The location of the primary tumor may influence outcome. Disease-free survival at 3 years appears to be 2% to 14% higher following surgery for tumors of the left than of the right colon. Some studies suggest a survival advantage for patients with colon versus rectal cancers.

As many as 3% of colorectal carcinomas arise before age 30 years, and only 11% have a predisposing condition such as FAP or UC. The prognosis is worse than for older patients and is particularly poor in the pediatric age group. Poor prognosis may be related to a higher percentage of more advanced cancers and mucinous adenocarcinomas in these younger patients. Patients with tumors demonstrating MSI, on the other hand, appear to have a better prognosis

Table 115–11 | **Pathologic, Molecular, and Clinical Features That May Affect Prognosis in Patients with Colorectal Cancer**

FEATURE OR MARKER	EFFECT ON PROGNOSIS
Pathologic	
Surgical-pathologic stage	
Depth of bowel wall penetration	Increased penetration diminishes prognosis
Number of regional nodes involved by tumor	1–4 nodes better than > 4 nodes
Tumor morphology/histology	
Degree of differentiation	Well differentiated better than poorly differentiated
Mucinous (colloid) or signet-ring-cell histology	Diminished prognosis
Scirrhous histology	Diminished prognosis
Venous invasion	Diminished prognosis
Lymphatic invasion	Diminished prognosis
Perineural invasion	Diminished prognosis
Local inflammation and immunologic reaction	Improved prognosis
Tumor morphology	Polypoid/exophytic better than ulcerating/infiltrating
Tumor DNA content	Increased DNA content (aneuploidy) diminishes prognosis
Tumor size	No effect in most studies
Molecular	
Loss of heterozygosity at chromosome 18q (*DCC, DPC4*)	Diminished prognosis
Loss of heterozygosity at chromosome 17p (p53)	Diminished prognosis
Loss of heterozygosity at chromosome 8p	Diminished prognosis
Increased labeling index for $p21^{WAF/CIP1}$ protein	Improved prognosis
Microsatellite instability	Improved prognosis
Mutation in *BAX* gene	Diminished prognosis
Clinical	
Diagnosis in asymptomatic patients	?Improved prognosis
Duration of symptoms	No demonstrated effect
Rectal bleeding as presenting symptom	Improved prognosis
Bowel obstruction	Diminished prognosis
Bowel perforation	Diminished prognosis
Tumor location	?Colon better than rectum ?Left colon better than right colon
Age less than 30 yr	Diminished prognosis
Preoperative CEA	Diminished prognosis with high CEA level
Distant metastases	Markedly diminished prognosis

CEA, carcinoembryonic antigen.

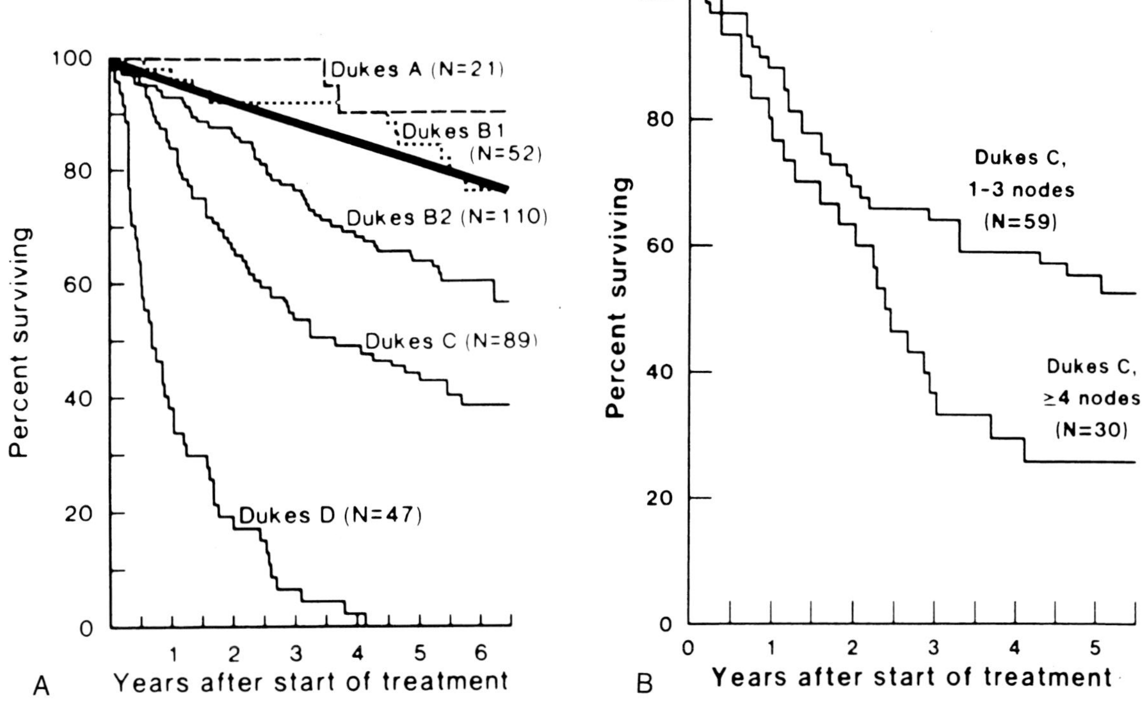

Figure 115–20. *A,* Survival probabilities according to Duke's stage as modified by Astler-Coller (Table 115–9) in patients undergoing potentially curative surgery for colorectal cancer. Expected survival among age- and sex-matched general population is indicated by the heavy line. *B,* Survival probabilities according to the number of nodes involved in patients with stage C colorectal carcinoma. (From Moertel CG, O'Fallon JR, Go VL, et al: The preoperative carcinoembryonic antigen test in the diagnosis, staging, and prognosis of colorectal cancer. Cancer 58:603, 1986.)

irrespective of patient age.[90, 91] Thus, whereas colorectal cancers occur at a younger age in those with HNPCC, these individuals have a better prognosis than those with microsatellite stable cancers.

Outcome is related to the preoperative serum carcinoembryonic antigen (CEA) level.[147, 155] Tumor recurrence is higher, and the estimated mean time to recurrence shorter, in patients with Dukes' B and C cancers who have high preoperative CEA levels. The preoperative CEA level may be of prognostic value only in patients with Dukes' C colorectal cancers who also have 4 or more involved lymph nodes (stage C2), but CEA level may not be indicative of survival probability in patients with Dukes' A and B lesions or Dukes' C lesions with fewer than 4 nodes involved. Expression of mucin-associated carbohydrate antigens other than CEA, such as sialyl Lewis^x, may also correlate with prognosis.[97, 99, 100] Expression of the carbohydrate-binding protein galectin-3 correlates with tumor progression in the colon and may confer a poor prognosis.[101]

Approximately one fourth of patients with colorectal cancer exhibit clinical evidence of hematogenous spread when initially seen, and half eventually develop metastases to a

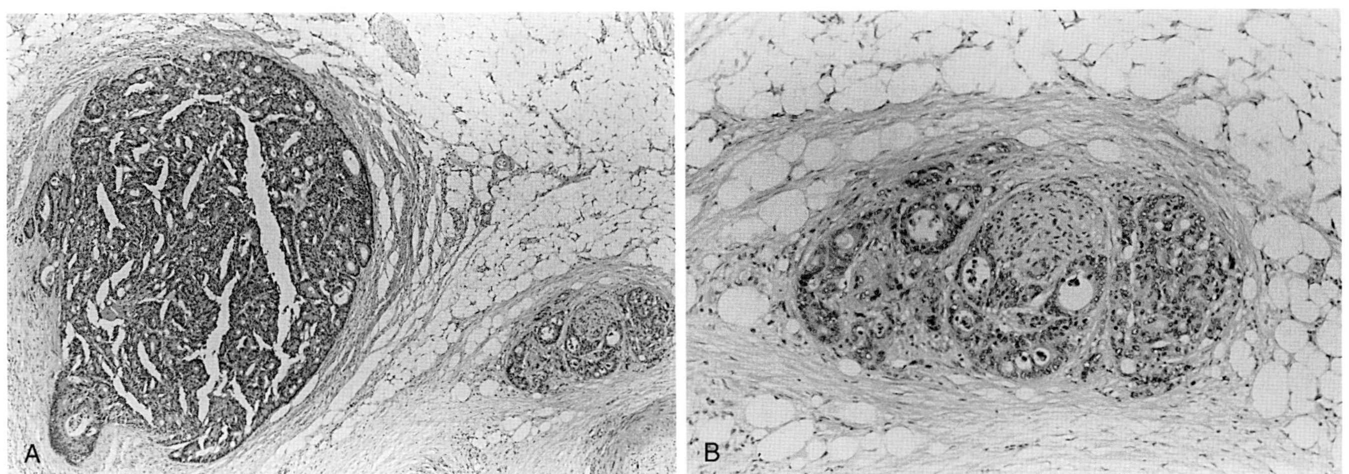

Figure 115–21. *A,* Pathologic features that may influence prognosis negatively include venous invasion (*left*) and perineural invasion (*right*). *B,* High-power view of perineural invasion by tumor.

distant site, usually the liver. These metastases carry a very poor prognosis at all times in the clinical course. The most important determinant of survival time for patients who present with liver metastases is the extent of hepatic involvement by tumor.

CLINICAL PRESENTATIONS

Adenocarcinomas of the colon and rectum grow slowly and may be present as long as 5 years before symptoms appear. However, persons with asymptomatic cancers often have occult blood loss from their tumors, and the bleeding rate increases with tumor size and degree of ulceration (Fig. 115–22).

Symptoms depend to some extent on the site of the primary tumor. Cancers of the proximal colon usually grow larger before they produce symptoms than do those of the left colon and rectum. Constitutional symptoms (fatigue, shortness of breath, angina) secondary to microcytic hypochromic anemia may be the principal presentation of right colon tumors. Less often, blood from right colon cancers is admixed with stool and appears as "mahogany feces." As a tumor grows, it produces vague abdominal discomfort or presents as a palpable mass. Obstruction is uncommon because of the large diameters of the cecum and ascending colon, although cecal cancers may block the ileocecal valve and cause distal small bowel obstruction.

The left colon has a narrower lumen than the proximal colon, and cancers of the descending and sigmoid colon often involve the bowel circumferentially and cause obstructive symptoms. Patients may present with colicky abdominal pain, particularly after meals, and a change in bowel habits. Constipation may alternate with increased frequency of defe-

Table 115–12 | **Differential Diagnosis of Colorectal Cancer**

Mass lesions
Benign tumors (mucosal and submucosal)
Diverticulosis
Inflammatory masses
Diverticulitis
Inflammatory bowel disease
Ischemia
Infections (tuberculosis, amebiasis, fungal infection)
Strictures
Inflammatory bowel disease (Crohn's colitis)
Ischemia
Radiation (late sequelae)
Rectal bleeding
Hemorrhoidal bleeding
Diverticulosis
Ulcerative colitis/Crohn's colitis
Infectious colitis
Ischemic colitis
Solitary rectal ulcer
Abdominal pain
Ischemia
Diverticulitis
Inflammatory bowel disease
Irritable bowel syndrome
Change in bowel habits
Inflammatory bowel disease
Infectious diarrhea
Medications (constipation or diarrhea)
Irritable bowel syndrome

This list includes common clinical situations that may be initially confused with signs or symptoms of colorectal cancer, but it is not meant to be inclusive.

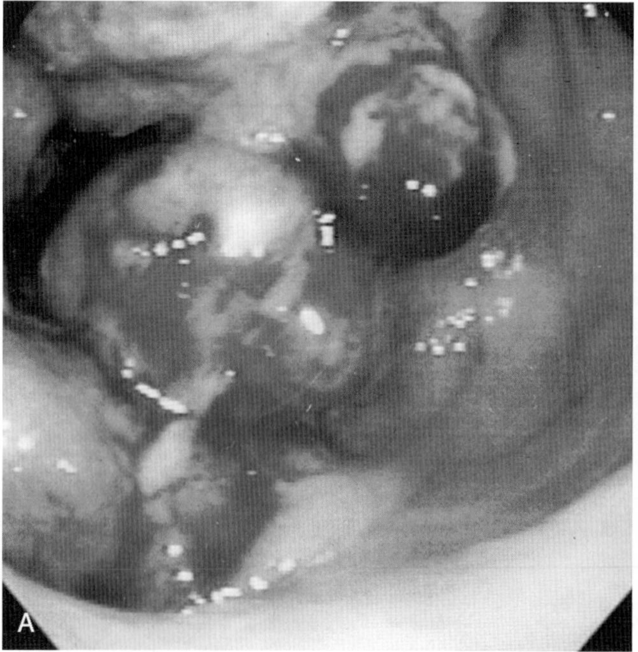

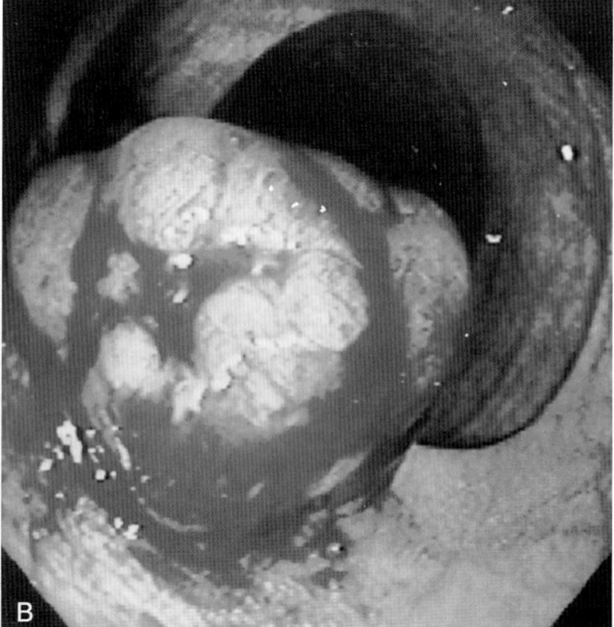

Figure 115–22. Colonoscopic view of bleeding carcinomas of the sigmoid colon (*A*) and cecum (*B*). Carcinomas of the colon often bleed intermittently. Patients may present with evidence of microcytic anemia or with red blood per rectum (hematochezia), depending on tumor site and amount of blood loss.

cation, as small amounts of retained stool move beyond the obstructing lesion. Hematochezia is present more often with distal lesions than with proximal ones, and bright red blood passed per rectum or coating the surface of the stool is common with cancers of the left colon and rectum. Rectal cancers also cause obstruction and changes in bowel habits, including constipation, diarrhea, and tenesmus. Rectal cancers may invade locally to involve the bladder, vaginal wall, or surrounding nerves, resulting in perineal or sacral pain, but this is a late occurrence.

Symptomatic patients with colorectal cancer are often misdiagnosed. Symptoms are ascribed to benign conditions such as diverticular disease (abdominal pain, bleeding, change in stool caliber), irritable bowel syndrome (abdominal pain, change in bowel habits), or hemorrhoids (rectal bleeding) (Table 115–12). Colorectal carcinoma should be considered when a patient—especially one older than 40 years—presents with hypochromic microcytic anemia or frank hematochezia and rectal bleeding. Too often, anemia in elderly people is ascribed to "chronic disease," only to be diagnosed later as a sign of advanced colorectal cancer. Abdominal pain—in any form—and bleeding also merit evaluation for cancer in this age group. Large bowel cancer may affect younger patients, particularly those with inflammatory bowel disease or a strong family history for colorectal and other cancers. Judicious evaluation of younger patients for colorectal cancer is therefore warranted when suggested by history and clinical presentation.

DIAGNOSIS AND SCREENING

Diagnosis When Colorectal Cancer Is Suspected

When colorectal cancer is suspected because of clinical signs and symptoms or when screening suggests the possibility of a large bowel tumor (discussed later), prompt endoscopic or radiographic diagnostic evaluation should be undertaken (Fig. 115–23). Colonoscopy is more accurate than air-contrast barium enema, especially for detecting small lesions such as adenomas less than 1 cm; up to half of adenomas larger than 1 cm may be missed by barium enema.[156–158] If colonoscopy is unavailable, technically difficult, or refused by the patient, an air-contrast barium enema should be performed following sigmoidoscopy. Air-contrast examinations are more accurate than full-column barium enemas, not only for diagnosing cancers but also for detecting small adenomas, which are often present intercurrently. Neoplasms in the rectum and sigmoid colon are sometimes difficult to diagnose radiologically, and proctosigmoidoscopy should be used as a complement to double-contrast enema imaging. Flexible sigmoidoscopy is superior to rigid sigmoidoscopy.

If a carcinoma is detected radiographically or by sigmoidoscopy, a full colonoscopic examination should be done because of the high incidence of synchronous lesions and the possible implications of the colonoscopic findings for the surgical treatment plan. As many as half the patients with proven cancers of the colon and rectum may harbor additional lesions, and for almost 10% the operative plan will have to be modified as a result of preoperative colonoscopy.

Principles of Screening

Cancer prevention may be categorized as primary or secondary. Primary prevention concerns the ability to identify genetic, biologic, and environmental factors that are etiologic or pathogenetic and to alter their effects on tumor development. Although several areas of study have been identified that may lead to primary prevention of large bowel cancer, available data do not yet provide a firm basis for the practical application of primary preventive measures. The goal of secondary prevention is to identify existing preneoplastic and early neoplastic lesions, symptomatic and asymptomatic, and to treat them thoroughly and expeditiously. The assumption is that early detection improves prognosis. In symptomatic patients it is important to minimize the delay in diagnosis. When the clinical setting suggests colorectal malignant disease (e.g., iron deficiency anemia in an elderly patient), prompt diagnostic evaluation should be undertaken. This approach pertains to individual patients and small groups seen in daily practice and is known as *case finding*. *Screening* pertains to large populations. Screening an asymptomatic

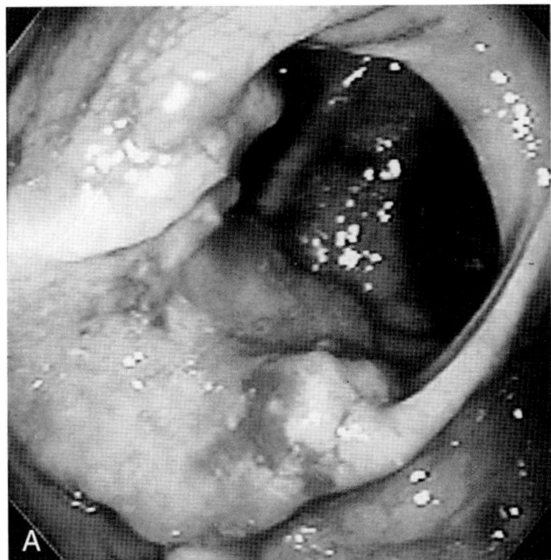

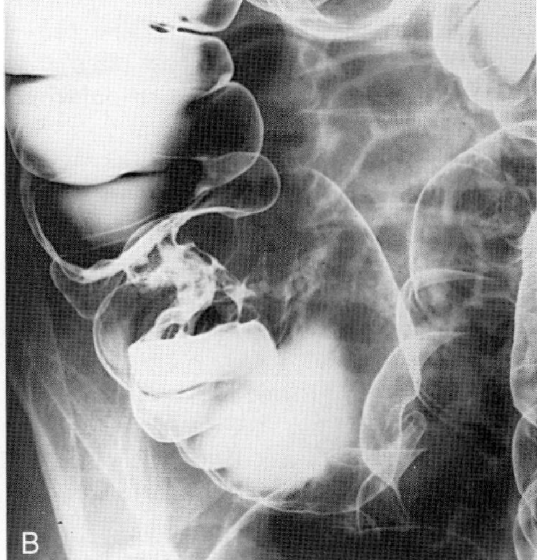

Figure 115–23. Carcinoma of the cecum infiltrating a cecal fold as seen by *(A)* colonoscopy and *(B)* air-contrast barium enema.

Table 115–13 | **Average-Risk Screening Guidelines**

SCREENING TOOL	USPSTF*	MULTIDISCIPLINARY EXPERT PANEL†	AMERICAN CANCER SOCIETY‡
FOBT	Recommended annually	Recommended annually	Recommended annually as an option
Flexible sigmoidoscopy	Recommended (periodicity unspecified)	Recommended every 5 yr	Recommended every 5 yr as an option
FOBT + flexible sigmoidoscopy	Recommended as an option	Recommended as an option	Annual FOBT plus flexible sigmoidoscopy every 5 yr recommended as an option
Colonoscopy	Insufficient evidence	Recommended as an option every 10 yr	Recommended as an option every 10 yr
Double-contrast barium enema	Insufficient evidence	Recommended as an option every 5–10 yr	Recommended as an option every 5 yr

*U.S. Preventive Services Task Force (reference 159).
†Reference 161. Endorsed by numerous medical and surgical societies.
‡Updated guidelines, 2001 (reference 121), provides menu of options rather than recommending any specific option in order to increase compliance with screening. Fecal occult blood testing (FOBT) should use take-home sample method. All positive tests should be followed up with colonoscopy.

population for any disease is worthwhile if (1) the disease represents a major health problem, (2) effective therapy is available if the disease is found, (3) a sensitive and specific screening test is available that is readily acceptable to patients and physicians, and (4) the screening test is cost effective.

Colorectal cancer fulfills the first two of these conditions, since it represents a major health problem, and localized lesions are curable by surgical resection. Furthermore, the prolonged natural history of colonic neoplasia affords time to detect and eliminate early neoplastic lesions before they reach an advanced, incurable stage. The challenge that remains is to develop effective, easily administered, and cost-effective screening tests for the disease. Current evidence indicates that screening for colorectal cancer reduces related mortality. This finding has resulted in a new recommendation by the United States Preventive Services Task Force: screening for colorectal cancer be performed in all persons aged 50 years and older by *annual* fecal occult blood testing (FOBT) or sigmoidoscopy, or both (periodicity not specified).[159] Although the American Cancer Society[119, 120] and the World Health Organization[160] currently advocate annual FOBT and flexible sigmoidoscopy *every 5 years*, the optimal interval for testing and the benefit of combined screening with these modalities remain to be determined.

Almost all major health-related agencies have endorsed screening for colorectal cancer (Table 115–13), but the key questions of "who, how, and how often" remain a source of debate. In 1997, clinical practice guidelines for colorectal cancer screening were published in a 48-page document and endorsed by several major agencies.[161] These Agency for Health Care Policy Research (AHCPR) guidelines set forth a variety of options for colorectal cancer screening (FOBT, sigmoidoscopy, colonoscopy, air contrast barium enema) and provided a lengthy rationale for each. The American Cancer Society followed shortly thereafter with its own set of guidelines for colorectal cancer screening and surveillance.[119] These guidelines provided recommendations in three major categories based on risk (average, moderate, and high). Moderate- and high-risk categories were further subdivided according to personal and family history of adenoma, carcinoma, or predisposing disease.

Average risk is defined as all people 50 years or older who do not fall into moderate- or high-risk categories. This category encompasses 70% to 80% of individuals in the American population. Annual FOBT plus flexible sigmoidoscopy every 5 years was recommended for this group. Colonoscopy every 10 years, or double-contrast barium enema (DCBE) every 5 to 10 years, was provided as an alternative screening modality.

In 2001, the American Cancer Society updated these recommendations to offer a broader set of screening choices for different levels of colorectal cancer risk.[121] This was to allow for greater flexibility in achieving screening goals, due to evidence showing little progress in improving colorectal cancer screening rates.[162] Screening options included FOBT annually, flexible sigmoidoscopy every 5 years, annual FOBT plus flexible sigmoidoscopy every 5 years (preferred to either alone), DCBE every 5 years, or colonoscopy every 10 years (see Table 115–13). Although each of the choices has inherent characteristics related to accuracy, prevention, potential costs, and risks, the concept is that any one of the tests is better than no test at all. Multiple options can be confusing, however, to both patients and physicians. Furthermore, the test options are not of equal efficacy, and such guidelines may lead to coverage of suboptimal testing by third-party payers.

The willingness of both patients and physicians to comply with recommendations for screening programs has a major impact on the effectiveness of colorectal cancer screening. Compliance by both potential screenees and physicians has historically been poor, and interventions to increase screening adherence have been disappointing.[163] The Year 2000 goals set forth by the National Cancer Institute in 1996 called for 50% of the population older than 40 years to have had FOBT tests within the prior 2 years, a goal that has not been met. Compliance rates are generally higher for FOBT than for sigmoidoscopy. Clinical trials report compliance rates of 50% to 80% for FOBT among volunteers,[164–173] but much lower rates (15% to 30%) are reported from community screening programs.[164, 172, 173] Data from the 1992 National Health Interview Survey indicated that only 17% of the population older than 49 years reported FOBT within the past year and 26% in the past 3 years, whereas the median adherence rate to programmatic offers of FOBT was 40% to 50%, depending on the type of population. Adherence to recommended follow-up testing after an initial positive FOBT result may also be lower in the community setting than in larger screening trials. Up to one third of people who test positive also may not respond to requests for follow-up. A recent analysis of diagnostic testing following positive FOBT in elderly medicine recipients[174] indicated that not only was compliance poor, but follow-up diagnostic testing was often inadequate or improper. Unfortunately, compliance is often poorer among elderly persons, who are at greatest risk for colon cancer, and among minorities[6] in whom mortality is high. Despite the availability of flexible sigmoidoscopy (FS), most elderly patients are reluctant to have this test because of cost, discomfort, and fear.

While most physicians agree in principle with guidelines for sigmoidoscopic screening, many do not follow them with all patients. Reluctance to perform what is perceived as an uncomfortable and invasive procedure in asymptomatic persons, requirements for training, and limitations of time and resources contribute to reluctance on the part of primary care physicians. Compliance is also extremely important in any determination of cost effectiveness.[164, 175]

Compliance with colorectal cancer screening has a major impact on the cost effectiveness of such programs. In one model, the cost per death prevented as the result of FOBT increased from $225,000 to $331,000 as compliance decreased from 100% to 50%.[164] FOBT is especially sensitive to the impact of compliance compared with other tests.[164, 175]

In the absence of firm clinical data indicating which screening strategy provides the best balance of sensitivity, specificity, logistic feasibility, and cost, various mathematical models have been employed to examine this issue.[156, 164, 175, 176] One cost analysis[156] compared five screening programs during a 10-year interval (for persons aged 55 to 65 years), including annual FOBT alone, FS every 5 years, FS and FOBT combined, one-time colonoscopy, and air-contrast barium enema. FOBT alone was the most cost-effective modality ($225,000 per death prevented at 100% compliance), but it prevented fewer cancer deaths than other programs and required the highest level of compliance to achieve a targeted mortality reduction. The addition of FS to FOBT resulted in a 2.2-fold increase in cancer prevention (22.5% versus 50%) but was more costly ($250,000 per death prevented). The cost effectiveness of FS alone was similar to that of FS plus FOBT, but their screening approach prevented fewer deaths. One-time colonoscopy ($274,000 per death prevented) had the greatest impact on colorectal cancer mortality (68% of cancers prevented), largely because of assumptions that cancer would be prevented in most patients undergoing polypectomy. Barium enema was not cost effective relative to other screening programs. Compliance was an important determinant of effectiveness for all the programs.

Another study suggests that screening elderly patients from age 65 years with annual FOBT plus FS every 3 years would cost approximately $43,000 per year of life gained.[156] This compares with annual breast cancer screening with mammography (approximately $34,500 per year of life gained) and with hemodialysis for end-stage renal disease (estimated at $36,000 per year of life gained). The cost effectiveness of three screening strategies (annual FOBT, sigmoidoscopy every 5 years, or colonoscopy every 10 years) was recently compared using a computer model of 100,000 persons 50 years of age.[175] This model takes into account the costs of follow-up events. Positive results on FOBT or adenomatous polyps found at sigmoidoscopy are worked up using colonoscopy. After polypectomy, colonoscopy is repeated every 3 years until no polyps are found. This study indicated that colonoscopy represented a cost-effective means of screening for colorectal cancer because it reduces mortality at relatively low incremental costs. Compliance rates render colonoscopy every 10 years the most cost-effective primary screening strategy for colorectal cancer, according to this study.

The use of screening modalities for detection of adenomatous polyps is discussed in Chapter 114. Table 115–14 presents some of the characteristics of tests used to diagnose and screen for colorectal neoplasms.

Table 115–14 | **Procedures for Diagnosing and Screening for Colorectal Polyps and Cancers**

Proportion of adenomatous polyps and cancers that can be detected by various instruments:	
Rigid sigmoidoscope	30%
60-cm flexible sigmoidoscope	55%
Colonoscope	95%
Air-contrast barium enema	92%
Single-column barium enema	85%
Random false-negative rates:	
FOBT	40%
Sigmoidoscopies*	15%
Colonoscopy	5%
Air-contrast barium enema	15%
Single-column barium enema	30%
Random false-positive rates:	
FOBT†	2%
Air-contrast barium enema	3.5%
Single-column barium enema	3%
Complications:‡	
Bleeding rate with diagnostic colonoscopy	0.15%
Bleeding rate with polypectomy	2%
Perforation rate with diagnostic colonoscopy	0.2%
Perforation rate with polypectomy	0.38%
Perforation rate with sigmoidoscopy	0.011%
Cost for each procedure in U.S. dollars:§	
FOBT	$3.50
Flexible sigmoidoscopy	$400.56
Colonoscopy	$695.95
Colonoscopy with polypectomy	$1003.76
Air-contrast barium enema	$118.86
Single-column barium enema	$159.77

*Rigid sigmoidoscopy may miss two to three times as many lesions as flexible sigmoidoscopy in examining the same bowel segment.

†A false-positive FOBT will lead to additional work-up and charges. This needs to be considered in assessing the cost of a false-positive FOBT.

‡Also see Chapter 30.

§Costs are based on average Medicare payments in 2000. These do not reflect actual charges at a given institution or the costs of resultant additional evaluation after a positive test.

FOBT, fecal occult blood test.

Results from Eddy DM, Nugent FW, Eddy JW, et al: Screening for colorectal cancer in a high-risk population. Results of a mathematical model. Gastroenterology 92:682, 1987; and Sonnenberg A, Delco F, Inadomi JM: Cost effectiveness of colonoscopy in screening for colorectal cancer. Ann Intern Med 133:573, 2000.

Screening Techniques

Fecal Occult Blood Testing

Qualitative chromogen tests, which rely on the oxidative conversion of a colorless compound to a colored one in the presence of the pseudoperoxidase activity of hemoglobin, have been standardized employing guaiac-impregnated paper and developing solutions (hydrogen peroxide in denatured

Table 115–15 | **Proper Performance of the Slide Guaiac Test for Fecal Occult Blood**

1. For three days before and during testing, patients should avoid:
   a. Rare red meat
   b. Peroxidase-containing vegetable/fruits (e.g., broccoli, turnip, cantaloupe, cauliflower, radish)
   c. The following medications:
      Iron supplements
      Vitamin C
      Aspirin and other NSAIDs
2. Two samples of each of three consecutive stools should be tested. (It is proper to sample areas of obvious blood.)
3. Slides should be developed within 4–6 days. Slides should not be rehydrated prior to developing (for average-risk screening). If rehydrated, red meat must have been avoided (otherwise, too many false-positives).

alcohol) and have been widely studied and utilized clinically (e.g., Hemoccult, Hemoccult II). These are commercially available, convenient, and inexpensive; however, their effectiveness in detecting occult blood in the stool depends on the degree of fecal hydration (increases sensitivity), amount of hemoglobin degradation during storage or by focal flora (decreases sensitivity), and the absence of interfering substances (e.g., ascorbic acid) that can either enhance or inhibit oxidation of the indicator dye.

Any food-containing compounds that have pseudoperoxidase or peroxidase activity (such as nonhuman hemoglobin in rare red meat and uncooked fruits and vegetables) can produce a positive reaction. Red meat and peroxidase-containing foods (broccoli, turnips, cauliflower, radishes, cantaloupes), therefore, should be avoided for 3 days before and during testing. Although a drop of water added to the slide before development (rehydration) increases sensitivity, this is not recommended for screening average-risk populations, as it gives too many false-positive results. If rehydration is considered, dietary restriction to exclude peroxidase- and heme-rich foods is especially important. Some studies report false-positive FOBT results in patients who took a supplemental iron preparation, but recent studies have reported few or no false-positive FOBTs in those patients. Recommendations for proper performance of these tests are listed in Table 115–15, and the advantages and limitations of FOBT with the Hemoccult-type slide guaiac tests are outlined in Table 115–16.

Colorectal cancers and adenomas bleed intermittently, and detection of fecal occult blood by Hemoccult test depends on the degree of blood loss. In general, 2 mL of blood in the stool is necessary to produce a positive result. Sampling multiple stool specimens is, therefore, likely to result in fewer false-negative evaluations. Sampling one specimen yields a 40% to 50% false-negative rate, which improves (i.e., false negatives decrease) progressively as more stools are sampled. Two samples of each of three consecutive (daily) stools should therefore be tested. Location of the lesion also affects the ability to detect a cancer by Hemoccult (Table 115–17). Right-sided cancers produce fewer false-negative tests than cancers elsewhere in the colon, since large bulky tumors bleed frequently. Potential "blind spots" of the Hemoccult test with high false-negative rates include the transverse and descending colon. Although the value of a positive FOBT performed in conjunction with a digital rectal examination has been disputed (because of potential trauma), one study did not demonstrate an increase in false-positive tests when the FOBT was performed in this manner.[161]

In studies that have examined the potential benefit of FOBT for detecting colorectal neoplasms in large populations, compliance has been in the range of 50% to 70%, although elderly patients—those at substantial risk for colon cancer—tend to be less compliant. The overall positivity rate ranges from 2% to 6% of those tested, and the positive predictive value is about 20% for adenomas and 5% to 10% for cancers. The majority of studies report that a large percentage of detected cancers are Dukes' A and B lesions.

Large controlled studies of Hemoccult testing of asymptomatic patients in the general population have been reported

Table 115–16 | **Advantages and Limitations of the Guaiac-Impregnated Slide Test for Fecal Occult Blood Testing**

ADVANTAGES
Readily available
Convenient
Inexpensive
Good patient compliance in motivated groups
DISADVANTAGES
Depends on degree of fecal hydration
Affected by storage (hemoglobin degradation)
Affected by tumor location (see Table 115–17)
FALSE-POSITIVE TESTS
Exogenous peroxidase activity
Red meat (nonhuman hemoglobin)
Uncooked fruits and vegetables (vegetable peroxidase; see Table 115–15)
Any source of gastrointestinal blood loss (epistaxis, gingival bleeding, upper GI tract pathology, hemorrhoids, and so on)
Medications
Topical iodine
Aspirin, nonsteroidal anti-inflammatory agents (induce upper GI bleeding)
FALSE-NEGATIVE TESTS
Storage of slides
Degradation of hemoglobin by colonic bacteria
Ascorbic acid (vitamin C) ingestion
Improper sampling/developing
Lesion not bleeding at time of stool collection

Table 115–17 | **Colorectal Cancer: Rate of Blood Loss and Detectability by Hemoccult Testing**

LOCATION	MEAN DAILY BLOOD LOSS* (mL)	FALSE-NEGATIVE HEMOCCULT (Standard Method)
Ascending colon and cecum	9.3	17
Transverse and descending colon	1.5	46
Sigmoid colon	1.9	36
Rectum	1.8	31
Overall		31

*Determined by injecting ^{51}Cr-labeled erythrocytes intravenously and measuring fecal excretion of label. Normal stool contains less than 1 mL of blood per day.

Data from Macrae F, St John DJ: Relationship between patterns of bleeding and Hemoccult sensitivity in patients with colorectal cancers or adenomas. Gastroenterology 82:891, 1982.

Table 115–18 | **Controlled Trials of Fecal Occult Blood Testing (FOBT) in Screening Asymptomatic Persons for Colorectal Cancer**[166–170, 177]

	MINNESOTA	NOTTINGHAM	GOTEBORG	FUNEN	NEW YORK
Study population	46,000 50–80 yr	152,850 50–74 yr	28,000 60–64 yr	61,933 45–74 yr	22,000 ≥40 yr
Study design	Random; annual vs. biennial control	Random	Random	Random; biennial vs. control	Allocation by month-assigned
Rehydration of test cards*	Yes—most	No	Yes—most	No	No
Compliance	Annual 75%; biennial 78%	50%		56%	
Positivity rate	2.4% (nonhydrated) 9.8% (rehydrated)	1st screen: 2.1% 2nd screen: 1.2%	1st screen: 1.9% (nonhydrated); 5.8% (rehydrated) 2nd screen: 4.8% (prev. rehydrated); 8.0% (prev. nonhydrated)	1st screen: 1.0% 2nd screen: 0.8% 3rd screen: 0.9% 4th screen: 1.3% 5th screen: 1.8%	Regular Attendees: 1.4% First time Screen: 2.6%
Positive predictive value for colorectal cancer	2.2% (rehydrated) 5.6% (nonhydrated)	1st round: 9.9% 2nd round: 11.9%	1st round: 5.0% (nonhydrated) 2nd round: 4.2% (rehydrated)	1st round: 17.7% 2nd round: 8.4%	10.7%
Colorectal cancer (CRC) mortality†	18-yr follow-up: 33% reduction for annual group; 21% reduction for biennial group; CRC mortality/1000: Annual: 9.46% [7.75–11.17] Biennial: 11.19% [9.39–12.99] Control: 14.09% [12.01–16.17] Mortality ratio: Annual 0.67 [0.51–0.83] Biennial 0.79 [0.62–0.97]	7.8-yr follow-up: 15% reduction in cumulative CRC mortality Mortality ratio: 0.85 [0.74–0.98]	Not yet available	10-yr follow-up: 18% reduction in CRC-related mortality in screened group Mortality ratio: 0.82 [0.68–0.99]	10 yr follow-up: 43% reduction in CRC mortality in screened group

*Hemoccult test cards were used—rehydrated or nonhydrated.
†Reductions in mortality are relative risk reductions. Data in brackets represent 95% confidence intervals.

from the United States,[167, 177] Great Britain,[166] and Scandinavia[168–170] (Table 115–18). These studies cite a rate of test positivity of 1% to 2.6% on first screen for nonhydrated slides and a predictive value for colonic neoplasms (adenomas plus carcinomas) of 22% to 58%. The positive predictive value for carcinomas alone is substantially less (5.6% to 18% for nonhydrated slides). Rehydration of slides with a drop of water before processing results in an increase in positivity and sensitivity but in a decrease in specificity and positive predictive value. Eighteen-year follow-up in the Minnesota trial[177] demonstrated a marked reduction in Dukes' stage D cancers in the screened groups in comparison with the control group. Long-term follow-up of patients tested with Hemoccult in a large group practice setting (Kaiser) has yielded similar results.[171] The predictive value of a positive test for colorectal carcinoma was 8% at 1 year, 10% at 2 years, and 11% at 4 years. Predictive value depends on what group is screened, and it may be increased in older age groups.

Mortality data are now available from the Minnesota Study, a randomized controlled trial that has provided the best evidence for the effectiveness of screening with FOBT.[167, 177] After 13 years of follow-up, data indicate a 33% reduction in colorectal cancer–associated mortality with annual screening, but an insignificant reduction of approximately 5% with biannual screening. Approximately 80% of samples were rehydrated, yielding a high positivity rate of 9.8% (compared with 2.4% for nonhydrated slides). This resulted in a 38% rate of colonoscopy, leading some to suggest that a substantial portion of the mortality reduction was due to chance detection through colonoscopy of nonbleeding cancers.[173] This has been refuted by the investigators, who find that only 6% to 11% of the mortality reduction was due to chance detection.

Results of 18 years of follow-up have recently been reported. Cumulative 18-year colorectal cancer mortality remains 33% lower in the annual group than in the control group. The group tested with biennial screening now demonstrates a 21% lower colorectal cancer mortality than the control group. Other randomized studies reported similar results. Data from Funen, Denmark, suggest an 18% decrease in colorectal cancer mortality during a ten-year study period,[168] and a recent update of data from Nottingham, UK, also indicates a 15% reduction in mortality at 7.8 years follow-up.[166] Data from New York suggest a 43% reduction in mortality in the screened group at 10 years.[160]

Methods that may decrease the false-positive rates of FOBT while maintaining or increasing sensitivity are currently being refined and compared for efficiency with Hemoccult-type slide tests. These include HemeSelect, an immunochemical test for human hemoglobin, and HemoQuant, a quantitative assay for fecal blood based on the fluorescence of heme-derived porphyrins. Hemoccult SENSA is a guaiac-based test similar to Hemoccult but has greater in vitro sensitivity. In one study, replicate stool samples with known lesions were tested with Hemoccult, Hemoccult SENSA,

HemoQuant, and HemeSelect. HemeSelect, the immunochemical test, was the most sensitive for detecting adenomas and carcinomas, while maintaining specificity.[178] The performance of Hemoccult, Hemoccult SENSA, and HemeSelect recently were tested prospectively in patients aged 50 years or older in a large managed-care setting.[179] Results of this study suggest that HemeSelect and a combination test in which HemeSelect is used to confirm positive Hemoccult SENSA provide more accurate results than Hemoccult in screening for colorectal cancer. In a cost effectiveness analysis of colorectal cancer screening in Japan, strategies that used an immunochemical test rather than a guaiac-based test were also found to be the most cost effective.[176]

Proctosigmoidoscopy

The benefit of proctosigmoidoscopy in screening programs for colorectal cancer was suggested by several uncontrolled studies that used the rigid proctosigmoidoscope. Those studies suggested that proctosigmoidoscopy in asymptomatic average-risk persons might detect early-stage cancers and that detection and removal of adenomas could result in a lower than expected frequency of rectosigmoid cancers in the screened population (see Chapter 114).

Two case-control studies provided strong evidence that sigmoidoscopy can reduce colorectal cancer mortality. A study from the Kaiser-Permanente Medical Care Program[180] compared 261 members who died of cancer of the rectum or distal colon with 868 age- and sex-matched control subjects. Only 8.8% of case subjects had undergone screening by rigid sigmoidoscopy, compared with 24.2% of controls. Rigid sigmoidoscopy had no effect on mortality in another group whose lesions were beyond the reach of the sigmoidoscope. Furthermore, the beneficial effect of sigmoidoscopy extended 10 years. This and a second case-control study[181] indicate that sigmoidoscopy can result in a 70% to 80% reduction in mortality from cancers within reach of the sigmoidoscope. Since approximately 50% of all colorectal cancers can be detected using the 60-cm flexible sigmoidoscope (see Fig. 115–3), these data suggest that periodic sigmoidoscopic screening could reduce overall colorectal cancer–related mortality by around one third. Because FS is superior to rigid instruments in detecting lesions, the flexible sigmoidoscope has replaced the rigid sigmoidoscope for colorectal cancer screening. A case-control study using FS and polypectomy[182] demonstrated a 60% reduction in colon cancer incidence associated with this procedure. Randomized, controlled trials are now under way to measure the effect of screening with FS on colorectal cancer mortality.[154] This procedure can be learned by nonphysicians and has been used successfully in screening programs that employ nurse practitioners.[183, 184]

Colonoscopy, Barium Enema, and Virtual Colonoscopy

Colonoscopy may well be the most effective tool for colorectal cancer screening, but data from prospective randomized trials are lacking. The National Polyp Study of polypectomy and surveillance strongly suggested a reduction in colorectal cancer mortality as the result of removing adenomatous polyps.[185] It has been argued that colonoscopy is preferable to sigmoidoscopy, since there may be a substantial incidence of proximal colonic cancers and advanced adenomas out of reach of the sigmoidoscopy.[186–190] Some of these individuals may not have distal findings on sigmoidoscopy that would trigger a subsequent colonoscopy. Two recent trials[189, 190] suggested that approximately 50% of individuals with advanced proximal neoplasms (adenoma >1 cm; adenoma with villous features or dysplasia; cancer) have no distal neoplasms. Less than 2% of those who did not have distal neoplasms, however, had an advanced proximal lesion.[189] Given the need for colonoscopic follow-up should FOBT or sigmoidoscopy be positive, colonoscopy may also prove to be cost effective.[175]

Air-contrast barium enema has been included as an option in a variety of screening guidelines. No studies, however, have directly addressed the effectiveness of barium enema for colon cancer screening. Several studies have indicated that the sensitivity of air-contrast barium enema is less than that of colonoscopy,[157, 158] especially for detecting lesions less than 1 cm.

"Virtual" colonoscopy involves the use of helical computed tomography (CT) to generate high-resolution, two-dimensional images of the abdomen and pelvis. Three-dimensional images of the colon can be reconstructed by computer generation off-line (Fig. 115–24).[191, 192] Virtual colonoscopy has the potential advantage of being a rapid and safe method of providing full structural evaluation of the entire colon. Low sensitivity and specificity and the need for rapid high-resolution helical CT scanners preclude its wide application for routine colorectal cancer screening at the moment. Improved software and techniques designed to improve the speed, accuracy, and reproducibility of results are emerging. Recognition of the importance of colorectal cancer screening has raised concerns over the ability of existing resources to handle the ensuing volume of expected procedures such as colonoscopy. Virtual colonoscopy using CT or magnetic resonance imaging could represent an alternate method with promise for the future.

Carcinoembryonic Antigen and Serologic Tumor Markers

A great deal of effort has been spent in search of serologic markers that would permit early detection and diagnosis of colorectal cancer. A variety of proteins, glycoproteins, and cellular and humoral substances have been studied as potential tumor markers, but none has been found to be specific for colorectal cancer. The most widely studied marker, carcinoembryonic antigen (CEA), may be useful in the preoperative staging and postoperative follow-up of patients with large bowel cancer, but it has a low predictive value for diagnosis in asymptomatic patients. The test's relatively low sensitivity and specificity combine to make it unsuitable for screening large asymptomatic populations. Several new protein and carbohydrate antigens are being examined, and such tests hold some promise in terms of specificity for preneoplastic and early neoplastic lesions in the colon.[97–101] How-

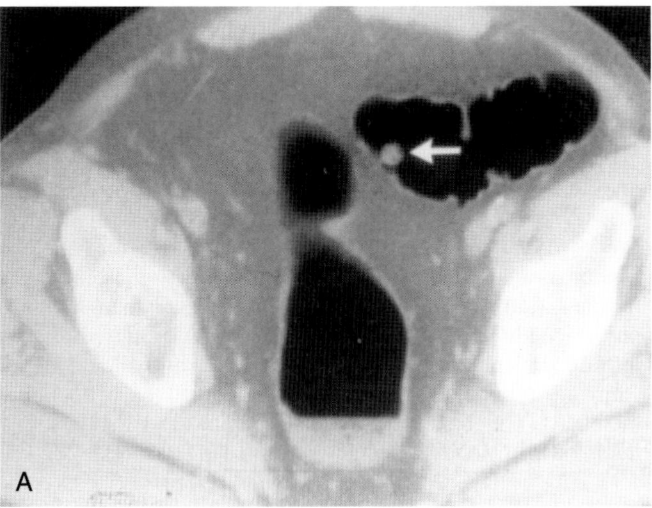

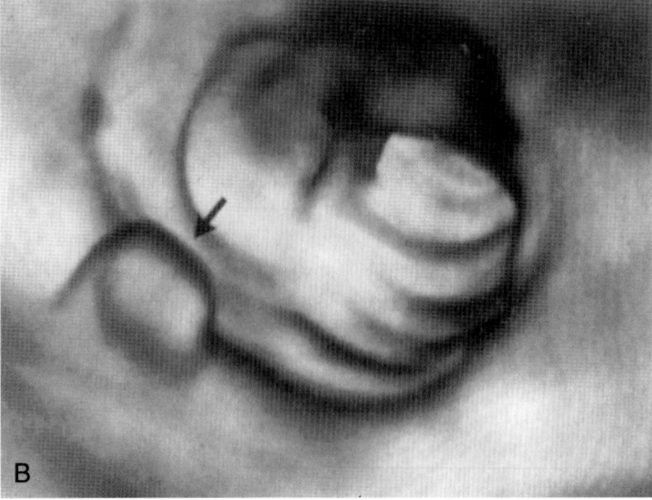

Figure 115–24. Virtual Colonoscopy. An 8-mm polyp identified on an axial two-dimensional CT image of the colon (*A, arrow*), and on an endoluminal three-dimensional reconstruction (*B*). (From Fenlon HM, Nunes DP, Schroy PC, et al: A comparison of virtual and conventional colonoscopy for the detection of colorectal polyps. N Engl J Med 341:1496, 1999.)

ever, their effectiveness for screening remains to be determined.

Genetic Testing

A great deal of knowledge has been accumulated recently about genetic alterations that occur during colon carcinogenesis (discussed earlier), but specific tests are not currently available for the majority of patients at risk for developing colorectal cancer (sporadic colorectal cancer). In a preliminary study, *ras* gene mutations could be identified in the stool of patients with adenomas and carcinomas.[193] More recently, the feasibility of detecting altered DNA in stool has been demonstrated using a multitarget assay panel of molecular markers.[194] Genetic testing is now a reality for families with FAP (see Chapter 114).[106] Testing for altered products of the *APC* gene allows for early and accurate identification of family members at risk who require intensive surveillance. Proper genetic counseling, however, must be incorporated into the screening process.[75, 195] Genetic testing for mutations in the *hMSH2* and *hMLH1* genes soon also may be introduced for family members of kindreds with HNPCC. This presents more difficulty than screening for FAP, since not all the genes involved have been identified, and the preferred method by which families should be screened has yet to be determined.[196, 197] An allele of *APC* designated I1307K[198] is relatively infrequent in the general population but common in the Jewish population of Ashkenazi descent. There is a modest increase in the relative risk for colorectal cancer in those with this allele, but the penetrance for colorectal cancer is low compared with carrier frequencies, and genetic testing for I1307K is not recommended.

Approach to Screening

Screening and case-finding approaches are different for patients in average-risk (older than age 50 years) and high-risk groups. The latter group includes patients with long-standing UC, previous colorectal cancer, previous adenomas, female genital cancer, familial polyposis, HNPCC, and familial colon cancer.

Average-Risk Group

Patients registered in a health care system should be categorized according to risk, so that appropriate screening can be added to other variables of medical evaluation. Relative risk should be assessed by family history and by personal history using questionnaires. A variety of options are available for screening average-risk individuals (50 years of age and older with no personal or family history of colorectal adenoma or carcinoma, and no personal history of inflammatory bowel disease). These have been discussed previously, including guidelines from various healthcare agencies (see Table 115–13). While yearly FOBT and flexible sigmoidoscopy every 5 years are individual options, it has been suggested that combining the two tests can increase the benefits of either test alone.[119, 199] The tests are complementary since FOBT has the potential for detecting occult blood from a lesion anywhere in the colon, whereas flexible sigmoidoscopy can detect bleeding and nonbleeding lesions distal to the splenic flexure. The combined approach was compared with sigmoidoscopy alone in a single study,[200] which showed a 20% advantage for earlier-stage diagnosis and survival compared with sigmoidoscopy alone.

Colonoscopy every 10 years has the advantage of examining the entire colon and rectum and providing the opportunity to biopsy or remove lesions should they be found. Growing evidence suggests that colonoscopy may be a cost-effective option with an acceptable risk profile.[175] Two trials are now under way to examine colonoscopy for average-risk screening. A diagnostic work-up is indicated for individuals with a positive FOBT or distal neoplasm (adenoma, carcinoma) found at sigmoidoscopy. Colonoscopy is the diagnostic modality of choice. If colonoscopy is unavailable, not feasible, or not desired by the patient, double-contrast barium enema alone or in combination with flexible sigmoidoscopy is an acceptable alternative for evaluation of a positive FOBT.

Screening should be accompanied by programs that educate patients and heighten physicians' awareness of the concepts and technology involved in screening, diagnosis, treatment, and follow-up. The popular misconceptions that colorectal cancer is an incurable disease and that surgical intervention invariably leads to an impaired life-style, owing to the colostomy, must be discredited.

High-Risk Groups

FAMILIAL ADENOMATOUS POLYPOSIS AND FAMILIAL CANCER. Screening of family members in kindreds with familial polyposis or Gardner's syndrome is discussed in Chapter 114. Screening should include genetic testing to detect abnormal (truncated) *APC* gene products if a diagnosis can be made by this method in one family member. Those who test positive should have annual or biannual FS, beginning at puberty, to assess for emergence of adenomas and to plan appropriate timing for colectomy. If genetic testing is unavailable, annual FS should begin at puberty. Genetic testing should always be combined with education and counseling of the individual as well as family members.

Patients with a family history of HNPCC must be examined colonoscopically, beginning at age 25 years, or at an age 5 years younger than that of the index case, since one cannot rely only on FOBT in these very-high-risk patients. A reasonable approach is to perform colonoscopy every 2 years.[201] The search is primarily for the scattered adenomas that antedate carcinomas in these syndromes, and, for detection, colonoscopy is more sensitive than radiography. Genetic testing for HNPCC, is now being introduced into clinical practice.[196, 202–205] Genetic testing should be accompanied by counseling of the individual and the family members. The benefits of colonoscopic surveillance in patients with HNPCC mutations are suggested by recent screening trials.[203, 206]

The approach to patients with a suggestive family history—for example, one first-degree relative with colon cancer—is not firmly established. Whether these patients should be monitored in the same way as average-risk patients or be screened more rigorously remains to be definitively determined. Some studies suggest that evidence supporting the

Table 115–19 | **Guidelines for the Early Detection of Cancer in People at Increased Risk or at High Risk**

RISK CATEGORY	AGE TO BEGIN	RECOMMENDATION	COMMENT
Increased Risk			
People with a single, small (< 1 cm) adenoma	3–6 years after the initial polypectomy	Colonoscopy*	If the examination is normal, the patient can thereafter be screened as per average risk guidelines.
People with large (1 cm +) adenoma, multiple adenomas, or adenomas with high-grade dysplasia or villous change	Within 3 yr after the initial polypectomy	Colonoscopy*	If normal, repeat examination in 3 years; if normal then, the patient can thereafter be screened as per average risk guidelines.
Personal history of curative-intent resection of colorectal cancer	Within 1 yr after cancer resection	Colonoscopy*	If normal, repeat examination in 3 years; if normal then, repeat examination every 5 years.
Either colorectal cancer or adenomatous polyps in any first-degree relative before age 60 yr, or in two or more first-degree relatives at any age (if not a hereditary syndrome)	Age 40 yr, or 10 yr before the youngest case in the immediate family	Colonoscopy*	Every 5–10 years. Colorectal cancer in relatives more distant than first-degree does not increase risk substantially above the average-risk group.
High Risk			
Family history of familial adenomatous polyposis (FAP)	Puberty	Early surveillance with endoscopy, and counseling to consider genetic testing	If the genetic test is positive, colectomy is indicated. These patients are best referred to a center with experience in the management of FAP.
Family history of hereditary non-polyposis colon cancer (HNPCC)	Age 21 yr	Colonoscopy and counseling to consider genetic testing	If the genetic test is positive or if the patient has not had genetic testing, every 1–2 years until age 40 years, then annually. These patients are best referred to a center with experience in the management of HNPCC.
Inflammatory bowel disease (chronic ulcerative colitis; Crohn's disease)	Cancer risk begins to be significant 8 yr after the onset of pancolitis, or 12–15 years after the onset of left-sided colitis	Colonoscopy with biopsies for dysplasia	Every 1–2 years. These patients are best referred to a center with experience in the surveillance and management of inflammatory bowel disease.

*If colonoscopy is unavailable, not feasible, or not desired by the patient, double-contrast barium enema (DCBE) alone, or the combination of flexible sigmoidoscopy and DCBE, is acceptable, alternated. Adding flexible sigmoidoscopy to DCBE may provide a more comprehensive diagnostic evaluation than DCBE alone in finding significant lesions. A supplementary DCBE may be needed if a colonoscopic examination fails to reach the cecum, and a supplementary colonoscopy may be needed if a DCBE identifies a possible lesion, or does not adequately visualize the entire colorectum.

From Smith RA, von Eschenbach AC, Wender R, et al: American Cancer Society Guidelines for early detection of cancer: Update of early detection guidelines for prostate, colorectal, and endometrial cancers. CA Cancer J Clin 1:51, 2001.

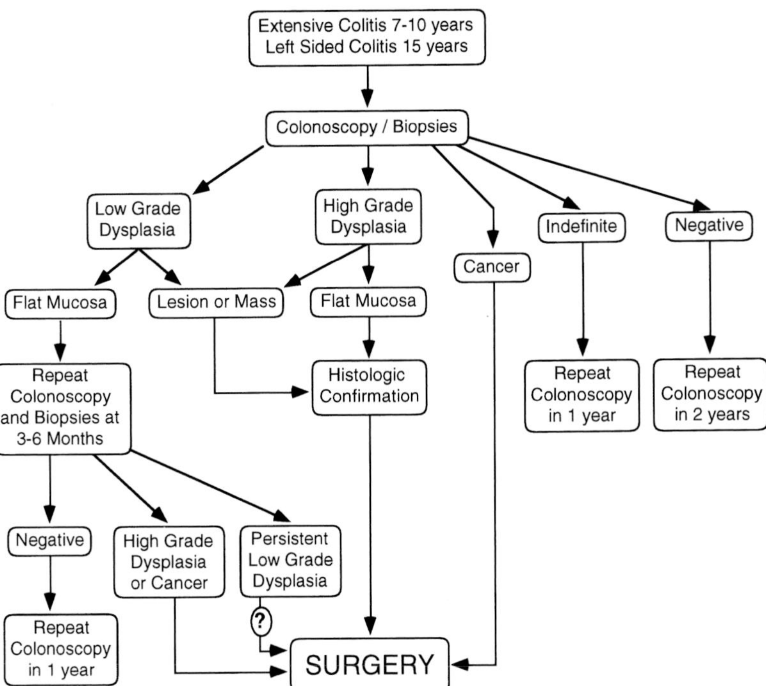

Figure 115–25. Algorithm for colonoscopic surveillance of patients with ulcerative colitis. Histologic confirmation refers to agreement by a second experienced pathologist that the biopsy meets the criteria for dysplasia as defined by the Inflammatory Bowel Disease Dysplasia Morphology Study Group.[134] (Modified from Ahnen DJ: Dysplasia and chronic ulcerative colitis. In Rustgi A [ed]: Gastrointestinal Cancers: Biology, Diagnosis, and Therapy. Philadelphia, JB Lippincott, 1995, p 399.)

use of colonoscopy as the first step in screening persons with one first-degree relative with colorectal cancer is insufficient, but other recent studies indicate that the risk may be sufficient to recommend colonoscopy, especially if adenoma or cancer in the index case occurred before age 60 years, or if two first-degree relatives have had an adenoma or cancer at any age.[112] The American Cancer Society recommends that if colorectal cancer or adenomatous polyps occurred in any first-degree relative before age 60 years, or in two or more first-degree relatives at any age, then colonoscopy should be performed every 5 to 10 years, beginning at age 40 years, or 10 years before the youngest case in the immediate family.[121] In those with more than two affected first-degree relatives, special care should be taken to exclude the diagnosis of HNPCC, and periodic colonoscopy is advised.

PRIOR ADENOMAS OR COLON CANCER. Table 115–19 lists the American Cancer Society (ACS) guidelines for screening, surveillance, and early detection of colorectal adenomas and cancer for individuals at increased risk or at high risk of disease, updated in 2001.[121] While the majority of the ACS guidelines are in keeping with those of other agencies, surveillance of individuals with a personal history of adenomatous polyps deserves mention. The ACS suggests that those whose index lesion is a single adenoma less than 1 cm should have a follow-up colonoscopy 3 to 6 years after the initial polypectomy. If the examination is normal, the patient can be screened as per average-risk guidelines. In those with a large (greater than 1 cm) adenoma, multiple adenomas, or adenomas with high-grade dysplasia or villous change, colonoscopy should be repeated within 3 years after the initial polypectomy. If normal, the examination should be repeated once again in 3 years. If it remains normal, then the patient can thereafter be screened as per average-risk guidelines. The guidelines for the latter group differ somewhat from previous ACS guidelines,[119] and what is often practiced (colonoscopy 3 years after removal of an adenoma; if negative, colonoscopy every 5 years). Whether these new guidelines will become standard practice remains to be determined. A discussion of surveillance of patients with a personal history of adenomas is provided in Chapter 114, and the reader is referred there for a more detailed discussion of surveillance in this group.

Patients who have had a large bowel cancer resected should have colonoscopy performed 6 months to 1 year after surgery, followed by colonoscopy in 3 years. If the results are negative, colonoscopy should then be performed every 5 years (see Table 115–19). Serum CEA levels should be measured at regular intervals since postoperative CEA determinations may be cost effective for detecting recurrent cancers. How long an asymptomatic patient who has had multiple negative examinations should be tested by various modalities is at present unclear. It should be noted that the above recommendations are to some extent "educated guesses," and not all are based on prospective randomized trials.

INFLAMMATORY BOWEL DISEASE. The appropriate surveillance schedule for patients with inflammatory bowel disease remains to be determined in long-term prospective trials. Colonoscopy combined with mucosal biopsy may be effective in detecting preneoplastic and early neoplastic lesions in patients with ulcerative colitis. The current recommendation is for colonoscopy every 1 or 2 years for patients who have had universal colitis for 8 years or left-sided ulcerative colitis for 12 to 15 years (see Table 115–19) (Fig. 115–25). Biopsies should be taken throughout the colon at 10-cm intervals, with special attention to areas that suggest a dysplasia-associated lesion or mass. Although this biopsy procedure examines the histology of only a small area of the colon, the short-term risk of carcinoma for patients with negative biopsy results is low. If dysplasia is high-grade or associated with a macroscopic lesion or mass, a recommendation should be given for colectomy. A histologic diagnosis of low-grade dysplasia merits endoscopic follow-up at short intervals—e.g., at 3 to 6 months—as does an "indeterminate" reading due to active inflammation. Colectomy has been advocated by some for confirmed low-grade dysplasia. Patients with Crohn's disease of the colon should be evaluated endoscopically as dictated by symptoms, and special attention should be paid to strictured areas. Recent studies suggest a role for surveillance colonoscopy.[137]

Insurance Coverage for Colorectal Cancer Screening

Based on evidence from several randomized trials, the Health Care Financing Administration (HCFA) decided to provide coverage for colon cancer screening procedures to medical beneficiaries beginning January 1, 1998. Coverage for average-risk individuals includes annual FOBT and flexible sigmoidoscopy every 4 years. Barium enema is included as an option every 4 years in place of flexible sigmoidoscopy, after written justification. Colonoscopy is covered every 2 years for "high-risk" individuals (family history of colorectal cancer, personal history of adenoma or carcinoma, history of inflammatory bowel disease, positivity for a recognized genetic marker of inherited colorectal cancer). After intense lobbying by several groups, Medicare will provide coverage for screening colonoscopy in average-risk individuals every 10 years or at an interval 4 years from a previous sigmoidoscopy. This bill was signed December 21, 2000, and coverage was initiated July 1, 2001. A bill is currently before Congress for legislation requiring private insurers to cover colorectal cancer screening for any participant or beneficiary over the age of 50 years or those under 50 years who are at high risk for developing colorectal cancer. The frequency of screenings would comply with current Medicare colorectal cancer screening regulations.

TREATMENT

Surgery

Surgical resection is the treatment of choice for most colorectal cancers. Preoperative colonoscopy should be performed, if possible, to rule out synchronous lesions, and serum CEA should be measured to inform staging and postoperative follow-up. CT is not indicated as a routine preoperative staging procedure. It can be valuable, however, for the evaluation of focal hepatic metastases if partial hepatectomy or regional hepatic artery infusion of chemotherapeutic agents is contemplated. CT is also useful for postoperative detection of pelvic recurrence in patients with rectosigmoid tumors. Transrectal ultrasonography is also of value in the preoperative assessment of patients with rectal cancer.

The goal of surgery is wide resection of the involved segment of bowel, together with removal of its lymphatic

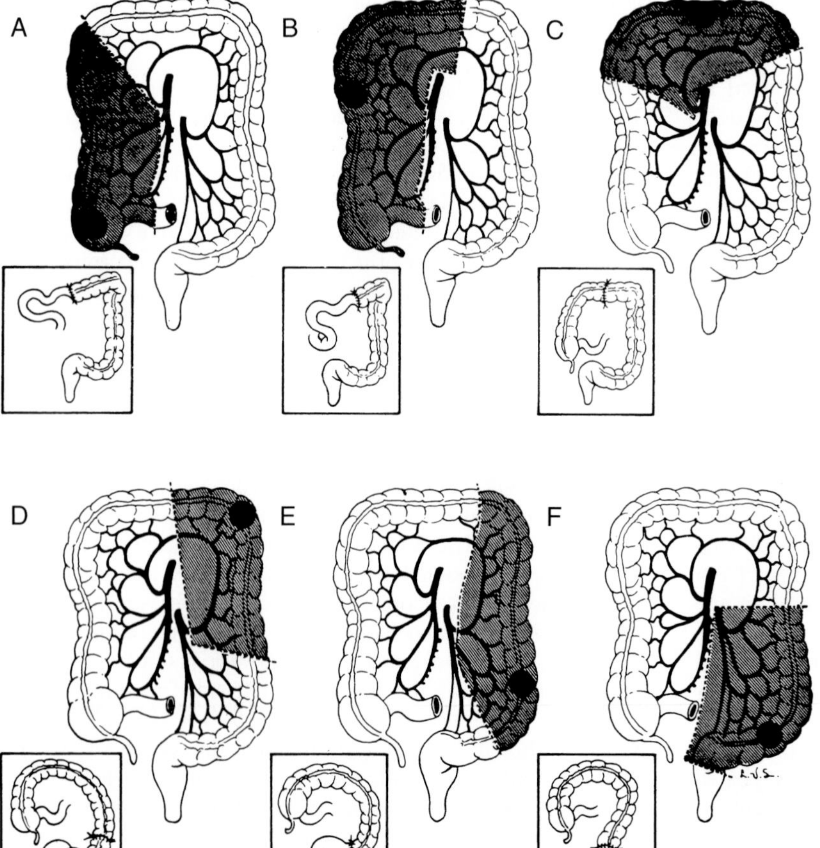

Figure 115–26. Surgical resection of colorectal cancer based on location of the primary tumor, blood supply, and lymphatic drainage. (From Schrock T: Large intestine. In Way LW [ed]: Current Surgical Diagnosis and Treatment, 10th ed. New York, Lange Medical Publishers, 1994.)

drainage vessels (Fig. 115–26). The extent of colonic resection is determined by the blood supply and distribution of regional lymph nodes. The resection should include a segment of colon at least 5 cm on either side of the tumor, although wider margins are often included because of obligatory ligation of the arterial blood supply. Extensive "superradical" colonic and lymph node resection does not increase survival over that associated with segmental resection, and it increases morbidity.

The approach toward rectal cancers depends on the location of the lesion. For lesions of the rectosigmoid and upper rectum, low anterior resection can be performed through an abdominal incision and primary anastomosis accomplished (Fig. 115–26*F*). Even for low rectal lesions, a sphincter-saving resection can be safely performed if a distal margin of at least 2 cm of normal bowel can be resected below the lesion—an end now facilitated by new end-to-end stapling devices. Tumor recurrence and survival are similar after sphincter-saving resections for rectal cancer versus abdominoperineal resection (APR), if a 2-cm distal margin can be preserved in the former. The inability to obtain an adequate distal margin, the presence of a large, bulky tumor deep within the pelvis, and extensive local spread of rectal cancer all dictate the need for APR in which the distal sigmoid, rectosigmoid, rectum, and anus are removed through a combined abdominal and perineal approach and a permanent sigmoid colostomy established.

In a patient with colorectal cancer, the primary tumor generally should be resected, even in the presence of distant metastases, to prevent obstruction or bleeding. In patients with advanced disease and multiple medical problems, repeated palliative fulguration of rectal tumors may be preferable to surgery. Newer modalities, such as laser photoablation, are being tested as alternative means of palliation in these patients. Polypoid carcinomas may be removed endoscopically by snare polypectomy techniques.

Several studies indicate that though the age and physiologic status of a patient may affect operative mortality, advanced age per se does not affect tumor-associated mortality after surgery. Therefore, resection of cancer should not be limited or denied on the basis of age alone.

POSTSURGICAL FOLLOW-UP. The incidence of recurrent colon cancer after surgical resection is high in persons who have serosal penetration or lymph node involvement by tumor. In addition, the incidence of metachronous (subsequent) colorectal cancer is 1.1% to 4.7%.[116–118] It is not clear how often, or by what means, a patient should be evaluated following an apparently successful resection for cure. Colonoscopy is beneficial in the detection and removal of synchronous and metachronous adenomatous polyps in the high-risk group. History and physical examination, combined with CEA determinations at regular intervals, may provide the highest cost-effective benefit for detecting recurrent cancers. The sensitivity for detecting early recurrences is about 61% using either CT or CEA, but CT can be especially useful in examining the pelvis for recurrence after resection of rectosigmoid tumors. CT portography is an accurate method for detecting liver metastases if liver resection is considered. Immunoscintigraphy after administration of radiolabeled monoclonal antibodies raised against various tumor antigens, including CEA, may provide clinically significant information in staging patients prior to surgery or in detection of recurrent disease,[207, 208] but use of this modality has not been standardized. The role of positron emission (PET) scanning is currently being evaluated.[209] MRI ultimately may produce the clearest delineation of hepatic metastases. Intraoperative ultrasonography (IOUS) is now being used to increase the ability to detect small and deep hepatic lesions that are not palpable during surgery.

Serial CEA determinations have been used to direct "second-look" surgical procedures. Measuring CEA levels at least every 2 months for the first 2 years after resection, and then every 4 months for the next 3 years, yields a small percentage of patients (about 5%) for whom CEA-directed second-look operations for recurrent carcinoma may be indicated. Survival following second-look procedures is high when surgeons have specialized training in oncologic surgery, but other surgeons have had more limited success, and long-term survival data are lacking. The concept of CEA-directed second-look laparotomy has been applied to resection of localized hepatic metastases.

SURGICAL RESECTION OF HEPATIC METASTASES. The most common site of distant metastases from colorectal cancer is the liver. Synchronous metastases to the liver are evident at initial presentation in 10% to 25% of patients with large bowel cancer, and 40% to 70% of those whose cancers disseminate have hepatic involvement. Some 70% to 80% of hepatic metastases appear within 2 years after primary resection. The uniformly poor prognosis for patients with untreated hepatic metastases underlies an aggressive approach.[210] Hepatic resection is therefore recommended for certain candidates with hepatic metastasis from colorectal cancer. Candidates for resection of hepatic lesions are those whose primary tumor has been resected with curative intent and in whom where is no evidence of extrahepatic disease. The extent of liver involvement that is deemed resectable varies from tumor involving one lobe of the liver to focal disease in multiple lobes. The percentage of "resectable" liver metastases therefore varies in different series from 4.5% to 11% (5% to 6% in most series).

Modern techniques of anatomic dissection and hemostasis have resulted in operative mortality of about 2% in highly trained hands.[211] Dissections along nonanatomic lines have permitted the resection of multiple lesions that might have previously been considered unresectable. Overall 5-year survival rates range from 20% to 34% in selected patients. The literature is difficult to interpret, however, because no uniform staging system is used, and prospective controls are lacking. Further, reported 2- and 3-year survival rates may not be valid, since recent data suggest that patients with unresected solitary liver lesions live at least 3 years. Long-term survival for those who undergo surgical resection of hepatic metastases depends on the absence of extrahepatic disease and adequate surgical margins.[210–215] In some series, the stage of the primary lesion is also a significant prognostic variable. It is not clear whether patients with a solitary focus of metastasis live longer after resection than those who undergo resection of multiple metastases in the same lobe. It is clear that patients with bilobar metastases are at increased risk for recurrence of metastasis in the liver after resection and that resection should not be attempted when more than four hepatic lesions are present. In patients whose tumor

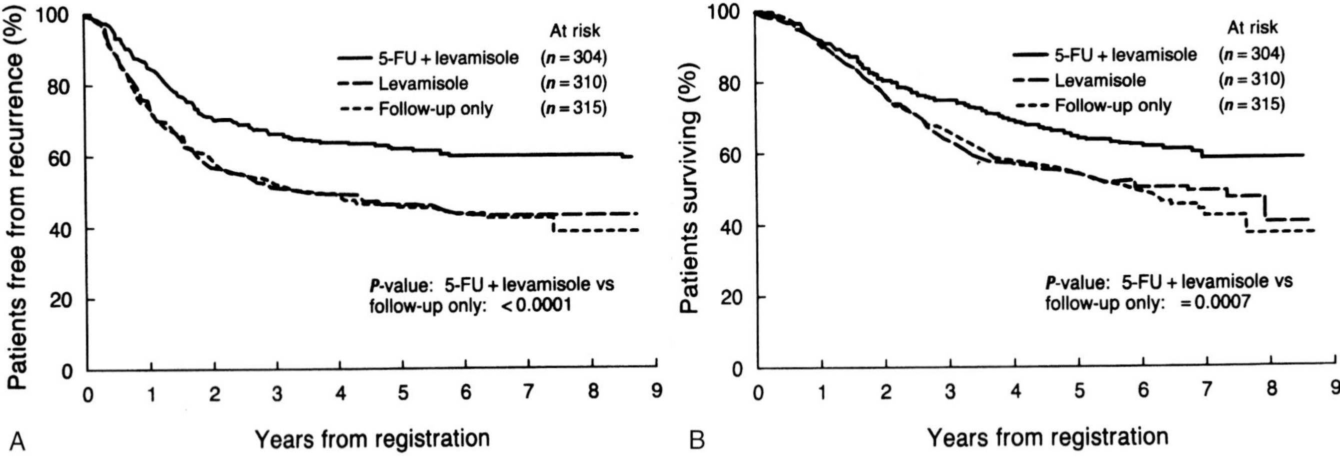

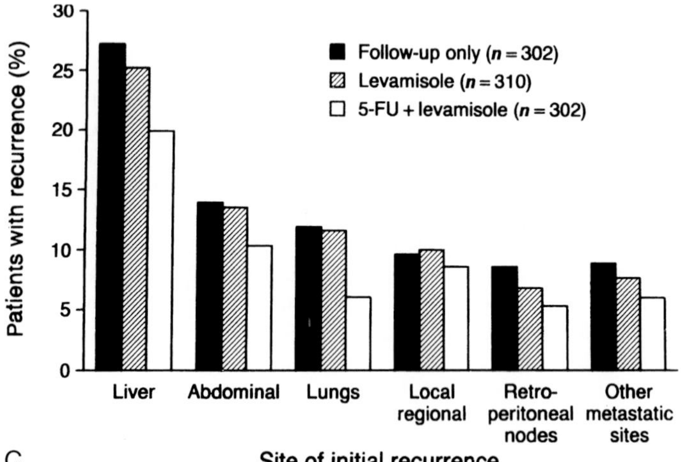

Figure 115–27. Adjuvant therapy of colon cancer in patients with Dukes' C (stage III) disease. Effects of therapy with levamisole and 5-fluorouracil (5-FU) on (*A*) tumor recurrence and (*B*) survival. *C*, Patterns of recurrence according to treatment arm. (From Moertel CG, Fleming TR, MacDonald JS, et al: Fluorouracil plus levamisole as effective adjuvant therapy after resection of stage III colon carcinoma: A final report. Ann Intern Med 122:321, 1995.)

recurs after hepatic resection, the liver is the initial site of recurrence in about 35%. Repeat hepatic resection for isolated metastases can result in long-term survival in selected persons.[213] Improved survival after pulmonary resection of metastatic colorectal cancer has also been reported.

Cryotherapy is a technique by which rapid freezing results in crystal formation and produces significant cellular damage and cell death. Tumors are frozen rapidly by means of a probe with intraoperative ultrasonographic guidance, so that malignant lesions can be ablated while the remaining liver tissue is preserved.[216] This is an alternative approach to treatment in patients whose liver metastases are unsuitable for surgical resection.

Chemotherapy

Adjuvant Chemotherapy

The prognosis for patients with colorectal cancer who undergo potentially curative surgery is strongly correlated with the stage of the primary tumor at surgery. Despite resection of all macroscopic tumor, patients whose primary tumor has penetrated the serosa or who have regional lymph node metastases at the time of surgery have high recurrence rates (see Table 115–9 and Fig. 115–27). Patients who undergo aggressive surgical resection of isolated hepatic metastases also have high tumor recurrence rates in the liver and elsewhere. An effective adjuvant program to eradicate microscopic tumor foci is clearly needed for such high-risk patients, who number 35,000 to 40,000 each year in the United States.[211] The principle behind such adjuvant therapy is that treatment is most effective when tumor burden is minimal and cell kinetics are optimal. Data from recent studies have now demonstrated delays in tumor recurrence and increases in survival for specific groups of patients with colon and rectal cancer who have received adjuvant therapy within 8 weeks of surgery, marking a major advance in the treatment of these diseases.

The major advance in the adjuvant treatment of colorectal cancer came with the results of trials that explored the combination of 5-fluorouracil (5-FU) and levamisole. A large study assessed the benefit of this regimen in 1296 patients with resected colon cancer that was either locally invasive (Dukes' B2; stage II) or had regional lymph node involvement (Dukes' C; stage III).[217] The majority of patients were treated in community practice. Therapy with 5-FU plus levamisole reduced the relative risk of cancer recurrence by 42%, and the overall death rate by 33% relative to surgery alone in patients with stage III disease. The results in patients with stage II disease were equivocal and too preliminary to allow firm conclusions to be drawn. Levamisole

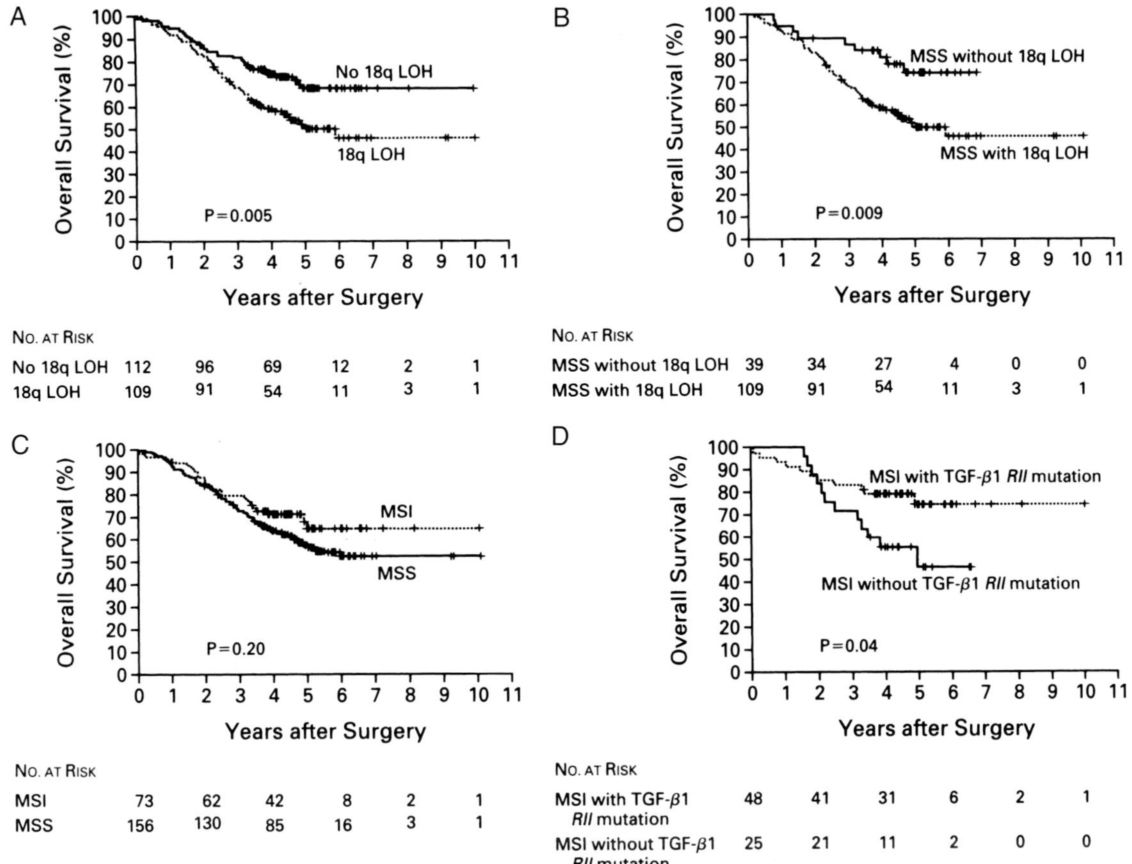

Figure 115–28. Molecular markers that predict a favorable outcome after adjuvant chemotherapy with 5-fluorouracil-based regimens. LOH, loss of heterozygosity; MSS, microsatellite stable; MSI, microsatellite instability; TGF-β1 RII, transforming growth factor β-1 receptor-II. (From Watanabe T, Wu T-T, Catalano PJ, et al: Molecular predictors of survival after adjuvant chemotherapy for colon cancer. N Engl J Med 344:1196, 2001.)

alone had no detectable effect, and its mechanism of action is not clearly understood. Updated data on all 929 eligible patients followed for 5 years or more confirm that 5-FU plus levamisole reduced recurrence rate by 40% and the death rate by 33%.[218] The major effect was on reduction in recurrence at distant sites, such as the liver and the lungs. Based on these data, patients with Dukes' C (stage III) colon cancer were offered adjuvant therapy with fluorouracil and levamisole.

The success of combinations of 5-FU and leucovorin for the treatment of advanced colorectal cancer led to the trial of this regimen in the adjuvant setting. Several trials suggested that this combination was successful in prolonging disease-free and overall survival.[219–221] This led to the direct comparison of 5-FU/levamisole versus 5-FU/leucovorin for the adjuvant treatment of colorectal cancer. Comparison of these two regimens in randomized clinical trials suggests a small advantage in disease-free and overall survival in favor of 5-FU plus leucovorin.[222, 223] Review of the combined data suggests that while 5-FU/levamisole given for 1 year is still considered an acceptable regimen, 5-FU/leucovorin given for 6 months after "curative" surgery is superior with regard to convenience and efficacy. 5-FU plus leucovorin should therefore be considered the new standard for adjuvant treatment of colorectal cancer. It is not clear whether patients with stage II, node-negative colon cancer should receive adjuvant chemotherapy, since the risk-benefit ratio has not been established.

Recent trials have included patients with modified Dukes' stages B2 and C disease. Anatomic or biologic features may, in the future, define subsets of patients with stage II colon cancer who will benefit from adjuvant therapy. Such features may include colloid, signet-ring, or poorly differentiated cancers, high preoperative CEA, aneuploid DNA content or high S phase, alterations in molecular markers, and the expression of certain tumor-associated antigens (e.g., sialyl-Tn, sialyl Lewis^x) or other genetic determinants (see section on Prognostic Factors). A recent analysis[79] indicated that retention of 18q alleles in microsatellite-stable cancers and mutation of the gene for *TGF-β1* in cancers with high levels of MSI indicate a favorable outcome after adjuvant therapy with fluorouracil-based regimens in patients with stage III colon cancer (Fig. 115–28). Other combined adjuvant chemotherapies for colon cancer are currently being studied, including those containing the oral 5-FU predrug UFTC (uracil, 5-FU, and tegafur), oxaliplatin, and irinotecan. Portal infusion of chemotherapeutic agents as adjuvant therapy reduces liver metastasis, but this approach remains investigational.[224]

Adjuvant therapy for rectal cancer should be considered separate from that for colon cancer, since patterns of failure are different. Complete pelvic extirpation is common for

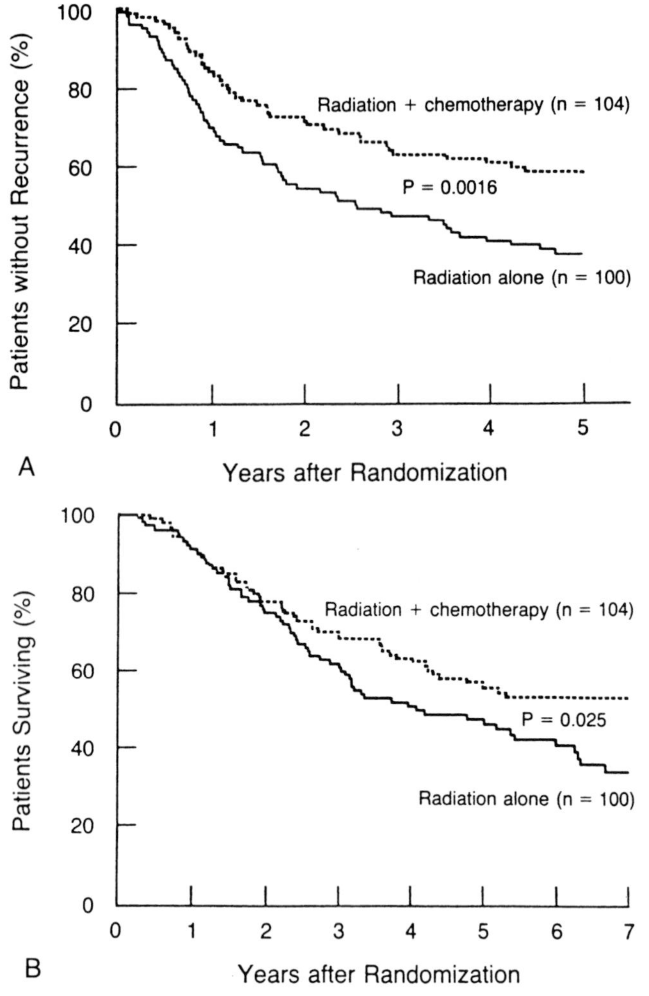

Figure 115–29. Combined modality adjuvant therapy of stages II and III rectal cancer. Effects of radiation and chemotherapy on (*A*) tumor recurrence and (*B*) survival. (From Krook JE, Moertel CG, Gunderson LL, et al: Effective adjuvant therapy for high-risk rectal carcinoma. N Engl J Med 324:709, 1991.)

patients with rectal cancer, since wide margins of resection may be difficult to obtain. Thus, local recurrence for stage II rectal cancer after primary resection approaches 25% to 30%, with a 50% or greater local recurrence rate in those with stage III tumors. Local recurrence is associated with significant morbidity, and patients with locally invasive rectal cancer are at high risk for systemic relapse. Studies during the past 2 decades have shown a significant decrease in local recurrence of rectal cancer in patients who receive moderate to high doses of preoperative and/or postoperative radiation (40 to 50 Gy), but with little impact on systemic recurrence and survival.

Combined adjuvant radiation and chemotherapy has been used to address this potential for local and systemic recurrence. Results of early, prospectively randomized designed trials to evaluate the efficacy of combined-modality adjuvant therapy in patients with modified Dukes' B2 and C (stage II and III) rectal cancer following curative surgery were encouraging. A trial by the North Central Cancer Treatment Group evolved from this earlier work and now strongly suggested that postsurgical combined-modality therapy decreases tumor relapse and improves survival over those with surgery alone or full-dose postoperative radiation therapy.[225] This trial randomized patients with stage II or stage III rectal cancer to receive postoperative radiation alone or radiation plus 5-FU and methyl-CCNU. After a median follow-up of more than 7 years, combined therapy significantly reduced local and overall recurrence and distant metastasis and improved patient survival over that compared with radiation alone (Fig. 115–29). Cancer-related deaths were reduced by 36% and the overall death rate by 29%. Combining protracted-infusion 5-FU with radiation therapy improved the effect of combined-treatment postoperative adjuvant therapy in patients with high-risk rectal cancer.[226] Based on these data, patients with resected rectal cancer with transmural extension (TNM stage II; Dukes' B2) or with positive lymph nodes (TNM stage III; Dukes' C) should be considered for such combined-modality therapy.

Subsequent intergroup trials have attempted to identify the optimal chemotherapeutic agents and the best method of delivery.[227] These trials have compared a variety of chemotherapeutic agents in combination with postoperative radiation as adjuvant treatment of rectal cancer. Regimens include 5-FU alone, 5-FU with leucovorin, 5-FU with levamisole, 5-FU with leucovorin and levamisole, and others. Comparisons have also included the relative benefits of continuous infusion 5-FU during pre-and postradiation therapy (RT) phases versus bolus 5-FU during the non-RT portion. Definitive results are still pending. Preoperative "neoadjuvant" therapy allows radiation to be delivered in a nonoperated abdomen, reducing the chance of postoperative complications such as adhesions and bowel damage. Higher doses of preoperative (versus postoperative) radiation can be delivered. Several trials are ongoing to evaluate the efficacy of pre- versus postoperative multimodality adjuvant therapy (radiation and chemotherapy) for rectal cancer. Accurate endorectal ultrasound and MRI staging has allowed the use of preoperative therapy without the unnecessary treatment of patients with early stage disease.

Chemotherapy for Advanced Disease

Results of existing systemic chemotherapy for disseminated colorectal cancer are disappointing: only modest proven efficacy is reported for the fluoropyrimidines (5-FU, 5-fluorodeoxyuridine), the nitrosoureas, and mitomycin C. A number of new agents, however, have recently shown promise in combination with 5-FU–based regimens.

By interacting with thymidylate synthetase and inhibiting the methylation of deoxyuridylic to thymidylic acid, 5-FU inhibits DNA synthesis. It has been administered as an oral agent, intravenously in bolus doses, or by continuous intravenous infusion, and is associated with a response rate of approximately 20% in most studies. Responses are often short-lived (4 to 5 months) and have not been associated with long-term survival. Toxicity of 5-FU includes myelosuppression, vomiting, diarrhea, and stomatitis and varies according to dose and mode of administration. Similar modest response rates have been reported for the nitrosoureas (10% to 15%) and mitomycin C (12% to 16%) given as single agents.

Although small pilot studies often report the superiority

of various combinations of chemotherapeutic agents for the management of metastatic disease, larger multicenter phase III trials often fail to demonstrate statistically significant benefit compared with 5-FU alone. A combination of 5-FU and high-dose intravenous leucovorin (tetrahydrofolate) has become standard therapy, because leucovorin potentiates the binding of 5-FU to thymidylate synthetase, and the combination is more effective than 5-FU alone.[226–231] Although response rates for this combined regimen have in most cases been superior to 5-FU alone (30% to 48% versus 11% to 13%), overall survival has not yet been convincingly demonstrated to be significantly prolonged. Enhanced toxicity from the combined regimen includes greater degrees of stomatitis and diarrhea. The optimal doses of 5-FU and leucovorin and the optimal mode of 5-FU administration (bolus versus infusion) remain to be determined, but intensive-course 5-FU plus low-dose leucovorin appears to have a superior therapeutic index, as well as lower cost and less toxicity, in comparison with weekly 5-FU plus high-dose leucovorin.[231] Continuous infusion 5-FU appears to be superior to bolus regimens in terms of response rates and toxicity.[232]

Methotrexate added to 5-FU, with or without leucovorin, is not uniformly superior to 5-FU alone, and toxicity is greater. Another therapy under investigation for advanced colon cancer combines 5-FU and recombinant interferon alfa-2a (IFN). Trials involving small groups of patients suggest that the addition of IFN to 5-FU enhances objective response rates (35% to 42% response) but also enhances toxicity. Irinotecan (CPT-11) is a potent inhibitor of topoisomerase I, a nuclear enzyme involved in the unwinding of DNA during replication. Weekly treatment with irinotecan plus 5-FU and leucovorin was recently demonstrated to be superior to a widely used regimen of 5-FU and leucovorin for metastatic colorectal cancer in terms of progression-free survival and overall survival.[233] Other drugs currently under investigation include topotecan and 9-aminocamptothecin, trimetrexate (an antifolate), tomudex (a thymidylate synthase inhibitor), oxaliplatin, and UFT (an oral 5-FU prodrug composed of a 1:4 fixed molar ratio of tegafur and uracil).[234]

Selective infusion of chemotherapeutic agents into the hepatic arterial system may be employed to treat hepatic metastases. This method delivers more concentrated drug into the tumor capillary bed than do conventional means.[210] The infusion catheter is usually implanted into the common hepatic artery via the gastroduodenal artery at the time of laparotomy. The development of implantable infusion pumps has led to increasing use of such therapy in major centers. Fluorinated pyrimidines, such as 5-FU and floxuridine (FUDR), have high hepatic extraction (80% to 95%), and it is felt that high concentrations of these drugs can be delivered with low systemic toxicity by direct hepatic arterial infusion. Floxuridine has received the most attention. Continuous hepatic arterial infusion of floxuridine to treat hepatic metastases from colorectal cancer in patients not previously treated may achieve response rates of 54% to 83%. Criteria for response vary, however, and it is still unclear whether an impact on survival will be observed.[210]

Randomized trials of systemic versus intrahepatic infusion of FUDR in patients with liver metastasis have shown significantly higher response rates for intrahepatic therapy,[210] but the impact on survival remains unclear. Complications of the procedure, which include arterial occlusion, local infection, and catheter leak, occur in a small number of patients. Morbidity of treatment consists of gastrointestinal tract inflammation and ulceration, hepatic injury with elevation in serum bilirubin and transaminases, and biliary ductal sclerosis, all of which may be substantial. It has been suggested that alternating hepatic intra-arterial FUDR and 5-FU may produce less toxicity than FUDR alone. Some investigators have combined hepatic artery occlusion or embolization with chemotherapeutic agents (chemoembolization) in an attempt to achieve better response rates in patients with extensive hepatic tumor.[235]

Immunotargeted Therapy and Immunotherapy

Recent advances in immunology, molecular biology, and imaging have led to the development of radiolabeled monoclonal antibodies that can be used in the detection of metastatic lesions from colorectal cancer (radioimmunodetection). These same antibodies can be linked to cytotoxic agents such as the A subunit of the plant toxin ricin, the toxin A

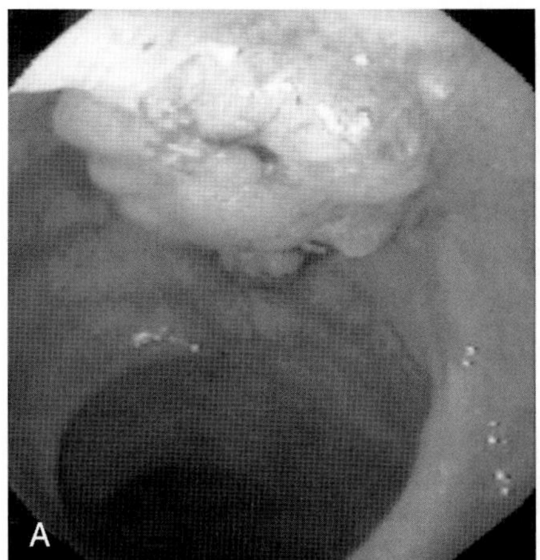

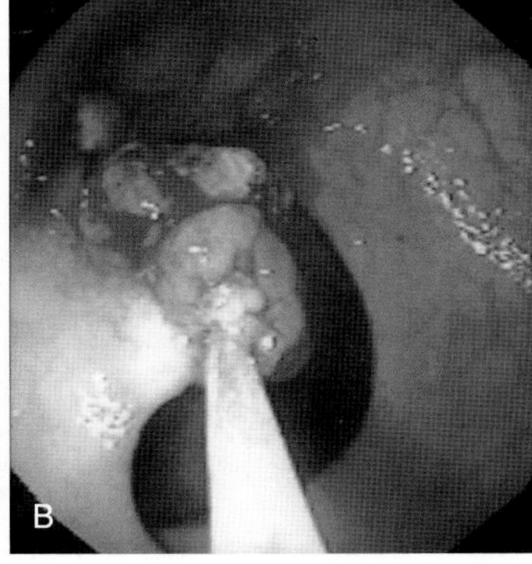

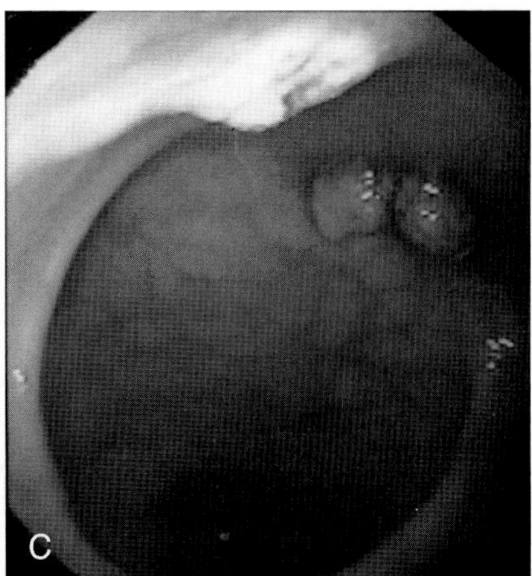

Figure 115–30. Removal of a polypoid carcinoma by snare cautery in a patient at high operative risk due to intercurrent illness. *A*, Polypoid carcinoma. *B*, Piecemeal removal by snare cautery. *C*, Site of former lesion after removal.

chain of diphtheria, lymphokine-activated killer cells, or chemotherapeutic agents for immunotargeted therapy.[236] Liposomes containing chemotherapeutic agents can be linked to monoclonal antibodies and delivered in a similar fashion. Most patients treated thus far with such therapy have had advanced disease, and further studies utilizing these agents in adjuvant therapy are needed.

Attempts to modulate the immune system of patients with metastatic disease have also been reported.[234] Immunostimulant therapy with agents such as interleukin-2 remains experimental, however, and may be associated with substantial toxicity. Dose adjustments and additional experience may make this a more viable approach in the future. Active specific immunotherapy with autologous tumor cell–bacille Calmette-Guérin (BCG) vaccines has also been attempted, but benefits have been modest and results are too preliminary to evaluate.

Radiation Therapy

Patients with rectal cancers whose lesions have penetrated the bowel wall or who have regional lymph nodes involved by tumor are at 40% to 50% risk for local recurrence following resection of the primary tumor. Radiation therapy is used preoperatively or postoperatively to decrease local recurrence in those with high-risk rectal and rectosigmoid cancers (Dukes' B2 and C lesions), or in a combined preoperative and postoperative "sandwich approach." It is also used to convert unresectable large tumors and those fixed to pelvic organs to resectable lesions. Radiation therapy occasionally may be useful for palliation of bleeding and pain due to advanced rectal disease. The possible advantages of radiation therapy must be balanced against its potential complications of radiation proctitis and small bowel damage (see Chapter 102).

Preoperative radiation reduces local recurrence in patients with rectal and rectosigmoid cancers, but there is no convincing evidence that it improves survival. Sphincter preservation is a major goal of preoperative therapy. When sphincter preservation is the goal, the use of preoperative therapy should be limited to those who are not technically able to undergo excision. Since preoperative radiation delays surgery and prevents adequate pathologic staging, postoperative radiotherapy may be preferable. Postoperative radiotherapy is generally restricted to patients at high risk for local recurrence of rectal cancer (penetration of the bowel wall, positive lymph nodes). Prospective but nonrandomized series show a substantial reduction in local recurrence for those receiving postoperative radiotherapy (6% to 8% for those receiving radiation versus 40% to 50% for those receiving surgery alone). A randomized study also demonstrated results favoring radiation (an overall reduction in local-regional recurrence from 25% to 16%).[227] Distant metastases remain a problem, however, and it is not clear whether survival is altered substantially. Given the recent demonstration of decreased recurrence and increased survival in patients with rectal cancer receiving combined postoperative radiation and chemotherapy, this would appear to be the treatment of choice for high-risk patients with transmural tumor extension or lymph node metastases.

Endoscopic Therapy

Endoscopic therapy using the neodymium-yttrium-aluminum-garnet (Nd:YAG) laser has been used to recanalize the rectum as palliative therapy in patients with obstructing rectal cancers who are poor surgical risks or who have advanced stages of malignant disease. Palliation generally has been satisfactory. Reported complications are bleeding and perforation, but they are fewer than would be anticipated after surgery in these high-risk patients. Electrofulguration using a heater probe device has also been reported under similar circumstances, but data are limited. Endoscopy with the use of snare cautery may also be used to remove polypoid lesions (Fig. 115–30), often in a piecemeal fashion.

Photodynamic therapy (PDT) also has been used to treat patients who are poor surgical risks. Patients are sensitized with a hematoporphyrin derivative, which is taken up by the tumor. Phototherapy is then performed using a tuneable dye laser and a flexible optical fiber, which can be inserted into the tumor. The number of patients treated in this manner has been small, and the method remains experimental.

OTHER MALIGNANT LARGE BOWEL TUMORS

Malignant tumors other than adenocarcinomas rarely originate in the large bowel. These include lymphomas, malignant carcinoid tumors, and leiomyosarcomas. In addition, lymphomas, leiomyosarcomas, malignant melanomas, and cancers of the breast, ovary, prostate, lung, stomach, and other organs can be metastatic to the colon (see Chapter 29). Malignant carcinoid tumors are discussed in Chapter 112 and lymphomas in Chapter 26. Carcinomas of the anal canal are discussed in Chapter 117.

REFERENCES

1. Greenlee RT, Hill-Harmon B, Murray T, et al: Cancer statistics 2001. CA Cancer J Clin 51:15, 2001.
2. Parkin DM, Pisani P, Ferlay J: Global cancer statistics. CA Cancer J Clin 49:33, 1999.
3. Ries L, Eisner M, Kosary C, et al: SEER Cancer Statistics Review, 1973–1977. Series. Bethesda, MD, National Cancer Institute, 2000.
4. Parkin DM, Whelen SL, Ferlay J, et al: Cancer Incidence in Five Continents (IARC Sci. Publ. No. 143). Series. Lyon, International Agency for Research on Cancer, 1997.
5. Weaver P, Harrison B, Eskander G, et al: Colon cancer in blacks. A disease with a worsening prognosis. J Natl Med Assoc 83:133, 1991.
6. Theuer CP, Wagner JL, Taylor TH, et al: Racial and ethnic colorectal cancer patterns affect the cost-effectiveness of colorectal cancer screening in the United States. Gastroenterology 120:848, 2001.
7. DeVesa S, Chow W: Variation in colorectal cancer incidence in the United States by subsite of origin. Cancer 71:3819, 1993.
8. Bufil JA: Colorectal cancer: Evidence for distinct genetic categories based on proximal or distal location. Ann Intern Med 113:779, 1990.
9. Cooper GS, Yuan Z, Landefeld S, et al: A national population-based study of incidence of colorectal cancer and age. Implications for screening older Americans. Cancer 75:775, 1995.
10. Demers RY, Severasa RK, Schottenfeld D, et al: Incidence of colorectal adenocarcinoma by anatomic subsite. Cancer 79:441, 1997.
11. Potter JD: Colorectal cancer: Molecules and populations. J Natl Cancer Inst 91:916, 1999.
12. Shike M, Winawer SJ, Greenwald PH: Primary prevention of colorectal cancer. Bull WHO 68:377, 1990.

13. Willet WC, Stamfer MJ, Colditz GA, et al: Relation of meat, fat and fiber intake to risk of colon cancer in a prospective study among women. N Engl J Med 323:1664, 1990.
14. Neugut AI, Garbowski GC, Lee WC, et al: Dietary risk factors for the incidence and recurrence of colorectal adenomatous polyps. A case-control study. Ann Intern Med 118:91, 1993.
15. Howe GR, Aronson KJ, Genito E, et al: The relationship between dietary fat intake and risk of colorectal cancer: Evidence from the combined analysis of 13 case-control studies. Cancer Causes Control 8:215, 1997.
16. Giovannucci E, Ascherio A, Rimm EB, et al: Physical activity, obesity and risk for colon cancer and adenoma in men. Ann Intern Med 122: 327, 1995.
17. Rao CV, Simi B, Wynn T-T, et al: Modulating effect of amount and types of dietary fat on colonic mucosal phospholipase A_2 phosphatidylinositol-specific phospholipase C activities, and cyclooxygenase metabolite formation during different stages of colon tumor promotion in male F344 rats. Cancer Res 56:532, 1996.
18. Glinghammar B, Rafter J: Colonic luminal contents induce cyclooxygenase 2 transcription in human colon carcinoma cells. Gastroenterology 120:401, 2001.
19. Giovanucci E, Rimm EB, Stampfer MJ, et al: Aspirin use and the risk of colorectal cancer and adenoma in male health professionals. Ann Intern Med 121:241, 1994.
20. Giovanucci E, Egan KM, Hunter DJ, et al: Aspirin and the risk of colorectal cancer in women. N Engl J Med 333:609, 1995.
21. Bresalier RS: In search of a better aspirin: Suppression of intestinal polyposis by targeted inhibition of cyclooxygenase-2. Gastroenterology 113:1039, 1997.
22. Oshima M, Dinchuk JE, Kargman SL, et al: Suppression of intestinal polyposis in $Apc^{\Delta 716}$ knockout mice by inhibition of cyclooxygenase 2 (COX-2). Cell 87:803, 1996.
23. Howe GR, Benitu E, Castelleto R, et al: Dietary intake of fiber and decreased risk of cancer of the colon and rectum: Evidence from combined analysis of 13 case-control studies. J Natl Cancer Inst 84: 1887, 1992.
24. Trock B, Lanza E, Greenwald P: Dietary fiber, vegetables, and colon cancer: Critical review and meta-analysis of the epidemiologic evidence. J Natl Cancer Inst 82:650, 1990.
25. Freudenheim JL, Grahm S, Horvath PJ, et al: Risks associated with source of fiber and fiber components in cancer of the colon and rectum. Cancer Res 50:3295, 1990.
26. Alberts DS, Martinez ME, Roe DJ, et al: Lack of effect of a high-fiber cereal supplement on the recurrence of colorectal adenomas. N Engl J Med 342:1156, 2000.
27. Schatzkin A, Lanza E, Corle D, et al: Lack of effect of a low-fat, high-fiber diet on the recurrence of colorectal adenomas. N Engl J Med 342:1149, 2000.
28. Kikendall JW, Bowen PE, Burgess MB, et al: Cigarettes and alcohol as independent risk factors for colonic adenomas. Gastroenterology 97:660, 1989.
29. World Cancer Research Fund (WCRF) Panel (Potter JD, Chair): Diet Nutrition and the Prevention of Cancer: A Global Perspective. Washington, DC, WCRF/American Institute of Cancer Research, 1997.
30. Baron JA, Sandler RS, Haile RW, et al: Folate intake, alcohol consumption, cigarette smoking, and risk of colorectal adenomas. J Natl Cancer Inst 90:57, 1998.
31. Bostick RM, Potter JD, Sellers TA, et al: Relation of calcium, vitamin D, and dairy food intake to incidence of colon cancer among older women: The Iowa Women's Health Study. Am J Epidemiol 137:1302, 1993.
32. Holt PR, Atillasoy EO, Gilman J, et al: Modulation of abnormal colonic epithelial cell proliferation and differentiation by low-fat dairy foods. A randomized controlled trial. JAMA 280:1074, 1998.
33. Pence BC: Role of calcium in colon cancer prevention: Experimental and clinical studies. Mutat Res 290:87, 1993.
34. Bautista D, Obrador A, Moreno V, et al: *Ki-ras* mutation modifies the protective role of dietary monosaturated fat and calcium on sporadic colorectal cancer. Cancer Epidemiol Biomarkers Prev 6:57, 1997.
35. Alberts DS, Ritenbaugh C, Strong JA, et al: Randomized double-blind, placebo-controlled study of wheat bran and calcium on fecal bile acids in patients with resected adenomas of the colon. J Natl Cancer Inst 88:81, 1996.
36. Kim KE, Brasitus TA: The role of vitamin D in normal and pathologic processes in the colon. Curr Opin Gastroenterol 17:72, 2001.
37. Sheng GG, Shao J, Sheng H, et al: A selective cyclooxygenase 2 inhibitor suppresses the growth of H-*ras*-transformed rat intestinal epithelial cells. Gastroenterology 113:1883, 1997.
38. He T-C, Chan TA, Vogelstein B, et al: PPARδ is an APC-regulated target of nonsteroidal anti-inflammatory drugs. Cell 99:335, 1999.
39. Taylor MT, Lawson KR, Ignatenko NA, et al: Sulindac sulfone inhibits K-*ras*-dependent cyclooxygenase-2 expression in human colon cancer cells. Cancer Res 60:6607, 2000.
40. Kargman S, O'Neill G, Vickers P, et al: Expression of prostaglandin G/H synthase-1 and -2 protein in human colon cancer. Cancer Res 55: 2556, 1995.
41. Hull MA, Fenwick SW, Chapple KS, et al: Cyclooxygenase-2 expression in colorectal cancer liver metastases. Clin Exp Metast 18:21, 2000.
42. Jacoby RF, Seibert K, Cole CE, et al: The cyclooxygenase-2 inhibitor celecoxib is a potent preventive and therapeutic agent in the min mouse model of adenomatous polyposis. Cancer Res 60:5040, 2000.
43. Oshima M, Murai(Hata) N, Kargman S, et al: Chemoprevention of intestinal polyposis in the $Apc^{\Delta 716}$ mouse by rofecoxib, a specific cyclooxygenase-2 inhibitor. Cancer Res 61:1733, 2001.
44. Reddy BS, Hirose Y, Lubet R, et al: Chemoprevention of colon cancer by specific cyclooxygenase-2 inhibitor, celecoxib, administered during different stages of carcinogenesis. Cancer Res 60:193, 2000.
45. Tsuji M, DuBois RN: Alterations in cellular adhesion and apoptosis in epithelial cells overexpressing prostaglandin endoperoxide synthase 2. Cell 83:493, 1995.
46. Lippman SM, Benner SE, Hong WK: Cancer chemoprevention. J Clin Oncol 12:851, 1994.
47. Janne PA, Mayer RJ: Chemoprevention of colorectal cancer. N Engl J Med 342:1960, 2000.
48. Lippman SM, Lee JJ, Sabichi AL: Cancer chemoprevention: Progress and promise. J Natl Cancer Inst 90:1514, 1998.
49. Fleischer D: Chromoendoscopy and magnification endoscopy in the colon. Gastrointest Endosc 49:S45, 1999.
50. Takayama T, Katsuki S, Takahashi Y, et al: Aberrant crypt foci of the colon as precursors of adenoma and cancer. N Engl J Med 339:1277, 1998.
51. McKeown-Eyssen GE, Bright-See E, Bruce WR, et al: A randomized trial of a low-fat high-fiber diet in the recurrence of colorectal polyps. J Clin Epidemiol 47:525, 1994.
52. Fuchs CS, Giovannucci EL, Colditz GA, et al: Dietary fiber and the risk of colorectal cancer and adenoma in women. N Engl J Med 340: 169, 1999.
53. Baron JA, Beach M, Mandel JS, et al: Calcium supplements for the prevention of colorectal adenomas. N Engl J Med 340:101, 1999.
54. Greenberg ER, Baron JA, Tosteson TD, et al: A clinical trial of antioxidant vitamins to prevent colorectal adenoma. N Engl J Med 331:141, 1994.
55. Giovannucci E, Stampfer MJ, Colditz GA, et al: Multivitamin use, folate, and colon cancer in women in the Nurses Health Study. Ann Intern Med 129:517, 1998.
56. Kim Y-I, Shirwadkar S, Choi S-W, et al: Effects of dietary folate on DNA strand breaks within mutation-prone exons of the *p53* gene in rat colon. Gastroenterology 119:151, 2000.
57. Grodstein F, Newcomb PA, Stampfer MJ: Postmenopausal hormone therapy and the risk of colorectal cancer: A review and meta-analysis. Am J Med 106:574, 1999.
58. Muscat JE, Stellman SD, Wynder EL: Nonsteroidal anti-inflammatory drugs and colorectal cancer. Cancer 74:1847, 1994.
59. Gann PH, Manson JE, Glynn RJ, et al: Low-dose aspirin and incidence of colorectal tumors in a randomized trial. J Natl Cancer Inst 85:1220, 1993.
60. Giardello FM, Hamilton SR, Krush AJ, et al: Treatment of colonic and rectal adenomas with sulindac in familial adenomatous polyposis. N Engl J Med 328:1313, 1993.
61. Steinbach G, Lynch PM, Phillips RKS, et al: The effect of celecoxib, a cyclooxygenase-2 inhibitor, in familial adenomatous polyposis. N Engl J Med 342:1946, 2000.
62. Risio M, Lipkin M, Cundelaresi G, et al: Correlations between rectal mucosal proliferation and the clinical pathological features of nonfamilial neoplasia of the large intestine. Cancer Res 51:1917, 1991.
63. Lichtenstein P, Holm NV, Verkasalo PK, et al: Environmental and heritable factors in the causation of cancer. N Engl J Med 343:78, 2000.

64. Chung DC: The genetic basis of colorectal cancer: Insights into critical pathways of tumorigenesis. Gastroenterology 119:854, 2000.
65. Grady WM, Markowitz S: Genomic instability and colorectal cancer. Curr Opin Gastroenterol 16:62, 2000.
66. Vogelstein B, Fearon ER, Hamilton SR, et al: Genetic alterations during colorectal tumor development. N Engl J Med 319:525, 1988.
67. Nishio E, Nakamura Y, Mioshi Y, et al: Mutations of 5q21 gene in FAP and colorectal cancer patients. Science 253:665, 1991.
68. Powell SM, Zilz N, Beazer-Barclay Y, et al: APC mutations occur early during colorectal tumorigenesis. Nature 359:235, 1992.
69. Boland CR, Sato J, Appelman HD, et al: Microallelotyping defines the sequence and tempo of allelic losses at tumor suppressor gene loci during colorectal cancer progression. Nature Med 1:907, 1995.
70. Laurent-Puig P, Olschwang S, Delattre O, et al: Survival and acquired genetic alterations in colorectal cancer. Gastroenterology 102:1136, 1992.
71. Jen J, Kim H, Piantadose S, et al: Allelic loss of chromosome 18q and prognosis in colorectal cancer. N Engl J Med 331:213, 1994.
72. Carethers JM, Hawn MT, Greenson JK, et al: Prognostic significance of allelic loss at chromosome 18q21 for stage II colorectal cancer. Gastroenterology 114:1188, 1998.
73. Kahlenberg MS, Stoler DL, Rodriguez-Bigas MA, et al: p53 Tumor suppressor gene mutations predict decreased survival of patients with sporadic colorectal carcinoma. Cancer 88:1814, 2000.
74. Shibata D, Reale MA, Lavin P, et al: The DCC protein and prognosis in colorectal cancer. N Engl J Med 335:1727, 1996.
75. Giardiello FM, Brensinger JD, Petersen GM, et al: The use and interpretation of commercial APC gene testing for familial adenomatous polyposis. N Engl J Med 336:823, 1997.
76. Korinek V, Barker N, Morin PJ, et al: Constitutive transcriptional activation by a β-catenin-Tcf complex in APC -/- colon carcinoma. Science 275:1784, 1997.
77. Morin PJ, Sparks AB, Korinek V, et al: Activation of β-catenin-Tcf signaling in colon cancer by mutations in β-catenin or APC. Science 275:1787, 1997.
78. Martinez-Lopez E, Abad A, Font A, et al: Allelic loss on chromosome 18q as a prognostic marker in stage II colorectal cancer. Gastroenterology 114:1180, 1998.
79. Watanabe T, Wu T-T, Catalano PJ, et al: Molecular predictors of survival after adjuvant chemotherapy for colon cancer. N Engl J Med 344:1196, 2001.
80. Takaku K, Oshima M, Miyoshi H, et al: Intestinal tumorigenesis in compound mutant mice of both *Dpc4* (*Smad4*) and APC genes. Cell 92:645, 1998.
81. Bresalier RS: Tumor progression in the intestine: *SMAD* about you. Gastroenterology 115:1598, 1998.
82. Yoshida BA, Sokoloff MM, Welch DR, et al: Metastasis-suppressor genes: A review and perspective of an emerging field. J Natl Cancer Inst 92:1717, 2000.
83. Chung DC, Rustgi AK: DNA mismatch repair and cancer. Gastroenterology 109:1685, 1995.
84. Parsons R, Guo-Min L, Longley MJ, et al: Hypermutability and mismatch repair deficiency in RER+ tumor cells. Cell 75:1227, 1993.
85. Fischel R, Lescoe MK, Rao MRS, et al: The human mutator gene homolog MSH2 and its association with hereditary nonpolyposis colon cancer. Cell 75:1027, 1993.
86. Peltomaki P, Aaltonen LA, Sistonen P, et al: Genetic mapping of a locus predisposing to human colorectal cancer. Science 260:810, 1993.
87. Leach FS, Niconides NC, Papadopoulos N, et al: Mutations of a mut S homolog in hereditary non-polyposis colorectal cancer. Cell 75: 1215, 1993.
88. Leach FS, Polyak K, Burrell M, et al: Expression of the human repair gene *hMSH2* in normal and neoplastic tissue. Cancer Res 56:235, 1996.
89. Grady WM, Myeroff LL, Swinler SE, et al: Mutational inactivation of transforming growth factor β receptor type II in microsatellite stable colon cancers. Cancer Res 59:320, 1999.
90. Gryfe R, Kim H, Hsieh ETK, et al: Tumor microsatellite instability and clinical outcome in young patients with colorectal cancer. N Engl J Med 342:69, 2000.
91. Watson P, Lin KM, Rodriguez-Bigas MA, et al: Colorectal carcinoma survival among hereditary nonpolyposis colorectal carcinoma family members. Cancer 83:259, 1998.
92. Carethers JM, Chauhan DP, Fink D, et al: Mismatch repair proficiency and in vitro response to 5-fluorouracil. Gastroenterology 117:123, 1999.
93. Hemminki A, Mecklin J-P, Jarvinen H, et al: Microsatellite instability is a favorable prognostic indicator in patients with colorectal cancer receiving chemotherapy. Gastroenterology 119:921, 2000.
94. Issa J-P: The epigenetics of colorectal cancer. Ann N Y Acad Sci 910:140, 2000.
95. Kane M, Loda M, Lipman J, et al: Methylation of the hMLH1 promoter correlates with lack of hMLH1 in sporadic tumors and mismatch repair-defective human tumor cell lines. Cancer Res 57:808, 1997.
96. Deng G, Chen A, Hong J, et al: Methylation of CpG in a small region of the hMLH1 promoter invariably correlates with the absence of gene expression. Cancer Res 59:2029, 1999.
97. Izkowitz SH, Bloom EJ, Kokal WA, et al: Sialosyl-Tn. A novel mucin antigen associated with prognosis in colorectal cancer patients. Cancer 66:1960, 1990.
98. Bresalier RS: The biology of colorectal cancer metastasis. Gastroenterol Clin North Am 25:805, 1996.
99. Bresalier RS, Ho SB, Schoeppner HL, et al: Enhanced sialylation of mucin-associated carbohydrate structures in colon cancer metastasis. Gastroenterology 24:338, 1996.
100. Sternberg LR, Byrd JC, Yunker CK, et al: Liver colonization by human colon cancer cells is reduced by antisense inhibition of MUC2 synthesis. Gastroenterology 116:363, 1999.
101. Bresalier RS, Mazurek N, Sternberg LR, et al: Expression of the β-galactoside binding protein gelectin-3 correlates with the metastatic potential of human colon cancer cells. Gastroenterology 115:287, 1998.
102. Rustgi AK: Hereditary gastrointestinal polyposis and nonpolyposis syndromes. N Engl J Med 331:1694, 1994.
103. Lynch HT, Smyrk TC, Watson P, et al: Genetics, natural history, tumor spectrum, and pathology of hereditary nonpolyposis colorectal cancer: An updated review. Gastroenterology 104:1535, 1993.
104. Rodriguiz-Bigas MD, Boland CR, Hamilton SR, et al: A National Cancer Institute workshop on hereditary nonpolyposis colorectal cancer syndrome: Meeting highlights and Bethesda guidelines. J Natl Cancer Inst 89:1758, 1997.
105. Mecklin JP: Frequency of hereditary colorectal cancer. Gastroenterology 93:1021, 1987.
106. Burt RW: Colon cancer screening. Gastroenterology 119:837, 2000.
107. Cannon-Albright LA, Skolnick MH, Bishop DT, et al: Common inheritance of susceptibility to colonic adenomatous polyps and associated colorectal cancers. N Engl J Med 319:533, 1988.
108. Leppert M, Burt R, Hughs JP, et al: Genetic analysis of an inherited predisposition to colon cancer in a family with a variable number of adenomatous polyps. N Engl J Med 322:404, 1990.
109. Neugut AI, Jacobson JS, Ahsan H, et al: Incidence and recurrence rates of colorectal adenomas: A prospective study. Gastroenterology 108:402, 1995.
110. Fuchs CS, Giovannucci EL, Colditz GA, et al: A prospective study of family history and the risk of colorectal cancer. N Engl J Med 331: 1669, 1994.
111. St John DJB, McDermott FT, Hopper JL, et al: Cancer risk in relatives of patients with common colorectal cancer. Ann Intern Med 118: 785, 1993.
112. Winawer SJ, Zauber AG, Gercles H, et al: Risk of colorectal cancer in families of patients with adenomatous polyps. N Engl J Med 334:82, 1996.
113. Atkin WS, Morson BC, Cuzick J: Long-term risk of colorectal cancer after excision of rectosigmoid adenomas. N Engl J Med 326:658, 1992.
114. O'Brien NJ, Winawar SJ, Zauber AG, et al: The National Polyp Study. Patient and polyp characteristics associated with high-grade dysplasia in colorectal adenomas. Gastroenterology 98:371, 1990.
115. Eide TJ: Risk of colorectal cancer in adenoma-bearing individuals within a defined population. Int J Cancer 38:173, 1986.
116. Langevin JM, Nivatvongs S: The true incidence of synchronous cancer of the large bowel. A prospective study. Am J Surg 197:330, 1984.
117. Pagana TJ, Ledesma EJ, Mittelman A, et al: The use of colonoscopy in the study of synchronous colorectal neoplasms. Cancer 55:356, 1984.
118. Heald RJ: Synchronous and metachronous carcinoma of the colon and rectum. Ann R Coll Surg Engl 72:172, 1990.
119. Byers T, Levin B, Rothenberger D, et al: American Cancer Society guidelines for screening and surveillance for early detection of colo-

rectal polyps and cancer: Update 1997. CA Cancer J Clin 47:154, 1997.
120. Burt R: Impact of family history on screening and surveillance. Gastrointest Endosc 49:541, 1999.
121. Smith RA, Von Eschenbach AC, Wender R, et al: American Cancer Society Guidelines for early detection of cancer: Update of early detection guidelines for prostate, colorectal and endometrial cancers. CA Cancer J Clin 1:51, 2001.
122. Hamilton SR, Liu B, Parsons RE, et al: The molecular basis of Turcot's syndrome. N Engl J Med 332:839, 1995.
123. Cohen PR, Kohn SR, Kurzrock R: Association of sebaceous gland tumors and internal malignancy: The Muir-Torre syndrome. Am J Med 90:606, 1991.
124. Giardiello FM, Brensinger JD, Tersmette AC, et al: Very high risk of cancer in familial Peutz-Jeghers syndrome. Gastroenterology 119:1447, 2000.
125. Provenzale D, Kowdley KU, Arora S, et al: Prophylactic colectomy or surveillance for chronic ulcerative colitis? A decision analysis. Gastroenterology 109:1188, 1995.
126. Nugent FW, Haggitt RC, Gilpin PA: Cancer surveillance in ulcerative colitis. Gastroenterology 100:1241, 1991.
127. Lennard-Jones JE, Melville DM, Morson BC, et al: Precancer and cancer in extensive ulcerative colitis: Findings among 401 patients over 22 years. Gut 31:800, 1990.
128. Ekbom A, Helmick C, Zack M, et al: Ulcerative colitis and colorectal cancer. A population-based study. N Engl J Med 323:1228, 1990.
129. Katzka I, Brody RS, Morris E, et al: Assessment of colorectal cancer risk in patients with ulcerative colitis: Experience from a private practice. Gastroenterology 85:22, 1983.
130. Nuako KW, Ahlquist DA, Mahoney DW, et al: Familial predisposition for colorectal cancer in chronic ulcerative colitis: A case-control study. Gastroenterology 115:1079, 1998.
131. Heuschen UA, Hinz U, Allemeyer EH, et al: Backwash ileitis is strongly associated with colorectal carcinoma in ulcerative colitis. Gastroenterology 120:841, 2001.
132. Hamilton SR: Colorectal carcinoma in patients with Crohn's disease. Gastroenterology 80:318, 1985.
133. Persson P-G, Karlen P, Bernell O, et al: Crohn's disease and cancer: A population-based cohort study. Gastroenterology 107:1675, 1994.
134. Riddell RH, Goldman H, Ransohoff DF, et al: Dysplasia in inflammatory bowel disease: Standardized classification with provisional clinical application. Hum Pathol 11:14, 1983.
135. Blackstone MO, Riddel RH, Rodgers BHG, et al: Dysplasia-associated lesion or mass (DALM) detected by colonoscopy in long-standing ulcerative colitis; An indication for surgery. Gastroenterology 80:366, 1981.
136. Willenbucher RF, Zelman SJ, Ferrel LD, et al: Chromosomal alteration in ulcerative colitis-related neoplastic progression. Gastroenterology 113:791, 1997.
137. Friedman S, Rubin PH, Bodian C, et al: Screening and surveillance colonoscopy in chronic Crohn's colitis. Gastroenterology 120:820, 2001.
138. Adanik HL, Meirik O, Gustavsson S, et al: Colorectal cancer after cholecystectomy: Absence of risk within 11–14 years. Gastroenterology 85:859, 1983.
139. Lagergren J, Ye W, Ekbom A: Intestinal cancer after cholecystectomy: Is bile involved in intestinal carcinogenesis? Gastroenterology (in press).
140. American Joint Committee on Cancer: Manual for Staging of Cancer, 5th ed. Philadelphia, JB Lippincott, 1997.
141. Wolmark N, Fisher B: An analysis of survival and treatment failure following abdominoperineal and sphincter-saving resection in Dukes' B and C rectal carcinoma. Ann Surg 204:480, 1986.
142. Gastrointestinal Tumor Study Group: Adjuvant therapy of colon cancer—results of a prospectively randomized trial. N Engl J Med 310: 737, 1984.
143. Wolmark N, Fisher ER, Wieand S, et al: The relationship of depth of penetration and tumor size to the number of positive nodes in Dukes' C colorectal cancer. Cancer 53:2707, 1984.
144. Rich T, Gunderson LL, Lew R, et al: Patterns of recurrences after potentially curable surgery. Cancer 52:1317, 1983.
145. Heiman TM, Szporn A, Bolnick K, et al: Local recurrence following surgical treatment of rectal cancer. Comparison of anterior and abdominoperineal resection. Dis Colon Rectum 29:862, 1986.
146. Wolmark N, Fisher B, Wieand HS: The prognostic value of the modifications of the Dukes' C class of colorectal cancer. Ann Surg 203:115, 1986.
147. Moertel CG, O'Fallon JR, Go VL, et al: The preoperative carcinoembryonic antigen test in the diagnosis, staging and prognosis of colorectal cancer. Cancer 58:603, 1986.
148. Wolmark N, Cruz I, Redmond CK, et al: Tumor size and regional lymph node metastasis in colorectal cancer. Cancer 51:1315, 1983.
149. Steinberg SM, Barwick KW, Stablein DM: Importance of tumor pathology and morphology in patients with surgically resected colon cancer. Cancer 58:1340, 1986.
150. Bresalier RS, Niv Y, Byrd JC, et al: Mucin production by human colonic carcinoma cells correlates with their metastatic potential in animal models of colon cancer metastasis. J Clin Invest 87:1037, 1991.
151. Giacchero A, Aste H, Baracchini P, et al: Primary signet-ring carcinoma of the large bowel. Cancer 56:1723, 1985.
152. Armitage NC, Ballantyne KC, Sheffield JP, et al: A prospective evaluation of the effect of tumor cell DNA content on recurrence in colorectal cancer. Cancer 67:2599, 1991.
153. Albe X, Vassilakos P, Helfer-Guarnori K, et al: Independent prognostic value of ploidy in colorectal cancer. A prospective study using image cytometry. Cancer 66:1168, 1990.
154. Prorok PC, Andriole GL, Bresalier RS, et al: Design of the prostate, lung, colorectal and ovarian (PLCO) cancer screening trial. Control Clin Trials 21:2495, 2000.
155. Bates SE: Clinical applications of serum tumor markers. Ann Intern Med 115:623, 1991.
156. Eddy DM, Nugent FW, Eddy JF, et al: Screening for colorectal cancer in a high risk population. Results of a mathematical model. Gastroenterology 92:682, 1987.
157. Rex DK, Rahmani EY, Haseman JH, et al: Relative sensitivity of colonoscopy and barium enema for detection of colorectal cancer in clinical practice. Gastroenterology 112:17, 1997.
158. Winawer SJ, Stewart ET, Zauber AG, et al: A comparison of colonoscopy and double-contrast barium enema for surveillance after polypectomy. N Engl J Med 342:1766, 2000.
159. U.S. Preventive Services Task Force: Guide to Clinical Preventative Services. Washington, DC, US Public Health Service, 1995, p 75.
160. Winawer SJ, St John DJ, Bond JH, et al: Prevention of colorectal cancer: Guidelines based on new data. Bull WHO 73:7, 1995.
161. Winawer SJ, Fletcher RH, Miller L, et al: Colorectal cancer screening: Clinical guidelines and rationale. Gastroenterology 112:594, 1997.
162. Centers for Disease Control: Screening for colorectal cancer—United States, 1997. Morb Mortal Wkly Rep 48:116, 1999.
163. Vernon SW: Participation in colorectal cancer screening: A review. J Natl Cancer Inst 89:1406, 1997.
164. Lieberman DA: Cost-effectiveness model for colon cancer screening. Gastroenterology 109:1781, 1995.
165. Toribara NW, Sleisenger MH: Screening for colorectal cancer. N Engl J Med 332:861, 1995.
166. Hardcastle JD, Chamberlain JO, Robinson MHE, et al: Randomized controlled trial of faecal-occult-blood screening for colorectal cancer. Lancet 348:1472, 1996.
167. Mandel JS, Bond JH, Curch TR, et al: Reducing mortality from colorectal cancer by screening for fecal occult blood. N Engl J Med 328:1365, 1993.
168. Kronborg O, Fenger C, Worm J, et al: Causes of death during the first 5 years of a randomized trial of mass screening for colorectal cancer with fecal occult blood test. Scand J Gastroenterol 27:47, 1992.
169. Kewenter J, Asztely M, Ergaras B, et al: A randomized trial of fecal occult blood testing for early detection of colorectal cancer: Results of screening and rescreening 51325 subjects. In Miller AB, et al (eds): Cancer Screening. Cambridge, UK, Cambridge University Press, 1991, p 116.
170. Kronborg O, Fenger C, Olsen J, et al: Randomized study of screening for colorectal cancer with faecal-occult-blood test. Lancet 348:1467, 1996.
171. Allison JE, Feldman RF, Tekawa IS: Hemoccult screening in detecting colorectal neoplasm: Sensitivity, specificity and predictive value. Long-term follow-up in a large practice setting. Ann Intern Med 112: 328, 1990.
172. Ahlquist DA: Occult blood screening: Obstacles to effectiveness. Cancer 70:1259, 1992.
173. Lang CA, Ransohoff D: Fecal occult blood screening for colorectal cancer. JAMA 271:1011, 1994.

174. Lurie JD, Welch HG: Diagnostic testing following fecal occult blood screening in the elderly. J Natl Cancer Inst 91:1641, 1999.
175. Sonnenberg A, Delco F, Inadomi JM: Cost-effectiveness of colonoscopy in screening for colorectal cancer. Ann Intern Med 133:573, 2000.
176. Shimbo T, Glick HA, Eisenberg JM: Cost-effectiveness of strategies for colorectal cancer screening in Japan. Int J Technol Assess Health Care 10:359, 1994.
177. Mandel JS, Church TR, Ederer F, et al: Colorectal cancer mortality: Effectiveness of biennial screening for fecal occult blood. J Natl Cancer Inst 91:434, 1999.
178. St John DJ, Young GP, Alexyeff MA, et al: Evaluation of new occult blood tests for detection of colorectal neoplasia. Gastroenterology 104: 1161, 1993.
179. Allison JE, Tekawa IS, Randsom LJ, et al: A comparison of fecal occult-blood tests for colorectal cancer screening. N Engl J Med 334: 155, 1996.
180. Selby JV, Friedman GD, Quesenberry CP, et al: A case-control study of screening sigmoidoscopy and mortality from colorectal cancer. N Engl J Med 326:653, 1992.
181. Newcomb PA, Norfleet RG, Surawicz TS, et al: Screening sigmoidoscopy and colorectal cancer mortality. J Natl Cancer Inst 84:1572, 1992.
182. Muller AD, Sonnenberg A: Prevention of colorectal cancer by flexible endoscopy and polypectomy. A case-control study of 32,702 veterans. Ann Intern Med 123:904, 1995.
183. Mawle WF: Screening for colorectal cancer by nurse endoscopists. N Engl J Med 330:183, 1994.
184. Schoenfeld PS, Case B, Kita J, et al: Effectiveness and patient satisfaction with screening flexible sigmoidoscopy performed by registered nurses. Gastrointest Endosc 49:158, 1999.
185. Winawer SJ, Zauber AG, Ho MN, et al: Prevention of colorectal cancer by colonoscopic polypectomy. N Engl J Med 329:1977, 1993.
186. Leard LE, Savides TJ, Ganiats TG: Patient preferences for colorectal cancer screening. J Fam Pract 45:211, 1997.
187. Rex DK, Chak A, Vasudeva R, et al: Prospective determination of distal colon findings in average-risk patients with proximal colon cancer. Gastrointest Endosc 49:727, 1999.
188. Schoen RE, Corle D, Cranston K, et al: Is colonoscopy needed for the nonadvanced adenoma found on sigmoidoscopy? Gastroenterology 115:533, 1998.
189. Imperiale TF, Wagner DR, Lin CY, et al: Risk of advanced proximal neoplasms in asymptomatic adults according to the distal colorectal findings. N Engl J Med 343:169, 2000.
190. Lieberman DA, Weiss DG, Bond JH, et al: Use of colonoscopy to screen asymptomatic adults for colorectal cancer. N Engl J Med 343: 162, 2000.
191. Fenlon HM, Nunes DP, Schroy PC, et al: A comparison of virtual and conventional colonoscopy for the detection of colorectal polyps. N Engl J Med 341:1496, 1999.
192. Chaoui AS, Barish MA: Virtual colonoscopy: A new tool for colorectal cancer screening. Curr Opin Gastroenterol 17:78, 2001.
193. Sidransky D, Tokino T, Hamilton SR, et al: Identification of *ras* oncogene mutations in the stool of patients with curable colorectal tumors. Science 256:103, 1992.
194. Ahlquist DA, Skoletsky JE, Boynton KA, et al: Colorectal cancer screening by detection of altered human DNA in stool: Feasibility of a multitarget assay panel. Gastroenterology 119:1219, 2000.
195. Kinney AY, DeVellis BM, Skrzynia C, et al: Genetic testing for colorectal carcinoma susceptibility. Focus group responses of individuals with colorectal carcinoma and first-degree relatives. Cancer 91:57, 2001.
196. Syngal S, Fox EA, Li C, et al: Interpretation of genetic tests for hereditary nonpolyposis colorectal cancer. JAMA 282:247, 1999.
197. Bresalier RS: Genetic testing for hereditary nonpolyposis colorectal cancer: Are we there yet? Gastroenterology 118:230, 2000.
198. Stern HS, Viertelhausen S, Hunter AGW, et al: APC I1307K increases risk of transition from polyp to colorectal carcinoma in Ashkenazi Jews. Gastroenterology 120:392, 2001.
199. Barnes CJ, Lee M: Chemoprevention of spontaneous intestinal adenomas in the adenomatous polyposis coli Min mouse model with aspirin. Gastroenterology 114:873, 1998.
200. Winawer SH, Flehinger BJ, Schothenfield D, et al: Screening for colorectal cancer with fecal occult blood testing and sigmoidoscopy. J Natl Cancer Inst 85:1311, 1993.
201. Jarvinen HJ, Mecklin J-P, Sistonen P: Screening reduces colorectal cancer rate in families with hereditary nonpolyposis colorectal cancer. Gastroenterology 108:1405, 1995.
202. Luce M, Marra G, Chauhan DP, et al: In vitro transcription/translation assay for the screening of hMLH1 and hMSH2 mutations in familial colon cancer. Gastroenterology 109:1368, 1995.
203. Syngal S, Weeks JC, Schrag D, et al: Benefits of colonscopic surveillance and prophylactic colectomy in patients with hereditary nonpolyposis colorectal cancer mutations. Ann Intern Med 129:787, 1998.
204. Wijnen JT, Vasen HFA, Kahn M, et al: Clinical findings with implications for genetic testing in families with clustering of colorectal cancer. N Engl J Med 339:511, 1998.
205. Aaltonen LA, Salovaara R, Kristo P, et al: Incidence of hereditary nonpolyposis colorectal cancer and the feasibility of molecular screening for the disease. N Engl J Med 338:1481, 1998.
206. Jarvinen HJ, Aarnio M, Mustonen H, et al: Controlled 15-year trial on screening for colorectal cancer in families with hereditary nonpolyposis colorectal cancer. Gastroenterology 118:829, 2000.
207. Moffat FL, Pilski CM, Hammershaimb L, et al: Clinical utility of external immunoscintigraphy with the IMMU-4 technetium −99m Fab′ antibody fragment in patients undergoing surgery for carcinoma of the colon and rectum: Results of a pivotal, phase III trial. J Clin Oncol 14:2295, 1996.
208. Wolff BG, Bolton J, Baum R: Radioimmunoscintigraphy of recurrent, metastatic or occult colorectal cancer with Tc99m88BV59H21-2V67-66 (HumaSPECT-Tc), a totally human monoclonal antibody: Patient management: Benefit from a phase III multicenter study. Dis Colon Rectum 41:553, 1998.
209. Delbeke D, Vitola JV, Scindler M, et al: Staging recurrent metastatic colorectal carcinoma with PET. J Natl Med 38:1196, 1997.
210. Kemeny NE, Ron IG: Liver metastases. Curr Treat Options Gastroenterol 2:49, 1999.
211. Vetto JT, Hughs KS, Rosenstein R, et al: Morbidity and mortality of hepatic resection for metastatic colorectal carcinoma. Dis Colon Rectum 33:408, 1990.
212. Scheele J, Stargl R, Altendorf-Hofmann A: Hepatic metastases from colorectal carcinoma: Impact of surgical resection on natural history. Br J Surg 77:1241, 1990.
213. Stone MD, Cady B, Jenkins RL, et al: Surgical therapy for recurrent liver metastases from colorectal cancer. Arch Surg 125:718, 1990.
214. Steele GD, Bledoy R, Mayer R, et al: Prospective evaluation of hepatic resection for colorectal carcinoma metastases to the liver: Gastrointestinal Tumor Study Group Protocol 6J84. J Clin Oncol 9: 1105, 1991.
215. Cady B, Stone MD, McDermott WV, et al: Technical and biological factors in disease-free survival after hepatic resection for colorectal cancer metastases. Arch Surg 127:561, 1992.
216. McCarthy TM, Kuhn JA: Cryotherapy for liver tumors. Oncology 12: 979, 1998.
217. Moertel CG, Fleming TR, MacDonald JS, et al: Levamisole and fluorouracil for adjuvant therapy of resected colon carcinoma. N Engl J Med 322:352, 1990.
218. Moertel CG, Fleming TR, MacDonald JE, et al: Fluorouracil plus levamisole as effective adjuvant therapy after resection of stage III colon carcinoma: A final report. Ann Intern Med 122:321, 1995.
219. Wolmark N, Rockette H, Fisher B: The benefit of leucovorin-modulated fluorouracil as postoperative adjuvant therapy for primary colon cancer: Results from the National Surgical Adjuvant Breast and Bowel Project Protocol C-03. J Clin Oncol 11:1879, 1993.
220. Francini G, Petrioli R, Lorenzin L, et al: Folinic acid and 5-fluorouracil as adjuvant chemotherapy in colon cancer. Gastroenterology 106: 899, 1994.
221. International Multicenter Pooled Analysis of Colon Cancer Trials (IMPACT) Investigators: Efficacy of adjuvant fluorouracil, leucovorin, and levamisole in Dukes' B and C carcinoma of the colon: Results from the National Adjuvant Breast and Bowel Project C-04. Lancet 345:939, 2000.
222. Wolmark N, Rockette H, Mamounas E, et al: Clinical trial to assess the relative efficacy of fluorouracil, fluorouracil and leucovorin, fluorouracil and levamisole, and fluorouracil, leucovorin, and levamisole in Dukes' B and C carcinoma of the colon: Results from the National Adjuvant Breast and Bowel Project C-04. J Clin Oncol 17:3553, 1999.
223. O'Connell MJ, Laurie JA, Kahn M, et al: Prospectively randomized trial of postoperative adjuvant chemotherapy in patients with high-risk colon cancer. J Clin Oncol 16:295, 1998.

224. Liver Infusion Meta-analysis Group: Portal vein chemotherapy for colorectal cancer: A meta-analysis of 4000 patients in 10 studies. J Natl Cancer Inst 89:497, 1997.
225. Krook JE, Moertel CG, Gunderson LL, et al: Effective adjuvant therapy for high-risk rectal carcinoma. N Engl J Med 324:709, 1991.
226. O'Connell MJ, Martenson JA, Wiand HS, et al: Improving adjuvant therapy for rectal cancer by combining protracted-infusion fluorouracil with radiation therapy after curative surgery. N Engl J Med 331:502, 1994.
227. Ajlouni M: The role of radiation in adjuvant treatment of rectal cancer. Curr Opin Gastroenterol 17:86, 2001.
228. Project ACCM: Modulation of fluorouracil by leucovorin in patients with advanced colorectal cancer: Evidence in terms of response rate. J Clin Oncol 10:856, 1992.
229. Doroshow JH, Multhauf P, Leong L, et al: Prospective randomized comparison of fluorouracil versus fluorouracil and high-dose continuous infusion leucovorin calcium for treatment of advanced measurable colorectal cancer in patients previously unexposed to chemotherapy. J Clin Oncol 8:491, 1990.
230. Poon MA, O'Connell MJ, Moertel CG, et al: Biochemical modulation of fluorouracil: Evidence of significant improvement of survival and quality of life in patients with advanced colorectal carcinoma. J Clin Oncol 7:1907, 1989.
231. Buroker TR, O'Connell MJ, Wieand HS, et al: Randomized comparison of two schedules of fluorouracil and leucovorin in the treatment of advanced colorectal cancer. J Clin Oncol 12:14, 1994.
232. Meta-analysis Group in Cancer: Efficacy of intravenous infusion of fluorouracil 1 compound with bolus administration in advanced colorectal cancer. J Clin Oncol 16:301, 1998.
233. Saltz LB, Cox JV, Blanke C, et al: Irinotecan plus fluorouracil and leucovorin for metastatic colorectal cancer. N Engl J Med 343:905, 2000.
234. Partyka S, Ajani J: Chemotherapy of colorectal cancer. Curr Treatment Options Gastroenterol 2:38, 1999.
235. Hafstrom L, Engaras B, Holmberg SB, et al: Treatment of liver metastases from colorectal cancer with hepatic artery occlusion, intraportal 5-fluorouracil infusion, and oral allopurinol. A randomized clinical trial. Cancer 74:2749, 1994.
236. Qi T, Moyana T, Bresalier RS, et al: Antibody targeted lymphokine-activated killer cells inhibit liver micrometastasis in severe combined immunodeficient mice. Gastroenterology 109:1950, 1995.

Chapter 116

Proctitis and Sexually Transmissible Intestinal Disease

Ronald Fried and Christina Surawicz

Sexually transmissible diseases (STDs) include viral, bacterial, protozoal, and helminthic infections. In some cases, malignant disease is a direct consequence of such infections. Sexual behavior is a major factor in the transmission of infectious disease; anal receptive sexual practices as well as manual and oral contact with a partner's anus may cause direct person-to-person transmission of infectious agents.

Following the acquired immunodeficiency syndrome (AIDS) epidemic, safer sex practices in male homosexuals altered epidemiologic patterns of sexually transmitted diseases. In STD clinics in Seattle and San Francisco, the number of reported cases of gonorrhea and syphilis fell dramatically from 1982 to 1988.[1] Reductions in the number of AIDS cases among men who have sex with men (MSM) also have been attributed to increasingly effective antiretroviral therapy since the mid-1990s. On the other hand, in San Francisco, more recent data from annual behavioral surveys among MSM (1994–1997) and from the STD surveillance program (1990–1997) have demonstrated increases in the frequency of unsafe sexual behavior and in rates of rectal gonorrhea among MSM.[2] In a study from Amsterdam in 1999, increases of 46% and 111% in the number of cases of gonorrhea and syphilis, respectively, were observed, compared with 1998. The largest increase was seen among MSM, in whom the number of diagnosed cases of anorectal gonorrhea in 1999 was twice as high as that in 1998, and the number of cases of syphilis was four times as high.[3] The increase in the frequency of unsafe sexual behavior may relate to a more casual attitude about AIDS, now that effective antiretroviral treatment is available. Promiscuity and the failure to use condoms remain important risk factors for STDs in both homosexuals and heterosexuals. Physicians and other health-care providers continue to have an important role in preventing STDs through education of those at risk.

This chapter considers gastrointestinal infections that are primarily sexually transmitted. Infectious diseases for which sexual contact is not the principal mode of transmission, such as viral hepatitis (Chapter 68) and infectious diarrhea (Chapter 96), are discussed extensively elsewhere in this book.

CLINICAL SYNDROMES

Sexually transmitted gastrointestinal syndromes can be grouped into one of four broad categories: proctitis, perianal disease, proctocolitis, and enteritis (Table 116–1). The enteritic syndrome consists of watery, nonbloody diarrhea, often accompanied by weight loss and abdominal pain. Many of the causative pathogens, such as *Giardia lamblia*, do not result in proctitis or proctocolitis. Proctitis is characterized by inflammation of the rectum, and proctocolitis is characterized by inflammation extending proximally in the colon. A careful and thorough sexual history may suggest which pathogens are likely to be involved in a given patient. Each clinical syndrome suggests specific pathogens, although sometimes a specific organism is not identified. In addition, multiple pathogens can be found in many cases.

In patients presenting with gastrointestinal complaints and a history of high-risk sexual behavior, the gastrointestinal manifestations of AIDS (discussed in Chapter 28) must be differentiated from other sexually acquired infections. Biliary tract disease in such persons is more likely to be a complication of HIV infection than of another sexually acquired infection. In persons with HIV infection, nonsexually transmitted infections also are common. Sexual practices that decrease the risk of HIV infection, such as fellatio, are, nevertheless, a significant risk for STDs.[4, 5]

Table 116–1 | **Common Sexually Transmitted Gastrointestinal Syndromes**

	PROCTITIS	PROCTOCOLITIS	ENTERITIS
Symptoms	Rectal pain, discharge, tenesmus	Symptoms of proctitis plus cramps, diarrhea	Diarrhea, cramps, bloating, nausea
Pathogen(s)	*Neisseria gonorrhoeae* *Chlamydia trachomatis* *Treponema pallidum* Herpes simpex virus	*Entamoeba histolytica* *Campylobacter jejuni* *Shigella flexneri* *Chlamydia trachomatis* (LGV*)	*Giardia lamblia*
Mode of Acquisition	Receptive anal intercourse	Direct or indirect fecal-oral contact	Direct or indirect fecal-oral contact
Anoscopic Findings	Rectal exudate ± friability	Rectal exudate, friability that may extend into the sigmoid colon	Normal

*Lymphogranuloma venereum strains.
From Rompalo AM: Diagnosis and treatment of sexually acquired proctitis and proctocolitis: An update. Clin Infect Dis 28(Suppl 1):S84–S90, 1999.

Proctitis and Perianal Disease

Proctitis is inflammation limited to the distal 15 cm of the rectum, as detected by flexible sigmoidoscopy. Sigmoidoscopic findings of proctitis include erythema and friable mucosa in the rectum. Infectious proctitis is often a result of anal-receptive intercourse, which can introduce pathogens.[6] The squamous epithelium of the anal canal can be infected by herpes simplex virus (HSV), syphilis, and human papilloma virus (HPV). Other pathogens can involve rectal mucosa more proximally.[7] The pathogens most frequently involved are *Neisseria gonorrhoeae, Chlamydia trachomatis* (non-lymphogranuloma venerum [LGV] types), HSV *type II*, and *Treponema pallidum*. Multiple pathogens may be found in the same person.

Symptoms of proctitis can include anorectal mucoid, mucopurulent, or bloody discharge; anal pain, itching, or burning; and tenesmus. When anal pain is severe, constipation is more common than diarrhea, although either can occur. Some pathogens cause perianal or anal lesions, and HSV II, *Chlamydia trachomatis*, and syphilis are the most common of these. Anal and buttock pain with HSV infection is caused by sacral neuralgia. Systemic symptoms and fever are uncommon, except in primary HSV and *Chlamydia trachomatis* LGV strain infections.

HSV infection may present with systemic viral symptoms like fever, chills, and malaise. The perianal symptoms can be severe and include anal pain and discharge, often with constipation because of the pain. Neural involvement by the virus also may explain the constipation, as well as difficulty in urination, impotence, and sacral paresthesias. Perianal vesicles are typical, as are pustules and ulcers, and can be associated with severe skin lesions on the buttocks.

Syphilis can cause anal mass lesions or ulcers. The chancre, which is the lesion of primary syphilis, can present as a perianal ulcer. These ulcers are typically painless and well demarcated, with indurated edges and a clean base. They typically occur 2 to 6 weeks after exposure. Other symptoms are itching, bleeding, discharge, constipation, and tenesmus. The lesions of secondary syphilis are usually painful and can present as an anorectal mass.[8] Such lesions also can cause painful defecation, thereby mimicking a fissure, fistula, or even perirectal abscess. Tender inguinal lymph nodes may be present.

Gonorrhea typically causes anal discharge that can be detected by anoscopic exam. Other symptoms are nonspecific and include itching, pain with defecation, rectal fullness, and constipation. Asymptomatic infections are common.

Both LGV and non-LGV immunotypes of *C. trachomatis* can cause proctitis and proctocolitis.[9] Typically, the non-LGV strains cause mild proctitis with rectal discharge, tenesmus, and anorectal pain. The LGV strains cause more severe inflammation, with intense anorectal pain, bloody mucoid discharge, and tenesmus. Symptoms can be chronic, lasting weeks to years, with complications such as strictures and fistulas that can mimic Crohn's disease.

In one of the earliest classic prospective studies of anorectal infections in homosexual men, the most common infectious causes of proctitis (in order of decreasing frequency) were HSV, *N. gonorrhoeae*, syphilis, and *C. trachomatis*.[10] This work, performed in Seattle, was published in 1981, just as the HIV epidemic was beginning. Since that time, safe sex practices have led to a decrease in the incidence of gastrointestinal STDs in the United States, although these disorders are still common in other areas of the world. For example, seroprevalence rates of HSV type II have dropped from 70% in the 1980s to 26% currently.[11] However, even in the United States some persons remain at high risk for STDs because they do not practice safe sex. A more recent study in Seattle documented that bacterial STDs are still common, and a 1998 study of STDs among MSM showed that during a follow-up period of 1 year, 31 men (5.7 per 100 person years) had 34 episodes of a symptomatic bacterial STD syndrome (urethritis, epididymitis, or proctitis).[5] In addition, the practice of oral sex, which has less risk of transmitting HIV, is still an important risk factor for rectal gonorrhea,[12] as well as for urethral gonorrhea and nonchlamydial nongonococcal urethritis.[4] Unprotected insertive anal sex also remains a major risk factor for anorectal infections.[5]

Routine evaluation of the patient with proctitis or perianal disease should include a test for syphilis (a Venereal Disease Research Laboratory [VDRL] antigen test), smears and culture for *N. gonorrhoeae*, and a rectal swab for *C. trachomatis*. Diarrhea can be present with proctitis but is more common with enteritis or proctocolitis. In that case, stool cultures for bacterial pathogens such as *Shigella* species and *Campylobacter* species and stool examinations for ova and parasites are indicated, and flexible sigmoidoscopy must be considered.

Human Papillomavirus, Warts, and Anal Cancer

Symptoms of perianal disease include pruritus, pain, and tenesmus. Perianal itching may be caused by *Enterobius vermicularis* (pinworm or threadworm) infestation. Human papillomavirus (HPV) causes warts, also known as condyloma acuminata. HPV infection is the most common sexually transmitted infection among MSM, and receptive anal intercourse is the most common mode of transmission. Typically the lesions are raised and pale. The warts can be present externally or internally in the anal canal as well as in the genital area. Warts can be present singly, in small clusters, or even in large exophytic masses. Symptoms of external warts include friability, itching, and bleeding. Internal warts are usually asymptomatic.

The increased frequency of anal cancer among HIV-positive homosexual men has been linked to HPV infection, as has cervical cancer in women.[13] There are over 60 strains of HPV, some of which have more oncogenic potential, specifically strains 16, 18, 45, and 46. HPV types 6 and 11 typically cause benign disease. Dysplastic lesions may be precursors of squamous cell anal cancers in men and cervical carcinoma in women. In patients with HIV infection, warts may be more extensive, resistant to treatment, and associated with anal squamous cell cancer and its presumed precursor, anal squamous intraepithelial lesion (ASIL).[14] With improved survival associated with highly active antiretroviral therapy (HAART), more cases of anal cancer can be expected; some authorities advocate screening all homosexual and bisexual men using anal cytology by rectal swab and anoscopy to look for anal cancer or its precursor ASIL, as is done for cervical cancer.[15, 16]

Proctocolitis

Proctocolitis is inflammation extending beyond 15 cm in the rectum. Common symptoms are those of proctitis, as just noted, but symptoms can also include watery or bloody diarrhea. Associated symptoms are abdominal cramps, left lower quadrant abdominal pain, and fever. Systemic symptoms can occur, including weight loss and anorexia. Enteric pathogens are the most likely cause, specifically *Entamoeba histolytica, Shigella*, and *Campylobacter*. In persons treated with antibiotics within the previous 2 months, antibiotic-associated colitis caused by *Clostridium difficile*, with or without pseudomembranes, also must be considered. *Shigella* infection causes predominantly distal colitis with watery or bloody diarrhea, tenesmus, and abdominal cramping. Other pathogens include *Chlamydia trachomatis* (LGV types), *Escherichia coli, Salmonella* species, and *Yersinia*. Enteric pathogens that can cause ileocolitis and a predominance of right-sided colonic symptoms are *Salmonella, Campylobacter*, and *E. coli* O157:H7 (see Chapters 96, 97, and 98).

Enteritis

Enteritis is inflammation or infection of the small intestine. The most common symptoms of enteritis are diarrhea that is usually watery rather than bloody, malabsorption, and weight loss. Abdominal pain, when present, is often periumbilical and crampy. Associated symptoms can include nausea, vomiting, anorexia, bloating, flatulence, and fever. Infectious enteritis usually results from oral ingestion of material that has been contaminated with feces; oral-anal sexual contact is an important risk factor. Usual causative organisms are the parasites *Giardia lamblia, E. histolytica*, and enteric bacterial pathogens. Multiple pathogens can be found in approximately 20% of cases. Diagnosis is made by stool culture and examination for ova and parasites (see Chapters 96 and 98).

Hepatic and Biliary Tract Diseases

Biliary tract involvement with sexually transmitted diseases is unusual, with two exceptions: gonococcal or chlamydial perihepatitis and biliary tract infections associated with HIV infection. Liver diseases associated with HIV infection are discussed in greater detail in Chapter 28.

Perihepatitis

Gonococcal or chlamydial infection of the cervix can extend to the surface of the liver; this entity has been called Fitz-Hugh–Curtis syndrome and is more common in sexually active women than in sexually inactive women. The organisms presumably travel from infected fallopian tubes through the peritoneal cavity to the liver surface. In some cases, symptoms of the initial pelvic inflammatory disease (pelvic pain and tenderness and vaginal discharge) may be absent.

Symptoms of perihepatitis include acute right upper abdominal pain with tenderness, guarding, and sometimes fever; nausea; vomiting; and arthralgias. The right upper quadrant pain may mimic hepatitis or cholecystitis; an acute presentation can also suggest a perforated viscus, such as peptic ulcer disease, appendicitis, or a subphrenic abscess. Sometimes pathognomonic evidence of disseminated gonococcal infection, such as the typical skin papules or pustules, can be seen on physical examination. Laboratory evaluation usually shows leukocytosis, an elevated erythrocyte sedimentation rate, and mild elevation of serum aminotransferase levels. Cervical cultures are usually positive for *N. gonorrhoeae* or *Chlamydia*, even if there is no visible cervical discharge. In rare cases, laparoscopy may be needed to make the diagnosis; typical findings are "violin string"-like filmy adhesions on the surface of the liver.

Biliary Tract Disease in Patients with HIV Infection

Cholangiopathy associated with HIV was first described in 1983, early in the HIV epidemic, when cryptosporidiosis was found in the biliary tree.[17, 18] Typical clinical symptoms are right upper quadrant pain, fever, and an elevated serum alkaline phosphatase level.[19] Jaundice is uncommon. Diarrhea is common because many of the pathogens infect the small bowel as well. On physical examination, right upper quadrant or epigastric tenderness is characteristic.

Table 116–2 | **Reported Pathogens in AIDS Cholangiopathy and Cholecystitis**

Cryptosporidium parvum
Microsporidium
a) Enterocytozoon bieneusi
b) Encephalitozoon intestinalis
c) Encephalitozoon cuniculi
Cyclospora cayetanesis
Cytomegalovirus
Mycobacterium avium complex
Isospora belli
Salmonella enteritidis
Salmonella typhimurium
Enterobacter cloacae
Campylobacter fetus
Candida albicans

From Wilcox CM, Monkemuller KE: Hepatobiliary diseases in patients with AIDS: Focus on AIDS cholangiopathy and gallbladder disease. Dig Dis Sci 16: 206, 1998.

Most patients with cholangiopathy have severe immunosuppression, with $CD4^+$ counts of less than 200/mm^3. Most cases are associated with opportunistic infections; cytomegalovirus (CMV) and *Cryptosporidium* are most common but *Microsporidium* also has been reported[20] (Table 116–2). Endoscopic retrograde cholangiopancreatography (ERCP) typically shows intrahepatic or extrahepatic changes (or both) of sclerosing cholangitis. Papillary stenosis is common as well.

DIAGNOSIS

History

Symptoms of proctitis include anal discharge or bleeding and anorectal pain or tenesmus. Diarrhea may be related to proctitis but more often indicates an enteric syndrome or proctocolitis. Careful and explicit history-taking concerning sexual preferences and practices is essential, and physicians should not be reluctant to ask such questions. Specifically, anal-receptive intercourse and oral or manual contact with the partner's anus are common ways for person-to-person transmission of pathogens to occur. The term *gay bowel syndrome*, which was used in the past, is misleading, because women also can acquire similar infections after heterosexual anal intercourse.

Physical Examination and Endoscopy

Physical examination, including anoscopy, helps classify patients with regard to the various gastrointestinal syndromes associated with STDs. Anoscopy identifies changes of the distal rectal mucosa and the anal canal and detects noninfectious diseases, such as an anal fissure or hemorrhoids. Anoscopy also allows one to obtain adequate specimens to identify sexually transmissible intestinal infections. Flexible sigmoidoscopy and colonoscopy help determine the extent of mucosal changes in the colon and obtain mucosal biopsies. The algorithm shown in Figure 116–1 provides a reasonable approach to the diagnostic evaluation of patients with gastrointestinal manifestations of STDs.

Rectal Swab

Rectal swabs are a simple means to detect anorectal infection caused by *N. gonorrhoeae* or *C. trachomatis*. A sterile cotton swab is passed through the anal canal and rotated a few times for 10 seconds. Swabs showing visible pus are more likely to yield positive cultures for *N. gonorrhoeae* than are swabs coated with feces. It is not clear whether the diagnostic yield is improved if swabs are taken through an anoscope or proctoscope. Swabs should be placed directly into appropriate transport media. A Gram stain that is positive for *N. gonorrhoeae* is diagnostic but misses approximately 50% of gonococcal infections.

Histology

Biopsy of specific anal or rectal lesions is usually indicated to determine whether they are inflammatory, infectious, or malignant. In cases of proctitis, biopsy specimens from the rectal mucosa often reveal nonspecific inflammatory changes. Some causative pathogens may be detected on hematoxylin and eosin stains or with additional techniques, such as immunofluorescence for HSV and immunohistology or in situ hybridization for CMV and HSV. Polymerase chain reaction (PCR) methodology is becoming increasingly useful for detecting some pathogens.

Serology

Serologic confirmation may be helpful for diagnosing infections caused by *C. trachomatis*, *T. pallidum*, and HSV and some cases of amebiasis. Diagnosis of acute infection by serologic testing is specific if an increase in antibody titer is observed over time.

SPECIFIC DISEASES

Bacterial Infections

Gonococcal Proctitis

In acute gonoccal proctitis, symptoms develop 5 to 7 days after exposure and typically include a mucopurulent rectal discharge, rectal bleeding, hematochezia, and anal dyspareunia. Severe tenesmus and constipation may occur. In most cases, however, the presentation is mild and nonspecific. Moreover, an asymptomatic carrier status is common. In one study, 53% of patients with positive cultures for *N. gonorrhoeae* had nonspecific or atypical symptoms.[21] In such cases proctoscopy may be unrevealing, or there may be evidence of a mild proctitis with erythema and friability, especially around the anorectal junction. Perirectal abscess or fistulas, rectal stricture, and septicemia are rare complications of anorectal gonorrhea.

Diagnosis is based on positive cultures from rectal swabs or a Gram stain that shows gram-negative intracellular diplococci. Rectal swabs should be placed directly on Thayer-Martin media or into special transport media, and a second swab should be smeared onto a microscope slide and examined by Gram stain. Swabs obtained through an anoscope

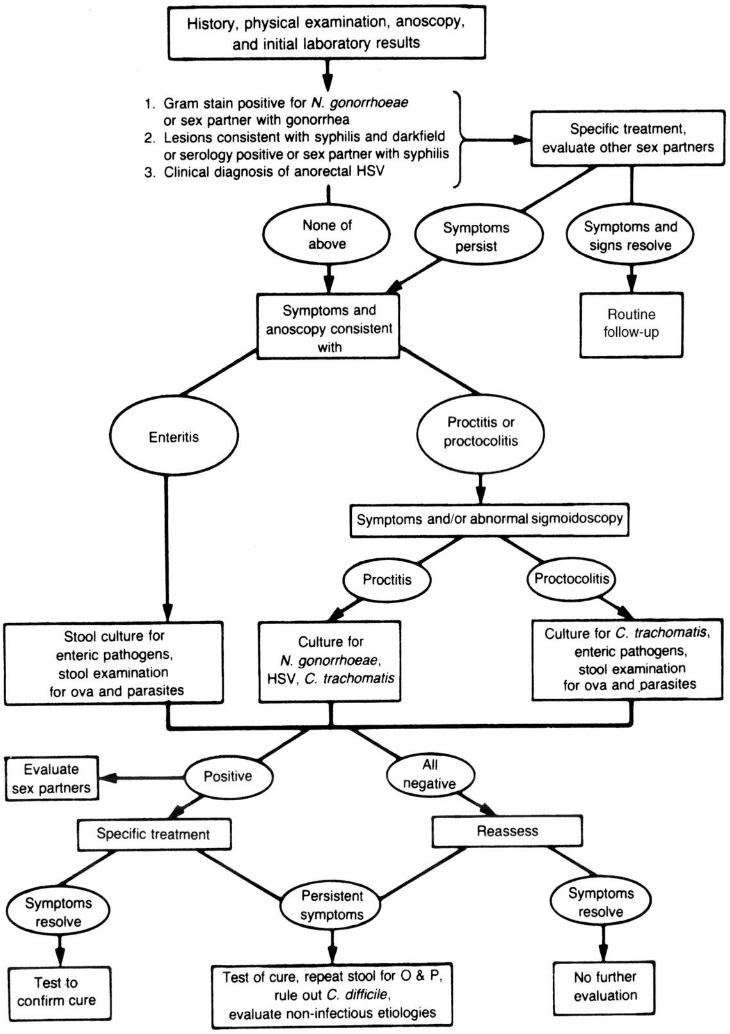

History, physical examination, anoscopy, and initial laboratory results

1. Gram stain positive for *N. gonorrhoeae* or sex partner with gonorrhea
2. Lesions consistent with syphilis and darkfield or serology positive or sex partner with syphilis
3. Clinical diagnosis of anorectal HSV

Specific treatment, evaluate other sex partners

None of above

Symptoms persist

Symptoms and signs resolve

Symptoms and anoscopy consistent with

Routine follow-up

Enteritis

Proctitis or proctocolitis

Symptoms and/or abnormal sigmoidoscopy

Proctitis

Proctocolitis

Stool culture for enteric pathogens, stool examination for ova and parasites

Culture for *N. gonorrhoeae*, HSV, *C. trachomatis*

Culture for *C. trachomatis*, enteric pathogens, stool examination for ova and parasites

Evaluate sex partners

Positive

All negative

Specific treatment

Reassess

Symptoms resolve

Persistent symptoms

Symptoms resolve

Test to confirm cure

Test of cure, repeat stool for O & P, rule out *C. difficile*, evaluate non-infectious etiologies

No further evaluation

Figure 116–1. Algorithm for evaluation of enteric symptoms following anal-receptive intercourse. HSV, herpes simplex virus; O & P, ova and parasites. (Reprinted, with permission, from Quinn TC, Stamm WE, Goodell SE, et al: The polymicrobial origin of intestinal infections in homosexual men. N Engl J Med 309:576–582, 1983.)

under direct visualization have a higher diagnostic yield than blind swabs.

DNA-based assays for detecting gonococci have been studied extensively in urogenital specimens, but their role in gonococcal proctitis is less clear. In a study from Edinburgh in 1995–1996, the sensitivity and specificity of the Gen-Probe PACE 2 assay for the detection of rectal and pharyngeal gonorrhea were assessed. The assay uses a chemiluminescent-labelled single-stranded DNA probe to detect gonococcal ribosomal RNA. Rectal swabs were collected from 161 homosexual men for culture on modified New York City medium and detection of gonococcal nucleic acid by the Gen-Probe assay. The Gen-Probe assay was not significantly more sensitive than rectal culture. Because the Gen-Probe assay may detect nucleic acid from nonviable gonococci, the clinical significance of a probe-positive, culture-negative specimen from a patient without culture evidence of gonorrhea at another site is uncertain. However, a positive Gen-Probe assay result does indicate exposure to the organism and could be important in ensuring appropriate notification of a partner who may have been infected.[22]

In a retrospective study from the same group of investigators in Edinburgh, the possible source of infection in homosexual men with rectal gonorrhea was identified in 46 of 155 cases. Although the urethra was the site of infection in 33 (72%) of the contacts, pharyngeal gonorrhea alone was identified in 9 (20%) men. In 25 of 26 cases, there was concordance in the serotype of *N. gonorrhoeae* between contacts with urethral gonorrhea and the index case of rectal gonorrhea. Eleven of twelve pharyngeal isolates were of the same serotype as the index case. This study supports the hypothesis that rectal gonorrhea can be acquired from the oropharynx. Because rectal infection is an independent risk factor for acquisition of HIV, screening for rectal and pharyngeal gonorrhea should be offered to MSM, even when there is no history of unprotected receptive anal intercourse.[23]

Treatment of anorectal gonorrhea is with cefixime, 400 mg once orally, or ceftriaxone, 125 mg once intramuscularly. Ciprofloxacin, 500 mg, or ofloxacin, 400 mg in a single oral dose, may be equally effective in patients with uncomplicated gonorrhea,[24] but the emergence of resistant strains has been a cause for concern.[25] Doxycycline, 100 mg orally twice daily for 7 days, or azithromycin, 1 g once orally, should be prescribed as well, because concurrent *Chlamydia* infection is common.[26] The persistence of symptoms despite eradication of gonococcal infection may be related to concomitant infection with *C. trachomatis*.

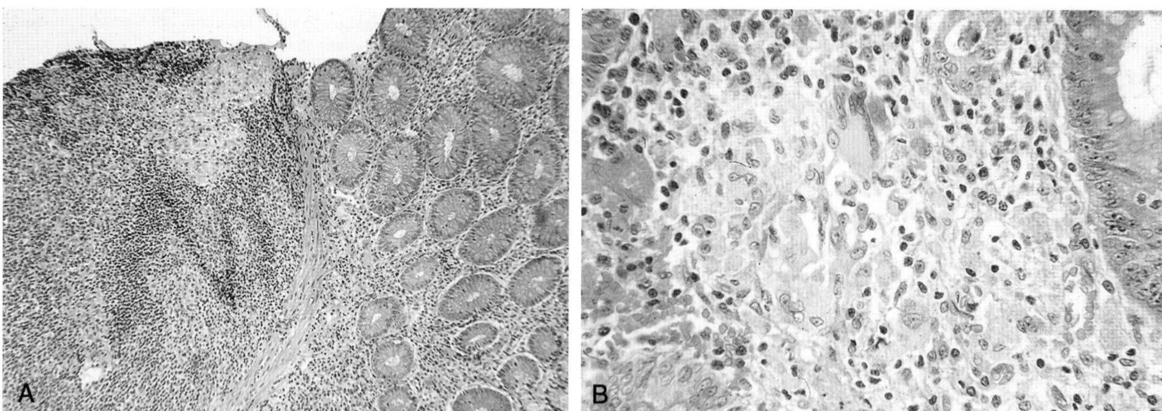

Figure 116–2. Histopathology of *Chlamydia trachomatis* proctitis in a homosexual man. On sigmoidoscopy the rectal mucosa was indurated and ulcerated. *A,* The low-power view shows granulomatous inflammation in the mucosa. *B,* A higher power view of the granuloma shows typical epithelioid cells and giant cells. (Hematoxylin and eosin stain.)

Chlamydial Proctitis

C. trachomatis, the agent of LGV, accounts for up to 20% of cases of proctitis in homosexual men.[10] LGV strains L1, L2, and L3 are responsible for most cases of proctitis. Patients infected with non-LGV strains of *Chlamydia* may be asymptomatic or only mildly symptomatic. Infection with LGV strains causes typical symptoms of proctitis, such as bloody or mucopurulent rectal discharge, diarrhea, and, less commonly, rectal pain, tenesmus, and obstipation. Diarrhea and fistula formation may occur, mimicking Crohn's disease. Chronic infection may lead to perirectal abscesses, fistulas, and rectal strictures. Tender, enlarged inguinal lymph nodes can be observed. An asymptomatic carrier state is found in 2% to 5% of cases. Anoscopy reveals friable rectal mucosa and a mucopurulent discharge.

Diagnosis is based on culture of the organisms from rectal swabs and a monoclonal antibody test for chlamydial antigen in infected cells. A Gram stain shows increased numbers of polymorphonuclear cells. Swabs should be placed directly in a transport medium containing 0.2 M sucrose-phosphate and then plated onto McCoy's cells. Rectal biopsies can show granulomatous inflammation with giant cells and crypt abscesses (Fig. 116–2). The organisms sometimes can be demonstrated in rectal biopsies by Giemsa stain. Serologic testing by a complement-fixation assay or microimmunofluorescent test is diagnostic if a fourfold rise in antibody titers is observed.

The treatment of choice is doxycycline, 100 mg orally twice daily for 7 days; erythromycin, 500 mg orally three times daily for 7 days; or tetracycline, 500 mg orally four times a day for 7 days. If an LGV strain is present, therapy should be extended for 21 days. Azithromycin, 1 g once orally, is effective for chlamydial urethritis and cervicitis and has been recommended for uncomplicated proctitis.

Anorectal Syphilis

The frequency of anorectal syphilis in homosexual men decreased during the 1980s because of safer sex practices. The disease is now as common in heterosexual men and women as in homosexual men. After sexual contact with an infected partner, a chancre forms in the perianal area, anal canal, or rectal mucosa. The chancre begins as a papule that later erodes to become an ulcer. The incubation period is usually 3 weeks, with a range of 10 to 90 days. *T. pallidum* penetrates a break in the skin or the intact mucosa. Perianal chancres are often painless, but lesions in the anal canal cause pain, possibly because of secondary infection. Primary syphilitic lesions in the anal canal can be mistaken for anal fissures or fistulas (Fig. 116–3). Enlarged, tender inguinal lymph nodes are often found. The chancre itself is indurated.

Syphilitic proctitis produces a purulent discharge. Endoscopically, anal or rectal ulcerations are observed, and diffuse involvement of the rectosigmoid has been reported (Fig. 116–4). Diagnosis is made by detection of the organism by darkfield microscopy in material taken from the base of the lesion. Serologic diagnosis depends on detecting antibodies to nontreponemal and treponemal antigens, including the VDRL and rapid plasma reagin (RPR) tests. These tests

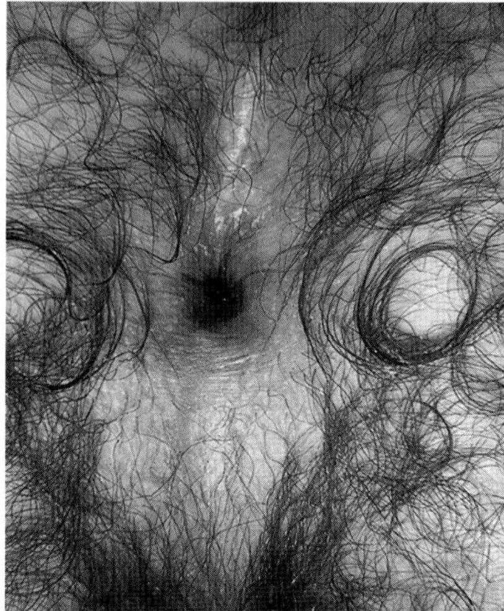

Figure 116–3. Anal inspection of a patient with perianal syphilis. Note the ulcer in the perianal area. This was a painful fissure associated with syphilis. (Courtesy of Dr. Steven Medwell, Seattle, Washington.)

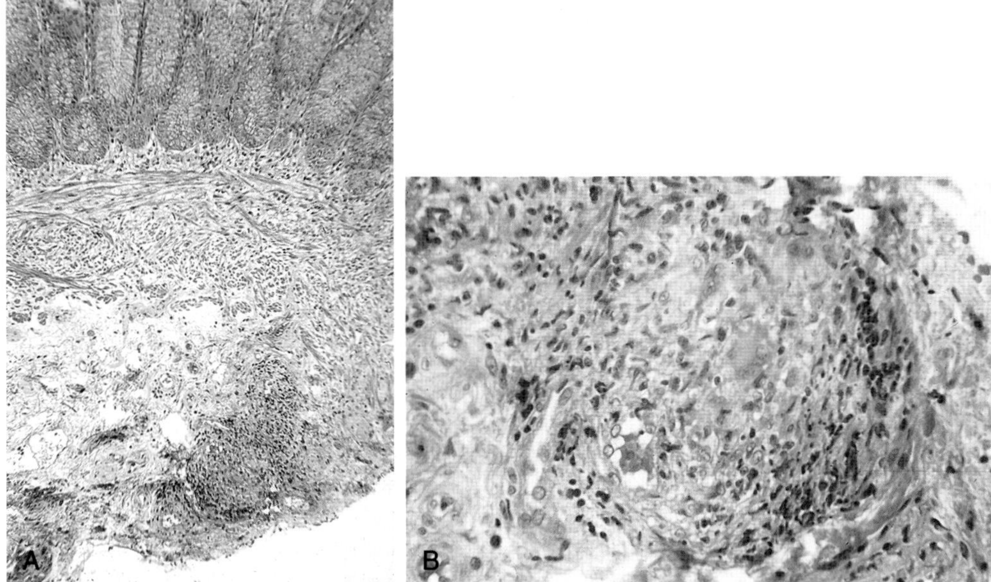

Figure 116–4. Histopathology of syphilis in a patient with secondary syphilis and an anorectal mass. *A,* On low-power examination, there is a granuloma around a vessel in the submucosa. *B,* A high-power view shows the granulomatous vasculitis associated with secondary syphilis. (Hematoxylin and eosin stain.)

become positive a few weeks after the infection. Positive tests should be confirmed with a fluorescent treponemal antibody-absorbed (FTA-ABS) test.

Treatment is with penicillin G, 2.4 million units once intramuscularly. All other therapies are less effective. In a person who is allergic to penicillin, desensitization to and treatment with penicillin is recommended. Alternatively, patients allergic to penicillin can be given doxycycline, 200 mg orally twice daily for 15 days, but close follow-up is essential. Table 116–3 lists other acceptable treatment regimens. Retesting for VDRL after 3 and 6 months to demonstrate a decrease in titer is necessary to confirm the success of treatment. For syphilis of more than 1 year's duration, patients should be treated with penicillin G, 2.4 million units intramuscularly weekly for 3 doses. All sexual contacts of infected patients should be treated as well.

Spirochetosis

Spirochetosis is the term used for colonic infestations of non-*T. pallidum* spirochetes. These organisms have been identified in colonic biopsy specimens and in stool for over a century, and debate over their pathogenicity continues. Nontreponemal spirochetes can be found in the colon, appendix, and rectum. The term *colorectal spirochetosis* may therefore be preferable to intestinal spirochetosis. Spirochetes can be detected by careful microscopic examination of colonic mucosal biopsy specimens that are stained with hematoxylin and eosin. Histologic features include a thickened (3 μm) blue band that coats the surface of the epithelial and goblet cells and extends a short distance into the crypts. Silver stains make the diagnosis of spirochetosis more apparent (Fig. 116–5). Because spirochetes generally do not cause inflammatory changes in the mucosa, they may be undetected if biopsies are not taken.

There are at least two different types of spirochetes. The larger *Spirochaeta eurygyrata* is 4 to 10 μm in length, 0.2 to 0.5 μm in diameter, and has irregular coils. The smaller organism is up to 6 μm in length and 0.2 μm in diameter, with regular coils. It has been termed *Brachyspira aalborgii* and *Treponema D 60*.

A case report by Harland and Lee[27] described spirochetes on the mucosal surface of a rectal biopsy from a homosexual man revived interest in these organisms. Subsequently, they have been documented in 2% to 8% of various populations from many countries, suggesting a worldwide distribution. The organism has been found in up to 44% of inflamed appendices, suggesting a possible role for the organisms in some cases of appendicitis.[28, 29] The highest rates of spirochetosis (between 5.9% and 35%, depending on the population studied) have been found in homosexual men. Some of these men had gastrointestinal symptoms, but others were asymptomatic; thus, it has been unclear whether the organism is a pathogen or a harmless commensal in immunocompetent persons.[30]

Symptoms of spirochetosis have included nausea, abdominal pain, diarrhea, perianal burning, pain, discharge, rectal bleeding, constipation, tenesmus, and malaise. Many case reports of persons with gastrointestinal symptoms and spirochetosis suggest that symptoms resolve with therapy. These reports suggest that in some cases either the spirochete was a pathogen, or other unidentified organisms that caused symptoms were eradicated with treatment.[31] However, in one Danish series of 15 patients with spirochetosis, diarrhea did not resolve after treatment with antibiotics.[32] Even if the organism is demonstrated to be invasive on histology, symptoms may improve without specific therapy.[33] In patients infected with HIV, spirochetosis may be more likely to be a pathogen, and therapy has been recommended. In non-HIV–infected persons, treatment with metronidazole, 500 mg three

Table 116–3 | **Treatment of Sexually Transmissible Anorectal Infections**

ORGANISMS	TREATMENT OF CHOICE	ALTERNATIVE THERAPY	COMMENTARY
Bacterial			
N. gonorrhoeae	Cefixime, 400 PO once, or ceftriaxone, 125 mg IM once, plus doxycycline, 100 mg PO bid for 7 days, or azithromycin, 1 g PO once	Ciprofloxacin, 500 mg PO once, or ofloxacin, 400 mg PO once, plus doxycycline, 100 mg PO bid for 7 days, or azithromycin, 1 g PO once	Concurrent infection with *C. trachomatis* is common Strains resistant to quinolones have been observed in Asian countries
C. trachomatis	Doxycycline, 100 mg PO bid for 14 days	Erythromycin, 500 mg PO qid for 14 days or azithromycin, 1 g PO once	Erythromycin preferred during pregnancy
C. trachomatis (LGV strains)	Doxycycline, 100 mg PO bid for 21 days	Tetracycline, 500 mg qid for 21 days	
T. pallidum	Penicillin G, 2.4 million U IM once, or doxycycline, 200 mg PO bid for 15 days In syphilis of more than 1 year's duration: Penicillin G, 2.4 million U IM weekly for 3 doses	Tetracycline, 500 mg qid for 14 days or ceftriaxone, 1 g/d IM or IV for 10 days	Treatment suggestions for primary and secondary syphilis only Re-examine after 3 and 6 months to confirm treatment success
Spirochetosis	Metronidazole, 500 mg tid for 10 days		Rarely indicated, because symptoms improve without therapy in most cases
Viral			
Herpes simplex virus	Acyclovir 400 mg PO tid for 7–10 days (initial episode) or valacyclovir 1 g PO bid for 7–10 days or famciclovir 250 mg PO tid for 7–10 days	For recurrences, acyclovir 400 mg PO tid for 5 days or valacyclovir 500 mg PO bid for 3–5 days or famciclovir 125 mg PO bid for 5 days	Topical application of acyclovir six times a day for 7 days may accelerate healing of lesions
Cytomegalovirus	Ganciclovir, 5 mg/kg IV q12h as induction therapy for 14–21 days, followed by maintenance treatment with ganciclovir, 5 g/kg IV q24h	Foscarnet, 60 mg/kg IV q8h as induction therapy for 14–21 days, followed by maintenance treatment with foscarnet, 90 mg/kg IV q24h	In immunocompromised patients
Parasitic			
Entamoeba histolytica	Metronidazole, 750 mg PO tid for 7–10 days plus iodoquinol, 650 mg/PO daily for 20 days	Metronidazole, 750 mg PO tid for 7–10 days plus Tinidazole 2 g/day for 3 days followed by iodoquinol 650 mg PO daily for 20 days	Asymptomatic carriers are treated with a luminal amebicide only (iodoquinol or paromomycin or diloxanide furoate) to prevent transmission
Enterobius vermicularis	Mebendazole, 100 mg PO once, repeat after 2 wk	Pyrantel, 11 mg/kg PO once, repeat after 2 and 4 wk	Household members and sexual contacts also should be treated

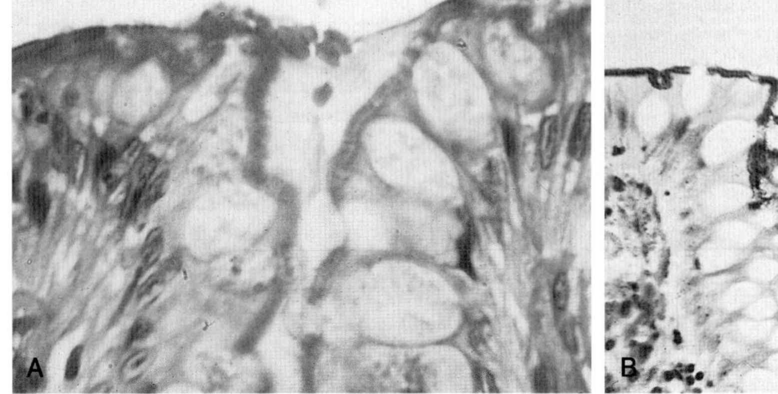

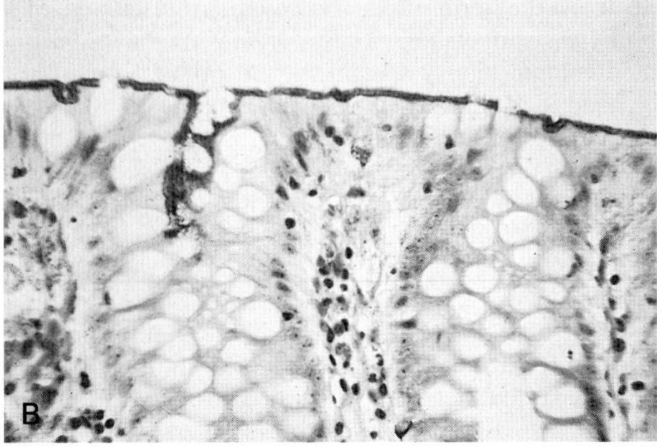

Figure 116–5. Histopathology of spirochetosis. *A,* Under high power, this colonoscopic mucosal biopsy shows a thick layer of spirochete organisms that coat the surface of the mucosa and the superficial portion of the crypt. (Hematoxylin and eosin stain.) *B,* The adjacent photomicrograph shows a silver stain with which the organisms are easier to detect.

times daily orally for 10 days, may be considered if no other cause of the person's symptoms is found.[34]

Viral Infections

Herpes Simplex Proctitis

HSV proctitis is associated with anal pain and tenesmus, discharge, and constipation. Infection is more commonly caused by HSV type 2 (90%) than by HSV type I (10%). Urinary retention and lower abdominal or buttock pain are common. Sexual transmission is by direct skin-to-skin contact through anal intercourse or oral-anal contact. Because of pain, anal examination may be possible only after application of local anesthesia. In the anal canal, the characteristic lesions are small, focal ulcerations or herpetic vesicles that are sometimes confluent (Fig. 116–6). Proctosigmoidoscopy may reveal ulcers and vesicles. Biopsy samples show acute and chronic inflammatory changes with focal microabscesses and superficial ulcerations (Fig. 116–7). In material taken from the ulcer base, multinucleated giant cells can be demonstrated by Giemsa stain.

The diagnosis of HSV proctitis is confirmed by direct immunofluorescent staining or by viral isolation from rectal swabs or biopsy specimens. PCR methodology is being used for diagnosis increasingly and is more sensitive than cultures. The diagnosis is confirmed by a fourfold rise in titer.

Treatment of mild HSV proctitis is symptomatic, with sitz baths, analgesics, application of ointments or suppositories that contain a local anesthetic, and acyclovir. Local glucocorticoids should be avoided. Oral acyclovir, 400 mg five times daily for 10 days, has been shown to be clinically efficacious compared with placebo and is recommended for severe disease.[35] Topical application of acyclovir six times a day for 7 days also may accelerate healing of lesions.[36] Famciclovir and valacyclovir have been studied extensively in urogenital herpes, but there are no data for HSV proctitis in immunocompetent persons. In HIV-positive patients with recurrent mucocutaneous (orolabial or genital) HSV infection, famciclovir, 500 mg twice daily for 7 days, is as effective as acyclovir, 400 mg five times a day, with the convenience of less frequent dosing.[37]

HIV-infected patients with severe mucocutaneous HSV infection should be treated with intravenous acyclovir (5 to 10 mg/kg every 8 hours) until clinical resolution.

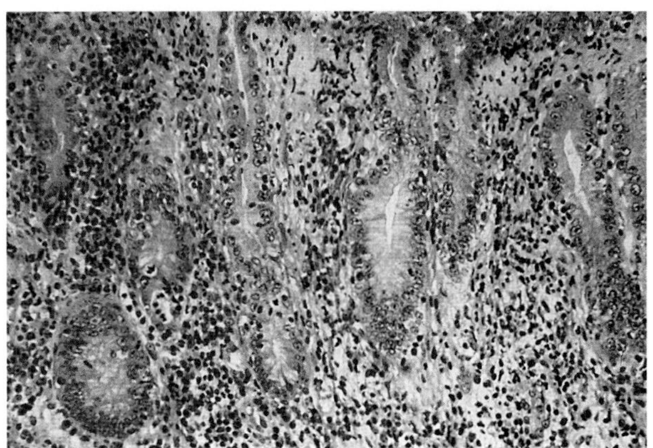

Figure 116–7. Histology of herpes simplex virus proctitis. Note the intense inflammation in the lamina propria associated with herpetic inflammation. (Hematoxylin and eosin stain.)

Human Papillomavirus Infection

Condylomata acuminata, or anal and genital warts, have been known since ancient times (Fig. 116–8). They are characterized by many small raised points, in contrast to the flat *condylomata lata* of secondary syphilis. Warts are caused by the human papillomavirus (HPV), the most common sexually transmitted viral infection in the United States.[38] HPV usually infects the basal cells of the squamous epithelium, but it also may infect transitional and cuboidal epithelium. Infectious viral particles are produced only by the completely differentiated cells of the upper epithelium, because cellular differentiation is necessary for the HPV growth cycle.[39] Infection with HPV can result in clinical or latent infection and in some cases may lead to the development of cancer[40] (Fig. 116–9).

Receptive anal intercourse is common in patients with anal warts, and, conceivably, coital trauma allows entry of latent virus in the anorectal region into the anal epidermis. Anal dysplasia has been demonstrated in 12% of homosexual men with internal warts.[41]

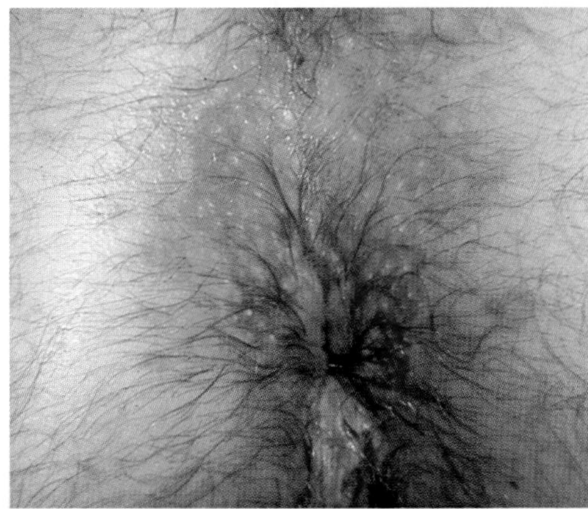

Figure 116–6. Anal examination of a patient with perianal herpes infection. Note the erythema, redness, and superficial ulceration. (Courtesy of Dr. Steven Medwell, Seattle, Washington.)

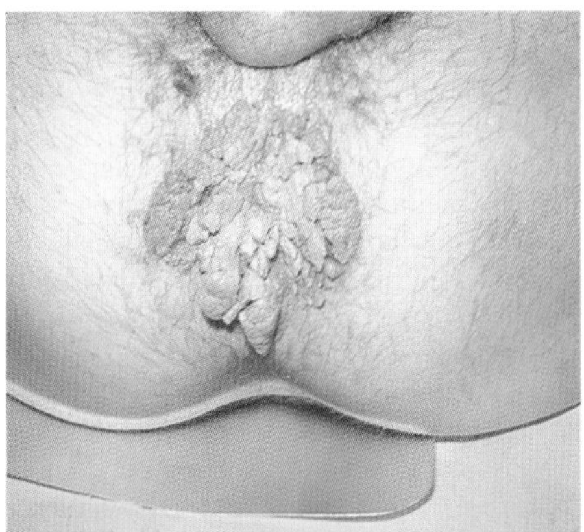

Figure 116–8. Perianal warts. Note the large accumulation of warts around the anus in a homosexual man. These warts are caused by human papillomavirus. (Courtesy of Dr. Steven Medwell, Seattle, Washington.)

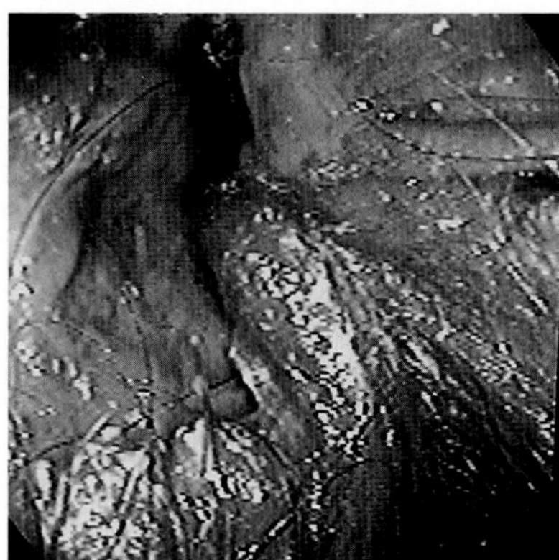

Figure 116–9. Anal cancer presenting as a painful anal ulcer that crosses the anal canal. The ulcer was found to be a squamous cell carcinoma in a man who was HIV positive.

Symptoms of condylomata acuminata include pruritus, bleeding, anal wetness, and pain, although warts are frequently asymptomatic. Large warts may interfere with defecation. On clinical examination, raised papillary lesions are seen on the vulva and the perianal region. In over 50% of affected men, condylomata acuminata extend into the anal canal.[42]

A variety of nucleic acid hybridization techniques are used to detect and type HPV infection. Exfoliated epithelial cell samples or tissue biopsies, either fresh or fixed, can be analyzed. The diagnosis of a condyloma acuminatum, however, is clinical. Visual inspection and anoscopy or colposcopy reveal the extent of the lesions and may determine the best therapeutic approach. Colposcopy also visualizes flat subclinical lesions on the cervix and the internal anal canal. The detection of HPV DNA and of HPV antibodies in the sera of patients has been described,[43] but the clinical significance of a positive result in the absence of a lesion and the relevance of persistent detection of HPV are not clear.

Of the more than 60 types of HPV, approximately 30 may be associated with anogenital diseases. Several types of HPV (16, 18, 45, 56) have oncogenic potential and are the causal agent of most genital tract squamous cell cancers in women.[44] HPV infection, mainly with types 16 and 18, also is related to anal squamous cell cancer in men.[45] The development of malignancy may depend on several cofactors, such as other STDs and smoking.[46, 47] Malignant transformation has been described in 30% of cases of giant anorectal condyloma acuminatum (Buschke-Loewenstein tumors). The course of giant anorectal condylomas associated with oncogenic HPV may be aggressive, and affected patients may benefit from early medical and surgical intervention.[48]

Immunosuppression confers an increased risk of developing HPV-related neoplasia. Anal dysplasia has been reported to be significantly more common in HIV-positive than in HIV-negative homosexual men.[41]

Treatment of external condylomata acuminata is often with topical agents. Single small perianal lesions may be treated with podophyllin in a 25% compound of tincture of benzoin. Treatment may require several sessions at weekly intervals. For more extensive disease, surgical excision or ablation with CO_2 laser, electrocautery, or cryosurgery is the treatment of choice.[49] With any of these approaches, recurrence is frequent. Intralesional interferon alpha may be a useful adjunct to surgical methods to decrease recurrence.[50] In a placebo-controlled study, the injection of interferon alpha, 500,000 IU, into four quadrants of the anal canal reduced the recurrence rate from 39% to 12% during a mean follow-up period of 3.8 months. This treatment is not widely used because of its toxicity and expense.

Because of the high rate of recurrence, frequent follow-up visits are recommended. Recurrence may result from latent infection, for which there is no effective therapy. It is not known whether the treatment of partners of affected persons or the use of condoms prevents reinfection.

Cytomegalovirus Proctocolitis

Serologic evidence of prior exposure to CMV is found in more than 90% of homosexual patients.[51] In immunocompetent persons, the infection rarely becomes symptomatic. Acute ulcerative proctocolitis has been reported.[52] Treatment is necessary if gastrointestinal manifestations occur because of immunosuppression (see later).

Parasitic Infections (Protozoa and Helminths)

(See also Chapters 98 and 99)

Amebiasis

The role of sexual transmission in parasitic infections is suggested by the high prevalence of *Giardia lamblia* and *Entamoeba histolytica* infections in homosexual men.[53] The presence of these parasites correlates with a history of anilingus to a greater degree than with travel to endemic areas. Symptoms of amebiasis are often nonspecific and can include bloating, abdominal cramping, and diarrhea. Many infected patients are asymptomatic. Unusual features in asymptomatic homosexual men who are infected with *E. histolytica* include the absence of serum antibodies and the presence of cysts, rather than trophozoites, in the stool. Long-term follow-up has suggested that symptomatic episodes in these infected patients are rare and that therapy is not required.[54] The only rationale for treatment would be to prevent transmission to others.

The diagnosis of amebiasis is based on the presence of amebic trophozoites in the stool. The sensitivity rate for diagnosis is 90% if three separate stool samples are taken. Serologic tests (enzyme-linked immunosorbent assay or indirect hemagglutination) may be helpful in diagnosing invasive disease[55] but can remain positive for as long as 10 years after an acute episode of amebiasis. Sigmoidoscopy may show nonspecific inflammatory changes, including erythema, edema, and friability. Shallow ulcers, covered with a yellowish exudate, can be found. Histologically, the inflammatory changes are nonspecific. Amebae can be found at the mucosal surface or in the adjacent exudate associated with an ulcer (Fig. 116–10).

The treatment of choice for invasive amebiasis is metronidazole 750 mg three times daily orally for 7 to 10 days plus iodoquinol, 650 mg daily orally for 20 days.[56] Instead of metronidazole, tinidazole, 2 g/day for 3 days, can be given. Asymptomatic carriers should be treated with a luminal amebicide (iodoquinol, paromomycin, or diloxanide furoate) to prevent transmission.

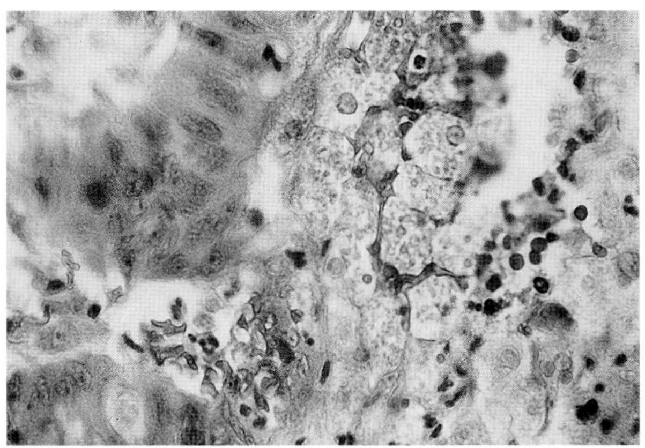

Figure 116–10. Histopathologic features of amebiasis in a rectal biopsy specimen from a patient with many amebic organisms present in the mucus on the surface of the mucosa.

Enterobius vermicularis

Enterobius vermicularis, called pinworm in the United States and threadworm in Great Britain, resides in the colon. Eggs are deposited by the female worm in the perianal area. Most infected persons remain asymptomatic, but severe pruritus may develop. Stool surveys of homosexual men have shown a low prevalence of *E. vermicularis*, but the true prevalence may be much higher, because the eggs are usually present only in the perianal area. Although pinworms usually cause only perianal symptoms, eosinophilic colitis also has been described.[57] The diagnosis is made by microscopic examination of a cellophane tape pressed against the unwashed skin of the perianal area.

The infection is treated with a single dose of mebendazole (Vermox), 100 mg orally. Household members and sexual contacts also should be treated to prevent reinfection, and the treatment should be repeated after 2 weeks. For recurrent pinworm infestation, a 3-month course of mebendazole (100 mg once a month) should be considered.

Giardia lamblia

Although water remains the most common mode of transmission of *G. lamblia*, there has been an increase in the number of person-to-person cases. *G. lamblia* causes symptoms of enteritis, including diarrhea, bloating, abdominal cramps, and nausea. Patients also may complain of eructation and bad breath. Single stool examinations are often negative, but the sensitivity rate of three consecutive stool tests approaches 95%. Enzyme immunoassays for the detection of *G. lamblia* antigen in stool have become commercially available. Antigen tests can be useful to detect *G. lamblia* and may replace microscopic examination in areas of high endemicity.[58] If giardiasis is suspected despite negative stool tests, upper endoscopy with duodenal biopsy should be performed.

Treatment is with metronidazole, 250 mg three times daily orally for 5 days, or tinidazole, 500 mg twice daily orally for 7 days or a single 2-g oral dose. Alternatively, especially for pregnant women who require treatment, paromomycin, a nonabsorbable aminoglycoside, 500 mg three times daily for 7 to 10 days, may be tried first and metronidazole used if initial treatment fails.

Anorectal Lesions and Proctocolitis in HIV-Infected Patients

HIV-infected patients with $CD4^+$ T-lymphocyte counts above 100/mm^3 are subject to the same infections as HIV-negative patients. When the count falls to less than 100/mm^3, the most common viral cause of colitis is CMV, which can cause a painful colitis or proctitis. Symptoms include crampy abdominal pain, diarrhea, bleeding, fever, and often tenesmus. The colitis can be focal or diffuse, and ulcers can occur. Because antibodies to CMV are commonly found in patients with high-risk sexual practices, serology is not helpful, and the diagnosis of colitis must be based on positive biopsies from the rectosigmoid or colonic mucosa (Fig. 116–11).

Treatment with ganciclovir, 5 mg/kg every 12 hours intravenously, is recommended. In a placebo-controlled, double-blind study of 62 patients, symptoms resolved during the first week of therapy with ganciclovir. Patients treated with ganciclovir also were able to maintain body weight, in contrast to controls.[59] Induction therapy is given for 14 to 21 days, followed by maintenance treatment with ganciclovir, 5 g/kg intravenously every 24 hours. If CMV infection is re-

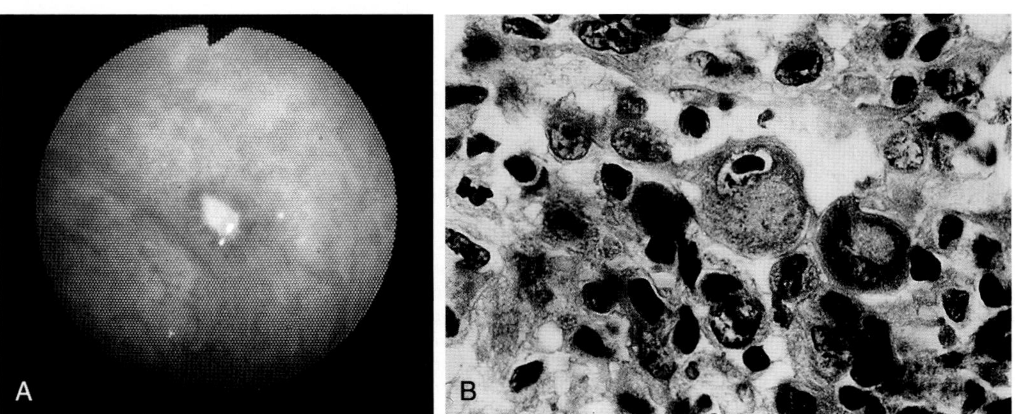

Figure 116–11. *A*, Endoscopic view of an isolated cytomegalovirus (CMV) ulcer in the colon. *B*, Corresponding histology shows the large CMV inclusion cell with a clear halo around it and the granular component of the CMV in the cytoplasm.

sistant to ganciclovir, foscarnet, 60 mg/kg intravenously every 8 hours, is given as induction therapy for 14 to 21 days, followed by maintenance treatment at a dose of 90 mg/kg intravenously every 24 hours. In an open-labeled study, foscarnet induced clinical remission in eight of ten patients with CMV colitis in whom ganciclovir therapy had failed.[60]

In patients with AIDS, viral infections (HSV and condylomata acuminata) tend to follow a more aggressive course. Treatment, however, is the same as in HIV-negative patients, although longer courses of therapy may be necessary.

Enteritis Syndromes in HIV-Infected Patients

The colon is a frequent site of gastrointestinal complications in patients with HIV infection, and these colonic disorders increase in frequency as immunodeficiency worsens. The most common clinical manifestations of colonic disease in patients with AIDS are diarrhea, lower gastrointestinal bleeding, and abdominal pain. Toxic megacolon, intussusception, typhlitis, idiopathic colonic ulcer, and pneumatosis intestinalis also have been described. In the HIV-infected patient with preserved immunity, the most common cause of colitis is bacterial, but as the degree of immunodeficiency worsens, opportunistic pathogens (CMV, protozoa, mycobacteria, fungi) and neoplasms become more frequent. The use of antibiotics and chemotherapeutic agents and frequent hospitalizations increase susceptibility to *Clostridium difficile* colitis. Endoscopy plays an integral role in the management of many colonic disorders in AIDS.[61] Since the introduction of highly active antiretroviral therapy (HAART), there appears to be have been a reduction in the incidence of many of these opportunistic disorders. In fact, gastrointestinal opportunistic disorders now seem to be uncommon in HIV-infected patients who undergo endoscopy, despite a low $CD4^+$ lymphocyte count, and this reduction in the frequency of such disorders appears to be associated with the use of HAART.[62]

Noninfectious Proctitis

Trauma to the anorectum may occur after insertion of foreign objects as well as the hand or forearm as part of sexual practices. Symptoms are similar to those associated with infectious causes of proctitis, and differentiation from infectious proctitis may be difficult. Polymorphonuclear leukocytes in Gram-stained smears from rectal swabs usually are absent in traumatic proctitis, which suggests an infectious cause. Secondary infection of traumatic proctitis with colonic pathogens may occur.

Treatment of traumatic proctitis is symptomatic, with sitz baths, ointment, or suppositories that contain a local anesthetic and softening of stools with bulk agents or stool softeners. Allergic proctitis may be caused by lubricants, including KY jelly.[63] Soaps, oil, or medicinal cream may irritate the rectal mucosa. Suppositories containing 5-aminosalicylic acid or glucocorticoids may accelerate healing and resolution of symptoms.

REFERENCES

1. Handsfield HH, Schwebke J: Trends in sexually transmitted diseases in homosexually active men in King County, Washington, 1980–1990. Sex Transm Dis 17:211, 1990.
2. Increases in unsafe sex and rectal gonorrhea among MSM—San Francisco, California, 1994–1997. MMWR Morb Mortal Wkly Rep 48:45–48, 1999.
3. Fennema JS, Cairo I, Coutinho RA: [Substantial increase in gonorrhea and syphilis among clients of Amsterdam Sexually Transmitted Diseases Clinic.] Ned Tijdschr Geneeskd 144: 602–603, 2000.
4. Lafferty WE, Hughes JP, Hansfield HH: Sexually transmitted diseases in MSM. Acquistion of gonorrhea and nongonococcal urethritis by fellatio and implications for STD/HIV prevention. Sex Transm Dis 24: 272–278, 1997.
5. Tabet SR, Krone MR, Paradise MA, et al: Incidence of HIV and sexually transmitted diseases (STD) in a cohort of HIV-negative men who have sex with men (MSM). AIDS 12:2041–2048, 1998.
6. Andrews H, Wyke J, Lane M, et al: Prevalence of sexually transmitted disease among male patients presenting with proctitis. Gut 29:332–335, 1988.
7. Rompalo AM: Diagnosis and treatment of sexually acquired proctitis and proctocolitis: An update. Clin Infect Dis 28(Suppl 1):S84–S90, 1999.
8. Quinn TC, Lukehart SA, Goodell S, et al: Rectal mass caused by *Treponema pallidum*: Confirmation by immunofluorescent staining. Gastroenterology 82:135–139, 1982.
9. Boisvert J-F, Koutsky LA, Suchland RJ, Stamm WE: Clinical features of *Chlamydia trachomatis* rectal infection by serovar among homosexually active men. Sex Transm Dis 26:392–398, 1999.
10. Quinn TC, Corey L, Chaffee RG, et al: The etiology of anorectal infections in homosexual men. Am J Med 71:395–406, 1981.
11. Fleming DT, McQuillan GM, Johnson RE, et al: Herpes simplex virus type 2 in the United States, 1976 to 1994. N Engl J Med 337:1105–1111, 1997.
12. McMillan A, Young H, Moyes A: Rectal gonorrhea in homosexual men: Source of infection. J STD AIDS 11:284–287, 2000.
13. Ryan DP, Compton CC, Mayer RJ: Carcinoma of the anal canal. N Engl J Med 342:792–800, 2000.
14. Palefsky JM: Anal squamous intraepithelial lesions in human immunodeficiency virus–positive men and women. Semin Oncol 27:471–479, 2000.
15. Palefsky JM: Anal squamous intrepithelial lesions: Relation to HIV and human papillomavirus infection. J AIDS 21:S42–S48, 1999.
16. Volberding P: Looking behind: Time for anal cancer screening. Am J Med 108:674–675, 2000.
17. Guarda LA, Stein SA, Cleraly KA, Ordoflez NG: Human cryptosporidiosis in the acquired immunodeficiency syndrome. Arch Pathol Lab Med 107:562–566, 1983.
18. Pitlik S, Fainstein V, Garza D, et al: Human cryptosporidiosis: Spectrum of disease: Report of six cases and review of the literature. Arch Intern Med 143:2269–2275, 1983.
19. Wilcox CM, Monkemuller KE: Hepatobiliary diseases in patients with AIDS: Focus on AIDS cholangiopathy and gallbladder disease. Dig Dis 16:206–213, 1998.
20. Willson R, Harrington R, Stuewart B, Fritsche T: Human immunodeficiency virus 1–associated necrotizing cholangitis caused by infection with Septata intestinalis. Gastroenterology 108:247–251, 1995.
21. Rompalo AM, Price CB, Roberts PL, et al: Potential value of rectal-screening cultures for *Chlamydia trachomatis* in homosexual men. J Infect Dis 153:888, 1986.
22. Young H, Anderson J, Moyes A, McMillan A: Non-cultural detection of rectal and pharyngeal gonorrhea by the Gen-Probe PACE 2 assay. Genitourin Med 43:59–62, 1997.
23. McMillan A, Young H, Moyes A: Rectal gonorrhoea in homosexual men: Source of infection. Int J STD AIDS 11:284–287, 2000.
24. Echols RM, Heyd A, O'Keeffe BJ, et al: Single-dose ciprofloxacin for the treatment of uncomplicated gonorrhea: A worldwide summary. Sex Transm Dis 21:345–352, 1994.
25. Gordon SM, Carlyn CJ, Doyle LJ, et al: The emergence of *Neisseria gonorrhoeae* with decreased susceptibility to ciprofloxacin in Cleveland, Ohio: Epidemiology and risk factors. Ann Intern Med 125:456–470, 1996.
26. 1998 guidelines for treatment of sexually transmitted diseases. Centers

for Disease Control and Prevention. MMWR Morb Mortal Wkly Rep 47(RR-1):1–111, 1998.
27. Harland WA, Lee FD: Intestinal spirochetosis. Brit Med J 3:718–719, 1967.
28. Lee FD, Kraszewski A, Godon J, et al: Intestinal spirochetosis. Gut 12: 126–133, 1971.
29. Henrik-Nielsen R, Lundbeck FA, Teglbjaerg PS, et al: Intestinal spirochetosis of the vermiform appendix. Gastroenterology 88:971–977, 1985.
30. Surawicz CM: Colorectal spirochetosis. In Surawicz CM, Owen RL (eds): Gastrointestinal and Hepatic Infections. Philadelphia. WB Saunders, 1995, pp 353–358.
31. Surawicz CM, Roberts PR, Rompalo A, et al: Intestinal spirochetosis in homosexual men. Am J Med 82:5878–5892, 1987.
32. Nielsen RH, Orholm M, Petersen JO, et al: Colorectal spirochetosis: Clinical significance of the infestation. Gastroenterology 85:62–67, 1983.
33. Padmanabhan V, Dahlstrom J, Maxwell L, et al: Invasive intestinal spirochetosis: A report of three cases. Pathology 28:283–286, 1996.
34. Cotton DWK, Kirkham N, Hicks DA: Rectal spirochaetosis. Br J Vener Dis 60:106–109, 1984.
35. Rompalo AM, Mertz GJ, Davis LG, et al: Oral acyclovir for treatment of first-episode Herpes simplex virus proctitis. JAMA 259:2879, 1988.
36. Corey L, Spear PG: Infections with herpes simplex viruses. N Engl J Med 314:686, 1986.
37. Romanowski B, Aoki FY, Martel AY, et al: Efficacy and safety of famciclovir for treating mucocutaneous herpes simplex infection in HIV-infected individuals. AIDS 14:1211–1217, 2000.
38. Stone KM: Epidemiologic aspects of genital HPV infection. Clin Obstet Gynecol 32:112–116, 1989.
39. Broker TR: Structure and genetic expression of papillomaviruses. Obstet Gynecol Clin North Am 14:329–348, 1987.
40. Syrjanen KJ: Epidemiology of human papillomavirus infections and their association with genital squamous cell cancer. APMIS 97:957–970, 1989.
41. Kiviat NB, Critchlow CW, Holmes KK, et al: Association of anal dysplasia and human papillomavirus with immunosuppression and HIV infection among homosexual men. AIDS 7:43–49, 1993.
42. Carr G, William DC: Anal warts in a population of gay men in New York City. Sex Transm Dis 4:56, 1977.
43. Gissmann L: Immunologic responses to human papillomavirus infection. Obstet Gynecol Clin North Am 23:625–639, 1996.
44. Munoz N, Bosch FX: HPV and cervical cancer: Review of case-control and cohort studies. In Munoz N, Bosch FX, Shah KV, et al (eds): The Epidemiology of Human Papillomavirus and Cervical Cancer, vol 119. Lyon, IARC Sci Pub, 1992, pp 251–261.
45. Vincent-Salomon A, de la Rochefordiere A, Salmon R, et al: Frequent association of human papillomavirus 16 and 18 DNA with anal squamous cell and basaloid carcinoma. Mod Pathol 9:614–620, 1996.
46. Daling JR, Weiss NS, Hislop TG, et al: Sexual practices, sexually transmitted diseases, and the incidence of anal cancer. N Engl J Med 317:973–977, 1987.
47. Daling JR, Sherman KJ, Hislop TG, et al: Cigarette smoking and the risk of anogenital cancer. Am J Epidemiol 135:180–189, 1992.
48. Kibrite A, Zeitouni NC, Cloutier R: Aggressive giant condyloma acuminatum associated with oncogenic human papilloma virus: A case report. Can J Surg 40:143–145, 1997.
49. Congilosi SM, Madoff RD: Current therapy for recurrent and extensive anal warts. Dis Colon Rectum 38:1101–1107, 1995.
50. Fleshner PR, Freilich MI: Adjuvant interferon for anal condyloma. Dis Colon Rectum 37:1255–1259, 1994.
51. Drew WL, Mintz L, Miner RC, et al: Prevalence of cytomegalovirus infection in homosexual men. J Infect Dis 143:188, 1981.
52. Diepersloot RJA, Kroes ACM, Visser W, et al: Acute ulcerative proctocolitis associated with primary cytomegalovirus infection. Arch Intern Med 150:1749, 1990.
53. Allason-Jones E, Mindel A, Sargeaunt P, et al: *Entamoeba histolytica* as a commensal intestinal parasite in homosexual men. N Engl J Med 315:353, 1986.
54. Allason-Jones E, Mindel A, Sargeaunt P, et al: Outcome of untreated infection with *Entamoeba histolytica* in homosexual men with and without HIV antibody. Br Med J 297:654, 1988.
55. Flores BM, Reed SL, Ravdin JI, et al: Serologic reactivity to purified recombinant and native 29-kilodalton peripheral membrane protein of pathogenic *Entamoeba histolytica*. J Clin Microbiol 31:1403–1407, 1993.
56. Drugs for parasitic infections. Med Lett 37:99, 1995.
57. Liu LX, Chi J, Upton MP, et al: Eosinophilic colitis associated with larvae of the pinworm *Enterobius vermicularis*. Lancet 346:410–412, 1995.
58. Maraha B, Buiting AG: Evaluation of four enzyme immunoassays for the detection of *Giardia lamblia* antigen in stool specimens. Eur J Clin Microbiol Infect Dis 19:485–487, 2000.
59. Dieterich DT, Kotler DP, Busch DF, et al: Ganciclovir treatment of cytomegalovirus colitis in AIDS: A randomized, double-blind, placebo-controlled multicenter study. J Infect Dis 167:278–282, 1993.
60. Dieterich DT, Poles MA, Dicker M, et al: Foscarnet treatment of cytomegalovirus gastrointestinal infections in acquired immunodeficiency syndrome patients who have failed ganciclovir induction. Am J Gastroenterol 88:542–548, 1993.
61. Monkemuller KE, Wilcox CM: Diagnosis and treatment of colonic disease in AIDS. Gastrointest Endosc Clin North Am 4:889–911, 1998.
62. Monkemuller KE, Bussian AH, Lazenby AJ, Wilcox CM: Special histologic stains are rarely beneficial for the evaluation of HIV-related gastrointestinal infections. Am J Clin Pathol 114:387–394, 2000.
63. Fisher AA, Brancaccio RR: Allergic contact sensitivity to propylene glycol in a lubricant jelly. Arch Dermatol 115:1451, 1979.

Chapter 117

Examination and Diseases of the Anorectum

Tracy Hull

ANATOMY

The functional anal canal is 3 to 4 cm long; it begins at the top of the anorectal ring (at the puborectalis sling) and extends down to the anal verge (anal orifice).[1] The top or upper anal canal is lined mostly with columnar epithelium; this is the continuation of the same type of tissue that lines the rectum. However, some squamous epithelium starts to be intermixed at about 1 cm above the dentate line. This change to squamous epithelium is gradual, and the area 1 to 1.5 cm proximal to the dentate line is termed the transitional zone.[2] The dentate line is located in the midanal canal and is seen as a wavy line. Distal to the dentate line, the tissue is squamous epithelium but is not like true skin, as it has no hair, sebaceous glands, or sweat glands. It is commonly referred to as anoderm. The anoderm is thin, pale, and delicate appearing. It looks like shiny, stretched skin. At the anal verge, the skin becomes thicker, and hair follicles begin to be seen[3] (Fig. 117–1).

Embryologically, the dentate line represents the junction between endoderm and ectoderm. Proximal to the dentate line, there is sympathetic and parasympathetic innervation; distally, the nerve supply is somatic.[3] Therefore, above the dentate line pain sensation is negligible—a biopsy can be done painlessly above the dentate line. However, below the dentate line anesthesia is needed to perform a biopsy.

The arterial supply to the anal area is from the superior hemorrhoidal artery (which is a continuation of the inferior mesenteric artery), the middle hemorrhoidal artery (from the hypogastric artery), and the inferior hemorrhoidal artery (a branch of the internal pudendal artery).[3] The venous drainage from the anal canal is by both the systemic and portal systems. The internal hemorrhoidal plexus drains into the superior rectal veins, which drain into the inferior mesenteric vein and then into the portal vein. The distal part of the anal canal drains via the external hemorrhoidal plexus through the middle rectal vein and pudendal vein into the internal iliac vein (the systemic circulation).[2]

The lymphatic drainage varies at the dentate line. Proximally, the lymphatic drainage accompanies the blood vessels to the inferior mesenteric and periaortic nodes.[1–3] Distal to the dentate line, the lymph nodes drain to the inguinal nodes. Therefore, inguinal adenopathy can be seen with inflammatory and malignant disease of the lower anal canal.

Immediately proximal to the dentate line, the mucosa appears to have 6 to 14 pleats. This configuration represents the funneling of the rectum as it narrows into the anal canal. The pleats are called the columns of Morgagni. Located at the base of the columns of Morgagni are anal crypts that lead to small rudimentary anal glands.[3] These glands may extend through the internal anal sphincter and, if blocked, lead to an anal abscess or fistula (see Fig. 117–1).

The muscles surrounding the anal canal are important for fecal continence. The internal anal sphincter is the thickened continuation of the circular smooth muscle of the rectum. This muscle is involuntary and composed of smooth muscle, which gives it a black hypoechoic appearance on anal ultrasound. The internal sphincter ends above the external sphincter.[3] The internal sphincter is important for continence but can be divided without leading to incontinence.

The external anal sphincter is composed of a voluntary sheet of skeletal muscle, which is arranged as a tube surrounding the internal sphincter. It appears as a broad cylinder with mixed echogenicity on anal ultrasound. Proximally, the external sphincter is fused with the puborectalis muscle, and distally, it ends slightly past the internal sphincter.[1, 3] Therefore, a groove can be palpated between the internal sphincter and external sphincter on digital examination (intersphincteric groove). The puborectalis is shaped like a U and forms a sling that goes behind the lower rectum and attaches to the pubis. Therefore, it is prominent laterally and posteriorly but absent anteriorly. The anorectal ring is palpable at the top of the anal canal, where the canal meets the rectum. It is composed of the puborectalis and the upper external and internal sphincters. The nerve supply to the external sphincter and puborectalis muscle is from the inferior rectal branch of the internal pudendal nerve (S2, S3, S4) and also from fibers of the fourth sacral nerve.[1, 3]

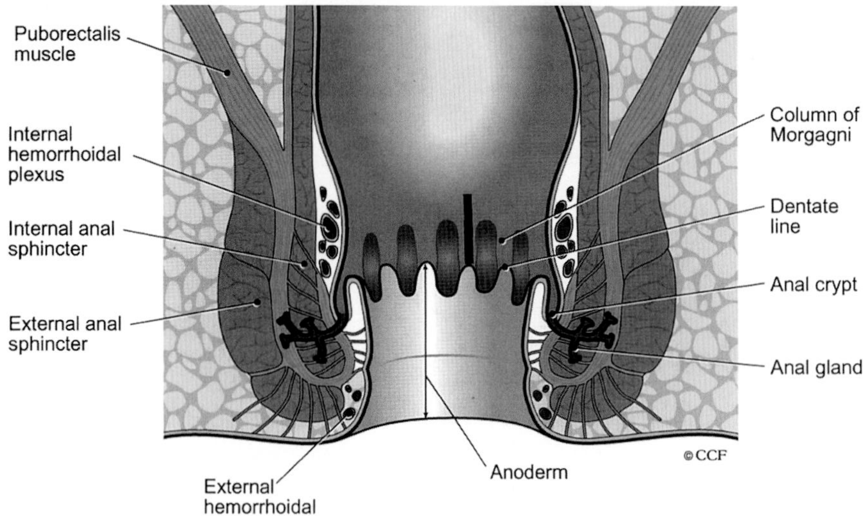

Figure 117–1. Anatomy of the anal region. The heavy vertical line denotes the transition zone that is located 1 to 1.5 cm proximal to the dentate line. (Reprinted with the permission of The Cleveland Clinic Foundation.)

EXAMINATION OF THE ANUS AND RECTUM

All routine comprehensive adult physical examinations should include a digital anal examination. When patients present with problems focused on the anorectal region or colon, a more comprehensive examination is indicated. Any examination of the anorectal region begins with a thorough history taking. This allows the patient to describe the symptoms and concerns, and the physician can develop a rapport with the patient that will help alleviate the patient's apprehension and embarrassment about the examination. It is important to remember that many patients delay coming to the physician, even when they have significant problems, out of fear and embarrassment. Therefore, when doing the examination, *explaining each step* along with a gentle touch, helps alleviate discomfort. It is equally important to avoid inducing excessive pain during the examination, particularly when looking for a fissure or anal abscess. Sometimes when the examination is too painful, performing it in the operating room under anesthesia is indicated.

Patients can be examined in the office in several positions. The most popular is probably the left lateral position. The patient is positioned on the examination table on his or her left side with the thighs and knees flexed. The buttocks project slightly beyond the edge of the examination table. An assistant is needed to retract the left buttock for optimal viewing.

In the knee-chest (or prone jackknife) position, the patient is on his or her knees with the shoulders and head on the examining table. In a variant of this position, the patient is placed on a special hydraulic table that has a shelf. The patient kneels on the shelf and drapes his or her chest over the main table. The table then is raised and tipped up, propelling the buttocks forward and in the air. This position allows the buttocks to splay apart for a clear view of the anus.

The dorsolithotomy position is the typical position used for the female gynecologic examination. It is also sometimes used to examine the anorectal region, particularly when looking for an anovaginal fistula.

During the examination, it is important to have all instruments available and have an assistant who additionally can help reassure the patient. Good lighting is essential to view the skin critically and to perform endoscopy of the anus and rectum.

Inspection

The examination next turns to inspecting the skin. In some cases, looking at the underwear will give a clue to the character of anal drainage or stool incontinence. As the buttocks are gently retracted, scars, dermatologic skin abnormalities, stool, pus, anal tags, warts, hemorrhoids, or lesions prolapsing from the anal canal are noted. The anus is inspected for gaping or scars, and the patient may be asked to squeeze to evaluate the movement of the anal muscles. Next, the patient may be asked to strain so that the anal area can be examined for abnormal descent below its resting level (perineal descent syndrome). Also, prolapse of the vagina, leakage of urine, prolapse of the rectum, or hemorrhoids should be noted during straining. In some instances, prolapse of the rectum may be seen only if the patient is placed on the toilet and asked to strain. Traction laterally on each side of the anal orifice with a gauze sponge will allow eversion of the distal anus for further inspection. This technique is particularly helpful in viewing a fissure without causing undo pain. Some examiners rub the perianal skin with a Q-tip to look for reflex contraction of the anal muscles (anocutaneous reflex) or check sensation with a pinprick. These maneuvers give a crude determination of sphincter innervation. The surrounding skin of the buttocks, perivaginal region, base of the scrotum, and up to the tip of the coccyx should be viewed. Adenopathy in the inguinal region may be seen when lesions are found distal to the dentate line.

Palpation

Next, using a gloved and lubricated index finger, the examiner palpates the anal canal and perianal skin. Slow insertion and gentle pressure are needed. The index finger is swept all around the anal canal. The tone is noted, as are any scars, masses, or tenderness. Internal hemorrhoids are not palpable unless they are thrombosed. If insertion of the index finger is too painful, an attempt to apply pressure with the insertion finger on the wall opposite the area of tenderness may allow insertion of the finger. If the examination is still too painful, an examination under anesthesia may be warranted.

Abnormalities sometimes appreciated in the anal canal include fistulous tracts, which feel like a cord or induration; the internal opening of a fistula, which may be appreciated as a knob of tissue in an otherwise smooth area of mucosa; cancers, which may be firm and hard; and ulcers, which feel uneven and craterous. The patient may be asked to squeeze on the examining finger to assess the external sphincter muscle. Palpation anteriorly in a woman may reveal a rectocele.

Palpation of the distal rectum allows the detection of polyps and cancers. Attention should be directed to the exact location of the lesion (i.e., anterior, posterior, right, left, or "in-between"), and its size, mobility, and character (i.e., soft, ulcerated, hard, or pedunculated). Lesions outside the rectal wall may also be appreciated. The cervix can be appreciated through the rectal wall in women, and the prostate should be examined in men. The character of the prostate should be noted, along with any hard nodularity that could represent cancer. Further studies are then ordered if needed. The mucosal wall should be assessed for its smoothness; in patients with proctitis, for example, the mucosa feels like sandpaper.

In some patients with unexplained anal pain, the levator muscles should be palpated to look for spasm or tenderness. Similarly, the coccyx should be palpated between the examining internal index finger and the index finger of the opposite hand pressed over the external skin at the level of the coccyx. This maneuver is done to look for pain with motion.

The contents of the rectum should be assessed regarding the character and amount of the stool. When the index finger is removed, any stool, blood, pus, or mucus should be noted.

Endoscopy

The decision to perform endoscopy depends on the findings on physical examination. Endoscopy is necessary for the exclusion of organic disease in patients with fecal incontinence, constipation, unexplained anal pain,[4] anemia, diarrhea, and rectal bleeding.

ANOSCOPY. Anoscopy allows visualization of the anal canal, dentate line, internal hemorrhoids, and distal rectum. This is the best method of viewing the anal canal. The anoscope is a metal or plastic tubular device with a beveled end. *An anoscope should NEVER be inserted or turned without the obturator in place.* Most adult anoscopes have a 2-cm diameter, but smaller ones are available. Fiberoptic light attachments give the optimal view; however, external lighting is used with some models.

The lubricated anoscope is inserted slowly as the examiner applies gentle pressure on the end of the obturator (to push the instrument in). The obturator is removed, and the anal canal region is examined. To rotate the anoscope while it is in the canal, the obturator is replaced and the scope is turned. The obturator is then removed again. The scope can be pulled slowly back to view the entire area from the upper anal canal to the anoderm. To reinsert the scope, the obturator again must be replaced. Internal hemorrhoids can be seen bulging above the dentate line or prolapsing downward. Internal fistulous openings may be viewed, particularly along the dentate line. When the external skin is compressed, pus may be seen to bubble from the internal opening of a fistula. Occasionally, the anoscope is needed to remove a low rectal polyp that cannot be removed through a flexible endoscope because of the low position of the polyp in the rectum or a difficult angulation on retroflexion of the endoscope.

RIGID PROCTOSCOPY. The rigid proctoscope is 25 cm long, but usually it cannot be passed to its full extent into the rectosigmoid. The diameter of the scope varies from 11 to 20 mm. The obturator is placed in the cylinder, and the instrument lubricated. With the thumb of the examiner on the obturator, the instrument is advanced gently through the anal canal. The obturator is then removed. The instrument requires fiberoptic light for visualization. Under direct vision (to avoid perforation), the scope is then advanced. The depth of insertion (usually from the anal verge) is noted. Examination is done during withdrawal of the instrument, usually while small puffs of air are supplied to keep the rectum from collapsing. The appearance of the mucosa is noted.

Usually a patient must have an enema before rigid proctoscopy for optimal visualization of the mucosa. Exceptions to this rule are patients with severe inflammation (proctitis) or with suspected infections, in which case stool will be collected for cultures or other tests.

In the modern era of fiberoptic and video sigmoidoscopes, there are still some instances when a rigid proctoscope is superior. The proctoscope can measure the exact distance of a rectal tumor from the anal verge. It also can give the precise location of a lesion on the wall of the rectum. Such measurements are highly inaccurate with flexible scopes and are important for planning operative strategies. The rigid proctoscope is sometimes quicker and easier to use than a flexible scope when evaluating the rectum and doing a biopsy or aspirating fecal contents. Rigid biopsy forceps can be placed through the proctoscope. Caution must be used when doing biopsies with the rigid forceps anteriorly above 7 to 10 cm. This area corresponds to the intra-abdominal colon above the peritoneal reflection, and care must be taken to avoid perforation into the abdominal cavity. The biopsy forceps used with flexible endoscopes also can be used through the rigid proctoscope.

FLEXIBLE SIGMOIDOSCOPY. The flexible sigmoidoscope is simply a shorter version of a colonoscope. It measures 60 cm in length. A formal bowel prepreparation used for colonoscopy usually is not done for flexible sigmoidoscopy; rather, two enemas are given before the examination. Sedation also is usually not used. As for colonoscopy, the lubricated tip of the sigmoidoscope is inserted and advanced under direct vision. The goal is to examine the left colon, which is reached 80% of the time.[5] Lesions can be biopsied, but polyps usually mandate full colonoscopy following a bowel preparation to exclude other polyps or cancer. The use of electrocautery is usually avoided during sigmoidoscopy, unless the preparation is optimal.

The exact role of flexible sigmoidoscopy is evolving. With the gradual shift of colorectal cancers to the more proximal colon over recent decades, flexible sigmoidoscopy is not adequate when a complete colonic examination is needed. However, flexible sigmoidoscopy can be used to enhance the diagnostic capability of barium enema, which at times fails to visualize the distal rectum optimally because of the balloon needed to distend the colon and infuse the barium. Lesions of the sigmoid seen on radiologic studies also can be evaluated by flexible sigmoidoscopy. Flexible sigmoidoscopy permits serial examinations of the activity of proctosigmoiditis in patients with inflammatory bowel disease and allows rectosigmoid biopsies to be done. It is also the preferred endoscopic tool for surveying family members at risk for familial adenomatous polyposis.

HEMORRHOIDS

Hemorrhoids are perhaps the most misunderstood anorectal problem for patients and many physicians alike. In clinical practice patients use the term hemorrhoid to describe almost any anorectal problem, from pruritus ani to cancer.[6] In fact, hemorrhoids are a normal part of human anatomy,[7, 8] in contrast to hemorrhoidal disease, which is manifested by prolapse, bleeding, and itching.[7] Hemorrhoids are dilated vascular channels located in three fairly constant locations—left lateral, right posterior, and right anterior. Internal hemorrhoids originate above the dentate line and are covered with rectal or transitional mucosa. External hemorrhoids are located closer to the verge and are covered with squamous epithelium. Traditionally, internal hemorrhoids have been classified into four grades: (1) first-degree hemorrhoids bleed with defecation; (2) second-degree hemorrhoids prolapse with defecation but return naturally to their normal position; (3) third-degree hemorrhoids prolapse through the anal canal at any time but especially with defecation and can be replaced manually; and (4) fourth-degree hemorrhoids are prolapsed permanently.[8]

Although the exact incidence of hemorrhoidal disease is unknown, 10% to 25% of the adult population is thought to be affected.[9] Symptoms seem to be more common in older individuals, with a peak in prevalence at 45 to 65 years.

Internal Hemorrhoids

It is speculated that internal hemorrhoids become symptomatic when the supporting structures become disrupted and the vascular anal cushions prolapse.[10] However, the exact pathogenesis is not clear. Hemorrhoids occur more frequently in people with constipation who have hard, infrequent stools.[11] Painless bleeding usually is seen on the toilet tissue or dripping into the toilet at the end of defecation. Sometimes the bleeding can be more substantial, and the blood can accumulate in the rectum with the passage of dark blood or clots.[8] When hemorrhoids prolapse, blood or mucus may stain a patient's underwear, and the mucus against the anal skin may lead to itching.[10]

The diagnosis of internal hemorrhoids is made with the beveled anoscope. The cushions can be seen to bulge into the anal lumen, or the tissue may prolapse out the anal canal. Hemorrhoids may be symptomatic only intermittently and may look entirely normal if the patient is over a "flare."

TREATMENT. Treatment is based on the grade. Grade 1 and some early grade 2 internal hemorrhoids usually respond to dietary manipulation, along with avoidance of medications that promote bleeding, such as nonsteroidal anti-inflammatory drugs (NSAIDs). A high-fiber diet with 25 to 30 g of daily fiber should be introduced gradually into the diet and accompanied by 6 to 8 glasses of fluid daily. Patients are encouraged to read the package regarding the amount of fiber per serving; for instance, a bowl of bran cereal can have 5 to 7 g of dietary fiber per serving.[12] Fiber supplementation with psyllium or hydrophilic colloid may be added to achieve the optimal amount of daily fiber.

Patients often are concerned that fiber supplementation will be "addictive" or that the package label calls the supplement a "laxative," and counseling about the goal of increasing the amount of dietary fiber helps them understand the importance of these agents. Fiber supplements can be started in a dose of 1 teaspoon daily for a week and then increased to 1 tablespoon daily so as to allow the digestive tract to adjust to the increase in fiber. Additionally, patients are urged to avoid straining during defecation and reading while on the toilet. Also, they should not defer the urge to defecate for long periods of time. They should be encouraged to wipe the anal area gently after defecation with a moist facial tissue or baby wipes. Excessive scrubbing when showering or bathing is discouraged. Most over-the-counter agents are not efficacious, even though many patients report some relief of their symptoms with use of these products.[11] Sometimes docusate sodium can be prescribed if the stool is hard and does not respond to increased intake of fiber and fluid. Laxative and enemas are rarely needed.[12] Even patients who require more aggressive treatment of their hemorrhoids should be advised to increase their dietary fiber and fluids and to avoid straining during defecation to prevent recurrence after treatment.

When dietary manipulation does not work, more aggressive treatment is needed. These measures can apply to grades 1, 2, and 3 internal hemorrhoids. Unless the patient has fourth-degree internal hemorrhoids, aggressive nonsurgical treatment is usually tried. (Most patients with fourth-degree hemorrhoids require surgical intervention.) Most treatments are designed to fix the vascular cushion to the underlying sphincter. Options include injection with a sclerosing agent, rubber band ligation, cryotherapy, infrared photocoagulation, electrocoagulation, and application of a heater probe. These procedures can be performed in the office, usually after the patient has received an enema to evacuate the rectum.

Sclerosing Agents. Injection therapy for hemorrhoids has been practiced for over 100 years. The goal is to inject an irritant into the submucosa above the internal hemorrhoid at the anorectal ring (the area that does not have somatic innervation) to create fibrosis and prevent prolapse.[13] Usually less than 1 mL is needed to create a raised area. Many substances have been used, but sterilized arachis oils containing 5% phenol are the most popular.[13] This approach is usually advocated for first- and second-degree hemorrhoids.

Sclerotherapy can produce a dull pain for up to 2 days after injection. A rare but severe complication is life-threatening pelvic sepsis, which can occur 3 to 5 days after injection and is usually manifested by any combination of perianal pain, perineal swelling, watery anal discharge, fever, leukocytosis, and other signs of sepsis. Prompt surgical intervention and intravenous antibiotics are mandatory.[13, 14] Approximately 75% of patients improve after second-degree hemorrhoids are treated by injection therapy.[15]

Rubber Band Ligation. Rubber band ligation has become the most common office procedure for the treatment of second- and third-degree hemorrhoids.[16] Generally, this approach cannot be used with first-degree hemorrhoids, because there is insufficient tissue to pull into the bander. Treatment of fourth-degree hemorrhoids is almost never appropriate with this method. Patients are usually asked to refrain from taking aspirin or NSAIDs for approximately 5 days before and after the treatment, to reduce the risk of bleeding. The rubber bands are placed on the rectal mucosa just proximal to the internal anal cushion. To avoid severe pain, bands are never placed on the external component, which is innervated by somatic fibers. There is disagreement as to how many bands should be placed at one time. Studies have shown that triple rubber band ligation is safe and effective at one sitting,[16] but many authorities believe that the severity of pain and risk of complications are less if one band is applied per visit.

Patients may experience discomfort after banding. Usually soaking in a sitz bath and taking acetaminophen are all that is required. Immediate severe pain usually signals that the band has been placed too close to the dentate line and must be removed. Patients are instructed to increase the fiber in their diet and employ the other noninvasive bowel habit modifications discussed previously. Success is reported in 75% of patients with first- (when band ligation can be used) and second-degree hemorrhoids and 65% of those with third-degree hemorrhoids. The technique usually is not used for fourth-degree hemorrhoids.[15]

There can be important complications from rubber band ligation. Bleeding when the band comes off in 4 to 7 days may be severe and may require intervention. Placing a large-caliber Foley catheter in the rectum, injecting the balloon with 25 to 30 mL or more of fluid, and pulling the balloon tight against the top of the anal ring can usually tamponade the bleeding. If this approach fails, epinephrine can be injected at the bleeding site, but sometimes a suture is required to stop the bleeding. A more serious complication is life-threatening sepsis. There have been five recorded deaths, two additional patients with life-threatening sepsis, and three cases of severe pelvic cellulitis following rubber band ligation of hemorrhoids.[14] The onset is usually 2 to 8 days after the banding in otherwise healthy people. New or increasing anal pain, sometimes radiating down the leg, or difficulty voiding may be the first indications of a life-threatening infection. Immediate intravenous antibiotics and surgical débridement are required.

Cryotherapy. Cryotherapy freezes the tissue, thereby destroying the hemorrhoidal plexus. Once a popular treatment, its use has declined because of the profuse, foul-smelling discharge resulting from necrosis of tissue. The procedure also can be painful, and healing can be prolonged.[17]

Infrared Photocoagulation. Infrared photocoagulation produces infrared radiation just proximal to the internal hemorrhoid plexus, thereby coagulating the tissue and leading to fibrosis. The device is applied for 1.5 sec in 2 to 3 sites proximal to the hemorrhoidal plexus. Reported results for first- and second-degree hemorrhoids are as good as those reported for rubber band ligation or sclerotherapy.[15] Pain and other complications are rare.

Electrocoagulation and Heater Probe. Use of thermal injury to fix the internal hemorrhoidal plexus is the basis for electrocoagulation and heater probe therapy. Both types of therapy compare favorably with rubber band ligation for the treatment of first- and second-degree hemorrhoids but have not gained popularity.

Surgical Treatments. Methods to reduce the internal anal sphincter pressure in patients with internal hemorrhoids have been advocated in the past. These methods include internal sphincterotomy and manual dilatation of the anus (Lord's procedure) and are based on the general finding of an increase in resting pressure in patients with hemorrhoids.[18] However, these procedures have not had widespread acceptance. One study of the Lord's procedure to treat second- and third-degree internal hemorrhoids with a median follow-up of 17 years found a nearly 40% recurrence rate and a 52% rate of incontinence.[19] Lateral internal sphincterotomy occasionally is performed if patients have both a fissure and extensive hemorrhoids at the time of surgery for hemorrhoids.

Hemorrhoidectomy is the surgical procedure of choice for fourth-degree and some third-degree hemorrhoids. Rarely is this treatment needed for first- or second-degree hemorrhoids. The procedure can be done with local, regional, or general anesthesia. Whether the edges of the mucosa are closed or left open after excision of the hemorrhoidal tissue is a matter of preference, as results and postoperative pain are similar with either approach.[20] In one of the few long-term studies of hemorrhoidectomy, recurrent hemorrhoids were found in 26% at a median follow-up of 17 years,[19] but only 11% of patients needed an additional procedure.

Postoperative pain is a major drawback of hemorrhoidectomy. In an effort to reduce postoperative pain, a new procedure has been introduced in which a circular stapler is used to staple the mucosa circumferentially just above the anorectal ring.[21] In preliminary studies, this new method has proved effective without the degree of postoperative pain seen with traditional excision.

Table 117–1 summarizes the treatment options for internal hemorrhoids.

External Hemorrhoids and Anal Tags

External hemorrhoids are visible on the anal verge and perianal skin. They actually are skin tags that represent residual redundant skin from previous episodes of edematous external hemorrhoids. They are easily seen when the buttocks are parted. They do not bleed because they are covered with squamous epithelium. They usually are seen in young and middle-aged adults and cause no symptoms, although many people are uncomfortable during anal wiping and when they feel the redundant tissue. Occasionally, external hemorrhoids interfere with perianal hygiene and cause itching and irritation. External hemorrhoids can cause acute pain from thrombosis.[10] The level of pain is variable, but patients may notice a rapidly increasing throbbing or burning pain accompanied by a new "lump" in the anal region. Sometimes the "lump" has a bluish discoloration caused by the clot. With time, a

Table 117–1 | **Treatment Options for Internal Hemorrhoids**

TYPE OF TREATMENT	GRADE FOR EACH TREATMENT	SUCCESS RATE	COMMENTS
Diet (increase in fiber and fluids) and habit modification	1 & 2	Unknown	Patients with all grades of hemorrhoids should follow these guidelines
Sclerosing agent	1 & 2	75%	Rare life-threatening sepsis
Rubber band ligation	2 & 3	65%–75%	Grade 1 hemorrhoids usually are too small for this treatment Rarely used for grades 1 & 4 Controversial as to how many pedicles to band at one treatment Rare life-threatening sepsis
Cryotherapy	N/A	N/A	Currently not used, terrible odor as tissue necrosis occurs
Infrared coagulation	1 & 2	Same as rubber band ligation	Rare complications
Electrocoagulation or heater probe	1 & 2	Same as rubber band ligation	Has not gained popularity in treatment
Surgical *anal dilatation*	N/A	N/A	No longer popular because of high risk of incontinence
Surgical *lateral internal sphincterotomy*	All	—	Used if an anal fissure is present and anal tone is increased
Surgical *hemorrhoidectomy*	3 & 4	>75% on 10-year follow-up	Postoperative pain is significant; circular stapled hemorrhoidectomy may be less painful

N/A, not applicable.

small area of necrosis may form over the lump and the clot is extruded. When this happens, old blood may emanate from the area.

The treatment of external hemorrhoids usually is with reassurance and proper anal hygiene, including delicate washing of the anal area and avoiding aggressive wiping with harsh toilet tissue. Rarely is resection done. Resection is painful, and, because of the swelling that accompanies any surgical excision, redundant tissue may persist after the patient has healed. The patient may feel the redundant tissue again and become upset about the "recurrence." When surgical excision is undertaken for internal hemorrhoids, as discussed earlier, any external component usually is excised at the same time.

The treatment of thrombosed hemorrhoids depends on the associated symptoms. With time, the pain associated with the acute thrombosis will subside. If the patient has minimal or moderate pain, sitz baths and analgesics are prescribed. For severe pain, the clot is enucleated under local anesthesia. Because of the high rate of recurrence with simple enucleation alone, some authorities recommend excising the entire thrombosis and overlying skin. This procedure also can be done in the office with scissors and local anesthesia.[10] The skin edges are left open to heal by secondary intention.

Table 117–2 summarizes the treatment options for external hemorrhoids.

SPECIAL CONSIDERATIONS. Large, edematous, shiny perianal skin tags should alert the physician to the possibility of Crohn's disease. The tags may have a bluish discoloration. Careful history taking is indicated and further testing needed if there is any suspicion that the tags are not ordinary. Surgical excision is avoided with Crohn's disease in almost every situation, because after surgery the patient usually is left with unhealed anal ulcers.

Patients who are infected with the human immunodeficiency virus (HIV) usually are treated as if they do not carry HIV, unless their immune status is significantly compromised. In a study of 11 HIV-positive men with a mean CD4+ count of 420/mm^3 and a mean follow-up of 6 months, no complications occurred after rubber band ligation of hemorrhoids, and symptoms improved in all 11.[22]

Pregnant women with problematic hemorrhoids usually are managed medically. Simply increasing the fiber and fluids and at times adding a stool softener is all that is needed. If a complication develops, such as acute prolapse with strangulation, surgical intervention in the operating room may be necessary.

ANAL FISSURE

An anal fissure is a longitudinal "cut" in the anoderm; it starts at the anal verge and can extend to the dentate line. Over 90% of anal fissures are located in the midposterior position of the anus. Ten percent are anterior. Any fissure not located in the anterior or posterior position should alert the physician to the possibility of other diagnoses, such as Crohn's disease.

The etiology of anal fissures is unknown. Using laser Doppler flowmetry, it has been shown that the posterior area of the anoderm is less well perfused than other areas of

Table 117–2 | **Treatment of External Hemorrhoids and Tags**

TREATMENT	INDICATION
Good hygiene	All patients
Reassurance	All patients
Surgical excision	Difficulty with cleanliness or itching unresponsive to conservative treatment
Surgical excision	Thrombosed hemorrhoid that is painful (usually in the acute phase less than 48 hr after occurrence) or recurrent thrombosed hemorrhoid in the same location

anoderm. There is speculation that increased tone in the internal sphincter muscle further reduces the blood flow, especially at the posterior midline.[23] Based on these findings, fissures are thought to represent ischemic ulceration.[24] Trauma during defecation is believed to initiate the formation of a fissure. The trauma can be the result of passage of a hard, constipated stool or explosive diarrhea.

Fissures are usually exquisitely tender, and the act of defecation is reported by patients to feel like passing razor blades. The history is classically one of *severe* pain during defecation. After defecation patients may experience continued pain or burning for up to several hours. Bright red blood may be seen on the toilet tissue. On examination, a tender, edematous skin tag may be seen just distal to the fissure. Simply spreading the buttocks usually increases the pain and leads to anal sphincter muscle spasm. *A digital examination causes inhumane pain, increases the spasm, and should be avoided.* Once the fissure is healed or the pain has lessened, an examination can be done to exclude other problems. If an examination is done and the anal canal is visualized, a hypertrophied anal papilla may be seen in patients with a chronic fissure. If the diagnosis is in doubt or the patient does not respond to treatment, an examination under anesthesia is indicated.

The differential diagnosis of anal fissure includes Crohn's disease, leukemic ulcer, tuberculosis ulcer, syphilis, cancer, and HIV-related anal ulcer.

Fissures can be acute or chronic. Acute fissures are simply a split or crack in the anoderm. In contrast, chronic fissures show signs of chronicity, with rolled edges, fibrosis of the edges, deep ulceration with exposure of the underlying internal sphincter muscle, enlargement of the tissue at Ihe dentate line (hypertrophied anal papilla), and edematous skin tags at the distal anal verge (Fig. 117–2).

Treatment of both acute and chronic anal fissures starts with dietary modification. As for hemorrhoids, patients are placed on a high-fiber diet with fiber supplements, and fluid intake is increased. Soaking in a sitz bath relaxes the sphincter and can provide some relief.[10] If needed, stool softeners are added. Acute fissures respond better than chronic fissures to these measures.

Treatment of fissures remained unchanged for most of the past 50 years.[25] However, recently several new treatment modalities have become popular. With the knowledge that nitric oxide (NO) mediates relaxation of the internal sphincter muscle,[23] NO donors such as nitroglycerin have been used to reduce anal pressure and improve blood flow to the anoderm. A pea-sized amount of 0.2% nitroglycerin ointment is applied to the anal area. Gradual escalation of the dose to three times daily reduces the chance of headaches (a major drawback of this treatment). In one study, 67% of fissures treated in this manner healed at 8 weeks, compared with 32% of those treated with placebo.[26] Recurrence was seen in 33% of patients at a median follow-up of 9 months. Unfortunately, headaches were reported by 72% of treated patients.

The injection of botulinum toxin A, which inhibits acetylcholine release, into the internal sphincter close to a fissure was first described by Jost and Schimrigk in 1993.[27] Since then, this modality has gained popularity as a treatment for chronic anal fissure. In a study from Italy, 73% of anal fissures were healed at 8 weeks,[28] with no recurrences at a mean of 16 months later. Botulinum toxin injection also has been compared with topical nitroglycerin ointment, and at 8 weeks fissures were healed in 96% of patients injected with botulinum toxin and 60% of those treated with nitroglycerin. In neither group was there a recurrence at a mean follow-up of 15 months.[29]

The optimal dose of botulinum toxin is unclear. It appears that injection of 20 units with a 27-gauge needle into the internal sphincter on each side of the fissure is optimal.[30] In one study, anterior injection of botulinum toxin was associated with earlier healing of a posterior fissure than was posterior injection.[31] No long-term complications have been reported in the literature. However, the cost of the treatment is not insignificant. A single 20-unit injection of botulinum toxin must be taken from a vial of 100 units, which costs $238. The toxin, when mixed, must be used within 4 hours, so that optimal utilization requires that four patients be treated within the 4 hours. The cost of botulinum toxin compares to a cost of nitroglycerin ointment for 6 weeks of only $6 to $10.[32] It has been suggested that, in an effort to

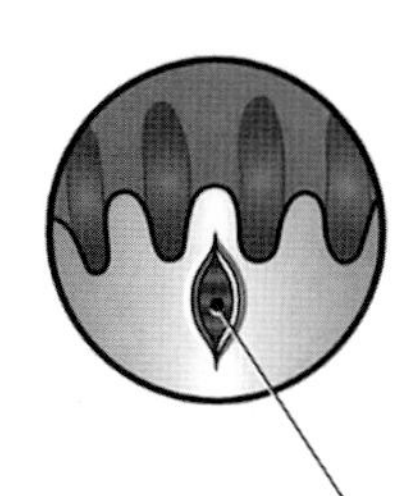

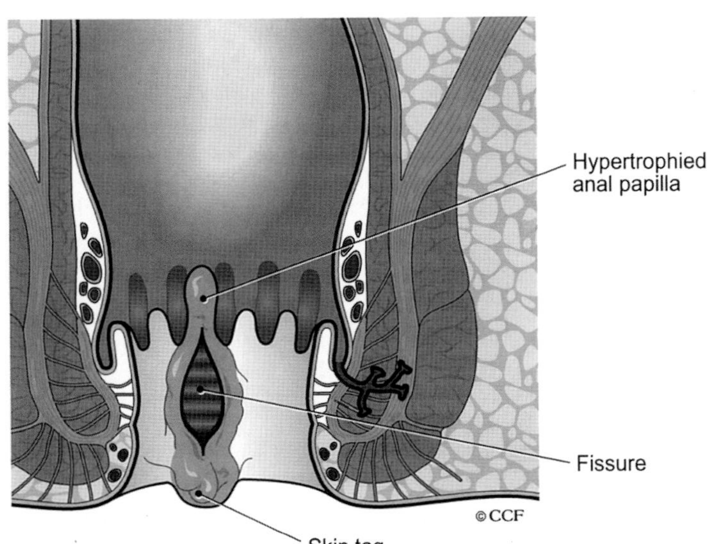

Figure 117–2. Acute and chronic anal fissure. An acute fissure is depicted on the left as simply a split in the anoderm. A chronic fissure can show signs of chronicity with rolled edges, fibrosis, hypertrophied anal papilla proximally, a tender distal skin tag, and exposed internal anal muscle. (Reprinted with the permission of The Cleveland Clinic Foundation.)

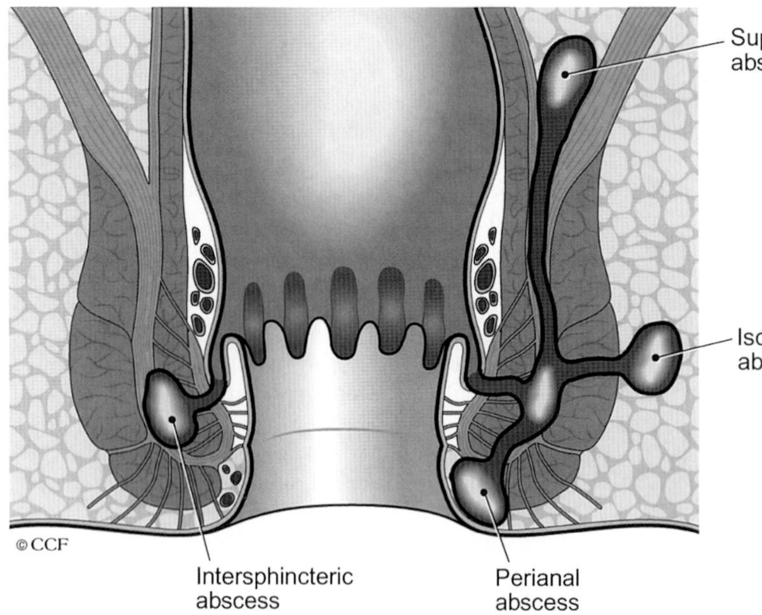

Figure 117–3. Classification of abscesses of the anal region based on the location of the abscess. (Reprinted with the permission of The Cleveland Clinic Foundation.)

contain costs, patients should be treated initially with nitroglycerin ointment, with botulinum toxin injection reserved for treatment failures.[32]

Oral nifedipine, 20 mg twice daily, has been reported to heal chronic anal fissures. In a pilot study, 9 of 15 (60%) fissures healed at 8 weeks. Ten of 15 patients experienced flushing, and 4 had mild headaches.[33] This treatment modality is currently under further study.

The standard treatment of chronic anal fissures has been surgery—lateral internal sphincterotomy. It remains the standard by which all other treatments must be measured. One long-term study found that among 2108 patients with anal fissures who underwent outpatient surgery with local anesthesia and intravenous sedation, the results were very good to excellent in 96% at a follow-up of 4 to 20 years. The rate of recurrent fissures was 1%. Permanent incontinence did not occur.[34] When performed correctly, lateral internal sphincterotomy still appears to be superior (and probably cheaper in the long-term) to any currently available medical treatment.

Patients requiring special consideration are postpartum women. In one study, painful fissures developed in 9% of 209 postpartum primigravid women. Anal sphincter hypertonia was not seen in these patients.[35] Therefore, in this setting, division of the anal sphincter may be detrimental. Twenty-seven of the 29 fissures healed with intensive medical treatment (which was not specified). The researchers felt that if surgical intervention is needed in a postpartum woman with an anal fissure, an advancement flap may be preferable to a lateral sphincterotomy.[36]

ANAL SEPSIS—ABSCESSES AND FISTULAS

Anorectal Abscesses

Almost all anorectal suppurative disease results from infection of the anal glands extending from the anal crypts (cryptoglandular), located along the dentate line at the base of the columns of Morgagni. An acute infection can cause an abscess and can lead to a chronic fistula-in-ano. Other causes include Crohn's disease, fissures that bore into the anal muscle, trauma, hematologic malignancies, tuberculosis, actinomycosis, foreign bodies, and anal surgery. The differential diagnosis also includes a pilonidal sinus, hidradenitis suppurativa, carcinoma, Bartholin's gland abscess, and lymphoma.

Because the anal glands terminate in the intersphincteric plane, abscesses originate in the intersphincteric space. They then can travel up, down, or circumferentially around the anus. Abscesses are classified according to where they extend to and cause pain, erythema, and swelling. They may be perianal, ischiorectal, intersphincteric, or supralevator (Fig. 117–3). The most common type is the perianal abscess (40% to 50%), and the least common type is the supralevator abscess (2% to 9%).[37]

As mentioned earlier, a diagnosis of anorectal abscess is based on typical symptoms and signs. Swelling, throbbing, and continuous pain are the most common symptoms. On examination, erythema or swelling may be seen. However, if the abscess is in the intersphincteric space, there may be no abnormal findings on the external skin. Nevertheless, a digital examination may be impossible because of pain, or a boggy area may be felt over the internal anal sphincter adjacent to the abscess. An ischiorectal abscess may produce pain in the buttock, but no abnormality may be appreciated on examination, because the ischiorectal space is potentially large, and the pus may move upward rather than toward the skin.[37] If the patient cannot be evaluated because the pain is severe or if no abnormality can be found on examination, the patient should undergo an examination under anesthesia. In elusive cases, an intra-anal ultrasound examination under anesthesia may be needed.

Treatment of an abscess in the perineal region requires incision and drainage. *Antibiotics alone are not adequate.* Failure to drain an abscess promptly can result in spread to adjacent spaces and some necrotizing infections, which can be mutilating and life-threatening. Small abscesses can be drained in the office. The external opening should be made as close to the anal sphincter complex as possible without injuring it. Therefore, if a fistula develops, the fistulous tract will be as short as possible. The incision should be large enough or made in a cruciate fashion so that it will not close over before the inflammatory process has resolved. Packing should not be used, but some surgeons prefer to place a small "mushroom" catheter (one end is shaped like a mushroom) into the cavity to facilitate drainage. Large or high abscesses require drainage in the operating room.

It usually is not necessary to culture the pus. Hospitalization and intravenous antibiotics are reserved for patients who are immunocompromised or diabetic or who have signs of systemic infection, such as high fever. Patients should be followed closely to ensure that the process resolves.

Anorectal Fistula-in-Ano

A fistula-in-ano is a tunnel that connects an internal opening with an external opening, usually on the perianal skin. The internal opening usually is at an anal crypt at the base of the columns of Morgagni at the dentate line. A fistulo-in-ano will develop in 50% patients who undergo incision and drainage of an abscess. Goodsall's rule can be used as a guide to find the internal opening of the fistula (Fig. 117–4). The rule states that when an imaginary line is drawn transversely through the center of the anus, external openings anterior to this line follow a radial (straight) path toward the anal canal and the diseased crypt; if the external opening is posterior to this line, the fistulous tract will curve and enter the anal canal in the posterior midline. Exceptions to the rule occur when an anterior opening curves around and is located in the posterior midline. In these cases, the external opening is usually several centimeters from the anal verge. This type of fistula is termed a horseshoe fistula because of its long, curved course. Because of the nature of the spaces around the anus, the fistulous tract can curve around and have an additional external opening anywhere along the tract on the opposite side.

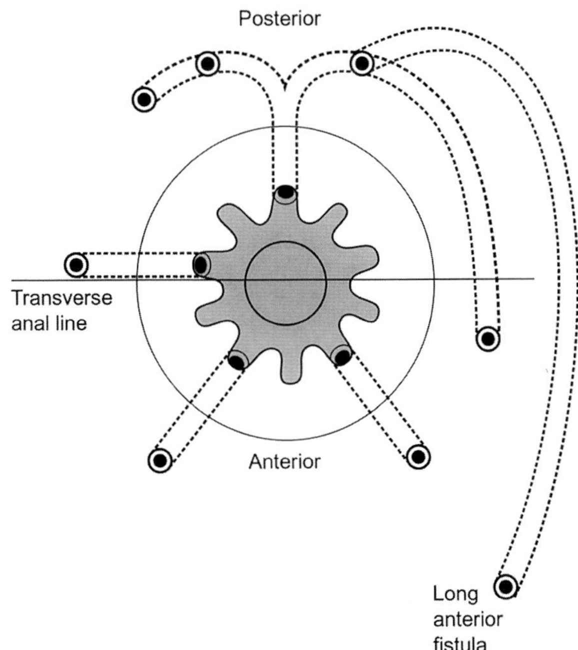

Figure 117–4. Goodsall's rule is a guide to finding the internal opening of a fistula-in-ano based on the location of the external opening and is important for surgical treatment. The rule states that when an imaginary line is drawn transversely through the center of the anus, external openings anterior to this line follow a radial (straight) path toward the anal canal and the diseased crypt. If the external opening is posterior to this line, the fistulous tract will curve and enter the anal canal in the posterior midline. Exceptions to the rule occur when an anterior opening curves around and tracks to the posterior midline. In these cases, the external opening is usually several centimeters from the anal verge.

The diagnosis of a fistula is made by seeing the drainage of blood, pus, and sometimes stool from the external opening. Some patients complain of perianal itching. If the tract seals over, pus may accumulate, and pain may develop. Long tracts can have secondary openings along their course. If the tract is chronic, it can be palpated as a cord under the skin. Pus sometimes may be expressed from the opening when the cord is palpated. Occasionally, anoscopy may reveal the internal opening of the fistula. Remembering Goodsall's rule can help the physician anticipate the probable location of the internal opening.

The differential diagnosis of fistula-in-ano is the same as for anal abscesses.

Treatment consists of surgical intervention. The course of the fistulous tract influences the type of surgical treatment (Fig. 117–5). The most common treatment is a fistulotomy, or unroofing of the tunnel. Fistulotomy must be approached with caution if the tract traverses a substantial portion of the sphincter, in which case division would threaten continence. However, most fistulas can be unroofed and the base curetted and allowed to heal from the bottom up. The cure rate for uncomplicated fistulas not associated with Crohn's disease approaches 100%. Controversy exists as to whether fistulotomy should be done if a tract is found at the time a primary abscess is drained.[38]

A fistula that involves a substantial portion of the anal sphincter requires special treatment to avoid incontinence. Transanal advancement flaps are the most common surgical repair for complex fistulas. Success rates vary from 68% to 75%.[39, 40] Rates of incontinence after a flap repair range from 10% to 35%.[40, 41]

Fibrin adhesive made from autologous blood or commercial fibrin sealant has been used to close anal fistulas. Success rates vary from 60% to 80%.[42, 43] The fistulous tract is aggressively curetted, and the fibrin product is injected via the external opening until it is seen to emerge in the anal canal. Some surgeons prefer to place a suture over the internal opening to seal it off so that the fibrin is not dislodged by stool as the fibrin solidifies. No complications have been reported with this method, and continence is not affected. Re-treatment for failures can be successful. The tract must be at least 1 cm long to allow sufficient length for the fibrin plug to adhere to the tract.

A seton is a rubber band–like material that is threaded through a fistula so that each end is tied loosely on the outside skin. Setons may be used to drain a fistulous tract before surgical repair to prevent the accumulation of pus. However, they can also be therapeutic if used as a cutting seton. With this approach, after the seton is placed, the skin alone (not the sphincter) is incised over the fistulous tract, and the seton is tightened gradually over several weeks so

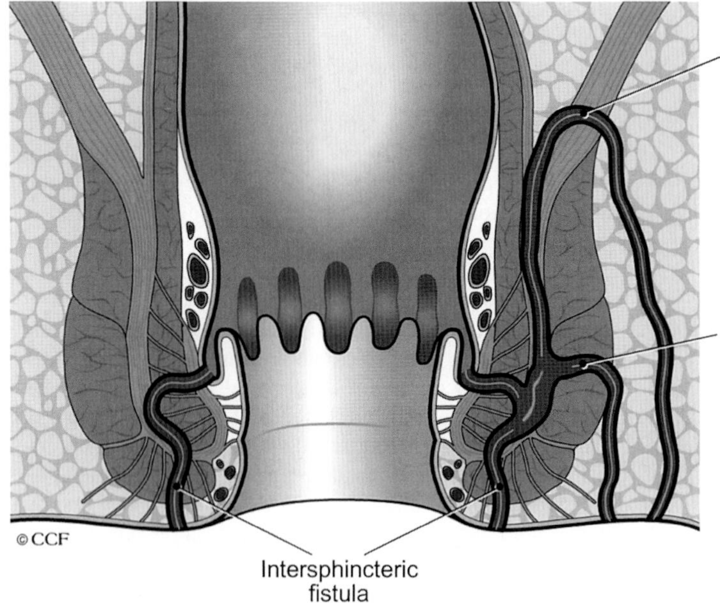

Figure 117–5. Classification of fistulas-in-ano. Fistulotomy is not appropriate for extrasphincteric fistulas because it would leave the patient incontinent. (Reprinted with the permission of The Cleveland Clinic Foundation.)

that it gradually cuts through the muscle. With gradual division of the muscle, the muscle will remain scarred in place and the ends will not spring back as they would when cut during a fistulotomy. This technique allows the fistulous tract to be unroofed gradually as the cut ends of the muscle scar close to their usual location, thereby minimizing the chance of incontinence.

SPECIAL FISTULAS

Several types of fistula deserve special mention. Fistulas due to Crohn's disease are not cryptoglandular in origin but may be related to increased lymphoid tissue in the intersphincteric plane. They do not follow Goodsall's rule and usually are complex, with curved, multiple tracts. Any unusual fistula or nonhealing fistulotomy site should raise the possibility of Crohn's disease. Anal disease may be the first manifestation of Crohn's disease. Anorectal abscesses and suppuration may be less tender in patients with Crohn's disease than in some patients with cryptoglandular fistulas.[44] Treatment is tailored to the overall activity of the Crohn's disease (see Chapter 103). The goal is to improve the patient's quality of life, and curing the Crohn's disease is not realistic nor may healing the fistula be possible. Therefore, before treatment is started, the patient's gastrointestinal tract should be evaluated. In patients with severe colonic or rectal disease, the placement of a loose seton or mushroom catheter in an anal fistula may decrease symptoms; the seton or catheter may be left in indefinitely.[44] Some patients improve simply with the addition of oral metronidazole with or without ciprofloxacin.[45] The immunosuppressant 6-mercaptopurine also has been used with some success. Whether therapy with infliximab, a chimeric antibody to tumor necrosis factor, improves the healing of these difficult fistulas remains to be determined.

Fibrin glue products also have been used to treat fistulas associated with Crohn's disease, but the rate of success is less than that in patients with non-Crohn's fistulas.[42]

Fistulotomy may be done for low fistulas with minimal anorectal involvement.[44] However, persistent nonhealing may be a problem. Advancement flaps have been used successfully to close Crohn's fistulas; there should be minimal anorectal involvement with Crohn's disease when this type of repair is attempted. Despite the array of approaches, some patients have severe perianal sepsis and require fecal diversion with an ileostomy. In many, proctectomy is later required because of persistent discomfort or other problems. In general, surgical repair must be used with caution in anal fistulas in patients with Crohn's disease, and chronic, indwelling, loose setons are preferred to control symptoms of sepsis while preserving anal function.

In women with Crohn's disease, anovaginal fistulas present additional challenges. Traditionally, proctectomy or long-term seton drainage have been the accepted methods of treatment. Most such fistulas are too short to be amenable to fibrin glue. Surgical treatment with various flap repairs has been successful. In one study of 35 women, the initial success rate in selected women was 54%, with 68% healing after multiple flap procedures.[46, 47]

Anovaginal fistulas not associated with Crohn's are also difficult to treat. Almost all are related to obstetric injury, with a few being cryptoglandular in origin. The local tissue is usually scarred and too rigid for successful treatment with advancement flaps. The anovaginal septum is usually very thin. Success is more likely if the sphincter is repaired in conjunction with repair of the fistula to give more tissue bulk to the anovaginal septum.[48]

Fistulas associated with radiation treatment, usually from cervical cancer, are also challenging. The first issue is to exclude recurrent cancer as the cause of the fistula. If the output of stool and gas per vagina is great, a stoma may be needed. A stoma also allows the tissue to soften, so additional treatment options can be evaluated. It may take up to 1 year for the area to become pliable enough for a reasonable attempt at surgical intervention to be undertaken. Repair with a flap can be attempted if the tissue looks normal and is pliable, but this is rarely the case. Resection of the rectum with anastomosis of the healthy colon to the anus at the dentate line can be successful (coloanal anastomosis). Interposition of the gracilis muscle between the wall of the anorectum and vagina brings healthy tissue to the area and can lead to healing.

ANAL CANCER

Anal cancers are infrequent, with an incidence rate of 0.9 per 100,000 population per year.[49] Approximately 3400 new cases were diagnosed in the United States in 2000.[50] The incidence has increased 2% to 3% every year in the U.S. since the early 1980s.[51] Anal cancer occurs with equal frequency in men and women. Almost 80% are squamous cell cancers, 16% are adenocarcinomas, and 4% are other types.[49] Adenocarcinomas of the anal canal behave like adenocarcinomas of the rectum and are treated as such. Patients undergo abdominal-perineal resection with pre- or postoperative chemoradiation therapy when the tumor is large or invasive or lymph nodes are positive for tumor.[52]

The nomenclature of squamous cell carcinoma has been confusing in the past. Tumors arising in the distal anal canal are usually keratinizing squamous cell carcinomas. Those arising in the transitional mucosa frequently are nonkeratinizing squamous cell carcinomas. In the past, the two nonkeratinizing subtypes were referred to as transitional-cell and cloacogenic. These two subtypes now are recognized as variants of squamous cell carcinoma that lack terminal differentiation. One type is composed of large cells, and the other is composed of small cells.[53] The behavior of keratinizing and nonkeratinizing squamous cell cancers is similar. Anal bleeding is the most common symptom (45%), followed by the sensation of a mass (30%) or no symptoms (20%).[53] The development of anal cancer has been associated with infection with human papillomavirus.[53]

ANAL MARGIN CANCERS. Cancers arising distal to the anal verge (anal margin) are considered skin cancers and treated as such. Small lesions (less than 4 cm^2) with no fixation to deeper tissues are excised widely. Treated patients are then followed closely for 5 years. If the disease recurs, chemoradiation therapy is started. Invasive squamous cell cancer of the anal margin is treated with chemoradiation therapy.

ANAL CANAL CANCERS. In the past, standard treatment of anal canal cancers was abdominal-perineal resection with a permanent colostomy. In 1974, Nigro and colleagues presented the results of combined radiation and chemotherapy and showed that cure was possible without abdominal-perineal resection.[54] This led to a regimen of external beam radiation with fluorouracil and mitomycin as the treatment of choice, with surgery reserved for residual cancer seen in the scar after treatment. Recently, cisplatin has been substituted for mitomycin in treatment trials, and complete response rates to combination treatment have been seen in 94% of patients. At a follow-up of 37 months, only 14% of patients required a colostomy for residual or recurrent disease.[53] Further studies are underway to confirm these results.

Patients with persistent or recurrent squamous cell carcinoma of the anal canal are treated with an abdominal-perineal resection. About 50% of patients who undergo surgery can be cured.[53] Success has also been reported with an additional boost of radiation therapy combined with cisplatin-based chemotherapy.[53]

MELANOMA. Melanoma is as deadly in the anal region as elsewhere. The cure rate is poor with any treatment, and many investigators have questioned the use of abdominal-perineal resection for anal melanoma. Most patients have regional or distant metastasis at presentation.[52] Thin lesions (less than 0.3 mm thick) are treated by wide local excision. The choice of treatment for lesions greater that 0.3 mm thick is debatable; either wide local excision or abdominal-perineal resection is considered, but the prognosis with either approach is poor. Inguinal lymph node dissection is reserved for palliation.[49]

BOWEN'S DISEASE. Anal intraepithelial neoplasia, also known as Bowen's disease, is a dysplastic condition of the epithelium of the anal canal and perianal skin. It is speculated that this condition can predispose to cancer, and surgical resection of the dysplastic epithelium has been recommended.[55] It is difficult to determine the extent of disease at surgery and thus difficult to achieve complete resection of the abnormal epithelium. It is also speculated that human papillomavirus is a predisposing factor,[56] and the virus will remain in the "normal" tissue that is not excised. Many authorities recommend that for patients with Bowen's disease (including HIV-positive patients), the best treatment option may be close observation, with regular biopsy of any suspicious areas to exclude invasive malignancy.[55, 57]

PAGET'S DISEASE (EXTRAMAMMARY). This is a rare intraepithelial mucinous adenocarcinoma appearing as an erythematous, eczematoid plaque. It probably arises from the dermal apocrine sweat glands. The disease is more common in women than men and presents as an intractable itch. Diagnosis is by biopsy, and wide local excision is the treatment if invasion is not found. For invasive cancer, abdominal-perineal resection is the treatment of choice.

ANAL WARTS

Anal warts, or condylomata acuminata, are caused by the human papillomavirus. There are over 70 types of papillomavirus, of which 30 types infect the anogenital tract. As stated earlier, it is speculated that most squamous cell cancers of the anal area are caused by this virus.[51] About 1% of sexually active people have anal warts. Condylomata are sexually transmitted, although nonsexual transmission may be possible.[58] Multiple treatment modalities exist (Table 117–3), but even when bulky lesions have resolved, the virus remains.

Podophyllin is a topical agent that is antimitotic. It requires repeated applications.[59] As a single agent, it results in cure rates of 50%.[59, 60] However, podophyllin cannot be used in the anal canal and is poorly absorbed by keratinized lesions, which are characteristic of longstanding warts. The drug can cause skin irritation (severe necrosis and scarring have been reported) and has been teratogenic in animals.

Trichloroacetic and dichloroacetic acid cause sloughing of tissue. These acids must be used with care to control the depth and size of the wound. They can be used in the anal canal. Cure rates of 75% have been reported.[59, 61]

Table 117–3 | **Treatment Options for Anal Warts**

TREATMENT	SUCCESS RATE	COMMENTS
Podophyllin	20%–50%	Repeat applications needed Skin irritation can occur Not used in anal canal Poorly absorbed by keratinized lesions (most chronic warts are keratinized)
Trichloroacetic or dichloroacetic acid	75%	Can be used in anal canal Careful usage required to control the size of slough
Cryotherapy	75%	Can be used in anal canal Careful evaluation required to limit the size of wound created Fumes contain the active virus
Topical 5-fluorouracil	50%–75%	Probably best used after surgical excision to decrease incidence of recurrence
Imiquimod	75% in women, 33% in men	Cannot be used in anal canal Works better in women than men
Surgical excision (usually combined with cautery)	63%–91%	Fumes contain the virus if cautery is used
Intralesional alpha-interferon injection	About 70%	Injected into base of up to five warts three times a week for 3–8 wk

Cryotherapy can be used in the anal canal. The depth and width of the wound must be monitored carefully. Success rates are similar to those associated with trichloroacetic acid.[59, 62]

Topical 5-fluorouracil (5-FU) penetrates the skin and is used in a 5% cream. Success rates have ranged from 50% to 75%. Perhaps the best use of topical 5-FU is its biweekly application after surgical removal of warts to decrease rates of recurrence, as compared with placebo.[59, 63]

Imiquimod cream is an immune response modifier that stimulates monocytes and macrophages to produce cytokines that affect cell growth and have an antiviral effect.[64] The cream is applied to the warts at bedtime three times a week for a total of 16 weeks. Imiquimod cannot be used for anal canal warts. The drug seems to work better for women than men, with one study reporting clearance of warts in 72% of women compared with 33% of men.[65] Few side effects have been reported, although local skin irritation is seen.

Surgical excision and cautery yields the highest success rate. Laser seems to offer no advantage over cautery. Cure rates of 63% to 91% are reported. Disadvantages include the need for local or other forms of anesthesia and the presence of bioactive human papillomavirus in cautery-induced fumes.[59, 66]

Alpha-interferon is approved by the Food and Drug Administration for injectional therapy of refractory condylomata acuminata. The dose is 1×10^6 units injected beneath a maximum of 5 lesions up to three times weekly for 3 to 8 weeks. Recurrence rates are 20% to 40%.[67] Topical interferon cream seems to be no better than placebo.[68]

Combined surgery, to eradicate the largest lesion, and topical or intralesional therapy may decrease recurrence rates.

Anogenital warts may affect immunocompromised patients, including those who are HIV-positive and transplant recipients. In these persons, the warts are more aggressive, recur earlier, and are more often dysplastic than in immunocompetent persons. In HIV-positive patients, dysplasia and histologic evidence of human papillomavirus can occur in the absence of gross warts.[69] Gross warts should be treated as just discussed. Topical 5-FU cream and serial examinations, rather than extensive excision, have been advocated in HIV-positive patients with dysplasia.[69] Excision is reserved for patients with obvious lesions of the skin. Anal cytology (the "anal Pap test") has been considered in this group of patients, but as yet there are no firm recommendations for its use.

Buschke-Löwenstein tumors are a rare variant of anal warts. These lesions appear as giant condylomas that grow rapidly and cause extensive destruction of surrounding tissue and local invasion. Treatment is by surgical excision, if possible. The lesions have also responded to radiation therapy.[70]

PRURITUS ANI

Pruritus ani is an itch localized to the anus and perianal skin. Pruritus ani is categorized as either idiopathic or secondary. Idiopathic pruritus ani is diagnosed when no underlying etiology is found. Secondary pruritus ani results from an underlying disorder, and specific treatment leads to resolution of symptoms. Because pruritus ani is poorly understood and an underlying premalignant lesion such as Bowen's disease or Paget's disease may be the cause of symptoms, all patients with pruritus ani deserve a thorough investigation. In one study, 52% of patients presenting to a colorectal clinic with a complaint of anal itching were found to have anorectal disease (most commonly hemorrhoids and anal fissure).[71] After treatment (both medical and surgical), only 10% of the patients still had symptoms. A further 11% of the patients had rectal cancer, and 6% had anal cancer. The itching resolved with treatment of the underlying cancer. Overall, 89% of patients responded to treatment, whereas 11% were refractory.[71]

Thorough history taking and a physical examination are the starting points for evaluating patients with anal itching. An examination of the rectum and sigmoid colon should be included. The pattern of irritation should be noted. Consideration should be given to a biopsy of any abnormal skin. Usually diet-induced pruritus is symmetrical, whereas infectious causes lead to an asymmetrical pattern of anal irritation. Leakage of stool or mucus because of fecal incontinence and leakage of mucus because of prolapse of the rectum or hemorrhoids can cause irritation and itching. Other causes include contact dermatitis, infections (such as a fungus), parasites, systemic diseases (diabetes mellitus), diet (coffee, cola, chocolate, milk, beer, and others), and some medications. It has been said that dietary factors, especially any form of coffee, may be the most common culprit.[72] Coffee acts as an irritant on the perianal skin.

Any underlying disorder should be treated. However, in many patients a cause of pruritus ani may not be identified. These patients should be advised to modify their habits. Most important is to convince the patient to stop "polishing" his or her anus. Frequently, the patient feels that the anal area is unclean, and he or she rubs the area vigorously, both for comfort and to try to clean the area more completely. Wiping gently with wet facial tissue or baby wipes is recommended. Avoiding soap and a washcloth in the shower may help. The patient should be instructed to use plain water and his or her hand to wash the perineum in the tub or shower. Creams or emulsifying ointments may be used instead of soap.[73] Perfumed soaps and astringents (such as witch hazel) should be avoided. A cotton ball placed by the anus and changed several times a day will absorb moisture and create a drier environment. A diet high in fiber with plenty of fluids (similar to the diet described for hemorrhoids) is recommended. Potential dietary culprits such as coffee, tea, and chocolate should be eliminated during this trial period. A limited amount of 1% hydrocortisone cream can be used. Patients should be warned that chronic use of hydrocortisone will thin the anal skin and may lead to more problems.

Most patients respond to this regimen. Relapse is common and may require re-education of the patient. The physician should be aware that a previously overlooked underlying problem may be the cause of the pruritus and should take a fresh look at a patient who relapses. Assistance from a dermatologist also may be helpful and should be considered initially.[73]

Intradermal injection of methylene blue has been used successfully for the treatment of intractable idiopathic pruritus ani that has not responded to any other measures.[74]

ANAL STENOSIS

Anal stenosis is a narrowing of the anal canal. The condition may develop gradually after anorectal surgery, usually radical hemorrhoidectomy. Surgeons have modified their surgical technique in an attempt to prevent this problem in the modern era. Other causes include chronic anal fissure, inflammatory bowel disease (especially Crohn's disease), cancer, irradiation,[75] chronic diarrheal disease, habitual use of laxatives (especially mineral oil), and infections (tuberculosis, lymphogranuloma venereum, syphilis, and others).

The treatment of anal stenosis depends on the degree of stenosis and associated symptoms. In mild stenosis, the examiner's finger can be placed just through the narrowing. Patients are placed on a high-fiber diet and bulking agents to produce stools that pass more easily. Additionally, the bulky stools provide natural dilatation. Gradual dilatation by the patient (usually daily in the shower) with a commercial medical dilator or a smooth white candle also can produce improvement.[76]

In moderate stenosis, more force is required to insert the index finger. Patients may respond to dietary changes and graded dilatations. The initial dilatation may need to be done under anesthesia. If improvement is insufficient, surgery is indicated. Release of a stricture or a sphincterotomy may suffice. However, some patients may require an advancement flap.[76]

In severe stenosis, even the tip of the examiner's fifth finger cannot be inserted into the anal canal. There is loss of the anoderm, and surgical intervention is needed to deliver healthy tissue into the anal canal to compensate for this loss. Various advancement flaps are successful, and the type used depends on the patient's anatomy and the surgeon's preference.[76]

UNEXPLAINED ANAL PAIN

Unexplained anal pain refers to pain in the anorectal region in the absence of an underlying anatomic abnormality. The diagnosis is based almost entirely on the patient's symptoms. Confusing nomenclature has further confused the issue.

Coccygodynia is a cramp or ache in the tailbone and typically results from trauma to the coccyx or arthritis. Movement of the coccyx can reproduce the pain. Treatment in the acute setting includes sitz baths, NSAIDs, and stool softeners.[77] Glucocorticoid injections have been used in an attempt to reduce the pain. Rarely, removal of the coccyx is necessary.[78]

Levator ani syndrome and proctalgia fugax are probably not the same entity. However, in the literature, the terms are often used interchangeably (incorrectly).

Levator ani syndrome seems to affect women less than 45 years of age. The episodes of pain are chronic or recurring and occur during 12 weeks in the preceding year, with each episode lasting 20 minutes or more.[79] The discomfort is described as a vague tenderness or aching sensation high in the rectum. It usually does not awaken the patient from sleep. The pain usually is worse after defecation and with sitting; walking or lying down seems to relieve the pain.[80] The symptoms have been attributed to spasm of the levator muscles. The physical examination may be normal, or the levator muscle may feel like a tight, tender band.[77]

Proctalgia fugax seems to occur in young men and "perfectionists." It is seen in early adulthood and subsides by middle age. The pain lasts seconds or minutes and then disappears. The pain is described as a sharp cramp or stabbing pain and may awaken the patient from sleep.[79, 80] The pathogenesis is thought to involve anal smooth muscle dysfunction.[80] Stressful events may trigger the pain. The frequency of proctalgia fugax may be increased in patients with other functional gastrointestinal complaints, such as unexplained abdominal pain, bloating, irritable bowel syndrome, and a sensation of incomplete evacuation. Physical examination is normal.[77, 79, 80]

Treatment of the levator ani syndrome and proctalgia fugax is controversial, and no single treatment works for all patients. Treatments for these disorders are grouped together, in part because of our incomplete understanding of the two conditions. Initial treatment is reassurance, sitz baths, perineal strengthening exercises, and regulation of bowel habits. These measures are usually effective.[77] Many other treatments have been proposed, including electrogalvanic stimulation,[81] levator massage, biofeedback,[82] drug therapies, acupuncture, and psychiatric evaluation.

In the past, the drug treatment of choice was a benzodiaz-

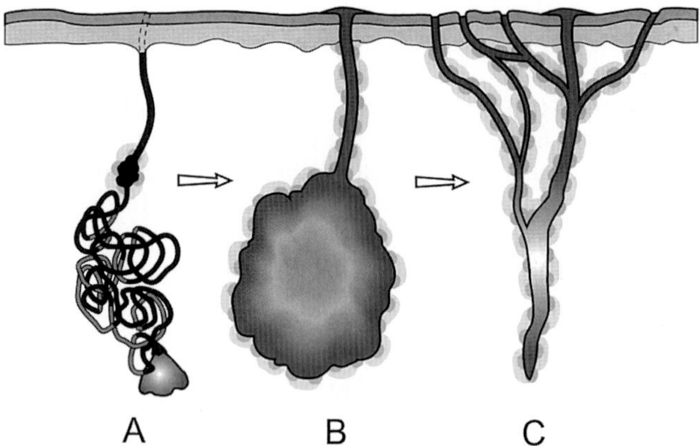

Figure 117–6. Hidradenitis suppurativa, an inflammatory disease of the apocrine sweat glands and adjacent connective tissue. *A,* The initiating event is occlusion of the apocrine duct by a keratinous plug. *B,* Bacteria are trapped beneath the keratinous plug and multiply to form an abscess, which can rupture into adjacent tissue. *C,* The end result is recurrent abscesses, chronic draining sinuses, and indurated scarred skin and subcutaneous tissues. Frequently, multiple tracts are interconnected and lead to the skin.

epine. However, because of their addictive potential and the chronic nature of these problems, the popularity of these drugs has declined. In the only randomized controlled trial for proctalgia fugax, a salbutamol inhaler was used successfully.[83] Two puffs at the onset of pain were reported to lead to rapid relief.

Clonidine, an α_2 agonist, relaxes smooth muscle and has been used successfully.[84] The dose is 150 μg twice daily for 3 days, tapered to 75 μg twice daily for 2 days, and then 75 μg daily for 2 days.

Diltiazem, a calcium antagonist, relaxes smooth muscle and also has been effective in a dose of 80 mg twice daily.[85]

Topical nitroglycerin, 0.2% or 0.3%, used at the onset of proctalgia fugax also has been used successfully.[86]

HIDRADENITIS SUPPURATIVA

Hidradenitis suppurativa is an inflammatory disease of the apocrine sweat glands and adjacent connective tissue. The initiating event is occlusion of the apocrine duct by a keratinous plug, leading in turn to ductal dilation and stasis. Secondary bacterial infection ensues. The infection can rupture into the surrounding soft tissue (Fig. 117–6). The chronic, cyclic nature of the disease ultimately leads to fibrosis and hypertrophic scarring of the skin. Commonly involved bacteria include *Streptococcus milleri, Staphylococcus aureus,* anaerobic streptococci, *Bacteroides* species,[87] *Escherichia coli, Klebsiella,* and *Proteus.*[88] The axilla is the most common site of disease, followed by the anogenital region. Clinical features include recurrent abscesses, chronic draining sinuses, and indurated, scarred skin and subcutaneous tissues. The spectrum of severity ranges from mild disease with spontaneous regression to severe involvement at multiple sites. Coexistent Crohn's disease occurs more frequently than expected, with a frequency of nearly 40% in one study.[89]

The diagnosis is based on the clinical presentation. Early symptoms include itching and erythema. Later, a firm, pea-sized nodule may be detected and may rupture spontaneously. The lesion heals with fibrosis but may recur adjacent to the original area. Over time, multiple abscesses and sinus tracts develop in the subcutaneous region to form a honeycomb-like pattern.[88] Discharge from the open areas may be serous or purulent.

Treatment consists initially of antibiotics active against *Staphylococcus.* Oral isotretinoin has been used successfully in mild cases.[90] Intralesional glucocorticoids, antiandrogen therapy,[88] and topical clindamycin[91] also have been used. Surgery is required for chronic disease. Apparent "cure" can be achieved by extensive excision of the involved area down to the soft tissue with wide margins. The area is then closed with a skin graft or left to granulate.[92] However, new lesions can develop in untreated skin and close follow-up is needed.

PILONIDAL DISEASE

Pilonidal disease is an acquired problem that affects young adults after puberty. It occurs in the intergluteal cleft and may be confused with fistula-in-ano. The prevailing theory of pathogenesis is that hair in the cleft, along with desquamated epithelium, is propelled into the base of the cleft, where the barbs of hair shafts prevent them from being expelled, thereby setting up a granulomatous reaction, which creates a sinus.[93] With movement, the buttocks exert a drilling effect on the hair, further driving them into the sinus. Further suppuration and abscess formation occur, with occlusion of the sinus by the accumulation of hair and debris. The unique hair distribution in affected persons is thought to play a role in the pathogenesis.[93] Free hair is found in the cyst or abscess cavity and also may be seen protruding from pits in the intergluteal deft. Symptoms may result from an acute abscess, chronic cyst, or draining sinuses. The diagnosis is made by identifying the abscess, which is characteristically several centimeters cephalad to the anus, or tiny openings in the intergluteal cleft over the sacrum (Fig. 117–7).

In mild cases, successful treatment has been achieved simply by shaving the hair on a regular basis (usually monthly) to prevent the hair from embedding in the intergluteal cleft. Any abscess requires immediate drainage. In pa-

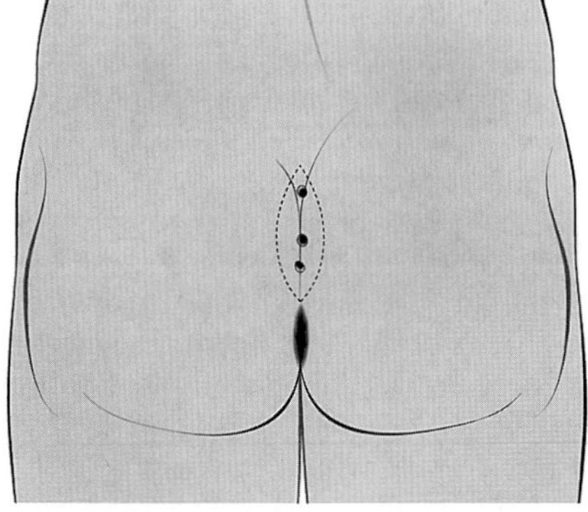
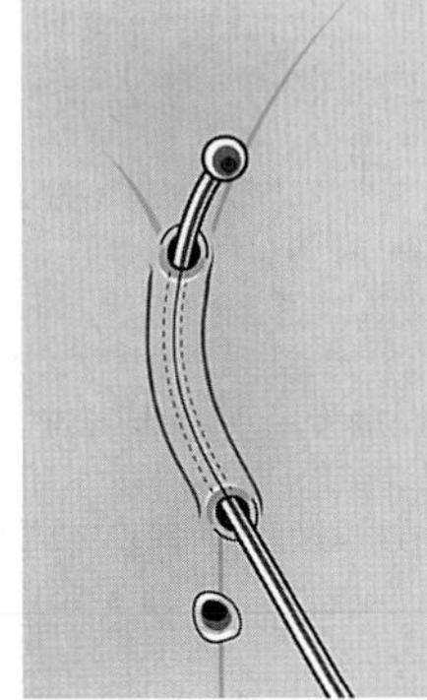

Figure 117–7. Pilonidal disease. On examination, there may be multiple pits or external openings in the intergluteal cleft proximal to the anus, as seen on the left. The openings frequently communicate with each other, as shown on the right. A probe can be passed between this network of tracts that communicate. One successful treatment option is to unroof all the tracts.

tients with chronic disease, more extensive surgical treatment is needed. This usually consists of unroofing all sinus tracts with marsupialization; excision of the area with or without closure of the skin edges; or creation of advancement flaps, musculocutaneous flaps, or some variant of these.[93–95] Afterwards, it is still necessary to shave the surrounding hair periodically to prevent recurrence. As with any other chronic draining fistula or sinus, squamous cell carcinoma may arise with longstanding disease.[96]

RECTAL FOREIGN BODY

Most foreign bodies in the rectum are not the result of oral ingestion. However, accidental ingestion of a toothpick or a fishbone may present as an abscess in the wall of the rectum or anus. More commonly, foreign bodies are placed into the rectum via the anus. Treatment (removal) often requires skill, trial and error, and luck to avoid a laparotomy. Most rectal foreign bodies are iatrogenic and result from sexual (erotic) stimulation or criminal assault. The history obtained from the patient is notoriously unreliable[97] as to what exactly the object is and how it was placed. If the patient indicates that the object was placed as a result of sexual assault, a full sexual assault examination is needed, including perianal brushings and sampling for sperm.[98] An abdominal radiograph is useful to determine the size and location of the foreign body. If free air is seen, a laparotomy is almost unavoidable.

To remove the object, relaxation and sedation are needed. If removal cannot be accomplished in the office or emergency room with local anesthesia, the patient should be taken to the operating room for regional or general anesthesia. An important principle in removing the object via the anus is that the rectum exerts a traction vacuum effect on the foreign body. Therefore, passage of a well-lubricated Foley catheter will break the air seal and aid in removal of the object. Imagination is needed at times to remove the object via the anus. Obstetric forceps and an obstetric vacuum extractor have been used with success.[99] When a vacuum extractor is used, it is important to make sure that no rectal mucosa becomes trapped in the extractor. Another innovative approach is to put plaster of Paris into the foreign body (if it is a hollow object) and place a string into the plaster of Paris. The entire concoction is allowed to harden, and the string is pulled out with the foreign body.[98] Having the patient in the lithotomy position allows pressure to be applied simultaneously over the lower abdomen to facilitate expulsion of the foreign body. After any foreign body has been removed from the anus, sigmoidoscopic examination is needed to rule out a perforation. If the sigmoidoscopic examination is negative, a water-soluble contrast enema study should be done as well to exclude a perforation, even if the foreign body does not look capable of causing injury.[100] The object that was used to place the foreign body in the rectum may have perforated the bowel.[100]

Laparotomy is reserved for cases of colonic perforation and objects that cannot be removed otherwise. After opening the abdomen, attempts still should be made to milk the object distally and expel it via the anus, by means of intra-abdominal manipulation. If this approach fails, a colotomy is done to retrieve the object. In many instances, simple closure of the colotomy is risky because of trauma from the attempts at removal and the additional trauma caused by the grinding of the object against the rectal wall. In these situations, a colostomy may be needed. Following removal of the object via laparotomy, other perforations that may have occurred when the object was inserted still must be excluded.

REFERENCES

1. Keighley MRB, Williams NS: Surgical anatomy. In Surgery of the Anus, Rectum and Colon, 2nd ed. Philadelphia, WB Saunders, 1997, p 7.
2. Godlewski G, Prudhomme M: Embryology and anatomy of the anorectum. Surg Clin North Am 80:319, 2000.
3. Jorge JMN, Wexner SD: Anatomy and physiology of the rectum and anus. Eur J Surg 163:723, 1997.
4. American Gastroenterological Association Medical Position Statement on Anorectal Testing Techniques. Gastroenterology 116:732, 1999.
5. DiSario JA, Sanowski RA: Sigmoidoscopy training for nurses and resident physicians. Gastrointest Endosc 39:29, 1993.
6. Orkin B, Young H: When are "hemorrhoids" really hemorrhoids? A prospective study. Dis Colon Rectum 43:A35, 2000.
7. Cirocco WC: A matter of semantics: Hemorrhoids are a normal part of human anatomy and differ from hemorrhoidal disease. Gastrointest Endosc 51:772, 2000.
8. Mazier WP: Hemorrhoids, fissures, and pruritus ani. Surg Clin North Am 74:1277, 1994.
9. Nelson RL, Abcarian H, Davis FG, et al: Prevalence of benign anorectal disease in a randomly selected population. Dis Colon Rectum 38:341, 1995.
10. Metcalf A: Anorectal disorders. Postgrad Med 98:81, 1995.
11. Pfenninger JL, Surrell J: Nonsurgical treatment options for internal hemorrhoids. Am Family Phys 52:821, 1995.
12. Orkin BA, Schwartz AM, Orkin M: Hemorrhoids: What the dermatologist should know. J Am Acad Dermatol 41:449, 1999.
13. Kaman L, Aggarwal S, Kumar R, et al: Necrotizing fasciitis after injection sclerotherapy for hemorrhoids. Dis Colon Rectum 42:419, 1999.
14. Barwell J, Watkins RM, Lloyd-Davies E, Wilkins DC: Life-threatening retroperitoneal sepsis after hemorrhoid injection sclerotherapy. Dis Colon Rectum 42:421, 1999.
15. MacRae HM, McLeod RS: Comparison of hemorrhoidal treatment modalities. A meta-analysis. Dis Colon Rectum 38:687, 1995.
16. Law W-L, Chu K-W: Triple rubber band ligation for hemorrhoids: Prospective, randomized trial of use of local anesthetic injection. Dis Colon Rectum 42:363, 1999.
17. Smith LE, Goodreau JJ, Fouty WJ: Operative hemorrhoidectomy versus cryodestruction. Dis Colon Rectum 22:10, 1979.
18. Loder PB, Kamm MA, Nicholls RJ, Phillips RKS: Haemorrhoids: Pathology, pathophysiology and aetiology. Br J Surg 81:946, 1994.
19. Konsten J, Baeten CGMI: Hemorrhoidectomy vs. Lord's method: 17-year follow-up of a prospective, randomized trial. Dis Colon Rectum 43:503, 2000.
20. Arbman G, Krook H, Haapaniemi S: Closed vs. open hemorrhoidectomy—is there any difference? Dis Colon Rectum 43:31, 2000.
21. Mehigan BJ, Monson JRT, Hartley JE: Stapling procedure for haemorrhoids versus Milligan-Morgan haemorrhoidectomy: Randomised controlled trial. Lancet 355:782, 2000.
22. Moore B, Fleshner P: Rubber band ligation for hemorrhoidal disease can be safely performed in select HIV-positive patients. Dis Colon Rectum 43:A32, 2000.
23. Schouten WR, Briel JW, Auwerda JJA, Boerma MO: Anal fissure: new concepts in pathogenesis and treatment. Scand J Gastroenterol 31 Suppl 218:78, 1996.
24. Schouten WR, Briel JW, Auwerda JJA, De Graaf EJR: Ischaemic nature of anal fissure. Br J Surg 83:63, 1996.
25. Lund JN, Scholefield JH: Aetiology and treatment of anal fissure. Br J Surg 83:1335, 1996.
26. Carapeti EA, Kamm MA, McDonald PJ, et al: Randomised controlled trial shows that glyceryl trinitrate heals anal fissures, higher doses are not more effective, and there is a high recurrence rate. Gut 44:727, 1999.

27. Madalinski MH: Nonsurgical treatment modalities for chronic anal fissure using botulinum toxin. Gastroenterology 117:516, 1999.
28. Maria G, Cassetta E, Gui D, et al: A comparison of botulinum toxin and saline for the treatment of chronic anal fissure. N Engl J Med 338:217, 1998.
29. Brisinda G, Maria G, Bentivoglio AR, et al: A comparison of injections of botulinum toxin and topical nitroglycerin ointment for the treatment of chronic anal fissure. N Engl J Med 341:65, 1999.
30. Maria G, Brisinda G, Bentivoglio AR, et al: Botulinum toxin injections in the internal anal sphincter for the treatment of chronic anal fissure. Long-term results after two different dosage regimens. Ann Surg 228:664, 1998.
31. Maria G, Brisinda G, Bentivoglio AR, et al: Influence of botulinum toxin site of injections on healing rate in patients with chronic anal fissure. Am J Surg 179:46, 2000.
32. Kaiser AM: Letter to the editor. N Engl J Med 341:1701, 1999.
33. Cook TA, Humphreys MMS, Mortensen NJM: Oral nifedipine reduces resting anal pressure and heals chronic anal fissure. Br J Surg 86: 1269, 1999.
34. Argov S, Levandovsky O: Open lateral sphincterotomy is still the best treatment for chronic anal fissure. Am J Surg 179:201, 2000.
35. Corby H, Donnelly VS, O'Herlihy C, O'Connell PR: Anal canal pressures are low in women with postpartum anal fissure. Br J Surg 84:86, 1997.
36. Nyam DCNK, Wilson RG, Stewart AJ, et al: Island advancement flaps in the management of anal fissures. Br J Surg 82:326, 1995.
37. Janicke DM, Pundt MR: Anorectal disorders. Emerg Med Clin North Am 14:757, 1996.
38. Cox SW, Senagore AJ, Luchtefeld MA, et al: Outcome after incision and drainage with fistulotomy for ischiorectal abscess. Am Surg 63: 686, 1997.
39. Ozuner G, Hull TL, Cartmill J, Fazio VW: Long-term analysis of the use of transanal rectal advancement flaps for complicated anorectal/vaginal fistulas. Dis Colon Rectum 39:10, 1996.
40. Schouten WR, Zimmerman DDE, Briel JW: Transanal advancement flap repair of transsphincteric fistulas. Dis Colon Rectum 42:1419, 1999.
41. Golub RW, Wise WM Jr, Kerner BA, et al: Endorectal mucosal advancement flap: The preferred method for complex cryptoglandular fistula-in-ano. J Gastrointest Surg 1:487, 1997.
42. Cintron JR, Park JJ, Orsay CP, et al: Repair of fistulas-in-ano using autologous fibrin tissue adhesive. Dis Colon Rectum 42:607, 1999.
43. Venkatesh KS, Ramanujam P: Fibrin glue application in the treatment of recurrent anorectal fistulas. Dis Colon Rectum 42:1136, 1999.
44. Sangwan YP, Schoetz DJ Jr, Murray JJ, et al: Perianal Crohn's disease. Dis Colon Rectum 39:529, 1996.
45. Solomon MJ, McLeod RS, O'Connor BI, et al: Combination ciprofloxacin and metronidazole in severe perianal Crohn's disease. Can J Gastroenterol 7:571, 1993.
46. Hull TL, Fazio VW: Surgical approaches to low anovaginal fistula in Crohn's disease. Am J Surg 173:95, 1997.
47. Hull TL, Fazio VW: Rectovaginal fistula in Crohn's disease. In Phillips RKS, Lunniss PJ (eds): Anal Fistula: Surgical Evaluation and Management. London, Chapman and Hall Medical, 1996, p 143.
48. Tsang CBS, Madoff RD, Wong WD, et al: Anal sphincter integrity and function influences outcome in rectovaginal fistula repair. Dis Colon Rectum 41:1141, 1998.
49. Spratt JS: Cancer of the anus. J Surg Oncol 74:173, 2000.
50. Greenlee RT, Murray T, Bolden S, et al: Cancer statistics. CA Cancer J Clin 50:7, 2000.
51. Franco EL: Epidemiology of anogenital warts and cancer. Obstet Gynecol Clin North Am 23:597, 1996.
52. Klas JV, Rothenberger DA, Wong WD, Madoff RD: Malignant tumors of the anal canal: The spectrum of disease, treatment, and outcomes. Cancer 85:1686, 1999.
53. Ryan DP, Compton CC, Mayer RJ: Carcinoma of the anal canal. N Engl J Med 342:792, 2000.
54. Nigro ND, Vaitkevicius VK, Considine B Jr: Combined therapy for cancer of the anal canal: A preliminary report. Dis Colon Rectum 17: 354, 1974.
55. Brown SR, Skinner P, Tidy J, et al: Outcome after surgical resection for high-grade anal intraepithelial neoplasia (Bowen's disease). Br J Surg 86:1063, 1999.
56. Sarmiento JM, Wolff BG, Burgart LJ, et al: Perianal Bowen's disease: Associated tumors, human papillomavirus, surgery, and other controversies. Dis Colon Rectum 40:912, 1997.
57. Cleary RK, Schaldenbrand JD, Fowler JJ, et al: Perianal Bowen's disease and anal intraepithelial neoplasia. Dis Colon Rectum 42:945, 1999.
58. Wikstrom A: Clinical and serological manifestations of genital human papillomavirus infection. Acta Derm Venereol Suppl (Stockh) 193:1, 1995.
59. Congilosi SM, Madoff RD: Current therapy for current and extensive anal warts. Dis Colon Rectum 38:1101, 1995.
60. Greene I: Therapy for genital warts. Dermatol Clin 10:253, 1992.
61. Swerdlow DB, Salvati EP: Condyloma acuminatum. Dis Colon Rectum 14:226, 1971.
62. Godley MJ, Bradbeer CS, Gellan M, Thin RN: Cryotherapy compared with trichloroacetic acid in treating genital warts. Genitourin Med 63: 390, 1987.
63. Krebs HB: Treatment of genital condylomata with topical 5-fluorouracil. Dermatol Clin 9:333, 1991.
64. Miller R, Birmachu E, Gerster J, et al: Imiquimod: Cytokine induction and antiviral activity. Int Antiviral News 3:111, 1995.
65. Schneider A, Sawada E, Gissmann L, Shah K: Human papillomaviruses in women with a history of abnormal Papanicolaou smears and their male partners. Obstet Gynecol 69:554, 1987.
66. King AR: Genital warts—therapy. Semin Dermatol 11:247, 1992.
67. Browder JF, Araujo OE, Myer NA, Flowers FP: The interferons and their use in condyloma acuminata. Ann Pharmacother 26:42, 1992.
68. Kraus SJ, Stone KM: Management of genital infection caused by human papillomavirus. Rev Infect Dis 12:S620, 1990.
69. Karamanoukian R, DeLaRosa J, Cosman B, et al: Conservative management of anal squamous dysplasia in patients with human immunodeficiency virus. Dis Colon Rectum 43:A5, 2000.
70. Sobrado CW, Mester M, Nadalin W, et al: Radiation-induced total regression of a highly recurrent giant perianal condyloma: Report of a case. Dis Colon Rectum 43:257, 2000.
71. Daniel GL, Longo WE, Vernava AM III: Pruritus ani: Causes and concerns. Dis Colon Rectum 37:670, 1994.
72. Friend WG: Pruritus ani. In Fazio VW (ed): Current Therapy in Colon and Rectal Surgery. Toronto, BC Decker, 1990, p 42.
73. Dasan S, Neill SM, Donaldson DR, Scott HJ: Treatment of persistent pruritus ani in a combined colorectal and dermatological clinic. Br J Surg 86:1337, 1999.
74. Farouk R, Lee PWR: Intradermal methylene blue injection for the treatment of intractable idiopathic pruritus ani. Br J Surg 84:670, 1997.
75. Aitola PT, Hiltunen K-M, Matikainen MJ: Y-V anoplasty combined with internal sphincterotomy for stenosis of the anal canal. Eur J Surg 163:839, 1997.
76. Liberman H, Thorson AG: Anal stenosis. Am J Surg 179:325, 2000.
77. Hull TL, Milsom JW: Pelvic floor disorders. Surg Clin North Am 74: 1399, 1994.
78. Wesselmann U, Burnett AL, Heinberg LJ: The urogenital and rectal pain syndromes. Pain 73:269, 1997.
79. Whitehead WE, Diamant E, Enck P, et al: Functional disorders of the anus and rectum. Gut 45(Suppl II):II-55, 1999.
80. Vincent C: Anorectal pain and irritation: Anal fissure, levator syndrome, proctalgia fugax, and pruritis ani. Prim Care 26:53, 1999.
81. Hull TL, Milsom JW, Church J, et al: Electrogalvanic stimulation for levator syndrome: How effective is it in the long term? Dis Colon Rectum 36:731, 1993.
82. Gilliland R, Heymen JS, Altomare DF, et al: Biofeedback for intractable rectal pain: Outcome and predictors of success. Dis Colon Rectum 40:190, 1997.
83. Eckardt VF, Dodt O, Kanzler G, Bernhard G: Treatment of proctalgia fugax with salbutamol inhalation. Am J Gastroenterol 91:686, 1996.
84. Swain R: Oral clonidine for proctalgia fugax. Gut 28:1039, 1987.
85. Boquet J: Diltiazem for proctalgia fugax. Lancet 8496:1493, 1986.
86. Lowenstein B, Cataldo PA: Treatment of proctalgia fugax with topical nitroglycerin: Report of a case. Dis Colon Rectum 41:667, 1998.
87. Parks RW, Parks TG: Pathogenesis, clinical features and management of hidradenitis suppurativa. Ann Royal Coll Surg Engl 79:83, 1997.
88. Brown TJ, Rosen T, Orengo IF: Hidradenitis suppurativa. South Med J 91:1107, 1998.
89. Church JM, Fazio VW, Lavery IC, et al: The differential diagnosis and comorbidity of hidradenitis suppurativa and perianal Crohn's disease. Int J Colorectal Dis 8:117, 1993.
90. Boer J, van Gemert MJP: Long-term results of isotretinoin in the treatment of 68 patients with hidradenitis suppurativa. J Am Acad Dermatol 40:73, 1999.

91. Jemec GBE, Wendelboe P: Topical clindamycin versus systemic tetracycline in the treatment of hidradenitis suppurativa. J Am Acad Dermatol 39:971, 1998.
92. Endo Y, Tamura A, Ishikawa O, Miyachi Y: Perianal hidradenitis suppurativa: Early surgical treatment gives good results in chronic or recurrent cases. Br J Dermatol 139:906, 1998.
93. Schoeller T, Wechselberger G, Otto A, Papp C: Definite surgical treatment of complicated recurrent pilonidal disease with a modified fasciocutaneous V-Y advancement flap. Surgery 121:258, 1997.
94. Spivak H, Brooks VL, Nussbaum M, Friedman I: Treatment of chronic pilonidal disease. Dis Colon Rectum 39:1136, 1996.
95. Rosen W, Davidson JSD: Gluteus maximus musculocutaneous flap for the treatment of recalcitrant pilonidal disease. Ann Plast Surg 37:293, 1996.
96. Abboud B, Ingea H: Recurrent squamous-cell carcinoma arising in sacrococcygeal pilonidal sinus tract: Report of a case and review of the literature. Dis Colon Rectum 42:525, 1999.
97. Mackinnon RPG: Removing rectal foreign bodies: Is the ventouse gender-specific [letter]? Med J Aust 169:670, 1998.
98. Fry RD: Anorectal trauma and foreign bodies. Surg Clin North Am 74:1491, 1994.
99. Johnson SO, Hartranft TH: Nonsurgical removal of a rectal foreign body using a vacuum extractor: Report of a case. Dis Colon Rectum 39:935, 1996.
100. Losanoff JE, Kjossev KT: Rectal "oven mitt:" the importance of considering a serious underlying injury. J Emerg Med 17:31, 1999.

Chapter 118

OTHER DISEASES OF THE COLON AND RECTUM

David Blumberg and Arnold Wald

RECTAL PROLAPSE

Etiology

Rectal prolapse, or procidentia, is a medical condition that is often misdiagnosed as prolapsed hemorrhoids. It is distinguished by its classic appearance of concentric radial folds and represents an intussusception of the rectum through the anal canal (Fig. 118–1). The extent of the prolapse may vary from involvement of the rectal mucosa only to involvement of the full thickness of the rectum and sigmoid colon. A number of pathophysiologic processes have been proposed to explain rectal prolapse. Regardless of etiology, common mechanisms include increased abdominal pressure, a traction effect of the intussusception, or decreased pelvic and perineal support of the rectum. Etiologies include chronic constipation, a colonic tumor, and a redundant sigmoid colon. A redundant sigmoid colon is present in many patients, but it is unclear whether the redundancy is the result of constipation or cause of prolapse. Lack of fixation of the rectum to the sacrum, a diastasis of the levator muscles, and a patulous anus also are seen in many patients with rectal prolapse and may be causes of this disorder. Rectal prolapse is often associated with prolapse of other pelvic organs such as the bladder and uterus, further implicating weakness in the pelvic floor as an etiology of prolapse. Neurologic diseases such as cauda equina syndrome and spinal cord lesions may lead to denervation of the pelvic floor with attendant pelvic floor weakness that results in prolapse. Schistosomiasis has been reported to be a common cause of rectal prolapse that affects young men in Egypt. Affected persons have reduced pelvic floor muscle mass and a shorter functional anal canal length during squeeze. Biopsies have revealed degenerative changes, with distortion of muscle fibers and deposition of immune complexes in the sarcolemmal membrane, blood vessels, and septa, suggesting an immunologic type of myopathy. Other unusual etiologies include prolapse associated with Marfan syndrome and Ehlers-Danlos syndrome.[1]

Clinical Features and Diagnosis

Patients with rectal prolapse commonly are elderly women, many of whom are nulliparous. They may be asymptomatic or present with rectal bleeding, a mass, pain, anal pruritus, constipation, or incontinence. Other rare but dramatic presentations include a gangrenous prolapse from incarceration and transanal evisceration of the small intestine through a defect in the wall of the prolapse.[2]

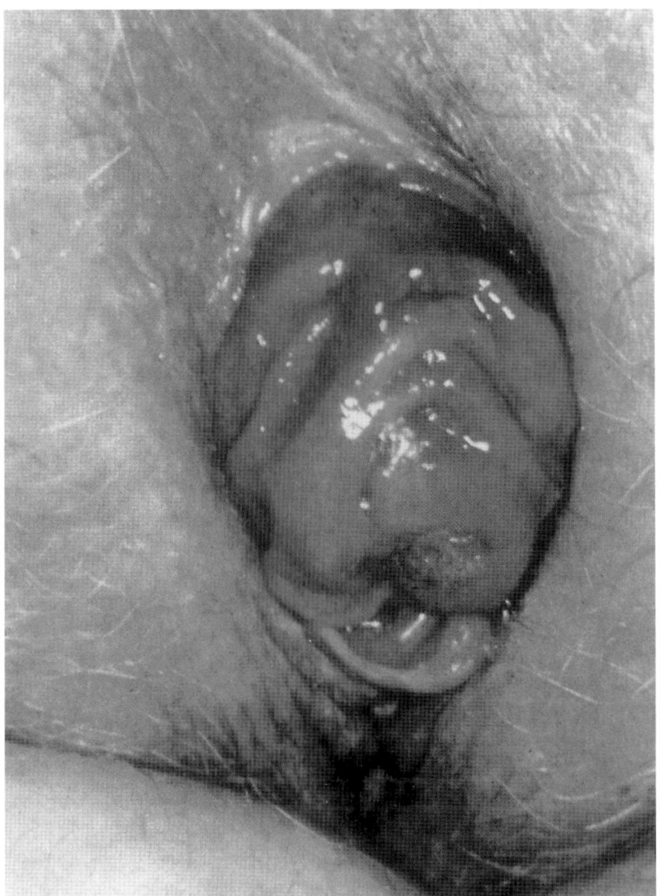

Figure 118–1. Gross appearance of rectal prolapse with protrusion of all layers of the rectum through the anus.

Demonstrating the prolapse is aided by having the patient strain while in a sitting position on a toilet. Digital rectal examination provides an assessment of anal sphincter tone and voluntary muscle contraction. Anoscopy is important in differentiating prolapse from internal hemorrhoids and anorectal tumors. Endoscopic examination of the colon is performed routinely to exclude an associated colorectal neoplasm. In one study, patients with rectal prolapse had a 5.7% frequency of associated colorectal cancer.[3] A complete pelvic floor examination is important because women may have multiple pelvic organ prolapse: bladder (cystocele), uterus (hysterocele), or rectum.[4]

Assessment of pudendal nerve terminal motor latency may be useful in predicting whether incontinence will improve with surgery.[5] The pudendal nerve may be injured from chronic traction by a rectal prolapse. With significant injury, denervation of the external sphincter muscle may occur and incontinence may persist even after repair of the rectal prolapse. Defecography may reveal an occult prolapse (Fig. 118–2) not seen on routine examination.[6] The defecogram is performed by administering a barium paste enema to the patient, which the patient evacuates under fluoroscopy. The defecogram also can determine whether the prolapse is contributing to obstruction of defecation, which will be visualized radiographically as incomplete evacuation of rectal contrast.

Treatment

Although correction of constipation and various perineal support devices may provide some relief for patients with rectal prolapse, surgery is the mainstay of therapy. Because of the varied proposed etiologies for this disorder, it is not surprising that there are over 50 different operations to repair rectal prolapse. In general, surgery for rectal prolapse is performed by either a transabdominal or a perineal approach. Transabdominal procedures are generally associated with the lowest recurrence rates but have the potential for greatest morbidity. Selection of the optimal procedure for a patient with rectal prolapse must take into account the morbidity and recurrence rate of the procedure and the patient's performance status. A transabdominal procedure is usually selected for younger patients who can tolerate more extensive surgery and who may benefit from a more durable procedure, whereas a perineal approach is best suited for frail and elderly patients.

The more common transabdominal approaches are anterior resection, rectopexy, and anterior resection with rectopexy. Anterior resection involves removal of the redundant rectosigmoid and may allow fixation of the rectum to the sacrum by formation of adhesions. Recurrence rates for anterior resection range from 7.3% to 8.9%.[7, 8] Serious postoperative complications are uncommon and include anastomotic leak, small bowel obstruction, ureteral injury, and pelvic bleeding. Rectopexy re-establishes fixation of the rectum to the sacrum and may be performed with direct suturing[9] or with Teflon, Marlex, or Vicryl mesh.[10] Recurrence rates after rectopexy are low, ranging from 3.7% to 9.6%. Unique and significant postoperative complications to this approach include mesh infection, rectal stricture, and rare intervertebral infections.[11–13] In a recent series examining 112 patients undergoing Ripstein rectopexy, in which the rectum is fixed to the sacrum with mesh, severe complications included 1 large bowel obstruction, 1 lethal fecaloma, and 2 rectovaginal fistulas caused by mesh erosion.[13] Combining rectosigmoid resection with rectopexy has been reported to result in the lowest recurrence rates, with only 2 of 102 patients experiencing recurrent prolapse in one series.[14] Of the ab-

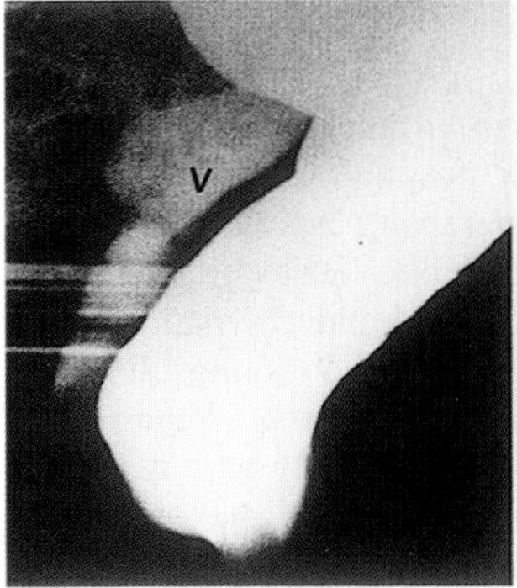

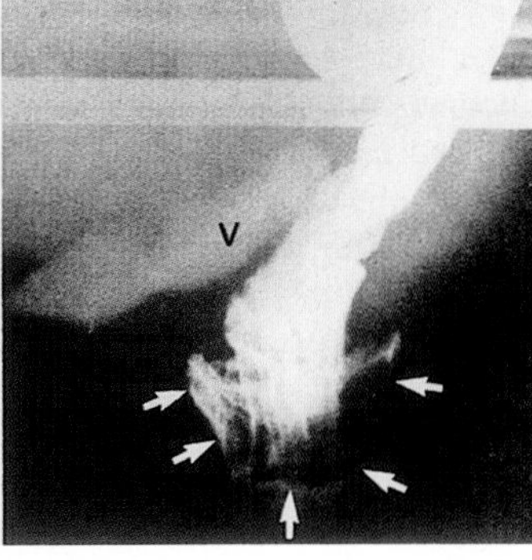

Figure 118–2. Barium defecogram of rectal intussusception. The *left panel* shows an apparently normal rectum prior to an attempt at defecation. In the *right panel,* attempted defecation leads to rectal intussusception *(arrows)* without visible protrusion through the anus. This condition is also known as occult rectal prolapse. V, vagina (identified with a radiocontrast-soaked tampon). (From Feldman M, Boland CR [eds]: Slide Atlas of Gastroenterology and Hepatology. Philadelphia, Current Medicine, 1996.)

dominal approaches for rectal prolapse repair, combined rectosigmoid resection and rectopexy seems to be the preferred procedure in patients with rectal prolapse associated with constipation. In one prospective study comparing surgical techniques, only 22% of patients who underwent combined rectosigmoid resection and rectopexy reported constipation postoperatively compared with 88% who underwent rectopexy alone.[15]

Recently, several series have documented successful laparoscopic repair of rectal prolapse by rectopexy, either alone or with rectosigmoid resection.[16–18] This approach has great potential to decrease the length of hospital stay and frequency of postoperative adhesions and associated small bowel obstructions. Although this approach appears to be safe, more long-term outcome data are needed to determine the efficacy of laparoscopic repairs for rectal prolapse.

Perineal approaches for repair of rectal prolapse are best suited for debilitated and elderly patients. These procedures have a relatively short operative time, may be performed under spinal anesthesia, and avoid the morbidities of an abdominal incision and pelvic dissection. The more commonly performed operations include the Altemeier procedure (perineal proctosigmoidectomy), Delorme procedure, and anal encirclement procedures. The Altemeier procedure consists of a full-thickness resection of the rectal prolapse performed through an incision made transrectally 1 to 2 cm above the dentate line. The resection may include the rectum as well as the sigmoid colon if there is redundancy of the sigmoid. Repair of levator muscle diastasis may be performed by plicating the muscles with nonabsorbable sutures, and this maneuver has been associated with improved continence.[19, 20] Altemeier and colleagues reported excellent results and a recurrence rate of only 2.8% with this procedure.[21] Others have had variable success, with recurrence rates ranging from 5.5% to 54%.[19, 20] A modification of the Altemeier technique that may decrease the recurrence rate was recently described in seven elderly patients by Yoshioka and colleagues, who used a perineal approach to perform a combined perineal proctosigmoidectomy with rectopexy, pelvic floor repair, and construction of an anastomosis with a colonic pouch.[22] There were no recurrences on follow-up.[22]

Although recurrence rates are generally higher with perineal repairs than abdominal repairs, there has been a recent trend toward performing perineal proctosigmoidectomies rather than abdominal repairs,[23] probably because patient outcomes are similar, and the perineal approach is less invasive and associated with a shorter hospital stay. In addition, the complication rate for perineal repairs is extremely low, with a 1.5% frequency of anastomotic leak, bleeding, or stricture.[23] In addition to the frail and elderly patient, the Altemeier procedure may be preferred in young, healthy patients because of its low morbidity. In young women who wish to avoid the potential hazard of infertility as a result of adhesion formation, the Altemeier procedure may be warranted even though it is associated with a higher recurrence rate than abdominal procedures. Similarly, in young men, the risk of autonomic denervation and impotence associated with pelvic surgery may be avoided by a perineal repair. The Altemeier procedure is also the procedure of choice when the prolapsed rectum is incarcerated and gangrenous.

The Delorme procedure also is performed via a transrectal approach. Unlike the Altemeier procedure, resection in a Delorme procedure involves only the mucosa of the rectal prolapse. After the mucosa is removed, the prolapsed muscular layers are plicated with sutures. This procedure is best suited for mucosal prolapse in a debilitated patient. Recurrence rates have been variable, ranging from 3% to 38%.[24–26] However, in series reporting low recurrence rates, functional results have been acceptable. In a recent series of 33 patients, overall results were good to excellent in 76% of patients, with alleviation of constipation in 89% and of rectal bleeding in 79% of cases.[25]

For the frail and debilitated patient, anal encirclement (synonymous with the Thiersch procedure) is the procedure of choice. The goal is to prevent the rectum from prolapsing through the anus by encircling the anus with a prosthesis to narrow it. The operation does not involve resection of the prolapse and may be performed under local anesthesia. The technique involves making two incisions around the anus and tunneling a mesh circumferentially around the anus to narrow it. Although simple with little surgical trauma, the procedure is associated with significant complications, including mesh breakage, mesh erosion into the rectum, and rectal stenosis.[27] Approximately 25% of patients ultimately require reoperation for one or more of these complications.[28]

SOLITARY RECTAL ULCER SYNDROME

The solitary rectal ulcer syndrome (SRUS) is a poorly understood syndrome first described, in 1969, by Madigan and Morson. SRUS is rare, with an estimated prevalence of one in 100,000 persons per year.[29] The syndrome is poorly named, because in some affected patients there is no ulcer, whereas in others multiple ulcers are found. In addition, some patients may have ulcers that are not confined to the rectum. The lesion, which may be an ulcer or polypoid mass, must be differentiated from an adenoma, cancer, inflammatory bowel disease, and colitis cystica profunda.

Etiology

The pathogenesis of SRUS is unclear but probably multifactorial. Two of the more common theories for its development implicate direct trauma or local ischemia as causes. In persons with constipation, removal of stool from the rectum by repetitive self-digitation may lead to direct trauma to the mucosa and formation of an ulcer.[30] However, many patients deny rectal digitation, and the ulcer often occurs in the midrectum, which is not generally reached by digitation.

Trauma secondary to constipation or hard stool impaction may be a potential mechanism for ulcer formation. Straining, constipation, and fecal impaction also may lead to ischemic injury with a resulting ulcer. Ischemia from the use of ergotamine suppositories also has been documented.[31] Radiation may induce SRUS via an ischemic mechanism.[32] Ischemia has been speculated to occur by (1) traction on the submucosal vessels; (2) replacement of blood vessels by the ingrowth of fibroblasts; (3) pressure necrosis of prolapsed mucosa by the anal sphincter; and (4) high intrarectal pressure generated by an obstructing rectal prolapse that causes venous congestion and ulceration.[33]

The histologic findings support an ischemic origin of this condition. Microscopically, there are obliteration of the lamina propria by fibromuscular proliferation, thickening of the

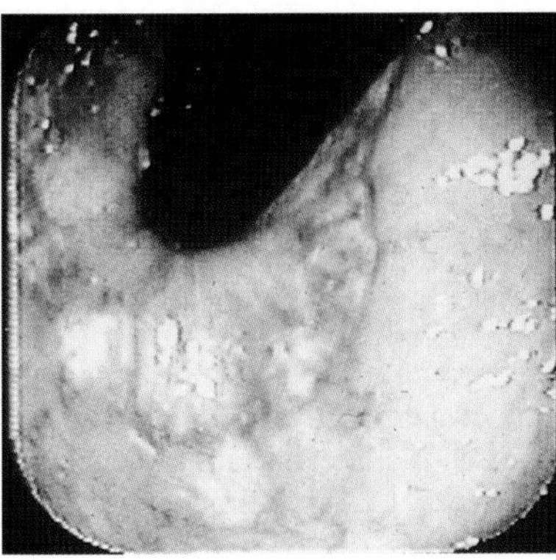

Figure 118–3. Endoscopic view of solitary rectal ulcer located approximately 10 cm from the anal verge in a patient with long-standing defecatory difficulty. (From Feldman M, Boland CR [eds]: Slide Atlas of Gastroenterology and Hepatology. Philadelphia, Current Medicine, 1996.)

muscularis mucosa, disordered arrangement of fibroblasts and muscle fibers between crypts, and diffuse collagen infiltration of the lamina propria. The diffuse fibrosis is demonstrated with connective tissue stains and helps differentiate SRUS from collagenous and ischemic colitis.

Rectal prolapse also may play a role in the pathogenesis of SRUS.[34] Between 13% and 94% of patients with SRUS have an associated rectal prolapse.[34, 35] Histologically, the features of SRUS are strikingly similar to those of mucosal prolapse, and some investigators have suggested that the two syndromes are identical.[36] Similar findings are noted when the mucosa overlying prolapsed ileostomies and colostomies is examined histologically.[37] It is believed that the associated rectal prolapse develops in patients with SRUS as a result of straining against a functional obstruction caused by nonrelaxation of the puborectalis during defecation. Normally the puborectalis, a muscle that encircles the anterior portion of the upper anal canal, relaxes to straighten the anorectal angle, thereby allowing defecation to occur (see Fig. 118–2). As many as 50% of patients with SRUS have electromyographic (EMG) studies documenting a failure to relax the puborectalis muscle or a paradoxical contraction of the muscle, or both.[38, 39] Rectal prolapse also may be related to overactivity of the external sphincter muscle with resulting functional obstruction in up to 70% of persons with this abnormality.[35] Once the rectum prolapses, wall stresses and underlying ischemia and ulceration may ensue.

Clinical Features and Diagnosis

SRUS affects men and women equally[40, 41] and often is described in young adults. Symptoms may include rectal bleeding, straining, constipation or diarrhea, incontinence, tenesmus, passage of mucus, and a sensation of incomplete defecation.[29, 35, 42] As many as 26% of patients may be asymptomatic.[35] The diagnosis is made by sigmoidoscopy. Classically, a single ulcer is seen on the anterior rectal wall 5 to 10 cm from the anal verge (Fig. 118–3). Other endoscopic appearances include a polypoid lesion in 25%, patches of hyperemic mucosa in 18%,[29] and multiple lesions in 30% of patients. Other diagnoses to consider when a solitary ulcer is visualized endoscopically include invasive cancer, Crohn's disease, mucosal erosions secondary to drugs such as nonsteroidal anti-inflammatory drugs (NSAIDs), and an infectious ulcer. Endoscopic biopsies help confirm the diagnosis.

The histologic features of SRUS include distortion of the colonic glands, fibrous replacement of the lamina propria, and diffuse excess collagen deposition, which can be demonstrated with connective tissue stains (Fig. 118–4).[43] Biopsies always should be taken to exclude a malignancy masquerading as SRUS. In addition, an underlying carcinoma may be present in association with SRUS.[44–46] Transrectal ultrasonography is useful to distinguish SRUS from other conditions such as invasive cancer. In SRUS, ultrasonography may reveal a thickened muscularis propria and marked thickening of the internal anal sphincter.[47, 48] Defecography frequently reveals an unrecognized rectal prolapse or nonrelaxation of the puborectalis muscle.[84, 49]

Treatment

Patients who are asymptomatic may not require treatment, and in some patients, symptoms may resolve spontaneously. For patients with significant symptoms, a variety of therapies have been tried. Because there are few controlled studies and SRUS may resolve spontaneously, it is difficult to make definitive recommendations for treatment. Several therapies thought to be beneficial include topical medications, behavior modification supplemented by fiber, biofeedback, and surgery.

Topical medications have had variable success in treating SRUS. Although glucocorticoids applied topically and sulfasalazine enemas are not efficacious,[29, 40] 5-aminosalicylate enemas have been reported anecdotally to be useful.[50] In one series, six patients treated with sucralfate enemas improved symptomatically.[51] Fibrin glue also has been used successfully for the treatment of SRUS. Fibrin glue may be beneficial because it stimulates the proliferation of fibroblasts and vessel growth. In one report, fibrin glue was applied topically to the ulcer in six patients and resulted in complete healing after 14 days.[52] At 1-year follow-up, there were no recurrences in these patients. The success rate of fiber in

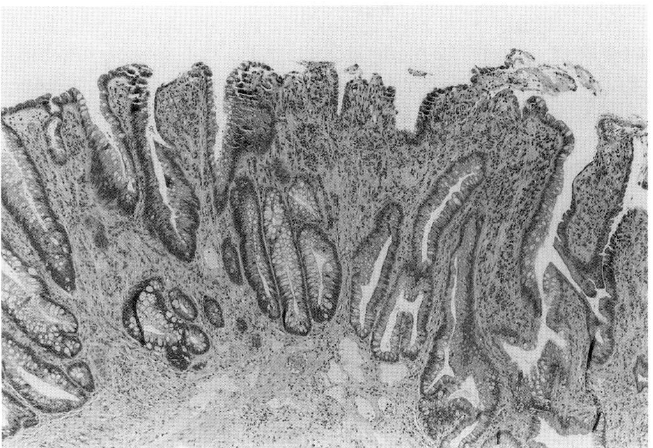

Figure 118–4. Low-power histologic view of solitary rectal ulcer. Regenerating branching glands are surrounded by smooth muscle that replaces the lamina propria. (Courtesy of Dr. Sidney Finkelstein, University of Pittsburgh Medical Center.)

treating SRUS has ranged from 19% to 70%.[29, 35] With behavior modification and dietary supplementation with fiber, in one study symptoms improved in 14 of 21 patients.[53] In more than 50% of the patients who improved symptomatically, the ulcer healed completely.

Biofeedback may be successful in selected patients with SRUS. Biofeedback includes correcting abnormal pelvic floor behavior, such as excessive straining with defecation, and encouraging patients to stop laxatives, suppositories, and enemas. In one prospective study, biofeedback was associated with improved symptoms in 13 patients with SRUS.[54] After biofeedback, the majority of patients had less straining and less need for manual disimpaction. Five of nine patients no longer relied on laxatives. Both the frequency of defecation and time required to defecate were reduced. Biofeedback may be particularly helpful for patients with SRUS associated with a nonrelaxing puborectalis muscle (NRPR). In one report of biofeedback, symptoms improved in patients with SRUS and NRPR; straining, bleeding, and mucus decreased, and defecation improved.[55]

Surgery also may be helpful in the management of some patients with SRUS. In one retrospective study of 21 patients from the Cleveland Clinic, surgery benefited approximately one third of patients. All patients were found to have an associated rectal prolapse. Eighteen underwent rectopexy, and three underwent sigmoid colectomy and rectopexy. Complete healing of the ulcer occurred in 28% of patients undergoing rectopexy and 33% of patients treated with resection and rectopexy.

In a second prospective study, defecography was used to determine the outcome in patients with SRUS. In 18 of 19 patients with SRUS and rectal prolapse on defecography, rectal prolapse disappeared completely after rectopexy.[56] In a retrospective study of 66 patients who underwent surgery for SRUS refractory to medical therapy (22 with internal rectal prolapses), resolution of or significant improvement in symptoms, sustained for at least 1 year postoperatively, was demonstrated in 27 of 49 who underwent rectopexy and 5 of 9 who underwent a Delorme procedure.[57] The researchers concluded that antiprolapse operations have a long-term success rate of about 55% to 60% in the treatment of SRUS. Clearly, diagnostic evaluation to identify an associated rectal prolapse seems useful in patients with SRUS to identify patients who may derive benefit from antiprolapse surgery.

For patients with SRUS, medical therapy appears to be a good first option. If medical therapy is not successful, biofeedback or surgery may be appropriate in selected patients. Antiprolapse operations may benefit patients with SRUS who demonstrate rectal prolapse and a relaxing pelvic floor on defecography. For patients with a nonrelaxing pelvic floor, medical therapy with biofeedback may decrease symptoms and permit easier defecation.

NONSPECIFIC COLONIC ULCERS

Benign nonspecific ulcers of the colon are uncommon, and the causes remain unknown. The most recent large review of the literature encompassed 127 patients and indicated that colonic ulcers occur at any age, with a peak incidence in the fourth and fifth decades and a slight female predominance.[58] The majority of ulcers occur in the proximal colon, virtually all are solitary and are located on the antimesenteric side of the colon, and most are round and sharply demarcated from relatively normal surrounding mucosa (Fig. 118–5).[58–60] Histologically, there is nonspecific acute and chronic inflammation.[58]

Pathogenesis

The causes of nonspecific colonic ulcers are unknown. Hypotheses that have been advanced, but with little or no supporting evidence, include ischemia, cecal diverticulosis,[61] and acid-peptic disease. Correlations with the use of drugs such as glucocorticoids, NSAIDs,[62, 63] oral contraceptives, and oxyphenbutazone have been suggested, but causation has not been established nor have such drugs been implicated in most of the ulcers reported. It is likely that no single causative agent explains all cases. There have been reports of associations with chronic renal failure and renal transplantation,[64] Churg-Strauss syndrome,[65] Wegener's granulomatosis,[66] Behçet's disease, essential mixed cryoglobulinemia,[67] and systemic lupus erythematosus; perhaps a mechanism common to all may exist, but none has been identified.

Clinical Features

The most frequent presenting symptoms have been abdominal pain and bleeding. Over one half of patients present with acute or chronic abdominal pain, often in the right lower abdomen and mimicking appendicitis.[58] One third have had lower gastrointestinal bleeding with hematochezia, and 16% present with an abdominal mass, most often when the ulcer is located in the left or sigmoid colon. A cecal ulcer should be suspected in a patient with gastrointestinal bleeding associated with a clinical picture consistent with appendicitis or in a patient with symptoms suggestive of pelvic inflamma-

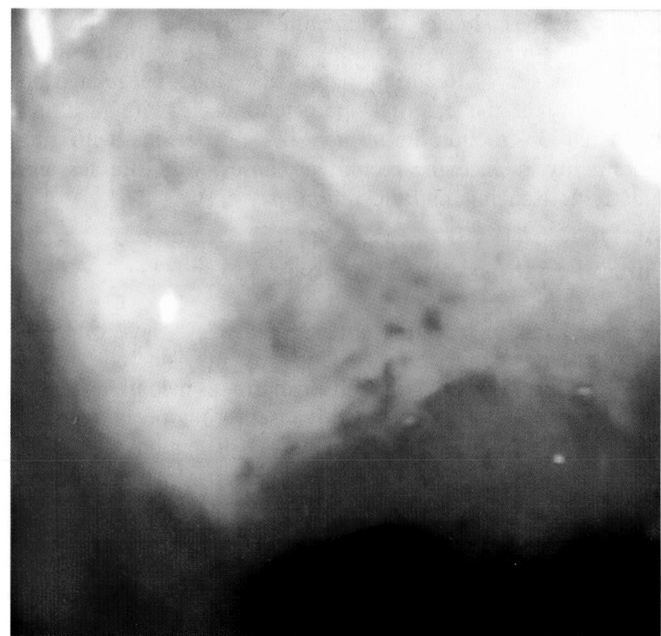

Figure 118–5. Endoscopic appearance of nonspecific ulcer of the colon.

tory disease, ovarian disease, or Crohn's disease in the absence of these diseases.

Diagnosis

Historically, nonspecific colonic ulcers were often diagnosed at laparotomy after complications occurred. In an early review, Barron described an 82% mortality rate without surgical intervention. With the advent of endoscopy, many colonic ulcers now may be diagnosed preoperatively and, in some cases, managed conservatively.

Colonoscopy is currently the diagnostic test of choice.[58, 68] Flexible sigmoidoscopy is inadequate because most colonic ulcers are beyond the reach of the instrument. Abnormalities have been described in up to 75% of air-contrast barium enemas[58] and include mucosal irregularities, intraluminal filling defects or narrowing, a mass effect, or localized colonic spasm (Fig. 118–6). However, the findings are nonspecific and diagnostically inferior to direct inspection by colonoscopy. Computed tomographic (CT) scans are most helpful in the presence of perforation or associated abscess formation.

The key to the diagnosis is the exclusion of diseases that are associated with ulceration; these include Crohn's disease, infections such as tuberculosis, *Entamoeba histolytica,* cytomegalovirus, and *Salmonella typhi* infections, stercoral ulcers, and SRUS. Neoplastic causes such as carcinoma, lymphoma, and amyloidosis[69] are distinguished on histologic grounds but may not be distinguishable from nonspecific colonic ulcers on the basis of endoscopic appearance alone.

Treatment

Surgery is recommended for patients with ulcers complicated by perforation, significant gastrointestinal bleeding, and intra-abdominal bleeding and those with persistent symptoms and failure of the ulcer to heal. However, in uncomplicated cases, a conservative, expectant approach has been advocated, with colonoscopy every 6 weeks to monitor healing.[68] The most common surgical procedures are local excision of the ulcer, oversewing of the ulcer if there is significant bleeding, and more extensive resections of the affected colon.[58, 70]

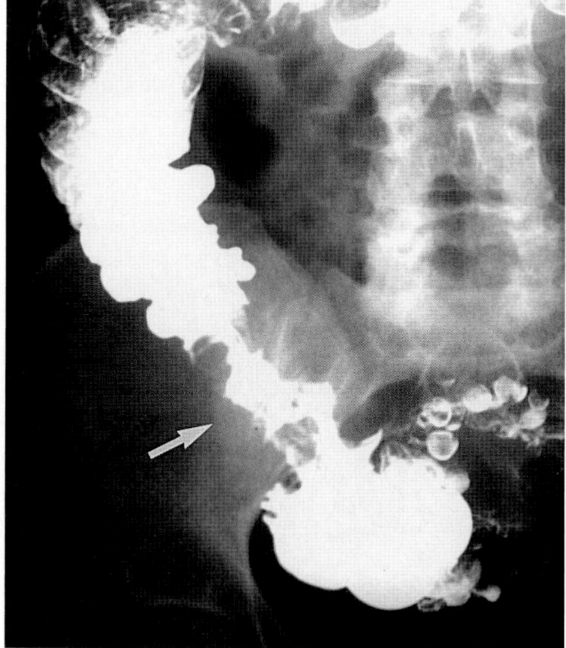

Figure 118–6. Nonspecific ulcer of the colon. Barium enema of the lesion shown in Figure 118–5 *(arrow)*. Initial diagnosis was carcinoma of the ascending colon.

DIEULAFOY-TYPE COLONIC ULCERATION

In 1897, Georges Dieulafoy first described massive gastrointestinal bleeding emanating from a relatively enlarged ("persistent calibre") submucosal artery by way of a minute mucosal ulcer at the most superficial point of the vessel.[71] Although originally described in the stomach and most commonly occurring in the gastric fundus, identical lesions have been described in other gastrointestinal organs, including the colon and rectum.[72–75] In the colon, Dieulafoy-type lesions appear to have a strong male predominance and have been reported in all age groups.

Histologically, colonic Dieulafoy-type lesions are identical to those found elsewhere in the gastrointestinal tract. The submucosal artery is tortuous and hypertrophic, curving toward the mucosa. Inflammation is absent, and the solitary mucosal ulceration extends no deeper than the upper submucosal layer.

The clinical picture is one of acute and massive bleeding, with hematochezia and hemodynamic changes. Colonoscopy can identify the lesion in some cases[75] but is often difficult or impossible, especially if bleeding continues or thorough cleansing of the colon cannot be accomplished. Selective mesenteric angiography is the diagnostic study of choice, and surgical resection has been the principal form of therapy. Even after angiographic detection of the bleeding site, precise localization of the lesion is frequently difficult, and more extended resection often is required. In some cases, colonic lesions appear as pseudopolyps,[73] and successful treatment with sclerotherapy or electrocautery may obviate the need for surgery.[76]

STERCORAL ULCER

Stercoral ulcers are a relatively uncommon cause of colonic ulcers and result from pressure necrosis of the mucosa by the direct effect of a fecal mass.[77] The ulcers are asymptomatic unless there is bleeding or perforation with resultant peritonitis.

Stercoral ulcers have been described in patients of all ages and both sexes.[78, 79] The predominant risk factors are constipation and conditions that cause or worsen constipation, such as residence in a nursing home or other chronic care facility, use of constipating medications, hypothyroidism, colonic strictures, and renal failure or transplantation. A recent review identified only 81 cases of stercoral perforation in the literature since the first published report in 1894. Stercoral ulcers accounted for 3.2% of all colonic perforations reported during a 5-year period in a single institution.[80] Most of the ulcers occur in the sigmoid colon or rectum, although ulcers in the more proximal colon have been reported.[77, 81]

As with nonspecific colonic ulcers, stercoral ulcers vary greatly in size and may be multiple. All occur on the antimesenteric side of the lumen where the colonic blood supply is poorest and presumably where the increased intraluminal pressure first exceeds the capillary perfusion pressure.[78] The ulcer margins are often irregular, conforming to the surface of the adjacent fecal mass.[80] Histologically, the mucosa is necrotic, with acute and chronic inflammatory changes.

Several factors help explain why the sigmoid colon is predisposed to stercoral ulcers. Fecal material becomes more dehydrated as it approaches the sigmoid, and the sigmoid and rectosigmoid are the narrowest segments of the colon. Fecalomas pass with greater difficulty and may become lodged in these areas, thus exerting prolonged pressure on the wall of the colon. Increased intraluminal pressure in this area may further compromise the colonic microcirculation, thereby resulting in pressure necrosis, ulceration, and perforation.

The definitive approach to stercoral ulcers is surgical resection with either primary reanastomosis (if there is no perforation) or resection with a colostomy.[78, 82] Resection with an end-colostomy and Hartmann's pouch or mucous fistula has been reported to have the lowest mortality of the various procedures and is advocated as the surgical procedure of choice.[82] Both peritoneal lavage to reduce fecal contamination after perforation and intraoperative colonic lavage to remove remaining scybala proximal to the perforation[81] have been recommended for optimal results.

LYMPHOCYTIC AND COLLAGENOUS COLITIS

Background

Lymphocytic and collagenous colitis are uncommon disorders characterized by chronic, watery diarrhea and histologic evidence of chronic mucosal inflammation in the absence of endoscopic or radiologic abnormalities of the colon. The two disorders are histologically distinct but have been grouped under the term "microscopic colitis." They differ principally by the presence or absence of a thickened collagenous band, which is located in the colonic subepithelium in collagenous colitis.

The term *collagenous colitis* was first used in 1976 by Lindstrom for a middle-aged woman in whom an evaluation for chronic diarrhea was normal except for colonic biopsies that showed a thickened band of subepithelial collagen and increased lymphocytes in the lamina propria.[83] Histologically, the findings resembled the subepithelial collagen deposits in small intestinal mucosa found in collagenous sprue. The term *microscopic colitis* was first used in 1980 by Read and associates, who described a group of patients with chronic diarrhea of unknown origin, a subset of whom had a normal colonoscopy but abnormal histopathology on biopsy.[84] Later review showed that most of these patients had collagenous colitis, but some had increased lymphocytes in the lamina propria in the absence of a thickened collagen band. The term *lymphocytic colitis* was proposed in 1989 by Lazenby and associates[85] as a more specific histopathologic definition to distinguish this entity from other patterns of microscopic colitis in which the presence of other cellular elements such as eosinophils and mast cells or neutrophils dominate.

Whether collagenous and lymphocytic colitis represent two ends of the spectrum of a single disorder or different entities remains uncertain, but their clinical presentations, evaluations, and treatments are similar.

Epidemiology

Both lymphocytic and collagenous colitis occur most commonly between ages 50 and 70 years, with a strong female predominance and frequent association with arthritis, celiac disease, and autoimmune disorders. In a large population-based study in Spain, the demographic features of both collagenous and lymphocytic colitis were similar; the disorders were found in 9.5 of every 100 patients with chronic watery diarrhea and normal-appearing mucosa on colonoscopy; the incidence rate of lymphocytic colitis was three times higher than that of collagenous colitis.[86] This last observation contrasts strikingly with published reports of more than 400 cases of collagenous colitis compared with more than 60 cases of lymphocytic colitis, a finding which suggests that there may be a publication bias. The overall mean annual incidence of both colitides was 4.2 per 100,000 inhabitants in Spain, similar to a previous epidemiologic study in Sweden[87] but almost twice as high as that of a French study. Although the incidence is clearly higher in older age groups, both entities have been reported in children, in whom the clinical presentation is similar to that of adults.[88]

Pathology

In both lymphocytic and collagenous colitis, there is a modest increase in mononuclear cells within the lamina propria and between crypt epithelial cells, consisting primarily of $CD8^+$ T lymphocytes, plasma cells, and macrophages.[85] There may be flattening of the surface epithelial cells, a mild decrease in the number of goblet cells, Paneth cell hyperplasia, and an increased number of intraepithelial lymphocytes, all of which are distinctive features of this disorder (Fig.

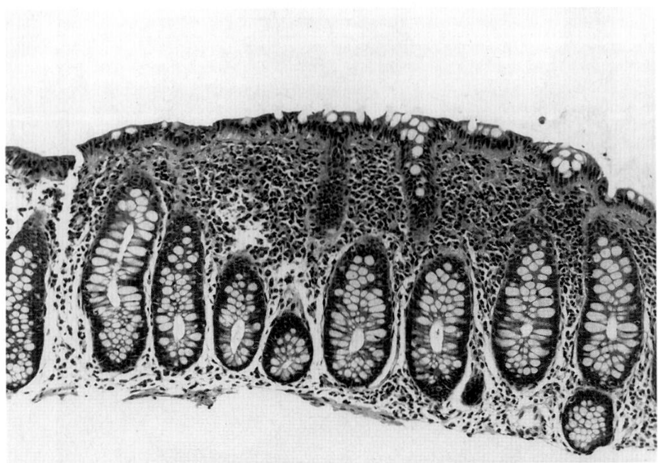

Figure 118–7. Histology of lymphocytic colitis. A chronic inflammatory infiltrate involves the superficial epithelium and lamina propria. (Courtesy of Dr. Sidney Finkelstein, University of Pittsburgh Medical Center.)

118–7). Neutrophils are not prominent, and cryptitis and crypt distortion are unusual.

In collagenous colitis, there is a thickened subepithelial collagen layer, which may be continuous or patchy (Fig. 118–8). In the normal colon, the width of this collagen band is less than 4 to 5 μm, whereas in collagenous colitis, it is greater than 10 μm and averages 20 to 60 μm.[89] In the normal colon, the subepithelial collagen band consists predominantly of type IV collagen, whereas in collagenous colitis, the band is reportedly composed of types I and III as well as fibronectin.[90] Although inflammatory changes occur diffusely throughout the colon, the characteristic collagen band thickening is highly variable, occurring in the cecum and transverse colon in over 80% of cases and in the rectum in less than 30% of cases. Although involvement of the left colon appears to be less intense than involvement of the right colon, multiple biopsies of the left colon above the rectosigmoid during flexible sigmoidoscopy are sufficient to make the diagnosis in approximately 90% of cases.[89] It is essential to emphasize that a diagnosis of collagenous colitis requires both mucosal inflammation and a thickened collagen band and that artifact resulting from poor orientation may give the mistaken appearance of a thickened basement membrane.[91]

Etiology and Pathogenesis

The cause of the two entities is unknown. The most widely held hypothesis is that they are inflammatory disorders arising from epithelial immune responses to luminal contents or epithelial antigens. This hypothesis has been supported by the regression of inflammation following diversion of the fecal stream and recurrence of inflammation following restoration of intestinal continuity in three patients.[92] The identity of the inciting factors is uncertain, although medications such as NSAIDs,[93, 94] bile salts, toxins, and infectious agents[95] have been postulated.

The strong association of arthritis with the microscopic colitides has raised the possibility that NSAIDs may play an etiologic role. One well-controlled study[96] found that chronic

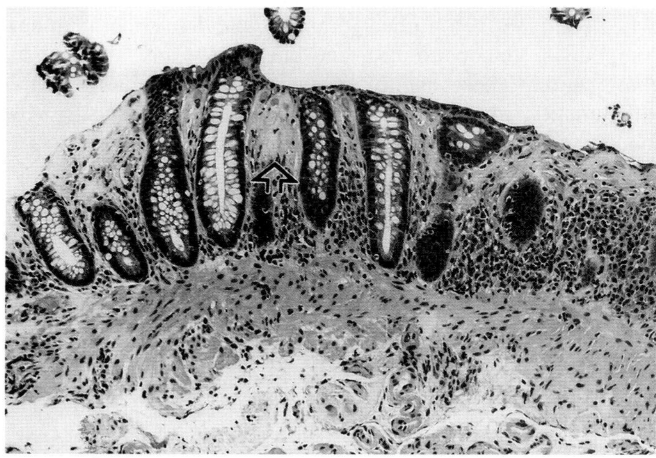

Figure 118–8. Histology of collagenous colitis. An extensive subepithelial deposition of collagen in colonic mucosa *(arrow)* is associated with a chronic inflammatory infiltrate in the lamina propria. (Courtesy of Dr. Sidney Finkelstein, University of Pittsburgh Medical Center.)

NSAID use occurred more frequently in patients with collagenous colitis than in age- and gender-matched controls (61% vs. 13%, $p < 0.02$), but this difference was not confirmed by another study.[97] One of the postulated mechanisms by which NSAIDs may damage the colon is by increasing colonic permeability to allow luminal antigens to enter the lamina propria and promote inflammation. Because many patients with collagenous or lymphocytic colitis have not used NSAIDs and because NSAID use in older adults is common and these disorders are uncommon, other causes, including genetic susceptibility, have been invoked. Genetic susceptibility is supported by the occurrence of collagenous colitis in several members of each of two families[98] and by different susceptibilities of inbred rat strains to indomethacin.[99]

Approximately 20% to 30% of patients with celiac disease have been reported to have lymphocytic colitis, raising the possibility of similar pathogenetic mechanisms.[100, 101] One report suggested that in 40% of patients with collagenous colitis, bowel biopsies were compatible with celiac disease,[102] but the frequency of celiac disease was only 2% in another larger series of patients with collagenous colitis.[103] Patients with collagenous and lymphocytic colitis do not respond to a gluten-free diet; neither collagenous nor lymphocytic colitis is associated with human leukocyte antigens (HLA) B8 and DR3, as is celiac disease; and $CD8^+$ T intraepithelial cells are predominant, in contrast to celiac disease.

However, because possible autoimmune disorders, such as arthritis and thyroid abnormalities, have been described in patients with collagenous and lymphocytic colitis, there have been continued efforts to associate both types of colitis with various autoimmune HLA haplotypes and serum markers. One small study showed that HLA-A1 antigens were expressed with increased frequency in lymphocytic but not collagenous colitis,[104] whereas another study showed similar abnormal expressions of HLA-DR antigens by mucosal epithelial cells in both conditions.[105] Whether such abnormalities are the cause or the result of these disorders is unknown. A recent study found that HLA-DQ2 or DQ1,3 genes were more frequent in patients with celiac disease and in patients with either lymphocytic or collagenous colitis than in controls.[106] Although gluten is most certainly not the inciting antigen in microscopic colitis, similar immune mechanisms may be involved in celiac disease and microscopic colitis.

The pathogenesis of the increased collagen band has been unclear, although it has been assumed that collagen synthesis is increased in collagenous colitis. However, in a recent study of patients with collagenous colitis, colonic biopsies exhibited decreased levels of interstitial collagenase, suggesting that reduced matrix degradation rather than increased production results in the accumulation of matrix proteins.[107]

The mechanism of diarrhea in both disorders is related to the severity of inflammation and not the extent or thickness of the collagen band. Perfusion studies have demonstrated defective active and passive absorption of sodium and chloride and reduced chloride-bicarbonate exchange in the colon[108]; two of six subjects had coexisting abnormalities of small intestine fluid and electrolyte absorption. Other investigators have correlated colonic fluid absorption with the severity of inflammation.[109] The finding of high luminal prostaglandin E_2 levels in one patient with active colonic chloride secretion suggests a potential role for soluble mediators produced by activated immune and mesenchymal cells,[110] as does a report that diarrhea was prevented by a histamine H_1 antagonist in a patient with microscopic colitis characterized by increased numbers of mast cells.[111] A recent study has suggested that bile acid malabsorption may contribute to diarrhea in patients with collagenous colitis[112] and that treatment with a bile acid–binding resin such as cholestyramine may lead to a reduction in diarrhea.[113] However, bile acids are unlikely to cause the histologic changes observed in collagenous colitis, and a reduction in diarrhea was not associated with a decrease in colitis.[114] Hormonal studies, including serum gastrin, vasoactive intestinal polypeptide, and urine 5-hydroxyindoleacetic acid levels, have been normal.[115]

Clinical and Laboratory Features

Patients with collagenous and lymphocytic colitis usually present with chronic watery diarrhea, with an average of eight stools each day, often nocturnally, ranging in volume from 300 to 1700 g per 24 hours,[108] and associated with occasional fecal incontinence, abdominal cramps, and a decrease in symptoms with fasting.[87] Nausea, weight loss, and fecal urgency also have been reported but are variable. Diarrhea is generally long-standing, lasting from months to years, with a fluctuating course of remissions and exacerbations. In one series of 172 patients, the median time from the onset of symptoms to diagnosis was 11 months,[103] whereas in another series of 31 patients the median time was 5.4 years.[97] Physical examination is usually unremarkable, and blood is not detected in the stool. Routine laboratory studies are also normal.

Examination of fresh stools showed fecal leukocytes in 55% of 116 patients with collagenous colitis.[103] Mild steatorrhea, mild anemia, low serum vitamin B_{12} levels, and hypoalbuminemia have been reported in variable numbers of patients but are not characteristic. Autoimmune markers that have been identified in patients with collagenous colitis include antinuclear antibodies (in up to 50%), antineutrophil cytoplasmic antibodies (pANCA) (in 14%), rheumatoid factor, and increased C_3 and C_4 complement levels.[109] Occasionally, autoantibodies have been found in lymphocytic colitis[116] but are not of diagnostic value.[109]

Colonoscopic examination is usually normal, but nonspecific abnormalities were reported in one study.[117] Findings included patchy edema, erythema, friability, and an abnormal vascular pattern. In the absence of control subjects, the specificity or reproducibility of such findings is uncertain.

Differential Diagnosis

Infectious agents should be excluded by testing the stool for enteric pathogens, ova, and parasites and *Clostridium difficile* toxin. Many patients are diagnosed with irritable bowel syndrome, a disorder that can be excluded by the abnormal colonic biopsies and the finding of increased stool volume, both of which are uncharacteristic of irritable bowel syndrome.

Other diseases can produce colitis but should be distinguishable on histologic grounds. Acute infectious colitis is characterized by neutrophilic inflammation and decreased intraepithelial lymphocytes. Eosinophilic enterocolitis of the mucosal type is characterized by eosinophilic infiltration, foreshortened crypts, inflammation of the deeper parts of the lamina propria, and absence of increased intraepithelial lymphocytes.[118] Amyloidosis has been mistaken for collagenous colitis,[119] but its distribution includes the basement membranes of the crypts and blood vessels as well as the epithelium; confirmation can be made by histochemical staining. Mild cases of ulcerative colitis and Crohn's disease should present no diagnostic confusion in view of the characteristic endoscopic and histologic findings and absence of increased intraepithelial lymphocytes. Hormone-producing tumors, surreptitious laxative abuse, and hyperthyroidism can be excluded on histopathologic grounds.

Treatment

There have been few controlled trials for either collagenous or lymphocytic colitis, and therapy is largely empirical. Evaluation of therapy is difficult, because both disorders usually exhibit a relapsing and remitting course over many years. No single agent works in all cases.

About one third of patients respond to antidiarrheal agents, such as loperamide or diphenoxylate with atropine, as well as bulk agents such as psyllium or methylcellulose; however, clinical response is not associated with improvement in inflammation or collagen thickness. In a recent open-label trial of 12 patients, bismuth subsalicylate, 8 chewable tablets per day for 8 weeks, resulted in resolution of diarrhea and reduction in stool weight within 2 weeks, and in 9 patients colitis resolved, with disappearance of the collagen band thickening.[120] Over a 7- to 28-month follow-up, nine patients remained well, two were well but required retreatment, and one had persistent diarrhea. Both collagenous and lymphocytic colitis responded with equal efficacy, and there were no side effects. Although the basis for its efficacy is unknown, bismuth subsalicylate possesses antidiarrheal, antibacterial, and anti-inflammatory properties, and bismuth enemas have been reported to be effective in ulcerative colitis[121] and chronic pouchitis.[122]

Other treatment trials for collagenous colitis and lymphocytic colitis have studied 5-aminosalicylate (mesalamine) compounds, glucocorticoids, and bile acid resins, alone or in combination. These agents appear to improve diarrhea and inflammation in some, but certainly not all, patients.[123] Although glucocorticoids given by either the oral or rectal route provide symptomatic improvement and decrease inflammation in over 80% of cases, relapse usually occurs quickly after the drug is stopped.[87, 124] Moreover, long-term use of glucocorticoids has undesirable effects, especially in older patients. The value of other immunosuppressants, such as azathioprine and 6-mercaptopurine, is uncertain.

A recent open-label study reported that budesonide was successful in treating collagenous colitis in seven patients.[125] Budesonide is a topically acting corticosteroid with both a high receptor-binding affinity in the mucosa and a high first-pass effect in the liver. When given in pH-modified release capsules in a dose of 3 mg three times daily, stool frequency decreased rapidly within 10 days. Improvement was maintained after a reduction in dose to 1 mg three times daily after 2 months. Regression of histologic changes was demonstrated in three patients, with no recurrence of diarrhea 7 to 15 months after treatment. In another study, three of five patients had a complete response and two had a partial response to budesonide.[126, 127] Successful treatment in one patient with lymphocytic colitis was also reported with oral beclomethasone dipropionate, another experimental corticosteroid with properties similar to those of budesonide.[127]

The only report of surgery for collagenous colitis involved nine patients who underwent ileostomy for disabling refractory collagenous colitis.[128] All had symptomatic and histologic remission. In patients in whom intestinal continuity was restored, the disease recurred. Of three patients who underwent proctocolectomy with ileal pouch–anal anastomosis, problematic diarrhea occurred. Surgery should be considered only as a last resort but appears to be effective in patients with disabling and refractory symptoms.

Based on available data, the treatment algorithm shown in Figure 118–9 is proposed.

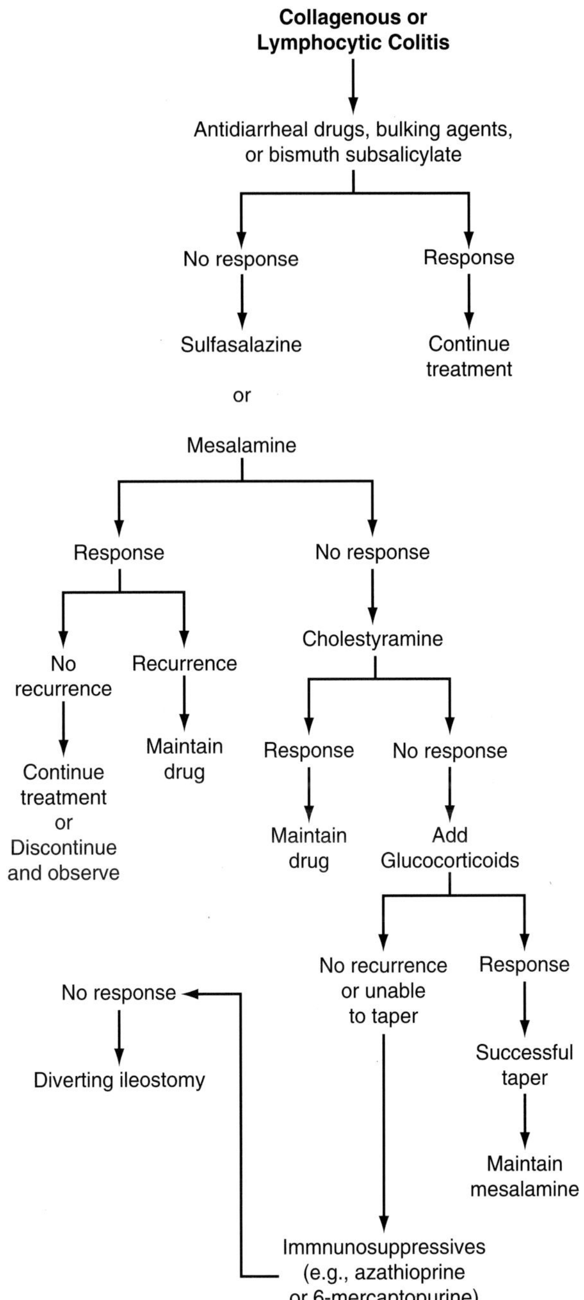

Figure 118–9. Approach to the treatment of collagenous or lymphocytic colitis.

DIVERSION COLITIS

Background and Epidemiology

Diversion colitis is an inflammatory process that occurs in segments of the colon and rectum that are bypassed after surgical diversion of the fecal stream. The entity was first reported in 1981 by Glotzer and associates in ten patients who had undergone ileostomy or colostomy for various indications other than inflammatory bowel disease (IBD).[128] Since then, diversion colitis has been found in patients who have undergone surgical diversion for any indication, including IBD[129]; indeed, diversion colitis has been reported to occur more commonly in patients with IBD (89%) than in those with carcinoma (23%) and other non-neoplastic conditions (50%).[130] The prevalence of diversion colitis has been underestimated because many patients are asymptomatic; however, histologic changes may occur in all patients within months of surgical diversion.

Pathology

A spectrum of histologic changes has been described, ranging from lymphoid follicular hyperplasia and mixed mononuclear and neutrophilic infiltration to severe inflammation with crypt abscesses, mucin granulomas, and Paneth cell metaplasia.[131, 132] However, large ulcers and transmural changes are absent, and crypt architecture is generally preserved. Endoscopic findings include erythema, friability, nodularity, edema, aphthous ulcerations, exudates, and frank bleeding, as in idiopathic IBD. After extended periods following diversion, inflammatory pseudopolyps, strictures, and aphthous ulcers may develop.

Pathogenesis

Diversion colitis appears to be caused largely by luminal nutrient deficiency of the colonic epithelium. The principal nutrient substrates of colonic epithelium are luminal short-chain fatty acids (SCFAs), which are metabolic products of carbohydrate and peptide fermentation by anaerobic bacteria.[133, 134] Roediger demonstrated that SCFAs are the major and preferred energy source for colonic epithelium and that the distal colon is more dependent on SCFAs for its metabolic needs than is the proximal colon.[134a] Butyrate supplies the bulk of oxidative energy to the distal colon, whereas acetate, glutamine, and ketones provide alternative sources of energy. Harig and associates demonstrated that the excluded segments of colon contain negligible amounts of SCFAs and that infusion of glucose results in no appreciable anaerobic fermentation.[135] Obligate anaerobes are reduced in number in the excluded colon, consistent with reduced SCFA production.[136] Moreover, instillation of enemas containing SCFAs resulted in disappearance of endoscopic changes within 4 to 6 weeks in four patients, whereas resolution of histologic abnormalities was slower but incomplete.

Although SCFA deficiency has been widely accepted as the cause of diversion colitis, other observations suggest that SCFA deficiency may not be the entire explanation for diversion colitis. First, studies in children indicate that SCFA enemas are not universally successful in treating diversion colitis.[137] Second, in germ-free rodents with surgical diversion and in patients receiving long-term parenteral nutrition or elimination diets (all circumstances in which luminal SCFA concentrations are low), mucosal atrophy rather than inflammation occurs.[138] Third, inflammation does not occur in urinary colon conduits, where the fecal stream is diverted, and urine does not contain measurable SCFAs.[139] Finally, in a prospective randomized double-blind study of 13 patients with diversion colitis, butyrate enemas given for 14 days provided no improvement in either endoscopic or histologic parameters.[140] In a subsequent study by the same group, administration of SCFAs did not affect the bacterial population in the excluded colon.[141] Other luminal elements besides SCFA deficiency must play a role, but the nature of such factors is unknown.

Diagnosis

The diagnosis of diversion colitis is based on the clinical picture, endoscopic findings, and histology. Diagnosis is relatively straightforward in a patient without preexisting IBD, but radiation colitis and ischemia should be considered in the appropriate clinical setting. Stool specimens for *Clostridium difficile* toxin, ova and parasites, and cultures are usually adequate to exclude other etiologies.

In patients with a preoperative diagnosis of Crohn's disease, diversion colitis must be distinguished from recurrent IBD. Colonoscopic findings such as linear ulcers and possibly strictures are said to favor Crohn's disease, as do transmural inflammation, marked crypt architectural abnormalities, and epithelioid granulomas.[129] Lymphoid hyperplasia occurs in both disorders but tends to be more prominent in diversion colitis.[142] If rectal involvement with Crohn's disease is absent prior to diversion, rectal inflammation is more likely to be caused by diversion than Crohn's disease.[129]

Treatment

The preferred treatment is surgical restoration of colonic continuity, which rapidly reverses symptoms and histologic changes. If symptoms are moderate to severe and reanastomosis is not feasible, SCFA enemas containing a mixture of 60 mmol of acetate, 30 mmol of propionate, and 40 mmol of butyrate with 22 mmol of sodium chloride per liter are administered into the anus or mucous fistula twice daily for 4 weeks and then decreased to once or twice weekly.[135] There are anecdotal reports that 5-aminosalicylate enemas are effective as well.[143]

CATHARTIC COLON

Cathartic colon is an infrequent and severe manifestation of chronic irritant laxative abuse. In 1943, Heilbrun first described radiographic abnormalities of the colon and terminal ileum associated with prolonged abuse of irritant cathartics.[144] Fewer than 50 cases have been reported in the literature, all in women with a duration of laxative abuse ranging from 10 to 70 years. However, it is important to emphasize that the term *cathartic colon* is based on barium enema characteristics and is not synonymous with prolonged use of laxatives or with laxative abuse. Indeed, misapplication of the term cathartic colon has led to inappropriate concerns over the chronic use of laxatives that, when used appropriately, are not associated with structural or functional damage to the colon. Nor is cathartic colon the inevitable consequence of chronic laxative abuse, which is associated with a variety of reversible symptoms as well as fluid and electrolyte abnormalities. In a review of 240 cases of chronic laxative abuse that were published in more than 70 reports, no case of cathartic colon was demonstrated.[145, 146]

Radiologic Features

Heilbrun originally described the following characteristics in his original case report: loss of haustrations, pseudostrictures, dilated colon and terminal ileum, and gaping of the ileocecal valve.[144] Similarities to the radiologic appearance of chronic ulcerative colitis were noted in this and subsequent studies.[147, 148] Characteristic changes are not always found throughout the colon, and there is a predilection for involvement of the right colon. Pathologic changes in resected specimens of cathartic colon have included mucosal atrophy, chronic inflammation with thickening of the muscularis mucosa, submucosal fatty infiltration, and mild fibrosis. However, irreversible strictures and degenerative changes in intestinal neurons are absent.[147] Neuronal changes have been found in patients with chronic laxative abuse, but these patients did not exhibit cathartic colon as defined here.[149]

Do Laxatives Damage the Colon?

The original suggestion that irritant laxatives, predominantly anthraquinones, damage the colon was based on studies in laboratory animals and in colons resected from laxative abusers.[150] Although mucosal atrophy and abnormalities of the enteric nervous system were described, the identities of the laxatives were not documented, nor was there information concerning preexisting conditions that may have resulted in chronic use of laxatives.

Subsequent studies have reported changes in colonic epithelial cells and the submucosa in patients with long-term laxative abuse, and both anthraquinones and bisacodyl have been implicated.[149] However, the nature and duration of laxative use and the inability to exclude preexisting conditions make the significance of these observations uncertain. Other studies in rodents and in chronically constipated women do not support the deleterious effect of anthraquinones on the ultrastructure of colonic nerves.[151, 152] Nor is there evidence to suggest that sennosides, bisacodyl, or related substances cause significant morphologic damage to the colonic enteric nervous system in either experimental animals or humans. Perhaps one or more laxatives that are no longer in use, such as podophyllin, may account for cases of cathartic colon, because no case of cathartic colon has been reported in persons who began to use or abuse irritant laxatives after 1960.[146]

Clinical Features

Habitual laxative users and abusers often complain of abdominal discomfort, bloating, fullness, or inability to defecate completely without using laxatives. In the more severe cases, electrolyte and fluid abnormalities such as hypokalemia and hypovolemia are associated with excessive thirst and weakness. Uncommonly, protein-losing enteropathy has been reported. All symptoms are reversible on withdrawal of laxatives or conversion to a more appropriate regimen of laxative use.

Treatment

Treatment of cathartic colon and symptoms of chronic laxative use is focused on reducing or eliminating irritant laxatives, substituting bulking or osmotic agents, and retraining the bowel. Although often thought to be irreversible, there is evidence that cathartic colon can partially or completely reverse after withdrawal of laxatives.[148] In severe or refractory cases, subtotal colectomy or proctocolectomy has been effective.

The cathartic colon is of historic interest and is unlikely to be identified in current clinical practice. There is no evidence that currently used laxatives can produce this entity. The term *cathartic colon* should not be confused with "chronic laxative abuse syndrome," nor should the term imply that current laxatives are dangerous if used chronically but appropriately.

(PSEUDO)MELANOSIS COLI

Melanosis coli is a brownish discoloration of the colonic mucosa caused by the accumulation of pigment in macrophages of the lamina propria (Fig. 118–10). First described in the early 19th century, the term *melanosis coli* was coined by Virchow in 1857, because the pigment was considered to be melanin or a melanin-like substance. Subsequently, the pigment proved to be more characteristic of lipofuscin, both histochemically and ultrastructurally,[153, 154] and the term *pseudomelanosis coli* is more accurate, but has not been widely adopted.

The association between pseudomelanosis coli and chronic use of anthraquinone laxatives is firmly established and is further supported by the development of characteristic pigmentation in laboratory animals after administration of anthraquinones.[155] Pseudomelanosis develops in over 70% of persons who use anthraquinone laxatives (cascara sagrada, aloe, senna, rhubarb, and frangula), often within 4 months of use, with an average of 9 months.[156] The condition is widely regarded as benign and reversible, and disappearance of the pigment generally occurs within 1 year of stopping laxatives.[157] However, pseudomelanosis can probably result from other factors or exposure to other laxatives and is not pathognomonic for anthraquinone use.

The pigment in pseudomelanosis coli is thought to originate from either macrophages or from organelles within epithelial cells after damage by anthraquinone laxatives, which cause cells to die by apoptosis. Such a sequence of damage has been demonstrated in guinea pigs exposed to anthraquinones.[158] Histologically, the number and size of macrophages within the lamina propria are increased, and the greatest amount of pigment is found in macrophages farthest from the lumen. Abnormalities of colonic epithelial cells are noted on electron microscopy but not light microscopy.[159]

Concern about a possible relationship between pseudomelanosis coli and the development of colonic neoplasms[160] has not been substantiated in a recent prospective case-control study.[161] Other confounding factors such as chronic constipation or dietary intake may account for an increased risk of colon cancer suggested by earlier studies. Colonic neoplasms lack pigment-containing macrophages and are easily identified in patients with melanosis coli.[162] Therefore, biopsies should be taken of any nonpigmented area of the colon in a patient with pseudomelanosis coli who undergoes colonoscopy.

CHEMICAL COLITIS

Damage to the colon has been reported after exposure to a number of rectally administered agents. The best known of these are soaps and detergents used as cleansing ene-

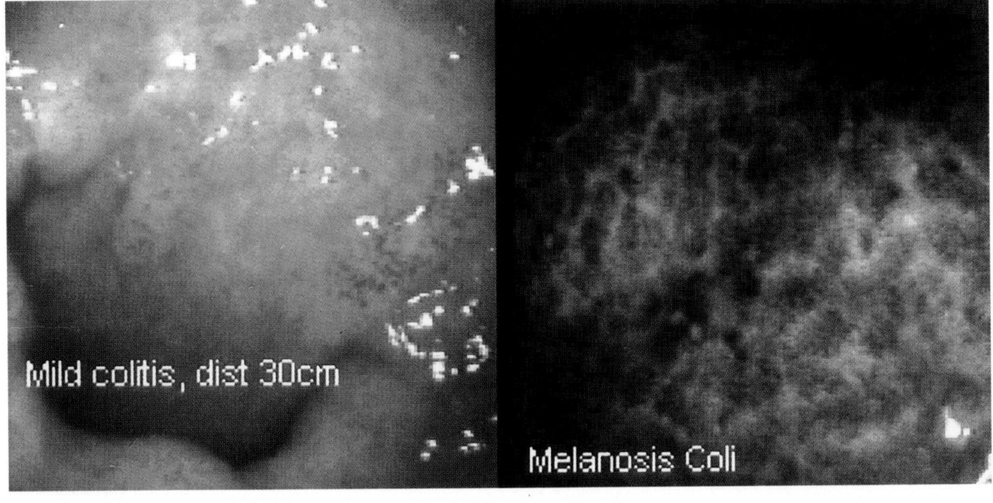

Figure 118–10. Colonoscopic view of melanosis coli associated with the chronic use of senna laxatives in a patient with ulcerative proctitis. There is little or no pseudomelanin pigment in the distal 30 cm of colon in the presence of active mild colitis *(left),* in contrast to the heavy pigmentation in the remaining colon *(right).* (Courtesy of Dr. Miguel Regueiro, University of Pittsburgh Medical Center.)

mas.[163,163] Other offending substances include hydrogen peroxide,[165] water-soluble contrast agents such as sodium diatrizoate (Hypaque, Gastrografin),[166] vinegar, potassium permanganate, herbal medications,[167] glutaraldehyde,[168] copper sulfate, and chloroxylenol (Dettol). Milder damage to the mucosa occurs after use of monobasic or dibasic sodium phosphate enemas[169] and bisacodyl suppositories. Colonic damage presumably occurs from a detergent, hypertonic, or direct toxic effect on the mucosa. The severity of the reaction depends on the type and concentration of the substance, the duration and extent of contact with the mucosa, and perhaps the presence of underlying colonic disease.

Soaps consist of a number of substances, including strong alkali, potash, phenol, and sodium and potassium salts of long-chain fatty acids. These agents produce liquefaction necrosis with mild to severe inflammation and saponification of the layers of the colon wall. Acute histologic changes include necrosis, leading, in more severe cases, to ulceration and formation of granulation tissue. Acute colitis may heal with fibrosis and scarring or progress to transmural necrosis and perforation. The severity of damage probably is related to the concentration of soap and duration of mucosal contact. Endoscopic findings have ranged from loss of the normal mucosal vascular pattern to mucosal sloughing and ulceration.

Hydrogen peroxide enemas are no longer frequently used, but at one time they were employed to relieve meconium ileus and remove fecal impactions. There are reports of severe damage associated with use of hydrogen peroxide, including severe colitis, pneumatosis coli, perforation, sepsis, and death. Within minutes of contact, diffuse mucosal emphysema occurs, and after about 1 hour, the colon may become ischemic and eventually ulcerated. A similar reaction has been reported after glutaraldehyde.[168]

Colitis has been reported following the use of several hyperosmolar water-soluble contrast materials that often are employed to opacify partial colon obstructions and to treat fecal impactions in adults.[166] Damage is believed to occur because of the hypertonicity of these agents, but the addition of Tween 80 may contribute to mucosal damage because of its detergent properties. Most reports of injury have occurred in the colon proximal to an obstruction and mainly in the right colon, suggesting that prolonged contact with these agents predisposes to mucosal injury.

Prevention and Treatment

Proper cleaning and rinsing of endoscopes are required to minimize exposure of the patient to injurious disinfecting chemicals. Protocols require strict adherence to proper maintenance and adjustments in the rinse cycle of disinfecting machines.[170] Forced air drying and rinsing of endoscope channels and the exterior of the instrument should assure a chemical-free procedure.

Patients and health care professionals should be admonished that soapsuds enemas should never be used. Rectal instillation of substances other than commercially available enemas for medicinal or ritualistic activities should be discouraged.

Treatment of chemical colitis is largely supportive, with intravenous fluids and broad-spectrum antibiotics. Surgery may be indicated in severe cases of bowel necrosis leading to gangrene or perforation. Most patients will recover completely after 4 to 6 weeks.

MALAKOPLAKIA

Malakoplakia is a rare chronic granulomatous disease first described by Michaelis and Gutmann in 1902.[171] The word *malakoplakia* is derived from the Greek "*malakos*" (soft) and "*plakos*" (plaque). The condition appears grossly as friable, yellow granulomas on the mucosa. Microscopically, coliform bacteria are located in the cytoplasm of macrophages in the muscularis propria (von Hansemann bodies), and calcified intracytoplasmic inclusion bodies (Michaelis-Gutmann bodies) are found.[172]

Malakoplakia may affect many organs, including lung, brain, adrenal glands, pancreas, and bone, but most commonly affects the genitourinary tract.[173] Colorectal malakoplakia was first described by Terner and Lattes in 1965.[174] As of 1995, only 85 cases of malakoplakia of the gastrointestinal tract had been documented.[175] The most common sites of colonic involvement are the rectum, sigmoid, and right colon, in descending order of frequency.[175]

Etiology

The pathogenesis of the disease is unknown. Proposed etiologies are an infection, immunosuppression, systemic illness, neoplasia, and genetic disorder. Evidence for an infectious etiology is based on the finding that some patients with malakoplakia have associated chronic infections. The presence of chronic infection was first described in the urologic form of malakoplakia in which more than 75% of patients were infected with *Escherichia coli*. This finding led to a belief that *Escherichia coli* might be a primary cause of malakoplakia. However, other organisms also have been isolated, including *Klebsiella*, *Proteus*, *Mycobacterium*, *Staphylococcus*, and fungi[176] suggesting that infection is not the primary cause of the disease.

Current evidence points to a defect in macrophage killing as the cause of malakoplakia. Nondigested microorganisms are found within the lysosomes of macrophages in affected persons. The macrophages from these patients show a decrease in cyclic guanosine monophosphate (cGMP), resulting in impaired bactericidal activity.[177] Peripheral blood monocytes also are found to have decreased bactericidal activity. The defect in macrophage dysfunction may be reversed with the addition of a cholinergic agonist, both in vitro and in vivo.[178]

An association between immunosuppression and malakoplakia also has been documented. Malakoplakia has been reported in patients receiving chemotherapy or immunosuppressive therapy for organ transplantation.[179] Reversal of both macrophage abnormalities and clinical symptoms occurred after discontinuation of glucocorticoids and azathioprine.[180] Malakoplakia has been reported in various immune deficient states such as primary hypogammaglobulinemia and the acquired immunodeficiency syndrome (AIDS).[181, 182] Malakoplakia also has been associated with chronic systemic diseases such as systemic lupus erythematosus, ulcerative colitis, and sarcoidosis.[175]

There have been a substantial number of cases to support a neoplastic etiology for malakoplakia. A review by Bates and colleagues in 1996 identified 19 cases of colorectal adenocarcinoma associated with malakoplakia.[183] Evidence for an etiologic role of the neoplasm was supported by the observation that malakoplakia was present only as a focal area adjacent to the tumor, in contrast to cases not associated with a neoplasm, in which multiple organs may be affected. A genetic etiology also has been suggested by one report of colonic malakoplakia that clustered in a family.[184]

Clinical Features and Diagnosis

Patients usually present with abdominal pain, diarrhea, hematochezia, and fever.[175] Physical findings include a palpable rectal mass, abdominal mass, and weight loss. Diagnosis is best made by colonoscopy and biopsy; these generally reveal three patterns of the disease:

1. Isolated rectosigmoid involvement. The lesions appear as yellowish plaques that may be sessile, polypoid, and ulcerated. The colonic lumen may be strictured, and intestinal fistulas may occur, suggesting a diagnosis of cancer or Crohn's disease;
2. Diffuse colonic involvement, which is characteristic of immunosuppressed patients;
3. Focal lesions, which may be associated with an adenomatous polyp or cancer.

Biopsy is essential to confirm the diagnosis and to exclude an underlying colonic malignancy (Fig. 118–11). The histology reveals the classic von Hansemann bodies (intracellular organisms) and Michaelis-Gutmann bodies (intracytoplasmic inclusion bodies). The histiocytes must be distinguished from those found in fungal disease, leprosy, Whipple's disease, reticulum cell sarcoma, and macrophages harboring *Mycobacterium avium* complex.[182]

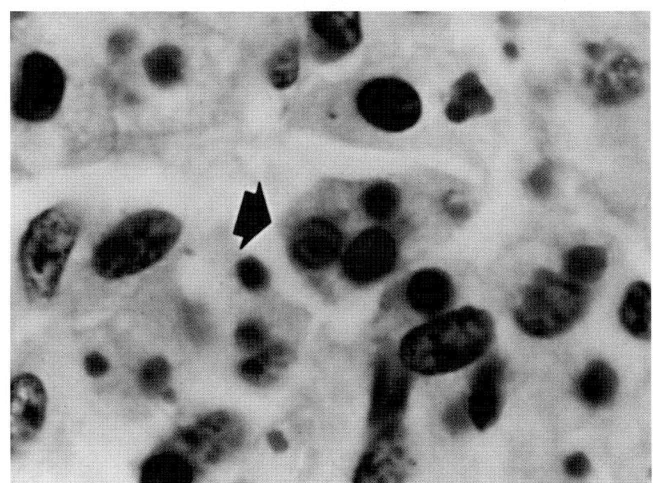

Figure 118–11. Malakoplakia, histology. Sheets of large pale histiocytes characterize the histologic change in malakoplakia. High-power view of one of these histiocytes *(arrow)* containing the characteristic dark, concentrically laminated Michaelis-Gutmann bodies. Hematoxylin-eosin stain; magnification, ×2000. (Courtesy of R. L. Goldman, M.D.)

Treatment

Patients with newly diagnosed malakoplakia should undergo a thorough medical evaluation to determine the presence of coexisting medical illnesses, malnutrition, or immunosuppressive medications. Tests of immune function and screening for bladder malakoplakia and colorectal cancer are prudent. Patients receiving immunosuppressive medications may improve after these medications are discontinued. Antibiotics such as trimethoprim-sulfamethoxazole and ciprofloxacin have been successful in treating malakoplakia.[185, 186] Both antibiotics appear to kill the bacteria associated with malakoplakia and can penetrate the defective host macrophages. Cholinergic agents also may be useful in treating children with malakoplakia.[178] Surgical resection of the involved colon is recommended for cases associated with carcinoma or severe bleeding.

PNEUMATOSIS COLI (PNEUMATOSIS CYSTOIDES INTESTINALIS)

The term *pneumatosis coli* is synonymous with pneumatosis cystoides intestinalis when the disorder is limited to the colon. The disease is uncommon and of undetermined etiology. It is characterized by multiple gas-filled cysts located in the submucosa and subserosa of the intestine. The majority of cases of pneumatosis cystoides intestinalis occur in the jejunum and ileum, with only 6% of cases involving the colon. There is a propensity for involvement of the left side of the colon.[187] Numerous conditions have been associated with pneumatosis cystoides intestinalis, including appendicitis, Crohn's disease[188] ulcerative colitis,[189] diverticular disease,[189, 190] necrotizing enterocolitis, pseudomembranous colitis,[191] ileus,[192] and sigmoid volvulus.[193] Pneumatosis also has been associated with nongastrointestinal conditions, including emphysema, collagen vascular diseases,[192, 194] transplantation,[194] AIDS,[195] glucocorticoid use, and chemotherapy.[192] In approximately 20% of cases, there are no associated medical conditions and pneumatosis is considered primary.[196]

Etiology

Several theories have been suggested to explain the large and varied number of conditions associated with pneumatosis cystoides intestinalis. Three of the more common theories are (1) the mechanical theory, (2) the pulmonary theory, and (3) the bacterial theory.

According to the mechanical theory, luminal gas enters the bowel wall through a defect in the intestinal mucosa. The mucosal defect may occur from direct trauma or increased intraluminal pressure. This hypothesis could account for reports of pneumatosis after sigmoidoscopy without biopsy[197]; with colitis, perforated duodenal ulcers, and jejunal diverticula; and after intestinal anastomoses. The absence of a connection between the mucosa and the cysts diminishes the plausibility of this theory.

According to the pulmonary theory, severe coughing in a patient with chronic obstructive lung disease leads to rupture of a pulmonary bleb, and the air from the ruptured bleb dissects through the mediastinum into the retroperitoneum and along the perivascular spaces to lodge in the subserosa of the intestine. The absence of gas in the mediastinum and the frequent finding of localized cysts argue against this theory.

The bacterial theory suggests that the cystic gas collections are the by-products of bacteria. This theory has been supported by clinical observations and laboratory experiments. Pneumatosis cystoides intestinalis has been observed in premature infants with necrotizing enterocolitis. In laboratory animals, pneumatosis coli also can be induced by injecting gas-forming bacteria into the bowel wall.[198] In addition to local invasion of the intestinal wall, bacteria may produce gas cysts by manufacturing large amounts of hydrogen gas as a result of the fermentation of carbohydrates. Levitt and Olsson theorized that the high hydrogen tension in the colonic lumen leads to rapid diffusion into an intramural gas bubble and may cause N_2, O_2, and CO_2 to diffuse from the circulation into the gas bubble.[199] According to their theory, the gas bubble enlarges if there is continued diffusion of hydrogen into it. Indeed, high hydrogen content in the cysts has been documented[200]; breath hydrogen levels, indicative of carbohydrate malabsorption, are increased in affected persons; and cysts regress in patients fed an elemental diet to decrease carbohydrate substrate for colonic bacteria.[201] Successful treatment with antibiotics[200, 202] and colonic washouts[200] also supports a bacterial etiology for pneumatosis coli. In one study, stools from patients with pneumatosis coli were demonstrated to lack two major hydrogen-consuming bacteria.[203] Because hydrogen is normally produced only in the colon and not in the small intestine, pneumatosis coli may differ from pneumatosis intestinalis with respect to pathogenic mechanisms.

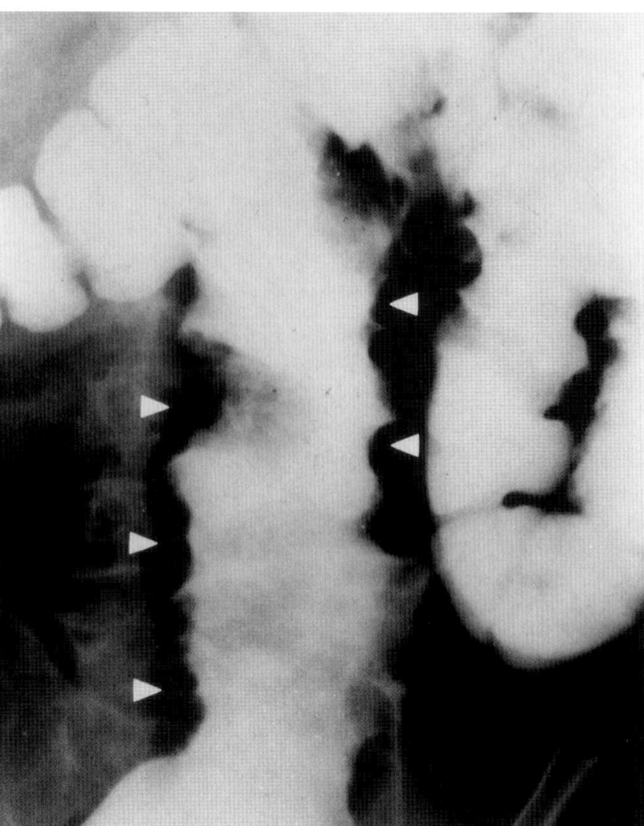

Figure 118–12. Single-contrast barium enema demonstrating the presence of gas-filled pockets in the wall of the colon, characteristic of pneumatosis coli *(arrows).* Gas in the bowel wall can be benign, as it was in this patient, or can be associated with underlying disease such as ischemia. (From Feldman M, Boland CR [eds]: Slide Atlas of Gastroenterology and Hepatology. Philadelphia, Current Medicine, 1996.)

Clinical Features and Diagnosis

The frequency of pneumatosis coli is highest in the 6th decade, with equal frequency in men and women.[196] In the majority of cases, pneumatosis is an unexpected finding on an abdominal radiograph. When symptoms occur, the most common are diarrhea (68%), mucus discharge (68%), rectal bleeding (60%), and constipation (48%).[196] Approximately 3% of patients present with a complication of pneumatosis coli, including pneumoperitoneum, volvulus, intestinal obstruction, intussusception, tension pneumoperitoneum, hemorrhage, and intestinal perforation.[204] Physical examination may detect an abdominal mass, and rectal examination may reveal the cystic lesions. A plain abdominal radiograph may identify radiolucent clusters along the bowel and pneumoperitoneum, if a cyst has ruptured. A markedly redundant sigmoid colon as well as the outline of the cysts may be seen on barium enema (Fig. 118–12).[196] Endoscopic examination with biopsy is necessary for definitive diagnosis, to exclude carcinoma, and to differentiate pneumatosis from familial adenomatosis polyposis.[205] The endoscopic appearance is of multiple cysts, which vary in size from a few millimeters to several centimeters (Fig. 118–13). On pathologic examination, the bowel is seen to have a characteristic honeycombed appearance, with no communication between the air spaces and the bowel lumen. The characteristic microscopic appearance is that of cystic spaces lined by large macrophages in the submucosa (Fig. 118–14).

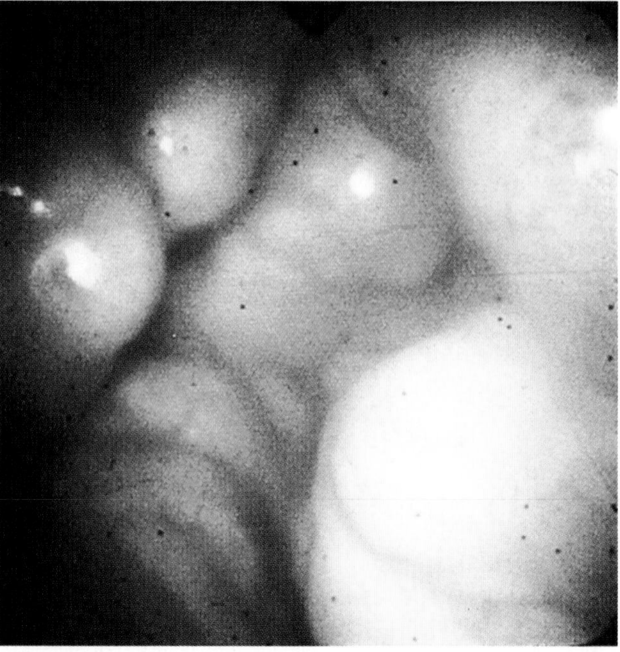

Figure 118–13. Colonoscopic view of pneumatosis coli demonstrating numerous gas-filled cysts in the submucosa.

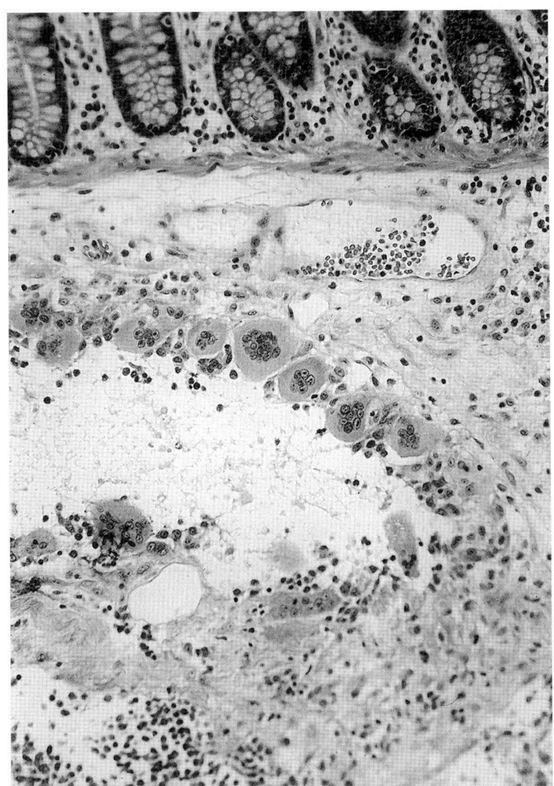

Figure 118–14. High-power histologic view of a gas-filled cyst in the submucosa lined by histiocytes and multinucleated giant cells in a patient with pneumatosis coli. Such cysts may also be present in the subserosa. (Courtesy of Edward Lee, M.D., Dallas, TX.)

Treatment

Because the natural history of pneumatosis is one of spontaneous regression in up to 50% of cases and because cysts may reappear after surgery, specific treatment is not recommended in asymptomatic individuals. Symptomatic patients may be treated successfully by breathing high-flow oxygen for several days. There have been a number of reports of dramatic responses with this approach.[190, 206] It appears that high oxygen levels lead to replacement of hydrogen within the cysts with a corresponding reduction in the size of the cysts. Because cysts may recur after oxygen therapy,[206] a minimum of 48 hours of oxygen therapy is recommended to maximize the success rate. Metronidazole also has been reported to be efficacious in treating pneumatosis coli, an observation which suggests that anaerobic bacteria play a role in the genesis of the disorder. Because cysts have been reported to recur after short courses of metronidazole,[202] treatment should continue until complete endoscopic resolution of the cysts is seen. In general, colonic resection is reserved for patients with complications such as intestinal obstruction and massive bleeding.

COLITIS CYSTICA PROFUNDA

Colitis cystica profunda is a rare disease characterized by mucin-filled cysts located in the submucosa of the large intestine (Fig. 118–15). The disease was first described in 1766 by Stark, who reported two cases associated with dysentery.[207] There are three patterns of disease: (1) localized with a polypoid lesion, (2) diffuse with multiple polypoid lesions, and (3) diffuse with a confluent sheet of cysts.

Etiology

The etiology of colitis cystica profunda is unknown, but several theories have been proposed. A possible congenital etiology is supported by several findings. In embryologic examinations, submucosal cysts have been found in multiple gastrointestinal locations. The occurrence of colitis cystica profunda in children and its association with other congenital conditions such as Peutz-Jeghers syndrome[208] also support a congenital origin for this disease. However, the absence of submucosal cysts in large autopsy series of infants and children reduces the plausibility of this etiology.

Colitis cystica profunda also has been associated with acquired diseases that predispose to ulceration and inflammation of the mucosa. These diseases include ulcerative colitis,[209] Crohn's disease,[210] and infectious colitis.[211] Submucosal cysts also have been reported in areas exposed to local trauma, such as an intestinal anastomosis or colostomy.[212] Studies in animals support an inflammatory origin. Hubmann reported that proctitis cystica profunda occurred in rats treated with irradiation.[213] Brynjolfsson and Haley described the occurrence of colitis cystica profunda at small bowel stomas.[213a]

Colitis cystica profunda also has been found in association with adenocarcinoma of the colon,[57, 183] suggesting a neoplastic etiology. Several cases of adenocarcinoma of the stomach associated with gastritis cystica profunda have been reported.[214] In some reports, there is strong evidence of a causal link between cancer and colitis cystica profunda, because the submucosal cysts are often found adjacent to the adenocarcinoma, whereas adjacent benign mucosa is devoid of submucosal cysts.

The localized form of colitis cystica profunda is associated with rectal prolapse and SRUS.[207] Mucosal prolapse has been found in 54% of patients with the localized form of the

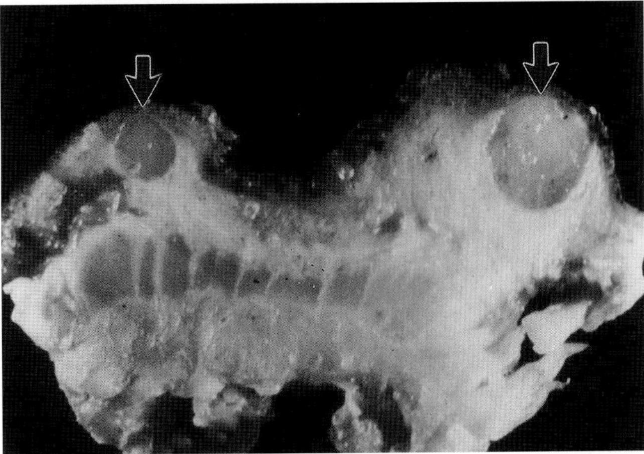

Figure 118–15. Gross resection specimen of colitis cystica profunda. Several submucosal cysts *(arrows)* are filled with mucinous material. (From Feldman M, Boland CR [eds]: Slide Atlas of Gastroenterology and Hepatology. Philadelphia, Current Medicine, 1996.)

disease. Trauma or ischemia caused by chronic traction on the mucosa and intramural vessels may play a role in the development of the submucosal cysts. Microscopic features of the localized form of the disease often include fibrosis of the lamina propria and hypertrophic muscle fibers, changes that are characteristic of SRUS.[215]

Clinical Features and Diagnosis

Colitis cystica profunda affects men and women equally. The most common symptoms are rectal bleeding, mucus discharge, and diarrhea.[207] Less common are tenesmus, abdominal pain, and rectal pain. Rarely, the patient may present with intestinal obstruction secondary to the cysts.[216] At endoscopy, the majority of lesions are located on the anterior rectal wall 6 to 7 cm from the anal verge. The lesions appear as polyps with overlying mucosa that may be normal, inflamed, or ulcerated. Endoscopy may disclose an associated rectal prolapse in some cases. The endoscopic appearance of the lesions may be indistinguishable from a variety of lesions, including adenocarcinoma, adenomatous polyps, submucosal lipoma, neurofibroma, inflammatory pseudopolyps of ulcerative colitis or Crohn's disease, pneumatosis coli, and endometriosis.[207] Barium enema may reveal radiolucent filling defects.[198] Transrectal ultrasound may be useful in differentiating this disease from cancer. Ultrasound reveals hypoechoic cysts that may be surrounded by intact submucosa, unlike invasive cancer.[217] Biopsy is necessary to differentiate this lesion from a variety of inflammatory (i.e., Crohn's disease, ulcerative colitis), neoplastic (i.e., adenocarcinoma, adenomatous polyps, colloid carcinoma) and infectious (i.e., amebiasis, herpes) conditions. On biopsy, the submucosa is seen to be thickened by the presence of the mucus-filled cysts (Fig. 118–16). The cysts usually communicate with the lumen through small openings in the mucosa. Although usually confined to the submucosa, cysts involving the muscularis propria and serosa have been reported. The surrounding connective tissue often shows chronic inflammation, and there may be extensive replacement of the lamina propria by fibroblasts.[215]

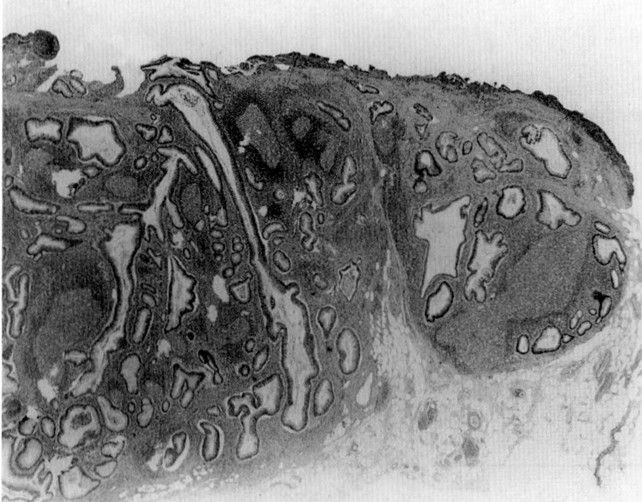

Figure 118–16. Low-power histologic view of colitis cystica profunda. There is extension of glandular mucosa into submucosal sites of previous injury with several submucosal cysts, some of which contain mucinous material. (Courtesy of Dr. Sidney Finkelstein, University of Pittsburgh Medical Center.)

Treatment

A high-fiber diet and bowel retraining have led to regression of this disease in a few cases.[218] Glucocorticoid enemas also have been used with some success.[207] However, the majority of patients have been treated with surgery. In patients with associated rectal prolapse, repair of the prolapse alone may treat the colitis cystica profunda successfully,[219] whereas for disease localized to the rectum, local excision through a transanal approach is efficacious.[200] When the disease is localized to the rectum but is circumferential, total excision may be accomplished by mucosal sleeve resection and coloanal pull-through.[220] More diffuse lesions have been removed with segmental resections. Segmental resection may be necessary for large obstructing lesions and for lesions that cause severe anemia from chronic blood loss, hypokalemia, and hypoalbuminemia. A diverting colostomy may lead to regression of this disease and may be the best option for the patient with significant comorbidities.

NEUTROPENIC ENTEROCOLITIS (TYPHLITIS)

Neutropenic enterocolitis (typhlitis) is a potentially life-threatening condition associated with neutropenia related to chemotherapy. The entity was described initially by Wagner in 1970 in children undergoing chemotherapy for leukemia.[221] The disease commonly affects the ileum and cecum and may result in intestinal perforation. The frequency in persons at risk varies from 1% to 46%.[222] Neutropenic enterocolitis has been described in patients with leukemias treated with cytosine arabinoside,[223] solid tumors treated with combination chemotherapy, organ transplants, and AIDS.[224–227]

Etiology

The etiology of neutropenic enterocolitis may be multifactorial. The initial injury is an ulceration of the bowel mucosa with no associated inflammatory response. Mucosal injury may occur secondary to leukemic infiltration, stasis of bowel contents, or mucosal ischemia from splanchnic vasoconstriction resulting from sepsis.[226, 228, 229] Certain drugs also may contribute to mucosal damage. Cytosine arabinoside can cause necrosis and delayed regeneration of intestinal glandular epithelium.[230] Vinca alkaloids used to treat leukemia also may contribute to cecal distention by damaging the myenteric plexus of the intestine. With mucosal injury in the setting of impaired host defenses, infectious colitis subsequently occurs. The infection is often polymicrobial; causative bacteria include *E. coli*, *Staphylococcus aureus*, *Clostridia septicum*, and *Klebsiella* species.[231] Fungal organisms such as *Aspergillus* and *Candida* also have been isolated.[231] In addition to transmural infection of the intestine, the cecum may become gangrenous and perforate as a result of increased distention and ischemia. The process may involve the ileum alone or both the ileum and cecum.[231]

Clinical Features and Diagnosis

The most common presentation is with fever, diarrhea, nausea, vomiting, and abdominal pain in a patient receiving antineoplastic drugs.[223, 232] Abdominal tenderness characteristically is localized to the right lower quadrant of the abdomen. Shock may occur as a result of bacteremia or intestinal perforation. On occasion, the sigmoid colon may be affected, further complicating the diagnosis.[233] Additionally, abdominal tenderness may be absent or masked by drugs such as prednisone. Alternatively, localized tenderness may progress rapidly to diffuse signs of peritonitis as a result of intestinal perforation. Neutropenia is noted, and blood cultures are positive in up to 50% of cases.[226, 231] The differential diagnosis includes appendicitis, pseudomembranous colitis, ischemic colitis, volvulus, diverticulitis, and drug-induced diarrhea.

The diagnostic work-up should include a radiologic evaluation to exclude other diseases, confirm the diagnosis, and determine the severity of illness. Abdominal radiographs may demonstrate dilated loops of small bowel with decreased air in the right lower quadrant and free intraperitoneal air if intestinal perforation has occurred (Fig. 118–17).[226] CT scans are most sensitive for establishing the diagnosis and help to exclude other conditions such as appendicitis and diverticulitis. The CT scan may reveal a thickened bowel wall, pneumatosis intestinalis, ascites, and free air.[234] Barium enema should be avoided because of the potential risk of perforation. Stool cultures for *C. difficile* toxin should be performed routinely to exclude pseudomembranous colitis.

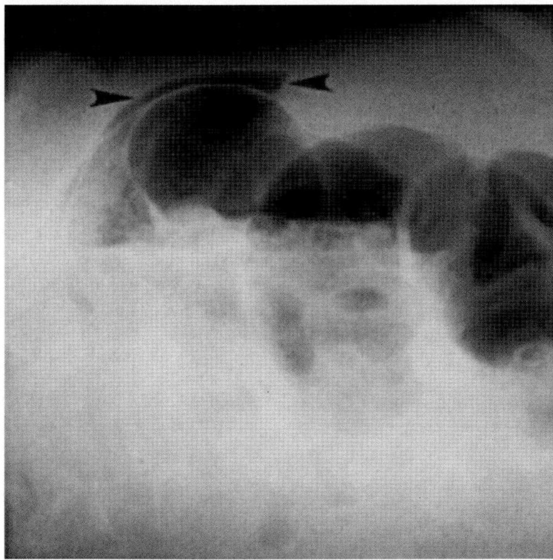

Figure 118–17. Neutropenic typhlitis, plain films. Left lateral decubitus radiograph in a patient with neutropenic typhlitis. The colon is dilated with a prominent intraluminal gas-fluid interface and free peritoneal air *(arrows)* resulting from cecal perforation. (From Hunger TB, Bjelland UJC: Gastrointestinal complications of leukemia and its treatment. AJR 142:513, 1984. Copyright American Roentgen Ray Society, 1984.)

Treatment

The management of neutropenic enterocolitis has varied. Approaches have included supportive measures alone, aggressive initial surgical resection, and combined medical and surgical treatment. Both successes and failures have been documented with all these approaches. In two studies, all patients treated medically recovered, whereas in another similar series, all patients managed medically died.[235] Clearly, successful management of patients with neutropenic enterocolitis needs to be individualized to optimize the outcome.

In general, medical management includes broad-spectrum antibiotics, nasogastric suction, and bowel rest. Fluid resuscitation with isotonic solutions is critical for maintaining renal perfusion in the face of decreased systemic vascular resistance from sepsis and intra-abdominal fluid sequestration. Close observation and serial abdominal and radiographic examinations are necessary to monitor the response to medical treatment. Antibiotics should have activity against enteric gram-negative organisms, gram-positive organisms, and anaerobes. Causative microorganisms include *Pseudomonas*, *S. aureus*, *E. coli*, and Group A *Streptococcus*.[231] For patients who do not respond to antibacterial agents, amphotericin should be considered, because fungemia is common.[231] Blood transfusions may be necessary because the diarrhea is often bloody. Granulocyte-macrophage colony–stimulating factor to correct the neutropenia appears to be a useful adjunct to medical therapy.[236] Early surgical intervention has been recommended in persons with a rapidly deteriorating course despite maximal medical therapy. Two series have shown a decreased mortality rate in patients with severe disease who are treated surgically compared with those treated medically.[235] For patients with complications such as frank gangrene, intestinal perforation, and shock despite vasopressor support, surgical intervention is mandatory.

Controversy surrounds the choice of an operation. Gangrenous or perforated bowel should be resected. When the bowel is edematous with no vascular compromise and no signs of perforation, successful management has included no resection,[237] intestinal diversion with no resection,[235] and resection of the involved bowel. If a resection is performed, construction of an ileostomy and mucous fistula may be the safest option, because the intestinal anastomosis may be prone to break down in patients with neutropenia.[238] Because recurrences of neutropenic enterocolitis are common when chemotherapy is restarted, right hemicolectomy is recommended before chemotherapy is resumed.[228]

ENDOMETRIOSIS

Endometriosis, defined as the presence of endometrial tissue outside the uterine cavity and musculature, was first described by von Rokitansky in 1860. Most often, these ectopic tissues lie in the vicinity of the uterus and reportedly occur in up to 15% of menstruating women and up to 30% of infertile women.[239] The initial description of nonpigmented endometriosis in 1986 resulted in a much higher prevalence of this disorder than appreciated previously.[240] In contrast to endometrial involvement of the female reproductive organs, gastrointestinal involvement is thought to be less common, usually asymptomatic, and clinically less important.[241] The most frequent intestinal organs involved are the rectosigmoid colon (96%), appendix (10%), and ileum (5%), with other organs involved uncommonly.[242] Nevertheless, intestinal endometriosis can mimic a wide variety of inflammatory, infectious, and neoplastic digestive disorders.[243]

Etiology and Pathogenesis

Several hypotheses have been advanced to explain the ectopic location of endometrial tissue.[244-246] The most commonly accepted is that of retrograde transportation of endometrial tissue, which then implants and grows on pelvic organs and the peritoneum. From these sites, more distant implants arise via hematogenous or lymphatic dissemination; further dissemination may occur during surgical interventions. A less accepted hypothesis, which has fewer supporting data, is that of endometrial metaplasia in which multipotential peritoneal mesothelial cells are induced by unknown factors to undergo metaplastic transformation to endometrial tissue.

Once implanted, endometrial tissue appears to be regulated by hormonal influences, so that estrogen promotes and progesterone inhibits growth. These cycles of growth and sloughing of tissues can lead to serosal irritation and progressive invasion of intestinal muscle with fibrosis and muscle hypertrophy. Thus, in some cases, pain may arise from nerve impingement or serosal inflammation, whereas obstruction may occur from luminal narrowing or intestinal kinking.

Clinical Features

Endometriosis is found almost exclusively in women of childbearing age, with clinical onset usually between the ages of 20 and 45 years.[242] Women who experience symptoms or who undergo surgery beyond menopause presumably have chronic fibrosis or exacerbations induced by exogenous estrogens.

Although most women with endometrial implants on intestinal structures have no symptoms, those with serosal implants may complain of localized tenderness, low backache, or abdominal pain. However, penetration of endometrial tissue into the bowel wall may produce constipation, diarrhea, and partial obstruction resulting in intermittent abdominal pain. Contrary to popular thinking, symptoms are not always cyclic and may not fluctuate with hormonal levels, nor are gastrointestinal symptoms necessarily associated with gynecologic symptoms. Rarely, hematochezia occurs when endometrial implants penetrate to the mucosa or when severe colonic fibrosis results in ischemia.[241]

Less common presentations occur with more proximal colonic or small intestinal involvement. These presentations include acute appendicitis caused by an obstructing endometrioma, small bowel intussusception, and volvulus.[243, 247]

Diagnosis

The clinical diagnosis of intestinal endometriosis may be difficult because often symptoms are nonspecific and there is no relationship between the symptoms and the menstrual cycle. However, endometriosis should always be considered in women with recurrent abdominal pain and bowel symptoms, especially if they are in their reproductive years and have gynecologic complaints. Diagnosis is especially difficult because irritable bowel syndrome is so common in women.

An important component of the evaluation is a careful pelvic examination that includes combined rectovaginal palpation. Finding tender nodules or irregularities in the cul-de-sac is highly suggestive of endometriosis. Because findings may vary considerably during the menstrual cycle, the pelvic examination should be performed immediately before and again after menstruation.

It is rare to see endometrial implants on the colonic mucosa except when there is hematochezia. Thus, colonoscopy is often normal except for areas of extrinsic compression or strictures with intact mucosa.[248] More helpful is an air-contrast barium enema, which will demonstrate submucosal polypoid masses or areas of noncircumferential narrowing of the lumen (Fig. 118–18). Diagnostic yield and accuracy may be enhanced by performance of these tests just before the onset of menses. Computed tomography (Fig. 118–19), ultrasonography, and magnetic resonance imaging have all been reported to assist with the diagnosis or assessment of the extent of endometrial involvement.[249] Endovaginal and transrectal ultrasonography also may be useful in detecting small endometrial implants.

The definitive diagnosis is often made by laparoscopy or laparotomy with biopsy and is especially useful in patients with intestinal implants without pelvic involvement. The ap-

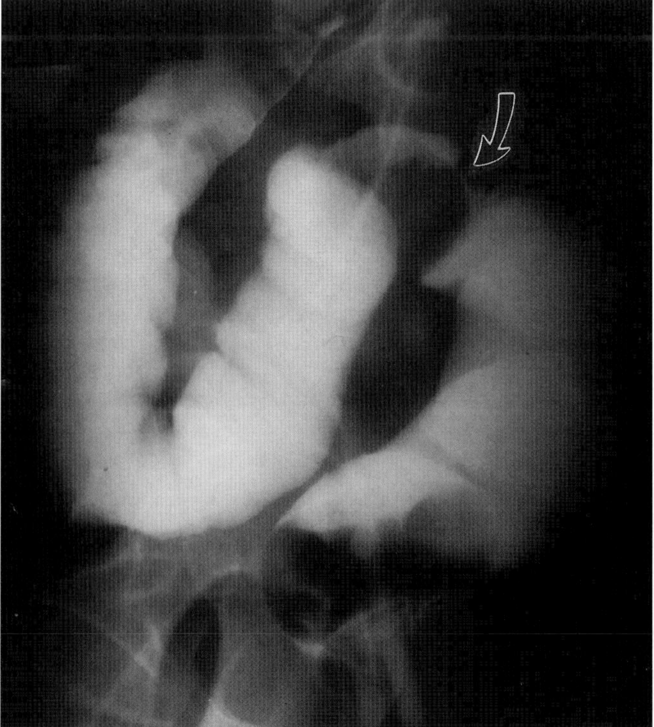

Figure 118–18. Single-contrast barium enema demonstrating a large nodular partially obstructing endometrioma in the rectosigmoid colon *(arrow)*. (Courtesy of Dr. Mark Peterson, University of Pittsburgh Medical Center.)

preciation that endometrial tissue may be nonpigmented has increased the yield of these procedures considerably.[240]

The differential diagnosis of intestinal endometriosis includes inflammatory disorders such as Crohn's ileitis and colitis, ulcerative colitis with stricture, diverticulitis, infectious diseases such as ileocolonic tuberculosis and schistosomiasis, benign and malignant neoplastic disorders, and colonic ischemia.[243] It is important to emphasize that no radiographic or imaging finding is pathognomonic of endometriosis, that mucosal abnormalities which permit positive biopsies are rare, and that tissue for a definitive diagnosis is usually obtained only at laparotomy (Fig. 118–20).

Treatment

In general, when a diagnosis of serosal intestinal endometriosis is made, hormonal therapy is often the first therapeutic option, similar to the standard approach to pelvic endometriosis.[250, 251] Low-dose estrogen-progestin compounds cause a pseudopregnancy state that results in decidualization of endometrial tissue and often relieves dysmenorrhea. However, their use in more severe disease is questionable, and they are generally not recommended for symptomatic intestinal disease.

The most effective agents currently available are the synthetic androgen danazol and the gonadotropin-releasing hormone (GnRH) agonists.[252, 253] Both act to decrease ovarian steroid synthesis by inhibiting pituitary release of follicle-stimulating hormone (FSH) and luteinizing hormone (LH). Although both are effective in decreasing pelvic pain associated with endometriosis and appear to decrease the size of endometrial implants, there are no studies of these agents in intestinal disease, and there is some concern that treatment may result in increased fibrosis and inadequate symptom resolution.[254, 255] Ablation of endometrial implants on surfaces that can be visualized laparoscopically can be accomplished using a laparoscopic carbon dioxide laser.[256]

For endometriosis that causes partial obstruction of the colon or small intestine, segmental resection of the involved area is considered to provide the best results and also serves to exclude an underlying carcinoma.[257, 260] Resection can be performed by laparoscopic techniques or by open surgery, according to available expertise. If the patient is postmenopausal or if future pregnancies are not wanted, hysterectomy and bilateral salpingo-oophorectomy can be done at the time of resective surgery to minimize the risk of symptomatic disease in the future. Similar surgery also can be performed in premenopausal women who have failed medical therapy and who have intractable symptoms.

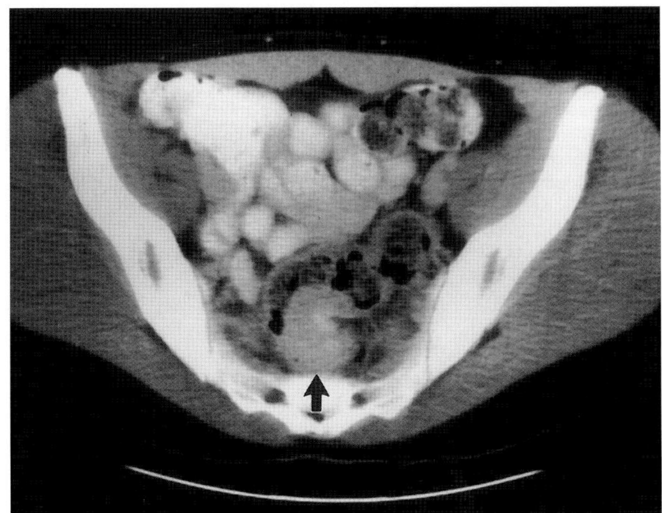

Figure 118–19. Computed tomographic scan of the same patient in Figure 118–18 showing the endometrial mass in the cul-de-sac *(arrow)* extending into the colon. (Courtesy of Dr. Mark Peterson, University of Pittsburgh Medical Center.)

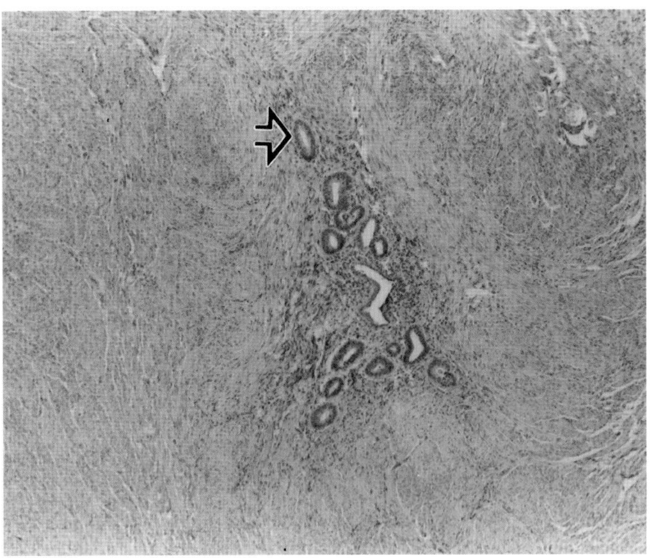

Figure 118–20. Histologic specimen showing a focus of endometrial glands *(arrow)* in the muscularis propria of the colon. (Courtesy of Dr. Sidney Finkelstein, University of Pittsburgh Medical Center.)

REFERENCES

1. Carley M, Schaffer J: Urinary incontinence and pelvic organ prolapse in women with Marfan or Ehlers-Danlos syndrome. Am J Obstet Gynecol 182:1021, 2000.
2. Gooley N, Kuhnke M, Eusebio E: Acute transanal ileal evisceration. Dis Colon Rectum 30:479, 1987.
3. Basson R: Association of rectal prolapse with colorectal cancer. Surgery 119:51, 1996.
4. Corman M, Veidenheimer M, Coller J: Managing rectal prolapse. Geriatrics 29:87, 1974.
5. Birnbaum E, Stamm L, Rafferty J, et al: Pudendal nerve terminal motor latency influences surgical outcome in treatment of rectal prolapse. Dis Colon Rectum 39:1215, 1996.
6. Agachan F, Pfeifer J, Wexner S: Defecography and proctography: Results of 744 patients. Dis Colon Rectum 39:899, 1996.
7. Wolff B, Dietzen C: Abdominal resectional procedures for rectal prolapse. Semin Colon Rectal Surg 2:184, 1991.
8. Cirocco W, Brown A: Anterior resection for the treatment of rectal prolapse: A 20-year experience. Am Surg 59:265, 1993.
9. Novell J, Osborne M, Winslet M, Lewis A: Prosepctive randomized trial of Ivalon sponge versus sutured rectopexy for full-thickness rectal prolapse. Br J Surg 81:904, 1994.
10. Winde G, Reers B, Nottberg H, et al: Clinical and functional results of abdominal rectopexy with absorbable mesh-graft for the treatment of complete rectal prolapse. Eur J Surg 159:301, 1993.
11. Keighley M, Fielding J, Alexander-Williams J: Results of Marlex mesh abdominal rectopexy for rectal prolapse in 100 consecutive patients. Br J Surg 70:229, 1983.
12. Tjandra J, Fazio V, Church J, et al: Ripstein procedure is an effective

treatment for rectal prolapse without constipation. Dis Colon Rectum 36:501, 1993.

13. Schultz IM, Mellgren AM, Dolk AM, et al: Long-term results and functional outcome after Ripstein rectopexy. Dis Colon Rectum 43:35, 2000.
14. Watts J, Rothenberger D, Buls J, et al: The management of procidentia: 30 years' experience. Dis Colon Rectum 28:96, 1985.
15. McKee R, Lauder J, Poon F, et al: A prospective randomized study of abdominal rectopexy with and without sigmoidectomy in rectal prolapse. Surg Gynecol Obstet 174:145, 1992.
16. Bruch H-PM, Herold AM, Schiedeck TM, Schwandner OM: Laparoscopic surgery for rectal prolapse and outlet obstruction. Dis Colon Rectum 42:1189, 1999.
17. Kessler H, Jerby B, Milsom J: Successful treatment of rectal prolapse by laparoscopic suture rectopexy. Surg Endosc 13:858, 1999.
18. Heah S, Hartley J, Hurley J, et al: Laparoscopic suture rectopexy without resection is effective treatment for full-thickness rectal prolapse. Dis Colon Rectum 43:638, 2000.
19. Ramanujam P, Venkatesh K, Fietz M: Perianal excision of rectal procidentia in elderly high-risk patients. Dis Colon Rectum 37:1027, 1994.
20. Williams J, Rothenberger D, Madoff R, Goldberg S: Treatment of rectal prolapse in the elderly by perineal rectosigmoidectomy. Dis Colon Rectum 35:830, 1992.
21. Altemeier W, Culbertson W, Schowengerdt C, Hunt J: Nineteen years' experience with one-stage perianal repair of rectal prolapse. Ann Surg 173:993, 1971.
22. Yoshioka K, Ogunbiyi O, Keighley M: Pouch perianal rectosigmoidectomy gives better functional results than conventional rectosigmoidectomy in elderly patients with rectal prolapse. Br J Surg 85:1525, 1998.
23. Kim D-S, Tsang C, Wong W, et al: Complete rectal prolapse. Evolution of management and results. Dis Colon Rectum 42:460, 1999.
24. Oliver G, Vachon D, Eisenstat T, et al: Delorme's procedure for complete rectal prolapse in severely debilitated patients: An analysis of 41 cases. Dis Colon Rectum 37:461, 1994.
25. Lieberman H, Hughes C, Dippolito A: Evaluation and outcome of the Delorme procedure in the treatment of rectal outlet obstruction. Dis Colon Rectum 43:188, 2000.
26. Watts A, Thompson M: Evaluation of Delorme's procedure as a treatment for full-thickness rectal prolapse. Br J Surg 87:218, 2000.
27. Hunt T, Fraser I, Maybury N: Treatment of rectal prolapse by sphincter support using Silastic rods. Br J Surg 72:491, 1985.
28. Heine J, Wong W: Rectal prolapse. In Mazier WP, Levien DH, Luchtefeld MA, Senagore AJ (eds): Surgery of the Colon, Rectum, and Anus. Philadelphia, WB Saunders, 1995, p 515.
29. Martin C, Parks T, Biggart J: Solitary rectal ulcer syndrome in Northern Ireland, 1971–1980. Br J Surg 68:744, 1981.
30. Thompson H, Hill D: Solitary rectal ulcer: Always a self-induced condition? Br J Surg 67:784, 1980.
31. Eckardt V, Kanzler G, Remmele W: Anorectal ergotism: Another cause of solitary rectal ulcers. Gastroenterology 91:1123, 1986.
32. Crowe J, Stellato T: Radiation-induced solitary rectal ulcer. Dis Colon Rectum 28:610, 1985.
33. Mackle E, Parks T: The pathogenesis and pathophysiology of rectal prolapse and solitary rectal ulcer syndrome. Clin Gastroenterol 15:985, 1986.
34. Kuijpers H, Schreve R, ten Cate Hoedmakers H: Diagnosis of functional disorders of defecation causing the solitary rectal syndrome. Dis Colon Rectum 29:126, 1986.
35. Tjandra J, Fazio V, Church J, et al: Clinical conundrum of solitary rectal ulcer. Dis Colon Rectum 35:227, 1992.
36. du Boulay C, Fairbrother J, Isaacson P: Mucosal prolapse syndrome—a unifying concept for solitary ulcer syndrome and related disorders. J Clin Pathol 36:1264, 1983.
37. Attenoos R, Billings P, Hughes L, Williams G: Ileostomy polyps, adenomas and adenocarcinomas. Gut 37:840, 1995.
38. Jones P, Lubowski D, Swash M, et al: Is paradoxical contraction of puborectalis muscle of functional importance? Dis Colon Rectum 30: 667, 1987.
39. Snooks S, Nicholls R, Henry M, et al: Electrophysiological and manometric assessment of the pelvic floor in the solitary rectal ulcer syndrome. Br J Surg 72:131, 1985.
40. Kennedy D, Hughes E, Masterson J: The natural history of benign ulcer of the rectum. Surg Gynecol Obstet 144:718, 1975.
41. Tandon R, Atmakuri S, Mehra N, et al: Is solitary rectal ulcer a manifestation of a systemic disease? J Clin Gastroenterol 12:286, 1990.
42. Lam T, Lubowski D, King D: Solitary rectal ulcer syndrome. Baillieres Clin Gastroenterol 6:129, 1992.
43. Malik A, Bhaskar K, Kochhar R, et al: Solitary rectal ulcer of the rectum—a histopathologic characterisation of 33 biopsies. Indian J Pathol Microbiol 33:216, 1990.
44. Tsuschida K, Okayama N, Miyata M: Solitary rectal ulcer syndrome accompanied by submucosal invasive carcinoma. Am J Gastroenterol 93:2235, 1998.
45. Li S, Hamilton S: Malignant tumors in the rectum simulating solitary rectal ulcer syndrome in endoscopic biopsy specimens. Am J Surg Pathol 22:106, 1998.
46. Mönkemuller K, Lewis J Jr, Ruiz F, et al: Association of solitary rectal ulcer syndrome and mucinous adenocarcinoma of the rectum. Am J Gastroenterol 91:2031, 1996.
47. Van Outryve M, Pelckmans P, Fierens H, Van Maercke Y: Transrectal ultrasound study of the pathogenesis of solitary rectal ulcer syndrome. Gut 34:1422, 1993.
48. Halligan S, Sultan A, Rottenberg G, Bartram C: Endosonography of the anal sphincters in solitary rectal ulcer syndrome. Int J Colorectal Dis 10:79, 1995.
49. Halligan S, Nicholls R, Bartram C: Proctographic changes after rectopexy for solitary rectal ulcer syndrome and preoperative predictive factors for a successful outcome. Br J Surg 82:314, 1995.
50. Malatjalian D, Williams C: 5-ASA therapy in solitary rectal ulcer syndrome. Report of three patients. Can J Gastroenterol 2:18, 1988.
51. Zagar S, Khuroo M, Mahajan R: Sucralfate retention enemas in solitary rectal ulcer. Dis Colon Rectum 34:455, 1991.
52. Ederle A, Bulighin G, Orlandi P, Pilati S: Endoscopic application of human fibrin sealant in the treatment of solitary recal ulcer syndrome. Endoscopy 24:736, 1992.
53. van den Brandt Gradel V, Huibregtse K, Tytgat G: Treatment of solitary rectal ulcer syndrome with high-fiber diet and abstention of straining at defecation. Dig Dis Sci 29:1005, 1984.
54. Vaizey C, Roy A, Kamm M: Prospective evaluation of the treatment of solitary rectal syndrome with biofeedback. Gut 41:817, 1997.
55. Kang Y, Kamm M, Nicholls R: Solitary rectal ulcer and complete rectal prolapse: One condition or two? Int J Colorectal Dis 10:87, 1995.
56. Halligan S, Nicholls R, Bartram C: Evacuation proctography in patients with solitary rectal ulcer syndrome: Anatomic abnormalities and frequency of impaired emptying and prolapse. AJR Am J Roentgenol 164:91, 1995.
57. Sitzler P, Kamm M, Nicholls R, McKee R: Long-term clinical outcome of surgery for solitary rectal ulcer syndrome. Br J Surg 85:1246, 1998.
58. Ona FV, Allende HD, Vivenio R, et al: Diagnosis and management of nonspecific colon ulcer. Arch Surg 117:888, 1982.
59. Barron ME: Simple, nonspecific ulcer of the colon. Arch Surg 17:375, 1928.
60. Khawaja FI, Vakil N: Colonoscopy as an aid in the diagnosis of nonspecific ulcers of the colon. Gastrointest Endosc 33:43, 1987.
61. Williams KL: Acute solitary ulcers and acute diverticulitis of caecum and ascending colon. Br J Surg 47:351, 1960.
62. Kaufman HL, Fischer AH, Carroll M, Becker JM: Colonic ulceration associated with nonsteroidal anti-inflammatory drugs. Review of three cases. Dis Colon Rectum 39(6):705, 1999.
63. Buchman AL, Schwartz MR: Colonic ulceration associated with the systemic use of nonsteroidal anti-inflammatory medication. J Clin Gastroenterol 22:224, 1996.
64. Mills B, Zuckerman G, Sicard G: Discrete colon ulcers as a cause of lower gastrointestinal bleeding and perforation in endstage renal disease. Surgery 89:548, 1981.
65. Shimamoto C, Hirata I, Ohshiba S, et al: Churg-Strauss syndrome (allergic granulomatous angiitis) with peculiar multiple colonic ulcers. Am J Gastroenterol 85:316, 1990.
66. Wilson RT, Dean PJ, Upshaw JD, Wruble LD: Endoscopic appearance of Wegener's granulomatosis involving the colon. Gastrointest Endosc 33:388, 1987.
67. Baxter R, Nino-Murcia M, Bloom RJ, Kosek J: Gastrointestinal manifestations of essential mixed cryoglobulinemia. Gastrointest Radiol 13: 160, 1988.
68. Blundell CR, Earnest DL: Idiopathic cecal ulcer: Diagnosis by colon-

oscopy followed by nonoperative management. Dig Dis Sci 25:494, 1980.
69. Hirata K, Sasaguri T, Kunoh M, et al: Solitary "amyloid ulcer" localized in the sigmoid colon without evidence of systemic amyloidosis. Am J Gastroenterol 92:356, 1997.
70. Shallman RW, Kuehner M, Williams GH, et al: Benign cecal ulcers. Dis Colon Rectum 28:732, 1985.
71. Dieulafoy P: Leçons clinique de l'Hotel-Dieu de Paris. Paris: Mason 2:1, 1897.
72. Franko E, Chardavoyne R, Wise L: Massive rectal bleeding from a Dieulafoy's-type ulcer of the rectum: A review of this unusual disease. Am J Gastroenterol 86:1545, 1991.
73. Gadenstatter M, Wetscher G, Crookes PF, et al: Dieulafoy's disease of the large and small bowel. J Clin Gastroenterol 27:169, 1998.
74. Nozae T, Kitamura M, Matsumata T, Sugimachi K: Dieulafoy-like lesions of colon and rectum in patients with chronic renal failure on long-term hemodialysis. Hepato-gastroenterology 46:3121, 1999.
75. Dy NM, Gostout CJ, Balm RK: Bleeding from the endoscopically identified Dieulafoy lesion of the proximal small intestine and colon. Am J Gastroenterol 90:108, 1995.
76. Abdulian JD, Santoro MJ, Chen YK, Collen MJ: Dieulafoy-like lesion of the rectum presenting with exsanguinating hemorrhage: Successful endoscopic therapy. Am J Gastroenterol 88:1939, 1993.
77. Lalla R, Enquist I, Oloumi M, Velez FJ: Stercoraceous perforation of the right colon. South Med J 82:80, 1989.
78. Serpell JW, Nicholls RJ: Stercoral perforation of the colon. Br J Surg 77:1325, 1990.
79. Gekas P, Schuster MM: Stercoral perforation of the colon: Case report and review of the literature. Gastroenterology 80:1054, 1981.
80. Maurer CA, Renzulli P, Mazzucchelli L, et al: Use of accurate diagnostic criteria may increase incidence of stercoral perforation of the colon. Dis Colon Rectum 43:991, 2000.
81. Serpell JW, Giddins SG, Nicholls RJ, Bradfield WJD: Stercoral perforation of the colon proximal to an end-colostomy. Postgrad Med J 67: 299, 1991.
82. Guyton DP, Evans D, Schreiber H: Stercoral perforation of the colon: Concepts of operative management. Am Surg 51:520, 1985.
83. Lindstrom CG: "Collagenous colitis" with watery diarrhea. A new entity. Pathol Eur 11:87, 1976.
84. Read NW, Krejs GJ, Read MG, et al: Chronic diarrhea of unknown origin. Gastroenterology 68:264, 1980.
85. Lazenby AJ, Yardley JH, Giardiello FM, et al: Lymphocytic ("microscopic") colitis: A comparative histopathologic study with particular reference to collagenous colitis. Hum Pathol 20:18, 1989.
86. Fernandez-Banares F, Salas A, Forne M, et al: Incidence of collagenous and lymphocytic colitis: A 5-year population-based study. Am J Gastroenterol 94:418, 1999.
87. Bohr J, Tysk C, Ericksson S, et al: Collagenous colitis: A retrospective study of clinical presentations and treatment in 163 patients. Gut 39:846, 1996.
88. Raclot G, Queneau PE, Ottignon Y, et al: Incidence of collagenous colitis: A retrospective study in the east of France. Gastroenterology 106:A23, 1994.
89. Tanaka M, Mazzoleni G, Riddell RH: Distribution of collagenous colitis: Utility of flexible sigmoidoscopy. Gut 33:65, 1992.
90. Flejou JF, Grimaud JA, Molas G, et al: Collagenous colitis: Ultrastructural study and collagen immunotyping of four cases. Arch Pathol Lab Med 108:977, 1984.
91. Lazenby AJ, Yardley JH, Giardiello FM, Bayless TM: Pitfalls in the diagnosis of collagenous colitis: Experience with 75 cases from a registry of collagenous-colitis at The Johns Hopkins Hospital. Hum Pathol 21:905, 1990.
92. Jarnerot G, Tysk C, Bohr J, Ericksson S: Collagenous colitis and fecal stream diversion. Gastroenterology 109:449, 1995.
93. Giardiello FM, Hansen FC, Lazenby AJ, et al: Collagenous colitis in setting of nonsteroidal anti-inflammatory drugs and antibiotics. Dig Dis Sci 35:257, 1990.
94. Bjarnason I, Hayllar J, MacPherson AJ, Russel AS: Side effects of nonsteroidal anti-inflammatory drugs on the small and large intestine in humans. Gastroenterology 104:1832, 1993.
95. Anderson T, Anderson JR, Tvede M, Franzmann MB: Collagenous colitis: Are bacterial cytotoxins responsible? Am J Gastroenterol 88: 375, 1993.
96. Riddell RH, Tanaka M, Mazzoleni G: Non-steroidal anti-inflammatory drugs as a possible cause of collagenous colitis: A case control study. Gut 33:683, 1992.
97. Goff JS, Barnett JL, Pelke T, Appelman HD: Collagenous colitis: Histopathology and clinical course. Am J Gastroenterol 92:57, 1997.
98. Van Tilburg AJP, Lam HGT, Seldenrijk CA, et al: Familial occurrence of collagenous colitis. J Clin Gastroenterol 12:279, 1990.
99. Sartor RB, Bender DE, Holt LC: Susceptibility of inbred rat strains to intestinal and extraintestinal inflammation induced by indomethacin. Gastroenterology 102:A690, 1992.
100. DuBois RN, Lazenby AJ, Yardley JH, et al: Lymphocytic enterocolitis in patients with "refractory sprue." JAMA 262:935, 1989.
101. Wolber R, Owen D, Freeman H: Colonic lymphocytosis in patients with celiac sprue. Hum Pathol 21:1092, 1990.
102. Armes J, Gee DC, Macrae FA, et al: Collagenous colitis: Jejunal and colorectal pathology. J Clin Pathol 45:784, 1992.
103. Zins BJ, Tremaine WJ, Carpenter HA: Collagenous colitis: Mucosal biopsies and association with fecal leukocytes. Mayo Clin Proc 70: 430, 1995.
104. Giardiello FM, Lazenby AJ, Yardley JH, et al: Increased HLA A1 and diminished HLA A3 in lymphocytic colitis compared to controls and patients with collagenous colitis. Dig Dis Sci 37:496, 1992.
105. Sylwestrowicz T, Kelly JK, Hwang WS, et al: Collagenous colitis and microscopic colitis: The watery diarrhea-colitis syndrome. Am J Gastroenterol 84:763, 1989.
106. Fine KD, Do K, Schulte K, et al: High prevalence of celiac sprue–like HLA-DQ genes and enteropathy in patients with the microscopic colitis syndrome. Am J Gastroenterol 95:1974, 2000.
107. Aigner T, Neureiter D, Muller S, et al: Extracellular matrix composition and gene expression in collagenous colitis. Gastroenterology 113: 136, 1997.
108. Bo-Linn GW, Vendrell DD, Lee E, Fordtran JS: An evaluation of the significance of microscopic colitis in patients with chronic diarrhea. J Clin Invest 75:1559, 1985.
109. Lee E, Schiller LR, Vendrell D, et al: Subepithelial collagen table thickness in colon specimens from patients with microscopic colitis and collagenous colitis. Gastroenterology 103:1790, 1992.
110. Rask-Madsen J, Grove O, Hansen MGJ, et al: Colonic transport of water and electrolytes in a patient with secretory diarrhea due to collagenous colitis. Dig Dis Sci 28:1141, 1983.
111. Baum CA, Bhatia P, Miner PB: Increased colonic mucosal mast cells associated with severe watery diarrhea and microscopic colitis. Dig Dis Sci 34:1462, 1998.
112. Giardiello FM, Bayless TM, Jessurun J, et al: Collagenous colitis: Physiologic and histopathologic studies in seven patients. Ann Intern Med 106:46, 1987.
113. Marteau P, Lavergne-Slove A, Lemann M, et al: Primary villous atrophy is often associated with microscopic colitis. Gut 41:561, 1997.
114. Ung K-A, Gillberg R, Kilander A, Abrahamsson H: Role of bile acids and bile acid binding agents in patients with collagenous colitis. Gut 46:170, 2000.
115. Tremaine WJ: Collagenous colitis and lymphocytic colitis. J Clin Gastroenterol 80:245, 2000.
116. Bohr J, Tysk C, Yang P, et al: Autoantibodies and immunoglobulins in collagenous colitis. Gut 30:73, 1996.
117. Richieri JP, Bonneau HP, Cano N, et al: Collagenous colitis: An unusual endoscopic appearance. Gastrointest Endosc 39:192, 1993.
118. Clouse RE, Alpers DH, Hockenbery DM, et al: Pericrypt eosinophilic enterocolitis and chronic diarrhea. Gastroenterology 103:168, 1992.
119. Garcia-Gonzales R, Fernandez FA, Garijo MF, Fernando V-BJ: Amyloidosis of the rectum mimicking collagenous colitis. Pathol Res Pract 194:731, 1998.
120. Fine KD, Lee EL: Efficacy of open label bismuth subsalicylate for the treatment of microscopic colitis. Gastroenterology 114:29, 1998.
121. Pullan RD, Ganesh S, Mani V, et al: Comparison of bismuth citrate and 5-aminosalicylic acid enemas in distal ulcerative colitis: A controlled trial. Gut 34:676, 1993.
122. Tremaine WJ, Sandborn WJ, Wolff BG, et al: Bismuth carbomer foam enemas for treatment-resistant active chronic pouchitis: A randomized, double-blind placebo-controlled trial. Gastroenterology 112:A1105, 1997.
123. Zins BJ, Sandborn WJ, Tremaine WJ: Collagenous and lymphocytic colitis: Subject review and therapeutic alternatives. Am J Gastroenterol 90:1394, 1995.
124. Sloth H, Bisgaard C, Grove A: Collagenous colitis: A prospective trial of prednisolone in six patients. J Intern Med 302:443, 1991.
125. Tromm A, Griga T, Mollman HW, et al: Budesonide for the treatment of collagenous colitis: First results of a pilot trial. Am J Gastroenterol 94:1871, 1999.

126. Delarive J, Saraga E, Dorta G, Blum A: Budesonide in the treatment of collagenous colitis. Digestion 59:364, 1998.
127. Rai RM, Hendrix TJ, Moskaluk C, et al: Treatment of idiopathic lymphocytic enterocolitis with oral beclomethasone dipropionate. Am J Gastroenterol 92:147, 1997.
128. Glotzer DJ, Glick ME, Goldman H: Proctitis and colitis following diversion of the fecal stream. Gastroenterology 24:211, 1981.
129. Korelitz BI, Cheskin LJ, Sohn N, Sommers SC: The fate of the rectal segment after diversion of the fecal stream in Crohn's disease: Its implications for surgical management. J Clin Gastroenterol 7:37, 1985.
130. Haas PA, Fox TA, Szilag EJ: Endoscopic examination of the colon and rectum distal to a colostomy. Am J Gastroenterol 85:850, 1990.
131. Yeong ML, Bethwaite PB, Prasad J, Isbister WH: Lymphoid follicular hyperplasia—a distinctive feature of diversion colitis. Histopathology 19:55, 1991.
132. Haque S, Eisen RN, West AB: The morphologic features of diversion colitis: Studies of a pediatric population with no other disease of the intestinal mucosa. Hum Pathol 24:211, 1993.
133. Cook SI, Sellin JH: Review article: Short chain fatty acids in health and disease. Aliment Pharmacol Ther 12:507, 1998.
134. Mortensen PB, Clausen MR: Short-chain fatty acids in the human colon: Relation to gastointestinal health and disease. Scand J Gastroenterol 216:132, 1996.
134a. Roediger WEW: Utilization of nutrients by isolated epithelial cells of the rat colon. Gastroenterology 83:424, 1982.
135. Harig JM, Soergel KH, Komorowski RA, Wood CM: Treatment of diversion colitis with short-chain fatty acid irrigation. N Engl J Med 320:23, 1989.
136. Neut C, Colombel JF, Guillemot F, et al: Impaired bacterial flora in human excluded colon. Gut 30:1094, 1989.
137. Ordein JJ, DiLorenzo CD, Flores A, Hyman PE: Diversion colitis in children with severe gastrointestinal motility disorders. Am J Gastroenterol 87:88, 1992.
138. Morin CL, Ling V, Bourassa D: Small intestinal and colonic changes induced by a chemically defined diet. Dig Dis Sci 25:123, 1980.
139. Tomasino RM, Morello V, Latteri MA, et al: Histological and histochemical changes in the colon mucosa after ureterosigmoidostomy or colon conduit. Eur Urol 15:248, 1988.
140. Guillemot F, Colombel JF, Neut C, et al: Treatment of diversion colitis by short chain fatty acids. Prospective and double blind study. Dis Colon Rectum 34:861, 1991.
141. Neut C, Guillemot F, Gowerrousseau C, et al: Treatment of diversion colitis by short chain fatty acids. Prospective and double blind study. Gastroenterol Clin Biol 19:871, 1995.
142. Geraghty JM, Talbot IC: Diversion colitis: Histological features in the colon and rectum after defunctioning colostomy. Gut 32:1020, 1991.
143. Sartor RB, Murphy ME, Rydzak E: Miscellaneous inflammatory and structural disorders of the colon. In Yamada T (ed): Textbook of Gastroenterology, 3rd ed. Philadelpina, Lippincott Williams & Wilkins, 1999, p 1857.
144. Heilbrun N: Roentgen evidence suggesting enterocolitis associated with prolonged cathartic abuse. Radiology 41:486, 1943.
145. Leng-Peschlow E: Senna and its rational use. Pharmacology 44(Suppl 1), 1992.
146. Muller-Lissner S: What has happened to the cathartic colon? Gut 39: 486, 1996.
147. Urso FP, Urso MJ, Lee CH: The cathartic colon: Pathological findings and radiological/pathological correlation. Radiology 116:557, 1975.
148. Campbell WL: Cathartic colon: Reversibility of roentgen changes. Dis Colon Rectum 26:445, 1983.
149. Rieman JF, Zimmerman W: Ultrastructural studies of colonic nerve plexuses in chronic laxative abuse. Gastroenterology 74:1085, 1978.
150. Smith B: Effect of irritant purgatives on the myenteric plexus in man and the mouse. Gut 139:43, 1969.
151. Dufour P, Gendre P: Ultrastructure of mouse intestinal mucosa and changes observed after long-term anthraquinone administration. Gut 15:1358, 1984.
152. Riecken EO, Zertz M, Ende C, et al: The effect of an anthraquinone laxative on colonic nerve tissue: A controlled trial in constipated women. Z Gastroenterol 28:660, 1990.
153. Ghadially FN, Walley VM: Pigments of the gastrointestinal tract: A comparison of light microscopic and electron microscopic findings. Ultrastruct Pathol 19:213, 1995.
154. Benavides SR, Morgante PE, Monserrat AJ, et al: The pigment of melanosis coli: A lectin histochemical study. Gastrointest Endosc 46: 131, 1997.
155. Walker NI, Bennett RE, Axelson RA: Melanosis coli: A consequence of anthraquinone-induced apoptosis of colonic epithelial cells. Am J Pathol 131:465, 1988.
156. Badiali D, Marcheggiano A, Pallone F, et al: Melanosis of the rectum in patients with chronic constipation. Dis Colon Rectum 28:241, 1985.
157. Speare GS: Melanosis coli: Experimental observations of its production and elimination in twenty-three cases. Am J Surg 82:631, 1951.
158. Mengs U, Rudolph RL: Light and electron-microscopic changes in the colon of the guinea pig after treatment with anthranoid and non-anthranoid laxatives. Pharmacology 47(Suppl 1):172, 1993.
159. Balazs M: Melanosis coli: Ultrastructural study in 45 patients. Dis Colon Rectum 29:839, 1986.
160. Van Gorkom BAP, DeVries EGE, Karrenbeld A, Kleibeulier JH: Review article: Anthranoid laxatives and their potential carcinogenic effects. Aliment Pharmacol Ther 13:443, 1999.
161. Nusko G, Schneider B, Wittekind C, Hahn EG: Anthranoid laxative use is not a risk factor for colorectal neoplasia: Results of a prospective case control study. Gut 46:651, 2000.
162. Morganstern L, Shemen L, Allen W, et al: Melanosis coli: Changes in appearance when associated with colonic neoplasia. Arch Surg 118:62, 1983.
163. Hardin RD, Tedesco FJ: Colitis after Hibiclens enema. J Clin Gastroenterol 8:572, 1986.
164. Pike BF, Phillippi PJ, Lawson EH Jr: Soap colitis. N Engl J Med 285: 217, 1971.
165. Bollen P, Goossens A, Hauser B, Vandenplas Y: Colonic ulcerations caused by an enema containing hydrogen peroxide. J Pediatr Gastroenterol Nutr 26:232, 1998.
166. Lutzger LG, Factor SM: Effects of some water-soluble contrast media on the colonic mucosa. Radiology 118:545, 1976.
167. Segal I, Tim LO, Hamilton DG, et al: Ritual-enema-induced colitis. Dis Colon Rectum 22:195, 1979.
168. Coche G, Izet T, Descombes P, et al. Chemical colitis caused by glutaraldehyde. J Radiol 78:215, 1997.
169. Chan A, Depew W, Vanner S: Use of oral sodium phosphate colonic lavage solution by Canadian colonoscopists: Pitfalls and complications. Can J Gastroenterol 11:334, 1997.
170. Jonas G, Mahoney A, Murray J, Gertler S: Chemical colitis due to endoscope cleaning solutions: A mimic of pseudomembranous colitis. Gastroenterology 95:1403, 1988.
171. Michaelis L, Gutmann C: Ueber Einschlusse in Blasentumoren. Z Clin Med 47:208, 1902.
172. Lewin K, Harell G, Lee A, Crowley L: An electron-microscopic study: Demonstration of bacilliform organisms in malacoplakic macrophages. Gastroenterology 66:28, 1974.
173. Long J, Althausen A: Malacoplakia: A 25-year experience with a review of the literature. J Urol 141:1328, 1989.
174. Terner J, Lattes R: Malacoplakia of colon and rectoperitoneum. Am J Clin Pathol 44:20, 1965.
175. Cipolletta L, Bianco M, Fumo F, et al: Malacoplakia of the colon. Gastrointest Endosc 41:225, 1995.
176. Stevens S, McClure J: The histochemical features of the Michaelis-Gutmann body and a consideration of the pathophysiological mechanisms of its formation. J Pathol 137:119, 1982.
177. Thorning D, Vaco R: Malacoplakia: Defect in digestion of phagocytosed material due to impaired vacuolar acidification? Arch Pathol 99: 456, 1975.
178. Abdou N, NaPombejara C, Sagawa A, et al: Malacoplakia: Evidence for monocyte lysosomal abnormality correctable by cholinergic agonist in vitro and in vivo. N Engl J Med 297:1413, 1977.
179. Streem S: Genitourinary malacoplakia in renal transplant recipients: Pathogenic, prognostic and therapeutic considerations. J Urol 132:10, 1984.
180. Biggar W, Crawford L, Cardella C, et al: Malacoplakia and immunosuppressive therapy. Reversal of clinical and leukocyte abnormalities after withdrawal of prednisone and azathioprine. Am J Pathol 119:5, 1985.
181. Mir-Madjlessi S, Tavassolie H, Kamalian N: Malakoplakia of the colon and recurrent colonic strictures in a patient with primary hypogammaglobulinemia: An association not previously described. Dis Colon Rectum 25:723, 1982.
182. Schwartz D, Ogden P, Blumberg H, et al: Pulmonary malakoplakia in a patient with the acquired immunodeficiency syndrome. Arch Pathol Lab Med 114:1267, 1990.
183. Bates A, Dev S, Baithun S: Malakoplakia and colorectal adenocarci-

noma. London, Department of Morbid Anatomy, London Hospital Medical College and Department of Histopathology, St Andrew's Hospital, 1996, p 171.
184. El-Mouzan M, Satti M, Al-Quorain A, El-Ageb A: Colonic malacoplakia—occurrence in a family. Report of cases. Dis Colon Rectum 31:390, 1988.
185. Maderazo E, Berlin B, Marhardt C: Treatment of malacoplakia with trimethoprim-sulfamethoxazole. Urology 13:70, 1979.
186. Van Furth R, Van't Wout J, Wertheimer P, Zwartendijk J: Ciprofloxacin for treatment of malacoplakia. Lancet 339:148, 1992.
187. Jamart J: Pneumatosis cystoides intestinalis: A statistical study of 919 cases. Acta Hepato-Gastroenterol 26:419, 1979.
188. John A, Dickey K, Fenwick J, et al: Pneumatosis intestinalis in Crohn's disease. Dig Dis Sci 37:813, 1992.
189. Galanduik S, Fazio V: Pneumatosis cystoides intestinalis. Dis Colon Rectum 29:358, 1986.
190. Holt S, Gilmour H, Buist T, et al: High flow oxygen therapy for pneumatosis coli. Gut 20:493, 1979.
191. Tak P, Van Duinen C, Bun P, et al: Pneumatosis cystoides intestinalis with intestinal pseudo-obstruction: Resolution after metronidazole. Dig Dis Sci 37:949, 1992.
192. Knetchle S, Davidoff A, Rice R: Pneumatosis intestinalis: Clinical management and surgical outcome. Ann Surg 212:160, 1990.
193. Moote D, Fried L, Le Brun G, Fraser D: Pneumatosis coli: Is there a relationship with sigmoid colon redundancy? Gastrointest Radiol 14: 79, 1989.
194. Sequeira W: Pneumatosis cystoides intestinalis in systemic sclerosis and other diseases. Semin Arthritis Rheum 19:269, 1990.
195. Collins C, Blanchard C, Cramp M, et al: Pneumatosis intestinalis occurring in association with cryptosporidiosis. Clin Radiol 46:410, 1992.
196. Gagliardi G, Thompson I, Hershman M, et al: Pneumatosis coli: A proposed pathogenesis based on study of 25 cases and review of the literature. Int J Colorectal Dis 11:11, 1996.
197. Marshak R, Linder A, McKlansky D: Pneumatosis cystoides coli. Gastrointest Radiol 2:85, 1977.
198. Stone H, Allen W, Smith RI, et al: Infantile pneumatosis intestinalis. J Surg Res 8:301, 1968.
199. Levitt M, Olsson S: Pneumatosis cystoides intestinalis and high breath H_2 excretion: Insights into the role of H_2 in this condition. Gastroenterology 108:1560, 1995.
200. Read N, Al-Janabi N, Cann P: Is raised breath hydrogen related to the pathogenesis of pneumatosis coli? Gut 25:839, 1984.
201. Van der Linden W, Marsell R: Pneumatosis cystoides coli associated with a high H_2 excretion. Scand J Gastroenterol 14:173, 1979.
202. Ellis B: Symptomatic treatment of primary pneumatosis coli with metronidazole. Br Med J 280:763, 1980.
203. Christl S, Gibson G, Murgatroyd P, et al: Impaired hydrogen metabolism in pneumatosis cystoides intestinalis. Gastroenterology 104:392, 1993.
204. Galandiuk S, Fazio V: Pneumatosis cystoides intestinalis: Review of the literature. Dis Colon Rectum 29:358, 1986.
205. Spigelman A, Williams C, Ansell J, et al: Pneumatosis coli: A source of diagnostic confusion. Br J Surg 77:155, 1990.
206. Miralbes M, Hinojosa J, Aconso J, Berenguer J: Oxygen therapy in pneumatosis coli. What is the minimum oxygen requirement? Dis Colon Rectum 26:458, 1983.
207. Guest CB, Reznick RK: Colitis cystica profunda: Review of the literature. Dis Colon Rectum 32:983, 1989.
208. Anderson N, Rivera E, Flores D: Peutz-Jeghers syndrome with cervical adenocarcinoma and enteritis cystica profunda. West J Med 141: 242, 1984.
209. Castleman B, McNeely BU: Case records of the Massachusetts General Hospital: Weekly clinicopathological exercises. N Engl J Med 286:147, 1972.
210. Aftalion B, Lipper S: Enteritis cystica profunda associated with Crohn's disease. Arch Pathol Lab Med 108:532, 1984.
211. Wayte D, Helwig E: Colitis cystica profunda. Am J Clin Pathol 48: 159, 1967.
212. Rosen Y, Vallant J, Yermakov V: Submucosal cysts at a colostomy site: Relationship to colitis cystica profunda and reopen of a case. Dis Colon Rectum 19:453, 1976.
213. Hubmann F: Proctitis cystica profunda and radiation fibrosis in the rectum of the female Wistar rat after x-irradiation: A histopathological study. J Pathol 138:193, 1982.
213a. Brynjolfsson G, Haley H: Experimental enteritis cystica in rats. Am J Clin Pathol 47:69, 1967.
214. Franzin G, Novelli P: Gastritis cystica profunda. Histopathology 5: 535, 1981.
215. Levin D: "Solitary" rectal ulcer syndrome. Are "solitary" rectal ulcer syndrome and "localized" colitis cystica profunda analogous syndromes caused by rectal prolapse? Gastroenterology 92:243, 1987.
216. Bentley E, Chandrasoma P, Cohen H, et al: Colitis cystica profunda presenting with complete intestinal obstuction and recurrence. Gastroenterology 89:1157, 1985.
217. Petritsch W, Hinterleitner T, Aichbichler B, et al: Endosonography in colitis cystica profunda and solitary rectal ulcer syndrome. 41:382, 1995.
218. Yale C, Balish E: Pneumatosis cystoides intestinalis. Dis Colon Rectum 19:107, 1976.
219. Stuart M: Proctitis cystica profunda: Incidence, etiology, and treatment. Dis Colon Rectum 27:153, 1984.
220. Guy P, Hall M: Colitis cystica profunda of the rectum treated by mucosal sleeve resection and colo-anal pullthrough. Br J Surg 75:289, 1988.
221. Wagner M, Rosenberg H, Ferbach D, Singleton E: Typhlitis: A complication of leukemia in childhood. AJR Am J Roentgenol 109:341, 1970.
222. Moir D, Bale P: Necropsy findings on childhood leukemia emphasizing neutropenic enterocolitis and cerebral calcification. Pathology 8: 247, 1976.
223. Shamberger R, Weinstein H, Delorey M, Levey R: The medical and surgical managment of typhlitis in children with acute nonlymphocytic (myelogenous) leukemia. Cancer 56:603, 1986.
224. Petruzzelli G, Johnson J, de Vries E: Neutropenic enterocolitis: A new complication of the head and neck cancer chemotherapy. Arch Otolaryngol Head Neck Surg 116:209, 1990.
225. Starnes H, Moore F, Mentzer S, et al: Abdominal pain in neutropenic cancer patients. Cancer 57:616, 1986.
226. Ettinghausen SE: Inflammatory disorders of the colon: Collagenous colitis, eosinophilic colitis, and neutropenic colitis. Surg Clin North Am 73:993, 1993.
227. Till M, Lee N, Soper W, Murphy R: Typhlitis in patients with HIV-1 infection. Ann Intern Med 116:998, 1992.
228. Keidan R, Fanning J, Gatenby R, Weese JL: Recurrent typhlitis. A disease resulting from aggressive chemotherapy. Dis Colon Rectum 32:206, 1989.
229. Paulino A, Kenney R, Forman E, Medeiros L: Typhlitis in a patient with acute lymphoblastic leukemia prior to the administration of chemotherapy. Am J Pediatr Hematol Oncol 16:348, 1994.
230. Slavin R, Dias M, Saral R: Cytosine arabinoside–induced gastrointestinal toxic alterations in sequential chemotherapeutic protocols. Cancer 42:1747, 1978.
231. Katz J, Wagner M, Gresik M, et al: Typhlitis: An 18-year experience and postmortem review. Cancer 65:1041, 1990.
232. Sloas M, Flynn P, Kaste S, Patrick C: Typhlitis in children with cancer: A thirty-year experience. Clin Infect Dis 17:484, 1993.
233. Abbasoglu O, Cakmakci M: Neutropenic enterocolitis in patients without leukemia. Surgery 113:113, 1993.
234. Vas W, Seeling R, Manhanta B, et al: Neutropenic colitis: Evaluation with computed tomography. CT J Comput Tomogr 12:211, 1988.
235. Moir C, Scudamore C, Benny W: Typhlitis: Selective surgical managment. Am J Surg 151:563, 1986.
236. Kouroussis C, Samonis G, Androulakis N, et al: Successful conservative treatment of neutropenic enterocolitis complicating taxane-based chemotherapy. Am J Clin Oncol (CCT) 23:309, 2000.
237. Mower W, Hawkins J, Nelson E: Neutropenic enterocolitis in adults with acute leukemia. Arch Surg 121:571, 1986.
238. Villar H, Warneke J, Peck M, et al: Role of surgical treatment in the management of complications of the gastrointestinal tract in patients with leukemia. Surg Gynecol Obstet 165:217, 1987.
239. Olive DL, Schwartz LB: Endometriosis; Medical progress. N Engl J Med 328:1759, 1993.
240. Jansen RP. Russel P: Nonpigmented endometriosis: Clinical, laparoscopic and pathological definition. Am J Obstet Gynecol 155:1154, 1986.
241. Zwas FR, Lyon DT: Endometriosis. An important condition in clinical gastroenterology. Dig Dis Sci 36:353, 1991.
242. Weed JC, Ray JE: Endometriosis of the bowel. Obstet Gynecol 69: 727, 1987.

243. Shah M, Tager D, Feller E: Intestinal endometriosis masquerading as common digestive disorders. Arch Intern Med 155:977, 1995.
244. Rock JA, Markham SM: Pathogenesis of endometriosis. Lancet 240: 1264, 1992.
245. Bontis JN, Vavilis DT: Etiopathology of endometriosis. Ann NY Acad Sci 816:305, 1997.
246. Oral E, Arici A: Pathogenesis of endometriosis. Obstet Gynecol Clin North Am 24:219, 1997.
247. Ferguson CM: Case records of the Massachusetts General Hospital. Weekly clinicopathological exercises. Case 28-1996. A 45-year-old woman with abdominal pain and a polypoid mass in the colon. N Engl J Med 335:807, 1996.
248. Bozdech JM: Endoscopic diagnosis of colonic endometriosis. Gastrointest Endosc 38:568, 1992.
249. St Ville EW, Jafri SZH, Madrazo BL, et al: Endorectal sonography in the evaluation of rectal and perirectal disease. AJR Am J Roentgenol 157:503, 1991.
250. Olive DL, Pritts EA: Treatment of endometriosis. N Engl J Med 345: 266, 2001.
251. Kettel LM, Hummel WP: Modern medical management of endometriosis. Obstet Gynecol Clin North Am 24:361, 1997.
252. Berquist IA: Hormonal regulation of endometriosis and the rationales and effects of gonadotropin-releasing hormone agonist treatment: A review. Hum Reprod 10:446, 1995.
253. Hornstein MD, Yuzpe AA, Burry KA, et al: Prospective randomized double-blind trial of 3 versus 6 months of nafarelin therapy for endometriosis-associated pelvic pain. Fertil Steril 63:955, 1995.
254. Hall LLH, Malone JM, Ginsburg KA: Flare-up of endometriosis induced by gonadotropin-releasing hormone agonist leading to bowel obstruction. Fertil Steril 64:1204, 1995.
255. Hajiar LR, Kim W, Nolan GH, et al: Intestinal and pelvic endometriosis presenting as a tumor and associated with tamoxifen therapy; Report of a case. Obstet Gynecol 82:642, 1993.
256. Sutton C, Hill D: Laser laparoscopy in the treatment of endometriosis. A 5-year study. Br J Obstet Gynaecol 97:181, 1990.
257. Cameron IC, Rogers S, Collins MC, Reed MW: Intestinal endometriosis: Presentation, investigation, and surgical management. Int J Colorectal Dis 10:83, 1995.
258. Tran KT, Kuijpers HC, Willemsen WN, Bulten H: Surgical treatment of symptomatic rectosigmoid endometriosis. Eur J Surg 162:139, 1996.
259. Nozhat C, Nezhat F, Pennington E: Laparoscopic treatment of infiltrative rectosigmoid colon and rectovaginal septum endometriosis by the technique of videolaparoscopy and the CO_2 laser. Br J Obstet Gynaecol 99:664, 1992.
260. Redwine DB, Koning M, Sharpe DR: Laparoscopically assisted transvaginal segmental resection of the rectosigmoid colon for endometriosis. Fertil Steril 65:198, 1996.

Section Eleven

VASCULATURE AND SUPPORTING STRUCTURES

Chapter 119

INTESTINAL ISCHEMIA

Lawrence J. Brandt and Scott J. Boley

Intestinal ischemia produces a broad spectrum of disorders, depending on the onset, duration, and cause of the injury; the area and length of bowel affected; the vessel involved; and the degree of collateral blood flow. Variability in these factors influences not only the presentation of the ischemic event but also its treatment and outcome. Ischemic injury may be acute or chronic; it may be caused by a disturbance in the arterial supply or venous drainage of the bowel and involve the small intestine, the colon, or both. Since the development and widespread use of colonoscopy, angiography, computed tomography (CT), and other imaging modalities, various types of ischemic injury to the gastrointestinal tract have been recognized and increasingly appreciated (Table 119–1; see also Tables 119–2 and 119–3). Our concepts of their pathogenesis, diagnosis, and management have been so altered since the 1980s that much of what has been written in the past is no longer applicable. In this chapter we describe the spectrum of ischemic damage to the gastrointestinal tract and discuss the management of these conditions in light of recent advances.

ANATOMY OF THE SPLANCHNIC CIRCULATION[1]

The celiac axis (CA), superior mesenteric artery (SMA), and inferior mesenteric artery (IMA) supply almost all of the blood flow to the digestive tract. There is marked variability of vascular anatomy among individuals, but typical patterns have emerged from anatomic dissections and abdominal angiography.

Celiac Axis (Fig. 119–1)

The CA arises from the anterior aorta and gives rise to three major branches: the left gastric artery; the common hepatic artery and its gastroduodenal, right gastroepiploic, and superior pancreaticoduodenal arterial branches; and the splenic artery with its pancreatic and left gastroepiploic arterial branches. The CA and its branches supply the stomach, duodenum, pancreas, and the liver.

Superior Mesenteric Artery (Fig. 119–2)

The SMA has its origin from the anterior aorta near the neck of the pancreas. It gives rise to four major vessels: the inferior pancreaticoduodenal, middle colic, right colic, and ileocolic arteries, as well as to a series of jejunal and ileal branches, all of which supply their named portions of intestine. These intestinal branches typically form a series of arcades, and from the terminal arcade, numerous straight vessels arise that enter the intestinal wall.

Inferior Mesenteric Artery (Fig. 119–3)

The IMA arises 3 to 4 cm above the aortic bifurcation close to the inferior border of the duodenum. It branches into the left colic artery and multiple sigmoid branches and terminates as the superior rectal artery. The IMA and its branches supply the large intestine from the distal transverse colon to the proximal rectum. The distal rectum is supplied by branches of the internal iliac (hypogastric) artery.

Table 119–1 | **Types and Approximate Incidences of Intestinal Ischemia**

TYPE	INCIDENCE (%)*
Colonic ischemia	75
Acute mesenteric ischemia	25
Focal segmental ischemia	5
Chronic mesenteric ischemia	5
Mesenteric venous thrombosis	Included in above

*Figures are approximations.

Collateral and Anastomotic Circulation

Abundant collateral circulation to the stomach, duodenum, and rectum accounts for the paucity of ischemic events in these organs. The major anastomosis between the CA and the SMA is formed from the superior pancreaticoduodenal branch of the CA and the inferior pancreaticoduodenal branch of the SMA. These vessels constitute the pancreaticoduodenal arcade and provide blood to the duodenum and the pancreas. The splenic flexure and sigmoid colon have limited anastomoses, and ischemic damage is more common in these locations. There are three paths of communication between the SMA and IMA: (1) the marginal artery of Drummond, which is closest to and parallel with the wall of the intestine; (2) the central anastomotic artery, a larger and more centrally placed vessel; and (3) the arc of Riolan, an artery in the base of the mesentery. In the presence of SMA or IMA occlusion, a large collateral termed the *meandering artery* may be identified angiographically and represents a dilated central anastomotic artery or arc of Riolan (Fig. 119–4).

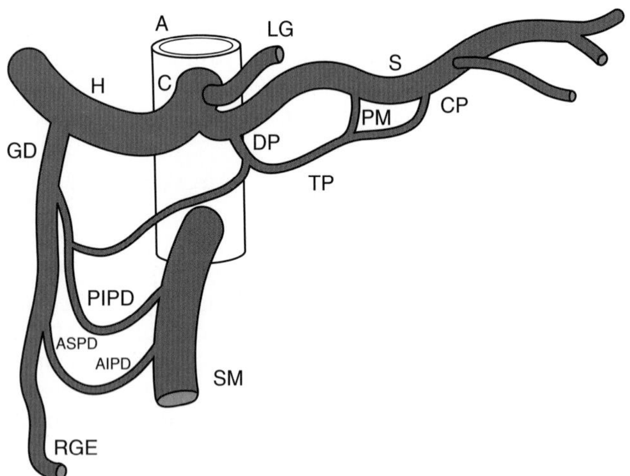

Figure 119–1. Diagram of typical celiac axis anatomy and branching pattern. A, aorta; C, celiac axis; H, hepatic artery; GD, gastroduodenal artery; LG, left gastric artery; S, splenic artery; DP, dorsal pancreatic artery; TP, transverse pancreatic artery; PM, pancreata magna; CP, caudal pancreatic artery; SM, superior mesenteric artery; PIPD, posterior inferior pancreaticoduodenal artery; ASPD, anterior superior pancreaticoduodenal artery; AIPD, anterior inferior pancreaticoduodenal artery; RGE, right gastroepiploic artery. (From Nebesar RA, Kornblith PL, Pollard JJ, Michels NA: Celiac and Superior Mesenteric Arteries: A Correlation of Angiograms and Dissections. Boston, Little, Brown, 1969.)

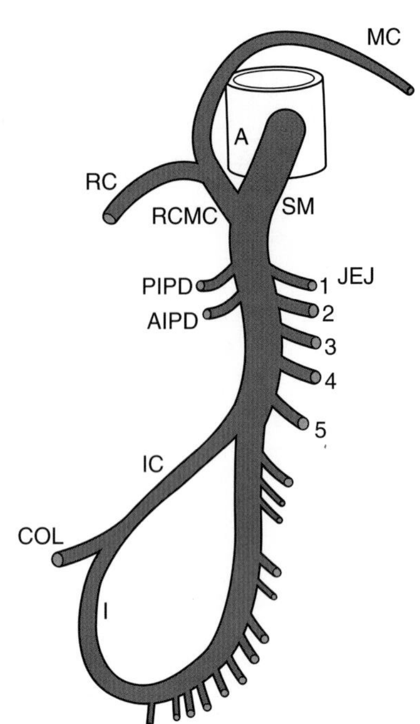

Figure 119–2. Diagram of typical superior mesenteric artery anatomy and branching pattern. A, aorta; MC, middle colic artery; RC, right colic artery; SM, superior mesenteric artery; PIPD, posterior inferior pancreaticoduodenal artery; AIPD, anterior inferior pancreaticoduodenal artery; JEJ, jejunal branches; IC, ileocolic artery; COL, colic branches; I, ileal branches. (From Nebesar RA, Kornblith PL, Pollard JJ, Michels NA: Celiac and Superior Mesenteric Arteries: A Correlation of Angiograms and Dissections. Boston, Little, Brown, 1969.)

PATHOPHYSIOLOGY AND PATHOLOGY OF MESENTERIC ISCHEMIA

Ischemic injury of the intestine results from deprivation of oxygen and nutrients necessary for cellular integrity. Remarkably, the bowel can tolerate a 75% reduction of mesenteric blood flow and oxygen consumption for 12 hours with no changes on light microscopy, because only one fifth of the mesenteric capillaries are open at any time.[2] Below a critical level of blood flow, however, oxygen consumption falls sharply because increased oxygen extraction can no longer compensate for diminished blood flow.

When a major vessel is occluded, collaterals open immediately in response to the drop in arterial pressure distal to the obstruction and remain open so long as pressure in the vascular bed distal to the obstruction remains below systemic pressure. After several hours of ischemia, however, vasoconstriction develops in the obstructed bed, elevating its pressure and reducing collateral flow. If sustained for a prolonged period, the vasoconstriction can become irreversible and persist after correction of the cause of the ischemic event. Such persistent vasoconstriction explains the operative findings of progressive bowel ischemia after cardiac function has been optimized and in the absence of arterial or venous obstruction.

Blood flow is affected by a variety of functional, humoral, local, and neural influences. The sympathetic nervous system, mainly via α-adrenergic receptors, is of primary importance in maintaining resting splanchnic arteriolar tone;

other vasoactive substances, including angiotensin II, vasopressin, and prostaglandins, also have been implicated in the pathogenesis of ischemic injury.

Ischemic damage results both from hypoxia during the period of ischemia and reperfusion injury when blood flow is re-established. Most injury from brief ischemia appears during reperfusion, but as the ischemic period lengthens, hypoxia becomes more detrimental than reperfusion.[3] Thus, the injury after 3 hours of ischemia and 1 hour of reperfusion is more severe than that after 4 hours of ischemia. Reperfusion injury has been attributed to many factors, including reactive oxygen radicals. When molecular oxygen is reduced in univalent steps, superoxide, hydrogen peroxide, and hydroxyl radicals are formed. These oxygen radicals damage an array of molecules found in tissues, including nucleic acids, membrane lipids, enzymes, and receptors; such widespread damage can result in cell lysis, impaired cell function, and necrosis on reperfusion of ischemic tissues.

A potent source of oxygen radicals in ischemic, reperfused tissue is the enzyme xanthine oxidase (XO), the rate-limiting enzyme in nucleic acid degradation. In nonischemic tissue, this enzyme exists as a dehydrogenase (XDH) that uses nicotinamide adenine dinucleotide rather than O_2 as the electron acceptor during purine oxidation; therefore, it does not produce oxygen radicals. During ischemia, XDH is converted to XO with production of reactive oxygen radicals. Inhibition of XO by allopurinol dramatically attenuates the epithelial cell necrosis and the increased microvascular permeability seen during reperfusion.

Neutrophils are another source of reactive oxygen metabolites. During reperfusion, XO-derived oxidants initiate the production and release of leukotriene B_4 and platelet-activating factor, which lead to neutrophil adherence and migration. The adherent leukocytes mediate microvascular injury by release of proteases and physical disruption of the endothelial barrier. Oxygen radical scavengers (superoxide dismutase, dimethyl sulfoxide), XO inhibitors, and agents that inhibit leukocyte adherence and migration have been shown experimentally to protect various organs against reperfusion injury but are not yet used clinically.[3]

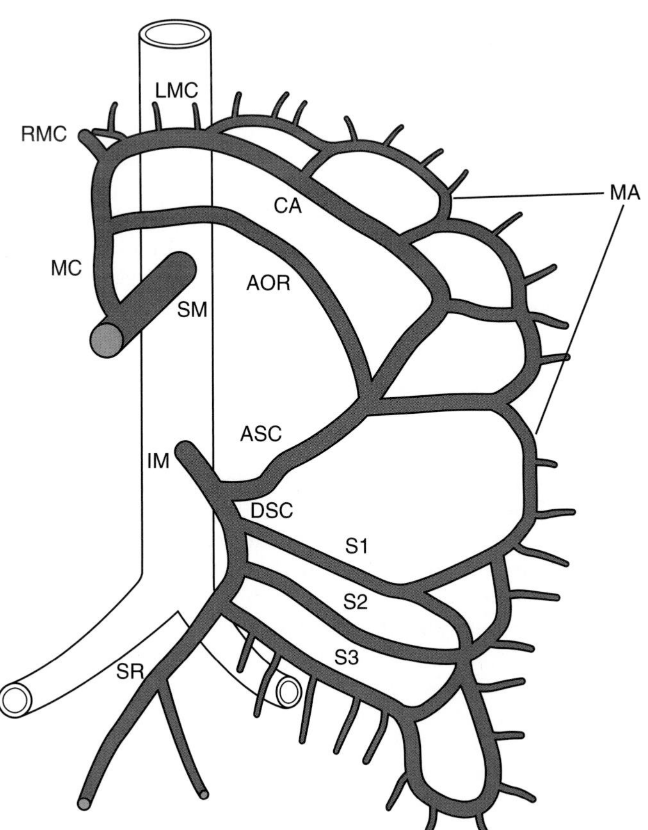

Figure 119–3. Diagram of typical inferior mesenteric artery anatomy and branching pattern. SM, superior mesenteric artery; MC, middle colic artery; RMC, right branch of middle colic artery; LMC, left branch of middle colic artery; AOR, arc of Riolan; CA, central artery; MA, marginal artery; IM, inferior mesenteric artery; ASC, ascending branch; DSC, descending branch; S1, S2, S3, sigmoid branches; SR, superior rectal artery. (From Nebesar RA, Kornblith PL, Pollard JJ, Michels NA: Celiac and Superior Mesenteric Arteries: A Correlation of Angiograms and Dissections. Boston, Little, Brown, 1969.)

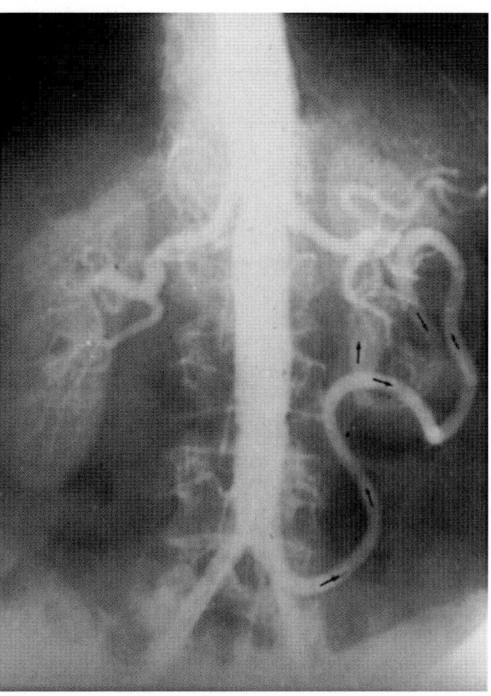

Figure 119–4. In this flush aortogram of a patient with superior mesenteric artery occlusion, the prominent meandering artery shows that collateral channels have been present for some time and that the occlusion is not acute. The *arrows* show the direction of flow from the inferior mesenteric artery to the superior mesenteric artery. (From Boley SJ, Brandt LJ, Veith FJ: Ischemic disorders of the intestines. Curr Probl Surg 15:29, 1978.)

ACUTE MESENTERIC ISCHEMIA

Intestinal ischemia can be classified as acute or chronic and of venous or arterial origin (Table 119–2). In the acute forms, intestinal viability is threatened, whereas in the chronic forms, blood flow is inadequate to support the functional demands of the intestine. Acute mesenteric ischemia (AMI) is much more common than the chronic type, and arterial disease is more frequent than venous disease. Arterial forms of AMI include SMA embolus (SMAE), nonoc-

Table 119–2 | **Causes and Approximate Incidences of Acute Mesenteric Ischemia**

CAUSE	INCIDENCE (%)
SMA embolus	50
Nonocclusive mesenteric ischemia	25
SMA thrombosis	10
Mesenteric venous thrombosis	10
Focal segmental ischemia	5

SMA, superior mesenteric artery.

clusive mesenteric ischemia (NOMI), SMA thrombosis (SMAT), and focal segmental ischemia (FSI). Acute mesenteric venous thrombosis (AMVT) and FSI caused by strangulation obstruction of the small intestine are the venous forms of AMI.

AMI results from inadequate blood flow to all or part of the small intestine and the right half of the colon. Regardless of the cause of the ischemic insult, the end results are similar—a spectrum of bowel injury that ranges from transient alteration of bowel function to transmural gangrene. Clinical manifestations vary with the extent of ischemic injury and, to a lesser degree, with its cause.

Incidence

AMI accounts for about 0.1% of admissions to our large tertiary care center. This figure has risen over the past 25 years, owing to increased recognition of the disorder, an aging population, and the widespread use of intensive care units with the salvage of patients who previously would have died from cardiovascular conditions but who now survive to develop AMI as a delayed consequence of their primary disease.

Most series of AMI reported in the late 1970s and early 1980s showed that SMAE was responsible for 40% to 50%, NOMI for 20% to 30%, and SMAT for 10% to 20% of cases. More recently, the incidence of NOMI has declined, likely because intensive care unit monitoring enables prompt correction of hypotension and blood volume deficits, and the widespread use of calcium channel blockers and other systemic vasodilators may protect the vascular bed from spasm. Today, SMAE is the most common cause of AMI.

Clinical Aspects

Early identification of AMI requires a high index of suspicion, especially in patients older than 50 years who have long-standing congestive heart failure (particularly if poorly controlled), cardiac arrhythmias, recent myocardial infarction, or hypotension. The development of sudden abdominal pain in a patient with any of these risk factors should suggest the diagnosis of AMI. A history of postprandial abdominal pain in the weeks to months preceding the acute onset of severe abdominal pain is associated only with SMAT.

Almost all patients with AMI have acute abdominal pain. The early pain of AMI is far more impressive than the early physical findings. Initially, the pain is severe, but the abdomen usually is flat, soft, and most often not tender or less tender than expected based on the magnitude of the pain. Sudden, severe abdominal pain accompanied by rapid and often forceful bowel evacuation, especially with minimal or no abdominal signs, strongly suggests SMAE. A more indolent and less striking onset is more typical of MVT, whereas with NOMI, appreciation of abdominal pain may be overshadowed by the precipitating disorders, such as hypotension, acute congestive heart failure, acute hypovolemia, or cardiac arrhythmias. Pain is absent in as many as 25% of patients with NOMI.

Unexplained abdominal distention or gastrointestinal bleeding may be the only indications of AMI when pain is absent, especially when due to NOMI. Distention, although absent early in the course of AMI, is often the first sign of intestinal infarction. The stool contains occult blood in 75% of patients. Right-sided abdominal pain associated with the passage of maroon or bright red blood in the stool, although characteristic of colonic ischemia, also may be seen with AMI, because the blood supply to both the right colon and small bowel originates from the SMA. Elderly patients with AMI have been reported to develop mental confusion acutely in as many as 30% of cases.[4] Patients who survive cardiopulmonary resuscitation and who then develop recurrent bacteremia or sepsis should be suspected of having had NOMI, which resulted in a segment of bowel with subacute ischemic injury, acting as a portal for bacterial translocation.[5]

Although abdominal findings early in the course of intestinal ischemia are minimal or absent, increasing tenderness, rebound tenderness, and muscle guarding reflect progressive loss of intestinal viability. Such abdominal findings strongly indicate the presence of infarcted bowel. The rate of progression from the onset of abdominal pain to intestinal infarction varies, not with the specific cause of ischemia, but with the severity of the ischemic insult; MVT generally has a more indolent course than do the arterial causes of AMI.

Laboratory Findings and Diagnostic Studies

On admission to the hospital, approximately 75% of patients with AMI have leukocytosis above 15,000 cells per cubic millimeter and about 50% have metabolic acidemia. Elevated levels of serum phosphate, amylase, D-lactate, and other enzymes have been noted, as have high peritoneal fluid amylase and intestinal alkaline phosphatase activity, but the sensitivity and specificity of these markers of intestinal ischemia have not been established.[6] Moreover, such serum markers, when elevated, usually indicate late-stage disease.

Plain radiographs of the abdomen usually are normal in AMI before infarction. Later on, formless loops of small intestine, ileus, or "thumbprinting" of the small bowel or right colon may develop (Fig. 119–5).

Duplex scanning and Doppler flowmetry have been of value in identifying portal and SMV thrombosis, and some instances of (proximal) SMA occlusion. SMA flow can be reproducibly determined by this method, but the wide range of normal SMA blood flow (from 300 to 600 mL per minute[7]) limits the value of this test. Moreover, only the proximal portions of the major vessels can be evaluated reliably by these techniques; the peripheral arterial tree cannot be well visualized.

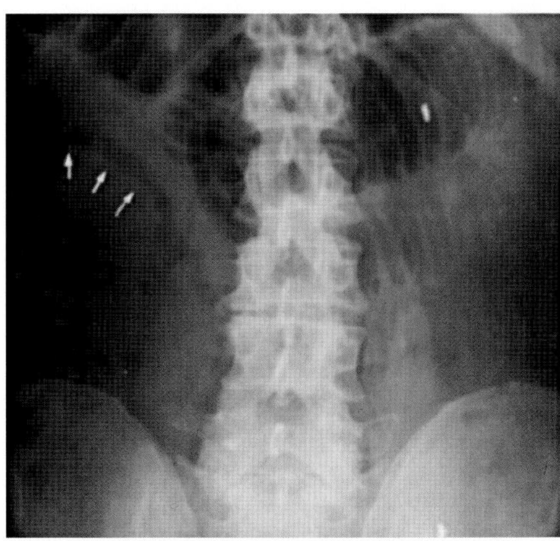

Figure 119–5. Plain film of the abdomen reveals ileus and a formless, fixed loop of small intestine *(arrows)* in a patient with acute mesenteric ischemia due to superior mesenteric artery embolus.

CT also has been used to identify arterial and venous thromboses as well as ischemic bowel. Findings on CT include bowel wall thickening, luminal dilation, and engorgement of mesenteric veins. Less common but more specific findings include intramural gas and mesenteric or portal venous gas (Fig. 119–6). Unfortunately, the early signs on CT are nonspecific and the late signs reflect necrotic bowel.[8] Therefore, abdominal CT and duplex ultrasonography cannot be recommended as first-line diagnostic studies in the evaluation of AMI.

Laparoscopy may be useful when angiography is contraindicated, but it can be misleading because early in ischemic injury, blood may be shunted to the serosa, giving a normal appearance to the outside of the bowel while the mucosa may be necrotic. Moreover, laparoscopy is potentially dangerous because SMA blood flow decreases when intraperitoneal pressure exceeds 20 mm Hg.

Selective mesenteric angiography, frequently with use of papaverine infusion, currently is the mainstay of diagnosis and initial treatment of both occlusive and nonocclusive forms of AMI and should be performed promptly if AMI is suspected.[9] Further details on angiography are described later in this chapter.

Diagnosis and Treatment

Our approach to the diagnosis and management of AMI is based on several observations. First, if the diagnosis is not made before intestinal infarction, the mortality rate is 70% to 90%. Second, the diagnosis of both the occlusive and nonocclusive forms of AMI can be made in most patients by angiography. Third, vasoconstriction, which may persist even after the cause of the ischemia is corrected, is the basis of NOMI and a contributing factor in the other forms of AMI. Finally, the vasoconstriction can be relieved by vasodilators infused into the SMA. The cornerstones of our approach, therefore, are the earlier and more liberal use of angiography and the incorporation of intra-arterial papaverine in the treatment of both occlusive AMI and NOMI.

Patients older than 50 years who have the risk factors previously described and younger patients, especially those with atrial fibrillation or vasculitis or any evidence of a coagulation disorder, who seek medical attention for sudden, severe abdominal pain that lasts longer than 2 hours should be suspected of having AMI. These patients should be managed according to the algorithm in Figure 119–7. Less absolute indications for inclusion into this protocol include unexplained acute abdominal distention, colonoscopic evidence of isolated right-sided colonic ischemia, or acidosis without an identifiable cause.

Initial management of patients suspected of having AMI includes resuscitation, abdominal plain films, and selective angiography. Resuscitation includes relief of acute congestive heart failure and correction of hypotension, hypovolemia, and cardiac arrhythmias. Broad-spectrum antibiotics are given immediately because of the high incidence of positive blood cultures in AMI and because they reduce the extent and severity of ischemic injury in experimental animals.

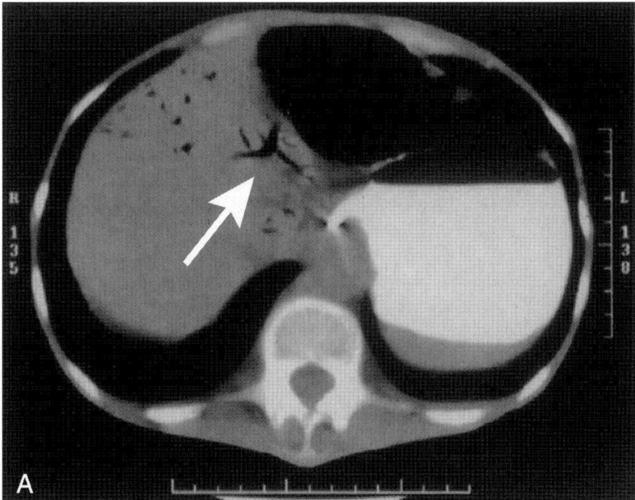

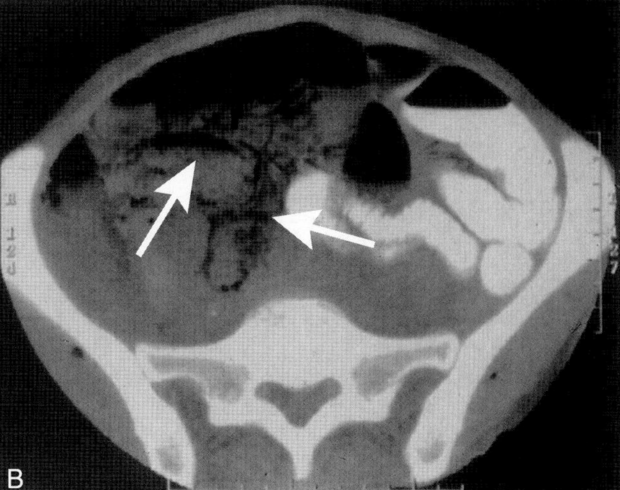

Figure 119–6. CT scans showing gas *(arrow)* in the portal veins *(A)* and gas *(arrows)* in the wall of the bowel, mesentery, and mesenteric vessels *(B)*. Pneumatosis is a late sign of ischemic injury, connotes bowel necrosis, and mandates exploration.

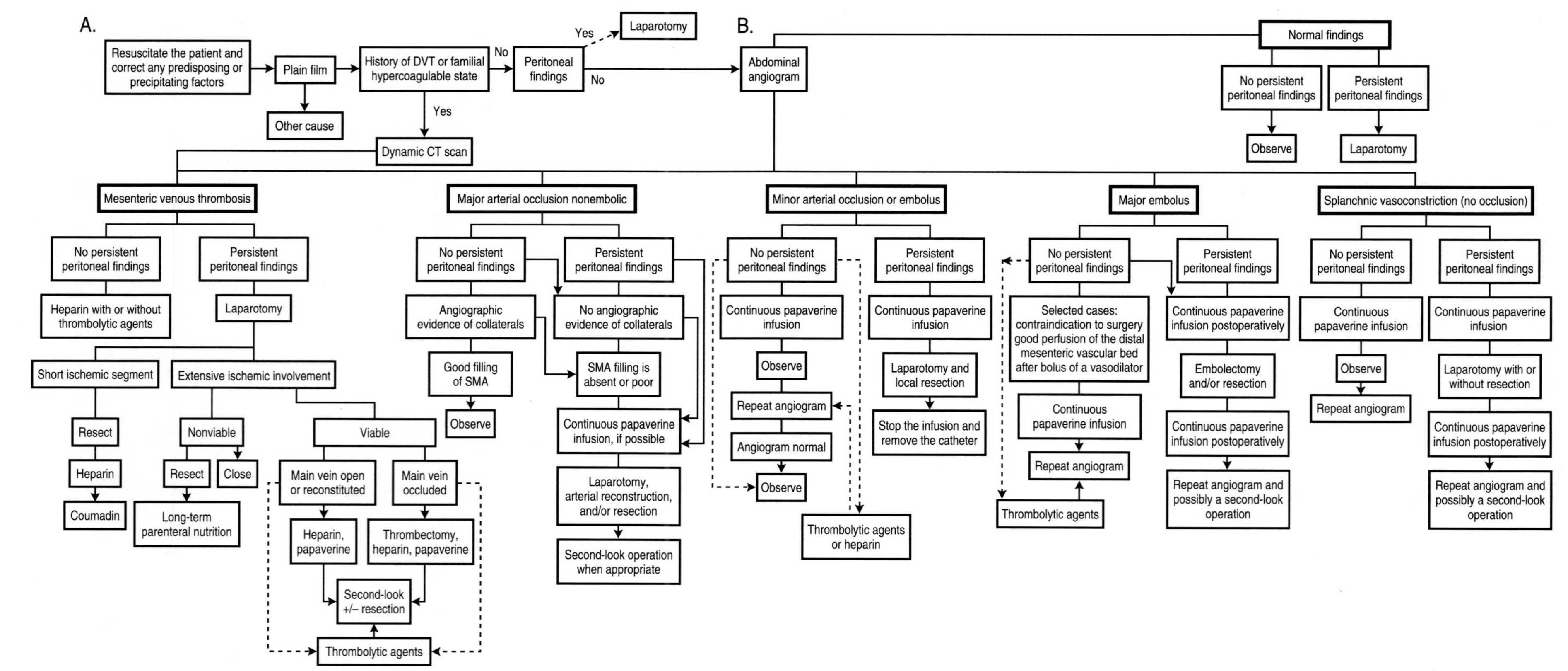

Figure 119–7. Algorithm for the diagnosis *(A)* and treatment *(B)* of intestinal ischemia. DVT, deep venous thrombosis; SMA, superior mesenteric artery. (From Brandt LJ, Boley SJ: AGA technical review on intestinal ischemia: American Gastrointestinal Association. Gastroenterology 118:954, 2000; corrected version in Gastroenterology 119:281, 2000.)

There are no randomized, controlled studies showing the benefit of antibiotics in AMI, and it is unlikely that such studies will ever be done. After resuscitation, plain films or CT scan of the abdomen are obtained, not to establish the diagnosis of AMI but rather to exclude other causes of abdominal pain. A normal plain film or CT scan does not exclude AMI; ideally, patients are studied before radiographic signs appear because these connote irreversibly damaged bowel. If no alternative diagnosis is made on these studies, selective SMA angiography is performed. Based on the angiographic findings and the presence or absence of peritoneal signs, the patient is treated according to the algorithm in Figure 119–7.

Even when the decision to operate has been based on clinical grounds, preoperative angiography should be performed to manage the patient properly at and after laparotomy. Relief of mesenteric vasoconstriction is essential to the treatment of emboli, thromboses, and the nonocclusive "low-flow" states. Infusion of papaverine through the angiography catheter in the SMA is used to relieve mesenteric vasoconstriction preoperatively and postoperatively. The papaverine (1 mg/mL) is infused by pump at a constant rate of 30 to 60 mg per hour; a more concentrated solution can be used if fluid restriction is necessary.

Although most of the papaverine infused into the mesenteric bed is cleared during one pass through the liver, blood pressure and cardiac rate and rhythm must be monitored constantly. Some patients with liver disease may exhibit a drop in blood pressure with this dose of papaverine, but the most common cause of hypotension during the papaverine infusion is catheter dislodgment. Patients who have a sudden drop in blood pressure should have the papaverine replaced with a saline or glucose solution and promptly undergo plain film imaging of the abdomen to confirm the catheter's location. If the catheter has come out of the SMA, it should be replaced and the papaverine restarted. The clinical and angiographic responses of the patient to the vasodilator determine the duration of therapy.

Laparotomy is performed in AMI to restore arterial flow obstructed by embolus or thrombosis or to resect irreparably damaged bowel. Embolectomy, thrombectomy, or arterial bypass precedes evaluation of intestinal viability, because bowel that initially appears infarcted may show surprising recovery after adequate blood flow is restored. In the operating room, intestinal viability can be assessed clinically, by qualitative or quantitative surface fluorescence or by Doppler ultrasonography.[10]

Short segments of bowel that are nonviable or questionably viable after revascularization are resected, and a primary anastomosis is performed. If extensive portions of the bowel are of questionable viability, only the clearly necrotic bowel is resected and re-exploration (second look) is planned for within 12 to 24 hours. The interval between the first and second operations is used both to allow better demarcation between viable and nonviable bowel and to attempt to improve intestinal blood flow using intra-arterial papaverine and maximizing cardiac output.

The use of anticoagulants in the management of AMI is controversial. Anticoagulation with heparin may cause intestinal or intraperitoneal hemorrhage and, except for MVT, should not be used routinely in the immediate postoperative period; 48 hours after embolectomy or arterial reconstruction, when thrombosis is frequent, anticoagulation is appropriate.

Specific Types of Acute Mesenteric Ischemia and Their Management

Superior Mesenteric Artery Emboli

Superior mesenteric artery emboli (SMAE) are responsible for 40% to 50% of AMI episodes. Emboli usually originate from a left atrial or ventricular mural thrombus. Many patients with SMAE have had previous peripheral artery emboli, and approximately 20% have synchronous emboli. SMAE lodge at points of normal anatomic narrowing, usually immediately distal to the origin of a major branch. Angiography typically reveals a rounded filling defect with nearly complete obstruction to flow. Mesenteric atherosclerosis is usually not as severe as in SMAT. Emboli proximal to the origin of the ileocolic artery are considered "major" emboli. "Minor" emboli are those that lodge in the SMA distal to the takeoff of the ileocolic artery or in the distal branches of the SMA (Fig. 119–8).

Various therapeutic approaches have been proposed for SMAE, depending on the presence or absence of peritoneal signs, whether the embolus is partially or completely occluding, and whether the embolus is in the SMA above the origin of the ileocolic artery (i.e., a major embolus) or more distally in the SMA or one of its branches (i.e., minor embolus). Therapy for SMAE has included surgical revascularization, intra-arterial perfusion with vasodilators or thrombolytic agents, and anticoagulation.[9] In the absence of peritoneal signs, minor SMA emboli have been treated successfully with all of these agents without the need for surgery. Patients with major emboli usually are explored after papaverine infusion is begun. Nonoperative therapy using just papaverine is employed if there are significant contraindications to surgery, no peritoneal signs, and adequate perfusion of the vascular bed distal to the embolus after a bolus of vasodilator into the SMA.

Exploratory laparotomy is mandatory when peritonitis is present; embolectomy and bowel resection are performed as necessary. If possible, intra-arterial papaverine is begun before surgery and is continued during surgery. If no second look is planned, infusion is continued for 12 to 24 hours postoperatively; persistent vasospasm is excluded by angiography before removal of the catheter (see Fig. 119–8). If a second operation is planned, the infusion is continued through the second procedure until vasoconstriction has been shown by angiography to have ceased. Recognition of persistent vasoconstriction has prompted some authorities to recommend routine use of intra-arterial papaverine in all patients with SMAE; the best survival rates are seen in patients treated in this way.[9]

Thrombolytic therapy using streptokinase, urokinase, or recombinant tissue plasminogen activator has been used in small series of patients with some success. Thrombolytic therapy is most likely to be successful when the embolus is partially occluding, or is minor, and the study is performed within 12 hours of the onset of symptoms.[9, 11]

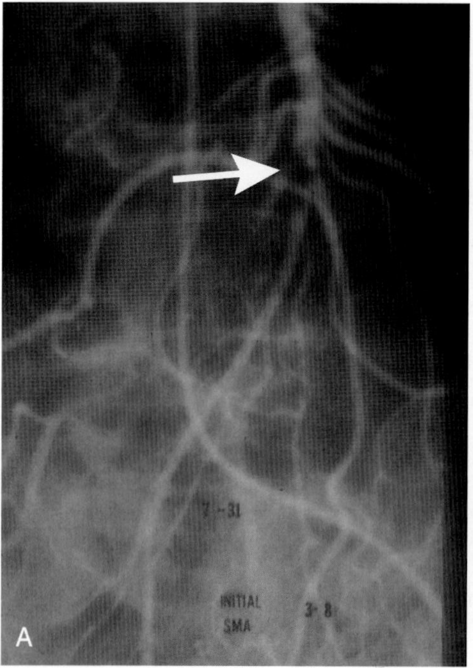

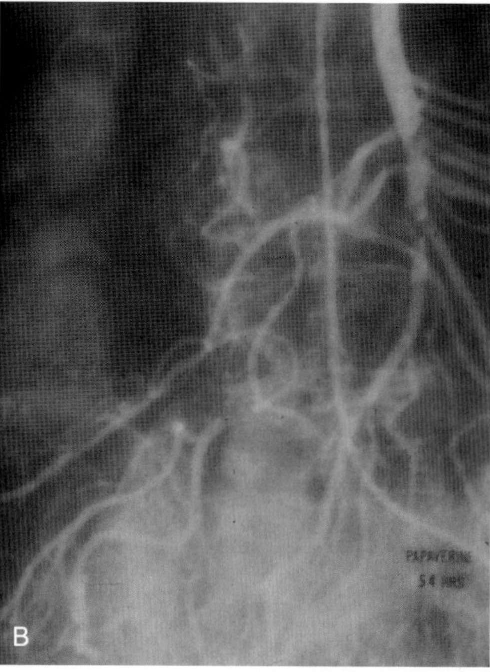

Figure 119–8. *A,* Superior mesenteric artery (SMA) angiogram from a 71-year-old man with abdominal pain shows an embolus occluding the SMA at the level of the origin of the right colic artery *(arrow).* Vasoconstriction is noted distal to the embolus. *B,* Repeat angiogram made 24 hours after SMA embolectomy and preoperative and postoperative papaverine infusions into the SMA. Vasodilation is seen, and all vessels are patent except for a distal jejunal branch.

Nonocclusive Mesenteric Ischemia

Nonocclusive mesenteric ischemia (NOMI) is responsible for 20% to 30% of AMI and usually is due to splanchnic vasoconstriction consequent to a preceding cardiovascular event, such as pulmonary edema, arrhythmias, and shock. AMI may appear hours to days after the event, and vasoconstriction, which initially is reversible, may persist even after the precipitating event has been corrected. Precipitating causes for NOMI include acute myocardial infarction, congestive heart failure, cirrhosis, and chronic renal failure—especially when dialysis is required.

NOMI is diagnosed by angiography using four reliable criteria: (1) narrowing of the origins of SMA branches; (2) irregularities in the intestinal branches; (3) spasm of the arcades; and (4) impaired filling of intramural vessels. Patients with these signs who are neither in shock nor on vasopressors and who do not have pancreatitis can be considered to have NOMI[12] (Fig. 119–9).

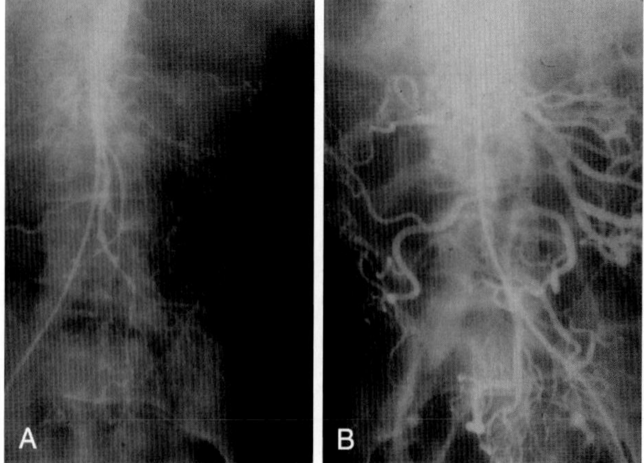

Figure 119–9. Patient with nonocclusive mesenteric ischemia (NOMI) following a bout of gastrointestinal hemorrhage and shock. *A,* Superior mesenteric artery angiogram shows the diffuse vasoconstriction of NOMI. *B,* Marked vasodilation is evident on the repeat study after 48 hours of an intra-arterial papaverine infusion. (From Brandt LJ, Boley SJ: Ischemic intestinal syndromes. Adv Surg 15:1–45, 1981.)

SMA infusion of papaverine is begun as soon as the diagnosis is made. Operation is performed if peritoneal signs are present, and the infusion is continued during and after exploration. Necrotic bowel is resected; it is better to leave bowel of questionable viability and perform a second-look operation than to perform massive enterectomy, because compromised but viable bowel often improves with supportive measures. The infusion is continued as for second-look operations following embolectomy.

When papaverine infusion is used as the only treatment for NOMI, in patients without signs of peritonitis, it is continued for 24 hours, and repeat angiography is performed 30 minutes after changing the papaverine to normal saline. The infusion is maintained and angiography repeated daily until there is no roentgenographic evidence of vasoconstriction and the patient's clinical findings resolve. Infusions, usually discontinued after 24 hours, have been given for as long as 5 days.

Acute Superior Mesenteric Artery Thrombosis

Acute superior mesenteric artery thrombosis (SMAT) occurs in areas of severe atherosclerotic narrowing, most often at the origin of the SMA. The acute ischemic episode is commonly superimposed on chronic mesenteric ischemia, and 20% to 50% of these patients have a history of postprandial abdominal pain and weight loss during the weeks to months preceding the acute event. Evidence of coronary, cerebrovascular, or peripheral arterial insufficiency is common.

SMAT is demonstrated on flush aortography, which usually shows occlusion of the SMA 1 to 2 cm from its origin. Some distal filling of the SMA via collaterals is common. Branches both proximal and distal to the obstruction may show localized or diffuse vasoconstriction. In patients with abdominal pain, no abdominal tenderness, and complete occlusion of the SMA on aortography, it is important, though difficult, to distinguish between acute thrombosis and longstanding, coincidental chronic occlusion. Prominent collaterals between the SMA and other major splanchnic vessels indicate chronic SMA occlusion. If there is good filling of the SMA, the occlusion is considered to be chronic and the abdominal pain unrelated to mesenteric vascular disease (see Fig. 119–4). The absence of collateral vessels or the presence of collaterals with inadequate filling of the SMA indicates an acute occlusion and demands prompt intervention. If possible, an angiographic catheter is placed in the proximal SMA, and papaverine infusion is begun before surgery is undertaken.

At surgery, necrotic bowel is resected and remaining bowel is revascularized. Papaverine infusion is continued throughout the operative period, and management is the same as for SMAE, including heparin. There are but few reports of use of thrombolytic agents or percutaneous angioplasty for SMAT.

Complications of Therapy

Complications of angiography and prolonged infusion of vasodilator drugs include transient acute tubular necrosis following angiography, local hematomas at the arterial puncture sites, dislodgment of catheters, and fibrin clots on the arterial catheter. Infusion for more than 5 days has not had significant systemic effects.

Results of Therapy

Although mortality rates of 70% to 90% are reported for AMI through the 1980s for patients diagnosed and treated conventionally, the suggested approach described earlier can reduce these catastrophic figures. The best survival is reported in series in which angiography has been used routinely in the management of AMI.[9, 13–17]

In our center, more than 50% of the patients with AMI treated according to our approach survived, and more than 75% have lost less than 1 m of intestine. The importance of early diagnosis is emphasized by the survival of 90% of patients who had AMI but no signs of peritonitis and who had angiography early in their course. Ideally, all patients with AMI should be studied when plain films of the abdomen are normal, before signs of an acute surgical abdomen and laboratory evidence of infarction appear. *Diagnosis before the occurrence of intestinal infarction is the most important factor in improving survival of patients with AMI.*

MESENTERIC VENOUS THROMBOSIS

Mesenteric venous thrombosis (MVT) occurs as an acute, subacute, or chronic disorder. It is only since the development of recent imaging techniques that these various forms of MVT have been recognized; previously, only acute MVT was known, and diagnosis was made at laparotomy or autopsy.

Incidence

In early studies, MVT was believed to be the major cause of AMI, but most of these cases probably represented NOMI. Today, only 5% to 10% of patients with AMI have MVT, and the reported mean age of these individuals is younger, 48 to 60 years, than of those with other forms of AMI.

Predisposing Conditions (Table 119–3)

Previously, a cause of MVT was identified in fewer than half of patients. The discoveries of the primary and secondary hypercoagulable states along with use of estrogens for contraception and hormone replacement have enabled identification of the cause in almost 90% of patients.[18, 19]

Pathophysiology

The location of the initial thrombus within the mesenteric venous circulation varies with the cause. MVT secondary to cirrhosis, neoplasm, or operative injury begins at the site of obstruction and extends peripherally, whereas thrombosis of hypercoagulable states starts in smaller branches and propagates into the major trunks. Intestinal infarction is rare unless the branches of the peripheral arcades and the vasa recta are involved. When collateral circulation is inadequate and venous drainage from a segment of bowel is compromised, the affected intestine becomes congested, edematous, cyanotic, and thickened with intramural hemorrhage. Serosanguineous peritoneal fluid heralds early hemorrhagic infarction. Arterial vasoconstriction can be marked, but pulsations

Table 119–3 | **Conditions Associated with Mesenteric Venous Thrombosis**

Hypercoagulable states
Antithrombin III deficiency
Protein C deficiency
Protein S deficiency
MTHF (methyltetrahydrofolate) deficiency
Factor V Leiden
Estrogens
Polycythemia vera
Thrombocytosis
Neoplasms
Peripheral deep venous thrombosis
Pregnancy
Portal hypertension
Cirrhosis
Congestive splenomegaly
After sclerotherapy of esophageal varices
Inflammation
Pancreatitis
Peritonitis (e.g., appendicitis, perforated viscus)
Inflammatory bowel disease
Pelvic or intra-abdominal abscess
Diverticulitis
Postoperative state or trauma
Blunt abdominal trauma
Splenectomy and other postoperative states
Other: decompression sickness

persist up to the bowel wall. The occurrence of transmural infarction may make it impossible to differentiate venous from arterial occlusion.

Clinical Features

MVT can have an acute, subacute (weeks to months), or chronic onset; except for late complications, the latter is asymptomatic. As many as 60% of patients have a history of peripheral vein thromboses.[20]

Acute MVT presents with abdominal pain in more than 90% of patients and, as with acute arterial ischemia, the pain initially is out of proportion to the physical findings. The mean duration of pain before admission is 5 to 14 days but may be more than 1 month in as many as 25% of individuals.[21] Other symptoms, including nausea and vomiting, occur in more than 50%. Lower gastrointestinal bleeding, bloody diarrhea, or hematemesis occurs in 15% and indicates bowel infarction. Fecal occult blood is found in more than half of instances during the course of MVT. Initial physical findings vary at different stages and with different degrees of ischemic injury, but guarding and rebound tenderness develop as bowel infarction evolves. Most patients have a temperature higher than 38°C, and 25% exhibit signs of septic shock.

Subacute MVT describes the condition in patients who have abdominal pain for weeks to months but no intestinal infarction. Subacute MVT can be due either to extension of thrombosis at a rate rapid enough to cause pain but that permits collaterals to develop, thus preventing infarction, or to acute thrombosis of venous drainage sufficient to permit recovery from ischemic injury. The diagnosis usually is made on imaging studies ordered to diagnose other conditions.

Nonspecific abdominal pain usually is the only symptom of subacute MVT, and findings of physical examination and laboratory tests are normal. Some patients who present with subacute MVT ultimately develop intestinal infarction; this blurs the distinction between the acute and subacute forms of MVT. At autopsy, coexistent new and old thromboses have been found in nearly half of the patients.

Chronic MVT is seen in patients who are asymptomatic at the time of thrombosis but who may develop gastrointestinal bleeding from varices.[22] Most patients bleed from gastroesophageal varices secondary to thrombosis of the portal or splenic vein, and they have physical findings of portal hypertension. Findings are absent if only the SMV is involved. Laboratory studies may show secondary hypersplenism with pancytopenia or thrombocytopenia.

Diagnosis

Acute Mesenteric Venous Thrombosis

The absence of specific symptoms, signs, or laboratory results and the typical variability in the course of the disease make it difficult to diagnose acute MVT preoperatively. Abdominal plain film signs of MVT are similar to those of other forms of AMI and almost always reflect the presence of infarcted bowel. Barium enemas are of little diagnostic value, because MVT rarely involves the colon. Characteristic findings on small bowel series include marked thickening of the bowel wall due to congestion and edema with separation of loops and "thumbprinting."

Selective mesenteric arteriography can establish a definitive diagnosis before bowel infarction, can differentiate venous thrombosis from arterial forms of ischemia, and can provide access for vasodilator therapy. Angiographic findings include thrombus in the SMV with partial or complete occlusion, failure to visualize the SMV or portal vein, slow or absent filling of the mesenteric veins, arterial spasm, failure of the arterial arcades to empty, reflux of contrast medium into the artery, and prolonged blush in the involved segment.[23]

Ultrasonography, CT, and magnetic resonance imaging (MRI) all have been used to demonstrate thrombi in the SMV and the portal vein.[24–26] CT can diagnose MVT in more than 90% of patients and is the diagnostic study of choice. Specific findings include thickening and enhancement of the bowel wall, enlargement of the SMV, a central lucency in the lumen of the vein (representing a thrombus), a sharply defined vein wall with a rim of increased density, and dilated collateral vessels in a thickened mesentery (Fig. 119–10). When MVT is diagnosed on CT, angiography may not be necessary, but in selected symptomatic patients it better delineates thrombosed veins and provides access for intra-arterial vasodilators. Esophagogastroduodenoscopy and

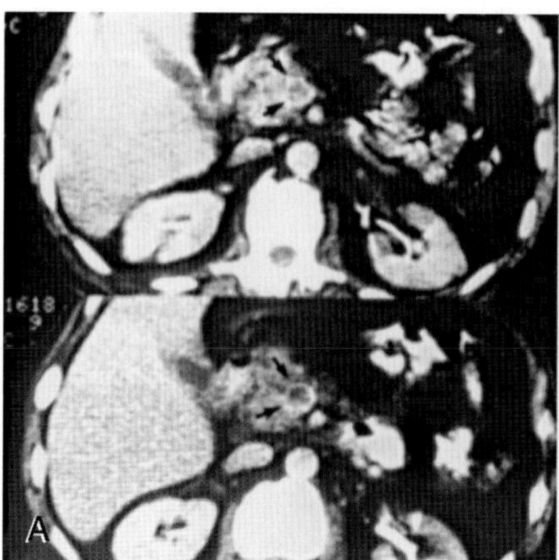

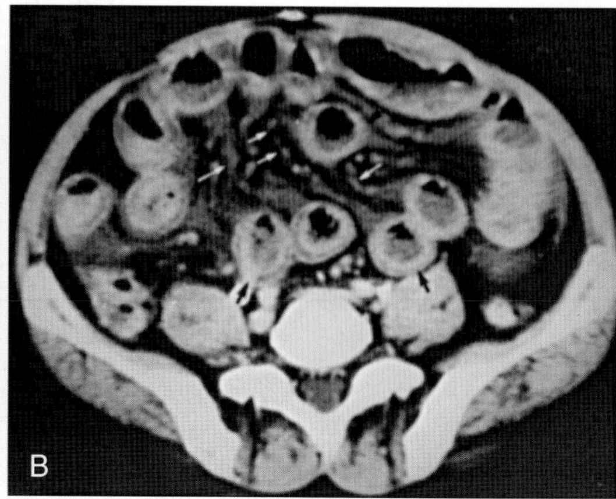

Figure 119–10. *A,* Abdominal CT with contrast agent demonstrates enlarged superior mesenteric vein with central lucency in the lumen, representing the thrombus. The vein wall is sharply defined with a rim of increased density surrounding the thrombus *(arrows). B,* Abdominal CT with contrast agent shows thickening and persistent enhancement of the bowel wall *(white arrows),* and dilated collateral vessels within a thickened mesentery *(black arrows).* (From Boley SJ, Brandt LJ: Ischemic disorders of the intestines. Surg Clin North Am 72:194, 1992.)

colonoscopy are rarely helpful, because the duodenum and colon are infrequently involved. As in other forms of AMI, laparoscopy may be useful when other studies are contraindicated.[27]

The diagnosis of MVT usually has been made at laparotomy, where its hallmarks are serosanguineous peritoneal fluid, dark red to blue-black edematous bowel, thickening of the mesentery, good arterial pulsations in the involved segment, and thrombi in cut mesenteric veins. At this stage, some degree of intestinal infarction invariably has occurred. When persons suspected to have AMI exhibit features suggesting MVT, contrast-enhanced CT is performed before SMA angiography. A history of deep vein thrombosis or a family history of an inherited coagulation defect prompts CT as the first imaging study.

Chronic Mesenteric Venous Thrombosis

Because chronic MVT is asymptomatic or presents as gastrointestinal bleeding, the diagnostic evaluation is directed toward determining the cause of the bleeding. Endoscopy and appropriate imaging studies should identify the cause and site of bleeding and the extent of thrombosis. Papaverine-enhanced selective SMA angiography may further delineate the anatomy.

Treatment

Acute Mesenteric Venous Thrombosis

Most patients with acute MVT initially are believed to have some form of AMI and are treated as discussed in the sections above and as outlined in the algorithm of Figure 119–7. If signs of infarction or impending infarction are present, surgery is performed and segments of infarcted bowel are removed. If long segments of questionably viable bowel are found, papaverine is infused and if arterial spasm is relieved and the SMV or portal vein is visualized, thrombectomy and/or a second look may be attempted to determine whether resection should be performed. Following surgery, heparin should be administered. In asymptomatic persons in whom the diagnosis is made on a CT scan done for other than abdominal pain, either no therapy or 3 to 6 months of anticoagulation is reasonable. In symptomatic individuals, treatment is determined by the presence or absence of peritoneal signs; signs of peritonitis mandate laparotomy and resection of infarcted bowel. Immediate heparinization for 7 to 10 days has been shown to diminish recurrence and progression of thrombosis and to improve survival.[19, 28, 29] In the absence of peritoneal signs, immediate heparinization followed by a 3- to 6-month course of warfarin may be all that is needed. A few case reports have documented the use of thrombolytic agents in the treatment of acute MVT.

Chronic Mesenteric Venous Thrombosis

Treatment of chronic MVT is aimed at controlling bleeding, usually from esophageal varices. Sclerotherapy, portosystemic shunts, devascularization procedures, and bowel resection all have a place in treating selected patients. No treatment is indicated for patients with asymptomatic chronic MVT.

Results of Therapy and Prognosis

Mortality associated with acute MVT is lower than that for other forms of AMI, varying from 20% to 50%. Recurrence rates of 20% to 25% fall to about 15% if heparin therapy is begun promptly. The natural history of chronic MVT is not known, but from postmortem studies it appears that almost 50% of patients with MVT have no bowel infarction and most have no symptoms.

FOCAL SEGMENTAL ISCHEMIA OF THE SMALL BOWEL

Vascular insults to short segments of small bowel produce a broad spectrum of clinical features without the life-threatening complications associated with more extensive ischemia. The causes of focal segmental ischemia (FSI) include atheromatous emboli, strangulated hernias, immune complex disorders and vasculitis, blunt abdominal trauma, segmental venous thrombosis, radiation therapy, and oral contraceptives, among others. With FSI there is usually adequate collateral circulation to prevent transmural infarction; the most common lesion is partial bowel wall necrosis with invasion by intestinal bacteria. Limited necrosis may present as acute enteritis, chronic enteritis, or a stricture. In the acute pattern, abdominal pain often simulates acute appendicitis. Physical findings are those of acute abdomen, and an inflammatory mass may be palpated. The chronic enteritis pattern may be indistinguishable from that of Crohn's disease and includes crampy abdominal pain, diarrhea, fever, and weight loss. The most common presentation is chronic small bowel obstruction with intermittent abdominal pain, distention, and vomiting. Bacterial overgrowth and protein-losing enteropathy also can occur. Treatment of FSI is resection of the involved bowel.

COLONIC ISCHEMIA

Colonic ischemia (CI) is a frequent disorder of the large bowel in older persons and is the most common form of intestinal ischemic injury. It comprises a spectrum (Table 119–4) including (1) reversible colopathy (submucosal or

Table 119–4 | **Types and Approximate Incidences of Colonic Ischemia**

TYPE	INCIDENCE (%)
Reversible colopathy	30–40
Transient colitis	15–20
Chronic ulcerating colitis	20–25
Stricture	10–15
Gangrene	15–20
Fulminant universal colitis	<5

intramural hemorrhage); (2) transient colitis; (3) chronic colitis; (4) stricture; (5) gangrene; and (6) fulminant, universal colitis. The initial presentation usually is the same among these types and does not necessarily predict the course of disease, with the exception of ischemia involving the ascending colon simultaneously with the small intestine. This latter pattern usually is caused by SMAE or NOMI, may have associated shock, and carries a mortality rate of more than 50%.[30, 31]

Pathophysiology and Causes

CI can result from alterations in the systemic circulation or anatomic or functional changes in the local mesenteric vasculature (Table 119–5). In most cases, no specific cause for the ischemia is identified, and such episodes are viewed as localized nonocclusive ischemia, perhaps secondary to small vessel disease. Abnormalities on angiography rarely correlate with clinical manifestations of disease, but age-related abnormalities in the splanchnic vessels, including narrowings of small vessels, tortuosity of the long colic arteries, and fibromuscular dysplasia of the superior rectal artery, may contribute to CI. The colon is particularly susceptible to ischemia, perhaps owing to its relatively low blood flow, its unique decrease in blood flow during periods of functional activity, and its sensitivity to autonomic stimulation. What triggers the episode of CI, however, usually is not known.

Incidence

The incidence of CI is underestimated, because many patients suffer only mild or transient damage and do not seek medical attention. Also, CI is frequently misdiagnosed and confused with other disorders, notably inflammatory bowel disease. In our tertiary care hospital, CI accounts for 1 in approximately 2000 hospital admissions and is seen in approximately 1 in 100 flexible sigmoidoscopies and colonoscopies. CI has no sex predilection, and more than 90% of patients with CI of noniatrogenic causes are older than 60 years. CI affecting young persons has been documented in case reports or series of a few patients and has been due to vasculitis, coagulation disorders, illicit use of cocaine, and iatrogenic causes, including a wide variety of medications such as estrogens, psychotropics, sumatriptan, and methamphetamine.

Pathology

Morphologic changes after CI vary with the duration and severity of the injury. The mildest injury is mucosal and submucosal hemorrhage and edema, with or without partial necrosis and ulceration of the mucosa. With more severe injury, chronic ulcerations, crypt abscesses, and pseudopolyps develop, changes that may mimic inflammatory bowel disease (Fig. 119–11)[32]; pseudomembranes also may be seen. Iron-laden macrophages and submucosal fibrosis are characteristic of ischemic injury. With severe ischemia, the muscularis propria is replaced by fibrous tissue, forming a stricture. The most severe form of ischemic damage causes transmural infarction.

Table 119–5 | **Causes of Colonic Ischemia**

Inferior mesenteric artery thrombosis
Arterial embolus
Cholesterol emboli
Cardiac failure or arrhythmias
Shock
Pheochromocytoma
Volvulus
Strangulated hernia
Amyloidosis
Pancreatitis
Vasculitis
Systemic lupus erythematosus
Polyarteritis nodosa
Rheumatoid vasculitis
Buerger's disease
Takayasu's arteritis
Kawasaki's disease
Hematologic disorders and coagulopathies
Sickle cell disease
Polycythemia vera
Paroxysmal nocturnal hemoglobinuria
Protein C and S deficiency
Antithrombin III deficiency
Activated protein C resistance
Prothombin 20210A mutation
Infection
Parasites (*Angiostrongylus costaricensis*)
Bacteria (*Escherichia coli* O157:H7)
Viruses (hepatitis B, cytomegalovirus)
Allergy
Trauma, blunt or penetrating
Ruptured ectopic pregnancy
Competitive long-distance running
Iatrogenic causes
Surgical
Aneurysmectomy
Aortoiliac reconstruction
Gynecologic operations
Exchange transfusions
Colon bypass
Lumbar aortography
Colectomy with inferior mesenteric artery ligation
Colonoscopy and barium enema examination
Medications and drugs
Digitalis
Estrogens
Progestins
Danazol
Vasopressin
Pseudoephedrine
Phenylephrine
Sumatriptan
Methamphetamine
Ergot
Gold
Psychotropic drugs
Nonsteroidal anti-inflammatory drugs
Oral saline laxatives
GoLYTELY
Glycerin enema
Interferon α
Flutamide
Penicillin
Immunosuppressive agents
Alosetron
Pit viper toxin
Cocaine

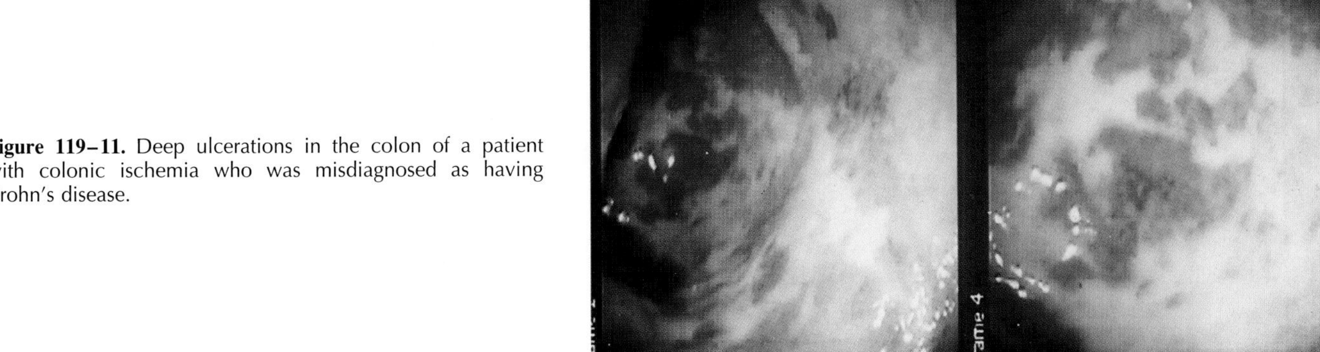

Figure 119–11. Deep ulcerations in the colon of a patient with colonic ischemia who was misdiagnosed as having Crohn's disease.

Clinical Presentation and Diagnosis

CI usually presents with sudden, crampy, mild, left lower abdominal pain, an urgent desire to defecate, and passage within 24 hours of bright red or maroon blood mixed with the stool. Bleeding is usually not sufficient to require transfusion. Mild to moderate abdominal tenderness usually is present over the involved segment of bowel.

The splenic flexure, descending colon, and sigmoid most commonly are affected (Fig. 119–12). Certain causes tend to affect particular segments: systemic low-flow states, the right colon; local nonocclusive ischemic injuries, the "watershed" areas (the splenic flexure and rectosigmoid); and ligation of the IMA, the sigmoid. The length of affected bowel also depends on the cause: atheromatous emboli involve short segments, and nonocclusive injuries involve longer portions of colon.

If CI is suspected and the patient has no signs of peritonitis and an unrevealing abdominal plain film, colonoscopy or the combination of sigmoidoscopy and a gentle barium enema should be performed on the unprepared bowel within 48 hours of the onset of symptoms. During colonoscopy and barium enema, examination care should be taken not to overdistend the colon, because high intraluminal pressure diminishes intestinal blood flow and may aggravate ischemic damage, particularly in patients with vasculitis.[33] Colonoscopy is preferable to barium studies because it is more sensitive in diagnosing mucosal abnormalities and biopsy specimens may be obtained.[34] Hemorrhagic nodules seen at colonoscopy represent bleeding into the submucosa and are equivalent to thumbprints on barium enema studies. (Fig. 119–13). Segmental distribution of these findings, with or without ulceration, is highly suggestive of CI, but the diagnosis of CI cannot be made conclusively in a single study unless mucosal gangrene is seen (Fig. 119–14).

The initial diagnostic study should be performed within 48 hours, because thumbprinting disappears within days as the submucosal hemorrhages are resorbed or the overlying mucosa sloughs. Studies performed 1 week after the initial study should reflect evolution of the injury—either normalization of the colon or replacement of the thumbprints with a segmental ulcerative colitis-type pattern (Fig. 119–15). Universal colonic involvement, however, favors true ulcerative colitis, whereas fistula formation suggests Crohn's disease. Occasionally, an abundant inflammatory response can produce heaping-up of mucosa and submucosa that resembles a stricture or neoplasm (Fig. 119–16).

At the time of symptom onset, colon blood flow typically has returned to normal, and, therefore, mesenteric angiography usually is not indicated. An exception to this rule is when the clinical presentation does not allow a clear distinction to be made between CI and AMI; then, administration of air during flexible sigmoidoscopy can be used to reveal

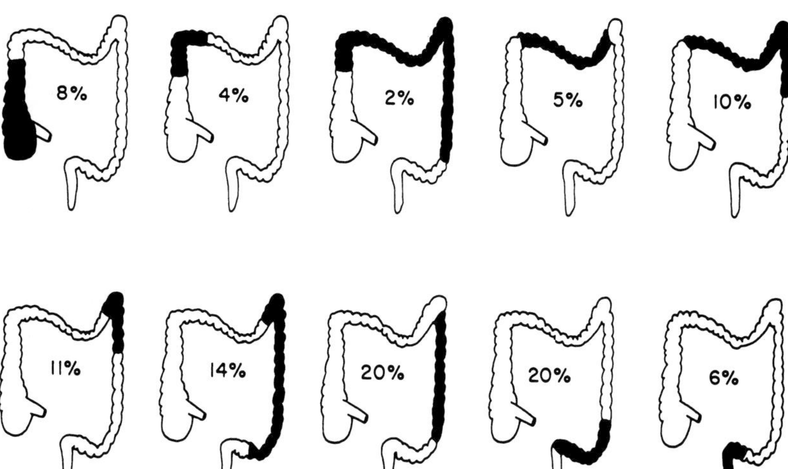

Figure 119–12. Schematic of patterns of colonic ischemia showing the percentage of involvement of each pattern from a total of 250 cases.

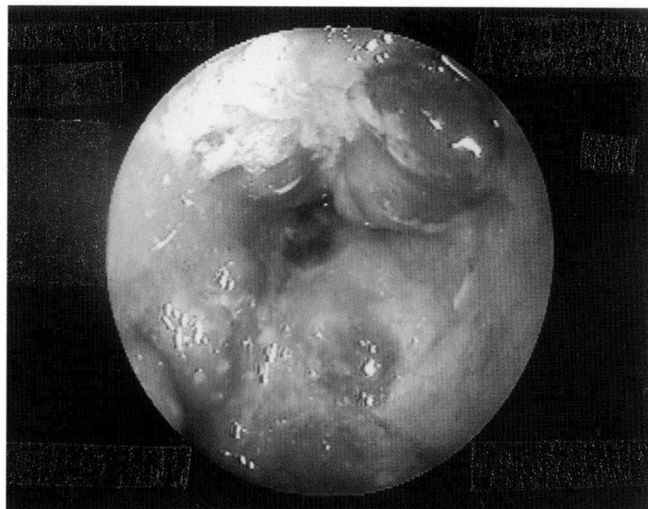

Figure 119–13. Colonoscopic equivalent of a "thumbprint," caused by submucosal hemorrhage and edema.

thumbprinting not otherwise visible on abdominal plain films. Thumbprinting isolated to the ascending colon suggests SMA disease and the need for angiography.

Clinical Course and Management

(Fig. 119–17)

When CI is diagnosed and physical examination does not suggest gangrene or perforation, the patient is treated expectantly. Parenteral fluids are administered and the bowel is placed at rest. Broad-spectrum antibiotics are given to "cover" the fecal flora, because in experimental models, antibiotics reduce the interval and severity of bowel damage. No randomized, controlled, blinded trials have been done to prove the validity of this recommendation. Cardiac failure and arrhythmias are treated, and medications that cause mesenteric vasoconstriction (e.g., digitalis and vasopressors) are withdrawn. If the colon appears distended, it is decompressed with a rectal tube. Serial radiographic or endoscopic evaluations of the colon and continued monitoring of the hemoglobin level, white blood cell count, and electrolyte levels are indicated until the patient's condition stabilizes.

Increasing abdominal tenderness, guarding, rebound tenderness, rising temperature, and paralytic ileus indicate colonic infarction and demand immediate laparotomy and colon resection. Mucosal injury may be extensive, despite normal-looking serosa, and the extent of resection should be guided by the distribution of disease as seen on preoperative studies rather than the appearance of the serosal surface of the colon at the time of operation.

In more than half of patients with CI, the disease is reversible. Generally, the symptoms of CI resolve within 48 hours and the colon heals in 1 to 2 weeks. With severe injury it may take 1 to 6 months for the colon to heal. The remaining patients with CI suffer irreversible damage—gangrene and perforation, segmental ulcerating colitis, stricture, or universal colitis.

Gangrene

Abdominal tenderness with fever and signs of peritonitis suggests infarction and the need for emergent laparotomy.

Segmental Ulcerating Colitis

Segmental ulcerating colitis may be seen with any of the following clinical patterns: asymptomatic but with recurrent fevers and sepsis; continuing or recurrent bloody diarrhea; and persistent or chronic diarrhea with protein-losing colopathy. Patients who are asymptomatic or minimally symptomatic but have endoscopic evidence of persistent disease should undergo follow-up colonoscopy to determine whether the colitis is healing, becoming chronic, or forming a stricture. Recurrent fever, leukocytosis, and septicemia suggest unhealed segmental colitis and, if found, mandates elective resection of the ischemic segment of bowel. Patients with persistent diarrhea, bleeding, or protein-losing colopathy of more than 2 weeks' duration are at high risk of perforation, and early resection is indicated. Patients who present with segmental ulcerating colitis are frequently misdiagnosed as having inflammatory bowel disease. Response to steroid therapy usually is poor and may be associated with an increased incidence of perforation. Some success has been achieved with fatty acid enemas (Dr. Lawrence Brandt, personal experience). Patients whose symptoms cannot be controlled medically should have a segmental resection, which usually is curative.

Ischemic Stricture

Ischemic strictures that produce no symptoms should be observed. Some disappear over 12 to 24 months with no therapy. Of course, resection is required for those that cause obstruction.

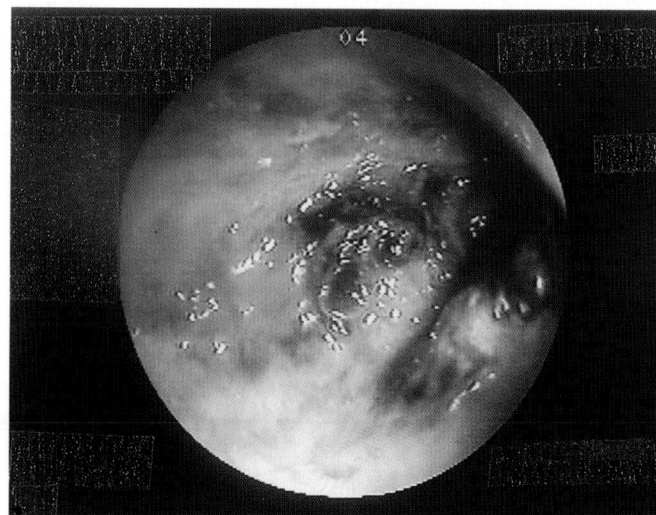

Figure 119–14. Colonoscopic demonstration of the characteristic appearance of mucosal gangrene. The necrotic epithelium appears black against the relatively healthy tissue.

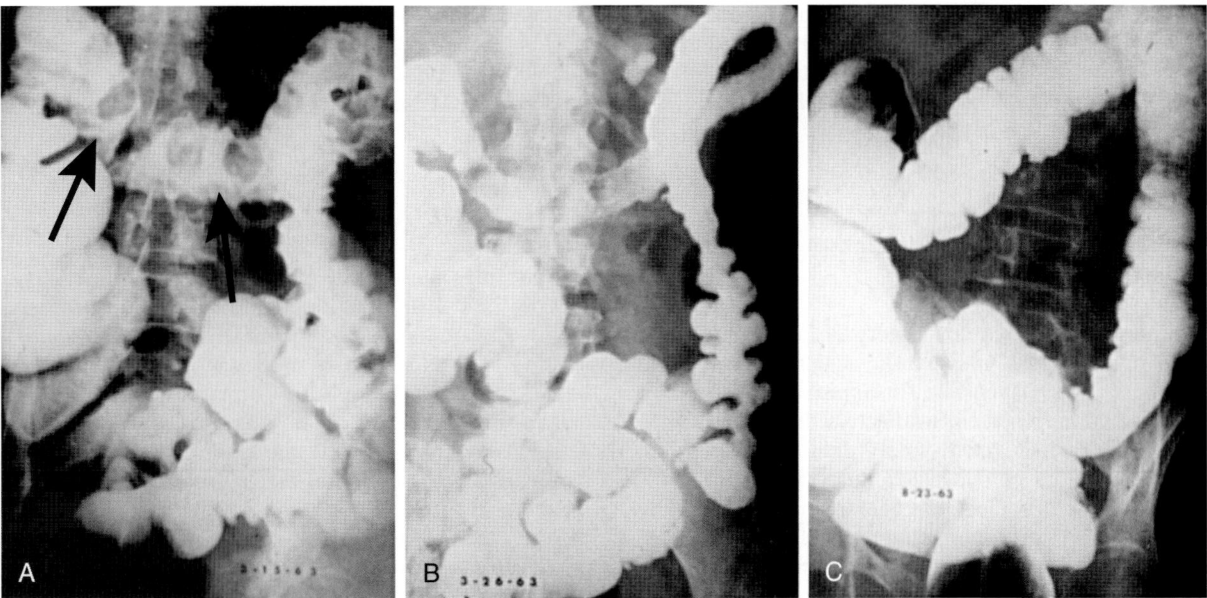

Figure 119–15. Ischemic changes in transverse colon and splenic flexure. *A,* Initial study shows dramatic thumbprints *(arrows)* throughout area of involvement. *B,* Eleven days later, the thumbprints are gone, and the involved colon has the typical appearance of segmental colitis. *C,* Five months after onset, there is complete return to normal. Patient was asymptomatic 3 weeks after her illness. (From Boley SJ, Schwartz SS: Colonic ischemia: Reversible ischemic lesions. In Boley SJ, Schwartz SS, Williams LF [eds]: Vascular Disorders of the Intestines. New York, Appleton-Century-Crofts, 1971, p 589.)

Universal Fulminant Colitis

Sudden onset of a "toxic universal colitis picture" with signs of peritonitis and a rapidly progressive course are typical of universal fulminant colitis, a rare variant of CI. Total abdominal colectomy with ileostomy usually is required.

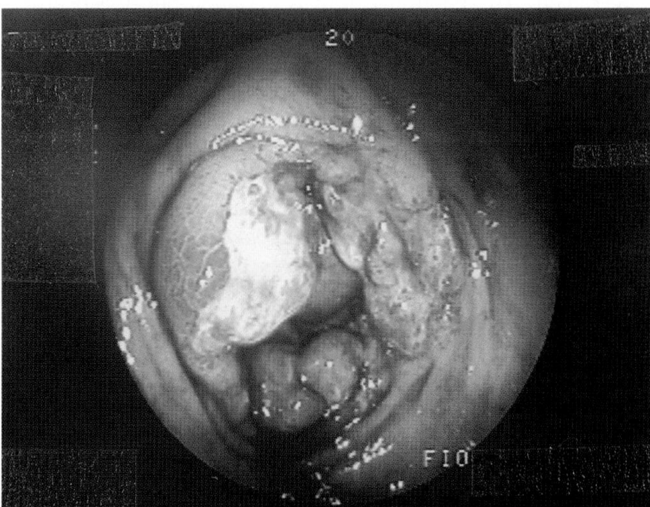

Figure 119–16. Colonoscopic photograph of colonic ischemia resembling neoplasia of the cecum in a patient with metastatic cancer treated with interleukin-2 and interferon-α. The inflamed, edematous mass was thought to be due to neoplasia both colonoscopically and on barium enema. The lesion spontaneously resolved after just 5 days. (From Sparano JA, Dutcher JP, Kaleya R, et al: Colonic ischemia complicating immunotherapy with interleukin-2 and interferon-alpha. Cancer 68: 1538–1544, 1991.)

Special Clinical Problems

Colonic Ischemia in Patients with Carcinoma of the Colon and Other Potentially Obstructive Lesions

Less than 10% of our patients with CI have a distal and potentially obstructing lesion or disorder. In half the cases,

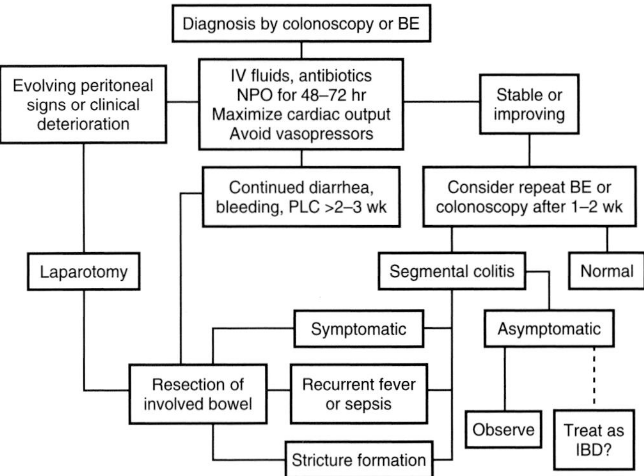

Figure 119–17. Management of colonic ischemia. Solid lines indicate accepted management plan; dashed line indicates alternative management plan. BE, barium enema; IBD, inflammatory bowel disease; IV, intravenous; NPO, nothing by mouth; PLC, protein-losing colopathy. (From Brandt LJ, Boley SJ: AGA technical review on intestinal ischemia: American Gastrointestinal Association. Gastroenterology 118:954, 2000.)

carcinoma of the colon is present, whereas in the remaining half, diverticulitis, volvulus, fecal impaction, postoperative stricture, prior ischemic stenosis, or radiation stricture is seen. Typically, the associated lesion is distal, and there is a segment of normal colon between the distal lesion and the proximal colitis (Fig. 119–18).

Colonic Ischemia Complicating Aortic Surgery

CI complicates elective aortic surgery in up to 7% and surgery for ruptured abdominal aortic aneurysms in up to 60% of cases.[35] CI is responsible for approximately 10% of the deaths after aortic replacement. Factors that contribute to postoperative CI include aneurysmal rupture, hypotension, operative trauma to the colon, hypoxemia, arrhythmias, prolonged cross-clamp time, and improper management of the IMA during aneurysmectomy. Tonometric determination of intramural pH of the sigmoid before and after cross-clamping the aorta has been used successfully to predict which patients will develop colonic ischemia after aneurysmectomy.[36]

Because postoperative CI is serious and difficult to diagnose early, colonoscopy should be performed within 2 to 3 days after surgery for a ruptured abdominal aortic aneurysm or in patients with a prolonged cross-clamping time, a patent IMA on preoperative aortography, nonpulsatile flow in the hypogastric arteries during surgery, or postoperative diarrhea. If CI is identified, oral feeding and liquids are stopped and antibiotic therapy is begun; clinical deterioration requires reoperation. At surgery, all ischemic colon must be resected.

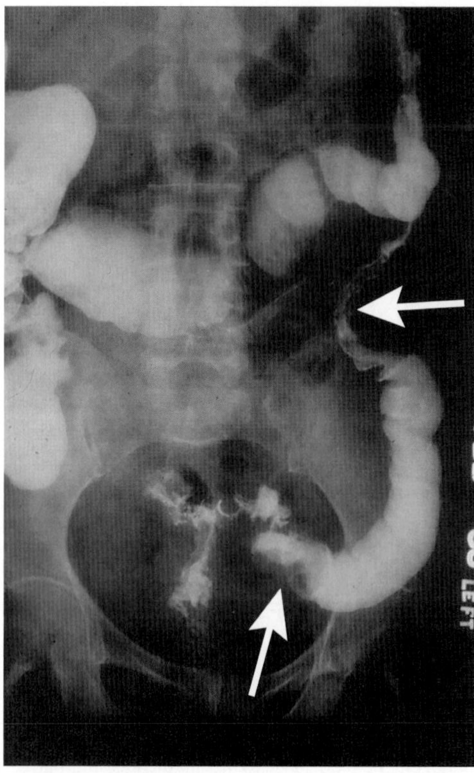

Figure 119–18. Barium enema demonstrating a narrowed segment of colonic ischemia *(upper arrow)* proximal to a carcinoma in the distal sigmoid *(lower arrow)*. The area of colon in between the lesion and the ischemic segment is normal. (From Boley SJ, Brandt LJ, Veith FJ: Ischemia disorders of the intestines. Curr Probl Surg 15:1–85, 1978.)

CHRONIC MESENTERIC ISCHEMIA (INTESTINAL ANGINA)

Chronic mesenteric ischemia (CMI) is uncommon, accounting for less than 5% of all intestinal ischemic diseases; it almost always is caused by mesenteric atherosclerosis. Abdominal pain is caused by ischemia in the small intestine as blood is "stolen" from this organ to meet the increased demand for gastric blood flow as food enters the stomach.[37] This observation explains the relatively rapid onset of abdominal pain so soon after eating, when food still remains in the stomach.

The cardinal clinical feature of CMI is abdominal cramping discomfort that usually occurs within 30 minutes after eating, gradually increases in severity, and then slowly resolves over 1 to 3 hours. Although minimal at first, abdominal pain progressively increases in severity over weeks to months. The association of pain with meals leads to fear of eating with resultant weight loss. Nausea, bloating, episodic diarrhea, and malabsorption or constipation may occur, but it is the weight loss and relation of the abdominal pain to the meals that characterize this syndrome. Early in the course of disease, if patients do not eat, they remain pain free; pain occurs only after eating or during a meal. Later, pain may become continuous, and this portends intestinal infarction. Physical findings are usually limited, but patients with advanced disease may appear cachectic. Many patients have evidence of cardiac, cerebral, or peripheral vascular disease. The abdomen typically remains soft and nontender even during painful episodes, although significant distention may be appreciated. An abdominal bruit is common but nonspecific.

Diagnosis of intestinal angina is difficult because of the vague nature of the complaints and the lack of a specific diagnostic test. Plain radiographs of the abdomen are usually normal, although vascular calcification may be present. Endoscopic inspection of the GI tract reveals it to be normal, and random biopsies of the upper tract may show only nonspecific abnormalities. Barium studies are normal or show nonspecific evidence of either malabsorption or a motility disturbance. A number of tests have been proposed to establish the presence of CMI, including duplex ultrasonography and MR angiography, but none have proven sufficiently sensitive and specific to be diagnostic. Elevated "peak systolic velocity" in the SMA and CA as determined by duplex ultrasonography indicates significant stenosis; this, however, does not establish the diagnosis of CMI.[38, 39] Duplex ultrasonography and MRI of the SMA and CA have been used to measure the effect of eating on mesenteric blood flow, all based on the principle that eating normally increases blood flow to the small intestine, whereas in CMI, this fails to occur. More experience with these provocative tests is needed before firm conclusions can be made. All are indirect measurements of an anatomic limitation of splanchnic blood flow and do not establish the presence or absence of intestinal ischemia.

In the absence of any specific, reliable diagnostic test, diagnosis is based on the clinical symptoms, the arteriographic demonstration of an occlusive process of the splanchnic vessels, and, to a great measure, the exclusion of other gastrointestinal disorders. Angiography should show occlusion of two or more splanchnic arteries to allow the diagnosis of CMI; however, such occlusions, even of all three vessels, do not by themselves make the diagnosis of CMI, because they may be present with no corresponding clinical symptoms. In most patients with CMI, at least two of the three splanchnic vessels either are completely obstructed or severely stenosed. In a large review of patients with CMI,[40] 91% had occlusion of at least two vessels and 55% had involvement of all three; 7% and 2% had isolated occlusion of the SMA and CA, respectively. There is no specific association between CMI and smoking

CMI is not considered to require urgent therapy, although acute complete occlusion of the blood supply may occur if thrombosis is superimposed on the already narrowed arteries. A patient with the typical pain of CMI and unexplained weight loss whose diagnostic evaluation has excluded other gastrointestinal disease (Fig. 119–19) and whose angiogram shows occlusive involvement of at least two of the three major arteries should undergo revascularization.

Surgical revascularization has been the method of therapy for most patients with CMI. Since the early 1980s, percutaneous transluminal mesenteric angioplasty (PTMA) alone or with stent insertion has been offered as alternative therapy but is reported only in small numbers of patients. Whether surgery or PTMA is better will be determined by their relative success in relieving symptoms and the durability of such relief. The results of surgical revascularization for CMI vary in different reports, depending on the nature of the operations used, the number of splanchnic vessels revascularized, and whether concurrent operations such as aortic reconstruction are performed.

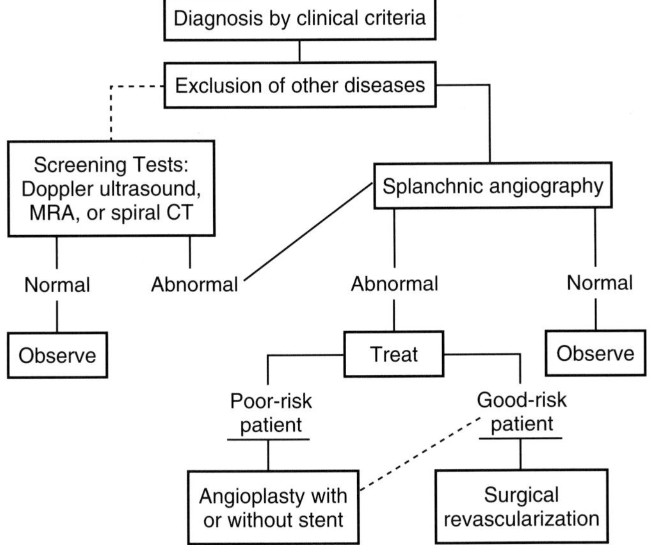

Figure 119–19. Management of chronic mesenteric ischemia. Solid lines indicate accepted management plan; dashed line indicates alternative management plan. CT, computed tomography; MRA, magnetic resonance angiography. (From Brandt LJ, Boley SJ: AGA technical review on intestinal ischemia: American Gastrointestinal Association. Gastroenterology 118:954, 2000.)

The true efficacy of surgical revascularization and PTMA is difficult to determine because of the varied criteria used by different investigators to define a successful outcome. Thus, some authors use graft or vessel patency rates, whereas others define success by relief of symptoms, recurrence rates, or long-term survival. A tabulation of 17 series of surgical revascularization for CMI totaling 614 patients yielded perioperative mortality rates that ranged from 0%[41] to 16%[42] and success rates and recurrence rates of 59%[43] to 100%[41, 44] and 0%[41, 42, 45] to 26.5%,[46] respectively.[9] Most recent series have reported mortality rates below 10%, success rates of more than 90%, and recurrence rates generally under 10%.[9] Several long-term studies have shown that patients surviving surgical revascularization have cumulative 5-year survival rates of approximately 80% to 90%.[9]

The initial success rates of PTMA are similar to those of surgical revascularization. The experience with PTMA is more limited but has been achieved in patients often considered too high risk for a surgical procedure. In 10 representative series of PTMA for CMI, and totaling 128 patients, clinical success rates (i.e., relief of symptoms) have varied from 63%[47] to 100%,[48] with little mortality.[9] Recurrence of symptoms, however, has been much higher than after surgical revascularization, varying from 10% to 67% in the larger series.[9] More recently, intraluminal stenting has been added to PTMA in an attempt to decrease the incidence of recurrent stenoses. Too few patients have been treated in this fashion to permit a conclusion as to its long-term value in managing patients with CMI.

Patients with CMI who are otherwise relatively healthy probably should be treated by surgical revascularization; poorer risk patients should have an initial attempt at PTMA with or without stenting to relieve symptoms. If, however, the use of stents proves to reduce the recurrence rates of PTMA close to those of surgical revascularization, PTMA may become the method of choice.

VASCULITIS OF THE SPLANCHNIC CIRCULATION[49] (see Chapter 29)

Inflammation and necrosis can affect splanchnic blood vessels of all sizes: arteries, veins, the vasa recta, arterioles, and venules. Symptoms depend on the size of the involved vessel. Polyarteritis nodosa and rheumatoid arthritis affect medium and large vessels and, clinically, may be indistinguishable from AMI, caused by emboli or thromboses, except for the associated systemic features such as renal failure, cutaneous nodules, or a positive rheumatoid factor.

The vasa recta and intramural arteries and arterioles may be affected in the systemic vasculitides. With vasculitis, the ischemic injury typically involves small segments of the intestine. Abdominal pain, fever, gastrointestinal bleeding, diarrhea, and intestinal obstruction are common. Ulceration and stricture formation are common, but with small vessel involvement perforation is less frequent.

Typically, vasculitis is caused by immune complex deposition in the wall of vessels, which leads to activation of the complement system and an inflammatory reaction; aneurysm formation, vessel rupture and bleeding, vascular occlusion, thrombosis, and/or fibrosis may ensue.

Polyarteritis Nodosa

Polyarteritis nodosa is a necrotizing vasculitis of medium- and small-sized arteries characterized by aneurysms at branch points. Abdominal symptoms are reported in up to half of patients with the disorder, most frequent of which is abdominal pain, usually from ischemia.[50] Involvement of the small bowel is most common, followed by lesions of colon, liver, and pancreas. Diagnosis is suggested by typical angiographic findings of aneurysms in the mesenteric, renal, and hepatic vasculature. Treatment with corticosteroids and cyclophosphamide or azathioprine has improved survival greatly.

Vasculitis resembling polyarteritis also is associated with hepatitis B and C virus infection.[51, 52] Fifty percent of patients with classic polyarteritis are hepatitis B surface antigen positive, but unlike classic polyarteritis, only small arteries are involved. Patients develop a polyarteritis picture following the viral infection, presumably from deposition of antigen-associated immune complexes on the vessel wall.

Allergic Granulomatous Angiitis (Churg-Strauss Syndrome)

Allergic granulomatous angiitis is a disorder that is typified by asthma, glomerulonephritis, eosinophilia, and granulomatous inflammation associated with antineutrophil cytoplasmic autoantibodies.[53] Necrotizing vasculitis affects small- and medium-sized vessels and involves the gastrointestinal tract in almost half the patients. As in other vasculitides, abdominal pain and bleeding secondary to ischemia are the usual manifestations. Glucocorticoid therapy usually is effective.

Hypersensitivity Vasculitis

Hypersensitivity vasculitis uncommonly (15%) affects the splanchnic vasculature, and, in contrast with necrotizing vasculitis, which involves arteries, it affects primarily the postcapillary venules. A large variety of causes are known to trigger this disorder, including infections (*Streptococcus*, *Staphylococcus*, hepatitis B virus, influenza virus, cytomegalovirus, mycobacteria, and rickettsiae), drugs, and chemicals.

Systemic Lupus Erythematosus

Systemic lupus erythematosus (SLE) affects the gastrointestinal system in about half of cases and may involve any of the hollow and solid gastrointestinal organs.[49] The most common symptoms are nausea, vomiting, and abdominal pain, but diarrhea, malabsorption, pseudo-obstruction, peritonitis, pancreatitis, protein-losing enteropathy, and ascites are also well-known occurrences. The systemic nature of the disorder makes differential diagnosis complicated, but vasculitis-induced ischemia underlies many of the presentations. The vasculitis typically involves small vessels and causes FSI and gastrointestinal bleeding, both of which are associated with high mortality rates if not diagnosed promptly.

Rheumatoid Arthritis

Rheumatoid vasculitis affects the gastrointestinal tract in approximately 10% of patients, usually those who have subcutaneous nodules and are seropositive for rheumatoid factor.[54] As with all vasculitides, ischemia manifests with abdominal pain, bleeding, perforation, and gangrene. Other diseases have been noted in association with rheumatoid arthritis, including atrophic gastritis, inflammatory bowel disease, collagenous colitis, and amyloidosis.

Henoch-Schönlein Purpura (see Chapter 29)

Henoch-Schönlein purpura typically affects children aged 4 to 7 years of age. It is characterized by IgA immune complexes deposited within the small vessels of the skin, gastrointestinal tract, joints, and kidneys and is often preceded by an upper respiratory infection. The classic clinical triad consists of palpable purpura (usually below the waist), arthritis (knees and ankles), and abdominal pain; the gastrointestinal tract is involved in up to 75% of patients.[55] Abdominal pain and gastrointestinal bleeding are most common and are caused by mucosal and submucosal hemorrhage; a submucosal hematoma may be the lead point of an intussusception. Gastrointestinal involvement may be documented by endoscopy[56] or by CT study.[57] The disease is usually self-limited, but the outlook may be less favorable in adults, in large measure because of the development of renal failure.

Behçet's Disease (see Chapter 29)

Behçet's disease is characterized by oral and genital ulcers, recurrent iritis or chorioretinitis, and skin lesions. It is most often seen in Eastern Mediterranean men and is strongly associated with the B51 allele. Small-vessel vasculitis accounts for much of the damage, but large-vessel involvement of both arteries and veins is not uncommon. Gastrointestinal disease, present in 50% of patients, typically affects the ileocecal area, although involvement of the esophagus and small intestine has been reported.[58] Attacks are recurrent and usually self-limited; they do not cause a chronic disorder, except for the uveitis. The most common gastrointestinal symptoms are abdominal pain, diarrhea, and bleeding; deep ulcers are responsible for the most common intestinal complications, severe bleeding, and perforation. Mortality is low in Behçet's disease; however, intestinal perforation is one of the common causes of death. Therapy with glucocorticoids, immunosuppressive agents, and colchicine has been tried, with varying success.

Köhlmeier-Degos Disease (Malignant Atrophic Papulosis)

Köhlmeier-Degos disease is a rare form of progressive occlusive vascular disease of young men that affects the small and medium-sized arteries, mainly those of the skin and intestine.[59] Typically, skin lesions are found on the trunk and upper extremities and look like porcelain-white, punctate scars with erythematous borders. The rash is followed, within months to years, by the development of abdominal pain and spontaneous intestinal perforation. Thrombosis of small and medium-sized vessels is found, without inflammatory cell infiltration. There is no known therapy for this disease, and it is generally fatal.

Takayasu's Disease

Takayasu's disease ("pulseless disease") is an idiopathic chronic inflammatory disorder that most often affects the aorta and its branches in young women of Asian heritage; the splanchnic vessels unusually are involved.[60] It leads ultimately to fibrotic occlusion of the involved vessels. Takayasu's disease rarely has been associated with Crohn's disease and ulcerative colitis, and in the serum of some of these patients, antibodies to both colonic mucosa and aorta have been detected. Treatment is large doses of glucocorticoids prior to reconstructive surgery, and the 5-year survival rate is higher than 90%.

Cogan's Syndrome

Cogan's syndrome is a rare disorder of young people characterized by vasculitis of the conjunctiva, cornea, and cochlea.[61] Although this vasculitis usually is localized, it is considered to be a hypersensitivity reaction to an unknown viral agent, and the disease can become disseminated. Three percent to 10% of patients develop gastrointestinal symptoms, with diarrhea and bloody stools. High-dose glucocorticoids—and occasionally cytotoxic agents—are required; perhaps vascular surgery also may be needed after inflammation is controlled.

Kawasaki's Disease

Kawasaki's disease, also called *infantile febrile mucocutaneous lymph node syndrome,* is a necrotizing vasculitis of medium-sized arteries.[62] It manifests as fever, rash on the palms and soles, desquamation, conjunctival congestion, "strawberry" tongue, and cervical lymphadenopathy in infants and children. Many have nausea, vomiting, abdominal pain, and diarrhea, and they may suffer ileus, small bowel obstruction, bleeding, and perforation. Death may be due to coronary artery aneurysms and myocardial infarction. Treatment is aspirin for the acute phase and large intravenous doses of gamma globulin for the prevention of coronary artery aneurysms.

Buerger's Disease

Also called *thromboangiitis obliterans,* Buerger's disease involves medium-sized and small peripheral arteries and veins, especially the infrapopliteal vessels; foot claudication and rubor are the most frequent symptoms. It is largely a disease of men, especially those who have smoked cigarettes from an early age, and typically has its onset in patients younger than 50 years of age; there is a distinct absence of other atherosclerotic risk factors. Intestinal involvement is unusual, but most common is involvement of the vessels supplying the small intestine.[63] In the acute lesions, inflammation spreads from the thrombus-endothelium interface through the vessel wall. Later, microabscesses, necrotizing granulomas, and multinucleated giant cells occur in the thrombus, after which the thrombus organizes and becomes occlusive. Intestinal involvement usually requires resection.

REFERENCES

1. Kornblith PL, Boley SJ, Whitehouse BS: Anatomy of the splanchnic circulation. Surg Clin North Am 72:1, 1992.
2. Boley SJ, Freiber W, Winslow PR, et al: Circulatory responses to acute reduction of superior mesenteric arterial flow. Physiologist 12:180, 1969.
3. Zimmerman BJ, Granger DN: Reperfusion injury. Surg Clin North Am 72:65, 1992.
4. Finucane PM, Arunachalam T, O'Dowd J, et al: Acute mesenteric infarction in elderly patients. J Am Geriatr Soc 37:355, 1989.
5. Gaussorgues P, Guerugniand PY, Vedrinne JM, et al: Bacteremia following cardiac arrest and cardiopulmonary resuscitation. Intensive Care Med 14:575, 1988.
6. Kurland B, Brandt LJ, Delany HM: Diagnostic tests for intestinal angina. Surg Clin North Am 72:85, 1992.
7. Qamar MI, Read AE, Skidmore R, et al: Transcutaneous Doppler ultrasound measurements of superior mesenteric artery blood flow in man. Gut 27:100, 1986.
8. Bartnicke BJ, Balfe DM: CT appearance of intestinal ischemia and intramural hemorrhage. Radiol Clin North Am 32:845, 1994.
9. Boley SJ, Spreyregen S, Siegelman SS, et al: Initial results from an aggressive roentgenological and surgical approach to acute mesenteric ischemia. Surgery 82:848, 1977.
10. Horgan PG, Gorey JF: Operative assessment of intestinal viability. Surg Clin North Am 72:143, 1992.
11. Schoenbaum SW, Pena C, Koenigsberg P, et al: Superior mesenteric artery embolism: Treatment with intraarterial urokinase. J Vasc Interv Radiol 3:485, 1992.
12. Siegelman SS, Sprayregen S, Boley SJ, et al: Angiographic diagnosis of mesenteric arterial vasoconstriction. Radiology 122:533, 1974.
13. Boley SJ, Feinstein FR, Sammartano R, et al: New concepts in the management of emboli of the superior mesenteric artery. Surg Gynecol Obstet 153:561, 1981.
14. Clark RA, Gallant TE: Acute mesenteric ischemia: Angiographic spectrum. AJR Am J Roentgenol 142:555, 1984.
15. Boos S: [Angiography of the mesenteric artery 1976–1991: A change in the indications during mesenteric circulatory disorders?]. Radiologe 32:154, 1992.
16. Bottger T, Schafer W, Weber W, et al: [Value of preoperative diagnosis in mesenteric vascular occlusion: A prospective study]. Langenbecks Arch Chir 375:278, 1990.
17. Czerny M, Trubel W, Claeys L, et al: [Acute mesenteric ischemia]. Zentralbl Chir 122:538, 1997.
18. Harward RTS, Green D, Bergan JJ, et al: Mesenteric venous thrombosis. J Vasc Surg 9:328, 1989.
19. Kaleya RN, Boley SJ: Mesenteric venous thrombosis. In Najarian JS, Delaney JP (eds) : Progress in Gastrointestinal Surgery. Chicago, Year Book, 1989, p 417.
20. Clavien PA, Durig M, Harder F: Venous mesenteric infarction: A particular entity. Br J Surg 75:252, 1988.
21. Font VE, Hermann RE, Longworth DL: Chronic mesenteric venous thrombosis: Difficult diagnosis and therapy. Cleve Clin J Med 56:823, 1989.
22. Warshaw AL, Gongliang J, Ottinger LW: Recognition and clinical implications of mesenteric and portal vein obstruction in chronic pancreatitis. Arch Surg 123:410, 1987.
23. Clark AZ, Gallant TE: Acute mesenteric ischemia: Angiographic spectrum. Am J Radiol 142:555, 1984.
24. Matos C, Van Gansbeke D, Zaleman M, et al: Mesenteric venous thrombosis: Early CT and ultrasound diagnosis and conservative management. Gastrointest Radiol 11:322, 1986.

25. Clavien PA, Huber O, Mirescu D, et al: Contrast-enhanced CT scan as a diagnostic procedure in mesenteric ischemia due to mesenteric venous thrombosis. Br J Surg 76:93, 1989.
26. Al Karawi MA, Quaiz M, Clark D, et al: Mesenteric vein thrombosis, non-invasive diagnosis and followup (US + MRI) and non-invasive therapy by streptokinase and anticoagulants. Hepatogastroenterology 37: 507, 1990.
27. Serreyn RF, Schoofs PR, Baetens PR, et al: Laparoscopic diagnosis of mesenteric venous thrombosis. Endoscopy 18:249, 1986.
28. Rhee RY, Gloviczki P, Mendonca CT, et al: Mesenteric venous thrombosis: Still a lethal disease in the 1990s. J Vasc Surg 20:688, 1994.
29. Grieshop RJ, Dalsing MC, Cikrit DF, et al: Acute mesenteric venous thrombosis: Revisited in a time of diagnostic clarity. Am Surg 57:573, 1991.
30. Sakai L, Keltner R, Kaminski D: Spontaneous and shock-associated ischemic colitis. Am J Surg 140:755, 1980.
31. Guttormson NL, Bubrick MP: Mortality from ischemic colitis. Dis Colon Rectum 26:462, 1983.
32. Brandt LJ, Boley SJ, Goldberg L, et al: Colitis in the elderly. Am J Gastroenterol 76:239, 1981.
33. Church JM: Ischemic colitis complicating flexible endoscopy in a patient with connective tissue disease. Gastrointest Endosc 41:181, 1995.
34. Scowcroft CW, Sanowski RA, Kozarek RA: Colonoscopy in ischemic colitis. Gastrointest Endosc 27:156, 1981.
35. Zelenock GB, Strodel WE, Knol JA, et al: A prospective study of clinically and endoscopically documented colonic ischemia in 100 patients undergoing aortic reconstructive surgery with aggressive colonic and direct pelvic revascularization, compared with historic controls. Surgery 106:771, 1989.
36. Schiedler MG, Cutler BS, Fiddian-Green RG: Sigmoid intramural pH for prediction of ischemic colitis during aortic surgery: A comparison with risk factors and inferior mesenteric artery stump pressures. Arch Surg 122:881, 1987.
37. Poole JW, Sammartano RJ, Boley SJ: Hemodynamic basis of the pain of chronic mesenteric ischemia. Am J Surg 153:171, 1987.
38. Moneta GL, Yeager RA, Dalman R, et al: Duplex ultrasound criteria for diagnosis of splanchnic artery stenosis or occlusion. J Vasc Surg 14:511, 1991.
39. Bowersox JC, Zwolak RM, Walsh DB, et al: Duplex ultrasonography in the diagnosis of celiac and mesenteric artery occlusive disease. J Vasc Surg 14:780, 1991.
40. Moawad J, Gewertz BL: Chronic mesenteric ischemia: Clinical presentation and diagnosis. Surg Clin North Am 77:357, 1997.
41. Wolf YG, Verstandig A, Sasson T, et al: Mesenteric bypass for chronic mesenteric ischermia. Cardiovasc Surg 6:34, 1998.
42. Van Damme H, Creemers E, Limet E: [Surgical treatment of chronic mesenteric ischemia]. Acta Gastroenterol Belg 52:406, 1989.
43. Sandmann W, Bohner H, Kneiemeyer HW, et al: [Chronic mesenteric ischemia]. Dtsch Med Wochenschr 119:979, 1994.
44. Johnston KW, Lindsay TF, Walker PM, et. al: Mesenteric arterial bypass grafts: Early and late results and suggested surgical approach for chronic and acute mesenteric ischemia. Surgery 118:1, 1995.
45. Moawad J, McKinsey JF, Wyble CW, et al: Current results of surgical therapy for chronic mesenteric ischemia. Arch Surg 132:613, 1997.
46. Hollier LH, Bernatz PE, Pairolero PC, et al: Surgical management of chronic intestinal ischemia: A reappraisal. Surgery 90:940, 1981.
47. Matsumoto AH, Tegtmeyer CJ, Fitzcharles EK, et al: Percutaneous transluminal angioplasty of visceral arterial stenoses: Results and long-term clinical follow-up. J Vasc Interv Radiol 6:165, 1995.
48. Roberts L Jr, Wertman DA, Mills SR, et al: Transluminal angioplasty of the superior mesenteric artery: An alternative to surgical revascularization. AJR Am J Roentgenol 141:1039, 1983.
49. Bailey M, Chapin W, Licht H, et al: The effects of vasculitis on the gastrointestinal tract and liver. Gastroenterol Clin North Am 27:747, 1998.
50. Bassel K, Harford W: Gastrointestinal manifestations of collagen-vascular disease. Semin Gastrointest Dis 6:228, 1995.
51. Deny P, Guillevin L, Bonacorsi S, et al: Association between hepatitis C virus and polyarteritis nodosa. Clin Exp Rheumatol 10:319, 1992.
52. Guillevin L, Lhote F, Cohen P, et al: Polyarteritis nodosa related to hepatitis B virus: A prospective study with long-term observation of 41 patients. Medicine 74:238, 1995.
53. Lhote F, Guillevin L: Polyarteritis nodosa, microscopic polyangiitis, and Churg-Strauss syndrome: Clinical aspects and treatment. Rheum Dis Clin North Am 21:911, 1995.
54. Scott DGI, Baco PA, Tribe CR: Systemic rheumatoid vasculitis: A clinical laboratory study of 50 cases. Medicine 60:288, 1981.
55. Robson WL, Leung AK: Henoch-Schonlein purpura. Adv Pediatr 41: 163, 1994.
56. Nakasone H, Hokama A, Fukuchi J, et al: Colonoscopic findings in an adult patient with Henoch-Schönlein purpura. Gastrointest Endosc 52: 392, 2000.
57. Jeong YK, Ha HK, Yoon CH, et al: Gastrointestinal involvement in Henoch-Schönlein syndrome: CT findings. Am J Roentgenol 168:965, 1997.
58. Lee RG: The colitis of Behçet's syndrome. Am J Surg Pathol 10:888, 1986.
59. Fruhwirth J, Mischinger HJ, Werkgartner G, et al: Köhlmeier-Degos disease with primary intestinal manifestation. Scand J Gastroenterol 10: 1066, 1997.
60. Sharma BK, Jain S, Sagar S: Systemic manifestations of Takayasu arteritis: The expanding spectrum. Int J Cardiol 54S:149, 1996.
61. Haynes G, Kaiser-Kupfer M, Mason P, et al: Cogan's syndrome. Medicine 59:426, 1980.
62. Kawasaki T: Clinical features of Kawasaki's syndrome. Acta Paediatr Jpn 25:79, 1983.
63. Lie JT: Visceral intestinal Buerger's disease. Int J Cardiol 66S:249, 1998.

Chapter 120

Vascular Lesions of the Gastrointestinal Tract

David A. Greenwald and Lawrence J. Brandt

Through the widespread use of endoscopy and angiography, vascular lesions of the gastrointestinal (GI) tract are being recognized with increasing frequency as a cause of GI hemorrhage. They may be solitary or multiple, isolated abnormalities, or part of a syndrome or systemic disorder (Table 120–1). In this chapter, we discuss a few of the more important vascular lesions that cause GI bleeding and that are representative of the spectrum of vascular lesions of the GI tract.

VASCULAR LESIONS

Vascular Ectasias (VEs)

Vascular ectasia of the colon, also referred to as angiodysplasia or less accurately as arteriovenous malformation or angioma, is a distinct clinical and pathologic entity.[1–4] It is the most common vascular abnormality of the GI tract and probably the most frequent cause of recurrent lower intestinal bleeding after age 60 years. Controversy exists concerning the nomenclature, behavior, and appropriate therapy of these lesions, but with increasing experience, there is growing consensus on these issues.[5] VEs are probably degenerative lesions associated with aging and, in contrast to congenital or neoplastic vascular lesions of the GI tract, are not associated with angiomas of the skin or other viscera. However, when patients with vascular lesions of the colon are aggressively studied with angiography or enteroscopy, concomitant lesions may be seen in the small intestine in approximately 10% of patients.[6, 7] VEs almost always are confined to the cecum or ascending colon, usually are multiple rather than single, and are smaller than 10 mm in diameter. They are seldom identified by the surgeon at operation or by the pathologist using standard techniques in the laboratory, but usually they can be diagnosed by angiography or colonoscopy (Figs. 120–1, 120–2, and 120–3).

Bleeding from cecal VEs was first shown in 1961 by intraoperative angiography and since then has become well recognized, especially after the introduction of selective angiography and colonoscopy for identifying the source of intestinal bleeding[8] (see Chapter 13). VEs and diverticulosis are the two most common causes of lower GI hemorrhage in elderly persons and often coexist (see Chapters 13 and 108). The problem of attributing bleeding to one or the other cause, when bleeding from the lesion is not demonstrated by endoscopy or by extravasation of contrast material on angiography, is compounded by the frequency of these disorders without bleeding in people over age 60 years. The prevalence of diverticulosis is estimated to be as high as 50% in the population older than age 60 years; mucosal VEs of the right colon can be found by injection studies of colons removed at surgery in more than 25% of patients in this same age range without any evidence of bleeding.[8] In large series of colonoscopies, VEs have been seen in 0.2% to 2.9% of "nonbleeding persons"[9, 10] and 2.6% to 6.2% of patients evaluated specifically for occult blood in the stool, anemia, or hemorrhage.[9–11] In the absence of a demonstrated site of hemorrhage, the only basis for determining whether an identified ectasia or diverticulosis is responsible for bleeding is the indirect evidence provided by the patient's course after resection or ablation of the suspected lesion.

There is no gender predilection for VEs, and most patients are older than 50 years. "Angiodysplasias" of the small bowel and in the left colon have been reported in adolescents,[12] but none of these reports bears histologic proof that these are the same vascular lesions as in older patients. In another report unaccompanied by histologic documentation, lesions were said to occur distal to the hepatic flexure in 46% of patients.[13] Limited review of tissue sections taken from supposed VEs in the small bowel or left colon has revealed totally different changes from those seen with VEs in the right colon. Histologic proof of the nature of vascular lesions is mandatory before categorizing them.

Table 120–1 | **Vascular Lesions of the Gastrointestinal Tract**

PRIMARY VASCULAR LESIONS
Aneurysms of the aorta and its branches
Blue rubber bleb nevus
Capillary phlebectasia
Congenital arteriovenous malformation
Dieulafoy's lesion
Glomus tumor
Hemangioendothelioma
Hemangioma
Hemangiomatosis
Hemangiopericytoma
Hemangiosarcoma
Hemorrhoids
Kaposi's sarcoma
Vascular ectasia (angiodysplasia)
DISEASES AND SYNDROMES WITH VASCULAR LESIONS
Dystrophic angiectasias
Ehlers-Danlos syndrome (Sack variant)
Hereditary hemorrhagic telangiectasia (Osler-Weber-Rendu disease)
Klippel-Trenaunay syndrome
Kohlmeier-Degos syndrome
Marfan's syndrome
Pseudoxanthoma elasticum
Scurvy
Systemic sclerosis (scleroderma, CREST)
Turner's syndrome (plexiform telangiectasias)
von Willebrand's disease
SYSTEMIC DISEASES ASSOCIATED WITH VASCULAR LESIONS
Portal hypertension
Varices
Spiders
Venous stars
Congestive gastropathy and colopathy
Watermelon stomach (GAVE)
Renal failure
Gastrointestinal telangiectasias
Watermelon stomach
Vasculitis (e.g., systemic lupus erythematosus, polyarteritis nodosa)
Miscellaneous
Inflammatory bowel disease
Radiation telangiectasia
Carcinoma telangiectatum

CREST, calcinosis, Raynaud's phenomenon, esophageal dysfunction, sclerodactyly, and telangiectasia [syndrome]; GAVE, gastric antral vascular ectasia.

Bleeding from VEs typically is recurrent and low grade, although approximately 15% of patients present with massive hemorrhage. The nature and degree of bleeding frequently vary in the same patient with different episodes, and patients may have bright red blood, maroon-colored stools, and melena on separate occasions. In 20% to 25% of episodes, only tarry stools are passed, and in 10% to 15% of patients, bleeding is evidenced solely by iron deficiency anemia, with stools that are intermittently positive for occult blood.[5] This spectrum reflects the varied rate of bleeding from the ectatic capillaries, venules, and, in advanced lesions, arteriovenous communications. In more than 90% of instances, bleeding stops spontaneously. In the past, as many as 30% of patients with VEs had had "blind" partial gastrectomy or left colon resection for presumed diverticular or idiopathic bleeding. With the advent of colonoscopy, the percentage of patients who have had previous operations has decreased, since most lesions are being identified and treated at the time of the first bleeding episode.

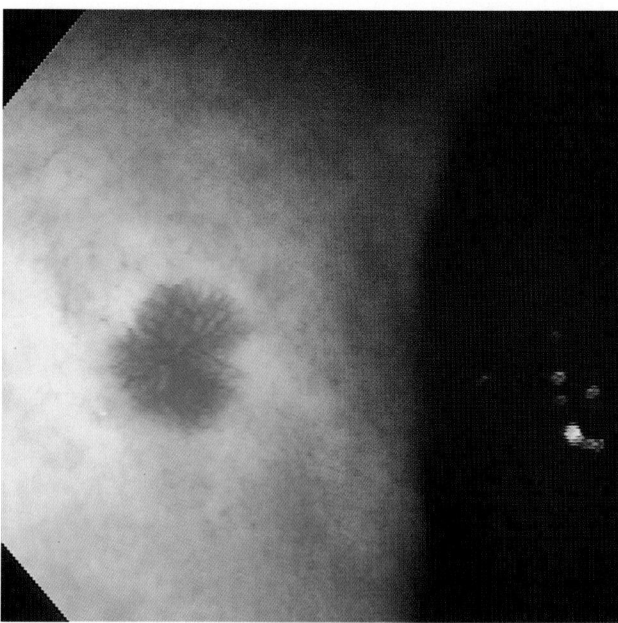

Figure 120–1. Vascular ectasia. This large ectasia has a characteristic pattern. The central blood vessel can be seen, with an emanating feathery appearance. (From Wilcox CM: Atlas of Clinical Gastrointestinal Endoscopy. Philadelphia, W.B. Saunders, 1995, p. 122.)

Approximately 50% of patients with bleeding VEs have evidence of cardiac disease, and as many as 25% have been reported to have aortic stenosis. The interrelationships of aortic stenosis, VE, and GI bleeding had been controversial. However, an elegant subject review and analysis of the available data in 1988 failed to find conclusive evidence to support such an association[14]; none of several subsequent

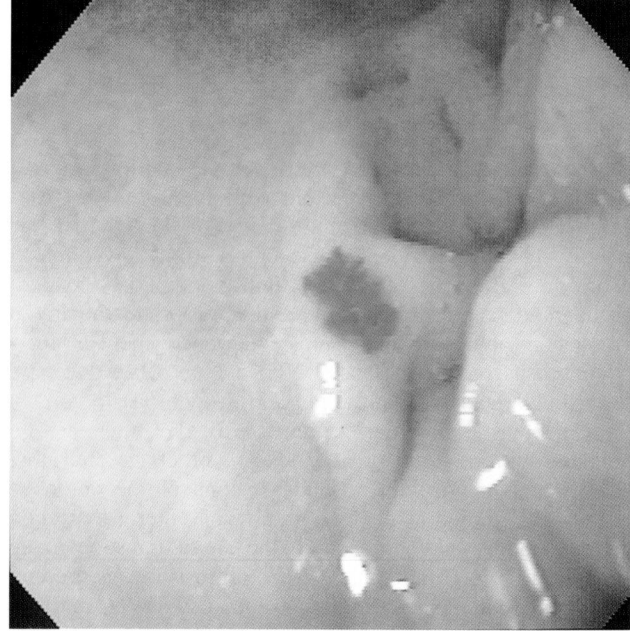

Figure 120–2. Vascular ectasia. Air has been withdrawn from the duodenal bulb to bring the ectasia closer, documenting the lack of depth and the characteristic frond-like appearance. (From Wilcox CM: Atlas of Clinical Gastrointestinal Endoscopy. Philadelphia, W.B. Saunders, 1995, p. 182.)

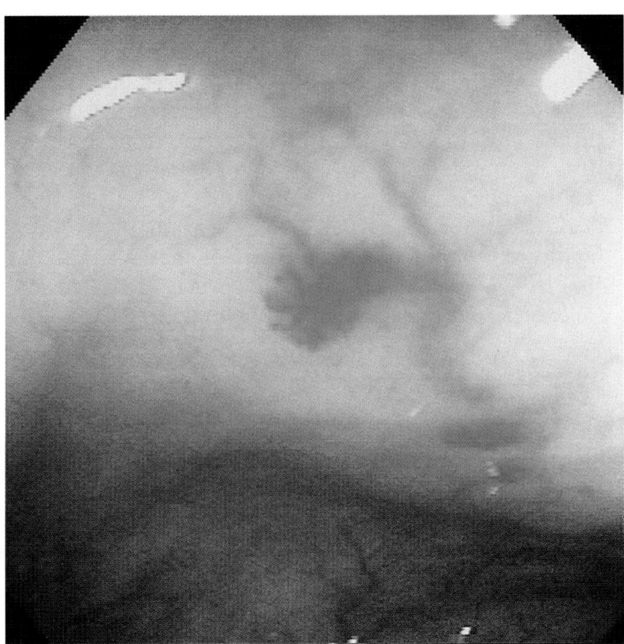

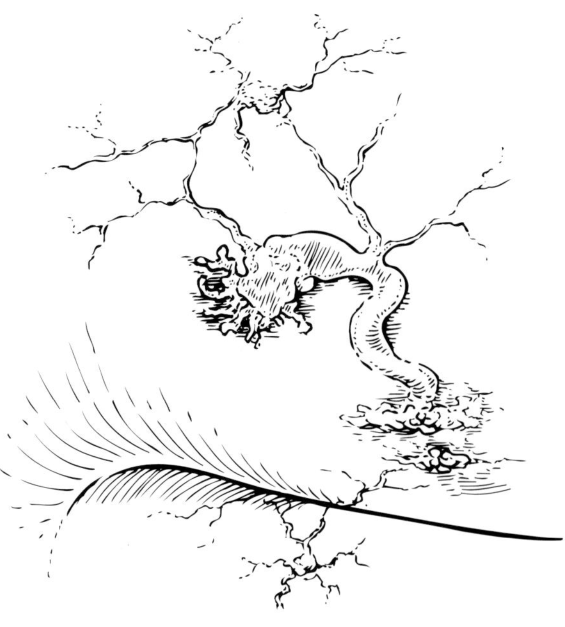

Figure 120–3. Vascular ectasias. A tuft of blood vessels resembles spider angioma in the cecum. A large draining vein is seen emanating from the ectasia. Several other vascular ectasias are noted proximally. (From Wilcox CM: Atlas of Clinical Gastrointestinal Endoscopy. Philadelphia, W.B. Saunders, 1995, p. 270.)

retrospective, uncontrolled studies[15, 16] or a prospective, controlled investigation[17] substantiates a causative role or association of aortic valve disease with colon VE. Replacement of the aortic valve for control of bleeding secondary to these vascular lesions is not indicated.

Pathology

Histologic identification of VEs is difficult unless special techniques are used.[1] Although usually less than one third of lesions are found by routine pathologic examination, almost all can be identified by injecting the colonic vasculature with silicone rubber, dehydrating the cells with increasing concentrations of alcohol, clearing the specimen with glycerol, and then viewing the specimen in a dissecting stereomicroscope[1] (Fig. 120–4). In a study utilizing these methods, 26 colons were analyzed and found to have one or more mucosal VEs measuring 1 mm to 1 cm in diameter. VEs were usually multiple, and in this study, all were located within the cecum and ascending colon; the most distal one was 23 cm from the ileocecal valve.[1]

Microscopically, mucosal VEs consist of dilated, distorted, thin-walled vessels that are lined by endothelium and, infrequently, by a small amount of smooth muscle. Structurally, they appear to be ectatic veins, venules, and capillaries. The earliest abnormality is the presence of dilated, tortuous, submucosal veins (Fig. 120–5), often in areas where mucosal vessels appeared normal. More extensive lesions show increasing numbers of dilated and deformed vessels traversing the muscularis mucosa and involving the mucosa until, in the most severe lesions, the mucosa is replaced by a maze of distorted, dilated vascular channels (see Fig. 120–5). Enlarged arteries and thick-walled veins occasionally are seen in advanced lesions in which the dilated arteriolar-capillary-venular unit has become a small arteriovenous fistula. Large, thick-walled arteries are more typical of congenital arteriovenous malformations.

Pathogenesis

The previously described studies using injection and clearing techniques indicated that VEs are degenerative lesions associated with aging and that they represent a unique clinical and pathologic entity.[1] That VEs are common acquired lesions associated with aging is supported by their frequent

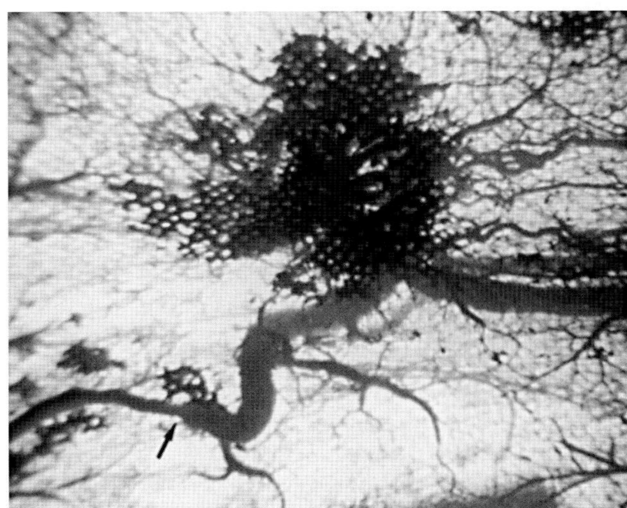

Figure 120–4. Transilluminated, cleared colon showing a mucosal ectasia surrounded by normal crypts with ectatic venules leading to a large, distended, tortuous, underlying submucosal vein. A sharp constriction (*arrow*) can be seen where the vein traverses the muscle layers. (From Boley SJ, Brandt LJ, Mitsudo S: Adv Intern Med 29:301, 1984, with permission.)

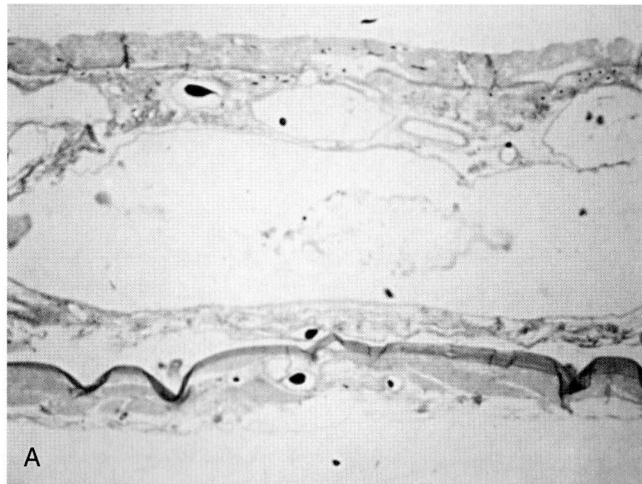

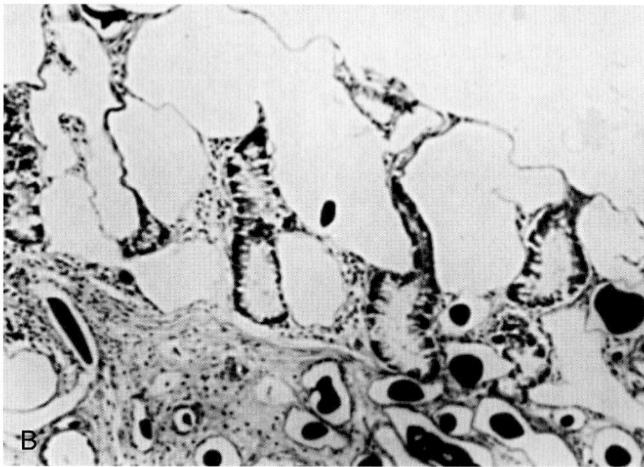

Figure 120–5. Histopathology of vascular ectasia. *A*, A large, distended vein completely filling the submucosa with a few dilated venules in the overlying mucosa. This is the hallmark of an early ectasia (Hematoxylin-eosin stain; magnification, ×50). (From Boley SJ, Brandt LJ, Mitsudo S: Adv Intern Med 29:301, 1984, with permission). *B*, An advanced lesion shows total disruption of the mucosa with replacement by ectatic vessels. Only one layer of endothelium separates the lumen of the cecum from those of the dilated vessels (Hematoxylin-eosin stain; magnification, ×50.)

identification both at colonoscopy in elderly people and in injected colons resected from older patients with no history of bleeding.[1, 6] The likely cause is partial, intermittent, low-grade obstruction of submucosal veins at the site where these vessels pierce the muscular layers of the colon. Repeated episodes of transiently elevated pressure during muscular contraction and distention of the cecum over many years ultimately result in dilation and tortuosity of the submucosal vein, and later, of the venules and capillaries of the mucosal units that drain into it. Finally, the capillary rings dilate, the precapillary sphincters lose their competency, and a small arteriovenous fistula is produced (Fig. 120–6). The latter is responsible for the "early-filling vein," which was the original angiographic hallmark of this lesion. Prolonged increased flow through the arteriovenous fistula can then produce alterations in the arteries supplying the area and in the extramural veins that drain it.

This concept of the cause of VEs is based upon (1) a prominent submucosal vein, either in the absence of any mucosal lesion, or underlying only a minute mucosal VE supplied by a normal artery; (2) dilation of the veins, starting where they traverse the muscularis propria (see Fig. 120–4); and (3) previous studies showing that venous flow in the bowel may be diminished by increases in colon motility, intramural tension, and intraluminal pressure.[18, 19] Following this logic, the prevalence of VEs in the right colon can be attributed to the greater tension in the cecal wall compared with that in other parts of the colon, according to LaPlace's principle: $T = \pi DP$ (where T is tension, D is diameter, and P is intraluminal pressure).

Management

Management of incidental (nonbleeding) VEs detected by colonoscopy is conservative. The natural history of colonic VE is benign in healthy, asymptomatic people, and the risk of bleeding is small.[20, 21] In such cases endoscopic therapy is not warranted.[22]

Management of bleeding VEs consists of three phases: (1) diagnosis, (2) conversion of the emergency situation to an elective one by control of the acute hemorrhage, and (3) definitive treatment of the VE by colonoscopic ablation or surgical removal. The diagnostic approach to colonic VEs is essentially the same as that to lower intestinal bleeding in general and includes radionuclide bleeding scans, colonoscopy, and angiography. Nuclide scans are used to determine whether a patient is actively bleeding, and if so, to localize the site (see Chapter 13). Although angiography previously had been the principal means of identifying VE as the source, colonoscopy currently is the preferred method (see Figs. 120–1, 120–2, and 120–3).

The endoscopist's ability to diagnose the specific nature of a vascular lesion is limited by the similar appearance of many disparate lesions. VEs, spider angiomas, hereditary hemorrhagic telangiectasia, angiomas, the focal hypervascularity of radiation colitis, ulcerative colitis, Crohn's disease, ischemic colitis, certain infections (e.g., syphilis, *Pneumocystis*), and hyperplastic and adenomatous polyps can all, on occasion, resemble each other (Table 120–2).

Because traumatic and endoscopic suction artifacts may resemble vascular lesions, all lesions must be evaluated immediately on insertion of the colonoscope, rather than during withdrawal. Pinch biopsy samples of vascular lesions obtained during endoscopy are usually nonspecific; therefore, the risk of performing biopsies of these abnormalities is not justified.

Because the appearance of vascular lesions is influenced by blood pressure, blood volume, and state of hydration, such lesions may not be evident in patients with severely reduced blood volumes or who are in shock; thus, accurate evaluation may not be possible until red cell and volume deficits are corrected. Cold water lavage of the colon, as is sometimes done to clean the luminal surface from debris during colonoscopy, may mask underlying VEs.[23] Meperidine also may diminish the prominence of some vascular abnormalities; its use should be minimized and its effects reversed by naloxone, in order to detect colonic vascular lesions more accurately. Use of naloxone can enhance the appearance of normal colonic vasculature in about 10% of patients and cause ectasias to appear (2.7%) or increase in

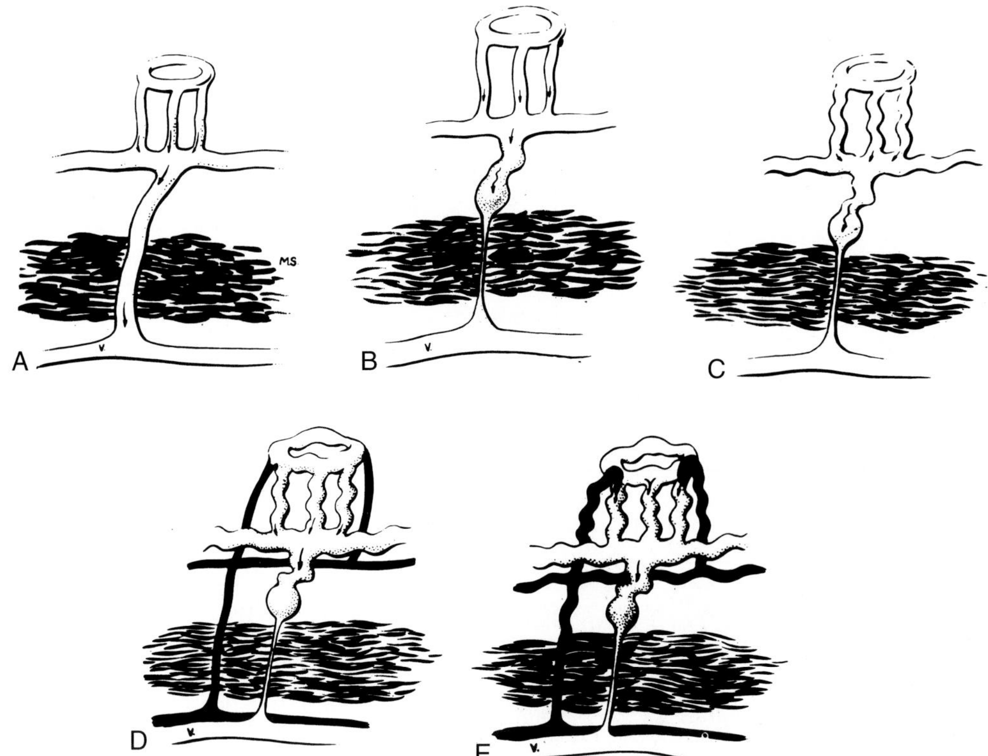

Figure 120–6. Proposed concept of the development of cecal vascular ectasias: Normal state of vein (v.) perforating muscular layers (*A*); with muscular contraction or increased intraluminal pressure, the vein is partially obstructed (*B*); after repeated episodes over many years, the submucosal vein becomes dilated and tortuous (*C*); later the veins and venules draining into the abnormal submucosal vein become similarly involved (*D*); ultimately the capillary ring becomes dilated, the precapillary sphincter becomes incompetent, and a small arteriovenous communication is present through the ectasia (*E*). (From Boley SJ, Sammartano RJ, Adams A, et al: On the nature and etiology of vascular ectasias of the colon: Degenerative lesions of aging. Gastroenterology 72:650, 1977, with permission.)

size (5.4%).[24] For these reasons, naloxone is an important adjunctive medication for patients undergoing evaluation for lower intestinal bleeding.

Angiography is used to determine the site and nature of lesions during active bleeding and can identify some vascular lesions even when bleeding has ceased. The three reliable angiographic signs that diagnose VEs are a densely opacified, slowly emptying, dilated, tortuous vein; a vascular tuft; and an early-filling vein (Fig. 120–7).[25] A fourth sign, extravasation of contrast material, identifies the site of bleeding when bleeding volume is at least 0.5 mL/min but does not contribute to the diagnosis of ectasia.

Table 120–2 | **Lesions Confused with Vascular Ectasias on Endoscopy**

VASCULAR
Arteriovenous malformations
Angiomas
Phlebectasias
Spiders
Telangiectases
Varices
Venous stars
NONVASCULAR
Trauma
Polyps
Adenomatous
Hyperplastic
Lymphoid
COLITIS
Inflammatory bowel disease
Ischemic
Infectious
Radiation

The slowly emptying vein persists late into the venous phase, after the other mesenteric veins have emptied. Vascular tufts are created by the ectatic venules that join the mucosal VE and the submucosal vein. They are seen best in the arterial phase, are usually located at the termination of a branch of the ileocolic artery, appear as small candelabra-like or oval clusters of vessels, and still are seen in the venous phase communicating with a dilated, tortuous, intramural vein. The early filling vein is one seen in the arterial phase within 4 to 5 seconds of injection (see Fig. 120–7). It is not a valid sign of a VE if vasodilators such as papaverine or tolazoline (Priscoline) have been used to enhance the study. Intraluminal extravasation of contrast material usually appears during the arterial phase of angiography and persists throughout the study. Extravasation identifies a site of active bleeding, but in the absence of other signs of VEs, it suggests another cause for the bleeding.

Bleeding can be controlled nonsurgically in most patients, avoiding the higher morbidity and mortality of emergency operation. Vasopressin infusions, either intravenously or intra-arterially through the angiographic catheter, successfully arrest hemorrhage from VE in more than 80% of patients in whom extravasation is demonstrated.[10] The intravenous route appears to be as effective as the intra-arterial route when the bleeding is in the left colon, but intra-arterial administration is more successful when the bleeding is from the right colon or small bowel. Infarction of the sigmoid colon and severe arterial spasm and ischemia of a leg have been seen following vasopressin infusions into the inferior mesenteric artery (IMA) given at the same rate as that used in the superior mesenteric artery (SMA). These complications may be avoided by infusing less than 0.4 unit/min (the dose of SMA infusions), recognizing the lesser blood flow of the IMA.

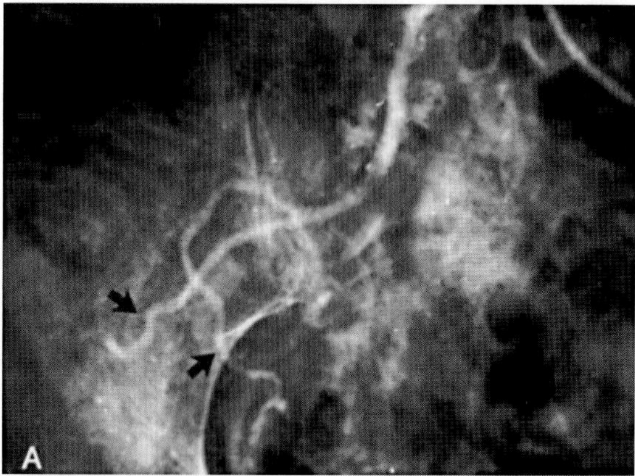

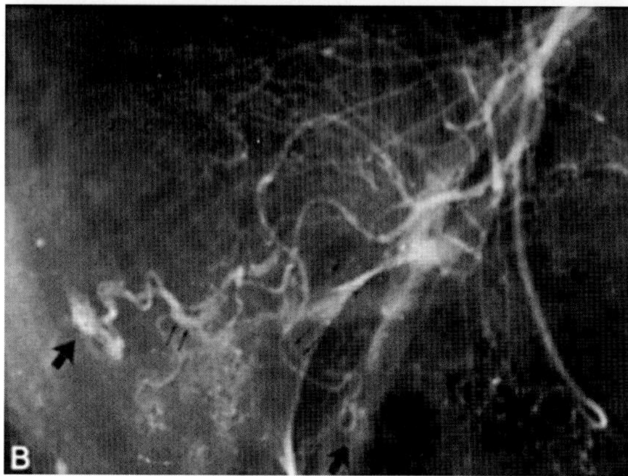

Figure 120–7. Angiography of vascular ectasia. *A,* Superior mesenteric artery arteriogram from a patient with vascular ectasias shows two densely opacified, slowly emptying, dilated, tortuous cecal veins *(arrows)* at 14 sec. Note the late visualization of the ileocolic vein after other veins have cleared. *B,* An arterial phase of the same arteriogram shows two vascular tufts *(large arrows)* and two early-filling veins *(small arrows)* at 6 sec. (From Boley SJ, Sprayregen S, Sammartano RJ, et al: The pathophysiologic basis for the angiographic signs of vascular ectasias of the colon. Radiology 125:615, 1977, with permission.)

Transcatheter embolization may stop lower intestinal bleeding, but colonic infarction and delayed stricture may follow this form of therapy.[26]

Hormonal therapy, usually with conjugated estrogens, has been used to treat patients with vascular lesions of the GI tract in an attempt to reduce or terminate bleeding.[27] The mechanisms by which such agents might work are not known, although procoagulant effects and endothelial injury are popular theories. The results of several prospective, controlled trials examining hormonal therapy have been divergent.[28–30] In a long-term observational study, combination hormonal therapy was shown to stop bleeding in patients with occult GI bleeding of obscure origin, likely to have resulted from small bowel angiodysplasias. No such study has been done for known colonic VEs.

Argon and Nd:YAG laser,[4, 7, 31, 32] endoscopic sclerosis,[33] monopolar[34] and bipolar[35] electrocoagulation, the heater probe,[35] and argon plasma coagulation (APC) all have been used to ablate vascular lesions throughout the GI tract and can be used to control active bleeding. Although none has been established as being superior, the heater probe and bipolar methods are used most often.[10] Recurrent bleeding from cecal VEs appears to be reduced after laser therapy or ablation via the heater probe or BICAP coagulators, but patients usually need more than one session of endoscopic hemostasis.[36] The main risks of thermal therapy for colonic VEs are severe delayed bleeding in 5% of patients and postcoagulation syndrome in 1.7% of patients.[35]

In preparation for endoscopic ablation of vascular lesions, aspirin and aspirin-containing drugs, nonsteroidal anti-inflammatory agents, anticoagulants, and antiplatelet agents should be withdrawn at least 1 week to 10 days before the procedure. Care should be taken not to distend the cecum fully, as the wall would be further thinned and the risk of perforation increased.

Right hemicolectomy remains the treatment of choice for a patient who has bled and whose right colon VE has been identified by either colonoscopy or angiography *if* (1) the bleeding continues, (2) an endoscopist experienced in transcolonoscopic ablation is not available, and (3) endoscopic ablation has been unsuccessful or is not feasible for technical reasons. In the latter two situations, right hemicolectomy is done as an elective procedure once active bleeding is controlled. The presence or absence of diverticulosis in the left colon does not alter the extent of colonic resection; only the right half of the colon is removed. It is important that the entire right half of the colon be removed to ensure that no VEs are left behind. Since 50% to 80% of bleeding diverticula are located in the right side of the colon, the risks of leaving left colon containing diverticula, which might be the source of the bleeding, are far outweighed by the increased morbidity and mortality of the more extensive subtotal colectomy. Recurrent bleeding can be expected in up to 20% of patients so treated. Subtotal colectomy should be performed only as a last resort—that is, when active colonic bleeding persists, the angiogram is completely normal, and colonoscopy either yields negative findings or is not helpful.

Hereditary Hemorrhagic Telangiectasia (Osler-Weber-Rendu Disease)

This autosomal dominant familial disorder is characterized by telangiectases of the skin and mucous membranes as well as recurrent GI bleeding.[37–39] The pathogenesis may relate to mutations of the endoglin and ALK-1 genes, which have an important role in determining the properties of endothelial cells during angiogenesis.[40] Lesions typically are noticed in the first few years of life, and recurrent epistaxis in childhood is characteristic of the disease. By age 10 years, about half of patients have had some GI bleeding. Severe hemorrhage is unusual before the fourth decade and has a peak incidence in the sixth decade. In most patients, bleeding presents as melena; bright red blood per rectum, epistaxis and hematemesis are less frequent. Bleeding is chronic and may be severe; patients may receive more than 50 transfusions in a lifetime. A family history of disease has been reported in 80% of patients with the disorder but is less common in those who bleed later in life. Telangiectases usually are present on the lips, oral and nasopharyngeal membranes, tongue, and periungual areas; lack of involvement of these sites casts suspicion on the diagnosis (Fig. 120–8, *A* and *B*).

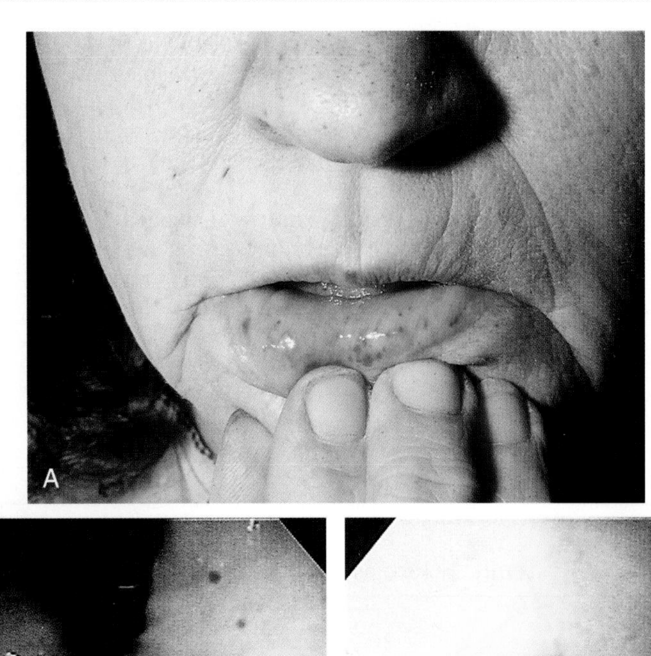

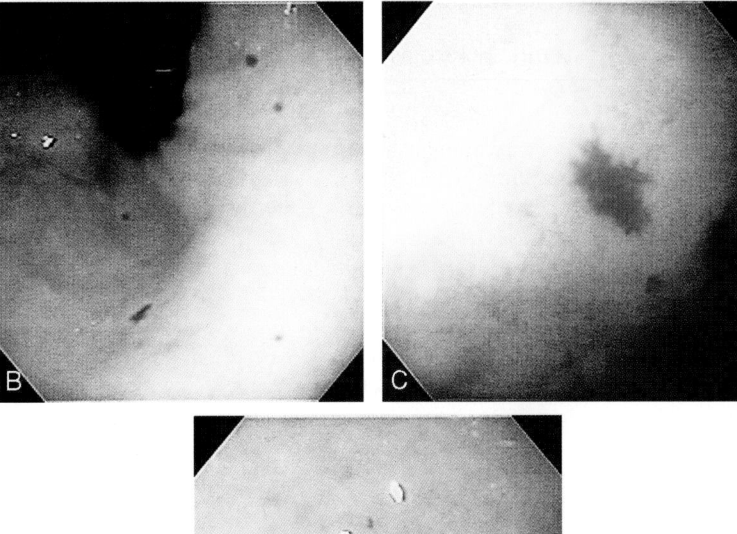

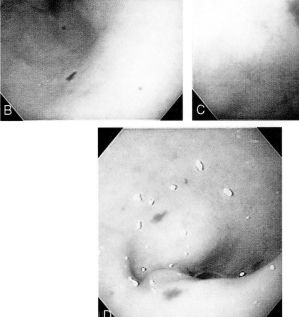

Figure 120–8. Vascular ectasias of Osler-Weber-Rendu disease. *A,* Multiple telangiectases on the nose and lips. *B–D.* Vascular ectasias of varying size and shape in the proximal gastric body *(B),* antrum *(C),* and duodenal bulb *(D).* (From Wilcox CM: Atlas of Clinical Gastrointestinal Endoscopy. Philadelphia, W.B. Saunders, 1995, p. 123.)

Vascular involvement of the liver is not uncommon in this disorder and frequently is asymptomatic; hepatic manifestations during the course of the disease are seen in 8% to 31% of patients. Typical clinical presentations of liver involvement are high-output heart failure due to right-to-left intrahepatic shunting, portal hypertension, and biliary tract disease.[41] Serious complications, including liver failure and the need for liver transplantation, have been reported. Telangiectases occur in the colon but are more common in the stomach and small bowel, where they also are more apt to cause significant bleeding.

Telangiectases are seen easily on endoscopy, although in the presence of severe anemia and blood loss they transiently may become less obvious or even invisible; with blood replacement, they become prominent again. Angiographic findings may be normal or may demonstrate arteriovenous communications, conglomerate masses of abnormal vessels, phlebectasia, and aneurysms.[42] Angiography may be misleading when it demonstrates multiple vascular abnormalities because some of these lesions have been shown to be in the mesentery rather than in the bowel.

Grossly, the telangiectases are the size of millet seeds and typically appear as cherry-red, smooth hillocks. Pathologically, the major changes involve the capillaries and venules, but arterioles also may be affected. Lesions consist of irregular, ectatic, tortuous blood spaces lined by a delicate single layer of endothelial cells and supported by a fine layer of fibrous connective tissue. No elastic lamina or muscular tissue is present in these vessels, so they cannot contract. This may explain why they tend to bleed. Arterioles show intimal proliferation and commonly have thrombi in them, suggesting vascular stasis. In contrast to the thinned venules of VEs, venules are abnormally thick in Osler-Weber-Rendu disease, have prominent, well-developed longitudinal muscles, and apparently play the major role in regulating blood flow in the telangiectasia.[43]

Many forms of treatment have been recommended for these and other vascular lesions, including estrogens,[28, 44] aminocaproic acid,[45] endoscopic ablation,[7, 32] and resection of involved bowel. Endoscopic ablation, including the use of the APC and thermal contact devices, appears most promising, may be performed during active bleeding or between bleeding episodes, and has reduced the urgency for resecting bowel. Long-term follow-up studies are needed to evaluate the ultimate efficacy of the various forms of therapy.

Progressive Systemic Sclerosis

(See also Chapter 29)

Vascular lesions are a prominent feature of progressive systemic sclerosis, especially in the CREST variant (calcinosis, Raynaud's phenomenon, esophageal dysmotility, scleroderma, and telangiectases).[46] Sites most frequently involved by these telangiectases are the hands, lips, tongue, and face, but gastric, intestinal, and colorectal lesions have been reported. These tiny lesions may be the source of occult or clinically significant bleeding and are best treated, if possible, by endoscopic electrocoagulation or laser photocoagulation.[47]

Gastric Antral Vascular Ectasia (Watermelon Stomach) and Portal Hypertensive Gastropathy (PHG)

Gastric antral vascular ectasia (GAVE), or the watermelon stomach, describes a vascular lesion of the antrum that consists of tortuous, dilated vessels radiating outward from the pylorus, like spokes from a wheel, and resembling the dark stripes on the surface of a watermelon.[48] This lesion causes both acute hemorrhage and chronic occult bleeding. Its cause is unknown, although it has been proposed that gastric peristalsis causes prolapse of the loose antral mucosa with consequent elongation and ectasia of the mucosal vessels[48] (Fig. 120–9). GAVE also has been thought to result from delayed gastric emptying as well as from humoral factors such as hypergastrinemia, prostaglandin E_2, proliferation of neuroendocrine cells containing 5-hydroxytryptamine (serotonin), and vasoactive intestinal polypeptide (VIP).

GAVE is seen particularly in middle-aged or older women and in association with achlorhydria, atrophic gastritis, cirrhosis, the CREST syndrome, and after bone marrow transplantation.[46, 49] The association of cirrhosis and portal hypertension in approximately 40% of reported cases of GAVE suggests that this lesion may be due to portal hypertension or veno-occlusive disease.[50] Microscopic features include dilated capillaries with focal thrombosis, dilated and tortuous submucosal venous channels, and fibromuscular hyperplasia of the muscularis mucosa.

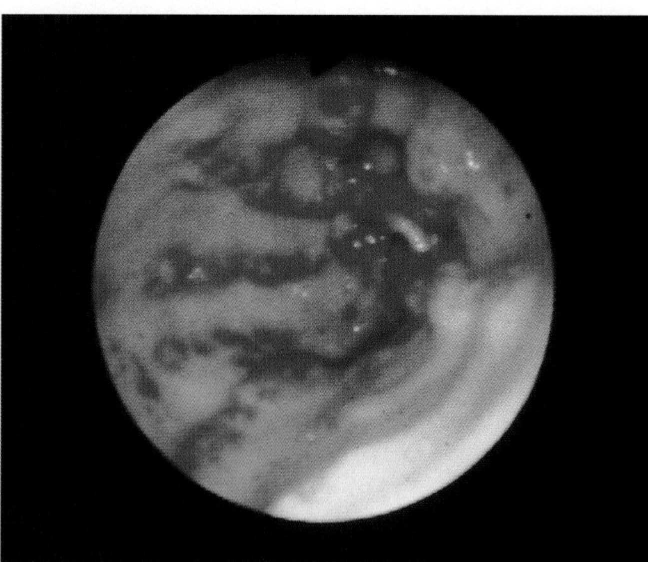

Figure 120–9. Endoscopic appearance of watermelon stomach.

Some researchers believe that GAVE and portal hypertensive gastropathy (PHG) are different manifestations of the same pathogenetic process, whereas others view them as separate entities with unique clinical and histologic features. PHG is characterized endoscopically by three distinct patterns: (1) fine red speckling of the mucosa; (2) superficial reddening, especially on the tips of the rugae; and, most commonly, (3) the presence of a mosaic pattern with red spots (snake-skin appearance) in the gastric fundus or body (Fig. 120–10). Histologically, the stomach in PHG contains dilated, tortuous, irregular veins in the mucosa and submucosa, sometimes with intimal thickening, usually in the absence of significant inflammation.[51] The presence of portal hypertension in a patient with GAVE and bleeding is more difficult to manage than GAVE alone since bleeding in the former instance is usually greater and more resistant to treatment than is the latter.[52]

Iron therapy, transfusions, and brief trials with corticosteroids have been used with limited success in attempts to diminish the bleeding episodes in GAVE; antrectomy often was required. Transendoscopic laser photocoagulation,[53] APC, and heater-probe therapy[54] are being used with increasing success to treat GAVE as well as sites of bleeding of PHG without GAVE. Transjugular intrahepatic portosystemic shunting (TIPS) offers another modality when GAVE is associated with portal hypertension or when bleeding due to PHG is not controlled by some type of coagulation therapy (see also Chapters 13 and 77).

Portal Colopathy

Portal colopathy is the term used to describe the vascular manifestations of portal hypertension in the colon. These include hemorrhoids, varices, and spider-like telangiectases. Mucosal lesions of portal colopathy typically resemble those seen in PHG and may have a diffuse, colitis-like appearance, including granularity, erythema, and friability. The lesions of portal colopathy are amenable to the same thermal therapies as for GAVE and PHG.[55]

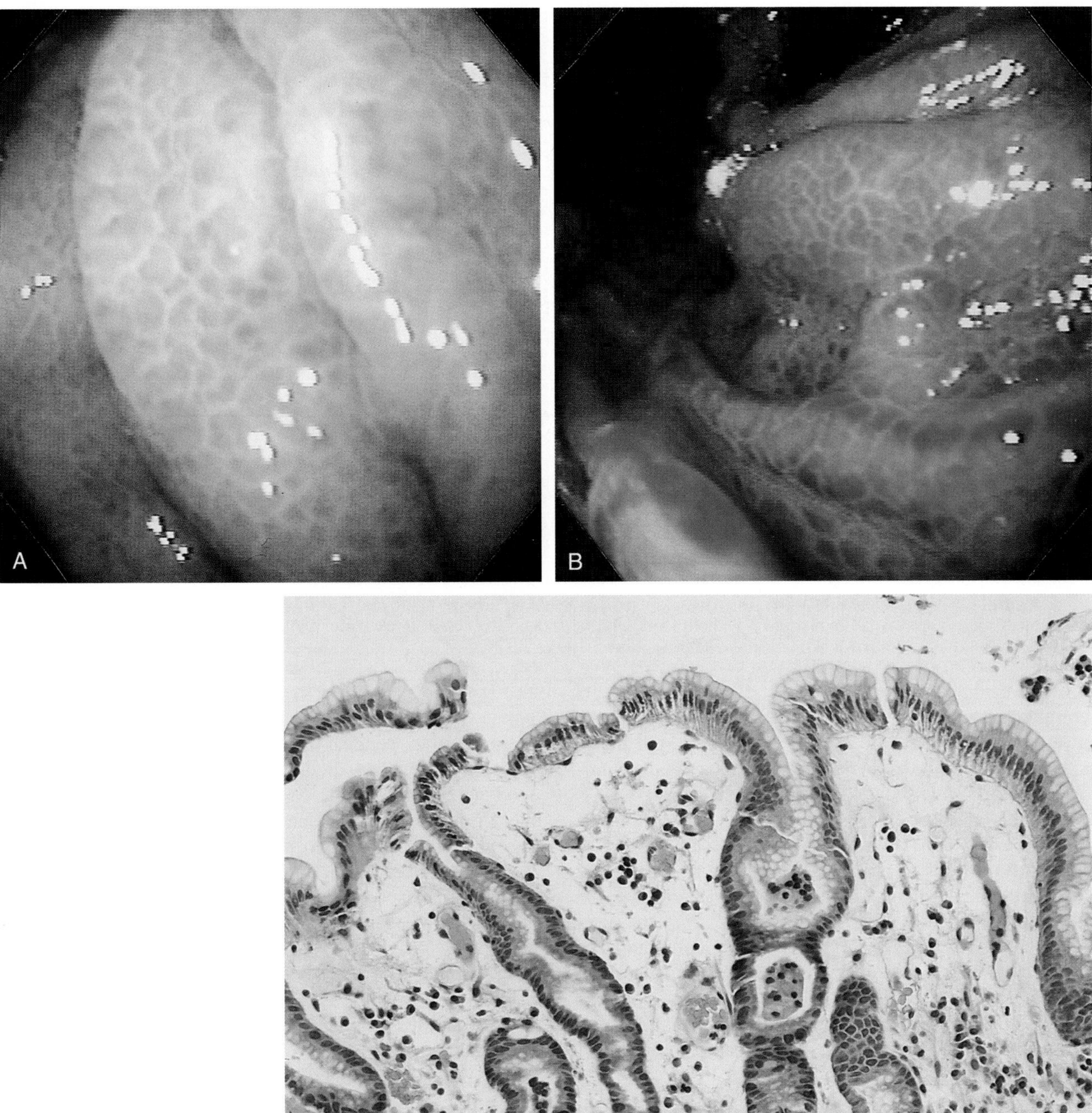

Figure 120–10. Portal hypertensive gastropathy. *A,* Mild disease is manifested by prominence of the areae gastricae, with areas of erythema and subepithelial hemorrhage. This appearance is not pathognomonic but may be noted with other disorders inducing mucosal edema, such as *H. pylori* gastritis. *B,* Severe gastropathy with diffuse subepithelial hemorrhage in a snake-skin pattern. *C,* Prominent edema of the lamina propria with multiple congested blood vessels. No histologic evidence of gastritis is seen. (From Wilcox CM: Atlas of Clinical Gastrointestinal Endoscopy. Philadelphia, W.B. Saunders, 1995, p. 109.)

Dieulafoy's Lesion (Exulceratio Simplex)

This vascular lesion is a rare cause of massive GI hemorrhage, usually from the stomach, but sometimes from the small or large bowel[56] (Fig. 120–11). It is twice as common in men as in women and presents at a mean age of 52 years. The vascular abnormality is the presence of arteries of persistent large caliber in the submucosa, and in some instances, the mucosa, typically with a small, overlying mucosal defect. Dieulafoy called the lesion "exulceratio simplex" because he thought it was the initial stage of a gastric ulcer. This lesion also has been called an *atherosclerotic aneurysm,* an inaccurate term since the caliber of the artery's walls is uniform throughout and shows no unusual degree of arteriosclerosis. It is believed that focal pressure from these large "caliber-persistent" vessels thins the overlying mucosa, leading to erosion of the exposed vascular wall and resultant hemorrhage. Massive hematemesis or melena typically is not preceded by any GI tract symptoms and usually is followed by intermittent and severe bleeding over several days. The

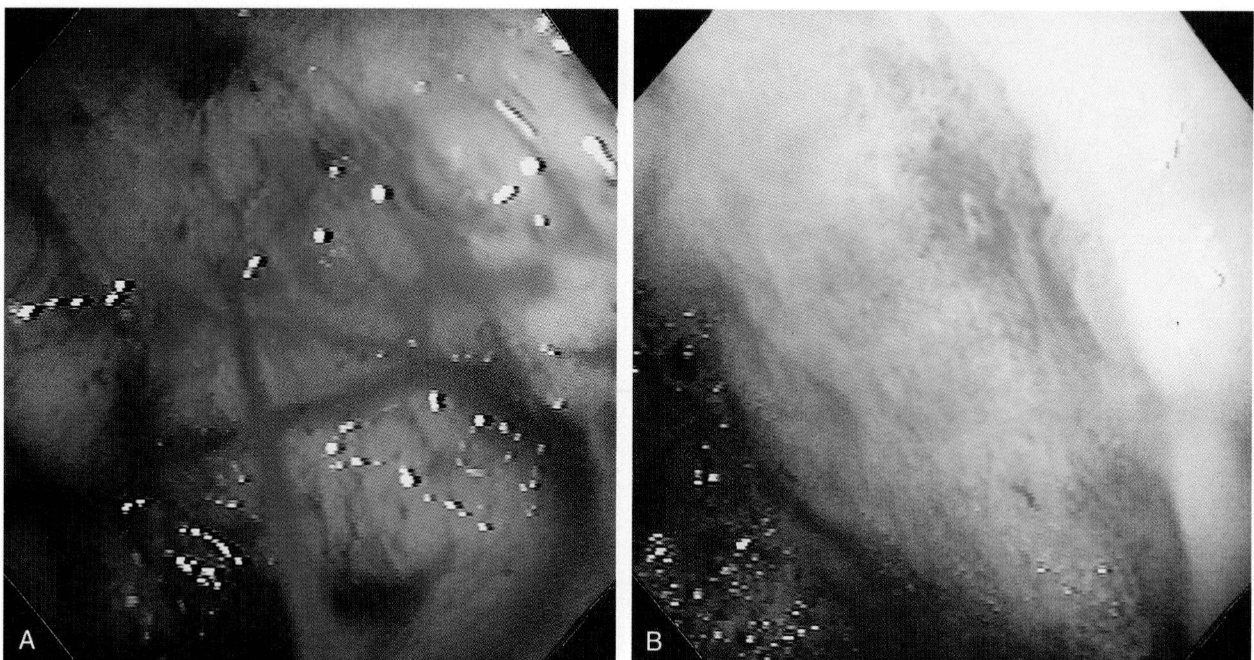

Figure 120–11. Dieulafoy's lesion. *A,* Arterial bleeding (spurting) just distal to the gastroesophageal junction. *B,* The bleeding point was a small defect without endoscopic evidence of ulceration. (From Wilcox CM: Atlas of Clinical Gastrointestinal Endoscopy. Philadelphia, W.B. Saunders, 1995, p. 122.)

most common site of bleeding is 6 cm distal to the cardioesophageal junction, where the arteries are largest, but many lesions have been reported in extragastric locations, including the esophagus, small bowel, and rectum.[57]

The mortality rate for elderly patients with this lesion has been high; nearly 80% before diagnostic endoscopy was available and more than 20% in cases reported between 1970 and 1986. The high mortality rate was due to the inability to localize the bleeding site and the frequent need for emergency gastric surgery. Current angiographic and endoscopic techniques to localize and treat bleeding lesions have led to an improvement in 30-day mortality, now reported to be 13%. Therapeutic approaches to bleeding Dieulafoy's lesions include injection therapy, heater probe, laser, APC, band ligation, and Hemoclip placement.[57, 58]

Hemangiomas

Hemangiomas are the second most common vascular lesion of the colon. Considered by some to be true neoplasms, they are generally thought to be hamartomas because most are present at birth. Colonic hemangiomas may be solitary or multiple lesions limited to the colon, or they may be part of diffuse GI or multisystem angiomatoses. Hemangiomas may be classified as cavernous, capillary, or mixed types. Most are small, ranging from a few millimeters to 2 cm, but larger lesions do occur, especially in the rectum.

Bleeding from colonic hemangiomas usually is slow, producing occult blood loss with anemia or melena. Hematochezia is less common, except in large, cavernous hemangiomas of the rectum, which may cause massive hemorrhage. Diagnosis is best established by endoscopy, including enteroscopy, since roentgenologic studies, including angiography, frequently are normal.

Hemangiomas are well circumscribed but not encapsulated. Grossly, *cavernous hemangiomas* appear as polypoid or moundlike, reddish-purple lesions on the mucosa. Histologically, numerous dilated, irregular, blood-filled spaces are seen within the mucosa and submucosa, sometimes extending through the muscular wall to the serosal surface. The vascular channels are lined by flat endothelial cells with flat or plump nuclei, and their walls are composed of fibrous tissue. *Capillary hemangiomas* are plaquelike or moundlike reddish-purple lesions composed of a proliferation of fine, closely packed, newly formed capillaries separated by very little stroma. The endothelial cells are large, usually hypertrophic, and in some areas, may form solid cords or nodules with ill-defined capillary spaces. Small hemangiomas that are solitary or few in number and can be approached endoscopically are locally ablated. Most large or multiple lesions require resection of either the hemangioma alone or the involved segment of colon.

Cavernous Hemangiomas of the Rectum

These solitary and extensive lesions involve much of the rectum with or without portions of the rectosigmoid and often cause massive hemorrhage. The diagnosis often can be suggested on plain films of the abdomen by the presence of phleboliths and by displacement or distortion of the rectal air column. On barium enema, the rectal lumen typically shows narrowing and rigidity, scalloping of the rectal wall, and widening of the presacral space. Endoscopically, elevated plum-red nodules or vascular congestion is seen; ulcers and proctitis also may be present. Angiography can demonstrate these lesions but seldom is necessary to establish the diagnosis.

Local measures to control the massive bleeding from rectal hemangiomas usually are effective only temporarily. Embolization and surgical ligation of major feeding vessels also have been used, but ultimately, excision of the rectum often is required.[59]

Diffuse Intestinal Hemangiomatosis

In this entity, numerous lesions, usually of the cavernous type, involve the stomach, small bowel, and colon; hemangiomas of the skin or soft tissues of the head and neck frequently are present. Bleeding or anemia in childhood usually leads to the diagnosis, which may be made by endoscopy and barium studies. Angiographic findings can be normal despite the numerous lesions. Surgical intervention may be required for continuous, slow bleeding or for intussusception. At operation, all identifiable lesions should be excised either through enterotomies or by limited bowel resections. Intraoperative endoscopy may be helpful in finding small lesions. Repeated operations may be necessary to control blood loss.[60]

Blue Rubber Bleb Nevus Syndrome (Cutaneous and Intestinal Cavernous Hemangiomas)

In 1860, an association between cutaneous vascular nevi, intestinal lesions, and GI bleeding was described, later named *blue rubber bleb syndrome* to distinguish it from other cutaneous vascular lesions (Fig. 120–12). A familial history is infrequent, although a few cases of autosomal dominant transmission have been reported.[61]

The lesions are distinctive; they are blue and raised, vary from 0.1 to 5.0 cm in diameter, and have a wrinkled surface. Characteristically, the contained blood can be emptied by direct pressure, leaving a wrinkled sac. The hemangiomas may be single or numerous and are usually found on the trunk, extremities, and face, but not on mucous membranes. They may involve any portion of the GI tract, but are most common in the small bowel. In the colon, they are more common distally. They are detected infrequently by barium or angiographic studies and are seen best by endoscopy. Microscopically, they are cavernous hemangiomas composed of clusters of dilated capillary spaces lined by cuboidal or flattened endothelium with connective tissue stroma. Resection of the involved segment of bowel is recommended for recurrent hemorrhage. Endoscopic laser coagulation may be dangerous because these lesions may involve the full thickness of the bowel wall; successful sclerotherapy and band ligation of GI tract lesions have been reported.

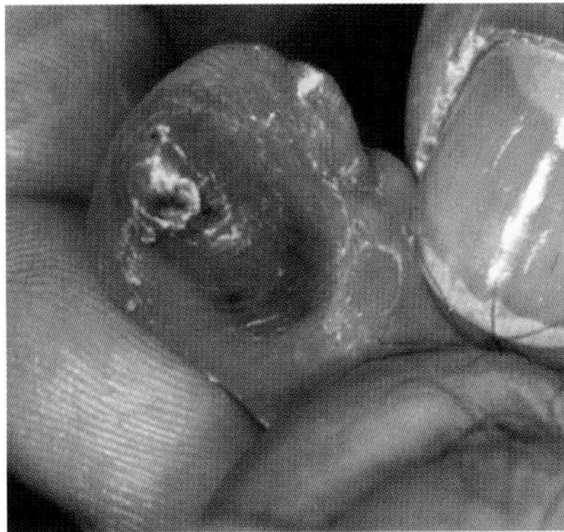

Figure 120–12. Fingertip lesion in the blue nevus syndrome.

Congenital Arteriovenous Malformations (AVMs)

AVMs are embryonic growth defects and are considered to be developmental anomalies, in contrast to vascular ectasias, which are acquired lesions (see earlier discussion of VEs). Although AVMs are found mainly in the extremities, they may occur anywhere in the vascular tree. In the colon, they may be small and resemble VEs, or they may involve a long segment of bowel. The most extensive lesions typically are in the rectum and sigmoid.

Histologically, AVMs are persistent congenital communications between arteries and veins located primarily in the submucosa, in contrast to VEs which are a manifestation of degeneration of submucosal veins. Characteristically, there is "arterialization" of the veins (i.e., tortuosity, dilation, and thick walls with smooth muscle hypertrophy and intimal thickening or sclerosis). In long-standing AVMs, the arteries are dilated with atrophic and sclerotic degeneration.

Angiography is the primary means of diagnosis. Early-filling veins in small lesions and extensive dilation of arteries or veins in large lesions are typical. Patients with significant bleeding from large AVMs should have resection of the involved segment; transendoscopic therapy may be beneficial for smaller lesions.

Klippel-Trenaunay-Weber Syndrome

In the initial description, this syndrome consisted of (1) a vascular nevus involving the lower limb, (2) varicose veins limited to the affected side and appearing at birth or in childhood, and (3) hypertrophy of all tissues of the involved limb, especially the bones.[62, 63] Subsequently, a variety of vascular lesions associated with the hypertrophic limb were described. Although the cause of bony elongation is controversial, one theory invokes in utero venous hypertension and stasis.[62] Edema of the involved leg is common, and if the thigh is involved, a variety of lymphatic abnormalities usually are present (e.g., chylous mesenteric cysts, chlyoperitoneum, and protein-losing enteropathy; see Chapter 25).

Symptomatic GI or genitourinary involvement is rare (prevalence about 1%) and manifests with hemorrhage. Bleeding may be recurrent and mild or severe, and usually is due to a rectal or vaginal hemangioma, localized rectovaginal varices caused by obstruction of the internal iliac system, or portal hypertension with varices. Physical examination is diagnostic, and various imaging techniques are used to define the anatomy and plan surgical repair. Plain films showing calcified pelvic phleboliths in a child suggest pelvic hemangiomatosis.

ABDOMINAL AORTIC ANEURYSM

About 95% of abdominal aortic aneurysms are atherosclerotic in origin; the remainder are caused by trauma, vasculitis, syphilis, or other infections (mycotic aneurysm).[64] Eighty-five percent of affected people are men and 15% are women. Abdominal aneurysms commonly are infrarenal and may be fusiform or saccular. The major complication of these aneurysms is rupture, which in untreated aneurysms is frequent, especially with larger lesions; the incidence of rupture correlates with size.[65]

Most abdominal aortic aneurysms are asymptomatic. The most common symptom is epigastric pain, often radiating through to the back, and severe pain may presage rupture. On physical examination, a pulsatile epigastric mass often is palpable. Distinguishing an aneurysm from an overlying abdominal mass with transmitted pulsations may be difficult; with an aneurysm, the pulsations are felt directly over the mass and displace the examining fingers laterally. A bruit may be present, but unless it is of recent onset, usually it is of no help in diagnosis.

Abdominal plain films may show a soft tissue mass with peripheral calcification in the region of the abdominal aorta. With large aneurysms, erosion of the lumbar vertebrae or displacement of surrounding viscera, including bowel, kidneys, and ureters, may be seen. Because plain film studies usually are not sufficiently sensitive to establish the presence or size of an aneurysm, ultrasonography and computed tomography (CT) have become the standard means of evaluation. These procedures are simple, safe, and very accurate in the diagnosis and sizing of aneurysms. Ultrasonography is less sensitive than CT in determining the extent of the aneurysmal process, but it is a useful screening procedure.[66] Angiography is used preoperatively to demonstrate aortic and vascular anatomy and thereby help the surgeon plan the appropriate operative procedure.

Rupture or "leakage" is associated with sudden onset or worsening of pain in the abdomen, flank, or back, but pain may be present for several weeks preceding overt rupture. Pain may be exacerbated by lying recumbent and is relieved by sitting or leaning forward. In one series, only 14% of patients referred for treatment of rupture had been known to have an aneurysm previously.[67]

Abdominal aortic aneurysms most commonly rupture into the retroperitoneal tissues that surround the aorta. Less commonly, the aneurysm may communicate with the peritoneal cavity, in which case shock develops rapidly. Patients whose aneurysm ruptures into the small intestine, most commonly the third portion of the duodenum, usually present with massive GI bleeding; bleeding may be intermittent, as clot alternately forms and is dislodged from the eroded bowel or fistulous opening. Indeed, many of these patients will have a "herald bleed" followed by massive hemorrhage several hours or days later.[68] Endoscopy is the most sensitive method for diagnosing this complication. Rarely, abdominal aneurysms rupture into the inferior vena cava.

Operative management of an abdominal aortic aneurysm usually consists of replacement of the aneurysm with a prosthetic graft, which may be done through a laparotomy or a groin incision by means of an endovascular graft.[69] In elective cases, preoperative angiography is useful for demonstrating other significant vascular disease (e.g., stenosis or occlusion of the splanchnic arteries) and may help avoid postoperative bowel ischemia. Elective open surgical repair carries a mortality of 2% to 8% and requires a hospital stay of 7 to 10 days; mortality increases sharply to 34% to 85% when the procedure is done as an emergency for rupture or impending rupture.[67, 69–70] Patients receiving endovascular grafts can be discharged earlier, but concerns about leakage and late rupture have been raised.[69, 71]

Aneurysms larger than 5 cm, symptomatic aneurysms, or enlarging aneurysms of any size should be resected electively in good-risk patients.[72] Patients whose condition contraindicates aneurysmectomy may be treated by inducing thrombosis in the aneurysm and restoring the circulation to the lower limbs and pelvis with an axillary bifemoral graft, or by nonsurgical endovascular graft placement.[71–73] Patients with asymptomatic and nonexpanding aneurysms 4 to 5 cm in diameter also should be regarded as candidates for elective aneurysmectomy, since the incidence of rupture for aneurysms of this size approximates 25%. Aneurysms that are not treated surgically should be followed ultrasonographically at 3- to 6-month intervals, with the expectation that their size will probably increase by an average of 0.40 to 0.50 cm per year[72]; thus, all eventually would reach a size that would mandate elective resection. Asymptomatic aneurysms smaller than 5 cm in diameter have a less than 10% risk of rupture and are not thought to require operation. Smaller aneurysms should be followed carefully by periodic ultrasonography or CT; an increase in size or the development of symptoms is an indication for resection.[74]

PARAPROSTHETIC ENTERIC AND AORTOENTERIC FISTULA

An uncommon but potentially catastrophic complication of aortic aneurysmectomy and other procedures in which vascular prostheses are placed in the retroperitoneum or abdomen is the formation of a fistula between the graft and the adjacent bowel, usually the third portion of the duodenum.[75, 76] The incidence of this complication is between 0.6% and 2.35%. Such fistulas develop as early as 21 days postoperatively, but in most cases, they are delayed beyond 2 years; in one case, an interval of 14 years was documented. This complication is thought to result from local conditions at the time of, or subsequent to, graft placement, including infection, damage to the duodenum or its blood supply during the dissection, and subsequent erosion of the duodenal wall by the graft. Newer surgical techniques, including the use of nonabsorbable sutures and antibiotics, strict hemostasis, and covering of suture lines with retroperitoneal tissue and peritoneum, as well as the increasing use of endovascular grafts, may reduce the incidence of fistula formation.

Clinically, such patients present with upper or lower GI bleeding that if untreated may be massive and rapidly fatal. Upper GI endoscopy is the procedure of choice for aiding diagnosis by excluding other obvious lesions. CT enhanced with intravenous contrast is the best method for accurate diagnosis. The most important clue to the diagnosis is awareness of the possibility in a patient with GI bleeding who has had an aortoiliac artery graft.

SUPERIOR MESENTERIC ARTERY SYNDROME

The third portion of the duodenum is cradled in an angle formed by the root of the superior mesenteric artery (SMA) and the wall of the aorta. Rarely, the SMA impinges on the duodenum, leading to intestinal obstruction, a condition referred to as the *superior mesenteric artery syndrome*.[77, 78] This term is felt by some to be confusing, as the condition is not one of vascular insufficiency. Symptoms may be acute or chronic and typically include episodic epigastric distress, vomiting, and, in severe cases, weight loss. The syndrome has been associated with immobilization in a body cast, rapid growth in children, and marked, rapid weight loss in adults, particularly young women. Barium studies may show an abrupt cut-off in the third portion of the duodenum with dilation proximally, particularly when the patient is supine.[79] Treatment approaches have included small feedings or a liquid diet. Symptoms typically improve after restoration of lost weight or removal of the body cast. Surgery is necessary only rarely, and duodenojejunostomy may relieve the symptoms (see Chapter 8).

CELIAC AXIS COMPRESSION SYNDROME (CACS)

Whether CACS is a cause of GI ischemia has been a subject of controversy ever since the description of postprandial pain and an epigastric bruit in a patient in whom angiography showed narrowing of the celiac axis caused by compression of a fibrotic celiac ganglion.[80] After release of the artery, the murmur and postprandial pain disappeared. Since that description, compression of the celiac axis by both the median arcuate ligament of the diaphragm and the celiac ganglion has been identified.

A major difficulty in determining the validity of the CACS, also sometimes referred to as Dunbar syndrome, arises from the different criteria used by various investigators to define it.[81, 82] At the least, clinical features that should be present to diagnose CACS include postprandial epigastric pain, diarrhea, weight loss, and an abdominal bruit that intensifies with expiration.

Compression of the celiac axis is demonstrated by lateral aortography or selective studies of the artery. Compression by the crural fibers of the diaphragm, the celiac ganglion, or both, produces a smooth, asymmetric narrowing of the superior aspect of the celiac axis and displaces it toward the SMA (Fig. 120–13). These findings are best shown during expiration.

The clinical significance of celiac axis narrowing on angiography has been questioned because it occurs with equal frequency in patients in whom intestinal angina is suspected, in those with GI diseases not primarily characterized by pain, and in those with miscellaneous problems that do not involve the alimentary tract. Because the anatomic lesion forming the basis for the syndrome is narrowing of the major artery to the upper abdominal viscera, the pain most frequently has been attributed to ischemia. This concept has persisted, despite clinical and experimental evidence that isolated compromise of the celiac axis is almost always compensated for by collateral circulation from either the SMA or the IMA.

A popular alternative theory to the ischemic origin of the pain in CACS is that the pain arises in the celiac ganglion itself, possibly secondary to pressure or throbbing by the compressed artery. The increased splanchnic blood flow and dilation of the artery that accompanies the ingestion of food may explain the relationship of pain to meals.

Operative approaches to CACS include division of the median arcuate ligament, with or without gangliectomy, or arterial reconstruction or bypass. Results of operations for CACS have varied as much as the criteria used to diagnose it. In the largest study of the long-term results of patients treated for CACS, Evans found that 83% of patients were asymptomatic 6 months after a decompression procedure, but only 41% remained asymptomatic 3 to 11 years later.[83] Furthermore, no correlation existed between the presenting symptoms and the results of surgery, and no clinical patterns emerged to identify those patients who might benefit from surgery. Additionally, of 12 patients treated nonoperatively, 9 remained free of pain at the time of Evans' report.

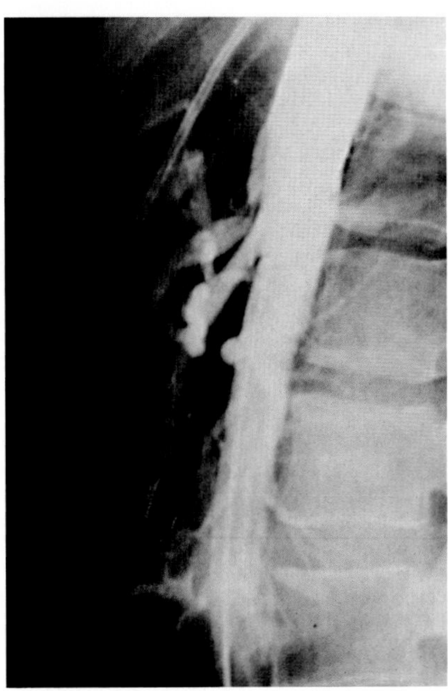

Figure 120–13. Lateral flush aortogram showing typical compression of the origin of the celiac axis with some poststenotic dilatation. The study is from a patient with no abdominal complaints related to this finding. (From Boley SJ, Brandt LJ, Veith FJ: Ischemic disorders of the intestines. Curr Probl Surg 15:1–85, 1978.)

The controversy concerning CACS continues. A small number of patients "with distressing abdominal pain not explained by customary diagnoses and not helped by customary management" are relieved by some aspect of the operations performed for celiac axis compression.[84] If only patients who fulfill the criteria previously described are operated on, unnecessary procedures should be kept to a minimum.

REFERENCES

1. Boley SJ, Sammartano RJ, Adams A, et al: On the nature and etiology of vascular ectasias of the colon: Degenerative lesions of aging. Gastroenterology 72:650, 1977.
2. Mitsudo S, Boley S, Brandt LJ, et al: Vascular ectasias of the colon. Hum Pathol 10:585, 1979.
3. Naveau S, Leger-Ravet MB, Houdayer C, et al: Nonhereditary colonic angiodysplasias: Histomorphometric approach to their pathogenesis. Dig Dis Sci 40:839, 1995.
4. Foutch PG: Angiodysplasia of the gastrointestinal tract. Am J Gastroenterol 88:807, 1993.
5. Boley SJ, Brandt LJ: Vascular ectasias of the colon—1986. Dig Dis Sci 31:26S, 1986.
6. Trudel JL, Fazio VW, Sivak MV: Colonoscopic diagnosis and treatment of arteriovenous malformations in chronic lower gastrointestinal bleeding: Clinical accuracy and efficacy. Dis Colon Rectum 31:107, 1988.

7. Gostout CJ, Bowyer BA, Ahlquist DA, et al: Mucosal vascular malformations of the gastrointestinal tract: Clinical observations and results of endoscopic Neodymium: Yttrium-Aluminum-Garnet laser therapy. Mayo Clin Proc 63:993, 1988.
8. Reinus JF, Brandt LJ: Vascular ectasias and diverticulosis: Common causes of lower GI bleeding. Gastroenterol Clin North Am 23:1, 1994.
9. Danesh BJ, Spiliadis C, Williams CB, et al: Angiodysplasia, an uncommon cause of colonic bleeding: Colonic evaluation of 1,050 patients with rectal bleeding and anemia. Int J Colon Dis 2:218, 1987.
10. Richter JM, Christensen MR, Colditz GA, et al: Angiodysplasia: Natural history and efficacy of therapeutic interventions. Dig Dis Sci 34: 1542, 1989.
11. Rockey DC: Gastrointestinal tract evaluation in patients with iron deficiency anemia. Semin Gastrointest Dis 10:53, 1999.
12. Hemingway AP, Allison DJ: Angiodysplasia and Meckel's diverticulum: A congenital association? Br J Surg 69:493, 1982.
13. Hochter WJ, Weingart W, Kunner E, et al: Angiodysplasia in the colon and rectum: Endoscopic morphology, localization and frequency. Endoscopy 17:182, 1985.
14. Imperiale TF, Ransohoff DF: Aortic stenosis, idiopathic gastrointestinal bleeding, and angiodysplasia: Is there an association? A methodologic critique of the literature. Gastroenterology 95:1670, 1988.
15. Mehta PM, Heinsimer JA, Bryg RJ, et al: Reassessment of the association between gastrointestinal arteriovenous malformations and aortic stenosis. Am J Med 86:275, 1989.
16. Oneglia C, Sabatini T, Rusconi C, et al: Prevalence of aortic valve stenosis in patients affected by gastrointestinal angiodysplasia. Eur J Med 2:75, 1993.
17. Bhutani MS, Gupta SC, Markert RJ, et al: A prospective controlled evaluation of endoscopic detection of angiodysplasia and its association with aortic valve disease. Gastrointest Endosc 42:398, 1995.
18. Semba T, Fujii Y: Relationship between venous flow and colonic peristalsis. Jpn J Physiol 20:408, 1970.
19. Chou CC, Dabney JM: Interrelation of ileal wall compliance and vascular resistance. Am J Dig Dis 12:1198, 1967.
20. Wilcox CM, Alexander LN, Clark WS: Prospective evaluation of the gastrointestinal tract in patients with iron deficiency anemia and no systemic or gastrointestinal signs or symptoms. Am J Med 103:405, 1997.
21. Foutch PG, Rex DK, Lieberman DA: Prevalence and natural history of colonic angiodysplasia among healthy asymptomatic people. Am J Gastroenterol 90:564, 1995.
22. Brandt LJ: A cecal angiodysplastic lesion is discovered during diagnostic colonoscopy performed for iron-deficiency anemia associated with stool positive for occult blood. What therapy would you recommend? Am J Gastroenterol 83:710, 1988.
23. Brandt LJ, Mukhopadhyay D: Masking of colon vascular ectasias by cold water lavage. Gastrointest Endosc 49:141, 1999.
24. Brandt LJ, Spinell MK: Ability of nalaxone to enhance the colonoscopic appearance of normal colon vasculature and colon vascular ectasias. Gastrointest Endosc 49:79, 1999.
25. Boley SJ, Sprayregen S, Sammartano RJ, et al: The pathophysiologic basis for the angiographic signs of vascular ectasias of the colon. Radiology 125:615, 1977.
26. Sniderman KW, Franklin J, Sos TA: Successful transcatheter gelfoam embolization of a bleeding cecal vascular ectasia. AJR Am J Roentgenol 131:157, 1978.
27. Granieri R, Mazzulla JP, Yarborough GW: Estrogen-progesterone therapy for recurrent gastrointestinal bleeding secondary to gastrointestinal angiodysplasia. Am J Gastroenterol 83:556, 1988.
28. van Cutsem E, Rutgeerts P, Vantrappen G: Treatment of bleeding gastrointestinal vascular malformations with oestrogen-progesterone. Lancet 335:953, 1990.
29. Lewis B, Salomon P, Rivera-MacMurray S, et al: Does hormonal therapy have any benefit for bleeding angiodysplasia? J Clin Gastroenterol 15:99, 1992.
30. Barkin JS, Ross BS: Medical therapy for chronic gastrointestinal bleeding of obscure origin. Am J Gastroenterol 93:1250, 1998.
31. Cello JP, Grendell JH: Endoscopic laser treatment for gastrointestinal vascular ectasias. Ann Intern Med 104:352, 1986.
32. Naveau S, Aubert A, Poynard AT, et al: Long-term results of treatment of vascular malformations of the gastrointestinal tract by Neodymium YAG laser photocoagulation. Dig Dis Sci 35:821, 1990.
33. Richter JM, Christensen MR, Colditz GA, et al: Angiodysplasia: Natural history and efficacy of therapeutic intervention. Dig Dis Sci 34: 1542, 1989.
34. Rogers BH: Endoscopic diagnosis and therapy of mucosal vascular abnormalities of the gastrointestinal tract occurring in elderly patients and associated with cardiac, vascular, and pulmonary disease. Gastrointest Endosc 26:134, 1980.
35. Jensen DM, Machicado GA: Colonoscopy for diagnosis and treatment of severe lower gastrointestinal bleeding: Routine outcomes and cost analysis. Gastroenterol Clin North Am 7:477, 1997.
36. Hutcheon DF, Kabelin J, Bulkley GB, et al: Effect of therapy on bleeding rates in gastrointestinal angiodysplasia. Am Surg 53:6, 1987.
37. Kjeldsen AD, Kjeldsen J: Gastrointestinal bleeding in patients with hereditary hemorrhagic telangiectasia. Am J Gastroenterol 95:415, 2000.
38. Guttmacher AE, Marchuk DA, White RI: Hereditary hemorrhagic telangiectasia. N Engl J Med 333:918, 1995.
39. Sharma VK, Howden CW: Gastrointestinal and hepatic manifestations of hereditary hemorrhagic telangiectasia. Dig Dis 16:169, 1998.
40. Azuma H: Genetic and molecular pathogenesis of hereditary hemorrhagic telangiectasia. J Med Invest 47:81, 2000.
41. Garcia-Tsao G, Korzenik JR, Young L: Liver disease in patients with hereditary hemorrhagic telangiectasia. N Engl J Med 343:931, 2000.
42. Halpern M, Turner AF, Citron BP: Hereditary hemorrhagic telangiectasia. An angiographic study of abdominal visceral angiodysplasias associated with gastrointestinal hemorrhage. Radiology 90:1143, 1968.
43. Martini GA: The liver in hereditary hemorrhagic teleangiectasia: An inborn error of vascular structure with multiple manifestations: A reappraisal. Gut 19:531, 1978.
44. Van Cutsam E, Rutgeerts P, Geboes K, et al: Estrogen-progesterone treatment of Osler-Weber-Rendu disease. J Clin Gastroenterol 10:676, 1988.
45. Saba HI, Morelli GA, Logrono LA: Brief report: Treatment of bleeding in hereditary hemorrhagic telangiectasia with aminocaproic acid. N Engl J Med 330:1789, 1995.
46. Sjogren RW: Gastrointestinal features of scleroderma. Curr Opin Rheumatol 8:569, 1996.
47. Duchini A, Sessoms SL: Gastrointestinal hemorrhage in patients with systemic sclerosis and CREST syndrome. Am J Gastroenterol 93:1453, 1998.
48. Jabbari M, Cherry R, Lough JO, et al: Gastric antral vascular ectasia: The watermelon stomach. Gastroenterology 87:1165, 1984.
49. Toyota M, Hinoda Y, Nakagawa N, et al: Gastric antral vascular ectasia causing severe anemia. J Gastroenterol 31:710, 1996.
50. Fisher NC: Gastric antral vascular ectasia and its relation to portal hypertension. Gut 46:441, 2000.
51. Payen JL, Cales P, Voigt JJ: Severe portal hypertensive gastropathy and antral vascular ectasia are distinct entities in patients with cirrhosis. Gastroenterology 108:138, 1995.
52. Brandt LJ: Gastric antral vascular ectasia: Is there to be a consensus? Gastrointest Endosc 44:355, 1996.
53. Bourke MJ, Hope RL, Boyd P: Endoscopic laser therapy for watermelon stomach. J Gastroenterol Hepatol 11:832, 1996.
54. Yamada M, Nishimura D, Hoshino H: Gastric antral vascular ectasia successfully treated by endoscopic electrocoagulation. J Gastroenterol 33:546, 1998.
55. Kozarek RA, Botoman VA, Bredfeldt JE, et al: Portal colopathy: Prospective study of colonoscopy in patients with portal hypertension. Gastroenterology 101:1192, 1991.
56. Fockens P, Tytgat GN: Dieulafoy's disease. Gastrointest Endosc Clin North Am 6:739, 1996.
57. Gadenstatter M, Wetscher G, Crookes PF: Dieulafoy's disease of the large and small bowel. J Clin Gastroenterol 27:169, 1998.
58. Norton ID, Peterson BT, Sorbi D: Management and long-term prognosis of Dieulafoy lesion. Gastrointest Endosc 50:762, 1999.
59. Tanaka N, Onda M, Seya T, et al: Diffuse cavernous hemangioma of the rectum. Eur J Surg 165:280, 1999.
60. Fremond B, Yazbeck S, Dubois J, et al: Intestinal vascular anomalies in children. J Pediatr Surg 6:873, 1997.
61. Oksuzoglu BC, Oksuzoglu G, Cakir U, et al: Blue rubber bleb nevus syndrome. Am J Gastroenterol 91:780, 1996.
62. Servelle M, Bastin R, Loygue J, et al: Hematuria and rectal bleeding in the child with Klippel and Trenaunay syndrome. Ann Surg 183:418, 1976.
63. Samuel M, Spitz L: Klippel-Trenaunay syndrome: Clinical features, complications and management in children. Br J Surg 82:757, 1995.
64. Estes JE: Abdominal aortic aneurysm. A study of 102 cases. Circulation 2:258, 1950.
65. Pierce GE: Abdominal aortic aneurysms. Surg Clin North Am 69:4, 1989.
66. Delin A, Ohlson H, Swendenborg J: Growth rates of abdominal aortic

aneurysms as measured by computed tomography. Br J Surg 7:530, 1985.
67. Ottinger LW: Ruptured arteriosclerotic aneurysms of the abdominal aorta. JAMA 233:147, 1975.
68. Champion MC, et al: Aortoenteric fistula: Incidence, presentation, recognition, and management. Ann Surg 195:314, 1982.
69. Ohki T, Veith FJ: Abdominal aortic aneurysms. Curr Treat Options Cardiovasc Med 1:19, 1999.
70. Hollier LA, Taylor LM, Ochner J: Recommended indications for operative treatment of abdominal aortic aneurysms. J Vasc Surg 15:1046, 1992.
71. Zarins CK, White RA, Schwarten D, et al: Aneurysm stent graft versus open surgical repair of abdominal aortic aneurysms: Multicenter prospective clinical trial. J Vasc Surg 29:292, 1999.
72. Nevitt MP, Ballard DJ, Hallet JW: Prognosis of abdominal aortic aneurysms: A population-based study. N Engl J Med 15;1009, 1989.
73. Seelig MH, Oldenberg WA, Hakaim AG, et al: Endovascular repair of abdominal aortic aneurysms: Where do we stand? Mayo Clin Proc 74: 999, 1999.
74. Guirguis EM, Barber GG: The natural history of abdominal aortic aneurysms. Am J Surg 162:481, 1991.
75. Bashir RM, al-Kiwas FH: Rare causes of occult small intestinal bleeding including aortoenteric fistulas, small bowel tumors and small bowel ulcers. Gastrointest Endosc Clin North Am 6:709, 1996.
76. Gozzetti G, et al: Aortoenteric fistulae: Spontaneous and after aorto-iliac operations. J Cardiovasc Surg 25:420, 1984.
77. Baltazar U, Dunn J, Floresguerra C, et al: Superior mesenteric artery syndrome: An unusual cause of intestinal obstruction. South Med J 93: 606, 2000.
78. Lee CS, Mangla JC: Superior mesenteric artery compression syndrome. Am J Gastroenterol 70:141, 1978.
79. Marchant EA, Alvear DT, Fagelman KM: True clinical entity of vascular compression of the duodenum in adolescence. Surg Gynecol Obstet 168:381, 1989.
80. Harjola PT: A rare obstruction of the celiac artery. Ann Chir Gynaecol Fenn 52:547, 1963.
81. Brandt LJ, Boley S: Celiac axis compression syndrome: A critical review. Am J Gastroenterol 23:633, 1978.
82. Szilagyi DE, Rian RL, Elliot JP, et al: The celiac artery compression syndrome: Does it exist? Surgery 6:849, 1972.
83. Evans WE: Long-term evaluation of the celiac band syndrome. Surgery 76:867, 1974.
84. Bech FR: Celiac artery compression syndromes. Surg Clin North Am 77:409, 1997.

Chapter 121

Surgical Peritonitis and Other Diseases of the Peritoneum, Mesentery, Omentum, and Diaphragm

Bruce A. Runyon and José Such

Ascites, ascites fluid analysis, spontaneous bacterial peritonitis (SBP), and surgical peritonitis in the setting of ascites are discussed in Chapter 78. This chapter deals with (1) surgical peritonitis in the absence of ascites, (2) other diseases of the peritoneum (including further details regarding peritoneal carcinomatosis), and (3) structural anomalies, tumors, and fibrosing processes involving the mesentery, omentum, and diaphragm. Finally, the role of laparoscopy in evaluating peritoneal diseases is discussed. Abdominal abscesses and fistulas are covered in Chapter 24.

ANATOMY AND PHYSIOLOGY

Gross Anatomy

The peritoneum is a membrane covered by a single sheet of mesothelial cells, with an estimated area of 1.7 m^2, similar to the total body surface area. The structure of the peritoneum is sealed in males and open to the exterior via the ostia of fallopian tubes in females. Usually the peritoneal space contains a few milliliters of sterile peritoneal fluid that may act as part of the local defense against bacteria, as well as a lubricant.

The peritoneum is divided into parietal and visceral components. The parietal peritoneum covers the anterior, lateral, and posterior abdominal walls, the inferior surface of the diaphragm, and the pelvis. A large portion of the surface of the intraperitoneal organs (stomach, jejunum, ileum, transverse colon, liver, and spleen) is covered by visceral peritoneum, whereas only the anterior aspect of the retroperitoneal organs (duodenum, left and right colon, pancreas, kidneys, and adrenals) is covered by visceral peritoneum. The intraperitoneal organs are suspended by thickened bands of peritoneum (i.e., the abdominal ligaments). The 11 ligaments and mesenteries identified by Meyers and colleagues are the coronary, gastrohepatic, hepatoduodenal, falciform, gastrocolic, duodenocolic, gastrosplenic, splenorenal, and phrenicocolic ligaments and the transverse mesocolon and small bowel mesentery (Fig. 121–1).[1] These ligamentous structures, which are apparent at laparotomy as well as on computed tomography (CT), subdivide the abdomen into interconnected compartments. Familiarity with the anatomy can be used to predict the route of spread of disease; for example, the gastrohepatic and gastrocolic ligaments allow a gastric tumor to spread to the liver and colon. The spread of infection within the peritoneal cavity is governed by the site of infection, the sites of fibrinous and fibrous adhesions, intraperitoneal pressure gradients, and the position of the patient. After leakage of visceral contents, dependent recesses (e.g., paracolic gutters, pelvis, lesser sac, and subhepatic and subphrenic spaces) tend to become sites of abscess formation.

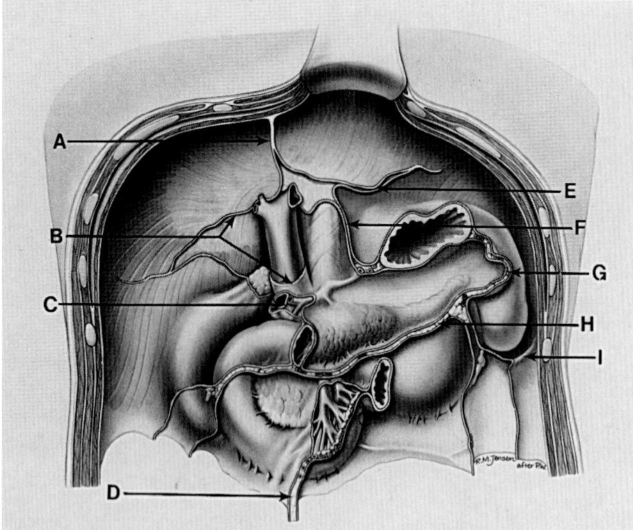

Figure 121–1. Peritoneal ligaments and mesenteries of the upper abdomen. *A*, Falciform ligament; *B*, right coronary ligament; *C*, hepatoduodenal ligament; *D*, root of small bowel mesentery; *E*, left triangular ligament; *F*, gastrohepatic ligament; *G*, gastrosplenic ligament; *H*, transverse mesocolon; *I*, phrenicocolic ligament. (From Meyers MA, Oliphant M, Berne AS, Feldberg MAM: The peritoneal ligaments and mesenteries: Pathways of intraabdominal spread of disease. Radiology 163:593–604, 1987.)

The mesentery is defined as a membranous bilayer of peritoneum that attaches an organ to the body wall. An omentum is a fold of peritoneum that connects the stomach with adjacent organs of the peritoneal cavity. The greater omentum spreads from the greater curvature of the stomach to the transverse colon. The lesser omentum joins the lesser curvature of the stomach to the liver, and it is called gastrohepatic omentum.

Microscopic Anatomy

The word *peritoneum* is derived from the Greek "*peri-*" meaning around and "*tonos*," meaning a stretching; therefore a stretching around. It is formed by a single layer of mesothelial cells. Mesothelium is, in turn, a simple squamous epithelium of mesodermal origin. An interesting phenomenon is the potential ability of its cells to be phagocytic. Mesothelial cells are covered by microvilli in their apical surface and are joined by intercellular gaps that allow rapid absorption of fluid and particulate matter from the peritoneal cavity.

Blood Supply and Innervation

The visceral peritoneum is supplied by the splanchnic blood vessels, and the parietal peritoneum by intercostal, subcostal, lumbar, and iliac vessels. The visceral peritoneum is supplied by visceral, nonsomatic sympathetic nerves (without pain receptors), and the parietal peritoneum by somatic nerves. This key difference explains the reason of easily localizable origin of parietal peritoneal pain, and the diffuse and obscure situation of visceral pain.

Physiology

Particles, solutes, and fluids are absorbed from the peritoneal cavity by two different routes. Particles smaller than 2 kd may be absorbed through peritoneal mesothelial venous pores and are directed to the portal circulation.[2] Particles larger than 3 kd are absorbed through peritoneal mesothelial lymphatic cells, entering the lymphatic thoracic duct and from there the systemic circulation.[2] This last route of absorption plays an important role in controlling abdominal infections, since it has a huge capacity of absorption. The anatomic structure of these large channels between the peritoneal cavity and the diaphragmatic vessels and the negative pressure of the thorax during inspiration make this mechanism extremely effective in the removal of bacteria and cells.

SURGICAL PERITONITIS

Surgical peritonitis is a severe clinical situation caused by the rupture of a viscus or abscess that allows free entry of bacteria into the peritoneal cavity. Leakage may be a massive or a slow process, depending on the underlying cause. Generalized and rapidly developing peritonitis is usually caused by a massive liberation of bacteria or their products into the peritoneal cavity; this is regularly followed by deterioration of hemodynamic parameters and shock.

Causes and Pathogenesis

Perforated peptic ulcer disease is the cause of about 40% of cases of generalized peritonitis requiring urgent surgery (ratio, about 3:1 duodenal-gastric).[3] These numbers are probably lower today, since eradication of *Helicobacter pylori* has reduced the number of patients with complicated peptic ulcer disease.[4] Other causes of overt peritonitis are appendicitis in about 20% of patients, gallbladder disease in about 15%, postoperative complications in about 10%, and others in 15%.[3]

A special form of peritonitis is Mediterranean fever, or familial paroxysmal polyserositis. This form of peritonitis will be discussed later, in "Peritonitis of Other Causes."

Other nonbacterial causes of peritonitis include leakage of blood into the peritoneal cavity due to rupture of a tubal pregnancy or ovarian cysts. Blood is highly irritating to the peritoneum and may cause abdominal pain similar to that found in septic peritonitis. Bile leakage into the peritoneal cavity can also cause signs and symptoms of peritonitis, although this can be rapidly followed by bacterial contamination and development of septic peritonitis.

Peritoneal Clearance of Bacteria

Once bacteria enter the peritoneal cavity, clearance of the offending microorganisms begins immediately. Within 6 minutes of intraperitoneal inoculation of bacteria in dogs, thoracic lymph becomes culture-positive. Twelve minutes later, bacteremia may be evident. This is probably important in patient survival, since blockade of the thoracic duct in an animal model of peritonitis decreases bacteremia episodes[5] but clearly increases mortality and induces liver necrosis. This appears to be directly related to the amount of endotoxin to which the liver is exposed.[6] Decades before it was known that the diaphragm was the predominant site of clearance of bacteria, Fowler, in 1900, proposed his head-up, pelvis-down position for prevention of absorption of toxins from infected peritoneal cavities. In the preantibiotic era, documentation of the delayed clearance of bacteria from experiments in infected dogs in the head-down position confirms the wisdom (in an attempt to prevent fatal bacteremia) of this positioning for patients with peritonitis.

Killing Mechanisms and Sequestration Mechanisms

In addition to mechanisms of bacterial clearance through the diaphragm, intraperitoneal defense mechanisms include cellular and humoral responses. Macrophages and neutrophils are attracted to the peritoneal cavity, and in this setting, microvilli of the mesothelial cell play a significant role in leukocyte migration into the peritoneal cavity, by providing the needed substrates for adhesion, intercellular adhesion molecule-1 (ICAM-1) and vascular cell adhesion molecule-1 (VCAM-1).[7]

The degree of cellular recruitment may be a key factor in a patient's survival, since a prolonged peritoneal inflammatory response has been observed to be adversely correlated with survival outcome in an animal model of peritonitis.[8] Humoral antibacterial agents are released into the peritoneal cavity, such as complement factors, fibronectin, and globulins. These opsonins coat bacteria and render them recognizable as foreign; then they are entrapped and killed by phagocytes.[9]

Sequestration mechanisms include fibrin trapping of bacteria, fibrinous adhesions, and omental loculation of foci of infection (Table 121–1).[10] It has been known since 1950 that bacteria are more readily destroyed on a surface than in a liquid medium. The microscopic and macroscopic networks of surfaces provided by fibrin and the omentum assist phagocytes in locating, trapping, ingesting, and killing bacteria. The volume of peritoneal fluid in which infection develops has a remarkable effect on mortality; 20% of rats inoculated with *Escherichia coli* diluted in 1 mL of saline die, whereas 75% of rats inoculated with the same number of viable bacteria diluted in 30 mL of saline die.[11] This phenomenon in part explains the risk of development of spontaneous bacterial peritonitis in relation to the ascitic fluid total protein concentration.[12] The more voluminous the ascitic fluid, the lower the concentration of proteins and opsonins, the less efficient the trapping of bacteria, and the higher the risk of an uncontrolled infection. Patients undergoing chronic ambulatory peritoneal dialysis frequently develop sclerosing encapsulating peritonitis, which may be a reaction to multiple episodes of bacterial infection, since the dilution of opsonins in these patients may contribute to the development of peritonitis.

Table 121–1 | **Peritoneal Defense Mechanisms**

REMOVAL MECHANISMS
Peritoneal clearance of bacteria through the diaphragm to the thoracic duct
LEUKOCYTE-ATTRACTING MECHANISMS
Microvilli of the mesothelial cell
ICAM-1 and VCAM-1
KILLING MECHANISMS
Macrophages
Neutrophils
Opsonins
Complement C3b
Immunoglobulin G (IgG)
Fibronectin
Mast cell–derived leukotrienes
SEQUESTRATION MECHANISMS
Fibrin trapping of bacteria
Formation of fibrinous adhesions
Omental loculation of foci of inflammation

ICAM, intercellular adhesion molecule; VCAM, vascular adhesion molecule.

Flora (See Chapter 78)

Although the flora of the gut, especially of the large bowel, is quite complicated, the numbers of types of organisms rapidly decrease after leakage of gut contents into the peritoneal cavity.[13] *E. coli*, enterococci, *Bacteroides fragilis*, and *Clostridia* organisms predominate. A recent study of infections associated with ruptured diverticulitis reported pure anaerobes in 15% of cases, aerobic bacteria only in 11%, and mixed aerobic and anaerobic flora in 74%; cultures from peritoneal abscesses detected anaerobic bacteria in 18%, aerobes alone in 5%, and mixed aerobic and anaerobic flora in 77%.[14]

Based on an animal model of monomicrobial and polymicrobial peritonitis with various combinations of bacteria, it is apparent that (1) *E. coli* is the organism most often responsible for death from this form of iatrogenic peritonitis, at least in part owing to its ability to cause bacteremia, and (2) combinations of anaerobes and facultative organisms lead to abscess formation.[15] As stated earlier, 77% of bacterial cultures from peritoneal abscesses are polymicrobial.[14] Other adjuvant substances, such as dead tissue, mucus, bile, hemoglobin, and barium, can act synergistically to increase mortality in surgical peritonitis through their ability to interfere with phagocytosis and killing of bacteria. These considerations form the basis for the treatment of surgical peritonitis, which is described later.

History

Clinical history and careful physical examination are the key factors in making a timely diagnosis of surgical peritonitis. In general, the sooner the diagnosis is made, the better the prognosis. Abdominal pain is the hallmark symptom of the problem. The exact details of the onset of pain can be helpful in drawing attention to the affected organ. The pain's character, location, area of radiation, change over time, and provocative and palliative factors are key pieces of information in assisting with the diagnosis. The pain of peritonitis can be reduced or even absent in elderly or very young patients, psychotic patients and patients receiving corticosteroids or analgesics, as well as in diabetics with advanced neuropathy and those under the influence of alcohol. Patients with cirrhosis and ascites may show no pain during episodes of spontaneous bacterial peritonitis, probably because the presence of ascites prevents the friction between visceral and parietal peritoneal surfaces. Peritoneal pain is usually associated with ileus, and therefore vomiting and a change in bowel habits are common symptoms about which to inquire.

Physical Examination

On examination, the patient with surgical peritonitis is usually immobile because any movement acutely worsens the pain. Fever of 100° to 101°F is expected, as is tachycardia and hypotension. Fever is a basic endogenous mechanism to help fight against infection. In fact, the increase in body temperature that is usually found during bacterial infections, including peritonitis, seems to be essential for optimal host defense against bacteria.[16] Gentle auscultation provides information about the degree of tenderness before palpation. The absence of bowel sounds in all four quadrants of the abdomen helps confirm suspected peritonitis. The absence of percussible hepatic dullness favors free air in the peritoneal cavity. Exquisite tenderness to percussion should lead to very gentle palpation. Overly vigorous palpation of a very tender abdomen may cause patients such pain that they are subsequently unable to cooperate for the remainder of the examination.

Palpation should begin farthest from the area that the patient identifies as the source of the most pain. Palpation of a truly boardlike abdomen is so impressive to the examiner that it cannot be forgotten. Lesser degrees of rigidity must be compared with this extreme end of the spectrum. Voluntary guarding in the presence of mild tenderness may be misinterpreted as rigidity by the inexperienced examiner if the patient is anxious and palpation too vigorous. It is usually not necessary to check for rebound tenderness to palpation if rebound tenderness is noted during auscultation or percussion. Often, rebound tenderness is evident when the examining bed is jarred. Analgesic administration should be avoided until physical exploration has been completed and a decision has been made. After this, it seems unethical not to alleviate pain in these patients (see Chapter 4, Acute Abdominal Pain).

Examining the rectum and pelvis can provide information about the possibility of abscesses in or near these areas. Checking for iliopsoas and obturator signs can be helpful in detecting retroperitoneal or pelvic collections.

Repeated physical examinations by the same examiner will provide evidence of progressive peritoneal irritation. This, together with imaging procedures and laboratory tests, will indicate the need for surgical intervention.

Laboratory Tests and Radiologic Assessment

The most common laboratory sign of peritonitis in an immunocompetent patient is an increased white blood cell count with left shift. The presence of circulating juvenile forms is a reflection of an increasing demand of white cells from the bone marrow. A low white blood cell count in the course of a bacterial infection associated at times with gram-negative septicemia may indicate the presence of an exhausted bone marrow, with a poorer prognosis. In addition, metabolic acidosis, hemoconcentration, and subsequent prerenal azotemia may be present. Free air may be detected on upright or decubitus abdominal films, but this finding may be only 60% sensitive in detecting gut perforation.[17] The absence of free air should not delay surgical intervention in an otherwise appropriate clinical setting. Ultrasound can be very helpful in demonstrating abscesses, bile duct dilatation, pancreatitis, and large fluid collections. CT scan may supplement the results of ultrasonography and can also identify periappendiceal processes, gut tumors, and lymph nodes that may not be detected with ultrasound.

Diagnosis

The diagnosis of surgical peritonitis is suspected based on the history, physical examination, and laboratory and radiologic tests and is confirmed at laparotomy when purulent fibrinous peritonitis is found. In patients who may not be able to provide a history, such as a confused elderly, inebreated, or psychotic patient, and in patients with an unreliable physical examination because of coma or some other problem, peritoneal lavage with 1 L of saline can be helpful in detecting peritonitis. If the effluent contains more than 500 WBC per cubic millimeter, an amylase or bilirubin level greater than the corresponding serum value, or bacteria on Gram's stain, there is approximately a 90% likelihood of surgical peritonitis.[18] Laparotomy is usually indicated in this setting.

Treatment

General

Fluid resuscitation and antibiotic therapy followed by urgent laparotomy are the mainstays of treatment of surgical peritonitis (Table 121–2). Rational administration of fluid requires frequent monitoring of physiologic parameters, including blood pressure (by arterial line if shock is present), pulse, central venous pressure or pulmonary capillary wedge pressure, and urine output, as well as hematocrit, WBC count, electrolytes, glucose, creatinine, and blood gases. Hypovole-

Table 121–2 | **Treatment of Surgical Peritonitis**

Resuscitation and maintenance of air flow
Intravenous fluids
Intravenous colloid
Hemodynamic monitoring
Central or pulmonary capillary wedge pressure
Urine output
Hematocrit, glucose, creatinine, electrolytes, blood gases
Gut decompression through nasogastric tube
Pressors as needed
No glucocorticoids
Broad-spectrum non-nephrotoxic antibiotics
Consideration of heparin, liposomal antibiotics, and neutralizing antibodies to proinflammatory cytokines in randomized clinical trials
Total parenteral nutrition
Surgical intervention

mia, hypotension, metabolic acidosis, hypoxia, and hemoconcentration from loss of plasma into the peritoneal cavity are expected. Transfer to an intensive care unit is usually required. Glucocorticoids have been shown not to provide benefit in the setting of septic shock.[19] Pressors (e.g., dopamine less than 5 μg/kg/min) may be needed, but the dose should be kept as low as possible, to prevent visceral vasoconstriction; renal perfusion is also compromised at higher rates of infusion. The gut is routinely decompressed by means of a nasogastric tube or a longer tube with low, intermittent suction.

Antibiotics and Other Therapeutic Approaches

In addition to these therapeutic measures, antibiotic therapy is required before, during, and after surgical intervention. The type of bacteria causing peritonitis depends in part on the clinical setting, i.e., community-acquired or nosocomial. Infections occurring in patients after long periods of hospitalization may include multiresistant pathogens and enterococci, whereas in community-acquired peritonitis, susceptible gram-negative bacilli, strict anaerobic bacteria, and enterococci are found. It has been shown in experimental models of peritonitis that there is bacterial synergism between aerobic and anaerobic pathogens.[20] Despite a large number of bacteria with different susceptibilities, it recently has been shown that monotherapy with a broad-spectrum beta-lactam is as effective as combination therapy with a beta-lactam and an aminoglycoside.[21]

New therapeutic strategies are emerging, including agents that modify bacterial adhesion characteristics and agents that affect the host's cytokines. Other experimental approaches to the treatment of peritonitis include the use of liposomal antibiotics[22] and the administration of low-dose heparin to reduce bacterial adherence and the risk of development of abscesses.[23] The existence of bacteria resistant to antibiotics is a common concern; the administration of low-solubility antibiotics delivered in fibrin may be efficacious against resistant bacteria.[24]

An explosive host inflammatory response against peritonitis may be harmful for the patient. The administration of neutralizing antibodies to TNF-alpha and IL-1-beta in microspheres may be effective in reducing this response.[25]

In animal models, antibiotics directed against gram-negative enteric organisms minimize mortality, and drugs effective against anaerobes prevent abscess formation.[26] The availability of broad-spectrum antibiotics, including beta-lactams and third- and fourth-generation cephalosporins, make it unnecessary to use aminoglycosides, thus avoiding the use of nephrotoxic drugs in patients who may have compromised renal function.[27] The coverage of all potential organisms is not necessary.[28] The flora of surgical peritonitis simplifies with time, even before initiation of antibiotics. Killing certain key species may change the microenvironment sufficiently to prevent growth and allow killing of other flora. Data-supported guidelines regarding optimal treatment have been hampered by suboptimal study design and nonuniform efficacy criteria in the controlled trials that have been performed.[28]

Surgical Intervention

Antibiotics help treat or prevent fatal bacteremia but do not cure most patients with surgical peritonitis unless laparotomy is performed. Neither free leakage of gut contents nor abscesses can be sterilized by antibiotics in the absence of drainage. Surgical intervention should take place as soon as possible after the patient is stabilized and resuscitated and antibiotics have been given. The aims of surgical treatment include source control, peritoneal toilet, and prevention of recurrent infection. Recent reports confirm the possibility of successful laparoscopic treatment of some forms of peritonitis.[29] Also, temporary therapeutic approaches, such as laparostomy, may become useful tools when control of the source of infection is not possible at the initial operation.[30] It has been suggested that a conservative surgical treatment supplemented with intraoperative lavage reduces the reoperation rate compared with standard treatment options and achieves a low mortality rate in patients with diffuse peritonitis.[30]

Preoperative and postoperative fluid and nutritional support are crucial to prompt wound healing and survival. Peritonitis has been compared with a 50% total body surface area burn, and calorie intake of 3000 to 4000 kcal per day may not even achieve a positive nitrogen balance.

Prognosis

Despite the modern approach to the diagnosis and treatment of surgical peritonitis, mortality remains high in certain subgroups of patients, especially elderly patients and patients who suffer organ failure before the development of peritonitis.[31] In general, peritonitis-related mortality may be as low as 14%,[30] with appendicitis and perforated duodenal ulcer at the low end of the spectrum (10%) and postoperative peritonitis mortality as high as 50%.[31]

PERITONITIS OF OTHER CAUSES

(Table 121–3)

Primary Peritonitis

Spontaneous bacterial peritonitis (SBP) or peritonitis without a known surgical source, is the most common cause of primary peritonitis. This occurs predominantly in patients with cirrhosis and ascites and is discussed in Chapter 78.

Table 121–3 | **Classification of Nonsurgical Peritonitis**

Spontaneous bacterial peritonitis
Secondary to chronic ambulatory peritoneal dialysis (CAPD)
Tuberculosis
Secondary to AIDS
Chlamydia
Gonococcal (Fitz-Hugh–Curtis)
Rare causes
Polyarteritis nodosa
Systemic lupus erythematosus
Scleroderma
Familial Mediterranean fever

AIDS, acquired immunodeficiency syndrome.

Primary peritonitis may also occur in patients with ascites due to nephrotic syndrome.[32] Primary peritonitis in the absence of cirrhosis or nephrosis is much less common and usually occurs in children.

Peritonitis in Ambulatory Peritoneal Dialysis

Continuous ambulatory peritoneal dialysis (CAPD) is a common treatment of renal failure.[33] Bacterial peritonitis occurs 1.4 times per patient-year of treatment.[34] The most common isolate in patients treated with CAPD is *Staphylococcus epidermidis* and other skin flora.[35] Other pathogens, such as fungi or *Mycobacterium tuberculosis*, are less frequently described in these patients. The most probable explanation for this high incidence of infection is inadvertent contamination of the indwelling catheter. Even with better patient education regarding sterile technique, peritonitis in this group of patients is a major source of morbidity and the largest single cause of patient failure on CAPD.[36] New technical maneuvers[37] or special management of insertion site[38] may decrease the incidence of infections in these patients.

Abdominal pain and tenderness are found in about 75% of patients, but fever is found in only about one third.[39] A consistent feature is cloudy effluent, noted in 98%.[39] The diagnosis is suspected on the basis of signs and symptoms and is confirmed by a total fluid WBC count greater than 100 neutrophils/mm^3, or the presence of organisms on Gram's stain. Treatment should be started immediately without waiting for the results of culture, similar to the empiric treatment of patients with cirrhosis and neutrocytic ascites.[40] Initial treatment of suspected CAPD peritonitis should cover the most frequently isolated bacteria. Vancomycin and second- or third-generation cephalosporins are good options. The intraperitoneal route of administration is probably the most effective.[39] The sensitivity of the organism isolated determines the subsequent antibiotic choice. Most of these patients are successfully treated on an outpatient basis without stopping dialysis. Prompt treatment ensures survival; however, recurrent infection is common and may lead to catheter removal or scarring of the peritoneum and poor dialysis exchange. Addition of heparin to the dialysis bag in cases of peritonitis may decrease the formation of fibrin and, thereby, the incidence of postinfection adhesions. However, these infections often require removal of the catheter.

Tuberculous Peritonitis

The number of patients with tuberculous peritonitis has increased in recent years, due in part to the development of this disease in patients with acquired immunodeficiency syndrome (AIDS) with a high rate of multiresistant strains of *M. tuberculosis* (Fig. 121–2*A*).[41]

Patients with this form of peritonitis, in the absence of cirrhosis, usually have ascites with high protein content, low glucose, and low serum-to-ascites albumin gradient.[42] Patients almost always have an elevated ascitic fluid WBC count and a lymphocyte predominance. The algorithm in evaluation of patients with high-lymphocyte count ascites includes cytologic evaluation of the fluid and consideration of laparoscopy.[42] Patients with lymphatic ascites and fever usually have tuberculosis, whereas afebrile patients usually have malignancy-related ascites. Cancer is the cause of ascites about ten times more frequently than is tuberculosis (see Chapter 78). If peritoneal carcinomatosis is present, the cytologic findings are positive more than 90% of the time, and the laparoscopy can be avoided.[43] If the cytology is

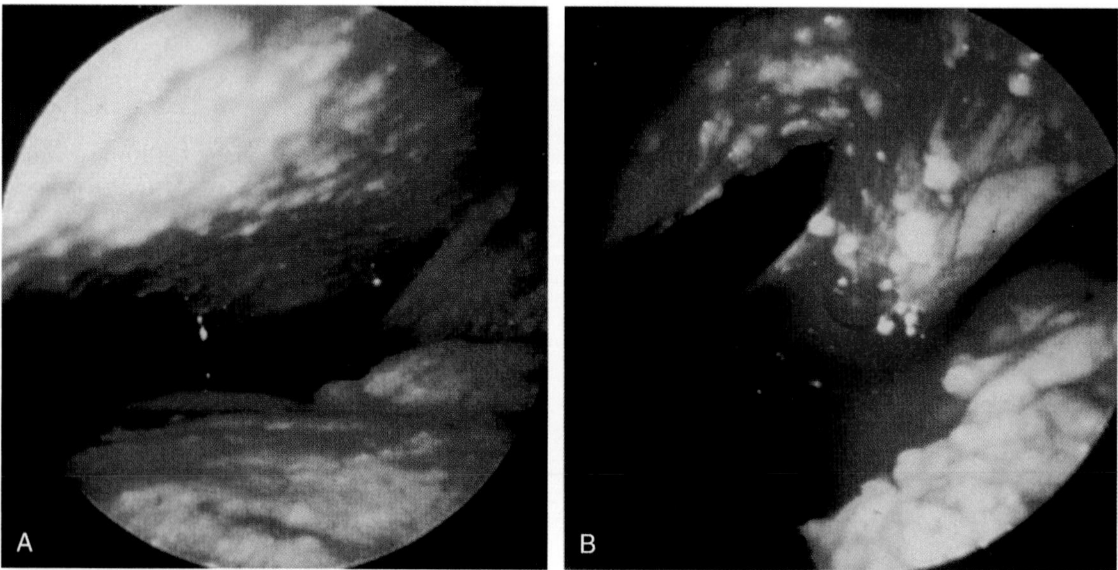

Figure 121–2. *A*, Laparoscopic appearance of tuberculous peritonitis with numerous small yellowish-white nodules present on the peritoneal surfaces. *B*, Peritoneal carcinomatosis as seen laparoscopically appears as larger white nodules of various sizes. (From Chu, CM, Lin, SM, Peng, SM, et al: The role of laparoscopy in the evaluation of ascites of unknown origin. Gastrointest Endosc 40:285, 1994.)

negative, laparoscopy is performed and is nearly 100% sensitive in detecting tuberculous peritonitis. Tuberculous peritonitis may also appear in a miliary form or as a pelvic mass with high levels of CA125, making the diagnosis difficult to distinguish from metastatic ovarian tumor in women.[44]

Treatment with isoniazid, rifampin, and pyrazinamide for 8 weeks, followed by isoniazid and rifampin for 4 months more, is considered adequate.[45] More drugs may be needed, depending on local susceptibility testing. More than half of patients with tuberculous peritonitis in the United States have underlying cirrhosis, usually alcohol-related,[46] whereas in Third World countries, peritoneal tuberculosis usually occurs in the absence of cirrhosis. The presence of cirrhosis affects the results of ascitic fluid tests, including reducing the sensitivity of adenosine deaminase to 30% (see Chapter 78).[46] Further, ascites may diminish or disappear with diuretics but fever usually persists, as does a high lymphocyte count. Since alcoholics are notoriously noncompliant, their antituberculous therapy must be supervised carefully by public health nurses as well as physicians. Erratic treatment leads to emergence of resistant strains.

Peritonitis Associated with Acquired Immunodeficiency Syndrome (AIDS)

(See Chapter 28)

Patients with acquired immunodeficiency syndrome may develop peritonitis through many different types of pathogens: bacteria (mono- or polymicrobial), viruses (cytomegalovirus, herpes, and others) and fungal organisms (*Histoplasma, Cryptococcus,* and *Coccidioides* organisms), parasites (*Pneumocystis carinii, Trypanosoma cruzi*), and mycobacteria (*M. tuberculosis* and *M. avium-intracellulare*). Also, neoplastic lesions, such as Kaposi's sarcoma and non-Hodgkin's lymphoma, may metastasize to the peritoneum. Like other forms of peritonitis, the common features of presentation are abdominal pain, anorexia, fever, and ascites, which typically has a high protein content. The diagnosis of a rare form of peritonitis sometimes leads to a diagnosis of AIDS[47] in a human immunodeficiency virus (HIV)-positive patient. The treatment of these opportunistic infections involving the peritoneum is generally medical (antibiotics, amphotericin B, ganciclovir, and so on), unless bowel involvement has led to gut perforation.

Chlamydia Peritonitis

Fitz-Hugh–Curtis syndrome, or perihepatitis, was originally thought to be due to the gonococcus. However, in recent years *Chlamydia* is increasingly implicated in perihepatitis.[48] *Chlamydia* perihepatitis occurs only in women, owing to seeding of bacteria from the fallopian tubes. Symptoms presenting in these patients include inflammatory ascites, pain in the right upper abdominal quadrant, fever, and a hepatic friction rub. If there is enough ascitic fluid to be clinically detectable, it has an elevated white cell count with a predominance of neutrophils and a high protein content, even in excess of 9.0 g/dL.[48] Laparoscopy is very helpful in confirming the diagnosis, revealing "violin strings" and "bridal veil" adhesions from the abdominal wall to the liver. Doxycycline is usually curative.

Fungal and Parasitic Peritonitis

Fungal peritonitis can be due to gut perforation into the peritoneal cavity, or it can be a complication of acquired immunodeficiency. Fungal peritonitis may be limited to the pelvis in cases of gynecologic dissemination; this may be treated with fluconazole.[49] The most common isolate is *Candida* spp., probably because routine blood culture media can detect *Candida.* Although infrequent, fungal peritonitis has been described in patients undergoing chronic ambulatory peritoneal dialysis.[50]

Although currently rare in the United States, peritoneal histoplasmosis, coccidioidomycosis, and cryptococcal infection are increasing in frequency in the setting of acquired immunodeficiency. Schistosomiasis, pinworms, ascariasis, strongyloidiasis, and amebiasis may also involve the peritoneal cavity (see Chapter 98).

Rare Causes of Peritonitis

Years ago, approximately 1 of every 1000 patients who underwent laparotomy developed fever and migratory abdominal pain 2 to 3 weeks postoperatively secondary to contamination of the peritoneum by glove powder starch. This is much less frequent today,[51] probably because starch has been replaced by other more inert lubricants. Connective tissue diseases lead to peritonitis as a manifestation of serositis in approximately 5% of patients with lupus and approximately 10% of patients with polyarteritis and scleroderma.[52] Treatment of the underlying disease usually controls the serositis (see Chapters 29 and 78).

Familial Mediterranean fever is an autosomal recessive hereditary disease that affects the peritoneum as well as other serous membranes. It is more frequently found in patients of Ashkenazi Jewish, Armenian, and Arabic ancestry. It is an aseptic form of recurrent peritonitis; no infectious agent has been observed to be related to this disease. Patients usually present with sporadic episodes of abdominal pain and fever, although other forms of serositis may be present, including synovitis and pleuritis. Treatment with colchicine appears to prevent attacks and can prevent fatal renal amyloidosis[53] (see Chapter 29).

PERITONEAL TUMORS

(Table 121–4)

Tumors Metastatic to the Peritoneum

Metastatic cancer is by far the most common peritoneal tumor (Fig. 121–2*B*). Although it is frequently assumed that tumors cause ascites only when malignant cells line the peritoneal cavity (i.e., peritoneal carcinomatosis), extraperitoneal tumors, including massive liver metastases, hepatocellular carcinoma with or without cirrhosis, malignant lymph node obstruction as in lymphoma, and Budd-Chiari syndrome with or without inferior vena cava obstruction, are

Table 121–4 | **Peritoneal Tumors**

Metastatic
Breast, lung, stomach
Pancreas, ovary
Sarcomas
Lymphomas
Pseudomyxoma peritonei
Mesothelioma
Pelvic lipomatosis
Benign peritoneal cysts

associated with ascites.[43] Ascitic fluid characteristics often allow their distinction,[43] which is important since each may require different treatment (see Chapter 78 for details of pathogenesis and ascitic fluid analysis).

Tissue of Origin

Tumors that preferentially metastasize to the peritoneum include the following adenocarcinomas: ovarian, stomach, colon, breast, pancreas, and lung, as well as lymphoma and other sarcomas (Fig. 121–3).

Clinical Presentation

Ascites usually appears in patients as evidence of advanced disease of a known tumor with a large burden, rather than as a primary manifestation of cancer. Weight loss, abdominal pain, and early satiety are common. The patients in general have a poor prognosis (see Prognosis later). Alternatively, ascites in a middle-aged woman without risk factors for liver disease may be the first manifestation of peritoneal spread of an ovarian cancer; the prognosis in this situation is better than that of nonovarian cancer (see Prognosis later).

Patients with malignancy-related ascites of recent onset usually tolerate its presence poorly, probably because of less compliance of the abdominal wall compared with patients with cirrhosis who have repeated episodes of ascites. As the malignancy progresses, the fluid component tends to be replaced by solid tumor, leading to bowel obstruction. Some common myths about peritoneal carcinomatosis are that the cytology is insensitive and that the fluid is frequently bloody (see Chapter 78).

Treatment

DIURETICS DO NOT WORK. Therapeutic paracentesis for symptomatic palliation is the mainstay of treatment for the majority of patients with peritoneal carcinomatosis. Although diuretics have been recommended for their treatment, this was based largely on supposition rather than hard data. A study of ascitic fluid volume and intravascular volume in patients with peritoneal carcinomatosis who lost weight taking large doses of diuretics demonstrated that the weight was lost at the expense of blood volume, not ascitic fluid volume.[54] The characteristics of the ascitic fluid may help direct diuretic use. In general, ascites with a high serum-ascites albumin gradient (≥1.1 g/dL) responds to diuretics.[54] Therefore, in cancer patients, diuretics should be reserved for those with edema or some specific indication other than peritoneal carcinomatosis.

SURGERY AND INTRAPERITONEAL CHEMOTHERAPY. Since the usual response to routine therapy is poor, new treatments have been suggested, such as peritonectomy combined with hyperthermic antiblastic perfusion.[55] In some instances this allows better survival for patients with extensive carcinomatosis who were no longer responsive to traditional therapies. The rationale for application of intraperitoneal chemotherapy is that its use would allow larger concentrations of drugs delivered to tumor cells. Other treatment options that are under investigation include gene therapy[56] and the use of angiogenesis inhibitors to reduce the ability of the peritoneal tumor to spread.[57] Also, systemic "antidotes" to certain drugs (e.g., leucovorin or methotrexate) could be administered to reduce toxicity further.

OVARIAN VERSUS NONOVARIAN CANCER. The results of treatment for ovarian cancer are the most encouraging. Surgical debulking and chemotherapy have led to long-term survival. Although most patients with ovarian cancer still require therapeutic paracentesis for relief of symptoms related to distention, new experimental approaches are emerging, including administration of inhibitors of vascular endothelial growth factor receptors, to control ascites formation and tumor growth.[58] However, no hard data regarding the usefulness of this approach in patients are available so far.

Prognosis

Prognosis is very poor in general for patients with peritoneal cancer.[59] In one large study, only 70% of patients survived 1 month, 25% survived 3 months, 12% survived 6 months,

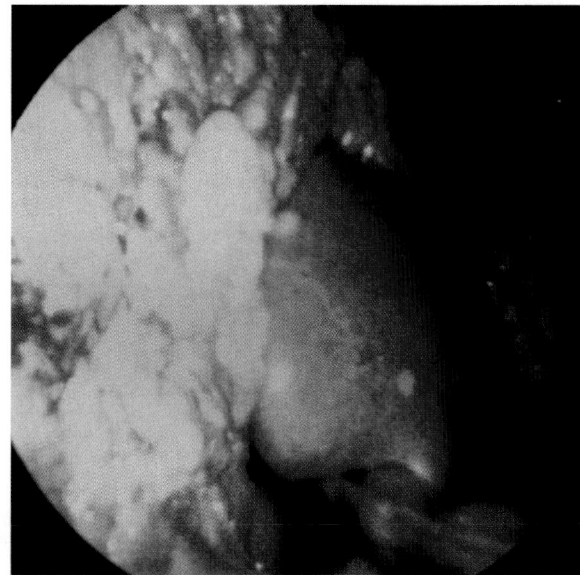

Figure 121–3. Laparoscopic appearance of non-Hodgkin's lymphoma in a patient infected with human immunodeficiency virus. The raised white irregular plaques are present over the visceral and parietal peritoneal surfaces. (From Jeffers LJ, Alzate I, Aguilar H, et al: Laparoscopic and histologic findings in patients with the human immunodeficiency virus. Gastrointest Endosc 40:160, 1994.)

and 4% survived longer than 1 year after diagnosis.[59] Their course involves recurrent and progressive bowel obstruction, malnutrition, and wasting prior to death. Hopefully some of the new therapeutic approaches—inhibitors of vascular endothelial growth factor receptors, gene therapy, intraperitoneal hyperthermic antiblastic perfusion—may increase life expectancy in these patients.

Pseudomyxoma Peritonei

Pseudomyxoma peritonei represents a rare (approximately 2 in 10,000 laparotomies) and special case in metastatic peritoneal tumors.[60] Seventy-five percent of these patients are women between 45 and 75 years of age. This tumor causes gelatinous implants on the peritoneum. The sites of origin of the tumor are ovary and appendix. Its degree of malignant potential is variable; about 50% of patients live 5 years.[60] Lymphatic or extraperitoneal spread of the tumor is rare. Presenting symptoms include painless abdominal distention and ovarian mass; mucin may accumulate intraperitoneally many years after resection of an ovarian mass.[60] Diagnosis is made when the jelly-like material is encountered at laparotomy or laparoscopy. Aggressive surgical debulking, with copious irrigation of the peritoneal cavity with warm dextrose solution, appears to be the treatment of choice.[60] Unfortunately, chemotherapy appears to be ineffective, and recurrence usually causes bowel obstruction, malnutrition, and death.

Mesothelioma

Sixty-five to seventy percent of these tumors arise in the pleura, and 25% in the peritoneum.[61] Most peritoneal mesotheliomas are malignant, are associated with asbestos exposure, and are usually detected 35 to 40 years after initial exposure. The families of asbestos workers are also at risk. Diagnosis is usually made at laparotomy or laparoscopy, but occasionally diagnostic malignant mesothelial cells are found on ascitic fluid analysis. Classic treatment options include surgical resection, radiation, and chemotherapy, or a combination. However, new therapeutic strategies are emerging based on gene therapy. The adenovirus-based transfer of the herpes simplex–thymidine kinase gene may cause the tumor to become sensitive to ganciclovir.[62]

Pelvic Lipomatosis

Normal fat deposits found in the perirectal and perivesical spaces may develop nonmalignant overgrowth and are recognized as a distinct clinicopathologic entity, pelvic lipomatosis. It occurs predominantly in black men (male-female ratio 18:1) between 20 and 60 years of age[63] and may cause hypertension, proliferative cystitis, urinary tract obstruction, and, occasionally, gastrointestinal symptoms. The abnormal proliferation of fat is accompanied by varying degrees of fibrous reaction. Transrectal ultrasound and CT are important in diagnosis, particularly in differentiating it from liposarcoma. The disease does not progress in most patients; however, in some, urinary obstruction will require diversion.

Benign Peritoneal Cysts

Benign peritoneal cysts are rare. Benign cystic mesotheliomas occur in adult women, are manifested by pain, and recur after resection. Benign cystic lymphangiomas affect young men, present as mass lesions, and seldom recur after resection.

DISEASES OF THE MESENTERY AND OMENTUM

(Table 121–5)

Diseases of the mesentery and omentum (in decreasing order of frequency) include hemorrhage, tumors, inflammatory and fibrotic conditions, and infarction. Abscesses are covered in Chapter 24.

Hemorrhage

Mesenteric and retroperitoneal bleeding and their complications are usually due to trauma or anticoagulants. In rare cases, aneurysms of the splanchnic arteries may rupture, leading to intraperitoneal hemorrhage. Traumatic hematomas may or may not require surgical intervention, depending on the site of the lesion and whether the trauma was blunt or penetrating.[64] Intraperitoneal bleeding may be a consequence of a previous surgical procedure, such as cytoreductive surgery for gynecologic cancer.[65] A special case of spontaneous hemoperitoneum is that found in patients with cirrhosis and hepatocellular carcinoma.

Symptoms usually are pain and obstructive effects of the hematoma mass. Diagnosis depends on a high index of suspicion and ultrasonography or CT, which demonstrates the collection of blood. An ultrasound-guided fine-needle aspiration may help in confirming the diagnosis. Treatment consists of discontinuation of anticoagulants in those being treated; in others it is dictated by the local or systemic symptoms of hemorrhage. In certain cases angiographic embolization may help treat intraperitoneal hemorrhage.[66]

Tumors

Tumors originating in the mesentery and omentum are rare and include soft tissue tumors (e.g., cysts, fibromas, sarcomas, desmoids) and tumors specific to this site, such as Castleman's disease and leiomyomatosis peritonealis dissem-

Table 121–5 | **Diseases of the Mesentery and Omentum**

Hemorrhage (from trauma, vascular ruptures, anticoagulants)
Intraperitoneal
Retroperitoneal
Mesenteric
Tumors
Mesenteric cysts
Solid tumors
Multifocal leiomyomas
Castleman's disease
Inflammatory and fibrotic conditions
Infarction of the omentum

inata. Most tumors are large when detected in this site because of the large potential space in which they can grow. They may also be detected incidentally when an imaging study is performed for an unrelated reason.

Mesenteric Cysts

Mesentric cysts are probably the most uncommon among these rare tumors (prevalence: 1 per 100,000 admissions).[67] A review of the English-language literature revealed only 139 such lesions as of 1986.[67] They occur in both children and adults. Symptoms include pain in 58% and distention in 50%. Some cases may present with fever and chills, and other are asymptomatic, being discovered incidentally and misdiagnosed before laparotomy.[68] These are typically large (13 cm), fluid-filled (2000 mL) lesions and, despite their size, are malignant in only 3% of cases and cause death in only 2%.[67] They are usually cured by complete excision.

Solid Tumors

Solid tumors appear to be next in decreasing order of frequency. Among mesenteric tumors, two thirds are benign, including fibromas, xanthogranulomas, lipomas, leiomyomas, capillary and cavernous hemangiomas, neurofibromas, and mesenchymomas. The malignant tumors include hemangiopericytomas, fibrosarcomas, liposarcomas, leiomyosarcomas, and malignant mesenchymomas. Solid tumors of the omentum are remarkably similar in histologic type and prevalence of malignancy.[69] Typical of mesenteric and omental tumors, symptoms include pain and distention from large lesions. Treatment is surgical resection. Prognosis is generally fair: About 18% of patients die of the tumor, overall, and the rate of 5-year survival for patients with malignant tumors is only 21%.[70]

Multifocal Leiomyomas

Multifocal leiomyomatous tumors are even less common, can be malignant, and can mimic peritoneal carcinomatosis. They may appear together with other leiomyomatous lesions[71] or endometriosis.[72] These lesions consist of small, rubbery nodules, appear to be hormone sensitive, develop during pregnancy or estrogen therapy, can cause pain or gut bleeding, and may regress with hormone withdrawal.

Castleman's Disease

Castleman's disease (giant lymph node hyperplasia) of the mesentery is an extraordinarily infrequent finding. Lesions in the abdomen usually occur in young women and frequently are associated with malabsorption of iron and iron deficiency. However, a variety of other diseases have been related to Castleman's disease, such as nephrotic syndrome,[73] pemphigus,[74] renal amyloidosis,[75] neuropathy,[76] and others. Surgical removal of the mass is usually successful, and prognosis is good.

Inflammatory and Fibrotic Conditions

Background

This subset of diseases of the mesentery and retroperitoneum is the most confusing, in part because of their rarity and because of overlapping clinical and histologic features. Most clinicians and pathologists never encounter an example. At least a dozen terms are used to describe the three basic diseases: *retractile mesenteritis, mesenteric panniculitis*, and *retroperitoneal fibrosis*. To add to the confusion, some cases have been reported with different names. These diseases could easily represent different aspects of the same spectrum of inflammation and scarring of these structures. Retractile mesenteritis was the name used in the first description of these diseases. This entity represents the fibrotic end of the spectrum and has also been known as sclerosing mesenteritis, multifocal subperitoneal sclerosis, fibromatosis, and desmoid tumor.[77] The inflammatory end of the spectrum has been called mesenteric panniculitis, mesenteric lipodystrophy, lipogranuloma of the mesentery, liposclerotic mesenteritis, mesenteric Weber-Christian disease, and systemic nodular panniculitis.[78] There have been attempts to subclassify this disease into diffuse, single, and multiple forms and to suggest an association with lymphoma.[78] Overlapping names such as sclerosing lipogranuloma, the well-documented progression and conversion of mesenteric panniculitis to retractile mesenteritis over a 12-year period, and the concurrence of sclerosing mesenteritis and retroperitoneal fibrosis all indicate that these are simply stages of one basic underlying process.

Although mesenteric panniculitis and retractile mesenteritis are usually manifested by abdominal pain, symptoms of gut obstruction, and a mass lesion,[79] cases associated with prolonged high-grade fever and autoimmune hemolytic anemia without abdominal symptoms have been described.[80] Retractile mesenteritis and mesenteric panniculitis are always idiopathic, but retroperitoneal fibrosis has a cause approximately 30% of the time, including drugs, malignancy, trauma, or inflammation.[81] Most of reported cases are drug induced (methysergide, ergotamine). The process of fibrosis may lead to ureteral or vascular obstruction.

Histologically, retractile mesenteritis and mesenteric panniculitis can both have inflammation with lymphocytes and neutrophils, fat necrosis, fibrosis, and calcification.[77] In contrast, only mesenteric panniculitis has multinucleate giant cells, cholesterol clefts, lipid-laden macrophages, and lymphangiectasia.[77] Retroperitoneal fibrosis consists of dense connective tissue, with or without inflammation.

Diagnosis and Treatment

These diseases have usually been diagnosed at laparotomy or autopsy in the past; however, noninvasive techniques such as CT scan or MRI may assist in preoperative diagnosis.[82, 83] Radiologic findings suggestive of mesenteric panniculitis have been found in 0.6% of patients in a large series of abdominal CT scans. There was a female predominance and an association with malignancy in 34 of 49 patients with radiologic features of mesenteric pannicultis.[83]

Treatment may be needed in patients with retractile mesenteritis if it obstructs the intestine. Treatment is usually surgical, but administration of progesterone has been reported to down-regulate fibrogenesis.[84]

The prognosis of patients with retroperitoneal fibrosis seems to be better than in the past. Successful treatment of this entity with immunosuppressives, such as azathioprine with steroids, has been reported.[85] In other cases, ureterolysis may be required.

Infarction of the Omentum

This omental disease has been reported predominantly in children and young adults, and it is usually diagnosed at laparotomy performed for suspected appendicitis.[86] If a diagnosis by imaging techniques (such as CT scan or MRI) is achieved preoperatively,[87] laparoscopic resection of the necrotic mass is curative.[88] However, the diagnosis is difficult and often delayed. We have seen a patient who was diagnosed at laparotomy with omental torsion several months after the onset of symptoms.

DISEASES OF THE DIAPHRAGM

(Table 121–6)

Hernias and Eventration

Diaphragmatic hernias consist of herniation of an abdominal organ through the diaphragm into the thorax. Theoretically, all intraperitoneal structures can undergo herniation, but intestinal hernias are the most common. Hernias of the diaphragm are congenital or acquired. Congenital defects in the sternocostal foramen of Morgagni or vertebrolumbar foramen of Bochdalek lead to hernias with these eponyms. These hernias have a prevalence of 1 per 2200 births. Morgagni hernias are small, rarely symptomatic, and usually diagnosed by lateral chest film followed by CT or barium swallow imaging. Although they may affect stomach, colon, or omentum, the rare bowel obstruction usually involves the colon. Bochdalek hernias are larger and more symptomatic and can cause lung hypoplasia, respiratory failure, and death in infants. These hernias are detected on chest film and confirmed on CT or barium swallow, and they frequently require surgical intervention, especially in young persons.

Traumatic hernias of the diaphragm may follow blunt or penetrating trauma. The most common injury is a large tear of the diaphragm from the esophageal hiatus to the costal attachments. This usually takes place on the left side. Although the defect occurs early, years may pass before a herniated viscus is detected. Usually it is the stomach, spleen, colon, or left lobe of liver. These hernias are manifested by vomiting, pain, and respiratory distress. Chest film, contrast studies, or CT is usually diagnostic in the appropriate historical setting.

Eventration is not a true hernia but consists of a localized weakness in the dome of the diaphragm that can lead to bulging of abdominal viscera into the thorax. This is usually an incidental finding on chest films, but symptomatic patients require surgical correction. These symptoms, including intermittent, severe chest pain or upper abdominal pain (particularly after meals or with physical exertion), are due to either paraesophageal hernia or gastric volvulus. Awareness of these associations is important to avoid mistaking the symptoms for angina pectoris or even myocardial infarction.

These conditions and hiatal and paraesophageal hernias are covered in Chapter 20.

Table 121–6 | **Diseases of the Diaphragm**

Hernias
Foramen of Morgagni
Foramen of Bochdalek
Traumatic
Eventration
Tumors

Tumors

Diaphragmatic tumors are usually of connective tissue origin and may be benign or malignant or may consist of simple cysts.[89, 90] They are detected by screening chest films or in evaluation of pleuritic chest pain.

Hiccups

Hiccups are quick inhalations that follow abrupt rhythmic involuntary contractions of the diaphragm and closure of the glottis. When they last only a few minutes, they are considered a form of physiologic myoclonus.[91] For hiccups of longer duration, home remedies include breath holding, sudden fright, rebreathing from a paper bag, eating dry granulated sugar, drinking cold liquids, and so on. Intractable hiccups last weeks or even longer, can be familial, and are usually due to diaphragmatic irritation, gastric distention, thoracic or central nervous system irritation or tumors, hyponatremia, or other metabolic derangements. Treatment includes pharmacologic agents, noninvasive phrenic nerve stimulation, or, rarely, phrenic nerve crushing. Drugs that have been reported to be successful include chlorpromazine, metoclopramide, quinidine, phenytoin, valproic acid, baclofen, sertraline, gabapentin, and nifedipine. The implantation of breathing pacemakers that control the diaphragmatic excursions may be an interesting approach for treatment of chronic hiccups.[92]

LAPAROSCOPY IN THE EVALUATION OF PERITONEAL DISEASES

General Considerations

Diagnostic laparoscopy, as first described by Kelling in 1901, is a safe and effective means of evaluating the abdominal cavity. Less invasive imaging techniques have reduced its necessity; however, it continues to have a role in the evaluation of liver and peritoneal diseases. While considered less invasive and generally well tolerated, possible complications include prolonged abdominal pain, vasovagal reaction, viscus perforation, bleeding (either from biopsy sites or within abdominal wall), splenic laceration, ascites fluid leakage, and postlaparoscopy fever.[91] It has been suggested recently that abdominal insufflation during laparoscopy could increase bacterial translocation, making the practice of laparoscopy dangerous in certain clinical settings, such as septic peritonitis.[93] These observations, however, are not uniformly accepted.[94]

Laparoscopy allows direct visualization of the liver surface, peritoneal lining, and mesentery for directed biopsies. The role of laparoscopy in the diagnosis of unusual causes of peritonitis and peritoneal tumors is discussed further in Chapter 78. (See Figures 121–2 and 121–3 for illustration of peritoneal tuberculosis, carcinomatosis, and lymphoma.)

Ascites of Unknown Origin

Clinical presentation, conventional laboratory examinations, and ascitic fluid analysis identify the cause of ascites in the majority of patients; however, occasionally these methods fail. Laparoscopy is a nonsurgical means of inspecting the peritoneal and liver surfaces and obtaining specimens for histology and culture. In the United States, occult cirrhosis and peritoneal malignancy account for the majority of cases.[91] In studies from Eastern countries, peritoneal malignancy is also the most common cause of unexplained ascites; however, tuberculous peritonitis accounts for an increasing number of cases (see Fig. 121–3).[95] In patients with HIV, peritoneal involvement may result from a variety of opportunistic infections and neoplasms (see earlier section, Peritonitis Associated with Acquired Immunodeficiency Syndrome). Non-Hodgkin's lymphoma (see Fig. 121–2) accounts for the majority of these peritoneal lesions revealed by laparoscopy, but *M. tuberculosis, M. avium-intracellulare*, and *P. carinii* are often revealed.[96]

REFERENCES

1. Meyers MA, Oliphant M, Berne AS, Feldberg MAM: The peritoneal ligaments and mesenteries: Pathways of intra-abdominal spread of disease. Radiology 163:593, 1987.
2. Kraft AR, Tomplins RK, Jesseph JE: Peritoneal electrolyte absorption: Analysis of portal, systemic venous, and lymphatic transport. Surgery 64:148, 1968.
3. Crawfurd E, Ellis H: Generalised peritonitis: The changing spectrum: A report of 100 consecutive cases. Br J Clin Pract 39:177, 1985.
4. Ng EK, Lam YH, Sung JJ, et al: Eradication of *Helicobacter pylori* prevents recurrence of ulcer after simple closure of duodenal ulcer perforation: Randomized controlled trial. Ann Surg 231:153, 2000.
5. Aydin M, Guler O, Yigit MF, et al: The effect on survival of thoracic duct ligation in experimental peritonitis. Hepatogastroenterology 46:308, 1999.
6. Guler O, Ugras S, Aydin M, et al: The effect of lymphatic blockage on the amount of endotoxin in portal circulation, nitric oxide synthesis, and the liver in dogs with peritonitis. Surg Today 29:735, 1999.
7. Liang Y, Sasaki K: Expression of adhesion molecules relevant to leukocyte migration on the microvilli of liver peritoneal mesothelial cells. Anat Rec 258:39, 2000.
8. Martineau L, Shek PN: Peritoneal cytokine concentrations and survival outcome in an experimental bacterial infusion model of peritonitis. Crit Care Med 28:788, 2000.
9. Runyon BA, Morrissey R, Hoefs JC, Wyle F: Opsonic activity of human ascitic fluid: A potentially important protective mechanism against spontaneous bacterial peritonitis. Hepatology 5:634, 1985.
10. Dunn DL, Barke RA, Knight NB, et al: Role of resident macrophages, peripheral neutrophils, and translymphatic absorption in bacterial clearance from the peritoneal cavity. Infect Immun 49:257, 1985.
11. Dunn DL, Barke RA, Ahrenholz DH, et al: The adjuvant effect of peritoneal fluid in experimental peritonitis: Mechanism and implications. Ann Surg 199:37, 1984.
12. Runyon BA: Low-protein-concentration ascitic fluid is predisposed to spontaneous bacterial peritonitis. Gastroenterology 91:1343, 1986.
13. Lorber B, Swenson RM: The bacteriology of intra-abdominal infections. Surg Clin North Am 55:1349, 1975.
14. Brook I, Frazier EH: Aerobic and anaerobic microbiology in intra-abdominal infections associated with diverticulitis. J Med Microbiol 49: 827, 2000.
15. Onderdonk AB, Bartlett JG, Louie T, et al: Microbial synergy in experimental intra-abdominal abscess. Infect Immun 13:22, 1976.
16. Jiang Q, Cross AS, Singh IS, et al: Febrile core temperature is essential for optimal host defense in bacterial peritonitis. Infect Immun 68:1265, 2000.
17. Lee PWR, Costen PDM, Wilson DH, Halsall AK: Pneumoperitoneum in perforated duodenal ulcer disease: A further look. Br J Clin Pract 31:108, 1977.
18. Lobbato V, Cioroiu M, LaRaja RD, et al: Peritoneal lavage as an aid to diagnosis of peritonitis in debilitated and elderly patients. Am Surg 51: 508, 1985.
19. Bone RC, Fisher CJ, Clemmer TP, et al: A controlled trial of high-dose methylprednisolone in the treatment of severe sepsis and septic shock. N Engl J Med 317:653, 1987.
20. Chalfine A, Carlet J: Antibiotic treatment of peritonitis. J Chir (Paris) 136:15, 1999.
21. Dupont H, Carbon C, Carlet J: Monotherapy with a broad-spectrum beta-lactam is as effective as its combination with an aminoglycoside in treatment of severe generalized peritonitis: A multicenter randomized controlled trial. Antimicrob Agents Chemother 44:2028, 2000.
22. Martineau L, Shek PN: Efficacy of liposomal antibiotic therapy in a rat infusion model of *Escherichia coli* peritonitis. Crit Care Med 27:1153, 1999.
23. Vela AR, Littleton JC, O'Leary JP: The effects of minidose heparin and low molecular weight heparin on peritonitis in the rat. Am Surg 65:473, 1999.
24. Woolverton CJ, Huebert K, Burkhart B, MacPhee M: Subverting bacterial resistance using high dose, low solubility antibiotics in fibrin. Infection 27:28, 1999.
25. Oettinger CW, D'Souza M, Milton GV: Targeting macrophages with microspheres containing cytokine-neutralizing antibodies prevents lethality in gram-negative peritonitis. J Interferon Cytokine Res 19:33, 1999.
26. Bartlett JG, Louie TJ, Gorbach SL, Onderdonk AB: Therapeutic efficacy of 29 antibiotic regimens in experimental intraabdominal sepsis. Rev Infect Dis 3:535, 1981.
27. Dupont H, Carbon C, Carlet J: Monotherapy with a broad-spectrum beta-lactam is as effective as its combination with an aminoglycoside in treatment of severe generalized peritonitis: A multicenter randomized controlled trial. Antimicrob Agents Chemother 44:2028, 2000.
28. Solomkin JS, Meakins JL, Allo MD, et al: Antibiotic trials in intra-abdominal infections: A critical evaluation of study design and outcome reporting. Ann Surg 200:29, 1984.
29. Kafih M, Fekak H, el Idrissi A, Zerouali NO: Perforated duodenal ulcer: Laparoscopic treatment of perforation and ulcerous disease. Ann Chir 125:24, 2000.
30. Seiler CA, Brugger L, Forssmann U, et al: Conservative surgical treatment of diffuse peritonitis. Surgery 127:178, 2000.
31. Bohnen J, Boulanger M, Meakins JL, McLean APH: Prognosis in generalized peritonitis. Arch Surg 118:285, 1983.
32. Chuang TF, Kao SC, Tsai CJ, et al: Spontaneous bacterial peritonitis as the presenting feature in an adult with nephrotic syndrome. Nephrol Dial Transplant 14:181, 1999.
33. Nolph KD, Lindblad AS, Novak JW: Continuous ambulatory peritoneal dialysis. N Engl J Med 318:1595, 1988.
34. Rubin J, Rogers WA, Taylor HM, et al: Peritonitis during continuous ambulatory peritoneal dialysis. Ann Intern Med 92:7, 1980.
35. Golden GT, Stevenson TR, Ritchie WP: Primary peritonitis in adults. South Med J 68:413, 1975.
36. Saklayen MG: CAPD peritonitis. Incidence, pathogens, diagnosis, and management. Med Clin North Am 74:997, 1990.
37. Kagawa K, Park S, Tokioka K, et al: Reduction of peritonitis with the rectus abdominis muscle flap in a CAPD patient. Pediatr Nephrol 14: 114, 2000.

38. Montenegro J, Saracho R, Aguirre R: Exit-site care with ciprofloxacin otologic solution prevents polyurethane catheter infection in peritoneal dialysis patients. Perit Dial Int 20:209, 2000.
39. Paterson PK, Matzke G, Keane WF: Current concepts in the management of peritonitis in patients undergoing continuous ambulatory peritoneal dialysis. Rev Infect Dis 9:604, 1987.
40. Such J, Runyon BA: Spontaneous bacterial peritonitis. Clin Infect Dis 27:669, 1998.
41. Hopewell PC: Impact of human immunodeficiency virus infection on the epidemiology, clinical features, management, and control of tuberculosis. Clin Infect Dis 15:540, 1992.
42. Runyon BA: Care of patients with ascites. N Engl J Med 330:337, 1994.
43. Runyon BA, Hoefs JC, Morgan TR: Ascitic fluid analysis in malignancy-related ascites. Hepatology 8:1104, 1988.
44. Geisler JP, Crook DE, Geisler HE, et al: The great imitator: Miliary peritoneal tuberculosis mimicking stage III ovarian carcinoma. Eur J Gynaecol Oncol 21:115, 2000.
45. Combs DL, O'Brien RJ, Geiter LJ: USPHS tuberculosis short-course chemotherapy trial 21: Effectiveness, toxicity, and acceptability: The report of final results. Ann Intern Med 112:397, 1990.
46. Hillebrand DJ, Runyon BA, Yasmineh WG, Rynders GP: Ascitic fluid adenosine deaminase insensitivity in detecting tuberculous peritonitis in the United States. Hepatology 24:1408, 1996.
47. Libbrecht E, Brissart N, Roger M, Fur A: Pneumococcal pelvioperitonitis revealing HIV seropositivity. Presse Med 29:246, 2000.
48. Lopez-Zeno JA, Keith LG, Berger GS: The Fitz-Hugh–Curtis syndrome revisited. J Reprod Med 30:567, 1985.
49. Mikamo H, Sato Y, Hayasaki Y, Tamaya T: Current status and fluconazole treatment of pelvic fungal gynecological infections. Chemotherapy 46:209, 2000.
50. Warady BA, Bashir M, Donaldson LA: Fungal peritonitis in children receiving peritoneal dialysis: A report of the NAPRTCS. Kidney Int 58: 384, 2000.
51. Malinger G, Ginath S, Zeidel L, et al: Starch peritonitis outbreak after introduction of a new brand of starch powdered latex gloves. Acta Obstet Gynecol Scand 79:610, 2000.
52. Matolo NM, Albo D: Gastrointestinal complications of collagen vascular diseases. Am J Surg 122:678, 1971.
53. Zemer D, Pras M, Sohar E, et al: Colchicine in the prevention and treatment of the amyloidosis of familial Mediterranean fever. N Engl J Med 314:1001, 1986.
54. Pockros PJ, Esrason KT, Nguyen C, et al: Mobilization of malignant ascites with diuretics is dependent on ascitic fluid characteristics. Gastroenterology 103:1302, 1992.
55. Cavaliere F, Di Filippo F, Botti C, et al: Peritonectomy and hyperthermic antiblastic perfusion in the treatment of peritoneal carcinomatosis. Eur J Surg Oncol 26:486, 2000.
56. Sumantran VN, Lee DS, Baker VV, et al: A bcl-x(S) adenovirus demonstrates therapeutic efficacy in an ascites model of human breast cancer. J Soc Gynecol Invest 7:184, 2000.
57. Yoshikawa T, Yanoma S, Tsuburaya A, et al: Angiogenesis inhibitor, TNP-470, suppresses growth of peritoneal disseminating foci. Hepatogastroenterology 47:298, 2000.
58. Xu L, Yoneda J, Herrera C, et al: Inhibition of malignant ascites and growth of human ovarian carcinoma by oral administration of a potent inhibitor of the vascular endothelial growth factor receptor tyrosine kinases. Int J Oncol 16:445, 2000.
59. Yamada S, Takeda T, Matsumoto K: Prognostic analysis of malignant pleural and peritoneal effusions. Cancer 51:136, 1983.
60. Mann WJ, Wagner J, Chumas J, et al: The management of pseudomyxoma peritonei. Cancer 66:1636, 1990.
61. McDonald AD, McDonald JC: Malignant mesothelioma in North America. Cancer 46:1650, 1980.
62. Hwang HC, Smythe WR, Elshami AA, et al: Gene therapy using adenovirus carrying the herpes simplex–thymidine kinase gene to treat in vivo models of human malignant mesothelioma and lung cancer. Am J Respir Cell Mol Biol 13:7, 1995.
63. Heyns CF. Pelvic lipomatosis: A review of its diagnosis and management. J Urol 146:267, 1991.
64. Feliciano DV: Management of traumatic retroperitoneal hematoma. Ann Surg 211:109, 1990.
65. Campagnutta E, Giorda G, De Piero G, et al: Different patterns of postoperative bleeding following cytoreductive surgery for gynecological cancer. Eur J Gynaecol Oncol 21:91, 2000.
66. Velmahos GC, Chahwan S, Falabella A, et al: Angiographic embolization for intraperitoneal and retroperitoneal injuries. World J Surg 24: 539, 2000.
67. Kurtz RJ, Heimann TM, Beck AR., et al: Mesenteric and retroperitoneal cysts. Ann Surg 203:109, 1986.
68. Yasoshima T, Mukaiya M, Hirata K, et al: A chylous cyst of the mesentery: Report of a case. Surg Today 30:185, 2000.
69. Stout AP, Hendry J, Pardie FJ: Primary solid tumors of the greater omentum. Cancer 16:231, 1963.
70. Schwartz RW, Reames M, McGrath PC, et al: Primary solid neoplasms of the greater omentum. Surgery 109:543, 1991.
71. Horiuchi K, Yabe H, Mukai M, et al: Multiple smooth muscle tumors arising in deep soft tissue of lower limbs with uterine leiomyomas. Am J Surg Pathol 22:897, 1998.
72. Herrero J, Kamali P, Kirschbaum M: Leiomyomatosis peritonealis disseminata associated with endometriosis: A case report and literature review. Eur J Obstet Gynecol Reprod Biol 76:189, 1998.
73. Keven K, Nergizoglu G, Ates K, et al: Remission of nephrotic syndrome after removal of localized Castleman's disease. Am J Kidney Dis 35:1207, 2000.
74. Wolff H, Kunte C, Messer G, et al: Paraneoplastic pemphigus with fatal pulmonary involvement in a woman with a mesenteric Castleman tumour. Br J Dermatol 140:313, 1999.
75. Moon WK, Kim SH, Im JG, et al: Castleman disease with renal amyloidosis: Imaging findings and clinical significance. Abdom Imaging 20:376, 1995.
76. Vingerhoets F, Kuntzer T, Delacretaz J, et al: Chronic relapsing neuropathy associated with Castleman's disease (angiofollicular lymph node hyperplasia). Eur Neurol 35:336, 1995.
77. Reske M, Nimiki H: Sclerosing mesenteritis: Report of two cases. Am J Clin Pathol 64:661, 1975.
78. Kipfer RE, Moertel CG, Dahlin DC. Mesenteric lipodystrophy. Ann Intern Med 80:582, 1984.
79. Parra-Davila E, McKenney MG, Sleeman D, et al: Mesenteric panniculitis: Case report and literature review. Am Surg 64:768, 1998.
80. Papadaki HA, Kouroumalis EA, Stefanaki K, et al: Retractile mesenteritis presenting as fever of unknown origin and autoimmune haemolytic anaemia. Digestion 61:145, 2000.
81. Higgins PM, Aber GM: Idiopathic retroperitoneal fibrosis: An update. Dig Dis 8:206, 1990.
82. Kronthal AJ, Kang YS, Fishman EK, et al: MR imaging in sclerosing mesenteritis. Am J Radiol 156:517, 1991.
83. Daskalogiannaki M, Voloudaki A, Prassopoulos P, et al: CT evaluation of mesenteric panniculitis: Prevalence and associated diseases. AJR Am J Roentgenol 174:427, 2000.
84. Mazure R, Fernandez J, Marty P, et al: Successful treatment of retractile mesenteritis with oral progesterone. Gastroenterology 114:1317, 1998.
85. Netzer P, Binek J, Hammer B: Diffuse abdominal pain, nausea and vomiting due to retroperitoneal fibrosis: A rare but often missed diagnosis. Eur J Gastroenterol Hepatol 9:1005, 1997.
86. al Husaini H, Onime A, Oluwole SF: Primary torsion of the greater omentum. J Natl Med Assoc 92:306, 2000.
87. Stella DL, Schelleman TG: Segmental infarction of the omentum secondary to torsion: Ultrasound and computed tomography diagnosis. Australas Radiol 44:212, 2000.
88. Gassner PE, Cox MR, Cregan PC: Torsion of the omentum: Diagnosis and resection at laparoscopy. Aust NZ J Surg 69:466, 1999.
89. Anderson L, Forrest J: Tumors of the diaphragm. AJR Am J Roentgenol 119:259, 1973.
90. Greenberg M, Maden V, Ataii E, et al: Intradiaphragmatic cyst: A diagnostic challenge. JAMA 230:1176, 1974.
91. Vargas C, Jeffers LJ, Bernstein D, et al: Diagnostic laparoscopy: A 5-year experience in a hepatology training program. Am J Gastroenterol 90:1258, 1995.
92. Dobelle WH: Use of breathing pacemakers to suppress intractable hiccups of up to thirteen years duration. ASAIO J 45:524, 1999.
93. Evasovich MR, Clark TC, Horattas MC, et al: Does pneumoperitoneum during laparoscopy increase bacterial translocation?. Surg Endosc 10: 1176, 1996.
94. Tug T, Ozbas S, Tekeli A, et al: Does pneumoperitoneum cause bacterial translocation? J Laparoendosc Adv Surg Tech A 8:401, 1998.
95. Chu C, Lin S, Peng S, et al: The role of laparoscopy in the evaluation of ascites of unknown origin. Gastrointest Endosc 40:285, 1994.
96. Jeffers LJ, Alzate I, Agulfer H, et al: Laparoscopic and histologic findings in patients with the human immunodeficiency virus. Gastrointest Endosc 40:160, 1994.

PSYCHOSOCIAL FACTORS IN GASTROINTESTINAL DISEASE

Chapter 122

A Biopsychosocial Understanding of Gastrointestinal Illness and Disease

Douglas A. Drossman

This chapter presents an integrated overview of how psychosocial factors relate to gastrointestinal function, disease susceptibility, and clinical illness and its outcomes, and it provides an integrated approach to the care of the patient with gastrointestinal illness. These factors are also discussed in other chapters of this textbook dealing with specific diseases.

A CONCEPTUALIZATION

Traditional Biomedical Model

In Western civilization, the traditional understanding of illness and disease* has been the *biomedical model*.[1, 2] This model adheres to two premises: First, any illness can be linearly reduced to a single etiology (reductionism). Therefore, identifying and modifying the underlying etiology are necessary and sufficient to explain the illness and ultimately lead to cure. The second premise is that an illness can be classified as either a disease or "organic" disorder, having objectively defined pathophysiology, or a "functional" disorder, with no specifically identifiable pathophysiology (dualism). This dichotomy presumes to distinguish medical (organic) from psychological (functional) illness or relegates functional illness to a condition with no etiology or treatment.

The limitations of this biomedical model are demonstrated when a patient's illness cannot be explained by evident medical disease, as in the following case example:

Case Study

Ms. L., a 42-year-old woman, presents to her new physician with a 20-year history of mid to lower abdominal pain with nausea and occasional vomiting. She states: "I can't live with this pain anymore." Her bowel function is normal, and her weight is stable. She is unable to work, she feels that the symptoms have taken over her life, and she perceives no sense of control over her symptoms or any ability to decrease them. There is a long-standing history of major losses and depression as well as sexual and physical abuse. She requests narcotics for pain relief and that the physician expeditiously "find the cause of the pain and remove it." The record shows frequent emergency department visits and several hospital admissions where diagnostic studies were negative and narcotics were given for pain relief. Previous studies, including upper gastrointestinal series with small bowel follow-through, colonoscopy, computed tomography of the abdomen, abdominal and pelvic ultrasonography, and laparoscopy, have been normal. A prior cholecystectomy did not document gallstones, and a hysterectomy was done several years earlier for endometriosis. On this occasion an upper endoscopy is done that shows normal mucosal morphology. The CLO test is positive for *Helicobacter pylori*, and she receives a 2-week course of antibiotics without benefit. The patient is then referred to a psychiatrist, who makes a diagnosis of post-traumatic stress dis-

*A semantic distinction is made between disease (abnormalities in structure and function of organs and tissues) and illness (the personal experience of ill health or bodily dysfunction). Illness is determined by current or previous disease, as well as psychosocial, familial, and cultural influences. As discussed, these terms cannot be conceptualized independently of each other.

order and major depression, along with the recommendation that other possible medical disease be excluded. On the next visit to the medical physician, the patient refuses further psychiatric care and requests referral to another medical center.

This example highlights several issues engendered by approaching the care of some illnesses from a biomedical perspective. First, for 20 years, Ms. L. has had no evidence of a structural ("organic") diagnosis to explain her symptoms, yet she still urges that further diagnostic studies be done to "find and fix" the problem. Initially, the physician accedes to this request by having an upper endoscopy performed. However, failure to find a specific structural etiology for medical symptoms is the rule rather than the exception in an ambulatory care setting. In a study involving 1000 ambulatory internal medicine patients,[3] of 567 new complaints, only 16% over a 3-year period were eventually found to have an organic cause (11% in the case of abdominal pain), and only an additional 10% were given a psychiatric diagnosis.

The patient in our case study has functional abdominal pain syndrome (see Chapter 5),[4, 5] one of 21 functional gastrointestinal disorders that comprise more than 40% of a gastroenterologist's practice.[6, 7] Because functional gastrointestinal disorders do not fit into a biomedical construct (i.e., they represent an "illness without evident disease"), they may not be accepted by adherents of this biomedical model[8] as legitimate. So both patients and physicians are at risk to pursue unneeded and costly diagnostic tests to find "the cause," thereby deflecting proper attention away from symptom management.

Second, this patient exhibits several psychosocial features, including major loss, depression, abuse history, and maladaptive thinking (i.e., "catastrophizing" and perceived inability to manage the symptoms) that adversely influence the clinical outcome and that are amenable to proper treatment.[9] However, from the biomedical perspective, patients and physicians tend to view psychosocial factors and conditions as separate from medical illness and may even stigmatize individuals having them.[10] Understandably, when the endoscopy is negative, only then does the physician refer the patient to the psychiatrist, and the patient is reluctant to address these issues in her care.

Third, there are difficulties evident in the physician-patient interaction. For example, the patient believes that narcotics will provide the needed relief, yet their repeated use may aggravate the symptoms ("narcotic bowel syndrome").[11] There is risk that these differing views with regard to narcotic use will interfere with the conduct of the visits that may focus on issues of prescribing narcotics rather than directing efforts toward more effective multicomponent treatment. In addition, the patient was clearly not satisfied with seeing the psychiatrist and requested referral to another medical facility. These behaviors relate to different levels of understanding of the illness and its treatment and to poor communication relating to these issues.

The limitations imposed in caring for patients from a biomedical perspective are highlighted in this case. They emphasize the need to educate physicians that (1) medical disorders are often inadequately explained by structural abnormalities; (2) psychosocial factors predispose to the onset and perpetuation of illness and disease, are part of the illness experience, and strongly influence the clinical outcome; and (3) successful understanding of these issues and proper management require an effective physician-patient relationship. This chapter addresses these issues by (1) presenting a framework to understand the integrative nature of psychosocial and biologic factors in all gastrointestinal disorders, and (2) offering techniques that can improve communication skills, build an effective physician-patient interaction, and ultimately produce a better outcome. To accomplish these goals we must first apply a different conceptual understanding of gastrointestinal illness and disease.

Biopsychosocial Model

The *biopsychosocial model* proposes that illness and disease result not from a single etiology but from simultaneously interacting systems at the cellular, tissue, organism, interpersonal, and environmental levels. Furthermore, psychosocial factors have direct physiologic and pathologic consequences and vice versa. For example, change at the subcellular level (e.g., development of human immunodeficiency virus infection or susceptibility to inflammatory bowel disease has the potential to affect organ function, the person, the family, and society. Similarly, a change at the interpersonal level, such as the death of a spouse, can affect psychological status, cellular immunity, and, ultimately, disease susceptibility.[12] It also explains why the clinical expression of biologic substrates (e.g., oncogene alteration) varies among patients in terms of its clinical expression and in the response to treatment. This biopsychosocial model is more consistent with emerging scientific data about the mechanisms of disease and clinical care and is assumed to be valid in this presentation.

Figure 122–1 provides the framework to understand the mutually interacting relationship of psychosocial and biologic factors in the clinical expression of illness and disease. Early life factors (e.g., genetic predisposition, early learning, and the cultural milieu) can influence the individual's later psychosocial environment, physiologic functioning, and expression of disease (pathology) and their reciprocal interaction via the brain-gut (central and enteric nervous systems

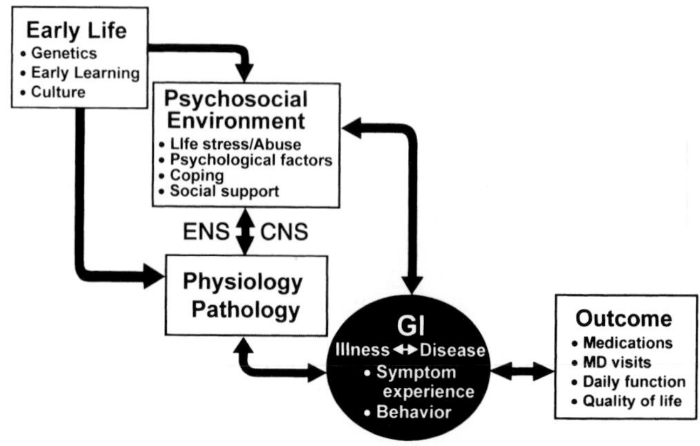

Figure 122–1. Systems (biopsychosocial) model of gastrointestinal (GI) illness. The relationships among early life, psychosocial environment, physiology and pathology, symptom experience and behavior, and outcome are presented as interacting systems. This figure serves as a template for the discussion in this chapter. See text for details.

[CNS/ENS]) axis. The product of this brain-gut interaction affects symptom experience and behavior and, ultimately, the clinical outcome. This diagrammatic representation serves as a reference point for the discussion that follows.

EARLY LIFE

Early Learning

Developmental Aspects

At or perhaps even before birth, a person's genetic composition (not discussed in this chapter) and interactions with the environment begin to affect later behaviors and susceptibility to illness. The earliest interactions are with feeding and elimination. According to psychoanalytic theory, situations of conflict arise early in which the child's innate impulses (e.g., to eat or defecate) confront external environmental (i.e., parental) constraints, and normal personality development involves successful resolution of these conflicts. The complex behaviors of feeding and elimination, sources of intense gratification to the infant, must gradually be controlled by the growing child according to the prevailing mores of family and society. To varying degrees during development, these adopted constraints remain in conflict with desires for immediate gratification. With increased motor control of these functions, the child can either defy or comply with environmental constraints by choosing to eat, resist eating, bite, defecate, or withhold stool. When and how these behaviors are displayed depend on the child's needs and the quality and intensity of the environmental controls. Behaviors learned during this period are considered pivotal in the child's personality and development and later interaction with the environment: the development of autonomy, of distinguishing right from wrong, and of disciplining impulses in a socially acceptable manner. Conversely, failure to resolve these early conflicts may make the adult vulnerable in situations that tax these character traits. Thus, the obstinate ("obstipation") person who withholds or resists when feeling controlled may have been influenced by unresolved interactions around control of elimination.

Several studies suggest that certain gastrointestinal disorders may be influenced by early learning difficulties. Case reports of patients with functional constipation,[13] psychogenic vomiting,[14] adult rumination (merycism),[15] and anorexia nervosa[16] who have undergone psychoanalysis report highly emotional and/or repressive interactions with parents over the processes of feeding and elimination, and this may contribute to later physiologic dysfunction. For example, children with functional constipation hold back stool to avoid painful defecation; in one study, adults who were told to voluntarily suppress the defecation urge for only 3 days had significantly reduced right-sided colonic transit.[17] Disorders of anorectal function (e.g., pelvic floor dyssynergia and encopresis) also may have resulted from learning difficulties relating to bowel habit.[18] Encopretic children may withhold stool out of a fear of the toilet, to struggle for control, or to receive attention from parents.[19] One study proposed that encopretic children were more likely than controls to have been toilet trained by coercive techniques, to have psychological difficulties, and to have poor rapport with their mothers.[20] Almy has shown that patients with irritable bowel syndrome (IBS) who have pain and constipation display aggressive or coping ("controlling") behaviors with increased (nonpropulsive) motor contractions, whereas patients with diarrhea display helplessness, defeat, and withdrawal ("giving up"), which is associated with decreased sigmoid contractions and more rapid transit.[21] Although these studies are methodologically limited owing to ascertainment bias and possible investigator bias and therefore require confirmation, survey data support the role of early conflict in symptom experience and reporting behavior.[22]

Conditioning

Early conditioning experiences may also influence physiologic functioning and, possibly, the development of psychophysiologic disorders.* Visceral functions such as the secretion of digestive juices and motility of the gallbladder, stomach, and intestine can be classically conditioned,† even by family interaction.[23]

Case Study

A young child wakes up on the day of a school examination with anxiety and "flight-fight" symptoms of tachycardia, diaphoresis, abdominal cramps, and diarrhea. The parent keeps the child home because of a "tummy ache" and allows him to stay in bed and watch television. Several days later, the symptoms recur when the child is about to go to school.

In this case, the parent focuses on the abdominal discomfort as an illness requiring school absence rather than a physiologic response to a distressing situation, and the child experiences relief through avoidance of the feared situation. Repetition of such events positively reinforces future psychophysiologic symptom responses or the child's attitudes and behaviors toward them ("illness modeling"). For example, patients with IBS recalled more parental attention toward their illnesses than those with IBS not seeking health care, they stayed home from school and saw physicians more often, and they received more gifts and privileges.[24]

Culture and Family

Social and cultural belief systems modify how a patient experiences illness and interacts with the health care system.[25] In a study at a New York City hospital in the 1950s, first- and second-generation Jews and Italians were observed to be more dramatic in their response to pain, whereas the

*Psychophysiologic reactions involve psychologically induced alterations in the function of target organs without structural change. They are often viewed as physiologic concomitants of an affect such as anger or fear, although the person is not always aware of the affect. The persistence of an altered physiologic state or the enhanced physiologic response to psychological stimuli is considered by some as a psychophysiologic disorder.

†Two types of learning systems exist that may affect gastrointestinal function. Classic conditioning, as described by Pavlov, involves linking a neutral food or unconditioned stimulus (sound of a bell) with a conditioned stimulus (food) that elicits a conditioned response (salivation). After several trials, the unconditioned stimulus is able to produce the conditioned response. Operant conditioning involves the development of a desired response through motivation and reinforcement. Playing basketball is one example: Accuracy improves through practice; the correct behavior is reinforced by the reward of scoring a basket.

Irish tended to deny their symptoms, and the "Old Americans" were most stoical. Furthermore, Italians were satisfied with relief of pain, whereas the Jewish patients needed to understand the meaning of the pain and its future consequences.[26] Many ethnic populations in Western countries, including African Americans, Asians, Hispanics, and Native Americans, maintain culturally derived beliefs about illness and its treatment. In fact, 70% to 90% of all self-recognized illnesses in these populations are managed outside traditional medical facilities, often with self-help groups or religious cult practitioners providing a substantial portion of the care.[27] One in three white patients see practitioners who use unconventional treatments (e.g., homeopathy, high colonic enemas, crystal healing) at a frequency that exceeds primary care visits, and most patients do not inform their physicians about this.[28] It is therefore important for the physician to inquire about the patient's beliefs relating to the onset, cause, clinical course, and desired or expected treatment, because these factors affect compliance and response to traditional treatments.

PSYCHOSOCIAL ENVIRONMENT

As the child moves into adulthood, genetics, culture, early learning, and other environmental influences are integrated into the individual's unique personality and behavioral style. These predisposing factors, in addition to intercurrent factors including life stress, one's current psychological state, including comorbid psychiatric diagnosis, and one's coping style and degree of social support, will in combination determine the physiologic functioning of the gut, susceptibility to and activity of disease, and the clinical outcome.

Life Stress and Abuse

Unresolved life stress (e.g., psychosocial trauma such as the loss of a parent; an abortion; a major, personal, catastrophic event or their anniversaries) or daily life stresses (e.g., a chronic illness) may influence the individual's illness in several ways: (1) to produce psychophysiologic effects (e.g., changes in motility, blood flow/secretion or sensation), thereby exacerbating symptoms; (2) to increase one's vigilance toward symptoms; and (3) to lead to maladaptive coping and greater illness behaviors and health care seeking. Despite numerous methodologic limitations in studying the relationship of such psychosocial factors to illness, disease, and its outcome, it is reasonably clear that such factors can clearly exacerbate functional gastrointestinal disorders[29, 30] and also symptoms of certain structural disorders such as inflammatory bowel disease.[31] Although the scientific evidence for such factors to be etiologic in the development of pathologic diseases (based on retrospective studies and psychoimmunologic mechanisms) is compelling, it is not fully established. Nevertheless, the negative impact of stressful life events on the psychological state and illness behaviors requires the physician to address them in the day-to-day care of all patients.

A history of physical or sexual abuse strongly influences the severity of gastrointestinal symptoms and the clinical outcome.[32] When compared with patients without abuse history, patients with abuse history seen in a referral gastroenterology clinic reported 70% more severe pain and 40% greater psychological distress, spent more days in bed in the previous 3 months, had almost twice as poor daily function, saw physicians more often, and underwent more surgical procedures. This explains the higher frequency of abuse history among patients with more severe or refractory painful gastrointestinal symptoms seen in referral practices, when compared with patients with milder symptoms seen in primary care settings.[33] So life stress and abuse history amplify the severity of the condition and are seen to a greater degree among patients with more severe clinical presentations.

Several possible mechanisms help explain the relationship of abuse history to poor outcome.[34] Patients with a history of abuse may (1) be susceptible to developing psychological conditions that increase perception of visceral input (central hypervigilance and somatization); (2) develop psychophysiologic (e.g., autonomic, humoral, immunologic) responses that affect gut motor or sensory function or inflammation; (3) develop peripheral and/or central sensitization from increased motility or physical trauma (visceral hyperalgesia/allodynia); (4) abnormally appraise and behaviorally respond to physical sensations of perceived threat (response bias); and (5) develop maladaptive coping styles leading to increased illness behavior and health care seeking (e.g., catastrophizing). Severe abuse can also alter brain function[35] and structure,[36] and this helps explain reported effects on memory, perception, pain modulation, and illness behaviors.

Psychological Factors

As shown in Figure 122–1, along with life stress and abuse, there is a "mix" of concurrent psychosocial factors that can influence gastrointestinal physiology and susceptibility to developing a pathologic condition and its symptomatic and behavioral expression, all of which affects the outcome. The psychological factors relate both to long-standing (also called "trait") features (e.g., personality and psychiatric diagnosis), and more modifiable "state" features (e.g., psychological distress and mood) amenable to psychological and psychopharmacologic interventions. In addition there are modulating ("buffering") effects of coping style and social support (discussed later).

Personality as an Etiologic Factor

Are there specific personalities associated with gastroenterologic disorders? During the psychoanalytically dominated era of psychosomatic medicine (1920 to 1955), certain psychological conflicts were believed to underlie the development of personalities that expressed specific "psychosomatic" disease (asthma, rheumatoid arthritis, ulcerative colitis, essential hypertension, neurodermatitis, thyrotoxicity, and duodenal ulcer).[37] In the biologically predisposed host, disease would develop when environmental stress was sufficient to activate the psychological conflict. For example, the activation of a conflict relating to an intensely dependent relationship with a controlling and dominating mother or other key figure was thought to produce or aggravate ulcerative colitis and explain the hypersensitivity of patients to rejection, reluctance to develop trusting relationships, and dependence on certain persons on whom they placed unrealistic demands.[38] Disruption of a key relationship, such as by marriage or the death of the dominant person, could activate or reactivate the disease.

The idea of personality features specifically relating to causation (albeit in the biologically predisposed host) of medical disease is simplistic. Currently, investigators view personality and other psychological traits as enablers or modulators of illness along with other contributing factors, such as life stress, the social environment, and coping.

Psychiatric Diagnosis

The co-occurrence of psychiatric diagnoses in patients with medical disorders (comorbidity) is common, and it aggravates the clinical presentation and outcome.[39] The most common psychiatric diagnoses seen among patients with chronic gastrointestinal disorders are depression (including dysthymia) and anxiety (including panic),[40] and these psychiatric disorders are often amenable to psychopharmacotherapy or psychological treatment.

An issue of clinical concern relates to when certain other psychiatric disorders and personality traits adversely affect an individual's experience and behavior to the point that they interfere with interactions involving family, social peers, and physicians. These can include *somatization disorder,* characterized by a fixed pattern of experiencing and reporting numerous physical complaints beginning early in life; *factitious disorder,* or possibly *Munchausen's syndrome,* in which patients surreptitiously simulate illness (e.g., ingesting laxatives, feigning symptoms of medical illness) to obtain certain effects (e.g., to receive narcotics, operations, and procedures); and *borderline personality disorder,* in which the individual develops unstable and intense (e.g., overly dependent) interpersonal relationships, experiences marked shifts in mood (e.g., depression, anger), and exhibits impulsive (e.g., suicidal, self-mutilating, sexual) behaviors. Physicians must recognize these patterns to avoid maladaptive interactions, maintain clear boundaries of medical care (e.g., not to overdo studies based on patient requests), and, when necessary, refer to a mental health professional skilled in the care of patients having these conditions. Standardized criteria for diagnosis of psychiatric and personality disorders are available.[41]

Psychological Distress

Even for healthy individuals, having an illness can cause psychological distress and lead to transient symptoms of anxiety, depression, and other mood disturbances. Psychological distress also impacts on the medical disorder and its outcome; it lowers pain threshold and influences health care seeking for patients with functional bowel disturbances[42, 43] and structural disease.[44, 45] For example, the higher frequency of depression and greater psychological distress among patients with Crohn's disease, when compared with those with ulcerative colitis, is attributed more to the severity of this disorder than to the diagnosis itself.

Psychosocial Awareness

An important clinical observation is the inverse association between having major psychosocial difficulties as related to illness exacerbation and severity and one's recognition or acknowledgment of them. For example, patients with IBS seeking health care, when compared with those with IBS who do not see physicians, report greater levels of psychological difficulties but also tend to deny a role for psychological factors in their illness. They do not recognize mood disturbances such as depression,[46] and they believe their illness to be more serious than those with structural disease and will see physicians more often for these physical complaints.[47]

This construct may develop early in life. The young child described earlier may not only learn to report somatic symptoms when distressed but also may not recognize or communicate the association with the stressful precipitants, because they are not addressed within the family. *Alexithymia* (from the Greek word meaning "absence of words for emotions") describes patients who have chronic difficulties recognizing and verbalizing emotions. It is believed that alexithymia develops in response to early traumatic experiences such as abuse, severe childhood illness, or deprivation. Patients with alexithymia may express strong emotions, such as anger or sadness in relation to their illness, but they know little about the psychological basis for these feelings and cannot link them with past experience or current illness.[48] This limits their ability to regulate emotions, to use coping strategies effectively, and to adjust to their chronic condition. Their tendency to communicate emotional distress through somatic symptoms and illness behavior rather than verbally appears to be associated with more frequent physician visits and a poorer prognosis.[49, 50]

Coping and Social Support

Coping and social support modulate the effects of life stress, abuse, and morbid psychological factors on the illness and its outcome. They can "buffer" (turn down) or enable (turn up) and amplify these effects. *Coping* is defined as "efforts, both action-oriented and intrapsychic, to manage (i.e., master, tolerate, minimize) environmental and internal demands and conflicts, which tax or exceed a person's resources."[51] In general, more emotion-based coping (e.g., denial), although possibly adaptive for acute overwhelming stresses, is not effective for chronic stressors, while problem-based coping strategies (e.g., seeking social support or reappraising the stressor) involve efforts to change one's response to the stressor and are more effective for chronic illness. One prospective study of gastrointestinal outpatients referred for all types of diagnoses found that a maladaptive emotional coping style, catastrophizing, along with the perceived inability to decrease symptoms, led to greater pain scores, more physician visits, and poorer functioning over the subsequent 1-year period.[52] Therefore, efforts made through psychological treatments to improve one's appraisal of the stress of illness and ability to manage symptoms are likely to improve health status and outcome.

Social support through family, church, community organizations, and other social networks can have similar effects of reducing the impact of various stressors on physical and mental illness, thereby improving one's ability to cope with the illness.[53] In one study, of 86 patients with metastatic breast cancer, a 1-year intervention of weekly supportive group therapy was undertaken, and both the treatment (n =

50) and control groups (n = 36) had routine oncologic care. At 10 years' follow-up, only 3 of the patients were alive, and death records were obtained for the other 83. Mean survival from the time of randomization and onset of intervention was 37 months in the treatment group compared with 19 months in the control group.

CENTRAL AND ENTERIC NERVOUS SYSTEMS: THE BRAIN-GUT AXIS

This section addresses both known and potential mechanisms for communication between the brain (psychosocial environment) and the gut (physiology and pathology) through the CNS/ENS (brain-gut axis) and its consequences on peripheral systems (e.g., motility, secretion, sensation, inflammation, symptoms, and clinical outcome). Much of this work has emerged only since the 1990s, and the findings support the biopsychosocial model used in clinical practice.

Stress and Gastrointestinal Function (Motility)

An observational relationship between "stress* and gastrointestinal function has been a part of the writings of poets and philosophers for centuries."[54] Healthy subjects commonly have abdominal discomfort or change in bowel function when upset or distressed,[55] a fact usually taken into account by clinicians when managing patients. Clinical reports and psychophysiologic studies in animals and humans support these observations. Cannon noted a cessation in bowel activity among cats reacting to a growling dog.[56] Beaumont observed changes in color of the mucosa and in secretory activity of a gastric pouch in response to psychological and physical stimuli in his patient with a traumatic fistula.[57] Pavlov first reported that psychic factors affect acid secretion via the vagus nerve in dogs with fistulas.[58] Studies of patients with gastric fistulas showed that different emotional make-ups produce distinct changes in gastric function.[59, 60] Gastric hyperemia and increased motility and secretion were linked to feelings of anger, intense pleasure, or aggressive behavior toward others. Conversely, mucosal pallor and decreased secretion and motor activity accompanied fear or depression, states of withdrawal ("giving-up behavior"), or disengagement from others.

Later studies showing the effects of experimental stress on physiologic functioning were reported in most all areas of the gastrointestinal tract. Complicated cognitive tasks produce (1) high-amplitude, high-velocity esophageal contractions[61]; (2) increased pancreatic chymotrypsin output[62]; and (3) a reduction of phase II and a prolongation of phase III activity of the migrating myoelectric complex in the small intestine.[63] Experimentally induced anger increases motor and spike potential activity in the colon, and this occurs to a greater degree in patients with functional bowel disorders.[64]

*Stress is difficult to understand and study; no definition is entirely satisfactory. The human organism functions in a constantly changing environment. Any influence on one's steady-state that requires adjustment or adaptation can be considered stress. The term *stress* is nonspecific and encompasses both the stimulus and its effects. The stimulus can be a biologic event such as infection, a social event such as a change of residence, or even a disturbing thought. Stress can be desirable or undesirable. Some stimuli, such as pain, sex, or threat of injury, often elicit a predictable response in animals and humans. In contrast, life events and many other psychological processes have more varied effects. For example, a change of jobs may be of little concern to one person yet be a crisis to another who perceives it as a personal failure. A stimulus may produce a variety of responses among persons or within the same person at different times. There may be no observable effect, a psychological response (anxiety, depression), physiologic changes (diarrhea, diaphoresis), disease onset (asthma, colitis), or any combination. A person's interpretation of events as stressful or not and his or her response depend on prior experience, attitudes, coping mechanisms, personality, culture, and biologic factors, including susceptibility to disease. The nonspecific nature of the term *stress* precludes its use as a distinct variable for research.

Brain-Gut Communication: The Role of Neurotransmitters

The richly innervated nerve plexus and neuroendocrine associations of the CNS and ENS provide the "hardwiring" for reciprocal activity between brain and gut. The mediation of these activities involves neurotransmitters and neuropeptides found in the CNS and gut: corticotropin-releasing factor (CRF), vasoactive intestinal polypeptide (VIP), 5-hydroxytryptamine and its congeners, substance P, nitric oxide, cholecystokinin, and the enkephalins, to name a few. These substances have integrated activities on gastrointestinal function and human behavior, depending on their location. For example, the stress hormone CRF[65] produces gastric stasis and an increased colonic transit rate in response to psychologically aversive stimuli. CRF is also involved in the communication between the immune and gastrointestinal systems. It has even been proposed that hypersecretion of CRF in the brain may contribute to stress-induced exacerbation of IBS. The administration of cholecystokinin increases gut motility and also elicits postprandial satiety in animals,[66] and the meal-associated release of this hormone may influence the clinical expression of bulimia nervosa.[67] The location of the enkephalins affects pain control, gastrointestinal motility, feeding activity,[68] emotional behavior, and immunity.[69] Finally, neurotransmitters (e.g., nitric oxide) can even increase the expression of protooncogenes (e.g., *cfos*) involved in the transcriptional control of genes that encode production of other neuropeptides (e.g., dynorphin), and this can lead to semipermanent changes in brain or gut function (e.g., visceral sensitization).[70]

Regulation of Visceral Pain (Disinhibition)

The brain and gut reciprocally affect the experience and regulation of visceral pain (see Chapter 5). Visceral signals are transmitted via ascending (e.g., spinothalamic and spinoreticular) pathways to the midbrain, thalamus, and cortex. The somatosensory cortex receives somatotypic information about the location and intensity of pain, whereas the limbic system (anterior cingulate cortex, insula, medial thalamus) is involved with the affective and motivational component of pain. This latter system has the potential to modulate the pain experience, via activation of descending regulatory pathways (e.g., the endorphin-mediated analgesic system) to the dorsal horn. This "gate control" system[71] can thus upregulate or down-regulate incoming visceral signals. This explains how emotional distress or early encoded painful experiences (e.g., childhood physical trauma) might increase ascending visceral signals from similar sites, thereby later producing more pain for a given visceral stimulus (hyperalgesia and allodynia), whereas psychological interventions (e.g., hypnosis, cognitive-behavioral treatment) or antidepressants can decrease the experience of the stimulus and reduce pain. Furthermore, repetitive stimuli in the gut, either mechanical or inflammatory, can lead to transient or prolonged changes in the spinal cord or higher brain centers that increase pain awareness to even normal afferent signals (visceral sensitization; see Chapter 5).

Effects of Stress on Immune Function and Disease Susceptibility

Stressful experiences can also affect peripheral immune function, and ultimately, susceptibility to disease; conversely, peripheral immune-inflammatory mediators can affect psychological functioning. The discipline of psychoneuroimmunology began in the 1970s when alterations of immune function were first documented in astronauts after splashdown.[72] Later in vitro experiments showed effects of acute stress on lymphoproliferative activity, interferon production, and DNA repair.[73, 74] Clinical studies showed that chronically distressed individuals (e.g., long-term caregivers of demented spouses) had impaired cellular immunity and higher frequencies of depression and respiratory infections compared with matched controls.[75] Another study found that persons in psychological distress had a higher frequency of respiratory infections after intranasal virus inoculation.[76] Behavioral interventions such as stress management treatment have been associated among patients with multiple myeloma with an increased number of natural killer cell activity, and this eventuated 6 years later in a significantly lower mortality and a trend toward fewer tumor recurrences when compared with the control group.[77]

The principal mediators of the stress immune response include the CRF and the locus coeruleus–norepinephrine systems in the CNS. These systems are influenced by numerous positive and negative feedback systems that allow for both behavioral and peripheral adaptations to stress.[78] The peripheral limb of the CRF system is the hypothalamic-pituitary-adrenal (HPA)-immune axis, a negative feedback system involved in psychoneuroimmunologic regulation. In the HPA system, inflammatory cytokines, primarily tumor necrosis factor-α, interleukin-1 (IL-1), and IL-6 liberated during inflammation, stimulate the paraventricular nucleus of the hypothalamus to secrete CRF. CRF stimulates the pituitary gland to release corticotropin, which, in turn, stimulates the adrenal glands to release glucocorticoids. Finally, the glucocorticoids suppress inflammation and cytokine production, thereby completing the negative feedback loop.[79]

It has been proposed that disruptions in the HPA system can lead to behavioral and systemic disorders from either increased reactivity (e.g., Cushing's syndrome, depression, susceptibility to infection), or decreased reactivity (adrenal insufficiency, rheumatoid arthritis, chronic fatigue, post-traumatic stress disorder), and that inflammatory gastrointestinal disorders (e.g., inflammatory bowel disease) may be affected through this stress-mediated system. Experimental data to support this hypothesis include the following:

1. In the eosinophilia-myalgia syndrome, a disorder associated with colonic inflammation, the ingestion of impure L-tryptophan suppresses hypothalamic expression of messenger RNA for CRF, thereby down-regulating HPA function and possibly leading to uncontrolled cytokine activity and increased systemic inflammation.[80]
2. Experimental colitis induced by streptococcal peptidoglycan-polysaccharide occurs in Lewis and Sprague-Dawley rats having genetically deficient HPA axis reactivity but not in Fischer or Buffalo rats having increased HPA axis reactivity.[81]
3. Stress may rekindle experimental colitis in previously conditioned rats.[82] Balb/c mice who recovered from dinitrobenzenesulfonic (DNBS) acid–induced colitis developed reactivation colitis only when stressed with a swimming challenge along with a subthreshold dose of DNBS acid compared with those mice given only the DNBS acid. The authors demonstrated this to be mediated through activation of CD4+ lymphocytes.

Other possible pathways for stress-induced activation of inflammatory bowel disease might involve cholinergically mediated increases in gut mucosal permeability, thereby allowing transmural migration of antigenic macromolecules,[83] or peripheral actions of CNS neuropeptides, including CRF and VIP on inflammation and immune function.[84]

The clinical evidence to support a role for stress in activation of human inflammatory bowel disease or, for that matter, other structural disorders is limited, perhaps because of methodologic difficulties. However, the evidence from clinical observational data is compelling and is supported by more recent, better designed studies that assess the effects of long-term stress. For example, in one study of 62 patients with ulcerative colitis followed prospectively for more than 5 years,[85] patients who scored high on long-term perceived stress had an increased risk of disease exacerbation; exacerbation was not associated with short-term perceived stress or disease extent, duration, or severity.

Post-infectious IBS

The long-held observation that a subgroup of patients with IBS develop their condition after an acute infectious gastroenteritis[86] may relate to brain-gut dysfunction. Postinfectious IBS appears to involve an interaction between the ability of the infection to induce dysmotility, inflammation, and visceral hypersensitivity[87] and the brain's ability to modulate these functions and to produce symptoms[88, 89] (see Chapter 5).

In a prospective study of 94 patients having no prior bowel symptoms who were hospitalized with acute gastroenteritis, 30% continued 3 months later to retain symptoms consistent with IBS. However, visceral hypersensitivity and dysmotility persisted in all subjects 3 months later whether or not bowel symptoms were present. Psychological disturbance occurring at the time of hospitalization 3 months earlier and an increased number of inflammatory cells and interleukin 1-β activity at 3 months distinguished those with IBS symptoms from those without symptoms.[89] Therefore, while both groups had altered gastrointestinal physiology post-infection, the psychological disturbance may have led to central "upregulation" of the visceral signals, thereby producing symptoms.

Cytokines and the Brain

Not only might stress have proinflammatory effects but also gut inflammation may reciprocally affect behavior via cytokine activation. Many of the behavioral features of chronic inflammatory diseases (e.g., fever, fatigue, anorexia, depression) called "sickness behavior" may result from the central effects of peripherally activated inflammatory cytokines.[90, 91] In rat studies of experimental colitis, the onset of the colitis had behavioral consequences, including an 80% reduction in food intake that may be mediated by the central effects of IL-1 activity.[92]

SYMPTOM EXPERIENCE AND BEHAVIOR

The product of the interacting effects of the brain and gut relates to the clinical expression of illness and disease, namely, the symptom experience and subsequent illness-related behaviors. The meaning of illness, the perceived effect of alterations in body image (e.g., colostomy), social acceptability, the degree of functional impairment and its implications at work and at home, and the likelihood of surgery or untimely death all must be dealt with by the patient. How well the patient adapts and the quality of the physician's involvement are crucial to the patient's psychological well-being and clinical course. Some chronically ill patients regress and become dependent. Their continued symptoms, restricted activity, and health care tax family, friends, and physician, all of whom may feel helpless to give enough emotional or medical assistance. Conversely, other patients may resist help to avoid acknowledging their imposed dependence. The family must then deal with feelings of guilt and anger, the expressions of which, though unavoidable, are not usually socially permitted. Often the physician carries the burden of such feelings of the patient and family and must reconcile them. In most instances, the problems are worked out and the patient establishes a pattern of coping. However, if the patient has difficulty coping psychologically with the illness, if the disorder is particularly incapacitating, or if the interpersonal family relationships are unstable, additional physician and ancillary effort will be required, such as psychological counseling, social service, and peer support groups.

OUTCOME

Measures of severity or activity of gastrointestinal disease are not sufficient to fully explain a patient's health status and its consequences. Early life conditioning and current psychological difficulties also influence a variety of outcome measures, including symptoms, health care seeking, quality of life,* and health care costs, in some instances more than disease-related factors.[93–95]

One study[96] assessed the possible effects of early life conditioning on health care visits and costs. The children of parents diagnosed with IBS had significantly more ambulatory care visits for all medical and for gastrointestinal symptoms, and outpatient health care costs were also higher than the comparison group of children having parents without IBS. Presumably, the parents with IBS were vigilant to, and responded more to, the gastrointestinal-nongastrointestinal symptoms of their children and more readily sought health care for them.

Other studies demonstrate the effects of psychosocial factors on symptom reporting and health care seeking. Among patients with gastroesophageal reflux disease,[97] many of the subjects, when given a stressful task, reported greater heartburn severity but without an increase in physiologic reflux. The authors proposed that anxiety related to the task amplifies normal intensity signals, which is then perceived as heartburn. In a survey of 997 subjects with inflammatory bowel disease, the number of physician visits was strongly influenced by psychosocial factors (psychological distress, perceived well-being, and physical functioning), whereas symptom severity was not found to significantly predict the number of physician visits.[45] Other important psychosocial predictors of adverse health outcome (e.g., symptom severity, phone calls, physician visits, daily function, and health-related quality of life) for functional or structural disorders include a history of sexual or physical abuse,[95] maladaptive illness beliefs,[98, 99] ineffective coping strategies (e.g., catastrophizing), and perceived inability to decrease symptoms.[52]

Health-Related Quality of Life is a global measure of the patient's perceptions, illness experience, and functional status. It incorporates social, cultural, psychological, and disease-related factors.

CLINICAL APPLICATIONS

The data relating the scientific and conceptual basis of psychosocial factors with gastrointestinal illness and disease require that the physician obtain, organize, and integrate psychosocial information to achieve optimal care. The recommendations offered in the following sections are particularly useful for patients with chronic illness or who have major psychosocial difficulties. More comprehensive discussions of technique and interview process are found elsewhere.[100, 101]

Obtaining the Data: The History

The physician's dialogue with the patient is the most important asset to the physician-patient relationship, diagnosis, and treatment and is often underutilized. Consider the information obtained in this office interview:

Doctor: *How can I help you?* (looking at chart)

Patient: *I developed a flare-up of my Crohn's, . . . the pain, nausea, and vomiting, . . . when I came back from vacation . . .* (pause) . . . (pensive) *I . . .*

Doctor: (interrupting) *Was the pain like what you had before?*

Patient: *Yes, . . . well, almost, . . . I think . . .*

Doctor: *Was it made worse by food?* (looks up)

Patient: *Yes.*

Doctor: *Did you have fever? or diarrhea?* (leaning forward)

Patient: *Well, yes, . . . I think, . . . I didn't take my temperature* (looks down)

Doctor: *So you had fever and diarrhea?*

Patient: *Uh, no, well, . . . they were a little loose, . . . I guess.*

The physician eventually diagnosed partial small bowel obstruction from Crohn's disease. However, some relevant information was not elicited, and because of the interruptions and leading questions, the accuracy of the information after the first question is uncertain. Furthermore, the nonverbal communication did not facilitate an effective physician-patient interaction.

The medical history should be obtained through a patient-centered, nondirective interview where the patient is encouraged to tell the story in his or her own way, so that the events contributing to the illness unfold naturally.[102] Open-ended questions are used initially to generate hypotheses, and additional information is obtained with facilitating expressions: "Yes?," "Can you tell me more?," repeating the patient's previous statements, head nodding, or even silent pauses with an expectant look. Avoid closed-ended (yes-no) questions at first, although they can be used later to further characterize the symptoms. Never use multiple choice or leading questions because the patient's desire to comply may bias the responses.

The traditional "medical" and "social" histories should not be separated, but elicited together, so the medical problem is described in the context of the psychosocial events surrounding the illness. The setting of symptom onset or exacerbation should always be obtained. At all times, the questions should communicate the physician's willingness to address both biologic and psychological aspects of the illness.

Doctor: *How can I help you?* (concerned, looking at patient)

Patient: *I developed a flare-up of my Crohn's, . . . the pain, nausea, and vomiting, . . . when I came back from vacation . . .* (pause)

Doctor: *Yes?*

Patient: *I was about to start my new position as floor supervisor, and thought I'd take vacation to get prepared . . . and then all this happened.*

Doctor: *Oh, I see . . .* (pause)

Patient: (continues) *I started getting that crampy feeling right here . . .* (points to lower abdomen) *. . . and then it got worse after eating. So I knew I'd be obstructed again if I didn't get in to see you.*

Doctor: *Hmmm . . . Any other symptoms?*

Patient: *Well, I felt warm, but I didn't take my temperature.*

Doctor: *What was your bowel pattern like?*

Patient: *They started getting loose when I was on vacation. Now they're slowing down. I haven't gone today.*

The number of verbal exchanges is the same, yet the patient offers more information. The clinical features are clearer, and additional knowledge of an association of symptoms with beginning a new job situation is obtained. This interview method also encourages patient self-awareness and provides for possible behavioral treatments (stress reduction techniques, job change, counseling) that may ameliorate future symptom flare-ups.

The historical information should be obtained from the perspective of the patient's understanding of the illness. Important questions to ask include, "What do you think is causing this problem?," "Why did it happen now?," "What kind of treatment do you think you should receive?," and "What do you fear most about your illness?"[103]

Evaluating the Data

The physician must assess the relative influences of the biologic, psychological, and social dimensions on the illness. It is unnecessary, and possibly countertherapeutic, to determine *whether* psychosocial *or* biologic processes are operative in an illness. Usually both are important and treatment is based on determining which is identifiable and remediable. A negative medical evaluation is not sufficient for making a psychosocial diagnosis. Table 122–1 lists several questions for the physician to consider in the assessment and evaluation of the patient.

Decision-Making in Diagnosis

Deciding which tests to order depends on the their clinical usefulness. Is it safe and cost-effective? Will the results make a difference in treatment? Patients who are persistent in their complaints or who challenge their physician's competence may tempt the physician to schedule unneeded studies or surgery out of uncertainty or just to "do something." This can be avoided by basing decisions on objective evaluation of data (e.g., blood in the stool, fever, abnormal serum chemistries) rather than solely by the patient's illness behavior.

The patient with persistent and unexplained abdominal pain is familiar to the gastroenterologist. The urge to further "work up" the patient with chronic abdominal pain must be tempered by the evidence that an adequate initial evaluation considerably reduces the likelihood of later finding an overlooked etiology (see Chapter 5). Here, the clinical approach is not medical diagnosis but psychosocial assessment and treatment of the chronic pain. Some factors associated with, or exacerbating, chronic pain symptoms include (1) a recent disruption in the family or social environment (e.g., child leaving home, argument); (2) major loss or anniversaries of losses (e.g., death of a family member or friend, hysterectomy or interference with the outcome of pregnancy); (3) a history of sexual or physical abuse; (4) the onset or worsening of depression or other psychiatric diagnosis; and (5) a "hidden agenda" (narcotic-seeking behavior, laxative abuse, attempt to obtain benefits due to disability). Although psychiatric consultation and treatment may be needed, it is also important for the medical physician to continue in the care and be vigilant to the development of new findings.

At times, decisions must be made with incomplete or

Table 122–1 | **Questions to Consider in the Clinical Evaluation of the Patient**

1. Does the patient have acute or chronic illness?
2. What is the patient's life history of illness?
3. Why is the patient coming now?
4. What are the patient's perceptions and expectations?
5. Does the patient exhibit abnormal illness behavior?
6. What is the impact of the illness?
7. Is there a concurrent psychiatric diagnosis?
8. Are there cultural or ethnic influences?
9. How does the family interact around the illness?
10. What are the patient's other psychosocial resources?
11. How far should I go in the work-up?
12. Should I call the psychiatric consultant?

nonspecific information. Particularly for chronic symptoms, when studies are unrevealing and the patient is clinically stable, it is wiser to tolerate the uncertainty in diagnosis and observe the patient for new developments over a period of time ("Don't just do something—stand there!"). Experienced physicians usually make diagnostic and treatment decisions based on the degree of change in the condition over weeks or months rather than on one or two occasions.

Psychiatric consultation should be considered when additional psychological data could clarify the illness or improve patient care. Examples include (1) identifying psychiatric diagnoses that would benefit from specific treatment (e.g., psychopharmacologic agents); (2) when the patient's level of psychosocial functioning is seriously impaired (e.g., inability to work); or (3) when invasive diagnostic or therapeutic strategies are being considered on the basis of patient complaints without clear indications from medical data.

Treatment Approach

Establish a Therapeutic Relationship

The physician establishes a therapeutic relationship when he or she (1) elicits and validates the patient's beliefs, concerns, and expectations; (2) offers empathy when needed; (3) clarifies patient misunderstandings; (4) provides education; and (5) negotiates the plan of treatment with the patient. This strategy must be individualized, because patients vary in the degree of negotiation and participation they require. The physician must be nonjudgmental, show interest in the patient's well-being, and be prepared to exercise effective communication skills.

Elicit, Evaluate, and Communicate the Role for Psychosocial Factors

A sensitive and nonjudgmental interview facilitates patient disclosure of psychosocial information. At times the patient may be unwilling or unable to discuss this information, particularly on the first visit or in the context of seeing the gastroenterologist for "medical" problems. Fear of disapproval and lack of trust often prevent the patient from sharing intimate thoughts and feelings, and this can be overcome by a good physician-patient relationship. When the patient is unwilling or unable to accept the role of psychosocial factors in illness, the physician can still obtain such information indirectly, by inference, and should not attempt to provide the patient with "insight." If asked whether the problem is "in my head," the physician explains that illness is rarely either mental or physical and that it is important to understand all factors, including the patient's feelings, indicating that many chronic conditions are associated with depression or unrealistic fears. Consistent with the biopsychosocial model of illness, it is not helpful to discuss psychosocial and biologic factors in terms of causation ("it's common for stress to cause your problems") or by exclusion ("the work-up is negative, it must be stress").

Reassurance

Patient fears and concerns require reassurance. However, if it is premature, inadequate, or inappropriate, it will be perceived as insincere or as a lack of thoroughness by the physician. Although the physician should respond to the patient's needs and requests empathically, this does not mean "going along" when it is not in the patient's best interest. For example, disability may be a disincentive in helping the patient reestablish "wellness" and return to gainful employment.

Recognize Patient Adaptations to Chronic Illness

Illness is associated with certain adaptations: increased attention and support, release from usual responsibilities, and possibly social and financial compensation. For some patients, more may be lost by giving up the state of illness than gained by wellness, and improvement may be slow. It can be advanced if help is also directed toward improving the psychosocial adjustment to the illness (e.g., improving coping strategies).

Reinforce Healthy Behaviors

Sometimes, complaints of physical distress are a maladaptive effort to communicate emotional distress or to receive attention.[105] The physician may unwittingly reinforce this behavior by (1) paying a great deal of attention to patient complaints to the exclusion of other aspects, (2) acting on each complaint by ordering diagnostic studies or giving prescriptive medication, or (3) assuming total responsibility for the patient's well-being. The patient minimizes personal responsibility for health care management by placing the responsibility with the physician, thus perpetuating the cycle of symptom recitation and passive interaction.

To encourage patients to take more responsibility for their care and a heightened sense of control, the physician offers a choice among several treatments (e.g., high-fiber diet and/or psyllium seed preparation for constipation) or designs an exercise program. The physician should limit discussion about symptoms (the "organ recital") to only satisfy medical concerns and focus on adaptations to the illness rather than the cure. I often find it best not to ask about the patient's symptom (e.g., "How is your pain?"), because that puts my attention to the patient having symptoms. Rather, I ask about the symptoms in the context of the patient's health-promoting behaviors (e.g., "What are you doing to manage your pain?").

Psychopharmacologic Medication

Psychopharmacologic medications are indicated for treatment of an associated primary psychiatric disorder but can also be used for patients with chronic gastrointestinal complaints for other reasons, including depressed mood associated with the medical condition, impaired daily functioning and quality of life, and management of persistent, painful symptoms.

The *tricyclic antidepressants* in relatively low dosages can reduce chronic pain[105] through peripheral and central mechanisms, including endorphin activation of corticofugal pain inhibitory pathways (see Chapter 5). They can also treat major and secondary depressive symptoms and panic attacks in full antidepressant dosages. The *selective serotonin-reup-*

take inhibitors are not as established as antinociceptive agents. However, they are often used in this fashion and are particularly helpful for psychiatric comorbid conditions, including major depression, panic disorder, and other high-anxiety conditions (e.g., obsessive-compulsive disorder, post-traumatic stress disorder, social phobia). The presence of any of these syndromes associated with deterioration in daily function (e.g. inability to work), or in "vegetative" activities such as poor appetite, weight loss, sleep disturbance, and decreased energy and libido (subserved by central brain monoamine function), is a reasonable indication for a therapeutic trial. They should be considered even if the patient denies feelings of sadness ("masked" depression). Treatment should be increased to full therapeutic levels over 2 to 3 weeks and maintained for 6 to 9 months. Poor clinical responses may be due to relatively low dosages.[106] *Anxiolytic agents*, particularly the benzodiazepines, are frequently used to ameliorate anxiety disorders or short-term acute anxiety, particularly if it is associated with stress-induced flare-ups of bowel disturbance. Their potential benefit should be balanced with the long-term risks of sedation, drug interactions, habituation, and withdrawal rebound. *Antipsychotic drugs* or neuroleptics include the phenothiazines (e.g., chlorpromazine), butyrophenones (e.g., haloperidol), and new classes of safer antipsychotic agents (e.g., clozapine, olanzapine) and are used primarily for treating disturbances of thought, perception, and behavior in psychotic patients. They may also treat acute episodes of agitation, alcohol withdrawal, or psychotic (somatic) delusional disorders presenting as a gastrointestinal disorder, but psychiatric consultation is recommended. *Opiate drugs* have little role in treating patients with chronic pain or psychosocial disturbance because of the their potential for abuse, dependency, and narcotic bowel syndrome.[107]

Psychotherapy and Behavioral Treatments

Adjunctive care by a psychiatrist, psychologist, or other mental health professional should be determined through an assessment of the personal, social, and economic hardship of the illness rather than identification of a specific psychiatric diagnosis. It is based on the likelihood of improved function, mood, or coping style to such intervention. The patient must see psychological care as relevant to personal needs rather than "to prove I'm not crazy."

Cognitive-behavioral treatment can be effective for patients with functional gastrointestinal symptoms, chronic pain, depression, and bulimia. It involves the patient in identifying stressors and thoughts that increase mental distress and in learning new ways of coping by restructuring these thoughts. *Interpersonal* or *dynamic psychotherapy* is recommended for patients motivated to address and adjust interpersonal difficulties associated with exacerbations of symptoms. For the patient who would benefit from peer support or who has interpersonal difficulties or limited finances, *group therapy* can be considered. *Crisis intervention* is designed to get the individual over a particularly difficult period in a few sessions. It can help the patient with chronic illness who experiences identifiable causes for recent deterioration in function. *Family* or *marital counseling* is indicated when difficulties in the family interaction interfere with health-promoting activities. Finally, other *behavioral treatments* (e.g., relaxation training, generalized biofeedback, meditation, hypnosis) are safe, noninvasive, and cost-effective methods designed to (1) reduce anxiety levels, (2) teach patients how to engage in health-promoting behaviors, (3) give patients greater responsibility and control of their health care, and (4) improve pain control.

Physician-Related Issues

The patient's psychosocial difficulties may affect the physician's needs, attitudes, and behaviors and, if unrecognized, adversely affect the patient's care. Physicians are uncomfortable making decisions in the face of diagnostic uncertainty, because it is assumed that greater knowledge will make the illness more treatable. Nonetheless, many clinical treatments are undertaken for symptoms or psychosocial concerns not based on a specific diagnosis, particularly for patients with unexplained complaints who urgently request a diagnosis. The physician risks overdoing the diagnostic evaluation or instituting unneeded or harmful treatments in such patients ("furor medicus"[108]). Alternatively, the physician may not believe that the complaints are legitimate, and patients will recognize this.

Awareness of the psychosocial dimensions of illness and their effects on the genesis of symptoms legitimizes the complaints and puts them into better perspective. Some interactions between patient and physician become conflicted. They may cause physicians to react with blame or stigmatization or to feel dissatisfied or "drained."[109] The physician must understand these behaviors in terms of the patient's psychological traits or the medical illness rather than as some personal failure. In our role as physicians, we may have expectations for rapid relief with displays of gratitude from patients. However, some patients will resist improvement and may be unable or unwilling to acknowledge the physician's efforts. Here, it is best to refocus the treatment from cure to improvement in daily function despite continued symptoms. Gratification can be obtained from the personal effort rather than from the patient's acknowledgment of gratitude. Finally, each physician must set personal limits in time and energy toward the care of patients who are particularly challenging. Factors such as limiting the length of office visits, allocating part of the care to other health care workers, and, when necessary, saying "no" all are important methods for achieving a balance between personal needs and benefit for the patient.

REFERENCES

1. Reading A: Illness and disease. Med Clin North Am 61:703, 1977.
2. Engel GL: The need for a new medical model: A challenge for biomedicine. Science 196:129, 1977.
3. Kroenke K, Mangelsdorff AD: Common symptoms in ambulatory care: Incidence, evaluation, therapy, and outcome. Am J Med 86:262, 1989.
4. Drossman DA: Chronic functional abdominal pain. Am J Gastroenterol 91:2270, 1996.
5. Thompson WG, Longstreth GF, Drossman DA, et al: Functional bowel disorders and functional abdominal pain. In Drossman DA, Talley NJ, Thompson WG, et al (eds): Rome II: Functional Gastrointestinal Disorders: Diagnosis, Pathophysiology, and Treatment, 2nd ed. McLean, VA, Degnon, 2000, pp 351–432.
6. Mitchell CM, Drossman DA: Survey of the AGA membership relating to patients with functional gastrointestinal disorders. Gastroenterology 92:1282, 1987.

7. Russo MW, Gaynes BN, Drossman DA: A National Survey of Practice Patterns of Gastroenterologists with Comparison to the Past Two Decades. J Clin Gastroenterol 29:343, 1999.
8. Christensen J: Heraclides or the physician. Gastroenterol Int 3:45, 1990.
9. Drossman DA, Creed FH, Olden KW, et al: Psychosocial aspects of the functional gastrointestinal disorders. In Drossman DA, Talley NJ, Thompson WG, et al (eds): Rome II: Functional Gastrointestinal Disorders: Diagnosis, Pathophysiology, and Treatment, 2nd ed. McLean, VA, Degnon, 2000, pp 157–245.
10. Drossman DA: Presidential address: Gastrointestinal illness and biopsychosocial model. Psychosom Med 60:258, 1998.
11. Rogers M, Cerda JJ: The narcotic bowel syndrome [editorial]. J Clin Gastroenterol 11:132, 1989.
12. Kiecolt-Glaser JK, Glaser R: Psychoneuroimmunology and health consequences: Data and shared mechanisms [review]. Psychosom Med 57:269, 1995.
13. Buxbaum E, Sodergren SS: A disturbance of elimination and motor development: The mother's role in the development of the infant. Psychoanal Study Child 32:195, 1977.
14. Hill OW: Psychogeneic vomiting. Gut 9:348, 1968.
15. Philippopoulos GS: The analysis of a case of merycism: Psychopathology-psychodynamics. Psychother Psychosom 22:364, 1973.
16. Drossman DA, Ontjes DA, Heizer WH: Anorexia nervosa. Gastroenterology 77:1115, 1979.
17. Klauser AG, Voderholzer WA, Heinrich CA, et al: Behavioral modification of colonic function: Can constipation be learned? Dig Dis Sci 35:1271, 1990.
18. Whitehead WE, Crowell MD, Schuster MM: Functional disorders of the anus and rectum. Semin Gastroenterol Dis 1:74, 1990.
19. Bemporad JR, Kresch RA, Asnes R: Chronic neurotic encopresis as a paradigm of a multifactorial psychiatric disorder. J Nerv Ment Dis 166:472, 1978.
20. Bellman M: Studies on encopresis. Acta Paediatr Scand 56:1, 1966.
21. Almy TP: Experimental studies on the irritable colon. Am J Med 10: 60, 1951.
22. Drossman DA, Creed FH, Olden KW, et al: Psychosocial aspects of the functional gastrointestinal disorders. Gut 45:II25, 1999.
23. Whitehead WE, Winget C, Fedoravicius AS, et al: Learned illness behavior in patients with irritable bowel syndrome and peptic ulcer. Dig Dis Sci 27:202, 1982.
24. Lowman BC, Drossman DA, Cramer EM, et al: Recollection of childhood events in adults with irritable bowel syndrome. J Clin Gastroenterol 9:324, 1987.
25. Rosen G, Kleinman A: Social science in the clinic: Applied contributions from anthropology to medical teaching and patient care. In Carr JE, Dengerink HA (eds): Behavioral Science in the Practice of Medicine. New York, Elsevier, 1983, pp 85–103.
26. Zborowski M: Cultural components in responses to pain. J Social Issues 8:16, 1952.
27. Kleinman A, Eisenberg L, Good B: Culture, illness, and care: Clinical lessons from anthropologic and cross-cultural research. Ann Intern Med 88:251, 1978.
28. Eisenberg DM, Kessler RC, Foster C, et al: Unconventional medicine in the United States. N Engl J Med 328:246, 1993.
29. Stermer E, Bar H, Levy N: Chronic functional gastrointestinal symptoms in Holocaust survivors. Am J Gastroenterol 86:417, 1991.
30. Creed FH, Craig T, Farmer RG: Functional abdominal pain, psychiatric illness, and life events. Gut 29:235, 1988.
31. Drossman DA: Psychosocial factors in ulcerative colitis and Crohn's disease. In Kirsner JB (ed): Inflammatory Bowel Disease, 5th ed. Philadelphia, WB Saunders, 1999, pp 342–357.
32. Drossman DA, Talley NJ, Olden KW, et al: Sexual and physical abuse and gastrointestinal illness: Review and recommendations. Ann Intern Med 123:782, 1995.
33. Longstreth GF, Wolde-Tsadik G: Irritable bowel–type symptoms in HMO examinees: Prevalence, demographics, and clinical correlates. Dig Dis Sci 38:1581, 1993.
34. Drossman DA: Irritable bowel syndrome and sexual/physical abuse history. Eur J Gastroenterol Hepatol 9:327, 1997.
35. Ringel Y, Drossman DA, Turkington TG, et al: Anterior cingulate cortex (ACC) dysfunction in subjects with sexual/physical abuse. Gastroenterology 118:A444, 2000.
36. Bremner JD, Randall P, Vermetten E, et al: Magnetic resonance imaging–based measurement of hippocampal volume in posttraumatic stress disorder related to childhood physical and sexual abuse—a preliminary report. Biol Psychiatry 41:23, 1997.
37. Alexander F: Psychosomatic Medicine: Its Principles and Applications. New York, WW Norton, 1950.
38. Engel GL: Studies of ulcerative colitis: III. The nature of the psychologic process. Am J Med 19:231, 1955.
39. Olden KW, Drossman DA: Psychologic and psychiatric aspects of gastrointestinal disease. Adv Gastroenterol 84:1313, 2000.
40. Drossman DA: Psychosocial factors in the care of patients with gastrointestinal disorders. In Yamada T (ed): Textbook of Gastroenterology, 3rd ed. Philadelphia, Lippincott-Raven, 1999, pp 638–659.
41. Diagnostic and Statistical Manual of Mental Disorders, 4th ed. Washington, DC, American Psychiatric Association, 1994, pp 1–886.
42. Whitehead WE, Bosmajian L, Zonderman AB, et al: Symptoms of psychologic distress associated with irritable bowel syndrome: Comparison of community and medical clinic samples. Gastroenterology 95:709, 1988.
43. Drossman DA, McKee DC, Sandler RS, et al: Psychosocial factors in the irritable bowel syndrome: A multivariate study of patients and nonpatients with irritable bowel syndrome. Gastroenterology 95:701, 1988.
44. Smith RC, Greenbaum DS, Vancouver JB, et al: Psychosocial factors are associated with health care seeking rather than diagnosis in irritable bowel syndrome. Gastroenterology 98:293, 1990.
45. Drossman DA, Leserman J, Mitchell CM, et al: Health status and health care use in persons with inflammatory bowel disease: A national sample. Dig Dis Sci 36:1746, 1991.
46. Toner BB, Garfinkel PE, Jeejeebhoy KN, et al: Self-schema in irritable bowel syndrome and depression. Psychosom Med 52:149, 1990.
47. Sandler RS, Drossman DA, Nathan HP, et al: Symptom complaints and health care–seeking behavior in subjects with bowel dysfunction. Gastroenterology 87:314, 1984.
48. Sifneos PE: The prevalence of "alexyithymic" characteristics in psychsomatic patients. Psychother Psychosom 22:255, 1973.
49. Lumley MA, Stettner L, Wehmer F: How are alexithymia and physical illness linked? A review and critique of pathways. J Psychosom Res 41:505, 1996.
50. Egan KJ, Katon WJ: Responses to illness and health in chronic pain patients and healthy adults. Psychosom Med 49:470, 1987.
51. Lazarus RS, Folkman S: Stress, Appraisal, and Coping. New York, Springer-Verlag, 1984, pp 1–445.
52. Drossman DA, Li Z, Leserman J, et al: Effects of coping on health outcome among female patients with gastrointestinal disorders. Psychosom Med 62:309, 2000.
53. Berkman LF: The relationship of social networks and social support to morbidity and mortality. In Cohen S, Syme SL (eds): Social Support and Health. New York, Academic Press, 1985, pp 241–277.
54. Hinkle LE: The concept of "stress" in the biological and social sciences. In Lipowski ZJ (ed): Psychosomatic Medicine: Current Trends and Clinical Applications. New York, Oxford University Press, 1977, pp 27–49.
55. Drossman DA, Sandler RS, McKee DC, et al: Bowel patterns among subjects not seeking health care: Use of a questionnaire to identify a population with bowel dysfunction. Gastroenterology 83:529, 1982.
56. Cannon WB: The movements of the intestine studied by means of roentgen rays. Am J Physiol 6:251, 1902.
57. Beaumont W: Experiments and observations on the gastric juice and the physiology of digestion. Plattsburgh, FP Auen, 1833.
58. Pavlov I: The Work of the Digestive Glands. London, C. Griffin, 1910.
59. Wolf S, Wolff HG: Human Gastric Function. London, Oxford University Press, 1943, pp 1–195.
60. Engel GL, Reichsman F, Segal HL: A study of an infant with gastric fistula: I. Behavior and the rate of total hydrochloric acid secretion. Psychosom Med 18:374, 1956.
61. Young LD, Richter JE, Anderson KO, et al: The effects of psychological and environmental stressors on peristaltic esophageal contractions in healthy volunteers. Psychophysiology 24:132, 1987.
62. Holtmann G, Singer MV, Kriebel R, et al: Differential effects of acute mental stress on interdigestive secretion of gastric acid, pancreatic enzymes, and gastroduodenal motility. Dig Dis Sci 34:1701, 1989.
63. Kellow JE, Langeluddecke PM, Eckersley GM, et al: Effects of acute psychologic stress on small intestinal motility in health and the irritable bowel syndrome. Scand J Gastroenterol 27:53, 1992.
64. Welgan P, Meshkinpour H, Beeler M: Effect of anger on colon motor

and myoelectric activity in irritable bowel syndrome. Gastroenterology 94:1150, 1988.

65. Tache Y, Martinez V, Million M, et al: Corticotropin-releasing factor and the brain-gut motor response to stress. Can J Gastroenterol 13(Suppl A):18A, 1999.
66. Smith GP: Satiety effect of gastrointestinal hormones. In Beers RF Jr, Bassett EG (eds): Polypeptide Hormones. New York, Raven Press, 1980, pp 413–420.
67. Geracioti TD Jr, Liddle RA: Impaired cholecystokinin secretion in bulimia nervosa. N Engl J Med 319:683, 1988.
68. Baile CA, McLaughlin CL, Della Fera MA: Role of cholecystokinin and opioid peptides in control of food intake. Physiol Rev 66:172, 1986.
69. Shavit Y, Terman GW, Martin FC, et al: Stress, opioid peptides, the immune system, and cancer. J Immunol 135:834s, 1985.
70. Coderre TJ, Katz J, Vaccarino AL, et al: Contribution of central neuroplasticity to pathological pain: Review of clinical and experimental evidence. Pain 52:259, 1993.
71. Melzack R, Wall P: Gate-control and other mechanisms. In Melzack R, Wall P (eds): The Challenge of Pain, 2nd ed. London, Pelican Books, 1988, pp 165–193.
72. Kimzey SL, Johnson PC, Ritzman SE, et al: Hematology and immunology studies: The second manned skylab mission. Aviat Space Environ Med 47:383, 1976.
73. Kiecolt-Glaser JK, Glaser R: Psychosocial moderators of immune function. Ann Behav Med 9:16, 1989.
74. Kiecolt-Glaser JK, Stephens RE, Lipetz PD, et al: Distress and DNA repair in human lymphocytes. J Behav Med 8:311, 1985.
75. Kiecolt-Glaser JK, Dura JR, Speicher CE, et al: Spousal caregivers of dementia victims: Longitudinal changes in immunity and health. Psychosom Med 53:345, 1991.
76. Cohen S, Tyrrell AJ, Smith AP: Psychological stress and susceptibility to the common cold. N Engl J Med 325:606, 1991.
77. Fawzy FI, Fawzy NW, Hyun CS, et al: Malignant melanoma: Effects of an early structured psychiatric intervention, coping, and affective state on recurrence and survival 6 years later. Arch Gen Psychiatry 50:681, 1993.
78. Chrousos GP: The hypothalamic-pituitary-adrenal axis and immune-mediated inflammation. N Engl J Med 332:1351, 1995.
79. Sternberg EM, Chrousos GP, Wilder RL, et al: The stress response and the regulation of inflammatory disease. Ann Intern Med 117:854, 1992.
80. De Schryver-Kecskemeti K, Bennert KW, Cooper GS, et al: Gastrointestinal involvement in L-tryptophan (L-Trp)-associated eosinophilia-myalgia syndrome (EMS). Dig Dis Sci 37:697, 1992.
81. Sartor RB, Cromartie WJ, Powell DW, et al: Granulomatous enterocolitis induced in rats by purified bacterial cell wall fragments. Gastroenterology 89:587, 1985.
82. Qiu BS, Vallance BA, Blennerhassett PA, et al: The role of CD4+ lymphocytes in the susceptibility of mice to stress-induced reactivation of experimental colitis. Nature Med 5:1, 1999.
83. Saunders PR, Hanssen NPM, Perdue MH: Cholinergic nerves mediate stress-induced intestinal transport abnormalities in Wistar-Kyoto rats. Am J Physiol 273:G486, 1997.
84. Ottoway CA: Role of the neuroendocrine system in cytokine pathways in inflammatory bowel disease. Aliment Pharmacol Ther 10:10, 1996.
85. Levenstein S, Prantera C, Varvo V, et al: Stress and exacerbation in ulcerative colitis: A prospective study of patients enrolled in remission. Am J Gastroenterol 95:1213, 2000.
86. Chaudhary NA, Truelove SC: The irritable colon syndrome: A study of the clinical features, predisposing causes, and prognosis in 130 cases. Q J Med 31:307, 1962.
87. Collins SM, Giovanni B, Vallance B: Stress, inflammation, and the irritable bowel syndrome. Can J Gastroenterol 13:47A, 1999.
88. Drossman DA: Mind over matter in the postinfective irritable bowel. Gut 44:306, 1999.
89. Gwee KA, Leong YL, Graham C, et al: The role of psychological and biological factors in post-infective gut dysfunction. Gut 44:400, 1999.
90. Sternberg EM: Perspectives series: Cytokines and the brain. J Clin Invest 100:2641, 1997.
91. Watkins LR, Maier SF, Goehler LE: Cytokine-to-brain communication: A review and analysis of alternative mechanisms. Life Sci 57: 1011, 1995.
92. McHugh K, Weingarten HP, Keenan C, et al: On the suppression of food intake in experimental models of colitis in the rat. Am J Physiol 264:R871, 1993.
93. Lundeen TF, George JM, Toomey TC: Health care system utilization for chronic facial pain. J Craniomandib Disord Facial Oral Pain 5:280, 1991.
94. Maxton DG, Whorwell PJ: Use of medical resources and attitudes to health care of patients with "chronic abdominal pain." Br J Med Econ 2:75, 1992.
95. Drossman DA, Li Z, Leserman J, et al: Health status by gastrointestinal diagnosis and abuse history. Gastroenterology 110:999, 1996.
96. Levy RL, Whitehead WE, Von Korff MR, et al: Intergenerational transmission of gastrointestinal illness behavior. Am J Gastroenterol 95:451, 2000.
97. Bradley LA, Richter JE, Pulliam TJ, et al: The relationship between stress and symptoms of gastroesophageal reflux: The influence of psychological factors. Am J Gastroenterol 88:11, 1993.
98. Drossman DA, Hu Y, Jia H, et al: The influence of psychosocial factors on health care utilization in patients with functional bowel disorders (FBD). Gastroenterology 118:A842, 2000.
99. Drossman DA, Hu Y, Jia H, et al: The influence of psychosocial factors on health status in patients with functional bowel disorders (FBD). Gastroenterology 118:A398, 2000.
100. Drossman DA: Psychosocial factors in the care of patients with gastrointestinal disorders. In Yamada T (ed): Textbook of Gastroenterology, 2nd ed. Philadelphia, JB Lippincott, 1995, pp 620–637.
101. Drossman DA: Psychosocial sound bites: Exercises in the patient-doctor relationship. Am J Gastroenterol 92:1418, 1997.
102. Lipkin M Jr: The medical interview and related skills. In Branch WT (ed): Office Practice of Medicine, 3rd ed. Philadelphia, WB Saunders, 1994, pp 970–986.
103. Drossman DA: Diagnosing and treating patients with refractory functional gastrointestinal disorders. Ann Intern Med 123:688, 1995.
104. Drossman DA: Struggling with the "controlling" patient. Am J Gastroenterol 89:1441, 1994.
105. Jackson JL, O'Malley PG, Tomkins G, et al: Treatment of functional gastrointestinal disorders with antidepressants: A meta-analysis. Am J Med 108:65, 2000.
106. Cakkues AL, Popkin MK: Antidepressant treatment of medical-surgical inpatients by nonpsychiatric physicians. Arch Gen Psychiatry 44: 157, 1987.
107. Sandgren JE, McPhee MS, Greenberger NJ: Narcotic bowel syndrome treated with clonidine. Ann Int Med 101:331, 1984.
108. DeVaul RA, Faillace LA: Persistent pain and illness insistence—a medical profile of proneness to surgery. Am J Surg 135:828, 1978.
109. Drossman DA: Challenges in the physician–patient relationship: Feeling "drained." Gastroenterology 121:1037, 2001.

INDEX

Note: Page numbers followed by f and t refer to figures and tables, respectively.